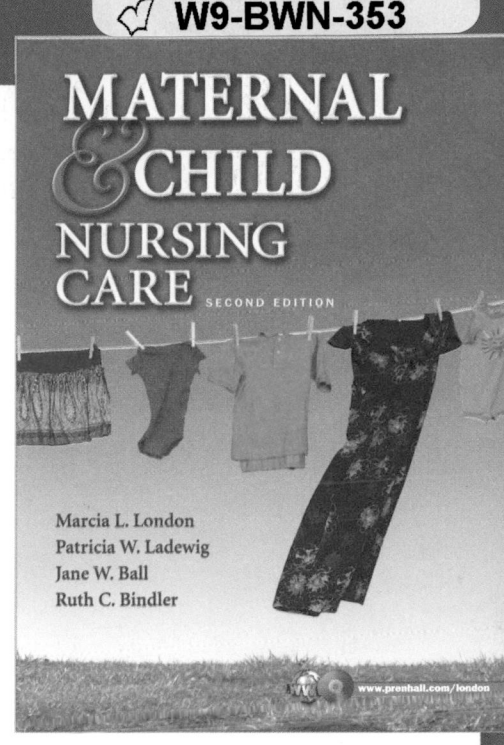

Dear Future Nurse:

As a nursing student, you have many demands on your time. During our conversations with students and faculty, we heard them say a lack of time is the number one problem facing students in this course, and we made it our primary concern in writing *Maternal & Child Nursing Care*. One way that we addressed this need is with a new tool called the Critical Concept Review at the end of each chapter. It links important concepts from the chapter to each learning objective. You can use the Critical Concept Review to focus and make the most of your study time.

If you attend class, study, and work hard, you will build the knowledge and skills you need to be successful in the classroom, in clinical, and on the NCLEX RN®. Here's how you can use this textbook to your benefit:

READ THE BOOK

Preparing for class by reading assigned pages beforehand helps you to get the most out of your classes and clinicals. It's the best way to start building your knowledge and skill base.

USE THE BOXES IN THE BOOK

Some students tell us they only read the boxes; some tell us they skip the boxes and read only the text. Your textbook is designed so that helpful information appears in a format that enhances your ability to comprehend and remember what you read. Take some time to review the Preface and familiarize yourself with the features of your book.

USE THE RESOURCES ACCOMPANYING THIS BOOK

A wealth of material accompanies this textbook to help you master the course content and apply the concepts using your critical thinking skills. Additionally, there are numerous opportunities to practice NCLEX-RN® questions and watch case studies, as well as many animations and videos that help bring the textbook concepts to life. Use the Student CD-ROM or the Companion Website at *www.prenhall.com/london* to access these valuable resources.

Nursing is a valuable and noble profession, and we applaud your desire to become a successful nurse. We wish you the best of luck as you embark on your life-long journey of rewards and successes in your nursing career.

Sincerely,

Marcia London   Patricia Ladewig   Jane Ball   Ruth Bindler

We keep your time in mind.

Preparing for the NCLEX-RN® is important to you, and we provide resources that help make your study time more effective.

Student CD-ROM—Your Student CD-ROM provides more than 550 questions to prepare you for the NCLEX-RN® exam. Review the rationales and assessment results to identify areas in which you need further study.

Prentice Hall Reviews & Rationales—These popular resources provide a core content and NCLEX-RN® review of maternal-newborn and pediatric nursing. The pre-tests, post-tests, and CD-ROMs guide you through a self-paced review.

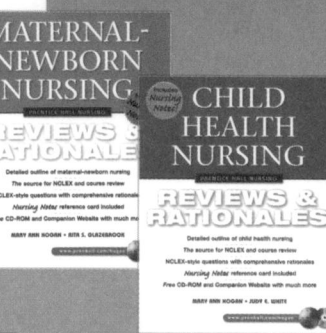

Prepare for NCLEX-RN® Exams

Prentice Hall offers instructors using *Maternal & Child Nursing Care* an online course management system to plan and administer your course online.

OneKey features everything you and your students need for out-of-class work, conveniently organized to match your syllabus:
- Interactive Modules
- Text and Image PowerPoint Presentations
- Animations
- Videos
- Case Studies

OneKey also provides course management in a separate section accessible only to instructors with tools to:
- Build online tests
- Create assignments
- Enter grades
- Post announcements
- Communicate with students

OneKey content is available in three platforms: BlackBoard, WebCT, and the reliable, easy-to-use CourseCompass platform. Please contact your Prentice Hall sales representative for a demonstration or go online to www.prenhall.com/nursing.

  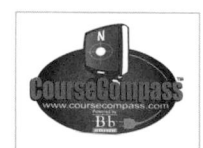

so little time...

Critical Thinking in Action—Applying the concepts you learned in class is what clinical time is all about. This case study introduces a client situation at the end of each chapter that continues on the Student CD-ROM, where it comes to life with videos and images. Experience the case as you decide what nursing actions are appropriate.

Clinical Skills Manual—Provides procedures with step-by-step instructions, rationales, and photographs to help you perform maternity and pediatric skills successfully.

Companion Website—A rich online resource to accompany your text, the Companion Website can help you apply your knowledge with chapter resources, such as objectives, audio glossary, chapter summary, additional NCLEX-RN® review, case studies, care plans, MediaLink applications, links to other resources, and more. It's a quick, easy way to review the important content from each chapter and test your knowledge.
www.prenhall.com/london

Prepare for Clinicals

Prepare for Course Exams

Prentice Hall Real Nursing Skills Series—Used for classroom instruction or packaged with the textbook, these CD-ROMs reduce student time in the lab and prepare students for the clinical setting. The **Maternal-Newborn** package contains 24 skills on 2 CD-ROMs, and the **Pediatrics** package contains 65 skills on 3 CD-ROMs. Ask your Prentice Hall sales representative for pricing and packaging information.

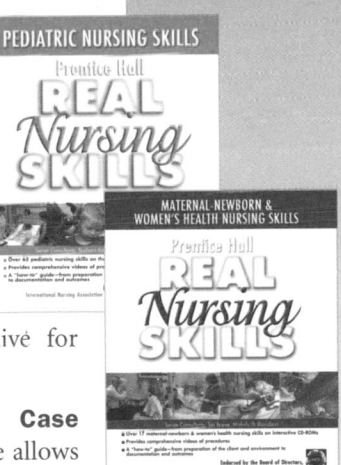

Prentice Hall Custom Nursing Case Studies—This unique online database allows you to select cases applicable to your course and student needs. Case studies are available for every nursing specialty, and with the searchable database, finding the right ones is quick and easy. Go to www.prenhall.com/nursingcases to start building your custom case study book today.

Test Generator—Equipped with TestGen 7.2, the Instructor Resource CD-ROM provides a test bank with more than 850 questions, including the new NCLEX-RN® alternate item formats, all written at the analysis or application cognitive level. You can search for test items by level, chapter, or topic and can preview answers, rationales, NCLEX-RN® Test Plan and the cognitive level for all questions. TestGen 7.2 can output either print or electronic tests.

Brief Contents

MATERNAL &CHILD NURSING CARE

SECOND EDITION

Marcia L. London, RNC, MSN, APRN, NNP
Senior Clinical Instructor & Director
of Neonatal Nurse Practitioner Option
Beth-El College of Nursing and Health Sciences
University of Colorado at Colorado Springs
Colorado Springs, Colorado

Patricia A. Wieland Ladewig, PhD, RN
Professor and Academic Dean
Rueckert-Hartman School for Health Professions
Regis University
Denver, Colorado

Jane W. Ball, RN, CPNP, DrPH
Executive Director
Emergency Medical Services for Children
National Resource Center, Children's National Medical Center
Washington, District of Columbia

Ruth C. Bindler, RNC, PhD
Associate Professor
Washington State University
Intercollegiate College of Nursing
Spokane, Washington

PEARSON

Prentice
Hall

Upper Saddle River, New Jersey 07458

Library of Congress Cataloging-in-Publication Data

Maternal & child nursing care / Marcia L. London . . . [et al.].—2nd ed.
   p. ; cm.
   Rev. ed. of: Maternal-newborn and child nursing. c2003
   Includes bibliographical references and index.
   ISBN 0-13-172394-4
   1. Maternity nursing. 2. Pediatric nursing.
   [DNLM: 1. Maternal-Child Nursing—methods. 2. Pediatric Nursing—
methods. WY 157.3 M42525 2006] I. Title: Maternal and child nursing care.
II. London, Marcia L. III. Maternal-newborn and child nursing.
   RG951.M3145 2006
   618.2'0231—dc22

                           2006004208

Publisher: Julie Levin Alexander
Assistant to Publisher: Regina Bruno
Editor-in-Chief: Maura Connor
Executive Editor: Pamela Lappies
Senior Managing Editor: Marilyn Meserve
Development: Elena Mauceri, Dynamic WordWorks, Inc.
Assistant Editor: Danielle Doller
Editorial Assistant: Joanna Satkowitz
Director of Production and Manufacturing: Bruce Johnson
Managing Production Editor: Patrick Walsh
Production Liaison: Nicholas Radhuber
Production Editor: Lynn Steines, Carlisle Publishing Services
Manufacturing Manager: Ilene Sanford
Design Director: Cheryl Asherman
Design Coordinator: Maria Guglielmo
Interior Designer: Wanda Espana
Cover Designer: Maria Guglielmo
Electronic Art Creation: Precision Graphics
Manager of Media Production: Amy Peltier
Senior Media Project Manager: John Jordan
New Media Project Manager: Stephen Hartner
New Media Production: Hector Grillone, Anne Lukens, Jody Small, Kate Stillings,
   Video Production Services; CD programming and design: Red Frog, Inc.
Director of Marketing: Karen Allman
Marketing Manager: Francisco Del Castillo
Marketing Coordinator: Michael Sirinides
Composition: Carlisle Publishing Services
Cover Printer: Phoenix Color Corp.
Printing and Binding: Quebecor World

Notice: Care has been taken to confirm the accuracy of information presented in this book. The authors, editors, and the publisher, however, cannot accept any responsibility for errors or omissions or for consequences from application of the information in this book and make no warranty, express or implied, with respect to its contents. The authors and publishers have exerted every effort to ensure that drug selections and dosages set forth in this text are in accord with current recommendations and practice at time of publication. However, in view of ongoing research, changes in government regulations, and the constant flow of information relating to drug therapy and drug reactions, the reader is urged to check the package inserts of all drugs for any change in indications of dosage and for added warnings and precautions. This is particularly important when the recommended agent is a new and/or infrequently employed drug.

Pearson Education, LTD.
Pearson Education Singapore, Pte. Ltd.
Pearson Education Canada, Ltd.
Pearson Education Japan
Pearson Education Australia PTY, Limited

Pearson Education North Asia Ltd.
Pearson Educación de Mexico, S.A. de C.V.
Pearson Education Malaysia, Pte. Ltd.
Pearson Education, Upper Saddle River, New Jersey

Permission was granted by Elsevier Science to reprint in our Nursing Care Plans the nursing intervention and outcome classifications (NIC and NOC), from McCloskey & Bulechek, *Nursing Interventions Classification* and Johnson et al., *Nursing Outcomes Classification*.

10 9 8 7 6
ISBN 0-13-172394-4

Marcia L. London Marcia L. London has been able to combine her two greatest passions by being both a nurse caring for children and families, and a teacher for almost 35 years. She received her BSN and school nurse certificate from Plattsburgh State University in Plattsburgh, New York. After graduation, she began her nursing career as a pediatric nurse at St. Luke's Hospital in New York City. She then moved to Pittsburgh, where she began her teaching career. Mrs. London accepted a faculty position at Pittsburgh's Children's Hospital Affiliate Program and received her MSN in pediatrics as a clinical nurse specialist from the University of Pittsburgh. Mrs. London began teaching at Beth-El School of Nursing and Health Science in 1974 after opening the first intensive care nursery at Memorial Hospital of Colorado Springs. She has served in many administrative and faculty positions at Beth-El, including coordinator for nursing care of children for 32 years. Mrs. London maintains her clinical skills working in an urgent care and after-hours clinic and doing undergraduate pediatric clinical supervision. She obtained her postmaster's neonatal nurse practitioner certificate in 1983 and subsequently developed the neonatal nurse practitioner (NNP) program and the master's NNP program at Beth-El. She is active nationally in neonatal nursing and was involved in the development of the Neonatal Nurse Practitioner Educational Program Guidelines. She has contributed five chapters to various neonatal nursing texts. Mrs. London is active in nurse practitioner education in general. She was involved in the revision of the Core Competency for Nurse Practitioners and Curriculum Guidelines for Nurse Practitioner Education, as a member of the Education Committee of the National Organization of Nurse Practitioner Faculties and participated as part of the Core Competency Validation Expert Panel. Mrs. London has also pursued her interest in college student learning by taking doctoral classes in higher education administration and adult learning at the University of Denver in Colorado. She feels fortunate to be involved in the education of her future colleagues. Her teaching philosophy is that, with support, students can achieve more than they may initially believe they are capable of achieving. Mrs. London and her husband have two sons and one dog (Reilly, daughter by proxy). Her two sons, Craig and Matthew, are involved in computer informatics, and media arts and animation and are more than willing to give Mom helpful hints.

Patricia A. Wieland Ladewig Patricia A. Wieland Ladewig received her BS from the College of Saint Teresa in Winona, Minnesota. After graduation, she worked as a pediatric nurse before joining the U.S. Air Force. After completing her tour of duty, she relocated to Florida, where she accepted a faculty position at Florida State University. There she embraced teaching as her calling. Over the years, she taught at several schools of nursing while earning her MSN in maternal-newborn nursing from Catholic University of America in Washington, D.C., and her PhD in higher education administration from the University of Denver in Colorado. In addition, she became a women's health nurse practitioner and maintained a part-time clinical practice. In 1988 Dr. Ladewig became the first director of the nursing program at Regis College in Denver and, in 1991, when the college became Regis University, she became dean of the Rueckert-Hartman School for Health Professions. Under her guidance, the Department of Nursing has added a graduate program and the school has added three departments: the Department of Physical Therapy, the Department of Health Services Administration and Management, and the Department of Health Care Ethics. Dr. Ladewig feels that teaching others to be excellent, caring nurses gives her the best of all worlds because it keeps her in touch with the profession she loves and enables her to help shape the future of the nursing profession. When not at work or writing textbooks, Pat and her husband, Tim, enjoy skiing, baseball games, and traveling. However, their greatest pleasure comes from their family: son Ryan, his wife, Amanda, and grandson Reed, and son Erik, his wife, Kedri, and granddaughter Emma.

Jane W. Ball Jane W. Ball graduated from the Johns Hopkins Hospital School of Nursing, and subsequently received a BS from the Johns Hopkins University. She worked in the surgical, emergency, and outpatient units of the Johns Hopkins Children's Medical and Surgical Center, first as a staff nurse and then as a pediatric nurse practitioner. This began her career as a pediatric nurse and advocate for children's health needs. Jane obtained both a master of public health and doctor of public health degree from the Johns Hopkins University Bloomberg School of Public Health with a focus on maternal and child health. After graduation she became the chief of child health services for the Commonwealth of Pennsylvania Department of Health. In this capacity she oversaw the state-funded well-child clinics and explored ways to improve education for the state's community health nurses. After relocating to Texas, she joined the faculty at the University of Texas at Arlington School of Nursing to teach community pediatrics to registered nurses returning to school for a BSN. During this time she became involved in writing her first textbook, *Mosby's Guide to Physical Examination*, which is currently in its sixth edition. After relocating to the Washington, D.C., area, she joined Children's National Medical Center to manage a federal project to teach instructors of emergency medical technicians from all states about the special care children need during an emergency. Exposure to the shortcomings of the emergency medical services system in the late 1980s with regard to pediatric care was a career-changing event. With federal funding, she developed educational curricula for emergency medical technicians and emergency nurses to help them provide improved care for children. A textbook entitled *Pediatric Emergencies, A Manual for Prehospital Providers* was developed from these educational ventures. For the past 14 years, she has managed the federally funded Emergency Medical Services for Children National Resource Center. As executive director, Dr. Ball directs the provision of consultation and resource development for state health agencies, health professionals, families, and advocates about successful methods to improve the healthcare system so that children get optimal emergency care in all healthcare settings.

Ruth C. McGillis Bindler Ruth Bindler received her BSN from Cornell University–New York Hospital School of Nursing in New York. She worked in oncology nursing at Memorial–Sloan Kettering Cancer Center in New York, and then moved to Wisconsin and became a public health nurse in Dane County. Thus began her commitment to work with children as she visited children and their families at home, and served as a school nurse for several elementary, middle, and high schools. Due to this interest in child healthcare needs, she earned her MS in child development from the University of Wisconsin. A move to Washington State was accompanied by a new job as a faculty member at the Intercollegiate Center for Nursing Education in Spokane, Washington. Dr. Bindler has been fortunate to be involved for over 30 years in the growth of this nursing education consortium, which is a combination of public and private universities and colleges and is now the Washington State University/Intercollegiate College of Nursing. She has taught theory and clinical courses in child health nursing, cultural diversity and health, graduate research, pharmacology, and assessment, as well as serving as lead faculty for child health nursing. Her first professional book, *Pediatric Medications*, was published in 1981, and she has continued to publish articles and books in the areas of pediatric medications and pediatric health. Research efforts are focused in the area of childhood obesity, type 2 diabetes, and cardiovascular risk factors in children. Ethnic diversity has been another theme in her work. She facilitates international and other diversity experiences for students and performs research with culturally diverse children. Dr. Bindler believes that her role as a faculty member has enabled her to learn continually, to foster the development of students in nursing, and to participate fully in the profession of nursing. In addition to teaching, research, publication, and leadership, she enhances her life by service in several professional and community activities, and by activities with her family.

Thank You!

W e are grateful to all the nurses, both clinicians and educators, who reviewed the manuscript of this text. Their insights, suggestions, and eye for detail helped us prepare a more relevant and useful book, one that focuses on the essential components of learning in the fields of maternal, newborn, and child health nursing.

Joan P. Anderson, MA, RN,
Suffolk County Community College

Jane L. Andrews, RNC, MSN,
Shasta Community College

Margaret Batson, RNC, MSN,
San Joaquin Delta College

Ann L. Bianchi, RN, MSN,
Calhoun Community College

Mary Beth Bohli, MSN, RN,
Onondaga Community College

Diana Breed-Williamson, RN, MSN,
Mesa Community College

Brenda S. Broussard, RN, MSN, CNM, WHNP,
University of Louisiana at Lafayette College of Nursing

Nancy Danou, RN, CPN, MSN,
Viterbo University

Katherine Tate Dewar, RN, MN, PNP,
Ohlone College

Pamela DiNapoli, RN, PhD,
University of New Hampshire

Mary Dooley, RN, MSN, ANP,
Onondaga Community College

Eileen Drabik, RN, MS,
Orange County Community College

Anna M. Drazenovic, MSN, RN, FNP,
Mesa Community College

Cynthia A. Dyson, MSN, RN, BC,
Charleston Southern University

Patricia Eads, BSN, MS,
Ivy Tech Community College

Patricia H. Economidis, MS, ARNP-BC,
Lake-Sumter Community College

Sandra B. Englert, BS, MSN,
Niagara County Community College

Bonnie Ewing, PhD, RN,
Adelphi University

Lisa Fernandez, RNC, MS, OGNP, ANP,
Suffolk County Community College

Heather H. Finley, MSN, RN,
Grambling, LA

Alison Fisher, MSN, RN,
Del Mar College

Denise Flynn, BSN, RN,
Keiser College

Lisa Fraine, RN, CNM, MS,
Cedarcrest College

Betty Drake Freund, MSN, RN, BC,
Kent State University

Jean H. Gardeski, MA, BSN, RN,
Bergen Community College

Carolyn M. Garzone, RN, MSN, ANP,
Bergen Community College

Shari Gholson, MSN, RN,
West Kentucky Community and Technical College

Sharon K. Hammond, RN, MSN,
McLennan Community College

Cynthia Hatcher, MSN, RN,
San Antonio College

Ramona Hunter, BSN,
Rush University

Karen A. Joho, RN, MS, BC,
Union County College

Helen W. Jones, PhD, RN, APN, BC,
Raritan Valley Community College

Mary F. King, RN, MS,
Phillips Community College of the University of Arkansas

Amy Knepp, NP-C, MSN, RN,
University of St. Francis

Darcus M. Kottwitz, RN, MSN,
Fort Scott Community College

Christine King Kuoni, MSN, RN,
San Antonio College

Maxine Lesser, ARNP-C, MSN, SANE-A,
Daytona Beach Community College

Cherie A. Mavissakalian, RN, MS,
Niagara Community College

Deborah M. Miller, RN, MSN,
Calhoun Community College

Susan M. Miovech, PhD, RNC,
Holy Family University

Kathy Mix, RN, MS,
Linn Benton Community College

Mary Neville, MSN, RN,
San Joaquin Delta College

Jan Jones Nolan, MS, RN,
Tulsa Community College

Jennifer Ortiz, RNC, MSN,
Suffolk Community College

Brenda L. Overton, MSN, RN,
Baltimore City Community College

Gena Porter-Lankist, ARNP, MSN,
Chipola College

Jill A. Price, RN, MSN,
Waukesha County Technical College

Christine M. Rosner, RN, PhD,
Holy Family University

Karen S. Randall, RN, MS,
Ivy Tech Community College

Lori Riden, MSN, RN,
Gateway Community College

Zepure Samawi, RN, MSN,
Saint Xavier University

Sheryl Sandahl, MPH, CNP, RN,
College of St. Scholastica

June M. Sanders, RN, MSN,
Bristol Community College

Joanne Burgess Schnell, PhD,
State University of New York

Susan Parnell Scholtz, RN, DNSc,
Moravian College

Terri Klasko Snow, RN, MSN, CPNP,
Shasta College

Claudia Stoffel, RN, MSN,
West Kentucky Community and Technical College

Shari Stoops, MSN, RNC, FNP-C,
Del Mar College

Mary Tanner, PhD, RN,
College of St. Scholastica

Sharon K. Tighe, EdD, MN, RN-C, ARNP,
Daytona Beach Community College

Michelle Tippitt, RN, BSN, MSN,
Phillips Community College of the University
of Arkansas, University of Phoenix

Loretta Wack, RN, BSN, MSN,
Blue Ridge Community College

Cheryl M. Ward-Simons, BSN, MA,
Orange County Community College

Marcie Weissner, MSN, BNC,
University of St. Francis

Kathryn L. Whitley, MSN,
Patrick Henry Community College

Susan J. Wroten, RN, BSN, MSN,
Pima Community College

Mindy Yoder, APRN, BC,
University of St. Francis

Dedication

Throughout the ages, nurses have made a difference—treating, healing, soothing, and caring.
And so we dedicate this book to nurses—

> For their wisdom, expertise, and compassion
> For their willingness to challenge the system when necessary
> For their ability to remain strong during times of difficulty and stress
> And for their unfailing commitment to the families they assist.

And to nursing students everywhere—

> For seeking to serve others when so many have become self-serving
> For committing their minds and talents to a proud profession
> For accepting the challenges posed by the changes in healthcare
> And for daring to envision a brighter tomorrow.

Then, too, as always, we honor our beloved families—

> David London, Craig and Matthew
> Timothy Ladewig, Ryan, Amanda, and Reed, Erik, Kedri, and Emma
> Ronald Ball
> Julian Bindler, Dana and her fiancé, Brady, and Ross

Preface

Faculty and students in today's maternity and pediatric nursing courses face a wide variety of issues and challenges. Courses are growing increasingly shorter, and clinical experiences are more limited. Time truly is precious for both students and faculty. The primary goal in this edition is to present key content in an accurate, readable format that helps students and faculty focus on what's important and helps students develop the skills and abilities they need now and in the future in an ever-changing healthcare environment. This is done through the new Critical Concept Review feature at the end of each chapter, through the illustrations and photographs that clarify concepts more efficiently than words can do, and through the accompanying Student CD-ROM, which depicts clinical situations and requires students to engage in critical thinking. In its structure, format, and delivery, this text provides a concise look at maternal-newborn, women's health, and pediatric nursing.

ORGANIZATION

The organization of the text also reflects a time-saving approach. As educators and nurses, we know how difficult it is to teach everything that students need to learn in so little time. Consequently, we sought to reduce duplication in the text by carefully integrating maternity and pediatric nursing topics. For example, Chapter 1 begins with introductory concepts important for maternal, newborn, and child nursing, such as family-centered care, cultural considerations, health promotion, community and home care, and legal and ethical considerations, as well as emerging areas such as cord blood banking, the Human Genome Project, and stem cell research. Later chapters focus on reproductive issues and women's health, pregnancy, birth processes, postpartum care, and newborn management, and then transition into the pediatric care chapters. The pediatric chapters also cover general issues first, beginning with introductory concepts followed by two chapters, Chapters 37 and 38, on health promotion for children ranging from infancy to adolescence. Chapters 39 through 57 cover the nursing care of children with various disorders, organized by body system. Throughout the text we have eliminated potentially conflicting information.

Students may notice a "voice" change within chapters. For example, within theory-based sections, we use "the nurse." Within the nursing management sections, however, we speak to the students directly in second person, e.g., "Assess . . ." or "Manage. . . ." This way, students have a very clear understanding of their responsibilities and can put themselves in the role of the nurse more easily.

IMPORTANT THEMES IN THIS EDITION

Central to this edition are several key themes that are increasingly evident in nursing care of childbearing and childrearing families.

Family-Centered Nursing Care

Nursing care for pregnant women and children is a family-centered process. The underlying philosophy of *Maternal & Child Nursing Care* is simple: We believe that family members are co-participants in care, whether this is related to pregnancy and childbirth or to care of the infant or child at any stage of development. Families experience the excitement and exhilaration of welcoming a healthy infant into their home, but they also experience sorrow and concern when a health problem occurs. Nurses play a pivotal role in helping families celebrate the normal life processes associated with birth, in promoting the health of the family and child, and in fostering the child's growth and development from infancy through adolescence. We are committed to providing a text that integrates the needs of families across the continuum from conception through adolescence.

Health Promotion

In this textbook, we subscribe to the paradigm that all childbearing and childrearing families and children need health promotion and health maintenance interventions, no matter where they seek healthcare or what health conditions they may be experiencing. Families may visit offices or other community settings, specifically to obtain health supervision care. Nurses may also integrate health promotion and health maintenance into the care for childbearing and childrearing families and children with acute and chronic illness in a variety of inpatient and outpatient settings. This textbook integrates health promotion and health maintenance content throughout, most visibly in three new chapters: Chapter 4, "Health Promotion for Women," Chapter 37, "Health Promotion and Health Maintenance for the Infant and Young Child," and Chapter 38,

"Health Promotion and Health Maintenance for the Older Child and Adolescent."

In addition, a new feature entitled **Health Promotion** summarizes the needs of children with specific chronic conditions, such as asthma or diabetes. These overviews teach the student to look at the child with a chronic illness like any other child, with health maintenance needs for prevention, education, and basic care.

Nursing Care in the Community

Most maternity and pediatric nursing care occurs in the community setting, especially since most children and pregnant women are healthy and have only episodic acute health conditions. Even women with high-risk pregnancies and children with serious chronic health conditions are receiving more care in their homes and in the community. This textbook integrates community and home care throughout, including information on long-term management of complex health conditions, which are especially challenging to manage in community settings.

Four chapters provide a theoretical perspective and important tools in caring for childbearing and childrearing families in the community setting: Chapter 10, "Antepartal Nursing Assessment," Chapter 11, "The Expectant Family: Needs and Care," Chapter 32, "Home Care of the Postpartum Family," and Chapter 39, "Nursing Considerations for the Child and Family in the Community." In addition, **Nursing Care in the Community** is a special heading used throughout this text. Because we consider home care to be one form of community-based care, it often has a separate heading under Nursing Care in the Community sections of Nursing Management.

Client Education

 Client education remains a critical element of effective nursing care, one that we emphasize in this text. Nurses teach their clients during all stages of pregnancy and the childbearing process, and during the child's health visits and care for specific conditions. Throughout the book, we include **Teaching Highlights** that present a special healthcare issue or problem and the related key teaching points for care by the family.

Critical Thinking

 Today's nurses must be able to think critically and problem solve effectively. Nurses are often faced with managing care for multiple families with diverse healthcare needs, and working collaboratively with other health professionals to enhance care.

To promote the development of critical thinking skills that will support nurses in challenging situations, **Thinking Critically** boxes provide brief scenarios that ask students to determine the appropriate response. Students can test their own decision-making skills by submitting answers to these questions via the Companion Website, where the feature also appears. The instructor can then grade their answers using the suggested answers provided in the Instructor's Manual, which is replicated on the Instructor's Resource CD-ROM. Students can access a variety of critical thinking exercises and case studies on the textbook's Companion Website at www.prenhall.com/london.

Another feature that emphasizes these skills is the **Critical Thinking in Action** feature. This case study introduces a client situation at the end of each chapter and continues on the Student CD-ROM, where it comes to life with videos and images. Students benefit from experiencing the case on the CD-ROM as they decide what nursing actions are appropriate.

The Instructor's Resource Manual has more suggestions for critical thinking exercises for both the classroom and clinicals.

Research and Evidence-Based Nursing Practice

 Healthcare professionals are increasingly aware of the importance of using evidence-based approaches as the foundation for planning and providing effective care. The approach of evidence-based practice draws on information from a variety of sources, including nursing research. To help nurses become more comfortable integrating new knowledge into their nursing practice, a brief discussion of evidence based practice is included in Chapter 1.

A new feature entitled **Evidence-Based Nursing** further enhances the approach of using research to determine nursing actions. It describes a particular problem or clinical question and investigates the evidence that suggests solutions to the problem. In these features, we provide an interpretation explaining the implications of the studies and then invite the student to apply critical thinking skills to further identify nursing care approaches.

Cultural Competence

 The influence of a family's culture on health beliefs and healthcare practices cannot be underestimated. Chapter 1 briefly introduces cultural issues relevant to maternity and child nursing care. Additionally, we devote a new chapter entirely to culture, Chapter 2, "Culture and the Family."

We also emphasize cultural competence throughout the text. We highlight specific cultural issues and their application to nursing care in the **Developing Cultural Competence** features.

Other New or Expanded Concepts in This Edition

Many other important concepts are emphasized throughout this text:

- **Assessment** is an essential and core role in the nursing process. Several chapters are dedicated to helping the student perform an assessment at each stage along the pregnancy continuum, initially of the fetus and newborn, and later through the stages of childhood.

- **Communication** is one of the most important skills that students need to learn. Effective communication is the very fiber of nursing practice. This book integrates communication skills in an applied manner where students can most benefit. It is an essential part of the **Nursing Process** and **Teaching Highlights** boxes.

- **Ensuring appropriate nutrition** during pregnancy, infancy, and childhood is important to promote growth, development, and health. A growing national focus on healthy nutrition patterns underscores the importance of this information. Chapters 12, 29, and 34 address nutrition for pregnant women, newborns, and children.

- **Pain** is now considered the fifth vital sign, and pain management is a priority in healthcare settings. All of the chapters in Unit IV, *Birth and the Family,* address pain assessment and management, as do five of the chapters (23, 24, 25, 28, and 32) in Unit V, *The Postpartal Childbearing Family and Newborn.* In Unit VI, Chapters 35, 40, and 41 address pain assessment and management, and it is the primary subject in Chapter 42, "Pain Assessment and Management in Children." We discuss applicable pain management when appropriate in other chapters, including each of the chapters in Unit VII, *Caring for Children with Alterations in Health Status.*

- **End-of-life care** has gained greater national prominence. Expanded focus on the care of the family and the child who is dying has been added to Chapter 41, "The Child with a Life-Threatening Illness and End-of-Life Care." Grief and loss associated with miscarriage is addressed in Chapter 15, "Pregnancy at Risk: Gestational Onset" and in Chapter 21, "Childbirth at Risk."

TOOLS THAT FOCUS STUDENT REVIEW TO MAXIMIZE TIME

Instructors and students both value learning aids that unify the objectives and concepts of a chapter as well as reinforce the overall themes in a text. In keeping with our theme of family-centered care, each chapter begins with a **Family Quote** that helps set the stage for content that follows from the family's perspective. This is followed by a list of **Learning Objectives** (new to this edition) and **Key Terms**

with page numbers to identify the place where the term first appears in the chapter. An **Audio Glossary** of these terms commonly used in the field of maternal-newborn and child nursing can be found on the Student CD-ROM and the Companion Website, with audio pronunciations of the terms as well as printed definitions.

Critical Concept Review

In this new edition, we responded to instructors' and students' requests by providing more opportunities for review. Each chapter ends with a **Critical Concept Review**, a

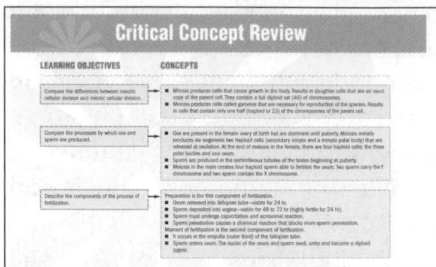

new feature designed to help students retain the most important concepts from a chapter in a short period of time. This visual tool isolates the essential content in a chapter by means of a flowchart that links **Learning Objectives** to their corresponding **Concepts**. Students save time by having the important concepts identified for them, allowing them to use more of their study time for reviewing the concepts themselves.

Critical Thinking in Action

Following the Critical Concept Review is a feature that challenges students to apply all concepts learned in that chapter. **Critical Thinking in Action** provides a real-life scenario with a series of critical thinking questions so that students can "practice" what they learned. To further enhance the true-to-life nature of the case study, the Student CD-ROM continues the exercise with a video enactment of the situation, followed by the critical thinking questions from the text as well as five short-answer questions. Not only can students review chapter content in an easy, quick-view format, but they can also apply the concepts used in preparation for clinical work.

EXPLORE MediaLink

EXPLORE MediaLink

The review section ends with a list of references and a section entitled EXPLORE MediaLink. This last section encourages students to use the additional chapter-specific NCLEX-RN® Review questions and other interactive exercises that appear on the accompanying Student CD-ROM and the Companion Website at www.prenhall.com/london. The MediaLink feature will further enhance the student's learning experience, build upon knowledge gained from this textbook, prepare students for the NCLEX-RN®, and foster critical thinking.

APPLICATION OF THE NURSING PROCESS

NURSING MANAGEMENT

The nursing process is emphasized throughout the nursing care chapters. The heading **Nursing Management** highlights nursing actions. In chapters with frequently seen or high-risk health issues or conditions, the expanded section on nursing management helps students understand and apply the nursing process more completely. The expanded section includes Nursing Assessment and Diagnosis, Planning and Implementation, and Evaluation.

In keeping with changing approaches to nursing care management, we feature **Nursing Care Plans** and **Clinical Pathways** throughout the text.

The **Nursing Care Plans** address nursing care for clients who have complications, such as a woman with preeclampsia or a child with otitis media. We designed this feature to help students approach care from the nursing process perspective. They integrate Nursing Diagnosis, Nursing Intervention Classifications (NIC), and Nursing Outcome Classifications (NOC). In this edition, we added 10 new Nursing Care Plans to help students better understand the conceptual approach that nurses employ in providing care for clients.

The **Clinical Pathways** describe nursing actions as they are integrated into care of other health professionals. They help students plan and manage care within normally anticipated time frames as the patient's health status improves. The plans and pathways help students become familiar with these two approaches to managing care so that they are better equipped for variations in clinical settings.

VISUALS THAT TEACH

The conviction that art can teach is evident throughout the book. There are hundreds of contemporary photographs of childbearing and childrearing families and children in healthcare and related settings throughout the textbook, as well as illustrations, all of which serve to display conditions, compare developmental stages, and depict concepts.

PATHOPHYSIOLOGY ILLUSTRATED

Pathophysiology Illustrated figures allow the student to see into the body and to visualize the causes and effects of conditions on childbearing women, newborns, and children. These unique drawings illustrate conditions on a cellular or organ level, and may also portray the step-by-step process of a disease. Drawings or photos with artistic overlays relate disease to its anatomic location and action.

AS CHILDREN GROW

As Children Grow illustrations help the student visualize the important anatomic and physiologic differences between a child and an adult. These features illustrate the important ways that a child's development influences healthcare needs and how the child progresses through developmental stages.

MORE FEATURES THAT HELP YOU USE THIS BOOK SUCCESSFULLY

On the foldout inside the front cover of this book, we show you how some of the features of the textbook and media can help you to be successful in this course. In addition, we offer the following features to further enhance the learning process and help you use this book successfully:

Nursing Practice features offer hands-on suggestions and clinical tips. These are placed at locations in the text that will help students apply them. They include topics such as legal and ethical considerations, nursing alerts, and home and community care considerations.

Complementary Care boxes present information about commonly used alternative and complementary measures to treat or provide comfort for various conditions.

Drug Guides for selected medications commonly used in maternal-newborn and child nursing guide students in correctly administering the medications and evaluating their actions. There are also tables of **Medications Used to Treat** certain health conditions, to provide an overview of the types of medications that can be used for a specific condition.

We highlight important **laboratory values** within the text as a tool for students to assess their patients' conditions—a critical precursor to determining appropriate nursing interventions. In addition, an appendix presents normal ranges for pregnant women, newborns, and children by age group.

Cross-reference icons ∞ help the student to easily locate related information in other chapters.

MEDIALINK Entry into practice application

MediaLink tabs with **CD-ROM** and **Skills** icons remind the student to use the Student CD-ROM or

Companion Website to find additional information or activities related to the concepts introduced on that page in the textbook. These resources enhance learning and provide an application beyond the textbook experience.

 Assessment Guides, found in the maternal-newborn chapters, assist students with diagnoses by incorporating physical assessment and normal findings, alterations and possible causes, as well as guidelines for nursing interventions.

 Clinical Manifestations tables help students understand the association between the pathophysiology and the signs and symptoms of a particular condition. In some cases, these tables present several similar conditions so that students can see the differentiation between conditions. In others, the tables include treatment for the clinical manifestations and conditions.

 Growth and Development boxes, found exclusively in the pediatric chapters, provide information about the different responses of children at various ages to health conditions.

MORE RESOURCES TO HELP YOU MANAGE YOUR TIME

To enhance the teaching and learning process, we developed the following resources to correlate with this textbook. The full complement of supplemental teaching materials is available to all qualified instructors from your Prentice Hall sales representative.

Student CD-ROM. Packaged with every copy of the textbook is a CD-ROM that includes many valuable learning supplements. Provided for each chapter are the following:

- *Objectives*—Learning goals are offered at the beginning of each chapter.

- *Audio Glossary*—The glossary reviews key terms from the textbook and presents correct pronunciation.

- *Nursing Skills Forms*—This feature provides step-by-step procedures and the rationales for specific actions for the care of pregnant women, newborns, and children.

- *NCLEX-RN® Review*—Written at the analysis and application levels, these questions emphasize the application of nursing care. Students can test their knowledge and gain immediate feedback through rationales for right and wrong answers.

- *Animations and Videos*—To help students understand and visualize difficult concepts, animations and videos appear where applicable.

- *Nursing in Action*—These brief video clips of real nurses and clients depict scenarios linked to chapter topics and are followed by questions to stimulate critical thinking.

- *Critical Thinking in Action*—Linked to the end-of-chapter Critical Thinking in Action feature in the text, these case studies are presented in video or graphic format, followed by questions that require the use of critical thinking skills.

- *Tools*—Resources to facilitate learning and aid in applying principles from the text are available for printing.

Companion Website and Syllabus Manager®. Faculty and students using this textbook may access the free Companion Website at www.prenhall.com/london. This Website serves as a text-specific, interactive online workbook for *Maternal & Child Nursing Care*. It includes modules for objectives, chapter outlines, an audio glossary with definitions, discussion questions with essay responses, research activities, NCLEX-RN® Review questions with automatic grading, links to other sites for student research and essay responses, additional nursing care plans and clinical pathways activities, and more. Instructors adopting this textbook for their courses have access to an online Syllabus Manager with a whole host of features that facilitate the students' use of this Companion Website as assigned homework and allow faculty to post their syllabi online for their students. For more information or a demonstration of Syllabus Manager, please contact your Prentice Hall sales representative.

Clinical Skills Manual. Also available is the *Clinical Skills Manual*, which describes a more comprehensive set of commonly performed maternal, newborn, women's health, and pediatric nursing skills. This colorful and highly visual manual clearly depicts the steps required to perform each skill and is formatted for easy use in the clinical setting. It includes both hospital-based and community-based skills. Marginal boxes emphasize material such as clinical tips and safety considerations. The protocols for performing skills contain rationales when needed to clarify recommended actions.

Instructor's Resource Manual. This effective teaching aid guides instructors on how to use *Maternal & Child Nursing Care* for their courses. It includes lecture suggestions, objectives, test questions, answers to the textbook's Thinking Critically exercises, a guide to the PowerPoint images and animations on the Instructor's Resource CD-ROM, and a guide to using the Companion Website and Syllabus Manager. Finally, it includes a test bank of items that follow the NCLEX-RN® format and are classified by cognitive level, nursing process step, and client needs.

Instructor's Resource CD-ROM. This CD-ROM has everything instructors need for classroom preparation. For each learning objective, it offers correlating lecture notes, numbered PowerPoint slides, and suggestions for classroom and clinical activities. With more than 100 animations and videos, the Instructor's Resource CD-ROM enables instructors to view and select resources to show in the classroom. Each chapter gives an overview of the homework to assign on the Student CD-ROM and the Companion Website. The Instructor's Resource CD-ROM also provides chapter-specific, integrated PowerPoint presentations with more than 2100 text slides and 1000 image slides all ready to go and integrated in the classroom.

Online Course Management Systems. Also added to this package are online course companions available for schools using Blackboard, WebCT, or Course Compass course management systems. For more information about adopting an online course management system to accompany *Maternal & Child Nursing Care*, please contact your Prentice Hall Health sales representative or go online to www.prenhall.com/demo.

Nursing is facing many new challenges: an ongoing nursing shortage, dramatic advances in healthcare knowledge, and natural and man-made disasters that create a critical need for skilled nurses. We believe that nursing is becoming reenergized, and is facing these issues and challenges with enthusiasm and commitment. Many people feel a strong desire to choose professions that make a difference—professions such as nursing. We, like you, know that expert nurses can have a tremendous impact on the lives of childbearing and childrearing families. Our goal in writing this text is to help prepare nurses with the skills and knowledge to make a difference—one family at a time.

Marcia L. London
Patricia W. Ladewig
Jane W. Ball
Ruth C. Bindler

Acknowledgments

Nursing is a dynamic, exciting healthcare profession. As curricula develop, many nursing programs have begun to offer nursing of childbearing families and nursing of children together in a single course. This combined format requires that faculty approach these two fields with a similar framework and philosophy, and with similar teaching methods, so that students can maximize learning. With this second edition, we have created a tool that will enable students to master these two critical areas of nursing—the care of childbearing families and the care of children. Creating a dynamic and integrated text would not be possible without the skill and dedication of a host of people.

We wish to acknowledge the contributions to the Complementary Care features in the textbook and on the Companion Website. These individuals brought their specialized knowledge to the project:

Faye Bailey, RN, BSN, C, CIMI
Carol Baldwin, PhD, RN, HNC
Karen Fontaine, RN, MSN, AASECT
Lynette Leeseberg Stamler, RN, PhD
Marilyn Joy Leeseberg, BA, MMT
Karen C. Haack, BMtrs
Sylvia M. Kubsch, RN, PhD
Geralyn Jadin, RN, BSN, C
Nicette Julevics, MC, ICCE
Kathryn Landon-Malone, PNP
John D. Mark, MD
Sunny Pendleton Mayor, BS
Suzi Cekarmis Schoon, DNS, RN
Ilene Spector, DO
Maria Luisa Urdaneta, RN, PhD
Sherry Warden, PhD, RN
Beverly Yates, ND

Claudia Stoffel, MSN, RN, contributed one of the pivotal features in the text, the Learning Outcomes and Concepts in the **Critical Concept Review**. Wendy Bowles, MSN, CPNP, and Joyce Stehle, RN, MSN, contributed the cutting-edge **Critical Thinking in Action** features that are also at the end of every chapter. Thank you, Claudia, Wendy, and Joyce, for creating such valuable tools for student success! For their reviews and suggestions to the Critical Thinking in Action vignettes on the Student CD-ROM, we wish to acknowledge the work done by Michael D. Aldridge, MSN, RN, CCRN, CNS, from the University of Texas at Austin, and Ann Bianchi, RN, MSN, ICCE, ICD, from Calhoun Community College.

We wish to express gratitude to the following individuals who contributed to the CD-ROM and Companion Website:

Marcia Gasper, RNC, MSN, EdD
East Stroudsburg University, East Stroudsburg, Pennsylvania

Rebecca Gesler, MSN, RN
Spalding University, Louisville, Kentucky

Susan M. Miovech, PhD, RNC
Holy Family University, Philadelphia, Pennsylvania

LaDonna Northington, DNS, RN, BC, CCRN
University of Mississippi, Jackson, Mississippi

Robin Wilkerson, PhD, RN
University of Mississippi, Jackson, Mississippi

We also wish to acknowledge the authors of the Instructor's Resource Manual:

Michael D. Aldridge, MSN, RN, CCRN, CNS
University of Texas at Austin

Mary Dowell, PhD
University of Mary Hardin–Baylor

Bernadette Dragich, PhD, APRN, BC
Bluefield State College

Yvette Rolle, MSN
Houston Community College

We would personally like to thank several people. At Prentice Hall, Maura Connor, editor-in-chief, first envisioned and supported the need for this textbook. Her creative, visionary enthusiasm is outstanding. This edition has been guided by Pamela Lappies, the new nursing editor, who merits our deepest thanks. She has been open, enthusiastic, and dedicated; she is always receptive to our ideas and encourages our development as authors. Our thanks also go to Julie Levin Alexander, our publisher. Julie is committed to excellence and creativity. She is the driving force behind the exciting changes occurring at Prentice Hall Health and is truly a creative futurist in publishing. We also wish to thank Maria Guglielmo, art director, for the striking design of the text; Nick Radhuber, production editor, for his calm coordination of the production of the manuscript; Danielle Doller, associate editor, for her carefully orchestrated work on the supplements; and Joanna Satkowitz, editorial assistant, for helping with the myriad details involved in preparing a manuscript of this size.

Operationally, this book exists in large part because of the tremendous dedication, patience, and skill of our developmental editor, Elena Mauceri. During the long months of hard work, Elena remained calm, focused, organized, and creative. She noted discrepancies, worked for continuity, pitched in everywhere, and earned the respect of all of us. She is truly amazing and we hope to work with her on future projects.

Special thanks to the people of Carlisle Communications, especially Lynn Steines, for coordinating production, and Joan Lyon, for her work as copyeditor. They are perceptive, organized, and skillful in all of the tasks of publishing.

Finally we all wish to thank our other co-authors. As four individuals, but two teams, we came together with our own ideas, writing styles, and vision for this book. We collaborated, argued, cajoled, and compromised. It was a challenging but rewarding process. Together we created a new and different text for maternal, newborn, and child health nursing, a book and associated learning aids that we hope will be a useful tool for legions of nursing students to come.

Marcia L. London
Patricia W. Ladewig
Jane W. Ball
Ruth C. Bindler

Special Features

DEVELOPING CULTURAL COMPETENCE

DRUG GUIDE

EVIDENCE-BASED NURSING

GROWTH AND DEVELOPMENT

THINKING CRITICALLY

Detailed Contents

UNIT IV
BIRTH AND THE FAMILY 393

UNIT V
THE POSTPARTAL CHILDBEARING FAMILY AND NEWBORN 565

UNIT VI
CARE AND NEEDS OF CHILDREN 887

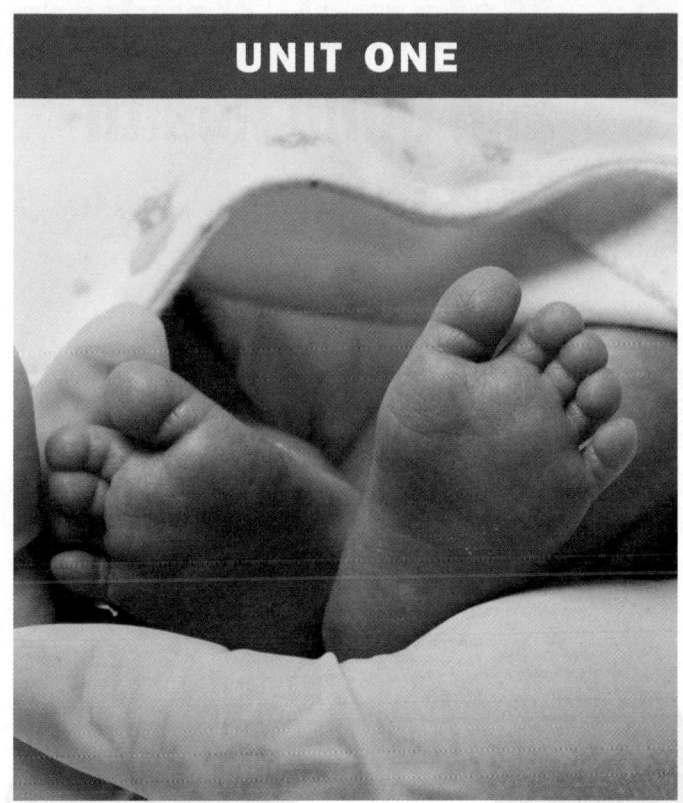

UNIT ONE

Family-Centered Care: Introductory Concepts

CHAPTER 1

Maternal, Newborn, and Child Health Nursing

My younger son turned 21 today—officially a man now. I remember so well the night he was born in a birthing room at our local hospital. I watched my husband rock our baby and talk to him just minutes after his birth. Over the years we sought emergency healthcare for our son several times—when he was diagnosed with asthma as a high school freshman, when he fell skateboarding and needed surgery to put three pins in his wrist, when he fell snowboarding and dislocated his shoulder. Active kids do get their share of bumps! It is easy to take good healthcare for granted, but we shouldn't. It can make all the difference.

—Marjorie, 47

LEARNING OBJECTIVES

- Identify the nursing roles available to maternal-newborn and pediatric nurses.

- Summarize the use of community-based nursing care in meeting the needs of childbearing and childrearing families.

- Summarize the current status of factors related to health insurance and access to healthcare.

- Define the following statistical terms relevant to healthcare: birth rate, infant mortality rate, neonatal mortality rate, and maternal mortality rate.

- Identify the goals for client safety developed by the Joint Commission on the Accreditation of Healthcare Organizations (JCAHO).

- Delineate significant legal and ethical issues that influence the practice of maternal-child nursing.

- Discuss the role of evidence-based practice in improving the quality of nursing care for childbearing families.

MEDIALINK

www.prenhall.com/london

CD-ROM
NCLEX-RN® Review

Companion Website
Audio Glossary
NCLEX-RN® Review
Case Study: Cord Blood Banking

S killed nurses care for people, care about people, and use their expertise to help people care for themselves. This is the essence of nursing. Most nurses experience special moments professionally, times in which they know that they have practiced the essence of nursing and, in doing so, have touched the lives of others. For nurses who work with childbearing families or with children and their families, the rewards that come from skilled nursing practice can be especially rich.

This chapter focuses on introductory concepts related to the nurse and childbearing families, infants, children, and adolescents.

NURSING ROLES IN MATERNAL-CHILD NURSING

Traditionally, **maternal-child nursing** refers to the care of women during pregnancy, birth, and postpartum, as well as the care of infants, children, and adolescents. However, this label is somewhat misleading because it fails to acknowledge clearly the consideration due to fathers, partners, and family members. As nurses who work with families quickly learn, a holistic, inclusive approach is crucial to effective nursing care.

The nursing process provides the framework for delivery of direct nursing care. The nurse assesses the client—whether childbearing woman, infant, child, or adolescent—and identifies the nursing diagnoses that describe the responses of the individual and family to the illness or injury. The nurse then implements and evaluates nursing care. This care is designed to meet specific physical and psychosocial needs. For children the care is tailored to the individual developmental stage, giving the child additional responsibility for self-care with increasing age.

Nurses play a major role in minimizing the psychologic and physical distress experienced by childbearing families and by children and their families. This often involves listening to concerns, being present during stressful or emotional experiences, and implementing strategies to help the individual and family members cope. Nurses can help families by suggesting ways to support their loved one in the hospital, in community settings, and in the home. Nurses also suggest ways to support families with informational resources, family support groups, referral for healthcare services, and, in some cases, respite care.

Client education is a major component of maternal child nursing. During pregnancy, nurses provide anticipatory guidance to prepare the woman and her partner, if he or she is involved, for the changes that each month brings. For example, the woman is taught self-care measures to relieve discomforts and learns to identify the warning signs that she should report. Both partners receive information on the psychologic changes of pregnancy that they may experience. Education for the laboring woman focuses on activities that help her deal successfully with a challenging experience—childbirth—whereas postpartum teaching addresses the needs of the woman and her newborn to prepare them for discharge.

In pediatric nursing, education is especially challenging because nurses must be prepared to work with children at various levels of understanding and to include family members in all aspects of care. As client educators, nurses help children adapt to the hospital setting and prepare them for procedures.

When a child is ill, most hospitals encourage a parent to stay with the child and to provide much of the direct and the supportive care. Nurses teach parents to watch for important signs and responses to therapies, to increase the child's comfort, and even to provide advanced care. Taking an active role during hospitalization helps prepare the parent to assume total responsibility for care after the child leaves the hospital. See "Developing

Cultural Competence" for guidelines about assessing and writing client education materials.

DEVELOPING CULTURAL COMPETENCE

LOWERING THE READING LEVEL OF CLIENT EDUCATION MATERIALS

Almost 25% of the adult population in the United States and Canada is functionally illiterate. Printed information to educate children and families about a health condition might be readily available, but they often are written at an 11th- or 12th-grade level. Most Internet consumer education information is written at a 10th-grade level. You need to evaluate each resource to determine the reading level before giving it to your client and his or her family. The average adult in the United States cannot read above an 8th-grade level, and Medicaid enrollees generally read at a 5th-grade level (Winslow, 2001). In addition the materials need to be evaluated for cultural appropriateness. Just because printed material may be available in the primary language of the client and family, do not assume that the family has reading skills in that language. The following are some tips for developing client education material with a lower reading level:

- Use short, familiar words with one or two syllables.
- Substitute simple language that defines a medical term rather than using the term.
- Use short sentences.
- Use active voice rather than passive voice.
- Use numerals rather than spelling out the number.

Nurses also serve as advocates, acting to safeguard and advance the interests of families. To be an effective advocate, the nurse must be aware of the individual's needs, the family's needs and resources, and the healthcare services available in the hospital and the community. The nurse can then assist the family to make informed choices about these services and to act in their best interests. Nurses must also ensure that the policies and resources of healthcare agencies meet the psychosocial needs of childbearing women and of children and their families.

Collaborative practice is a comprehensive model of healthcare that uses a multidisciplinary team of health professionals to provide high-quality, cost-effective care. In maternal-newborn settings the team generally includes certified nurse-midwives (see later discussion), physicians, nurse practitioners, nurses, and other health specialists such as pharmacists, lactation consultants, or childbirth educators. Similarly, the multidisciplinary team assembled when a child has a significant health problem or handicapping condition may include physicians, nurses, social workers, physical and occupational therapists, and other specialists. Their goal is to create an interdisciplinary plan designed to meet the child's medical, nursing, developmental, educational, and psychoso-

cial needs. Because nurses spend large amounts of time providing nursing care for the client and family, they often are better informed than other healthcare professionals about the family's wishes and resources. As a member of the team, the nurse serves as an advocate to ensure that the plan of care considers the family's wishes and contains appropriate services.

Case management is a process of coordinating the delivery of healthcare services in a manner that focuses on both quality and cost outcomes. This is often a collaborative practice with other healthcare providers designed to promote continuity of care. The nurse case manager has control over the use of healthcare resources that are considered appropriate for the client's condition and links the client and family to these services. The goal is to help the individual and family have the best healthcare outcome and decrease fragmentation of care, while controlling the cost of healthcare services. In maternal-child nursing, case management is often used for a complicated high-risk pregnancy, for the care of a hospitalized child, and for long-term care of chronic conditions.

Discharge planning is a form of case management. Effective discharge planning promotes a smooth, rapid, and safe transition into the community and improves the results of treatment begun in the hospital. To be a discharge planner, the nurse needs to know about community medical resources, appropriate home care agencies, educational interventions, and services reimbursed by the individual's health plan or other financial resources.

In addition, several advanced-practice roles are available to maternal-child nurses with additional education. *Nurse practitioners (NPs),* who have specialized education in a master's degree program or a certificate program, often provide ambulatory care services to pregnant women, newborns, children, adolescents, and families. NPs focus on physical and psychosocial assessments, including history, physical examination, and certain diagnostic tests and procedures. They make clinical judgments and begin appropriate treatments, seeking physician consultation when necessary. *Clinical nurse specialists (CNSs)* have a master's degree and specialized knowledge and competence in a specific clinical area. They often are found on mother-baby units, on pediatric units, and in intensive care units assisting staff to provide excellent, evidence-based care. The **certified nurse-midwife (CNM)** is educated in the two disciplines of nursing and midwifery and is certified by the American College of Nurse-Midwives. The CNM is prepared to manage independently the care of women at low risk for complications during pregnancy, birth, and the postpartum period, as well as the care of healthy newborns (Figure 1–1).

FAMILY-CENTERED MATERNAL-CHILD CARE

Contemporary childbirth is family centered—that is, characterized by an emphasis on the family and the family's choices

◉ FIGURE 1–1

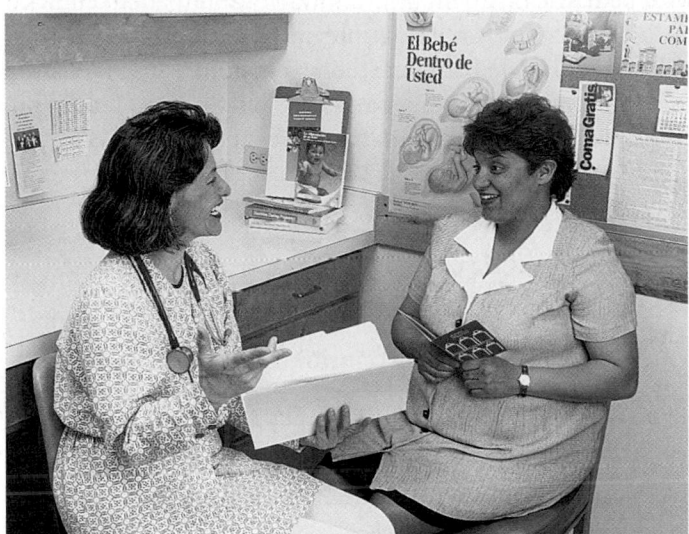

A certified nurse-midwife confers with her client.

about their birth experience. Consequently, today the concept of family-centered childbirth is accepted and encouraged. Fathers and partners are active participants, not simply bystanders; siblings are encouraged to visit and meet the newest family member, and they may even attend the birth.

New definitions of family are evolving. For example, the family of a single mother may include her mother, her sister, another relative, a close friend, a lesbian partner, or the father of the child. Many cultures also recognize the importance of extended families, and several family members may provide care and support.

The family can make choices about the place of birth (hospital, birthing center, or home), the primary caregiver (physician, CNM, or even lay midwife), the approaches to childbirth (Lamaze, Bradley, and so forth), and birth-related experiences (position for birth, use of analgesia and anesthesia, and methods of childbirth preparation, for example) as well as breastfeeding and childcare choices.

In pediatric settings, *family-centered care* is designed to meet the emotional, social, and developmental needs of children and families seeking healthcare. The importance of the family in helping the child recover from illnesses and injuries is recognized. Families are considered partners in the child's care, learning about the child's condition and participating in decisions regarding the child's care. Thus families gain greater confidence and competence in caring for their children, which has become even more important as families play an ever-increasing role in providing care for children's healthcare problems. The key elements of family-centered care are provided in Table 1–1.

TABLE 1–1 ⁜ Elements of Family-Centered Care

Elements

The family at the center: Incorporate into policy and practice the recognition that the family is the constant in a child's life, while the service systems and support personnel within those systems fluctuate, and that the illness or injury of a child affects all members of the family system.

Family-professional collaboration: Facilitate family-professional collaboration at all levels of hospital, home, and community care for:
Care of an individual child
Program development, implementation, evaluation, and evolution
Policy formation

Family-professional communication: Exchange complete and unbiased information between families and professionals in a supportive manner at all times.

Cultural diversity of families: Incorporate into policy and practice the recognition and honoring of cultural diversity, strengths, and individuality within and across all families, including ethnic, racial, spiritual, social, economic, educational, and geographic diversity.

Coping differences and support: Recognize and respect different methods of coping and implementing comprehensive policies and programs that provide families with the developmental, educational, emotional, spiritual, environmental, and financial supports needed to meet their diverse needs.

Family-centered peer support: Encourage and facilitate family-to-family support and networking.

Specialized service and support systems: Ensure that hospital, home, and community service and support systems for children needing specialized health and developmental care and their families are flexible, accessible, and comprehensive in responding to diverse family-identified needs.

Holistic perspective of family-centered care: Appreciate families as families and children as children, recognizing that they possess a wide range of strengths, concerns, emotions, and aspirations beyond their need for specialized health and developmental services and support.

Used with permission from Lewandowski, L. A., & Tesler, M. D. (Eds.). (2003). Family-centered care: Putting it into action. *The SPN/ANA Guide to Family-Centered Care.* Washington, DC: American Nurses Association.

CONTEMPORARY CHILDBIRTH

In the early 1990s, women who gave birth vaginally remained in the hospital for about 3 days. This provided time for nurses to assess the family's knowledge and skill and to complete essential teaching. In the late 1990s, in an effort to control costs, discharge within 12 to 24 hours after birth became the norm. This practice did not necessarily cause problems for women with supportive families, thorough prenatal preparation, and adequate resources for necessary follow-up care. However, because early discharge severely limits the time available for client teaching, women with little knowledge, experience, or support were often inadequately prepared to care for themselves and their newborn infants. Fortunately, the negative impact of this practice gained recognition nationwide and resulted in legislation that provides for a postpartum stay of up to 48 hours following a vaginal birth and up to 96 hours following a cesarean birth at the discretion of the mother and her healthcare provider.

The place of birth is an important decision. As discussed in Chapter 8, ∞ birthing centers and special "homelike" labor-delivery-recovery-postpartum (LDRP) rooms in hospitals have become increasingly popular. Some women choose to give birth at home, although healthcare professionals do not generally recommend this approach. Most professionals are concerned that, in the event of an unanticipated complication, delay in receiving emergency care might jeopardize the well-being or even the life of the mother or her infant. Consequently, the majority of home births are attended by direct-entry midwives (lay midwives) who are not RNs. In the past, training as a lay midwife followed an apprenticeship model, with a more senior midwife teaching a younger one. Today only a few midwives gain their training in that way. Many more women are choosing to complete a direct-entry midwifery education program and may take a certification exam to become a *certified midwife (CM)*. Accreditation for both CNMs and CMs is offered through the American College of Nurse-Midwives (Camacho, 2003).

CONTEMPORARY CARE OF CHILDREN

More than 79.4 million children age 19 years or younger live in the United States. They account for 28% of the population (U.S. Census Bureau, 2003). At one time children were valued primarily as laborers. Over the past century, however, the unique needs and qualities of children have been recognized. In today's society, children are considered to have special value; they are vulnerable and need protection.

Pediatric nursing is a specialized area of nursing that focuses on caring for children. Pediatric nurses function in many different settings. Within the hospital, acute care may be provided in the emergency department, observation or short-stay unit, post-anesthesia unit, intensive care unit, general pediatric inpatient unit, and various outpatient clinics.

The hospital stay is now integrated into a continuum that allows children to complete therapy at home, at school, or in other community settings. Pediatric nurses assist families in making the transition from the acute hospital setting to

- The home, for a short recuperation or long-term management.
- A rehabilitation center or long-term care hospital.
- A nurse-managed home care or hospice program.

Managing the child's transition from acute care to another setting involves planning the discharge, implementing interdisciplinary plans, ensuring that the family understands the aspects of care they need to provide, helping the family to develop an emergency care plan in the event their child has an unexpected healthcare crisis, and collaborating with a broad range of healthcare professionals.

Pediatric nurses also work in several other healthcare settings, including the following:

- In *pediatricians' offices* and health centers, nurses assess children, provide telephone counseling, and support and counsel families about growth and development and nutrition.
- In *clinic settings,* nurses assess children, assist with medical procedures, provide nursing care, and educate families to ensure the continuous management of the child's healthcare problem (Figure 1–2 ●).
- In *home health agencies,* nurses provide home care to children with acute and chronic conditions. Children may need medical treatment and nursing care for

● **FIGURE 1–2**

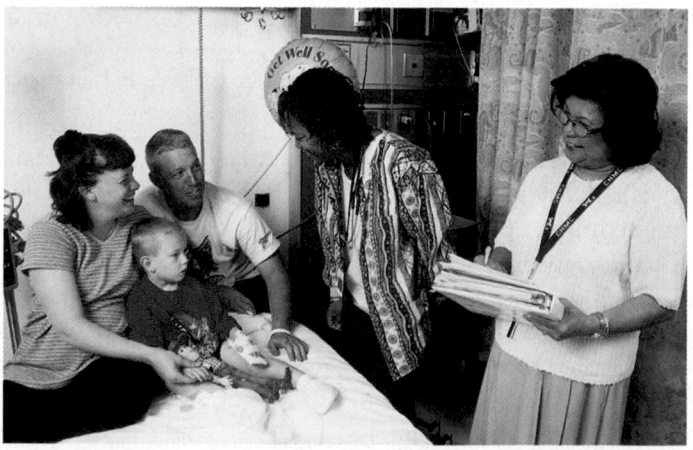

Children need to be involved actively in decisions regarding their care when appropriate. Here, the family and staff come together to discuss the child's care in a positive and honest manner.

acute, self-limited, chronic, and terminal conditions. Care may involve visits for specific interventions such as medication administration or "private duty" care (one-on-one nursing care).

■ In *rehabilitation centers,* nurses provide inpatient and ambulatory care to help restore children to an optimal state and plan for discharge management of chronic conditions.

■ In *schools,* nurses assess children, monitor their health status, and provide health education to teachers and children. Many children who are assisted by technology or have chronic conditions attend school as required by the Individuals with Disabilities Education Act (IDEA). Individual school health plans are developed, implemented, and evaluated by the school nurse.

MATERNAL-CHILD CARE IN THE COMMUNITY

Primary care is the focus of much attention as caregivers search for a new, more effective direction for healthcare. Primary care includes a focus on health promotion, illness prevention, and individual responsibility for one's own health. These services are best provided in community-based settings. Third-party payers and managed care organizations are beginning to recognize the importance of primary care in containing costs and maintaining health. Community-based healthcare systems providing primary care and some secondary care are becoming available in schools, workplaces, homes, churches, clinics, transitional care programs, and other ambulatory settings.

The growth and diversity of managed care plans offer both opportunities and challenges for women's and children's healthcare. The potential exists for managed care organizations to work with consumers to provide a model for coordinated and comprehensive well-woman and well-child care that includes improved delivery of screening and preventive services. One challenge that managed care organizations face is how to relate to essential community providers of care, such as family-planning clinics, women's health centers, and well-child centers that offer a unique service or serve groups of women and children with special needs (adolescents, women and children with disabilities, and ethnic or racial minorities).

Community-based care remains an essential element of healthcare for uninsured or underinsured individuals, as well as for individuals who benefit from programs such as Medicare, Medicaid, or state-sponsored health-related programs. Whereas some of these programs, such as those offered through public health departments, are broad based, others, such as parenting classes for adolescents, are geared to the needs of a specific population.

Community-based care is also part of a trend initiated by consumers, who are asking for a seamless system of family-centered, comprehensive, coordinated healthcare, health education, and social services. This seamless system requires coordination as clients move from primary care services to acute care facilities and then back into the community. Nurses can assume this care management role and perform an important service for individuals and families.

Maternal-child nurses are especially sensitive to these changes in healthcare delivery because the vast majority of healthcare provided to childbearing and childrearing families takes place outside of hospitals in clinics, offices, and community-based organizations. In addition, maternal-child nurses offer specialized services such as childbirth preparation classes, sibling classes, and parenting classes.

Home Care

Providing healthcare in the home is an especially important dimension of community-based nursing care. Shorter hospital stays end in the discharge of individuals who still require support, assistance, and teaching. Home care helps fill this gap. Home care also enables infants, children, and women to remain at home with conditions that formerly would have required hospitalization.

Nurses are major providers of home care services. Home care nurses perform direct nursing care and also supervise unlicensed assistive personnel who provide less skilled levels of service. In a home setting, nurses use their skills in assessment, intervention, communication, teaching, problem solving, and organization to meet the needs of childbearing and childrearing families. They also play a major role in coordinating services from other providers, such as physical therapists or lactation consultants.

Postpartum and newborn home visits help ensure a satisfactory transition from the birthing center to the home. This trend is a positive method of meeting the needs of childbearing families and hopefully will become standard practice. See Chapter 32 ∞ for discussion of home care and guidance about making a home visit. Information on home care is also provided as appropriate throughout this text.

Many children with severe chronic illnesses can be treated at home rather than by continued hospitalization. After studies in the 1980s found that home healthcare was substantially less expensive than hospital care, Congress amended laws to permit payment of home care services with federal funds, such as through Medicaid. In 1998 more than 400,000 children under 18 years were discharged by hospitals to a home care program. Nearly 300,000 of these were children under 6 years of age (National Center for Health Statistics, 2004). Some families have regained control over their lives by creating intensive care units in their homes. Children with conditions considered fatal 10 years ago are thriving with home care and are participating in family, community, and school life.

COMPLEMENTARY THERAPIES

Interest in complementary and alternative medicine (CAM) therapies continues to grow nationwide and affects the care of childbearing and childrearing families. CAM includes a wide array of therapies, such as acupuncture, acupressure, therapeutic touch, biofeedback, massage therapy, meditation, herbal therapies, and homeopathic remedies. Concepts related to the use of CAM by families are presented in more detail in Chapter 2 ∞ and in special boxed features throughout the text.

ACCESS TO HEALTHCARE

In the year 2002, healthcare expenditures in the United States were $1.6 trillion, a 9.3% increase over the previous year. The healthcare share of the gross domestic product (GDP) was 14.9%, a significant increase over previous years (Cowan, Catlin, Smith et al., 2004). Despite this increase in spending, however, not all pregnant women and children in the United States have access to healthcare. In 2003, 15.6% of the population (45 million people) were

without health insurance. For people living in poverty, Medicaid is the most prevalent form of insurance, covering 12.4% of people (35.6 million), including pregnant women who fall into specified income categories (DeNavas-Walt, Proctor, & Mills, 2004).

For women who become pregnant, early prenatal care is one of the most important approaches available to reduce adverse pregnancy outcomes. In 2002, 83.4% of pregnant women in the United States began prenatal care in the first trimester. However, these percentages vary significantly among groups, with black, Hispanic, and Native American women less likely to receive early and adequate prenatal care than white and Asian women (National Center for Health Statistics, 2004).

In 2003, 8.4 million children, 11.4% of all those below 18 years of age, had no health insurance. Not surprisingly, children living in poverty were more likely to be uninsured (19.2%) than the general population of children (DeNavas-Walt et al. 2004). See Figure 1–3 ◉. Most of these children had difficulty obtaining the most basic preventive healthcare, including immunizations.

Efforts to provide universal access to healthcare for children continue to grow. Congress passed legislation to create the State Children's Health Insurance Program (SCHIP) in 1997 to enable more children to obtain access to essential healthcare services. States are allocated federal funds to encourage enrollment of children living with families whose income is up to 200% of the federal poverty level (Smith, Wise, Chavkin et al., 2000). Children enrolled must be provided with health benefits coverage that is substantially equal to the benefits coverage in the federal or state employee benefits plan or the plan of the largest health maintenance organization in the state. As of the end of September 2002, 5.3 million children were enrolled (Centers for Medicare and Medicaid Services, 2003). Many pregnant adolescents are also served in these state programs.

CULTURALLY COMPETENT CARE

The population of the United States daily becomes more diverse. Currently over one third of all children less than 20 years of age are from families of minority populations. Thus, it is vitally important that a nurse who cares for women and for children recognizes the importance of a family's cultural values and beliefs, which may be quite different from those of the nurse.

Specific elements that contribute to a family's value system include the following:

- Religion and social beliefs
- Presence and influence of the extended family, as well as socialization within the ethnic group
- Communication patterns

◉ **FIGURE 1–3**

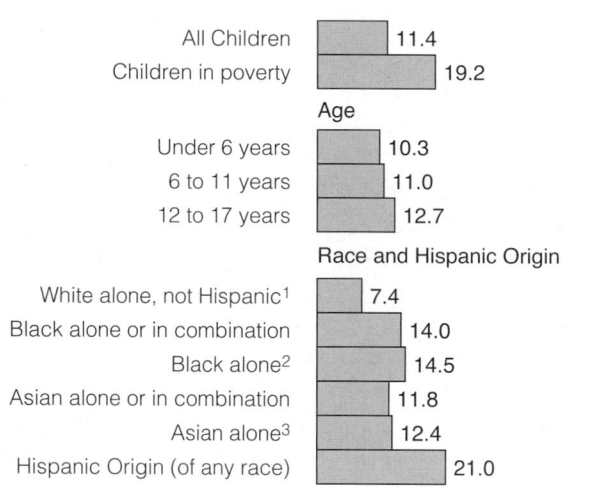

¹ The 2003 CPS asked respondents to choose one or more races. White alone refers to people who reported White and did not report any other race. The use of this single-race population does not imply that it is the preferred method of presenting or analyzing data. The Census Bureau uses a variety of approaches. More than one race was reported for about 4% of children in Census 2000.
² Black alone refers to people who reported Black and did not report any other race category.
³ Asian alone refers to people who reported Asian and did not report any other race category.
Note: For discussion of statistically significant differences between groups, see text.
Source: U.S. Census Bureau, Current Population Survey, 2004 Annual Social and Economic Supplement.

Uninsured children by race, Hispanic origin, and age: 2003.

Courtesy of DeNavas-Walt, C., Proctor, B. D., & Mills, R. J. (2004). Income, poverty, and health insurance coverage in the United States: 2003. Washington, DC: U.S. Census Bureau.

- Beliefs and understanding about the concepts of health and illness
- Permissible physical contact with strangers
- Education

DEVELOPING CULTURAL COMPETENCE

CULTURAL CONFLICTS

Conflicts can occur within a family when traditional rituals and practices of the family's elders do not conform with current healthcare practices. Nurses need to be sensitive to the potential implications for the child's healthcare, especially after the child is discharged from the hospital. When cultural values are not part of the nursing care plan, parents may be forced to decide whether the family's beliefs should take priority over the healthcare professional's guidance.

When the family's cultural values are incorporated into the care plan, the family is more likely to accept and comply with the needed care, especially in the home care setting. It is important for nurses to avoid imposing personal cultural values on the families and children in their care. By learning about the values of the different ethnic groups in the community—their religious beliefs that have an impact on healthcare practices, their beliefs about common illnesses, and their specific healing practices—nurses can develop an individualized nursing care plan for each child and family.

Because of the importance of culturally competent care, this topic is discussed in more depth in Chapter 2 ∞ and throughout the book as well.

STATISTICAL DATA AND MATERNAL-CHILD CARE

Health-related statistics provide an objective basis for projecting client needs, planning the use of resources, and determining the effectiveness of specific treatments. Although these statistics support no conclusions about why some phenomenon has occurred, they do identify certain trends and high-risk target groups. The following sections discuss descriptive statistics that are particularly important to maternal-child healthcare.

BIRTH RATE

Birth rate refers to the number of live births per 1000 people. Worldwide birth rates vary dramatically, as Table 1–2 demonstrates. In the United States in 2002, the birth rate of 13.9 reflected the steady pattern of decrease seen for the past several years. Most encouraging, the birth rate for teens decreased for the 11th straight year to 43 births per 1000 females 15 to 19 years of age. This was the lowest birth rate for

TABLE 1–2 ✤ Estimated Live Birth Rates and Infant Mortality Rates in Selected Countries, 2005

Country	Birth Rate	Infant Mortality Rate
Afghanistan	47.0	163.1
Argentina	16.2	15.2
Australia	12.3	4.7
Canada	10.8	4.8
China	13.1	24.2
Egypt	23.3	32.6
Ethiopia	38.6	95.3
France	12.2	4.3
Iraq	32.5	50.3
Japan	9.5	3.3
Mexico	21.0	20.9
United Kingdom	10.8	5.2
United States	14.1	6.5

Data from *The World Fact Book, 2005.* Washington, DC. The Central Intelligence Agency.

that group in more than six decades. Increasing birth rates for women 35 to 39 years of age (42.4 per 1000) and for women 40 to 44 years of age (8.2 per 1000) reflect an emerging trend (National Center for Health Statistics, 2004). This may be occurring as women delay childbearing and may also be related to other societal factors such as remarriage and the decision of the couple to have a child together.

The statistics do raise questions. For example: What is the impact of cultural differences and changing societal values on birth rates? Do birth rates change when access to information on contraception increases? What role does government policy, such as China's legislation limiting births to one child per family, play?

MATERNAL MORTALITY

The **maternal mortality rate** is the number of deaths from causes related to or aggravated by pregnancy or the management of pregnancy during the pregnancy cycle (including the 42-day postpartum period) per 100,000 live births. In 2002, 357 women died of pregnancy-related causes, a decrease of 42 deaths from the 2001 total, which is a rate of 8.9. However, for black women in the United States, the rate of death (24.9) was more than 4 times the rate for white women (6.0) (Kochanek, Murphy, Anderson et al., 2004).

Factors influencing the long-term decrease in maternal mortality include the increased use of hospitals and specialized healthcare personnel by maternity clients, the establishment of care centers for high-risk mothers and infants, the prevention and control of infection with antibiotics and improved techniques, the availability of blood products for transfusions, and the lowered rates of anesthesia-related deaths.

INFANT MORTALITY

The **infant mortality rate** is the number of deaths of infants under 1 year of age per 1000 live births in a given population (Figure 1–4 ⦿). In 2002 the U.S. infant mortality rate increased to 7.0 infant deaths compared to the 2001 rate of 6.8. (*Neonatal mortality* is the number of deaths of infants less than 28 days of age per 1000 live births, *perinatal mortality* includes both neonatal deaths and *fetal deaths* per 1000 live births, and fetal death is death in utero at 20 weeks or more gestation.) This rate increase was concentrated in the neonatal period, especially during the first week of life. Not surprisingly, two key predictors of infant health—the percentage of infants born preterm (before 37 completed weeks' gestation) and the per-

centage of low-birth-weight (less than 2500 g) infants—also increased in 2002 (Kochanek et al., 2004).

The U.S. infant mortality rate continues to be an area of concern because the United States ranks low in infant mortality rankings among industrialized nations. Healthcare professionals, policy makers, and the public continue to stress the need for better prenatal care, coordination of health services, and provision of comprehensive maternal-child services in the United States. In the United States, the leading causes of infant mortality are as follows: (1) congenital malformations and chromosomal abnormalities, (2) disorders related to prematurity and low birth weight, (3) sudden infant death syndrome (SIDS), (4) newborn affected by maternal complications, (5) umbilical cord and placental complications, (6) accidents, (7) respiratory distress of the newborn, (8) bacterial sepsis, (9) circulatory system diseases, and (10) intrauterine hypoxia and birth asphyxia (Kochanek et al., 2004).

Disparities in infant mortality exist among racial and ethnic groups, with highest rates among black and American Indian mothers. Infant mortality also increases as the mother's education level decreases. In 2001, for example, non-Hispanic white infants born to mothers with less than a high school education had a mortality rate more than twice that of infants of mothers with more than a high school education (National Center for Health Statistics, 2004).

Table 1–2 identifies estimated infant mortality rates for selected countries for 2005. As the data indicate, the range is dramatic among the countries listed. Information about birth rates and mortality rates is limited for some countries because of a lack of organized reporting mechanisms. The information raises many concerns such as access to healthcare during pregnancy and after birth and about standards of living, nutrition, and sociocultural factors.

PEDIATRIC MORTALITY

Children have different healthcare problems than adults, and the problems may depend on the age and development of the child. The most common cause of death for children between 1 and 14 years of age is unintentional injury. For children age 1 to 4 years, congenital malformations, cancer, homicide, and diseases of the heart round out the top five causes of death. For children ages 5 to 14, cancer is the second leading cause of death, followed by congenital malformations, homicide, and suicide (National Center for Health Statistics, 2004). In 2001, motor vehicle crashes were the major cause of unintentional injury in all children ages 1 to 14. In children 1 to 4, this was followed by drowning, fires and burns, and firearms. In children 5 to 14 years, firearms and drowning were essentially tied for second place (Health Resources and Services Administration, 2003).

Unintentional injury continues to be the leading cause of death in adolescents 15 through 19 years. Homicide, sui-

⦿ **FIGURE 1–4**

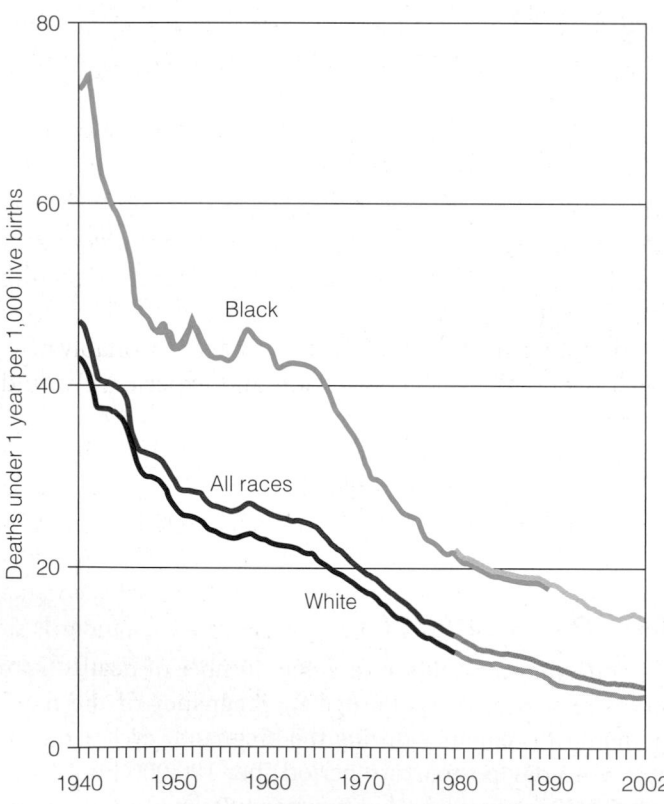

Notes: Infant deaths are classified by race of decedent. For 1940–90, live births are classified by race of parents and for 1980–2001, by race of mother. See "Technical Notes."

Infant mortality rates by race: United States, 1940–2002.

cide, cancer, and heart disease are other major causes of death. Of all deaths from unintentional and intentional injury, motor vehicle crashes are the leading cause, followed by firearms, suffocation, drowning, and poisoning.

PEDIATRIC MORBIDITY

Morbidity—an illness or injury that limits activity, requires medical attention or hospitalization, or results in a chronic condition—also varies according to the age of the child. In 2000 there were 3.4 million hospital discharges for children in the United States between 1 and 21 years of age, an average of 4 discharges per 100 children. This represents a 38% decrease in overall hospitalizations for children between 1 and 14 years of age between 1985 and 2000 (Health Resources and Services Administration, 2003). Respiratory diseases are the leading cause of hospitalization in children between 1 and 9 years of age, accounting for 33% of hospital discharges in this age group. Although injury is a leading cause of death in children 1 to 14 years of age, it accounted for only 9% of hospital discharges in 2000. Mental disorders were the leading cause of hospitalization in children between 10 and 14 years of age. Pregnancy and childbirth was the leading cause of hospitalization for adolescents between 15 and 21 years of age, followed by hospitalization for mental disorders.

In 2003 chronic illnesses and impairments limited the activities of 8% of children between 5 and 17 years of age; however, this rate varied by sex. Males (10%) had more activity limitations than females (6%). Children who have activity limitations are more likely to have one or more chronic conditions with duration of 3 months or more, miss more days from school, and often have higher medical costs (Federal Interagency Forum on Child and Family Statistics, 2005).

IMPLICATIONS FOR NURSING PRACTICE

Nurses can use statistics in a number of ways. For example, they can use statistical data to:

- Determine populations at risk.
- Assess the relationship between specific factors.
- Help establish databases for specific client populations.
- Determine the levels of care needed by particular client populations.
- Evaluate the success of specific nursing interventions.
- Determine priorities in caseloads.
- Estimate staffing and equipment needs of hospital units and clinics.
- Apply for funding to support health needs.

Nurses who use this information are better prepared to promote the health needs of maternal-newborn clients and their families.

In the report *Healthy People 2010*, the U.S. government established updated objectives to improve pregnancy outcome and the health of women, infants, children, and young adults. These objectives focus on improving pregnancy outcomes, reducing the incidence of death and disability from the major causes of death, and so forth. Federal funding is available to healthcare organizations for the development of programs aimed at reducing the number of deaths from these factors in specific high-risk groups. For a complete listing of *Healthy People 2010* objectives, visit the Companion Website at *http://www.prenhall.com/london*.

LEGAL CONSIDERATIONS IN MATERNAL-CHILD NURSING

SCOPE OF PRACTICE

The *scope of practice* is defined as the limits of nursing practice set forth in state statutes. Although some state practice acts continue to limit nursing practice to the traditional responsibilities of providing client care related to health maintenance and disease prevention, most state practice acts cover expanded practice roles that include collaboration with other health professionals in planning and providing care, physician-delegated diagnosis and prescriptive privilege, and the delegation of direct care tasks to other specified licensed and unlicensed personnel. A nurse must function within the scope of practice or risk being accused of practicing medicine without a license.

STANDARDS OF NURSING CARE

Standards of care establish minimum criteria for competent, proficient delivery of nursing care. Such standards are designed to protect the public and are used to judge the quality of care provided. Legal interpretation of actions within standards of care is based on what a reasonably prudent nurse with similar education and experience would do in similar circumstances.

The American Nurses Association (ANA) has published standards of practice for maternal-child health. ANA and the Society of Pediatric Nurses (2003) collaborated on the development of standards for pediatric clinical nursing practice. The ANA and the National Association of Neonatal Nurses also recently published the scope and standards of practice for neonatal nursing (2004). Specialty organizations such as the Association of Women's Health, Obstetric and Neonatal Nurses (AWHONN) continue to set the standards of professional nursing practice in the care of women and newborns (2003). Specialty organizations such as the Association of Operating Room Nurses (AORN) have also developed standards for specialty practice.

Agency policies, procedures, and protocols also provide appropriate guidelines for care standards. For example,

MEDIALINK Standards of Practice

GROWTH AND DEVELOPMENT

By 7 or 8 years of age, a child is able to understand concrete explanations about informed consent for research participation. By age 11, a child's abstract reasoning and logic are advanced. By age 14, an adolescent can weigh options and make decisions regarding consent as capably as an adult.

clinical practice guidelines and critical pathways are comprehensive interdisciplinary care plans for a specific condition that describe the sequence and timing of interventions that should result in expected client or patient outcomes. Clinical practice guidelines or critical pathways are adopted within a healthcare setting to reduce variation in care management, to limit costs of care, and to evaluate the effectiveness of care. The Joint Commission on Accreditation of Healthcare Organizations (JCAHO), a nongovernmental agency that audits the operation of hospitals and healthcare facilities, has also contributed to the development of nursing standards.

Some standards carry the force of law; others, although not legally binding, carry important legal significance. Any nurse who fails to meet appropriate standards of care invites allegations of negligence or malpractice. However, any nurse who practices within the guidelines established by an agency, or follows local or national standards, is assured that clients are provided with competent nursing care, which decreases the potential for litigation.

CLIENT/PATIENT SAFETY

JCAHO has identified patient safety as an important responsibility of healthcare providers and has established seven goals as requirements for accreditation in 2005. See "Nursing Practice" for a list of these goals.

NURSING PRACTICE

The 2005 National Patient Safety Goals established by JCAHO's International Center for Patient Safety are as follows:

- Improve the accuracy of patient identification.
- Improve the effectiveness of communication among caregivers.
- Improve the safety of using medications.
- Improve the safety of using infusion pumps.
- Reduce the risk of healthcare-associated infections.
- Accurately and completely reconcile medications across the continuum of care.
- Reduce the risk of patient harm resulting from falls.

Source: http://www.jcipatientsafety.org

Infants and children are at a higher risk for medical error than other patients and also may be more vulnerable to harm from errors made. Most errors in medical care within hospitals are "systems" errors related to equipment, complex procedures, fragmented care, and lack of standardized procedures. Reasons for the increase in medical errors among children include the following:

- Medication dosage calculations are more complex. Dosages are based upon weight, whereas adults are given standard doses.
- Many drug preparations require dilution to achieve the small dosage required by infants.
- Medications not yet approved by the U.S. Food and Drug Administration (FDA) for use in children are sometimes prescribed.
- Young children cannot communicate well if they are having a reaction to the medication.
- Critically ill and injured children do not have the reserves to deal with an overdose of medication like a healthy, older child or adult.

Limited English proficiency may also be a potential source of medical error for childbearing women and children. In such cases a risk exists for errors in interpretation—either of what the health professional says or what the family member says. Even when using a hospital interpreter, errors such as omitting instructions on dose, frequency, and duration of medications have potential clinical consequences (Flores, Laws, Mayo et al., 2003). Healthcare facilities are actively working to implement strategies that will reduce medical errors in all child patients.

INFORMED CONSENT

Informed consent is a legal concept that protects a person's right to autonomy and self-determination by specifying that no action may be taken without that individual's prior understanding and freely given consent. Although this policy is usually enforced for such major procedures as surgery or regional anesthesia, it pertains to any nursing, medical, or surgical intervention. To touch a person without consent (except in an emergency) constitutes battery. Consent is not informed unless the client, or parent in the case of a child, understands the usual procedures, their rationales, and any associated risks.

The person, usually the physician, who is ultimately responsible for the treatment or procedure should provide the information necessary to obtain informed consent. In such cases the nurse's role is to witness the client's signature (or the parent's signature for a child) giving consent. The nurse may also serve as a witness if parents give verbal consent by telephone. If the nurse determines that the individual does not understand the procedure or risks, the nurse must notify the physician, who must then provide additional information to ensure that the consent is informed. The nurse also responds to questions asked by adult clients or by parents and children. Anxiety, fear, pain, and medications that alter consciousness may influence an individual's ability to give informed consent. An oral consent is legal, but written consent is easier to defend in a court of law.

Children under 18 or 21 years of age, depending on state law, can legally give informed consent in the following circumstances:

- When they are minor parents of the child client
- When they are **emancipated minors** (self-supporting adolescents under 18 years of age, not subject to parental control). In most states, a pregnant teen is considered emancipated.
- When they are adolescents between 16 and 18 years of age seeking birth control, mental health counseling, or substance abuse treatment (Dickey & Deatrick, 2000)

Mature minors (14- and 15-year-old adolescents who are able to understand treatment risks) can give consent for treatment or refuse treatment in some states.

Refusal of a treatment, medication, or procedure after appropriate information is provided also requires that the individual sign a form releasing the doctor and clinical facility from liability resulting from the effects of such a refusal. Jehovah's Witnesses' refusal of blood transfusions is an example of such refusal.

Nurses are responsible for educating clients about any nursing care. Before each nursing intervention, the maternal-child nurse lets the individual and/or family know what to expect, thus ensuring cooperation and obtaining consent. Afterward the nurse documents the teaching and the learning outcomes in the person's record. The importance of clear, concise, and complete nursing records cannot be overemphasized. These records are evidence that the nurse obtained consent, performed prescribed treatments, reported important observations to the appropriate staff, and adhered to acceptable standards of care.

Because children are not considered competent to make healthcare decisions, parents, as the legal custodians of minor children, are customarily requested to give informed consent on behalf of a child. Both children and parents must understand that they have the right to refuse treatment at any time. In an emergency, consent for treatment to preserve life or limb is not required. When parents are divorced, some states limit the parental rights to give informed consent to the parent with custody. When parents have joint custody, in most cases either may give consent. Proxy consent can be granted in writing by the parent to another adult so that children can obtain

healthcare when needed (Berger & Committee on Medical Liability, 2003).

Parents or guardians have absolute authority to make choices about their child's healthcare except in specific cases:

- When the child and parents do not agree on major treatment options
- When the parents' choice of treatment does not permit lifesaving treatment for the child
- When there is a potential conflict of interest between the child and parents, such as with suspected child abuse or neglect
- When the parents are incapacitated and cannot make a decision (e.g., critically injured in the same motor vehicle crash) (Dickey & Deatrick, 2000)

In some cases the court may be requested to appoint a proxy decision maker for the child or to determine that the child is capable of making a major treatment decision.

Children should become more actively involved in decision making about treatment procedures as their reasoning skills develop. Children too young to give informed consent can be given age-appropriate information about their condition and asked about their care preferences. Their parents, however, make ultimate decisions about their care.

With regard to children's participation in research, federal guidelines state that children 7 years of age and older must receive information about a research project and give assent (the voluntary agreement to participate in a research project or to accept treatment) before they are enrolled. Children should be given adequate time to ask questions and be told that they have the right to refuse to participate in the study (Lindeke, Hauck, & Tanner, 2000; U.S. Department of Health and Human Services, 1983). The number of children asked to participate in research is expected to increase because of new FDA regulations requiring manufacturers to assess the safety and effectiveness of new drugs and biologic products in pediatric patients associated with the Best Pharmaceuticals for Children Act of 2003 (Lewin & Dale, 2003; U.S. Food and Drug Administration, 1998).

RIGHT TO PRIVACY

The *right to privacy* is the right of a person to keep his or her person and property free from public scrutiny. To protect this right for clients and families, only those responsible for their care should conduct an examination or discuss their case.

The right to privacy is protected by state constitutions, statutes, and common law. The ANA, the National League for Nursing (NLN), and JCAHO have adopted professional standards protecting the privacy of clients. Healthcare agencies should also have written policies dealing with client privacy. The Health Insurance Portability and Accountability Act of 1996 (HIPPA), which was fully implemented in 2002, also has a provision to guarantee the security and privacy of health information.

Laws, standards, and policies about privacy specify that information about clients' treatment, condition, and prognosis can be shared only by health professionals responsible for their care. Information considered vital statistics (name, age, occupation, and so on) may be revealed legally, but is often withheld because of ethical considerations. The client should be consulted as to what information may be released and to whom.

Children and Confidentiality

Concerns about privacy and the fear of disclosure of sensitive information to parents is a major reason why adolescents do not seek healthcare (Ford, Bearman, & Moody, 1999). When the child is an emancipated or mature minor, many states permit healthcare providers to provide birth control and treatment for sexually transmitted infections including HIV/AIDS, pregnancy, and substance abuse without informing the child's parents (Dickey & Deatrick, 2000).

NURSING PRACTICE

Breaching confidentiality is a potential problem for adolescents, who are just learning whom they can trust in the healthcare system. Make sure you openly discuss the limits of confidentiality for such things as mandatory reporting requirements with the client and family. Inadvertent disclosure of personal information may lead to psychologic, social, or physical harm in some clients.

PATIENT SELF-DETERMINATION ACT

The federal Patient Self-Determination Act directs healthcare institutions to inform hospitalized patients about their rights, which include expressing a preference for treatment options and making **advance directives** (writing a living will or authorizing a durable power of attorney for healthcare decisions on the individual's behalf). Nurses often discuss these issues with clients and their families. Minor children and their parents should also be informed of their rights. Adolescents with serious acute or chronic conditions with a higher risk of death should be encouraged to talk with their parents about their healthcare wishes and to prepare advance directives jointly (Dickey & Deatrick, 2000).

Do not resuscitate (DNR) orders have become more common for children with terminal illnesses in which no further treatments are possible or desired. In many cases these children are cared for at home or in a hospice program, but some still attend school. Implementation of

DNR orders for such children then becomes a community issue, to ensure that resuscitation measures are not initiated by any emergency care provider when the child has a life-threatening event. State health policies must be developed so children with these signed orders are easily identified and appropriate documentation of the orders is on file.

ETHICAL ISSUES IN MATERNAL-CHILD NURSING

Although ethical dilemmas confront nurses in all areas of practice, those related to pregnancy, birth, newborns, and children seem especially difficult to resolve.

MATERNAL-FETAL CONFLICT

Until fairly recently the fetus was viewed legally as a nonperson. Mother and fetus were viewed as one complex client—the pregnant woman—of which the fetus was an essential part. However, advances in technology have permitted the physician to treat the fetus and monitor fetal development. The fetus is increasingly viewed as a client separate from the mother, although treatment of the fetus necessarily involves the mother. Thus the medical emphasis has shifted from one of unity to one of duality (Hornstra, 1999). This focus on the fetus intensified in 2002 when President George W. Bush announced that "unborn children" would qualify for government healthcare benefits. This move was designed to promote prenatal care, but it represented the first time that any U.S. federal policy had defined childhood as starting at conception.

Most women are strongly motivated to protect the health and well-being of their fetus. In some instances, however, women have refused interventions on behalf of the fetus, and forced interventions have occurred. These include forced cesarean birth, coercion of mothers who practice high-risk behaviors such as substance abuse to enter treatment, and, perhaps most controversial, mandated experimental in utero therapy or surgery in an attempt to correct a specific birth defect. These interventions infringe on the autonomy of the mother. They may also be detrimental to the baby if, as a result, maternal bonding is hindered, the mother is afraid to seek prenatal care, or the mother is herself harmed by the actions taken (Hornstra, 1999). Attempts have also been made to criminalize the behavior of women who fail to follow a physician's advice or who engage in behaviors (such as substance abuse) that are considered harmful to the fetus. This raises two thorny questions: (1) What practices should be monitored? and (2) Who will determine when the behaviors pose such a risk to the fetus that the courts should intervene?

The American College of Obstetricians and Gynecologists (ACOG) Committee on Ethics (2004) and the American Academy of Pediatrics (AAP) Committee on Bioethics (1999) both affirm the fundamental right of pregnant women to make informed, uncoerced decisions about medical interventions. ACOG and AAP also recognize that cases of maternal-fetal conflict involve two clients, both of whom deserve respect and treatment. Such cases are best resolved by using internal hospital mechanisms, including counseling, the intervention of specialists, and consultation with an institutional ethics committee. Court intervention should be considered a last resort, appropriate only in extraordinary circumstances.

ABORTION

Since the 1973 Supreme Court decision in *Roe v. Wade*, elective abortion has been legal in the United States. Abortion can be performed until the period of viability. After that time, abortion is permissible only when the life or health of the mother is threatened. Before viability the rights of the mother are paramount; after viability the rights of the fetus take precedence.

Personal beliefs, cultural norms, life experiences, and religious convictions shape people's attitudes about abortion. Ethicists have thoughtfully and thoroughly argued positions supporting both sides of the question. Nevertheless, few issues spark the intensity of response seen when the issue of abortion is raised.

At present the decision about abortion is to be made by the woman and her physician. Nurses (and other caregivers) have the right to refuse to assist with the procedure if abortion is contrary to their moral and ethical beliefs. However, if a nurse works in an institution where abortions may be performed, the nurse may be dismissed for refusing. To avoid being placed in a situation contrary to personal ethical values and beliefs, it is important to identify the practices of an institution before going to work there. A nurse who refuses to participate in an abortion because of moral or ethical beliefs has a responsibility to ensure that someone with similar qualifications is available to provide appropriate care for the client. Clients must never be abandoned, regardless of a nurse's beliefs.

INTRAUTERINE FETAL SURGERY

Intrauterine fetal surgery, an example of therapeutic research, is a therapy for anatomic lesions that can be corrected surgically and are incompatible with life if not treated. The procedure involves opening the uterus during the second trimester (before viability), performing the planned surgery, and replacing the fetus in the uterus. The risks to the fetus are substantial, and the mother is committed to cesarean births for this and subsequent pregnancies (because the upper, active segment of the uterus is entered). The parents must be informed of the experimental nature

of the treatment, the risks of the surgery, the commitment to cesarean birth, and alternatives to the treatment.

As in other aspects of maternity care, caregivers must respect the pregnant woman's autonomy. The procedure involves health risks to the woman, and she retains the right to refuse any surgical procedure. Healthcare providers must be careful that their zeal for new technology does not lead them to focus unilaterally on the fetus at the expense of the mother.

REPRODUCTIVE ASSISTANCE

Assisted reproductive technology (ART) is the term used to describe highly technologic approaches used to produce pregnancy. *In vitro fertilization* and *embryo transfer (IVF-ET)*, a therapy offered to selected infertile couples, is perhaps the best known ART technique.

Some legislative efforts have been made to address consumer concerns about ART. In the United States, the federal Fertility Clinic Success Rate and Certification Act (FCSRCA) of 1992 requires standardized reporting of pregnancy success rates associated with ART programs and addresses issues related to laboratory quality. To help ensure data accuracy, a validation process, which includes site visits to a portion of reporting clinics, is completed.

Slightly more than one third of pregnancies that result from ART are multiple pregnancies. Multiple pregnancy occurs because the use of ovulation-inducing medications typically triggers the release of multiple eggs, which, when fertilized, produce multiple embryos that are then implanted. Multiple pregnancy increases the risk of miscarriage, preterm birth, and neonatal morbidity and mortality. It also increases the mother's risk of complications, including cesarean birth. To help prevent a high-level multiple pregnancy, the American Society for Reproductive Medicine has issued guidelines to limit the number of embryos transferred. This practice raises ethical considerations about the handling of the unused embryos. However, when a multiple pregnancy does occur, the physician may suggest that the woman abort some of the embryos to give the remaining embryos a better chance for survival. Clearly this procedure raises ethical concerns about the sacrifice of some so that the remainder can survive (ACOG, 2002).

Surrogate childbearing is another approach to infertility. Surrogate childbearing occurs when a woman agrees to become pregnant for a childless couple. She may be artificially inseminated with the male partner's sperm or a donor's sperm or may receive a gamete transfer, depending on the infertile couple's needs. If fertilization occurs, the woman carries the fetus to term and releases the infant to the couple after birth.

These methods of resolving infertility raise ethical issues about candidate selection, responsibility for a child born with a congenital defect, and religious objections to artificial conception. Other ethical questions include the following: What should be done with surplus fertilized oocytes? To whom do frozen embryos belong? Who is liable if a woman or her offspring contracts HIV from donated sperm? Should children be told about their conception?

EMBRYONIC STEM CELL RESEARCH

Human stem cells can be found in embryonic tissue and in the primordial germ cells of a fetus. Research has demonstrated that in tissue cultures these cells can be made to differentiate into other types of cells such as blood, nerve, or heart cells, which might then be used to treat problems such as diabetes, Parkinson and Alzheimer diseases, spinal cord injury, or metabolic disorders. The availability of specialized tissue or even organs grown from stem cells might also decrease society's dependence on donated organs for organ transplants (National Institutes of Health, 2004).

The ethical questions and dilemmas associated with embryonic stem cell research are staggering and complex. The following are two of the most pressing issues to be considered (Roche & Grodin, 2000):

- What moral status should be attached to the human embryo? How should an embryo be viewed? With full status as a person? As a cluster of undifferentiated cells with no moral status? As having status somewhere in between—that is, beyond mere cells and deserving of special respect?

- What sources of embryonic tissue are acceptable for research? Is it ever ethical to create embryos solely for stem cell research? Is there justification for using embryos remaining after fertility treatments?

Equally significant, advancements in stem cell research play a major role in the rapidly approaching convergence of reproductive and genetic technologies with all of their related ethical dilemmas, as the following discussion suggests.

THE HUMAN GENOME PROJECT

The *Human Genome Project* is an international, multidisciplinary effort to explore and map all human genetic material. In 2003 the mapping of the human genome was completed, 2 years ahead of schedule. It revealed that there are between 30,000 and 40,000 human genes, a significantly lower number than previously estimated. Currently researchers and scientists are exploring future directions for the field of genomics (National Human Genome Research Institute, 2004). As more genetic information becomes available, questions arise about the ethical use and protection of such information. Other emerging issues include

the question of payment for genetic testing; appropriate counseling following testing; confidentiality; qualifications of individuals engaged in testing, counseling, and interventions; mandated testing; and the right to refuse to receive information about genetic findings.

CORD BLOOD BANKING

Cord blood, taken from a newborn's umbilical cord at birth and stored or "banked," may play a role in combating leukemia, certain other cancers, and immune and blood system disorders. This is possible because cord blood, like bone marrow and embryonic tissue, contains regenerative stem cells, which can replace diseased cells in the affected individual.

Ethical issues associated with cord blood banking include the following (Smith & Thomson, 2000):

- Who owns the blood? The donor? The parents? Private blood banks? Society?

- How will informed consent be obtained and by whom?

- How will confidentiality be ensured? The family must understand that, if they choose to donate, the mother will be asked to provide a blood sample and a detailed history about her health and infectious disease status.

- How will obligations to notify the family and donor be addressed if testing of the blood reveals infectious diseases or genetic disorders?

- How will the harvested blood be allocated to ensure fairness and availability to individuals from all races, ethnic groups, and income levels?

MAKING TREATMENT DECISIONS FOR CHILDREN

Technology makes it possible to sustain the lives of children who previously would have died, thus creating many ethical issues. Problems may develop because physicians, nurses, and parents have differing opinions about treatments for an infant or child with a serious or fatal condition. Nurses often face ethical dilemmas when providing care to such a child, especially as they witness parents struggling to decide among treatment options. Ethical issues in pediatrics are often more complex because most children lack the capacity to make or to participate in medical decisions that directly affect them.

When making treatment decisions in pediatrics, healthcare professionals need to determine whether their responsibility is limited to the child or includes the interests of the parents. The healthcare institution's ethics committee often plays a role in resolving conflicts about treatment decisions. Courts should make ethical decisions only when healthcare professionals and parents are unable to agree about providing or withholding treatment.

TERMINATING LIFE-SUSTAINING TREATMENT

Federal "Baby Doe" regulations were developed to protect the rights of infants with severe defects. Parents of such infants are usually the ultimate decision makers about the child's care. They may want to terminate treatment because of the tremendous social, emotional, and financial burden they face (Schrode, 2000). Physicians may believe treatment will help the child and improve the quality of life (sometimes defined as a meaningful existence or an ability to develop human relationships). Federal regulations require a formalized ethical decision-making process before physicians accept or reject a parent's wishes.

Justifications for withholding, withdrawing, or limiting therapy include the following:

■ The treatment in question has a poor rate of success.

■ The burdens of the treatment outweigh the benefits, or the quality of life is poor after treatment.

■ The burdens of the disease outweigh the benefits of continued survival, or the quality of life is poor before the treatment (Cassidy & Fleischman, 1996).

Each of these conditions is considered according to the individual beliefs of the members of the ethics committee and their perceptions of the value of specific interventions for an individual child. Treatment to save the infant's life is often elected if it has the potential for improving the quality of life as well. Physicians are not obligated to offer interventions that cause extreme pain and suffering when there is no potential benefit or only limited potential benefit. Treatments that only prolong life represent a misuse of expensive healthcare resources.

ORGAN TRANSPLANTATION ISSUES

The death of a child can benefit another child through organ transplantation. The National Organ Transplant Act (PL 98-507) generated laws, regulations, and guidelines for organ collection and transplantation. For example, the transplant team cannot provide care to the potential donor. In addition the institution has specific requirements to approach family members when brain death is suspected or confirmed to request organ donation.

Regulations are important because too few organs are available for people needing transplantation. The limited supply of organs has created numerous ethical issues:

■ Which individuals on a waiting list should receive the organs available?

■ Should families be permitted to pay donor families for organs?

■ Should the family's ability to pay for an organ transplant give a child higher priority for an organ?

■ What are the brain death and non-heartbeating criteria for children that enable organ collection to proceed?

IMPLICATIONS FOR NURSING PRACTICE

The complex ethical issues facing maternal-child nurses have many social, cultural, legal, and professional ramifications. Ethical decisions in maternal-child nursing are often complicated by moral obligations to more than one client. Straightforward solutions to the ethical dilemmas encountered in caring for children and childbearing families are often, quite simply, not available.

Nurses must learn to anticipate ethical dilemmas, clarify their own positions related to the issues, understand the legal implications of the issues, and develop appropriate strategies for ethical decision making. To accomplish these tasks, they can read about bioethical issues, participate in discussion groups, attend courses and workshops on ethical topics pertinent to their areas of practice, and serve on ethics committees.

EVIDENCE-BASED PRACTICE IN MATERNAL-CHILD NURSING

Evidence-based practice—that is, nursing care in which all interventions are supported by current, valid research evidence—is emerging as a force in healthcare. It provides a useful approach to problem solving and decision making and to self-directed, client-centered, lifelong learning. Evidence-based practice builds on the actions necessary to transform research findings into clinical practice by also considering other forms of evidence that can be useful in making clinical practice decisions. These other forms of evidence may include statistical data, quality measurements, risk management measures, and information from support services such as infection control.

As practicing clinicians, nurses need to meet two basic competencies related to evidence-based practice. Nurses need to (1) recognize which clinical practices are supported by good evidence, which practices have conflicting findings as to their effect on client outcomes, and which practices have no evidence to support their use; and (2) use data in their clinical work. In truth, market pressures are also a force in the use of evidence-based practice because they are forcing nurses and other healthcare providers to evaluate routines to improve efficiencies and provide better outcomes for clients.

Nurses need to know what data are being tracked where they work and how care practices and outcomes are improved as a result of quality improvement initiatives. However, there is more to evidence-based practice than simply knowing what is being tracked and how the results are being used. Competent, effective nurses learn to question the very basis of their clinical work.

Throughout this text we have provided *snapshots* of evidence-based practice related to childbearing women and families, such as the one on page 34. We believe that these snapshots will help you understand the concept more clearly. We also expect that these examples may challenge you to question the usefulness of some of the routine care you ob-serve in clinical practice. That is the impact of evidence-based practice—it moves clinicians beyond practices of "habit and opinion" to practices based on high-quality, current science.

Critical Concept Review

LEARNING OBJECTIVES

CONCEPTS

Identify the nursing roles available to the maternal-newborn and pediatric nurses.	→

1. Registered nurse:
   ■ Provide nursing care to both inpatient and outpatient women with childbearing or reproductive issues as well as newborns and children.
2. Nurse practitioner:
   ■ Provide ambulatory care services to expectant families and to children.
   ■ Provide care in some acute care, high-risk units such as neonatal intensive care units.
   ■ Focus on physical and psychosocial assessments and order diagnostic tests and procedures.
   ■ Make clinical judgments and order appropriate care.
3. Certified nurse-midwife:
   ■ Manage the care of a woman who is at low risk for complications during pregnancy and childbirth.

Summarize the use of community-based nursing care in meeting the needs of childbearing and childrearing families.

Community-based care is important in meeting the needs of the childbearing and childrearing family because the vast majority of care takes place outside of hospitals:
1. Clinics.
2. Offices.
3. Community-based organizations.
4. Private homes.

Summarize the current status of factors related to health insurance and access to healthcare.

1. Community-based care remains an essential element of healthcare for uninsured or underinsured individuals, as well as for individuals who benefit from programs such as Medicare, Medicaid, or state-sponsored, health-related programs.
2. Healthcare insurers are beginning to recognize the importance of primary care in containing costs and maintaining health.

Define the following statistical terms relevant to healthcare: birth rate, infant mortality rate, neonatal mortality rate, and maternal mortality rate.

1. Birth rate:
   ■ Number of live births per 1000 people.
2. Infant mortality rate:
   ■ Number of deaths of infants under 1 year of age per 1000 live births in a given population.
3. Neonatal mortality rate:
   ■ Number of deaths of infants less than 28 days of age per 1000 live births.
4. Maternal mortality rate:
   ■ Number of deaths from any cause during the pregnancy cycle per 100,000 live births.

Identify the goals for client safety developed by the Joint Commission on the Accreditation of Healthcare Organizations (JCAHO).

2005 National Patient Safety Goals established by JCAHOs International Center for Patient Safety are:
1. Improve the accuracy of patient identification.
2. Improve the effectiveness of communication among caregivers.
3. Improve the safety of using medications.
4. Improve the safety of using infusion pumps.
5. Reduce the risk of healthcare-associated infections.
6. Accurately and completely reconcile medications across the continuum of care.
7. Reduce the risk of patient harm resulting from falls.

LEARNING OBJECTIVES

CONCEPTS

Delineate significant legal and ethical issues that influence the practice of maternal-child nursing.

→

1. Abortion can legally be performed until the fetus reaches the age of viability. The decision to have an abortion is made by a woman in consultation with her physician.
2. *Assisted reproductive technology (ART)* is the term used to describe highly technologic approaches used to produce pregnancy.
3. Cord blood banking provides the opportunity to have stem cells available to treat a variety of cancers and blood disorders. Its growing popularity has revealed several ethical issues.
4. Federal "Baby Doe" regulations were developed to protect the rights of infants with severe defects.

Discuss the role of evidence-based practice in improving the quality of nursing care for childbearing families.

→

1. Evidence-based practice refers to clinical practice based on research findings and other available data.
2. Evidence-based practice increases nurses' accountability to integrate current knowledge and research into practice and results in better client outcomes.

CRITICAL THINKING IN ACTION

*View the **Critical Thinking in Action** video in Chapter 1 of the CD-ROM. Then, answer the questions that follow.*

You are working as a prenatal nurse in a local clinic. Before entering a client's room, you review the chart for pertinent information such as cultural background, significant family members, weeks of gestation, test results, birth plan, and education for health promotion. You greet each client and family members by name and ask how they are coping with the pregnancy. Depending on the trimester of the pregnancy, you review the discomforts or concerns of the mother/family and what they may expect. You examine the mother, including fundal height, fetal heart rate and fetal position if appropriate, maternal blood pressure, weight gain, and urine analysis. With each client, you discuss the community resources available such as prenatal classes, lactation consultants, and prenatal exercise/yoga classes. Based upon the information you obtain, you might refer the mother to social services or the WIC program as appropriate. At the end of the clinic session, you review the clients with the collaborating physician.

1. How would you define the terms *family* and *family-centered care*?
2. Describe how the nursing process provides the framework for the delivery of direct nursing care.
3. How would you describe the concept of community-based care?
4. How would you describe culturally competent care?

MEDIALINK

www.prenhall.com/london

■ NCLEX-RN® Review, case studies, and other interactive resources for this chapter can be found on the Companion Website at http://www.prenhall.com/london. Click on "Chapter 1" to select the activities for this chapter.

Home > Chapter 1 > MediaLink

MediaLinks

- **SCHIP program information**
  Linking the Nation's Children to Health Insurance.
- **CMS State Children's Health Insurance Program (SCHIP)**
  The Centers for Medicare & Medicaid Services (CMS) is a federal agency within the U.S. Department of Health and Human Services.
- **CMS – Medicaid**
  Centers for Medicare & Medicaid Services.
- **CMS – HIPAA**
  The Health Insurance Portability and Accountability Act of 1996.
- **America's Children**
  America's Children – a report that includes detailed information on a set of key indicators of child well-being.
- **Biotechnics.net**
  Great source for information on medical ethics.
- **National Center for Youth Law**
  Ethics – a private, nonprofit law office serving the legal needs of children and their families.
- **Adolescent Health Confidentiality Toolkit**
  Ethics – a licensed health plan providing affordable health coverage to low- and middle-income residents living in San Francisco.

■ For animations, more NCLEX-RN®Review questions, and an audio glossary, access the accompanying CD-ROM in this textbook.

REFERENCES

American Academy of Pediatrics, Committee on Bioethics. (1999). Fetal therapy—Ethical considerations (RE9817). *Pediatrics, 103*(5), 1061–1063.

American College of Obstetricians and Gynecologists (ACOG). (2002). *Nonselective embryo reduction: Ethical guidelines for the obstetrician-gynecologist* (Committee opinion). Washington, D.C.: Author.

American College of Obstetricians and Gynecologists, Committee on Ethics. (2004). *Parent choice: Maternal-fetal relationship* (Opinion No. 214). Washington, DC: Author.

American Nurses Association. (1998). *Standards of clinical nursing practice* (2nd ed.). Washington, DC: American Nurses Publishing.

American Nurses Association and the National Association of Neonatal Nurses. (2004). *Neonatal nursing: Scope and standards of practice.* Washington, DC: American Nurses Association.

American Nurses Association and the Society of Pediatric Nurses. (2003). *Scope and standards of pediatric nursing practice.* Washington, DC: American Nurses Association.

Association of Women's Health, Obstetric and Neonatal Nurses. (2003). *Standards for professional nursing practice in the care of women and newborns* (6th ed.). Washington, DC: Author.

Baird, P. A. (1996). New reproductive technologies: The Canadian perspective. *Women's Health Issues, 6*(3), 156–166.

Berger, J. E., & Committee on Medical Liability. (2003). Consent by proxy for nonurgent pediatric care. *Pediatrics, 112*(5), 1186–1195.

Camacho, K. (2003). Innovations in midwifery education. *Journal of Midwifery and Women's Health, 48*(6), 393–397.

Cassidy, R. C., & Fleischman, A. R. (1996). *Pediatric ethics—From principles to practice.* Amsterdam: Harwood Academic Publishers.

Centers for Medicare and Medicaid Services. (2003). *State Children's Health Insurance Program.* Retrieved July 7, 2003, from http://www.cms.gov/schip/schip02.pdf

Cowan, C., Catlin, A., Smith, M. A., & Sensenig, A. (2004). National health expenditures, 2002. *Health Care Financing Review, 25*(4), 143–147.

DeNavas-Walt, C., Proctor, B. D., & Mills, R. J. (2004). *Income, poverty, and health insurance coverage in the United States: 2003.* Washington, DC: U.S. Census Bureau.

Dickey, S. B., & Deatrick, J. (2000). Autonomy and decision making for health promotion in adolescence. *Pediatric Nursing, 26*(5), 461–467.

Federal Interagency Forum on Child and Family Statistics. (2005). *America's Children: Key national indicators of well-being, 2005.* Washington, D.C.: U.S. Government Printing office.

Flores, G., Laws, M. B., Mayo, S. J., Zuckerman, B., Abreu, M., Medina, L., & Hardt, E. J. (2003). Errors in medical interpretation and their potential clinical consequences in pediatric encounters. *Pediatrics, 111*(1), 6–14.

Ford, C. A., Bearman, P. S., & Moody, J. (1999). Foregone health care among adolescents. *Journal of the American Medical Association, 282*(23), 2227–2234.

Health Care Finance Administration. (2000). *The state children's health insurance program (SCHIP).* Baltimore, MD: Centers for Medicare and Medicaid Services.

Health Resources and Services Administration. (2003). *Child Health USA, 2003.* Rockville, MD: U.S. Department of Health and Human Services.

Hornstra, D. (1999). A realistic approach to maternal-fetal conflict. *Neonatal Intensive Care, 12*(2), 24–31.

Kochanek, K. D., Murphy, S. L., Anderson, R. N., & Scott, C. (2004). Deaths: Final data for 2002. *National Vital Statistics Reports, 53*(5), 1–16.

Lewin, L., & Dale, J. (2003). Research considerations with children and adolescents. *Journal of Pediatric Health Care, 17*(5), 268–270.

Lindeke, L. L., Hauck, M. R., & Tanner, M. (2000). Practical issues in obtaining child assent for research. *Journal of Pediatric Nursing, 15*(2), 99–104.

Maiese, D. R. (2001). Monitoring women's health through performance measures. *Title V Today, 3*(1), 6–7.

Maternal and Child Health Bureau. (1995). *Child health USA '94* (DHHS Publication No. HRSA-MCH-95-1). Washington, DC: Government Printing Office.

Melnyk, B. M., Fineout-Overholt, E., Stone, P., & Ackerman, M. (2000). Evidence-based practice: The past, the present, and recommendations for the millennium. *Pediatric Nursing, 26*(1), 77–80.

Merritt, T. A., Palmer, D., Bergman, D. A., & Shiono, P. H. (1997). Clinical practice guidelines in pediatric and newborn medicine. Implications for their use in practice. *Pediatrics, 99*(1), 100–114.

National Center for Health Statistics. (2004). *Health, United States, 2004.* Hyattsville, MD: Author.

National Human Genome Research Institute. (2004). *About the Human Genome Project.* Retrieved March 13, 2004, from http://www.genome.gov/10001772

National Institutes of Health. (2004). *Stem cell basics.* Retrieved March 13, 2004, from http://stemcells.nih.gov/infoCenter/stemCellBasics.asp

Roche, P. A., & Grodin, M. A. (2000). The ethical challenge of stem cell research. *Women's Health Issues, 10*(3), 136–139.

Sackett, D. L., Straus, S. E., Richardson, W. S., Rosenberg, W., & Haynes, R. B. (2000). *Evidence-based medicine: How to practice and teach EBM.* Edinburgh, Scotland: Churchill Livingstone.

Schrode, K. (2000). Baby Doe and the Baby Doe regulations. *Children's National Medical Center Pediatric Ethicscope, 11*(1), 1–4.

Smith, F. O., & Thomson, B. G. (2000). Umbilical cord blood collection, banking, and transplantation: Current status and issues relevant to perinatal caregivers. *Birth, 27*(2), 127–135.

Smith, L. A., Wise, P. H., Chavkin, W., Romero, D., & Zuckerman, B. (2000). Implications in welfare reform for child health: Emerging challenges for clinical practice and policy. *Pediatrics, 106*(5), 1117–1125.

U.S. Census Bureau. (2003). *United States: General demographic characteristics: 2003.* Retrieved May 29, 2005, from http://www.Factfinder.census. gov

U.S. Department of Health and Human Services. (1983). *Protection of human subjects: Code of federal regulations* (45 CFR No. 46, Subpart D). Washington, DC: Author.

U.S. Department of Health and Human Services. (2000). *Healthy people 2010* (Conference Edition). Washington, DC: Author.

U.S. Food and Drug Administration. (1998, December 2). Regulations requiring manufacturers to assess the safety and effectiveness of new drugs and biological products in pediatric patients. *Federal Register, 63*(231), 66631– 66672.

Wilcox, L. S., & Marks, J. S. (1996). Regulating assisted reproductive technologies: Public health, consumer protection, and public resources. *Women's Health Issues, 6*(3), 175–180.

Winslow, E. H. (2001). Patient education materials: Care patients read them or are they ending up in the trash? *American Journal of Nursing, 101*(10), 33–38.

Culture and the Family

My parents came here from China when I was three. They wanted the chance to make a better life and they wanted another child. Needless to say, although I have always felt loved and cherished, I know how thrilled they were when my brother was born. Sometimes I feel as though I am walking a line between their ways and the ways I have learned growing up in this country. My husband is Chinese but he, too, grew up here. We are expecting our second baby in a few months. We talk often about which Chinese ways we want to retain and which new ways make more sense. I am not sure that my parents will understand, however. To them the old ways are always best.

—Li Wei, 29

LEARNING OBJECTIVES

- Distinguish among several different types of families.

- Identify the stages of a family life cycle.

- Identify prevalent cultural norms related to childbearing and childrearing.

- Summarize the importance of cultural competency in providing nursing care.

- Discuss the use of a cultural assessment tool as a means of providing culturally sensitive care.

- Identify key considerations in providing spiritually sensitive care.

- Distinguish between *complementary* and *alternative therapies.*

- Identify the benefits and risks of complementary and alternative therapies.

- Discuss complementary therapies appropriate for the nurse to use with childbearing and childrearing families.

MediaLink   www.prenhall.com/london

CD-ROM

NCLEX-RN® Review
Audio Glossary

Companion Website

NCLEX-RN® Review
MediaLink Applications:
    Critical Thinking: Examine Your Cultural Influences
    Cultural Assessment Tools
Audio Glossary

Individuals do not live in isolation. Their values, beliefs, behaviors, decisions, attitudes, and biases are shaped by many factors, including their families, their culture, and their religious beliefs. Nurses who provide effective, holistic care recognize this reality and seek to learn about and care for the entire family.

This chapter begins with a brief discussion of family types, functioning, and assessment. It then addresses the impact of culture on the family and concludes with a brief examination of some of the complementary and alternative therapies a family might use.

THE FAMILY

The U.S. Census Bureau defines a **family** as individuals who are joined together by marriage, blood, adoption, or residence in the same household. More broadly, however, bonds of emotional closeness, sharing, and support generally characterize families.

Within families, members are guided by a common set of values that bind them together. These family values are greatly influenced by external factors, including cultural background, social norms, education, environmental influences, socioeconomic status, and beliefs held by peers, coworkers, political and community leaders, and other individuals outside the family unit. Because of the influence of these external factors, a family's values may change considerably over the years.

TYPES OF FAMILIES

Various types of families—both traditional and nontraditional—exist in contemporary American society. The following list identifies common types of family structure:

- The *nuclear family* consists of a husband provider, a wife who stays home, and children. Although the nuclear family was once the norm in the United States, it is no longer the most common type of family.

- In the *dual-career/dual-earner family,* both parents work, either by choice or necessity. Today, two thirds of all two-parent families are this type. Dual-career families have to address issues related to child care, household chores, and spending time together.

- The *childless family* is a growing trend. While as many as 10% of couples experience infertility problems, 5% of married couples are voluntarily without children.

- In *extended families* a couple shares household and childrearing responsibilities with parents, siblings, or other relatives. Multigenerational arrangements of this sort are more common in non-U.S. cultures and in working-class families.

- An *extended kin network family* is a specific form of an extended family in which two nuclear families of primary or unmarried kin live in close proximity to each other. The family shares a social support network, chores, goods, and services. This type of family model is common in the Latino community.

- Although rare in the past, the *single-parent family* is becoming increasingly common. In the traditional single-parent family, the head of the household is widowed, divorced, abandoned, or separated. In the nontraditional single-parent family, the head of the household, most

● **FIGURE 2–1**

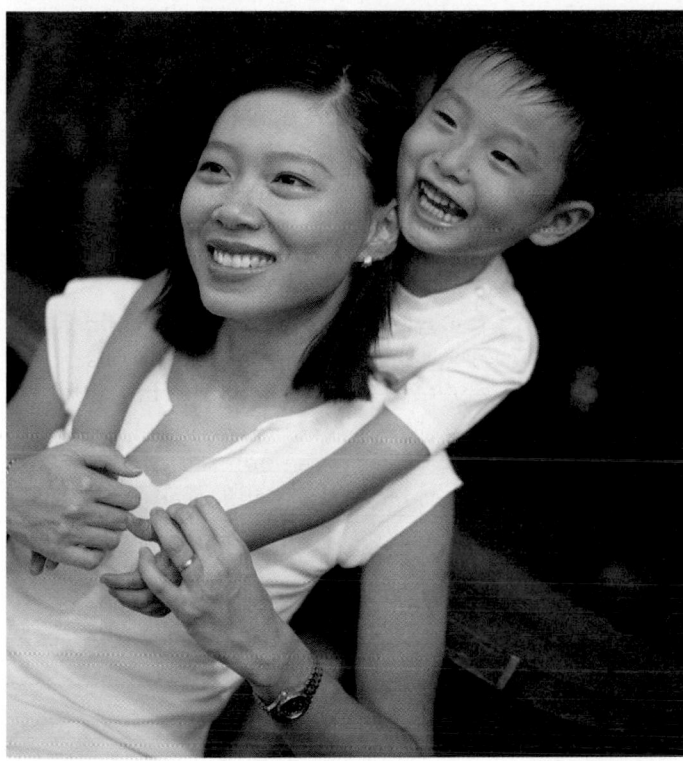

Single-parent families account for nearly one third of all U.S. families. What types of challenges do single-parent families face?

Used with permission from Joyce Choo/CORBIS.

often the mother, was never married. Some single-parent families are established by choice and have good support. Other single-parent families often face difficulties because the sole parent may lack social and emotional support, need assistance with childrearing issues, and face financial strain (Figure 2–1 ●).

■ A *stepfamily* consists of a biologic parent with children and a new spouse who may or may not have children. This family structure has become increasingly common because of high rates of divorce and remarriage. These families are also known as *remarried, reconstituted,* or *blended families.* Stepfamily models have both strengths and challenges. Stepfamilies have fewer financial issues and may actually offer a child a new support person and role model. Also, marriage provides a new opportunity for a successful relationship for the parents; however, the relationship between stepparents and stepchildren can be strained. Stresses can include discipline issues, adjustment problems, role ambiguity, strain with the other biologic parent, and communication issues.

■ A *binuclear family* is a post-divorce family in which the biologic children are members of two nuclear households, both that of the father and that of the mother. The children alternate between the two homes, and both parents have equal responsibility and legal rights, regardless of where the children live. The binuclear family model enables both parents to be involved in a child's upbringing and provides additional support and role models from extended family members.

■ A *nonmarital heterosexual cohabiting family* describes a heterosexual couple who may or may not have children and who live together outside of marriage. This may include never-married individuals as well as divorced or widowed persons. While some individuals choose this model for personal reasons, others do so for financial reasons or to seek companionship.

■ *Gay and lesbian families* include those in which two or more people who share a same-sex orientation live together (with or without children), and those in which a gay or lesbian single parent rears a child. Small studies that have evaluated children reared by gay and lesbian couples found that the children show no significant differences from children reared in other types of families (American Academy of Pediatrics, 2002). Children raised in gay and lesbian families may face unique issues in interacting with peers and in revealing their parents' sexual orientation.

NURSING PRACTICE

It is important to establish which parent has legal custody, current visitation policies, and other variables (restraining orders, supervised visitation, etc.) when communicating information to parents about their children. Certain legal issues may prohibit the nurse from sharing some information with the noncustodial parent.

FAMILY DEVELOPMENT FRAMEWORKS

Family development refers to the dynamics or changes that a family experiences over time, including changes in relationships, communication patterns, roles, and interactions. Although each family is unique, developmental frameworks describe typical stages in family life. For example, Duvall (1977) developed an eight-stage family life cycle that describes the developmental process that each family encounters. This model is based on the nuclear family (Table 2–1). The oldest child serves as a marker for the family's developmental stages except in the last two stages when children are no longer present. Couples with more than one child may find themselves in overlapping stages with developmental advances occurring simultaneously.

TABLE 2–1 ✤ The Eight-Stage Family Life Cycle

Stage I	Beginning families	Marriage between partners, identification as partners, establishing goals for future, interaction and building relationships with kin.
Stage II	Childbearing families	Birth of first child, new role as parents, integrating new family member into existing family.
Stage III	Families with preschool children	Establishing family network, socialization of children, reinforcing independence in children when separating from parents.
Stage IV	Families with school-age children	Facilitating peer relationships while maintaining family dynamics, adjusting to outside influences.
Stage V	Families with teenagers	Increase in children's independence and autonomy; parents' concerns shift to aging parents, careers, and marital relationship.
Stage VI	Families launching young adults	Readjustment of marital relationship; parents and children establish separate identities outside the family unit.
Stage VII	Middle-aged parents	Renewed marital relationship, new outside interests, fewer family responsibilities, new roles as grandparents and as in-laws, increased concern for aging parents, death, and disability of older generation.
Stage VIII	Retirement and old age	End of career, shift to retirement, maintain functioning during the aging process, maintain marital relationship, adjust to potential loss of spouse, friends, and siblings, prepare for eventual death.

Adapted with permission from Duvall, Elizabeth M. *Marriage and Family Development,* 5th ed. Published by Allyn and Bacon, Boston, MA. Copyright © 1977 by Pearson Education. Friedman, M. M. (2003). *Family Nursing: Research, Theory, and Practice* (5th ed.). Upper Saddle River, NJ Pearson Education.

Other family development models have been developed to address the stages and developmental tasks facing the unattached young adult, the gay and lesbian family, those who divorce, and those who remarry. For further information on this topic, refer to textbooks on families and on developmental psychology.

FAMILY ASSESSMENT

The nurse's understanding of a family's structure helps provide insight into the family's support system and needs. A *family assessment* is a collection of data about the family's type and structure, current level of functioning, support system, sociocultural background, environment, and needs.

To obtain an accurate and concise family assessment, the nurse needs to establish a trusting relationship with the woman or child, and the family. Data are best collected in a comfortable, private environment, free from interruptions.

Basic information should include the following:

- Name, age, sex, and family relationship of all people residing in the household.
- Family type, structure, roles, and values.
- Cultural associations, including cultural norms and customs related to childbearing, childrearing, and infant feeding.

- Religious affiliations, including specific religious beliefs and practices related to childbearing.
- Support network, including extended family, friends, and religious and community associations.
- Communication patterns, including language barriers.

The nurse also gathers information about the health of individual family members because health status can have a major impact on family functioning. When possible it is helpful to have information about the family's home environment as well. In many cases this information is gathered during client interviews. However, a home visit provides far more data about family relationships, roles, needs, and preparation for a new baby. See Chapter 39 for more information about family assessment. ∞

CULTURAL INFLUENCES AFFECTING THE FAMILY

When caring for families, it is critical to consider the influence of culture, which may affect how a family responds to health-related issues. **Culture** can be defined as the thoughts, communication, actions, beliefs, values, attitudes, and practices that are accepted by a racial, ethnic, religious, or social group and passed on from one generation to the next (Office of Minority Health, 2001). Culture is characterized by certain key elements, including the following:

- *Culture is based upon shared values and beliefs, and expected behaviors.* Each culture identifies and articulates its shared values and beliefs. Expected behaviors and roles emerge that are consistent with those values and beliefs. This belief system suggests what preventive health measures and treatment for diseases are sought and accepted. It may also state the importance of children, of the family, of other individuals, and of the collective group, all of which can influence the choices people in the culture make regarding health.

- *Culture is learned and dynamic.* A child is born into a culture and starts learning the beliefs and practices of the group from birth. Children who are members of two cultural groups, such as African and immigrant, learn about both groups as they grow and develop. Immigrants may face challenges when integrating the rules of the dominant culture. Children who have family members from two or more cultural groups integrate parts of the world view from each group. Therefore, although culture is connected with groups, each individual's manifestation of his or her own cultural background will be unique. Culture evolves and adapts as new members are born into or join the group, and as the surrounding social and physical environments change. For example, as first-generation immigrants enter a new country, they generally closely follow the cultural patterns of their native lands. As their children grow, the youth maintain some of the family cultural patterns but begin to incorporate some of the new culture (Figure 2–2 ●).

- *Culture is integrated into life and uses symbols.* Culture is integrated through social institutions such as schools, friendships, families, and occupation. This provides a variety of opportunities for learning about one's culture. The sense of integration may be disrupted or harder to maintain as individuals move frequently and as cultures intertwine with each other. Symbols are an important way that many cultures communicate with each other and with the outside world. Language, dress, music, tools, and nonverbal gestures are symbols a culture uses to display and transmit the culture.

Race refers to a group of people who share biologic similarities such as skin color, bone structure, and genetic traits. Examples of races include white (sometimes called Caucasian or European American in the United States), black (sometimes called African American in the United

● **FIGURE 2–2**

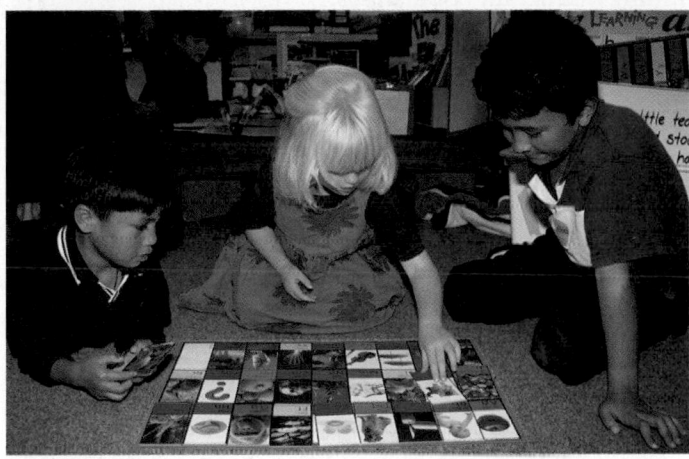

Preschoolers from various cultural backgrounds play together. How can nurses partner with families to assist children to understand and respect cultural differences?

States), Hispanic, Natives (such as Native Americans, Alaskan Native, Hawaiian Native, and First Nation people of Canada), and Asian.

Ethnicity is a social identity that is associated with shared behaviors and patterns. These include family structure, religious affiliation, ancestry or national origin, language, dress, foods and eating habits, and health behaviors. Examples of ethnic groups include Hmong, Jews, and Irish Americans. Even the mainstream or majority of groups usually identify with an ethnic group. Some beliefs and practices are common among certain ethnic groups, but it is important to avoid **stereotyping** individuals, assuming that all members of a group have the same characteristics. The nurse should assess the woman or child and family to see which characteristics common to a group are possessed by the client rather than assume that because individuals identify themselves as a specific ethnicity they must practice certain customs.

Acculturation is the process by which people adapt to a new cultural norm. When a group completely changes their cultural identity to become part of the majority culture, **assimilation** occurs.

Acculturation frequently occurs when people leave their country of origin and immigrate to a new country. Often acculturation is associated with improved health status and health behaviors, especially if the immigration is associated with improved socioeconomic status, which leads to better nutrition and access to healthcare. This is frequently true for people who immigrate to the United States from a developing country. On the other hand, health sometimes declines with acculturation. For example, obesity is a problem that is growing rapidly within the United States and particularly among immigrant populations.

FAMILY ROLES AND STRUCTURE

A family's roles and organization are largely dependent upon cultural influence. The family structure defines acceptable roles and behavior of family members. For example, culture may determine who has authority (head of household) and is the primary decision maker for other members of the family. Additionally the role of decision maker may change according to specific decisions. In some cultures, decisions regarding the family's healthcare are primarily the responsibility of the female, while other decisions are male dominated. Family dominance patterns may be *patriarchal,* as may be seen in Appalachian cultures; *matriarchal,* as may be seen in African-American cultures; or more *egalitarian,* as may be seen in European-American cultures. Nurses need to be alert for roles and functions in families since teaching may need to be directed to those responsible for decision making in order to promote health for all family members.

Culture also defines gender roles, the role of the elderly, and the role of the extended family. For example, Native Americans may consult tribal elders (considered part of the extended family) before agreeing to medical care for a pregnant woman or for a child. In some cultures, major decisions for the family, including a child's healthcare, include input from grandparents and other extended family members (Figure 2–3 ●). Grandparents may serve as fos-

● **FIGURE 2–3**

Many cultures value the input of grandparents and other elders in the family or group. In this multigenerational family, the grandmother's guidance is highly valued and significantly influences the family's childrearing practices.

ter parents or assume responsibility for the care of the children in the family, particularly if both parents work.

Family goals are also determined by cultural values and practices, as are family member roles and childbearing and childrearing practices and beliefs.

TEACHING HIGHLIGHTS

INCLUDING GRANDPARENTS AND CULTURAL HEALTH PRACTICES IN THE TEACHING PLAN

When you care for a family in which the grandparents play a key role in decision making, be sure that they are present if you are teaching something that is important for the family to understand and act upon if necessary. This might include, for example, signs of illness in the newborn that need immediate follow-up.

If a specific cultural health practice is important to the family and will not cause harm, such as prayer, chanting, or specific foods, respect the family's beliefs and develop a teaching plan that includes those practices. Respecting their values improves the likelihood that the newly recommended healthcare actions will be accepted.

HEALTH BELIEFS

The three views of health described by Andrews, Boyle, and Carr (2003) are magico-religious, scientific, and holistic. Many people ascribe to a view that combines more than one of these belief systems, but it is helpful to examine them separately.

In the *magico-religious belief view,* health and illness are determined by supernatural forces such as God, gods, magic, spirits, or fate. A miscarriage, for example, or the illness of a pregnant woman or of a child may be perceived as a punishment for actions. Children of preschool age usually have this view of illness; some adults also believe that higher or supernatural powers determine health and illness. It is wise to ask both children and their families what they think caused an illness or how they believe they can stay well. People who believe in this paradigm may gain comfort from prayer, healing rituals, and faith healing. Young children who believe that they have caused their own illness because of their developmental level (usually preschool and early school age) can be expressly told that it was not something they did that caused the illness in order to decrease their feelings of guilt.

The *scientific or biomedical health belief* assumes that physiology explains all illness and life itself (Andrews et al., 2003). Biochemical reactions and the genomic code are used to explain all health states. Illness is always caused by viruses, bacteria, or damage to the body in this framework. This approach is often called "Western medicine." Families who hold this view expect a traditional Western medical intervention, such as medication, treatment, or surgery, to treat the specific health problem. Within this belief system, it is very difficult to understand certain health conditions. Families may struggle to "explain" an illness by wondering if the child was exposed to something harmful during fetal life or has been exposed to something in the environment. A reason for the condition is needed to understand it.

Most physicians, nurses, and other healthcare professionals adhere primarily to the biomedical or scientific theories to explain and treat illnesses. However, certain therapies such as therapeutic touch, biofeedback, and other nontraditional methods that are more common in a holistic health paradigm are gaining popularity within these professions. For the family with this belief system, health professionals sometimes need to emphasize that certain conditions have no known cause, and should suggest treatments other than traditional Western medicine if other approaches may be helpful.

Balance and harmony of the body and nature are important concepts in the *holistic health belief*. It is believed that illness results when the natural balance or harmony is disturbed. Infections and other illnesses gain entry into the body when it is not in balance. This health belief is most common in Eastern world views and in Native American people. Increasingly the ideas of holism are being integrated into Western healthcare and combined with other approaches. An example of integration of approaches is use of a medication or radiation for illness in combination with adequate rest and a diet that is designed to increase immune function.

An associated holistic health belief is the *equilibrium model of health*. It is based on the concept of balance between light and dark, heat and cold. Some Eastern philosophies focus on the notion of *yin* and *yang*. Yin represents the female, passive principle—darkness, cold, wetness—whereas yang is the masculine, active principle—light, heat, and dryness. When the two are combined, they are all that can be. The hot-cold classification is seen in cultures in Latin America, the Near East, and Asia.

Some Mexican Americans, for example, may consider illness to be an excess of either hot or cold. To restore health, imbalances are often corrected by the proper use of foods, medications, or herbs (Table 2–2). These substances are also classified as hot or cold. For example, an illness attributed to an excess of cold is treated with hot foods or medications. The classification of foods is not always consistent, but it conforms to a general structure of traditional knowledge. Certain foods, spices, herbs, and medications are perceived to cool or heat the body. These perceptions do not necessarily correspond to the actual temperature; some hot dishes are said to have a cooling quality.

HEALTHCARE PRACTITIONERS

The family seeking care for the child may choose one or a combination of magico-religious, holistic, or biomedical healthcare providers. The use of *folk healers* varies according to the culture. Though the healer's role and position in the community differ among cultures, healers do share commonalities. Healers speak the language of the cultural group, use common methods of communication for the culture, and live in the same community. They most often conduct healing in their homes or the homes of the patients. Cost is usually reasonable for the family, or some type of bartering may be common (Roy, Torrez, & Dale, 2004).

Mexican Americans and some Latino cultures may seek healing by a *curandero* (male healer) or *curandera* (female healer), who deals with all levels of illness, from minor colds to cancer (Spector, 2004). The curandero's treatment is holistic and may include use of herbs, laying on of hands, massaging the afflicted area, cleansing the body with herbs, preparing an amulet to be worn, burning a candle with a specific prayer printed on the candle jar, or calling the spirit of a saint to bless the individual. Essential to the curandero and the family is the faith the family has in the curandero's abilities. Families may combine curanderismo (Hispanic medical system) with a Western approach for some conditions.

TABLE 2–2 ❖ Hot and Cold Conditions and Foods

Hot Conditions	Cold Foods Used to Treat Hot Conditions	Cold Conditions	Hot Foods Used to Treat Cold Conditions
Diarrhea	Barley water	Cancer	Beef
Fever	Chicken	Earaches	Cheese
Gastrointestinal disturbances	Dairy products	Headaches	Eggs
Infection	Dried fruits	Musculoskeletal conditions	Grains
Kidney problems	Fish	Pneumonia	Liquor
Sore throats	Fresh fruits		Onions
	Fresh vegetables		Spicy foods
	Goat meat		Vitamins

Data from Purnell, L. D. (2003). *Mexican Americans*. In L. D. Purnell & B. J. Paulanka (Eds.), *Transcultural health care: A culturally competent approach* (2nd ed.). Philadelphia: F. A. Davis.

For example, a child with seizures may be given medications for the disorder obtained from Western care and may be fed a tea that the healer believes will treat the condition.

African Americans often combine Western and traditional beliefs about illness. Some believe in spirits as causes of illness and may use powders, oils, and ceremony to maintain health.

Native Americans may seek healing from a shaman, healer, or medicine man or woman. Because Native Americans believe in the balance of nature and a state of harmony, they seek advice to identify what they have done to disrupt their body harmony. The healer will then prescribe the required treatment for restoration of balance and harmony. Teas, other herbal products, sweats, smudges, meditation, and other approaches are common. Returning to one's family, home, and roots may produce a sense of balance.

IMPACT OF RELIGION AND SPIRITUALITY

The terms *religion* and *spirituality* mean different things to different people. Many people view religion, which is sometimes termed "faith-based belief," as an organized system that shares a common set of beliefs and practices about the significance, cause, and purpose of life and the universe. Religion is usually centered on the belief in or worshipping of a supreme being (such as God). **Spirituality** refers to an individual's concern with the spirit or soul and may also include his or her experience with and interpretation of a transcendent power.

A family's religious beliefs, affiliation, and practices can deeply influence their experiences and attitudes toward healthcare, childbearing, and childrearing. Members of certain religious groups such as Christian Scientists may attempt to avoid all medical interventions, whereas others such as Jehovah's Witnesses may refuse specific interventions, such as blood transfusions. Roman Catholics may refuse contraception. In most cases, families gain comfort from acknowledgment of and respect for their religious beliefs and practices in the healthcare setting. However, the agnostic (one who has doubts about the existence of a transcendent being) or the atheist (one who believes that there is no higher power) may be offended if care providers assume that references to God or to a higher power will be comforting.

A religious or spiritual history is often completed when a woman is admitted to a clinic or labor setting or when a child is admitted to the hospital. The assessment can include questions about current spiritual beliefs and practices and preferences for religious rituals. Whenever possible the nurse should attempt to accommodate religious rituals and practices requested by the family.

Considering the diversity of religious beliefs, it is not unusual for nurses to encounter childbearing families whose beliefs conflict with their own. This is not problematic as long as the nurse avoids attempts to influence the family's decision making. For example, a nurse who does not believe in baptism should avoid revealing this to a Catholic seeking baptism for her stillborn infant. Nurses should also examine their religious beliefs related to genetic screening procedures, use of assisted reproductive technology to achieve pregnancy, abortion, use of technology to support life in a severely compromised newborn or a terminally ill child, and even less dramatic issues such as methods of contraception, circumcision, infant feeding, and disciplinary practices for children.

Although spirituality and faith-based belief are generally positive in supporting families to maintain and restore health, at times they can have potentially negative effects for children. Certain groups may blame individuals for their own illnesses, and children may develop guilt as a result. If prejudice toward or denigration of other groups occurs, unhealthy responses may interfere with the child's healthy development. Abuse may result from parental religious beliefs about corporal punishment and discipline. If lifesaving treatments are denied by a religious group, courts may intervene to ensure care for the child. Children involved in cult groups may suffer emotional and psychologic harm. Adolescents who are homosexual may be the target of negative feedback and response from their religious community. This may lead them to avoid healthcare that could be potentially beneficial.

The three most common faith traditions in the United States are Christianity, Judaism, and Islam (Fosarelli, 2003) (Figure 2–4 ●). Although adherence to a religious tradition is predominant in the United States, it should not be assumed that all individuals believe in or practice organized religion. The nurse should always ask the family if they follow a faith tradition and if they would like a leader from that faith to visit when in the hospital. Adolescents

● **FIGURE 2–4**

Today very few communities are limited to one culture. The children in this multicultural choir are representative of the changes in demographics of many Western countries. Even though they may differ in cultural background, a common thread is found in their religious preference.

may follow different faith traditions than their parents and should be asked the question individually.

Collaboration between the healthcare team and family is essential to providing care congruent with the child and family's expectations. Although spirituality is important for many families, it is often overlooked as a healing strategy. Illness and injury may cause the family to turn to spiritual guidance as a method of understanding and coping. The trust in a higher being or purpose provides meaning for many children, supporting them as they deal with health problems (Elkins & Cavendish, 2004). The nurse must respect the family's view and avoid being judgmental toward their beliefs. Partnering with the child and family to incorporate their traditional practices and beliefs with prescribed therapies will help to ensure the delivery of safe and effective care for the child.

In many institutions, nurses can ask to be reassigned to a different client if their religious beliefs are in conflict because of healthcare being provided or refused by the client and family; however, if other personnel are not available, it is the nurse's responsibility to provide sensitive, appropriate, and nonjudgmental care to that client.

CHILDBEARING PRACTICES

Children are generally valued all over the world, not only for the joy they bring, but also because they ensure continuation of the family and cultural values. This valuing of children may manifest itself in different ways, however. Families in the United States and many Western countries commonly have only one or two children out of a desire to provide the children with the best home and education they can afford and to spend as much free time with them as possible. In contrast, in many cultures throughout the world, it is common to have as many children as possible.

In some cultures a woman who gives birth achieves a higher status, especially if the child is male. This is especially true in the traditional Chinese culture and in some Middle Eastern cultures. In the western United States, people of the Mormon faith view motherhood as the most important aspect of a woman's life, comparable with the male role of priesthood (Faust, 2000). In Mexican-American society and among many other Latino groups, having children is evidence of the male's virility and is a sign of manliness or *machismo,* a desired trait.

Culture may also influence attitudes and beliefs about contraception. For example, many Muslims from the Middle East do not practice contraception because children are highly valued and it is believed that the traditional role of women is to bear children. In Chinese society, on the other hand, where state policy limits the number of children a couple can have, contraception is common.

Health values and beliefs are also important in understanding reactions and behavior. Certain behaviors can be expected if a culture views pregnancy as a sickness, whereas other behaviors can be expected if the culture views pregnancy as a natural occurrence. For example, because Native Americans, African Americans, and Mexican Americans generally view pregnancy as a natural and desirable condition, prenatal care may not be a priority. Although many cultures view pregnancy as a natural occurrence, it may also be seen as a time of increased vulnerability. In Orthodox Judaism, for example, it is a man's responsibility to procreate, but it is a woman's right, not her obligation, to do so. This is because, according to Orthodox Jewish law, the health of the mother, both physically and mentally, is of primary concern, and she should never be obliged to do something that threatens her life (Bodo & Gibson, 1999a). Individuals of many cultures take certain protective precautions based on their beliefs. For example, many Southeast Asian women fear that they will have a complicated labor and birth if they sit in a doorway or on a step. Thus, they tend to avoid areas near doors in waiting rooms and examining rooms (Mattson, 1995).

In the Mexican-American culture, the concept of *mal aire,* or bad air, is sometimes related to evil spirits. It is thought that air, especially night air, might enter the body and cause harm. Preventive measures, such as keeping the windows closed or covering the head, are used. Some Latinos may place a raisin on the cord stump of a newborn to prevent drafts from entering the body (Murray & Zentner, 2001). For many Vietnamese women, lifting the arms above the head is believed to increase the risk of preterm birth. Vietnamese women also are discouraged from sitting or lying down for lengthy periods because doing so might permit the baby to become too large (Bodo & Gibson, 1999b).

A **taboo** is a behavior or thing that is to be avoided. Many cultures, including those found in the United States, have taboos centered on the unborn baby or newborn that are meant to ensure that the baby will survive. In developing countries, mortality rates among infants and young children are extremely high; thus, certain traditions focus on preventing early death. For example, it is common among Muslims to avoid naming babies until they are born and to ensure that the first words a baby hears are from God (Purnell & Paulanka, 2003). Taboos also arise from the belief that a pregnant woman has evil powers. As a result, pregnant women are sometimes prohibited from taking part in certain activities with other people.

NURSING PRACTICE

When offering your clients fluids, ask if they would prefer them hot, warm, or iced. This can help ensure that proper hydration is maintained and cultural beliefs are supported.

CHILDREARING PRACTICES

In some families children are expected to take on responsibilities early and may be expected to take on tasks such as management of their own chronic disease and nutritional intake. In other families, children are given long periods to grow up and are not expected to manage healthcare needs. Directing teaching to a child with diabetes in the second type of family may not be appropriate.

Nurses often provide information and ask about developmental milestones for children. It is commonly expected that children are weaned by around 1 year and toilet trained at about 2 years of age. However, there may be variations in family goals and it is not unusual that families accomplish these tasks with children at younger or older ages. The nurse should ask about the norms in the family and whether the child is following expectations of the parents. As long as the child is progressing in motor, language, and social tasks, some variation is expected due to cultural norms.

Views about alternative lifestyles such as sexual orientation and single parenting are also established by the family's values and beliefs. Understanding such values assists the nurse in providing sensitive care. Some examples of childrearing practices common to particular cultures are listed in Table 2–3.

CULTURE AND NURSING CARE

Healthcare providers are often unaware of the cultural characteristics they themselves demonstrate. Without cultural awareness, caregivers tend to project their own cultural responses onto foreign-born clients; clients from different socioeconomic, religious, or educational groups; or clients from different regions of the country. This projection leads care providers to assume that the clients are demonstrating a specific behavior for the same reason that they themselves would. Moreover, healthcare providers often fail to realize that medicine has its own culture, which has been dominated historically by traditional middle-class values and beliefs.

Ethnocentrism is the conviction that the values and beliefs of one's own cultural group are the best or only acceptable ones. It is characterized by an inability to understand the beliefs and worldview of another culture. To a certain extent, everyone is guilty of ethnocentrism, at least some of the time. Thus, the nurse who values stoicism during labor

---

TABLE 2–3 ✛ Childrearing Practices of Selected Cultures

Culture	Childrearing Practices	Culture	Childrearing Practices
African American	Children may be raised by grandparent (typically grandmother) Children are expected to demonstrate respectfulness, conformity to rules, obedience, and good behavior May use belly band or coin on umbilicus to prevent protrusion of umbilicus	Chinese American	Family may lavish resources on child Children typically depend on family for all needs and may not be expected to earn their own money as adolescents Male children are often more valued than female children Children may be taught to avoid displaying their emotions/feelings Children are expected to assist parents in the home (chores) High educational achievement is expected
Amish	Children are expected to continue with the Amish tradition Grandparents often provide care to children Family may not seek prenatal care Children are expected to follow the rules as prescribed by the church district		
Appalachian	Large families are common Strict parenting practices Grandparents frequently provide care to children	Mexican American	Children are closely protected and are not encouraged to leave the home Godparents are included in care of the child; considered "co-parents" Children are expected to demonstrate respect for parents and elder family members Discipline may include physical punishment
Arab American	Father is typically the disciplinarian The child's character is considered a reflection of the family's influence Aggression toward parents and authority is strongly disapproved Discipline may include physical punishment and shaming Preference may be noted toward male children	Navajo Indian	Children's name may not be revealed until their first laugh Infants may be kept in a cradleboard to protect them Grandmothers frequently are responsible for toilet training, disciplining, and weaning Older children may be taught to be stoic and uncomplaining

Data from Purnell, L. D., & Paulanka, B. J. (Eds.). (2003). *Transcultural health care: A culturally competent approach* (2nd ed.). Philadelphia: F. A. Davis.

may be uncomfortable with the more vocal response of some Latin American women. Another nurse may be disconcerted by a Southeast Asian woman who believes that pain is something to be endured rather than alleviated and who is intent on maintaining self-control in labor.

Healthcare providers sometimes believe that if members of other cultures do not share Western values and beliefs, they should adopt them. For example, a nurse who believes strongly in equality of the sexes may find it difficult to remain silent if a woman from a Middle Eastern culture defers to her husband in decision making. It is important to remember that pressure to defy cultural values and beliefs can be stressful and anxiety provoking for these women.

To address issues of cultural diversity in the provision of healthcare, emphasis is being placed on developing **cultural competence**—that is, the skills and knowledge necessary to appreciate, respect, and effectively work with individuals from different cultures. It requires self-awareness, awareness and understanding of cultural differences, and the ability to adapt clinical skills and practices as needed by integrating them into the family's belief system.

DEVELOPING CULTURAL COMPETENCE

CULTURE SHOCK

The experience that people have in attempting to understand or adapt to a culture that is fundamentally different from their own culture is known as culture shock. Feelings of discomfort, powerlessness, anxiety, and disorientation are common. Immigrants to the United States and Canada may experience culture shock when differences or conflicts arise between their own values, beliefs, and customs and the ways of their new surroundings. The nurse should assess childbearing women, children, and their families who have recently immigrated for indications of culture shock. Referring the family to counseling or support from representatives of the family's culture, such as a translator or community group, may be helpful.

CULTURALLY INFLUENCED RESPONSES

The nurse can begin developing cultural competence by becoming knowledgeable about the cultural differences and practices of various groups. Nurses who are knowledgeable of differences and who take them into account in planning and providing nursing care will be far more effective caregivers than those who do not.

Biologic Differences

Genetic and physical differences occur among cultural groups and can lead to disparity in needs and care. Blacks are more likely to experience hypertension, strokes, obesity, diabetes, and sickle cell anemia. Thalassemia, another type of anemia, is most common in Mediterranean people. Blacks and Native Americans tend to have higher rates of tuberculosis than the general population. On the other hand, blacks have higher bone mass than whites and lower rates of osteoporosis. Whites have high rates of obesity and heart disease. Whites from certain geographic origins are more likely to manifest cystic fibrosis, celiac disease, and Crohn disease. Hispanics have high rates of diabetes and lactose intolerance. Asians and Native Americans often do not metabolize alcohol readily and are more prone to either injury after alcohol ingestion or to alcohol abuse. Otitis media, or infection of the middle ear, is common in Native American and Alaskan Native children. Diabetes, liver disease, and injuries are common in Native American groups (Spector, 2004). Metabolism of certain drugs is also linked to genetics in certain groups.

Nurses must understand other genetic characteristics in order to perform culturally competent nursing assessments and interventions. Differences in skin color and tone may make cyanosis, pallor, and jaundice difficult to recognize and describe. Mongolian spots are darkened skin on the lower back and buttocks of some babies with dark skin tones. Variations in texture of hair require different approaches to hygiene among various racial groups.

Communication Patterns

Communication is the method by which members of cultural groups share information and preserve their beliefs, values, norms, and practices. To ensure effective care, it is essential for families to be able to communicate with nurses and other healthcare providers. This becomes an issue when the family does not speak the language of the health professionals. In such cases it is best if the healthcare facility provides translators. Often children are most likely to speak both the language of the parents and of the healthcare providers and may appear to be likely translators. However, experts recommend that they never be used to translate in healthcare situations due to the confidentiality needs of both parent and child. Signs, posted literature, and brochures should also be available in the languages of the families served.

NURSING PRACTICE

Speaking and reading may not occur in the same language. For example, an immigrant may read and speak fluently in his or her primary language and speak but not read the language of the new country. The immigrant's child may read and speak the language of the present country and speak but not read the native language of the family. Always ask about both reading and speaking preferences.

Critical Thinking: Examine Your Cultural Influences

Language can also affect health literacy skills. A large number of instructions are given in writing. Examples include prescriptions and directions on medication bottles, signs hanging in health facilities, consent forms for procedures and surgery, insurance forms, directions for techniques or procedures, future appointment dates, and health promotion materials. Nurses need to verify what the client and family can read and whether alternative methods are needed. Nurses can verbally give the information and provide paper and pencil so that the family can write it down in their own language. Translation services should be available in all healthcare settings.

Variations in communication among cultures are reflected in their word meaning, voice inflection and quality, and verbal styles. Culture influences not only the manner in which feelings are expressed, but also which verbal and nonverbal expressions of communication are considered appropriate. An individual's willingness to discuss certain topics or to express or conceal certain thoughts and feelings is also influenced by the cultural norms. For example, Native Americans and people of Asian descent may feel it is appropriate to remain quiet when experiencing pain, whereas people of Italian, Jewish, and Latino descent may feel that it is best to express pain more vocally.

Use of names varies among cultural groups. Assuming that each person wishes to be called by a first name can be disrespectful. Address family members respectfully, usually using terms such as Mr., Mrs., and Ms. If the person has a title such as doctor, judge, or senator, it should be used. The nurse should ask what the person prefers to be called and record this in the health record for future reference. In some cultures such as Korean, Cambodian, and Filipino, the first name used is actually the family name. Asking for the "family name" rather than the "last name" may clarify this practice.

Nonverbal Communication. Nonverbal communication patterns may hinder or help communication. For example, gestures and body language may be misunderstood or misinterpreted. Similarly eye contact has different meanings among cultures. European Americans, for example, value eye contact with communication and interpret this as a sign of sincerity and interest. In other cultures, such as Asian and Native American, sustained eye contact may be considered rude or disrespectful.

Silence may also be considered a sign of respect in some cultures. Among those groups, offering an immediate response to a question may be viewed as being disrespectful since an instant reply could indicate that no thought was given to the matter. Nurses should watch for patterns in various cultures and alter their approach to be more congruent. For example, many nurses commonly nod and say "yes" or "oh, I see" when a health client is speaking. This may seem disruptive to some cultures. If the listener is silent and does not use such patterns of agreement, the nurse should alter his or her response to match more closely the acceptable method of communication for the family. Silence and quiet listening can be perceived as positive approaches.

Touch. The appropriateness of touch varies with each culture. For example, an Asian may consider touching an unfamiliar person of the opposite gender to be inappropriate, whereas touch between men and women may be viewed as appropriate by another culture. Adults commonly feel that it is acceptable to touch children of all ages, but this may not be accurate. It is best to look for responses from the family to touch and progress accordingly.

Space. Depending on an individual's specific culture, the use of space has different meanings. Space, as defined in this context, refers to the relationship between the individual and other persons and objects in the environment. Cultures may have specific spatial preferences, such as personal distance and social distance. Some cultures tend to prefer close contact with less space since they use touch as a form of communication. The nurse should be alert for how close a childbearing woman or a child comes to other individuals and try to maintain this space during interactions. Nursing procedures often cause the space barrier to be broken. Nurses need to touch clients to take vital signs, administer injections, change dressings, and the like. This does not mean that close touch is appropriate at all times. It is essential to tell all clients before touching them for procedures so they understand what is happening.

Time Orientation

Time orientation can vary significantly among cultures. Cultural groups may place emphasis on the events of the past, those events that occur in the present, or those events that will occur in the future. Time is also influenced by development. Young children sometimes do not understand the use of clocks, the importance ascribed to being "on time," or other time orientations.

Cultures that are oriented predominantly to the past may want to begin healthcare encounters with lengthy descriptions of past healthcare treatments, family history of diseases, or individual past experiences with health. There may be little interest in learning methods of adapting to or maintaining a new plan of care.

For cultures that are oriented predominantly to the present, little consideration may be given to either the past or the future. For example, adolescents commonly focus on the present, and may not engage in preventive health practices for long-term health. Short-term goals often provide more incentive to adolescents.

Cultures that are oriented predominantly to the future, such as European American, may not focus on what is important at the present time. For example, the family focusing on the future may focus on the dreams they had for a child's education or sports performance and have trouble setting present goals for treatment of a disease such as juvenile rheumatoid arthritis. One commonly hears that it was a big adjustment to learn to "take one day at a time." Not living up to the family's expectation for their future success may be difficult for a child who has developed an illness that has a chronic course.

Time also refers to punctuality about schedules and appointments. In the United States and Canada, the predominant culture respects promptness and considers time valuable and not to be wasted. Other cultures may not reflect this same concern for time. This may be manifested by a family's inability to follow timed medication schedules or treatments, or to show up as scheduled for an appointment. In these cases it is not intended as a sign of disrespect.

Nutrition

Nutritional practices begin even before birth as many cultural groups have beliefs that determine foods that are healthy to eat or should be avoided during pregnancy. Nutritional habits and patterns vary among cultures and are related to both religious practices and health beliefs. Certain cultures and religions have restrictions on or prescriptions about specific foods and preparation methods. Ritualistic behaviors involving eating and drinking, for example on special occasions and holidays, are observed by most cultures. Many religions recommend fasts during specific holy seasons, such as Lent for Roman Catholics, Yom Kippur for Jews, and Ramadan for Muslims. However, in most cases, small children, pregnant women, the elderly, and sick individuals are not required to fast.

Some cultures value large size or may associate a healthy child with being "large." Other cultures value slimness and look down upon obese individuals. Both of these views influence family eating patterns and expectations for the child; the child's self-esteem can therefore be influenced. The U.S and Canadian cultures honor being slim in the media but reinforce eating and large size by the availability of fast food and positive image of large sports stars such as some football players, resulting in confusion in the minds of some youth.

Nutrition may also be essential to the culture's practices for health promotion and care during illness. Health problems associated with specific cultures that may require dietary changes are also identified. Nutrition can be closely related to environmental situations, and families with few resources may not be able to obtain or eat cultural foods due to access or financial issues. Nutrition plays a powerful role in maintaining health, so resources for nutritious and desired foods may be needed.

NURSING MANAGEMENT

Mattson and Smith (2004) suggest that care providers conduct a cultural assessment to glean information about health practices based on the client's beliefs, values, and customs. This kind of assessment might include questions such as the following:

- Who in the family must be consulted before decisions are made about a person's care?
- Does the client, or do the parents of a child, see primarily in the present or do they have a futuristic time orientation?
- What type of health provider is most appropriate for (or preferred by) the woman, the child, or the family?
- Does the family have beliefs or traditions that may affect the plan of care?

Several cultural assessment tools are available to assist the nurse in gathering this information. These tools are becoming increasingly common at healthcare agencies as providers act in response to the expectation of culturally competent care. The nurse who respects cultural diversity is an asset to the childbearing and childrearing family as they adjust to their new role. Establishing a trusting relationship enables the nurse to assist the family in meeting educational needs.

The use of North American Nursing Diagnosis Association (NANDA) nursing diagnoses to describe situations specifically related to culture may in itself be culturally biased because the foci of these diagnoses are based on Western cultural beliefs. For example, the nurse may apply diagnoses such as "noncompliance" or "impaired verbal communication" to the child and family; however, that could be construed as culturally biased. Is someone who speaks a different language "impaired" in communication?

Specific nursing diagnoses are dependent upon the reason the family seeks contact with healthcare professionals, ranging from a pregnancy to a child's health promotion and health maintenance (e.g., immunizations) to the care of a chronic or terminally ill child. Examples include the following:

- *Ineffective Therapeutic Regimen Management* related to mistrust of healthcare personnel
- *Fear* related to separation from support system in stressful situation such as hospitalization
- *Spiritual Distress* related to discrepancy between spiritual beliefs and prescribed treatment
- *Interrupted Family Processes* related to a shift in family roles due to illness

The planning and implementation of nursing care for the culturally diverse family depends specifically on the findings of the previous assessments. Nurses need to partner with the family to establish a safe, effective, and desirable plan of care. Nurses can ensure access to an interpreter if needed and evaluate whether the match with a particular interpreter is appropriate for the child and family.

EVIDENCE-BASED NURSING

INVESTIGATING CULTURE AND HEALTHCARE BARRIERS

Clinical Question

What barriers to providing accessible healthcare exist among ethnically diverse families with children?

Evidence

A review of several studies of families from minority populations revealed that cost and the need for additional information are two factors influencing a family's access to healthcare.

An interview with 62 Haitian family members about care for their school-age children revealed that the major reason for not obtaining care was cost. About 42% of the children did not have healthcare coverage because families did not believe they were eligible for care, could not get transportation to the office to complete applications for care, lacked knowledge about programs available, were opposed to the detailed questions asked on forms, or had general distrust of government (Schantz, Charron, & Folden, 2003).

In another study of immigrants, Korean children were examined for completion of the hepatitis B vaccination series. Perception that hepatitis B was a serious disease was an incentive for completion of the series, while difficulty paying the cost was a major barrier to completion (Kim, 2004).

A study was conducted with 42 family members of Latino children and 42 family members of European Americans with special healthcare needs. Both groups cited frustrations in care related to access to rehabilitation, and lack of integration of care within the school system. Latino families often cited need for more information and access to a support group, while European-American families cited a need for referral to day care and respite care resources (Gannotti, Kaplan, Handwerker, & Groce, 2004).

Implications

When cost is a factor, nurses need to refer families to sources for healthcare services and then follow up to be sure the families were able to access care. Referrals to neighborhood clinics and giving instructions for transportation to the health setting are important for many families. A need for information is another theme among most groups. Explaining why an immunization is needed as well as providing information about the child's condition are important nursing roles. Referring the family to others from the same group and assisting them in navigating complex systems such as school and social services may also be necessary.

Critical Thinking

What is the process that immigrant families in your state or province must follow to secure healthcare for their children? How would you help to guide someone through this process?

What cultural groups are common in your community? Do you speak their language? If not, what measures should you take to ensure that they understand the teaching offered in clinical settings? What type of support groups will be helpful for families when they have a child with special healthcare needs?

References

Gannotti, M. E., Kaplan, L. C., Handwerker, W. P., & Groce, N. E. (2004). Cultural influences on health care use: Differences in perceived unmet needs and expectations of providers by Latino and Euro-American parents of children with special health care needs. *Journal of Developmental and Behavioral Pediatrics, 25,* 156-165.

Kim, Y. O. R. (2004). Access to hepatitis B vaccination among Korean American children in immigrant families. *Journal of Health Care for the Poor and Underserved, 15,* 170-174.

Schantz, S., Charron, S. A., & Folden, S. L. (2003). Health seeking behaviors of Haitian families for their school aged children. *Journal of Cultural Diversity, 10,* 62-68.

Recognizing the influence of culture on one's beliefs, values, and healthcare practices is essential for the nurse to deliver culturally competent care. The nurse who develops his or her own techniques in assessing the influence of culture on the pregnant woman or the child and family and who incorporates that information into an individualized plan of care demonstrates appropriate strategies for delivering culturally sensitive care.

Culturally competent nurses find effective ways to partner with the family to assist them in determining how they can incorporate prescribed therapies with their healthcare practices. Ensure that the woman herself or the child and family understand the problem or illness, treatment, and health promotion activities. Apply culturally sensitive techniques when dispelling any cultural myths.

Nurses can also collaborate with a multidisciplinary team including social workers and language specialists to assist the family with barriers to care such as transportation, financial issues, remote access, and any other barriers to effective healthcare.

COMPLEMENTARY AND ALTERNATIVE THERAPIES AND THE FAMILY

Through the latter part of the 20th century in the United States, it was rare for European-American childbearing families to consult anyone except their obstetrician for advice about their pregnancy, birth, and postpartum. Similarly, most childrearing families closely followed the advice of their pediatrician about all aspects of child care. Though such clients are still encountered today, nurses are more likely to care for families who integrate other types of practitioners and therapies with traditional Western medicine.

A **complementary therapy** may be defined as an adjunct to conventional medical treatment that has been through rigorous scientific testing that shows that it has some reliability. Although complementary therapies were absent from clinics and hospitals until the last few decades, therapies such as acupuncture, acupressure, and massage therapy are now often used with conventional medical care, and many health insurance plans cover at least a portion of the cost of such therapies.

In contrast, an **alternative therapy** is generally considered a substance or procedure that is used in place of conventional biomedical care. It usually has not undergone rigorous scientific testing in this country, although it might have been thoroughly tested in other countries. Alternative therapies are not usually available in conventional clinics and hospitals, and their costs are not typically covered under most health insurance policies. For example, research studies indicating the benefits of magnet therapy in treating some chronic conditions such as carpal tunnel syndrome have been conducted in India, Japan, and Russia; however, researchers in the United States are only beginning to study the effects of magnet therapy. Thus, this therapy is still considered experimental and would be classified as an alternative therapy.

The dramatic increase in complementary and alternative therapies that began in the final decade of the 20th century was probably the result of a combination of several factors:

- Increased consumer awareness of the limitations of conventional Western medicine
- Increased international travel
- Increased media attention
- Advent of the Internet

In this new century, it seems clear that Western healthcare will see an ever-increasing integration between conventional medicine and complementary therapies. Some obvious examples of this new integration in perinatal settings include the acceptance of certain herbal teas for antepartum discomforts; the use of massage, Reiki, or therapeutic touch during the first stage of labor; music during childbirth; and the increased emphasis on skin-to-skin mother-to-baby bonding in the immediate postpartum period.

Further evidence of this increased integration is the establishment in 1992 of the Office of Alternative Medicine (OAM) at the National Institutes of Health. The OAM was mandated by Congress to promote research into complementary and alternative therapies and dissemination of information to consumers. In 1998 the OAM was incorporated into a new National Center for Complementary and Alternative Medicine (NCCAM) with an expanded mission and increased funding. Many studies of complementary and alternative therapies are currently under way at NCCAM, which can be accessed at *http://nccam.nih.gov*.

BENEFITS AND RISKS

Complementary and alternative therapies undisputedly have many benefits for women and children. Many complementary and alternative therapies emphasize prevention and wellness, and place a higher value on holistic healing than on physical cure. Many are noninvasive, have few side effects, and are more affordable and available than conventional therapies.

However, many of these remedies have associated risks that must be considered thoughtfully before a decision is made to use them. These risks include lack of standardization, lack of regulation and research substantiating safety and effectiveness (particularly in children), inadequate training and certification of some healers, and financial and health risks of unproven methods.

TYPES OF COMPLEMENTARY AND ALTERNATIVE THERAPIES

Numerous forms of complementary and alternative therapies are available. Only a few of the most commonly used approaches are presented here.

Homeopathy

Homeopathy is best understood in contrast to conventional Western medicine, which is also called *allopathic medicine*. The term *allopathy* is derived from the Greek words *allos* meaning different and *pathos* meaning suffering. Thus, allopathic medicine uses remedies that produce effects differing from—or in opposition to—those of the disease being treated. For example, conventional healthcare practitioners may prescribe an anti-inflammatory to reduce swelling, or an antibiotic for infection.

The term *homeopathy* is derived from the Greek word *homos* meaning the same. Thus, it is often described as a healing system that uses like to cure like; that is, homeopathic remedies are minute dilutions of substances that, if ingested in larger amounts, would produce effects *similar* to the symptoms of the disorder being treated. For example, *Cantharis vesicatoria* is a species of beetle (commonly called Spanish fly) whose poison causes, among other symptoms, burning pains and a frantic urge to urinate (Lockie & Geddes, 2000). Homeopathic *Cantharis* is a minute dilution of this toxin and is thus a remedy of choice for women suffering from cystitis.

Naturopathy

Naturopathy is commonly referred to as *natural medicine*. It is more precisely defined as a healing system that employs various natural means of preventing and treating human disease. Many naturopathic physicians are eclectic, employing a variety of therapies in their practice. These might include clinical nutrition, botanical medicine, homeopathy, acupuncture, hydrotherapy, physiotherapy, and counseling for lifestyle modification. Certain medications, treatments, and immunizations may be refused in this approach (Atwood, 2003).

Traditional Chinese Medicine

Traditional Chinese medicine (TCM) developed more than 3000 years ago in the Chinese culture and then gradually spread with modifications to other Asian countries. The underlying focus of TCM is prevention, although diagnosis and treatment of disease also play an important role.

TCM seeks to ensure the balance of energy, which is called *chi* or *qi* (pronounced "chee"). Chi is the invisible flow of energy in the body that maintains health and energy and enables the body to carry out its physiologic functions. Chi flows along certain pathways or meridians.

Another important concept in TCM is that of *yin* and *yang* (discussed earlier), opposing internal and external forces that, together, represent the whole.

TCM includes the following therapeutic techniques:

- *Acupuncture* uses very fine (hairlike) stainless steel needles to stimulate specific acupuncture points, depending on the client's medical assessment and condition.

- *Acupressure* (Chinese massage) uses pressure from the fingers and thumbs to stimulate pressure points.

- *Herbal therapy* is an important part of TCM, but it is sometimes difficult to locate a skilled herbalist because there are relatively few in the United States and other English-speaking countries.

- *Qigong* (pronounced "chee-goong") is a self-discipline that involves the use of breathing, meditation, self-massage, and movement. Typically practiced daily, the movements are nontiring and are designed to stimulate the flow of chi.

- *Tai chi* (pronounced "ty chee") is a form of martial art. It originally focused on physical fitness and self-defense, but it is currently used to improve health as well (Fontaine, 2005).

- *Moxibustion* involves the application of heat from a small piece of burning herb called *moxa*. When applied to the appropriate acupoint, the heat is believed to regulate the flow of chi (Shealy, 1999).

Mind-Based Therapies

Biofeedback is a method used to help individuals learn to control their physiologic responses based on the concept that the mind controls the body. An individual is hooked up to a system of highly sensitive instruments that relay information about the body back to that person. Currently biofeedback has more than 150 applications for disease prevention and the restoration of health. The effectiveness of biofeedback has been proven in countless studies, and it is now considered a conventional therapy more than a complementary one.

Hypnosis, whether guided by a trained hypnotherapist or induced through self-hypnosis, is a state of great mental and physical relaxation during which a person is very open to sug-gestions. In this state the individual is able to modify body responses. Pregnant women who receive hypnosis before childbirth have reported shorter, less painful labors and births.

Visualization is a complementary therapy in which a person goes into a relaxed state and focuses on or "visualizes" soothing or positive scenes such as a beach or a mountain glade. Visualization helps reduce stress and encourage relaxation.

Guided imagery is a state of intense, focused concentration used to create compelling mental images. It is sometimes considered a form of hypnosis. Guided imagery is useful in imagining a desired effect such as weight loss or in mentally rehearsing a new procedure or activity.

Chiropractic

Chiropractic, the third largest independent health profession in the United States (behind medicine and dentistry), is based on concepts of manipulation to address health problems that are thought to be the result of abnormal nerve transmissions (subluxation) caused by misalignment of the spine. Chiropractors also stress the importance of proper nutrition and regular exercise to good health. Chiropractic is widely available, and popular demand has earned it a higher level of insurance coverage than most other alternative therapies.

Massage Therapy

Massage has been used for centuries as a form of therapy. *Massage therapy* involves the manipulation of the soft tissues of the body to reduce stress and tension, increase circulation, diminish pain, and promote a sense of well-being. Different techniques have been developed, including Swedish massage, shiatsu massage, rolfing, and trigger point massage. Most forms use techniques such as pressing, kneading, gliding, circular motion, tapping, and vibrational strokes.

Certain massage therapists specialize in massage for women during pregnancy. Massage is often helpful as women adapt to the discomforts of their changing bodies. Certified nurse-midwives often use perineal massage prior to labor to stretch the muscles of the perineum around the vaginal opening and thereby prevent tearing of the tissues during childbirth. During labor, massage of the back and buttocks by the nurse, labor coach, or *doula* can help the woman relax and may help decrease her discomfort.

Infant massage is also growing in popularity in the United States, and many parents have learned to massage their infants and young children (Figure 2–5 ●). Massage also plays a role in therapy for children with a variety of conditions, including eczema.

Herbal Therapies

Herbal therapy or herbal medicine has been used since ancient times to treat illnesses and ailments. Like vitamins and minerals, herbs are a form of dietary supplement, but

FIGURE 2-5

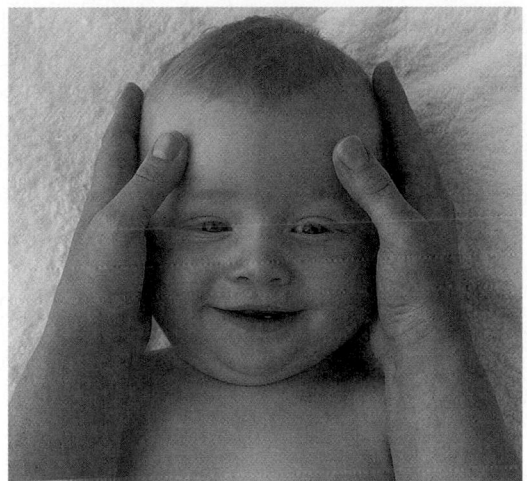

Infant massage.

thcy are often used to treat the symptoms of specific ailments rather than simply to enhance overall health. Well-known herbal remedies include, for example, ginger, rosemary, ginseng, ginkgo, chamomile, oil of evening primrose, *Echinacea*, garlic, lemon balm, and black cohosh.

Currently about 1500 botanical substances are sold in the United States as dietary supplements or as part of traditional ethnic medications. However, herbal formulations are not subject to U.S. Food and Drug Administration (FDA) premarket testing for safety and effectiveness (National Toxicology Program, 2003). Thus, these products can be sold over the counter with only little control over quality or potency. (The FDA does have the authority to pull a product off the market if it is proven to be dangerous.) Consequently most of what is known about herbs comes from Europe, where they have been studied for some time. Herbal products from Germany, France, England, and Australia are reasonably safe because in these countries, herbs are regulated as if they were drugs (Graedon & Graedon, 2001).

The use of herbs during pregnancy is an especially important consideration for nurses working with childbearing families. Pregnant women interested in using herbs are best advised to follow basic principles (Belew, 1999):

1. Avoid the use of any herbs, even tonic herbs, during the first trimester, whenever possible.

2. Avoid highly concentrated extracts because the risk of side effects tends to be higher than with whole plant extracts.

In addition, pregnant women need to avoid certain categories of herbs such as abortifacient (abortion-inducing) herbs, herbs that induce menstruation, nervous system stimulants, stimulant laxatives, and so forth.

Lists identifying common herbs that women are advised to avoid or use with caution during pregnancy and lactation are available. Caution is the key focus for childbearing families and children. NCCAM (2004) states specifically, "Women who are pregnant or nursing should be especially cautious about using herbal supplements, since these products can act like drugs. This caution also applies to treating children with herbal supplements" (p. 2).

DEVELOPING CULTURAL COMPETENCE

HERBALISM

The World Health Organization estimates that 80% of the earth's population depends on plants to treat common ailments. Herbalism is an essential part of traditional Indian, Asian, Native American, and naturopathic medicines. Many homeopathic remedies are also developed from herbs (Balch & Balch, 2000).

Therapeutic Touch

Therapeutic touch is a complementary therapy meant to be used with conventional medical care. It was developed in the early 1970s by Dr. Delores Krieger, a nursing professor at New York University, and Dora Kunz, a clairvoyant healer. Therapeutic touch is grounded in the belief that people are a system of energy with a self-healing potential. The therapeutic touch practitioner, often a nurse, can unite his or her energy field with that of the client's, directing it in a specific way to promote well-being and healing. Proponents of therapeutic touch believe that a strong desire to help the recipient is essential as is a conscious use of self to act as a link between the universal life energy and the other person (Fontaine, 2005).

Like many other conventional and complementary therapies, therapeutic touch should be applied cautiously to pregnant women, newborns, and children by trained providers (Figure 2–6).

Other Types of Complementary and Alternative Therapies

This discussion only touched on some of the most common forms of complementary and alternative therapies. Other examples include ayurveda (the traditional medicine of India), meditation, craniosacral therapy, reflexology, hydrotherapy, Hatha yoga, regular physical exercise, aromatherapy, color and light therapy, music and sound therapies, magnetic therapy, and Reiki, to name a few. Readers interested in these therapies are referred to specialty texts.

○ **FIGURE 2–6**

During pregnancy, therapeutic touch is often helpful in easing pain and reducing anxiety.

Used with permission from Nurse Healers–Professional Associates International, *the official organization for Therapeutic Touch, http://www.therapeutic_touch.org.*

NURSING CARE OF THE FAMILY USING COMPLEMENTARY THERAPIES

Research suggests that the people most likely to use complementary and alternative medicine are middle-aged, female, and affluent. Significantly, 80% of the people who use CAM also use conventional medicine. However, 70% do not discuss their use of CAM with their traditional care provider (Murphy, Kronenberg, & Wade, 1999).

The reality that families may use CAM and not reveal it raises some concern. Certain CAM modalities such as biofeedback, acupuncture, aromatherapy, and massage are not likely to cause adverse effects. However, the possibility exists that there might be interactions between herbal therapies and other medications prescribed by the care provider. Complications might also develop from the use of vitamin supplements.

The ANA Code of Ethics (2001) mandates that the nurse must promote and protect the health, safety, and rights of clients. Nurses need to become knowledgeable about CAM to be able to maximize its benefits and to protect pregnant women and children from any possible harm. The use of CAM in the care of children must be addressed because lim-

ited research with this age group exists and developmental variations might influence efficacy and safety. Although many CAM therapies may have been proven effective in adults, they may have little effect on children or even be harmful.

Nurses who create a climate of respect and openness tend to be more effective in gathering information about a family's use of complementary or alternative therapies. The following recommendations may be useful to nurses in taking a history (Cady, 2002; Vincler & Nicol, 1997):

- Ask questions that are direct and nonjudgmental in seeking information about the client's use of CAM. Identify what the perceived benefits are to the pregnant woman or child.

- Ask questions about specific therapies, including the use of herbal therapy and homeopathy. Because many people consider herbs to be natural substances and because they are often sold as dietary supplements, clients may not think to mention them.

- Avoid making negative or disparaging comments about CAM. Such comments send the message that CAM is not desirable and may discourage people from disclosing their use of CAM therapies.

In working with childbearing and childrearing families, or indeed with any clients, nurses who use CAM therapies should choose methods that are within the scope of nursing practice in their state and not limited by the licensure of other providers (such as massage therapists). Nurses are also best advised to use CAM therapies that are considered somewhat mainstream and that are supported by evidence about their safety and effectiveness (Gaydos, 2001). For example, nurses working with a pregnant woman might use acupressure wristbands for the treatment of nausea. Other therapies nurses often employ include progressive relaxation, exercise and movement, therapeutic touch, visualization and guided imagery, prayer, meditation, music therapy, massage, storytelling, aromatherapy, and journaling.

Nurses who use complementary modalities should document their use within the context of nursing practice. This is most effective when the modality is identified as an intervention to address a specific nursing diagnosis or identified client need (Frisch, 2001). Thus, music therapy might be used for a child to help address the identified nursing diagnosis of "acute pain."

Nurses have a role in conducting and supporting research on CAM. Because of the variety of CAM therapies in use, research is needed in a host of areas. The results of research on CAM can be found in professional journals and at the National Institutes of Health (NIH) Web site. As the evidence supporting the use of certain interventions grows, nurses and other healthcare providers are incorporating the results as part of their evidence-based practice.

Critical Concept Review

LEARNING OBJECTIVES	CONCEPTS
Distinguish among several different types of families.	1. Nuclear families consist of a mother, father, and children. 2. Dual-career/dual-earner families make up the majority of contemporary families in the United States. 3. Childless families are a growing trend in American culture. 4. Extended family members can play an active role in family life, decision making, and family roles. 5. Single-parent families account for almost a third of all U.S. families, and stepparent and binuclear families are increasingly common. 6. Nonmarital heterosexual cohabitating family is often chosen for financial reasons or for companionship. 7. Gay and lesbian families have children who show no significant differences from children raised in more traditional families.
Identify the stages of a family life cycle.	1. Stage I: Beginning families. 2. Stage II: Childbearing families. 3. Stage III: Families with preschool children. 4. Stage IV: Families with school-age children. 5. Stage V: Families with teenagers. 6. Stage VI: Families launching young adults. 7. Stage VII: Middle-aged parents. 8. Stage VIII: Retirement and old age.

Identify prevalent cultural norms related to childbearing and childrearing.	Childbearing and childrearing are influenced by the following cultural norms:
	1. Status of the family unit:
	  ■ Pregnancy may elevate the status of both the man and the woman depending upon the culture.
	2. Contraception:
	  ■ Culture may prohibit the use of contraception or may determine the type used.
	3. View of pregnancy:
	  ■ May be seen as an honor.
	  ■ May be viewed as a sickness.
	  ■ May determine the responsibilities of the mother or father.
	4. Existence of taboos.
	5. Equilibrium model of health:
	  ■ Health is restored by the use of heat or cold.
	  ■ May influence the way the mother is cared for during labor and the way the infant is treated at birth.

Summarize the importance of cultural competency in providing nursing care.	The nurse who provides culturally competent care: 1. Recognizes the importance of the childbearing family's value system. 2. Acknowledges that differences occur among people. 3. Seeks to respect and respond to ethnic diversity in a way that leads to mutually desirable outcomes.
Discuss the use of a cultural assessment tool as a means of providing culturally sensitive care.	A cultural assessment tool provides information of health practices based on: 1. Client beliefs. 2. Client values. 3. Client customs.
Identify key considerations in providing spiritually sensitive care.	To provide spiritually sensitive care, the nurse should: 1. Determine the current spiritual and religious beliefs and practices that will affect the mother and baby. 2. Accommodate these practices where possible. 3. Examine one's own spiritual or religious beliefs to be more aware and able to provide nonjudgmental care.

(continued)

LEARNING OBJECTIVES

CONCEPTS

Distinguish between *complementary* and *alternative therapies.*

1. A complementary therapy is an adjunct to conventional medical treatment that has been through rigorous scientific testing, which shows that it has some reliability.
2. An alternative therapy is usually considered a distance or procedure that has not undergone rigorous scientific testing in this country, although it might have been thoroughly tested in other countries.

Identify the benefits and risks of complementary and alternative therapies.

1. CAM therapies have several benefits. Many of them emphasize prevention and wellness, place a higher value on holistic healing than on physical cure, are noninvasive, and have few side effects. In addition, many are more affordable and available than conventional therapies.
2. Risks of CAM therapies include lack of standardization, lack of regulation and research substantiating safety and effectiveness, inadequate training and certification of some healers, and financial and health risks of unproven methods.

Discuss complementary therapies appropriate for the nurse to use with childbearing and childrearing families.

Nurses may use the following CAM therapies:
1. Guided imagery.
2. Acupressure.
3. Prayer.
4. Music therapy.
5. Massage.
6. Story telling.
7. Exercise and movement.
8. Mediation.
9. Aromatherapy.
10. Journaling.

CRITICAL THINKING IN ACTION

View the **Critical Thinking in Action** video in Chapter 2 of the CD-ROM. Then, answer the questions that follow.

While working in an inner-city clinic for adolescents, you meet a new client, a 14-year-old Latina girl named Juanita. She is accompanied by her parents. None of them speak English. Through a translator, Juanita tells you that she recently moved here with her parents. They have brought her here today because she has a sore throat. The curandero they took her to see prescribed the herbal remedy

Echinacea, but her throat is still sore. The rapid test you perform for strep throat is positive and the nurse practitioner prescribes an antibiotic.

1. According to the national standards for culturally and linguistically appropriate services in healthcare set by the government, what are examples of important standards of care you as the nurse can provide in the care of this adolescent?
2. How can you, as the nurse, take steps to achieve cultural competence?
3. How would you, as the nurse, be able to address some of the disparities that can exist when this client comes to the clinic?
4. What are some examples of common food preferences in the Latino-American culture?

MEDIALINK

www.prenhall.com/london

- NCLEX-RN® Review, case studies, and other interactive resources for this chapter can be found on the Companion Website at http://www.prenhall.com/london. Click on "Chapter 2" to select the activities for this chapter.

Critical Thinking

Examine cultural patterns of your family that you learned as a young child, particularly as they relate to health beliefs and practices. Identify how you were socialized to the culture and how your experience differed from others around you as you grew up. Reflect on the manner in which your background might affect the nursing care you provide.

This activity contains 2 questions.

1. *How does the information you learned about your cultural heritage*
[Hint] *affect the way you anticipate working with families from other cultural traditions?*

To create paragraphs in your essay response, type <p> at the beginning of the paragraph, and </p> at the end.

- For animations, more NCLEX-RN® Review questions, and an audio glossary, access the accompanying CD-ROM in this textbook.

REFERENCES

American Academy of Pediatrics Committee on Psychosocial Aspects of Child and Family Health. (2002). Coparent and second parent adoption by same-sex parents. *Pediatrics, 109*(3), 339–340.

American Nurses Association. (2001). *Code of ethics.* Washington, DC: Author. http://nursingworld/ org/readroom/fsdemogrpt.htm. Retrieved February 7, 2005.

Andrews, M. M., Boyle, J. S., & Carr, T. J. (2003). *Transcultural concepts in nursing care* (4th ed.). Philadelphia: Lippincott Williams & Wilkins.

Atwood, K. C. (2003). Naturopathy: A critical appraisal. *Medscape General Medicine, 5*(4). Retrieved May 10, 2004, from http://www.medscape.com/viewarticle/465994

Balch, P. A., & Balch, J. F. (2000). *Prescription for Nutritional Healing* (3rd ed.). New York: Penguin Putnam.

Belew, C. (1999). Herbs and the childbearing woman: Guidelines for midwives. *Journal of Nurse-Midwifery, 44*(3), 231–246.

Bodo, K., & Gibson, N. (1999a). Childbirth customs in Orthodox Jewish traditions. *Canadian Family Physician, 45,* 682–686.

Bodo, K., & Gibson, N. (1999b). Childbirth customs in Vietnamese traditions. *Canadian Family Physician, 45,* 690–697.

Cady, R. (2002). Are there legal issues of concern for nurses when patients use complimentary (sic) and alternative medicine? *MCN. American Journal of Maternal Child Nursing, 27*(2), 119.

Duvall, E. M. (1977). *Marriage and family development* (5th ed.). New York: Harper Row.

Elkins, M., & Cavendish, R. (2004). Developing a plan for pediatric spiritual care. *Holistic Nursing Practice, 18,* 179–184.

Faust, J. E. (2000). *Womanhood: The highest place of honor.* Salt Lake City, UT: The Church of Jesus Christ Latter-day Saints

Fontaine, K. L. (2005). *Healing practices: Alternative therapies for nursing practice* (2nd ed.). Upper Saddle River, NJ: Prentice-Hall Health.

Fosarelli, P. (2003). Children and the development of faith: Implications for pediatric practice. *Contemporary Pediatrics, 20,* 85–98.

Frisch, N. C. (2001). Nursing as a context for alternative/complementary modalities. *Online Journal of Issues in Nursing, 6*(2). Retrieved June 19, 2001 from http://www. nursingworld.org.ojin/ topic15/tpc15_2.htm

Gannotti, M. E., Kaplan, L. C., Handwerker, W. P., & Groce, N. E. (2004). Cultural influences on health care use: Differences in perceived unmet needs and expectations of providers by Latino and Euro-American parents of children with special health care needs. *Journal of Developmental and Behavioral Pediatrics, 25,* 156–165.

Gaydos, H. L. (2001). *Complementary and alternative therapies in nursing education: Trends and issues.* Retrieved June 19, 2001, from http://www. nursingworld.org.ojin/topic15/tpc15_5.htm

Graedon, J., & Graedon, T. (2001). *The people's pharmacy guide to home and herbal remedies.* New York: St. Martin's Triffin.

Kim, Y. O. R. (2004). Access to hepatitis B vaccination among Korean American children in immigrant families. *Journal of Health Care for the Poor and Underserved, 15,* 170–174.

Lockie, A., & Geddes, N. (2000). *Complete guide to homeopathy: The principles and practice of treatment homeopathy.* New York: DK Publishing.

Mattson, S. (1995). Culturally sensitive perinatal care for Southeast Asians. *Journal of Obstetric, Gynecologic, and Neonatal Nursing, 24*(4), 335–341.

Mattson, S., & Smith, J. E. (2004). *Core curriculum for maternal-newborn nursing* (3rd ed.). Philadelphia: Saunders.

Mayo Clinic. (2002). *Using herbal supplements wisely.* Retrieved September 2, 2002, from http://www.mayoclinic.com

Murphy, P. A., Kronenberg, F., & Wade, C. (1999). Complementary and alternative medicine in women's health. Developing a research agenda. *Journal of Nurse-Midwifery, 44,* 192–204.

Murray, M., & Pizzorno, P. (2001). *Encyclopedia of natural medicine.* Rocklin, CA: Prima.

Murray, R. B., & Zentner, J. P. (2001). *Health promotion strategies through the lifespan* (7th ed.). Upper Saddle River, NJ: Prentice-Hall.

National Center for Complementary and Alternative Medicine (NCCAM). (2004). Herbal supplements: Consider safety, too. *Get the Facts.* Retrieved June 16, 2005, from http://nccam.nih. gov/health/supplement-safety/index.htm

National Toxicology Program. (2003). Herbal medicines. *NTP Fact Sheet—Year 2003.* Retrieved June 16, 2005, from http://ntp-server.niehs.nih.gov

Office of Minority Health. (2001). *National standards for chronically and linguistically appropriate services in health care.* Washington, DC: U.S. Department of Health and Human Services.

Purnell, L. D., & Paulanka, B. J. (2003). *Transcultural healthcare: A culturally competent approach* (2nd ed.). Philadelphia: F.A. Davis.

Roy, L. C., Torrez, C., & Dale, J. C. (2004). Ethnicity, traditional health beliefs, and health-seeking behavior: Guardians' attitudes regarding their children's medical treatment. *Journal of Pediatric Health Care, 18,* 22–30.

Schantz, S., Charron, S. A., & Folden, S. L. (2003). Health seeking behaviors of Haitian families for their school aged children. *Journal of Cultural Diversity, 10,* 62–68.

Shealy, N. (Consulting Ed.). (1999). *The complete illustrated encyclopedia of alternative healing therapies.* Boston: Elements Books Limited.

Spector, R. E. (2004). *Cultural diversity in health and illness* (6th ed.). Upper Saddle River, NJ: Pearson Prentice Hall.

Vincler, L., & Nicol, M. (1997). When ignorance isn't bliss: What healthcare practitioners and facilities should know about complimentary (sic) and alternative medicine. *American Health Lawyers Association, Journal of Health Law, 30*(3), 160.

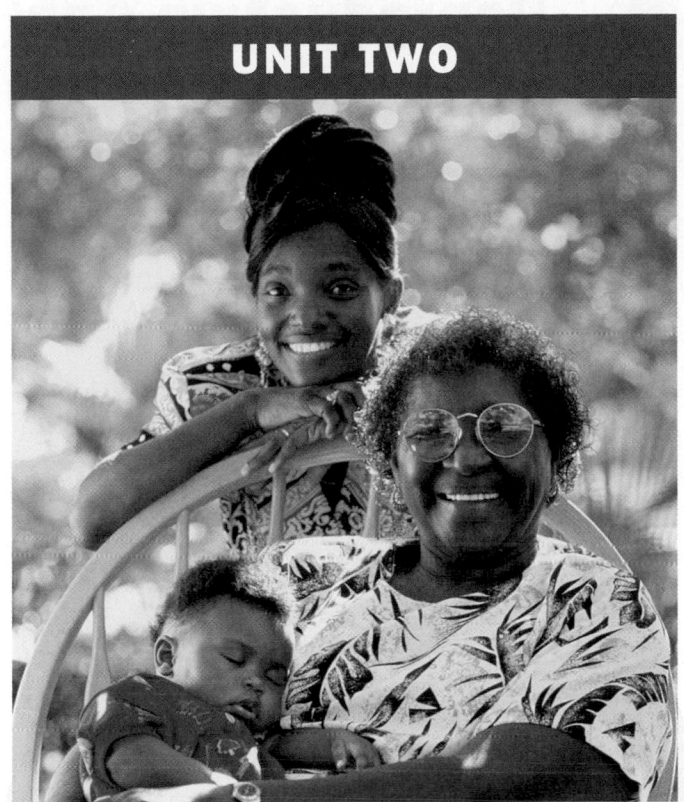

UNIT TWO

The Reproductive Years and Beyond

Reproductive Anatomy and Physiology

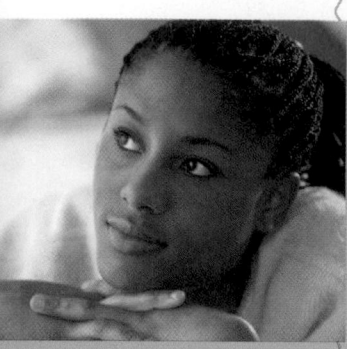

At my last "female checkup" at the clinic, the nurse told me about their free family-planning classes. So I went to one with a friend, and I learned so much about my body and about men's bodies. I thought I knew all there was to know about that stuff—but I guess not. My boyfriend, Jontau, has been looking at the handouts they gave me, and asking me questions. I think he's completely amazed at how our bodies work. I know I am.

—Sheena, 16

LEARNING OBJECTIVES

- Identify the structures and functions of the female and male reproductive systems.

- Summarize the actions of the hormones that affect reproductive functioning.

- Identify the two phases of the ovarian cycle and the changes that occur in each phase.

- Describe the phases of the menstrual cycle, their dominant hormones, and the changes that occur in each phase.

- Discuss the significance of specific female reproductive structures during childbirth.

- Identify the functions of specific male reproductive structures for reproduction.

MEDIALINK www.prenhall.com/london

CD-ROM
NCLEX-RN® Review
Audio Glossary
Activity: Female Reproductive System
Activity: Ovulation
Activity: Male Reproductive System
Animations:
   3-D Female Pelvis
   3-D Male Pelvis

Companion Website
NCLEX-RN® Review
MediaLink Applications:
   Case Study: Sex Education for Teens
   Care Plan Activity: Irregular Menses in a Client
      with Anxiety

Understanding childbearing requires more than understanding sexual intercourse or the process by which the female and male sex cells unite. The nurse must also become familiar with the structures and functions that make childbearing possible and the phenomena that initiate it. This chapter presents the anatomic, physiologic, and sexual aspects of the female and male reproductive systems. Beginning on page 72, Chapter 4 discusses the psychosocial aspects of human sexuality. ∞

The female and male reproductive organs are homologous; that is, they are fundamentally similar in structure and function. The primary functions of both female and male reproductive systems are to produce sex cells and transport them to locations where their union can occur. The sex cells, called *gametes*, are produced by specialized organs called *gonads*. A series of ducts and glands within both male and female reproductive systems contributes to the production and transport of the gametes.

Although the genetic sex of an embryo is determined at fertilization, the male and female reproductive systems are undifferentiated for about the first 8 weeks of gestation. This undifferentiated period is followed by a period of rapid, dramatic changes as the reproductive organs differentiate into recognizable structures (Figure 3–1 ●).

PUBERTY

The term **puberty** refers to the developmental period between childhood and attainment of adult sexual characteristics and functioning. Generally boys mature physically about 2 years later than girls. The age at onset and progress of puberty vary widely, physical changes overlap, and the sequence of events can vary from person to person. (For a detailed discussion of physical changes associated with puberty, see Chapters 33 and 34. ∞) This diversity results from each individual's response to hormonal stimulation.

PHYSIOLOGY OF ONSET

Puberty is initiated by the maturation of the hypothalamic-pituitary-gonad complex (the *gonadostat*) and input from the central nervous system. The process, which begins during fetal life, is sequential and complex.

The central nervous system releases a neurotransmitter that stimulates the hypothalamus to synthesize and release **gonadotropin-releasing hormone (GnRH)** (Ferin, 2003). GnRH is transmitted to the anterior pituitary, where it causes the synthesis and secretion of the gonadotropins **follicle-stimulating hormone (FSH)** and **luteinizing hormone (LH)** (Figure 3–2 ●).

Although the gonads do produce small amounts of *androgens* (male sex hormones) and *estrogens* (female sex hormones) before the onset of puberty, FSH and LH stimulate increased secretion of these hormones. Androgens and estrogens influence the development of secondary sex characteristics. FSH and LH stimulate the processes of spermatogenesis and maturation of ova.

Other hormones are involved in the onset of puberty. Although less direct, their action is essential. Abnormally high or low levels of adrenocorticotropic hormone (ACTH), thyroid hormone, or growth hormone (GH) can disrupt the onset of normal puberty (see Chapter 56 for a detailed discussion ∞) (Ferin, 2003). The maturation process which begins during fetal life continues through puberty and childbearing years. The external and internal female reproductive organs develop and mature in response to estrogen and progesterone.

Undifferentiated

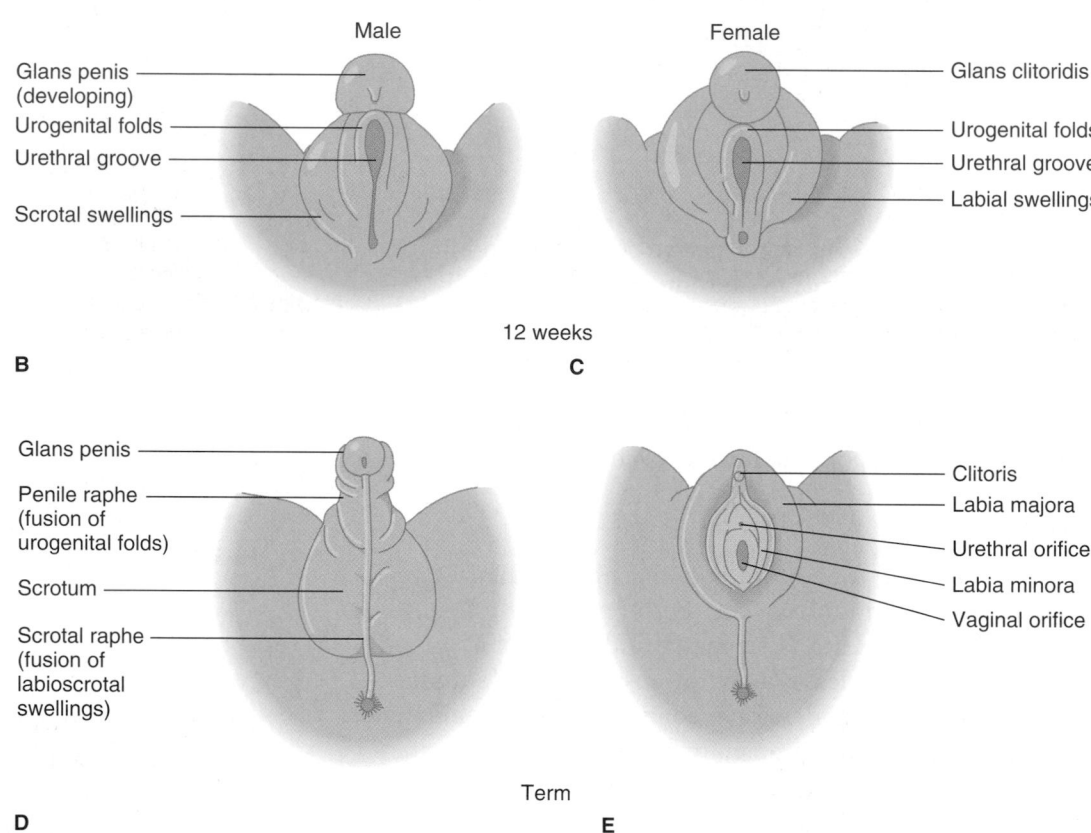

Sexual differentiation. **A,** At 7 weeks' gestation, male and female genitalia are identical (undifferentiated). **B** and **C,** By 12 weeks' gestation, noticeable differentiation begins to occur. **D** and **E,** Differentiation continues until birth but is almost complete at term.

FEMALE REPRODUCTIVE SYSTEM

The *female reproductive system* consists of the external and internal genitals and the accessory organs of the breasts. Because of its importance to childbearing, the bony pelvis is also discussed in this chapter.

EXTERNAL GENITALS

All the external reproductive organs except the glandular structures can be directly inspected. The appearance of the external genitalia varies greatly among women. Heredity, age, race, and the number of children a woman has borne influence the size, color, and shape of her external organs. The female external genitals, also referred to as the **vulva**, include the following structures (Figure 3–3 ●):

- Mons pubis
- Labia majora
- Labia minora
- Clitoris

● **FIGURE 3-2**

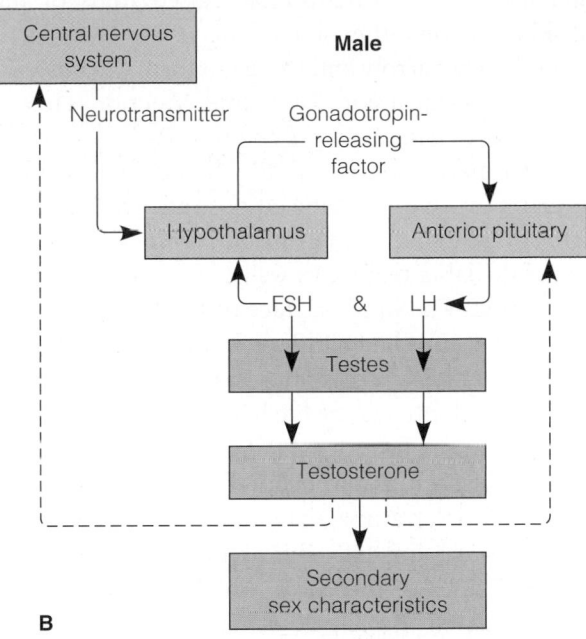

A

B

Physiologic changes leading to onset of puberty. **A,** In females, and **B,** in males. Solid lines illustrate stimulation of hormone production, and broken lines illustrate inhibition. Through a neurotransmitter the central nervous system stimulates the hypothalamus, which in turn produces a gonadotropin-releasing factor that causes the anterior pituitary to produce gonadotropins (FSH or LH). These hormones stimulate specific structures in the gonads to secrete steroid hormones (estrogen, progesterone, or testosterone). The rise in pituitary hormone production increases hypothalamus activity. Elevated steroid hormone levels stimulate the central nervous system and pituitary gland to inhibit hormone production.

■ Urethral meatus and opening of the paraurethral (Skene's) glands

■ Vaginal vestibule (vaginal orifice, vulvovaginal glands, hymen, and fossa navicularis)

■ Perineal body

Although they are not true parts of the female reproductive system, the urethral meatus and perineal body are considered here because of their proximity and relationship to the vulva. The vulva has a generous supply of blood and nerves. As a woman ages, estrogen secretions decrease, causing the vulvar organs to atrophy and become subject to a variety of lesions.

Mons Pubis

The mons pubis is a softly rounded mound of subcutaneous fatty tissue beginning at the lowest portion of the anterior abdominal wall (see Figure 3–3). Also known as the mons veneris, this structure covers the front portion of the symphysis pubis after puberty. The mons pubis is covered with pubic hair, typically with the hairline forming a transverse line across the lower abdomen. The hair is short in all women. It can vary from sparse and fine in Asian women to heavy, coarse, and curly in women of African descent. The mons pubis protects the pelvic bones, especially during coitus.

● **FIGURE 3-3**

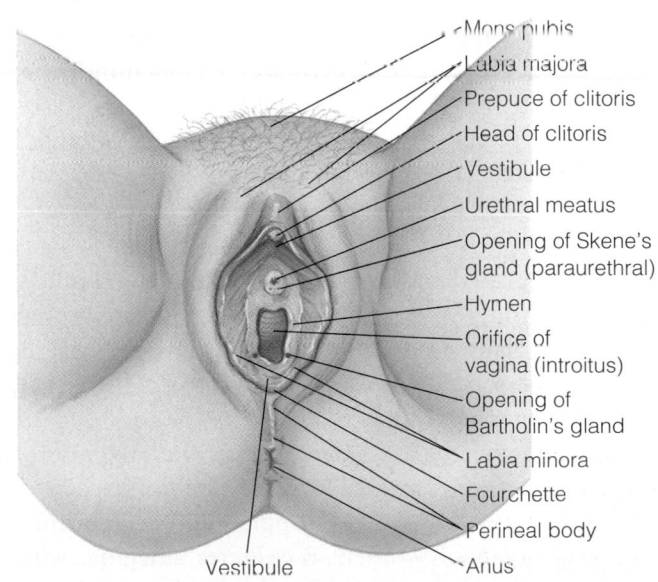

Female external genitals, longitudinal view.

Labia Majora

The *labia majora* are longitudinal, raised folds of pigmented skin, one on either side of the vulvar cleft. As the pair descend, they narrow and merge to form the posterior junction of the perineal skin. Their chief function is to protect the structures lying between them.

The labia majora are covered by hair follicles and sebaceous glands, with underlying adipose and muscle tissue. The dartos muscle sheet is responsible for the wrinkled appearance of the labia majora as well as for their sensitivity to heat and cold. The inner surface of the labia majora in women who have not had children is moist and looks like mucous membrane, whereas after many births it is more skinlike. With each pregnancy the labia majora become less prominent. Because of the extensive venous network in the labia majora, varicosities may occur during pregnancy, and obstetric or sexual trauma may cause hematomas. The labia majora share an extensive lymphatic supply with the other structures of the vulva, which can facilitate the spread of cancer in the female reproductive organs. Because of the nerves supplying the labia majora (from the first lumbar and third sacral segment of the spinal cord), certain regional anesthesia blocks will affect them and cause numbness.

Labia Minora

The *labia minora* are soft folds of skin within the labia majora that converge near the anus, forming the fourchette. Each labium minus has the appearance of shiny mucous membrane, moist and devoid of hair follicles. The labia minora are rich in sebaceous glands, which lubricate and waterproof the vulvar skin and provide bactericidal secretions. Because the sebaceous glands do not open into hair follicles but open directly onto the surface of the skin, sebaceous cysts commonly occur in this area. Vulvovaginitis in this area is very irritating because the labia minora have many tactile nerve endings. The labia minora increase in size at puberty and decrease after menopause because of changes in estrogen levels.

Clitoris

The *clitoris*, located between the labia minora, is about 5 to 6 mm long and 6 to 8 mm across. Its tissue is essentially erectile. The glans of the clitoris is partly covered by a fold of skin called the *prepuce*, or clitoral hood. This area resembles an opening to an orifice and may be confused with the urethral meatus. Accidental attempts to insert a catheter in this area produce extreme discomfort. The clitoris has rich blood and nerve supplies and is the primary erogenous organ of women. It secretes smegma, which along with other vulval secretions has a unique odor that may be sexually stimulating to the male.

Urethral Meatus and Paraurethral Glands

The urethral meatus is located 1 to 2.5 cm beneath the clitoris in the midline of the vestibule; it often appears as a puckered, slitlike opening. At times the meatus is difficult to visualize because of the presence of blind dimples or small mucosal folds. The paraurethral glands, or *Skene's glands*, open into the posterior wall of the urethra close to its opening (see Figure 3–3). Their secretions lubricate the vaginal opening, facilitating sexual intercourse.

Vaginal Vestibule

The vaginal vestibule is a boat-shaped depression enclosed by the labia majora and visible when they are separated. The vestibule contains the vaginal opening, or *introitus*, which is the border between the external and internal genitals.

The *hymen* is a thin, elastic collar or semicollar of tissue that surrounds the vaginal opening. The appearance changes during the woman's lifetime. The hymen is essentially avascular. For thousands of years, some societies have perpetuated the belief that the hymen covers the vaginal opening and is a sign of virginity. However, modern studies of female genital anatomy have revealed that the hymen surrounds rather than entirely covers the vaginal opening, and can be torn not only through sexual intercourse but also through strenuous physical activity, masturbation, menstruation, or the use of tampons, thus dispelling old beliefs.

External to the hymen at the base of the vestibule are two small papular elevations containing the openings of the ducts of the *vulvovaginal (Bartholin's) glands*. They lie under the constrictor muscle of the vagina. These glands secrete a clear, thick, alkaline mucus that enhances the viability and motility of the sperm deposited in the vaginal vestibule. These gland ducts can harbor *Neisseria gonorrhoeae* and other bacteria, which can cause pus formation and abscesses in the Bartholin's glands.

The vestibular area is innervated mainly by the perineal nerve from the sacral plexus. The area is not sensitive to touch generally; however, the hymen contains numerous free nerve endings as receptors to pain.

Perineal Body

The **perineal body** is a wedge-shaped mass of fibromuscular tissue found between the lower part of the vagina and the anus. The superficial area between the anus and the vagina is referred to as the *perineum*.

The muscles that meet at the perineal body are the external sphincter ani, both levator ani (the superficial and deep transverse perineal), and the bulbocavernosus. These muscles mingle with elastic fibers and connective tissue in an arrangement that allows a remarkable amount of stretching. During the last part of labor, the perineal body thins out until it is just a few centimeters thick. This tissue is the site of the possible episiotomy or lacerations during childbirth (see Chapter 22 for more information ∞).

FEMALE INTERNAL REPRODUCTIVE ORGANS

The female internal reproductive organs are the vagina, uterus, fallopian tubes, and ovaries (Figure 3–4 ●). These are target organs for estrogenic hormones, and they play a unique part in the reproductive cycle. Certain internal reproductive organs can be palpated during vaginal examination and assessed with various instruments.

Vagina

The **vagina** is a muscular and membranous tube that connects the external genitals with the uterus. It extends from the vulva to the uterus in a position nearly parallel to the plane of the pelvic brim. The vagina is often called the birth

canal because it forms the lower part of the pelvis through which the fetus must pass during birth.

Because the cervix of the uterus projects into the upper part of the anterior wall of the vagina, the anterior wall is approximately 2.5 cm shorter than the posterior wall. Measurements range from 6 to 8 cm for the anterior wall and from 7 to 10 cm for the posterior wall.

In the upper part of the vagina, which is called the vaginal vault, there is a recess or hollow around the cervix. This area is called the vaginal *fornix*. Since the walls of the vaginal vault are very thin, various structures can be palpated through the walls, including the uterus, a distended bladder, the ovaries, the appendix, the cecum, the colon, and the ureters. The upper fourth of the vagina is separated from the rectum by the pouch of Douglas (sometimes referred to as the cul-de-sac of Douglas). This deep pouch or recess is posterior to the cervix. When a woman lies on her

● **FIGURE 3–4**

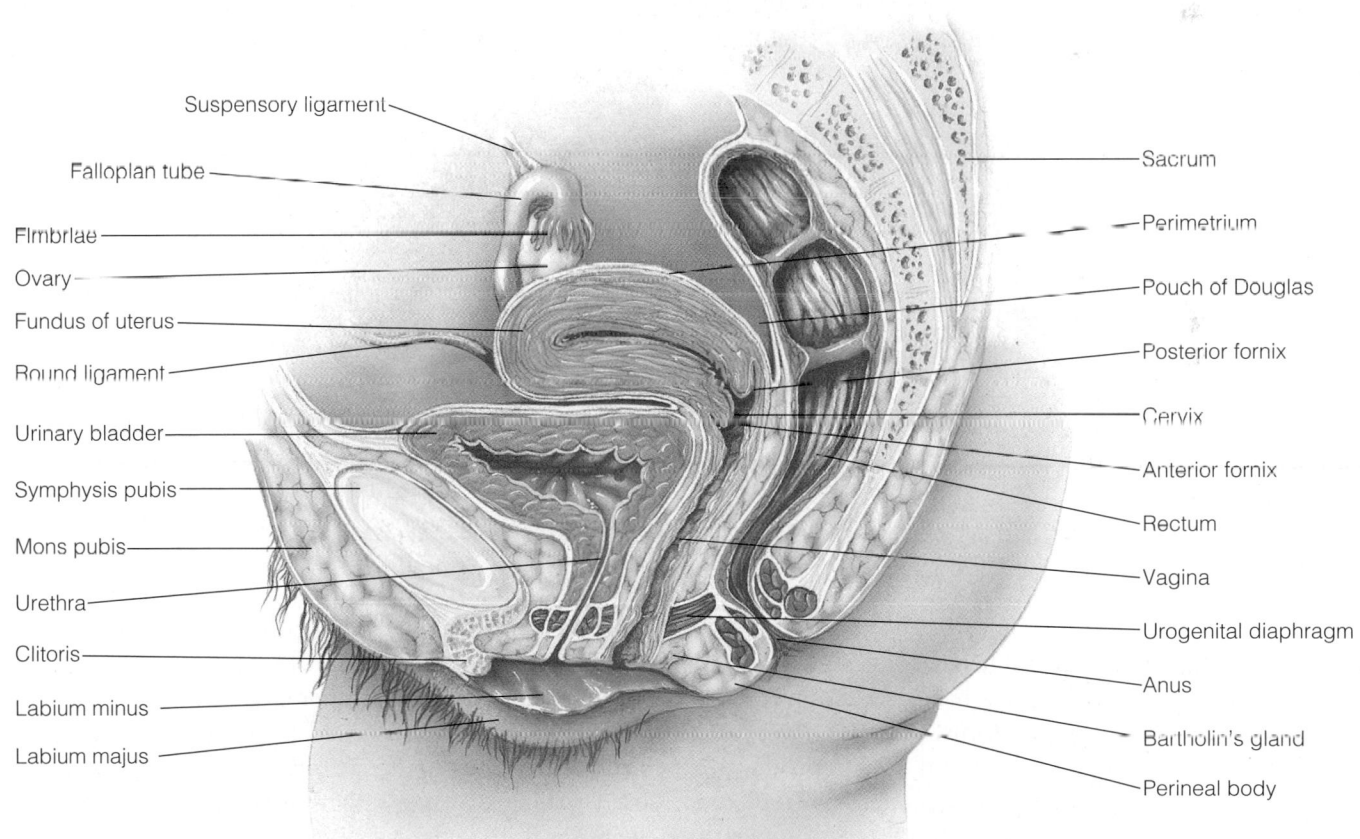

Female internal reproductive organs.

back after intercourse, the space in the fornix permits the pooling of semen. The collection of a large number of sperm near the cervix at or near the time of ovulation increases the chances of pregnancy.

The walls of the vagina are covered with ridges, or rugae, crisscrossing each other. These rugae allow the vaginal tissues to stretch enough for the fetus to pass through during childbirth.

During a woman's reproductive life, an acidic vaginal environment is normal (pH 4 to 5). Secretion from the vaginal epithelium provides a moist environment. The acidic environment is maintained by a symbiotic relationship between lactic acid–producing bacilli (Döderlein's bacillus or lactobacillus) and the vaginal epithelial cells. These cells contain glycogen, which is broken down by the bacilli into lactic acid. The amount of glycogen is regulated by the ovarian hormones. Any interruption of this process can destroy the normal self-cleaning action of the vagina. Such interruption may be caused by antibiotic therapy, douching, or use of perineal sprays or deodorants. (See Chapter 4 for more information on comfort issues for women. ∞) The acidic vaginal environment is normal only during the mature reproductive years and in the first days of life when maternal hormones are operating in the infant. A relatively neutral pH of 7.5 is normal from infancy until puberty and after menopause.

The vagina's blood supplies are extensive. The pudendal nerve supplies what relatively little somatic innervation there is to the lower third of the vagina. Thus, sensation during sexual excitement and coitus is reduced in this area, as is vaginal pain during the second stage of labor.

The vagina has three functions:

- To serve as the passage for sperm and for the fetus during birth
- To provide passage for the menstrual products from the uterine endometrium to the outside of the body
- To protect against trauma from sexual intercourse and infection from pathogenic organisms

Uterus

As the core of reproduction and hence continuation of the human race, the **uterus**, or womb, has been endowed with a mystical aura. Numerous customs, taboos, mores, and values have evolved about women and their reproductive function. Although scientific knowledge has replaced much of this folklore, remnants of old ideas and superstitions persist. To provide effective care, nurses must be cognizant of their own attitudes and beliefs, as well as those of their clients.

The uterus is a hollow, muscular, thick-walled organ shaped like an upside-down pear (Figure 3–5 ◉). It lies in the center of the pelvic cavity between the base of the bladder and the rectum and above the vagina. It is level with or slightly below the brim of the pelvis, with the external opening of the cervix (external os) about the level of the ischial spines. The uterus of the mature woman weighs about 40 to 70 g and is approximately 6 to 8 cm long and 1 to 2.5 cm thick (Monga & Sanborn, 2004).

The body of the uterus can move freely forward or backward. Only the cervix is anchored laterally. Thus, the position of the uterus can vary, depending on a woman's posture and musculature, number of children borne, bladder and rectal fullness, and even normal respiratory patterns. Generally the uterus bends forward, forming a sharp angle with the vagina. There is a bend in the area of the isthmus of the uterus; from there the cervix points downward. The uterus is said to be anteverted when it is in this position. The anteverted position is considered normal.

Four pairs of ligaments (i.e., the cardinal, uterosacral, round, and broad) support the uterus. Single anterior and posterior ligaments also support the uterus.

The uterus is divided into two major parts, an upper triangular portion called the **corpus** or uterine body and a lower cylindric portion called the cervix. The upper two thirds of the uterus (the corpus or uterine body) is composed mainly of a smooth muscle layer (myometrium). The lower third is the cervix or neck. The rounded uppermost (dome-shaped top) portion of the corpus that extends above the points of attachment of the fallopian tubes is called the **fundus**. The elongated portion of the uterus where the fallopian tubes enter is called the cornua.

The isthmus is that portion of the uterus between the internal cervical os and the endometrial cavity. The isthmus

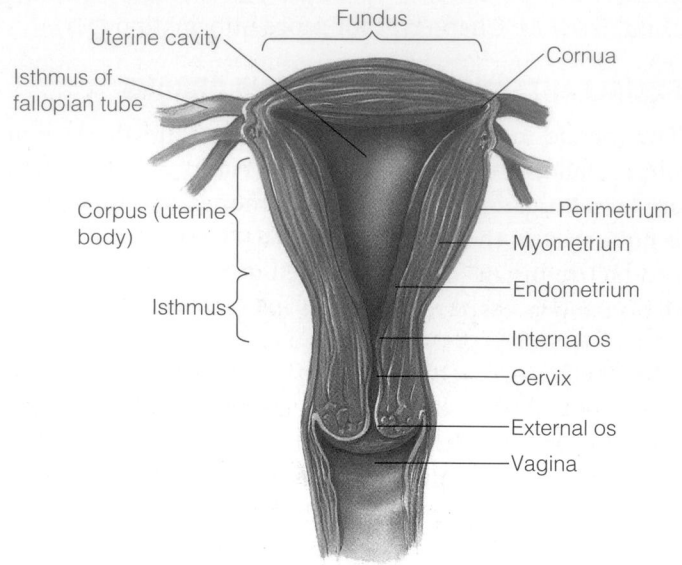

Structures of the uterus.

is about 6 mm above the uterine opening of the cervix (the internal os), and it is in this area that the uterine lining changes into the mucous membrane of the cervix; it joins the corpus to the cervix. The isthmus takes on importance in pregnancy because it becomes the lower uterine segment. With the cervix, it is a passive segment and not part of the contractile uterus. At birth this thin lower segment, situated behind the bladder, is the site for lower segment cesarean births (see Chapter 22 for more information ∞).

The blood and lymphatic supplies to the uterus are extensive. Innervation of the uterus is entirely by the autonomic nervous system (Figure 3–6 ◉). Even without an intact nerve supply, the uterus can contract adequately for birth; for example, women who are hemiplegic have adequate uterine contractions.

The function of the uterus is to provide a safe environment for fetal development. The uterine lining is cyclically prepared by steroid hormones for implantation of the embryo, a process known as **nidation**. Once the embryo is implanted, the developing fetus is protected until it is expelled.

◉ **FIGURE 3–6**

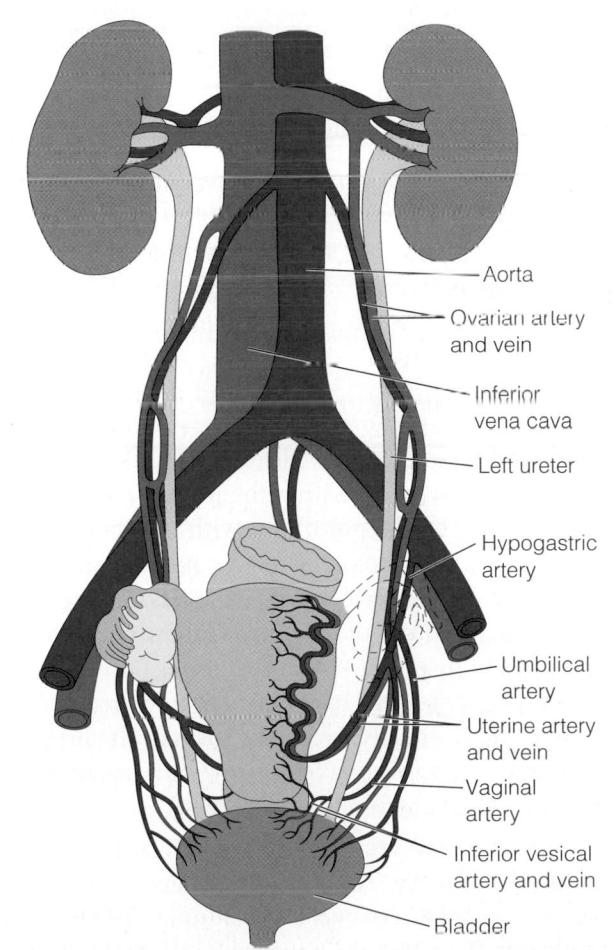

Aorta

Ovarian artery and vein

Inferior vena cava

Left ureter

Hypogastric artery

Umbilical artery

Uterine artery and vein

Vaginal artery

Inferior vesical artery and vein

Bladder

Pelvic blood supply.

Both the body of the uterus and the cervix are changed permanently by pregnancy. The body never returns to its prepregnant size, and the external os changes from a circular opening of about 3 mm to a transverse slit with irregular edges.

Uterine Corpus. The uterine corpus is made up of three layers. The outermost layer is the *serosal layer*, or **perimetrium**, which is composed of peritoneum. The middle layer is the *muscular uterine layer*, or **myometrium**. This muscular uterine layer is continuous with the muscle layers of the fallopian tubes and the vagina. This continuity helps these organs present a unified reaction to various stimuli—ovulation, orgasm, or the deposit of sperm in the vagina. These muscle fibers also extend into the ovarian, round, and cardinal ligaments and minimally into the uterosacral ligaments, which helps explain the vague but disturbing pelvic "aches and pains" reported by many pregnant women.

The myometrium has three distinct layers of uterine (smooth) involuntary muscles (Figure 3–7 ◉). The outer layer, found mainly over the fundus, is made up of longitudinal muscles that cause cervical effacement and expel the fetus during birth. The thick middle layer is made up of interlacing muscle fibers in figure-eight patterns. These muscle fibers surround large blood vessels, and their contraction produces a hemostatic action (a tourniquet-like action on blood vessels to stop bleeding after birth). The inner muscle layer is composed of circular fibers that form sphincters at the fallopian tube attachment sites and at the internal os. The internal os sphincter inhibits the expulsion of the uterine contents during pregnancy but stretches in labor as cervical dilatation occurs. An incompetent cervical os can be caused by a torn, weak, or absent sphincter at the internal os. The sphincters at the fallopian tubes prevent menstrual blood from flowing backward into the fallopian tubes from the uterus. Although each layer of muscle has been discussed as having a unique function, the uterine musculature actually works as a whole. The uterine contractions of labor are responsible for the dilatation of the cervix and provide the major force for the passage of the fetus through the pelvis and vaginal canal at birth.

The *mucosal* layer, or **endometrium**, of the uterine corpus is the innermost layer. This single layer is composed of columnar epithelium, glands, and stroma. From menarche to menopause, the endometrium undergoes monthly degeneration and renewal in the absence of pregnancy. As it responds to the governing hormonal cycle and prostaglandin influence, the endometrium varies in thickness from 0.5 to 5 mm. The glands of the endometrium produce a thin, watery, alkaline secretion that keeps the uterine cavity moist. This endometrial milk not only helps sperm travel to the fallopian tubes but also nourishes the developing embryo before it implants in the endometrium (see Chapter 7 for more information ∞).

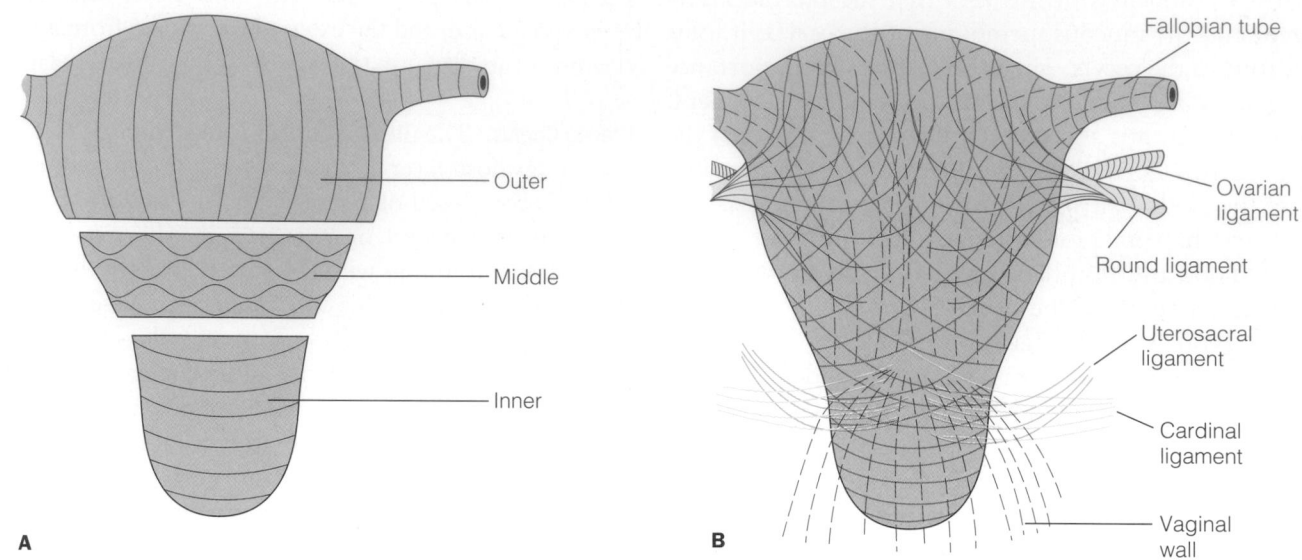

Uterine muscle layers. **A,** Muscle fiber placement. **B,** Interlacing of uterine muscle layers.

The blood supply to the endometrium is unique. Some of the blood vessels are not sensitive to cyclic hormonal control, whereas others are extremely sensitive to it. These differing responses allow part of the endometrium to remain intact while other endometrial tissue is shed during menstruation. When pregnancy occurs and the endometrium is not shed, the reticular stromal cells surrounding the endometrial glands become the decidual cells of pregnancy. The stromal cells are highly vascular, channeling a rich blood supply to the endometrial surface.

Cervix. The narrow neck of the uterus is the **cervix**. It meets the body of the uterus at the internal os and descends about 2.5 cm to connect with the vagina at the external os (see Figure 3–5). Thus, it provides a protective entrance for the body of the uterus. The cervix is divided by its line of attachment into the vaginal and supravaginal areas. The vaginal cervix projects into the vagina at an angle of from 45 to 90 degrees. The *supravaginal cervix* is surrounded by the attachments that give the uterus its main support: the uterosacral ligaments, the transverse ligaments of the cervix (Mackenrodt's ligaments), and the pubocervical ligaments.

The vaginal cervix appears pink and ends at the external os. The cervical canal appears rosy red and is lined with columnar ciliated epithelium, which contains mucus-secreting glands. Most cervical cancer begins at this *squamocolumnar junction*. The specific location of the junction varies with age and number of pregnancies. Elasticity is the chief characteristic of the cervix. Its ability to stretch is due to the high fibrous and collagenous content of the supportive tissues and also to the vast number of folds in the cervical lining.

The cervical mucus has three functions:

- To lubricate the vaginal canal
- To act as a bacteriostatic agent
- To provide an alkaline environment to shelter deposited sperm from the acidic vagina

At **ovulation**, cervical mucus is clearer, thinner, more profuse, and more alkaline than at other times.

Uterine Ligaments

The uterine ligaments support and stabilize the various reproductive organs. The ligaments shown in Figure 3–8 ● are described as follows:

1. The **broad ligament** keeps the uterus centrally placed and provides stability within the pelvic cavity. It is a double layer that is continuous with the abdominal peritoneum. The broad ligament covers the uterus anteriorly and posteriorly and extends outward from the uterus to enfold the fallopian tubes. The round and ovarian ligaments are at the upper border of the broad ligament. At its lower border, it forms the cardinal ligaments. Between the folds of the broad ligament are connective tissue, involuntary muscle, blood and lymph vessels, and nerves.

2. The **round ligaments** help the broad ligament keep the uterus in place. The round ligaments arise from the sides of the uterus near the fallopian tube insertions. They extend outward between the folds of the broad ligament, passing through the inguinal ring and canals and eventually fusing with the connective

FIGURE 3–8

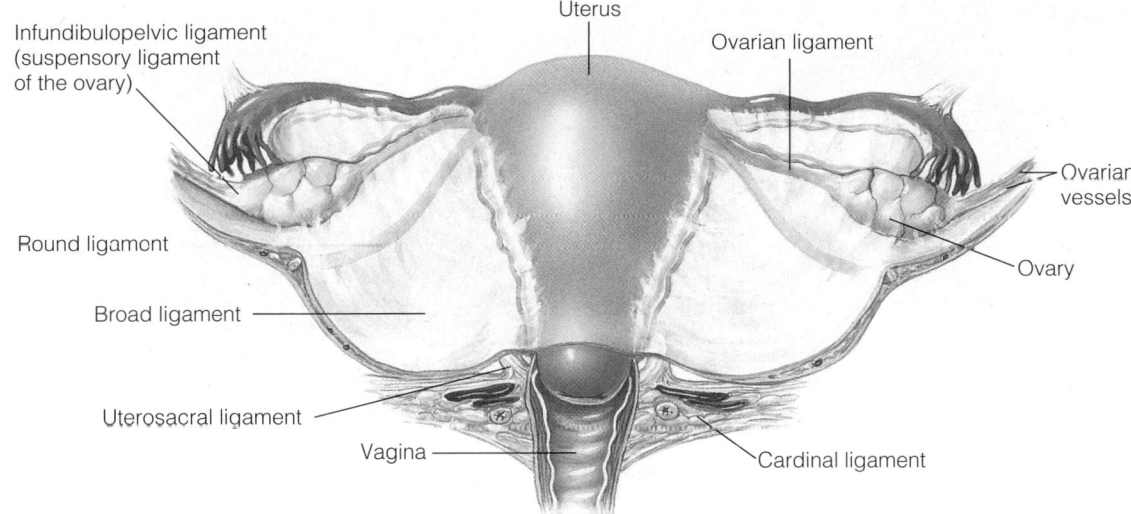

Infundibulopelvic ligament
(suspensory ligament
of the ovary)

Uterus

Ovarian ligament

Ovarian
vessels

Round ligament

Ovary

Broad ligament

Uterosacral ligament

Vagina

Cardinal ligament

Uterine ligaments.

tissue of the labia majora. Made up of longitudinal muscle, the round ligaments enlarge during pregnancy. During labor the round ligaments steady the uterus, pulling downward and forward so that the presenting part of the fetus is moved into the cervix.

3. The **ovarian ligaments** anchor the lower pole of the ovary to the cornua of the uterus. They are composed of muscle fibers that allow the ligaments to contract. This contractile ability influences the position of the ovary to some extent, thus helping the fimbriae of the fallopian tubes to "catch" the ovum as it is released each month.

4. The **cardinal ligaments** are the chief uterine supports and suspend the uterus from the side walls of the true pelvis. These ligaments, also known as Mackenrodt's or transverse cervical ligaments, arise from the sides of the pelvic walls and attach to the cervix in the upper vagina. These ligaments prevent uterine prolapse and also support the upper vagina.

5. The **infundibulopelvic ligament** suspends and supports the ovaries. Arising from the outer third of the broad ligament, the infundibulopelvic ligament contains the ovarian vessels and nerves.

The **uterosacral ligaments** provide support for the uterus and cervix at the level of the ischial spines. Arising on each side of the pelvis from the posterior wall of the uterus, the uterosacral ligaments sweep back around the rectum and insert on the sides of the first and second sacral vertebrae. The uterosacral ligaments contain smooth muscle fibers, connective tissue, blood and lymph vessels, and

nerves. They also contain sensory nerve fibers that contribute to dysmenorrhea (painful menstruation) (see Chapter 4 for more information ∞).

Fallopian Tubes

The two **fallopian tubes**, also known as the oviducts or uterine tubes, arise from each side of the uterus and reach almost to the sides of the pelvis, where they turn toward the ovaries (Figure 3–9 ●). Each tube is approximately 8 to 13.5 cm long. A short section of each fallopian tube is inside the uterus; its opening into the uterus is only 1 mm in diameter. The fallopian tubes link the peritoneal cavity with the uterus and vagina. This linkage increases a woman's biologic vulnerability to disease processes.

Each fallopian tube may be divided into three parts: the isthmus, the ampulla, and the infundibulum, or fimbria. The **isthmus** is straight and narrow, with a thick muscular wall and an opening (lumen) 2 to 3 mm in diameter. It is the site of tubal ligation, a surgical procedure to prevent pregnancy (see Chapter 5 for more information ∞).

Next to the fallopian tube isthmus is the curved **ampulla**, which comprises the outer two thirds of the tube. Fertilization of the secondary oocyte by a spermatozoon usually occurs here. The ampulla ends at the fimbria, which is a funnel-shaped enlargement with many projections, called **fimbriae**, reaching out to the ovary. The longest of these, the fimbria ovarica, is attached to the ovary to increase the chances of intercepting the ovum as it is released.

The wall of the fallopian tube is made up of four layers: peritoneal (serous), subserous (adventitial), muscular, and mucous tissues. The peritoneum covers the tubes. The subserous layer contains the blood and nerve supply, and

● **FIGURE 3–9**

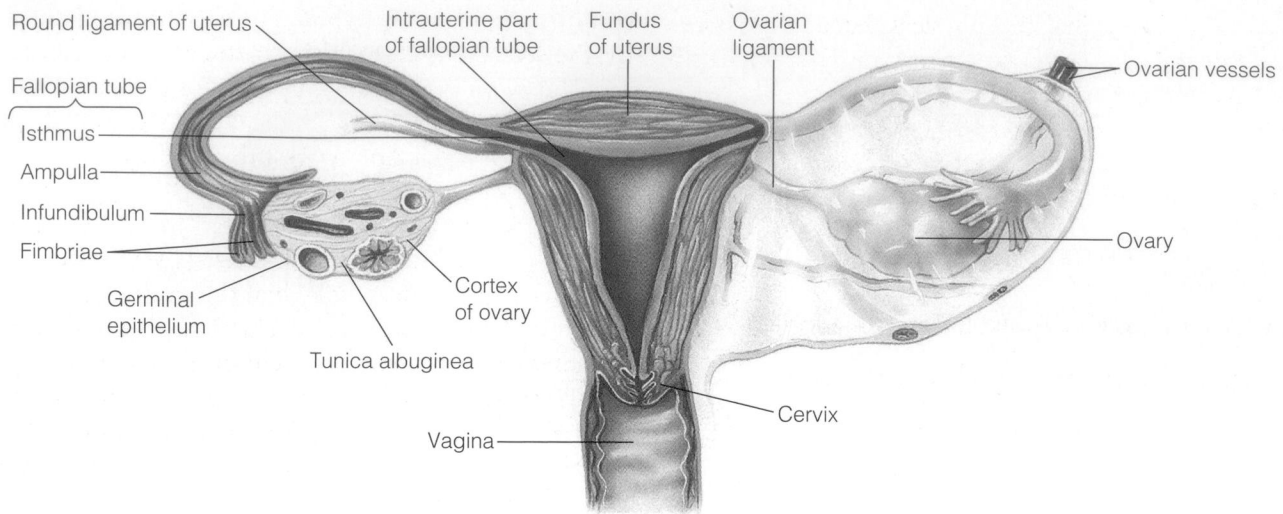

Fallopian tubes and ovaries.

the muscular layer is responsible for the peristaltic movement of the tube. The mucosal layer, immediately next to the muscular layer, is composed of ciliated and nonciliated cells, with the number of ciliated cells more abundant at the fimbria. Nonciliated cells secrete a protein-rich, serous fluid that nourishes the ovum. The constantly moving tubal cilia propel the ovum toward the uterus. Because the ovum is a large cell, this ciliary action is needed to assist the tube's muscular layer peristalsis. Any malformation or malfunction of the tubes can result in infertility, ectopic pregnancy, or even sterility.

A rich blood and lymphatic supply serves each fallopian tube. Thus, the tubes have an unusual ability to recover from an inflammatory process.

The fallopian tubes have three functions:

- To provide transport for the ovum from the ovary to the uterus (transport time through the fallopian tubes varies from 3 to 4 days)
- To provide a site for fertilization
- To serve as a warm, moist, nourishing environment for the ovum or zygote (fertilized egg) (See Chapter 7 for further discussion. ∞)

Ovaries

The **ovaries** are two almond-shaped structures just below the pelvic brim. One ovary is located on each side of the pelvic cavity. Their size varies among women and with the stage of the menstrual cycle. Each ovary weighs approximately 6 to 10 g and is 1.5 to 3 cm wide, 2 to 5 cm long, and 1 to 1.5 cm thick. The ovaries of girls are small, but they become larger after puberty and then decrease in size following menopause. They also change in appearance from a dull white, smooth-surfaced organ to a pitted gray organ over time as the woman ages. The pitting is caused by scarring due to ovulation.

The ovaries are held in place by the broad, ovarian, and infundibulopelvic ligaments. There is no peritoneal covering for the ovaries. Although this lack of covering assists the mature ovum to erupt, it also allows easier spread of malignant cells from cancer of the ovaries. A single layer of cuboidal epithelial cells, called the germinal epithelium, covers the ovaries. The ovaries are composed of three layers: the tunica albuginea, the cortex, and the medulla. The *tunica albuginea* is dense and dull white and serves as a productive protective layer. The *cortex* is the main functional part because it contains ova, graafian follicles, corpora lutea, the degenerated corpora lutea (corpora albicantia), and degenerated follicles. The *medulla* is completely surrounded by the cortex and contains the nerves and the blood and lymphatic vessels.

The ovaries are the primary source of two important hormones: the estrogens and progesterone. **Estrogens** are associated with those characteristics contributing to femaleness, including breast alveolar lobule growth and duct development. The ovaries secrete large amounts of estrogen, while the adrenal cortex (extraglandular sites) produces minute amounts of estrogen in nonpregnant women.

Progesterone is often called the *hormone of pregnancy* because its effects on the uterus allow pregnancy to be maintained. The placenta is the primary source of progesterone during pregnancy. This hormone also inhibits the action of prolactin, thereby preventing lactation during pregnancy (Lawrence & Lawrence, 2004). The interplay between the ovarian hormones and other hormones such as follicle-stimulating hormone (FSH) and luteinizing hormone (LH) is responsible for the cyclic changes that allow pregnancy. The hormonal and physical changes that occur during the female reproductive cycle are discussed in depth later in this chapter.

Between the ages of 45 and 55, a woman's ovaries secrete decreasing amounts of estrogen. Eventually, ovulatory activity ceases and menopause occurs.

BONY PELVIS

The female bony pelvis has two unique functions:

- To support and protect the pelvic contents
- To form the relatively fixed axis of the birth passage

Because the pelvis is so important to childbearing, its structure must be understood clearly.

Bony Structure

The pelvis is made up of four bones: two innominate bones, the sacrum, and the coccyx. The pelvis resembles a bowl or basin; its sides are the innominate bones, and its back is the sacrum and coccyx. Lined with fibrocartilage and held tightly together by ligaments (Figure 3–10 ⬤), the four bones join at the symphysis pubis, the two sacroiliac joints, and the sacrococcygeal joints.

The innominate bones, popularly known as the hip bones, are made up of three separate bones: the ilium, ischium, and pubis. These bones fuse to form a circular cavity, the *acetabulum*, which articulates with the femur.

The *ilium* is the broad, upper prominence of the hip. The *iliac crest* is the margin of the ilium. The **ischial spines**, the foremost projection nearest the groin, is the site of attachment for ligaments and muscles.

The *ischium*, the strongest bone, is under the ilium and below the acetabulum. The L-shaped ischium ends in a marked protuberance, the ischial tuberosity, on which the weight of a seated body rests. The ischial spines arise near the junction of the ilium and ischium and jut into the pelvic cavity. The shortest diameter of the pelvic cavity is between the ischial spines. The ischial spines serve as reference points during labor to evaluate the descent of the fetal head into the birth canal (see Chapter 17 and Figure 17–7 for more information ∞).

The **pubis** forms the slightly bowed front portion of the innominate bone. Extending medially from the acetabulum to the midpoint of the bony pelvis, each pubis meets the other to form a joint called the **symphysis pubis**. The triangular space below this junction is known as the pubic arch. The fetal head passes under this arch during birth. The symphysis pubis is formed by heavy fibrocartilage and the superior and inferior pubic ligaments. The mobility

⬤ **FIGURE 3-10**

Innominate bone
Right sacroiliac joint
Sacroiliac ligament
Sacrospinous ligament
Ischial spine
Sacrotuberous ligament
Sacrum
Iliopectineal eminence
Coccyx
5th lumbar vertebra
Sacral promontory
Sacral body
Iliopectineal line
Symphysis pubis

Pelvic bones with supporting ligaments.

of the inferior ligament increases during a first pregnancy and to a greater extent in subsequent pregnancies.

The sacroiliac joints also have a degree of mobility that increases near the end of pregnancy as the result of an upward, gliding movement. The pelvic outlet may be increased by 1.5 to 2 cm in the squatting, sitting, and dorsal lithotomy positions. These relaxations of the joints are induced by the hormones of pregnancy.

The *sacrum* is a wedge-shaped bone formed by the fusion of five vertebrae. On the anterior upper portion of the sacrum is a projection into the pelvic cavity known as the **sacral promontory**. This projection is another obstetric guide in determining pelvic measurements. (See Chapter 10 for more information on pelvic measurements. ∞)

The small triangular bone last on the vertebral column is the coccyx. It articulates with the sacrum at the sacrococcygeal joint. The coccyx usually moves backward during labor to provide more room for the fetus.

Pelvic Floor

The muscular *pelvic floor* of the bony pelvis is designed to overcome the force of gravity exerted on the pelvic organs. It acts as a buttress to the irregularly shaped pelvic outlet, thereby providing stability and support for surrounding structures.

Deep fascia, the levator ani, and coccygeal muscles form the part of the pelvic floor known as the **pelvic di-aphragm**. The components of the pelvic diaphragm function as a whole, yet they are able to move over one another. This feature provides an exceptional capacity for dilatation during birth and return to prepregnancy condition following birth. Above the pelvic diaphragm is the **pelvic cavity**; below and behind it is the perineum.

The levator ani muscle makes up the major portion of the pelvic diaphragm and consists of four muscles: the iliococcygeus, pubococcygeus, puborectalis, and pubovaginalis. The ileococcygeal muscle, a thin muscular sheet underlying the sacrospinous ligament, helps the levator ani support the pelvic organs. Muscles of the pelvic floor are shown in Figure 3–11 ● and discussed in Table 3–1.

Pelvic Division

The pelvic cavity is divided into the false pelvis and the true pelvis (Figure 3–12A ●). The **false pelvis**, the portion above the pelvic brim, or linea terminalis, supports the weight of the enlarged pregnant uterus and directs the presenting fetal part into the true pelvis.

The **true pelvis** is the portion that lies below the linea terminalis. The bony circumference of the true pelvis is made up of the sacrum, coccyx, and innominate bones and represents the bony limits of the birth canal. The relationship between the true pelvis and the fetal head is of paramount importance: the size and shape must be adequate for normal fetal passage during labor and at birth.

● FIGURE 3–11

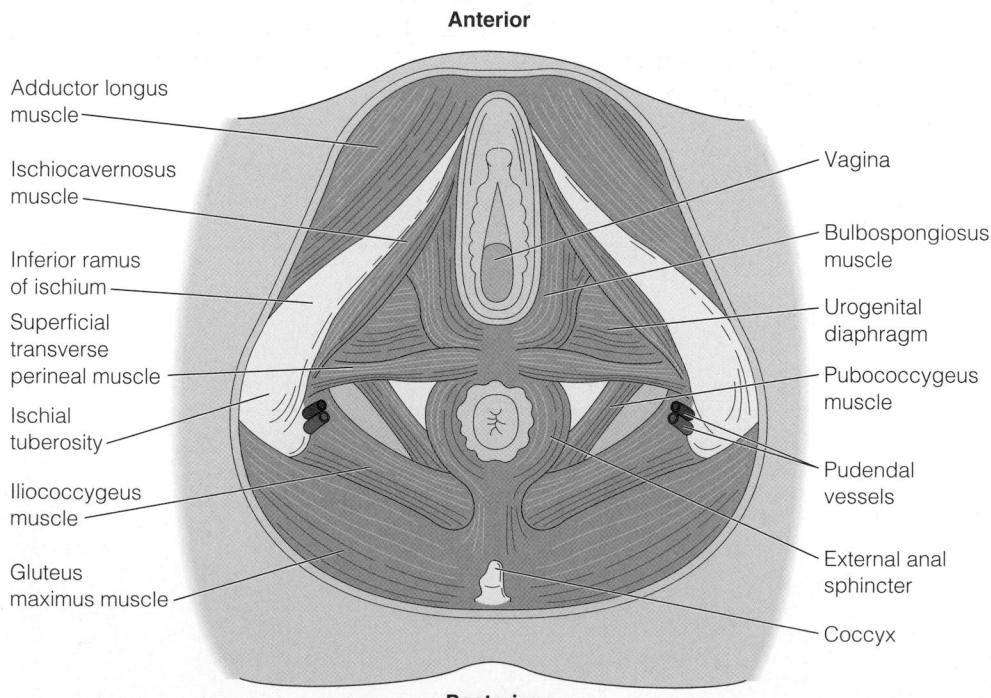

Muscles of the pelvic floor. (The puborectalis, pubovaginalis, and coccygeal muscles cannot be seen from this view.)

TABLE 3–1 ✤ Muscles of the Pelvic Floor

Muscle	Origin	Insertion	Innervation	Action
Levator ani	Pubis, lateral pelvic wall, and ischial spine	Blends with organs in pelvic cavity	Inferior rectal, second and third sacral nerves, plus anterior rami of third and fourth sacral nerves	Supports pelvic viscera; helps form pelvic diaphragm
Iliococcygeus	Pelvic surface of ischial spine and pelvic fascia	Central point of perineum, coccygeal raphe, and coccyx		Assists in supporting abdominal and pelvic viscera
Pubococcygeus	Pubis and pelvic fascia	Coccyx		
Puborectalis	Pubis	Blends with rectum; meets similar fibers from opposite side		Forms sling for rectum, just posterior to it, raises anus
Pubovaginalis	Pubis	Blends into vagina		Supports vagina
Coccygeus	Ischial spine and sacrospinous ligament	Lateral border of lower sacrum and upper coccyx	Third and fourth sacral nerves	Supports pelvic viscera; helps form pelvic diaphragm, flexes and abducts coccyx

The true pelvis consists of three parts: the inlet, the pelvic cavity, and the outlet (Figure 3–12B ●). Each part has distinct measurements that aid in evaluating the adequacy of the pelvis for childbirth. (See Chapter 10 for more information. ∞)

The **pelvic inlet** is the upper border of the true pelvis and is typically rounded. Its size and shape are determined by assessing three anteroposterior diameters. The **diagonal conjugate** extends from the subpubic angle to the middle of the sacral promontory and is typically 12.5 cm. The diagonal conjugate can be measured manually during a pelvic examination. The **obstetric conjugate** extends from the middle of the sacral promontory to an area approxi-

mately 1 cm below the pubic crest. Its length is estimated by subtracting 1.5 cm from the length of the diagonal conjugate (Figure 3–13 ●). The fetus passes through the obstetric conjugate, and the size of this diameter determines whether the fetus can move down into the birth canal in order for engagement to occur. The true (anatomic) conjugate, or **conjugate vera**, extends from the middle of the sacral promontory to the middle of the pubic crest (superior surface of the symphysis). One additional measurement, the **transverse diameter**, helps determine the shape of the inlet. The transverse diameter is the largest diameter of the inlet and is measured by using the linea terminalis as the point of reference.

● **FIGURE 3–12**

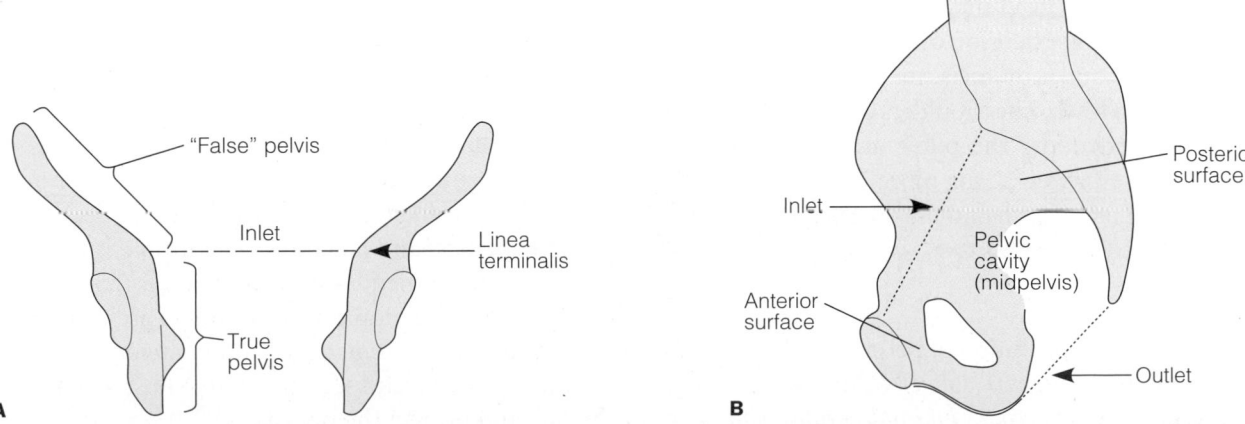

Female pelvis. **A,** The false pelvis is a shallow cavity above the inlet; the true pelvis is a deeper portion of the cavity below the inlet. **B,** The true pelvis consists of the inlet, cavity (midpelvis), and outlet.

● **FIGURE 3–13**

Pelvic planes: coronal section and diameters of the bony pelvis.

The pelvic cavity (canal) is a curved canal with a longer posterior than anterior wall. A change in the lumbar curve can increase or decrease the tilt of the pelvis and can influence the process of labor because the fetus has to adjust itself to this curved path as well as to the different diameters of the true pelvis (see Figure 3–12B).

The **pelvic outlet** is at the lower border of the true pelvis. The size of the pelvic outlet can be determined by assessing the *transverse diameter*, which is also called the bi-ischial, or intertuberous, diameter. This diameter extends from the inner surface of one ischial tuberosity to the other. The pubic arch is also part of the pelvic cavity. The pubic arch has great importance because the fetus must pass under it during birth. If it is narrow, the baby's head may be pushed backward toward the coccyx, making extension of the head difficult. This situation, known as outlet dystocia, may require the use of forceps or a cesarean birth. The shoulders of a large baby may also become wedged under the pubic arch, making birth more difficult (see Chapter 22 for more information ∞). The clinical assessment of each of these obstetric diameters is discussed further in Chapter 10. ∞

Pelvic Types

The Caldwell-Moloy classification of pelves is widely used to differentiate bony pelvic types (Caldwell & Moloy, 1933). The four basic types are *gynecoid, android, anthropoid,* and *platypelloid* (see Figure 17–1 in Chapter 17 ∞). Each type has a characteristic shape, and each shape has implications

for labor and birth. (See Chapter 10 and Chapter 17 for more information. ∞)

BREASTS

The **breasts**, or *mammary glands*, considered accessories of the reproductive system, are specialized sebaceous glands (Figure 3–14 ●). They are conical and symmetrically placed on the sides of the chest. The greater pectoral and anterior serratus muscles underlie each breast. Suspending the breasts are fibrous tissues, called *Cooper's ligaments*, that extend from the deep fascia in the chest outward to just under the skin covering the breast. Frequently the left breast is larger than the right. In different racial groups, breasts develop at slightly different levels in the pectoral region of the chest.

In the center of each mature breast is the **nipple**, a protrusion about 0.5 to 1.3 cm in diameter. The nipple is composed mainly of erectile tissue, which becomes more rigid and prominent during the menstrual cycle, sexual excitement, pregnancy, and lactation. The nipple is surrounded by the heavily pigmented **areola**, which is 2.5 to 10 cm in diameter. Both the nipple and the areola are roughened by small papillae called *tubercles of Montgomery*. As an infant suckles, these tubercles secrete a fatty substance that helps lubricate and protect the breasts.

The breasts are composed of glandular, fibrous, and adipose tissue. The glandular tissue is arranged in a series of 15

FIGURE 3–14

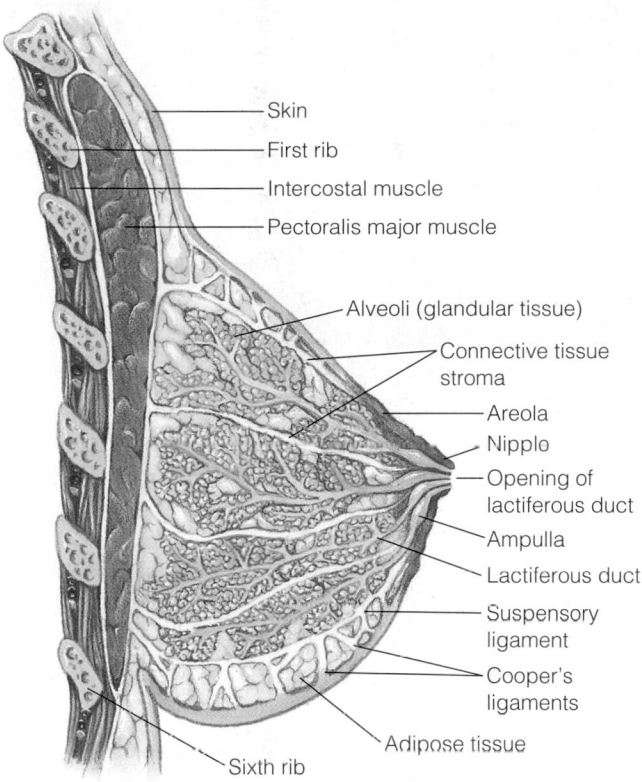

Skin
First rib
Intercostal muscle
Pectoralis major muscle
Alveoli (glandular tissue)
Connective tissue stroma
Areola
Nipple
Opening of lactiferous duct
Ampulla
Lactiferous duct
Suspensory ligament
Cooper's ligaments
Adipose tissue
Sixth rib

Anatomy of the breast: sagittal view of left breast.

to 24 lobes separated by fibrous and adipose tissue. Each lobe is made up of several lobules composed of many alveoli clustered around tiny ducts. The lining of these ducts secretes the various components of milk. The ducts from several lobules merge to form the *larger lactiferous ducts* and join to form the lactiferous sinuses, which serve as reservoirs for milk collection and open on the surface of the nipple. The biologic function of the breasts is to provide nourishment and protective maternal antibodies to infants through the lactation process. They are also a source of pleasurable sexual sensation.

FEMALE REPRODUCTIVE CYCLE

The **female reproductive cycle** is composed of the ovarian cycle, during which ovulation occurs, and the uterine cycle, during which menstruation occurs. These two cycles take place simultaneously (Figure 3–15 ●).

EFFECTS OF FEMALE HORMONES

After menarche a female undergoes a cyclic pattern of ovulation and menstruation, which is disrupted only by pregnancy, for a period of 30 to 40 years. This cycle is an orderly process under neurohormonal control. Each month one oocyte matures, ruptures from the ovary, and enters the fal-

lopian tube. The ovary, vagina, uterus, and fallopian tubes are major target organs for female hormones.

The ovaries produce mature gametes and secrete hormones. Ovarian hormones include the estrogens, progesterone, and testosterone. The ovary is sensitive to FSH and LH. The uterus is sensitive to estrogen and progesterone. The relative proportion of these hormones to each other controls the events of both ovarian and menstrual cycles.

Estrogens

Estrogens are hormones that are associated with characteristics contributing to "femaleness." The major estrogenic effects are due primarily to three classic estrogens: estrone, β-estradiol, and estriol. The major estrogen is β-estradiol.

Estrogens control the development of the female secondary sex characteristics: breast development, widening of the hips, and deposits of tissue (fat) in the buttocks and mons pubis. Estrogens also assist in the maturation of the ovarian follicles and cause the endometrial mucosa to proliferate following menstruation. The amount of estrogens is greatest during the proliferative (follicular or estrogenic) phase of the menstrual cycle. Estrogens also cause the uterus to increase in size and weight because of increased glycogen, amino acids, electrolytes, and water. Blood supply is expanded as well. Under the influence of estrogens, myometrial contractility increases in both the uterus and the fallopian tubes, and uterine sensitivity to oxytocin increases. Estrogens inhibit FSH production and stimulate LH production.

Estrogens have effects on many hormones and other carrier proteins, such as contributing to the increased amount of protein-bound iodine in pregnant women and women who use oral contraceptives containing estrogen. Estrogens may increase libidinal feelings in humans. They decrease the excitability of the hypothalamus, which may cause an increase in sexual desire.

Progesterone

Progesterone is secreted by the **corpus luteum** and is found in greatest amounts during the secretory (luteal or progestational) phase of the menstrual cycle. It decreases uterine motility and contractility caused by estrogens, thereby preparing the uterus for implantation after the ovum is fertilized. The endometrial mucosa is in a ready state as a result of estrogenic influence. Progesterone causes the uterine endometrium to further increase its supply of glycogen, arterial blood, secretory glands, amino acids, and water. This hormone is often called the hormone of pregnancy because its effects on the uterus allow pregnancy to be maintained. Under the influence of progesterone, the vaginal epithelium proliferates and the cervix secretes thick, viscous mucus. Breast glandular tissue increases in size and complexity. Progesterone also prepares the breasts for lactation.

● **FIGURE 3–15**

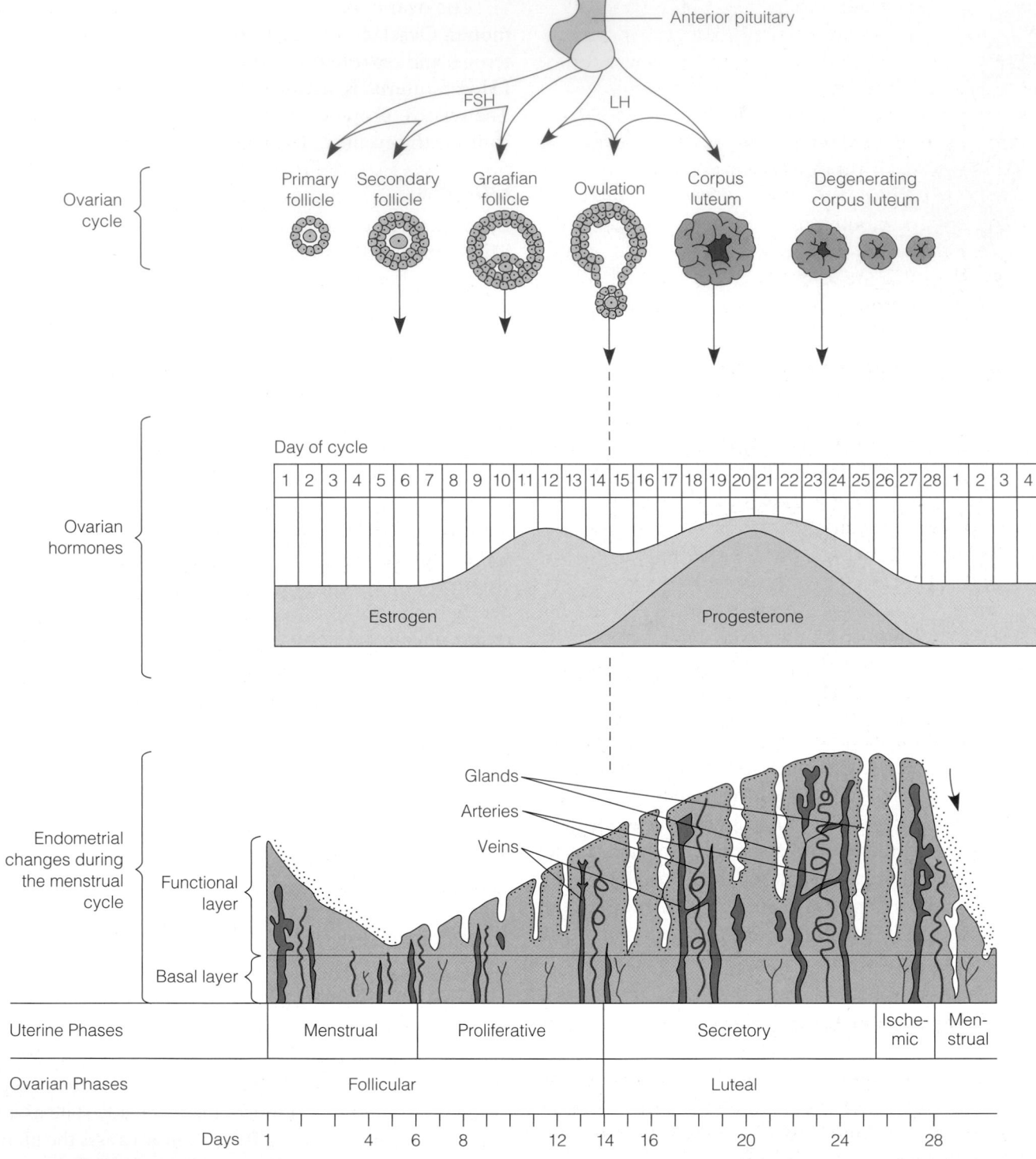

Female reproductive cycle: interrelationships of hormones with the four phases of the uterine cycle and the two phases of the ovarian cycle in an ideal 28-day cycle.

The temperature rise of about 0.3°C to 0.6°C (0.5°F to 1°F) that accompanies ovulation and persists throughout the secretory phase of the menstrual cycle is due to progesterone.

Prostaglandins

Prostaglandins (PGs) are oxygenated fatty acids produced by the cells of the endometrium and are also classified as hormones. Prostaglandins have varied action in the body. The two primary types of prostaglandins are group E and F. Generally, PGE relaxes smooth muscles and is a potent vasodilator; PGF is a potent vasoconstrictor and increases the contractility of muscles and arteries. Although their primary actions seem antagonistic, their basic regulatory functions in cells are achieved through an intricate pattern of reciprocal events.

Prostaglandin production increases during follicular maturation, is dependent on gonadotropins, and seems to be critical to follicular rupture (Ferin, 2003). Extrusion of the ovum, resulting in follicular swelling and increased contractility of the smooth muscle in the theca layer of the mature follicle, is thought to be caused by $PGF_2\alpha$. Significant amounts of PGs are found in and around the follicle at the time of ovulation.

NEUROHUMORAL BASIS OF THE FEMALE REPRODUCTIVE CYCLE

The female reproductive cycle is controlled by complex interactions between the nervous and endocrine systems and their target tissues. These interactions involve the hypothalamus, anterior pituitary, and ovaries.

The hypothalamus secretes gonadotropin-releasing hormone (GnRH) to the pituitary gland in response to signals received from the central nervous system. This releasing hormone is often called both luteinizing hormone releasing hormone (LHRH) and follicle-stimulating hormone–releasing hormone (FSHRH) (Blackburn, 2003).

In response to GnRH, the anterior pituitary secretes the gonadotropic hormones FSH and LH. FSH is primarily responsible for the maturation of the ovarian follicle. As the follicle matures, it secretes increasing amounts of estrogen, which enhance the development of the follicle (Ferin, 2003). (This estrogen is also responsible for the building or proliferation phase of the endometrium after it is shed during menstruation.)

Final maturation of the follicle cannot come about without the action of LH. The anterior pituitary's production of LH increases six- to tenfold as the follicle matures. The peak production of LH can precede ovulation by as much as 12 hours (Blackburn, 2003).

The LH is also responsible for the "luteinizing" of the theca and granulosa cells of the ruptured follicle. As a result, estrogen production is reduced and progesterone secretion continues. Thus, estrogen levels fall a day before ovulation; tiny amounts of progesterone are in evidence. Ovulation takes place following the rapid growth of the follicle, as the sustained high level of estrogen diminishes and progesterone secretion begins.

The ruptured follicle undergoes rapid change, complete luteinization is accomplished, and the mass of cells becomes the corpus luteum. The lutein cells secrete large amounts of progesterone with smaller amounts of estro-

gen. (Concurrently the excessive amounts of progesterone are responsible for the secretory phase of the uterine cycle.) The corpus luteum also secretes significant amounts of inhibin A. On day 7 or 8 following ovulation, the corpus luteum begins to involute, losing its secretory function. The production of both progesterone and estrogen is severely diminished. The anterior pituitary responds with increasingly large amounts of FSH; a few days later, LH production begins. New follicles become responsive to another ovarian cycle and begin maturing.

OVARIAN CYCLE

The ovarian cycle has two phases: the *follicular phase* (days 1 to 14) and the *luteal phase* (days 15 to 28 in a 28-day cycle). Figure 3–16 ☉ depicts the changes that the follicle undergoes during the ovarian cycle. In women whose menstrual cycles vary, usually only the length of the follicular phase varies, because the luteal phase is of fixed length. During the follicular phase, the immature follicle matures as a result of FSH. Within the follicle the oocyte grows.

A mature **graafian follicle** appears on about the 14th day under dual control of FSH and LH. It is a large structure, measuring about 5 to 10 mm. The mature follicle produces increasing amounts of estrogen. In the mature graafian follicle, the cells surrounding the antral cavity are granulosa cells. The mass of granulosa cells surrounding the oocyte and follicular fluid is called the cumulus oophorus. In the fully mature graafian follicle, the zona pellucida, a thick elastic capsule, develops around the oocyte.

☉ **FIGURE 3–16**

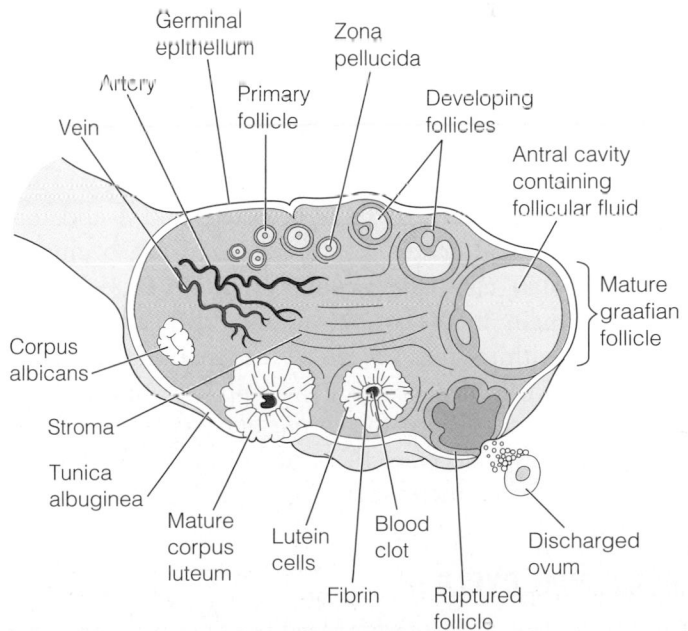

Various stages of development of the ovarian follicles.

Just before ovulation the mature oocyte completes its first meiotic division (see Chapter 7 for a description of meiosis ∞). As a result of this division, two cells are formed: a small cell called a *polar body*, and a larger cell called the *secondary oocyte*. The secondary oocyte matures into the ovum (see Figure 7–2).

As the graafian follicle matures and enlarges, it comes close to the surface of the ovary. The ovary surface forms a blisterlike protrusion 10 to 15 mm in diameter, and the follicle walls become thin. The secondary oocyte, polar body, and follicular fluid are pushed out. The ovum is discharged near the fimbria of the fallopian tube and is pulled into the tube to begin its journey toward the uterus.

In some women ovulation is accompanied by midcycle pain known as *mittelschmerz*. This pain may be caused by a thick tunica albuginea or by a local peritoneal reaction to the expelling of the follicular contents. Vaginal discharge may increase during ovulation, and a small amount of blood (midcycle spotting) may be discharged as well.

The body temperature increases about 0.3°C to 0.6°C (0.5°F to 1°F) 24 to 48 hours after the time of ovulation. It remains elevated until the day before menstruation begins. There may be an accompanying sharp basal body temperature drop before the increase. These temperature changes are useful clinically to determine the approximate time ovulation occurs (Blackburn, 2003).

Generally the ovum takes several minutes to travel through the ruptured follicle to the fallopian tube opening. The contractions of the tube's smooth muscle and its ciliary action propel the ovum through the tube. The ovum remains in the ampulla, where, if it is fertilized, cleavage can begin. The ovum is thought to be fertile for only 6 to 24 hours. It reaches the uterus 72 to 96 hours after its release from the ovary.

The luteal phase begins when the ovum leaves its follicle. Under the influence of LH, the corpus luteum develops from the ruptured follicle. Within 2 or 3 days, the corpus luteum becomes yellowish and spherical and increases in vascularity. If the ovum is fertilized and implants in the endometrium, the fertilized egg begins to secrete **human chorionic gonadotropin (hCG)**, which is needed to maintain the corpus luteum. If fertilization does not occur, within about a week after ovulation the corpus luteum begins to degenerate, eventually becoming a connective tissue scar called the *corpus albicans*. With degeneration comes a decrease in estrogen and progesterone. This allows for an increase in LH and FSH, which trigger the hypothalamus.

MENSTRUAL CYCLE

Menstruation is cyclic uterine bleeding in response to cyclic hormonal changes. Menstruation occurs when the ovum is not fertilized; it begins about 14 days after ovulation in a 28-day cycle. The menstrual discharge, also referred to as the *menses*, or *menstrual flow*, is composed of blood mixed with fluid, cervical and vaginal secretions, bacteria, mucus, leukocytes, and other cellular debris. The menstrual discharge is dark red and has a distinct odor.

Menstrual parameters vary greatly among individuals. Generally, menstruation occurs approximately every 29 days but varies from 21 to 35 days. Some women normally have longer cycles, which can skew standard calculations of the estimated date of birth (EDB). Emotional and physical factors such as illness, excessive fatigue, stress or anxiety, and vigorous exercise programs can alter the cycle interval. The duration of menses is from 2 to 8 days, with the blood loss averaging 25 to 60 mL and the loss of iron averaging 0.5 to 1 mg daily.

A review of the endometrium and its arterial blood supply provides further understanding of the menstrual process (Figure 3–17 ⊙). Blood flow from the spiral arterioles in the superficial endometrium is reduced, leading to a lack of blood and oxygen, which in turn produces tissue death (necrosis) and discharge of the superficial endometrium (menses). At the same time, the straight arterioles provide the basal endometrium with sufficient blood flow to maintain this layer of the endometrium and the endometrial glands (or seeds) that are responsible for the generation of the endometrium in the next female reproductive or menstrual cycle (see Figure 3–15). Bleeding is controlled by vasospasm of the straight basal arterioles, resulting in coagulative necrosis at the vessel tips.

The uterine (menstrual) cycle has four phases: menstrual, proliferative, secretory, and ischemic. Menstruation occurs during the *menstrual phase*. Some endometrial areas are shed, while others remain. Some of the remaining tips of the endometrial glands begin to regenerate. The endometrium is in a resting state following menstruation. Estrogen levels are low, and the endometrium is 1 to 2 mm deep. During this part of the cycle, the cervical mucosa is scanty, viscous, and opaque.

The *proliferative phase* begins when the endometrial glands enlarge, becoming twisted and longer in response to increasing amounts of estrogen. The blood vessels become prominent and dilated, and the endometrium increases in thickness six- to eightfold. This gradual process reaches its peak just before ovulation. The cervical mucosa becomes thin, clear, watery, and more alkaline, making the mucosa more favorable to spermatozoa. As ovulation nears, the cervical mucosa shows increased elasticity, called *spinnbarkeit*. At ovulation the mucus will stretch more than 5 cm. The cervical mucosa pH increases from below 7.0 to 7.5 at the time of ovulation. On microscopic examination the mucosa shows a characteristic ferning pattern (see Figure 6–3 ∞). This fern pattern is a useful aid in assessing ovulation time.

● FIGURE 3–17

Endometrial gland ("seed")

Radial artery

Spiral (coiled) arteriole

Straight arteriole

Uterine artery

Arcuate artery

Radial artery

Myometrium

Endometrium

Blood supply to the endometrium (cross-sectional view of the uterus).

The *secretory phase* follows ovulation. The endometrium, under estrogenic influence, undergoes slight cellular growth. Progesterone, however, causes such marked swelling and growth that the epithelium is warped into folds. The amount of tissue glycogen increases. The glandular epithelial cells begin to fill with cellular debris, become twisted, and dilate. The glands secrete small quantities of endometrial fluid in preparation for a fertilized ovum. The vascularity of the entire uterus increases greatly, providing a nourishing bed for implantation. If implantation occurs the endometrium, under the influence of progesterone, continues to develop and become even thicker (see Chapter 7 for a discussion of implantation ∞).

If fertilization does not occur, the *ischemic phase* begins. The corpus luteum begins to degenerate, and as a result both estrogen and progesterone levels fall. Areas of necrosis appear under the epithelial lining. Extensive vascular changes also occur. Small blood vessels rupture, and the spiral arteries constrict and retract, causing a deficiency of blood in the endometrium, which becomes pale. This ischemic phase is characterized by the escape of blood into the stromal cells of the uterus. The menstrual flow begins, thus beginning the menstrual cycle again. After menstruation the basal layer remains, so that the tips of the glands can regenerate the new functional endometrial layer. For further discussion, see Table 3–2.

MALE REPRODUCTIVE SYSTEM

The primary reproductive functions of the male genitals are to produce and transport sex cells (sperm) through and eventually out of the male genital tract and into the female genital tract. The external and internal genitals of the male reproductive system are shown in Figure 3–18 ●.

TABLE 3–2 ✢ Summary of Female Reproductive Cycle

Ovarian Cycle

Follicular phase (days 1–14): Primordial follicle matures under influence of FSH and LH up to the time of ovulation.

Luteal phase (days 15–28): Ovum leaves follicle; corpus luteum develops under LH influence and produces high levels of progesterone and low levels of estrogen.

Menstrual Cycle

Menstrual phase (days 1–6): Estrogen levels are low; cervical mucus is scant, viscous, and opaque.

Proliferative phase (days 7–14): Estrogen peaks just prior to ovulation. Cervical mucus at ovulation is clear, thin, watery, alkaline, and more favorable to sperm; shows ferning pattern; and has spinnbarkeit greater than 5 cm. Just before ovulation, body temperature may drop slightly, then at ovulation body temperature rises sharply and remains elevated under influence of progesterone.

Secretory phase (days 15–26): Estrogen drops sharply, and progesterone dominates.

Ischemic phase (days 27–28): Both estrogen and progesterone levels drop.

EXTERNAL GENITALS

The two external reproductive organs are the penis and scrotum. The *penis* is an elongated, cylindric structure consisting of a body, called the *shaft,* and a cone-shaped end, called the *glans.* The penis lies in front of the scrotum.

Penis

The shaft of the penis is made up of three longitudinal columns of erectile tissue: the paired *corpora cavernosa* and the *corpus spongiosum.* These columns are covered by dense

FIGURE 3-18

Vas deferens
Symphysis pubis
Corpus cavernosum
Corpus spongiosum
Epididymis
Scrotum
Testis
Glans
Urethra

Ampulla of vas deferens
Seminal vesicle
Ejaculatory duct
Rectum
Prostate
Prostatic urethra
Bulbourethral (Cowper's) gland

Male reproductive system, sagittal view.

fibrous connective tissue and then enclosed by elastic tissue. The penis is covered by a thin outer layer of skin.

The corpus spongiosum contains the urethra and becomes the glans at the distal end of the penis. The urethra widens within the glans and ends in a slitlike opening, located in the tip of the glans, called the *urethral meatus*. A circular fold of skin arises just behind the glans and covers it. Known as the *prepuce*, or *foreskin*, it may be removed by the surgical procedure of circumcision (see Chapter 28 ∞). If the corpus spongiosum does not surround the urethra completely, the urethral meatus may occur on the ventral aspect of the penile shaft (hypospadias) or on the dorsal aspect (epispadias).

The penis is innervated by the pudendal nerve. Sexual stimulation causes the penis to elongate, thicken, and stiffen, a process called *erection*. The penis becomes erect when its blood vessels become engorged, a consequence of parasympathetic nerve stimulation. If sexual stimulation is intense enough, the forceful and sudden expulsion of semen occurs through the rhythmic contractions of the penile muscles. This phenomenon is called *ejaculation*.

The penis serves both the urinary and the reproductive systems. Urine is expelled through the urethral meatus. The reproductive function of the penis is to deposit sperm in the vagina so that fertilization of the ovum can occur.

Scrotum

The *scrotum* is a pouchlike structure that hangs in front of the anus and behind the penis. Composed of skin and the *dartos muscle*, the scrotum shows increased pigmentation and scattered hairs. The sebaceous glands open directly onto the scrotal surface; their secretion has a distinct odor. Contraction of the dartos and cremasteric muscles shortens the scrotum and draws it closer to the body, thus wrinkling its outer surface. The degree of wrinkling is greatest in young men and at cold temperatures and is least in older men and at warm temperatures.

Inside the scrotum are two lateral compartments. Each compartment contains a testis with its related structures. Because the left spermatic cord grows longer, the left testis and its scrotal sac hang lower than on the right. A ridge (raphe) on the external scrotal surface marks the position of the medial septum and continues anteriorly on the urethral surface of the penis, disappearing in the perineal area.

The function of the scrotum is to protect the testes and the sperm by maintaining a temperature lower than that of the body. Spermatogenesis cannot occur if the testes fail to descend and thus remain at body temperature. Because it is sensitive to touch, pressure, temperature, and pain, the scrotum defends against potential harm to the testes.

MALE INTERNAL REPRODUCTIVE ORGANS

The male internal reproductive organs include the gonads (testes or testicles), a system of ducts (epididymides, vas deferens, ejaculatory duct, and urethra), and accessory glands (seminal vesicles, prostate gland, bulbourethral glands, and urethral glands). See Table 3–3.

Testes

The *testes* are a pair of oval, compound glandular organs contained in the scrotum. In the sexually mature male, they

TABLE 3–3 ❖ Summary of Male Reproductive Organ Functions

The testes house seminiferous tubules and gonads.
- Seminiferous tubules contain sperm cells in various stages of development and undergoing meiosis.
- Sertoli's cells nourish and protect spermatocytes (phase between spermatids and spermatozoa).
- Leydig's cells are the main source of testosterone.
- Epididymides provide an area for maturation of sperm and a reservoir for mature spermatozoa.
- The vas deferens connects the epididymis with the prostate gland, then connects with ducts from the seminal vesicle to become an ejaculatory duct.
- Ejaculatory ducts provide a passageway for semen and seminal fluid into the urethra.
- Seminal vesicles secrete yellowish fluid rich in fructose, prostaglandins, and fibrinogen. This provides nutrition that increases the motility and fertilizing ability of sperm. Prostaglandins also aid fertilization by making the cervical mucus more receptive to sperm.
- The prostate gland secretes thin, alkaline fluid containing calcium, citric acid, and other substances. Alkalinity counteracts acidity of ductus and seminal vesicle secretions.
- Bulbourethral (Cowper's) glands secrete alkaline, viscous fluid into semen aiding in neutralization of acidic vaginal secretions.

are the site of spermatozoa production and the secretion of several male sex hormones.

Each testis is 4 to 6 cm long, 2 to 3 cm wide, and 3 to 4 cm thick and weighs about 10 to 15 g. Each is covered by an outer serous membrane and an inner capsule that is tough, white, and fibrous. The connective tissue sends projections inward to form septa, dividing the testis into 250 to 400 lobules. Each lobule contains one to three tightly packed, convoluted *seminiferous tubules* containing sperm cells in all stages of development.

The seminiferous tubules are surrounded by loose connective tissue that houses abundant blood and lymph vessels and *interstitial (Leydig's) cells*. The interstitial cells produce testosterone, the primary male sex hormone. The tubules also contain *Sertoli's cells*, which nourish and protect the spermatocytes. The seminiferous tubules come together to form 20 to 30 straight tubules, which in turn form an anastomotic network of thin-walled spaces, the *rete testis*. The rete testis forms 10 to 15 efferent ducts that empty into the duct of the epididymis.

Most of the cells lining the seminiferous tubules undergo **spermatogenesis**, a process of maturation in which spermatocytes become spermatozoa. (Chapter 7, on page 158, further discusses the process of spermatogenesis. ∞) Sperm production varies among and within the tubules, with cells in different areas of the same tubule undergoing different stages of spermatogenesis. The sperm are eventu-

ally released from the tubules into the epididymis, where they continue to mature.

Like the female reproductive cycle, the process of spermatogenesis and other functions of the testes are the result of complex neural and hormonal controls. The hypothalamus secretes releasing factors that stimulate the anterior pituitary to release the gonadotropins, FSH and LH. These hormones cause the testes to produce testosterone, which maintains spermatogenesis, increases sperm production by the seminiferous tubules, and stimulates production of seminal fluid.

Testosterone is the most prevalent and potent of the testicular hormones. It is also responsible for the development of secondary male characteristics and certain behavioral patterns. The effects of testosterone include structural and functional development of the male genital tract, emission and ejaculation of seminal fluid, distribution of body hair, promotion of growth and strength of long bones, increased muscle mass, and enlargement of the vocal cords. The action of testosterone on the central nervous system is thought to produce aggressiveness and sexual drive. The action of testosterone is constant, not cyclic like that of the female hormones. Its production is not limited to a certain number of years, but it is thought to decrease with age.

The testes have two primary functions:

- To serve as the site of spermatogenesis
- To produce testosterone

Epididymis

The *epididymis* (plural, *epididymides*) is a duct about 5.6 m long, although it is convoluted into a compact structure about 3.75 cm long. An epididymis lies behind each testis. It arises from the top of the testis, courses downward, and then passes upward, where it becomes the vas deferens.

The epididymis provides a reservoir where maturing spermatozoa can survive for a long period. When discharged from the seminiferous tubules into the epididymis, the sperm are immotile and incapable of fertilizing an ovum. The spermatozoa remain in the epididymis for 2 to 10 days. As the sperm move along the convoluted path of the epididymis, they become both motile and fertile.

Vas Deferens and Ejaculatory Ducts

The *vas deferens*, also known as the *ductus deferens*, is about 40 cm long and connects the epididymis with the prostate. One vas deferens arises from the posterior border of each testis. It joins the spermatic cord and weaves over and between several pelvic structures until it meets the vas deferens from the opposite side. Each vas deferens terminus expands to form the *terminal ampulla*. It then unites with the seminal vesicle duct (a gland) to form the ejaculatory duct, which enters the prostate gland and ends in the prostatic urethra. The ejaculatory ducts serve as passageways for semen and fluid secreted by the seminal vesicles. The main function of the vas deferens is to rapidly squeeze the sperm from their storage sites (the epididymis and distal part of the vas deferens) into the urethra.

Urethra

The male urethra is the passageway for both urine and semen. The urethra begins in the bladder and passes through the prostate gland, where it is called the *prostatic urethra*. The urethra emerges from the prostate gland to become the *membranous urethra*. It terminates in the penis, where it is called the penile urethra. In the penile urethra, goblet secretory cells are present, and smooth muscle is replaced by erectile tissue.

Accessory Glands

The male accessory glands secrete a unique and essential component of the total seminal fluid in an ordered sequence.

The *seminal vesicles* are two glands composed of many lobes. Each vesicle is about 7.5 cm long. They are situated between the bladder and the rectum, immediately above the base of the prostate. The epithelium lining the seminal vesicles secretes an alkaline, viscid, clear fluid rich in high-energy fructose, prostaglandins, fibrinogen, and amino acids. During ejaculation this fluid mixes with the sperm in the ejaculatory ducts. This fluid helps provide an environment favorable to sperm motility and metabolism.

The *prostate gland* encircles the upper part of the urethra and lies below the neck of the bladder. Made up of several lobes, it measures about 4 cm in diameter and weighs 20 to 30 g. The prostate is made up of both glandular and muscular tissue. It secretes a thin, milky, alkaline fluid containing high levels of zinc, calcium, citric acid, and acid phosphatase. This fluid protects the sperm from the acidic environment of the vagina and the male urethra, which could be spermicidal.

The *bulbourethral (Cowper's) glands* are a pair of small, round structures on either side of the membranous urethra. The glands secrete a clear, thick, alkaline fluid rich in mucoproteins that becomes part of the semen. This secretion also lubricates the penile urethra during sexual excitement and neutralizes the acid in the male urethra and vagina, thereby enhancing sperm motility.

The *urethral (Littre's) glands* are tiny mucus-secreting glands found throughout the membranous lining of the penile urethra. Their secretions add to those of the bulbourethral glands.

FIGURE 3–19

Schematic representation of a mature spermatozoon.

Semen

The male ejaculate, *semen or seminal fluid*, is made up of spermatozoa and the secretions of all the accessory glands. The seminal fluid transports viable and motile sperm to the female reproductive tract. Effective transportation of sperm requires adequate nutrients, an adequate pH (about 7.5), a specific concentration of sperm to fluid, and an optimal osmolarity.

A spermatozoon is made up of a *head* and a *tail*. The tail is divided into the middle piece and end piece (Figure 3–19 ●). The head's main components are the *acrosome* and *nucleus*. The head carries the male's haploid number of chromosomes (23), and it is the part that enters the ovum at fertilization (see Chapter 7 ∞). The tail, or flagellum, is divided into the middle and end piece and is specialized for motility.

Sperm may be stored in the male genital system for up to 42 days, depending primarily on the frequency of ejaculations. The average volume of ejaculate following abstinence for several days is 2 to 5 mL but may vary from 1 to 10 mL. Repeated ejaculation results in decreased volume. Once ejaculated, sperm can live only 2 or 3 days in the female genital tract.

Critical Concept Review

LEARNING OBJECTIVES

CONCEPTS

Identify the structures and functions of the female and male reproductive systems.

Female reproductive system:
1. Ovaries
   - Produce female germ cells and female sex hormones.
2. Fallopian tubes
   - Capture the ovum.
   - Allow transport of the ovum to the uterus.
3. Uterus
   - Implantation site for the fertilized ovum.
4. Cervix
   - Connection between the vagina and the uterus.
   - Protective portal for the body of the uterus.
5. Vagina
   - Passageway from the external genitals to the uterus.
   - Provides for discharge of menstrual products out of the body.

Male reproductive system:
1. Testes
   - Produce male germ cells and male sex hormones.
2. Epididymis, vas deferens, and ejaculatory duct
   - Transport spermatozoa outside the body.
3. Accessory glands
   - Produce secretions necessary for sperm nutrition, survival, and transport.
4. Penis
   - Reproductive organ of intercourse.

Summarize the actions of the hormones that affect reproductive functioning.

1. Estrogen:
   - Controls development of female secondary sex characteristics.
   - Assists in the maturation of the ovarian follicles.
   - Causes endometrial mucosa to proliferate following menstruation.
   - Causes uterus to increase in size and weight.
   - Increases myometrial contractility in both the uterus and fallopian tubes.
   - Increases uterine sensitivity to oxytocin.
   - Inhibits FSH production.
   - Stimulates LH production.
2. Progesterone:
   - Decreases uterine motility and contractility.
   - Causes uterine endometrium to increase its supply of glycogen, arterial blood, secretory glands, amino acids, and water.
   - Vaginal epithelium proliferates.
   - Cervix secretes thick, viscous mucus.
   - Increases breast glandular tissue, both in size and in complexity.
   - Prepares breasts for lactation.
3. Prostaglandins:
   - Necessary for follicular rupture.

Identify the two phases of the ovarian cycle and the changes that occur in each phase.

1. Follicular phase:
   - Primordial follicle matures under the influence of FSH and LH until ovulation occurs.
2. Luteal phase:
   - Ovum leaves the follicle.
   - Corpus luteum develops under the influence of LH.
   - Corpus luteum produces high levels of progesterone and low levels of estrogen.

(continued)

LEARNING OBJECTIVES

CONCEPTS

Describe the phases of the menstrual cycle, their dominant hormones, and the changes that occur in each phase.

→

1. Menstrual phase:
   - Shedding of the endometrial lining.
   - Low estrogen levels.
2. Proliferative phase:
   - Enlargement of the endometrial glands under influence of estrogen.
   - Changes in cervical mucus; peak at ovulation.
   - Increasing estrogen levels.
3. Secretory phase:
   - Follows ovulation.
   - Influenced primarily by progesterone.
   - Increase in vascularity of the uterus to make ready for possible implantation.
4. Ischemic phase:
   - Decreasing levels of estrogen and progesterone.
   - Degeneration of the corpus luteum.
   - Constriction of the spiral arteries.
   - Escape of blood into the stromal cells of the endometrium.

Discuss the significance of specific female reproductive structures during childbirth.

→

1. Ischial spines:
   - Serve as a reference point during labor to evaluate the descent of the fetal head.
2. Pubic arch (symphysis pubis):
   - Fetal head passes under this arch during birth.
3. False pelvis:
   - Serves to support the weight of the enlarged pregnant uterus and direct the presenting fetal part into the true pelvis.
4. True pelvis:
   - Shape and size must be adequate for normal fetal passage.
   - Fetus must change its position to move through the diameter of the true pelvis.
5. Pelvic cavity:
   - Can influence the length of labor.

Identify the functions of specific male reproductive structures for reproduction.

→

1. Penis:
   - Deposits sperm in the vagina so fertilization of the ovum can occur.
2. Scrotum:
   - Protects the testes and sperm by maintaining a temperature lower than the body.
3. Testes:
   - Serve as a site for spermatogenesis.
   - Produce testosterone.
4. Epididymis:
   - Provides a reservoir for maturing spermatozoa.
5. Vas deferens:
   - Rapidly squeeze the sperm from their storage sites into the urethra.
6. Ejaculatory duct:
   - Passageway for semen and fluid secreted by the seminal vesicles.
7. Urethra:
   - Passageway for both urine and semen.
8. Seminal fluid:
   - Provides environment favorable to sperm mobility and metabolism.
   - Transports viable and mobile sperm to the female reproductive tract.

CRITICAL THINKING IN ACTION

View the Critical Thinking in Action video in Chapter 3 of the CD-ROM. Then, answer the questions that follow.

You are working in the OB/GYN clinic when Sally Smith, a 17-year-old teenager, comes in complaining of irregular menses. She believes her periods are really "messed up" and interfering with her active schedule. She wants them to be more regular and asks you for birth control. She tells you that she is a member of the swimming team and is a senior in high school. She says she is planning to start community college next year to obtain an associate degree in computer technology. You assess Sally's history as follows: menarche began at age 12; periods occur every 28 to 32 days. She usually experiences cramping in the first 2 days and the flow lasts 4 to 5 days. She uses an average of 4 to 5 tampons a day during her period. She has never been hospitalized, has no prior medical problems, and is up to date on her immunizations except for meningitis.

1. Based on your knowledge of menstruation, how would you describe Sally's menstrual cycle?
2. What is your primary goal in discussing Sally's menstrual cycle with her?
3. What information would you give Sally relating to her menstrual cycle?
4. What important request does Sally have?
5. Sally expresses problems dealing with the cramping she experiences with the first 2 days of her menses. What would you suggest to Sally to cope with the discomfort?

MEDIALINK
www.prenhall.com/london

- NCLEX-RN® Review, case studies, and other interactive resources for this chapter can be found on the Companion Website at http://www.prenhall.com/london. Click on "Chapter 3" to select the activities for this chapter.

- For animations, more NCLEX-RN® Review questions, and an audio glossary, access the accompanying CD-ROM in this textbook.

REFERENCES

Blackburn, S. T. (2003). *Maternal, fetal, & neonatal physiology: A clinical perspective* (2nd ed.). St. Louis, MO: Saunders.

Caldwell, W. E., & Moloy, H. C. (1933). Anatomical variations in the female pelvis and their effect on labor with a suggested classification [Historical article]. *American Journal of Obstetrics and Gynecology, 26,* 479–505.

Ferin, M. (2003). The hypothalamus-hypophyseal-ovarian axis and the menstrual cycle. In J. J. Sciarri (Ed.), *Gynecology and obstetrics* (Vol. 5, chap. 6, pp. 1–21). Philadelphia: Lippincott Williams & Wilkins.

Lawrence, R. M., & Lawrence, R. A. (2004). The breast and the physiology of lactation. In R. K. Creasy & R. Resnik (Eds.), *Maternal-fetal med-*

icine: Principles and practice (5th ed.). Philadelphia: Saunders.

Monga, M., & Sanborn, B. M. (2004). Biology and physiology of the reproductive tract and control of myometrial contraction. In R. K. Creasy & R. Resnik (Eds.), *Maternal-fetal medicine: Principles and practice* (5th ed.). Philadelphia: Saunders.

CHAPTER 4

Health Promotion for Women

I am 58 now, an early baby boomer. I am astonished at the changes that have occurred in women's healthcare in my lifetime. I remember that my mom was shocked when our family doctor taught me to do a breast exam when I turned 18. What a farsighted man. Information on sexually transmitted infections was not as generally available. AIDS was beyond our imagination. Contraceptive options were more limited although the pill was gaining in popularity. Menopause seemed like the end of life—menopausal women were old. Today more and more of us women are becoming savvy healthcare consumers. We have more information, we have treatment options, we decide our own care. I think this is the most exciting change of all!

—Alice

LEARNING OBJECTIVES

- Summarize information that women may need to implement effective self-care measures for dealing with menstruation.

- Contrast dysmenorrhea and premenstrual syndrome.

- Compare the advantages, disadvantages, and effectiveness of the various methods of contraception available today.

- Delineate basic gynecologic screening procedures indicated for well women.

- Discuss the physical and psychologic aspects of menopause.

- Explain the cycle of violence and its application to battered women, including pregnant women.

- Delineate the nurse's role in working with women who have experienced intimate partner violence or rape.

MEDIALINK www.prenhall.com/london

CD-ROM
NCLEX-RN® Review
Audio Glossary
Skill 2-2: Assisting with a Pelvic Examination
Animation: Oral Contraceptive
Spousal Abuse Video

Companion Website
NCLEX-RN® Review
Case Study
Thinking Critically

A woman's healthcare needs change throughout her lifetime. As a young girl she needs health teaching about menstruation, sexuality, and personal responsibility. As a teen she needs information about reproductive choices and safe sexual activity. During this time she should also be introduced to the importance of healthcare practices such as breast self-examination and regular Pap smears. The mature woman may need to be reminded of these self-care issues and prepared for the physical changes that accompany childbirth and aging. By educating women about their bodies, their healthcare choices, and their right to be knowledgeable consumers, nurses can help women assume responsibility for the healthcare they receive. This chapter provides information about selected aspects of women's healthcare with an emphasis on conditions typically addressed in a community-based setting.

NURSING CARE IN THE COMMUNITY

Women's health refers to a holistic view of women and their health-related needs within the context of their everyday lives. It is based on the awareness that a woman's physical, mental, and spiritual status are interdependent and affect her state of health or illness. The woman's view of her situation, her assessment of her needs, her values, and her beliefs are valid and important factors to be incorporated into any healthcare intervention.

Nurses can work with women to provide health teaching and information about self-care practices in schools, during routine examinations in a clinic or office, at senior centers, at meetings of volunteer organizations, through classes offered by local agencies or schools, or in the home. This community-based focus is the key to providing effective nursing care to women of all ages.

In reality the vast majority of women's healthcare is provided outside of acute care settings. Nurses oriented to community-based care are especially effective in recognizing the autonomy of each individual and in dealing with clients holistically. This holistic approach is important in addressing not only physical problems but also major health issues such as violence against women, which may go undetected unless care providers are alert for signs of it. See "Developing Cultural Competence."

THE NURSE'S ROLE IN ADDRESSING ISSUES OF SEXUALITY

Because sexuality and its reproductive implications are such intrinsic and emotion-laden parts of life, people have many concerns, problems, and questions about sex roles, behaviors, education, inhibitions, morality, and

KEY TERMS

Amenorrhea, 74

Breast self-examination (BSE), 86

Cervical cap, 79

Coitus interruptus, 77

Combined oral contraceptives (COCs), 82

Condom, 77

Date rape, 95

Depo-Provera, 83

Diaphragm, 78

Domestic violence, 92

Dysmenorrhea, 74

Emergency contraception, 84

Fertility awareness methods, 75

Hormone replacement therapy (HRT), 89

Intimate partner violence, 92

Intrauterine device (IUD), 81

Mammogram, 86

Menopause, 88

Osteoporosis, 89

Perimenopause, 89

Premenstrual syndrome (PMS), 74

Rape, 94

Sexual assault, 94

Spermicides, 77

Sterilization, 84

Subdermal implants, 83

Tubal ligation, 84

Vasectomy, 84

related areas such as family planning. The reproductive implications of sexual intercourse must also be considered. Some people desire pregnancy; others wish to avoid it. Health factors are another consideration. The increase in the incidence of sexually transmitted infections, especially HIV/AIDS and herpes, has caused many people to modify their sexual practices and activities. Women frequently ask questions or voice concerns about these issues to the nurse in a clinic or ambulatory setting. Thus, the nurse may need to assume the role of counselor or educator on sexual and reproductive matters.

Nurses who assume this role must recognize their own feelings, values, and attitudes about sexuality so they can be more sensitive when they encounter the values and beliefs of others. Nurses need to have accurate, up-to-date information about anatomy and physiology and about topics related to sexuality, sexual practices, and common gynecologic problems. In addition, when a woman is accompanied by her partner, it is important that the nurse be sensitive to the dynamics of the relationship between the two.

TAKING A SEXUAL HISTORY

Nurses are often responsible for taking a woman's initial history, including her gynecologic and sexual history. For the interview to be its most useful, the nurse must have effective communication skills and should conduct the interview in a quiet, private place free of distractions. It is important to phrase questions in a sensitive and nonjudgmental manner and to assure the woman of strict confidentiality.

Opening the discussion with a brief explanation of the purpose of such questions is often helpful. For example, the nurse might say, "As your nurse, I'm interested in all aspects of your well-being. Often women have concerns or questions about sexual matters, especially when they are pregnant (or starting to be sexually active). I will be asking you some questions about your sexual history as part of your general health history."

It may be helpful to use direct eye contact as much as possible unless the nurse knows it is culturally unacceptable to the woman. The nurse should do little, if any, writing during the interview, especially if the woman seems ill at ease or is discussing very personal issues. Beginning with general questions such as, "What brings you here today?" before progressing to more sensitive topics will provide an opportunity for the woman to develop trust with the nurse. Open-ended questions are often useful in eliciting information. For example, "What, if anything, would you change about your sex life?" will elicit more information than "Are you happy with your sex life now?" The nurse needs to clarify terminology and proceed from easier topics to those that are more difficult to discuss.

Throughout the interview the nurse should be alert to body language and nonverbal cues. It is important that the nurse not assume that the client is heterosexual. Some women are open about lesbian relationships; others are more reserved until they develop a sense of trust in their caregivers.

After completing the sexual history, the nurse assesses the information obtained. If there is a problem that requires further medical tests and assessments, the nurse refers the woman to a nurse practitioner, certified nurse-midwife, physician, or counselor as necessary. In many instances the nurse alone will be able to develop a nursing diagnosis and then plan and implement therapy. The nurse must be realistic in making assessments and planning interventions. It requires insight and skill to recognize when a woman's problem requires interventions that are beyond a nurse's preparation and ability. In such situations it is essential that the nurse makes appropriate referrals.

MENSTRUATION

Girls today begin to learn about puberty and menstruation at a young age. Unfortunately, the source of their "education" is sometimes their peers or the media; thus, the information is often incomplete, inaccurate, and sensationalized. Nurses who work with young girls and adolescents recognize this and are working hard to provide accurate health teaching and to correct misinformation about *menarche* (the onset of menses) and the menstrual cycle.

Cultural, religious, and personal attitudes about menstruation are part of the menstrual experience and often reflect negative attitudes toward women. Currently in the Western world, there are few customs associated with menstruation. In many cultures, sexual intercourse during menses is a common practice. Physiologically, it is not generally contraindicated. For most couples the decision is one of personal preference. (The physiology of menstruation is discussed in Chapter 3. ∞)

COUNSELING THE PREMENSTRUAL GIRL ABOUT MENARCHE

Many young women find it embarrassing to discuss menstruation, both because of the taboos associated with the subject and because of their immaturity. However, the most critical factor in successful adaptation to menarche is the adolescent's level of preparedness. Information should be given to premenstrual girls over time rather than all at once. This allows them to absorb information and develop questions.

The following basic information is helpful for young clients:

- *Cycle length.* Cycle length is determined from the first day of one menses to the first day of the next menses.

Initially a female's cycle length is about 29 days, but the normal length may vary from 21 to 35 days. As a woman matures, cycle length often shortens to a median of 25+ days just before menopause. Cycle length frequently varies by a day or two from one cycle to the next, although greater normal variations may also occur.

- *Amount of flow.* The average flow is approximately 25 to 60 mL per period. Usually women characterize the amount of flow in terms of the number of pads or tampons used. Flow is often heavier at first and lighter toward the end of the period.
- *Length of menses.* Menses usually lasts from 2 to 8 days, although this may vary.

The nurse should make it clear that variations in age at menarche, length of cycle, and duration of menses are normal, because girls may worry if their experience varies from that of their peers. It also is helpful to acknowledge the negative aspects of menstruation (messiness, cramping, embarrassment) while stressing its positive role as a symbol of maturity and womanhood.

EDUCATIONAL TOPICS

Pads and Tampons

Since early times women have made pads and tampons from cloth or rags, which required washing but were reusable. Commercial tampons were introduced in the 1930s.

Today adhesive-stripped minipads and maxipads and flushable tampons are readily available. However, the deodorants and increased absorbency that manufacturers have added to both pads and tampons may prove harmful. The chemical used to deodorize can create a rash on the vulva and damage the tender mucous lining of the vagina. Excessive or inappropriate use of tampons can produce dryness or even small sores or ulcers in the vagina.

Because the use of superabsorbent tampons has been linked to the development of toxic shock syndrome (TSS), women should avoid using them (see Care of the Woman with Toxic Shock Syndrome in Chapter 5 ∞). They should use regular absorbency tampons only for heavy menstrual flow (during the first 2 or 3 days of the period), not during the whole period, and change them every 3 to 6 hours. Because *Staphylococcus aureus*, the causative organism of TSS, is frequently found on the hands, a woman should wash her hands before inserting a fresh tampon and should avoid touching the tip of the tampon when unwrapping it or before insertion.

In the absence of a heavy menstrual flow, tampons absorb moisture, leaving the vaginal walls dry and subject to injury. The absorbency of regular tampons varies. If the tampon is hard to pull out or shreds when removed, or if the vagina becomes dry, the tampon is probably too absorbent.

A woman may want to use tampons only during the day and switch to pads at night to avoid vaginal irritation. She should avoid using tampons on the last, spotty days of her period and should never use them for midcycle spotting or leukorrhea. If a woman experiences vaginal irritation, itching, or soreness or notices an unusual odor while using tampons, she should stop using them or change brands or absorbencies to see if that helps.

Vaginal Spray, Douching, and Cleansing

Vaginal sprays are unnecessary and can cause infections, itching (pruritis), burning, vaginal discharge, rashes, and other problems. If a woman chooses to use a spray, she needs to know that these sprays are for external use only and should never be applied to irritated or itching skin or used with pads.

Although douching is sometimes used to treat vaginal infections, douching as a hygiene practice is unnecessary since the vagina cleanses itself. Douching washes away the natural mucus and upsets the vaginal ecology, which can make the vagina more susceptible to infection. Perfumed douches can cause allergic reactions, and too frequent use of an undiluted or strong douche solution can cause irritation or even tissue damage. Propelling water up the vagina may also erode the antibacterial cervical plug and force bacteria and germs from the vagina into the uterus. Women should avoid douching during menstruation because the cervix is dilated to permit the downward flow of menstrual fluids from the uterine lining. Douching may force tissue back up into the uterine cavity, which could contribute to endometriosis.

The mucous secretions that bathe the vagina are odor-free while they are in the vagina; odor develops only when they mingle with perspiration and are exposed to the air. Keeping one's skin clean and free of bacteria with plain soap and water is the most effective method of controlling odor. A soapy finger or soft washcloth should be used to wash gently between the vulvar folds. Bathing is as important during menses as at any other time. A long, leisurely soak in a warm tub promotes menstrual blood flow and relieves cramps by relaxing the muscles.

Keeping the vulva fresh throughout the day means keeping it dry and clean. A woman can ensure adequate ventilation by wearing cotton panties and clothes loose enough to permit the vaginal area to "breathe." After using the toilet, a woman should always wipe herself from front to back and, if necessary, follow up with a moistened paper towel or toilet paper. If an unusual odor persists despite these efforts, it may be a sign that something is awry. Certain conditions such as vaginitis produce a foul-smelling discharge.

ASSOCIATED MENSTRUAL CONDITIONS

A variety of menstrual irregularities have been identified. An abnormally short duration of menstrual flow is termed *hypomenorrhea;* an abnormally long one is called *hypermenorrhea.* Excessive, profuse flow is called *menorrhagia,* and bleeding between periods is known as *metrorrhagia.* Infrequent and too frequent menses are termed *oligomenorrhea* and *polymenorrhea,* respectively. An *anovulatory cycle* is one in which ovulation does not occur. (*Note:* Anovulatory cycles often occur during the first year after menarche and during the perimenopause, the period around the time of menopause.) Generally menstrual irregularities should be investigated to rule out disease.

Amenorrhea

Amenorrhea, the absence of menses, is classified as primary or secondary. Primary amenorrhea exists if menstruation has not been established by 16 years of age or within 4 years of breast development. Secondary amenorrhea exists when an established menses (of longer than 3 months) ceases for at least 6 months.

Primary amenorrhea necessitates a thorough assessment of the young woman to determine its cause. Possible causes include congenital obstructions, Turner syndrome, congenital absence of the uterus, testicular feminization (external genitals appear female but uterus and ovaries are absent and testes are present), or absence or imbalance of hormones. Treatment depends on the causative factors. Some causes are not correctable.

Secondary amenorrhea is caused most frequently by pregnancy. Additional causes include lactation, hormonal imbalances, poor nutrition (anorexia nervosa, obesity, and fad dieting), ovarian lesions, strenuous exercise (associated with long-distance runners, dancers, and other athletes with low body fat ratios), debilitating systemic diseases, stress of high intensity or long duration, stressful life events, a change in season or climate, use of oral contraceptives, use of the phenothiazine and chlorpromazine group of tranquilizers, and syndromes such as Cushing and Sheehan. The causative factors dictate treatment. The nurse can explain that once the underlying condition has been corrected—for example, when sufficient body weight is gained—menses will resume. Athletes and women who participate in strenuous exercise routines may be advised to increase their caloric intake or reduce their exercise levels for a month or two to see whether a normal cycle ensues. If it does not, medical referral is indicated.

Dysmenorrhea

Dysmenorrhea, or painful menstruation, occurs at or a day before the onset of menstruation and disappears by the end of menses. Dysmenorrhea is classified as primary or secondary. Primary dysmenorrhea is defined as cramps without underlying disease. Prostaglandins F_2 and $F_{2\alpha}$, which are produced by the uterus in higher concentrations during menses, are the primary cause. They increase uterine contractility and decrease uterine artery blood flow, causing ischemia. The end result is the painful sensation of cramps. Dysmenorrhea typically disappears after a first pregnancy and does not occur if cycles are anovulatory. Treatment of primary dysmenorrhea includes combined oral contraceptives, which block ovulation; prostaglandin inhibitors (such as ibuprofen, aspirin, and naproxen), which act as prostaglandin inhibitors; and self-care measures such as regular exercise, rest, heat, and good nutrition. Biofeedback has also been used with some success.

Secondary dysmenorrhea is associated with pathology of the reproductive tract and usually appears after menstruation has been established. Conditions that most frequently cause secondary dysmenorrhea include endometriosis; residual pelvic inflammatory disease; anatomic anomalies such as cervical stenosis, imperforate hymen, and uterine displacement; ovarian cysts; and the presence of an intrauterine device. Because primary and secondary dysmenorrhea may coexist, accurate differential diagnosis is essential for appropriate treatment.

Some nutritionists suggest that vitamins B and E help relieve the discomforts associated with menstruation. Vitamin B_6 may help relieve the premenstrual bloating and irritability some women experience. Vitamin E, a mild prostaglandin inhibitor, may help decrease menstrual discomfort. Avoiding salt can decrease discomfort from fluid retention.

Heat is soothing and promotes increased blood flow. Any source of warmth, from sipping herbal tea to soaking in a hot tub or using a heating pad, may be helpful during painful periods. Massage can also soothe aching back muscles and promote relaxation and blood flow.

Regular exercise can ease menstrual discomfort and help prevent cramps and other menstrual complaints. Aerobic exercises such as jogging, cycling, swimming, and fast-paced walking are especially helpful. Persistent discomfort should be medically evaluated.

Premenstrual Syndrome

Premenstrual syndrome (PMS) refers to a symptom complex associated with the luteal phase of the menstrual cycle (2 weeks prior to the onset of menses). The symptoms must, by definition, occur between ovulation and the onset of menses. They repeat at the same stage of each menstrual cycle and include some or all of the following:

- *Psychologic:* irritability, lethargy, depression, low morale, anxiety, sleep disorders, crying spells, hostility
- *Neurologic:* classic migraine, vertigo, syncope
- *Respiratory:* rhinitis, hoarseness, and occasionally asthma

- *Gastrointestinal:* nausea, vomiting, constipation, abdominal bloating, craving for sweets
- *Urinary:* retention, oliguria
- *Dermatologic:* acne
- *Mammary:* swelling and tenderness

Most women experience only some of these symptoms. The symptoms usually are most pronounced 2 or 3 days before the onset of menstruation and subside as menstrual flow begins, with or without treatment. *Premenstrual dysphoric disorder* (PMDD) is a diagnosis that may be applied to a subgroup of women with PMS whose symptoms are primarily mood related and severe.

The exact cause of PMS is unknown, although a variety of theories have been put forth to explain it. These include, for example, hormone imbalance, nutritional deficiency, prostaglandin excess, and endorphin deficiency. PMS may also be related to serotonin because serotonin levels in women with PMS fall after ovulation (Hudson, 2002).

Nursing Management. The nurse can help the woman identify specific symptoms and develop healthy behavior. After assessment, counseling for PMS may include advising the woman to restrict her intake of foods containing methylxanthines such as chocolate, cola, and coffee; restrict her intake of alcohol, nicotine, red meat, and foods containing salt and sugar; increase her intake of complex carbohydrates and protein; and increase the frequency of meals. For women whose primary symptoms are psychologic, supplementation with B-complex vitamins, especially B$_6$, may decrease anxiety and depression. Vitamin E supplements may help reduce breast tenderness. Supplementation with 1200 mg calcium daily may help relieve certain symptoms, including negative mood, food cravings, water retention, and pain (Hudson, 2002).

A program of aerobic exercise such as fast walking, jogging, and aerobic dancing is generally beneficial. In addition to vitamin supplements, pharmacologic treatments for PMS include diuretics and prostaglandin inhibitors. Serotonin agents such as fluoxetine hydrochloride (Prozac) and sertraline hydrochloride (Zoloft) may help relieve symptoms of PMDD. For women who are not planning a pregnancy, low-dose combined oral contraceptives, which suppress ovulation, are often helpful.

A woman benefits a great deal from an empathetic relationship with a healthcare professional to whom she feels free to voice concerns. Encourage the woman to keep a diary to help identify life events associated with PMS. Self-care groups and self-help literature both help women feel they have control over their bodies. Some women use complementary therapies such as homeopathic remedies or herbs. It is important that women using such alternatives seek advice from knowledgeable, experienced homeopaths or herbalists.

CONTRACEPTION

The decision to use a method of contraception may be made individually by a woman (or, in the case of vasectomy, by a man) or jointly by a couple. The decision may be motivated by a desire to avoid pregnancy, to gain control over the number of children conceived, or to determine the spacing of future children. In choosing a specific method, consistency of use outweighs the absolute reliability of the given method.

Decisions about contraception should be made voluntarily, with full knowledge of available choices, advantages, disadvantages, effectiveness, side effects, contraindications, and long-term effects. Many outside factors influence this choice, including cultural practices, religious beliefs, attitudes and personal preferences, cost, effectiveness, misinformation, practicality of method, and self-esteem. Different methods of contraception may be appropriate at different times for individuals or couples.

FERTILITY AWARENESS METHODS

Fertility awareness methods, also known as *natural family planning*, are based on an understanding of the changes that occur throughout a woman's ovulatory cycle. All these methods require periods of abstinence and recording of certain events throughout the cycle; cooperation of the partners is important.

Fertility awareness methods are free, safe, and acceptable to many whose religious beliefs prohibit other methods. They provide an increased awareness of the body, involve no artificial substances or devices, encourage a couple to communicate about sexual activity and family planning, and are useful in helping a couple plan a pregnancy.

On the other hand, these methods require extensive initial counseling to be used effectively. They may interfere with sexual spontaneity; they require extensive maintenance of records for several cycles before beginning to use them; they may be difficult or impossible for women with irregular cycles to use; and, although theoretically they should be very reliable, in practice they may not be as reliable in preventing pregnancy as other methods.

The *basal body temperature (BBT)* method to detect ovulation requires that a woman take her BBT every morning upon awakening (before any activity) and record the readings on a temperature graph. To do this she uses a BBT thermometer, which shows tenths of a degree rather than the two tenths shown on standard thermometers. She may also use tympanic thermometry (an "ear thermometer"). After 3 to 4 months of recording temperatures, a woman with regular cycles should be able to predict when ovulation will occur. The method is based on the fact that the temperature sometimes drops just before ovulation and almost always rises and remains elevated for several days after. The temperature rise occurs in response to the increased progesterone levels that occur in the second half of the cycle. Figure 4–1 ● shows a sample BBT chart. To avoid conception the couple abstains from intercourse on the day of the temperature rise and for 3 days after. Because the temperature rise does not occur until after ovulation, a woman who had intercourse just before the rise is at risk of pregnancy. To decrease this risk, some couples abstain from intercourse for several days before the *anticipated* time of ovulation and then for 3 days after.

The *calendar,* or *rhythm, method* is based on the assumptions that ovulation tends to occur 14 days (plus or minus 2 days) before the start of the next menstrual period, sperm are viable for 48 to 72 hours, and the ovum is viable for 24 hours. To use this method, the woman must record her menstrual cycles for 6 to 8 months to identify the shortest and longest cycles. The first day of menstruation is the first day of the cycle. The fertile phase is calculated from 18 days before the end of the shortest recorded cycle through 11 days from the end of the longest recorded cycle. For example, if a woman's cycle lasts from 24 to 28 days, the fertile phase would be calculated as day 6 through day 17. Once this information is obtained, the woman can identify the fertile and infertile phases of her cycle. For effective use of this method, she must abstain from intercourse during the fertile phase. The calendar method is the least reliable of the fertility awareness methods and has largely been replaced by other, more scientific approaches.

The *cervical mucus method,* sometimes called the *ovulation method* or the *Billings method,* involves the assessment of cervical mucus changes that occur during the menstrual cycle. The amount and character of cervical mucus change because of the influence of estrogen and progesterone. At the time of ovulation, the mucus (estrogen-dominant mucus) is clearer, more stretchable (a quality called *spinnbarkeit*), and more permeable to sperm. It also shows a characteristic fern pattern when placed on a glass slide and allowed to dry (see Figure 6–3, page 129 ∞). During the luteal phase, the cervical mucus is thick and sticky (progesterone-dominant mucus) and forms a network that traps sperm, making their passage more difficult.

To use the cervical mucus method, the woman abstains from intercourse for the first menstrual cycle. Each day she assesses her cervical mucus for amount, feeling of slipperiness or wetness, color, clearness, and spinnbarkeit, as she becomes familiar with varying characteristics.

The peak day of wetness and clear, stretchable mucus is assumed to be the time of ovulation. To use this method correctly, the woman should abstain from intercourse from the time she first notices that the mucus is becoming clear, more elastic, and slippery until 4 days after the last wet mucus (ovulation) day. Because this method evaluates the effects of hormonal changes, it can be used by women with irregular cycles.

The *symptothermal method* consists of various assessments made and recorded by the couple. These include information regarding cycle days, coitus, cervical mucus changes, and secondary signs such as increased libido, abdominal bloating, *mittelschmerz* (midcycle abdominal pain), and BBT. Through the various assessments, the couple learns to recognize signs that indicate ovulation. This combined approach tends to improve the effectiveness of fertility awareness as a method of birth control.

● **FIGURE 4–1**

Sample basal body temperature chart.

SITUATIONAL CONTRACEPTIVES

Abstinence can be considered a method of contraception, and, partly because of changing values and the increased risk of infection with intercourse, it is gaining increased acceptance.

Coitus interruptus, or *withdrawal,* is one of the oldest and least reliable methods of contraception. This method requires that the male withdraw from the female's vagina when he feels that ejaculation is impending. He then ejaculates away from the external genitalia of the woman. Failure tends to occur for two reasons: (1) this method demands great self-control on the part of the man, who must withdraw just as he feels the urge for deeper penetration with impending orgasm, and (2) some pre-ejaculatory fluid, which can contain sperm, may escape from the penis during the excitement phase prior to ejaculation. The fact that the quantity of sperm in this pre-ejaculatory fluid is increased after a recent ejaculation is especially significant for couples who engage in repeated episodes of intercourse within a short period of time. Couples who use this method should be aware of postcoital contraceptive options in case the man fails to withdraw in time.

Douching after intercourse is an ineffective method of contraception and is not recommended. It may actually facilitate conception by pushing sperm farther up the birth canal.

SPERMICIDES

Spermicides, available as creams, jellies, foams, vaginal film, and suppositories, are inserted into the vagina before intercourse. They destroy sperm or neutralize vaginal secretions and thereby immobilize sperm. Spermicides that effervesce in a moist environment offer relatively rapid protection, and coitus may take place immediately after they are inserted. Suppositories may require up to 30 minutes to dissolve and will not offer protection until they do so. The woman should be instructed to insert these spermicide preparations high in the vagina and maintain a supine position.

Spermicides are minimally effective when used alone, but their effectiveness increases in conjunction with a diaphragm or condom. The major advantages of spermicides are their wide availability and low toxicity. Skin irritation and allergic reactions to spermicides are the primary disadvantages. Spermicides do not offer protection against the organisms that cause gonorrhea and chlamydia, or against the human immunodeficiency virus (HIV), which causes acquired immunodeficiency syndrome (AIDS) (Centers for Disease Control and Prevention [CDC], 2002).

BARRIER METHODS OF CONTRACEPTIVES

Barrier methods of contraception prevent the transport of sperm to the ovum, immobilize sperm, or are lethal against sperm.

Male and Female Condoms

The male **condom** offers a viable means of contraception when used consistently and properly (Figure 4–2). Acceptance has been increasing as a growing number of men

● **FIGURE 4–2**

A B

A, Unrolled condom with reservoir tip. *B,* Correct use of a condom.

are assuming responsibility for regulation of fertility. The condom is applied to the erect penis, rolled from the tip to the end of the shaft, before vulvar or vaginal contact. A small space must be left at the end of the condom to allow for collection of the ejaculate, so that the condom will not break at the time of ejaculation. If the condom or vagina is dry, a water-soluble lubricant such as K-Y jelly should be used to prevent irritation and possible condom breakage.

Couples should be careful when removing the condom after intercourse. For optimal effectiveness the man should withdraw his penis from the woman's vagina while it is still erect and hold the condom rim to prevent spillage. If after ejaculation the penis becomes flaccid while still in the vagina, the man should hold onto the edge of the condom while withdrawing to avoid spilling semen and to prevent the condom from slipping off.

The effectiveness of male condoms is largely determined by their use. The condom is small, disposable, and inexpensive; it has no side effects, requires no medical examination or supervision, and offers visual evidence of effectiveness. Most condoms are made of latex, although polyurethane and silicone rubber condoms are available for individuals allergic to latex. All condoms, except natural "skin" condoms, made from lamb's intestines, offer protection against both pregnancy and sexually transmitted infections (STIs). Breakage, displacement, perineal or vaginal irritation, and dulled sensation are possible disadvantages.

The male condom is becoming increasingly popular because of the protection it offers from infections. For women, sexually transmitted infection increases the risk of pelvic inflammatory disease (PID) and resultant infertility. Many women are beginning to insist that their sexual partners use condoms, and many women carry condoms with them.

The *Reality female condom* (Figure 4–3 ●) is a thin polyurethane sheath with a flexible ring at each end. The inner ring, at the closed end of the condom, serves as the means of insertion and fits over the cervix like a diaphragm. The second ring remains outside the vagina and covers a portion of the woman's perineum. It also covers the base of the man's penis during intercourse. Available over the counter and designed for onetime use, the condom may be inserted up to 8 hours before intercourse. The inner sheath is prelubricated but does not contain spermicide and is not designed to be used with a male condom. Data on its effectiveness against pregnancy are still limited, although the female condom is slightly less reliable than the diaphragm, male condom, vaginal sponge, and cervical cap (Sobrero, 2002). Because it also covers a portion of the vulva, it probably provides better protection than other methods against some pathogens. High cost, noisiness during intercourse, and the cumbersome feel of the device make acceptability a problem for some couples.

Diaphragm and Cervical Cap

The **diaphragm** (Figure 4–4 ●) is used with spermicidal cream or jelly and offers a good level of protection from conception. The woman must be fitted with a diaphragm and instructed in its use by trained personnel. The diaphragm should be rechecked for correct size after each childbirth and whenever a woman has gained or lost 15 lb or more.

The diaphragm must be inserted before intercourse, with approximately 1 teaspoon (or 1.5 inches from the tube) of spermicidal jelly placed around its rim and in the cup. This chemical barrier supplements the mechanical barrier of the diaphragm. The diaphragm is inserted through the vagina and covers the cervix. The last step in insertion is to push the edge of the diaphragm under the symphysis pubis, which may result in a "popping" sensation. When fitted properly and correctly in place, the diaphragm should not cause discomfort to the woman or her partner. Correct placement of the diaphragm can be checked by touching the cervix with a fingertip through the cup. The cervix feels like a small, firm, rounded structure and has a consistency similar to that of the tip of the nose. The center of the diaphragm should be over the cervix. If more than 4 hours elapse between insertion of the diaphragm and intercourse, additional spermicidal cream or jelly should be used. It is necessary to leave the diaphragm in place for at least 6 hours after coitus. The diaphragm should then be removed, cleaned with mild soap and water, and allowed to air dry before it is stored in its case. If intercourse is desired again within the 6 hours, another type of contraception must be used or additional spermicidal jelly placed in the vagina with an applicator, taking care not to disturb the placement of the diaphragm. Periodically the diaphragm should be held up to the light and inspected for tears or holes.

Some couples feel that the use of a diaphragm interferes with the spontaneity of intercourse. The nurse can suggest that the partner insert the diaphragm as part of foreplay. The woman can then easily verify the placement herself.

Diaphragms are an excellent contraceptive method for women who are lactating, who cannot or do not wish to use the pill (oral contraceptives), who are smokers over age 35, or who wish to avoid the increased risk of PID associated with intrauterine devices.

Women who object to manipulating their genitals to insert the diaphragm, check its placement, and remove it may find this method unsatisfactory. It is not recommended for women with a history of urinary tract infection, because pressure from the diaphragm on the urethra may interfere with complete bladder emptying and lead to recurrent urinary tract infections. Women with a history of toxic shock syndrome should not use diaphragms or any of

FIGURE 4–3

A, The female condom. To insert the condom: **B,** Remove condom and applicator from wrapper by pulling up on the ring. **C,** Insert condom slowly by gently pushing the applicator toward the small of the back. **D,** When properly inserted, the outer ring should rest on the folds of skin around the vaginal opening, and the inner ring (closed end) should fit loosely against the cervix.

the barrier methods because they are left in place for prolonged periods. For the same reason, the diaphragm should not be used during a menstrual period or if a woman has abnormal vaginal discharge.

The **cervical cap** (Figure 4–5 ●) is a cup-shaped device, used with spermicidal cream or jelly, that fits snugly over the cervix and is held in place by suction. Effectiveness rates and method of insertion are similar to those for the diaphragm. Although the cap may be left in place for up to 48 hours, most caregivers recommend that it not be left in

place for more than 24 hours. Advantages, disadvantages, and contraindications are similar to those associated with the diaphragm. The cervical cap may be more difficult to fit because of limited size options. It also tends to be more difficult for women to insert and remove.

Lea's shield is a reusable, silicone rubber device shaped like an elliptic bowl. It is similar to the cervical cap but contains a centrally located valve that permits the passage of cervical secretions and air. It can be used for up to 24 hours with a single application of spermicide. The device has

Inserting the diaphragm. **A,** Apply jelly to the rim and center of the diaphragm. **B,** Insert the diaphragm. **C,** Push the rim of the diaphragm under the symphysis pubis. **D,** Check placement of the diaphragm. Cervix should be felt through the diaphragm.

⊙ **FIGURE 4–5**

A cervical cap.

been available over the counter in Germany, Austria, and Switzerland for over a decade because one size fits virtually all women. In the United States, when the manufacturer elects to market it, the device will be available by prescription only (Nelson, Linn, Derman, & Strickland, 2003).

Vaginal Sponge

The *vaginal sponge* is again available in the United States. It is a pillow-shaped, soft, absorbent synthetic sponge containing spermicide that is available over the counter. It is made with a concave or cupped area on one side that fits over the cervix. It has a loop for easy removal. The sponge is moistened thoroughly with water before insertion to activate the spermicide and then inserted into the vagina with the cupped side against the cervix (Figure 4–6 ⊙). It should be left in place for 6 hours following intercourse and may be worn for up to 24 hours, then removed and discarded.

Advantages include the following: professional fitting is not required, it may be used for multiple acts of coitus for up

FIGURE 4–6

The contraceptive sponge is moistened well with water and inserted into the vagina with the concave portion positioned over the cervix.

FIGURE 4–7

The Mirena Intrauterine System, which releases levonorgestrel gradually, may be left in place for up to 5 years.

Used with permission from Berlex Laboratories, Inc.

to 24 hours, one size fits all, and it acts as both a barrier and a spermicide. Disadvantages include cost (about $30 for a 12-pack), problems associated with removing it, and irritation or allergic reactions. Research indicates that the sponge is less effective than the diaphragm at preventing pregnancy, and women using the sponge are more likely than diaphragm users to stop using their method of contraception (Kuyoh, Toroitich-Ruto, Grimes, Schulz et al., 2003).

Intrauterine Devices

The **intrauterine device (IUD)** is designed to be inserted into the uterus by a qualified healthcare provider and left in place for an extended period, providing continuous contraceptive protection. Traditionally the IUD was believed to act by preventing the implantation of a fertilized ovum. Thus, the IUD was considered an abortifacient (abortion-causing) method. This belief is not accurate. IUDs truly are contraceptives; they trigger a spermicidal type reaction in the body, thereby preventing fertilization. The IUD is also known to have local inflammatory effects on the endometrium.

Advantages of the IUD include high rate of effectiveness, continuous contraceptive protection, no coitus-related activity, and relative inexpensiveness over time. Possible adverse reactions to the IUD include discomfort to the wearer, increased bleeding during menses, PID, perforation of the uterus, intermenstrual bleeding, dysmenorrhea, and expulsion of the device.

Two IUDs are currently available in the United States. The copper T380A (ParaGard) is highly effective and can be left in place for up to 10 years. The levonorgestrel-releasing intrauterine system (LNG-IUS) (Mirena), which releases levonorgestrel gradually, is comparable in effectiveness to the copper T and may be left in place for up to 5 years

(Figure 4–7). The primary advantage of the LNG-IUS is that it produces diminished periods or even amenorrhea, which women welcome once they are advised that the absence of menses is safe and not an indication of pregnancy.

IUDs are recommended only for women who have at least one child and are in a monogamous relationship, because these women have the lowest risk of developing a pelvic infection. It is not recommended for women with multiple sexual contacts, because they are at higher risk for sexually transmitted infections.

The IUD is inserted into the uterus with its string or tail protruding through the cervix into the vagina. It may be inserted during a menstrual period or during the 4- to 6-week postpartum check. After insertion the clinician instructs the woman to check for the presence of the string once a week for the first month and then after each menses. She is told that she may have some cramping or bleeding intermittently for 2 to 6 weeks and that her first few menses may be irregular. Follow-up examination is suggested 4 to 8 weeks after insertion.

Women with IUDs should contact their healthcare providers if they are exposed to an STI or if they develop the following warning signs: late period, abnormal spotting or bleeding, pain with intercourse, abdominal pain, abnormal discharge, signs of infection (fever, chills, and malaise), or missing string. If the woman becomes pregnant with an IUD in place, the device is generally removed if the string is visible.

HORMONAL CONTRACEPTION

Hormonal contraceptives are available in a variety of forms. They may be progestin-only hormones, most often using a synthetic form of progesterone called progestin, or a combination of estrogen and a progestin.

Combined Estrogen-Progestin Approaches

Combined hormonal approaches work by inhibiting the release of an ovum, by creating an atrophic endometrium, and by maintaining thick cervical mucus that slows sperm transport and inhibits the process that allows sperm to penetrate the ovum.

Combined Oral Contraceptives. Combined oral contraceptives **(COCs)**, also called *birth control pills*, are typically a combination of the hormones estrogen and progesterone. COCs are safe, highly effective, and rapidly reversible. Many COCs are available. The pill is taken daily for 21 days, typically beginning on the Sunday after the first day of the menstrual cycle. In most cases menses occurs 1 to 4 days after the last pill is taken. Seven days after taking her last pill, the woman restarts the pill. Thus the woman always begins the pill on the same day. Some companies offer a 28-day pack with seven "blank" pills so that the woman never stops taking a pill. The pill should be taken at approximately the same time each day—usually upon arising or before retiring in the evening.

Recently discussion has focused on "extended" or continuous use of COCs (without the 7 contraception-free days). When COCs are taken all the time, women have far fewer bleeding days and often cease having periods. The continuous approach also makes it easier for some women to use COCs correctly because they do not have to think about whether to take a pill. Research indicates that there is no increase in pathologic changes or adverse side effects with continuous use (Zite, Gilliam, & Darney, 2004). Seasonale, the first extended-cycle COC approved by the U.S. Food and Drug Administration (FDA), is now available by prescription. Seasonale is a 91-day regimen in which a woman takes an active tablet daily for 84 consecutive days followed by 7 days of inactive tablets during which the woman has a period. Using Seasonale a woman has only 4 periods a year. Pregnancy prevention rates and risks are comparable to those of other COCs (Reuters Health Information, 2003).

Although they are highly effective when taken correctly, COCs may produce a variety of side effects, which may be either progesterone or estrogen related (Table 4–1). The use of low-dose (35 mcg or less estrogen) preparations has reduced many of the side effects. The newer 20-mcg pills have even fewer side effects, but they may result in less contraceptive effectiveness.

Contraindications to the use of COCs include pregnancy, previous history of thrombophlebitis or thromboembolic disease, acute or chronic liver disease of cholestatic type with abnormal function, presence of estrogen-dependent carcinomas, undiagnosed uterine

TABLE 4–1 ✤ Side Effects Associated with Oral Contraceptives

Estrogen Effects	Progestin Effects
Alterations in lipid metabolism	Acne, oily skin
Breast tenderness, engorgement; increased breast size	Breast tenderness; increased breast size
Cerebrovascular accident	Decreased libido
Changes in carbohydrate metabolism	Decreased high-density lipoprotein (HDL) cholesterol levels
Chloasma (Melasma)	
Fluid retention; cyclic weight gain	Depression
Headache	Fatigue
Hepatic adenomas	Hirsutism
Hypertension	Increased appetite; weight gain
Leukorrhea, cervical erosion, ectopia	Increased low-density lipoprotein (LDL) cholesterol levels
Nausea	Oligomenorrhea, amenorrhea
Nervousness, irritability	Pruritus
Telangiectasia	Sebaceous cysts
Thromboembolic complications—thrombophlebitis, pulmonary embolism	

bleeding, heavy smoking, gallbladder disease, hypertension, diabetes, and hyperlipidemia. In addition, women with the following relative contraindications who use COCs need to be monitored frequently: migraine headaches, epilepsy, depression, oligomenorrhea, and amenorrhea. Women who choose this method of contraception should be fully advised of its potential side effects.

COCs also have some important noncontraceptive benefits. Many women experience relief of uncomfortable menstrual symptoms. Cramps are lessened, flow is decreased, and cycle regularity is increased. Mittelschmerz is eliminated, and the incidence of functional ovarian cysts is decreased. More important, there is a substantial reduction in the incidence of ectopic pregnancy, ovarian cancer, endometrial cancer, iron deficiency anemia, and benign breast disease. In addition, COCs are considered a good solution to the physiologic problems some women experience during the perimenopause. Because of the increased risk of myocardial infarction (heart attack), women over age 35 who smoke should not take COCs.

The woman using COCs should contact her healthcare provider if she becomes depressed, becomes jaundiced, develops a breast lump, or experiences any of the following warning signs: severe abdominal pain, severe chest pain or shortness of breath, severe headaches, dizziness, changes in vision (vision loss or blurring), speech problems, or severe leg pain.

Another oral contraceptive is the progesterone-only pill, also called the *minipill*. It is used primarily by women who have a contraindication to the estrogen component of the combination pills, such as history of thrombophlebitis, but are strongly motivated to use this form of contraception. The major problems with this preparation are amenorrhea or irregular spotting and bleeding patterns.

Other Combined Hormonal Methods. Hormones can now be administered transdermally using a *contraceptive skin patch* called Ortho Evra, which releases a combination of norelgestromin and ethinyl estradiol. The patch is roughly the size of a silver dollar, but square. The woman applies the patch to the abdomen, buttocks, trunk, or upper outer arm and wears it continuously for 1 week. This routine is followed for 3 weeks; no patch is applied for the fourth week. During the treatment free week, the woman menstruates. The patch is highly effective in women who weigh less than 198 lb. The patch is as safe and reliable as COCs and has a better rate of compliance.

NuvaRing vaginal contraceptive ring (manufactured by Organon), another form of low-dose, sustained-release hormonal contraceptive, is a flexible soft ring that the woman inserts into her vagina (Figure 4–8). The ring is

FIGURE 4–8

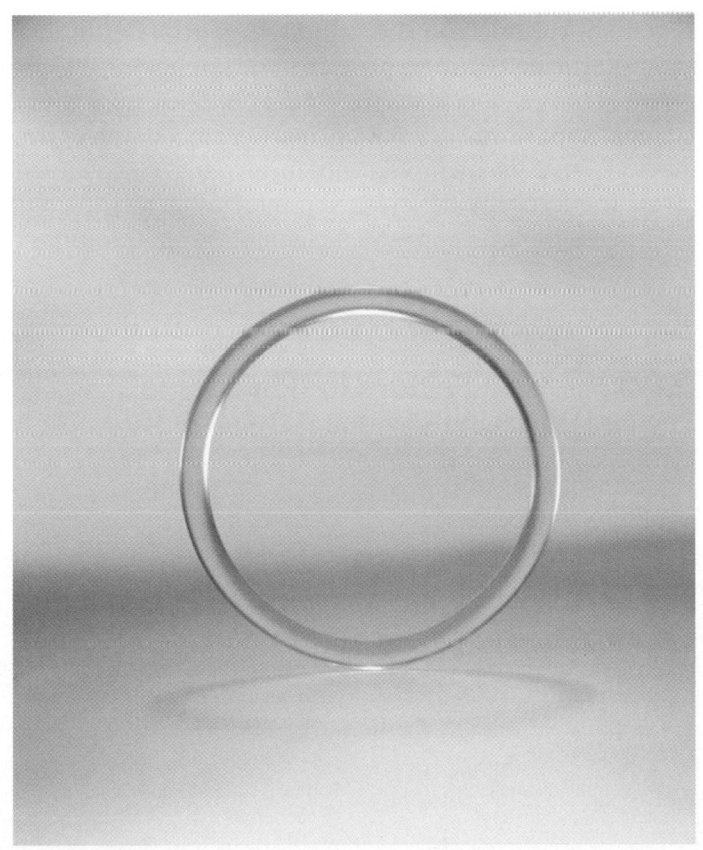

The NuvaRing vaginal contraceptive ring.
Courtesy of Organon, Inc.

left in place for 3 weeks and then removed for 1 week to allow for withdrawal bleeding. One size fits virtually all women. The ring is highly effective and has minimal side effects. The ring can be worn during intercourse and is comfortable for both the woman and her partner. However, the woman should be advised to use a backup form of contraceptive for one week if she removes the ring from her vagina for more than 3 hours (Zite et al., 2004).

Lunelle, an injectable combination of medroxyprogesterone acetate (MPA) and estradiol cypionate (E_2C), is administered every 28 to 30 days (not to exceed 33 days) intramuscularly. Lunelle is a highly effective contraceptive that has a side-effect pattern similar to that of COCs. Lunelle was withdrawn from the U.S. market in 2002.

Long-Acting Hormonal Contraceptives

Subdermal implants are not currently available in the United States. Norplant is a system consisting of six Silastic capsules containing levonorgestrel, a progestin, which are implanted in the woman's arm. It is available in over 50 countries worldwide. Norplant prevents ovulation in most women. It also stimulates the production of thick cervical mucus, which inhibits sperm penetration. Norplant provides effective, continuous contraception separate from the act of coitus. In other words, the woman does not have to insert a device or barrier for each act of intercourse. Possible side effects include spotting, irregular bleeding or amenorrhea, an increased incidence of ovarian cysts, weight gain, headaches, fluid retention, acne, mood changes, and depression.

U.S. distribution of Norplant was voluntarily suspended by its manufacturer, Wyatt Pharmaceuticals. Wyatt has received FDA approval for a two-rod version of Norplant called Jadelle, which is used in many countries, but the company has no plans to market Jadelle in the United States. A single-rod, highly effective system called Implanon, manufactured by Organon, is used by 1 million European women. It may become available in the United States in the near future (Zite et al., 2004).

Depot-medroxyprogesterone acetate (DMPA) (**Depo-Provera**), another long-acting progestin, suppresses ovulation for 3 months when given as a single injection of 150 mg. DMPA provides levels of progesterone high enough to block the luteinizing hormone (LH) surge, thereby suppressing ovulation. It also thickens the cervical mucus to block sperm penetration. Side effects include menstrual irregularities, headache, weight gain, breast tenderness, and depression. Prolonged use has been associated with significant, long-term loss of bone density, and many physicians have stopped prescribing it because of this. It should not be used for long-term birth control (longer than 2 years) unless other methods of birth control are not adequate. Return of fertility may be delayed for an average of 9 months.

EMERGENCY POSTCOITAL CONTRACEPTION

Emergency contraception is indicated when a woman is worried about pregnancy because of unprotected intercourse or possible contraceptive failure (e.g., broken condom, slipped diaphragm, or too long a time between DMPA injections). Two product kits, Preven, a combined hormonal approach (levonorgestrel/ethinyl estradiol), and Plan B, a progestin-only approach (levonorgestrel), are now FDA approved for emergency contraception.

Though sometimes called the "morning-after pill," the phrase is misleading because the woman actually takes a dose as soon after intercourse as possible and a second dose 12 hours later. This regimen must be started within 72 hours after unprotected intercourse; the earlier the treatment is started, the greater the effectiveness.

OPERATIVE STERILIZATION

Operative **sterilization** refers to surgical procedures that permanently prevent pregnancy. Before sterilization is performed on either partner, the physician provides a thorough explanation of the procedure to both. Each needs to understand that sterilization is not a decision to be taken lightly or entered into when psychologic stresses, such as separation or divorce, exist. Even though both male and female procedures are theoretically reversible, the permanency of the procedure should be stressed and understood.

Male sterilization is achieved through a relatively minor procedure called a **vasectomy**. This procedure involves surgically severing the vas deferens in both sides of the scrotum. Following vasectomy it takes about 4 to 6 weeks and 6 to 36 ejaculations to clear the remaining sperm from the vas deferens. During that period the couple is advised to use another method of birth control and to bring in two or three semen samples for a sperm count. The man is rechecked at 6 and 12 months to ensure that fertility has not been restored by recanalization. Side effects of a vasectomy include pain, infection, hematoma, sperm granulomas, and spontaneous reanastomosis (reconnecting).

Vasectomies can sometimes be reversed by using microsurgery techniques. Restored fertility, as measured by subsequent pregnancy, ranges from 30% to 76%, depending primarily on the length of time between vasectomy and reversal (Pollack & Barone, 2000).

Female sterilization is most frequently accomplished by **tubal ligation**. The tubes are located through a small subumbilical incision or by minilaparotomy techniques and are crushed, ligated, electrocoagulated, banded, or plugged (in the newer, reversible procedures). Tubal ligation may be done at any time. However, the postpartum period is an ideal time to perform a tubal ligation because the tubes are somewhat enlarged and easily located.

Complications of female sterilization procedures include coagulation burns on the bowel, bowel perforation, pain, infection, hemorrhage, and adverse anesthesia effects. Reversal of a tubal ligation depends on the type of procedure performed. With microsurgical techniques a pregnancy rate of 44% to 81% is possible (DeLeon & Peters, 2000).

MALE CONTRACEPTION

The vasectomy and the condom, discussed previously, are currently the only forms of male contraception available in the United States. Hormonal contraception for men has yet to be developed, although studies are under way.

NURSING MANAGEMENT

In most cases the nurse who provides information and guidance about contraceptive methods works with the female partner, because most contraceptive methods are female oriented. Because men can purchase condoms without seeing a healthcare provider, counseling and interaction with a nurse are required only with vasectomy. As a nurse, you can play an important role in helping a woman choose a method of contraception acceptable to her and to her partner.

In addition to completing a history and assessing for any contraindications to specific methods, spend time with a woman learning about her lifestyle, personal attitudes about particular contraceptive methods, religious beliefs, personal biases, and plans for future childbearing, before helping the woman select a particular contraceptive method. Once the method is chosen, help the woman learn to use it effectively. Table 4–2 summarizes factors to consider in choosing an appropriate method of contraception.

TABLE 4–2 ✤ **Factors to Consider in Choosing a Method of Contraception**

Effectiveness of method in preventing pregnancy	Lifestyle: How frequently does client have intercourse?
Safety of the method: Are there inherent risks?	Does she have multiple partners?
Does it offer protection against STIs or other conditions?	Does she have ready access to medical care in the event of complications?
Client's age and future childbearing plans	Is cost a factor?
Any contraindications in client's health history	Partner's support and willingness to cooperate
Religious or moral factors influencing choice	Personal motivation to use method
Personal preferences, biases	

TEACHING HIGHLIGHTS

USING A METHOD OF CONTRACEPTION

- Discuss factors a woman should consider in choosing a method of contraception (see Table 4–2). Note that different methods may be appropriate at different times in a woman's life.
- Review the woman's reasons for choosing a particular method and confirm the absence of any contraindications to specific methods.
- Give a step-by-step description of the correct procedure for using the method chosen. Provide opportunities for questions.
- If a technique is to be learned, such as charting BBT or inserting a diaphragm, demonstrate and then have the woman do a return demonstration as appropriate.
(*Note:* If certain aspects are beyond your level of expertise, such as fitting a cervical cap, review the content about its use and confirm that the woman understands what she is to do.)
- Provide information on what the woman should do if unusual circumstances arise (for example, she misses a pill or forgets a morning temperature). These can be presented in a written handout as well.
- Stress warning signs that may require immediate action by the woman and explain why these signs indicate a risk. (These should also be covered in the handout.)
- Arrange to talk with the woman again soon, either by phone or at a return visit, to see if she has any questions or has encountered any problems.

Also review any possible side effects and warning signs related to the method chosen and counsel the woman about what action to take if she suspects she is pregnant. In many cases the nurse is involved in telephone counseling of women who call with questions and concerns about contraception. Thus, it is vital to be knowledgeable about this topic and have resources available to find answers to less common questions. "Teaching Highlights: Using a Method of Contraception" provides guidelines for helping women use a method of contraception effectively.

CLINICAL INTERRUPTION OF PREGNANCY

Although abortion was legalized in the United States in 1973, controversy over moral and legal issues continues. Many people are opposed to abortion for religious, ethical, or personal reasons. Others feel that access to a safe, legal abortion is every woman's right. A number of physical and psychosocial factors influence a woman's decision to seek an abortion. Some situations may involve lack of knowledge about contraceptive options, contraceptive failure, rape, or incest.

Mifepristone (Mifeprex), originally called RU-486, may be used to induce a medical abortion during the first

7 weeks of pregnancy (up to 49 days following conception). Mifepristone blocks the action of progesterone, thereby altering the endometrium. After the length of the woman's gestation is confirmed, she takes a dose of mifepristone. Two days later she returns to her caregiver and takes a dose of the prostaglandin misoprostol, which induces contractions that expel the embryo/fetus. About 12 days after taking the misoprostol, the woman is seen a third time to confirm that the abortion was successful.

Surgical abortion in the first trimester is technically easier and safer than abortion in the second trimester. It may be performed by dilation and curettage (D&C), minisuction, or vacuum curettage. Second-trimester abortion may be done using dilation and evacuation (D&E), hypertonic saline, systemic prostaglandins, and intrauterine prostaglandins.

Nursing Management

Important aspects of nursing care for a woman who decides to have an abortion include providing information about the methods of abortion and associated risks; counseling regarding available alternatives to abortion and their implications; encouraging verbalization by the woman; providing counseling and emotional support before, during, and after the procedure; monitoring vital signs, intake, and output; providing for physical comfort and privacy throughout the procedure; and health teaching about self-care, the importance of the postabortion checkup, and contraception review.

HEALTH PROMOTION FOR WOMEN

Health care providers and consumers alike are becoming increasingly aware of the importance of activities that promote health and prevent illness, including lifestyle choices. In addition, the value of regular screenings to detect any health problems early cannot be overemphasized. Health screening recommendations vary by age. General screening and immunization guidelines for women can be found on the Companion Website.

This section focuses on some of the most commonly used screening procedures: breast self-examination and breast examination by a trained healthcare provider, mammography, Pap smear, and pelvic examination.

BREAST EXAMINATION

Like the uterus, the breast undergoes regular cyclic changes in response to hormonal stimulation. Each month, in rhythm with the cycle of ovulation, the breasts become engorged with fluid in anticipation of pregnancy, and the woman may experience sensations of tenderness, lumpiness, or pain. If conception does not occur, the accumulated fluid drains away via the lymphatic network. *Mastodynia* (premenstrual swelling

THINKING CRITICALLY

Monique Hermann, age 37, was divorced 3 years ago. Her only son, now 19, is away at college. Recently, with some trepidation, Monique began dating, and she is now enjoying an active social life. She is being seen today for advice about contraception, which had not been an issue during her marriage because her husband had had a vasectomy. She reports that she is a little nervous about becoming sexually active because until this point her husband had been her only sexual partner. She is very attracted to two different men but does not prefer one over the other at this point. She states that she wants a reliable method that would permit her to have intercourse at any time without having to take action beforehand because she thinks that would be embarrassing for her. Similarly she is not interested in the patch, which is visible. She is not willing to consider a tubal ligation. She is a nonsmoker who drinks occasionally. She has no known contraindications to any available methods. Which methods of contraception might be appropriate for Monique?

and tenderness of the breasts) is common. It usually lasts for 3 to 4 days before the onset of menses, but the symptoms may persist throughout the month.

After menopause, adipose breast tissue atrophies and is replaced by connective tissue. Elasticity is lost, and the breasts may droop and become pendulous. The recurring breast engorgement associated with ovulation ceases. If estrogen replacement therapy is used to counteract other symptoms of menopause, breast engorgement may resume.

Monthly **breast self-examination (BSE)** is the best method for detecting breast masses early. A woman who knows the texture and feel of her own breasts is far more likely to detect changes that develop. Thus, it is important for a woman to develop the habit of doing routine BSE as early as possible, preferably as an adolescent. Women at high risk for breast cancer are especially encouraged to be attentive to the importance of early detection through routine BSE.

The effectiveness of BSE is determined by the woman's ability to perform the procedure correctly. She should do a BSE on a regular monthly basis about 1 week after each menstrual period, when the breasts are typically not tender or swollen. After menopause she should perform BSE on the same day each month (as chosen by the woman). See "Teaching Highlights: Breast Self-Examination."

Clinical breast examination by a trained healthcare provider, such as a physician, nurse practitioner, or nurse-midwife, is an essential element of a routine gynecologic examination. Experience in differentiating among benign, suspicious, and worrisome breast changes lets the caregiver reassure the woman if the findings are normal or move forward with additional diagnostic procedures or referral if the findings are suspicious or worrisome.

MAMMOGRAPHY

A **mammogram** is a soft-tissue x-ray of the breast without the injection of a contrast medium. It can detect lesions in the breast before they can be felt and has gained wide acceptance as an effective screening tool for breast cancer. Currently the American Cancer Society recommends that all women age 40 and over have an annual mammogram. The National Cancer Institute and the American College of Obstetricians and Gynecologists (ACOG) recommend mammograms every 1 to 2 years for women ages 40 to 49 and annually for all women age 50 and older.

PAP SMEAR AND PELVIC EXAMINATION

The Papanicolaou test (*Pap smear*), a form of cervical cytology testing, has helped dramatically decrease the incidence of death from cervical cancer. Its purpose is to detect cellular abnormalities by examining a smear containing cells from the cervix and the endocervical canal. A newer test, the *ThinPrep Pap smear,* is proving even more effective than the traditional Pap smear in detecting abnormalities. In this test, no slide is prepared. Instead the cervical cells, gathered in the same way as for the Pap smear, are transferred directly to a vial of preservative fluid, thereby preserving the entire specimen.

NURSING PRACTICE

Whenever you teach about pelvic examination and Pap smear, be sure the woman understands that she should not douche for at least 24 hours beforehand. Douching can interfere with the accuracy of the Pap smear. Occasionally a caregiver will specifically request that a woman use a douche before a Pap smear; douching should only be done in this circumstance.

For best test results, also advise women to avoid intercourse and the use of other female hygiene products and spermicidal agents immediately before a specimen is obtained. Specimens should not be obtained during menstruation or when visible cervicitis exists.

The pelvic examination lets the healthcare provider assess a woman's vagina, uterus, ovaries, and lower abdominal area. It is often performed after the Pap smear but may also be performed without a Pap for diagnostic purposes. Women sometimes perceive the pelvic examination as uncomfortable and embarrassing. The negative feelings may cause women to delay having yearly gynecologic examinations, and this avoidance may pose a threat to life and health.

To make the pelvic examination less threatening and thus improve health-seeking behavior, caregivers can offer the woman a mirror to watch the procedure, point out anatomic parts to her, and position and drape her to allow eye-to-eye contact with the practitioner.

TEACHING HIGHLIGHTS

BREAST SELF-EXAMINATION

Begin by discussing the risk factors associated with breast cancer and the use of BSE in breast cancer detection. Then describe and demonstrate the correct procedure for BSE.

1. Timing—Instruct the woman to perform BSE on a monthly basis. Be specific based on whether she is premenopausal, pregnant, postmenopausal, or postmenopausal receiving hormone therapy.
2. Inspection—Instruct the woman to inspect her breasts by standing or sitting in front of a mirror. She should inspect them in three positions: both arms relaxed at her sides, both arms raised straight over her head, and both hands placed on her hips while she leans forward (Figure 4–9). In these positions she should do the following:

   ■ Note size and symmetry of the breasts. Some size difference between breasts is normal. Breasts may vary but the variations should remain constant during rest or movement—note abnormal contours.

■ Note shape and direction of breasts. Breasts can be rounded or pendulous with some variation between breasts. Breasts should point slightly laterally.

■ Observe for color and venous patterns. Check for redness or inflammation. A blue hue with a marked venous pattern that is focal or unilateral may indicate an area of increased blood supply due to tumor. Symmetric venous patterns are normal.

■ Observe for thickening or edema. Skin edema is seen as thickened skin with enlarged pores ("orange peel"). It may indicate blocked lymph drainage due to tumor.

■ Note the surface of the skin. Skin dimpling, puckering, or retraction when the hands are pressed together or against the hips suggests malignancy. Striae (stretch marks) are normal.

■ Note nipple size, shape, and direction. Long-standing nipple inversion is normal, but an inverted nipple previously capable of erection is suspicious. Note any deviation, flattening, or broadening of the nipples.

■ Check for rashes, ulcerations, or discharge.

● **FIGURE 4–9**

Both arms relaxed at sides

Both hands on hips while leaning forward

C

Both arms stretched above the head

A

B

Positions for inspection of the breasts.

(continued)

TEACHING HIGHLIGHTS—continued

3. Palpation—Instruct the woman to palpate (feel) her breasts as follows:
   - Lie down. Put one hand behind your head. With the other hand, fingers flattened, gently feel your breast. Press lightly (Figure 4–10A).
   - Figure 4–10B shows you how to check each breast. Begin as you see in B and follow the arrows, feeling gently for a lump or thickening. Remember to feel all parts of each breast, including the "tail" of tissue near the armpit. Repeat the process on the second breast.
   - Now repeat the same process on each breast sitting up, with your hand still behind your head (Figure 4–10C).

   - Squeeze the nipple between your thumb and forefinger. Look for any discharge—clear, bloody, or milky (Figure 4–10D).
4. Take the woman's hand and help her identify her "normal bumps" (e.g., mammary ridge, ribs, nodularity in the upper, outer quadrants).
5. Determine whether she has any questions about her findings during this examination. If she has questions, palpate the area and attempt to identify whether it is normal.
6. If a breast model is available, give the woman the opportunity to palpate it and identify the lumps.
7. Provide her with a monthly reminder such as an American Cancer Society shower card.

● FIGURE 4–10

With one hand behind your head, flatten your fingers and press lightly on your breast, feeling gently for a lump or thickening.

A

Check each breast in a circular manner, feeling all parts of the breast.

B

Repeat the same procedure sitting up with your hand still behind your head.

C

Squeeze your nipple between your thumb and forefinger; look for any clear or bloody discharge.

D

Procedure for breast self-examination.

Caregivers can encourage the woman to participate by asking questions and giving feedback.

Nurse practitioners, certified nurse-midwives, and physicians all perform pelvic examinations. Nurses assist the practitioner and the woman during the examination. See "Skill 2–2: Assisting with a Pelvic Examination" in the Clinical Skills Manual, **SKILLS** as well as the accompanying CD-ROM.

MENOPAUSE

Menopause, the time when menses cease, is a time of transition for a woman, marking the end of her reproductive abilities. *Climacteric,* or *change of life* (often used synonymously with menopause), refers to the psychologic and physical alterations that occur around the time of menopause. Today the median age at menopause is 51.3 years, and the average life span of a woman in the United States is over 80 years. Thus the average woman will live one third of her life after menopause. A woman's psychologic adaptation to menopause and the climacteric is multifactorial. She is influenced by her own expectations and knowledge, physical well-being, family views, marital stability, and sociocultural expectations. As the number of women reaching menopause increases, the negative emotional connotations society once attached to menopause are diminishing, enabling menopausal women to cope more effectively and even encouraging them to view menopause as a time of personal growth.

Perimenopause is the term applied to the period preceding menopause, usually about 2 to 8 years, when ovarian function wanes and hormonal deficiencies begin to produce symptoms. Contraception remains a concern during perimenopause. Combined oral contraceptives are becoming increasingly popular among healthy nonsmokers because many women also benefit from the noncontraceptive effects, including regulation of menses, relief of symptoms of estrogen deficiency, and a decreased risk of endometrial and ovarian cancers. Other contraceptive options for perimenopausal women include the contraceptive patch, the vaginal ring, IUDs, progestin-only methods, and barrier methods such as condoms, diaphragm, cervical cap, and spermicides.

The physical characteristics of menopause are linked to the shift from a cyclic to a noncyclic hormonal pattern. The age at onset may be influenced by nutritional, cultural, or genetic factors. The onset of menopause occurs when estrogen levels become so low that menstruation stops.

Generally, ovulation ceases 1 to 2 years before menopause, but individual variations exist. Atrophy of the ovaries occurs gradually. Follicle-stimulating hormone levels rise, and less estrogen is produced. Menopausal symptoms include atrophic changes in the vagina, vulva, and urethra and in the trigonal area of the bladder.

Many menopausal women experience a vasomotor disturbance commonly known as *hot flashes,* a feeling of heat arising from the chest and spreading to the neck and face. The hot flashes are often accompanied by sweating and sleep disturbances. These episodes may occur as often as 20 to 30 times a day and generally last 3 to 5 minutes. Some women also experience dizzy spells, palpitations, and weakness. Many women find their own most effective ways to deal with the hot flashes. Some report that using a fan or drinking a cool liquid helps relieve distress; others seek relief through hormone replacement therapy. In addition, many women use complementary therapies (see later discussion).

The uterine endometrium and myometrium atrophy, as do the cervical glands. The uterine cavity constricts. The fallopian tubes and ovaries atrophy extensively. The vaginal mucosa becomes smooth and thin, and the rugae disappear, leading to loss of elasticity. As a result, intercourse can be painful, but this problem may be overcome by using lubricating gel. Dryness of the mucous membrane can lead to burning and itching. The vaginal pH level increases as the number of Döderlein's bacilli decreases.

Postmenopausal women can still be multiorgasmic. Some women find that their sexual interest and activity improve as the need for contraception disappears and personal growth and awareness increase. Other women experience a decrease in libido at this time. Vulvar atrophy occurs late, and the pubic hair thins, turns gray or white, and may ultimately disappear. The labia shrink and lose their heightened pigmentation. Pelvic fascia and muscles atrophy, resulting in decreased pelvic support. The breasts become pendulous and decrease in size and firmness.

Long-range physical changes may include **osteoporosis**, a decrease in the bony skeletal mass. This change is thought to be associated with lowered estrogen and androgen levels, lack of physical exercise, and a chronic low intake of calcium. Moreover, the estrogen deprivation that occurs in menopausal women may significantly increase their risk of coronary heart disease. Loss of protein from the skin and supportive tissues causes wrinkling. Postmenopausal women frequently gain weight, which may be due to excessive caloric intake or to lower caloric need with the same level of intake.

CLINICAL THERAPY

Hormone Replacement Therapy

Hormone replacement therapy (HRT), usually involving estrogen with or without a progestin, had for years been the treatment of choice for relieving menopausal symptoms, especially hot flashes, night sweats, and urogenital symptoms. HRT has also been recognized as very effective in preventing the development of osteoporosis. Nevertheless in 2002 the advisability of HRT was called into question because of the results of the Women's Health Initiative (WHI) study, which suggested that the risks of HRT outweigh the benefits, especially for long-term use, because of the slightly increased risk of breast cancer, thromboembolic disease, and stroke (Writing Group for the Women's Health Initiative Investigations, 2002).

Furthermore the beneficial effect of long-term estrogen use in reducing the incidence of Alzheimer disease (AD) was called into question by the Women's Health Initiative Memory Study (WHIMS), which found a 105% increase in AD with estrogen use (Shumaker, Legault, Rapp et al., 2003). However, the WHIMS study participants were all 65 years or older when they began therapy. Thus, it is likely that those women already had brain changes related to AD (Gambrell, 2004). Other research about AD risk indicates that the age when estrogen is initiated is crucial. When estrogen is begun at menopause and used for more than 10 years, there is a reduction of up to 83% in lifetime risk (Gambrell, 2004; Zandi, Carlson, Plassman et al., 2002).

Consequently the picture about HRT is somewhat clouded. Currently HRT is recognized as the most effective short-term (1 to 2 years) therapy for women who experience severe menopausal symptoms. However, women considering HRT should clearly understand the associated risks so that they can make an informed decision about using it. HRT is not indicated for the prevention of coronary heart disease, and women at risk of osteoporosis should explore alternative treatments (see later discussion).

When estrogen is given alone, it can produce endometrial hyperplasia and increase the risk of endometrial cancer. Thus, in women who still have a uterus, estrogen is opposed by giving a progestin, often Provera, continuously or sequentially. Current research focuses on using lower doses of estrogen (less than 0.625 mg/day); consideration has also been given to using lower doses or less frequent administration of progestins to minimize progestin exposure (Hackley & Rousseau, 2004). Although most women prefer to take estrogen orally, some choose the transdermal estrogen skin patch. Estrogen may also be given by injection. For women experiencing decreased libido, combination estrogen-testosterone preparations are available.

A thorough history, physical examination including Pap smear, and baseline mammogram are indicated before starting HRT. An initial endometrial biopsy is indicated for women with an increased risk of endometrial cancer; biopsy is also indicated if excessive, unexpected, or prolonged vaginal bleeding occurs. Women taking estrogen should be advised to stop immediately if they develop headaches, visual changes, signs of thrombophlebitis, or chest pain.

Complementary and Alternative Therapies

For women who do not wish to take HRT or who have medical contraindications to it, a variety of approaches have been proposed as alternative or complementary treatment or preventive measures for the discomforts of the perimenopausal and postmenopausal years. These include diet and nutrition, specifically a high-fiber, low-fat diet with supplements of vitamins D and E. *Phytoestrogens* (plant substances with estrogen properties) have been used by many women, but recent research has shown that they do not improve hot flashes or other menopausal symptoms (Krebs, Ensrud, MacDonald, & Wilt, 2004). Phytoestrogens are found in a number of foods, especially soy products (see "Complementary Care: Phytoestrogens"). Some women have tried herbal remedies such as dong quai and black cohosh, which have been used in traditional Chinese medicine for years but have not yet been well studied. Weight-bearing exercises such as walking, jogging, tennis, and low-impact aerobics help increase bone mass and

COMPLEMENTARY CARE

PHYTOESTROGENS

Phytoestrogens are naturally occurring plant sterols that have an estrogen-like effect. Herbs that contain phytoestrogen include ginseng, agnus castus, beth root, black cohosh, dong quai, fenugreek, licorice, red sage, sarsaparilla, and wild Mexican yam. Phytoestrogens are also found in soy products such as soy milk and tofu. Currently the effectiveness of the herbs and soy is receiving considerable study as more and more women elect to use alternative approaches to treat their menopausal symptoms. A recent study concluded that phytoestrogens in soy and red clover extracts do not improve hot flashes or other menopausal symptoms (Krebs, Ensrud, MacDonald, & Wilt, 2004).

decrease the risk of osteoporosis. Exercise also improves cholesterol profiles and contributes to overall health. Stress management and relaxation techniques such as biofeedback, meditation, yoga, visualization, and massage may provide a sense of well-being. Some women also use homeopathic remedies and herbal treatments for symptom relief.

Prevention and Treatment of Osteoporosis

Osteoporosis is more common in women who are middle-aged or older. In fact, in the United States, 13% to 18% of women age 50 and older have osteoporosis (ACOG, 2004). Risk factors associated with osteoporosis include European American or Asian heritage; small-boned, thin build; low body weight (less than 127 lb); family history of osteoporosis; lack of regular weight-bearing exercise; never pregnant; early onset of menopause; consistently low intake of calcium; cigarette smoking; moderate to heavy alcohol intake; and the use of certain medications such as anticonvulsants, corticosteroids, or lithium.

Bone mineral density (BMD) testing is useful in identifying individuals who are at risk for osteoporosis. ACOG (2004) recommends BMD testing for the following:

- All postmenopausal women age 65 or older
- Postmenopausal women with a fracture
- Postmenopausal women under age 65 with one or more risk factors

A variety of conditions, including malabsorption syndrome, cancer, cirrhosis of the liver, chronic use of cortisone, and rheumatoid arthritis, can cause secondary arthritis, which resembles osteoporosis. If these causes have been eliminated, treatment for osteoporosis is initiated.

Prevention of osteoporosis is a primary goal of care. Women are advised to maintain an adequate calcium intake. Women over age 50 should have a daily calcium intake of 1200 mg. Most women require supplements to achieve this level. They should also have a daily vitamin D intake of 400 to 800 IU. Women are also advised to participate regularly in exercise, to consume only modest quantities of alcohol and caffeine, and to stop smoking. Alcohol and smoking have a negative effect on the rate of bone resorption. Women's height should be measured at each visit, because a loss of height is often an early sign that vertebrae are being compressed because of reduced bone mass. See "Evidence-Based Nursing: Prevention of Osteoporosis."

The effectiveness of estrogen in preventing osteoporosis is well documented. However, because of the increased risks associated with long-term use of hormone replacement therapy, other pharmacologic agents are being used more frequently to prevent and treat osteoporosis. These include the following (Davidson, 2003):

- *Bisphosphonates* are calcium regulators that act by inhibiting bone resorption and increasing bone mass. Alendronate (Fosamax) and risedronate (Actonel) are the two most commonly prescribed.

- *Selective estrogen receptor modulators (SERMs)* such as raloxifene (Evista) preserve the beneficial effects of estrogen, including its protection against osteoporosis, but do not stimulate uterine or breast tissue.

- *Calcitonin* is a calcium regulator that may inhibit bone loss. Generally administered as a nasal spray, although it is also available as an injection, its value is less clear than that of the other medications listed.

NURSING MANAGEMENT

Most menopausal women deal well with this developmental phase of life, although some women may need counseling to adjust successfully. Nurses and other health professionals can help menopausal women achieve high-level functioning at this time in life. Of major importance is the nurse's ability to understand and provide support for the woman's views and feelings. Use an empathetic approach in counseling, health teaching, and providing physical care.

Explore the question of the woman's comfort during sexual intercourse. In counseling, it may be appropriate to say, "After menopause many women notice that their vagina seems drier and intercourse can be uncomfortable. Have you noticed any changes?" This gives the woman information and may open discussion. Then go on to explain that dryness and shrinking of the vagina can be addressed by use of a water-soluble jelly. Use of estrogen, orally or in vaginal creams, may also be indicated. Increased frequency of intercourse will maintain some elasticity in the vagina. When assessing the menopausal woman, address the question of sexual activity openly but tactfully, because the woman may have been socialized to be reticent in discussing sex.

EVIDENCE-BASED NURSING

PREVENTION OF OSTEOPOROSIS

Clinical Question
What value does exercise have as an intervention to prevent osteoporosis in postmenopausal women?

Evidence
A team of nine medical experts examined 18 randomized controlled trials that met strict criteria for methodological soundness. Additional content experts were consulted in developing the final systematic review. The value of exercise as an intervention for the prevention of postmenopausal bone loss is a controversial subject, and this systematic review evaluated objective evidence about its efficacy. The reviewers concluded that exercise is effective in increasing bone mass density of the spine, hip, and wrist of postmenopausal women.

Implications
Aerobic exercises, weight-bearing activity (fast walking), and resistance exercises were all effective in increasing the bone mass density of the spine in postmenopausal women. Walking was effective in increasing bone mass density of the hip. As would be expected, walking had no effect on bone mass density of the wrist, but aerobic exercises had a positive effect. All of the exercise activities were equally effective, so the best advice may be to recommend an exercise regimen that is most similar

to normal activities of daily living, (i.e., a walking program). In these studies, exercise programs were not compared to "no exercise at all," but rather to normal activity, so exercise in addition to normal activities of daily living is required to have a beneficial effect. It is also necessary to stick to an exercise program for the long term, as the evidence demonstrated slowing of bone loss after one year or longer of an exercise program.

You should encourage postmenopausal women to use a variety of exercises to prevent the loss of bone mass density during menopause. Although any exercise—aerobic, resistance, or weight bearing—is effective, a walking program may be the most practical. Continue to encourage exercise as a long-term activity as menopause progresses.

Critical Thinking
For your clients who cannot bear weight, what exercise would you recommend to prevent the loss of bone mass density? How can you encourage postmenopausal women to stick with an exercise program?

Reference
Bonaiuti, D., Shea, B., Iovine, R., Negrini, S., Robinson, V., Kemper, H. S., et al. (2003). Exercise for preventing and treating osteoporosis in postmenopausal women (Cochrane Review). *The Cochrane Library, Issue 3.* Oxford: Update Software.

The crucial need of women in the perimenopausal period of life is for adequate information about the changes taking place in their bodies and their lives. Supplying that information provides both a challenge and an opportunity for nurses.

VIOLENCE AGAINST WOMEN

Violence against women is a major health concern, one that costs the healthcare system millions of dollars and thousands of lives. Violence affects women of all ages, races, ethnic backgrounds, socioeconomic levels, educational levels, and walks of life. Two of the most common forms of violence are domestic violence and rape. Often people not only accept these forms of violence but also shift the blame for the violence to the women themselves by asking questions such as, "How did she make him so mad?" "Why does she stay?" "What was she doing out so late?" and "Why did she dress that way?"

Violence against women is also a major health concern. In addition to causing injuries, associated physical and mental health outcomes, and fatalities, violence costs the healthcare system millions of dollars annually. In response to this epidemic, healthcare providers are becoming more knowledgeable about actions they should take to identify women at risk, implement preventive measures, and provide effective care.

DOMESTIC VIOLENCE

Domestic violence is defined as collective methods used to exert power and control by one individual over another in an adult domestic or intimate relationship. It is also termed **intimate partner violence**. This section focuses on domestic violence experienced by women in heterosexual relationships, although gay and lesbian individuals do experience domestic violence in their relationships as well.

Domestic violence is staggeringly common in the United States, although the incidence has decreased significantly in the last decade. Currently it accounts for 20% of violent crimes against women (Rennison, 2003). Worldwide as many as one in three women will be the victim of violence or sexual coercion at some point in her life (State of the World Population, 2000).

The woman may be married to her abuser, or she may be living with, dating, or divorced from him. Domestic violence takes many forms, including verbal attacks, insults, intimidation, threats, emotional abuse, social isolation, economic deprivation, intellectual derision, ridicule, stalking, and physical attacks and injury. Physical battering includes slapping, kicking, shoving, punching, forms of torture, attacks with objects or weapons, and sexual assault. Women who are physically abused can also suffer psychologic and emotional abuse.

Cycle of Violence

In an effort to explain the experience of battered women, Walker (1984) developed the theory of the *cycle of violence*. Battering takes place in a cyclic fashion through three phases:

1. In the *tension-building phase*, the batterer demonstrates power and control. This phase is characterized by anger, arguing, blaming the woman for external problems, and possibly minor battering incidents. The woman may blame herself and believe she can prevent the escalation of the batterer's anger by her own actions.

2. The *acute battering incident* is typically triggered by some external event or internal state of the batterer. It is an episode of acute violence distinguished by lack of control, lack of predictability, and major destructiveness. The cycle of violence can be interrupted before the acute battering incident if proper interventions take place.

3. The *tranquil, loving phase* is sometimes termed the honeymoon period. This phase may be characterized by extremely kind and loving behavior on the part of the batterer as he tries to make up with the woman, or it may simply be manifested as an absence of tension and violence. Without intervention this phase will end and the cycle of violence will continue. Over time the violence increases in severity and frequency.

Characteristics of Battered Women

Battered women often hold traditional views of sex roles. Many were raised to be submissive, passive, and dependent and to seek approval from male figures. Some battered women were exposed to violence between their parents, whereas others first experienced it from their partners. Many battered women do not work outside the home. As part of the manipulation of batterers, they are isolated from family and friends and totally dependent on their partners for their financial and emotional needs.

Women with physically abusive partners nearly always experience psychologic abuse as well and have been told repeatedly by their batterers that the family's problems are all their fault. Many believe their batterers' insults and accusations. As these women become more isolated, they find it harder to judge who is right. Eventually they fully believe in their inadequacy, and their low self-esteem reinforces their belief that they deserve to be beaten. Battered women often feel a pervasive sense of guilt, fear, and depression. Their sense of hopelessness and helplessness reduces their problem-solving ability. Battered women may also experience a lack of support from family, friends, and their religious community.

Characteristics of Batterers

Batterers come from all backgrounds. They often have feelings of insecurity, socioeconomic inferiority, powerlessness, and helplessness that conflict with their assumptions of male supremacy. Emotionally immature and aggressive men have a tendency to express these overwhelming feelings of inadequacy through violence. Many batterers feel undeserving of their partners, yet they blame and punish the very women they value.

Battered women often describe their husbands or partners as lacking respect toward women in general, having come from homes where they witnessed abuse of their mothers or were themselves abused as children, and having a hidden rage that erupts occasionally. Batterers accept traditional macho values, yet when they are not angry or aggressive, they appear childlike, dependent, seductive, manipulative, and in need of nurturing. They may be well respected in the community. This dual personality of batterers reflects the conflict between their belief that they must live up to their macho image and their feelings of inadequacy in the role of husband or provider. Combined with low frustration tolerance and poor impulse control, their pervasive sense of powerlessness leads them to strike out at life's inequities by abusing women.

DEVELOPING CULTURAL COMPETENCE

LATINA WOMEN WHO ARE VICTIMS OF ABUSE

To provide nursing care to Latina women who are victims of abuse, consider the following:

- Culturally it is often difficult for Latina women to seek help outside their families.
- Some Latina women who experience abuse may perceive it as their lot in life because of the concept of marianismo or the myth of martyrdom, which says that it is a woman's duty to sacrifice all for her family, even her own health and well-being (Mattson & Rodriguez, 1999).
- Language can be a powerful barrier to effective communication. Thus, it is important to have Spanish-speaking nurses and personnel available.
- Similarly, assessment tools should be translated into Spanish.
- Latina clients are often receptive to questions about how to screen other women for abuse. When asked, the woman's desire to help another may lead her to relate her own experiences of abuse (Barcelone de Mendoza, 2001).
- Have information available about appropriate community resources including individual and family counseling services in Spanish, shelters with bilingual staff, low-cost services, and the like.
- Community-run interventions designed to raise awareness and provide education can be especially effective if they are culturally sensitive and respectful of differences and individuality.

NURSING MANAGEMENT

Nurses often come in contact with abused women but fail to recognize them, especially if their bruises are not visible. Women at high risk for battering often have a history of alcohol or drug abuse, child abuse, or abuse in the previous or present relationship. Other possible signs of abuse include expressions of helplessness and powerlessness; low self-esteem revealed by the woman's dress, appearance, and the way she relates to healthcare providers; signs of depression evidenced by fatigue, hopelessness, and somatic problems such as headache, insomnia, chest pain, back pain, or pelvic pain; and possible suicide attempts. In addition, the abused woman may have a history of missed or frequently changed appointments, perhaps because she had signs of abuse that kept her from coming in or because her partner prevented it.

Because female partner abuse is so prevalent, many caregivers now advocate *universal screening of all female clients at every health encounter.* Screening should be done privately, with only the caregiver and client present, in a safe and quiet place. Specific language leads to higher disclosure rates. Possible screening questions include the following (ACOG, 1999):

1. Has your partner or anyone close to you ever threatened to hurt you?

2. During the past year, have you been kicked, hit, choked, or hurt physically?

3. Has your partner or anyone else ever forced you to have sex?

During the screening, assure the woman that her privacy will be respected (Figure 4–11 ●). It is essential to remain

● **FIGURE 4–11**

Screening for domestic violence should be done privately.

nonjudgmental. Create a warm, caring climate conducive to sharing, and demonstrate a willingness to talk about violence. A battered woman may interpret your willingness to discuss violence as permission for her to discuss it as well.

When a woman seeks care for an injury, be alert to the following cues of abuse:

- Hesitation in providing detailed information about the injury and how it occurred
- Inappropriate affect for the situation
- Delayed reporting of symptoms
- Pattern of injury consistent with abuse, including multiple injury sites involving bruises, abrasions, and contusions to the head (eyes and back of the neck), throat, chest, abdomen, or genitals
- Inappropriate explanation for the injuries
- Lack of eye contact
- Signs of increased anxiety in the presence of the possible batterer, who frequently does much of the talking

When a battered woman comes in for treatment, she needs to feel safe physically and secure in talking about her injuries and problems. If a man is with her, ask or tell him to remain in the waiting room while the woman is examined. A battered woman also needs to regain a sense of predictability by knowing what to expect and how she can interact. Provide sufficient information about what to expect in terms the woman can understand.

In providing care, let the woman work through her story, problems, and situation at her own pace. Reassure the woman that she is believed and that her feelings are reasonable and normal. Anticipate the woman's ambivalence (due to her fear and possible love-hate relationship with her batterer), but also respect the woman's capacity to change and grow when she is ready. The woman may need help identifying specific problems and developing realistic ideas for reducing or eliminating those problems. In all interactions, stress that no one should be abused and that the abuse is not the woman's fault.

Nursing Care in the Community

Inform any woman suspected of being in an abusive situation of the services available in the community. A battered woman may need the following:

- Medical treatment for injuries
- Temporary shelter to provide a safe environment for her and her children
- Counseling to raise her self-esteem and help her understand the dynamics of violence
- Legal assistance for a restraining order, protection, or prosecution

- Financial assistance to obtain shelter, food, and clothing
- Job training or employment counseling
- An ongoing support group with counseling

If the woman returns to an abusive situation, encourage her to develop an exit plan for herself and her children, if any. As part of the plan, she should pack a change of clothing for herself and her children, including toiletries and an extra set of car and house keys. She should store these items away from the house with a friend or relative. If possible she should have money, identification papers (driver's license, social security card, and birth certificates for herself and her children), checkbook, savings account information, other financial information (such as mortgage papers, automobile papers, and pay stubs), court papers or orders, and information about the children to help her enroll them in school. She should also plan where she will go, regardless of the time of day. Ensure that the woman has a planned escape route and emergency telephone numbers she can call, including local police, a phone hotline, and a women's shelter if one is available in the community.

Working with battered women is challenging, and many healthcare providers feel frustrated and impotent when the women repeatedly return to their abusive situations. Nurses must realize that they cannot rescue battered women; battered women must decide on their own how to handle their situations. Effective nurses provide battered women with information that empowers them in decision making and supports their decisions, knowing that incremental assistance over the years may be the only alternative until the battered women are ready to explore other options.

SEXUAL ASSAULT AND RAPE

Broadly, **sexual assault** is involuntary sexual contact with another person. The National Crime Victimization Survey defines **rape** as forced sexual intercourse, including both physical force as well as psychologic coercion. Forms of forced sexual intercourse include vaginal, anal, or oral penetration by the offender(s) (Rape, Abuse, and Incest National Network [RAINN], 2003a).

Research indicates that one in six American women over age 12 has been the victim of sexual assault or rape. However, the incidence of sexual assault is down by half since 1993. In 2002 there were 247,730 reported sexual assaults and rapes, compared to 485,000 in 1993. Experts attribute this dramatic decline to two trends (RAINN, 2003b):

1. *Tough-on-crime policies with longer sentences and three-strike laws.* All types of criminals commit rapes, and rapists often commit other forms of crime.
2. *Generational changes.* Over three fourths of rape survivors are under 30 years of age and have grown

up knowing that "no means no." These young women are more cautious about potentially risky situations and more willing to express their wishes forcefully.

Even more encouraging, in 2002 over half (53.7%) of sexual assaults and rapes were reported to the police (Rennison & Rand, 2003). This change is probably related to increased media attention and greater societal openness about the subject.

No woman of any age or ethnicity is immune. However, statistics indicate that young, unmarried women, women who are unemployed or have a low family income, and students have the highest incidence of sexual assault or attempted assault.

Why do men rape? Of the many theories put forth, none provides a completely satisfactory explanation. So few assailants are actually caught and convicted that a clear characteristic of the assailant has not been developed. However, rapists tend to be emotionally weak and insecure and may have difficulty maintaining interpersonal relationships. Many assailants also have trouble dealing with the stresses of daily life. Such men may become angry and overcome by feelings of powerlessness. They then commit a sexual assault as an expression of power or anger.

Acquaintance rape, which occurs when the assailant is someone with whom the victim has had previous nonviolent interaction, is the most common form of rape. In fact, in 69% of the cases of rape or sexual assault, the assailant is known (Rennison & Rand, 2003). One type of acquaintance rape, **date rape**, which occurs between a dating couple, is an increasing problem on high school and college campuses. In some cases an assailant uses alcohol or other drugs to sedate his intended victim. One drug, flunitrazepam (Rohypnol), has gained notoriety as a date rape drug because it frequently produces amnesia in its victims. In date rape situations, the male is usually determined to have sex and will do whatever he feels necessary if denied.

Responses to Sexual Assault

Sexual assault is a *situational crisis*. It is a traumatic event that the survivor cannot be prepared to handle because it is unforeseen. Following an assault the victim generally experiences a cluster of symptoms, described by Burgess and Holmstrom (1979) as the *rape trauma syndrome*, which last far beyond the rape itself. These phases are described in Table 4–3. Although the phases of response are listed individually, they often overlap, and individual responses and their duration may vary. A fourth phase—integration and recovery—has also been suggested (Holmes, 1998).

Research suggests that survivors of sexual assault may exhibit high levels of post-traumatic stress disorder, the same disorder that developed in many of the veterans of the Vietnam War. Post-traumatic stress disorder is marked by varying degrees of intensity. Assault victims with this disorder often require lengthy, intensive therapy to regain a sense of trust and feeling of personal control.

Care of the Sexual Assault Survivor

Survivors of sexual assault often enter the healthcare system by way of the emergency department. Thus, the emergency department nurse is often the first person to counsel them. Because the values, attitudes, and beliefs of the caregiver necessarily affect the competence and focus of the care, it is essential that nurses clearly understand their feelings about sexual assault and assault survivors and resolve any conflicts that may exist. In many communities a specially trained sexual assault nurse examiner (SANE) coordinates the care

TABLE 4–3 ✤ Phases of Recovery Following Sexual Assault

Phase	Response
Acute phase (disorganization)	Fear, shock, disbelief, desire for revenge, anger, anxiety, guilt, denial, embarrassment, humiliation, helplessness, dependence, self-blame, wide variety of physical reactions, lost or distorted coping mechanisms
Outward adjustment phase (denial)	Survivor appears outwardly composed, denying and repressing feelings (e.g., she returns to work, buys a weapon); refuses to discuss the assault; denies need for counseling
Reorganization	Survivor makes many life adjustments, such as moving to a new residence or changing her phone number; uses emotional distancing; may engage in risky sexual behaviors; may experience sexual dysfunction, phobias, flashbacks, sleep disorders, nightmares, anxiety; has a strong urge to talk about or resolve feelings; may seek counseling or remain silent
Integration and recovery	Time of resolution; survivor begins to feel safe and be comfortable trusting others; places blame on assailant; may become an advocate for others

of survivors of sexual assault, gathers necessary forensic evidence, and is then available as an expert witness when assailants are tried for the crime.

The first priority in caring for a survivor of a sexual assault is to create a safe, secure milieu. Admission information is gathered in a quiet, private room. The woman should be reassured that she is safe and not alone. The nurse assesses the survivor's appearance, demeanor, and ways of communicating for the purpose of planning care. Initially the woman is evaluated to determine the need for emergency care. Obtaining a careful, detailed history is essential. After the woman has received any necessary emergency care, a forensic chart and kit are completed.

NURSING PRACTICE

Strive to listen nonjudgmentally. Impartial listening can often make the difference in a victim's readiness to disclose the full details of the assault and can also assist her in the recovery process.

The woman is given a thorough explanation of the procedures to be carried out and signs a consent form for the forensic examination and collection of materials. Sexual assault kits contain all the necessary supplies for collecting and labeling evidence. The woman's clothing is collected and bagged, swabs of stains and secretions are taken, hair samples and any fingernail scrapings are collected, blood samples are drawn, tissue swabs are obtained, and photographs are taken. Vaginal and rectal examinations are performed, along with a complete physical examination for trauma. The woman is offered prophylactic treatment for sexually transmitted infections. If the assailant's HIV status is not known, the woman may be offered postexposure prophylaxis with HIV antiviral medications. In such cases, consultation with an HIV specialist is advised (CDC, 2002). The woman is also questioned about her menstrual cycle and contraceptive practices. If she could become pregnant as a result of the rape, she is offered postcoital contraceptive therapy.

Throughout the experience the nurse acts as the sexual assault survivor's advocate, providing support without usurping decision making. The nurse need not agree with all the survivor's decisions but should respect and defend her right to make them.

The family members and friends on whom the survivor calls also need nursing care. The reactions of the family will depend on the values to which they ascribe. Many families or mates blame the survivor for the assault and feel angry with her for not having been more careful. They may also incorrectly view the assault as a sexual act rather than an act of violence. They may feel personally wronged and see the survivor as devalued or unclean. Their reactions may compound the survivor's crisis. By spending some time with family members before their first interaction with the survivor, the nurse can perhaps reduce their anxiety and absorb some of their frustrations, sparing the woman further trauma.

Sexual assault counseling, provided by qualified nurses or other counselors, is a valuable tool in helping the survivor come to terms with her assault and its impact on her life. In counseling, the woman is encouraged to explore and identify her feelings and determine appropriate actions to resolve her problems and concerns. The counselor must avoid reinforcing the prevalent myth that the assault was somehow the woman's fault. The fault lies with the assailant. The counselor also plays an important role in emphasizing that the loss of control the woman experienced during the rape was temporary and that the woman can regain a feeling of control over life.

Prosecution of the Assailant

Legally, sexual assault is considered a crime against the state, and prosecution of the assailant is a community responsibility. The survivor, however, must begin the process by reporting the assault and pressing charges against her assailant. In the past, the police and the judicial system were notoriously insensitive in dealing with survivors. However, many communities now have classes designed to help officers work effectively with sexual assault survivors or have special teams to carry out this important task.

Many women who have sought to use the judicial process have had such a traumatic experience that they refer to it as a second assault. The woman may be asked repeatedly to describe the experience in intimate detail, and her reputation and testimony may be attacked by the defense attorney. In addition, publicity may intensify her feelings of humiliation, and, if her assailant is released on bail or found not guilty, she may fear retaliation.

The nurse acting as a counselor needs to be aware of the judicial sequence to anticipate rising tension and frustration in the survivor and her support system. The woman needs consistent, effective support at this crucial time.

Critical Concept Review

LEARNING OBJECTIVES

CONCEPTS

Summarize information that women may need to implement effective self-care measures for dealing with menstruation.

→

For effective self-care the woman may need information about:
1. Choice of sanitary protection:
   - Pads.
   - Tampons.
2. Use of vaginal sprays.
3. Douching practices.
4. Comfort measures:
   - Proper nutrition.
   - Exercise.
   - Use of heat and massage.

Contrast dysmenorrhea and premenstrual syndrome.

→

1. Dysmenorrhea:
   - Begins at onset of menstruation and disappears by the end of menstruation.
   - Treated with oral contraceptives, NSAIDs, or prostaglandin inhibitors.
   - Self-care measures include improved nutrition, exercise, heat application, and extra rest.
2. Premenstrual syndrome:
   - Symptoms are associated with the luteal phase (2 weeks prior to onset of menses).
   - Pronounced symptoms begin 2–3 days before onset of menstruation and subside as menstruation starts.
   - Symptoms disappear with or without treatment.
   - Treatment includes the use of progesterone agonists and prostaglandin inhibitors.
   - Self-care measures include use of vitamin B and E supplements, calcium, avoidance of sodium and caffeine, and increased aerobic exercise.

Compare the advantages, disadvantages, and effectiveness of the various methods of contraception available today.

→

1. Fertility awareness methods:
   - Advantages: Natural and noninvasive.
   - Disadvantages: Requires extensive initial counseling for effectiveness. Requires couple to practice abstinence during parts of each month.
   - Effectiveness: In practice, it may be less reliable than other methods.
2. Barrier contraceptives:
   - Advantages: Easy to use with no side effects. Condoms prevent spread of most venereal diseases.
   - Disadvantages: Some types must be fitted by a nurse practitioner or physician. Must be placed prior to intercourse. Must be used with spermicides.
   - Effectiveness: Excellent when used correctly.
3. Spermicides:
   - Advantages: Inexpensive and easy to obtain.
   - Disadvantages: Must be applied prior to intercourse. Considered "messy" by many people.
   - Effectiveness: Minimally effective when used alone.
4. Intrauterine devices:
   - Advantages: Effective for up to 5 years (Mirena) or 10 years (ParaGard) without removal.
   - Disadvantages: May cause cramping and bleeding for first 3–6 months. Woman must check for proper placement after each menses. Does not protect from STIs. May predispose woman to PID.
   - Effectiveness: Very effective while in place.
5. Hormonal contraceptives:
   - Advantages: Menstrual symptoms are lessened. Menstruation is very predictable.
   - Disadvantages: May increase chance of blood clots. Should not be used by anyone who smokes, has a heart condition, or has previous history of thromboembolic disease. Does not protect from STIs.
   - Effectiveness: Highly effective when used correctly.
6. Sterilization:
   - Advantages: Permanent form of birth control. No additional costs once procedure is completed.
   - Disadvantages: Considered nonreversible. Requires general anesthesia for the woman and local anesthesia for the man. Vasectomy does not produce immediate sterility; semen sample must be clear before other form of contraception is stopped. Does not protect against STIs.
   - Effectiveness: Considered completely effective.

(continued)

LEARNING OBJECTIVES	CONCEPTS
Delineate basic gynecologic screening procedures indicated for well women.	1. Breast examination (yearly). 2. Mammography: Recommended every 1–2 years after age 40 and annually for women age 50 or older. 3. Pap smear and pelvic examination (yearly).
Discuss the physical and psychologic aspects of menopause.	1. Physical aspects of menopause: ■ Ovulation ceases 1–2 years prior to menopause. ■ Gradual atrophy of ovaries. ■ FSH levels rise. ■ Less estrogen is produced. ■ Atrophic changes of vagina, vulva, urethra, and bladder. ■ Vasomotor disturbances such as "hot flashes." ■ Atrophy of uterine endometrium and myometrium, and fallopian tubes. ■ Constriction of uterine cavity. ■ Vaginal tissue becomes smooth, thins, and loses elasticity. ■ Thinning of pubic hair. ■ Decreased pelvic support. ■ Decrease in breast firmness. ■ Possible development of osteoporosis. ■ Increased risk of coronary heart disease. 2. Psychologic aspects of menopause: ■ Possible helpless feelings at physical changes. ■ Fatigue from lack of sleep due to hot flashes. ■ Decreased libido. ■ Possible increase in enjoyment of sexual intercourse due to lack of worry about pregnancy.
Explain the cycle of violence and its application to battered women, including pregnant women.	Cycle of violence: 1. Tension-building phase: ■ Batterer demonstrates power and control. 2. Acute battering incident: ■ Triggered by an external event or internal state of batterer. ■ Episode of acute violence. 3. Tranquil phase: ■ Kind and loving behavior on part of batterer as way to make up for violence. Application to battered women: 1. Woman may have been raised to be submissive, passive, and dependent. 2. Develop a sense of hopelessness. 3. Incidents may increase during pregnancy.
Delineate the nurse's role in working with women who have experienced intimate partner violence or rape.	The nurse's role includes the following: 1. Create a safe, secure milieu. 2. Obtain a careful, detailed history. 3. Complete a forensic chart and kit. 4. Explain all procedures. 5. Act as the survivor's advocate.

CRITICAL THINKING IN ACTION

View the **Critical Thinking in Action** video in Chapter 4 of the CD-ROM. Then, answer the questions that follow.

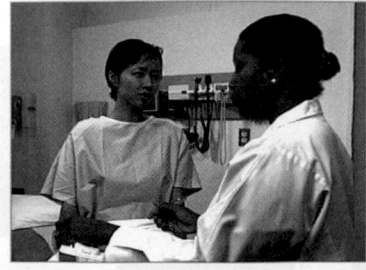

You are working at a local clinic when Joy Lang, age 20, presents for her first pelvic exam. You obtain the following GYN history: menarche age 12, menstrual cycle 28–30 days lasting 4–5 days, heavy one day, then lighter. She tells you that she needs to use superabsorbent tampons on the first day of her period and then she switches to a regular absorbency tampon for the remaining days. She confirms that she changes the tampon every 6 to 8 hours, never leaving it in overnight. She denies premenstrual syndrome, dysmenorrhea, or medical problems and says that she is not taking any medication on a regular schedule. She tells you that she recently got married, but would like to wait before getting pregnant. She'd like to discuss birth control methods. Joy tells you that doctors make her nervous and she admits to being anxious about her first pelvic exam.

1. What steps would you take to reduce Joy's anxiety relating to the pelvic exam?
2. What position is best to relax Joy's abdominal muscles for the pelvic exam?
3. What precaution should be taken when obtaining a Pap smear?
4. Explain the purpose of the Pap smear.
5. What factors do you include in a discussion of the type of birth control that Joy could practice?

MEDIALINK

www.prenhall.com/london

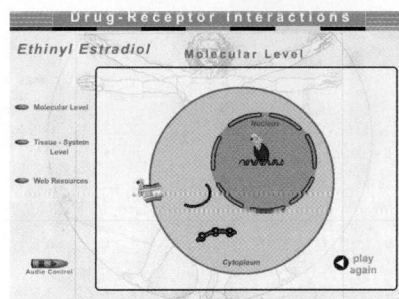

- NCLEX-RN® Review, case studies, and other interactive resources for this chapter can be found on the Companion Website at http://www.prenhall.com/london. Click on "Chapter 4" to select the activities for this chapter.

- For animations, more NCLEX-RN® Review questions, and an audio glossary, access the accompanying CD-ROM in this textbook.

REFERENCES

American Cancer Society. (2004). *Chronological history of ACS recommendations on early detection of cancer.* Retrieved April 4, 2004, from http://www.cancer.org

American College of Obstetricians and Gynecologists. (1999). *Domestic violence* (ACOG Educational Bulletin No. 257). Washington, DC: Author.

American College of Obstetricians and Gynecologists. (2003). *Benefits and risks of sterilization* (ACOG Practice Bulletin No. 46). Washington, DC: Author.

American College of Obstetricians and Gynecologists. (2004). *Osteoporosis* (ACOG Practice Bulletin No. 50). Washington, DC: Author.

Barcelone de Mendoza, V. (2001). Culturally appropriate care for pregnant Latina women who are victims of domestic violence. *Journal of Obstetric, Gynecologic, and Neonatal Nursing, 30*(6), 579–588.

Burgess, A. W., & Holmstrom, L. L. (1979). *Rape: Crisis and recovery.* Englewood Cliffs, NJ: Prentice-Hall.

Centers for Disease Control and Prevention (CDC). (2002, May 10). Sexually transmitted diseases guidelines 2002. *Morbidity and Mortality Weekly Report, 51* (RR-6).

Davidson, M. R. (2003). Contraceptive update. *Clinician Review, 13*(6), 52–59.

DeLeon, F. D., & Peters, A. J. (2000). Reversal of female sterilization. In J. J. Sciarra (Ed.), *Gynecology and obstetrics* (Vol. 6, chap. 46, pp. 1–6). Philadelphia: Lippincott Williams & Wilkins.

Endicott, J., Bardack, L., Grady-Weliky, T. A., Ling, F. W., & Schmidt, P. J. (2000). An update on premenstrual dysphoric disorder. *Female Patient, 25*(2), 45–56.

Gambrell, R. D. (2004). The Women's Health Initiative Reports: Critical review of the findings. *Female Patient, 29*(11), 23–29, 54.

Hackley, B., & Rousseau, M. E. (2004). Managing menopause symptoms after the Women's Health Initiative. *Journal of Midwifery and Women's Health, 49*(2), 87–95.

Holmes, M. M. (1998). The clinical management of rape in adolescents. *Contemporary OB/GYN, 43*(5), 62–78.

Hudson, T. (2002). Premenstrual syndrome, part 1. *Female Patient, 27*(5), 47–49.

Krebs, E. E., Ensrud, K. E., MacDonald, R., & Wilt, T. J. (2004). Phytoestrogens for treatment of menopausal symptoms: A systematic review. *Obstetrics and Gynecology, 104*(4), 824–836.

Kuyoh, M. A., Toroitich-Ruto, C., Grimes, D. A., Schulz, K. F., & Gallo, M. F. (2003). Sponge versus diaphragm for contraception: A Cochrane review. *Contraception, 67*, 15–18.

Mattson, S., & Rodriguez, E. (1999). Battering in pregnant Latinas. *Issues in Mental Health Nursing, 20*, 405–422.

Nelson, A. L., Linn, E., Derman, R. J., & Strickland, J. L. (2003). Contraception update, part 1. *Female Patient, 28*(11), 42–51.

Nelson, A. L., & Zieman, M. (2003). Emergency contraception: What's new. *Female Patient, 28*(12), 58–59.

Pollack, A. E., & Barone, M. A. (2000). Reversing vasectomy. In J. J. Sciarra (Ed.), *Gynecology and obstetrics* (Vol. 6, chap. 48, pp. 1–5). Philadelphia: Lippincott Williams & Wilkins.

Rape, Abuse, and Incest National Network. (2003a). *Facts about sexual assault.* Retrieved December 6, 2003, from http://www.rainn.org

Rape, Abuse, and Incest National Network. (2003b). *RAINN News: New report shows dramatic increase in willingness to report rape to the police.* Retrieved December 6, 2003, from http://www.rainn.org/news/ncvs2002.html

Rennison, C. M. (2003, February). *Intimate partner violence, 1993–2001.* Washington, DC: Bureau of Justice Statistics, U.S. Department of Justice.

Rennison, C. M., & Rand, M. R. (2003, August). *Crime victimization, 2002. Findings from the National Crime Victimization Survey.* Washington, DC: Bureau of Justice Statistics, U.S. Department of Justice.

Reuters Health Information. (2003). *Extended oral contraceptive formulation approved by FDA.* Retrieved September 18, 2003, from http://www.medscape.com/viewarticle/461076_print

Shumaker, S. A., Legault, C., Rapp, S. R., Thal, D., Wallace, R. B., Ockene, J. K., et al. (2003). Estrogen plus progestin and the incidence of dementia and mild cognitive impairment in postmenopausal women: The Women's Health Initiative Memory Study: A randomized controlled trial. *Journal of the American Medical Association, 289*(20), 2651–2662.

Sobrero, A. J. (2002). Use and effectiveness of barrier and spermicidal contraceptive methods. In J. J. Sciarra (Ed.), *Gynecology and Obstetrics 2002.* (Vol 6, chap. 17). Philadelphia: Lippincott Williams and Wilkins.

State of the world Population. (2000). *Ending violence against women and girls.* New York: United Nations Population Fund. http://www.unfpa.org/5wp 2000

Walker, L. (1984). *The battered woman syndrome.* New York: Springer.

Wallach, M., & Grimes, D. A. (2000). *Modern oral contraception: Update from the Contraception Report.* Totowa, NJ: Emron.

Writing Group for the Women's Health Initiative Investigations. (2002). Risks and benefits of estrogen plus progestin in healthy postmenopausal women: Principal results from the Women's Health Initiative randomized controlled trial. *Journal of the American Medical Association, 288*, 321–333.

Zandi, P. P., Carlson, M. C., Plassman, B. L., Welsh-Bohmer, K. A., Mayer, L. S., Steffens, D. C., et al. (2002). Hormone replacement therapy and incidence of Alzheimer's disease in older women: The Cache County Study. *Journal of the American Medical Association, 288*(17), 2123–2129.

Zite, N., Gilliam, M., & Darney, P. (2004). Contraception choices for 2004. *Contemporary OB/GYN, 49*(2), 30–44.

CHAPTER 5

Common Gynecologic Problems

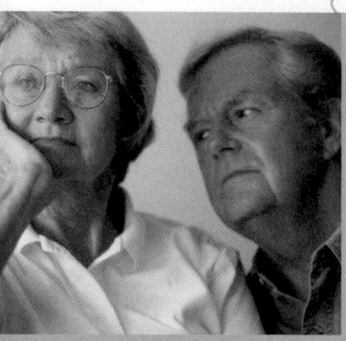

I was 53 when I learned that I had human papillomavirus infection. My first reaction was denial. I had been a virgin when I married and always thought I had the world's best marriage. When I confronted my husband of 30 years, I learned that he had been unfaithful to me with three different women over the course of our marriage. At first I was ready to walk away. But my husband begged for a second chance, we saw a counselor for almost 6 months, and eventually rebuilt our life together. Many women would call me a fool but I know that, for me, it was important to save something I had committed to—for better or for worse—and to practice the forgiveness so many preach but fail to follow.

—Leonora

LEARNING OBJECTIVES

- Contrast the common benign breast disorders.
- Discuss the signs and symptoms, medical therapy, and implications for fertility of endometriosis.
- Identify the risk factors, treatment options, and nursing interventions for a woman with toxic shock syndrome.
- Compare vulvovaginal candidiasis and bacterial vaginosis.
- Describe the common sexually transmitted infections.

- Summarize the health teaching a nurse needs to provide to a woman with a sexually transmitted infection.
- Relate the implications of pelvic inflammatory disease (PID) for future fertility to its pathology, signs and symptoms, and treatment.
- Identify the implications of an abnormal finding during a pelvic examination.
- Contrast cystitis and pyelonephritis.

The contemporary woman is likely to encounter various major or minor gynecologic or urinary problems during her lifetime. Some may be minor and easily treated; others may be more serious. This chapter provides information about a variety of gynecologic conditions, with an emphasis on problems commonly addressed in community-based settings.

CARE OF THE WOMAN WITH A BENIGN DISORDER OF THE BREAST

This section deals with the most common breast disorders women encounter. For information on breast cancer, consult a medical-surgical nursing textbook.

FIBROCYSTIC BREAST CHANGES

Fibrocystic breast changes, the most common of the benign breast disorders, are most prevalent in women 30 to 50 years of age. *Fibrosis* is a thickening of the normal breast tissue. Cyst formation that may accompany fibrosis is considered a later change in the condition. Fibrocystic breast changes are probably caused by an imbalance in estrogen and progesterone that distorts the normal changes of the menstrual cycle. The symptoms often increase as the woman approaches menopause and generally decrease after menopause. However, if a postmenopausal woman is treated with hormone replacement therapy (HRT), the cyclic breast changes may resume. Only women whose fibrocystic breast changes are accompanied by certain cellular changes (usually found incidentally when a biopsy is done) have an increased risk of developing cancer.

The woman often reports pain, tenderness, and swelling that occur cyclically and are most pronounced just before menses. Physical examination may reveal only mild signs of irregularity, or the breasts may feel dense, with areas of irregularity and nodularity. Women often refer to this irregularity as "lumpiness." Some women may also have expressible nipple discharge. Although unilateral discharge and serosanguineous discharge are the most worrisome findings, all breast discharge should be investigated further.

If the woman has a large, fluid-filled cyst, she may experience a localized painful area as the capsule containing the accumulated fluid distends coincident with her cycle. However, if small cysts form, the woman may experience not a solitary tender lump but a diffuse tenderness. A cyst may often be differentiated from a malignancy because a cyst is more mobile and tender and is not associated with skin retraction (pulling) in the surrounding tissue.

Mammography, sonography, palpation, and fine-needle aspiration are used to confirm fibrocystic breast changes. Often, fine-needle aspiration is the treatment as well, affording relief from the tenderness or pain. Treatment of palpable cysts is conservative; invasive procedures such as biopsy are used only if the diagnosis is questionable.

Women with mild symptoms may benefit from restricting sodium intake and taking a mild diuretic during the week before the onset of menses. This counteracts fluid retention, relieves pressure in the breast, and helps decrease the pain. In other cases a mild analgesic is necessary. In severe cases the hormone inhibitor danazol is often helpful, although it can cause undesirable side effects.

Some researchers suggest that methylxanthines (found in caffeine products, such as coffee, tea, colas, and chocolate, and in some medications) may contribute to the development of fibrocystic breast changes and that limiting

KEY TERMS

Colposcopy, 112

Dyspareunia, 103

Endometriosis, 103

Fibrocystic breast changes, 101

Hysterectomy, 117

Pelvic inflammatory disease (PID), 111

Sexually transmitted infection (STI), 107

Toxic shock syndrome (TSS), 104

Urinary tract infection (UTI), 114

intake of these substances will help decrease fibrocystic changes. Other research fails to demonstrate a clear association between methylxanthines and fibrocystic breast changes. Additional medical therapies that are helpful in varying degrees include combined oral contraceptives (COCs), progestins, bromocriptine, and the antiestrogen medication tamoxifen (although this is an "off-label" use for it). All of these therapies work on the principle of estrogen suppression and progesterone stimulation or augmentation. Oil of evening primrose may also be effective.

OTHER BENIGN BREAST DISORDERS

Fibroadenoma is a common benign tumor seen in women in their teens and early twenties. It has not been significantly associated with breast cancer. Fibroadenomas are freely movable, solid tumors that are well defined, sharply delineated, and rounded, with a rubbery texture. They are asymptomatic and nontender.

If there are any disquieting features to the appearance of a lump, fine-needle biopsy or excision of the mass may be indicated. Caution is exercised when deciding on biopsy because excision of the mass in a young girl may interfere with normal breast development. Watchful observation and possible surgical excision are the only treatments for fibroadenomas. Surgery is often deferred, but when advisable because of severe symptoms or concerns about malignancy, it ends the treatment.

Intraductal papillomas, most often occurring during the menopausal years, are tumors growing in the terminal portion of a duct or, sometimes, throughout the duct system within a section of the breast. They are typically benign but have the potential to become malignant. Although relatively uncommon, they are the most frequent cause of nipple discharge in women who are not pregnant or lactating.

The majority of papillomas present as solitary nodules. These small, ball-like lesions may be detected on mammography but often are nonpalpable. A papilloma is often frightening to the woman, because her primary symptom is a discharge from the nipple that may be serosanguineous or brownish green due to old blood. The location of the papilloma within the duct system and its pattern of growth determine whether nipple discharge will be present.

If the woman reports a nipple discharge, the breast should be milked to obtain fluid. The fluid obtained is sent for a Pap smear. The diagnosis is confirmed if papilloma cells are present. The lesion must be excised and histologically examined because of the difficulty in differentiating between a benign papilloma and a papillary carcinoma. Treatment for benign intraductal papilloma is excision with follow-up care.

Duct ectasis (comedomastitis), an inflammation of the ducts behind the nipple, commonly occurs during or near the onset of menopause and is not associated with malignancy. The condition typically occurs in women who have borne and breastfed children. It is characterized by a thick, sticky nipple discharge and by burning pain, pruritus, and inflammation. Nipple retraction may also be noted, especially in postmenopausal women. Treatment is conservative, with drug therapy aimed at symptomatic relief. The major central ducts of the breast occasionally have to be excised.

NURSING MANAGEMENT

NURSING ASSESSMENT AND DIAGNOSIS

During the period of diagnosis of any breast disorder, the woman may be anxious about a possible change in body image or a diagnosis of cancer. Use therapeutic communication to assess the significance the woman places on her breasts; her current emotional status, coping mechanisms used during periods of stress, knowledge and beliefs about cancer; and other variables that may influence her coping and adjustment.

Nursing diagnoses that may apply to a woman with a benign disorder of the breast include the following:

- *Health-Seeking Behaviors: Information about Diagnostic Procedures for Breast Disorders* related to an expressed desire to understand procedures
- *Anxiety* related to threat to body image

PLANNING AND IMPLEMENTATION

During the prediagnosis period, clarify misconceptions and encourage the woman to express her anxiety. Once a diagnosis is made, ensure that the woman understands her condition, its association to breast malignancy, and the treatment options. Also point out that frequent professional breast examinations and regular mammograms help detect any abnormalities and that the woman who practices monthly breast self-examination, follows her caregiver's advice, and is examined regularly has taken action to protect her health.

EVALUATION

Expected outcomes of nursing care include the following:

- The woman is able to discuss her fears, concerns, and questions during the period of diagnosis.
- The diagnosis is made quickly and accurately, and treatment is initiated if indicated.

CARE OF THE WOMAN WITH ENDOMETRIOSIS

Endometriosis, a condition characterized by the presence of endometrial tissue outside the endometrial cavity, occurs in about 8% to 10% of women of childbearing age (Conversations with Colleagues, 2002–2003). Endometriosis has been found almost everywhere in the body, including the vagina, lungs, cervix, central nervous system, and gastrointestinal tract. The most common location, however, is the pelvis. This tissue responds to the hormonal changes of the menstrual cycle and bleeds in a cyclic fashion. The bleeding results in inflammation, scarring of the peritoneum, and formation of adhesions.

Endometriosis may occur at any age after puberty, but it is most common in women between ages 20 and 45. The exact cause of endometriosis is unknown. Leading theories include retrograde menstrual flow and inflammation of the endometrium, hereditary tendency, and a possible immunologic defect.

The most common symptom of endometriosis is pelvic pain, which is often dull or cramping. Usually the pain is related to menstruation and is thought to be dysmenorrhea by the affected woman. **Dyspareunia** (painful intercourse) and abnormal uterine bleeding are other common signs. The condition is often diagnosed when the woman seeks evaluation for infertility. Bimanual examination may reveal a fixed, tender, retroverted uterus and palpable nodules in the cul-de-sac. Diagnosis is confirmed by laparoscopy.

Treatment may be medical, surgical, or a combination of the two. During the laparoscopic examination, any visible implants of endometrial tissue are removed using excision, endocoagulation, electrocautery, or laser vaporization. Surgery is effective in relieving pain symptoms, at least for a time. In women with minimal disease and symptoms, treatment includes observation, analgesics, and nonsteroidal anti-inflammatory drugs (NSAIDs). If the woman does not currently desire pregnancy, she may be started on a COC, often in combination with an NSAID. The COC creates a pseudopregnancy state with decreased menstrual bleeding. If the COC does not relieve symptoms, therapy with medroxyprogesterone acetate (MPA), danazol, or a gonadotropin-releasing hormone (GnRH) agonist may be indicated.

MPA causes endometrial tissue to atrophy, thereby decreasing symptoms. It is administered intramuscularly every 3 months, and the effectiveness of treatment is evaluated every 3 to 6 months. Side effects include weight gain, bloating, acne, headaches, emotional lability, and irregular bleeding.

Danazol is a testosterone derivative that suppresses GnRH and has high-androgen and low-estrogen effects that inhibit the growth of the endometrium. It suppresses ovulation and causes amenorrhea. However, Danazol has some significant side effects including hirsutism, vaginal bleeding, acne, oily skin, weight gain, reduced libido, voice changes and hoarseness, clitoral enlargement, and decreased breast size.

GnRH agonists such as nafarelin acetate (given as a metered nasal spray twice daily) and leuprolide acetate (Lupron) (given once a month as an intramuscular injection) are gaining popularity. Many women tolerate them better than danazol, and their results in treating endometriosis are comparable. GnRH agonists suppress the menstrual cycle through estrogen antagonism. This may result in the hypoestrogen side effects of hot flashes, vaginal dryness, decreased libido, pain in muscles and joints, and loss of bone density. These side effects can be reduced by adding an oral progestin or a combination of low-dose estrogen and progestin (Winkel, 2003). (*Note:* The estrogen dose should be comparable to that used for symptoms of menopause. COC estrogen levels are too high for add-back therapy.)

In more advanced cases, surgery may be done to remove endometrial implants and break up adhesions. If severe dyspareunia or dysmenorrhea are symptoms, the surgeon may perform a presacral neurectomy. In advanced cases in which childbearing is not an issue, treatment may be a hysterectomy (removal of the uterus) with bilateral salpingo-oophorectomy (removal of the fallopian tubes and ovaries).

NURSING MANAGEMENT

NURSING ASSESSMENT AND DIAGNOSIS

The nurse needs to know the symptoms of endometriosis and elicit an accurate history. If a woman is being treated for endometriosis, assess the woman's understanding of the condition, its implications, and the treatment alternatives.

Nursing diagnoses that may apply to a woman with endometriosis include the following:

- *Acute Pain* related to peritoneal irritation secondary to endometriosis
- *Ineffective Individual Coping* related to depression secondary to infertility

PLANNING AND IMPLEMENTATION

Be available to explain the condition, its symptoms, treatment alternatives, and prognosis. Help the woman evaluate treatment options and make appropriate choices. If the woman begins taking medication, review the dosage, schedule, possible side effects, and any warning signs. A woman with endometriosis is often advised to avoid delaying pregnancy because of the risk of infertility. The woman may wish to discuss the implications of this decision on her life choices, relationship with her partner, and personal preferences. Be a nonjudgmental listener and help the woman consider her options.

EVALUATION

Expected outcomes of nursing care include the following:

- The woman is able to discuss her condition, its implications for fertility, and her treatment options.
- After considering the alternatives, the woman chooses appropriate treatment options.

CARE OF THE WOMAN WITH TOXIC SHOCK SYNDROME

Toxic shock syndrome (TSS) is primarily a disease of women at or near menses or during the postpartum period. The causative organism is *Staphylococcus aureus.* The use of superabsorbent tampons was once related to an increased incidence of TSS. That incidence has declined. Occluding the cervical os with a contraceptive device such as a diaphragm or cervical cap during menses may also increase the risk of TSS (McGregor, 2000).

Early diagnosis and treatment are important in preventing death. The most common signs of TSS include fever (often greater than 38.9°C [102°F]); rash on the trunk initially followed by desquamation of the skin, especially the palms and soles, which usually occurs 1 to 2 weeks after the onset of symptoms; hypotension; and dizziness. Systemic symptoms often include vomiting, diarrhea, severe myalgia, and inflamed mucous membranes (oropharyngeal, conjunctival, or vaginal). Disorders of the central nervous system, including alterations in consciousness, disorientation, and coma, may also occur.

Women with TSS are generally hospitalized and given supportive therapy, including intravenous fluids to maintain blood pressure. Severe cases may require renal dialysis, administration of vasopressors, and intubation. Broadspectrum antibiotic therapy (including antistaphylococcal agents) is initiated immediately until septicemia is excluded as a diagnosis; antibiotic therapy also reduces the risk of recurrence (McGregor, 2000).

NURSING MANAGEMENT

Nurses play a major role in helping educate women about preventing the development of TSS. It is crucial that women understand the importance of avoiding prolonged use of tampons. Women who choose to continue using tampons may reduce their risk of TSS by alternating them with pads and avoiding overnight use of tampons. Women should avoid the use of tampons for 6 to 8 weeks after childbirth. Women who use diaphragms or cervical caps

should not leave them in place for prolonged periods and should not use them during the postpartum period or when they are menstruating. Also, help make women aware of the signs and symptoms of TSS so that they will seek treatment promptly if symptoms occur.

CARE OF THE WOMAN WITH A VAGINAL INFECTION

Vaginitis is the most common reason women seek gynecologic care. Symptoms of vaginitis or vulvovaginitis may include increased vaginal discharge, vulvar irritation, pruritus, foul odor, and pain when urine touches irritated vulvar tissue. It may be caused by an infection or by an alteration of normal flora, as in the case of bacterial vaginosis or *Candida albicans.*

BACTERIAL VAGINOSIS

Bacterial vaginosis (BV) is more prevalent among sexually active women, but it is not considered a sexually transmitted infection. BV is an alteration of normal vaginal bacterial flora that results in the loss of hydrogen peroxide-producing lactobacilli, which are normally the main vaginal flora. With the loss of this natural defense, bacteria such as *Gardnerella*, mycoplasmas, and anaerobes overgrow in large numbers, causing vaginitis. The cause of this overgrowth is not clear, although tissue trauma and sexual intercourse are sometimes identified as contributing factors (Mayeaux, 2003).

The infected woman often notices an excessive amount of thin, watery, white or gray vaginal discharge with a foul odor described as "fishy." The characteristic "clue" cell is seen on a wet-mount preparation (Figure 5–1 ●). The addition of 10% potassium hydroxide (KOH) solution to the vaginal secretions, called a "whiff" test, releases a strong, fishy odor. The vaginal pH is usually greater than 4.5.

The nonpregnant, symptomatic woman is generally treated with metronidazole (Flagyl) orally or as a vaginal cream. (See "Drug Guide: Metronidazole.") If metronidazole is prescribed, the woman and her partner should be cautioned to avoid alcohol while taking it; the combination has an effect similar to that of alcohol and disulfiram (Antabuse)—abdominal pain, flushing, and tremors. Alternatively, clindamycin (Cleocin) vaginal cream may be used, although it is slightly less effective (Centers for Disease Control and Prevention [CDC], 2002).

Until recently, metronidazole was avoided during pregnancy because of its potential teratogenic effects. However, the CDC (2002) reported that multiple studies failed to document a relationship between metronidazole use in pregnancy and teratogenesis in the newborn. Currently the recommended treatment for pregnant women with BV is either oral metronidazole or oral clindamycin.

● FIGURE 5–1

Depiction of the clue cells characteristically seen in bacterial vaginosis. Unlike normal epithelial cells, which appear translucent and have a clear border, clue cells are desquamated epithelial cells with bacteria adhering to them. The presence of the bacteria makes the cell appear to be speckled with black dots. The borders are also obscured because of the bacteria.

BV during pregnancy may be a factor in premature rupture of the membranes and preterm birth. Treatment of male sexual partners has not been effective in preventing recurrence (CDC, 2002).

VULVOVAGINAL CANDIDIASIS

Vulvovaginal candidiasis (VVC), also called moniliasis or yeast infection, is one of the most common forms of vaginitis that women experience. Recurrences are frequent for some women. *Candida albicans* is the fungal species responsible for most vaginal yeast infections. Factors that contribute to VVC are the use of COCs, immunosuppressants, and antibiotics, which destroy normal bacteria that usually keep the yeast cells in check. Other factors are frequent douching, pregnancy, and diabetes mellitus.

DRUG GUIDE

METRONIDAZOLE (FLAGYL)

Overview of Action
Metronidazole is an antiprotozoal and antibacterial agent. It possesses direct trichomonacidal and amebicidal activity against *T. vaginalis* and *E. histolytica*. Metronidazole is active in vitro against most obligate anaerobes but does not appear to possess any clinically relevant activity against facultative anaerobes or obligate aerobes. It is used in the treatment of various infections caused by organisms that are sensitive to this drug. It is used predominantly to treat the following infections in women: *T. vaginalis*, bacterial vaginosis, endometritis, endomyometritis, tubo-ovarian abscess, and postsurgical vaginal cuff infection.

Route, Dosage, Frequency
Trichomoniasis—1-day treatment: 2 g orally in a single dose; 7-day treatment: 500 mg orally twice a day for 7 consecutive days (CDC, 2002).

Amebiasis—Adults: 750 mg orally three times a day for 5–10 days; children: 35–50 mg/kg/24 hours orally divided into three doses for 10 days.

Bacterial vaginosis—500 mg orally twice a day for 7 consecutive days or one full applicator of metronidazole gel 0.75% intravaginally, once daily for 5 days (CDC, 2002).

Contraindications
Blood dyscrasias

Breastfeeding women (drug secreted in breast milk)

Impaired kidney or liver function

Active CNS disease

Side Effects
Convulsive seizures	Weakness
Peripheral neuropathy	Insomnia

Nausea/vomiting	Cystitis
Headache	Reversible neutropenia and
Anorexia	thrombocytopenia
Diarrhea	Flattening of the T wave on ECG
Epigastric distress	Polyuria
Abdominal cramping	Incontinence
Constipation	Pelvic pressure
Metallic taste in mouth	Proliferation of *Candida* in the
Dizziness	vagina and mouth
Vertigo	Joint pains
Uncoordination	Decreased libido
Ataxia	Dryness in the mouth, vulva,
Confusion	and vagina
Irritability	Dyspareunia
Dysuria	Depression

Nursing Considerations
1. Inform woman about potential side effects.
2. Stress the importance of contraceptive compliance during course of treatment.
3. Obtain baseline renal and liver function tests as ordered.
4. Teach woman about the signs, symptoms, and treatment of vulvovaginal candidiasis.
5. Counsel the woman to avoid alcoholic beverages while taking the medication.
6. If the woman is taking oral contraceptives, a backup nonhormonal contraceptive method is recommended during treatment.
7. Take thorough history to rule out the woman's exposure to this medication within the last 6 weeks.
8. Teach woman to monitor the signs and symptoms of her infection.
9. Encourage cooperation with the entire course of treatment.

The woman with VVC often complains of thick, curdy vaginal discharge, severe itching, dysuria, and dyspareunia. A male sexual partner may experience a rash or excoriation of the skin of the penis and possibly pruritus. The male may be symptomatic and the female asymptomatic.

On physical examination the woman's labia may be swollen and excoriated if pruritus has been severe. A speculum examination reveals thick, white, tenacious cheeselike patches adhering to the vaginal mucosa. Diagnosis is confirmed by microscopic examination of the vaginal discharge; hyphae and spores are usually seen on a wet-mount preparation (Figure 5–2 ●).

Treatment of VVC includes intravaginal butoconazole, miconazole, tioconazole, terconazole, clotrimazole, or nystatin suppositories, cream, or tablets. Single-dose and short-course (3 days) approaches are effective for 80% to 90% of women with uncomplicated VVC. Oral fluconazole, 150 mg in a single dose, is also effective for uncomplicated VVC (Gelber & Nyirjesy, 2005). If the vulva is also affected, the cream is applied topically. Some of the topical medications are available over the counter. They are indicated for women with a history of yeast infections who clearly recognize the symptoms.

Treatment of the male partner is generally not necessary unless candidal balanitis (inflammation of the glans penis) is present or if the man's partner has recurrent infection. Then treatment with a topical antifungal medication is indicated (CDC, 2002).

If a woman experiences recurrent VVC (four or more symptomatic episodes in one year), she should be tested for an elevated blood glucose level to determine whether a diabetic or prediabetic condition is present. Women at high risk for sexually transmitted infections should also be

tested for HIV. Recurrent infection is then treated with an intensive regimen of oral and local agents for 7 to 14 days followed by maintenance antifungal therapy. Pregnant women with VVC are treated only with topical azole preparations applied for 7 days (CDC, 2002). Infection at the time of birth may cause *thrush* (a mouth infection) in the newborn.

NURSING PRACTICE

To distinguish among the common types of vaginitis and their treatments, it is useful to remember the following:

Vulvovaginal candidiasis (moniliasis)

Cause: *Candida albicans*

Appearance of discharge: Thick, curdy, like cottage cheese

Diagnostic test: Slide of vaginal discharge (treated with potassium hydroxide) shows characteristic hyphae and spores

Treatment: Clotrimazole vaginal cream or suppositories

Bacterial vaginosis (Gardnerella vaginalis vaginitis)

Cause: *Gardnerella vaginalis*

Appearance of discharge: Gray, milky

Diagnostic test: Slide of vaginal discharge shows characteristic "clue" cells

Treatment: Metronidazole

Trichomoniasis

Cause: *Trichomonas vaginalis*

Appearance of discharge: Greenish white and frothy

Diagnostic test: Saline slide of vaginal discharge shows motile flagellated organisms

Treatment: Metronidazole

NURSING MANAGEMENT

NURSING ASSESSMENT AND DIAGNOSIS

The nurse should suspect VVC if a woman complains of intense vulvar itching and a curdy, white discharge. Because pregnant women with diabetes mellitus are especially susceptible to this infection, be alert for symptoms in these women. In some areas, nurses are trained to do speculum examinations and wet-mount preparations and can confirm the diagnosis themselves. In most cases, however, the nurse who suspects a vaginal infection reports it to the woman's healthcare provider.

Nursing diagnoses that might apply to the woman with VVC include the following:

- *Risk for Impaired Skin Integrity* related to scratching secondary to discomfort of the infection

● **FIGURE 5–2**

The hyphae and spores of *Candida albicans,* the fungus responsible for vulvovaginal candidiasis.

Courtesy of Centers for Disease Control and Prevention.

■ *Health-Seeking Behaviors: Information about Yeast Infection* related to an expressed desire to learn about ways of preventing VVC

PLANNING AND IMPLEMENTATION

If the woman is experiencing discomfort because of pruritus, recommend gentle bathing of the vulva with a weak sodium bicarbonate solution. If a topical treatment is being used, the woman will need to bathe the area before applying the medication.

Also discuss with the woman the factors that contribute to the development of VVC and suggest ways to prevent recurrences, such as wearing cotton underwear and avoiding vaginal powders or sprays that may irritate the vulva. Stress the importance of completing the course of medication even during menses. Some women report that the addition of yogurt to the diet or the use of activated culture of plain yogurt as a vaginal douche helps prevent recurrence by maintaining high levels of lactobacilli.

EVALUATION

Expected outcomes of nursing care include the following:

■ The woman's symptoms are relieved, and the infection is cured.

■ The woman is able to identify self-care measures to prevent further episodes of VVC.

CARE OF THE INDIVIDUAL WITH A SEXUALLY TRANSMITTED INFECTION

The occurrence of **sexually transmitted infection (STI)**, or *sexually transmitted disease (STD)*, has increased over the past few decades. In fact, vaginitis and STIs are the most common reasons for outpatient, community-based treatment of women.

Children and adolescents can also become infected with sexually transmitted organisms through sexual experimentation, sexual play, molestation, and sexual abuse. Adolescents are considered an at-risk population because of their inexperience and lack of knowledge about STIs. They may disregard the importance of using barrier protection, may have multiple sexual partners, may have sex frequently, and often do not seek medical treatment until symptoms are well advanced. The adolescent who acquires an STI has a 40% chance of acquiring another STI within a year, especially if gonorrhea is the first infection (Stamm & McGregor, 2001). Of the 15 million new STI cases each year, approximately 25% occur in adolescents (CDC, 2002). The most frequently diagnosed STIs are chlamydia, genital herpes (herpes simplex type 2), gonorrhea, genital warts (human papillomavirus), trichomoniasis, and syphilis.

Additional information, including specifics as to which STIs must be reported, can be found on the Companion Website. For more detailed information on the specific signs, symptoms, and treatment of males with STIs, consult a medical-surgical nursing textbook.

TRICHOMONIASIS

Trichomoniasis is an infection caused by *Trichomonas vaginalis*, a microscopic motile protozoan that thrives in an alkaline environment. Most infections are acquired through sexual intimacy. Transmission by shared bath facilities, wet towels, or wet swimsuits may be possible. Trichomoniasis is often linked with increased rates of other STIs, including gonorrhea and HIV/AIDS (Schwebke, 2003).

In females, symptoms of trichomoniasis include a yellow-green, frothy, odorous discharge frequently accompanied by inflammation of the vagina and cervix, dysuria, and dyspareunia. Visualization of *T. vaginalis* under the microscope on a wet-mount preparation of vaginal discharge confirms the diagnosis (Figure 5–3 ●). Most males are asymptomatic, although a few may have nongonococcal urethritis (NGU).

Treatment for trichomoniasis is metronidazole (Flagyl) administered in a single 2-g dose for both male and female sexual partners; a 7-day regimen is also available (CDC, 2002). Partners should avoid intercourse until both are cured.

Pregnant women with trichomoniasis may be at increased risk for premature rupture of the membranes, preterm birth, and low birth weight. Pregnant women who are symptomatic should be treated with a single 2-g dose of metronidazole (CDC, 2002).

● **FIGURE 5 3**

Microscopic appearance of *Trichomonas vaginalis*.
Courtesy of Centers for Disease Control and Prevention.

CHLAMYDIAL INFECTION

Chlamydial infection, caused by *Chlamydia trachomatis,* is the most common bacterial STI in the United States. A strain of chlamydia is responsible for trachoma, the world's leading cause of preventable blindness.

In males, chlamydia is a major cause of NGU. In females it can cause infections similar to those that occur with gonorrhea. It can infect the fallopian tubes, cervix, urethra, and Bartholin's glands. Pelvic inflammatory disease, infertility, and ectopic pregnancy are associated with chlamydia. The newborn of a woman with untreated chlamydia is at risk of developing ophthalmia neonatorum, which responds to erythromycin ophthalmic ointment prophylaxis at birth. The newborn may also develop chlamydia pneumonia.

Both males and females may be asymptomatic. In females, symptoms of chlamydia include a thin or purulent discharge, burning and frequency of urination, and lower abdominal pain. Diagnosis is often made after treatment of a male partner for NGU or in a symptomatic woman with a negative gonorrhea culture. Laboratory detection is now simpler because antigen detection, deoxyribonucleic acid (DNA) probe assays, and polymerase chain reaction (PCR) tests have become available. Treatment is a single dose of azithromycin orally or doxycycline orally twice daily for 7 days. Sexual partners are also treated; couples should abstain from intercourse for 7 days (CDC, 2002). Pregnant women are treated with erythromycin ethylsuccinate or amoxicillin, although neither is highly effective (CDC, 2002). Preliminary data on azithromycin, a category B drug, indicate that it is safe during pregnancy, and many clinicians prescribe it.

GONORRHEA

Gonorrhea is an infection caused by the bacteria *Neisseria gonorrhoeae.* If a nonpregnant woman contracts the disease, she is at risk of developing pelvic inflammatory disease. If a woman becomes infected after the third month of pregnancy, the mucous plug in the cervix will prevent the infection from ascending, and it will remain localized in the urethra, cervix, and Bartholin's glands until the membranes rupture. Then it can spread upward.

Often women with gonorrhea are asymptomatic. Thus, it is routine to screen for this infection using a cervical culture during the initial prenatal examination. For women at high risk, the culture may be repeated during the last month of pregnancy. Cultures of the urethra, throat, and rectum may also be required for diagnosis, depending on the body orifices used for intercourse.

In females the most common symptoms of gonorrheal infection include a purulent, greenish yellow vaginal discharge, dysuria, and urinary frequency. Some women also develop inflammation and swelling of the vulva. The cervix may appear swollen and eroded and may secrete a foul-smelling discharge in which gonococci are present. In males, urethritis, or inflammation of the urethra, is the cardinal symptom. This is marked by burning during urination and the presence of discharge from the urethra.

Treatment for nonpregnant women consists of antibiotic therapy with cefixime, ciprofloxacin, or levofloxacin orally (or ceftriaxone intramuscularly) plus doxycycline or azithromycin administered orally. This combined approach provides dual treatment for gonorrhea and chlamydia because the two infections often occur together. Additional treatment may be required if the cultures remain positive 7 to 14 days after completion of treatment. All sexual partners must also be treated or the woman may become reinfected. Pregnant women should be treated with ceftriaxone intramuscularly or cefixime orally. This treatment is combined with erythromycin or amoxicillin to address the risk of coinfection with chlamydia (CDC, 2002).

Women should be informed of the need for reculture to verify cure and the need for abstinence or condom use until cure is confirmed. Both sexual partners should be treated if either has a positive test for gonorrhea.

HERPES GENITALIS

Herpes infections are caused by the herpes simplex virus (HSV). Two types of herpes infections can occur: HSV-1 (the cold sore), which can cause genital herpes through oral-genital contact, and HSV-2, which is usually associated with genital infections. The clinical symptoms and treatment of both types are the same. At least 50 million people in the United States have been diagnosed with genital HSV-2 infection—*herpes genitalis* (CDC, 2002).

The primary episode of herpes genitalis is characterized by the development of single or multiple blisterlike vesicles. In males these usually occur on the penis or anal area. In females the vesicles occur in the genital area and sometimes affect the vaginal walls, cervix, urethra, and anus. The vesicles may appear within a few hours to 20 days after exposure and rupture spontaneously to form painful, open, ulcerated lesions. Inflammation and pain secondary to the presence of herpes lesions can cause difficult urination and urinary retention. Inguinal lymph node enlargement may be present. Flulike symptoms and genital pruritus or tingling also may be noticed. Primary episodes usually last the longest and are the most severe. Lesions heal spontaneously in 2 to 4 weeks.

After the lesions heal, the virus enters a dormant phase, residing in the nerve ganglia of the affected area. Some individuals never have a recurrence, whereas others have regular recurrences. Recurrences are usually less severe than the initial episode and seem to be triggered by emotional stress, menstruation, ovulation, pregnancy, frequent or vigorous intercourse, poor health status or a generally run-down physical condition, tight clothing, or overheating. Although good diagnostic tests are available to detect HSV-2 infection, it is estimated that 80% to 90% of HSV infections are undiagnosed (Morrow, 2003). Diagnosis is most often made on the basis of the clinical appearance of the lesions, Pap smear or culture of the lesions, and PCR identification.

No known cure for herpes exists. The recommended treatment of the first clinical episode of genital herpes is oral acyclovir, valacyclovir, or famciclovir. These same medications, in somewhat different dosages, are also recommended for recurrent herpes infection and for daily suppression therapy for people who have frequent recurrences. Because there is more documented information on use of acyclovir during pregnancy, it may be administered orally to pregnant women with first-episode genital herpes or severe recurrent herpes. Its use in the third trimester may reduce the incidence of cesarean births by decreasing the incidence of recurrences at term (CDC, 2002).

Keeping the genital area clean and dry, wearing loose clothing, and wearing cotton underwear or none at all help promote healing. If herpes is present in the genital tract of a woman during childbirth, it can have a devastating effect on the newborn. See Chapter 15 for more information. ∞

SYPHILIS

Syphilis is a chronic STI caused by the spirochete *Treponema pallidum*. Syphilis is divided into early and late stages. During the early stage (primary), a chancre appears at the site where the *T. pallidum* organism entered the body. Symptoms include slight fever, loss of weight, and malaise. The chancre persists for about 4 weeks and then disappears. In 6 weeks to 6 months, secondary symptoms appear. Skin eruptions called condylomata lata, which resemble wartlike plaques and are highly infectious, may appear on the vulva. Other secondary symptoms are acute arthritis, enlargement of the liver and spleen, nontender enlarged lymph nodes, iritis, and a chronic sore throat with hoarseness.

Syphilis may also be transmitted transplacentally. When infected in utero, the newborn exhibits secondary-stage symptoms of syphilis. Transplacentally transmitted syphilis may cause intrauterine growth restriction, preterm birth, and stillbirth. As a result of the disease's impact on the fetus in utero, serologic testing of every pregnant woman is recommended; some state laws require it. Testing is done at the initial prenatal screening and repeated in the third trimester. Blood studies in early pregnancy may be negative if the woman has only recently contracted the infection.

Diagnosis of syphilis is made by dark-field examination for spirochetes. Blood tests such as the Venereal Disease Research Laboratory (VDRL) test, the rapid plasma reagin (RPR) test, or the more specific fluorescent treponemal antibody absorption (FTA-ABS) test are commonly done.

For nonpregnant and pregnant women with syphilis of less than a year's duration, the CDC (2002) recommends 2.4 million units of benzathine penicillin G administered intramuscularly in a single dose. If syphilis is of long (more than a year) duration, 2.4 million units of benzathine penicillin G is given intramuscularly once a week for 3 weeks. For nonpregnant women allergic to penicillin, doxycycline or tetracycline can be given. The pregnant woman who is allergic to penicillin should be desensitized to penicillin and then treated with it (CDC, 2002). Maternal serologic testing may remain positive for 8 months, and the newborn may have a positive test for 3 months.

CONDYLOMATA ACUMINATA (VENEREAL WARTS)

The infection *condylomata acuminata*, also called *venereal warts*, is a relatively common sexually transmitted condition caused by the human papillomavirus (HPV). Often an individual seeks medical care after noticing single or multiple soft, grayish pink, cauliflower-like lesions on the penis or in the genital area (Figure 5–4 ●). In women the moist, warm environment of the genital area is conducive to the growth of the warts, which may be present on the vulva, vagina, cervix, and anus. The incubation period following exposure is 3 weeks to 3 years.

● **FIGURE 5–4**

Condylomata acuminata on the vulva.

Used with permission from Ken Greer/Visuals Unlimited.

Because condylomata sometimes resemble other lesions and malignant transformation is possible, all atypical, pigmented, and persistent warts should be biopsied and treatment should be instituted promptly. The CDC does not specify a treatment of choice for genital warts but recommends that treatment be determined based on client preference, available resources, and experience of the health care provider. Client-applied therapies include podofilox solution or gel or imiquimod cream. Provider-administered therapies include cryotherapy with liquid nitrogen or cryoprobe; trichloroacetic acid (TCA); bichloroacetic acid (BCA); intralesional interferon; surgical removal by tangential scissor excision, shave excision, or curettage; or laser surgery (CDC, 2002). Imiquimod, podophyllin, and podofilox are not used during pregnancy because they are thought to be teratogenic and in large doses have been associated with fetal death.

Certain forms of HPV have been linked to cervical cancer. Women with HPV infections should have frequent Pap smears to monitor cervical cellular changes. Sex partners are probably infected but do not require treatment unless large lesions are present. The use of male or female condoms may reduce the risk of transmitting the virus to an uninfected partner.

ACQUIRED IMMUNODEFICIENCY SYNDROME

Acquired immunodeficiency syndrome (AIDS) is a fatal disorder caused by the human immunodeficiency virus (HIV). Medical-surgical texts more fully describe care of people with HIV/AIDS. However, because HIV/AIDS has profound implications for the pregnant woman's fetus, AIDS is discussed in more detail in Chapter 14. ∞

NURSING MANAGEMENT

NURSING ASSESSMENT AND DIAGNOSIS

Nurses need to become adept at taking a thorough history and identifying people at risk for STIs. Risk factors include multiple sexual partners, a partner's involvement with other partners, high-risk sexual behaviors such as intercourse without barrier contraception or anal intercourse, partners with high-risk behaviors, treatment with antibiotics while taking oral contraceptives, and young age at onset of sexual activity. Be alert for signs and symptoms of STIs and be familiar with diagnostic procedures if an STI is suspected.

When children or adolescents have a possible STI, the nurse usually encounters them and their families in the emergency department, outpatient clinic, or nursing unit. Because adolescents are often afraid of the consequences of reporting symptoms, it is important to develop good assessment skills, particularly when asking questions about

sexual activity, partners, and the possibility of abuse. When a child or adolescent is diagnosed with one STI, it is important to screen for others because these diseases may coexist. Adolescents who are symptomatic may postpone care because of their discomfort with examinations and cultures. Routine screening of sexually active adolescents is recommended because many have subclinical infections or are asymptomatic.

NURSING PRACTICE

- When a child is found to have an STI, the law requires that a report be made to social services and the local health department and that an investigation take place.
- When a child younger than 10 years of age is found to have gonorrhea or another STI, consider the possibility of sexual abuse.
- Whenever anorectal symptoms are found in a child, suspect molestation.

Although each STI has certain distinctive characteristics, the following complaints warrant further investigation: presence of a sore or lesion on the penis or vulva, increased vaginal discharge, malodorous vaginal discharge, urethral discharge (males), burning with urination, dyspareunia, bleeding after intercourse, and pelvic pain. In many instances a woman is asymptomatic but may report symptoms in her partner, especially painful urination or urethral discharge. It is often helpful to ask the woman whether her partner is experiencing any symptoms.

Nursing diagnoses that may apply when an STI is diagnosed include the following:

- *Interrupted Family Processes* related to the effects of a diagnosis of STI on the couple's relationship
- *Health-Seeking Behaviors: Information on Preventing STIs* related to an expressed desire to prevent infection

PLANNING AND IMPLEMENTATION

Provide the client who has an STI with information about the infection, methods of transmission, implications for pregnancy or future fertility, and the importance of thorough treatment, including treatment of the partner if indicated. The person should also understand the need to abstain from sexual activity, if necessary, during treatment.

Some STIs such as trichomoniasis or chlamydia may cause a woman concern but, once diagnosed, are rather easily treated. Other STIs may be simple to treat medically but may carry a stigma and be emotionally difficult to accept. Stress prevention with all clients and encourage them to require partners, especially new partners, to use condoms. See "Teaching Highlights: Preventing STIs and Their Consequences."

As a nurse, you can be especially helpful in encouraging a client to explore feelings about the diagnosis. People may, for example, experience anger or feel betrayed by a partner, they may feel guilt or see their diagnosis as a form of punishment, or they may feel concern about the long-term implications for future childbearing or ongoing intimate relationships. Opportunities to discuss personal feelings in a nonjudgmental environment can be very helpful. Offer suggestions about support groups, if indicated, and assist the person in planning for future sexual activity.

An attitude of acceptance and matter-of-factness conveys the message that the individual is an acceptable person who happens to have an infection. See "Teaching Highlights" for key information about STIs.

EVALUATION

Expected outcomes of nursing care include the following:

- The infection is identified and cured, if possible; if not, supportive therapy is provided.
- The individual and partner can describe the infection, its method of transmission, its implications, and the therapy.
- The person copes successfully with the impact of the diagnosis on self-concept.

TEACHING HIGHLIGHTS

PREVENTING STIs AND THEIR CONSEQUENCES

The risk of contracting an STI increases with the number of sexual partners. Because of the extended time between infection with HIV and evidence of infection, intercourse with an individual exposes a female or male to all the other sexual partners of that individual for the past 5 or more years. In light of this risk, it is important to take the following actions:

- Plan ahead and develop strategies to refuse sex (especially important for adolescents who may be less confident about saying "no" to casual sexual encounters). Abstinence is the best method of preventing STIs.
- Limit the number of sexual contacts and practice mutual monogamy with an uninfected partner.
- The condom is the best contraceptive method currently available (other than abstinence) for protection from STIs. Use one for every act of vaginal or anal intercourse. Other contraceptives such as the diaphragm, cervical cap, and spermicides also offer some protection against STIs.
- Plan strategies for negotiating condom use with a partner. Do not assume that a sexually experienced partner knows how to practice safe sex.
- Reduce high-risk behaviors. Use of recreational drugs and alcohol can increase sexual risk taking.
- Refrain from oral sex if your partner has active sores in the mouth, on the genitals, or around the anus.
- Refrain from sexual interaction when signs and symptoms of an STI are present.
- Seek care as soon as you notice symptoms and make sure your partner gets treatment if indicated. Absence of symptoms or disappearance of symptoms does not mean that treatment is unnecessary if you suspect an STI. Take all prescribed medications completely.
- The presence of a genital infection may lead to an abnormal Pap smear. Women with certain infections should have more frequent Pap smears according to a schedule recommended by their caregiver. Ask your healthcare provider if you need more frequent Paps.

CARE OF THE WOMAN WITH PELVIC INFLAMMATORY DISEASE

Pelvic inflammatory disease (PID) occurs in approximately 1% of women between ages 15 and 39, although sexually active young women between 15 and 24 have the highest infection rate (Scott & Hasik, 2001). The disease is more common in women who have had multiple sexual partners, a history of PID, early onset of sexual activity, a recent gynecologic procedure, or an IUD. It usually produces a tubal infection (salpingitis) that may or may not be accompanied by a pelvic abscess. However, perhaps the greatest problem of PID is postinfection tubal damage, which is closely associated with infertility.

The organisms most frequently identified with PID are *Chlamydia trachomatis* and *Neisseria gonorrhoeae*. Symptoms of PID include bilateral sharp, cramping pain in the lower quadrants, fever, chills, purulent vaginal discharge, irregular bleeding, malaise, nausea, and vomiting. However, it is also possible to be asymptomatic and have normal laboratory values.

Diagnosis is based on examination, cultures for gonorrhea and chlamydia, a complete blood count with differential, and an RPR or VDRL to test for syphilis. Physical examination usually reveals direct abdominal tenderness with palpation, adnexal tenderness, and cervical and uterine tenderness with movement (chandelier sign). A palpable mass is evaluated with ultrasound. Laparoscopy may confirm the diagnosis and enable the examiner to obtain cultures from the fallopian tubes and directly from the fluid of the cul-de-sac of Douglas.

The decision to hospitalize is based on clinical judgment. Inpatient treatment includes intravenous fluids, pain medications, and intravenous antibiotics—often either cefoxitin or cefotetan, plus doxycycline or clindamycin plus gentamicin (CDC, 2002). Outpatient therapy usually includes ofloxacin plus metronidazole orally. Other antibiotic combinations may also be used. In addition, supportive therapy is often indicated for severe symptoms. The sexual partner should be treated. If the woman has an IUD, it is generally removed 24 to 48 hours after antibiotic therapy is started.

NURSING MANAGEMENT

NURSING ASSESSMENT AND DIAGNOSIS

Be alert to factors in a woman's history that put her at risk for PID. Question the woman who has an IUD about possible symptoms, such as aching pain in the lower abdomen, foul-smelling discharge, malaise, and the like. The woman who is acutely ill will have obvious symptoms, but a low-grade infection is more difficult to detect.

Nursing diagnoses that may apply to a woman with PID include the following:

- *Acute Pain* related to peritoneal irritation
- *Health-Seeking Behaviors: Information about the Possible Effects of PID on Fertility* related to a request for specific information

PLANNING AND IMPLEMENTATION

The nurse plays a vital role in helping to prevent or detect PID. Accordingly, spend time discussing risk factors related to this infection. The woman who uses an IUD for contraception and has multiple sexual partners needs to understand clearly the risk she faces. Discuss signs and symptoms of PID and stress the importance of early detection.

The woman who develops PID should be counseled on the importance of completing her antibiotic treatment and of returning for follow-up evaluation. She should also understand the possibility of decreased fertility following the infection.

EVALUATION

Expected outcomes of nursing care include the following:

- The woman describes her condition, her therapy, and the possible long-term implications of PID on her fertility.
- The woman completes her course of therapy and the PID is cured.

CARE OF THE WOMAN WITH AN ABNORMAL FINDING DURING PELVIC EXAMINATION

ABNORMAL PAP SMEAR RESULTS

As discussed in Chapter 4, a Papanicolaou (Pap) smear is a test done to screen for the presence of cellular anomalies of the cervix and endocervical canal. Although the Pap smear is useful in detecting a variety of abnormalities, it has had its greatest impact on the detection of cervical cancer. The *Bethesda system* (Table 5–1) has become the most widely used system in the United States for reporting Pap smear results. Early detection of abnormalities allows changes to be treated before cells reach the precancerous or cancerous stage. Notification of an abnormal Pap smear usually causes anxiety for a woman, so it is important that she be told in a caring way. The woman needs accurate, complete information about the meaning of the results and the next steps to be taken. She should also be given time to ask questions and express her concerns.

Diagnostic or therapeutic procedures used in cases of abnormalities include repetition of the Pap test using the ThinPrep method rather than a smear, Pap tests at shorter intervals, colposcopy and endocervical biopsy, cryotherapy, laser conization, or large loop excision of the transformation zone (LLETZ). Management is based on the specific report.

Colposcopy has become a common second step in many cases of abnormal Pap smears. The examination, done in an office or clinic, permits more detailed visualization of the cervix in bright light, using a high-magnification microscope. The cervix can be visualized directly and again following application of acetic acid. The acetic acid causes abnormal epithelium to assume a characteristic white appearance. The colposcope can also be used to obtain a directed biopsy.

OVARIAN MASSES

Ovarian masses may be palpated during the pelvic examination. Between 70% and 80% of ovarian masses are benign. More than 50% are functional cysts, occurring most commonly in women 20 to 40 years of age. Functional cysts are rare in women who take oral contraceptives. Ovarian cysts usually represent physiologic variations in the menstrual cycle. Dermoid cysts (cystic teratomas) and endometriomas, or "chocolate cysts," are common types of ovarian masses. No relationship exists between ovarian masses and ovarian cancer. However, ovarian cancer is the most fatal of all cancers in women because it is difficult to diagnose and often has spread throughout the pelvis before it is detected.

Many women with a benign ovarian mass are asymptomatic; the mass may be noted on a routine pelvic examination. Others experience a sensation of fullness or cramping in the lower abdomen (often unilateral), dyspareunia, irregular bleeding, or delayed menstruation. Diagnosis is made on the basis of a palpable mass with or without tenderness and other related symptoms. Radiography or ultrasonography may be used to assist in the diagnosis.

TABLE 5–1 ✤ The Bethesda System for Classifying Pap Smears

Specimen Type

Indicate conventional smear (Pap smear) vs. liquid based vs. other

Specimen Adequacy

Satisfactory for evaluation *(describe presence or absence of endocervical/transformation zone component and any other quality indicators, e.g., partially obscuring blood inflammation, etc.)*

Unsatisfactory for evaluation . . . *(specify reason)*

Specimen rejected/not processed *(specify reason)*

Specimen processed and examined, but unsatisfactory for evaluation of epithelial abnormality because of *(specify reason)*

General Categorization (optional)

Negative for intraepithelial lesion or malignancy.

Epithelial cell abnormality. See Interpretation/Result *(specify 'squamous' or 'glandular' as appropriate)*

Other: See Interpretation/Result *(e.g., endometrial cells in a woman ≥40 years of age).*

Automated Review

If case examined by automated device, specify device and result.

Ancillary Testing

Provide a brief description of the test methods and report the result so that it is easily understood by the clinician.

Interpretation/Result

Negative for intraepithelial lesion or malignancy
(when there is no cellular evidence of neoplasia, state this in the General Categorization above and/or in the Interpretation/Result section of the report, whether or not there are organisms or other nonneoplastic findings)

ORGANISMS:

Trichomonas vaginalis

Fungal organisms morphologically consistent with *Candida* spp.

Shift in flora suggestive of bacterial vaginosis.

Bacteria morphologically consistent with *Actinomyces* spp.

Cellular changes associated with herpes simplex virus.

OTHER NON-NEOPLASTIC FINDINGS *(Optional to report list not inclusive).*

Reactive cellular changes associated with

—inflammation (includes typical repair)

—radiation

—intrauterine contraceptive device (IUD)

Glandular cells status posthysterectomy

Atrophy

Other

Endometrial cells (in a woman ≥40 years of age) (Specify if negative for squamous intraepithelial lesion)

Epithelial cell abnormalities
SQUAMOUS CELL

Atypical squamous cells

—of undetermined significance (ASC-US)

—cannot exclude HSIL (ASC-H)

Low-grade squamous intraepithelial lesion (LSIL)

—encompassing HPV/mild dysplasia/CIN-1

High-grade squamous intraepithelial lesion (HSIL)

—encompassing: moderate and severe dysplasia CIS/CIN-2 and CIN-3

—with features suspicious for invasion *(if invasion is suspected)*

Squamous cell carcinoma

GLANDULAR CELL

Atypical

—endocervical cells *(NOS or specify in comments)*

—endometrial cells *(NOS or specify in comments)*

—glandular cells *(NOS or specify in comments)*

Atypical

—endocervical cells, favor neoplastic

—glandular cells, favor neoplastic

Endocervical adenocarcinoma in situ

Adenocarcinoma

—endocervical

endometrial

—extrauterine

—not otherwise specified (NOS)

Other malignant neoplasms (specify)

Educational Notes and Suggestions (optional)

Suggestions should be concise and consistent with clinical follow-up guidelines published by professional organizations (references to relevant publications may be included).

Courtesy of National Cancer Institute.

The woman is often kept under observation for a month or two because most cysts resolve on their own and are harmless. Oral contraceptives may be prescribed for 1 to 2 months to suppress ovarian function. If this regimen is effective, a repeat pelvic examination should be normal. If the mass is still present after 60 days of observation and oral contraceptive therapy, a diagnostic laparoscopy or la-

parotomy may be considered. Tubal or ovarian lesions, ectopic pregnancy, cancer, infection, or appendicitis also must be ruled out before a diagnosis can be confirmed.

Surgery is not always necessary but is considered if the mass is larger than 6 to 7 cm in circumference; if the woman is over 40 years of age with an adnexal mass, a persistent mass, or continuous pain; or if the woman is taking oral contraceptives. Surgical exploration is also indicated when a palpable mass is found in an infant, a young girl, or a postmenopausal woman.

Women taking oral contraceptives should be informed of their preventive effect against ovarian masses. Women may need clear explanations about why the initial therapy is observation. A discussion of the origin and resolution of ovarian cysts may clarify this treatment plan. If a surgical treatment removes or impairs the function of one ovary, the woman needs to be assured that the remaining ovary can be expected to take over ovarian functioning and that pregnancy is still possible if desired.

UTERINE MASSES

Fibroid tumors, or *leiomyomas,* are among the most common benign disease entities in women and are the most common reason for gynecologic surgery. Between 20% and 50% of women develop leiomyomas by age 40. The potential for cancer is minimal. Leiomyomas are more common in women of African heritage.

Fibroid tumors vary in size from 1 to 2 cm to the size of a 10-week fetus. Frequently the woman is asymptomatic. Lower abdominal pain, fullness or pressure, menorrhagia, metrorrhagia, or increased dysmenorrhea may occur, particularly with large tumors. Ultrasonography revealing masses or nodules can assist and confirm the diagnosis. Leiomyoma is also considered a possible diagnosis when masses or nodules involving the uterus are palpated on a pelvic examination.

The majority of these masses require no treatment and will shrink after menopause. Close observation for symptoms or an increase in size of the uterus or the masses is the only management most women need. Routine pelvic examinations every 3 to 6 months are recommended unless new symptoms appear.

If a woman notices symptoms, or pelvic examination reveals that the mass is increasing in size, therapies include uterine fibroid embolization (a non-surgical technique in which tiny plastic particles are injected into the artery supplying blood to the tumor), magnetic resonance guided focused ultrasound (a procedure that uses high-intensity ultrasound waves to destroy the fibroid tissue); or surgery (myomectomy, dilation and curettage, or hysterectomy). The choice of surgery depends on the age and reproductive status of the woman and the significance of the noted changes (Society of Interventional Radiology, 2005).

Endometrial cancer, most commonly a disease of postmenopausal women, has a high rate of cure if detected early. The hallmark sign is vaginal bleeding in postmenopausal women not treated with hormone replacement therapy. Diagnosis is made by endometrial biopsy, transvaginal ultrasound, or posthysterectomy pathology examination of the uterus. The treatment is total abdominal hysterectomy and bilateral salpingo-oophorectomy. Radiation therapy may also be indicated, depending on the stage of the cancer.

NURSING MANAGEMENT

Pelvic examinations and Pap smears are not done by nurses except those with special training. In most cases, nursing assessment is directed toward an evaluation of the woman's understanding of the findings and their implications and her psychosocial response.

The woman needs accurate information on etiology, symptomatology, and treatment options. Encourage her to report symptoms and keep appointments for follow-up examination and evaluation. The woman needs realistic reassurance if her condition is benign; she may require counseling and effective emotional support if a malignancy is likely. If the management plan includes surgery, she may need the nurse's support in obtaining a second opinion and making her decision about treatment.

CARE OF THE WOMAN WITH A URINARY TRACT INFECTION

A **urinary tract infection (UTI)** is defined as significant bacteriuria in the presence of symptoms. Approximately 50% to 70% of women experience a UTI in their lifetime, and 20% to 30% will have recurrent infection (Dwyer & O'Reilly, 2002). Bacteria usually enter the body by way of the urethra. The organisms are capable of migrating against the downward flow of urine. The shortness of the female urethra facilitates the passage of bacteria into the bladder. Other conditions associated with bacterial entry are relative incompetence of the urinary sphincter, frequent enuresis (bed-wetting) before adolescence, and urinary catheterization. Wiping from back to front after urination may transfer bacteria from the anorectal area to the urethra. Voluntarily suppressing the desire to urinate is a predisposing factor. Retention overdistends the bladder and can lead to an infection. A relationship also exists between recurring UTI and coitus. General poor health or lowered resistance to infection can increase a woman's susceptibility to UTI.

Asymptomatic bacteriuria (ASB) (bacteria in the urine actively multiplying without accompanying clinical symptoms) is a condition that becomes especially significant if the woman is pregnant. About 30% to 40% of pregnant women with untreated ASB go on to develop cystitis or pyelonephritis (Lentz, 2000). ASB is almost always caused by a single organism, typically *Escherichia coli.* Other commonly found causative organisms include *Klebsiella* and *Proteus.* A woman who has had a UTI is susceptible to recurrent infection. If a pregnant woman develops an acute UTI, especially with a high temperature, amniotic fluid infection may develop and retard the growth of the placenta.

LOWER URINARY TRACT INFECTION (CYSTITIS)

Because UTIs are ascending, it is important to recognize and diagnose a lower UTI early to avoid the sequelae associated with an upper UTI. Symptoms of frequency, pyuria, and dysuria without bacteriuria may indicate urethritis caused by *Chlamydia trachomatis;* it has become a common pathogen in the genitourinary system.

When cystitis develops, the initial symptom is often dysuria, specifically at the end of urination. Urgency and frequency also occur. Cystitis is usually accompanied by a low-grade fever (38.3°C [101°F] or lower), and hematuria is occasionally seen. Urine specimens usually contain an abnormal number of leukocytes and bacteria. Diagnosis is made with a urine culture.

NURSING PRACTICE

To avoid contamination of a clean-catch urine specimen in a woman with a suspected UTI, you might try having her place a cotton ball or gauze square just inside her vagina. After she obtains the urine specimen and closes the container, she then removes the cotton ball or gauze square and discards it in the appropriate trash receptacle.

Treatment depends on the causative organism. The Infectious Diseases Society of America (Lugg, 2003) recommends oral trimethoprim-sulfamethoxazole (TMP-SMX) for 3 days as standard therapy to prevent the development of resistance to other, stronger antibiotics. In communities with a high resistance to TMP-SMX, fluoroquinolones may be used. (For treatment options during pregnancy, see Table 15–5 in Chapter 15.) Phenazopyridine ∞ (Pyridium), a bladder analgesic, may also be prescribed to treat the dysuria.

NURSING MANAGEMENT

NURSING ASSESSMENT AND DIAGNOSIS

During each visit, note any complaints from the woman of dysuria or other urinary difficulties. If any concerns arise, obtain a clean-catch urine specimen from the woman.

Nursing diagnoses that may apply to a woman with a lower UTI include the following:

■ *Acute Pain* related to dysuria secondary to the UTI

■ *Health-Seeking Behaviors: Information about Self-Care Measures to Prevent UTI* related to an expressed desire to prevent recurrence

---

TEACHING HIGHLIGHTS

PREVENTING CYSTITIS

Following is information for women about ways to avoid cystitis:

■ If you use a diaphragm for contraception, try changing methods or using another size of diaphragm.

■ Avoid bladder irritants such as alcohol, caffeine products, and carbonated beverages.

■ Increase fluid intake, especially water, to a minimum of six to eight glasses per day.

■ Make regular urination a habit; avoid long waits.

■ Practice good genital hygiene, including wiping from front to back after urination and bowel movements.

■ Be aware that vigorous or frequent sexual activity may contribute to urinary tract infection.

■ Urinate before and after intercourse to empty the bladder and cleanse the urethra.

■ Complete medication regimens even if symptoms decrease.

■ Do not use medication left over from previous infections.

■ Drink cranberry juice to acidify the urine. This has been found to relieve symptoms in some cases.

PLANNING AND IMPLEMENTATION

Make sure the woman is aware of good hygiene practices, since most bacteria enter through the urethra after having spread from the anal area. See "Teaching Highlights: Preventing Cystitis." Reinforce instructions or answer questions about the prescribed antibiotic, the amount of liquids to take, and the reasons for these treatments. Cystitis usually responds rapidly to treatment, but follow-up urinary cultures are important.

EVALUATION

Expected outcomes of nursing care include the following:

■ The woman implements self-care measures to help prevent cystitis.

■ The woman can identify the signs, symptoms, therapy, and complications of cystitis.

■ The woman's infection is cured.

UPPER URINARY TRACT INFECTION (PYELONEPHRITIS)

Pyelonephritis (inflammatory disease of the kidneys) is less common but more serious than cystitis and is often preceded by lower UTI. It is more common during the latter part of pregnancy or early postpartum and poses a serious threat to maternal and fetal well-being. Women with symptoms of pyelonephritis during pregnancy have an increased risk of preterm birth and of intrauterine growth restriction.

Acute pyelonephritis has a sudden onset, with chills, high temperature of 39.6°C to 40.6°C (103°F to 105°F), and flank pain (either unilateral or bilateral). The right side is almost always involved if the woman is pregnant because the large bulk of intestines to the left pushes the uterus to the right, putting pressure on the right ureter and kidney. Nausea, vomiting, and general malaise may ensue. With accompanying cystitis, the woman may experience frequency, urgency, and burning with urination.

Edema of the renal parenchyma or ureteritis with blockage and swelling of the ureter may lead to temporary suppression of urinary output. This is accompanied by severe colicky (spastic, intense) pain, vomiting, dehydration, and ileus of the large bowel. Women with acute pyelonephritis generally have increased diastolic blood pressure, positive fluorescent antibody titer (FA test), low creatinine clearance, significant bacteremia in urine culture, pyuria, and presence of white blood cell casts.

Often the woman is hospitalized and started on intravenous antibiotics. In the case of obstructive pyelonephritis, a blood culture is necessary. The woman is kept on bed rest. After the sensitivity report is received, the antibiotic is changed as necessary. If signs of urinary obstruction occur or continue, the ureter may be catheterized to establish adequate drainage.

With appropriate drug therapy, the woman's temperature should return to normal. The pain subsides and the urine shows no bacteria within 2 to 3 days. Follow-up urinary cultures are needed to determine that the infection has been eliminated completely.

NURSING MANAGEMENT

NURSING ASSESSMENT AND DIAGNOSIS

During a woman's visit, obtain a sexual and medical history to identify whether she is at risk for UTI. A clean-catch urine specimen is evaluated for evidence of ASB.

Nursing diagnoses that may apply to a woman with an upper UTI include the following:

- *Acute Pain* related to dysuria, systemic discomforts, or renal pain secondary to UTI
- *Fear* related to the possible long-term effects of the disease

Give the woman information to help her recognize the signs of UTI. Also discuss hygiene practices, the advantages of wearing cotton underwear, and the need to void frequently to prevent urinary stasis. Stress the importance of maintaining a good fluid intake. Drinking cranberry juice daily and taking 500 mg of vitamin C help acidify the urine and may help prevent recurrence of infection. Women with

a history of UTI find it helpful to drink a glass of fluid before sexual intercourse and to void afterward.

EVALUATION

Expected outcomes of nursing care include the following:

- The woman completes her prescribed course of antibiotic therapy.
- The woman's infection is cured.
- The woman incorporates preventive self-care measures into her daily regimen.

PELVIC RELAXATION

A *cystocele* is the downward displacement of the bladder, which appears as a bulge in the anterior vaginal wall. Genetic predisposition, childbearing, obesity, and increased age are factors that may contribute to cystocele. Symptoms of stress incontinence are most common, including loss of urine with coughing, sneezing, laughing, or sudden exertion. Vaginal fullness, a bulging out of the vaginal wall, or a dragging sensation may also be noticeable.

If pelvic relaxation is mild, Kegel exercises help restore tone. The exercises involve contraction and relaxation of the pubococcygeal muscle (see Perineal Exercises in Chapter 11 for more information) ∞. Women have found these exercises helpful before and after childbirth in maintaining vaginal muscle tone. Estrogen may improve the condition of vaginal mucous membranes, especially in menopausal women. Vaginal pessaries or rings may be used if surgery is undesirable or impossible or until surgery can be scheduled. Surgery may be considered for cystoceles considered moderate to severe.

The nurse may instruct the woman in the use of Kegel exercises. Information on causes and contributing factors and discussion of possible alternative therapies greatly help the woman.

A *rectocele* may develop when the posterior vaginal wall is weakened. The anterior wall of the rectum can then sag forward, ballooning into the vagina, pushing the weakened posterior wall of the vagina in front of it. When the woman strains to have a bowel movement, a pocket of rectum develops that traps stool, and constipation results. To defecate, a woman with a rectocele may find it necessary to press the tissue between the vagina and rectum, which elevates the rectocele.

Diagnosis is based on history and physical examination. Decisions about treatment are based on the size of the rectocele, the presence and severity of symptoms, and the woman's individual situation, including her overall health. Surgery is often indicated.

Uterine prolapse occurs when the uterus protrudes downward (drops) into the upper vagina, pulling the vagina with it. The extent of the prolapse is determined by the location of the cervix in the vagina. In severe cases the uterus may prolapse below the vaginal introitus. The woman may report a "dragging" sensation in her groin and a backache over the sacrum, which is caused by pulling on the uterosacral ligaments. Typically these symptoms are relieved when the woman lies down. As with cystocele, conservative treatment includes the use of topical or systemic estrogen and vaginal pessaries. Surgery for uterine prolapse often involves hysterectomy and repair of the prolapsed vaginal walls.

CARE OF THE WOMAN REQUIRING A HYSTERECTOMY

Hysterectomy is the surgical removal of the uterus. In the United States, it is the most common nonpregnancy-related surgical procedure that women undergo (Kim & Lee, 2001). Removal of the uterus through a surgical incision is called a *total abdominal hysterectomy (TAH)*, and removal of both fallopian tubes and ovaries is called a *bilateral salpingo-oophorectomy (BSO)*. When both procedures are performed at the same time it is called a TAH-BSO. When the uterus is removed through the vagina, it is termed a *total vaginal hysterectomy (TVH)*.

Abdominal hysterectomy is the usual treatment for several conditions, including cancer of the cervix, endometrium, or ovary; large fibroids; severe endometriosis; chronic PID; and adenomyosis. TAH is preferred when cancer is expected because it permits easier exploration of the abdomen. It is also helpful when large uterine masses are present.

Vaginal hysterectomy is generally done for pelvic relaxation, abnormal uterine bleeding, or small fibroids. Advantages of vaginal hysterectomy include earlier ambulation, less postoperative pain, less anesthesia and operative time, less blood loss, no visible scar, and a shorter hospital stay. The major disadvantage is the increased risk of trauma to the bladder.

NURSING CARE MANAGEMENT

NURSING ASSESSMENT AND DIAGNOSIS

Preoperatively the nurse needs to identify the woman's physiologic and psychologic needs as she approaches surgery. Additionally it is important to evaluate her learning needs in relation to the surgery and its implications postoperatively. In assessing the woman, consider her age, her culture and educational level, the attitudes of her part-

○ **FIGURE 5–5**

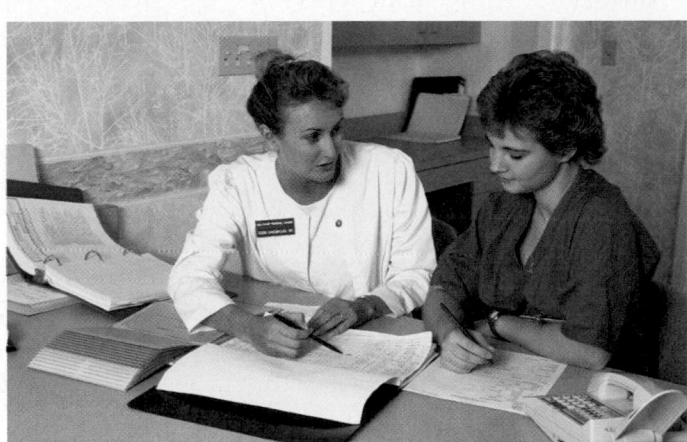

The nurse provides information for the woman during preoperative teaching.

ner and family, her preoperative status, and whether the hysterectomy is being performed because of a cancer diagnosis. The significance of her reproductive health to her self-image is also a consideration.

Nursing diagnoses that may apply to a woman having a hysterectomy include the following:

- *Deficient Knowledge* related to a lack of information about preoperative routines, postoperative activities, and expected postoperative changes
- *Fear* related to the risk of possible surgical complications

NURSING PLAN AND IMPLEMENTATION

Preoperative teaching should include information about the procedure, expected preparation, type of anesthesia to be used, possible risks and complications, postoperative care routines, and expected recovery time (Figure 5–5 ○).

Routine postoperative care includes monitoring of physiologic and emotional responses and implementation of nursing interventions to ensure physical well-being and comfort. The woman should be aware of possible complications and when to follow up with her surgeon. Follow up with the woman regarding any psychosocial implications discussed preoperatively, such as support at home and potential for sadness or depression related to perception of changed sexuality or self-image.

EVALUATION

Expected outcomes of nursing care include the following:

- The woman can discuss the reasons for her hysterectomy and the type of procedure performed, the alternatives, and aspects of self-care following surgery.

■ The woman has an uneventful recovery without complications.

■ The woman participates in decision making about her care.

■ The woman can identify available resources if she has physical or emotional concerns in the postoperative period.

Critical Concept Review

LEARNING OBJECTIVES	CONCEPTS
Contrast the common benign breast disorders.	1. Fibrocystic breast changes: ■ May be caused by an imbalance in progesterone and estrogen. ■ Breasts have increased tenderness and swelling before beginning of menses. ■ Sodium and caffeine restriction may help. 2. Fibroadenoma: ■ Freely movable solid benign tumor. ■ Asymptomatic and nontender. ■ Surgically removed if malignancy is suspected. 3. Intraductal papilloma: ■ Tumor within the ductal system of the breast. ■ Potentially malignant. ■ Most frequent cause of nipple discharge. ■ Must be surgically removed. 4. Duct ectasis (comedomastitis): ■ Inflammation of duct behind the nipple. ■ Occurs during or near menopause. ■ Treatment is symptom relief or surgical removal.
Discuss the signs and symptoms, medical therapy, and implications for fertility of endometriosis.	1. Signs and symptoms: ■ Pelvic pain. ■ Dyspareunia. ■ Abnormal uterine bleeding. 2. Treatment: ■ Surgical removal of visible endometrial tissue. ■ Oral contraceptives. ■ Hormonal therapy. ■ Surgical removal of uterus and ovaries in severe cases if childbearing is not an issue. 3. Implications for fertility: ■ Pregnancy must be delayed until oral contraceptive or hormonal therapy is over, due to suppression of the menstrual cycle.
Identify the risk factors, treatment options, and nursing interventions for a woman with toxic shock syndrome.	1. Risk factors: ■ Use of superabsorbent tampons. ■ Use of cervical cap or diaphragm during menses. 2. Treatment options: ■ IV fluids for hydration. ■ Broad-spectrum antibiotics. 3. Nursing interventions: ■ Instruct women about proper use of superabsorbent tampons, cervical caps, and diaphragms. ■ Instruct women not to use tampons for first 6–8 weeks after childbirth.

LEARNING OBJECTIVES

CONCEPTS

Compare vulvovaginal candidiasis and bacterial vaginosis.

1. Vulvovaginal candidiasis:
   - Most common form of vaginitis.
   - Related to use of oral contraceptives, immunosuppressants, and antibiotics.
   - Thick, curdy, white vaginal discharge.
   - Severe itching, dysuria, and dyspareunia.
   - Treated topically or systemically with antifungal drugs.
2. Bacterial vaginosis:
   - Caused by an alteration in normal vaginal bacterial flora.
   - Most common cause of vaginal discharge or odor.
   - Thin vaginal discharge with a "fishy" smell.
   - Treated with metronidazole (Flagyl).

Describe the common sexually transmitted infections.

1. Trichomoniasis:
   - Yellow-green, frothy, odorous discharge.
   - Causes vaginal itching.
   - Both partners are treated with metronidazole (Flagyl).
2. Chlamydial infection:
   - May cause disease in newborn.
   - Often asymptomatic.
   - Both partners are treated with doxycycline or azithromycin.
3. Gonorrhea:
   - May cause pelvic inflammatory disease.
   - Often asymptomatic.
   - Purulent, green-yellow discharge, dysuria, and urinary frequency.
   - Both partners are treated with antibiotics.
4. Herpes genitalis:
   - Cannot be cured.
   - Recurrences may be triggered by physical or emotional stress.
   - Treatment with antiviral medication may decrease length of outbreak.
   - May cause fatal fetal infection if herpes lesion is present in genital tract during childbirth.
5. Syphilis:
   - Testing for disease is required during pregnancy.
   - Treated with penicillin.
6. Human papillomavirus (HPV)/condylomata acuminata:
   - Genital warts.
   - Certain forms of HPV have been linked to cervical cancer.
   - Treatment is removal of warts by chemical or surgical means.
7. Acquired immunodeficiency syndrome (AIDS):
   - Fatal disorder caused by the human immunodeficiency virus (HIV).
   - Has profound implications for the fetus if infected woman is pregnant.

Summarize the health teaching a nurse needs to provide to a woman with a sexually transmitted infection.

The nurse must provide the woman with information about:
1. The infection.
2. Methods of transmission of the infection.
3. Implications of the infection on present pregnancy, future fertility, and general health.
4. Importance of completion of treatment.
5. Treatment of both partners.
6. Need for abstinence until treatment is completed.

Relate the implications of pelvic inflammatory disease (PID) for future fertility to its pathology, signs and symptoms, and treatment.

1. Pathology:
   - Often caused by chlamydia or gonorrhea.
   - Infection may cause scarring of fallopian tubes, preventing union of sperm and ova.
2. Signs and symptoms:
   - Chills and fever.
   - Purulent vaginal discharge.
   - Irregular vaginal bleeding.
   - Nausea and vomiting.
3. Treatment:
   - Antibiotics (IV or PO).
   - Treatment of sexual partner.

(continued)

LEARNING OBJECTIVES

CONCEPTS

Identify the implications of an abnormal finding during a pelvic examination.

1. Abnormal Pap smear results:
   - May indicate abnormal cervical cells or cervical malignancy.
2. Ovarian masses:
   - May indicate cysts or malignancy.
   - Cysts are often observed closely unless they cause symptoms.
3. Uterine abnormalities:
   - Fibroid tumors are most common.
   - May be observed or removed depending upon symptoms of woman.

Contrast cystitis and pyelonephritis.

1. Cystitis:
   - Infection of lower urinary tract.
   - Often causes dysuria, urgency, and frequency.
   - Treated is with PO antibiotics.
2. Pyelonephritis:
   - Infection of upper urinary tract.
   - May be preceded by lower urinary tract infection.
   - Sudden onset of chills, high temperature, and flank pain.
   - May also have dysuria, urgency, and frequency.
   - More serious than cystitis.
   - Treated is with IV or PO antibiotics.

CRITICAL THINKING IN ACTION

View the **Critical Thinking in Action** video in Chapter 5 of the CD-ROM. Then, answer the questions that follow.

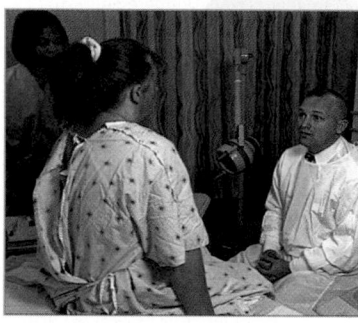

Linda Knoll, 35 years old, presents to you at the GYN clinic for her annual physical and pelvic exam. You obtain the following menstrual history: LMP 8 days ago. Periods occur every 29 days and last 5 days. She tells you that she uses superabsorbent tampons during the first 2 days of her period and then changes to regular absorbency tampons for the duration, and that she currently has an IUD in place for contraception. She tells you that her husband has been complaining for the last few months that she seems irritable, tense, and moody near "that time of the month." Linda admits that she doesn't feel well before her period and describes having low pelvic discomfort, breast tenderness, "bloating," and some constipation. She seems to cry easily 2 to 3 days before her period. She has noticed this pattern over the last 4 or 5 months. You recognize these symptoms as related to premenstrual syndrome (PMS). Linda asks you if these changes are due to female hormones.

1. How would you answer Linda's question concerning female hormones?
2. After reviewing Linda's diet with her, what would you recommend to help?
3. Linda has an IUD in place. What other type of contraceptive might help reduce the symptoms of PMS?
4. What other activities can you suggest to help Linda reduce PMS symptoms?
5. What should you tell Linda about using tampons during heavy menstrual flow?

MEDIALINK

www.prenhall.com/london

- NCLEX-RN® Review, case studies, and other interactive resources for this chapter can be found on the Companion Website at http://www.prenhall.com/london. Click on "Chapter 5" to select the activities for this chapter.

Case Study
A young woman is brought to the Emergency Department by her mother with a fever of 101 degrees Fahrenheit, a rash that has quickly spread to her palms and the soles of her feet, and dizziness.
This activity contains 3 questions.

1. What further assessment data is important for the nurse to gather?
[Hint]

To create paragraphs in your essay response, type <p> at the beginning of the paragraph, and </p> at the end.

- For animations, more NCLEX-RN® Review questions, and an audio glossary, access the accompanying CD-ROM in this textbook.

REFERENCES

American College of Obstetricians and Gynecologists. (1999). *Medical management of endometriosis* (ACOG Practice Bulletin No. 11). Washington, DC: Author.

A simpler cure for pelvic infections. (1997, April). *Health,* p. 18.

Centers for Disease Control and Prevention. (2002). Sexually transmitted diseases treatment guidelines 2002. *Mortality and Morbidity Weekly Report, 51*(RR-6), 1–84.

Conversations with Colleagues. (2002–2003). Endometriosis sufferers risk other diseases. *AWHONN Lifelines, 6*(6), 502–504.

Dwyer, P., & O'Reilly, J. (2002). Recurrent urinary tract infections in the female. *Current Opinion in Obstetrics and Gynecology, 14*(5), 537–543.

Eschenbach, D. A. (2000). Infectious vaginitis. In J. J. Sciarra (Ed.), *Gynecology and obstetrics* (Vol. 1, chap. 40, pp. 1–17). Philadelphia: Lippincott Williams & Wilkins.

Gelber, S. E., & Nyirjesy, P. (2005). Update on vulvovaginal candidiasis *The Female Patient, 30*(5), 36–42.

Hammerschlag, M. R. (1999). New diagnostic methods for chlamydial infection in women. *Medscape Women's Health, 4*(5), 1–7.

Kim, K. H., & Lee, K. A. (2001). Symptom experience in women after hysterectomy. *Journal of Obstetric, Gynecologic, and Neonatal Nursing, 30*(5), 472–480.

Lauver, D. R., Baggot, A., & Kruse, K. (1999). Women's experiences in coping with abnormal Papanicolaou results and follow-up colposcopy. *Journal of Obstetric, Gynecologic, and Neonatal Nursing, 28*(3), 283–290.

Lentz, G. M. (2000). Urinary tract infections in obstetrics and gynecology. In J. J. Sciarra (Ed.), *Gynecology and obstetrics* (Vol. 2.). Philadelphia: Lippincott Williams & Wilkins.

Lugg, J. A. (2003). U.S. and European guidelines for antimicrobial treatment of uncomplicated acute bacterial cystitis in women: How to benefit from both. *Infectious Urology, 16*(3), 59–64.

Mayeaux, E. J. (2003). Bacterial vaginosis: Diagnosis and therapy. *The Female Patient, 28*(8), 21–26.

McGregor, J. A. (2000). Toxic shock syndrome. In J. J. Sciarra (Ed.), *Gynecology and obstetrics* (Vol. 1, chap. 43, pp. 1–9). Philadelphia: Lippincott Williams & Wilkins.

Morrow, R. A. (2003, April). Diagnosis: Infections and the nature of disease. *The Female Patient, 28* (Suppl.), 3–7.

Schwebke, J. R. (2003, February). Diagnosis and treatment of vaginal infections. *The Female Patient, 28* (Suppl.), 8–11.

Scott, L. D., & Hasik, K. J. (2001). The similarities and differences of endometritis and pelvic inflammatory disease. *Journal of Obstetric, Gynecologic, and Neonatal Nursing, 30*(3), 332–341.

Society of Interventional Radiology. (2005). Uterine treatment options. Retrieved September 2, 2005 from www.sirweb.org

Stamm, C. A., & McGregor, J. A. (2001). Diagnosing and treating STDs in young women. *Contemporary Pediatrics 18*(2), 53–57.

Thomason, J. L., & Scaglione, N. J. (1999). Bacterial vaginosis. *Contemporary OB/GYN, 44*(6), 15–24.

Winkel, C. A. (2003). Looking for a better way to manage endometriosis-related pain. *Contemporary OB/GYN, 48*(4), 44–56.

CHAPTER 6

Special Reproductive Issues for Families

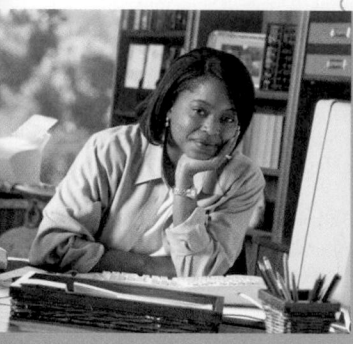

As we sat in the in vitro clinic waiting room, I felt great apprehension. For 4 years we had been unable to conceive. I'd been through two surgeries, dozens of blood tests, and hormone drugs that made me irrational and emotional. It was difficult at times—I blamed myself, felt out of control, and had surprisingly painful reactions to seeing mothers with babies. We were on the brink of the most expensive infertility treatment—the last resort for most infertile couples. Was this the right thing to do?

—Samantha, 38

LEARNING OBJECTIVES

- Identify the essential components of fertility.

- Describe the elements of the preliminary investigation of infertility.

- Summarize the indications for the tests and associated treatments, including assisted reproductive technologies, that are done in an infertility workup.

- Explore the couple's psychologic reactions related to infertility issues.

- Describe the nurse's role as counselor, educator, and advocate for couples during infertility evaluation and treatment.

- Discuss the indications for preconceptual chromosomal analysis and prenatal testing.

- Identify the characteristics of autosomal dominant, autosomal recessive, and X-linked (sex-linked) recessive disorders.

- Compare prenatal and postnatal diagnostic procedures used to determine the presence of genetic disorders.

- Explore the emotional impact on a couple undergoing genetic testing or coping with the birth of a baby with a genetic disorder, and explain the nurse's role in supporting the family undergoing genetic counseling.

MEDIALINK www.prenhall.com/london

CD-ROM
Audio Glossary
NCLEX-RN® Review
Activity: Ovulation
Skill 2–5: Assisting During Amniocentesis

Companion Website
Thinking Critically
NCLEX-RN® Review
MediaLink Applications:
    Case Study: Infertility
    Care Plan: Infertile Couple

M ost couples who want children are able to conceive them without difficulty. Pregnancy and childbirth usually take their normal course, and a healthy baby is born without problems. But some less fortunate couples are unable to fulfill their dream of having the desired baby because of infertility or genetic problems.

This chapter explores two particularly troubling reproductive problems: the inability to conceive and the risk of bearing babies with genetic abnormalities.

INFERTILITY

Infertility is defined as lack of conception despite unprotected sexual intercourse for at least 12 months (Kakarla & Bradshaw, 2003). It has a profound emotional, psychologic, and economic impact on both the affected couples and society. *Sterility* is the term applied when there is an absolute factor preventing reproduction. **Subfertility** is used to describe a couple that has difficulty conceiving because both partners have reduced fertility.

Approximately 16% of couples in their reproductive years are infertile in the United States (Klock, 2004). Public perception is that the incidence of infertility is increasing, but in fact there has been no significant change in the proportion of infertile couples in the United States. What has changed is the composition of the infertile population; the infertility diagnosis has increased in the age group 25 to 44 years because of delayed childbearing and the entry of the baby boom cohort into this age range in Western society.

The perception that infertility is on the rise may be related to the following factors:

- The deferring of pregnancy and then the desire to have a family shortly after marriage
- The increase in assisted reproduction techniques
- The increase in availability and use of infertility services
- The increase in insurance coverage of some ethnic groups for diagnosis of and treatment for infertility
- The increased number of childless women over age 35 seeking medical attention for infertility

ESSENTIAL COMPONENTS OF FERTILITY

Understanding the elements essential for normal fertility can help the nurse identify the many factors that may cause infertility. The components necessary for normal fertility are correlated with possible causes of deviation in Table 6–1. In addition, adequate reproductive hormones must be present.

With intricacies of timing and environment playing such a crucial role, it is an impressive natural phenomenon that the majority of couples in the United States are able to conceive. The remaining couples experience infertility due to a male factor (40%), a female factor (40%), or either an unknown cause (unexplained infertility) or a problem with both partners (20%) (Klock, 2004). Professional intervention can help approximately 65% of infertile couples achieve pregnancy (Klock, 2004).

Couples should be referred for infertility evaluation if they have been unable to conceive after at least 1 year of attempting to achieve pregnancy. If the woman is over age 35, it may be appropriate to refer the couple after only 6 to 9 months of unprotected intercourse without conception. At age 25, when couples are the most fertile, the average length of time needed to

KEY TERMS

Autosomes, 138

Basal body temperature (BBT), 126

Chromosomes, 138

Endometrial biopsy, 128

Ferning capacity, 128

Gamete intrafallopian transfer (GIFT), 136

Genotype, 142

Hysterosalpingography (HSG), 130

Infertility, 123

In vitro fertilization (IVF), 135

Karyotype, 139

Laparoscopy, 130

Mendelian (single-gene) inheritance, 142

Monosomies, 139

Mosaicism, 139

Nonmendelian (multifactorial) inheritance, 142

Pedigree, 142

Phenotype, 142

Postcoital test or Huhner test, 130

Spinnbarkeit, 128

Subfertility, 123

Therapeutic insemination, 134

Transvaginal ultrasound, 128

Trisomies, 139

Tubal embryo transfer (TET), 136

Zygote intrafallopian transfer (ZIFT), 136

TABLE 6–1 ✢ Possible Causes of Infertility

Necessary Norms	Deviations from Normal
Female	
Favorable cervical mucus	Cervicitis, cervical stenosis, use of coital lubricants, antisperm antibodies (immunologic response)
Clear passage between cervix and tubes	Myomas, adhesions, adenomyosis, polyps, endometritis, cervical stenosis, endometriosis, congenital anomalies (e.g., septate uterus, diethylstilbestrol [DES] exposure)
Patent tubes with normal motility	Pelvic inflammatory disease, peritubal adhesions, endometriosis, intrauterine device, salpingitis (e.g., chlamydia, recurrent sexually transmitted infections), neoplasm, ectopic pregnancy, tubal ligation
Ovulation and release of ova	Primary ovarian failure, polycystic ovarian disease, hypothyroidism, pituitary tumor, lactation, periovarian adhesions, endometriosis, premature ovarian failure, hyperprolactinemia, Turner syndrome
No obstruction between ovary and tubes	Adhesions, endometriosis, pelvic inflammatory disease
Endometrial preparation	Anovulation, luteal phase defect malformation, uterine infection, Asherman syndrome
Male	
Normal semen analysis	Abnormalities of sperm or semen, polyspermia, congenital defect in testicular development, mumps after adolescence, cryptorchidism, infections, gonadal exposure to x-rays, chemotherapy, smoking, alcohol abuse, malnutrition, chronic or acute metabolic disease medications (e.g., morphine, ASA, ibuprofen), cocaine use, marijuana use, constrictive underclothing, heat
Unobstructed genital tract	Infections, tumors, congenital anomalies, vasectomy, strictures, trauma, varicocele
Normal genital tract secretions	Infections, autoimmunity to semen, tumors
Ejaculate deposited at the cervix	Premature ejaculation, impotence, hypospadias, retrograde ejaculation (e.g., diabetic), neurologic cord lesions, obesity (inhibiting adequate penetration)

achieve conception is 5.3 months. In about 25% of cases, conception occurs within the first month of unprotected intercourse (Johnson, 2003).

INITIAL INVESTIGATION: PHYSICAL AND PSYCHOSOCIAL ISSUES

The earliest and least intrusive infertility testing approach is used first. Extensive testing for infertility is avoided until data confirm that the timing of intercourse and length of coital exposure have been adequate. The nurse provides information about the most fertile times to have intercourse during the menstrual cycle. Teaching the couple the signs and timing of ovulation and most effective times for intercourse within the cycle may solve the problem (Table 6–2). Primary assessment, including a comprehensive history and physical examination for any obvious causes of infertility, is done before a costly, time-consuming, and emotionally trying investigation is initiated.

During the first visit for the preliminary investigation, the nurse explains the basic infertility workup. The basic investigation for the couple depends on the individuals' history and usually includes assessment of ovarian function, cervical mucosal adequacy and receptivity to sperm,

sperm adequacy, tubal patency, and the general condition of the pelvic organs. Since about 40% of infertility is related to a male factor, a semen analysis should be one of the

TABLE 6–2 ✢ Fertility Awareness

- Avoid douching and artificial lubricants. Prevent alteration of pH of vagina and introduction of spermicidal agents.
- Promote retention of sperm. The male superior position with the female remaining recumbent for at least 1 hour after intercourse maximizes the number of sperm reaching the cervix.
- Avoid leakage of sperm. Elevate the woman's hips with a pillow after intercourse. Avoid getting up to urinate for 1 hour after intercourse.
- Maximize the potential for fertilization. Have intercourse one to three times per week at intervals no less than 48 hours.
- Avoid emphasizing conception during sexual encounters to decrease anxiety and potential sexual dysfunction.
- Maintain adequate nutrition and reduce stress. Stress reduction techniques and good nutritional habits increase sperm production.
- Explore other methods to increase fertility awareness, such as home assessment of cervical mucus and basal body temperature (BBT) recordings.
- Seek counsel and advice from a valued friend or family member.
- Consider incorporating culturally appropriate methods to enhance fertility.

first diagnostic tests done before moving on to more invasive diagnostic procedures involving the woman.

The mutual desire to have children is a cornerstone of many marriages. A fertility problem is a deeply personal, emotion-laden area in a couple's life. The self-esteem of one or both partners may be threatened if the inability to conceive is perceived as a lack of virility or femininity (Klock, 2004). It is never easy to discuss one's sexual activity, especially when potentially irreversible problems with fertility exist. The nurse can provide comfort to couples by offering a sympathetic ear, a nonjudgmental approach, and appropriate information and instructions throughout the diagnostic and therapeutic process. Because counseling includes discussion of very personal matters, nurses who are comfortable with their own sexuality are able to establish rapport and elicit relevant information from couples with fertility problems.

The first interview should involve both partners and include a comprehensive history and physical examination. Table 6–3 lists the items in a complete infertility physical workup and laboratory evaluation for both partners.

TABLE 6–3 ❖ Initial Infertility Physical Workup and Laboratory Evaluation

Female	Male
Physical Examination	**Physical Examination**
Assessment of height, weight, blood pressure, temperature, and general health status	General health (assessment of height, weight, blood pressure)
Endocrine evaluation of thyroid for exophthalmos, lid lag, tremor, or palpable gland	Endocrine evaluation (e.g., presence of gynecomastia)
Optic fundi evaluation for presence of increased intracranial pressure, especially in oligomenorrheal or amenorrheal women (possible pituitary tumor)	Visual fields evaluation for bitemporal hemianopia
	Abnormal hair patterns
Reproductive features (including breast and external genital area)	**Urologic Examination**
Physical ability to tolerate pregnancy	Presence or absence of phimosis
Pelvic Examination	Location of urethral meatus
Papanicolaou smear	Size and consistency of each testis vas deferens and epididymis
Culture for gonorrhea if indicated and possibly chlamydia or mycoplasma culture (opinions vary)	Presence of varicocele
Signs of vaginal infections	**Rectal Examination**
Shape of escutcheon (e.g., does pubic hair distribution resemble that of a male?)	Size and consistency of prostate with microscopic evaluation of prostate fluid for signs of infection
Size of clitoris (enlargement caused by endocrine disorders)	Size and consistency of seminal vesicles
Evaluation of cervix; old lacerations, tears, erosion, polyps, condition and shape of os, signs of infections, cervical mucus (evaluate for estrogen effect of spinnbarkeit and cervical ferning)	**Laboratory Examination**
	Complete blood count
Bimanual Examination	Sedimentation rate, if indicated
Size, shape, position, and motility of uterus	Serology
Presence of congenital anomalies	Urinalysis
Presence of endometriosis	Rh factor and blood grouping
Evaluation of adnexa ovarian size, cysts, fixations, or tumors	Semen analysis
Rectovaginal Examination	If indicated, testicular biopsy, buccal smear, Hormonal assays, FSH, LH, prolactin
Presence of retroflexed or retroverted uterus	
Presence of rectouterine pouch masses	
Presence of possible endometriosis	
Laboratory Examination	
Complete blood count	
Sedimentation rate, if indicated	
Serology	
Urinalysis	
Rh factor and blood grouping	
If indicated, thyroid function tests, prolactin levels, glucose tolerance test, hormonal assays including estradiol, LH, progesterone, FSH, dehydroepiandrosterone (DHEA), androstendione, testosterone, 17 α-hydroxy progesterone (17-OHP).	

Flow chart for management of the infertile couple.

Figure 6–1 ● outlines the historical database, diagnostic tests usually performed, and healthcare interventions used in cases of infertility.

ASSESSMENT OF THE WOMAN'S FERTILITY

After a thorough history and physical examination, both partners may undergo tests to identify causes of infertility. A thorough female evaluation includes assessment of the hypothalamic-pituitary axis in terms of ovulatory function, as well as structure and function of the cervix, uterus, fallopian tubes, and ovaries. (See Chapter 4 for an in-depth discussion of the fertility cycle. ∞)

Evaluation of Ovulatory Factors

Ovulation problems account for approximately 15% of infertility causes. (See Chapter 3 for more information on female reproductive cycle characteristics. ∞)

Basal Body Temperature Recording. One basic test of ovulatory function is the **basal body temperature (BBT)** recording, which aids in identification of follicular and luteal phase abnormalities. At the initial visit, the nurse instructs the woman in the technique of recording BBT on a special form. The woman is instructed to begin a new chart on the first day of every monthly cycle. The temperature can be taken with a standard oral or rectal thermometer calibrated by tenths of a degree, making slight temperature changes readily apparent. A special kind of thermometer (BBT) may be used to measure temperatures only between 35°C and 37.8°C (96°F and 100°F). In addition to the traditional glass and mercury thermometer, tympanic thermometry, which provides a reading in only a few seconds, may also be a valid method. Computerized or digitalized BBT devices ("the Rabbit," Fertil-A-Chron) are being developed to identify the fertile period more accurately at home (Moghissi, 2003).

The woman records daily variations on the temperature graph. The temperature graph shows a typical biphasic pattern during ovulatory cycles, whereas in anovulatory cycles it remains monophasic. The woman uses the readings on the temperature graph to detect ovulation and direct timing of intercourse (Figure 6–2).

Basal temperature for females in the preovulatory phase is usually below 36.7°C (98°F). As ovulation approaches, production of estrogen increases and at its peak may cause a slight drop, then a rise, in the basal temperature. The slight drop in temperature before ovulation is often difficult to capture on the BBT chart. After ovulation there is a surge of luteinizing hormone (LH), which stimulates production of progesterone. Since progesterone is thermogenic (produces heat), it causes a 0.3°C to 0.6°C (0.5°F to 1°F) sustained rise in basal temperature during the second half of the menstrual cycle (luteal phase). Immediately before or coincident with the onset of menses, the temperature falls below 98°F. These changes in the basal temperature create the typical biphasic pattern. Figure 6–2B shows a biphasic ovulatory BBT chart. Temperature elevation does not predict the day

FIGURE 6-2

A

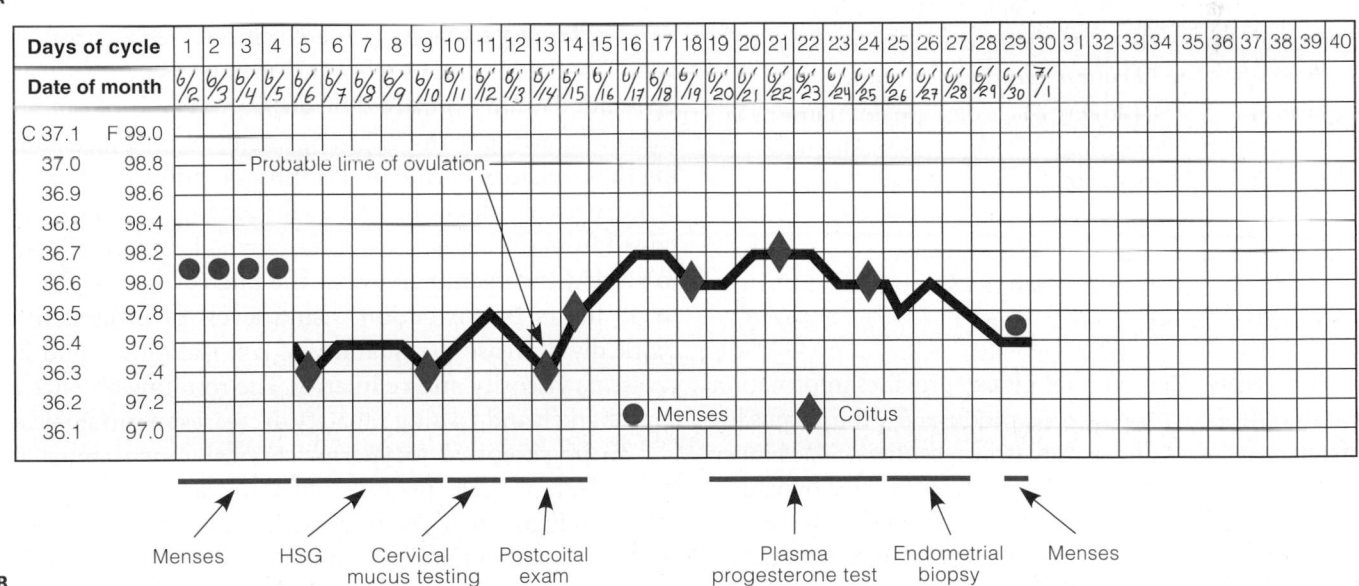

B

A, A monophasic, anovulatory basal body temperature (BBT) chart. **B,** A biphasic BBT chart illustrating probable time of ovulation, the different types of testing, and the time in the cycle that each would be performed.

of ovulation, but it does provide supportive evidence of ovulation about a day after it has occurred. Actual release of the ovum probably occurs 24 to 36 hours before the first temperature elevation (estrogen peak).

Based on serial BBT charts, the clinician might recommend sexual intercourse *every other day* beginning 3 to 4 days prior to and continuing for 2 to 3 days after the expected time of ovulation. (See "Teaching Highlights: Methods of Determining Ovulation.")

Hormonal Assessments of Ovulatory Function. Hormonal assessments of ovulatory function fall into the following categories:

1. **Gonadotropin levels (FSH, LH).** Baseline hormonal assessment of FSH and LH provides valuable information about normal ovulatory function. Measured on cycle day 3, FSH is the single most valuable test of ovarian reserve and function. FSH should always be measured, particularly in women over age 35, to predict the potential for successful treatment with ovulation-induction treatment cycles. LH levels may be measured early in the cycle to rule out androgen excess disorders, which disrupt normal follicular development and oocyte maturation. Daily sampling of LH at midcycle can detect the LH surge. The day of the LH surge is believed to be the day of maximum fertility. Urine LH ovulation prediction kits are also available for home use to better time postcoital testing, insemination, and coitus (Moghissi, 2003).

2. **Progesterone assays.** Progesterone levels furnish the best evidence of ovulation and corpus luteum functioning. Serum levels begin to rise with the LH surge and peak about 8 days later. A level of 3 ng/mL 3 days after the LH surge confirms ovulation (Johnson, 2003). On day 21 (7 days postovulation) a level of 10 ng/mL or higher indicates an adequate luteal phase. Hormonal assessment may also be conducted for prolactin, thyroid-stimulating hormone, and androgen (testosterone, dehydroepiandrosterone [DHEAS], and androstenedione) levels.

Endometrial Biopsy. **Endometrial biopsy** provides information about the effects of progesterone produced by the corpus luteum after ovulation and endometrial receptivity. The biopsy is performed not earlier than 10 to 12 days after ovulation (usually day 22 or 23 of menstrual cycle) and involves removing a sample of endometrium with a small pipette attached to suction (Varney, Kriebs, & Gegor, 2004). The woman should be informed that some pelvic discomfort, cramping, and vaginal spotting are normal during and following the procedure. The onset of menses following biopsy should be disclosed for accurate interpretation of the biopsy report. A dysfunction may exist if the endometrial lining does not show the expected amount of secretory tissue for that day of the woman's menstrual cycle. A repeat biopsy is indicated to confirm luteal phase dysfunction. Serum progesterone assay may also be used in conjunction with endometrial biopsy to confirm luteal phase dysfunction.

Transvaginal Ultrasound. **Transvaginal ultrasound** is the method of choice for follicular monitoring of women undergoing induction cycles, for timing ovulation for insemination and intercourse, for retrieving oocytes for in vitro fertilization, and for monitoring early pregnancy. The use of a transvaginal color flow Doppler to investigate uterine blood flow may in the future help the endocrinologist evaluate the adequacy of the developing follicle, further assess oocyte maturity and endometrial development and patterns, and improve the diagnosis of luteal phase defects (Pierson & Olatunbosum, 2004).

Evaluation of Cervical Factors

The mucous cells of the endocervix consist predominantly of water. As ovulation approaches, the ovary increases its secretion of estrogen and produces changes in the cervical mucus. The amount of mucus increases 10-fold, and the water content rises significantly.

At ovulation, mucus elasticity (**spinnbarkeit**) increases and viscosity decreases. Excellent spinnbarkeit exists when the mucus can be stretched 8 to 10 cm or longer. Mucus elasticity is determined by using two glass slides (see Figure 6–3A ○) or by grasping some mucus at the external os and stretching it through the vagina toward the introitus. (See "Teaching Highlights: Methods of Determining Ovulation.")

The **ferning capacity** (crystallization) (see Figure 6–3B and C) of the cervical mucus also increases as ovulation approaches. Ferning is caused by decreased levels of salt and water interacting with the glycoproteins in the mucus during the ovulatory period and is thus an indirect indication of estrogen production. To test for ferning, mucus is obtained from the cervical os, spread on a glass slide, allowed to air dry, and examined under the microscope. Within 24 to 48 hours postovulation, rising levels of progesterone markedly decrease the quantity of cervical mucus and increase its viscosity and cellularity. The resulting absence of spinnbarkeit and ferning capacity decreases sperm survival.

To be receptive to sperm, cervical mucus must be thin, clear, watery, profuse, alkaline, and acellular. As shown in Figure 6–4 ○, the mazelike microscopic mucoid strands align in a parallel manner to allow for easy sperm passage. The mucus is termed *inhospitable* if these changes do not occur.

Cervical mucus inhospitable to sperm survival can have several causes, some of which are treatable. For example, estrogen secretion may be inadequate for development

TEACHING HIGHLIGHTS

METHODS OF DETERMINING OVULATION

The basal body temperature (BBT) method relies on assessing the woman's temperature pattern. Describe the expected findings with a biphasic ovulatory cycle (see Figure 6–2), and stress the need to monitor BBT for 3 to 4 months to establish a pattern. BBT can be used to time intercourse if pregnancy is desired or as a method of natural family planning. Describe the timing of intercourse to achieve or avoid pregnancy.

Procedure for Measuring BBT

- Using a BBT thermometer, the woman chooses one site (oral, vaginal, or rectal), which she uses consistently.
- The woman takes her temperature for 5 minutes every day before getting out of bed, and before starting any activity, including smoking.
- She then immediately records the result on a special BBT chart, and connects the temperature dots for each day to form a graph.
- She then shakes the thermometer down in preparation for use the next day.

Certain situations can disturb body temperature such as large alcohol intake, sleeplessness, fever, warm climate, jet lag, shift work, or the use of an electric blanket.

Cervical Mucus Method

Cervical mucus characteristics change throughout a woman's menstrual cycle, and the quality of the mucus can be used to predict ovulation (Figure 6–3).

Procedure for Assessing Cervical Mucus Changes

- Every day when she uses the bathroom, the woman checks her vagina, either by dabbing the vaginal opening with toilet paper or by putting a finger in the opening.
- She notes the wetness (presence of mucus), collects some mucus, determines its color and consistency, and records her findings on a chart. For discussion of mucus characteristics, see page 128.
- She washes her hands before and after the procedure.

Stress that the presence and consistency of the mucus are altered by vaginal infection, vaginal medications, spermicides, lubricants, douching, sexual arousal, and semen.

● FIGURE 6–3

A

B

C

A, Spinnbarkeit (elasticity). ***B,*** Ferning pattern. ***C,*** Lack of ferning.

Note (B) Courtesy of Lavena Porter OB/GYN NP. (C) Used with permission from Speroff, L., et al. (1994). Clinical gynecologic endocrinology and infertility (5th ed., p. 818). Baltimore: Williams & Wilkins.

● **FIGURE 6-4**

Sperm passage through cervical mucus. **_A,_** Appearance at the time of ovulation with channels favoring efficient sperm penetration and migration upward. **_B,_** Unfavorable mazelike configuration found at other times during the menstrual cycle.

Used with permission from Corson, S. (1998). Conquering infertility: A guide for couples (4th ed., p. 16). Vancouver, BC: EMIS-Canada.

of receptive mucus. Cone biopsy, electrocautery, or cryosurgery of the cervix may remove large numbers of mucus-producing glands, creating a "dry cervix" that decreases sperm survival. Treatment with clomiphene citrate may have harmful effects on cervical mucus due to its antiestrogenic properties. Therapy with supplemental estrogen for approximately 6 days before expected ovulation encourages the formation of suitable spinnbarkeit. However, intrauterine insemination (IUI) is more often the most appropriate therapy to overcome these obstacles. When mucosal hostility to sperm is due to cervical infection, antimicrobial therapy may be effective.

The cervix can also be the site of secretory immunologic reactions in which antisperm antibodies are produced, causing agglutination or immobilization of sperm. The most widely used serum-sperm bioassay to detect specific classes of antibodies in serum and seminal fluid is immunobead testing (IBT)(Kipersztok, Kim, Morris et al., 2003). The treatment for antisperm antibodies may include intrauterine insemination of the man's washed sperm to bypass the cervical factor.

The **postcoital test**, also called the **Huhner test**, is performed 1 or 2 days before the expected date of ovulation as determined by previous BBT charts, the length of prior cycles, or a urinary LH kit. This examination evaluates the cervical mucus, sperm motility, sperm-mucus interaction, and the sperm's ability to negotiate the cervical mucus barrier. The couple can have intercourse 2 to 8 hours before the examination. If the results are abnormal, the test should be repeated at the optimal time of 2 to 3 hours after intercourse. A small plastic catheter attached to a 10-mL syringe is placed in the cervix. Mucus is aspirated from the endocervical canal, measured, and examined microscopically for signs of infection, spinnbarkeit, ferning, number and

motility of active spermatozoa per high-power field (HPF), and number of sperm with poor or no motility. The focus of the postcoital examination on the timing of intercourse may promote sexual difficulties in some infertile couples.

Evaluation of Uterine Structures and Tubal Patency

Tubal patency tests are usually done after BBT evaluation, semen analysis, and other less invasive tests. Tubal patency and uterine structure are usually evaluated by hysterosalpingography. Other invasive tests of tubular function are laparoscopy and hysteroscopy. Hysteroscopy may be performed earlier in the evaluation if the woman's history suggests possible tubal or adhesive disease or uterine abnormalities.

Hysterosalpingography. **Hysterosalpingography (HSG)**, or hysterogram, involves an instillation of a radiopaque substance into the uterine cavity. As the substance fills the uterus and fallopian tubes and spills into the peritoneal cavity, it is viewed with x-ray techniques. This procedure can reveal tubal patency and any distortions of the uterine cavity. In addition the oil-based dye and injection pressure used in HSG may have a therapeutic effect. This effect may be caused by the flushing of debris, breaking of adhesions, or induction of peristalsis by the instillation.

The HSG should be performed in the proliferative phase of the cycle to avoid interrupting an early pregnancy. This timing also avoids the lush secretory changes in the endometrium that occur after ovulation, which may prevent the passage of the dye through the tubes and present a false picture of cornual obstruction. HSG causes moderate discomfort. The pain is referred from the peritoneum (which is irritated by the subdiaphragmatic collection of gas) to the shoulder. The cramping may be decreased if the radiopaque dye is warmed to body temperature before instillation. Women can take an over-the-counter prostaglandin synthesis inhibitor (such as ibuprofen) 30 minutes before the procedure to decrease the pain, cramping, and discomfort. HSG can also cause recurrence of pelvic inflammatory disease, so prophylactic antibiotics are recommended to prevent infection that could be triggered by the procedure (Johnson, 2003).

Hysteroscopy. *Hysteroscopy* allows the physician to further evaluate any areas of suspicion within the uterine cavity or fallopian tubes revealed by the HSG. It is often done in conjunction with a laparoscopy, but it can be done independently and does not require general anesthesia. A fiberoptic instrument is inserted into the uterus for further evaluation of polyps, fibroids, or structural variations (Johnson, 2003).

Laparoscopy. **Laparoscopy** enables direct visualization of the pelvic organs and is usually done 6 to 8 months after the HSG unless symptoms suggest the need for earlier evaluation. Diagnostic laparoscopy is an outpatient procedure requiring the use of general anesthesia. Generally a three-puncture approach is used; entry is made through the umbilical area, and supporting instruments are inserted in two suprapubic incisions. The peritoneal cavity is distended with carbon dioxide gas so that the pelvic organs can be directly visualized with a fiberoptic instrument. Tube patency can be assessed by instillation of dye into the uterine cavity through the cervix. The pelvis is evaluated for endometriosis, adhesions, organ fixations, pelvic inflammatory disease, tumors, and cysts. The intraperitoneal gas is usually manually expressed at the end of the procedure. In routine preanesthesia instructions, the woman is told that she may have some discomfort from organ displacement and shoulder and chest pain caused by gas in the abdomen. She should be informed that she can resume normal activities as tolerated after 24 hours. Using postoperative pain medication and assuming a supine position may help relieve discomfort caused by any remaining gas.

ASSESSMENT OF THE MAN'S FERTILITY

If the man's history indicates the need, he may be referred to a urologist for testing. A semen analysis of sperm quality, quantity, and motility is the single most important initial diagnostic study of the man. It should be done early in the couple's evaluation, before invasive testing of the woman. Although a postcoital test can provide information about sperm viability, it does not provide sufficient information about normal seminal parameters.

To obtain adequate results, the specimen is collected after 2 to 3 days of abstinence, usually by masturbation to avoid contamination or loss of any ejaculate. If the man has difficulty producing sperm by masturbation, special medical-grade condoms are available to collect the sperm during intercourse. Regular latex and nonlatex condoms should not be used, because they contain agents that impair the motility of sperm, and sperm can be lost in the condom (Hopps & Schlegel, 2003). Most lubricants also are spermicidal and should not be used unless approved by the andrology laboratory.

Both seasonal and incidental variability may be seen in count and motility in successive semen analyses from the same person. Thus, a repeat semen analysis may be required to assess the man's fertility potential adequately; a minimum of two separate analyses is recommended for confirmation. In cases in which a known testicular insult has occurred (infection, high fevers, or surgery), a repeat analysis may not be done for at least 2.5 months to allow for new sperm maturation.

Sperm analysis provides information about sperm motility and morphology and a determination of the absolute number of spermatozoa present (Table 6–4). Although low numbers and motility may indicate compromised fertility, other parameters, such as morphology, motion patterns, and

TABLE 6–4 ✤ **Normal Semen Analysis**	
Factor	**Value**
Volume	> 2 mL
pH	7 to 8
Total sperm count	> 20 million/mL
Liquefaction	Complete in 1 hour
Motility	50% or greater forward progression
Normal forms	30% or greater
Round cells	< 5 million/mL
White cells	< 1 million/mL

Courtesy of the World Health Organization. (1993). *The WHO laboratory manual for the examination of human semen and sperm-cervical mucus interaction* (3rd ed.). Geneva, Switzerland: Author.

progression, are important prognostic indicators. Values previously thought to indicate subfertility may in fact be compatible with normal fertility when morphology, motion patterns, and progression factors are considered. An infertile specimen is one that has fewer than 20 million sperm per milliliter, less than 50% motility at 6 hours, or less than 30% normal sperm forms (Hassan & Killick, 2003). Some studies have indicated that the quality of sperm decreases with increased age. For example, fathers older than 50 years have infants at increased risk for trisomy.

A variety of environmental factors can affect male fertility. Causes of increased scrotal heat, such as jockey shorts, hot tubs, or occupations requiring long hours of sitting, are thought to decrease fertility potential, but there are no clinical studies to substantiate this belief. Heavy use of marijuana, alcohol, or cocaine within 2 years of testing can depress sperm count and testosterone levels; cigarette smoking may depress sperm motility (Zitzmann, Rolf, Nordoff et al., 2003). Neurologic ejaculatory dysfunction can be associated with the use of drugs such as alpha-blockers, for example: phentolamine, methyldopa, guanethidine, and reserpine. Lead and pesticide exposure can also reduce sperm count (Hopps & Schlegel, 2003).

Spermatozoa have been shown to possess intrinsic antigens that can provoke male immunologic infertility. Immunologic infertility is especially apparent following vasectomy reversals or genital trauma, such as testicular torsion, in which autoimmunity to sperm (the man produces antibodies to his sperm) develops. Research indicates that it is the actual presence of antibodies on the spermatozoal surface (not just the presence of antibodies in the serum) that affects sperm function and thus leads to subfertility. Antisperm antibodies can be screened for by the immunobead binding test (Kipersztok, Kim, Morris et al., 2003). Treatment for antisperm antibodies is directed toward preventing the formation of antibodies or arresting the underlying mechanism that compromises sperm function. Therapies such as immunosuppression with corticosteroids have not proved effective. The treatment of choice for clinically significant antisperm antibodies is in vitro fertilization or intrauterine insemination.

METHODS OF INFERTILITY MANAGEMENT

Methods of managing infertility include pharmacologic agents, therapeutic insemination, in vitro fertilization, and other assisted reproductive techniques.

Pharmacologic Agents

The pharmacologic treatments chosen depend on the specific cause of infertility.

Clomiphene Citrate. If a woman has normal ovaries, a normal prolactin level, and an intact pituitary gland, *clomiphene*

citrate (Clomid or Serophene) is often used (see "Drug Guide: Clomiphene Citrate" on page 134). This medication induces ovulation in 80% of women by actions at both the hypothalamic and ovarian levels; 40% of these women will become pregnant. Approximately 8% of women develop multiple-gestation pregnancies, almost exclusively twins (Johnson, 2003). Clomid works by stimulating the hypothalamus to secrete more GnRH, which increases the secretion of LH and FSH. These stimulate follicular growth and facilitate the release of ova.

The woman can assess the presence of ovulation and possible response to clomiphene citrate therapy by doing BBT and urinary LH tests. The woman should be knowledgeable about side effects and call her healthcare provider if they occur. When visual disturbances (flashes, blurring, or spots) occur, bright lighting should be avoided. This side effect disappears within a few days or weeks after discontinuation of therapy. Hot flashes may be due to the antiestrogenic properties of clomiphene citrate. The woman can obtain some relief by increasing intake of fluids and using fans.

Human Menopausal Gonadotropins. Therapy using *human menopausal gonadotropins (hMG)*, which include *menotropins* (Pergonal, Humegon, and Repronex) and *urofollitropin* (Fertinex), is indicated as a first line of therapy for anovulatory infertile women with low to normal levels of gonadotropins (FSH and LH) and as a second line of therapy in women who fail to ovulate or conceive with clomiphene citrate therapy and in women undergoing assisted reproduction to induce superovulation. Menotropin is a combination of FSH and LH, and urofollitropin is a further purified form and contains only FSH. Because hMG is inactive, it must be given by intramuscular injection. Immediately prior to injection, the powder is reconstituted with diluent. Recombinant FSH is available which is homogenous and free of contaminants by proteins (unlike urinary menotropins) and thus allows for subcutaneous administration. Preparations using recombinant LH are now being tested.

Gonadotropin therapy requires close observation by use of serum estradiol levels and ultrasound. Monitoring of follicle development is necessary to minimize the risk of multiple pregnancy and to avoid ovarian hyperstimulation. The daily dose of medication given is titrated based on serum estradiol and ultrasound findings. When follicle maturation has occurred, human chorionic gonadotropin (hCG) may be administered by intramuscular injection to stimulate ovulation. The couple is advised to have intercourse 24 to 36 hours after hCG administration and for the next 2 days. Women who elect to have hMG medication usually have passed through all other forms of management without conceiving. Strong emotional support and

EVIDENCE-BASED NURSING

ORAL (ANTIESTROGENS) VERSUS INJECTABLE (GONADOTROPINS) OVULATION STIMULANTS FOR TREATMENT OF SUBFERTILITY

Problem

A diagnosis of *unexplained subfertility* is assigned to couples with normal results on a standard infertility workup. Some women with documented ovulation may experience subtle defects in ovulatory function that are not detected by standard tests. The rationale for treating these women with superovulation is that it may overcome such subtle defects or that by increasing the number of eggs available, the likelihood of pregnancy is increased. Couples who are unresponsive to clomiphene or with unexplained infertility usually respond to stimulation with human gonadotropins, which have been routinely administered by either intramuscular or subcutaneous injections.

Evidence

Three gynecologists conducted a systematic review of randomized controlled trials comparing the effectiveness of oral versus injectable ovulation stimulants for the treatment of unexplained subfertility. Both desirable and detrimental outcomes were evaluated. Five high-quality randomized controlled trials representing 231 couples with unexplained subfertility were reviewed as a basis for conclusions. The evidence suggests that oral agents are neither inferior nor superior to injectable agents in the treatment of unexplained subfertility (Athaullah, Proctor, & Johnson, 2003). Information about the harm of each type of agent was less definitive. More research is needed to clearly identify the relative risks of oral versus injectable ovulation stimulants.

Implications

There was not a significant difference in the chances of a pregnancy and successful live birth when oral agents were compared to injectable agents for the treatment of unexplained subfertility. Detrimental outcomes miscarriage, ovarian hyperstimulation syndrome, and discontinued cycles—were also statistically the same between the two types of agents. There was no difference in the rate of multiple births.

The choice of an ovulation stimulant is based on a thorough assessment of the reasons for subfertility. However, when the fertility problem is unexplained, you can counsel couples that oral agents have been demonstrated to be as effective as injectable agents in producing desired outcomes and avoiding detrimental ones. Injections may be difficult to obtain, so oral agents may provide a more convenient treatment regimen for the subfertile couple.

Critical Thinking

After reading the full article cited below, review the indications for each type of ovulation induction agent. In which cases are oral agents inappropriate? What assessments would differentiate subfertility—for which these agents appear equally effective—from infertility?

Reference

Athaullah, N., Proctor, M., & Johnson, N. P. (2003). Oral versus injectable ovulation induction agents for unexplained subfertility (Cochrane Review). *The Cochrane Library, 4,* Chichester, UK: John Wiley & Sons.

---

thorough education are needed because of the numerous office visits and injections. Often the male partner is instructed, with return demonstration, to administer the daily injections.

Bromocriptine. High prolactin levels may impair the glandular production of FSH and LH or block their action on the ovaries. When hyperprolactinemia accompanies anovulation, the infertility may be treated with *bromocriptine* (Parlodel). This medication acts directly on the prolactin-secreting cells in the anterior pituitary. It inhibits the pituitary's secretion of prolactin, thus preventing suppression of the pulsatile secretion of FSH and LH. Thus, normal menstrual cycles are restored and ovulation is induced by allowing FSH and LH production. If treatment is successful, the tests of ovulatory function will indicate that ovulation is occurring with a normal luteal phase. Bromocriptine should be discontinued if pregnancy is suspected or at the anticipated time of ovulation because of its possible teratogenic effects. Side effects include nausea, diarrhea, dizziness, headache, and fatigue, which can be attributed to the dopaminergic action of bromocriptine. To minimize side effects for women who are extremely sensitive, treatment may be initiated with a

dose of 1.25 mg, slowly building tolerance toward the usual dose of 2.5 mg given twice daily. An intravaginal preparation may also be used to decrease the occurrence of side effects (Johnson, 2003).

Other Pharmacologic Agents. Pharmacologic treatments for endometriosis-related infertility use danazol (Danocrine), oral contraceptives or oral medroxyprogesterone acetate, and gonadotropin-releasing hormone (GnRH) agonists. (See Chapter 5 for more information on the management and care of endometriosis. ∞) Treatment of luteal phase defects may include the use of progesterone to augment luteal phase progesterone levels. Ovulation induction agents, such as clomiphene citrate or menotropins, may be used to augment proliferative phase FSH production in the developing follicle, as women with luteal phase defects have been found to have decreased FSH production in the proliferative phase. This is associated with a decline in luteal phase progesterone and estrogen production and is manifested by an out-of-phase endometrial biopsy. It is also common to use progesterone supplementation in conjunction with these ovulation induction agents if the drug alone does not correct the luteal phase. Occasionally, hCG therapy may be used in the luteal phase to stimulate corpus luteum production of progesterone.

DRUG GUIDE

CLOMIPHENE CITRATE (CLOMID, MILOPHENE, SEROPHENE) PREGNANCY CATEGORY: X

Overview of Action
Clomid stimulates follicular growth by stimulating the release of FSH and LH. Ovulation is expected to occur 5 to 9 days after the last dose. Used when anovulation is caused by hypothalamic dysfunction, luteal phase dysfunction, or oligo-ovulation, and for in vitro fertilization protocols.

Route, Dosage, Frequency
Administered orally. First course: 50 mg/day for 5 days; start on fifth day of cycle following start of spontaneous or induced bleeding (with progestin) or at any time in a woman who has had no recent uterine bleeding (Wilson, Shannon, & Stang, 2005). If ovulation does not occur, a second course of 100 mg/day for 5 days should be given. If ovulation does not occur after 3 courses of therapy, further treatment is not recommended and the woman should be reevaluated.

Contraindications
Presence of ovarian enlargement, polycystic ovary syndrome, liver disease, visual problems, pregnancy.

Interactions: Herbal: Black cohosh may antagonize infertility treatments (Wilson et al., 2005).

Side Effects
Antiestrogenic effects may cause decrease in cervical mucus production and endometrial lining development. Other side effects include vasomotor flushes; abdominal distention and ovarian enlargement secondary to follicular growth (bloating) and multiple corpus luteum formation; pain, soreness, breast discomfort; nausea and vomiting, visual symptoms (spots, flashes); headaches; dryness or loss of hair; multiple pregnancies.

Nursing Considerations
Determine if couple has been advised to have sexual intercourse every other day for 1 week beginning 5 days after the last day of medications.

Instruct the couple on use of the BBT chart to assess whether ovulation has occurred, or instruct on the use of urinary LH kits to predict the onset of LH surge. Also inform couple that ultrasound, plasma progesterone, and postcoital test may be done. Remind couples that if the woman does not have a period, she must be checked for the possibility of pregnancy before another trial of Clomid is started.

Therapeutic Insemination

Therapeutic insemination has replaced the previously used term *artificial insemination* and involves depositing semen at the cervical os or in the uterus by mechanical means. *Therapeutic donor insemination (TDI)* is the current term for use of donor semen, and *therapeutic husband insemination (THI)* is the current term for use of the husband's semen.

THI is generally indicated for such seminal deficiencies as oligospermia (low sperm count), asthenospermia (decreased motility), and teratospermia (low percentage, abnormal morphology); for anatomic defects accompanied by inadequate deposition or penetration of semen such as hy-pospadias (congenital abnormal male urethral opening on the underside of the penis); and for ejaculatory dysfunction, such as retrograde ejaculation (Kakarla & Bradshaw, 2003). THI is also indicated in cases of unexplained infertility and some cases of female factor infertility, such as scant or inhospitable mucus, persistent cervicitis, or cervical stenosis. IUI, with or without ovulation induction therapy, is an option for many couples before more aggressive treatments such as in vitro fertilization are employed.

TDI is considered in cases of azoospermia (absence of sperm), severe oligospermia or asthenospermia, inherited male sex-linked disorders, and autosomal dominant disorders. In the past several years, indications for donor insemination have expanded to include single women or lesbians desirous of pregnancy. Some states have specified the parental rights of single women and donors, but most are silent on the issue. Seminal fluid contains high levels of prostaglandins, which can cause nausea, severe cramps, abdominal pain, and diarrhea when absorbed by the uterine lining. Therefore, sperm preparation for IUI involves washing sperm from the seminal plasma.

Intra Cytoplasmic sperm injection (ICSI), microsurgical epididymal sperm aspiration (MESA), percutaneous epididymal sperm aspiration (PESA), and testicular sperm aspiration (TESA) are procedures that address severe male factor infertility. ICSI is a microscopic procedure to inject a single sperm into the outer layer of an ovum so that fertilization will occur. MESA, PESA, and TESA involve the retrieval of sperm from the gonadal tissue of men who have azoospermia (Figure 6–5 ●). PESA and TESA are replacing MESA as the preferred techniques for retrieval of sperm because they are not surgical procedures.

TDI has become more complicated and expensive in the past decade because of the need for strict screening and processing procedures to prevent transmission of a genetic defect or sexually transmitted infection to the offspring or recipient. Guidelines have been established that include mandatory medical (genetic) and infectious disease screening of both donor and recipient, the need for informed consent from all parties, the need to limit the number of pregnancies per donor, and the need for accurate means of record keeping. Because of the risk of transmitting infectious diseases, donated sperm must be frozen and quarantined for 6 months from the time of acquisition, and the donor must be retested before sperm can be released for use.

Numerous factors need to be evaluated before TDI is performed. Has every possible effort been made to diagnose and treat the cause of the male infertility? Do tests indicate normal fertility and sperm-ovum transport in the woman? Has the couple discussed this option with an infertility counselor to explore the issues of secrecy, disclosure, and potential feelings of loss the couple (particularly the male

FIGURE 6–5

Assisted reproductive techniques.

partner) may feel about not having a genetic child? Are there any religious constraints? After making the decision, the couple should allow themselves time to further access their concerns and explore their feelings individually and together to ensure that this option is acceptable to both.

In Vitro Fertilization

The **in vitro fertilization (IVF)** procedure is selectively used in cases in which infertility has resulted from tubal factors, mucus abnormalities, male infertility, unexplained infertility, male and female immunologic infertility, and cervical factors. In IVF a woman's eggs are collected from her ovaries, fertilized in the laboratory, and placed into her uterus after normal embryo development has begun. If the procedure is successful, the embryo continues to develop in the uterus, and pregnancy proceeds naturally.

The potential for a successful pregnancy with IVF is maximized when three to four embryos (rather than one) are placed in the uterus. For this reason, fertility drugs are used to induce ovulation prior to the process. Follicular development and oocyte maturity are monitored frequently with ultra-

sound and hormonal assays. Monitoring usually begins around cycle day 5, and medications are titrated according to individual response. When follicles appear mature, hCG is given to stimulate final egg maturation and control the induction of ovulation. Egg retrieval is performed approximately 35 hours later on an outpatient basis. Once the eggs are fertilized and progress to the embryo stage, the embryos are placed in the uterus. After the procedure the woman is advised to engage in only minimal activity for 12 to 24 hours, and progesterone supplementation is prescribed.

Success with IVF depends on many factors, but especially the woman's age and the specific indication. Women have a good chance of achieving pregnancy with an average of three cycles of IVF. Many couples find the emotional, physical, and financial costs of going beyond three cycles too great. Clinical birth rates reported by the Society of Assisted Reproductive Technology (SART) in 1999 were 31.1% per embryo transfer for women regardless of age or indication (American Society for Reproductive Medicine, 2002). The increase in maternal and neonatal morbidity associated with IVF because of the rates of multiple gestation remains an issue. Differences in transfer (TET). In these procedures eggs are retrieved and incubated with the man's sperm. However, the eggs are transferred back to the woman's body at a much earlier stage of cell division than in IVF and, as in GIFT, are placed in the fallopian tube or tubes and not the uterus. In TET the placement is done at the embryo stage. These procedures allow fertilization to be documented, which is not possible with GIFT, and the pregnancy rate is theoretically increased when the fertilized ovum is placed in the fallopian tube.

When considering IVF and the transfer procedures, several factors must be weighed. IVF success rates approximate those that have been achieved with the GIFT procedure, and IVF is a much less invasive and costly procedure. For these reasons, GIFT and other tubal procedures have lost some acceptance and IVF techniques are more often used. However, GIFT may be more acceptable to adherents of some religions, since fertilization does not occur outside the woman's body.

Several new reproductive technologies can help families with genetic problems or infertile women who are unable to carry a pregnancy. The diagnosis of genetic disorders via *blastomere analysis* before implantation gives couples the option of forgoing the attempt to establish a pregnancy and thereby avoiding a difficult decision about terminating an affected pregnancy (Simpson, 2002). *Assisted embryo hatching* is a micromanipulation procedure that has proved to be an effective adjunct therapy in IVF (Zhang & Xu, 2003). IVF using a *gestational surrogacy* allows infertile women who are genetically sound but unable to carry a pregnancy to exercise the option of having their own biologic child. Other technologies involve oocyte donation and cryopreservation of the embryo.

successful IVF may exist between various ethnic groups (Sharara & McClamrock, 2000).

Other Assisted Reproductive Techniques

Other assisted reproductive techniques include procedures for transfer of gametes, zygotes, or embryos; cryopreservation of embryos; IVF using donor oocytes; micromanipulation techniques; and use of a gestational surrogacy as described later in this chapter (Kashyap & Davis, 2003).

Gamete intrafallopian transfer (GIFT) involves the retrieval of oocytes by laparoscopy; immediate placement of the oocytes in a catheter with washed, motile sperm; and placement of the gametes into the fimbriated end of the fallopian tube. Fertilization occurs in the fallopian tube as with normal conception (in vivo) rather than in the laboratory (in vitro). The fertilized egg then travels through the fallopian tube to the uterus for implantation as in normal reproduction.

From the GIFT technology evolved procedures such as **zygote intrafallopian transfer (ZIFT)** and **tubal embryo**

Adoption

Infertile couples consider various alternatives for resolving their infertility; adoption is one option that will be considered at several points during the treatment process. As couples begin to consider adoption, an important aspect of this exploration is reading magazines, books, and informational Web sites, such as the National Adoption Information Clearinghouse; attending adoption support groups and conferences; and meeting with adoptive parents to discuss their experiences with adoption.

The adoption of an infant in the United States can be difficult and frustrating, often involving long waiting periods, continued setbacks, and high costs. Thus, many couples seek international adoption or consider adopting older children, children with disabilities, or children of mixed parentage because the adoption process in such cases is quicker and more children are available. Nurses in the community can assist couples considering adoption by providing information on community resources for adoption and support through the adoption process. Couples need support if they remain or choose to be childless. Informational books, Web sites such as Childless by Choice, and support groups such as San Francisco RESOLVE's "living without children" are available to those who remain or choose to be childless.

Pregnancy after Infertility

The feeling of being infertile does not necessarily disappear with pregnancy. Although there may be initial ecstasy, couples may face a whole new arena of fear and anxiety, and the parents-to-be often do not know where they "fit in." They may feel a great sense of isolation because those who have had no trouble conceiving cannot relate to the physical and emotional pain they endured to achieve the pregnancy. Contact with their past support system of other infertile couples may vanish when peers learn they have resolved their infertility problems. Although the desperation to become pregnant may have superseded the couple's ability to acknowledge their concerns about undergoing various treatments or procedures, questions about the repeated cycle of fertility drugs or the achievement of pregnancy through IVF technology or cryopreservation may now arise. The expectant couple may be very concerned about the potential of these treatments to adversely affect the fetus (Johnson, 2003). Couples may need reassurance throughout the pregnancy to allay these anxieties. The nurse can assist couples who conceive after infertility by acknowledging their past experiences of infertility treatment; validating their fears and anxieties as they face childbirth classes, birth, and parenting issues; and providing support and education about what to anticipate physically and emotionally throughout the pregnancy. These interventions will go a long way toward normalizing the experience for the couple.

NURSING MANAGEMENT

Infertility therapy taxes a couple's financial, physical, and emotional resources. Treatment can be costly, and often insurance coverage is limited. Years of effort and numerous evaluations and examinations may take place before conception occurs, if it occurs at all. In a society that values children and considers them to be the natural result of marriage, infertile couples face a myriad of tensions and discrimination.

Clinic nurses need to be constantly aware of the emotional needs of the couple confronting infertility evaluation and treatment. Often an intact marriage will become stressed with intrusive infertility procedures and treatments. Constant attention to temperature charts and instructions about their sex life from a person outside the relationship naturally affect the spontaneity of a couple's interactions.

Tests and treatments may heighten feelings of frustration or anger between partners. The need to share this intimate area of a relationship, especially when one or the other

is identified as "the cause" of infertility, may precipitate feelings of guilt or shame. Infertility often becomes a central focus for role identity, especially for women (Klock, 2004).

The couples may experience feelings of loss of control, feelings of reduced competency and defectiveness, loss of status and ambiguity as a couple, a sense of social stigma, stress on the marital and sexual relationship, and strained relationships with healthcare providers. The nurse's role can be summarized as that of counselor, educator, and advocate.

Tasks of the infertile couple and appropriate nursing interventions are summarized in Table 6–5. Throughout the evaluation process, nurses play a key role in lessening the stress these couples must endure by providing resources and accurate information about what is entailed in treatment and what physical, emotional, and financial demands the couple can anticipate throughout the process (Klock, 2004).

The nurse's ability to assess and respond to emotional and educational needs is essential to give infertile couples a sense of control (Hammond, 2001). An assessment tool such as an infertility questionnaire (Table 6–6) may be helpful. Extensive and repeated explanations and written instruction may be necessary because the couple's anxiety often overwhelms their ability to retain all the information given. It is important to use a nursing framework that recognizes the multidimensional needs of the infertile individual or couple within physical, social, psychologic, spiritual, and environmental contexts.

Infertility may be perceived as a loss by one or both partners. Affected individuals have described this as loss of their relationship with spouse, family, or friends; their health; their status or prestige; their self-esteem and self-confidence; their security; and the potential child. One such loss alone may lead to depression, but in many cases

TABLE 6–5 ✤ Tasks of the Infertile Couple

Tasks	Nursing Interventions
Recognize how infertility affects their lives and express feelings (may be negative toward self or mate)	Supportive: help to understand and facilitate free expression of feelings
Grieve the loss of potential offspring	Help to recognize feelings
Evaluate reasons for wanting a child	Help to understand motives
Decide about management	Identify alternatives; facilitate partner communication

Used with permission from Sawatzky, M. (1981). Tasks of the infertile couple. *Journal of Obstetric, Gynecologic, and Neonatal Nursing, 10,* 132.

TABLE 6–6 ❖ Infertility Questionnaire

Self-Image

1. I feel bad about my body because of our inability to have a child.
2. Since our infertility, I feel I can do anything as well as I used to.
3. I feel as attractive as before our infertility.
4. I feel less masculine/feminine because of our inability to have a child.
5. Compared with others, I feel I am a worthwhile person.
6. Lately, I feel I am sexually attractive to my wife/husband.
7. I feel I will be incomplete as a man/woman if we cannot have a child.
8. Having an infertility problem makes me feel physically incompetent.

Guilt/Blame

1. I feel guilty about somehow causing our infertility.
2. I wonder if our infertility problem is due to something I did in the past.
3. My spouse makes me feel guilty about our problem.
4. There are times when I blame my spouse for our infertility.
5. I feel I am being punished because of our infertility.

Sexuality

1. Lately, I feel I am able to respond to my spouse sexually.
2. I feel sex is a duty, not a pleasure.
3. Since our infertility problem, I enjoy sexual relations with my spouse.
4. We have sexual relations for the purpose of trying to conceive.
5. Sometimes I feel like a "sex machine," programmed to have sex during the fertile period.
6. Impaired fertility has helped our sexual relationship.
7. Our inability to have a child has increased my desire for sexual relations.
8. Our inability to have a child has decreased my desire for sexual relations.

Note: The questionnaire is scored on a Likert scale, with responses ranging from "strongly agree" to "strongly disagree." Each question is scored separately, and the mean score is determined for each section (Self-Image, Guilt/Blame, and Sexuality). The total mean score is then divided by 3. A final mean score of greater than 3 indicates distress.

Used with permission from Bernstein, J., Potts, N., & Mattox, J. H., (1985). Assessment of psychological dysfunction associated with infertility. *Journal of Obstetric, Gynecologic, and Neonatal Nursing, 14* (Suppl.), 64S, Table 1. Washington, DC: Author. © 1985 by the Association of Women's Health, Obstetric and Neonatal Nurses. All rights reserved.

the crisis of infertility evokes feelings of all these losses (Klock, 2004). Each couple passes through several stages of feelings, not unlike those identified by Kübler-Ross: surprise, denial, anger, isolation, guilt, grief, and resolution.

The impact of these feelings on the couple and how fast they move into resolution, if ever, may depend on the cause and on the duration of treatment. Each partner may progress through the stages at different rates (Klock, 2004). Nonjudgmental acceptance and a professional, caring attitude on the nurse's part can go far in dissipating the negative emotions the couple may experience while going through these stages.

This is also a time when the nurse may assess the couple's relationship: Are both partners able and willing to communicate verbally and share feelings? Are the partners mutually supportive? The answers to such questions may help the nurse to identify areas of strength and weakness and to construct an appropriate plan of care.

Referral to mental health professionals is helpful when the emotional issues become too disruptive in the couple's relationship or life. The couple should be aware of infertility support and education organizations such as RESOLVE (National Infertility Association), which may help meet some of their needs and validate their feelings. Finally, individual or group counseling with other infertile couples may help the couple resolve feelings brought about by their own difficult situation.

GENETIC DISORDERS

Even when conception has been achieved, families can have special reproductive concerns. The desired and expected outcome of any pregnancy is the birth of a healthy, "perfect" baby. Parents experience grief, fear, and anger when they discover that their baby has been born with a defect or a genetic disease. Such an abnormality may be evident at birth or may not appear for some time. The baby may have inherited a disorder from one parent, or both, creating guilt and strife within the family.

Regardless of the type or scope of the problem, parents will have many questions: "What did I do?" "What caused it?" "Will it happen again?" The nurse must anticipate the couple's questions and concerns and guide, direct, and support the family. To do so, the nurse must have a basic knowledge of genetics and genetic counseling. Professional nurses can help expedite this questioning process if they understand the principles involved and can direct the family to the appropriate resources.

CHROMOSOMES AND CHROMOSOMAL ANALYSIS

All hereditary material is carried on tightly coiled strands of DNA known as **chromosomes**. The chromosomes carry the *genes,* the smallest units of inheritance (see Chapter 7 for more information ∞). The *Human Genome Project* has made remarkable advances toward determining the exact DNA sequence of the human gene and the precise genes that are associated with certain abnormalities such as fragile X syndrome and cystic fibrosis, as discussed in greater detail later in this chapter (Prosen & Hogge, 2004).

All *somatic (body) cells* contain 46 chromosomes, which is the *diploid* number; the sperm and egg contain 23 chromosomes, or the *haploid* number (see Chapter 7 for more information ∞). There are 23 pairs of homologous chromosomes (a matched pair of chromosomes, one inherited from each parent); 22 of the pairs are **autosomes** (nonsex chromosomes), and one pair is made up of the sex chromosomes, X and Y. A normal female has a 46,XX chromosome constitution; a normal male has a 46,XY chromosome constitution (Figures 6–6 ⊙ and 6–7 ⊙).

The **karyotype**, or pictorial analysis of these chromosomes, is usually obtained from specially treated and stained peripheral blood lymphocytes. Placental tissue taken from a site near the insertion of the cord and deep enough to include chorion can also be sent for karyotyping of the fetus.

⊙ **FIGURE 6–6**

Normal female karyotype.

Courtesy of David Peakman, Reproductive Genetics Center, Denver, CO.

⊙ **FIGURE 6–7**

Normal male karyotype.

Courtesy of David Peakman, Reproductive Genetics Center, Denver, CO.

Chromosomal abnormalities can occur in either the autosomes or the sex chromosomes and can be divided into two categories: abnormalities of number and abnormalities of structure. Even small alterations in chromosomes can cause problems, especially those associated with delayed growth and development. Because some of these problems can be passed on to other offspring, in many cases chromosomal analysis is appropriate even if clinical manifestations are mild.

Abnormalities of Chromosome Number

Abnormalities of chromosome number are most commonly seen as trisomies, monosomies, and mosaicism. In all three cases, the abnormality is most often caused by nondisjunction, a failure of paired chromosomes to separate during cell division. If nondisjunction occurs in either the sperm or the egg before fertilization, the resulting zygote (fertilized egg) will have an abnormal chromosome makeup in all of the cells (trisomy or monosomy). If nondisjunction occurs after fertilization, the developing zygote will have cells with two or more different chromosome makeups, evolving into two or more different cell lines (mosaicism).

Trisomies are the product of the union of a normal gamete (egg or sperm) with a gamete that contains an extra chromosome. The individual will have 47 chromosomes and is trisomic (has three copies of the same chromosome) for whichever chromosome is extra (Table 6–7). Down syndrome (formerly called mongolism) is the most common trisomy abnormality seen in children (Figure 6–8 ⊙). The presence of the extra chromosome 21 produces distinctive clinical features (Figure 6–9 ⊙). Although children born with Down syndrome have a variety of physical ailments, advances in medical science have extended their life expectancy.

Two other common trisomies are trisomy 18 and trisomy 13. The prognosis for both trisomies 13 and 18 is extremely poor. Most children (70%) die within the first 3 months of life secondary to complications related to respiratory and cardiac abnormalities. However, 10% survive the first year of life; therefore, the family needs to plan for the possibility of long-term care of a severely affected infant and for family support.

Monosomies occur when a normal gamete unites with a gamete that is missing a chromosome. In this case the individual has only 45 chromosomes and is said to be monosomic. Monosomy of an entire autosomal chromosome is incompatible with life.

Mosaicism occurs after fertilization and results in an individual who has two different cell lines, each with a different chromosomal number. Mosaicism tends to be more common in the sex chromosomes than in the autosomes; when it occurs in the autosomes, it is most common in those with Down syndrome. A person with many classic signs of

TABLE 6–7 ✛ **Chromosomal Syndromes**

Altered Chromosome: 21	Characteristics
Genetic defect: trisomy 21 (Down syndrome) (secondary nondisjunction or 14/21 unbalanced translocation) Incidence: average 1 in 700 live births, incidence variable with age of woman (Figure 6-9)	Central nervous system (CNS): mental retardation; hypotonia at birth Head: flattened occiput; depressed nasal bridge; mongoloid slant of eyes; epicanthal folds; white specking of the iris (Brushfield spots); protrusion of the tongue; high, arched palate; low-set ears Hands: broad, short fingers; abnormalities of finger and foot; dermal ridge patterns (dermatoglyphics); transverse palmar crease (simian line) Other: congenital heart disease

Altered Chromosome: 18	Characteristics
Genetic defect: trisomy 18 Incidence: 1 in 3,000 live births	CNS: mental retardation; severe hypotonia Head: prominent occiput; low-set ears; corneal opacities; ptosis (drooping eyelids) Hands: third and fourth fingers overlapped by second and fifth fingers; abnormal dermatoglyphics; syndactyly (webbing of fingers) Other: congenital heart defects; renal abnormalities; single umbilical artery; gastrointestinal tract abnormalities; rocker-bottom feet; cryptorchidism; various malformations of other organs

Altered Chromosome: 13	Characteristics
Genetic defect: trisomy 13 Incidence: 1 in 5,000 live births	CNS: mental retardation; severe hypotonia; seizures Head: microcephaly; microphthalmia and/or coloboma (keyhole-shaped pupil); malformed ears; aplasia of external auditory canal; micrognathia (abnormally small lower jaw); cleft lip and palate Hands: polydactyly (extra digits); abnormal posturing of fingers; abnormal dermatoglyphics Other: congenital heart defects; hemangiomas; gastrointestinal tract defects; various malformations of other organs

Altered Chromosome: 5P	Characteristics
Genetic defect deletion of short arm of chromosome 5 (cri du chat, or cat cry syndrome) Incidence: 1 in 20,000 live births	CNS: severe mental retardation; a catlike cry in infancy Head: microcephaly; hypertelorism (widely spaced eyes); epicanthal folds; low-set ears Other: failure to thrive; various organ malformations

Altered Chromosome: XO (Sex Chromosome)	Characteristics
Genetic defect: only one X chromosome in female (Turner syndrome) Incidence: 1 in 300–7,000 live female births (Figure 6-10)	CNS: no intellectual impairment; some perceptual difficulties Head: low hairline; webbed neck Trunk: short stature; cubitus valgus (increased carrying angle of arm); excessive nevi (congenital discoloration of skin due to pigmentation); broad, shieldlike chest with widely spaced nipples; puffy feet; no toenails Other: fibrous streaks in ovaries; underdeveloped secondary sex characteristics; primary amenorrhea; usually infertile; renal anomalies; coarctation of the aorta

Altered Chromosome: XXY (Sex Chromosome)	Characteristics
Genetic defect: extra X chromosome in male (Klinefelter syndrome) Incidence: 1 in 1,000 live male births, approximately 1%–2% of institutionalized males	CNS: mild mental retardation Trunk: occasional gynecomastia (abnormally large male breasts); eunuchoid body proportions (lack of male muscular and sexual development) Other: small, soft testes; underdeveloped secondary sex characteristics: usually sterile

FIGURE 6-8

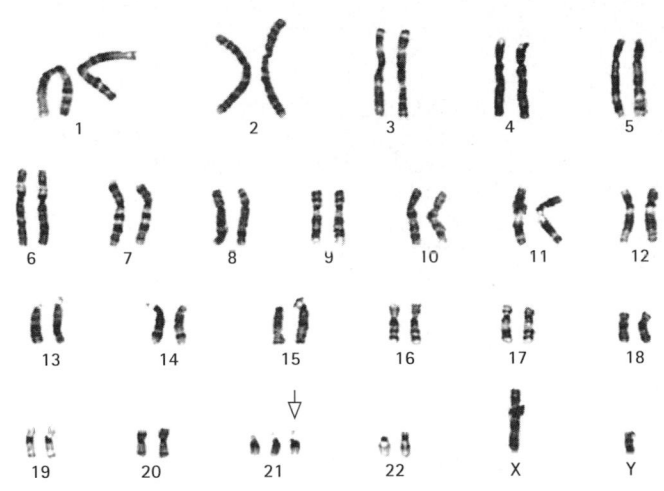

Karyotype of a male who has trisomy 21, Down syndrome. Note the extra 21 chromosome.

Courtesy of David Peakman, Reproductive Genetics Center, Denver, CO.

FIGURE 6-9

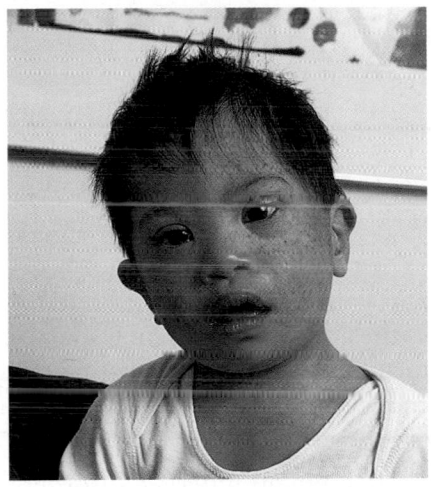

A boy with Down syndrome.

Down syndrome but with normal or near-normal intelligence should be investigated for the possibility of mosaicism.

Abnormalities of Chromosome Structure

Abnormalities of chromosome structure involve only parts of the chromosome and occur in two forms: translocation and deletions or additions. Some children born with Down syndrome have an abnormal rearrangement of chromosomal material known as a *translocation*. Clinically, the two types of Down syndrome are indistinguishable; the only way to distinguish them is to do a chromosome analysis.

The translocation occurs when the carrier parent has 45 chromosomes, usually with one chromosome fused to another. For example, a common translocation is one in which a particle of chromosome 14 breaks and fuses to chromosome 21. The parent has one normal 14, one normal 21, and one 14/21 chromosome. Since all the chromosomal material is present and functioning normally, the parent is clinically normal. This individual is known as a *balanced translocation carrier*. When a person who is a balanced translocation carrier has a child with a partner who has a structurally normal chromosome constitution, the child can have a normal number of chromosomes, be a carrier, or have an extra chromosome 21. Such a child has an *unbalanced translocation* and has Down syndrome.

Structure abnormality is also caused by *additions* or *deletions* of chromosomal material. Any portion of a chromosome may be lost or added, generally leading to some adverse effect. Depending on how much chromosomal material is involved, the clinical effects may be mild or severe. Many types of additions and deletions have been described, such as the deletion of the short arm of chromosome 5 (cri du chat, or cat cry, syndrome) or the deletion of the long arm of chromosome 18 (see Table 6-7).

Abnormalities of the Sex Chromosomes

To better understand abnormalities of the sex chromosomes, the nurse should know that in a female, at an early embryonic stage, one of the two normal X chromosomes becomes inactive. The inactive X chromosome forms a dark staining area known as the *Barr body*. The typical female has one Barr body, since one of her two X chromosomes has been inactivated. The typical male has no Barr bodies because he has only one X chromosome.

The most common sex chromosome abnormalities are Turner syndrome in females (45, XO with no Barr bodies present; see Figure 6–10 ⬤) and Klinefelter syndrome in males (47, XXY with one Barr body present). See Table 6–7 for clinical descriptions of these abnormalities and Chapter 56 for nursing management. ∞ The mosaic form of the XO chromosome is associated with daughters of women who took the drug diethylstilbestrol (DES) during pregnancy. The fertility of women with the mosaic form of the XO chromosome may not be impaired; however, there is a higher percentage of uterine malformation and hormonal difficulty associated with it and therefore a high degree of miscarriage.

MODES OF INHERITANCE

Many inherited diseases are produced by an abnormality in a single gene or pair of genes. In such instances the chromosomes are grossly normal. The defect is at the gene level. Some of these gene defects can be detected by technologies such as DNA and biochemical assays. The two major categories of

● FIGURE 6–10

Infant with Turner syndrome at 1 month of age. Note prominent ears.

Used with permission from Lemli, L., & Smith, D. W. (1963). The XO syndrome: A study of the differentiated phenotype in 25 patients. Journal of Pediatrics, 63, 577.

● FIGURE 6–11

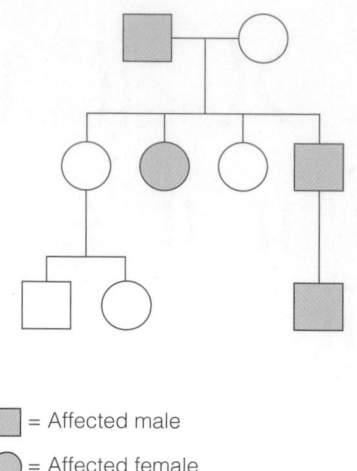

■ = Affected male

● = Affected female

Autosomal dominant pedigree. One parent is affected. Statistically, 50% of offspring will be affected, regardless of sex.

inheritance are **mendelian (single-gene) inheritance** and **nonmendelian (multifactorial) inheritance**. Each single-gene trait is determined by a pair of genes working together. These genes are responsible for the observable expression of the traits (e.g., blue eyes, dark skin), referred to as the **phenotype**. The total genetic makeup of an individual is referred to as the **genotype** (pattern of the genes on the chromosomes).

One of the genes for a trait is inherited from the mother, the other from the father. A person who has two identical genes at a given locus is *homozygous* for that trait. A person is *heterozygous* for a particular trait when he or she has two different *alleles* (alternate forms of the same gene) at a given locus on a pair of homologous chromosomes.

The best-known modes of single-gene inheritance are autosomal dominant, autosomal recessive, and X-linked (sex-linked) recessive. There is also an X-linked dominant mode of inheritance, which is less common, and the now identified mode of inheritance, fragile X syndrome.

Autosomal Dominant Inheritance

A person is said to have an autosomal dominantly inherited disorder if the disease trait is heterozygous; that is, the

abnormal gene overshadows the normal gene of the pair to produce the trait. It is essential to remember that in autosomal dominant inheritance, the following occurs:

1. An affected person generally has an affected parent. Thus, the family **pedigree** (graphic representation of a family tree) usually shows multiple generations with the disorder.
2. An affected person has a 50% chance of passing on the abnormal gene to each of his or her children (Figure 6–11 ●).
3. Males and females are equally affected, and a father can pass the abnormal gene on to his son. This is an important principle when distinguishing autosomal dominant disorders from X-linked disorders.
4. Autosomal dominant inherited disorders have varying degrees of presentation. This is an important factor when counseling families concerning autosomal dominant disorders. A parent with a mild form of the disease may have a child with a more severe form.

Some common autosomal dominant inherited disorders are Huntington disease, polycystic kidney disease, neurofibromatosis (von Recklinghausen disease), and achondroplastic dwarfism.

Autosomal Recessive Inheritance

In an autosomal recessive inherited disorder, the person must have two abnormal genes to be affected. A *carrier* is heterozygous for the abnormal gene and clinically normal. It is not until two people mate and pass on the same abnor-

FIGURE 6–12

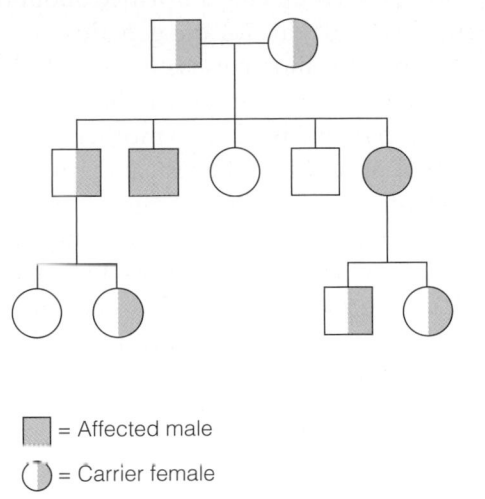

= Affected male

= Carrier female

Autosomal recessive pedigree. Both parents are carriers. Statistically, 25% of offspring are affected, regardless of sex.

FIGURE 6–13

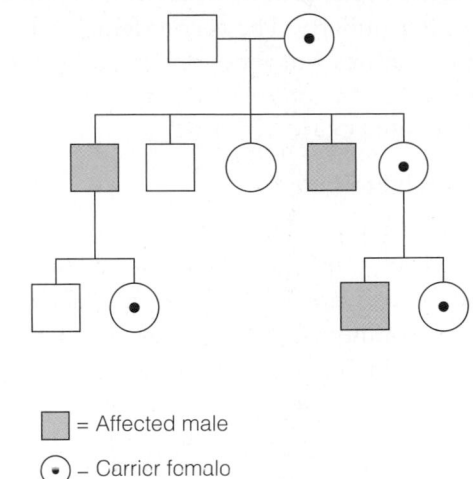

= Affected male

= Carrier female

X-linked recessive pedigree. The mother is the carrier. Statistically, 50% of male offspring are affected, and 50% of female offspring are carriers.

mal gene that affected children may appear. It is essential to remember that in autosomal recessive inheritance, the following occurs:

1. An affected person may have clinically normal parents, but both parents are carriers of the abnormal gene (Figure 6–12 ⬤).
2. With two carrier parents, there is a 25% chance that the abnormal gene will be passed on to any of their offspring. Each pregnancy has a 25% chance of resulting in an affected child.
3. If a child of two carrier parents is clinically normal, there is a 50% chance that he or she is a carrier of the gene.
4. Both males and females are equally affected.
5. There is an increased history of consanguineous matings (mating of close relatives).

Some common autosomal recessive inherited disorders are cystic fibrosis, phenylketonuria, (PKU), galactosemia, sickle cell anemia, Tay-Sachs disease, and most metabolic disorders.

X-Linked Recessive Inheritance

X-linked, or sex-linked, disorders are those for which the abnormal gene is carried on the X chromosome. Thus an X-linked disorder is manifested in a male who carries the abnormal gene on his X chromosome. His mother is considered to be a carrier when the normal gene on one X chromosome overshadows the abnormal gene on the other X chromosome. It is essential to remember that in X-linked recessive inheritance, the following occurs:

1. There is no male-to-male transmission. Affected males are related through the female line (Figure 6–13 ⬤).
2. There is a 50% chance that a carrier mother will pass the abnormal gene to each of her sons, who will thus be affected. There is a 50% chance that a carrier mother will pass the normal gene to each of her sons, who will thus be unaffected. Finally, there is a 50% chance that a carrier mother will pass the abnormal gene to each of her daughters, who will become carriers.
3. Fathers affected with an X-linked disorder cannot pass the disorder to their sons, but all their daughters become carriers of the disorder.

Common X-linked recessive disorders are hemophilia, Duchenne muscular dystrophy, and color blindness.

X-Linked Dominant Inheritance

X-linked dominant disorders are rare, the most common being vitamin D–resistant rickets and now the recognized fragile X syndrome. When X-linked dominant inheritance does occur, the pattern is similar to that of X-linked recessive inheritance except that heterozygous females are affected. It is essential to remember that in X-linked dominant inheritance, there is no male-to-male transmission. Affected fathers will have affected daughters but no affected sons.

Fragile X Syndrome

Fragile X syndrome is a common inherited form of mental retardation second only to Down syndrome among all causes of moderate mental retardation in males. Fragile X syndrome is a central nervous system disorder linked to a "fragile" site on the X chromosome. It is characterized by moderate mental retardation, large protuberant ears, and large testes after puberty. The carrier females do not have the abnormal features, but about one third are mildly mentally retarded. (See Chapter 54 for management and nursing care discussion. ∞)

Multifactorial Inheritance

Many common congenital malformations, such as cleft palate, heart defects, spina bifida, dislocated hips, clubfoot, and pyloric stenosis, are caused by an interaction of many genes and environmental factors. They are, therefore, multifactorial in origin. It is essential to remember that in multifactorial inheritance the following occurs:

1. The malformations may vary from mild to severe. For example, spina bifida may range in severity from mild (spina bifida occulta) to more severe (myelomeningocele). It is believed that the more severe the defect, the greater the number of genes present for that defect.

2. There is often a sex bias. For example, pyloric stenosis is more common in males, whereas cleft palate is more common in females. When a member of the less commonly affected sex shows the condition, a greater number of genes must usually be present to cause the defect.

3. In the presence of environmental influences (such as seasonal changes, altitude, irradiation, chemicals in the environment, or exposure to toxic substances), fewer genes are needed to manifest the disease in the offspring.

4. In contrast to single-gene disorders, there is an additive effect in multifactorial inheritance. The more family members who have the defect, the greater the risk that the next pregnancy will also be affected (Prosen & Hogge, 2004).

Although most congenital malformations are multifactorial traits, a careful family history should always be taken, since cleft lip and palate, certain congenital heart defects, and other malformations occasionally can be inherited as autosomal dominant or recessive traits. Other disorders thought to be within the multifactorial inheritance group are diabetes, hypertension, some heart diseases, and mental illness.

PRENATAL DIAGNOSTIC TESTS

Parent-child and family-planning counseling have become a major responsibility of professional nurses. (See Chapter 8 and Chapter 12 for discussion of preconception counseling and impact on maternal nutrition. ∞) To be effective counselors, nurses must have the most up-to-date information about prenatal diagnosis. Appropriate counseling

should occur before prenatal screening is done. It is essential that couples be completely informed about the known and potential risks of each of the genetic diagnostic procedures. The prescreening counseling should include the conditions detectable by the screen, diagnostic test available if the screen is positive, risk to mother and child of the test performed, accuracy of the test, and limitations of the test (Evans, Bui, & Yaron, 2003). Nurses must recognize the emotional impact on the family of a decision to have or not have a genetic diagnostic procedure. The ability to diagnose certain genetic diseases has enormous implications for the practice of preventive health care. Several methods are available for prenatal diagnosis, although some are still experimental.

Genetic Ultrasound

Ultrasound may be used to assess the fetus for genetic or congenital problems. With ultrasound, one can visualize the fetal head for abnormalities in size, shape, and structure (see Chapter 16 for more information on ultrasound technology ∞). Craniospinal defects (anencephalus, microcephaly, hydrocephalus), thoracic malformations (diaphragmatic hernia), gastrointestinal malformations (omphalocele, gastroschisis), renal malformations (dysplasia or obstruction), and skeletal malformations (caudal regression, conjoined twins) are only some of the disorders that have been diagnosed in utero by ultrasound. Screening by ultrasound for congenital anomalies is best done at 18 to 20 weeks, when fetal structures have developed completely. With the addition of fetal nuchal translucency measurement at 10 to 13 weeks, there is a high correlation with fetal chromosome abnormalities. There is no information documenting harm to the fetus or long-term effects from exposure to ultrasound. However, complete safety is not guaranteed; therefore, the practitioner and the parents must evaluate the risks against the benefits on an individual basis.

Genetic Amniocentesis

The major method of prenatal diagnosis is genetic amniocentesis (Figure 6–14 ● and Skill 2–5).

The indications for genetic amniocentesis include the following:

1. **Maternal age 35 or older at the time of birth.**
   Women age 35 or older are at greater risk for having children with chromosomal abnormalities (see Chapter 12 for more information ∞). Chromosomal abnormalities due to maternal age include trisomy 21, trisomy 13, trisomy 18, XXX, or XXY. The risk of having a live-born infant with a chromosome problem is 1 in 200 for a 35-year-old woman; the risk for trisomy 21 is 1 in 365. At age 45 the risks are 1 in 20 and 1 in 40, respectively (Verp, 2004).

FIGURE 6–14

A, Genetic amniocentesis for prenatal diagnosis is done at 14 to 16 weeks' gestation. **B,** Chorionic villus sampling is done at 8 to 10 weeks, and the cells are karyotyped within 48 to 72 hours.

2. **Previous child born with a chromosomal abnormality.** Young couples who have had a child with a trisomy 21, 18, or 13 have an approximately 1% to 2% risk of a future child having a chromosomal abnormality.

3. **Parent with balanced translocation (chromosomal abnormality).** A woman who carries a balanced 14/21 translocation has a risk of approximately 10% to 15% that her children will be affected with the unbalanced translocation of Down syndrome; if the father is the carrier, there is a 2% to 5% risk.

4. **Mother carrying an X-linked disease.** In families in which the woman is a known or possible carrier of an X-linked disorder such as hemophilia A or B, or Duchenne muscular dystrophy, options may include genetic amniocentesis, chorionic villus sampling (CVS), or percutaneous umbilical blood sampling (PUBS). For a known female carrier, the risk of an

affected male fetus is 50%. DNA testing may make it possible to distinguish affected males from nonaffected males in some disorders. In disorders in which female carriers can be distinguished from noncarriers, only the carrier females would be offered prenatal diagnosis.

5. **Parents carrying an inborn error of metabolism that can be diagnosed in utero.** Metabolic disorders detectable in utero include argininosuccinicaciduria, cystinosis, Fabry disease, galactosemia, Gaucher disease, homocystinuria, Hunter syndrome, Hurler syndrome, Krabbe disease, Lesch-Nyhan syndrome, maple syrup urine disease, metachromatic leukodystrophy, methylmalonic aciduria, Niemann-Pick disease, Pompe disease, Sanfilippo syndrome, and Tay-Sachs disease.

6. **Both parents carrying an autosomal recessive disease.** When both parents are carriers of an

autosomal recessive disease, there is a 25% risk *for each pregnancy* that the fetus will be affected. Diagnosis is made by testing the cultured amniotic fluid cells (enzyme level, substrate level, product level, or DNA) or the fluid itself. Autosomal recessive diseases identified by amniocentesis are hemoglobinopathies such as sickle cell anemia, thalassemia, and cystic fibrosis.

7. **Family history of neural tube defects.** Genetic amniocentesis is available to couples who have had a child with neural tube defects or who have a family history of these conditions, which include anencephaly, spina bifida, and myelomeningocele. Neural tube defects are usually multifactorial traits.

Percutaneous Umbilical Blood Sampling and Chorionic Villus Sampling

Percutaneous umbilical blood sampling (PUBS) is a technique used for obtaining blood that allows for rapid chromosome diagnosis, genetic studies, or transfusion for Rh isoimmunization or hydrops. Chorionic villus sampling (CVS) is used in selected regional centers, and its diagnostic capability is similar to that of amniocentesis. Its advantages are that diagnostic information is available at 8 to 10 weeks' gestation and that products of conception are tested directly. (See Chapter 16 for more information. ∞)

Alpha-Fetoprotein (AFP)

The maternal circulation or amniotic fluid is tested for alpha-fetoprotein (AFP). The maternal serum AFP (MSAFP) level is elevated in cases of infants with open neural tube defects, anencephaly, omphalocele, and gastroschisis; fetal death; vaginal bleeding; or multiple gestations (Jenkins & Wapner, 2004). Low MSAFP level has been associated with Down syndrome. MSAFP testing is done at 15 to 22 weeks' gestation (Jenkins & Wapner, 2004). Ultrasound and amniocentesis are offered to clients with low or high MSAFP levels. Inaccurate dating is the most common cause for abnormal AFP; therefore, ultrasound dating is very important. With high MSAFP levels, normal amniotic fluid AFP, and normal ultrasound, there is an increased risk for preterm labor, perinatal death, and intrauterine growth restriction.

Implications of Prenatal Diagnostic Testing

It is imperative that counseling precede any procedure for prenatal diagnosis. Many questions and points must be considered if the family is to reach a satisfactory decision. See Table 6–8 and "Developing Cultural Competence: Genetic Screening Recommendations for Various Ethnic and Age Groups." With the advent of diagnostic techniques such as amniocentesis and CVS, couples at risk who would not

TABLE 6–8 ✤ Couples Who May Benefit from Prenatal Diagnosis
Women age 35 or over at time of birth
Couples with a balanced translocation (chromosomal abnormality)
Family history of known or suspected mendelian genetic disorder (e.g., cystic fibrosis, hemophilia A and B, Duchenne muscular dystrophy)
Couples with a previous child with chromosomal abnormality
Couples in which either partner or a previous child is affected with, or in which both partners are carriers for, a diagnosable metabolic disorder
Family history of birth defects or mental retardation (e.g., neural tube defects, congenital heart disease, cleft lip or palate)
Ethnic groups at increased risk for specific disorders (see "Developing Cultural Competence: Genetic Screening Recommendations for Various Ethnic and Age Groups")
Couples with history of two or more first-trimester spontaneous abortions
Women with an abnormal maternal serum alpha-fetoprotein (MSAFP or AFP3) test
Women with a teratogenic risk secondary to an exposure or maternal health condition (e.g., diabetes)

otherwise have additional children can decide to conceive. Following prenatal diagnosis a couple can decide not to have a child with a genetic disease. For many couples, prenatal diagnosis is not selected because abortion is not an option for them. The decision about whether to use prenatal diagnosis can only be made by the family. Even when termination is not an option, prenatal diagnosis can give parents an opportunity to prepare for the birth of a child with special needs, to contact the families of children with similar problems, or to access support services before the birth.

Every pregnancy has a 3% to 4% risk of resulting in an infant with a birth defect. When an abnormality is detected or suspected before birth, an attempt is made to determine the diagnosis by assessing the family health history (via the pedigree) and the pregnancy history and by evaluating the fetal anomaly or anomalies via ultrasound. Experts on a specific disorder are consulted, and healthcare professionals can then present the parents with options.

Treatment of prenatally diagnosed disorders may begin during the pregnancy, thus possibly preventing irreversible damage. For example, a mother carrying a fetus with galactosemia may follow a galactose-free diet. In light of the philosophy of preventive healthcare, information that can be obtained prenatally should be made available to all couples who are expecting a baby or who are contemplating pregnancy.

Postnatal Diagnosis

Questions about genetic disorders (cause, treatment, and prognosis) are most often first discussed in the newborn nursery or during the infant's first few months of life. When a child is born with anomalies, has a stormy newborn period, or does not progress as expected, a genetic evaluation may be warranted. An accurate diagnosis and an optimal treatment plan incorporate the following:

- Complete and detailed history to determine whether the problem is prenatal (congenital), postnatal, or familial in origin
- Thorough physical examination, including dermatoglyphics analysis (Figure 6–15 ⦿)
- Laboratory analysis, which includes chromosome analysis; enzyme assay for inborn errors of metabolism; DNA studies (both direct and by linkage); and antibody titers for infectious teratogens, such as toxoplasmosis, rubella, cytomegalovirus, and herpesvirus (TORCH syndrome) (see Chapter 15 for more information on these tests ∞).

To make an accurate diagnosis, the geneticist consults with other specialists and reviews the current literature before arriving at a diagnosis and plan of action. The Human Genome Project has significant implications for the identification and management of inherited disorders. Once genes have been identified, it will be possible to detect their presence in carriers and lead to better genetic counseling. New genetic material might be inserted into cells to provide important missing information (gene transfer) as may be possible in cystic fibrosis, or medications can be specifically designed to target the disease on a molecular level (Hamilton & Wynshaw-Boris, 2004).

However, concerns have been voiced about ethical considerations with genetic research. What guidelines are needed to protect children and families so that genetic testing does not lead to discrimination in future employment or health insurance? Who should be tested for genetic diseases, and who should have access to the results? Since children cannot yet give informed consent for genetic testing (see Chapter 1 for more information on informed consent ∞), it is recommended that children and adolescents should have genetic testing *only* when medical treatment could help if the disease is identified, or when another family member's health might benefit from the knowledge and the child will not be harmed by the testing (American Academy of Pediatrics, Committee on Genetics, 2000; Drenkard & Ferguson, 2002). When genetic testing is performed, counseling about the results must be made available. Some nurses are acquiring additional education that enables them to work in the growing field of genetics and health care (Tinkle & Cheek, 2002).

MEDIALINK Human Genome Project

NURSING PRACTICE

The explosion in knowledge and clinical therapy related to genetics will offer challenges to those in healthcare. Just because a genetic test for a disease exists, should it be done on all newborns? What might be the potential harmful uses of information obtained about someone's genetic information? What forms of disadvantage and discrimination might occur if someone was known to carry a gene for breast cancer, a neurologic disease, or Alzheimer's disease? The rapidly advancing technology demands a focus on the ethical aspects of use of genetic tests and information. The Ethical, Legal, and Social Implications (ELSI) Program of the National Human Genome Research Institute has been established to explore these issues (American Academy of Pediatrics, 2000; Giarelli & Jacobs, 2000)

⦿ FIGURE 6–15

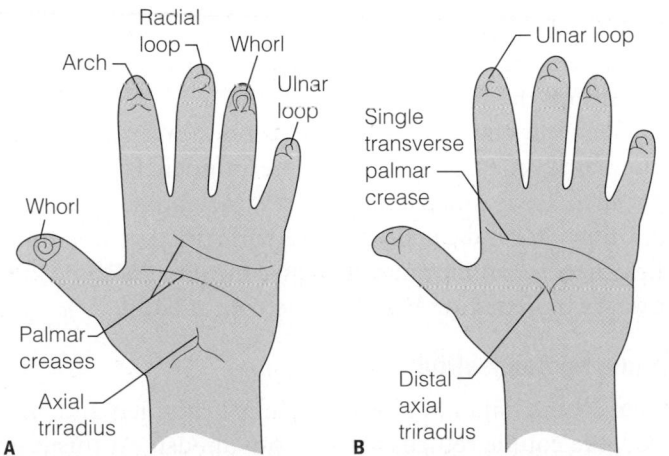

Dermatoglyphic patterns of the hands in **A,** a normal individual, and **B,** a child with Down syndrome. Note the single transverse palmar crease, distally placed axial triradius, and increased number of ulnar loops.

GENETIC COUNSELING

Genetic counseling is a communication process in which a genetic counselor, physician, or specially trained and certified nurse tries to provide a family with the most complete and accurate information about the occurrence or the risk of recurrence of a genetic disease in that family (Pagon, Hanson, Neufeld-Kaiser, & Covington, 2001). Genetic counseling is an appropriate course of action for any family wondering, "Will it happen again?"

Referral

Genetic counseling referral is advised for any of the following categories:

1. **Congenital abnormalities, including mental retardation.** Any couple who has a child or a relative with a congenital malformation may be at increased risk and should be so informed. If mental retardation

of unidentified cause has occurred in a family, there may be an increased risk of recurrence. In some cases the genetic counselor will identify the cause of a malformation as a teratogen (see Chapter 11 for more information ∞). The family should be aware of teratogenic substances so they can avoid exposure during any subsequent pregnancy.

2. **Familial disorders.** Families should be told that certain diseases may have a genetic component and that the risk of their occurrence in a particular family may be higher than that in the general population. Such disorders as diabetes, heart disease, cancer, and mental illness fall into this category.

3. **Known inherited diseases.** Families may know that a disease is inherited but not know the mechanism or the specific risk for them. An important point to remember is that family members who are not at risk for passing on a disorder should be as well informed as family members who are at risk.

4. **Metabolic disorders.** Any family at risk for having a child with a metabolic disorder or biochemical defect should be referred. Because most inborn errors of metabolism are inherited in an autosomal recessive manner, a family may not be identified as being at risk until the birth of an affected child. Carriers of the sickle cell trait can be identified before they conceive a child, and the risk of having an affected child can be determined. Prenatal diagnosis of an affected fetus is available on an experimental basis only.

5. **Chromosomal abnormalities.** As discussed previously, any couple who has had a child with a chromosomal abnormality may be at increased risk of having another child similarly affected. This group includes families in which there is concern about a possible translocation.

After a couple has been referred to the genetics clinic, they are sent a form requesting information on the health status of various family members. This information assists the genetic counselor in creating the family pedigree.

The pedigree and history facilitate identification of other family members who might also be at risk for the same disorder (Figure 6–16 ●). The couple being counseled may wish to notify relatives at risk so that they, too, can begin genetic counseling. When done correctly, the family history and pedigree can be powerful tools for determining a family's risk.

Initial Session

The counselor gathers additional information about the pregnancy, the affected child's growth and development, and the family's understanding of the problem. The coun-

Screening pedigree. Arrow indicates the nearest family member affected with the disorder being investigated. Basic data have been recorded. Numbers refer to the ages of the family members.

selor also elicits information concerning ethnic background and family origin. Many genetic disorders are more common among certain ethnic groups or in particular geographic areas (see "Developing Cultural Competence: Genetic Screening Recommendations for Various Ethnic and Age Groups").

Generally the child undergoes a physical examination. Other family members may also be examined. If laboratory tests such as chromosomal analyses, metabolic studies, or viral titers are indicated, they are performed at this time. The genetic counselor may then give the parents some preliminary information based on the data at hand.

Follow-Up Counseling

When all the data have been carefully examined and analyzed, the couple returns for a follow-up visit. At this time the genetic counselor gives the parents all the information available, including the medical facts, diagnosis, probable course of the disorder, and any available management; the inheritance pattern for this particular family and the risk of

DEVELOPING CULTURAL COMPETENCE

GENETIC SCREENING RECOMMENDATIONS FOR VARIOUS ETHNIC AND AGE GROUPS

Background of Population at Risk	Disorder	Screening Test	Definitive Test
Ashkenazic Jewish, French-Canadians, Cajuns	Tay-Sachs disease	Decreased serum hexosaminidase-A	CVS* or amniocentesis for hexosaminidase-A assay
African; Hispanic from Caribbean, Central America, or South America; Arabs, Egyptians; Asian Indians	Sickle cell anemia	Presence of sickle cell hemoglobin; confirmatory hemoglobin electrophoresis	CVS or amniocentesis for genotype determination; direct molecular studies
Greek, Italian	Beta-thalassemia	Mean corpuscular volume < 80%; confirmatory hemoglobin electrophoresis	CVS or amniocentesis for genotype determination (direct molecular studies or indirect RFLP[†] analysis)
Southeast Asian (Vietnamese, Loatian, Cambodian), Filipino	Alpha-thalassemia	Mean corpuscular volume < 80%; confirmatory hemoglobin electrophoresis	CVS or amniocentesis for genotype determination (direct molecular studies)
Women over age 35 (all ethnic groups)	Chromosomal trisomies	None	CVS or amniocentesis for cytogenetic analysis
Women of any age (all ethnic groups; particularly suggested for women from British Isles, Ireland)	Neural tube defects and selected other anomalies	Maternal serum alpha-fetoprotein (MSAFP).	Amniocentesis for amniotic fluid, alpha-fetoprotein, and acetylcholinesterase assays
Ashkenazic Jewish	Gaucher disease	Decreased glucocerebrosidase	CVS
Caucasians (Northern Europeans, Celtic population), Ashkenazic Jewish	Cystic fibrosis	Delta F508 amino acid mutation	CVS or amniocentesis for genotype determination; definitive diagnosis for all fetuses not possible

*Chorionic villus sampling.

[†]Restriction fragment length polymorphism.

recurrence; and the options or alternatives for dealing with the risk of recurrence. The remainder of the counseling session is spent discussing the course of action that seems appropriate to the family in view of the risk and family goals (Pagon et al., 2001). For couples who desire to become parents or who want a subsequent child, options include prenatal diagnosis, early detection and treatment, and, in some cases, adoption, artificial insemination, and delayed childbearing.

The couple may consider therapeutic donor insemination (TDI), discussed earlier in this chapter. This alternative is appropriate, for example, if the male partner has an autosomal dominant disorder; TDI would decrease to zero the risk of having an affected child (if the sperm donor is not at risk) because the child would not inherit any genes from the affected parent. If the man has an X-linked disorder and does not wish to continue the gene in the family (all his daughters would be carriers), TDI is an alternative to terminating all pregnancies with a female fetus. If the man is a carrier for a balanced translocation and if termination of pregnancy is against family ethics, TDI is the most appropriate alternative. If both parents are carriers of

an autosomal recessive disorder, TDI lowers the risk to a very low level or to zero if a carrier test is available. Finally, TDI may be appropriate if the couple is at high risk for a multifactorial disorder.

Couples who are young and at risk may decide to delay childbearing for a few years. These couples may find in a few years that prenatal diagnosis is available or that a disease can be detected and treated early to prevent irreversible damage.

When the parents have completed the counseling sessions, the counselor sends them and their certified nurse-midwife or physician a letter detailing the contents of the sessions. The parents keep this document for reference. See Table 6–9 for a list of nursing responsibilities in genetic counseling.

Nursing Care Management

In both prospective and retrospective genetic counseling, timely nursing intervention is a crucial factor. During annual examinations and other clinical appointments, the nurse should interview all women of childbearing age to determine any family history or other risk factors for genetic disorders. If the woman is planning to conceive, genetic

TABLE 6–9 ✢ Nursing Responsibilities in Genetic Counseling

Identify families at risk for genetic problems.

Determine how the genetic problem is perceived and what information is desired before proceeding.

Assist families in acquiring accurate information about the specific problem.

Act as a liaison between the family and the genetic counselor.

Assist the family in understanding and dealing with information received.

Provide information on support groups.

Aid families in coping with this crisis.

Provide information about known genetic factors.

Assure continuity of nursing care to the family.

counseling should be encouraged prior to discontinuation of contraception.

The nurse has a key role in preventing recurrence. One cannot expect a couple who has just learned that their child has a birth defect or Down syndrome to take in any information concerning future risks. However, the couple should never be "put off" from genetic counseling for so long that they conceive another affected child because of lack of information. The perinatal nursing team frequently has the first contact with the family who has a newborn with a congenital abnormality. At the birth of an affected child, the nurse can inform the parents that genetic counseling is available before they attempt to have another child.

After genetic counseling, the nurse with the appropriate knowledge of genetics is in an ideal position to help couples review what has been discussed during the counseling sessions and to answer any additional questions they might have. As families return to daily living, the nurse can provide helpful information on the day-to-day aspects of caring for a child, answer questions as they arise, support parents in their decisions, and refer families to other health and community agencies.

The family may return to the genetic counselor a number of times to ask questions and express concerns, especially if the couple is considering having more children, or if siblings want information about their affected brother or sister. It is most desirable for the nurse working with the family to attend many or all of these counseling sessions. Because the nurse has already established a rapport with the couple, she or he can act as a liaison between the family and the genetic counselor. Hearing directly what the genetic counselor says helps the nurse clarify the issues for the family, which in turn helps them formulate questions. Many genetic centers have found the public health nurse to be the ideal health professional to provide such follow-up care.

Nurses must be careful not to assume a diagnosis, determine carrier status or recurrence risks, or provide genetic counseling without adequate information and training. Inadequate, inappropriate, or inaccurate information may be misleading or harmful. Healthcare professionals need to learn the appropriate referral systems and options for care in their region.

Critical Concept Review

LEARNING OBJECTIVES	CONCEPTS
Identify the essential components of fertility.	Female: 1. Cervical mucus must be favorable. 2. Fallopian tubes must be patent. 3. Ovaries must produce and release ova in a regular, cyclic fashion. 4. Endometrium must be prepared for implantation of the blastocyst. 5. Adequate reproductive hormones must be present. Male: 1. Testes must produce adequate numbers of sperm. 2. Unobstructed genital tract. 3. Genital tract secretions must be normal. 4. Ejaculated sperm must reach cervix.

LEARNING OBJECTIVES

CONCEPTS

Describe the elements of the preliminary investigation of infertility.

1. Information about most fertile times for intercourse.
2. Explanation of basic infertility workup.
3. Basic assessments:
   - Ovarian function.
   - Cervical mucus adequacy.
   - Receptivity to sperm.
   - Sperm adequacy.
   - Tubal patency.
   - General condition of pelvic organs.
   - Semen analysis.
4. Complete physical examination of both partners.
5. Laboratory examination:
   - CBC.
   - UA.
   - Hormonal assays.

Summarize the indications for the tests and associated treatments, including assisted reproductive technologies, that are done in an infertility workup.

1. If lack of ovarian function is suspected:
   - Basal body temperature recording.
   - Hormonal assessments.
   - Endometrial biopsy.
   - Transvaginal ultrasound.
2. If cervical problems are suspected:
   - Ferning capacity of cervical mucus.
   - Postcoital test.
3. If tubal or uterine problems are suspected:
   - Hysterosalpingography.
   - Hysteroscopy.
   - Laparoscopy.
4. If male's fertility is suspected:
   - Semen analysis.
   - Screening for antisperm antibodies.
5. Pharmacologic intervention is prescribed if ovarian or endometrial function is abnormal.
6. Therapeutic insemination is indicated for low or abnormal sperm counts or structural defects in the male reproductive tract.
7. In vitro fertilization (IVF) is used when infertility has resulted from tubal factors, mucus abnormalities, male infertility, female immunologic infertility, and cervical factors.

Explore the couple's psychologic reactions related to infertility issues.

1. Development of lack of spontaneity of sexual intercourse.
2. Feelings of loss of control.
3. Feelings of reduced competency.
4. Loss of status and ambiguity as a couple.
5. Sense of social stigma.
6. Stress on marital and sexual relationship.
7. Strained relationship with healthcare providers.

Describe the nurse's role as counselor, educator, and advocate for couples during infertility evaluation and treatment.

1. Support the couple and help them to understand and facilitate the free expressions of feelings.
2. Help the couple to recognize feelings.
3. Help the couple to understand motives.
4. Help the couple identify alternatives, and facilitate partner communication.

Discuss the indications for preconceptual chromosomal analysis and prenatal testing.

1. Women who are of advanced maternal age.
2. Family history of a chromosomal disorder, birth defects, or mental retardation.
3. Previous child with chromosomal disorder.
4. Ethnic group with history of chromosomal disorders.
5. Couples with a history of two or more first-trimester spontaneous abortions.
6. Women with an abnormal serum alpha-fetoprotein test.

(continued)

LEARNING OBJECTIVES

CONCEPTS

Identify the characteristics of autosomal dominant, autosomal recessive, and X-linked (sex-linked) recessive disorders.	1. Autosomal dominant disorder:
	  ■ An affected parent has a 50% chance of having an affected child with each pregnancy.
	2. Autosomal recessive disorders:
	  ■ Both parents must be carriers.
	  ■ Each offspring has a 25% chance of having the disease and a 50% chance of being a carrier.
	3. X-linked recessive disorders:
	  ■ No male-to-male transmission.
	  ■ Effects limited to males.
	  ■ 50% chance a carrier mother will pass abnormal gene to her son.
	  ■ 50% chance the daughter of a carrier mother will be a carrier.
	  ■ 100% chance that daughter of an affected father will be a carrier.

Compare prenatal and postnatal diagnostic procedures used to determine the presence of genetic disorders.	1. Prenatal diagnostic tests:
	  ■ Invasive procedure performed on mother, though it may affect the fetus.
	  ■ Genetic ultrasound.
	  ■ Serum alpha-fetoprotein tests.
	  ■ Genetic amniocentesis.
	  ■ Chorionic villus sampling.
	  ■ Percutaneous umbilical blood sampling.
	2. Postnatal diagnostic tests:
	  ■ Physical examination and laboratory analysis is performed on the newborn.

Explore the emotional impact on a couple undergoing genetic testing or coping with the birth of a baby with a genetic disorder, and explain the nurse's role in supporting the family undergoing genetic counseling.	1. Emotional impact:
	  ■ Concern for infant's survival and possible lifelong difficulties.
	  ■ Fear of results of testing.
	  ■ Blame for infant's disorder.
	2. The nurse's role:
	  ■ Help families to acquire adequate information and understand this information.
	  ■ Act as a liaison between family and genetic counselor.
	  ■ Provide information about support groups.
	  ■ Provide continuity of care to the family.

CRITICAL THINKING IN ACTION

*View the **Critical Thinking in Action** video in Chapter 6 of the CD-ROM. Then, answer the questions that follow.*

Marie Neives, age 19, presents while you are working at a Planned Parenthood Clinic. She is there for a GYN exam and tells you that she is sexually active with her boyfriend but doesn't want to become pregnant. Since she lives at home with her parents, she does not want to use "the pill" because her mother might find out. Marie tells you she has a family history of sickle cell anemia and is concerned that she will pass the disease on. Marie asks you for information concerning fertility awareness. You obtain a menstrual history as follows: menarche age 12, cycle every 28 days x 5 days, dysmenorrhea the first 2 days with moderate flow. She has had one sexual partner. She states her boyfriend doesn't like to use condoms and that she has been lucky so far in not getting pregnant. You assist the nurse practitioner with a physical and pelvic exam. The results show that Marie is essentially healthy. The nurse practitioner asks you to review with Marie the basal body temperature (BBT) method of fertility awareness.

1. Explore with Marie "natural family planning." How would you explain this to her?
2. Briefly explain why the basal body temperature (BBT) method can predict ovulation.
3. How would you describe to Marie the procedure for obtaining BBT?
4. After figuring out her menstruation cycle, to avoid conception when would you tell Marie to abstain from unprotected intercourse?

MEDIALINK   www.prenhall.com/london

- NCLEX-RN® Review, case studies, and other interactive resources for this chapter can be found on the Companion Website at http://www.prenhall.com/london. Click on "Chapter 6" to select the activities for this chapter.

- For animations, more NCLEX-RN® Review questions, and an audio glossary, access the accompanying CD-ROM in this textbook.

REFERENCES

American Academy of Pediatrics, Committee on Genetics. (2000). Molecular genetic testing in pediatric practice: A subject review. *Pediatrics, 106,* 1494–1497.

American Society for Reproductive Medicine. (2002). Assisted reproductive technology in the United States: 1999 results generated from the American Society for Reproductive Medicine/Society for Assisted Reproductive Technology Registry. *Fertility and Sterility, 78*(5), 918–931.

Athaullah, N., Proctor, M., & Johnson, N. P. (2003). Oral versus injectable ovulation induction agents for unexplained subfertility (Cochrane Review). *The Cochrane Library, 4,* Chichester, UK: John Wiley & Sons.

Chang, R., Chung, P. H., & Rosenwaks, Z. (2002). Role of acupuncture in the treatment of female infertility. *Fertility and Sterility, 78*(6), 1149–1153.

Chen, J. C., Chen, L. D., Tsauer, W., Tsai, C. C., Chen, B. C., & Chen, Y. J. (2001). Effect of Ginsenoside Rb2 and Rc on inferior human sperm motility in vitro. *American Journal of Chinese Medicine, 29*(1), 155–160.

Drenkard, K., & Ferguson, S. (2002). Genetic testing and discrimination: Case example—Virginia. *Pediatric Nursing, 28*(1), 71–73.

Evans, M. I., Bui, The-Hung, & Yaron, Y., (2003). Biochemical screening. In J. J. Sciarri (Ed.), *Gynecology and obstetrics* (Vol. 3, chap. 114, pp.1–8). Hagerstown, MD: Harper & Row.

Giarelli, E., & Jacobs, L. A. (2000). Issues related to the use of genetic material and information. *Oncology Nursing Forum, 27,* 459–467.

Gurfinkel, E., Cedenho, A. P., Yamamura, Y., & Srougi, M. (2003). Effects of acupuncture and moxa treatment in patients with semen abnormalities. *Asian Journal of Andrology, 5,* 345–348.

Hamilton, B. A., & Wynshaw-Boris, A. (2004). Basic genetics and patterns of inheritance. In R. K. Creasy & R. Resnik (Ed.), *Maternal-fetal medicine: Principles and practice* (5th ed., pp. 3–36). Philadelphia: Saunders.

Hammond, K. (2001). How to help an infertile couple. *Nurse Practitioner, 26*(Supp.1), 1–15.

Hassan, M. A. M., & Killick, S. R. (2003). Effect of male age on fertility: Evidence for the decline in male fertility with increasing age. *Fertility and Sterility, 79*(3), 1520–1527.

Hopps, C. V., & Schlegel, P. N. (2003). Evaluation of the male in infertility. In J. J. Sciarri (Ed.), *Gynecology and obstetrics* (Vol. 5, chap. 63, pp. 1–14). Philadelphia: Lippincott Williams & Wilkins.

Inhorn, M. C. (2002). "Local" confronts the "Global": Infertile bodies and the new reproductive technology in Egypt. In M. C. Inhorn & F. Van Balen (Eds.), *Infertility around the globe: New thinking on childlessness, gender, and reproductive technologies.* Berkeley and Los Angeles: University of California Press.

Jenkins, T. M., & Wapner, R. J. (2004). Prenatal diagnosis of congenital disorders. In R. K. Creasy & R. Resnik (Eds.), *Maternal-fetal medicine: Principles and practice* (5th ed., pp. 235–280). Philadelphia: Saunders.

Johnson, J. V. (2003). Infertility. In J. R. Scott, R. S. Gibbs, B. Y. Karlan, & A. F. Haney (Eds.), *Danforth's obstetrics and gynecology* (9th ed., pp. 685–695). Philadelphia: Lippincott Williams & Wilkins.

Kahn, S. M. (2002). Rabbis and reproduction: The uses of new reproductive technologies among Ultraorthodox Jews in Israel. In M. C. Inhorn & F. Van Balen (Eds.), *Infertility around the globe: New thinking on childlessness, gender, and reproductive technologies.* Berkeley and Los Angeles: University of California Press.

Kakarla, N., & Bradshaw, K. (2003). Evaluation and management of the infertile couple. In J. J. Sciarri (Ed.), *Gynecology and obstetrics* (Vol. 5, chap. 50, pp. 1–18). Hagerstown, MD: Harper & Row.

Kashyap, S., & Davis, O. K. (2003). In vitro fertilization. In J. J. Sciarri (Ed.), *Gynecology and obstetrics* (Vol. 5, chap. 97, pp. 1–18). Hagerstown, MD: Harper & Row.

Kipersztok, S., Kim, B. D., Morris, L., Drury, K. C., Williams, R. S., & Rhoton-Viasak, A. (2003). Validity of a rapid assay for antisperm antibodies in semen. *Fertility and Sterility, 79*(3), 522–528.

Klock, S. C. (2004). Psychological issues related to infertility. In J. J. Sciarri (Ed.), *Gynecology and obstetrics* (Vol. 6, chap. 74, pp. 1–8). Philadelphia: Lippincott Williams & Wilkins.

Kridli, S. A. (2002). Health beliefs and practices among Arab women. *MCN. American Journal of Maternal Child Nursing, 27*(3), 178–182.

Moghissi, K. S. (2003). Documentation of ovulation. In J. J. Sciarri (Ed.), *Gynecology and obstetrics* (Vol. 5, chap. 54, pp. 1–14). Philadelphia: Lippincott Williams & Wilkins.

Pagon, R. A., Hanson, N. B., Neufeld-Kaiser, W., & Covington, M. L. (2001). Genetic consultation. *Western Journal of Medicine, 174*(6), 397–399.

Paulus, W. E., Zhang, M., Strehler, E., El-Danasouri, I., & Sterzik, K. (2002). Influence of acupuncture on the pregnancy rate in patients who undergo assisted reproduction therapy. *Fertility and Sterility, 77*(4), 721–724.

Pierson, R. A., & Olatunbosum, O. A., (2004).Transvaginal ultrasonography and the evaluation of female infertility. In J. J. Sciarri (Ed.), *Gynecology and obstetrics* (Vol. 5, chap. 55, pp. 1–12). Philadelphia: Lippincott Williams & Wilkins.

Prosen, T., & Hogge, W. A. (2004). Molecular and mendelian disorders. In J. J. Sciarri (Ed.), *Gynecology and obstetrics* (Vol. 3, chap. 115, pp. 1–13). Philadelphia: Lippincott Williams & Wilkins.

Purnell, L. D., & Paulanka, B. J. (2005). *Guide to culturally competent health care.* Philadelphia: F. A. Davis.

Sharara, F. I., & McClamrock, H. D. (2000). Differences in in vitro fertilization (IVF) outcome between white and black women in an inner-city, university-based IVF program. *Fertility and Sterility, 73*(6), 1170–1173.

Simpson, J. L. (2002). Genetic counseling and prenatal diagnosis. In S. G. Gabbe, J. R. Niebyl, &

J. L. Simpson (Eds.), *Obstetrics: Normal and problem pregnancies* (4th ed., pp. 187–219). Philadelphia: Churchill Livingstone.

Sinclair, S. (2000). Male infertility: Nutritional and environmental considerations. *Alternative Medicine Review, 5*(1), 28–38.

Tinkle, M. B., & Cheek, D. J. (2002). Human genomics: Challenges and opportunities. *Journal of Obstetric, Gynecologic, and Neonatal Nursing, 31*(2), 178–187.

Varney, H., Kriebs, J. M., & Gegor, C. L. (2004). *Varney's midwifery* (4th ed.). Boston: Jones & Bartlett.

Verp, M. S. (2004). Antenatal diagnosis of chromosomal abnormalities. In J. J. Sciarri (Ed.), *Gynecology and obstetrics* (Vol. 3, chap. 113, pp. 1–17). Philadelphia: Lippincott Williams & Wilkins.

White, A. R. (2003). A review of controlled trials of acupuncture for women's reproductive health care. *Journal of Family Planning and Reproductive Health Care, 29*(4), 233–236.

Wilson, B. A., Shannon, M. T., & Stang, C. L. (2005). *Prentice Hall nurse's drug guide—2005*. Upper Saddle River, NJ: Pearson Education.

Zhang, J. X., & Xu, K. (2003). Intracytoplasmic sperm injection and other micromanipulation techniques for assisted reproduction. In J. J. Sciarri (Ed.), *Gynecology and obstetrics* (Vol. 5, chap. 102, pp. 1–17). Philadelphia: Lippincott Williams & Wilkins.

Zitzmann, M., Rolf, C., Nordhoff, V., Schrader, G., Rickert-Fohring, M., Gassner, P., et al. (2003). Male smokers have a decreased success rate for in vitro fertilization and intracytoplasmic sperm injection. *Fertility and Sterility, 79* (Supp. 3), 1550–1554.

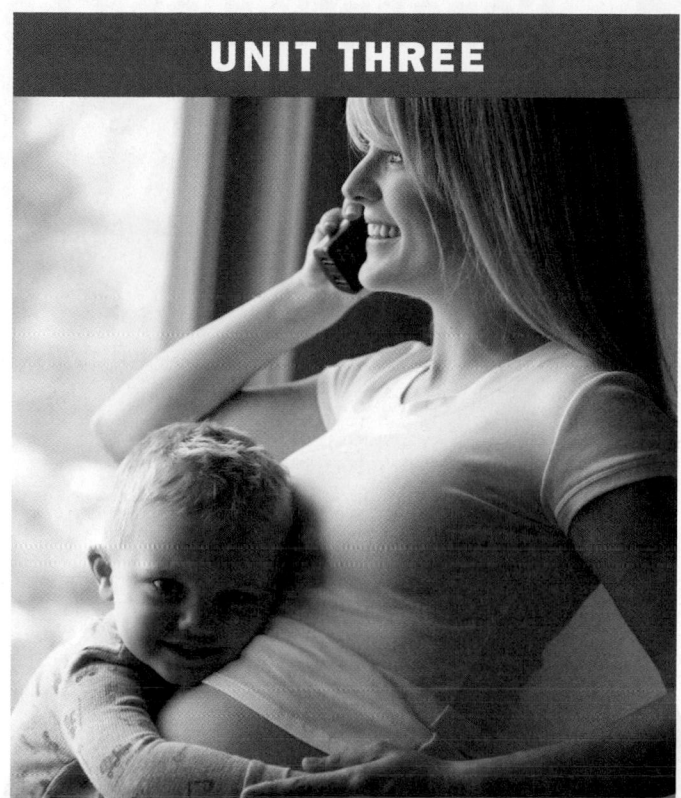

Pregnancy and Family

Conception and Fetal Development

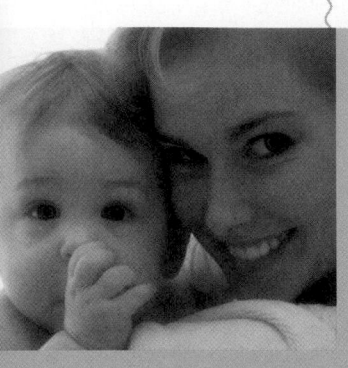

My friends tease me when I say this, but I know the moment my son was conceived. My husband and I had both been so busy at work, but finally we planned a getaway weekend. It was wonderful. We got back some of the magic as we took long walks and talked. Until that weekend, whenever we discussed having children it was always "maybe someday."

On the second night, we decided to skip the diaphragm for the first time. Our lovemaking seemed so special and magical—a true reflection of the emotional closeness we had recaptured. We are convinced that Michael is the result of that night together.

—Michelle, 29

LEARNING OBJECTIVES

- Compare the differences between meiotic cellular division and mitotic cellular division.

- Compare the processes by which ova and sperm are produced.

- Describe the components of the process of fertilization.

- Describe in order of increasing complexity the structures that form during the cellular multiplication and differentiation stages of intrauterine development.

- Describe the development, structure, and functions of the placenta and umbilical cord during intrauterine life.

- Identify the differing processes by which fraternal (dizygotic) and identical (monozygotic) twins are formed.

- Summarize the significant changes in growth and development of the fetus at 4, 6, 12, 16, 20, 24, 28, 36, and 40 weeks' gestation.

MEDIALINK

www.prenhall.com/london

CD-ROM

Animations:
 Conception
 Cell Division
 Oogenesis
 Spermatogenesis
 Oogenesis and Spermatogenesis Compared
 Matching Oogenesis and Spermatogenesis
 Placenta Formation
 Embryonic Heart Formation and Circulation
 Fetal Circulation

Companion Website

Audio Glossary
Thinking Critically
Additional NCLEX-RN® Review
MediaLink Applications:
 Case Study: Teaching about Pregnancy
 Care Plan Activity: Client Fearful of Multiple
  Gestation

The human genome contains, by current estimate, about 50,000 *genes*. Each gene is a unit of genetic information (Hamilton & Wynshaw-Boris, 2004). Genes are encoded in the deoxyribonucleic acid (DNA) that makes up the chromosomes in the nucleus of each cell. These chromosomes, which determine the structure and function of organ systems and traits, are biochemical substances. How then does each person become unique? The answer lies in the physiologic mechanisms of heredity, the processes of cellular division, and the environmental factors that influence human development from the moment of conception. This chapter explores the processes involved in conception and fetal development—the basis of human uniqueness.

CELL DIVISION

Each human begins life as a single cell called a fertilized ovum or zygote. This single cell reproduces itself, and each resulting cell also reproduces itself in a continuing process. The new cells are similar to the cells from which they came. Cells are reproduced by either mitosis or meiosis, two different but related processes.

Mitosis is a process of cell division that results in daughter cells that are exact copies of the original cell. They are identical to the parent cell and to each other. These cells contain a full set of chromosomes or genetic material and are called diploid because of this. Mitosis makes growth and development possible, and in mature individuals it is the process by which the somatic (body) cells continue to divide and replace themselves.

Meiosis is a process of cell division that leads to the development of eggs and sperm needed to produce a new organism. Unlike cells produced during mitosis, the cells produced during meiosis contain only half the genetic material or number of chromosomes (the haploid number).

MITOSIS

During mitosis, the cell undergoes several changes ending in cell division. As the last phase of cell division nears completion, a furrow develops in the cell cytoplasm, which divides it into two *daughter cells,* each with its own nucleus. These daughter cells are identical to the parent cell. They have the same **diploid number of chromosomes** (46) and the same genetic makeup as the cell from which they came. When a cell with 46 chromosomes goes through mitosis, the result is two identical cells, each with 46 chromosomes.

MEIOSIS

Meiosis is a special type of cell division that produces reproductive cells called **gametes** (sperm and ova). These cells are different from other somatic (body) cells because they contain half the genetic material of the parent cell—only 23 chromosomes, the **haploid number of chromosomes**.

Meiosis consists of two successive cell divisions. In the first division, the chromosomes replicate. Next a pairing takes place between homologous chromosomes (Sadler, 2004). Instead of separating immediately, as in mitosis, the chromosomes become closely intertwined. At each point of contact, there is a physical exchange of genetic material between the chromatids (the arms of the chromosomes). New combinations are provided by the newly formed chromosomes; these combinations account for the wide variation of traits in people (e.g., hair or eye color). The chromosome pairs then separate, and the members of the pair move to opposite sides of the cell. (In contrast, during mitosis the chromatids of each chromosome separate and move to opposite poles.) The cell divides, forming two daughter cells, each with 23 double-structured chromosomes—the same amount of DNA as a normal somatic cell. In the second division, the chromatids of each chromosome separate and move to opposite poles of each of the daughter cells. Cell division occurs, resulting in the formation of four cells, each containing 23 single chromosomes (the haploid number of chromosomes). These daughter cells contain only half the DNA of a normal somatic cell (Sadler, 2004) (see Table 7–1).

Mutations may occur during the second meiotic division. If two of the chromatids do not move apart rapidly enough when the cell divides, the still-paired chromatids are carried into one of the daughter cells and eventually form an extra chromosome. This condition, *autosomal nondisjunction* (chromosomal mutation), is harmful to the offspring if fertilization occurs. Another type of chromosomal mutation can occur if chromosomes break during meiosis. If the broken segment is lost, the result is a shorter chromosome; this situation is known as *deletion*. If the broken segment becomes attached to another chromosome, a harmful mutation called a *translocation* is the result. (See Chapter 6 for discussion of the implications of translocation and autosomal nondisjunction.∞)

TABLE 7–1 ✤ Comparison of Meiosis and Mitosis

Meiosis

Purpose

Produce reproductive cells (gametes). Reduction of chromosome number by half (from diploid [46] to haploid [23]), so that when fertilization occurs the normal diploid number is restored. Introduces genetic variability.

Cell division

Two-stage reduction.

Number of daughter cells

Four daughter cells, each containing one half the number of chromosomes as the mother cell, or 23 chromosomes. Nonidentical to original cell.

Mitosis

Purpose

Produce cells for growth and tissue repair. Cell division characteristic of all somatic cells.

Cell division

One-stage cell division.

Number of daughter cells

Two daughter cells identical to the mother cell, each with the diploid number (46 chromosomes).

GAMETOGENESIS

Gametogenesis is the process of cell division that produces sex cells, which are called gametes. These cells are unique in that they contain only half the genetic material of a typical body cell. The female gamete, called an ovum, and the male gamete, called a sperm, unite during fertilization, resulting in a zygote with a complete set of genetic material (46 chromosomes)—half of it from the mother and half from the father.

OOGENESIS

Oogenesis is the process that produces the female gamete, called an ovum (egg). As discussed in Chapter 3, ∞ the ovaries begin to develop early in the fetal life of the female. All the ova that the female will produce in her lifetime are present at birth. The ovary gives rise to oogonial cells, which develop into oocytes. Meiosis (cell replication by division) begins in all oocytes before the female fetus is born but stops before the first division is complete and remains in this arrested phase until puberty. During puberty, the mature primary oocyte continues through the first meiotic division in the graafian follicle of the ovary.

The first meiotic division produces two cells of unequal size with different amounts of cytoplasm but with the same number of chromosomes. One of these cells is the *secondary oocyte,* and the other is a minute *polar body.* Both the secondary oocyte and the polar body contain 22 double-structured autosomal chromosomes and one double-structured sex chromosome (X).

At the time of ovulation, a second meiotic division begins immediately and proceeds as the oocyte moves down the fallopian tube. Division is again not equal, and the secondary oocyte moves into the metaphase stage of cell division, where its meiotic division is arrested until and unless the oocyte is fertilized.

When the secondary oocyte completes the second meiotic division after fertilization, the result is a mature ovum with the haploid number of chromosomes and virtually all the cytoplasm. In addition the second polar body (also haploid) forms at this time. The first polar body has also divided in two, producing two additional polar bodies. Thus, at the completion of meiosis, four haploid cells have been produced: the three polar bodies, which eventually disintegrate, and one ovum (Sadler, 2004) (Figure 7–1 ◉).

SPERMATOGENESIS

During puberty the production of the male gamete, or sperm, begins. This process is called spermatogenesis. The spermatogonium (primordial germ cell) begins with a

● **FIGURE 7–1**

Primordial germ cells

Oogonium
(diploid)
(44XX)

Chromosomal
replication

Primary
oocyte
46 chromosomes
(44XX)

Resting state --------------------- } First meiotic
division

Secondary oocyte
23 chromosomes
(22X)

First polar body
23 chromosomes
(22X)

Fertilization - - - - - - - - - - - -

Second
meiotic
division

Polar
bodies

Ovum
(haploid)

Second
polar body

A

Primordial germ cells

Spermatogonium
(diploid) (44XX or 44XY)

Mitotic division

Primary spermatocyte
46 chromosomes
(44XY)
} First meiotic
division

Secondary spermatocytes
(haploid) 23 chromosomes
(22X or Y)
} Second meiotic
division

Spermatids
(haploid)
(22X or Y)

Sperm cells
(spermatozoa)
(haploid)
(22X or Y)

B

Gametogenesis involves meiosis within the ovary and testis. **A,** During meiosis, each oogonium produces a single haploid ovum once some cytoplasm moves into the polar bodies. **B,** Each spermatogonium produces four haploid spermatozoa.

complete set of genetic material—the diploid number of chromosomes. This cell replicates before it enters the first meiotic division, during which it is called the *primary spermatocyte.* During this first meiotic division, the spermatogonium forms two cells called *secondary spermatocytes,* each of which contains 22 double-structured autosomal chromosomes and either a double-structured X sex chromosome or a double-structured Y sex chromosome. During the second meiotic division, they divide to form four spermatids, each with the haploid number of chromosomes.

The spermatids undergo a series of changes during which they lose most of their cytoplasm and become sperm (spermatozoa) (see Figure 7–1). The nucleus becomes compacted into the head of the sperm, which is covered by a cap called an *acrosome* that is, in turn, covered by a plasma membrane. A long tail is produced from one of the centrioles.

THE PROCESS OF FERTILIZATION

When an ovum and a sperm unite, a fertilized ovum or **zygote** is created. This zygote begins life as a single cell with a complete set of genetic material, 23 chromosomes from the mother's ovum and 23 chromosomes from the father's sperm for a total of 46 chromosomes.

PREPARATION FOR FERTILIZATION

The mature ovum and spermatozoa have only a brief time to unite. Ova are considered fertile for about 12 to 24 hours after ovulation. Sperm can survive in the female reproductive tract for 48 to 72 hours but are believed to be healthy and highly fertile for only about 24 hours (De Jonge, 2000).

The ovum's cell membrane is surrounded by two layers of tissue. The layer closest to the cell membrane is called the *zona pellucida.* It is a clear, noncellular layer

MEDIALINK Animation: Spermatogenesis

whose thickness influences the fertilization rate. Surrounding the zona pellucida is a ring of elongated cells, called the *corona radiata* because they radiate from the ovum like the gaseous corona around the sun. These cells are held together by hyaluronic acid. The ovum has no power of movement of its own.

During ovulation, high estrogen levels facilitate fertilization by increasing peristalsis within the fallopian tubes, which helps move the ovum through the tube toward the uterus. The high estrogen levels also cause a thinning of the cervical mucus, easing passage of the sperm through the cervix, into the uterus, and up the fallopian tube.

Actual fertilization takes place in the ampulla (outer third) of the fallopian tube. In a single ejaculation, the male deposits approximately 200 million to 500 million spermatozoa in the vagina, of which only hundreds of sperm actually reach the ampulla (Sadler, 2004). Fructose in the semen, secreted by the seminal vesicles, is the energy source for the sperm. The spermatozoa propel themselves up the female tract by the flagellar movement of their tails. Transit time from the cervix into the fallopian tube can be as short as 5 minutes but usually takes an average of 2 to 7 hours after ejaculation (Sadler, 2004). Prostaglandins in the semen may increase uterine smooth muscle contractions, which help transport the sperm. The fallopian tubes have a dual ciliary action that facilitates movement of the ovum toward the uterus and movement of the sperm from the uterus toward the ovary.

The sperm must undergo two processes before fertilization can occur: capacitation and the acrosomal reaction. **Capacitation** is the removal of the plasma membrane overlying the spermatozoa's acrosomal area and the loss of seminal plasma lipids, proteins. If the glycoprotein coat is not removed, the sperm will not be able to fertilize the ovum (Sadler, 2004). Capacitation occurs in the female reproductive tract (aided by uterine enzymes) and is thought to take about 7 hours.

The **acrosomal reaction** follows capacitation. The acrosome caps of the sperms surrounding the ovum release their enzymes (hyaluronidase, a protease called acrosin, and trypsin-like substances). These enzymes break down the hyaluronic acid that holds the elongated cells of corona radiata together (Sadler, 2004). Hundreds of acrosomes must rupture to clear enough hyaluronic acid for even a single sperm to penetrate the ovum successfully.

At the moment of penetration by a fertilizing sperm, the zona pellucida undergoes a reaction that prevents additional sperm from entering a single ovum. This is known as the *block to polyspermy*. This cellular change is mediated by release of materials from the cortical granules, organelles found just below the ovum's surface, and is called the *cortical reaction* (Figure 7–2 ●).

THE MOMENT OF FERTILIZATION

After the sperm enters the ovum, a chemical signal prompts the secondary oocyte to complete the second meiotic division, forming the nucleus of the ovum and ejecting the second polar body. Then the nuclei of the ovum and sperm swell and approach each other. The true moment of **fertilization** occurs as the nuclei unite. Their individual nuclear membranes disappear, and their chromosomes pair up to produce the diploid zygote. Since each nucleus contains a haploid number of chromosomes (23), this union restores the diploid number (46). The zygote contains a new combination of genetic material that results in an individual different from either parent or anyone else.

It is also at the moment of fertilization that the sex of the zygote is determined. The two chromosomes of the 23rd pair (the sex chromosomes)—either XX or XY—determine the sex of an individual. X chromosomes are larger and bear more genes than the Y chromosome. Females have two X chromosomes, and males have an X and a Y chromosome. The mature ovum produced by oogenesis can have only one type of sex chromosome—an X. Spermatogenesis produces two sperm with an X chromosome and two sperm with a Y chromosome. When each gamete contributes an X chromosome, the resulting zygote is female. When the ovum contributes an X and the sperm contributes a Y chromosome, the resulting zygote is male. As discussed in Chapter 6 ∞, certain traits are termed *sex-linked* because they are controlled by the genes on the X sex chromosome. Two examples of sex-linked traits are color blindness and hemophilia.

PREEMBRYONIC DEVELOPMENT

The first 14 days of development, starting the day the ovum is fertilized (conception), are called the preembryonic stage, or the stage of the ovum. Development after fertilization can be divided into two phases: cellular multiplication and cellular differentiation. These phases are characterized by rapid cellular multiplication and differentiation, and the establishment of the embryonic membranes and primary germ layers. Development of both the endometrium and embryo must be synchronized for implantation to succeed (Groll & Lessey, 2003). These phases and the process of implantation (nidation), which occurs between them, are discussed next.

CELL MULTIPLICATION

Cellular multiplication begins as the zygote moves through the fallopian tube toward the cavity of the uterus. This transport takes 3 days or more and is accomplished mainly by a weak fluid current in the fallopian tube, resulting from the beating action of the ciliated epithelium that lines the tube.

FIGURE 7-2

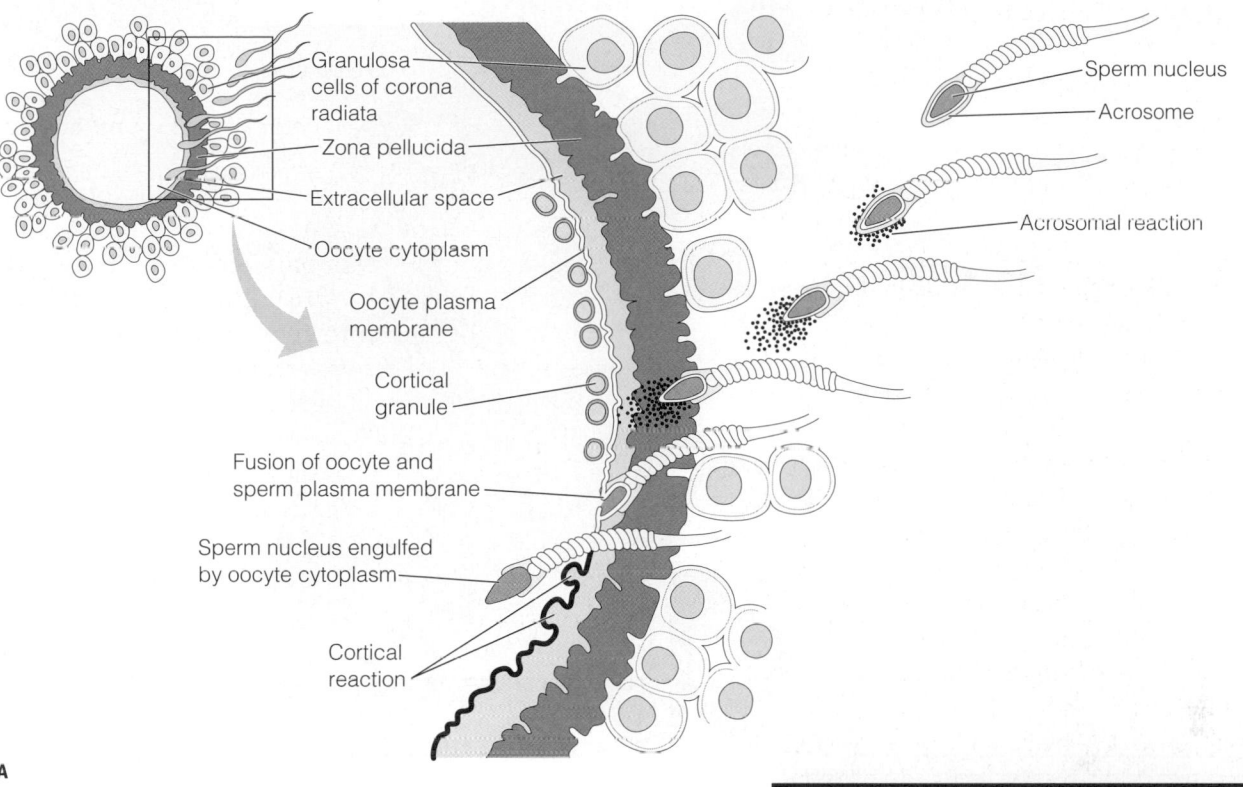

A

B

Sperm penetration of an ovum. **A,** The sequential steps of oocyte penetration by a sperm are depicted moving from top to bottom. **B,** Scanning electron micrograph of a human sperm surrounding a human ovum (750×). The smaller spherical cells are granulosa cells of the corona radiata.

Scanning electron micrograph used with permission from Nilsson, L. (1990). A child is born. New York: Dell Publishing.

The zygote now enters a period of rapid mitotic divisions, called **cleavage**, during which it divides into two cells, four cells, eight cells, and so on. These cells, called *blastomeres,* are so small that the developing cell mass is only slightly larger than the original zygote. The blastomeres are held together by the zona pellucida, which is under the corona radiata. The blastomeres eventually form a solid ball of 12 to 16 cells called the **morula**.

As the morula enters the uterus, two things happen: the intracellular fluid in the morula increases, and a central cavity forms within it. Inside this cavity is an inner solid mass of cells called the **blastocyst**. The outer layer of cells that surrounds the cavity and replaces the zona pellucida is the **trophoblast**. Eventually the trophoblast develops into one of the embryonic membranes, the **chorion**. The blastocyst develops into a double layer of cells called the

FIGURE 7-3

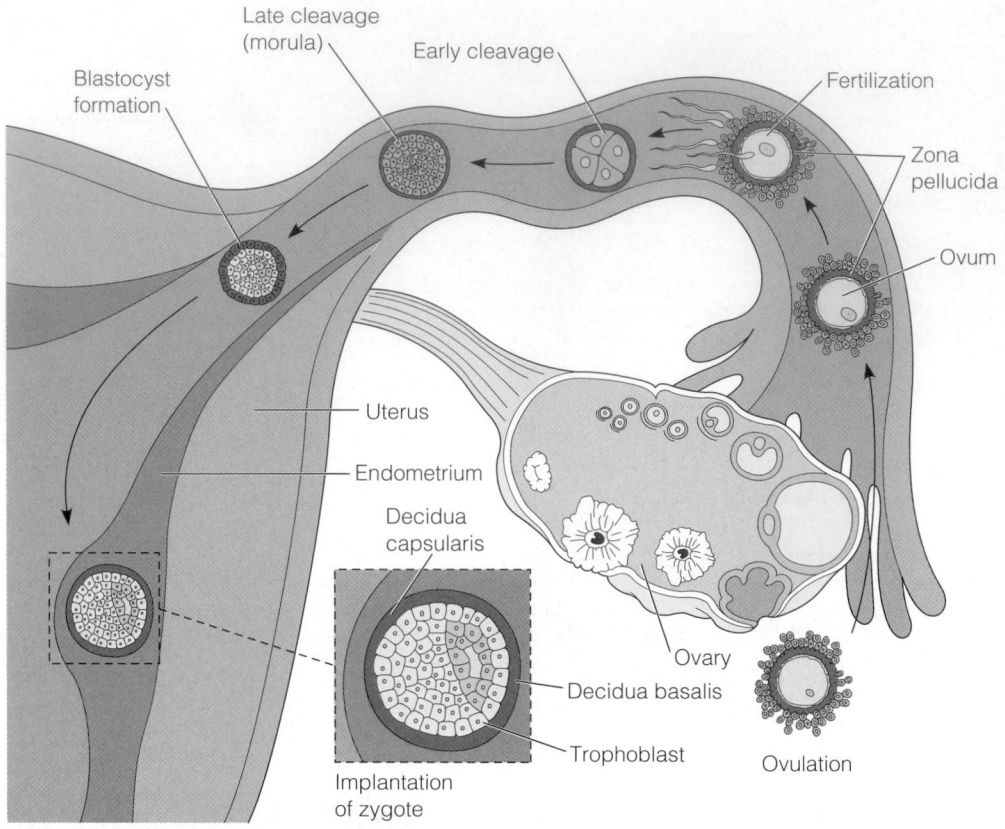

During ovulation the ovum leaves the ovary and enters the fallopian tube. Fertilization generally occurs in the outer third of the fallopian tube. Subsequent changes in the fertilized ovum from conception to implantation are depicted.

embryonic disc, from which the embryo and the amnion (embryonic membrane) will develop. The journey of the fertilized ovum to its destination in the uterus is illustrated in Figure 7–3 ◉.

One early pregnancy factor (EPF), an immunosuppressant protein, is secreted by the trophoblastic cells. EPF appears in the maternal serum within 24 to 48 hours after fertilization and forms the basis of a pregnancy test during the first 10 days of development (Moore & Persaud, 2003).

IMPLANTATION (NIDATION)

While floating in the uterine cavity, the blastocyst is nourished by the uterine glands, which secrete a mixture of lipids, mucopolysaccharides, and glycogen. The trophoblast attaches itself to the surface of the endometrium for further nourishment. The most frequent site of attachment is the upper part of the posterior uterine wall. Between days 7 and 10 after fertilization, the zona pellucida disappears and the blastocyst implants itself by burrowing into the uterine lining. It penetrates down toward the maternal capillaries until it is completely covered (Liu, 2004). The lining of the uterus thickens below the implanted blas-

tocyst, and the cells of the trophoblast grow down into the thickened lining, forming processes called chorionic villi.

Under the influence of progesterone, the endometrium increases in thickness and vascularity in preparation for implantation and nutrition of the ovum. After implantation the endometrium is called the *decidua.* The portion of the decidua that covers the blastocyst is called the **decidua capsularis.** The portion directly under the implanted blastocyst is the **decidua basalis,** and the portion that lines the rest of the uterine cavity is the **decidua vera (parietalis)** (Benirschke, 2004b). The maternal part of the placenta develops from the decidua basalis, which contains large numbers of blood vessels (see magnified insert in Figure 7–3). The chorionic villi (discussed shortly) in contact with the decidua basalis will form the fetal portion of the placenta.

CELL DIFFERENTIATION

Primary Germ Layers

About the 10th to 14th day after conception, the homogeneous mass of blastocyst cells differentiates into the primary germ layers (Figure 7–4 ◉). These three layers, the **ectoderm**, **mesoderm**, and **endoderm**, are formed at the

○ FIGURE 7–4

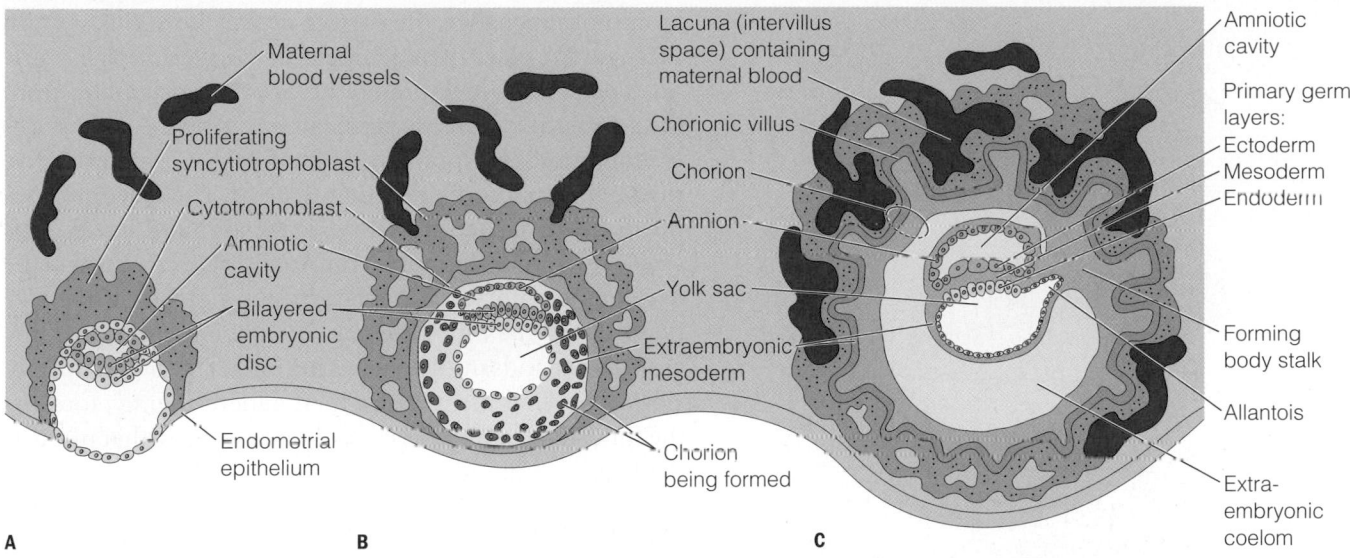

Formation of primary germ layers. **A,** Implantation of a 7 1/2-day blastocyst in which the cells of the embryonic disc are separated from the amnion by a fluid-filled space. The erosion of the endometrium by the syncytiotrophoblast is ongoing. **B,** Implantation is completed by day 9, and extraembryonic mesoderm is beginning to form a discrete layer beneath the cytotrophoblast. **C,** By day 16 the embryo shows all three germ layers, a yolk sac, and an allantois (an outpouching of the yolk sac that forms the structural basis of the body stalk, or umbilical cord). The cytotrophoblast and associated mesoderm have become the chorion, and chorionic villi are developing.

same time as the embryonic membranes. All tissues, organs, and organ systems develop from these primary germ cell layers (Table 7–2). For example, differentiation of the endoderm results in the formation of the epithelium lining the respiratory and digestive tracts (Figure 7–5 ○).

Embryonic Membranes

The **embryonic membranes** begin to form at the time of implantation (Figure 7–6 ○). These membranes protect and support the embryo as it grows and develops inside the uterus. The first and outermost membrane to form is the chorion. This thick membrane develops from the trophoblast and has many fingerlike projections called *chorionic villi* on its surface. These chorionic villi can be used for early genetic testing of the embryo at 8 to 11 weeks' gestation by chorionic villi sampling (see Chapter 16 ∞). As pregnancy progresses, the chorionic villi begin to degenerate, except for those just under the embryo, which

TABLE 7–2 ✛ Derivation of Body Structures from Primary Cell Layers

Ectoderm	Mesoderm	Endoderm
Epidermis	Dermis	Respiratory tract epithelium
Sweat glands	Wall of digestive tract	Epithelium (except nasal), including pharynx, tongue, tonsils, thyroid, parathyroid, thymus, tympanic cavity
Sebaceous glands	Kidneys and ureter (suprarenal cortex)	
Nails	Reproductive organs (gonads, genital ducts)	
Hair follicles	Connective tissue (cartilage, bone, joint cavities)	Lining of digestive tract
Lens of eye	Skeleton	Primary tissue of liver and pancreas
Sensory epithelium of internal and external ear, nasal cavity, sinuses, mouth, anal canal	Muscles (all types)	Urethra and associated glands
Central and peripheral nervous systems	Cardiovascular system (heart, arteries, veins, blood, bone marrow)	Urinary bladder (except trigone)
Nasal cavity	Pleura	Vagina (parts)
Oral glands and tooth enamel	Lymphatic tissue and cells	
Pituitary gland	Spleen	
Mammary glands		

◉ FIGURE 7–5

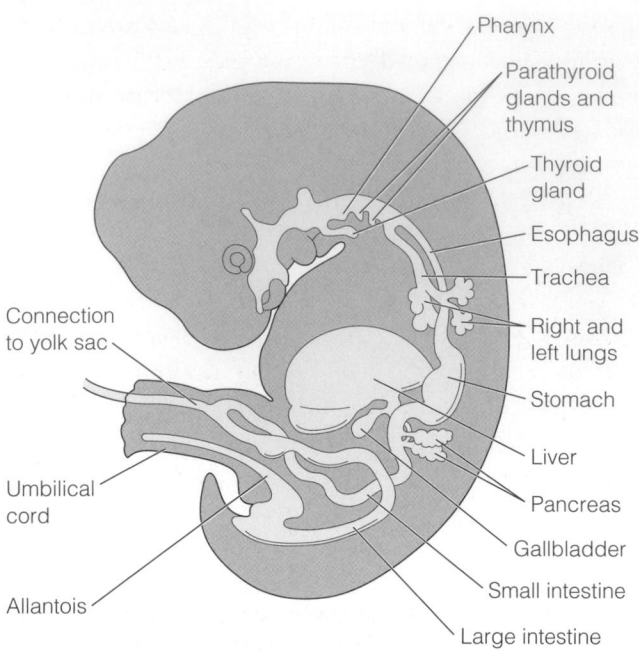

Pharynx

Parathyroid glands and thymus

Thyroid gland

Esophagus

Trachea

Right and left lungs

Stomach

Liver

Pancreas

Gallbladder

Small intestine

Large intestine

Connection to yolk sac

Umbilical cord

Allantois

5-week embryo

Endoderm differentiates to form the epithelial lining of the digestive and respiratory tracts and associated glands.

◉ FIGURE 7–6

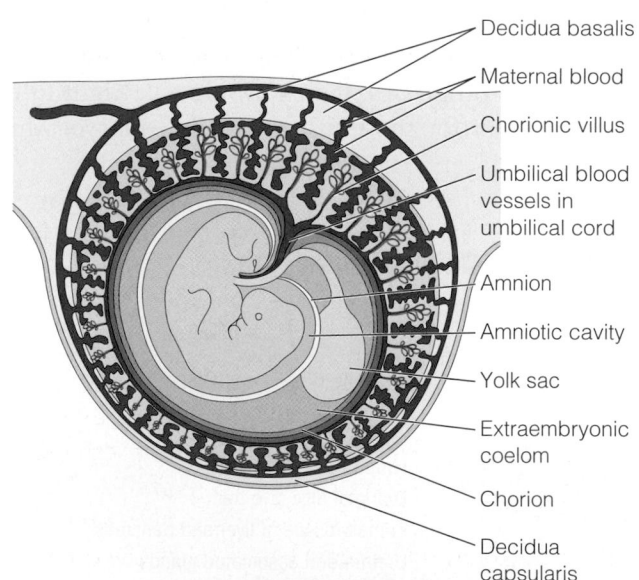

Decidua basalis

Maternal blood

Chorionic villus

Umbilical blood vessels in umbilical cord

Amnion

Amniotic cavity

Yolk sac

Extraembryonic coelom

Chorion

Decidua capsularis

Early development of primary embryonic membranes. At 4 1/2 weeks, the decidua capsularis (placental portion enclosing the embryo on the uterine surface) and decidua basalis (placental portion encompassing the elaborate chorionic villi and maternal endometrium) are well formed. The chorionic villi lie in blood-filled intervillous spaces within the endometrium. The amnion and yolk sac are well developed.

grow and branch into depressions in the uterine wall, forming the fetal portion of the placenta. By the fourth month of pregnancy, the surface of the chorion is smooth except at the place of attachment to the uterine wall.

The second membrane, the amnion, originates from the ectoderm, a primary germ layer, during the early stages of embryonic development. The **amnion** is a thin protective membrane that contains amniotic fluid. The space between the membrane and the embryo is the amniotic cavity. This cavity surrounds the embryo and yolk sac, except where the developing embryo (germ-layer disc) attaches to the trophoblast via the umbilical cord. As the embryo grows, the amnion expands until it comes in contact with the chorion. These two fetal membranes then adhere slightly, forming the fluid-filled amniotic sac, or **bag of waters**, that protects the floating embryo.

Amniotic Fluid

The primary functions of **amniotic fluid** are to:

- Act as a cushion to protect against mechanical injury.
- Help control the embryo's temperature (relies on mother to release heat).
- Permit symmetric external growth and development of the embryo-fetus.
- Act as an extension of fetal extracellular space (hydropic infants have increased amniotic fluid).
- Prevent adherence of the amnion to the embryo-fetus (decreases chance of amniotic band syndrome) to allow freedom of movement so that the embryo-fetus can change position (flexion and extension), thus aiding in musculoskeletal development.
- Allow the umbilical cord to be relatively free of compression.
- Act as a wedge during labor.
- Provide fluid for analysis to determine fetal health and maturity.

Amniotic fluid is slightly alkaline and contains albumin, uric acid, creatinine, lecithin, sphingomyelin, bilirubin, vernix, leukocytes, epithelial cells, enzymes, and fine hair called **lanugo**. The amount of amniotic fluid at 10 weeks is about 30 mL, and it increases to 350 mL at 20 weeks. After 20 weeks the volume ranges from 700 to 1000 mL. The amniotic fluid volume is constantly changing as the fluid moves back and forth across the placental membrane. As the pregnancy continues, the fetus contributes to the volume of amniotic fluid by excreting urine. The fetus swallows up to 600 mL every 24 hours, and about 400 mL of amniotic fluid flows out of the fetal lungs each day (Gilbert & Brace, 1993). See Chapter 21 for an in-depth discussion of alterations in amniotic fluid volume. ∞

Yolk Sac

In humans the yolk sac is small and functions early in embryonic life. It develops as a second cavity in the blastocyst on about day 8 or 9 after conception. It forms primitive red blood cells during the first 6 weeks of development, until the embryo's liver takes over the process. As the embryo develops, the yolk sac is incorporated into the umbilical cord, where it can be seen as a degenerated structure after birth.

Umbilical Cord

As the placenta is developing, the **umbilical cord** is also being formed from the amnion. The *body stalk,* which attaches the embryo to the yolk sac, contains blood vessels that extend into the chorionic villi. The body stalk fuses with the embryonic portion of the placenta to provide a circulatory pathway from the chorionic villi to the embryo. As the body stalk elongates to become the umbilical cord, the vessels in the cord decrease to one large vein and two smaller arteries. About 1% of umbilical cords have only two vessels, an artery and a vein; this condition may be associated with congenital malformations primarily of the renal, gastrointestinal, and cardiovascular systems. A specialized connective tissue known as **Wharton's jelly** surrounds the blood vessels in the umbilical cord. This tissue, plus the high blood volume pulsating through the vessels, prevents compression of the umbilical cord in utero. The umbilical cord has no sensory or motor innervation, so cutting the cord after birth is not painful. At term (38 to 42 weeks' gestation), the average cord is 2 cm (0.8 in.) across and about 55 cm (22 in.) long. The cord can attach itself to the placenta in various sites. Central insertion into the placenta is considered normal. (See Chapter 21 for a discussion of the various attachment sites. ∞)

Umbilical cords appear twisted or spiraled. This is most likely caused by fetal movement. A true knot in the umbilical cord rarely occurs; if it does, the cord is usually long. More common are so-called false knots, caused by the folding of cord vessels. A nuchal cord exists when the umbilical cord encircles the fetal neck.

TWINS

Twins occur in approximately 1 in 80 pregnancies, and triplets occur in 1 in 8,000 pregnancies. Fraternal twins have been reported to occur more often among black women than among white women and more often among white women than among women of Asian origin (Moore & Persaud, 2003). Among all groups, as parity (having given birth to a viable infant) increases, so does the chance for multiple births.

Twins may be either fraternal or identical (Figure 7–7 ⬤). If twins are fraternal, they are dizygotic, which means they arise from two separate ova fertilized by two separate spermatozoa. There are two placentas, two chorions, and two amnions; however, the placentas sometimes fuse and appear to be one. Despite their birth relationship, fraternal twins are no more similar to each other than they would be to siblings born singly. They may be of the same or different sex.

Dizygotic twinning increases with maternal age up to about age 35 and then decreases abruptly. The chance of dizygotic twins increases with parity, in conceptions that occur in the first 3 months of marriage, and also with coital frequency. The chance of dizygotic twinning decreases during periods of malnutrition and during winter and spring for women living in the Northern Hemisphere. Studies indicate that dizygotic twins occur in certain families, perhaps because of genetic factors that result in elevated serum gonadotropin levels and thus double ovulation (Benirschke, 2004a).

Identical, or monozygotic, twins develop from a single fertilized ovum. They are of the same sex and have the same genotype (appearance). Identical twins usually have a common placenta (see Figure 7–7). Monozygosity is not affected by environment, race, physical characteristics, or fertility.

Monozygotic twins originate from division of the fertilized ovum at different stages of early development, after the zygote consists of thousands of cells. Complete separation of the cellular mass into two parts is necessary for twin formation. The number of amnions and chorions present depends on the timing of the division:

1. If division occurs within 3 days of fertilization (before the inner cell mass and chorion are formed), two embryos, two amnions, and two chorions will develop. This dichorionic-diamniotic situation occurs about 20% to 30% of the time, and there may be two distinct placentas or a single fused placenta.

2. If division occurs about 5 days after fertilization (when the inner cell mass is formed and the chorion cells have differentiated but those of the amnion have not), two embryos develop with separate amniotic sacs. These sacs will eventually be covered by a common chorion; thus, there will be a monochorionic-diamniotic placenta.

3. If the amnion has already developed, approximately 7 to 13 days after fertilization, division results in two embryos with a common amniotic sac and a common chorion (a monochorionic-monoamniotic placenta). This type occurs about 1% of the time (Benirschke, 2004a).

Monozygotic twinning is considered a random event and occurs in approximately 3.5 per 1,000 live births (Benirschke, 2004a). The survival rate of monozygotic twins is 10% lower than that of dizygotic twins, and congenital anomalies are more prevalent. Both twins may have the same malformation.

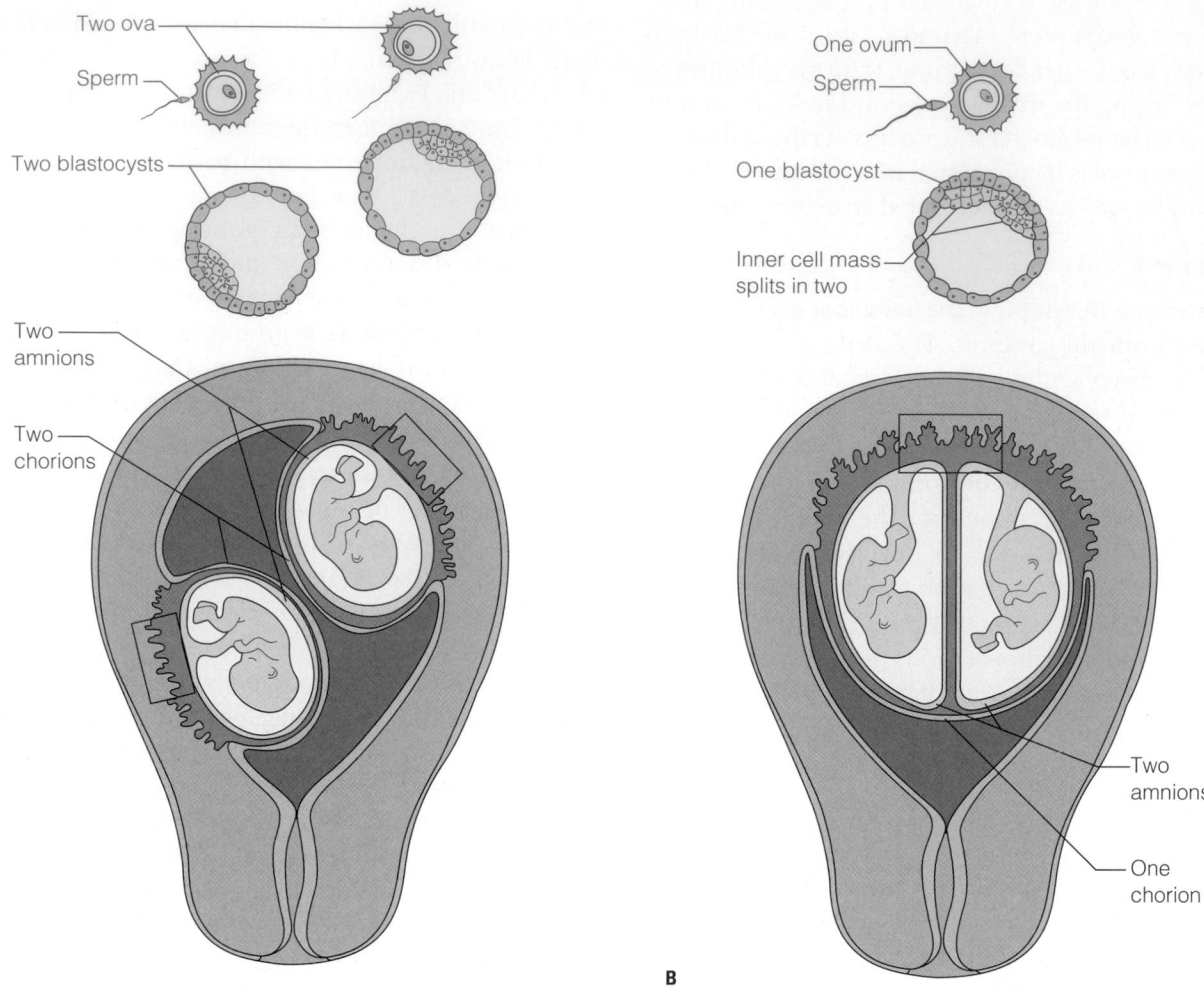

Two ova

Sperm

Two blastocysts

Two amnions

Two chorions

One ovum

Sperm

One blastocyst

Inner cell mass splits in two

Two amnions

One chorion

A

B

A, Formation of fraternal twins. (Note separate placentas.) **B,** Formation of identical twins.

DEVELOPMENT AND FUNCTIONS OF THE PLACENTA

The **placenta** is the means of metabolic and nutrient exchange between the embryonic and maternal circulations. Placental development and circulation do not begin until the third week of embryonic development. The placenta develops at the site where the embryo attaches to the uterine wall. Expansion of the placenta continues until about the 20th week, when it covers approximately one half of the internal surface of the uterus. After 20 weeks' gestation, the placenta becomes thicker but not wider. At 40 weeks' gestation, the placenta is about 15 to 20 cm (5.9 to 7.9 in.) in diameter and 2.5 to 3 cm (1 to 1.2 in.) in thickness. It weighs about 400 to 600 g (14 to 21 oz).

The placenta has two parts: the maternal and fetal portions. The maternal portion consists of the decidua basalis and its circulation. Its surface is red and fleshlike. The fetal portion consists of the chorionic villi and their circulation. The fetal surface of the placenta is covered by the amnion, which gives it a shiny, gray appearance (Figures 7–8 ● and 7–9 ●).

Development of the placenta begins with the chorionic villi. The trophoblastic cells of the chorionic villi form spaces in the tissue of the decidua basalis. These spaces fill with maternal blood, and the chorionic villi grow into them. As the chorionic villi differentiate, two trophoblastic layers appear: an outer layer called the *syncytium* (consisting of syncytiotrophoblasts), and an inner layer known as the *cytotrophoblast* (see Figure 7–4). The cytotrophoblast thins out and disappears about the fifth month, leaving only a single layer of syncytium covering the chorionic villi. The syncytium is in direct contact with the maternal blood in the intervillous spaces. It is the functional layer of the placenta and secretes the placental hormones of pregnancy.

A third, inner layer of connective mesoderm develops in the chorionic villi, forming *anchoring villi*. These anchoring villi eventually form the septa (partitions) of the placenta. The

FIGURE 7–8

Maternal side of placenta (Dirty Duncan).

septa divide the mature placenta into 15 to 20 segments called **cotyledons** (subdivisions of the placenta made up of anchoring villi and decidual tissue). In each cotyledon the *branching villi* form highly complex vascular systems. The exchange of gases and nutrients takes place across these vascular systems.

Exchange of substances across the placenta is minimal during the first 3 to 5 months of development because the villous membrane is initially too thick, which limits how permeable it is. As the villous membrane thins, placental permeability increases (until about the last month of pregnancy, when permeability begins to decrease as the placenta ages). In the fully developed placenta, fetal blood in

FIGURE 7–9

Fetal side of placenta (Shiny Shultz).

the villi and maternal blood in the intervillous spaces are separated by three to four thin layers of tissue.

PLACENTAL CIRCULATION

After implantation of the blastocyst, the cells distinguish themselves into fetal cells and trophoblastic cells. The proliferating trophoblast successfully invades the decidua basalis of the endometrium, first opening the uterine capillaries and later opening the larger uterine vessels. The chorionic villi are an outgrowth of the blastocystic tissue. As these villi continue to grow and divide, the fetal vessels begin to form. The intervillous spaces in the decidua basalis develop as the endometrial spiral arteries are opened.

By the fourth week, the placenta has begun to function as a means of metabolic exchange between embryo and mother. The completion of the maternal-placental-fetal circulation occurs about 17 days after conception, when the embryonic heart begins functioning (Moore & Persaud, 2003). By 14 weeks the placenta has grown in thickness as a result of growth in the length and size of the chorionic villi and accompanying expansion of the intervillous space.

In the fully developed placenta's umbilical cord, fetal blood flows through the two umbilical arteries to the capillaries of the villi, becomes oxygen enriched, and then flows back through the umbilical vein into the fetus (Figure 7–10). Late in pregnancy, a soft, blowing sound (*funic souffle*) can be heard over the area of the umbilical cord. The sound is synchronous with the fetal heartbeat and fetal blood flow through the umbilical arteries.

Maternal blood, rich in oxygen and nutrients, moves from the arcuate artery to the radial artery to the uterine spiral arteries and then spurts into the intervillous spaces. These spurts are produced and controlled by the maternal blood pressure. The blood is directed toward the chorionic plate, and as the spurt loses pressure, it becomes lateral (spreads out). Fresh blood enters continuously and exerts pressure on the contents of the intervillous spaces, pushing blood toward the exits in the basal plate. The blood then drains through the uterine and other pelvic veins. If vasoconstriction of the uterine arteries occurs as in preeclampsia, intrauterine growth restriction can occur (see further discussion in Chapter 30 ∞). A *uterine souffle*, timed precisely with the mother's pulse, is also heard just above the mother's symphysis pubis during the last months of pregnancy. This souffle is caused by the augmented blood flow entering the dilated uterine arteries.

Braxton Hicks contractions (see Chapter 17 ∞) are believed to facilitate placental circulation by enhancing the movement of blood from the center of the cotyledon through the intervillous space. Placental blood flow is enhanced when the woman is lying on her left side because the vena cava is not compromised. Some evidence exists that lying on either side can enhance blood flow.

○ FIGURE 7–10

Vascular arrangement of the placenta. Arrows indicate the direction of blood flow. Maternal blood flows through the uterine arteries to the intervillous spaces of the placenta and returns through the uterine veins to maternal circulation. Fetal blood flows through the umbilical arteries into the villous capillaries of the placenta and returns through the umbilical vein to the fetal circulation.

PLACENTAL FUNCTIONS

Placental exchange functions occur only in those fetal vessels in intimate contact with the covering syncytial membrane. The syncytium villi have brush borders containing many microvilli, which greatly increase the exchange rate between maternal and fetal circulation (Sadler, 2004).

The placental functions, many of which begin soon after implantation, include fetal respiration, nutrition, and excretion. To carry out these functions, the placenta is involved in metabolic and transfer activities. In addition it has endocrine functions and special immunologic properties.

Metabolic Activities

The placenta continuously produces glycogen, cholesterol, and fatty acids for fetal use and hormone production. The placenta also produces numerous enzymes required for fetoplacental transfer, breaks down certain substances such as epinephrine and histamine, and stores glycogen and iron.

Transport Function

The placental membranes actively control the transfer of a wide range of substances by four major mechanisms (Bawdon & Hnat, 2003):

1. *Simple diffusion* moves substances from an area of higher concentration to an area of lower concentration. Substances that move across the placenta by simple diffusion include water, oxygen, carbon dioxide, electrolytes (sodium and chloride), anesthetic gases, and drugs. Insulin and steroid hormones originating from the adrenals and thyroid hormones also cross the placenta, but at a very slow rate. The rate of oxygen transfer across the placental membrane is greater than that allowed by simple diffusion, indicating that oxygen is also transferred by some type of facilitated diffusion transport. Unfortunately, many substances of abuse, such as cocaine, cross the placenta via simple diffusion.

2. *Facilitated transport* involves a carrier system to move molecules from an area of greater concentration to an area of lower concentration at a more rapid rate than by simple diffusion. Molecules such as glucose, galactose, and some oxygen are transported by this method. The glucose level in the fetal blood is ordinarily 20% to 30% lower than the glucose level in the maternal blood because the fetus metabolizes glucose rapidly. This lower level, in turn, causes rapid transport of additional glucose from the maternal blood into the fetal blood.

3. *Active transport* can work against a concentration gradient and allows molecules to move from areas of

lower concentration to areas of higher concentration. Amino acids, calcium, iron, iodine, water-soluble vitamins, and glucose are transferred across the placenta this way. The measured amino acid content of fetal blood is greater than that of maternal blood, and calcium and inorganic phosphate occur in greater concentration in fetal blood than in maternal blood (Blackburn, 2003).

Other modes of transfer also exist. *Pinocytosis* is important for transferring large molecules such as albumin and gamma globulin. Materials are engulfed by ameba-like cells, forming plasma droplets.

4. *Hydrostatic* and *osmotic pressures* allow the bulk flow of water and some solutes. Fetal red blood cells pass into the maternal circulation through breaks in the placental membrane, particularly during labor and birth. Certain cells, such as maternal leukocytes, and microorganisms, such as viruses (e.g., the human immunodeficiency virus [HIV], which causes acquired immunodeficiency syndrome [AIDS]) and the bacterium *Treponema pallidum,* which causes syphilis, can also cross the placental membrane under their own power (Moore & Persaud, 2003). Some bacteria and protozoa infect the placenta by causing lesions and then entering the fetal blood system.

Reduction of the placental surface area, as with abruptio placentae (partial or complete premature separation of an abnormally implanted placenta), lessens the area that is functional for exchange. Placental diffusion distance also affects exchange. In conditions such as diabetes and placental infection, edema of the villi increases the diffusion distance, thus increasing the distance the substance has to be transferred. Blood flow alteration changes the transfer rate of substances. Decreased blood flow in the intervillous space is seen in labor and with certain maternal diseases such as preeclampsia. Mild fetal hypoxia increases the umbilical blood flow, but severe hypoxia results in decreased blood flow.

As the maternal blood picks up fetal waste products and carbon dioxide, it drains back into the maternal circulation through the veins in the basal plate. Fetal blood is hypoxic by comparison; it therefore attracts oxygen from the mother's blood. Affinity for oxygen increases as the fetal blood gives up its carbon dioxide, which also decreases its acidity.

Endocrine Functions

The placenta produces hormones vital to survival of the fetus. These include human chorionic gonadotropin (hCG); human placental lactogen (hPL); and two steroid hormones, estrogen and progesterone.

The hormone hCG is similar to luteinizing hormone (LH) and prevents the normal involution of the corpus luteum at the end of the menstrual cycle. If the corpus luteum stops functioning before the 11th week of pregnancy, spontaneous abortion occurs. The hCG also causes the corpus luteum to secrete increased amounts of estrogen and progesterone.

After the 11th week, the placenta produces enough progesterone and estrogen to maintain pregnancy. In the male fetus, hCG also exerts an interstitial cell-stimulating effect on the testes, resulting in the production of testosterone. This small secretion of testosterone during embryonic development is the factor that causes male sex organs to grow. Human chorionic gonadotropin may play a role in the trophoblast's immunologic capabilities (ability to exempt the placenta and embryo from rejection by the mother's system). This hormone is used as a basis for pregnancy tests (see Chapter 9 ∞).

Human chorionic gonadotropin is present in maternal blood serum 8 to 10 days after fertilization, just as soon as implantation has occurred, and is detectable in maternal urine at the time of missed menses. It reaches its maximum level at 50 to 70 days' gestation and begins to decrease as placental hormone production increases.

Progesterone is a hormone essential for pregnancy. It increases the secretions of the fallopian tubes and uterus to provide appropriate nutritive matter for the developing morula and blastocyst. It also appears to aid in ovum transport through the fallopian tube (Liu, 2004). Progesterone causes decidual cells to develop in the uterine endometrium, and it must be present in high levels for implantation to occur. Progesterone also decreases the contractility of the uterus, thus preventing uterine contractions from causing spontaneous abortion.

Prior to stimulation by hCG, the production of progesterone by the corpus luteum reaches a peak about 7 to 10 days after ovulation. Implantation occurs at about the same time as this peak. At 16 days after ovulation, progesterone reaches a level between 25 and 50 mg per day and continues to rise slowly in subsequent weeks. After 10 weeks the placenta (specifically, the syncytiotrophoblast) takes over the production of progesterone and secretes it in tremendous quantities, reaching levels of more than 250 mg per day late in pregnancy.

By 7 weeks the placenta produces more than 50% of the estrogens in the maternal circulation. *Estrogens* serve mainly a proliferative function, causing enlargement of the uterus, breasts, and breast glandular tissue. Estrogens also have a significant role in increasing vascularity and vasodilation, particularly in the villous capillaries toward the end of pregnancy. Placental estrogens increase markedly toward the end of pregnancy, to as much as 30 times the daily production in the middle of a normal monthly menstrual cycle. The primary estrogen secreted by the placenta is different from that secreted by the ovaries. The placenta secretes mainly *estriol,* whereas the ovaries secrete primarily *estradiol.*

The placenta cannot synthesize estriol by itself. The fetal adrenal glands provide essential precursors that are transported to the placenta for the final conversion to estriol.

The hormone hPL, also called human chorionic somatomammotropin (hCS), is similar to human pituitary growth hormone; hPL stimulates certain changes in the mother's metabolic processes. These changes ensure that more protein, glucose, and minerals are available for the fetus. Secretion of hPL can be detected by about 4 weeks after conception.

Immunologic Properties

The placenta and embryo are transplants of living tissue within the same species and are therefore considered *homografts*. Unlike other homografts, the placenta and embryo appear exempt from immunologic reaction by the host. The most recent data suggest that the placental hormones (progesterone and hCG) suppress cellular immunity during pregnancy. One theory suggests that trophoblastic tissue is immunologically inert. It may contain a cell coating that masks transplantation antigens, repels sensitized lymphocytes, and protects against antibody formation.

DEVELOPMENT OF THE FETAL CIRCULATORY SYSTEM

The circulatory system of the fetus has several unique features that, by maintaining the blood flow to the placenta, provide the fetus with oxygen and nutrients, while removing carbon dioxide and other waste products.

Most of the blood supply bypasses the fetal lungs, since they do not carry out respiratory gas exchange. The placenta assumes the function of the fetal lungs by supplying oxygen and allowing the fetus to excrete carbon dioxide into the maternal bloodstream. Figure 7–11 ● shows the fetal circulatory system. The blood from the placenta flows through the umbilical vein, which enters the abdominal wall of the fetus at the site that, after birth, is the umbilicus (belly button). As umbilical venous blood approaches the liver, a small portion of the blood enters the liver sinusoids and mixes with blood from the portal circulation and then enters the inferior vena cava via hepatic veins. Most of the umbilical vein's blood flows through the **ductus venous** directly into the inferior vena cava by bypassing the liver. This blood then enters the right atrium, passes through the **foramen ovale** into the left atrium, and pours into the left ventricle, which pumps it into the aorta. Some blood returning from the head and upper extremities by way of the superior vena cava is emptied into the right atrium and passes through the tricuspid valve into the right ventricle. This blood is pumped into the pulmonary artery, and a small amount passes to the lungs for nourishment only. The larger portion of blood passes from the pulmonary artery through the **ductus arteriosus** into the descending aorta, bypassing the lungs. Finally, blood returns to the placenta through the two umbilical arteries, and the process is repeated.

The fetus obtains oxygen via diffusion from the maternal circulation because of the gradient difference of PO_2 of 50 mm Hg in maternal blood in the placenta to 30 mm Hg PO_2 in the fetus. At term the fetus receives oxygen from the mother's circulation at a rate of 20 to 30 mL per minute (Sadler, 2004). Fetal hemoglobin facilitates obtaining oxygen from the maternal circulation, because it carries as much as 20% to 30% more oxygen than adult hemoglobin. For further discussion, see Chapter 23. ∞

Fetal circulation delivers the highest available oxygen concentration to the head, neck, brain, and heart (coronary circulation) and a lesser amount of oxygenated blood to the abdominal organs and the lower body. This circulatory pattern leads to cephalocaudal (head-to-tail) development in the fetus.

EMBRYONIC AND FETAL DEVELOPMENT

Pregnancy is calculated to last an *average* of 10 lunar months: 40 weeks, or 280 days. This period of 280 days is calculated from the onset of the last normal menstrual period to the time of birth. Estimated date of birth (EDB), sometimes referred to as the estimated date of delivery (EDD), is usually calculated by this method. Most fetuses are born within 10 to 14 days of the calculated date of birth. The fertilization age (or postconception age) of the fetus is calculated to be *about* 2 weeks less: 266 days (38 weeks), or 9.5 calendar months. This latter measurement is more accurate because it measures time from the fertilization of the ovum, or conception. The basic events of organ development in the embryo and fetus are outlined in Table 7–3. The time periods in the table are **postconception age periods**. During the period from fertilization to the end of the embryonic period (8 weeks), age is often expressed in days but can be given in weeks. During the fetal period (ninth week until birth), age is given in weeks (Moore & Persaud, 2003). For detailed discussion of the development of each body system, see Chapter 23; ∞ the foldout poster in the middle of the book summarizes fetal development.

Human development follows three stages. The preembryonic stage consists of the first 14 days of development after the ovum is fertilized, the embryonic stage covers the period from day 15 until approximately the end of the eighth week, and the fetal stage extends from the end of the eighth week until birth.

EMBRYONIC STAGE

The stage of the **embryo** starts on day 15 (the beginning of the third week after conception) and continues until approximately the eighth week, or until the embryo reaches a

● **FIGURE 7–11**

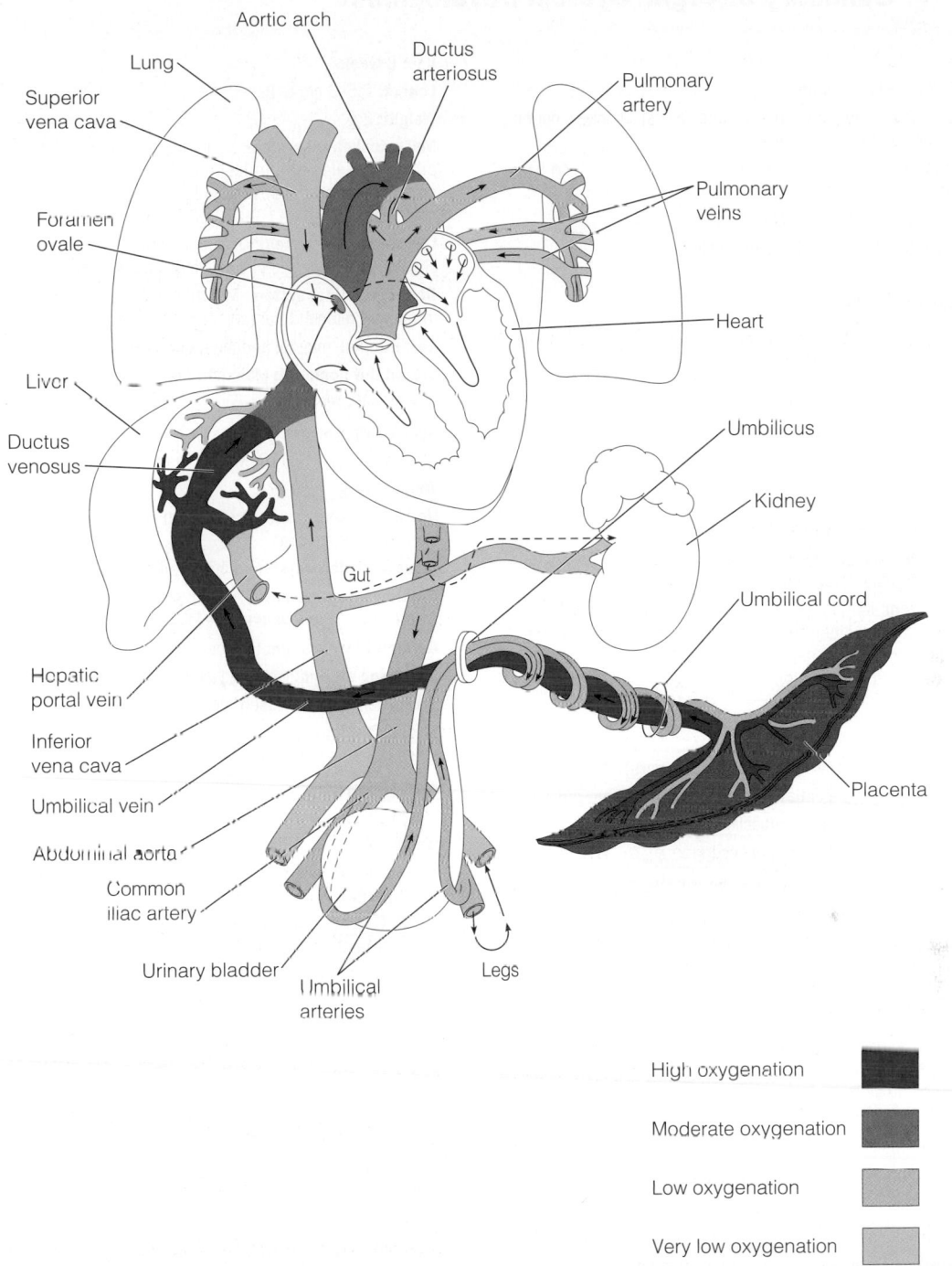

High oxygenation

Moderate oxygenation

Low oxygenation

Very low oxygenation

Fetal circulation. Blood leaves the placenta and enters the fetus through the umbilical vein. After circulating through the fetus, the blood returns to the placenta through the umbilical arteries. The ductus venosus, the foramen ovale, and the ductus arteriosus allow the blood to bypass the fetal liver and lungs.

crown-to-rump (C–R) length of 3 cm (1.2 in.). This length is usually reached about 56 days after fertilization (the end of the eighth gestational week). During the embryonic stage, tissues differentiate into essential organs and the main external features develop (Figure 7–12 ●). The embryo is the most vulnerable to teratogens during this period.

Three Weeks

In the third week, the embryonic disc becomes elongated and pear shaped, with a broad cephalic end and a narrow caudal end. The ectoderm has formed a long cylindric tube for brain and spinal cord development. The gastrointestinal tract, created from the endoderm, appears as another

TABLE 7–3 ✢ Summary of Organ System Development

Age: 2–3 weeks
Length: 2 mm C–R (Crown-to-Rump)
Nervous system: Groove forms along middle back as cells thicken; neural tube forms from closure of neural groove.
Cardiovascular system: Beginning of blood circulation; tubular heart begins to form during third week.
Gastrointestinal system: Liver begins to function.
Genitourinary system: Formation of kidneys beginning.
Respiratory system: Nasal pits forming.
Endocrine system: Thyroid tissue appears.
Eyes: Optic cup and lens pit have formed; pigment in eyes.
Ear: Auditory pit is now enclosed structure.

Age: 4 weeks
Length: 4–6 mm C–R
Weight: 0.4 g
Nervous system: Anterior portion of neural tube closes to form brain; closure of posterior end forms spinal cord.
Musculoskeletal system: Noticeable limb buds.
Cardiovascular system: Tubular heart beats at 28 days, and primitive red blood cells circulate through fetus and chorionic villi.
Gastrointestinal system: Mouth: formation of oral cavity; primitive jaws present; esophagotracheal septum begins division of esophagus and trachea. Digestive tract: stomach forms; esophagus and intestine become tubular; ducts of pancreas and liver forming.

Age: 5 weeks
Length: 8 mm C–R
Weight: Only 0.5% of total body weight is fat (to 20 weeks).
Nervous system: Brain has differentiated and cranial nerves are present.
Musculoskeletal system: Developing muscles have innervation.
Cardiovascular system: Atrial division has occurred.

Age: 6 weeks
Length: 12 mm C–R
Musculoskeletal system: Bone rudiments present; primitive skeletal shape forming; muscle mass begins to develop; ossification of skull and jaws begins.
Cardiovascular system: Chambers present in heart; groups of blood cells can be identified.
Gastrointestinal system: Oral and nasal cavities and upper lip formed; liver begins to form red blood cells.
Respiratory system: Trachea, bronchi, and lung buds present.
Ear: Formation of external, middle, and inner ear continues.
Sexual development: Embryonic sex glands appear.

Age: 7 weeks
Length: 18 mm C–R
Cardiovascular system: Fetal heartbeats can be detected.
Gastrointestinal system: Mouth: tongue separates; palate folds. Digestive tract: stomach attains final form.
Genitourinary system: Separation of bladder and urethra from rectum.
Respiratory system: Diaphragm separates abdominal and thoracic cavities.
Eyes: Optic nerve formed; eyelids appear, thickening of lens.
Sexual development: Differentiation of sex glands into ovaries and testes begins.

Age: 8 weeks
Length: 2.5–3 cm C–R
Weight: 2 g
Musculoskeletal system: Digits formed; further differentiation of cells in primitive skeleton; cartilaginous bones show first signs of ossification; development of muscles in trunk, limbs, and head; some movement of fetus now possible.
Cardiovascular system: Development of heart essentially complete; fetal circulation follows two circuits—four extraembryonic and two intraembryonic.
Gastrointestinal system: Mouth: completion of lip fusion. Digestive tract: rotation in midgut; anal membrane has perforated.
Ear: External, middle, and inner ear assuming final forms.
Sexual development: Male and female external genitals appear similar until end of ninth week.

Age: 10 weeks
Length: 5–6 cm C–H (Crown-to-Heel)
Weight: 14 g
Nervous system: Neurons appear at caudal end of spinal cord; basic divisions of brain present.
Musculoskeletal system: Fingers and toes begin nail growth.
Gastrointestinal system: Mouth: separation of lips from jaw; fusion of palate folds. Digestive tract: developing intestines enclosed in abdomen.
Genitourinary system: Bladder sac formed.
Endocrine system: Islets of Langerhans differentiated.
Eyes: Eyelids fused closed; development of lacrimal duct.
Sexual development: Males: production of testosterone and physical characteristics between 8 and 12 weeks.

Age: 12 weeks
Length: 8 cm C–R; 11.5 cm C–H
Weight: 45 g
Musculoskeletal system: Clear outlining of miniature bones (12–20 weeks); process of ossification is established throughout fetal body; appearance of involuntary muscles in viscera.
Gastrointestinal system: Mouth: completion of palate. Digestive tract: appearance of muscles in gut; bile secretion begins; liver is major producer of red blood cells.
Respiratory system: Lungs acquire definitive shape.
Skin: Pink and delicate.
Endocrine system: Hormonal secretion from thyroid; insulin present in pancreas.
Immunologic system: Appearance of lymphoid tissue in fetal thymus gland.

Age: 16 weeks
Length: 13.5 cm C–R; 15 cm C–H
Weight: 200 g
Musculoskeletal system: Teeth beginning to form hard tissue that will become central incisors.
Gastrointestinal system: Mouth: differentiation of hard and soft palate. Digestive tract: development of gastric and intestinal glands; intestines begin to collect meconium.
Genitourinary system: Kidneys assume typical shape and organization.
Skin: Appearance of scalp hair; lanugo present on body; transparent skin with visible blood vessels; sweat glands developing.
Eye, ear, and nose: Formed.
Sexual development: Sex determination possible.

Note: Age refers to postconception age or postfertilization age.

TABLE 7–3 ✤ Summary of Organ System Development—continued

Age: 18 weeks

Musculoskeletal system: Teeth beginning to form hard tissue (enamel and dentin) that will become lateral incisors.

Cardiovascular system: Fetal heart tones audible with fetoscope at 16–20 weeks.

Age: 20 weeks

Length: 19 cm C–R; 25 cm C–H

Weight: 435 g (6% of total body weight is fat)

Nervous system: Myelination of spinal cord begins.

Musculoskeletal system: Teeth beginning to form hard tissue that will become canine and first molar. Lower limbs are of final relative proportions.

Gastrointestinal system: Fetus actively sucks and swallows amniotic fluid; peristaltic movements begin.

Skin: Lanugo covers entire body; brown fat begins to form; vernix caseosa begins to form.

Immunologic system: Detectable levels of fetal antibodies (IgG type).

Blood formation: Iron is stored and bone marrow is increasingly important.

Age: 24 weeks

Length: 23 cm C–R; 28 cm C–H

Weight: 780 g

Nervous system: Brain looks like mature brain.

Musculoskeletal system: Teeth are beginning to form hard tissue that will become the second molar.

Respiratory system: Respiratory movements may occur (24–40 weeks). Nostrils reopen. Alveoli appear in lungs and begin production of surfactant; gas exchange possible.

Skin: Reddish and wrinkled, vernix caseosa present.

Immunologic system: IgG levels reach maternal levels.

Eyes: Structurally complete.

Age: 28 weeks

Length: 27 cm C–R; 35 cm C–H

Weight: 1200–1250 g

Nervous system: Begins regulation of some body functions.

Skin: Adipose tissue accumulates rapidly; nails appear; eyebrows and eyelashes present.

Eyes: Eyelids open (28–32 weeks).

Sexual development: Males; testes descend into inguinal canal and upper scrotum.

Age: 32 weeks

Length: 31 cm C–R; 38–43 cm C–H

Weight: 2000 g

Nervous system: More reflexes present.

Age: 36 weeks

Length: 35 cm C–R; 42–48 cm C–H

Weight: 2500–2750 g

Musculoskeletal system: Distal femoral ossification centers present.

Skin: Pale; body rounded, lanugo disappearing, hair fuzzy or woolly; few sole creases; sebaceous glands active and helping to produce vernix caseosa (36–40 weeks).

Ears: Earlobes soft with little cartilage.

Sexual development: Males: scrotum small and few rugae present; descent of testes into upper scrotum to stay (36–40 weeks). Females: labia majora and minora equally prominent.

Age: 38 weeks

Length: 40 cm C–R; 48–52 cm C–H

Weight: 3200+ g (16% of total body weight is fat)

Respiratory system: At 38 weeks, lecithin-sphingomyelin (L/S) ratio approaches 2:1 (indicates decreased risk of respiratory distress from inadequate surfactant production if born now).

Skin: Smooth and pink; vernix present in skinfolds; moderate to profuse silky hair; lanugo hair on shoulders and upper back; nails extend over tips or digits; creases cover sole.

Ears: Earlobes firmer due to increased cartilage.

Sexual development: Males: rugous scrotum. Females: labia majora well developed and minora small or completely covered.

Note: Age refers to postconception age or postfertilization age.

Data from Sadler, I. W. (2004). *Langman's medical embryology* (9th ed.). Philadelphia: Lippincott Williams & Wilkins.

---

tubelike structure communicating with the yolk sac. The most advanced organ is the heart. At 3 weeks a single tubular heart forms just outside the body cavity of the embryo.

Four to Five Weeks

During days 21 to 32, *somites* (a series of mesodermal blocks) form on either side of the embryo's midline. The vertebrae that form the spinal column will develop from these somites. Prior to 28 days, arm and leg buds are not visible, but the tail bud is present. The pharyngeal arches—which will form the lower jaw, hyoid bone, and larynx—develop at this time. The pharyngeal pouches appear; these pouches will form the eustachian tube and cavity of the middle ear, the tonsils, and the parathyroid and thymus glands. The primordia of the ear and eye are also present. By the end of 28 days, the tubular heart is beating at a reg-

ular rhythm and pushing its own primitive blood cells through the main blood vessels.

During the fifth week, the optic cups and lens vessels of the eye form and the nasal pits develop. Partitioning in the heart occurs with the dividing of the atrium. The embryo has a marked C-shaped body, accentuated by the rudimentary tail and the large head folded over a protuberant trunk (Figure 7–13 ●). By day 35 the arm and leg buds are well developed, with paddle-shaped hand and foot plates. The heart, circulatory system, and brain show the most advanced development. The brain has differentiated into five areas, and 10 pairs of cranial nerves are recognizable.

Six Weeks

At 6 weeks the head structures are more highly developed and the trunk is straighter than in earlier stages. The upper

● **FIGURE 7–12**

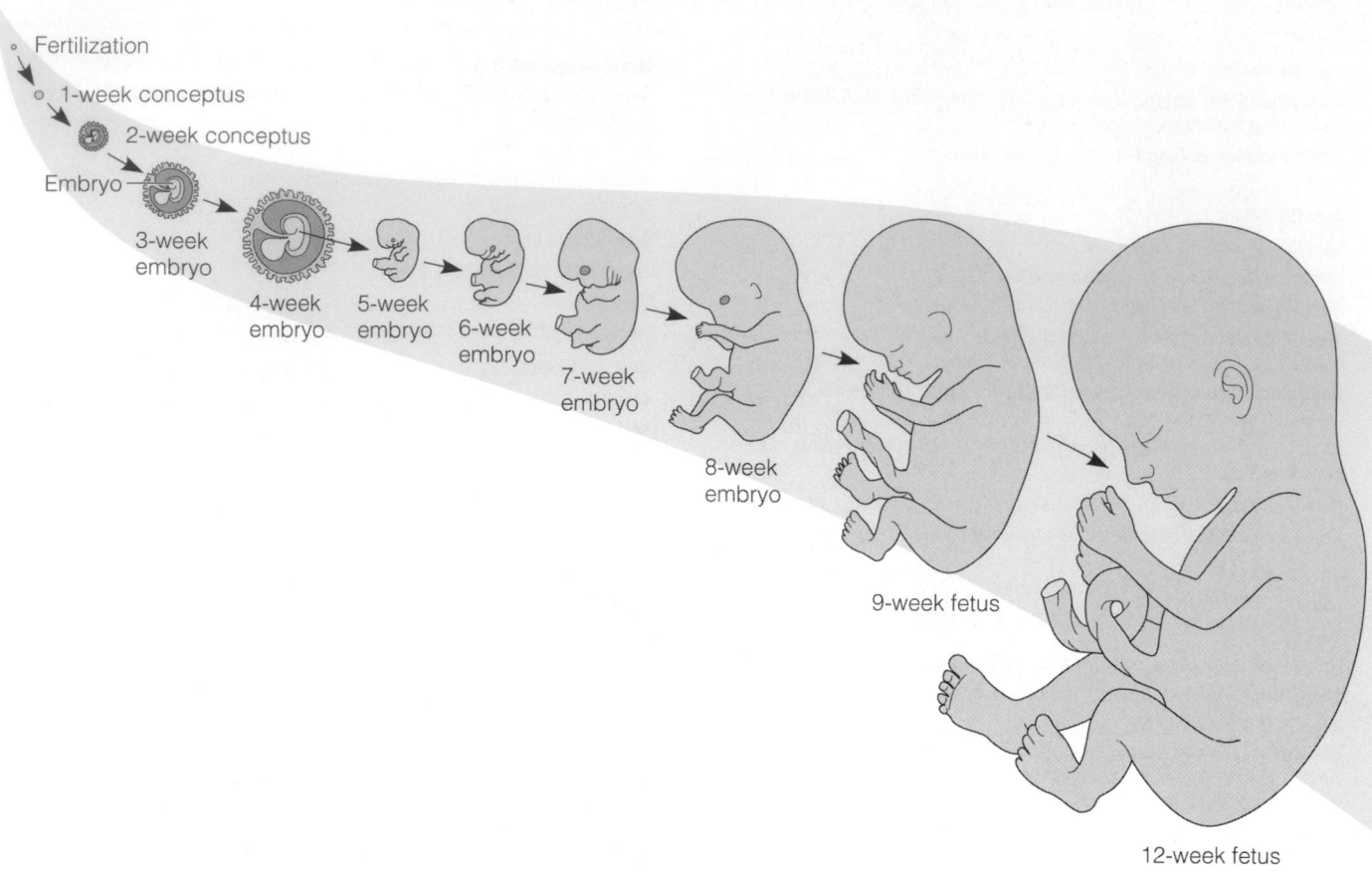

- Fertilization
- 1-week conceptus
- 2-week conceptus
- Embryo
- 3-week embryo
- 4-week embryo
- 5-week embryo
- 6-week embryo
- 7-week embryo
- 8-week embryo
- 9-week fetus
- 12-week fetus

The actual size of a human conceptus from fertilization to the early fetal stage. The embryonic stage begins in the third week after fertilization; the fetal stage begins in the ninth week.

and lower jaws are recognizable, and the external nares are well formed. The trachea has developed, and its caudal end is divided for beginning lung formation. The upper lip has formed, and the palate is developing. The ears are developing rapidly. The arms have begun to extend ventrally across the chest, and both arms and legs have digits, although they may still be webbed. There is a slight elbow bend in the arms, which are more advanced in development than the legs. Beginning at this stage, the prominent tail will recede. The heart has most of its definitive characteristics, and fetal circulation begins to be established. The liver starts to produce blood cells.

Seven Weeks

At 7 weeks the head of the embryo is rounded and nearly erect (Figure 7–14 ●). The eyes have shifted and are closer together, and the eyelids are beginning to form. Prior to this time the rectal and urogenital passages

formed one tube that ended in a blind pouch; they now separate into two tubular structures. The intestines enter the extraembryonic coelom in the area of the umbilical cord (called umbilical herniation) (Moore & Persaud, 2003). The beginnings of all essential external and internal structures are present.

Eight Weeks

At 8 weeks the embryo is approximately 3 cm (1.2 in.) long C–R and clearly resembles a human being. Facial features continue to develop. The eyelids begin to fuse. Auricles of the external ears begin to assume their final shape, but they are still set low (Moore & Persaud, 2003). External genitals appear, but the embryo's sex is not clearly discernible, and the rectal passage opens with the perforation of the anal membrane. The circulatory system through the umbilical cord is well established. Long bones are beginning to form, and the large muscles are capable of contracting.

● FIGURE 7–13

The embryo at 5 weeks. The embryo has a marked C-shaped body and a rudimentary tail.

Used with permission from Petit Format/Nestle/Science Source/Photo Researchers, Inc.

● FIGURE 7–14

The embryo at 7 weeks. The head is rounded and nearly erect. The eyes have shifted forward and closer together, and the eyelids begin to form.

Used with permission from Petit Format/Nestle/Science Source/Photo Researchers, Inc.

FETAL STAGE

By the end of the eighth week, the embryo is sufficiently developed to be called a **fetus**. Every organ system and external structure that will be found in the full-term newborn is present. The remainder of gestation is devoted to refining structures and perfecting function.

Nine to Twelve Weeks

By the end of the ninth week, the fetus reaches a C–R length of 5 cm (2 in.) and weighs about 14 g (0.5 oz). The head is large and comprises almost half of the fetus's entire size (Figure 7–15 ●). At 12 weeks the fetus reaches 8 cm (3.2 in.) C–R and weighs about 45 g (1.6 oz). The face is well formed, with the nose protruding, the chin small and receding, and the ear acquiring a more adult shape. The eyelids close at about the 10th week and will not begin to reopen until about the 26th week. Some movement of the lips suggestive of the sucking reflex has been observed at 3 months. Tooth buds appear for all 20 of the child's first teeth (baby teeth). The limbs are long and slender, with well-formed digits. The fetus can curl the fingers toward the palm and begins to make a tiny fist. The legs are still shorter and less developed than the arms. The urogenital tract completes its development, well-differentiated genitals appear, and the kidneys begin to produce urine. Red blood cells are produced primarily by the liver. Spontaneous movements of the fetus occur. Fetal heart rates can be ascertained by electronic devices between 8 and 12 weeks. The rate is 120 to 160 beats per minute.

Thirteen to Sixteen Weeks

This is a period of rapid growth. At 13 weeks the fetus weighs 55 to 60 g (1.9 to 2.1 oz) and is about 9 cm (3.6 in.) in C–R length. Lanugo, or fine hair, begins to develop, especially on the head. Blood vessels are clearly visible beneath the trans-

● FIGURE 7–15

The fetus at 9 weeks. Every organ system and external structure is present.

Used with permission from Nilsson, L. (1990). A child is born. New York: Dell Publishing.

parent skin. More muscle tissue and body skeleton have developed and hold the fetus more erect (Figure 7–16 ◉). Active movements are present; the fetus stretches and exercises its arms and legs. It makes sucking motions, swallows amniotic fluid, and produces meconium in the intestinal tract. By the beginning of week 16, skeletal ossification is clearly identifiable.

Twenty Weeks

The fetus doubles its C–R length and now measures 19 cm (8 in.) long. Fetal weight is between 435 and 465 g (15.2 and 16.3 oz). Lanugo covers the entire body and is especially prominent on the shoulders. Subcutaneous deposits of brown fat, which has a rich blood supply, make the skin less transparent. Nipples appear over the mammary glands. The head is covered with fine, woolly hair, and the eyebrows and eyelashes are beginning to form. Muscles are well developed, and the fetus is active (Figure 7–17 ◉). The mother feels fetal movement known as quickening. The fetal heartbeat is audible through a fetoscope. Quickening and fetal heartbeat can help in validating the estimated date of birth.

Twenty-Four Weeks

The fetus at 24 weeks reaches a crown-to-heel (C–H) length of 28 cm (11.2 in.). It weighs about 780 g (1 lb, 10 oz). The hair on the head is growing long, and eyebrows and eyelashes have formed. The eye is structurally com-

◉ FIGURE 7–17

The fetus at 20 weeks weighs 435 to 465 g and measures about 19 cm. Subcutaneous deposits of brown fat make the skin a little less transparent. "Woolly" hair covers the head, and nails have developed on the fingers and toes.

Used with permission from Nilsson, L. (1990). A child is born. New York: Dell Publishing.

◉ FIGURE 7–16

The fetus at 14 weeks. During this period of rapid growth, the skin is so transparent that blood vessels are visible beneath it. More muscle tissue and body skeleton have developed, and they hold the fetus more erect.

Used with permission from Nilsson, L. (1990). A child is born. New York: Dell Publishing.

plete and will soon open. The fetus has a reflex hand grip (grasp reflex) and, by the end of 6 months, a startle reflex. Skin covering the body is reddish and wrinkled, with little subcutaneous fat. Skin on the hands and feet has thickened, with skin ridges on palms and soles forming distinct foot- and fingerprints. The skin over the entire body is covered with **vernix caseosa**, a protective cheese-like, fatty substance secreted by the sebaceous glands. The alveoli in the lungs are just beginning to form.

Twenty-Five to Twenty-Eight Weeks

At 6 months the fetal skin is still red, wrinkled, and covered with vernix caseosa. The brain is developing rapidly, and the nervous system is complete enough to provide some degree of regulation of body functions. The eyelids can open and close under neural control. Nails are present on the fingers and toes. In the male fetus, the testes begin to descend into the scrotal sac. Respiratory and circulatory systems have developed; even though the lungs are still physiologically immature, they are sufficiently developed to provide gas exchange. A fetus born at this time will require immediate and prolonged intensive care to survive and then to decrease the risk of major handicap. The fetus at 28 weeks is about 35 to 38 cm (14 to 15 in.) long C–H and weighs 1200 to 1250 g (2 lb, 10.5 oz to 2 lb, 12 oz).

Twenty-Nine to Thirty-Two Weeks

At 30 weeks the pupillary light reflex is present (Moore & Persaud, 2003). The fetus is gaining weight from an increase in body muscle and fat and weighs about 2000 g (4 lb, 6.5 oz), with a length of about 38 to 43 cm (15 to 17 in.), by 32 weeks of age. The central nervous system has matured enough to direct rhythmic breathing movements and partially control body temperature; however, the lungs are not yet fully mature. Bones are fully developed but soft and flexible. The fetus begins storing iron, calcium, and phosphorus. In males the testicles may be located in the scrotal sac but are often still high in the inguinal canals.

Thirty-Five to Thirty-Six Weeks

The fetus begins to get plump, and less wrinkled skin covers the deposits of subcutaneous fat. Lanugo begins to disappear, and the nails reach the edge of the fingertips. By 35 weeks of age, the fetus has a firm grasp and exhibits spontaneous orientation to light. By 36 weeks of age, the weight is usually 2500 to 2750 g (5 lb, 12 oz to 6 lb, 11.5 oz), and the C–H length of the fetus is about 42 to 48 cm (16 to 19 in.). An infant born at this time has a good chance of surviving but may require some special care, especially if there is intrauterine growth restriction.

Thirty-Eight to Forty Weeks

The fetus is considered full term 38 to 40 weeks after conception. The C–H length varies from 48 to 52 cm (19 to 21 in.), with males usually longer than females. Generally, males also weigh more than females. The weight at term is about 3000 to 3600 g (6 lb, 10 oz to 7 lb, 15 oz) and varies in different ethnic groups. The skin has a smooth, polished look. The only lanugo left is on the upper arms and shoulders. The hair on the head is no longer woolly but is coarse and about 1 inch long. Vernix caseosa is present, with heavier deposits remaining in the creases and folds of the skin. The body and extremities are plump with good skin turgor, and the fingernails extend beyond the fingertips. The chest is prominent but still a little smaller than the head, and mammary glands protrude in both sexes. The testes are in the scrotum or palpable in the inguinal canals.

As the fetus enlarges, amniotic fluid diminishes to about 500 mL or less, and the fetal body mass fills the uterine cavity. The fetus assumes what is called its *position of comfort,* or lie. The head is generally pointed downward, following the shape of the uterus (and possibly because the head is heavier than the feet). The extremities, and often the head, are well flexed. After 5 months, feeding and sleeping patterns as well as activity patterns become established, so at term the fetus has its own body rhythms and individual style of response. See Table 7–4 for important developmental milestones.

TABLE 7–4 ✤ Fetal Development: What Parents Want to Know

4 weeks:	The fetal heart begins to beat.
8 weeks:	All body organs are formed.
8–12 weeks:	Fetal heart tones can be heard by Doppler device.
16 weeks:	Baby's sex can be seen. Although thin, the fetus looks like a baby.
20 weeks:	Heartbeat can be heard with fetoscope. Mother feels movement (quickening). Baby develops a regular schedule of sleeping, sucking, and kicking. Hands can grasp. Baby assumes a favorite position in utero. Vernix (lanolin-like covering) protects the body, and lanugo (fine hair) keeps oil on skin.
24 weeks:	Weighs 1 lb, 10 oz. Activity is increasing. Fetal respiratory movements begin.
28 weeks:	Eyes begin to open and close. Head hair, eyebrows, and eyelashes present. Baby can breathe at this time. Surfactant needed for breathing at birth is formed. Baby is two thirds its final size.
32 weeks:	Baby has fingernails and toenails. Subcutaneous fat is being laid down. Baby appears less red and wrinkled.
38+ weeks:	Baby fills total uterus. Baby gets antibodies from mother.

FACTORS INFLUENCING EMBRYONIC AND FETAL DEVELOPMENT

Factors that may affect embryonic development include the quality of the sperm or ovum from which the zygote was formed, the genetic code established at fertilization, and the adequacy of the intrauterine environment. If the environment is unsuitable before cellular differentiation occurs, all the cells of the zygote are affected. The cells may die, which causes spontaneous abortion, or growth may be slowed, depending on the severity of the situation. When differentiation is complete and the fetal membranes have formed, an injurious agent has the greatest effect on those cells undergoing the most rapid growth. Thus, the time of injury is critical in the development of anomalies.

Because organs are formed primarily during embryonic development, the growing organism is considered most vulnerable to harmful agents during the first months of pregnancy. Any agent—such as a drug, virus, or radiation—that can cause development of abnormal structures in an embryo is called a **teratogen**. Chapter 11 discusses the effects of specific teratogenic agents on the developing fetus. ∞

Adequacy of the maternal environment is also important during the periods of rapid embryonic and fetal development. Maternal nutrition can affect brain development. The period of maximum brain growth and myelination begins with the fifth lunar month before birth and continues during the first 6 months after birth, when there is a twofold increase in myelination (Volpe, 2000). Amino acids, glucose, and fatty acids are considered to be the primary dietary factors in brain growth. A subtle type of damage that affects the associative capacity of the brain, possibly leading to learning disabilities, may be caused by nutritional deficiency at this stage. Vitamins and folic acid supplements taken prior to conception can reduce the incidence of neural tube defects (Chacko, Anding, Kozinetz, Grover, & Smith, 2003). Maternal nutri-

THINKING CRITICALLY

Melodie Chong, in her third week of pregnancy, develops a fever of 101°F but refuses to take any medication because she is afraid that drugs will harm her baby. Is she correct?

tion may also predispose offspring to the development of adult coronary heart disease, hypertension, and diabetes in babies who were small or disproportionate at birth. (Maternal nutrition is discussed in depth in Chapter 13. ∞)

Another prenatal influence on the intrauterine environment is maternal hyperthermia associated with sauna or hot tub use. Studies of the effects of maternal hyperthermia (temperature over 104°F) during the first trimester have raised concern about spontaneous abortion, possible central nervous system defects, and failure of neural tube closure. Maternal substance abuse also affects the intrauterine environment and is discussed in Chapter 14 and Chapter 15. ∞

Critical Concept Review

LEARNING OBJECTIVES

CONCEPTS

Compare the differences between meiotic cellular division and mitotic cellular division.	▪ Mitosis produces cells that cause growth in the body. Results in daughter cells that are an exact copy of the parent cell. They contain a full diploid set (46) of chromosomes. ▪ Meiosis produces cells called gametes that are necessary for reproduction of the species. Results in cells that contain only one half (haploid or 23) of the chromosomes of the parent cell.
Compare the processes by which ova and sperm are produced.	▪ Ova are present in the female ovary at birth but are dominant until puberty. Meiosis initially produces via oogenesis two haploid cells (secondary oocyte and a minute polar body) that are released at ovulation. At the end of meiosis in the female, there are four haploid cells: the three polar bodies and one ovum. ▪ Sperm are produced in the seminiferous tubules of the testes beginning at puberty. ▪ Meiosis in the male creates four haploid sperm able to fertilize the ovum. Two sperm carry the Y chromosome and two sperm contain the X chromosome.
Describe the components of the process of fertilization.	Preparation is the first component of fertilization. ▪ Ovum released into fallopian tube—viable for 24 hr. ▪ Sperm deposited into vagina—viable for 48 to 72 hr (highly fertile for 24 hr). ▪ Sperm must undergo capacitation and acrosomal reaction. ▪ Sperm penetration causes a chemical reaction that blocks more sperm penetration. Moment of fertilization is the second component of fertilization. ▪ It occurs in the empulla (outer third) of the fallopian tube. ▪ Sperm enters ovum. The nuclei of the ovum and sperm swell, unite and become a diploid zygote.

LEARNING OBJECTIVES

CONCEPTS

| Describe in order of increasing complexity the structures that form during the cellular multiplication and differentiation stages of intrauterine development. |

Cellular multiplication:
- Rapid mitotic division (cleavage).
- Blastomeres grow to morula (solid ball of 12 to 16 cells).
- Morula divides into a solid mass (blastocyst) surrounded by an outer layer of cells (trophoblast).
- Implantation occurs in 7 to 10 days.

Cellular differentiation:
- At 10 to 14 days of age, blastocyst differentiates into three primary germ layers (ectoderm, mesoderm, and endoderm) from which all tissues, organs, and organ systems develop.
- Embryonic membranes form at implantation and include the chorion and the amnion.
- Amniotic fluid is created when the amnion and chorion grow and connect and form the amniotic sac and produce fluid.
- Amniotic fluid cushions the fetus against mechanical injury, controls the embryo's temperature, allows symmetrical growth, permits freedom of movement, and prevents adherence to the amnion.
- Yolk sac develops as part of the blastocyst and produces primitive red blood cells. It is soon incorporated into the umbilical cord.
- After implantation, the endometrium is called the deciduas. Decidua capsularis is the portion that covers the blastocyst. Decidua basalis is the portion that is directly under the blastocyst.

| Describe the development, structure, and functions of the placenta and umbilical cord during intrauterine life. |

Umbilical cord:
- Develops from amnion. Contains two arteries and one vein and is surrounded by Wharton's jelly, which protects the vessels.
- Function is to provide a circulatory pathway to the embryo.

Placenta:
- Develops at site of embryonic attachment to the uterus and is composed of two parts, the maternal side and the fetal side. The placenta is made up of 15 to 20 segments called cotyledons.
- Serves as endocrine (production of hPL, hCG, estrogen, and progesterone), metabolic and immunologic functions for the fetus. It acts as the fetus's respiratory organ, is an organ of excretion, and aids in the exchange of nutritents.

| Identify the differing processes by which fraternal (dizygotic) and identical (monozygotic) twins are formed. |

Identical twins:
- Develop from a single fertilized egg. Both fetuses are same sex with same characteristics.
- Single placenta.

Fraternal twins:
- Develop from two separate ova fertilized by two separate sperm.
- Two placentas.

| Summarize the significant changes in growth and development of the fetus at 4, 6, 12, 16, 20, 24, 28, 36, and 40 weeks' gestation. |

- 4 weeks: 4 to 6 mm C–R, brain formed from anterior neural tube, limb buds seen, heart begins to beat.
- 6 weeks: 12 mm C–R, primitive skeletal shape, chambers in heart, respiratory system begins, ear formation begins.
- 12 weeks: 8 cm C–R, ossification of skeleton begins, liver produces red cells, palate complete in mouth, skin pink, thyroid hormone present, and insulin present in pancreas.
- 16 weeks: 13.5 cm C–R, teeth begin to form, meconium begins to collect in intestines, kidneys assume shape, hair present on scalp. Sex can be determined.
- 20 weeks: 19 cm C–R, myelination of spinal cord begins. Suck and swallow begins, lanugo covers body, vernix begins to form.
- 24 weeks: 23 cm C–R, respiratory movement and surfactant production begins, brain appears mature.
- 28 weeks: 27 cm C–R, nervous system begins regulation of some functions, adipose tissue accumulates rapidly. Nails, eyebrows and eyelids are present. Eyes open and close.
- 36 weeks: 35 cm C–R, earlobes soft with little cartilage, few sole creases.
- 40 weeks: 40 cm C–R, adequate surfactant, vernix in skin folds and lanugo on shoulders, earlobes firm, and sex apparent.

CRITICAL THINKING IN ACTION

View the **Critical Thinking in Action** *video in Chapter 7 of the CD-ROM. Then, answer the questions that follow.*

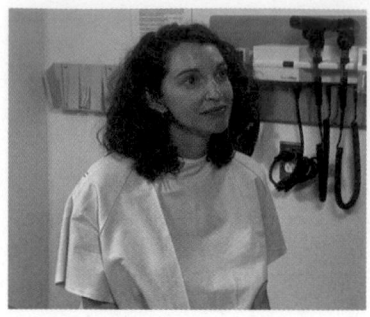

You are working at the local clinic when Frances, a 28-year-old G2 P1001 at 11 weeks' gestation, comes into the office. Frances tells you that early in the first trimester, her husband experienced a flulike syndrome and that he was later diagnosed with cytomegalovirus (CMV) pneumonia. She tells you that his physician found an enlarged supraclavicular lymph node and an ulcer on one tonsil. Laboratory testing revealed elevated liver enzymes. Further testing led to the discovery of positive cytomegalovirus (CMV) IgM levels. She has come today with symptoms including night sweats, persistent sore throat, joint pain, headache, vomiting, and fatigue. You obtain vital signs of temperature 99°F, pulse 90, respirations 14, BP 110/70. Her physical exam is normal; no lymphadenopathy are present. Her weight gain is 2 lb even with nausea and some vomiting. She is worried that her husband's illness could be related to her current symptoms.

1. How would you respond to Frances's concern?
2. Frances asks you if her baby is formed. How would you discuss the three stages of development?
3. Frances asks when her baby is most vulnerable for abnormal growth or structure. How would you answer?
4. Frances asks what stage her baby is in. What would you tell her?

MEDIALINK www.prenhall.com/london

- NCLEX-RN® Review, case studies, and other interactive resources for this chapter can be found on the Companion Website at http://www.prenhall.com/london. Click on "Chapter 7" to select the activities for this chapter.

- For animations, more NCLEX-RN® Review questions, and an audio glossary, access the accompanying CD-ROM in this textbook.

REFERENCES

Bawdon, R. E., & Hnat, M. (2003). Placental transmission of antibiotics. In J. J. Sciarra & T. J. Watkins (Eds.), *Gynecology and obstetrics* (Vol. 3, chap. 34, pp. 1–9). Philadelphia: Lippincott Williams & Wilkins.

Benirschke, K. (2004a). Multiple gestation: The biology of twinning. In R. K. Creasy & R. Resnik (Eds.), *Maternal-fetal medicine: Principles and practice* (5th ed.). Philadelphia: Saunders.

Benirschke, K. (2004b). Normal early development. In R. K. Creasy & R. Resnik (Eds.), *Maternal-fetal medicine: Principles and practice* (5th ed.). Philadelphia: Saunders.

Blackburn, S. T. (2003). *Maternal, fetal, & neonatal physiology: A clinical perspective* (2nd ed.). St. Louis, MO: Saunders.

Chacko, M. R., Anding, R., Kozinetz, C. A., Grover, J. L., & Smith, P. B. (2003). Neural tube de-

fects: Knowledge and preconceptional prevention practices in minority young women. *Pediatrics, 112* (3), 536–542.

De Jonge, C. J. (2000). Egg transport and fertilization. In J. J. Sciarra & T. J. Watkins (Eds.), *Gynecology and obstetrics* (Vol. 5, chap. 46, pp. 1–7). Philadelphia: Lippincott Williams & Wilkins.

Gilbert, W. M., & Brace, R. A. (1993). Amniotic fluid volume and normal flows to and from the amniotic cavity. *Seminars in Perinatology, 17*(3), 150–157.

Groll, J. M., & Lessey, B. A. (2003). Implantation. In J. J. Sciarra & T. J. Watkins (Eds.), *Gynecology and obstetrics* (Vol. 5, chap. 47, pp. 1–23). Philadelphia: Lippincott Williams & Wilkins.

Hamilton, B. A., & Wynshaw-Boris, A. (2004). Basic genetics and patterns of inheritance. In

R. K. Creasy & R. Resnik (Eds.), *Maternal-fetal medicine: Principles and practice* (5th ed.). Philadelphia: Saunders.

Liu, J. H. (2004). Endocrinology of pregnancy. In R. K. Creasy & R. Resnik (Eds.), *Maternal-fetal medicine: Principles and practice* (5th ed.). Philadelphia: Saunders.

Moore, K. L., & Persaud, T. V. N. (2003). *The developing human: Clinically oriented embryology* (7th ed.). Philadelphia: Saunders.

Sadler, T. W. (2004). *Langman's medical embryology* (9th ed.). Philadelphia: Lippincott Williams & Wilkins.

Volpe, J. J. (2000). *Neurology of the newborn* (4th ed.). Philadelphia: Saunders.

Preparation for Parenthood

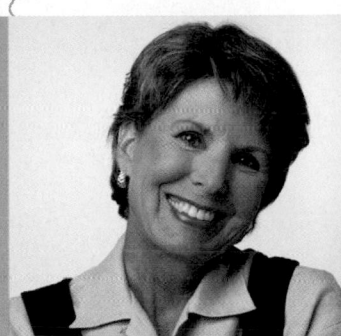

We took our childbirth education classes with seven other couples. Our instructor, who was a nurse, was great—warm and funny but very knowledgeable. After we all had given birth, she had everyone over to her house for a "reunion." We lined the babies up together on the sofa and took a picture. They leaned against each other, topsy-turvy. It was hilarious. My son is now 23 but I still love that picture of him. What memories it triggers of such a very special time!

—*Trish, 47*

LEARNING OBJECTIVES

- Provide a rationale for preconception counseling.

- Delineate the many issues related to pregnancy, labor, and birth that require decision making by the parents.

- Describe the types of antepartal education programs available to expectant couples and their families.

- Compare methods of childbirth preparation.

- Identify ways in which the nurse conveys respect for client individuality in preparing for childbirth.

MEDIALINK

www.prenhall.com/london

CD-ROM

Audio Glossary
NCLEX-RN® Review

Companion Website

Care Plan: Preconception Counseling
Case Study: Preparing for Pregnancy
Further Information about Parteras
NCLEX-RN® Review

As pregnancy progresses, expectant parents begin to look forward to their birth experience and the challenges of parenthood. This is a time for plans and decisions. Where will the birth be? Who do they wish to be present? How will they prepare themselves for this experience?

Today's professional nurse can assist a pregnant woman or expectant couple, if the partner is involved, to make the choices that are part of pregnancy and birth. For first-time parents, the decisions may seem numerous and complicated, and the nurse has a unique opportunity to help them establish a pattern of decision making that will serve them well in their years as parents.

PRECONCEPTION COUNSELING

One of the first questions a couple should ask themselves is whether they wish to have children. This decision involves consideration of each person's goals, expectations of the relationship, and desire to be a parent. Sometimes one person wishes to have a child, but the other does not. In such situations, an open discussion is essential to reach a mutually acceptable decision.

Couples who wish to have children need to decide about the timing of pregnancy. When do they believe it would be best to become parents? For couples who have religious beliefs that do not support contraception or who feel that fertility planning is unnatural, planning the timing of the pregnancy is unacceptable and irrelevant. These couples can still take steps to ensure that they are in the best possible physical and mental health when pregnancy occurs.

PRECONCEPTION HEALTH MEASURES

The nurse begins by teaching the couple about known or suspected health risks. The nurse advises the woman who smokes to cease smoking if possible or to limit her cigarette intake to less than half a pack per day. Because of the hazards of secondhand smoke, it is helpful for the woman to avoid environments where secondhand smoke is common and to ask her partner to refrain from smoking around her. Although the effects of caffeine are less clearly understood, the woman is advised to avoid or limit her intake of caffeine. Alcohol, social drugs, and street drugs pose a real threat to the fetus. A woman who uses any prescription or over-the-counter medications needs to discuss the implications of their use with her healthcare provider. It is best to avoid using any medication if possible. Because of the possible teratogenic effects of environmental hazards, the nurse urges the couple contemplating pregnancy to determine whether they are exposed to any environmental hazards at work or in their community.

Physical Examination

It is wise for both partners to have a physical examination to identify any health problems so that they can be corrected if possible. These problems might include medical conditions such as high blood pressure, diabetes, or obesity; problems that threaten fertility, such as certain sexually transmitted infections; or conditions that keep the individual from achieving optimal health, such as anemia or colitis. If the family history indicates previous genetic disorders, or if the couple is planning pregnancy when the woman is over age 35, the healthcare provider may suggest that the couple consider genetic counseling. In addition to the history and physical examination, the woman may have a variety of laboratory tests. (See "Assessment Guide: Initial Prenatal Assessment" in Chapter 10. ∞) The woman is advised to have a dental examination and any necessary dental work done prior to concep-

COMPLEMENTARY CARE

AYURVEDA AND PRECONCEPTION LIFESTYLE

Ayurveda is an ancient system of natural and medical healing that originated in India. *Ayur* means "life" and *veda* means "science." It includes a wide range of modalities, including the use of diet, herbs, massage, exercise, music therapy, aromatherapy, meditation, and yoga, among others. Ayurvedic practitioners believe that these modalities should be practiced not only during pregnancy, but also prior to conception for optimal maternal and fetal health.

Ayurvedic practitioners recommend that both the mother and the father take part in a healthy lifestyle prior to conception. Some of the preconception lifestyle recommendations include:

- Avoiding stress and overwork.
- Avoiding alcohol, tobacco, and drugs.
- Avoiding meat and dairy products, and eating primarily a vegetarian diet.
- Striving for a positive emotional relationship between the man and woman.

For more information see Chapter 44, "Complementary Care: Ayurvedic Treatment of the Common Cold." ∞

---

tion to avoid exposure to x-rays and the risk of infection while she is pregnant.

Nutrition

Prior to conception it is advisable for the woman to be at an average weight for her body build and height. The woman is advised to follow a nutritious diet that contains ample quantities of all the essential nutrients. Some nutritionists advocate emphasizing the following nutrients: calcium, protein, iron, B-complex vitamins, vitamin C, and magnesium. Folic acid supplementation prior to conception is recommended to decrease the risk of neural tube defects. Intake of certain vitamins in megadoses can cause severe fetal problems and should be avoided. See Chapter 12 for further discussion of nutrition. ∞

Exercise

A woman is advised to continue her present pattern of exercise or to establish a regular exercise plan beginning at least 3 months before she attempts to become pregnant. An exercise routine that she enjoys and maintains will provide the best results. Exercise that includes some aerobic conditioning and some general muscle toning improves the woman's circulation and general health. Once an exercise program is well established, the woman is generally encouraged to continue it during pregnancy.

CONTRACEPTION

A woman who uses hormonal contraception, such as combined oral contraceptives, the NuvaRing, the Ortho Evra patch, or Depo-Provera, is advised to stop using the hormonal birth control method and have two or three normal menses before attempting to conceive. This waiting period allows the natural hormonal cycle to return and facilitates dating the subsequent pregnancy. A woman using an intrauterine device is advised to have it removed and to wait 1 month before attempting to conceive. During the waiting period, she can use barrier methods of contraception (condoms, diaphragm, or cervical cap with spermicides).

CONCEPTION

Most preconception recommendations focus on helping the couple attain their best possible health state so that they do not enter pregnancy with unnecessary risks. Conception is a personal and emotional experience. Even if a couple is prepared, they may feel some ambivalence. Ambivalence is a normal response, but they may need reassurance that the feeling will pass. A couple may get so caught up in preparation and in their efforts to "do things right" that they lose sight of the pleasure they derive from each other and their lives together and cease to value the joy of spontaneity in their relationship. It is often helpful for the healthcare provider to remind an overly zealous couple to take pleasure in the present moment.

Healthcare providers can assist the couple to achieve conception by identifying the woman's most fertile period. The nurse can also educate the woman about possible signs of ovulation (presence of ovulatory mucus, changes in the woman's temperature, and the presence of mittelschmerz [ovulation-related pain]). These factors are discussed in Chapter 3. ∞

CHILDBEARING DECISIONS

Once the couple has conceived, they should begin exploring their options for a healthcare provider and birth setting, as well as labor support and sibling preparation, if appropriate. These decisions are influenced by a variety of factors.

DEVELOPING CULTURAL COMPETENCE

BIRTH CHOICES

Sometimes nurses make the mistake of assuming that a pregnant woman will make the same decisions about the birth experience as the nurse would have. However, the choices a woman and her family make are influenced by many factors, including ethnic background, culture, and religious beliefs. These factors may profoundly influence decisions such as care provider (male or female), birth setting, labor support person(s), use of medications for analgesia, position during birth, saving the placenta, dietary practices immediately postpartum, and a host of other issues. There is no one right way to give birth.

CARE PROVIDER

One of the first decisions facing expectant parents is the selection of a healthcare provider. The nurse assists them by explaining the various options and outlining what can be expected from each. Expectant parents should have a thorough understanding of the differences of educational preparation, skill level, general philosophy, and characteristics of practice of certified nurse-midwives, obstetricians, family practice physicians, and direct entry (lay) midwives. The nurse can encourage expectant parents to investigate the care provider's credentials, education and training, philosophy of childbirth, fee schedule or insurance plans accepted, availability to new clients, and on-call coverage issues. They can often get this information by telephoning the provider's office. The nurse can help the expectant parents develop a list of questions for their first visit to a care provider to help determine compatibility. These questions might include the following:

- Who is in practice with you, or who covers for you when you are unavailable?

- How do your partners' philosophies compare with yours?

- How do you feel about my partner, other support person, or other children coming to the prenatal visits?

- What are your feelings about _____ (fill in special desires for the birth event, such as different positions assumed during labor, episiotomy, induction of labor, other people present during the birth, breastfeeding immediately after the birth, no separation of infant and parents following birth, and so on)?

- If a cesarean birth is necessary, could my partner be present?

- Are you familiar with _____ (fill in complementary or alternative forms of healthcare that may be used currently if applicable)? How will this practice affect my plan of care?

Choosing a care provider is just one of the decisions pregnant women and couples make. A method that has helped many couples make these choices is a **birth preference plan**. By writing down preferences, prospective parents identify aspects of the childbearing experience that are most important to them (Figure 8–1 ○). Used as a tool for communication among the expectant parents, the healthcare provider, and the healthcare professionals at the birth setting, the written plan identifies options that are available as well as those that are not.

The birth plan also helps pregnant women and couples set priorities. Using the plan, they identify areas that they want to incorporate into their own birth experience. They can then discuss the document at a visit with their prospective care provider and use it as a basis for communicating their needs and wishes during the childbirth experience.

○ **FIGURE 8–1**

Sample Birth Plan

Choice	Choice
Care provider:	Position during birth:
Certified nurse-midwife	On side
Obstetrician	Hands and knees
Family physician	Kneeling
Direct entry midwife	Squatting
Birth setting:	Birthing chair
Hospital:	Birthing bed
Birthing room	Other:
Delivery room	Family present (siblings)
Birth center	Filming of birth (videotaping)
Home	Photography of birth
Support during labor and birth:	Use of LeBoyer Method
Partner present	Episiotomy
Doula present	No sterile drapes
During labor:	Partner to cut umbilical cord
Ambulate as desired	Hold baby immediately after birth
Shower if desired	Breastfeed immediately after birth
Wear own clothes	No separation after birth
Use hot tub	Save the placenta
Use own rocking chair	Collect cord blood for banking
Have perineal prep	Newborn care:
Have enema	Eye treatment for the baby
Membranes:	Vitamin K injection
Rupture naturally	Heptovac injection
Amniotomy if needed	Breastfeeding
Labor stimulation if needed	Formula feeding
Medication:	Pacifier use
Identify type desired	Glucose water
Fluids or ice as desired	Circumcision
Music during labor and birth	Postpartum care:
Massage	Short stay
Therapeutic touch	48-hour stay after vaginal birth
Healing touch	Home visits after discharge
	Home doula
	Other:

Birth preference sheet. The columns list the various choices that a couple may consider during their childbirth experience. Once the couple has considered each of the choices, they can circle the items they desire.

Expectant parents also need to consider the qualities they want in a care provider for the newborn. They may want to visit several before the birth to select someone who will meet their needs and those of their child.

Pregnant women and couples will make many more choices. Some are explored in Table 8–1. Although many birth experiences are very close to the desired experience, at times expectations cannot be met. This may be because of the unavailability of some choices in the community, limitations set by insurance providers, or unexpected problems during pregnancy or birth. It is important for the nurse to help expectant parents keep sight of what is realistic for their situation while also acting as an advocate for them.

BIRTH SETTING

The nurse can help expectant parents choose a birth setting by suggesting they tour facilities and talk with nurses there

TABLE 8–1 ✤ Benefits and Risks of Some Consumer Decisions During Pregnancy, Labor, and Birth

Issue	Benefits	Risks
Breastfeeding	■ No additional expense ■ Contains maternal antibodies ■ Decreases incidence of infant otitis media, vomiting, diarrhea, hospitalizations during the first year of life, and allergies ■ Easier to digest than formula ■ Immediately after birth, promotes uterine contractions and decreases incidence of postpartum hemorrhage ■ Promotes maternal-infant bonding	■ Transmission of maternal infections such as HIV to newborn ■ Irregular ovulation and menses can cause false sense of security and nonuse of hormonal contraceptives ■ Increased nutritional requirement in mother ■ Limitation of birth control options in the postpartum period
Perineal prep	■ May decrease risk of infection ■ Facilitates episiotomy repair	■ Nicks can be portal for bacteria ■ Discomfort as hair grows back
Enema	■ May facilitate labor ■ Increases space for infant in pelvis ■ May increase strength of contractions ■ May prevent contamination of sterile field	■ Increases discomfort and anxiety
Ambulation during labor	■ Comfort for laboring woman ■ May assist in labor progression by ■ Stimulating contractions ■ Allowing gravity to help descent of fetus ■ Giving sense of independence and control	■ Cord prolapse with rupture of membranes unless engagement has occurred ■ Birth of infant in undesirable locations (hallways, outdoors, waiting area) ■ Inability to monitor fetal heart rate
Electronic fetal monitoring	■ Helps evaluate fetal well being ■ Helps identify fetal stress ■ Useful in diagnostic testing ■ Helps evaluate labor progress	■ Supine postural hypotension ■ Intrauterine perforation (with internal uterine pressure device) ■ Infection (with internal monitoring) ■ Decreases personal interaction with mother because of attention paid to the machine ■ Mother is unable to ambulate or change her position freely
Whirlpool (jet hydrotherapy)	■ Increased relaxation ■ Decreased anxiety ■ Stimulation of labor ■ Provides pain relief ■ Slight decrease in blood pressure ■ Increased diuresis ■ Decreased incidence of vacuum and forceps births ■ Increased pain threshold ■ Higher satisfaction with birth ■ Decreased use of pain medication	■ May slow contractions if used before active labor is established ■ Possible risk of infection if membranes are ruptured ■ Slight increase in maternal temperature and pulse in tub ■ Hypothermia ■ Increases fetal heart rate by 10–20 beats per minute (Ieschendorf & Evans, 2000)
Analgesia	■ Maternal relaxation facilitates labor	■ All drugs reach the fetus in varying degrees and with varying effects
Episiotomy	■ Decreases irregular tearing of perineum ■ Easier to repair for practitioner	■ Increased pain after birth and for 1–3 months following birth ■ Dyspareunia ■ Infection ■ Increased frequency of third- and fourth-degree lacerations (Low, Seng, Murtland et al., 2000)

as well as with friends or acquaintances who are recent parents. However, the choice of healthcare provider may largely determine the birth setting. Questions that expectant parents might ask of new parents include the following:

- What kind of care and support did you receive during labor?

- If the setting has both labor and delivery rooms and birthing rooms, was a birthing room available when you wanted it?

- Were you encouraged to be mobile during labor or do what you wanted to do (walking, sitting in a rocking chair, sitting in a whirlpool bath, standing in a shower, and so on)? If not, were there reasonable circumstances that prevented you from doing so?

- Were you encouraged to be involved in your plan of care and kept well informed of progress or proposed changes?

- Was your labor partner or coach treated well?

- Were your birth preferences respected? Did you share them with the facility before the birth? If something did not work, why do you think there were problems?

- During labor, did the nurse offer or suggest a variety of comfort measures?

- How were medications handled during labor? Were you comfortable with this arrangement?

- Were siblings welcomed in the birth setting? After the birth?

- Was the nursing staff helpful after the baby was born? Did you receive self-care and infant care information? Did you have a choice about what information was provided?

LABOR SUPPORT

Another important choice the expectant family faces is how active a support role the father or partner wants to take during labor and birth. Although many partners are comfortable acting as the primary physical and emotional support for the laboring woman, some partners are not. Studies have found that many men are discouraged when the comfort measures they learned in childbirth classes do not seem to work in labor, and some feel that the classes do not offer valuable information (Lee & Schmied, 2001). In lieu of the partner, other options for labor support include asking a friend or family member to attend the birth and help with comfort needs, contacting a local childbirth advocate group for a volunteer referral, or hiring a specialized childbirth support person, known as a **doula**.

The doula attends to the needs of the childbearing family. Specially trained to assist with births and provide support to new parents and family members, the doula is an adjunct to the health care team. Doulas have a role in providing labor support, offering support and encouragement, building a good team relationship, helping the laboring woman cover gaps in her care, and encouraging good communication among the woman and her family and caregivers. In a managed care environment in which nursing staff are often stretched thinly, a doula can be an asset to the nurse by attending to the many comfort needs of the laboring mother and her family (Gilliland, 2002).

DEVELOPING CULTURAL COMPETENCE

PARTERAS

The increasing numbers of Mexican Americans living in the United States make it important for nurses to become familiar with the use of *parteras* by many members of this population. Parteras are one of several types of *curanderas* (traditional healers) found in Latino communities. Parteras or direct-entry midwives—not to be confused with certified nurse-midwives—are usually women in their 40s or older who are themselves mothers or grandmothers. They have learned their skills from their mothers or other respected elder women.

Traditionally, it is a cultural preference that a pregnant woman be attended by a partera and give birth at home or in a birthing center. The partera stays with the expectant mother all through active labor. Parteras are trained to do perineal massage and manual stretching of muscles and soft tissues of the birth canal, instead of episiotomies. They do not conduct vaginal examinations. The partera uses no medicines, no forceps, no episiotomy, no stitches, no oxytocins, and no breaking of the amniotic membrane to hasten birth. Parteras acknowledge the body/mind/soul and spiritual connection of the client (Arizága, 1999).

Not all women wishing to have their babies at home assisted by a partera are able to do so. U.S. midwifery laws prohibit the partera from accepting as clients women who are severely overweight, diabetic, hypertensive, or anemic, or who have been told by a physician that they have a medical problem that would make home birth unsafe.

SIBLING PARTICIPATION IN THE BIRTH

Some expectant parents may wish to have their other children present at the birth. Children who will attend a birth can be prepared through books, audiovisual materials, use of models, discussion, and sibling classes. Nurses can assist parents with sibling preparation by helping them understand the stresses a child may experience. For example, the child may become frightened if the laboring mom is irritable and visibly showing discomfort, feel left out when there is a new child to love, or feel disappointed if a brother is born when a sister was expected.

During the birth it is important that a sibling have his or her own support person whose sole responsibility is tending to the child's needs. The support person needs to be familiar to the child; warm, sensitive, and flexible;

knowledgeable about the birth process; and comfortable with sexuality and birth. This person must be prepared to interpret what is happening for the child and to intervene when necessary. For example, the support person needs to be prepared to remove the child from the birthing room at the child's request or if the situation warrants that action.

Siblings should be allowed to react to the birth in whatever manner they choose, as long as it is not disruptive. They should understand that they can stay or leave the room as they choose. They should also feel free to ask questions and express feelings.

Siblings who are present at birth tend to have feelings of interest and the desire to nurture "our" baby, as opposed to jealousy and rivalry directed at "Mom's" baby. The mother does not disappear mysteriously into the hospital and return with a demanding outsider. Instead, the family attending the birth together finds a new opportunity for closeness and growth by sharing in the birth of a new member.

CLASSES FOR FAMILY MEMBERS DURING PREGNANCY

Prenatal education programs provide important opportunities to share information about pregnancy and childbirth and to enhance the parents' decision-making skills (Figure 8–2 ●). The content of each class is generally directed by the overall goals of the program. The nurse who knows the types of prenatal programs available in the community can direct expectant parents to programs that meet their special needs and learning goals.

From the expectant parents' point of view, class content is best presented in chronology with the pregnancy.

● **FIGURE 8–2**

In a group setting with a nurse-instructor, expectant parents share information about pregnancy and childbirth.

Photographer: © Elena Dorfman.

TABLE 8–2 ✛ **Possible Content of Classes for Childbirth Preparation**
Early Classes (First Trimester)
Early gestational changes
Self-care during pregnancy
Fetal development, environmental dangers for the fetus
Sexuality in pregnancy
Birth settings and types of care providers
Nutrition, rest, and exercise suggestions
Relief measures for the common discomforts of pregnancy
Psychologic changes in pregnancy
Information for getting pregnancy off to a good start
Danger signs that warrant immediate medical attention
Feeding choices/benefits of breastfeeding
Later Classes (Second and Third Trimesters)
Preparation for birth process
Postpartum self-care
Birth choices (episiotomy, medications, fetal monitoring, perineal prep, enema, etc.)
Relaxation techniques
Breathing techniques
Infant stimulation
Newborn safety issues, such as car seats and sleeping positions
Alternative therapies in pregnancy and labor
Adolescent Preparation Classes
Stresses specific to adolescents
Newborn care
Health dangers for the baby
Weight gain issues and nutrition
How to recognize when baby is ill
Baby care: Physical and emotional
Sexuality
Peer relationships
Breastfeeding Programs
Advantages and disadvantages
Medical benefits of breastfeeding
Maternal nutrition
Techniques of breastfeeding
Methods of breast preparation
Involvement of fathers in feeding process
Cultural considerations

Thus, prenatal classes are often divided into early and late classes (Table 8–2).

EARLY CLASSES: FIRST TRIMESTER

Early prenatal classes often include prepregnant women and couples as well as those in early pregnancy. The classes cover early gestational changes; self-care during pregnancy; fetal development and environmental dangers for the fetus; sexuality in pregnancy; birth settings and types of care providers; nutrition, rest, and exercise suggestions; common discomforts of pregnancy and relief measures; psychologic changes in pregnancy for the woman and man; methods of coping with stress; and the benefits of following a healthful lifestyle. Early classes provide information about factors that place the woman at risk for preterm labor or other adverse pregnancy-related conditions, as well as how to recognize symptoms of possible problems and what to do if they occur. Early classes should also present information about breastfeeding and formula-feeding. Most women have made their infant feeding decision before the sixth month of pregnancy.

LATER CLASSES: SECOND AND THIRD TRIMESTERS

The later classes focus on preparation for the birth, including birth choices (episiotomy, medications, fetal monitoring, epidural, and so forth), postpartum self-care, infant care and feeding, and newborn safety issues. Since many expectant parents purchase a car seat before the birth of their child, later classes should also include information about the importance of car seats, how they work, and how to select an approved car seat.

Childbirth preparation classes are an ideal time to incorporate infant stimulation concepts. These concepts help develop parenting skills and enhance prenatal and neonatal bonding. Tactile, vestibular, and auditory stimulation can be explained. As the uterine wall thins during the pregnancy, the mother and father are better able to feel the baby, and the fetus can sense the parents' stroking and patting through the abdominal wall. **Abdominal effleurage** (a light stroking movement made over the abdominal wall with the fingertips) can provide tactile stimulation to the fetus. The pelvic-tilt exercise provides vestibular stimulation through movement of the fetus. Rocking in a rocking chair is also a comfortable way to provide both relaxation for the expectant woman and vestibular stimulation for the fetus. Playing music can provide auditory stimulation. Classical music is found to stimulate the fetus.

ADOLESCENT PARENTING CLASSES

Adolescents have special learning needs during pregnancy. Areas of concern for teens focus on how to be a good parent, how to care for a new baby, health dangers to the baby, and healthful foods to eat during pregnancy. Teens also need to learn how to recognize when the baby is sick, protect the baby from accidents, and make the baby feel happy and loved. Pregnant teens are often eager to hear more about the birth process (especially ways to cope with pain during the birth process), the personal health of the mother, the discomforts and life changes that accompany pregnancy, and sexuality.

BREASTFEEDING PROGRAMS

Programs offering information on breastfeeding are increasing. For many years a primary source of information has been **La Leche League**, a nonprofit organization that promotes breastfeeding. Certified lactation educators; clinical lactation consultants; and nurses at birthing centers, hospitals, and health clinics can also provide information. Expectant parents learn positioning and techniques of breastfeeding, advantages and disadvantages, and methods of breast pumping and milk storage. The father's support and encouragement of the mother is vital, so it is important to include him in the educational programs and decision making. Some fathers may feel ambivalent or resentful about breastfeeding and need opportunities in the prenatal period to discuss and share feelings and experiences.

SIBLING PREPARATION: ADJUSTMENT TO A NEWBORN

The birth of a new sibling is a significant event in a child's life. Attendance at sibling preparation classes can enhance positive adjustment (Figure 8–3 ⦿). The classes usually fo-

⦿ **FIGURE 8–3**

It is especially important that siblings be well prepared when they are going to be present for the birth. However, all siblings can benefit from information about birth and the new baby ahead of time.

NURSING PRACTICE

Many states now mandate car seats for infants and young children. Advise parents of community resources available for inspecting the installation of car seats. Many police departments and fire stations have car-seat inspection clinics that are conducted within the community. Some fire stations have set hours when parents can bring in their car seat and have it installed free of charge. Remind new parents that newborns should be in a rear-facing position until the age of 12 months.

cus on reducing the child's anxiety, giving the child opportunities to express feelings and concerns, and encouraging realistic expectations of the newborn. Parents learn strategies to prepare the child for the birth and help the child cope with a new family member.

Sibling preparation can be addressed through a formal class or in a less formal way by providing a booklet for parents that addresses issues affecting both parents and children.

CLASSES FOR GRANDPARENTS

Grandparents are an important source of support and information for prospective and new parents. They are often included in the birthing process. Prenatal programs for grandparents can be a valuable source of information about current beliefs and practices in childbearing. The most useful content may include changes in birthing and parenting practices and helpful tips for being a supportive grandparent. Grandparents who will be integral members of the labor and birth team need information about that role.

EDUCATION OF THE FAMILY HAVING CESAREAN BIRTH

Cesarean birth is an alternative method of birth. However, because the need for a cesarean birth is rarely known in advance, specific classes covering this alternative are uncommon. Since one out of every four or five births is by cesarean, preparation for this possibility should be an integral part of every childbirth education curriculum.

Class content should cover what the parents can expect to happen during a cesarean birth, what they might feel, and what choices are available. All pregnant women and couples should be encouraged to discuss with their certified nurse-midwife or physician the progression of events if a cesarean birth becomes necessary.

When expectant parents are anticipating a repeat cesarean birth, they have time to plan and prepare. Many birthing units provide preparation classes for repeat cesarean birth. Parents who have had previous negative experiences need an opportunity to describe what contributed to their feelings. They should be encouraged to identify what they would like to change and to list interventions that would make the experience more positive. Those who have had positive experiences require reassurance that their needs and desires will be met in a similar manner. All parents should be encouraged to air any fears or anxieties.

A specific concern of the woman facing a repeat cesarean is anticipation of pain. She needs reassurance that subsequent cesarean births are often less painful than the

first. In addition, planned cesarean births involve less fatigue than unplanned procedures because they are not preceded by a long, strenuous labor. Providing this information will help the woman cope more effectively with stressful stimuli, including pain.

PREPARATION FOR PARENTS DESIRING VAGINAL BIRTH AFTER CESAREAN BIRTH (VBAC)

Parents who have had a cesarean birth and are now anticipating a vaginal birth have unique needs. Because they may have unresolved questions and concerns about the last birth, it is helpful to begin the series of classes with an informational session. The nurse can supply information about the criteria necessary to attempt a trial of labor and identify decisions to be made regarding the birth experience. Some childbirth educators suggest that parents prepare two birth plans: one for vaginal birth and one for cesarean birth. Preparing birth plans seems to give parents some sense of control over the birth experience and tends to increase the positive aspects of the experience.

CHILDBIRTH PREPARATION METHODS

Childbirth preparation classes are usually taught by certified childbirth educators. Various types of childbirth preparation are available. Vital to each method is the educational component, which helps alleviate fear. The classes vary in coverage of subjects related to the maternity cycle, but all teach relaxation and coping techniques, as well as what to expect during labor and birth. Most classes also feature exercises to relax and condition muscles and breathing exercises for use in labor. The greatest differences among the methods lie in the theories of why they work and in the specific comfort techniques and breathing patterns they teach.

DEVELOPING CULTURAL COMPETENCE

CHILDBIRTH ATTENDANCE

Women from Latino cultures typically want their partner with them during labor. These women generally prefer both emotional and physical support, such as verbal reassurance, hand-holding, or assistance with ambulation. The woman may also want female relatives present during the labor and birth to provide additional support.

On the other hand, in most Middle Eastern countries, childbirth is exclusively attended by women. A woman in labor is commonly surrounded by female relatives and friends. It is customary for the husband to be excluded from the birthing area or delivery room.

Childbirth preparation offers several advantages. Most important is that judicious use of analgesics and anesthetics optimizes the baby's health. Another advantage is the satisfaction of the parents, for whom childbirth becomes a shared and profound emotional experience. In addition, each method has been shown to shorten labor. All nurses should know how these techniques differ, so that they can support each birth experience effectively.

PROGRAMS FOR PREPARATION

Some antepartal classes, specifically oriented to preparation for labor and birth, have a name associated with a theory of pain reduction in childbirth. The most common methods of this type are the **Lamaze** (psychoprophylactic), Kitzinger (sensory-memory), Bradley (partner-coached childbirth), and HypnoBirthing (deep relaxation). Table 8–3 identifies characteristics of each method.

TABLE 8–3 ✤ Summary of Selected Childbirth Preparation Methods

Method	Purpose or Philosophy	Goals	Techniques	Class Content
Bradley	To have the best, safest, and most rewarding birth experience possible.	■ Natural childbirth. ■ Active participation of the husband as coach. ■ Excellent nutrition. ■ Breastfeeding, beginning at birth.	■ Working in harmony with the body using breath control and deep abdominopelvic breathing (Bradley, 1974) ■ Promoting general body relaxation (Bradley, 1974)	■ Nutrition ■ Coach's role ■ Introduction to stages of labor ■ Birth planning ■ Variations and complications of labor ■ Postpartum preparation ■ Advanced first- and second-stage techniques ■ Preparation for the new family
Lamaze	Childbirth education empowers women to make informed choices in health care, to assume responsibility for their health, and to trust their inner wisdom.	■ Birth is normal, natural, and healthy. ■ The experience of birth profoundly affects women and their families. ■ Women's inner wisdom guides them through birth. ■ Women have the right to give birth free from routine medical interventions.	■ Disassociation relaxation ■ Controlled muscular relaxation ■ Breathing patterns	■ Nutrition ■ Gestational changes ■ Labor and birth techniques for easing pain ■ Breathing techniques ■ Positioning during labor
Kitzinger	■ Sheila Kitzinger campaigns for women to have the information they need to make choices about childbirth. ■ She is a strong believer in the benefits of home birth for women who are not at high risk.	■ Uses sensory memory to help the woman understand and work with her body in preparation for birth.	■ Uses chest breathing in conjunction with abdominal relaxation ■ Incorporates elements of the Stanislavsky method of acting in a way to teach relaxation	■ Antenatal care ■ Birth plans ■ Therapeutic touch during labor ■ Post-traumatic stress following childbirth ■ Breastfeeding
HypnoBirthing	Eliminate fear and experience birth in a stress-free, calm, and gentle environment that most resembles nature's own design.	■ With both mind and body relaxed, the muscles of the uterus work in complete neuromuscular harmony. ■ When in a relaxed state, the body releases endorphins, the body's natural anesthesia.	■ Relaxation techniques ■ Deep breathing ■ Slow breathing ■ Breathing the baby down ■ Maintaining comfort and eliminating pain	■ HypnoBirthing philosophy ■ Rapid, progressive relaxation/deepening techniques for transition ■ Visualizations for labor ■ Composing a birth plan ■ Early signs of labor ■ Birthing companion's integral role in labor ■ Pushing techniques ■ Postnatal bonding of parents with baby

Developing maternal confidence is a major component of childbirth education. The Council of Childbirth Education Specialists encourages education that focuses on the interconnectedness of the mind and spirit. Once that is understood, coping strategies, stress reduction, and relaxation techniques are taught (Castor, 2003). Childbirth preparation programs typically have an educational component aimed at eliminating fear and teaching coping techniques. The programs teach relaxation techniques, conditioning exercises, and breathing patterns to use during labor. They differ primarily in the theories of why they work and in the specific breathing and relaxation patterns they teach.

Another prominent organization that provides educational resources and certification for educators is the International Childbirth Education Association (ICEA). This organization does not advocate a particular method of childbirth preparation but rather promotes a philosophy of "freedom of choice based on knowledge of alternatives" (International Childbirth Education Association, 2000). Many expectant parents find this approach consistent with their own desires to experience birth as informed healthcare consumers. ICEA educators often teach a combination of techniques designed to meet individual needs.

BODY-CONDITIONING EXERCISES

Some body-conditioning exercises, such as the pelvic tilt, pelvic rock, and Kegel exercises, are taught in childbirth preparation classes. Other exercises strengthen the abdominal muscles for the expulsive phase of labor. (See Chapter 11 for a description of recommended exercises. ∞)

RELAXATION EXERCISES

Relaxation during labor allows the woman to conserve energy and the uterine muscles to work more efficiently. Without practice it is difficult to relax the whole body in the midst of intense uterine contractions. Progressive relaxation exercises such as those taught to induce sleep can be helpful during labor. "Teaching Highlights: Touch Relaxation" provides information on one approach.

An additional exercise specific to Lamaze is disassociation relaxation. The woman is taught to become familiar with the sensation of contracting and relaxing the voluntary muscle groups throughout her body. She then learns to contract a specific muscle group and relax the rest of her body. The exercise conditions the woman to relax uninvolved muscles while the uterus contracts, creating an active relaxation pattern.

The relaxation techniques described are most effective if the woman practices them daily both alone and with her support person. During a practice session, the partner begins by checking the woman's neck, shoulders, arms, and legs for relaxation. As tense areas are found, the

TEACHING HIGHLIGHTS

TOUCH RELAXATION

Touch relaxation technique often combines patterned abdominal breathing with focused relaxation. It may be used to achieve relaxation of specific body parts or for general body relaxation.

Goals

The woman learns to release tension in the areas that her partner touches. The partner learns to watch his or her partner carefully and becomes attuned to tense, tightened muscles.

Technique

- The partner gently touches the woman's brow.
- The woman uses abdominal breathing. As she breathes in through her nose, her abdomen rises, and as she breathes out through her mouth, her abdomen falls. As each breath is released, she lets all tightness and tension flow out with the breath.
- The partner continues to lightly touch her brow until relaxation is felt. The partner may want to provide quiet encouragement such as, "You are doing fine, you are releasing the tension in your forehead." After at least five breaths, the partner may touch the woman's shoulders and repeat the pattern described earlier.
- The partner moves on to the arms, chest, abdomen, thighs, and calves. The last aspect is to breathe in, let the whole body relax and go limp, and slowly release the breath. It will be helpful at the end of each labor contraction to let the body go limp and release all tension.
- As the couple practices, it is important for the woman to relax each part of her body. When she is in labor, it will not be possible to go through the whole body; however, the woman can indicate what would be most helpful (e.g., touch her shoulder during each contraction). The partner can also be alert for signs of muscle tension and tightening. As the partner and woman practice touch relaxation, they may want to make the situation more realistic. They could decide that uterine contractions are occurring every 5 minutes and are lasting for 30 seconds. A clock will help the partner keep track of time. The partner can indicate that a contraction is beginning and suggest the woman begin her breathing. To help her focus, the partner may touch her shoulder or hand. In some instances, it is helpful for the partner to breathe along with the woman. Each couple can determine what works best for them.

helper encourages the woman to relax those body parts. By gentle touch and verbal cues, the woman learns to respond to her own perceptions of tense muscles and also to the suggestion from others. Relaxation may also be promoted by cutaneous stimulation. One type commonly used prior to the transitional phase of labor is abdominal effleurage (Figure 8–4 ●). This light abdominal stroking can relieve mild to moderate pain but not intense pain.

○ **FIGURE 8–4**

A   B

Effleurage is light stroking of the abdomen with the fingertips. **A,** Starting at the symphysis, the woman lightly moves her fingertips up and around in a circular pattern. **B,** An alternative approach involves using one hand in a figure-eight pattern. This light stroking can also be done by the support person.

BREATHING TECHNIQUES

Breathing techniques are a key element of most childbirth preparation programs. They help keep the mother and her unborn baby adequately oxygenated, and help the mother relax and focus her attention appropriately. Breathing techniques are best taught during the final trimester of pregnancy. The nurse then supports the mother's use of breathing techniques during labor. Breathing techniques are described in Chapter 19. ∞

NURSING PRACTICE

Identify the methods of childbirth preparation commonly used in your area and learn the basics of their approaches to relaxation and breathing. Then practice these methods so that you can support a laboring couple more effectively.

PREPARATION FOR CHILDBIRTH THAT SUPPORTS INDIVIDUALITY

Childbirth educators stress the value of individuality when providing information to expectant parents. The goal is to encourage women to incorporate their own natural responses into coping with the pain of labor and birth. Self-care activities that may be used include vocalization or "sounding" to relieve tension in pregnancy and labor, massage (light touch) to facilitate relaxation, use of warm water for showers or bathing during labor, visualization (imagery), relaxing music, subdued lighting, and the use of a birthing ball (see Chapter 19 ∞).

Nurses need to encourage expectant mothers and couples to make the birth a personal experience. A woman might choose to bring items from home that help create a more personal birthing space. These items might include warm socks, extra pillows, bath powder, lotion, or a favorite blanket. She may wish to bring photos of special people or places. Many expectant parents enjoy listening to tapes of favorite music or watching favorite home videos. Such personalization of the birth experience may give expectant parents feelings of increased serenity and empowerment.

Critical Concept Review

LEARNING OBJECTIVES	CONCEPTS

Provide a rationale for preconception counseling.	Preconception counseling is designed to: ■ Teach the client about environmental and lifestyle hazards that could affect conception and pregnancy. ■ Identify any health problems that could impede a successful pregnancy. ■ Advise the client about contraception and fertility.
Delineate the many issues related to pregnancy, labor, and birth that require decision making by the parents.	Couples are faced with the need to make decisions about issues such as: ■ Choice of a healthcare provider. ■ Birth experience plan. ■ Choice of birth setting. ■ Choice of support person during labor. ■ Choice of who should be present during the birth, such as other family members and siblings.
Describe the types of antepartal education programs available to expectant couples and their families.	A broad range of classes are available, including: ■ Description of each stage of pregnancy. ■ Childbirth preparation. ■ Preparation for a cesarean birth. ■ Breastfeeding. ■ Sibling preparation. ■ Grandparent role preparation.
Compare methods of childbirth preparation.	There are many different methods to prepare clients for childbirth. They all emphasize measures that help to decrease anxiety and pain. The childbirth methods discussed in this chapter are: ■ Lamaze: uses breathing patterns, controlled muscular relaxation techniques (psychoprophylactic). ■ Bradley: partner-coached childbirth. ■ Kitzinger: sensory-memory techniques. ■ HypnoBirthing: deep relaxation techniques.
Identify ways in which the nurse conveys respect for client individuality in preparing for childbirth.	Nurses convey respect during childbirth preparation by: ■ Emphasizing the uniqueness of each birth experience. ■ Providing the client with tools such as breathing and relaxation to choose the best childbirth methods.

CRITICAL THINKING IN ACTION

*View the **Critical Thinking in Action** video in Chapter 8 of the CD-ROM. Then, answer the questions that follow.*

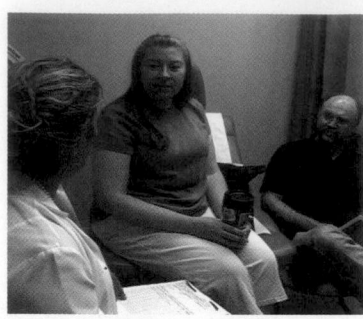

Terry Dole, a 38-year-old G1 P0000, at 6 weeks' gestation, presents to you at the OB clinic for her first prenatal visit with the certified nurse-midwife (CNM). One of the first decisions facing Terry is the selection of a healthcare provider. The midwife explains the various options available to Terry at the clinic related to the differences in educational preparation, skill level, practice characteristics, and general philosophy of CNMs and obstetricians. Terry tells you that she has been married for 6 years and works as a massage therapist. You obtain the following data: BP 110/70, temperature 97.0°F, pulse 76, respirations 12, weight 140 lb, height 5'7. The physical and pelvic exams are essentially normal. The CNM asks you to teach Terry about birth plans.

1. Discuss the advantages of a birth plan.
2. Discuss the disadvantages of a birth plan.
3. Explain the role of a doula.
4. What gender differences are there in moving toward parenthood?

MEDIALINK

www.prenhall.com/london

- NCLEX-RN® Review, case studies, and other interactive resources for this chapter can be found on the Companion Website at http://www.prenhall.com/london. Click on "Chapter 8" to select the activities for this chapter.

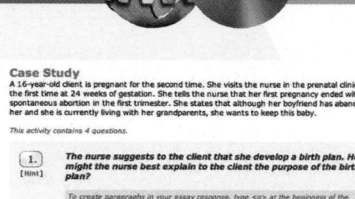

- For animations, more NCLEX-RN® Review questions, and an audio glossary, access the accompanying CD-ROM in this textbook.

REFERENCES

Arizága, G. (1999). Curanderismo as holistic medicine. In G. Cajeta (Ed.), *A people's ecology: Explorations in sustainable living* (pp. 210–233). Santa Fe, NM: Clear Light.

Bradley, R. A. (1974). *Husband-coached childbirth.* New York: Harper Row.

Castor, C. R. (2003). *Council of Childbirth Education Specialists teaching notes.* Williamsburg, VA: Council of Childbirth Education Specialists. Retrieved July 24, 2003, from http://www.councilces.org

Gilliland, A. L. (2002). Beyond holding hands: The modern role of the professional doula. *Journal of Obstetric, Gynecologic, and Neonatal Nursing, 31*(6), 762–769.

International Childbirth Education Association. (2000). ICEA philosophy statement. *International Journal of Childbirth Education, 15*(1).

Lee, J., & Schmied, V. (2001). Fathercraft: Involving men in antenatal education. *British Journal of Midwifery, 9*(9), 559–561.

Low, L. K., Seng, J. S., Murtland, T. L., & Oakley, D. (2000). Clinician-specific episiotomy rates: Impact on perineal outcomes. *Journal of Nurse-Midwifery and Women's Health, 45*(2), 87–91.

Steinberg, D., & Beal, M. W. (2003). Homeopathy and women's health care. *Journal of Obstetric, Gynecologic, and Neonatal Nursing, 32*(2), 207–214.

Teschendorf, M., & Evans, C. P. (2000). Hydrotherapy during labor: An example of developing a practice policy. *American Journal of Maternal-Child Nursing, 25*(4), 198–203.

Wolcott, H. D., & Conry, J. A. (2000). Normal labor. In A. T. Evans & K. R. Niswander (Eds.), *Manual of obstetrics* (6th ed., pp. 392–424). Philadelphia: Lippincott Williams & Wilkins.

Physical and Psychologic Changes of Pregnancy

Our son and his wife just told us they are pregnant. I am going to be a grandfather! I have tried to be a good father, to give my boy love, to teach him to respect others, to show him what it means to be a real man, someone a family can count on. Guess time will tell if the lessons took—I'm betting they have.

—Patrick, 52

LEARNING OBJECTIVES

- Identify the anatomic and physiologic changes that occur during pregnancy.

- Relate these anatomic and physiologic changes to the signs and symptoms that develop in the woman.

- Compare subjective (presumptive), objective (probable), and diagnostic (positive) changes of pregnancy.

- Contrast the various types of pregnancy tests.

- Discuss the emotional and psychologic changes that commonly occur in a woman, her partner, and her family during pregnancy.

- Summarize cultural factors that may influence a family's response to pregnancy.

MEDIALINK www.prenhall.com/london

CD-ROM

Audio Glossary
NCLEX-RN® Review

Companion Website

Care Plan: Preparing Siblings for New Baby
Case Study: Prenatal Education
Thinking Critically
NCLEX-RN® Review

Pregnancy is divided into three trimesters, each a 3-month period. Each trimester brings predictable changes for both the mother and the fetus. How does pregnancy affect the woman physically and psychologically? How does it affect her family, including siblings, partner, and grandparents? This chapter describes these physical and psychologic changes and the responses of the entire family to pregnancy. It also presents the various cultural factors that can affect a pregnant woman's well-being. Subsequent chapters build on this information in describing effective approaches to planning and providing care.

ANATOMY AND PHYSIOLOGY OF PREGNANCY

REPRODUCTIVE SYSTEM

Uterus

Before pregnancy the uterus is a small, almost solid, pear-shaped organ measuring approximately $7.5 \times 5 \times 2.5$ cm and weighing about 60 g (2 oz). At the end of pregnancy, it measures about $28 \times 24 \times 21$ cm and weighs approximately 1100 g; its capacity has also increased from about 10 mL to 5000 mL (5 L) or more (Cunningham, Leveno, Bloom et al., 2005). The change is primarily due to the enlargement (hypertrophy) of the preexisting myometrial cells as a result of the stimulating influence of estrogen and the distention caused by the growing fetus. Only a limited increase in cell number (hyperplasia) occurs. The fibrous tissue between the muscle bands increases markedly, which adds to the strength and elasticity of the muscle wall. The enlarging uterus, developing placenta, and growing fetus require additional blood flow to the uterus. By the end of pregnancy, one sixth of the total maternal blood volume is contained within the vascular system of the uterus.

Braxton Hicks contractions, which are irregular, generally painless contractions of the uterus, occur intermittently throughout pregnancy. They may be felt through the abdominal wall beginning about the fourth month of pregnancy. In later months these contractions become uncomfortable and may be confused with true labor contractions.

NURSING PRACTICE

Beginning early in pregnancy, have the woman feel her uterus periodically so that she becomes familiar with the size and the way it feels. As her pregnancy progresses, she then will be more likely to identify Braxton Hicks contractions and preterm labor, if it occurs.

Cervix

Estrogen stimulates the glandular tissue of the cervix, which increases in cell number and becomes hyperactive. The endocervical glands secrete a thick, sticky mucus that accumulates and forms the **mucous plug**, which seals the endocervical canal and prevents the ascent of organisms into the uterus. This mucous plug is expelled when cervical dilatation begins. The hyperactivity of the glandular tissue also increases the normal physiologic mucorrhea, at times resulting in profuse discharge. Increased cervical vascularity also causes both the softening of the cervix (Goodell's sign) and its bluish discoloration (Chadwick's sign).

Ovaries

The ovaries stop producing ova during pregnancy, but the corpus luteum continues to produce hormones until about weeks 6 to 8. The progesterone, which the corpus luteum secretes until about the seventh week of pregnancy, maintains the endometrium until the placenta assumes the task. The corpus luteum then begins to disintegrate slowly.

Vagina

Estrogen causes a thickening of the vaginal mucosa, a loosening of the connective tissue, and an increase in vaginal secretions (leukorrhea). These secretions are thick, white, and acidic (pH 3.5 to 6.0). The acid pH helps prevent bacterial infection but favors the growth of yeast organisms. Thus, the pregnant woman is more susceptible to monilial infection than usual.

The supportive connective tissue of the vagina loosens throughout pregnancy. By the end of pregnancy, the vagina and perineal body are sufficiently relaxed to permit passage of the infant. Because blood flow to the vagina is increased, the vagina may show the same blue-purple color (Chadwick's sign) as the cervix.

Breasts

Estrogen and progesterone cause many changes in the mammary glands. The breasts enlarge and become more nodular as the glands increase in size and number in preparation for lactation. Superficial veins become more prominent, the nipples become more erectile, and the areolae darken. Montgomery's follicles (sebaceous glands) enlarge, and striae (reddish stretch marks that slowly turn silver after childbirth) may develop.

Colostrum, an antibody-rich yellow secretion, may leak or be expressed from the breasts during the last trimester. Colostrum gradually converts to mature milk during the first few days after childbirth.

RESPIRATORY SYSTEM

Many respiratory changes occur to meet the increased oxygen requirements of a pregnant woman. The volume of air breathed each minute increases 30% to 40%. In addition, progesterone decreases airway resistance, permitting a 15% to 20% increase in oxygen consumption, as well as increases in carbon dioxide production and in the respiratory functional reserve.

As the uterus enlarges, it presses upward and elevates the diaphragm. The subcostal angle increases, so that the rib cage flares. The anteroposterior diameter increases, and the chest circumference expands by as much as 6 cm; as a result there is no significant loss of intrathoracic volume. Breathing changes from abdominal to thoracic as pregnancy progresses, and descent of the diaphragm on inspi-

ration becomes less possible. Some hyperventilation and difficulty in breathing may occur.

Nasal stuffiness and epistaxis (nosebleeds) may also occur because of estrogen-induced edema and vascular congestion of the nasal mucosa.

CARDIOVASCULAR SYSTEM

Blood volume progressively increases beginning in the first trimester, increases rapidly in the second trimester, and slows in the third. It peaks near term (when the baby is due), at about 40% to 45% above nonpregnant levels. This increase is due to increases in both erythrocytes and plasma.

During pregnancy, blood flow increases to organ systems with an increased workload. Thus, blood flow increases to the uterus and kidneys, whereas hepatic and cerebral flow remains unchanged. Cardiac output begins to increase early in pregnancy and remains elevated throughout gestation.

The pulse may increase by as many as 10 to 15 beats per minute at term. The blood pressure decreases slightly, reaching its lowest point during the second trimester. It gradually increases to near prepregnant levels by the end of the third trimester.

The enlarging uterus puts pressure on pelvic and femoral vessels, interfering with returning blood flow and causing stasis of blood in the lower extremities. This condition may lead to dependent edema and varicosity of the veins in the legs, vulva, and rectum (hemorrhoids) in late pregnancy. This increased blood volume in the lower legs may also make the pregnant woman prone to postural hypotension.

When the pregnant woman lies supine, the enlarging uterus may press on the vena cava, thus reducing blood flow to the right atrium, lowering blood pressure, and causing dizziness, pallor, and clamminess. The enlarging uterus may also press on the aorta and its collateral circulation (Cunningham et al., 2005). This condition is called **supine hypotensive syndrome**. It may also be referred to as **vena caval syndrome** or **aortocaval compression** (Figure 9–1 ⬤). It can be corrected by having the woman lie on her side or by placing a pillow or wedge under her right hip.

The total erythrocyte (red blood cell) volume increases by about 30% in women who receive iron supplementation but only about 18% without iron supplementation. This increase in erythrocytes is necessary to transport the additional oxygen required during pregnancy. However, the increase in plasma volume during pregnancy averages about 50%. Because the plasma volume increase (50%) is greater than the erythrocyte increase (30%), the hematocrit, which measures the concentration of red blood cells in the plasma, decreases slightly. This decrease is referred to as the **physiologic anemia of pregnancy** (pseudoanemia).

● FIGURE 9–1

Vena caval syndrome. The gravid uterus compresses the vena cava when the woman is supine. This reduces the blood flow returning to the heart and may cause maternal hypotension.

Iron is necessary for hemoglobin formation, and hemoglobin is the oxygen-carrying component of erythrocytes. Thus, the increase in erythrocyte levels results in an increased need for iron by the pregnant woman. Even though the gastrointestinal absorption of iron is moderately increased during pregnancy, it is usually necessary to add supplemental iron to the diet to meet the expanded red blood cell and fetal needs.

Leukocyte production increases slightly to an average of 5000 to 12,000/mm³. During labor and early postpartum, these levels may reach 25,000/mm³ or higher (Cunningham et al., 2005).

Both fibrin and plasma fibrinogen levels increase during pregnancy. Although the blood-clotting time of the pregnant woman does not differ significantly from that of the nonpregnant woman, clotting factors VII, VIII, IX, and X increase; thus, pregnancy is a somewhat hypercoagulable state. These changes, coupled with venous stasis in late pregnancy, increase the pregnant woman's risk of developing venous thrombosis.

GASTROINTESTINAL SYSTEM

Nausea and vomiting are common during the first trimester because of elevated human chorionic gonadotropin (hCG) levels and changed carbohydrate metabolism. Gum tissue may soften and bleed easily. The secretion of saliva may increase and even become excessive (ptyalism).

Elevated progesterone levels cause smooth muscle relaxation, resulting in delayed gastric emptying and decreased peristalsis. As a result the pregnant woman may complain of bloating and constipation. These symptoms are aggravated as the enlarging uterus displaces the stomach upward and the intestines laterally and posteriorly. The cardiac sphincter also relaxes, and heartburn (pyrosis) may occur due to reflux of acidic secretions into the lower esophagus. Hemorrhoids frequently develop in late pregnancy from constipation and from pressure on vessels below the level of the uterus.

The emptying time of the gallbladder is prolonged during pregnancy as a result of smooth muscle relaxation from progesterone. This, coupled with the elevated levels of cholesterol in the bile, can predispose the woman to gallstone formation.

URINARY TRACT

During the first trimester, the enlarging uterus is still a pelvic organ and presses against the bladder, producing urinary frequency. This symptom decreases during the second trimester, when the uterus becomes an abdominal organ and pressure against the bladder lessens. Frequency reappears during the third trimester, when the presenting part descends into the pelvis and again presses on the bladder, reducing bladder capacity, contributing to hyperemia, and irritating the bladder.

The ureters (especially the right ureter) elongate and dilate above the pelvic brim. The glomerular filtration rate rises by as much as 50% beginning in the second trimester and remains elevated until birth. To compensate for this increase, renal tubular reabsorption also increases. However, glycosuria is sometimes seen during pregnancy because of the kidneys' inability to reabsorb all the glucose filtered by the glomeruli. Glycosuria may be normal or may indicate gestational diabetes, so it always warrants further testing.

SKIN AND HAIR

Changes in skin pigmentation commonly occur during pregnancy. They are thought to be stimulated by increased estrogen, progesterone, and α-melanocytic-stimulating hormone levels. Pigmentation of the skin increases primarily in areas that are already hyperpigmented: the areolae, the nipples, the vulva, and the perianal area. The skin in the middle of the abdomen may develop a pigmented line, the **linea nigra**, which usually extends from the pubic area to the umbilicus or higher (Figure 9–2 ●). Facial **chloasma (melasma gravidarum)**, also known as the "mask of pregnancy," a darkening of the skin over the forehead and around the eyes, may develop. Melasma is more prominent in dark-haired women and is aggravated by exposure to the sun. Fortunately, it fades or becomes less prominent soon after childbirth when the hormonal influence of pregnancy subsides. The sweat and sebaceous glands are often hyperactive during pregnancy. **Striae** (**striae gravidarum** when they result from pregnancy), or stretch marks, are reddish, wavy streaks that may appear on the abdomen, thighs, buttocks, and breasts. They result from reduced connective tissue strength due to elevated adrenal steroid levels.

FIGURE 9–2

Linea nigra.

Vascular spider nevi, small, bright-red elevations of the skin radiating from a central body, may develop on the chest, neck, face, arms, and legs. They may be caused by increased subcutaneous blood flow in response to elevated estrogen levels.

The proportion of hair in the growing phase increases during pregnancy compared to the number of hair follicles in the resting or dormant phase. After birth the number of hair follicles in the resting phase increases sharply, and the woman may notice increased hair shedding beginning 1 to 4 months postpartum. Practically all hair is replaced within 6 to 12 months, however (Cunningham et al., 2005).

MUSCULOSKELETAL SYSTEM

No demonstrable changes occur in the teeth of pregnant women. The dental caries that sometimes accompany pregnancy are probably caused by inadequate oral hygiene and dental care, especially if the woman has problems with bleeding gums or nausea and vomiting.

The joints of the pelvis relax somewhat because of hormonal influences. The result is often a waddling gait. As the pregnant woman's center of gravity gradually changes, the lumbar spinal curve becomes accentuated (lordosis), and her posture changes (Figure 9–3). This posture change compensates for the increased weight of the uterus anteriorly and frequently results in low backache.

Pressure of the enlarging uterus on the abdominal muscles may cause the rectus abdominis muscle to separate, producing **diastasis recti**. If the separation is severe and muscle tone is not regained postpartally, subsequent pregnancies will not have adequate support and the woman's abdomen may appear pendulous.

FIGURE 9–3

| 12 weeks | 20 weeks | 28 weeks | 36 weeks | 40 weeks |

Postural changes during pregnancy. Note the increasing lordosis of the lumbosacral spine and the increasing curvature of the thoracic area.

METABOLISM

Most metabolic functions increase during pregnancy because of the increased demands of the growing fetus and its support system. For a detailed discussion of nutrient, vitamin, and mineral metabolism, see Chapter 12. ∞

Weight Gain

The recommended weight gain for women of normal weight before pregnancy is 25 to 35 lb (11.4 to 15.9 kg); for women who are overweight, the recommended gain is 15 to 25 lb (6.8 to 11.4 kg). Underweight women are advised to gain the weight needed to reach their ideal weight plus 25 to 35 lb (11.4 to 15.9 kg) (Mattson & Smith, 2000). The average pattern of weight gain is 3.5 to 5 lb (1.6 to 2.3 kg) during the first trimester and 12 to 15 lb (5.5 to 6.8 kg) during each of the last two trimesters. Adequate nutrition and weight gain are important during pregnancy (see Chapter 11 for more discussion ∞).

Water Metabolism

Increased water retention, a basic alteration of pregnancy, is caused by several interrelated factors. The increased level of steroid sex hormones affects sodium and fluid retention. The lowered serum protein also influences fluid balance, as do increased intracapillary pressure and permeability. The extra water is needed for the fetus, the placenta, amniotic fluid, and the mother's increased blood volume, interstitial fluids, and enlarged organs.

Nutrient Metabolism

The fetus makes its greatest protein and fat demands during the second half of pregnancy, doubling in weight during the last 6 to 8 weeks. Protein (contributing nitrogen) must be stored during pregnancy to maintain a constant level within the breast milk and to avoid depletion of maternal tissues. Carbohydrate needs also increase, especially during the second and third trimesters. Fats are more completely absorbed during pregnancy, and the level of free fatty acids increases in response to human placental lactogen (hPL). The levels of lipoproteins and cholesterol also increase. Because of these changes, increased levels of dietary fat or reduced carbohydrate production may lead to ketonuria in the pregnant woman.

ENDOCRINE SYSTEM

Thyroid

The thyroid gland often enlarges slightly during pregnancy because of increased vascularity and hyperplasia of glandular tissue. Estrogen increases its capacity to bind thyroxine, resulting in an increase in serum protein-bound iodine. The basal metabolic rate increases by as much as 20% to 25% during pregnancy. However, within a few weeks after birth, all thyroid function returns to normal limits.

COMPLEMENTARY CARE

HERBS DURING PREGNANCY

Pharmaceutical companies have not included pregnant women in their studies of drug safety, claiming excessive costs and other research problems. As a result, very few over-the-counter or prescription drugs can claim to be safe for pregnant women and breastfeeding mothers. The same can be said for herbal medicines. Although herbs have been researched extensively in Europe, Asia, and Australia, there has been little clinical research done in the United States on the use of herbs in pregnancy. However, this is beginning to change. Future chapters of this text include recent research that has been conducted on the use of various herbal treatments in pregnancy. Every pregnant or breastfeeding woman must be extremely cautious about everything she ingests—foods, liquids, medications, and herbs. If a problem warrants intervention, she and her primary healthcare provider should discuss the benefits and risks of all treatments, synthetic and natural.

Pituitary

Pregnancy is made possible by the hypothalamic stimulation of the anterior pituitary gland, which in turn produces follicle-stimulating hormone (FSH), which stimulates ovum growth, and luteinizing hormone (LH), which brings about ovulation. Stimulation of the pituitary also prolongs the ovary's corpus luteal phase, which maintains the endometrium in case conception occurs. Prolactin, another anterior pituitary hormone, is responsible for initial lactation.

The posterior pituitary secretes vasopressin (antidiuretic hormone) and oxytocin. Vasopressin causes vasoconstriction, which results in increased blood pressure; it also helps regulate water balance. Oxytocin promotes uterine contractility and stimulates ejection of milk from the breasts (the letdown reflex) in the postpartum period.

Adrenals

During pregnancy, circulating cortisol, which regulates carbohydrate and protein metabolism, increases in response to increased estrogen levels. Cortisol blood levels return to normal within 1 to 6 weeks postpartum. The adrenals secrete increased levels of aldosterone by the early part of the second trimester. This increase in aldosterone in a normal pregnancy may be the body's protective response to the increased sodium excretion associated with progesterone (Cunningham et al., 2005).

Pancreas

The pregnant woman has increased insulin needs, and the pancreatic islets of Langerhans, which secrete insulin, are stressed to meet this increased demand. Any marginal pancreatic function quickly becomes apparent, and the woman may show signs of gestational diabetes.

Hormones in Pregnancy

Human Chorionic Gonadotropin. The trophoblast secretes hCG in early pregnancy. This hormone stimulates progesterone and estrogen production by the corpus luteum to maintain the pregnancy until the placenta is developed sufficiently to assume that function.

Human Placental Lactogen. Also called human chorionic somatomammotropin, hPL is produced by the syncytiotrophoblast. Human placental lactogen is an antagonist of insulin; it increases the amount of circulating free fatty acids for maternal metabolic needs and decreases maternal metabolism of glucose to favor fetal growth.

Estrogen. Secreted originally by the corpus luteum, estrogen is produced primarily by the placenta as early as the seventh week of pregnancy. Estrogen stimulates uterine development to provide a suitable environment for the fetus. It also helps develop the ductal system of the breasts in preparation for lactation.

Progesterone. Also produced initially by the corpus luteum and then by the placenta, progesterone plays the greatest role in maintaining pregnancy. It maintains the endometrium and inhibits spontaneous uterine contractility, preventing early spontaneous abortion. Progesterone also helps develop the acini and lobules of the breasts in preparation for lactation.

Relaxin. Relaxin is detectable in the serum of a pregnant woman by the time of the first missed menstrual period. Relaxin inhibits uterine activity, diminishes the strength of uterine contractions, aids in the softening of the cervix, and has the long-term effect of remodeling collagen. Its primary source is the corpus luteum, but small amounts are believed to be produced by the placenta and uterine decidua.

Prostaglandins in Pregnancy

Prostaglandins are lipid substances that can arise from most body tissues but occur in high concentrations in the female reproductive tract and are present in the decidua during pregnancy. The exact functions of prostaglandins during pregnancy are still unknown, although it has been proposed that they are responsible for maintaining reduced placental vascular resistance. Decreased prostaglandin levels may contribute to preeclampsia-eclampsia. Prostaglandins are also believed to play a role in the complex biochemistry that initiates labor.

SIGNS OF PREGNANCY

Many of the changes women experience during pregnancy are used to diagnose the pregnancy itself. They are called the subjective, or presumptive, changes; the objective, or probable, changes; and the diagnostic, or positive, changes of pregnancy.

SUBJECTIVE (PRESUMPTIVE) CHANGES

The subjective changes of pregnancy are the symptoms the woman experiences and reports. Because they can be caused by other conditions, they cannot be considered proof of pregnancy (Table 9–1). Several subjective signs can be diagnostic clues when other signs and symptoms of pregnancy are also present.

Amenorrhea, or the absence of menses, is the earliest symptom of pregnancy. Missing more than one menstrual period, especially in a woman whose cycle is ordinarily regular, is an especially useful diagnostic clue.

Nausea and vomiting in pregnancy (NVP) occur frequently during the first trimester. Because these symptoms often occur in the early part of the day, they are commonly

TABLE 9–1 ❖ Differential Diagnosis of Pregnancy—Subjective Changes

Subjective Changes	Possible Alternative Causes
Amenorrhea	Endocrine factors: early menopause; lactation; thyroid, pituitary, adrenal, ovarian dysfunction
	Metabolic factors: malnutrition, anemia, climatic changes, diabetes mellitus, degenerative disorders, long-distance running
	Psychologic factors: emotional shock, fear of pregnancy or sexually transmitted infection, intense desire for pregnancy (pseudocyesis), stress
	Obliteration of endometrial cavity by infection or curettage
	Systemic disease (acute or chronic), such as tuberculosis or malignancy
Nausea and vomiting	Gastrointestinal disorders
	Acute infections such as encephalitis
	Emotional disorders such as pseudocyesis or anorexia nervosa
Urinary frequency	Urinary tract infection
	Cystocele
	Pelvic tumors
	Urethral diverticula
	Emotional tension
Breast tenderness	Premenstrual tension
	Chronic cystic mastitis
	Pseudocyesis
	Hyperestrogenism
Quickening	Increased peristalsis
	Flatus ("gas")
	Abdominal muscle contractions
	Shifting of abdominal contents

referred to as **morning sickness**. In reality the symptoms may occur at any time and can range from a mere distaste for food to severe vomiting. Women who experience NVP often have a more favorable pregnancy outcome than those who do not.

Excessive fatigue may be noted within a few weeks after the first missed menstrual period and may persist throughout the first trimester.

Urinary frequency is experienced during the first trimester as the enlarging uterus presses on the bladder.

Changes in the breasts are frequently noted in early pregnancy. These changes include tenderness and tingling sensations, increased pigmentation of the areola and nipple, and changes in Montgomery's glands. The veins also become more visible and form a bluish pattern beneath the skin.

Quickening, or the mother's perception of fetal movement, occurs about 18 to 20 weeks after the last menstrual period in a woman pregnant for the first time but may occur as early as 16 weeks in a woman who has been pregnant before. Quickening is a fluttering sensation in the abdomen that gradually increases in intensity and frequency.

NURSING PRACTICE

Some women suggest that it is easiest to imagine the fluttering associated with quickening by letting the outer tips of the eyelashes brush a finger and then imagining that same sensation deep inside the abdomen.

OBJECTIVE (PROBABLE) CHANGES

An examiner can perceive the objective changes that occur in pregnancy. Because these changes can have other causes, they do not confirm pregnancy (Table 9–2).

Changes in the pelvic organs—the only physical changes detectable during the first 3 months of pregnancy—are caused by increased vascular congestion. These changes are noted on pelvic examination. As noted earlier, there is a softening of the cervix called **Goodell's sign**. **Chadwick's sign** is a bluish, purple, or deep-red discoloration of the mucous membranes of the cervix, vagina, and vulva (some sources consider this a presumptive sign). **Hegar's sign** is a softening of the isthmus of the uterus, the area between the cervix and the body of the uterus (Figure 9–4 ⊙). **McDonald's sign** is an ease in flexing the body of the uterus against the cervix.

General enlargement and softening of the body of the uterus can be noted after the eighth week of pregnancy. The fundus of the uterus is palpable just above the symphysis pubis at about 10 to 12 weeks' gestation and at the level of the umbilicus at 20 to 22 weeks' gestation (Figure 9–5 ⊙).

TABLE 9–2 ✤ Differential Diagnosis of Pregnancy—Objective Changes	
Objective Changes	**Possible Alternative Causes**
Changes in pelvic organs	Increased vascular congestion
Goodell's sign	Estrogen-progestin oral contraceptives
Chadwick's sign	Vulvar, vaginal, cervical hyperemia
Hegar's sign	Excessively soft walls of nonpregnant uterus
Uterine enlargement	Uterine tumors
Enlargement of abdomen	Obesity, ascites, pelvic tumors
Braxton Hicks contractions	Hematometra, pedunculated, submucous, and soft myomas
Uterine souffle	Large uterine myomas, large ovarian tumors, or any condition with greatly increased uterine blood flow
Pigmentation of skin	Estrogen-progestin oral contraceptives
Chloasma (melasma)	Melanocyte hormonal stimulation
Linea nigra	
Nipples/areolae	
Abdominal striae	Obesity, pelvic tumor
Ballottement	Uterine tumors/polyps, ascites
Pregnancy tests	Increased pituitary gonadotropins at menopause, choriocarcinoma, hydatidiform mole
Palpation for fetal outline	Uterine myomas

Enlargement of the abdomen during the childbearing years is usually regarded as evidence of pregnancy, especially if it is continuous and accompanied by amenorrhea. *Braxton Hicks contractions* can be palpated most commonly after the 28th week. As the woman approaches the end of pregnancy, these contractions may become uncomfortable. They are often called *false labor*.

Uterine souffle may be heard when the examiner auscultates the abdomen over the uterus. It is a soft, blowing sound that occurs at the same rate as the maternal pulse and is caused by the increased uterine blood flow and blood pulsating through the placenta. It is sometimes confused with the funic souffle, a soft, blowing sound of blood pulsating through the umbilical cord. The funic souffle occurs at the same rate as the fetal heart rate.

Changes in pigmentation of the skin are common in pregnancy. The nipples and areolae may darken, and the linea nigra may develop. Facial melasma (chloasma) may become noticeable, and striae may appear.

The fetal outline may be identified by palpation in many pregnant women after 24 weeks' gestation.

○ FIGURE 9–4

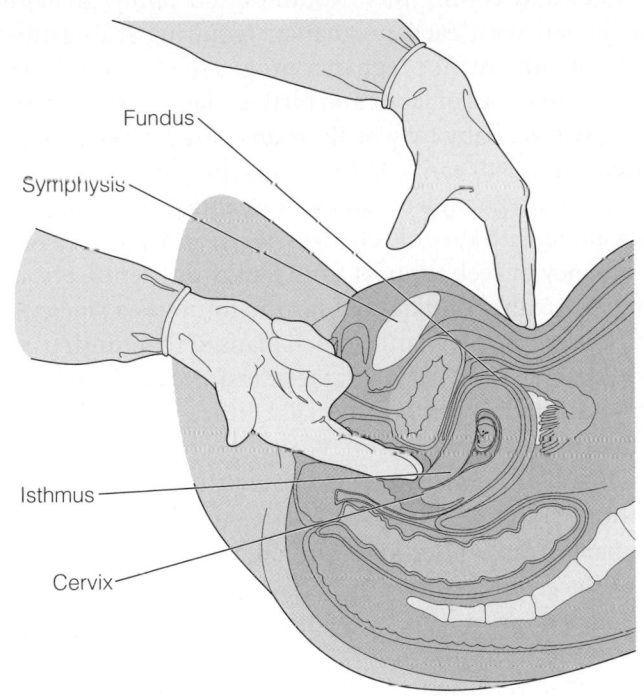

Fundus

Symphysis

Isthmus

Cervix

Hegar's sign, a softening of the isthmus of the uterus, can be determined by the examiner during a vaginal examination.

○ FIGURE 9–5

Approximate height of the fundus at various weeks of pregnancy.

THINKING CRITICALLY

At 33 weeks' gestation, Elena Martinez, G2P1, who is 5 feet 4 inches tall and weighs 144 lb (prepregnancy weight of 120 lb), is examined by her certified nurse-midwife. At that time her fundal height is measured as 33 cm. Because of a vacation trip, she is not seen again by her midwife until 36 weeks' gestation. At that time her fundus measures 35 cm and she weighs 147 lb. Elena asks if there is something wrong with her baby's growth. What is your assessment?

Ballottement is the passive fetal movement elicited when the examiner inserts two gloved fingers into the vagina and pushes against the cervix. This action pushes the fetal body up, and, as it falls back, the examiner feels a rebound.

Pregnancy tests detect the presence of hCG in the maternal blood or urine. These are not considered a positive sign of pregnancy because other conditions can cause elevated hCG levels.

Clinical Pregnancy Tests

A variety of assay techniques are available to detect hCG during early pregnancy.

Hemagglutination-inhibition test (Pregnosticon R test), an immunoassay, is based on the fact that no clumping of cells occurs when the urine of a pregnant woman is added to the hCG-sensitized red blood cells of sheep.

Latex agglutination test (Gravindex and Pregnosticon Slide tests), also an immunoassay, is based on the fact that latex particle agglutination is inhibited in the presence of urine containing hCG.

The two tests just described are done on the woman's first early morning urine because it is adequately concentrated. The tests become positive within 10 to 14 days after the first missed period.

Several pregnancy tests are done on maternal serum, including the following:

- β-*subunit radioimmunoassay (RIA)* uses an antiserum with specificity for the β-subunit of hCG in maternal blood. This very accurate pregnancy test has generally been replaced clinically by the technically simpler immunoradiometric assay.

- *Immunoradiometric assay (IRMA)* (Neocept, Pregnosis) uses a radioactive antibody to identify the presence of hCG in the serum. This test can detect very low concentrations of hCG and requires only about 30 minutes to perform.

- *Enzyme-linked immunosorbent assay (ELISA)* (Model Sensichrome, Quest Confidot) does not use radioisotopes but a substance that results in a color change after binding. The test is sensitive and quick. It can detect hCG levels as early as 7 to 9 days after ovulation and conception, which is 5 days before the first missed period (Buster & Carson, 2002).

■ *Fluoroimmunoassay (FIA)* (Opus hCG, Stratus hCG) uses an antibody tagged with a fluorescent label to detect serum hCG. The test, which takes about 2 to 3 hours to perform, is extremely sensitive and is used primarily to identify and follow hCG concentrations.

Over-the-Counter Pregnancy Tests

Home pregnancy tests are available over the counter at a reasonable cost. These enzyme immunoassay tests, performed on urine, are quite sensitive and detect even low levels of hCG. Most of the current kits can detect a pregnancy as early as the first day of the missed period. If the results are negative, the woman should repeat the test in 1 week if she has not started her period.

DIAGNOSTIC (POSITIVE) CHANGES

The positive signs of pregnancy are completely objective, cannot be confused with a pathologic state, and offer conclusive proof of pregnancy.

The *fetal heartbeat* can be detected with an electronic Doppler device as early as weeks 10 to 12 of pregnancy.

Fetal movement is actively palpable by a trained examiner after about the 20th week of pregnancy.

Visualization of the fetus by ultrasound examination confirms a pregnancy. The gestational sac can be observed by 4 to 5 weeks' gestation (2 to 3 weeks after conception). Fetal parts and fetal movement can be seen as early as 8 weeks' gestation. Transvaginal ultrasound has been used to detect a gestational sac as early as 10 days after implantation (Cunningham et al., 2005).

PSYCHOLOGIC RESPONSE OF THE EXPECTANT FAMILY TO PREGNANCY

Pregnancy is a turning point in a family's life, and thus it is accompanied by stress and anxiety, whether the pregnancy is desired or not. For beginning families, pregnancy is the transition period from childlessness to parenthood. If the pregnancy results in the birth of a child, the couple enters a new, irreversible stage of their life together. The expectant couple may be unaware of the physical, emotional, and cognitive changes of pregnancy and may anticipate no problems from such a normal event. Thus, they may be confused and distressed by new feelings and behaviors that are essentially normal.

If the expectant woman is married or has a stable partner, she no longer is only a mate but must also assume the role of mother. Her partner, too, will soon be a parent. Career goals and mobility may be affected, and the couple's relationship takes on a different meaning to them and their families and community. Routines and family dynamics are altered with each pregnancy, requiring readjustment and realignment. As pregnancy progresses, the couple must face the anxieties of labor and birth and must also deal with fears that the baby may be ill or disfigured. Classes in prepared childbirth can help the couple prepare.

If the pregnant woman has no stable partner, she must deal alone with the role changes, fears, and adjustments of pregnancy or seek support from family or friends. She also faces the reality of planning for the future as a single parent. Even if the pregnant woman plans to relinquish her infant, she must still deal with the adjustments of pregnancy. This adjustment can be especially difficult without a good support system.

In most pregnancies, finances are an important consideration. Traditional lore relegates to the father the role of primary breadwinner, and indeed finances are often a very real concern for fathers. In today's society, however, even pregnant women with stable partners recognize the financial impact of a child and may feel concern about financial issues. For the single mother, finances may be a major source of concern.

Decisions about financial matters need to be made at this time. Will the woman work during her pregnancy and return to work after her child is born? If so, who will provide child care? Couples may also need to decide about the division of domestic tasks. Any differences of opinion must be discussed openly and resolved so that the family can meet the needs of its members.

Pregnancy can be viewed as a developmental stage with its own distinct developmental tasks. For a couple it can be a time of support or conflict, depending on the amount of adjustment each is willing to make to maintain the family's equilibrium. Most pregnant women turn to their partners as their primary source of social support. In particular, a woman needs support from her partner that affirms that she is valued and that her baby will be welcomed and accepted (Logsdon, 2000–2001).

During a first pregnancy, the couple plans together for the child's arrival, collecting information on how to be parents. At the same time, each continues to participate in some separate activities with friends or family members. The availability of a social support network is an important factor in psychosocial well-being during pregnancy. The social network is often a major source of advice for the pregnant woman. However, both sound and unsound information may be conveyed.

During pregnancy, the expectant mother and father both face significant changes and must deal with major psychosocial adjustments (Table 9–3). Other family members, especially other children of the woman or couple and the grandparents-to-be, must also adjust to the pregnancy.

TABLE 9–3 ✣ Parental Reactions to Pregnancy

First Trimester	Second Trimester	Third Trimester
Mother's Reactions	**Mother's Reactions**	**Mother's Reactions**
Informs father secretively or openly.	Remains regressive and introspective, projects all problems with authority figures onto partner, may become angry as if lack of interest is sign of weakness in him.	Experiences more anxiety and tension, with physical awkwardness.
Feels ambivalent toward pregnancy, anxious about labor and responsibility of child.	Continues to deal with feelings as a mother and looks for furniture as something concrete.	Feels much discomfort and insomnia from physical condition.
Is aware of physical changes, daydreams of possible miscarriage.	May have other extreme of anxiety and wait until ninth month to look for furniture and clothes for baby.	Prepares for birth, assembles layette, picks out names.
Develops special feelings for and renewed interest in her own mother, with formation of a personal identity.	Feels movement and is aware of fetus and incorporates it into herself.	Dreams often about misplacing baby or not being able to give birth, fears birth of deformed baby.
	Dreams that partner will be killed, telephones him often for reassurance.	Feels ecstasy and excitement, has spurt of energy during last month.
	Experiences more distinct physical changes; sexual desires may increase or decrease.	
Father's Reactions	**Father's Reactions**	**Father's Reactions**
Differ according to age, parity, desire for child, economic stability.	If he can cope, will give her extra attention she needs; if he cannot cope, will develop a new time-consuming interest outside of home.	Adapts to alternative methods of sexual contact.
Acceptance of pregnant woman's attitude or complete rejection and lack of communication.	May develop a creative feeling and a "closeness to nature."	Becomes concerned over financial responsibility.
Is aware of his own sexual feelings, may develop more or less sexual arousal.	May become involved in pregnancy and buy or make furniture.	May show new sense of tenderness and concern, treats partner like doll.
Accepts, rejects, or resents mother-in-law.	Feels for movement of baby, listens to heartbeat, or remains aloof, with no physical contact.	Daydreams about child as if older and not newborn, dreams of losing partner.
May develop new hobby outside of family as sign of stress.	May have fears and fantasies about himself being pregnant, may become uneasy with this feminine aspect in himself.	Renewed sexual attraction to partner.
	May react negatively if partner is too demanding, may become jealous of physician and of physician's importance to partner and her pregnancy.	Feels he is ultimately responsible for whatever happens.

For some, pregnancy is more than a developmental stage; it is a crisis. *Crisis* can be defined as a disturbance or conflict in which the individual cannot maintain a state of equilibrium. Pregnancy can be considered a maturational crisis, since it is a common event in the normal growth and development of the family. During such a crisis, the individual or family is in disequilibrium. Egos weaken, usual defense mechanisms are not effective, unresolved material from the past reappears, and relationships shift. If the crisis is not resolved, it will result in maladaptive behaviors in one or more family members and possible disintegration of the family. Families that are able to resolve a maturational crisis will return successfully to normal functioning and can even strengthen the bonds in the family relationship.

THE MOTHER

Pregnancy alters body image and also necessitates a reordering of social relationships and changes in roles of family members. The way each woman meets the stresses of pregnancy is influenced by her emotional makeup, her sociologic and cultural background, and her acceptance or rejection of the pregnancy. However, many women manifest similar psychologic and emotional responses during pregnancy, including ambivalence, acceptance, introversion, mood swings, and changes in body image.

A woman's attitude toward her pregnancy can be a significant factor in its outcome. Even if the pregnancy is planned, there is an element of surprise at first. Many women commonly experience feelings of ambivalence during early pregnancy. This ambivalence may be related to feelings that the timing is somehow wrong; worries about the need to modify existing relationships or career plans; fears about assuming a new role; unresolved emotional conflicts with the woman's own mother; and fears about pregnancy, labor, and birth. These feelings may be more pronounced if the pregnancy is unplanned or unwanted. Indirect expressions of ambivalence include complaints about considerable physical discomfort, prolonged or frequent depression, significant dissatisfaction with changing body shape, excessive mood swings, and difficulty accepting the life changes resulting from the pregnancy.

Women who view their pregnancy as unwanted are more likely to delay prenatal care and to experience complications. The support and opinion of the woman's current partner, even if he is not the father of the child, has a major impact on pregnancy wantedness. Financial and emotional support from the partner are essential to the woman's positive attitude (Kroelinger & Oths, 2000). Involving the partner in the prenatal care may help promote a supportive attitude.

Conflicts about adapting to pregnancy are no more pronounced for older pregnant women (age 35 and over) than for younger ones. Moreover, older pregnant women tend to be less concerned about the normal physical changes of pregnancy and are confident about handling issues that arise during pregnancy and parenting. This difference may result because mature pregnant women have more experience with problem solving. However, mature pregnant women may have fewer pregnant peers and thus may have fewer people with whom to share concerns and expectations.

Pregnancy produces marked changes in a woman's body within a relatively short period. Pregnant women experience changes in body image because of physical alterations and may feel a loss of control over their bodies during pregnancy and later during childbirth. These perceptions are related to a certain extent to personality factors, social network responses, and attitudes toward pregnancy. Although changes in body image are normal, they can be stressful for the woman. Explanation and discussion of the changes may help both the woman and her partner deal with the stress associated with this aspect of pregnancy.

First Trimester

During the first trimester, feelings of disbelief and ambivalence are paramount. The woman's baby does not seem real, and she focuses on herself and her pregnancy. She may experience one or more of the early symptoms of pregnancy, such as breast tenderness or morning sickness, which are unsettling and at times unpleasant.

During this time, the expectant mother begins to exhibit some characteristic behavioral changes. She may become increasingly introspective and passive. She may be emotionally labile, with characteristic mood swings from joy to despair. She may fantasize about a miscarriage and

feel guilt because of these fantasies. She may worry that these thoughts will harm the baby in some way.

Second Trimester

During the second trimester, quickening occurs. This perception of fetal movement helps the woman think of her baby as a separate person, and she generally becomes excited about the pregnancy even if earlier she was not. The woman becomes increasingly introspective as she evaluates her life, her plans, and her child's future. This introspection helps the woman prepare for her new mothering role. Emotional lability, which may be unsettling to her partner, persists. In some instances the partner may react by withdrawing. This withdrawal is especially distressing to the woman, because she needs increased love and affection. Once the couple understands that these behaviors are characteristic of pregnancy, they are easier to accept; however, they may be sources of stress to some extent throughout pregnancy.

As pregnancy becomes more noticeable, the woman's body image changes. She may feel great pride, embarrassment, or concern. Generally women feel best during the second trimester, which is a relatively tranquil time.

Third Trimester

In the third trimester, the woman feels pride about her pregnancy and anxiety about labor and birth. Physical discomforts increase, and the woman is eager for the pregnancy to end. She experiences increased fatigue, her body movements are awkward, and her interest in sexual activity may decrease. The woman tends to be concerned about the health and safety of her unborn child and may worry that she will not cope well during childbirth. Toward the end of this period, there is often a surge of energy as the woman prepares a "nest" for the infant. Many women report bursts of energy, during which they vigorously clean and organize their homes.

Psychologic Tasks of the Mother

Rubin (1984) identified four major tasks that the pregnant woman undertakes to maintain her intactness and that of her family and to incorporate her new child into the family system. These tasks form the foundation for a mutually gratifying relationship with her infant:

1. *Ensuring safe passage through pregnancy, labor, and birth.* The pregnant woman feels concern for both her unborn child and herself. She looks for competent maternity care to provide a sense of control. She may seek information from literature, observation of other pregnant women and new mothers, and discussion with others. She often engages in self-care activities related to diet, exercise, alcohol consumption, and so forth. In the third trimester, she becomes more aware of external threats in the environment—a toy on the stairs, the awkwardness of an escalator—that pose a

threat to her well-being. Sleep becomes more difficult and she longs for birth even though it, too, is frightening.

2. *Seeking acceptance of this child by others.* The birth of a child alters a woman's primary support group (her family) and her secondary affiliative groups. The woman slowly and subtly alters her network to meet the needs of her pregnancy. In this adjustment the woman's partner is the most important figure. The partner's support and acceptance help form a maternal identity. If there are other children in the home, the mother also works to ensure their acceptance of the coming child. The woman without a partner looks to others such as a family member or friend for this support.

3. *Seeking commitment and acceptance of herself as mother to the infant (binding-in).* During the first trimester, the child remains a rather abstract concept. With quickening, however, the child begins to become a real person, and the mother begins to develop bonds of attachment. The mother experiences movement of the child within her in an intimate, exclusive way, and bonds of love form. The mother develops a fantasy image of her ideal child. This binding-in process, characterized by its strong emotional component, motivates the pregnant woman to become competent in her role and provides satisfaction for her in the role of mother.

4. *Learning to give of oneself on behalf of one's child.* Childbirth involves many acts of giving. The man "gives" a child to the woman; she in turn "gives" a child to him. Life is given to an infant; a sibling is given to older children of the family. The woman begins to develop a capacity for self-denial and learns to delay immediate personal gratification to meet the needs of another. Baby showers and gifts are acts of giving that increase the mother's self-esteem and help her recognize the separateness and needs of the coming baby.

Accomplishment of these tasks helps the pregnant woman develop her self-concept as mother. The expectant mother who was well nurtured by her own mother may view her as a role model and emulate her; the woman who views her mother as a "poor mother" may worry that she will make similar mistakes (Lederman & Miller, 1998). A woman's self-concept as a mother expands with actual experience and continues to grow through subsequent childbearing and child rearing.

THE FATHER

For the expectant father, pregnancy is a psychologically stressful time because he, too, must make the transition from nonparent to parent or from parent of one or more to parent of two or more. Research indicates that most men handle the transition to fatherhood well, and generally any anxieties they feel resolve over time. However, the anxieties they have are sometimes missed prenatally because most attention is devoted to the expectant mother (Buist, Morse, & Durkin, 2003).

Initially, expectant fathers may feel pride in their virility, which pregnancy confirms, but also have many of the same ambivalent feelings as expectant mothers. The extent of ambivalence depends on many factors, including the father's relationship with his partner, his previous experience with pregnancy, his age, his economic stability, and whether the pregnancy was planned.

In adjusting to his role, the expectant father must first deal with the reality of the pregnancy and then gain recognition as a parent from his partner, family, friends, coworkers, and society—and from his baby as well. The expectant mother can help her partner adjust if she has a definite sense of the experience as their pregnancy and their infant, and not her pregnancy and her infant.

The expectant father must establish a fatherhood role, just as the woman develops a motherhood role. Fathers who are most successful at this task generally like children, are excited about the prospect of fatherhood, are eager to nurture a child, and have confidence in their ability to be a parent. They also share the experiences of pregnancy and birth with their partners. (See Table 9–3.)

First Trimester

After the initial excitement attending the announcement of the pregnancy, an expectant father may begin to feel left out. He may be confused by his partner's mood changes. He might resent the attention she receives and her need to modify their relationship as she experiences fatigue and possibly a decreased interest in sex. He might also be concerned about what kind of father he will be. During this time, his child is a "potential" baby. Fathers often picture interacting with a child of 5 or 6 years, not a newborn. The pregnancy itself may seem unreal until the woman shows more physical signs.

Second Trimester

The father's role in the pregnancy is still vague in the second trimester, but his involvement may increase as he watches and feels fetal movement and listens to the fetal heartbeat during a prenatal visit. Like expectant mothers, expectant fathers need to confront and resolve some of their conflicts about the parenting they received. A father needs to sort out which behaviors of his own father he wants to imitate and which he wants to avoid.

Evidence suggests that the father-to-be's anxiety is lessened if both parents agree on the paternal role the man is to assume. For example, if both see his role as that of breadwinner, the man's stress is low. However, if the man views his role as that of breadwinner and the woman expects him to be actively involved in child care, his stress increases. Thus, the ability of the couple to negotiate a mutually agreeable role for the man may provide a significant coping mechanism for the expectant father (Diemer, 1997).

As the woman's appearance begins to change, her partner may have several reactions. Her appearance may decrease his sexual interest, or it may have the opposite effect. Because of the variety of emotions both partners may feel, communication and acceptance remain important.

Third Trimester

If the couple's relationship has grown through effective communication of their concerns and feelings, the third trimester is often a rewarding time. They may attend childbirth classes and make concrete preparations for the arrival of the baby. If the father has developed a detached attitude about the pregnancy, however, it is unlikely he will become a willing participant, even though his role becomes more obvious.

Concerns and fears may recur. The father may worry about hurting the unborn baby during intercourse or become concerned about labor and birth. He may also wonder what kind of parents he and his partner will be.

Couvade

Couvade has traditionally referred to the observance of certain rituals and taboos by the male to signify the transition to fatherhood. This observance affirms his psychosocial and biophysical relationship to the woman and child. More recently the term has been used to describe the unintentional development of physical symptoms such as fatigue, increased appetite, difficulty sleeping, depression, headache, or backache by the partner of a pregnant woman. Men who demonstrate couvade syndrome tend to have a higher degree of paternal role preparation and be involved in more activities related to this preparation.

SIBLINGS

Bringing a new baby home often marks the beginning of sibling rivalry. The siblings view the baby as a threat to the security of their relationships with their parents. Parents who recognize this potential problem early in pregnancy and begin constructive actions can minimize the problem of sibling rivalry.

Preparation of the young child begins several weeks before the anticipated birth. Because they do not have a clear concept of time, young children should not be told too early about the pregnancy. From the toddler's point of view, several weeks is an extremely long time. The mother may let the child feel the baby moving in her uterus, explaining that the uterus is "a special place where babies grow." The child can help the parents put the baby clothes in drawers or prepare the baby's room.

Consistency is important in dealing with young children. They need reassurance that certain people, special things, and familiar places will continue to exist after the new baby arrives. The crib is often an important though transient object in a child's life. If it is to be given to the new baby, the parents should thoughtfully help the older child adjust to this change. Any move from crib to bed or from one room to another should precede the baby's birth by several weeks or more. If the new baby will share a room with siblings, the parents must also discuss this situation with the older child or children.

Some parents advocate cosleeping (one or both parents sleeping with the baby or young child), and then the crib is less of an issue. Cosleeping, common in many non-Western cultures, is attracting more support in the United States. Opinion varies sharply about the advantages and risks of the practice, especially in light of an American Academy of Pediatrics policy statement (2000) recommending against cosleeping because of the increased risk of sudden infant death syndrome (SIDS). See the discussion in Chapter 32. ∞ Parents who choose to cosleep must make decisions about the sleeping arrangements of other siblings following the birth of the baby.

If the child is ready, toilet training is most effective several months before or after the baby's arrival. It is not unusual for an older, toilet-trained child to regress to wetting or soiling because of the attention the newborn gets for such behavior. The older, weaned child may want to breast feed or drink from the bottle again after the baby arrives. If the new mother anticipates these behaviors, they will be less frustrating during her early postpartum days.

Pregnant women may find it helpful to bring their children on a prenatal visit to the certified nurse-midwife or physician to give them an opportunity to listen to the fetal heartbeat. Such a visit helps make the baby seem more real to the children.

If siblings are school-age children, pregnancy should be viewed as a family affair. Teaching should be suitable to the child's level of understanding and may be supplemented with appropriate books. Taking part in family discussions, attending sibling preparation classes, feeling fetal movement, and listening to the fetal heartbeat help the school-age child take part in the experience of pregnancy and not feel like an outsider.

Older children or adolescents may appear to have sophisticated knowledge but may have many misconceptions about pregnancy and birth. The parents should make opportunities to discuss their concerns and involve the children in preparations for the new baby.

Even after birth, siblings need to feel that they are taking part. Having siblings visit their mother and the new baby at the hospital or birthing center will help. After the baby comes home, siblings can share in "showing off" the new baby.

Sibling preparation is essential, but other factors are equally important. These factors include how much parental attention the new arrival receives, how much attention the older child receives after the baby comes home, and how well the parents handle regressive or aggressive behavior.

GRANDPARENTS

The first relatives told about a pregnancy are usually the grandparents. The expectant grandparents often become increasingly supportive of the couple, even if conflicts previously existed. But it can be difficult for even sensitive grandparents to know how deeply to become involved in the childrearing process.

Because grandparenting can occur over a wide expanse of years, people's response to this role can vary considerably. Younger grandparents leading active lives may not demonstrate as much interest as the young couple would like. In other cases, expectant grandparents may give advice and gifts unsparingly. For grandparents, conflict may be related to the expectant couple's need to feel in control of their lives, or it may stem from events signaling changing roles in the grandparents' own lives (e.g., retirement, financial concerns, menopause, or death of a friend). Some parents of expectant couples may already be grandparents with a developed style of grandparenting. This influences their response to the pregnancy.

Because childbearing and childrearing practices have changed, family cohesiveness is promoted by effective communication and frank discussion between young couples and interested grandparents about the changes and the reasons for them. Classes for grandparents may provide information about changes in birth and parenting practices. These classes help familiarize grandparents with new parents' needs and may offer suggestions for ways in which the grandparents can support the childbearing couple.

CULTURAL VALUES AND PREGNANCY

Cultures have a universal tendency to create ceremonial rituals or rites around important life events. The rituals and customs of a group are a reflection of the group's values. Thus, the identification of cultural values is useful in predicting reactions to pregnancy. An understanding of male and female roles, family lifestyles, religious values, or the meaning of children in a culture may explain reactions of joy or shame.

Generalization about cultural characteristics or values is difficult because not every individual in a culture may display these characteristics. Just as variations are seen between cultures, variations are also seen within cultures. For example, because of their exposure to the American culture, a third-generation Cambodian-American family might have very different values and beliefs from those of a Cambodian family that has recently immigrated to the United States. For this reason, the nurse needs to supplement a general knowledge of cultural values and practices with a complete assessment of the individual's values and practices. "Developing Cultural Competence: Providing Effective Prenatal Care to Families of Different Cultures" summarizes the key actions a nurse can take to become more culturally aware.

DEVELOPING CULTURAL COMPETENCE

PROVIDING EFFECTIVE PRENATAL CARE TO FAMILIES OF DIFFERENT CULTURES

Nurses who are interacting with expectant families from a different culture or ethnic group can provide more effective, culturally sensitive nursing care by

- Critically examining their own cultural beliefs.
- Identifying personal biases, attitudes, stereotypes, and prejudices.
- Making a conscious commitment to respect the values and beliefs of others.
- Using sensitive, current language when describing others' cultures.
- Learning the rituals, customs, and practices of the major cultural and ethnic groups with whom they have contact.
- Including cultural assessment and assessment of the family's expectations of the healthcare system as a routine part of prenatal nursing care.
- Incorporating the family's cultural practices into prenatal care as much as possible.
- Fostering an attitude of respect for and cooperation with alternative healers and caregivers whenever possible.
- Providing for the services of an interpreter if language barriers exist.
- Learning the language (or at least several key phrases) of at least one of the cultural groups with whom they interact.
- Recognizing that ultimately it is the woman's right to make her own healthcare choices.
- Evaluating whether the woman's healthcare beliefs have any potential negative consequences for her health.

Cultural assessment is an important aspect of prenatal care. The nurse needs to identify the prospective parents' main beliefs, values, and behaviors about pregnancy and childbearing. This includes information about ethnic background, amount of affiliation with the ethnic group, patterns of decision making, religious preference, language, communication style, and common etiquette practices. The nurse can also explore the woman's (or family's) expectations of the healthcare system. Once this information is gathered, the nurse can then plan and provide care that is appropriate and responsive to family needs. See Chapter 2 for more detail on these topics. ∞

Critical Concept Review

LEARNING OBJECTIVES

CONCEPTS

Identify the anatomic and physiologic changes that occur during pregnancy.

- Uterus: Increased amounts of estrogen and growing fetus cause enlargement in size and weight, strength, elasticity, and vascularity.
- Cervix: Hyperplasia occurs (increase in cell number) due to increased estrogen level. Mucous plug forms to prevent organisms from entering uterus.
- Vagina: Increased thickness of mucosa, increased vaginal secretions to prevent bacterial infections. Connective tissue relaxes. Caused by increased estrogen level.
- Breasts: Estrogen and progesterone cause an increase in size and number of mammary glands; nipples more erectile, areolae darken, colostrum produced in last trimester.
- Respiratory system: Increasing levels of progesterone cause increased volume of air, deceased airway resistance, increased anteroposterior diameter. Thoracic breathing occurs as uterus enlarges.
- Cardiovascular system: Cardiac output increases, blood volume increases. Increased size of uterus interferes with blood return from lower extremities. Increased level of red cells to increase oxygen delivery to cells. Clotting factors increase. Caused by increased level of estrogen and progesterone.
- Gastrointestinal system: Delayed gastric emptying and decreased peristalsis. Caused by increased progesterone levels.
- Genitourinary system: Glomerular filtration rate and renal tubular reabsorption increase as a result of increased blood volume.
- Skin and hair: Increased skin pigmentation caused by increased estrogen and progesterone.
- Musculoskeletal: Relaxation of joints caused by increased estrogen and progesterone.

Relate these anatomic and physiologic changes to the signs and symptoms that develop in the woman.

- Uterus: Increased strength and elasticity allows uterus to contract and expel fetus during labor.
- Cervix: Mucous plug expelled as labor begins. Increased vascularity may cause bleeding after vaginal examinations.
- Vagina: Acid pH increases chance of vaginal yeast infections.
- Breasts: Increase in size causes soreness. Colostrum may be expressed during the third trimester.
- Respiratory system: Increased size of uterus may cause shortness of breath. Increased vascularity may cause nasal stuffiness and nosebleeds.
- Cardiovascular system: Decreased blood return from lower extremities may cause varicose veins and hemorrhoids. Pressure on the vena cava by the enlarged uterus may cause dizziness and decreased blood pressure.
- Gastrointestinal system: Nausea and vomiting and constipation caused by increased estrogen level and slow peristalsis and motility.
- Genitourinary system: Increased size of uterus, pressure on bladder, increased blood volume and glomerular filtration rate cause increased urination.
- Skin and hair: Increased skin pigmentation causes linea nigra and chloasma (melasma).

Compare subjective (presumptive), objective (probable), and diagnostic (positive) changes of pregnancy.

Subjective (presumptive) changes:
- Amenorrhea
- Nausea and vomiting
- Fatigue
- Urinary frequency
- Breast changes
- Quickening

Objective (probable) changes:
- Goodell's and Chadwick's sign
- Hegar's and McDonald's sign
- Enlargement of the abdomen
- Braxton Hicks contractions
- Uterine souffle
- Skin pigmentation changes
- Pregnancy tests

Diagnostic (positive) changes:
- Fetal heartbeat
- Fetal movement
- Visualization of the fetus

LEARNING OBJECTIVES

CONCEPTS

Contrast the various types of pregnancy tests.

→
- Urine tests: Detect hCG during early pregnancy.
- Serum tests: Also may detect hCG but may detect presence earlier than urine tests.
- Home (OTC) tests: Urine tests designed to detect hCG.

Discuss the emotional and psychologic changes that commonly occur in a woman, her partner, and her family during pregnancy.

→
Mother:
- First trimester: Disbelief and ambivalence.
- Second trimester: Quickening helps mother to view fetus as separate from herself.
- Third trimester: Anxiety about labor and birth. Nesting (bursts of energy) occurs.
- Rubin identified four tasks:
     Ensuring safe passage through pregnancy, labor, and birth
     Seeking acceptance of this child by others
     Seeking commitment and acceptance of herself as mother to infant
     Learning to give of oneself on behalf of one's child

Father/partner:
- First trimester: May feel left out. Disbelief.
- Second trimester: Begins to decide which behaviors of own father he wants to imitate or discard.
- Third trimester: Anxiety about labor and birth.

Family:
- Siblings' reaction depends upon age of siblings, but preparation is essential.
- Grandparents are usually supportive and excited about the birth.

Summarize cultural factors that may influence a family's response to pregnancy.

→
- Cultural assessment should be done to determine the beliefs, wishes, and traditions of the family. Factors such as religious preference, language, and communication style will affect the family's plans for the pregnancy.

CRITICAL THINKING IN ACTION

View the **Critical Thinking in Action** video in Chapter 9 of the CD-ROM. Then, answer the questions that follow.

Twenty-two-year-old Jean Simmons is an aerobic instructor, G0, P0000 in her first trimester of pregnancy. She presents to you at the local clinic complaining of frequent nausea, urinary frequency, and fatigue. You obtain her vital signs as: BP 108/60, temperature 97°F, pulse 68, respirations 12, weight 125 lb, height 64 inches. Her urine tests negative for ketones, albumin, leukocytes, and sugar. You note that Jean has lost 3 lb since her last visit. You assist the certified nurse midwife with a physical exam, the findings of which are essentially normal. Jean says that while she knows it could become an issue, she would like to continue working as an aerobic instructor for as long as she possibly can during the pregnancy. You identify Jean's complaints as normal discomforts of pregnancy, and proceed with prenatal education.

1. What advice would you suggest to cope with the nausea of pregnancy?
2. What advice might you suggest to cope with urinary frequency?
3. What teaching would be important relating to exercise in pregnancy?
4. What symptoms related to exercise should Jean report to her physician?

MEDIALINK www.prenhall.com/london

- NCLEX-RN® Review, case studies, and other interactive resources for this chapter can be found on the Companion Website at http://www.prenhall.com/london. Click on "Chapter 9" to select the activities for this chapter.

Case Study

A client arrives at the prenatal clinic for initial workup. She is a G1P0 and is 24 years old. The client is extremely excited and scared about this pregnancy, and has lots of questions. She is approximately 12 weeks gestation at this time.

This activity contains 3 questions.

1. The client has basic questions related to what type of changes can she expect over the next few months. What type of topics and information should be presented to alleviate her concerns?

To create paragraphs in your essay response, type <p> at the beginning of the paragraph, and </p> at the end.

- For animations, more NCLEX-RN® Review questions, and an audio glossary, access the accompanying CD-ROM in this textbook.

REFERENCES

American Academy of Pediatrics. (2000). Policy statement: Changing concepts of sudden infant death syndrome: Implications for infant sleep environment and sleep position. *Pediatrics, 105*(3), 650–656.

Beckman, C. R. B., & Dysart, D. (2000). The challenge of multicultural medical care. *Contemporary OB/GYN, 45*(12), 12–33.

Buist, A., Morse, C. A., & Durkin, S. (2003). Men's adjustment to fatherhood: Implications for obstetric health care. *Journal of Obstetric, Gynecologic, and Neonatal Nursing, 32*(2), 172–180.

Buster, J. E., & Carson, S. A. (2002). Endocrinology and diagnosis of pregnancy. In S. G. Gabbe, J. R. Niebyl, & J. L. Simpson (Eds.), *Obstetrics: Normal and problem pregnancies* (4th ed.). New York: Churchill Livingstone.

Cunningham, F. G., Leveno, K. J., Bloom, S. L., Hauth, J. C., Gilstrap, L. C., III, & Wenstrom, K. D. (2005). *Williams obstetrics* (22nd ed.). New York: McGraw-Hill.

Diemer, G. A. (1997). Expectant fathers: Influence of perinatal education on stress, coping, and spousal relations. *Research in Nursing & Health, 20*(4), 281–293.

Kroelinger, C. D., & Oths, K. S., (2000). Partner support and pregnancy wantedness. *Birth, 27*(2), 112–119.

Lederman, R., & Miller, D. S. (1998). Adaptations to pregnancy in three different ethnic groups: Latin-American, African-American, and Anglo-American. *Canadian Journal of Nursing Research, 30*(3), 37–51.

Logsdon, M. C. (2000–2001). Helping hands: Exploring the cultural implications of social support during pregnancy. *AWHONN Lifelines, 4*(6), 29–32.

Mattson, S., & Smith, J. E. (2000). *Core curriculum for maternal-newborn nursing* (2nd ed.). Philadelphia: Saunders.

Rubin, R. (1984). *Maternal identity and the maternal experience.* New York: Springer.

Sorenson, D. S., & Schuelke, P. (1999). Fantasies of the unborn among pregnant women. *MCN. American Journal of Maternal Child Nursing, 24*(2), 92–97.

Antepartal Nursing Assessment

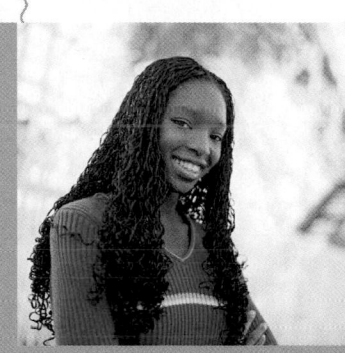

I'm 16—just got my license—so it was weird telling my friends that my mom is pregnant. I was embarrassed (and a little jealous) at first but now I kind of like the idea of having a baby sister. Mom had an amniocentesis because she is 37, so we know it's a girl. My mom has been great about including me and telling me what is going on. I've gone to a couple of her prenatal appointments so I got to hear the heartbeat and I saw the baby moving on ultrasound. I'm surprised by how interesting I am finding everything. Don't laugh, but I think I might like to be a nurse-midwife someday.

—*Krista, 16*

LEARNING OBJECTIVES

- Summarize the essential components of a prenatal history.

- Define common obstetric terminology found in the history of maternity clients.

- Identify factors related to the father's health that are generally recorded on the prenatal record.

- Describe areas that should be evaluated as part of the initial assessment of psychosocial and cultural factors related to a woman's pregnancy.

- Describe the normal physiologic changes one would expect to find when performing a physical assessment of a pregnant woman.

- Compare the methods most commonly used to determine the estimated date of birth.

- Develop an outline of the essential measurements that can be determined by clinical pelvimetry.

- Delineate the possible causes of abnormal findings during the initial or subsequent prenatal examination.

- Relate the components of the subsequent prenatal history and assessment to the progress of pregnancy.

MEDIALINK

www.prenhall.com/london

CD-ROM

Audio Glossary
NCLEX-RN® Review

Companion Website

Thinking Critically
NCLEX-RN® Review
Case Study: Initial Prenatal Assessment
Care Plan Activity: Initial Assessment of Primigravida

How can the registered nurse (RN) caring for a pregnant woman establish an environment of comfort and open communication with each antepartal visit? Including the family in the prenatal visits, such as inviting siblings to listen to the fetal heartbeat, is one way. The RN may complete many areas of prenatal assessment. Advanced practice nurses such as certified nurse-midwives (CNMs) and nurse practitioners are able to perform complete antepartal assessments. This chapter focuses on the prenatal assessments completed initially and at subsequent visits to provide optimum care for the childbearing family.

INITIAL CLIENT HISTORY

The course of a pregnancy depends on a number of factors, including the woman's prepregnancy health, presence of disease states, emotional status, and past healthcare. A thorough history helps determine the status of a woman's prepregnancy health.

DEFINITION OF TERMS

The following terms are used in recording the history of maternity clients:

Gestation: the number of weeks of pregnancy since the first day of the last menstrual period

Abortion: birth that occurs before the end of 20 weeks' gestation

Term: the normal duration of pregnancy (38 to 42 weeks' gestation)

Antepartum: time between conception and the onset of labor; usually used to describe the period during which a woman is pregnant; used interchangeably with *prenatal*

Intrapartum: time from the onset of true labor until the birth of the infant and placenta

Postpartum: time from the delivery of the placenta and membranes until the woman's body returns to a nonpregnant condition

Preterm or **premature labor:** labor that occurs after 20 weeks' but before completion of 37 weeks' gestation

Postterm labor: labor that occurs after 42 weeks' gestation

Gravida: any pregnancy, regardless of duration, including present pregnancy

Nulligravida: a woman who has never been pregnant

Primigravida: a woman who is pregnant for the first time

Multigravida: a woman who is in her second or any subsequent pregnancy

Para: birth after 20 weeks' gestation regardless of whether the infant is born alive or dead

Nullipara: a woman who has had no births at more than 20 weeks' gestation

Primipara: a woman who has had one birth at more than 20 weeks' gestation, regardless of whether the infant was born alive or dead

Multipara: a woman who has had two or more births at more than 20 weeks' gestation

Stillbirth: an infant born dead after 20 weeks' gestation

The terms *gravida* and *para* are used in relation to pregnancies, not to the number of fetuses. Thus twins, triplets, and so forth count as one pregnancy and one birth.

The following examples illustrate how these terms are applied in clinical situations:

1. Jean Sanchez has one child born at 38 weeks' gestation and is pregnant for the second time. At her initial prenatal visit, the nurse indicates her obstetric history as "gravida 2 para 1 ab 0." Jean Sanchez's present pregnancy terminates at 16 weeks' gestation. She is now "gravida 2 para 1 ab 1."

2. Tracy Hopkins is pregnant for the fourth time. At home she has a child who was born at term. Her second pregnancy ended at 10 weeks' gestation. She then gave birth to twins at 35 weeks. One twin died soon after birth. At her antepartal assessment, the nurse records her obstetric history as "gravida 4 para 2 ab 1."

To provide comprehensive data, a more detailed approach is used in some settings. Using the detailed system, gravida keeps the same meaning, but the meaning of para changes because the detailed system counts each infant born rather than the number of pregnancies carried to viability (Varney, Kriebs, & Gegor, 2004). For example, triplets count as one pregnancy but three babies.

A useful acronym for remembering the system is TPAL:

T: number of term infants born—that is, the number of infants born after 37 weeks' gestation or more

P: number of preterm infants born—that is, the number of infants born after 20 weeks' but before the completion of 37 weeks' gestation

A: number of pregnancies ending in either spontaneous or therapeutic abortion

L: number of currently living children

Using this approach the nurse would have initially described Jean Sanchez (see the first example) as "gravida 2 para 1001." Following Jean's spontaneous abortion, she would be "gravida 2 para 1011." Tracy Hopkins would be described as "gravida 4 para 1212" (Figure 10–1 ●). Occasionally a fifth digit is added to indicate the number of pregnancies that ended in multiple births (Varney et al., 2004). Using the five-digit system, Tracy Hopkins would be gravida 4 para 12121.

CLIENT PROFILE

The history is essentially a screening tool to identify factors that may place the mother or fetus at risk during the pregnancy. The following information is obtained for each pregnant woman at the first prenatal assessment:

1. Current pregnancy
   - First day of last normal menstrual period (LMP). Is she sure of the dates or uncertain? Do her cycles normally occur every 28 days, or do her cycles tend to be longer?
   - Presence of cramping, bleeding, or spotting since LMP
   - Woman's opinion about the time when conception occurred and when infant is due
   - Woman's attitude toward pregnancy (Is this pregnancy planned? Wanted?)
   - Results of pregnancy tests, if completed
   - Any discomforts since LMP such as nausea, vomiting, urinary frequency, fatigue, or breast tenderness

2. Past pregnancies
   - Number of pregnancies
   - Number of abortions, spontaneous or induced
   - Number of living children
   - History of previous pregnancies, length of pregnancy, length of labor and birth, type of birth (vaginal, forceps or vacuum-assisted birth, or cesarean), type of anesthesia used (if any), woman's perception of the experience, and complications (antepartal, intrapartal, and postpartal)
   - Neonatal status of previous children: Apgar scores, birth weights, general development, complications, and feeding patterns (breast milk or formula)
   - Loss of a child (miscarriage, elective or medically indicated abortion, stillbirth, neonatal death, relinquishment, or death after the neonatal period). What was the experience like for her? What coping skills helped? How did her partner, if involved, respond?
   - If Rh negative, was medication received after birth to prevent sensitization?
   - Prenatal education classes and resources (books)

● **FIGURE 10–1**

Name	Gravida	Term	Preterm	Abortions	Living Children
Jean Sanchez	2	1	0	1	1
Tracy Hopkins	4	1	2	1	2

The TPAL approach provides detailed information about the woman's pregnancy history.

3. Gynecologic history
- Date of last Pap smear; any history of abnormal Pap smear
- Previous infections: vaginal, cervical, tubal, or sexually transmitted
- Previous surgery
- Age at menarche
- Regularity, frequency, and duration of menstrual flow
- History of dysmenorrhea
- Sexual history
- Contraceptive history (If birth control pills were used, did pregnancy occur immediately following cessation of pills? If not, how long after?)

4. Current medical history
- Weight
- Blood type and Rh factor, if known
- General health, including nutrition, normal dietary practices, and regular exercise program (type, frequency, and duration)
- Any medications presently being taken (including prescription, nonprescription, homeopathic, or herbal medications) or taken since the onset of pregnancy
- Previous or present use of alcohol, tobacco, or caffeine (Ask specifically about the amounts of alcohol, cigarettes, and caffeine [specify coffee, tea, colas, or chocolate] consumed each day.)
- Illicit drug use or abuse (Ask about specific drugs such as cocaine, crack, and marijuana.)
- Drug allergies and other allergies
- Potential teratogenic insults to this pregnancy such as viral infections, medications, x-ray examinations, surgery, or cats in the home (possible source of toxoplasmosis)
- Presence of disease conditions such as diabetes, hypertension, cardiovascular disease, renal problems, or thyroid disorder
- Record of immunizations (especially rubella)
- Presence of any abnormal symptoms

5. Past medical history
- Childhood diseases
- Past treatment for any disease condition (Any hospitalizations? History of hepatitis? Rheumatic fever? Pyelonephritis?)
- Surgical procedures
- Presence of bleeding disorders or tendencies (Has she received blood transfusions?)

6. Family medical history
- Presence of diabetes, cardiovascular disease, cancer, hypertension, hematologic disorders, tuberculosis, or preeclampsia-eclampsia
- Occurrence of multiple births

- History of congenital diseases or deformities
- Occurrence of cesarean births and cause, if known

7. Religious, spiritual, and cultural history
- Does the woman wish to specify a religious preference on her chart? Does she have any religious beliefs or practices that might influence her healthcare or that of her child, such as prohibition against receiving blood products, dietary considerations, or circumcision rites?
- What practices are important to maintain her spiritual well-being?
- Might practices in her culture or that of her partner influence her care or that of her child?

8. Occupational history
- Occupation
- Physical demands (Does she stand all day, or are there opportunities to sit and elevate her legs? Any heavy lifting?)
- Exposure to chemicals or other harmful substances
- Opportunity for regular meals and breaks for nutritious snacks
- Provision for maternity or family leave

9. Partner's history
- Presence of genetic conditions or diseases
- Age
- Significant health problems
- Previous or present alcohol intake, drug use, or tobacco use
- Blood type and Rh factor
- Occupation
- Educational level; methods by which he learns best
- Attitude toward the pregnancy

10. Personal information about the woman
- Age
- Educational level; methods by which she learns best
- Race or ethnic group (to identify need for prenatal genetic screening and racially or ethnically related risk factors)
- Housing; stability of living conditions
- Economic level
- Acceptance of pregnancy
- Any history of emotional or physical deprivation or abuse of herself or children or any abuse in her current relationship (Ask specifically whether she has been hit, slapped, kicked, or hurt within the past year or since she has been pregnant. Is she afraid of her partner or anyone else? If yes, of whom is she afraid? [It is important to ask only when she is alone.])
- History of emotional problems
- Support systems available to her

- Personal preferences about the birth (expectations of both the woman and her partner, presence of others, and so on) (For more information see Chapter 8. ∞)
- Plans for care of child following birth
- Feeding preference for the baby (breast milk or formula?)

OBTAINING DATA

A questionnaire is used in many instances to obtain information. The woman should complete the questionnaire in a quiet place with a minimum of distractions. The nurse can get further information in an interview, which allows the pregnant woman to clarify her responses to questions and gives the nurse and client the opportunity to develop rapport.

The partner can be encouraged to attend the prenatal examinations. The partner is often able to contribute to the history and may use the opportunity to ask questions or express concerns.

HIGH-RISK SCREENING

Risk factors are any findings that suggest the pregnancy may have a negative outcome, for either the woman or her unborn child. Screening for risk factors is an important part of the prenatal assessment. Many risk factors can be identified during the initial assessment; others may be detected during subsequent prenatal visits. It is important to identify high-risk pregnancies early so that appropriate interventions can be started promptly. Not all risk factors threaten a pregnancy equally; thus, many agencies use a scoring sheet to determine the degree of risk. Information must be updated throughout pregnancy as necessary. Any pregnancy may begin as low risk and change to high risk because of complications.

Table 10–1 identifies the major risk factors currently recognized. The table also identifies maternal and fetal or newborn implications if the risk is present in the pregnancy.

INITIAL PRENATAL ASSESSMENT

The prenatal assessment focuses on the woman holistically by considering physical, cultural, and psychosocial factors that influence her health. The establishment of the nurse-client relationship is a chance to develop an atmosphere conducive to interviewing, support, and education. Because many women are excited and anxious at the first antepartal visit, the initial psychosocial-cultural assessment is general.

As part of the initial psychosocial-cultural assessment, discuss with the woman any religious or spiritual, cultural, or socioeconomic factors that influence the woman's expectations of the childbearing experience. It is especially helpful to be familiar with common practices of the members of various religious and cultural groups who reside in the community.

After obtaining the history, prepare the woman for the physical examination. The physical examination begins with assessment of vital signs; then the woman's body is examined. The pelvic examination is performed last.

Before the examination the woman should provide a clean urine specimen. When her bladder is empty, the woman is more comfortable during the pelvic examination and the examiner can palpate the pelvic organs more easily. After the woman empties her bladder, the nurse should ask her to disrobe and give her a gown and sheet or some other protective covering.

Increasing numbers of nurses, such as CNMs, nurse practitioners, and other nurses in advanced practice, are prepared to perform complete physical examinations. The nurse who is not an advanced practitioner assesses the woman's vital signs, explains the procedures to allay apprehension, positions her for examination, and assists the examiner as necessary.

NURSING PRACTICE

In a clinic or office setting, gowns and goggles for the healthcare provider are usually not necessary because splashing of body fluids is unlikely. Gloves are worn for procedures that involve contact with body fluids such as drawing blood for lab work, handling urine specimens, and conducting pelvic examinations.

Thoroughness and a systematic procedure are the most important considerations when performing the physical portion of an antepartal examination. See "Assessment Guide: Initial Prenatal Assessment." To promote completeness, the assessment guide is organized in three columns that address the areas to be assessed (and normal findings), the variations or alterations that may be observed, and nursing responses to the data. Certain organs and systems are assessed concurrently with others during the physical portion of the examination.

Nursing interventions based on assessment of the normal physical and psychosocial changes of pregnancy, evaluation of the cultural influences associated with pregnancy, and mutually defined client teaching and counseling needs are discussed further in Chapter 11. ∞

THINKING CRITICALLY

Karen Blade, a 23-year-old, G1P0, is 10 weeks pregnant when she sees you for her first prenatal examination. She has been experiencing some mild nausea and fatigue but otherwise is feeling well. She asks you about continuing with her routine exercises (walking 3 miles a day and lifting light weights). She also asks about using the heated pool and a hot tub. What should you tell her?

MEDALINK Case Study: Initial Prenatal Assessment

TABLE 10–1 ✤ Prenatal High-Risk Factors

Factor	Maternal Implications	Fetal or Neonatal Implications
Social and Personal		
Low income level and/or low educational level	Poor antenatal care Poor nutrition ↑ risk preecalmpsia	Low birth weight Intrauterine growth restriction (IUGR)
Poor diet	Inadequate nutrition ↑ risk anemia ↑ risk of preeclampsia	Fetal malnutrition Prematurity
Living at high altitude	↑ hemoglobin	Prematurity IUGR ↑ hemoglobin (polycythemia)
Multiparity >3	↑ risk antepartum or postpartum hemorrhage	Anemia Fetal death
Weight <45.5 kg (100 lb)	Poor nutrition Cephalopelvic disproportion Prolonged labor	IUGR Hypoxia associated with difficult labor and birth
Weight >91 kg (200 lb)	↑ risk hypertension ↑ risk cephalopelvic disproportion ↑ risk diabetes	↓ fetal nutrition ↑ risk macrosomia
Age < 16	Poor nutrition Poor antenatal care ↑ risk preeclampsia ↑ risk cephalopelvic disproportion	Low birth weight ↑ fetal demise
Age > 35	↑ risk preeclampsia ↑ risk cesarean birth	↑ risk congenital anomalies ↑ chromosomal aberrations
Smoking one pack/day or more	↑ risk hypertension ↑ risk cancer	↓ placental perfusion →↓ O$_2$ and nutrients available Low birth weight IUGR Preterm birth
Use of addicting drugs	↑ risk poor nutrition ↑ risk of infection with IV drugs ↑ risk HIV, hepatitis C	↑ risk congenital anomalies ↑ risk low birth weight Neonatal withdrawal Lower serum bilirubin
Excessive alcohol consumption	↑ risk poor nutrition Possible hepatic effects with long-term consumption	↑ risk fetal alcohol syndrome
Preexisting Medical Disorders		
Diabetes mellitus	↑ risk preeclampsia, hypertension Episodes of hypoglycemia and hyperglycemia ↑ risk cesarean birth	Low birth weight Macrosomia Neonatal hypoglycemia ↑ risk congenital anomalies ↑ risk respiratory distress syndrome
Cardiac disease	Cardiac decompensation Further strain on mother's body ↑ maternal death rate	↑ risk fetal demise ↑ prenatal mortality
Anemia: hemoglobin <9 g/dL (white) <29% hematocrit (white) <8.2 g/dL hemoglobin (black) <26% hematocrit (black)	Iron-deficiency anemia Low energy level Decreased oxygen-carrying capacity	Fetal death Prematurity Low birth weight
Hypertension	↑ vasospasm ↑ risk central nervous system irritability → convulsions ↑ risk cerebrovascular accident ↑ risk renal damage	↓ placental perfusion → low birth weight Preterm birth

A Day in the Life of a Nurse-Midwife

TO ME, PREGNANCY IS A WONDERFUL, normal experience—part of the cycle of life. That's why I love the fact that I can participate in all aspects of it, from pregnancy through birth and into the postpartal period. My practice enables me to ensure that a family's childbirth experience incorporates their personal beliefs and meets their expectations as much as possible. Come along with me for a day.

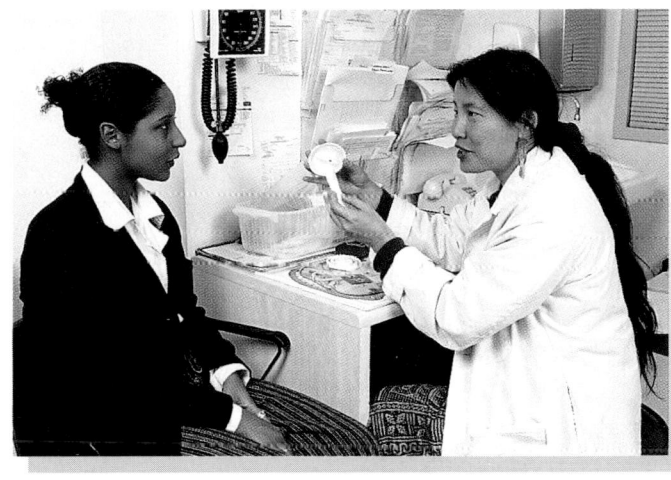

Cherrene has come for contraceptive information. I find it helpful to use models and examples during the discussion.

Dianne and her family come together for every appointment. We all enjoy listening to the fetal heartbeat.

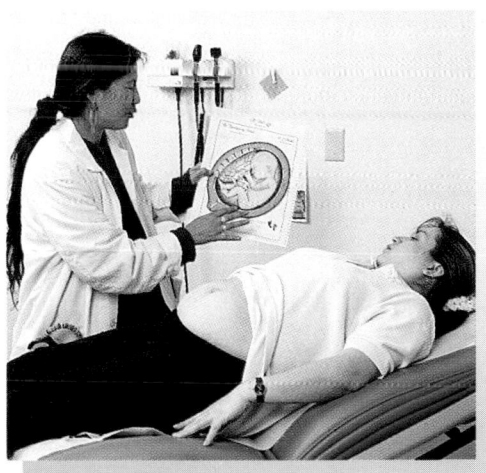

Gretchen's pregnancy is progressing well. She asks what her baby looks like now. I like to use a visual device as I talk with her about her baby's development.

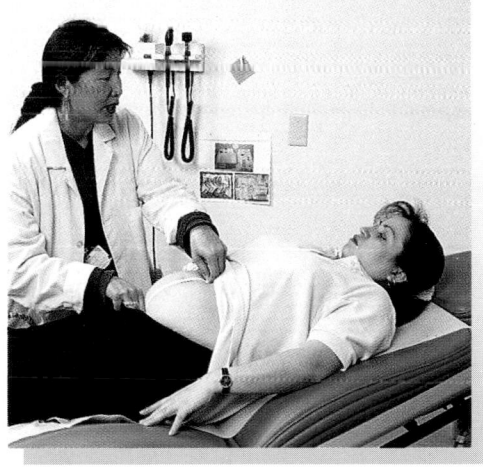

I measure the height of the fundus to determine if the baby is growing as expected. Gretchen and I talk about the impact of her nutrition, exercise, and healthy lifestyle habits on her baby and the outcome of her pregnancy.

Development is rapid; heart begins to pump blood; limb buds are well developed. Facial features and major divisions of the brain are discernible. Ears develop from skin folds; tiny bones and muscles are formed beneath the thin skin.

Embryo becomes a fetus, its beating heart discernible by ultrasound. Assumes a more human shape as lower body develops. At week 12, first movements begin. Sex is determinable. Kidneys produce urine.

Musculoskeletal system has matured; nervous system begins to exert control. Blood vessels rapidly develop. Fetal hands can grasp; legs kick actively. All organs begin to mature and grow. Fetus weighs about 7 oz (½ lb). FHT discernible with Doppler. Pancreas produces insulin.

Morning sickness, may persist to 12 weeks. Uterus changes from pear to globular shape. Hegar's, Goodell's and Piskacek's signs appear. Cervix flexes; leukorrhea increases. Surprise and ambivalence about pregnancy may occur. No noticeable weight gain.

Chadwick's sign appears. Uterus rises above pelvic brim by 12 weeks. Braxton Hicks contractions may begin and continue throughout pregnancy. Potential for urinary tract infection (UTI) increases and exists throughout pregnancy. Weight gain of about 2½ to 4 lb during first trimester.

Placenta now fully functioning and producing hormones.

Fundus halfway between symphysis and umbilicus. Woman gains slightly less than 1 lb per wk for remainder of pregnancy. May feel more energetic. BPD measurement on ultrasound. Vaginal secretions increase. Itching, irritation, malodor suggest infection. Woman may begin wearing maternity clothes. Pressure on bladder lessens and urinary frequency decreases.

Eat dry crackers before arising; try frequent small, dry, low-fat meals with fluids taken between meals. Avoid use of hot tubs, saunas, and steam rooms throughout pregnancy.

Discuss attitudes toward pregnancy. Discuss value of early pregnancy classes that focus on what to expect during pregnancy. Provide information about childbirth preparation classes.

Adequate fluid intake and frequent voiding (every 2 hr while awake) help prevent UTI. Also helpful to void following intercourse. Wipe from front to rear.

Discuss nutrition and appropriate weight gain. Stress value of regular physical exercise, especially non-weightbearing activities or walking. Discuss possible effects of pregnancy on sexual relationship.

Daily shower or bath and thorough drying of vulva helpful; avoid douching during pregnancy. Consult caregiver if infection suspected; use only prescribed medications.

Review danger signs of pregnancy. Discuss infant feeding options; provide information on the value of breast-feeding. Provide information about clothing, shoes.

MATERNAL-FETAL DEVELOPMENT

0

1

FETAL DEVELOPMENT

The sperm fertilizes the ovum, which then divides and burrows into the uterus.

From the embryonic disk (ecto-derm, entoderm, mesoderm), the first body segments appear that will eventually become the spine, brain, and spinal cord. Heart, blood circulation, and digestive tract take shape. Embryo is less than a quarter-inch long.

MATERNAL CHANGES

Mother misses first period; breasts become tender, may enlarge. Chronic fatigue and urin-ary frequency be-gin, may persist for three or more months. hCG in urine and serum 9 days after conception.

CLIENT TEACHING/ ANTICIPATORY GUIDANCE

Supportive bra may ease discom-fort. Increased rest and relaxation necessary now and throughout pregnancy. Increase fluids during the day; decrease fluid intake only at night to help prevent nocturia; sleep on side to decrease pressure on bladder. Avoid using any medi-cations unless prescribed. Avoid use of social drugs; check with caregiver before using any OTC preparations.

Darnell and Ayisha are expecting their first baby. Ayisha calls to tell me her labor has begun, and I meet them at the birth center. After the electronic fetal monitor is applied, we talk about the fetal heart tracing. I want to be sure they understand the monitor and have the opportunity to ask questions.

I do an exam to see how labor is progressing and share my findings with them.

During the active phase of Ayisha's labor, Darnell lovingly provides comfort and support.

It's time to push. Ayisha wants to stand and is most comfortable on the bed. Darnell stands behind her and provides support. I continue to talk with them and provide encouragement. After an hour of pushing, baby Kinshasa is born.

While I'm at the birth center, I check in on Alisa and Richard. Their baby, Lydia Rose, was born 6 hours ago. Alisa has asked for help with breast-feeding. Baby Lydia is a sleepy little one and needs encouragement to latch on and begin feeding.

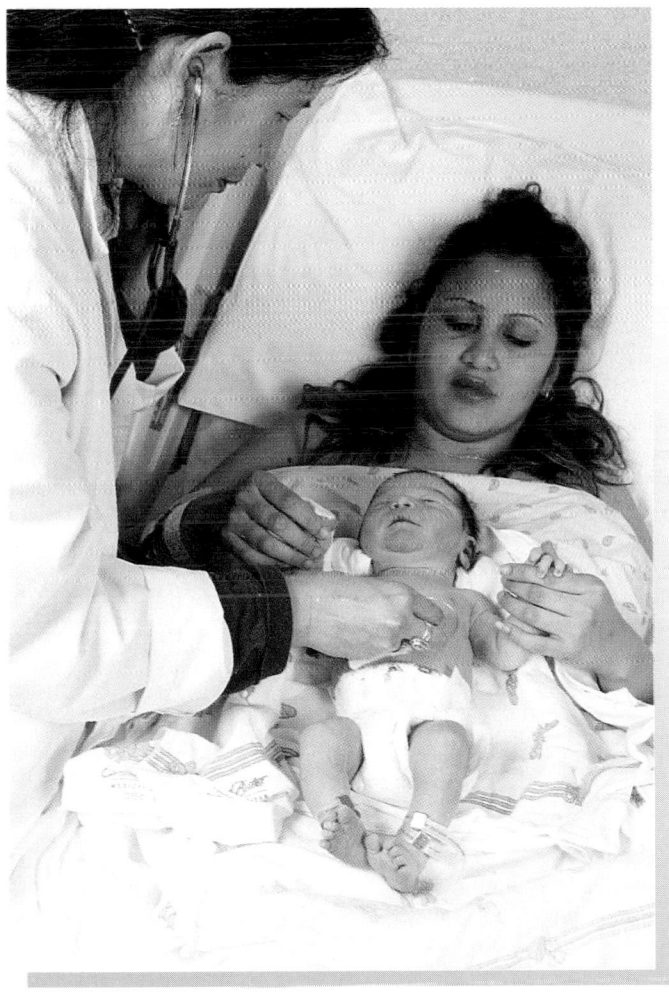

After baby Lydia has finished nursing, I do a physical assessment. I prefer to do an assessment in the room with the parents. It is such a wonderful opportunity for them to learn about their baby.

Brown fat deposits are developing beneath the skin to insulate the baby following birth. Baby has grown to about 15–17 in. Begins storing iron, calcium, and phosphorus.

The entire uterus is occupied by the baby, thus restricting its activity. Maternal antibodies are transferred to the baby. This provides immunity for about 6 months until the infant's own immune system can take over.

Illustrations by Charles W. Hoffman, MA, AMI

Fundus reaches xyphoid process; breasts full and tender. Urinary frequency may return. Swollen ankles and sleeping problems may develop. Dyspnea may develop.

The fetus descends deeper into the mother's pelvis (lightening). The placenta is nearly 4 times as thick as it was 20 weeks ago, weighing nearly 20 oz. Mother is eager for birth, may have final burst of energy. Backaches, urinary frequency increase. Braxton Hicks contractions intensify as cervix and lower uterine segment prepare for labor. Couple may tour labor and delivery area.

Wear well-fitting supportive bra. Elevate legs once or twice daily for an hour or so. Sleep on left side if possible. Use naturally occurring diuretics such as 2 tbsp lemon juice in 1 cup water or a generous serving of watermelon if available. Avoid most diuretics unless specifically prescribed. Maintain proper posture; use extra pillows at night for severe dyspnea. Following culture and personal preference, may begin preparing nursery now.

Review signs of labor. Discuss plans for other children (if any), transportation to agency.

Continue pelvic tilt exercises. Wear low-heeled shoes or flats. Avoid heavy lifting. Sleep on side to relieve bladder pressure. Urinate frequently. Avoid all analgesics except acetominophen. Pack suitcase for delivery.

Discuss postpartum period including decisions such as circumcision, rooming-in. Discuss common postpartum discomforts; mention postpartum blues. Discuss family planning methods, infant care. Stress need for adequate rest postpartally. Provide support, especially if baby is overdue.

Vernix protects the body; fine hair (lanugo) covers the body and keeps the oil on the skin. Eyebrows, eyelashes, and head hair develop. Fetus develops a regular schedule of sleeping, sucking and kicking.

Skeleton develops rapidly as bone-forming cells increase activity. Respiratory movements begin. Fetus weighs about 1 lb, 10 oz.

Fetus can breathe, swallow, regulate temperature. Surfactant forms in lungs. Eyes begin open and close. Baby is ⅔ the size it will be at birth.

Fundus reaches level of umbilicus. Breasts begin secreting colostrum. Amniotic sac holds about 400mL fluid. Faintness and dizziness may occur, especially with sudden position changes Varicose veins may begin to develop. Woman experiences fetal movement, and pregnancy may suddenly seem more "real." Areola darken. Nasal stuffiness may develop. Leg cramps may begin to occur. Constipation may develop.

Fundus above umbilicus. Backache and leg cramps may begin. Skin changes can include striae gravidarum, chloasma, linea negra, acne, redness on palms of hands and soles of feet. Nosebleeds can occur. May experience abdominal itching as uterus enlarges, will continue until end of pregnancy.

Fundus halfway between umbilicus and xyphoid process. May develop hemorrhoids. Thoracic breathing replaces abdominal breathing. Fetal outline palpable. May be tired of pregnancy and eager for the mothering role. Heartburn may begin to occur. May begin taking childbirth preparation classes with partner or support person.

Sit with feet elevated when possible; rise slowly and carefully. Avoid pressure on lower thighs. Support stockings may be helpful. Cool-air vaporizer may help. Eat foods containing fiber, such as raw fruits, vegetables, cereals with bran; drink liquids and exercise frequently.

Discuss breast care. Discuss dorsiflexion of foot to relieve cramps; heat to affected muscle.

Assure woman that skin changes generally subside soon after birth. Discuss specific exercises such as pelvic tilt to help strengthen back and abdominal muscles, and stress importance of good body mechanics. Reiterate importance of avoiding medications, caffeine, alcohol and smoking.

Woman may choose to apply petroleum jelly in nostrils to relieve nosebleeds. Cool vaporizer may also help. Lanolin-based cream can relieve itching. Mild soap can remove excess oil associated with acne.

Avoid constipation; use sitz baths, gentle reinsertion of hemorrhoids with a fingertip as necessary. Topical anesthetic agents may offer relief of hemorrhoids. Stool softeners may be prescribed by caregiver. Elevate legs and assume sidelying position when resting. Eat small, more frequent meals; avoid fatty food lying down after eating. Maalox or mylanta may be helpful; Avoid sodium bicarbonate. Discuss expectations about labor and delivery, caring for an infant.

Alisa is fascinated with baby Lydia's tiny fingers and toes. I love being with parents as they explore their baby. Each new baby is such a wonder. . . such a miracle.

Now my attention turns to Alisa. As part of my assessment, I check the position and tone of her fundus. All is well. I head home after a busy, but rewarding, day.

TABLE 10–1 ✜ Prenatal High-Risk Factors—continued

Factor	Maternal Implications	Fetal or Neonatal Implications
Preexisting Medical Disorders—*continued*		
Thyroid disorder	↑ infertility	↑ spontaneous abortion
Hypothyroidism	↓ basal metabolic rate, goiter, myxedema	↑ risk congenital goiter
Hyperthyroidism	↑ risk postpartum hemorrhage ↑ risk preeclampsia Danger of thyroid storm	Mental retardation → cretinism ↑ incidence congenital anomalies ↑ incidence preterm birth ↑ tendency to thyrotoxicosis
Renal disease (moderate to severe)	↑ risk renal failure	↑ risk IUGR ↑ risk preterm birth
Diethylstilbestrol (DES) exposure	↑ infertility, spontaneous abortion ↑ cervical incompetence	↑ spontaneous abortion ↑ risk preterm birth
Obstetric Considerations		
Previous Pregnancy		
Stillborn	↑ emotional or psychologic distress	↑ risk IUGR ↑ risk preterm birth
Habitual abortion	↑ emotional or psychologic distress ↑ possibility diagnostic workup	↑ risk abortion
Cesarean birth	↑ possibility repeat cesarean birth	↑ risk preterm birth ↑ risk respiratory distress
Rh or blood group sensitization	↑ financial expenditure for testing	Hydrops fetalis Icterus gravis Neonatal anemia Kernicterus Hypoglycemia
Large baby	↑ risk cesarean birth ↑ risk gestational diabetes	Birth injury Hypoglycemia
Current Pregnancy		
Rubella (first trimester)		Congenital heart disease Cataracts Nerve deafness Bone lesions Prolonged virus shedding
Rubella (second trimester)		Hepatitis Thrombocytopenia
Cytomegalovirus		IUGR Encephalopathy
Herpes virus type 2	Severe discomfort Concern about possibility of cesarean birth, fetal infection	Neonatal herpes virus type 2 2% hepatitis with jaundice Neurologic abnormalities
Syphilis	↑ incidence abortion	↑ fetal demise Congenital syphilis
Abruptio placenta and placenta previa	↑ risk hemorrhage Bed rest Extended hospitalization	Fetal or neonatal anemia Intrauterine hemorrhage ↑ fetal demise
Preeclampsia or eclampsia	See hypertension	↓ placental perfusion → low birth weight
Multiple gestation	↑ risk postpartum hemorrhage ↑ risk preterm labor	↑ risk preterm birth ↑ risk fetal demise
Elevated hematocrit >41% (white) >38% (black)	Increased viscosity of blood	Fetal death rate 5 times normal rate
Spontaneous premature rupture of membranes	↑ uterine infection	↑ risk preterm birth ↑ fetal demise

ASSESSMENT GUIDE

INITIAL PRENATAL ASSESSMENT

PHYSICAL ASSESSMENT/ NORMAL FINDINGS	ALTERATIONS AND POSSIBLE CAUSES*	NURSING RESPONSES TO DATA†
Vital Signs		
Blood pressure (BP): ≤ 135/85 mm Hg	High BP (essential hypertension; renal disease; pregestational hypertension, apprehension or anxiety associated with pregnancy diagnosis, exam, or other crises; preeclampsia if initial assessment not done until after 20 weeks' gestation)	BP > 140/90 requires immediate consideration; establish woman's BP; refer to physician if necessary. Assess woman's knowledge about high BP; counsel on self-care and medical management.
Pulse: 60–90 beats/min; rate may increase 10 beats/min during pregnancy	Increased pulse rate (excitement or anxiety, cardiac disorders)	Count for 1 full minute; note irregularities.
Respirations: 16–24 breaths/min (or pulse rate divided by four); pregnancy may induce a degree of hyperventilation; thoracic breathing predominant	Marked tachypnea or abnormal patterns	Assess for respiratory disease.
Temperature: 36.2–37.6°C (97–99.6°F)	Elevated temperature (infection)	Assess for infection process or disease state if temperature is elevated; refer to physician or CNM.
Weight		
Depends on body build	Weight < 45 kg (100 lb) or > 91 kg (200 lb); rapid, sudden weight gain (preeclampsia)	Evaluate need for nutritional counseling; obtain information on eating habits, cooking practices, foods regularly eaten, income limitations, need for food supplements, pica and other abnormal food habits. Note initial weight to establish baseline for weight gain throughout pregnancy.
Skin		
Color: Consistent with racial background; pink nail beds	Pallor (anemia); bronze, yellow (hepatic disease; other causes of jaundice)	The following tests should be performed: complete blood count (CBC), bilirubin level, urinalysis, and blood urea nitrogen (BUN).
	Bluish, reddish, mottled; dusky appearance or pallor of palms and nail beds in dark skinned women (anemia)	If abnormal, refer to physician.
Condition: Absence of edema (slight edema of lower extremities is normal during pregnancy)	Edema (preeclampsia); rashes, dermatitis (allergic response)	Counsel on relief measures for slight edema. Initiate preeclampsia assessment; refer to physician.
Lesions: Absence of lesions	Ulceration (varicose veins, decreased circulation)	Further assess circulatory status; refer to physician if lesion is severe.
Spider nevi common in pregnancy	Petechiae, multiple bruises, ecchymosis (hemorrhagic disorders; abuse)	Evaluate for bleeding or clotting disorder. Provide opportunities to discuss abuse if suspected.
Moles	Change in size or color (carcinoma)	Refer to physician.
Pigmentation: Pigmentation changes of pregnancy include linea nigra, striae gravidarum, melasma		Assure woman that these are normal manifestations of pregnancy and explain the physiologic basis for the changes.
Café-au-lait spots	Six or more (Albright syndrome or neurofibromatosis)	Consult with physician.
Nose		
Character of mucosa: Redder than oral mucosa; in pregnancy nasal mucosa is edematous in response to increased estrogen, resulting in nasal stuffiness (rhinitis of pregnancy) and nosebleeds	Olfactory loss (first cranial nerve deficit)	Counsel woman about possible relief measures for nasal stuffiness and nosebleeds (epistaxis); refer to physician for olfactory loss.

*Possible causes of alterations are identified in parentheses.

†This column provides guidelines for further assessment and initial nursing intervention.

ASSESSMENT GUIDE—continued

INITIAL PRENATAL ASSESSMENT

PHYSICAL ASSESSMENT/ NORMAL FINDINGS	ALTERATIONS AND POSSIBLE CAUSES*	NURSING RESPONSES TO DATA†
Mouth		
May note hypertrophy of gingival tissue because of estrogen	Edema, inflammation (infection); pale in color (anemia)	Assess hematocrit for anemia; counsel regarding dental hygiene habits. Refer to physician or dentist if necessary. Routine dental care appropriate during pregnancy (no x-ray studies, no nitrous anesthesia).
Neck		
Nodes: Small, mobile, nontender nodes	Tender, hard, fixed, or prominent nodes (infection, carcinoma)	Examine for local infection; refer to physician.
Thyroid: Small, smooth, lateral lobes palpable on either side of trachea; slight hyperplasia by third month of pregnancy	Enlargement or nodule tenderness (hyperthyroidism)	Listen over thyroid for bruits, which may indicate hyperthyroidism. Question woman about dietary habits (iodine intake). Ascertain history of thyroid problems; refer to physician.
Chest and Lungs		
Chest: Symmetric, elliptic, smaller anteroposterior (AP) than transverse diameter	Increased AP diameter, funnel chest, pigeon chest (emphysema, asthma, chronic obstructive pulmonary disease [COPD])	Evaluate for emphysema, asthma, pulmonary disease (COPD).
Ribs: Slope downward from nipple line	More horizontal (COPD)	Evaluate for COPD. Evaluate for fractures.
	Angular bumps	Consult physician.
	Rachitic rosary (vitamin C deficiency)	Consult nutritionist.
Inspection and palpation: No retraction or bulging of intercostal spaces (ICS) during inspiration or expiration; symmetric expansion.	ICS retractions with inspiration, bulging with expiration; unequal expansion (respiratory disease)	Do thorough initial assessment. Refer to physician.
Tactile fremitus	Tachypnea, hyperpnea, Cheyne-Stokes respirations (respiratory disease)	Refer to physician.
Percussion: Bilateral symmetry in tone	Flatness of percussion, which may be affected by chest wall thickness	Evaluate for pleural effusions, consolidations, or tumor.
Low-pitched resonance of moderate intensity	High diaphragm (atelectasis or paralysis), pleural effusion	Refer to physician.
Auscultation: Upper lobes—bronchovesicular sounds above sternum and scapulas; equal expiratory and inspiratory phases	Abnormal if heard over any other area of chest	Refer to physician.
Remainder of chest: Vesicular breath sounds heard; inspiratory phase longer (3:1)	Rales, rhonchi, wheezes; pleural friction rub; absence of breath sounds; bronchophony, egophony, whispered pectoriloquy	Refer to physician.
Breasts		
Supple; symmetric in size and contour; darker pigmentation of nipple and areola; may have supernumerary nipples, usually 5–6 cm below normal nipple line	"Pigskin" or orange-peel appearance, nipple retractions, swelling, hardness (carcinoma); redness, heat, tenderness, cracked or fissured nipple (infection)	Encourage monthly self-examination; instruct woman how to examine her own breasts.
Axillary nodes unpalpable or pellet sized	Tenderness, enlargement, hard node (carcinoma); may be visible bump (infection)	Refer to physician if evidence of inflammation.

*Possible causes of alterations are identified in parentheses.

†This column provides guidelines for further assessment and initial nursing intervention.

(continued)

☀ ASSESSMENT GUIDE—continued

INITIAL PRENATAL ASSESSMENT

PHYSICAL ASSESSMENT/ NORMAL FINDINGS	ALTERATIONS AND POSSIBLE CAUSES*	NURSING RESPONSES TO DATA†
Breasts *(continued)*		
Pregnancy changes: 1. Size increase noted primarily in first 20 weeks. 2. Become nodular. 3. Tingling sensation may be felt during first and third trimester; woman may report feeling of heaviness. 4. Pigmentation of nipples and areolae darkens. 5. Superficial veins dilate and become more prominent. 6. Striae seen in multiparas. 7. Tubercles of Montgomery enlarge. 8. Colostrum may be present after 12th week. 9. Secondary areola appears at 20 weeks, characterized by series of washed-out spots surrounding primary areola. 10. Breasts less firm, old striae may be present in multiparas.		Discuss normalcy of changes and their meaning with the woman. Teach and/or institute appropriate relief measures. Encourage use of supportive, well-fitting brassiere.
Heart		
Normal rate, rhythm, and heart sounds ***Pregnancy changes:*** 1. Palpitations may occur due to sympathetic nervous system disturbance. 2. Short systolic murmurs that increase in held expiration are normal due to increased volume.	Enlargement, thrills, thrusts, gross irregularity or skipped beats, gallop rhythm or extra sounds (cardiac disease)	Complete an initial assessment. Explain normalcy of pregnancy-induced changes. Refer to physician if indicated.
Abdomen		

Normal appearance, skin texture, and hair distribution; liver nonpalpable; abdomen nontender
 Pregnancy changes:
 1. Purple striae may be present (or silver striae on a multipara) as well as linea nigra.
 2. Diastasis of the rectus muscles late in pregnancy.
 3. Size: Flat or rotund abdomen; progressive enlargement of uterus due to pregnancy.
    10–12 weeks: Fundus slightly above symphysis pubis.
    16 weeks: Fundus halfway between symphysis and umbilicus.
    20–22 weeks: Fundus at umbilicus.
    28 weeks: Fundus three finger breadths above umbilicus.
    36 weeks: Fundus just below ensiform cartilage.
 4. Fetal heart rate: 110–160 beats/min may be heard with Doppler at 10–12 weeks' gestation; may be heard with fetoscope at 17–20 weeks.
	Muscle guarding (anxiety, acute tenderness); tenderness, mass (ectopic pregnancy, inflammation, carcinoma)
	
	 Size of uterus inconsistent with length of gestation (intrauterine growth restriction [IUGR], multiple pregnancy, fetal demise, hydatidiform mole)
	
	 Failure to hear fetal heartbeat with Doppler (fetal demise, hydatidiform mole)
		Assure woman of normalcy of diastasis. Provide initial information about appropriate prenatal and postpartum exercises. Evaluate woman's anxiety level. Refer to physician if indicated.
		
		 Reassess menstrual history regarding pregnancy dating. Evaluate increase in size using McDonald's method. Use ultrasound to establish diagnosis.
		
		 Refer to physician. Administer pregnancy tests. Use ultrasound to establish diagnosis.

*Possible causes of alterations are identified in parentheses.

†This column provides guidelines for further assessment and initial nursing intervention.

ASSESSMENT GUIDE—continued

INITIAL PRENATAL ASSESSMENT

PHYSICAL ASSESSMENT/ NORMAL FINDINGS	ALTERATIONS AND POSSIBLE CAUSES*	NURSING RESPONSES TO DATA†
Abdomen (continued)		
5. Fetal movement palpable by a trained examiner after the 18th week.	Failure to feel fetal movements after 20 weeks' gestation (fetal demise, hydatidiform mole)	Refer to physician for evaluation of fetal status.
6. Ballottement: During fourth to fifth month fetus rises and then rebounds to original position when uterus is tapped sharply.	No ballottement (oligohydramnios)	Refer to physician for evaluation of fetal status.
Extremities		
Skin warm, pulses palpable, full range of motion; may be some edema of hands and ankles in late pregnancy; varicose veins may become more pronounced; palmar erythema may be present	Unpalpable or diminished pulses (arterial insufficiency); marked edema (preeclampsia)	Evaluate for other symptoms of heart disease; initiate follow-up if woman mentions that her rings feel tight. Discuss prevention and self-treatment measures for varicose veins; refer to physician if indicated.
Spine		
Normal spinal curves: Concave cervical, convex thoracic, concave lumbar	Abnormal spinal curves; flatness, kyphosis, lordosis	Refer to physician for assessment of cephalopelvic disproportion (CPD).
In pregnancy, lumbar spinal curve may be accentuated	Backache	May have implications for administration of spinal anesthetics; see Chapter 20 for relief measures.∞
Shoulders and iliac crests should be even	Uneven shoulders and iliac crests (scoliosis)	Refer very young women to a physician; discuss back-stretching exercise with older women.
Reflexes		
Normal and symmetric	Hyperactivity, clonus (preeclampsia)	Evaluate for other symptoms of preeclampsia.
Pelvic Area		
External female genitals: Normally formed with female hair distribution; in multiparas, labia majora loose and pigmented; urinary and vaginal orifices visible and appropriately located	Lesions, hematomas, varicosities, inflammation of Bartholin's glands; clitoral hypertrophy (masculinization)	Explain pelvic examination procedure. Encourage woman to minimize her discomfort by relaxing her hips. Provide privacy.
Vagina: Pink or dark pink, vaginal discharge odorless, nonirritating; in multiparas, vaginal folds smooth and flattened; may have episiotomy scar	Abnormal discharge associated with vaginal infections	Obtain vaginal smear. Provide understandable verbal and written instructions about treatment for woman and partner, if indicated.
Cervix: Pink color; os closed except in multiparas, in whom os admits fingertip	Eversion, reddish erosion, nabothian or retention cysts, cervical polyp; granular area that bleeds (carcinoma of cervix); lesions (herpes, human papilloma virus [HPV]); presence of string or plastic tip from cervix (intrauterine device [IUD] in uterus)	Provide woman with a hand mirror and identify genital structures for her; encourage her to view her cervix if she wishes. Refer to physician if indicated. Advise woman of potential serious risks of leaving an IUD in place during pregnancy; refer to physician for removal.
Pregnancy changes:		
1–4 weeks' gestation: Enlargement in anteroposterior diameter		
4–6 weeks' gestation: Softening of cervix (Goodell's sign), softening of isthmus of uterus (Hegar's sign); cervix takes on bluish coloring (Chadwick's sign)	Absence of Goodell's sign (inflammatory conditions, carcinoma)	Refer to physician.

*Possible causes of alterations are identified in parentheses.

†This column provides guidelines for further assessment and initial nursing intervention.

(continued)

ASSESSMENT GUIDE—continued

INITIAL PRENATAL ASSESSMENT

PHYSICAL ASSESSMENT/ NORMAL FINDINGS	ALTERATIONS AND POSSIBLE CAUSES*	NURSING RESPONSES TO DATA†
Pelvic Area (continued)		
8–12 weeks' gestation: Vagina and cervix appear bluish violet in color (Chadwick's sign)		
Uterus: Pear shaped, mobile; smooth surface	Fixed (pelvic inflammatory disease [PID]); nodular surface (fibromas)	Refer to physician.
Ovaries: Small, walnut shaped, nontender (ovaries and Fallopian tubes are located in the adnexal areas)	Pain on movement of cervix (PID); enlarged or nodular ovaries (cyst, tumor, tubal pregnancy, corpus luteum of pregnancy)	Evaluate adnexal areas; refer to physician.
Pelvic Measurements		
Internal measurements: 1. Diagonal conjugate at least 11.5 cm (Figure 10-5)	Measurement below normal	Vaginal birth may not be possible if deviations are present.
2. Obstetric conjugate estimated by subtracting 1.5-2 cm from diagonal conjugate	Disproportion of pubic arch	
3. Inclination of sacrum	Abnormal curvature of sacrum	
4. Motility of coccyx; external intertuberosity diameter > 8 cm	Fixed or malposition of coccyx	
Anus and Rectum		
No lumps, rashes, excoriation, tenderness; cervix may be felt through rectal wall	Hemorrhoids, rectal prolapse; nodular lesion (carcinoma)	Counsel about appropriate prevention and relief measures; refer to physician for further evaluation.
Laboratory Evaluation		
Hemoglobin: 12–16 g/dL; women residing in areas of high altitude may have higher levels of hemoglobin	<11 g/dL (anemia)	Note: Wear gloves when drawing blood. Hemoglobin < 12 g/dL requires nutritional counseling; < 11 g/dL requires iron supplementation.
ABO and Rh typing: Normal distribution of blood types	Rh negative	If Rh negative, check for presence of anti-Rh antibodies. Check partner's blood type; if partner is Rh positive, discuss with woman the need for antibody titers during pregnancy, management during the intrapartal period, and possible need for Rh immune globulin. (See Chapter 15 ∞).
Complete blood count (CBC)		
Hematocrit: 38%–47% physiologic anemia (pseudoanemia) may occur	Marked anemia or blood dyscrasias	Perform CBC and Schilling differential cell count.
Red blood cells (RBC): 4.2-5.4 million/microliter		
White blood cells (WBC): 5000-12,000/microliter	Presence of infection; may be elevated in pregnancy and with labor	Evaluate for other signs of infection.
Differential Neutrophils: 40%–60%		
Bands: up to 5%		
Eosinophils: 1%–3%		
Basophils: up to 1%		
Lymphocytes: 20%–40%		
Monocytes: 4%–8%		

*Possible causes of alterations are identified in parentheses.

†This column provides guidelines for further assessment and initial nursing intervention.

ASSESSMENT GUIDE—continued

INITIAL PRENATAL ASSESSMENT

PHYSICAL ASSESSMENT/ NORMAL FINDINGS	ALTERATIONS AND POSSIBLE CAUSES*	NURSING RESPONSES TO DATA†
Laboratory Evaluation (*continued*)		
Syphilis tests: Serologic tests for syphilis (STS), complement fixation test, veneral disease research laboratory (VDRL) test—nonreactive	Positive reaction STS—tests may have 25%–45% incidence of biologic false-positive results; false results may occur in individuals who have acute viral or bacterial infections, hypersensitivity reactions, recent vaccinations, collagen disease, malaria, or tuberculosis	Positive results may be confirmed with the fluorescent treponemal antibody-absorption (FTA-ABS) test; all tests for syphilis give positive results in the secondary stage of the disease; antibiotic tests may cause negative test results.
Gonorrhea culture: Negative	Positive	Refer for treatment.
Urinalysis (u/a): Normal color, specific gravity; pH 4.6–8.0	Abnormal color (porphyria, hemoglobinuria, bilirubinemia); alkaline urine (metabolic alkalemia, *Proteus* infection, old specimen)	Repeat u/a; refer to physician.
Negative for protein, red blood cells, white blood cells, casts	Positive findings (contaminated specimen, kidney disease)	Repeat u/a; refer to physician.
Glucose: Negative (small degree of glycosuria may occur in pregnancy)	Glycosuria (low renal threshold for glucose, diabetes mellitus)	Assess blood glucose level; test urine for ketones.
Rubella titer: Hemagglutination-inhibition (HAI) test—1:10 or above indicates woman is immune	HAI titer < 1:10	Immunization will be given on postpartum or within 6 weeks after childbirth. Instruct woman whose titers are < 1:10 to avoid children who have rubella.
Hepatitis B screen for hepatitis B surface antigen (HbsAg); negative	Positive	If negative, consider referral for hepatitis B vaccine. If positive, refer to physician. Infants born to women who test positive are given hepatitis B immune globulin soon after birth followed by first dose of hepatitis B vaccine.
HIV screen: Offered to all women; encouraged for those at risk; negative	Positive	Refer to physician.
Illicit drug screen: Offered to all women; negative	Positive	Refer to physician.
Sickle-cell screen for clients of African descent: Negative	Positive; test results would include a description of cells	Refer to physician.
Pap smear: Negative	Test results that show atypical cells	Refer to physician. Discuss with the woman the meaning of the findings and the importance of follow-up.

CULTURAL ASSESSMENT	VARIATIONS TO CONSIDER*	NURSING RESPONSES TO DATA†
Determine the woman's fluency in English.	Woman may be fluent in a language other than English.	Work with a knowledgeable translator to provide information and answer questions.
Ask the woman how she prefers to be addressed.	Some women prefer informality; others prefer to use titles.	Address the woman according to her preference. Maintain formality in introducing oneself if that seems preferred.
Determine customs and practices regarding prenatal care:	Practices are influenced by individual preference, cultural expectations, or religious beliefs.	Honor a woman's practices and provide for specific preferences unless they are contraindicated because of safety.
■ Ask the woman if there are certain practices she expects to follow when she is pregnant.	Some women believe that they should perform certain acts related to sleep, activity, or clothing.	Have information printed in the language of different cultural groups that live in the area.
■ Ask the woman if there are any activities she cannot do while she is pregnant.	Some women have restrictions or taboos they follow related to work, activity, sexual, environmental, or emotional factors.	

*Possible causes of alterations are identified in parentheses.

†This column provides guidelines for further assessment and initial nursing intervention.

(continued)

ASSESSMENT GUIDE—continued

INITIAL PRENATAL ASSESSMENT

CULTURAL ASSESSMENT	VARIATIONS TO CONSIDER*	NURSING RESPONSES TO DATA†
■ Ask the woman whether there are certain foods she is expected to eat or avoid while she is pregnant. Determine whether she has lactose intolerance. ■ Ask the woman whether the gender of her caregiver is of concern. ■ Ask the woman about the degree of involvement in her pregnancy that she expects or wants from her support person, mother, and other significant people. ■ Ask the woman about her sources of support and counseling during pregnancy.	Foods are an important cultural factor. Some women may have certain foods they must eat or avoid; many women have lactose intolerance and have difficulty consuming sufficient calcium. Some women are comfortable only with a female caregiver. A woman may not want her partner involved in the pregnancy. For some the role falls to the woman's mother or a female relative or friend. Some women seek advice from a family member, *curandera*, tribal healer, and so forth.	Respect the woman's food preferences, help her plan an adequate prenatal diet within the framework of her preferences, and refer to a dietitian if necessary. Arrange for a female caregiver if it is the woman's preference. Respect the woman's preferences about her partner or husband's involvement; avoid imposing personal values or expectations. Respect and honor the woman's sources of support.

Psychologic Status

Excitement and/or apprehension, ambivalence	Marked anxiety (fear of pregnancy diagnosis, fear of medical facility) Apathy; display of anger with pregnancy diagnosis	Establish lines of communication. Active listening is useful. Establish trusting relationship. Encourage woman to take active part in her care. Establish communication and begin counseling. Use active listening techniques.

Educational Needs

May have questions about pregnancy or may need time to adjust to reality of pregnancy		Establish educational, supporting environment that can be expanded throughout pregnancy.

Support Systems

Can identify at least two or three individuals with whom woman is emotionally intimate (partner, parent, sibling, friend)	Isolated (no telephone, unlisted number); cannot name a neighbor or friend whom she can call upon in an emergency; does not perceive parents as part of her support system	Institute support system through community groups. Help woman to develop trusting relationship with healthcare professionals.

Family Functioning

Emotionally supportive Communications adequate Mutually satisfying Cohesiveness in times of trouble	Long-term problems or specific problems related to this pregnancy, potential stressors within the family, pessimistic attitudes, unilateral decision making, unrealistic expectations of this pregnancy or child	Help identify the problems and stressors, encourage communication, and discuss role changes and adaptations.

Economic Status

Source of income is stable and sufficient to meet basic needs of daily living and medical needs	Limited prenatal care; poor physical health; limited use of healthcare system; unstable economic status	Discuss available resources for health maintenance and the birth. Institute appropriate referral for meeting expanding family's needs—food stamps and so forth.

Stability of Living Conditions

Adequate, stable housing for expanding family's needs	Crowded living conditions; questionable supportive environment for newborn	Refer to appropriate community agency. Work with family on self-help ways to improve situation.
	*Possible causes of alterations are identified in parentheses.	†This column provides guidelines for further assessment and initial nursing intervention.

DETERMINATION OF DUE DATE

Childbearing families generally want to know the "due date," or the date around which childbirth will occur. Historically the due date has been called the estimated date of confinement (EDC). However, the concept of confinement is rather negative, and some caregivers avoid it by referring to the due date as the estimated date of delivery (EDD). Childbirth educators often stress that babies are not "delivered" like a package; they are born. In keeping with a view that emphasizes the normality of the process, the authors of this text refer to the due date as the **estimated date of birth (EDB)**.

To calculate the EDB, it is helpful to know the date of the LMP. However, some women have episodes of irregular bleeding or fail to keep track of menstrual cycles. Thus, other techniques also help to determine how far along a woman is in her pregnancy—that is, at how many weeks' gestation she is. Techniques include evaluating uterine size, determining when quickening occurs, and auscultating fetal heart rate with a Doppler device or ultrasound.

NÄGELE'S RULE

The most common method of determining the EDB is **Nägele's rule**, which uses 280 days as the mean length of pregnancy. To use this method, begin with the first day of the LMP, subtract 3 months, and add 7 days. For example:

First day of LMP	November 21
Subtract 3 months	− 3 months
	August 21
Add 7 days	+ 7 days
EDB	August 28

It is simpler to change the months to numeric terms:

November 21 becomes	11–21
Subtract 3 months	− 3
	8–21
Add 7 days	+ 7
EDB	8–28

A gestation calculator or wheel lets the caregiver calculate the EDB even more quickly (Figure 10–2 ●).

Nägele's rule may be a fairly accurate determiner of the EDB if the woman has a history of menses every 28 days, remembers her LMP, and was not taking oral contraceptives before becoming pregnant.

However, Nägele's rule is not foolproof. A delay in ovulation affects the formula Nägele's rule uses to determine the EDB.

Ovulation usually occurs 14 days *before* the onset of the next menses, not 14 days after the previous menses. Consequently, if a woman's cycle is irregular, or more than 28 days long, the time of ovulation may be delayed. If a woman has been using oral contraceptives, ovulation may

● FIGURE 10–2

The EDB wheel can be used to calculate the due date. To use it, place the "last menses began" arrow on the date of the woman's LMP. Then read the EDB at the arrow labeled 40. In this case the LMP is September 8, and the EDB is June 17.

be delayed several weeks following her last menses. Then, too, a postpartum woman who is breastfeeding may resume ovulating but be amenorrheic for a time, making calculation based on LMP impossible.

UTERINE ASSESSMENT

Physical Examination

When a woman is examined in the first 10 to 12 weeks of her pregnancy and her uterine size is compatible with her menstrual history, uterine size may be the single most important clinical method for dating her pregnancy. In many cases, however, women do not seek maternity care until well into their second trimester, when it becomes much more difficult to evaluate specific uterine size. In obese women it is difficult to determine uterine size early in a pregnancy because the uterus is more difficult to palpate.

Fundal Height

Fundal height may be used as an indicator of uterine size, although this method is less accurate late in pregnancy. A centimeter tape measure is used to measure the distance abdominally from the top of the symphysis pubis to the top of the uterine fundus (McDonald's method) (Figure 10–3 ●). Fundal height in centimeters correlates well with weeks of gestation between 22 to 24 weeks and 34 weeks. Thus, at 26 weeks'

● **FIGURE 10-3**

A cross-sectional view of fetal position when McDonald's method is used to assess fundal height.

gestation, fundal height is probably about 26 cm. If the woman is very tall or very short, fundal height will differ. To be most accurate, fundal height should be measured by the same examiner each time. The woman should have voided within one-half hour of the examination and should lie in the same position each time. In the third trimester, variations in fetal weight decrease the accuracy of fundal height measurements.

A lag in progression of measurements of fundal height from month to month and week to week may signal intrauterine growth restriction (IUGR). A sudden increase in fundal height may indicate twins or hydramnios (excessive amount of amniotic fluid).

ASSESSMENT OF FETAL DEVELOPMENT

Quickening

Fetal movements felt by the mother, called quickening, may indicate that the fetus is nearing 20 weeks' gestation. However, quickening may be experienced between 16 and 22 weeks' gestation, so this method is not completely accurate.

Fetal Heartbeat

The ultrasonic Doppler device (Figure 10–4 ●) is the primary tool for assessing fetal heartbeat. It can detect fetal heartbeat, on average, at 8 to 12 weeks' gestation. If an ul-

trasonic Doppler is not available, a fetoscope may be used, although in current practice it is seldom necessary. The fetal heartbeat can be detected by fetoscope as early as week 16 and almost always by 19 or 20 weeks' gestation.

● **FIGURE 10-4**

Listening to the fetal heartbeat with a Doppler device.

Ultrasound

In the first trimester, ultrasound scanning can detect a gestational sac as early as 5 to 6 weeks after the LMP, fetal heart activity by 6 to 7 weeks, and fetal breathing movement by 10 to 11 weeks of pregnancy. Crown-to-rump measurements can be made to assess fetal age until the fetal head can be visualized clearly. Biparietal diameter (BPD) can then be used. BPD measurements can be made by approximately 12 to 13 weeks and are most accurate between 20 and 30 weeks, when rapid growth in the biparietal diameter occurs. (See Chapter 14 ∞ for discussion of fetal ultrasound scanning.)

ASSESSMENT OF PELVIC ADEQUACY (CLINICAL PELVIMETRY)

The pelvis can be assessed vaginally to determine whether its size is adequate for a vaginal birth. This procedure, clinical pelvimetry, is performed by physicians or by advanced practice nurses such as CNMs or nurse practitioners. For a detailed description of clinical pelvimetry, refer to a nurse-midwifery text. This section provides basic information about the assessment of the inlet and outlet (see Figures 10–5 ● and 10–6 ●), which were described in Chapter 3. ∞

● **FIGURE 10–5**

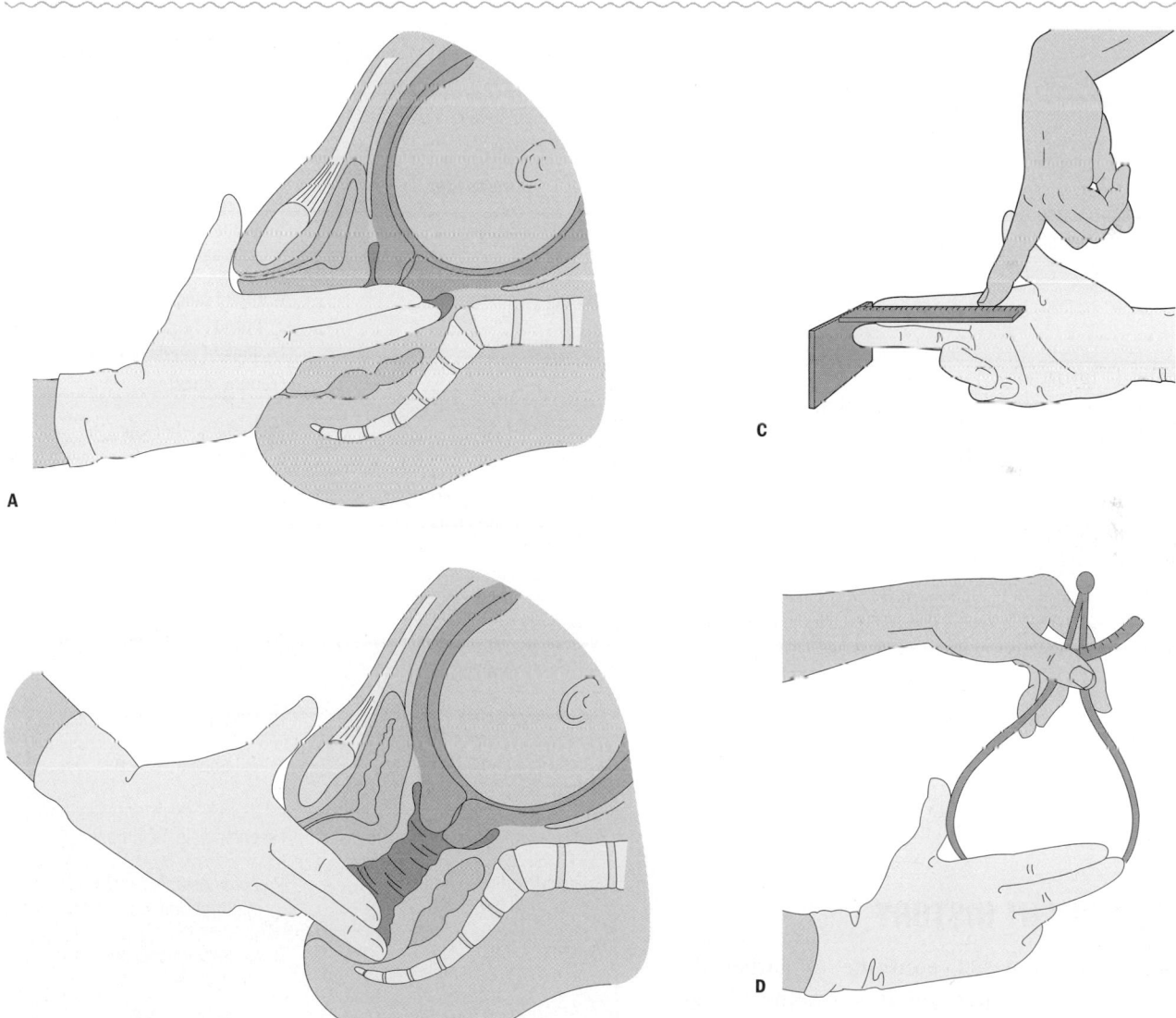

Manual measurement of inlet and outlet. **A,** Estimation of the diagonal conjugate, which extends from the lower border of the symphysis pubis to the sacral promontory. **B,** Estimation of the anteroposterior diameter of the outlet, which extends from the lower border of the symphysis pubis to the tip of the sacrum. **C** and **D,** Methods that may be used to check the manual estimation of anteroposterior measurements.

● FIGURE 10-6

Use of a closed fist to measure the outlet. Most examiners know the distance between their first and last proximal knuckles. If they do not, they can use a measuring device.

1. Pelvic inlet (Figure 10–5)
   - **Diagonal conjugate** (the distance from the lower posterior border of the symphysis pubis to the sacral promontory) at least 11.5 cm
   - **Obstetric conjugate** (a measurement approximately 1.5 cm smaller than the diagonal conjugate) 10 cm or more
2. Pelvic outlet (Figures 10–5 and 10–6)
   - Anteroposterior diameter, 9.5 to 11.5 cm
   - Transverse diameter (bi-ischial or intertuberous diameter), 8 to 10 cm

The pelvic cavity (midpelvis) cannot be accurately measured by clinical examination. Examiners estimate its adequacy. However, that discussion is also beyond the scope of this text.

SUBSEQUENT CLIENT HISTORY

At subsequent prenatal visits, continue to gather data about the course of the pregnancy to date and the woman's responses to it. Also ask about the adjustment of the support person and of other children, if any, in the family. As pregnancy progresses, inquire about the preparations the family has made for the new baby.

Ask specifically whether the woman has experienced any discomfort, especially the kinds of discomfort that are often seen at specific times during a pregnancy. Inquire about physical changes that relate directly to the pregnancy, such as fetal movement. Also ask about the danger signs of pregnancy (Table 10–2).

Other pertinent information includes any exposure to contagious illnesses, medical treatment and therapy prescribed for nonpregnancy problems since the last visit, and any prescription or over-the-counter medications that were not prescribed as part of the woman's prenatal care.

Periodic prenatal examinations offer a chance to assess the childbearing woman's psychologic needs and emotional status. If the woman's partner attends the antepartal

TABLE 10–2 ✤ Danger Signs in Pregnancy

The woman should report the following danger signs in pregnancy immediately:

Danger Sign	Possible Cause
Sudden gush of fluid from vagina	Premature rupture of membranes
Vaginal bleeding	Abruptio placentae, placenta previa
	Lesions of cervix or vagina "Bloody show"
Abdominal pain	Premature labor, abruptio placentae
Temperature above 38.3°C (101°F) and chills	Infection
Dizziness, blurring of vision, double vision, spots before eyes	Hypertension, preeclampsia
Persistent vomiting	Hyperemesis gravidarum
Severe headache	Hypertension, preeclampsia
Edema of hands, face, legs, and feet	Preeclampsia
Muscular irritability, convulsions	Preeclampsia, eclampsia
Epigastric pain	Preeclampsia, ischemia in major abdominal vessel
Oliguria	Renal impairment, decreased fluid intake
Dysuria	Urinary tract infection
Absence of fetal movement	Maternal medication, obesity, fetal death

COMPLEMENTARY CARE

YOGA DURING PREGNANCY

The following advice is important for women who practice yoga during pregnancy (Fontaine, 2005):

- During pregnancy, some yoga poses or positions are contraindicated. In particular, pregnant women should avoid those poses that put pressure on the uterus as well as any extreme stretching positions.
- Because of the changed center of gravity that occurs as pregnancy progresses, women need to be especially careful to maintain balance when doing stretching.
- Pregnant women should avoid stomach-lying for any poses. After 20 weeks' gestation, women should lie on their left side rather than on their back for floor positions.
- Pregnant women should immediately stop any pose that is uncomfortable.
- Warning signs that indicate the need to contact the physician or certified nurse-midwife immediately include the following: dizziness, extreme shortness of breath, sudden swelling, vaginal bleeding.

visits, they can also be a time to identify the partner's needs and concerns. The woman should have sufficient time to ask questions and air concerns. If a nurse provides the time and demonstrates genuine interest, the woman will be more at ease bringing up questions that she may believe are silly or has been afraid to verbalize.

Be sensitive to religious or spiritual, cultural, and socioeconomic factors that may influence a family's response to pregnancy, as well as to the woman's expectations of the healthcare system. One way to avoid stereotyping clients is simply to ask each woman about her expectations for the antepartal period. Although many women's responses may reflect what are thought to be traditional norms, other women will have decidedly different views or expectations that represent a blending of beliefs or cultures. During the antepartal period, it is also essential to begin assessing the readiness of the woman and her partner (if possible) to assume their responsibilities as parents successfully.

SUBSEQUENT PRENATAL ASSESSMENT

The "Assessment Guide: Subsequent Prenatal Assessment" provides a systematic approach to the regular

EVIDENCE-BASED NURSING

GUIDELINES FOR PREVENTION OF PERINATAL GROUP B STREPTOCOCCAL DISEASE

Clinical Question

How can we effectively screen and treat pregnant women who have colonized for perinatal group B streptococcus (GBS)?

Evidence

Four experts from the National Center for Infectious Diseases revised its 1996 guideline, using input and consultation from 26 infectious disease practitioners from a variety of settings. After reviewing clinical trials and public health cohort studies, these experts concluded that risk-based screening is no longer acceptable to prevent perinatal GBS.

Implications

All pregnant women should be screened between 35 and 37 weeks' gestation for vaginal and rectal GBS colonization. Collection of specimens for culture may be conducted in an outpatient setting either by the woman, with instruction, or by the healthcare provider. If a woman is identified as a GBS carrier, chemoprophylaxis should be started at the time of labor or when membranes rupture. Antimicrobial agents should not be used before the intrapartum period to treat GBS colonization. Doing so has not been found to prevent neonatal disease and may have adverse consequences.

An exception is made if the GBS has been identified in the woman's urine. In this case, chemoprophylaxis should be started earlier because urinary concentration indicates a heavy colonization. Increased risk of giving birth to an infant with early-onset GBS disease warrants use of the

drug during pregnancy, even with the risk of complications. If a woman has previously given birth to an infant with invasive GBS disease, she should get chemoprophylaxis during the intrapartum period as well.

Only if the colonization status of the mother is unknown should the decision about chemoprophylaxis during labor be based on assessment of risk, rather than on cultures. Risks that would indicate treatment include premature gestation, prolonged rupture of the membranes, or a temperature greater than $38\,^\circ C$.

You should encourage women to be screened for GBS during late pregnancy. Clients need information about when to expect that preventive antimicrobial prophylaxis will be initiated. (Client resources and brochures are available from the Centers for Disease Control Web site at www.cdc.gov) In most cases, prophylaxis is started when the woman is in labor but may be initiated earlier if heavy colonization is confirmed. Prevention of neonatal disease is a primary focus.

Critical Thinking

How will you respond to the questions mothers have about the safety of antimicrobial prophylaxis during labor? Earlier in the pregnancy? What assessments would indicate to you that a mother can expect the use of antimicrobials during labor?

Reference

Centers for Disease Control and Prevention. (2002). Prevention of perinatal group B streptococcal disease: Revised guidelines from CDC. *MMWR Recommendations and Reports, 51*(RR-11), 1–22.

ASSESSMENT GUIDE

SUBSEQUENT PRENATAL ASSESSMENT

PHYSICAL ASSESSMENT/ NORMAL FINDINGS	ALTERATIONS AND POSSIBLE CAUSES*	NURSING RESPONSES TO DATA†
Vital Signs		
Temperature: 36.2–37.6°C (97–99.6°F)	Elevated temperature (infection)	Evaluate for signs of infection. Refer to physician.
Pulse: 60–90/min Rate may increase 10 beats/min during pregnancy	Increased pulse rate (anxiety, cardiac disorders)	Note irregularities. Assess for anxiety and stress.
Respiration: 16–24/min	Marked tachypnea or abnormal patterns (respiratory disease)	Refer to physician.
Blood pressure: ≤ 135/85 (falls in second trimester)	> 140/90 or increase of 30 mm systolic and 15 mm diastolic (preeclampsia)	Assess for edema, proteinuria, and hyperreflexia. Refer to physician. Schedule appointments more frequently.
Weight Gain		
First trimester: 1.6–2.3 kg (3.5–5 lb)	Inadequate weight gain (poor nutrition, nausea, IUGR)	Discuss appropriate weight gain.
Second trimester: 5.5–6.8 kg (12–15 lb)	Excessive weight gain (excessive caloric intake, edema, preeclampsia)	Provide nutritional counseling. Assess for presence of edema or anemia.
Third trimester: 5.5–6.8 kg (12–15 lb)		
Edema		
Small amount of dependent edema, especially in last weeks of pregnancy	Edema in hands, face, legs, and feet (preeclampsia)	Identify any correlation between edema and activities, blood pressure, or proteinuria. Refer to physician if indicated.
Uterine Size		
See "Assessment Guide: Initial Prenatal Assessment" for normal changes during pregnancy	Unusually rapid growth (multiple gestation, hydatidiform mole, hydramnios, miscalculation of EDB)	Evaluate fetal status. Determine height of fundus (page 227). Use diagnostic ultrasound.
Fetal Heartbeat		
120–160/min Funic souffle	Absence of fetal heartbeat after 20 weeks' gestation (maternal obesity, fetal demise)	Evaluate fetal status.
Laboratory Evaluation		
Hemoglobin: 12–16 g/dL Pseudoanemia of pregnancy	< 11 g/dL (anemia)	Provide nutritional counseling. Hemoglobin is repeated at 7 months' gestation. Women of Mediterranean heritage need a close check on hemoglobin because of possibility of thalassemia.
Quad marker screen: Blood test performed at 15–20 weeks' gestation. Evaluates four factors—maternal serum alpha-fetoprotein (MSAFP), unconjugated estriol (UE), hCG, and inhibin-A: normal levels	Elevated MSAFP (neural tube defect, underestimated gestational age, multiple gestation). Lower than normal MSAFP (Down syndrome, trisomy 18). Higher than normal hCG and inhibin-A (Down syndrome). Lower than normal UE (Down syndrome).	Recommended for all pregnant women; especially indicated for women with any of the following risk factors: age 35 and over, family history of birth defects, previous child with a birth defect, insulin-dependent diabetes prior to pregnancy (Cleveland Clinic, 2005). If quad screen abnormal, further testing such as ultrasound or amniocentesis may be indicated.
	*Possible causes of alterations are identified in parentheses.	†This column provides guidelines for further assessment and initial nursing intervention.

ASSESSMENT GUIDE—continued

SUBSEQUENT PRENATAL ASSESSMENT

PHYSICAL ASSESSMENT/ NORMAL FINDINGS	ALTERATIONS AND POSSIBLE CAUSES*	NURSING RESPONSES TO DATA†
Laboratory Evaluation *(continued)*		
Triple screen—Screening test gradually being replaced by quad screen. Tests MSAFP, UE, and hCG but not inhibin-A	See quad screen.	Refer to physician. See quad screen.
Indirect Coombs test done on Rh negative women: Negative (done at 28 weeks' gestation)	Rh antibodies present (maternal sensitization has occurred)	If Rh negative and unsensitized, Rh immune globulin given (see page 362 in Chapter 15 ∞). If Rh antibodies present, Rh immune globulin not given; fetus monitored closely for isoimmune hemolytic disease. Discuss implications of GDM. Refer for a diagnostic 100 g oral glucose tolerance test.
50 g 1-hour glucose screen (done between 24 and 28 weeks' gestation)	Plasma glucose level > 140 mg/dL (gestational diabetes mellitus [GDM]) *Note:* Some facilities use level > 130 mg/dL, which identifies 90% of women with GDM (American Diabetes Association, 2000)	
Urinalysis: See "Assessment Guide: Initial Prenatal Assessment" for normal findings	See "Assessment Guide: Initial Prenatal Assessment" for deviations	Repeat urinalysis at 7 month's gestation. Repeat dipstick test at each visit.
Protein: Negative	Proteinuria, albuminuria (contamination by vaginal discharge, urinary tract infection, preeclampsia)	Obtain dipstick urine sample. Refer to physician if deviations are present.
Glucose: Negative	Persistent glycosuria (diabetes mellitus)	Refer to physician.
Note: Glycosuria may be present due to physiologic alterations in glomerular filtration rate and renal threshold		
Screening for Group B streptococcus (GBS): Rectal and vaginal swabs obtained at 35–37 weeks' gestation for all pregnant women (Centers for Disease Control and Prevention [CDC], 2002).	Positive culture (maternal infection)	Explain maternal and fetal/neonatal risks (see page 369 in Chapter 15 ∞). Refer to physician or CNM for therapy.

CULTURAL ASSESSMENT	VARIATIONS TO CONSIDER*	NURSING RESPONSES TO DATA†
Determine the mother's (and family's) attitudes about the sex of the unborn child.	Some women have no preference about the sex of the child; others do. In many cultures, boys are especially valued as firstborn children.	Provide opportunities to discuss preferences and expectations; avoid a judgmental attitude to the response.
Ask about the woman's expectations of childbirth. Will she want someone with her for the birth? Whom does she choose? What is the role of her partner?	Some women want their partner present for labor and birth; others prefer a female relative or friend. Some women expect to be separated from their partner once cervical dilation has occurred (Andrews & Boyle, 1998).	Provide information on birth options but accept the woman's decision about who will attend.
Ask about preparations for the baby. Determine what is customary for the woman.	Some women may have a fully prepared nursery; others may not have a separate room for the baby.	Explore reasons for not preparing for the baby. Support the mother's preferences and provide information about possible sources of assistance if the decision is related to a lack of resources.

*Possible causes of alterations are identified in parentheses.   †This column provides guidelines for further assessment and initial nursing intervention.

(continued)

ASSESSMENT GUIDE—continued

SUBSEQUENT PRENATAL ASSESSMENT

PSYCHOSOCIAL ASSESSMENT	VARIATIONS TO CONSIDER*	NURSING RESPONSES TO DATA†
Expectant Mother		
Psychologic status	Increased stress and anxiety	Encourage woman to take an active part in her care.
First trimester: Incorporates idea of pregnancy; may feel ambivalent, especially if she must give up desired role; usually looks for signs of verification of pregnancy, such as increase in abdominal size or fetal movement	Inability to establish communication; inability to accept pregnancy; inappropriate response or actions; denial of pregnancy; inability to cope	Establish lines of communication. Establish a trusting relationship. Counsel as necessary. Refer to appropriate prefessional as needed.
Second trimester: Baby becomes more real to woman as abdominal size increases and she feels movement; she begins to turn inward, becoming more introspective		
Third trimester: Begins to think of baby as separate being; may feel restless and may feel that time of labor will never come; remains self-centered and concentrates on preparing place for baby		
Educational needs		
Self-care measures and knowledge about the following:	Inadequate information	Provide information and counseling.
Health promotion		
Breast care		
Hygiene		
Rest		
Exercise		
Nutrition		
Relief measures for common discomforts of pregnancy		
Danger signs in pregnancy (See Key Facts to Remember on p. 217)		
Sexual activity: Woman knows how pregnancy affects sexual activity	Lack of information about effects of pregnancy and/or alternative positions during sexual intercourse	Provide counseling.
Preparation for parenting: Appropriate preparation	Lack of preparation (denial, failure to adjust to baby, unwanted child)	Counsel. If lack of preparation is due to inadequacy of information, provide information.
Preparation for childbirth **Client aware of the following:**		If couple chooses particular technique, refer to classes (see page 190 in Chapter 8 ∞ for description of childbirth preparation techniques). Encourage prenatal class attendance. Educate woman during visits based on current physical status. Provide reading list for more specific information.
1. Prepared childbirth techniques		
2. Normal processes and changes during childbirth		
3. Problems that may occur as a result of drug and alcohol use and of smoking	Continued abuse of drugs and alcohol; denial of possible effect on self and baby	Review danger signs that were presented on initial visit.
Woman has met other physician or nurse-midwife who may be attending her birth in the absence of primary caregiver	Introduction of new individual at birth may increase stress and anxiety for woman and partner	Introduce woman to all members of group practice.

*Possible causes of alterations are identified in parentheses.

†This column provides guidelines for further assessment and initial nursing intervention.

ASSESSMENT GUIDE—continued

SUBSEQUENT PRENATAL ASSESSMENT

PSYCHOSOCIAL ASSESSMENT	VARIATIONS TO CONSIDER*	NURSING RESPONSES TO DATA†
Expectant Father		
Impending labor **Client knows signs of impending labor:** 1. Uterine contractions that increase in frequency, duration, and intensity 2. Bloody show 3. Expulsion of mucous plug 4. Rupture of membranes	Lack of information	Provide appropriate teaching, stressing importance of seeking appropriate medical assistance.
Psychologic status **First trimester:** May express excitement over confirmation of pregnancy and of his virility; concerns move toward providing for financial needs; energetic, may identify with some discomforts of pregnancy and may even exhibit symptoms	Increasing stress and anxiety; inability to establish communication; inability to accept pregnancy diagnosis; withdrawal of support; abandonment of the mother	Encourage expectant father to come to prenatal visits. Establish lines of communication. Establish trusting relationship.
Second trimester: May feel more confident and be less concerned with financial matters; may have concerns about wife's changing size and shape, her increasing introspection		Counsel. Let expectant father know that it is normal for him to experience these feelings.
Third trimester: May have feelings of rivalry with fetus, especially during sexual activity; may make changes in his physical appearance and exhibit more interest in himself; may become more energetic; fantasizes about child but usually imagines older child; fears mutilation and death of woman and child		Include expectant father in pregnancy activities as he desires. Provide education, information, and support. Increasing numbers of expectant fathers are demonstrating desire to be involved in many or all aspects of prenatal care, education, and preparation.

*Possible causes of alterations are identified in parentheses.

†This column provides guidelines for further assessment and initial nursing intervention.

physical examinations the pregnant woman should undergo for optimal antepartal care and also provides a model for evaluating both the pregnant woman and the expectant father, if he is involved in the pregnancy.

NURSING PRACTICE

When assessing blood pressure, have the pregnant woman sit up with her arm resting on a table so that her arm is at the level of her heart. Expect a decrease in blood pressure from baseline during the second trimester because of typical physiologic changes. If the decrease does not occur, evaluate further for signs of preeclampsia.

The recommended frequency of antepartal visits in an uncomplicated pregnancy is as follows:

- Every 4 weeks for the first 28 weeks' gestation
- Every 2 weeks until 36 weeks' gestation
- After week 36, every week until childbirth

During the subsequent antepartal assessments, most women demonstrate ongoing psychologic adjustment to pregnancy. However, some women may exhibit signs of possible psychologic problems such as the following:

- Increasing anxiety
- Inability to establish communication
- Inappropriate responses or actions
- Denial of pregnancy
- Inability to cope with stress
- Intense preoccupation with the sex of the baby
- Failure to acknowledge quickening
- Failure to plan and prepare for the baby (e.g., living arrangements, clothing, and feeding methods)
- Indications of substance abuse

If the woman's behavior indicates possible psychologic problems, the nurse can provide ongoing support and counseling and also refer the woman to appropriate professionals.

Critical Concept Review

LEARNING OBJECTIVES	CONCEPTS
Summarize the essential components of a prenatal history.	A detailed prenatal history includes the following: ■ Details of current pregnancy (such as LMP). ■ History of past pregnancies. ■ Gynecologic history (such as last Pap and contraceptive use). ■ Current medical history (such as weight, prescription medications, chronic diseases). ■ Past medical history (past surgeries). ■ Family medical history (cancer or diabetes). ■ Religious, spiritual, and cultural history. ■ Occupational history (physical demands of present job). ■ Partner's history (genetic conditions, blood type). ■ Demographic information about woman (age, educational level, and ethnic background).
Define common obstetric terminology found in the history of maternity clients.	■ Terms about the number of pregnancies and births: gravida, parity, and TPAL. ■ Terms that denote the phase of pregnancy: ante-, intra-, and postpartum. ■ Terms that denote age and developmental status of fetus at birth: prematurity, postmaturity, and term (see page 214).
Identify factors related to the father's health that are generally recorded on the prenatal record.	Father's health details to be recorded: ■ History of chronic illness in father or immediate family member. ■ Blood type and Rh factor. ■ Present use of alcohol, tobacco, or recreational drugs. ■ Occupation. ■ Age.
Describe areas that should be evaluated as part of the initial assessment of psychosocial and cultural factors related to a woman's pregnancy.	■ Language preference. ■ Determine how woman should be addressed. ■ Determine food customs and preferences. ■ Determine significant people to woman, and degree of involvement of these persons. ■ Psychologic status. ■ Educational needs. ■ Support system. ■ Family functioning. ■ Economic status. ■ Stability of living conditions.
Describe the normal physiologic changes one would expect to find when performing a physical assessment of a pregnant woman.	Vital signs: ■ Pulse may increase by 10 beats/min. ■ Respiration may be increased, and thoracic breathing predominant. ■ Temperature and blood pressure within normal limits. Weight: ■ Varies, but should be proportional to the gestational age of the fetus. Skin: ■ Linea nigra. ■ Striae gravidarum. ■ Melasma. ■ Spider nevi. Nose: ■ Nasal stuffiness. Mouth: ■ Gingival hypertrophy.

LEARNING OBJECTIVES   ## CONCEPTS

Neck:
- Small, nontender nodes.
- Slight hyperplasia of thyroid in third trimester.

Chest and lungs:
- Transverse diameter greater than anteroposterior diameter.

Breasts:
- Increasing size.
- Pigmentation of nipples and areolae.
- Tubercles of Montgomery enlarge.
- Colostrum appears in third trimester.

Abdomen:
- Progressive enlargement by Doppler.
- Fetal heart rate heard by Doppler at approximately 12 weeks' gestation.

Extremities:
- Possible edema late in pregnancy.

Spine:
- Lumbar spinal curve may be accentuated.

Pelvic area:
- Vagina without significant discharge.
- Cervix closed.
- Uterus shows progressive growth.

Laboratory tests:
- Physiologic anemia may occur (hematocrit).
- Small degree of glycosuria may occur.

Compare the methods most commonly used to determine the estimated date of birth.

Nägele's rule:
- Date of LMP minus 3 months plus 7 days.
- Accurate only if woman has 28-day cycles.

Physical examination:
- Uterine size.

Fundal height:
- Measurement should be made from the top of the symphysis pubis to the top of the uterine fundus.

Ultrasound:
- BPD.

Develop an outline of the essential measurements that can be determined by clinical pelvimetry.

These measurements are estimates to determine probable adequacy of the pelvis to allow a vaginal birth:
- Pelvic inlet:
  - Diagonal conjugate (should be at least 11.5 cm).
  - Obstetric conjugate (should be 10 cm or more).
- Pelvic outlet:
  - Anteroposterior diameter (should be 9.5 to 11.5 cm).
  - Transverse diameter (should be 8 to 10 cm).

Delineate the possible causes of abnormal findings during the initial or subsequent prenatal examination.

Vital signs:
- Elevations may be due to infection.
- Blood pressure elevation may be due to preeclampsia.

Weight:
- Less than expected weight gain may be due to inadequate nutrition.
- More than expected weight gain may be due to preeclampsia.

Skin:
- Pallor due to anemia.
- Edema due to decreased venous return or preeclampsia.
- Petechiae or bruises may be due to bleeding disorders or physical abuse.

Nose and mouth:
- Pale mucous membrane may be due to anemia.
- Inflamed gingival tissue.

(continued)

LEARNING OBJECTIVES

CONCEPTS

Delineate the possible causes of abnormal findings during the initial or subsequent prenatal examination.—*continued*	**Neck:** ■ Tender, hard, fixed nodes may be due to infection or cancer. ■ Enlarged thyroid may be due to hyperthyroidism. **Chest and lungs:** ■ Abnormal lung sounds may be due to infection or asthma. ■ Increased respiration may be due to pleural effusion or collapsed lung.
Delineate the possible causes of abnormal findings during the initial or subsequent prenatal examination (*continued*)	**Breasts:** ■ Hard nodes may be due to cancer. ■ Nipple discharge may be due to cancer or infection. ■ Redness, tenderness may be due to infection. **Heart:** ■ Abnormal rhythm, extra sounds may be due to normal changes of pregnancy but also may indicate cardiac disease. **Abdomen:** ■ Tenderness, mass, or guarding may indicate ectopic pregnancy, cancer, infection, or obstruction. ■ Failure to hear fetal heart tones may be due to death of fetus or hydatidiform mole. **Extremities:** ■ Edema may be due to preeclampsia. ■ Lack of pulses may be due to arterial insufficiency. **Spine:** ■ Abnormal spinal curves may be due to scoliosis or normal changes of expanding abdomen. **Reflexes:** ■ Hyperactivity may be due to preeclampsia. **Pelvic area:** ■ Lesions of the external genitalia may be due to sexually transmitted disease. ■ Varicose veins may be due to poor venous return. ■ Vaginal discharge may indicate infection. ■ Lesions of the cervix may be due to erosion, polyp, or human papillomavirus. **Pelvic measurements:** ■ Measurements below normal may indicate an inability to have a vaginal birth. **Rectum and anus:** ■ Hemorrhoids may be due to poor venous return. **Laboratory tests:** ■ Low hemoglobin and hematocrit may indicate anemia. ■ High white count may indicate infection. ■ Positive tests for sexually transmitted disease may indicate presence of these diseases. ■ Urine with elevated white cells may indicate infection. ■ Urine with presence of glucose may indicate gestational diabetes. ■ Elevated blood glucose may indicate gestational diabetes. ■ Tests may indicate the presence of hepatitis B or human immunodeficiency virus (HIV).
Relate the components of the subsequent prenatal history and assessment to the progress of pregnancy.	At each visit the woman will be assessed for: ■ Vital signs. ■ Weight gain. ■ Edema. ■ Uterine size. ■ Fetal heartbeat. ■ Urinalysis. ■ Blood tests for alpha, fetoprotein, glucose. ■ Vaginal swab for group B streptococcus. ■ Expected psychologic stage of pregnancy.

CRITICAL THINKING IN ACTION

*View the **Critical Thinking in Action** video in Chapter 10 of the CD-ROM. Then, answer the questions that follow.*

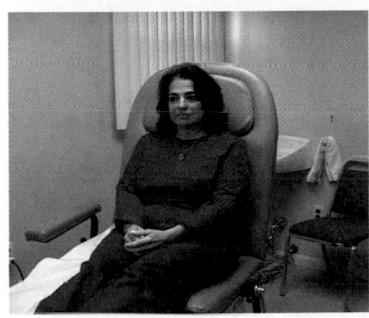

Wendy Stodard, age 40, G3, P0020 comes to the obstetrician's office where you are working for a prenatal visit. Wendy has experienced two spontaneous abortions followed by a D & C at 14 and 15 weeks' gestation during the previous year. She has a history of *Chlamydia trachomatis* infection 3 years ago, which was treated with azithromycin. She is at 10 weeks' gestation. Wendy tells you that she is afraid of losing this pregnancy as she did previously. She says that she has been experiencing some mild nausea, breast tenderness, and fatigue, which did not occur with her other pregnancies. You assist the obstetrician with an ultrasound. The gestational sac is clearly seen, fetal heartbeat is observed, and crown-to-rump measurements are consistent with gestational age of 10 weeks. The pelvic exam demonstrates a closed cervix, and positive Goodell's, Hegar's, and Chadwick's signs. You discuss with Wendy the signs of a healthy pregnancy.

1. What signs are reassuring with this pregnancy?
2. What symptoms should be reported to the obstetrician immediately?
3. What is the frequency of antepartal visits?

MEDIALINK   www.prenhall.com/london

- NCLEX-RN® Review, case studies, and other interactive resources for this chapter can be found on the Companion Website at http://www.prenhall.com/london. Click on "Chapter 10" to select the activities for this chapter.

Care Plan
A 40-year-old businesswoman has entered the birthing center where you work. She is a primigravida arriving at the center for her initial history and physical. The pregnancy is the result of artificial insemination, and at this time the father is not included in the expected pregnancy process. Develop a plan of care to include the teaching aspects for use with this individual. Fill in the appropriate elements of the Care Plan for the client in the boxes below.

This activity contains 3 questions.

1. **Assessment and Diagnosis**

To create paragraphs in your essay response, type <p> at the beginning of the paragraph, and </p> at the end.

- For animations, more NCLEX-RN® Review questions, and an audio glossary, access the accompanying CD-ROM in this textbook.

REFERENCES

American College of Obstetricians and Gynecologists. (2000). *Planning your pregnancy and birth* (3rd ed.). Washington, DC: Author.

American Diabetes Association. (2000). Position statement: Gestational diabetes mellitus. *Diabetes Care, 23*(Suppl. 1), 1–6.

Andrews, M. M., & Boyle, J. S. (1998). *Transcultural concepts in nursing care* (2nd ed.). Glenview, IL: Scott, Foresman/Little, Brown.

Centers for Disease Control and Prevention. (2002). Prevention of perinatal group B streptococcal disease: Revised guidelines from CDC. *MMWR Recommendations and Reports, 51*(RR-11), 1–22.

Cleveland Clinic. (2005). Quad screen, Retrieved September 2, 2005 from www.cchs.net/health/health-info/docs/0300/0386.asp? index-4695

Cunningham, F. G., Leveno, K. J., Bloom, S. L., Hauth, J. C., Gilstrap, L. C., III, &

Wenstrom, K. D. (2005). *Williams obstetrics* (22nd ed.). New York: McGraw-Hill.

Jontaine, K. L. (2005). *Healing practices: alternative therapies for nursery* (2nd ed.). Upper Saddle River, NJ: Prentice Hall.

Varney, H., Kriebs, J. M., & Gegor, C. L. (2004). *Varney's midwifery* (4th ed.). Sudbury, MA: Jones & Bartlett.

The Expectant Family: Needs and Care

We have what I guess you would call a blended family. I have two college-age sons from my first marriage, and my wife has a 12-year-old boy. She is expecting our first child now. Because she is 38, she had an amniocentesis done and we know that this baby is a girl. How excited we all are! I don't think anything could have done more to unite us as a new family. Now if we can just agree on a name.

—Ricardo, 46

LEARNING OBJECTIVES

- Describe actions that the nurse can take to help maintain the well-being of the expectant father and siblings during a family's pregnancy.

- Explain the causes of the common discomforts of pregnancy.

- Identify appropriate relief measures for the common discomforts of pregnancy.

- Discuss the basic information that a nurse should provide to the expectant family to enable them to carry out appropriate self-care.

- Delineate some of the concerns that an expectant couple might have about sexual activity.

- Summarize the medical risks and special concerns of the older expectant woman and her partner.

MEDIALINK   www.prenhall.com/london

CD-ROM

Audio Glossary
NCLEX-RN® Review

Companion Website

Additional NCLEX-RN® Review
Case Study: First Trimester Client
Thinking Critically

From the moment a woman finds out she is pregnant, she faces a future marked by dramatic changes—changes in her appearance, in her relationships, and in her psychologic state. In coping with these changes, she and her loved ones need to make adjustments in their daily lives.

Nurses caring for pregnant women need an up-to-date understanding of pregnancy to be effective in implementing the nursing process as they plan and provide care. With this in mind, Chapter 9 provided a database for the nurse by presenting material related to the normal physical, social, cultural, and psychologic changes of pregnancy. Chapter 10 then used that database to begin discussing nursing care management by focusing on assessment. This chapter further addresses nursing care management as it relates to the needs of the expectant woman and her loved ones.

NURSING CARE DURING THE PRENATAL PERIOD

NURSING DIAGNOSIS DURING PREGNANCY

The nurse may see a pregnant woman only once every 3 to 4 weeks during the first several months of her pregnancy. Therefore, a written care plan or clinical path that incorporates the database, nursing diagnoses, and client goals is essential to ensure continuity of care.

The nurse can anticipate that, for many women with a low-risk pregnancy, certain nursing diagnoses will be made more frequently than others. The diagnoses will, of course, vary from woman to woman and according to the time in the pregnancy. After formulating an appropriate diagnosis, the nurse and woman establish related goals to guide the nursing plan and interventions.

PLANNING AND IMPLEMENTATION DURING PREGNANCY

Once nursing diagnoses have been identified, the next step is to establish priorities of nursing care. Sometimes priorities of care are based on the most immediate needs or concerns expressed by the woman. For example, during the first trimester, when she is experiencing nausea or is concerned about sexual intimacy with her partner, the woman is not likely to want to hear about labor and birth. At other times, priorities may develop from findings during a prenatal examination. For example, a woman who is showing signs of preeclampsia (a pregnancy complication discussed in Chapter 15 ∞) may feel physically well and find it hard to accept the nurse's emphasis on the need for frequent rest periods. It then becomes the responsibility of medical and nursing professionals to help the woman and her family to understand the significance of a problem and to plan interventions to deal with it.

Nursing Care in the Community

Prenatal care, especially for women with low-risk pregnancies, is community based, typically in a clinic or a private office. The healthcare community recognizes the value of providing a primary care nurse in these settings to coordinate holistic care for each childbearing family. The nurse in a clinic or health maintenance organization may be the only source of continuity for the woman, who may see a different physician or certified nurse-midwife at each visit. The nurse can be extremely effective in working with the expectant family by answering questions; providing complete information about pregnancy, prenatal healthcare activities, and community resources; and supporting the healthcare activities of the woman and her family. Communities often have a wealth of services and educational opportunities available for pregnant women and their families, and the knowledgeable nurse can help expectant mothers to assess and access these services.

Throughout the prenatal period, the nurse shares information with the family, both verbally and through written materials. The nurse also provides anticipatory guidance to help the family plan for changes that will occur after childbirth. The nurse encourages the expectant couple to identify and discuss issues that could be sources of postpartum stress. Issues to be addressed beforehand may include the sharing of infant and household chores, help in the first few days after childbirth, options for babysitting to allow the mother (and couple) some free time, the mother's return to work after the baby's birth, and sibling rivalry. Couples resolve these issues in different ways, but postpartum adjustment tends to be easier for couples who address the issues than for couples who do not confront and resolve them.

Home Care. Home care can be of benefit to any pregnant woman, but it is especially effective in removing barriers for women who have difficulty accessing healthcare. These barriers may include lack of locally available healthcare facilities, problems with transportation to the facility, or schedule conflicts with available appointment times because of employment hours or family responsibilities.

In-home nursing assessments vary according to the experience and preparation of the nurse and include current history, vital signs, weight, urine screen, physical activity, dietary intake, reflexes, tests of fetal well-being, and cervical examinations, if indicated. Once the assessments are completed, the nurse can determine the level of follow-up home care or telephone contact needed. See Chapter 31 ∞ for further discussion of home care of the childbearing family.

Currently, home care is most often used for women with prenatal complications that can be managed without hospitalization if effective nursing assessment and care are provided in the home.

CARE OF THE EXPECTANT FATHER AND SIBLINGS

The well-being of the pregnant woman is intertwined with the well-being of those to whom she is closest. Thus, the nurse also addresses the needs of the woman's family. Although the expectant father is often involved in the pregnancy, his presence cannot be assumed. If he is not part of the family structure, it is important to assess the woman's support system to determine which significant people in her life will play a major role during this childbearing experience.

Anticipatory guidance of the expectant father, if he is involved in the pregnancy, is a necessary part of any plan of care. He may need information about the anatomic, phys-

iologic, and emotional changes that occur for the expectant mother and father during and after pregnancy; the couple's sexuality and sexual response; and the reactions that he is experiencing. He may wish to express his feelings about the sex of the child, his ability to parent, and other topics.

If it is culturally acceptable to the couple and personally acceptable to the expectant father, refer the couple to expectant parents' classes. These classes provide valuable information about pregnancy and childbirth, using a variety of teaching strategies such as discussion, films, demonstrations with educational models, and written handouts. Some classes even give the father the opportunity to get a "feel" for pregnancy by wearing a pregnancy simulator (Figure 11–1 ◉). Such classes also offer the couple an opportunity to gain support from other couples.

The nurse assesses the father's intended degree of participation during labor and birth and his knowledge of what to expect. If the couple prefers that his participation be minimal or restricted, support their decision. With this type of consideration and collaboration, the father is less apt to develop feelings of alienation, helplessness, and guilt during the pregnancy. As the couple's relationship is strengthened and the father's self-esteem is raised, he is better able to provide physical and emotional support to his partner during labor and birth.

In the plan for prenatal care, the nurse also incorporates a discussion about the negative feelings older children may develop. Parents may be distressed to see an older child regress to "babyish" behavior or become aggressive toward the newborn. Parents who are unprepared for the

◉ **FIGURE 11–1**

The Empathy Belly® is a pregnancy simulator that allows men and women to experience some of the symptoms of pregnancy. The "belly," which weighs 33 lb, produces symptoms such as shortness of breath, bladder pressure, shift in the center of gravity with resulting waddling gait, increased lordosis and backache, and fatigue. It also can simulate fetal kicking movements.
Used with permission from Birthways Childbirth Resource Center.

older child's feelings of anger, jealousy, and rejection may respond inappropriately in their confusion and surprise. The nurse emphasizes that open communication between parents and children (or acting out feelings with a doll if the child is too young to verbalize) helps children master their feelings. Children may feel less neglected and more secure if they know that their parents are willing to help with their anger and aggressiveness.

The nurse also addresses the couple's expectations of the grandparents and encourages the couple to explore ways of dealing with any conflicts that may arise over child-rearing approaches. Couples resolve these issues in different ways. However, postpartum adjustment is easiest for couples who acknowledge potential problems and develop strategies to address them beforehand.

CULTURAL CONSIDERATIONS IN PREGNANCY

As discussed in Chapter 2, actions during pregnancy are often determined by cultural beliefs. Table 11–1 presents

---

TABLE 11–1 ✤ Cultural Beliefs and Practices During Pregnancy

Here are a few examples of cultural beliefs and practices related to pregnancy. It is important not to make assumptions about a client's beliefs, because cultural norms vary greatly within a culture and from generation to generation. The nurse should observe the client carefully and take the time to ask questions. Clients will benefit greatly from the nurse's increased awareness of their cultural beliefs and practices.

Belief or Practice	Nursing Consideration
Home Remedies Pregnant women of Native American background may use herbal remedies. An example is the dandelion, which contains a milky juice in its stem believed to increase breast milk flow in mothers who choose to breastfeed (Spector, 2004). Clients of Chinese descent may drink ginseng tea for faintness after childbirth or as a sedative when mixed with bamboo leaves. Some people of African heritage may use self medication for pregnancy discomforts—for example, laxatives to prevent or treat constipation (Spector, 2004).	Find out what medications and home remedies your client is using and counsel your client regarding overall effects. It is common for individuals to avoid telling healthcare workers about home remedies; the client may feel her use of home remedies will be judged unfavorably. Phrase your questions in a sensitive, accepting way.
Nutrition Some women of Italian background may believe that it is necessary to satisfy desires for certain foods in order to prevent congenital anomalies. Also, they may believe that they must eat food that they smell, or else the fetus will move "inside," which will result in a miscarriage. Pregnant women of African descent may continue the tradition of eating clay, dirt, or starch, which they believe will benefit the mother and fetus (Spector, 2004). To practice *Tae Kyo,* a set of rules for safe childbirth, pregnant women of Korean descent may practice food taboos by eating particular high-quality foods and avoiding other foods believed to cause an unhealthy fetus (Choi, 1995).	Discuss the woman's beliefs and practices in regard to nutrition during pregnancy. Obtain a diet history from her. Discuss the importance of a well-balanced diet during pregnancy, with consideration of the client's cultural beliefs and practices. In some cases, you might want to suggest remedies that may be more effective—for example, eating high-fiber foods to reduce constipation. If the home remedy is not harmful, there is no reason to ask a client to discontinue this practice.
Alternative Healthcare Providers Pregnant women of Mexican background may choose to seek out the care of a *partera* (midwife) for prenatal and intrapartal care. A *partera* speaks their language, shares a similar culture, and can help pregnant women give birth at home or in a birthing center instead of a hospital. Some people in Hispanic-American communities may use the *curandero,* the folk healer. The *curandero* frequently uses herbs, massage, and religious artifacts for treatment (Spector, 2004).	Discuss the variety of choices of healthcare providers available to the pregnant woman. Contrast the benefits and risks of different settings for prenatal care and birth. Provide reassurance that the goal of healthcare during pregnancy and birth is a healthy outcome for mother and baby, with respect for the specific cultural beliefs and practices of the client.
Exercise Pregnant women of Italian descent may fear changing their body position in certain ways because they believe doing so may cause the fetus to develop abnormally (Spector, 2004). Some people of European, African, and Mexican descent believe that reaching over the head during pregnancy can harm the baby.	Ask your client whether there are any activities she is afraid to do because of the pregnancy. Assure her that reaching over her head will not harm the baby and evaluate other activities related to their effect on the pregnancy.
Spirituality Native Americans of the Navajo tribe may meet with the medicine man 2 months prior to birth, feeling that the prayers will ensure a safe birth and healthy baby. Some people of European background may tend to pay more attention to spirituality in their life to alleviate fears and ensure a safe birth.	Encourage the use of support systems and spiritual aids that provide comfort for the mother.

activities encouraged or forbidden by some specific cultures. The table is not meant to be all-inclusive, nor is it meant to imply that all members of a given culture hold these beliefs. Rather it offers a few examples of cultural activities that may be important to some women during the prenatal period.

In working with clients of other cultures, health professionals should be open to and respectful of other beliefs. Culturally competent nurses recognize that each childbearing family, shaped by culture and life experience, has expectations of both its members and the healthcare system during pregnancy and birth.

Language barriers often pose a challenge in providing effective prenatal nursing care. When possible, it is important to have an interpreter—family member, friend, or staff person—present at prenatal visits so that the nurse can provide basic information about pregnancy and prenatal care. The nurse should also give the woman opportunities to ask questions or express concerns. It is essential to have printed material available in the woman's language. See "Nursing Care Plan: Language Barriers at First Prenatal Visit."

DEVELOPING CULTURAL COMPETENCE

NATIVE AMERICAN CULTURES

In caring for pregnant women of Native American descent, it is helpful to consider the following general points (Cesario, 2001):

- Because there are more than 500 federally recognized tribes in the United States, it is difficult to summarize common cultural characteristics of Native Americans.
- Many Native American tribes are matrilineal. Women are respected and heeded in decision making, and the children belong to the clan of their mother.
- Three-generation extended families are common, and the grandparents, aunts, and uncles often assume primary responsibility for discipline and education of the children. Thus, it is important to learn whether a new mother will be the primary caregiver for her infant.
- Many tribes are "present oriented," viewing events such as childbearing as part of the rhythms of life. Thus, during pregnancy a Native American woman is often focused on the pregnancy itself and not on issues that will follow such as contraception or childrearing practices. This has implications for the focus of the teaching a nurse offers.

COMMON DISCOMFORTS OF PREGNANCY

The common discomforts of pregnancy result from physiologic and anatomic changes and are fairly specific to each of the three trimesters. Table 11–2 identifies the common discomforts of pregnancy, their possible causes, and self-care measures that often help relieve the discomfort.

NURSING PRACTICE

At each prenatal visit, focus your teaching on changes or possible discomforts the woman might encounter during the coming month and the next trimester. If the pregnancy is progressing normally, spend a few minutes describing her baby at this stage of development.

FIRST TRIMESTER

Nausea and Vomiting

Nausea and vomiting of pregnancy (NVP) are early, common symptoms occurring in 70% to 85% of pregnant women (American College of Obstetricians and Gynecologists [ACOG], 2004). These symptoms appear sometime after the first missed menstrual period and usually cease by the fourth missed menstrual period. Some women develop an aversion to specific foods, many experience nausea when they get up in the morning, and others experience nausea throughout the day or in the evening.

The exact cause of NVP is unknown, but it is thought to be multifactorial. An elevated human chorionic gonadotropin (hCG) level is believed to be a major factor, but changes in carbohydrate metabolism, fatigue, and emotional factors may also play a role.

In addition to common self-care measures (see "Complementary Care: Ginger and Acupressure for Morning Sickness") and the use of acupressure wristbands (Figure 11–2 ●), some women find pyridoxine (vitamin B_6) or pyridoxine plus doxylamine (Unisom), an over-the-counter antihistamine, helpful in reducing symptoms. Antihistamine H_1 receptor blockers, benzamines, and phenothiazines are considered safe and effective for treating refractory cases. In severe cases, methylprednisolone, a steroid, may be used, but as a last resort, because it poses a potential risk to the fetus (ACOG, 2004).

The nurse should advise a woman to contact her healthcare provider if she vomits more than once a day or shows signs of dehydration such as dry mouth and concentrated urine. In such cases the physician or certified nurse-midwife might order an antiemetic. However, antiemetics should be avoided if possible during this time because of possible harmful effects on embryo development.

Urinary Frequency

Urinary frequency, a common discomfort of pregnancy, occurs early in pregnancy and again during the third trimester because the enlarging uterus puts pressure on the bladder. Although frequency is considered normal during the first and third trimesters, advise the woman to tell her healthcare provider about signs of bladder infection such as pain, burning with voiding, or blood in the urine. Fluid

NURSING CARE PLAN

LANGUAGE BARRIERS AT FIRST PRENATAL VISIT

Intervention	Rationale	Expected Outcome

1. Nursing Diagnosis: Ineffective Health Maintenance related to alteration in verbal and written communication skills.

Intervention	Rationale	Expected Outcome
NIC Intervention: Effective communication: Developing and providing prenatal instruction for a non-English-speaking client.		**NOC Outcome:** Effective communication occurs. The client will gain an understanding of basic prenatal information as evidenced by using hand gestures, by pointing to pictures on posters and translated phrases on handouts, and through an interpreter, if one is available.

Goal: Client will demonstrate understanding of health information received during prenatal visits.

Intervention	Rationale	Expected Outcome
■ If no interpreter is available, refer to posters with pictures to explain routine care and procedures during the prenatal examination. ■ Provide handouts and brochures about prenatal care in the woman's native language.	■ Posters put words into verbal images and are helpful in communicating information. ■ Translated handouts provide information that the client can refer to at home. This reinforces information discussed during the visit and helps the family understand what the woman will experience during the pregnancy and at each visit.	
■ Use teaching models to demonstrate procedures. Teaching models may include plastic pelvis, knitted uterus, fetal model, breast model, birth control devices, ultrasound equipment, and so forth. ■ Schedule an interpreter for subsequent prenatal visits.	■ Visual aids help to communicate information during the examination. ■ If a family member cannot translate the health information to the client, an independent translator is essential to ensure that information is accurately provided. When an interpreter is used (especially a family member), the nurse should be sure that the interpreter is translating information received from the woman and not simply answering the questions for her.	
■ Refer the woman to prenatal classes taught in her own language, if available. ■ Involve other members of the healthcare team in planning and providing care.	■ Prenatal classes taught in the woman's language enable her to receive health information that is easily understood, which will provide a better understanding of what she should expect during pregnancy, birth, and postpartum. Prenatal classes may also provide a social outlet for clients. ■ Cultures vary in language, nonverbal expression, dietary habits, use of time, spatial expectations, and so forth. Use of medication and blood products may also be influenced by cultural beliefs. Social workers who are familiar with the client's cultural beliefs, for example, may help the client adjust to different healthcare practices while providing suggestions to ensure prenatal care that is more in line with the woman's cultural beliefs. Dietitians may help the woman plan meals that are aligned with her cultural practices while meeting the nutritional needs of pregnancy.	

TABLE 11–2 ✛ **Self-Care Measures for Common Discomforts of Pregnancy**

Discomfort	Influencing Factors	Self-Care Measures
First Trimester		
Nausea and vomiting	Increased levels of human chorionic gonadotropin Changes in carbohydrate metabolism Emotional factors Fatigue	Avoid odors or causative factors. Eat dry crackers or toast before arising in morning. Have small but frequent meals. Avoid greasy or highly seasoned foods. Take dry meals with fluids between meals. Drink carbonated beverages.
Urinary frequency	Pressure of uterus on bladder in both first and third trimesters	Void when urge is felt. Increase fluid intake during the day. Decrease fluid intake only in the evening to decrease nocturia.
Fatigue	Specific causative factors unknown May be aggravated by nocturia due to urinary frequency	Plan time for a nap or rest period daily. Go to bed earlier. Seek family support and assistance with responsibilities so that more time is available to rest.
Breast tenderness	Increased levels of estrogen and progesterone	Wear well-fitting, supportive bra.
Increased vaginal discharge	Hyperplasia of vaginal mucosa and increased production of mucus by the endocervical glands due to the increase in estrogen levels	Promote cleanliness by daily bathing. Avoid douching, nylon underpants, and pantynose; cotton underpants are more absorbent; powder can be used to maintain dryness if not allowed to cake.
Nasal stuffiness and nosebleed (epistaxis)	Elevated estrogen levels	May be unresponsive, but cool air vaporizer may help; avoid use of nasal sprays and decongestants.
Ptyalism (excessive, often bitter salivation)	Specific causative factors unknown	Use astringent mouthwashes, chew gum, or suck hard candy.
Second and Third Trimesters		
Heartburn (pyrosis)	Increased production of progesterone, decreasing gastrointestinal motility and increasing relaxation of cardiac sphincter, displacement of stomach by enlarging uterus, thus regurgitation of acidic gastric contents into the esophagus	Eat small and more frequent meals. Use low-sodium antacids. Avoid overeating, fatty and fried foods, lying down after eating, and sodium bicarbonate.
Ankle edema	Prolonged standing or sitting Increased levels of sodium due to hormonal influences Circulatory congestion of lower extremities Increased capillary permeability Varicose veins	Practice frequent dorsiflexion of feet when prolonged sitting or standing is necessary. Elevate legs when sitting or resting. Avoid tight garters or restrictive bands around legs.
Varicose veins	Venous congestion in the lower veins that increases with pregnancy Hereditary factors (weakening of walls of veins, faulty valves) Increased age and weight gain	Elevate legs frequently. Wear supportive hose. Avoid crossing legs at the knees, standing for long periods, garters, and hosiery with constrictive bands.

TABLE 11–2 ❖ Self-Care Measures for Common Discomforts of Pregnancy—continued

Discomfort	Influencing Factors	Self-Care Measures
Second and Third Trimesters		
Hemorrhoids	Constipation (see following discussion) Increased pressure from gravid uterus on hemorrhoidal veins	Avoid constipation. Apply ice packs, topical ointments, anesthetic agents, warm soaks, or sitz baths; gently reinsert into rectum as necessary.
Constipation	Increased levels of progesterone, which cause general bowel sluggishness Pressure of enlarging uterus on intestine Iron supplements Diet, lack of exercise, and decreased fluids	Increase fluid intake, fiber in the diet, and exercise. Develop regular bowel habits. Use stool softeners as recommended by physician.
Backache	Increased curvature of the lumbosacral vertebrae as the uterus enlarges Increased levels of hormones, which cause softening of cartilage in body joints Fatigue Poor body mechanics	Use proper body mechanics. Practice the pelvic-tilt exercise. Avoid uncomfortable working heights, high-heeled shoes, lifting heavy loads, and fatigue.
Leg cramps	Imbalance of calcium/phosphorus ratio Increased pressure of uterus on nerves Fatigue Poor circulation to lower extremities Pointing the toes	Practice dorsiflexion of feet to stretch affected muscle. Evaluate diet. Apply heat to affected muscles. Arise slowly from resting position.
Faintness	Postural hypotension Sudden change of position causing venous pooling in dependent veins Standing for long periods in warm area Anemia	Avoid prolonged standing in warm or stuffy environments. Evaluate hematocrit and hemoglobin.
Dyspnea	Decreased vital capacity from pressure of enlarging uterus on the diaphragm	Use proper posture when sitting and standing. Sleep propped up with pillows for relief if problem occurs at night.
Flatulence	Decreased gastrointestinal motility leading to delayed emptying time Pressure of growing uterus on large intestine Air swallowing	Avoid gas-forming foods. Chew food thoroughly. Get regular daily exercise. Maintain normal bowel habits.
Carpal tunnel syndrome	Compression of median nerve in carpal tunnel of wrist Aggravated by repetitive hand movements	Avoid aggravating hand movements. Use splint as prescribed. Elevate affected arm.

intake should never be decreased to prevent frequency. The woman needs to maintain an adequate fluid intake—at least 2000 mL (eight to ten 8-oz glasses) per day. Also, encourage her to empty her bladder frequently (about every 2 hours while awake).

Fatigue

Marked fatigue is so common in early pregnancy that it is considered a presumptive sign of pregnancy. It is aggra-vated if the woman cannot sleep through the night because of urinary frequency. Typically it resolves after the end of the first trimester.

Breast Tenderness

Sensitivity of the breasts occurs early and continues throughout the pregnancy. Increased levels of estrogen and progesterone contribute to soreness and tingling of the breasts and increased sensitivity of the nipples.

FIGURE 11–2

Acupressure wristbands are sometimes used to help relieve nausea during early pregnancy.

COMPLEMENTARY CARE

GINGER AND ACUPRESSURE FOR MORNING SICKNESS

Ginger and acupressure are among the most frequently used alternative therapies for the nausea and vomiting of morning sickness.

Ginger

Ginger is widely used in traditional Chinese medicine but without contraindications in pregnancy (Blumenthal, 2003). Many clinical trials have confirmed the effectiveness and safety of ginger (Blumenthal, 2003; Keating & Chez, 2002; Portnoi et al., 2004; Smith et al., 2004). As with any substance ingested during pregnancy, ginger should be used with caution; in most of the safety trials, the dosage did not exceed 1 g of dried root daily.

Ginger has the potential to interact with anticoagulants and antihypertensives, so women on either of these medications should avoid ginger (Tiran, 2003). Ginger is available in many forms, including capsules, candied, syrup, or as a tea.

Acupressure

Acupressure, like acupuncture, is a therapy based on the ancient philosophy of traditional Chinese medicine. Acupressure involves the application of pressure using fingers or thumbs to stimulate and balance the body's healing energy, known by the Chinese as *chi*. A specific acupressure point that relieves nausea is located on the forearm, three finger-widths above the wrist closest to the palm, toward the elbow. The point is pressed firmly for 30 seconds every couple of minutes. A motion sickness wristband (brand names include Sea-Band and Acuband) can be purchased that puts gentle pressure on this acupressure point (Roscoe & Matteson, 2002; Steele, French, Gatherer-Boyles, Newman, & Leclaire, 2001).

Increased Vaginal Discharge

Increased whitish vaginal discharge, called **leukorrhea**, is common in pregnancy. It occurs as a result of hyperplasia of the vaginal mucosa and increased mucus production by the endocervical glands. The increased acidity of the secretions encourages the growth of *Candida albicans*, so the woman is more susceptible to monilial vaginitis.

Nasal Stuffiness and Epistaxis

Once pregnancy has progressed somewhat, elevated estrogen levels may produce edema of the nasal mucosa, which results in nasal stuffiness, nasal discharge, and obstruction. *Epistaxis* (nosebleeds) may also result. Cool air vaporizers and normal saline nasal sprays may help, but the problem is often unresponsive to treatment. Women experiencing these problems find it difficult to sleep and may resort to using medicated nasal sprays and decongestants. Such interventions may provide initial relief but can actually increase nasal stuffiness over time. Pregnant women should avoid using any medications, if possible.

Ptyalism

Ptyalism is a rare discomfort of pregnancy in which excessive, often bitter saliva is produced. The cause is unknown, and effective treatments are limited.

SECOND AND THIRD TRIMESTERS

The discomforts discussed in this section usually do not appear until the third trimester in primigravidas but may occur earlier with each succeeding pregnancy.

Heartburn (Pyrosis)

Heartburn is the regurgitation of acidic gastric contents into the esophagus. It creates a burning sensation in the esophagus and sometimes leaves a bad taste in the mouth. Heartburn during pregnancy appears to be primarily a result of the displacement of the stomach by the enlarging uterus. The increased production of progesterone in pregnancy, decreased gastrointestinal motility, and relaxation of the cardiac (esophageal) sphincter also contribute to heartburn.

Liquid forms of low-sodium antacids are often most effective in providing relief. However, many women prefer chewable antacids such as TUMS. The nurse should advise women that antacids containing aluminum may cause constipation, and antacids containing magnesium can cause diarrhea. The nurse should also let women know that they should avoid sodium bicarbonate (baking soda) and Alka-Seltzer because they may lead to electrolyte imbalance.

If maternal heartburn is severe, not relieved by antacids, and accompanied by gastrointestinal reflux, an antisecretory agent (H₂ blocker) such as ranitidine (Zantac), cimetidine (Tagamet), or omeprazole (Losec) may be

○ **FIGURE 11-3**

Swelling and discomfort from varicosities can be decreased by lying down with the legs and one hip elevated (to avoid compression of the vena cava).

helpful. To date they have not been linked with an excessive risk of birth defects.

Ankle Edema

Most women experience ankle edema in the last part of pregnancy because of the increasing difficulty of venous return from the lower extremities. Prolonged standing or sitting and warm weather increase the edema. It is also associated with varicose veins. Ankle edema becomes a concern only when accompanied by hypertension or proteinuria or when the edema is not postural in origin.

Varicose Veins

Varicose veins are a result of weakening of the walls of veins or faulty functioning of the valves. Poor circulation in the lower extremities predisposes people to varicose veins in the legs and thighs, as does prolonged standing or sitting. The pregnant uterus puts pressure on the pelvic veins, preventing good venous return, so it may aggravate existing problems or contribute to obvious changes in the veins of the legs (Figure 11–3 ○).

Surgical correction of varicose veins is not generally recommended during pregnancy. The nurse should advise the woman that treatment may be needed after she gives birth because the problem will be aggravated by a succeeding pregnancy.

Although less common, varicosities in the vulva and perineum may also develop. They produce aching and a sense of heaviness. Wearing two sanitary pads inside the underpants sometimes provides support for vulvar varicosities. A woman may relieve uterine pressure on the pelvic veins by resting on her side. Blocks placed under the foot of her bed to elevate it slightly may also help.

Flatulence

Flatulence results from decreased gastrointestinal motility, leading to delayed emptying, and from pressure on the large intestine by the growing uterus. Air swallowing may also contribute to the problem.

Hemorrhoids

Hemorrhoids are varicosities of the veins in the lower rectum and the anus. During pregnancy the gravid uterus presses on the veins and interferes with venous circulation. In addition the straining that accompanies constipation is frequently a contributing cause of hemorrhoids.

Some women may not be bothered by hemorrhoids until the second stage of labor, when the hemorrhoids appear as they push. These hemorrhoids usually become asymptomatic a few days after childbirth. Symptoms of hemorrhoids include itching, swelling, pain, and bleeding. Women who have had hemorrhoids before pregnancy will probably experience difficulties with them during pregnancy.

Some women find relief by gently reinserting the hemorrhoid. The woman lies on her side, places some lubricant on her finger, and presses against the hemorrhoids, pushing them inside. She holds them in place for 1 to 2 minutes and then gently withdraws her finger. The anal sphincter should then hold them inside the rectum. The woman will find it especially helpful if she can maintain a side-lying (Sims) position for a time, so this method is best done before bed or prior to a daily rest period.

Constipation

Conditions that predispose the pregnant woman to constipation include general bowel sluggishness caused by increased progesterone and steroid metabolism; displacement of the intestines, which increases with growth of the fetus; and the oral iron supplements most pregnant women need. In severe or preexisting cases of constipation, the woman may need stool softeners, mild laxatives, or suppositories as recommended by her healthcare provider.

Backache

Many pregnant women experience backache, due primarily to exaggeration of the lumbosacral curve that occurs as the uterus enlarges and becomes heavier. Maintaining good posture and using proper body mechanics throughout pregnancy can help prevent backache. Advise the pregnant woman to avoid bending over at the waist to pick up objects and to bend from the knees instead (Figure 11–4 ●). She should place her feet 12 to 18 inches apart to maintain body balance. If the woman uses work surfaces that require her to bend, advise her to adjust the height of the surfaces.

Leg Cramps

Leg cramps are painful muscle spasms in the gastrocnemius muscles. They occur most often after the woman has gone to bed at night but may occur at other times. Extension of the foot can often cause leg cramps. The nurse should warn the pregnant woman not to extend the foot during childbirth preparation exercises or during rest periods. The exact cause of leg cramps is not known, but pressure of the enlarged uterus on pelvic nerves or blood vessels leading to the legs may be a contributing factor

● **FIGURE 11–4**

When picking up objects from floor level or lifting objects, the pregnant woman must use proper body mechanics.

COMPLEMENTARY CARE

PHYSICAL MODALITIES FOR RELIEF OF BACKACHE AND OTHER PREGNANCY-RELATED MUSCULAR PAIN

Massage Therapy for Low Back Pain

Massage often helps relieve the low back pain associated with pregnancy. During the first 4 months of pregnancy, the body should be massaged with a gentle, soft touch. The best position for lumbar massage is with the woman sitting on a stool, resting her arms on a table, and leaning her forehead against her arms. The person doing the massage kneels on the floor behind her, which enhances the ability to apply an effective amount of pressure to the back muscles.

Yoga

Many women find that the regular practice of yoga builds and tones muscles, increases flexibility, improves endurance, and promotes a state of relaxation. One of the many applications of yoga is in pregnancy and childbirth. In fact, many of the techniques taught in childbirth classes, such as focus, relaxation, and systematic breathing, have their roots in yoga. The gentle stretching of the poses helps ease the muscle aches of pregnancy and strengthens the muscles that will be used during childbirth. The breathing techniques may lessen the shortness of breath that often accompanies advanced pregnancy.

Yoga practiced while pregnant is slightly different from regular yoga in that some poses are contraindicated. These poses are the extreme stretching positions and any position that puts pressure on the uterus. Full forward bends will probably be uncomfortable for both woman and baby. A woman's center of balance has shifted completely, and thus she must be careful with balance poses. Pregnant women should never lie on the stomach for any pose. If any pose feels uncomfortable, the woman should stop at once. If she experiences dizziness, sudden swelling, extreme shortness of breath, or vaginal bleeding, she should see her midwife or doctor immediately.

Reflexology for Sciatica

Reflexology is a field of therapy that uses specific touch techniques to stimulate "reflex points and areas" on the feet, hands, and ears. Reflexologists believe that each of these points corresponds to a specific part of the body. The growing baby can put pressure on the large sciatic nerve. The pressure inflames the nerve, causing severe lower back pain that radiates into the legs. Reflexology may provide significant symptom relief (Mollart, 2003). The reflex points for the sciatic nerve are on the heel. A woman in her second or third trimester can press gently and release with her thumbs to stimulate first one whole heel, then the other. Each heel can be worked for a minute or two twice a day until the pain is gone.

Women who are in the first trimester of pregnancy should not have reflexology that stimulates the uterine points on the hands, feet, or ears. In general it is best for pregnant women to receive reflexology that uses light, gentle pressure.

(Varney, Kriebs, & Gegor, 2004), especially during the third trimester.

Stretching provides immediate relief of the muscle spasm. With the woman lying on her back, another person presses the woman's knee down to straighten her leg while pushing her foot toward her leg. The woman may also stand and put her foot flat on the floor. Massage and warm packs can alleviate the discomfort of leg cramps (Figure 11–5 ●). A diet that includes daily portions of both calcium and phosphorus may help prevent leg cramps.

Faintness

Many pregnant women occasionally feel faint, especially in warm, crowded areas. Faintness is caused by a combination of changes in the blood volume and postural hypotension due to pooling of blood in the dependent veins. Sudden change of position or standing for prolonged periods can also cause this sensation, and the woman may faint.

If a woman begins to feel faint from prolonged standing or from being in a stuffy room, she should sit down and lower her head between her knees. If this procedure does not help, she should ask someone to help her to an area where she can lie down and get fresh air. The nurse should advise the woman that when getting up from a resting position, it is important to move slowly. Women whose jobs

● **FIGURE 11–5**

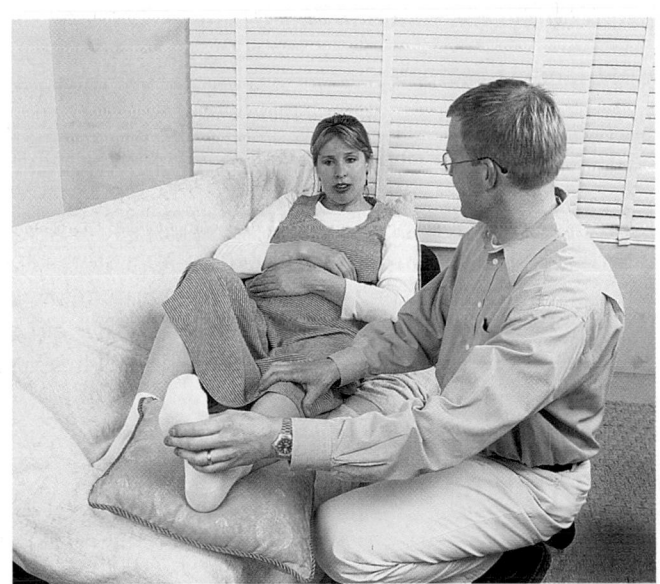

The expectant father can help relieve the woman's painful leg cramps by flexing her foot and straightening her leg.

require standing in one place for long periods should march in place regularly to increase venous return from the legs.

Shortness of Breath (Dyspnea)

Shortness of breath occurs as the uterus rises into the abdomen and causes pressure on the diaphragm. This problem worsens in the last trimester because the enlarged uterus presses directly on the diaphragm, decreasing vital capacity. The primigravida experiences considerable relief from shortness of breath in the last few weeks of pregnancy, when **lightening** occurs, and the fetus and uterus move down in the pelvis. Because the multigravida does not usually experience lightening until labor, she tends to feel short of breath throughout the latter part of her pregnancy.

Difficulty Sleeping

Many physical factors in late pregnancy may make sleeping difficult. The enlarged uterus may make it difficult to find a comfortable position for sleep, and an active fetus may aggravate the problem. Other discomforts of pregnancy such as urinary frequency, shortness of breath, and leg cramps may also make it hard to sleep.

Round Ligament Pain

As the uterus enlarges during pregnancy, the round ligaments stretch and hypertrophy as the uterus rises up in the abdomen, causing pain. The woman may feel concern when she first experiences round ligament pain, because it is often intense and causes a "grabbing" sensation in the lower abdomen and inguinal area. The nurse should warn the pregnant woman of this possible discomfort. Once it has been determined that the cause of the pain is not a medical complication such as appendicitis, the woman may find that applying a heating pad to the abdomen brings relief.

Carpal Tunnel Syndrome

Carpal tunnel syndrome, characterized by numbness and tingling of the hand near the thumb, occurs in about one fourth of pregnant women (Cunningham et al., 2005). It is caused by compression of the median nerve in the carpal tunnel of the wrist. The syndrome is aggravated by repetitive hand movements such as typing and may disappear following childbirth. Treatment usually involves splinting and avoiding aggravating movements, but surgery may be needed in severe cases if more conservative approaches are not effective.

PROMOTION OF SELF-CARE DURING PREGNANCY

FETAL ACTIVITY MONITORING

Many healthcare providers encourage pregnant women to monitor their unborn child's well-being by regularly assessing fetal activity beginning at 28 weeks' gestation. Vigorous activity generally provides reassurance of fetal well-being, but a marked decrease in activity or cessation of movement may indicate a problem that needs immediate evaluation. Fetal activity is affected by fetal sleep, sound, time of day, blood glucose levels, cigarette smoking, and some illicit drugs such as crack and cocaine. At times a healthy fetus may be minimally active or inactive. A variety of methods for tracking fetal activity have been developed. They focus on having the woman keep a **fetal movement record (FMR)** using a technique such as the Cardiff Count-to-Ten method. An FMR is noninvasive and lets the pregnant woman monitor and record movements easily and without expense. See "Teaching Highlights: Assessing Fetal Activity."

BREAST CARE

Whether the pregnant woman plans to formula-feed or breastfeed her infant, support of the breasts is important to promote comfort, retain breast shape, and prevent back strain, particularly if the breasts become large and pendulous. The sensitivity of the breasts in pregnancy is often relieved by good support.

A well-fitting, supportive brassiere has the following qualities:

- The straps are wide and do not stretch (elastic straps soon lose their tautness with the weight of the breasts and frequent washing).
- The cups hold all breast tissue comfortably.
- The brassiere has tucks or other devices that allow it to expand and accommodate the enlarging chest circumference.
- The brassiere supports the nipple line approximately midway between the elbow and shoulder but is not pulled up in the back by the weight of the breasts.

Cleanliness of the breasts is important, especially as the woman begins producing colostrum. Colostrum that crusts on the nipples can be removed with warm water. The nurse should advise the woman planning to breastfeed not to use soap on her nipples because of its drying effect.

Nipple preparation, generally begun during the third trimester, helps prevent soreness during the first few days of breastfeeding. Nipple preparation promotes the distribution of the natural lubricants produced by Montgomery's tubercles and helps develop the protective layer of skin over the nipple. Women who are planning to breastfeed can begin by going braless when possible and by exposing their nipples to sunlight and air. Rubbing the nipples removes protective oils and is best avoided, but rolling the nipple—grasping it between thumb and forefinger and gently rolling it for a short time each day—helps prepare

TEACHING HIGHLIGHTS

ASSESSING FETAL ACTIVITY

- Explain that fetal movements are first felt around 18 weeks' gestation. From that time the fetal movements get stronger and easier to detect. A slowing or stopping of fetal movement may be an indication that the fetus needs some attention and evaluation.
- Explain the procedure for the Cardiff Count-to-Ten method or for the daily fetal movement record. For both methods, advise the woman to:
  - Keep a daily record of fetal movement, beginning at about 27 weeks' gestation.

- Try to begin counting at about the same time each day, about 1 hour after a meal if possible.
- Lie quietly in a side-lying position.
- Using the Cardiff card, have the woman place an X for each fetal movement until she has recorded 10. Movement varies considerably, but most women feel fetal movement at least 10 times in 3 hours (see Figure 11–6).
- Using the daily fetal movement record, have the woman count three times a day for 20 to 30 minutes each session. If

● FIGURE 11–6

Fetal movement assessment method: the Cardiff Count-to-Ten scoring card (adaptation).

(continued)

TEACHING HIGHLIGHTS—continued

there are fewer than 3 movements in a session, have the woman count for 1 hour or more.

- Explain when to contact the care provider:
  - If there are fewer than 10 movements in 3 hours
  - If overall the fetus's movements are slowing, and it takes much longer each day to note 10 movements
  - If there are no movements in the morning
  - If there are fewer than 3 movements in 8 hours
- Describe procedures and demonstrate how to assess fetal movement. Sit beside the woman and show her how to place her hand on the fundus to feel fetal movement.
- Provide a written teaching sheet for the woman's use at home.
- Demonstrate how to record fetal movements on the Cardiff Count-to-Ten scoring card or on the daily fetal movement record.

- Watch the woman fill out the record as examples are provided. Encourage her to complete the record each day and bring it with her to each prenatal visit. Assure her that the record will be discussed at each prenatal visit, and questions may be addressed at that time if desired.
- Provide the woman with a name and phone number in case she has further questions.
- Evaluate learning by having the woman explain the method and by asking the woman to fill the card in using a fictitious situation. At each prenatal visit, the expectant mother's record is reviewed. This provides another opportunity for evaluation of learning and for questions and clarification.

---

for breastfeeding. However, the nurse should advise women with a history of preterm labor not to use this technique because nipple stimulation triggers the release of oxytocin. See Chapter 16 ∞ for further discussion of the effects of nipple stimulation on contractions.

Nipple rolling is more difficult for women with flat or inverted nipples, but it can still be useful in preparing for breastfeeding. Breast shields designed to correct inverted nipples can be worn during pregnancy. The shields appear to be the only available measure that offers help to some women with inverted nipples (Figure 11–7 ●). For further discussion of inverted nipples, see Chapter 26. ∞

Oral stimulation of the nipple by the woman's partner during sex play is also an excellent technique for toughening the nipple in preparation for breastfeeding. The nurse should encourage couples who enjoy this stimulation to continue it throughout the pregnancy, except when the woman has a history of preterm labor, as discussed earlier.

CLOTHING

Clothing in pregnancy is generally an important factor in the woman's feelings about herself and her appearance. Clothes should be loose and nonconstricting. Maternity clothing can be expensive and is worn for a relatively short time, so women may economize by wearing regular clothing, sharing clothes with friends, sewing their own garments, or buying used maternity clothes.

High-heeled shoes tend to aggravate back discomfort by increasing the curvature of the lower back. Women who experience backache or have problems with balance do best to avoid them. Shoes should fit properly and feel comfortable.

BATHING

Hygiene is important because perspiration and mucoid vaginal discharge increase during pregnancy. Keep in

● **FIGURE 11–7**

This breast shield is designed to increase the protractility of inverted nipples. Worn the last 3 to 4 months of pregnancy, it exerts gentle pulling pressure at the edge of the areola, gradually forcing the nipple through the center of the shield. It may be used after childbirth if still necessary.

mind, however, that cultural norms often influence bathing and cleansing practices. A pregnant woman may choose to cleanse only some portions of her body regularly or may elect to take showers or tub baths. Advise women to be careful in the tub because balance becomes a problem in late pregnancy. Rubber mats and hand grips are important safety devices. Vasodilation due to warm water may cause the woman to feel faint when she gets out of the tub, so she may need assistance, especially during the last trimester.

EMPLOYMENT

In general, women with low-risk pregnancies can continue working until the start of labor. However, studies of women employed outside the home during pregnancy and those who do not work show distinct differences. Pregnant women whose jobs require prolonged standing have a higher incidence of preterm birth (Cunningham et al., 2005). Similarly, women who engage in strenuous physical activity during pregnancy tend to have babies with lower birth weight, possibly because of decreased placental blood flow (Rao et al., 2003).

Overfatigue, excessive physical strain, fetotoxic hazards in the environment, and medical or obstetric complications are the major deterrents to certain types of employment during pregnancy. In the second half of pregnancy, women whose occupations involve balance should make adjustments as needed.

Fetotoxic hazards are always a concern to the expectant couple. The pregnant woman (or the woman contemplating pregnancy) who works in industry should contact her company physician or nurse about possible hazards in her work environment and should do her own reading and research on environmental hazards as well. Her partner can also find out how hazards in his workplace might affect his sperm.

TRAVEL

Pregnant women without complications can travel as usual. Pregnant women should avoid travel if they have a history of bleeding or preeclampsia or if multiple births are anticipated.

Travel by automobile can be tiring, aggravating many of the discomforts of pregnancy. The pregnant woman needs frequent opportunities to get out of the car and walk. (A good pattern is to stop every 2 hours and walk around for about 10 minutes.) She should wear both lap and shoulder belts; the lap belt should fit snugly and be positioned under the abdomen and across the upper thighs. Seat belts help save the lives of expectant mothers and fetuses (Cunningham et al., 2005). Fetal death in car accidents is sometimes caused by placental separation (abruptio placentae) as a result of uterine distortion.

Shoulder belts decrease the risk of traumatic flexion of the woman's body, making placental separation less likely.

As pregnancy progresses, long-distance trips are best taken by plane or train. Remind near-term women who travel to think about the availability of medical care at the destination.

ACTIVITY AND REST

Exercise during pregnancy helps maintain maternal fitness and muscle tone, leads to improved self-image, promotes regular bowel function, increases energy, improves sleep, relieves tension, helps control weight gain, and is associated with improved postpartum recovery. A woman with an uncomplicated pregnancy can and should continue normal participation in exercise. The woman can check with her certified nurse-midwife or physician about strenuous sports such as skiing and horseback riding. The skilled sportswoman should not usually be discouraged from participating in these activities if her pregnancy is uncomplicated. However, pregnancy is not the appropriate time to learn a new or strenuous sport.

Certain conditions contraindicate exercise. These conditions include rupture of the membranes, preeclampsia, incompetent cervix or cerclage placement, persistent vaginal bleeding, risk factors for preterm labor or a history of preterm labor in the prior or current pregnancy, placenta previa after 26 weeks' gestation, and chronic medical conditions that might be negatively affected by vigorous exercise such as significant heart disease (ACOG, 2002).

The following guidelines are helpful in counseling pregnant women about exercise. Even mild to moderate exercise is beneficial during pregnancy. Regular exercise—at least 30 minutes of moderate exercise daily or at least most days—is preferred (ACOG, 2002). After the first trimester, women should avoid exercising in the supine position. In most pregnant women, the supine position is associated with decreased cardiac output. Because uterine blood flow is reduced during exercise as blood is shunted from the visceral organs to the muscles, the remaining cardiac output is further decreased. Similarly, women should also avoid standing motionless for prolonged periods (ACOG, 2002).

Because decreased oxygen is available for aerobic exercise during pregnancy, women should modify the intensity of their exercise based on their symptoms, should stop when they become fatigued, and should avoid exercising to the point of exhaustion. Non-weight-bearing exercises such as swimming and cycling are recommended because they decrease the risk of injury and provide fitness with comfort.

As pregnancy progresses and the center of gravity changes, especially in the third trimester, women should avoid exercises in which the loss of balance could pose a risk to mother or fetus. Similarly, women should avoid any type of exercise that might result in even mild abdominal trauma.

A normal pregnancy requires an additional 300 kcal per day. Women who exercise regularly during pregnancy should be careful to ensure that their diet is adequate.

To avoid overheating, especially during the first trimester, pregnant women who exercise should wear clothing that is comfortable and loose, drink plenty of fluids, and avoid the prolonged overheating that can come from vigorous exercise in hot, humid weather. Hyperthermia may have teratogenic effects on the fetus (Heffernan, 2000). For the same reason, pregnant women are advised to avoid hot tubs and saunas.

Women should avoid reaching their maximum physical effort during pregnancy. As a general rule, their pulse rates should not exceed 140 beats per minute (Shrock, 2000).

The woman should wear a supportive bra and appropriate shoes when exercising. She should also warm up and stretch to help prepare the joints for activity and cool down with a period of mild activity to help restore circulation and avoid pooling of blood. A moderate, rhythmic exercise routine involving large muscle groups such as swimming, cycling, or brisk walking is best. Jogging or running is acceptable for women already conditioned to these activities as long as they avoid exercising at maximum effort and overheating.

When exercising, pregnant women should be alert for warning signs such as pain of any kind, decreased or absent fetal movement, difficulty walking, dizziness, headache, muscle weakness, dyspnea before exertion, uterine contractions, vaginal bleeding, or fluid loss from the vagina (ACOG, 2002; Clapp, 2001). The woman should stop exercising if these symptoms occur and modify her exercise program. If the symptoms persist, the woman should contact her caregiver.

During pregnancy, adequate rest is important for both physical and emotional health. Women need more sleep,

● FIGURE 11–8

Position for relaxation and rest as pregnancy progresses.

particularly in the first and last trimesters, when they tire easily. Without enough rest, pregnant women have less resilience. Finding time to rest during the day may be difficult for women who work outside the home or who have small children. The nurse can help the expectant mother examine her daily schedule to develop a realistic plan for short periods of rest and relaxation.

Sleeping becomes more difficult during the last trimester because of the enlarged abdomen, increased frequency of urination, and greater activity of the fetus. Finding a comfortable position becomes difficult. Figure 11–8 ● shows a position most pregnant women find comfortable. Women can also prepare for sleep with progressive relaxation techniques similar to those taught in prepared childbirth classes.

EXERCISES TO PREPARE FOR CHILDBIRTH

Certain exercises help strengthen muscle tone in preparation for birth and promote more rapid restoration of muscle tone after birth. A few of the more common body-conditioning exercises for pregnancy are discussed here.

The **pelvic tilt**, or pelvic rocking, helps prevent or reduce back strain as it strengthens abdominal muscles. To do the pelvic tilt, the pregnant woman lies on her back and puts her feet flat on the floor. This flexes the knees and helps prevent strain or discomfort. She decreases the curvature in her back by pressing her spine toward the floor. With her back pressed to the floor, the woman tightens her abdominal muscles as she tightens and tucks in her buttocks. The woman can also do the pelvic tilt on her hands and knees (Figure 11–9 ●), while sitting in a chair, or while standing with her back against a wall. The woman should maintain the body alignment that results when the pelvic tilt is done correctly as much as possible throughout the day.

● FIGURE 11–9

A

B

C

D

A, Starting position when the pelvic tilt is done on hands and knees. The back is flat and parallel to the floor, the hands are below the head, and the knees are directly below the buttocks. *B,* A prenatal yoga instructor offers pointers for proper positioning for the first part of the tilt: head up, neck long and separated from the shoulders, buttocks up, and pelvis thrust back, allowing the back to drop and release on an inhaled breath. *C,* The instructor helps the woman assume the correct position for the next part of the tilt. It is done on a long exhalation, allowing the pregnant woman to arch her back, drop her head loosely, push away from her hands, and draw in the muscles of her abdomen to strengthen them. In this position the pelvis and buttocks are tucked under, and the buttock muscles are tightened. *D,* Proper posture. The knees are slightly bent but not locked, and the pelvis and buttocks are tucked under, thereby lengthening the spine and helping support the weighty abdomen. With her chin tucked in, this woman's neck, shoulders, hips, knees, and feet are all in a straight line perpendicular to the floor. Her feet are parallel. This is also the starting position for doing the pelvic tilt while standing.

NURSING PRACTICE

Doing the pelvic rock on hands and knees may aggravate back strain. Teach women with a history of minor back problems to do the pelvic rock only in the standing position.

Abdominal Exercises

A basic exercise to increase abdominal muscle tone is tightening abdominal muscles with each breath. It can be done in any position, but it is best learned while lying supine. With knees flexed and feet flat on the floor, the woman expands her abdomen and slowly takes a deep breath. Exhaling slowly, she gradually pulls in her abdominal muscles until they are fully contracted. She relaxes for a few seconds and then repeats the exercise.

Partial sit-ups strengthen abdominal muscle tone and are done according to individual comfort levels. A partial sit-up must be done with the knees flexed and the feet flat on the floor to avoid strain on the lower back. The woman stretches her arms toward her knees as she slowly pulls her head and shoulders off the floor to a comfortable level (if she has poor abdominal muscle tone, she may not be able to pull up very far). She then slowly returns to the starting position, takes a deep breath, and repeats the exercise. To strengthen the oblique abdominal muscles, she repeats the process but stretches the left arm to the side of her right knee, returns to the floor, takes a deep breath, and then reaches with the right arm to the left knee.

Women can do these exercises approximately five times in a sequence and repeat the sequence at other times during the day as desired. It is important to do the exercises slowly to prevent muscle strain and overtiring.

Perineal Exercises

Perineal muscle tightening, also called **Kegel exercises**, strengthens the pubococcygeus muscle and increases its elasticity (Figure 11–10 ●). The woman can feel the specific muscle group to be exercised by stopping urination midstream. Doing Kegel exercises while urinating is discouraged, however, because this practice has been associated with urinary stasis and urinary tract infection.

Childbirth educators sometimes use the following technique to teach Kegel exercises. They tell the woman to think of her perineal muscles as an elevator. When she relaxes, the elevator is on the first floor. To do the exercises,

she contracts, bringing the elevator to the second, third, and fourth floors. She keeps the elevator on the fourth floor for a few seconds, and then gradually relaxes the area. If the exercise is properly done, the woman does not contract the muscles of the buttocks and thighs. Kegel exercises can be done at almost any time. Some women use ordinary events—for instance, stopping at a red light or talking on the telephone—as a cue to remember to do the exercise.

Inner Thigh Exercises

The nurse can advise the pregnant woman to assume a cross-legged sitting position whenever possible. This "tailor sit" stretches the muscles of the inner thighs in preparation for labor and birth.

SEXUAL ACTIVITY

Because of the physiologic, anatomic, and emotional changes of pregnancy, couples usually have many questions and concerns about sexual activity during pregnancy. Often these questions are about possible injury to the baby or the woman during intercourse and about changes in the desire each partner feels for the other.

In the past, couples were often warned to avoid sexual intercourse during the last 6 to 8 weeks of pregnancy to prevent complications such as infection or premature rupture of the membranes. However, these fears seem to be unfounded. In a healthy pregnancy, there is no medical reason to limit sexual activity. Intercourse is contraindicated for medical reasons such as multiple pregnancy, threatened abortion, incompetent cervix, a partner with sexually transmitted infection, or a maternal history of miscarriage following orgasm (Shrock, 2000). Most healthcare providers

● **FIGURE 11–10**

 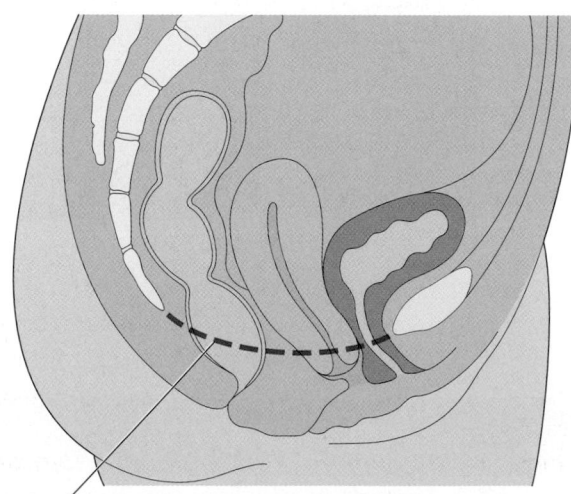

Pubococcygeus muscle with good tone

Pubococcygeus muscle with poor tone

Kegel exercises. The woman learns to tighten the pubococcygeus muscle, which improves support to the pelvic organs.

also advise against intercourse when the membranes are ruptured and in women with a history of preterm labor.

The expectant mother may experience changes in sexual desire and response. Often these changes are related to the various discomforts that occur throughout pregnancy. For instance, during the first trimester, fatigue or nausea and vomiting may decrease sexual desire. During the second trimester, many of these discomforts are lessened and sexual satisfaction increases. During the third trimester, interest in sex may again decrease as the woman becomes more uncomfortable and tired. Shortness of breath, urinary frequency, leg cramps, and decreased mobility may also lessen sexual desire and activity. If they are not already doing so, the couple should consider coital positions other than male superior, such as side-by-side, female superior, and vaginal rear entry.

Sexual activity does not have to include intercourse. Many of the nurturing and sexual needs of the pregnant woman can be satisfied by cuddling, kissing, and being held. The warm, sensual feelings that accompany these activities can be an end in themselves. Her partner, however, may choose to masturbate more frequently than before.

Many factors in pregnancy also affect the sexual desires of men. The man's previous relationship with the partner, acceptance of the pregnancy, attitudes toward the partner's change of appearance, and concern about hurting the expectant mother or baby can all play a role. Some men find it difficult to view their partners as sexually appealing while they are adjusting to the concept of them as mothers. Other men find their partners' pregnancies arousing and experience feelings of increased happiness, intimacy, and closeness.

The expectant couple should be aware of their changing sexual desires, the normality of these changes, and the importance of communicating these changes to each other so that they can make nurturing adaptations. It is important that the couple feel free to express concerns about sexual activity. Use a relaxed manner when responding to questions and giving anticipatory guidance. See "Teaching Highlights: Sexual Activity During Pregnancy."

DENTAL CARE

Proper dental hygiene is important in pregnancy. In fact, research suggests a link between periodontal disease in pregnant women and preterm birth and low-birth-weight infants (Carl, Roux, & Matacale, 2000). In spite of such discomforts as nausea and vomiting, gum hypertrophy, and heartburn, it is important for pregnant women to maintain regular oral hygiene.

Encourage the pregnant woman to have a dental checkup early in her pregnancy. General dental repair and extractions can be done during pregnancy, preferably in the second trimester and under local anesthetic (Carl et al., 2000). The woman should inform her dentist

TEACHING HIGHLIGHTS

SEXUAL ACTIVITY DURING PREGNANCY

In starting a discussion about sexual activity during pregnancy, universal statements that give permission, such as "Many couples experience changes in sexual desire during pregnancy. What kind of changes have you experienced?" are often effective.

In your teaching, explain the following points to the woman and her partner:

- The pregnant woman may experience changes in desire during the course of pregnancy. During the first trimester, discomforts such as nausea, fatigue, and breast tenderness may make intercourse less desirable for many women. In the second trimester, as symptoms decrease, desire may increase. In the third trimester, discomfort and fatigue may lead to decreased desire in the woman.

- Men may notice changes in their level of desire, too. This may be related to feelings about their partner's changing appearance, their belief about the acceptability of sexual activity with a pregnant woman, or concern about hurting the woman or fetus. Some men find the changes of pregnancy erotic; others must adjust to the notion of their partners as mothers.

- The woman may notice that orgasms are much more intense during the last weeks of pregnancy and may be followed by cramping.

- Because of the pressure of the enlarging uterus on the vena cava, the woman should not lie flat on her back for intercourse after about the fourth month. If the couple prefer that position, a pillow should be placed under her right hip to displace the uterus. Alternative positions such as side-by-side, female superior, or vaginal rear entry may become necessary as her uterus enlarges.

- Sexual activities that both partners enjoy are generally acceptable. It is not advisable for couples who favor anal sex to go from anal penetration to vaginal penetration because of the risk of introducing *Escherichia coli* into the vagina.

- Alternative methods of expressing intimacy and affection such as cuddling, holding and stroking each other, and kissing may help maintain the couple's feelings of warmth and closeness. If the man feels desire for further sexual release, his partner may help him masturbate to ejaculation, or he may prefer to masturbate in private.

- Sexual intercourse is contraindicated once the membranes are ruptured or if bleeding is present. Women with a history of preterm labor may be advised to avoid intercourse because the oxytocin that is released with orgasm stimulates uterine contractions and may trigger preterm labor. Because oxytocin is also released with nipple stimulation, fondling the breasts may also be contraindicated in those cases.

Stress the importance of open communication so that the couple feel comfortable expressing their feelings, preferences, and concerns. Deal with any specific questions about the physical and psychologic changes that the couple may have.

of her pregnancy so that she is not exposed to teratogenic substances. Dental x-ray examinations and extensive dental work need to be delayed until after the birth when possible.

IMMUNIZATIONS

Immunizations with attenuated live viruses, such as rubella vaccine, should not be given in pregnancy because of the teratogenic effect of the live viruses on the developing embryo. Vaccinations using killed viruses may be used, however.

COMPLEMENTARY AND ALTERNATIVE THERAPIES

As discussed in Chapter 2, many women use complementary and alternative medicine (CAM) such as homeopathy, herbal medicine, acupressure and acupuncture, biofeedback, therapeutic touch, massage, and chiropractic as part of a holistic approach to their healthcare. However, they often do not report use of alternative approaches to their healthcare provider. Thus, nurses working with pregnant women and childbearing families need to develop a general understanding of the more commonly used therapies to be able to answer basic questions and to provide resources as needed.

Nurses caring for pregnant women can develop printed materials describing the use of homeopathic remedies and herbs during pregnancy and identifying those that may present a risk. It is especially important that women choosing these complementary approaches consult someone who is knowledgeable, well trained, and experienced in the specific therapy and that they buy their herbs or homeopathic remedies from reputable manufacturers.

TERATOGENIC SUBSTANCES

Substances that adversely affect the normal growth and development of the fetus are called teratogens (see Chapter 3 ∞). Many substances are known or suspected teratogens, including, for example, certain medications, psychotropic drugs, and alcohol. The harmful effects of others, such as some pesticides or exposure to x-rays in the first trimester of pregnancy, have also been documented. It is essential to provide pregnant women with information about recognized teratogens and environmental risks.

Medications

The use of medications during pregnancy, including prescriptions, over-the-counter drugs, and herbal remedies, is of great concern because maternal drug exposure is thought to account for at least 10% of all birth defects (Black & Hill, 2003). Many pregnant women need medication to treat infections, allergies, or other pathologic processes. In these situations the problem can be complex. Care providers do not prescribe known teratogenic agents and can usually replace them with safer medications. However, even when a woman is highly motivated to avoid taking any medications, she may have taken potentially teratogenic medications before her pregnancy was confirmed, especially if she has an irregular menstrual cycle.

The fetus is at highest risk for gross abnormalities during the first trimester of pregnancy, when fetal organs are first developing. The classic period of teratogenesis in a woman with a 28-day cycle extends from day 31 after the last menstrual period (17 days after fertilization) to day 71 (57 days after fertilization) (Niebyl, 2002). Many factors influence teratogenic effects, including the type of teratogen and the dose, the stage of embryo development, and the genetic sensitivity of the mother and fetus. For example, the commonly prescribed acne medication isotretinoin (Accutane) is associated with a high incidence of spontaneous abortion and congenital malformations if taken early in pregnancy.

To provide information for healthcare providers and clients, the U.S. Food and Drug Administration has developed the following classification system for medications administered during pregnancy:

Category A: Controlled studies in women have demonstrated no associated fetal risk. Few drugs fall into this category.

Category B: Animal studies show no risk, but there are no controlled studies in women, or animal studies indicate a risk, but controlled human studies fail to demonstrate a risk. The penicillins fall into this category.

Category C: Either (1) no adequate animal or human studies are available or (2) animal studies show teratogenic effects, but no controlled studies in women are available. Many drugs fall into this category, which, because of the lack of information, is a problematic one for caregivers. Epinephrine, beta-blockers, and zidovudine (a drug used to decrease perinatal transmission of HIV) fall into this category.

Category D: Evidence of human fetal risk exists, but the benefits of the drug in certain situations are thought to outweigh the risks. Examples of drugs in this category include tetracycline, vincristine, lithium, and hydrochlorothiazide.

Category X: The demonstrated fetal risks clearly outweigh any possible benefit. Examples of drugs in this category include isotretinoin (Accutane), the acne medication, which can cause multiple central nervous system, facial, and cardiovascular anomalies.

If a woman has taken a drug in category D or X, she should be informed of the risks associated with that drug and of her alternatives. A woman who has taken a drug in the safer categories can be reassured (Cunningham et al., 2005).

Although the first trimester is the critical period for teratogenesis, some medications are known to have a teratogenic effect when taken in the second and third trimesters. For example, tetracycline taken in late pregnancy is commonly associated with staining of teeth in children and has been shown to depress skeletal growth, especially in premature infants. Sulfonamides taken in the last few weeks of pregnancy are known to compete with bilirubin attachment of protein-binding sites, increasing the risk of jaundice in the newborn.

Pregnant women need to avoid all medication—prescribed, homeopathic, or over-the-counter—if possible. If no alternative exists, it is wisest to select a well-known medication rather than a newer drug whose potential teratogenic effects may not be known. When possible the oral form of a drug should be used, and it should be prescribed in the lowest possible therapeutic dose for the shortest time possible. Caution is the watchword for nurses caring for pregnant women who have been taking medications. It is essential that pregnant women check with their certified nurse-midwives or physicians about any herbs or medications they were taking when pregnancy began and about any nonprescription drugs they are thinking of using. The advantage of using a particular medication must outweigh the risks. Any medication with possible teratogenic effects is best avoided.

Tobacco

Infants of mothers who smoke during pregnancy have a higher incidence of low birth weight than infants of mothers who do not smoke. For women with a twin pregnancy, this effect is even more pronounced (Pollack, Lantz, & Frohna, 2000). Smoking during pregnancy has also been associated with an increased risk of spontaneous abortion, IUGR, preterm birth, premature rupture of the membranes, placenta previa, abruptio placentae, and higher morbidity (Kuczkowski, 2003). The risk is related to the number of cigarettes smoked. Smoking has also been linked to an increased risk of cleft lip and palate in the newborn (Chung, Kowalski, Kim, & Buchman, 2000). The specific mechanism of smoking's effect on the fetus is not known. However, the main ingredients in cigarette smoke that account for adverse effects in the fetus are carbon monoxide and nicotine, because they decrease the availability of oxygen to maternal and fetal tissues.

Currently about 15% to 29% of women smoke during pregnancy. This rate has declined steadily since 1989—a positive trend (ACOG, 2000b). Women who smoke tend to stop smoking or at least reduce their intake once pregnancy is confirmed. Unfortunately, a majority of women who quit smoking during pregnancy resume following childbirth, although this percentage is lower for women who quit early in pregnancy. Any decrease in smoking during pregnancy most likely improves fetal outcome, and researchers continue to explore approaches designed to help women quit smoking. Pregnancy may be a difficult time for a woman to stop smoking, but the nurse should encourage her to reduce the number of cigarettes she smokes daily. The perceived need to protect her unborn child may increase her motivation.

Alcohol

Fetuses of women who drink heavily are at increased risk of developing **fetal alcohol syndrome** (see Chapter 25 ∞). This syndrome, which is characterized by growth restriction, facial anomalies, and central nervous system dysfunction of varying severity, is the major cause of mental retardation in the United States (Cunningham et al., 2005). Moreover, in pregnancies complicated by heavy alcohol use, the overall perinatal mortality is 18% (Kuczkowski, 2003).

The effects of moderate drinking during pregnancy are unclear. Research indicates an increased incidence of lowered birth weight and some neurologic effects, such as attention deficit disorder. Evidence suggests that the risk of teratogenic effects increases proportionately with increased average daily intake of alcohol. Although an occasional drink during pregnancy does not carry any known risk, no safe level of drinking during pregnancy has been identified; thus, healthcare providers recommend that pregnant women abstain from all alcohol during pregnancy. In most cases once a woman becomes aware of her pregnancy, she decreases her consumption of alcohol. However, the alcohol consumed after conception and before pregnancy is diagnosed remains a cause for concern.

Assessment of alcohol intake is a major part of every woman's medical history. The nurse should ask questions in a direct, nonjudgmental manner. All women need to be counseled about the role of alcohol in pregnancy. If heavy consumption is involved, the nurse should refer the pregnant woman immediately to an alcoholic treatment program. Counselors in these programs need to know about a woman's pregnancy before drug therapy is suggested, since certain drugs may be harmful to the developing fetus. For example, the drug disulfiram (Antabuse), often used in conjunction with alcohol treatment, is suspected to be a teratogenic agent.

Caffeine

Current research offers no evidence that caffeine has teratogenic effects in humans nor is it linked to IUGR, low birth weight, or preterm birth. An increased risk of decreased birth weight has been found in infants of mothers who consume at least 600 mg of caffeine daily (about six 10-oz cups of coffee). Until more definitive data are available, nurses can advise women about common sources of caffeine, including coffee, tea, colas, and chocolate, and suggest that they moderate their daily caffeine intake.

Marijuana

The prevalence of marijuana use raises many concerns about its effect on the fetus, but no teratogenic effects of marijuana use during pregnancy have yet been documented (Cunningham et al., 2005). Research on marijuana use in pregnancy is difficult, however, because it is an illegal drug. Unreliability of reporting, lack of a representative population, inability to determine strength or composition of the marijuana used (including the presence of herbicides), and use of other drugs at the same time all complicate the research being done.

Cocaine

A woman who uses cocaine during pregnancy is at increased risk for acute myocardial infarction, cardiac arrhythmias, ruptured ascending aorta, seizures, cerebrovascular accidents, hyperthermia, bowel ischemia, and sudden death (Cunningham et al., 2005). Cocaine use during pregnancy has been related to abruptio placentae, preterm birth, fetal distress, low birth weight, neonatal withdrawal, sudden infant death syndrome (SIDS), and developmental delays as a toddler (Blatt, Meguid, & Church, 2000). Several congenital anomalies have also been linked to maternal cocaine use, including genitourinary anomalies, congenital heart defects, limb reduction defects, and central nervous system anomalies (Cunningham et al., 2005).

As the number of women of childbearing age using cocaine increases, healthcare providers must be alert to early signs of cocaine use. It is often difficult for a nurse or physician to face the fact that a client is using cocaine, but ongoing alertness and an open, nonjudgmental approach are important in early detection. Urine screening for cocaine is valuable, but because cocaine is metabolized rapidly, the drug screen is negative within 24 to 48 hours after cocaine use. Thus, it is probable that many expectant mothers who use cocaine are not identified.

EVALUATION

Throughout the antepartal period, evaluation is an ongoing and essential part of effective nursing care. In evaluating the effectiveness of the interactions, try creative solutions that are logical and carefully thought out. Creative solutions are especially important in dealing with families from other cultures. If a practice is important to a woman and not harmful, the culturally competent nurse will not discourage it.

Be alert for situations that require referral for further evaluation. For example, a woman who has gained 4 lb in a single week does not require counseling about nutrition; she needs further assessment for preeclampsia. The nurse who has a sound knowledge of theory will recognize this need and act immediately.

Throughout the course of pregnancy, certain criteria determine the quality of care. In essence, nursing care has been effective if the following occur:

- The common discomforts of pregnancy are quickly identified and are relieved or lessened effectively.
- The woman is able to discuss the physiologic and psychologic changes of pregnancy.
- The woman uses self-care measures, if needed, during pregnancy.
- The woman avoids substances and situations that pose a risk to her or her child's well-being.
- The woman seeks regular prenatal care.

CARE OF EXPECTANT PARENTS OVER AGE 35

Today an increasing number of women are choosing to have their first baby after age 35. In the United States, birth rates for women between the ages of 35 and 39 (41 births per 1,000 women) and between 40 and 44 (8 per 1,000) are the highest in more than three decades (Martin et al., 2003). Many factors have contributed to this trend, including the following:

- The availability of effective birth control methods
- The expanded roles and career options available for women
- The increased number of women getting advanced education, pursuing careers, and delaying parenthood until they are established professionally
- The increased incidence of later marriage and second marriage
- The high cost of living, which causes some young couples to delay childbearing until they are more secure financially
- The increased number of women in this older reproductive age group due to the baby boom between 1946 and 1964
- The increased availability of specialized fertilization procedures, which may help women previously considered infertile

There are advantages to having a first baby after age 35. Single women or couples who delay childbearing until they are older tend to be well educated and financially secure. Usually their decision to have a baby was deliberately and thoughtfully made (Figure 11–11 ●). Because of their greater life experiences, they also are more aware of the realities of having a child and what it means to have a baby at their age. Many of the women have experienced fulfillment in their careers and feel secure enough to take on the added responsibility of a child. Some women are ready to make a change in their lives,

● FIGURE 11-11

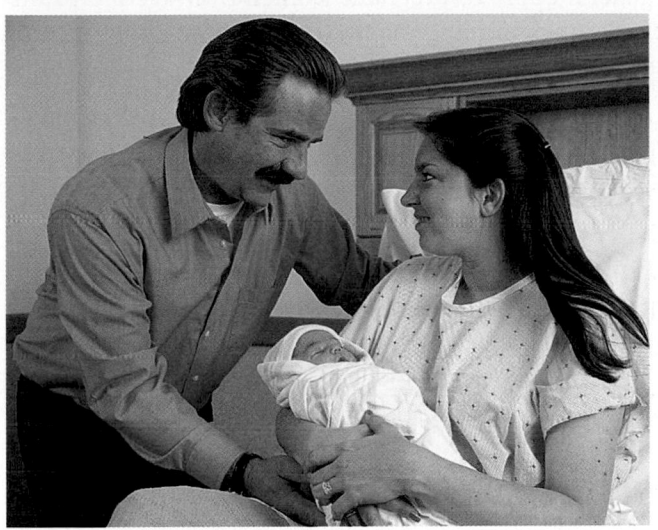

For many older couples, the decision to have a child may be very rewarding.

wanting to stay home with a new baby. Those who plan to continue working typically can afford good child care.

MEDICAL RISKS

In the United States, the risk of fetal death has declined dramatically over the past 30 years for women of all ages. However, the risk of fetal death is significantly higher for women over age 35 and even higher for women age 40 and older. This is true regardless of a woman's parity, the time at which she begins prenatal care, and her level of education (Callaghan & Berg, 2003).

Women over age 35, especially those over age 40, are more likely to have chronic medical conditions that can complicate a pregnancy. Preexisting medical conditions such as hypertension or diabetes probably play a more significant role than age in maternal well-being and the outcome of pregnancy. The incidence of low-birth-weight infants and preterm births is higher among women age 35 and older (Tough et al., 2002). In addition, placenta previa, abruptio placentae, spontaneous abortion, macrosomia, and congenital malformations occur more frequently in pregnant women over 35 (Cunningham et al., 2005). For women over age 50 with singleton pregnancies, the risk of low-birth-weight, preterm, and very preterm babies is triple that of younger women, and the risk of small-for-gestational-age infants and fetal mortality is double that of younger women (Salihu, Shumpert, Slay et al., 2003).

The cesarean birth rate is also increased in pregnant women over age 35. This may be related both to pregnancy complications and to increased concern by the woman and her physician about the pregnancy outcome (Cunningham et al., 2005).

The risk of conceiving a child with Down syndrome increases with age, especially over age 35. Amniocentesis is routinely offered to all women over age 35 to permit the early detection of several chromosomal abnormalities, including Down syndrome. Genetic testing is not routinely offered to couples in whom there is only advanced paternal age, because there is not enough evidence to determine a paternal age at which to start genetic testing. However, advanced paternal age affects autosomal dominant inherited diseases, such as neurofibromatosis, achondroplasia, and Marfan syndrome.

Multiple marker screening tests are available to help identify women at increased risk for Down syndrome and trisomy 18. The *quadruple screen* (quad screen) is a safe, useful screening test performed on the mother's serum between weeks 15 and 20 of pregnancy. The test is used to detect levels of specific serum markers—alpha fetoprotein (AFP), human chorionic gonadotropin (hCG), unconjugated estriol (UE), and inhibin A (a placental hormone). The quad test has generally replaced the triple screen, which did not include inhibin-A testing. If test results reveal higher than normal AFP levels, it could indicate a fetal neural tube defect, a multiple gestation, or a pregnancy that is farther along than believed. Lower than normal AFP could indicate that the woman is at risk for Down syndrome or trisomy 18. Higher than normal levels of hCG and inhibin A and lower than normal UE may also indicate that a woman is at increased risk of having a baby with Down syndrome. If the screening results are not in the normal range, follow-up testing using ultrasound and amniocentesis is often indicated (Cleveland Clinic, 2004).

Research is also focusing on new screening approaches for Down syndrome. One study, called FASTER (First and Second Trimester Evaluation of Risk), includes first-trimester ultrasound assessment of the thickness of the fetal nuchal fold (called *nuchal translucency* [NT]) combined with a serum screen of pregnancy-associated plasma protein A (PAPP-A). These tests are combined with a second-trimester quad screen. This combined protocol is more effective in identifying Down syndrome than the quad test alone, but the NT evaluation requires a skilled ultrasonographer and specialized training (Dolan, 2004).

SPECIAL CONCERNS OF EXPECTANT PARENTS OVER AGE 35

No matter what their age, most expectant parents have concerns about the well-being of the fetus and their ability to parent. Expectant parents over age 35 often have additional concerns about their age, especially the closer they are to age 40. Some couples are concerned about whether they will have enough energy to care for a new baby. Of greater concern is their ability to deal with the needs of the child as they age.

The financial concerns of the older couple are usually different from those of the younger couple. The older couple is generally more financially secure, but when their "baby" is ready for college, the older couple may be close to retirement and might not have the means to provide for their child. The older couple may also be forced to face their own mortality. Certainly the realization of one's mortality is not uncommon in midlife, but older expectant parents may confront the issue earlier as they consider what will happen as their child grows.

Older couples facing pregnancy in a late or second marriage or after therapy for infertility may find themselves somewhat isolated socially. They may feel different because they are often the only couple in their peer group expecting their first baby. In fact, many of their peers are likely to be parents of adolescents or young adults and may be grandparents as well.

Older couples who already have children may respond quite differently to learning that the woman is pregnant, depending on whether the pregnancy was planned or unexpected. Other factors influencing their response include their children's, family's, and friends' attitudes toward the pregnancy; the impact on their lifestyle; and the financial implications of having another child. Sometimes couples who had previously been married to other mates will choose to have a child together. *Blended families* are formed when "her" children, "his" children, and "their" children come together as a new family group.

Healthcare professionals may treat older expectant parents differently than they would a younger couple. They may offer older women more medical procedures, such as amniocentesis and ultrasound, than younger women. They may also discourage an older woman from using a birthing room or birthing center even if she is healthy because her age is considered to put her at risk.

The woman who has delayed pregnancy may be concerned about the limited amount of time that she has to bear children. When pregnancy does not occur as quickly as she had hoped, the older woman may become increasingly anxious as time slips away on her "biological clock." When an older woman becomes pregnant but has a spontaneous abortion, her grief for the loss of her unborn child is exacerbated by anxiety about ability to conceive again in the time remaining to her.

NURSING MANAGEMENT

NURSING ASSESSMENT AND DIAGNOSIS

In working with a woman in her late 30s or 40s who is pregnant, make the same assessments as are indicated in caring for any woman who is pregnant. Assess physical status, the woman's understanding of pregnancy and its changes, the couple's attitudes about the pregnancy and their expectations of the impact a baby will have on their lives, their health teaching needs, the degree of support the woman has, and her knowledge of infant care.

The nursing diagnoses applicable to pregnant women in general apply to pregnant women over age 35. Examples of other nursing diagnoses that may apply include the following:

- *Decisional Conflict* related to unexpected pregnancy
- *Moderate Anxiety* related to uncertainty about fetal well-being

PLANNING AND IMPLEMENTATION

Once an older couple has made the decision to have a child, respect and support the couple in this decision. As with any client, discuss risks, identify concerns, and promote strengths. Do not make the woman's age an issue. It is helpful in promoting a sense of well-being to treat the pregnancy as normal unless the woman has specific health risks.

As the pregnancy continues, identify and discuss concerns the woman may have related to her age or to specific health problems. The older woman who has made a conscious decision to become pregnant often has carefully thought through potential problems and may actually have fewer concerns than a younger woman or one with an unplanned pregnancy.

Childbirth education classes are important in promoting adaptation to the event of childbirth for expectant parents of any age. However, older expectant parents often feel uncomfortable in classes in which most of the participants are much younger. Consequently, classes for expectant parents over age 35 are now available in many communities.

Women who are over age 35 and having their first baby tend to be better educated than other healthcare consumers. These clients frequently know the kind of care and services they want and may be assertive in their interactions with the healthcare system. You should not be intimidated by these individuals and should not assume that anticipatory guidance and support are not needed. Instead, support the couple's strengths and be sensitive to their individual needs.

In working with older expectant couples or an older single woman, the nurse should be sensitive to special needs. A particularly difficult issue these couples face is the possibility of bearing an unhealthy child or a child with a genetic disorder. As discussed previously, a quad screening test, also called multiple marker screen, is useful in assessing for Down syndrome. Because of the risk of Down syndrome in these families, amniocentesis is often suggested.

For couples who agree to amniocentesis, the first few months of pregnancy are a difficult time. Amniocentesis cannot be done until week 14 of pregnancy, and the chromosomal studies take roughly 2 weeks to complete. Their fear that the fetus is at risk may delay the successful completion of the psychologic tasks of early pregnancy.

You can support couples who decide to have amniocentesis by providing information and answering questions about the procedure and by providing comfort and emotional support during the amniocentesis. If the results indicate that the fetus has Down syndrome or another genetic abnormality, ensure that the couple has complete information about the condition, its range of possible manifestations, and its developmental implications.

EVALUATION

Expected outcomes of nursing care include the following:

- The woman and her partner are knowledgeable about the pregnancy and express confidence in their ability to make appropriate healthcare choices.

- The expectant parents (and their children) are able to cope with the pregnancy and its implications for the future.

- The woman receives effective healthcare throughout her pregnancy and during birth and the postpartum period.

- The woman and her partner develop skills in child care and parenting.

Critical Concept Review

LEARNING OBJECTIVES

CONCEPTS

Describe actions that the nurse can take to help maintain the well-being of the expectant father and siblings during a family's pregnancy.

1. Father:
   - Provide information about expected changes (physical and emotional) during pregnancy.
   - Encourage the father to express feelings about pregnancy and other related topics such as feeding, ability to parent, and sexual activity.
   - Refer the couple to parenting classes for information about labor and birth. Also provide for support from other couples in the same situation.
   - Assess father's intended level of participation during labor and birth.
2. Siblings:
   - Discuss the possible negative feelings of siblings that may take place at the birth of a new child.
   - Teach parents to use open communication during the transition time.

Explain the causes of the common discomforts of pregnancy.

1. In the first trimester:
   - Nausea and vomiting are caused by increased levels of hCG as well as changes in carbohydrate metabolism.
   - Urinary frequency is caused by pressure of the uterus on the bladder.
   - Fatigue may be caused by urinary frequency at night.
   - Breast tenderness is caused by increased estrogen and progesterone.
   - Increased vaginal discharge is caused by cervical hyperplasia and increased production of mucus by the endocervical gland.
   - Nasal stuffiness and epistaxis are caused by increased estrogen levels.
2. In the second and third trimesters:
   - Heartburn is caused by increased levels of progesterone as well as decreased gastric motility, increased relaxation of cardiac sphincter, and increased size of uterus which displaces the stomach.
   - Ankle edema is caused by prolonged sitting or standing, slow venous return, increased capillary permeability, and increased level of sodium.
   - Varicose veins are caused by venous congestion and weight gain.
   - Hemorrhoids are caused by constipation and slow venous return of blood.
   - Constipation is caused by slow peristalsis due to increased level of progesterone. Constipation is also caused by decreased fluids, decreased exercise, increased level of iron, and pressure of the uterus on the intestines.
   - Backache is caused by increased lumbosacral vertebrae curve due to enlarging uterus.
   - Leg cramps are caused by an imbalance of calcium and phosphorus, fatigue, and poor lower extremity circulation.

(continued)

LEARNING OBJECTIVES

CONCEPTS

Explain the causes of the common discomforts of pregnancy.—*continued*

- Faintness is caused by a sudden change of position which precipitates postural hypotension.
- Dyspnea is caused by decreased vital capacity due to increasing size of uterus.
- Flatulence is caused by decreased gastric motility and air swallowing.
- Carpal tunnel syndrome is caused by compression of median nerve precipitated by edema.

Identify appropriate relief measures for the common discomforts of pregnancy.

1. In the first trimester:
   - For nausea and vomiting: avoid odors and eat dry crackers before arising in a.m. Drink fluids between meals and avoid greasy foods.
   - For urinary frequency: increase fluid intake during day and decrease in the evening.
   - For fatigue: plan rest periods and ask for help from family or support persons.
   - For breast tenderness: wear a well-supporting bra.
   - For increased vaginal discharge: bathe daily and wear cotton underwear.
   - For nasal stuffiness and epistaxis: use cool mist vaporizer.
2. In the second and third trimester:
   - For heartburn: eat small, frequent meals, avoid overeating and lying down after eating.
   - For ankle edema: elevate legs while sitting or standing and dorsiflex feet frequently.
   - For varicose veins: elevate legs as much as possible and wear support hose.
   - For hemorrhoids: avoid constipation, use ice packs or sitz baths as necessary.
   - For constipation: increase fluid and fiber in diet. Develop regular bowel habits.
   - For backache: use good body mechanics and practice pelvic tilt exercises.
   - For leg cramps: apply heat to affected muscles and dorsiflex feet.
   - For faintness: change positions slowly, avoid standing for long periods of time.
   - For dyspnea: use good posture to sit and stand, and sleep in a semi-Fowler's position.
   - For flatulence: chew food completely and avoid gas-forming foods.
   - For carpal tunnel syndrome: avoid repetitive hand movement and elevate arm as needed.

Discuss the basic information that a nurse should provide to the expectant family to enable them to carry out appropriate self-care.

1. Fetal activity monitoring:
   - Cardiff Count-to-Ten Method: Lie quietly in the same position for 20–30 minutes each time. Should feel at least 10 fetal movements in 3 hours.
2. Breast care:
   - Wear a bra with good support and fit.
   - If breastfeeding, avoid soap on the nipples.
3. Nipple preparation:
   - Go braless to toughen nipples.
   - Roll nipple to prepare for breastfeeding. (Should be avoided in women who have had previous preterm labor.)
   - Have partner orally stimulate the nipple during sexual activity to help prepare nipple.
4. Clothing:
   - Should be loose and nonconstricting.
   - Wear low-heeled, comfortable, well-fitting shoes.
5. Bathing (be aware of cultural norms):
   - Be careful to avoid falls or feelings of faintness.
   - Shower may be easiest way to bathe in third trimester.
6. Employment:
   - Women with low-risk pregnancy can work until labor begins.
   - Workplace should be assessed for fetotoxic hazards.
7. Travel:
   - Avoid travel if woman has history of complications or has a multiple pregnancy.
   - With car travel, stop every 2 hours and walk. Position the seat belt under the abdomen.
8. Activity and rest:
   - Maintain regular exercise in uncomplicated pregnancy.
   - Avoid supine position.
   - Drink fluids and make sure to eat adequate amount of calories.
   - Avoid exercise during hot and humid weather.
   - Stop exercising with any suspicions of complications.
   - Plan for more sleep and regular rest periods.
   - Instruct in exercises to prepare for childbirth, including the pelvic tilt, partial sit-up, Kegel exercises, and the cross-legged sitting ("tailor sit") position.

LEARNING OBJECTIVES

CONCEPTS

9. Dental care:
    - Maintain regular dental checkups.
    - Dental work should be done in the second trimester.
    - Delay dental x-rays until after baby is born.
10. Immunizations:
    - Avoid live virus vaccines.
11. Complementary and alternative therapies:
    - The nurse should develop understanding of most common ones.
    - The nurse should provide printed information about risks and benefits of homeopathic remedies and herbs.
12. Medications:
    - Avoid all OTC medications.
    - Take only medications approved by healthcare provider.
13. Substances to avoid during pregnancy:
    - All of the following should be avoided completely or decrease the amount of substance used: tobacco, alcohol, marijuana, and cocaine.
    - Caffeine has not been proven to impact pregnancy so women should be advised concerning common sources of caffeine and advised to moderate its use.

Delineate some of the concerns that an expectant couple might have about sexual activity.

1. Traditional positions for intercourse may be uncomfortable; consider alternative positions
2. Sexual desire may change during pregnancy.
3. Partners need to communicate feelings and needs.
4. Intercourse is contraindicated in:
    - Multiple pregnancy.
    - Threatened abortion.
    - Incompetent cervix.
    - Sexually transmitted infection.
    - Miscarriage following orgasm.
    - Rupture of membranes.
    - Preterm labor.

Summarize the medical risks and special concerns of the older expectant mother and her partner.

1. Medical risks:
    - Fetal death risk is increased for all women older than 35.
    - Mother is more likely to have chronic medical conditions such as diabetes and hypertension that could pose a risk to the fetus.
    - Increased risk for cesarean birth.
    - Increased risk for Down syndrome and all autosomal dominant inherited disorders.
2. Special concerns:
    - Parents' ability to meet needs of child.
    - Not doing same things as peers, which could lead to social isolation.
    - Concern that "biological clock" continues to tick.
    - Fear of own mortality.

CRITICAL THINKING IN ACTION

View the **Critical Thinking in Action** video in Chapter 11 of the CD-ROM. Then, answer the questions that follow.

Thirty-seven-year-old Cathy Sommers, G1, P0000, presents to you, with her husband, at the OB physician's office at 32 weeks' gestation. Cathy tells you that she and her husband are practicing lawyers with their own firm. The couple delayed starting a family because it has been important to them to advance their careers and establish their firm. Cathy had an amniocentesis at 18 weeks' gestation because of her advanced maternal age, and the results ruled out chromosomal abnormalities. The couple knows that the baby is a boy and are anticipating a vaginal birth. Cathy tells you that she is experiencing more fatigue, leg cramps, and shortness of breath when climbing stairs. The physical exam including a negative Homans' sign is within normal limits with the exception of slight ankle edema. Her weight is 150 lb, temperature 98.6°F, pulse 88, respirations 16, BP 126/70. You discuss pregnancy discomforts in the third trimester with Cathy and her husband.

1. What measures can you suggest to cope with fatigue?
2. Discuss measures to decrease leg cramps.
3. Discuss the physiologic changes underlying dyspnea.
4. Review Braxton Hicks contractions.

MEDIALINK
www.prenhall.com/london

- NCLEX-RN® Review, case studies, and other interactive resources for this chapter can be found on the Companion Website at http://www.prenhall.com/london. Click on "Chapter 11" to select the activities for this chapter.

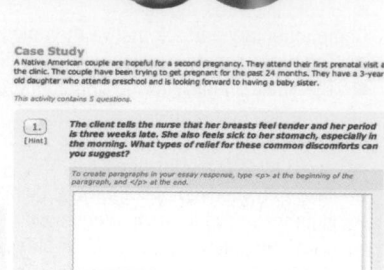

- For animations, more NCLEX-RN® Review questions, and an audio glossary, access the accompanying CD-ROM in this textbook.

REFERENCES

American College of Obstetricians and Gynecologists. (2000a). *Planning your pregnancy and birth* (3rd ed.). Washington, DC: Author.

American College of Obstetricians and Gynecologists. (2000b). *Smoking cessation during pregnancy* (ACOG Educational Bulletin No. 260). Washington, DC: Author.

American College of Obstetricians and Gynecologists. (2002). *Exercise during pregnancy and the postpartum period* (ACOG Technical Bulletin No. 267). Washington, DC: Author.

American College of Obstetricians and Gynecologists. (2004). *Diagnosis and treatment of nausea and vomiting in pregnancy* (ACOG Practice Bulletin No. 52). Washington, DC: Author.

Baer, J. S., Sampson, P. D., Barr, H. M., Connor, P. D., & Streissguth, A. P. (2003). A 21-year longitudinal analysis of the effects of prenatal alcohol exposure on young adult drinking. *Archives of General Psychiatry, 60*(4), 377–385.

Belew, C. (1999). Herbs and the childbearing woman: Guidelines for midwives. *Journal of Nurse-Midwifery, 44*(3), 231–246.

Black, R. A., & Hill, D. A. (2003). Over-the-counter medications in pregnancy. *American Family Physician, 67*(12), 2517–2524.

Blatt, S. D., Meguid, V., & Church, C. C. (2000). Prenatal cocaine: What's known about outcomes? *Contemporary OB/GYN, 45*(9), 67–81.

Blumenthal, M. (2003). Ginger as an antiemetic during pregnancy. *Alternative Therapies in Health and Medicine, 9,* 19–21.

Bracken, M. B., Triche, E. W., Belanger, K., Hellenbrand, K., & Leaderer, B. P. (2003). Association of maternal caffeine consumption with decrements in fetal growth. *American Journal of Epidemiology, 157*(5), 456–466.

Callaghan, W. M., & Berg, C. J. (2003). Pregnancy-related mortality among women aged 35 years and older, United States, 1991–1997. *Obstetrics and Gynecology, 102*(5, Pt. 1), 1015–1021.

Carl, D. L., Roux, G., & Matacale, R. (2000). Exploring dental hygiene and perinatal outcomes. *AWHONN Lifelines, 4*(1), 22–27.

Cesario, S. K. (2001). Care of the Native American woman: Strategies for practice, education, and research. *Journal of Obstetric, Gynecologic, and Neonatal Nursing, 30*(1), 13–19.

Chez, R. A., & Niebyl, J. (2000). Management of nausea and vomiting in pregnancy: Traditional therapies. *Contemporary OB/GYN, 45*(3), 130–136.

Choi, E. C. (1995). A contrast of mothering behaviors in women from Korea and the United States. *Journal of Obstetric, Gynecologic, and Neonatal Nursing, 24*(4), 363–369.

Chung, K. C., Kowalski, C. P., Kim, H. M., & Buchman, S. R. (2000). Maternal cigarette smoking during pregnancy and the risk of having a child with cleft lip/palate. *Plastic and Reconstructive Surgery, 105*(2), 485–491.

Clapp, J. F., III. (2001). Recommending exercise during pregnancy. *Contemporary OB/GYN, 46*(1), 30–40.

Cleveland Clinic. (2004). *Quad marker screen.* Retrieved April 10, 2004, from http://www.cchs.net/health/health-info/docs/0300/ 0386.asp?index=4698

Cunningham, F. G., Gant, N. F., Leveno, K. J., Gilstrap, L. C., III, Hauth, J. C., & Wenstrom, K. D. (2001). *Williams obstetrics* (21st ed.). New York: McGraw-Hill.

Davies, G. A., Wolfe, L. A., Mottola, M. F., MacKinnon, C., Arsenault, M. Y., Bartellas, E., et al. (2003). SOGC Clinical Practice Obstetrics Committee, Canadian Society for Exercise Physiology Board of Directors. Exercise in pregnancy and the postpartum period. *Journal of Obstetrics and Gynaecology of Canada, 25,* 516–529.

Dolan, S. (2004). New approaches to screening for Down syndrome. *Medscape Ob/Gyn and Women's Health, 9*(1). Retrieved April 2, 2004, from http://www.medscape.com/viewarticle/469782_print

Eisenberg, D. M., Davis, R. B., Ettner, S. L., Appel, S., Wilkey, S., Van Rompey, M., et al. (1998). Trends in alternative medicine use in the United States, 1990–1997. *Journal of the American Medical Association, 280,* 1569–1575.

Fontaine, K. L. (2000). *Healing practices: Alternative therapies for nursing.* Upper Saddle River, NJ: Prentice Hall.

Heffernan, A. E. (2000). Exercise and pregnancy in primary care. *Nurse Practitioner, 25*(3), 42–60.

Hoyert, D. L., Danel, I., & Tully, P. (2000). Maternal mortality, United States and Canada, 1982–97. *Birth, 27*(1), 4–11.

Jackson, E. A. (2001). Is ginger root effective for decreasing the severity of nausea and vomiting in early pregnancy? *Journal of Family Practice, 50*(8), 720.

Jackson, M. T. (2003). Prenatal yoga: What you need to know. *Female Patient, 28*(2), 66–70.

Keating, A., & Chez, R. A. (2002). Ginger syrup as an antiemetic in early pregnancy. *Alternative Therapies in Health and Medicine, 8*(5), 89–91.

Kuczkowski, K. M. (2003). Tobacco and ethanol use in pregnancy: Implications for obstetric and anesthetic management. *Female Patient, 28*(4), 16–22.

Lie, D. (2004). *Ginger helpful for nausea and vomiting of pregnancy. Medscape CME offering.* Retrieved January 13, 2004, from http://www.medscape.com/viewarticle/466746_print

Martin, J. A., Hamilton, B. E., Sutton, P. D., Ventura, S. J., Menacker, F., & Munson, M. L. (2003). Births: Final data for 2002. *National Vital Statistics Reports, 52*(10), 1–114.

Mollart, L. (2003). Single-blind trial addressing the differential effects of two reflexology techniques versus rest, on ankle and foot oedema in late pregnancy. *Complementary Therapies in Nursing and Midwifery, 9*(4), 203–208.

Niebyl, J. R. (2002). Drugs in pregnancy and lactation. In S. G. Gabbe, J. R. Niebyl, & J. L. Simpson (Eds.), *Obstetrics: Normal and problem pregnancies*

(4th ed., pp. 221–250). New York: Churchill Livingstone.

Orleans, C. T., Barker, D. C., Kaufman, N. J., & Marx, J. F. (2001). Helping pregnant smokers quit: Meeting the challenge of the next decade. *Western Journal of Medicine, 174*(4), 276–281.

Pittler, M. H., & Ernst, E. (2002). Horse chestnut seed extract for chronic venous insufficiency (Cochrane Review). *The Cochrane Library, 2.* Oxford: Update Software.

Pollack, H., Lantz, P. M., & Frohna, J. G. (2000). Maternal smoking and adverse birth outcomes among singletons and twins. *American Journal of Public Health, 90*(3), 395–400.

Portnoi, G., Chng, L.A., Karimi-Tabesh, L., Koren, G., Tan, M. P., & Einarson, A. (2004). Prospective comparative study of the safety and effectiveness of ginger for the treatment of nausea and vomiting in pregnancy. *American Journal of Obstetrics and Gynecology, 189*(5), 1374–1377.

Rao, S., Kanade, A., Margetts, B. M., Yajnik, C. S., Lubree, H., Rege, S., et al. (2003). Maternal activity in relation to birth size in rural India. The Pune Maternal Nutrition Study. *European Journal of Clinical Nutrition, 57*(4), 531–542.

Roscoe, J. A., & Matteson, S. E. (2002). Acupressure and acustimulation bands for control of nausea: A brief review. *American Journal of Obstetrics and Gynecology, 186*(5), S244–247.

Salihu, H. M., Shumpert, M. N., Slay, M., Kirby, R. S., & Alexander, G. R. (2003). Childbearing beyond maternal age 50 and fetal outcomes in the United States. *Obstetrics and Gynecology, 102*(5, Pt. 1), 1006–1014.

Shrock, P. (2000). Exercise and physical activity during pregnancy. In J. J. Sciarra (Ed.), *Gynecology and obstetrics* (Vol. 2, chap. 8, pp. 1–17). Philadelphia: Lippincott Williams & Wilkins.

Smith, C., Crowther, C., Willson, K., Hotham, N., & McMillian, V. (2004). A randomized controlled trial of ginger to treat nausea and vomiting in pregnancy. *Obstetrics and Gynecology, 103*(4), 630–645.

Spector, R. E. (2004). *Cultural diversity in health and illness* (6th ed.). Upper Saddle River, NJ: Prentice-Hall Health.

Strandberg, T. E., Andersson, S., Jarvenpaa, A. L., & McKeigue, P. M. (2002). Preterm birth and licorice consumption during pregnancy. *American Journal of Epidemiology, 156*(9), 803–805.

Steele, N. M., French, J., Gatherer-Boyles, J., Newman, S., & Leclaire, S. (2001). Effect of acupressure by Sea-Bands on nausea and vomiting of pregnancy. *Journal of Obstetric, Gynecologic, and Neonatal Nursing, 30*(1), 61–70.

Tiran, D. (2003). The use of herbs by pregnant and childbearing women: A risk-benefit assessment. *Complementary Therapies in Nursing and Midwifery, 9,* 176–181.

Tough, S. C., Newburn-Cook, C., Johnston, D. W., Svenson, L. W., Rose, S., & Belitok, J. (2002). Delayed childbearing and its impact on population rate changes in lower birth weight, multiple births, and preterm delivery. *Pediatrics, 109*(3), 399–403.

Varney, H., Kriebs, J. M., & Gegor, C. L. (2004). *Varney's midwifery* (4th ed.). Sudbury, MA: Jones & Bartlett.

Windridge, K. C., & Berryman, J. C. (1999). Women's experiences of giving birth after 35. *Birth, 26*(1), 16–23.

Maternal Nutrition

When I was young I thought nutrition was boring. Now that I am pregnant I find it endlessly fascinating. I realize how important good nutrition is for me, for my husband, and for the well-being of our child. My mother just laughs and reminds me about the times I resisted her efforts to help me develop better eating habits. Oh well, it is just another example of how smart our parents get as we get older!

—Maria, 26

LEARNING OBJECTIVES

- Delineate recommended levels of weight gain during pregnancy.

- Identify the role of specific nutrients in the diet of the pregnant woman.

- Compare nutritional needs during pregnancy, the postpartum period, and lactation with nonpregnant requirements.

- Plan adequate prenatal vegetarian diets based on the nutritional requirements of pregnancy.

- Describe ways in which various physical, psychosocial, and cultural factors can affect nutritional intake and status.

- Compare recommendations for weight gain and nutrient intakes in the pregnant adolescent with those for the mature pregnant adult.

- Discuss basic factors a nurse should consider when offering nutritional counseling to a pregnant adolescent.

- Compare nutritional counseling issues for breastfeeding and formula-feeding mothers.

MEDIALINK www.prenhall.com/london

CD-ROM
NCLEX-RN® Review
Audio Glossary

Companion Website
NCLEX-RN® Review
Case Study: Maternal Weight Gain
Thinking Critically
Care Plan Activity: Maternal Nutrition

A woman's nutritional status before and during pregnancy can significantly influence her health and that of her fetus. In most prenatal clinics and offices, nurses offer nutritional counseling directly or work closely with the nutritionist in providing nutritional assessment and teaching. This chapter focuses on the nutritional needs of a normal pregnant woman. Special sections consider the nutritional needs of the pregnant adolescent and the woman after giving birth.

Fetal growth occurs in three overlapping stages: (1) growth by increase in cell number, (2) growth by increases in cell number and cell size, and (3) growth by increase in cell size alone. Nutritional problems that interfere with cell division may have permanent consequences. If the nutritional deficit occurs when cells are mainly enlarging, the changes are usually reversible when normal nutrition resumes.

Growing fetal and maternal tissues require increased quantities of essential dietary components. These are listed in the **dietary reference intakes (DRIs)** as either the recommended dietary allowance (RDA) or adequate intake (AI). An RDA is the daily dietary intake that is considered sufficient to meet the nutritional requirements of nearly all individuals in a specific life stage and gender group. An AI is a value cited for a nutrient when there is not sufficient data to calculate an estimated average requirement. Women can get most of the recommended nutrients by eating a well-balanced diet each day. The basic food groups and recommended amounts during pregnancy and lactation are presented in Table 12–1.

MATERNAL WEIGHT GAIN

Maternal weight gain is an important factor in fetal growth and infant birth weight. Optimal weight gain depends on the woman's weight for height (body mass index) and her prepregnant nutritional state. An adequate weight gain indicates an adequate caloric intake. However, it does not ensure that the woman has a good diet nutritionally. The pregnant woman must maintain the nutritional quality of her diet as her weight gain progresses.

The Institute of Medicine (1992) recommends optimum ranges of weight gain, as follows:

- Underweight woman: 28 to 40 lb (12.5 to 18 kg)
- Normal-weight woman: 25 to 35 lb (11.5 to 16 kg)
- Overweight woman: 15 to 25 lb (7 to 11.5 kg)
- Obese woman: ≤15 lb (≤7 kg)

The average maternal weight gain is distributed as follows:

11 lb (5 kg)	Fetus, placenta, amniotic fluid
2 lb (0.9 kg)	Uterus
4 lb (1.8 kg)	Increased blood volume
3 lb (1.4 kg)	Breast tissue
5 to 10 lb (2.3 to 4.5 kg)	Maternal stores

The pattern of weight gain is important. For a normal-weight woman, the ideal pattern of weight gain during pregnancy is a gain of 3.5 to 5 lb (1.6 to 2.3 kg) during the first trimester, followed by a gain of about 1 lb (0.5 kg) per week during the second and third trimesters. A normal-weight woman who is expecting twins should gain about 1.5 lb per week during the second and third trimesters of her pregnancy (Brown & Carlson, 2000).

Calorie, 273
Dietary reference intakes (DRIs), 271
Folic acid, 273
Kilocalorie, 273
Lactase deficiency (lactose intolerance), 281
Lacto-ovovegetarians, 278
Lactovegetarians, 278
Pica, 282
Vegans, 278

TABLE 12–1 ✤ Daily Food Plan for Pregnancy and Lactation

Food Group	Nutrients Provided	Food Source	Recommended Daily Amount During Pregnancy	Recommended Daily Amount During Lactation
Dairy products	Protein; riboflavin; vitamins A, D, and others; calcium; phosphorus; zinc; magnesium	Milk—whole, 2%, skim, dry, buttermilk Cheeses—hard, semisoft, cottage Yogurt—plain, low-fat Soybean milk—canned, dry	Four (8 oz) cups (five for teenagers) used plain or with flavoring, in shakes, soups, puddings, custards, cocoa Calcium in 1 cup milk equivalent to 1 1/2 cups cottage cheese, 1 1/2 oz hard or semisoft cheese, 1 cup yogurt, 1 1/2 cups ice cream (high in fat and sugar)	Four (8 oz) cups (five for teenagers); equivalent amount of cheese, yogurt, and so forth
Meat and meat alternatives	Protein; iron; thiamine, niacin, and other vitamins; and minerals	Beef, pork, veal, lamb, poultry, animal organ meats, fish, eggs; legumes; nuts, seeds, peanut butter, grains in proper vegetarian combination (vitamin B_{12} supplement needed)	Three servings (one serving = 2 oz), combination in amounts necessary for same nutrient equivalent (varies greatly)	Two servings
Grain products, whole grain or enriched	B vitamins; iron; whole grain also has zinc, magnesium, and other trace elements; provides fiber	Breads and bread products such as cornbread, muffins, waffles, hotcakes, biscuits, dumplings, cereals, pastas, rice	Six to 11 servings daily: one serving = one slice bread, 3/4 cup or 1 oz dry cereal, 1/2 cup rice or pasta	Same as for pregnancy
Fruits and fruit juices	Vitamins A and C; minerals; raw fruits for roughage	Citrus fruits and juices, melons, berries, all other fruits and juices	Two to four servings (one serving for vitamin C): one serving = one medium fruit, 1/2–1 cup fruit, 4 oz orange or grapefruit juice	Same as for pregnancy
Vegetables and vegetable juices	Vitamins A and C; minerals; provides roughage	Leafy green vegetables; deep yellow or orange vegetables such as carrots, sweet potatoes, squash, tomatoes; green vegetables such as peas, green beans, broccoli; other vegetables such as beets, cabbage, potatoes, corn, lima beans	Three to five servings (one serving of dark green or deep yellow vegetable for vitamin A): one serving = 1/2–1 cup vegetable, two tomatoes, one medium potato	Same as for pregnancy
Fats	Vitamins A and D; linoleic acid	Butter, cream cheese, fortified table spreads; cream, whipped cream, whipped toppings; avocado, mayonnaise, oil, nuts	As desired in moderation (high in calories): one serving = 1 tbsp butter or enriched margarine	Same as for pregnancy
Sugar and sweets		Sugar, brown sugar, honey, molasses	Occasionally, if desired	Same as for pregnancy
Desserts		Nutritious desserts such as puddings, custards, fruit whips, and crisps; other rich, sweet desserts and pastries	Occasionally, if desired	Same as for pregnancy
Beverages	Fluid	Coffee, decaffeinated beverages, tea, bouillon, carbonated drinks	As desired, in moderation	Same as for pregnancy
Miscellaneous		Iodized salt, herbs, spices, condiments	As desired	Same as for pregnancy

Note: The pregnant woman should eat regularly, three meals a day, with nutritious snacks of fruit, cheese, milk, or other foods between meals if desired. (More frequent but smaller meals are also recommended.) Four to 6 (8 oz) glasses of water and a total of 8 to 10 (8 oz) cups total fluid intake should be consumed daily. Water is an essential nutrient.

Pregnancy is not a time for dieting, and severe dieting during pregnancy can result in maternal ketosis, a threat to fetal well-being. In 2005 the traditional Food Pyramid, which had formed the basis for nutritional guidance for years, was replaced by new *Dietary Guidelines for Americans 2005*. These guidelines encourage people to eat fewer calories, to make wiser food choices, and to be more active (U.S. Department of Health and Human Services and U.S. Department of Agriculture, 2005). As part of this change, the concept of a personalized food pyramid based on age, weight, and activity level was introduced as MyPyramid (Figure 12–1 ●). People can access a Web site—*http://www.mypyramid.gov*—enter information about themselves, and receive a general nutrition plan. Counseling the pregnant woman to eat according to the new guidelines places less emphasis on the amount of her weight gain and more on the quality of her diet and on her activity level.

NURSING PRACTICE

Weight varies with time of day, amount of clothing, inaccurate scale adjustment, or weighing error. Do not overemphasize a single weight, but pay attention to the overall pattern of weight gain.

NUTRITIONAL REQUIREMENTS

The RDA for almost all nutrients increases during pregnancy, although the amount of increase varies with each nutrient. These increases reflect the additional requirements of both the mother and the developing fetus.

Folic acid and iron are the only nutritional supplements generally recommended during pregnancy. An adequate diet can usually meet the increased need for other vitamins and minerals. To avoid possible deficiencies, however, many healthcare professionals still recommend a daily vitamin supplement.

CALORIES

The term **calorie** (cal) designates the amount of heat required to raise the temperature of 1 g of water 1°C. The **kilocalorie** (kcal) is equivalent to 1000 cal and is the unit used to express the energy value of food.

The RDA for energy requirements during pregnancy is as follows: no increase during the first trimester but an increase of 300 kcal/day during the second and third trimesters. Prepregnant weight, height, maternal age, health status, and activity level all influence caloric needs, and weight should be monitored regularly during the pregnancy. See "Teaching Highlights: Adding 300 kcal During Pregnancy."

● **FIGURE 12-1**

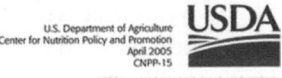

"MyPyramid: Steps to a Healthier You" identifies the basic food groups and provides guidance about healthful eating. Grains, vegetables, fruits, and dairy products are emphasized, with slightly less emphasis on protein. The narrow yellow bar is designated for fats, sugar, and salt. People are encouraged to have most of their fat intake come from fish, nuts, and vegetable oils while limiting solid fats like butter, margarine, shortening, and lard. The emphasis is also placed on limiting added sugars, which contribute calories but few, if any, nutrients.

Courtesy of the U.S. Department of Agriculture; U.S. Department of Health and Human Services.

TEACHING HIGHLIGHTS

ADDING 300 KCAL DURING PREGNANCY

- The notion of "eating for two" may result in overeating.
- The additional 300 kcal/day recommended during pregnancy can be achieved by adding two milk servings and one serving of meat or alternative.
- The MyPyramid guide (see Figure 12-1) is helpful in planning healthy meals. It is designed to represent the food groups needed to make a balanced diet.
- A balanced diet includes the following:
  1. Grains: Six to eleven servings (one serving = 1 slice bread, 1/2 hamburger roll, 1 oz dry cereal, 1 tortilla, 1/2 cup pasta, rice, grits)
  2. Fruits: Two to four servings; one should be a good source of vitamin C (one serving = 1 medium-sized piece of fruit, 1/2 cup juice)
  3. Vegetables: Three to five servings (one serving = 1 cup raw vegetable, 1 cup green leafy vegetable, 1/2 cup cooked vegetable)
  4. Dairy: Two to three servings (one serving = 1 cup milk or yogurt, 1.5 oz hard cheese, 2 cups cottage cheese, 1 cup pudding made with milk)

  5. Meats and alternatives: Two to three servings (one serving = 2 oz cooked lean meat, poultry, or fish; 2 eggs; 1/2 cup cottage cheese; 1 cup cooked legumes [kidney, lima, garbanzo, or soybeans, split peas]; 6 oz tofu; 2 oz nuts or seeds; 4 tbsp peanut butter)
- Not all foods that are nutritionally equivalent have the same number of calories; it is important to consider that when making food choices.
- Consider using low-fat milk, lean cuts of meat, or fish broiled or baked instead of fried.
- Foods can be combined. For example, 1 cup spaghetti with a 2-oz meatball would count as 1 serving meat, 3/4 cup spaghetti = 1 grain, and 1/4 cup tomato sauce = 1/2 serving vegetable.
- Use a calorie-counting guide to compare the calories in a variety of foods that are equivalent, such as 2 oz beef and 2 oz fish or 1 cup low-fat milk and 1 cup whole milk.

CARBOHYDRATES

Carbohydrates provide the body's main source of energy as well as the fiber necessary for proper bowel functioning. If the total caloric intake is not adequate, the body uses protein for energy. Protein then becomes unavailable for growth needs. In addition, protein breakdown leads to ketosis.

The carbohydrate and caloric needs of the pregnant woman increase, especially during the last two trimesters. Carbohydrate intake promotes weight gain and growth of the fetus, placenta, and other maternal tissues. Dairy products, fruits, vegetables, and whole-grain cereals and breads all contain carbohydrates and other important nutrients.

PROTEIN

Protein supplies the amino acids required for the growth and development of maternal tissues, such as the uterus and breasts, and to meet fetal needs. This is especially important during the last half of pregnancy, when fetal growth is greatest.

The protein requirement for a pregnant woman is 60 g/day, an increase of 14 g over nonpregnant levels. Animal products such as meat, fish, poultry, and eggs provide high-quality protein. Dairy products are also important protein sources. A quart of milk supplies 32 g of protein, more than half the average daily protein requirement. A woman can incorporate milk into her diet in a variety of dishes, including soups, puddings, custards, sauces, and yogurt. Beverages such as hot chocolate and milk-and-fruit

drinks can also be included, but they are high in calories. Various kinds of hard and soft cheeses and cottage cheese are excellent protein sources, although cream cheese is considered a fat source only. Women who have allergies to milk, are lactose intolerant, or practice vegetarianism may find soy milk acceptable. It can be used in cooked dishes or as a beverage. Tofu, or soybean curd, can replace cottage cheese.

FAT

Fats are valuable sources of energy for the body. Fats are more completely absorbed during pregnancy, resulting in a marked increase in serum lipids, lipoproteins, and cholesterol, and decreased elimination of fat through the bowel. Fat deposits in the fetus increase from about 2% at midpregnancy to almost 12% at term. However, fat requirements are unchanged during pregnancy and should account for about 30% of daily caloric intake, of which less than 10% should be saturated fat.

MINERALS

Calcium and Phosphorus

Calcium and phosphorus are involved in the mineralization of fetal bones and teeth and acid-base buffering. The body absorbs and uses calcium more efficiently during pregnancy. Some calcium and phosphorus are required early in pregnancy, but most fetal bone calcification occurs during the last 2 to 3 months. Teeth begin to form at about

COMPLEMENTARY CARE

ESSENTIAL FATTY ACIDS

The essential fatty acids (EFAs) are important for the development of the central nervous system of the fetus. The omega-3 fatty acids are of particular importance in the American diet, including their derivative, docosahexaenoic acid (DHA). Maternal dietary intake of DHA during pregnancy and breastfeeding enhances infant attention and visual development (Agostoni & Verduci, 2003; Smuts, Borod, Peeples, & Carlson, 2003). Studies have also shown that an intake of omega-3 fatty acids during pregnancy may lower the risk of preterm birth (Olsen & Secher, 2002; Smuts, Huang et al., 2003; Villar et al., 2003).

The best sources of omega-3 fatty acids are flaxseeds and their oil, and fish oils (but see the information regarding fish consumption under "Mercury in Fish" later in this chapter). Another source includes eggs that have been enriched with omega-3 fatty acids, which can now be purchased in grocery stores.

8 weeks' gestation and are formed by birth. The 6-year molars begin to calcify just before birth.

The identified AI for calcium for the pregnant or lactating woman, age 19 or older, is 1000 mg/day. It is 1300 mg/day for pregnant women under age 19. If calcium intake is low, fetal needs will be met at the mother's expense by demineralization of bone.

A diet that includes 4 cups of milk or an equivalent dairy alternative will provide sufficient calcium. Smaller amounts of calcium are supplied by legumes, nuts, dried fruits, and dark green leafy vegetables (such as kale, cabbage, collards, and turnip greens).

The RDA for phosphorus is 700 mg/day for the pregnant or lactating woman age 19 and older. It is 1250 mg/day for pregnant women under 19 years. Because phosphorus is so widely available in foods, the daily requirement is readily supplied through calcium- and protein-rich foods.

Iodine

Iodine is an essential part of the thyroid hormone thyroxine. The thyroid gland may become enlarged if iodine is not replaced by adequate dietary intake or an additional supplement. Moreover, cretinism may occur in the infant if the mother has a severe iodine deficiency. Pregnant women can meet the iodine allowance of 220 mcg/day by using iodized salt. When salt is restricted, the physician may prescribe an iodine supplement.

Sodium

Sodium is essential for proper metabolism and the regulation of fluid balance. Sodium intake in the form of salt is never entirely restricted during pregnancy, even when hypertension is present. The pregnant woman may season food to taste during cooking but should avoid using extra salt at the table. She can avoid excessive intake by eliminating salty foods such as potato chips, ham, sausages, and sodium-based seasonings.

Zinc

Zinc is needed for protein metabolism and the synthesis of DNA and RNA. It is essential for normal fetal growth and development as well as milk production during lactation. The RDA during pregnancy is 11 mg/day for women age 19 and older. This increases to 12 mg during lactation. Sources include meats, shellfish, poultry, whole grains, and legumes.

Magnesium

Magnesium is essential for cellular metabolism and structural growth. The RDA for pregnancy is 350 mg/day for women age 19 to 30. Good sources include milk, whole grains, dark green vegetables, nuts, and legumes.

Iron

Iron requirements increase during pregnancy because of the growth of the fetus and placenta and the increased maternal blood volume. Anemia in pregnancy is mainly caused by low iron stores, although it may also be caused by inadequate intake of other nutrients, such as vitamins B_6 and B_{12}, folic acid, ascorbic acid, copper, and zinc. Iron deficiency anemia is generally defined as a decrease in the oxygen-carrying capacity of the blood. Anemia leads to a significant reduction in hemoglobin in the volume of packed red cells per deciliter of blood (hematocrit) or in the number of erythrocytes. Iron deficiency anemia is associated with a higher incidence of preterm birth and low-birth-weight infants (Salzberg, 2002).

Fetal demands for iron further contribute to symptoms of anemia in the pregnant woman. The fetal liver stores iron, especially during the third trimester. The infant needs this stored iron during the first 4 months of life to compensate for the normally inadequate levels of iron in breast milk and non-iron-fortified formulas.

To prevent anemia the woman must balance iron requirements and intake. Adequate iron intake is a problem for nonpregnant women and a greater one for pregnant women. By carefully choosing foods high in iron, the woman can increase her daily iron intake considerably. Lean meats, dark green leafy vegetables, eggs, and whole-grain and enriched breads and cereals are the usual food sources of iron. Other iron sources include dried fruits, legumes, shellfish, and molasses.

Iron absorption is usually higher for animal products than for vegetable products. However, the woman can increase absorption of iron from nonmeat sources by combining them with meat or a food rich in vitamin C. The RDA for iron during pregnancy is 27 mg/day, but this intake is almost impossible to achieve through diet alone. Thus, the pregnant woman should take a supplement of simple iron salt, such as ferrous gluconate, ferrous fumarate, or ferrous sulfate. A daily supplement of 30 mg elemental iron is recommended by most healthcare providers beginning at the first prenatal visit. Unfortunately, iron supplements often cause gastrointestinal discomfort, especially if taken on an empty stomach. Taking the iron supplement after a meal may help reduce this discomfort. Iron supplements may also cause constipation, so an adequate fluid intake is important in pregnancy.

VITAMINS

Vitamins are organic substances needed for life and growth. They are found in small amounts in specific foods and generally cannot be synthesized by the body in adequate amounts.

Vitamins are grouped according to solubility. Vitamins A, D, E, and K dissolve in fat; vitamin C and the B-complex vitamins dissolve in water. An adequate intake of all vitamins is essential during pregnancy; however, several are required in larger amounts to fulfill specific needs.

Fat-Soluble Vitamins

The fat-soluble vitamins, A, D, E, and K, are stored in the liver and thus are available if the dietary intake becomes inadequate. The major complication related to these vitamins is not deficiency but toxicity due to overdose. Unlike water-soluble vitamins, excess amounts of vitamins A, D, E, and K are not excreted in the urine. Symptoms of vitamin toxicity include nausea, gastrointestinal upset, dryness and cracking of the skin, and loss of hair.

Vitamin A is involved in the growth of epithelial cells, which line the entire gastrointestinal tract and make up the skin. It also plays a role in the metabolism of carbohydrates and fats. Without vitamin A the body cannot synthesize glycogen, and the body's ability to handle cholesterol is also affected. In addition the protective layer of tissue surrounding nerve fibers does not form properly if vitamin A is lacking.

Probably the best known function of vitamin A is its effect on vision in dim light. A person's ability to see in the dark depends on the eye's supply of retinol, a form of vitamin A. Adequate vitamin A prevents night blindness. Vitamin A is associated with the formation and development of healthy eyes in the fetus. The RDA for vitamin A is 770 mcg/day for pregnant women age 19 and older.

Although routine supplementation with vitamin A is not recommended, supplementation with 5000 international units is indicated for women whose dietary intake may be inadequate, such as strict vegetarians and recent emigrants from countries where deficiency of vitamin A is endemic (American College of Obstetricians and Gynecologists [ACOG], 1998). Rich sources of vitamin A include deep green, deep orange, and yellow vegetables; animal sources include egg yolk, cream, butter, and fortified margarine and milk.

Vitamin D is best known for its role in the absorption and use of calcium and phosphorus in skeletal development. To supply the needs of the developing fetus, the pregnant woman should have a vitamin D intake of 5 mcg/day. Main food sources of vitamin D include fortified milk, margarine, butter, and egg yolks. Drinking a quart of milk daily provides the vitamin D needed during pregnancy. Exposure to the ultraviolet rays of sunlight is also an important source of vitamin D. However, season, time of day, latitude, smog, cloud cover, and sunscreens affect ultraviolet ray exposure. (*Note:* It is still important to use sunscreens routinely.) For example, the average amount of sunlight in Boston and in points further north is insufficient to produce significant synthesis of vitamin D from November through February. Thus, it is vital for people with limited sun exposure to consume a diet that contains good sources of vitamin D (National Institutes of Health, 2002).

Excessive intake of vitamin D usually comes from high-potency vitamin preparations, not from the diet. Overdoses during pregnancy can cause hypercalcemia, or high blood calcium levels, due to withdrawal of calcium from the skeletal tissue. Symptoms of toxicity include excessive thirst, loss of appetite, vomiting, weight loss, irritability, and high blood calcium levels.

The major function of vitamin E, or tocopherol, is antioxidation. Vitamin E takes on oxygen, thus preventing another substance from undergoing chemical change. For example, vitamin E helps spare vitamin A by preventing its oxidation in the intestinal tract and in the tissues. It decreases the oxidation of polyunsaturated fats, thus helping to retain the flexibility and health of the cell membrane. For this reason, vitamin E affects the health of all cells in the body.

Vitamin E is also involved in certain enzymatic and metabolic reactions. It is essential for the synthesis of nucleic acids required in the formation of red blood cells in the bone marrow. Vitamin E is useful in treating certain types of muscular pain and intermittent claudication, in surface healing of wounds and burns, and in protecting lung tissue from the damaging effects of smog. These functions may help explain the abundant claims and cures attributed to vitamin E, many of which have not been scientifically proved.

The recommended intake of vitamin E for pregnant women is unchanged at 15 mg/day. The vitamin E requirement varies with the polyunsaturated fat content of the diet. Vitamin E is widely distributed in foodstuffs, especially vegetable fats and oils, whole grains, greens, and eggs. Excessive intake of vitamin E has been associated with abnormal coagulation in the newborn.

Vitamin K, or menadione (as used synthetically in medicine), is essential for the synthesis of prothrombin, so its function is related to normal blood clotting. It is synthesized in the intestinal tract by the *Escherichia coli* bacteria normally found in the large intestine. However, the body's need for vitamin K is not totally met by synthesis. Green leafy vegetables are excellent sources. The RDA for vitamin K does not increase during pregnancy.

Intake of vitamin K is usually adequate in a well-balanced prenatal diet. Problems may arise if an illness is present that results in malabsorption of fats or if antibiotics are used for an extended period, which would inhibit vitamin K synthesis by destroying intestinal *E. coli.*

Water-Soluble Vitamins

Water-soluble vitamins are excreted in the urine. Since only small amounts are stored, adequate amounts must be consumed daily. During pregnancy the concentration of water-soluble vitamins in the maternal serum falls, whereas high concentrations are found in the fetus.

The RDA for vitamin C (ascorbic acid) increases in pregnancy from 75 to 85 mg. Vitamin C's major function is to aid in the formation and development of connective tissue and the vascular system. Ascorbic acid is essential to the formation of collagen, which binds cells together. If the collagen begins to disintegrate because of a lack of ascorbic acid, cell functioning is disturbed and cell structure breaks down, resulting in muscular weakness, capillary hemorrhage, and eventual death. These are symptoms of scurvy, the disease caused by vitamin C deficiency. Infants fed mainly cow's milk become deficient in vitamin C, and they are the main group that develops these symptoms. Surprisingly, newborns of women who have taken megadoses of vitamin C may have a rebound form of scurvy.

Maternal plasma levels of vitamin C progressively decrease during pregnancy, with values at term being about half those found at midpregnancy. It appears that ascorbic acid concentrates in the placenta; levels in the fetus are 50% or more above maternal levels.

A nutritious diet should meet the pregnant woman's needs for vitamin C without additional supplementation. Common food sources of vitamin C include citrus fruit, tomatoes, cantaloupe, strawberries, potatoes, broccoli, and other leafy greens. Ascorbic acid is readily destroyed by water and oxidation. Therefore, foods containing vitamin C must be stored and cooked properly.

The B vitamins include thiamine (B_1), riboflavin (B_2), niacin, folic acid, pantothenic acid, vitamin B_6, and vitamin B_{12}. These vitamins serve as vital coenzyme factors in many reactions such as cell respiration, glucose oxidation, and energy metabolism. The quantities needed increase as caloric intake increases to meet the metabolic and growth needs of the pregnant woman.

The thiamine requirement increases from the prepregnant level of 1.1 mg/day to 1.4 mg/day. Sources include pork, milk, potatoes, and enriched breads and cereals.

Riboflavin deficiency is manifested by cheilosis (fissures and cracks of the lips and corners of the mouth) and other skin lesions. During pregnancy, women may excrete less riboflavin and still require more because of increased energy and protein needs. An additional 0.3 mg/day, to 1.4 mg/day, is recommended for pregnant women age 19 and older. Sources include milk, eggs, enriched breads, and cereals.

Niacin intake should increase 4 mg/day during pregnancy to 18 mg/day. Sources of niacin include meat, fish, poultry, whole grains, enriched breads, cereals, and peanuts.

Folic acid, or folate, is required for normal growth, reproduction, and lactation and prevents the macrocytic, megaloblastic anemia of pregnancy. Megaloblastic anemia due to folate deficiency is rarely found in the United States, but it does occur.

Even more significantly, an inadequate intake of folic acid has been associated with neural tube defects (NTDs) (spina bifida, meningomyelocele) in the fetus or newborn. Although these defects are considered multifactorial (see Chapter 7 ∞), the Centers for Disease Control and Prevention (CDC) estimates that 50% to 70% of spina bifida and anencephaly could be prevented by adequate intake of folic acid (CDC, 2005). Consequently experts recommend that all women of childbearing age (15 to 45 years) consume 400 mcg of folic acid daily because half of all U.S. pregnancies are unplanned and NTDs occur very early in pregnancy (3 to 4 weeks after conception), before most women realize they are pregnant (National Center on Birth Defects and Developmental Disabilities, 2004). The best food sources of folates are fresh green leafy vegetables, liver, peanuts, and whole-grain breads and cereals. Folic acid can be made inactive by oxidation, ultraviolet light, and heating. It can easily be lost during improper storage and cooking. To prevent unnecessary loss, foods should be stored covered to protect them from light, cooked with only a small amount of water, and not overcooked. See "Evidence-Based Nursing: Folate Supplementation in Pregnancy."

No allowance has been set for pantothenic acid in pregnancy, but 5 mg/day is considered a safe, adequate intake. Sources include meats, egg yolk, legumes, and whole-grain cereals and breads.

Vitamin B_6 (pyridoxine) is associated with amino acid metabolism; thus, a higher-than-average protein intake requires increased pyridoxine intake. The RDA for vitamin B_6 during pregnancy is 1.9 mg/day, an increase of 0.6 mg over the allowance for nonpregnant women. Generally the slightly increased need can be supplied by dietary sources, which include wheat germ, yeast, fish, liver, pork, potatoes, and lentils.

Vitamin B_{12}, or cobalamin, is the cobalt-containing vitamin found only in animal sources. Women of reproductive age rarely have a B_{12} deficiency. Vegans (see later discussion on vegetarian diets) can develop a deficiency, however, so it is essential that their dietary intake be supplemented with this vitamin. The RDA during pregnancy

EVIDENCE-BASED NURSING

FOLATE SUPPLEMENTATION IN PREGNANCY

Clinical Question

What are the effects of prenatal folate supplementation on neonatal neural tube defects?

Evidence

Two experts in obstetrics assessed the quality of randomized controlled trials involving 6,425 women. The review was specific to the effects of folate supplements on neonatal neural tube defects. The evidence is clear and compelling that prenatal folate supplementation has a strong protective effect against neural tube defects.

Implications

Prenatal folate supplementation significantly reduces the risk of neonatal neural tube defects. The reduction in risk is the same for mothers who have never had a baby with a defect and for those with a previously affected infant. The evidence supporting prevention of recurrent defects is so strong that offering routine folate supplementation of *0.4 mg (400 mcg)* per day is widely accepted as public health policy. Supplemental folate was not associated with an increase in miscarriage, ectopic pregnancy, or stillbirth.

There is uncertainty as to whether counseling about modifying the diet to include foods rich in folate—as opposed to supplementation—consistently results in an adequate daily dosage of folate. Dietary strategies appear to be most helpful when initiated at least 2 months prior to conception. There was no information provided about the risks of overconsumption of folate during pregnancy.

All women who have a previous fetus or newborn with a diagnosed neural tube defect need to be given information about the risk of recurrence in subsequent pregnancies, and advised to routinely take *4 mg per day (4000 mcg)* of a folate supplement. Encourage all women who are considering pregnancy to increase their dietary intake of foods rich in folate, ideally at least 2 months before conception. Add a caution, though, that dietary intake alone may not be enough during pregnancy, and recommend folate supplementation. You can reassure women that folate supplements do not appear to present any increased risks for the fetus.

Critical Thinking

What dietary modifications can you recommend that would help women increase their consumption of naturally occurring folate? How can you incorporate these recommendations into your counseling of all women of childbearing age?

Reference

Lumley, J., Watson, L., Watson, M., & Bower, C. (2003). Periconceptional supplementation with folate and/or multivitamins for preventing neural tube defects (Cochrane Review). In: *The Cochrane Library,* Issue 4. Chichester, UK: John Wiley & Sons.

---

is 2.6 mcg/day, an increase of 0.2 mcg. A deficiency may be due to a congenital inability to absorb vitamin B_{12}, resulting in pernicious anemia. Infertility is a complication of this type of anemia.

FLUID

Water is essential for life, and it is found in all body tissues. It is necessary for many biochemical reactions. It also serves as a lubricant, as a medium of transport for carrying substances in and out of the body, and as an aid in temperature control. A pregnant woman should consume at least 8 to 10 (8-oz) glasses of fluid each day, of which 4 to 6 glasses should be water. Because of their sodium content, diet sodas should be consumed in moderation. Caffeinated beverages have a diuretic effect, which is counterproductive to increasing fluid intake.

VEGETARIANISM

Vegetarianism is the dietary choice of many people for religious, health, or ethical reasons. There are several types of vegetarians. **Lacto-ovovegetarians** include milk, dairy products, and eggs in their diet. **Lactovegetarians** include dairy products but no eggs in their diets. **Vegans** are

COMPLEMENTARY CARE

NUTRITIONAL CONTENT OF HERBS

Several herbs are good sources of various vitamins and minerals. Like other "whole" foods, herbs contain all the necessary nutrients and enzymes to increase bioavailability versus isolated substances (such as in vitamin and mineral supplements).

Dandelion root and herb: Contains high concentrations of vitamins A and C, beta-carotene, and potassium (Blumenthal, 2000; Kemper, 1999).

Oat straw: Rich in calcium and magnesium, plus iron, manganese, and zinc (Blumenthal, 2000; Skidmore-Roth, 2004). Note that this is the same plant from which we derive oatmeal.

Raspberry leaf: Contains vitamin C and naturally chelated iron (Skidmore-Roth, 2004).

It is best to advise pregnant women interested in using herbs to follow three basic principles: (1) if at all possible, avoid the use of herbs, even tonic herbs, during the first trimester (with the exception of ginger in amounts less than 1 g daily); (2) avoid standardized or highly concentrated extracts because the risk of side effects tends to be higher than with whole plant extracts; and (3) do not take essential oils internally (Belew, 1999).

THINKING CRITICALLY

Jaya Singh, a 28-year-old, G1P0, is 14 weeks pregnant. The rate and total amount of her weight gain during the first trimester have been consistent with recommendations. She has gained an average of 0.5 kg (1 lb) per week during both of the past 2 weeks. Her appetite is good, and she consumes three meals per day and snacks between meals on occasion.

Jaya has altered her diet because she is concerned about excessive weight gain. She told you that she has decreased her intake from the bread and dairy groups in order to limit her calorie intake. Because she has omitted most dairy products, she has increased her consumption of salads and broccoli to provide calcium sources.

A diet history revealed the following:

Grain	3-4 servings, mainly cereal and rice
Fruit	2-4 servings, fresh fruit
Vegetables	3-5 servings, salads, peas, corn, broccoli
Meat	4-5 servings, beef, pork, chicken
Dairy	occasionally cheese, ice cream, pudding
Fats, oils, sweets	occasionally salad dressings, margarine, desserts
Beverages	8-10 servings, soda, juices, water

After assessing her diet history, what is your evaluation of Jaya's diet? How would you counsel her?

"pure" vegetarians who will not eat any food from animal sources.

The expectant mother who is vegetarian must eat the proper combination of foods to obtain adequate nutrients. If her diet allows, a woman can obtain ample and complete proteins from dairy products and eggs. An adequate, pure vegan diet contains protein from unrefined grains (brown rice, whole wheat), legumes (beans, split peas, lentils), nuts in large quantities, and a variety of cooked and fresh vegetables and fruits. Complete proteins can be obtained by eating different types of plant-based proteins such as beans and rice, peanut butter on whole-grain bread, and whole-grain cereal with soy milk, either in the same meal or over the day. Seeds may provide adequate protein in the vegetarian diet if the quantity is large enough. Obtaining sufficient calories to ensure adequate weight gain may be difficult because vegan diets tend to be high in fiber and therefore filling. Figure 12–2 depicts the vegetarian food pyramid.

A daily supplement of 1 mg of vitamin B_{12} is necessary because vegans use no animal products. If the woman uses soy milk, only partial supplementation may be needed. If she uses no soy milk, she needs daily supplements of 1200 mg of calcium and 10 mcg of vitamin D.

Because the best sources of iron and zinc are animal products, vegan diets may also be low in these minerals. In addition a high fiber intake may reduce mineral (calcium, iron, and zinc) bioavailability. Nurses need to emphasize the use of foods containing these nutrients. A vegetarian food group guide appears in Table 12–2.

FIGURE 12-2

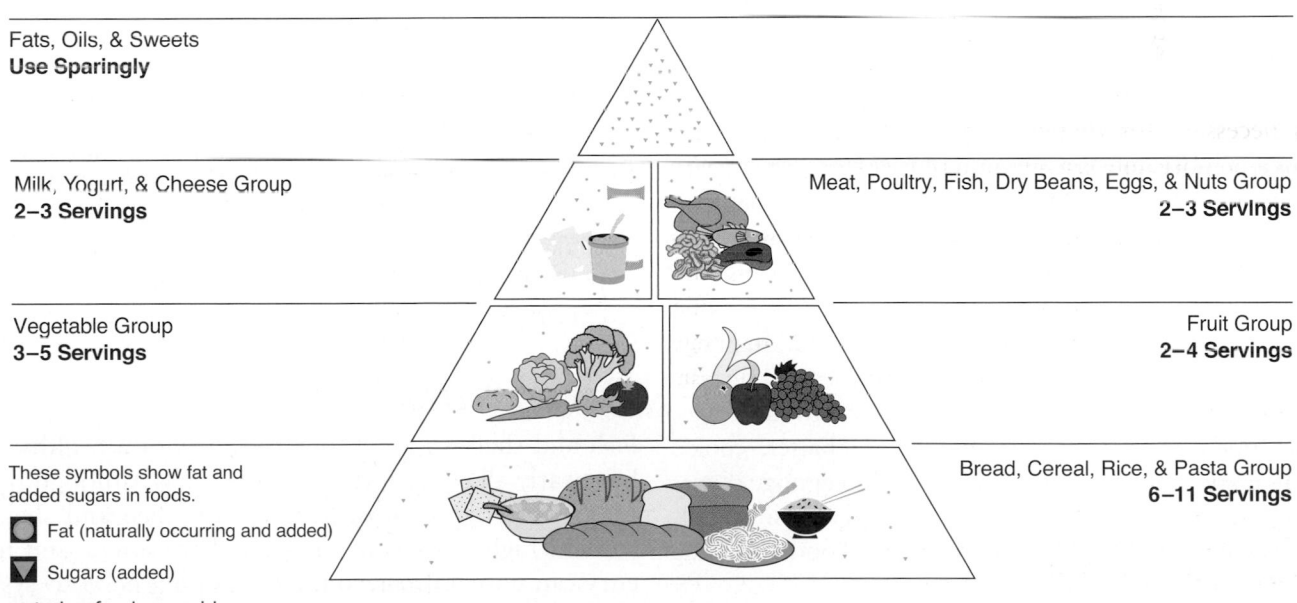

The vegetarian food pyramid.

Adapted with permission from the Health Connection, 55 West Oak Ridge Drive, Hagerstown, MD 21740-7390.

TABLE 12–2 ✤ Vegetarian Food Groups

Food Group	Mixed Diet	Lacto-ovovegetarian	Lactovegetarian	Vegan
Grain	Bread, cereal, rice, pasta	Bread, cereal, rice, pasta	Bread, cereal, rice, pasta	Bread, cereal, rice, pasta
Fruit	Fruit, fruit juices	Fruit, fruit juices	Fruit, fruit juices	Fruit, fruit juices
Vegetable	Vegetables, vegetable juices	Vegetables, vegetable juices	Vegetables, vegetable juices	Vegetables, vegetable juices
Dairy and dairy alternatives	Milk, yogurt, cheese	Milk, yogurt, cheese	Milk, yogurt, cheese	Fortified soy milk, rice milk
Meat and meat alternatives	Meat, fish, poultry, eggs, legumes, tofu, nuts, nut butters	Eggs, legumes, tofu, nuts, nut butters	Legumes, tofu, nuts, nut butters	Legumes, tofu, nuts, nut butters

FACTORS INFLUENCING NUTRITION

It is important to consider the many factors that affect a client's nutrition. What are the age, lifestyle, and culture of the pregnant woman? What food beliefs and habits does she have? What a person eats is determined by availability, economics, and symbolism. These factors and others influence the expectant mother's acceptance of dietary recommendations.

COMMON DISCOMFORTS OF PREGNANCY

Gastrointestinal functioning can be altered at times during pregnancy, resulting in discomforts such as nausea, vomiting, heartburn, and constipation. Although these changes can be uncomfortable for the woman, they are seldom a major problem. These discomforts and dietary modifications that may provide relief are discussed in Chapter 11. ∞

SALMONELLA AND *LISTERIA* INFECTION

The pregnant woman's immune system is somewhat weakened during pregnancy, As a result, pregnant women and their fetuses are at high risk for foodborne illnesses, which can cause miscarriage, serious health problems, or even maternal death.

Because of the risk of *Salmonella* contamination in raw eggs, pregnant women are advised to avoid eating or tasting foods that may contain raw or lightly cooked eggs. These foods include, for example, cake batter, cookie dough made with raw eggs, homemade eggnog, sauces made with raw eggs such as Caesar salad dressing, hollandaise sauce, and homemade ice cream (Food and Drug Administration [FDA], 2005).

Listeria monocytogenes is another bacterium that poses a threat to an expectant mother and her fetus. *Listeria* is especially challenging because the organism can be found in refrigerated, ready-to-eat foods such as unpasteurized milk and dairy products, meat, poultry, and seafood. To prevent listeria infection (listeriosis) pregnant women should be advised to do the following (FDA, 2005):

- Maintain refrigerator temperature at 40°F (4°C) or below and the freezer at 0°F (−18°C).
- Refrigerate or freeze prepared foods, leftovers, and perishables within 2 hours after eating or preparation.
- Do not eat hot dogs and luncheon meats unless they are reheated until they are steaming hot.
- Avoid soft cheeses such as feta, brie, Camembert, blue-veined cheeses, queso fresco or queso blanco (a soft cheese often used by Hispanic women in their cooking) unless the label clearly states that they are made with pasteurized milk.
- Do not eat refrigerated patés or meat spreads, foods that contain raw (unpasteurized) milk, or drink unpasteurized milk.
- Avoid eating refrigerated smoked seafood such as salmon, trout, cod, tuna, or mackerel unless it is in a cooked dish such as a casserole. Canned or shelf-stable patés, meat spreads, and smoked seafood are considered safe to eat.

MERCURY IN FISH

Fish and shellfish are important parts of a healthy diet, but nearly all contain traces of mercury. Although this is not a concern for most people, some fish and shellfish contain higher levels of mercury than others, and mercury can pose a threat to the developing nervous system of an unborn baby or a young child. Because of this, the U.S. government issued the following guidelines for women who are pregnant or who may become pregnant, breastfeeding mothers, and young children (U.S. Department of Health and Human Services and U.S. Environmental Protection Agency, 2004):

- Do not eat swordfish, shark, tilefish, or king mackerel because these fish contain high levels of mercury.

- Eat up to 12 oz/week (two average meals) of a variety of shellfish and fish that are lower in mercury. (Commonly eaten fish that are lower in mercury include canned light tuna, shrimp, salmon, catfish, and pollack. Albacore [white] tuna has more mercury than canned light tuna, so only 6 oz/week of albacore tuna is recommended.)

- Check local advisories about the mercury content of fish caught locally by family and friends. If no information is available, limit fish caught in local areas to 6 oz/week and avoid consuming additional fish that week.

- Note, however, that fish oil supplements are available which have been lab tested for mercury. It is important to check labels for this lab certification when purchasing fish oil supplements.

LACTASE DEFICIENCY (LACTOSE INTOLERANCE)

Some individuals have difficulty digesting milk and milk products. This condition, known as **lactase deficiency (lactose intolerance)**, results from an inadequate amount of the enzyme lactase, which breaks down the milk sugar lactose into smaller digestible substances.

Lactase deficiency is found in most adults of African, Mexican, Native American, Ashkenazic Jewish, and Asian descent and, indeed, in many other adults worldwide. People of northern European heritage are usually not affected. Symptoms include abdominal distention, discomfort, nausea, vomiting, loose stools, and cramps.

In counseling pregnant women who might be intolerant of milk and milk products, be aware that even one glass of milk can produce symptoms. Milk in cooked form, such as custards, is sometimes tolerated, as are cultured or fermented dairy products such as buttermilk, some cheeses, kefir, and yogurt. Lactase deficiency need not be a problem for pregnant women because the enzyme is available over the counter in tablets or drops. Lactase-treated milk is also available commercially in some grocery stores.

CULTURAL, ETHNIC, AND RELIGIOUS INFLUENCES

Cultural, ethnic, and religious backgrounds determine people's experiences with food and influence food preferences and habits (Figure 12–3 ⊙). People of different nationalities are accustomed to eating different foods because of the kinds of foodstuffs available in their countries of ori-

⊙ FIGURE 12–3

Food preferences and habits are affected by cultural factors.

gin. The way food is prepared varies, depending on the customs and traditions of the ethnic and cultural group. In addition, the laws of certain religions forbid the use of some foods and direct the preparation and serving of meals. (See "Developing Cultural Competence.")

DEVELOPING CULTURAL COMPETENCE

KOSHER DIETS

The kosher diet followed by many Jewish people forbids the eating of pig products and shellfish. Certain cuts of meat from sheep and cattle are allowed as are fish with fins and scales. In addition, many Jews believe that meat and milk should not be mixed and eaten at the same meal.

In each culture certain foods have symbolic meaning. Generally these symbolic foods are related to major life experiences such as birth, death, or developmental milestones. Although generalizations have been made about the food practices of ethnic and religious groups, there are many variations. The extent to which people continue to eat traditional ethnic foods and follow food-related ethnic customs is affected by their exposure to other cultures and the availability, quality, and cost of traditional foods.

When working with pregnant women from any ethnic background, it is important to understand the impact of the woman's cultural beliefs on her eating habits and to identify any beliefs she may have about food and pregnancy. Talking with the client can help determine the level of influence that traditional food customs exert. It is then possible to give dietary advice in a way that is meaningful to the woman and her family.

PSYCHOSOCIAL FACTORS

Various psychosocial factors may influence a woman's food choices. The sharing of food has long been a symbol of friendliness, warmth, and social acceptance in many cultures. Some foods and food practices are associated with status. Some foods are prepared "just for company"; others are served only on special occasions or holidays.

Socioeconomic level may be a determinant of nutritional status. Poverty-level families cannot afford the same foods that higher income families can. Thus, pregnant women with low incomes are frequently at risk for poor nutrition.

Knowledge about the basic components of a balanced diet is essential. Often educational level is related to economic status, but even people on very limited incomes can prepare well-balanced meals if they know enough about nutrition.

The expectant mother's attitudes and feelings about her pregnancy influence her nutritional status. For example, foods may be used as a substitute for the expression of emotions, such as anger or frustration, or as a way of expressing feelings of joy. The woman who is depressed or does not wish to be pregnant may manifest these feelings in loss of appetite or overindulgence in certain foods.

EATING DISORDERS

Two serious eating disorders, anorexia nervosa and bulimia nervosa, affect millions of men and women, although they develop most commonly in adolescent girls and young women. Both conditions are psychologic disorders that can have a major impact on physiologic well-being.

Anorexia nervosa is an eating disorder characterized by an extreme fear of weight gain and fat. People with this problem have distorted body images and perceive themselves as fat even when they are extremely underweight. Their dietary intake is very restrictive in both variety and quantity. They may also engage in excessive exercise to prevent weight gain.

Bulimia is characterized by bingeing (secretly consuming large amounts of food in a short time) and purging. Self-induced vomiting is the most common method of purging; laxatives or diuretics may also be used. Individuals with bulimia nervosa often maintain normal or near-normal weight for their height, so it is difficult to know whether bingeing and purging occur.

Individuals with anorexia nervosa do not often become pregnant because of the physiologic changes that affect their reproductive systems. Women with bulimia can become pregnant. Their self-induced vomiting may produce many of the same complications as hyperemesis gravidarum (see Chapter 15 ∞). In both anorexia nervosa and bulimia, a multidisciplinary approach to treatment, involving medical, nursing, psychiatric, and dietetic practitioners, is indicated. Pregnant women with eating disorders need to be closely monitored and supported throughout their pregnancies.

PICA

Pica is the persistent eating of substances, such as soil or clay, powdered laundry starch or corn starch, soap, baking powder, ice, freezer frost, burned matches, or ashes, that are not ordinarily considered edible or nutritionally valuable. In the United States, pica is more common among economically disadvantaged women, women of African-American descent, women who practiced pica before pregnancy, women whose culture encourages pica as important for fertility, and women who have family members who also practice pica (Corbett, Ryan, & Weinrich, 2003).

Iron deficiency anemia is the most common concern in pica. Eating laundry starch or certain types of clay may contribute to iron deficiency because they interfere with iron absorption. The ingestion of large quantities of clay could fill the intestine and cause fecal impaction; eating starch may be associated with excessive weight gain.

Assessment for pica is an important part of a nutritional history. However, a woman may be embarrassed about her cravings or reluctant to discuss them for fear of criticism. Using a nonjudgmental approach, give the woman information that can help her decrease or eliminate this practice.

NUTRITIONAL CARE OF THE PREGNANT ADOLESCENT

Nutritional care of the pregnant adolescent is of particular concern to healthcare professionals. Many adolescents are nutritionally at risk because of a variety of complex emotional, social, and economic factors. Important nutrition-related factors to assess in pregnant adolescents include low prepregnant weight, low weight gain during pregnancy, young age at menarche, smoking, excessive prepregnant weight, anemia, unhealthy lifestyle (drugs or alcohol use), chronic disease, and history of an eating disorder.

The nutritional needs of adolescents are generally estimated by using the DRI for nonpregnant teenagers (ages 11 to 14 or 15 to 18) and adding nutrient amounts recommended for all women. If she is mature (more than 4 years since menarche), the pregnant adolescent's nutritional needs approach those reported for pregnant adults. However, adolescents who become pregnant less than 4 years after menarche are at risk due to their physiologic and anatomic immaturity. They are more likely than older adolescents to still be growing, which can affect the fetus's development. Thus, young adolescents (age 14 and under) need to gain more weight than older adolescents (18 years and older) to produce babies of equal size.

In determining the optimal weight gain for the pregnant adolescent, add the recommended weight gain for an adult pregnancy to that expected during the postmenarcheal year in which the pregnancy occurs. If the teenager is underweight, additional weight gain is recommended to bring her to a normal weight for her height.

SPECIFIC NUTRIENT CONCERNS

Caloric needs of pregnant adolescents vary widely. Major factors in determining caloric needs include whether growth has been completed and the physical activity level of the individual. Figures as high as 50 kcal/kg have been suggested for young, growing teens who are very active physically. A satisfactory weight gain usually confirms an adequate caloric intake.

An inadequate iron intake is a major concern with the adolescent diet. Iron needs are high for the pregnant teen due to the requirement for iron by the enlarging maternal muscle mass and blood volume. Iron supplements are definitely indicated.

Calcium is another important nutrient for pregnant adolescents. Inadequate intake of calcium is often a problem in this age group. Adequate calcium intake is necessary to support normal growth and development of the fetus as well as growth and maintenance of calcium stores in the adolescent. An extra serving of dairy products is usually suggested for teenagers. Calcium supplementation is indicated for teens who dislike milk, unless they consume enough other dairy products or significant calcium sources.

Because folic acid plays a role in cell reproduction, it is also an important nutrient for pregnant teens. As previously indicated, a supplement is usually recommended for pregnant females of all ages.

Other nutrients and vitamins must be considered when evaluating the overall nutritional quality of the teenager's diet. Nutrients that have frequently been found to be deficient in this age group include zinc and vitamins A, D, and B_6. Eating a wide variety of foods—especially fresh and lightly processed foods—helps the teen get adequate amounts of trace minerals, fiber, and other vitamins.

DIETARY PATTERNS

Healthy adolescents often have irregular eating patterns. Many skip breakfast, and most tend to be frequent snackers. Teens rarely follow the traditional three-meals-a-day pattern. Their day-to-day intake often varies drastically, and they eat food combinations that may seem bizarre to adults. Despite these practices, adolescents usually achieve a better nutritional balance than most adults would expect.

In assessing the diet of the pregnant adolescent, it is important to consider the eating pattern over time, not simply a single day's intake. Once the pattern is identified, counseling can be directed toward correcting deficiencies.

COUNSELING ISSUES

Counseling about nutrition and healthy eating practices is an important element of care for pregnant teenagers. Nurses can effectively provide this counseling in a community setting. It may be individualized, involve other teens, or provide a combination of both approaches. If an adolescent's family member does most of the meal preparation, it may be useful to include that person in the discussion if the adolescent agrees. Involving the expectant father in counseling may also be helpful. Clinics and schools often offer classes and focused activities designed to address this topic.

The pregnant teenager's understanding of nutrition will influence not only her well-being but also that of her child. However, teens tend to live in the present, and counseling that stresses long-term changes may be less effective than more concrete approaches. In many cases, group classes are effective, especially those with other teens.

POSTPARTUM NUTRITION

Nutritional needs change following childbirth. Nutrient requirements vary depending on whether the mother decides to breastfeed. An assessment of postpartum nutritional status is necessary before nutritional guidance is given.

POSTPARTUM NUTRITIONAL STATUS

Postpartum nutritional status is determined based on the new mother's weight, hemoglobin and hematocrit levels, clinical signs, and dietary history. As mentioned previously, an ideal weight gain during pregnancy is 25 to 35 lb (11.5 to 16 kg). After birth there is a weight loss of approximately 10 to 12 lb. Additional weight loss is most rapid during the next few weeks as the body adjusts to the end of pregnancy. The mother's weight then begins to stabilize. This weight stabilization may take 6 months or longer. The mother's weight should be considered in terms of ideal weight, prepregnancy weight, and weight gain during pregnancy. Refer women who want information about weight reduction to a dietitian.

Hemoglobin and erythrocyte levels should return to normal within 2 to 6 weeks after childbirth. Iron supplements are generally continued for 2 to 3 months following childbirth to build stores depleted by pregnancy.

Constipation is a common problem following birth. To prevent it the woman should maintain a high fluid intake, which helps keep the stool soft. Dietary sources of fiber, such as whole grains, fruits, and vegetables, also help prevent constipation.

It is important to get specific information on dietary intake and eating habits directly from the woman. Visiting the mother during mealtimes provides an opportunity for unobtrusive nutritional assessment. Which foods has the woman selected? Is her diet nutritionally sound? A comment focusing on a positive aspect of her meal selection may initiate a discussion of nutrition.

Notify the dietitian about any woman whose cultural or religious beliefs require specific foods so that appropriate meals can be prepared for her. Also consider referring women with unusual eating habits or numerous questions about good nutrition to the dietitian. In addition, providing literature on nutrition ensures that the woman has a source of information at home.

NUTRITIONAL CARE OF FORMULA-FEEDING MOTHERS

After birth the formula-feeding mother's dietary requirements return to prepregnancy levels. If the mother has a good understanding of nutritional principles, it is sufficient to advise her to reduce her daily caloric intake by about 300 kcal and to return to prepregnancy levels for other nutrients.

If the mother has a limited understanding of nutrition, now is the time to teach her the basic principles and the importance of a well-balanced diet. Her eating habits and dietary practices will eventually be reflected in the diet of her child.

If the mother has gained excessive weight during pregnancy (or perhaps was overweight before pregnancy) and wishes to lose weight, a referral to the dietitian is appropriate. The dietitian can design weight reduction diets to meet nutritional needs and food preferences. Weight loss goals of 1 to 2 lb/week are usually suggested.

In addition to meeting her own nutritional needs, the new mother is usually interested in learning how to provide for her infant's nutritional needs. A discussion of infant feeding that includes topics such as selecting infant formulas, formula preparation, and vitamin and mineral supplementation is appropriate and generally well received.

NUTRITIONAL CARE OF BREASTFEEDING MOTHERS

A breastfeeding woman needs increased nutrients. Table 12–1 provides a sample daily food guide for lactating women. It is especially important for the breastfeeding mother to consume sufficient calories, because inadequate caloric intake can reduce milk volume. However, milk quality generally remains unaffected. The breastfeeding mother should increase her calories by about 200 kcal over her pregnancy requirement, or 500 kcal over her prepregnancy requirement. This results in a total of about 2500 to 2700 kcal/day for most women.

Because protein is an important ingredient in breast milk, an adequate intake while breastfeeding is essential. An intake of 65 g/day during the first 6 months of breastfeeding and 62 g/day during the second 6 months is recommended. As in pregnancy, it is important to consume adequate nonprotein calories to prevent the use of protein as an energy source.

Calcium is an important ingredient in milk production. Requirements during lactation remain the same as during pregnancy—an increase of 1000 mg/day. If the intake of calcium from food sources is not adequate, calcium supplements are recommended.

> ## NURSING PRACTICE
>
> Explain to breastfeeding mothers that liquids are especially important during lactation, because inadequate fluid intake may decrease milk volume. Encourage them to drink at least 8 to 10 (8-oz) glasses of fluid daily, including water, juice, milk, and soups.

Iron is not a principal mineral component of milk; thus, the needs of lactating women are not substantially different from those of nonpregnant women. However, supplementation for 2 to 3 months after childbirth is advisable to replenish maternal stores depleted by pregnancy.

In addition to counseling breastfeeding mothers on how to meet their increased nutrient needs, the nurse should discuss a few issues related to infant feeding. For example, many mothers are concerned about how specific foods they eat will affect their babies during breastfeeding. Generally the breastfeeding mother need not avoid any foods except those to which she might be allergic. Occasionally, however, some breastfeeding mothers find that their babies are affected by certain foods. Onions, turnips, cabbage, chocolate, spices, and seasonings are commonly listed as offenders. The best advice to give the breastfeeding mother is to avoid those foods she suspects cause distress in her infant. For the most part, however, she should be able to eat any nourishing food she wants without fear that her baby will be affected. For further discussion of successful infant feeding, see Chapter 29. ∞

NURSING MANAGEMENT

NURSING ASSESSMENT AND DIAGNOSIS

In order to plan an optimal diet with each woman, it is essential to assess nutritional status. The woman's chart and a client interview provide information about (1) the woman's height and weight, as well as her weight gain during pregnancy; (2) pertinent laboratory values, especially hemoglobin and hematocrit; (3) clinical signs that have possible nutritional implications, such as constipation, anorexia, or heartburn; and (4) dietary history to evaluate the woman's views on nutrition as well as her specific nutrient intake.

While gathering data, seek information about psychologic, cultural, and socioeconomic factors that may influence food intake. Also use the opportunity to discuss important aspects of nutrition within the context of the family's needs and lifestyle. A nutritional questionnaire is often useful in gathering and recording important facts. This information can be used to develop an intervention plan to fit the woman's individual needs. The sample questionnaire shown in Figure 12–4 ● has been filled in to demonstrate this process.

Once information is obtained, begin to analyze the information, formulate appropriate nursing diagnoses, and, with the woman, develop goals and desired outcomes. For a woman during the first trimester, for example, the diagnosis may be *Imbalanced Nutrition: Less than Body Requirements related to nausea and vomiting*. If a woman has excessive weight gain, the diagnosis might be *Imbalanced Nutrition: More Than Body Requirements related to excessive caloric intake*. Be specific in addressing issues such as inadequate intake of nutrients, including iron, calcium, or folic acid; problems with nutrition because of a limited food budget; problems related to physiologic alterations, including anorexia, heartburn, or nausea; and behavioral problems related to excessive dieting, binge eating, and so on. At other times the diagnosis *health-seeking behaviors* may seem most appropriate, especially if the woman asks for information about nutrition.

PLANNING AND IMPLEMENTATION

After determining the nursing diagnosis, plan an approach to address any nutritional deficiencies or improve the overall quality of the diet. To be truly effective, this plan must be made in cooperation with the woman. The following example demonstrates ways to plan with the woman based on the nursing diagnosis:

- Nursing Diagnosis: *Imbalanced Nutrition: Less than Body Requirements related to low intake of calcium*
- Goal: The woman will increase her daily intake of calcium to the minimum DRI level.
- Implementation:
  1. Plan with the woman how to add more milk or dairy products to the diet (specify amounts).
  2. Encourage the use of other calcium sources such as leafy greens and legumes.
  3. Plan for the addition of powdered milk in cooking and baking.

4. If none of the preceding options are realistic or acceptable, consider the use of calcium supplements.

Most families can benefit from guidance about food purchasing and preparation. Advise women to plan food purchases thoughtfully by preparing general menus and a list before shopping. It is also helpful to monitor sales, compare brands, and be cautious when purchasing convenience foods, which tend to be expensive. Other techniques for keeping food costs down without jeopardizing quality include buying food in season, using bulk foods when appropriate, using whole-grain or enriched products, buying lower grade eggs (grading has no relation to the egg's nutritional value but indicates color of the shell, delicacy of flavor, and so forth), and avoiding foods from specialty shops and foods in elaborate packaging.

Nursing Care in the Community

Food is a significant portion of a family's budget, and meeting nutritional needs may be a challenge for families on limited incomes. Community-based services offered through clinics, local agencies, schools, and volunteer organizations address these needs. Increasingly nurses play an important role in managing such community-based services, especially services focusing on client education. Most communities offer special assistance to qualifying families to meet their nutritional needs. The Food Stamp Program provides stamps or coupons for participating households whose net monthly income is below a specified level. These stamps can be used to purchase food for the household each month.

The Special Supplemental Food Program for Women, Infants, and Children (WIC) is designed to assist pregnant or breastfeeding women with low incomes and their children under 5 years of age. The program provides food assistance, nutrition education, and referrals to healthcare providers. The food distributed, including dried beans and peas, peanut butter, eggs, cheese, milk, fortified adult and infant cereals, juice, and iron-fortified formula, is designed to provide good sources of iron, protein, and certain vitamins and minerals for people with an inadequate diet.

EVALUATION

Once a plan has been developed and implemented, work with the woman to identify ways of evaluating its effectiveness. This may involve keeping a food journal, writing out weekly menus, returning for weekly weigh-ins, and the like. If anemia is a special problem, periodic hematocrit assessments are also indicated. Refer women with serious nutritional deficiencies to a dietitian.

● **FIGURE 12–4**

NUTRITIONAL QUESTIONNAIRE

Name Susan Longmont   **Date** 5-18-06

Age 20

Ethnic group Caucasian

Religion Protestant

Gravida 1   **Para** 0   **EDB** 1-9-07

Age of youngest child? NA

Birth weights of previous children? NA

Usual nonpregnant weight 119   **Present weight** 125

Weight gain during last pregnancy? NA

Vitamin or herbal supplements? none

Current medications? aspirin for headache

Do you smoke? yes   **How much per day?** 1-1½ packs

Have you ever had anorexia or bulimia?   **Please describe the circumstances.**

Eating patterns:

1. How many meals per day? 2   **when** 12:30 pm   6:30 pm

2. How many snacks per day? 3   **when** 10:30 am   4:00 pm   10:00 pm

3. What other foods are important to your usual diet? chocolate and candy bars

4. Amount per day 4 bars/week

5. Do you have any different food preferences now? no

6. Do you eat nonfoods such as:

                             Amount

    laundry starch   no   NA

    ice   yes   10 cubes/day

    other (name)   no   NA

7. What foods do you dislike or do not eat? spinach and dried beans

8. For added information complete a typical daily intake (24-hour recall is suggested).

Do you have special problems in food preparation such as:

1. Physical disability   yes   no ✓   Explain

2. Cooking appliances   yes   no ✓   Explain

3. Refrigeration of food   yes   no ✓   Explain

Who does the meal planning? I do.   **shopping?** We both do.

cooking? I do most of the time but my husband likes to help.

Are there transportation problems? We have only one car but we go in the evening.

Financial situation: My husband is working and going to school.

I am not working.   **Food Stamps** yes   **WIC** no

Do you have any previous nutritional problems? No. I have never paid much attention

to food before, but now I have lots of questions.

Are there any problems with this pregnancy? Nausea Yes, in the morning.

Constipation No   **Other** NA

Assessment by the nurse following the completion of the questionnaire.

Basic estimated nutrient and caloric value of typical daily intake.

Please circle one of the following:

Protein intake was   low   (adequate)   high

Caloric intake was   low   adequate   (high)

Calcium intake was   (low)   adequate   high

Iron intake was   (low)   adequate   high

Vitamin C intake was   low   (adequate)   high

Sample nutritional questionnaire used in nursing management of a pregnant woman.

Critical Concept Review

LEARNING OBJECTIVES

CONCEPTS

Delineate recommended levels of weight gain during pregnancy.	Weight gain recommendations are dependent upon the woman's prepregnancy weight: ■ Underweight: 28–40 lb (12.5 to 18 kg) ■ Normal weight: 25–35 lb (11.5 to 16 kg) ■ Overweight: 15–25 lb (7 to 11.5 kg) ■ Obese: ≤15 lb (≤7 kg)

Identify the role of specific nutrients in the diet of the pregnant woman.

1. Carbohydrates: the body's primary source of energy. Promotes weight gain and growth of the fetus and placenta.
2. Protein: supplies needed amino acids for growth of tissue.
3. Fat: source of maternal energy; also promotes fetal fat deposits.
4. Calcium and phosphorus: promotes mineralization of fetal bones and teeth.
5. Iodine: promotes fetal thyroid gland function.
6. Sodium: regulates fluid balance and metabolism in the mother.
7. Zinc: promotes growth of fetus and sufficient lactation.
8. Magnesium: promotes cellular metabolism and bone mineralization.
9. Iron: prevents maternal anemia and contributes to fetal and infant stores of iron.
10. Vitamins: maintain good maternal health. Folic acid, taken prior to conception, may prevent neural tube defects in the fetus.

Compare nutritional needs during pregnancy, the postpartum period, and lactation with nonpregnant requirements.

1. During pregnancy and lactation, nutritional requirements increase significantly from nonpregnant requirements:
   - Calories in second and third trimester increase by 300 kcal/day, and during lactation, by another 200 kcal/day.
   - Protein increases by 14 mg to 60 g/day.
   - Calcium requirements for the pregnant or lactating woman increase to 1000–1300 mg/day depending upon the age of the woman.
   - Magnesium increases to 350 mg/day.
   - Iron increases to 27 mg/day. (It is very difficult to eat enough iron-rich foods in the regular diet, so iron supplements are commonly prescribed.)
   - Iodine increases to 220 mcg/day.
   - Zinc increases to 11 mg/day during pregnancy and 12 mg/day during lactation.
   - Vitamin A increases to 770 mcg/day.
   - Vitamin D increases to 5 mcg/day.
   - Vitamin C increases from 75 to 85 mg/day.
   - Thiamine increases from 1.1 mg to 1.4 mg/day.
   - Riboflavin increases from 1.1 mg to 1.4 mg/day.
   - Niacin increases from 14 to 18 mg/day.
   - Pantothenic acid increases to 5 mg/day.
   - Vitamin B_{12} increases from 2.4 to 2.6 mcg/day.
   - Fluid needs increase to 8–10 glasses of noncaffeinated beverages/day.
2. For nonbreastfeeding mothers, during the postpartum period, nutritional requirements return to prepregnancy levels.

Plan adequate prenatal vegetarian diets based on the nutritional requirements of pregnancy.

1. There are different types of vegetarian diets, which differ in the types of animal-based products that are eaten.
2. Vegans do not eat any animal-based products, but can obtain protein from beans, rice, peanut butter, soy products, and seeds. Most vegans need additional supplementation of vitamins B_{12} and D, and calcium.
3. Vegetarians' daily food requirements are:
   - 6–11 servings of whole grains, cereal, pasta, and rice.
   - 2–4 servings of fruit.
   - 3–5 servings of vegetables.
   - 2–3 servings of legumes, nuts, seeds, and meat alternatives.
   - 2–3 servings of milk products (unless vegan).

(continued)

LEARNING OBJECTIVES

CONCEPTS

Describe ways in which various physical, psychosocial, and cultural factors can affect nutritional intake and status.	1. Nausea, vomiting, constipation, and heartburn can limit a woman's intake of nutritional foods especially during the first trimester. 2. Lactose intolerance may cause diarrhea or bloating after intake of dairy products. 3. Cultural, ethnic, and religious influences may prohibit use of certain foods that are needed for adequate nutrition. 4. Socioeconomic level may limit amounts of nutritional foods available to the woman. 5. Lack of knowledge about proper nutrition may limit the woman's ability to prepare nutritional foods. 6. Clients with eating disorders may have nutritional and electrolyte imbalances due to starvation or vomiting. 7. Pica may result in iron deficiency anemia.
Compare recommendations for weight gain and nutrient intakes in the pregnant adolescent with those for the mature pregnant adult.	1. Weight gain: add recommended weight gain of the adult pregnancy to the expected gain of the adolescent. 2. Nutrient needs: adolescent needs more iron, calcium, and folic acid than the adult pregnant woman.

Discuss basic factors a nurse should consider when offering nutritional counseling to a pregnant adolescent.	1. Basic factors to consider:
	  ■ Number of years since adolescent reached menarche.
	  ■ Whether growth has been completed.
	  ■ Most adolescents have irregular eating patterns.
	  ■ Adolescent may not be the one who regularly prepares meals, so the individual who prepares meals should be included in nutritional counseling.
	  ■ Teens are present, not future, oriented which impacts nutritional counseling.

Compare nutritional counseling issues for breastfeeding and formula-feeding mothers.	1. Formula-feeding mothers:
	  ■ Eat a well-balanced diet.
	  ■ Dietary requirements are the same as before pregnancy.
	  ■ Weight loss of 1–2 lb/week is acceptable.
	2. Breastfeeding mothers:
	  ■ Calorie requirements increase by 200 kcal/day over needs during pregnancy.
	  ■ Need 2500–2700 kcal/day.
	  ■ Need 65 g/day of protein.
	  ■ Need 1000 mg/day of calcium.
	  ■ Should avoid foods that irritate the infant.

CRITICAL THINKING IN ACTION

*View the **Critical Thinking in Action** video in Chapter 12 of the CD-ROM. Then, answer the questions that follow.*

Sandra Hill is a 17-year-old at 19 weeks' gestation with her first pregnancy. She presents to you accompanied by her mother. Her mother tells you that Sandra is an active teenager who plays sports and has been taking dance lessons for 5 years. She maintains a "B+" in school. Sandra voices concern about potential weight gain during pregnancy. She tells you that this was not a planned pregnancy and she has ambivalent feelings about it. You become concerned as she tells you that she has reduced her caloric intake over the last few months to try to keep her weight down and camouflage her pregnancy. You do a nutritional assessment and find that she is deficient in calcium, iron, and protein. Sandra seems to have irregular eating patterns and she admits to often skipping breakfast. She asks why she has to gain so much weight when you explain the nutritional needs of her baby during the pregnancy.

1. Discuss weight distribution in pregnancy.
2. Discuss foods that will increase calcium, protein, and iron in her diet.
3. Explain why folate supplementation is important.
4. What criteria will measure adequate caloric intake during pregnancy?

- NCLEX-RN® Review, case studies, and other interactive resources for this chapter can be found on the Companion Website at http://www.prenhall.com/london. Click on "Chapter 12" to select the activities for this chapter.

- For animations, more NCLEX-RN® Review questions, and an audio glossary, access the accompanying CD-ROM in this textbook.

REFERENCES

Agostoni, C., & Verduci, E. (2003). DHA in pregnancy benefits child development. *Pediatric Research, 54*(3), 292–293.

American College of Obstetricians and Gynecologists. (1996). *Nutrition and women* (ACOG Educational Bulletin No. 229). Washington, DC: Author.

American College of Obstetricians and Gynecologists. (1998). *Vitamin A supplementation during pregnancy* (ACOG Committee Opinion No. 196). Washington, DC: Author.

Belew, C. (1999). Herbs and the childbearing woman: Guidelines for midwives. *Journal of Nurse-Midwifery, 44*(3), 231–246.

Blumenthal, M. (2000). *Herbal medicine: Expanded Commission E Monographs.* Austin, TX: American Botanical Council.

Brown, J. E., & Carlson, M. (2000). Nutrition and multifetal pregnancy. *Journal of the American Dietetic Association, 100*(3), 343–348.

Centers for Disease Control and Prevention. (1998, April 3). Recommendations to prevent and control iron deficiency in the United States. *Morbidity and Mortality Weekly Reports, 47*(RR-3), 1–36.

Centers for Disease Control and Prevention. (2005). *Folic acid: Public health service recommendations.* Retrieved September 2, 2005, from http://www.cdc.gov/ncbddd/folicacid/health_recomm.htm

Corbett, R. W., Ryan, C., & Weinrich, S. P. (2003). Pica in pregnancy. *MCN. American Journal of Maternal Child Nursing, 28*(3), 183–189.

Doyle, W. (1998). Nutrition and pregnancy. *Nursing Times, 94*(Suppl. 16), 22–28.

Fabi, R. (2003). Food pyramid redesigned to slim U.S. waistline. *Reuters Health Information.* Retrieved September 18, 2003, from http://www.medscape.com/viewarticle/461294_print

Food and Drug Administration (FDA). (2005). *Food safety for motors-to-be: Educator's resource guide.* College Park, MD: Center for Food Safety and Applied Nutrition.

Gallagher, J. (2004). Omega 3 oils and pregnancy. *Midwifery Today: International Midwife, 69*, 26–31.

Institute of Medicine, Subcommittee for a Clinical Application Guide. (1992). *Nutrition during pregnancy and lactation: An implementation guide.* Washington, DC: National Academy Press.

Institute of Medicine, Subcommittee on Dietary Intake and Nutrient Supplements During Pregnancy, Committee on Nutrition Status During Pregnancy and Lactation, Food and Nutrition Board. (1990). *Nutrition during pregnancy: Weight gain and nutrient supplements.* Washington, DC: National Academy Press.

Kemper, K. J. (1999, November). Longwood Herbal Task Force and the Center for Holistic Pediatric Education and Research: Monograph on Dandelion (*Taraxacum offinalis*).

Moss, N., & Carver, K. (1998). The effect of WIC and Medicaid on infant mortality in the United States. *American Journal of Public Health, 88*(9), 1354–1361.

National Center on Birth Defects and Developmental Disabilities. (2004). *Birth defects.* Retrieved April 26, 2004, from http://www.cdc.gov/ncbddd/bd/mp.htm

National Institutes of Health. (2002). *Facts about dietary supplements: Vitamin D.* Retrieved April 24, 2004, from http://www.cc.nih.gov/ccc/supplements/vitd.html

Olsen, S. F., & Secher, N. J. (2002). Low consumption of seafood in early pregnancy as a risk factor for preterm delivery: Prospective cohort study. *British Medical Journal, 324*(7335), 447.

Reifsnider, E., & Gill, S. L. (2000). Nutrition for the childbearing years. *Journal of Obstetric, Gynecologic, and Neonatal Nursing, 29*(1), 43–55.

Salzberg, H. S. (2002). Nutrition in pregnancy. In J. J. Sciarra (Ed.), *Gynecology and obstetrics* (Vol. 2, chap. 7). Philadelphia: Lippincott Williams & Wilkins.

Skidmore-Roth, L. (2001). *Mosby's handbook of herbs & natural supplements.* St. Louis, MO: Mosby.

Smuts, C. M., Borod, E., Peeples, J. M., & Carlson, S. E. (2003). High-DHA eggs: Feasibility as a means to enhance circulating DHA in mother and infant. *Lipids, 38*(4), 407–414.

Smuts, C. M., Huang, M., Mundy, D., Plasse, T., Major, S., & Carlson, S. E. (2003). A randomized trial of docosahexaenoic acid supplementation during the third trimester of pregnancy. *Obstetrics and Gynecology, 101*(3), 469–479.

U.S. Department of Health and Human Services and U.S. Department of Agriculture. (2005). *Dietary Guidelines for Americans 2005.* Washington, DC: U.S. Government Printing Office.

U.S. Department of Health and Human Services and U.S. Environmental Protection Agency. (2004). *What you need to know about mercury in fish and shellfish.* Retrieved April 24, 2004, from http://www.cfsan.fda.gov/~dms/admehg3.html

Villar, J., Merialdi, M., Gulmezoglu, A. M., Abalos, E., Carroli, G., Kulier, R., & de Onis, M. (2003). Nutritional interventions during pregnancy for the prevention or treatment of maternal morbidity and preterm delivery: An overview of randomized controlled trials. *Journal of Nutrition, 133*(5, Suppl. 2), 1606S–1625S.

Willett, W. C. (2001). Food pyramids: What should you really eat. Reprinted from *Eat, drink, and be healthy* by Walter C. Willett. New York: Simon & Schuster. Retrieved April 24, 2004, from http://www.hsph.harvard.edu/nutritionsource/pyramids.html

Willett, W. C., & Stampfer, M. (2002, September 17). *Rebuilding the food pyramid.* Retrieved May 3, 2003, from http://www.sciam.com

I was a child when I had my daughter—just 16—and so afraid. I was one of the lucky ones though. My parents were wonderfully supportive and I went to a special teen clinic for my pregnancy. The nurses really taught me a lot about my body and about taking care of my baby. With help and encouragement from Mom and Dad, I got by. Last spring, at age 28 I graduated with a degree in nursing. I wanted a job with real security and opportunity, but more important, I want to give something back, to give others a little of the support I received.

—Joanna, 29

LEARNING OBJECTIVES

- Define the scope of the problem of adolescent pregnancy.

- Summarize factors contributing to adolescent pregnancy.

- Discuss the physical, psychologic, and sociologic risks a pregnant adolescent faces.

- Delineate characteristics of the fathers of children of adolescent mothers.

- Discuss the range of reactions of the adolescent's family and social network to her pregnancy.

- Formulate a plan of care to meet the needs of a pregnant adolescent.

- Describe successful community approaches to prevention of adolescent pregnancy.

MEDIALINK www.prenhall.com/london

CD-ROM

NCLEX-RN® Review
Audio Glossary

Companion Website

NCLEX-RN® Review
MediaLink Applications:
    Case Study: Adolescent Pregnancy
    Care Plan Activity: Adolescent Pregnancy
Thinking Critically

Pregnancy is an especially challenging time if the expectant mother is an adolescent. In the United States each year about 900,000 teenage girls (ages 15 to 19) become pregnant, and most of these pregnancies are unplanned. Of these pregnancies, about 51% end in live births, 35% are terminated by therapeutic abortion, and about 14% end in miscarriage or stillbirth (Klein & The Committee on Adolescence, 2005). More than half the teens who give birth keep their babies. Very few adolescents give up their babies for adoption.

The U.S. birth rate (number of births per 1000 women) for adolescents ages 15 to 19 has dropped 33% since 1991 from 61.8 per 1000 females to a historic low of 41.7 births in 2003 (Hamilton, Martin, & Sutton, 2004). This continuing decline is encouraging. Nevertheless, the United States continues to have one of the highest levels of adolescent childbearing among industrialized nations (National Campaign to Prevent Teen Pregnancy, 2004). The incidence of sexual activity among teens in many other countries is as high as it is in the United States. These countries may have lower adolescent pregnancy rates because of family influences, a greater openness about sexuality, better access to contraceptives, and a more comprehensive approach to sex education.

Research suggests that adolescent girls in the United States who have never had sex and who abstain do so for many reasons. The three most common reasons are fear of pregnancy, fear of acquiring a sexually transmitted infection, and a belief that sex is not right for someone their age (younger adolescents) or that they want to wait until marriage (older adolescents). Sexually experienced girls who abstain also cite fear of pregnancy and fear of a sexually transmitted infection as their primary reasons (Loewenson, Ireland, & Resnick, 2004).

This chapter explores the issue of adolescent pregnancy and the role of the nurse in meeting the special needs and concerns of pregnant adolescents and their families. It concludes with a discussion of efforts to prevent adolescent pregnancy.

OVERVIEW OF THE ADOLESCENT PERIOD

PHYSICAL CHANGES

Puberty—that period during which an individual becomes capable of reproduction—is a maturational process that can last from 1.5 to 6 years. The major physical changes of puberty include a growth spurt, weight change, and the appearance of secondary sexual characteristics. Menarche, or the time of the first menstrual period, usually occurs in the last half of this maturational process, with the average age between 12 and 13. The initial menstrual cycles are usually irregular and often anovulatory, although they are not always so. Thus, contraception is important for all sexually active adolescents.

PSYCHOSOCIAL DEVELOPMENT

Many writers have described the developmental tasks of adolescence, based on a variety of classic theories. The following are major developmental tasks of this period (Steinberg, 2002):

- Developing a sense of identity
- Gaining autonomy and independence
- Developing intimacy in a relationship
- Developing comfort with one's own sexuality
- Developing a sense of achievement

Early adolescence, 292
Late adolescence, 292
Middle adolescence, 292

Resolution of these tasks is a developmental process that occurs over time. Although average ages for the completion of tasks have been identified, these ages are somewhat arbitrary and are affected by many factors, including culture, religion, and socioeconomic status.

In **early adolescence** (age 14 and under) the teen still sees authority in the parents. However, he or she begins the process of gaining independence from the family by spending more time with friends. Conformity to peer group standards is important. The adolescent in this phase is very egocentric and is a concrete thinker, with only minimal ability to see him- or herself in the future or to foresee the consequences of his or her behavior. Teens perceive their locus of control as external; that is, their destinies are controlled by others such as parents and school authorities.

Middle adolescence (ages 15 to 17 years) is the time for challenging; experimenting with drugs, alcohol, and sex is a common avenue for rebellion. Middle adolescents seek independence and turn increasingly to their peer groups. They begin to move from concrete thinking to formal operational thought but are not yet able to anticipate the long-term implications of all their actions. These years are often a time of great turmoil for the family as the adolescent struggles for independence and challenges the family's values and expectations.

In **late adolescence** (ages 18 to 19 years) teens are more at ease with their individuality and decision-making ability. They can think abstractly and anticipate consequences. Late adolescents are capable of formal operational thought. They learn to solve problems, to conceptualize, and to make decisions. These abilities help them see themselves as having control, which leads to the ability to understand and accept the consequences of their behavior.

FACTORS CONTRIBUTING TO ADOLESCENT PREGNANCY

SOCIOECONOMIC AND CULTURAL FACTORS

Poverty is a major risk factor for adolescent pregnancy. Adolescents who do not have access to middle-class opportunities tend to maintain their pregnancies, because they see pregnancy as their only option for adult status; 85% of births to unmarried teens occur to those from poor or low-income families (Alan Guttmacher Institute, 2002). Not surprisingly, research indicates that the more time high-school students spend without adult supervision, the greater their level of sexual activity.

In the United States, the adolescent birth rate is higher among African-American and Hispanic teens than among white teens. However, pregnancy rates in these groups are declining. Since 1991 the pregnancy rate for black teens

ages 15 to 17 has been cut in half (Martin et al., 2003). To some degree, the higher teenage pregnancy rate in these groups reflects the impact of poverty, as a disproportionately higher number of African-American and Hispanic youths live in poverty.

Low educational achievement is another major risk factor for adolescent pregnancy. Teenage girls who participate in after-school activities are less likely to be sexually experienced than girls who do not participate (Cohen, Farley, Taylor et al., 2002). Similarly, compared with other teens, teens with future goals (i.e., college or job) tend to use birth control more consistently; if they become pregnant, they are also more likely to have abortions.

The younger the teen when she first gets pregnant, the more likely she is to have another pregnancy in her teens. Moreover, the likelihood of repeat pregnancies increases when the teen is living with her sexual partner and has dropped out of school. Daughters and sisters of women who had a baby in their early teens tend to have intercourse earlier and are at higher risk for teen pregnancy themselves (Short & Rosenthal, 2003).

Internationally, adolescent women are more likely to welcome a pregnancy in a country in which Islam is the predominant religion, where large families are desired, where social change is slow in coming, and where most childbearing occurs within marriage. Early pregnancy is less desired in countries in which the reverse is true.

DEVELOPING CULTURAL COMPETENCE

IMPACT OF EDUCATION ON MARRIAGE AND CHILDBEARING

Throughout the world, the higher a woman's educational level, the more likely she is to delay marriage and childbirth.

HIGH-RISK BEHAVIORS

Among adolescents there is great peer pressure to become sexually active during the teen years. Premarital sexual activity is commonplace, and teenage pregnancy is more socially acceptable today than it was in the past. In fact, by their late teen years, at least three fourths of all males and females have had sexual intercourse, and over two thirds of sexually experienced adolescents have had two or more partners (Alan Guttmacher Institute, 2002). Sexual innuendo permeates every aspect of the popular media, but issues of sexual responsibility are commonly ignored.

High-risk sexual behaviors—for example, multiple partners and lack of contraceptive use—are of concern. Research indicates that young people 15 to 24 years of age comprise 25% of the sexually experienced population in the United States. However, they account for 48% of the new cases of sexually transmitted infections (STIs). This is particularly worrisome because many STIs, including human immunodeficiency virus (HIV), are asymptomatic. Thus, apparently healthy young people who are infected may not seek healthcare (Weinstock, Berman, & Cates, 2004).

Statistics have demonstrated an increased use of condoms among the adolescent population, probably because of the tremendous educational efforts related to HIV (National Campaign to Prevent Teen Pregnancy, 2000). Nevertheless, adolescents remain inconsistent contraceptive users. Contraceptive use is more consistent in situations in which teens discuss contraception before having sex, when they have waited a longer time after starting a relationship to have sex with that person, and when they use dual methods of contraception (Manlove, Ryan, & Franzetta, 2003).

Many teens lack accurate and adequate knowledge about contraceptive options. This is a common topic of sex education programs; however, debate continues about the appropriateness of such programs in schools. Proponents advocate early sex education to provide teens with the knowledge they need to avoid unwanted pregnancy and the risk of STIs. Opponents feel that sex education is the responsibility of parents and worry that sex education in the schools will promote sexual activity. However, a review of research on sex education reveals that it does not increase initiation of sexual activity at an earlier age (Doniger, Adams, Utter, & Riley, 2001). Other factors affecting the use of contraception include access or availability, cost of supplies, and concern about confidentiality.

PSYCHOSOCIAL FACTORS

Family dysfunction and poor self-esteem are also major risk factors for adolescent pregnancy. Some young teenagers deliberately plan to get pregnant. The adolescent girl may use pregnancy for various subconscious or conscious reasons: to punish her parents, to escape from an undesirable home situation, to gain attention, or to feel that she has someone to love and to love her. Pregnancy may also be a young woman's form of acting out.

More teens who become pregnant, compared with teens who have not been pregnant, have been physically, emotionally, or sexually abused. In fact, maltreatment of any kind is a high-risk contributor to early teen pregnancy (Montgomery, 2003).

Teenage pregnancy can result from an incestuous relationship. In the very young adolescent, incest or sexual abuse should be suspected as a possible cause of pregnancy.

EVIDENCE-BASED NURSING

SCREENING FOR SEXUALLY TRANSMITTED INFECTIONS DURING PREGNANCY

Clinical Question

How are adolescents screened for sexually transmitted infections during pregnancy?

Evidence

In conjunction with the Agency for Healthcare Research and Quality, the Centers for Disease Control assembled a large group of medical experts and consultants from a variety of disciplines to develop guidelines for screening for sexually transmitted infections (STIs). The final guideline was based on controlled trials, population health studies, and expert opinion. This guideline was particularly important for practitioners working with adolescents because the highest rates of many STIs occur among this age group. Intrauterine or perinatally transmitted STIs can have serious effects for teens, their partners, and their fetuses.

Implications

At the first prenatal visit, several screening tests for STIs should be conducted. All women should be offered voluntary human immunodeficiency virus (HIV) testing. If refused, the tests should be reoffered in the third trimester and at birth. Serologic tests are indicated early in the pregnancy for syphilis, for hepatitis B surface antigen, and for hepatitis C antibodies. Tests for *Chlamydia trachomatis* and *Neisseria gonorrhoeae* should also be done at the first prenatal visit.

Routine cultures for herpes simplex virus are not indicated if there are no active lesions in the third trimester, even for women with a history of recurrent genital herpes. Prophylactic cesarean birth is not indicated for women who do not have active genital herpes lesions at the onset of labor.

When working with pregnant teens, you should address any lack of awareness of the consequences of STIs for these mothers, and offer guidance to help teens develop healthy sexual behaviors. Make sure the teen knows the rationale for and importance of screening tests for STIs both early in pregnancy and at childbirth. Encourage teens to be screened for HIV as well.

Critical Thinking

What assessments would indicate that you are working with an adolescent at high risk for STIs? What will be your teaching plan for pregnant adolescents relative to screening for STIs? How can you help teens develop healthy sexual behaviors?

Reference

Centers for Disease Control and Prevention. (2002, May 10). Special populations: Sexually transmitted diseases treatment guidelines. *MMWR Recommendations and Reports, 51*(RR-6), 5–7.

Teenage pregnancy could also be caused by other nonvoluntary sexual experiences such as acquaintance rape.

RISKS TO THE ADOLESCENT MOTHER

PHYSIOLOGIC RISKS

Adolescents over age 15 who receive early, thorough prenatal care are at no greater risk during pregnancy than women over age 20. Unfortunately, adolescents typically begin prenatal care later in pregnancy than any other age group (Montgomery, 2003). Thus, risks for pregnant adolescents include preterm births, low-birth-weight infants, cephalopelvic disproportion, iron deficiency anemia, and preeclampsia and its sequelae. In the adolescent age group, prenatal care is the critical factor that most influences pregnancy outcome.

Teens ages 15 to 19 have a high incidence of STIs, including herpesvirus, syphilis, and gonorrhea. The incidence of chlamydial infection is also increased in this age group. The presence of such infections during a pregnancy greatly increases the risk to the fetus. Other problems seen in adolescents are cigarette smoking and drug use. By the time pregnancy is confirmed, the fetus may already have been harmed by these substances.

PSYCHOLOGIC RISKS

The major psychologic risk to the pregnant adolescent is the interruption of her developmental tasks. Adding the tasks of pregnancy to her developmental tasks creates a huge amount of psychologic work, the completion of which will affect the adolescent's and her newborn's futures. Table 13–1 suggests typical behaviors of the adolescent when she becomes aware of her pregnancy. In reviewing these behaviors, the nurse should realize that other factors may influence individual response.

TABLE 13–1 ✣ Initial Reaction to Awareness of Pregnancy

Age	Adolescent Behavior	Nursing Implications
Early adolescent (14 and under)	Fears rejection by family and peers. Enters healthcare system with an adult, most likely mother (parents still seen as locus of control). Value system closely reflects that of parents, so teen turns to parents for decisions or approval of decisions. Pregnancy probably not result of intimate relationship. Is self-conscious about normal adolescent changes in body. Self-consciousness and low self-esteem likely to increase with rapid breast enlargement and abdominal enlargement of pregnancy.	Be nonjudgmental in approach to care. Focus on needs and concerns of adolescent, but if parent accompanies daughter, include parent in plan of care. Encourage both to express concerns and feelings regarding pregnancy and options: abortion, maintaining pregnancy, adoption. Be realistic and concrete in discussing implications of each option. During physical exam of adolescent, respect increased sense of modesty. Explain in simple and concrete terms physical changes that are produced by pregnancy versus puberty. Explain each step of physical exam in simple and concrete terms.
Middle adolescent (15–17 years)	Fears rejection by peers and parents. Unsure in whom to confide. May seek confirmation of pregnancy on own with increased awareness of options and services, such as over-the-counter pregnancy kits and Planned Parenthood. If in an ongoing, caring relationship with partner (peer), may choose him as confidant. Economic dependence on parents may determine if and when parents are told. Future educational plans and perception of parental support or lack of support are significant factors in decision regarding termination or maintenance of the pregnancy. Possible conflict between parental and own developing value system.	Be nonjudgmental in approach to care. Reassure the adolescent that confidentiality will be maintained. Help adolescent identify significant individuals in whom she can confide to help make a decision about the pregnancy. Be aware of state laws regarding requirement of parental notification if abortion intended. Also be aware of state laws regarding requirements for marriage: usually, minimum age for both parties is 18; 16- and 17-year-olds are, in most states, allowed to marry only with consent of parents. Encourage adolescent to be realistic about parental response to pregnancy.
Late adolescent (18–19 years)	Most likely to confirm pregnancy on own and at an earlier date due to increased acceptance and awareness of consequences of behavior. Likely to use pregnancy kit for confirmation. Relationship with father of baby, future educational plans, and personal value system are among significant determinants of decision about pregnancy.	Be nonjudgmental in approach to care. Reassure the adolescent that confidentiality will be maintained. Encourage adolescent to identify significant individuals in whom she can confide. Refer to counseling as appropriate. Encourage adolescent to be realistic about parental response to pregnancy.

SOCIOLOGIC RISKS

Being forced into adult roles before completing adolescent developmental tasks causes a series of events that may result in prolonged dependence on parents, lack of stable relationships with the opposite sex, and lack of economic and social stability. Many teenage mothers drop out of school during their pregnancy. Many never complete their education. Lack of education reduces the quality of jobs available to them. Childbearing at an early age is a strong predictor of need for public assistance, especially in lower socioeconomic groups and when the pregnant teen's family does not support her (National Campaign to Prevent Teen Pregnancy, 2004).

Adolescent mothers frequently fail to establish a stable family, especially if they have a second child while still in their teens. Their family structure tends to be single parent and matriarchal, often the same type in which the adolescents themselves were raised. Some pregnant adolescents choose to marry the father of the baby, who may also be a teenager. Unfortunately, the majority of adolescent marriages end in divorce. This fact should not be surprising because pregnancy and marriage interrupt the adolescents' childhood and basic education. Lack of maturity in dealing with an intimate relationship also contributes to marital breakdown.

The increased incidence of maternal complications, preterm birth, and low-birth-weight babies among teen mothers also affects society because many of these mothers are on welfare. The need for increased financial support for good prenatal care and nutritional programs remains critical.

Table 13–2 identifies the early adolescent's response to the developmental tasks of pregnancy. Middle and older adolescents respond differently, reflecting their progression through developmental tasks. In addition to her

TABLE 13–2 ❖ The Early Adolescent's Response to the Developmental Tasks of Pregnancy

Stage	Developmental Tasks of Pregnancy	Early Adolescent's Response to Pregnancy	Nursing Implications
First trimester	Pregnancy confirmation. Seeks early prenatal care as a confirmation tool. Begins to evaluate her diet and general health habits. Initial ambivalence common. Usually supportive partner.	May delay confirmation of pregnancy until late part of first trimester or later. Reasons for delay may include lack of awareness that she is pregnant, fear of confiding in anyone, and denial. Rapid enlargement and sensitivity of breasts are embarrassing and frightening to early adolescent—may be perceived as changes of puberty. If confiding in mother, may be experiencing family turmoil in response to pregnancy.	Explain physiologic changes of pregnancy versus those associated with puberty. Explain that ambivalence is normal with any pregnancy, but recognize it as a much greater concern with adolescent pregnancy. Emphasize need for good nutrition as important for her well-being as much as infant's (prevention of preeclampsia and anemia). Use simple explanations and lots of audiovisual aids. Have adolescent listen to fetal heart rate with Doppler.
Second trimester	Changes in physical appearance begin, and fetal movement is experienced, causing pregnancy to be experienced as a reality. Begins wearing maternity clothes to accommodate the physical changes. As a result of quickening, she perceives her fetus as a real baby and begins preparing for the maternal role and new relationships with her partner and members of her family.	Some teenagers may delay validation of pregnancy until now, with family turmoil occurring at this time. Abdominal enlargement and quickening may be perceived as loss of control over body image. May try to maintain prepregnant weight and wear restrictive clothing to control and conceal changing body. Becomes dependent on her own mother for support. Egocentric; unable to develop a maternal role at this time.	Continue to discuss importance of good nutrition and adequate weight gain as noted above. Discuss ways of utilizing common teenage clothing (large sweatshirts, blouses) to promote comfort but preserve adolescent image to some degree. Discuss plans being made for baby, continued educational plans, and role of teen's parents.
Third trimester	At end of second trimester, begins to view fetus as separate from self. Buys baby clothes and supplies. Prepares a place for the baby. Realistic about what baby is like. Prepares to give birth to infant. Anxiety increases as labor and birth approach and has concerns about well-being of fetus.	May focus on "wanting it to be over." May have trouble individuating fetus. May have fantasies, dreams, or nightmares about childbirth. Natural fears of labor and birth greater than with older primigravida. Probably has not been in a hospital, and may associate this with negative experiences.	Assess whether adolescent is preparing for baby by buying supplies and preparing a place in the home. Childbirth education is important. Provide hospital tour. Assess for discomforts of pregnancy, such as heartburn and constipation. Adolescent may be uncomfortable mentioning these and other problems.

maturational level, the amount of nurturing the pregnant adolescent receives is a critical factor in the way she handles pregnancy and motherhood.

RISKS FOR HER CHILD

Children of adolescent parents are at a disadvantage in many ways because teens are not developmentally or economically prepared to be parents. In general, children of teenage mothers are found to be at a developmental disadvantage compared with children whose mothers were older at the time of their birth. Many factors contribute to these differences, especially the adverse social and economic conditions many teenage mothers face. These factors result in high rates of family instability, disadvantaged neighborhoods, and high rates of behavior problems. In addition these children have an increased risk of academic problems, substance abuse, behavioral disorders, depression, and early sexual activity. Children born to adolescent mothers also have higher rates of abuse and neglect, and are more likely to become adolescent parents themselves (Klein & The Committee on Adolescence, 2005).

PARTNERS OF ADOLESCENT MOTHERS

Almost half of the fathers of infants of adolescent mothers are 20 years of age or older. Regardless of age, however, the poorer the man's education, the greater the risk that he will father the child of an adolescent, possibly because he is seeking an intellectual and emotional equal. Often the older partners of pregnant adolescents are similar to adolescent fathers socioeconomically. They have experienced early school failure, are unemployed, and are no more likely than adolescent fathers to support the mother. Adult paternity also tends to be higher when the teenage mother was born outside the United States. This difference may reflect cultural norms.

Adolescent males tend to become sexually active at an earlier age than females, and they have more sexual partners in their teenage years (Marcell, Raine, & Eyre, 2003). When the father is an adolescent, he too has uncompleted developmental tasks for his age group and is no better prepared psychologically than his female counterpart to deal with the consequences of pregnancy. Consequently the adolescent who attempts to assume his responsibility as a father faces many of the same psychologic and sociologic risks as the adolescent mother. The mother and father are generally from similar socioeconomic backgrounds and have similar educational levels.

Adolescent fathers tend to achieve less formal education than older fathers, and they enter the workforce earlier. They tend to pursue less prestigious careers and have less job satisfaction. They often marry at a younger age than older fathers and have more children.

Although they may not be married, many adolescent couples have meaningful relationships. The male partners may be very involved in the pregnancy and may be present for the birth. Healthcare providers should support the adolescent father in his decision to assume responsibility, but recognize that he probably does not understand the physical and psychologic changes his partner is experiencing. The young man will need education about pregnancy, childbirth, child care, and parenting. It is also important to ensure that the pregnant adolescent has the opportunity to decide for herself whether she wants the father to participate in her healthcare. The lack of responsibility shown by some unmarried fathers has caused a shift in cultural and community attitudes. Fathers are included on birth certificates far more frequently today than in the past. This inclusion helps ensure the fathers' rights and encourages them to meet their responsibilities to their children. In addition, legal paternity gives children access to military and social security benefits and to medical information about their fathers.

In some situations the pregnant adolescent may not want to identify or contact the father of the baby, and the male may not readily acknowledge paternity. Those situations include rape, exploitative sexual relations, incest, and casual sexual relations. If healthcare providers suspect any of the first three causes, further investigation into the situation is important for the well-being of the pregnant adolescent, and referral to other resources should be made as appropriate.

Although the adolescent father may have been included in the healthcare of the young woman throughout the pregnancy, it is not unusual for her to want her mother as her primary support person during labor and birth. Younger adolescents are especially likely to choose their mothers for this role. It is important to support the pregnant adolescent's wishes and to acknowledge and support the adolescent father's wishes as appropriate.

As a part of counseling, the nurse should assess the young man's stressors, his support systems, his plans for involvement in the pregnancy and childbearing, and his future plans. He should be referred to social services for counseling about his educational and vocational future. When the father is involved in the pregnancy, the young mother feels less deserted, more confident in her decision making, and better able to discuss her future.

REACTIONS OF FAMILY AND SOCIAL NETWORK TO ADOLESCENT PREGNANCY

The reactions of families and support groups to adolescent pregnancy vary widely. In families that foster children's educational and career goals, adolescent pregnancy is often a shock. Anger, shame, and sorrow are common reactions. The majority of pregnant adolescents from these families are likely to choose abortion, with the exception of teens whose cultural and religious beliefs prevent them from seeking abortions.

In populations in which adolescent pregnancy is more prevalent and more socially acceptable, family and friends may be more supportive of the adolescent parents. In many cases the teen's friends and mother are present at the birth. The expectant parents may also have friends who are already teen parents. Some male partners of these adolescent mothers see pregnancy and the birth of a baby as signs of adult status and increased sexual prowess—a source of pride.

The mother of the pregnant adolescent is usually among the first to be told about the pregnancy. She typically becomes involved with decision making, especially with the young adolescent, about issues such as maintaining the pregnancy, abortion, and dealing with the father-to-be and his family.

Once the pregnant adolescent decides how to proceed, it is often her mother who helps the teen access healthcare and accompanies her to her first prenatal visit. If the pregnancy is maintained, the mother may participate in prenatal care and classes and can be an excellent source of support for her daughter. She should be encouraged to participate if the mother-daughter relationship is positive. If the baby's father is involved in the pregnancy, he and the pregnant adolescent's mother may be able to work together to support the teenage mother. The nurse can update the pregnant adolescent's mother on childbearing practices to clarify any misconceptions she might have. During labor and birth, the mother may be a key figure for her daughter, offering reassurance and instilling confidence in the teen.

The younger the adolescent when she gives birth, the more she needs her mother's support. Children of adolescent parents experience more negative outcomes, including more aggressive behavior at a younger age, when the adolescent is in constant conflict with her mother and becomes less involved in parenting.

NURSING MANAGEMENT

NURSING ASSESSMENT AND DIAGNOSIS

Establish a knowledge base to plan interventions for the adolescent mother-to-be and family. Areas of assessment include history of family and personal physical health, developmental level and impact of pregnancy, and emotional and financial support. Also assess the family and social support network and the father's degree of involvement in the pregnancy.

As with all pregnant women, it is important to have information on general physical health. This may be the first time the adolescent has ever provided a health history. Consequently it may be helpful to ask specific questions

and give examples if the young woman appears confused about a question. The teen's mother may be best able to answer questions about family history because the adolescent is often unaware of this information.

Assess the following areas: family and personal health history, medical history, menstrual history, obstetric and gynecologic history, and substance abuse history. It is also important to assess the maturational level of each person. The adolescent's development level and the impact of pregnancy are reflected in the degree of recognition of the realities and responsibilities involved in teenage pregnancy and parenting. Also assess the mother's self-concept (including body image), her relationship with the significant adults in her life, her attitude toward her pregnancy, and her coping methods in the situation, as well as the teen's knowledge of, attitude toward, and anticipated ability to care for the coming baby.

Ask specifically about dating violence. Teens are not likely to reveal dating violence unless they are asked about it. Because of social pressures to date or to be in an intimate relationship, some girls tolerate dating violence; others misinterpret a partner's controlling or coercive behavior as evidence of his love. Adolescent girls are at increased risk if their family uses violence to resolve conflict (Seimer, 2004).

The socioeconomic status of the pregnant adolescent often places the baby at risk throughout life, beginning with conception. It is essential to assess family and social support systems, as well as the extent of financial support available.

The nursing diagnoses applicable to pregnant women in general apply to the pregnant adolescent. Other nursing diagnoses are influenced by the adolescent's age, support systems, socioeconomic situation, health, and maturity. Examples of nursing diagnoses specific to the pregnant adolescent may include the following:

- *Health-Seeking Behaviors: Information about Child Care* related to expressed desire to parent effectively
- *Imbalanced Nutrition: Less than Body Requirements* related to poor eating habits
- *Risk for Situational Low Self-Esteem* related to unanticipated pregnancy

PLANNING AND IMPLEMENTATION

Nursing Care in the Community

Nurses who work with adolescent girls can help them by providing information and guidance that enables each teen to make choices that are based on and lead to the attainment of four goals (Short & Rosenthal, 2003):

- Developing a positive attitude about her body and its physical changes
- Accepting and feeling comfortable about desire, arousal, and sexual feelings

- Feeling comfortable about sexual behavior
- Practicing safer-sex behaviors (for sexually experienced adolescents)

If pregnancy occurs, early, thorough prenatal care is the strongest and most critical determinant for reducing risk for the adolescent mother and her newborn. The nurse needs to understand the special needs of the adolescent mother to meet this challenge successfully.

Many new and innovative community-based programs have evolved to provide care for high-risk clients and their partners throughout the childbearing experience and beyond. In addition, family planning clinics and clinics offering reproductive health services are beginning to offer male clinics to encourage young men to be more responsible for their own health and that of their partners (Raine, Marcell, Rocca, & Harper, 2003). Nurses in community-based agencies can help adolescents access the healthcare system as well as social services and other support services (e.g., food banks and the Special Supplemental Nutrition Program for Women, Infants, and Children [WIC]). These nurses are also involved extensively in counseling and client teaching.

Issue of Confidentiality. Most states in the United States have passed legislation that confirms the right of some minors to assume the rights of adults; they are then called *emancipated minors*. An adolescent may be considered emancipated if he or she is self-supporting and living away from home, married, pregnant, a parent, or in the military service. The pregnant adolescent, even if very young, is generally considered emancipated and has the right and responsibility to consent to healthcare for herself and, later, for her child. If she is considered emancipated, she is entitled to confidentiality in her dealings with healthcare providers. Only with her agreement can other adults, including her parents, be included in communication.

Development of a Trusting Relationship with the Pregnant Adolescent. The first visit to the clinic or caregiver's office may make the young woman feel anxious and vulnerable. Making this first experience as positive as possible for the young woman will encourage the adolescent to return for follow-up care and to cooperate with her caregivers and will help her recognize the importance of healthcare for her and her baby. Developing a trusting relationship with the pregnant adolescent is essential. Honesty, respect, and a caring attitude promote self-esteem.

Depending on the adolescent's age, this may be her first pelvic examination, an anxiety-provoking experience for any woman. Provide explanations during the procedure. A gentle and thoughtful examination technique will help the young woman to relax.

Promotion of Self-Esteem and Problem-Solving Skills. Assist the adolescent in her decision-making and problem-solving skills so that she can proceed with her developmental tasks and begin to assume responsibility for her life and that of her newborn. Many adolescents are not aware of the legally available options to deal with an unplanned pregnancy. In an open, nonjudgmental way, without imposing personal values, educate the teen about her alternatives: terminating the pregnancy, maintaining the pregnancy and parenting the infant, or relinquishing the infant for adoption. The nurse can also provide information about community resources available to help with each alternative. Once the teen has decided on a course of action, healthcare providers should respect her decision and support her efforts to achieve her goals.

If the adolescent chooses to continue her pregnancy, describe what she can expect over the prenatal period and provide an explanation and rationale for each procedure as it occurs. This overview fosters the adolescent's understanding and gives her some control (Figure 13–1 ●).

Early adolescents tend to be egocentric and oriented to the present. They may not think it is important that their health and habits affect the fetus. Thus, it is often helpful to emphasize how these practices affect the teens themselves.

● **FIGURE 13–1**

The nurse gives this young mother an opportunity to listen to her baby's heartbeat.

Early adolescents also need help in problem solving and in visualizing the future so they can plan effectively.

Middle adolescents are developing the ability to think abstractly and can recognize that actions may have long-term consequences. They may not yet have acquired assertive communication skills, however, and may be reluctant to ask questions. Therefore, ask teens directly if they have questions. Middle adolescents can absorb more detailed health teaching and apply it.

Late adolescents can think abstractly, plan for the future, and function in a manner comparable to older pregnant women. They can also handle complex information and apply it.

Promotion of Physical Well-Being. Baseline weight and blood pressure measurements are valuable in assessing weight gain and predisposition to preeclampsia. Encourage the adolescent to take part in her care by measuring and recording her own weight. Use this time as an opportunity for assisting the young woman in problem solving. Encourage her to ask herself the following questions: "Have I gained too much or too little weight?" "What influence does my diet have on my weight?" "How can I change my eating habits?"

Also introduce the subject of nutrition during measurement of baseline and subsequent hemoglobin and hematocrit values. Because the adolescent is at risk for anemia, she needs education about the importance of iron in her diet. Indeed, basic education about nutrition is a critical component of care for pregnant teens.

Preeclampsia-eclampsia is the most prevalent medical complication of pregnant adolescents. Blood pressure readings of 140/90 mm Hg are not acceptable as the determinant of preeclampsia in adolescents. Women ages 14 to 20 years without evidence of high blood pressure usually have diastolic readings between 50 and 66 mm Hg. Gradual increases from the prepregnant diastolic readings, along with excessive weight gain, must be evaluated as precursors to preeclampsia. Establishment of baseline readings is one reason early prenatal care is vital to management of the pregnant adolescent.

THINKING CRITICALLY

A MOTHER CONSIDERING ADOPTION

Rachel Kalaras is an 18-year-old G1P0 who is 16 weeks pregnant when she arrives for her prenatal visit. When discussing her plans for the pregnancy, Rachel indicates that she is considering adoption. She has not discussed this plan with anyone but is seeking information about the process of relinquishment. What should you consider in discussing this issue with Rachel?

Adolescents have an increased incidence of STIs. The initial prenatal examination should include gonococcal and chlamydial cultures; wet-mount prep for *Candida, Trichomonas,* and *Gardnerella;* and tests for syphilis. Although today's teens are knowledgeable about HIV/AIDS, they know much less about other STIs, especially with regard to symptoms and risk reduction, so education is important. If the adolescent's history indicates that she is at increased risk for HIV, she should be given information about it and offered HIV screening.

Discuss substance abuse with the adolescent. It is important to review the risks associated with the use of tobacco, caffeine, drugs, and alcohol. The young woman should be aware of how these substances affect both her and her fetus's development.

Ongoing care should include the same assessments that an older pregnant woman receives. Pay special attention to evaluating fetal growth by determining when quickening occurs and by measuring fundal height, fetal heart rate, and fetal movement. If there is a question of size-date discrepancy by 2 cm either way when assessing fundal height, an ultrasound is warranted to establish fetal age so that instances of intrauterine growth restriction can be detected early.

Promotion of Family Adaptation. Assess the family situation during the first prenatal visit and find out the level of involvement the adolescent wants from each of her family members and the father of the child, as well as her perception of their present support. If the mother and daughter agree, the mother should be included in the client's care. Also help the teen's mother assess and meet her daughter's needs. Some adolescents become more dependent during pregnancy, and some become more independent. The mother can ease and encourage her daughter's self-growth by understanding how best to respond to and support the adolescent.

The adolescent's relationship with her father is also affected by her pregnancy. Provide information to the adolescent's father and encourage his involvement to whatever degree is acceptable to both daughter and father.

The father of the adolescent's infant should not be forgotten in promoting the family's adaptation to the pregnancy. He should be included in prenatal visits, classes, health teaching, and the birth itself to the extent that he wishes and that is acceptable to the teenage mother. He should also have the opportunity to express his feelings and concerns and to have his questions answered.

Facilitation of Prenatal Education. School systems attempt to meet prenatal education needs in many ways. The most effective method appears to be mainstreaming the pregnant adolescent in academic classes with her peers and adding classes appropriate to her needs during pregnancy and postpartum. Classes about growth and development beginning with the newborn and early infancy periods can help teenage parents to develop realistic expectations of their infants and may help decrease child abuse. Mainstreaming is an ideal way to help teens complete their education while learning the skills they need to cope. Vocational guidance in this setting is also beneficial as they plan for their futures.

Most childbirth educators believe that prenatal classes with other teens are best, even though they can be challenging to teach (Figure 13–2 ●). The pregnant teen may be accompanied by her mother, her boyfriend, or her girlfriends. Those who bring girlfriends may bring a different one each time, and giggling and side conversations may occur. Such activity reflects the short attention span of the teen and is fairly typical. Thus, to keep the attention of the participants, it is important to use a variety of teaching strategies including audiovisual aids, demonstrations, and games.

Goals for prenatal classes may include some or all of the following:

- Providing anticipatory guidance about pregnancy
- Preparing participants for labor and birth
- Helping participants identify the problems and conflicts of teenage pregnancy and parenting
- Promoting increased self-esteem
- Providing information about available community resources
- Helping participants develop adaptive coping skills

Although parenting topics are sometimes included in prenatal classes for adolescents, teens may not retain the information because they tend to be present oriented. Parenting skills are crucial, but adolescents generally are not ready to learn about these skills until birth makes the newborn—and thus parenting—a reality.

● **FIGURE 13–2**

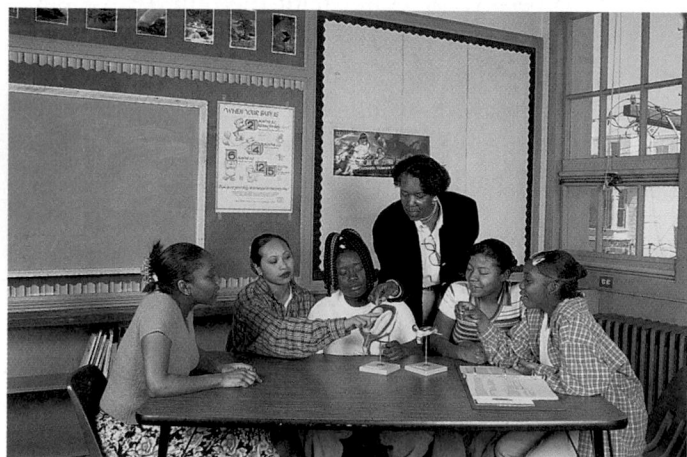

Young adolescents may benefit from prenatal classes designed for them.

Hospital-Based Nursing Care

The adolescent's mother is often present during the teen's labor and birth. The father of the baby may also be involved. Close girlfriends may arrive soon after the teen is admitted. At admission, ask the teen who will be her primary support person in labor and who she wants involved in the labor and birth. This information may also be included on her prenatal record.

The adolescent in labor has the same care needs as any pregnant woman. However, she may require more sustained care. Be readily available and answer questions simply and honestly, using lay terminology. Also help the adolescent's support people understand their roles in assisting the teen. If the father of the baby is involved, encourage him, at his own level of comfort, to play an active role in all phases of the birth process, perhaps by supporting the teen's relaxation techniques, feeding her ice chips, timing her contractions, and coaching her with her breathing. Recommend hand-holding, back rubs, and supportive touching.

During the postpartum period, most teens do not foresee that they will become sexually active in the near future and are often adamant that they will not become pregnant again for a long time. However, the statistics demonstrate a different reality. Consequently, predischarge teaching should include information about the resumption of ovulation and the importance of contraception. It is especially helpful to provide this information to both the adolescent mother and her sexual partner. Encourage the couple to use condoms and spermicide until they choose another method of birth control. Additional effective contraceptive options for adolescents include combined oral contraceptives, the contraceptive patch, and NuvaRing (vaginal ring). Implanted rods such as Norplant are also a good choice in countries where the rods are available, although teens tend to dislike the associated side effects. Intrauterine devices (IUDs) are not recommended for adolescents (Graydanus, Patel, & Rimsza, 2001), and many teens are not comfortable with a diaphragm. See the discussion of contraceptive options in Chapter 4. ∞

As part of discharge planning, ensure that the teen is aware of community resources available to assist her and her family. Postpartum classes, especially with peers, can be particularly beneficial. Such classes address a variety of topics, including postpartum adaptation, infant and child development, and parenting skills.

EVALUATION

Expected outcomes of nursing care include the following:

- A trusting relationship is established with the pregnant adolescent.
- The adolescent is able to use her problem-solving abilities to make appropriate choices.

- The adolescent follows the recommendations of the healthcare team and receives effective healthcare throughout her pregnancy, the birth, and the postpartum period.

- The adolescent, her partner (if he is involved), and their families are able to cope successfully with the effects of the pregnancy.

- The adolescent is able to discuss pregnancy, prenatal care, and childbirth.

- The adolescent develops skill in child care and parenting.

PREVENTION OF ADOLESCENT PREGNANCY

In 1996 the National Campaign to Prevent Teen Pregnancy was founded. The group's purpose is to reduce teenage pregnancy one third by 2005 (National Campaign to Prevent Teen Pregnancy, 2000). The National Campaign is a private, nonprofit organization made up of a broad spectrum of religious, political, social, human services, health, and academic organizations. The Association of Women's Health, Obstetric and Neonatal Nurses (AWHONN) is one of the many professional organizations that joined this group and made a commitment to focus on adolescent pregnancy prevention. Not surprisingly, the task forces have found that adolescent pregnancy is a multifaceted problem with no easy answers. The best approach is local and is based on strong, community-wide involvement with a variety of programs directed at the multiple causes of the problem.

One of the major problems in local communities continues to be intense conflict among different groups about how to approach adolescent pregnancy prevention. Some groups believe that abstinence is the only answer, whereas others believe that abstinence programs do not work with the many teens who are already sexually active. The latter groups believe that sex education and easy availability of contraception are the answers. Many parents advocate an "abstinence-plus" approach that stresses abstinence as the best approach but includes information on condoms and contraception for those teens who do not abstain.

Recent research suggests that only 7% of people in the United States believe that sex education should not be provided in schools. Moreover, controversy about the type of sex education offered in schools seems to have decreased. Nearly three fourths (74%) of principals surveyed state that they have not had any recent discussions or debate (in school board, Parent-Teacher Association, or other public meetings) about what should be taught (National Public Radio [NPR], Kaiser Family Foundation, and John F. Kennedy School of Government, 2004).

Research suggests that programs to address societal problems and give teens hope for a different future are more effective than programs narrowly focused on teen sexual activity (Aquiline & Bragadottir, 2000). In teen populations with job accessibility and education, easy, confidential access to sex education and contraception is also important in reducing teen pregnancy rates.

After visiting communities that have launched programs to prevent adolescent pregnancy, members of the National Campaign concluded that adults must agree to disagree and individual groups must be encouraged to move ahead with their different programs. This conclusion reflects a recognition that the cause of adolescent pregnancy varies from one community to another and thus a variety of approaches are needed. For instance, in inner-city areas, where there are high rates of poverty, low self-esteem, school failure, early behavioral problems, and delinquent behaviors, it is critical to offer programs that promote self-esteem, deal with these social ills, and provide hope for these youth.

The National Campaign's task forces have also identified characteristics shared by all successful programs, regardless of the type of offering or community. Effective adolescent pregnancy prevention programs are long term and intensive. They also involve adolescents in program planning, include good role models from the same cultural and racial backgrounds, and focus on the adolescent male.

Survey data from a representative sample of teens and adults provide some additional interesting insights (National Campaign to Prevent Teen Pregnancy, 2004):

- Parents tend to underestimate their influence on their adolescents. Teens report that their parents, and not their friends, have the most influence on the teens' decisions about sex. However, a preponderance of teens also report that it would be easier to deal with issues related to sexuality and teen pregnancy if they could have more honest, open conversations with their parents.

- Teens' expressed attitudes about sexual activity reflect more cautious values and attitudes than generally believed. Teens report that their values, morals, religious beliefs, and concern for their future influence their decisions about sex more than concerns about becoming pregnant or developing a sexually transmitted infection.

- Almost all the adults and teens surveyed said that society should give teens a strong message that they should not have sex until they are at least out of high school.

- The majority of both groups advocate a message stressing abstinence while also providing information about contraception. They rejected the notion that such an approach sends a "mixed message."

- Teens want more information about sexuality, abstinence, and contraception.

- Teens tend to overestimate the percentage of their classmates and peers who have had sex.

Critical Concept Review

LEARNING OBJECTIVES	CONCEPTS
Define the scope of the problem of adolescent pregnancy.	1. The adolescent pregnancy rate is 41.7 per 1000 females. This rate has been declining and is at historic lows. 2. Despite the decline, the United States continues to have one of the highest levels of adolescent childbearing among industrialized nations.
Summarize factors contributing to adolescent pregnancy.	1. Many factors contribute to the high teenage pregnancy rate: ■ Earlier age at first experience with sexual intercourse. ■ Lack of knowledge about conception. ■ Lack of easy access to contraception. ■ Lessened stigma associated with adolescent pregnancy in some populations. ■ Poverty. ■ Early school failure. ■ Early childhood sexual abuse.
Discuss the physical, psychologic, and sociologic risks a pregnant adolescent faces.	1. Physical risks: ■ Preterm birth. ■ Low birth weight of infant. ■ Cephalopelvic disproportion of mother. ■ Iron deficiency anemia. ■ Preeclampsia. 2. Psychologic risks: ■ Interruption of the developmental tasks of adolescence. 3. Sociologic risks: ■ More likely to drop out of school. ■ Need for public assistance. ■ Low-paying employment. ■ Single parenthood. ■ Increased domestic violence.
Delineate characteristics of the fathers of children of adolescent mothers.	1. Fathers of children of adolescent mothers: ■ 50% are greater than 20 years of age. ■ Generally from same socioeconomic and educational level as adolescent mother. ■ Often have experienced early school failure.
Discuss the range of reactions of the adolescent's family and social network to her pregnancy.	1. Families with high educational and career goals for their children experience: ■ Anger. ■ Shock. ■ Shame. ■ Sorrow. 2. Teen often chooses abortion unless cultural or religious beliefs prohibit this. 3. Teen receives more support from family and friends where adolescent pregnancy is more common and more socially acceptable. 4. Some adolescent fathers may view pregnancy as: ■ Sign of adult status. ■ Sign of increased sexual prowess. 5. The mother of the adolescent usually provides the most support.

LEARNING OBJECTIVES

CONCEPTS

Formulate a plan of care to meet the needs of a pregnant adolescent.

1. Nursing care of the pregnant adolescent includes:
   - Obtaining consent for care.
   - Developing a trusting relationship with the adolescent.
   - Promoting self-esteem and problem-solving skills in the adolescent.
   - Promoting the physical health of the adolescent, especially with information concerning:
     - Regular prenatal visits.
     - Signs of complications.
     - Sexually transmitted diseases.
     - Substance abuse.
     - Promoting family adaptation.
     - Facilitating prenatal education.

Describe successful community approaches to prevention of adolescent pregnancy.

1. Effective adolescent pregnancy prevention programs:
   - Are long term and intensive.
   - Involve adolescents in program planning.
   - Include good role models from the same cultural and racial backgrounds.
   - Include a focus on the adolescent male.

CRITICAL THINKING IN ACTION

View the **Critical Thinking In Action** video in Chapter 13 of the CD-ROM. Then, answer the questions that follow.

Sixteen-year-old Linda Perez and her mother present to you at the OB clinic for Linda's first prenatal visit. You determine that Linda is 20 weeks pregnant. Her weight is 135 lb, height 5'4", T 98°F, P 80, R 14, BP 100/64. You assess that Linda's mother has type 2 diabetes, and that her siblings are healthy. Linda admits to having one sexual partner and says she has never been hospitalized. Her immunizations are up to date and she's never used tobacco or recreational drugs. To date, the father of the baby is not involved. Mrs. Perez is clearly upset over the fact that Linda's pregnancy is so far advanced without her knowledge. Linda is very quiet and speaks only when questioned directly. You do your best to try to establish a trusting relationship with Linda and her mother by providing an atmosphere where issues can be discussed.

1. What psychologic factors contribute to teenage pregnancy?
2. Explore reasons why teenagers delay prenatal care.
3. Linda's mother asks you what factors facilitate adolescent pregnancies.
4. You assess that Linda has some anxiety concerning the birth process. She states she is not interested in prenatal classes because she is single and does not want to have natural childbirth. Your best response would be:

MEDIALINK

www.prenhall.com/london

- NCLEX-RN® Review, case studies, and other interactive resources for this chapter can be found on the Companion Website at http://www.prenhall.com/london. Click on "Chapter 13" to select the activities for this chapter.

Care Plan
A 15-year-old high school student is in the 18th week of her pregnancy, but has not yet told her parents. She is still trying to wear her regular clothes and limit her eating in an attempt to stay slim. Develop a Care Plan to help the teenager address the related developmental tasks of pregnancy and improve her response to her pregnancy. Fill in the appropriate elements of the Care Plan for the client in the boxes below.

This activity contains 3 questions.

1.   Assessment and Diagnosis

To create paragraphs in your essay response, type <p> at the beginning of the paragraph, and </p> at the end.

- For animations, more NCLEX-RN® Review questions, and an audio glossary, access the accompanying CD-ROM in this textbook.

REFERENCES

Alan Guttmacher Institute. (2002). Sexual and reproductive health: Women and men. *Facts in brief.* Washington, DC: Author.

Aquiline, M., & Bragadottir, H. (2000). Adolescent pregnancy: Teen perspectives on prevention. *MCN. American Journal of Maternal Child Nursing, 25*(4), 192–197.

Cohen, D. A., Farley, T. A., Taylor, S. N., Martin, D. H., & Schuster, M. A. (2002). When and where do youths have sex? The potential role of adult supervision. *Pediatrics, 110*(6), e66.

Doniger, A., Adams, E., Utter, C. A., & Riley, J. S. (2001). Impact evaluation of the "not me, not now" abstinence-oriented adolescent pregnancy prevention communication program, Monroe County, New York. *Journal of Health Communication, 6*(1), 45–60.

Glass, N., Fredland, N., Campbell, J., Yonas, M., Sharps, P., & Kub, J. (2003). Adolescent dating violence: Prevalence, risk factors, health outcomes, and implications for clinical practice. *Journal of Obstetric, Gynecologic, and Neonatal Nursing, 32*(2), 227–238.

Graydanus, D., Patel, D., & Rimsza, M. (2001). Contraception in the adolescent: An update. *Pediatrics, 107*(3), 526–573.

Hamilton, B. E., Martin, J. A., & Sutton, P. D. (2004). Births: Preliminary data for 2003. *National Vital Statistics Reports, 53* (9), 1–18.

Klein, J. D., & The Committee on Adolescence. (2005). Adolescent pregnancy: Current trends and issues. *Pediatrics, 116*, 281–286.

Loewenson, P. R., Ireland, M., & Resnick, M. D. (2004). Primary and secondary sexual abstinence in high school students. *Journal of Adolescent Health, 34*(3), 209–215.

Manlove, J., Ryan, S., & Franzetta, K. (2003). Patterns of contraceptive use within teenagers' first sexual relationships. *Perspectives on Sexual and Reproductive Health, 35*(6), 246–255.

Marcell, A. V., Raine, T., & Eyre, S. L. (2003). Where does reproductive health fit into the lives of adolescent males? *Perspectives on Sexual and Reproductive Health, 35*(4), 180–186.

Martin, J. A., Hamilton, B. E., Sutton, P. D., et al. (2003). Birth: Final data for 2002. *National Vital Statistics Reports, 52*(10), 1–114.

Montgomery, K. S. (2003). Nursing care for pregnant adolescents. *Journal of Obstetric, Gynecologic, and Neonatal Nursing, 32*(2), 249–257.

National Campaign to Prevent Teen Pregnancy. (2000). *Fact sheet report.* Washington, DC: Author.

National Campaign to Prevent Teen Pregnancy. (2004). *Survey slices: Highlights from the National Campaign's 2003 Annual Survey.* Retrieved January 22, 2004, from http://www.teenpregnancy.org

National Public Radio [NPR], Kaiser Family Foundation, and John F. Kennedy School of Government. (2004). *NPR/Kaiser/Kennedy School Poll: Sex education in America.* Retrieved April 18, 2004, from http://www.kff.org

Preventing teenage pregnancy. (2002, June 10). U.S. Department of Health and Human Services press release. Retrieved October 20, 2002, from http://www.hhs.gov/news/press/2002press/teenpreg.html

Raine, T., Marcell, A. V., Rocca, C. H., & Harper, C. C. (2003). The other half of the equation: Serving young men in a young women's reproductive health clinic. *Perspectives on Sexual and Reproductive Health, 35*(5), 208–214.

Scheiman, L., & Zeoli, A. M. (2003). Adolescents' experiences of dating and intimate partner violence: "Once is not enough." *Journal of Midwifery and Women's Health, 48*(3), 226–228.

Seimer, B. S. (2004). Intimate violence in adolescent relationships. *MCN. American Journal of Maternal Child Nursing, 29*(3), 117–121.

Short, M. B., & Rosenthal, S. L. (2003). Helping teenaged girls make wise sexual decisions. *Contemporary OB/GYN, 48*(5), 84–95.

Singh, S., & Darroch, J. E. (2000). Adolescent pregnancy and childbearing: Levels and trends in developed countries. *Family Planning Perspectives, 32*(1), 14–23.

Steinberg, L. (2002). *Adolescence* (6th ed.). New York: McGraw-Hill.

Weinstock, H., Berman, S., & Cates, W. (2004). Sexually transmitted diseases among American youth: Incidence and prevalence estimates, 2000. *Perspectives on Sexual and Reproductive Health, 36*(1), 6–10.

Pregnancy at Risk: Pregestational Problems

When I learned I had gestational diabetes I felt panicky. My grandmother died of diabetes and it has always scared me. However, by taking each day as it came, cooperating with my doctors and nurses, and watching my diet, I did fine and gave birth to a beautiful 7 pound 10 ounce daughter. One good thing has come of the experience—I'm no longer so terrified of developing diabetes. I have become far more careful about taking care of myself, and I now think of diabetes as a chronic disease to be controlled.

—*Ayisha, 34*

LEARNING OBJECTIVES

- Summarize the effects of alcohol and illicit drugs on the childbearing woman and her fetus/newborn.

- Relate the pathology and clinical treatment of diabetes mellitus in pregnancy to the implications for nursing care.

- Discriminate among the types of anemia associated with pregnancy regarding signs, treatment, and implications for pregnancy.

- Discuss acquired immunodeficiency syndrome (AIDS), including care of the pregnant woman who has tested positive for the human immunodeficiency virus (HIV), fetal/neonatal implications, and ramifications for the childbearing family.

- Describe the effects of various heart disorders on pregnancy, including their implications for nursing care.

- Delineate the effects of selected pregestational medical conditions on pregnancy.

MEDIALINK

www.prenhall.com/london

CD-ROM

NCLEX-RN® Review
Audio Glossary

Companion Website

NCLEX-RN® Review
MediaLink Applications:
    Case Study: Client with Gestational Diabetes
    Care Plan: Woman with Diabetes Mellitus
    Care Plan Activity: Antepartal Client at Risk
Thinking Critically

For some women, pregnancy may become a life-threatening event because of potential or existing complications. These complications can be the result of factors such as age, parity, blood type, socioeconomic status, psychologic health, or preexisting chronic illnesses. This chapter focuses on women with pregestational medical disorders and their possible effects on the pregnancy.

CARE OF THE WOMAN WITH SUBSTANCE ABUSE PROBLEMS

Substance abuse occurs when a person experiences difficulties with work, family, social relations, and health as a result of alcohol or drug use. In general the rate of illicit drug use among pregnant women is significantly less than the rate among nonpregnant women. Approximately 3% of pregnant women ages 15 to 44 report having used an illicit drug in the past month as compared to 9% of nonpregnant women. However, illicit drug use varies significantly by age with higher rates among women ages 15 to 25 (6.8%) than among women ages 26 to 44 (0.5%) (Substance Abuse and Mental Health Services Administration [SAMHSA], 2004). See Figure 14–1 ●.

Drugs that are commonly misused include tobacco, alcohol, cocaine, marijuana, amphetamines, barbiturates, hallucinogens, club drugs, heroin, and other narcotics. (Tobacco is discussed in Chapter 11 as a teratogenic substance. ∞) Polydrug use involving multiple substances such as alcohol, tobacco, and illicit drugs is fairly common and contributes to

● **FIGURE 14–1**

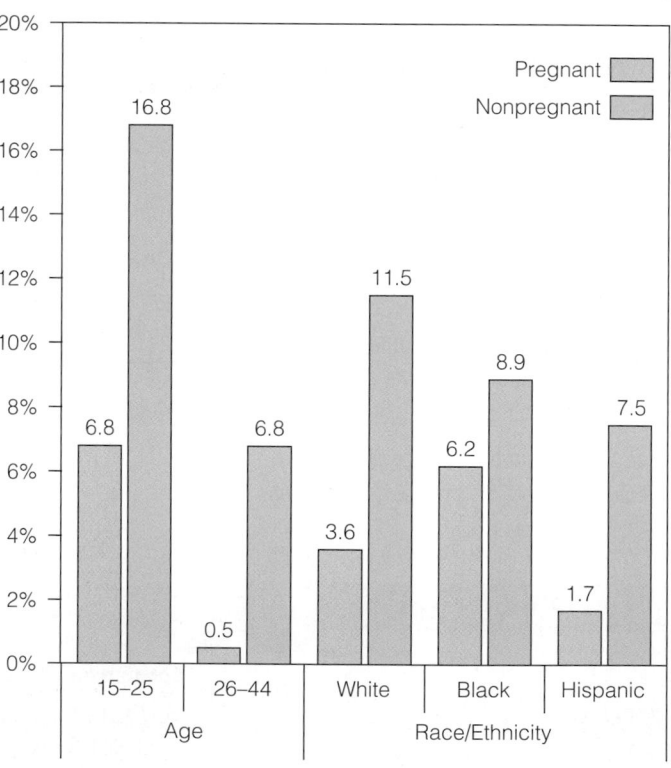

Percentages of past month illicit drug use among women ages 15 to 44, by pregnancy status, age, and race/ethnicity: 2002.

Data from the National Survey on Drug Use and Health (NSDUH) Report. *(2004). Pregnancy and substance use. Washington, DC: Office of Applied Sciences, Substance Abuse and Mental Health Services Administration.*

the risks a pregnant woman faces. Table 14–1 identifies common addictive drugs and their effects on the fetus or newborn.

Drug use during pregnancy, particularly in the first trimester, may have a negative effect on the health of the woman and the growth and development of the fetus. Unfortunately, prenatal drug use may be the most frequently missed diagnosis in all of maternity care. Physicians and nurses may fail to ask women about drug and alcohol use because of their own lack of knowledge, discomfort, or biases. Often substance-abusing women wait until late in pregnancy to seek healthcare. Moreover, the substance-abusing woman who seeks early prenatal care may not vol-untarily reveal her addiction, so healthcare providers should be alert for a history or physical signs that might indicate substance abuse.

NURSING PRACTICE

Keep in mind that at least 1 of 10 women in the United States, regardless of socioeconomic status or ethnic background, is currently abusing a substance. If you consider that possibility with every woman, you will ask the important questions about drug use and be alert for signs of substance abuse.

TABLE 14–1 ✣ Possible Effects of Selected Drugs of Abuse or Addiction on Fetus and Neonate

Maternal Drug	Effect on Fetus and Neonate
Depressants	
Alcohol	Mental retardation, microcephaly, midfacial hypoplasia, cardiac anomalies, intrauterine growth restriction (IUGR), potential teratogenic effects, fetal alcohol syndrome (FAS), fetal alcohol effects (FAE)
Narcotics	
Heroin	Withdrawal symptoms, convulsions, death, IUGR, respiratory alkalosis, hyperbilirubinemia
Methadone	Fetal distress, meconium aspiration; low birth weight; with abrupt termination of the drug, severe withdrawal symptoms, neonatal death
Barbiturates	Neonatal depression, increased anomalies; teratogenic effect (?); withdrawal symptoms, convulsions, hyperactivity, hyperreflexia, vasomotor instability
Phenobarbital	Bleeding (with excessive doses)
"T's and Blues" (combination of the following)	
Talwin (narcotic)	Safe for use in pregnancy; depresses respiration if taken close to time of birth
Amytal (barbiturate)	See barbiturates
Tranquilizers	
Phenothiazine derivatives	Withdrawal, extrapyramidal dysfunction, delayed respiratory onset, hyperbilirubinemia, hypotonia or hyperactivity, decreased platelet count
Diazepam (Valium)	Hypotonia, hypothermia, low Apgar score, respiratory depression, poor sucking reflex, possible cleft lip
Antianxiety drugs	
Lithium	Congenital anomalies, especially Ebstein anomaly; lethargy and cyanosis in the newborn
Stimulants	
Amphetamines	
Amphetamine sulfate (Benzedrine)	Generalized arthritis, learning disabilities, poor motor coordination, transposition of the great vessels, cleft palate
Dextroamphetamine sulfate (Dexedrine)	Congenital heart defects, hyperbilirubinemia
Cocaine	Cerebral infarctions, microcephaly, learning disabilities, poor state organization, decreased interactive behavior, central nervous system (CNS) anomalies, cardiac anomalies, IUGR, genitourinary anomalies, sudden infant death syndrome (SIDS)
Nicotine (half to one pack cigarettes/day)	Increased rate of spontaneous abortion, increased incidence of placental abruption, small for gestational age (SGA), cleft lip and palate, SIDS
Psychotropics	
PCP ("angel dust")	Flaccid appearance, poor head control, impaired neurologic development
LSD	Chromosomal breakage?
Marijuana	IUGR, SIDS

Providing effective prenatal care to chemically dependent women is often challenging for clinicians. However, pregnancy is a time when most women are receptive to caring interventions.

SUBSTANCES COMMONLY ABUSED DURING PREGNANCY

Alcohol

Alcohol is a central nervous system (CNS) depressant and a potent teratogen. The incidence of alcohol abuse is highest among women ages 20 to 40 years although alcoholism is also seen in teenagers. Alcohol use among pregnant women tends to decrease by trimester. Chronic abuse of alcohol can undermine maternal health by causing malnutrition (especially folic acid and thiamine deficiencies), bone marrow suppression, increased incidence of infections, and liver disease.

The effects of alcohol on the fetus may result in a group of signs known as *fetal alcohol syndrome (FAS)*. The syndrome has characteristic physical and mental abnormalities that vary in severity. (See discussion in Chapter 25. ∞) There is no final answer to how much alcohol a woman can safely drink during pregnancy. Consequently the expectant woman should avoid alcohol completely. Even low levels of alcohol cannot be recommended (Cunningham, Leveno, Bloom et al., 2005).

As a result of alcohol dependence, a woman may have withdrawal seizures in the intrapartal period as early as 12 to 48 hours after she stops drinking. Delirium tremens may occur in the postpartal period, and the newborn may suffer a withdrawal syndrome. Nurses in the maternal-newborn unit must be aware of the manifestations of alcohol abuse so they can prepare for the woman's special needs. Care includes sedation to decrease irritability and tremors, seizure precautions, intravenous (IV) fluid therapy for hydration, and preparation for an addicted newborn. Although high doses of sedatives and analgesics may be necessary for the woman, caution is advised because these medications can cause fetal depression.

Breastfeeding generally is not contraindicated, although alcohol is excreted in breast milk. Excessive alcohol consumption may intoxicate the infant and inhibit the maternal letdown reflex. Discharge planning for the alcohol-addicted mother and newborn needs to be correlated with the social service department of the hospital.

Cocaine and Crack

Nearly 3% of pregnant women use illicit drugs such as cocaine, marijuana, Ecstasy, other amphetamines, and heroin (March of Dimes, 2005). Cocaine use during pregnancy tends to affect between 1% and 5% of newborns (Wilson & Thorp, 2003). Cocaine acts at the nerve terminals to prevent the reuptake of dopamine and norepi-

nephrine, which in turn results in vasoconstriction, tachycardia, and hypertension. Placental vasoconstriction decreases blood flow to the fetus. The onset of cocaine effects occurs rapidly, but the euphoria lasts only about 30 minutes. Euphoria and excitement are usually followed by irritability, depression, pessimism, fatigue, and a strong desire for more cocaine. This pattern often leads the user to take repeated doses to sustain the effect. Cocaine metabolites may be present in the urine of a pregnant woman for as long as 4 to 7 days after use.

Cocaine can be taken by IV injection or by snorting the powdered form. *Crack*, a form of freebase cocaine that is made up of baking soda, water, and cocaine mixed into a paste and microwaved to form a rock, can be smoked. Smoking crack leads to a quicker, more intense high because the drug is absorbed through the large surface area of the lungs.

The cocaine user is difficult to identify prenatally. Because cocaine is illegal, many women are reluctant to admit that they use it. The nurse may recognize subtle signs of cocaine use, including mood swings and appetite changes, and withdrawal symptoms such as depression, irritability, nausea, lack of motivation, and psychomotor changes.

Major adverse maternal effects of cocaine use include seizures and hallucinations, pulmonary edema, cerebral hemorrhage, respiratory failure, and heart problems. Women who use cocaine have an increased incidence of spontaneous abortion, abruptio placentae, preterm birth, and stillbirth.

Fetal exposure to cocaine increases the risk of intrauterine growth restriction (IUGR), small head circumference, cerebral infarctions, altered brain development, shorter body length, malformations of the genitourinary tract, and lower Apgar scores. Newborns exposed to cocaine in utero may have neurobehavioral disturbances, marked irritability, an exaggerated startle reflex, labile emotions, and an increased risk of sudden infant death syndrome (SIDS). (See Chapter 30 for further discussion. ∞)

Cocaine crosses into breast milk and may cause symptoms in the breastfeeding infant, including extreme irritability, vomiting, diarrhea, dilated pupils, and apnea. Thus, women who continue to use cocaine after childbirth should avoid breastfeeding.

Marijuana

Marijuana is the most widely used illicit drug among women, both pregnant and nonpregnant (SAMHSA, 2004). More than 25% of women of reproductive age admit to current or past marijuana use (Wilson & Thorp, 2003). Marijuana use is associated with impaired coordination, memory, and critical thinking ability. As a result, the pregnant woman or new mother who uses marijuana may be at risk if she tries to perform tasks that require complex mental activities (Reedy & Brucker, 2004). To date, there is no strong evidence that marijuana has teratogenic effects on the fetus. However, its risks are dose related, with an increased risk of IUGR and SIDS in infants born to heavy users (Wilson & Thorp, 2003). In reality the impact of heavy marijuana use on pregnancy is difficult to evaluate because of the variety of social factors that may influence the results.

MDMA (Ecstasy)

Methylenedioxymethamphetamine (MDMA), better known as Ecstasy, is the most commonly used of a group of drugs referred to as *club drugs,* so called because they have become popular among adolescents and young adults who frequent dance clubs and "raves." Other club drugs include flunitrazepam (Rohypnol), gamma hydroxybutyrate (GHB), and ketamine hydrochloride. Phencyclidine (PCP) and LSD are sometimes classified as club drugs as well.

MDMA is taken by mouth, usually as a tablet. It produces euphoria and feelings of empathy for others. It has been widely perceived as a "safe" drug because of a relatively low incidence of adverse reactions. However, adverse responses are very unpredictable and the incidence is growing (Gowing, Henry-Edwards, Irvine, & Ali, 2002). Deaths have occurred among users.

Little is yet known about the effects of MDMA on pregnancy. However, the timing of Ecstasy use by the pregnant woman during fetal brain development may be a critical issue (Cockey, 2001). Infants exposed to Ecstasy in utero may experience some of the same risks as infants exposed to other amphetamines during pregnancy, including the possibility of withdrawal-like symptoms such as drowsiness, jitteriness, and breathing problems (March of Dimes, 2005).

Heroin

Heroin is an illicit CNS depressant narcotic that alters perception and produces euphoria. It is an addictive drug that is generally administered IV. Pregnancy in women who use heroin is considered high risk because of the increased incidence in these women of poor nutrition, iron deficiency anemia, and preeclampsia. Women addicted to heroin also have a higher incidence of sexually transmitted infections because many rely on prostitution to support their drug habit.

The fetus of a heroin-addicted woman is at increased risk for IUGR, meconium aspiration, and hypoxia. The newborn frequently shows signs of heroin addiction such as restlessness; shrill, high-pitched cry; irritability; fist sucking; vomiting; and seizures. Signs of withdrawal usually appear within 72 hours and may last for several days. (See discussion in Chapter 30. ∞)

Methadone

Methadone is the most commonly used therapy for women dependent on opioids such as heroin. Methadone blocks withdrawal symptoms and reduces or eliminates the craving for narcotics. Dosage should be individualized at the lowest possible therapeutic level. Methadone crosses the placenta and has been associated with preeclampsia, placental problems, and abnormal fetal presentation.

Prenatal exposure to methadone may result in reduced head circumference and lower birth weight. The newborn may experience withdrawal symptoms that are often more severe and longer lasting than those associated with heroin, possibly because of the longer half-life of methadone.

CLINICAL THERAPY

A team approach to the care of the pregnant woman with substance abuse problems ensures the management necessary to provide safe labor and birth for the woman and her child.

The management of drug addiction may include hospitalization if necessary to start detoxification. "Cold turkey" withdrawal is not advisable during pregnancy because of the possible risk to the fetus. Maintenance and support therapy are best individualized to the woman's history and condition. Urine screening is also done regularly throughout pregnancy if the woman has a known or suspected substance abuse problem. This testing helps to identify the type and amount of drug being abused.

NURSING MANAGEMENT

NURSING ASSESSMENT AND DIAGNOSIS

Because of the prevalence of substance abuse, it is important to screen all pregnant women for substance abuse during the health history. Several simple screening tools are available. In addition, be alert for clues in the history or appearance of the woman that suggest substance abuse. If abuse is suspected, ask direct questions, beginning with less threatening questions about use of tobacco, caffeine, and over-the-counter medications. Then progress to questions about alcohol intake and finally to questions focusing on past and current use of illegal drugs. A matter-of-fact, nonjudgmental approach is more likely to elicit honest responses.

When assessing a woman with a known substance abuse problem, focus on the woman's general health status, with specific attention to nutritional status, susceptibility to infections, and evaluation of all body systems. Also assess the woman's understanding of the impact of substance abuse on herself and on her pregnancy.

Nursing diagnoses that may apply to a woman at risk because of substance abuse include the following:

- *Imbalanced Nutrition: Less than Body Requirements* related to inadequate food intake secondary to substance abuse
- *Risk for Infection* related to use of inadequately cleaned syringes and needles secondary to IV drug use

- *Risk for Ineffective Health Maintenance* related to a lack of information about the impact of substance abuse on the fetus

PLANNING AND IMPLEMENTATION

Prevention of substance abuse during pregnancy is the ideal nursing goal and is best accomplished through education. Unfortunately, many women who abuse substances do not receive regular healthcare and may not seek care until they are far along in pregnancy.

Thus it is important to focus on ongoing assessment and client teaching. Consider providing information about the relationship between substance abuse and existing health problems and the implications for the woman's unborn child. Establishing a relationship of trust and support helps ensure the woman's cooperation. If possible, discuss strategies to help the woman quit (addiction treatment programs, 12-step programs, individual counseling) and suggest a referral for more in-depth assessment by a specialist.

Preparation for labor and birth should be part of prenatal planning. Nonnarcotic psychologic support and careful explanation of the labor process may help relieve the woman's fear, tension, and discomfort. If pain medication is necessary, it should not be withheld; the notion that it will contribute to further addiction is mistaken. Preferred methods of pain relief include the use of psychoprophylaxis and regional blocks such as epidurals or local anesthetics such as pudendal block and local infiltration. Immediate intensive care should be available for the newborn, who is often depressed, small for gestational age (SGA), and premature. (For care of the addicted newborn, see Chapter 30. ∞)

EVALUATION

Expected outcomes of nursing care include the following:

- The woman is able to describe the impact of her substance abuse on herself and her unborn child.
- The woman gives birth to a healthy infant.
- The woman accepts a referral to social services (or another appropriate community agency) for follow-up care after discharge.

CARE OF THE WOMAN WITH DIABETES MELLITUS

Diabetes mellitus (DM), an endocrine disorder of carbohydrate metabolism, results from inadequate production or use of insulin. Insulin, produced by the β-cells of the islets of Langerhans in the pancreas, lowers blood glucose levels by enabling glucose to move from the blood into muscle and adipose tissue cells. In the United States, over 8 million women have pregestational diabetes, and it occurs in 1% of pregnancies (American College of Obstetricians and Gynecologists [ACOG], 2005).

CARBOHYDRATE METABOLISM IN NORMAL PREGNANCY

In early pregnancy the rise in serum levels of estrogen, progesterone, and other hormones stimulates increased insulin production by the maternal pancreas and increased tissue response to insulin. Thus, an anabolic (building-up) state exists during the first half of pregnancy, with storage of glycogen in the liver and other tissues.

In the second half of pregnancy, placental secretion of human placental lactogen (hPL) and prolactin (from the decidua), as well as elevated cortisol and glycogen levels, cause increased resistance to insulin and decreased glucose tolerance. This decreased effectiveness of insulin results in a catabolic (destructive) state during fasting periods, such as during the night or after meal absorption. Because increasing amounts of circulating maternal glucose and amino acids are diverted to the fetus, maternal fat is metabolized much more readily during fasting periods than in a nonpregnant woman. As a result of this lipolysis (maternal metabolism of fat), ketones may be present in the urine.

The delicate system of checks and balances between glucose production and glucose use is stressed by the growing fetus, who derives energy from glucose taken solely from maternal stores. This stress is known as the *diabetogenic effect of pregnancy*. Thus, any preexisting disruption in carbohydrate metabolism is augmented by pregnancy, and any diabetic potential may precipitate gestational diabetes mellitus.

PATHOPHYSIOLOGY OF DIABETES MELLITUS

In DM the pancreas fails to produce insulin or does not produce enough insulin to allow necessary carbohydrate metabolism. Without adequate insulin, glucose does not enter the cells and they become energy depleted. Blood glucose levels remain high (hyperglycemia), and the cells break down their stores of fats and protein for energy. Protein breakdown results in a negative nitrogen balance; fat metabolism causes ketosis.

These pathologic developments cause the four cardinal signs and symptoms of DM: polyuria, polydipsia, polyphagia, and weight loss. Polyuria (frequent urination) results because water is not reabsorbed by the renal tubules due to the osmotic activity of glucose. Polydipsia (excessive thirst) is caused by dehydration from polyuria. Polyphagia (excessive hunger) is caused by tissue loss and a state of starvation, which results from the inability of the cells to use the blood

TABLE 14–2 ✣ Etiologic Classification of Diabetes Mellitus

I. Type 1 diabetes* (β-cell destruction, usually leading to absolute insulin deficiency)
   A. Immune mediated
   B. Idiopathic
II. Type 2 diabetes* (may range from predominantly insulin resistance with relative insulin deficiency to a predominantly secretory defect with insulin resistance)
III. Other specific types[†]
IV. Gestational diabetes mellitus

*Patients with any form of diabetes may require insulin treatment at some stage of their disease. Such use of insulin does not classify the client.

[†]The more detailed classification, which can be found in medical-surgical texts and the original source, provides eight subcategories of type.

Adapted from the 1999 Report of the Expert Committee on the Diagnosis and Classification of Diabetes Mellitus. *Diabetes Care*, Suppl. 5.

TABLE 14–3 ✣ White's Classification of Diabetes in Pregnancy

Class	Criterion
A	Chemical diabetes
B	Maturity onset (age over 20 years), duration under 10 years, no vascular lesions
C_1	Age 10 to 19 years at onset
C_2	10 to 19 years' duration
D_1	Under 10 years at onset
D_2	Over 20 years' duration
D_3	Benign retinopathy
D_4	Calcified vessels of legs
D_5	Hypertension
E	No longer sought
F	Nephropathy
G	Many failures
H	Cardiopathy
R	Proliferating retinopathy
T	Renal transplant (added by Tagatz and colleagues of the University of Minnesota)

Used with permission from White, P. (1978). Classification of obstetric diabetes. *American Journal of Obstetrics and Gynecology, 130*, 228.

glucose. Weight loss (seen with marked hyperglycemia) is due to the use of fat and muscle tissue for energy.

CLASSIFICATION

States of altered carbohydrate metabolism have been classified in several ways. Table 14–2 shows the classification of DM based on its cause. This classification contains four main categories: type 1 diabetes, type 2 diabetes, other specific types, and gestational diabetes mellitus. Type 1 diabetes develops because of β-cell destruction and generally results in an absolute insulin deficiency. Type 2 diabetes, which is the most common form, results from a combination of insulin secretory defect and insulin resistance (Caughron & Smith, 2002).

Table 14–3 shows White's classification of diabetes in pregnancy. This classification is useful for describing the extent of the disease.

Gestational diabetes mellitus (GDM) is defined as any degree of glucose intolerance that has its onset or is first diagnosed during pregnancy. It complicates about 7% of all pregnancies. Women who are markedly obese, have a prior history of GDM, have glycosuria, or have a strong family history of diabetes are at high risk (American Diabetes Association [ADA], 2004a). The woman may remain asymptomatic or may have a mild form of the disease. Diagnosis of GDM is very important, however, because even mild diabetes causes increased risk for perinatal morbidity and mortality. Furthermore, many women with GDM progress over time to overt type 1 or type 2 diabetes mellitus.

INFLUENCE OF PREGNANCY ON DIABETES

Pregnancy can affect diabetes significantly because the physiologic changes of pregnancy can drastically alter insulin requirements. Pregnancy may also alter the progress of vascular disease secondary to DM. Pregnancy can affect diabetes in the following ways:

- DM may be difficult to control because insulin requirements are changeable.

- During the first trimester, the need for insulin frequently decreases. Levels of hPL, an insulin antagonist, are low; fetal needs are minimal; and the woman may consume less food because of nausea and vomiting.

- Nausea and vomiting may cause dietary fluctuations and increase the risk of hypoglycemia, formerly called insulin shock.

- Insulin requirements begin to rise in the second trimester as glucose use and glucose storage by the woman and fetus increase. Insulin requirements may double or quadruple by the end of pregnancy as a result of placental maturation and hPL production.

- Increased energy needs during labor may require increased insulin to balance IV glucose.

- Usually an abrupt decrease in insulin requirement occurs after passage of the placenta and the resulting loss of hPL in maternal circulation.

- A decreased renal threshold for glucose leads to a higher incidence of glycosuria.

- The risk of ketoacidosis, which may occur at lower serum glucose levels in the pregnant woman with DM than in the nonpregnant woman with diabetes, increases.

- The vascular disease that accompanies DM may progress during pregnancy.

- Hypertension may occur, contributing to vascular changes.

- Nephropathy may result from renal impairment, and retinopathy may develop.

INFLUENCE OF DIABETES ON PREGNANCY OUTCOME

The pregnancy of a woman who has diabetes carries a higher risk of complications, especially perinatal mortality and congenital anomalies. Tight metabolic control (glucose between 70 and 120 mg/dL) reduces this risk. New techniques for monitoring blood glucose level, delivering insulin, and monitoring the fetus also help reduce perinatal mortality.

Maternal Risks

The prognosis for the pregnant woman with gestational, type 1, or type 2 diabetes without significant vascular damage is positive. However, diabetic pregnancy still carries a higher risk of complications than normal pregnancy.

Hydramnios, or an increase in the volume of amniotic fluid, occurs in 10% to 20% of pregnant women with diabetes. It is thought to be a result of excessive fetal urination because of fetal hyperglycemia (Dashe, Nathan, McIntire, et al., 2000). Premature rupture of membranes and onset of labor may occasionally be a problem with hydramnios.

Preeclampsia-eclampsia occurs more often in diabetic pregnancies than in normal pregnancies, especially when vascular changes already exist.

Hyperglycemia can lead to *ketoacidosis* as a result of the increase in ketone bodies (which are acidic) released in the blood from the metabolism of fatty acids. Decreased gastric motility and the anti-insulin effects of hPL also predispose the woman to ketoacidosis. Ketoacidosis usually develops slowly but, if untreated, can lead to coma and death for mother and fetus.

Pregnancy can also worsen *retinopathy* in women with diabetes. However, good control of blood glucose levels lessens the impact. Hence, women with preexisting diabetes should be referred to an ophthalmologist for evaluation during pregnancy.

The pregnant woman with diabetes is also at increased risk for monilial vaginitis and urinary tract infections because of increased glycosuria, which contributes to a favorable environment for bacterial growth.

Fetal-Neonatal Risks

Many of the problems of the newborn result directly from high maternal plasma glucose levels. In the presence of untreated maternal ketoacidosis, the risk of fetal death increases dramatically.

The incidence of *congenital anomalies* in diabetic pregnancies is 5% to 10% and is the major cause of death of infants born to women with diabetes. Research suggests that this increased incidence is related to multiple factors including high glucose levels in early pregnancy (Schaefer-Graf, Buchanan, Xiang et al., 2000). Most anomalies involve the heart, central nervous system, and skeletal system. One anomaly, *sacral agenesis,* appears almost exclusively in infants of diabetic mothers. In sacral agenesis, the sacrum and lumbar spine fail to develop and the lower extremities develop incompletely. Preconception counseling and strict diabetes control before conception help reduce the incidence of congenital anomalies.

Characteristically, infants of diabetic mothers on insulin therapy (or White's classes A, B, and C; see Table 14–3) are large for gestational age (LGA) as a result of the high maternal levels of blood glucose, from which the fetus derives its glucose. These elevated levels continually stimulate the fetal islets of Langerhans to produce insulin. This hyperinsulin state causes the fetus to use the available glucose, which leads to excessive growth (known as **macrosomia**) and fat deposits. If born vaginally the macrosomic infant is at increased risk for shoulder dystocia and traumatic birth injuries; thus, cesarean birth may be indicated.

Once the umbilical cord is cut after birth, the generous maternal blood glucose supply stops. However, continued islet cell hyperactivity leads to high insulin levels and depleted blood glucose (hypoglycemia) in 2 to 4 hours. Macrosomia can be significantly reduced by strict maternal blood glucose control.

Infants of mothers with advanced diabetes (vascular involvement) may demonstrate IUGR, which occurs because vascular changes in the mother decrease the efficiency of placental perfusion and the fetus is not as well sustained.

Respiratory distress syndrome appears to result from high levels of fetal insulin, which inhibit some fetal enzymes necessary for surfactant production. *Polycythemia* (excessive number of red blood cells) in the newborn is mainly due to the diminished ability of glycosylated hemoglobin in the mother's blood to release oxygen. *Hyperbilirubinemia* is a direct result of the inability of immature liver enzymes to metabolize the increased bilirubin resulting from the polycythemia.

CLINICAL THERAPY

All pregnant women, regardless of risk factors, should be screened for gestational diabetes toward the end of the second trimester (24 to 28 weeks) using a 1-hour, 50-g oral glucose tolerance test (GTT). Women with risk factors (age over 40; family history of diabetes in a first-degree relative; a prior macrosomic, malformed, or stillborn infant; obesity; hypertension; or glycosuria) should be screened earlier in pregnancy (ACOG, 2001a).

To do the 1-hour GTT, the woman drinks a 50-g oral glucose solution at any time during the day and provides a blood sample 1 hour later. If the plasma glucose level exceeds 140 mg/dL (some agencies use 130 mg/dL as the cutoff), a 3-hour oral GTT is necessary (ADA, 2004a).

To do this test, the woman eats a high-carbohydrate (at least 150 g carbohydrate daily) diet for 3 days before her scheduled test. She then drinks a 100-g oral glucose solution in the morning after an overnight fast. Plasma glucose levels are determined fasting and at 1, 2, and 3 hours. Gestational diabetes is diagnosed if two or more of the following values are equaled or exceeded:

Fasting	95 mg/dL
1 hour	180 mg/dL
2 hours	155 mg/dL
3 hours	140 mg/dL

If only one value is elevated, many clinicians recommend exercise and nutrition counseling and then either repeat the 3-hour oral GTT in 1 month or perform periodic glucose monitoring (ACOG, 2001a).

Laboratory Assessment of Long-Term Glucose Control

Measurement of glycosylated hemoglobin levels provides information about the long-term (previous 4 to 8 weeks) control of hyperglycemia. The test measures the percentage of glycohemoglobin in the blood. Glycohemoglobin, or HbA_{1c}, is the hemoglobin to which a glucose molecule is attached. Because glycosylation is a rather slow and essentially irreversible process, the test is not reliable for screening for gestational diabetes or for close daily control. Women with abnormal HbA_{1c} values greater than 10% are at most risk of having an infant with a malformation (Cunningham et al., 2005).

ANTEPARTAL MANAGEMENT OF DIABETES MELLITUS

To ensure an optimally healthy mother and newborn, good prenatal care using a team approach must be a top priority. The woman with gestational diabetes may find the diagnosis shocking and upsetting. She needs clear explanations and teaching to gain her cooperation in ensuring a good outcome. The nurse-educator plays a major role in this counseling. The woman with pregestational diabetes needs to understand what changes she can expect during pregnancy; she should receive such teaching in preconception counseling. In addition, preconception care focuses on stringent blood glucose control prior to conception and during the first trimester. Stringent glucose control during this period helps reduce the rate of infant malformations significantly (ADA, 2004b).

Dietary Regulation

The pregnant woman with diabetes needs to increase her caloric intake by about 300 kcal/day. During the first trimester, she generally requires about 30–35 kcal/kg of ideal body weight. During the second and third trimesters, she needs about 35 kcal/kg of ideal body weight. Approximately 40% to 50% of the calories should come from complex, high-fiber carbohydrates, 20% from protein, and 30% to 40% from fats (ACOG, 2005). The food is divided among three meals and three snacks. The bedtime snack is the most important and should include both protein and complex carbohydrates to prevent nighttime hypoglycemia. A nutritionist should work out meal plans with the woman based on the woman's lifestyle, culture, and food preferences. The woman needs to be familiar with the use of food exchanges so she can plan her own meals.

Glucose Monitoring

Glucose monitoring is essential to determine the need for insulin and to assess glucose control. Many physicians have the woman come in for weekly assessment of her fasting glucose levels and one or two postprandial levels. In addition, frequent self-monitoring of glucose levels is paramount in maintaining good glucose control. Self-monitoring is discussed on page 319.

Insulin Administration

Many women with gestational diabetes need insulin to maintain normal glucose levels. Those with pregestational diabetes typically have type 1 diabetes and are already on insulin. In either case, human insulin should be used because it is the least likely to cause an allergic reaction. Insulin is given either in multiple injections or by continuous subcutaneous infusion. Multiple injections are more common and generally produce excellent results. Most women receive a combination of intermediate and regular insulin. Some clinicians have moved away from the use of regular human insulin, replacing it with a fast-acting human analogue called lispro, which is associated with better glucose control. Often a four-dose approach is used, with regular insulin, insulin lispro, or insulin aspart taken before each meal and NPH or Lente insulin added before breakfast and at bedtime (ACOG, 2005). Other clinicians vary the NPH and regular insulin patterns slightly but still prefer a four-dose approach.

Oral hypoglycemics have not been well studied in pregnancy and are rarely used because most cross the placenta, and may be teratogenic. However, glyburide does not cross the placenta and has been used to treat GDM. At present, ACOG (2005) recommends that the use of oral hypoglycemics be limited and individualized pending further study.

Evaluation of Fetal Status

Information about the well-being, size, and maturation of the fetus is important for planning the course of pregnancy and the timing of birth. In pregnancies complicated by diabetes, the fetus is at increased risk of neural tube defects such as spina bifida, so maternal serum alpha-fetoprotein (MSAFP) screening is done at 16 to 20 weeks' gestation.

Ultrasound is done at 18 weeks to determine gestational age and detect anomalies. It is then repeated at 28 weeks to monitor fetal growth for IUGR or macrosomia. Some agencies do *fetal biophysical profiles* (ultrasound evaluations of fetal well-being that assess fetal breathing movements, fetal activity, reactivity, muscle tone, and amniotic fluid volume) as part of an ongoing evaluation of fetal status.

Daily maternal evaluation of *fetal activity* is begun at about 28 weeks. Nonstress testing (NST) is usually begun weekly at 28 weeks and increased to twice weekly at 32 weeks' gestation. If the NST is nonreactive, a fetal biophysical profile or *contraction stress test* is performed. (For an explanation of these tests, see Chapter 16. ∞) If the woman requires hospitalization for complications or to control blood glucose levels, NSTs may be done weekly.

INTRAPARTAL MANAGEMENT OF DIABETES MELLITUS

During the intrapartal period, medical therapy focuses on the following:

- **Timing of birth.** Most pregnant women with diabetes, regardless of the type, are allowed to go to term, with spontaneous labor. Some clinicians opt to induce labor in a woman at term to avoid problems related to an aging placenta. Cesarean birth may be indicated if signs of fetal distress exist. Birth before term may be indicated for some diabetic women with vascular changes, poor glucose control, a prior stillbirth, and worsening hypertension (ACOG, 2005). To determine fetal lung maturity, amniotic fluid (obtained by amniocentesis) is evaluated for lecithin/sphingomyelin (L/S) ratio and the presence of phosphatidylglycerol (see "phosphatidylglycerol" in Chapter 16. ∞) Preterm induced birth, often by cesarean, is considered if prenatal testing indicates that the fetus is deteriorating.

- **Labor management.** Frequently, maternal insulin requirements decrease dramatically during labor.

● FIGURE 14–2

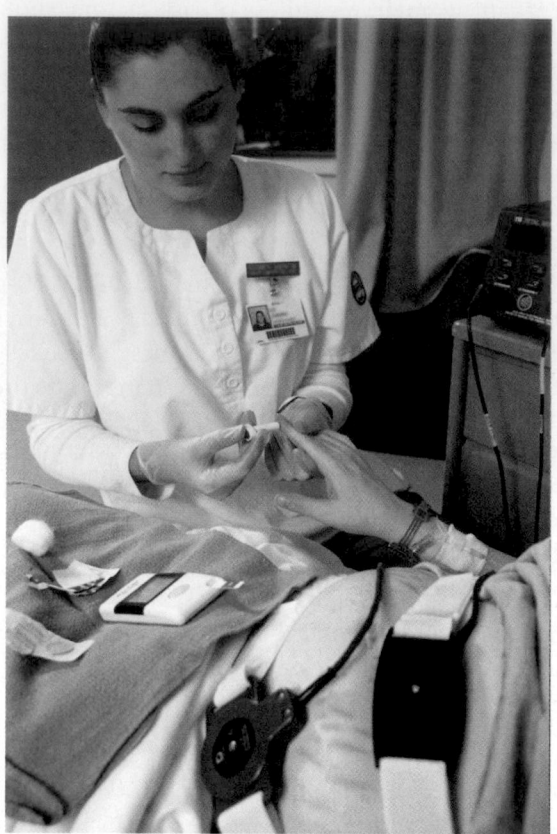

During labor the nurse closely monitors the blood glucose levels of the woman with diabetes mellitus.

Consequently maternal glucose levels are measured hourly to determine insulin need (Figure 14–2 ●). The primary goal in controlling maternal glucose levels intrapartally is to prevent neonatal hypoglycemia (Curet, 2000). Often two IV lines are used, one with a 5% dextrose solution and one with a saline solution. The saline solution is then available for piggybacking insulin or if a bolus is needed. Because insulin clings to plastic IV bags and tubing, the tubing should be flushed with insulin before the prescribed amount is added. During the second stage of labor and the immediate postpartal period, the woman may not need additional insulin. The IV insulin is discontinued at the end of the third stage of labor.

POSTPARTAL MANAGEMENT OF DIABETES MELLITUS

Generally maternal insulin requirements fall significantly during the postpartal period because, with placental separation, hormone levels fall and the anti-insulin effect ceases. For the first 24 hours postpartum, women with pre-existing diabetes typically require very little insulin. They are usually managed with a sliding scale specifying dosage based on blood glucose levels. Afterward a more regular insulin dosage pattern can be reestablished. Women with mild diabetes not requiring insulin often have sufficient glucose control and do not require any therapy while they are hospitalized. Antihyperglycemics are contraindicated during breastfeeding. Consequently a breastfeeding woman with diabetes that is not controlled by diet alone may need insulin for a time (Kjos, 2000).

Women with GDM who did not require insulin during pregnancy generally do not need it during the postpartum period. Clinicians routinely discontinue insulin for women with GDM following childbirth and then monitor blood glucose levels. If elevated glucose levels develop, oral anti-hyperglycemic agents may be tried if the woman is not breastfeeding (Curet, 2000). The woman should be re-assessed 6 weeks postpartum to determine whether her glucose levels are normal. If the levels are normal, she should be reassessed at a minimum of 3-year intervals (ADA, 2004a).

The establishment of parent-child relationships is a high priority during the postpartum. Therefore, if the newborn requires a special care nursery, the parents need ongoing information, support, and encouragement to visit and be involved in the newborn's care.

The nurse should encourage breastfeeding as beneficial to both mother and baby. Calorie needs increase during lactation to 500 to 800 kcal above prepregnant requirements, and insulin must be adjusted accordingly. Home blood glucose monitoring should continue for the woman with type 1 diabetes.

The woman and her partner, if he is involved, should also receive information on family planning. Barrier methods of contraception (diaphragm, cervical cap, condom) used with a spermicide are safe, effective, economical, and the method of choice for insulin-dependent diabetic women. The use of combined oral contraceptives (COCs) by women with diabetes is somewhat controversial. Many physicians who prescribe low-dose COCs to women with diabetes restrict them to women who have no vascular disease and do not smoke. The progesterone-only pill may also be used as may Depo-Provera. As discussed in Chapter 4 in "Long-Acting Hormonal Contraceptives," Depo-Provera has been associated with long-term loss of bone density and many caregivers have stopped prescribing it. ∞ Many couples who have completed their families choose elective sterilization.

NURSING MANAGEMENT

"Nursing Care Plan: The Woman with Diabetes Mellitus" addresses nursing management.

NURSING ASSESSMENT AND DIAGNOSIS

Whether diabetes has been diagnosed before pregnancy occurs or the diagnosis is made during pregnancy (GDM),

careful assessment of the disease process and the woman's understanding of diabetes is important. Thorough physical examination—including assessment for vascular complications of the disease, any signs of infectious conditions, and urine and blood testing for glucose—is essential on the first prenatal visit. Follow-up visits are usually scheduled twice a month during the first two trimesters and once a week during the last trimester.

Assessment provides information about the woman's ability to cope with the combined stress of pregnancy and diabetes and to follow a recommended regimen of care. Determine the woman's knowledge about diabetes and self-care before developing a teaching plan.

Nursing diagnoses that may apply to the pregnant woman with diabetes include the following:

- *Risk for Imbalanced Nutrition: More than Body Requirements* related to imbalance between intake and available insulin
- *Risk for Injury* related to possible complications secondary to hypoglycemia or hyperglycemia
- *Interrupted Family Processes* related to the need for hospitalization secondary to DM

PLANNING AND IMPLEMENTATION

For the woman with preexisting diabetes, a nurse and a physician may provide prepregnancy counseling using a team approach. Ideally they see the couple before pregnancy so that the DM can be evaluated. The outlook for pregnancy is good if the diabetes is of recent onset without vascular complications, provided that glucose levels can be controlled.

For women with GDM, nursing care focuses heavily on client education about the condition, its implications, and its management.

Nursing Care in the Community

In many cases, women with GDM are stabilized in the hospital and necessary teaching for self-care is begun. Women with preexisting diabetes may also require hospitalization for stabilization of their diabetes. In either case the majority of ongoing teaching and supervision of pregnant women with diabetes is then carried out by nurses in clinics, community agencies, and the women's homes.

Effective Insulin Use. Ensure that the woman and her partner understand the purpose of insulin, the types of insulin to be used, and the correct procedure for administering it. Remember that regular (short-acting) insulin should be given about 30 minutes before a meal, but insulin lispro should be taken immediately before eating (ACOG, 2005). Instruct the woman's partner about insulin administration in case it becomes necessary for the partner to give it. For some highly motivated women whose glucose levels are not

NURSING CARE PLAN

THE WOMAN WITH DIABETES MELLITUS

Intervention	Rationale	Expected Outcome
1. Nursing Diagnosis: Risk for Altered Nutrition: Less than Body Requirements related to poor carbohydrate metabolism		
NIC Intervention: **Nutrition management:** Assistance with or provision of a balanced dietary intake of foods and fluids		**NOC Outcome:** **Nutritional status:** Extent to which nutrients are available to meet metabolic needs
Goal: Client will maintain adequate nutrition throughout pregnancy.		
■ Emphasize importance of regular prenatal visits for assessment of weight gain, blood sugar levels, fetal heart tones, urine ketones, and fundal height measurement. ■ Coordinate care with a dietitian to assist client in meal planning and educate client on the daily caloric needs of pregnancy. ■ Instruct client on signs and symptoms of hyperglycemia: polyphagia, nausea, hot flushes, polydipsia, polyuria, fruity breath, abdominal cramps, rapid deep breathing, headache, weakness, drowsiness, and general malaise. Instruct client on signs and symptoms of hypoglycemia: hunger, clammy skin, irritability, slurred speech, seizures, tachycardia, headache, pallor, sweating, disorientation, shakiness, blurred vision, and, if untreated, coma or convulsions. ■ Instruct client on management of hyperglycemia and hypoglycemia. ■ Include family members in meal planning.	■ Regular follow-up and assessment of weight, blood sugar levels, fetal heart tones, urine ketones, and fundal height will promote a healthy pregnancy and outcome, as well as allow for modifications in the treatment regimen if necessary. ■ A daily intake of high-quality foods promotes fetal growth and controls maternal glucose levels. ■ Maintaining a euglycemic state throughout pregnancy aids in preventing diabetic complications and promotes a positive pregnancy outcome. ■ Gives the family member a sense of involvement and an understanding of the importance of adequate nutrition in pregnancy.	■ The client will maintain adequate nutrition as evidenced by adequate weight gain, controlled blood sugar levels, verbalization of understanding of personal treatment regimen, and appropriate fetal growth and development during pregnancy. ■ Client will recognize signs and intervene appropriately.
2. Nursing Diagnosis: Risk for Fetal Injury related to possible complications associated with altered tissue perfusion secondary to maternal diagnosis of diabetes mellitus		
NIC Intervention: **High-risk pregnancy care:** Identification and management of a high-risk pregnancy to promote healthy outcomes for mother and baby		**NOC Outcome:** **Risk control:** Actions to eliminate or reduce actual, personal, and modifiable health threats
Goal: Uncomplicated birth of a healthy newborn.		
■ Assess fetal heart tones for reassuring variability and accelerations.	■ Reassuring fetal heart rate variability and accelerations are interpreted as adequate placental oxygenation.	■ The fetus will not exhibit signs and symptoms of altered tissue perfusion as evidenced by positive fetal activity, reassuring fetal heart rate patterns, a biophysical profile score between 8 and 10, negative CST, L/S ratio indicating fetal lung maturity, and a reactive nonstress test.

NURSING CARE PLAN—continued

THE WOMAN WITH DIABETES MELLITUS

Intervention	Rationale	Expected Outcome
■ Instruct mother on how to lie in a left recumbent position after eating and record how many fetal movements she feels in an hour.	■ More than five fetal kicks in an hour are indicative of fetal well-being.	
■ **Collaborative:** Perform oxytocin challenge test (OCT)/contraction stress test (CST) and nonstress tests as determined by physician.	■ Fetal surveillance testing assesses fetal well-being and adequate placental perfusion.	
■ Prepare client for frequent ultrasound assessments.	■ Ultrasonography is indicated at 8, 12, 18, 28, and 36–38 weeks per physician's orders to confirm gestational age and fetal well-being.	
■ Prepare client for amniocentesis procedure.	■ A sample of amniotic fluid contains two phospholipids (lecithin/sphingomyelin) that can be used to detect fetal lung maturity and enables medical personnel to prepare for a potential preterm birth.	
■ Assist physician with biophysical profile assessment.	■ Helps assure fetal well-being and a positive fetal outcome.	

3. Nursing Diagnosis: Health-seeking Behaviors: Information about the effects of blood sugar on pregnancy related to an expressed desire to maintain stable blood glucose levels

NIC Intervention:		NOC Outcome:
Health education: Developing and providing instruction and learning experiences to facilitate voluntary adaptation of behavior conducive to health in individuals, families, groups, or communities		**Health-seeking behavior:** Actions to promote optimal wellness, recovery, and rehabilitation

Goal: The client and her family will verbalize the importance of maintaining blood sugar within prescribed ranges during pregnancy.

■ Assess the client and family's cognitive level and develop a teaching strategy that will facilitate learning at that level.	■ Behavior changes occur when teaching strategies are appropriate for the client and family's cognitive level.	■ The client and family members will verbalize understanding of the effects of blood sugar fluctuations on pregnancy as evidenced by asking questions and seeking health information when necessary. The client adheres to personal treatment regimen throughout pregnancy.
■ Teach blood glucose monitoring, insulin administration, and predicted insulin needs throughout pregnancy, and then have client and family members repeat the discussion.	■ Basic understanding of the relationship between blood sugar levels and how insulin needs change throughout pregnancy will foster compliance with prescribed regimen.	
■ Emphasize the importance of maintaining a healthy diet and exercise program during pregnancy. Encourage client and family to develop a sample diabetic diet and exercise regimen that is appropriate for pregnancy while present in the clinic or hospital and evaluate for appropriateness.	■ Involves the client and her family members in her care, and the evaluation method promotes positive reinforcement and a time for modifications of regimen if necessary.	
■ Emphasize the importance of prenatal care for the purpose of maternal and fetal surveillance.	■ Frequent prenatal visits allow for modifications in regimen and promote a healthy pregnancy outcome.	

(continued)

NURSING CARE PLAN—continued

THE WOMAN WITH DIABETES MELLITUS

Intervention	Rationale	Expected Outcome
4. Nursing Diagnosis: Risk for Infection related to increased levels of glucose in urine		
NIC Intervention: **Infection control:** Minimizing the acquisition and transmission of infectious agents		**NOC Outcome:** **Knowledge: Infection control:** Extent of understanding conveyed about prevention and control of infection
Goal: The client will have no urinary tract infections (UTIs) during pregnancy.		
■ Encourage client to utilize preventive measures to prevent UTIs: increasing intake of water and cranberry juice, wearing cotton underwear, wiping perineum from front to back, voiding frequently, and voiding before and immediately after sexual intercourse. ■ Instruct client on the signs and symptoms of UTIs: urinary frequency, dysuria, cloudy urine, hematuria, lower back pain, and foul-smelling urine. **Collaborative:** ■ Instruct client on how to obtain a clean-catch urine sample and send to lab for culture and sensitivity per physician's orders. ■ Administer prescribed antibiotic therapy and teach client about medication, adverse effects, and appropriate dosage. ■ Encourage client to drink 8–10 glasses of water each day.	■ Utilizing preventive measures decreases the likelihood of client acquiring a UTI. ■ Client will be aware of signs and symptoms of UTIs and report to physician for immediate intervention. ■ A clean-catch urine sample will contain bacteria if a UTI is present. ■ Antibiotic therapy is the appropriate treatment for a UTI. Compliance increases when a client fully understands medication regimen. ■ Increased fluid intake assists in flushing bacteria out of the urinary tract system.	■ Client will remain free of UTIs during pregnancy as evidenced by verbalizing and complying with appropriate preventive measures, increasing fluid intake, and negative urine samples during prenatal visits.
5. Nursing Diagnosis: Anxiety related to unfamiliarity with diagnosis		
NIC Intervention: **Anxiety reduction:** Minimizing apprehension, dread, foreboding, or uneasiness related to an unidentified source of anticipated danger		**NOC Outcome:** **Anxiety control:** Ability to eliminate or reduce feelings of apprehension and tension from an unidentifiable source
Goal: The client expresses less anxiety.		
■ Assess client's level of anxiety (mild-1, moderate-2, or severe-3) and have client verbalize causes of anxiety. ■ Share information on diabetes care such as nutrition, exercise, and glucose control in a clear and concise manner. ■ Instruct client on anxiety-reducing techniques such as imagery, breathing exercises, and massage used in pregnancy. ■ Refer client to a diabetes support group.	■ Verbalization of anxiety provokers encourages expression of feelings and questions. ■ Accurate information gives the client a sense of control and comfort. ■ Gives client the tools necessary for decreasing anxiety. ■ A support group allows clients with similar problems to express concerns and share information with each other.	■ The client demonstrates appropriate coping strategies as evidenced by utilizing resources efficiently and verbalizing feelings of anxiety and the ways to deal with them.

THINKING CRITICALLY

GLUCOSE INTOLERANCE

Patti Chang, a 35-year-old G3P2, is a well-educated, active Chinese-American woman with no history of glucose intolerance. Her two children were born healthy at 36 weeks' gestation. She receives the usual 50-g glucose tolerance test at 26 weeks' gestation, and her plasma level is 160 mg/dL. She seems irritated and frustrated when her obstetrician tells her that it would be best to perform a 3-hour fasting glucose tolerance test. After the physician leaves the room, Patti asks you the following questions: "Will the glucose hurt my baby? What will the treatment be?" How will you answer the questions? Why does Patti seem so upset?

NURSING PRACTICE

It is essential to have a woman with GDM who is learning to test her blood glucose do a finger stick while you watch. For many women, actually sticking their finger can be a challenge to overcome. In addition this observation enables you to verify that correct technique is used.

well controlled with multiple injections, the continuous infusion pump may improve glucose control.

Teach the woman how and when to monitor her blood glucose level, the desired range of blood glucose levels, and the importance of good control (Figure 14–3). Most women use a glucose meter to monitor blood sugar level because the meter is more accurate. Teach the woman to follow the manufacturer's directions exactly; to wash her hands thoroughly before puncturing her finger; to touch the blood droplet, not her finger, to the test pad on the strip; and to store the test strips as directed and discard them after the expiration date. Clients with diabetes need to keep a record of each blood sugar reading. Specific record sheets are available for this purpose.

Planned Exercise Program. Regardless of the type of diabetes, unless otherwise medically contraindicated, exercise is important for the woman's overall well-being. If she is used to a

regular exercise program, encourage her to continue. Advise the woman to exercise after meals when blood sugar levels are high, to wear diabetic identification, to carry a simple sugar such as hard candy (because of the possibility of exercise-induced hypoglycemia), to monitor her blood glucose levels regularly, and to avoid injecting insulin into an extremity that will soon be used during exercise.

If the woman has not been following a regular exercise plan, encourage her to begin gradually. Due to alterations in metabolism with exercise, the woman's blood glucose should be well controlled before she begins an exercise program.

Teaching for Self-Care. Using the information gained during the nursing assessment of the pregnant woman with diabetes, provide appropriate teaching to the woman and her family so that she can meet her own healthcare needs as much as possible.

- *Glucose monitoring.* Home monitoring of blood glucose levels is the most accurate and convenient method to determine insulin dose and assess control. Women learn self-monitoring techniques that they perform four to six times a day according to a specified schedule. They then regulate their insulin dosage based on blood glucose values and anticipated activity level. Women are encouraged to maintain blood glucose levels in normal ranges as follows: fasting (before eating or taking insulin), 70 to 100 mg/dL; 2 hours after each meal, less than 120 mg/dL (ADA, 2004b).

- *Symptoms of hypoglycemia and ketoacidosis.* The pregnant woman with diabetes must recognize symptoms of changing glucose levels and take appropriate action by immediately checking her capillary blood glucose level. If it is less than 65 to 70 mg/dL, she should take 20 g of carbohydrate, wait 20 minutes, and then retest her glucose level. She can obtain the necessary carbohydrate by drinking about a cup of skim milk, 1/2 cup orange or apple juice, or 1/2 cup cola, or by eating 1 tablespoon honey or brown sugar (Cleveland Clinic, 2003). Many people overtreat their symptoms by continuing to eat, but doing so can cause rebound hyperglycemia. The woman should carry a snack at all times and should have other fast sources of glucose (simple carbohydrates) at hand to treat an insulin

FIGURE 14–3

The nurse teaches the pregnant woman with gestational diabetes mellitus how to do home glucose monitoring.

reaction when milk or juice is not available. Family members also learn how to inject glucagon in case food does not work or is not feasible (e.g., in the presence of severe morning sickness).

■ *Smoking.* Smoking has harmful effects on both the maternal vascular system and the developing fetus and is contraindicated for both pregnancy and diabetes.

■ *Travel.* Insulin can be kept at room temperature while traveling. Insulin supplies should be kept with the traveler and not packed in the baggage. Special meals can be arranged by notifying most airlines a few days before departure. The woman should wear a diabetic identification bracelet or necklace and should check with her physician for any instructions or advice before traveling.

■ *Support groups.* Many communities have diabetes support groups or education classes that are helpful to women with newly diagnosed diabetes.

■ *Cesarean birth.* Chances for a cesarean birth increase if the pregnant woman is diabetic. The possibility should be anticipated; caregivers may suggest enrollment in cesarean birth preparation classes. The couple may prefer simply to discuss cesarean birth with the nurse and their obstetrician and read some books on the topic.

Hospital-Based Nursing Care

Hospitalization may become necessary during the pregnancy to evaluate blood glucose levels and adjust insulin dosages. In such cases, monitor the woman's status and provide teaching so that she is knowledgeable about her condition and its management. See "Care Plan: Woman with Diabetes Mellitus" starting on page 316.

During the intrapartum period, continue to monitor the woman's status, maintain her IV fluids, remain alert for signs of hypoglycemia, and provide the care indicated for any woman in labor. If a cesarean birth becomes necessary, provide appropriate care, as described in Chapter 22. ∞

EVALUATION

Expected outcomes of nursing care include the following:

■ The woman is able to discuss her condition and its possible impact on her pregnancy, labor and birth, and postpartum period.

■ The woman participates in developing a healthcare regimen to meet her needs and follows it throughout her pregnancy.

■ The woman avoids developing hypoglycemia or hyperglycemia.

■ The woman gives birth to a healthy newborn.

■ The woman is able to care for her newborn.

CARE OF THE WOMAN WITH ANEMIA

Anemia indicates inadequate levels of hemoglobin (Hb) in the blood. During pregnancy, anemia is defined as hemoglobin less than 10 g/dL (Cunningham et al., 2005). The common anemias of pregnancy are due either to insufficient hemoglobin production related to nutritional deficiency in iron or folic acid during pregnancy or to hemoglobin destruction in an inherited disorder such as sickle cell anemia. Table 14–4 describes these common anemias.

CARE OF THE WOMAN WITH HIV INFECTION

Human immunodeficiency virus (HIV) infection is one of today's major health concerns. It leads to a progressive disease that ultimately results in **acquired immunodeficiency syndrome (AIDS).** Women account for about 18% of cases in the United States. Certain groups—IV drug users; prostitutes; women whose current or previous sexual partners have been bisexual, have abused IV drugs, have hemophilia, or have tested positive for HIV; and women from countries where heterosexual transmission is common—are at increased risk for HIV infection (Centers for Disease Control and Prevention [CDC], 2003).

In the United States, heterosexually acquired infections account for 35% of all new HIV cases. Worldwide, however, the majority of HIV infections results from heterosexual contact (Hall, Lee, Glynn et al., 2004). Today an estimated 40 million people are living with HIV/AIDS. Of these, 2.5 million are children younger than 15 years of age (CDC, 2004).

DEVELOPING CULTURAL COMPETENCE

ETHNICITY AND AIDS INCIDENCE

Although less than one fourth of U.S. women are African American or Latina, these groups account for three quarters of all female AIDS cases (CDC, 2003).

PATHOPHYSIOLOGY OF HIV AND AIDS

HIV-1, which causes most cases of AIDS worldwide, typically enters the body through blood, blood products, or other body fluids such as semen, vaginal fluid, and breast milk. HIV affects specific T cells, thereby decreasing the body's immune responses. This makes the affected person susceptible to opportunistic infections such as *Pneumocystis carinii,* which causes a severe pneumonia, candidiasis, cytomegalovirus, tuberculosis, and toxoplasmosis.

Once infected with the virus, the individual develops antibodies that can be detected with the enzyme-linked immunosorbent assay (ELISA) and confirmed with the

TABLE 14–4 ✢ Anemia and Pregnancy

Condition	Brief Description	Maternal Implications	Fetal/Neonatal Implications
Iron deficiency anemia	Condition caused by inadequate iron intake resulting in hemoglobin levels below 11 g/dL. To prevent this, most women are advised to take supplemental iron during pregnancy.	Pregnant woman with this anemia tires easily, is more susceptible to infection, has increased chance of preeclampsia-eclampsia and postpartal hemorrhage, and cannot tolerate even minimal blood loss during birth. Healing of episiotomy or incision may be delayed.	Risk of low birth weight, prematurity, stillbirth, and neonatal death increases in women with severe iron deficiency anemia (maternal Hb less than 6 g/dL). Fetus may be hypoxic during labor due to impaired uteroplacental oxygenation.
Sickle cell anemia	Recessive autosomal disease in which normal adult hemoglobin, hemoglobin A, is abnormally formed. It occurs primarily in people of African descent and occasionally in people of Southeast Asian or Mediterranean descent (i.e., Greeks, Italians, Arabs, and Turks) (ACOG, 2000b). The disease is characterized by sickling of the RBCs in the presence of decreased oxygenation. Condition may be marked by crisis with profound anemia, jaundice, high temperature, infarction, and acute pain. Crisis is treated by rehydration with intravenous fluids, administration of oxygen, antibiotics, and analgesics. The fetus is monitored throughout.	Pregnancy may aggravate sickle cell anemia and bring on a vaso-occlusive crisis. Maternal mortality is rare but there is a significant risk of maternal infection, often urinary tract infection or pulmonary infection, because of impaired immune functioning (Cunningham et al., 2005). Congestive heart failure or acute renal failure may also occur. The goal of treatment is to reduce anemia and maintain good health. Because the woman maintains her hemoglobin levels by intense erythropoiesis, additional folic acid supplements (1 mg/day) are necessary. Maternal infections are treated promptly because dehydration and fever can trigger sickling and crisis. Oxygen supplementation is used throughout labor, and IV fluids are given to maintain hydration. Fetal heart rate is monitored closely. Antiembolism stockings are indicated postpartally.	Abortion, fetal death, and prematurity may occur. IUGR is also a characteristic finding in newborns of women with sickle cell anemia.
Folic acid deficiency anemia	Folic acid deficiency is the most common cause of megaloblastic anemia. In the absence of folic acid, immature RBCs fail to divide, become enlarged (megaloblastic), and are fewer in number. Increased folic acid metabolism during pregnancy and lactation can result in deficiency. Because the condition is difficult to diagnose, the best approach is prevention. All women who could become pregnant should take a multivitamin containing 400 mcg daily (generally found in prenatal vitamins) before conception and through at least the first trimester of pregnancy. The condition is treated with 1 mg folate daily (see Chapter 12). ∞	Folate deficiency is the second most common cause of anemia in pregnancy. Severe deficiency increases the risk that the mother may need a blood transfusion following birth due to anemia. She also has an increased risk of hemorrhage due to thrombocytopenia and is more susceptible to infection. Folic acid is readily available in foods such as fresh leafy green vegetables, red meat, fish, poultry, and legumes, but it is easily destroyed by overcooking or cooking with large quantities of water.	Maternal folic acid deficiency has been associated with an increased risk of neural tube defects (NTDs) such as spina bifida, meningomyelocele, and anencephaly in the newborn. Adequate folic acid intake can reduce the incidence of NTDs by 50% to 70% (CDC, 2005). Women who have already had one baby with a NTD are generally advised to take a larger dose of folic acid daily.

Western blot test. Antibodies can be detected in most individuals within 6 months after exposure, but in rare circumstances the latent period is longer. An asymptomatic period lasting from a few months to as long as 17 years (with a median length of 10 years) follows seroconversion (CDC, 2002). The majority of infected pregnant women fall into this category.

The diagnosis of AIDS is made when a person is HIV positive and has one of several specific opportunistic infections.

MATERNAL RISKS

AIDS-defining diseases that are more common in women than in men include wasting syndrome, esophageal candidiasis, and herpes simplex virus disease. Non-AIDS-defining gynecologic disorders, such as candidiasis or cervical pathology, are prevalent among women in all stages of HIV.

Many women who are HIV positive choose to avoid pregnancy because of the risk of infecting the fetus and the possibility of dying before the child is raised. Women who become pregnant should be advised that pregnancy is not believed to accelerate the progression of HIV/AIDS, that the use of antiretroviral (ARV) therapy during pregnancy significantly reduces the risk of transmitting the HIV-1 to the fetus, and that most medications used to treat HIV can be taken during the pregnancy.

FETAL-NEONATAL RISKS

HIV/AIDS may develop in infants whose mothers are seropositive, usually due to perinatal transmission. Perinatal transmission occurs transplacentally, at birth when the infant is exposed to maternal blood and vaginal secretions, and via breast milk. In the United States in 1994 there was a 21% mother-to-child transmission rate of HIV infection during pregnancy. Today the transmission rate is less than 2% because of the availability of ARV therapy, the use of elective cesarean birth when appropriate, and formula-feeding rather than breastfeeding (U.S. Public Health Service Task Force, 2003).

Following birth, infants often have a positive antibody titer, which reflects the passive transfer of maternal antibodies and does not indicate HIV infection. For further discussion of the infant who is HIV positive, see Chapter 27. ∞

CLINICAL THERAPY

CDC guidelines state that HIV screening should be part of prenatal care for all women, with the understanding that a woman can "opt out" of screening should she so choose (CDC, 2003). If the results are positive, the Western blot test is used to confirm the diagnosis. Women who test positive should be counseled about the implications of the diagnosis for themselves and their fetus to ensure an informed reproductive choice.

Established guidelines for pregnant women with HIV infection indicate that healthcare providers should (U.S. Public Health Service Task Force, 2003):

- Provide clinical evaluation of the HIV disease stage.
- Assess the degree of immunodeficiency as determined by a $CD4^+$ count.
- Evaluate the risk of disease progression as determined by the level of plasma HIV-1 RNA, which provides information about the viral load (amount of virus present in the body).
- Document history of prior or current ARV therapy.
- Discuss known or unknown risks and benefits of therapy during pregnancy.
- Develop strategies for the long-term evaluation and management of the mother and her infant.

- Provide counseling about risk factors for perinatal transmission. Cigarette smoking, illicit drug use, and unprotected sexual intercourse with multiple partners during pregnancy are associated with increased risk; thus, discontinuing these practices is advised. HIV-positive women should not breastfeed because HIV can be transmitted via breast milk.

Combination ARV therapy suppresses viral replication, helps preserve immune function, and reduces the development of resistance. ARV therapy usually consists of two nucleoside analogues reverse transcriptase inhibitors and a protease inhibitor. Zidovudine (ZDV) is perhaps the best known of the nucleoside analogues. It continues to form a cornerstone of therapy. (See "Evidence-Based Nursing: Use of Antiretroviral Drugs in Pregnant Women Who Are HIV-1 Infected.")

Pregnant women who are currently on ARV therapy should continue their provider-recommended regimen and should receive regular, careful monitoring for pregnancy complications and possible toxicities. Because the fetus is most susceptible to teratogenic effects during the first 10 weeks of pregnancy, and the risks of ARV therapy are not well known, women in the first trimester might elect to delay therapy until after 12 weeks' gestation. To reduce the risk of perinatal transmission, all pregnant women with HIV infection should be offered the three-part ZDV prophylaxis regimen beginning after the first trimester. This regimen includes (1) oral ZDV daily, (2) intravenous ZDV during labor and until birth, and (3) oral ZDV for the infant starting 8 to 12 hours after birth and continuing for 6 weeks (U.S. Public Health Service Task Force, 2003).

The woman infected with HIV should be evaluated and treated for other sexually transmitted infections and for conditions occurring more commonly in women with HIV, such as tuberculosis, cytomegalovirus, toxoplasmosis, and cervical dysplasia. If there is no history of hepatitis B, she should receive the hepatitis vaccine, as well as the pneumococcal vaccine and an annual flu shot. In addition to routine prenatal laboratory tests, a platelet count and a complete blood count with differential should be obtained at the first prenatal visit and repeated each trimester to identify anemia, thrombocytopenia, and leukopenia, which are associated with both HIV infection and antiviral therapy.

At each prenatal visit, asymptomatic, HIV-infected women are monitored for early signs of complications, such as weight loss in the second or third trimesters or fever. The clinician inspects the mouth for signs of infections such as thrush (candidiasis) or hairy leukoplakia; the lungs are auscultated for signs of pneumonia; and the lymph nodes, the liver, and the spleen are palpated for signs of enlargement.

EVIDENCE-BASED NURSING

USE OF ANTIRETROVIRAL DRUGS IN PREGNANT WOMEN WHO ARE HIV-1 INFECTED

Clinical Question

What antiretroviral therapy is most effective during pregnancy for the woman with HIV-1 infection?

Evidence

The Public Health Service assembled a task force to study evidence about the use of antiretroviral drugs during pregnancy. The group based their final recommendations on randomized controlled trials, epidemiologic studies, cohort trials, and meta-analyses. The guideline includes recommendations for counseling women who are HIV-1 infected preconception and for drug treatment during pregnancy and immediately postpartum. It is possible to prevent perinatal transmission of HIV to the newborn with adherence to a drug regimen for both mother and baby.

Implications

Women who are HIV-1 infected should receive counseling about effective contraception to avoid an unplanned pregnancy. The counseling should include information about the risks of transmission of the mother's infection to her baby.

When a pregnancy does occur, adherence to a treatment program for mothers who are HIV-1 infected should continue. Antiretroviral therapy should include agents that are effective in reducing the risk of perinatal HIV-1 transmission, and avoid agents with potential toxicity for the developing fetus. The recommended drug is zidovudine, given orally during the prenatal period, intravenously during the intrapartum period, and orally to the newborn after birth. Dosage should be carefully monitored

to attain a stable, maximally suppressed maternal viral load during the pregnancy. Monitoring for side effects that may represent a threat to the developing fetus (e.g., hyperglycemia, anemia, hepatic toxicity) should be part of the routine prenatal care for these mothers. Immunizations for prophylaxis of opportunistic infections are indicated and pose no threat to the fetus. Mothers should be counseled to maintain optimum nutrition during the prenatal period.

Less is known about the effects of combination antiretroviral therapy on the developing fetus. More intensive fetal monitoring should be considered for mothers who have received combination therapy during their pregnancy.

Ongoing assessment of fetal condition during the third trimester, including evaluation of fetal anatomy and growth, should be part of the care plan for mothers using combination therapy. Other nursing interventions—including counseling about nutrition, immunizations, and recognition of side effects—are indicated for these mothers.

Critical Thinking

How can you encourage mothers who are HIV-1 infected to adhere to their therapeutic regimen? What assessments would help you evaluate the well-being of an infant after birth to a mother who is HIV-1 infected?

Reference

U.S. Public Health Service Task Force. (2003, September 22). *Recommendations for use of antiretroviral drugs in pregnant HIV-1 infected women for maternal health and interventions to reduce prenatal HIV-1 transmission in the United States.* Rockville, MD: Author.

Each trimester the woman should have a visual examination and examination of the retina to detect such complications as toxoplasmosis.

In addition to routine prenatal testing, the woman who is HIV positive should be assessed regularly for serologic changes indicating that HIV/AIDS is progressing. This assessment includes the absolute CD4$^+$ lymphocyte count, which provides the number of helper T4 cells. When the CD4$^+$ count reaches a level of 200/mm^3 or lower, opportunistic infections are more likely to develop.

A pregnancy complicated by HIV infection, even if asymptomatic, is considered high risk, and the fetus is monitored closely. Weekly nonstress testing is begun at 32 weeks' gestation, and serial ultrasounds are done to detect IUGR. Biophysical profiles are also indicated (see Chapter 16 ∞). Invasive procedures such as amniocentesis are avoided when possible to prevent the contamination of a noninfected fetus.

Intrapartum care is similar to that for all pregnant women, although strict adherence to universal precautions is crucial to avoid nosocomial infection. To prevent exposure of an uninfected infant to HIV during labor and birth,

invasive procedures such as vaginal examinations following rupture of membranes, fetal scalp electrode monitoring, fetal scalp sampling, and vacuum extraction should be done only after carefully examining the risks and benefits (ACOG, 2000b).

Because cesarean birth appears to reduce the risk of transmission of HIV vertically from mother to baby, it is recommended for mothers whose viral load as measured by HIV RNA is greater than 1000 copies/mL (U.S. Public Health Service Task Force, 2003). If HIV status is unknown when a woman begins labor, most large centers are able to produce HIV test results within 45 minutes. If the test is positive, ARV therapy is started as soon as possible and the labor management precautions discussed previously should be followed (CDC, 2004).

Women who are HIV positive are at increased risk for complications such as intrapartal or postpartal hemorrhage, postpartal infection, poor wound healing, and infections of the genitourinary tract. Thus, they need careful monitoring and appropriate therapy as indicated. Research suggests that breastfeeding increases the risk of HIV transmission to the newborn. Consequently the

GARLIC SUPPLEMENTS INTERFERE WITH HIV MEDICATION

Garlic has been well regarded as a natural way of combating elevated cholesterol levels. This has made it attractive to many HIV-positive individuals on combination drug therapy because increased cholesterol is a side effect of treatment. However, research has revealed that garlic supplements may actually interfere with the effectiveness of the HIV medication saquinavir, a protease inhibitor, which is usually prescribed in combination with other HIV medications.

The study was conducted with nine healthy, HIV-negative volunteers. Blood analysis revealed that the blood concentrations of saquinavir decreased by over 50% when the volunteers took garlic caplets twice daily for 3 weeks. Moreover, even after a 10-day period with no garlic, the participants' blood levels were about 35% lower than the expected baseline.

At present, researchers do not know what impact the garlic supplements would have on a combined medication regimen but they do recommend that individuals on saquinavir *avoid* taking garlic supplements.

Data from National Institutes of Health News Release. (2001, December 5). Retrieved November 17, 2002, from http://www.nih.gov/news

Piscitelli, S. C., et al. (2001, December 3). The effect of garlic supplements on the pharmacokinetics of saquinavir. *Clinical Infectious Diseases* electronic edition.

HIV-positive woman should be cautioned against breastfeeding her infant.

NURSING MANAGEMENT

"Nursing Care Plan: The Woman with HIV Infection" addresses nursing management.

NURSING ASSESSMENT AND DIAGNOSIS

A woman who tests positive for HIV may be asymptomatic or may present with any of the following signs or symptoms: fatigue, anemia, malaise, progressive weight loss, lymphadenopathy, diarrhea, fever, neurologic dysfunction, cell-mediated immunodeficiency, or evidence of Kaposi's sarcoma (purplish, reddish brown lesions either externally or internally). If a woman tests positive for HIV or is involved in a relationship that places her at high risk, assess the woman's knowledge level about the disease, its implications for her and her fetus, and self-care measures the woman can take.

Examples of nursing diagnoses that might apply for a pregnant woman who tests positive for HIV include the following:

■ *Risk for Ineffective Health Maintenance* related to lack of information about HIV/AIDS and its long-term implications for the woman and her unborn child

■ *Risk for Infection* related to altered immunity secondary to HIV infection

■ *Compromised Family Coping* related to the implications of a positive HIV test in one of the family members

PLANNING AND IMPLEMENTATION

Nursing Care in the Community

Women need to understand that HIV/AIDS is a fatal disease. HIV infection can be avoided if women practice safe sex, including insisting that their partners wear a latex condom for each act of intercourse and avoiding sharing IV drug needles. Women at high risk for HIV/AIDS should be offered premarital and prepregnancy screening for HIV antibodies (ACOG, 2001b).

In monitoring the asymptomatic pregnant woman who is HIV positive, be alert for nonspecific symptoms such as fever, weight loss, fatigue, persistent candidiasis, diarrhea, cough, skin lesions, and behavior changes. These may be signs of developing symptomatic HIV infection. Laboratory findings such as increased viral load; decreased hemoglobin, hematocrit, and CD4 lymphocytes; elevated erythrocyte sedimentation rate (ESR); and abnormal complete blood count, differential, and platelets may indicate complications such as infection or progression of the disease.

Education about optimal nutrition and maintenance of wellness is important; review the information frequently with the woman. Give her information about her ZDV prophylaxis and the importance of following the established regimen for herself during pregnancy and for her newborn after birth.

Hospital-Based Nursing Care

Nurses who deal with childbearing families are exposed frequently to blood and body fluids and need to pay careful attention to the *universal precautions* addressed in introductory nursing courses as a preparation for clinical practice. Protocols have been established for postexposure treatment of a healthcare worker who experiences a needlestick or exposure to body fluids of a person with positive or unknown HIV status. The effectiveness of the therapy, usually a combined drug approach, depends on starting rapidly. Thus, such exposure should be reported immediately.

NURSING CARE PLAN

THE WOMAN WITH HIV INFECTION

Intervention	Rationale	Expected Outcome
1. Nursing Diagnosis: Risk for Infection related to inadequate defenses (leukopenia, suppressed inflammatory response) secondary to HIV-positive status		
NIC Intervention: **Infection control:** Minimizing the acquisition of infection		**NOC Outcome:** **Risk control:** Actions taken to eliminate or reduce risk of exposure to infection
Goal: Client will remain free of opportunistic infection during the course of pregnancy.		
▪ Obtain a complete health history and physical examination during first prenatal visit.	▪ A complete health history will help determine risk factors for the development of opportunistic infections, and a physical examination will assist in identifying any underlying problem symptoms or illnesses that may compromise the pregnancy or complicate the treatment of HIV.	▪ Client will remain free of opportunistic infection as evidenced by CD4[†] lymphocyte count within normal limits; no complaints of chills, fever, or sore throat; normal weight gain throughout pregnancy.
▪ Educate the woman as to the signs and symptoms of infection.	▪ Early recognition of signs and symptoms of infection will allow for immediate treatment, which may decrease the severity of the infection. Signs and symptoms of infections include fever, weight loss, fatigue, persistent candidiasis, diarrhea, cough, and skin lesions (Kaposi's sarcoma and hairy leukoplakia in the mouth).	
▪ Obtain nutritional history and monitor weight gain at each prenatal visit.	▪ The HIV-infected woman needs to maintain optimal nutritional intake. A compromised nutritional status may affect maternal and fetal well-being. Depleted reserves of protein and iron may decrease the client's ability to fight infection, thereby making her more susceptible to opportunistic infections.	
▪ **Collaborative:** Monitor the absolute CD4$^+$ T lymphocyte count, erythrocyte sedimentation rate (ESR), complete blood count (CBC) with differential, and hemoglobin and hematocrit (H & H) at each prenatal visit.	▪ Lab results provide information about the woman's immune system and the potential for disease progression. Opportunistic infections are more likely to occur when the CD4$^+$ T lymphocyte count drops below a level of 200/mm^3. ESR can rise above 20 mm/hr with anemia and with acute and chronic inflammation. CBC with differential and platelet count helps identify anemia, thrombocytopenia, and leukopenia. H & H can also identify anemia.	
2. Nursing Diagnosis: Risk for Ineffective Health Maintenance related to lack of information about HIV/AIDS and its long-term implications for the woman, her unborn child, and her family		
NIC Intervention: **Health information:** Providing instruction and learning experiences to facilitate the woman's understanding of her condition and to enhance her self-care activities		**NOC Intervention:** **Health-promoting behavior:** Actions to promote optimal wellness and a healthy pregnancy and birth

(continued)

NURSING CARE PLAN—continued

THE WOMAN WITH HIV INFECTION

Intervention	Rationale	Expected Outcome
Goal: The client and her family will verbalize the importance of following her medication regimen and of regular prenatal care.		
■ Assess the client's and family's level of understanding of HIV infection, its methods of spread, and the long-term implications. ■ Explain the risks of mother-to-child transmission of HIV infection. ■ Describe antiretroviral therapy. Include the regimen prescribed, its purposes, and the procedures for taking it. ■ Discuss signs the woman should be alert for, including fever, fatigue, weight loss, persistent candidiasis, diarrhea, cough, skin lesions, and behavior changes.	■ Knowledge of the woman's (and her family's) level of understanding about her HIV infection forms a starting point for further health teaching. ■ In untreated women the risk of transmission is 21%. That risk has been reduced dramatically because of the availability of antiretroviral therapy, the use of cesarean birth when indicated, and formula-feeding rather than breastfeeding. ■ ARV therapy approaches vary based on the health status of the individual woman and whether she is currently on ARV therapy. Generally it includes oral ZDV daily, IV ZDV during labor and until birth, and ZDV therapy for the infant for 6 weeks following birth. ■ These symptoms may indicate that the woman is developing symptomatic HIV infection.	■ Woman will actively seek information about her condition, her treatment regimen, and her pregnancy and will cooperate with her caregivers.

3. Nursing Diagnosis: Compromised Family Coping related to the implications of positive maternal HIV status on fetal/neonatal well-being and long-term family functioning

NIC Intervention: **Emotional support:** Provision of reassurance, acceptance, and encouragement during times of stress		**NOC Outcome:** **Family coping:** Family actions to manage stressors that tax family resources
Goal: Family is able to manage stressors related to the maternal diagnosis.		
■ Assess ability and readiness of family to learn about HIV and its long-term implications. ■ Provide woman and her family with accurate, reliable information about her diagnosis, its prognosis for her and for her baby, and the immediate and long-term implications for her care. ■ Assess interactions between the woman and her family. Be alert for potentially destructive behaviors. ■ Assist family in realistically identifying the needs of the woman and family unit. **Collaborative:** Explore available community resources and family support systems.	■ Readiness is a key element in the teaching-learning process. ■ Fear and anxiety will lessen when the woman and her family understand her health status and the implications of the HIV diagnosis and can then plan for the future. ■ If the HIV diagnosis was not expected, the couple may have to deal with issues of blame, concerns about mortality, and worries about the status of the baby. If the HIV diagnosis was known, concerns may focus on fetal/neonatal well-being. In either case, negative responses can lead to destructive behaviors. ■ Once needs are identified realistically, it is possible to plan interventions to meet the needs. ■ Because HIV is a long-term condition, the family may require ongoing assistance.	■ Family members actively participate in the treatment plan, are involved in planning for labor and birth in light of a positive HIV status, and are able to express unresolved feelings about the diagnosis.

Teaching for Self-Care

The psychologic implications of HIV/AIDS for the child-bearing family are staggering. The woman is faced with the knowledge that she and her newborn, if infected, have a decreased life expectancy. If her infant is not infected, she must face the possibility that others will raise her child. She must also face the reality that she can only hope to lengthen her life by carefully following an expensive, exacting medical regimen. The couple must deal with the impact of the illness on the partner, who may or may not be infected, and on other children. The woman and her family may feel fearful, helpless, angry, and isolated.

It is important to preserve confidentiality and the woman's right to privacy. Help ensure that the woman receives complete, accurate information about her condition and ways she might cope. Teach about transmission prevention using language the woman and her partner understand. In addition, ensure that the woman is referred to a comprehensive program that includes social services, psychologic support, and appropriate healthcare.

EVALUATION

Expected outcomes of nursing care include the following:

- The woman discusses the implications of her HIV infection (or diagnosis of AIDS), its implications for her unborn child and for herself, the method of transmission, and the treatment options.

- The woman uses information about social services (or other agency referral) for follow-up assistance and counseling.

- The woman begins to verbalize her feelings about her condition and its implications for her and her family.

CARE OF THE WOMAN WITH HEART DISEASE

Pregnancy results in increased cardiac output, heart rate, and blood volume. The normal heart is able to adapt to these changes without difficulty. The woman with heart disease, however, has decreased cardiac reserve, making it more difficult for her heart to handle the higher workload of pregnancy.

Cardiac disease complicates about 1% of pregnancies (Cunningham et al., 2005). The pathology found in a pregnant woman with heart disease varies with the type of disorder. The more common conditions are discussed briefly here.

Congenital heart defects have become more common in pregnant women as improved surgical techniques enable females born with heart defects to live to childbearing age. Congenital heart defects most commonly seen in pregnant women include atrial septal defect, ventricular septal defect, patent ductus arteriosus, coarctation of the aorta, and tetralogy of Fallot.

For women with congenital heart disease, the impact of pregnancy depends on the specific defect. If the heart defect has been surgically repaired and no evidence of heart disease remains, the woman may undertake pregnancy with confidence. Because of the risk of subacute bacterial endocarditis, even in cases where the defect was corrected surgically, antibiotic prophylaxis is often recommended at the time of birth. Women with congenital heart disease who experience cyanosis should be counseled to avoid pregnancy because the risk to mother and fetus is high.

Rheumatic fever, which may develop in untreated group A β-hemolytic streptococcal infections, is an inflammatory connective tissue disease that can involve the heart, joints, central nervous system, skin, and subcutaneous tissue. Once it occurs, rheumatic fever can recur; it is serious primarily because of the permanent damage it can do to the heart—rheumatic heart disease. Fortunately, rheumatic heart disease has declined rapidly in the past half century, primarily because of the availability of antibiotics for treatment.

Rheumatic heart disease results when recurrent inflammation from bouts of rheumatic fever causes scar tissue to form on the valves. The scarring results in stenosis (failure of the valve to open completely), regurgitation due to failure of the valve to close completely, or a combination of both, thereby increasing the workload of the heart. Although mitral valve stenosis is most common, the aortic and tricuspid valves may also be affected.

The increased blood volume of pregnancy, coupled with the pregnant woman's need for increased cardiac output, stresses the heart of a woman with mitral stenosis and increases her risk of developing congestive heart failure. Even the woman who has no symptoms at the onset of her pregnancy is at risk.

Mitral valve prolapse (MVP) is usually asymptomatic and commonly found in women of childbearing age. The condition is more common in women than in men and seems to run in families. In MVP the mitral valve leaflets tend to prolapse into the left atrium during ventricular systole because the chordae tendineae that support them are long, stretched, and thin. This produces a characteristic systolic click on auscultation. In more pronounced cases of MVP, mitral valve regurgitation occurs, producing a systolic murmur.

Women with MVP usually tolerate pregnancy well. Most women require assurance that they can continue with normal activities. A few women experience symptoms—primarily palpitations, chest pain, and dyspnea—which are often due to arrhythmias. They are usually treated with propranolol hydrochloride (Inderal). Limiting caffeine intake also helps decrease palpitations. Prophylactic antibiotics at the time of birth to prevent bacterial endocarditis are not usually necessary for women whose only sign of MVP is a systolic click. Antibiotics are recommended, however, for women with mitral valve regurgitation, valvular damage, or other risk factors (Cunningham et al., 2005).

Peripartum cardiomyopathy is a dysfunction of the left ventricle that occurs in the last month of pregnancy or the first 5 months postpartum in a woman with no previous history of heart disease. The cause is unknown, but the mortality rate is as high as 18% to 56% (Martin & Foley, 2002). The symptoms are similar to those of congestive heart failure: dyspnea, orthopnea, fatigue, cough, chest pain, palpitations, and edema. The woman may have an enlarged heart, tachycardia, rales, and a third heart sound. Treatment includes digoxin, diuretics, vasodilators as necessary, anticoagulants, sodium restriction, and strict bed rest. The condition may resolve with bed rest as the heart gradually returns to normal size. Subsequent pregnancy is strongly discouraged because the disease tends to recur during pregnancy.

CLINICAL THERAPY

The primary goal of clinical therapy is early diagnosis and ongoing management of the woman with cardiac disease. Echocardiogram, chest x-ray, auscultation of heart sounds, and sometimes cardiac catheterization are essential for establishing the type and severity of the heart disease. The severity of the disease can also be determined by the individual's ability to perform ordinary physical activity. The following classification of functional capacity has been standardized by the Criteria Committee of the New York Heart Association (1994):

- **Class I.** Asymptomatic. No limitation of physical activity.
- **Class II.** Slight limitation of physical activity. Asymptomatic at rest; symptoms occur with ordinary physical activity.
- **Class III.** Marked limitation of physical activity. Comfortable at rest but symptomatic during less-than-ordinary physical activity.
- **Class IV.** Inability to carry on any physical activity without discomfort. Even at rest the person experiences symptoms of cardiac insufficiency or anginal pain; discomfort increases with any physical activity.

Women in classes I and II usually experience a normal pregnancy and have few complications, whereas those in classes III and IV are at risk for more severe complications. Because anemia increases the work of the heart, it should be diagnosed early and treated if present. Infections, even if minor, also increase cardiac workload and should be treated. As pregnancy progresses the woman's activity should be limited to minimize cardiac workload. Similarly, weight gain may also be restricted.

Drug Therapy

The pregnant woman with heart disease may need drug therapy in addition to the iron and vitamin supplements ordinarily prescribed to maintain health during pregnancy. Antibiotics, usually penicillin if not contraindicated by allergy, are used during pregnancy to prevent recurrent bouts of rheumatic fever and subsequent heart valve damage. Antibiotics are also recommended during labor and the early postpartum period to prevent bacterial endocarditis in women with either acquired or congenital disease. If the woman develops coagulation problems, the anticoagulant heparin may be used. Heparin is safest for the fetus because it does not cross the placenta. The thiazide diuretics and furosemide (Lasix) may be used to treat congestive heart failure if it develops. Digitalis glycosides and common antiarrhythmic drugs may be used to treat cardiac failure and arrhythmias. These agents cross the placenta but have no reported teratogenic effect.

LABOR AND BIRTH

Spontaneous natural labor with adequate pain relief is usually recommended for women in classes I and II. Special attention should be given to the prompt recognition and treatment of any signs of heart failure (Figure 14–4 ⬤). Those in classes III and IV may have labor induced and may need to be hospitalized before the onset of labor for cardiac stabilization. They also require invasive cardiac monitoring during labor.

Use of low forceps provides the safest method of birth, with lumbar epidural anesthesia to reduce the stress of pushing. Cesarean birth is used only if fetal or maternal indications exist, not on the basis of heart disease alone.

NURSING MANAGEMENT

NURSING ASSESSMENT AND DIAGNOSIS

Assess the stress of pregnancy on the heart's functioning during every antepartal visit. Note the category of functional capacity assigned to the woman; take the woman's pulse, respirations, and blood pressure; and compare the findings with the normal values expected during pregnancy. Then determine the woman's activity level, including rest, and any changes in the pulse and respirations since previous visits. Identify and evaluate other factors that would increase strain on the heart. These factors might include anemia, infection, anxiety, lack of a support system, and household and career demands.

The following signs and symptoms, if they are progressive, indicate congestive heart failure:

- Cough (frequent, with or without blood-stained sputum [hemoptysis])
- Dyspnea (progressive, on exertion)

● FIGURE 14-4

When a woman with heart disease begins labor, the nursing students and instructor monitor her closely for signs of congestive heart failure.

- Edema (progressive, generalized, including extremities, face, eyelids)
- Heart murmurs (heard on auscultation)
- Palpitations
- Rales (auscultated in lung bases)
- Weight gain (related to fluid retention)

Progressiveness of the cycle is the critical factor because some of these same signs and symptoms are seen to a minor degree in a pregnancy without cardiac problems.

Nursing diagnoses that might apply to the pregnant woman with heart disease include the following:

- *Decreased Cardiac Output:* easy fatigability
- *Impaired Gas Exchange* related to pulmonary edema secondary to cardiac decompensation
- *Fear* related to the effects of the maternal cardiac condition on fetal well-being

PLANNING AND IMPLEMENTATION

Nursing care is directed toward maintaining a balance between cardiac reserve and cardiac workload.

Antepartal Nursing Care

The priority of nursing action varies based on the severity of the disease process and the individual needs of the woman determined by the nursing assessment. Ensure that the woman and her family thoroughly understand her condition and its management and that they recognize signs of potential complications; this level of understanding will decrease their anxiety. Providing thorough explanations, using printed material, and giving frequent opportunities to ask questions and discuss concerns lets the woman better meet her own healthcare needs and seek assistance appropriately.

As part of health teaching, explain the purposes of the required dietary and activity changes. A diet high in iron, protein, and essential nutrients but low in sodium, with adequate calories to ensure normal weight gain, best meets the nutrition needs of the woman with cardiac disease. To help preserve her cardiac reserves, the woman may need to restrict her activities. In addition, 8 to 10 hours of sleep, with frequent daily rest periods, are essential. Because upper respiratory infections may tax the heart and lead to decompensation, the woman must avoid contact with sources of infection.

During the first half of pregnancy, the woman is seen approximately every 2 weeks to assess cardiac status. During the second half of pregnancy, the woman is seen weekly. These assessments are especially important between weeks 28 and 30, when the blood volume reaches its maximum. If symptoms of cardiac decompensation occur, prompt medical intervention is indicated to correct the cardiac problem.

Intrapartal Period

Labor and birth exert tremendous stress on the woman and her fetus. This stress could be fatal to the fetus of a woman with cardiac disease, because the fetus may be receiving a decreased oxygen and blood supply. Thus, the intrapartal care of a woman with cardiac disease is aimed at reducing physical exertion and the accompanying fatigue.

Evaluate maternal vital signs frequently to determine the woman's response to labor. A pulse rate greater than 100 beats per minute or respirations greater than 25 per minute may indicate the onset of cardiac decompensation and require further evaluation. Auscultate the woman's lungs frequently for evidence of rales and carefully observe for other signs that she is developing decompensation.

To ensure cardiac emptying and adequate oxygenation, encourage the laboring woman to assume either a semi-Fowler's or side-lying position, with her head and shoulders elevated. Oxygen by mask, diuretics to reduce fluid retention, sedatives and analgesics, prophylactic antibiotics, and digitalis may also be used as indicated by the woman's status. Remain with the woman to support her. It is essential to keep the woman and her family informed of labor progress and management plans, collaborating with them to fulfill their wishes for the birth experience as much as possible. Maintain an atmosphere of calm to lessen the anxiety of the woman and her family.

Continuous electronic fetal monitoring provides ongoing assessment of the fetal response to labor. To prevent overexertion and the accompanying fatigue, encourage the woman to sleep and relax between contractions and give her emotional support and encouragement. Epidural anesthesia is often used to decrease exertion. During pushing, encourage the woman to use shorter, more moderate open-glottis pushing, with complete relaxation between pushes. Forceps or vacuum extraction may be used if pushing is too difficult. Monitor vital signs closely during the second stage.

Postpartal Period

The postpartal period is a significant time for the woman with cardiac disease. As extravascular fluid returns to the bloodstream for excretion, cardiac output and blood volume increase. This physiologic adaptation places great strain on the heart and may lead to decompensation, especially in the first 48 hours after birth.

To detect any possible problems, the woman may remain in the hospital postpartally longer than the low-risk woman. Monitor her vital signs frequently, and assess for signs of decompensation. She stays in the semi-Fowler's or side-lying position, with her head and shoulders elevated, and begins a gradual, progressive activity program. Appropriate diet and stool softeners facilitate bowel movement without undue strain.

Give the woman opportunities to discuss her birth experience and help her deal with any feelings or concerns that distress her. Encourage maternal-infant attachment by providing frequent opportunities for the mother to interact with her child.

No evidence exists that breastfeeding stresses the heart. Thus, the only concern about breastfeeding for women with cardiovascular disease is related to medications the mother may be taking. These should be evaluated for the likelihood of passing into the milk or affecting lactation.

Assist the breastfeeding mother to a comfortable side-lying position, with her head moderately elevated, or to a semi-Fowler's position. To conserve the mother's energy, position the newborn at the breast and be available to burp the baby and reposition him or her at the other breast.

In addition to providing the normal postpartal discharge teaching, ensure that the woman and her family understand the signs of possible problems from her heart disease or other postpartal complications. Work with the woman and her family to plan an activity schedule. Visiting nurse referrals may be necessary, depending on the woman's health status.

EVALUATION

Expected outcomes of nursing care include the following:

- The woman participates in developing an appropriate healthcare regimen and follows it throughout her pregnancy.
- The woman gives birth to a healthy infant.
- The woman avoids congestive heart failure, thromboembolism, and infection.
- The woman is able to identify signs and symptoms of possible postpartum complications.
- The woman is able to care effectively for her newborn infant.

OTHER MEDICAL CONDITIONS AND PREGNANCY

A woman with a preexisting medical condition needs to be aware of the possible impact of pregnancy on her condition, as well as the impact of her condition on the successful outcome of her pregnancy. Table 14–5 discusses some less common medical conditions in relation to pregnancy.

TABLE 14–5 ✛ Less Common Medical Conditions and Pregnancy

Condition	Brief Description	Maternal Implications	Fetal/Neonatal Implications
Rheumatoid arthritis	Chronic inflammatory disease believed to be caused by a genetically influenced antigen-antibody reaction. Symptoms include fatigue, low-grade fever, pain and swelling of joints, morning stiffness, pain on movement. Treated with salicylates, physical therapy, and rest. Corticosteroids used cautiously if not responsive to above.	Usually there is remission of rheumatoid arthritis symptoms during pregnancy, often with a relapse postpartum. Anemia may be present due to blood loss from salicylate therapy. Mother needs extra rest, particularly to relieve weight-bearing joints, but needs to continue range-of-motion exercises. If in remission, may stop medication during pregnancy.	Possibility of prolonged gestation and longer labor with heavy salicylate use. Possible teratogenic effects of salicylates.
Epilepsy	Chronic disorder characterized by seizures; may be idiopathic or secondary to other conditions, such as head injury, metabolic and nutritional disorders such as phenylketonuria (PKU) or vitamin B_6 deficiency, encephalitis, neoplasms, or circulatory interferences. Treated with anticonvulsants.	Vast majority of pregnancies in women with seizure disorders are uneventful and have an excellent outcome. Women with more frequent seizures before pregnancy may have exacerbations during pregnancy, but this may be related to nausea and vomiting, lack of cooperation with drug regimen, or sleep deprivation. During pregnancy the woman should continue to be treated with the medication that best controls her seizures. Folic acid therapy should be started prior to conception if possible. Folic acid and vitamin D are indicated throughout pregnancy (Crawford, 2001). Because pregnant women with epilepsy who take antiepileptic drugs (AED) are at increased risk for hemorrhagic disease of the newborn, the American Academy of Neurology recommends that they take vitamin K 10 mg/day orally beginning at 36 weeks' gestation. The newborn should also receive the standard injection of vitamin K after birth (Kandula, Liberato, & Harden, 2004).	Infants of women with epilepsy have at least twice the risk of congenital anomalies such as heart defects and cleft palate when compared to women without epilepsy although this risk has decreased with the advent of newer AEDs such as lamotrigine (Lamictal). The goals of therapy are to maintain seizure control while minimizing fetal exposure to AEDs. When possible the woman is maintained on single drug therapy at the lowest possible dose. To achieve this drug levels are monitored closely. This is especially important because blood levels of AEDs can be altered significantly because of maternal hormones and pregnancy-related physiologic changes such as increased cardiac output (Morrell, 2004).
Hepatitis B	Hepatitis B, caused by the hepatitis B virus (HBV), is a major, growing health problem. Groups at risk include those from areas with a high incidence (primarily developing countries), illegal IV drug users, prostitutes, homosexuals, those with multiple sex partners, or occupational exposure to blood, although many infected people have no identifiable source of infection. HBV transmission is blood borne, primarily sexually and perinatally transmitted. Because of the dramatic increase and the difficulty of vaccinating high-risk individuals before they become infected, the CDC now recommends (1) testing all pregnant women for the presence of hepatitis B surface antigen (HBsAg) and post exposure prophylaxis of at-risk infants; (2) routine vaccination of all newborns; (3) universal vaccination of children age 11–12 years who have not previously received the vaccine; (4) vaccination of adolescents and adults at high risk for infection (CDC, 2002).	Hepatitis B does not usually affect the course of pregnancy. However, chronic HBV carriers have a great potential for infecting others when exposure to blood and body fluids occurs. In addition, chronic carriers may develop long-term sequelae, such as chronic liver disease and liver cancer. Approximately 5000 deaths are caused annually by liver disease associated with chronic HBV infection. It is now recommended that all pregnant women be tested for the presence of HBsAg. A woman who is negative may be given the hepatitis B vaccine.	Perinatal transmission most often occurs at or near the time of childbirth. More important, the risk of becoming a chronic carrier of the HBV is inversely related to the age of the individual at the time of initial infection (Shiraki, 2000). Therefore, infants infected perinatally have the highest risk of becoming chronically infected if not treated. Recommendations now include routine vaccination of all neonates born to HBsAg-negative women and immunoprophylaxis to all newborns of HBsAg-positive women.

(continued)

TABLE 14–5 ✤ Less Common Medical Conditions and Pregnancy—continued

Condition	Brief Description	Maternal Implications	Fetal/Neonatal Implications
Hyperthyroidism (thyrotoxicosis)	Enlarged, overactive thyroid gland; increased T_4:TBG ratio and increased BMR. Symptoms include muscle wasting, tachycardia, excessive sweating, and exophthalmos. Treatment by antithyroid drug propylthiouracil (PTU) while monitoring free T_4 levels. Surgery used only if drug intolerance exists.	Mild hyperthyroidism is not dangerous. Increased incidence of preeclampsia and postpartum hemorrhage if not well controlled. Serious risk related to thyroid storm characterized by high fever, tachycardia, sweating, and congestive heart failure. Now occurs rarely. When diagnosed during pregnancy, may be transient or permanent.	Neonatal thyrotoxicosis is rare. Even low doses of antithyroid drug in mother may produce a mild fetal/neonatal hypothyroidism; higher dose may produce a goiter or mental deficiencies. Fetal loss not increased in euthyroid women. If untreated, rates of abortion, intrauterine death, and stillbirth increase. Breastfeeding contraindicated for women on antithyroid medication because it is excreted in the milk (may be tried by woman on low dose if neonatal T_4 levels are monitored).
Hypothyroidism	Characterized by inadequate thyroid secretions (decreased T_4:TBG ratio), elevated TSH, lowered BMR, and enlarged thyroid gland (goiter). Symptoms include lack of energy, excessive weight gain, cold intolerance, dry skin, and constipation. Treated by thyroxine replacement therapy.	Long-term replacement therapy usually continues at same dosage during pregnancy as before. Weekly nonstress test (NST) after 35 weeks' gestation.	If mother untreated, fetal loss 50%; high risk of congenital goiter or true cretinism. Therefore, newborns are screened for T_4 level. Mild TSH elevations present little risk because TSH does not cross the placenta.
Maternal phenylketonuria (PKU) (hyperphenylalaninemia)	Inherited recessive single gene anomaly causing a deficiency of the liver enzyme needed to convert the amino acid phenylalanine to tyrosine, resulting in high serum levels of phenylalanine. Brain damage and mental retardation occur if not treated early.	Low phenylalanine diet is mandatory before conception and during pregnancy. The woman should be counseled that her children will either inherit the disease or be carriers, depending on the zygosity of the father for the disease. Treatment at a PKU center is recommended.	Risk to fetus if maternal treatment not begun preconception. In untreated women, increased incidence of fetal mental retardation, microcephaly, congenital heart defects, and growth retardation. Fetal phenylalanine levels are approximately 50% higher than maternal levels.
Multiple sclerosis	Neurologic disorder characterized by destruction of the myelin sheath of nerve fibers. The condition occurs primarily in young adults, more commonly in females, and is marked by periods of remission; progresses to marked physical disability in 10 to 20 years.	Associated with remission during pregnancy, but with slightly increased relapse rate postpartum (Haas, 2000). Rest is important; help with child care should be planned. Uterine contraction strength is not diminished, but because sensation is frequently lessened, labor may be almost painless.	Increased evidence of a genetic predisposition. Therefore, reproductive counseling is recommended.
Systemic lupus erythematosus (SLE)	Chronic autoimmune collagen disease, characterized by exacerbations and remissions; symptoms range from characteristic rash to inflammation and pain in joints, fever, nephritis, depression, cranial nerve disorders, and peripheral neuropathies.	Women are generally advised that SLE should be in remission for at least 5–7 months before conceiving. However, many women disregard this advice. Women with SLE are at increased risk for diabetes, urinary tract infections, preeclampsia, and premature rupture of the membranes. Clinical management during pregnancy is often complicated by the fact that many of the medications used in SLE are contraindicated during pregnancy. Thus cure is best managed by a rheumatology/obstetrics team approach. Pospartally, oral contraceptives have been associated with lupus flares and are best avoided. Better contraceptive options include barrier contraceptive methods, an IUD, or sterilization (Petri, 2003).	Increased incidence of spontaneous abortion, stillbirth, prematurity, and IUGR. Infants born to women with SLE may have characteristic skin rash, which disappears as the infant metabolizes the maternal immunoglobulin. Congenital heart block occurs in about 2% of cases of neonatal SLE. This condition can be diagnosed prenatally using four-chamber fetal cardiac ultrasonography. At birth some newborns receive a pacemaker while others do not require immediate treatment although they may require a pacemaker later in their childhood (Petri, 2003).
Tuberculosis (TB)	Infection caused by *Mycobacterium tuberculosis*; inflammatory process causes destruction of lung tissue, increased sputum, and coughing. Associated primarily with poverty and malnutrition and may be found among refugees from countries where TB is prevalent. Treated with isoniazid and either ethambutol or rifampin or both.	The incidence of tuberculosis has begun to increase significantly since the late 1980s, and it is increasingly associated with HIV infection. If TB is inactive due to prior treatment, relapse rate is no greater than for nonpregnant women. When isoniazid is used during pregnancy, the woman should take supplemental pyridoxine (vitamin B_6). Extra rest and limited contact with others is required until disease becomes inactive.	If maternal TB is inactive, mother may breastfeed and care for her infant. If TB is active, newborn should not have direct contact with mother until she is noninfectious. Isoniazid crosses the placenta, but most studies show no teratogenic effects. Rifampin crosses the placenta. Possibility of harmful effects still being studied.

Critical Concept Review

LEARNING OBJECTIVES	CONCEPTS
Summarize the effects of alcohol and illicit drugs on the childbearing woman and her fetus/newborn.	1. Substance abuse (either drugs or alcohol) not only is detrimental to the mother's health but also may have profound, lasting effects on the fetus.
Relate the pathology and clinical treatment of diabetes mellitus in pregnancy to the implications for nursing care.	1. The key point in the care of the pregnant woman with diabetes is scrupulous maternal plasma glucose control. This is best achieved by home blood glucose monitoring, multiple daily insulin injections, and a careful diet.
Discriminate among the types of anemia associated with pregnancy regarding signs, treatment, and implications for pregnancy.	1. Anemia indicates inadequate levels of hemoglobin in the blood. 2. Signs include fatigue, paleness, and lack of energy. 3. Iron deficiency anemia is the most common form of anemia. Treatment is done through iron replacement by diet, iron supplement, or both. 4. Other forms of anemia include folic acid deficiency, sickle cell anemia, and thalassemia. 5. Implications for the infant include low birth weight, prematurity, and stillbirth.
Discuss acquired immunodeficiency syndrome (AIDS), including care of the pregnant woman who has tested positive for the human immunodeficiency virus (HIV), fetal/neonatal implications, and ramifications for the childbearing family.	1. HIV infection, which is transmitted via blood and body fluids, may also be transmitted vertically from the mother to the fetus. 2. Vertical transmission of HIV infection has been reduced dramatically with the administration of ZDV to the mother prenatally and during labor, and to the newborn. 3. Nurses should employ blood and body fluid precautions in caring for all women to avoid potential spread of infection.
Describe the effects of various heart disorders on pregnancy, including their implications for nursing care.	1. Cardiac disease during pregnancy requires careful assessment, limitation of activity, and reporting signs of impending cardiac decompensation by both client and nurse.
Delineate the effects of selected pregestational medical conditions on pregnancy.	1. All women with chronic medical conditions require increased vigilance of their condition during pregnancy. 2. Most chronic medical conditions will have some effect on the mother because pregnancy increases the stress on the mother's body. 3. Many chronic medical conditions in the mother increase risks to the newborn, such as premature birth, low birth weight, and growth retardation.

CRITICAL THINKING IN ACTION

View the **Critical Thinking in Action** video in Chapter 14 of the CD-ROM. Then, answer the questions that follow.

Jane Adams, a 23-year-old, G3 P2, at 37 weeks' gestation, presents to you in the birthing unit complaining of "vaginal pressure" but no contractions. You assess her and find that her history includes being HIV positive for 2 years, second-trimester cocaine and marijuana use, missed appointments, anemia (Hct 28%), and a positive syphilis serology. Jane tells you that she has other children and that they are being cared for by her mother, who has legal custody of them. You admit Jane and place her on the fetal monitor for evaluation of fetal well-being and contraction patterns. The monitor shows you that the fetal heart rate baseline is 120 to 130 with no decelerations; contractions are mild and irregular lasting 20 to 30 seconds. You obtain vital signs of BP 130/88, temperature 97.0°F - 88- 14. A vaginal exam determines that Jane is 7 cm dilated at

+1 station with intact membranes. She asks you if being HIV positive will affect her labor.

1. Discuss the prophylactic regimen for the prevention of HIV transmission to the fetus during labor.
2. Discuss the transmission of HIV to the fetus during pregnancy and birth.
3. Identify the emotional impact of HIV infection or other STIs on the woman.
4. On postpartum day 2, you inform Jane that her infant is HIV antibody positive. How would you clarify the results?

MediaLink www.prenhall.com/london

- NCLEX-RN® Review, case studies, and other interactive resources for this chapter can be found on the Companion Website at http://www.prenhall.com/london. Click on "Chapter 14" to select the activities for this chapter.

MediaLinks

- **Screening for Substance Abuse in Pregnancy**
  This 19-page document written by the National Center for Education in Maternal and Child Health provides the healthcare worker a useful screening tool to determine substance abuse during pregnancy.
- **Antepartum Fetal Surveillance**
  The American Academy of Family Physicians offers the American College of Obstetrics and Gynecology guidelines, indications, and recommendations for tests of fetal well-being.
- **Diabetes in Pregnancy**
  The American Diabetes Association offers practical advice to the pregnant Type II diabetic patient.
- **Pregnancy and Diabetes**
  Lifeclinic offers a comprehensive guide for the diabetic patient planning a pregnancy.
- **Anemia in Pregnancy**
  An article written by a certified nurse-midwife for the Maternity Center Association about anemia in pregnancy. Includes appropriate recipes to build iron stores.
- **AIDS in pregnancy**
  This site offers information about the providing care to the patient with AIDS during the antepartum, intrapartum, and postpartum periods.

- For animations, more NCLEX-RN® Review questions, and an audio glossary, access the accompanying CD-ROM in this textbook.

REFERENCES

American College of Obstetricians and Gynecologists. (2000a). *Genetic screening for hemoglobinopathies* (ACOG Committee Opinion No. 238). Washington, DC: Author.

American College of Obstetricians and Gynecologists. (2000b). *Scheduled cesarean delivery and the prevention of vertical transmission of HIV infection* (ACOG Committee Opinion No. 234). Washington, DC: Author.

American College of Obstetricians and Gynecologists. (2001a). *Gestational diabetes* (ACOG Practice Bulletin No. 30). Washington, DC: Author.

American College of Obstetricians and Gynecologists. (2001b). *Human immunodeficiency virus: Ethical guidelines for obstetricians and gynecologists* (ACOG Committee Opinion No. 255). Washington, DC: Author.

American College of Obstetricians and Gynecologists. (2005). *Pregestational diabetes mellitus* (ACOG Practice Bulletin No. 60). Washington, DC. Author.

American Diabetes Association. (2004a). Position statement: Gestational diabetes mellitus. *Diabetes Care, 27* (Suppl. 1), S88–S90.

American Diabetes Association. (2004b). Position statement: Preconception care of women with diabetes. *Diabetes Care, 27* (Suppl. 1), S76–S78.

Broening, H. W., Morford, L. L., Inman-Woods, S. L., Fukumura, M., & Vorhees, C. V. (2001). 3, 4-methylenedioxymethamphetamine (Ecstasy)-inducing learning and memory impairments depend on the age of exposure during early development. *Journal of Neuroscience, 21*(9), 3228–3235.

Caughron, K. F., & Smith, E. L. (2002). Diabetes mellitus. Selected guidelines. *Medscape.* Retrieved March 29, 2002, from http://www.medscape.com/viewarticle/426920_print

Centers for Disease Control and Prevention. (2002). Sexually transmitted diseases treatment guidelines 2002. *Morbidity and Mortality Weekly Report, 51* (RR-6), 1–79.

Centers for Disease Control and Prevention. (2003). *HIV/AIDS Surveillance Report 2002, 14,* 1–48.

Centers for Disease Control and Prevention. (2004). *Rapid HIV testing of women in labor and delivery.* Retrieved February 20, 2004, from http://www.cdc.gov/hiv/pubs/rt-women.htm

Centers for Disease Control and Prevention. (2005). Folic acid: Public Health Service recommendations. Retrieved September 2, 2005, from http://www.cdc.gov/ncbddd/folicacid/health_recomm.htm

Cleveland Clinic. (2003). *Hypoglycemia.* Retrieved February 3, 2003, from http://www.clevelandclinic.org/health/health-info/docs/0000/0098.asp

Cockey, C. D. (2001). On the edge. Prenatal ecstasy use and long-term memory loss. *AWHONN Lifelines, 5*(4), 23.

Crawford, P. (2001). Epilepsy and pregnancy. *Seizure, 10*(3), 212–219.

Criteria Committee of the New York Heart Association. (1994). *Nomenclature and criteria for diagnosis of diseases of the heart and great vessels* (9th ed.). Dallas, TX: American Heart Association.

Cunningham, F. G., Leveno, K. L., Bloom, S. L., Hauth, J. C., Gilstrap, L. C., III, & Wenstrom, K. D. (2005). *Williams' obstetrics* (22nd ed.). New York: McGraw-Hill.

Curet, L. B. (2000). Obstetric management of diabetes in pregnancy. In J. J. Sciarra (Ed.), *Maternal and fetal medicine* (Vol. 3, chap. 14, pp. 1–10). Philadelphia: Lippincott Williams & Wilkins.

Dashe, J. S., Nathan, L., McIntire, D. D., & Levano, K. (2000). Correlation between amniotic fluid glucose concentration and amniotic fluid volumes in pregnancy complicated by diabetes. *American Journal of Obstetrics and Gynecology, 182*(4), 901–904.

Farrell, M. (2003). Improving the care of women with gestational diabetes. *MCN. American Journal of Maternal Child Nursing, 28*(5), 301–305.

Friedman, J. M., & Polifka, J. E. (1996). *The effects of drugs on the fetus and nursing infant.* Baltimore: Johns Hopkins University Press.

Gowing, L. R., Henry-Edwards, S. M., Irvine, R. J., & Ali, R. L. (2002). The health effects of ecstasy: A literature review. *Drugs and Alcohol Review, 21*(1), 53–62.

Haas, J. (2000). High dose IVIG in the postpartum period for prevention of exacerbations in MS. *Multiple Sclerosis, 6*(Suppl. 2), 518–520.

Hall, H. I., Lee, L. M., Glynn, M. K., & Song, R. (2004, February 20). Heterosexual transmission of HIV— 29 states, 1999–2002. *Morbidity and Mortality Weekly Report, 53*(6), 125–129.

Jovanovic, L. (2000). Role of diet and insulin treatment of diabetes in pregnancy. *Clinical Obstetrics and Gynecology, 43*(1), 46–55.

Kandula, P., Liberato, B., & Harden, C. L. (2004). Pregnancy, contraception, and epilepsy: What are the risks? *Female Patient, 29*(5), 31–35.

Kjos, S. L. (2000). Postpartum care of the woman with diabetes. *Clinical Obstetrics and Gynecology, 43*(1), 75–82.

Landon, M. B. (2000). Obstetric management of pregnancies complicated by diabetes mellitus. *Clinical Obstetrics and Gynecology, 43*(1), 65–74.

March of Dimes. (2005). *Illicit drug use during pregnancy. For professionals and researchers.* Retrieved September 3, 2005, from http://www.marchofdimes.com

Martin, S. R., & Foley, M. R. (2002). Adult-onset heart disease in pregnancy. *Contemporary OB/GYN, 47*(11), 74–92.

Mersereau, P. W. (2000). Preventing neural tube defects: A national campaign. *Small Talk, 12*(2), 1–5.

Morrell, M. J. (2004). Epilepsy and pregnancy: Minimizing the risks. *Contemporary OB/GYN, 49*(1), 51–70.

Petri, M. (2003). Pregnancy in the lupus patient. *Female Patient, 28*(4), 12–15.

Reedy, N. J., & Brucker, M. C. (2004). Substance abuse. In H. Varney, J. M. Kriebs, & C. L. Gegor (Eds.), *Varney's midwifery* (4th ed., pp. 313–334). Sudbury, MA: Jones & Bartlett.

Schaefer-Graf, U. M., Buchanan, T. A., Xiang, A., Songster, G., Montoro, M., & Kjos, S. L. (2000). Patterns of congenital anomalies and relationship to initial maternal fasting glucose levels in pregnancy complicated by type 2 and gestational diabetes. *American Journal of Obstetrics and Gynecology, 182*(2), 313–320.

Shiraki, K. (2000). Perinatal transmission of hepatitis B virus and its prevention. *Journal of Gastroenterology and Hepatology, 15*(Suppl.), 11–15.

Sinclair, B. P. (1999–2000). HIV and women: Understand your responsibilities; reduce your risk. *AWHONN Lifelines, 3*(6), 35–38.

Substance Abuse and Mental Health Services Administration (SAMHSA). (2003). *Overview of findings from the 2002 National Survey on Drug Use and Health.* Rockville, MD: Office of Applied Studies, NHSDA Series H-21, DHHS Publication No. SMA 03–3774.

Substance Abuse and Mental Health Services Administration (SAMHSA). (2004). Pregnancy and substance use. *The NSDUH Report.* Retrieved May 11, 2004, from http://www.drugabusestatistics.samhsa.gov

U.S. Public Health Service Task Force. (2003). *Recommendations for use of antiretroviral drugs in pregnant HIV-1 infected women for maternal health and to reduce perinatal HIV-1 transmission in the United States.* Rockville, MD: Author.

Varney, H., Kriebs, J. M., & Gegor, C. L. (2004). *Varney's midwifery* (4th ed.). Sudbury, MA: Jones & Bartlett.

Wang, E. C. (1999). Methadone treatment during pregnancy. *Journal of Obstetric, Gynecologic, and Neonatal Nursing, 28*(6), 615–622.

Wilson, J. K., & Thorp, J. M., Jr. (2003). Substance abuse in pregnancy. In J. J. Sciarra (Ed.), *Gynecology and obstetrics* (Vol. 2, chap. 33). Philadelphia: Lippincott Williams & Wilkins.

Pregnancy at Risk: Gestational Onset

> *When we decided to have children we were so excited, so ready. I never expected that I would have two miscarriages. I can't tell you how hard that was to handle. Even today, with two healthy children, I remember the pain, the loss, the sense of failure, and I grieve for the children we will never know.*
> —*Jasmine, 36*

LEARNING OBJECTIVES

- Contrast the etiology, medical therapy, and nursing interventions for the various bleeding problems associated with pregnancy.

- Identify the medical therapy and nursing interventions indicated in caring for a woman with an incompetent cervix.

- Discuss the medical therapy and nursing care of a woman with hyperemesis gravidarum.

- Delineate the nursing care needs of a woman experiencing premature rupture of the membranes or preterm labor.

- Describe the development and course of hypertensive disorders associated with pregnancy.

- Explain the cause and prevention of hemolytic disease of the newborn secondary to Rh incompatibility.

- Compare Rh incompatibility to ABO incompatibility with regard to occurrence, treatment, and implications for the fetus or newborn.

- Summarize the effects of surgical procedures on pregnancy and explain ways in which pregnancy may complicate diagnosis.

- Discuss the impact of trauma due to an accident on the pregnant woman or her fetus.

- Explain the needs and care of the pregnant woman who experiences abuse.

- Describe the effects of infections on the pregnant woman and her unborn child.

MEDIALINK www.prenhall.com/london

CD-ROM

NCLEX-RN® Review
Skill 2–3: Assessing Deep Tendon Reflexes and Clonus
Skill 2–4: Administration of Rh Immune Globulin (RhIgG) (RhoGAM, HypRho-D)
Animation: Early Premature Labor
Audio Glossary

Companion Website

NCLEX-RN® Review
MediaLink Applications:
    Case Study: Client with Preclampsia
    Care Plan Activity: Client at Risk for Preterm Labor
Case Study

I n some pregnancies, problems arise that place the woman and her unborn child at risk. Regular prenatal care helps detect these complications quickly so that effective care can be provided. This chapter focuses on problems that develop during pregnancy, that is, problems with a *gestational onset*.

CARE OF THE WOMAN WITH A BLEEDING DISORDER

During the first and second trimesters, the major cause of bleeding is abortion. **Abortion** is the expulsion of the fetus prior to viability, which is considered to be 20 weeks' gestation or weight of less than 500 g. Definitions vary somewhat according to state reporting laws (Cunningham, Leveno, Bloom et al., 2005). Abortions are either *spontaneous* (occurring naturally) or *induced* (occurring as a result of medical or surgical means). Because the term *abortion* may have a negative connotation, spontaneous abortion is often called **miscarriage**.

Other complications that can cause bleeding in the first half of pregnancy are ectopic pregnancy and gestational trophoblastic disease. In the second half of pregnancy, particularly in the third trimester, the two major causes of bleeding are placenta previa and abruptio placentae. (See Chapter 21 for more information. ∞) Regardless of the cause of bleeding, however, the nurse has certain general responsibilities in providing nursing care.

GENERAL PRINCIPLES OF NURSING INTERVENTION

Spotting is relatively common during pregnancy and usually occurs following sexual intercourse or exercise because of trauma to the highly vascular cervix. However, the woman is advised to report any spotting or bleeding that occurs during pregnancy so that it can be evaluated.

It is often the nurse's responsibility to make the initial assessment of bleeding. In general the following nursing measures are indicated:

- Monitor blood pressure and pulse frequently.

- Observe the woman for behaviors indicative of shock, such as pallor, clammy skin, perspiration, dyspnea, or restlessness.

- Count and weigh pads to assess amount of bleeding over a given time period; save any tissue or clots expelled.

- If pregnancy is of 12 weeks' gestation or beyond, assess fetal heart tones with a Doppler.

- Prepare for intravenous (IV) therapy. There may be standing orders to begin IV therapy on clients who are bleeding.

- Prepare equipment for examination and have oxygen available.

- Collect and organize all data, including antepartal history, onset of bleeding episode, and laboratory studies (hemoglobin, hematocrit, hormonal assays) for analysis.

- Notify other members of the healthcare team, including the physician or nurse-midwife, operating room staff if a surgical procedure is planned, and so forth.

- Obtain an order to type and crossmatch for blood if evidence of significant blood loss exists.

- Assess coping mechanisms of the woman in crisis. Give emotional support to enhance her coping abilities by continuous, sustained presence; by clear explanation of procedures; and by communicating her status to her family. Prepare the woman for possible fetal loss. Assess her expressions of anger, denial, silence, guilt, depression, or self-blame.

■ Assess the family's response to the situation.

SPONTANEOUS ABORTION (MISCARRIAGE)

The incidence of first-trimester spontaneous abortion is about 10% to 12% for clinically recognized pregnancies, but the number may be higher overall. The likelihood of recurrent miscarriage is thought to be 25% to 30% (Simpson, 2002).

A majority of early miscarriages are related to chromosomal abnormalities. Other causes include teratogenic drugs, faulty implantation due to abnormalities of the female reproductive tract, a weakened cervix, placental abnormalities, chronic maternal diseases, endocrine imbalances, and maternal infections. Research does not support the belief that accidents and psychic trauma are primary causes of spontaneous abortion.

Classification

Spontaneous abortions are subdivided into the following categories:

■ **Threatened abortion** (Figure 15–1 ◉). The embryo or fetus is jeopardized by unexplained bleeding, cramping, and backache. The cervix is closed. Bleeding may persist for days. It may be followed by partial or complete expulsion of the embryo or fetus, placenta, and membranes (sometimes called the "products of conception").

■ **Imminent abortion** (Figure 15–1B). Bleeding and cramping increase. The internal cervical os dilates. Membranes may rupture. The term *inevitable abortion* also applies.

■ **Complete abortion.** All the products of conception are expelled.

■ **Incomplete abortion** (Figure 15–1C). Some of the products of conception are retained, most often the placenta. The internal cervical os is dilated slightly.

■ **Missed abortion.** The fetus dies in utero but is not expelled. Uterine growth ceases, breast changes regress, and the woman may report a brownish vaginal discharge. The cervix is closed. If the fetus is retained beyond 6 weeks, the breakdown of fetal tissues results in the release of thromboplastin, and disseminated intravascular coagulation (DIC) may develop.

■ **Recurrent (habitual) abortion.** Abortion occurs consecutively in three or more pregnancies.

■ **Septic abortion.** Infection is present. It may occur with prolonged, unrecognized rupture of the membranes, pregnancy with an intrauterine device

◉ **FIGURE 15–1**

A   B   C

Types of spontaneous abortion. *A,* Threatened. The cervix is not dilated, and the placenta is still attached to the uterine wall, but some bleeding occurs. *B,* Imminent. The placenta has separated from the uterine wall, the cervix has dilated, and the amount of bleeding has increased. *C,* Incomplete. The embryo or fetus has passed out of the uterus, but the placenta remains.

(IUD) in place, or attempts by unqualified individuals to end a pregnancy.

Clinical Therapy

Pelvic cramping and backache are reliable indicators of potential spontaneous abortion. These symptoms are usually absent in bleeding caused by polyps, ruptured cervical blood vessels, or cervical erosion. Ultrasound scanning may be used to detect the presence of a gestational sac or fetal heartbeat if the cause of bleeding is unclear. Results of human chorionic gonadotropin (hCG) levels are not particularly helpful because hCG levels fall slowly after fetal death and therefore cannot confirm a live embryo or fetus. Hemoglobin and hematocrit are obtained to assess blood loss. Blood is typed and crossmatched for possible replacement needs.

The therapy prescribed for the pregnant woman with bleeding is bed rest, abstinence from sex, and perhaps sedation. If bleeding persists and abortion is imminent or incomplete, the woman may be hospitalized, IV therapy or blood transfusions may be started to replace fluid, and dilation and curettage (D&C) or suction evacuation is performed to remove the remainder of the products of conception. If the woman is Rh negative and not sensitized, Rh immune globulin (RhoGAM) is given within 72 hours (see discussion on Rh alloimmunization beginning on page 361 in this chapter).

In missed abortions the products of conception usually are expelled spontaneously. Diagnosis is based on history, pelvic examination, and a negative pregnancy test and may be confirmed by ultrasound if necessary. If this does not occur within 4 to 6 weeks after embryo or fetal death, hospitalization is necessary. If in the first trimester, D&C or suction evacuation is done. In the second trimester, labor is induced or dilation and evacuation (D&E) may be used.

NURSING MANAGEMENT

NURSING ASSESSMENT AND DIAGNOSIS

Assess the woman's vital signs, amount and appearance of any bleeding, level of comfort, and general physical health. If the pregnancy is 10 to 12 weeks or more, determine fetal heart rates with a Doppler. It is also important to assess the responses of the woman and her family to this crisis, their coping mechanisms, and their ability to comfort each other.

Examples of nursing diagnoses that may apply include the following:

- *Acute Pain* related to abdominal cramping secondary to threatened abortion
- *Anticipatory Grieving* related to expected loss of unborn child

PLANNING AND IMPLEMENTATION

Nursing Care in the Community

If a woman in her first trimester of pregnancy begins cramping or spotting, she is often evaluated on an outpatient basis. Provide analgesics for pain relief if the woman's cramps are severe, and explain what is occurring throughout the process.

Feelings of shock or disbelief are normal. Couples who approached the pregnancy with joy and excitement now feel grief, sadness, and possibly anger. Because many women, even with planned pregnancies, feel some ambivalence initially, guilt is also a common emotion. These feelings may be even stronger for women who were negative about their pregnancies. The women may even believe that the miscarriage is a punishment for some wrongdoing.

Offer psychologic support to the woman and her family by encouraging them to talk about their feelings, allowing them the privacy to grieve, and listening sympathetically to their concerns about this pregnancy and future ones. To help decrease feelings of guilt or blame, inform the woman and her family about the causes of miscarriage. Refer them to other healthcare professionals for additional help as necessary. The grieving period following a miscarriage usually lasts 6 to 24 months. Many couples can be helped during this period by an organization or support group established for parents who have lost a fetus or newborn.

Hospital-Based Nursing Care

A woman with an incomplete or missed abortion may need a D&C or other procedure, which is typically done on an outpatient basis. Barring any complications, the woman can return home a few hours after the procedure. Monitor the woman's condition closely and provide instruction for self-care. Administer Rh immune globulin if it is indicated.

EVALUATION

Expected outcomes of nursing care include the following:

- The woman is able to explain spontaneous abortion, the treatment measures employed in her care, and long-term implications for future pregnancies.

- The woman suffers no complications.

- The woman and her partner begin verbalizing their grief and acknowledge that the grieving process lasts several months.

ECTOPIC PREGNANCY

Ectopic pregnancy (EP) is the implantation of the fertilized ovum in a site other than the endometrial lining of the uterus. It has many causes, including tubal damage from pelvic inflammatory disease (PID), previous tubal surgery, congenital anomalies of the tube, endometriosis, previous EP, presence of an IUD, and in utero exposure to diethylstilbestrol (DES).

The incidence of EP has increased in the past several years, from 4.5 per 1000 pregnancies in 1970 to 19.7 per 1000 pregnancies in 2000 (Gracia & Barnhart, 2001). Although incidence has increased, mortality rates have declined almost 90% due to better diagnostic techniques that allow detection before tubal rupture.

EP occurs when the fertilized ovum is prevented or slowed in its passage through the tube and thus implants before it reaches the uterus, usually in the ampulla of the fallopian tube. "Pathophysiology Illustrated: Ectopic Pregnancy" identifies other implantation sites.

Initially symptoms of pregnancy may be present, including amenorrhea, breast tenderness, and nausea. The hormone hCG is present in the blood and urine. As the pregnancy progresses, the chorionic villi grow into the tube wall or implantation site and establish a blood supply.

PATHOPHYSIOLOGY ILLUSTRATED

Ectopic Pregnancy

Various implantation sites in ectopic pregnancy. The most common site is within the fallopian tube, hence the name "tubal pregnancy."

When the embryo outgrows this space, the tube ruptures and there is bleeding into the abdominal cavity. This bleeding irritates the peritoneum, causing the characteristic symptoms of sharp, one-sided pain, syncope, and referred shoulder pain. The woman may also have lower abdominal pain. Vaginal bleeding occurs when the embryo dies and the decidua sloughs.

Physical examination usually reveals adnexal (area over each ovary and fallopian tube) tenderness. An adnexal mass is palpable about half the time. Bleeding tends to be slow and chronic, and the abdomen gradually becomes rigid and very tender. With bleeding into the abdominal cavity, pelvic examination is very painful, and a mass of blood may be palpated in the lower abdomen. Laboratory tests may reveal low hemoglobin and hematocrit levels and rising leukocyte levels.

Clinical Therapy

Diagnosis of EP begins with an assessment of menstrual history, including the date of the last menstrual period, followed by a pelvic examination to identify any pelvic masses and tenderness. A serum progesterone level is drawn. A viable intrauterine pregnancy can be diagnosed with 97.5% sensitivity if the progesterone level is 25 ng/mL or higher, whereas a serum progesterone lower than 5 ng/mL indicates a nonviable pregnancy. Transvaginal ultrasound is indicated for levels between 5 ng/mL and 25 ng/mL (Simpson, 2002). Serum β-hCG levels are drawn and reassessed in 48 hours if necessary. A woman with EP tends to have abnormally low hCG levels. In a normal pregnancy, hCG levels double every 48 to 72 hours. Nondoubling hCG levels occur in EP. If the β-hCG levels are above 1500 milli-international units/mm, transvaginal ultrasound is used to check for a uterine pregnancy or an adnexal mass. Confirming a uterine pregnancy nearly eliminates the diagnosis of EP.

Treatment may be medical or surgical. Methotrexate is used for the woman who desires future pregnancy if her ectopic pregnancy is unruptured and of 4 cm size or less and if her condition is stable. In addition there must be no fetal heart motion and the woman must have no evidence of a blood disorder or kidney or liver disease. Methotrexate, a folic acid antagonist that interferes with DNA synthesis and cell multiplication, is given intramuscularly (IM). As an outpatient the woman is monitored for increasing abdominal pain because a primary consideration is differentiating between the transient abdominal pain that indicates successful methotrexate therapy and the abdominal pain associated with a ruptured ectopic pregnancy. Serum β-hCG titers are also monitored regularly. Typically the hCG levels increase for 1 to 4 days and then decrease. If they do not, the woman may need a second dose of methotrexate or surgery (Cunningham et al., 2005).

If surgery is indicated and the woman desires future pregnancies, treatment involves salpingostomy via a laparoscope. With this method an incision is made lengthwise and the products of conception are gently removed. The surgical incision is left open and allowed to close naturally. If the tube is ruptured or if future childbearing is not an issue, laparoscopic salpingectomy (removal of the tube) is performed, leaving the ovary in place unless it is damaged. With both medical and surgical therapies for EP, the Rh negative nonsensitized woman is given Rh immune globulin to prevent sensitization.

DEVELOPING CULTURAL COMPETENCE

COMPLICATIONS OF PREGNANCY

- The incidence of ectopic pregnancy is higher for nonwhite women than for whites in every age category.
- The incidence of preeclampsia is also related to genetic predisposition. Women of African-American descent are at higher risk.
- Until recently, researchers thought that the incidence of GTD was significantly higher in women of Asian ancestry. However, population-based studies show that the incidence of GTD in most of the world is similar to that found in the United States—about 1 in 1000 pregnancies (Cunningham et al., 2005).

NURSING MANAGEMENT

NURSING ASSESSMENT AND DIAGNOSIS

When the woman with a suspected ectopic pregnancy is admitted to the hospital, assess the appearance and amount of vaginal bleeding and monitor vital signs for developing shock. Assess the woman's emotional state and coping abilities, and determine the couple's informational needs. Determine the woman's level of pain, which can be significant. If surgery is necessary, complete the appropriate ongoing assessments postoperatively.

Nursing diagnoses that may apply for a woman with EP include the following:

- *Acute Pain* related to abdominal bleeding secondary to tubal rupture
- *Anticipatory Grieving* related to expected pregnancy loss
- *Health-Seeking Behaviors: Request for Information about Treatment of Ectopic Pregnancy and its Long-Term Implications* related to stated unfamiliarity with the condition

PLANNING AND IMPLEMENTATION

Nursing Care in the Community

Women with EP are often seen initially in a clinic or office setting. Be alert to the possibility of EP if a woman presents with complaints of abdominal pain and lack of menses for 1 to 2 months. A woman receiving medical treatment using methotrexate is followed as an outpatient. Advise the woman that some abdominal pain is common following the injection, but generally it is mild and lasts only 24 to 48 hours. More severe pain might indicate treatment failure and should be evaluated. The woman should also report heavy vaginal bleeding, dizziness, or tachycardia. Stress the need to return for follow-up hCG testing.

Hospital-Based Nursing Care

Once a diagnosis of EP is made and surgery is scheduled, start an IV as ordered and begin preoperative teaching. Immediately report signs of developing shock. If the woman experiences severe abdominal pain, administer analgesics and evaluate their effectiveness.

Regardless of the treatment used, the woman and her family will need emotional support during this difficult time. Their feelings and responses to this crisis are generally similar to those that occur in cases of spontaneous abortion; similar nursing actions are required.

EVALUATION

Expected outcomes of nursing care include the following:

- The woman is able to explain ectopic pregnancy, treatment alternatives, and implications for future childbearing.
- The woman and her caregivers detect possible complications early and manage them successfully.
- The woman and her partner are able to begin verbalizing their loss.

GESTATIONAL TROPHOBLASTIC DISEASE

Gestational trophoblastic disease (GTD) is the pathologic proliferation of trophoblastic cells (the trophoblast is the outermost layer of embryonic cells). It includes hydatidiform mole, invasive mole (chorioadenoma destruens), and choriocarcinoma, a form of cancer.

Hydatidiform mole (molar pregnancy) is a disease in which (1) abnormal development of the placenta occurs, resulting in hydropic vesicles (a fluid-filled, grapelike cluster); and (2) the trophoblastic tissue proliferates. The disease results in the loss of the pregnancy and the possibility, though remote, of developing choriocarcinoma, a form of cancer, from the trophoblastic tissue.

Molar pregnancies are classified into two types, complete and partial, both of which meet the previously mentioned criteria. A *complete mole* develops from an ovum containing no maternal genetic material, an "empty egg," which is fertilized by a normal sperm. The embryo dies

very early, no circulation is established, the hydropic vesicles are avascular, and no embryonic tissue is found. Choriocarcinoma seems to be associated exclusively with the complete mole.

The *partial mole* usually has a triploid karyotype (69 chromosomes). Most often a normal ovum with 23 chromosomes is fertilized by two sperm (dispermy) or by a sperm that has failed to undergo the first meiotic division and therefore contains 46 chromosomes. There may be a fetal sac or even a fetus with a heartbeat. The fetus has multiple anomalies and little chance for survival. Often partial moles are recognized only after miscarriage, and they may go unnoticed even then.

Invasive mole (chorioadenoma destruens) is similar to a complete mole, but it involves the uterine myometrium. Treatment is the same as for complete mole.

Clinical Therapy

Initially the clinical picture is similar to that of pregnancy. However, classic signs soon appear. Vaginal bleeding occurs almost universally. It is often brownish due to liquefaction of the uterine clot, but it may be bright red. Uterine enlargement greater than expected for gestational age is a classic sign, present in about 50% of cases. In the remainder of cases, the uterus is appropriate or small for the gestational age. If hydropic vesicles are passed, they are diagnostic (Figure 15–2 ○). With a partial mole, the vesicles are often smaller and may not be noticed. Because serum hCG levels are higher with molar pregnancy than

● **FIGURE 15–2**

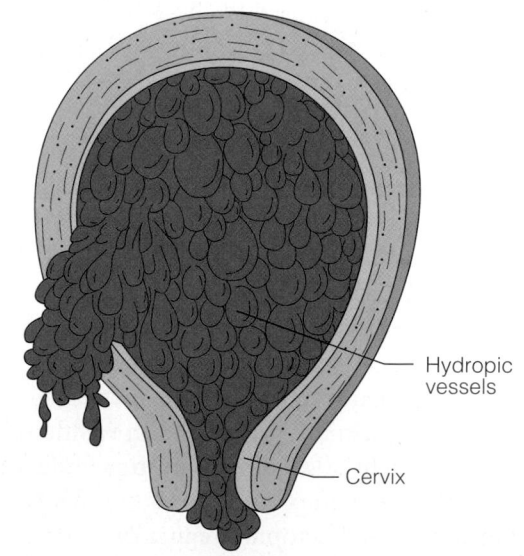

Hydatidiform mole. A common sign is vaginal bleeding, often brownish (the characteristic "prune juice" appearance) but sometimes bright red. In this figure, some of the hydropic vessels are being passed. This occurrence is diagnostic for hydatidiform mole.

with normal pregnancy, the woman may experience hyperemesis gravidarum. Anemia occurs frequently due to blood loss and poor nutrition secondary to hyperemesis. Symptoms of preeclampsia prior to 24 weeks' gestation strongly suggest a molar pregnancy. No fetal heart tones are heard, and no fetal movement is palpated. Transvaginal ultrasound is used for diagnosis.

Therapy begins with suction evacuation of the mole and curettage of the uterus to remove all fragments of the placenta. Early evacuation decreases the possibility of other complications. If the woman is older and has completed her childbearing, or if there is excessive bleeding, hysterectomy may be the treatment of choice to reduce the risk of choriocarcinoma.

Because of the risk of choriocarcinoma, the woman treated for hydatidiform mole should receive extensive follow-up therapy. Follow-up care includes a baseline chest x-ray to detect lung metastasis and a physical examination including a pelvic examination. Serum β-hCG levels are monitored weekly until the woman has normal titers for 3 consecutive weeks. Titers are then monitored monthly for 6 months, followed by every 2 months for 6 months more (Copeland & Landon, 2002). The woman should avoid pregnancy during that time because the elevated hCG levels associated with pregnancy would cause confusion about whether cancer had developed.

Continued high or rising hCG titers are abnormal. If they occur, a D&C is performed and the tissue is examined. If cancer cells are found, treatment at a center specializing in GTD is advised. Chemotherapy is started using methotrexate alone or with other chemotherapy agents. If, after a year of monitoring, the hCG serum titers are within normal limits, a couple may be assured that a normal pregnancy can be anticipated, with a low risk of recurring hydatidiform mole.

NURSING MANAGEMENT

NURSING ASSESSMENT AND DIAGNOSIS

Observe for symptoms of hydatidiform mole at each antepartal visit. The classic symptoms are found more frequently with the complete mole. Before evacuation the partial mole may be difficult to distinguish from a missed abortion. If a molar pregnancy is diagnosed, assess the woman's (or the couple's) understanding of the condition and its implications.

Nursing diagnoses that may apply include the following:

- *Fear* related to the possible development of choriocarcinoma
- *Anticipatory Grieving* related to the loss of the pregnancy secondary to GTD

PLANNING AND IMPLEMENTATION

Nursing Care in the Community

When a molar pregnancy is suspected, the woman needs emotional support. Answer questions about the condition and explain what ultrasound and other diagnostic procedures will entail. If a molar pregnancy is diagnosed, support the parents as they deal with their grief about the lost pregnancy. Healthcare counselors, a member of the clergy, or a professional counselor may also be of help.

Hospital-Based Nursing Care

When the woman is hospitalized for removal of the mole, monitor vital signs and vaginal bleeding for signs of hemorrhage. Determine the presence of abdominal pain and evaluate the woman's emotional state and coping ability. Have typed and crossmatched blood available for surgery. Administer oxytocin as ordered to keep the uterus contracted and to prevent hemorrhage. If the woman is Rh negative and not sensitized, give Rh immune globulin to prevent antibody formation.

Stress the importance of follow-up visits. Advise the woman to delay another pregnancy until the follow-up program is completed.

EVALUATION

Expected outcomes of nursing care include the following:

- The woman has a smooth recovery following successful evacuation of the mole.
- The woman is able to explain GTD and its treatment, follow-up, and long-term implications for pregnancy.
- The woman and her partner are able to begin talking about their grief at the loss of their anticipated child.
- The woman can discuss the importance of follow-up care and indicates her willingness to cooperate with the regimen.

CARE OF THE WOMAN WITH AN INCOMPETENT CERVIX

Incompetent cervix refers to the premature dilatation of the cervix, usually in the fourth or fifth month of pregnancy. It is associated with repeated second-trimester abortions. Possible causes include cervical trauma, infection, congenital cervical or uterine anomalies, or increased uterine volume (as with a multiple gestation).

Diagnosis is based on a positive history of repeated, relatively painless and bloodless second-trimester abortions. Serial pelvic examinations early in the second trimester reveal progressive effacement and dilatation of

● FIGURE 15–3

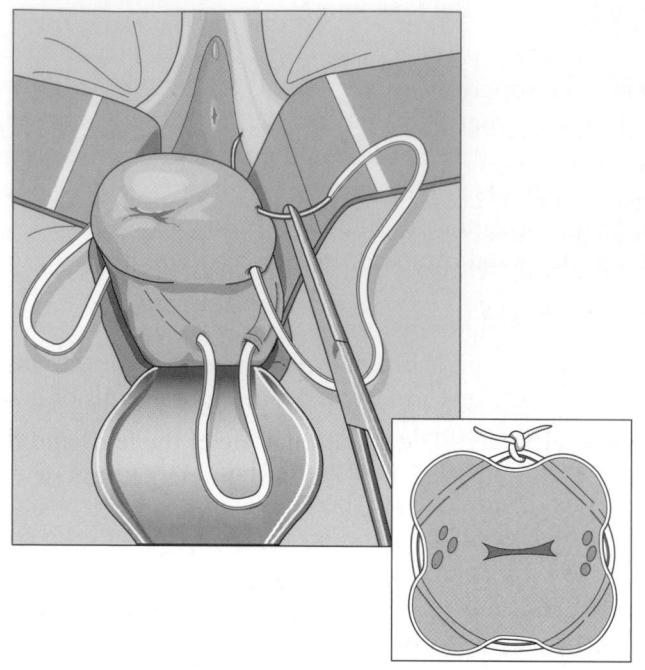

A cerclage or purse-string suture is inserted in the cervix to prevent preterm cervical dilatation and pregnancy loss. After placement the string is tightened and secured anteriorly.

the cervix and bulging of the membranes through the cervical os. If incompetent cervix is suspected, serial ultrasound provides information on dilatation of the internal cervical os before a dilated external os is detected.

Incompetent cervix is managed surgically with a Shirodkar procedure (cerclage)—or a modification of it by McDonald—which reinforces the weakened cervix by encircling it at the level of the internal os with suture material (Figure 15–3 ●). A purse-string suture is placed in the cervix in the first trimester or early in the second trimester. Once the suture is in place, a cesarean birth may be planned (to prevent repeating the procedure in subsequent pregnancies), or the suture may be cut at term and vaginal birth permitted. Recent research questions the effectiveness of cerclage in preventing late miscarriage or preterm birth (American College of Obstetricians and Gynecologists [ACOG], 2003).

The woman must understand the importance of contacting her physician immediately if her membranes rupture or labor begins. The physician can remove the suture to prevent possible complications.

CARE OF THE WOMAN WITH HYPEREMESIS GRAVIDARUM

Hyperemesis gravidarum, a relatively rare condition, is excessive vomiting during pregnancy. Clinicians now view hyperemesis as the far end of a continuum of nausea and vomiting of pregnancy. It may be mild at first, but true hyperemesis may progress to a point at which the woman not only vomits everything she swallows but also retches between meals.

Although the exact cause of hyperemesis is unclear, increased levels of hCG may play a role. Women with a history of migraine headaches, motion sickness, sickness related to oral contraceptives, and a family or personal history of hyperemesis are at increased risk. Other variables that may relate to hyperemesis include transient hyperthyroidism due to the effect of hCG on the thyroid-stimulating hormone (TSH) receptor, *Helicobacter pylori* infection, and psychologic factors, although research suggests that psychologic findings may be a *response* to hyperemesis gravidarum rather than a cause (Goodwin, 2004). In severe cases, hyperemesis causes dehydration, which leads to fluid-electrolyte imbalance and alkalosis from loss of hydrochloric acid. Hypovolemia, hypotension, tachycardia, increased hematocrit and blood urea nitrogen (BUN), and decreased urine output can also occur. If untreated, metabolic acidosis may develop. Severe potassium loss may disrupt cardiac functioning. Starvation causes muscle wasting and severe protein and vitamin deficiencies. Fetal or embryonic death may result, and the woman may suffer irreversible metabolic changes or death.

CLINICAL THERAPY

The goals of treatment include control of vomiting and dehydration, restoration of electrolyte balance, and maintenance of adequate nutrition. If the woman does not respond to standard approaches to the control of nausea and vomiting in pregnancy (see Chapter 11 ∞), she may require IV fluids on an outpatient basis. If her symptoms do not improve, hospitalization may be indicated. Initially the woman is given nothing by mouth (NPO), and IV fluids are administered. Potassium chloride is often added to the IV to prevent hypokalemia. Thiamine and pyroxidine (vitamin B_6) may be replaced to correct deficiencies and prevent peripheral neuropathy. Antiemetics may also be administered. Typically the woman remains NPO for 48 hours. If her condition does not improve, total parenteral nutrition may be needed. She then begins controlled oral feedings.

NURSING MANAGEMENT

NURSING ASSESSMENT AND DIAGNOSIS

When a woman is hospitalized for control of vomiting, assess the amount and character of any emesis, intake and output, fetal heart rate, signs of jaundice or bleeding, and her emotional state.

Nursing diagnoses that may apply include the following:

- *Imbalanced Nutrition: Less than Body Requirements* related to persistent vomiting secondary to hyperemesis

- *Fear* related to the effects of hyperemesis on fetal well-being

PLANNING AND IMPLEMENTATION

Nursing Care in the Community

Parenteral therapy provided at home in collaboration with a physician and a registered dietitian is sometimes used to enable the woman to remain in her home. This therapy also gives an opportunity to observe family interactions and evaluate the home environment. This assessment helps determine the pregnant woman's level of support, any significant stressors in her life, and her understanding of nutrition and self-care measures.

Hospital-Based Nursing Care

Nursing care is supportive and directed at maintaining a relaxed, quiet environment away from food odors or offensive smells. Once oral feedings resume, food needs to be attractively served. Oral hygiene is important because the mouth is dry and may be irritated from vomitus. Monitor weight regularly. In some cases emotional factors have appeared to play a role, although that remains controversial. Nevertheless, psychotherapy may sometimes be recommended. With proper treatment, prognosis is favorable.

EVALUATION

Expected outcomes of nursing care include the following:

- The woman is able to explain hyperemesis gravidarum, its therapy, and its possible effects on her pregnancy.

- The woman's condition is corrected and complications are avoided.

CARE OF THE WOMAN WITH PREMATURE RUPTURE OF MEMBRANES

Premature rupture of membranes (PROM) is spontaneous rupture of the membranes prior to the onset of labor. *Preterm PROM (PPROM)* is the rupture of membranes occurring before 37 weeks' gestation. PROM is associated with infection, previous history of PROM, hydramnios, multiple pregnancy, urinary tract infection, amniocentesis, placenta previa, abruptio placentae, trauma, incompetent cervix, bleeding during pregnancy, and maternal genital tract anomalies.

Maternal risk of infection increases as does the risk of abruptio placentae (discussed in Chapter 21 ∞). Fetal-newborn implications include risk of respiratory distress syndrome (with PROM), fetal sepsis due to ascending pathogens, malpresentation, prolapse of the umbilical cord, and increased perinatal morbidity and mortality.

CLINICAL THERAPY

A sterile speculum examination is done to detect the presence of amniotic fluid in the vagina. If fluid is not obviously pooling, the diagnosis can be confirmed with nitrazine paper (which turns deep blue) and a microscopic examination (ferning test). Digital examination increases the risk of infection and is not recommended unless a management plan has been developed.

Fetal well-being is assessed through a fetal heart rate tracing or biophysical profile, and the gestational age of the fetus is calculated. The gestational age of the fetus and the presence or absence of infection guide treatment for PROM. If maternal signs of infection are evident, antibiotic therapy (usually by IV infusion) is started immediately, and the fetus is born vaginally or by cesarean regardless of the gestational age. Prophylactic antibiotics are often administered for the first 48 hours while awaiting culture results. On admission to the nursery, the newborn is assessed for sepsis and placed on antibiotics. (For further information about the newborn with sepsis, see Chapter 28. ∞)

Management of PROM in the absence of infection and gestation of less than 37 weeks is usually conservative. The woman is hospitalized on bed rest. On admission, complete blood cell count (CBC), C-reactive protein, and urinalysis are obtained. Continuous electronic fetal monitoring may be ordered at the beginning of treatment but usually is discontinued after a few hours, unless the fetus is estimated to be very low birth weight. Regular nonstress tests (NSTs) or biophysical profiles are used to monitor fetal well-being. (These tests are discussed in Chapter 16. ∞) Maternal blood pressure, pulse, and temperature and fetal heart rate (FHR) are assessed every 4 hours. Regular laboratory evaluations are done to detect maternal infection. Vaginal examinations are avoided to decrease the chance of infection. As the gestation approaches 34 weeks, fetal lung maturity studies are indicated. [AAP]

After initial treatment and observation, if leaking of fluid ceases, some women (typically those with sufficient amniotic fluid, no infection, and cervical dilatation less than 4 cm) may be followed at home, although this is controversial. The woman is advised to continue bed rest (with bathroom privileges), monitor her temperature and pulse four times a day, keep a fetal movement chart, and have weekly NSTs. She is advised to contact her physician and return to the hospital if she has a fever, uterine tenderness or contractions, increased leakage of fluids, decreased fetal movement, or foul-smelling vaginal discharge.

Maternal corticosteroid administration to promote fetal lung maturity and prevent respiratory distress syndrome remains controversial because of possible harmful effects on

DRUG GUIDE

BETAMETHASONE (CELESTONE SOLUSPAN)

Overview of Maternal-Fetal Action

Studies have provided ample evidence that glucocorticoids such as betamethasone are capable of inducing pulmonary maturation and decreasing the incidence of respiratory distress syndrome in preterm infants. The mechanism by which corticosteroids accelerate fetal lung maturity is unclear, but it is related to the stimulation of enzyme activity by the drug. The enzyme is required for biosynthesis of surfactant by the type II pneumocytes. Surfactant is of major importance to the proper functioning of the lung in that it decreases the surface tension of the alveoli. Glucocorticoids also increase the rate of glycogen depletion, which leads to thinning of the interalveolar septa and increases the size of the alveoli. The thinning of the epithelium brings the capillaries into closer proximity with the air spaces and improves oxygen exchange.

Route, Dosage, Frequency

Prenatal maternal intramuscular injections of 12 mg of betamethasone are given once a day for 2 days. Dexamethasone may also be given in doses of 6 mg every 12 hours for four doses (NIH Consensus Development Panel, 2001). To obtain maximum results, birth should be delayed for at least 24 hours after completing the first round of treatment. The effect of corticosteroids may be transient. Currently, it is suggested that repeat courses of corticosteroids should not be used routinely.

Contraindications

Inability to delay birth

Adequate L/S ratio

Presence of a condition that necessitates immediate birth (e.g., maternal bleeding)

Presence of maternal infection, diabetes mellitus (relative contraindication)

Gestational age greater than 34 completed weeks

Maternal Side Effects

Increased risk for infection has not been supported in large studies. There may, however, be some increase in the incidence of infection in women with premature rupture of the membranes. Maternal hyperglycemia may occur during corticosteroid administration. Clients with type 1 diabetes may require insulin infusions for several days to prevent ketoacidosis. Corticosteroids possibly may increase the risk of pulmonary edema, especially when used concurrently with tocolytics (Iams, 2002; NIH Consensus Development Panel, 2001).

Effects on Fetus/Newborn

Lowered cortisol levels at birth, but rebound occurs by 2 hours of age

Hypoglycemia

Increased risk of neonatal sepsis

Animal studies have shown serious fetal side effects such as reduced head circumference, reduced weight of the fetal adrenal and thymus glands, and decreased placental weight. Human studies have not shown these effects, however.

Nursing Considerations

Assess for presence of contraindications.

Provide education regarding possible side effects.

Administer betamethasone deep into gluteal muscle, avoiding injection into deltoid (high incidence of local atrophy). (Dexamethasone may be administered IM or IV.)

Periodically evaluate BP, pulse, weight, and edema.

Assess lab data for electrolytes and blood glucose.

Although concomitant use of betamethasone and tocolytic agents has been implicated in increased risk of pulmonary edema, the betamethasone has little mineral corticoid activity; therefore, it probably doesn't add significantly to the salt and water retention effects of beta-adrenergic agonists. Other causes of noncardiogenic pulmonary edema should also be investigated if pulmonary edema develops during administration of betamethasone to a woman in preterm labor.

---

the fetus and mother. Currently a single course of betamethasone is recommended for women with PROM prior to 30 weeks' gestation, if there is no intra-amniotic infection. Repeat courses of corticosteroids should not be routinely used (National Institutes of Health [NIH] Consensus Development Panel, 2001). (See "Drug Guide: Betamethasone.")

NURSING MANAGEMENT

NURSING ASSESSMENT AND DIAGNOSIS

Determining the length of time the membranes have been ruptured is a major part of the intrapartum assessment. Ask the woman when her membranes ruptured and when labor began, because the risk of infection may be directly related to the time involved. Observe the mother for signs and symptoms of infection by reviewing her white blood cell count, her temperature, her pulse rate, and the character of her amniotic fluid. Check her hydration status. When a preterm or cesarean birth is anticipated, evaluate the childbirth preparation and coping abilities of the woman and her partner.

Nursing diagnoses that may apply to a woman with PROM include the following:

- *Risk for Infection* related to premature rupture of membranes

- *Impaired Gas Exchange in the Fetus* related to compression of the umbilical cord secondary to prolapse of the cord

- *Risk for Ineffective Individual Coping* related to unknown outcome of the pregnancy

TEACHING HIGHLIGHTS

AMNIOTIC MEMBRANES

To help a laboring woman and her family understand how the amniotic membranes provide protection, use a color chart that shows a side view of the fetus in the uterus with the membranes intact. Ask the couple to visualize what would happen if the membranes rupture. They will be able to see that pathogens have direct access to the uterus, increasing the risk of infection. They will also see that, when the membranes rupture and the fluid escapes, the cord could "wash out" with the fluid and become trapped between the pelvis and fetal head, causing cord compression.

TABLE 15–1 ✤ Risk Factors for Spontaneous Preterm Labor

Multiple gestation	Cervical shortening <1 cm
DES exposure	Uterine irritability
Known cervical incompetence	Age (<18 or >35)
Polyhydramnios	Low socioeconomic status
Uterine anomaly	Cigarettes—more than 10/day
Cervix dilated > 1 cm at 32 weeks	Substance abuse
	Low maternal weight
Second-trimester abortion	Poor weight gain
Fetal abnormality	More than 2 first-trimester abortions
Febrile illness	
Bleeding after 12 weeks	Non-white race
History of pyelonephritis or other maternal infection	Cervical cerclage in situ
	In vitro fertilization (singleton or multiple gestation)
Maternal medical disease	
Previous preterm birth	STD (trichomoniasis, chlamydia)
Previous preterm labor with term birth	Anemia
	Abdominal trauma
Abdominal surgery during second or third trimester	Foreign body (IUD)
History of cone biopsy	Bacterial vaginosis, E. coli (ascending intrauterine infection)
Uteroplacental ischemia	
Stress	Periodontal disease
Inadequate prenatal care	

PLANNING AND IMPLEMENTATION

Focus nursing actions on the woman, her partner, and the fetus. Report signs of infection to the certified nurse-midwife or physician. Evaluate uterine activity and fetal response to the labor but do not do vaginal examinations unless absolutely necessary. Encourage the woman to rest on her left side to promote optimal uteroplacental perfusion. Use comfort measures to help her rest and relax. Ensure that the woman is well hydrated, particularly if her temperature is elevated.

Educate the woman and her partner, if he is involved, about the implications of PROM and all treatment methods. Address side effects and alternative treatments. Explain that although the membranes are ruptured, amniotic fluid continues to be produced.

Psychologic support for the couple is critical. Listen empathetically, relay accurate information, and provide explanations as needed. Preparing the couple for a cesarean birth, a preterm newborn, and the possibility of fetal or newborn demise may be necessary.

EVALUATION

Expected outcomes of nursing care include the following:

- The woman's risk of infection and cord prolapse decreases.
- The couple is able to discuss the implications of PROM and all treatments and alternative treatments.
- The pregnancy is maintained without trauma to the mother or fetus.

CARE OF THE WOMAN AT RISK DUE TO PRETERM LABOR

Labor that occurs between 20 and 37 completed weeks of pregnancy is called **preterm labor (PTL)**. Prematurity continues to be the number-one perinatal and neonatal problem in the United States, with 11.6% of all live births

occurring prematurely (March of Dimes Birth Defects Foundation, 2003). Often PTL is related to multiple risk factors; only rarely is there a single cause. Table 15–1 presents a list of risk factors for spontaneous preterm labor.

Maternal implications of preterm labor include psychologic stress related to the baby's condition and physiologic stress related to medical treatment for preterm labor.

Fetal-neonatal implications include increased morbidity and mortality, especially due to respiratory distress syndrome, increased risk of trauma during birth, and maturational deficiencies (fat storage, heat regulation, immaturity of organ systems).

CLINICAL THERAPY

Women at risk for preterm labor are taught to recognize the symptoms associated with it and, if any symptoms are present, to notify their certified nurse-midwife or physician immediately. Though often difficult to diagnose because many of the symptoms are common in normal pregnancy, prompt diagnosis is necessary to stop preterm labor before it progresses to the point at which intervention will be ineffective. Research suggests that the strongest predictors of preterm birth include cervicovaginal fibronectin, abnormal cervical length on ultrasound, history of previous preterm birth, and the presence of bacterial vaginosis infection (discussed later in this chapter) (Iams, 2002).

EVIDENCE-BASED NURSING

PRETERM BIRTH PREVENTION

Clinical Question

How can the nurse provide education, monitoring, and intervention for the prevention of preterm birth?

Evidence

The Institute for Clinical Systems Improvement assembled an expert team of physicians and advanced practice nurses to review the literature and develop recommendations for the prevention of preterm birth. The group developed a clinical practice algorithm supported by annotated recommendations and research references. The evidence revealed that only 50% of women who give birth prematurely come from identified high-risk groups. As a result these recommendations focus on education and intervention to mediate risk factors in all pregnant women as opposed to weighted risk assessment.

Implications

Early confirmation of pregnancy is desirable because it allows for early mediation of risk factors for preterm birth. All women should be educated about the risk factors associated with preterm labor, and risk status should be monitored at each prenatal visit. Manageable or modifiable preterm birth risk factors should be identified, and interven-

tions applied to reduce or remove risk factors that can be changed. Modifiable risk factors include family stress, domestic abuse, tobacco and alcohol use, sexually transmitted infections, and poor nutritional status. Women should be educated about modifiable risk factors for preterm birth during early prenatal visits, and changes in status should be monitored. Nonmodifiable risk factors should also be monitored, including previous preterm birth, multiple gestation, inflammation, decidual hemorrhage, and pathologic distention of the uterus. Maternal illnesses associated with preterm birth (e.g., hypertension, diabetes, cardiac and renal disease) should be managed effectively to minimize the risk of preterm birth. The signs and symptoms of preterm birth should be reviewed at each prenatal visit so that early intervention is possible.

Critical Thinking

How can you help women modify risk factors that are behavior or lifestyle based? What teaching plan will help you educate women to differentiate signs of preterm labor from those expected in a normal pregnancy?

Reference

Institute for Clinical Systems Improvement. (2003, July). *Preterm birth prevention. Healthcare guidelines* (8th ed.). Bloomington, MN: Author.

Fetal fibronectin (fFN) is a protein normally found in the fetal membranes and decidua. It is found in the cervicovaginal fluid in early pregnancy but is not usually present in significant quantities between 18 and 36 weeks' gestation. A positive fFN test (fFN found in the cervicovaginal fluid) during this time puts the woman at increased risk for preterm birth. Conversely, a negative fFN in a woman with preterm contractions is associated with a very low risk of birth within 7 days (Giles, Bisits, Knox et al., 2000). The test is over 99% accurate for predicting no preterm birth within 7 days. The procedure for collecting a sample is similar to that of the Pap smear; results can be available within 1 hour.

The length of the cervix can be measured fairly reliably after 16 weeks' gestation using an ultrasound probe inserted into the vagina. A cervix that is shorter than expected may be useful in assisting a physician to identify the need for a cerclage to prevent preterm birth because of incompetent cervix. In general, cervical length less than 25 mm prior to term is abnormal (AAP & ACOG, 2002).

Diagnosis of preterm labor is confirmed if the pregnancy is between 20 and 37 weeks and if there are documented uterine contractions (four in 20 minutes or eight in 1 hour), documented cervical change, or cervical dilatation of greater than 1 cm or cervical effacement of 80% or more (AAP & ACOG, 2002). The goal of clinical therapy is to prevent the preterm birth of a compromised infant. Attempts to prevent labor are not indicated if one or more of the following conditions are present: severe preeclampsia or eclampsia, chorioamnionitis, hemorrhage, maternal cardiac disease, poorly controlled diabetes mellitus or thyrotoxicosis, severe abruptio placentae, fetal anomalies incompatible with life, fetal death, acute fetal distress, or fetal maturity.

The initial management of preterm labor is directed toward maintaining good uterine blood flow, detecting uterine contractions, and quieting the fetus. The mother is asked to lie on her side to increase profusion, and an IV infusion is started to promote maternal hydration. Maternal laboratory studies, including CBC, C-reactive protein, vaginal cultures, and urine cultures, are completed.

Tocolysis is the use of medications in an attempt to stop labor. Drugs currently used as tocolytics include the β-adrenergic agonists (also called β-mimetics), magnesium sulfate, prostaglandin synthetase inhibitors, and calcium channel blockers. The β-mimetics (ritodrine [Yutopar] and terbutaline sulfate [Brethine]) and magnesium sulfate are the most widely used tocolytics. Ritodrine is approved by the U.S. Food and Drug Administration (FDA) for tocolysis; however, it is much less frequently used than terbutaline, which is not approved by the FDA for this use.

Although tocolytic drugs suppress uterine contractions and allow pregnancy to continue, they may cause maternal side effects; the most serious is maternal pulmonary edema. Reducing the dose and duration of therapy sometimes reduces the side effects.

Because it is effective and has fewer side effects than the β-mimetics, magnesium sulfate administered IV is often the initial drug of choice for therapy. Therapy with magnesium sulfate is indicated in women with cardiopulmonary disease, diabetes, or infection. In all other cases, the selection of magnesium sulfate or β-mimetics depends on the experience of the health care providers. For magnesium sulfate the recommended loading dose is 4 to 6 g IV in 100 mL of IV fluid using an infusion pump over 15 to 20 minutes, followed by a maintenance dose of 1 to 4 g/hr titrated to response and side effects (Cunningham et al., 2005). The therapy is continued for 12 to 24 hours at the lowest rate that maintains cessation of contractions.

Side effects with the loading dose may include flushing, a feeling of warmth, headache, nystagmus, nausea, and dizziness. Other side effects include lethargy, sluggishness, and pulmonary edema (see "Drug Guide: Magnesium Sulfate"). Fetal side effects may include hypotonia and lethargy that persists for 1 or 2 days following birth.

One calcium channel blocker, nifedipine, is becoming increasingly popular as a tocolytic because it is easily administered orally or sublingually and has few serious maternal side effects. It decreases smooth muscle contractions by blocking the slow calcium channels at the cell surface. The most common side effects are related to arterial vasodilation and include hypotension, tachycardia, facial flushing, and headache. Nifedipine may be coadministered with the β-mimetics. However, it should not be used with magnesium because both drugs block calcium, and simultaneous administration has been implicated in serious maternal side effects related to low calcium levels.

Prostaglandin synthesis inhibitors such as indomethacin (Indocin) are being used for tocolysis in selected instances. However, potential fetal side effects, such as constriction of the ductus arteriosus, have been reported, especially in pregnancies at 32 weeks' gestation and beyond. Consequently, indomethacin use is limited to pregnancies less than 32 weeks' gestation; the duration of therapy should be less than 72 hours, if possible (Vermillion & Scardo, 2000).

The NIH Consensus Development Panel (2001) recommends that corticosteroids (typically betamethasone or dexamethasone) be administered antenatally to women at risk for preterm birth because of their beneficial effect on fetal lung maturation. Women who are candidates for tocolysis are candidates for antenatal corticosteroids, regardless of fetal gender, race, or availability of surfactant therapy for the newborn, especially between 24 and 34 weeks' gestation. (See "Drug Guide: Betamethasone.")

Research trials have shown that progesterone therapy may be effective in reducing the incidence of preterm birth, at least in certain high-risk populations (Da Fonseca, Bittar, Carvalho, & Zugaib, 2003; Meis, Klebanoff, Thom et al., 2003). Currently experts are evaluating whether this therapy should become an accepted part of clinical practice.

NURSING MANAGEMENT

NURSING ASSESSMENT AND DIAGNOSIS

During the antepartal period, identify the woman at risk for preterm labor by noting the presence of predisposing factors. During the intrapartal period, assess the progress of labor and the physiologic impact of labor on the mother and fetus.

Nursing diagnoses that may apply to the woman with preterm labor include the following:

- *Fear* related to risk of early labor and birth
- *Ineffective Individual Coping* related to need for constant attention to pregnancy

PLANNING AND IMPLEMENTATION

Nursing Care in the Community

Once the woman at risk for preterm labor has been identified, teach her about the importance of recognizing the onset of labor (see "Teaching Highlights: Preterm Labor").

Periodic home visits by a home care nurse are an important part of care. During these visits, complete physical assessments similar to those done in the hospital and assess the woman's emotional state. Provide information about support groups and other community resources for women at risk for preterm birth.

Increasing the woman's awareness of the subtle symptoms of preterm labor is an important teaching objective. The signs and symptoms of preterm labor include the following:

- Uterine contractions that occur every 10 minutes or less, with or without pain
- Mild menstrual-like cramps felt low in the abdomen
- Pelvic pressure that feels like the baby pressing down
- Rupture of membranes
- Constant or intermittent low, dull backache
- A change in the vaginal discharge (an increase in amount, a change to more clear and watery, or a pinkish tinge)
- Abdominal cramping with or without diarrhea

Also teach the woman to evaluate contraction activity once or twice a day. She does so by lying down tilted to one side with a pillow behind her back for support. The woman places her fingertips on the fundus of the uterus, which is above the umbilicus (navel). She checks for contractions (hardening or tightening in the uterus) for about 1 hour. It is important for the pregnant woman to know that uterine contractions occur occasionally throughout the pregnancy.

DRUG GUIDE

MAGNESIUM SULFATE
PREGNANCY RISK CATEGORY: B

Overview of Obstetric Action

Magnesium sulfate acts as a central nervous system depressant by decreasing the quantity of acetylcholine released by motor nerve impulses and thereby blocking neuromuscular transmission. This action reduces the possibility of convulsion, which is why magnesium sulfate is used in the treatment of preeclampsia. Because magnesium sulfate secondarily relaxes smooth muscle, it may decrease the blood pressure, although it is not considered an antihypertensive. Magnesium sulfate may also decrease the frequency and intensity of uterine contractions; as a result it is also used as a tocolytic in the treatment of preterm labor.

Route, Dosage, Frequency

Magnesium sulfate is generally given IV to control dosage more accurately and prevent overdosage. An occasional physician still prescribes IM administration. However, it is painful and irritating to the tissues and does not permit the close control that IV administration does. The IV route allows for immediate onset of action. It must be given by infusion pump for accurate dosage.

For Treatment of Preterm Labor

Loading dose: 4 to 6 g magnesium sulfate in 100-mL solution administered over a 15 to 20-minute period (Cunningham et al., 2005).

Maintenance dose: 1 to 4 g/hr via infusion pump

For Treatment of Preeclampsia

Loading dose: 6 g magnesium sulfate administered over a 20-minute period

Maintenance dose: 2 g/hr via infusion pump (Sibai, 2002)

Note: Magnesium sulfate is excreted via the kidneys. Because women in preterm labor typically have normal renal function, they generally require higher levels of magnesium to achieve a therapeutic range than women who have preeclampsia and may have compromised renal function. Maintenance dose may need to be adjusted based on serum magnesium levels.

Maternal Contraindications

Diagnosed maternal myasthenia gravis is the only absolute contraindication to the administration of magnesium sulfate. A history of myocardial damage or heart block is a relative contraindication to use of the drug because of the effects on nerve transmission and muscle contractility. Extreme care is necessary in administration to women with impaired renal function because the drug is eliminated by the kidneys, and toxic magnesium levels may develop quickly.

Maternal Side Effects

Most maternal side effects are dose related. Lethargy and weakness related to neuromuscular blockade are common. Sweating, a feeling of warmth, flushing, and nasal congestion may be related to periph-eral vasodilation. Other common side effects include nausea and vomiting, constipation, visual blurring, headache, and slurred speech. Signs of developing toxicity include depression or absence of reflexes, oliguria, confusion, respiratory depression, circulatory collapse, and respiratory paralysis. Rapid administration of large doses may cause cardiac arrest.

Effects on Fetus/Newborn

The drug readily crosses the placenta. Some authorities suggest that transient decrease in fetal heart rate variability may occur; others report that no change occurred. In general, magnesium sulfate therapy does not pose a risk to the fetus. Occasionally, the newborn may demonstrate neurologic depression or respiratory depression, loss of reflexes, and muscle weakness. Ill effects in the newborn may actually be related to fetal growth retardation, prematurity, or perinatal asphyxia.

Nursing Considerations

1. Monitor the blood pressure closely during administration.
2. Monitor maternal serum magnesium levels as ordered (usually every 6 to 8 hours). Therapeutic levels are in the range of 4.8 to 9.6 mg/dL. Reflexes often disappear at serum magnesium levels of 8 to 12 mg/dL; respiratory depression occurs at levels of 15 to 17 mg/dL; cardiac arrest occurs at levels above 30 mg/dL (Sibai, 2002).
3. Monitor respirations closely. If the rate is less than 12/min, magnesium toxicity may be developing, and further assessments are indicated. Many protocols require stopping the medication if the respiratory rate falls below 12/min.
4. Assess knee jerk (patellar tendon reflex) for evidence of diminished or absent reflexes. Loss of reflexes is often the first sign of developing toxicity. Also note marked lethargy or decreased level of consciousness and hypotension.
5. Determine urinary output. Output less than 30 mL/hr may result in the accumulation of toxic levels of magnesium.
6. If the respirations or urinary output fall below specified levels or if the reflexes are diminished or absent, no further magnesium should be administered until these factors return to normal.
7. The antagonist of magnesium sulfate is calcium. Consequently, an ampule of calcium gluconate should be available at the bedside. The usual dose is 1 g given IV over a period of about 3 minutes.
8. Monitor fetal heart tones continuously with IV administration.
9. Continue magnesium sulfate infusion for approximately 24 hours after birth as prophylaxis against postpartum seizures if given for preeclampsia-eclampsia.
10. If the mother has received magnesium sulfate close to birth, the newborn should be closely observed for signs of magnesium toxicity for 24 to 48 hours.

Note: Protocols for magnesium sulfate administration may vary somewhat according to agency policy. Consequently, individuals are referred to their own agency protocols for specific guidelines.

TEACHING HIGHLIGHTS

PRETERM LABOR

- Describe the dangers of preterm labor, especially the risk of prematurity in the infant, and all the potential problems.
- Explain that many of the early symptoms of labor, such as backache and increased bloody show, may be subtle initially.
- Summarize self-care measures (see Table 15–2) the woman can take to prevent preterm labor.
- Teach the woman how to palpate for uterine contractions. Demonstrate and ask for a return demonstration.

If they occur every 10 minutes for 1 hour, however, the cervix could begin to dilate, and labor could begin.

Ensure that the woman knows when to report signs and symptoms. If contractions occur every 10 minutes (or more frequently) for 1 hour, if any of the other signs and symptoms are present for 1 hour, or if clear fluid begins leaking from the vagina, the woman should telephone her physician or certified nurse-midwife and make arrangements to be checked for ongoing labor. When a woman is at risk for preterm labor, she may have many episodes of contractions and other signs or symptoms. Thus, the woman's call must be taken seriously. If she is treated positively, she will feel freer to report problems as they arise.

Preventive self-care measures are also very important. They are described in Table 15–2.

Hospital-Based Nursing Care

Supportive nursing care is important to the woman in preterm labor during hospitalization. Promote bed rest, monitor vital signs, measure intake and output, monitor the fetal heart rate continuously, and monitor uterine contractions. Having the woman lie on her left side facilitates maternal-fetal circulation. Keep vaginal examinations to a minimum. If tocolytic agents are being administered, monitor the mother and fetus closely for any adverse effects.

Whether preterm labor is arrested or proceeds, the woman and her partner, if he is involved, experience intense psychologic stress. Provide emotional support to help decrease the anxiety associated with the risk of a preterm newborn. Also recognize the stress of prolonged bed rest and of lack of sexual contact and help the couple find satisfactory ways of dealing with those stresses. Empathetically assist the couple to express their feelings, which commonly include guilt and anxiety, and identify and implement coping mechanisms. Keep the couple informed about the labor progress, the treatment regimen, and the status of the fetus. In the event of imminent vaginal or cesarean birth, offer the couple brief but ongoing explanations to prepare them for the actual birth process and the events following the birth.

TABLE 15–2 ✤ Self-Care Measures to Prevent Preterm Labor

Rest two or three times a day lying on your left side.

Drink 2 to 3 quarts of water or fruit juice each day. Avoid caffeine drinks. Filling a quart container and drinking from it will eliminate the need to keep track of numerous glasses of fluid.

Empty your bladder at least every 2 hours during waking hours.

Avoid lifting heavy objects. If small children are in the home, work out alternatives for picking them up, such as sitting on a chair and having them climb onto your lap.

Contact your healthcare provider if you experience menstrual-like cramping, unusual low back pain, unusual vaginal discharge, increased pelvic pressure, or more than 5 uterine contractions in 1 hour (whether painful or not).

Pace necessary activities to avoid overexertion.

Sexual activity may need to be modified or avoided.

Try to focus on 1 day or 1 week at a time rather than on longer periods of time.

If on bed rest, get dressed each day and rest on a couch rather than becoming isolated in the bedroom.

Find pleasurable ways to help compensate for limitations of activities and boost the spirits.

Prepared in consultation with Susan Bennett, RN, ACCE, Coordinator of the Prematurity Prevention Program, University of Washington Medical Center.

EVALUATION

Expected outcomes of nursing care include the following:

- The woman is able to discuss the cause, identification, and treatment of preterm labor.
- The woman states that she feels comfortable in her ability to cope with her situation and has resources to call on.
- The woman can describe appropriate self-care measures and can identify characteristics that need to be reported to her caregiver.
- The woman successfully gives birth to a healthy infant.

CARE OF THE WOMAN WITH A HYPERTENSIVE DISORDER

A number of hypertensive disorders can occur during pregnancy. The following classification is recommended by the NIH (2000):

- Preeclampsia-eclampsia
- Chronic hypertension
- Chronic hypertension with superimposed preeclampsia or eclampsia
- Gestational (or transient) hypertension

PREECLAMPSIA AND ECLAMPSIA

Preeclampsia, the most common hypertensive disorder in pregnancy, occurs in 2% to 7% of nulliparous women. For women who have a twin pregnancy, the rate is much higher (14%) as it is for those who had preeclampsia in a previous pregnancy (18%) (Coppage & Sibai, 2004). Preeclampsia is defined as gestational hypertension with a blood pressure of 140/90 or higher on two occasions at least 6 hours apart accompanied by proteinuria. Previously edema was included in the definition but was removed because it is such a common finding in pregnancy. However, sudden onset of severe edema warrants close evaluation to rule out preeclampsia or other pathologic processes such as renal disease (Higgins & de Swiet, 2001).

Preeclampsia, typically categorized as mild or severe, is a progressive disorder. In its most severe form, **eclampsia**, (generalized seizures or coma) develops. Most often preeclampsia occurs in the last 10 weeks of gestation, during labor, or in the first 48 hours after childbirth. Although birth of the fetus and removal of the placenta is the only known cure for preeclampsia, it can be controlled with early diagnosis and careful management. Preeclampsia is seen more often in teenagers and in women over age 35, especially if they are primigravidas. Women with a history of preeclampsia are at increased risk, as are women with GTD, Rh incompatibility, diabetes, and a large placental mass (as in multiple gestation).

Pathophysiology of Preeclampsia

The cause of preeclampsia-eclampsia remains unknown, despite decades of research. Preeclampsia affects all the major systems of the body. The following pathophysiologic changes are associated with the disease:

- In normal pregnancy the lowered peripheral vascular resistance and the increased maternal resistance to the pressor effects of angiotensin II result in lowered blood pressure. In preeclampsia, blood pressure begins to rise after 20 weeks' gestation, probably in response to a gradual loss of resistance to angiotensin II. This response has been linked to the ratio between the prostaglandins prostacyclin and thromboxane. Prostacyclin is a potent vasodilator. It is decreased in preeclampsia, often several weeks before symptoms develop. This changes the ratio between the two prostaglandins, allowing the potent vasoconstriction and platelet-aggregating effects of thromboxane to dominate. These hormones are produced partially by the placenta, which helps explain the reversal of the condition when the placenta is removed and why the incidence is increased when there is a larger than normal placental mass.

- Nitric oxide, a potent vasodilator, plays a role in the pregnant woman's resistance to vasopressors. Decreased nitric oxide production in women with preeclampsia may contribute to the development of hypertension.

- The loss of normal vasodilation of uterine arterioles and the concurrent maternal vasospasm result in decreased placental perfusion (see "Pathophysiology Illustrated: Preeclampsia"). The effect on the fetus may be growth restriction, decrease in fetal movement, and chronic hypoxia or fetal distress.

- In preeclampsia, normal renal perfusion is decreased. With a reduction of the glomerular filtration rate, serum levels of creatinine, BUN, and uric acid begin to rise from normal pregnant levels, while urine output decreases. Sodium is retained in increased amounts, which results in increased extracellular volume, increased sensitivity to angiotensin II, and edema. Stretching of the capillary walls of the glomerular endothelial cells allows the large protein molecules, primarily albumin, to escape in the urine, decreasing serum albumin levels. The decreased serum albumin concentration causes decreased plasma colloid osmotic pressure. This lowered pressure results in a further movement of fluid to the extracellular spaces, which also contributes to the development of edema.

- The decreased intravascular volume causes increased viscosity of the blood and a corresponding rise in hematocrit.

HELLP syndrome (**h**emolysis, **e**levated **l**iver enzymes, and low **p**latelet count) is sometimes associated with severe preeclampsia. Women who experience this multiple-organ-failure syndrome have high morbidity and mortality rates, as do their offspring.

The hemolysis that occurs is termed *microangiopathic hemolytic anemia*. It is thought that red blood cells are fragmented during passage through small, damaged blood vessels. Elevated liver enzymes occur from blood flow that is obstructed by fibrin deposits. Hyperbilirubinemia and jaundice may also be seen. Liver distention causes epigastric pain. Thrombocytopenia (platelet count less than 100,000/mm^3) is a frequent finding in preeclampsia. It occurs when platelets aggregate at the sites of vascular damage associated with vasospasm. Symptoms may include nausea, vomiting, flulike symptoms, or epigastric pain.

The mother's condition should be assessed and stabilized, especially if her platelet counts are very low. Platelet transfusions are indicated for platelet counts below 20,000/mm^3. The fetus is also assessed, using a nonstress test and biophysical profile. Once HELLP syndrome is diagnosed and the woman's condition is stable, birth of the child is indicated.

Maternal Risks

Central nervous system changes associated with preeclampsia-eclampsia are hyperreflexia, headache, and

PATHOPHYSIOLOGY ILLUSTRATED

Preeclampsia

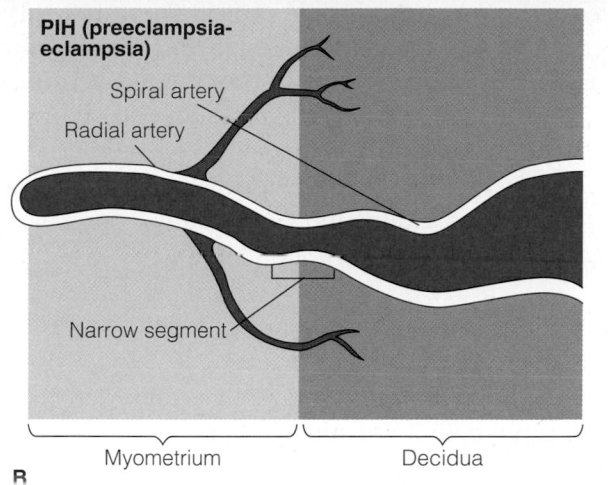

A, In a normal pregnancy, the passive quality of the spiral arteries permits increased blood flow to the placenta.
B, In preeclampsia vasoconstriction of the myometrial segment of the spiral arteries occurs.

seizures. Hyperreflexia may be due to increased intracellular sodium and decreased intracellular potassium levels. Cerebral vasospasm causes headaches, and cerebral edema and vasoconstriction are responsible for seizures. There is also increased risk for renal failure, abruptio placentae, DIC, ruptured liver, and pulmonary embolism.

Fetal-Neonatal Risks

Infants of women with preeclampsia tend to be small for gestational age (SGA). The cause is related specifically to maternal vasospasm and hypovolemia, which result in fetal hypoxia and malnutrition. In addition the newborn may be premature because of the necessity for early birth. At birth the newborn may be oversedated because of medications given to the mother. The newborn may also have hypermagnesemia due to treatment of the woman with large doses of magnesium sulfate.

Clinical Therapy

Clinical Manifestations and Diagnosis

Mild Preeclampsia. Women with mild preeclampsia may exhibit few if any symptoms. The blood pressure is elevated to 140/90 mm Hg or higher, 1+ proteinuria may occur, and liver enzymes may be elevated minimally. Although no longer considered a diagnostic sign of preeclampsia, edema may be present.

Severe Preeclampsia. Severe preeclampsia may develop suddenly. Blood pressure is 160/110 mm Hg or higher on two occasions at least 6 hours apart while the woman is on bed rest. Proteinuria of 5 g or higher is found in a 24-hour urine collection while a dipstick urine protein measurement is 3+ to 4+ on two random samples obtained at least 4 hours apart. Other characteristic symptoms include visual or cerebral disturbances (frontal headaches, blurred vision, scotomata [spots before the eyes]), cyanosis or pulmonary edema, epigastric or right upper quadrant pain, impaired liver function, thrombocytopenia or evidence of hemolysis or both, and intrauterine fetal growth restriction (AAP & ACOG, 2002). Other signs or symptoms may include nausea, vomiting, irritability, hyperreflexia, and retinal edema (retinas appear wet and glistening), with narrowed segments on the retinal arterioles when examined with an ophthalmoscope. Epigastric pain is often the sign of impending convulsion and is thought to be caused by increased vascular engorgement of the liver.

Eclampsia. Eclampsia, characterized by a grand mal convulsion, may occur before labor, during labor, or early in the postpartal period. Some women experience only one seizure; others have several.

Antepartal Management. The clinical therapy for preeclampsia depends on the severity of the disease.

Home Care of Mild Preeclampsia. For some women with mild preeclampsia, home care is an option. The woman monitors her blood pressure, weight, and urine protein daily. Weight gains of 1.4 kg (3 lb) in 24 hours or 1.8 kg (4 lb) in a 3-day period are generally a cause for concern. Remote NSTs are performed on a daily to biweekly basis. Nursing contact varies from daily to weekly, depending on physician request. It is extremely important to advise the woman to report to the doctor if she develops signs of worsening preeclampsia.

Hospital Care of Mild Preeclampsia. The woman is placed on bed rest, primarily on her left side, to decrease pressure on the vena cava, thereby increasing venous return, circulatory volume, and placental and renal perfusion. Her diet should be well balanced and moderate to high in protein (80 to 100 g/day, or 1.5 g/kg/day) to replace protein lost in the urine. Sodium intake should be moderate, not to exceed 6 g/day. Excessively salty foods should be avoided, but sodium restriction and diuretics are no longer used in treating preeclampsia.

To achieve a safe outcome for the fetus, tests to evaluate fetal status are done more frequently as preeclampsia progresses. The following tests are used:

- Fetal movement record
- Nonstress test
- Ultrasonography every 3 or 4 weeks for serial determination of growth
- Biophysical profile
- Serum creatinine determinations
- Amniocentesis to determine fetal lung maturity
- Doppler velocimetry beginning at 30 to 32 weeks to screen for fetal compromise

Severe Preeclampsia In severe cases, birth may be the treatment of choice for both mother and fetus, even if the fetus is immature. Other medical therapies for severe preeclampsia include the following:

- **Bed rest.** Bed rest must be complete. Stimuli that may bring on a seizure should be reduced.

- **Diet.** A high-protein, moderate-sodium diet is given as long as the woman is alert and has no nausea or indication of impending seizure.

- **Anticonvulsants.** Magnesium sulfate is the treatment of choice for convulsions. Its depressant action on the central nervous system reduces the possibility of seizure (see "Drug Guide: Magnesium Sulfate").

- **Fluid and electrolyte replacement.** The goal of fluid intake is to achieve a balance between correcting hypovolemia and preventing circulatory overload. Fluid intake may be oral or supplemented with IV therapy. IV fluids may be started "to keep lines open" in case they are needed for drug therapy even when oral intake is adequate. Electrolytes are replaced as indicated by daily serum electrolyte levels.

- **Corticosteroids.** Betamethasone or dexamethasone is often administered to the woman whose fetus has an immature lung profile. Corticosteroids may also have a beneficial effect in women with HELLP syndrome (Magann & Martin, 2000).

- **Antihypertensives.** These medications are most commonly used. Antihypertensive therapy is generally given for diastolic blood pressures of 105 to 110 mm Hg or higher. Hydralazine (Apresoline) is the medication most commonly used. Methyldopa is often used for long-term control of mild to moderate hypertension in pregnancy because it is safe and effective. Labetalol is used as a second-line IV drug but should be avoided in women with asthma or congestive heart failure.

Eclampsia. An eclamptic seizure requires immediate, effective treatment. A bolus of 4 to 6 g magnesium sulfate is given IV over 5 minutes to control convulsions. A sedative such as diazepam or amobarbital is used only if the seizures are not controlled by magnesium sulfate. Phenytoin (Dilantin) may be used for seizure prevention. The lungs are auscultated for pulmonary edema. The woman is observed for circulatory and renal failure and signs of cerebral hemorrhage. Furosemide (Lasix) may be given for pulmonary edema; digitalis may be given for circulatory failure. Intake and output are monitored hourly.

The woman is observed for signs of labor. She is also checked every 15 minutes for evidence of vaginal bleeding and abdominal rigidity, which might indicate abruptio placentae. While she is comatose, she is positioned on her side with the side rails up.

Because of the severity of her condition, the woman is often cared for in an intensive care unit. Invasive hemodynamic monitoring of either central venous pressure or pulmonary artery wedge pressure may be started using a Swan-Ganz catheter. When the condition of the woman and the fetus are stabilized, induction of labor is considered, because birth is the only known cure for preeclampsia-eclampsia. The woman and her partner should be given a careful explanation about her status and that of her unborn child and the treatment they are receiving. Plans for further treatment and for birth must be discussed with them.

Intrapartal Management. Labor may be induced by IV oxytocin when there is evidence of fetal maturity and cervical readiness. In very severe cases, cesarean birth may be necessary even if the fetus is immature.

COMPLEMENTARY CARE

NUTRITIONAL INTERVENTIONS FOR PREECLAMPSIA

Several nutritional supplements may help to prevent preeclampsia. Fish oils and vitamins C and E have shown promise and are being tested further to confirm their benefit. The antioxidant qualities of these supplements are believed to play a role in reducing the oxidative stress that is present in preeclampsia (Zhang et al., 2002). Moreover, calcium supplementation during pregnancy has been shown to reduce the incidence of preeclampsia and hypertension (Villar et al., 2003).

Assessment for signs of worsening preeclampsia continues. The woman may receive IV oxytocin and magnesium sulfate simultaneously. Infusion pumps should be used, and bags and tubing must be carefully labeled.

Analgesics may be used to decrease discomfort, or the woman may have an epidural block. Birth in the Sims' or semisitting position should be considered. If the lithotomy position is used, a wedge should be placed under the right buttock to displace the uterus. The wedge should also be used if birth is by cesarean. Oxygen is administered to the woman during labor if the need is indicated by fetal response to the contractions.

A pediatrician or neonatal nurse practitioner must be available to care for the newborn at birth. This caregiver must be informed of all amounts and times of medication the woman has received during labor.

Postpartal Management. The woman with preeclampsia usually improves rapidly after giving birth, although seizures can still occur during the first 48 hours postpartum. When the hypertension is severe, the woman may continue to receive antihypertensives or magnesium sulfate postpartally.

NURSING MANAGEMENT

See "Nursing Care Plan: The Woman with Preeclampsia" for information on nursing care.

NURSING ASSESSMENT AND DIAGNOSIS

Take and record the blood pressure during each antepartal visit. If the blood pressure rises, or if the normal decrease in blood pressure expected between 8 and 28 weeks of pregnancy does not occur, the woman should be followed closely. Also check the woman's urine for proteinuria at each visit.

If hospitalization becomes necessary, assess the following:

■ **Blood pressure.** Assess every 1 to 4 hours, or more frequently if indicated by medication or other changes in the woman's status.

■ **Temperature.** Take every 4 hours, or every 2 hours if elevated.

■ **Pulse and respirations.** Determine pulse rate and respirations along with blood pressure.

■ **Fetal heart rate.** Check the fetal heart rate with the blood pressure, or monitor continuously with the electronic fetal monitor if the situation indicates.

■ **Urinary output.** Measure every voiding. The woman frequently has an indwelling catheter. In this case, urine output can be assessed hourly. Output should be 700 mL or greater in 24 hours, or at least 30 mL/hr.

■ **Urine protein.** Evaluate urinary protein hourly if an indwelling catheter is in place or with each voiding. Readings of 3+ or 4+ indicate loss of 5 g or more of protein in 24 hours.

■ **Urine specific gravity.** Check specific gravity of the urine hourly or with each voiding. Readings over 1.040 correlate with oliguria and proteinuria.

■ **Weight.** Weigh the woman daily at the same time. She should be wearing the same robe or gown and slippers. Weighing may be omitted if the woman is to maintain strict bed rest.

■ **Pulmonary edema.** Observe the woman for coughing. Auscultate the lungs for moist respirations.

■ **Deep tendon reflexes.** Assess the woman for evidence of hyperreflexia in the brachial, wrist, patellar, or Achilles' tendons (Table 15–3). The patellar reflex is the easiest to assess. Clonus is assessed by vigorously dorsiflexing the foot while the knee is held in a fixed position (Figure 15–4 ●). Normally no clonus is present. If it is present, it is measured as beats and recorded as such. See Skill 2–3 in the Clinical Skills Manual **SKILLS** as well as on the CD-ROM that accompanies this text.

■ **Placental separation.** Assess hourly for vaginal bleeding and uterine rigidity.

■ **Headache.** Ask about the existence and location of any headache.

■ **Visual disturbance.** Ask about any visual blurring or changes or scotomata. The results of the daily funduscopic examination should be recorded on the chart.

■ **Epigastric pain.** Ask about any epigastric pain. It is important to differentiate it from simple heartburn, which tends to be familiar and less intense.

■ **Laboratory blood tests.** Daily tests of hematocrit to measure hemoconcentration; BUN, creatinine, and uric acid levels to assess kidney function; clotting studies for signs of thrombocytopenia or DIC; liver enzymes; and electrolyte levels are all indicated. Magnesium levels are monitored regularly in women receiving magnesium sulfate.

■ **Level of consciousness.** Observe the woman for alertness, mood changes, and any signs of impending convulsion.

■ **Emotional response and level of understanding.** Carefully assess the woman's emotional response so that support and teaching can be planned accordingly.

In addition assess the effects of any medications administered. Become familiar with the more commonly used medications and their purpose, implications, and associated untoward or toxic effects.

NURSING CARE PLAN

THE WOMAN WITH PREECLAMPSIA

Intervention	Rationale	Expected Outcome
1. Nursing Diagnosis: Deficient Fluid Volume related to fluid shift from intravascular to extravascular space secondary to vasospasm		
NIC Intervention: **Fluid management:** Promotion of fluid balance and prevention of complications related to fluid shifts		**NOC Outcome:** **Fluid balance:** Balance of fluid in the intracellular and extracellular compartments of the body
Goal: Client is restored to normal fluid volume levels.		
■ Encourage woman to lie in the left lateral recumbent position.	■ The left lateral recumbent position decreases pressure on the vena cava, thereby increasing venous return, circulatory volume, and placental and renal perfusion. Angiotensin II levels are decreased when there is improved renal blood flow, which helps to promote diuresis and lower blood pressure.	■ The signs and symptoms of preeclampsia will diminish as evidenced by decreased blood pressure, urine protein levels of zero, and a return of the deep tendon reflexes to normal.
■ Assess blood pressure every 1 to 4 hours as necessary.	■ Frequent monitoring will assess for progression of the disorder and allow for early intervention to ensure maternal and fetal health and well-being.	
■ Monitor urine for volume and proteinuria every shift or every hour per agency protocol.	■ Monitoring provides information to assess renal perfusion. Proteinuria is the last cardinal sign of preeclampsia to appear. As the disorder worsens, the capillary walls of the glomerular endothelial cells stretch, allowing protein molecules to pass into the urine. Normally urine does not contain protein. Reading of 3+ and 4+ indicate loss of 5 g or more protein in 24 hours. Urinary output decreases when there is a reduction of the glomerular filtration rate. Urinary output that falls below 30 mL per hour or less than 700 mL in a 24-hour period should be reported.	
■ Assess deep tendon reflexes and clonus.	■ Hyperreflexia may occur as preeclampsia worsens. Eliciting deep tendon reflexes provides information about CNS status and is also used to assess for magnesium sulfate toxicity. Reflexes are graded on a scale of 0 to 4+ using the Deep Tendon Reflex Rating Scale. A rating of 4+ is abnormal and indicates hyperreflexia. A rating of 0 or no response is also abnormal and is seen with high maternal serum magnesium levels. Clonus, an abnormal finding, is present if the foot "jerks" or taps the examiner's hand, at which time the examiner counts the number of taps or beats. The presence of clonus indicates a more pronounced hyperreflexia and is indicative of CNS irritability.	

NURSING CARE PLAN—continued

THE WOMAN WITH PREECLAMPSIA

Intervention	Rationale	Expected Outcome
■ Assess for edema.	■ Edema develops as fluid shifts from the intravascular to the extravascular spaces. Edema is assessed either by weight gain (more than 3.3 16/month in the second trimester or more than 1.1 16/week in the third trimester) or by assessing for pitting edema (assessed by using finger pressure to a swollen area, usually the lower extremities, and grading on a scale of 1+ to 4+).	
■ Administer magnesium sulfate per infusion pump as ordered.	■ As preeclampsia worsens, the risk of an eclamptic seizure increases. Magnesium sulfate is the treatment of choice for seizures because of its CNS depressant action. As a secondary effect, magnesium sulfate relaxes smooth muscles and may therefore decrease the blood pressure.	
■ Assess for magnesium sulfate toxicity.	■ Side effects of magnesium sulfate are dose related. Therapeutic levels are in the range of 4.8–9.6 mg/dL. As maternal serum magnesium levels increase, toxicity may occur. Signs of toxicity include decreased or absent DTRs, urine output below 30 mL/hr, respirations below 12, and confusion.	
■ Provide a balanced diet that includes 80–100 g/day or 1.5 g/kg/day of protein.	■ A diet rich in protein is necessary to replace protein that is excreted in the urine.	

2. Nursing Diagnosis: Risk for Injury to the Fetus related to uteroplacental insufficiency secondary to vasospasm

NIC Intervention:		NOC Outcome:
High-risk pregnancy care: Identification and management of preeclampsia to promote healthy outcomes for mother and baby		**Risk control:** Actions to manage signs and symptoms of preeclampsia and thereby reduce fetal risk

Goal: The fetus avoids complications related to uteroplacental insufficiency.

■ Instruct client to count fetal movements 3 times a day for 20 to 30 minutes.	■ Fetal activity provides reassurance of fetal well-being. Decrease in fetal movement or cessation of movement may indicate fetal compromise.	■ The fetus will have an adequate supply of oxygen and nutrients as evidenced by absence of signs of fetal distress and fetal diagnostic test results within normal limits.
■ Encourage client to rest in the left lateral recumbent position.	■ Lying in the left lateral recumbent position decreases pressure on the vena cava, which increases venous return, circulatory volume, and placental and renal perfusion. Blood flow to the fetus is increased, thereby reducing the risk of fetal hypoxia and malnutrition.	
■ **Collaborative:** Assist with serial ultrasounds.	■ Maternal vasospasm and hypovolemia result from preeclampsia, which may lead to SGA newborns. Ultrasound provides assessment of fetal growth by measuring the biparietal diameter of the fetal head or the fetal femur length.	

(continued)

THE WOMAN WITH PREECLAMPSIA

Intervention	Rationale	Expected Outcome
■ Perform nonstress test as ordered.	■ A nonstress test is performed to assess the fetal heart rate in response to fetal movement. Accelerations of fetal heart rate with fetal movement may indicate the fetus has adequate oxygenation and an intact central nervous system. (Refer to Chapter 16 ∞ for interpretation of NST results.)	
■ Describe for the woman the purposes of a biophysical profile (BPP).	■ Preeclampsia or eclampsia places the woman at risk for uteroplacental insufficiency due to the loss of normal vasodilation of uterine arterioles and maternal vasospasm. This results in decreased uteroplacental perfusion, which may lead to fetal hypoxia. A BPP is one assessment tool used to evaluate fetal well-being. Providing explanation of the diagnostic test helps relieve anxiety and ensures the woman understands what the test evaluates and what the results mean. See discussion of BPP in Chapter 16. ∞	
■ Assist with amniocentesis to obtain lecithin/sphingomyelin (L/S) ratio.	■ Women with preeclampsia may give birth before term. Amniotic fluid may be analyzed to determine the maturity of the fetal lungs. An L/S ratio of 2:1 or greater indicates fetal lung maturity and is usually achieved by 35 weeks' gestation.	
■ Explain the purpose of Doppler flow studies.	■ Doppler flow studies (umbilical velocimetry) help to assess placental function and sufficiency. Uteroplacental insufficiency is a risk for a woman with preeclampsia. (See Chapter 16. ∞)	

3. Nursing Diagnosis: Risk for Ineffective Health Maintenance related to deficient knowledge about new diagnosis (preeclampsia)

NIC Intervention:		NOC Outcome:
Disease process teaching: Assisting the woman to understand information related to the diagnosis of preeclampsia		**Knowledge:** Treatment regimen: Extent of understanding conveyed about treatment regimen for preeclampsia

Goal: The woman will describe the condition and treatment regimen.

■ Assess the woman and family's understanding of preeclampsia and its implications for pregnancy.	■ This assessment provides information about the woman's cognitive level and her understanding of her diagnosis. Behavior changes occur when teaching strategies are appropriate for the woman and family's cognitive level.	■ Woman will demonstrate understanding of preeclampsia and its implications as evidenced by verbalization of basic condition, signs and symptoms of progression, importance of sufficient rest in side-lying position, and need to follow prescribed diet.
■ Provide information about the disease process, impact on maternal well-being, risks of progression, implications for the fetus, and dangers of eclampsia.	■ Basic understanding of the condition and its implications is necessary for the woman to understand the treatment plan. A woman who shows signs of early preeclampsia often feels well and may have difficulty accepting the need to rest.	
■ Emphasize the importance of self-monitoring for signs that her condition is worsening and the importance of regular prenatal care for the purpose of maternal and fetal surveillance.	■ The woman should be able to identify signs of disease progression, including evidence of increasing edema, decreased urine output, signs of cerebral disturbance (frontal headache, blurred vision, scotomata), epigastric or right upper quadrant pain, nausea or vomiting, and increased irritability.	

Rating	Assessment
4+	Hyperactive; very brisk, jerky, or clonic response; abnormal
3+	Brisker than average; may not be abnormal
2+	Average response; normal
1+	Diminished response; low normal
0	No response; abnormal

TABLE 15–3 ✣ Deep Tendon Reflex Rating Scale

● **FIGURE 15–4**

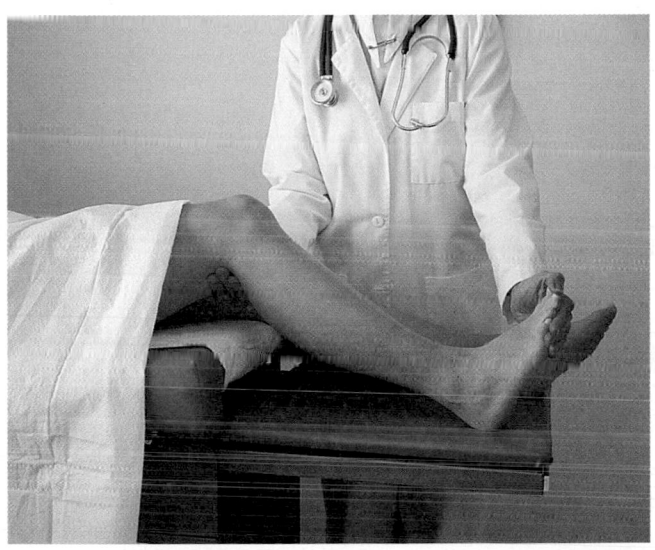

To elicit clonus, with the knee flexed and the leg supported, sharply dorsiflex the foot, hold it momentarily, and then release it. Normally the foot returns to its usual position of plantar flexion. Clonus is present if the foot "jerks" or taps against the examiner's hand. If so, the number of taps or beats of clonus is recorded.

Examples of nursing diagnoses that might apply include the following:

- *Deficient Fluid Volume* related to fluid shift from intravascular to extravascular space secondary to vasospasm
- *Risk for Injury* related to the possibility of seizure secondary to cerebral vasospasm or edema

PLANNING AND IMPLEMENTATION

Nursing Care in the Community

A woman with preeclampsia may fear losing her fetus, worry about her personal relationship with her other children and her personal and sexual relationship with her partner, be concerned about finances, and feel bored and a little resentful if she faces prolonged bed rest. If she has small children, she may have trouble providing for their care. Help couples identify and discuss these concerns. Offer information and explanations if certain aspects of therapy cause difficulty. Refer the woman and her family to community resources such as support groups or homemaker services as appropriate.

The woman needs to know which symptoms are significant and should be reported at once. Usually the woman with mild preeclampsia is seen once or twice weekly, but she may need to come in earlier than her next appointment if symptoms indicate that her condition is progressing.

Hospital-Based Nursing Care

The development of severe preeclampsia is a cause for increased concern about the prognosis for the woman and her fetus. Explain medical therapy and its purpose and offer honest, hopeful information. Keep the couple informed of fetal status and discuss other concerns the couple may express. Provide as much information as possible and seek other sources of information or aid for the family as needed. Offer to contact a member of the clergy or hospital chaplain for additional support if the couple so chooses.

Maintain a quiet, low-stimulus environment for the woman. She should be in a private room in a quiet location where she can be watched closely. Limit visitors to close family members or main support persons. The woman should maintain the left lateral recumbent position most of the time, with side rails up for her protection.

Avoid unlimited phone calls because the phone ringing unexpectedly may be too jarring. To avoid a sense of isolation, however, some women find it preferable to limit calls to a certain time of day. Bright lights and sudden loud noises may precipitate seizures in the woman with severe preeclampsia.

NURSING PRACTICE

When caring for a woman with preeclampsia who is receiving IV magnesium sulfate, it is imperative that you follow protocols for monitoring blood levels of magnesium. You are probably already aware of the common signs of increasing magnesium levels, such as diminished reflexes and decreased respiratory rate. However, you can also watch for some subtle clues that may suggest either the therapeutic or toxic range. When a woman's magnesium level is in the therapeutic range, she usually has some slurring of speech, awkwardness of movement, and decreased appetite. If the woman begins to have difficulty swallowing and begins to drool, she may be approaching the toxic range.

Monitor the effectiveness of medications administered. Be alert for signs of untoward effects or developing toxic levels.

The occurrence of a convulsion is frightening to any family members who may be present, although the woman will not be able to recall it when she becomes conscious. Therefore, it is essential to offer explanations to the family members and the woman herself later.

A grand mal seizure has both a tonic phase, marked by pronounced muscular contraction and rigidity, and a clonic phase, marked by alternate contraction and relaxation of the muscles, which causes the woman to thrash about wildly. When the tonic phase of the contraction begins, turn the woman to her side (if she is not already in that position) to aid circulation to the placenta. Turn her head face down to allow saliva to drain from her mouth. Attempting to insert a padded tongue blade is no longer advocated in many facilities; in others, it is used if it can be inserted without force because it may prevent injury to the woman's mouth. The side rails should be padded or a pillow put between the woman and each side rail.

After 15 to 20 seconds, the clonic phase starts. When the thrashing subsides, intensive monitoring and therapy begin. An oral airway is inserted, the woman's nasopharynx is suctioned, and oxygen is administered by nasal catheter. Fetal heart tones are monitored continuously. Monitor maternal vital signs every 5 minutes until they are stable, then every 15 minutes.

Nursing Management During Labor and Birth. Keep the woman positioned on her left side as much as possible. Carefully monitor both the woman and the fetus throughout labor. Note the progress of labor and remain alert for signs of worsening preeclampsia or its complications.

During the second stage of labor, encourage the woman to push in the side-lying position if possible. If she is unable to do so comfortably or effectively, she can be helped to a semisitting position for pushing and can then resume the lateral position between contractions. Birth is in the side-lying position or in the lithotomy position with a wedge placed under the woman's right hip. Encourage a family member or other support person to stay with the woman as much as possible. Keep the woman and her support person informed of the progress and plan of care. Whenever possible, respect their wishes concerning the birth experience.

Nursing Management During the Postpartal Period. Because the woman with preeclampsia is hypovolemic, even normal blood loss can be serious. Assess the amount of vaginal bleeding and observe the woman for signs of shock. Monitor blood pressure and pulse every 4 hours for 48 hours. Check hematocrit daily. Assess the woman for any further signs of preeclampsia. Measure intake and output. Normal postpartum diuresis helps eliminate edema and is a favorable sign.

Postpartum depression can develop after such a difficult pregnancy. To help prevent it, provide opportunities for frequent maternal-infant contact and encourage family members to visit. The couple may have many questions, so be available for discussion. Give the couple family-planning information. Oral contraceptives may be used if the woman's blood pressure has returned to normal by the time they are prescribed (usually 4 to 6 weeks after birth).

EVALUATION

Expected outcomes of nursing care include the following:

- The woman is able to explain preeclampsia-eclampsia, its implications for her pregnancy, the treatment regimen, and possible complications.

- The woman suffers no eclamptic seizures.

- The woman and her caregivers detect early evidence of increasing severity of the preeclampsia or possible complications so that treatment measures can be instituted.

- The woman gives birth to a healthy newborn.

CHRONIC HYPERTENSIVE DISEASE

Chronic hypertension exists when the blood pressure is 140/90 mm Hg or higher before pregnancy or before the 20th week of gestation, or when hypertension persists 42 days following childbirth. The cause of chronic hypertension has not been determined. In most women the disease is mild.

The goals of care are to prevent the development of preeclampsia and to ensure normal growth of the fetus. The woman is seen regularly for prenatal care (every 2 weeks until 28 weeks and then weekly until birth). The woman is taught the importance of daily rest periods in the left lateral recumbent position and also learns to monitor her blood pressure at home. Sodium is limited to about 2.4 g/day.

Antihypertensive medication is generally used only for women with blood pressure over 160/110. The drug of choice is methyldopa (Aldomet). Twenty-four-hour urines, serum creatinine, uric acid, hematocrit, and ultrasound examinations are repeated at least once in the second and third trimesters.

Nursing care is directed at providing information so that the woman can meet her healthcare needs. Provide information about her diet, the need for regular rest, her medications, the need for blood pressure control, and any procedures used to monitor the well-being of her fetus.

CHRONIC HYPERTENSION WITH SUPERIMPOSED PREECLAMPSIA

Preeclampsia develops in about 25% of women previously found to have chronic hypertension (NIH, 2000). Close monitoring and careful management are indicated if the following signs develop: (1) elevations of systolic blood pressure 30 mm

Hg above the baseline or diastolic blood pressure 15 to 20 mm Hg above the baseline, on two occasions at least 6 hours apart; (2) proteinuria; and (3) edema occurring in the upper half of the body. A woman with chronic hypertension who develops superimposed preeclampsia often progresses quickly to eclampsia, sometimes before 30 weeks of pregnancy.

GESTATIONAL HYPERTENSION

Gestational hypertension is characterized by hypertension occurring for the first time after midpregnancy without proteinuria. It is called transient hypertension if preeclampsia does not develop and if the blood pressure returns to normal within 12 weeks following childbirth.

DISSEMINATED INTRAVASCULAR COAGULATION

Disseminated intravascular coagulation (DIC) occurs more often in pregnancies complicated by preeclampsia, abruptio placentae, intrauterine fetal demise, amniotic fluid embolism, maternal liver disease, and septic abortion (Celik Gezginc, Altinteppe et al., 2003; Tank, Nadanwar, & Mayadeo, 2002). Although DIC is not considered a component of severe preeclampsia, eclampsia, or HELLP syndrome, it can occur as a complication when any of these conditions exist (Celik et al., 2003).

DIC occurs when there is an overactivation of the normal clotting process. In most instances, tissue factor entering the circulation is the primary trigger for DIC (Osterud & Bjorklid, 2001). When this occurs there is an imbalance between the coagulation and the fibrinolytic systems. This mechanism leads to hemorrhage and shock. During these events, clots are being formed and fibrin is being deposited into the microcirculation, resulting in cell or tissue damage. This triggers further coagulation, which eventually depletes the plasma clotting factors. These fibrin clots can lead to intravascular obstruction and infarctions. In addition the fibrinolytic system is activated, which results in the formation of fibrin-fibrinogen degradation products or fibrin split products. The release of these products decreases platelet functioning and further inhibits coagulation (Blackburn, 2003).

DIC is diagnosed when thrombocytopenia, low fibrinogen levels, and elevated fibrin split products are found in the laboratory findings. Serial platelet and serum fibrin degradation product counts are performed to monitor the mother's hematologic status. Supportive measures and reversing the causative factors are the primary interventions used to manage DIC (Letsky, 2001).

CARE OF THE WOMAN AT RISK FOR RH ALLOIMMUNIZATION

The Rh blood group is present on the surface of erythrocytes of most of the population. When it is present, a person is said to be Rh positive. Those without the factor are Rh negative. If an Rh-negative individual is exposed to Rh-positive blood, an antigen-antibody response occurs, and the person forms anti-Rh agglutinin and is said to be sensitized. Subsequent exposure to Rh-positive blood can then cause a serious reaction that results in agglutination and hemolysis of red blood cells (RBCs). Rh alloimmunization (sensitization), also called *isoimmunization,* most often occurs when an Rh-negative woman carries an Rh-positive fetus, either to term or to termination by miscarriage or induced abortion. It can also occur if an Rh-negative nonpregnant woman receives an Rh-positive blood transfusion.

The red blood cells from the fetus invade the maternal circulation, thereby stimulating the production of Rh antibodies. Because this transfer of RBCs usually occurs at birth, the first child is not affected. In a subsequent pregnancy, however, Rh antibodies cross the placenta and enter the fetal circulation, causing severe hemolysis. The destruction of fetal RBCs causes anemia in the fetus (Figure 15–5 ●).

FETAL-NEONATAL RISKS

Although maternal sensitization can now be prevented by administration of **Rh immune globulin** (**RhoGAM**, or RhIgG), sensitization still occurs and infants still die of Rh hemolytic disease. If treatment is not initiated, the anemia resulting from this disorder can cause marked fetal edema, called **hydrops fetalis**. Congestive heart failure may result; marked jaundice (called *icterus gravis*), which can lead to neurologic damage (*kernicterus*), is also possible. This severe hemolytic syndrome is known as **erythroblastosis fetalis**.

SCREENING FOR RH INCOMPATIBILITY AND SENSITIZATION

At the first prenatal visit, healthcare providers (1) take a history of previous sensitization, abortions, blood transfusions, or children who developed jaundice or anemia during the newborn period; (2) determine maternal blood type (ABO) and Rh factor and do a routine Rh antibody screen; and (3) identify other medical complications such as diabetes, infections, or hypertension. When assessment identifies an Rh-negative woman who may be pregnant with an Rh-positive fetus, an antibody screen (indirect Coombs' test) is done to determine if the woman is sensitized (has developed alloimmunization) to the Rh antigen. The indirect Coombs' test measures the number of antibodies in the maternal blood.

Negative antibody titers and a negative indirect Coombs' test can identify the fetus not at risk. However, the titers cannot reliably point out the fetus in danger, since titer level does not correlate with the severity of the disease. Antibody titers are determined periodically throughout the pregnancy. If the maternal antibody titer is 1:16 or greater, a delta optical density (ΔOD) analysis of the amniotic fluid

Rh alloimmunization sequence. *A,* Rh-positive father and Rh-negative mother. *B,* Pregnancy with Rh-positive fetus. Some Rh-positive blood enters the mother's bloodstream. *C,* As the placenta separates, the mother is further exposed to the Rh-positive blood. *D,* Anti-Rh-positive antibodies (triangles) are formed. *E,* In subsequent pregnancies with an Rh-positive fetus, Rh-positive red blood cells are attacked by the anti-Rh-positive maternal antibodies, causing hemolysis of the red blood cells in the fetus.

is performed. This ΔOD analysis measures the amount of pigment from the breakdown of RBCs and can determine the severity of the hemolytic process.

Ultrasound should be done at 14 to 16 weeks to determine gestational age. Then serial ultrasounds and amniotic fluid analysis can be used to follow fetal progress. Ascites and subcutaneous edema are signs of severe fetal involvement. Other indicators of the fetal condition include an increase in fetal heart size and hydramnios.

CLINICAL THERAPY

The goals of clinical management are the early identification and treatment of maternal conditions that predispose to hemolytic disease, evaluation of the Rh-sensitized woman, treatment for the affected newborn, and prevention of Rh sensitization if none is present.

Antepartal Management

Since transplacental hemorrhage is possible during pregnancy, an antibody screen is performed on an Rh-negative woman at 28 weeks' gestation. If she has no antibody titer, she is given an IM injection of 300 mcg Rh immune globulin (RhoGAM, HypRho-D). (*Note:* A new form of human Rh immune globulin—Rhophylac—is also available and can be administered either intravenously or intramuscularly.) The Rh immune globulin provides passive antibody protection against Rh antigens. This "tricks" the body,

which does not then produce antibodies of its own (active immunity). As discussed later, Rh immune globulin is also given postpartally.

When the woman is Rh negative and not sensitized and the father is Rh positive or unknown, Rh immune globulin is also given after each abortion (whether spontaneous or induced), ectopic pregnancy, hydatidiform mole, chorionic villus sampling (CVS), amniocentesis, placenta previa with bleeding, blunt trauma to the abdomen, external cephalic version, suspected abruption, or stillbirth. When CVS is performed or if abortion or ectopic pregnancy occurs in the first trimester, a smaller (50 mcg) dose of Rh immune globulin (MICRhoGAM or Mini-Gamulin Rh) may be used; however, many clinical agencies no longer stock the lower dose preparation, which costs about the same as the standard dose (Moise, 2004). A full 300-mcg dose is used after the first trimester.

Rh immune globulin is not given to the newborn or the father. It should not be given to a previously sensitized woman. However, sometimes after birth or an abortion the results of the blood test do not clearly show whether the mother is already sensitized to the Rh antigen. In such cases the Rh immune globulin is given; it will cause no harm (Table 15–4). (The treatment of the newborn is discussed in Chapter 27. ∞)

Two primary interventions can help the fetus whose blood cells are being destroyed by maternal antibodies:

TABLE 15–4 ✤ Rh Alloimmunization

When trying to work through Rh problems, remember the following:
- A potential problem exists when an Rh-negative mother and an Rh-positive father conceive a child who is Rh positive.
- In this situation, the mother may become sensitized or produce antibodies to her fetus's Rh-positive blood.

The following tests are used to detect sensitization:
- Indirect Coombs' test—done on the mother's blood to measure the number of Rh-positive antibodies.
- Direct Coombs' test—done on the infant's blood to detect antibody-coated Rh-positive red blood cells.

Based on the results of these tests, the following may be done:
- If the mother's indirect Coombs' test is negative and the infant's direct Coombs' test is negative, the mother is given Rh immune globulin within 72 hours of birth.
- If the mother's indirect Coombs' test is positive and her Rh-positive infant has a positive direct Coombs' test, Rh immune globulin is not given; in this case the infant is carefully monitored for hemolytic disease.
- It is recommended that Rh immune globulin be given at 28 weeks antenatally to decrease possible transplacental bleeding concerns.

Rh immune globulin is also administered after each abortion (spontaneous or therapeutic), ectopic pregnancy, or amniocentesis.

early birth and intrauterine transfusion. Both carry risks. Ideally, birth should be delayed until fetal maturity is confirmed at about 36 to 37 weeks.

New technology, available in some clinical facilities, enables clinicians to use a Doppler to measure peak systolic middle cerebral artery (MCA) velocity in the fetus. The increased fetal cardiac output and decreased blood viscosity seen in fetal anemia result in increased MCA blood flow velocity. MCA Dopplers can be done starting as early as 18 weeks' gestation but are unreliable after 35 weeks. The test is valuable because it reduces the need for invasive diagnostic procedures such as amniocentesis (Moise, 2004).

Ultrasound can also be used to detect ascites and subcutaneous edema, which are signs of severe fetal involvement. Other indicators of the fetal condition include an increase in fetal heart size and hydramnios.

If ΔOD indicates severe anemia or if fetal hydrops is present, percutaneous umbilical blood sampling (PUBS) (see Chapter 16 ∞) is performed to determine fetal hematocrit. If the hematocrit is low (generally below 30%), the fetus is given an intrauterine blood transfusion. Severely sensitized fetuses may require birth at 32 to 34 weeks.

Postpartal Management

The Rh-negative mother who has no antibody titer (indirect Coombs' test negative, nonsensitized) and has given birth to an Rh-positive fetus (direct Coombs' test negative) is given an injection of Rh immune globulin within 72 hours of childbirth so she does not have time to produce antibodies to fetal cells that entered her bloodstream when the placenta separated. Rh immune globulin provides her with temporary passive immunity, which prevents the development of permanent active immunity (antibody formation).

NURSING MANAGEMENT

NURSING ASSESSMENT AND DIAGNOSIS

As part of the initial prenatal history, ask the mother if she knows her blood type and Rh factor. Many women are aware that they are Rh negative and that this status has implications for pregnancy. Ask the woman if she has ever received Rh immune globulin, if she has had any previous pregnancies and their outcomes, and if she knows her partner's Rh factor. If the partner is Rh negative, there is no risk to the fetus, who will also be Rh negative. If the woman does not know what Rh type she is, intervention begins after the initial laboratory data are obtained. Plan care based on the findings.

If the woman becomes sensitized during her pregnancy, nursing assessment focuses on the knowledge and coping skills of the woman and her family. After birth, review data about the Rh type of the fetus. If the newborn is Rh positive, the mother is Rh negative, and no sensitization has occurred, it is necessary to administer Rh immune globulin.

Nursing diagnoses that might apply include the following:

- *Health-seeking Behaviors: Information about Rh Immune Globulin* related to an expressed need to understand the implications of being Rh negative and pregnant
- *Ineffective Coping* related to depression secondary to the development of indications of the need for fetal exchange transfusion

PLANNING AND IMPLEMENTATION

During the antepartal period, explain the mechanisms involved in alloimmunization (isoimmunization) and answer any questions the woman and her partner have. It is imperative that the woman understand the importance of receiving Rh immune globulin after every miscarriage, abortion, or ectopic pregnancy. In addition, explain the purpose of the Rh immune globulin administered at 28 weeks' gestation if the woman is not sensitized.

If the woman is sensitized to the Rh factor, it poses a threat to any Rh-positive fetus she carries. Provide emotional support to the family to help the members deal with their concern and any feelings of guilt about the infant's condition. If an intrauterine transfusion becomes necessary, provide support while also assuming responsibility as part of the healthcare team. During labor, when caring for an Rh-negative woman who has not been sensitized, ensure that the woman's blood is assessed for any antibodies and also has been crossmatched for Rh immune globulin. The postpartum nurse is usually responsible for administering the Rh immune globulin IM if the newborn is Rh positive. See Skill 2–4 in the Clinical Skills Manual as well as on the CD-ROM that accompanies this text. **SKILLS**

EVALUATION

Expected outcomes of nursing care include the following:

- The woman is able to explain the process of Rh sensitization and its implications for her unborn child and for subsequent pregnancies.

- If the woman has not been sensitized, she is able to discuss the importance of receiving Rh immune globulin when necessary and cooperates with the recommended dosage schedule.

- The woman gives birth to a healthy newborn.

- If complications develop for the fetus or newborn, they are detected quickly and therapy is instituted.

CARE OF THE WOMAN AT RISK DUE TO ABO INCOMPATIBILITY

In addition to the Rh antigen, human red blood cells may present one or more of the antigens of the ABO group, namely A or B. People with these antigens are then said to have type A, type B, or type AB blood. People whose blood cells present neither A nor B antigens have type O blood. In most cases ABO incompatibility is limited to type O mothers with a type A, B, or AB fetus. Group O infants, because they have no antigenic sites on the red blood cells, are never affected regardless of the mother's blood type. The incompatibility occurs as a result of the interaction of antibodies present in maternal serum and the antigen sites on the fetal red blood cells.

Anti-A and anti-B antibodies are naturally occurring; that is, women are naturally exposed to the A and B antigens through the foods they eat and through exposure to infection by gram-negative bacteria. As a result, some women have high serum anti-A and anti-B titers even before they become pregnant for the first time. Once they become pregnant, the maternal serum anti-A and anti-B antibodies cross the placenta and produce hemolysis of the fetal red blood cells. With ABO incompatibility, the first infant is often involved, and no relationship exists between the appearance of the disease and repeated sensitization from one pregnancy to the next.

Unlike Rh incompatibility, antepartal treatment is never warranted. As part of the initial assessment, however,

note whether the potential for an ABO incompatibility exists (type O mother and type A or B father). This alerts healthcare providers so that, following birth, the newborn can be assessed carefully for the development of hyperbilirubinemia (see Chapter 28 ∞).

CARE OF THE WOMAN REQUIRING SURGERY DURING PREGNANCY

A nonobstetric surgical condition—most commonly appendicitis, cholecystitis, pancreatitis, or bowel obstruction—complicates about 1 in 500 pregnancies (Angelini, 2003). Elective surgery should be delayed until the postpartum, but essential surgery can generally be done during pregnancy. Surgery poses some risks, however. The incidence of miscarriage is increased for women who have surgery in the first trimester. There is also an increased incidence of fetal mortality and of low-birth-weight (less than 2500 g) infants. When surgery is necessary, the incidence of preterm labor and intrauterine growth restriction increases.

Although general preoperative and postoperative care is similar for pregnant and nonpregnant women, special considerations must be kept in mind whenever the surgical client is pregnant. The early second trimester is the best time to operate because there is less risk of miscarriage or early labor, and the uterus is not so large as to block the surgical site. If a chest x-ray is done, the fetus should be shielded from radiation.

To prevent uterine compression of major blood vessels while the woman is supine, the caregiver must place a wedge under the woman's right hip to tilt the uterus during both surgery and recovery. The decreased intestinal motility and delayed gastric emptying that occur in pregnancy increase the risk of vomiting when anesthetics are given and during the postoperative period. Thus, a nasogastric tube is usually inserted before a pregnant woman has major surgery. An indwelling urinary catheter prevents bladder distention, decreases risk of injury to the bladder, and permits monitoring of output.

Pregnancy causes increased secretions of the respiratory tract and engorgement of the nasal mucous membrane, often making breathing through the nose difficult. Consequently, pregnant women often need an endotracheal tube to maintain an airway during surgery. Caregivers must guard against maternal hypoxia. During surgery, uterine circulation decreases, and fetal oxygenation may be reduced quickly. Fetal heart rate must be monitored electronically during and after surgery. Blood loss is also monitored throughout the procedure and following it.

Postoperatively encourage the woman to turn, breathe deeply, and cough regularly and to use any ventilation therapy, such as incentive spirometry, to avoid developing pneumonia. The pregnant woman is at increased risk for thrombophlebitis, so apply antiembolism stockings, encourage leg exercises while the woman is in bed, and have her ambulate as soon as possible.

Discharge teaching is very important. The woman and her family should understand what to expect regarding activity level, discomfort, diet, medications, and any special considerations. In addition, they should know the warning signs they need to report to the physician immediately.

CARE OF THE WOMAN SUFFERING TRAUMA FROM AN ACCIDENT

Trauma complicates 6% to 7% of pregnancies and is the leading nonobstetric cause of maternal death. When major blunt trauma to the mother occurs in the second or third trimester, the risk of fetal loss is 40% to 50%. Abruptio placentae (see Chapter 21 ∞) is the leading cause of fetal death when the mother's injuries are not fatal (Ludmir & Stubblefield, 2002). Motor vehicle accidents are the most common cause of blunt trauma, accounting for 60% to 80% of cases; another 10% to 12% of cases involve pregnant pedestrians hit by a car (Divekar & Keith, 2004). Falls and direct assaults account for most of the remaining cases. (Domestic violence is discussed in the next section.)

Late in pregnancy, when balance and coordination are affected, the woman may fall. Her protruding abdomen is vulnerable to a variety of minor injuries. The fetus is usually well protected by the amniotic fluid, which distributes the force of a blow equally in all directions, and by the muscle layers of the uterus and abdominal wall. In early pregnancy, while the uterus is still in the pelvis, it is shielded from blows by the surrounding pelvic organs, muscles, and bones.

Trauma that causes concern includes blunt trauma, penetrating abdominal injuries such as knife and gunshot wounds, and the complications of maternal shock, premature labor, and spontaneous abortion. Maternal mortality most often occurs from head trauma or hemorrhage. Uterine rupture is a rare but life-threatening complication of trauma. It may result from strong deceleration forces in an automobile accident, with or without seat belts. Traumatic separation of the placenta can occur; it causes a high rate of fetal mortality. Premature labor, often following rupture of membranes during an accident, is another serious hazard to the fetus. Premature labor can begin even if the woman is not injured. To help prevent trauma from automobile accidents, all pregnant women should wear both lap seat belts and shoulder harnesses.

Treatment of major injuries during pregnancy focuses initially on lifesaving measures for the woman. Such measures include establishing an airway, controlling external bleeding, and administering IV fluid to alleviate shock. The woman must be kept on her left side to prevent further hypotension. Oxygen is administered at 100%. Fetal heart rate and fetal movement are monitored. Exploratory surgery may be necessary following abdominal trauma to determine the extent of injuries. If the fetus is near term and the uterus has been damaged, cesarean birth is indicated. If the fetus is still immature, the uterus can often be repaired, and the pregnancy continues until term.

In cases of trauma in which the mother's life is not directly threatened, fetal monitoring for a minimum of 4 hours is suggested if there are no contractions, vaginal bleeding, uterine tenderness, or leaking amniotic fluid. Monitoring for 24 hours is recommended if the woman has experienced major trauma or shows signs of obstetric complications such as uterine bleeding, persistent contractions, premature rupture of the membranes, or abnormal fetal heart rate patterns (Divekar & Keith, 2004). Abruptio placentae may occur following a blow to the abdomen. Increased uterine irritability in the first few hours after trauma helps identify women who may be at risk for this potentially catastrophic complication.

CARE OF THE BATTERED PREGNANT WOMAN

Domestic violence, most often the intentional injury of a woman by her partner, often begins or increases during pregnancy. The incidence of abuse during pregnancy ranges from 4% to 8% (AAP & ACOG, 2002). Physical abuse may result in loss of pregnancy, preterm labor, low-birth-weight infants, and fetal death. Abused women have higher rates of complications such as anemia, infection, low weight gain, and first- and second-trimester bleeding (McFarlane, Parker, Soeken, Silva, & Reed, 1999).

The first step toward helping the battered woman is to identify her. Asking every woman about abuse at various times during pregnancy is crucial because a woman may not disclose abuse until she knows her caregivers better. ACOG (1999a) recommends screening for abuse at the first prenatal visit, at least once each trimester, and then again during the postpartum period.

Chronic psychosomatic symptoms can also be an indicator of abuse. The woman may have nonspecific or vague complaints. It is important to assess old scars around the head, chest, arms, abdomen, and genitalia. Any bruising or evidence of pain is also evaluated. Be especially alert for signs of bruising or injury to the woman's breasts, abdomen, or genitalia because these areas are common targets of violence during pregnancy. Other indicators include a decrease in eye contact; silence when the partner is in the room; and a history of nervousness, insomnia, drug overdose, or alcohol problems. Frequent visits to the emergency department and a history of accidents without understandable causes are possible indicators of abuse.

The goals of treatment are to identify the woman at risk, to increase her decision-making abilities to decrease the risk for further abuse, and to provide a safe environment for the woman and her unborn child. An environment that is private, accepting, and nonjudgmental is necessary so the woman can express her concerns. She needs to be aware of community resources available to her, such as emergency shelters; police, legal, and social services; and counseling. Ultimately it is the woman's decision to either seek assistance or return to old patterns.

Because abuse often begins during pregnancy, it may be a new, unexpected experience for the woman, one she believes is an isolated incident. She needs to know that battering may continue after childbirth and may extend to the child as well. This is an important time to provide information and establish a trusted link for the woman with a health professional. (For further discussion see Chapter 5. ∞)

CARE OF THE WOMAN WITH A PERINATAL INFECTION AFFECTING THE FETUS

Fetal infection may develop at any time during pregnancy. In general, perinatal infections are most likely to cause harm when the embryo is exposed during the first trimester when organ development is occurring. Infections that occur later in pregnancy create other concerns such as growth restriction, preterm birth, and neurologic changes. This section addresses several of the most commonly occurring viral and parasitic infections that may have an impact on the fetus if acquired during pregnancy.

TOXOPLASMOSIS

Toxoplasmosis is caused by the protozoan *Toxoplasma gondii*. It is barely noticeable in adults, but, when contracted in pregnancy, it can profoundly affect the fetus. The pregnant woman may contract the organism by eating raw or undercooked meat, by drinking unpasteurized goat's milk, or by contact with the feces of infected cats, either through the cat litter box or by gardening in areas frequented by cats.

Fetal-Neonatal Risks

The likelihood of fetal infection increases with each trimester of pregnancy, but the risk of serious impact on the fetus decreases. Thus, maternal infection contracted during the first trimester is associated with the lowest incidence of fetal infection but the highest risk of severe fetal disease or death. Maternal infection that occurs before conception is rarely associated with congenital effects (Lopez, Dietz, Wilson, Navin, & Jones, 2000). Most infants born with congenital toxoplasmosis are asymptomatic at birth but develop symptoms later. The infection may vary from mild to severe. In mild cases, retinochoroiditis (inflammation of the retina and choroid of the eye) may be the only recognizable damage, and it and other manifestations may not appear until adolescence or young adulthood. Severe neonatal disorders associated with congenital infection include convulsions, coma, microcephaly, and hydrocephalus. The infant with a severe infection may die soon after birth. Survivors are often blind, deaf, and severely retarded. Treatment of the mother can reduce the incidence of fetal infection by 60% (ACOG, 2000).

Clinical Therapy

Diagnosis can be made by serologic testing of antibody titers, specifically *Toxoplasma*-specific antibodies IgG and IgM using the indirect fluorescent antibody (IFA) test. The indirect hemagglutination test (IHAT) or the Sabin-Feldman dye test can also be used to establish the diagnosis. Ultrasound may be useful in detecting signs of fetal infection such as ascites, microcephaly, and fetal growth restriction (ACOG, 2000).

If diagnosis can be established by physical findings, history, and blood tests, the woman may be treated with sulfadiazine and pyrimethamine. This combination should not be started until after the first trimester because of the teratogenic effects of pyrimethamine. Infants born with congenital toxoplasmosis are treated aggressively using a combination of sulfadiazine, pyrimethamine, and leucovorin for 1 year (Duff, 2002). Such treatment reduces but does not completely prevent the late problems such as retinochoroiditis often seen with the disease.

NURSING MANAGEMENT

NURSING ASSESSMENT AND DIAGNOSIS

The incubation period for the disease is 10 days. The woman with acute toxoplasmosis may be asymptomatic, or she may develop myalgia, malaise, rash, splenomegaly, and enlarged posterior cervical lymph nodes. Symptoms usually disappear in a few days or weeks.

Nursing diagnoses that might apply include the following:

- *Risk for Ineffective Health Maintenance* related to lack of knowledge about ways in which a pregnant woman can contract toxoplasmosis

- *Anticipatory Grieving* related to potential effects on infant of maternal toxoplasmosis

PLANNING AND IMPLEMENTATION

During the antepartal period, discuss methods of preventing toxoplasmosis. The woman must understand the importance of avoiding poorly cooked or raw meat, especially pork, beef, lamb, and, in the Arctic region, caribou. Fruits and vegetables should be washed. She should avoid contact with the cat litter box and have someone else clean it frequently, since it takes approximately 48 hours for a cat's feces to become infectious. Stress the importance of wearing gloves when gardening and of avoiding garden areas frequented by cats.

EVALUATION

Expected outcomes of nursing care include the following:

- The woman is able to discuss toxoplasmosis, its methods of transmission, the implications for her fetus, and measures she can take to avoid contracting it.
- The woman implements health measures to avoid contracting toxoplasmosis.
- The woman gives birth to a healthy newborn.

RUBELLA

The effects of rubella (German measles) on the fetus and newborn are great because rubella causes a chronic infection that begins in the first trimester of pregnancy and may persist for months after birth.

Fetal-Neonatal Risks

The period of greatest risk for the effects of rubella on the fetus is the first trimester. The most common clinical signs of congenital infection include congenital cataracts, sensorineural deafness, and congenital heart defects, particularly patent ductus arteriosus. Other abnormalities, such as mental retardation or cerebral palsy, may become evident in infancy. Diagnosis in the newborn can be made in the presence of these conditions and with an elevated rubella IgM antibody titer at birth. Infants born with congenital rubella syndrome are infectious and should be isolated.

The *expanded rubella syndrome* relates to effects that may develop for years after the infection. These include an increased incidence of type 1 diabetes mellitus, sudden hearing loss, glaucoma, and a slow, progressive form of encephalitis.

Clinical Therapy

The best therapy for rubella is prevention. Live attenuated vaccine is available and should be given to all children. Women of childbearing age should be tested for immunity and vaccinated if susceptible once it is established that they are not pregnant.

As part of the prenatal laboratory screen, the woman is evaluated for rubella using hemagglutination inhibition (HAI), a serology test. The presence of a 1:16 titer or greater is evidence of immunity. A titer less than 1:8 indicates susceptibility to rubella. Because the vaccine is made with attenuated virus, pregnant women are not vaccinated. However, it is considered safe for newly vaccinated children to have contact with pregnant women.

If a woman becomes infected during the first trimester, therapeutic abortion is a legally available alternative.

NURSING MANAGEMENT

NURSING ASSESSMENT AND DIAGNOSIS

A woman who develops rubella during pregnancy may be asymptomatic or may show signs of a mild infection including a maculopapular rash, lymphadenopathy, muscular achiness, and joint pain. The presence of IgM antirubella antibody is diagnostic of a recent infection. These titers remain elevated for approximately 1 month after infection.

Nursing diagnoses that may apply to the woman who develops rubella early in her pregnancy include the following:

- *Ineffective Family Coping* due to an inability to accept the possibility of fetal anomalies secondary to maternal rubella exposure
- *Risk for Ineffective Health Maintenance* related to lack of knowledge about the importance of rubella immunization before becoming pregnant

PLANNING AND IMPLEMENTATION

Support is vital for the couple considering abortion due to a diagnosis of rubella. Such a decision may trigger a crisis for the couple. The parents need objective data to understand the possible effects on their unborn fetus and the long-term prognosis.

EVALUATION

Expected outcomes of nursing care include the following:

- The woman is able to describe the implications of rubella exposure during the first trimester of pregnancy.
- If exposure occurs in a woman who is not immune, she is able to identify her options and make a decision about continuing her pregnancy that is acceptable to her and her partner.
- The nonimmune woman receives the rubella vaccine during the early postpartal period.
- The woman gives birth to a healthy infant.

CYTOMEGALOVIRUS

Cytomegalovirus (CMV) causes both congenital and acquired infections referred to as cytomegalic inclusion disease (CID). This virus can be transmitted by asymptomatic pregnant women across the placenta to the fetus or by the cervical route during birth.

In the United States, over half of adults have antibodies for CMV. The virus can be found in virtually all body fluids. It can be passed between humans by any close contact, such as kissing, breastfeeding, and sexual intercourse. Asymptomatic CMV infection is particularly common in children and gravid women. It is a chronic, persistent infection in that the individual may shed the virus continually over many years. The cervix can harbor the virus, and an ascending infection can develop after birth. Although the virus is usually innocuous in adults and children, it may be fatal to the fetus.

Accurate diagnosis in the pregnant woman depends on the presence of CMV in the urine, a rise in IgM levels, and identification of the CMV antibodies within the serum IgM fraction. At present no treatment exists for maternal CMV or for the congenital disease in the newborn.

CMV is the most frequent cause of viral infection in the human fetus, infecting 0.5% to 2.5% of all newborns (Azam, Vial, Fawer, et al, 2001). Of these about 5% to 18% have overt symptoms at birth and 30% of severely affected infants die; 80% of the surviving infants develop severe neurologic problems, eye abnormalities, or hearing loss (Duff, 2002). Subclinical infections in the newborn may produce mental retardation and hearing loss, sometimes not recognized for several months, or learning disabilities not seen until childhood.

For the fetus, this infection can result in (1) extensive tissue damage that leads to fetal death; (2) survival with microcephaly, hydrocephaly, cerebral palsy, or mental retardation; or (3) survival with no damage at all. The infected newborn is often small for gestational age. The principal tissues and organs affected are the blood, brain, and liver. However, virtually all organs are potentially at risk.

HERPES SIMPLEX VIRUS

Herpes simplex virus (HSV-1 or HSV-2) infection can cause painful lesions in the genital area. Lesions may also develop on the cervix. (This condition and its implications for nonpregnant women are discussed in Chapter 5. ∞)

Fetal-Neonatal Risks

Primary infection poses the greatest risk to both the mother and her infant. Primary infection has been associated with spontaneous abortion, low birth weight, and preterm birth. Transmission to the fetus almost always occurs after the membranes rupture and the virus ascends or during birth through an infected birth canal. Transplacental infection is rare. Approximately 40% of all infants born vaginally to a mother experiencing a primary genital HSV infection develop some form of herpes infection. If antiviral therapy is not used, almost half of these infants will die, while 35% to 40% will experience severe problems such as microcephaly, mental retardation, seizures, retinal dysplasia, apnea, and coma (Duff, 2002).

The infected infant is often asymptomatic at birth but develops symptoms of fever (or hypothermia), jaundice, seizures, and poor feeding after an incubation period of 2 to 12 days. Approximately half of infected infants develop the characteristic vesicular skin lesions. Infants who show signs of neonatal herpes should be evaluated promptly and treated with intravenous acyclovir. Dosage is calculated based on the infant's weight; treatment length varies based on the extent of the infection (Centers for Disease Control and Prevention [CDC], 2002).

Clinical Therapy

The vesicular lesions of herpes have a characteristic appearance, and they rupture easily. Definitive diagnosis is made by culturing active lesions.

ACOG (1999b) recommends antiviral therapy for women with primary HSV infection during pregnancy to decrease viral shedding and promote healing. Women with recurrent infection may also benefit from antiviral therapy. Three medications are available for that purpose: acyclovir, valacyclovir, and famciclovir. Acyclovir has been shown to be effective and safe during pregnancy, but it is not as well absorbed as the other two drugs.

If no evidence of genital infection exists, vaginal birth is preferred. However, if the woman has any signs of active genital lesions or prodromal symptoms of infection such as vulvar pain or burning, cesarean birth is indicated. The woman with active HSV infection and ruptured membranes should also give birth by cesarean as soon as the necessary healthcare providers and equipment can be assembled (Duff, 2002).

HSV has not been found in breast milk. Present experience shows that breastfeeding is acceptable if there are no herpes lesions on the mother's breasts and if she washes her hands well to prevent any direct transfer of the virus.

NURSING MANAGEMENT

NURSING ASSESSMENT AND DIAGNOSIS

During the initial prenatal visit, it is important to learn whether the woman or her partner have had previous herpes infections. If so, ongoing assessment is indicated as pregnancy progresses.

Nursing diagnoses that may apply include the following:

- *Sexual Dysfunction* related to unwillingness to engage in sexual intercourse secondary to the presence of active herpes lesions
- *Ineffective Individual Coping* related to depression secondary to the risk to the fetus if herpes lesions are present at birth

PLANNING AND IMPLEMENTATION

Client education about this fast-spreading disease is crucial. Inform women of the association of HSV infection with spontaneous abortion, newborn mortality and morbidity, and the possibility of cesarean birth. A woman needs to inform all healthcare providers of her infection. She should also know of the possible association of genital herpes with cervical cancer and the importance of a yearly Pap smear.

The woman who acquired HSV infection as an adolescent may be devastated as a mature adult who wants to have a family. Counseling that allows her to express the negative feelings she may have about the infection may help. Literature may also help and is available from Planned Parenthood and public health agencies. The American Social Health Association has established the HELP program to provide information on genital herpes and has a quarterly journal, *The Helper*, for clients with HSV infection.

EVALUATION

Expected outcomes of nursing care include the following:

- The woman is able to describe her infection with regard to its method of spread, therapy and comfort measures, implications for her pregnancy, and long-term implications.
- The woman gives birth to a healthy infant.

GROUP B STREPTOCOCCAL INFECTION

Group B streptococcus (GBS) is a bacterial infection found in the lower gastrointestinal or urogenital tracts. Women may transmit GBS to their fetus in utero or during childbirth. GBS is one of the major causes of early-onset neonatal infection, occurring in 1 to 2 per 1000 live births (Duff, 2002). Newborns become infected in one of two ways: by vertical transmission from the mother during birth or from horizontal transmission from colonized nursing personnel or colonized infants. GBS causes severe, invasive disease in infants. In newborns the majority of cases occur within the first week of life and are thus designated as early-onset disease. Late-onset disease occurs one week or more after birth.

Early-onset GBS is often characterized by signs of serious illness, including pneumonia and overwhelming septicemia. Late-onset GBS often manifests as meningitis or pneumonia. Long-term neurologic complications are common in both types of GBS.

Risk factors for GBS neonatal sepsis include preterm labor, maternal intrapartum fever, prolonged rupture of the membranes, previous birth of an infected infant, and GBS bacteriuria in the current pregnancy. Guidelines for the detection and preventive treatment of newborns at risk include the following (Schrag, Gorwitz, Fultz-Butts, & Schuchat, 2002):

- All pregnant women should be screened for both vaginal and rectal GBS colonization at 35 to 37 weeks' gestation.
- Women identified as GBS carriers should receive antibiotic prophylaxis at the onset of labor or the rupture of membranes.
- Women with GBS in their urine in any concentration should receive intrapartal antibiotic prophylaxis because such women typically have heavy colonization with GBS and thus have an increased risk of giving birth to a newborn with early-onset disease. These women do not need vaginal and rectal cultures at 35 to 37 weeks because therapy is already indicated
- Women who have already given birth to a newborn with invasive GBS disease should receive intrapartal antibiotic prophylaxis. Culture-based screening is not necessary for them.
- If the results of GBS screening are not known when labor begins, prophylaxis is indicated for women with any of the following risk factors: gestation less than 37 weeks, membranes ruptured 16 hours or more, or temperature 100.4°F (38.0°C) or higher.

Intrapartum antibiotic therapy is recommended as follows: initial dose of penicillin G, 5 million units IV followed by 2.5 million units IV every 4 hours until childbirth. Alternatively, ampicillin 2 g initial dose IV followed by 1 g IV every 4 hours until childbirth may be used. Women at high risk for an anaphylactic reaction to penicillin because of marked allergy may be treated with clindamycin or erythromycin.

OTHER INFECTIONS IN PREGNANCY

Table 15–5 summarizes other urinary tract, vaginal, and sexually transmitted infections that contribute to risk

TABLE 15–5 ✢ Infections That Put Pregnancy at Risk

Condition and Causative Organism	Signs and Symptoms	Treatment	Implications for Pregnancy
Urinary Tract Infections (UTI)			
Asymptomatic bacteriuria (ASB): *Escherichia, Klebsiella, Proteus* most common	Bacteria present in urine on culture with no accompanying symptoms.	Oral sulfonamides early in pregnancy, ampicillin and nitrofurantoin (Furadantin) in late pregnancy. Antibody sensitivity results will guide the selection of an appropriate antibiotic.	Women with ASB in early pregnancy may go on to develop cystitis or acute pyelonephritis by third trimester if not treated. Oral sulfonamides taken in the last few weeks of pregnancy may lead to neonatal hyperbilirubinemia and kernicterus.
Cystitis (lower UTI): Causative organisms same as for ASB	Dysuria, urgency, frequency; low-grade fever and hematuria may occur. Urine culture (clean catch) shows ↑ leukocytes. Presence of 10^5 (100,000) or more colonies bacteria per mL urine.	Same.	If not treated, infection may ascend and lead to acute pyelonephritis.
Acute pyelonephritis: Causative organisms same as for ASB	Sudden onset. Chills, high fever, flank pain. Nausea, vomiting, malaise. May have decreased urine output, severe colicky pain, dehydration. Increased diastolic BP, positive fluorescent antibody (FA) test, low creatinine clearance. Marked bacteremia in urine culture, pyuria, WBC casts.	Hospitalization; IV antibiotic therapy. Other antibiotics safe during pregnancy include carbenicillin, methenamine, cephalosporins. Catheterization if output is ↓. Supportive therapy for comfort. Follow-up urine cultures are necessary.	Increased risk of premature birth and intrauterine growth restriction (IUGR). These antibiotics interfere with urinary estriol levels and can cause false interpretations of estriol levels during pregnancy.
Vaginal Infections			
Vulvovaginal candidiasis (yeast infection): *Candida albicans*	Often thick, white, curdy discharge, severe itching, dysuria, dyspareunia. Diagnosis based on presence of hyphae and spores in a wet-mount preparation of vaginal secretions.	Intravaginal insertion of miconazole, butoconazole, or other topical azole preparation, clotrimazole suppositories at bedtime for 1 week. Cream may be prescribed for topical application to the vulva if necessary (CDC, 2002).	If the infection is present at birth and the fetus is born vaginally, the fetus may contract thrush.
Bacterial vaginosis: *Gardnerella vaginalis*	Thin, watery, yellow-gray discharge with foul odor often described as "fishy." Wet-mount preparation reveals "clue cells." Application of potassium hydroxide (KOH) to a specimen of vaginal secretions produces a pronounced fishy odor.	Metronidazole 250 mg PO TID × 7 days or clindamycin 800 mg PO BID × 7 days (CDC, 2002).	CDC (2002) reports that multiple studies have failed to demonstrate a teratogenic effect from metronidazole.
Trichomoniasis: *Trichomonas vaginalis*	Occasionally asymptomatic. May have frothy greenish gray vaginal discharge, pruritus, urinary symptoms. Strawberry patches may be visible on vaginal walls or cervix. Wet-mount preparation of vaginal secretions shows motile flagellated trichomonads.	Single 2-g dose of metronidazole orally (CDC, 2002).	Increased risk for PROM, preterm birth, and low birth weight.

TABLE 15–5 ✤ Infections That Put Pregnancy at Risk—continued

Condition and Causative Organism	Signs and Symptoms	Treatment	Implications for Pregnancy
Sexually Transmitted Infections			
Chlamydial infection: *Chlamydia trachomatis*	Women are often asymptomatic. Symptoms may include thin or purulent discharge, urinary burning and frequency, or lower abdominal pain. Lab test available to detect monoclonal antibodies specific for *Chlamydia*.	Although nonpregnant women are treated with tetracycline, it may permanently discolor fetal teeth. Thus, pregnant women are treated with erythromycin or amoxicillin followed by repeat culture in 3 weeks (CDC, 2002).	Infant of woman with untreated chlamydial infection may develop newborn conjunctivitis, which can be treated with erythromycin eye ointment (but not silver nitrate). Infant may also develop chlamydial pneumonia. May be responsible for premature labor and fetal death.
Syphilis: *Treponema pallidum*, a spirochete	Primary stage: chancre, slight fever, malaise. Chancre lasts about 4 weeks, then disappears. Secondary stage: occurs 6 weeks to 6 months after infection. Skin eruptions (condyloma latal) also symptoms of acute arthritis, liver enlargement, iritis, chronic sore throat with hoarseness. Diagnosed by blood tests such as VDRL, RPR, FTA, ABS. Dark-field examination or spirochetes may also be done.	For syphilis less than 1 year in duration: 2.4 million units benzathine penicillin G IM. For syphilis of more than 1 year's duration: 2.4 million units benzathine penicillin G once a week for 3 weeks. Sexual partners should also be screened and treated (CDC, 2002).	Syphilis can be passed trans-placentally to the fetus. If untreated, one of the following can occur: second-trimester abortion, stillborn infant at term, congenitally infected infant, uninfected live infant.
Gonorrhea: *Neisseria gonorrhoeae*	Majority of women asymptomatic; disease often diagnosed during routine prenatal cervical culture. If symptoms are present they may include purulent vaginal discharge, dysuria, urinary frequency, inflammation, and swelling of the vulva. Cervix may appear eroded.	Nonpregnant women are treated with cefixime orally or ceftriaxone IM plus doxycycline. Pregnant women are treated with ceftriaxone plus erythromycin (CDC, 2002). Some practitioners use azithromycin to treat possible coinfection with chlamydia. All sexual partners are also treated.	Infection at time of birth may cause ophthalmia neonatorum in the newborn.
Condyloma acuminata: caused by a papovavirus	Soft, grayish pink lesions on the vulva, vagina, cervix, or anus.	Podophyllin not used during pregnancy. Trichloroacetic acid, liquid nitrogen, or cryotherapy CO_2 laser therapy done under colposcopy is also successful (CDC, 2002).	Possible teratogenic effect of podophyllin. Large doses have been associated with fetal death.

during pregnancy. (These are described in more detail in Chapter 6. ∞) Spontaneous abortion is frequently the result of a severe maternal infection. Some evidence links infection and prematurity. If the pregnancy is carried to term in the presence of infection, the risk of maternal and fetal morbidity and mortality increases. Thus, it is essential to maternal and fetal health that infection be diagnosed and treated promptly.

THINKING CRITICALLY

Your friend Jena Yoo, G1P0, is 6 months' pregnant and mentions to you that she is developing symptoms of a bladder infection. She has had several bladder infections over the past few years and feels she has warded off others by increasing her fluid intake and drinking acidic juices. Jena tells you that she plans to use the same approach this time because she just had her prenatal appointment last week. She assures you that if symptoms persist, she will discuss it with her care provider at her next prenatal visit. What advice would you give her?

Critical Concept Review

LEARNING OBJECTIVES	CONCEPTS

Contrast the etiology, medical therapy, and nursing interventions for the various bleeding problems associated with pregnancy.

→

1. Several health problems associated with bleeding arise from the pregnancy itself:
   - Spontaneous abortion.
   - Ectopic pregnancy.
   - Gestational trophoblastic disease.
2. The nurse needs to be alert to early signs of these situations:
   - Guard the woman against heavy bleeding and shock.
   - Facilitate the medical treatment.
   - Provide educational and emotional support.

Identify the medical therapy and nursing interventions indicated in caring for a woman with an incompetent cervix.

→

1. Medical therapy for incompetent cervix:
   - Placement of a cerclage to hold the cervix closed.
2. Nursing care:
   - Monitor the woman for premature labor.
   - Teach the woman signs of premature labor.

Discuss the medical therapy and nursing care of a woman with hyperemesis gravidarum.

→

1. Treatment of hyperemesis gravidarum is aimed at:
   - Controlling the vomiting.
   - Correcting fluid and electrolyte imbalance.
   - Correcting dehydration.
   - Improving nutritional status.
2. Nursing care includes:
   - Maintain a relaxed, quiet environment.
   - Monitor weight.
   - Vigilant oral hygiene.

Delineate the nursing care needs of a woman experiencing premature rupture of the membranes (PROM) or preterm labor.

→

1. PROM nursing care focuses on prevention of infection such as limiting vaginal exams and changing the bed pads frequently.
2. Nursing care during preterm labor focuses on administration of tocolytics and monitoring for progression of labor.

Describe the development and course of hypertensive disorders associated with pregnancy.

→

1. Hypertension may exist before pregnancy or, more often, may develop during pregnancy.
2. Preeclampsia can lead to growth retardation for the fetus.
3. Untreated preeclampsia may lead to seizures and death of the mother and infant.
4. It is important to educate the mother about the disease process. This may help motivate her to maintain the required rest periods in the left lateral recumbent position.
5. Antihypertensive and anticonvulsive drugs may be used.

Explain the cause and prevention of hemolytic disease of the newborn secondary to Rh incompatibility.

→

1. Rh incompatibility can occur when an Rh-negative woman and an Rh-positive partner conceive a child who is Rh positive.
2. Use of Rh immune globulin has greatly decreased the incidence of severe complications due to Rh incompatibility because the drug "tricks" the body into thinking antibodies have been produced in response to the Rh antigens.

LEARNING OBJECTIVES

CONCEPTS

Compare Rh incompatibility to ABO incompatibility with regard to occurrence, treatment, and implications for the fetus or newborn.

→

1. ABO incompatibility occurs when the mother has type O blood and the infant has A, B, or AB.
2. Unlike Rh incompatibility, no treatment exists to prevent the occurrence.
3. It creates hyperbilirubinemia in the infant, which is treated with phototherapy.

Summarize the effects of surgical procedures on pregnancy and explain ways in which pregnancy may complicate diagnosis.

→

1. During surgery, a wedge is placed under the mother's hip to prevent compressing vessels while the mother is supine.
2. Pregnancy may hinder diagnosis because of the risk x-rays pose to the developing fetus.
3. Surgery increases the risk of miscarriage, preterm labor, and growth retardation in the fetus.

Discuss the impact of trauma due to an accident on the pregnant woman or her fetus.

→

1. Trauma during pregnancy increases the risk of bleeding due to the increased blood volume of the mother.
2. The types of trauma that are of most concern are blunt trauma, penetrating injuries, and gunshot wounds.
3. Treatment centers on lifesaving measures to the mother.
4. Mother and fetus should be monitored after an accident even if no injury is apparent.

Explain the needs and care of the pregnant woman who experiences abuse.

→

1. The nurse needs to be alert for signs of abuse, including bruising or injury to the breasts, abdomen, or genitalia.
2. The woman should be given information about female partner abuse and about community resources available to assist her.

Describe the effects of infections on the pregnant woman and her unborn child.

→

1. Toxoplasmosis, rubella, cytomegalovirus, herpes, GBS, and other perinatal infections pose a grave threat to the fetus.
2. Prevention is the best therapy.
3. There is no known treatment for rubella or CMV, but antimicrobial drugs are available for toxoplasmosis, herpes, and GBS.

CRITICAL THINKING IN ACTION

*View the **Critical Thinking in Action** video in Chapter 15 of the CD-ROM. Then, answer the questions that follow.*

Carol Smith, a 40-year-old, single, G2, P0010 presents to you while you are working in the birthing unit, at 32 weeks' gestation. Her chief complaint is severe headache, nausea, and trouble seeing. She describes "blackened areas" in her visual fields bilaterally. Her prenatal record reveals long-term substance abuse, depression, and hypertension currently treated with nifedipine 60 mg by mouth once in the morning. You note that she has had two prenatal visits with this pregnancy. You determine her blood pressure to be 170/110; deep tendon reflexes are 3+, clonus negative. She has general edema and 3+ proteinuria. You place Carol on the external fetal monitor to observe for fetal well-being and any contractions. You position her on her left side with her head elevated and use pillows for comfort. You observe that the fetal heart rate is 143–148 with decreased long-term variability. No fetal heart rate decelerations or accelerations are noted. The uterus is soft, and no contractions are palpated or noted on the fetal monitor. Carol asks you why she should stay on her left side.

1. How would you explain the importance of the left side-lying position when on bed rest?
2. You administer nifedipine 10 mg sublingual and a loading dose of magnesium sulfate 4 gm IV piggyback to the main IV line of Ringer's lactate. What findings would indicate that Carol has therapeutic levels of magnesium?
3. What signs of magnesium toxicity should you monitor Carol for?
4. Carol asks if magnesium sulfate will affect her infant. How would you answer her?
5. Which signs of premature labor would you ask Carol to notify you of if she experiences?

MEDIALINK

www.prenhall.com/london

- NCLEX-RN® Review, case studies, and other interactive resources for this chapter can be found on the Companion Website at http://www.prenhall.com/london. Click on "Chapter 15" to select the activities for this chapter.

28-36 weeks

Birth weight under 1 kg

- For animations, more NCLEX-RN® Review questions, and an audio glossary, access the accompanying CD-ROM in this textbook.

REFERENCES

American Academy of Pediatrics (AAP) and American College of Obstetricians and Gynecologists (ACOG). (2002). *Guidelines for prenatal care* (5th ed.). Elk Grove Village, IL: Author.

American College of Obstetricians and Gynecologists. (1999a). *Domestic violence* (ACOG Educational Bulletin No. 257). Washington, DC: Author.

American College of Obstetricians and Gynecologists. (1999b). *Management of herpes in pregnancy* (ACOG Practice Bulletin No. 8). Washington, DC: Author.

American College of Obstetricians and Gynecologists. (2000). *Perinatal viral and parasitic infections* (ACOG Practice Bulletin No. 20). Washington, DC: Author.

American College of Obstetricians and Gynecologists. (2003). *No evidence that cerclage procedure is effective in preventing preterm birth* (ACOG News Release). Retrieved April 4, 2004, from http://www.acog.org/from_home/publications/press_releases/nr08-29-03-2.cfm

Angelini, D. J. (2003). Obstetric triage revisited: Update on non-obstetric surgical conditions in pregnancy. *Journal of Midwifery and Women's Health, 48*(2), 111–118.

Azam, A., Vial, Y., Fawer, C., Zuffrey, J., & Hohlfeld, P. (2001). Prenatal diagnosis of congenital cytomegalovirus infection. *Obstetrics and Gynecology, 97*(3), 443–448.

Blackburn, S. T. (2003). *Maternal, fetal, and neonatal physiology: A clinical perspective* (2nd ed.). St. Louis, MO: Saunders.

Celik, C., Gezginc, K., Altintepe, L., Tonbul, H. Z., Yaman, S. T., Akyurek, C., & Turk, S. (2003). Results of the pregnancies with HELLP syndrome. *Renal Failure, 25*(4), 613–618.

Centers for Disease Control and Prevention (CDC). (2002). Sexually transmitted diseases treatment guidelines 2002. *Morbidity and Mortality Weekly Report, 51*(RR-6), 1–84.

Copeland, L. J., & Landon, M. B. (2002). Malignant diseases and pregnancy. In S. G. Gabbe, J. R. Niebyl, & J. L. Simpson (Eds.), *Obstetrics:*

Normal and problem pregnancies (4th ed., pp. 1255–1281). New York: Churchill Livingstone.

Coppage, K. H., & Sibai, B. M. (2004). Preeclampsia and eclampsia. In J. J. Sciarri (Ed.), *Gynecology and obstetrics* (Vol. 3, chap. 7, pp. 1–18). Philadelphia: Lippincott Williams & Wilkins.

Cunningham, F. G., Leveno, K. J., Bloom, S. L., Hauth, J. C., Gilstrap, L. C., III, & Wenstrom, K. D. (2005). *Williams obstetrics* (22nd ed.). New York: McGraw-Hill.

Da Fonseca, E. B., Bittar, R. E., Carvalho, M. H., & Zugaib, M. (2003). Prophylactic administration of progesterone by vaginal suppository to reduce the incidence of spontaneous preterm birth in women at increased risk: A randomized placebo-controlled double-blind study. *American Journal of Obstetrics and Gynecology, 188*(2), 419–424.

Divekar, P., & Keith, L. G. (2004). Pregnancy outcome in motor vehicle accidents. *The Female Patient, 29*(2), 11–23.

Duff, P. (2002). Maternal and perinatal infection. In S. G. Gabbe, J. R. Niebyl, & J. L. Simpson (Eds.), *Obstetrics: Normal and problem pregnancies* (4th ed., pp. 1293–1345). New York: Churchill Livingstone.

Giles, W., Bisits, A., Knox, M., Madsen, G., & Smith, R. (2000). The effect of fetal fibronectin testing on admissions to a tertiary maternal fetal medicine unit and cost savings. *American Journal of Obstetrics and Gynecology, 182*(2), 439–443.

Goodwin, T. M. (2004). A practical approach to hyperemesis gravidarum. *Contemporary OB/GYN, 49*(6), 47–62.

Gracia, C. R., & Barnhart, K. T. (2001). Diagnosing ectopic pregnancy: Decision analysis comparing six strategies. *Obstetrics and Gynecology, 97*(3), 464–470.

Guinn, D., & Lee, M. J. (2000). Multiple courses of antenatal corticosteroids: New concerns. *Contemporary OB/GYN, 45*(2), 63–69.

Higgins, J. R., & de Swiet, M. (2001). Blood-pressure measurement and classification in pregnancy. *Lancet, 357,* 131–135.

Iams, J. (2002). Preterm birth. In S. G. Gabbe, J. R. Niebyl, & J. L. Simpson (Eds.), *Obstetrics:*

Normal and problem pregnancies (4th ed., pp. 755–826). New York: Churchill-Livingstone.

Jackson, M., & Branch, D. W. (2002). Alloimmunization in pregnancy. In S. G. Gabbe, J. R. Niebyl, & J. L. Simpson (Eds.), *Obstetrics: Normal and problem pregnancies* (4th ed., pp. 893–929). New York: Churchill-Livingstone.

Letsky, E. A. (2001). Disseminated intravascular coagulation. *Best Practice and Research. Clinical Obstetrics and Gynaecology, 15*(4), 623–644.

Lopez, A., Dietz, V. J., Wilson, M., Navin, T. R., & Jones, J. L. (2000, March 31). Preventing congenital toxoplasmosis. *Morbidity and Mortality Weekly Report, 49*(RR-02), 57–75.

Ludmir, J., & Stubblefield, P. G. (2002). Surgical procedures in pregnancy. In S. G. Gabbe, J. R. Niebyl, & J. L. Simpson (Eds.), *Obstetrics: Normal and problem pregnancies* (4th ed., pp. 607–651). Philadelphia: Churchill Livingstone.

Magann, E. F., & Martin, J. N. (2000). Critical care of HELLP syndrome with corticosteroids. *American Journal of Perinatology, 7*(8), 417–422.

March of Dimes Birth Defects Foundation. (2003). March of Dimes updates: Taking action against prematurity. *Contemporary OB/GYN, 48*(2), 92–104.

McFarlane, J., Parker, B., Soeken, K., Silva, C., & Reed, S. (1999). Severity of abuse before and during pregnancy for African American, Hispanic, and Anglo women. *Journal of Nurse-Midwifery, 44*(2), 139–144.

Meis, P. J., Klebanoff, M., Thom, E., Dombrowski, M. P., Sibai, B., Moawad, A. H., et al. (2003). Prevention of recurrent preterm delivery by 17 alpha-hydroxyprogesterone caproate. *New England Journal of Medicine, 348*(24), 2379–2385.

Moise, K. J. (2004). Rh disease: It's still a threat. *Contemporary OB/GYN, 49*(5), 34–48.

National Institutes of Health (NIH). (2000). *Working group report on high blood pressure in pregnancy.* Retrieved December 8, 2002, from http://www.nhlbi.nih.gov/health/prof/heart/hbp/hbp-preg.htm

National Institutes of Health (NIH) Consensus Development Panel. (2001). Antenatal corticosteroids revisited: Repeat courses—National Institutes of Health Consensus Development Conference Statement, August 17–18, 2000. *Obstetrics and Gynecology, 98*(1), 144–150.

Norwitz, E. R. (2002). Emergency cerclage: What do the data *really* show? *Contemporary OB/GYN, 47*(10), 48–66.

Osterud, B., & Bjorklid, E. (2001). The tissue factor pathway in disseminated intravascular coagulation. *Seminars in Thrombosis and Hemostasis, 27*(6), 605–617.

Schrag, S., Gorwitz, R., Fultz-Butts, K., & Schuchat, A. (2002, August 16). Prevention of perinatal group B streptococcal disease: Revised guidelines from the CDC. *MMWR Recommendations and Report, 51*(RR-11), 1–22.

Sibai, B. M. (2002). Hypertension. In S. G. Gabbe, J. R. Niebyl, & J. L. Simpson (Eds.), *Obstetrics: Normal and problem pregnancies* (4th ed., pp. 945–1004). Philadelphia: Churchill Livingstone.

Simpson, J. L. (2002). Fetal wastage. In S. G. Gabbe, J. R. Niebyl, & J. L. Simpson (Eds.), *Obstetrics: Normal and problem pregnancies* (4th ed., pp. 729–753). New York: Churchill Livingstone.

Skidmore-Roth, L. (2003). *Mosby's Handbook of herbs and natural supplements.* St. Louis, MO: Elsevier.

Soto, C. (2002). Toxoplasmosis in pregnancy. *Clinician Reviews, 12*(6), 51–56.

Tank, P. D., Nadanwar, Y. S., & Mayadeo, N. M. (2002). Outcome of pregnancy with severe liver disease. *International Journal of Gynaecology and Obstetrics, 76*(1), 27–31.

Vermillion, S. T., & Scardo, J. A. (2000). Using indomethacin as a tocolytic. *Contemporary OB/GYN, 45*(7), 102–108.

Villar, J., Merialdi, M., Gulmezoglu, A. M., Abalos, E., Carroli, G., Kulier, R., & de Onis, M. (2003). Nutritional interventions during pregnancy for the prevention or treatment of maternal morbidity and preterm delivery: An overview of randomized controlled trials. *Journal of Nutrition, 133* (5, Suppl. 2), 1606S–1625S.

Zhang, C., Williams, M. A., King, I. B., Dashow, E. E., Sorensen, T. K., Frederick, I. O., et al. (2002). Vitamin C and the risk of preeclampsia—results from dietary questionnaire and plasma assay. *Epidemiology, 13*(4), 409–416.

Assessment of Fetal Well-Being

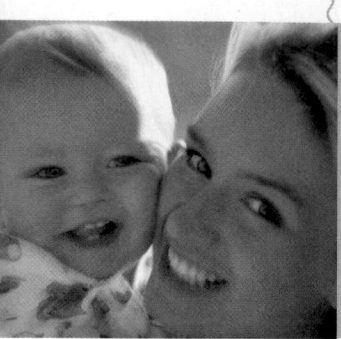

My first pregnancy was so tenuous that I didn't know from one moment to the next how it would end. I hoped for our baby's safety, but in the end the baby died. When I became pregnant the next time, I was very nervous. Being able to see the baby on ultrasound helped me so much. I knew then that our baby was alive and growing.

—*Sharon, 29*

LEARNING OBJECTIVES

- Identify pertinent information to be discussed with the woman regarding her own assessment of fetal activity and methods of recording fetal activity.

- Identify indications and interpret findings for ultrasound examination during pregnancy.

- Compare and contrast the procedure and information obtained from Doppler velocity, nonstress test, contraction stress test, and biophysical profile tests.

- Discuss the use of amniocentesis as a diagnostic tool.

- Describe the tests that can be done on amniotic fluid.

- Identify the advantages and disadvantages of chorionic villus sampling (CVS).

MEDIALINK

www.prenhall.com/london

CD-ROM

NCLEX-RN® Review
Skill 2-5: Assisting During Amniocentesis
Skill 2-8: Biophysical Profile (BPP)
Audio Glossary

Companion Website

NCLEX-RN® Review
MediaLink Applications:
   Case Study: Client Undergoing Contraction Stress
    Test
   Care Plan Activity: Assessment of Fetal Well-Being

The past few decades have produced a notable increase in the number of techniques used to assess fetal well-being. From the relatively simple maternal assessment of fetal movement to more complex diagnostic tests guided by ultrasound, each technique is used to obtain accurate and helpful data about the growing fetus. For example, specialized diagnostic tests can provide information about the normal growth of the fetus, the presence of congenital anomalies, the location of the placenta, and fetal lung maturity (Table 16–1). At times just one test is done, and in other circumstances a combination of testing is needed.

Some of these assessment techniques pose risks to the fetus and possibly to the pregnant woman, and the risk to both should be considered before the decision to perform the test is made. The healthcare provider must be certain that the advantages outweigh the potential risks and added expense. In addition the diagnostic accuracy and applicability of these tests may vary. Certainly not all high-risk pregnancies require the same tests. Conditions that indicate a pregnancy at risk include the following:

- Maternal age less than 16 or more than 35 years
- Chronic maternal hypertension, preeclampsia, diabetes mellitus, or heart disease
- Presence of Rh alloimmunization
- A maternal history of unexplained stillbirth
- Suspected intrauterine growth restriction (IUGR)
- Pregnancy prolonged past 42 weeks' gestation
- Multiple gestation
- Maternal history of preterm labor
- Previous cervical incompetence

See Chapter 9 for further discussion of prenatal at-risk factors and Chapters 14 and 15 for descriptions of various conditions that may threaten the successful completion of pregnancy. ∞

Nursing care for the woman who is undergoing diagnostic testing focuses on outcomes to ensure that she understands the reasons for the test, understands the test results, and has had support during the test (Table 16–2). Other objectives include completing the tests without complication and ensuring that the safety of the mother and her unborn child has been maintained.

MATERNAL ASSESSMENT OF FETAL ACTIVITY

Clinicians generally agree that vigorous fetal activity provides reassurance of fetal well-being and that marked decrease in activity or cessation of movement may indicate possible fetal compromise (or even death) requiring immediate follow-up. The technique is typically used to monitor fetal well-being from week 28 to week 38.

Fetuses spend approximately 10% of their time making gross body movements. Fetal movements are directly related to the infant's sleep-wake cycle and vary from the maternal sleep-wake cycle. The typical active fetal period lasts 40 minutes and peaks between 9:00 p.m. and 1:00 a.m. in response to maternal hypoglycemia (Moses, 2003). In women with a multiple gestation, daily fetal movements are significantly higher. After 38 weeks the fetus spends 75% of its time in a quiet sleep or active sleep state. Other factors affecting fetal movement include sound, cigarette smoking, and drugs (Varney, Kriebs, & Gegor, 2004).

The expectant mother's perception of fetal movements and her commitment to completing a fetal movement record may vary. When a woman

TABLE 16–1 ✥ Summary of Screening and Diagnostic Tests

Goal	Test	Timing
To validate the pregnancy	Ultrasound: gestational sac volume	5 and 6 weeks after last menstrual period by endovaginal ultrasound
To determine how advanced the pregnancy is	Ultrasound: crown–rump length	6 to 10 weeks' gestation
	Ultrasound: biparietal diameter, femur length, abdomen circumference	13 to 40 weeks' gestation
To identify normal growth of the fetus	Ultrasound: biparietal diameter	Most useful from 20 to 30 weeks' gestation
	Ultrasound: head/abdomen ratio	13 to 40 weeks' gestation
	Ultrasound: estimated fetal weight	About 24 to 40 weeks' gestation
To detect congenital anomalies and problems	Ultrasound	18 to 40 weeks' gestation
	Chorionic villus sampling	8 to 12 weeks' gestation
	Amniocentesis	16 to 18 weeks' gestation
	Fetoscopy	18 weeks' gestation
	Percutaneous blood sampling	Second and third trimesters
	Triple test or quadruple test	About 10 weeks' gestation
To localize the placenta	Ultrasound	Usually in third trimester or before amniocentesis
To assess fetal status	Biophysical profile	Approximately 28 weeks to birth
	Maternal assessment of fetal activity	About 28 weeks to birth
	Nonstress test	Approximately 28 weeks to birth
	Contraction stress test	After 28 weeks
To diagnose cardiac problems	Fetal echocardiography	Second and third trimesters
To assess fetal lung maturity	Amniocentesis	33 to 40 weeks
	L/S ratio	33 weeks to birth
	Phosphatidylglycerol	33 weeks to birth
	Phosphatidylcholine	33 weeks to birth
To obtain more information about breech presentation	Ultrasound	Just before labor is anticipated or during labor

understands the purpose of the assessment, how to complete the form, whom to call with questions, and what to report, and has the opportunity for follow-up during each visit, she generally views completing the fetal movement record as an important activity. The nurse is available to answer questions and clarify areas of concern. (See further discussion and "Teaching Highlights: Assessing Fetal Activity," in Chapter 11. ∞)

NURSING PRACTICE

Families undergoing fetal testing experience a wide range of emotions based on personal expectations, past experiences, fears, and cultural norms. Encouraging the family to verbalize concerns, ask questions, and express any apprehensions or fears can help put the family at ease.

ULTRASOUND

Valuable information about the fetus may be obtained from **ultrasound** testing. Intermittent ultrasonic waves (high-frequency sound waves) are transmitted by an alternating current to a transducer, which is applied to the woman's abdomen. The ultrasonic waves deflect off tissues within the woman's abdomen, showing structures of varying densities (Figures 16–1 ● and 16–2 ●).

Diagnostic ultrasound has several advantages. It is noninvasive, painless, and nonradiating to both the woman and the fetus, and it has no known harmful effects to either. Serial studies (several ultrasound tests done over a span of time) may be done for assessment and comparison. Soft-tissue masses (such as tumors) can be differentiated, the fetus can be visualized, fetal growth can be followed (especially in the presence of multiple gestation),

TABLE 16–2 ✤ Sample Nursing Approaches to Pretest Teaching

Assess whether the woman knows the reason the screening or diagnostic test is being recommended.
Examples:
"Has your doctor or nurse-midwife told you why this test is necessary?"
"Sometimes tests are done for many different reasons. Can you tell me why you are having this test?"
"What is your understanding about what the test will show?"

Provide an opportunity for questions.
Examples:
"Do you have any questions about the test?"
"Is there anything that is not clear to you?"

Explain the test procedure, paying particular attention to any preparation the woman needs prior to the test.
Example:
"The test that has been ordered for you is designed to . . ." (Add specific information about the particular test. Give the explanation in simple language.)

Validate the woman's understanding of the preparation.
Example:
"Tell me what you will have to do to get ready for this test."

Give permission for the woman to continue to ask questions if needed.
Example:
"I'll be with you during the test. If you have any questions at any time, please don't hesitate to ask."

cervical length and impending cervical incompetence can be detected, and a number of potential problems can be averted. In addition the ultrasonographer or physician obtains results immediately (Jasper, 2004).

Future research in fetal well-being will be generated and enhanced by the use of *four-dimensional ultrasound.*

◉ FIGURE 16–1

Ultrasound scanning permits visualization of the fetus in utero.

◉ FIGURE 16–2

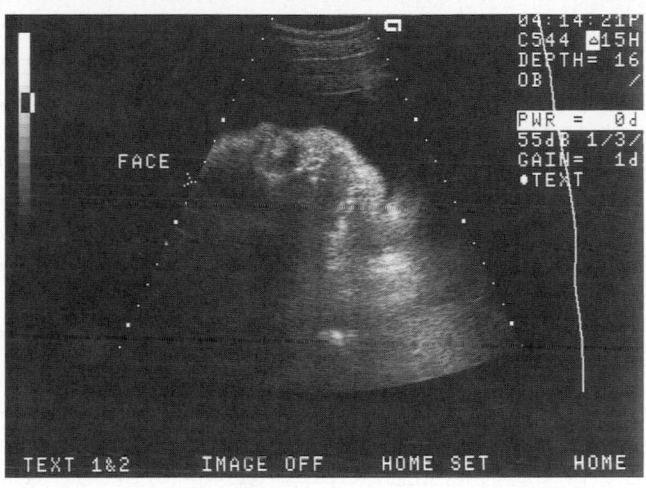

Ultrasound of fetal face.

Four-dimensional ultrasound combines the components of three-dimensional ultrasound with a fourth dimension, time, because it monitors live action. The technology produces images of photolike quality, allowing healthcare providers to better visualize fetal structures and providing better guidance during invasive intrauterine procedures such as amniocentesis and chorionic villus sampling (discussed later in this chapter). It is believed that this new technology will produce more accurate fetal growth and weight assessments.

PROCEDURES

The two most common methods of ultrasound scanning are transabdominal and transvaginal.

Transabdominal Ultrasound

In the transabdominal approach, the transducer is moved across the woman's abdomen. The woman is often scanned with a full bladder; when the bladder is full, the examiner can assess other structures, especially the vagina and cervix, in relation to the bladder. The ability to see the lower portion of the uterus and cervix is particularly important when vaginal bleeding is noted and placenta previa is the suspected cause. The woman is advised to drink 1 to 1.5 quarts of water approximately 2 hours before the examination, and she is asked to refrain from emptying her bladder. If the bladder is not sufficiently filled, she is asked to drink three to four 8-oz glasses of water and is rescanned 30 to 45 minutes later.

Mineral oil or a transmission gel is spread generously over the woman's abdomen, and the sonographer slowly moves a transducer over the abdomen to obtain a picture of the contents of the uterus. Ultrasound testing takes 20 to 30 minutes. The woman may feel discomfort due to pressure applied over a full bladder. If the woman lies on her back during the test, shortness of breath can develop. This may be relieved by elevating her upper body during the test or position on side with towel under hip to prevent vena caval compression.

Transvaginal Ultrasound

The transvaginal approach uses a probe inserted into the vagina. Once inserted, the transvaginal probe is close to the structures being imaged and so produces a clearer, more defined image. The improved images obtained by transvaginal ultrasound have enabled sonographers to identify structures and fetal characteristics earlier in pregnancy (Varney et al., 2004). Internal visualization can also be used as a predictor for preterm birth in high-risk cases (Berghella, Talucci, & Desai, 2003). Use of the ultrasound to detect shortened cervical length or funneling (a cone-shaped indentation in the cervical os) is helpful in predicting preterm labor, especially in women who have a history of preterm birth (Berghella et al., 2003).

After the procedure is fully explained to the woman, she is prepared in the same manner as for a pelvic examination: in the lithotomy position, with appropriate drapes to provide privacy, and a female attendant in the room. It is important that her buttocks are at the end of the table so that, once inserted, the probe can be moved in various directions. A small, lightweight vaginal transducer is covered with a specially fitted sterile sheath, a condom, or one finger of a glove. Ultrasound coupling gel is then applied to both the inside and the outside of the covering, making insertion into the vagina easier and providing a medium for enhancing the ultrasound image. The transvaginal procedure can be accomplished with an empty bladder, and most women do not feel discomfort during the examination. The probe is smaller than a speculum, so insertion is usually completed with ease. The woman may feel the movement of the probe during the examination as various structures are imaged. Some women may want to insert the probe themselves to enhance their comfort, whereas others would feel embarrassed even to be asked. The certified nurse-midwife, physician, or ultrasonographer offers the choice based on personal rapport with the woman.

CLINICAL APPLICATIONS

Ultrasound testing can be of benefit in the following ways (Varney et al., 2004):

- **Early identification of pregnancy.** Pregnancy may be detected as early as the fifth or sixth week after the last menstrual period (LMP).

- **Observation of fetal heartbeat and fetal breathing movements (FBMs).** FBMs have been observed as early as week 11 of gestation.

- **Identification of more than one embryo or fetus.**

- **Measurement of the biparietal diameter of the fetal head or the fetal femur length.** These measurements help determine the gestational age of the fetus and identify IUGR.

- **Clinical estimations of birth weight.** This assessment helps to identify macrosomia (infants greater than 4000 g at birth). Macrosomia has been identified as a predictor of birth-related trauma and is a risk factor for both maternal and fetal morbidity.

- **Detection of fetal anomalies such as anencephaly and hydrocephalus.**

- **Examination of nuchal translucency in the first trimester to assess for Down syndrome and other fetal structural anomalies.** Nuchal translucency describes an area in the back of the fetal neck that is measured via ultrasound during the first trimester of pregnancy. Fetuses with a nuchal translucency measurement of greater than 3 mm are at risk for certain birth defects, including trisomies 13, 18, and 21.

- **Examination of fetal cardiac structures (echocardiography).**

- **Identification of amniotic fluid index (AFI).** The maternal abdomen is divided into quadrants. The umbilicus is used to divide the upper and lower sections, and the linea nigra divides the right and left sections. The vertical diameter of the largest amniotic fluid pocket in each quadrant is measured. All measurements are totaled to obtain the AFI in centimeters. Women with an AFI of more than 20 cm are considered to have hydramnios, and women with less than 5 cm at term are considered to have oligohydramnios. An AFI between 5 and 20 cm is considered normal. After 39 weeks the amniotic fluid begins to decline (Gabbe, Niebyl, & Simpson, 2003). Both hydramnios and oligohydramnios are associated with increased risk to the fetus.

- **Location of the placenta.** The placenta is located before amniocentesis to avoid puncturing the placenta. Ultrasound is also used to determine the presence of placenta previa.

- **Placental grading.** As the fetus matures, the placenta calcifies. These changes can be detected by ultrasound and graded according to the degree of calcification (Jasper, 2004).

- **Detection of fetal death.** Inability to visualize the fetal heart beating and the separation of the bones in the fetal head are signs of fetal death.

- **Determination of fetal position and presentation.**
- **Accompanying procedures.** Amniocentesis, chorionic villus sampling, intrauterine procedures, and other procedures will be discussed shortly.

RISKS OF ULTRASOUND

Ultrasound has been used clinically for over 40 years, and to date no clinical studies verify harmful effects to the mother or the fetus or newborn. The use of ultrasound in pregnancy has spanned nearly three generations. Many pregnant clients themselves received diagnostic ultrasound in utero with no adverse effect.

NURSING MANAGEMENT

It is important to ascertain whether the woman understands why the ultrasound is being suggested. The nurse provides an opportunity for the woman to ask questions, and acts as an advocate if there are questions or concerns that need to be addressed before the ultrasound examination. The nurse can also inform women that the use of ultrasound is variable. Although ultrasounds are considered routine in most areas, variables that affect its use include availability, cost, provider perception of need, maternal history or risk factors, and insurance coverage issues. Explain the preparation needed and ensure that adequate preparation is done. After the test is completed, assist with clarifying or interpreting test results for the woman and her partner.

DOPPLER BLOOD FLOW STUDIES (UMBILICAL VELOCIMETRY)

Umbilical velocimetry, a noninvasive ultrasound test, measures blood flow changes that occur in maternal and fetal circulation in order to assess placental function. An ultrasound beam, like that provided by the pocket Doppler (a handheld ultrasound device), is directed at the umbilical artery (in some cases a maternal vessel such as the arcuate artery can also be used). The signal is reflected off the red blood cells moving within the vessels and creates a "picture" (waveform) that looks like a series of waves (Figures 16–3 ● and 16–4 ●). The highest velocity peak of the waves is the systolic measurement, and the lowest point is the diastolic velocity. To interpret the waveforms, the systolic (S) peak is divided by the end-diastolic (D) component. This calculation is called the S/D ratio. The normal S/D ratio is below 2.6 by 26 weeks' gestation and below 3 at term. A decrease in uteroplacental perfusion (because of narrowing of the vessels) causes an increase in placental bed resistance and a decrease in diastolic flow, resulting in an elevated S/D ratio

(Jasper, 2004). Elevations of 3 and above are considered abnormal. Doppler blood flow studies are helpful in assessing and managing pregnancies with suspected uteroplacental insufficiency before asphyxia occurs (Jasper, 2004).

● **FIGURE 16–3**

Serial studies of the umbilical artery velocity waveforms in a normal pregnancy from one client.

○ **FIGURE 16-4**

Two examples of abnormal umbilical artery velocity waveforms taken from a client with intrauterine growth restriction.

Used with permission from Cundiff, J. L., Haubrich, K. L., & Hinzman, N. G. (1990). Umbilical artery Doppler flow studies during pregnancy. Journal of Obstetric, Gynecologic, and Neonatal Nursing, *19(6), 475–481 (fig. 4, p. 478). Washington, DC: Author. © 1990 by the Association of Women's Health, Obstetric and Neonatal Nurses (AWHONN). All rights reserved.*

Doppler blood flow studies are relatively easy to obtain. The woman lies supine with a wedge under the left hip (to promote uteroplacental perfusion). Warmed transducer gel is applied to the abdomen, and a pulsed-wave Doppler device is used to ascertain the blood flow. The Doppler flow study takes about 15 to 20 minutes. Doppler flow studies can be initiated at 16 to 18 weeks' gestation and are then scheduled at regular intervals for women at risk.

NONSTRESS TEST

The **nonstress test (NST),** a widely used method of evaluating fetal status, may be used alone or as part of a more comprehensive diagnostic assessment called a *biophysical profile (BPP).* The nonstress test is based on the knowledge that when the fetus has adequate oxygenation and an intact central nervous system, there are accelerations of the fetal heart rate (FHR) with fetal movement (FM). An NST requires an electronic fetal monitor to observe and record these fetal heart rate accelerations (see discussion of acceleration in Chapter 18. ∞) A nonreactive NST is fairly consistent in identifying at-risk fetuses. The advantages of the NST are as follows:

■ It is quick to perform, permits easy interpretation, and is inexpensive.

■ It can be done in an office or clinic setting.

■ There are no known side effects.

The disadvantages of the NST include the following:

■ It is sometimes difficult to obtain a suitable tracing.

■ The woman has to remain relatively still for at least 20 minutes.

PROCEDURE FOR NST

The test can be done with the woman in a reclining chair or in bed in a semi-Fowler's or side-lying position (Jasper, 2004). An electronic fetal monitor is used to obtain a tracing of the FHR and FM. The nurse places the monitor under the woman's clothing. Privacy should be provided. The examiner puts two elastic belts on the woman's abdomen. One belt holds a device that detects uterine or fetal movement; the other belt holds a device that detects the FHR. As the NST is done, each fetal movement is documented, so that associated or simultaneous FHR changes can be evaluated.

INTERPRETATION OF NST RESULTS

Women with a high-risk factor will probably begin having NSTs at 30 to 32 weeks' gestation and at frequent intervals for the remainder of the pregnancy. The results of the NST are interpreted as follows:

■ **Reactive test.** A reactive NST shows at least two accelerations of FHR with fetal movements of 15 beats per minute, lasting 15 seconds or more, over 20 minutes (Figure 16–5 ●). This is the desired result (Table 16–3).

■ **Nonreactive test.** In a nonreactive test, the reactive criteria are not met. For example, the accelerations are not as much as 15 beats per minute or do not last 15 seconds (Figure 16–6 ●).

● **FIGURE 16-5**

Example of a reactive nonstress test (NST). Accelerations of 15 beats per minute lasting 15 seconds with each fetal movement (FM). Top of strip shows FHR; bottom of strip shows uterine activity tracing. Note that FHR increases (above the baseline) at least 15 beats and remains at that rate for at least 15 seconds before returning to the former baseline.

TABLE 16–3 ✢ **Nonstress Test**

Diagnostic Value	Results
Demonstrates fetus's ability to respond to its environment by acceleration of FHR with movement.	■ Reactive test: Accelerations (at least two) of 15 beats/min above the baseline, lasting 15 sec in a 20-min window, are present, indicating fetal well-being. ■ Nonreactive test: Accelerations are not present, indicating that the fetus is sick or asleep. ■ Unsatisfactory test: Data cannot be interpreted or there was inadequate fetal activity.

■ **Unsatisfactory test.** An NST is unsatisfactory if the data cannot be interpreted or there was inadequate fetal activity.

It is important that anyone who performs the NST understand the significance of any decelerations of the FHR during testing. If decelerations are noted, the certified nurse-midwife or physician should be notified for further evaluation of fetal status. (See Chapter 18 for further discussion of FHR decelerations. ∞)

CLINICAL MANAGEMENT

The clinical management of potential nonreassuring fetal status may vary somewhat among clinicians, depending on the clinical judgment of the care provider. One commonly used protocol is as follows: If the NST is reactive in less than 30 minutes, the test is concluded and rescheduled as indicated by the high-risk condition that is present; if it is nonreactive, the test time is extended for 30 minutes until the results are reactive, and then the test is rescheduled as indicated. It is estimated that 80% to 90% of nonreactive NSTs are due to fetal sleep states. If the FHR remains nonreactive for longer than 30 minutes, the test is typically repeated after the woman eats or the fetus is stimulated via vibroacoustic stimulation, a foot massage, or palpation. Such measures often awaken a fetus so a reactive NST can be obtained. If a reactive test is not obtained within 40 minutes, additional testing (such as diagnostic ultrasound and biophysical profile) or immediate birth is considered; if the NST is nonreactive and spontaneous decelerations of the FHR are present, diagnostic ultrasound and biophysical profile are performed and birth is recommended (Figure 16–7 ◉). Many testing guidelines vary in frequency, recommending a retest either once or twice a week, depending upon the at-risk condition that exists. In some situations, such as preterm premature rupture of membranes, testing may be done daily (Varney et al., 2004).

NURSING MANAGEMENT

Evaluate the woman's understanding of the NST and the possible results. Review the reasons for the NST and the procedure before beginning the test. Administer the NST, interpret the results, and report the findings to the certified nurse-midwife or physician and the expectant mother.

◉ **FIGURE 16–6**

Example of a nonreactive NST. There are no accelerations of FHR with FM. Baseline FHR is 130 beats per minute. The tracing of uterine activity is on the bottom of the strip.

○ **FIGURE 16-7**

NST management scheme.

Used with permission from Devoe, L. D. (1989). Nonstress and contraction stress testing. In R. Depp, D. A. Eschenbach, & J. J. Sciarri (Eds.), Gynecology and obstetrics (Vol. 3, p. 9, fig. 5). Philadelphia: Lippincott.

NURSING PRACTICE

If a nonstress test fails to become reactive, a 3-minute foot massage has been shown to stimulate the fetus and increase fetal activity. It also helps the woman to relax during the test.

FETAL ACOUSTIC STIMULATION TEST AND VIBROACOUSTIC STIMULATION TEST

Acoustic (sound) and vibroacoustic (vibration and sound) stimulation of the fetus can be used as an adjunct to the NST. A handheld, battery-operated device is applied to the woman's abdomen over the area of the fetal head. This device generates a low-frequency vibration and a buzzing sound that are intended to induce movement and associated accelerations of FHR in fetuses with a nonreactive NST and in fetuses with decreased variability of FHR during labor. (See discussion of variability in Chapter 18. ∞) A burst of a sound is given over the fetal head; if no accelerations occur, it is then repeated up to three times (Jasper, 2004). Whether the fetus responds more to the vibration or

to the sound is not known. Two FHR accelerations of 15 beats per minute, lasting 15 seconds, in a 20-minute period indicate a reactive test. Advantages of the fetal acoustic stimulation test (FAST) and the vibroacoustic stimulation test (VST) are as follows:

- Both are noninvasive techniques that are easy to perform.
- Results are rapidly available.
- Time for the NST is shortened.

BIOPHYSICAL PROFILE

The **biophysical profile (BPP)** is a comprehensive assessment of five biophysical variables:

1. Fetal breathing movement
2. Fetal movements of body or limbs
3. Fetal tone (extension and flexion of extremities)
4. Amniotic fluid volume (visualized as pockets of fluid around the fetus)
5. Reactive FHR with activity (reactive NST)

The first four variables are assessed by ultrasound scanning; FHR reactivity is assessed with the NST. By combining these

MediaLink Skill 2–8: Biophysical Profile

TABLE 16–4 ❖ Criteria for Biophysical Profile Scoring

Component	Normal (score = 2)	Abnormal (score = 0)
Fetal breathing movements	≥ 1 episode of rhythmic breathing lasting ≥ 30 sec within 30 min	≤ 30 sec of breathing in 30 min
Gross body movements	≥ 3 discrete body or limb movements in 30 min (episodes of active continuous movement considered as single movement)	≤ 2 movements in 30 min
Fetal tone	≥ 1 episode of extension of a fetal extremity with return to flexion, or opening or closing of hand	No movements or extension/flexion
Nonstress test	≥ 2 accelerations of ≥ 15 beats/min for ≥ 15 sec in 20 min	0 or 1 acceleration in 20 min
Amniotic fluid volume	Single vertical pocket > 2 cm	Largest single vertical pocket ≤ 2 cm

five assessments, the BPP helps to either identify the compromised fetus or confirm the healthy fetus. Specific criteria for normal and abnormal assessments are presented in Table 16–4. A score of 2 is assigned to each normal finding, and 0 to each abnormal one, for a maximum score of 10. The absence of a specific activity is difficult to interpret, since it may be indicative of central nervous system (CNS) depression or simply the resting state of a healthy fetus. Scores of 8 (with normal amniotic fluid) and 10 are considered normal. Such scores have the least chance of being associated with a compromised fetus unless a decrease in the amount of amniotic fluid is noted, in which case the infant's birth may be indicated (Varney et al., 2004).

The BPP is indicated when there is risk of placental insufficiency or fetal compromise because of the following:

- Intrauterine growth restriction (IUGR)
- Maternal diabetes mellitus
- Maternal heart disease
- Maternal chronic hypertension
- Maternal preeclampsia or eclampsia
- Maternal sickle cell anemia
- Suspected fetal postmaturity (more than 42 weeks' gestation)
- History of previous stillbirths
- Rh sensitization
- Abnormal estriol excretion
- Hyperthyroidism
- Renal disease
- Nonreactive NST

CONTRACTION STRESS TEST

The **contraction stress test (CST)** is a means of evaluating the respiratory function (oxygen and carbon dioxide exchange) of the placenta. It enables the healthcare team to identify the fetus at risk for intrauterine asphyxia by observing the response of the FHR to the stress of uterine contractions (spontaneous or induced). During contractions, intrauterine pressure increases. Blood flow to the intervillous space of the placenta is reduced momentarily, thereby decreasing oxygen transport to the fetus. A healthy fetus usually tolerates this reduction well and maintains a steady heart rate. If the placental reserve is insufficient, fetal hypoxia, depression of the myocardium, and a decrease in FHR occur.

In many areas the CST has given way to the biophysical profile and has limited use today. It is still used in areas where the availability of other technology is reduced (such as during night shifts) or limited (such as at small community hospitals or birthing centers). It may also be used as an adjunct to other forms of fetal assessment.

The CST is contraindicated in third-trimester bleeding from placenta previa or marginal abruptio placentae, previous cesarean with classic incision (vertical incision in the fundus of the uterus), premature rupture of the membranes, incompetent cervix, anomalies of the maternal reproductive organs, history of preterm labor (if being done prior to term), or multiple gestation.

PROCEDURE

The critical component of the CST is the presence of uterine contractions. They may occur spontaneously (which is unusual prior to the onset of labor), or they may be induced (stimulated) with oxytocin (Pitocin) administered intravenously (also known as an oxytocin challenge test). A natural method of obtaining oxytocin is through the use of breast stimulation (either via nipple self-stimulation or application of an electric breast pump); the posterior pituitary produces oxytocin in response to stimulation of the breasts or nipples.

An electronic fetal monitor is used to provide continuous data about the fetal heart rate and uterine contractions.

After a 15-minute baseline recording of uterine activity and FHR, the tracing is evaluated for evidence of spontaneous contractions. If three spontaneous contractions of good quality and lasting 40 to 60 seconds occur in a 10-minute window, the results are evaluated, and the test is concluded. If no contractions occur or they are insufficient for interpretation, oxytocin is administered intravenously or the breasts are stimulated via self-stimulation or application of an electric breast pump to produce contractions of good quality. (See Chapter 22 ∞ for more information on nursing care management of oxytocin induction.)

INTERPRETATION OF CST RESULTS

The CST is classified as follows:

- **Negative.** A negative CST shows three contractions of good quality lasting 40 or more seconds in 10 minutes without evidence of late decelerations. This is the desired result. It implies that the fetus can handle the hypoxic stress of uterine contractions.

- **Positive.** A positive CST shows repetitive persistent late decelerations with more than 50% of the contractions (Figure 16–8 ◉). This is not a desired result. The hypoxic stress of the uterine contraction causes a slowing of the FHR. The pattern will not improve and will most likely get worse with additional contractions.

- **Equivocal or suspicious.** An equivocal or suspicious test has nonpersistent late decelerations or decelerations associated with hyperstimulation (contraction frequency of every 2 minutes or duration of longer than 90 seconds). When this test result occurs, more information is needed.

CLINICAL APPLICATION

A negative CST implies that the placenta is functioning normally, fetal oxygenation is adequate, and the fetus will probably be able to withstand the stress of labor. If labor does not occur in the ensuing week, further testing is done.

A positive CST with a nonreactive NST presents evidence that the fetus will not likely withstand the stress of labor. Although a negative CST is reliable in predicting fetal status, a positive result needs to be verified. As many as one third of fetuses with positive CSTs may tolerate labor without any further signs of a nonreassuring fetal tracing (Varney et al., 2004). (See Table 16–5.)

NURSING MANAGEMENT

Ascertain the woman's understanding of the CST, the reasons for the test, and the possible results before the test begins. Written consent is required in some settings. In this case the certified nurse-midwife or physician is responsible for fully informing the woman about the test. Administer the CST, interpret the results, and report the findings to the certified nurse-midwife or physician and the pregnant woman. In some settings the presence of the certified nurse-midwife or physician is required since there is a risk of initiating labor or hypertonic uterine contractions. Throughout the procedure, perform critical assessments and provide continual reassurance to the woman and her support person.

◉ **FIGURE 16–8**

Example of a positive contraction stress test (CST). Repetitive late decelerations occur with each contraction. Note that there are no accelerations of FHR with three fetal movements (FM). The baseline FHR is 120 beats per minute. Uterine contractions (bottom half of strip) occurred four times in 12 minutes.

TABLE 16–5 ✤ Contraction Stress Test

Diagnostic Value	Results
Demonstrates reaction of FHR to stress of uterine contraction.	▪ **Negative test:** Stress of uterine contraction shows three contractions of good quality lasting 40 or more seconds in 10 minutes without evidence of late decelerations. ▪ **Positive test:** Stress of uterine contraction shows repetitive persistent late deceleration with more than 50% of the uterine contractions. ▪ **Equivocal or suspicious:** Nonpersistent late decelerations or decelerations associated with hyperstimulation.

positions and to identify adequate pockets of amniotic fluid. The skin is then cleaned with a povidone-iodine (Betadine) solution. The use of a local anesthesia at the needle insertion site is optional. A 22-gauge needle is then inserted into the uterine cavity, and amniotic fluid is withdrawn (Figure 16–9 ◉). After 15 to 20 mL of fluid has been removed, the needle is withdrawn and the site is assessed for streaming (movement of fluid), which is an indication of bleeding. The fetal heart rate and maternal vital signs are then assessed. Rh immune globulin is given to all Rh-negative women. The analysis of amniotic fluid provides valuable information about fetal status. Amniocentesis is a fairly simple procedure, although complications do occur rarely (less than 1% of cases). See "Clinical Skill 2–5: Assisting During Amniocentesis" for nursing interventions during amniocentesis in the Clinical Skills Manual as well as on the CD-ROM that accompanies this text. SKILLS

AMNIOTIC FLUID ANALYSIS

Amniocentesis is a procedure used to obtain amniotic fluid for testing. During an amniocentesis the physician scans the uterus using ultrasound to identify the fetal and placental

DIAGNOSTIC USES OF AMNIOCENTESIS

A number of studies can be performed on amniotic fluid. These tests can provide information about genetic disorders (see Chapter 7 ∞), fetal health, and fetal lung maturity.

◉ **FIGURE 16–9**

Amniocentesis. The woman is scanned by ultrasound to determine the placental site and to locate a pocket of amniotic fluid. Then the needle is inserted into the uterine cavity to withdraw amniotic fluid.

EVIDENCE-BASED NURSING

ULTRASOUND FOR FETAL ASSESSMENT IN EARLY PREGNANCY

Clinical Question (Problem)

Ultrasound is generally applied in pregnancy when maternal complications arise (e.g., bleeding) or when a fetus is suspected of being at risk for malformation or inappropriate growth. Because some pregnancies may result in adverse outcomes even without risk factors, it has been suggested that routine ultrasound could prove beneficial.

What are the advantages of early pregnancy ultrasound screening?

Evidence

An expert reviewer evaluated nine clinical trials for a systematic review. Study authors were contacted for additional information. The evidence supports routine ultrasound in early pregnancy for accurate assessment of gestational age, earlier detection of multiple pregnancies, and detection of clinically unsuspected fetal malformations at a time when termination of the pregnancy is an option.

The quality of ultrasound evaluation is dependent on the skill of the technician who conducts the ultrasound examination and the expertise of the professional interpreting the result. Mistakes may result in both false-positive and false-negative outcomes, so careful balancing of the risks and benefits of routine early ultrasound is necessary. When compared with risk-based ultrasound examinations, routine early ultrasound examination results in earlier diagnosis of twin pregnancies, a reduced incidence of the induction of labor for postterm pregnancy, and earlier recognition of fetal abnormalities in otherwise healthy pregnancies. Early detection of fetal abnormalities was associated with an increase in the rate of pregnancy terminations and a subsequent reduction in perinatal morbidity. No short- or long-term adverse events were identified in children as a result of prenatal exposure to ultrasound.

The benefits of early detection of twin pregnancies were not clear, as these studies did not demonstrate an associated improvement in fetal outcome. The optimal timing of the examination was not addressed. Earlier examination (less than 18 weeks' gestation) provided the most accurate assessment of fetal age, while later examination (18 to 22 weeks) resulted in better inspection of fetal anatomy. The financial costs of implementing routine early ultrasound examination may be a major consideration, particularly in developing countries.

Implications

Women who are pregnant should weigh the benefits of early ultrasound examination against the personal and financial costs. Educate women about what can be revealed by an early ultrasound examination, but caution them that early identification of some conditions does not necessarily translate into better outcomes. You can reassure the woman that early ultrasound will not harm her baby in either the short or long term. Early identification of fetal malformations is only of benefit if the mother intends to terminate the pregnancy if a defect is found.

Critical Thinking

How can you help pregnant women balance the personal costs and benefits of early ultrasound examination? What assessments might tell you that a woman would benefit from an early ultrasound examination?

Reference

Neilson, J. P. (2003). Ultrasound for fetal assessment in early pregnancy (Cochrane Review). In *The Cochrane Library*, Issue 4. Chichester, UK: John Wiley & Sons.

Evaluation of Fetal Health

Concentrations of certain substances in amniotic fluid provide information about the health status of the fetus. For example, the **triple test** (triple screen) assesses for appropriate levels of alpha-fetoprotein (AFP), human chorionic gonadotrophin (hCG), and unconjugated estriol (UE$_3$). The triple test is the most widely used test to screen for Down syndrome (trisomy 21), trisomy 18, and neural tube defects (NTDs). Although this test can be performed by analyzing the amniotic fluid, it is also commonly performed by drawing a sample of maternal blood (see Chapter 7 ∞). The **quadruple screen**, which adds measurement of the substance Diameric Inhibin-A, is a more sensitive and accurate detector of trisomy 21 and will replace the triple screen as the standard in the near future.

NURSING PRACTICE

When offering expectant parents the option of the triple test, clarify that the test is only used to screen for disorders and is not a diagnostic test. The triple test is accurate in detecting 60% of Down syndrome fetuses and 80% to 90% of fetuses affected with a neural tube defect. Of the women who screen positive (indicating a possible problem with the fetus), 90% will have an infant without any anomalies. Make sure the woman understands that the testing is typically offered to all pregnant women in most settings but is not mandatory.

Evaluation of Fetal Maturity

Because gestational age, birth weight, and the rate of development of organ systems do not necessarily correspond, amniotic fluid may also be analyzed to determine the maturity of the fetal lungs.

Lecithin/Sphingomyelin (L/S) Ratio. The alveoli of the lungs are lined with a substance called **surfactant**, which is composed of phospholipids. Surfactant lowers the surface tension of the alveoli when the newborn exhales. When a newborn with mature pulmonary function takes its first breath, a tremendously high pressure is needed to open the lungs. By lowering the alveolar surface tension, surfactant stabilizes the alveoli, and a certain amount of air always remains in the alveoli during expiration. Thus, when the infant exhales, the lungs do not collapse. An infant born before synthesis of surfactant is complete is unable to maintain lung stability. Each breath requires the same effort as the first. This results in underinflation of the lungs and the development of respiratory distress syndrome (RDS).

Fetal lung maturity can be ascertained by determining the **lecithin/sphingomyelin (L/S) ratio**; lecithin and sphingomyelin are two components of surfactant. Early in pregnancy the sphingomyelin concentration in amniotic fluid is greater than the concentration of lecithin, and so the L/S ratio is low (lecithin levels are low and sphingomyelin levels are high). At about 32 weeks' gestation, sphingomyelin levels begin to fall and the amount of lecithin begins to increase. By 35 weeks' gestation, an L/S ratio of 2:1 (also reported as 2.0) is usually achieved in the normal fetus. A 2:1 L/S ratio indicates that the risk of RDS is very low (Ross, 2002). Under certain conditions of stress (a physiologic problem in the mother, placenta, or fetus), the fetal lungs mature more rapidly.

Phosphatidylglycerol. **Phosphatidylglycerol (PG)** is another phospholipid in surfactant. PG is not present in the fetal lung fluid early in gestation. It appears when fetal lung maturity has been attained, at about 35 weeks' gestation. Since the presence of PG is associated with fetal lung maturity, when it is present the risk of RDS is low. PG determination is also useful in blood-contaminated specimens. Since PG is not present in blood or vaginal fluids, its presence is reliable in predicting lung maturity (Ross, 2002). See Table 16–6.

Lamellar Body Count. **Lamellar body count (LBC)** are present in amniotic fluid when phosphatidylglycerol (PG) is present (Jasper, 2004). When the LBC is over 35,000 counts/µL, probable lung maturity is assumed. The laboratory analysis for LBC is considerably less costly than tests discussed previously and can usually be performed at the acute care facility rather than a reference laboratory (Ross, 2002).

NURSING MANAGEMENT

Assist the physician during the amniocentesis and support the woman undergoing the procedure. Although the physi-

TABLE 16–6 ✤ Lecithin/Sphingomyelin (L/S) Ratio and Phosphatidylglycerol (PG)	
Diagnostic Value	**Results**
Provides information to help determine fetal lung maturity.	■ An L/S ratio of 2:1 and presence of PG correlate with 35 weeks' gestation. ■ An L/S ratio lower than 2:1, an absence of PG, or both, may indicate underinflation of lungs and an increased risk for development of respiratory distress syndrome.

cian has explained the procedure in advance so that the woman can give informed consent, the woman is likely to be apprehensive both about the amniocentesis itself and about the information it may reveal. She may become anxious during the procedure and need additional emotional support. Provide support by further clarifying the physician's instructions or explanations, by relieving the woman's physical discomfort when possible, and by responding verbally and physically to the woman's need for reassurance.

Obtain maternal blood pressure, temperature, pulse, and respirations, and FHR baseline data prior to the procedure and then monitor these parameters every 15 minutes during the procedure. Assist with the real-time ultrasound to assess needle position during the amniocentesis. Real-time ultrasound is used to identify fetal parts and locate pockets of amniotic fluid.

Following the amniocentesis, reiterate explanations given by the physician and provide opportunities for questions. Review the experience with the woman and explain self-care measures. Monitor the woman's blood pressure, pulse, and respirations, and the FHR. The woman's fundus is monitored with an external fetal heart monitor for 20 to 30 minutes after the amniocentesis. If the woman develops supine hypotension, initiate a treatment plan to increase venous return and cardiac output such as lying on her left side. The women's blood type and need for Rh immune globulin is determined. Prior to discharge the woman should understand the side effects that are to be reported to her primary care provider.

Reportable side effects of an amniocentesis include the following:

■ Unusual fetal hyperactivity or lack of movement

■ Vaginal discharge—clear drainage or bleeding

- Uterine contractions or abdominal pain
- Fever or chills

The woman is encouraged to engage in only light activity for 24 hours after amniocentesis to decrease uterine irritability. She is also encouraged to increase her fluid intake to increase uteroplacental circulation and thereby replace the amniotic fluid.

CHORIONIC VILLUS SAMPLING

Chorionic villus sampling (CVS) involves obtaining a small sample of chorionic villi from the developing placenta. CVS is performed in some medical centers for first-trimester diagnosis of genetic, metabolic, and deoxyribonucleic acid (DNA) studies. CVS can be performed either transabdominally or transcervically.

The advantages of this procedure are early diagnosis and short waiting time for results. Whereas amniocentesis is not done until at least 16 weeks' gestation, CVS is performed between 10 and 12 weeks. Risks of CVS include failure to obtain tissue, rupture of membranes, leakage of amniotic fluid, bleeding, intrauterine infection, maternal tissue contamination of the specimen, and

Rh alloimmunization. CVS testing has a higher rate of spontaneous abortion than amniocentesis (0.5% to 1%). Other complications include fetal limb defects and a low incidence of abnormalities of the fetal face and jaw (March of Dimes, 2003).

Because CVS testing is performed so early in pregnancy, it cannot detect neural tube defects. Women who desire testing for neural tube defects would need a triple or quadruple test after 15 weeks. This is a major disadvantage of the test since women with an abnormal MSAFP test indicating an increased risk of neural tube defects may require an amniocentesis, subjecting the fetus again to the risk of an invasive procedure.

NURSING PRACTICE

When explaining genetic testing options to expectant parents, inform the mother that even if a CVS shows no chromosomal abnormality, it cannot screen for neural tube defects. Women who have a normal CVS and an abnormal triple screen test should be offered amniocentesis. Women with risk factors for neural tube defects may want to consider amniocentesis instead of CVS since it screens for both types of disorders.

Critical Concept Review

LEARNING OBJECTIVES

CONCEPTS

LEARNING OBJECTIVES	CONCEPTS

Identify pertinent information to be discussed with the woman regarding her own assessment of fetal activity and methods of recording fetal activity.	1. Pertinent information to be discussed with the woman:
	  ■ The purpose of the assessment.
	  ■ How to complete the form.
	  ■ Whom to call with questions.
	  ■ What to report.
	2. Provide the opportunity for follow-up during each visit.

Identify indications and interpret findings for ultrasound examination during pregnancy.	1. Ultrasound offers a valuable means of assessing intrauterine fetal growth because the growth can be followed over a period of time. 2. It is noninvasive and painless. 3. It allows the certified nurse-midwife or physician to study the gestation serially. 4. It is nonradiating to both the woman and her fetus. 5. It has no known harmful effects.

LEARNING OBJECTIVES

CONCEPTS

Compare and contrast the procedure and information obtained from Doppler velocity, nonstress test, contraction stress test, and biophysical profile tests.	

1. Doppler blood flow studies are used to assess placental function and sufficiency.
   - It is noninvasive. The woman lies supine and the Doppler is placed on the abdomen.
2. A nonstress test is based on the knowledge that the FHR normally increases in response to fetal activity and to sound stimulation.
   - The woman is attached to an electronic fetal monitor for approximately 20 minutes. She is required to lie still during the test.
   - Desired result Is a reactive test.
3. A contraction stress test evaluates respiratory function of the placenta.
   - The woman is attached to an electronic fetal monitor and contractions are stimulated. This evaluates the ability of the fetus to handle contractions. The procedure may precipitate labor prematurely.
   - Desired result is a negative test.
4. A biophysical profile includes five variables:
   - Fetal breathing movement.
   - Fetal body movement.
   - Fetal tone.
   - Amniotic fluid volume.
   - Fetal heart rate reactivity.

   Biophysical profile is a combination of an ultrasound and a nonstress test to assess a fetus at risk for intrauterine compromise.

Discuss the use of amniocentesis as a diagnostic tool.	

1. Amniocentesis assesses amniotic fluid for the presence of genetic disorders, fetal health status, and evaluation of fetal maturity.

Describe the tests that can be done on amniotic fluid.	

1. The triple test and quadruple screen measure substances contained in the amniotic fluid that provide information regarding the presence of fetal anomalies such as neural tube defects and Down syndrome.
2. The lecithin/sphingomyelin ratio, presence of phosphatidylglycerol, and level of lamellar body counts can be assessed to determine fetal lung maturity.

Identify the advantages and disadvantages of chorionic villus sampling (CVS).	

1. Advantages:
   - Early detection of fetal disorders.
   - Decreased waiting time for results.
2. Disadvantages:
   - Increased risk of injury to fetus.
   - Inability to detect neural tube defects.
   - Potential for repeated invasive procedures.

CRITICAL THINKING IN ACTION

*View the **Critical Thinking in Action** video in Chapter 16 of the CD-ROM. Then, answer the questions that follow.*

Patricia Adams is a 20-year-old, married, G2, P0010 at 36 weeks' gestation with gestational diabetes. She presents to you during her prenatal visit with a complaint of decreased fetal movement for the "last day or so." Her OB history includes a 13 lb weight gain, hematocrit of 29%, diastolic BP ranging 80–96 mm Hg, and 1+ proteinuria. A 19-week ultrasound demonstrated no fetal anatomic defects. A hemoglobin A_1c at 23 weeks was 5.8%. Patricia has had weekly NST since 28 weeks' gestation. You place Patricia on the fetal monitor for a NST. You obtain vital signs of T 97°F, P 88, R 14, BP 130/88. After 30 minutes you observe that the fetal heart rate baseline is 160–165, long-term variability is decreased, and repetitive variable decelerations are occurring. No contractions are noted. The fetus is very active. You notify the physician of the fetal heart rate baseline and unsatisfactory NST. The physician orders a biophysical profile (BPP) for fetal well-being. You describe and explain the biophysical profile test to Patricia.

1. How would you describe and explain the biophysical profile test?
2. To heighten Patricia's awareness of fetal movement, how would you instruct her to do a daily fetal movement record (FMR)?
3. Explain when Patricia should contact her care provider.
4. Discuss the significance of fetal movement.
5. Explore factors that decrease fetal movements.

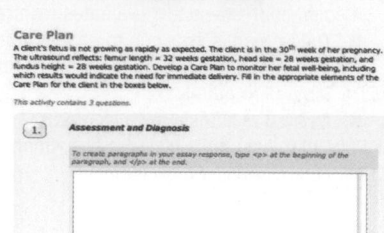

MEDIALINK

www.prenhall.com/london

■ NCLEX-RN® Review, case studies, and other interactive resources for this chapter can be found on the Companion Website at http://www.prenhall.com/london. Click on "Chapter 16" to select the activities for this chapter.

■ For animations, more NCLEX-RN® Review questions, and an audio glossary, access the accompanying CD-ROM in this textbook.

REFERENCES

Berghella, V., Talucci, M., & Desai, A. (2003). Does transvaginal sonographic measurement of cervical length before 14 weeks predict preterm delivery in high-risk pregnancies? *Ultrasound in Obstetrics and Gynecology, 21*(2), 140–144.

Gabbe, S. G., Niebyl, J. R., & Simpson, J. L. (2003). *Obstetrics: Normal and problem pregnancies pocket companion.* New York: Churchill Livingstone.

Jasper, M. L. (2004). Antepartum fetal assessment. In S. Mattson & J. E. Smith (Eds.), *Core cur-riculum for maternal-newborn nursing* (3rd ed., pp. 161–200). St. Louis, MO: Elsevier-Saunders.

March of Dimes. (2003). *Chorionic villus sampling.* Retrieved July 7, 2004, from http:// www. marchofdimes.com

Moses, S. (2003). *Family practice notebook: Fetal movement count.* Retrieved July 15, 2003, from http://www.fpnotebook.com/OB54.htm

Ross, G. (2002). Decreased laboratory testing for lecithin-to-sphingomyelin ratio and phos-phatidylglycerol after fetal lung maturity assessment from lamellar body count in amniotic fluid. *Journal of the American Osteopathic Association, 102*(8), 423–428.

Varney, H., Kriebs, J. M., & Gegor, C. L. (2004). *Varney's midwifery.* Boston: Jones & Bartlett.

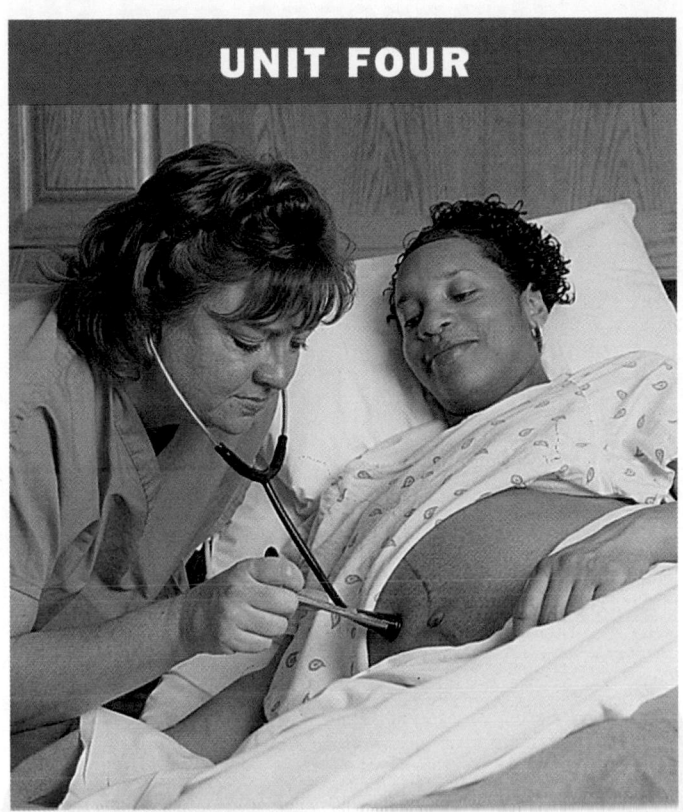

UNIT FOUR

Birth and the Family

Processes and Stages of Labor and Birth

I think experts refer to us as a blended family. I have two sons, ages 12 and 9, from a previous marriage. They live part-time with us and part-time with their father. My husband has a 15-year-old daughter who lives with her mother. Here I am, 6 months pregnant with our first child together. It has been quite the time, getting used to the idea of a baby and trying to include our children in the pregnancy. They have all heard the heartbeat and felt the baby move. My sons are pretty blasé about it. I didn't know how Jack's daughter would respond but she has been great. Maybe this new baby will help us all grow closer together. I sure hope so.

—Letetia, 34

LEARNING OBJECTIVES

- Examine the five critical factors that influence labor.
- Describe the physiology of labor.
- Discuss premonitory signs of labor.
- Differentiate between false and true labor.
- Describe the physiologic and psychologic changes occurring in each of the stages of labor.
- Summarize maternal systemic responses to labor.
- Explore fetal responses to labor.

MEDIALINK www.prenhall.com/london

CD-ROM

NCLEX-RN® Review
Animations:
    Rupturing Membranes
    Vaginal Birth
    Placenta Delivery
Videos:
    Fetal Lie
    First Stage of Labor and Transition
    Second Stage of Labor
    Third Stage of Labor
Audio Glossary

Companion Website

NCLEX-RN® Review
Case Study
Thinking Critically
MediaLink Applications:
    Case Study: Client in First Stage of Labor
    Care Plan Activity: Client in Uncomplicated Labor
    Care Plan Activity: Labor Progress

In the final weeks of pregnancy, both mother and baby begin to prepare for birth. The onset of labor begins a remarkable change in the relationship between the woman and her baby. In those hours and moments, the birth process may seem to carry all the power in the universe. The mother-to-be and her partner may feel stretched beyond their normal limits of concentration, purpose, endurance, and pain as they work to bring forth a precious new life.

This chapter focuses on the processes and stages of labor. Subsequent chapters describe intrapartum assessment and nursing care.

CRITICAL FACTORS IN LABOR

Five factors are important in the process of labor and birth: the passage, the fetus, the relationship between the passage and the fetus, the physiologic forces of labor, and the psychosocial considerations. Abnormalities that affect any component of these critical forces can alter the outcome of labor and jeopardize both the expectant woman and her baby. These factors are described in this section and summarized in Table 17–1. (Complications are discussed in Chapter 21. ∞)

THE BIRTH PASSAGE

The true pelvis, which forms the bony canal through which the fetus must pass, is divided into three sections: the inlet, the pelvic cavity (midpelvis), and

---

TABLE 17–1 ✤ Critical Factors in Labor

The birth passage
- Size of the pelvis (diameters of the pelvic inlet, midpelvis or pelvic cavity, and outlet)
- Type of pelvis (gynecoid, android, anthropoid, platypelloid, or a combination)
- Ability of the cervix to dilate and efface and ability of the vaginal canal and the external opening of the vagina (the introitus) to distend

The fetus
- Fetal head (size and presence of molding)
- Fetal attitude (flexion or extension of the fetal body and extremities)
- Fetal lie
- Fetal presentation (the part of the fetal body entering the pelvis first in a single- or multiple-gestation pregnancy)
- Placenta (implantation site)

The relationship between the passage and the fetus
- Engagement of fetal presenting part
- Station (location of fetal presenting part within the maternal pelvis)
- Fetal position (relationship of the presenting part to one of the four quadrants of the maternal pelvis)

Primary forces of labor
- Frequency, duration, and intensity of uterine contractions as the fetus moves through the birth passage
- Effectiveness of the maternal pushing effort
- Duration of labor

Psychosocial considerations
- Physical preparation for childbirth
- Sociocultural values and beliefs
- Previous childbirth experience
- Support from significant others
- Emotional status

● FIGURE 17–1

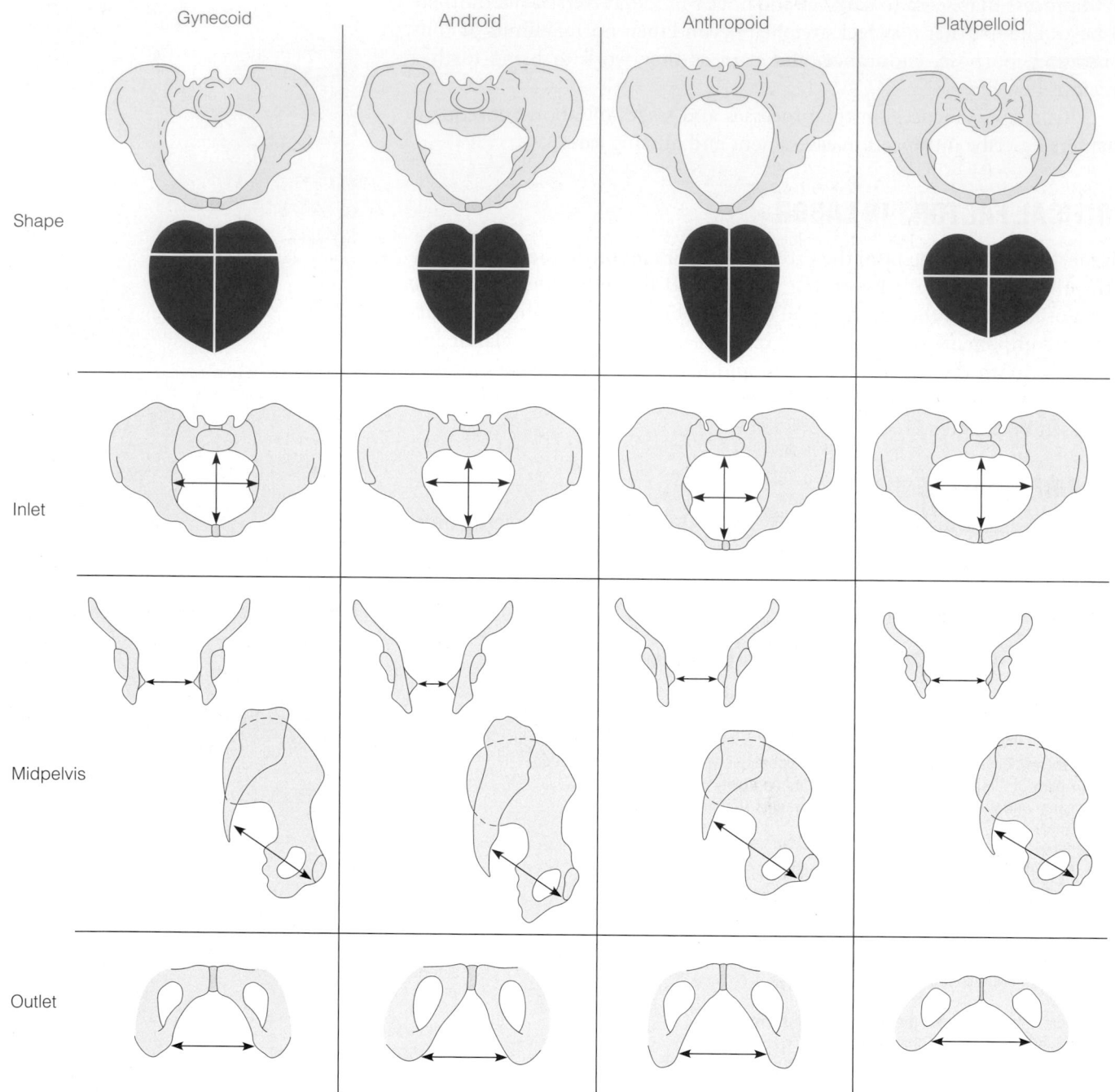

Comparison of Caldwell-Moloy pelvic types.

the outlet. (See Chapter 4 for discussion of the pelvis and Chapter 10 for assessment techniques. ∞)

The Caldwell-Moloy classification of pelvises is widely used to differentiate bony pelvis types. The four classic types of pelvis are *gynecoid, android, anthropoid,* and *platypelloid* (Caldwell & Moloy, 1933) (Figure 17–1 ●). The gynecoid, or female, pelvis is most common. All diameters of the gynecoid are adequate for childbirth. Implica-

tions of each type of pelvis for childbirth are summarized in Table 17–2.

THE FETUS

Fetal Head

The fetal skull (cranium) has three major parts: the face, the base of the skull, and the vault of the cranium (roof).

TABLE 17–2 ✦ Implications of Pelvic Type for Labor and Birth

Pelvic Type	Pertinent Characteristics	Implications for Birth
Gynecoid	Inlet rounded with all inlet diameters adequate Midpelvis diameters adequate with parallel side walls Outlet adequate	Favorable for vaginal birth
Android	Inlet heart-shaped, with short posterior sagittal diameter Midpelvis diameters reduced Outlet capacity reduced	Not favorable for vaginal birth Descent into pelvis is slow Fetal head enters pelvis in transverse or posterior position, with arrest of labor frequent
Anthropoid	Inlet oval in shape, with long anteroposterior diameter Midpelvis diameters adequate Outlet adequate	Favorable for vaginal birth
Platypelloid	Inlet oval in shape, with long transverse diameters Midpelvis diameters reduced Outlet capacity inadequate	Not favorable for vaginal birth Fetal head engages in transverse position Difficult descent through midpelvis Frequent delay of progress at outlet of pelvis

Note: Description of pelvic shape is exaggerated for easier comprehension.

The bones of the face and cranial base are well fused and essentially fixed. The base of the cranium is composed of the two temporal bones, each with a sphenoid and ethmoid bone. The bones composing the vault are the two frontal bones, the two parietal bones, and the occipital bone (Figure 17–2 ●). These bones are not fused, so this portion of the head can adjust in shape as the presenting part passes through the narrow portions of the pelvis. The cranial bones overlap under pressure of the powers of labor and the demands of the unyielding pelvis. This overlapping is called **molding**. Once the head (the least compressible and largest part of the fetus) has been born, the birth of the rest of the body is rarely delayed.

The **sutures** of the fetal skull are membranous spaces between the cranial bones. The intersections of the cranial sutures are called **fontanelles**. These sutures allow for molding of the fetal head and help the clinician to identify the position of the fetal head during vaginal examination. The important sutures of the cranium are as follows (see Figure 17–2):

- **Frontal (mitotic) suture:** located between the two frontal bones; becomes the anterior continuation of the sagittal suture
- **Sagittal suture:** located between the parietal bones; divides the skull into left and right halves; runs anteroposteriorly, connecting the two fontanelles
- **Coronal sutures:** located between the frontal and parietal bones; extend transversely left and right from the anterior fontanelle

- **Lambdoidal suture:** located between the two parietal bones and the occipital bone; extends transversely left and right from the posterior fontanelle

The anterior and posterior fontanelles are clinically useful (along with the sutures) in identifying the position of the

● FIGURE 17–2

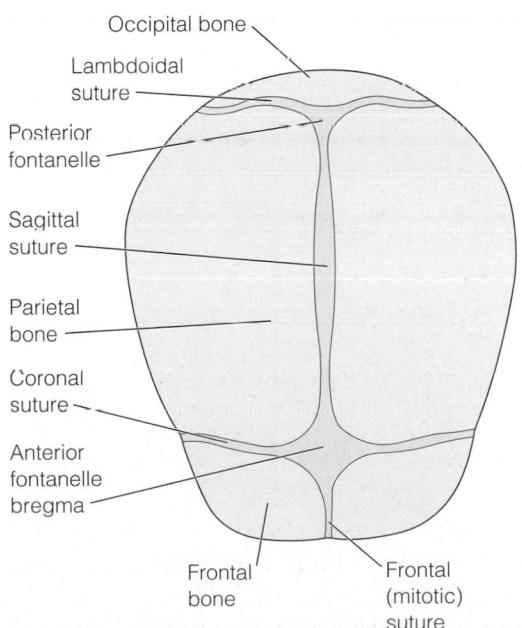

Superior view of the fetal skull.

● **FIGURE 17-3**

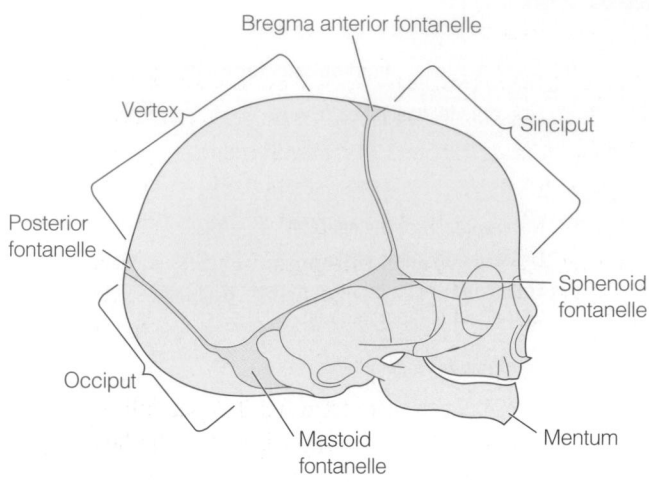

Lateral view of the fetal skull, identifying the landmarks that have significance during birth.

fetal head in the pelvis and in assessing the status of the newborn after birth. The anterior fontanelle is diamond shaped and measures about 2 by 3 cm. It permits growth of the brain by remaining unossified for as long as 18 months. The posterior fontanelle is much smaller and closes within 8 to 12 weeks after birth. It is shaped like a small triangle and marks the meeting point of the sagittal suture and the lambdoidal suture.

Following are several important landmarks of the fetal skull (Figure 17-3 ●):

- **Mentum:** fetal chin
- **Sinciput:** anterior area known as the brow

- **Bregma:** large diamond-shaped anterior fontanelle
- **Vertex:** area between the anterior and posterior fontanelles
- **Posterior fontanelle:** intersection between posterior cranial sutures
- **Occiput:** area of the fetal skull occupied by the occipital bone, beneath the posterior fontanelle

The diameters of the fetal skull vary considerably within normal limits. Some diameters shorten and others lengthen as the head is molded during labor. Fetal head diameters are measured between the various landmarks on the skull. For example, the suboccipitobregmatic diameter is the distance from the undersurface of the occiput to the center of the bregma, or anterior fontanelle. Typical fetal skull measurements are given in Figure 17-4 ●.

Fetal Attitude and Fetal Lie

Fetal attitude refers to the relation of the fetal parts to one another. The normal attitude of the fetus is one of moderate flexion of the head, flexion of the arms onto the chest, and flexion of the legs onto the abdomen (Figure 17-5 ●).

Fetal lie refers to the relationship of the cephalocaudal axis (spinal column) of the fetus to the cephalocaudal axis of the woman. The fetus may assume either a longitudinal or a transverse lie. A *longitudinal lie* occurs when the cephalocaudal axis of the fetus is parallel to the woman's spine. A *transverse lie* occurs when the cephalocaudal axis of the fetus is at a right angle to the woman's spine.

Fetal Presentation

Fetal presentation is determined by fetal lie and by the body part of the fetus that enters the pelvic passage first.

● **FIGURE 17-4**

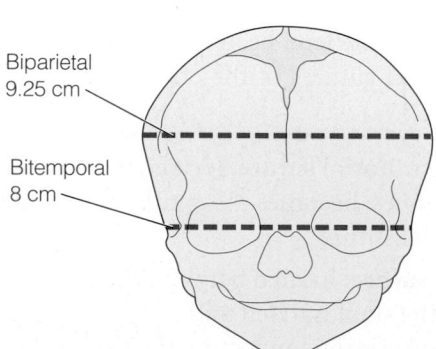

A, Typical anteroposterior diameters of the fetal skull. When the vertex of the fetus presents and the fetal head is flexed with the chin on the chest, the smallest anteroposterior diameter (suboccipitobregmatic) enters the birth canal. **B,** Transverse diameters of the fetal skull.

● **FIGURE 17–5**

Fetal attitude. The attitude (or relationship of body parts) of this fetus is normal. The head is flexed forward, with the chin almost resting on the chest. The arms and legs are flexed.

This portion of the fetus is referred to as the **presenting part**. Fetal presentation may be cephalic, breech, or shoulder. Cephalic presentation, in which the fetal head presents itself to the passage, occurs in approximately 97% of term births. When this presentation occurs, labor and birth are likely to proceed normally. Breech and shoulder presentations are associated with difficulties during labor, and labor does not proceed as expected; therefore, they are called **malpresentations** (see Chapter 21 for discussion ∞).

The cephalic presentation can be further classified according to the degree of flexion or extension of the fetal head (attitude).

■ In *vertex presentation,* the most common presentation, the fetal head is completely flexed onto the chest, and the smallest diameter of the fetal head (suboccipitobregmatic) presents to the maternal pelvis (Figure 17–6A ●). The occiput is the presenting part.

■ In *military presentation,* the fetal head is neither flexed nor extended. The occipitofrontal diameter presents to the maternal pelvis (Figure 17–6B ●); the top of the head is the presenting part.

■ In *brow presentation,* the fetal head is partially extended. The occipitomental diameter, the largest anteroposterior diameter, is presented to the maternal pelvis (Figure 17–6C ●); the sinciput is the presenting part (see Figure 17–3).

■ In *face presentation,* the fetal head is completely extended. The submentobregmatic diameter presents to the maternal pelvis (Figure 17–6D ●); the face is the presenting part.

Breech presentations occur in 3% of term births. These presentations are classified according to the attitude of the fetus's hips and knees. In all variations of the breech presentation, the sacrum is the landmark to be noted.

In *complete breech,* the fetal knees and hips are both flexed; the thighs are on the abdomen, and the calves are on

● **FIGURE 17–6**

| A | Suboccipitobregmatic diameter | B | Occipitofrontal diameter | C | Occipitomental diameter | D | Submentobregmatic diameter |

Cephalic presentation. **A,** Vertex presentation. Complete flexion of the head allows the suboccipitobregmatic diameter to present to the pelvis. **B,** Military (median vertex) presentation with no flexion or extension. The occipitofrontal diameter presents to the pelvis. **C,** Brow presentation. The fetal head is in partial (halfway) extension. The occipitomental diameter, which is the largest diameter of the fetal head, presents to the pelvis. **D,** Face presentation. The fetal head is in complete extension, and the submentobregmatic diameter presents to the pelvis.

the posterior aspect of the thighs. The buttocks and feet of the fetus present to the maternal pelvis. (Refer to Chapter 21, Figure 21–7. ∞)

In *frank breech*, the fetal hips are flexed, and the knees are extended. The buttocks of the fetus present to the maternal pelvis.

In *footling breech*, the fetal hips and legs are extended, and the feet of the fetus present to the maternal pelvis. In a single footling, one foot presents; in a double footling, both feet present.

A shoulder presentation is also called a *transverse lie*. Most frequently the shoulder is the presenting part and the acromion process of the scapula is the landmark to be noted. However, the fetal arm, back, abdomen, or side may present in a transverse lie. (See Chapter 21. ∞)

RELATIONSHIP OF MATERNAL PELVIS AND PRESENTING PART

Engagement

Engagement of the presenting part occurs when the largest diameter of the presenting part reaches or passes through the pelvic inlet (Figure 17–7 ◉). Engagement can be determined by vaginal examination. In primigravidas, engagement occurs approximately 2 weeks before term. Multiparas, however, may experience engagement several weeks before the onset of labor or during the process of labor. Engagement confirms the adequacy of the pelvic inlet. Engagement does not, however, indicate whether the midpelvis and outlet are also adequate.

Station

Station refers to the relationship of the presenting part to an imaginary line drawn between the ischial spines of the maternal pelvis. In a normal pelvis, the ischial spines mark the narrowest diameter through which the fetus must pass. These spines are not sharp protrusions that harm the fetus but blunted prominences at the midpelvis. The ischial spines as a landmark have been designated as zero station (Figure 17–8 ◉). If the presenting part is higher than the ischial spines, a negative number is assigned, noting centimeters above zero station. Positive numbers indicate that the presenting part has passed the ischial spines. Station −5 is at the pelvic inlet, and station +4 is at the outlet. If

◉ **FIGURE 17–7**

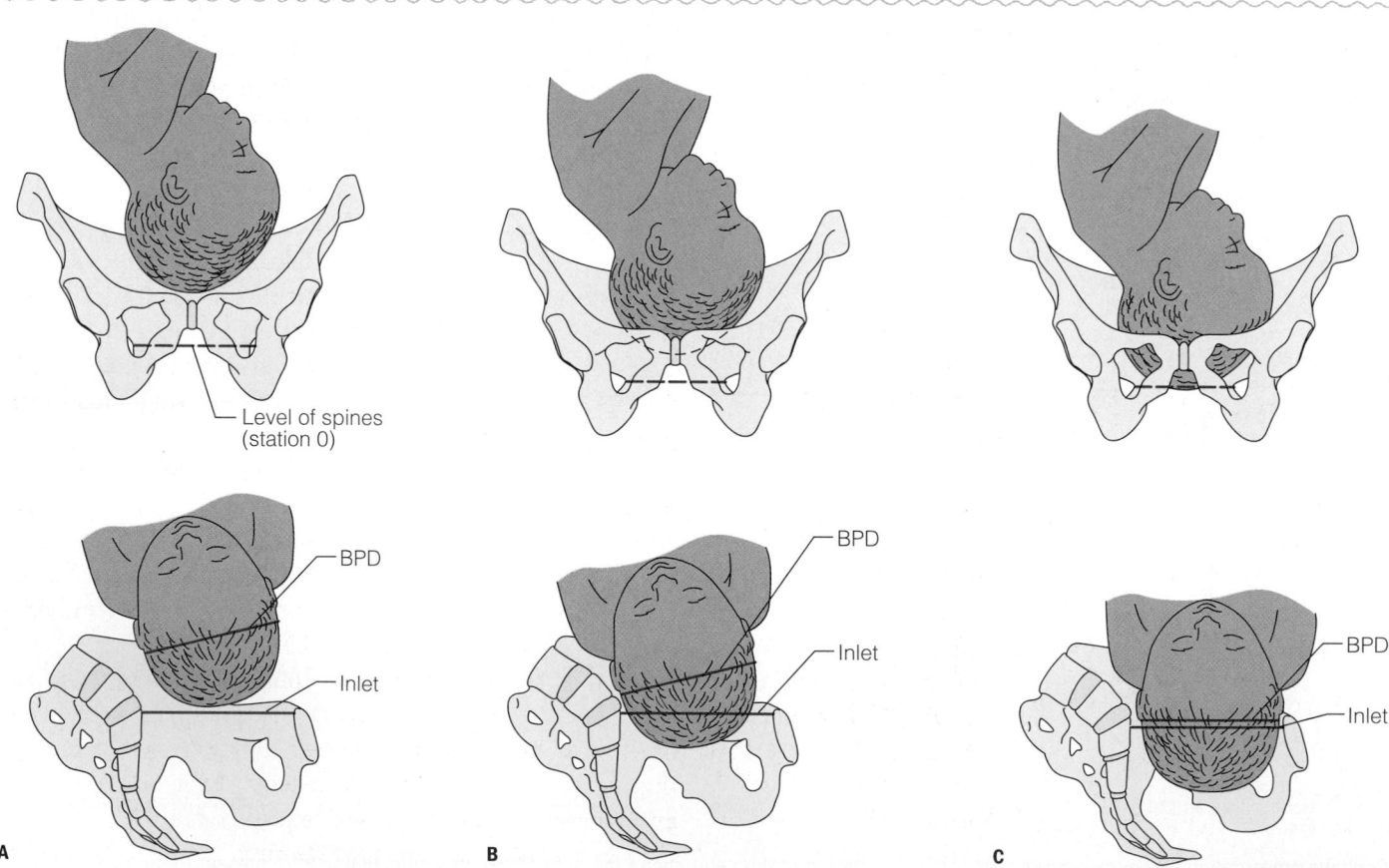

Process of engagement in cephalic presentation. **A,** Floating. The fetal head is directed down toward the pelvis but can still easily move away from the inlet. **B,** Dipping. The fetal head dips into the inlet but can be moved away by exerting pressure on the fetus. **C,** Engaged. The biparietal diameter (BPD) of the fetal head is in the inlet of the pelvis. In most instances the presenting part (occiput) is at the level of the ischial spines (zero station).

● FIGURE 17–8

cm
−5
−4
−3
−2
−1
0 ←→ Spine
+1
+2
+3
+4
+5

Measuring the station of the fetal head while it is descending. In this view the station is −2/−3.

the presenting part can be seen at the woman's perineum, birth is imminent. During labor the presenting part should move progressively from the negative stations to the mid-pelvis at zero station and into the positive stations. If the presenting part fails to descend in the presence of strong contractions, there may be disproportion between the maternal pelvis and fetal presenting part.

Fetal Position

Fetal position refers to the relationship of a designated landmark on the presenting fetal part to the front, sides, or back of the maternal pelvis. The landmark on the fetal presenting part is related to four imaginary quadrants of the pelvis: left anterior, right anterior, left posterior, and right posterior. These quadrants designate whether the presenting part is directed toward the front, back, left, or right of the passage. The landmark chosen for vertex presentations is the occiput, and the landmark for face presentations is the mentum. In breech presentations the sacrum is the designated landmark, and the acromion process on the scapula is the landmark in shoulder presentations. If the landmark is directed toward the side of the pelvis, fetal position is designated as *transverse*, rather than anterior or

posterior. Three notations are used to describe the fetal position:

1. Right (R) or left (L) side of the maternal pelvis
2. The landmark of the fetal presenting part: occiput (O), mentum (M), sacrum (S), or acromion process (A)
3. Anterior (A), posterior (P), or transverse (T), depending on whether the landmark is in the front, back, or side of the pelvis

The abbreviations of these notations help the health care team communicate the fetal position. Thus when the fetal occiput is directed toward the back and to the left of the birth passage, the abbreviation used is LOP (left occiput posterior). The term *dorsal* (D) is used when denoting the fetal position in a transverse lie; it refers to the fetal back. For example, RADA indicates that the acromion process of the scapula is directed toward the woman's right, and the fetus's back is anterior. The most frequently occurring positions are illustrated in Figure 17–9 ●. The most common fetal position is occiput anterior. When this position occurs, labor and birth are likely to proceed normally. Positions other than occiput anterior are more frequently associated with problems during labor; therefore, they are called *malpositions*. (See Chapter 21. ∞)

Assessment techniques to determine fetal position include inspection and palpation of the maternal abdomen and vaginal examination. They are discussed in Chapter 18. ∞

THE PHYSIOLOGIC FORCES OF LABOR

Primary and secondary forces work together to achieve birth of the fetus, the fetal membranes, and the placenta. The *primary force* is uterine muscular contractions, which cause the complete effacement and dilatation of the cervix. The *secondary force* is the use of abdominal muscles to push during the second stage of labor. The pushing adds to the primary force after full dilatation.

In labor, uterine contractions are rhythmic but intermittent. Between contractions a period of relaxation occurs. This allows uterine muscles to rest and provides relief for the laboring woman. It also restores uteroplacental circulation, which is important to fetal oxygenation and adequate circulation in the uterine blood vessels.

Each contraction has three phases: (1) *increment*, the building up of the contraction (the longest phase); (2) *acme*, or the peak of the contraction; and (3) *decrement*, or the letting up of the contraction. The terms *frequency, duration, and intensity* are used to describe uterine contractions during labor. **Frequency** refers to the time between the beginning of one contraction and the beginning of the next contraction. **Duration** is measured from the beginning of a contraction to the completion of that same contraction (Figure 17–10 ●). **Intensity** refers to the strength of the

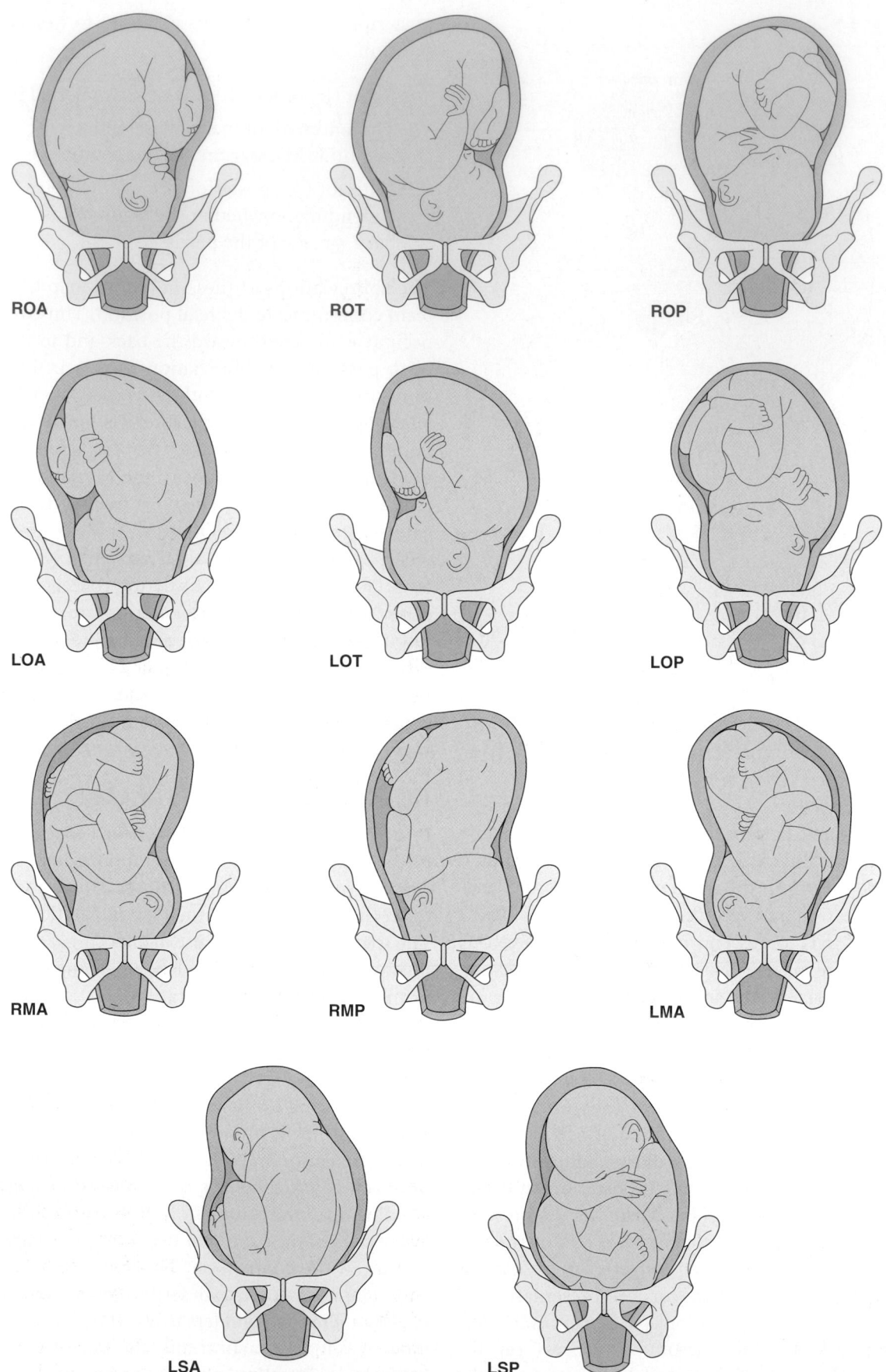

ROA ROT ROP

LOA LOT LOP

RMA RMP LMA

LSA LSP

Categories of presentation.

● FIGURE 17–10

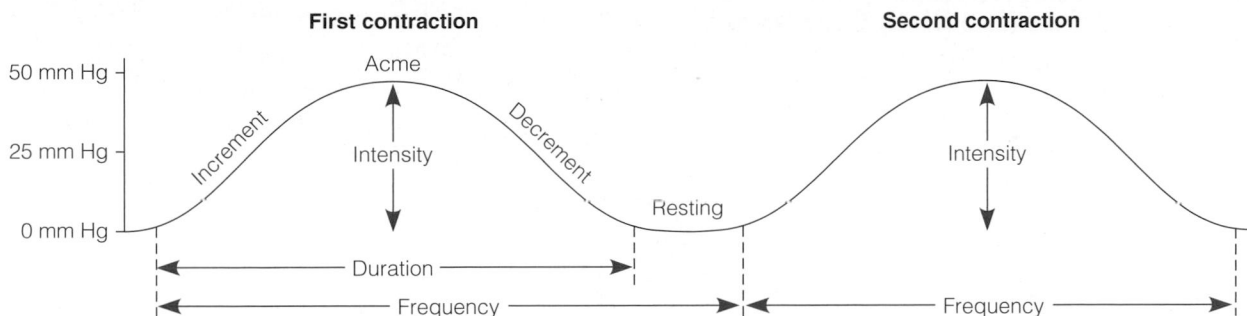

Characteristics of uterine contractions.

contraction during acme. In most instances, intensity is estimated by palpating the uterine fundus during a contraction, but it may be measured directly with an intrauterine catheter. When estimating intensity by palpation, the nurse determines whether it is mild, moderate, or strong by judging the amount of indentability of the uterine wall during the acme of a contraction. If the uterine wall can be indented easily, the contraction is considered mild. Strong intensity exists when the uterine wall cannot be indented. Moderate intensity falls somewhere between. When intensity is measured with an intrauterine catheter, the normal resting pressure in the uterus (between contractions) averages 10 to 12 mm Hg. During acme the intensity ranges from 25 to 40 mm Hg in early labor, 50 to 70 mm Hg in active labor, 70 to 90 mm Hg during transition, and 70 to 100 mm Hg while the woman is pushing in the second stage (Varney, Kriebs, & Gegor, 2004). (See Chapter 18 for further discussion of assessment techniques. ∞)

At the beginning of labor, contractions are usually mild, last about 30 seconds, and occur about every 5 to 7 minutes. As labor progresses, the duration of contractions increases to about 60 seconds, intensity increases, and frequency is every 2 to 3 minutes. Contractions are involuntary; the laboring woman cannot control their duration, frequency, or intensity.

After the cervix is completely dilated, the maternal abdominal muscles contract as the woman pushes. This pushing action (called *bearing down*) aids in the expulsion of the fetus and placenta. If the cervix is not completely dilated, however, bearing down can cause cervical edema (which retards dilatation), possible tearing and bruising of the cervix, and maternal exhaustion.

PSYCHOSOCIAL CONSIDERATIONS

The final critical factor influencing labor outcome is the parents' psychosocial readiness. Similar psychosocial factors affect the mother and the father. Both are making a transition to a new role, and both have expectations of themselves during the labor and birth experience.

Although many expectant mothers and fathers attend childbirth preparation classes, they still tend to be concerned about what labor will be like, whether they will be able to perform the way they expect, whether the discomfort and pain will be more than the mother expects or can cope with, and whether the father can provide helpful support. Every woman is uncertain about what her labor will be like. A woman approaching her first labor faces a totally new experience, whereas the woman who has given birth before knows that each labor is unique and different. Most women wonder if they will live up to their expectations for themselves; whether they will be injured through laceration, episiotomy, or cesarean incision; and whether loved ones will be supportive. They must also deal with concerns about loss of control of body functions, emotional responses to an unfamiliar situation, and reactions to the pain associated with labor.

Various factors influence a woman's reaction to the physical and emotional challenge of labor (Table 17–3). Her accomplishment of the tasks of pregnancy, usual coping mechanisms in response to stressful life events, support system, preparation for childbirth, and cultural influences are all significant factors.

Pregnant women mentally prepare for labor through meaningful actions and imaginary rehearsal. The actions frequently consist of "nesting behavior" (housecleaning, decorating the nursery) and a "psyching up" for the labor, which varies depending on the woman's self-confidence, self-esteem, and previous experiences with stress. Specific actions to prepare for labor may focus on becoming better informed and prepared. Just as a woman tries on the maternal role during pregnancy, fantasizing about labor seems to help her understand and become better prepared for it. Fantasies about the excitement of the baby's birth and the sharing of the experience are positive forms of preparation.

TABLE 17–3 ✤ Factors Associated with a Positive Birth Experience

Motivation for the pregnancy

Attendance at childbirth education classes

A sense of competence or mastery

Self-confidence and self-esteem

Positive relationship with mate

Perception of maintaining control during labor

Support from mate or other person during labor

Not being left alone in labor

Trust in the medical and nursing staff

Having personal control of breathing patterns, comfort measures

Choosing a physician or certified nurse-midwife who has a similar philosophy of care

Receiving clear information regarding procedures

COMPLEMENTARY CARE

MUSIC DURING CHILDBIRTH

The therapeutic use of music to help with pain management is becoming increasingly popular. Browning (2001) conducted a study with a group of primiparas to determine the value of music as a tool in reducing the pain of labor and birth. During their pregnancy, study participants chose preferred music and listened to it daily. They also received information about focused listening. During labor all the women used the music to help distract themselves from the pain or from their current situation, and all of them found that the music assisted with relaxation.

The following suggestions are useful in using music in labor (Browning, 2001):

1. Have the woman select the music herself, preferably during pregnancy.
2. Have her listen to it daily when she is in a relaxed state. That way she will begin associating the music with a pleasant activity and will develop a conditioned response to it in labor.
3. Several different tapes should be made to provide variety and avoid boredom during labor.
4. Make a special tape of music that has particular significance for the couple and use it during the birth. Consider having lullabies on the other side of the tape. These can be played for the newborn after birth.
5. Let the mother's response to the music be the guide to its use.

Many women fear the pain of contractions. They not only see the pain as threatening but also associate it with a loss of control over their bodies and emotions. It is important to realize that the discomfort and stresses of labor are an expected part of the process. Assurances that labor is progressing normally can go a long way toward reducing anxiety and thereby reducing pain. Women are likely to feel empowered and better able to cope with labor if they recognize that maintaining control is not important or perhaps even possible. A wide variety of coping techniques to assist both the laboring woman and her partner are discussed in Chapter 19 and Chapter 20. ∞ The laboring woman's support system may also influence the course of labor and birth. Although some women prefer not to have a support person or family member with them, for many women the presence of the father and other significant persons (especially the nurse) tends to have a positive effect. A labor partner's presence at the bedside provides a means to enhance communication and to demonstrate feelings of love. Communication needs may include talking and the use of affectionate and understanding words from the partner. Showing love may take the form of holding hands, hugging, or touching.

How the woman views the birth experience in hindsight may have implications for mothering behaviors. It appears that any activities by the expectant mother or by healthcare providers that enhance the birth experience are beneficial to the mother-baby connection. The father's experience of childbirth and his opportunities for bonding may have important implications for fathering as well.

THE PHYSIOLOGY OF LABOR

POSSIBLE CAUSES OF LABOR ONSET

The process of labor usually begins between the 38th and the 42nd week of gestation, when the fetus is mature and ready for birth. The exact cause of labor onset is not clearly understood. However, some important aspects have been identified: progesterone relaxes smooth muscle tissue, estrogen stimulates uterine muscle contractions, and connective tissue loosens to permit the softening, thinning, and eventual opening of the cervix (Blackburn, 2003). Currently, researchers are focusing on several promising areas of research about labor onset.

Progesterone Withdrawal Hypothesis

Progesterone, produced by the placenta, relaxes uterine smooth muscle by interfering with the conduction of impulses from one cell to the next. During pregnancy, progesterone exerts a quieting effect and the uterus generally does not have coordinated contractions. Toward the end of gestation, biochemical changes decrease the availability of progesterone to myometrial cells and may be associated with an antiprogestin that inhibits the relaxant effect but allows other progesterone actions such as lactogenesis. With the decreased availability of progesterone, estrogen is better able to stimulate contractions (Blackburn, 2003).

Prostaglandin Hypothesis

Although the exact relationship between prostaglandin and the onset of labor is not yet known, the effect is clinically demonstrated by the successful induction of labor after vaginal application of prostaglandin E. Preterm labor may be stopped by using an inhibitor of prostaglandin synthesis (Meadows, Eis, Brockman, & Myatt, 2003).

The amnion and decidua are the focus of research on the source of prostaglandins. Once prostaglandin is produced, stimuli for its synthesis may include rising levels of estrogen, decreased availability of progesterone, and increased levels of oxytocin, platelet-activating factor, and endothelin-1 (Pressman, Cavanaugh, & Woods, 2002; Rabl, Joura, Yucel, & Egarter, 2002).

Corticotropin-Releasing Hormone

Corticotropin-releasing hormone (CRH) has a possible role in labor onset. It increases during pregnancy, with a sharp increase at term. Plasma CRH increases prior to preterm labor, and CRH levels are elevated in multiple gestation. CRH is also known to stimulate the synthesis of prostaglandin F and prostaglandin E by amnion cells (McGrath & Smith, 2001).

MYOMETRIAL ACTIVITY

In true labor the muscles of the upper uterine segment shorten and exert a longitudinal pull on the cervix with each contraction, causing effacement. **Effacement** is the drawing up of the internal os and the cervical canal into the side walls of the uterus. The cervix changes progressively from a long, thick structure to one that is tissue-paper thin (Figure 17–11 ⦿). In primigravidas, effacement usually occurs before dilatation.

The uterus elongates with each contraction, decreasing the horizontal diameter. This elongation causes a

⦿ **FIGURE 17–11**

Effacement of the cervix in the primigravida. **A,** Beginning of labor. There is no cervical effacement or dilatation. The fetal head is cushioned by amniotic fluid. **B,** Beginning cervical effacement. As the cervix begins to efface, more amniotic fluid collects below the fetal head. **C,** Cervix about one half effaced and slightly dilated. The increasing amount of amniotic fluid exerts hydrostatic pressure. **D,** Complete effacement and dilatation.

straightening of the fetal body, pressing the upper portion against the fundus and thrusting the presenting part down toward the lower uterine segment and the cervix. The pressure exerted by the fetus is called the *fetal axis pressure*. As the uterus elongates, the longitudinal muscle fibers are pulled upward over the presenting part. This action and the hydrostatic pressure of the fetal membranes cause cervical dilatation. The cervical os and cervical canal widen from less than 1 cm to approximately 10 cm, allowing birth of the fetus. When the cervix is completely dilated and retracted up into the lower uterine segment, it can no longer be palpated. At the same time, the round ligament pulls the fundus forward, aligning the fetus with the bony pelvis.

MUSCULATURE CHANGES IN THE PELVIC FLOOR

The levator ani muscle and fascia of the pelvic floor draw the rectum and vagina upward and forward with each contraction, along the curve of the pelvic floor. As the fetal head descends to the pelvic floor, the pressure of the presenting part causes the perineal structure, which was once 5 cm in thickness, to thin to less than 1 cm. The anus everts, exposing the interior rectal wall as the fetal head descends forward (Cunningham, Leveno, Bloom et al., 2005).

PREMONITORY SIGNS OF LABOR

Most primigravidas and many multiparas experience the following signs and symptoms of impending labor.

Lightening

Lightening describes the effects that occur when the fetus begins to settle into the pelvic inlet (engagement). With fetal descent the uterus moves downward, and the fundus no longer presses on the diaphragm, which allows breathing to become easier. However, with increased downward pressure of the presenting part, the woman may notice the following:

- Leg cramps or pains due to pressure on the nerves that pass through the obturator foramen in the pelvis
- Increased pelvic pressure
- Increased venous stasis, leading to edema in the lower extremities
- Increased vaginal secretions resulting from congestion of the vaginal mucous membranes

Braxton Hicks Contractions

Before the onset of labor, *Braxton Hicks contractions* (the irregular, intermittent contractions that have been occurring throughout the pregnancy) may become uncomfortable. The pain seems to be focused in the abdomen and groin but may feel like the "drawing" sensations experienced by some women with dysmenorrhea. When these contractions are strong enough for the woman to believe she is in labor, she is said to be in *false labor*. False labor is uncomfortable and may be exhausting. Since the contractions can be fairly regular, the woman has no way of knowing if they are true labor.

Cervical Changes

Considerable change occurs in the cervix during the prenatal and intrapartal period. At the beginning of pregnancy, the cervix is rigid and firm, and it must soften so it can stretch and dilate to allow the fetus passage. This softening of the cervix is called *ripening*.

As term approaches, collagen fibers in the cervix are broken down by certain enzymes. As the fibers change, their ability to bind together decreases, while the water content of the cervix increases. All these changes result in a weakening and softening of the cervix.

Bloody Show

During pregnancy, cervical secretions accumulate in the cervical canal to form a barrier called a *mucous plug*. With softening and effacement of the cervix, the mucous plug is often expelled, resulting in a small amount of blood loss from the exposed cervical capillaries. The resulting pink-tinged secretions are called **bloody show**. Bloody show is considered a sign that labor will begin within 24 to 48 hours. Vaginal examination that includes manipulation of the cervix may also result in a blood-tinged discharge, which may be confused with bloody show.

Rupture of Membranes

In about 12% of women at term, the amniotic membranes rupture before the onset of labor. This is called *rupture of membranes (ROM)*. After the membranes rupture, 80% of these women experience onset of labor within 24 hours. If membranes rupture and labor does not begin spontaneously within 12 to 24 hours, labor may be induced to decrease the risk of infection. Labor is induced only if the pregnancy is near term (Varney et al., 2004).

When the membranes rupture, the amniotic fluid may be expelled in large amounts. If engagement has not occurred, there is danger of the umbilical cord washing out with the fluid (prolapsed cord). In addition the open pathway into the uterus increases the risk of infection. Because of these risks, when the membranes rupture, the woman is advised to call her certified nurse-midwife or physician and proceed to the hospital or birthing center. In some instances the fluid is expelled in small amounts and may be confused with episodes of urinary incontinence associated with urinary urgency, coughing, or sneezing. The discharge should be checked to determine its source and the appropriate action. (See Chapter 18 for assessment techniques. ∞)

MEDIALINK Animation: Rupturing Membranes

Sudden Burst of Energy

Some women report a sudden burst of energy approximately 24 to 48 hours before labor. The cause of the energy spurt is unknown. In prenatal teaching it is important to warn prospective mothers not to overexert themselves during this energy burst to avoid being overtired when labor begins.

NURSING PRACTICE

Encourage expectant mothers who experience a sudden burst of energy to eat small, frequent nutritious meals during this period, and to rest. Encourage the pregnant woman to have her significant other or a friend do chores and activities that she feels are essential to complete before the baby arrives.

Other Signs

Additional premonitory signs include the following:

- Weight loss of 1 to 3 lb resulting from fluid loss and electrolyte shifts produced by changes in estrogen and progesterone levels
- Diarrhea, indigestion, or nausea and vomiting just before onset of labor

The causes of these signs are unknown.

DIFFERENCES BETWEEN TRUE AND FALSE LABOR

The contractions of true labor produce progressive dilatation and effacement of the cervix. They occur regularly and increase in frequency, duration, and intensity. The discomfort of true labor contractions usually starts in the back and radiates around to the abdomen. The pain is not relieved by ambulation (in fact, walking may intensify the pain).

The contractions of false labor do not produce progressive cervical effacement and dilatation. Classically, they are irregular and do not increase in frequency, duration, and intensity. The contractions may be perceived as a hardening or "balling up" without discomfort, or discomfort may occur mainly in the lower abdomen and groin. The discomfort may be relieved by ambulation, changes of position, drinking a large amount of water, or a warm shower or tub bath (Varney et al., 2004). Many times the only way to differentiate accurately between true and false labor is to assess dilatation. The woman must feel free to come in for accurate assessment of labor and should be counseled not to feel foolish if the labor is false. She can be reassured that false labor is common and that it often cannot be distinguished from true labor except by vaginal examination (Table 17–4).

TABLE 17–4 ✣ Comparison of True and False Labor

True Labor	False Labor
Contractions occur at regular intervals.	Contractions are irregular.
Interval between contractions gradually shortens.	Usually no change.
Contractions increase in duration and intensity.	Usually no change.
Discomfort begins in back and radiates around to abdomen.	Discomfort is usually in abdomen.
Intensity usually increases with walking.	Walking has no effect on or lessens contractions.
Cervical dilatation and effacement are progressive.	No change.

STAGES OF LABOR AND BIRTH

The labor process is divided into phases and stages of labor. These represent theoretic separations in the process. A laboring woman does not usually experience distinct differences from one stage to the next.

The *first stage* begins with the onset of true labor and ends when the cervix is completely dilated to 10 cm. The *second stage* begins with complete dilatation and ends with the birth of the baby. The *third stage* begins with the birth of the baby and ends with the expulsion of the placenta. Some clinicians identify a *fourth stage*. During this stage, which lasts 1 to 4 hours after expulsion of the placenta, the uterus contracts to control bleeding at the placental site (Varney et al., 2004).

FIRST STAGE

The first stage of labor is divided into the *latent, active,* and *transition* phases. Each phase of labor is characterized by physical and psychologic changes.

Latent Phase

The *latent phase* starts with the beginning of regular contractions, which are usually mild. The woman feels able to cope with the discomfort. She may be relieved that labor has finally started. Although she may be anxious, she is able to recognize and express those feelings of anxiety. The woman is often talkative and smiling and is eager to talk about herself and answer questions. Excitement is high, and her partner or other support person is often as elated as she is.

Uterine contractions become established during the latent phase and increase in frequency, duration, and intensity.

They may start as mild contractions lasting 15 to 20 seconds with a frequency of 10 to 20 minutes and progress to moderate ones lasting 30 to 40 seconds with a frequency of 5 to 7 minutes. As the cervix begins to dilate, it also effaces, although little or no fetal descent is evident. For a woman in her first labor (nullipara), the latent (or early) phase of the first stage of labor averages 8.6 hours but should not exceed 20 hours. The latent phase in multiparas averages 5.3 hours but should not exceed 14 hours.

At the beginning of labor, the amniotic membranes bulge through the cervix in the shape of a cone. **Spontaneous rupture of membranes (SROM)** generally occurs at the height of an intense contraction with a gush of fluid out of the vagina. In many instances the membranes are ruptured by the certified nurse-midwife or physician, using an instrument called an *amnihook*. This procedure is called *amniotomy*, or **artificial rupture of membranes (AROM)**.

Active Phase

When a woman enters the early *active phase*, her anxiety tends to increase as she senses the intensification of contractions and pain. She begins to fear a loss of control and may use a variety of coping mechanisms. Some women show decreased ability to cope and a sense of helplessness. Women who have support people and family available may feel greater satisfaction and less anxiety than those without support. During this phase the cervix dilates from about 3 to 4 cm, to 8 cm. Fetal descent is progressive. Cervical dilatation averages 1.2 cm/hr in nulliparas and 1.5 cm/hr in multiparas.

Transition Phase

The *transition phase* is the last part of the first stage of labor. When the woman enters transition, she may show significant anxiety. She becomes acutely aware of the increasing force and intensity of the contractions. She may become restless, frequently changing position. By the time the woman enters the transition phase, she is inner directed and often tired. She may fear being left alone at the same time the support person may be feeling the need for a break. The nurse should reassure the woman that she will not be left alone. It is important to be available as relief support at this time and to keep the woman informed about where her labor support people are, if they leave the room.

During the active and transition phases, contractions become more frequent and longer in duration, and they increase in intensity. By the end of the active phase, contractions have a frequency of 2 to 3 minutes, duration of 60 seconds, and strong intensity. During transition, contractions have a frequency of about every 2 minutes, duration of 60 to 90 seconds, and strong intensity. Cervical dilatation slows as it progresses from 8 to 10 cm, and the rate of fetal descent dramatically increases. The average

COMPLEMENTARY CARE

VISUALIZATION FOR CHILDBIRTH

Visualization uses the power of the mind to influence psychologic and physiologic states. Guided imagery is a specific form of visualization that uses a leader or audiotape to paint a picture in the mind of a pleasant scene that stimulates natural healing responses, alleviates anxiety, promotes relaxation, or brings about changes in attitude and behavior. For example, visualization can prepare a pregnant woman to handle the different stages of labor and birth. During pregnancy a woman can imagine her unborn baby, sleeping and floating inside of her. During the early stage of labor, a woman can imagine her labor contractions as hugs to the baby or waves in the ocean crashing to shore (Kilson, 2002). The calm in between waves can be used as analogies of rest for the laboring woman and unborn baby. In the second stage of labor, images of a rose bud blossoming into a flower can be used to assist cervical dilatation. Images of a playground slide can help in bringing the baby down, crowning, and the actual birth itself. The third stage of labor is also receptive to visualization techniques that help the mother expel the placenta while relaxing and regaining control.

Many benefits of visualization are a direct result of decreased stress. Deep relaxation counters the effects of stress by arousing the parasympathetic nervous system, resulting in decreases in heart rate, respiratory rate, oxygen consumption, blood pressure, muscle tension, and gastric acidity.

rate of descent is 1.6 cm/hr and at least 1 cm/hr in nulliparas; the average rate is 5.4 cm/hr and at least 2.1 cm/hr in multiparas. The transition phase does not usually last longer than 3 hours for nulliparas or longer than 1 hour for multiparas.

As dilatation approaches 10 cm, the woman may feel increased rectal pressure and an uncontrollable desire to bear down, the amount of bloody show may increase, and the membranes may rupture (if it has not already occurred). The woman may also fear that she will be "torn open" or "split apart" by the force of the contractions. With the peak of a contraction, she may experience a sensation of pressure so great that it seems to her that her abdomen will burst open with the force. The nurse should inform the woman that what she is feeling is normal. The woman may doubt her ability to cope with labor and may become apprehensive, irritable, and withdrawn. She may be terrified of being left alone, though she does not want anyone to talk to or touch her. However, with the next contraction she may ask for verbal and physical support. Other characteristics of this phase may include the following:

- Increasing bloody show
- Hyperventilation, as the woman increases her breathing rate

- Generalized discomfort, including low backache, shaking and cramping in legs, and increased sensitivity to touch
- Increased need for partner's or nurse's presence and support
- Restlessness
- Increased apprehension and irritability
- Difficulty understanding directions
- A sense of bewilderment, frustration, and anger at the contractions
- Requests for medication
- Hiccuping, belching, nausea, or vomiting
- Beads of perspiration on the upper lip or brow
- Increasing rectal pressure and an urge to bear down

The woman in this phase is anxious to "get it over with." She may be amnesic and sleep between her frequent contractions. Her support persons may start to feel helpless and may turn to the nurse for increased help as their efforts to alleviate her discomfort seem less effective.

SECOND STAGE

The second stage of labor begins with complete cervical dilatation and ends with birth of the infant. The second stage is usually completed within 2 hours after the cervix becomes fully dilated for primigravidas; the stage averages 15 minutes for multiparas. Contractions continue with a frequency of about every 2 minutes, duration of 60 to 90 seconds, and strong intensity. Descent of the fetal presenting part continues until it reaches the perineal floor.

As the fetal head descends, the woman usually has the urge to push because of pressure of the fetal head on the sacral and obturator nerves. As she pushes, contraction of the maternal abdominal muscles exerts intra-abdominal pressure. As the fetal head continues its descent, the perineum begins to bulge, flatten, and move anteriorly. The amount of bloody show may increase. The labia begin to part with each contraction. Between contractions the fetal head appears to recede. With succeeding contractions and maternal pushing effort, the fetal head descends farther. **Crowning** occurs when the fetal head is encircled by the external opening of the vagina (introitus), and it means birth is imminent.

The woman may feel some relief that the acute pain she felt during the transition phase is over (Table 17–5). She may also be relieved that the birth is near and she can push. Some women feel a sense of purpose that they can be actively involved. Others, particularly those without childbirth preparation, may become frightened and fight each contraction. Such behavior may be disconcerting to the woman's support persons. The woman may feel she has lost her ability to cope and become embarrassed, or she may demonstrate extreme irritability toward the staff or her supporters as she attempts to regain control over forces against which she feels helpless. Most women feel acute, increasingly severe pain and a burning sensation as the perineum distends.

DEVELOPING CULTURAL COMPETENCE

PRESENCE OF THE FATHER

The presence of the father during labor and at birth, although common in countries such as the United States, Canada, and Australia, is not a universal norm. Rather it is strongly influenced by cultural practices. The father is not present at the birth in many countries, including Algeria, Brazil, China, Ethiopia, and Korea. Similarly, Orthodox Jews do not allow men to attend the labor and birth (Spector, 2004).

TABLE 17–5 ✤ Characteristics of Labor

	FIRST STAGE			SECOND STAGE
	Latent Phase	**Active Phase**	**Transition Phase**	
Nullipara	8.6 hr	4.6 hr	3.6 hr	Up to 3 hr
Multipara	5.3 hr	2.4 hr	Variable	0–30 min
Cervical dilatation	0–3 cm	4–7 cm	8–10 cm	
Contractions				
Frequency	Every 3–30 min	Every 2–3 min	Every 1½–2 min	Every 1½–2 min
Duration	20–40 sec	40–60 sec	60–90 sec	60–90 sec
Intensity	Begin as mild and progress to moderate; 25–40 mm Hg by intrauterine pressure catheter (IUPC)	Begin as moderate and progress to strong; 50–70 mm Hg by IUPC	Strong by palpation; 70–90 mm Hg by IUPC	Strong by palpation; 70–100 mm Hg by IUPC

EVIDENCE-BASED NURSING

POSITIONING DURING THE SECOND STAGE OF LABOR

Clinical Question

What maternal positions support and facilitate the second stage of labor?

Evidence

The Association of Women's Health, Obstetric and Neonatal Nurses (AWHONN) assembled an expert team to evaluate the evidence and develop a clinical practice guideline for nursing management of the second stage of labor. The final guideline was based on clinical trials and expert opinion. In this guideline, various maternal positions are recognized as helpful during the second stage of labor.

Implications

Assessment of the woman's knowledge about and preference for a specific position during the second stage of labor is important. The woman's ability to maintain effective alternative and upright positions should also be observed. Assist the woman in using an upright position during the second stage of labor whenever possible. Maintaining an upright position during labor has been shown to decrease the duration of the second stage, minimize intensity of pain, decrease the incidence of perineal trauma, and increase satisfaction with the birthing experience.

If the woman is unable to maintain the upright position for the second stage of labor, you can encourage lateral positioning instead. Help the woman to change positions frequently, especially if there is lack of descent of the fetal head. However, if rapid fetal descent occurs, help the woman maintain a lateral position, and avoid sitting or squatting positions. In general the lithotomy or semirecumbent positions are not helpful and should be avoided.

An upright position during labor may also increase the pelvic diameter, although the evidence is less strong on this point. Upright positioning aids—such as birthing balls, cushions, squat bars, and birthing stools—may be helpful, but the evidence is primarily anecdotal. Changing maternal positioning—such as lying on one's side or resting on hands and knees with a side-to-side pelvic rock—may facilitate rotation if fetal position is occiput posterior.

Critical Thinking

What assessments would tell you that you should discourage a sitting or squatting position? What maternal and fetal assessments will you use during the second stage of labor to ensure that proper positioning is maintained? How will you determine a mother's preference for a specific position during this stage?

Reference

Association of Women's Health, Obstetric and Neonatal Nurses (AWHONN). (2000, January 29). *Nursing management of the second stage of labor. Evidence-based clinical practice guideline.* Washington, DC: Author.

Spontaneous Birth (Vertex Presentation)

As the fetal head distends the vulva with each contraction, the perineum becomes extremely thin and the anus stretches and protrudes. With time the head extends under the symphysis pubis and is born. When the anterior shoulder meets the underside of the symphysis pubis, a gentle push by the mother aids in the birth of the shoulders. The body then follows (Figure 17–12 ●). (Birth of a fetus in other than a vertex presentation is discussed in Chapter 21. ∞)

Positional Changes of the Fetus

For the fetus to pass through the birth canal, the fetal head and body must adjust to the passage by certain positional changes. These changes, called **cardinal movements** or mechanisms of labor, are described in the order in which they occur (Figure 17–13 ●).

Descent. Descent occurs because of four forces: (1) pressure of the amniotic fluid, (2) direct pressure of the uterine fundus on the breech, (3) contraction of the abdominal muscles, and (4) extension and straightening of the fetal body. The head enters the inlet in the occiput transverse or oblique position because the pelvic inlet is widest from side to side. The

sagittal suture is an equal distance from the maternal symphysis pubis and sacral promontory.

Flexion. Flexion occurs as the fetal head descends and meets resistance from the soft tissues of the pelvis, the muscles of the pelvic floor, and the cervix. As a result of the resistance, the fetal chin flexes downward onto the chest.

Internal Rotation. The fetal head must rotate to fit the diameter of the pelvic cavity, which is widest in the anteroposterior diameter. As the occiput of the fetal head meets resistance from the levator ani muscles and their fascia, the occiput rotates—usually from left to right—and the sagittal suture aligns in the anteroposterior pelvic diameter.

Extension. The resistance of the pelvic floor, and the mechanical movement of the vulva opening anteriorly and forward, assist with extension of the fetal head as it passes under the symphysis pubis. With this positional change, the occiput, then brow and face, emerge from the vagina.

Restitution. The shoulders of the fetus enter the pelvic inlet obliquely and remain oblique when the head rotates to the anteroposterior diameter through internal rotation. Because of this rotation, the neck becomes twisted. Once the head is born and is free of pelvic resistance, the neck un-

● FIGURE 17–12

A

B

C

D

E

F

The birth sequence.

© Stella Johnson (www.stellajohnson.com)

○ **FIGURE 17–13**

Mechanisms of labor. **A** and **B,** Descent. **C,** Internal rotation. **D,** Extension. **E,** External rotation.

twists, turning the head to one side (restitution), and aligns with the position of the back in the birth canal.

External Rotation. As the shoulders rotate to the anteroposterior position in the pelvis, the head turns farther to one side (external rotation).

Expulsion. After the external rotation, and through the pushing efforts of the laboring woman, the anterior shoulder meets the undersurface of the symphysis pubis and slips under it. As lateral flexion of the shoulder and head occurs, the anterior shoulder is born before the posterior shoulder. The body follows quickly.

THIRD STAGE

Placental Separation

After the infant is born, the uterus contracts firmly, decreasing its capacity and the surface area of placental attachment. The placenta begins to separate because of this decreased surface area. As separation occurs, bleeding results in the formation of a hematoma between the placental tissue and the remaining decidua. This hematoma speeds the separation process. The membranes are the last to separate. They are peeled off the uterine wall as the placenta descends into the vagina. Signs of placental separation usually appear about 5 minutes after the birth of

the newborn. These signs are (1) a globular-shaped uterus, (2) a rise of the fundus in the abdomen, (3) a sudden gush or trickle of blood, and (4) further protrusion of the umbilical cord out of the vagina.

Placental Delivery

When the signs of placental separation appear, the woman may bear down to aid in placental expulsion. If this fails and the certified nurse-midwife or physician has ascertained that the fundus is firm, gentle traction may be applied to the cord while pressure is exerted on the fundus. The weight of the placenta as it is guided into the placental collection pan aids in the removal of the membranes from the uterine wall. A placenta is considered to be retained if 30 minutes have elapsed from completion of the second stage of labor.

If the placenta separates from the inside to the outer margins, it is expelled with the fetal (shiny) side presenting (Figure 17–14 ○). This is known as the Schultze mechanism of placental delivery or, more commonly, "shiny Schultze." If the placenta separates from the outer margins inward, it rolls up and presents sideways with the maternal surface expelled first. This is known as the Duncan mechanism and is commonly called "dirty Duncan" because the placental surface is rough. (Interventions for the third stage are discussed in Chapter 19. ∞)

FIGURE 17–14

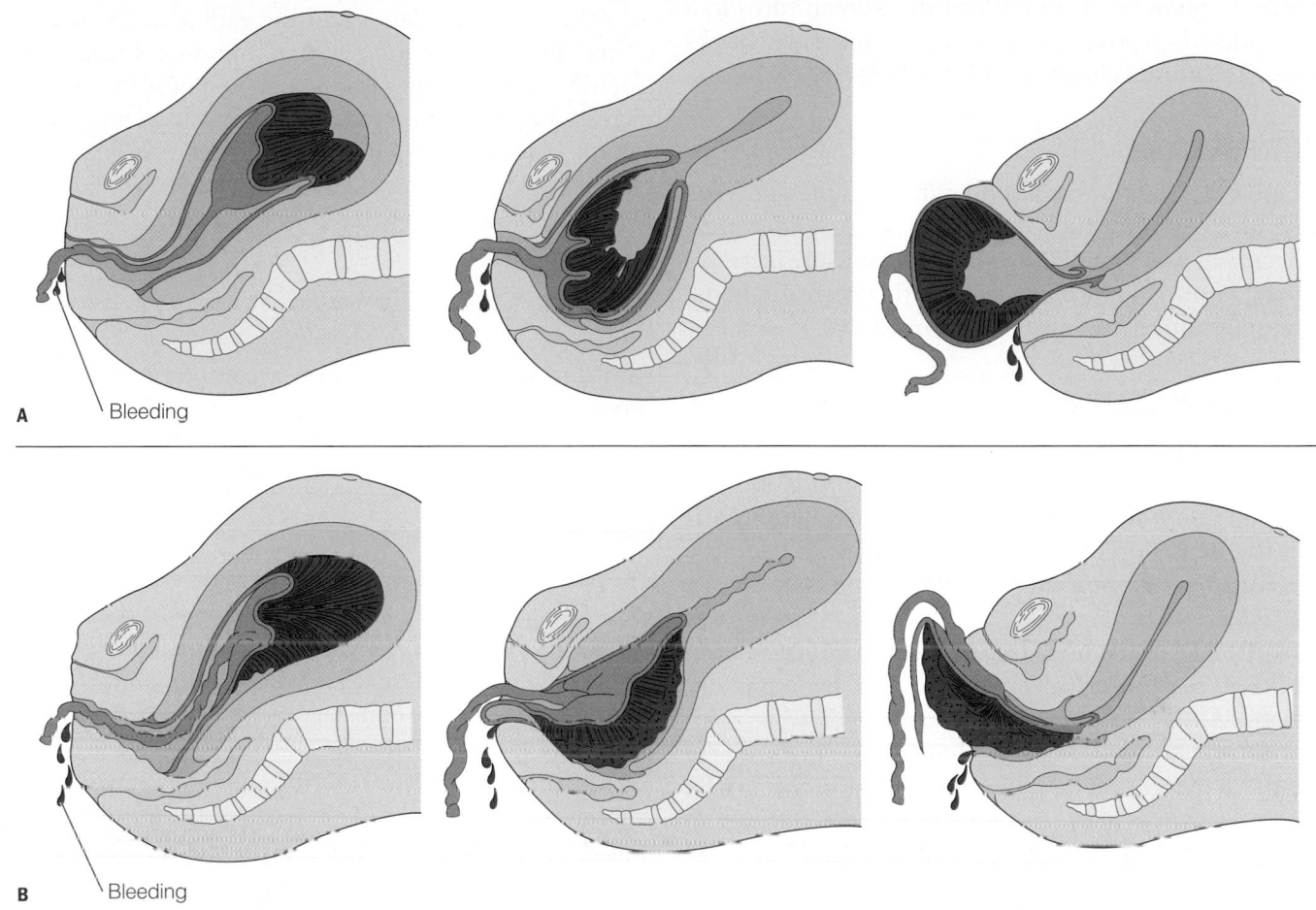

A   Bleeding

B   Bleeding

Placental separation and expulsion. **A,** Schultze mechanism. **B,** Duncan mechanism.

FOURTH STAGE

The fourth stage of labor is the time, from 1 to 4 hours after birth, during which physiologic readjustment of the mother's body begins. With the birth, hemodynamic changes occur. Blood loss ranges from 250 to 500 mL. With this blood loss and removal of the weight of the pregnant uterus from the surrounding vessels, blood is redistributed into venous beds. This results in a moderate drop in both systolic and diastolic blood pressure, increased pulse pressure, and moderate tachycardia (Cunningham et al., 2005).

The uterus remains contracted in the midline of the abdomen. The fundus is usually midway between the symphysis pubis and umbilicus. Its contracted state constricts the vessels at the site of placental implantation. Immediately after expulsion of the placenta, the cervix is widely spread and thick.

Nausea and vomiting usually cease. The woman may be thirsty and hungry. She may experience a shaking chill, which is thought to be associated with the ending of the physical exertion of labor. The bladder is often hypotonic due to trauma during the second stage or the administration of anesthetics that decrease sensations. Hypotonic bladder can lead to urinary retention.

MATERNAL SYSTEMIC RESPONSE TO LABOR

The process of labor and birth affects almost all maternal physiologic systems.

CARDIOVASCULAR SYSTEM

Uterine contractions and the pain, anxiety, and apprehension a laboring woman experiences stress her cardiovascular system. With each contraction, 300 to 500 mL of blood volume is forced back into the maternal circulation, which results in an increase in cardiac output of as much as 31% (Easterling, Carr, & Brateng, 2001). Cardiac output increases more as the laboring woman experiences pain with uterine contractions and her anxiety and apprehension increase.

Maternal position also affects cardiac output. In the supine position, cardiac output lowers, heart rate increases, and stroke volume decreases. When the woman turns to a lateral (side-lying) position, cardiac output increases (Blackburn, 2003; Lanni, Tillinghast, & Silver-Helayne, 2002).

BLOOD PRESSURE

As a result of increased cardiac output, blood pressure rises during uterine contractions. In the first stage, systolic pressure increases by 35 mm Hg and diastolic pressure increases by about 25 mm Hg. There may be further increases in the second stage during pushing (Blackburn, 2003).

RESPIRATORY SYSTEM

Oxygen demand and consumption increase when labor begins because of the presence of uterine contractions. As anxiety and pain from contractions increase, hyperventilation frequently occurs. With hyperventilation there is a fall in $PaCO_2$, and respiratory alkalosis results (Li, Zhang, & Xu, 2002).

By the end of the first stage, most women have developed a mild metabolic acidosis compensated by respiratory alkalosis. As they push in the second stage of labor, their $PaCO_2$ levels may rise along with blood lactate levels (due to muscular activity), and mild respiratory acidosis occurs. By the time the baby is born (end of second stage), the woman has metabolic acidosis uncompensated for by respiratory alkalosis. The changes in acid-base status that occur in labor are quickly reversed in the fourth stage because of changes in women's respiratory rates. Acid-base levels return to pregnancy levels by 24 hours after birth, and to nonpregnant values a few weeks after birth (Blackburn, 2003).

RENAL SYSTEM

During labor there is an increase in maternal renin, plasma renin activity, and angiotensinogen. This elevation is thought to be important in the control of uteroplacental blood flow during birth and the early postpartal period. Structurally the base of the bladder is pushed forward and upward when engagement occurs. The pressure from the presenting part may impair blood and lymph drainage from the base of the bladder, leading to edema (Cunningham et al., 2005).

GASTROINTESTINAL SYSTEM

During labor, gastric motility and absorption of solid food are reduced. Gastric emptying time is prolonged, and gastric volume (amount of contents that remain in the stomach) remains increased, regardless of the time the last meal was taken. Some narcotics also delay gastric emptying time and add to the risk of aspiration if general anesthesia is used.

IMMUNE SYSTEM AND OTHER BLOOD VALUES

The white blood cell (WBC) count increases to 25,000 to 30,000/mm³ during labor and the early postpartum. The change in WBC count is mostly due to increased neutrophils resulting from a physiologic response to stress. The increased WBC count makes it difficult to identify an infection. Maternal blood glucose levels decrease because the body uses glucose as an energy source during contractions. Decreased blood glucose levels lead to a decrease in insulin requirements.

PAIN

Pain during labor comes from a complexity of physical causes. Each woman will experience and cope with pain differently. Multiple factors affect a woman's reaction to labor pain.

Causes of Pain During Labor

The pain associated with the first stage of labor is unique in that it accompanies a normal physiologic process. Even though perception of the pain of childbirth varies among women, there is a physiologic basis for discomfort during labor. Pain during the first stage of labor arises from (1) dilatation of the cervix, which is the primary source of pain; (2) stretching of the lower uterine segment; (3) pressure on adjacent structures; and (4) hypoxia of the uterine muscle cells during contraction (Blackburn, 2003). The areas of pain include the lower abdominal wall and the areas over the lower lumbar region and the upper sacrum.

During the second stage of labor, discomfort is due to (1) hypoxia of the contracting uterine muscle cells, (2) distention of the vagina and perineum, and (3) pressure on adjacent structures. The area of pain increases as shown in Figures 17–15 ● and 17–16 ●.

Pain during the third stage results from uterine contractions and cervical dilatation as the placenta is expelled. This stage of labor is short, and after it anesthesia is needed primarily for episiotomy repair.

Factors Affecting Response to Pain

Many factors affect the individual's perception of and response to pain. For example, childbirth preparation classes may reduce the need for analgesia during labor. People tend to respond to painful stimuli in the way that is acceptable in their culture. In some cultures it is natural to communicate pain, no matter how mild, whereas members of other cultures stoically accept pain. Fatigue and sleep deprivation may also influence response to pain. The tired woman has less energy and ability to use such strategies as distraction or imagination to deal with pain. As a result she may lose her ability to cope with labor and choose analgesics or other medications to relieve the discomfort.

● FIGURE 17–15

Distribution of labor pain during the later phase of the first stage and early phase of the second stage. The darkest colored areas indicate the location of the most intense pain, moderate color indicates moderate pain, and lighter color indicates mild pain. The uterine contractions, which at this stage are very strong, produce intense pain.

Used with permission from Bonica, J. J. (1972). Principles and practice of obstetric analgesia and anesthesia (p. 109). Philadelphia: Davis.

● FIGURE 17–16

Distribution of labor pain during the later phase of the second stage and actual birth. The perineal component is the primary cause of discomfort. Uterine contractions contribute much less to the level of pain.

Used with permission from Bonica, J. J. (1972). Principles and practice of obstetric analgesia and anesthesia (p. 109). Philadelphia: Davis.

The woman's previous experience with pain and her anxiety level also affect her ability to manage current and future pain. Those who have had experience with pain seem more sensitive to painful stimuli than those who have not. Unfamiliar surroundings and events can increase anxiety, as does separation from family and loved ones. Anticipation of discomfort and questions about whether she can cope with the contractions may also increase anxiety.

Both attention and distraction influence the perception of pain. When pain sensation is the focus of attention, the perceived intensity is greater. A sensory stimulus such as a back rub can be a distraction that focuses the woman's attention on the stimulus rather than the pain.

FETAL RESPONSE TO LABOR

When the fetus is healthy, the mechanical and hemodynamic changes of normal labor have no adverse effects. Certain physiologic responses do occur, however.

- **Heart rate changes.** Early fetal heart rate decelerations can occur with intracranial pressures of 40 to 55 mm Hg, as the head pushes against the cervix. This early deceleration is believed to be due to hypoxic depression of the central nervous system, which is under vagal control. The absence of head compression decelerations in some fetuses during labor is explained by a threshold reached more gradually in the presence of intact membranes and lack of maternal resistance. These early decelerations are harmless in a normal fetus.

- **Acid-base status in labor.** Blood flow is decreased to the fetus at the peak of each contraction, which leads to a slow decrease in pH. During the second stage of labor, as uterine contractions become longer and stronger and the woman holds her breath to push, the fetal pH decreases more rapidly. The base deficit increases, and fetal oxygen saturation drops about 10% (Blackburn, 2003).

- **Hemodynamic changes.** The adequate exchange of nutrients and gases in the fetal capillaries and intervillous spaces depends in part on the fetal blood pressure. Fetal blood pressure protects the normal fetus during the anoxic periods caused by the contracting uterus during labor. The fetal and placental reserve is usually enough to see the fetus through these anoxic periods unharmed (Blackburn, 2003).

- **Fetal sensation.** Beginning at about 37 or 38 weeks' gestation, the fetus is able to experience sensations of light, sound, and touch. The full-term fetus is able to hear music and the maternal voice. Even in utero the fetus is sensitive to light and will move away from a bright light source. The term baby is aware of pressure sensations during labor such as the touch of the care provider during a vaginal examination or pressure on the head as a contraction occurs. Although the fetus may not be able to process this input, the fetus is experiencing labor as the woman labors.

Critical Concept Review

LEARNING OBJECTIVES	CONCEPTS
Examine the five critical factors that influence labor.	1. Birth passage: ■ The ability of the pelvis and cervix to accommodate the passage of the fetus. 2. Fetus: ■ The ability of the fetus to complete the birth process. 3. Relationship between the passage and the fetus: ■ The position of the fetus in relation to the pelvis. 4. Physiologic forces of labor: ■ Characteristics of contractions and the effectiveness of expulsion methods. 5. Psychosocial considerations: ■ Understanding and preparing for the childbirth experience. ■ Amount of support from others. ■ Present emotional status. ■ Beliefs and values.

LEARNING OBJECTIVES

CONCEPTS

Describe the physiology of labor.

1. Progesterone causes relaxation of smooth muscle tissue.
2. Estrogen causes stimulation of uterine muscle contractions.
3. Connective tissue loosens and permits the softening, thinning, and opening of the cervix.
4. Muscles of the upper uterine segment shorten and cause the cervix to thin and flatten.
5. Fetal body is straightened as the uterus elongates with each contraction.
6. Pressure of the fetal head causes cervical dilatation.
7. Rectum and vagina are drawn upward and forward with each contraction.
8. During the second stage, the anus everts.

Discuss premonitory signs of labor.

1. Lightening:
   - Fetus descends into the pelvic inlet.
2. Braxton Hicks contractions:
   - Irregular, intermittent contractions that occur during pregnancy.
   - Cause more discomfort closer to onset of labor.
3. Cervical changes:
   - Cervix begins to soften and weaken (ripening).
4. Bloody show:
   - Loss of the cervical mucous plug.
   - Causes blood-tinged discharge.
5. Rupture of membranes:
   - If membranes rupture prior to the onset of labor, there is a good chance labor will begin within 24 hours.
6. Sudden burst of energy:
   - Known as nesting.
   - Usually occurs 24–48 hours before the start of labor.
7. Other signs:
   - Loss of 1–3 pounds.
   - Diarrhea, indigestion, nausea, and vomiting may occur prior to the onset of labor.

Differentiate between false and true labor.

True labor is characterized by:
1. Contractions that occur at regular intervals and increase in duration and intensity.
2. Discomfort that begins in the back and radiates to the front of the abdomen.
3. Walking intensifies contractions.
4. Resting or relaxing in warm water does not decrease the intensity of contractions.
5. Contractions that produce cervical dilatation.
False labor is characterized by:
1. Irregular contractions that do not increase in duration or intensity.
2. Contractions that are not affected or lessened by walking, rest, or warm water.
3. Discomfort that is felt primarily in the abdomen.
4. Contractions that produce no effect on cervix.

Describe the physiologic and psychologic changes occurring in each of the stages of labor.

1a. Latent phase *physiologic* changes:
   - Regular, mild contractions begin and increase in intensity and frequency.
   - Cervical effacement and dilatation begins.
1b. Latent phase *psychologic* changes:
   - Relief that labor has begun.
   - High excitement with some anxiety.
2a. Active phase *physiologic* changes:
   - Contractions increase in intensity, frequency, and duration.
   - Cervical dilatation increases from 4–7 cm.
   - Fetus begins to descend into the pelvis.
2b. Active phase *psychologic* changes:
   - Fear of loss of control.
   - Anxiety increases.
   - Possible decrease in coping skills.
3a. Transition phase *physiologic* changes:
   - Contractions continue to increase in intensity, duration, and frequency.
   - Cervix dilates from 8–10 cm.
   - Fetus descends rapidly into the birth passage.
   - Woman may experience rectal pressure.
   - Woman may experience nausea, vomiting, or both.

LEARNING OBJECTIVES

CONCEPTS

Describe the physiologic and psychologic changes occurring in each of the stages of labor.—continued

3b. Transition phase *psychologic* changes:
  - Increased feelings of anxiety.
  - Irritability.
  - Eager to complete birth experience.
  - Need to have support person or nurse at bedside.

4a. Second stage *physiologic* changes:
  - Begins with complete cervical dilatation and ends with the birth of the infant.
  - Woman pushes due to pressure of fetal head on sacral and obturator nerves.
  - Woman uses intra-abdominal pressure.
  - Perineum begins to bulge, flatten, and move anteriorly as fetus descends.

4b. Second stage *psychologic* changes:
  - May feel a sense of purpose.
  - May feel out of control, frightened, and irritable.

5a. Third stage *physiologic* changes:
  - Placental separation: uterus contracts and the placenta begins to separate.
  - Placental expulsion: woman bears down and expels the placenta. Physician may put slight traction on the cord to assist the expulsion of the placenta.

5b. Third stage *psychologic* changes:
  - Woman may feel relief at the completion of the birth.
  - Woman is usually focused on welfare of the infant and may not recognize that placental expulsion is occurring.

6a. Fourth stage *physiologic* changes:
  - Woman experiences increased pulse and decreased blood pressure due to redistribution of blood from uterus and blood loss.
  - Uterus remains contracted and is located between umbilicus and symphysis pubis.
  - Woman may experience a shaking chill.
  - Urine may be retained due to decreased bladder tone and possible trauma to the bladder.

6b. Fourth stage *psychologic* changes:
  - May experience euphoria and be energized at birth of child.
  - May be thirsty and hungry.

Summarize maternal systemic responses to labor.

1. Cardiovascular changes:
  - Increase in cardiac output.
2. Blood pressure:
  - Rises with each contraction.
  - May rise further with pushing.
3. Respiratory system:
  - Increase in oxygen demand and consumption.
  - Mild respiratory acidosis usually occurs by time of birth.
4. Renal system:
  - Increase in renin, plasma renin activity, and angiotensinogen.
  - Edema may occur at base of bladder due to pressure of fetal head.
5. Gastrointestinal system:
  - Gastric motility decreased.
  - Gastric emptying is prolonged.
  - Gastric volume remains increased.
6. Immune system and other blood values:
  - WBC count increases.
  - Blood glucose decreases.
7. Pain:
  - In the first stage: arises from dilatation of cervix, stretching of lower uterine segment, pressure, and hypoxia of uterine muscle cells during contractions.
  - In the second stage: arises from hypoxia of contracting uterine muscle cells, distention of the vagina and perineum, and pressure.
  - In the third stage: arises from contractions and dilatation of cervix as placenta is expelled.

Explore fetal responses to labor.

1. Labor may cause no adverse effects in the healthy fetus.
2. FHR may decrease as the head pushes against the cervix.
3. Blood flow decreases to the fetus at the peak of each contraction, leading to a decrease in pH.
4. Further decrease of pH occurs during pushing due to the woman holding her breath.

CRITICAL THINKING IN ACTION

*View the **Critical Thinking in Action** video in Chapter 17 of the CD-ROM. Then, answer the questions that follow.*

Ann Nelson, a 28-year-old, G2, P0010 at 41 weeks' gestation, is admitted to the birthing unit where you are working. She is here for cervical ripening and induction of labor due to postdate pregnancy and decreased amniotic fluid volume. A review of her prenatal chart reveals a pertinent history of infertility (Clomid-induced pregnancy) and asthma (treated with inhalers on a PRN basis). The Doppler picks up a fetal heart rate of 120 bpm. You place Ann on the electronic fetal monitor and obtain the following data: BP 126/76, T 98°F, P 82, R 16; vaginal exam reveals a 20% effaced cervix, 1 cm dilatation in the posterior position, and vertex at −2 station. The fetal monitor shows a fetal heart rate baseline of 120 to 128 with occasional variable decelerations, accelerations to 140 with fetal activity. No contractions are noted on the monitor or palpated. Ann asks you what to expect with "cervical ripening" using prostaglandin gel.

1. Discuss the action of prostaglandin gel.
2. Ann asks you why cervical ripening and induction of labor are recommended for her and her baby. How would you best respond to her?
3. Ann asks how she will know if she is getting contractions. How would you answer her?
4. Discuss the difference between mild, moderate, and strong contractions.
5. Describe the latent phase of labor.

MEDIALINK   www.prenhall.com/london

- NCLEX-RN® Review, case studies, and other interactive resources for this chapter can be found on the Companion Website at http://www.prenhall.com/london. Click on "Chapter 17" to select the activities for this chapter.

- For animations, more NCLEX-RN® Review questions, and an audio glossary, access the accompanying CD-ROM in this textbook.

REFERENCES

Beckmann, C. R. B., & Dysart, D. (2000). The challenge of multicultural medical care. *Contemporary OB/GYN, 45*(12), 12-33.

Blackburn, S. T. (2003). *Maternal, fetal, and neonatal physiology: A clinical perspective* (2nd ed.). Philadelphia: Saunders.

Browning, C. A. (2001). Using music during childbirth. *Birth, 27*(4), 272-276.

Caldwell, W. E., & Moloy, H. C. (1933). Anatomical variation in the female pelvis and their effect on labor with a suggested classification. *American Journal of Obstetrics and Gynecology, 26*, 479-487.

Cunningham, F. G., Leveno, K. J., Gilstrap, L. C., Bloom, S. L., Hauth, J. C., & Wenstrom, K. D. (2005). *Williams obstetrics* (22nd ed.). New York: McGraw-Hill.

Dumas, L. (2002). Focus groups to reveal parents' needs for prenatal education. *Journal of Perinatal Education, 11*(3), 1-9.

Easterling, T., Carr, D., & Brateng, D. (2001). Treatment of hypertension in pregnancy: Effect of atenolol on maternal disease, preterm delivery and maternal growth. *Obstetrics and Gynecology, 98*(3), 427-433.

Kilson, K. (2002). *Preparing for guided imagery.* Retrieved September 12, 2004, from http://home.earthlink.net/~kkdombi/whatindexa.html

Lanni, S., Tillinghast, J., & Silver-Helayne, M. (2002). Hemodynamic changes and baroreflex gain in supine hypotension syndrome. *American Journal of Obstetrics and Gynecology, 187*, 1636-1641.

Lee, J., & Schmied, V. (2001). Fathercraft: Involving men in antenatal education. *British Journal of Midwifery, 9*(9), 559-561.

Li, S., Zhang, S., & Xu, S. (2002). Effect of oxygen inhalation during labor on the qualities of delivery. *Chinese Nursing Research, 16*(1), 22-23.

Locksmith, G., & Duff, P. (2001). Infection, antibiotics, and preterm delivery. *Seminars in Perinatology, 25*(5), 295-309.

McGrath, S., & Smith, R. (2001). Corticotropin-releasing hormone and parturition. *Clinical Endocrinology, 55*(5), 593-595.

Meadows, J. W., Eis, A. L., Brockman, D. E., & Myatt, L. (2003). Expression and localization of prostaglandin E synthase isoforms in human fetal membranes in term and preterm labor. *Journal of Clinical Endocrinology and Metabolism, 88*(1), 433-439.

Pressman, E. K., Cavanaugh, J. L., & Woods, J. R. (2002). Physical properties of the chorioamnion throughout gestation. *American Journal of Obstetrics and Gynecology, 187*(3), 672-675.

Rabl, M., Joura, E. A., Yucel, Y., & Egarter, C. (2002). A randomized trial of vaginal prostaglandin E2 for induction of labor: Insert vs. tablet. *Journal of Reproductive Medicine, 47*(2), 115-119.

Spector, R. E. (2004). *Cultural diversity in health and illness* (6th ed). Upper Saddle River, NJ: Pearson/Prentice-Hall.

Varney, H., Kriebs, J. M., & Gegor, C. L. (2004). *Varney's midwifery* (4th ed.). Boston: Jones & Bartlett.

Intrapartal Nursing Assessment

It was strange. After months of waiting for my baby's birth, labor took me by surprise. I wasn't quite ready to move from being pregnant to being a mother. Not that I had any choice!

—*Tammy, 23*

LEARNING OBJECTIVES

- Discuss high-risk screening and intrapartal assessment of maternal physical and psychosociocultural factors.

- Summarize methods used to evaluate the progress of labor.

- Describe auscultation of fetal heart rate.

- Delineate the procedure for performing Leopold's maneuvers and the information that can be obtained.

- Differentiate between baseline and periodic changes in fetal heart rate monitoring and describe the appearance and significance of each.

- Outline steps to be performed in the systematic evaluation of fetal heart rate tracings.

- Identify nonreassuring fetal heart rate patterns and appropriate nursing responses.

- Discuss nursing care of the family undergoing electronic fetal monitoring.

- Delineate the indications for fetal blood sampling and identify related pH values.

- Describe how fetal oxygen saturation ($FSpO_2$) monitoring uses pulse oximetry to monitor fetal oxygenation within the fetal blood to determine if hypoxia is occurring.

MEDIALINK

www.prenhall.com/london

CD-ROM

Skill 3–1: Performing an Intrapartal Vaginal Examination
Skill 3–3: Performing Leopold's Maneuvers
Skill 3–4: Auscultation of Fetal Heart Rate
Skill 3–5: External Electronic Fetal Monitoring
Skill 3–6: Electronic Fetal Monitoring
Audio Glossary
NCLEX-RN® Review

Companion Website

Thinking Critically
NCLEX-RN® Review
MediaLink Applications:
    Case Study: Maternal Assessment during Labor
    Care Plan Activity: Client with Decelerations

The physiologic events during labor call for many adaptations by the mother and the fetus. Thus, frequent and accurate assessments are crucial. The woman's partner or chosen support person is also an integral part of the childbirth experience. In nursing practice the traditional assessment techniques of observation, palpation, and auscultation are augmented by the judicious use of technology such as ultrasound and electronic monitoring. These tools may provide more detailed information for assessment. However, the technology only provides data; it is the nurse who monitors the mother and her baby.

MATERNAL ASSESSMENT

HISTORY

Obtain a brief oral history when the woman is admitted to the birthing area. Each agency has its own admission forms, but they usually include the following information:

- Woman's name and age
- Last menstrual period (LMP) and estimated date of birth (EDB)
- Attending physician or certified nurse-midwife (CNM)
- Personal data: blood type; Rh factor; results of serology testing; prepregnant and present weight; allergies to medications, foods, or other substances; prescribed and over-the-counter medications taken during pregnancy; and history of drug and alcohol use and smoking during the pregnancy
- History of previous illness, such as tuberculosis, heart disease, diabetes, and so forth
- Problems in the prenatal period, such as elevated blood pressure, bleeding problems, recurrent urinary tract infections, other infections
- Pregnancy data: gravida, para, abortions, and perinatal deaths
- The method chosen for infant feeding
- Type of prenatal education classes (childbirth education classes)
- Woman's preferences about labor and birth, such as no episiotomy, no analgesics or anesthetics, or the presence of the father or others at the birth
- Pediatrician or family practice physician
- Additional data: history of special tests such as nonstress test (NST), biophysical profile (BPP), or ultrasound; history of any preterm labor; onset of labor; amniotic fluid membrane status; and brief description of previous labor and birth
- Onset of labor
- Status of amniotic membranes (Are they intact or ruptured? If ruptured, time of rupture, color of fluid, and odor.)

The psychosocial history is a critical component of intrapartal nursing assessment. Because of the prevalence of domestic violence in society, the nurse needs to consider the possibility that the woman may have experienced abuse at some time in her life. The following screening questions should be asked universally when the woman is alone so that she can answer freely (American College of Obstetricians and Gynecologists [ACOG], 1999):

1. Has anyone close to you ever threatened to harm you?
2. Have you ever been hit, slapped, kicked, choked, or otherwise physically hurt by someone? If yes, by whom? Total number of times?

3. Has anyone, including your partner, ever forced you to have sex?

4. Are you afraid of your partner or anyone you mentioned?

NURSING PRACTICE

Many nurses have difficulty asking questions about domestic violence, sexual abuse, and drug or alcohol use during pregnancy. However, this information is necessary to provide the best nursing care possible. To create a relationship of trust in which the client feels safe answering uncomfortable questions, the following tips may be helpful:

- Explore your own beliefs and values.
- Use open-ended questions.
- Be receptive to the answers.
- Be accepting of others' life experiences.

THINKING CRITICALLY

You are the birthing center nurse and you have reason to suspect that Lynn Ling, who has just been admitted in labor, may be in an abusive relationship. How could you set up an interview so that the partner would leave the room (and take any accompanying children) without feeling that you are possibly increasing the risk to the woman? What communication techniques would you use to encourage Lynn to reveal if her partner is abusive?

INTRAPARTAL HIGH-RISK SCREENING

Screening for intrapartal high-risk factors is an integral part of assessing the normal laboring woman. As the history is obtained, note the presence of any factors that may be associated with a high-risk condition. For example, the woman who reports a physical symptom such as intermittent bleeding needs further assessment to rule out abruptio placentae or placenta previa before the admission process continues. It is also important to recognize the implications of a high-risk condition for the laboring woman and her fetus. For example, if there is an abnormal fetal presentation, labor may be prolonged, prolapse of the umbilical cord is more likely, and the possibility of a cesarean birth is increased.

Although physical conditions are major factors that increase risk in the intrapartal period, sociocultural variables such as poverty, nutrition, the amount of prenatal care, cultural beliefs about pregnancy, and communication patterns may also precipitate a high-risk situation. In addition, women who suffer from post-traumatic stress disorder may be at increased risk for some pregnancy complications (Seng et al., 2001). Other risk factors include smoking, drug use, and consumption of alcohol during pregnancy (Davidson, 2002).

Begin gathering data about sociocultural factors as the woman enters the birthing area. Observe the communication pattern between the woman and her support person or people and their responses to admission questions and initial teaching. If the woman and those supporting her do not speak English and translators are not available among the birthing unit staff, the course of labor and the ability of caregivers to interact and provide support and education are affected. The couple must receive information in their primary language to make informed decisions. Communication may also be affected by cultural practices such as beliefs about when to speak, who should ask questions, or whether it is acceptable to let others know about discomfort.

Table 18–1 provides a partial list of intrapartal risk factors to keep in mind during the intrapartal assessment.

TABLE 18–1 ❖ Intrapartal High-Risk Factors

Factor	Maternal Implications	Fetal-Neonatal Implications
Abnormal presentation	↑ Incidence of cesarean birth ↑ Incidence of prolonged labor	↑ Incidence of placenta previa Prematurity ↑ Risk of congenital abnormality Neonatal physical trauma ↑ Risk of intrauterine growth restriction (IUGR)
Multiple gestation	↑ Uterine distention → ↑ risk of postpartum hemorrhage ↑ Risk of cesarean birth ↑ Risk of preterm labor	Low birth weight Prematurity ↑ Risk of congenital anomalies Feto-fetal transfusion
Hydramnios	↑ Discomfort ↑ Dyspnea ↑ Risk of preterm labor Edema of lower extremities	↑ Risk of esophageal or other high-alimentary-tract atresias ↑ Risk of CNS anomalies (myelocele)

TABLE 18–1 ✤ Intrapartal High-Risk Factors—continued

Factor	Maternal Implications	Fetal-Neonatal Implications
Oligohydramnios	Maternal fear of "dry birth"	↑ Incidence of congenital anomalies ↑ Incidence of renal lesions ↑ Risk of IUGR ↑ Risk of fetal acidosis ↑ Risk of cord compression Postmaturity
Meconium staining of amniotic fluid	↑ Psychologic stress due to fear for baby	↑ Risk of fetal asphyxia ↑ Risk of meconium aspiration ↑ Risk of pneumonia due to aspiration of meconium
Premature rupture of membranes	↑ Risk of infection (chorioamnionitis) ↑ Risk of preterm labor ↑ Anxiety Fear for the baby Prolonged hospitalization ↑ Incidence of tocolytic therapy	↑ Perinatal morbidity Prematurity ↑ Birth weight ↑ Risk of respiratory distress syndrome Prolonged hospitalization
Induction of labor	↑ Risk of hypercontractility of uterus ↑ Risk of uterine rupture Length of labor if cervix not ready ↑ Anxiety	Prematurity if gestational age not assessed correctly Hypoxia if hyperstimulation occurs
Abruptio placentae/placenta previa	Hemorrhage Uterine atony ↑ Incidence of cesarean birth	Fetal hypoxia/acidosis Fetal exsanguination ↑ Perinatal mortality
Failure to progress in labor	Maternal exhaustion ↑ Incidence of augmentation of labor ↑ Incidence of cesarean birth	Fetal hypoxia/acidosis Intracranial birth injury
Precipitous labor (<3 hours)	Perineal, vaginal, cervical lacerations ↑ Risk of postpartum hemorrhage	Tentorial tears
Prolapse of umbilical cord	↑ Fear for baby Cesarean birth	Acute fetal hypoxia/acidosis
Fetal heart aberrations	↑ Fear for baby ↑ Risk of cesarean birth, forceps, vacuum Continuous electronic monitoring and intervention in labor	Tachycardia, chronic asphyxic insult, bradycardia, acute asphyxic insult Chronic hypoxia Congenital heart block
Uterine rupture	Hemorrhage Cesarean birth for hysterectomy ↑ Risk of death	Fetal anoxia Fetal hemorrhage ↑ Neonatal morbidity and mortality
Postdates (>42 weeks)	↑ Anxiety ↑ Incidence of induction of labor ↑ Incidence of cesarean birth ↑ Use of technology to monitor fetus ↑ Risk of shoulder dystocia	Postmaturity syndrome ↑ Risk of fetal-neonatal mortality and morbidity ↑ Risk of antepartum fetal death ↑ Incidence or risk of large baby
Diabetes	↑ Risk of hydramnios ↑ Risk of hypoglycemia or hyperglycemia ↑ Risk of preeclampsia-eclampsia	↑ Risk of malpresentation ↑ Risk of macrosomia ↑ Risk of IUGR ↑ Risk of respiratory distress syndrome ↑ Risk of congenital anomalies
Preeclampsia-eclampsia	↑ Risk of seizures ↑ Risk of stroke ↑ Risk of HELLP	↑ Risk of small-for-gestational-age baby ↑ Risk of preterm birth ↑ Risk of mortality
AIDS/STI	↑ Risk of additional infections	↑ Risk of transplacental transmission

INTRAPARTAL PHYSICAL AND PSYCHOSOCIOCULTURAL ASSESSMENT

A physical examination is part of the admission procedure and part of the ongoing care of the woman. Although the intrapartal physical assessment is not as complete and thorough as the initial prenatal physical examination (see Chapter 10 ∞), it does involve assessment of some body systems and the actual labor process. See "Assessment Guide: Intrapartal—First Stage of Labor" for a framework to use when examining the laboring woman.

The physical assessment portion includes assessments performed immediately on admission as well as ongoing assessments. When labor is progressing very quickly, there may not be time for a complete nursing assessment. In that case the critical physical assessments include maternal vital signs, labor status, fetal status, and laboratory findings. The cultural assessment portion provides a starting point for this increasingly important aspect of assessment. Individualized nursing care can best be planned and implemented when the values and beliefs of the laboring woman are known and honored. It is sometimes challenging to achieve a balance between cultural awareness and the risk of stereotyping because cultural responses are influenced by so many factors. Nurses are most effective when they combine an awareness of the major cultural values and beliefs of a specific group with the recognition that individual differences have an impact. "Developing Cultural Competence" provides examples of selected beliefs of some Native American women.

DEVELOPING CULTURAL COMPETENCE

The following list provides a few examples of the beliefs and taboos of some Native American women related to childbirth (Cesario, 2001):

■ If a pregnant woman eats the feet of animals, her infant will be born feet first.

■ If a pregnant woman eats an animal's tail, her infant will get stuck in the birth canal.

■ Weaving or tying knots during pregnancy will cause umbilical cord complications.

■ If the woman naps during labor it may cause a change in the desired sex of her infant.

■ A lengthy labor may result if a woman is exposed to cold during pregnancy because cold causes the woman's bag of waters to freeze, thereby holding the infant back.

■ When the infant's cord is being cut following birth, the mother should bite on a white pebble. This ensures that the infant's teeth will be white and strong.

The final section of the assessment guide addresses psychosocial factors. The laboring woman's psychosocial status is an important part of the total assessment. The woman has previous ideas, knowledge, and fears about childbearing. By assessing her psychosocial status, the nurse can meet the woman's needs for information and support.

While performing the intrapartal assessment, it is crucial to follow the Centers for Disease Control and Prevention (CDC) guidelines to prevent exposure to body substances. Provide information about the precautions in a factual manner.

METHODS OF EVALUATING LABOR PROGRESS

The nurse assesses the woman's contractions and cervical dilatation and effacement to evaluate labor progress.

Contraction Assessment

Uterine contractions may be assessed by palpation or continuous electronic monitoring.

Palpation. Assess contractions for frequency, duration, and intensity by placing one hand on the uterine fundus. It is important to keep the hand relatively still because excessive movement may stimulate contractions or cause discomfort. Determine the frequency of the contractions by noting the time from the beginning of one contraction to the beginning of the next. If contractions begin at 7:00, 7:04, and 7:08, for example, their frequency is every 4 minutes. To determine contraction duration, note the time when tensing of the fundus is first felt (beginning of contraction) and again as relaxation occurs (end of contraction). During the acme of the contraction, intensity can be evaluated by estimating the indentability of the fundus. Assess at least three successive contractions to provide enough data to determine the contraction pattern. See Table 18–2 for a review of characteristics in different phases of labor.

NURSING PRACTICE

Many experienced nurses note that mild contractions are similar in consistency to the tip of the nose, moderate contractions feel more like the chin, and with strong contractions, there is little indentability, much like the forehead. When palpating a woman's uterus during a contraction, compare the consistency to your nose, chin, and forehead to determine the intensity.

This is also a good time to assess the laboring woman's perception of pain. For example, how does she describe the pain? What is her affect? Is this contraction more uncomfortable than the last one? Note and chart the woman's affect and response to the contractions.

Electronic Monitoring of Contractions.. Electronic monitoring of uterine contractions provides continuous data. In many birth settings, electronic monitoring is routine for high-risk clients

ASSESSMENT GUIDE

INTRAPARTAL—FIRST STAGE OF LABOR

PHYSICAL ASSESSMENT/ NORMAL FINDINGS	ALTERATIONS AND POSSIBLE CAUSES*	NURSING RESPONSES TO DATA†
Vital Signs		
Blood pressure (BP): <130 systolic and <85 diastolic in adult 18 years of age or older or no more than 15–20 mm Hg rise in systolic pressure over baseline BP during early pregnancy	High BP (essential hypertension, preeclampsia, renal disease, apprehension or anxiety) Low BP (supine hypotension)	Evaluate history of preexisting disorders and check for presence of other signs of preeclampsia. Do not assess during contractions; implement measures to decrease anxiety and reassess. Turn woman on her side and recheck BP. Provide quiet environment. Have O₂ available.
Pulse: 60–90 beats per minute (bpm)	Increased pulse rate (excitement or anxiety, cardiac disorders, early shock)	Evaluate cause, reassess to see if rate continues; report to physician.
Respirations: 14–22/minute (or pulse rate divided by 4)	Marked tachypnea (respiratory disease), hyperventilation in transition phase	Assess between contractions; if marked tachypnea continues, assess for signs of respiratory disease.
Pulse oximeter (if used) 95% or greater	Hyperventilation (anxiety)	Encourage slow breaths if woman is hyperventilating.
Temperature: 36.2–37.6°C (98–99.6°F)	>90%; hypoxia, hypotension, hemorrhage	Apply O₂; notify physician
	Elevated temperature (infection, dehydration, prolonged rupture of membranes, epidural regional block)	Assess for other signs of infection or dehydration.
Weight		
25–35 lb greater than prepregnant weight	Weight gain >35 lb (fluid retention, obesity, large infant, diabetes mellitus, preeclampsia), weight gain <15 lb (SGA, substance abuse, psychosocial problems).	Assess for signs of edema. Evaluate pattern from prenatal record.
Lungs		
Normal breath sounds, clear and equal	Rales, rhonchi, friction rub (infection), pulmonary edema, asthma	Reassess; refer to physician.
Fundus		
At 40 weeks' gestation located just below xiphoid process	Uterine size not compatible with estimated date of birth (SGA, large for gestational age [LGA], hydramnios, multiple pregnancy, placental/fetal anomalies, malpresentation)	Reevaluate history regarding pregnancy dating. Refer to physician for additional assessment.
Edema		
Slight amount of dependent edema	Pitting edema of face, hands, legs, abdomen, sacral area (preeclampsia)	Check deep tendon reflexes for hyperactivity; check for clonus; refer to physician.
Hydration		
Normal skin turgor, elastic	Poor skin turgor (dehydration)	Assess skin turgor; refer to physician for deviations.
Perineum		
Tissues smooth, pink color (see Prenatal Initial Physical Assessment Guide, Chapter 10) ∞	Varicose veins of vulva, herpes lesions, genital warts	Exercise care while doing a perineal prep; note on client record need for follow-up in postpartal period; reassess after birth; refer to physician/CNM.

*Possible causes of alterations are placed in parentheses.

†This column provides guidelines for further assessment and initial nursing intervention.

(continued)

ASSESSMENT GUIDE—continued

INTRAPARTAL—FIRST STAGE OF LABOR

PHYSICAL ASSESSMENT/ NORMAL FINDINGS	ALTERATIONS AND POSSIBLE CAUSES*	NURSING RESPONSES TO DATA†
Perineum (continued)		
Clear mucus; may be blood tinged with earthy or human odor	Profuse, purulent, foul-smelling drainage	Suspected gonorrhea or chorioamnionitis; report to physician/CNM; initiate care to newborn's eyes; notify neonatal nursing staff and pediatrician.
Presence of small amount of bloody show that gradually increases with further cervical dilatation	Hemorrhage	Assess BP and pulse, pallor, diaphoresis; report any marked changes. (*Note:* Gaping of vagina or anus and bulging of perineum are signs that suggest the onset of the second stage of labor.) Follow universal precautions.
Labor Status		
Uterine contractions: regular pattern	Failure to establish a regular pattern, prolonged latent phase Hypertonicity Hypotonicity Dehydration	Evaluate whether woman is in true labor; ambulate if in early labor. Evaluate client status and contractile pattern. Obtain a 20-minute EFM strip. Notify physician or CNM. Provide hydration.
Cervical dilatation: progressive cervical dilatation from size of fingertip to 10 cm (see Skill 3–1 in the Clinical Skills Manual, as well as the CD-ROM that accompanies this text) **SKILLS**	Rigidity of cervix (frequent cervical infections, scar tissue, failure of presenting part to descend)	Evaluate contractions, fetal engagement, position, and cervical dilatation. Inform client of progress.
Cervical effacement: progressive thinning of cervix (see Skill 3–1) **SKILLS**	Failure to efface (rigidity of cervix, failure of presenting part to engage); cervical edema (pushing effort by woman before cervix is fully dilated and effaced, trapped cervix)	Evaluate contractions, fetal engagement, and position. Notify physician or CNM if cervix is becoming edematous; work with woman to prevent pushing until cervix is completely dilated. Keep vaginal exams to a minimum.
Fetal descent: progressive descent of fetal presenting part from station 25 to 14 (see Skill 3–1) **SKILLS**	Failure of descent (abnormal fetal position or presentation, macrosomic fetus, inadequate pelvic measurement)	Evaluate fetal position, presentation, and size. Evaluate maternal pelvic measurements.
Membranes: may rupture before or during labor	Rupture of membranes more than 12–24 hours before initiation of labor	Assess for ruptured membranes using Nitrazine test tape before doing vaginal exam. Follow universal precautions. Instruct woman with ruptured membranes to remain on bed rest if presenting part is not engaged and firmly down against the cervix. Keep vaginal exams to a minimum to prevent infection. When membranes rupture in the birth setting, **immediately assess FHR** to detect changes associated with prolapse of umbilical cord (FHR slows).
Findings on Nitrazine test tape: Membranes probably intact Yellow pH 5.0 Olive pH 5.5 Olive green pH 6.0 Membranes probably ruptured Blue-green pH 6.5 Blue-gray pH 7.0 Deep blue pH 7.5	False-positive results may be obtained if large amount of bloody show is present, previous vaginal examination has been done using lubricant, or tape is touched by nurse's fingers.	Assess fluid for consistency, amount, odor, assess FHR frequently. Assess fluid at regular intervals for presence of meconium staining. Follow universal precautions while assessing amniotic fluid. Teach woman that amniotic fluid is continually produced (to allay fear of "dry birth"). Teach woman that she may feel amniotic fluid trickle or gush with contractions. Change chux pads often.

*Possible causes of alterations are placed in parentheses.

†This column provides guidelines for further assessment and initial nursing intervention.

ASSESSMENT GUIDE—continued

INTRAPARTAL—FIRST STAGE OF LABOR

PHYSICAL ASSESSMENT/ NORMAL FINDINGS	ALTERATIONS AND POSSIBLE CAUSES*	NURSING RESPONSES TO DATA[†]
Labor Status *(continued)*		
Amniotic fluid clear, with earthy or human odor, no foul-smelling odor	Greenish amniotic fluid (fetal stress) Bloody fluid (abruptio placentae)	Assess FHR; do vaginal exam to evaluate for prolapsed cord; apply fetal monitor for continuous data; report to physician/CNM.
	Strong or foul odor (amnionitis)	Take woman's temperature and report to physician/CNM.
Fetal Status		
FHR: 110–160 bpm	<110 or >160 bpm (nonreassuring fetal status); abnormal patterns on fetal monitor: decreased variability, late decelerations, variable decelerations, absence of accelerations with fetal movement	Initiate interventions based on particular FHR pattern.
Presentation: Cephalic, 97% Breech, 3%	Face, brow, breech, or shoulder presentation	Report to physician/CNM; after presentation is confirmed as face, brow, breech, or shoulder, woman may be prepared for cesarean birth.
Position: left occiput anterior (LOA) most common	Persistent occipital posterior (OP) position; transverse arrest	Carefully monitor maternal and fetal status. Reposition mother to sidelying or hands and knees to promote rotation of fetal head.
Activity: fetal movement	Hyperactivity (may precede fetal hypoxia)	Carefully evaluate FHR; apply fetal monitor.
	Complete lack of movement (fetal distress or fetal demise)	Carefully evaluate FHR; apply fetal monitor. Report to physician or CNM.
Laboratory Evaluation		
Hematologic tests **Hemoglobin:** 12–16 g/dL	<11 g/dL (anemia, hemorrhage)	Evaluate woman for problems due to decreased oxygen-carrying capacity caused by lowered hemoglobin.
Complete blood count (CBC) **Hematocrit:** 38%–47% **Red blood cell count (RBC):** 4.2–5.4 million/mm^3 **White blood cell count (WBC):** 4,500–11,000/mm^3, although leukocytosis to 20,000/mm^3 is not unusual **Platelets:** 150,000–400,000/mm^3	Presence of infection or blood dyscrasias, loss of blood (hemorrhage, disseminated intravascular coagulation [DIC])	Evaluate for other signs of infection or for petechiae, bruising, or unusual bleeding.
Serologic testing Serologic test for syphilis (STS) or Venereal Disease Research Laboratory (VDRL) test: nonreactive	Positive reaction (Chapter 10, Initial Prenatal Physical Assessment Guide) ∞	For reactive test, notify newborn nursery and pediatrician.
Rh factor	Rh-positive fetus in Rh-negative woman	Assess prenatal record for titer levels during pregnancy. Obtain cord blood for direct Coombs' at birth.
Urinalysis **Glucose:** negative	Glycosuria (low renal threshold for glucose, diabetes mellitus)	Assess blood glucose level; test urine for ketones; ketonuria and glycosuria require further assessment of blood sugar levels.[‡]
Ketones: negative	Ketonuria (starvation ketosis)	

*Possible causes of alterations are placed in parentheses.

[†]This column provides guidelines for further assessment and initial nursing intervention.

[‡]Glycosuria should not be discounted. The presence of glycosuria necessitates follow-up.

(continued)

ASSESSMENT GUIDE—continued

INTRAPARTAL—FIRST STAGE OF LABOR

PHYSICAL ASSESSMENT/ NORMAL FINDINGS	ALTERATIONS AND POSSIBLE CAUSES*	NURSING RESPONSES TO DATA†
Laboratory Evaluation *(continued)*		
Proteins: negative	Proteinuria (urine specimen contaminated with vaginal secretions, fever, kidney disease); proteinuria of 2+ or greater found in uncontaminated urine may be a sign of ensuing preeclampsia	Instruct woman in collection technique; incidence of contamination from vaginal discharge is common. Report any increase in proteinuria to physician/CNM.
Red blood cells: negative	Blood in urine (calculi, cystitis, glomerulonephritis, neoplasm)	Assess collection technique (may be bloody show).
White blood cells: negative	Presence of white blood cells (infection in genitourinary tract)	Assess for signs of urinary tract infection.
Casts: none	Presence of casts (nephrotic syndrome)	

CULTURAL ASSESSMENT§	VARIATIONS TO CONSIDER	NURSING RESPONSES TO DATA†
Cultural influences determine customs and practices regarding intrapartal care	Individual preferences may vary.	
Ask the following questions: Who would you like to remain with you during your labor and birth?	She may prefer only her partner/significant other to remain or may also want family and/or friends.	Provide support for her wishes by encouraging desired people to stay. Provide information to others (with the woman's permission) who are not in the room.
What would you like to wear during labor?	She may be more comfortable in her own clothes.	Offer supportive materials such as chux pad if needed to protect her own clothing. Avoid subtle signals to the woman that she should not have chosen to remain in her own clothes. Have other clothing available if the woman desires. If her clothing becomes contaminated, it will be simple to place it in a plastic bag. The nurse can soak soiled clothing in cool water. The nurse needs to remember to wear disposable gloves and a plastic apron if splashing is anticipated.
What activity would you like during labor?	She may want to ambulate most of the time, stand in the shower, sit in the Jacuzzi (see "Complementary Care: Hydrotherapy" in Chapter 17 ∞), sit in a chair or on a stool, remain on the bed, and so forth.	Support the woman's wishes; provide encouragement and complete assessments in a manner so her activity and positional wishes are disturbed as little as possible.
What position would you like for the birth?	She may feel more comfortable in lithotomy with stirrups and her upper body elevated, or side-lying or sitting in birthing bed, or standing, or squatting, or on hands and knees.	Collect any supplies and equipment needed to support her in her chosen birthing position. Provide information to the coach regarding any changes that may be needed based on the chosen position.
Is there anything special you would like?	She may want the room darkened or to have curtains and windows open, music playing (see "Complementary Care: Music During Childbirth" in Chapter 17 ∞), a Leboyer birth, certain scents (see "Complementary Care: Aromatherapy in Childbirth" in this chapter), her coach to cut the umbilical cord, to save a portion of the umbilical cord, to save the placenta, to videotape the birth, and so forth.	Support requests and communicate requests to any other nursing or medical personnel (so requests can continue to be supported and not questioned). If another nurse or physician does not honor the request, act as advocate for the woman by continuing to support her unless her desire is truly unsafe.

§These are only a few suggestions. We do not mean to imply that this is a comprehensive cultural assessment; rather, it is a tool to encourage cultural sensitivity.

*Possible causes of alterations are placed in parentheses.

†This column provides guidelines for further assessment and initial nursing intervention.

ASSESSMENT GUIDE—continued

INTRAPARTAL—FIRST STAGE OF LABOR

CULTURAL ASSESSMENT§	VARIATIONS TO CONSIDER	NURSING RESPONSES TO DATA†
Ask the woman if she would like fluids and ask what temperature she prefers.	She may prefer clear fluids other than water (tea, clear juice). She may prefer iced, room-temperature, or warmed fluids.	Provide fluids as desired.
Observe the woman's response when privacy is difficult to maintain and her body is exposed.	Some women do not seem to mind being exposed during an exam or procedure; others feel acute discomfort.	Maintain privacy and respect the woman's sense of privacy. If the woman is unable to provide specific information, the nurse may draw from general information regarding cultural variation: a Southeast Asian woman may not want any family member in the room during exams or procedures. Her partner may not be involved with coaching activities during labor or birth. Saudi women may need to remain covered during the labor and birth and avoid exposure of any body part. The husband may need to be in the room but remain behind a curtain or screen so he does not view his wife at this time.
If the woman is to breastfeed, ask if she would like to feed her baby immediately after birth.	She may want to feed her baby right away or may want to wait a little while.	

Preparation for Childbirth

Woman has some information regarding process of normal labor and birth.	Some women do not have any information regarding childbirth.	Add to present information base.
Woman has breathing and/or relaxation techniques to use during labor.	Some women do not have any method of relaxation or breathing to use, and some do not desire them.	Support breathing and relaxation techniques that client is using; provide information if needed.

Response to Labor

Latent phase: relaxed, excited, anxious for labor to be well established	May feel unable to cope with contractions because of fear, anxiety, or lack of information	Provide support and encouragement; establish trusting relationship.
Active phase: becomes more intense, begins to tire Transitional phase: feels tired, may feel unable to cope, needs frequent coaching to maintain breathing patterns	May remain quiet and without any sign of discomfort or anxiety, may insist that she is unable to continue with the birthing process	Provide support and coaching if needed.
Coping mechanisms: ability to cope with labor through utilization of support system, breathing, relaxation techniques	May feel marked anxiety and apprehension, may not have coping mechanisms that can be brought into this experience, or may be unable to use them at this time.	Support coping mechanisms if they are working for the woman; provide information and support if she exhibits anxiety or needs alternative to present coping methods.
	Survivors of sexual abuse may demonstrate fear of IVs or needles, may recoil when touched, may insist on a female caregiver, may be very sensitive to body fluids and cleanliness, and may be unable to labor lying down.	Encourage participation of coach or significant other if a supportive relationship seems apparent. Establish rapport and a trusting relationship. Provide information that is true and offer your presence.

Anxiety

Some anxiety and apprehension is within normal limits	May show anxiety through rapid breathing, nervous tremors, frowning, grimacing, clenching of teeth, thrashing movements, crying, increased pulse and blood pressure.	Provide support, encouragement, and information. Teach relaxation techniques; support controlled breathing efforts. May need to provide a paper bag to breathe into if woman says her lips are tingling. Note FHR.

§These are only a few suggestions. We do not mean to imply that this is a comprehensive cultural assessment; rather, it is a tool to encourage cultural sensitivity.

†This column provides guidelines for further assessment and initial nursing intervention.

(continued)

ASSESSMENT GUIDE—continued

INTRAPARTAL—FIRST STAGE OF LABOR

CULTURAL ASSESSMENT§	VARIATIONS TO CONSIDER	NURSING RESPONSES TO DATA†
Sounds During Labor		
	Some women are very quiet; others moan or make a variety of noises.	Provide a supportive environment. Encourage woman to do what is right for her.
Support System		
Physical intimacy between mother and father (or mother and support person); caretaking activities such as soothing conversation, touching	Some women would prefer no contact; others may show clinging behaviors.	Encourage caretaking activities that appear to comfort the woman; encourage support to the woman; if support is limited, the nurse may take a more active role.
Support person stays in close proximity	Limited interaction may come from a desire for quiet.	Encourage support person to stay close (if this seems appropriate).
Relationship between mother and father (or support person): involved interaction	The support person may seem to be detached and maintain little support, attention, or conversation.	Support interactions; if interaction is limited, the nurse may provide more information and support.
		Ensure that coach or significant other has short breaks, especially prior to transition.

§These are only a few suggestions. We do not mean to imply that this is a comprehensive cultural assessment; rather, it is a tool to encourage cultural sensitivity.

†This column provides guidelines for further assessment and initial nursing intervention.

---

and women having oxytocin-induced labor; other facilities monitor all laboring women.

Electronic monitoring may be done externally with a device placed against the maternal abdomen, or internally with an **intrauterine pressure catheter**. When monitoring by external means, the portion of the monitoring equipment called a tocodynamometer, or "toco," is positioned against the fundus of the uterus and held in place with an elastic belt (Figure 18–1 ●). The toco contains a flexible disk that responds to pressure. When the uterus contracts,

TABLE 18–2 ✣ Contraction and Labor Progress Characteristics

Contraction Characteristics

Latent phase:	Every 10–30 min × 30 sec; mild, progressing to Every 5–7 min × 30–40 sec; moderate
Active phase:	Every 2–5 min × 40–60 sec; moderate to strong
Transition phase:	Every 1½–2 min × 60–90 sec; strong

Labor Progress Characteristics

Primipara:	1.2 cm/hr dilatation 1 cm/hr descent < 2 hr in second stage
Multipara:	1.5 cm/hr dilatation < 2 cm/hr descent < 1 hr in second stage

● FIGURE 18–1

Woman in labor with external monitor applied. The tocodynamometer placed on the uterine fundus is recording uterine contractions. The lower belt holds the ultrasonic device that monitors the fetal heart rate. The belts can be adjusted for comfort.

COMPLEMENTARY CARE

AROMATHERAPY IN CHILDBIRTH

Aromatherapy is the use of aromas for physical, mental, and emotional healing. The primary sources of healing aromas are essential oils distilled from herbs and flowers. Essential oils are volatile, which means that their molecules quickly evaporate into the environment. When you inhale an essential oil molecule, its active components react with the olfactory membrane in your nose, which is directly linked to the limbic system and hypothalamus in the brain. These two areas play a crucial role in regulating your emotions, mind, and body (Gottlieb, 2003).

Essential oils can also be applied directly to the skin. Because the oil is not only inhaled but also absorbed into the bloodstream, the effect can be doubled (Gottlieb, 2003). Essential oils are quite potent and can irritate the skin, so they should be diluted with a carrier oil such as sesame or sweet almond oil before being used on the skin. The fragrance

of the essential oil in the carrier oil does not have to be intense to be effective. In fact, the more intense the odor, the less pleasant it becomes.

For a few days before the expected due date and during labor, jasmine or lavender oil can be massaged into the abdomen and lower back using long, smooth movement and fairly firm pressure. The woman may find small circular movements of the lower back to be soothing. Both jasmine and lavender strengthen contractions and provide some analgesia. If the woman complains of feeling hot during labor, a few drops of lavender can be added to cool water, which is then used to sponge her face and body.

Women should not use essential oils during the first 3 months of pregnancy, since many oils contain thujone, a chemical that has been shown to have an abortive effect (Gottlieb, 2003).

---

the fundus tightens and the change in pressure against the toco is amplified and transmitted to the electronic fetal monitor. The monitor displays the uterine contraction as a pattern on graph paper.

External monitoring provides a continuous recording of the frequency and duration of uterine contractions and

is noninvasive. However, it does not accurately record the intensity of the uterine contraction, and it is difficult to obtain an accurate fetal heart rate (FHR) in some women, such as those who are very obese, those who have hydramnios (an abnormally large amount of amniotic fluid), or those whose fetus is very active. In addition the belt may

MediaLink Case Study: Maternal Assessment during Labor

EVIDENCE-BASED NURSING

FETAL HEART RATE ASSESSMENTS

Clinical Question

What fetal heart rate assessments will best assure fetal well-being during the intrapartum period?

Evidence

The Institute for Clinical Systems Improvement assembled an expert team of physicians and advanced practice nurses to evaluate research evidence and develop a clinical algorithm. The resulting practice guideline provides recommendations for action as well as supporting research resources. Evaluation of fetal status with either intermittent auscultation or continuous electronic fetal monitoring is effective when labor is not high risk. Continuous electronic fetal monitoring is indicated in all high-risk situations and in low-risk situations when 1:1 nursing staff is not available.

Implications

Fetal well-being can be monitored with either intermittent auscultation or continuous electronic fetal monitoring in low-risk situations. Nurse auscultatory monitoring consists of auscultating with a fetoscope or ultrasound device during a contraction and for 30 seconds after the contraction every 15 minutes during the active stage of labor and every 5 minutes during the second stage of labor. Close nurse monitoring with a high nurse-to-client ratio provides comparable outcomes to electronic monitoring and results in personalized high-quality obstetric care. In high-risk situations, continuous electronic fetal monitoring is indicated.

Regardless of method, monitoring should allow for early recognition and intervention in fetal heart rate patterns that indicate potential fetal stress. These include late decelerations, variable decelerations, prolonged deceleration, severe tachycardia or bradycardia, or a sinusoidal pattern. When a nonreassuring fetal heart rate pattern is detected, remedial techniques such as changes in maternal position, IV fluid bolus, oxygen administration, and discontinuing oxytocics may help the fetus revert to a normal heart rate pattern. If the nonreassuring fetal heart rate pattern continues, clinically appropriate interventions should be instituted, including continuous electronic fetal monitoring. Persistent nonreassuring tracings indicate the need for immediate birth. It is the responsibility of every member of the healthcare team to evaluate risk during labor and intervene appropriately. Electronic fetal monitoring is not a substitute for well-trained nurses and appropriate obstetric staffing.

Critical Thinking

What maternal signs and symptoms might indicate a need for immediate auscultation of fetal heart rate? If a nonreassuring heart rate pattern is detected, what will be your assessments and interventions?

Reference

Institute for Clinical Systems Improvement. (2002, October). Intrapartum fetal heart rate management. *Healthcare Guidelines. General Implementation.* Bloomington, MN: Author.

● FIGURE 18–2

To gauge cervical dilatation, the nurse places the index and middle fingers against the cervix and determines the size of the opening. Before labor begins, the cervix is long (approximately 2.5 cm), the sides feel thick, and the cervical canal is closed, so an examining finger cannot be inserted. During labor the cervix begins to dilate, and the size of the opening progresses from 1 cm to 10 cm in diameter.

bother the woman if it requires frequent readjustment when she changes position.

Internal intrauterine monitoring provides the same data and also provides accurate measurement of uterine contraction intensity (the strength of the contraction and the actual pressure within the uterus). After membranes have ruptured, the certified nurse-midwife or physician inserts the intrauterine pressure catheter into the uterine cavity and connects it by a cable to the electronic fetal monitor. A small micropressure device located in the tip of the catheter measures the pressure within the uterus in the resting state and during each contraction. Internal electronic monitoring is used when it is imperative to have accurate intrauterine pressure readings to evaluate the stress on the uterus.

In addition it is important to evaluate the woman's labor status by palpating the intensity and resting tone of the uterine fundus during contractions.

Cervical Assessment

Cervical dilatation and effacement are evaluated directly by vaginal examination (see Skill 3–1 in the *Clinical Skills Manual* as well as the CD-ROM that accompanies this

● FIGURE 18–3

Palpating the presenting part (portion of the fetus that enters the pelvis first). *A,* Left occiput anterior (LOA). The occiput (area over the occipital bone on the posterior part of the fetal head) is in the left anterior quadrant of the woman's pelvis. When the fetus is LOA, the posterior fontanelle (located just above the occipital bone and triangular in shape) is in the upper left quadrant of the maternal pelvis. *B,* Left occiput posterior (LOP). The posterior fontanelle is in the lower left quadrant of the maternal pelvis. *C,* Right occiput anterior (ROA). The posterior fontanelle is in the upper right quadrant of the maternal pelvis. *D,* Right occiput posterior (ROP). The posterior fontanelle is in the lower right quadrant of the maternal pelvis. *Note:* The anterior fontanelle is diamond shaped. Because of the roundness of the fetal head, only a portion of the anterior fontanelle can be seen in each of the views, so it appears to be triangular in shape.

● **FIGURE 18–4**

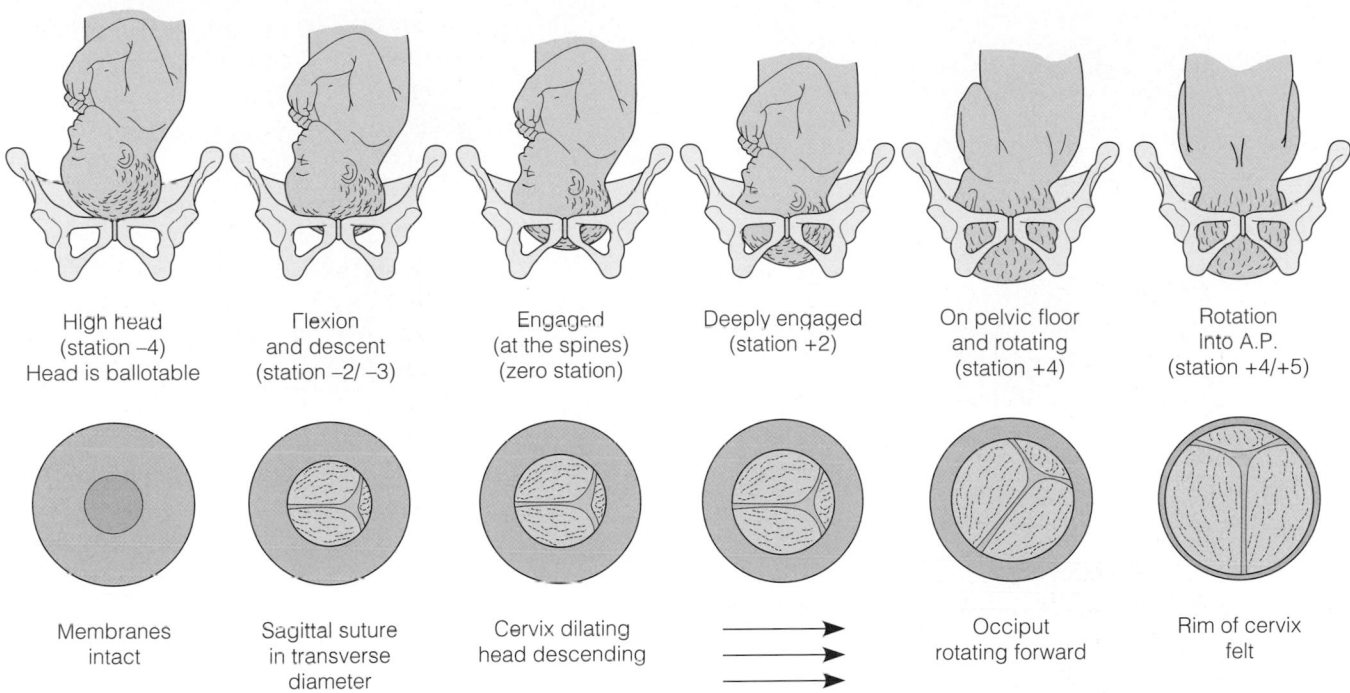

| High head (station –4) Head is ballotable | Flexion and descent (station –2/ –3) | Engaged (at the spines) (zero station) | Deeply engaged (station +2) | On pelvic floor and rotating (station +4) | Rotation into A.P. (station +4/+5) |

| Membranes intact | Sagittal suture in transverse diameter | Cervix dilating head descending | | Occiput rotating forward | Rim of cervix felt |

Top: The fetal head progressing through the pelvis. *Bottom:* The changes the nurse will detect on palpation of the occiput through the cervix while doing a vaginal examination.

Used with permission from Myles, M. F. (1975). Textbook for midwives (p. 246), by permission of the publisher: Churchill-Livingstone.

text). **SKILLS** The vaginal examination can also provide information about membrane status, characteristics of amniotic fluid, fetal position, and station. See Figures 18–2 ●, 18–3 ●, and 18–4 ●.

FETAL ASSESSMENT

FETAL POSITION AND PRESENTATION

Fetal position and presentation are determined by inspecting the woman's abdomen, palpating it, performing a vaginal examination, and auscultating FHR. Ultrasound may also be used.

Inspection

Observe the woman's abdomen for size and shape. Assess the lie of the fetus by noting whether the uterus projects up and down (longitudinal lie) or left to right (transverse lie).

Palpation: Leopold's Maneuvers

Leopold's maneuvers are a systematic way to evaluate the maternal abdomen. Frequent practice increases the examiner's skill in determining fetal position by palpation. Leopold's maneuvers may be difficult to perform on an obese woman or on a woman who has excessive amniotic

fluid (hydramnios). Before performing Leopold's maneuvers, have the woman (1) empty her bladder and (2) lie on her back with her feet on the bed and her knees bent. (See Figure 18–5 ● for technique. Also see Clinical Skills Manual that accompanies this text. **SKILLS**)

Vaginal Examination and Ultrasound

During a vaginal examination, the examiner can palpate the presenting part if the cervix is dilated. The examination also provides information about the position of the fetus and the degree of flexion of its head (in cephalic presentations). Visualization by ultrasound is used when the fetal position cannot be determined by abdominal palpation.

AUSCULTATION OF FETAL HEART RATE

The handheld Doppler ultrasound or the fetoscope is used to auscultate the FHR between, during, and immediately after uterine contractions. Instead of listening haphazardly over the woman's abdomen for the FHR, it is useful to perform Leopold's maneuvers first. Leopold's maneuvers not only indicate the probable location of the FHR but also help determine the presence of multiple fetuses, fetal lie, and fetal presentation. The FHR is heard most clearly at the fetal back (Figure 18–6 ●). Thus, in a cephalic presentation, the FHR is best heard in the lower quadrant of the maternal abdomen. In a breech presentation, it is heard at

● **FIGURE 18-5**

First maneuver

A

Second maneuver

B

Third maneuver

C

Fourth maneuver

D

Leopold's maneuvers for determining fetal position and presentation. **A,** First maneuver: Facing the woman, palpate the upper abdomen with both hands. Note the shape, consistency, and mobility of the palpated part. The fetal head is firm and round and moves independently of the trunk. The buttock feels softer, and it moves with the trunk. **B,** Second maneuver: Moving the hands on the pelvis, palpate the abdomen with gentle but deep pressure. The fetal back, on one side of the abdomen, feels smooth, and the fetal extremities on the other side feel knobby. **C,** Third maneuver: Place one hand just above the symphysis. Note whether the part palpated feels like the fetal head or the breech and whether it is engaged. **D,** Fourth maneuver: Facing the woman's feet, place both hands on the lower abdomen and move hands gently down the sides of the uterus toward the pubis. Note the cephalic prominence or brow.

or above the level of the maternal umbilicus. In a transverse lie, FHR may be heard best just above or just below the umbilicus. As the presenting part descends and rotates through the pelvic structure during labor, the location of the FHR tends to descend and move toward the midline.

After the FHR is located, it is usually counted for 30 seconds and multiplied by 2 to obtain the number of beats per minute (bpm). Check the woman's pulse against the fetal sounds. If the rates are the same, readjust the Doppler or fetoscope. Occasionally listen for a full minute, through and just after a contraction, to detect any abnormal heart rate, espe-

cially if the FHR is over 160 bpm (tachycardia), under 110 bpm (bradycardia), or irregular. If the FHR is irregular or has changed markedly from the last assessment, listen for a full minute through and immediately after a contraction (see Skill 3–4 in the *Clinical Skills Manual* as well as the CD-ROM that accompanies this text SKILLS and Table 18–3 for guidelines on how often to auscultate the FHR).

Intermittent auscultation has been found to be as effective as the electronic method for fetal surveillance. A growing number of healthcare professionals, doctors and nurses alike, are beginning to question the widespread use

● **FIGURE 18-6**

LSA
LOP
RSA
LOA
ROP
ROA

A

Location of FHR
in LOA position

B

Location of FHR in relation to the more commonly seen fetal positions.

of a technology that has not proven its overall worth (Carr & Schott, 2002).

ELECTRONIC MONITORING OF FETAL HEART RATE

Electronic fetal monitoring produces a continuous tracing of the FHR, which allows visual assessment of many characteristics of the FHR (see Skill 3–6 in the *Clinical Skills Manual* as well as the CD-ROM that accompanies this text). SKILLS

Indications for Electronic Monitoring

If one or more of the following factors are present, the FHR and contractions are monitored by electronic fetal monitoring:

TABLE 18–3 ❖ Frequency of Auscultation: Assessment and Documentation

Low-Risk Women	High-Risk Women
First stage of labor:	First stage of labor:
q1 hr in latent phase	q30 min in latent phase
q30 min in active phase	q15 min in active phase
Second stage of labor: q15 min	Second stage of labor: q5 min

Labor Events

Assess FHR prior to:

Initiation of labor-enhancing procedures (e.g., artificial rupture of membranes)

Periods of ambulation

Administration of medications

Administration or initiation of analgesia or anesthesia

Assess FHR following:

Rupture of membranes

Recognition of abnormal uterine activity patterns, such as increased basal tone or tachysystole

Evaluation of oxytocin (maintenance, increase, or decrease of dosage)

Administration of medications (at time of peak action)

Expulsion of enema

Urinary catheterization

Vaginal examination

Periods of ambulation

Evaluation of analgesia and/or anesthesia (maintenance, increase, or decrease of dosage)

Note: From Feinstein, N. F., Sprague, A., & Trepanier, M. J. (2000). Fetal heart rate auscultation. Washington DC: AWHONN, p. 27. © Association of Women's Health, Obstetric and Neonatal Nurses. All rights reserved.

- Previous history of a stillborn (fetus dies in the uterus) at 38 or more weeks' gestation

- Presence of a complication of pregnancy (e.g., preeclampsia-eclampsia, placenta previa, abruptio placentae, multiple gestation, prolonged or premature rupture of membranes)

- Induction of labor (labor that is begun as a result of some type of intervention such as an intravenous infusion of oxytocin [Pitocin])

- Preterm labor (gestation less than 37 completed weeks)

- Decreased fetal movement

- Nonreassuring fetal status

- Meconium staining of amniotic fluid (meconium has been released into the amniotic fluid by the fetus, which may indicate a problem)

- Trial of labor following a previous cesarean birth (Bujold & Gauthier, 2002)

MEDIALINK Skill 3-6: Electronic Fetal Monitoring

● **FIGURE 18–7**

Light blinks with each fetal heartbeat

Knob to regulate sound volume

Digital display of FHR

Graph paper

"Toco" monitors uterine contractions

Ultrasound device

Electronic fetal monitoring by external technique. The tocodynamometer ("toco") is placed over the uterine fundus. The toco provides information that can be used to monitor uterine contractions. The ultrasound device is placed over the area of the fetal back. This device transmits information about the FHR. Information from both the toco and the ultrasound device is transmitted to the electronic fetal monitor. The FHR is displayed in a digital display (as a blinking light), on the special monitor paper, and audibly (by adjusting a button on the monitor). The uterine contractions are displayed on the special monitor paper as well.

Methods of Electronic Monitoring of FHR

External monitoring of the fetus is usually accomplished by ultrasound. A transducer, which emits continuous sound waves, is placed on the maternal abdomen. When the transducer is placed correctly, the sound waves bounce off the fetal heart and are picked up by the electronic monitor. The actual moment-by-moment FHR is displayed graphically on a screen (Figure 18–7 ●). In some instances the monitor may track the maternal heart rate instead of the fetal heart rate. Avoid this error by comparing the maternal pulse to the FHR.

Recent advances in technology have led to the development of new ambulatory methods of external monitoring. Using a telemetry system, a small, battery-operated transducer transmits signals to a receiver connected to the monitor. This system, held in place with a shoulder strap, allows the woman to ambulate, helping her to feel more comfortable and less confined during labor. In contrast the system depicted in Figure 18–7 requires the woman to remain close to the electrical power source for the monitor.

Internal monitoring requires an internal spiral electrode. To place the spiral electrode on the fetal occiput, the amniotic membranes must be ruptured, the cervix must be dilated at least 2 cm, the presenting part must be down against the cervix, and the presenting part must be known (that is, the examiner must be able to detect the actual part of the fetus that is down against the cervix). If all these factors are present, the labor and birth nurse, the physician, or the certified nurse-midwife inserts a sterile internal spiral electrode into the vagina and places it against the fetal presenting part. The spiral electrode is rotated clockwise until it is attached to the presenting part. Wires that extend from the spiral electrode are attached to a leg plate (which is placed on the woman's thigh) and then attached to the electronic fetal monitor. This method of monitoring the FHR provides more accurate continuous data than external monitoring, because the signal is clearer and movement of the fetus or the woman does not interrupt it (Figure 18–8 ●). The FHR tracing at the top of Figure 18–9 ● was obtained by internal monitoring with a spiral electrode; the uterine contraction tracing at the bottom of the figure was obtained by external monitoring with a toco.

● **FIGURE 18–8**

B

C

Technique for internal, direct fetal monitoring. **A,** Spiral electrode. **B,** Attaching the spiral electrode to the scalp. **C,** Attached spiral electrode with the guide tube removed.

Baseline Fetal Heart Rate

The **baseline rate** refers to the average FHR observed during a 10-minute period of monitoring. Normal FHR (baseline rate) ranges from 110 to 160 bpm. There are two abnormal variations of the baseline rate—those above 160 bpm (tachycardia) and those below 110 bpm (bradycardia). Another change affecting the baseline is called *variability,* a change in FHR over a few seconds to a few minutes.

Fetal tachycardia is a sustained rate of 161 bpm or above. *Marked tachycardia* is 180 bpm or above. Causes of tachycardia include the following (Menihan & Zottoli, 2001):

- Early fetal hypoxia, which leads to stimulation of the sympathetic system as the fetus compensates for reduced blood flow

- Maternal fever, which accelerates the metabolism of the fetus

- Maternal dehydration

- Beta-sympathomimetic drugs such as ritodrine, terbutaline, atropine, and isoxsuprine, which have a cardiac stimulant effect

- Amnionitis (fetal tachycardia may be the first sign of developing intrauterine infection)

- Maternal hyperthyroidism (thyroid-stimulating hormones may cross the placenta and stimulate FHR)

- Fetal anemia (the heart rate is increased to improve tissue perfusion)

Tachycardia is considered an ominous sign if it is accompanied by late decelerations, severe variable decelerations, or decreased variability. If tachycardia is associated with

● **FIGURE 18–9**

Normal FHR pattern obtained by internal monitoring. Note normal FHR, 140 to 158 bpm, presence of long- and short-term variability, and absence of deceleration with adequate contractions. The bottom portion depicts uterine contractions obtained by external monitoring. Each dark vertical line marks 1 minute, and each small rectangle represents 10 seconds. The contraction frequency is about every 2 1/2 minutes, and the duration of the contractions is 50 to 60 seconds. Arrows on the bottom of tracing indicate beginnings of uterine contractions.

maternal fever, treatment may include antipyretics, antibiotics, or both.

Fetal bradycardia is a rate less than 110 bpm during a 10-minute period or longer. Causes of fetal bradycardia include the following (Menihan & Zottoli, 2001):

- Late (profound) fetal hypoxia (depression of myocardial activity)
- Maternal hypotension, which results in decreased blood flow to the fetus
- Prolonged umbilical cord compression; fetal baroreceptors are activated by cord compression and this produces vagal stimulation, which results in decreased FHR
- Fetal arrhythmia, which is associated with complete heart block in the fetus
- Uterine hyperstimulation
- Abruptio placentae
- Uterine rupture
- Vagal stimulation in the second stage (since this does not involve hypoxia, the fetus can recover)

Bradycardia may be a benign or an ominous sign. If average long-term variability exists, the bradycardia is considered benign. When bradycardia is accompanied by decreased long-term variability and late decelerations, it is considered a sign of nonreassuring fetal status (Menihan & Zottoli, 2001).

Variability

Baseline variability is a measure of the interplay (the push-pull effect) between the sympathetic and parasympathetic nervous systems. There are two types of fetal heart variability. **Short-term variability (STV)** is the beat-to-beat change in FHR. It represents fluctuations of the baseline. STV can only be measured via internal (scalp electrode) means and is classified as either present or absent. **Long-term variability (LTV)** is the waviness or rhythmic fluctuations (called cycles) of the FHR tracing, which occur three to five times per minute (Figure 18–10 ●).

Fetal heart rate variability is defined as follows (Garite, 2002):

- **Absent:** amplitude undetectable
- **Minimal:** amplitude greater than undetectable, and 5 bpm or less
- **Moderate:** amplitude 6 to 25 bpm
- **Marked:** amplitude greater than 25 bpm

⊙ FIGURE 18-10

A

B

←1 minute→

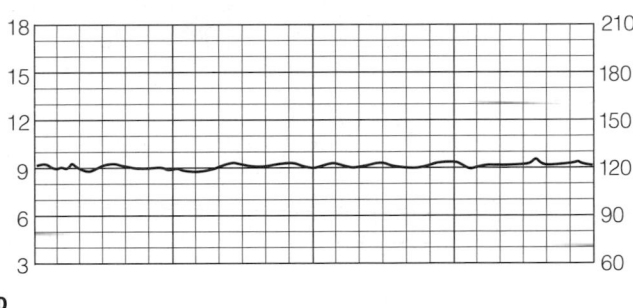

C

D

Variability. **A,** Marked variability. **B,** Moderate variability. **C,** Minimal variability. **D,** Absent variability.

The most important aspect of LTV is that even in the presence of abnormal or questionable FHR patterns, if the variability is normal, the fetus is not suffering from cerebral asphyxia.

Causes of decreased variability include the following (Menihan & Zottoli, 2001):

- Hypoxia and acidosis (decreased blood flow to the fetus)
- Administration of drugs such as meperidine hydrochloride (Demerol), diazepam (Valium), or hydroxyzine (Vistaril), which depress the fetal central nervous system
- Fetal sleep cycle (during fetal sleep, LTV is decreased; fetal sleep cycles usually last for 20 to 30 minutes)
- Fetus of less than 32 weeks' gestation (fetal neurologic control of heart rate is immature)
- Fetal anomalies affecting the heart, central nervous system, or autonomic nervous system
- Previous neurologic insult
- Tachycardia

Causes of increased variability include the following (Menihan & Zottoli, 2001):

- Early mild hypoxia (variability increases as a result of compensatory mechanism)
- Fetal stimulation or activity (stimulation of autonomic nervous system because of abdominal palpation,

maternal vaginal examination, application of spiral electrode on fetal head, or acoustic stimulation)

- Alteration in placental blood flow

If it does not appear to be associated with a fetal sleep cycle or the administration of drugs, absent variability is a warning sign of nonreassuring fetal status. It is especially ominous if absent or minimal variability is accompanied by late decelerations, explained shortly.

External electronic fetal monitoring is not an adequate method to assess STV. If decreased variability is noted on monitoring, application of a spiral electrode should be considered to obtain more accurate information.

Accelerations

Accelerations are transient increases in the FHR normally caused by fetal movement. When the fetus moves, the heart rate increases, just as the heart rates of adults increase during exercise. Often, accelerations accompany uterine contractions, usually due to fetal movement in response to the pressure of the contractions. Accelerations of this type are thought to be a sign of fetal well-being and adequate oxygen reserve. The accelerations with fetal movement form the basis for nonstress tests (see Chapter 16. ∞)

Decelerations

Decelerations are periodic decreases in FHR from the normal baseline. They are categorized as early, late, and variable

● **FIGURE 18-11**

FHR pattern	Early deceleration	Late deceleration	Variable deceleration
	Head compression (HC)	Uteroplacental insufficiency (UPI)	Umbilical cord compression (CC)
Shape	Waveform consistently uniform inversely mirrors contraction	Waveform uniform; shape reflects contraction	Waveform variable, generally sharp drops and returns
Onset	Just prior to or early in contraction	Late in contraction	Abrupt with fetal insult; not related to contraction
Lowest level	Consistently at or before midpoint of contraction	Consistently after the midpoint of the contraction	Variable around midpoint
Range	Usually within normal range of 120–160 beats/min	Usually within normal range of 120–130 beats/min	Not usually within normal range
Ensemble	Can be single or repetitive	Occasional, consistent, gradually increase—repetitive	Variable—single or repetitive

Types and characteristics of early, late, and variable decelerations.

Used with permission from Hon, E. (1976). An introduction to fetal heart rate monitoring (2nd ed., p. 29). Los Angeles: University of Southern California School of Medicine.

according to the time of their occurrence in the contraction cycle and their waveform (Figure 18–11 ●). When the fetal head is compressed, cerebral blood flow is decreased, which leads to central vagal stimulation and results in early deceleration. The onset of early deceleration occurs before the onset of the uterine contraction. This type of deceleration is of uniform shape, is usually considered benign, and does not require intervention.

Late deceleration is caused by uteroplacental insufficiency resulting from decreased blood flow and oxygen transfer to the fetus through the intervillous spaces during uterine contractions. The onset of the deceleration occurs after the onset of a uterine contraction and is of a uniform shape that tends to reflect associated uterine

contractions. The late deceleration pattern is considered a nonreassuring sign but does not necessarily require immediate childbirth.

Variable decelerations occur if the umbilical cord becomes compressed, thus reducing blood flow between the placenta and fetus. The resulting increase in peripheral resistance in the fetal circulation causes fetal hypertension. The fetal hypertension stimulates the baroreceptors in the aortic arch and carotid sinuses, which slow the FHR. The onset of variable decelerations varies in timing with the onset of the contraction, and the decelerations are variable in shape. This pattern requires further assessment. Nursing interventions for late and variable decelerations in FHR are presented in Table 18–4.

TABLE 18–4 ✤ Guidelines for Management of Variable, Late, and Prolonged Deceleration Patterns

Pattern	Nursing Interventions
Variable decelerations Isolated or occasional Moderate	Report findings to physician or CNM and document in chart. Provide explanation to woman and partner. Change maternal position to one in which FHR pattern is most improved. Discontinue oxytocin if it is being administered and other interventions are unsuccessful. Perform vaginal examination to assess for prolapsed cord or change in labor progress. Monitor FHR continuously to assess current status and for further changes in FHR pattern.
Variable decelerations Severe and uncorrectable	Give oxygen if indicated. Report findings to physician or CNM and document in chart. Provide explanation to woman and partner. Prepare for probable cesarean birth. Follow interventions listed above. Prepare for vaginal birth unless baseline variability is decreasing or FHR is progressively rising—then cesarean, forceps, or vacuum birth is indicated. Assist physician with fetal scalp sampling if ordered. Prepare for cesarean birth if scalp pH shows acidosis or downward trend.
Late decelerations	Give oxygen if indicated. Report findings to physician or CNM and document in chart. Provide explanation to woman and partner. Monitor for further FHR changes. Maintain maternal position on left side. Maintain good hydration with IV fluids (normal saline or lactated Ringer's). Discontinue oxytocin if it is being administered and late decelerations persist despite other interventions. Administer oxygen by face mask at 7 to 10 L/min. Monitor maternal blood pressure and pulse for signs of hypotension; possibly increase flow rate of IV fluids to treat hypotension. Follow physician's orders for treatment for hypotension if present. Increase IV fluids to maintain volume and hydration (normal saline or lactated Ringer's). Assess labor progress (dilatation and station). Assist physician with fetal blood sampling: If pH stays above 7.25, physician will continue monitoring and resample; if pH shows downward trend (between 7.25 and 7.2) or is below 7.2, prepare for birth by most expeditious means.
Late decelerations with tachycardia or decreasing variability	Report findings to physician or CNM and document in chart. Maintain maternal position on left side. Administer oxygen by face mask at 7 to 10 L/min. Discontinue oxytocin if it is being administered. Assess maternal blood pressure and pulse. Increase IV fluids (normal saline or lactated Ringer's). Assess labor progress (dilatation and station). Prepare for immediate cesarean birth. Explain plan of treatment to woman and partner. Assist physician with fetal blood sampling (if ordered).
Prolonged decelerations	Perform vaginal examination to rule out prolapsed cord or to determine progress in labor status. Change maternal position as needed to try to alleviate decelerations. Discontinue oxytocin if it is being administered. Notify physician or CNM of findings and initial interventions and document in chart. Provide explanation to woman and partner. Increase IV fluids (normal saline or lactated Ringer's). Administer tocolytic if hypertonus noted and ordered by physician or CNM. Anticipate normal FHR recovery following deceleration if FHR previously normal. Anticipate intervention if FHR previously abnormal or deceleration lasts > 3 minutes.

A *sinusoidal pattern* appears similar to a waveform. The characteristics of this pattern include absence of variability and the presence of a smooth, wavelike shape. Typically there are no periods during which the heart rate appears normal (Menihan & Zottoli, 2001). This pattern is associated with Rh alloimmunization, fetal anemia, severe fetal hypoxia, or a chronic fetal bleed. It may also occur with the administration of medications such as meperidine (Demerol) or butorphanol tartrate (Stadol). When it appears in association with medication, the pattern is usually temporary and is commonly referred to as *pseudosinusoidal* (Menihan & Zottoli, 2001).

NURSING PRACTICE

The presence of repetitive early decelerations may be a sign of advanced dilatation or the beginning of the second stage of labor. If the monitoring strip shows recurring early decelerations, ask the laboring woman if she is experiencing any pressure. Pressure that occurs only with the contractions typically indicates advanced dilatation. Intense pressure that does not change or ease up when the contractions cease may indicate the beginning of the second stage. A vaginal examination may be performed to establish the dilatation.

Psychologic Reactions to Electronic Monitoring

Responses to electronic fetal monitoring can be varied and complex. Many women have little knowledge of monitoring unless they have attended a prenatal class that dealt with this subject. Some women react to electronic monitoring positively, viewing it as a reassurance that "the baby is OK." They may also feel that the monitor helps identify problems that develop in labor. Other women may have ambivalent or even negative feelings about the monitor. They may think that the monitor is interfering with a natural process, and they do not want the intrusion. Some women may find that the equipment, wires, and sounds increase their anxiety. The discomfort of lying in one position and fear of injury to the baby are other objections.

Nursing Responsibilities

A key strength of technology is its ability to explain and possibly predict health patterns or problems. However, this advantage has the potential to dehumanize the nurse-client relationship. Therefore, it is important to recognize that every encounter with the childbearing family offers an opportunity to provide education and empowerment to the laboring woman and her partner. Helping to provide information when needed, answering questions, and encouraging the woman to make decisions establishes a trusting nurse-client relationship.

Technology has been advancing at a rapid rate in the labor and birthing arena, and each new development challenges nurses to understand, include, and balance technology with holistic nursing practice. Before using the electronic fetal monitor, explain the reason for its use and the information that it can provide. After applying the monitor, record basic information on the monitor strip. Newer fetal monitors have an attached keyboard that records typed entries directly onto the monitor strip. In facilities that have not yet begun using the keyboards, record data in ink directly on the monitor strip. These data should include the date, client's name, physician or certified nurse-midwife's name, hospital identification number, age, gravida, para, estimated date of birth, membrane status, and maternal vital signs. As the monitor strip runs and care is provided, occurrences during labor should be recorded not only in the medical record but also on the monitor strip. This information helps the healthcare team assess current status and evaluate the tracing.

Note the following information on the tracing (American Academy of Pediatrics [AAP] & ACOG, 2002):

- Vaginal examination (dilatation, effacement, station, position)
- Amniotomy or spontaneous rupture of membranes, color and amount of amniotic fluid, presence of any odor
- Maternal vital signs
- Maternal position in bed and changes of position
- Application of spiral electrode or intrauterine pressure catheter
- Medications given
- Oxygen administration
- Maternal behaviors (emesis, coughing, hiccups)
- Fetal scalp stimulation or fetal scalp blood sampling
- Vomiting
- Pushing
- Administration of anesthesia blocks

If the monitor does not automatically add the time on the strip at specific intervals, include the time when recording any information on the strip. If more than one nurse is adding information to the monitor strip, it is essential to initial each note. The tracing is considered a legal part of the woman's medical record and is submissible as evidence in court.

The laboring woman needs to feel that what is happening to her is the central focus. Acknowledge this need by always speaking to and looking at the woman when entering the room, before looking at the monitor.

Evaluation of FHR Tracings

It is important to use a systematic approach in evaluating FHR tracings. Evaluation of the electronic monitor tracing begins by looking at the uterine contraction pattern:

- Determine the uterine resting tone.
- Assess the contractions: What is the frequency? What is the duration? What is the intensity (if internal monitoring)?

The next step is to evaluate the FHR tracing:

- Determine the baseline: Is the baseline within the normal range? Is there evidence of tachycardia? Is there evidence of bradycardia?
- Determine FHR variability: Is STV present or absent? Is LTV average? Minimal? Absent? Moderate? Marked?
- Determine if a sinusoidal pattern is present.
- Determine if there are periodic changes: Are accelerations present? Do they meet the criteria for a reactive nonstress test? Are decelerations present? Are they uniform in shape? If so, determine if they are early or late decelerations. Are they nonuniform in shape? If so, determine whether they are variable decelerations.

After evaluating the FHR tracing for the factors just listed, classify the tracing as reassuring (normal) or nonreassuring (worrisome). Reassuring patterns contain normal parameters and do not require additional treatment or intervention.

Characteristics of reassuring FHR patterns include the following.

- Baseline rate is 110 to 160 bpm.
- STV is present.
- LTV ranges from three to five cycles per minute. Periodic patterns consist of accelerations with fetal movement, and early decelerations may be present.

Nonreassuring patterns may indicate that the fetus is becoming stressed and intervention is needed. Characteristics of nonreassuring patterns include the following:

- Severe variable decelerations (FHR drops below 70 bpm for longer than 30 to 45 seconds and is accompanied by rising baseline or decreasing variability or slow return to baseline)
- Late decelerations of any magnitude
- Absence of variability (no STV or LTV present)
- Prolonged deceleration (a deceleration that lasts 60 to 90 seconds or more)
- Severe (marked) bradycardia (FHR baseline of 70 bpm or less)

Nonreassuring patterns may require continuous monitoring and more involved treatment and intervention (see Table 18–4).

It is vital to provide information to the laboring woman about the FHR pattern and the interventions, if necessary, that will help her fetus. Most women are aware that some-

thing is happening. Sharing information with them provides reassurance that a potential or actual problem is identified and that they are active participants in the interventions. Occasionally a problem arises that requires immediate intervention. In that case it may be helpful to say something like, "It is important for you to turn on your left side right now because the baby is having a little difficulty. I'll explain what is happening in just a few moments." This type of response lets the woman know that although an action needs to be accomplished rapidly, information will soon be provided. In the haste to act quickly, nurses and other caregivers must not forget that it is the woman's body and her baby.

SCALP STIMULATION TEST

When there is a question about fetal status, a scalp stimulation test can be used before the more invasive fetal blood sampling. In this test the examiner applies pressure to the fetal scalp by gently stroking or massaging it for 15 seconds while doing a vaginal examination. The fetus who is not in any stress or distress responds with an acceleration of the FHR of at least 15 bpm for at least 15 seconds (Varney, Kriebs, & Gegor, 2004).

Fetal vibroacoustic stimulation using a handheld artificial larynx applied to the maternal abdomen may also be used to assess fetal status. As with scalp stimulation, fetal heart rate accelerations in response are a sign of fetal well-being (Varney et al., 2004).

FETAL SCALP BLOOD SAMPLING

When nonreassuring or confusing FHR patterns are noted, additional information about the acid-base status of the fetus is needed. This information may be obtained by **fetal blood sampling**. The physician or CNM usually draws the blood sample from the fetal scalp but may obtain it from the fetal buttocks if the fetus is in the breech position (Cunningham et al., 2005).

Before fetal blood can be sampled, the membranes must be ruptured, the cervix must be dilated at least 2 to 3 cm, and the presenting part must not be above − 2 station. Sampling is not done when FHR patterns are ominous. It is contraindicated in acute emergencies and in cases of vaginal bleeding. In these instances, birth by the most expeditious means is indicated.

Normal fetal pH values during labor are above 7.25; 7.2 to 7.25 is considered borderline, warranting further sampling. Values below 7.2 are nonreassuring and necessitate birth without delay (Cunningham et al., 2005).

The more information that is available from FHR monitoring, the less need there is for fetal blood sampling. This adjunctive procedure is indicated only when FHR patterns are not interpretable, are worsening, or are suggestive of high risk. Fetal blood sampling may prevent unnecessary cesarean birth.

FETAL OXYGEN SATURATION (FSpO₂) MONITORING

Fetal arterial oxygen saturation (FSpO₂) is a direct method used to determine fetal oxygenation levels. An intrauterine device is placed adjacent to the fetal cheek or temple, maintaining constant contact with the fetal skin. Using pulse oximetry, the monitor displays fetal oxygenation saturation as a percentage of oxygen within the fetal blood. Levels of 40% to 70% are considered reassuring. Levels less than 30% indicate hypoxia and require immediate birth. Levels between 30% and 40% indicate mild acidosis and require continuous monitoring and assessment (Menihan & Zottoli, 2001).

$FSpO_2$ monitoring can be used when the fetus is in a vertex presentation, the membranes are ruptured, the cervix is at least 2 cm dilated, the station is − 1 or lower, and the pregnancy is at least 36 weeks' gestation age or more (Menihan & Zottoli, 2001). Use of $FSpO_2$ monitoring allows labor to continue despite a nonreassuring tracing if fetal oxygen levels are within normal range.

CORD BLOOD ANALYSIS AT BIRTH

In cases where significant abnormal FHR patterns have been noted, meconium-stained amniotic fluid is present, or the infant is depressed at birth, umbilical cord blood may be analyzed immediately following the birth to determine if acidosis is present. AAP and ACOG (2002) recommend performing cord blood analysis in cases in which the Apgar score is below 7 at 5 minutes of age.

The cord is clamped before the infant takes the first breath. A small amount of blood is aspirated with a syringe from one of the umbilical arteries. If the cord blood will not be analyzed immediately, a heparinized syringe should be used. Normal fetal blood pH should be above 7.25 (AAP & ACOG, 2002). Lower levels indicate acidosis and hypoxia. Many practitioners obtain cord blood analysis to minimize medicolegal exposure.

Critical Concept Review

LEARNING OBJECTIVES

CONCEPTS

Discuss high-risk screening and intrapartal assessment of maternal physical and psychosociocultural factors.

→

1. High-risk screening is completed to determine if there are any factors present that may be associated with a high-risk condition.
2. Maternal physical factors include:
   ■ Vital signs.
   ■ Labor status.
   ■ Fetal status.
   ■ Laboratory findings.
3. Cultural assessment:
   ■ Individual beliefs and preferences.
4. Psychosocial factors:
   ■ Childbearing fears.
   ■ Childbearing knowledge and fantasies.
   ■ Previous history of psychological disorders.

Summarize methods used to evaluate the progress of labor.

→

Progress of labor is evaluated by:
1. Assessment of strength and frequency of contractions:
   ■ Hand palpation.
   ■ Electronic monitoring.
   ■ External and internal pressure catheters.
2. Cervical assessment:
   ■ Evaluated directly by vaginal examination.

LEARNING OBJECTIVES   ## CONCEPTS

Describe auscultation of fetal heart rate.

1. Location of fetal heart rate:
   - Heard best at the fetal back.
2. Assessment may be intermittent:
   - Handheld Doppler ultrasound auscultates the FHR between, during, and after a contraction.
   - Fetoscope may be used.
3. Most assessment is continuous:
   - External.
   - Internal scalp electrode.

Delineate the procedure for performing Leopold's maneuvers and the information that can be obtained.

Leopold's maneuvers evaluate the position, presentation and lie of the fetus by palpation of the woman's abdomen:
1. Woman empties her bladder and lies on her back with her knees flexed.
2. The practitioner palpates the abdomen gently but deeply using the palms of the hands.
3. One hand is held steady while the other explores one side of the abdomen, then the action of the hands is switched.

Differentiate between baseline and periodic changes in fetal heart rate monitoring and describe the appearance and significance of each.

Baseline fetal heart rate:
1. Average FHR observed during a 10-minute period of monitoring.
2. Should be between 110–160 bpm.
3. Baseline changes of the FHR include tachycardia, bradycardia, and variability.
Periodic changes:
1. Accelerations:
   - Usually caused by fetal movement.
   - Reassuring sign of fetal well-being when it occurs during a contraction.
2. Decelerations:
   - Early deceleration occurs before a contraction and usually requires no intervention.
   - Later deceleration occurs during and after a contraction and indicates insufficient blood flow to the fetus. It is a nonreoccuring sign.
   - Variable decelerations occur due to umbilical cord compression and require further assessment.
   - Sinusoidal pattern appears when there are no periods of normal fetal heart rate. It is associated with Rh problems, fetal anemia, severe fetal hypoxia, or a chronic fetal bleed.

Outline steps to be performed in the systematic evaluation of fetal heart rate tracings.

1. Evaluate the uterine contraction pattern.
2. Determine the baseline FHR.
3. Determine FHR variability.
4. Determine if a sinusoidal pattern is present.
5. Determine if there are periodic changes.

Identify nonreassuring fetal heart rate patterns and appropriate nursing responses.

1. Severe variable decelerations.
2. Late decelerations of any magnitude.
3. Absence of variability.
4. Prolonged deceleration.
Nursing responses include:
1. Notify the physician or CNM.
2. Administer maternal oxygen.
3. Turn mother to the left side.
4. Discontinue oxytocin if being administered.
5. Monitor FHR continuously.
6. Provide explanation to the mother and partner.

Discuss nursing care of the family undergoing electronic fetal monitoring.

1. Explain the use of EFM.
2. Look at mother prior to looking at monitor.
3. Record pertinent data on monitor strip.

(continued)

LEARNING OBJECTIVES

CONCEPTS

Learning Objective	Concept
Delineate the indications for fetal blood sampling and identify related pH values.	Fetal blood is sampled when: 1. Nonreassuring or confusing FHR are noted. 2. Acid-base information is needed. Related pH values: 1. Values greater than 7.25 are normal. 2. Values of 7.2–7.25 are borderline and require further assessment. 3. Values less than 7.2 necessitate birth without delay.
Describe how fetal oxygen saturation ($FSpO_2$) monitoring uses pulse oximetry to monitor fetal oxygenation within the fetal blood to determine if hypoxia is occurring.	A fetal oxygen saturation ($FSpO_2$) monitor is placed adjacent to the fetal cheek or temple and must be in constant contact with the fetal skin. 1. Monitoring $FSpO_2$ allows labor to continue despite a nonreassuring FHR tracing. 2. Levels of 40–70% are considered reassuring. 3. Levels less than 30% indicate hypoxia and require immediate birth. 4. Levels between 30% and 40% indicate mild acidosis and require continuous monitoring and assessment.

CRITICAL THINKING IN ACTION

*View the **Critical Thinking in Action** video in Chapter 18 of the CD-ROM. Then, answer the questions that follow.*

Cindy Bell, a 20-year-old gravida 2, para 1 at 40 weeks' gestation, presents to you in the birthing unit with contractions every 5 to 7 minutes. She is accompanied by her husband. Spontaneous rupture of membranes occurred 2 hours prior to admission. Cindy tells you that the fluid was colorless and clear. You orient Cindy and her family to the birthing room and perform a physical assessment, documenting the following data: vital signs are normal. A vaginal exam demonstrates the cervix is 75% effaced, 4 cm dilated with a vertex at − 1 station in the LOP position. You place Cindy on an external fetal monitor. The fetal heart rate baseline is 140–147 with accelerations to 156; no decelerations are noted. Contractions are 5–6 minutes apart, moderate intensity and lasting 40 to 50 seconds. Cindy states she would like to stay out of bed as long as possible because lying down seems to make the contractions more painful, especially in her back.

1. Discuss the benefits of ambulation in labor.
2. Cindy would like her daughter to be present for the baby's birth. What would you discuss with her about the impact of having a young sibling present during labor and birth?
3. What fetal heart rate assessment will best ensure fetal well-being during the period Cindy is ambulating?
4. When a nonreassuring fetal heart pattern is detected, what remedial nursing intervention is carried out?
5. What are indications for continuous fetal monitoring in labor?

MEDIALINK

www.prenhall.com/london

- NCLEX-RN® Review, case studies, and other interactive resources for this chapter can be found on the Companion Website at http://www.prenhall.com/london. Click on "Chapter 18" to select the activities for this chapter.

Case Study

The nurse is assigned to care for Della Williams, a G3P1 laboring client. Ms. Williams presents at term to the birthing center with her partner and her 2-year-old daughter. Ms. Williams is an insulin-controlled diabetic, with a history of a stillborn.

This activity contains 5 questions.

1. What questions would the nurse ask Ms. Williams to assess her safety and abuse issues?
[Hint]

To create paragraphs in your essay response, type <p> at the beginning of the paragraph, and </p> at the end.

- For animations, more NCLEX-RN® Review questions, and an audio glossary, access the accompanying CD-ROM in this textbook.

REFERENCES

American Academy of Pediatrics & American College of Obstetricians and Gynecologists. (2002). *Guidelines for perinatal care* (5th ed.).Washington, DC: Author.

American College of Obstetricians and Gynecologists. (1995). *Fetal heart rate patterns: Monitoring, interpretation, and management* (ACOG Technical Bulletin No. 207). Washington, DC: Author.

American College of Obstetricians and Gynecologists. (1999). *Vaginal birth after previous cesarean delivery* (ACOG Practice Bulletin No. 5). Washington, DC: Author.

Bujold, E., & Gauthier, R. J. (2002). Neonatal morbidity associated with uterine rupture: What are the risk factors? *American Journal of Obstetrics and Gynecology, 186*(2), 311–314.

Callister, L. C. (2001). Culturally competent care of women and newborns: Knowledge, attitude, and skills. *Journal of Obstetric, Gynecologic, and Neonatal Nursing, 30*(2), 209–215.

Carr, C. A., & Schott, A. (2002). Differences in evidence-based care in midwifery practice and education. *Journal of Nursing Scholarship, 34*(2), 153–158.

Cesario, S. K. (2001). Care of the Native American Woman: Strategies for practice, education, and research. *Journal of Obstetric, Gynecologic, and Neonatal Nursing, 30*(1), 13–18.

Cunningham, F. G., Leveno, K. J., Bloom, S. L., Hauth, J. C., Gilstrap III, L. C., & Wenstrom, K. D. (2005). *Williams obstetrics* (22nd ed.). New York: McGraw-Hill.

Davidson, M. R. (2002). Outcomes of high-risk women cared for by certified nurse-midwives. *Journal of Midwifery and Women's Health, 47*(1), 46–49.

Garite, T. J. (2002). Intrapartum fetal evaluation. In S. G. Gabbe, J. R. Niebyl, & J. L. Simpson (Eds.) *Obstetrics: Normal and problem pregnancies.* (4th ed.). Churchill Livingstone.

Gottlieb, B. (2003). *Alternative cures.* Emmaus, PA: Rodale Books.

Menihan, C. A., & Zottoli, E. K. (2001). *Electronic fetal monitoring: Concepts and application.* Philadelphia: Lippincott.

Seng, J. S., Oakley, D. J., Samselle, C. M., Killion, C., Graham-Bermann, S., & Liberzon, I. (2001). Posttraumatic stress disorder and pregnancy complications. *Obstetrics and Gynecology, 97*(1), 17–22.

Varney, H., Kriebs, J. M., & Gegor, C. L. (2004). *Varney's midwifery* (4th ed.). Sudbury, MA.: Jones & Bartlett.

CHAPTER 19

The Family in Childbirth: Needs and Care

For as long as I can remember, I have been fascinated with birth. Currently, I am a labor and delivery nurse at our town's only hospital. I'm still fascinated with birth but a little nervous, too. You see, I was just admitted in early labor with my first child. Before I got here I worried that I would be a "bad" patient or that I would lose my cool. How silly I was. All that matters is that my baby is healthy and that I am able to take care of him effectively. (Yes. We know it is a boy!)

—*Amanda, 31*

LEARNING OBJECTIVES

- Identify the database to be created from information obtained when a woman is admitted to the birthing area.

- Review the nursing care provided at admission.

- Discuss nursing interventions to meet the psychologic, social, physiologic, and spiritual needs of the woman during each stage of labor.

- Compare methods of promoting comfort during the first and second stages of labor.

- Summarize the immediate needs of the newborn following birth.

- Discuss the unique needs of the adolescent during birth.

- Delineate management of a precipitous birth.

MEDIALINK

www.prenhall.com/london

CD-ROM

Skill 4–2: Evaluating Lochia
Skill 5–1: Performing Nasal Pharyngeal Suctioning
Skill 5–2: Assigning Newborn Apgar Scores
Animation: Placental Delivery
Audio Glossary
NCLEX-RN® Review
Videos
    Fourth Stage of Labor
    Newborn Assessment

Companion Website

Complementary Care: Doula Information
Thinking Critically
NCLEX-RN® Review
MediaLink Applications
    Case Study: Labor and Birth
    Care Plan Activity: Presence of Extended Family

It is time for a child to be born. The parents are about to undergo one of the most meaningful and stressful events of their lives. The adequacy of their preparation for childbirth, including the coping mechanisms, communication, and support systems that they have established, will be put to the test. Like Amanda, the childbearing woman may feel that her psychologic and physical limits are about to be challenged. These events may be even more challenging for the single woman, especially if she lacks a strong support system.

Family-centered care is a model of care based on the philosophy that physical, sociocultural, spiritual, and economic needs of the family are combined and considered collectively when planning care for the childbearing family (Association of Women's Health, Obstetric and Neonatal Nurses [AWHONN], 2003b). To reflect the consumer demand for family-centered care, most birthing centers now have **birthing rooms**, single rooms where the woman and her partner or other family members will stay for the labor, birth, recovery, and possibly the postpartum period. These rooms may be called *labor, delivery, recovery, and postpartum (LDRP) rooms* or *single-room maternity care (SRMC)*.

The birthing room atmosphere is more relaxed than a traditional labor room, and families seem to feel more comfortable in it. Not having to be transferred from one area to another for birth helps the laboring woman create her own space to labor in and enhances the family's involvement. Birthing rooms usually have beds that can be adapted for birth by removing a small section near the foot. The room's decor is designed to produce a homelike atmosphere in which families can feel both safe and at ease.

The previous two chapters provided information about physiologic and psychologic changes during labor and birth and needed nursing assessments. This chapter focuses on nursing care during labor and birth. See "Clinical Pathway: For Intrapartal Stages."

NURSING DIAGNOSIS DURING LABOR AND BIRTH

When devising a plan of care for the intrapartal period, the nurse can develop a general plan that encompasses the total process, from the beginning of labor through the fourth stage, or a more specific plan for each stage of labor and birth. A general plan presents an overview of the whole process, whereas a plan of care that gives nursing diagnoses for each stage is a chance to identify more specific nursing care.

Examples of appropriate nursing diagnoses may include the following:

- *Fear* related to uncertainty about the outcome of the birth process
- *Acute Pain* related to uterine contractions, cervical dilatation, and fetal descent
- *Health-seeking Behaviors: Information About the Fetal Monitor* related to an expressed desire to understand equipment used
- *Readiness for Enhanced Family Processes* related to opportunity to incorporate newborn into the family

NURSING CARE DURING ADMISSION

During prenatal visits, instruct the woman to come to the birthing unit if any of the following occur:

- Rupture of membranes (ROM)
- Regular, frequent uterine contractions (nulliparas, 5 minutes apart for 1 hour; multiparas, 6 to 8 minutes apart for 1 hour)

CLINICAL PATHWAY

FOR INTRAPARTUM STAGES

CATEGORY	FIRST STAGE	SECOND AND THIRD STAGES	FOURTH STAGE BIRTH TO 1 HOUR PAST BIRTH
Referral	Review prenatal record Advise physician/CNM of admission	Labor record for first stage	Report to recovery room nurse **EXPECTED OUTCOMES** Appropriate resources identified and utilized
Assessments	Admission assessments: Ask about problems since last prenatal visit; labor status (contraction frequency and duration), membrane status (intact or ruptured); coping level; support; woman's desires during labor and birth; ability to verbalize needs; laboratory testing (blood and UA) Intrapartum assessments: cervical assessment: from 1 to 10 cm dilatation; nullipara (1.2 cm/h), multipara (1.5 cm/h) Cervical effacement: from 0% to 100% Fetal descent: progressive descent from −4 to +4 Membrane assessment: intact or ruptured; when ruptured, Nitrazine positive, fluid clear, no foul odor Comfort level: woman states she is able to cope with contractions Behavioral characteristics: facial expressions, tone of voice, and verbal expressions are consistent with comfort level and ability to cope Latent phase: ■ BP, P, R q1h if in normal range (BP≤135/85 or not >30 mm Hg systolic or 15 mm Hg diastolic over baseline; pulse 60–90; respirations 16–24/min, quiet, easy) ■ Temp q4h unless >37.6°C (99.6°F) or membranes ruptured then q2h ■ Uterine contractions q30min (contractions q5–10 min, 15–40 sec, mild intensity) ■ FHR q60min (for low-risk women) and q30min (for high-risk women) if reassuring (reassuring FHR has: baseline 110–160, STV and LTV present, accelerations with fetal movement, no late decelerations); if nonreassuring, position on side, start O₂, assess for hypotension, monitor continuously, notify physician/CNM *Active phase:* ■ BP, P, R q1h if WNL ■ Temp as above ■ Uterine contractions q15–30min: contractions q2–5 min, 40–60 sec, moderate to strong ■ FHR q30min (for low-risk women) and q15min (for high-risk women) if reassuring; if nonreassuring institute interventions and continuous electronic monitoring	Second-stage assessments: ■ BP, P, R q5–15 min ■ Uterine contractions palpated continuously ■ FHR q15min (for low-risk women) and q5min (for high-risk women) if reassuring; if nonreassuring, monitor continuously Fetal descent: descent continues to birth Comfort level: woman states she is able to cope with contractions and pushing Behavioral characteristics: response to pushing, facial expressions, verbalization Third-stage assessments: ■ BP, P, R q5min ■ Uterine contractions, palpate occasionally until placenta is expelled, fundus maintains tone, and contraction pattern continues to expulsion of placenta Newborn assessments: ■ Assess Apgar score of newborn ■ Respirations: 30–60, irregular ■ Apical pulse: 110–160 and somewhat irregular ■ Temperature: Skin temp above 36.5°C (97.8°F) ■ Umbilical cord: two arteries, one vein (if one artery, assess for anomalies and urine output) ■ Gestational age: 38–42 weeks	Immediate postbirth assessments of mother q15min for 1h: ■ BP: <135/85; should return to prelabor level ■ Pulse: slightly lower than in labor; range is 60–90 ■ Respirations: 16–24/min; easy; quiet ■ Temperature: 36.2–37.6°C (97–99.6°F) ■ Fundus firm, in midline, at the umbilicus ■ Lochia rubra; moderate amount; <2 pad/hr; no free flow or passage of clots with massage ■ Perineum: sutures intact; no bulging or marked swelling; minimal bruising may be present; no c/o severe pain or rectal pain ■ Bladder nondistended; spontaneous void of >100 mL clear, straw-colored urine; bladder nondistended following voiding ■ If hemorrhoids present, no tenseness or marked engorgement; <2 cm diameter Comfort level: pain <3 on scale of 1 to 10 Energy level: awake and able to hold newborn Newborn assessments if newborn remains with parents: ■ Respirations: 30–60; irregular ■ Apical pulse: 110–160 and somewhat irregular ■ Temperature: skin temperature above 36.5°C (97.8°F); skin feels warm to touch ■ Skin color noncyanotic ■ Mucus: small amount, clear, easily suctioned with bulb syringe without skin color change ■ Behavioral: newborn opens eyes widely if room is slightly darkened ■ Movements rhythmic; no hand tremors present **EXPECTED OUTCOMES** Findings indicate normal progression with absence of complications

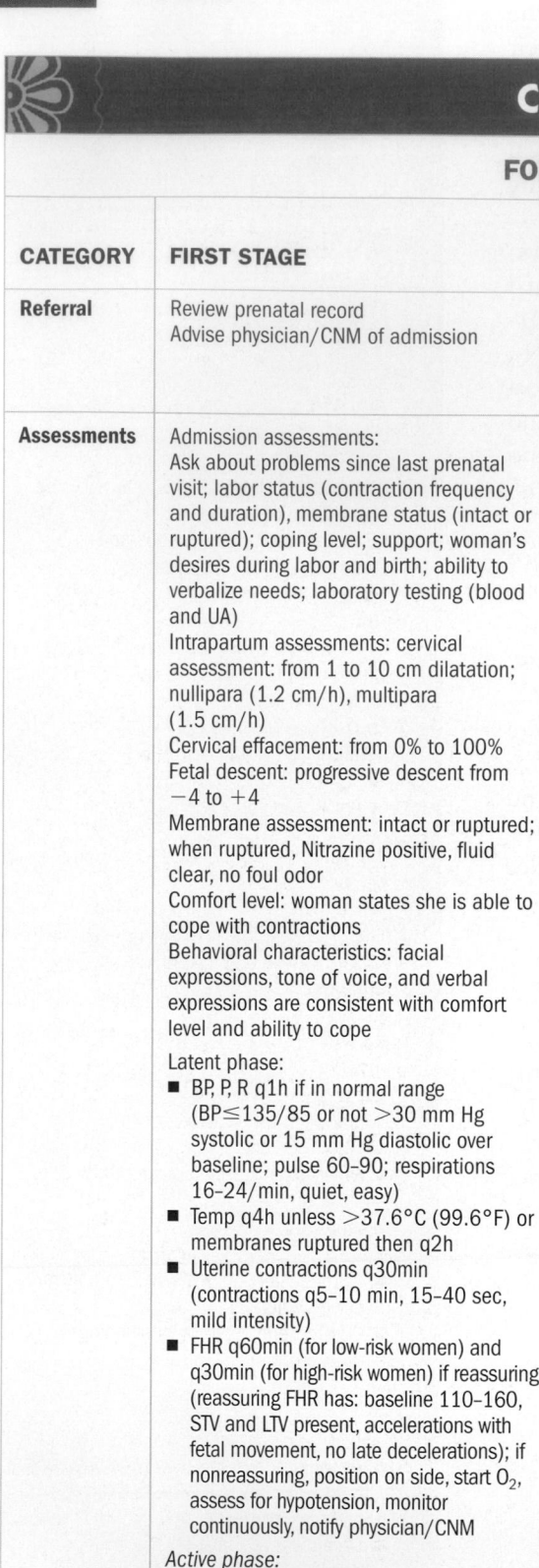

CLINICAL PATHWAY—continued

FOR INTRAPARTUM STAGES

CATEGORY	FIRST STAGE	SECOND AND THIRD STAGES	FOURTH STAGE BIRTH TO 1 HOUR PAST BIRTH
Assessments *(continued)*	*Transition:* ■ BP, P, R, q30min ■ Uterine contractions q15min: contractions q1/2–2 min, 60–90 sec, strong ■ FHR q15min if nonreassuring, see above		
Teaching/ psychosocial	**Establish rapport** Orient to environment, expected assessments, and procedures Answer questions and provide information Orient to EFM if used Teach relaxation, visualization, and breathing pattern if needed Explain comfort measures available Assume advocacy role for woman/family during labor and birth	Orient to expected assessments and procedures Answer questions and provide information Explain comfort measures available Continue advocacy role	Explain immediate assessments and care after this first hour Teach self-massage of fundus and expected findings Instruct to call for assistance if mother desires to get OB Begin newborn teaching; bulb syringe, positioning; maintaining warmth Assist parents in exploring their newborn Assist with first breastfeeding experience **EXPECTED OUTCOMES** Client and partner verbalize/demonstrate understanding of teaching
Nursing care management and report	Straight cath prn if bladder distended If regional block administered monitor BP, FHR, sensation per protocol Provide continuing status reports to physician/CNM Perform sterile vaginal examination as indicated	Straight cath prn if bladder distended Continue monitoring VS, FHR, and sensation if regional block has been given	Straight cath if bladder distended and women unable to void Monitor return of motor ability and sensation if regional block has been given Weigh perineal pads if lochia flow >1 saturated pad in 15 min, presence of boggy uterus and clots; ↑BP, ↓P **EXPECTED OUTCOMES** ■ Maternal/fetal well-being maintained and supported ■ Mother and newborn experience safe labor and birth ■ Family participates in process as desired
Activity	Encourage ambulation unless contraindicated Maintain bed rest immediately after administration of IV pain medication, or following regional block Woman rests comfortably between contractions	Position comfortably for birth Woman rests comfortably between pushing efforts and while awaiting expulsion of placenta	Position of comfort **EXPECTED OUTCOMES** ■ Activity maintained as desired unless contraindicated ■ Comfort enhanced by positioning/ movement
Comfort	Institute comfort measures: ambulation, frequent position change, effleurage, focal point, patterned-paced breathing, visualization, therapeutic touch, back rub, moist cloths to face, holding hand, words of encouragement, changing underpad, shower, whirlpool, staying with the woman/family, warmed blanket at back, sacral pressure Offer pain medication or administer if requested Assist with administration of regional block	Institute comfort measures: ■ Second stage: cool cloth to forehead, encouragement, coaching, help support legs while pushing, position of comfort for pushing and birth ■ Third stage: cool cloth to forehead, assist parents to see newborn, position mother to hold newborn, provide encouragement	Institute comfort measures: ■ Perineal discomfort: gently cleanse and apply ice pack; position to decrease pressure on perineum ■ Uterine discomfort: palpate fundus gently ■ Hemorrhoids: ice pack ■ General fatigue: position of comfort, encourage rest ■ Administer pain medication PRN **EXPECTED OUTCOMES** ■ Optimal comfort level maintained ■ Active reduction of pain/discomfort achieved

(continued)

CLINICAL PATHWAY—continued

FOR INTRAPARTUM STAGES

CATEGORY	FIRST STAGE	SECOND AND THIRD STAGES	FOURTH STAGE BIRTH TO 1 HOUR PAST BIRTH
Nutrition	Ice chips and clear fluids Evaluate for signs of dehydration	Ice chips and clear fluids	Regular diet if assessments are WNL Encourage fluids **EXPECTED OUTCOMES** Nutritional needs met
Elimination	Voids at least q2h; urine clear, straw-colored, negative for protein Bladder nondistended May have bowel movement Monitor I & O with IVs	May void spontaneously with pushing May pass stool with pushing	Voids spontaneously **EXPECTED OUTCOMES** Urinary bladder and bowel function unimpaired
Medications	Administer pain medication per woman's request	Local infiltration of anesthetic agent for birth by physician/CNM Pitocin 10–20 units IM, IVP per IV tubing, or added to IV fluids	Continue Pitocin infusion Administer pain medication PRN **EXPECTED OUTCOMES** Comfort enhanced by pain-relieving techniques, administration of analgesia agent, or an analgesic or anesthetic block
Discharge planning	Evaluate knowledge of labor and birth process Evaluate support system and need for referral after birth		Provide information if mother to be moved from LDR room Provide opportunity for parents to ask questions regarding newborn Evaluate knowledge of normal postpartum, newborn care **EXPECTED OUTCOMES** Mother and newborn transferred to low-risk postpartum and newborn care
Family involvement	Identify available support person(s) Recognize possible impact of culture on responses Observe interaction between woman and partner Create moment alone with woman to identify possible abuse Assess current parenting skills	Provide opportunities for woman and support person(s) to watch newborn assessments Perform newborn assessment on mother's abdomen/chest if possible	Provide opportunity for parents to be with baby Encourage skin-to-skin contact Darken room to encourage eye-to-eye contact Provide quiet time for new family Parenting: demonstrates early culturally expected parenting behaviors **EXPECTED OUTCOMES** Incorporation of newborn into family Family verbalizes comfort with newborn care
Date			

CNM, certified nurse-midwife; BP, blood pressure; FHR, fetal heart rate; STV, short-term variability; LTV, long-term variability; WNL, within normal limits; VS, vital signs; EFM, electronic fetal monitoring; IV, intravenous; I & O, intake & output; IM, intramuscularly; IVP, intravenous push; LDR, labor, delivery, and recovery; OB, out of bed; UA, urinary analysis; PRN, as needed; c/o, complains of.

- Vaginal bleeding
- Decreased fetal movement

The woman in labor and her partner or support person(s) tend to be concerned about arriving at the birth center in time for the birth. Sometimes the labor is advanced and birth is imminent, but usually the woman is in early labor at admission. If time permits and the family is not familiar with what will occur during labor, provide necessary infor-

mation. (See "Teaching Highlights: What to Expect During Labor.")

The way the maternity nurse greets the woman and her partner influences the course of the woman's hospital stay. The sudden environmental change and the sometimes impersonal and technical aspects of admission can produce significant stress. If women and their families are greeted in a brusque, harried manner, they are less likely to look to the nurse for support. A calm, pleasant manner indicates to the

TEACHING HIGHLIGHTS

WHAT TO EXPECT DURING LABOR

Describe aspects of the admission process:

- Abbreviated history
- Physical assessment (maternal vital signs, fetal heart rate, contraction status, status of membranes)
- Assessment of uterine contractions (frequency, duration, intensity)
- Orientation to surroundings
- Introductions to other staff
- Determination of the woman's and support person's expectations of the nurse

Present aspects of ongoing physical care, such as when to expect assessment of maternal vital signs, fetal heart rate, and contractions.

If an electronic fetal monitor is used, describe how it works and the information it provides. Orient the woman to sights and sounds of the monitor.

Explain what "normal" data look like and what characteristics are being watched for.

Be sure to note that assessments will increase as the labor progresses, especially during the transition phase, to help keep the mother and baby safe by noting any changes from the normal course.

Explain the vaginal examination and the information it can provide.

Review comfort techniques that may be used in labor and ascertain what the woman thinks will promote comfort.

Review breathing techniques the woman has learned so that you can support her technique.

Review comfort and support measures such as positioning, back rub, effleurage, touch, distraction techniques, and ambulation.

If the woman is in early labor, offer her a tour of the birthing area.

Have printed materials available for reference, especially for the partner or support person.

If time permits, a brief video describing procedures may be helpful.

woman that she is important. It helps to instill a sense of confidence in the staff's ability to provide quality care during this critical time.

Following the initial greeting, escort the woman to the birthing room and provide a quick yet thorough orientation to the facility, including the location of the restrooms, public phones, and nurse-call or emergency-call system. These simple steps can go a long way toward helping the woman and her partner feel more at ease. Explain the monitoring equipment or other unfamiliar technology and make every effort to make the environment less frightening for the laboring woman and her support person(s).

Some women prefer that their partner remain with them during the admission process, and others prefer to have the partner wait outside. While helping the woman undress and get into a hospital gown, begin to develop rap-

port and establish a nursing database. The experienced labor and birth nurse can obtain essential information about the woman and her pregnancy within a few minutes after admission, initiate any immediate interventions needed, and establish individualized priorities.

The woman may be facing a number of unfamiliar procedures that seem routine for healthcare providers. Remember that all women have the right to determine what happens to their bodies. The woman's informed consent should be obtained prior to any procedure that involves touching her.

If indicated, assist the woman into bed. A side-lying or semi-Fowler's position rather than a supine position is most comfortable and avoids supine hypotensive syndrome (vena caval syndrome). After obtaining the essential information from the woman and her records, begin the intrapartal assessment. (Chapter 18 considers intrapartal maternal assessment in depth. ∞) Once the assessment is complete, it is possible to make effective nursing decisions about intrapartal care, such as the following:

- Should ambulation, bed rest, or a combination of both be encouraged?
- Is more frequent or continuous electronic fetal monitoring needed?
- What does the woman want during her labor and birth?
- Is a support person available?
- What special needs do this woman and her partner have?

Auscultate the fetal heart rate (FHR). (See Chapter 18 ∞) Determine the woman's blood pressure, pulse, respirations, and oral temperature and assess contraction frequency, duration, and intensity (possibly while gathering other data). Before the vaginal examination, inform the woman about the procedure and its purpose; afterward, report the findings. If signs of advanced labor exist (frequent contractions, an urge to bear down, and so on), a vaginal examination must be done immediately. If there are signs of excessive bleeding or if the woman reports episodes of painless bleeding in the last trimester, suspect placenta previa. *Do not do a vaginal examination, and notify the physician or certified nurse-midwife (CNM) immediately.*

Results of FHR assessment, uterine contraction evaluation, and the vaginal examination help determine whether the rest of the admission process can proceed at a leisurely pace or whether additional interventions are required. For example, a FHR of less than 110 beats per minute on auscultation indicates that a fetal monitor should be applied immediately to obtain additional data. The woman's vital signs can be assessed once the monitor is in place.

After obtaining admission data, collect a clean voided midstream urine specimen. The woman with intact membranes may collect her specimen in the bathroom. If the membranes are ruptured and the presenting part is not engaged, the woman generally remains in bed to avoid prolapse of the umbilical cord. Views vary about the wisdom of ambulation once the membranes are ruptured. The decision is generally based on history and physical findings (for example, history of precipitous labors, indications for continuous fetal monitoring, presence of meconium), clinician orders, the woman's desires, agency policy, and safety concerns.

Use a dipstick to test the woman's urine for the presence of protein, ketones, and glucose before sending the sample to the laboratory. This procedure is especially important if edema or elevated blood pressure is noted on admission. Proteinuria of 1+ or more may be a sign of impending preeclampsia. Glycosuria (sugar in the urine) is found frequently in pregnant women because of the increased glomerular filtration rate in the proximal tubules and the inability of these tubules to increase reabsorption of glucose. However, it may also be associated with gestational diabetes, so do not discount it. While the woman is collecting the urine specimen, gather the equipment needed for any procedures ordered by the CNM or physician.

Laboratory tests are done during early admission. Hemoglobin and hematocrit values help determine the oxygen-carrying capacity of the circulatory system and the woman's ability to withstand blood loss at birth. Elevation of the hematocrit may reveal hemoconcentration of blood, which occurs with edema or dehydration. A low hemoglobin, in the absence of other evidence of bleeding, suggests anemia. Blood may be typed and crossmatched if the woman is in a high-risk category. Platelets are also evaluated because low platelets can lead to bleeding problems. Additional serologic testing may be performed as indicated. HIV testing should be offered to all women who have not been previously screened (Centers for Disease Control and Prevention [CDC], 2003).

In many hospitals the admission process also includes signing an informed consent for treatment and providing information about advance directives. In all cases an identification bracelet is attached to the expectant mother's wrist.

Depending on how rapidly labor is progressing, notify the CNM or physician before or after completing the admission procedures. The report should include the following information: parity, cervical dilatation and effacement, station, presenting part, status of the membranes, contraction pattern, FHR, vital signs that are not in the normal range, any significant prenatal history, the woman's birth preferences, and her reaction to labor.

Enter a nursing admission note into the computer or the charting system. The admission note should include the reason for admission, the date and time of the woman's arrival and notification of the CNM or physician, the condition of the woman and her baby, and labor and membrane status (American Academy of Pediatrics [AAP] & American College of Obstetricians and Gynecologists [ACOG], 2002).

NURSING CARE DURING THE FIRST STAGE OF LABOR

After completing the nursing assessment and diagnosis steps, create a plan of care to achieve identified nursing goals. For instance, if the woman and her support person did not have the opportunity to attend childbirth preparation classes, the nursing goal would be to provide desired information. To accomplish this goal, the nurse would assess the current level of the couple's understanding and then plan to provide brief explanations as labor progresses.

INTEGRATION OF FAMILY EXPECTATIONS

Families come into the birth setting with basic expectations that they will not be harmed and that the labor and birth will be safe for the mother and baby. In addition, women look for the following from their nurses:

- Emotional support, which includes sustained presence of the nurse, praise, encouragement, reassurance, and companionship
- Comfort measures such as the use of touch, provision of ice chips and fluids, massage, assistance with care, and a bath or shower
- Information and advice, which includes offering information about procedures, interventions as they occur, and reports of labor progress
- Advocacy to help the woman and her partner achieve their goals, hopes, and dreams for their labor and birth experience
- Support of the partner, including encouragement, praise for his or her efforts, an opportunity for rest breaks, and role modeling

INTEGRATION OF CULTURAL BELIEFS

Knowledge of values, customs, and practices of different cultures is as important during labor as it is in the prenatal period. Without this knowledge a nurse is less likely to understand a family's behavior and may attempt to impose personal values and beliefs on them. As cultural sensitivity increases, so does the likelihood of providing high-quality care.

The following sections briefly present a few possible cultural responses to labor. It is difficult to present even such a limited discussion in a clear, nonjudgmental way, because once a statement is made it may appear stereotypic, and of course no statement of a specific behavior can accurately reflect the preference of all people in a group. An individual example of a birthing practice will never be pertinent to all women in a given group. General information about any culture or belief system needs to be viewed as background to help caregivers meet each individual's needs and desires. Culture is also discussed in Chapter 2. ∞

Modesty

Modesty is an important consideration for women regardless of culture. However, some women may be more uncomfortable than others with the degree of exposure needed for certain procedures during labor and the birth process. Some women may be particularly uncomfortable when men are present and feel more comfortable with women; others may be uncomfortable with exposure of personal body parts regardless of the gender of the caregivers. The nurse should be alert to the woman's responses to examinations and procedures and provide the draping and privacy the woman needs. It is more prudent to assume that embarrassment will occur with exposure and take measures to provide privacy than to assume that it will not matter to the woman if she is exposed during procedures.

Pain Expression

The manner in which a woman chooses to deal with the discomfort of labor varies widely. Some women seem to turn inward and remain very quiet during the whole process. They speak only to ask others to leave the room or cease conversation. Others may be very vocal, with behaviors such as counting out loud, moaning quietly, crying, or use of loud vocalization. They may also turn from side to side or change positions frequently.

In many Asian cultures, it is important for individuals to act in a way that will not bring shame on the family. Therefore, the Korean woman may not express pain outwardly for fear of shaming herself or her family, and Filipina women say it is best to lie quietly. Silence is valued in Chinese society, so a woman of that heritage is usually quiet and stoic to avoid dishonoring herself or her family. Hispanic women are encouraged to be patient and not to cry out or the "uterus will rise up." European Americans demonstrate a wide variety of behaviors in response to pain, from silence to shouting. It is important to support a woman's individual expression, whatever it may be (as long as harm is not done to another), in order to enhance the birthing experience for mother, baby, and family.

Cultural Beliefs: Some Examples

Hmong women from Laos report that squatting during childbirth is common in their culture. During labor they may want to be active and move about. The husband is frequently present and actively involved in providing comfort. Traditionally, the woman prefers that the amniotic membranes not be ruptured until just before birth. It is

thought that the escape of fluid at this time makes the birth easier. During labor the woman usually prefers only "hot" foods and warm water to drink (St. Hill, Lipson, Ibrahim et al., 2003). As soon as the baby is born, the family may request that a soft-boiled egg be given to the mother to restore her energy.

Vietnamese women usually maintain self-control and may even smile throughout labor. They may prefer to walk about during labor and to give birth in a squatting position. The woman may avoid drinking cold water and prefer fluids at room temperature. The newborn is protected from praise to prevent jealousy (St. Hill et al., 2003).

Latina women have identified expectations of their partners during labor and birth such as wanting their partners to stay with them and to reassure them that everything will be all right. As they labor, the women want their partners to show their love and to speak using affectionate words.

Muslim women may have their husband, a female friend or relative, or a male relative with them during childbirth. Family support is important but does not preclude the importance of the nurse's presence. The woman may want to retain her head covering (*khimar*) and may prefer to wear two long-sleeved gowns to enhance modesty. It is important for a female nurse, physician, or CNM to perform examinations whenever possible.

Maternity nurses can provide culturally sensitive care by first becoming acquainted with the beliefs and practices of the various subcultures in their communities. In the birthing situation, the truly effective nurse supports the family's cultural practices as long as it is safe to do so.

PROVISION OF CARE IN THE FIRST STAGE OF LABOR

Latent Phase

As discussed in Chapter 18, it is important to assess the physical well-being of the woman and her fetus. ∞ Monitor maternal temperature every 4 hours unless the temperature is over 37.5°C (99.6°F); in such cases take it every hour. Monitor blood pressure, pulse, and respirations every hour.

THINKING CRITICALLY

GENDER-SPECIFIC CARE PREFERENCE

Fatima Al Ahala is a 22-year-old, G1 who presents in labor. Fatima and her husband Samir are from Pakistan. The couple has stated that they can accept care only from female providers. The couple is being attended by a female nurse-midwife, and the backup physician is also a female. When her labor intensifies, Fatima requests an epidural. The only anesthesiologist available is a male physician. What actions can you take to help this family meet their cultural preferences?

If the woman's blood pressure is over 140/90 mm Hg or her pulse is more than 100, notify the CNM or physician and reevaluate the blood pressure and pulse more frequently. Palpate uterine contractions for frequency, intensity, and duration. Auscultate the FHR every 60 minutes for low-risk women and every 30 minutes for high-risk women as long as it remains between 110 and 160 beats per minute and is reassuring. Auscultate the FHR throughout one contraction and for about 15 seconds after the contraction to ensure that there are no decelerations. If the FHR baseline is not in the 110 to 160 range or if decelerations are heard, continuous electronic monitoring is recommended (Table 19–1).

Offer the woman fluids in the form of clear liquids or ice chips frequently, unless complications exist that may result in a cesarean birth. Some certified childbirth educators advise the woman to bring lollipops to help combat the dryness that occurs with some of the labor breathing patterns. Avoiding both liquids and solids during labor, which was once a standard of practice, is becoming controversial. Current guidelines suggest avoiding solid foods for 6 to 8 hours prior to an elective cesarean birth; however, modest amounts of clear liquids are recommended for women experiencing a normal labor (ACOG, 2002). Previously it was believed that eating should be avoided because it can lead to vomiting due to the decreased gastric emptying time. Although vomiting is a concern during the first stage of labor, many women have more energy and tolerate labor better with oral intake. If vomiting does occur, provide oral care and reassurance.

Active Phase

During the active phase, contractions have a frequency of 2 to 5 minutes, a duration of 40 to 60 seconds, and a moderate to strong intensity. Palpate contractions every 15 to 30 minutes. As the contractions become more frequent and intense, vaginal exams assess cervical dilatation and effacement and fetal station and position. During the active phase, the cervix dilates from 4 to 7 cm, and vaginal discharge and bloody show increase. Monitor maternal blood pressure, pulse, and respirations every hour for low-risk women (unless elevated, as previously noted) and every 30 minutes for high-risk women. Auscultate the FHR every 30 minutes for low-risk women and every 15 minutes for high-risk women (AWHONN, 2003a).

A woman who has been ambulatory up to this point may wish to sit in a chair or on a bed. If the woman wants to lie on the bed, encourage her to assume a side-lying position, help her into a comfortable position, and place pillows to support her body. To increase comfort, offer a back rub or effleurage or place a cool cloth on the woman's forehead or across her neck. Because vaginal discharge increases, change the chux pad frequently. Washing the perineum with warm soap and water removes secretions and increases comfort. During such procedures it is essential to wear disposable gloves to avoid exposure to vaginal discharge.

TABLE 19–1 ❖ Nursing Assessments in the First Stage

Phase	Mother	Fetus
Latent	Blood pressure, respirations each hour if in normal range Temperature every 4 hours unless over 37.5 °C (99.6 °F) or membranes ruptured, then every hour Uterine contractions every 30 minutes	Fetal heart rate (FHR) every 60 minutes for low-risk women and every 30 minutes for high-risk women if normal characteristics present (average variability, baseline in the 110–160 beats per minute range, without late or variable decelerations). Note fetal activity. If electronic fetal monitor in place, assess for reactive nonstress test (NST).
Active	Blood pressure, pulse, respirations every hour if in normal range Uterine contractions every 15 to 30 minutes	FHR every 30 minutes for low-risk women and every 15 minutes for high-risk women if normal characteristics are present.
Transition	Blood pressure, pulse, respirations every 30 minutes Uterine contractions at least every 15 minutes	FHR every 30 minutes for low-risk women and every 15 minutes for high-risk women if normal characteristics are present.

If the amniotic membranes have not ruptured previously, they may do so during this phase. When the membranes rupture, note the color, odor, and consistency of the amniotic fluid and the time of rupture, and immediately note the FHR on the monitor if one is being used. If the woman is not on a monitor, auscultate FHR. The fluid should be clear, with no odor. Fetal stress leads to intestinal and anal sphincter relaxation, and meconium may be released into the amniotic fluid, which turns the fluid greenish brown. Whenever meconium-stained fluid is present, apply an electronic monitor to assess the FHR continuously. Note the time of rupture because medical practice suggests that birth should occur within 24 hours of the rupture of membranes.

Prolapse of the umbilical cord is a possible risk when membranes rupture and the fetus is not engaged because the amniotic fluid coming through the cervix might wash the umbilical cord out through the cervix. With each contraction the cord would then become trapped between the presenting part and the maternal pelvis. The FHR is auscultated because a drop in the rate might indicate an undetected prolapsed cord. Immediate intervention is necessary to remove pressure on a prolapsed umbilical cord (see Chapter 21 ∞). (See Table 19–2 for additional deviations from normal.)

Transition

During transition the contraction frequency is every 1½ to 2 minutes, duration is 60 to 90 seconds, and intensity is strong. Cervical dilatation increases from 8 to 10 cm, effacement is complete (100%), and there is usually a heavy amount of bloody show. Palpate contractions at least every 15 minutes. Sterile vaginal examinations may be done

TABLE 19–2 ❖ Deviations from Normal Labor Process Requiring Immediate Intervention

Problem	Immediate Action
Woman admitted with vaginal bleeding or history of painless vaginal bleeding	Do not perform vaginal examination. Assess fetal heart rate (FHR). Evaluate amount of blood loss. Evaluate labor pattern. Notify physician or certified nurse-midwife (CNM) immediately.
Presence of greenish or brownish amniotic fluid	Continuously monitor FHR. Evaluate dilatation of cervix and determine if umbilical cord is prolapsed. Evaluate presentation (vertex or breech). Maintain woman on complete bed rest on left side. Notify physician or CNM immediately.
Absence of FHR and fetal movement	Notify physician or CNM. Provide truthful information and emotional support to laboring couple. Remain with the couple.
Prolapse of umbilical cord	Relieve pressure on cord manually. Continuously monitor FHR; watch for changes in FHR pattern. Notify physician or CNM. Assist woman into knee-chest position or place in Trendelenburg position. Administer oxygen.

Woman admitted in advanced labor; birth imminent	Prepare for immediate birth.
	 Obtain critical information:
	     Estimated date of birth (EDB)
	     History of bleeding problems
	     History of medical or obstetric problems
	     Past or present use or abuse of prescription, over-the-counter (OTC), or illicit drugs
	     Problems with this pregnancy
	     FHR and maternal vital signs
	     Whether membranes are ruptured and how long since rupture
	     Blood type and Rh
	 Direct another person to contact physician or CNM.
	 Do not leave woman alone.
	 Provide support to couple.
	 Put on gloves.

more frequently because this stage of labor usually is accompanied by rapid change. Take the maternal blood pressure, pulse, and respirations at least every 30 minutes, and auscultate FHR every 15 minutes.

Comfort measures are important in this phase of labor, but continual assessment is required to intervene appropriately. The woman may rapidly change from wanting a back rub and other hands-on care to wanting to be left completely alone. The support person and the nurse need to follow her cues and change interventions as needed. Because the woman is breathing more rapidly, increase her comfort by offering small spoonfuls of ice chips to moisten her mouth or offer an emollient for her dry lips. Encourage the woman to rest between contractions. If analgesics have been administered, a quiet environment enhances the quality of rest between contractions. Awaken the woman just before a contraction begins so that she can begin patterned breathing.

Some women have difficulty coping during this time and need help with their breathing. Either the support person or the nurse can breathe along with the woman during each contraction to help her maintain her pattern. It is helpful to encourage the woman and to assure her that she is doing a good job. The woman will begin to feel increased rectal pressure as the fetal presenting part moves down the birth canal. To help prevent cervical edema, encourage the woman to refrain from pushing until the cervix is completely dilated.

The end of transition and the beginning of the second stage may be indicated by a change in the woman's voice or the sounds she is making. As the fetus moves down and she feels increased pressure and a bearing-down sensation, her voice tends to deepen. A moan during a contraction takes on a more guttural quality.

PROMOTION OF COMFORT IN THE FIRST STAGE

The first step in planning care is to talk with the woman and her partner or support person to identify their goals. Usually the woman or couple is concerned with discomfort, so it is helpful to identify factors that may contribute to discomfort. These factors include uncomfortable positions, diaphoresis, continual leaking of amniotic fluid, a full bladder, a dry mouth, anxiety, and fear. Nursing interventions can minimize the effects of these factors. These interventions are described later in this section.

There are many responses to pain. As the intensity of the contraction increases with the progress of labor, the woman becomes less aware of the environment and may have difficulty hearing and understanding verbal instructions. The pattern of coping with labor contractions varies from the use of highly structured breathing techniques to turning inward. Low moaning that begins deep in the throat, rocking or swaying, facial grimacing, and using loud vocalizations are all effective means of dealing with the power of labor

and birth. Some women feel that making sounds helps them cope and do the work of labor, whereas others make loud sounds only as they lose their perception of control.

The most frequent physiologic manifestations of pain are increased pulse and respiratory rates, dilated pupils, increased blood pressure, and muscle tension. In labor these reactions are transitory because the pain is intermittent. Increased muscle tension is most significant because it may impede the progress of labor. Women in labor often tighten skeletal muscles voluntarily during a contraction and remain motionless. This method of dealing with the contractions may actually increase the level of discomfort because of muscular tension, but the women may believe it is the only acceptable way to cope with the pain.

A woman generally wants touching, massage, effleurage (see Chapter 8 ∞), and other forms of physical contact during the first part of labor, but when she moves into the transition phase, she may rebuff all efforts and pull away. Women may provide verbal and nonverbal signs such as crying, moaning, and beseeching the coach or nurse to hold their hand or rub their back. They may reach out and grasp the support person or indicate their anxiety or fear through eye contact. However, some women are uncomfortable with being touched at all, regardless of the phase of labor. It is important to confirm the woman's preferences and to meet each family on its own terms, always keeping in mind that this is their experience.

Many nurses like to incorporate touch into their nursing care, and they readily respond to the woman's needs. As the nurse and woman or couple work together to increase comfort during contractions, a ritual of supportive measures begins to develop. The nurse watches for cues and nonverbal behaviors and asks for feedback from the woman. As labor progresses, the nurse and couple use their prior experience and growing rapport to change comfort measures as needed. A decrease in the intensity of discomfort is one of the goals of nursing support during labor. Nursing measures used to decrease pain include the following:

- Ensuring general comfort
- Providing information to decrease anxiety
- Using specific supportive relaxation techniques
- Encouraging controlled breathing
- Administering pharmacologic agents as ordered by the physician or CNM

General Comfort

General comfort measures are of great importance during labor. By relieving minor discomforts, the nurse helps the woman optimize her ability to cope with pain. Encourage the woman to ambulate as long as there are no contraindications, such as vaginal bleeding or rupture of membranes

FIGURE 19-1

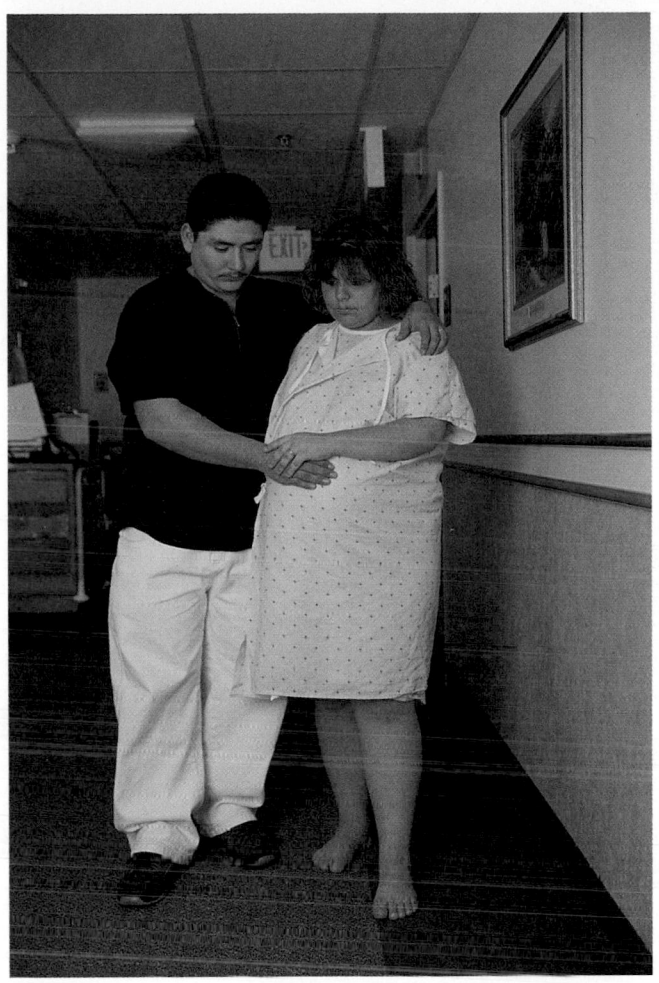

Woman and her partner walking in the hospital during labor.

Pillows may be placed under each arm and under the knees to provide further support. Because a pregnant woman is at increased risk for thrombophlebitis, excessive pressure behind the knee and calf should be avoided. Assess pressure points frequently.

Back rubs and frequent changes of position contribute to comfort and relaxation. Wearing socks or slippers may alleviate cold feet, just as adjusting the room's thermostat can offset excessive warmth. Attention to such details allows the woman to focus on the more important issues of giving birth.

Diaphoresis and the constant leaking of amniotic fluid can dampen the woman's gown and bed linen. Fresh, smooth, dry bed linen promotes comfort. To avoid having to change the bottom sheet following rupture of the membranes, replace chux pads at frequent intervals (following body substance isolation precautions). Keep the woman's perineal area as clean and dry as possible to promote comfort and to prevent infection.

A full bladder adds to the discomfort during a contraction and may prolong labor by interfering with the descent of the fetus. The bladder should be kept as empty as possible. Even if the woman is voiding, urine may be retained because of the pressure of the fetal presenting part. To detect a full bladder, palpate directly over the symphysis pubis. Some regional analgesia procedures contribute to the inability to void, and catheterization may be necessary. Encourage the woman to empty her bladder every 1 to 2 hours.

Family members also need to be encouraged to maintain their own comfort. Because they are paying attention to the laboring woman, they may forget their own needs. It may be necessary to encourage them to take breaks, to eat and drink, and to rest.

before the fetus is engaged in the pelvis. Ambulation can increase comfort and aid in fetal descent (Figure 19-1 ●).

Even if the woman prefers not to walk around, upright positions such as sitting in a rocker or leaning against a wall or bed can enhance comfort. If she stays in bed, encourage the woman to assume positions that she finds comfortable (Figure 19-2 ●). A side-lying position is generally the most advantageous for the laboring woman, although frequent position changes seem to achieve more efficient contractions. It is important to support all body parts, with the joints kept slightly flexed. For instance, when the woman is in a side-lying position, pillows may be placed against her chest and under the uppermost arm. Place a pillow or folded bath blanket between her knees to support the uppermost leg and relieve tension or muscle strain. A pillow placed at the woman's midback also helps provide support. If the woman is more comfortable on her back, elevate the head of the bed to relieve the pressure of the uterus on the vena cava.

Handling Anxiety

A woman's anxiety as she begins labor is related to a combination of factors inherent to the process. A moderate amount of anxiety about the pain enhances the woman's ability to deal with it. In contrast, an excessive degree of anxiety decreases her ability to cope. Women in the latent phase of labor who have increased anxiety about safety and their ability to cope are much more likely to describe their pain as unbearable.

To decrease anxiety not related to pain, give information (which eases fear of the unknown), establish rapport with the couple (which helps them preserve their personal integrity), and express confidence in the couple's ability to work with the labor process. It is important to demonstrate genuine concern for the laboring woman. Remaining with the woman as much as possible conveys a caring attitude and dispels fears of abandonment. Praise for breathing, relaxation, and pushing efforts not only encourages repetition of the behavior but also decreases anxiety about the ability to cope with labor.

⊙ FIGURE 19–2

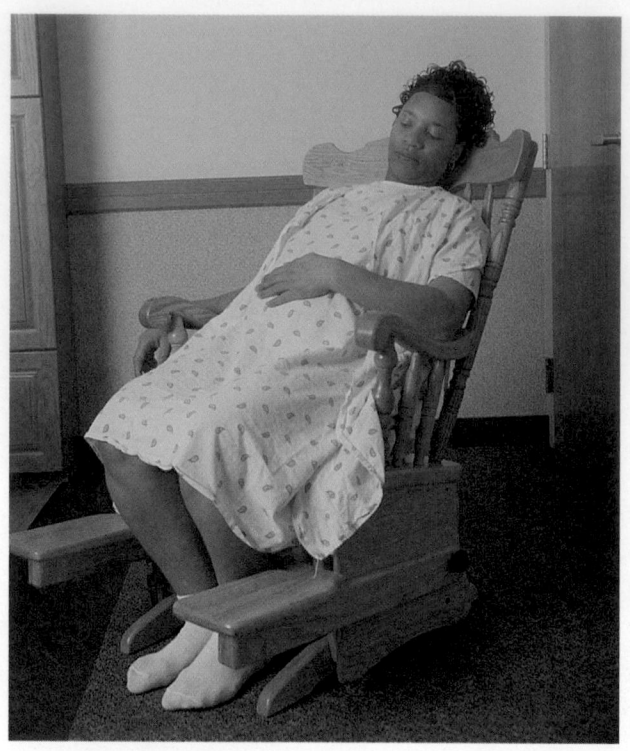

The laboring woman is encouraged to choose a comfortable position. The nurse modifies assessments and intervention as necessary.

TEACHING HIGHLIGHTS

ANXIETY ABOUT VAGINAL EXAMINATION

If a woman is experiencing severe fear or anxiety about a vaginal examination, advise her to slowly count to 10 during the examination while continually wiggling her toes. This source of distraction may lessen her fear and anxiety. It also enables the woman to have a sense of control.

Client Teaching

Providing truthful information about the nature of the discomfort that will occur during labor is important. Stressing the intermittent nature and maximum duration of the contractions can be most helpful. The woman can cope with pain better when she knows that a period of relief will follow. Describing the type of discomfort and specific sensations that will occur as labor progresses helps the woman

recognize these sensations as normal and expected when she does experience them.

Descriptions of sensations are best accompanied by information on specific comfort measures. Some women experience the urge to push during transition, when the cervix is not fully dilated and effaced. Panting can control this sensation (it is difficult to pant and bear down at the same time). If time permits, explain the purpose of panting and have the woman practice before the technique is needed.

Thorough orientation and explanation of surroundings, procedures, and equipment being used also decrease anxiety, thereby reducing pain. Being attached to an electronic monitor can produce fear because equipment of this type is associated with critically ill people. Explain beeps, clicks, and other strange noises and give a simplified explanation of the monitor strip, emphasizing that the use of the fetal monitor provides a way to assess the well-being of the fetus during labor. It helps to show the woman and her partner or support person how the monitor can identify the beginnings of contractions. At the onset of each contraction, encourage the woman to begin her breathing technique to lessen her perception of pain.

Labor and childbirth may be a critical time for the woman with a history of childhood sexual abuse or rape. All women entering the healthcare arena need to be evaluated for a history of sexual abuse or rape. However, a woman may or may not be able to address this issue with the nurse, because sharing such personal information with a stranger is difficult. It is especially important to be alert for nonverbal cues, such as unexplained anxiety, unrelenting pain, or fear during vaginal examinations, and to be prepared to offer additional teaching and relaxation support to help offset the woman's anxiety.

Supportive Relaxation Techniques

Tense muscles increase resistance to the descent of the fetus and contribute to maternal fatigue. This fatigue increases pain perception and decreases the woman's ability to cope with the pain. Comfort measures, massage, water therapy (see "Complementary Care: Water Therapy During Labor"), techniques for decreasing anxiety, and client teaching can contribute to relaxation. Adequate sleep and rest are also important. Encourage the laboring woman to use the periods between contractions for rest and relaxation. A prolonged prodromal phase of labor may have kept her awake. Moreover, a woman beginning labor is naturally excited, making it difficult for her to sleep even if her contractions are mild and infrequent.

Distraction helps increase relaxation and ability to cope with discomfort. During early labor, conversation or activities such as light reading or playing cards or other games serve as distractions. It may be helpful to have the woman concentrate on a pleasant experience she has had in the past. Other techniques include the use of a specific visual or mental focal point, breathing techniques, counting or humming, or visualization.

Touch is another type of distraction (Figure 19–3). Although some women regard touching as an invasion of privacy or threat to their independence, many want to touch and be touched during a painful experience. Nurses can make themselves available to the woman who desires touch by placing a hand on the side of the bed within the woman's reach. The person who needs touch will reach out for contact. (See "Complementary Care: Intuitive Touch.")

Mild to moderate abdominal discomfort during contractions may be relieved or lessened by effleurage. Firm pressure on the lower back or sacral area may relieve back pain associated with labor. To apply firm pressure, place a hand or a rolled, warmed towel or blanket in the small of the woman's back. In addition to the measures just described,

COMPLEMENTARY CARE

WATER THERAPY DURING LABOR

Centuries old, water immersion in hot springs, and more recently in Jacuzzis and spas, is used all over the world to promote relaxation. Current evidence supports hydrotherapy in labor as an effective method for pain management during the first stage of labor. Studies have shown a significant reduction in pain and the use of analgesia among women who are immersed in water during the first stage of labor (Benfield, 2002; Cluett, Nikodem, McCandlish et al., 2004).

Water immersion offers both psychologic and physiologic benefits. Physiologically, water provides the right counterpressure and support for the stretching tissues. The studies cited above have shown no adverse outcomes on labor duration, operative birth, or neonatal outcomes.

Some women may choose to labor *and* give birth in a water environment. Several studies have reported adverse neonatal and maternal effects of water births, such as neonatal and maternal sepsis due to contaminated water. In addition, infants may require more resuscitation measures in water births (Pinette, Wax, & Wilson, 2004). Infection control measures should be followed in any water birth; a sanitized tub is extremely important. Only women with low-risk pregnancies should consider this option, and they should be made aware of the possible risks.

enhance the woman's relaxation by providing encouragement and support for her controlled breathing techniques.

Breathing Techniques

Breathing techniques may help the laboring woman. Used correctly they increase the woman's pain threshold, permit relaxation, enhance the woman's ability to cope with the uterine contractions, and allow the uterus to function more efficiently.

● FIGURE 19–3

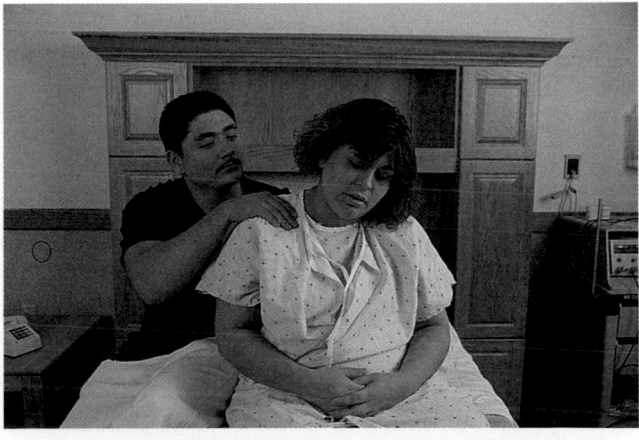

The woman's partner provides support and encouragement during labor.

COMPLEMENTARY CARE

INTUITIVE TOUCH

Intuitive touch is the nurse's intentional use of physical contact with the woman with the intent of helping to slow down and regulate the breathing pattern. This type of touch has also been referred to as purposeful, affective, comforting, or empathetic touch (Bottorff, 1993; Snyder & Nojima, 1998). (*Note:* Therapeutic touch, a complementary therapy that focuses on energy fields, is a different process. See discussion in Chapter 2. ∞)

Evidence suggests that touch induces the relaxation response, which is mediated through the neuroendocrine and sympathetic nervous systems. Deep relaxation results in decreased heart rate, respiratory rate and volume, oxygen consumption, blood pressure, skeletal muscle tension, and gastric acidity and motility, and it increases peripheral blood flow and the activity of natural killer cells.

A variety of techniques can be used. These include hand-holding; stroking or patting of a woman's arm, face, or legs; placing one hand on her shoulder; putting an arm around her shoulders; and hugging. To implement intuitive touch, use long, slow, up-and-down strokes on the woman's limbs. You do not need special training to use this intervention; all that is needed is the intention to help regulate the breathing pattern and the willingness to use a little time to achieve this goal.

Many women learn patterned-paced breathing during childbirth preparation classes. This type of controlled breathing often has three levels. The woman tends to begin with the first level and then proceed to the next when she feels the need. Regardless of the level of breathing used, a cleansing breath begins and ends each pattern. A cleansing breath involves only the chest. It consists of inhaling through the nose and exhaling through pursed lips (Table 19–3).

First Pattern. The first pattern may also be called slow, deep breathing or slow-paced breathing. During the breathing movements, only the chest moves. The woman inhales slowly through her nose. She moves her chest up and out during the inhalation. She exhales through pursed lips. The breathing rate is 6 to 9 breaths a minute.

Second Pattern. The second pattern is also called shallow or modified-paced breathing. The woman begins with a cleansing breath and at the end of the cleansing breath pushes out a short breath. She then inhales and exhales through the mouth at a rate of about 4 breaths every 5 seconds. This pattern can be altered into a more rapid rate that does not exceed 2 to 2 1/2 breaths every second.

Third Pattern. The third pattern is also called pant-blow or patterned-paced breathing. It is similar to modified-paced breathing except the breathing is punctuated every few breaths by a forceful exhalation through pursed lips. A pat-

tern of 4 breaths may be used to begin. All breaths are kept equal and rhythmic. As the contraction becomes more intense, the woman may adjust the pattern as needed to 3:1, 2:1, and finally 1:1.

If the woman has not learned a controlled breathing technique, teaching her may be difficult when she is admitted in active labor. In this instance, teach abdominal and pant-pant-blow breathing (see Table 19–3). In abdominal breathing the woman moves the abdominal wall upward as she inhales and downward as she exhales. This method tends to lift the abdominal wall off the contracting uterus and thus may provide some pain relief. The breathing is deep and rhythmic. As transition approaches, the woman may feel the need to breathe more rapidly. To avoid breathing too rapidly, the woman can use the pant-pant-blow breathing pattern.

Hyperventilation is the result of an imbalance of oxygen and carbon dioxide (i.e., too much carbon dioxide is exhaled, and too much oxygen remains in the body). Hyperventilation may occur when a woman breathes very rapidly over a prolonged period. The signs and symptoms of hyperventilation are tingling or numbness in the tip of the nose, lips, fingers, or toes; dizziness; spots before the eyes; or spasms of the hands or feet (carpal-pedal spasms). If hyperventilation occurs, encourage the woman to slow her breathing rate and take shallow breaths. With instruction and encouragement, many women are able to change their breathing to correct the problem. It may also help to count out loud for the woman so she can pace her breathing during contractions. If the signs and symptoms continue or become more severe (they progress from numbness to spasms), the woman can breathe into a paper surgical mask or a paper bag until symptoms go away. Breathing into a mask or bag causes rebreathing of carbon dioxide. During this time remain with the woman to reassure her.

In some instances, analgesics or regional anesthetic blocks may be used to increase comfort and relaxation during labor. (See Chapter 18. ∞) Table 19–4 summarizes labor progress, possible responses of the laboring woman, and support measures.

Role of the Doula

Throughout the first stage of labor, assess and support the interactions between the woman and her support person or partner. In the absence of a partner, or when the partner wants a less active role in the support of the laboring woman, it is becoming more common for women to employ a paid care provider, often called a **doula**, who has experience in caring for laboring women. The doula typically has received special training and may even be certified. The role of the doula is to enhance the comfort and decrease the anxiety of the laboring woman. A doula can be a valuable advocate to the laboring woman and her family, as well as an

TABLE 19–3 ✣ Nursing Support of Patterned-Paced Breathing

Determine which breathing method the woman (couple) has learned. Provide encouragement as needed in maintaining breathing pattern. Provide support to the labor coach and assist as needed.

Lamaze Breathing Pattern Levels

First level (slow paced)

Pattern begins and ends with a cleansing breath (in through the nose and out through pursed lips as if cooling a spoonful of hot food). While inhaling through the nose and exhaling through pursed lips, slow breaths are taken, moving only the chest. The rate should be approximately 6–9/minute or 2 breaths/15 seconds. The coach or nurse may assist by reminding the woman to take a cleansing breath, and then the breaths could be counted out if needed to maintain pacing. The woman inhales as someone counts "one one thousand, two one thousand, three one thousand, four one thousand." Exhalation begins and continues through the same count.

Second level (modified paced)

Pattern begins and ends with a cleansing breath. Breaths are then taken in and out silently through the mouth at approximately 4 breaths/5 seconds. The jaw and entire body need to be relaxed. The rate can be accelerated to 2–2½ breaths/second. The rhythm for the breaths can be counted out as "one and two and one and two and. . ." with the woman exhaling on the numbers and inhaling on "and."

Third level (pattern paced)

Pattern begins and ends with a cleansing breath. All breaths are rhythmic, in and out through the mouth. Exhalations are accompanied by a "hee" or "hoo" sound in a varying pattern, 2:1, which begins as 3:1 (hee hee hee hoo) and can change to 2:1 (hee hee hoo) or 1:1 (hee hoo) as the intensity of the contraction changes. The rate should not be more rapid than 2–2½ breaths/second. The rhythm of the breaths would match a "one and two and . . ." count.

Abdominal Breathing Pattern Cues

The abdomen moves outward during inhalation and downward during exhalation. The rate remains slow, with approximately 6–9 breaths/minute.

Quick Method

When the woman has not learned a particular method and is in the active phase of labor, the nurse may teach her a combination of two patterns. Abdominal breathing may be used until labor is more advanced. Then a more rapid pattern consisting of two short blows from the mouth followed by a longer blow can be used. (This pattern is called "pant-pant-blow" even though all exhalations are a blowing motion.)

First level for use during uterine contractions (The level begins and ends with a cleansing breath [CB].)

CB — CB
|← 45 seconds →|

Second level

CB — CB
|← 60 seconds →|

Third level (Darkened spike represents "hoo.")

CB — CB
|← 60–90 seconds →|

Breathing sequence for abdominal breathing.

|← 60 seconds →|

Pant-pant-blow breathing pattern

|← 60 seconds →|

asset to the labor nurse. For example, the doula might support the woman by helping identify the beginning of each contraction and encouraging her as she breathes through it.

NURSING CARE DURING THE SECOND STAGE OF LABOR

The second stage is reached when the cervix is fully dilated (10 cm). The contractions continue as in the transition phase. Assess maternal pulse and blood pressure and FHR every 5 to 15 minutes. Once the second stage is reached, the labor nurse remains with the woman continually and does not generally leave the room.

As the woman pushes during the second stage, she may make a variety of sounds. A low-pitched, grunting sound ("uhhh") usually indicates that the woman is working with the pushing. The nurse who feels comfortable with maternal sounds and stays sensitive to changes in the sounds may be able to detect if the woman is losing her ability to cope. For instance, if the woman feels afraid of the sensations produced by her pushing effort, her sound may change to a high-pitched cry or whimper, and the nurse can then provide extra

TABLE 19–4 ✤ Normal Progress. Psychologic Characteristics, and Nursing Support During the First and Second Stages of Labor

Phase	Cervical Dilatation	Uterine Contractions	Woman's Response	Support Measures
Stage 1 Latent phase	1–4 cm	Every 10–20 minutes, 15–20 seconds' duration Mild intensity *progressing to* Every 5–7 minutes, 30–40 seconds' duration Moderate intensity	Usually happy, talkative, and eager to be in labor Exhibits need for independence by taking care of own bodily needs and seeking information	Establish rapport on admission and continue to build during care. Assess information base and learning needs. Be available to consult regarding breathing technique if needed; teach breathing technique if needed and in early labor. Orient family to room, equipment, monitors, and procedures. Encourage woman and partner to participate in care as desired. Provide needed information. Assist woman into position of comfort; encourage frequent change of position; encourage ambulation during early labor. Offer fluids or ice chips. Keep couple informed of progress. Encourage woman to void every 1 to 2 hours. Assess need for an interest in using visualization to enhance relaxation, and teach if appropriate.
Active phase	4–7 cm	Every 2–3 minutes, 40–60 seconds' duration Moderate to strong intensity	May experience feelings of helplessness Exhibits increased fatigue and may begin to feel restless and anxious as contractions become stronger Expresses fear of abandonment Becomes more dependent because she is less able to meet her needs	Encourage woman to maintain breathing patterns. Provide quiet environment to reduce external stimuli. Provide reassurance, encouragement, support; keep couple informed of progress. Promote comfort by giving back rubs, sacral pressure, cool cloth on forehead, assistance with position changes, support with pillows, effleurage. Provide ice chips, ointment for dry mouth and lips. Encourage to void every 1 to 2 hours. Offer shower, whirlpool, or warm bath if available.
Transition phase	8–10 cm	Every 2 minutes, 60–75 seconds' duration Strong intensity	Tires and may exhibit increased restlessness and irritability May feel she cannot keep up with labor process and is out of control Physical discomforts Fear of being left alone May fear tearing open or splitting apart with contractions	Encourage woman to rest between contractions. If she sleeps between contractions, wake her at beginning of contraction so she can begin breathing pattern (increases feeling of control). Provide support, encouragement, and praise for efforts. Keep couple informed of progress; encourage continued participation of support persons. Promote comfort as listed earlier but recognize that many women do not want to be touched when in transition. Provide privacy. Provide ice chips, ointment for lips. Encourage to void every 1 to 2 hours.
Stage 2	Complete	Every 2 minutes	May feel out of control, helpless, panicky	Assist woman in pushing efforts. Encourage woman to assume position of comfort. Provide encouragement and praise her efforts. Keep couple informed of progress. Provide ice chips. Maintain privacy as woman desires.

support. During the second stage, the woman may interpret rectal pressure as a need to move her bowels. The instinctive response is to resist and to tighten muscles rather than bear down (push). A sensation of splitting apart also occurs in the latter part of the second stage, and the woman may fear the urge to push. The woman who expects these sensations and understands that bearing down contributes to progress at this stage is more likely to do so effectively.

When the urge to bear down becomes uncontrollable and pushing begins, the nurse can help by encouraging the woman and by assisting with positioning (Figure 19–4 ●). The woman may want to be supported with pillows in a semi-reclining position, be side-lying, position herself on her hands and knees, or use a squatting bar. Most women spontaneously push very effectively in response to messages from their body. However, in some settings sustained, forceful pushing is believed to be necessary. In that case, when the contraction begins, the woman is told to take a cleansing breath or two, then to take a third large breath and hold it while pushing down with her abdominal muscles (called the Valsalva maneuver). A more natural approach that lets the mother wait to bear down until she feels an urge to push may shorten the pushing phase, reducing the incidence of physiologic stress in the mother and acidosis in the newborn. This technique may also decrease the incidence of instrument births and damage to maternal perineal tissue (Roberts, 2002).

A nullipara is usually prepared for birth when perineal bulging is noted. A multipara usually progresses far more quickly, so she may be prepared for the birth when the cervix is dilated 7 to 8 cm. As the birth approaches, the woman's partner or support person also prepares for the birth.

Monitor the woman's blood pressure and the FHR between contractions, and palpate the contractions until the birth. Continue to assist the woman in her pushing efforts, keep both the woman and the coach informed of procedures and progress, and support them both throughout the birth.

NURSING PRACTICE

Birth is imminent if the woman shows the following changes:
- Bulging of the perineum
- Uncontrollable urge to bear down
- Increased bloody show

PROMOTION OF COMFORT IN THE SECOND STAGE

Most of the comfort measures used during the first stage remain appropriate at this time. Applying cool cloths to the face and forehead may help cool the woman involved in the intense physical exertion of pushing. The woman may feel hot and want to remove some covers. Care still needs to be taken to provide privacy even though covers are removed. Encourage the woman to rest and relax all muscles during the periods between contractions. With the support person(s), help the woman into a pushing position with each contraction. Sips of fluids or ice chips may relieve dry mouth. Continually provide encouragement and positive reinforcement.

ASSISTING DURING BIRTH

In addition to assisting the woman and her partner, the nurse also assists the physician or CNM in preparing for the birth. The physician or CNM dons a sterile gown and gloves and may place sterile drapes over the woman's abdomen and legs. An episiotomy may be done just before the actual birth if needed. (See the discussion of episiotomy in Chapter 22 ∞.)

Shortly before the birth, the birthing room or delivery room is prepared with the equipment and materials that may be needed. Family members do not need to change into other clothing if the birth occurs in a birthing room; they don a disposable scrub suit or scrubs provided by the facility if the birth is to occur in a delivery room or surgery suite. Thorough handwashing is required of the nurses and CNM or physician. Nurses who will be in direct contact with the mother at the time of birth need to wear protective clothing such as an apron or gown with a splash apron, disposable gloves, and eye covering. The CNM or physician also needs to wear a plastic apron or a gown with a splash apron, eye covering, and sterile gloves.

If the laboring woman is to give birth in a location other than the birthing room (such as in the case of a cesarean birth), she is moved on her bed or a cart shortly before

● **FIGURE 19–4**

The nurse provides encouragement and support during pushing efforts.

birth. To ensure the woman's safety, the side rails should be raised into a locked position. It is important that the woman move from one bed to another between contractions. During the contraction the woman feels increased discomfort and may be involved in pushing efforts. Take care to preserve her privacy during the transfer. The labor bed or transfer cart must be carefully braced against the delivery table to ensure the woman's safety during the transfer.

Even though there are differences in the delivery room setting, the family can still be together during the birth. Encourage family members to participate, because the delivery room environment may seem intimidating. The family member may hesitate to continue providing support because of fear of interfering or being in the way.

Maternal Birthing Positions

Until modern times the upright posture for birth was considered normal in most societies. Women chose to squat, kneel, stand, or sit for birth. The recumbent position (lithotomy) became more usual in the Western world because of the convenience it offers in applying technology. The lithotomy position has thus become the conventional manner in which North American women give birth in hospitals. In seeking alternative positions, consumers and professionals alike are refocusing on the comfort of the laboring woman rather than on the convenience of the CNM or physician (Figure 19–5 ● and Table 19–5).

The woman is typically positioned for birth on a bed with leg supports, in a squatting position, or perhaps on her hands and knees. If a birthing bed is used, the back is elevated 30 to 60 degrees to help the woman bear down. Stirrups, if needed and used, are padded to avoid pressure. If helping the woman place her legs in the stirrups, lift both legs simultaneously to avoid strain on abdominal, back, and perineal muscles. Adjust the stirrups to fit the woman's legs. The feet are supported in the stirrup holders. The height and angle of the stirrups are adjusted so there is no pressure on the backs of the knees or the calves, which might cause discomfort and

● FIGURE 19–5

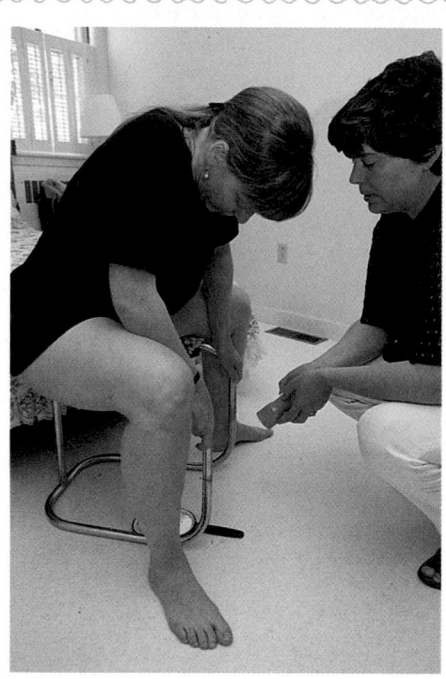

Birthing positions. **A,** Side-lying (also known as left lateral Sims') position. **B,** Using a birthing stool. **C,** Using a birthing bar.

B, © *Stella Johnson (www.stellajohnson.com).*

TABLE 19-5 ✤ Comparison of Birthing Positions

Position	Advantages	Disadvantages	Nursing Actions
Sitting on birthing stool	Gravity aids descent and expulsion of infant. Does not compromise venous return from lower extremities. Woman can view birth process.	It is difficult to provide support for the woman's back.	Encourage woman to sit in a position that increases her comfort.
Semi-Fowler's	Does not compromise venous return from lower extremities. Woman can view birth process.	If legs are positioned wide apart, relaxation of perineal tissues is decreased.	Assess that upper torso is evenly supported. Increase support of body by changing position of bed or using pillows as props.
Left lateral Sims'	Does not compromise venous return from lower extremities. Increases perineal relaxation and decreases need for episiotomy. Appears to prevent rapid descent.	It is difficult for the woman to see the birth.	Adjust position so that the upper leg lies on the bed (scissor fashion) or is supported by the partner or on pillows.
Squatting	Size of pelvic outlet is increased. Gravity aids descent and expulsion of newborn. Second stage may be shortened.	It may be difficult to maintain balance while squatting.	Help woman maintain balance. Use a birthing bar if available.
Sitting in birthing bed	Gravity aids descent and expulsion of the fetus. Does not compromise venous return from lower extremities. Woman can view the birth process. Leg position may be changed at will.		Ensure that legs and feet have adequate support.
Hands and knees	Increases perineal relaxation and decreases need for episiotomy. Increases placental and umbilical blood flow and decreases fetal distress. Improves fetal rotation. Better able to assess the perineum. Better access to fetal nose and mouth for suctioning at birth. Facilitates birth of infant with shoulder dystocia.	Woman cannot view birth. There is decreased contact with birth attendant. Caregivers cannot use instruments. There may be increased maternal fatigue.	Adjust birthing bed by dropping the foot down. Supply extra pillows for increased support.

postpartal vascular problems. When stirrups are not used for the birth, the woman's legs may be placed in stirrups after the birth to enhance visibility if a perineal repair is needed.

Cleansing the Perineum

After the woman has been positioned for the birth, her vulvar and perineal areas are cleansed to increase her comfort and to remove any bloody discharge. Depending on agency protocol or on physician or CNM orders, perineal cleansing methods range from use of soapy water to aseptic technique. Once the cleansing is completed, the woman returns to the desired birthing position.

Continued Labor Support

Both the woman's partner and the nurse who has been with the woman during the labor continue to provide support during contractions. The woman is encouraged to push with each contraction and, as the fetal head emerges, is asked to take shallow breaths or to pant to prevent pushing. While supporting the head, the physician or certified nurse-midwife assesses whether the umbilical cord is around the fetal neck and removes it if it is, then suctions the mouth and nose with a bulb syringe. The mouth is suctioned first to prevent reflex inhalation of mucus when the nostrils are touched with the bulb syringe tip. The woman is encouraged to push again as the rest of the newborn's body is born. Figure 19–6 ● depicts a birth.

NURSING CARE DURING THE THIRD AND FOURTH STAGES OF LABOR

INITIAL CARE OF THE NEWBORN

The CNM or physician places the newborn on the mother's abdomen, which promotes attachment, or in the radiant-heated unit. The newborn is maintained in a modified Trendelenburg position. In this position, gravity aids drainage of mucus from the nasopharynx and trachea. Dry the newborn immediately and help keep the infant warm by placing warmed blankets over the newborn or by placing the newborn in skin-to-skin contact with the mother. If the newborn is in a radiant-heated unit, he or she is dried, placed on a dry blanket, and left uncovered. Because radiant heat warms the outer surface of objects, a newborn wrapped in blankets will receive no benefit from the unit.

Suction the newborn's nose and mouth with a bulb syringe as needed. Most immediate care of the newborn can be done while the newborn is in the parent's arms or in the radiant-heated unit.

Apgar Scoring System

The Apgar scoring system (Table 19–6) evaluates the physical condition of the newborn at birth. The newborn is rated 1 minute after birth and again at 5 minutes and receives a total score (**Apgar score**) ranging from 0 to 10 based on the following assessments:

1. *Heart rate* is auscultated or palpated at the junction of the umbilical cord and skin. This is the most important assessment. A heart rate above 100 is scored as 2, a heart rate below 100 receives a 1, and a score of 0 is assigned if there is no heartbeat. A newborn heart rate of less than 100 beats per minute indicates the need for immediate resuscitation.

2. *Respiratory effort* is the second most important Apgar assessment. Complete absence of respirations is termed apnea (scored 0). A vigorous cry indicates adequate respirations and is scored as 2, whereas a slow, irregular respiratory effort receives a 1.

3. *Muscle tone* is determined by evaluating the degree of flexion and resistance to straightening of the

extremities. A normal newborn's elbows and hips are flexed, with the knees positioned up toward the abdomen (scored as 2). Some flexion of the extremities is scored as 1, while a flaccid infant receives a 0.

4. *Reflex irritability* is evaluated by stroking the baby's back along the spine or by flicking the soles of the feet. A cry merits a full score of 2. A grimace is 1 point, and no response is 0.

5. *Skin color* is inspected for cyanosis and pallor. Generally, newborns have blue extremities, with a pink body, which merits a score of 1. This condition is termed *acrocyanosis* and is present in many normal newborns at 1 minute after birth. A totally pink newborn scores a 2, and a totally cyanotic, pale infant scores 0. Newborns with darker skin are not pink in color. Their skin color is assessed for pallor and acrocyanosis.

A score of 8 to 10 indicates a newborn in good condition who requires only nasopharyngeal suctioning and perhaps some oxygen near the face (called "blow-by" oxygen). If the Apgar score is below 8, resuscitative measures may be needed. (See the discussion in Chapter 27. ∞)

Care of Umbilical Cord

If the physician or CNM has not placed some type of cord clamp on the newborn's umbilical cord, the nurse does so. Before applying the cord clamp, examine the cut end of the cord for the presence of two arteries and one vein. The umbilical vein is the largest vessel, and the arteries are seen as smaller vessels. Record the number of vessels on the birth and newborn records. The cord is clamped approximately 1/2 to 1 inch from the abdomen to allow room between the abdomen and clamp as the cord dries. Abdominal skin must not be clamped, because this will cause necrosis of the tissue. The most common type of cord clamp is the plastic Hollister cord clamp (Figure 19–7 ●). The Hollister clamp is removed in the nursery about 24 hours after the cord has dried.

Cord Blood Collection for Banking

A growing number of parents are arranging for cord blood banking with individual cord blood registries (see discussion in Chapter 1 ∞). These registries provide the parents with a special container for the cord blood, which they bring with them to the birth. The parents should have received directions from the registry about the storage and care of the container prior to the birth. Immediately after the newborn's umbilical cord is clamped and cut and the placenta is expelled, the CNM or physician withdraws blood from the remaining umbilical cord and the placenta and places it in the special container. The

FIGURE 19-6

A birthing sequence.

TABLE 19–6 ✤ The Apgar Scoring System

	SCORE		
Sign	**0**	**1**	**2**
Heart rate	Absent	Slow—below 100	Above 100
Respiratory effort	Absent	Slow—irregular	Good crying
Muscle tone	Flaccid	Some flexion of extremities	Active motion
Reflex irritability	None	Grimace	Vigorous cry
Color	Pale blue	Body pink, blue extremities	Completely pink

Data from Apgar, V. (1968, August). The newborn (Apgar) scoring system, reflections and advice. *Pediatric Clinics of North America, 13,* 645.

cord blood remains with the mother until it is picked up by the cord blood registry.

Physical Assessment of the Newborn

The nurse performs an abbreviated systematic physical assessment in the birthing area to detect any abnormalities (Table 19–7). First, note the size of the newborn and the contour and size of the head in relationship to the rest of the body. The newborn's posture and movements indicate tone and neurologic functioning.

Inspect the skin for discoloration, presence of vernix caseosa and lanugo, and signs of trauma and desquamation (peeling of skin). Vernix caseosa is a white, cheesy substance found normally on newborns. It is absorbed within 24 hours after birth. Vernix is abundant on preterm infants and absent on postterm newborns. Fine hair (lanugo) is often seen on preterm newborns' shoulders, foreheads, backs, and cheeks. Desquamation is seen in postterm newborns.

Observe the nares (nostrils) for flaring and, as the newborn cries, inspect the palate for cleft palate. Look for mucus in the nose and mouth, and remove it with a bulb syringe as needed. Inspect the chest for respiratory rate and the presence of retractions. If retractions are present, assess the newborn for grunting or stridor. A normal respiratory rate is 30 to 60 per minute. Auscultate the lungs bilaterally for breath sounds. Absence of breath sounds on one side could mean pneumothorax. Rales may be heard immediately after birth because a small amount of fluid may remain in the lungs; this fluid will be absorbed. Rhonchi indicate aspiration of oral secretions. If there is excessive mucus or respiratory distress, suction the newborn with a mucus trap. (See Figure 19–8 ● as well as Skill 4–2 in the Clinical Skills Manual and the CD-ROM that accompanies this text. **SKILLS**) Note and record elimination of urine or meconium on the newborn record.

Newborn Identification

Place two ID bands on the newborn—one on the wrist and one on the ankle. The bands must fit snugly so they will not be lost. To ensure correct identification, while still in the birthing or delivery room, give the mother and her partner each a band that matches that of the baby. The bands allow access to the infant care areas and must not be removed until the infant is discharged.

Some facilities now use an umbilical cord clamp that includes an infant security alarm. The cord clamp and

● **FIGURE 19–7**

Hollister cord clamp. **A,** Clamp is positioned 1/2 to 1 inch from the abdomen and then secured. **B,** Cut cord. The one vein and two arteries can be seen. **C,** Plastic device for removing clamp after cord has dried. After the cord is cut, the nurse grasps the Hollister clamp on either side of the cut area and gently separates it.

TABLE 19–7 ✣ Initial Newborn Evaluation

Assess	Normal Findings
Respirations	Rate 36–60, irregular No retractions, no grunting
Apical pulse	Rate 120–160 and somewhat irregular
Temperature	Skin temp above 36.5°C (97.8°F)
Skin color	Body pink with bluish extremities
Umbilical cord	Two arteries and one vein
Gestational age	Should be 38–42 weeks to remain with parents for extended time
Sole creases	Sole creases that involve the heel

In general, expect scant amount of vernix on upper back, axilla, groin; lanugo only on upper back; ears with incurving of upper 2/3 of pinnae and thin cartilage that springs back from folding; male genitals—testes palpated in upper or lower scrotum; female genitals—labia majora larger, clitoris nearly covered

In the following situations, newborns should generally be stabilized rather than remaining with parents in the birth area for an extended period of time:

- Apgar less than 8 at 1 minute and less than 9 at 5 minutes or baby requires resuscitation measures (other than whiffs of oxygen)
- Respirations below 30 or above 60, with retractions and/or grunting
- Apical pulse below 120 or above 160 with marked irregularities
- Skin temperature below 36.5°C (97.8°F)
- Skin color pale blue or circumoral pallor
- Baby less than 38 or more than 42 weeks' gestation
- Baby very small or very large for gestational age
- Congenital anomalies involving open areas in the skin (meningomyelocele)

● FIGURE 19–8

To clear secretions from the newborn's nose or oropharynx, a DeLee mucus trap (shown here) or other suction device is used. One end of the suction tubing is connected to low suction, and the other end of the tubing is inserted 3 to 5 inches into the newborn's nose or mouth. Suction is applied as the tubing is pulled out. The process is repeated for as long as fluid is aspirated.

alarm are left in place until the mother and baby are discharged home. The alarm sounds if the infant is removed from the hospital unit or if the cord clamp or alarm is cut or disengaged (Figure 19–9 ●).

Additional hospital security measures are now commonplace in maternity settings. This includes mandating that all staff wear appropriate identification at all times. Parents are instructed that individuals without appropriate identification should not be allowed to remove their infant under any circumstances. The nurse also advises the parents to place the infant on the side of the bed away from the window, and to have the baby returned to the nursery whenever the mother naps or showers and no other family member is present.

Many hospitals also footprint the newborn and fingerprint the mother. To prepare the newborn for footprinting, wipe the soles of both of the newborn's feet to remove any vernix caseosa. Once used for security purposes, fingerprinting and footprinting of infants is now performed to provide a souvenir for the new parents.

DELIVERY OF THE PLACENTA

After birth the certified nurse-midwife or physician prepares for the delivery of the placenta. The following signs suggest placental separation:

1. The uterus rises upward in the abdomen.
2. As the placenta moves downward, the umbilical cord lengthens.
3. A sudden trickle or spurt of blood appears.
4. The shape of the uterus changes from a disk to a globe.

While waiting for these signs, palpate the uterus to check for ballooning caused by uterine relaxation and subsequent bleeding into the uterine cavity. After the placenta has separated, the woman may be asked to bear down to aid delivery of the placenta.

Oxytocics are frequently given at the time of the delivery of the placenta, so the uterus will contract and bleeding will be minimized. Oxytocin (Pitocin), 10 to 20 units, may be added to an intravenous (IV) infusion, or 10 units may be given intramuscularly. Some physicians order methylergonovine maleate (Methergine), 0.2 mg administered intramuscularly, or carboprost tromethamine (Hemabate), 250 mcg/mL administered intramuscularly. In addition to administering the ordered medications, it is essential to assess and record maternal blood pressure before and after administration of oxytocics. For further information, refer

FIGURE 19–9

Umbilical alarm in place on a newborn infant.

to "Drug Guide: Oxytocin" (in Chapter 22) and "Drug Guide: Methylergonovine Maleate" (in Chapter 30 ∞). After expulsion of the placenta, the CNM or physician inspects the placental membranes to make sure they are intact and that all cotyledons are present. If there is a defect or a part missing from the placenta, a manual uterine examination is done. On the birth record, note the time of delivery of the placenta.

After the placenta is expelled, the physician or CNM inspects the vagina and cervix for lacerations and makes any necessary repairs. The episiotomy may be repaired if it has not been done previously (see Chapter 22 ∞).

ENHANCING ATTACHMENT

The first few hours and even minutes after birth are an important period for the attachment of mother and infant. If this period of contact can occur during the first hour after birth, the newborn will be in the quiet state and able to interact with parents by looking at them. Newborns also turn their heads in response to a spoken voice. (For further discussion of newborn states, see Chapter 23. ∞)

The first parent-newborn contact may be brief (a few minutes), to be followed by a more extended contact after uncomfortable procedures (expulsion of the placenta and suturing of the episiotomy) are completed. When the newborn is returned to the mother, help her begin breastfeeding if she so desires. The baby may seek out the mother's breast, and early contact between the two can greatly affect breastfeeding success. Even if the newborn does not actively nurse, he or she can lick, taste, and smell the mother's skin. This activity by the newborn stimulates the maternal release of prolactin, which promotes the onset of lactation.

Darkening the birthing room by turning out most of the lights causes newborns to open their eyes and gaze around. This in turn enhances eye-to-eye contact with the parents. (*Note:* If the physician or CNM needs a light source, the spotlight can be left on.) Treatment of the newborn's eyes may also be delayed. Many parents who establish eye contact with the newborn are content to quietly gaze at their infant. Others may show more active involvement by touching or inspecting the newborn. Some mothers talk to their babies in a high-pitched voice, which seems to be soothing to newborns. Some couples verbally express amazement and pride when they see they have produced a beautiful, healthy baby. Their verbalization enhances feelings of accomplishment and ecstasy.

Both parents need to be encouraged to do whatever they feel most comfortable doing. Some parents prefer only limited contact with the newborn immediately after birth and instead want private time together in a quiet environment. In spite of the current zeal for providing immediate attachment opportunities, nursing personnel need to be aware of parents' wishes. The desire to delay interaction with the newborn does not necessarily imply a decreased ability of the parents to bond with their newborn. (For further discussion of parent-newborn attachment, see Chapter 28. ∞)

PROVISION OF CARE IN THE FOURTH STAGE

The period of 1 to 4 hours immediately following the expulsion of the placenta, during which the mother's condition stabilizes, is often referred to as the fourth stage of labor and birth. This is actually the initial recovery period.

After childbirth it is critical that the uterine fundus stay well contracted to clamp off uterine blood vessels at the placental site and thereby prevent hemorrhaging. Consequently palpate the uterine fundus at frequent intervals for the first 4 hours to ensure that it remains firmly contracted. Normally the fundus is located in the midline and at or below the umbilicus. Palpate the fundus (Figure 19–10 ●) but do not massage it unless it is soft (boggy). When a uterus becomes boggy, pooling of blood occurs within it, causing clots. Anything left in the

DRUG GUIDE

CARBOPROST TROMETHAMINE (HEMABATE)

Pregnancy Risk Category: D

Overview of Action

Carboprost tromethamine (Hemabate) is used to reduce blood loss secondary to uterine atony. It stimulates myometrial contractions to control postpartum hemorrhaging that is unresponsive to usual techniques. Carboprost tromethamine can also be used to induce labor in women desiring an elective termination of a pregnancy. The drug is also used to induce labor in cases of intrauterine fetal death and hydatidiform mole (Wilson, Shannon, & Stang, 2006).

Route, Dosage, Frequency

In cases of immediate postpartum hemorrhage, the usual intramuscular dose is 250 mcg (1 mL) which can be repeated every 1½ to 3½ hours if uterine atony persists. The dosage can be increased to 500 mcg (2 mL) if uterine contractility is inadequate after several doses of 250 mcg. The total dosage should not exceed 12 mg. The maximum duration of use is 48 hours (Wilson et al., 2006).

Contraindications

The drug is contraindicated in women with active cardiac, pulmonary, or renal disease. It should not be administered during pregnancy or in women with acute pelvic inflammatory disease. It should be used with caution in women with asthma, adrenal disease, hypotension, hypertension, diabetes mellitus, epilepsy, fibroids, cervical stenosis, or previous uterine surgery (Wilson et al., 2006).

Side Effects

The most common side effects are nausea and diarrhea. Fever, chills, and flushing can occur. Headache, muscle, joint, abdominal, or eye pain can also occur (Wilson et al., 2006).

Nursing Considerations

1. The injection should be given in a large muscle. Aspiration should be performed to avoid injection into a blood vessel which can result in bronchospasm, tetanic contractions, and shock.

2. After administration, monitor uterine status and bleeding carefully.

3. Report excess bleeding to the physician/CNM.

4. Check vital signs routinely, observing for an increase in temperature, elevated pulse, and decreased blood pressure.

5. Breastfeeding should be delayed for 24 hours after administration (Wilson et al., 2006).

---

uterus prevents it from contracting effectively. Thus, if the uterus becomes boggy or appears to rise in the abdomen, massage the fundus until firm; then with one hand supporting the uterus at the symphysis pubis, use the other hand to exert steady pressure on the fundus to express retained clots. The uterus is very tender at this time so all palpation and massage must be done as gently as possible.

In some women the uterus becomes so relaxed that it cannot be found when palpation is attempted. In this case, place one hand in the midline of the abdomen at about the level of the umbilicus and begin to make kneading motions. This motion generally stimulates the uterus to contract, and it then feels like a firm, hard object.

Wash the woman's perineum with gauze squares and warmed solution and dry the area well with a towel before placing the maternity pad. If stirrups have been used, remove both of the woman's legs from the stirrups at the same time to avoid muscle strain. Encourage the woman to move her legs gently up and down in a bicycle motion. The woman remains in the same bed or is transferred to a recovery room bed. Help her don a clean gown and offer her something to drink.

During the recovery period, it is essential to monitor maternal vital signs closely. Check the maternal blood pressure at 5- to 15-minute intervals to detect any changes. Blood pressure should return to the prelabor level due to an increased volume of blood returning to the maternal circulation from the uteroplacental shunt. Pulse rate should be slightly lower than it was during labor. Baroreceptors cause a vagal response, which slows the pulse. A rise in blood pressure may be a response to oxytocic drugs or may be caused by preeclampsia. A lowered blood pressure and a rising pulse rate may reflect blood loss (Table 19–8).

Also monitor the woman's temperature. Frequently, women have tremors in the immediate postpartum period, possibly caused by a difference in internal and external body temperatures (higher temperature inside the body than outside). Another theory is that the woman is reacting to the fetal cells that have entered the maternal circulation at the placental site. A heated bath blanket placed next to the woman is helpful and can be replaced as often as the mother desires.

Inspect the bloody vaginal discharge for amount and chart it as minimal, moderate, or heavy and with or without clots. This discharge, lochia rubra, should be bright red. A soaked perineal pad contains approximately 100 mL of blood. If the perineal pad becomes soaked in a 15-minute period or if blood pools under the buttocks, continuous observation is necessary (see Skill 5–1 in the Clinical Skills Manual, as well as in the CD-ROM that accompanies this text **SKILLS**). When the fundus is firm, a continuous trickle of blood may signal laceration of the vagina or cervix or an unligated vessel in the episiotomy.

MediaLink · Skill 5–1: Performing Nasal Pharyngeal Suctioning

⊙ FIGURE 19–10

Suggested method of palpating the fundus of the uterus during the fourth stage. The left hand is placed just above the symphysis pubis, and gentle downward pressure is exerted. The right hand is cupped around the uterine fundus.

TABLE 19–8 ❖	**Maternal Adaptations Following Birth**
Characteristic	**Normal Finding**
Blood pressure	Returns to prelabor level
Pulse	Slightly lower than in labor
Uterine fundus	In the midline at the umbilicus or one to two finger-breadths below the umbilicus
Lochia	Red (rubra), small to moderate amount (from spotting on pads to 1/4–1/2 of pad covered in 15 minutes)
	Does not exceed saturation of one pad in first hour
Bladder	Nonpalpable
Perineum	Smooth, pink, without bruising or edema
Emotional state	Wide variation, including excited, exhilarated, smiling, crying, fatigued, verbal, quiet, pensive, and sleepy

If the fundus rises and displaces to the right, it is important to consider two factors:

1. As the uterus rises, the uterine contractions become less effective and increased bleeding may occur.

2. The most common cause of uterine displacement is bladder distention.

Palpate the bladder to determine whether it is distended. The bladder fills rapidly with the extra fluid volume returned from the uteroplacental circulation (and with any fluid received intravenously during labor and birth). The postpartal woman may not realize that her bladder is full because trauma to the bladder and urethra during childbirth and the use of regional anesthesia decrease bladder tone and the urge to void.

Use a variety of measures to help the mother to void. Place a warm towel across the lower abdomen or pour warm water over the perineum to relax the urinary sphincter and facilitate voiding. If the woman is unable to void, catheterization is necessary.

The perineum is inspected for edema and hematoma formation. An ice pack often reduces the swelling and alleviates the discomfort of an episiotomy.

The couple may be tired, hungry, and thirsty. Some agencies serve the couple a meal. The tired mother will probably drift off into a welcome sleep. The partner can also be encouraged to rest, since the supporting role is physically and mentally tiring. If the mother is not in a birthing room, she is usually transferred from the birthing unit to the postpartal or mother-baby area after 2 hours or more, depending on agency policy and whether the following criteria are met:

- Stable vital signs
- No bleeding
- Undistended bladder
- Firm fundus
- Sensations fully recovered from any anesthetic agent received during birth

SUPPORT OF THE ADOLESCENT DURING BIRTH

As with all women, each adolescent in labor is different. Assess what each teen brings to the experience by considering the following:

- Has the young woman received prenatal care?
- What are her attitudes and feelings about the pregnancy?
- Who will attend the birth and what is the person's relationship to her?
- What preparation has she had for the experience?
- What are her expectations and fears regarding labor and birth?

- How has her culture influenced her?
- What are her usual coping mechanisms?
- Does she plan to keep the newborn?

Adolescent women are at highest risk for pregnancy and labor complications and must be assessed carefully. Fetal well-being is established by fetal monitoring. Be especially alert for any physiologic complications of labor. The young woman's prenatal record is carefully reviewed for risks, and she is screened for preeclampsia, cephalopelvic disproportion, anemia, drugs ingested during pregnancy, sexually transmitted infections, and size-date discrepancies.

The support role of the nurse depends on the young woman's support system during labor. The adolescent may not be accompanied by someone who will stay with her during childbirth, or she may have her mother, the father of the baby, or a close friend as her labor partner. Regardless of whether the teen has a support person, it is important to establish a trusting relationship with her. In this way it is possible to help the teen understand what is happening to her. Establishing rapport without recrimination for possible inappropriate behavior is essential. The adolescent given positive reinforcement for "work well done" will leave the experience with increased self-esteem, despite the emotional problems that may accompany her situation. If a support person accompanies the adolescent, that person also needs encouragement and support. Explain changes in the young woman's behavior and describe ways the support person can be of help.

The adolescent who has taken childbirth education classes is generally better prepared for labor than the adolescent who has not. However, the younger the adolescent, the less she may be able to participate actively in the process, even if she has taken prenatal classes. See Figure 19–11 ●.

The very young adolescent (age 14 and under) has fewer coping mechanisms and less experience to draw on than her older counterparts. Because her cognitive development is incomplete, the younger adolescent may have fewer problem-solving capabilities. She may be more threatened by the experience, and she may be more vulnerable to stress and discomfort.

The very young adolescent needs someone to rely on at all times during labor. She may be more childlike and dependent than older teens. Instructions and explanations should be simple and concrete. During the transition phase, the young teenager may become withdrawn and unable to express her need to be nurtured. Touch, soothing encouragement, and measures to provide comfort help her maintain control and meet her needs for dependence. During the second stage of labor, the young adolescent may feel as if she is losing control and may reach out to those around her. It is important to remain calm and give clear, simple directions to help the teen cope with feelings of helplessness.

● FIGURE 19–11

An adolescent mother receives breastfeeding assistance in the immediate postpartum period.

The middle adolescent (age 15 to 17 years) often attempts to remain calm and unflinching during labor. Nevertheless, a caring attitude still helps the young woman. Many older adolescents believe that they "know it all," but they may be no more prepared for childbirth than their younger counterparts. Positive reinforcement and a nonjudgmental manner will help them save face. If the adolescent has not taken childbirth preparation classes, she may require preparation and explanations. The older teenager's (age 18 to 19) response to the stresses of labor, however, is similar to that of the adult woman.

Even if the adolescent is planning to relinquish her newborn, she should be given the option of seeing and holding the infant. She may be reluctant to do this at first, but the mother's grieving process is facilitated if she sees the infant. However, seeing or holding the newborn should be the young woman's choice. (See Chapter 22 for further discussion of the relinquishing mother and the adolescent parent. ∞)

NURSING CARE DURING PRECIPITOUS BIRTH

Occasionally labor progresses so rapidly that the maternity nurse is faced with the task of managing the actual birth of the baby. This is called a **precipitous birth**. The attending nurse has the primary responsibility for providing a physically and psychologically safe experience for the woman and her baby. A woman whose certified nurse-midwife or physician is not present may feel disappointed, frightened, abandoned, angry, and cheated. She may fear what is going to happen and feel that everything is out of her control. In working with the woman, the nurse provides support by keeping her informed about the labor progress and assuring her that the nurse will stay with her.

If birth is imminent, the nurse must not leave the mother alone. The nurse can direct auxiliary personnel to contact the CNM or physician and retrieve the emergency birth pack ("precip pack"), which should be readily accessible to birthing rooms. A typical pack contains the following items:

- A small drape that can be placed under the woman's buttocks to provide a sterile field
- A bulb syringe to clear mucus from the newborn's mouth
- Two sterile clamps (Kelly or Rochester) to clamp the umbilical cord before applying a cord clamp
- Sterile scissors to cut the umbilical cord
- A sterile umbilical cord clamp, either Hesseltine or Hollister
- A baby blanket to wrap the newborn in after birth
- A package of sterile gloves

As the materials are being gathered, the nurse must remain calm; the woman is reassured by the composure of the nurse and feels that the nurse is competent. At all times during the birth, the nurse provides suggestions such as when to maintain a controlled breathing pattern and when to push, supports the woman's efforts, and provides reassurance.

The nurse assists in the precipitous birth as follows: The woman is encouraged to assume a comfortable position. If time permits, the nurse scrubs his or her hands with soap and water and puts on sterile gloves. Sterile drapes are placed under the woman's buttocks. The nurse may place an index finger inside the lower portion of the vagina and the thumb on the outer portion of the perineum and gently massage the area to help stretch perineal tissues and prevent perineal lacerations. This procedure is called "ironing the perineum."

When the infant's head crowns, the nurse instructs the woman to pant, which decreases her urge to push. The nurse checks whether the amniotic sac is intact. If it is, the nurse tears the sac so the newborn will not breathe in amniotic fluid with the first breath.

With one hand the nurse applies gentle pressure against the fetal head to prevent it from popping out rapidly. The nurse does not hold the head back forcibly. Rapid birth of the head may result in tears in the woman's perineal tissues. The rapid change in pressure within the fetal head may cause subdural or dural tears. The nurse supports the perineum with the other hand and allows the head to be born between contractions.

As the woman continues to pant, the nurse inserts one or two fingers along the back of the fetal head to check for the umbilical cord. If there is a nuchal cord (umbilical cord around the neck), the nurse bends his or her fingers like a fish hook, grasps the cord, and pulls it over the baby's head. It is important to check that the cord is not wrapped around the neck more than one time. If the cord is tightly looped and cannot be slipped over the baby's head, two clamps are placed on the cord, the cord is cut between the clamps, and the cord is unwound.

Immediately after birth of the head, the nurse suctions the baby's mouth, throat, and nasal passages. The nurse then places one hand on each side of the head and exerts gentle downward traction until the anterior shoulder passes under the symphysis pubis. Then gentle upward traction aids the birth of the posterior shoulder. The nurse then instructs the woman to push gently so that the rest of the body can be born quickly. The newborn must be supported as he or she emerges.

The newborn is held at the level of the uterus to facilitate blood flow through the umbilical cord. The combination of amniotic fluid and vernix makes the newborn very slippery, so the nurse must be careful to avoid dropping the baby. The nose and mouth of the newborn are suctioned again, using a bulb syringe. The nurse then dries the newborn to prevent heat loss. As soon as the nurse determines that the newborn's respirations are adequate, the infant can be placed on the mother's abdomen. The newborn's head should be slightly lower than the body to aid drainage of fluid and mucus. The weight of the newborn on the mother's abdomen stimulates uterine contractions, which aid in placental separation. The umbilical cord should not be pulled. The nurse is alert for signs of placental separation (slight gush of dark blood from the vagina, lengthening of the cord, or a change in uterine shape from discoid to globular). When these signs are present, the nurse tells the mother to push so that the placenta can be delivered. The nurse inspects the placenta to determine whether it is intact.

The nurse checks the firmness of the uterus. The fundus may be gently massaged to stimulate contractions and decrease bleeding. Putting the newborn to breast also stimulates uterine contractions through release of oxytocin from the pituitary gland.

The umbilical cord may now be cut. The nurse places two sterile Kelly clamps approximately 1 to 3 inches from the newborn's abdomen. The cord is cut between the Kelly clamps with sterile scissors. The nurse places a sterile umbilical cord clamp adjacent to the clamp on the newborn's cord, between the clamp and the newborn's abdomen. The clamp must not be placed snugly against the abdomen, because the cord will dry and shrink.

The nurse cleanses the area under the mother's buttocks and inspects her perineum for lacerations. Bleeding from lacerations may be controlled by pressing a clean perineal pad against the perineum and instructing the woman to keep her thighs together.

If the CNM or physician's arrival is delayed or if the newborn is having respiratory distress, the newborn should be transported immediately to the nursery. The newborn must be properly identified before he or she leaves the birth area. The nurse notes and places on a birth record the following information:

- Position of fetus at birth
- Presence of cord around neck or shoulder (nuchal cord)
- Time of birth
- Apgar scores at 1 and 5 minutes after birth
- Gender of newborn
- Time of expulsion of placenta
- Method of placental expulsion
- Appearance and intactness of placenta
- Mother's condition

- Any medications given to mother or newborn (per agency protocol)

EVALUATION

Evaluation determines the effectiveness of nursing care. As a result of comprehensive nursing care during the intrapartal period, the following outcomes may be anticipated:

- The mother's physical and psychologic well-being has been maintained and supported.
- The baby's physical and psychologic well-being has been protected and supported.
- The couple have had input into the birth process and have participated as much as they desired.
- The mother and her baby have had a safe birth.

Critical Concept Review

LEARNING OBJECTIVES

CONCEPTS

Identify the database to be created from information obtained when a woman is admitted to the birthing area.	Information obtained during admission is used to develop a clinical pathway for the four stages of labor: 1. Prenatal information. 2. Current assessments. 3. Expected teaching. 4. Nursing care expected for each stage. 5. Expected activity level. 6. Proposed comfort measures. 7. Elimination and nutritional needs. 8. Level of family involvement.
Review the nursing care provided at admission.	The nursing care at admission focuses on providing an orientation to the unit and obtaining an overall physical assessment of the mother that focuses on the well-being of the mother and fetus: 1. Assess the maternal vital signs and FHR. 2. Perform a vaginal exam to determine stage of cervical dilatation and state of membranes. 3. Determine frequency and intensity of contractions. 4. Review systems such as respiratory and neurological. 5. Assess any recent symptoms experienced by the woman. 6. Assess the woman's understanding of the labor process and identification of the woman's support system.
Discuss nursing interventions to meet the psychologic, social, physiologic, and spiritual needs of the woman during each stage of labor.	First stage of labor: 1. Establish rapport with the woman and support person. 2. Discuss expectations of labor and birth. 3. Provide for privacy. 4. Discuss individual expression of pain and discomfort.

(continued)

LEARNING OBJECTIVES	CONCEPTS

Discuss nursing interventions to meet the psychologic, social, physiologic, and spiritual needs of the woman during each stage of labor.—continued

Second stage of labor:
1. Provide as much privacy as possible.
2. Encourage the woman and support person to decide who should be present at the birth.
3. Provide praise and encouragement of progress.

Third and fourth stages of labor:
1. Encourage the woman and support person to hold and look at infant as much as possible.
2. Teach the woman the care to be performed after the baby is born.
3. Provide the woman with food and fluids as allowed.

Compare methods of promoting comfort during the first and second stages of labor.

Comfort measures common to the first and second stages of labor include:
1. Assist the woman to reduce anxiety.
2. Teach the woman about what to expect during the labor experience.
3. Promote relaxation techniques.
4. Instruct in appropriate controlled breathing pattern.
5. Give instruction to the woman's support person.

Comfort measures specific to the first stage of labor:
1. Administer pharmacologic agents as ordered by the physician or certified nurse-midwife.
2. Assist with the placement of an epidural for pain control.

Comfort measures specific to the second stage of labor:
1. Help the woman find an effective pushing pattern.
2. Support the woman's attempt to rest between pushes.

Summarize the immediate needs of the newborn following birth.

Immediate care of the newborn includes:
1. Maintain respiration.
2. Promote warmth.
3. Prevent infection.
4. Provide accurate identification.

Discuss the unique needs of the adolescent during birth.

The adolescent is unique in that she has developmental needs as well as physical needs that must be addressed.

Delineate management of a precipitous birth.

1. A precipitous birth is one that occurs rapidly without a physician or certified nurse-midwife in attendance.
2. The nurse attends to the woman, guides the infant's passage through the birth canal, clamps the umbilical cord, and immediately transports the infant to the nursery for care.
3. The nurse focuses care on the woman and the expulsion of the placenta and contraction of the uterus.

CRITICAL THINKING IN ACTION

View the **Critical Thinking in Action** video in Chapter 19 of the CD-ROM. Then, answer the questions that follow.

Anita Grey, a 22-year-old primigravida at 40 weeks' gestation, is admitted by you to the birthing center in labor. Anita was sent from her physician's office after being evaluated at her prenatal visit. While in the office, she was assessed to be 4 cm dilated, 100% effaced, vertex at 0 station with bulging membranes. She tells you that her husband is on his way to the birthing center and that she is anxious for him to arrive. A review of her prenatal record shows no complications affecting this pregnancy. Anita's vital signs are within normal limits. You assess the fetal heart rate and contraction pattern with the fetal monitor and observe a fetal heart rate of 140 to 150 bpm with accelerations to 160s. Contractions are every 3 to 4 minutes × 30 seconds of moderate intensity by palpation. Anita seems to be tolerating the contractions well, but still seems anxious about her husband's arrival.

1. What steps can you take to reduce the stress and anxiety of the laboring woman and her family?
2. When you notify the physician/midwife, what pertinent information should the report contain?
3. What support measures can you give in the active phase of labor?
4. What measures can be used to decrease discomfort/pain as labor progresses?
5. What observations reflect the physiologic manifestations of pain?

MEDIALINK www.prenhall.com/london

- NCLEX-RN® Review, case studies, and other interactive resources for this chapter can be found on the Companion Website at http://www.prenhall.com/london. Click on "Chapter 19" to select the activities for this chapter.

- For animations, more NCLEX-RN® Review questions, and an audio glossary, access the accompanying CD-ROM in this textbook.

REFERENCES

American Academy of Pediatrics & American College of Obstetricians and Gynecologists. (2002). *Guidelines for perinatal care* (5th ed.). Washington, DC: Author.

American College of Obstetricians and Gynecologists. (2002). *Obstetric analgesia and anesthesia* (ACOG Practice Bulletin No. 36). Washington, DC: Author.

Association of Women's Health, Obstetric and Neonatal Nurses (AWHONN). (2003a). *Fetal heart rate monitoring: Principles and practice* (3rd ed.). Dubuque, IA: Kendall Hunt.

Association of Women's Health, Obstetric and Neonatal Nurses (AWHONN) (2003b). *Standards for professional nursing practice in the care of women and newborns* (6th ed.). Washington, DC: Author.

Benfield, R. D. (2002). Hydrotherapy in labor. *Journal of Nursing Scholarship, 34*(4), 347–352.

Bottorff, J. (1993). The use and meaning of touch in caring for patients with cancer. *Oncology Nursing Forum, 20*, 531–538.

Centers for Disease Control and Prevention (CDC). (2003, April 18). Advancing HIV prevention: New strategies for a changing epidemic, United States, 2003. *Morbidity and Mortality Weekly Report, 52*(15), 329–332.

Cluett, E. R., Nikodem, V. C., McCandlish, R. E., & Burns, E. E. (2004). Immersion in water in pregnancy, labour and birth. *Cochrane Database of Systematic Reviews, 2*, CD000111.

Kim, S. W., Nam, S. W., Lee, S. K., Kim, K. S., & Kim, J. K. (1999). The effects of electrostimulation on acupuncture loci upon duration of labor in primipara. *Kyunghee Medicine, 15*(2), 198–202.

Pinette, M. G., Wax, J., & Wilson, E. (2004). The risks of underwater birth. *American Journal of Obstetrics and Gynecology, 190*(5), 1211–1215.

Putnam, F. W. (2003). Ten-year research update review: Child sexual abuse. *Journal of the American Academy of Child and Adolescent Psychiatry, 42*(3), 269–278.

Rennisson, C. M. (2002). *Rape and sexual assault: Reporting to police and medical personnel, 1992–2000.* Washington, DC: Department of Justice.

Roberts, J. (2002). The "push" for evidence: Management of the second stage. *Journal of Midwifery and Women's Health, 47*(1), 2–15.

Soet, J. E., Brack, G. A., & Dilorio, C. (2003). Prevalence and predictors of women's experience of psychological trauma during childbirth. *Birth, 30*(1), 36–46.

St. Hill, P. F., Lipson, J. G., Ibrahim, A., & Meleis, A. F. (2003). *Caring for women cross-culturally.* Philadelphia: F. A. Davis.

Snyder, M., & Nojima, Y. (1998). Purposeful touch. In M. Snyder and R. Lindquist, *Complementary/alternative therapies in nursery* (3rd ed., pp. 149–158). New York: Springs Publishing.

Wilson, B. A., Shannon, M. T., & Stang, C. L. (2006). *Nurse's drug guide: 2006.* Upper Saddle River, NJ: Prentice Hall.

Pharmacologic Pain Relief

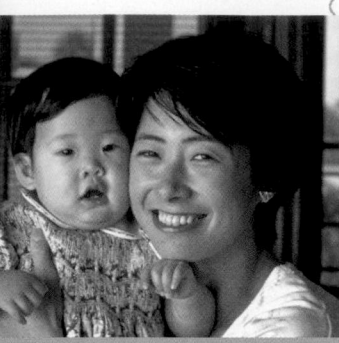

We had attended our classes and practiced through the last few weeks, but I was not ready for the amount of discomfort that I felt during my labor. I've always been able to handle pain much better, but this pain was very different. I had hoped to go through all of labor and birth without medications, but we had talked about it and I knew that if I felt I needed something, it would be all right. My nurse was also helpful and supportive of my decision. She helped me feel that I was making a good decision and that I wasn't failing somehow.

—*Kyung-aie, 36*

LEARNING OBJECTIVES

- Describe the use of systemic drugs to promote pain relief during labor.

- Compare the major types of regional analgesia and anesthesia, including area affected, advantages, disadvantages, techniques, and nursing implications.

- Discuss the possible complications of regional anesthesia.

- Describe the nursing care related to general anesthesia.

- Delineate the major complications of general anesthesia.

MEDIALINK

www.prenhall.com/london

CD-ROM

NCLEX-RN® Review
Video: Epidural Placement
Audio Glossary

Companion Website

NCLEX-RN® Review
MediaLink Applications:
　　Case Study: Pain Relief Therapies during Birth
　　Care Plan Activity: Client with an Epidural
Thinking Critically
Complementary Care: Acupressure Information

Childbearing women experience varying levels of pain and other demanding sensations during labor and birth. As discussed in Chapter 19, ∞ nursing interventions directed toward pain relief begin with psychologic measures such as providing information, support, and encouragement. Measures to promote physical comfort include back rubs, showers, ambulation, whirlpools (Jacuzzi), and the application of cool cloths. Some laboring women need no further interventions.

For other women the progression of labor brings increasing pain that interferes with their ability to cope. These women may elect to use pharmacologic agents such as systemic drugs, regional nerve blocks (epidural, spinal, or combined epidural-spinal), and local anesthetic blocks (pudendal and perianal) to decrease discomfort, increase relaxation, and reestablish their ability to participate more effectively in the labor and birth experience. The methods are not all mutually exclusive, and any of them may be used in combination with other nonpharmacologic comfort measures.

There is a good deal of peer pressure on expectant parents to have the "ideal" birth experience. They may plan a natural childbirth, and the need for analgesia may make them feel inadequate and guilty. The nurse has a special role in helping a woman and her partner to accept alterations in the original plan and to recognize the unique qualities of their birth experience. Reassurance that accepting analgesia for discomfort is not a failure can help maintain the woman's self-esteem. The emphasis should be on achieving a healthy, satisfying outcome for the family.

SYSTEMIC DRUGS

The goal of pharmacologic analgesia during labor is to provide maximum pain relief at minimum risk for the mother and fetus. To reach this goal, clinicians must consider a number of factors, including the following:

All systemic drugs used for pain relief during labor cross the placental barrier by simple diffusion, but some drugs cross more readily than others.

Drug action in the body depends on the rate at which the substance is metabolized by liver enzymes and excreted by the kidneys.

High drug doses may remain in the fetus for long periods because fetal liver enzymes and kidney excretion are inadequate for metabolizing analgesic agents.

COMPLEMENTARY CARE

LABOR DOULAS

Labor doulas are sometimes hired by women who want to avoid pharmacologic pain relief methods during labor and birth. The role of the doula is to provide continuous labor support and to be an advocate for the woman and her family. A doula often meets the woman at her home during labor prior to admission to the hospital setting. A doula specializes in assisting the woman to maintain comfort and control throughout the labor and birth.

DEVELOPING CULTURAL COMPETENCE

CULTURAL INFLUENCE ON RESPONSES TO PAIN

A woman's cultural background may influence her responses to pain. Following are generalizations of how some cultures perceive pain and pain responses:

- Mexican-American women may moan rhythmically and massage their thighs and abdomen when in pain.
- Haitian women may prefer massage, movement, and position changes to increase comfort.
- Filipino women may lie quietly because they believe that noise and activity increase labor pain.
- Black, Puerto Rican, and Middle Eastern women are often verbally expressive of pain.
- Native American women may be viewed as stoic, using meditation, self-control, and traditional herbs.
- Thai women's silent but restless behavior can reflect high levels of pain.
- Japanese, Chinese, Vietnamese, Laotian, and other women of Asian descent may feel that crying out during labor is shameful.
- Samoan women may believe no verbal response is allowed.

NURSING CARE MANAGEMENT

Analgesic drugs provide pain relief for the laboring woman but also affect the fetus and the labor process. Pain medication given too early may prolong labor and depress the fetus; if given too late, it is of minimal use to the woman and may lead to respiratory depression in the newborn. The nurse assesses the mother and fetus and also evaluates the contraction pattern before administering prescribed systemic medications.

Maternal assessment parameters include the following:

- The woman is willing to receive medication after being advised about it.
- Vital signs are stable.
- Contraindications (such as specific drug allergy, respiratory compromise, or current drug dependence) are not present.

Fetal assessment parameters include the following:

- The fetal heart rate (FHR) baseline is between 110 and 160 beats per minute, and no late decelerations or nonreassuring FHR patterns are present.
- Short-term and long-term variability are present.
- The fetus exhibits normal movement, and accelerations are present with fetal movement.
- The fetus is at term.

Assessment of labor includes the following:

- Contraction pattern is well established.
- The cervix is dilating.
- There is progressive descent of the fetal presenting part.

If normal parameters are absent, the nurse may need to complete further assessments with the physician or certified nurse-midwife (CNM).

Before administering the medication, the nurse once again ascertains whether the woman has a history of any drug reactions or allergies and provides information about the medication (see Table 20–1). After giving the medication, the nurse records the drug name, dose, route, and site, and the woman's blood pressure (BP) and pulse, on the FHR monitor strip and on the woman's records. If the woman is alone, side rails should be raised to provide safety. The nurse assesses the FHR for possible adverse effects of the medication.

When an analgesic medication is administered by intramuscular or subcutaneous route, it takes a few minutes for the effect to be felt. The nurse can continue with other supportive measures to enhance comfort, such as ensuring a quiet environment, providing a back rub or cool cloth, assisting with relaxation and visualization exercises, or providing therapeutic touch until the woman feels the effect of the medication. Often, continued reassurance and verbal praise have a calming effect. When the medication begins to take effect, the woman may sleep between contractions. This short period of rest helps her relax and can restore her energy. When an intravenous route is ordered by the physician or CNM, the effect of the drug will be felt within a few minutes, so if any change of position is necessary or if the woman needs to void, the nurse may suggest that these activities be completed before the drug administration. Some women may be so uncomfortable that they do not want anything except the medication. In this case, administering the medication first would be more helpful for the woman.

TABLE 20–1 ✣ What Women Need to Know about Pain Relief Medications

Before receiving medications, the woman should understand the following:

- Type of medication administered
- Route of administration
- Expected effects of medication
- Potential adverse maternal effects
- Implications for fetus or newborn
- Safety measures needed (e.g., remain in bed with side rails up)

NARCOTIC ANALGESICS

Narcotic analgesic agents that are injected into the circulation have their primary action at sites in the brain, activating the neurons to the spinal cord.

Butorphanol Tartrate (Stadol)

Butorphanol tartrate (Stadol) is a synthetic agonist-antagonist narcotic analgesic agent that can be given by the intramuscular (IM) or intravenous (IV) route. Its onset of action is rapid after IV injection, peak analgesia occurs in 30 to 60 minutes, and the duration is from 3 to 4 hours (Wilson, Shannon, & Stang, 2005). The recommended initial dose is 2 mg administered IM every 3 to 4 hours. If it is given IV, the dosage is reduced. Respiratory depression of both the mother and the fetus or newborn can occur. The effects of butorphanol can be reversed with naloxone (Narcan). Butorphanol should not be used for women with a known opiate dependency and should be used with caution if drug dependence is suspected because it may precipitate withdrawal (Wilson et al., 2005).

Urinary retention following administration of butorphanol is not common but does occur. Therefore, the nurse should be alert for bladder distention when a woman has received butorphanol for analgesia during labor, has IV fluids infusing, and receives regional anesthesia for the birth. Butorphanol needs to be protected from light and stored at room temperature (Wilson et al., 2005).

Nalbuphine Hydrochloride (Nubain)

Like butorphanol, nalbuphine hydrochloride (Nubain) is a synthetic agonist-antagonist narcotic analgesic and may precipitate drug withdrawal if the woman is physically dependent on narcotics. It also crosses the placenta to the fetus and can cause a nonreassuring fetal heart rate and neonatal respiratory depression (Wilson et al., 2005). Nalbuphine may be given by the intramuscular, subcutaneous, or intravenous route. It is most frequently given by the intravenous route in the birth setting. The usual dose for adults is 10 to 20 mg (Wilson et al., 2005). If given intravenously, onset of action occurs in 2 to 3 minutes, peak of action occurs in 15 to 20 minutes, and duration is 3 to 6 hours. When given by the IV route, nalbuphine may be given directly into the tubing of a running IV infusion; 10 mg should be administered over 3 to 5 minutes (Wilson et al., 2005). Adverse effects in the woman include respiratory depression, drowsiness, dizziness, crying, blurred vision, nausea, diaphoresis, and urinary urgency (Wilson et al., 2005). See "Drug Guide: Nalbuphine Hydrochloride (Nubain)."

ANALGESIC POTENTIATORS

The use of **analgesic potentiators**, also known as *ataractics*, can decrease anxiety and increase the effectiveness of analgesics when given simultaneously. These drugs, which are classified as tranquilizers, have no specific properties that decrease pain; however, they do work

---

DRUG GUIDE

NALBUPHINE HYDROCHLORIDE (NUBAIN)

Overview of Action

Nubain is a synthetic narcotic analgesic with agonist and weak antagonist properties. Analgesic properties are equal to that produced by morphine. Nubain's potency is 3 to 4 times greater than pentazocine. The incidence of respiratory depression that occurs is equivalent to morphine.

Dosage Route

Nubain is indicated for moderate to severe pain. Adults: 10-20 mg every 3-6 hours prn subcutaneous IM/IV.

Maternal Contraindications

Hypersensitivity or allergy to nalbuphine hydrochloride.

Maternal Side Effects

Sedation; clammy, sweaty skin; dry mouth; bitter taste in mouth; nausea and vomiting; dizziness; vertigo; nervousness; restlessness; depression; crying; euphoria; dysphoria; confusion; hallucinations; unusual dreams; distortion of body image; numbness; tingling sensations; headache; miosis; hypertension; hypotension; bradycardia; tachycardia; flushing; abdominal cramps; dyspnea; asthma; speech difficulty; and urinary urgency.

Nursing Considerations

Assess client's sensitivity to narcotics on admission.

Inform woman of potential side effects.

Monitor and evaluate analgesic effect. Ask client about comfort level and notify anesthesiologist of inadequate pain relief.

Observe for symptoms of hypersensitivity: pruritus, urticaria, or burning sensation.

May produce an allergic response in clients with sulfite sensitivity.

If allergic reaction (urticaria, edema, or respiratory difficulties) occurs, administer naloxone or diphenhydramine per physician order.

Assess respiratory rate prior to administration. Notify healthcare provider if respirations less than 12 per minute.

Monitor urinary output and assess bladder for distention. Assist client to void.

Assist client with ambulation after administration.

Counsel client that use with alcohol or other central nervous system depressants may increase medication effects.

Prolonged use with abrupt discontinuation can result in symptoms consistent with narcotic withdrawal.

well to potentiate the effects of narcotic analgesics without increasing unwanted side effects. This enhancement enables the woman to receive a smaller dose of the narcotic being administered. These drugs can also be used to manage unpleasant side effects, such as nausea or vomiting, associated with the administration of narcotic analgesics. Commonly used analgesic potentiators include promethazine (Phenergan), hydroxyzine (Vistaril), propiomazine (Largon), promazine (Sparine), and metoclopramide (Reglan). The main side effect associated with these medications is sedation. Sedation may be helpful in promoting rest in women who have had a prolonged labor or who have had little sleep; however, the effect may be undesirable to other women.

OPIATE ANTAGONIST: NALOXONE (NARCAN)

Since naloxone is an antagonist with little or no agonistic effect, it exhibits little pharmacologic activity in the absence of narcotics. Naloxone can be used to reverse the mild respiratory depression that follows administration of small doses of opiates. The drug is useful for respiratory depression caused by fentanyl, morphine, and meperidine, as well as butorphanol tartrate and nalbuphine hydrochloride. Naloxone is the drug of choice when the depressant is unknown because it will cause no further depression (Wilson et al., 2005). An initial dose of 0.4 to 2 mg may be administered to the laboring woman. Naloxone may be given to the newborn if needed after birth (Wilson et al., 2005). (See "Drug Guide: Naloxone Hydrochloride (Narcan)" in Chapter 28. ∞)

When naloxone is given, other resuscitative measures may be indicated, and trained personnel should be readily available. The duration of the drug's effect is shorter than

---

THINKING CRITICALLY

COUNSELING THE WOMAN ON USE OF ANALGESIA

Luisa Silva, a 33-year-old G1P0, is 32 weeks' pregnant. She is trying to decide whether she should accept any analgesia during her labor. She has finished childbirth education classes and wants an unmedicated labor and birth. She says, "I want to do this on my own, but I'm afraid it may be too much. Will it be OK if I need to take something?" What will you tell her?

---

that of the analgesic drug for which it is acting as an antagonist, so the nurse must be alert to the return of respiratory depression and the need for repeated doses. Naloxone should be given with caution in women with known or suspected opiate dependency because it may precipitate severe withdrawal (Wilson et al., 2005).

REGIONAL ANESTHESIA AND ANALGESIA

Regional anesthesia is the temporary loss of sensation produced by injecting an anesthetic agent (called a *local*) into direct contact with nervous tissue. Loss of sensation happens because the local agents stabilize the cell membrane, which prevents initiation and transmission of nerve impulses. The regional anesthetic blocks most commonly used in childbirth include the epidural, spinal, and combined epidural-spinal blocks. Epidural blocks may be used for analgesia during labor and vaginal birth and for anesthesia during cesarean birth.

An epidural relieves pain associated with the first stage of labor by blocking the sensory nerves supplying the uterus. Pain associated with the second stage of labor and with birth can be alleviated with epidural, combined epidural-spinal, and pudendal blocks (Figure 20–1 ●).

Until the last few years, the same anesthetic agents used for regional epidurals were also used to produce **regional analgesia** (pain relief to a body region) during labor. This practice was problematic because the anesthetic agents used alter the transmission of impulses to the bladder, making voiding difficult. The agents also interfere with blood pressure stability and leg movement. The descent of the fetus may be slowed because of the woman's decreased ability to push during the second stage of labor (Fraser, Cayer, Soeder et al., 2002). To address these difficulties, regional analgesia is now obtained by injecting a narcotic such as fentanyl along with only a small amount of local anesthetic agent. Recent studies have determined that the new drug combinations relieve the woman's pain while minimizing the side effects just mentioned (Segal, 2002).

COMPLEMENTARY CARE

ACUPRESSURE FOR LABOR PAIN

Acupressure can lessen pain during the first stage of labor (Chung, Hung, Kuo et al., 2003). The acupressure point for labor and birth is found in the webbing between the thumb and index finger. This point should never be stimulated during pregnancy since it stimulates uterine contractions. The mother places her right thumb on the back of her left hand and her right index finger on the front of the left hand at the acupressure point. She can rub the point to stimulate labor and squeeze the point to decrease labor pain. Another acupressure point is found between the inner ankle bone and the Achilles' tendon. Squeezing for 1 minute on each ankle reduces labor pain. See the Companion Website at http://www.prenhall.com/london for more information on acupressure, including an interview with a labor and delivery nurse on her use of acupressure to relieve labor pain.

EVIDENCE-BASED NURSING

HYDROTHERAPY IN LABOR

Clinical Question

Is hydrotherapy an effective way to manage pain during labor?

Evidence

Thirty-three studies using a variety of research methodologies were reviewed. While the range of study designs and protocols made it difficult to generate definitive recommendations, several important findings were evident. Intervention with hydrotherapy (defined in this review as a bath or whirlpool) was associated with a reduction in pain and anxiety through maternal relaxation, although the exact mechanism of this action was not determined. A trend toward decreased use of analgesia in women undergoing hydrotherapy was noted. Maternal bathing in labor was not associated with adverse neonatal or maternal effects. Neonatal Apgar scores were unaffected by hydrotherapy, and neither maternal nor neonatal infections increased.

Study findings indicated support for using hydrotherapy to manage rapid pain and anxiety in early stages of labor. Effects were seen quickly after instituting hydrotherapy, but were short acting. Most mothers used hydrotherapy for no more than 1 hour. Hydrotherapy was associated with increases in fetal heart rate acceleration and increased fetal movement, both of which are signs of fetal well-being.

In one study, elevated maternal bathing temperatures were associated with an increased need for neonatal resuscitation, although this finding was not confirmed. There may be adverse effects of hydrotherapy for women with prolonged rupture of the membranes. No clear evidence exists that bathing increases cervical dilatation, hastens fetal descent, shortens labor, or decreases operative delivery rates.

Implications

You can support the mother who chooses hydrotherapy for relaxation during early labor without concern that it will cause adverse effects, as long as she has not had prolonged rupture of membranes. The nurse should carefully monitor water temperature. Recommended water temperature is 98.6°F (37°C). Levels of pain should be assessed routinely, as hydrotherapy appears to be a short-acting pain relief measure.

Critical Thinking

What assessments of maternal labor might indicate that hydrotherapy would be an effective intervention? What assessments would you identify as contraindications for its use? What assessments would you carry out during hydrotherapy to avoid any adverse effects?

Reference

Benfield, R. (2002). Hydrotherapy in labor. *Journal of Nursing Scholarship, 34*(4), 347–352.

The intrathecal injection of narcotics results in another type of regional analgesia. In this case the narcotic is injected into the subarachnoid space. Fentanyl citrate and preservative-free morphine are the most commonly used drugs. The woman's pain is usually relieved, but she may experience urinary retention, pruritus, nausea, and vomiting (Mayberry, Clemmens, & De, 2002).

Nursing care during administration of regional analgesia is directed toward helping the woman void prior to the injection, assisting her with positioning during and after the procedure, monitoring and assessing vital signs and respiratory status, monitoring analgesic effect, and determining fetal well-being. Reassurance and thorough explanations help decrease anxiety and fear. Additional measures may be needed to address pruritus, nausea and vomiting, and urinary retention.

As with other procedures, the woman needs to know how the block is given, the expected effect on her and the fetus, advantages and disadvantages, and possible complications. Many women discuss possible anesthetic blocks with their care provider at some point in the pregnancy. If they have not, it is important to give them an opportunity to ask questions and obtain information before receiving the block while in labor.

DEVELOPING CULTURAL COMPETENCE

RUSSIAN CULTURE PAIN RELIEF METHODS

In Russia, pain medication typically is not given to laboring women. While some complementary pain relief methods, such as massage and water therapy, are used, traditional customs are also incorporated. These include tying and untying knots, locking and unlocking doors, and placing the father's clothing under the laboring woman.

ANESTHETIC AGENTS FOR REGIONAL BLOCKS

Local anesthetic agents block the conduction of nerve impulses from the periphery to the central nervous system by preventing the propagation of an action potential from the source of pain (Aveline, El Metaoua, Masmoudi et al., 2002). The types of nerve fibers are differentially sensitive to the various anesthetic agents. In general, the smaller the fiber, the more sensitive it is to local agents. For example, it is possible to block the small C and A delta fibers, which transmit pain and temperature, without blocking the larger A alpha, A beta, and A gamma fibers, which continue to maintain a sense of pressure, muscle tone, position sense, and motor function.

● FIGURE 20-1

Schematic diagram showing pain pathways and sites of interruption. **A,** Lumbar epidural block: the dark area demonstrates peridural (epidural) space and nerves affected, and the gray tube represents a continuous plastic catheter. **B,** Pudendal block: relief of perineal pain. **C,** Lumbar sympathetic (spinal) block: relief of uterine pain only.

Used with permission from Bonica, J. J. (1972). Principles and practice of obstetric analgesia and anesthesia (pp. 492, 512, 521, 614). Philadelphia: Davis.

Absorption of local anesthetics depends primarily on the vascularity of the area of injection. The agents themselves contribute to increased blood flow by causing vasodilation. High concentrations of drugs cause greater vasodilation. Good maternal physical condition or a high metabolic rate aids absorption. Malnutrition, dehydration, electrolyte imbalance, and cardiovascular and pulmonary problems increase the potential for toxic effects. The pH of tissues affects the rate of absorption, which has implications for fetal complications such as acidosis. The addition of vasoconstrictors such as epinephrine delays absorption and prolongs the anesthetic effect. Epinephrine decreases uteroplacental blood flow, making it an undesirable additive in many situations. The breakdown of local anesthetics in the body is accomplished by the liver and plasma esterase, and the resulting substance is eliminated by the kidneys. It is important to use the weakest concentration and the smallest amount necessary to produce the desired results.

TYPES OF LOCAL ANESTHETIC AGENTS

Three types of local anesthetic agents are currently available: esters, amides, and opiates. The ester type includes procaine hydrochloride (Novocain), chloroprocaine hydrochloride (Nesacaine), and tetracaine hydrochloride (Pontocaine). Esters are rapidly metabolized; therefore, toxic maternal levels are not as likely to be reached, and placental transfer to the fetus is prevented.

Amide types include lidocaine hydrochloride (Xylocaine), mepivacaine hydrochloride (Carbocaine), and bupivacaine hydrochloride (Marcaine). Amide types are more powerful and longer acting agents. They readily cross the placenta, can be measured in the fetal circulation, and affect the fetus for a prolonged period.

Opioids are used with epidural blocks for labor. Some of the agents used include morphine, fentanyl, butorphanol, and meperidine. When only opioids are used epidurally, rather than in combination with another type of agent, the amount of pain relief is not as effective, especially toward the end of labor; therefore, a combination of opioids and a low dose of local are given (Bowes & Thorp, 2004).

ADVERSE MATERNAL REACTIONS TO ANESTHETIC AGENTS

Reactions to local anesthetic agents range from mild symptoms to cardiovascular collapse. Mild reactions include palpitations, tinnitus, apprehension, confusion, and a metallic taste in the mouth. Moderate reactions include more severe degrees of mild symptoms plus nausea and vomiting, hypotension, and muscle twitching, which may progress to convulsions. Severe reactions are sudden loss of consciousness, coma, severe hypotension, bradycardia, respiratory depression, and cardiac arrest. Anesthetic agents should not be used unless an IV line is in place.

The preferred treatment for a mild toxic reaction is administration of oxygen and IV injection of a short-acting barbiturate to diminish anxiety.

NEONATAL NEUROBEHAVIORAL EFFECTS OF ANESTHESIA AND ANALGESIA

Many studies have focused on the neurobehavioral effects on the newborn of pharmacologic agents used during labor and birth. Although analgesic and anesthetic agents may alter the behavioral and adaptive function of the newborn, physiologic factors such as hunger, degree of hydration, and time within the sleep-wake cycle may also exert an influence (Fisk, Gitau, Teixeira et al., 2001).

EPIDURAL BLOCK

A lumbar **epidural block** involves injection of an anesthetic agent into the epidural space to provide pain relief throughout labor. The epidural space, a potential space between the dura mater and the ligamentum flavum, is accessed through the lumbar area (Figure 20–2 ●). The epidural is most frequently used as a continuous block to provide analgesia and anesthesia from active labor through episiotomy repair (Figure 20–3 ●).

Epidurals have become a relatively common method of analgesia and anesthesia during labor and birth in the United States. It is estimated that 50% of all women in the United States receive an epidural during their labor (National Institutes of Health [NIH], 2001). An epidural can be given as soon as active labor is established (Hughes, Levinson, Rosen et al., 2002). Some insurance providers have limited women's access to epidural anesthesia; however, the American College of Obstetricians and Gynecologists (ACOG) believes that a woman's request is sufficient justification for providing an epidural (ACOG & ASA, 2000).

Advantages

The epidural block relieves discomfort during labor and birth, and the woman is fully awake and a part of the birth process. The continuous epidural allows different blocking for each stage of labor, so that the fetus is able to descend and rotate in the maternal pelvis; many times the woman's urge to bear down is preserved.

Disadvantages

The most common complication of an epidural block is maternal hypotension, which is generally prevented by administering intravenous fluid prior to epidural placement, left uterine displacement, and maternal positioning on her side. In some instances, labor progress and fetal descent may be slowed, and pushing efforts in the second stage may be less effective due to a decrease in sensation. The average increase in the length of labor is approximately 25

minutes. There does not appear to be an increase in forceps or vacuum use related to epidural anesthesia (Bowes & Thorp, 2004). Delay in return of bladder sensation may result in the need for catheterization during labor and in the fourth stage.

Contraindications

The absolute contraindications for epidural block are client refusal, infection at the site of the needle puncture, maternal problems with blood coagulation (coagulopathies), specific drug allergy to the agent being used, and hypovolemic shock (Hughes et al., 2002).

● **FIGURE 20–2**

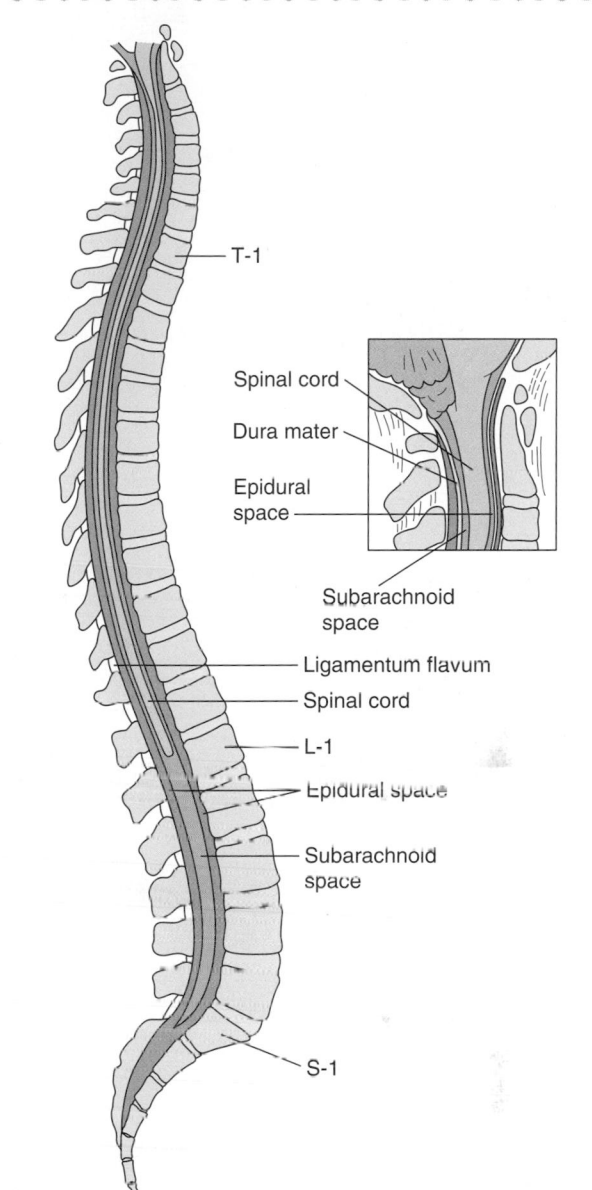

T-1

Spinal cord
Dura mater
Epidural space
Subarachnoid space
Ligamentum flavum
Spinal cord
L-1
Epidural space
Subarachnoid space
S-1

The epidural space is between the dura mater and the ligamentum flavum, extending from the base of the skull to the end of the sacral canal.

FIGURE 20–3

L-4

L-5

S-1

Subarachnoid space
Dura mater
Epidural space
Spinal cord
Ligamentum flavum
Spread of anesthetic solution

A

B   C   D

Technique for lumbar epidural block. **A,** Proper position of insertion. **B,** Needle in the ligamentum flavum. **C,** Tip of needle in epidural space. **D,** Force of injection pushing dura away from tip of needle.

Used with permission from Bonica, J. J. (1972). Principles and practice of obstetric analgesia and anesthesia (p. 631). Philadelphia: Davis.

Nursing Care Management

Assessment of the woman's knowledge level about an epidural block is essential. Before providing information, the nurse determines the woman's current knowledge and evaluates factors related to learning, such as primary language spoken, ability to hear and interpret information, and the presence of anxiety. Although the nurse is an integral person in providing information, the anesthesiologist is the essential person to provide information to obtain written informed consent.

NURSING PRACTICE

Advise the woman to identify when uterine contractions are occurring. Reassure her that the anesthesiologist will administer the injection between contractions when she is comfortable. Provide encouragement and reposition the woman as needed after a contraction occurs, since it is common for the woman to slouch during intense uterine contractions.

In preparation for the epidural, the nurse encourages the woman to empty her bladder, because the block may interfere with her ability to void. The nurse assesses maternal blood pressure, pulse, and respirations and FHR to determine that normal parameters are present and to establish a baseline. Continuous electronic fetal monitoring to assess fetal status and frequent monitoring of maternal blood pressure and pulse for hypotension are essential. An intravenous infusion is usually begun with an 18-gauge plastic indwelling catheter. A large-gauge catheter is used so that IV fluids can be administered quickly if hypotension occurs. A bolus of 500 to 1000 mL of IV fluid is given before beginning the epidural block to decrease the incidence of hypotension.

Either of two positions can be used to achieve epidural placement: side-lying or sitting. If the side-lying position is used, the nurse assists the woman to move to the edge of the bed, where the mattress is firmer and provides more support. The woman's head is supported with a small pillow so it remains in alignment with the spine. A pillow may also be placed in front of her chest to provide support for her upper arm. Her back needs to remain straight, with the shoulders square. Her legs are bent and her knees kept together so that the upper hip does not roll forward and cause the spine to twist.

The block may also be given with the woman in a sitting position, with her back arched and her feet supported on a stool. The nurse typically stands directly in front of the woman with hands placed on the woman's shoulders. The woman is encouraged to arch her back and push back toward the anesthesiologist. After positioning, the nurse continues to provide support and tries to ensure that the woman does not move during the procedure. After the needle and catheter are placed, the woman is assisted into a reclining position.

Maternal vital signs are assessed frequently per protocol until the block wears off. The blood pressure can be monitored by a mechanical blood pressure device or by the nurse directly. The vital signs are recorded on the fetal monitor strip, the client record, or both. The nurse encourages the woman to maintain a side-lying position to maximize uteroplacental blood flow and to change her position (from side to side) frequently to increase circulation, promote comfort, and avoid a one-sided block. The nurse assesses the woman's ability to lift her legs and her level of sensation every 30 minutes to monitor the effects of the nerve block.

NURSING PRACTICE

An important assessment following the administration of regional blocks, such as the epidural, is the location and degree of lost sensation. Landmarks (called dermatomes) can be used to measure and document where these sensory levels begin and end. Some useful tips include the following:

- Use dermatome level charts.
- Use a cool alcohol prep pad to check for areas and levels of sensation.
- Assess dermatome levels approximately every 30 minutes.
- Evaluate the level of anesthesia. The anesthesia level is too high if the patient reports numbness in her chest, face, or tongue or any difficulty breathing. Be alert for statements such as "I feel like I can't take a full breath" or "My tongue feels funny."

The nurse assesses the woman's bladder for distention frequently because the epidural block lessens the urge to urinate. During the second stage of labor, the woman with an epidural block may need assistance with pushing. The nurse may need to tell the woman when contractions begin and give extra assistance by holding her legs during pushing efforts. The woman's legs need to be protected from pressure applied to them while sensation is diminished. If

the woman has little or no control of her legs, stirrups may be needed to avoid injury.

The most common side effect of epidural regional block is hypotension. The risk can be minimized by a preload fluid bolus of crystalloid solution (Bowes & Thorp, 2004). If hypotension occurs the nurse increases the IV flow rate (to increase intravascular volume and raise the blood pressure), ensures or verifies left uterine displacement (to increase circulation), and administers oxygen (to improve oxygenation). If blood pressure is not restored in 1 to 2 minutes, ephedrine, 5 to 10 mg IV, is administered (Hughes et al., 2002). After the ephedrine is administered, the blood pressure is continually monitored and the maternal and fetal responses are recorded.

The epidural may cause elevation of maternal temperature (pyrexia). Pyrexia may be confused with maternal infection and frequently results in additional testing of the newborn to rule out infection (Bowes & Thorp, 2004).

Headache (which may occur with spinal blocks) is not a side effect of epidural anesthesia because the dura mater of the spinal canal has not been penetrated and there is no leakage of spinal fluid. Therefore, lying flat for a prescribed number of hours after birth is not necessary. Motor control of the legs is weak but not totally absent after birth. Return of complete sensation and the ability to control the legs are essential before ambulation is attempted. Recovery may take several hours, depending on the anesthetic agent and the dose given.

To assess sensation the nurse touches various parts of the woman's legs and abdomen bilaterally to determine if the touch can be felt. The nurse can evaluate motor control by asking the woman to raise her knees, to lift her feet (one at a time) off the bed, or to dorsiflex her foot. Even though assessments may indicate that sensation and motor control have returned, the nurse needs to be ready to support the woman's weight as she stands and quickly return her to bed if motor control is inadequate. In addition, blood pressure assessments help the nurse determine the safety of ambulation. The nurse assesses blood pressure while the woman is lying down, then sitting in the bed. As long as blood pressure values remain stable (no evidence of orthostatic hypotension), a standing blood pressure is assessed. It is advisable to have additional assistance when the woman stands for the first time, to maintain safety.

CONTINUOUS EPIDURAL INFUSION

Epidural anesthesia may be given with a continuous infusion pump. Some of the benefits include good to excellent analgesia, infrequent nausea, minimal sedation, decreased anxiety, earlier mobilization, retained cough reflex, decreased risk of deep vein thrombosis, decreased myocardial oxygen demand, and ease of administration.

Obviously, ease of administration does not imply lack of need for close observation. Malfunctioning equipment with subsequent overdose is always a possibility. Fortunately,

MediaLink Care Plan Activity: Client with an Epidural

infusion pumps designed specifically for use in epidural anesthesia have safety factors incorporated. Continuous epidural infusions should be administered with the same precautions used for intermittent injections.

Some of the potential problems of epidural infusions include breakthrough pain, sedation, nausea and vomiting, pruritus, and hypotension. Breakthrough pain may occur at any time during the epidural infusion but usually occurs when the infusion rate of the agent is below the recommended therapeutic rate. It may also occur when the infusion pump rate is altered or the integrity of the epidural line is broken. When breakthrough pain occurs, the nurse checks the integrity of the epidural infusion line and notifies the anesthesiologist or nurse anesthetist. There may be standing orders for treatment of breakthrough pain, but it is best to inform the anesthesiologist of any problems that occur. Often, breakthrough pain can be corrected with a bolus dose of medication. In rare circumstances the epidural itself may need to be replaced.

General sedation and resulting respiratory depression may occur from the systemic effect of the epidural agents as they are absorbed into the circulation. The respiratory rate, along with the quality of respirations, should be assessed no less frequently than every 15 to 30 minutes. The nurse should notify the anesthetist of any significant decreases in respiratory rate or respiratory pattern change. If respiratory rate decreases below 14 respirations per minute, naloxone may be given to counteract the effect of the anesthetic agent; typically respirations then return to a normal rate.

Nausea and vomiting can occur at any time during or after epidural infusion. The nurse should give an antiemetic if one is ordered and notify the anesthesiologist. The nausea and vomiting can make the woman very uncomfortable, and the infusion rate of the epidural may need to be decreased or terminated to alleviate this discomfort. Nausea and vomiting can sometimes occur as a result of transition rather than a direct side effect of the epidural infusion.

Pruritus (itching and rash) may occur at any time during the epidural infusion. It usually appears first on the face, neck, or torso and is usually the result of the agent in the epidural infusion. Treatment generally involves administration of diphenhydramine hydrochloride (Benadryl). If no standing order exists, the nurse notifies the anesthetist and identifies the problem. The epidural infusion may need to be decreased or terminated.

Hypotension may occur from hypovolemia or from the effect of the epidural. Treatment involves administering oxygen by mask, administering a bolus of crystalloid fluid, and notifying the anesthetist. Standing orders for treatment of hypotension are usually graded in terms of the degree of hypotension. The epidural infusion may have to be terminated and the woman placed in the Trendelenburg position.

EPIDURAL NARCOTIC ANALGESIA AFTER BIRTH

To provide analgesia for approximately 24 hours after the birth, the anesthesiologist may inject an opioid, such as morphine sulfate (Duramorph), into the epidural space immediately after the birth. The analgesic effect begins approximately 30 to 60 minutes after the injection. The side effects include pruritus, nausea and vomiting, and urinary retention. The onset seems to occur early, and it resolves within 14 to 16 hours after the birth. (See "Drug Guide: Postpartum Epidural Morphine" in Chapter 30. ∞)

SPINAL BLOCK

In a **spinal block**, a local anesthetic agent is injected directly into the spinal fluid in the spinal canal to provide anesthesia for cesarean birth and occasionally for vaginal birth. The technique of administration varies depending on whether the spinal block is being given for a cesarean or vaginal birth (Figure 20–4 ●).

Advantages

The advantages of spinal block are immediate onset of anesthesia, relative ease of administration, a need for smaller drug volume, and maternal compartmentalization of the drug.

Disadvantages

The primary disadvantage of spinal block is blockade of sympathetic nerve fibers, resulting in a high incidence of hypotension; maternal hypotension may lead to alterations in the fetal heart rate and fetal hypoxia. In addition uterine tone is maintained, which makes intrauterine manipulation difficult.

Contraindications

Contraindications for spinal block include severe hypovolemia (regardless of the cause), central nervous system disease, infection over the puncture site, allergy to local anesthetic agents, coagulation problems, and client refusal.

Nursing Care Management

If an intravenous infusion is not already in place, it is started with a 16- to 18-gauge plastic catheter, and a bolus of 500 to 1000 mL is infused rapidly. The nurse assesses maternal vital signs and the FHR to establish a baseline and then positions the woman in a sitting position (or a side-lying position). The woman sits on the side of the bed or operating room table and places her feet on a stool. The woman places her arms between her knees or up around the nurse's shoulders, places her head to her chest, and arches her back to widen the intervertebral spaces. The nurse supports the woman in this position and palpates the uterus to identify the beginning of uterine contractions (if

FIGURE 20–4

Level of anesthesia for cesarean birth

Level of anesthesia for vaginal birth

Levels of spinal anesthesia for vaginal and cesarean births.

Reprinted with permission from Ross Laboratories, Columbus, OH. From Clinical Education Aid No. 17.

labor is present). The physician injects the anesthetic agent between contractions. If the anesthetic agent is injected during a contraction, the level of anesthesia obtained is higher and may compromise respirations.

The woman remains in a sitting position for 30 seconds and then returns to a lying position, with a rolled towel or blanket under her right hip to displace the uterus from the vena cava. The nurse monitors maternal blood pressure and pulse frequently per protocol or physician's order. The blood pressure is also reassessed when the woman is moved after birth, because movement may lower blood pressure.

If the spinal block is being used during vaginal birth, the nurse monitors uterine contractions and instructs the woman to bear down during a contraction. The block may reduce the woman's ability to push, although the new combinations of medications tend to decrease this side effect. Sometimes the birth may be assisted with forceps or vacuum extractor (see Chapter 22 ∞).

After birth the temporary motor paralysis of the woman's legs continues. The nurse needs to exercise caution when moving the woman from the birthing bed (or operating room table) to protect her from injury. The woman remains in bed for 6 to 12 hours following the block; she may not regain sensation and control of her bladder for 8 to 12 hours and may need to be catheterized. An indwelling bladder catheter is usually inserted before surgery for women undergoing cesarean birth.

COMBINED SPINAL-EPIDURAL BLOCK

Spinal anesthesia may be combined with an epidural block. The combined spinal-epidural (CSE) block can be used for labor analgesia and for cesarean birth. The anesthetic and analgesic agents used differ according to the purpose of the CSE block. A CSE is accomplished by inserting an epidural needle into the epidural space. A narrow-gauge atraumatic (24- to 27-gauge pencil point) needle is inserted through the epidural needle, through the dura, and into the cerebral spinal fluid. A small amount of local anesthetic agent, opioid, or both is injected, and the atraumatic needle is withdrawn. An epidural catheter is then threaded through the epidural needle and into the epidural space. The epidural needle is removed, and the epidural catheter is secured.

An advantage of CSE block is that the spinal (intrathecal) anesthetic or analgesic agent has a faster onset than medications that are injected into the epidural space. Most drugs are used in low dose, so spinal analgesia may be given in early labor to assist in alleviating labor pain. The epidural is activated when active labor begins (Hughes et al., 2002). Another advantage of a CSE block is that laboring women can ambulate after the CSE is placed.

NURSING PRACTICE

Advise women with a CSE in place always to have assistance during ambulation to prevent falls.

PUDENDAL BLOCK

A **pudendal block**, administered by a transvaginal method, intercepts signals to the pudendal nerve (Figure 20–5 ●). The pudendal block provides perineal anesthesia for the latter part of the first stage of labor, the second stage, birth, and episiotomy repair. The pudendal block relieves the pain of perineal distention and typically relieves pain in the

● FIGURE 20–5

A, Pudendal block by the transvaginal approach. **B,** Area of perineum affected by pudendal block.

● FIGURE 20–6

Technique of local infiltration for episiotomy and repair.

Used with permission from Bonica, J. J. (1972). Principles and practice of obstetric analgesia and anesthesia (p. 505). Philadelphia: Davis.

lower vagina, vulva, and perineum but not the discomfort of uterine contractions (Bowes & Thorp, 2004).

Advantages of the pudendal block are ease of administration and absence of maternal hypotension. It also may be used to decrease the discomfort of low forceps or vacuum-assisted birth. Because a pudendal block does not alter maternal vital signs or FHR, additional assessments are not necessary. The nurse explains the procedure and answers any questions.

The disadvantages of the pudendal block include possible broad ligament hematoma, perforation of the rectum, and trauma to the sciatic nerve. A moderate dose of anesthetic agent has minimal ill effects on the course of labor, but the urge to push may decrease.

LOCAL INFILTRATION ANESTHESIA

Local infiltration anesthesia is accomplished by injecting an anesthetic agent into the intracutaneous, subcutaneous, and intramuscular areas of the perineum (Figure 20–6 ●). It is generally used at the time of birth, both in preparation for an episiotomy if one is needed and for the episiotomy

repair. Women who have followed some type of prepared childbirth method and want minimal analgesia and anesthesia usually do not object to local anesthesia for the episiotomy or laceration repair. The administration procedure is technically uncomplicated and is practically free from complications.

A disadvantage of local infiltration is that large amounts of local anesthetic must be used to infuse the tissues. Although any local anesthetic may be used, chloroprocaine hydrochloride (Nesacaine), lidocaine hydrochloride (Xylocaine), and mepivacaine hydrochloride (Carbocaine) are the agents of choice because of their capacity for diffusion. Because local anesthetic agents have no effect on maternal vital signs or FHR, additional assessments are unnecessary.

GENERAL ANESTHESIA

Occasionally, **general anesthesia** (induced unconsciousness) may be needed for cesarean birth and for surgical intervention with some complications. The method used to achieve general anesthesia is usually a combination of IV injection and inhalation of anesthetic agents.

NURSING PRACTICE

Some women may wake from general anesthesia with an awareness of events that occurred during a cesarean birth. A small number of women experience unpleasant thoughts or nightmares as a result. If a woman expresses anxiety or states she has unpleasant memories of the birth, the nurse should encourage her to discuss her feelings and the experiences she remembers. The anesthesiologist and physician should be notified so they can establish a therapeutic dialogue with the woman. Some women may have to be referred for counseling to prevent or treat post-traumatic stress disorder.

COMPLICATIONS OF GENERAL ANESTHESIA

A primary danger of general anesthesia is fetal depression. Most general anesthetic agents reach the fetus in about 2 minutes. The depression in the fetus is directly proportional to the depth and duration of the anesthesia. The poor fetal metabolism of general anesthetic agents is similar to that of analgesic agents administered during labor. General anesthesia is not advocated when the fetus is considered to be at high risk, particularly in preterm birth. Infants whose mothers receive general anesthesia suffer more respiratory depression than those whose mothers have received epidural anesthesia (Hughes et al., 2002).

The majority of general anesthetic agents cause some degree of uterine relaxation. They may also cause vomiting and aspiration. Since pregnancy results in decreased gastric motility, and the onset of labor halts the process almost entirely, food eaten hours earlier may remain undigested in the stomach. The nurse must find out when the laboring woman last ate and record this information on the client's chart and on her anesthesia record. Even when food and fluids have been withheld, the gastric juice produced during fasting is highly acidic and can cause chemical pneumonitis if aspirated.

NURSING CARE MANAGEMENT

Prophylactic antacid therapy to reduce the acidic content of the stomach before general anesthesia is common practice. A nonparticulate antacid (such as Bicitra) is often used. Cimetidine (Tagamet) has also been suggested by some anesthesiologists.

Before induction of anesthesia, the nurse places a wedge under the woman's right hip to displace the uterus and prevent vena caval compression in the supine position. The woman should also be preoxygenated with 3 to 5 minutes of 100% oxygen. Intravenous fluids are started so that access to the intravascular system is immediately available.

During the process of rapid induction of anesthesia, the nurse applies cricoid pressure to occlude the esophagus and prevent possible aspiration; the esophagus is occluded by depressing the cricoid cartilage 2 to 3 cm posteriorly. Cricoid pressure is maintained until the anesthesiologist has placed the endotracheal tube and indicates that the pressure can be released. Figure 20–7 ● shows the appropriate technique.

It should be noted that this discussion of obstetric analgesia and anesthesia applies only to a healthy woman and fetus. Pain relief during labor and birth for women with high-risk conditions, such as preterm labor, preeclampsia, blood disorders, or diabetes mellitus, requires skilled decision making, close observation, and awareness of all the potential threats to both the woman and her baby.

● **FIGURE 20–7**

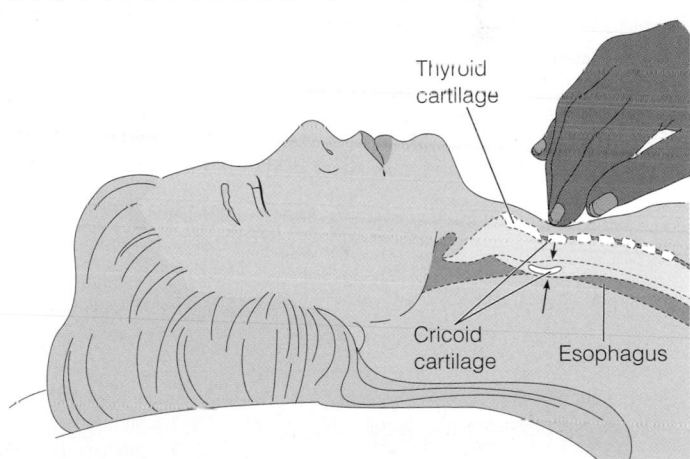

Proper position for fingers in applying cricoid pressure until a cuffed endotracheal tube is placed by the anesthesiologist or nurse anesthetist. The cricoid cartilage is depressed 2 to 3 cm posteriorly so that the esophagus is occluded.

Critical Concept Review

LEARNING OBJECTIVES

CONCEPTS

Describe the use of systemic drugs to promote pain relief during labor.

1. The goal is to provide maximum pain relief with minimum risk to the mother and fetus.
2. After complete assessment, an analgesia agent is generally administered when cervical change has occurred.
3. Drugs may cause fetal respiratory depression at birth if given too late in labor.
4. Maternal and fetal vital signs must be stable before systemic drugs may be administered.
5. Naloxone (Narcan) should be available at birth to treat respiratory depression in the newborn.

Compare the major types of regional analgesia and anesthesia, including area affected, advantages, disadvantages, techniques, and nursing implications.

1. Epidural:
   - Injection of anesthetic agent into the epidural space.
   - Produces little or no feeling to the area from the uterus downward.
   - Pushing during second stage of labor may be impaired due to lack of sensation.
   - Hypotension is the most common side effect.
   - May preload with crystalloid solution bolus.
   - Woman may need urinary catheterization due to the loss of bladder sensation.
   - Assess sensation motor control, and orthostatic blood pressure.
2. Continuous epidural analgesia:
   - Provides good analgesia.
   - Produces less nausea and provides a greater ability to cough.
   - May produce breakthrough pain, sedation, and respiratory depression.
   - Itching and hypotension are side effects.
3. Spinal block:
   - A local anesthetic agent is injected directly into spinal canal. The level of anesthesia is dependent upon level of administration. May be administered higher for cesarean birth or lower for vaginal birth.
   - The onset of anesthesia is immediate.
   - Side effects include maternal hypotension, which can lead to fetal hypoxia.
   - Requires frequent blood pressure monitoring with changes in position.
   - Indwelling urinary catheter is usually needed due to decreased bladder sensation and tone.
   - Woman's legs must be protected from injury for 8–12 hours after birth of baby due to decreased movement and sensation.
4. Pudendal block:
   - Local anesthesia is injected directly into the pudendal nerve which produces anesthesia to the lower vagina, vulva, and perineum.
   - Only produces pain relief at the end of labor.
   - Has no effect on fetus or the progress of labor.
   - May cause hematoma, perforation of the rectum, or trauma to the sciatic nerve.
5. Local infiltration anesthesia:
   - Local anesthesia is injected into the perineum prior to an episiotomy.
   - Provides pain relief only for the episiotomy incision.
   - There is no effect on maternal or fetal vital signs.
   - Requires large amounts of local anesthetic agents.

Discuss the possible complications of regional anesthesia.

Regional anesthesia administered per spinal or epidural route has similar possible complications:
1. Maternal hypotension.
2. Bladder distention.
3. Inability to push during second stage of labor.
4. Severe headache with spinal anesthesia.
5. Elevated temperature with epidural anesthesia.
6. Possible neurologic damage.

LEARNING OBJECTIVES

CONCEPTS

| Describe the nursing care related to general anesthesia. | → | The nurse should:
1. Assess when the mother ate or drank last.
2. Administer prescribed premedications such as an antacid.
3. Place a wedge under the mother's right hip to displace the uterus and prevent vena cava compression.
4. Provide oxygen prior to the start of the surgery.
5. Ensure that IV access is established.
6. Assist the anesthesiologist by applying cricoid pressure during the placement of the endotracheal tube. |

| Delineate the major complications of general anesthesia. | → | Major complications of general anesthesia are:
1. Fetal depression.
2. Uterine relaxation.
3. Vomiting.
4. Aspiration. |

CRITICAL THINKING IN ACTION

View the **Critical Thinking in Action** video in Chapter 20 of the CD-ROM. Then, answer the questions that follow.

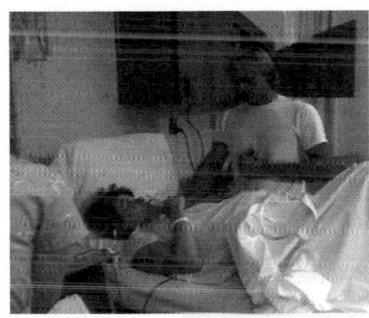

Sandra, a 26-year-old G1 P0000, is in active labor when she presents to you at the birthing center. She has been in labor for 5 hours and is clearly tired and seems to be having difficulty coping with the pain. Her contractions are occurring every 2 to 4 minutes lasting 50 to 60 seconds, and are moderate to strong in intensity. You assess the fetal heart rate of 120 to 130 with early decelerations; moderate long-term variability is present. Sandra's vital signs are stable and her laboratory results are within normal limits. She is requesting an epidural analgesia for pain control. A vaginal exam demonstrates the cervix is 100% effaced, 6 cm dilated with the vertex at 0 station in the LOT position. You notify the physician of Sandra's wish for pain relief and labor progress. You review the client's record for written consent for regional analgesia and assist the anesthesiologist with the procedure.

1. Discuss the advantages of regional analgesia.
2. Describe the nursing responsibility during the administration of regional analgesia.
3. Discuss the side effects of regional analgesia.
4. What are the absolute contraindications for an epidural block?
5. How do you assist Sandra with the second stage of labor when she cannot feel her contractions?

MEDIALINK   www.prenhall.com/london

- NCLEX-RN® Review, case studies, and other interactive resources for this chapter can be found on the Companion Website at http://www.prenhall.com/london. Click on "Chapter 20" to select the activities for this chapter.

- For animations, more NCLEX-RN® Review questions, and an audio glossary, access the accompanying CD-ROM in this textbook.

REFERENCES

American College of Obstetricians and Gynecologists (ACOG) & American Society of Anesthesiologists (ASA). (2000). *Pain relief during labor* (Committee Opinion No. 231). Washington, DC: ACOG.

Aveline, C., El Metaoua, S., Masmoudi, A., Boelle, P. Y., & Bonnet, F. (2002). The effect of clonidine on the minimum local analgesic concentrations of epidural ropivacaine during labor. *Anesthesia and Analgesia, 95*(3), 735–740.

Bowes, W. A., & Thorp, J. M. (2004). Clinical aspects of normal and abnormal labor. In R. K. Creasy & R. Resnik (Eds.), *Maternal-fetal medicine: Principles and practice* (5th ed., chap. 36, pp. 671–705). Philadelphia: Saunders.

Chung, U. L., Hung, L. C., Kuo, S. C., & Huang, C. L. (2003). Effects of L14 and BL 67 acupressure on labor pain and uterine contractions in the first stage of labor. *Journal of Nursing Research, 11*(4), 251–260.

Fisk, N. M., Gitau, R., Teixeira, J. M., Giannakoulopoulos, X., Cameron, A. D., & Glover, V. A. (2001). Effect of direct fetal opioid analgesia on fetal hormonal and hemodynamic stress response to intrauterine needling. *Anesthesiology, 95,* 828–835

Fraser, W. D., Cayer, M., Soeder, B. M., Turcot, L., & Marcoux, S. (2002). Risk factors for difficult delivery in nulliparas with epidural analgesia in second stage. *Obstetrics and Gynecology, 99,* 409–418.

Hughes, S. C., Levinson, G., Rosen, M. A., & Shnider, S. M. (2002). *Shnider and Levinsons' anesthesia for obstetrics* (4th ed.). Philadelphia: Lippincott Williams and Wilkins.

Mayberry, L. J., Clemmens, D., & De, A. (2002). Epidural analgesia side effects, cointerventions, and care of women during childbirth: A systematic review. *American Journal of Obstetrics and Gynecology, 186*(5), S81–S93.

National Institutes of Health. (2001, August 9). *NIH News Release: Epidural pain relief during labor does not increase chance of C-section.* Bethesda, MD: Author.

Segal, S. (2002). Epidural analgesia and the progress and outcome of labor and delivery. *International Anesthesiology Clinics, 40*(4), 13–26.

Wilson, B. A., Shannon, M. T., & Stang, C. L. (Eds.). (2005). *Prentice Hall nurse's drug guide: 2005.* Upper Saddle River, NJ: Pearson Education.

Childbirth at Risk

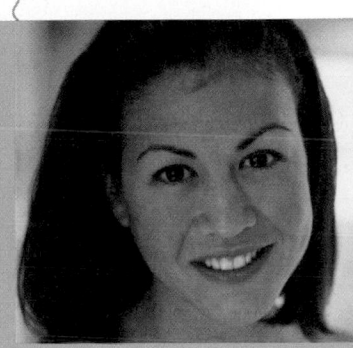

We arrived at the birthing unit with such wonderful plans for the birth of our first baby. I was able to do my breathing with the assistance of my husband and the nurse. Then suddenly my baby's heart rate dropped. It lasted for about 20 seconds but it felt like a lifetime. The nurse helped me to my side, and just stayed with us while we waited and watched the fetal monitor. There were no further problems, but I will never forget that moment.
—Yolanda, 26

LEARNING OBJECTIVES

- Compare and contrast hypertonic and hypotonic labor patterns, including the risks, clinical therapy, and nursing care management.

- Describe the possible impact of postterm pregnancy on the childbearing family.

- Relate the various types of fetal malposition and malpresentation to the possible associated problems.

- Discuss the identification, management, and care of fetal macrosomia.

- Delineate the nursing care for the woman with more than one fetus.

- Summarize the nursing care indicated for nonreassuring fetal status.

- Compare and contrast abruptio placentae and placenta previa, including implications for the mother and fetus and nursing care.

- Identify variations that may occur with or in the umbilical cord and insertion into the placenta.

- Contrast the identification, management, and nursing care of women with amniotic fluid embolus, hydramnios, and oligohydramnios.

- Delineate the effects of pelvic contractures on labor and birth.

- Identify common complications of the third and fourth stages of labor.

- Discuss perinatal loss, including etiology, diagnosis, and the nurse's role in facilitating the family's grief work.

- Describe the psychologic factors that may be accelerated secondary to complications during labor and birth.

MEDIALINK   www.prenhall.com/london

CD-ROM

NCLEX-RN® Review
Audio Glossary
Skill 3–9: Care of the Woman with a Cord Prolapse

Companion Website

MediaLink Applications:
    Case Study: Client with Hemorrhage
    Care Plan Activity: Prevention of Cord Prolapse
Thinking Critically

Successful completion of a pregnancy requires the harmonious functioning of the five critical factors discussed in the Critical Factors in Labor section in Chapter 17: the birth passage, the fetus, the relationship between the passage and the fetus, the forces of labor, and psychosocial considerations. ∞ Disruptions in any of these components may cause dystocia (abnormal or difficult labor). The most common of these disruptions are discussed in this chapter.

CARE OF THE WOMAN WITH DYSTOCIA RELATED TO DYSFUNCTIONAL UTERINE CONTRACTIONS

Dystocia, or difficult labor, may be due to a wide variety of problems, the most common of which is dysfunctional (or uncoordinated) uterine contractions. These uncoordinated contractions result in a prolonged labor. Contractions that result in a more normal progression of labor tend to be moderate to strong when palpated and occur regularly (two to four contractions in 10 minutes in early labor and four to five per 10 minutes in later phases). Dysfunctional contractions are typically irregular in strength, timing, or both. These irregular uterine contractions often arrest cervical dilatation.

HYPERTONIC LABOR PATTERNS

A normal contraction pattern is shown in Figure 21–1A ●. In hypertonic labor patterns, ineffectual uterine contractions of poor quality occur in the latent phase of labor, and the resting tone of the myometrium increases. Contractions usually become more frequent, but their intensity may decrease (Figure 21–1B). The contractions are painful but ineffective in dilating and effacing the cervix, and a prolonged latent phase may result.

Risks of Hypertonic Labor

Maternal risks of hypertonic labor include the following:

- Increased discomfort due to uterine muscle cell anoxia
- Fatigue as the pattern continues and no labor progress results
- Stress on coping abilities
- Dehydration and increased incidence of infection if labor is prolonged

  Fetal-neonatal risks include the following:

- Nonreassuring fetal status because contractions and increased resting tone interfere with the uteroplacental exchange
- Prolonged pressure on the fetal head, which may result in cephalhematoma, caput succedaneum, or excessive molding (Figure 21–2 ●)

CLINICAL THERAPY

Management of hypertonic labor may include bed rest and sedation to promote relaxation and reduce pain. Often pharmacologic intervention to promote sedation will stop these contractions. If the hypertonic pattern continues and develops into a prolonged latent phase, oxytocin (Pitocin) infusion or amniotomy may be considered (see Care of the Women During Labor Induction in Chapter 22 ∞). These methods are instituted only

● **FIGURE 21–1**

A

B

C

Comparison of labor patterns. **A,** Normal uterine contraction pattern. In this example, contraction frequency is every 3 minutes; duration is 60 seconds. The baseline resting tone is below 10 mm Hg. **B,** Hypertonic uterine contraction pattern. Note that the contraction frequency is every 1 1/2 minutes, duration is 90 seconds. The baseline resting tone is 10 mm Hg. **C,** Hypotonic uterine contraction pattern. In this example, the contraction frequency is every 7 minutes (with some uterine activity between contractions), duration is 50 seconds, and intensity increases approximately 25 mm Hg during contractions.

after cephalopelvic disproportion (CPD) and fetal malpresentation have been ruled out. If the maternal pelvic diameters are less than average, or if the fetus is particularly large or is in a malpresentation or malposition, CPD is said to be present. In such cases, labor is not stimulated because vaginal birth is not possible. Instead a cesarean birth will be performed.

NURSING MANAGEMENT

NURSING ASSESSMENT AND DIAGNOSIS

As part of the labor assessment, evaluate the relationship between the intensity of the pain being experienced and the degree to which the cervix is dilating and effacing. Also note whether anxiety is negatively affecting labor progress. Evidence of increasing frustration and discouragement on the part of the mother and her partner may indicate the need to provide some additional information or assurance.

Nursing diagnoses that may apply to the woman in hypertonic labor include the following:

■ *Fatigue* related to inability to relax and rest secondary to a hypertonic labor pattern

■ *Acute Pain* related to the woman's inability to relax secondary to hypertonic uterine contractions

■ *Ineffective Individual Coping* related to ineffectiveness of breathing techniques to relieve discomfort

■ *Anxiety* related to slow labor progress

FIGURE 21–2

Effects of labor on the fetal head. **A,** Caput succedaneum formation. The presenting portion of the scalp area is encircled by the cervix during labor, causing swelling of the soft tissue. **B,** Molding of the fetal head in cephalic presentations: (1) occiput anterior, (2) occiput posterior, (3) brow, (4) face.

PLANNING AND IMPLEMENTATION

A key nursing responsibility is to provide comfort and support to the laboring woman and her partner. The woman experiencing a hypertonic labor pattern will probably be very uncomfortable because of the increased force of contractions. Her anxiety level and that of her partner may be high. Work to reduce the woman's discomfort and promote a more effective labor pattern.

Suggest supportive measures such as a change of position: left lateral side-lying, high Fowler's, or on her knees in the bed with her arms up around the top of the bed while it is in high Fowler's, rocking in a rocking chair, sitting up, and walking. It may be helpful to offer soothing measures such as a quiet environment, use of music the woman finds calming, back rubs, therapeutic touch, and visualization, as well as comfort measures such as mouth care, change of linens, effleurage, and relaxation exercises. The use of tub baths or a warm shower can help promote comfort and uterine relaxation. If sedation is ordered, ensure that the environment is conducive to relaxation. The labor partner may also need assistance in helping the woman cope. A calm, understanding approach offers the woman and her partner further support. Providing information about the cause of the hypertonic labor pattern and assuring the woman that she is not overreacting to the situation are important nursing actions.

Client education is key for the woman experiencing hypertonic labor. She needs information about the dysfunctional labor pattern and the possible implications for her and her baby. Information will help relieve anxiety and thereby increase relaxation and comfort. Explain treatment options and offer opportunities to ask questions.

EVALUATION

Expected outcomes of nursing care include the following:

- The woman has increased comfort and decreased anxiety.
- The woman and her partner are able to cope with the labor.
- The woman experiences a more effective labor pattern.

HYPOTONIC LABOR PATTERNS

A hypotonic labor pattern usually develops in the active phase of labor, after labor has been well established. Hypotonic labor is characterized by fewer than two to three contractions in a 10-minute period (see Figure 21–1C).

Hypotonic labor may occur when the uterus is over-stretched from a twin gestation, or in the presence of a large fetus, hydramnios, or grand multiparity. Bladder or bowel distention and CPD may also be associated with this pattern.

Risks of Hypotonic Labor

Maternal implications of hypotonic labor patterns include the following risks:

- Maternal exhaustion
- Stress on coping abilities
- Postpartum hemorrhage from insufficient uterine contractions following birth
- Intrauterine infection if labor is prolonged

Fetal-neonatal implications include the following:

- Nonreassuring fetal status due to prolonged labor pattern
- Fetal sepsis from pathogens that ascend from the birth canal

THINKING CRITICALLY

FETAL HEART RATE TRACING

A fetal heart rate (FHR) tracing demonstrates the following: baseline heart rate of 140 with variability of 6 to 10 bpm. When you compare the FHR with the uterine contractions, you note that there is a slowing of the FHR at the time of the contraction and that the FHR tracing looks like the contraction curve, but it is upside down. Based on this tracing, what would you do?

Clinical Therapy

Improving the quality of the uterine contractions while ensuring a safe outcome for the woman and her baby are the goals of therapy. Uterine contractions can be stimulated in several ways, including the use of Pitocin, amniotomy, or stimulation of the nipples, which causes the release of oxytocin. Before initiating treatment for hypotonic labor, the physician or certified nurse-midwife (CNM) validates the adequacy of pelvic measurements and completes tests to establish gestational age if fetal maturity is in question. After CPD, fetal malpresentation, and fetal immaturity have been ruled out, Pitocin may be given intravenously (IV) via an infusion pump to improve the quality of uterine contractions. Intravenous fluid is useful to maintain adequate hydration and prevent maternal exhaustion. Amniotomy may be used to stimulate the labor process. The application of an electric breast pump or manual stimulation of the nipples may help strengthen uterine contractions, and is an excellent starting point for women who want an unmedicated birth.

Some physicians support the use of **active management of labor (AMOL)**, a process whereby labor is managed from the beginning with amniotomy, timed cervical examinations are performed, and augmentation of labor with IV administration of Pitocin is begun if a specified level of progress is not met. Supporters of AMOL contend that it is a preventive treatment that reduces the chance for protracted labor and decreases the cesarean birth rate (Dudley, 2003). Opponents argue that the use of AMOL increases the incidence of infection (because of frequent vaginal examinations), necessitates the use of additional interventions, and increases the incidence of instrument-assisted births.

An improvement in the quality of uterine contractions is demonstrated by noticeable progress in the labor. If the labor pattern does not become effective or if other complications develop, further interventions, including cesarean birth, may be necessary.

NURSING MANAGEMENT

NURSING ASSESSMENT AND DIAGNOSIS

Assessment of contractions (for frequency, intensity, and duration), maternal vital signs, and FHR provides data to evaluate maternal-fetal status. Also be alert for signs and symptoms of infection and dehydration. Because of the stress associated with a prolonged labor, observe the woman and her partner's success in implementing coping mechanisms.

Nursing diagnoses that may apply to the woman in hypotonic labor include the following:

- *Acute Pain* related to uterine contractions secondary to dysfunctional labor
- *Ineffective Individual Coping* related to unanticipated discomfort and slow progress in labor
- *Health-Seeking Behaviors* related to lack of information about dysfunctional labor

PLANNING AND IMPLEMENTATION

Nursing measures to promote maternal-fetal physical well-being include frequent monitoring of contractions, maternal vital signs, and FHR. If amniotic membranes are ruptured, assess for the presence of meconium (dark green or black stool expelled from the fetal large intestine). The presence of meconium in the amniotic fluid makes close observation of fetal status more critical because it often indicates that the fetus is experiencing some form of stress. An intake and output record provides a way of determining maternal hydration or dehydration. Encourage the woman to void every 2 hours, and check her bladder for distention. Because labor may be prolonged, continue to monitor the woman for signs of infection (elevated temperature, chills, foul-smelling amniotic fluid, and fetal tachycardia). Vaginal examinations should be kept to a minimum to decrease the risk of introducing an infection.

Clients experiencing a hypotonic labor pattern require emotional support. Help the woman and her partner to cope with the frustration of a lengthy labor process. Combine a warm, caring approach with techniques to reduce anxiety and discomfort.

The teaching plan must include information regarding the dysfunctional labor process and implications for the mother and baby. Disadvantages of and alternatives to treatment also need to be discussed and understood.

EVALUATION

Expected outcomes of nursing care include the following:

- The woman maintains comfort during labor.
- The woman understands the type of labor pattern that is occurring and the treatment plan.

CARE OF THE WOMAN EXPERIENCING PRECIPITOUS LABOR

Precipitous labor lasts less than 3 hours and results in rapid birth. Contributing factors in precipitous labor are multiparity, large pelvis, previous precipitous labor, and a small fetus in a favorable position. One or more of these factors, plus strong contractions, result in a rapid descent of the infant through the birth canal (Smith, 2004).

Precipitous labor and precipitous birth are not the same. A precipitous birth is an unexpected, sudden, and often unattended birth. (See Nursing Care During Precipitous Birth in Chapter 19. ∞)

RISKS OF PRECIPITOUS LABOR

Maternal risks of precipitous labor include the following:

- Loss of coping abilities
- Lacerations of the cervix, vagina, and perineum due to rapid descent and birth of the fetus
- Postpartum hemorrhage due to undetected lacerations or inadequate uterine contractions after birth

Fetal-neonatal implications include the following:

- Nonreassuring fetal status or hypoxia from decreased uteroplacental circulation due to intense uterine contractions
- Cerebral trauma from rapid descent through the birth canal
- Pneumothorax from rapid descent through the birth canal

Clinical Therapy

Any woman with a history of precipitous labor requires close monitoring in the last few weeks of pregnancy. If the cervix softens and begins to dilate, the woman may be scheduled for immediate induction of labor.

NURSING MANAGEMENT

NURSING ASSESSMENT AND DIAGNOSIS

During the intrapartum nursing assessment, identify a woman at increased risk of precipitous labor (e.g., a previous history of precipitous or short labor places the woman at risk). During labor the presence of one or both of the following factors may indicate potential problems:

- Accelerated cervical dilatation (more than 2 cm/hr in multigravidas and more than 1.2 cm/hr in primigravidas) and fetal descent
- Intense uterine contractions with little uterine relaxation between contractions

Nursing diagnoses that may apply to the woman with precipitous labor include the following:

- *Risk for Injury* related to rapid labor and birth
- *Acute Pain* related to rapid labor process

PLANNING AND IMPLEMENTATION

If the woman has a history of precipitous labor, monitor her closely and keep an emergency birth pack at hand. Stay in constant attendance if possible and promote comfort and rest by assisting the woman to a comfortable position, providing a quiet environment, and administering sedatives as needed. Give information and support before and after the birth.

To avoid possible precipitous labor and hyperstimulation of the uterus during Pitocin administration, be alert to the dangers of Pitocin overdosage (see "Drug Guide: Oxytocin" in Chapter 22 ∞). If the woman receiving Pitocin develops an accelerated labor pattern, the Pitocin is discontinued immediately, and the woman is turned on her left side to improve uterine perfusion. Oxygen may be administered to increase the available oxygen in the maternal circulating blood, which in turn increases the amount available for exchange at the placental site. The fetus is monitored for signs of hypoxia and other indications of nonreassuring fetal status.

EVALUATION

Expected outcomes of nursing care include the following:

- The woman and her baby are closely monitored during labor, and a safe birth occurs.
- The woman maintains optimal comfort.

CARE OF THE WOMAN WITH POSTTERM PREGNANCY

A **postterm pregnancy** is one that *extends more than 294 days or 42 weeks past the first day of the last menstrual period (LMP).* It is important to distinguish between the terms *postdate,* which means that the pregnancy has gone beyond the estimated date of birth (EDB), and *postterm,* which indicates that the pregnancy has gone at least 1 day beyond 42 complete weeks from the last menstrual period. The actual incidence of postterm pregnancies is relatively small, with a range of 4% to 14%. The number of postterm pregnancies fell from 10.3% to 2.7% when ultrasound biometric criteria is used rather than the LMP criteria to determine gestational age (Resnik & Resnik, 2004). The cause of true postterm pregnancy is unknown, but it seems to occur more frequently in primigravidas and women over age 35 (Blackburn, 2003).

RISKS OF POSTTERM PREGNANCY

Maternal risks associated with postterm pregnancy include the following (Blackburn, 2003):

- Probable labor induction
- Increased risk for large-for-gestational-age (LGA) infant
- Increased incidence of forceps-assisted, vacuum-assisted, or cesarean birth
- Increased psychologic stress as the due date passes and concern for the baby increases

Fetal risks include the following (Blackburn, 2003):

- Decreased perfusion from the placenta
- Oligohydramnios (decreased amount of amniotic fluid), which increases the risk of cord compression
- Meconium aspiration (aspiration of meconium-stained amniotic fluid by the fetus at the time of birth), which is more likely if oligohydramnios and thick meconium are present

Some fetuses continue to grow beyond the 42nd week of pregnancy and can be excessively large at birth (macrosomia). In other cases the intrauterine environment becomes unfavorable for growth, and at birth the infant has lost muscle mass and subcutaneous fat. The macrosomic fetus is at risk for birth trauma, whereas the small-for-gestational-age (SGA) fetus is at risk for nonreassuring fetal status during labor because there is often associated oligohydramnios (Resnik & Resnik, 2004).

Clinical Therapy

When the 40th week of gestation is completed and birth has not occurred, most practitioners begin using the nonstress test (NST) and biophysical profile (BPP) (especially the amniotic fluid volume portion of the BPP) as assessment tools. These tests may be done two to three times a week to help evaluate fetal well-being (Resnik & Resnik, 2004). If at any time the fetal assessment tests indicate a problem, interventions are initiated to accomplish the birth.

NURSING MANAGEMENT

NURSING ASSESSMENT AND DIAGNOSIS

When the woman is admitted into the birthing area, ongoing assessments of fetal well-being begin as soon as the postterm condition has been verified. Identify reassuring FHR characteristics and evaluate for the presence of nonreassuring patterns, such as nonperiodic variable decelerations (which may indicate cord compression), so that corrective actions can be taken. When the amniotic membranes rupture, assess the fluid for meconium. In addition, assess the woman's knowledge about the condition, implications for her baby, risks, and possible interventions.

Nursing diagnoses that may apply to the woman with postterm pregnancy include the following:

- *Health-Seeking Behaviors* related to lack of information about postterm pregnancy
- *Fear* related to the unknown outcome for the baby
- *Ineffective Individual Coping* related to anxiety about the status of the baby

PLANNING AND IMPLEMENTATION

Nursing Care in the Community

If the woman has not been assessing fetal movement every day, teach her how to do so. It is vital to stress the importance of identifying inadequate fetal movement and immediately contacting her healthcare provider. (See Fetal Activity Monitoring in Chapter 11 ∞ for further discussion of techniques to detect fetal movement.)

Client education about the postterm pregnancy is another important nursing responsibility. Address the implications and associated risks for the baby, as well as possible treatment plans. The woman and her partner need opportunities to ask questions and clarify information.

Hospital-Based Nursing Care

Promoting fetal well-being requires careful assessment of the response of the fetus during labor. If oligohydramnios exists, a continuous FHR tracing is obtained and evaluated frequently. Variable decelerations are often associated with oligohydramnios, because the decreased amount of fluid may allow compression of the umbilical cord. If the fetus is macrosomic, careful assessment of labor progress (contraction characteristics, progressive cervical dilatation, and fetal descent) is also needed.

Emotional support is a key nursing intervention for women with pregnancies that extend past the due date. Women experiencing postterm pregnancy frequently feel increased stress and anxiety and have difficulty coping. Encouragement, support, and recognition of the woman's anxiety are helpful strategies.

EVALUATION

Expected outcomes of nursing care include the following:

- The woman has knowledge about the postterm pregnancy.

- The woman and her partner feel supported and able to cope with the postterm pregnancy.

- Fetal status is maintained, any abnormalities are quickly identified, and supportive measures are initiated.

CARE OF THE WOMAN AND FETUS AT RISK DUE TO FETAL MALPOSITION

The *occiput posterior (OP) position* is the most common fetal malposition. When the fetus is OP, the occiput of the fetal head is directed toward the back of the maternal pelvis. During labor, 87% of OP fetuses rotate to an occiput anterior (OA) position (Polo, Chang, Herrera et al., 2003).

A variation of OP called the **persistent occiput posterior (POP) position** occurs in 5% of labors. In this case the fetus enters the birth canal, descends, and is born in the OP position. Lack of rotation can be due to poor contractions, abnormal flexion of the head, incomplete rotation, inadequate maternal pushing efforts usually related to epidural anesthesia, or a large fetus. Labor may be prolonged; however, most POP fetuses are born without the aid of forceps.

RISKS OF FETAL MALPOSITION

Maternal risks related to the POP position include the following:

- Risk of third- or fourth-degree perineal lacerations during birth

- Risk of extension of a midline episiotomy

Fetal implications do not include an increased mortality risk unless labor is prolonged or additional interventions such as forceps-assisted, vacuum-assisted, or cesarean birth are required.

CLINICAL THERAPY

Clinical treatment focuses on close monitoring of maternal and fetal status and labor progress to determine whether vaginal or cesarean birth is the safer method. A cesarean birth is chosen if maternal or fetal problems make a vaginal birth unwise or if CPD is present. Although the majority of POP fetuses are born vaginally, in some cases forceps-assisted birth may be necessary. The forceps can be used to deliver the fetus while it is still in the occiput posterior position or to rotate the occiput to an anterior position (called Scanzoni's maneuver). A rotation from left occiput posterior (LOP) or right occiput posterior (ROP) to an anterior position may be accomplished with a vacuum assistance device. (See Chapter 22 for further discussion of forceps and vacuum. ∞)

NURSING MANAGEMENT

NURSING ASSESSMENT AND DIAGNOSIS

Signs and symptoms of a POP position include complaints of intense back pain by the laboring woman, a dysfunctional labor pattern, hypotonic labor (the fetal head does not put adequate pressure on the cervix), arrest of dilatation, or arrest of fetal descent. The back pain is caused by the fetal occiput compressing the sacral nerves. Further assessment may reveal a depression in the maternal abdomen above the symphysis. FHR is typically heard far laterally on the abdomen. On vaginal examination the physician or CNM finds the wide, diamond-shaped anterior fontanelle in the anterior portion of the pelvis. This fontanelle may be difficult to feel because of molding of the fetal head.

Nursing diagnoses that may apply to women with POP position fetuses include the following:

- *Acute Pain* related to back discomfort secondary to the OP position

- *Ineffective Individual Coping* related to unanticipated discomfort and slow progress in labor

PLANNING AND IMPLEMENTATION

Changing maternal posture has been used for many years to enhance rotation of OP or occiput transverse (OT) to OA. A number of position changes may be tried. For instance, the woman may be asked to lie on one side and then asked to move to the other side as the fetus begins to rotate. This side-lying position may promote rotation; it also enables the support person to apply counterpressure on the sacral area to decrease discomfort. A knee-chest position provides a downward slant to the vaginal canal, directing the fetal head downward on descent. A hands-and-knees position is often effective in rotating the fetus. In addition to maintaining a hands-and-knees position on the bed, the woman may try pelvic rocking, and the support person may firmly stroke the abdomen. The stroking begins over the fetal back and swings around to the other side of the abdomen. After the fetus has rotated, the woman lies in a Sims' position on the side opposite the fetal back.

EVALUATION

Expected outcomes of nursing care include the following:

- The woman's discomfort is decreased.
- The coping abilities of the woman and her partner are strengthened.

CARE OF THE WOMAN AND FETUS AT RISK DUE TO FETAL MALPRESENTATION

In a normal presentation, the occiput is the presenting part (Figure 21–3A ○). Fetal malpresentations include brow, face, breech, shoulder (transverse lie), and compound presentation.

BROW PRESENTATION

In a brow presentation, the forehead of the fetus becomes the presenting part. In the military presentation, the fetal head is between flexion and extension (Figure 21–3B ○), whereas in the occipitomental presentation, the fetal head enters the birth canal with the widest diameter of the head (approximately 13.5 cm) foremost (Figure 21–3C ○).

The brow presentation occurs more often in multiparas than in nulliparas and is thought to be due to lax abdominal and pelvic musculature. Many brow presentations spontaneously convert to face or occipital presentations (Bowes & Thorp, 2004). Brow presentations are the least common types of abnormal presentations.

Risks of Brow Presentation

Maternal implications of brow presentation include increased risk of the following:

- Longer labor due to ineffective contractions and slow or arrested fetal descent
- Cesarean birth if brow presentation persists

Fetal-neonatal risks include increased mortality because of cerebral and neck compression and damage to the trachea and larynx (Bowes & Thorp, 2004). In addition, facial edema, bruising, and exaggerated molding of the newborn's head may be observed.

Clinical Therapy

If a brow presentation fails to convert to occipital or face presentation, cesarean birth is indicated in most cases (Bowes & Thorp, 2004). If a vaginal birth is attempted, the woman is closely monitored for CPD and will probably need an episiotomy. Right mediolateral (RML) or left mediolateral (LML) episiotomy is preferable, because the more common midline episiotomy has the risk of extending into the anus and rectum (fourth-degree laceration).

○ FIGURE 21–3

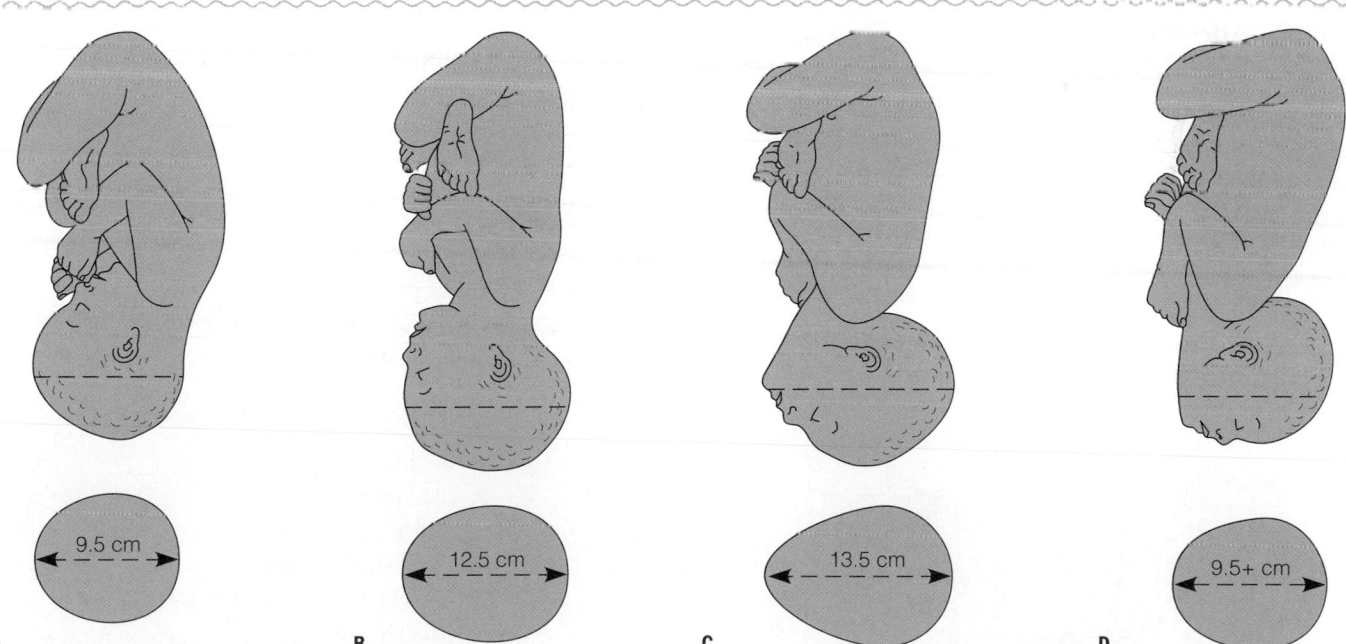

9.5 cm | 12.5 cm | 13.5 cm | 9.5+ cm

A   B   C   D

Types of cephalic presentations. **A,** The occiput is the presenting part because the head is flexed and the fetal chin is against the chest. The largest anteroposterior (AP) diameter that presents and passes through the pelvis is approximately 9.5 cm. **B,** Military presentation. The head is neither flexed nor extended. The presenting AP diameter is approximately 12.5 cm. **C,** Brow presentation. The largest diameter of the fetal head (approximately 13.5 cm) presents in this situation. **D,** Face presentation. The AP diameter is 9.5 cm.

Used with permission from Danforth, D. N., & Scott, J. R. (Eds.). (1990). Obstetrics and gynecology (5th ed., p. 170, fig. 8–9). New York: Lippincott.

NURSING MANAGEMENT

NURSING ASSESSMENT AND DIAGNOSIS

A brow presentation can be detected on vaginal examination (with ultrasound or x-ray confirmation) by palpation of the diamond-shaped anterior fontanelle on one side and orbital ridges and root of the nose on the other side.

Nursing diagnoses that may apply to a woman with a brow presentation include the following:

- *Health-Seeking Behaviors* related to lack of information about the possible maternal-fetal effects of brow presentation
- *Risk for Injury* to the fetus related to pressure on fetal structures secondary to brow presentation

PLANNING AND IMPLEMENTATION

Closely observe the woman for labor problems and the fetus for signs of hypoxia as evidenced by late decelerations and bradycardia.

Also provide emotional support to the family. Explain the fetal position to the woman and her support person or interpret what the physician or CNM has told them. Stay close at hand to reassure the couple, inform them of any changes, and assist them with labor-coping techniques. In face and brow presentations, the newborn's face may be edematous. The couple may need help in beginning the attachment process because of the newborn's facial appearance. After the infant is inspected for any abnormalities, the pediatrician and nurse can assure the couple that the facial edema is only temporary and will subside in 3 or 4 days and that the molding will be much less visible in a few days (even though completion of the process takes several weeks).

EVALUATION

Expected outcomes of nursing care include the following:

- The woman and her partner understand the implications and associated problems of brow presentation.
- The mother and her baby have a safe labor and birth.

FACE PRESENTATION

In a face presentation, the face of the fetus is the presenting part (Figure 21–3D ● and Figure 21–4 ●). The fetal head is hyperextended even more than in the brow presentation. Face presentation occurs most frequently in multiparas, in preterm birth, and in the presence of anencephaly. The incidence of face presentation is about 1 in 600 births.

Risks of Face Presentation

Maternal risks related to face presentation include the following:

- Increased risk of CPD and prolongation of labor
- Increased risk of infection (with prolonged labor)
- Cesarean birth if fetal chin is posterior (mentum posterior)

Fetal-neonatal risks include the following:

- Cephalhematoma

● **FIGURE 21–4**

Mechanism of birth in face (mentoanterior) position. **A,** The submentobregmatic diameter at the outlet. **B,** The fetal head is born by the movement of flexion.

FIGURE 21–5

Face presentation. Mechanism of birth in mentoposterior position. Fetal head is unable to extend farther. The face becomes impacted.

■ Edema of the face and throat if the fetal chin is anterior (mentum anterior)

■ Pronounced molding of the head

Clinical Therapy

A vaginal birth may be anticipated if no CPD is present, the chin (mentum) is anterior, the labor pattern is effective, and the fetal status is reassuring. Many mentum posterior presentations spontaneously convert to anterior in the late stages of labor. If the mentum remains posterior, a vaginal birth is not possible and a cesarean birth is necessary (Figure 21–5 ●).

NURSING MANAGEMENT

NURSING ASSESSMENT AND DIAGNOSIS

When performing Leopold's maneuvers, the back of the fetus is difficult to outline, and a deep furrow can be palpated between the hard occiput and the fetal back (Figure 21–6 ●). Fetal heart tones are audible on the side where the fetal feet are palpated. It may be difficult to determine by vaginal examination whether a breech or face is presenting, especially if facial edema is already present. During the vaginal examination, palpation of the saddle of the nose and the gums should be attempted. When assessing engagement, remember that the face has to be deep within the pelvis before the biparietal diameters have entered the inlet.

Nursing diagnoses that may apply to the woman with a fetus in face presentation include the following:

■ *Fear* related to unknown outcome of the labor and a possible instrument-assisted or cesarean birth

FIGURE 21–6

A

B

Face presentation. **A,** Palpation of the maternal abdomen with the fetus in right mentum posterior (RMP) position. **B,** Vaginal examination may permit palpation of facial features of the fetus.

■ *Risk for Injury to the Newborn's Face* related to edema secondary to the birth process

PLANNING AND IMPLEMENTATION

Nursing interventions are the same as those indicated for the brow presentation.

EVALUATION

Expected outcomes of nursing care include the following:

■ The woman and her partner understand the implications and associated problems of face presentation.

■ The mother and her baby have a safe labor and birth.

BREECH PRESENTATION

The exact cause of breech presentation (Figure 21–7 ●) is unknown. This malpresentation occurs in about 3% to 4% of labors and is frequently associated with preterm birth, placenta previa, hydramnios, multiple gestation, uterine anomalies (such as bicornuate uterus), and fetal anomalies (especially anencephaly and hydrocephaly) (Bowes & Thorp, 2004).

Risks of Breech Presentation

The maternal implication of breech presentation is a likelihood of cesarean birth. Fetal-neonatal implications include the following (Bowes & Thorp, 2004):

■ Higher perinatal morbidity and mortality rates

■ Increased risk of prolapsed cord, especially in incomplete breeches, because space is available between the cervix and presenting part

● **FIGURE 21–7**

Breech presentation. **A,** Frank breech. **B,** Incomplete (footling) breech. **C,** Complete breech in left sacral anterior (LSA) position. **D,** On vaginal examination the nurse may feel the anal sphincter. The tissue of the fetal buttocks feels soft.

■ Increased risk of cervical cord injuries due to hyperextension of the fetal head during vaginal birth

■ Increased risk of birth trauma (especially of the head) during either vaginal or cesarean breech birth

Clinical Therapy

Current clinical therapy is directed toward converting the breech presentation to a cephalic presentation prior to the beginning of labor. Therefore, an external cephalic version (ECV) may be attempted at 36 to 38 weeks' gestation as long as the woman is not in labor. (See Chapter 22 ∞ for discussion of external version.) Opinions differ about the best method of birth for the fetus in a breech presentation. When the fetus is still in breech presentation and labor occurs, the method of birth varies depending on gestational age, presence of other fetuses, estimated fetal weight, type of breech, and physician preference.

NURSING MANAGEMENT

NURSING ASSESSMENT AND DIAGNOSIS

Frequently it is the nurse who first recognizes a breech presentation. On palpation the firm fetal head is felt in the uterine fundus and the wider sacrum in the lower part of the abdomen. If the sacrum has not descended, ballottement causes the entire fetal body to move. Furthermore, FHR is usually auscultated above the umbilicus. Passage of meconium into the amniotic fluid due to compression of the fetus's intestinal tract is common.

If membranes are ruptured, be particularly alert for a prolapsed umbilical cord, especially in footling breeches, because there is space between the cervix and presenting part through which the cord can slip. If the infant is small and the membranes rupture, the danger is even greater. The risk of a prolapsed umbilical cord is one reason any woman with ruptured membranes should not ambulate until a full assessment, including vaginal examination, has been performed.

Nursing diagnoses that may apply to a woman with a breech presentation include the following:

■ *Impaired Gas Exchange in the Fetus* related to interruption in umbilical blood flow secondary to compression of the cord

■ *Health-Seeking Behaviors* related to lack of information about the implications and associated complications of breech presentation for the mother and fetus

PLANNING AND IMPLEMENTATION

During labor, promote maternal-fetal physical well-being by frequently assessing fetal and maternal status. Since the fetus is at increased risk for prolapse of the cord, agency protocols may call for continuous fetal monitoring. If the head is not completely engaged, continuous monitoring is warranted and the woman should maintain complete bed rest. Provide teaching and information about the breech presentation and the nursing care needed.

As many as 90% of infants in breech presentations are born by cesarean birth. Most physicians perform cesarean births in consideration of the increased fetal risks associated with breech vaginal birth. Most breech vaginal births are performed on multiparous women with a proven pelvis (prior birth of a normal or large size fetus without difficulty). The nurse assists with the vaginal birth by including Piper forceps (used to guide the after-coming fetal head) in the birth table setup. The nurse may assist the physician if forceps are needed for the birth. If the family and physician or CNM decide on a cesarean birth, assist as with any cesarean birth. Breech births commonly occur in the operating room with a "double setup" in place. If difficulties arise with the birth, the room is already prepared for a cesarean birth so the procedure can be performed quickly.

EVALUATION

Expected outcomes of nursing care include the following:

- The woman and her partner understand the implications and associated problems of breech presentation.
- Major complications are recognized early and corrective measures are instituted.
- The mother and baby have a safe labor and birth.

TRANSVERSE LIE (SHOULDER PRESENTATION) OF A SINGLE FETUS

A transverse lie occurs in approximately 1 in 300 term births (Bowes & Thorp, 2004). Maternal conditions associated with a transverse lie are grand multiparity with relaxed uterine muscles, preterm fetus, abnormal uterus, excessive amniotic fluid, placenta previa, and contracted pelvis (Figure 21–8 ◉).

Clinical Therapy

The management of shoulder presentation depends on the gestational age. If discovered before term, the management is expectant (watchful), because some fetuses may change presentation without intervention. When a shoulder presentation is still evident at 37 completed weeks of gestation, an external cephalic version (ECV) attempt (followed, if successful, by induction of labor) is recommended, because the associated risk of prolapsed cord is significant. Intrapartum ECV is often successful in early labor and can reduce the need for cesarean birth. If it is unsuccessful, cesarean birth is indicated.

◉ FIGURE 21–8

Scapula
Ribs
Humerus
Acromion process

B

Transverse lie. **A,** Shoulder presentation. **B,** On vaginal examination the nurse may feel the acromion process as the fetal presenting part.

Nursing Management

The nurse can identify a transverse lie by inspection and palpation of the abdomen, by auscultation of FHR, and by vaginal examination. On inspection the woman's abdomen appears widest from side to side as a result of the long axis of the infant's body lying parallel to the ground and across the mother's uterus.

COMPLEMENTARY CARE

MOXIBUSTION TO PROMOTE VERSION IN BREECH PRESENTATIONS

Traditional Chinese medicine uses the herb mugwort in the form of moxa to promote version in a breech presentation. Moxa is a system of treatment, often combined with acupuncture, in which an herb is dried, rolled into cones (like incense cones), and placed on certain meridian points of the body. The moxa is then lit and allowed to burn close to the skin, hence the *bustion* component of the name. The heat and pungency of mugwort stimulates the point, and it is believed that the energy moves through the body and increases fetal activity.

The meridian point that is used in moxibustion to promote version in breech presentation is acupoint BL 67, located beside the outer corner of the fifth toenail. Treatment may take from 7 days to 2 weeks. In a recent clinical study, moxibustion was found to be an effective modality in the management of breech presentation (Neri, Airola, Contu et al., 2004).

On palpation no fetal part is felt in the fundal portion of the uterus or above the symphysis. The head may be palpated on one side and the breech on the other. Fetal heart rate is usually auscultated just below the midline of the umbilicus. If a presenting part is palpated on vaginal examination, it is the ridged thorax or possibly an arm compressed against the chest.

Assist in the interpretation of the fetal presentation and provide information and support to the couple. The nurse also assesses maternal and fetal status frequently, and prepares the woman for a cesarean birth (see Chapter 22 ∞).

COMPOUND PRESENTATION

A compound presentation is one in which there are two presenting parts, such as the occiput and fetal hand or the complete breech and fetal hand. Most compound presentations resolve themselves spontaneously, but others require additional manipulation at birth.

CARE OF THE WOMAN AND FETUS AT RISK DUE TO MACROSOMIA

Fetal **macrosomia** is defined as a newborn weight of more than 4000 g at birth. Some sources suggest that the fetus not be considered macrosomic unless it weighs 4500 g or more and that considerations of ethnic grouping be incorporated as well (Sokol & Blackwell, 2003). The condition is more common among male infants, offspring of large parents, mothers with diabetes who had a previous infant who weighed more than 4000 g, and in cases of grand multiparity and postterm gestation (Sokol & Blackwell, 2003).

RISKS OF MACROSOMIA

Maternal implications of macrosomia include increased risk of the following:

- CPD
- Dysfunctional labor
- Soft-tissue laceration during vaginal birth
- Postpartum hemorrhage

Fetal-neonatal implications include increased risk of the following:

- Meconium aspiration
- Asphyxia
- Shoulder dystocia, in which, after birth of the head, the anterior shoulder fails to deliver either spontaneously or with gentle traction (unresolved shoulder dystocia can lead to fetal death)
- Upper brachial plexus injury and fractured clavicles

CLINICAL THERAPY

The occurrence of maternal and fetal problems associated with excessively large infants may be lessened somewhat by identifying macrosomia before the onset of labor. If a large fetus is suspected, the maternal pelvis should be evaluated carefully. Fetal size can be estimated by palpating the crown-to-rump length of the fetus in utero and by ultrasound or x-ray pelvimetry. Clinical studies have demonstrated that palpation and ultrasound are equally effective assessments of fetal weight. Routine use of ultrasound to predict fetal weight is not recommended (Sokol & Blackwell, 2003). When the uterus appears excessively large, either hydramnios, an oversized fetus, or multiple gestation must be considered as the possible cause.

When fetal weight is estimated to be 4500 g or more, a cesarean birth is usually planned. The best method of birth for an estimated fetal weight of 4000 to 4500 g is debatable. The discussion centers primarily on the incidence of shoulder dystocia during vaginal birth and the difficulty in accurately estimating the fetal weight. Unexpected shoulder dystocia during vaginal birth can be a grave problem. As an emergency measure, the physician or CNM may ask the nurse to assist the woman into the McRoberts maneuver (sharp flexion of the thighs toward the hips and abdomen) or to apply gentle suprapubic pressure in an attempt to aid in the birth of the fetal shoulders. Fundal pressure should never be used since it can further wedge the anterior shoulder under the symphysis pubis.

NURSING MANAGEMENT

Assist in identifying women who are at risk for carrying a large fetus and those who exhibit signs of macrosomia. Because these women are prime candidates for dystocia and its complications, frequently assess the FHR for indications of nonreassuring fetal status and evaluate the rates of cervical dilatation and fetal descent.

Apply the fetal monitor for continuous fetal evaluation. Early decelerations (caused by fetal head compression) could mean size disproportion at the bony inlet. Report any sign of labor dysfunction or nonreassuring fetal status to the physician or CNM immediately. Lack of fetal descent is another indicator that should alert the nurse to the possibility that the infant is too large for a vaginal birth.

The nurse provides support for the laboring woman and her partner and information about the implications of macrosomia and possible associated problems. During the birth, continue to provide support and encouragement to the woman or the couple.

Inspect macrosomic newborns after birth for cephalhematoma, Erb's palsy, and fractured clavicles, and inform the nursery staff of any problems so that the newborn can be closely monitored for cerebral, neurologic, and motor problems.

In a woman with a macrosomic fetus, the uterus has been stretched farther than it would have been with an average-sized fetus. The overstretching may lead to contractile problems during labor or after birth. After birth the overstretched uterus may not contract well (uterine atony) and will feel boggy (soft). In this case, uterine hemorrhage is likely. The fundus of the uterus is massaged to stimulate contraction; IV or IM Pitocin may be needed. Monitor maternal vital signs closely for deviation suggestive of shock.

CARE OF THE WOMAN WITH MULTIPLE GESTATION

In part due to advances in infertility treatments, the incidence of twins in the United States now accounts for 3% of all live births in the United States. The incidence of triplets and higher order multiples (more than three fetuses) has also increased. Incidence of spontaneous twins varies but is highest in African Americans, women of greater age and parity, and women who are tall and overweight. The incidence is low in the Asian population (Malone & D'Alton, 2004). The physiology of multiple gestation is discussed as "twins" in Chapter 7. ∞

During the prenatal period, visualization of two gestational sacs at 5 to 6 weeks, fundal height greater than expected for the length of gestation, and auscultation of heart rates that differ by at least 10 beats per minute are the most likely clues to multiple-gestation pregnancies. In addition, the alpha-fetoprotein level is usually elevated in twin or multiple-gestation pregnancies, and many women experience severe nausea and vomiting (due to elevated levels of the human chorionic gonadotropin [hCG] hormone) (Blackburn, 2003).

MATERNAL IMPLICATIONS

During pregnancy the woman may experience physical discomfort such as shortness of breath, dyspnea on exertion, backaches, and pedal edema. Other associated problems include urinary tract infections, preeclampsia, preterm labor, and placenta previa (Blackburn, 2003). Complications during labor include abnormal fetal presentations, uterine dysfunction, prolapsed cord, and hemorrhage at birth or shortly after (Blackburn, 2003).

FETAL-NEONATAL IMPLICATIONS

The perinatal mortality rate is approximately 10 times greater for twins than for a single fetus, and the morbidity rate is 5 times higher (Malone & D'Alton, 2004). The perinatal mor-

tality rate for monoamniotic siblings has been estimated to be as high as 50% to 60% (Malone & D'Alton, 2004). Fetal problems include decreased intrauterine growth rate for each fetus, increased incidence of fetal anomalies, increased risk of prematurity and its associated problems, abnormal presentations, and an increase in cerebral palsy (Blackburn, 2003). Twins are more likely to have long-term disabilities when compared to children who were singleton births.

CLINICAL THERAPY

Once the presence of twins has been detected, preventing and treating problems that infringe on the development and birth of normal fetuses is the most significant clinical goal. Prenatal visits are more frequent for women with twins than for those with one fetus. Women with multiple-gestation pregnancies need to understand the nutritional implications of multiple fetuses, the assessment of fetal activity, the signs of preterm labor, and the danger signs of pregnancy.

Serial ultrasounds are used to assess the growth of each fetus and provide early recognition of intrauterine growth restriction (IUGR). Some physicians believe that bed rest in the lateral position enhances uteroplacental-fetal blood flow and decreases the risk of preterm labor. Others question the value of bed rest for the prevention of periodic uterine contractions, which seem to precede preterm labor. More recent strategies include work leave, lifestyle modifications, and pelvic rest.

Testing usually begins at 30 to 34 weeks' gestation and may include NST, BPP, and Doppler ultrasound to assess umbilical blood waveforms (Malone & D'Alton, 2004). A reactive NST is associated with good fetal outcome if birth occurs within 1 week of the testing. The NST is done every 3 to 7 days until birth or until results become nonreactive. The BPP is also accurate in assessing fetal status with twin pregnancies. A biophysical profile of 8 or better for each fetus is considered reassuring, and weekly or biweekly BPPs and NSTs continue until birth (Malone & D'Alton, 2004).

Intrapartum management requires careful attention to maternal and fetal status. The mother should have an IV with a large-bore needle in place. Anesthesia and cross-matched blood should be readily available. The twins are monitored by continuous dual electronic fetal monitoring.

The decision about method of birth, which depends on a variety of factors, may not be made until labor occurs. The presence of maternal complications such as placenta previa, abruptio placentae, or severe preeclampsia usually indicates the need for cesarean birth. Fetal factors such as severe IUGR, preterm birth, fetal anomalies, nonreassuring fetal status, and unfavorable fetal position or presentation also require cesarean birth.

Any combination of presentations and positions can occur with multiple births. Figure 21–9 ● shows some

● FIGURE 21–9

A   B   C

D   E   F

Twins may be in any of these presentations while in utero.

possible presentations of twins. When the presenting fetus is in a nonvertex position, cesarean birth is usually indicated (Malone & D'Alton, 2004).

NURSING MANAGEMENT

Nursing Care in the Community

During pregnancy the woman may need counseling about diet and daily activities. Help her plan meals to meet her increased needs. A daily intake of 4000 kcal (minimum) and 135 g of protein is recommended for optimal weight gain and fetal growth. A prenatal vitamin and 1 mg of folic acid should also be taken daily. A weight gain of 40 to 50 lb, with a 15- to 20-lb weight gain by 20 weeks, has been recommended for women with multiple-gestation pregnancy (Malone & D'Alton, 2004).

Counseling about daily activities may include encouraging the woman to plan frequent rest periods during the day. The rest period is most effective if the woman rests in a side-lying position (which increases uteroplacental blood flow) and elevates her lower legs and feet to reduce edema. Back discomfort may be relieved by pelvic rocking, maintaining good posture, consistent use of a pregnancy belt to support the abdomen and lower back, and using good body mechanics when lifting objects and moving about.

Hospital-Based Nursing Care

During labor the FHRs of the siblings are monitored continuously by electronic fetal monitor (EFM). Electronic monitoring equipment now makes it possible to monitor the fetuses simultaneously. They are monitored throughout labor and vaginal birth or up to the time of abdominal incision if a cesarean is done.

The nurse must prepare to receive two or more newborns instead of one. This means duplicating everything, including resuscitation equipment, radiant warmers, and newborn identification papers and bracelets. Two or more physicians or nurses should be available for newborn resuscitation.

CARE OF THE WOMAN AND FETUS IN THE PRESENCE OF NONREASSURING FETAL STATUS

When the oxygen supply is insufficient to meet the physiologic needs of the fetus, a nonreassuring fetal status may result. This status may be transient or chronic, and may be prompted by a variety of factors. The most common are cord compression and uteroplacental insufficiency, possibly caused by preexisting maternal or fetal disease or placental abnormalities. If the resulting hypoxia persists and metabolic acidosis occurs, the situation could cause permanent damage to or be life threatening for the fetus.

The most common initial signs of nonreassuring fetal status are meconium-stained amniotic fluid and ominous FHR patterns such as persistent late decelerations (regardless of the depth of deceleration), persistent severe variable decelerations (especially if the return to baseline is prolonged), and prolonged decelerations. When these patterns are detected, **intrauterine resuscitation** (corrective measures used to optimize the oxygen exchange within the maternal-fetal circulation) should be started without delay. Treatment of maternal hypotension involves having the woman turn to a left lateral position (right lateral may also be tried), beginning an IV infusion or increasing the flow rate if an infusion is already in place, or, if cord prolapse is suspected, having the woman assume a knee-chest position. Position changes that result in an increase in the fetal heart rate should be maintained. A vaginal examination should be performed to attempt to detect a prolapsed cord. Uterine activity can be decreased by discontinuing IV Pitocin administration or administering a tocolytic agent (such as terbutaline) to decrease contraction frequency and intensity. Oxygen is also administered to the woman via facial mask.

Caregivers can obtain additional information about the condition of the fetus by fetal scalp blood sampling, fetal scalp stimulation, or fetal acoustic stimulation (see Fetal Acoustic Stimulation Test and Vibroacoustic Stimulation Test in Chapter 16 ∞). The management scheme for nonreassuring fetal status is illustrated in Figure 21–10 ⊙.

MATERNAL IMPLICATIONS

Indications of nonreassuring fetal status greatly increase the psychologic stress of a laboring woman and her family members. Professional staff members may become so involved in assessing fetal status and initiating corrective measures that they fail to provide the woman and her partner with explanations and emotional support. It is imperative to offer both. In many instances, if birth is not imminent, the woman must undergo cesarean birth. This method of birth may be a source of fear and frustration, too, if the couple prepared for a shared vaginal birth experience.

CLINICAL THERAPY

Treatment centers on improving the blood flow to the fetus by correcting maternal hypotension, decreasing the intensity and frequency of contractions if present, providing IV fluids to the woman as needed, administering oxygen, and gathering further information about fetal status. Fetal response to intrauterine resuscitation measures dictates subsequent actions.

NURSING MANAGEMENT

The nurse reviews the woman's prenatal history and notes the presence of any conditions (such as preeclampsia, diabetes, renal disease, or IUGR) that may be associated with decreased uteroplacental-fetal blood flow. When the membranes rupture, assess the FHR immediately and note the characteristics of the amniotic fluid. As labor progresses, be especially alert to suspicious changes in the FHR. At all times, encourage and support maternal positioning that maximizes utero-placental-fetal blood flow.

CARE OF THE WOMAN AND FETUS AT RISK DUE TO PLACENTAL PROBLEMS

The most common types of placental problems are abruptio placentae, placenta previa, and abnormalities in placental formation and structure. Because the placenta is highly vascular, problems are usually associated with maternal and possibly fetal hemorrhage. Abruptio placentae is a major emergency in labor and birth and requires rapid, effective interventions. Although placenta previa is primarily an antepartum problem, it is presented here for the sake of comparison. Table 21–1 identifies causes and sources of hemorrhage.

ABRUPTIO PLACENTAE

Abruptio placentae is the premature separation of a normally implanted placenta from the uterine wall. Premature separation is considered a catastrophic event because of the severity of the resulting hemorrhage. The incidence of abruptio placentae is approximately 1 in 100 births and occurs more frequently in pregnancies complicated by hypertension and cocaine abuse. The risk of recurrence is much higher than for the general population (Yeo, Ananth, & Vintzileos, 2004).

The cause of abruptio placentae is largely unknown. Theories have been proposed relating its occurrence to decreased blood flow to the placenta through the sinuses during the last trimester. Excessive intrauterine pressure caused by hydramnios or multiple-gestation pregnancy, maternal hypertension, cigarette smoking, alcohol ingestion, increased maternal age and parity, trauma, domestic

◯ FIGURE 21–10

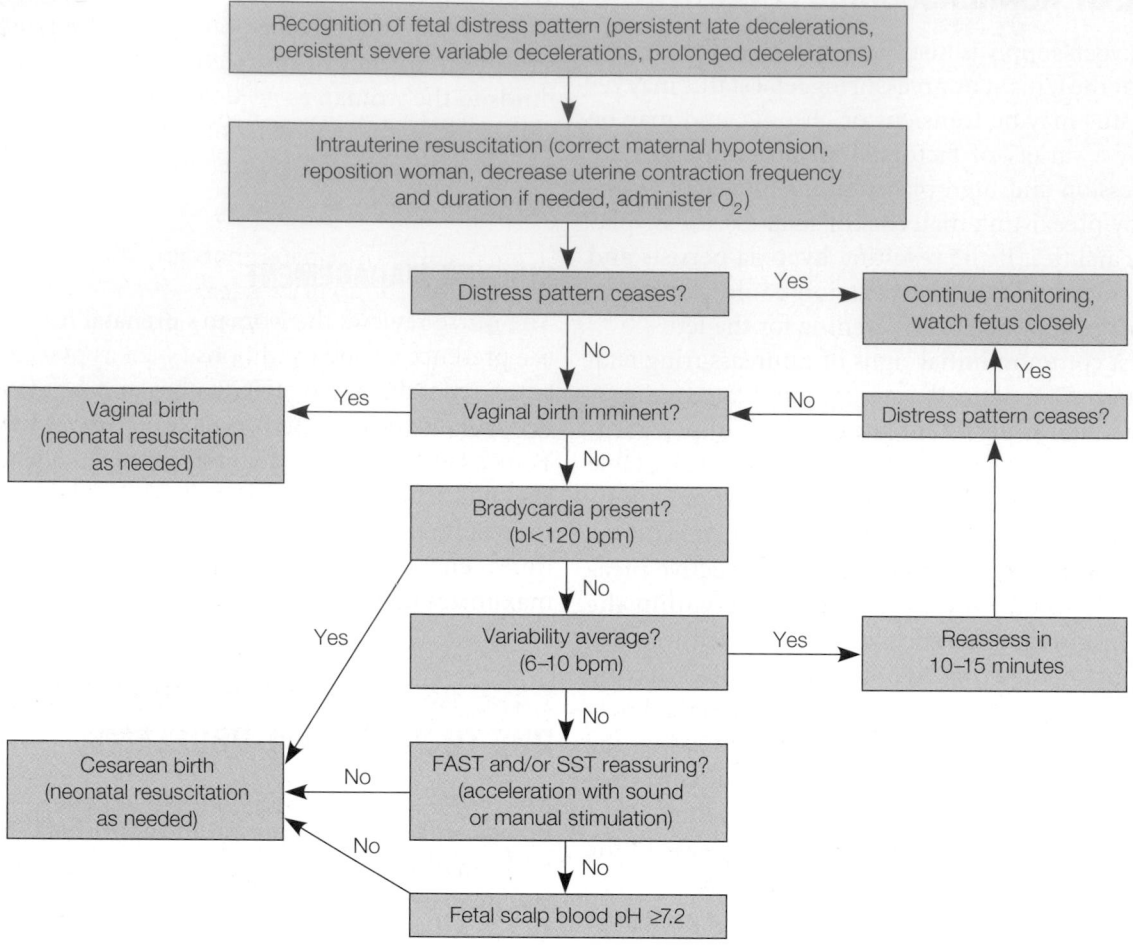

Intrapartum management of nonreassuring fetal status.

Note: bl = baseline; FAST = fetal acoustic stimulation test; SST = scalp stimulation test. Used with permission from Zuspan, F. P., & Quilligan, E. J. Handbook of obstetrics, gynecology, and primary care. Copyright 1998, Mosby. Reprinted with permission from Elsevier Science.

violence and abuse, nonvertex presentation, and sudden changes in intrauterine pressure (as with amniotomy) have been suggested as contributing factors (Sheiner, Shoham-Vardi, Hallak et al., 2003).

Abruptio placentae is subdivided into three types (Figure 21–11 ◯):

- **Marginal.** The placenta separates at its edges, the blood passes between the fetal membranes and the uterine wall, and the blood escapes vaginally (also called marginal sinus rupture).

- **Central.** The placenta separates centrally, and the blood is trapped between the placenta and the uterine wall. Entrapment of the blood results in concealed bleeding.

- **Complete.** Massive vaginal bleeding is seen in the presence of total separation.

In severe cases of central abruptio placentae, the blood invades the myometrial tissues between the muscle fibers.

This occurrence accounts for the uterine irritability that is a significant sign of abruptio placentae. If hemorrhage continues, eventually the uterus turns entirely blue because the muscle fibers are filled with blood. After birth the uterus contracts poorly. This condition is known as *Couvelaire uterus* and frequently necessitates hysterectomy.

Maternal Implications

As a result of the damage to the uterine wall and the retroplacental clotting with central abruption, large amounts of thromboplastin are released into the maternal blood supply. This thromboplastin triggers the development of disseminated intravascular coagulation (DIC) and resultant hypofibrinogenemia. Fibrinogen levels, which are ordinarily elevated in pregnancy, may drop in minutes to the point at which blood will no longer coagulate (Blackburn, 2003). Postpartum problems depend in large part on the severity of the intrapartum bleeding, coagulation defects (DIC),

TABLE 21–1 ❖ Causes and Sources of Hemorrhage

Causes and Sources	Signs and Symptoms
Antepartum Period	
Abortion	Vaginal bleeding
	Intermittent uterine contractions
	Rupture of membranes
Placenta previa	Painless vaginal bleeding after seventh month
Abruptio placentae	
Partial	Vaginal bleeding: no increase in uterine pain
Severe	Vaginal bleeding may or may not be present
	Extreme tenderness of abdominal area
	Rigid, boardlike abdomen
	Increase in size of abdomen
Intrapartum Period	
Placenta previa	Bright-red vaginal bleeding
Abruptio placentae	Same signs and symptoms listed earlier
Uterine atony in stage 3	Bright-red vaginal bleeding
	Ineffectual contractility
Postpartum Period	
Uterine atony	Boggy uterus
	Dark vaginal bleeding
	Presence of clots
Retained placental fragments	Boggy uterus
	Dark vaginal bleeding
	Presence of clots
Lacerations of cervix or vagina	Firm uterus
	Bright red blood

hypofibrinogenemia, and time between separation and birth. Moderate to severe hemorrhage results in hemorrhagic shock, which may prove fatal to the mother if it is not rapidly reversed. In the postpartum period, women with this disorder are at risk for hemorrhage and renal failure due to shock, vascular spasm, intravascular clotting, or a combination of these factors.

Fetal-Neonatal Implications

The combined perinatal mortality and morbidity associated with abruptio placentae ranges from 20% to 40% with a mortality rate of 12% (Yeo et al., 2004). In severe cases in which most of the placenta has separated, the infant mortality rate is near 100%. In less severe separation, fetal outcome depends on the level of maturity and the length of time to birth. The most serious complications in the newborn arise from preterm labor, anemia, and hypoxia. If fetal hypoxia progresses unchecked, irreversible brain damage or fetal demise may result. Thorough assessment and prompt action on the part of the health team can improve both fetal and maternal outcomes.

Clinical Therapy

Because of the risk of DIC, evaluating the results of coagulation tests is imperative. In DIC, fibrinogen levels and platelet counts usually decrease; prothrombin times and partial thromboplastin times are normal to prolonged. If the values are not markedly abnormal, serial testing may be helpful in establishing an abnormal trend indicative of coagulopathy. Another test determines levels of fibrin-degradation products; these values rise with DIC.

After establishing the diagnosis, immediate priorities are maintaining the cardiovascular status of the mother and developing a plan for the birth of the fetus. The birth

● **FIGURE 21–11**

A   B   C

Abruptio placentae. **A,** Marginal abruption with external hemorrhage. **B,** Central abruption with concealed hemorrhage. **C,** Complete separation.

method selected depends on the condition of the woman and fetus and the speed in which the birth will occur; in many circumstances, cesarean birth will be the safest option.

If the separation is mild and the pregnancy is near term, labor may be induced and the fetus born vaginally with as little trauma as possible. If rupture of membranes and Pitocin infusion by pump do not initiate labor, a cesarean birth is required. A long delay would raise the risk of increased hemorrhage, with resulting hypofibrinogenemia.

Supportive actions to decrease the risk of DIC include typing and crossmatching for blood transfusions (at least 4 units), evaluating the clotting mechanism, and providing intravenous fluids (Yeo et al., 2004).

In cases of moderate to severe placental separation, a cesarean birth is done concurrently with treatment of hypofibrinogenemia by intravenous infusion of cryoprecipitate or plasma. Vaginal birth is impossible with a Couvelaire uterus, because the uterus would not contract properly in labor, and a hysterectomy is often needed.

The hypovolemia that accompanies severe abruptio placentae is life threatening. If the fetus is alive, emergency cesarean birth is the method of choice. With a stillborn fetus, vaginal birth is preferable if bleeding has stabilized, unless maternal shock from hemorrhage has already occurred. Central venous pressure (CVP) monitoring may be needed to evaluate intravenous fluid replacement. A normal CVP of 5 to 12 cm H_2O is the goal (Poole, 2004). The CVP is evaluated hourly, and results are communicated to the physician. Elevations of CVP may indicate fluid overload and pulmonary edema. Laboratory testing is ordered to provide ongoing data regarding hemoglobin, hematocrit, and coagulation status. The hematocrit is maintained through the administration of packed red blood cells or whole blood. Measures are taken to stimulate labor to prevent DIC. An amniotomy may be performed, and Pitocin is given to hasten birth. Progressive dilatation and effacement usually occur.

Nursing Management

Electronic monitoring of the uterine contractions and resting tone between contractions provides information about the labor pattern and effectiveness of the Pitocin induction. Since uterine resting tone is frequently increased with abruptio placentae, it must be evaluated frequently for further increase. Abdominal girth measurements may be ordered hourly and are obtained by placing a tape measure around the maternal abdomen at the level of the umbilicus. Another method of evaluating uterine size, which increases as more bleeding occurs at the site of abruption, involves placing a mark at the top of the uterine fundus; the distance from the symphysis pubis to the mark may be measured hourly. Overdisten-

tion of the uterus can lead to a ruptured uterus, another life-threatening complication.

NURSING PRACTICE

The amount of bleeding per vagina is no guide to the degree of placental separation.

PLACENTA PREVIA

In **placenta previa** the placenta is implanted in the lower uterine segment rather than the upper portion of the uterus. This implantation may be on a portion of the lower segment or over the internal cervical os. As the lower uterine segment contracts and dilates in the later weeks of pregnancy, the placental villi are torn from the uterine wall, thus exposing the uterine sinuses at the placental site. Bleeding begins, but because its amount depends on the number of sinuses exposed, initially it may be either scanty or profuse (Figure 21–12 ●).

Placenta previa has been previously categorized as being total (the internal os is completely covered), partial (the internal os is partially covered), marginal (the edge of the placenta is covered), or low-lying (the placenta is implanted in the lower uterine segment in close proximity to but not covering the os). With the advent of diagnostic ultrasonography, a new classification of placenta previa is being proposed. The new classification system includes placenta previa (placenta covers part or all of the internal cervical os in the third trimester), marginal previa (edge of the placenta is within 2 to 3 cm of the internal cervical os but does not

● **FIGURE 21–12**

A   B

Classification of placenta previa. **A,** Marginal placental implantation. **B,** Placenta previa.

cover it), and low-lying placenta (reserved for those situations in which the exact relationship of placenta to the cervical os has not been determined) (Clark, 2004; Poole, 2004).

The cause of placenta previa is unknown. It occurs in about 4 in every 1000 births. Women with a previous history of placenta previa have an increased risk of developing another previa in future pregnancies. Other factors associated with placenta previa are multiparity, increasing age, placenta accreta, defective development of blood vessels in the decidua, a large placenta, smoking and cocaine use in pregnancy, previous cesarean section or abortion, and male fetus (Faiz & Ananth, 2003).

Fetal-Neonatal Implications

The prognosis for the fetus depends on the extent of placenta previa. In cases of a marginal previa or a low-lying placenta, the woman may be allowed to labor. Changes in the FHR and meconium staining of the amniotic fluid may be apparent. In a profuse bleeding episode, the fetus is compromised and suffers some hypoxia. FHR monitoring is imperative when the woman is admitted, particularly if a vaginal birth is anticipated, because the presenting part of the fetus may obstruct the flow of blood from the placenta or umbilical cord. If nonreassuring fetal status occurs, cesarean birth is indicated. Women who are diagnosed with a complete or partial previa will undergo a cesarean birth since the risk of intrapartum hemorrhage is high. After birth, blood sampling should be done to determine whether the intrauterine bleeding episodes of the woman have caused anemia in the newborn.

Clinical Therapy

The goal of medical care is to identify the cause of bleeding and to provide treatment that will ensure birth of a mature newborn. Indirect diagnosis is made by localizing the placenta through tests that require no vaginal examination, such as the ultrasound scan. Vaginal examinations should never be performed on a woman with bleeding since the examiner's fingers could perforate the placenta if cervical dilatation has occurred. If placenta previa is ruled out, a vaginal examination can be performed with a speculum to determine the cause of bleeding (such as cervical lesions).

The differential diagnosis of placental or cervical bleeding takes careful consideration. Table 21–2 provides a comparison of the signs and symptoms of placenta previa and abruptio placentae. Partial separation of the placenta may also present with painless bleeding, and true placenta previa may not demonstrate overt bleeding until labor begins, thus confusing the diagnosis.

Care of the woman with painless late-gestation bleeding depends on (1) the week of gestation during which the first bleeding episode occurs and (2) the amount of bleed-

TABLE 21–2 ✥ **Differential Signs and Symptoms of Placenta Previa and Abruptio Placentae**

	Placenta Previa	Abruptio Placentae
Onset	Quiet	Sudden
Bleeding	External	External or concealed
Color of blood	Bright red	Dark venous
Anemia	= Blood loss	> Apparent blood loss
Shock	= Blood loss	> Apparent blood loss
Toxemia	Absent	May be present
Pain	Only during labor	Severe and steady
Uterine tenderness	Absent	Present
Uterine tone	Soft and relaxed	Firm to stony hard
Uterine contour	Normal	May enlarge and change shape
Fetal heart tones	Usually present	Present or absent
Engagement	Absent	May be present
Presentation	May be abnormal	No relationship

Data from Oxorn, H. (1986). Human labor and birth (5th ed., p. 507). Norwalk, CT: Appleton & Lange.

ing (Figure 21–13 ⦿). If the pregnancy is less than 37 weeks' gestation, expectant management is used to delay birth until about 37 weeks' gestation to allow the fetus to mature. Expectant management involves stringent regulation of the following:

1. Bed rest with bathroom privileges as long as the woman is not bleeding
2. No vaginal examinations
3. Monitoring blood loss, pain, and uterine contractility
4. Evaluating FHR with an external fetal monitor
5. Monitoring maternal vital signs
6. Complete laboratory evaluation: hemoglobin, hematocrit, Rh factor, and urinalysis
7. Intravenous fluid (lactated Ringer's solution)
8. Two units of crossmatched blood available for transfusion

If frequent, recurrent, or profuse bleeding persists, or if fetal well-being appears threatened, a cesarean birth may be performed.

● **FIGURE 21-13**

Management of placenta previa.

Data from Barker, R. K., Fields, D. H., & Kaufman, S. A. (1990). Quick reference to OB-GYN procedures (3rd ed.). New York: Lippincott/Harper & Row.

NURSING MANAGEMENT

NURSING ASSESSMENT AND DIAGNOSIS

Assessment of the woman with placenta previa must be ongoing to prevent or treat complications that are potentially lethal to the mother and fetus. Painless, bright-red vaginal bleeding is the most accurate diagnostic sign of placenta previa. If this sign develops during the last 3 months of pregnancy, placenta previa should always be considered until ruled out by ultrasound examination. The first bleeding episode is generally scanty. If no vaginal examinations are performed, it often subsides spontaneously. However, each subsequent hemorrhage is more profuse.

The uterus remains soft, and if labor begins, it relaxes fully between contractions. The FHR usually remains stable unless profuse hemorrhage and maternal shock occur. As a result of the placement of the placenta, the fetal presenting part is often unengaged, and transverse lie is common.

Assess blood loss, pain, and uterine contractility both subjectively and objectively. Maternal vital signs and the results of blood and urine tests provide additional data about the woman's condition. Evaluate the FHR with continuous external fetal monitoring. Another pressing nursing responsibility is to observe and verify the family's ability to cope with the anxiety associated with an unknown outcome.

Nursing diagnoses that may apply include the following:

- *Fluid Volume Deficit* related to hypovolemia secondary to excessive blood loss

- *Risk for Impaired Gas Exchange of the Fetus* related to decreased blood volume and maternal hypotension

- *Anxiety* related to concern for own personal status and the baby's safety

PLANNING AND IMPLEMENTATION

Monitor the woman and her fetus to determine the status of the bleeding and the responses of the mother and baby. Vital signs, intake and output, and other pertinent assessments must be made frequently. Use the electronic monitor tracing to evaluate fetal status. Have a whole-blood setup ready for IV infusion and establish a patent IV line before caregivers undertake any intrusive procedures. Monitor maternal vital signs every 15 minutes in the absence of hemorrhage and every 5 minutes with active hemorrhage. Connect the external tocodynamometer to the maternal abdomen to monitor uterine activity continuously.

Providing emotional support for the family is an important nursing care goal. During active bleeding, direct the assessments and management toward physical support. However, emotional aspects need to be addressed simultaneously. Explain the assessments and treatment measures needed. Make time for questions, and act as an advocate in obtaining information for the family. Offer emotional support by staying with the family and using touch.

Promoting neonatal physiologic adaptation is another important nursing responsibility. Check the newborn's hemoglobin, cell volume, and erythrocyte count immediately and then monitor them closely. The newborn may require oxygen, administration of blood, and admission into a special care nursery. See "Nursing Care Plan: Hemorrhage in the Third Trimester."

EVALUATION

Expected outcomes of nursing care include the following:

- The cause of hemorrhage is recognized promptly and corrective measures are taken.
- The woman's vital signs remain in the normal range.
- Any other complications are recognized and treated early.
- The family understands what has happened and the implications and associated problems of placenta previa.
- The woman and her baby have a safe labor and birth.

OTHER PLACENTAL PROBLEMS

Other problems of the placenta are presented in Table 21–3. Nursing care of the woman with bleeding is addressed fully in "Nursing Care Plan: Hemorrhage in the Third Trimester."

CARE OF THE WOMAN AND FETUS WITH A PROLAPSED UMBILICAL CORD

A **prolapsed umbilical cord** results when the umbilical cord precedes the fetal presenting part. When this occurs, pressure is placed on the umbilical cord as it is trapped between the presenting part and the maternal pelvis. Consequently the vessels carrying blood to and from the fetus are compressed (Figure 21–14 ●). Prolapse of the cord may occur with rupture of the membranes if the presenting part is not well engaged in the pelvis.

MATERNAL IMPLICATIONS

Although a prolapsed cord does not directly precipitate physical alterations in the woman, her immediate concern for the baby creates enormous stress. The woman may need to deal with some unusual interventions, a cesarean birth, and, in some circumstances, the death of her baby.

● **FIGURE 21–14**

Prolapse of the umbilical cord.

FETAL-NEONATAL IMPLICATIONS

Compression of the cord results in decreased blood flow and leads to nonreassuring fetal status. If labor is under way, the cord is compressed further with each contraction. If the pressure on the cord is not relieved, the fetus will die.

CLINICAL THERAPY

Preventing prolapse of the cord is the preferred medical approach. A laboring woman with a confirmed rupture of membranes will be kept horizontal, usually in bed, until the fetal head is well engaged and the risk of a prolapse is significantly decreased. If a prolapse occurs, relieving the compression on the cord is critical to fetal outcome. The medical and nursing team must work together to facilitate birth.

Bed rest is indicated for all laboring women with a history of ruptured membranes, until engagement with no cord prolapse has been documented. Furthermore, with spontaneous rupture of membranes or amniotomy, the FHR should be auscultated for at least a full minute and at the beginning and end of contractions for several contractions. If fetal bradycardia is detected on auscultation, a vaginal examination is performed to rule out cord prolapse. In the presence of cord prolapse, electronic monitor tracings show severe, moderate, or prolonged variable decelerations with baseline bradycardia.

If a loop of cord is discovered, the examiner's gloved fingers must remain in the vagina to provide firm pressure on the fetal head (to relieve compression) until the physician or CNM arrives. This is a lifesaving measure. The mother is given oxygen via face mask, and the FHR is monitored to determine whether the cord compression is adequately relieved.

The force of gravity can be employed to relieve umbilical cord compression. The woman assumes the knee-chest

(text continues on page 522)

MEDIALINK Care Plan Activity: Prevention of Cord Prolapse

NURSING CARE PLAN

HEMORRHAGE IN THE THIRD TRIMESTER

Intervention	Rationale	Expected Outcome
1. Nursing Diagnosis: High Risk for Fluid Volume Deficit related to excessive vascular loss during pregnancy		
NIC Intervention: **Fluid management:** Promotion of fluid balance and prevention of complications resulting from abnormal or undesired fluid levels		**NOC Outcome:** **Fluid balance:** Balance of water in the intracellular and extracellular compartments of the body
Goal: Patient will not experience signficant fluid volume deficit during the third trimester of pregnancy.		
■ Monitor vital signs (i.e., temperature—normal range is 96.8–100.4 °F, pulse—normal is 60–80, respirations—normal is 12–20, blood pressure—normal range is 110/70 to 138/88, central venous pressure—normal range is 5–10 mm H_2O). Compare present blood pressure with woman's baseline blood pressure. Note pulse pressure.	■ Any deviations in a patient's baseline vital signs could indicate intravascular fluctuations.	■ The patient will show signs of adequate fluid volume during pregnancy as evidenced by vital signs within normal limits, capillary refill < 3 seconds, adequate sensorium, and urine output > 30 mL/hr.
■ Instruct patient on initiating pad counts. Teach patient how to weigh pads and chux, with each gram = to approximately 1 mL of blood loss. ■ Report amount of blood loss within a specific period of time (e.g., 50 mL of bright-red blood on pad in 20 minutes).	■ The combination of weighing and counting pads and chux assists medical personnel in determining patient blood loss.	
■ Monitor urinary output hourly and measure urine specific gravity (normal: 1.010–1.025).	■ A decrease in urinary output (< 30 ml/hr) and an increase in specific gravity suggest dehydration and a need for an increase in fluid intake.	
■ Palpate bilateral peripheral pulses (normal: equal and strong) and note capillary refill (normal: < 3 seconds). Also, assess skin color and temperature (normal: pink, warm, dry, and intact).	■ Helps determine signs of circulatory loss or hypovolemic shock that include weak pulses, capillary refill > 3 seconds, skin color that is cyanotic or pallor, and skin temperature that is cool and clammy.	
■ Assess mental status at frequent intervals.	■ Excessive blood loss can lead to changes in mentation.	
■ Assess patient for signs and symptoms of disseminated intravascular coagulation.	■ Provides vital information on maternal status.	
■ Instruct patient on importance of strict bed rest and avoidance of any sexual activity that may lead to orgasm.	■ Bleeding may cease with limited activity. Pressure on the abdomen and orgasms can stimulate uterine activity, thereby causing bleeding.	
■ Monitor fetal status and uterine activity by continuous fetal monitoring.	■ May determine origin of bleeding and fetal well-being.	
Collaborative: Collect and review blood work: complete blood count (CBC), type and crossmatch, Rh titer, fibrinogen levels, platelet count, activated partial thromboplastin time (APTT), prothrombin time (PT), and hCG levels.	■ Determines blood loss and need for intervention if blood work is abnormal.	
■ Administer appropriate isotonic IV solutions and blood products (e.g., plasma expanders, whole blood, serum albumin, or packed red blood cells) as ordered by physician.	■ Reverses shock symptoms by increasing blood volume.	
■ Insert Foley catheter.	■ Close monitoring of urinary output will aid in determining adequate renal perfusion.	

HEMORRHAGE IN THE THIRD TRIMESTER

Intervention	Rationale	Expected Outcome
2. Nursing Diagnosis: Risk for Ineffective Tissue Perfusion (uteroplacental) related to hypovolemia secondary to excessive maternal blood loss		
NIC Intervention: **Electronic fetal monitoring:** Electronic evaluation of fetal heart rate response to movement, external stimuli, or uterine contractions during antepartum testing		**NOC Outcome:** **Circulation status:** Extent to which blood flows unobstructed, unidirectionally, and at an appropriate pressure through large vessels of the systemic and pulmonary circuits
Goal: The fetus will have no evidence of hypoxia during pregnancy.		
■ Assess maternal vital signs. ■ Monitor fetal heart tones continuously, assessing for variability, accelerations, and decelerations, and record. ■ Encourage patient to adhere to a strict lateral-lying bed rest regimen. ■ Assess fundal height. ■ Assess labor progression by determining cervical dilatation and effacement if contractions are present. **Collaborative:** ■ Perform scalp stimulation to assess fetal accelerations. ■ Assess amniotic fluid for meconium. ■ Assist physician during ultrasonography and amniocentesis for lecithin/sphingomyelin [LS] ratio sample.	■ Closely monitoring maternal physiologic status and circulatory status will assist in determining if an episode of bleeding has occurred and allow for interventions to protect maternal and fetal well-being. ■ Continuous electronic fetal monitoring will aid in detecting signs of fetal hypoxia and allow time for appropriate intervention. ■ Promotes good placental/fetal oxygen exchange because pressure on the inferior vena cava is relieved. ■ Determines an approximate gestational age. ■ This provides information on maternal labor status. ■ FHR acceleration is considered 15 beats above the baseline lasting for 15 seconds and is indicative of fetal well-being. ■ Impaired gas exchange relaxes fetal intestinal motility, causing expulsion of meconium into amniotic fluid. ■ Determines viability and alerts appropriate medical personnel of fetal age if birth is imminent.	■ Fetus will demonstrate adequate tissue perfusion as evidenced by fetal heart tones that remain within 120–160 bpm, long-term variability and short-term variability present, positive periodic changes (no variable or late decelerations), and fetal scalp blood pH > 7.25.
3. Nursing Diagnosis: Fear/Anxiety related to personal and fetal well-being secondary to third-trimester hemorrhage		
NIC Intervention: **Anxiety reduction:** Minimizing apprehension, dread, foreboding, or uneasiness related to an unidentified source of anticipated danger		**NOC Outcome:** **Fear control:** Ability to eliminate or reduce disabling feelings of alarm aroused by an identifiable source
Goal: The patient will verbalize a decrease in fear and anxiety.		
■ Maintain frequent contact with patient and family members. ■ Provide patient with accurate, reliable information concerning diagnosis and prognosis. ■ Allow patient and family members to verbalize origination of fears. ■ Explain all procedures in an easy-to-understand, nonthreatening manner, and allow patient and family members to ask questions.	■ Establishes trust with patient and family members, and so the patient will not feel alone or abandoned. ■ Fear and anxiety will lessen when patient is informed of health status and is allowed to make decisions based on present situation. ■ Recognizing the origination of fear gives the patient and family the appropriate tool to begin the process of developing coping strategies for dealing with the fears. ■ Accurate information prepares patient and family members for the impending procedures, thereby reducing fear of the unknown.	■ The patient will actively seek information about diagnosis and prognosis. ■ The patient and family members develop appropriate coping strategies that decrease fear and anxiety.

TABLE 21–3 ❖ Placental and Umbilical Cord Variations

Placental Variation	Maternal Implications	Fetal-Neonatal Implications
Succenturiate Placenta One or more accessory lobes of fetal villi will develop on the placenta.	Postpartum hemorrhage from retained lobe	None, as long as all parts of the placenta remain attached until after birth of the fetus
Circumvallate Placenta A double fold of chorion and amnion form a ring around the umbilical cord, on the fetal side of the placenta.	Increased incidence of late abortion, antepartum hemorrhage, and preterm labor	Intrauterine growth restriction, prematurity, fetal death
Battledore Placenta The umbilical cord is inserted at or near the placental margin.	Increased incidence of preterm labor and bleeding	Prematurity, nonreassuring fetal status
Velamentous Insertion of the Umbilical Cord The vessels of the umbilical cord divide some distance from the placenta in the placental membranes.	Hemorrhage if one of the vessels is torn	Nonreassuring fetal status, hemorrhage

position or the bed is adjusted to the Trendelenburg position, and the woman is transported to the delivery or operating room in this position (Figure 21–15 ◉). The nurse must remember that the cord may be occultly prolapsed with an actual loop extending into the vagina or lying alongside the presenting part. It may be pulsating strongly or so weakly that it is difficult to determine upon palpation of the cord whether the fetus is alive.

NURSING MANAGEMENT

Because there are few outward signs of cord prolapse, each pregnant woman is advised to call her physician or CNM when the membranes rupture and to go to the office, clinic, or birthing facility. A sterile vaginal examination determines if there is danger of cord prolapse. If the presenting part is well engaged, the risk of cord prolapse is minimal, and the woman

● FIGURE 21–15

Knee-chest position is used to relieve cord compression during cord prolapse emergency.

may ambulate as desired. If the presenting part is not well engaged, bed rest is recommended to prevent cord prolapse.

Because cord prolapse can be associated with fetal death, some physicians and CNMs insist that bed rest be maintained after rupture of membranes regardless of fetal engagement. This can lead to conflict if the laboring woman and her partner do not hold the same opinions. Ease this situation by helping the physician or CNM and the couple communicate.

During labor any alteration of the FHR or the presence of meconium in the amniotic fluid indicates the need to assess for cord prolapse. Vaginal birth is possible with prolapsed cord if the cervix is completely dilated and pelvic measurements are adequate.

If these conditions are not present, cesarean birth is the method of choice. The woman is transported to the operating room, and the examiner continues to relieve the pressure on the cord until the infant is born.

CARE OF THE WOMAN AND FETUS AT RISK DUE TO AMNIOTIC FLUID-RELATED COMPLICATIONS

AMNIOTIC FLUID EMBOLISM

In the presence of a small tear in the amnion or chorion high in the uterus, a small amount of amniotic fluid may leak into the chorionic plate and enter the maternal system as an **amniotic fluid embolism**. The fluid can also enter at areas of placental separation or cervical tears. Under pressure from the contracting uterus, the fluid is driven into the maternal circulation and then the maternal lungs. The more debris in the amniotic fluid (such as meconium), the greater the maternal problems. This condition frequently occurs during or after the birth when the woman has had a difficult, rapid labor.

Maternal Implications

The woman with an amniotic fluid embolism experiences sudden onset of respiratory distress, circulatory collapse, acute hemorrhage, and cor pulmonale as the embolism blocks the vessels of the lungs. She exhibits dyspnea and cyanosis leading to hemorrhagic shock and coma. Birth must be facilitated immediately to obtain a live fetus.

Clinical Therapy

Any woman exhibiting chest pain, dyspnea, cyanosis, frothy sputum, tachycardia, hypotension, and massive hemorrhage requires the cooperation of every member of the health team if her life is to be saved. Medical interventions are supportive. Recovery is contingent on return of the mother's cardiovascular and respiratory stability. If necessary a cesarean birth is performed.

Nursing Management

In the absence of the physician or CNM, the nurse administers oxygen under positive pressure until medical help arrives. An intravenous line is quickly established. If respiratory and cardiac arrest occurs, initiate cardiopulmonary resuscitation (CPR) immediately.

Ready the equipment necessary for blood transfusion and for the insertion of the CVP line. As the blood volume is replaced, using fresh whole blood to provide clotting factors, the CVP must be monitored frequently. In the presence of cor pulmonale, fluid overload could easily occur.

HYDRAMNIOS

Hydramnios (also called polyhydramnios) occurs when there is more than 2000 mL of amniotic fluid or amniotic fluid index of 20 cm or greater (Jasper, 2004). The exact cause of hydramnios is unknown; however, it is associated with major congenital anomalies (Laughlin & Knuppel, 2003). In addition to the fetal implications, the maternal implications include significantly increased incidence of cesarean birth.

During the second half of the pregnancy, the fetus begins to swallow and inspire amniotic fluid and to urinate, which contributes to the amount of amniotic fluid present. In cases of hydramnios, no pathology has been found in the amniotic epithelium. However, hydramnios is associated with fetal malformations that affect the fetal swallowing mechanism and neurologic disorders in which the fetal meninges are exposed in the amniotic cavity. This condition is also found in cases of anencephaly, in which the fetus is thought to urinate excessively due to overstimulation of the cerebrospinal centers. When monozygotic twins manifest hydramnios, it is because the twin with the increased blood volume urinates excessively. The weight of the placenta has been found to be increased in some cases of hydramnios, indicating that increased functioning of the placental tissue may be a factor.

There are two types of hydramnios: chronic and acute. In the chronic type, the fluid volume gradually increases and is a problem of the third trimester. Most cases are of this variety. In acute cases, the volume increases rapidly over a period of a few days. The acute type is usually diagnosed between 20 and 24 weeks' gestation.

Maternal Implications

When the amount of amniotic fluid is 3000 mL or more, the woman experiences shortness of breath and edema in the lower extremities from compression of the vena cava. Milder forms of hydramnios occur more frequently and are associated with minimal symptoms. Hydramnios is associated with maternal disorders such as diabetes and Rh sensitization and with multiple-gestation pregnancies.

If the amniotic fluid is removed rapidly before birth, abruptio placentae can result from too sudden a change in the size of the uterus. Because of overdistention of uterine muscles, uterine dysfunction can occur in the intrapartum period, and the incidence of postpartum hemorrhage increases.

Fetal-Neonatal Implications

Fetal malformations and preterm birth are common with hydramnios; thus, the perinatal mortality rate is fairly high. Prolapsed cord can occur when the membranes rupture, a further complication for the fetus. The incidence of malpresentations also increases.

Clinical Therapy

Hydramnios is managed with supportive treatment unless the intensity of the woman's distress and symptoms dictates otherwise. If the accumulation of amniotic fluid is severe enough to cause maternal dyspnea and pain, hospitalization and removal of the excessive fluid are required. Fluid can be removed vaginally or by amniocentesis. The dangers of performing the technique vaginally are prolapsed cord and the inability to remove the fluid slowly. If amniocentesis is performed, it should be done with the aid of sonography to prevent inadvertent damage to the fetus and placenta. The fluid should be removed slowly to prevent abruption.

Nursing Management

Hydramnios should be suspected when the fundal height increases out of proportion to the gestational age. As the amount of fluid increases, the nurse may have difficulty in palpating the fetus and auscultating the FHR. In more severe cases, the maternal abdomen appears extremely tense and tight on inspection. On sonography, large spaces can be seen between the fetus and the uterine wall.

When amniocentesis is performed, it is vital to maintain sterile technique to prevent infection. Offer support to the couple by explaining the procedure to them.

If the fetus has been diagnosed with a congenital defect in utero or is born with a defect, the family needs psychologic support. Collaborate with social services to offer the family this additional help.

OLIGOHYDRAMNIOS

Oligohydramnios, in which the amount of amniotic fluid is severely reduced and concentrated, is a rare maternal finding. Many researchers agree that less than 500 mL of amniotic fluid at term and/or amniotic fluid index of less than 5 cm is considered oligohydramnios (Jasper, 2004). The exact cause of this condition is unknown. It is found in cases of postmaturity, with IUGR secondary to placental insufficiency, and in fetal conditions associated with major renal malformations, including renal aplasia with dysplastic kidneys and obstructive lesions of the lower urinary tract, and is associated with poor lung development (Laughlin & Knuppel, 2003). If oligohydramnios occurs in the first part of pregnancy, there is a danger of fetal adhesions (one part of the fetus may adhere to another part).

Maternal Implications

Labor can be dysfunctional, and progress is slow.

Fetal-Neonatal Implications

During the gestational period, fetal skin and skeletal abnormalities may occur because fetal movement is impaired as a result of reduced amniotic fluid volume. Because there is less fluid available for the fetus to use during fetal breathing movements, pulmonary hypoplasia may develop. During the labor and birth, the oligohyramnios reduces the cushioning effect for the umbilical cord, and cord compression is more likely to occur. Decreased amniotic fluid also contributes to fetal head compression.

Clinical Therapy

During the antepartum period, oligohydramnios may be suspected when the uterus does not increase in size according to the dates, the fetus is easily palpated and outlined by the examiner, and the fetus is not ballotable. The fetus can be assessed by biophysical profiles, nonstress tests, and serial ultrasounds. During labor the fetus is monitored by continuous EFM to detect cord compression, which is indicated by variable decelerations. Some clinicians advocate the use of an amnioinfusion (a transcervical instillation of 500 mL of warmed sterile saline, followed by a continuous infusion rate of 100 to 200 mL/hr) after membranes have ruptured to decrease the frequency and severity of variable decelerations in the FHR during labor (Parer & Nageotte, 2004). The infusion of saline provides more fluid for the umbilical cord to float in and thereby lessens or prevents cord compression.

Nursing Management

Continuous electronic fetal monitoring is an important part of the assessment during the labor and birth. Evaluate the EFM tracing for the presence of variable decelerations or other nonreassuring signs (such as increasing or decreasing baseline, decreased variability, or presence of late decelerations). If variable decelerations are noted, the woman's position can be changed (to relieve pressure on the umbilical cord), and the physician or CNM should be notified. After the birth, the newborn is evaluated for signs of congenital anomalies, pulmonary hypoplasia, and postmaturity.

CARE OF THE WOMAN WITH CEPHALOPELVIC DISPROPORTION

The birth passage includes the maternal bony pelvis, beginning at the pelvic inlet and ending at the pelvic outlet, and the maternal soft tissues within these anatomic areas. A contracture (narrowed diameter) in any of the described areas can result in **cephalopelvic disproportion (CPD)** if the fetus is larger than the pelvic diameters. Abnormal fetal presentations and positions occur in CPD as the fetus moves to accommodate its passage through the maternal pelvis.

The gynecoid and anthropoid pelvic types are usually adequate for vertex birth, but the android and platypelloid types are predisposed to CPD. Certain combinations of types also can result in pelvic diameters inadequate for vertex birth. (See Chapter 17 or a description of pelvic types and their implications for childbirth. ∞)

TYPES OF CONTRACTURES

The pelvic inlet is contracted if the shortest anterior-posterior diameter is less than 10 cm or the greatest transverse diameter is less than 12 cm. The anterior-posterior diameter may be approximated by measuring the diagonal conjugate, which in the contracted inlet is less than 11.5 cm. Clinical and x-ray pelvimetry are used to determine the smallest anterior-posterior diameter through which the fetal head must pass.

The treatment goal is to allow the natural forces of labor to push the biparietal diameter of the fetal head beyond the potential interspinous obstruction. Although forceps may be used, they cause difficulty because pulling on the head destroys flexion, and the space is further diminished. A bulging perineum and crowning indicate that the obstruction has been passed.

An interischial tuberous diameter of less than 8 cm constitutes an outlet contracture. Outlet and midpelvic contractures frequently occur simultaneously. Whether vaginal birth can occur depends on the woman's interischial tuberous diameters and the fetal posteriosagittal diameter.

MATERNAL IMPLICATIONS

Labor is prolonged in the presence of CPD. Membrane rupture can result from the force of the unequally distributed contractions being exerted on the fetal membranes. In obstructed labor, in which the fetus cannot descend, uterine rupture can occur. With delayed descent, necrosis of maternal soft tissues can result from pressure exerted by the fetal head. Eventually necrosis can cause fistulas from the vagina to other nearby structures. Difficult, forceps-assisted births can also result in damage to maternal soft tissue.

FETAL-NEONATAL IMPLICATIONS

If the membranes rupture and the fetal head has not entered the inlet, there is a danger of cord prolapse. Excessive molding of the fetal head can result. Traumatic, forceps-assisted birth can damage the fetal skull and central nervous system.

CLINICAL THERAPY

Fetopelvic relationships can be assessed by comparing pelvic measurements obtained by a manual examination before labor and by computed tomography (CT). An estimated weight of the fetus is obtained by ultrasound measurements.

When the pelvic diameters are borderline or questionable, a trial of labor (TOL) may be advised. In this process the woman continues to labor, and careful, frequent assessments of cervical dilatation and fetal descent are made. As long as there is continued progress, the TOL continues. If progress ceases, the decision for a cesarean birth is made.

NURSING MANAGEMENT

The adequacy of the maternal pelvis for a vaginal birth should be assessed both during and before labor. During the intrapartum assessment, the size of the fetus and its presentation, position, and lie must also be considered. (See Fetal Assessment in Chapter 18 ∞ for intrapartum assessment techniques.)

The nurse should suspect CPD when labor is prolonged, cervical dilatation and effacement are slow, and engagement of the presenting part is delayed. The couple may need support in coping with the stresses of this complicated labor. Keep the couple informed of what is happening and explain the procedures being used. This knowledge reassures the couple that measures are being taken to resolve the problem.

Nursing actions during the TOL are similar to care during any labor except that cervical dilatation and fetal descent are assessed more frequently. Both contractions and the fetus should be monitored continuously. Report any signs of nonreassuring fetal status to the physician or CNM immediately.

The mother may be positioned in a variety of ways to increase the pelvic diameters. Sitting or squatting increases the outlet diameters and may be effective when there is failure of, or slow, fetal descent. Changing from one side to the other or maintaining a hands-and-knees position may assist the fetus in the occiput posterior position to change to an occiput anterior position. The mother may instinctively want to assume one of these positions. If not, the nurse may encourage a change of position.

CARE OF THE WOMAN AT RISK DUE TO COMPLICATIONS OF THE THIRD AND FOURTH STAGES OF LABOR

Common complications of the third and fourth stages of labor include retained placenta, lacerations, and placenta accreta.

RETAINED PLACENTA

Retention of the placenta beyond 30 minutes after birth is termed **retained placenta**. It occurs in 2% to 3% of all vaginal births. Bleeding as a result of a retained placenta can be excessive. If placenta expulsion does not occur, a manual removal of the placenta by the physician or CNM is attempted. In women who do not have an epidural in place, intravenous sedation may be required because of the discomfort caused by the procedure. Failure to retrieve the placenta via manual removal usually necessitates surgical removal by curettage. If the woman does not have an epidural in place, the procedure can be performed under general anesthesia. Retained placenta may be a symptom of an accreta, increta, or percreta (to be discussed shortly).

LACERATIONS

Lacerations of the cervix or vagina may be indicated when bright-red vaginal bleeding persists in the presence of a well-contracted uterus. The incidence of lacerations is higher when the childbearing woman is young or a nullipara, has an epidural, has forceps-assisted birth and an episiotomy, and has not done perineal massage or preparation during pregnancy. Vaginal and perineal lacerations are often categorized in terms of degree, as follows:

■ First-degree laceration is limited to the fourchette, perineal skin, and vaginal mucous membrane.

■ Second-degree laceration involves the perineal skin, vaginal mucous membrane, underlying fascia, and

muscles of the perineal body; it may extend upward on one or both sides of the vagina.

■ Third-degree laceration extends through the perineal skin, vaginal mucous membranes, and perineal body and involves the anal sphincter; it may extend up the anterior wall of the rectum.

■ Fourth-degree laceration is the same as third-degree but extends through the rectal mucosa to the lumen of the rectum; it may be called a third-degree laceration with a rectal wall extension.

PLACENTA ACCRETA

The chorionic villi attach directly to the myometrium of the uterus in *placenta accreta*. Two other types of placental adherence are *placenta increta*, in which the myometrium is invaded, and *placenta percreta*, in which the myometrium is penetrated. The adherence itself may be total, partial, or focal, depending on the amount of placental involvement. The incidence of placenta accreta is 10% to 25% in the presence of placenta previa (Clark, 2004). It is the most common type, accounting for 80% of adherent placentas.

The primary complication with placenta accreta is maternal hemorrhage and failure of the placenta to separate following birth of the infant. An abdominal hysterectomy may be necessary, depending on the amount and depth of involvement.

CARE OF THE FAMILY EXPERIENCING PERINATAL LOSS

Perinatal loss is death of a fetus or infant from the time of conception through the end of the newborn period 28 days after birth. Spontaneous abortion (miscarriage) in the antepartum period was discussed beginning in Chapter 15; ∞ this section discusses intrauterine fetal death (IUFD) after 20 weeks' gestation, often referred to as stillbirth or fetal demise.

COMMON CAUSES OF PERINATAL LOSS

The incidence of fetal death after 20 weeks in the United States is 6.8 per 1000 total births, accounting for 50% of all perinatal deaths (fetal and neonatal) (Magann, Chauhan, Bofill et al., 2002). Over 80% of stillbirths occur before term, with more than 50% occurring before 28 weeks' gestation (Cunningham et al., 2005). The cause may be unknown, or it may result from any of a number of physiologic maladaptations, including preeclampsia or eclampsia, abruptio placentae, placenta previa, diabetes, congenital anomalies, renal disease, cord accidents, fetal growth restriction, and alloimmunization. Perinatal loss associated with birth defects can occur if the fetus is exposed to teratogens late in pregnancy (Blackburn, 2003) (Table 21–4).

TABLE 21-4 ✣ Factors Associated with Perinatal Loss

Fetal Factors

Chromosomal disorders

Birth defects, not chromosomal in nature

Anencephaly, open neural tube defects, isolated hydrocephalus, congenital heart defects

Nonimmune hydrops

Infections

Complications of multiple gestations

Maternal Factors

Prolonged pregnancy

Diabetes

Chronic hypertension

Preeclampsia-eclampsia

Advanced maternal age

Hereditary thrombophilias

Antiphospholipid syndrome

Uterine rupture

Rh disease

Ascending bacteria from the vagina

Placental and Other Factors

Placenta previa

Abruptio placentae

Cord accident

Premature rupture of membranes

Unknown factors

Perinatal loss in industrialized countries has declined in recent years as early diagnosis of congenital anomalies and advances in genetic testing techniques have increased the use of elective termination (Liu, Joseph, & Wen, 2002). Surprisingly, other reproductive advances have increased the incidence of fetal death. It appears fetal death occurs more frequently in monochorionic twins and twins conceived by assisted reproductive technologies (Skeie, Froen, Vege et al., 2003). Certain genetic testing procedures such as amniocentesis and chorionic villus sampling (CVS) can actually cause fetal loss (Papp & Papp, 2003).

In developing countries, infection plays a significant role in fetal deaths, accounting for 10% to 25% of all fetal demises (Goldenberg & Thompson, 2003). Ascending bacterial organisms include *Escherichia coli*, group B streptococci, and *Ureaplasma urealyticum*. These infections can occur either before or after the membranes have ruptured, resulting in fetal demise. Viral causes of fetal demise include parvovirus and coxsackievirus. *Toxoplasma gondii*, *Listeria monocytogenes*, and the organisms that cause leptospirosis, Q fever, and Lyme disease have also been identified as causative factors for still-

birth. Untreated syphilis is associated with a high stillborn rate as are malaria infections when contracted for the first time by the mother during pregnancy (Goldenberg & Thompson, 2003). These infections carry a much higher morbidity and mortality rate in developing countries.

Paternal causes of fetal death are also being examined. One recent study determined that paternal exposure to pesticides resulted in a high rate of fetal anomalies and fetal deaths (Regidor, Ronda, Garcia et al., 2004).

Certain maternal conditions can also be associated with higher rates of fetal death. Past maternal exposure to certain bacterial and viral antigens can produce an autoimmune response that can result in fetal death (Blackwell, Romero, Chaiworapongsa et al., 2003). Women with aquired and immune thrombophilia have higher rates of miscarriage and fetal demise than those without hematologic alterations (Alonso, Soto, Urgelles et al., 2002). Women who lack the endothelial cell protein C receptor are more prone to thrombosis within the placenta, resulting in an increased incidence of fetal loss (Gu, Crawley, Ferrell et al., 2002).

MATERNAL PHYSIOLOGIC IMPLICATIONS

Prolonged retention of the dead fetus may lead to the development of disseminated intravascular coagulation (DIC), also called consumption coagulopathy, in the mother. After the release of thromboplastin from the degenerating fetal tissues into the maternal bloodstream, the extrinsic clotting system is activated, triggering the formation of multiple tiny blood clots. Fibrinogen and factors V and VII are subsequently depleted, and the woman begins to display symptoms of DIC. Fibrinogen levels begin a linear descent 3 to 4 weeks after the death of the fetus and continue to decrease in the absence of appropriate medical intervention.

Besides DIC, other adverse outcomes can occur if the onset of labor and subsequent birth are delayed. Women with prolonged retention of a dead fetus are more prone to infection. A resulting infection can cause endometritis or sepsis. The longer the pregnancy continues, the higher the incidence of maternal infection.

Although immediate induction is routinely performed, there may be situations in which induction is delayed, such as maternal refusal or the presence of a multiple gestation. In these cases, fibrinogen levels are monitored weekly or biweekly to recognize and prevent progressive coagulopathy from occurring (Lindsey, 2002).

CLINICAL THERAPY

When fetal death has occurred, abdominal x-ray examination may reveal Spalding's sign, an overriding of the fetal cranial bones. In addition, maternal estriol levels fall. Diagnosis of IUFD is confirmed by absence of heart action on ultrasound. Without medical intervention, most women have spontaneous labor within 2 weeks of fetal death. The once common practice of waiting for the onset of labor has largely been abandoned in recent years since the risks of complications increase with delaying the birth. In 25% of all fetal deaths, the cause remains unknown even after autopsy. The specific cause is more difficult to identify if the time since the death is prolonged. Prompt birth increases the ability to identify the cause of death.

In modern practice, most women with a diagnosed fetal demise are given the option of waiting a few days or scheduling an induction procedure immediately. Most women will elect for an induction within a day or two of the final diagnosis. The mode of induction is dependent upon the gestational age of the fetus, the readiness of the cervix, and previous mode of birth. In women who have had a previous cesarean birth, a repeat cesarean may be performed since the use of Pitocin or prostaglandin agents can increase the risk of a uterine rupture. Women with an unfavorable cervix may be given vaginal prostaglandin agents, misoprostol, or laminaria tents. Women less than 28 weeks' gestation are typically given prostaglandin E_2 (PGE_2) 20 mg vaginal suppositories every 4 to 6 hours or oral or vaginal misoprostol 200 mcg every 4 to 6 hours until spontaneous labor occurs (Lindsey, 2002). Since PGE_2 suppositories can cause severe vomiting and diarrhea, women are commonly pretreated with antiemetic and antidiarrheal preparations to prevent or lessen these unpleasant side effects (Lindsey, 2002). *Laminara tents* are made from the stems of brown seaweed which are cut, shaped, dried, sterilized, and packaged in specific sizes. Laminara work by drawing water out of the cervical tissue, allowing the cervix to soften and dilate. They are commonly used to dilate the cervix in preterm gestations when induction is warranted.

POSTBIRTH EVALUATION

Identifying the causative factor of fetal loss assists many families in progressing through the grieving process. Information obtained from a postmortem examination or postmortem studies can provide vital information related to the cause of the fetal death, the possibility for reoccurrence, and closure for the couple. The types of studies and tests performed depend on the parents' past history, medical history, and preferences for the depth of testing desired. Chromosome studies should be considered if the couple has a history of other second- or third-trimester losses or if either parent has a suspected balanced translocation or mosaic chromosomal pattern (Lindsey, 2002).

If an intra-amniotic infection is the suspected cause, cultures of both the placenta and the fetus should be obtained. If specific infections are being considered, both IgM and IgG antibodies should be drawn to determine if an acute infectious process has occurred.

All stillborn infants should have a careful visual inspection at the time of birth for obvious defects or abnormalities. The placenta and membranes should also be closely examined, and the placenta should be sent to pathology for further testing. The umbilical cord should be inspected for true knots, a velamentous insertion, lack of Wharton's jelly, or a short cord to determine if a cord accident was the cause. If a specific cause is suspected, blood tests and x-rays can be performed (Lindsey, 2002). An autopsy is the best mechanism to determine the cause of death; however, in the event that the parents decline an autopsy, magnetic resonance imaging (MRI) can also provide detailed information (Lindsey, 2002).

Most practitioners perform a CBC and antibody screen upon admission. Since diabetes is a causative factor, a random or postpartum glucose level can be obtained to rule out this cause. Additional maternal factors can also be evaluated. Additional tests that may be performed are listed in Table 21–5.

PHASES OF GRIEF

Grief is an individual's total response to a loss, including physical symptoms, thoughts, feelings, functional limitations, and spiritual reactions. It may be manifested by certain behaviors and rituals of **mourning**, such as weeping or visiting a gravesite, which help the person experience, accept, and adjust to the loss. The period of adjustment to loss is known as **bereavement**.

Although enough similiarity among individuals exists to identify some common phases in the course of grief, the process is "more fluid than an ordering of discrete phases would seem to imply" (Kay, Roman, & Schulte, 1997, p. 8). The behaviors that couples exhibit while mourning may be associated with the five stages of grieving described by Kubler-Ross (1969). Often the first stage is *denial* of the death of the fetus. Even when the initial healthcare

TABLE 21–5 ✣ Tests to Determine Cause of Fetal Loss

Fetal Testing	Maternal Testing
Fetal blood tests and x-rays	Diabetes testing
Autopsy or MRI	CBC with platelet count
Placental studies	Kleihauer-Betke test
Chromosomal studies (if indicated)	Abnormal antibody testing (lupus anticoagulant, anticardiolipin antibodies)
	TSH levels
	Infectious disease testing (rubella, syphilis, malaria, toxoplasmosis, cytomegalovirus)
	Hereditary thrombophilia testing
	Toxicology testing

provider suspects fetal demise, the couple is hoping that a second opinion may be different. Some couples may not be convinced of the death until they see and hold the stillborn infant after birth. The second stage is *anger,* resulting from feelings of loss, loneliness, and perhaps guilt. The anger may be projected at significant others and healthcare team members, or it may be absent when the death is sudden and unexpected. The mother may attempt to identify a specific event that caused the death and may blame herself. *Bargaining,* the third stage, may or may not be present, depending on the couple's preparation for the death of the fetus. If the death is unanticipated, the couple may not have time for bargaining. When the death is expected, such as in the case of a known lethal congenital anomaly, bargaining is more commonly seen. It is marked by the couple making mental trade-offs in exchange for the fetus being healthy. In the fourth stage, *depression* is evidenced by preoccupation, weeping, and withdrawal. Changing hormonal levels in the first 24 to 48 hours after birth may compound the depression and associated grief. The final stage, *acceptance,* occurs when resolution occurs. This stage is highly individualized and may take months to years to complete.

NURSING PRACTICE

No matter who you are or how much nursing experience you have, when an expectant family is in pain because of their loss, and you feel you do not know the right thing to say, "I'm so sorry, I don't know what to say" is a start.

NURSING MANAGEMENT

NURSING ASSESSMENT AND DIAGNOSIS

Cessation of fetal movement reported by the mother to the nurse is frequently the first indication of fetal death. It is followed by a gradual decrease in the signs and symptoms of pregnancy. Fetal heart tones are absent, and fetal movement is no longer palpable. Once fetal demise is established, assess the family members' ability to adapt to their loss. Open communication between the mother, her partner, and the healthcare team members contributes to a realistic understanding of the medical condition and its associated treatments. Discuss prior experiences the family has had with loss and what they feel were their perceived coping abilities at that time. Identifying the family's social supports and resources is also important.

Perinatal loss may also occur in the intrapartum period as a result of an intrapartum complication, such as an unresolved shoulder dystocia, prolapsed umbilical cord, abruptio placentae, or other complication. In such emergency situations, healthcare team members often focus on the physical needs of the mother and an attempt to save the fetus's life. Commonly, it is not until the infant is born that the family is advised that a perinatal death has occurred. Thus, the parents are faced with the sudden and completely unanticipated death of their infant. The most common reaction is protest or disbelief.

Although the physician or CNM informs the family of the death, the nurse continues one-on-one care with the family, providing both physical and emotional support throughout this crucial period. Assist the family in the grief process and explore their immediate wishes for viewing and holding their deceased child.

Nursing diagnoses that may apply include the following (Wilkinson, 2005):

- *Anticipatory Grieving* related to imminent loss of a child
- *Powerlessness* related to lack of control in current situational crisis
- *Ineffective Denial* related to the unexpected death of the fetus
- *Compromised Family Coping* related to the death of a child/unresolved feelings regarding perinatal loss
- *Interrupted Family Processes* related to fetal demise
- *Hopelessness* related to sudden, unexpected fetal loss
- *Risk for Spiritual Distress* related to intense suffering secondary to unexpected fetal loss

PLANNING AND IMPLEMENTATION

Most facilities have an established protocol to follow in the event of perinatal death. It typically provides a holistic focus for family-centered nursing care. It is important that the entire healthcare team is notified so multidisciplinary care can be initiated. When fetal death has been confirmed before admission, the entire staff on the unit is informed so they can avoid making inappropriate remarks. Many facilities have a symbol, such as a card with a leaf or a cluster of flowers, that is placed on the mother's door so all staff members are aware of the loss.

Preparing the Family for the Birth

Upon arrival to the facility, the couple with a known or suspected fetal demise should immediately be placed in a private room. When possible the woman should be in a room that is farthest away from other laboring women. Take care not to leave the couple in the waiting room with other expectant parents or visitors waiting for news from other women in labor.

The couple should be allowed to remain together as much as they wish. Provide privacy as needed and maintain a supportive environment. Give the couple complete information about what to expect and what will happen. Encourage and answer questions. Stay with the couple so they do not feel alone and isolated; however, continuously assess cues from the couple that they want to be alone. Some couples may want outside support, such as family members or friends, to be present during the labor. Facilitate the couple's wishes.

When possible the same nurse should provide care for the couple so a therapeutic relationship can be established. As the relationship develops, provide solace by listening to the couple without offering explanations. Also provide ongoing opportunities for the couple to ask questions. It is not uncommon for the family to ask the same questions repeatedly. This is part of the initial grief process. Provide clear explanations and straightforward answers. Also arrange for other members of the multidisciplinary team to interact with the family. If a grief counselor is available, arrange an initial interaction with the couple. Some families may desire to see a spiritual advisor. Offer to contact the hospital chaplain or another cleric for them. A social worker is commonly involved. Coordinate members of the multidisciplinary team so a comprehensive plan of care can be initiated.

Explain details of the plan of care and allow the family to ask questions and make decisions for their labor and birth preferences. Review the availability of anesthesia and analgesia. The woman typically can have pain medication whenever she desires. Facilitate the participation of the woman and her partner in the labor and birth process.

It is important to remember that, in contrast to a typical birth experience, the birth of a stillborn infant marks both the beginning and the end. It is imperative that the couple and family have all wishes and preferences respected. The family may be overwhelmed and may have difficulty making decisions in this period. Assist the couple in exploring their feelings and help them to make decisions about who is present and what rituals will occur during and following the birth. Examples of birth preferences include the following:

- Use of music, dimmed lighting, or other environmental preferences
- Laboring or birthing in a specific position
- Having the infant placed on the mother's chest immediately after birth
- Allowing the father to cut the umbilical cord
- Presence of other family members or friends at the birth

Sometimes couples worry that others may view their preferences as "strange" or "wrong." Reassure the family that it is their experience and that there are no right or wrong feelings or wishes.

The couple may have waves of overwhelming grief, disbelief, or sadness. Encourage the couple to experience the grief that they feel. It is not uncommon for one partner to attempt to put on a "brave front," feeling that by showing grief he or she will make the other partner feel worse. It is also not uncommon for partners to have intense feelings that they are unable to share. Encourage partners to express their emotions freely to the extent they are able. Help them understand that they may each experience different feelings.

Supporting the Family in Viewing the Stillborn Infant

Advocates of seeing the stillborn infant believe that viewing assists in dispelling denial and enables the couple to progress to the next step in the grieving process. If they choose to see their stillborn infant, prepare the couple for what they will see by saying "she is going to feel cold," "he is going to be blue," or other appropriate statements. If the parents have shared with you the name they had chosen for their baby, use that name in discussing the baby, for example, "Jessie's face is bruised." Another common practice is to wrap the infant in a blanket or apply a hat to cover birth defects. This allows the parents an opportunity to view the infant before seeing the birth defect. Most parents will eventually remove the covering to inspect the infant; however, applying a covering allows them time to adjust to the appearance at their own pace.

Some families will hold their infant for a short time before returning him or her to the nurse, whereas others will wish to spend a great deal of time with their infant. Allow the infant to remain with the family for as long as the family desires. Some parents may elect to bathe or dress their stillborn baby; support them in their choice. Some couples may want other family members, friends, or their other children to see the infant. Act as an advocate to ensure that the family's wishes are respected.

Providing Discharge Care

Most facilities prepare a remembrance box or package for the family to take home. This typically consists of a photograph taken of the infant or the family, a card with the baby's footprints, a crib card, identification band, a lock of hair, and possibly a blanket or clothing worn by the infant. In the event that the couple declines the package, it is common for the hospital to retain these items for a specific period in case they change their minds.

After the birth, give the option of an early discharge (as early as 6 to 8 hours after the birth) to the couple. Facility protocol will dictate where mothers are transferred after a perinatal loss. Some hospitals have the women remain on the labor and delivery unit; others give the mother the option of choosing a postpartum room or one on a medical unit. If the mother is transferred to a postpartum room, select a room for her that is far away from other rooms and the newborn nursery. It is imperative that all staff members, as well as student nurses, are notified of the mother's status.

Include information on the grief process in discharge information. Prepare the couple to return home by stressing that others may not know what to say, and that even loved ones may make inappropriate comments because they do not know how to respond to grief and loss. This can prepare the couple for the reactions of others. If there are siblings, each will usually progress through age-appropriate grieving. Provide the parents with information about normal mourning reactions, both psychologic and physiologic.

When caring for a family suffering from a perinatal loss, it is important to remember that the nurse experiences many of the same grief reactions as the parents of a stillborn infant. It is important to have colleagues and family members available for counseling and support.

Facilitating the Family's Grief Work

The parents of a stillborn infant suffer a devastating experience that precipitates an intense emotional trauma. During pregnancy the couple has already begun the attachment process, which now must be terminated through the grieving process. Facilitating the family's grief work is thus a critical nursing intervention—one that requires skill, sensitivity, and compassion.

Following discharge, some families may need closure of the intrapartum event in order to continue the grief work. A consultation can be scheduled with the practitioner who cared for them during the pregnancy and birth. Families may also wish to read the results of tests performed during the intrapartum period and the autopsy report. Provide a copy of the medical record to the couple and encourage them to ask questions, express their feelings, and ask for clarification.

Families are routinely referred for counseling services after a perinatal loss has occurred. A counselor who specializes in perinatal issues can provide expertise and assist the couple in their grieving. Partners should be allowed to verbalize fears and concerns about future pregnancies. When appropriate, also provide referrals to genetic counselors, religious support persons, and social service agencies.

Besides referral information, the woman should receive scheduled, follow-up phone calls to assess the family's functioning and their progress with grief work. Use these follow-up phone calls to provide pertinent information and identify additional resources for the family.

As the grief process ensues, encourage families to implement cultural, religious, or social customs that will assist them in grieving and mourning. Advise the family that certain upcoming milestones, such as holidays, future birthdays, baby showers, Mother's Day, Father's Day, and other social events may trigger their grief. The family can better cope with these events if they are adequately prepared.

Referring the Family to Community Services

Although most facilities have an established protocol for families experiencing perinatal loss, more comprehensive intervention programs are being established in communities to assist these families. Community support groups that focus on perinatal loss can provide an important support network and resources. Specialized groups, such as those focused on early pregnancy loss, stillbirth, and perinatal loss associated with specific congenital anomalies, allow families the opportunity to interact with peers who have lost infants under similar circumstances. Provide the group name, contact person (if possible), and phone number. Also provide materials such as the book *When Hello Means Goodbye* by Schwiebert and Kirk (1985).

Internet technology has allowed large numbers of individuals to share resources and information, and participate in online support groups. Internet resources can be effective for all families and may be the only resources available for families in rural, underserved areas.

Specialized community outreach programs are another resource that can provide assistance to grieving families; some provide early counseling to parents whose fetus has a known lethal congenital anomaly. In perinatal hospice programs, parents are given the opportunity to explore options, such as elective termination or waiting for the onset of spontaneous labor or a medically indicated induced labor. For families wishing to continue their pregnancies, the program typically assigns a multidisciplinary team who provides compassionate care, ongoing counseling, referral to support groups, and spiritual guidance (Calhoun, Napolitano, Terry et al., 2003).

Care of the Couple Who Has Experienced Loss in a Previous Pregnancy

Couples who have had previous perinatal loss typically enter a subsequent pregnancy with conflicting feelings and may experience ambivalence, fear, and anxiety. Many times, their past experience is relived when another pregnancy occurs. Some couples conceive soon after a loss while others wait years. Some couples enter a subsequent pregnancy with grief work largely completed while others are still experiencing unresolved grief.

The nurse caring for a couple who has had a previous loss needs to be kind, compassionate, and patient. Couples need specific information and clear explanations of all prenatal information. Make referrals to genetic counselors when appropriate. Some couples may wish to have a consultation with a perinatologist. If unresolved grief issues are present or the family experiences extreme anxiety, counseling may be beneficial.

Interventions to decrease anxiety can help the couple tremendously. At the first visit, an early ultrasound can be performed to verify the presence of the fetal heart. In early pregnancy, women may be fearful when first-trimester pregnancy symptoms begin to resolve. It may be helpful for these women to come in for weekly visits for a period of time simply to hear the fetal heartbeat. This intervention may continue to be helpful until the woman begins to feel fetal movement. Throughout the pregnancy, the office or clinic nurse can play a key role by providing reassurance and answer questions that the woman may have.

Women with a previous loss typically receive additional antepartum testing throughout the pregnancy. Ultrasounds can be used to provide reassurance and assess fetal growth and development, placental functioning, and cord variations. Nonstress testing and biophysical profiles can be performed weekly after 32 weeks to ensure fetal well-being. Fetal kick counts should be initiated at 28 weeks and continue until the birth occurs. Women with a previous loss should give birth at their expected date of birth or when the pregnancy is at term and should not go over their due date, since placental functioning can decline in postdate pregnancies.

EVALUATION

Expected outcomes of nursing care for the family experiencing perinatal loss include the following:

- Family members express their feelings about the death of their baby.

- Family members participate in the decision making regarding preferences for the labor, birth, and the immediate postpartum period.

- Family members participate in the decision of whether to see their baby and other decisions about the baby.

- The family has resources available for continued support.

- Family members know the community resources available and have names and phone numbers to use if they choose.

- The family is moving into and through the grieving process.

CARE OF THE WOMAN WITH A PSYCHOLOGIC DISORDER

The onset of labor is a time of mixed emotions. Joy, excitement, happiness, fear of the unknown, and anxiety related to pain may all occur. These reactions are expected and pose no health risk in women with adequate coping mechanisms. In contrast, laboring women with **psychologic disorders** face additional emotional challenges and require additional nursing support in the intrapartum period.

The prevalence of psychologic disorders among adults in the United States is 22.1% (National Institute of Mental Health, 2002). Psychologic disorders are characterized by alterations in thinking, mood, or behavior. Although many such disorders can affect labor and birth, only the most common are discussed here. Since an in-depth discussion of psychologic disorders is beyond the scope of this text, students are encouraged to consult a mental-health nursing textbook for further reference. Postpartum psychologic disorders are discussed in Chapter 25. ∞

The psychologic disorders that most commonly affect pregnant women are depression, bipolar disorder, anxiety, phobias, obsessive-compulsive disorder, post-traumatic stress disorder, and schizophrenia. These disorders may manifest themselves in different ways during the birth process; however, all require the nurse to provide compassionate and consistent nursing care.

MATERNAL IMPLICATIONS

Depression can reduce the woman's ability to concentrate or process information being provided by healthcare team members. The labor process may feel overwhelming to her, and she may feel hopelessness about the outcome of her labor. Women with bipolar disorder experience the symptoms of depression during the depressive phase, but if labor occurs during a manic phase, the woman may be hyperexcitable. Anxiety disorders may cause the laboring woman to experience physical symptoms such as chest pain, shortness of breath, faintness, fear, or even terror. In general, laboring women with psychologic disorders tend to exhibit behaviors characteristic of their disorder, but these behaviors may be somewhat exaggerated.

CLINICAL THERAPY

The goal of clinical therapy is to provide strategies that will help decrease the anxiety of the woman and her partner, keep her oriented to reality, and promote optimal functioning while in labor. The woman should be oriented to her new environment. All questions and concerns should be addressed promptly. When needed, pharmacologic measures such as sedatives, analgesics, or antianxiety medications may be ordered.

NURSING MANAGEMENT

The nurse uses therapeutic communication and sharing of information to allay anxiety for both the woman and her support person. Consistent care enables the woman to adjust to a new environment and begin to establish a relationship with her nurse.

NURSING ASSESSMENT AND DIAGNOSIS

Unless birth is imminent or severe complications exist, begin the assessment by reviewing the woman's background. Factors such as age, marital and socioeconomic status, culture, methods of coping, support system, and understanding of the labor process contribute to the woman's psychologic response to labor. Ask the woman if she has ever been diagnosed with a psychologic disorder. If the woman has, also ask her if she is currently receiving any treatment, including medications or psychotherapy.

Assess the woman for objective cues indicating a psychologic disorder. Monotone replies or flat affect may indicate depression. Women with schizophrenia may lack orientation to person, time, and place. Objective cues indicating acute anxiety or signs of panic attack include tachycardia and hyperventilation.

As labor progresses, remain alert to the woman's verbal and nonverbal behavior responses to the pain and anxiety of labor. The woman who is too quiet and compliant, is disoriented, is agitated and seems uncooperative, or is experiencing acute anxiety symptoms may require further appraisal for psychologic disorders. These rare circumstances require one-on-one nursing care. A consultation with a psychiatrist is often warranted.

Nursing diagnoses that may apply to the woman with a psychologic disorder include the following:

- *Anxiety* related to stress of the labor process, unfamiliar environment, and unknown care providers.
- *Fear* related to unknown outcome of labor and invasive medical procedures.
- *Acute Pain* related to increased anxiety and stress
- *Ineffective Individual Coping* related to increased anxiety and stress

NURSING PLAN AND IMPLEMENTATION

The primary nursing interventions center on providing support to the laboring woman and her partner or family.

Families that have had the opportunity to attend prenatal classes may benefit from encouragement as they employ some of the coping techniques they have learned (see Chapter 8 ∞). If the woman begins to lose her ability to cope or her orientation to reality, assist her in regaining control and orientation by explaining where she is, why she is there, and what is currently happening. Provide reassurance, decrease stimuli, and acknowledge her fears, concerns, and symptoms.

The nurse's ability to help the woman and her partner cope with the stress of labor is directly related to the rapport they have established. By employing a calm, caring, confident, nonjudgmental approach, you may be able not only to acknowledge the anxiety or other emotions the woman is feeling but also to identify the source of the distress. Once the causative factors are known, implement appropriate interventions such as offering information, comfort measures, touch, or therapeutic communication. Some women with severe psychologic disorders may have excessive symptoms during their labor and birth. Although providing emotional support is imperative, focus your care of these women on maintaining a safe environment and ensuring maternal and fetal well-being. Pharmacologic interventions may be necessary for excessive symptoms.

EVALUATION

Expected outcomes of nursing care include the following:

- The woman experiences a decrease in physiologic and psychologic stress and an increase in physical and psychologic comfort.
- The woman remains oriented to person, time, and place.
- The woman uses effective coping mechanisms to manage her stress and anxiety in labor.
- The woman is able to verbalize feelings about her labor.
- The woman's and her family's fear is decreased.

Critical Concept Review

LEARNING OBJECTIVES

CONCEPTS

Compare and contrast hypertonic and hypotonic labor patterns, including the risks, clinical therapy, and nursing care management.

Hypertonic labor patterns:
1. Characterized by increased frequency but decreased effectiveness of contraction in effacing and dilating the cervix. Usually leads to a prolonged latent phase.
2. May cause mother to become fatigued and have difficulty coping with stress of labor.
3. Pattern may cause prolonged pressure on the fetal head.
4. Clinical therapy may involve sedation, pain medication, and bed rest. Pitocin may be given only if CPD and fetal malpresentation are ruled out.
5. Nursing management includes decreasing environmental stimuli, decreasing anxiety, and promoting comfort.

Hypotonic labor patterns:
1. Characterized by fewer than 2–3 contractions in a 10-minute period during the active phase of labor.
2. Mother may experience fatigue and coping difficulties.
3. Mother is at risk for intrauterine infection and postpartal hemorrhage.
4. Fetus is at risk for sepsis.
5. Clinical therapy includes assessment of adequacy of pelvic measurement and fetal maturity; the use of Pitocin or nipple stimulation once CPD and fetal malpresentation are ruled out.
6. Nursing management includes close monitoring for signs and symptoms of infection and dehydration, and keeping vaginal exams to a minimum.

Describe the possible impact of postterm pregnancy on the childbearing family.

Postterm pregnancy may result in an increased possibility of:
1. Probable labor induction.
2. Forceps or vacuum-assisted or cesarean birth.
3. Decreased perfusion to the placenta.
4. Decreased amount of amniotic fluid and possible cord compression.
5. Increased possibility of meconium aspiration.
6. Increased risk for macrosomia or a loss of fat and muscle mass resulting in small-for-gestational age (SGA).

Relate the various types of fetal malposition and malpresentation to the possible associated problems.

1. Occiput posterior position:
   - Baby is face up instead of face down as it enters the vagina.
   - May prolong labor.
   - Baby is usually able to be born vaginally but may need forceps assistance to turn baby.
2. Brow presentation:
   - Forehead of the fetus becomes the presenting part.
   - May cause labor to be prolonged.
   - Cesarean birth necessary if brow presentation persists.
3. Face presentation:
   - Face of the fetus is the presenting part.
   - Vaginal birth may be possible, but cesarean birth remains a significant possibility.
4. Breech presentation:
   - Fetal buttocks or foot/feet are the presenting part.
   - 90% of breech presentations result in cesarean birth.
5. Transverse lie:
   - Fetal shoulder is the presenting part.
   - Fetus must be born by cesarean.

Discuss the identification, management, and care of fetal macrosomia.

1. Identification of fetal macrosomia is conducted through:
   - Palpation of fetus in utero.
   - Ultrasound of fetus.
   - X-ray pelvimetry.

LEARNING OBJECTIVES   CONCEPTS

2. Management of fetal macrosomia involves the following:
- Cesarean birth performed if fetus is greater than 4500 g.
- Continuous fetal monitoring if labor is allowed to progress.
- Notification of physician for early decelerations, labor dysfunction, or nonreassuring fetal status.
3. Care of newborn with macrosomia requires:
- Assessment of newborn for cephalhematoma, Erb's palsy, and fractured clavicles.
4. Care of the mother after birth of newborn with macrosomia requires:
- Fundal massage to prevent maternal hemorrhage from overstretched uterus.
- Close monitoring of vital signs.

Delineate the nursing care for the woman with more than one fetus.

Care of the woman with more than one fetus includes:
1. Frequent assessment of the fetal heart tones of each fetus.
2. Education of the mother about signs and symptoms of preterm labor.
3. Encouraging the mother to rest frequently.
4. Prior to birth, preparation of equipment needed to care for each individual newborn.

Summarize the nursing care indicated for nonreassuring fetal status.

Nursing actions (intrauterine resuscitation) include:
1. Turn the woman to left lateral position to treat hypotension.
2. Begin or increase IV flow rate.
3. Perform vaginal exam to check for cord prolapse.
4. Have woman assume knee-chest position if cord prolapse is suspected.
5. Discontinue Pitocin or administer a tocolytic agent to decrease contraction frequency and intensity.
6. Administer oxygen.
7. Notify physician.
8. Obtain additional information about fetus by fetal scalp blood sampling or fetal acoustical stimulation.

Compare and contrast abruptio placentae and placenta previa, including implications for the mother and fetus and nursing care.

Abruptio placentae:
1. Condition in which the placenta prematurely separates from the uterine wall.
2. May result in severe hemorrhage.
3. May cause death to mother, fetus, or both.
4. May lead to clotting disorders in the mother.
5. Nursing care involves frequent assessment of uterine tone and measurement of abdominal girth.

Placenta previa:
1. Condition in which the placenta implants in the lower segment of the uterus. It may partially or completely cover the cervical os.
2. Bleeding occurs as the cervix begins to dilate. Bleeding may be mild to severe, depending upon how much of the placenta covers the cervical os.
3. Fetus may develop hypoxia, anemia, or both from bleeding episode.
4. Nursing care involves assessing blood loss, pain, and uterine contractions.
5. The nurse should NEVER perform a vaginal examination if placenta previa is suspected.

Identify variations that may occur with or in the umbilical cord and insertion into the placenta.

1. Prolapse umbilical cord:
- Umbilical cord precedes fetal presenting part, placing pressure on cord and diminishing blood flow to the fetus.
- Bedrest is recommended if engagement has not occurred and membranes have ruptured.
- Assess for nonreassuring fetal status.
2. Succenturiate placenta:
- One or more accessory lobes of fetal villi will develop on the placenta, possibly causing postpartal hemorrhage.
3. Circumvallate placenta:
- A double fold of chorion and amnion form a ring around the umbilical cord on the fetal side of the placenta, increasing the risk of late abortion, antepartal hemorrhage, and preterm labor. It may also cause IUGR, prematurity, and fetal death.

(continued)

LEARNING OBJECTIVES	CONCEPTS

Identify variations that may occur with or in the umbilical cord and insertion into the placenta.—Continued

→

4. Battledore placenta:
   - The umbilical cord is inserted at or near the placental margin, which may increase the chance of preterm labor and bleeding. It may also cause prematurity and nonreassuring labor status.
5. Velamentous insertion of the umbilical cord:
   - The vessels of the umbilical cord divide some distance from the placenta in the placental membranes; this may cause hemorrhage if one of the vessels is torn, if nonreassuring fetal status is present or hemorrhage in the fetus occurs.

Contrast the identification, management, and nursing care of women with amniotic fluid embolus, hydramnios, and oligohydramnios.

→

Amniotic fluid embolism:
1. Caused by a small tear in the chorion or amnion high in the uterus, which may allow amniotic fluid to enter the maternal circulatory system.
2. Usually occurs during or after birth.
3. The woman experiences sudden symptoms of respiratory distress leading to severe hemorrhage.
4. This disorder is life threatening, so medical management and nursing care is aimed at delivering lifesaving treatments such as CPR and transfusion until the woman is stabilized.

Hydramnios:
1. In this condition, the woman has greater than 2000 mL of amniotic fluid.
2. Associated with fetal swallowing and neurologic disorders.
3. Also associated with maternal gestational diabetes, Rh disorders, and multiple-gestation pregnancies.
4. Woman may experience shortness of breath and lower extremity edema.
5. Amniocentesis may be performed to remove some of the excess fluid.
6. The nurse monitors the mother for complications of the amniocentesis and supports the family if fetal disorders are the cause of the excess fluid.

Oligohydramnios:
1. In this condition the amount of amniotic fluid is reduced and concentrated.
2. Often found with some renal fetal disorders, fetal postmaturity, and placental insufficiency.
3. May cause fetal respiratory and skeletal abnormalities.
4. May cause prolonged labor.
5. Amnioinfusion may be used during labor to help to cushion the fetus and umbilical cord.
6. The nurse must continuously monitor the labor pattern for any sign of fetal distress.

Delineate the effects of pelvic contractures on labor and birth.

→

1. Labor is usually prolonged in the presence of CPD.
2. Vaginal birth may be possible depending upon the type of CPD.
3. Woman may increase pelvic diameter during labor by squatting, sitting, rolling from side to side, or maintaining a knee-chest position.
4. CPD may make cesarean birth the only available method of birth.

Identify common complications of the third and fourth stages of labor.

→

The most common complications are:
1. Retained placenta:
   - If not expelled, the placenta must be manually removed from uterus.
2. Lacerations:
   - Suspected when there is bright-red bleeding in the presence of a contracted uterus.
   - Usually repaired immediately after birth of child.
3. Placenta accreta:
   - In this condition, the chorionic villi attach directly to the myometrium of the uterus.
   - May result in maternal hemorrhage and failure of the placenta to separate from the uterus.
   - May result in the need for hysterectomy at time of birth.

Discuss perinatal loss, including etiology, diagnosis, and the nurse's role in facilitating the family's grief work.

→

1. Perinatal loss results from three factors:
   - Fetal factors: The fetus has or develops a disorder that is incompatible with life.
   - Maternal factors: The mother has a disorder such as diabetes or preeclampsia that creates a hostile environment for the fetus.
   - Placental or other factors: Certain conditions such as abruptio placentae or cord accident cut off blood supply to the fetus, leading to death.
2. Diagnosis may be made when the mother notices lack of movement in the fetus or at a regularly scheduled physician's visit when a fetal heart tone cannot be found.

LEARNING OBJECTIVES

CONCEPTS

3. Nursing care involves supporting the family through the grief work:
   - Assist the family through the labor and birth.
   - Provide for the woman's physical needs after the birth.
   - Encourage family members to express and share their thoughts and feelings about the loss.
   - Give the family an opportunity to view, hold, and name the infant.
   - Prepare items for the family to keep to remember the infant.
   - Provide opportunities for religious or spiritual counseling and cultural practices.
   - Visit or phone the family after discharge to assist in closure.
   - Make referrals to appropriate perinatal loss counseling services if indicated.

Describe the psychologic factors that may be accelerated secondary to complications during labor and birth.

→ Psychologic disorders such as depression and acute anxiety may have a profound effect on labor, particularly when complications occur that might jeopardize the mother or fetus.

CRITICAL THINKING IN ACTION

*View the **Critical Thinking in Action** video in Chapter 21 of the CD-ROM. Then, answer the questions that follow.*

June Dice, a 25-year-old G3, P1011, is admitted to you in labor and delivery at 38 weeks with a moderate amount of dark red vaginal bleeding. June's prenatal history is significant for late prenatal care (20 weeks' gestation by ultrasound) and cocaine abuse. An ultrasound is done upon admission which demonstrates a marginal placenta abruption. You place June on the fetal monitor and observe a fetal heart rate baseline of 146 to 155 with accelerations to 166 with fetal movement. There are occasional mild variable decelerations with a quick return to baseline. Contraction pattern is interpreted as an irritable uterus. An intravenous infusion with Ringer's lactate is started with a #18 intracath. June's vital signs are within normal limits. Her hematocrit is 29%. You assist the physician with a vaginal exam to rupture membranes and insert a fetal scalp electrode and intrauterine pressure catheter. A small amount of light yellow-green amniotic fluid is observed. The exam shows June is 4 cm dilated, 50% effaced, vertex at -1 station. You follow protocol and start an oxytocin induction/augmentation. June is asking why oxytocin is needed.

1. Explain the goal of labor induction/augmentation in response to June's question.
2. Explain potential risk factors associated with oxytocin induction of labor.
3. You observe a nonreassuring fetal heart rate of 144 to 150 with decreased variability, and persistent late decelerations with each contraction. What interventions would you immediately take?
4. What supportive actions are taken to decrease the risk of hypofibrinogenemia?
5. What complications might be present in the newborn at birth?

MEDIALINK

www.prenhall.com/london

- NCLEX-RN® Review, case studies, and other interactive resources for this chapter can be found on the Companion Website at http://www.prenhall.com/london. Click on "Chapter 21" to select the activities for this chapter.

NY Times

The College Times is a new site from NYTimes.com. Click here and it will take you directly to the latest information related to Nursing. Students and faculty can access a number of additional resources, including career planning information for students and instructional resources for faculty. In addition, students and faculty can also sign up to receive free e-mail alerts when new articles related to their specific areas of study are published on NYTimes.com.

- For animations, more NCLEX-RN® Review questions, and an audio glossary, access the accompanying CD-ROM in this textbook.

REFERENCES

Alonso, A., Soto, I., Urgelles, M. F., Corte, J. R., Rodriquez, M. J., & Pinto, C. R. (2002). Acquired and inherited thrombophilia in women with unexplained fetal losses. *American Journal of Obstetrics & Gynecology, 187*(5), 1337–1342.

Blackburn, S. T. (2003). *Maternal, fetal, & neonatal physiology: A clinical perspective* (2nd ed.). Philadelphia: Saunders.

Blackwell, S., Romero, R., Chaiworapongsa, T., Refuerzo, J., Gervasi, M. T., Yoshimatsu, J., et al. (2003). Unexplained fetal death is associated with changes in the adaptive limb of the maternal immune response consistent with prior antigenic exposure. *Journal of Maternal-Fetal & Neonatal Medicine, 14*(4), 241–246.

Bowes, W. A., & Thorp, J. M. (2004). Clinical aspects of normal and abnormal labor. In R. K. Creasy & R. Resnik (Eds.), *Maternal-fetal medicine* (5th ed., pp. 671–705). Philadelphia: Saunders.

Calhoun, B. C., Napolitano, P., Terry, M., Bussey, C., & Hoeldtke, N. J. (2003). Perinatal hospice: Comprehensive care for the family of the fetus with a lethal condition. *Journal of Reproductive Medicine, 48*(5), 343–348.

Clark, S. L. (2004). Placenta previa and abruptio placentae. In R. K. Creasy & R. Resnik (Eds.), *Maternal-fetal medicine* (5th ed., pp. 707–722). Philadelphia: Saunders.

Cunningham, F. G., Leveno, K. J., Bloom, S. L., Hauth, J. C., Gilstrap, L. C., & Wenstrom, K. D. (2005). Diseases and injuries of the fetus and newborn. *Williams obstetrics* (22nd ed. pp. 649–691). New York: McGraw-Hill.

Dudley, D. J. (2003). Complications of labor. In J. R. Scott, R. S. Gibbs, B. Y. Karlan, & A. F. Haney (Eds.), *Danforth's obstetrics and gynecology* (9th ed., pp. 397–419). Philadelphia: Lippincott Williams & Wilkins.

Faiz, A. S., & Ananth, C. V. (2003). Etiology and risk factors for placenta previa: An overview and meta-analysis of observational studies. *Journal of Maternal-Fetal & Neonatal Medicine, 13*(3), 175–190.

Goldenberg, R. L., & Thompson, C. (2003). The infectious origins of stillbirth. *American Journal of Obstetrics & Gynecology, 189*(3), 861–873.

Gu, J. M., Crawley, J. T., Ferrell, G., Zhang, F., Li, W., Esmon, N. L., & Esmon, C. T. (2002). Disruption of the endothelial cell protein C receptor gene in mice causes placental thrombosis and early embryonic lethality. *Journal of Biological Chemistry, 277*(45), 4335–4343.

Jasper, M. L. (2004). Antepartum fetal assessment. In S. Mattson & J. E. Smith (Eds.), *Core curriculum for maternal-newborn nursing* (3rd ed., pp. 161–200). St. Louis, MO: Elsevier Saunders.

Kay, J., Roman, B., & Schulte, H. M. (1997). Pregnancy loss and the grief process. In J. R. Woods & J. L. Esposito (Eds.), *Loss during pregnancy or in the newborn period: Principles of care with clinical cases and analyses* (pp. 5–36). Pittman, NJ: Jannetti Publications.

Kubler-Ross, E. (1969). *On death and dying.* New York: MacMillian.

Laughlin, D., & Knuppel, R. A. (2003). Maternal-placental-fetal unit: Fetal and early neonatal physiology. In A. H. DeCherney & L. Nathan (Eds.), *Current obstetric & gynecologic: Diagnosis & treatment* (9th ed., pp.163–191). New York: Lange Medical Books/McGraw-Hill.

Lindsey, J. L. (2002). *Evaluation of fetal death. E-medicine.* Retrieved May 13, 2004, from http://www.emedicine.com/med/topic3235.htm#section~bibliography

Liu, S., Joseph, K. S., & Wen, S. W. (2002). Trends in fetal and infant deaths caused by congenital anomalies. *Seminars in Perinatology, 26*(4), 268–276.

Magann, E. F., Chauhan, S. P., Bofill, J. A., Waddell, D., Rust, O. A., & Morrison, J. C. (2002). *Maternal morbidity and mortality associated with intrauterine fetal demise: Five year experience at a tertiary referral hospital.* Presented at the 70th annual meeting, Central Association of Obstetrics and Gynecologists, Maui, HI.

Malone, F. D., & D'Alton, M. E. (2004). Multiple gestation: Clinical characteristics and management. In R. K. Creasy & R. Resnik (Eds.), *Maternal-fetal medicine* (5th ed., pp. 513–536). Philadelphia: Saunders.

National Institute of Mental Health. (2002). *Do you suffer from a mental disorder?* Rockville, MD: Author.

Neri, I., Airola, G., Contu, G., Allais, G., Facchinetti, F., & Benedetto, C. (2004). Acupuncture plus moxibustion to resolve breech presentation: A randomized controlled study. *Journal of Maternal-Fetal & Neonatal Medicine, 15*(4), 247–252.

Papp, C., & Papp, Z. (2003). Chorionic villus sampling and amniocentesis: What are the risks in current practice? *Current Opinion in Obstetrics and Gynecology, 15*(2), 159–165.

Parer, J. T., & Nageotte, M. P. (2004). Intrapartum fetal surveillance. In R. K. Creasy &

R. Resnik (Eds.), *Maternal-fetal medicine* (5th ed., pp. 403–429). Philadelphia: Saunders.

Polo, A., Chang, L., Herrera, E., & Pernoll, M. L. (2003). Complications of labor and delivery. In A. H. DeCherney & L. Nathan (Eds.), *Current obstetric & gynecologic: Diagnosis & treatment* (9th ed., pp. 466–476). New York: Lange Medical Books/McGraw-Hill.

Poole, J. H. (2004). Hypertensive disorders in pregnancy. In S. Mattson & J. E. Smith (Eds.), *Core curriculum for maternal-newborn nursing* (3rd ed., pp. 554–592). St. Louis, MO: Elsevier Saunders.

Regidor, E., Ronda, E., Garcia, A. M., & Dominguez, V. (2004). Paternal exposure to agricultural pesticides can cause specific fetal death. *Occupational & Environmental Medicine, 61*(4), 334–339.

Resnik, J. L., & Resnik, R. (2004). Post-term pregnancy. In R. K. Creasy & R. Resnik (Eds.), *Maternal-fetal medicine* (5th ed., pp. 663–669). Philadelphia: Saunders.

Schwiebert, P., & Kirk, P. (1985). *When hello means goodbye.* Eugene, OR: Health Sciences University.

Sheiner, E., Shoham-Vardi, I., Hallak, M., Hadar, A., Gortzak-Uzan, L., Katz, M., et al. (2003). Placental abruption in term pregnancies: Clinical significance and obstetric risk factors. *Journal of Maternal-Fetal & Neonatal Medicine, 13*(1), 45–49.

Skeie, A., Froen, J. F., Vege, A., & Stray-Pedersen, B. (2003). Cause and risk of stillbirth in twin pregnancies: A retrospective audit. *Acta Obstetricia et Gynecologica Scandinavica, 82*(11), 1010–1016.

Smith, K. V. (2004). Normal childbirth. In S. Mattson & J. E. Smith (Eds.), *Core curriculum for maternal-newborn nursing* (3rd ed., pp. 271–303). St. Louis, MO: Elsevier Saunders.

Sokol, R. J., & Blackwell, S. C. (2003). Abnormal labor: Diagnosis and management. In J. J. Sciarri (Ed.), *Gynecology and obstetrics* (Vol. 2, chap. 73, pp. 1–15). Philadelphia: Lippincott Williams & Wilkins.

Wilkinson, J. M. (2005). *Nursing diagnosis handbook* (8th ed.). Upper Saddle River, NJ: Prentice Hall.

Yeo, L., Ananth, C. V., & Vintzileos, A. M. (2004). Placental abruption. In J. J. Sciarri (Ed.), *Gynecology and obstetrics* (Vol. 2, chap. 50, pp. 1–26). Philadelphia: Lippincott Williams & Wilkins.

Birth-Related Procedures

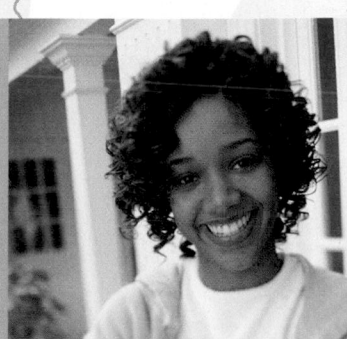

With our first baby, all of a sudden I had to have a cesarean. Everything happened so fast but our son was OK, and that's all that mattered. With our second baby, I wanted to try a vaginal birth. Even though I wanted to, I was afraid. I don't know what I would have done without my nurse. She stayed with me the whole time and kept giving me support. She explained what was happening and gave encouragement. I felt safe. I had a beautiful baby girl after 8 hours of labor.

—*Marianne, 22*

LEARNING OBJECTIVES

- Examine the methods and purpose of external and internal version.

- Discuss the use of amniotomy in current maternal-newborn care.

- Compare methods for inducing labor, explaining their advantages and disadvantages.

- Identify at least two indications for amnioinfusion.

- Describe the types of episiotomy performed and the associated nursing interventions.

- Summarize the indications for and risks of forceps-assisted birth.

- Discuss the use of vacuum extraction to assist birth.

- Explain the indications for cesarean birth, impact on the family unit, preparation and teaching needs, and associated nursing care.

- Discuss vaginal birth following cesarean birth.

MEDIALINK

www.prenhall.com/london

CD-ROM

NCLEX-RN® Review
Video: Vacuum Extractor
Cesarean Birth Videos
Skill 3–7: Assisting with Monitoring of Women
   Undergoing Induction of Labor with Pitocin and
   Cervical Reopening Agents
Audio Glossary

Companion Website

NCLEX-RN® Review
MediaLink Applications:
   Case Study: Client Undergoing Labor Induction
   Care Plan Activity: Client with Pitocin for Labor
     Augmentation
Thinking Critically

Generally women are aware of the possible need for an obstetric procedure during their labor and birth. However, some women expect to have a "natural" experience and do feel disappointed, angry, or even guilty when an unanticipated procedure is needed. This conflict between expectation and the need for intervention presents a challenge to maternity nurses. The nurse provides information about any procedure to help the woman and her partner understand what is proposed, the anticipated benefits and possible risks, and any alternatives.

CARE OF THE WOMAN DURING VERSION

Version, or turning the fetus, is a procedure used to change the fetal presentation by abdominal or intrauterine manipulation. The most common type of version is **external cephalic version (ECV)**, in which the fetus is changed from a breech to a cephalic presentation by external manipulation of the maternal abdomen (Figure 22–1 ●). A less common type of version, called **podalic version**, is used only with the second fetus during a vaginal twin birth and only if the twin does not descend readily or if the heart rate is nonreassuring. In a podalic version, medication is used to relax the uterus. The obstetrician places a hand inside the uterus, grabs the fetus's feet, and draws them down through the cervix.

CRITERIA FOR EXTERNAL VERSION

If breech or shoulder presentation (transverse lie) is detected in the later weeks of pregnancy, an external version may be attempted. Before the external version is begun, an ultrasound is used to locate the placenta and to confirm fetal presentation.

The following criteria should be met prior to performing external version:

- The pregnancy is 36 or more weeks' gestation. A version may result in complications that require immediate birth by cesarean (Kish & Collea, 2003).

- A nonstress test (NST) obtained immediately before the version is reactive. A reactive NST indicates fetal well-being.

- The fetal breech is not engaged. Once the presenting part is engaged it is difficult, if not impossible, to do a version.

CONTRAINDICATIONS FOR EXTERNAL VERSION

Contraindications include the following (Kish & Collea, 2003):

- Maternal problems, such as uterine anomalies, uncontrolled preeclampsia, or third-trimester bleeding

- Complications of pregnancy, such as rupture of membranes, oligohydramnios, hydramnios, or placenta previa

- Previous cesarean birth or other significant uterine surgery

- Multiple gestation

- Nonreassuring fetal heart rate (FHR) or other evidence of uteroplacental insufficiency

- Fetal abnormalities, such as intrauterine growth restriction (IUGR) or nuchal cord

External (or cephalic) version of the fetus. A new technique involves pressure on the fetal head and buttocks so that the fetus completes a "backward flip" or "forward roll."

Before the external version begins, an intravenous line may be established to administer medications in case of difficulty. The woman receives terbutaline subcutaneously to relax the uterus. The version is discontinued in the presence of severe maternal pain or significant fetal bradycardia or decelerations.

NURSING PRACTICE

Because the ECV procedure can be uncomfortable, encourage the woman to take slow, deep breaths. Using distraction and speaking in a calm, reassuring voice can help decrease fear and anxiety.

NURSING CARE MANAGEMENT

On admission the nurse begins a thorough assessment by verifying that there are no contraindications to the version procedure. Maternal vital signs and a reactive NST are obtained. This initial assessment period provides an ideal time for educating the woman and her partner and for addressing their concerns. They can be encouraged to express

their understanding and expectations of the procedure. At the same time, the possibility of failure of the EVC and slight risk of cesarean birth if the FHR becomes nonreassuring should also be discussed. Explaining what will happen in either of these circumstances will better prepare the woman and her partner in case intervention becomes necessary. While the physician is ultimately responsible for obtaining informed consent, it is also the nurse's role to ensure that the woman understands the procedure and has the opportunity to ask questions and voice her concerns or fears.

Throughout the procedure the nurse continues to monitor maternal blood pressure, pulse, and comfort level frequently (because the mother may experience pain during the procedure). Fetal well-being is ascertained before, intermittently during, and for (at least) 30 minutes after the procedure, using electronic fetal monitoring (EFM), ultrasound, or both. The nurse also assesses maternal-fetal response to the tocolytic. Aftercare instructions, which may include maternal monitoring for contractions and fetal movement (fetal kick counts), are provided as well.

CARE OF THE WOMAN DURING AMNIOTOMY

Amniotomy is the artificial rupture of the amniotic membranes (AROM). It is probably the most common invasive procedure in obstetrics. Because the amniotomy requires that an instrument, called an amnihook, be inserted through the cervix, at least 2 cm of cervical dilatation is required.

The amniotomy may be performed in hope of starting (inducing) labor. Amniotomy is successful as a means of inducing labor in 88% of cases (Gabbe, Niebyl, & Simpson, 2002). It can be used any time during the first stage to augment labor (accelerate the progress). An amniotomy done after 3 cm of cervical dilatation shortens the length of labor by 0.8 to 2.3 hours (Gabbe et al., 2002). Amniotomy manipulates both hormones and mechanical factors to stimulate labor. Upon rupturing the membranes, natural prostaglandins are released which stimulate uterine contractions. The escape of amniotic fluid allows the presenting part to descend and place direct pressure on the cervix, thus resulting in an acceleration of dilatation.

Amniotomy may also be done during labor to apply an internal fetal heart monitoring electrode to the scalp, to insert an intrauterine pressure catheter, or to obtain a fetal scalp blood sample for acid-base determination and fetal pH monitoring. In addition, amniotomy allows assessment of the color and composition of amniotic fluid. Amniotomy performed when the presenting part is not well applied to the cervix increases the risk of umbilical cord prolapse. See Care of the Woman and Fetus with a Prolapsed Umbilical Cord in Chapter 21. ∞

AROM PROCEDURE

While performing a vaginal examination, the physician or certified nurse-midwife (CNM) introduces an amnihook into the vagina and makes a small tear in the amniotic membrane, which allows amniotic fluid to escape.

NURSING PRACTICE

Prior to the AROM procedure, place several layers of disposable pads under the woman's buttocks and a folded towel between the woman's legs. The towel readily absorbs the fluid released during the procedure and prevents soiling of the bed linens. After the procedure, remove the towel as well as all layers of absorbent pads that have been soiled. Several clean absorbent pads should be placed under the woman's buttocks since amniotic fluid will continue to leak from the vagina. This increases the woman's comfort.

NURSING CARE MANAGEMENT

The nurse explains the AROM procedure to the woman and then assesses fetal presentation, position, and station. Amniotomy is usually delayed until engagement has occurred. The woman is asked to assume a semireclining position and is draped to provide privacy. The FHR is assessed just before and immediately after the amniotomy, and the two FHR assessments are compared. If there are marked changes, the nurse should check for prolapse of the cord (see Care of the Woman and Fetus with a Prolapsed Umbilical Cord in Chapter 21 ∞). The amniotic fluid is inspected for amount, color, odor, and the presence of meconium or blood. While wearing disposable gloves, the nurse cleanses and dries the perineal area and changes the underpads. Because there is now an open pathway for organisms to ascend into the uterus, the number of vaginal examinations must be kept to a minimum to reduce the chance of introducing an infection. The woman's temperature is monitored a minimum of every 2 hours. The nurse needs to provide information regarding the expected effects of the amniotomy. It is important for the woman to know that amniotic fluid is constantly produced, because some may worry that they will experience a "dry birth."

NURSING PRACTICE

Advise the woman that prostaglandin agents commonly cause uterine stimulation after insertion. Review the signs of labor that warrant further assessment after discharge home. Teach the woman the difference between common reactions to the prostaglandin agents (such as cramping, uterine irritability, and gel leakage) versus the true signs of labor (strong regular contractions, rupture of membranes) prior to leaving the hospital.

CARE OF THE WOMAN DURING CERVICAL RIPENING

Cervical ripening is softening and effacing of the cervix. It may be used for the pregnant woman at or near term when there is a medical or obstetric indication for induction of labor. Pharmacologic methods of cervical ripening include prostaglandin agents and Cytotec.

PROSTAGLANDIN AGENTS

The most commonly used ripening agent is Prepidil gel, which contains 0.5 mg dinoprostone, a prostaglandin E_2 (PGE_2) agent. It is placed intracervically. A similar agent called Cervidil is packaged as a 2-cm square vaginal insert that resembles a thin piece of cardboard. It releases 10 mg of dinoprostone at a rate of 0.3 mg per hour over 12 hours. Prostaglandin agents have been demonstrated to cause cervical ripening, to shorten labor, and to lower requirements for Pitocin during labor induction (Tenore, 2003). Prostaglandin agents are typically used when labor induction is indicated, but not urgent, such as maternal gestational diabetes, postdates, or large-for-gestational-age fetuses who warrant birth occurring in the near future. For example, a woman who is over 41 weeks but has a very unfavorable cervix may be given prostaglandin gel to ripen her cervix before a Pitocin induction is scheduled.

When prostaglandin gel is used in a hospital birthing unit, it is recommended that an obstetrician be available in case an emergency cesarean birth is needed (American College of Obstetricians and Gynecologists [ACOG], 1999a). Complications such as hyperstimulation and nonreassuring fetal status typically occur in the first hour after administration of the gel and peak at 4 hours. See "Drug Guide: Dinoprostone (Prepidil) Vaginal Gel" for additional information.

The nurse should monitor the woman for approximately 2 hours (depending on agency protocol) after the gel is administered. If the fetal heart rate remains unchanged during the initial 2-hour assessment and uterine activity has not become regular, the woman may be discharged once appropriate follow-up instructions and warning signs are provided to her. An induction is scheduled in the near future.

MISOPROSTOL (CYTOTEC)

Misoprostol (Cytotec) is a synthetic PGE_1 analogue that some agencies use to ripen the cervix and induce labor. It is available in a tablet form that is inserted vaginally. During the 1990s, when Cytotec was widely used for cervical ripening and labor induction, several reports associated its use with higher rates of uterine rupture. The drug manufacturer subsequently issued a statement that the drug should

DRUG GUIDE

DINOPROSTONE (PREPIDIL) VAGINAL GEL

Pregnancy Risk Category: C

Overview of Maternal-Fetal Action

Dinoprostone is a naturally occurring form of prostaglandin E_2. Dinoprostone can be used at term to ripen the cervix and can stimulate the smooth muscle of the uterus to enhance uterine contractions. Prepidil can be administered endocervically (Wilson, Shannon, & Stang, 2006).

Route, Dosage, Frequency

The gel contains 0.5 mg of dinoprostone. The gel is placed in the posterior fornix of the vagina, and the client is kept supine for 2 hours but then may ambulate. Continuous electronic monitoring is typically used for 1 to 2 hours after administration.

Contraindications

- Client with known sensitivity to prostaglandins
- Presence of nonreassuring fetal status
- Unexplained bleeding during pregnancy
- Strong suspicion of cephalopelvic disproportion
- Client already receiving Pitocin
- Client with six or more previous term pregnancies
- Client who is not anticipated to be able to give birth vaginally

Dinoprostone vaginal gel should be used with CAUTION in clients with ruptured membranes, a fetus in breech presentation, presence of glaucoma, or history of asthma (Wilson et al., 2006). Prepidil should not be used for women with a previous uterine scar since uterine rupture can occur (ACOG, 2004).

Maternal Side Effects

Uterine hyperstimulation with or without nonreassuring fetal status has occurred in a very small number (2.8% to 4.7%) of clients. Greater than or equal to 1% of clients have experienced fever, nausea, vomiting, or diarrhea (Wilson et al., 2006).

Effects on Fetus or Newborn

Nonreassuring fetal heart rate pattern.

Nursing Considerations

- Assess for presence of contraindications.
- Monitor maternal vital signs, cervical dilatation and effacement carefully, and for excessive vaginal bleeding and cramping pain.
- Monitor fetal status for presence of reassuring fetal heart rate pattern (baseline 110 to 160 bpm, presence of short-term variability, average variability, presence of accelerations with fetal movement, absence of late or variable decelerations).
- Remove vaginal insert if uterine hyperstimulation, sustained uterine contractions, nonreassuring fetal status, or any other maternal adverse reactions occur.
- Monitor for exacerbation of joint pain and limitation due to its effect on the inflammatory process.

not be used for inducing labor in pregnant women (Tenore, 2003). Many hospitals responded by discontinuing use of the drug; however, it is still used in some agencies. After a careful review of the literature and current

studies, ACOG (2000b) issued the following recommended guidelines for Cytotec administration:

- Use only during the third trimester for cervical ripening or labor induction.
- One fourth tablet or 25 mcg should be the initial dosage.
- Recurrent administration should not exceed dosing intervals of more than 3 to 6 hours.
- Pitocin should not be administered less than 4 hours after the last Cytotec dose.

Absolute contraindications for the use of Cytotec include the following (ACOG, 1999b):

- Presence of uterine contractions three times in 10 minutes
- Significant maternal asthma
- History of previous cesarean birth or other uterine scar
- Bleeding during the pregnancy
- Presence of placenta previa
- Nonreassuring fetal heart rate tracing

NURSING CARE MANAGEMENT

Physicians, CNMs, and birthing room nurses who have had special education and training may administer agents for cervical ripening. The woman and her support person are provided information about the procedure, and any questions are answered. Baseline maternal vital signs are assessed, and an electronic fetal monitor is applied. The EFM tracing should indicate minimal or absent uterine activity, a reassuring FHR pattern, and a reactive NST. If uterine contractions are not occurring regularly, the ripening agent is inserted into the vagina. Prepidil can be administered every 6 hours. If prescribed, Cytotec is administered every 3 to 6 hours until adequate cervical change occurs (Tenore, 2003). The nurse instructs the woman to lie supine with a right hip wedge for a specified time (usually at least 1 hour). The woman can then assume any comfortable position. The nurse monitors the woman for uterine hyperstimulation and FHR abnormalities (changes in baseline rate, variability, presence of decelerations) for at least 2 hours following insertion (Tenore, 2003). During administration of PGE_2, if nausea and vomiting are present or contractions occur more frequently than every 2 minutes (or last longer than 75 seconds), the gel is removed.

CARE OF THE WOMAN DURING LABOR INDUCTION

ACOG defines **labor induction** as the stimulation of uterine contractions before the spontaneous onset of labor, with or without ruptured fetal membranes, for the purpose of accomplishing birth. Induction may be indicated in the presence of the following (ACOG, 1999a):

- Diabetes mellitus
- Renal disease
- Preeclampsia
- Premature rupture of membranes (PROM)
- History of rapid labor (precipitous labor and birth)
- Chorioamnionitis
- Postterm gestation
- Mild abruptio placentae without evidence of nonreassuring fetal status
- Intrauterine fetal demise (IUFD)
- Intrauterine fetal growth restriction (IUGR)
- Alloimmunization

All contraindications to spontaneous labor and vaginal birth are contraindications to the induction of labor. Relative maternal contraindications include but are not limited to the following (ACOG, 1999a):

- Client refusal
- Placenta previa or vasa previa
- Transverse fetal lie
- Prior classic uterine incision (vertical incision in the upper portion of the uterus)
- Active genital herpes infection
- Some instances of positive maternal human immunodeficiency virus (HIV) status

LABOR READINESS

Before induction is attempted, appropriate assessment must indicate that both the woman and the fetus are ready for the onset of labor. This includes evaluation of fetal maturity and cervical readiness.

Fetal Maturity

The gestational age of the fetus is best evaluated by accurate maternal menstrual dating and early ultrasounds. Amniotic fluid studies also provide valuable information in assessing fetal lung maturity (see Amniotic Fluid Analysis in Chapter 16 for additional information ∞).

Cervical Readiness

The findings on vaginal examination help determine whether cervical changes favorable for induction have occurred. Bishop (1964) developed a prelabor scoring system that is helpful in predicting the potential success of induction (Table 22–1). Components evaluated are cervical dilatation, effacement, consistency, and position, as well as the station of the fetal presenting part. A score of 0, 1, 2, or 3 is given to each assessed characteristic. The higher the total score for all the criteria, the more likely that labor will occur. The lower the total score, the higher the failure rate. A favorable cervix is the most important criterion for a successful induction (Tenore, 2003). The presence of a cervix that is anterior, soft, 50% effaced, and dilated at least 2 cm, with the fetal head at −1 to +1 station or lower (Bishop score of 8 or 9), is favorable for successful induction (Tenore, 2003). If the cervix is unfavorable, a method of cervical ripening may be tried.

METHODS OF INDUCING LABOR

When the cervix is favorable, the most frequently used methods of induction are amniotomy (discussed previously), stripping the amniotic membranes, intravenous Pitocin infusion, and complementary methods.

TABLE 22–1 ❖ Prelabor Status Evaluation Scoring System

Factor	ASSIGNED VALUE			
	0	1	2	3
Cervical dilatation	Closed	1–2 cm	3–4 cm	5 cm or more
Cervical effacement	0%–30%	40%–50%	60%–70%	80% or more
Fetal station	−3	−2	−1,0	+1, or lower
Cervical consistency	Firm	Moderate	Soft	
Cervical position	Posterior	Midposition	Anterior	

Used with permission from the American College of Obstetricians and Gynecologists. Bishop, E. H. (1964). Pelvic scoring for elective inductions. Obstetrics and Gynecology, 24, 266.

COMPLEMENTARY CARE

Evening primrose oil is a natural substance that is extracted from the plant's seeds. It has been widely used for centuries by midwives as a means of softening the cervix, vagina, and perineum to facilitate the onset of labor. Evening primrose oil contains a fatty acid called gamma linolenic acid, which is converted into a prostaglandin compound (Gallagher, 2004). Prostaglandins play a key role in ripening the cervix so labor can begin. Women can be advised to begin evening primrose oil supplementation during the 36th week of pregnancy. The recommended dose is 2500 mg per day taken either orally or vaginally until birth. Side effects are rare but can include headaches, nausea, or skin rashes. Women who experience side effects should be counseled to discontinue the supplement unless advised otherwise by their physician or CNM (Midwifery Today E-News, 2002).

Stripping the Membranes

A nonpharmacologic method of induction frequently used by physicians and CNMs is *stripping* (or *sweeping*) *the amniotic membranes*. The practitioner inserts a gloved finger into the internal os and rotates it 360 degrees twice, separating the amniotic membranes that are lying against the lower uterine segment. This is thought to release prostaglandins that stimulate uterine contractions. Although the procedure is not 100% effective, if labor is initiated, it typically begins within 48 hours.

Oxytocin (Pitocin) Infusion

Administration of oxytocin (Pitocin) is an effective method of initiating uterine contractions to induce labor and may also be used to enhance ineffective contractions (*labor augmentation*). A primary line of 1000 mL of electrolyte solution (e.g., lactated Ringer's solution) is started intravenously. Ten units of Pitocin are added to a secondary line of intravenous (IV) fluid so the resulting mixture will contain 10 mU/mL of Pitocin (1 mU/min, or 6 mL/hr), and the prescribed dose can be calculated easily. After the primary infusion is started, the Pitocin solution is piggybacked into the primary tubing port closest to the catheter insertion. The infusion is then administered using an infusion pump to control the flow rate precisely. The rate of infusion is based on physician or CNM protocol and careful assessment of the contraction pattern. The goal for induction is to achieve stable contractions every 2 to 3 minutes that last 40 to 60 seconds. The uterus should relax to full baseline resting tone between each contraction. Progress is determined by changes in the effacement and dilatation of the cervix and station of the presenting part.

Pitocin induction is not without some associated risks, including hyperstimulation of the uterus, resulting in uterine contractions that are too frequent or too intense, with an increased resting tone. Hypertonic contractions may lead to decreased placenta perfusion and nonreassuring fetal status. Other risks include uterine rupture and water intoxication (Wilson et al., 2006).

Complementary Methods

In addition to the medical (allopathic) methods just discussed, a variety of more natural, noninvasive methods may also be used. These methods include sexual intercourse; self or partner nipple or breast stimulation; the use of herbs, castor oil, or enemas; acupuncture; and mechanical dilatation of the cervix with balloon catheters (Tenore, 2003). The cautions and contraindications are the same as those for medical induction of labor.

Although not frequently presented in medical (allopathic) or nursing texts, the natural methods can be effective, although some of them may not have undergone as rigorous scientific research as pharmacologic agents. Many certified nurse-midwives and their clients desire a less medical approach to birth and want to use natural methods whenever possible. It is important for basic nursing students, nurses, and consumers to be aware of all aspects of pregnancy care.

Sexual intercourse is a logical method of inducing cervical ripening and uterine contractions; female orgasm stimulates contractions, and male ejaculate contains a rich source of prostaglandins. Penetration during intercourse can also stimulate the lower uterine segment and cause uterine contractions. Breast and nipple stimulation, which are often part of lovemaking, cause the production of endogenous oxytocin, which in turn stimulates the uterus to contract (Tenore, 2003).

Herbal preparations and other homeopathic solutions have not been scientifically studied to the same extent as other natural methods. The caregiver needs a thorough personal knowledge or ongoing consultation with a homeopathic physician to safely recommend the use of these approaches during late pregnancy (Tenore, 2003).

Castor oil has been used for many years but has not been frequently studied as a method of labor induction. The mechanism by which castor oil stimulates uterine contractions is not understood. Some practitioners consider it to be an old-fashioned, nonuseful substance, whereas others have noted that it is especially effective for primigravidas.

NURSING CARE MANAGEMENT

Aspects to address during client teaching about induction of labor include the purpose, the procedure itself, nursing care that will be provided, assessments, comfort measures, and a review of breathing techniques that may be used during labor. Regardless of the induction method used, close

DRUG GUIDE

OXYTOCIN (PITOCIN)

Overview of Obstetric Action

Oxytocin (Pitocin) exerts a selective stimulatory effect on the smooth muscle of the uterus and blood vessels. Pitocin affects the myometrial cells of the uterus by increasing the excitability of the muscle cell, increasing the strength of the muscle contraction, and supporting propagation of the contraction (movement of the contraction from one myometrial cell to the next). Its effect on the uterine contraction depends on the dosage used and on the excitability of the myometrial cells. During the first half of gestation, there is little excitability of the myometrium, and the uterus is fairly resistant to the effects of oxytocin. However, from midgestation on, the uterus responds increasingly to exogenous IV oxytocin. Cautious use of diluted Pitocin administered IV at term results in a slow rise of uterine activity.

The circulatory half-life of Pitocin is 3 to 5 minutes. It takes approximately 40 minutes for a particular dose of Pitocin to reach a steady-state plasma concentration (Wilson et al., 2006).

The effects of Pitocin on the cardiovascular system can be pronounced. Blood pressure initially may decrease but after prolonged administration increase by 30% above the baseline. Cardiac output and stroke volume increase. With doses of 20 milliunits/min or above, Pitocin exerts an antidiuretic effect decreasing free water exchange in the kidney and markedly decreasing urine output.

Pitocin is used to induce labor at term and to augment uterine contractions in the first and second stages of labor. It may also be used immediately after birth to stimulate uterine contraction and thereby control uterine atony.

Route, Dosage, Frequency

For induction of labor: Add 10 units of Pitocin (1 mL) to 1000 mL of intravenous solution. (The resulting concentration is 10 milliunits Pitocin per 1 mL of intravenous fluid.) Using an infusion pump, administer IV, starting at 0.5 to 1 milliunit/min and increase by 1 to 2 milliunits/min every 40 to 60 minutes. Alternatively, start at 1 to 2 milliunits/min and increase by 1 milliunit/min every 15 minutes until a good contraction pattern (every 2 to 3 minutes and lasting 40 to 60 seconds) is achieved.

Maternal Contraindications

- Severe preeclampsia-eclampsia
- Cephalopelvic disproportion
- Malpresentation or malposition of the fetus, cord prolapse
- Preterm infant
- Rigid, unripe cervix; total placenta previa
- Presence of nonreassuring fetal status

Maternal Side Effects

Hyperstimulation of the uterus results in hypercontractility, which in turn may cause the following:

- Abruptio placentae
- Impaired uterine blood flow, leading to fetal hypoxia
- Rapid labor, leading to cervical lacerations
- Rapid labor and birth, leading to lacerations of cervix, vagina, or perineum; uterine atony; fetal trauma
- Uterine rupture
- Water intoxication (nausea, vomiting, hypotension, tachycardia, cardiac arrhythmia) if Pitocin is given in electrolyte-free solution or at a rate exceeding 20 milliunits/min; hypotension with rapid IV bolus administration postpartum

Effect on Fetus or Newborn

- Fetal effects are primarily associated with the presence of hypercontractility of the maternal uterus. Hypercontractility decreases the oxygen supply to the fetus, which is reflected by irregularities or decrease in fetal heart rate (FHR).
- Hyperbilirubinemia (Wilson et al., 2006).
- Trauma from rapid birth

Nursing Considerations

- Explain induction or augmentation procedure to client.
- Apply fetal monitor and obtain 15- to 20-minute tracing and NST to assess FHR before starting IV Pitocin.

---

observation and accurate, ongoing assessments are mandatory to provide safe, optimal care for both woman and fetus. A qualified clinician should be readily accessible to manage any complications that may occur.

As contractions are established, vaginal examinations are done to evaluate cervical dilatation, effacement, and station. The frequency of vaginal examinations primarily depends on the woman's parity, her comfort level, and strength of her contractions. In evaluating the need for analgesia, a vaginal examination should be performed to avoid giving the medication too early and increasing the risk of prolonging labor and to identify advanced dilatation and imminent birth.

Pitocin induction protocols recommend obtaining baseline data (maternal temperature, pulse, respirations, blood pressure), a 20- to 30-minute EFM recording demonstrating a reassuring FHR, a reactive NST, and the contraction status before the induction is started. The fetal monitor provides continuous data.

Before each increase of the Pitocin infusion rate, the nurse assesses the following:

- Maternal blood pressure, pulse, respirations, and temperature
- Contraction status, including frequency, duration, intensity, and resting tone

DRUG GUIDE—continued

OXYTOCIN (PITOCIN)

- For induction or augmentation of labor, start with primary IV and piggyback secondary IV with Pitocin and infusion pump.
- Ensure continuous monitoring of the fetus and uterine contractions.
- The maximum rate is 40 milliunits/min (ACOG, 1999a). Not all protocols recommend a maximum dose. When indicated, the maximum dose is generally between 16 and 40 milliunits/min. Protocols may vary from one agency to another.

  0.5 milliunit/min = 3 mL/hr
  1 milliunit/min = 6 mL/hr
  1.5 milliunits/min = 9 mL/hr
  2 milliunits/min = 12 mL/hr
  4 milliunits/min = 24 mL/hr
  6 milliunits/min = 36 mL/hr
  8 milliunits/min = 48 mL/hr
  10 milliunits/min = 60 mL/hr
  12 milliunits/min = 72 mL/hr
  15 milliunits/min = 90 mL/hr
  18 milliunits/min = 108 mL/hr
  20 milliunits/min = 120 mL/hr

- Assess FHR, maternal blood pressure, pulse, frequency and duration of uterine contractions, and uterine resting tone before each increase in the Pitocin infusion rate.
- Record all assessments and IV rate on monitor strip and on client's chart.
- Record Pitocin infusion rate in milliunit/min and mL/hr (e.g., 0.5 milliunit/min [3 mL/hr]).
- Record on monitor strip all client activities (such as change of position, vomiting), procedures done (amniotomy, sterile vaginal examination), and administration of analgesic agents to allow for interpretation and evaluation of tracing.
- Assess cervical dilatation as needed.

- Provide nursing comfort measures.
- Discontinue IV Pitocin infusion and infuse primary solution when (1) nonreassuring fetal status is noted (bradycardia, late or variable decelerations), (2) uterine contractions are more frequent than every 2 minutes, (3) duration of contractions exceeds more than 60 seconds, or (4) insufficient relaxation of the uterus between contractions or a steady increase in resting tone is noted (ACOG, 1999a). In addition to discontinuing IV Pitocin infusion, turn client to side. If nonreassuring fetal status is present, administer oxygen by tight face mask at 7 to 10 L/min; notify physician or CNM.
- Maintain intake and output record.

  For augmentation of labor:

  Prepare and administer IV Pitocin as for labor induction. Increase rate until labor contractions are of good quality. The flow rate is gradually increased every 30 to 60 minutes (Smith, 2004). In some settings or in a situation when limited fluids may be administered, a more concentrated solution may be used. When 10 units Pitocin are added to 500 mL IV solution, the resulting concentration is 1 milliunit/min = 3 mL/hr. If 10 units Pitocin are added to 250 mL IV solution, the concentration is 1 milliunit/min = 1.5 mL/hr.

  For administration after expulsion of placenta:

- Give one dose of 10 units Pitocin (1 ml) intramuscularly or add to IV fluids for continuous infusion.
- Apply nursing comfort measures.
- Monitor uterus for firmness and early detection of uterine bogginess.
- Monitor uterine placement to detect presence of a full bladder.
- Monitor lochia to detect signs of uterine bogginess and excessive bleeding.
- Notify physician or CNM immediately if uterine bogginess or excessive bleeding continues.

- FHR baseline, variability, and reactivity, noting the presence of accelerations, any decelerations, or bradycardia

For additional information about nursing interventions during use of Pitocin, see "Drug Guide: Oxytocin (Pitocin)" and "Clinical Pathway for Induction of Labor."

CARE OF THE WOMAN DURING AMNIOINFUSION

Amnioinfusion (AI) is a technique by which warmed, sterile normal saline or Ringer's lactate solution is introduced into the uterus through an intrauterine pressure catheter (IUPC). Amnioinfusion can be used intrapartum to increase the volume of fluid in cases of oligohydramnios, in which cord compression causes FHR deceleration and nonreassuring fetal status. It provides an extra cushion of fluid that relieves pressure on the umbilical cord and promotes increased perfusion to the fetus. AI is also used to dilute moderate to heavy meconium released in utero; when used for meconium dilution, AI has resulted in a significant decrease of meconium below the cords (aspiration of meconium below the vocal cords that results from inhalation of meconium when the infant takes its initial breath). At birth, if the infant inhales any meconium present in the

CLINICAL PATHWAY

CLINICAL PATHWAY FOR INDUCTION OF LABOR

CATEGORY	IMMEDIATE CARE	OUTCOMES
Referral	Review prenatal record Advise certified nurse-midwife (CNM) or physician of admission Anesthesia	**EXPECTED OUTCOMES** Appropriate resources identified and utilized
Assessments	Previous pregnancies, present pregnancy, and childbirth preparation Estimated gestational age of the fetus Assess woman's feelings regarding induction as well as knowledge base regarding the induction process Assess knowledge of breathing techniques; if woman does not have a method to use, teach breathing techniques before starting oxytocin infusion	**EXPECTED OUTCOMES** Potential and actual complications identified
Teaching/psychosocial	Provide emotional support through teaching and answering all questions	**EXPECTED OUTCOMES** Woman verbalizes or demonstrates understanding of information given
Nursing care management and reports	Examination of pregnant uterus (Leopold's maneuvers to determine fetal size and position) Vaginal examination to evaluate cervical readiness: <ul><li>Ripe cervix feels soft to the examining finger, is located in a medial to anterior position, is more than 50% effaced, and is 2-3 cm dilated</li><li>Unripe cervix feels firm to the examining finger, is long and thick, is perhaps in a posterior position, and is dilated little or not at all</li></ul>Presence of contractions Membranes intact or ruptured Maternal vital signs and a 20-minute baseline fetal monitoring strip prior to induction to determine fetal well-being Diagnostic studies: <ul><li>Fetal maturity tests (lecithin/sphingomyelin [L/S] ratio, creatinine concentrations, ultrasonography), NST, CST, BPP</li><li>Maternal blood studies (complete blood count [CBC], hemoglobin, hematocrit, blood type, Rh factor)</li><li>Urinalysis</li></ul>Monitor for nausea, vomiting, hypotension, tachycardia, cardiac arrhythmias, headache, mental confusion, decreased urinary output Monitor FHR by continuous electronic fetal monitoring; do not start infusion or advance rate (if induction has already begun) if FHR is not in range of 110–160 bpm, if decelerations are present, or if variability decreases Evaluate and document maternal BP and pulse before beginning induction and then before each increase in infusion rate; do not advance infusion rate in presence of maternal hypertension or hypotension or radical changes in pulse rate If the woman becomes hypotensive: <ul><li>Keep her on her side; may change to other side</li><li>Discontinue oxytocin infusion</li><li>Increase rate of primary IV line</li><li>Monitor FHR</li><li>Notify physician</li><li>Assess for cause of hypotension</li></ul>Evaluate and document contraction frequency, duration, and intensity prior to each increase in infusion rate Discontinue oxytocin infusion if: <ul><li>Contractions are more frequent than every 2 minutes</li><li>Contraction duration exceeds 90 seconds</li><li>Uterus does not relax between contractions</li></ul>	**EXPECTED OUTCOMES** Progression of labor and birth without difficulty Potential and actual complications minimized

BP, blood pressure; bpm, beats per minute; BPP, biophysical profile; CBC, complete blood count; CST, contraction stress test; FHR, fetal heart rate; I&O, intake and output; IV, intravenous; NST, nonstress test; prn, as needed; WNL, within normal limits

CLINICAL PATHWAY—continued

CLINICAL PATHWAY FOR INDUCTION OF LABOR

CATEGORY	IMMEDIATE CARE	OUTCOMES
Nursing care management and reports—continued	Increase oxytocin IV infusion rate every 20 minutes until adequate contractions are achieved. Do not exceed an infusion rate of 20–40 mL/min. (*Note:* Protocols directing how often oxytocin is increased may vary from 15 to 60 minutes. See ACOG, 1999a, for guidelines and refer to institutional protocols.) Check infusion pump to ensure oxytocin is infusing. Check whether pump is on, chamber refills and empties, level of fluid in IV bottle becomes lower. If problem is found, correct and restart infusion at beginning dose. Check main IV site frequently. Check piggyback connection to primary tubing to ensure solution is not leaking. Evaluate cervical dilatation by vaginal examination as indicated. Monitor FHR continuously (normal range is 110–160 bpm). In episodes of bradycardia (<110 bpm) lasting for more than 30 seconds, administer oxygen by face mask at 7–10 L/min. Stop oxytocin infusion. Position woman on left side if quick recovery of FHR does not occur. Carefully evaluate fetal tachycardia (>160 bpm). Sustained tachycardia may necessitate discontinuation of oxytocin infusion. Assess for presence of meconium staining. Notify physician.	
Activity	Ambulate until 5–10 cm. dilated, then bed Position woman in left lateral or semi-Fowler's position Encourage her to avoid supine position	**EXPECTED OUTCOMES** Activity individualized for woman
Comfort	Provide support to woman as she uses breathing techniques Encourage use of effleurage, back rub, and other supportive measures Assess need for analgesia or anesthesia	**EXPECTED OUTCOMES** Optimal comfort level maintained
Nutrition	IV or lactated Ringer's solution Ice chips, clear fluids	**EXPECTED OUTCOMES** Nutritional and hydration needs met
Elimination	Encourage voiding every 2 hours; monitor and record intake and output	**EXPECTED OUTCOMES** Intake and output WNL
Medications	Start primary IV as ordered Administer oxytocin in electrolyte solution (piggyback oxytocin onto primary IV at closest site to IV needle insertion) Pain medications prn	**EXPECTED OUTCOMES** Induction or augmentation of labor occurs within expected parameters
Discharge planning/ home care	Photo packet Birth certificate worksheet Sibling visitation Car seat	**EXPECTED OUTCOMES** Individualized discharge teaching completed
Family involvement	Family visitation policy per institutional protocol Encourage significant other to stay close and assist the woman with breathing techniques	**EXPECTED OUTCOMES** Family or support person involvement maximized
Date		

amniotic fluid, serious breathing problems and pneumonia may result. Amnioinfusion may also be indicated for preterm labor with premature rupture of membranes.

NURSING CARE MANAGEMENT

The nurse is often the first person to detect changes in fetal heart rate associated with cord compression or to observe meconium-stained amniotic fluid. When cord compression is suspected, the immediate intervention is to assist the laboring woman to another position. If this intervention is not successful in restoring the FHR, an amnioinfusion may be considered.

The nurse helps administer the AI, assess the woman's vital signs and contraction status, and monitors the fetal heart rate by continuous EFM. It is important to provide ongoing information to the laboring woman and her partner and to answer questions as they arise. Comfort measures and positioning are vital because the woman is now on bed rest. Frequent changing of disposable underpads and perineal care are also needed because of constant leakage of fluid from the vagina. The nurse ensures that fluids that are infused into the uterus are being adequately expelled. Fluid expulsion is evaluated by counting sanitary pads and visual observation during perineal care.

CARE OF THE WOMAN DURING AN EPISIOTOMY

An **episiotomy** is a surgical incision of the perineal body to enlarge the outlet. The second most common procedure in maternal-child care, the episiotomy has long been thought to minimize the risk of lacerations of the perineum and the overstretching of perineal tissues (Webb & Culhane, 2002). Though very common, the routine use of episiotomy has been seriously questioned for several years. Research suggests that (1) an episiotomy when combined with instrumentation (forceps or vacuum extraction) makes it more likely that the woman will have deep perineal tears and (2) perineal lacerations heal more quickly than deep perineal tears (Dandolu, Chatwani, Harmanli et al., 2005; Varney, Kriebs, & Gegor, 2004). In clinical practice, research has shown that the incidence of major perineal trauma (extension to or through the anal sphincter) is more likely to happen if a midline episiotomy is done (Varney et al., 2004). A repeat of the perineal trauma is likely to occur with subsequent births when instrumentation is combined with the episiotomy (Dandolu, et al., 2005). Additional complications associated with episiotomy are blood loss, infection, pain, and perineal discomfort that may continue for days or weeks past birth, including painful intercourse.

FACTORS THAT PREDISPOSE WOMEN TO EPISIOTOMY

Overall factors that place a woman at increased risk for episiotomy are primigravid status, large or macrosomic fetus, occiput posterior position, use of forceps or vacuum extractor, and shoulder dystocia.

Other factors that may be mitigated by nurses and physicians or CNMs include the following:

- Use of lithotomy and other recumbent positions (causes excessive and uneven stretching of the perineum)
- Encouraging or requiring sustained breath holding during second-stage pushing (causes excessive and rapid perineal stretching, can adversely affect blood flow in mother and fetus, and requires woman to be responsive to caregiver directions rather than her own urges to push spontaneously)
- Arbitrary time limit placed by the physician or CNM on length of second stage

PREVENTIVE MEASURES

Following are some general tips that may help reduce the incidence of routine episiotomies:

- Kegel exercises throughout pregnancy to improve vaginal tone
- Perineal massage during pregnancy
- Natural pushing during labor, and avoiding the lithotomy position or pulling back on legs (which tightens the perineum)

- Side-lying position for pushing, which helps slow birth and diminish tears

- Warm or hot compresses on the perineum and firm counterpressure.

- Encouraging a gradual expulsion of the infant at the time of birth by encouraging the mother to "push, take a breath, push, take a breath," thereby easing the infant out slowly.

EPISIOTOMY PROCEDURE

The two types of episiotomy in current practice are midline and mediolateral (Figure 22–2 ●). Just before birth when approximately 3 to 4 cm of the fetal head is visible during a contraction, the episiotomy is performed using sharp scissors with rounded points (Varney et al., 2004). The midline incision begins at the bottom center of the perineal body and extends straight down the midline to the fibers of the rectal sphincter. The mediolateral incision begins in the midline of the posterior fourchette and extends at a 45-degree angle downward to the right or left.

The episiotomy is usually performed with regional or local anesthesia but may be done without anesthesia in emergency situations. It is generally proposed that as crowning occurs, the distention of the tissues causes numbing. Repair of the episiotomy (episiorrhaphy) and any lacerations is completed during the period between birth of the newborn and before expulsion of the placenta or after expulsion of the placenta. Adequate anesthesia must be given for the repair.

NURSING CARE MANAGEMENT

The woman needs to be supported during the episiotomy and the repair because she may feel some pressure or pulling or tugging sensations. In the absence of adequate anesthesia, she may feel pain. Placing a hand on her shoulder and talking with her can provide comfort and distraction from the repair process. If the woman is having more discomfort than she can comfortably handle, the nurse needs to act as an advocate in communicating the woman's needs to the physician or CNM. At all times the woman

● **FIGURE 22–2**

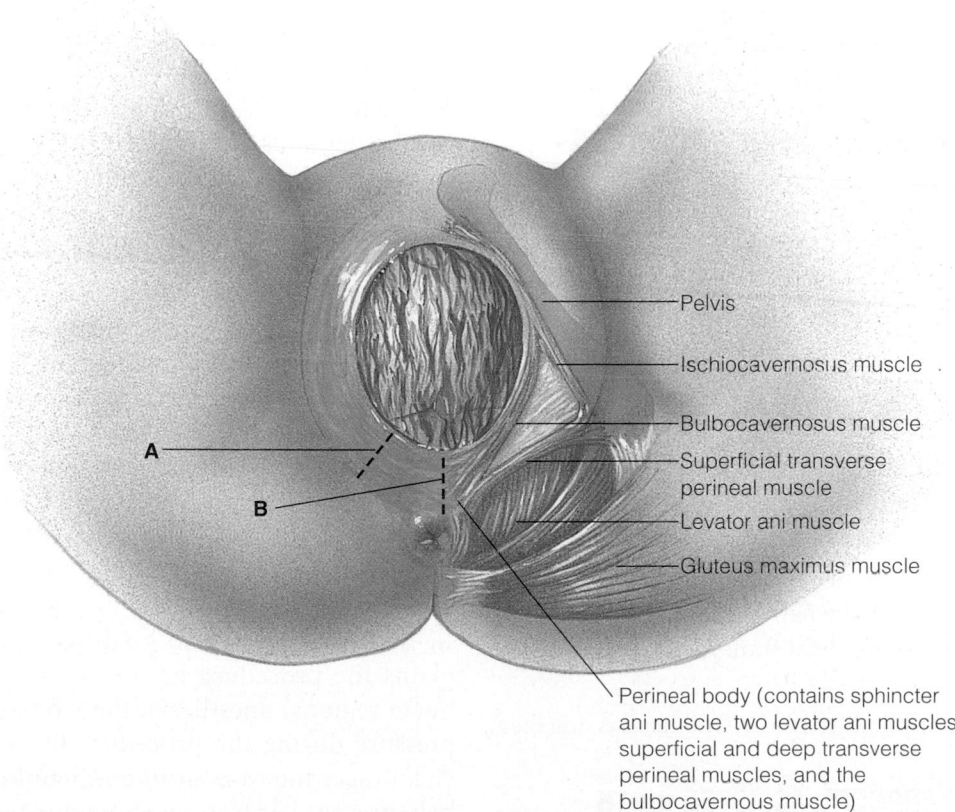

Pelvis

Ischiocavernosus muscle

Bulbocavernosus muscle

Superficial transverse perineal muscle

Levator ani muscle

Gluteus maximus muscle

Perineal body (contains sphincter ani muscle, two levator ani muscles, superficial and deep transverse perineal muscles, and the bulbocavernous muscle)

The two most common types of episiotomy are midline and mediolateral. **A,** Right mediolateral. **B,** Midline.

needs to be the one who decides whether the amount of discomfort she is experiencing is tolerable. She should never be told, "This doesn't hurt." She is the person experiencing the discomfort, and her evaluation needs to be respected.

The type of episiotomy is recorded on the birth record. This information should also be included in a report to subsequent caregivers so that adequate assessments can be made and relief measures instituted.

Comfort measures may begin immediately after birth with the application of an ice pack to the perineum. For optimal effect the ice pack should be applied for 20 to 30 minutes and removed for at least 20 minutes before being reapplied. The nurse assesses the perineal tissues frequently to prevent injury from the ice pack. The episiotomy site should be inspected every 15 minutes during the first hour after the birth for redness, swelling, tenderness, and hematomas. As part of postpartum care, the mother will need instruction in perineal hygiene care, self-care, and comfort measures.

It is important for nurses to recognize that perineal pain continues for a period of time and may be significant. This pain should not be discounted. Women who experience prolonged perineal pain tend to have problems with breastfeeding and depression and are reluctant to reestablish sexual activity.

Nursing advocacy is needed to promote selective rather than routine episiotomy. It is imperative that each nurse stay current regarding new information and research in order to maintain current practice standards.

CARE OF THE WOMAN DURING FORCEPS-ASSISTED BIRTH

Forceps are surgical instruments designed to assist in the birth of a fetus by providing either traction or the means to rotate the fetal head to an occiput anterior position. In medical literature and practice, **forceps-assisted birth** is also known as instrumental delivery or operative vaginal delivery. Three categories of forceps application exist:

1. Outlet forceps are applied when the fetal skull has reached the perineum, the fetal scalp is visible, and the sagittal suture is not more than 45 degrees from the midline.

2. Low forceps are applied when the leading edge (presenting part) of the fetal skull is at a station of +2 or more.

3. Midforceps are applied when the fetal head is engaged.

INDICATIONS FOR FORCEPS-ASSISTED BIRTH

Forceps may be indicated in the presence of any condition that threatens the mother or fetus and that can be relieved by birth. Conditions that put the woman at risk include heart disease, pulmonary edema, infection, and exhaustion. Fetal conditions include premature placental separation and nonreassuring fetal status. Forceps may be used to shorten the second stage of labor and assist the woman's pushing effort or when regional anesthesia has affected the woman's motor innervation and she cannot push effectively. Before forceps are used, the following conditions must be met (Gilstrap, Cunningham, & Van-Dorsten, 2002):

- The cervix must be completely dilated and the exact position and station of the fetal head known.

- Membranes must be ruptured to allow a firm grasp on the fetal head, which must be engaged and in vertex or face presentation.

- The type of pelvis should be known, because certain pelvic types do not permit rotation.

- The maternal bladder should be empty and adequate anesthesia given.

- No degree of cephalopelvic disproportion can be present.

NEONATAL AND MATERNAL RISKS

Some newborns may develop a small area of ecchymosis or edema along the sides of the face as a result of forceps application. Facial lacerations can also occur. Caput succedaneum or cephalhematoma (with subsequent hyperbilirubinemia) may occur, as may transient facial paralysis. Although rare, cerebral hemorrhages have also been reported.

Maternal risks include possible lacerations of the birth canal, extensions of a midline episiotomy into the anus, increased bleeding, bruising, and perineal edema.

NURSING CARE MANAGEMENT

By using ongoing assessment, the nurse may note the variables associated with an increased rate of instrument-assisted or operative birth. Nursing care measures could then be directed toward variables that may reduce the incidence of these factors. For example, labor dystocia may be corrected by changing maternal position, ambulation, use of breast or nipple stimulation, and frequent bladder emptying. FHR abnormalities may be improved by position changes, increased fluid intake, or adequate oxygen exchange.

If a forceps-assisted birth is required, the nurse explains the procedure briefly to the woman. With adequate regional anesthesia, the woman should feel some pressure during the procedure but no pain. The nurse encourages the woman to use breathing techniques that help prevent her from pushing during application of the forceps (Figure 22–3 ●). The nurse monitors contractions and advises the physician when one is present be-

● **FIGURE 22–3**

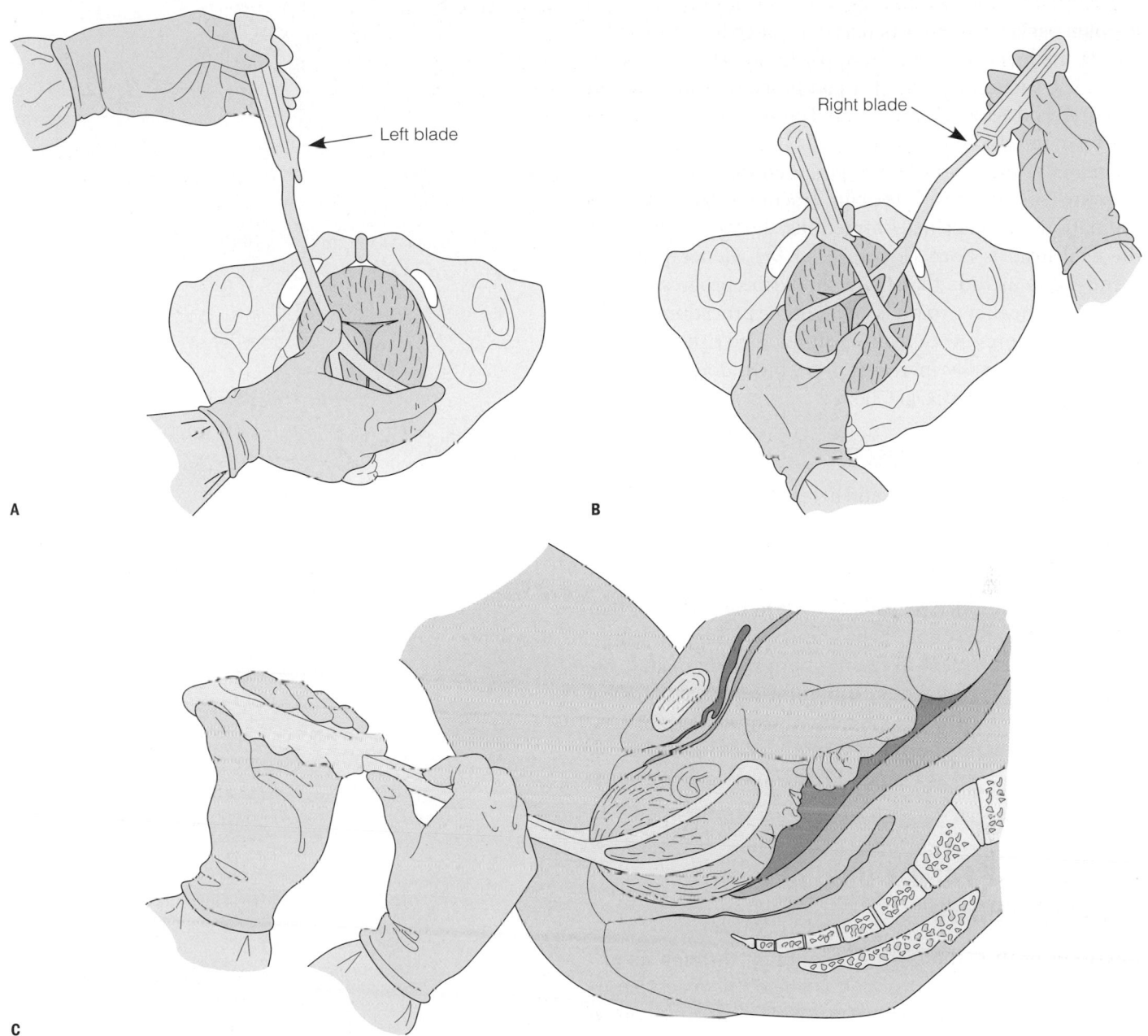

Application of forceps in occiput anterior (OA) position. *A,* The left blade is inserted along the left side wall of the pelvis over the parietal bone. *B,* The right blade is inserted along the right side wall of the pelvis over the parietal bone. *C,* With correct placement of the blades, the handles lock easily. During uterine contractions, traction is applied to the forceps in a downward and outward direction to follow the birth canal.

cause traction is only applied with a contraction. With each contraction the physician provides traction on the forceps as the woman pushes. The nurse reinforces to the woman that she needs to push while traction is being applied, explaining that the combined efforts help with the birth of the fetus. It is not uncommon to observe mild fetal bradycardia as traction is being applied to the forceps. This bradycardia results from head compression and is temporary.

Immediately following birth the newborn is assessed for facial edema, bruising, caput succedaneum, cephalhematoma, and any sign of cerebral edema. In the fourth stage, the nurse assesses the woman for perineal swelling, bruising, hematoma, excessive bleeding, and hemorrhage. In the postpartum period, it is important to assess for signs of infection if lacerations occurred during the procedure. The nurse provides an opportunity for questions and reiterates explanations provided.

CARE OF THE WOMAN DURING VACUUM-ASSISTED BIRTH

Vacuum-assisted birth is an obstetric procedure used to facilitate the birth of a fetus by applying suction to the fetal head. The vacuum extractor is composed of a soft suction cup attached to a suction bottle (pump) by tubing. The suction cup, which comes in various sizes, is placed against the fetal occiput, and the pump is used to create negative pressure (suction) inside the cup. Traction is applied in coordination with uterine contractions, descent occurs, and the fetal head is born (Figure 22–4 ●). General recommendations include that there should be progressive descent with the first two pulls and that the procedure should be limited to prevent cephalhematoma. The risk of cephalhematoma generally increases if the birth does not occur within 6 minutes (ACOG, 2000a).

NURSING CARE MANAGEMENT

The nurse keeps the woman and her partner informed about what is happening during the procedure. If adequate regional anesthesia has been administered, the woman feels only pressure during the procedure. The nurse assesses FHR by continuous EFM. The parents need to be reassured that the caput (chignon) on the baby's head will disappear within 2 to 3 days. Assessment of the newborn should include inspection and continued observation for cephalhematomas, intracerebral hemorrhage, and retinal hemorrhages (ACOG, 2000a). Since infants born via vacuum are at increased risk for jaundice, careful assessment of the infant's skin color is also needed.

CARE OF THE FAMILY DURING CESAREAN BIRTH

Cesarean birth is the birth of the infant through an abdominal and uterine incision. It is one of the oldest surgical procedures known. Until the 20th century, cesarean procedures were primarily used in an attempt to save the fetus of a dying woman. As the maternal and perinatal morbidity and mortality rates associated with cesarean birth steadily decreased throughout the 20th century, the proportion of cesarean births increased.

Beginning in the early 1970s, the cesarean rate rose steadily for almost two decades. In 1989, in an effort to contain healthcare costs, the number of cesarean births began to decline. But in 2002, the number of cesarean births performed in the United States reached an all-time high of 26.1% (Hamilton, Martin, & Sutton, 2003).

Cesarean birth rates differ dramatically in other parts of the world. Worldwide, cesarean birth is the least common in Bolivia (5%) and Peru (7%), and the most common in Brazil

● **FIGURE 22–4**

A

B

C

Vacuum extractor traction. **A,** The cup is placed on the fetal occiput and suction is created. Traction is applied in a downward and outward direction. **B,** Traction continues in a downward direction as the fetal head begins to emerge from the vagina. **C,** Traction is maintained to lift the fetal head out of the vagina.

and Chile (40%). Other countries with low cesarean birth rates include Austria (12.4%), the Netherlands (9.2%), Norway (12.5%), and Sweden (12%). In Thailand the rate of cesarean birth has increased by 64% in the last 5 years, with 31% of all births being cesareans (Bowes & Thorp, 2004).

The increasing rate in the United States is linked to a rise in repeat cesarean births fueled by concerns regarding the risk of uterine rupture with a vaginal birth after a previous cesarean birth. There is also an increase in requests from women for cesarean births so that they can avoid the pain of labor and vaginal birth. The trend increased further when some medical literature stated that vaginal births could result in pelvic floor damage during the birth process (Odibo & Macones, 2003). There is also an emerging trend to "schedule" birth into busy routines to meet specific needs of the parents, such as coordinating work projects, arranging for babysitting of older children, or arranging for relatives who live in other geographic locations to travel to be present for the birth itself.

Many other factors have contributed to the rise in the cesarean birth rate and need to be considered in any discussion about decreasing the rate. These factors include an increased use of epidural anesthesia, increased physician scheduling of cesarean births for personal convenience, policy statements from professional organizations encouraging cesarean birth, political pressure from malpractice insurance carriers who attempt to dictate practice standards, and fear of litigation (Young, 2003).

INDICATIONS

Commonly accepted indications for cesarean birth include complete placenta previa, cephalopelvic disproportion, placental abruption, active genital herpes, umbilical cord prolapse, failure to progress in labor, nonreassuring fetal status, previous classic incision on the uterus (either previous cesarean birth or myomectomy), benign and malignant tumors that obstruct the birth canal, and cervical cerclage. Indications that are more controversial include breech presentation, previous cesarean birth, major congenital anomalies, and severe Rh alloimmunization.

MATERNAL MORTALITY AND MORBIDITY

Cesarean births have a higher maternal mortality rate than vaginal births. Whereas approximately 2.1 per 100,000 women die during a vaginal birth, mortality is 5.9 per 100,000 for women who undergo an elective cesarean birth. Women who undergo an emergency cesarean birth face a significantly higher incidence of death, 18.2 per 100,000 (Hannah, 2004). Perinatal morbidity is often associated with infection, reaction to anesthesia, blood clots, and bleeding problems.

In addition to the complications associated with cesarean birth, there are risks that increase maternal mortality and morbidity in subsequent pregnancies. Women who have had a previous cesarean birth have an increased risk of bleeding problems in future pregnancies. The risk of placenta previa in subsequent pregnancies is 5.2 per 1000. Abruptio placentae occurs in 11.5 per 1000 of subsequent pregnancies. There is also an increase in fetal demise and in neonatal respiratory distress and the need for oxygen administration in fetuses whose mothers have previously given birth via cesarean (Hannah, 2004).

SKIN INCISIONS

The skin incision for a cesarean birth is either transverse (Pfannenstiel) or vertical and is not indicative of the type of incision made into the uterus. The transverse incision is made across the lowest and narrowest part of the abdomen. Since the incision is made just below the pubic hairline, it is almost invisible after healing. The limitation of this type of skin incision is that it does not allow for extension of the incision if needed. This incision is used when time is not of the essence (e.g., with failure to progress and stable fetal and maternal status), because it usually requires more time to make and repair.

The vertical incision is made between the navel and the symphysis pubis. This type of incision is quicker and is therefore preferred in cases of nonreassuring fetal status when rapid birth is indicated, with preterm or macrosomic infants, or when the woman is significantly obese (Lanneau, Muffley, & Magann, 2004). Time factors, client preference, previous vertical skin incision, or physician preference determine the type of skin incision.

UTERINE INCISIONS

The type of uterine incision depends on the need for the cesarean. The choice of incision affects the woman's opportunity for a subsequent vaginal birth and her risks of a ruptured uterine scar with a subsequent pregnancy.

The two major locations of uterine incisions are in the lower uterine segment and in the upper segment of the uterine corpus. The lower uterine segment incision most commonly used is a transverse incision (Figure 22–5 ●). The lower uterine segment incision is preferred for the following reasons:

- The lower segment is the thinnest portion of the uterus and involves less blood loss.
- It requires only moderate dissection of the bladder from underlying myometrium.
- It is easier to repair, although repair takes longer.
- The site is less likely to rupture during subsequent pregnancies.

⬤ FIGURE 22–5

A   B   C

Uterine incisions for a cesarean birth. **A,** This transverse incision in the lower uterine segment is called a Kerr incision. **B,** The Sellheim incision is a vertical incision in the lower uterine segment. **C,** This view illustrates the classic uterine incision that is done in the body (corpus) of the uterus. The classic incision was commonly used in the past but is associated with increased risk of uterine rupture in subsequent pregnancies and labor.

- There is a decreased chance of adherence of bowel or omentum to the incision line.

Disadvantages are as follows:

- It takes longer to make a transverse incision.
- It is limited in size because of the presence of major vessels on either side of the uterus.
- It has a greater tendency to extend laterally into the uterine vessels.
- The incision may stretch and become a thin window, but it usually does not create problems clinically until subsequent labor ensues.

The lower uterine segment vertical incision is preferred for multiple gestation, abnormal presentation, placenta previa, nonreassuring fetal status, and preterm and macrosomic fetuses. Disadvantages of this incision are as follows:

- The incision may extend downward into the cervix.
- More extensive dissection of the bladder is needed to keep the incision in the lower uterine segment; hemostasis and closure are more difficult.
- The vertical incision carries a higher risk of rupture with subsequent labor. Once a vertical incision is performed, future births need to be via cesarean.

One other incision, the classic incision, was the method of choice for many years but is used infrequently now. This vertical incision was made into the upper uterine segment.

More blood loss resulted and it was more difficult to repair. Most importantly, it carried an increased risk of uterine rupture with subsequent pregnancy, labor, and birth because the upper uterine segment is the most contractile portion of the uterus.

DEVELOPING CULTURAL COMPETENCE

TRANSLATING OPERATIVE REPORTS

Women from other countries who have had a previous cesarean birth typically have a vertical skin incision; however, the skin incision does not provide data on the type of uterine incision that was performed. Careful explanation should be provided and an operative report should be obtained when possible. Operative reports in other languages need to be translated by personnel familiar with medical terminology. In the event an operative report cannot be obtained, which is common, a thorough explanation regarding the need for a repeat cesarean should be provided.

ANALGESIA AND ANESTHESIA

There is no perfect anesthesia for cesarean birth. Each has its advantages, disadvantages, possible risks, and side effects. Goals for analgesia and anesthesia administration include safety, comfort, and emotional satisfaction for the client (see Spinal Block and Combined Spinal-Epidural Block in Chapter 20 ∞).

NURSING CARE MANAGEMENT

Preparation for Cesarean Birth

Because one of every four births is a cesarean, preparation for this possibility should be an integral part of all prenatal education. Pregnant women and their partners should be encouraged to discuss the possibility of a cesarean birth with their physician or CNM and at the same time discuss their specific needs and desires under those circumstances. Their preferences may include the following:

- Participating in the choice of anesthetic
- Father (or significant other) being present during the procedures and birth
- Father (or significant other) being present in the recovery or postpartum room
- Audio recording and/or taking pictures of the birth
- Delayed instillation of eyedrops to promote eye contact between parent and infant in the first hours after birth
- Physical contact or holding the infant while in the operating and/or recovery room (by the father if the mother cannot hold the newborn)
- Breastfeeding in the recovery area within the first hour of birth

Information that couples need about cesarean birth includes the following:

- What preparatory procedures to expect
- Description or viewing of the operating room
- Types of anesthesia for birth and analgesia available postpartum
- Sensations that may be experienced
- Roles of significant others
- Interaction with newborn
- Immediate recovery phase
- Postpartum phase

Preparing the woman and her family for birth involves more than the procedures of establishing an intravenous line, instilling a urinary indwelling catheter, and performing an abdominal prep. As discussed previously, good communication skills are essential in preparing the woman and her support person. The use of therapeutic touch and direct eye contact (if culturally acceptable and possible) assist the woman in maintaining a sense of control and lessen anxiety.

If the cesarean birth is scheduled and not an emergency, the nurse has ample time for preoperative teaching. The context in which this information is relayed should be birth oriented rather than surgery oriented. This pro-vides an opportunity for the woman to express her concerns, ask questions, and develop a relationship with the nurse.

In preparation for surgery, the woman is given nothing by mouth. To reduce the likelihood of serious pulmonary damage if gastric contents are aspirated, antacids may be administered within 30 minutes of surgery. If epidural anesthesia is used, the nurse may assist with the procedure, monitor the woman's blood pressure and response, and continue EFM. An abdominal and perineal prep is done, and an indwelling catheter is inserted to prevent bladder distention. An intravenous line is started with a large-bore needle to permit blood administration if it becomes necessary. Preoperative medication may be ordered. The pediatrician should be notified and preparation made to receive the new baby. The nurse ensures that the infant warmer is working and that resuscitation equipment is available.

The nurse assists in positioning the woman on the operating table. Fetal heart rate is assessed before surgery and during preparation because fetal hypoxia can result from the supine position. The operating room table is adjusted so it slants slightly to one side, or a hip wedge (folded blanket or towels) is placed under the right hip to tip the uterus slightly and reduce compression of blood vessels. The uterus should be displaced 15 degrees from the midline. This helps relieve the pressure of the heavy uterus on the vena cava and lessens the incidence of vena cava compression and maternal supine hypotension. The suction should be in working order and the uterine collection bag should be positioned under the operating room table to obtain proper drainage. Ausculation or EFM of the fetal heart rate is continued until immediately prior to the procedure. A last-minute check is done to ensure that the fetal scalp electrode has been removed if the fetus was internally monitored.

The nurse continues to provide reassurance and describe the various procedures being performed along with a rationale to ease anxiety and give the woman a sense of control.

NURSING PRACTICE

Women undergoing elective cesarean birth can be taught many aspects of postoperative teaching prior to their birth experience. Important components of client education that can be emphasized prior to birth include dealing with postoperative discomfort, splinting the incision to decrease pain, frequent deep breathing and coughing, and the importance of early ambulation. Women who receive this information prior to the birth are more apt to remember it when it is reviewed in the early postpartum period.

Preparation for Repeat Cesarean Birth

When a couple is anticipating a repeat cesarean birth, they have a general understanding of what will occur, which can help them make informed choices about their birth experience. Couples who have had previous negative experiences need an opportunity to describe what they felt. They can be encouraged to identify what they would like to be different and to list options that would make the experience more positive. Those who have already had positive experiences need reassurance that their needs and desires will be met in a similar manner. In addition an opportunity should be provided to discuss any fears or anxieties.

The positive aspects of a repeat cesarean birth should be emphasized. For women who previously labored and then had an unexpected cesarean birth, the experience may be perceived as negative. Positive aspects that should be emphasized include participation in selecting birth date, lack of fatigue related to labor, ability to prepare and make arrangements for other children, and ability for other family members or friends to be present at the hospital during or immediately after birth if desired by the couple.

Preparation for Emergency Cesarean Birth

When the need for a cesarean birth emerges suddenly, the period preceding surgery must be used to its greatest advantage. It is imperative that caregivers use their most effective communication skills in supporting the couple. The nurse describes what the couple may anticipate during the next few hours. Asking the couple, "What questions or concerns do you have about the decision?" gives them an opportunity for clarification. The nurse can prepare the woman in stages, giving her information and the rationale for interventions before beginning any procedure. It is essential to tell the woman (1) what is going to happen, (2) why it is being done, and (3) what sensations she may experience. This allows the woman to be informed and to consent to the procedure, which gives her a sense of control and reduces her feelings of helplessness.

Supporting the Father or Partner

Every effort should be made to include the father or partner in the birth experience. When attending the cesarean birth, the partner wears protective coverings similar to those worn by others in the operating suite. A stool can be placed beside the woman's head so that the partner can sit nearby to provide physical touch, visual contact, and verbal reassurance.

To promote participation of the father who chooses not to be in the operating suite, the nurse can do the following:

- Allow the father to be nearby, where he can hear the newborn's first cry.

- Encourage the father to carry or accompany the infant to the nursery for the initial assessment.

- Involve the father in postpartum care in the recovery room.

In some emergency circumstances, a support person may not be permitted in the operating room. In these situations the support person should receive a thorough explanation of what is happening and why, be advised when the staff will return to provide information, know the expected length of time for the procedure, and be reassured that the mother is receiving the care she and the baby need. Since this exclusion is stressful for family members, staff should try to provide information as soon as possible after providing emergency care to the mother.

IMMEDIATE POSTNATAL RECOVERY PERIOD

After the birth the nurse assesses the Apgar score and completes the same initial assessment and identification procedures used for vaginal births. Infant identification bands must be placed on the infant and the mother (as well as the third person, if present) prior to removing the infant from the operating room. Every effort should be made to assist the parents in bonding with their infant. If the mother is awake, one of her arms can be freed to enable her to touch and stroke the infant. The newborn may be placed on the mother's chest or held in an *en face* position. If physical contact is not possible, the nurse can provide a running narrative so the mother knows what is happening with her baby. The nurse assists the anesthesiologist or nurse anesthetist with raising the mother's head so she can see her infant immediately after birth. The parents can be encouraged to talk to the baby, and the father can hold the baby until he or she is taken to the nursery.

The nurse caring for the postpartum woman assesses the mother's vital signs every 5 minutes until they are stable, then every 15 minutes for an hour, then every 30 minutes until she is discharged to the postpartum unit. The nurse should remain with the woman until she is stable.

The nurse evaluates the dressing and perineal pad every 15 minutes for at least an hour. The fundus should be gently palpated to determine whether it is remaining firm; it may be palpated by placing a hand to support the incision. Intravenous Pitocin is usually administered to promote the contractility of the uterine musculature. If the woman has been under general anesthesia, she should be positioned on her side to facilitate drainage of secretions, turned, and assisted with coughing and deep breathing every 2 hours for at least 24 hours. If she has received a spinal or epidural anesthetic, the level of anesthesia is checked every 15 minutes until full sensation has returned. It is important for the nurse to monitor intake and output and to observe the urine for bloody tinge, which could mean surgical trauma to the bladder. The physician prescribes medication to relieve the mother's pain and nausea, and it is administered as needed.

NURSING PRACTICE

Bonding can be promoted by encouraging the mother to hold or breastfeed her infant during the recovery time period. If the infant has been moved to a separate area, such as the nursery, encourage maternal participation by allowing the support person to visit the infant and report back to the mother. The support person can take digital pictures or bring back the blanket that was used to wrap up the baby immediately after the birth. Frequent updates from the nurse such as "Your baby is doing just fine" provide reassurance to the mother if separation is necessary.

CARE OF THE WOMAN UNDERGOING VAGINAL BIRTH AFTER CESAREAN (VBAC)

Vaginal birth after cesarean (VBAC) has been the subject of debate for years. In the late 1990s there was an increasing trend to have a trial of labor and attempt VBAC in cases where the previous cesarean birth was necessitated by a nonrecurring indication (such as umbilical cord pro-lapse, breech, placenta previa, or nonreassuring fetal status). This trend was influenced by consumer demand and studies that have supported VBAC as a viable alternative to repeat cesarean.

Recent media reports identifying risks of VBAC (discussed shortly) have reintroduced the debate regarding its safety. At the same time, trends in counseling women to have an elective, repeat cesarean birth are driving rates of cesarean birth to an all-time high in the United States. Clearly, greater consumer awareness and more research into the risks and benefits are needed.

The ACOG (2004) guidelines state that the following aspects need to be considered for VBAC:

- A woman with one previous cesarean birth and a low transverse uterine incision may be counseled and encouraged to attempt VBAC.
- A clinically adequate pelvis is a requirement for VBAC.
- A classic or T uterine incision is a contraindication to VBAC.
- A woman with two previous cesareans who has also had a previous vaginal birth may attempt VBAC.
- It must be possible to perform a cesarean within 30 minutes.

EVIDENCE-BASED NURSING

VAGINAL BIRTH AFTER CESAREAN BIRTH

Clinical Question

When can a mother safely give birth vaginally when a previous cesarean birth has been performed?

Evidence

The Institute for Clinical Systems Improvement, a nonprofit collaboration of healthcare organizations, assembled a work group of medical experts and nurse-midwives to develop a guideline for vaginal birth after cesarean (VBAC). The group conducted a systematic review of the research evidence and solicited expert opinions to develop the final guideline. They concluded that VBAC is a safe option for carefully screened mothers in facilities equipped to provide special services for labor management.

Conditions that were suspected of increasing the risk of problems with VBAC, but which have not been supported by research evidence, include a previous postcesarean infection and a known overdistended uterus (e.g., twin pregnancy). Some maternal conditions are not clearly contraindicated but may increase risk during VBAC. These include two or more previous cesarean births, a history of failure to progress during labor, preterm birth, and prepregnancy weight of more than 300 lb.

Implications

At the first prenatal visit, a woman desiring VBAC should be carefully screened for contraindications. These include a previous classic incision, any other incision that deeply penetrates the upper uterus, or any fetal contraindication to vaginal birth. Those mothers who do not have contraindications need careful and thorough education about the risks and benefits associated with VBAC. For those mothers who elect to attempt VBAC, you should encourage the selection of a birthing facility that provides specialized labor management, including a team capable of performing a cesarean birth if it is ultimately indicated. The selected birthing facility should also have capability for intermittent or continuous electronic fetal heart monitoring, and a team capable of responding to obstetric emergencies. While left to the provider's discretion, intravenous access and availability of blood products is recommended.

You can discuss VBAC options in appropriate patients who have no contraindication. Provide patient education about the risks and benefits of this procedure. When a VBAC is planned, ensure that appropriate fetal monitoring is available, and consult with the obstetrician about maintaining a venous access line and having blood available. Be alert for any signs of nonreassuring fetal status or maternal complications.

Critical Thinking

What assessments would indicate that you should not encourage a mother to pursue VBAC? What signs and symptoms will you assess to determine if there are fetal or maternal indications for cesarean birth, even when a VBAC has been planned?

Reference

Institute for Clinical Systems Improvement. (2002, October). *Vaginal birth after cesarean* (pp. 1–23). Bloomington, MN: Author.

- A physician, adequate staff, anesthesia, and facilities must be readily available throughout active labor to perform a cesarean birth if needed.

The most common risks associated with failed VBAC births are hemorrhage, uterine scar separation or uterine rupture, hysterectomy, surgical injuries, infant death, and neurologic complications. It should be noted that these complications occur as a result of a uterine rupture.

The incidence of uterine rupture is 0.6% of all trials of labor when the mother has had a previous cesarean birth. Women who go into spontaneous labor have a much lower incidence of uterine rupture than women who undergo Pitocin induction. Prostaglandin agents should not be used in women attempting a VBAC due to the increased risk of uterine rupture. The incidence of uterine rupture in women who receive a prostaglandin agent is as high as 24.5 per 1000 (Odibo & Macones, 2003). Conservative policies, such as awaiting spontaneous labor, avoiding prostaglandin agents, and avoiding elective inductions, can assist in reducing the incidence of uterine rupture.

Women who have a successful VBAC have lower incidence of infection, less blood loss, fewer blood transfusions, and shorter hospital stays. Healthcare costs are considerably lower for women who have a VBAC than for those who have repeat cesarean birth (Odibo & Macones, 2003).

Research shows a close correlation between maternal weight and success for VBAC (Odibo & Macones, 2003). Mothers who weigh less than 200 lb were much more likely to have a subsequent vaginal birth (81%) compared to women over 300 lb (13%) (Odibo & Macones, 2003).

NURSING CARE MANAGEMENT

The nursing care of a woman undergoing VBAC varies according to institutional protocols. Generally a saline lock is inserted in case IV access is needed or an intravenous infusion of fluids is started. Continuous EFM is used, and clear fluids may be taken. A woman at higher risk may require additional precautionary measures such as internal monitoring after the membranes have ruptured. The nurse should take care to ensure that the woman and her partner feel safe but not unduly restricted by the VBAC status.

Supportive and comfort measures are very important. The woman may be excited about this opportunity to experience labor and vaginal birth, or she may be hesitant and frightened about the possibility of complications. The presence of the nurse is important in providing information and encouragement for the laboring woman and her partner.

Critical Concept Review

LEARNING OBJECTIVES

CONCEPTS

Examine the methods and purpose of external and internal version.

1. An external version (cephalic version) may be done after 36 weeks' gestation to change a breech presentation to a cephalic presentation.
   - Physician applies external manipulation to the maternal abdomen.
   - Fetal part must not be engaged.
   - NST performed to establish fetal well-being.
   - Tocolytic given during procedure to relax uterus.
2. Internal version (podalic version) is used to turn a second twin during a vaginal birth.
   - Used only if second fetus does not descend readily and heartbeat is not reassuring.
   - Physician reaches into uterus and grabs feet of fetus and pulls them down through cervix.
   - A tocolytic is given to relax uterus.

Discuss the use of amniotomy in current maternal-newborn care.

1. There are several reasons an amniotomy (artificial rupture of the amniotic membranes) is used:
   - To induce labor.
   - To accelerate labor.
   - To apply an internal fetal monitor or insert an intrauterine pressure catheter.
2. Risks include prolapse cord and infection.

LEARNING OBJECTIVES   CONCEPTS

LEARNING OBJECTIVES	CONCEPTS
Compare methods for inducing labor, explaining their advantages and disadvantages.	1. Cervical ripening: 　■ May hasten the beginning of labor or shorten the course of labor. 　■ May cause hyperstimulation of the uterus. 2. Stripping the membranes: 　■ May not induce labor; if labor is initiated, it typically begins within 48 hours. 　■ May cause bleeding. 3. Pitocin infusion: 　■ Usually effective at producing contractions. 　■ May cause hyperstimulation of uterus.
Identify at least two indications for amnioinfusion.	1. To increase volume of fluid in maternal oligohydramnios. 2. To dilute moderate to heavy meconium released in utero. 3. To delay labor during preterm labor with premature rupture of membranes. 4. To provide fluid cushion and relieve cord compression.
Describe the types of episiotomy performed and the associated nursing interventions.	1. There are two types of episiotomy used: 　■ Midline. 　■ Mediolateral. 2. During the episiotomy the nurse supports the woman, explaining the procedure. 3. After the birth: 　■ Place an ice pack to the perineum. 　■ Inspect the perineum frequently. 　■ Instruct the woman in perineal hygiene, self-care, and comfort measures.
Summarize the indications for and risks of forceps assisted birth.	Indications: 1. To shorten the second stage of labor. 　■ Used in the presence of nonreassuring fetal status and premature placental separation. 2. To assist woman's pushing effort. 　■ Used in the presence of maternal exhaustion, or when regional anesthesia impairs woman's ability to push effectively. Risks: 1. Newborn bruising, facial edema, facial lacerations, cephalhematoma, and transient facial paralysis. 2. Woman may experience vaginal lacerations, increased bleeding, bruising, and perineal edema.
Discuss the use of vacuum extraction to assist birth.	Vacuum extractor assists birth by applying suction to the fetal head. 1. May cause cephalhematoma. 2. Increases risk for jaundice.
Explain the indications for cesarean birth, impact on the family unit, preparation and teaching needs, and associated nursing care.	1. Most common indications for cesarean birth are: 　■ Nonreassuring fetal status. 　■ Lack of labor progression. 　■ Maternal infection. 　■ Pelvic size disproportion. 　■ Placenta previa. 　■ Previous cesarean birth. 2. Couples should be encouraged to participate in as many choices as possible concerning the surgical birth. 3. Preparation for cesarean birth requires: 　■ Establishing IV lines. 　■ Placing an indwelling catheter. 　■ Performing an abdominal prep. 4. Teaching needs include: 　■ What to expect before, during, and after birth. 　■ Role of significant others. 　■ Interaction with newborn.

(continued)

LEARNING OBJECTIVES

CONCEPTS

Explain the indications for cesarean birth, impact on the family unit, preparation and teaching needs, and associated nursing care.—Continued

→

5. Associated nursing care:
   - Routine postpartal care including fundal checks.
   - Care of incision.
   - Monitoring intake and output.
   - Assessment of respiratory system and returning bowel sounds.
   - Assessment of maternal pain level and provision of pain relief.

Discuss vaginal birth following cesarean birth.

→

1. Most common risks are:
   - Hemorrhage.
   - Uterine rupture.
   - Infant death.
2. Nursing care:
   - Continuous EFM.
   - Internal monitoring.
   - IV fluid.
3. Prostaglandin agents induction should be avoided if possible.

CRITICAL THINKING IN ACTION

*View the **Critical Thinking in Action** video in Chapter 22 of the CD-ROM. Then, answer the questions that follow.*

Betsy Jones, a 28-year-old G1 P0 is at 39 weeks' gestation, and her husband present to you in the labor suite for an external cephalic version procedure by her obstetrician. You introduce yourself and review her prenatal record for any significant risk factors or contraindications to the version procedure. Her prenatal chart is significant in that the fetus has been in a persistent frank breech position. You encourage Betsy and her husband to express their understanding and expectations of the procedure. You discuss certain criteria to be met prior

to the procedure and obtain vital signs as follows: T 98.8 °F, P 88, R 14, BP 110/80, urine screening negative for sugar, albumin, and ketones. You place Betsy on the external electronic fetal monitor which demonstrates a fetal heart rate baseline of 140 to 152 with moderate long-term variability. There are no contractions observed by the monitor or Betsy. After explaining how to record fetal movement on the monitor, you proceed with an NST.

1. Explain the contraindications to the version procedure.
2. Discuss the criteria that should be met prior to performing external version.
3. How would you explain to Betsy and her husband what to expect during the version procedure?
4. What support would you give Betsy during the procedure?
5. Explain postversion discharge teaching.

MEDIALINK

www.prenhall.com/london

- NCLEX-RN® Review, case studies, and other interactive resources for this chapter can be found on the Companion Website at http://www.prenhall.com/london. Click on "Chapter 22" to select the activities for this chapter.

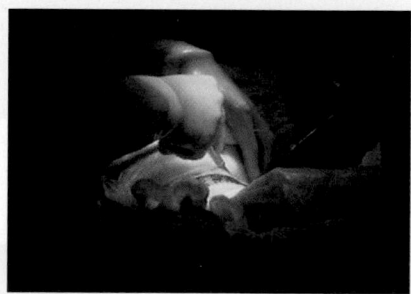

- For animations, more NCLEX-RN® Review questions, and an audio glossary, access the accompanying CD-ROM in this textbook.

REFERENCES

American College of Obstetricians and Gynecologists. (1999a). *Induction of labor* (ACOG Practice Bulletin No. 10). Washington, DC: Author.

American College of Obstetricians and Gynecologists (ACOG) Committee on Practice. (1999b). *Induction of labor with misoprostol.* ACOG Committee Opinion No. 228. Washington, DC: Author.

American College of Obstetricians and Gynecologists. (2000a). *Operative vaginal delivery* (ACOG Practice Bulletin No. 17). Washington, DC: Author.

American College of Obstetricians and Gynecologists. (2000b). *Response to Searle's warning on misoprostol* (ACOG Committee Opinion No. 248). Washington, DC: Author.

American College of Obstetricians and Gynecologists. (2004). *Vaginal birth after previous cesarean delivery* (ACOG Practice Bulletin No. 54). Washington, DC: Author.

Bishop, E. H. (1964). Pelvic scoring for elective inductions. *Obstetrics and Gynecology, 24,* 266.

Bowes, W. A., & Thorp, J. M. (2004). Clinical aspects of normal and abnormal labor. In R. K. Creasy & R. Resnik (Eds.), *Maternal fetal medicine: Principles and practice* (5th ed., pp. 671–705). Philadelphia: Saunders.

Dandolu, V., Chatwani, A. J., Harmanli, O., Floro, C., Gaughan, J. P., & Hernandez, E. (2005). Risk factors for obstetrical anal sphincter lacerations. *International Urogynecology Journal and Pelvic Floor Dysfunction* (16), 2. Retrieved on May 24, 2005, from http://www.ncbi.nlm.nih.gov/ent

Dandolu, V., Gaughan, J. P., Chatwani, A. J., Harmanli, O., Mabine, B., & Hernandez, E. (2005). Risk of reoccurrence of anal sphincter lacerations. *Obstetrics and Gynecology, 105*(4), 831–835.

Gabbe, S. G., Niebyl, J. R., & Simpson, J. L. (2002). *Obstetrics: Normal and problem pregnancies* (4th ed.). London: Churchill Livingstone.

Gallagher, S. (2004). Omega 3 oils and pregnancy. *Midwifery Today with International Midwife,* Spring (69), 26–31.

Gilstrap, L. C., Cunningham, F. G., & VanDorsten, J. P. (2002). *Operative obstetrics* (2nd ed.). New York: McGraw-Hill Professional.

Hamilton, B. E., Martin, J. A., & Sutton, P. D. (2003). Births: Preliminary data for 2002. *National Vital Statistics Reports, 5*(11), 1–20. Hyattsville, MD: National Center for Health Statistics.

Hannah, M. E. (2004). Planned elective cesarean: A reasonable choice for some women? *Canadian Medical Association Journal, 170*(5), 813–814.

Institute for Clinical Systems Improvement. (2002, October). *Vaginal birth after cesarean* (pp. 1–23). Bloomington, MN: Author.

Kish, K., & Collea, J. V. (2003). Malpresentation and cord prolapse. In A. H. DeCherney & L. Nathan (Eds.), *Current obstetrics & gynecologic diagnosis & treatment* (9th ed., pp. 369–386). New York: McGraw-Hill Companies.

Lanneau, G. S., Muffley, P., & Magann, E. F. (2004). Cesarean birth: Surgical techniques. In J. J. Sciarri (Ed.), *Gynecology and obstetrics* (Vol. 2, chap. 74, pp. 1–21). Philadelphia: Lippincott Williams & Wilkins.

Midwifery Today E-News. (2002). Herbs. *Midwifery Today Forums, 1,* 44. Retrieved July 20, 2004, from http://www.midwiferytoday.com/cnews

Odibo, A. O., & Macones, G. A. (2003). Current concepts regarding vaginal birth after cesarean delivery. *Current Opinions in Obstetrics and Gynecology, 15*(6), 479–482.

Smith, K. V. (2004). Normal childbirth. In S. Mattson & J. E. Smith (Eds.), *AWHONN core curriculum for maternal-newborn nursing* (3rd ed., pp. 271–302). St. Louis, MO: Elsevier Saunders.

Tenore, J. L. (2003). Methods for cervical ripening and induction of labor. *American Family Physician, 67,* 2123–2128.

Varney, H., Kriebs, J. M., & Gegor, C. L. (2004). *Varney's midwifery* (4th ed.). Boston: Jones & Bartlett.

Walker, R., Turnbull, D., & Wilkinson, C. (2002). Strategies to address global cesarean section rates: A review of the evidence. *Birth, 29*(1), 28–39.

Webb, D. A., & Culhane, J. F. (2002). Hospital variation in episiotomy use and the risk of perineal trauma during childbirth. *Birth, 29*(2), 132–136.

Wilson, B. A., Shannon, M. T., & Stang, C. L. (Eds.). (2006). *Nursing drug guide: 2006.* Upper Saddle River, NJ: Prentice-Hall.

Young, D. (2003). The push against vaginal birth. *Birth, 30*(3), 149–152.

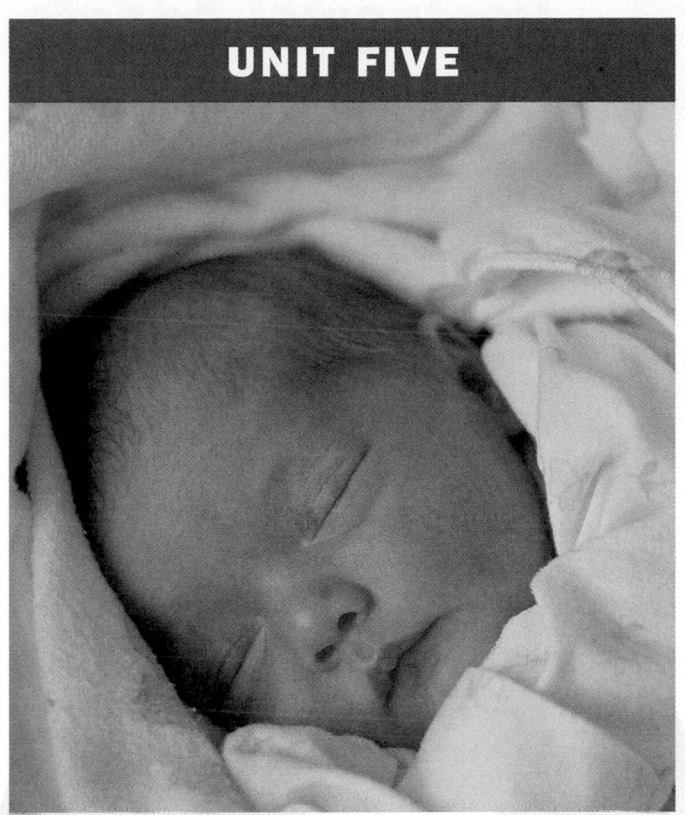

The Postpartal Childbearing Family and Newborn

Postpartal Adaptation and Nursing Assessment

I acutely felt the fatigue and sense of loss of the relationship with my baby that I had during pregnancy. But then the wonderful part happened with the reuniting with my new daughter. Holding her, having her latch on to my breast to get nourishment, and her looking into my eyes to say "hello Mom."

—*Susan, 34*

LEARNING OBJECTIVES

- Describe the basic physiologic changes that occur in the postpartal period as a woman's body returns to its prepregnant state.

- Discuss the psychologic adjustments that normally occur during the postpartal period.

- Summarize the factors that influence the development of parent-infant attachment.

- Delineate the physiologic and psychosocial components of a normal postpartal assessment.

- Discuss the physical and developmental tasks that the mother must accomplish during the postpartal period.

MEDIALINK www.prenhall.com/london

CD-ROM

NCLEX-RN® Review
Skill 4–1: Assessing the Uterine Fundus Following Vaginal Birth
Skill 4–2: Evaluating Lochia
Skill 4–3: Postpartum Perineal Assessment
Video: Postpartum Assessment
Nursing in Action: Postpartum Assessment
Audio Glossary

Companion Website

NCLEX-RN® Review
MediaLink Applications:
    Case Study: Mother-Infant Bonding
    Case Study: Woman Recovering from Cesarean Birth
Thinking Critically

The **puerperium**, or postpartal period, is when the woman adjusts physically and psychologically to the process of childbirth. It begins immediately after birth and continues for approximately 6 weeks, or until the body has returned to a near prepregnant state. This chapter describes the physiologic and psychologic changes that occur postpartally and the basic aspects of a thorough postpartal assessment. How can the nurse help the woman adjust to these changes?

POSTPARTAL PHYSICAL ADAPTATIONS

Comprehensive nursing assessment is based on a sound understanding of the normal anatomic and physiologic processes of the puerperium. These processes involve the reproductive organs and other major body systems.

REPRODUCTIVE SYSTEM

Involution of the Uterus

The term **involution** is used to describe the rapid reduction in size and the return of the uterus to a nonpregnant state. Following separation of the placenta, the decidua of the uterus is irregular, jagged, and varied in thickness. The spongy layer of the decidua is cast off as lochia, while the inner layer forms the basis for the development of new endometrium. Except at the placenta attachment site, this process takes about 3 weeks. The placenta site can take up to 6 to 7 weeks to completely heal (Blackburn, 2003). Bleeding from the larger uterine vessels of the placenta site is controlled by compression of the retracted uterine muscle fibers. The clotted blood is gradually absorbed by the body. Some of these vessels are eventually obliterated and replaced by new vessels with smaller lumens.

Rather than forming a fibrous scar in the decidua, the placenta site heals by a process of exfoliation. In this process the site is undermined by the growth of the endometrial tissue both from the margins of the site and from the fundi of the endometrial glands left in the basal layer of the site. The infarcted superficial tissue then becomes necrotic and is sloughed off (Blackburn, 2003). Exfoliation is a very important aspect of involution. If healing of the placenta site left a fibrous scar, the area available for future implantation would be limited, as would the number of possible pregnancies.

The uterus gradually decreases in size as the cells grow smaller and the hyperplasia of pregnancy reverses. Protein material in the uterine wall is broken down and absorbed. Factors that slow uterine involution include prolonged labor, anesthesia or excessive analgesia, difficult birth, grand multiparity, a full bladder, and incomplete expulsion of all of the placenta or fragments of the membranes. Factors that enhance involution include an uncomplicated labor and birth, complete expulsion of the placenta or membranes, breastfeeding, and early ambulation.

Changes in Fundal Position

Immediately following the expulsion of the placenta, the uterus contracts to the size of a large grapefruit. The **fundus**, or top portion of the uterus, is situated in the midline midway between the symphysis pubis and the umbilicus (Figure 23–1 ●). The walls of the contracted uterus are in close proximity, and the uterine blood vessels are firmly compressed by the myometrium. Within 6 to 12 hours after birth, the fundus of the uterus rises to the level of the umbilicus.

● FIGURE 23–1

Involution of the uterus. ***A,*** Immediately after expulsion of the placenta, the top of the fundus is in the midline and approximately halfway between the symphysis pubis and the umbilicus. ***B,*** About 6 to 12 hours after birth, the fundus is at the level of the umbilicus. The height of the fundus then decreases about one finger-breadth (approximately 1 cm) each day.

A fundus that is above the umbilicus and is boggy (feels soft and spongy rather than firm and well contracted) is associated with excessive uterine bleeding. As blood collects and forms clots within the uterus, the fundus rises; firm contractions of the uterus are interrupted, causing a **boggy uterus (uterine atony).** When the fundus is higher than expected on palpation and is not in the midline (usually deviated to the right), distention of the bladder should be suspected and the bladder should be emptied immediately and the uterus remeasured (Figure 23–2 ●). If the woman is unable to void, in-and-out catheterization of the bladder may be required.

After birth the top of the fundus remains at the level of the umbilicus for about half a day. On the first postpartum day, the top of the fundus is located about 1 cm below the umbilicus. The top of the fundus descends approximately one finger-breadth per day until it descends into the pelvis on the 10th day.

If the mother is breastfeeding, endogenous oxytocin released by the posterior pituitary in response to suckling hastens involution of the uterus. Barring complications,

● FIGURE 23–2

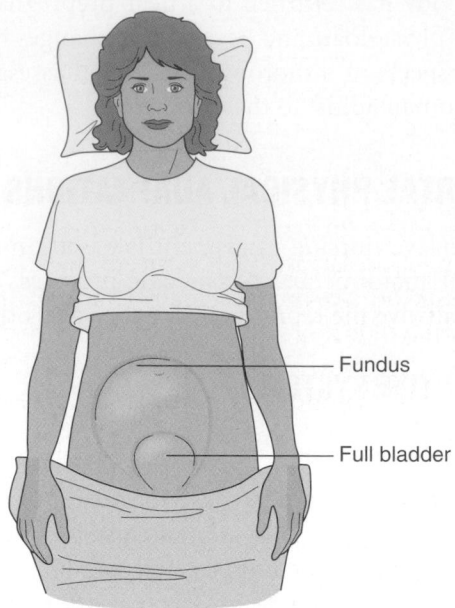

The uterus becomes displaced and deviated to the right when the bladder is full.

the uterus approaches its prepregnant size and location by 5 to 6 weeks.

Lochia

The uterus rids itself of the debris remaining after birth through a discharge called **lochia,** which is classified according to its appearance and contents. **Lochia rubra** is dark red. It occurs for the first 2 to 3 days and contains epithelial cells, erythrocytes, leukocytes, shreds of decidua, and occasionally fetal meconium, lanugo, and vernix caseosa. Lochia should not contain large (plum-sized) clots; if it does the cause should be investigated without delay. **Lochia serosa** is a pinkish color. It follows from about the 3rd until the 10th day. Lochia serosa is composed of serous exudate, shreds of degenerating decidua, erythrocytes, leukocytes, cervical mucus, and numerous microorganisms. Gradually the red blood cell component decreases, and **lochia alba,** a creamy or yellowish discharge, persists for an additional week or two. This final discharge is composed primarily of leukocytes, decidual cells, epithelial cells, fat, cervical mucus, cholesterol crystals, and bacteria. When the lochia flow stops, the cervix is considered closed, and chances of infection ascending from the vagina to the uterus decrease.

Like menstrual discharge, lochia flow has a musty, stale odor that is not offensive. Foul-smelling lochia or used perineal pads suggest infection and should be assessed promptly. Assessments should include a white blood cell count with differential, and checks for uterine tenderness and fever.

The total volume of lochia is about 225 mL, and the amount gradually declines with each passing day (Blackburn, 2003). The amount of discharge is greater in the morning due to pooling in the vagina and uterus while the mother lies sleeping. The amount of lochia may also be increased by exertion or breastfeeding. Multiparous women usually have more lochia than first-time mothers. Women who undergo a cesarean birth typically have less lochia than women who give birth vaginally (Blackburn, 2003).

Evaluation of lochia is necessary not only to determine the presence of hemorrhage but also to assess uterine involution. The type, amount, and consistency of lochia determine the stage of healing of the placenta site, and a progressive change from bright red at birth to dark red to pink to white or clear discharge should occur. Persistent discharge of lochia rubra or a return to lochia rubra indicates subinvolution or late postpartal hemorrhage (see Late Postpartal Hemorrhage in Chapter 25 ∞).

Cervical Changes

Following birth the cervix is flabby and formless and may appear bruised. The external os is markedly irregular and closes slowly. It admits two fingers for a few days following birth, but by the end of the first week it admits only a fingertip.

The shape of the external os is permanently changed by the first childbearing. The characteristic dimplelike os of the nullipara changes to the lateral slit (fish-mouth) os of the multipara. After significant cervical laceration or several lacerations, the cervix may appear lopsided.

Vaginal Changes

Following birth the vagina appears edematous and may be bruised. Small superficial lacerations may be evident, and the rugae are obliterated. The apparent bruising is due to pelvic congestion and will quickly disappear. The hymen, torn and jagged, heals irregularly, leaving small tags called the carunculae myrtiformes.

The size of the vagina decreases and rugae return within 3 weeks, facilitating the gradual return to smaller, although not nulliparous, dimensions. By 6 weeks the non-lactating woman's vagina usually appears normal. The lactating woman is in a hypoestrogenic state because of ovarian suppression, and her vaginal mucosa may be pale and without rugae; the effects of the lowered estrogen level may lead to dyspareunia (painful intercourse). Tone and contractility of the vaginal orifice may be improved by perineal tightening exercises such as Kegel's (see Perineal Exercises in Chapter 11 ∞). The labia majora and labia minora are more flaccid in the woman who has borne a child than in the nullipara.

Perineal Changes

During the early postpartal period, the soft tissue in and around the perineum may appear edematous with some bruising. If an episiotomy is present, the edges should be drawn together. Occasionally ecchymosis occurs, which may delay healing. Initial healing of the episiotomy or laceration occurs in 2 to 3 weeks after the birth, although complete healing may take up to 4 to 6 months (Blackburn, 2003). Perineal discomfort may be present during this time.

Recurrence of Ovulation and Menstruation

The return of ovulation and menstruation varies for each postpartal woman. Menstruation generally returns between 6 and 10 weeks after birth; 50% of the first cycles are anovulatory. The return of ovulation is directly associated with a rise in the serum progesterone level. Overall, 65% of non-lactating mothers resume menstruation by 12 weeks and 90% within 6 months following birth (Blackburn, 2003).

The return of ovulation and menstruation in breastfeeding mothers is usually prolonged. It is associated with the length of time the woman breastfeeds and whether formula supplements are used. If a mother breastfeeds for less than 1 month, the return of menstruation and ovulation is similar to that of the nonbreastfeeding mother. In women who exclusively breastfeed, menstruation is usually delayed for at least 3 months. Suckling by the infant typically results in alterations in the gonadotropin-releasing hormone (GnRH) production, which is thought to be the cause of amenorrhea (Blackburn, 2003).

However, since ovulation precedes menstruation, breastfeeding is not a reliable means of contraception. Approximately 5% to 15% of breastfeeding women become pregnant unintentionally prior to the onset of their first menstrual period (Blackburn, 2003).

ABDOMEN

Following birth the stretched abdominal wall appears loose and flabby, but it responds to exercise within 2 to 3 months. In the grand multipara, in the woman in whom overdistention of the abdomen has occurred, or in the woman with poor muscle tone before pregnancy, the abdomen may fail to regain good tone and will remain flabby. **Diastasis recti abdominis**, a separation of the abdominal muscle, may occur with pregnancy, especially in women with poor abdominal muscle tone (Figure 23–3 ●). If diastasis occurs, part of the abdominal wall has no muscular support but is formed only by skin, subcutaneous fat, fascia, and peritoneum. If rectus muscle tone is not regained, support may be inadequate during future pregnancies, and subsequent midline abdominal pain may occur. Inadequate support may result in a pendulous abdomen and increased

● **FIGURE 23–3**

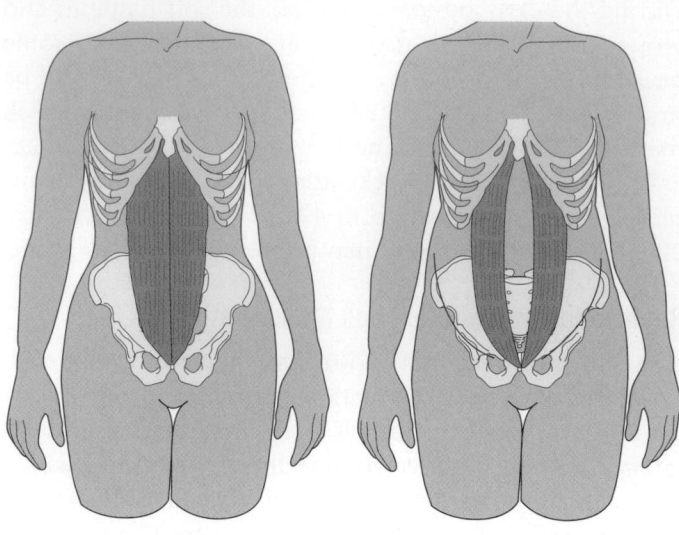

Normal location of rectus muscles of the abdomen

Diastasis recti: separation of the rectus muscles

Diastasis recti abdominis, a separation of the musculature, commonly occurs after pregnancy.

maternal backache. Fortunately, diastasis responds well to exercise, and abdominal muscle tone can improve significantly.

Striae (stretch marks), caused by stretching and rupture of the elastic fibers of the skin, are red to purple at the time of birth. These marks gradually fade after a time but remain visible.

LACTATION

During pregnancy, breast development in preparation for lactation results from the influence of both estrogen and progesterone. After birth the interplay of maternal hormones leads to milk production. (For further details, see Physiology of the Breasts and Lactation in Chapter 29. ∞)

GASTROINTESTINAL SYSTEM

Hunger following birth is common, and the mother may enjoy a light meal. She may also be quite thirsty and may drink large amounts of fluid. This helps replace fluids lost in labor, in the urine, and through perspiration.

A spontaneous bowel movement may not occur for 2 to 3 days after childbirth because of the lingering effects of progesterone and decreased abdominal muscle tone. Women who have had an episiotomy may tend to delay elimination for fear of increasing their pain or in the belief that their stitches will be torn if they bear down. The mother often anticipates discomfort during a bowel movement because of perineal tenderness as a result of an episiotomy, lacerations, or hemorrhoids. In resisting or

delaying the bowel movement, the woman may cause increased constipation and more pain when bowel elimination finally occurs.

The woman with a cesarean birth may receive clear liquids shortly after surgery; once bowel sounds are present, her diet is quickly advanced to solid food. The woman may experience some initial discomfort from flatulence; it is relieved by early ambulation and antiflatulent medications. It may take a few days for the bowel to regain its tone, especially if general anesthesia was used. The woman who has had a cesarean or a difficult birth may especially benefit from stool softeners.

URINARY TRACT

The postpartal woman has an increased bladder capacity, swelling and bruising of the tissue around the urethra, decreased sensitivity to fluid pressure, and a decreased sensation of bladder filling. Consequently she is at risk for overdistention, incomplete bladder emptying, and a buildup of residual urine. Women who have had an anesthetic block have inhibited neural functioning of the bladder and are more susceptible to bladder distention, difficulty voiding, and bladder infections.

Puerperal diuresis causes rapid filling of the bladder. Thus, adequate bladder elimination is an immediate concern. Urinary stasis increases the chances that a urinary tract infection will develop. A full bladder may also increase the tendency toward uterine relaxation by displacing the uterus and interfering with contractility, all of which may lead to hemorrhage. In the absence of infection, the dilated ureters and renal pelves return to prepregnant size by the end of the sixth week.

VITAL SIGNS

A maternal temperature of up to 38°C (100.4°F) may occur after childbirth as a result of the exertion and dehydration of labor. After the first 24 hours, the woman should be afebrile, and a temperature of 38°C (100.4°F) or greater suggests infection. (See discussion in Chapter 25. ∞)

Blood pressure readings should remain stable after childbirth but may be altered slightly. A decrease may indicate physiologic readjustment to decreased intrapelvic pressure, or it may be related to uterine hemorrhage. Orthostatic hypotension, as indicated by feelings of faintness or dizziness immediately after standing up, can develop in the first 48 hours as a result of abdominal engorgement that may occur after birth. A low or decreasing blood pressure may reflect hypovolemia secondary to hemorrhage, but it is a late sign. Blood pressure elevations may result from excessive use of oxytocin or vasopressor medications. Because preeclampsia can persist into or occur first in the postpartum period, routine evaluation of blood pressure is needed. If a woman complains of headache, hypertension must be ruled out before analgesics are administered.

Puerperal bradycardia with rates of 50 to 70 beats per minute commonly occurs during the first 6 to 10 days of the postpartal period. It may be related to decreased cardiac effort, the decreased blood volume following placental separation and contraction of the uterus, and increased stroke volume. Tachycardia occurs less frequently and is related to increased blood loss or difficult, prolonged labor and birth.

BLOOD VALUES

Blood values should return to the prepregnant state by the end of the postpartal period. Pregnancy-associated activation of coagulation factors may continue for variable amounts of time after birth. This condition, in conjunction with trauma, immobility, or sepsis, predisposes the woman to thromboembolism.

NURSING PRACTICE

During the first few hours after birth, the woman may have some orthostatic hypotension; it will cause her to have a lower blood pressure reading in a sitting position. For the most accurate reading, measure her blood pressure with her in the same position each time, preferably lying on her back with her arm at her side.

Nonpathologic leukocytosis often occurs during labor and in the immediate postpartum period, with white blood cell (WBC) counts of 25,000 to 30,000/mm³. WBC values typically return to normal levels by the end of the first postpartum week (Blackburn, 2003). Leukocytosis combined with the normal increase in erythrocyte sedimentation rate may obscure the diagnosis of acute infection at this time. Hemoglobin and hematocrit levels may be difficult to interpret in the first 2 days after birth because of the changing blood volume. This loss in blood in the first 24 hours accounts for half of the red blood cell (RBC) volume gained during the course of the pregnancy. In general a decrease of two percentage points from the hematocrit at admission to the birthing unit indicates a blood loss of 500 mL (Varney, Kriebs, & Gegor, 2004). In the first few days after birth, blood volume further decreases as a result of diuresis. After 3 to 4 days, mobilization of interstitial fluid leads to a slight increase in plasma volume. This hemodilution leads to a decrease in hemoglobin, hematocrit, and plasma protein by the end of the first postpartum week. Decreases in plasma volume reach nonpregnant levels by 4 to 6 weeks postpartum (Blackburn, 2003).

Platelet levels typically fall as a result of placental separation. They then begin to increase by the third to fourth postpartum day, gradually returning to normal by the sixth postpartum week. Fibrinolytic activity typically returns to normal during the hours following birth. The hemostatic system as a whole reaches its normal pregnant status by 3 to 4 weeks postpartum; however, the diameter of deep veins can take up to 6 weeks to return to prepregnant levels (Blackburn, 2003). This is why there is a prolonged risk of thromboembolism in the first 6 weeks following birth.

CARDIOVASCULAR CHANGES

The cardiovascular system undergoes dramatic changes during birth that can result in cardiovascular instability due to an increase in the cardiac output. The cardiac output typically stabilizes and returns to pregnancy levels within an hour following birth (Blackburn, 2003). Maternal hypervolemia typically occurs immediately following birth since the maternal circulation has an increase in blood volume that no longer travels through the placenta. Maternal hypervolemia acts to protect the mother from excessive blood loss. Cardiac output declines by 30% in the first 2 weeks and reaches normal levels by 6 to 12 weeks (Blackburn, 2003).

Diuresis in the first 2 to 5 days assists to decrease the extracellular fluid and results in a weight loss of 3 kg. Failure to diurese in the immediate postpartum period can lead to pulmonary edema and subsequent cardiac problems. This is seen more commonly in women with a history of preeclampsia or preexisting cardiac problems (Blackburn, 2003).

NEUROLOGIC CHANGES AND CONDITIONS

Neurologic problems and disorders can predispose women to higher rates of morbidity and mortality during pregnancy and in the postpartum period. Headaches are the most common neurologic symptoms encountered by postpartal women. It is estimated that up to 40% of postpartal women develop headaches within the first week following birth (Browne & Birnbach, 2003). There may be an increased incidence in headache if the woman had spinal or epidural anesthesia. Migraine headaches, although less frequent during pregnancy, tend to resume in the postpartum period (Shehata & Okosun, 2004). Women with epilepsy are at a 1% to 2% risk of having a seizure in the immediate postpartum period (Tatum, Liporace, Benbadis et al., 2004). It is nine times more likely that a woman will have a seizure during labor or in the first 24 hours after birth than it is during the pregnancy (Shehata & Okosun, 2004). Women with multiple sclerosis (MS) and Guillain-Barré syndrome are more likely to have symptoms in the postpartum period than during pregnancy (Wiertlewski, Magot, Drapier et al., 2004). Myasthenia gravis (autoimmune disease) affects the neuromuscular junctions. The increase in symptoms during pregnancy is variable; however, the first month of pregnancy and the first month of the postpartum period is the most critical (Shehata & Okosun, 2004).

WEIGHT LOSS

An initial weight loss of about 10 to 12 lb occurs as a result of the birth of the infant and expulsion of the placenta and amniotic fluid. Puerperal diuresis accounts for the loss of an additional 5 lb during the early puerperium. By the sixth to eighth week after birth, many women have returned to approximately prepregnant weight if they gained the average 25 to 30 lb. Women often express concern about the slow pace of their postpartum weight loss. Multiparas tend to be more positive than primiparas, probably because the multipara's previous experience has prepared her for the fact that the body does not immediately return to a prepregnant state.

POSTPARTAL CHILL

Frequently the mother experiences intense tremors that resemble shivering from a chill immediately after birth. Several theories have been offered to explain this shivering: the result of a sudden release of pressure on the pelvic nerves after birth, a response to a fetus-to-mother transfusion that occurred during placental separation, a reaction to maternal adrenaline production during labor and birth, or a reaction to epidural anesthesia. If not followed by fever, this chill is of no clinical concern, but it is uncomfortable for the woman. The nurse can increase the woman's comfort by covering her with a warmed blanket and reassure her that the shivering is a common, self-limiting situation. If she allows herself to go with the shaking, the shivering will last a short time. Some women may also find a warm drink helpful. Later in the puerperium, chill and fever indicate infection and require further evaluation.

POSTPARTAL DIAPHORESIS

The woman experiences greatly increased perspiration as the body eliminates excess fluid and waste products via the skin during the puerperium. Diaphoretic (sweating) episodes frequently occur at night, and the woman may awaken drenched with perspiration. This perspiration is not significant clinically, but the mother should be protected from chilling.

AFTERPAINS

Afterpains, caused by intermittent uterine contractions, are more common in multiparas than in primiparas. Although the uterus of the primipara usually remains consistently contracted, the lost tone of the multiparous uterus results in alternate contraction and relaxation. This phenomenon also occurs if the uterus has been markedly distended, as with a multiple-gestation pregnancy or hydramnios, or if clots or placental fragments were retained. These afterpains may cause the mother severe discomfort for 2 to 3 days after birth. The administration of oxytocic agents stimulates uterine contraction and increases the discomfort of the afterpains. Because endogenous oxytocin is released when the infant suckles, breastfeeding also increases the frequency and severity of the afterpains. The breastfeeding mother may find it helpful to take a mild analgesic approximately 1 hour before feeding her infant. The nurse can assure the mother that the prescribed analgesics are not harmful to the newborn and help improve the quality of the breastfeeding experience. An analgesic such as ibuprofen is also helpful at bedtime if the afterpains interfere with the mother's rest.

POSTPARTAL PSYCHOLOGIC ADAPTATIONS

The postpartal period is a time of readjustment and adaptation for the entire childbearing family, but especially for the mother. The woman experiences a variety of responses as she adjusts to a new family member, postpartum discomforts, changes in her body image, and the reality that she is no longer pregnant.

TAKING IN AND TAKING HOLD

During the first day or two after birth, the woman tends to be passive, somewhat dependent, and is focused on self. She follows suggestions, hesitates to make decisions, and is still rather preoccupied with her needs. She may have a great need to talk about her perceptions of her labor and birth. Talking helps her work through the process, sort out the reality from her fantasized experience, and clarify anything that she did not understand. Food and sleep are major needs. In her early work, Rubin (1961) labeled this the *taking-in period.*

By the second or third day after birth, the new mother is ready to resume control over her life and shifts her focus to her infant. She may be concerned about controlling her body functions such as elimination. If she is breastfeeding, she may worry about the quality of her milk and her ability to feed her baby. If her baby spits up after a feeding, she may view it as a personal failure. She may also feel that the nurse handles her baby more proficiently than she does. She requires assurance that she is doing well as a mother. Rubin labeled this the *taking-hold period* (1961). Today's mothers seem to be more independent and adjust more rapidly, exhibiting behaviors of "taking in" and "taking hold" in shorter time periods than those previously identified.

EVIDENCE-BASED NURSING

EARLY SKIN-TO-SKIN CONTACT FOR MOTHERS AND INFANTS

Clinical Question

Early skin-to-skin contact involves placing the naked newborn baby prone on the mother's bare chest. Contact is considered early if it occurs within 24 hours of the birth. What are the benefits of early skin-to-skin contact between mothers and their newborn infants?

Evidence

Seventeen studies, involving 806 women and their healthy babies, were evaluated by four experts for this systematic review. Separating women from their newborn babies is a uniquely Western feature of the childbirth experience and may have some harmful effects. Breastfeeding is widely shown to have beneficial effects and may be related to maternal-infant attachment. These reviewers documented the effects of skin-to-skin contact on breastfeeding behaviors and attachment, and found beneficial effects on both.

Mothers with early skin-to-skin contact are twice as likely to breastfeed, and continue for more than a month longer than those who do not have this contact. Timing appears to be important in enhancing breastfeeding success. Most infants are very alert in the first 2 hours after birth and will generally self attach to the nipple correctly at approximately 55 minutes after birth. Before 30 minutes the infant may only lick the nipple; after 2 hours the infant will become sleepy. Maternal affection and attachment behaviors are increased when early skin-to-skin contact occurs.

There is no negative effect on the infant's temperature when appropriate nursing care measures are taken (e.g., the infant is thoroughly dried and covered across the back with a prewarmed blanket, and the head is covered with a cap).

In some of the studies reviewed, the infant's heart rate and respiratory rate were lower after skin-to-skin contact, but no other physiologic outcomes were affected. The lower cardiorespiratory values may be due to the calming effect of the maternal contact, and they were associated with no bad outcomes.

Implications

You should encourage early skin-to-skin contact between mothers and their newborn babies. Contact between 30 minutes and 2 hours after birth is most effective in enhancing successful breastfeeding behaviors. Make sure the infant is kept warm and dry. Otherwise, there are no limitations on frequency and duration of skin-to-skin contact.

Critical Thinking

What measures must you institute to ensure control of infection in early skin-to-skin contact? What precautions will you take to ensure the infant does not become cold?

Reference

Anderson, G. C., Moore, E., Hepworth, J., & Bergman, N. (2003). Early skin-to-skin contact for mothers and their healthy newborn infants (Cochrane Review). In *The Cochrane Library*, Issue 4. Chichester, UK: John Wiley & Sons.

MATERNAL ROLE ATTAINMENT

Maternal role attainment is the process by which a woman learns mothering behaviors and becomes comfortable with her identity as a mother. Formation of a maternal identity occurs with each child a woman bears. As the mother grows to know this child and forms a relationship, the mother's maternal identity gradually, systematically evolves and she "binds in" to the infant (Rubin, 1984).

Maternal role attainment often occurs in four stages (Mercer, 1995):

1. The *anticipatory stage* occurs during pregnancy. The woman looks to role models, especially her own mother, for examples of how to mother.

2. The *formal stage* begins when the child is born. The woman is still influenced by the guidance of others and tries to act as she believes others expect her to act.

3. The *informal stage* begins when the mother begins to make her own choices about mothering. The woman begins to develop her own style of mothering and finds ways of functioning that work well for her.

4. The *personal stage* is the final stage of maternal role attainment. When the woman reaches this stage, she is comfortable with the notion of herself as mother.

In most cases, maternal role attainment occurs within 3 to 10 months after birth. Social support, the woman's age and personality traits, the marital relationship, presence of underlying anxiety or depression, the woman's previous childcare skills, the temperament of her infant, and the family's socioeconomic status all influence the woman's success in attaining the maternal role (Porter & Hsu, 2003).

The postpartum woman faces a number of challenges as she adjusts to her new role:

- For many women, finding time for themselves is one of the greatest challenges. It is often difficult for the new mother to find time to read a book, talk to her partner, or even eat a meal without interruption.

- Women also report feelings of incompetence because they have not mastered all aspects of the mothering role. Often they are unsure of what to do in a given situation.

- The next greatest challenge involves fatigue resulting from sleep deprivation. The demands of nighttime care are tremendously draining, especially if the woman has other children.

- Another challenge faced by the new mother involves the feeling of responsibility that having a child brings.

Women experience a sense of lost freedom, an awareness that they will never again be quite as carefree as they were before becoming mothers.

■ For women with older children, finding time for them is a challenge. Many women feel guilty because the new baby takes up so much of their time. Sibling rivalry or ill feelings about the baby from other children can put additional stress on the mother.

■ Mothers sometimes cite the infant's behavior as a challenge, especially when the child is about 8 months old. Stranger anxiety develops, the infant begins crawling and getting into things, teething may cause fussiness, and the baby's tendency to put everything in his or her mouth requires constant vigilance by the parent.

Postpartum nurses need to be aware of the long-term adjustments and stresses that the childbearing family faces as its members adjust to new and different roles. Nurses can help by providing anticipatory guidance about the realities of being a parent and by giving the postpartal family parenting literature for reference at home. Ongoing parenting groups give parents an opportunity to discuss problems and become comfortable in new roles.

POSTPARTUM BLUES

The **postpartum blues** consist of a transient period of depression that occurs during the first few days of the puerperium in 70% of all postpartal women (Varney et al., 2004). It may be manifested by tearfulness, anorexia, difficulty in sleeping, and a feeling of letdown. These mood changes frequently occur while the woman is still hospitalized, but may occur at home as well. Changing hormone levels are certainly a factor; psychologic adjustments, an unsupportive environment, and insecurity also have been identified as potential causes. In addition, fatigue, discomfort, and overstimulation may play a part. The postpartum blues usually resolve naturally within 10 to 14 days, but if they persist or symptoms worsen, the woman may need evaluation for postpartum blues (see Adjustment Reaction with Expressed Mood in Chapter 25 ∞).

IMPORTANCE OF SOCIAL SUPPORT

The psychologic outcomes of the postpartal period are far more positive when the parents have access to a support network. Women and their partners may find that family relationships become increasingly important, but the increased family interaction can be a source of stress. The new parents may also have increasing contact with other parents of small children while contact with coworkers declines. Of great concern are women and their partners who have no family or friends with whom to form a social network. Isolation at a time when the woman feels an increased need for support can result in tremendous stress and is often a contributing factor in situations of postpartum depression, child neglect, or abuse. New mother support groups are helpful for women who lack a social support system.

DEVELOPMENT OF FAMILY ATTACHMENT

A mother's first interaction with her infant is influenced by many factors, including her involvement with her family of origin, her relationships, the stability of her home environment, the communication patterns she has developed, and the degree of nurturing she received as a child. These factors have shaped the person she has become. Certain personal characteristics are also important:

■ **Level of trust.** What level of trust has this mother developed in response to her life experiences? What is her philosophy of childrearing? Will she be able to treat her infant as a unique individual with changing needs that should be met as much as possible?

■ **Level of self-esteem.** How much does she value herself as a woman and as a mother? Does she feel generally able to cope with the adjustments of life?

■ **Capacity for enjoying herself.** Is the mother able to find pleasure in everyday activities and human relationships?

■ **Adequacy of knowledge about childbearing and childrearing.** What beliefs about the course of pregnancy, the capacities of newborns, and the nature of her emotions influence her behavior at first contact with her infant and later? What is her previous experience with infants/children?

■ **Prevailing mood or usual feeling tone.** Is the woman predominantly content, angry, depressed, or anxious? Is she sensitive to her own feelings and those of others? Will she be able to accept her own needs and to obtain support in meeting them?

■ **Reactions to the present pregnancy.** Was the pregnancy planned? Did it go smoothly? Were there ongoing life events that enhanced her pregnancy or depleted her reserves of energy? How were other life roles changed due to her pregnancy and motherhood?

By the time of birth, each mother has developed an emotional orientation of some kind to the baby based on these factors.

INITIAL MATERNAL ATTACHMENT BEHAVIOR

New mothers demonstrate a fairly regular pattern of maternal behaviors at first contact with a normal newborn. In

FIGURE 23–4

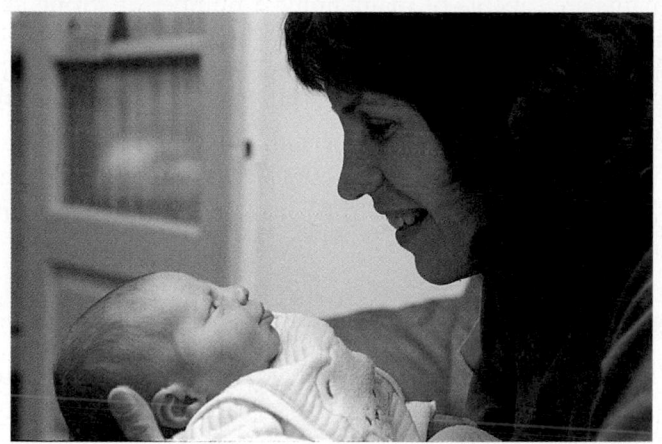

The mother has direct face-to-face and eye-to-eye contact in the en face position.

© Stella Johnson (www.stellajohnson.com)

a progression of touching activities, the mother proceeds from fingertip exploration of the newborn's extremities toward palmar contact with larger body areas and finally to enfolding the infant with the whole hand and arms. The time taken to accomplish these steps varies from minutes to days. The mother increases the proportion of time spent in the **en face** position (Figure 23–4 ⊙). She arranges herself or the newborn so that she has direct face-to-face and eye-to-eye contact. There is an intense interest in having the infant's eyes open. When the infant's eyes are open, the mother characteristically greets the newborn and talks in high-pitched tones to him or her.

In most instances the mother relies heavily on her senses of sight, touch, and hearing in getting to know what her baby is really like. She tends also to respond verbally to any sounds emitted by the newborn, such as cries, coughs, sneezes, and grunts. The sense of smell may be involved as well.

While interacting with her newborn, the mother may be experiencing shock, disbelief, or denial. She may state, "I can't believe she's finally here" or "I feel like he is a stranger." However, feelings of connectedness between the newborn and the rest of the family can be expressed in positive or negative terms: "She's got your cute nose, Daddy" or "Oh, no! He looks just like the first one, and he was an impossible baby." A mother's facial expressions or the frequency and content of her questions may demonstrate concerns about the infant's general condition or normality, especially if her pregnancy was complicated or if a previously born baby was not healthy.

During the first few days after her child's birth, the new mother applies herself to the task of getting to know her baby. This is termed the *acquaintance phase*. If the infant gives clear behavioral cues about needs, the infant's re-

sponses to mothering will be predictable, and this will make the mother feel effective and competent. Other behaviors that make an infant more attractive to caretakers are smiling, grasping a finger, breastfeeding eagerly, and being easy to console.

NURSING PRACTICE

Newborns that require immediate care in a special care or intensive care nursery are sometimes taken from their parents immediately after birth. The separation can interfere with the normal attachment process. The parents should be brought to the nursery as soon as possible to interact with their infant and should be allowed to hold and care for their infant as much as possible. If the infant is in an incubator and cannot be held, encourage the parents to stroke the infant's hand, foot, or cheek. Provide reassurance that this will not hurt the infant and is in fact beneficial.

During this time the newborn is also becoming acquainted. Within a few days after birth, infants show signs of recognizing recurrent situations and responding to changes in routine. To the extent that their mother is their world, they are actively acquainting themselves with her.

During the *phase of mutual regulation*, mother and infant seek to deal with the degree of control to be exerted by each partner in their relationship. In this phase of adjustment, a balance is sought between the needs of the mother and the needs of the infant. The most important consideration is that each should obtain a good measure of enjoyment from the interaction. During the mutual adjustment phase, negative maternal feelings are likely to surface or intensify. Because "everyone knows that mothers love their babies," these negative feelings often go unexpressed and are allowed to build up. If they are expressed, the response of friends, relatives, or healthcare personnel is often to deny the feelings to the mother: "You don't mean that." Some negative feelings are normal in the first few days after birth, and the nurse should be supportive when the mother vocalizes these feelings.

When mutual regulation arrives at the point where both mother and infant primarily enjoy each other's company, reciprocity has been achieved. **Reciprocity** is an interactional cycle that occurs simultaneously between mother and infant. It involves mutual cuing behaviors, expectancy, rhythmicity, and synchrony. The mother develops a new relationship with an individual who has a unique character and evokes a response entirely different from the fantasy response of pregnancy. When reciprocity is synchronous, the interaction between mother and infant is mutually gratifying and is sought and initiated by both partners.

DEVELOPING CULTURAL COMPETENCE

In some cultures there may be little involvement of the father in new-born care. In the Muslim culture, for example, emphasis on childrearing and infant care activities is on the mother and female relatives. Nurses need to be aware of cultural differences when evaluating a father's interaction with his newborn.

Father-Infant Interactions

In Western cultures, commitment to family-centered maternity care has fostered interest in understanding the feelings and experiences of the new father. Evidence suggests that the father has a strong attraction to his newborn and that the feelings he experiences are similar to the mother's feelings of attachment (Figure 23–5 ●). The characteristic sense of absorption, preoccupation, and interest in the infant demonstrated by fathers during early contact is termed **engrossment.** Differences in involvement still exist among fathers in Western culture, and may be influenced by factors other than culture (i.e., previous experience with paternal role, exposure to male/father role models).

● **FIGURE 23–5**

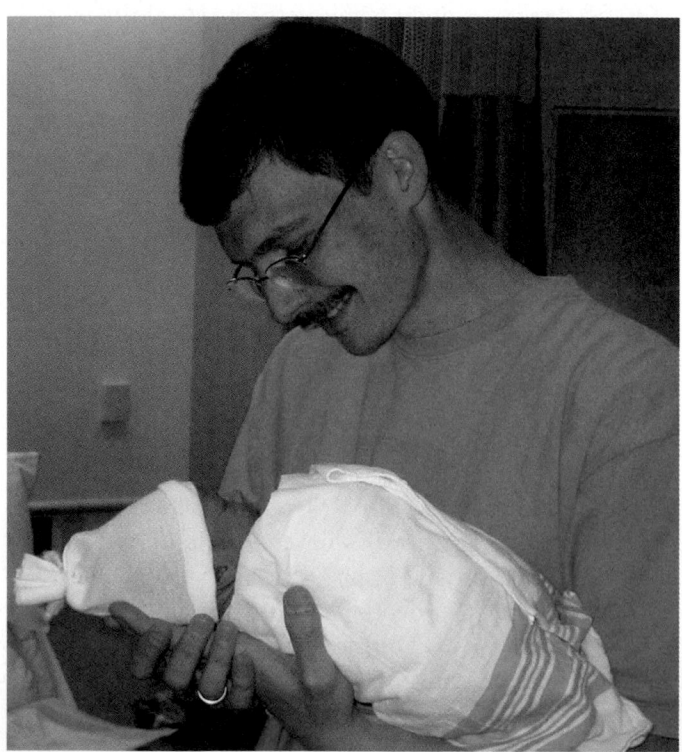

The father experiences strong feelings of attraction during engrossment.

Siblings and Others

Infants are capable of maintaining a number of strong attachments without loss of quality. These attachments may include siblings, grandparents, aunts, and uncles. The social setting and personality of the individual seem to be significant factors in the development of multiple attachments. The advent of open visiting hours and rooming-in permits siblings and grandparents to participate in the attachment process.

CULTURAL INFLUENCES IN THE POSTPARTAL PERIOD

The new mother's culture and personal values also influence her beliefs about her postpartal care. Her expectations about food, fluids, rest, hygiene, medications and relief measures, support and counsel, and other aspects of her life are influenced by the beliefs and values of her family and cultural group. Sometimes a new mother's wishes differ from what the physician or nurse expects.

Nurses belong to a particular ethnoculture and also share in the culture of healthcare. As part of the healthcare cultural group, nurses may take on some practices that support the general beliefs of that group, such as offering food in the recovery period after birth, providing iced fluids, expecting the woman to ambulate as soon as possible, and assuming the woman will want to shower and perhaps wash her hair soon after giving birth. It is important for nurses to recognize that they are approaching their client's care from their own perspective and that, to individualize care for each mother, they need to offer and support individual choices.

Although describing particular practices of differing cultural groups always involves some generalization, it is helpful for nurses to understand some of the possible differences in beliefs and practices. The woman of European heritage may expect to eat a full meal and have large amounts of iced fluids after the birth, in the belief that the food restores energy and the fluids help replace fluid lost during the labor. She may want to ambulate shortly after the birth and shower, wash her hair, and put on a fresh gown. She may expect a short stay in the hospital and may or may not be interested in educational classes.

In contrast, some cultures emphasize certain postpartal routines or rituals for mother and baby that are designed to restore the harmony, or the hot-cold balance, of the body. Some women of Hispanic, African, and Asian cultures may avoid cold after birth. This prohibition includes cold air, wind, and all water (even if heated). However, some traditional Mexican women may avoid eating "hot" foods such as pork just after the birth of a baby (considered a "hot" experience). It is important to note that individuals may define hot and cold conditions and foods differently. The nurse should ask each woman what she can eat and what foods she thinks would be helpful for healing. The nurse may encourage family members to bring preferred foods and beverages from home. For more detailed discussion of the hot-cold balance concept, see Chapter 2, Culture and the Family. ∞

In many cultures the extended family plays an essential role during the puerperium. The grandmother is often the primary helper to the mother and newborn. She brings wisdom and experience, allowing the new mother time to rest and giving her ready access to someone who can help with problems and concerns as they arise. It is important to ensure access for all family members during the postpartal period. Visiting rules may be broadened to allow family members to have access to the mother and newborn. These practices show respect and foster a blending of old and new behaviors to meet the goals of all concerned (Cesario, 2001).

POSTPARTAL NURSING ASSESSMENT

Comprehensive care is based on a thorough assessment that identifies individual needs or potential problems. See "Assessment Guide: Postpartal—First 24 Hours after Birth."

RISK FACTORS

Ongoing assessment and client education during the puerperium are designed to meet the needs of the childbearing family and to detect and treat possible complications. Table 23–1 identifies factors that may place the new mother at risk during the postpartal period. The nurse uses this knowledge during the assessment and is particularly alert for possible complications associated with identified risk factors.

PHYSICAL ASSESSMENT

There are several principles to remember in preparing for and completing the assessment of the postpartum woman:

- Select a time that will provide the most accurate data. Palpating the fundus when the woman has a full bladder, for example, may give false information about the progress of involution. Ask woman to void prior to assessment.
- Record the findings as clearly as possible.
- Perform the procedures as gently as possible to avoid unnecessary discomfort.
- Explain the purpose of regular assessment.

The physical assessment is an excellent opportunity for client teaching. For example, when assessing the breasts of a lactating woman, the nurse can discuss breast care, breast

TABLE 23–1 ✤ Postpartal High-Risk Factors	
Factor	**Maternal Implication**
Preeclampsia	↑ Blood pressure ↑ CNS irritability ↑ Need for bed rest › ↑ risk thrombophlebitis
Diabetes	Need for insulin regulation Episodes of hypoglycemia or hyperglycemia ↓ Healing
Cardiac disease	↑ Maternal exhaustion
Cesarean birth	↑ Healing needs ↑ Pain from incision ↑ Risk of infection ↑ Length of hospitalization
Overdistention of uterus (multiple gestation, hydramnios)	↑ Risk of hemorrhage ↑ Risk of anemia ↑ Stretching of abdominal muscles ↑ Incidence and severity of afterpains
Abruptio placentae, placenta previa	Hemorrhage → anemia ↓ Uterine contractility after birth → ↑ infection risk
Precipitous labor (<3 hours)	↑ Risk of lacerations to birth canal › hemorrhage
Prolonged labor (>24 hours)	Exhaustion ↑ Risk of hemorrhage Nutritional and fluid depletion ↑ Bladder atony or trauma
Difficult birth	Exhaustion ↑ Risk of perineal lacerations ↑ Risk of hematomas ↑ Risk of hemorrhage → anemia
Extended period of time in stirrups at birth	↑ Risk of thrombophlebitis
Retained placenta	↑ Risk of hemorrhage ↑ Risk of infection

milk production, the letdown reflex, and breast self-examination. A new mother may be very receptive to instruction on postpartal abdominal tightening exercises when the nurse assesses the woman's fundal height and diastasis. The assessment is also an excellent time to provide information about the body's postpartal physical and anatomic changes as well as danger signs to report (Table 23–2).

Because the time new mothers spend in the postpartum unit is often limited, the nurse needs to use every available opportunity for client education about self-care. One

TABLE 23–2 ✤ Common Postpartal Concerns

Several postpartal occurrences cause special concern for mothers. The nurse will frequently be asked about the following events.

Source of Concern	Explanation
Gush of blood that sometimes occurs when she first arises	Due to normal pooling of blood in vagina when the woman lies down to rest or sleep; gravity causes blood to flow out when she stands
Night sweats	Normal physiologic occurrence that results as body attempts to eliminate excess fluids that were present during pregnancy; may be aggravated by plastic mattress pad
Afterpains	More common in multiparas; due to contractions

of the best opportunities comes during the normal postpartal assessment. To assist nurses in recognizing these opportunities, examples of client teaching during the assessment are provided throughout the following discussion.

Vital Signs

The physical assessment may be organized in a variety of ways. Many nurses begin by assessing vital signs because the findings are more accurate when they are obtained with the woman at rest. In addition, establishing whether the vital signs are within the expected normal range will help determine if other assessments are needed. For instance, if the temperature is elevated, consider the time since birth and gather information to determine whether the woman is dehydrated or an infection is developing.

Temperature elevations (less than 38°C [100.4°F]) due to normal processes should last for only 24 hours. Evaluate any elevation of temperature in light of associated signs and symptoms and carefully review the woman's history to identify other factors, such as premature rupture of membranes or prolonged labor, which might increase the incidence of infection in the genital tract.

Alterations in vital signs may indicate complications; assess them at regular intervals. The blood pressure should remain stable, but the pulse often shows a characteristic slowness that is no cause for alarm. Pulse rates return to prepregnant norms very quickly unless complications arise.

Inform the woman of the results of the vital signs assessment and provide information about the normal changes in blood pressure and pulse. This may be an opportunity to determine whether the mother knows how to assess her own and her infant's temperature and how to read a thermometer.

Auscultation of Lungs

Breath sounds should be clear. Women who have been treated for preterm labor or preeclampsia are at higher risk for pulmonary edema (see Care of Woman, with a Hypertensive Disorder in Chapter 15 for further discussion ∞).

NURSING PRACTICE

An easy way to remember the components specific to the postpartal examination is to remember the term BUBBLEHE: B-breast, U-uterus, B-bladder, B-bowel, L-lochia, E-episiotomy/laceration, H-Homans/hemorrhoids, and E-emotional.

Breasts

Before examining the breasts, don gloves and then assess the fit and support of the woman's bra. If appropriate, offer information about how to select a supportive bra. A properly fitting bra supports the breasts and helps maintain breast shape by limiting stretching of supporting ligaments and connective tissue. If the mother is breastfeeding, the straps of the bra should be cloth, not elastic, and easily adjustable. The back should be wide and have at least three rows of hooks to adjust for fit. Traditional nursing bras have a fixed inner cup and a separate half cup that can be unhooked for breastfeeding while the cup continues to support the breast. Purchasing a nursing bra one size too large during pregnancy will usually result in a good fit because the breasts increase in size with milk production.

Then ask the woman to remove her bra so the breasts can be examined. Note the size and shape of the breasts and any abnormalities, reddened areas, or engorgement. Lightly palpate the breasts for softness, slight firmness associated with filling, firmness associated with engorgement, warmth, and tenderness. Assess the nipples for fissures, cracks, soreness, and inversion. Teach the woman the characteristics of the breast and explain how to recognize and manage problems such as fissures and cracks.

Assess the nonbreastfeeding mother for evidence of breast discomfort, and institute relief measures if necessary. (See discussion of lactation suppression in the nonbreastfeeding mother in Chapter 24. ∞) Breast assessment findings for a lactating woman may be recorded as follows: breasts soft, filling, no evidence of nipple tenderness or cracking.

Abdomen and Fundus

Before examination of the abdomen, the woman should void. This practice ensures that a full bladder is not displacing the uterus or causing any uterine atony; if atony is present, other causes must be investigated.

ASSESSMENT GUIDE

POSTPARTAL—FIRST 24 HOURS AFTER BIRTH

PHYSICAL ASSESSMENT/ NORMAL FINDINGS	ALTERATIONS AND POSSIBLE CAUSES*	NURSING RESPONSES TO DATA†
Vital Signs		
Blood pressure (BP): Should remain consistent with baseline BP during pregnancy.	High BP (preeclampsia, essential hypertension, renal disease, anxiety).	Evaluate history of preexisting disorders and check for other signs of preeclampsia (edema, proteinuria).
	Drop in BP (may be normal; uterine hemorrhage).	Assess for other signs of hemorrhage ($\uparrow$ pulse, cool clammy skin).
Pulse: 50–90 beats/minute. May be bradycardia of 50–70 beats/minute.	Tachycardia (difficult labor and birth, hemorrhage).	Evaluate for other signs of hemorrhage ($\downarrow$ BP, cool clammy skin).
Respirations: 16–24/minute.	Marked tachypnea (respiratory disease).	Assess for other signs of respiratory disease.
Temperature: 36.2–38°C (98–100.4°F)	After first 24 hours, temperature of 38°C (100.4°F) or above suggests infection.	Assess for other signs of infection; notify physician or certified nurse-midwife.
Breasts		
General appearance: Smooth, even pigmentation, changes of pregnancy still apparent; one may appear larger.	Reddened area (mastitis).	Assess further for signs of infection.
Palpation: Depending on postpartal day, may be soft, filling, full, or engorged.	Palpable mass (caked breast, mastitis).	Assess for other signs of infection: If blocked duct, consider heat, massage, position change for breastfeeding.
	Engorgement (venous stasis).	Assess for further signs.
	Tenderness, heat, edema (engorgement, caked breast, mastitis).	Report mastitis to physician or certified nurse-midwife.
Nipples: Supple, pigmented, intact; become erect when stimulated.	Fissures, cracks, soreness (problems with breastfeeding), not erectile with stimulation (inverted nipples).	Reassess technique; recommend appropriate interventions.
Abdomen		
Musculature: Abdomen may be soft, have a "doughy" texture; rectus muscle intact.	Separation in musculature (diastasis recti abdominis).	Evaluate size of diastasis; teach appropriate exercises for decreasing the separation.
Fundus: Firm, midline; following expected process of involution.	Boggy (full bladder, uterine bleeding, deviation from midline).	Massage until firm; assess bladder and have woman void if needed; attempt to express clots when firm.
		If bogginess remains or recurs, report to physician or certified nurse-midwife.
May be tender when palpated.	Constant tenderness (infection).	Assess for evidence of endometritis.
Lochia		
Scant to moderate amount, earthy odor; no clots.	Large amount, clots (hemorrhage).	Assess for firmness, express additional clots; begin peripad count.
	Foul-smelling lochia (infection).	Assess for other signs of infection; report to physician or certified nurse-midwife.
Normal progression: First 1–3 days: rubra.	Failure to progress normally or return to rubra from serosa (subinvolution).	Report to physician or certified nurse-midwife.
Following rubra: Days 3–10: serosa (alba seldom seen in hospital).		
	*Possible causes of alterations are identified in parentheses.	†This column provides guidelines for further assessment and initial nursing intervention.

(continued)

ASSESSMENT GUIDE—continued

POSTPARTAL—FIRST 24 HOURS AFTER BIRTH

PHYSICAL ASSESSMENT/ NORMAL FINDINGS	ALTERATIONS AND POSSIBLE CAUSES*	NURSING RESPONSES TO DATA†
Perineum		
Slight edema and bruising in intact perineum.	Marked fullness, bruising, pain (vulvar hematoma).	Assess size; apply ice glove or ice pack, analgesic and anesthetic sprays; report to physician or certified nurse-midwife.
Episiotomy: No redness, edema, ecchymosis, or discharge, edges well approximated.	Redness, edema, ecchymosis, discharge, or gaping stitches (infection).	Encourage sitz baths; review perineal care, appropriate wiping techniques.
Hemorrhoids: None present; if present, should be small and nontender.	Full, tender, inflamed hemorrhoids.	Encourage sitz baths, side-lying position; Tucks pads, anesthetic ointments, manual replacement of hemorrhoids, stool softeners, increased fluid intake.
Costovertebral Angle (CVA) Tenderness		
None.	Present (kidney infection).	Assess for other symptoms of urinary tract infection (UTI); obtain clean-catch urine sample; report to physician or certified nurse-midwife.
Lower Extremities		
No pain with palpation; negative Homans' sign.	Positive findings (thrombophlebitis).	Report to physician or certified nurse-midwife.
Elimination		
Urinary output: Voiding in sufficient quantities at least every 4–6 hours; bladder not palpable.	Inability to void (urinary retention). Urgency, frequency, dysuria (UTI).	Employ nursing interventions to promote voiding; if not successful, obtain order for catheterization. Report symptoms of UTI to physician or certified nurse-midwife.
Bowel elimination: Should have normal bowel movement by second or third day after birth.	Inability to pass feces or hard, small amount of stool (constipation due to fear of pain from episiotomy, hemorrhoids, perineal trauma).	Encourage fluids, ambulation, roughage in diet; sitz baths to promote healing of perineum; obtain order for stool softener.

CULTURAL ASSESSMENT‡	VARIATIONS TO CONSIDER	NURSING RESPONSES TO DATA†
Determine customs and practices regarding postpartum care.	Individual preference may include:	Provide for specific request if possible.
Ask the mother whether she would like fluids and ask what temperature she prefers.	· Room-temperature or warmed fluids rather than iced drinks.	If woman is unable to provide specific information, the nurse may draw from general information regarding cultural variation.
Ask the mother what foods or fluids she would like.	· Special foods or fluids to hasten healing after childbirth.	Mexican women may want food and fluids that restore hot-cold balance to the body. Women of European background may ask for iced fluids.
Ask the mother whether she would prefer to be alone during breastfeeding.	Some women may be hesitant to have someone with them when their breast is exposed.	Provide privacy as desired by mother.

‡These are only a few suggestions. It is not our intent to imply and this is a comprehensive cultural assessment.	*Possible causes of alterations are identified in parentheses.	†This column provides guidelines for further assessment initial nursing intervention.

ASSESSMENT GUIDE—continued

POSTPARTAL—FIRST 24 HOURS AFTER BIRTH

PSYCHOSOCIAL ASSESSMENT/ NORMAL FINDINGS	VARIATIONS TO CONSIDER*	NURSING RESPONSES TO DATA†
Psychologic Adaptation		
During first 24 hours: Passive; preoccupied with own needs; may talk about her labor and birth experience; may be talkative, elated, or very quiet.	Very quiet and passive; sleeps frequently (fatigue from long labor; feelings of disappointment about some aspect of the experience; may be following cultural expectation).	Provide opportunities for adequate rest; provide physical comfort measures; provide nutritious meals and snacks that are consistent with what the woman desires to eat and drink; provide opportunities to discuss birth experience in nonjudgmental atmosphere if the woman desires to do so.
Usually by 12 hours; beginning to assume responsibility; some women eager to learn; easily feel overwhelmed.	Excessive weepiness, mood swings, pronounced irritability (postpartum blues; feelings of inadequacy; culturally prescribed behavior).	Explain postpartum blues; provide supportive atmosphere; determine support available for mother; consider referral for evidence of profound depression.
Attachment		
En face position; holds baby close; cuddles and soothes; calls by name; identifies characteristics of family members in infant; may be awkward in providing care.	Continued expressions of disappointment in sex, appearance of infant; refusal to care for infant; derogatory comments; lack of bonding behaviors (difficulty in attachment, following expectations of cultural/ethnic group).	Provide reinforcement and support for infant caretaking behaviors; maintain nonjudgmental approach and gather more information if caretaking behaviors are not evident.
Initially may express disappointment over sex or appearance of infant but within 1-2 days demonstrates attachment behaviors.		
Client Education		
Demonstrates basic understanding of self-care activities and infant care needs; can identify signs of complications that should be reported.	Unable to demonstrate basic self-care and infant care activities (knowledge deficit; postpartum blues; following prescribed cultural behavior and will be cared for by grandmother or other family member).	Identify predominant learning style. Determine whether woman understands English and provide interpreter if needed; provide reinforcement of information through conversation and through written material (remember that some women and their families may not be able to understand written materials because of language difficulties or inability to read); provide information regarding infant care skills that are culturally consistent; give woman opportunity to express her feelings and demonstrate skills taught; consider social service home referral for women who have no family or other support, are unable to take in information about self-care and infant care, and demonstrate no caretaking activities.
	*Possible causes of alterations are identified in parentheses. and initial nursing action.	†This column provides guidelines for further assessment

MᴇᴅɪᴀLɪɴᴋ ● Skill 4–1: Assessing the Uterine Fundus Following Vaginal Birth

Check the relationship of the fundus to the umbilicus and also assess the firmness of the fundus. Measure the top of the fundus in finger-breadths above, below, or at the umbilicus (Figure 23–6 ●). See Skill 4–1 in the *Clinical Skills Manual* as well as the accompanying CD-ROM for more information. **SKILLS**

Note whether the fundus is in the midline or displaced to either side of the abdomen. If not midline, the uterus po-

sition should be located. Because the most common cause of displacement is a full bladder, this finding requires further assessment. Measure urine output for the next few hours until normal elimination status is established. Record the results of the assessment. Fundal height is recorded in finger-breadths (e.g., "2 FB ↓ U; 1 FB ↑ U"). Determine whether the fundus is firm. If it is not firm, lightly massage the abdomen until the fundus is firm. If

● FIGURE 23–6

Measurement of descent of fundus for the woman with vaginal birth. The fundus is located two finger-breadths below the umbilicus. Always support the bottom of the uterus during any assessment of the fundus.

massage was necessary, record the intervention response as "Uterus Boggy → firm with light massage." While completing the assessment, teach the woman about fundal position. The mother can be assisted in gently massaging her fundus to determine firmness. It is important to support the bottom of the uterus during the massage process and palpation to prevent prolapsing it. Correlate the position and firmness of the fundus with lochial flow.

In the woman who has had a cesarean birth, the abdominal incision is exquisitely tender. Therefore, palpate the fundus with extreme care and also inspect the abdominal incision for approximation (absence of separation between edges of incision), bleeding, and any signs of infection, including drainage, foul odor, edema, or redness. Also document whether internal sutures, steri-strips, or staples are intact. During the assessment, teach the woman about her incision. Review characteristics of normal healing, incision care, and discuss signs of infection.

Lochia

Evaluate the lochia, including character, amount, odor, and the presence of clots. Disposable gloves must be worn when assessing the perineum and lochia. Nurses may put on the gloves before beginning the assessment, just before assessing the abdomen and fundus, or when they are ready to assess the perineum and lochia. During the first 1 to 3 days after birth, the lochia should be rubra. A few small clots are normal and occur as a result of blood pooling in the vagina. However, the passage of numerous or large clots is abnormal, and the cause should be investigated immediately. After 2 to 3 days, the lochia flow becomes serosa.

Lochia should never exceed a moderate amount, such as four to eight partially saturated perineal pads daily, with an average of six. However, because this number is influenced by an individual woman's pad-changing practices, as well as the absorbency of the pad, ask about the length of time the current pad has been in use, whether the amount

is normal compared to her typical menstrual period, and whether any clots were passed before this examination, such as during voiding. If heavy bleeding is reported but not seen, ask the woman to put on a clean perineal pad and then reassess the woman's pad in 1 hour (Figure 23–7 ●). When a more accurate assessment of blood loss is needed, the perineal pads can be weighed, with 1 g considered the approximate equivalent of 1 mL of blood. See Skill 4–2 in the *Clinical Skills Manual* as well as the accompanying CD-ROM for more information. **SKILLS**

Clots and heavy bleeding may be caused by uterine relaxation (atony), retained placental fragments, or rarely, an unknown cervical laceration (seen as heavy bleeding but

● FIGURE 23–7

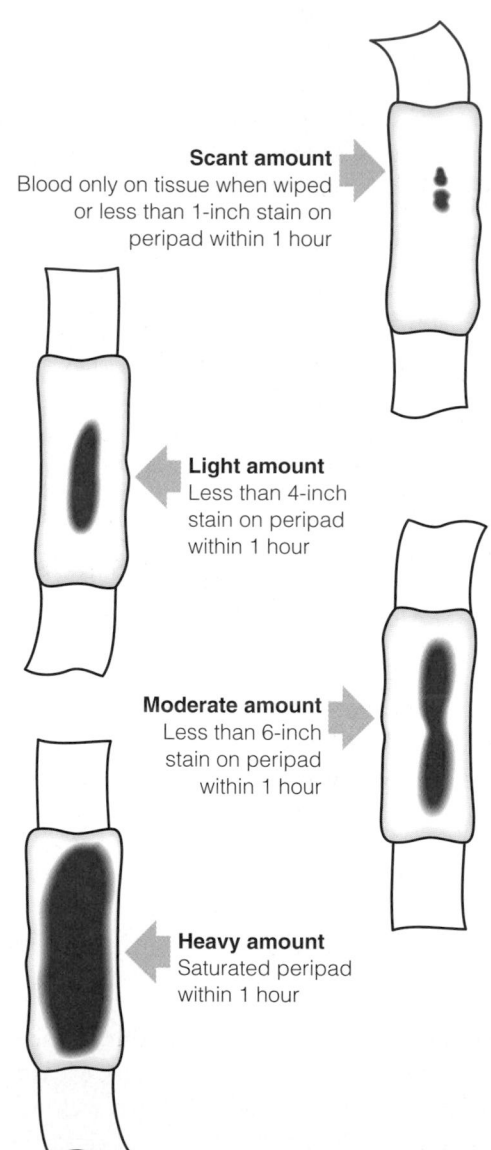

Scant amount
Blood only on tissue when wiped or less than 1-inch stain on peripad within 1 hour

Light amount
Less than 4-inch stain on peripad within 1 hour

Moderate amount
Less than 6-inch stain on peripad within 1 hour

Heavy amount
Saturated peripad within 1 hour

Suggested guideline for assessing lochia volume.

Used with permission from Jacobson, H. (1985, May-June). A standard for assessing lochia volume. Maternal-Child Nursing.

with firm fundus) that may require further assessment (see Table 23–3). Because of the evacuation of the uterine cavity during cesarean birth, women with such surgery usually have less lochia after the first 24 hours than mothers who give birth vaginally. If the woman is at increased risk for bleeding or is actually experiencing heavy flow of lochia rubra, the physician may also order methylergonovine maleate (Methergine). See "Drug Guide: Methylergonovine Maleate (Methergine)" in Chapter 24. ∞

The odor of the lochia is nonoffensive and never foul. If a foul odor is present, so is an infection. The amount of lochia is documented first, followed by character. For example:

- Lochia: moderate rubra
- Lochia: small rubra/serosa

Client teaching during assessment of the lochia may center on normal changes, effect of position changes, that can be expected in the amount and color of the flow. Review hygienic measures if appropriate and the need to notify nurse regression flow pattern (color, amount). Approach the teaching of hygienic practices delicately and with the goals of promoting comfort, enhancing tissue healing, and preventing infection. Avoid value-laden statements about the need for cleanliness or control of body odor.

Perineum

Inspect the perineum with the woman lying in a Sims' position. Lift the buttock to expose the perineum and anus.

If an episiotomy was done or a laceration required suturing, assess the wound and evaluate the state of healing by observing for ecchymosis and approximation. After 24

hours some edema may still be present, but the skin edges should be approximated (glued together) so that gentle pressure does not separate them. Gentle palpation should elicit minimal tenderness, and there should be no hard areas suggesting infection. Ecchymosis interferes with normal healing, as does infection. Hematomas sometimes occur, although these are considered abnormal.

Foul odors associated with drainage indicate infection. Also observe the incision for warmth, redness, tenderness, edema, and separation. Next assess whether hemorrhoids are present around the anus. If present, they are assessed for size, number, and pain or tenderness (Figure 23–8 ◉). See Skill 4–3 in the *Clinical Skills Manual* as well as the accompanying CD-ROM for more information. **SKILLS**

During the assessment, talk with the woman to determine the effectiveness of her comfort measures and provide teaching about the episiotomy. Some women do not thoroughly understand what and where an episiotomy is, and they may believe that the stitches must be removed as with other types of surgery. Frequently when women fear that the stitches must be removed manually, they are afraid to ask about them. While explaining the findings of the assessment, provide information about the episiotomy, its location, and the signs that are being assessed. This is an opportunity to casually add that the sutures are special and will dissolve slowly over the next few weeks as the tissues heal. By the time the sutures are dissolved, the tissues are strong and the incision

TABLE 23–3 ✤ Changes in Lochia That Cause Concern

Change	Possible Problem	Nursing Action
Presence of clots	Inadequate uterine contractions that allow bleeding from vessels at the placental site.	Assess location and firmness of fundus. Assess voiding pattern. Record and report findings.
Persistent lochia rubra	Inadequate uterine contractions; retained placental fragments; infection; undetected cervical laceration.	Assess location and firmness of fundus. Assess activity pattern. Assess for signs of infection. Record and report findings.

Intact perineum with hemorrhoids.

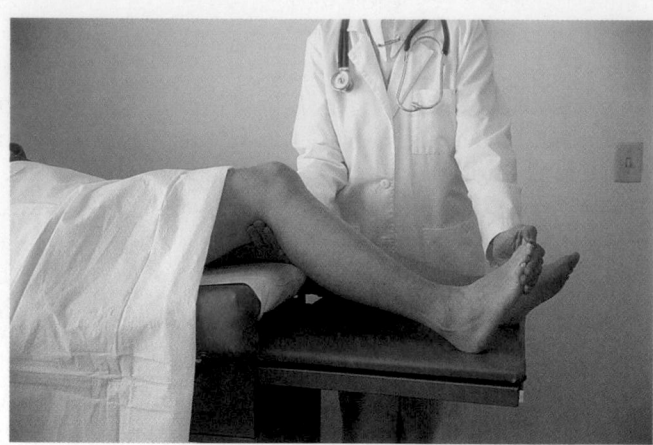

Homans' sign: With the woman's knee flexed, the nurse dorsiflexes the foot. Pain in the foot or leg is a positive Homans' sign.

Photographer: Elena Dorfman.

edges will not separate. This is also an opportunity to teach comfort measures (see Relief of Perineal Discomfort in Chapter 24 for more information ∞) and reinforce the need to consult with a healthcare provider prior to using OTC medications/supplements if nursing.

An example of documention of a perineal assessment might be: Midline episiotomy; no edema, tenderness, or ecchymosis present. Skin edges are approximated. Woman reports that a sitz bath and Tucks pads are controlling discomfort.

Lower Extremities

Postpartal women are at increased risk for *thrombophlebitis*, thrombus formation, and inflammation involving a vein (see Care of the Woman with Postpartal Thromboembolic Disease in Chapter 25 ∞). If thrombophlebitis occurs, the most likely site is in the woman's legs. To assess for it, her legs should be stretched out straight and relaxed with the knees flexed. Grasp the woman's foot and sharply dorsiflex it. No discomfort or pain should be present. The second leg is as-

sessed in the same way. If pain is elicited, notify the certified nurse-midwife or physician that the woman has a positive Homans' sign (Figure 23–9 ●). The pain is caused by inflammation of the vessel. Also evaluate the legs for edema by comparing both legs, since usually only one leg is involved. Any areas of redness, tenderness, and increased skin temperature are also noted.

Some facilities have discontinued performing a Homans' sign in the nursing assessment, stating it is not diagnostic and could lead to an embolus if the clot is dislodged during assessment. Although assessment of the Homans' sign is not diagnostic, supporters advocate its use as a screening tool. There are no published reports of an embolus occurring as a result of performing a Homans' sign. In the event of a positive Homans' sign, diagnosis is made by compression or duplex ultrasonography. Low-dose heparin therapy is used in postpartum women who develop a deep vein thrombosis (Drife, 2003).

Early ambulation is an important aspect in the prevention of thrombophlebitis. Most women are able to be up shortly after birth. The cesarean birth client requires range of motion exercises until she is ambulating more freely.

Client teaching associated with assessment of the lower extremities focuses on the signs and symptoms of thrombophlebitis. In addition, review self-care measures to promote circulation and measures to prevent thrombophlebitis, such as ambulation and avoiding pressure behind the knees, such as crossing the legs.

Elimination

During the hours after birth, carefully monitor a new mother's bladder status. A boggy uterus, a displaced uterus, or a palpable bladder are signs of bladder distention and re-

COMPLEMENTARY CARE

LYSINE

Lysine, an essential amino acid, has been identified as a supplement that decreases the incidence of pain following an episiotomy. Lysine is available as a supplement. The recommended adult dosage is 12 mg/kg of body weight per day. It is also present in dietary sources, including meat, cheese, fish, eggs, soybeans, and nuts.

quire nursing intervention. Encourage the postpartal woman to void every 4 to 6 hours. Assess the bladder for distention until the woman demonstrates complete emptying of the bladder with each voiding. The nurse may employ techniques to facilitate voiding, such as helping the woman out of bed to void or pouring warm water on the perineum. The physician will order a catheterization when the bladder is distended and the woman cannot void or when no voiding has occurred in 8 hours. The cesarean birth mother may have an indwelling catheter inserted prophylactically. Make the same assessments in evaluating bladder emptying once the catheter is removed.

During the physical assessment, ask the woman about the adequacy of her fluid intake, whether she feels she is emptying her bladder completely when she voids, and any signs of urinary tract infection (UTI) she may be experiencing.

Also ask about her intestinal elimination and any concerns she may have about it. Many mothers fear that the first bowel movement will be painful and possibly even damaging if an episiotomy has been done. Stool softeners may be ordered to increase bulk and moisture in the fecal material and to allow more comfortable and complete evacuation. Constipation is avoided to prevent pressure on sutures, which may increase discomfort. To enhance bowel elimination and help the woman reestablish her normal bowel pattern, encourage ambulation, increased fluid intake (up to 2000 mL/day or more), and additional fresh fruits and roughage in her diet.

During the assessment, provide information about postpartum diuresis and explain why the woman may be emptying her bladder so frequently. The need for additional fluid intake with suggestions of specific amounts may be helpful. The woman should drink at least eight 8-oz glasses of water or juice per day in addition to other fluids. Breastfeeding mothers will have a higher requirement (see Chapter 12 ∞). Discuss signs of urinary retention and overflow voiding and review symptoms of urinary tract infection if it seems an appropriate moment for teaching. Also review methods of assisting bowel elimination and provide opportunities for the woman to ask questions.

Rest and Sleep Status

Physical fatigue often affects other adjustments and functions of the new mother. The mother requires energy to make the psychologic adjustments to a new infant and to assume new roles. Fatigue is often a highly significant factor in a new mother's apparent disinterest in her newborn. Frequently the woman is so tired from a long labor and birth that everything seems to be an effort.

To avoid inadvertently classifying a very tired mother as one with a potential attachment problem, the nurse should do a psychologic assessment on more than one occasion. After a nap the new mother is often far more receptive to her baby and her surroundings. As part of the postpartal assessment, evaluate the amount of rest a new mother is getting. If the woman reports difficulty sleeping at night, try to determine the cause. If it is simply the strange environment, a warm drink and back rub may prove helpful. Appropriate nursing measures are indicated if the woman is bothered by normal postpartal discomforts such as afterpains, diaphoresis, or episiotomy or hemorrhoidal pain. See Chapter 24 for more detailed discussion of comfort/pain relief measures. ∞

Encourage a daily rest period and schedule hospital activities to allow time for napping. Also provide information about the fatigue new mothers experience and strategies to promote rest/sleep at home; and the impact it can have on a woman's emotions and sense of control.

Nutritional Status

Postpartal nutritional status is primarily determined based on information provided by the mother and on direct assessment. During pregnancy the daily recommended dietary allowances call for increases in calories, protein, and most vitamins and minerals. After birth the nonbreastfeeding mother's dietary requirements return to prepregnancy levels, whereas the lactating mother's requirements increase.

Visiting the mother during mealtime provides an opportunity for unobtrusive nutritional assessment and counseling. Advise the nonbreastfeeding mother about the need to reduce her caloric intake by about 300 kcal and to return to prepregnancy levels for other nutrients. The breastfeeding mother, however, should increase her caloric intake by about 200 kcal over the pregnancy requirements, or a total of 500 kcal over the nonpregnant requirement. Basic discussion often proves helpful, followed by referral as needed. In all cases, literature on nutrition should be provided so that the woman will have a source of information after discharge.

Inform the dietitian of any mother who is a vegetarian, has food allergies or lactose intolerance, or whose cultural or religious beliefs require specific foods. Appropriate meals can then be prepared for her. Many women, especially those who gained excessive weight, are interested in losing weight after birth. The dietitian can design weight reduction diets to meet nutritional needs and food preferences. The nurse may also refer women with unusual eating habits or numerous questions about good nutrition to the dietitian.

New mothers are advised that it is common practice to prescribe iron supplements for 3 months after birth. The hematocrit is then checked at the postpartal visit to detect any anemia.

PSYCHOLOGIC ASSESSMENT

During the first several postpartal weeks, the new mother must accomplish certain physical and developmental tasks:

- Restoring physical condition
- Developing competence in caring for and meeting the needs of her infant
- Establishing a relationship with her new child
- Adapting to altered lifestyles and family structure resulting from the addition of a new member

Adequate assessment of the mother's psychologic adjustment is an integral part of postpartal evaluation. This assessment focuses on the mother's general attitude, feelings of competence, available support systems, and caregiving skills. It also evaluates her fatigue level, sense of satisfaction, and ability to accomplish her developmental tasks.

Some new mothers have little or no experience with newborns and may feel totally overwhelmed. They may show these feelings by asking questions and reading all available material or by becoming passive and quiet because they simply cannot deal with their feelings of inadequacy. Avoid inaccurately concluding that the woman is disinterested, withdrawn, or depressed by asking the new mother questions about her plans and previous experience in a supportive, nonjudgmental way.

Problem clues might include excessive continued fatigue, marked depression, excessive preoccupation with physical status or discomfort, evidence of low self-esteem, lack of support systems, marital problems, inability to care for or nurture the newborn, and current family crises (illness, unemployment, and so on). These characteristics frequently indicate a potential for maladaptive parenting, which may lead to child abuse or neglect (physical, emotional, or intellectual) and cannot be ignored. Referrals to public health nurses or other available community resources may provide greatly needed assistance and alleviate potentially dangerous situations.

ASSESSMENT OF EARLY ATTACHMENT

A nurse in any of the various postpartal settings can periodically observe and note progress toward attachment. The assessment should include both parents when possible; however, in this section, these behaviors focus primarily on the mother's attachment process. As discussed previously, research shows that fathers experience similar attachment feelings to those experienced by mothers. The following questions can be addressed in the course of nurse-client interaction:

- Is the mother attracted to her newborn? To what extent does she seek face-to-face contact and eye contact? Has she progressed from fingertip touch, to palmar contact,

to enfolding the infant close to her own body? Is attraction increasing or decreasing? If the mother does not exhibit increasing attraction, why not? Do the reasons lie primarily within her, in the baby, or in the environment?

- Is the mother inclined to nurture her infant? Is she progressing in her interactions with her infant?
- Does the mother act consistently? If not, is the source of unpredictability within her or her infant?
- Is her mothering consistently carried out? Does she seek information and evaluate it objectively? Does she develop solutions based on adequate knowledge of valid data? Does she evaluate the effectiveness of her maternal care and adjust appropriately?
- Is she sensitive to the newborn's needs as they arise? How quickly does she interpret her infant's behavior and react to cues? Does she seem happy and satisfied with the infant's responses to her efforts? Is she pleased with feeding behaviors? How much of this ability and willingness to respond is related to the baby's nature and how much to her own?
- Does she seem pleased with her baby's appearance and sex? Is she experiencing pleasure in interaction with her infant? What interferes with the enjoyment? Does she speak to the baby frequently and affectionately? Does she call him or her by name? Does she point out family traits or characteristics she sees in the newborn?
- Are there any cultural factors that might modify the mother's response? For instance, is it customary for the grandmother to assume most of the childcare responsibilities while the mother recovers from childbirth?

Once these questions are addressed and the facts are assembled, combine the information with personal intuition and knowledge to answer three more unspoken questions: Is there a problem in attachment? What is the problem? What is its source? Then devise a creative approach to the problem as it presents itself in the context of a unique, developing mother-infant relationship.

DISCHARGE ASSESSMENT AND FOLLOW-UP

The final discharge assessment should include a physical examination and appropriate discharge teaching that includes both maternal and newborn care guidelines. The mother's laboratory values are examined. If the mother was nonimmune to rubella, a rubella vaccine is administered prior to discharge. Rh-negative mothers whose infants are Rh positive need RhoGAM before they go home. If either is given, document this in the mother's chart. If referrals, such as social service programs, support groups, lactation consultant, or a pediatrician, are needed, provide before the family leaves the facility.

Some obstetricians, nurse-midwives, and nurse practitioners see postpartal women 1 to 2 weeks after birth in addition to the routine 6-week checkup. This extra visit provides an opportunity for physical assessment as well as evaluation of the mother's psychologic and informational needs. Postdischarge care for the postpartal woman may be accomplished by home visits or follow-up phone calls. A home visit 1 to 3 days after discharge provides opportunities for further assessment and teaching. (See discussion of postpartum home care in Chapter 32. ∞)

The follow-up telephone call is usually made by a nurse from the postpartal unit of the agency where the mother gave birth. It is made soon after discharge and is designed to provide assessment and care if necessary, to reinforce knowledge and provide additional teaching, and to make referrals if indicated. Alternatively, a follow-up phone call from a nurse from the physician or nurse-midwife's office can provide new mothers with a source of support and an opportunity to ask questions. Women who appear to be having adjustment problems should be scheduled for an appointment for further evaluation.

In ideal situations a family approach involving the father, infant, other siblings, and grandparents permits a total evaluation and provides an opportunity for all family members to ask questions and express concerns. Such an approach also promotes diagnosis and treatment of disturbed family patterns to prevent future problems of neglect or abuse.

Critical Concept Review

LEARNING OBJECTIVES

CONCEPTS

Describe the basic physiologic changes that occur in the postpartal period as a woman's body returns to its prepregnant state.

1. Uterus is at the level of umbilicus within a few hours after childbirth. Decreases by about one finger breadth per day.
2. Placental site heals by a process of exfoliation, so no scar formation occurs.
3. Lochia flow progresses from rubra to serosa to alba.
4. Ovarian function and menstruation return in approximately 6–12 weeks in the nonlactating mother.
5. Breasts begin milk production.
6. Intestines are sluggish for a few days, leading to constipation, but return to prepregnant state within a week.
7. Postpartum diuresis occurs, bladder tone is decreased, and bladder takes approximately 6 weeks to return to prepregnant state.
A higher than usual boggy uterus, which deviates to the side, usually indicates a full bladder.
8. Bradycardia is normal for the first 6–10 days.
9. Hemostatic system reaches prepregnant state in 3–4 weeks. WBC count is often elevated. Activation of clotting factors predisposes to thrombus formation.

Discuss the psychologic adjustments that normally occur during the postpartal period.

1. Psychologic adjustment includes:
   - Taking-in.
   - Taking-hold.
   - Maternal role attainment.
   - Possibility of postpartum blues.

Summarize the factors that influence the development of parent-infant attachment.

1. Parent-infant attachment is influenced by:
   - Involvement with woman's own family.
   - Stability of relationships and home environment.
   - Mother's ability to trust.
   - Mother's level of self-esteem.
   - Mother's ability to enjoy herself.
   - Mother's knowledge of expectations of childbearing and child rearing.
   - Positive reaction to present pregnancy.

(continued)

LEARNING OBJECTIVES

CONCEPTS

Delineate the physiologic and psychosocial components of a normal postpartal assessment.

1. Systematic postpartal assessment includes:
   - Vital signs.
   - Breast examination.
   - Assessment of fundus, incision, episiotomy, and perineum.
   - Assessment of lochia in terms of type, quantity, and characteristics.
   - Assessment of bladder and bowels.
   - Assessment of lower extremities.
   - Psychologic assessment.
     - Expected phase of adjustment to parenthood.
     - Expected level of attachment to infant.
   - Client education concerning self-care.

Discuss the physical and developmental tasks that the mother must accomplish during the postpartal period.

1. The woman's physical condition returns to a nonpregnant state.
2. The woman gains competence and confidence in herself as a parent.

CRITICAL THINKING IN ACTION

*View the **Critical Thinking in Action** video in Chapter 23 of the CD-ROM. Then, answer the questions that follow.*

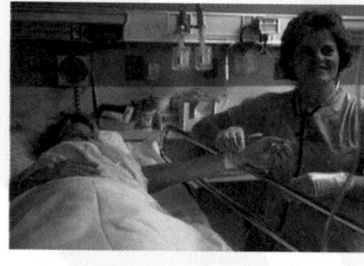

Janet Burns, a 25-year-old G3 P3, is 2 hours past a low forceps vaginal birth with a right medial lateral episiotomy of a live 8 pound baby boy. You obtain vital signs of BP 118/70, T 98.8°F, P 76, R 14. You observe the fundus is +1 finger above the umbilicus and slightly to the right. Her episiotomy is slightly ecchymotic and well approximated without edema or discharge. Ice has been applied to the episiotomy for the last 20 minutes. Lochia rubra is present and a pad was saturated in 90 minutes. Janet has an intravenous of Ringer's lactate with 10 units of Pitocin infusing at 100 mL/hr in her lower left arm and is complaining of moderate abdominal cramping. Janet's baby is sleeping peacefully in the bassinet next to her bed. She tells you that she is very tired and requests some pain medication so she can sleep for a while.

1. What nursing assessment is of immediate concern?
2. Discuss care of her episiotomy and perineum.
3. What other self-care measures could you advise?
4. Discuss postpartal occurrences that may cause special concern for the mother.
5. Janet expressed concern about her episiotomy healing. What information can you offer?

MEDIALINK

www.prenhall.com/london

- NCLEX-RN® Review, case studies, and other interactive resources for this chapter can be found on the Companion Website at http://www.prenhall.com/london. Click on "Chapter 23" to select the activities for this chapter.

- For animations, more NCLEX-RN® Review questions, and an audio glossary, access the accompanying CD-ROM in this textbook.

REFERENCES

Blackburn, S. T. (2003). *Maternal, fetal, & neonatal physiology: A clinical perspective* (2nd ed.). Philadelphia: Saunders.

Browne, I. M., & Birnbach, D. J. (2003). Neurocysticercosis: A new differential in the diagnosis of postdural puncture headache. *Anesthesia & Analgesia, 97*(2), 580–582.

Cesario, S. K. (2001). Care of the Native American woman: Strategies for practice, education, and research. *Journal of Obstetric, Gynecologic, and Neonatal Nursing, 30*(1), 13–18.

Drife, J. (2003). Thromboembolism. *British Medical Bulletin. Pregnancy: Reducing maternal death and disability, 67,* 177–190.

Mercer, R. T. (1995). *Becoming a mother.* New York: Springer.

Porter, C., & Hsu, H. C. (2003). First time mothers' perceptions of efficacy during the transition to motherhood: Links to infant temperament. *Journal of Family Psychology, 17*(1), 54–64.

Rubin, R. (1961). Puerperal change. *Nursing Outlook, 9,* 753.

Rubin, R. (1984). *Maternal identity and the maternal experience.* New York: Springer.

Shehata, H. A., & Okosun, H. (2004). Neurological disorders in pregnancy. *Current Opinion in Obstetrics & Gynecology, 16*(2), 117–122.

Tatum, W., Liporace, J., Benbadis, S., & Kaplan, P. (2004). Updates on the treatment of epilepsy in women. *Archives of Internal Medicine, 164*(2), 137–145.

Varney, H., Kriebs, J. M., & Gegor, C. L. (2004). *Varney's midwifery* (4th ed.). Sudbury, MA: Jones & Bartlett.

Wiertlewski, S., Magot, A., Drapier, S., Malinovsky, J. M., & Pereon, Y. (2004). Worsening of neurologic symptoms after epidural anesthesia for labor in a Guillain-Barré patient. *Anesthesia and Analgesia, 98*(3), 825–827.

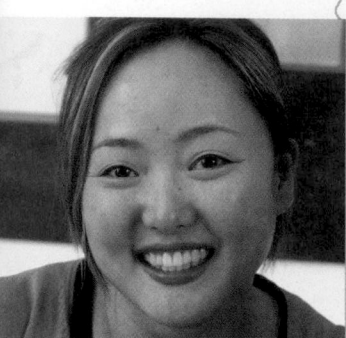

CHAPTER 24

The Postpartum Family: Needs and Care

More than anything else that happened after my baby was born, I was surprised by the fatigue I felt. In the first few weeks I spent every minute that my baby slept cleaning, doing laundry, and the like. Then, during my checkup, the nurse–midwife told me that I had to rest when my baby slept. What a difference that made. Suddenly I was less overwhelmed and more able to enjoy being a mother.

—*Mai Ling, 26*

LEARNING OBJECTIVES

- Relate the use of nursing diagnoses to the findings of the "normal" postpartum assessment and analysis.

- Delineate strategies for promoting family learning during the early postpartum period.

- Discuss appropriate nursing interventions to promote maternal comfort and well-being.

- Describe the nurse's role in promoting maternal rest and helping the mother gradually resume an appropriate level of activity.

- Identify client teaching topics for promoting postpartal family wellness.

- Compare the postpartal nursing needs of the woman who experienced a cesarean birth with the needs of a woman who gave birth vaginally.

- Summarize the nursing needs of the childbearing adolescent during the postpartal period.

- Describe possible approaches to sensitive, holistic nursing care for the woman who relinquishes her newborn.

- Delineate criteria and teaching topics related to postpartum discharge.

MEDIALINK

www.prenhall.com/london

CD-ROM
NCLEX-RN® Review
Audio Glossary

Companion Website
NCLEX-RN® Review
Medialink Applications:
    Case Study: Perineal Discomfort
    Discharge Teaching Checklist
Thinking Critically

The best postpartum care is family centered; incorporates the family's needs, desires, and values as much as possible; and disrupts the family unit as little as possible. This approach uses the family's resources to support an early and smooth adjustment to the newborn by all family members. Nursing care during this time is aimed at meeting individual and family needs. Goals are formulated after careful assessment, consultation with the woman and her family, and consideration of factors that could influence the outcome of care.

Chapter 23 provides a thorough discussion of postpartum assessment. ∞ How can the nurse use the remaining steps of the nursing process effectively to plan and provide care? This chapter provides that information, in addition to describing the specific nursing responses to the mother's physical needs and the family's psychosocial needs. See "Clinical Pathway: For the Postpartum Period."

NURSING CARE DURING THE EARLY POSTPARTUM PERIOD

For most postpartal women, physical recovery goes smoothly and is considered a healthy process. Because of this perception, caregivers too often assume that the woman and her family have no real needs and that no care plan is needed. Nothing could be further from the truth. Every member of the family has needs, although the needs may not be obvious, especially if they are psychologic or educational.

NURSING DIAGNOSIS

The postpartum family's needs, which should be identified during assessment, are the basis for developing nursing diagnoses. Many nurses have suggested that nursing diagnoses are difficult to make in a wellness setting because of their emphasis on "problems." Nurses involved in the effort to formulate standardized diagnoses recognize this difficulty and continue working to develop nursing diagnoses more congruent with wellness settings.

Many agencies that use nursing diagnoses prefer to use only the NANDA list. Consequently, physiologic alterations form the basis of many postpartum diagnoses. Examples of such diagnoses include the following:

- *Constipation* related to fear of tearing stitches or pain
- *Acute Pain* related to perineal edema or episiotomy

Fortunately, diagnoses have now been developed that focus on the positive aspects of childbirth and parenting. Examples of these diagnoses include the following:

- *Health-Seeking Behaviors: Information about Infant Care* related to an expressed desire to improve parenting skills
- *Readiness for Enhanced Family Coping* related to successful adjustment to new baby

After completing the assessment and diagnosis steps of the nursing process, the nurse identifies expected outcomes and selects nursing interventions that will help the family meet the expected outcomes.

PLANNING AND IMPLEMENTATION

Nursing management is individualized to meet the needs of each woman and her newborn. The plan of care needs to consider the baby's schedule, as well as the physical and psychologic well-being of each family member. An important component of nursing care is client teaching, which must be individualized to

Continuous epidural infusion (CEI), 606

Mother-baby care or couplet care, 604

Patient-controlled analgesia (PCA), 606

CLINICAL PATHWAY

FOR THE POSTPARTUM PERIOD

CATEGORY	FIRST 4 HOURS	4–8 HOURS PAST BIRTH	8–24 HOURS PAST BIRTH
Referral	**VB:** Report from labor nurse if applicable **CB:** Report from OR recovery nurse	Lactation consultation as needed **CB:** Respiratory therapist as needed	Home nursing, WIC referral if indicated **EXPECTED OUTCOMES** Referrals made
Assessments	**VB:** Postpartum assessments q30 min × 2, q1h × 2, then q4h. Includes ■ Fundus firm, midline, at or below umbilicus ■ Lochia rubra <1 pad/hr; no free flow or passage of clots with massage ■ Bladder: voids large amounts of urine spontaneously; bladder not palpable following voiding ■ Perineum: sutures intact; no bulging or marked swelling; no c/o severe pain. Minimal bruising may be present. If hemorrhoids present, no tenseness or marked engorgement; <2 cm diameter ■ Breasts: soft, colostrum present **Vital Signs:** ■ BP WNL: no hypotension; not 30 mm Hg systolic or 15 mm Hg diastolic over baseline ■ Temperature: <38°C (100.4°F) ■ Pulse: bradycardia normal, consistent with baseline ■ Respirations: 12–20/min; quiet, easy Comfort level: <3 on scale of 1–10 **CB:** Postpartum cesarean assessment q15min × 4, q30min × 4, q1h per protocol; all assessment parameters for VB included, as well as ■ Surgical dressing over incision clean and dry or with minimal drainage ■ Foley catheter in place, urine color and amount noted ■ IV: no swelling, pain, or redness at insertion site; infusing at prescribed rate ■ Bowel sounds: present, decreased, or minimal ■ LOC: alert and oriented, easily aroused if dozing ■ LOS: sensation WNL for anesthesia or analgesia type administered ■ Pulse ox: WNL ■ Input and output: WNL	**VB:** Continue postpartum assessment q4h × 2, then q8h Breast: evaluate nipple status; should be no evidence of cracks or bruising Observe feeding technique with newborn Vital signs assessment q8h; all WNL; report temperature >38°C (100.4°F) Assess Homans' sign q8h Continue assessment of comfort level **CB:** Continue cesarean assessments per protocol, including all assessments covered in VB; as well as ■ Determine if woman passing flatus ■ Determine if bowel sounds present	Continue postpartum assessment per protocol Breasts: nipples should remain free of cracks, fissures, bruising Feeding technique with newborn: should be good or improving Vital signs assessment q8h; all WNL; report temperature >38°C (100.4°F) Continue assessment of comfort level **EXPECTED OUTCOMES** Vital signs medically acceptable, voids qs, postpartum assessment WNL; comfort level <3 on a 1–10 scale, involution of uterus in process, demonstrates and verbalizes appropriate newborn feeding techniques

Information is included for both vaginal birth (VB) and cesarean birth (CB). However, since many of the nursing care interventions are the same for either, specific interventions or suggestions related to vaginal birth are designated VB, and those specific to cesarean are designated CB.

ADL, activities of daily living; BP, blood pressure; CB, cesarean birth; CNM, certified nurse-midwife; c/o, complains of; DC, discontinue; LDR, labor, delivery, and recovery; LOC, level of consciousness; LOS, level of sensation; OOB, out of bed; OR, operating room; prn, as needed; VB, vaginal birth; WNL, within normal limits.

CLINICAL PATHWAY—continued

FOR THE POSTPARTUM PERIOD

CATEGORY	FIRST 4 HOURS	4–8 HOURS PAST BIRTH	8–24 HOURS PAST BIRTH
Teaching/ psychosocial	Explain postpartum assessments Teach self-massage of fundus and expected findings; rationale for fundal massage Instruct to call for assistance first time OOB and prn Demonstrate perineal care, surgigator, sitz bath prn Explain comfort measures Begin newborn teaching; bulb suctioning, positioning, feeding, diaper change, cord care Orient to room if transferred from LDR room Provide information on early postpartum period Assess mother-infant attachment **CB:** Teach turn-cough and deep breathing exercise Explain importance of moving around in bed and moving legs up and down Demonstrate splinting of abdomen for increased comfort with movement Discuss plan of care related to cesarean recovery; activity and ambulation recommendations, advancement of diet, incision care, schedule for IV and Foley catheter removal Provide information about PCA, pain medications, and alternative measures for pain management	Discuss psychologic changes of postpartum period; facilitate transition through tasks of taking on maternal role Discuss perineal care/hygiene; encourage use of supportive brassiere for breast- or bottle-feeding Stress need for frequent rest periods Continue newborn teaching: soothing/comforting techniques, swaddling; return demonstrations indicate woman's understanding Provide opportunities for questions and review, reinforce previous teaching Breastfeeding: nipple care: air-drying, lanolin; proper latch-on technique; tea bags Formula-feeding: supportive bra, ice bags, breast binder Assess mother-infant attachment Stress need for movement and ambulation Discuss incision healing Explain benefit of a regular schedule of medications for pain to optimize comfort	Reinforce previous teaching, complete teaching evaluation Discuss involution; anticipated physical changes in first 2 weeks postpartum; postpartum exercises; need to limit visitors Discuss postpartum nutrition; balanced diet **Breastfeeding:** ■ Increase calories by 500 kcal over non-pregnant state (200 kcal over pregnant intake) ■ Explain milk production, letdown reflex, use of supplements, breast pumping, and milk storage **Formula-feeding:** ■ Return to nonpregnant caloric intake ■ Explain formula preparation and storage Discuss birth control options, sexuality Discuss sibling rivalry and plan for supporting siblings at home Discuss pets; suggestions for improving acceptance of infant by pets **EXPECTED OUTCOMES** Mother verbalizes teaching comprehension Positive bonding and emotional behaviors observed
Nursing care management and reports	**VB:** Ice pack to perineum to decrease swelling and increase comfort Straight catheter prn × 1 if distended or voiding small amounts If continues unable to void or only voids small amounts, insert Foley catheter and notify CNM or physician **CB:** Implement input and output regimen Maintain IV as ordered Medicate for pain Begin providing ice chips when bowel sounds are present	Sitz baths prn If woman Rh negative and infant Rh positive, Rh immune globulin workup; obtain consent; complete teaching Determine rubella status Obtain consent for rubella vaccine if indicated; explain purpose, procedure, implications of vaccine **CB:** Advance diet as ordered and tolerated Assist with perineal care and ADLs Obtain hematocrit and hemaglobin Discontinue Foley catheter when woman can ambulate to BR Discontinue of heplock IV when woman can tolerate oral fluids, or as ordered Maintain incision care as ordered	Continue sitz baths prn May shower if ambulating without difficulty DC buffalo cap (heparin lock) if present Administer rubella vaccine as indicated **EXPECTED OUTCOMES** Using sitz bath; voids qs; lab work WNL; performs ADL without sequelae
Activity	**VB:** Assistance when OOB first time, then prn Ambulate ad lib Rests comfortably between assessments **CB:** Assistance with movement in bed, to include leg exercises and sitting upright	Encourage rest periods Ambulate ad lib; may leave birthing unit after notifying staff of plan to ambulate off unit **CB:** Advance movement to include hanging legs over edge of bed and brief standing	Up ad lib **CB:** Assist woman to ambulate as soon as possible **EXPECTED OUTCOMES** Ambulates ad lib

(continued)

CLINICAL PATHWAY—continued

FOR THE POSTPARTUM PERIOD

CATEGORY	FIRST 4 HOURS	4–8 HOURS PAST BIRTH	8–24 HOURS PAST BIRTH
Comfort	Institute comfort measures: ■ Perineal discomfort: peri-care; sitz baths, topical analgesics ■ Hemorrhoids: sitz baths, topical analgesics, digital replacement of external hemorrhoids; side-lying or prone position ■ Afterpains: prone with small pillow under abdomen; warm shower or sitz baths; ambulation ■ Administer pain medication _____ **CB:** Implement PCA or pain medication schedule as ordered	Continue with pain management techniques Offer alternative pain management options: distraction with music, television, visitors; massage; warmed blankets or towels to affected area; using breathing techniques when infant latches on to breast or during cramping until medication's action is felt	Continue with pain management techniques **EXPECTED OUTCOMES** Comfort level <3 on 1–10 scale Verbalizes alternative pain management options
Nutrition	**VB:** Regular diet Fluid ≥2000 mL/day **CB:** Begin sips and chips when bowel sound present or per protocol	Continue diet and fluids **CB:** Advance diet to clear liquids as tolerated or per protocol	Continue diet and fluids **CB:** Advance diet as tolerated **EXPECTED OUTCOMES** Regular diet/fluids tolerated
Elimination	Voiding large amounts straw-colored urine **CB:** A minimum of 30 mL qh clear urine output in Foley catheter	Voiding large quantities May have bowel movement **CB:** A minimum of 30 mL qh clear urine output in Foley catheter	Same **EXPECTED OUTCOMES** Voiding qs; passing flatus or bowel movement
Medications	Pain medications as ordered Methergine 0.2 mg q4h po if ordered Stool softener _____ Tucks pad prn, perineal analgesic spray	Continue meds Lanolin to nipples prn; tea bags to nipples if tender; heparin flush to buffalo cap/heplock (if present) q8h or as ordered May take own prenatal vitamins	Continue medications RhoGAM and rubella vaccine administered if indicated **EXPECTED OUTCOMES** Vaccines administered; pain controlled
Discharge planning/ home care	Evaluate knowledge of normal postpartum and newborn care Evaluate support systems	Discuss typical newborn schedule; plan for periods of rest Birth certificate paperwork completed Evaluate plans for transporting newborn; car seat available **CB:** Evaluate for physical help at home	Review discharge instruction sheet/checklist Describe postpartum warning signs and when to call CNM or physician Provide prescriptions; gift packs given appropriate for formula- or breastfeeding Arrangements for baby pictures as desired Postpartum and newborn visits scheduled **EXPECTED OUTCOMES** Discharged home; mother verbalizes postpartum warning s/s, follow-up appointment times and dates
Family involvement	Identify available support persons Assess family perceptions of birth experience Parenting: demonstrates culturally expected early parenting behaviors	Involve support persons in care, teaching; answer questions Evidence of parental bonding behaviors present	Continue to involve support persons in teaching, involve siblings as appropriate. Plans made for providing support to mother following discharge **EXPECTED OUTCOMES** Evidence of parental bonding behavior; support persons verbalize understanding of woman's need for rest, good nutrition, fluids, and emotional support
Date			

the learning ability and readiness of the parents. As part of the teaching role, the nurse discusses desired outcomes and goals with the mother and family members. Interventions can then be designed to achieve optimal health promotion.

PROMOTION OF MATERNAL COMFORT AND WELL-BEING

The nurse can promote maternal physical well-being by monitoring uterine status, vital signs, cardiovascular status, elimination patterns, nutritional needs, sleep and rest, and support and educational needs. In addition the woman may need medications to promote comfort, treat anemia, provide immunity to rubella, and prevent development of antigens (in the nonsensitized Rh-negative woman).

MONITORING UTERINE STATUS

Complete an assessment of the uterus as discussed in Chapter 23. ∞ The assessment interval is usually every 15 minutes for the first hour after childbirth, every 30 minutes for the next hour, and then hourly for approximately 2 more hours. After that, monitor uterine status every 8 hours or more frequently if problems arise such as bogginess, positioning out of midline, heavy lochia flow, or the presence of clots (Table 24–1). When the uterus is firmly contracted, uterine blood vessels are compressed by the myometrium, and bleeding is controlled. Occasionally, however, a woman needs medications to maintain this contracted state. See "Drug Guide: Oxytocin (Pitocin)" in Chapter 22 ∞ and "Drug Guide: Methylergonovine Maleate (Methergine)" in this chapter. Monitor amount, consistency, color, and odor of the lochia on an ongoing basis (Table 24–2).

RELIEF OF PERINEAL DISCOMFORT

Before selecting a method to help relieve perineal discomfort, assess the perineum to determine the degree of edema and so on. It is also important to ask the woman if she believes any special measures will be particularly effective and

TABLE 24–1 ❖ Position of the Uterine Fundus Following Birth

Immediately after birth: The top of the fundus is in the midline about midway between the symphysis pubis and umbilicus.

Six to twelve hours after birth: The top of the fundus is in the midline and at the level of the umbilicus.

One day after birth: The top of the fundus is in the midline and one finger-breadth below the umbilicus.

Second day after birth and thereafter: The top of the fundus remains in the midline and descends about one finger-breadth per day.

TABLE 24–2 ❖ Changes in Lochia That Cause Concern

Change	Possible Problem	Nursing Action
Presence of clots	Inadequate uterine contractions that allow bleeding from vessels at the placental site	Assess location and firmness of fundus. Massage if boggy, then express clots. Assess voiding pattern. Record and report findings.
Persistent lochia rubra	Inadequate uterine contractions; retained placental fragments; infection	Assess location and firmness of fundus. Massage if boggy. Assess activity pattern. Assess for signs of infection. Record and report findings.

to offer her choices when possible. Wear disposable gloves while applying all relief measures and complete handwashing before and after using the gloves. At all times it is essential to remember good hygiene practices, such as moving from the front (area of the symphysis pubis) to the back (area around the anus) of the perineum. Avoiding contamination between the anal area and the urethral/vaginal area is vital to prevent infection.

Ice Pack

If an episiotomy is done at the time of birth, an ice pack is generally applied to the perineum to reduce edema and provide numbing of the tissues, which promotes comfort. In some agencies, chemical ice bags are used. Folding both ends toward the middle usually activates these ice bags. To make an inexpensive ice bag, fill a disposable glove with ice chips or crushed ice and then tape the top of the glove to close it. To protect the perineum from burns caused by contact with such an ice pack, rinse the glove under running water to remove any powder and then wrap it in an absorbent towel or washcloth before placing it against the perineum. For best results the ice pack is applied for approximately 20 minutes and then removed for about 10 minutes. Usually ice packs are needed for the first 24 hours. Provide information about the purpose of the ice pack, as well as anticipated effects, benefits, and possible problems, and explain how to make an ice pack for home use if edema is present and early discharge is planned.

Sitz Bath

The warmth of the water in the sitz bath provides comfort, decreases pain, and promotes circulation to the tissues.

DRUG GUIDE

METHYLERGONOVINE MALEATE (METHERGINE)

Overview of Action

Methylergonovine maleate (Methergine) is an ergot alkaloid that stimulates smooth muscle tissue. Because the smooth muscle of the uterus is especially sensitive to this drug, it is used postpartally to stimulate the uterus to contract in order to decrease blood loss by clamping off uterine blood vessels and to promote the involution process. In addition the drug has a vasoconstrictive effect on all blood vessels, especially the larger arteries. This may result in hypertension, particularly in a woman whose blood pressure is already elevated.

Route, Dosage, and Frequency

Methergine has a rapid onset of action and may be given orally or intramuscularly.

Usual IM dose: 0.2 mg following expulsion of the placenta. The dose may be repeated every 2–4 hours if necessary.

Usual oral dose: 0.2 mg every 4 hours (six doses).

Maternal Contraindications

Pregnancy, hepatic or renal disease, cardiac disease, hypertension, or preeclampsia contraindicate this drug's use. Methylergonovine maleate must be used with caution during lactation (Wilson, Shannon, & Stang, 2006).

Maternal Side Effects

Hypertension, nausea, vomiting, headache, bradycardia, dizziness, tinnitus, abdominal cramps, palpitations, dyspnea, chest pain, and allergic reactions may be noted.

Effects on Fetus or Newborn

Because Methergine has a long duration (3 hours [Wilson et al., 2006]) and action and can thus produce tetanic contractions, it **should never be used during pregnancy or in labor,** when it may result in a sustained uterine contraction that may cause amniotic fluid embolism (increased pressure in uterus may allow entry of amniotic fluid under the edge of the placenta and thus entry into the maternal venous system), uterine rupture, cervical and perineal lacerations (resulting from tetanic contractions and rapid birth of the baby), and hypoxia and intracranial hemorrhage in the baby (because of tetanic contractions, which severely decrease the maternal-placental-fetal blood flow, or uterine rupture, which causes cessation of blood flow to the unborn baby) (Wilson et al., 2006).

Nursing Considerations

- Monitor fundal height and consistency and the amount and character of the lochia.
- Assess the blood pressure before and routinely throughout drug administration.
- Observe for adverse effects or symptoms of ergot toxicity (ergotism) such as nausea and vomiting, headache, muscle pain, cold or numb fingers and toes, chest pain, and general weakness (Wilson et al., 2006).
- Provide client/family teaching regarding importance of not smoking during Methergine administration (nicotine from cigarettes leads to constricted vessels and may lead to hypertension) and signs of toxicity.

NURSING PRACTICE

You may be surprised by how quickly the postpartum woman shows signs of bladder distention, possibly as soon as 1 to 2 hours after childbirth. It results because of normal postpartum diuresis. You can help prevent overdistention by palpating the woman's bladder frequently and encouraging her to void. When attempting to void for the first time after vaginal birth, some mothers may feel the urge to urinate but are unable to begin the flow of urine. Possible interventions include letting her hear running water by turning water on in the sink or tub, running warm water in the sink and having her place one hand in the water, or placing her feet in a basin of warm water.

portant for the woman to have a clean, unused towel to pat dry her perineum after the sitz bath and to have a clean perineal pad to apply. Be alert during the first sitz bath because the warm, moist heat and warm environment may cause the woman to faint. Place a call bell well within reach and check on the woman frequently to maintain safety. Signs that she may feel faint include expressed feelings of dizziness, a floaty or spacy feeling, or difficulty hearing.

Cool sitz baths have gained popularity because they are effective in reducing perineal edema and in reducing the response of nerve endings, which cause perineal discomfort (Varney, Kriebs, & Gegor, 2004). In administering a cool sitz bath, have the woman start with the water at room temperature and add ice according to the woman's comfort. Since women may have different preferences, it is best to offer the woman a choice of either a warm or cold sitz bath. Provide information about the purpose and use of the sitz bath; anticipated effects, benefits, and possible problems; and safety measures to prevent injury from fainting, slipping, or excessive water temperature. Home

This promotes healing and reduces the incidence of infection (Figure 24–1 ●). Sitz baths may be ordered three times a day (tid) and as needed (prn). Prepare the sitz bath by cleaning the sitz bath equipment and adding water at 102°F to 105°F (38.9°C to 40.6°C). Encourage the woman to remain in the sitz bath for about 20 minutes. It is im-

◉ FIGURE 24–1

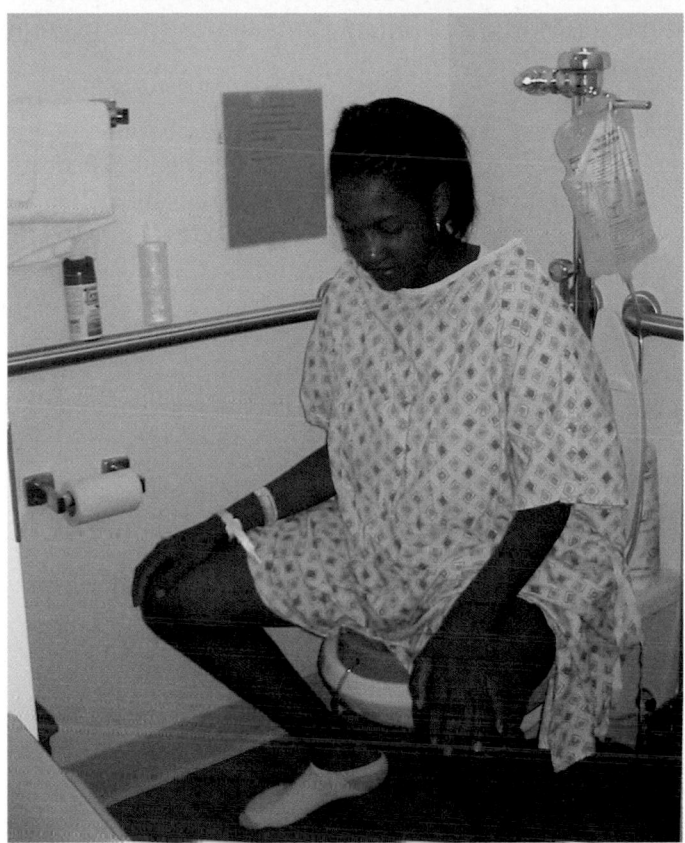

A sitz bath promotes healing and provides relief from perineal discomfort during the initial weeks following birth.

use of sitz baths may be recommended for the woman with an extensive episiotomy, and the woman may use a portable sitz bath or her bathtub. It is important to emphasize that in using a bathtub the woman draws only 4 to 6 inches of water, assesses the temperature, and uses the water only for the sitz and not for bathing. If the woman takes a tub bath, she should release the water, have a helper clean the tub, and draw new water prior to the sitz bath to prevent infection. See "Teaching Highlights: Perineal Inspection."

☀ TEACHING HIGHLIGHTS

PERINEAL INSPECTION

After the mother completes the sitz bath, teach her to inspect the perineal area for burns (that could be related to using water that is too hot), edema, and approximation by using a handheld mirror. If the mother routinely inspects the area, she will be aware of changes that may indicate an infection, such as redness, poor approximation, drainage, or odor.

Topical Agents

Topical anesthetics such as Dermoplast aerosol spray and Americaine spray may be used to relieve perineal pain. Advise the woman to apply the anesthetic after a sitz bath or perineal care. Witch hazel compresses may be used to relieve perineal pain and edema. Nupercainal ointment or Tucks pads may be ordered for relief of hemorrhoidal pain. Provide information about the spray or topical agent. The woman needs to understand the purpose, use, anticipated effects and benefits, and possible problems associated with the product. It is important to emphasize the need for the woman to wash her hands before and after using the topical treatments.

Perineal Care

Perineal care after each elimination cleanses the perineum and helps promote comfort. Many agencies provide "peri-bottles" that the woman can use to squirt warm tap water over her perineum following elimination. To cleanse her perineum, the woman should use moist antiseptic towelettes or toilet paper in a blotting (patting) motion and should be taught to start at the front (area just under the symphysis pubis) and proceed toward the back (area around the anus) to prevent contamination from the anal area. Similarly she should apply the perineal pad from front to back (place the front portion against the perineum first).

Demonstrate how to cleanse the perineum and assist the woman as necessary. Many women have never used perineal pads and will need help in using them during the postpartum period. The pad needs to be placed snugly against the perineum but should not produce pressure. If the pad is worn too loosely, it may rub back and forth, irritating perineal tissues and causing contamination between the anal and vaginal areas (for information regarding the care of the perineum following an episiotomy, see "Teaching Highlights: Episiotomy Care").

RELIEF OF HEMORRHOIDAL DISCOMFORT

Some mothers experience hemorrhoidal pain after giving birth. Relief measures include sitz baths, topical anesthetic ointments, rectal suppositories, or witch hazel pads applied directly to the anal area. The woman may be taught to replace external hemorrhoids digitally in her rectum. She may also find it helpful to maintain a side-lying position when possible and to avoid prolonged sitting. Encourage the woman to maintain an adequate fluid intake. Administer stool softeners to ensure greater comfort with bowel movements. The hemorrhoids usually disappear a few weeks after birth if the woman did not have them before her pregnancy.

RELIEF OF AFTERPAINS

Afterpains are the result of intermittent uterine contractions. A primipara may not have afterpains because her uterus is able to maintain a contracted state. Multiparous women and those who have had a multiple-gestation pregnancy or hydramnios frequently have discomfort from afterpains as the uterus contracts intermittently. Breastfeeding women are also more likely to have afterpains than bottle-feeding women because of the release of oxytocin when the infant suckles.

For relief the woman can lie prone, with a small pillow under her lower abdomen. The discomfort may feel intensified for about 5 minutes but then diminishes greatly if not completely. The prone position applies pressure to the uterus and thus stimulates contractions. When the uterus maintains a constant contraction, the afterpains cease. Additional nursing interventions include a sitz bath (for warmth), ambulation, or administration of an analgesic. An analgesic administered an hour before breastfeeding helps promote comfort and enhances maternal-infant interaction (Table 24–3).

Provide information about the cause of afterpains and methods to decrease discomfort. Explain any medications that are ordered, including their expected effect, benefits, and possible side effects, and any special considerations such as the possibility of dizziness or sleepiness with particular medications.

RELIEF OF DISCOMFORT FROM IMMOBILITY AND MUSCLE STRAIN

Discomfort may be caused by immobility. The woman who has been in stirrups for any length of time may experience muscular aches from such positioning. Moreover, depending on the effort they exerted in pushing during labor, women often experience joint pains and muscular pain in both arms and legs.

Early ambulation helps reduce the incidence of complications such as constipation and thrombophlebitis. It also helps promote a feeling of general well-being. Provide information about ambulation and the importance of monitoring signs of dizziness or weakness. Assist the woman the first few times she gets up during the postpartum period. Fatigue, effects of medications, loss of blood, and lack of food intake may cause feelings of dizziness or faintness when she stands up. Because this may be a problem during the woman's first shower, it is important to remain in the room, check the woman frequently, and have a chair close by in case she becomes faint. During this first shower, explain use of the emergency call button in the bathroom and tell the woman that if she becomes faint during a future shower, she should sit down and call for help.

RELIEF OF DISCOMFORT FROM POSTPARTUM DIAPHORESIS

Postpartum diaphoresis (excessive perspiration) may cause discomfort for new mothers. Offering a fresh, dry gown and changing the bed linens will enhance comfort. Some women may feel refreshed by a shower. It is important to consider cultural practices and realize that some women of Hispanic or Asian cultural background may prefer not to shower in the first few days following birth. Because diaphoresis may also increase thirst, offer fluids regularly, considering cultural practices. Women of western European background may prefer iced water, whereas Asian women may prefer water at room temperature. It is important to ascertain the woman's wishes rather than operate solely from personal values. Provide information about the normality of diaphoresis and methods to increase comfort.

SUPPRESSION OF LACTATION IN THE NONBREASTFEEDING MOTHER

For the woman who chooses not to breastfeed, lactation may be suppressed by mechanical inhibition. Although signs of engorgement do not usually appear until the second or third postpartum day, prevention of engorgement is best accomplished when the woman begins mechanical inhibition of lactation as soon as possible after birth. Ideally prevention involves having the woman begin wearing a supportive, well-fitting bra within 6 hours after birth. She wears the bra continuously until lactation is suppressed (usually about 5 to 7 days) and removes it only for showers. The bra provides support and eases the discomfort that can occur with tension on the breasts because of fullness. Ice packs should be applied

TABLE 24–3 ✛ Essential Information for Common Postpartum Drugs

Empirin #3 (325 mg aspirin and 30 mg codeine)

Drug class: Narcotic analgesic.

Dose/Route: Usual adult dose: 1–2 tablets PO every 4 hours prn.

Indication: For relief of mild to moderate pain.

Adverse Effects: Aspirin: Nausea, dyspepsia, epigastric discomfort, dizziness.

Codeine: Respiratory depression, apnea, light-headedness, dizziness, nausea, sweating, dry mouth, constipation, facial flushing, suppression of cough reflex, ureteral spasm, urinary retention, pruritus.

Nursing Implications: Determine whether woman is sensitive to aspirin or codeine; has history of impaired hepatic or renal function.

Monitor bowel sounds, respiration, urine output.

Administer with food or after meals if gastrointestinal upset occurs; encourage woman to drink one full glass (240 mL) with the tablet to reduce the risk of the tablet lodging in the esophagus.

Client Teaching: Inform client about name of drug, expected action, possible side effects, that it is secreted in breast milk (Note: Some physicians and certified nurse-midwives may avoid ordering this medication for breastfeeding mothers), and review safety measures (assess for dizziness, use side rails, call for assistance when getting out of bed and ambulating, report to nurse any signs of adverse effects); ask if she has any questions.

Nursing Diagnoses Related to Drug Therapy:
Deficient Knowledge related to lack of information about the drug therapy.

Risk for Injury related to dizziness secondary to effect of drug.

Percocet (325 mg acetaminophen and 5 mg oxycodone)

Drug Class: Narcotic analgesic

Drug/Route: 1–2 tablets PO every 4 hours prn.

Indication: For moderate to moderately severe pain. Can be used in aspirin-sensitive women.

Adverse Effects: Acetaminophen: Hepatotoxicity, headache, rash, hypoglycemia.

Oxycodone: Respiratory depression, apnea, circulatory depression, euphoria, facial flushing, constipation, suppression of cough reflex, ureteral spasm, urinary retention.

Nursing Implications: Determine whether woman is sensitive to acetaminophen or codeine; has bronchial asthma, respiratory depression, convulsive disorder.

Observe woman carefully for respiratory depression if given with barbiturates or sedative/hypnotics. Consider that women who have undergone cesarean birth may have depressed cough reflex, so teaching and encouragement to deep breathe and cough are needed.

Monitor bowel sounds, urine and bowel elimination.

Client Teaching: Teaching should include name of drug, expected effect, possible adverse effects, that drug is secreted in the breast milk, and encouragement to report any signs of adverse effects immediately.

Nursing Diagnoses Related to Drug Therapy:
Ineffective Breathing Pattern related to respiratory depression.

Constipation related to slowed gastrointestinal activity.

Rubella Virus Vaccine, Live (Meruvax 2)

Dose/Route: Single dose vial, inject subcutaneously in outer aspect of the upper arm.

Indication: Stimulate active immunity against rubella virus.

Adverse Effects: Burning or stinging at the injection site; about 2–4 weeks later may have rash, malaise, sore throat, or headache.

Nursing Implications: Determine whether woman has sensitivity to neomycin (vaccine contains neomycin); is immunosuppressed, or has received blood transfusions (not to be administered within 3 months of blood transfusion, plasma transfusion, or serum immune globulin).

Note: If a woman is to receive both RhoGAM and rubella, there is a possibility that the formation of antibodies to rubella may be suppressed by the RhoGAM injection. Most physicians will go ahead and order both injections and retest for maternal rubella immune status in about 3 months (Varney et al., 2004).

Client Teaching: Name of drug, expected effect, possible adverse effects, possible comfort measures to use if adverse effects occur, rubella titer will be assessed in about 3 months. Instruct woman to *avoid pregnancy for 3 months following vaccination.* Provide information regarding contraceptives and their use.

Nursing Diagnoses Related to Drug Therapy:
Health-Seeking Behavior: information about contraception related to an expressed desire to avoid pregnancy following rubella vaccination.

Pain related to rash and malaise.

(continued)

over the axillary area of each breast for 20 minutes four times daily. This practice, too, should begin soon after birth. Ice is also useful in relieving discomfort if engorgement occurs.

Advise the woman to avoid any stimulation of her breasts by her baby, herself, breast pumps, or her partner until the sensation of fullness has passed (usually about 5 to 7 days). Such stimulation increases milk production and delays suppression. Heat is avoided for the same reason. Encourage the mother to let shower water flow over her back rather than her breasts.

TABLE 24–3 ✣ **Essential Information for Common Postpartum Drugs**—continued

RhoGAM (RH Immune Globulin Specific for D Antigen)

Dose/Route: Postpartum: One vial IM within 72 hours of birth. Antepartum: One vial microdose RhoGAM IM at 28 weeks in Rh-negative women; after amniocentesis, spontaneous or therapeutic abortion, or ectopic pregnancy.

Indication: Prevention of sensitization to the Rh factor in Rh-negative women and to prevent hemolytic disease in the newborn in subsequent pregnancies. Mother must be Rh negative, not previously sensitized to Rh factor. Infant must be Rh positive, direct antiglobulin negative.

Adverse Effects: Soreness at injection site.

Nursing Implications: Confirm that criteria for administration are present. Ensure correct vial is used for the client (each vial is crossmatched to the specific woman and must be carefully checked). Inject entire contents of vial.

Client Teaching: Name of drug, expected action, possible side effects; report soreness at injection site to nurse; woman should carry information regarding Rh status and dates of RhoGAM injections with her at all times; explain use of RhoGAM with subsequent pregnancies.

Nursing Diagnoses Related to Drug Therapy:

Pain related to soreness at injection site.

Health-Seeking Behavior related to information about future need for Rh immune globulin regarding an expressed desire to understand the long-term implications of her Rh-negative status

Ambien (Zolpidem tartrate)

Drug Class: Hypnotic, sedative

Dose/Route: 5–10 mg PO at bedtime.

Indication: Promote sleep.

Adverse Effects: Dizziness, daytime drowsiness, diarrhea, drugged feelings, amnesia.

Nursing Implications: Determine if woman has compromised respiratory function. Monitor respirations, blood pressure, pulse. Modify environment to increase relaxation and promote sleep. Monitor for drug interaction if woman is taking other CNS depressants.

Client Teaching: Name of drug, expected effect, possible adverse effects, safety measures (side rails, use call bell, ask for assistance when out of bed); medication is secreted in breast milk.

Nursing Diagnoses Related to Drug Therapy:

Risk for Injury related to possible ataxia or vertigo.

Altered Thought Processes related to drug-induced confusion.

Knowledge Deficit related to lack of information about drug therapy.

Health-Seeking Behavior

Some mothers may inquire about suppression medications used in the past for nonbreastfeeding mothers. Because of concerns related to side effects, these medications are no longer used. Mechanical rather than pharmacologic methods are now employed.

PHARMACOLOGIC INTERVENTIONS

Pharmacologic preparations, including pain medications, vaccinations, and Rh immune globulin, are frequently administered in the postpartal period (see Table 24–3).

Rubella Vaccine

Women who have a rubella titer of less than 1:10, or test antibody negative on the enzyme-linked immunosorbent assay (ELISA), are usually given rubella vaccine in the postpartum period (Varney et al., 2004). Ensure that the woman understands the purpose of the vaccine and the need to avoid becoming pregnant in the next 3 months. To ensure that the woman understands, obtain an informed consent before giving the vaccine. Because avoiding pregnancy is so important, counseling about contraception is suggested.

Rh Immune Globulin

All Rh-negative women who meet specific criteria should receive Rh immune globulin (RhoGAM) within 72 hours after childbirth to prevent sensitization from the fetomaternal transfusion of Rh-positive fetal red blood cells. (For further discussion see Chapter 15. ∞) The Rh-negative woman needs to understand the implications of her Rh-negative status in future pregnancies. It is important to provide opportunities for her and her partner to ask questions.

RELIEF OF EMOTIONAL STRESS

The birth of a child, with the changes in role and the increased responsibilities it produces, is a time of emotional stress for the new mother. During the early postpartum period, the mother may be emotionally labile, and mood swings and tearfulness are common. Initially the mother may repeatedly discuss her experiences of labor and birth. This allows the mother to integrate her experiences. If she believes that she did not cope well with labor, she may have feelings of inadequacy and may benefit from reassurance that she did well. Some women feel that they did not have any perception of time during the labor and birth and want to know how long it really lasted, or they may not remember the entire experience. In this case it is helpful to talk with the woman and provide the information that she is missing and wants.

During this time the new mother must also adjust to the loss of her fantasized child and accept the child she has borne. This task may be more difficult if the child is not of the desired sex or if he or she has birth defects.

Immediately after the birth (the taking-in period) the mother is focused on bodily concerns and may not be fully ready to learn about personal and infant care. Following this initial dependent period, the mother typically becomes concerned about her ability to be a successful parent (the taking-hold period). During this time the mother needs reassurance that she is effective. She also tends to be receptive to teaching and demonstration designed to help her in mothering successfully. The depression, weepiness, and "let-down feeling" that characterize the postpartum blues are often a surprise for the new mother. Provide reassurance that these feelings are normal, an explanation about why they occur, and a supportive environment so that she can cry if she wishes without feeling guilty.

PROMOTION OF MATERNAL REST AND ACTIVITY

Following childbirth, some women feel exhausted and in need of rest. Other women may be euphoric and full of energy, ready to relive and recount the experience of birth repeatedly. Provide a period for airing of feelings and then encourage a period of rest.

Physical fatigue often affects other adjustments and functions of the new mother. For example, fatigue can reduce milk flow, thereby increasing problems with establishing breastfeeding. Energy is also needed to adjust to a new infant and to assume new roles. Encourage rest by or-

ganizing care activities to avoid frequent interruptions for the woman. It is helpful for the new mother to know that fatigue may persist for several weeks or even months.

Although most new mothers feel tired, if they have perceived the pregnancy and birth as a natural process, they tend to view themselves as healthy and well. However, some mothers view the postpartal period as a time for needed recuperation. In many non-Western cultures, the 40 days following the birth is a time of recovery when female relatives or friends assist the new mother in her daily activities. In the Middle East, for example, female relatives and friends stay and care for the house, tend to meals, and care for other children. This is also the custom in India, where it is believed that the mother and new baby need protection from evil spirits as well as from exposure to illness, since they are both considered vulnerable during this time (Kim-Godwin, 2003).

In Mexico this period lasts only 20 days. During the first 7 days, nonhousehold members are not permitted to visit or enter the home. The mother gradually increases activity after the first week. The end of the postpartum period is marked by a *sobada*, a massage performed by the midwife on the 20th day after birth (Kim-Godwin, 2003).

RESUMPTION OF ACTIVITIES

Ambulation and activity may gradually increase after birth. The new mother should avoid heavy lifting, excessive stair

---

EVIDENCE-BASED NURSING

PELVIC MUSCLE FUNCTION

Clinical Question

What postpartum exercises can help a new mother regain pelvic muscle function?

Evidence

The Association of Women's Health, Obstetric and Neonatal Nurses (AWHONN) assembled an expert team to study the evidence and develop a practice guideline for the prevention of incontinence in women. Part of the guideline was devoted to retraining of the pelvic floor muscles after birth. Pelvic floor muscle exercises should be taught during pregnancy and the postpartum period. Attention to rebuilding the strength of these muscles can prevent future health problems such as stress incontinence and cystocele.

Implications

A daily minimum of 30 to 45 pelvic floor contractions is recommended. These may be done as a set or divided into two or three sets, based on the woman's preference. The contractions should gradually build in duration until each contraction is held for 10 seconds. Ten seconds of relaxation should follow each contraction. Women should be instructed on how to do a contraction, by lifting up and drawing in of the perivaginal

and anal sphincter muscles. The mother should check for effectiveness either digitally, during sexual intercourse, or by attempting to stop the flow of urine. (This last test of effectiveness should be done no more than weekly.) Women should be encouraged to aim for a high level of concentrated effort with each contraction, but avoid bearing down or using the buttocks muscles.

You should begin teaching women about pelvic muscle training during pregnancy, and continue through the postpartal period. Provide reassurance that increased pelvic floor muscle strength, as evidenced by ability to sustain an effective contraction for at least 10 seconds, develops over time and is effective in preventing future urinary problems.

Critical Thinking

What is the best time to begin teaching about pelvic floor exercises? How can you help women stick with a pelvic floor exercise program after the baby is born?

Reference

Association of Women's Health, Obstetric and Neonatal Nurses (AWHONN). (2000, January 27). *Continence for women. Evidence-based practice guideline.* Washington, DC: Author.

climbing, and strenuous activity. One or two daily naps are essential and are most easily achieved if the mother sleeps when her baby does.

By the second week at home, the woman may resume light housekeeping. Although it is customary to delay returning to work for 6 weeks, most women are physically able to resume practically all activities by 4 to 5 weeks. Delaying the return to work until after the final postpartum examination minimizes the possibility of problems.

POSTPARTUM EXERCISES

Encourage the woman to begin simple exercises while in the birthing unit and to continue them at home. Inform her that increased lochia or pain means she should reevaluate her activity and make necessary alterations. Most agencies provide a booklet describing suggested postpartum activities. (Exercise routines vary for women undergoing cesarean birth or tubal ligation after childbirth.) (See Figure 24–2 ● for a description of some commonly used exercises.)

PROMOTION OF EFFECTIVE PARENT LEARNING

Meeting the educational needs of the new mother and her family is an important nursing responsibility. Each woman's educational needs vary based on her age, background, experience, and expectations. Because the mother is in the postpartum area for a brief period, it is difficult to address all individual characteristics and informational needs.

Assess the learning needs of the new mother through observation and tactfully phrased questions. For example, "What plans have you made for handling things when you get home?" may elicit a response of several words and may provide the opportunity for some information sharing and guidance. Some agencies also use checklists of common concerns for new mothers. The woman can check the concerns that are of interest to her.

Plan and implement teaching in a logical, nonthreatening way based on knowledge and respect of the family's cultural values and beliefs. Unless an activity would be

THINKING CRITICALLY

READY TO GO HOME?

You walk in and find Dana Sullivan, a 29-year-old G2P2, crying 48 hours after a repeat cesarean birth. She states, "I'm not ready to go home. With my first baby they made me go home after 2 days. Can they make me again?" How would you respond?

harmful, most cultural customs can be supported and encouraged. Postpartum units use a variety of approaches to teaching, including handouts, formal classes, videotapes, and individual interaction. Some facilities offer a hotline service so that new mothers can call with questions and concerns.

Regardless of the teaching technique, timing is important. The new mother becomes more receptive to teaching after the first 24 to 48 hours, when she is ready to assume responsibility for her own care and that of her newborn. Unfortunately, many women are discharged during the first 48 hours after birth. Consequently, many units provide printed material for new mothers to consult if questions arise at home. Timing is also important for new fathers, who are more likely to attend teaching sessions if they are scheduled in the late afternoon or early evening (Figure 24–3 ●).

Teaching should include information on role change and psychologic adjustments as well as skills. Anticipatory guidance can help prepare new parents for the many changes they will experience with a new family member.

Information is also essential for women with specialized educational needs such as the mother who has had a cesarean birth, the parents of twins, the parents of an infant with congenital anomalies, and so on. Nurses who are attuned to these individual problems can begin providing guidance as soon as possible. Evaluation may take several forms: return demonstrations, question-and-answer sessions, and even formal evaluation tools. Follow-up phone calls after discharge provide additional evaluative information and continue the helping process for the family.

Postpartum exercises (see facing page). Begin with 5 repetitions two or three times daily and gradually increase to 10 repetitions. First day: **A,** Abdominal breathing. Lying supine, inhale deeply using the abdominal muscles. The abdomen should expand. Then exhale slowly through pursed lips, tightening the abdominal muscles. **B,** Pelvic rocking. Lying supine with arms at sides, knees bent, and feet flat, tighten abdomen and buttocks and attempt to flatten back onto floor. Hold for a count of 10, then arch the back, causing the pelvis to "rock." On second day add the following: **C,** Chin to chest. Lying supine with no pillow and legs straight, raise head and attempt to touch chin to chest. Slowly lower head. **D,** Arm raises. Lying supine, arms extended perpendicular to the body, raise arms until hands touch. Lower slowly. On fourth day add the following: **E,** Knee rolls. Lying supine with knees bent, feet flat, and arms extended to the side, roll knees slowly to one side, keeping shoulders flat. Return to original position and roll to opposite side. **F,** Buttocks lift. Lying supine, arms at sides, knees bent, and feet flat, slowly raise the buttocks and arch the back. Return slowly to starting position. On sixth day add the following: **G,** Abdominal tighteners. Lying supine, knees bent, and feet flat, slowly raise the head toward the knees. Arms should extend along either side of the legs. Return slowly to original position. **H,** Knee to abdomen. Lying supine, arms at sides, bend one knee and thigh until foot touches buttocks. Straighten leg and lower it slowly. Repeat with other leg. After 2 to 3 weeks, more strenuous exercises such as side leg raises may be added as tolerated. Kegel exercises, begun antepartally, should be done many times daily during postpartum to restore vaginal and perineal tone.

● FIGURE 24–2

A

B

C

D

E

F

G

H

● FIGURE 24–3

The nurse provides educational information to both parents.

PROMOTION OF FAMILY WELLNESS

The promotion of family wellness involves several considerations, including a satisfactory maternity experience, the need for follow-up care for mother and infant, and birth control. The new or expanding family may also need information about adjustment of siblings and resuming sexual relations.

Today most facilities support family-centered care called **mother-baby care or couplet care**. It provides increased opportunities for parent-child interaction because the newborn shares the mother's unit and they are cared for together. Mother-baby care enables the mother to have time to bond with her baby and learn to care for him or her in a supportive environment. It is especially conducive to a hunger-demand feeding schedule for both breast- and formula-feeding babies. It also allows the father, siblings, and friends to help with the care of the new baby.

Mother-baby unit policies must be flexible enough to permit the mother to return the baby to the nursery if she finds it necessary because of fatigue or physical discomfort. Some mother-baby units also return the newborns to a central nursery at night so the mothers can get more rest. Mother-baby care provides excellent opportunities for family bonds to grow because the father, mother, newborn, and often siblings can begin functioning as a family unit immediately.

For new fathers, research suggests that interactions with their newborns and with nurses are important aspects of their postpartal experience. Nurses can encourage a couple in terms of mutual support and encourage them to tune in to their infant's cues by adopting an attitude of discovery in their interactions with their baby. Nurses can also support fathers by offering support, acknowledging the father's experience, and reinforcing the father's belief in his own capacities and strengths (deMontigny & Lacharité, 2004).

REACTIONS OF SIBLINGS

Sibling visits help meet the needs of both the siblings and their mother. A visit to the mother-baby unit reassures children that their mother is well and still loves them. It also provides an opportunity for the children to become familiar with the new baby. For the mother the pangs of separation are lessened as she interacts with her children and introduces them to the newest family member (Figure 24–4 ●).

Although the parents have prepared their children for the presence of a new brother or sister, the actual arrival of the baby in the home requires some adjustments. If small children are waiting at home, it is helpful if the father carries the infant inside so that the mother's arms are free to hug her older children. Many mothers bring a doll home with them for an older child. Caring for the doll alongside the mother or father helps the child to identify with the parents. This identification helps decrease anger and the need to regress for attention.

Parents may also provide supervised times when older children can hold the new baby and perhaps even help with a bottle-feeding. The older children feel a sense of accomplishment and learn tenderness and caring—qualities appropriate for both males and females. The nurse can help the parents come up with ways to show the other children that they, too, are valued and have their own places in the family.

SEXUAL ACTIVITY AND CONTRACEPTION

Typically, couples resume sexual intercourse once the episiotomy has healed and the lochial flow has stopped (usu-

● FIGURE 24–4

The sister of this newborn becomes acquainted with the new family member during a nursing assessment.

© Stella Johnson (www.stellajohnson.com)

ally by the end of the third week). Because this occurs prior to the scheduled 6-week postpartum examination, family-planning information should be made available before discharge. Unfortunately, because of in-hospital time restraints, this subject may be overlooked. (For a more detailed discussion on resumption of sexual activity, see Chapter 32. ∞ Specific contraceptive methods are discussed in detail in Chapter 3. ∞)

PROMOTION OF PARENT-INFANT ATTACHMENT

Nursing interventions to enhance the quality of parent-infant attachment should be designed to promote feelings of well-being, comfort, and satisfaction. Following are some suggestions for ways of promoting this:

- Determine the childbearing and childrearing goals of the infant's mother and father and support them whenever possible in planning care for the family. This includes giving the parents choices about their labor and birth and their initial time with their new infant.

- Postpone eye prophylaxis for 1 hour after birth to facilitate eye contact between parents and their newborn (eye ointment clouds the newborn's vision and makes eye contact difficult for the baby).

- Provide time and as much privacy as possible for the new family to become acquainted. Allow siblings to visit throughout the postpartal stay if requested by the parents.

- Arrange the healthcare setting so that the individual nurse-client relationship can be developed. A primary nurse can develop rapport and assess the mother's strengths and needs.

- Use anticipatory guidance from conception through the postpartum period to prepare the parents for expected problems of adjustment.

- Include parents in any nursing intervention, planning, and evaluation. Give choices whenever possible.

- Initiate and support measures to alleviate fatigue in the parents.

- Help parents identify, understand, and accept both positive and negative feelings related to the overall parenting experience.

- Support and assist parents in determining the personality and unique needs of their infant.

The beginnings of parent-newborn attachment may be observed in the first few hours after birth. Continued assessments may occur during the postpartum stay and in home visits after discharge. In assessing attachment it is important to remember that cultural values, beliefs, and practices will direct childcare activities and self-care practices. For example, some women of Mexican-American and South-

east Asian descent may deflect compliments directed toward their baby because of their belief that compliments may attract the attention of evil spirits. Some women treat the umbilical stump by placing a coin or belly band over it. People in many countries, for example, Greece, Iran, Italy, and Malaysia, often place amulets on the baby or in the crib for protection (Spector, 2004). (See Table 24–4 for behaviors related to parent-infant attachment.)

DEVELOPING CULTURAL COMPETENCE

POSTPARTAL CULTURAL TIPS FOR SOUTHEAST ASIAN WOMEN

The following information applies to many women from Southeast Asia during the postpartum period:

- Childbirth gives the woman increased status in her community.
- The female support system of relatives, especially the mother, mother-in-law, and sisters, is of special importance during postpartum for information on self-care and activities to avoid as well as assistance with household chores.
- The postpartum is viewed as a time for rest, often bed rest, for a month or more. During that time the woman is expected to do little except breastfeed.
- The newborn should be shielded from compliments because they may attract the attention of evil spirits (Spector, 2004).
- Because of the blood loss associated with childbirth, the body is in a "cold" state afterward. To regain balance the woman should have "hot" drinks and foods (warm water, rice, boiled chicken, and so forth). She should also avoid baths and showers, which cool the body (Davis, 2001).

NURSING CARE FOLLOWING CESAREAN BIRTH

After a cesarean birth, the new mother has postpartum needs similar to those of women who have given birth vaginally. Because she has undergone major abdominal surgery, the woman's nursing care needs are also similar to those of other surgical clients.

PROMOTION OF MATERNAL PHYSICAL WELL-BEING

The chances of pulmonary infection are increased because of immobility after the use of narcotics and sedatives and because of the altered immune response in postoperative clients. Therefore, encourage the woman to cough and deep breathe every 2 to 4 hours while awake until she is ambulating frequently. In addition, encourage leg exercises every 2 hours until the woman is ambulating. These exercises increase circulation, help prevent thrombophlebitis, and also aid intestinal motility by tightening abdominal muscles.

Monitor and manage the woman's pain during the postpartum period. Sources of pain include incisional

TABLE 24–4 ❖ Parent Attachment Behaviors

Assessment Area	Attachment	Behavior Requiring Assessment and Information
Caretaking	Talks with baby Demonstrates and seeks eye-to-eye contact Touches and holds baby Changes diapers when needed Baby is clean Clothing is appropriate for room temperature Feeds baby as needed and baby is gaining weight Positions baby comfortably and checks on baby	Does not refer to baby Completes activities without addressing the baby or looking at the baby Lack of interaction Does not recognize need for or demonstrate concern for baby's comfort Feeding occurs intermittently Baby does not gain weight Waits for baby to cry and then hesitates to respond
Perception of the baby	Has knowledge of expected child development Understands that the baby is dependent and cannot meet parent's needs Accepts sex and characteristics of child	Has unrealistic expectations of the baby's abilities and behaviors Expects love and interaction from the baby Believes that the baby will fulfill parent's needs Is strongly distressed over sex of baby or feels that some aspect of the baby is unacceptable
Support	Has friends who are available for support Seems to be comfortable with being a parent Has realistic beliefs of parent role	Is alone or isolated Is on edge, tense, anxious, and hesitant with the baby Demonstrates difficulty incorporating parenting with own wants and needs

Note: These are a few of the behaviors that may be associated with attachment. It is vitally important for the nurse to observe the parents on more than one occasion and to take into consideration individual characteristics, values, beliefs, and customs.

pain, gas pain, referred shoulder pain, periodic uterine contractions (afterbirth pains), and pain from voiding, defecation, or constipation. Nursing interventions are oriented toward preventing or alleviating pain or helping the woman cope with pain. Implement the following measures:

- Administer analgesics as needed, especially during the first 24 to 72 hours after childbirth. Use of analgesics relieves the woman's pain and enables her to be more mobile and active.

- Promote comfort through proper positioning, back rubs, oral care, and the reduction of noxious stimuli such as noise and unpleasant odors.

- Encourage visits by significant others, including the newborn. These visits distract the woman from the painful sensations and help reduce her fear and anxiety.

- Encourage the use of breathing, relaxation, and distraction (e.g., stimulation of cutaneous tissue) techniques taught in childbirth preparation class.

Epidural analgesia administered just after the cesarean birth is an effective method of pain relief for most women in the first 24 hours following birth (see "Drug Guide: Postpartum Epidural Morphine").

The physician may order **patient-controlled analgesia (PCA)**. With this approach the woman is given a bolus of analgesia, usually morphine or meperidine, at the beginning of therapy. Using a special intravenous (IV) pump system, the woman presses a button to self-administer small doses of the medication as needed. For safety the pump is preset with a time lockout so that the woman cannot deliver another dose until a specified period of time has elapsed. The frequent, smaller doses help the woman experience rapid pain relief without grogginess and a drugged feeling and also avoid the discomfort associated with injections.

Another technique of pain control that is sometimes used is the **continuous epidural infusion (CEI)** technique, in which the epidural catheter is left in place following the cesarean birth, and medication is continually administered via an electric pump. The device also has a button which the woman can depress if additional pain relief is needed. Fentanyl is the most commonly used drug for CEI (Hughes, Levinson, & Rosen, 2002). Hourly nursing assessments for women with a CEI in place include vital signs, level of pain, amount of drug received, and amount of self-administration. Inspect the tubing to ensure connections are maintained since movement by the woman in bed could disrupt the line. The epidural site should also be assessed to ensure the catheter has not been displaced.

Many physicians also order a nonsteroidal anti-inflammatory drug (NSAID) in addition to the previously mentioned agents once the woman is tolerating

DRUG GUIDE

POSTPARTUM EPIDURAL MORPHINE

Overview of Obstetric Action

Epidural morphine is used to provide relief of pain associated with cesarean birth, extensive episiotomies (mediolaterals), or third- and fourth-degree lacerations. Epidural morphine pain relief results directly from its effect on the opiate receptors in the spinal cord (it depresses pain impulse transmission). Morphine binds opiate receptors, thereby altering both the perception of and emotional response to pain. Women experience little or no discomfort or pain during recovery and for up to 24 hours afterward. There is no motor or sympathetic block or associated hypotension. Onset of analgesia is slower, but duration is longer.

Route, Dosage, and Frequency

Morphine (5–7.5 mg) is injected through a catheter into the epidural space, providing pain relief for about 24 hours (Wilson et al., 2006).

Maternal Contraindications

Allergy to morphine, narcotic addiction, chronic debilitating respiratory disease, infection at the injection site, or administration of parenteral corticosteroids in past 14 days (Wilson et al., 2006).

Maternal Side Effects

Late-onset respiratory depression (rare but may occur 8–12 hours after administration), nausea and vomiting (occurring between 4 and 7 hours after injection), itching (begins within 3 hours and lasts up to 10 hours), urinary retention, and, rarely, somnolence. Side effects can be managed with naloxone.

Neonatal Effects

No adverse effects since medication is injected after birth of baby.

Nursing Considerations

- Obtain history: sensitivity (allergy) to morphine, presence of any contraindications.

- Assess orientation, reflexes, skin color, texture, breath sounds, presence of lesions or infection over area of lumbar spine, voiding pattern, urinary output within normal limits (Wilson et al., 2006).
- Monitor and evaluate analgesic effect. Ask client about comfort level and notify anesthesiologist of inadequate pain relief.
- Check catheter for obvious knots, breaks, and leakage at insertion site and catheter hub.
- Assess for pruritus (scratching and rubbing, especially around face and neck).
- Administer comfort measures for narcotic-induced pruritus, such as lotion, back rubs, cool/warm packs, or diversional activities. If the itching can be tolerated, naloxone should be avoided, especially since it counteracts the pain relief.
- If allergic reaction (urticaria, edema, or respiratory difficulties) occurs, administer naloxone or diphenhydramine per physician order.
- Provide comfort measures for nausea/vomiting, such as frequent oral hygiene or gradual increase of activity; administer naloxone, trimethobenzamide (Tigan), or metoclopramide HCl per physician order.
- Assess postural blood pressure and heart rate before ambulation.
- Assist client with her first ambulation and then as needed.
- Assess respiratory function every hour for 24 hours, then q2–8 hr as needed. Also assess level of consciousness and mucous membrane color. May need to monitor client via apnea monitor for 24 hours.
- Monitor urinary output and assess bladder for distention. Assist client to void.

---

oral fluids well. NSAIDs assist with decreasing inflammation and do not have the negative side effects associated with many narcotics, such as sedation and constipation.

If a general anesthetic was used, abdominal distention may produce marked discomfort for the woman during the first few postpartum days. Measures to prevent or minimize abdominal distention include leg exercises, abdominal tightening, ambulation, avoiding carbonated or very hot or cold beverages, avoiding the use of straws, and providing a high-protein, liquid diet for the first 24 to 48 hours, until bowel sounds return. Medical intervention for gas pain includes using rectal suppositories and enemas to stimulate passage of flatus and stool and encouraging the woman to lie on her left side. Lying on the left side allows the gas to rise from the descending colon to the sigmoid colon so that it can be expelled more readily. Nurses can minimize discomfort and promote satisfaction as the mother assumes the activities of her new role. Assistance in

assuming comfortable positions when holding or breastfeeding the infant will do much to increase the mother's sense of competence and comfort.

The cesarean birth mother usually does extremely well postoperatively. Most women are ambulating by the day after the surgery. Usually by the second postpartum day, the incision can be covered with plastic wrap so the woman can shower, which seems to provide a mental as well as physical lift. Most women are discharged by the third day after birth.

PROMOTION OF PARENT-INFANT INTERACTION AFTER CESAREAN BIRTH

Many factors associated with cesarean birth may hinder successful maternal-infant interaction. These factors include the physical condition of the mother and newborn and maternal reactions to stress, anesthesia, and medications. The mother and her infant may be separated after birth because of birthing unit routines, prematurity, or neonatal complications. A healthy infant born by uncomplicated cesarean is no more fragile than one born vaginally. However, some agencies automatically place cesarean birth infants in the high-risk nursery for a time. This practice may cause anxiety for the parents and interfere with early parent-infant interaction.

Signs of depression, anger, or withdrawal may indicate a grief response to the loss of the fantasized birth experience. Fathers as well as mothers may experience feelings of "missing out," guilt, or even jealousy toward another couple who had a vaginal birth. The cesarean birth couple may need the opportunity to tell their story repeatedly to work through these feelings. Thus, it is important to provide factual information about the situation and support the couple's effective coping behaviors.

By the second or third day, the cesarean birth mother moves into the "taking-hold period" and is usually receptive to learning how to care for herself and her infant. Emphasize home management and encourage the mother to let others assume responsibility for housekeeping and cooking. Fatigue not only prolongs recovery but also interferes with breastfeeding and mother-infant interaction.

The presence of the father or significant other during the birth process positively influences the woman's perception of the birth event. His or her presence reduces the woman's fears, enhances her sense of control, and enables the couple to share feelings and respond to one another with touch and eye contact. Later they have the opportunity to relive the experience and fill in any gaps or missing pieces. The presence of the father or significant other is especially valuable if the mother has had general anesthesia. He or she can take pictures, hold the baby, and foster the discovery process by directing the mother's attention to the details of the newborn.

The reactions to a cesarean birth depend on how the woman defines that experience. Her reality is what she perceives it to be. If the woman's attitude is more positive than negative, successful resolution of subsequent stressful events is more likely. Often the mothering role is perceived as an extension of the childbearing role. Inability to fulfill expected childbearing behavior (vaginal birth) may lead to parental feelings of role failure and frustration. It is important to help families alter their negative definitions of cesarean birth and to encourage positive perceptions.

NURSING CARE OF THE POSTPARTAL ADOLESCENT

The adolescent mother has special postpartal needs, depending on her level of maturity, support system, and cultural background. The nurse needs to assess maternal-infant interaction, roles of support people, plans for discharge, knowledge of childrearing, and plans for follow-up care. It is

important that a community health service contact the adolescent shortly after discharge.

Contraception counseling is an essential part of teaching. The incidence of repeat pregnancies during adolescence is high. The younger the adolescent, the more likely she is to become pregnant again. (See Chapter 13 ∞ for discussion of adolescent pregnancy.)

The nurse has many opportunities to teach the teen about her newborn in the postpartum unit. As a role model, the manner in which the nurse handles the newborn greatly influences the young mother. The father should be included in as much of the teaching as possible.

A newborn examination done at the bedside gives the teen information about her baby's health and shows her possible positions for holding a baby. The nurse can also use this time to provide information about newborn and infant behavior. Parents who have some idea of what to expect from their infant are less frustrated with the newborn's behavior.

The adolescent mother appreciates positive feedback about her newborn and her developing maternal responses. Praise and encouragement increase her confidence and self-esteem. Group classes for adolescent mothers should include information about infant care skills, taking the baby's temperature, clearing the nose and mouth, growth and development, infant feeding, well-baby care, and danger signals in the ill newborn.

Ideally, teenage mothers should visit adolescent clinics, for assessment of the mother and newborn, for several years after birth. In this way the adolescent's enrollment in classes on parenting, need for vocational guidance, and school attendance can be supported and followed closely. School systems offering classes for young mothers are an excellent way of helping adolescents finish school and learn how to parent at the same time.

NURSING CARE OF THE WOMAN WHO RELINQUISHES HER BABY

Sometimes a woman is unable to parent her baby. The woman may be single, an adolescent, or economically restricted, or the pregnancy may be the result of incest or rape. She may feel that she is not emotionally ready for the responsibilities of parenthood. Her partner may strongly disapprove of the pregnancy. These and many other reasons may cause the woman to continue to reject her pregnancy. An emotional crisis arises as she attempts to resolve the problem. She may choose to have an abortion, to carry the fetus to term and parent the baby, or to have the baby and relinquish it for adoption.

A mother's decision to relinquish her infant is an extremely difficult one. There are social pressures against giving up one's child. Some women may want to prove to themselves that they can manage on their own by keeping their baby. The mother who chooses to let her child be adopted usually experiences intense ambivalence. These feelings may heighten just before birth and upon seeing her baby. After childbirth the mother needs to complete a grieving process to work through her loss.

The mother who decides to relinquish the child has usually made considerable adjustments in her lifestyle to give birth to this child. She may not have told friends and relatives about the pregnancy and so she may lack an extended support system. During the prenatal period, the nurse can help the woman by encouraging her and providing opportunities to express her grief, loneliness, guilt, and other feelings.

When the relinquishing mother is admitted to the birthing unit, the nurse should be informed about the mother's decision to relinquish the baby. The nurse needs to respect any special requests for the birth and encourage the woman to express her emotions. After the birth the mother should have access to the baby; she will decide whether she wants to see the newborn. Seeing the newborn often aids the grieving process. When the mother sees her baby, she may feel strong attachment and love. The nurse needs to assure the woman that these feelings do not mean that her decision to relinquish the child is a wrong one; relinquishment is often a painful act of love (Arms, 1990).

Postpartum nursing care also includes arranging ongoing care for the relinquishing mother. Some mothers may request an early discharge or a transfer to another medical unit. When possible the nurse supports these requests.

PREPARATION FOR DISCHARGE

Ideally, preparation for discharge begins the moment a woman enters the birthing unit to give birth. Nursing efforts should be directed toward assessing the parents' knowledge, expectations, and beliefs and then providing anticipatory guidance and teaching accordingly. Prior to discharge assess the mother's physical and psychologic condition, the newborn's adjustment to extrauterine life, and the family's overall adjustment. In general, ensure that the following criteria are assessed and met:

- Normal vital signs
- Appropriate involution of the uterus
- Appropriate amount of lochia without evidence of infection
- Knowledge of signs of infection
- Episiotomy or laceration well approximated with a decrease in edema or bruising
- Ability to perform perineal care and apply medications to perineal or anal area if ordered

---

> ### TABLE 24–5 ✢ Signs of Postpartum Complications
>
> After discharge, a woman should contact her physician or certified nurse-midwife if any of the following develop:
>
> - Sudden, persistent, or spiking fever
> - Change in the character of the lochia—foul smell, return to bright-red bleeding, excessive amount, passage of large clots
> - Evidence of mastitis, such as breast tenderness, reddened areas, malaise
> - Evidence of thrombophlebitis, such as calf pain, tenderness, redness
> - Evidence of urinary tract infection, such as urgency, frequency, burning on urination
> - Continued severe or incapacitating postpartum depression

- Ability to void and to pass flatus (some facilities' criteria may include having a bowel movement prior to discharge)
- Ability to take fluids and foods without difficulty
- Ability to care for self and newborn
- Has received rubella vaccine or Rh immune globulin if indicated

Since teaching is one of the primary responsibilities of the postpartum nurse, many agencies have elaborate teaching programs and videos. Before the actual discharge, spend time with the parents to determine if they have any last-minute questions. In general, discharge teaching includes at least the following information:

- The signs of possible complications (Table 24–5) and encouragement for the woman to contact her caregiver if she develops any of them.
- Review of literature the woman has received explaining recommended postpartum exercises, the need for adequate rest, the need to avoid overexertion initially, and the recommendation to abstain from sexual intercourse until lochia has ceased. The woman may take either a tub bath or shower and may continue sitz baths at home. If the family desires information about birth control methods, the nurse can provide such information at this time.
- The phone number of the mother-baby unit and encouragement to call if she has any questions or concerns.
- Information on local agencies or support groups, such as La Leche League and Mothers of Twins, that might be of particular assistance to the new mother.
- Information geared to the specific nutritional needs of breastfeeding or formula-feeding mothers. If the mother has been receiving vitamins or iron

supplements, the nurse encourages her to continue until the first postpartum examination.

- Information about when to schedule the first appointment for her postpartum examination and for her newborn's first well-baby examination.

- The procedure for obtaining copies of her infant's birth certificate.

- How to provide basic care for the infant, when to anticipate that the cord will fall off, when the infant can have a tub bath, when the infant will need his or her first immunizations, and so on. Parents should also be comfortable feeding and handling the baby and should be aware of basic safety considerations, including the need to use a car seat whenever the infant is in a car.

- The signs and symptoms that indicate possible problems in the infant and who the parents should contact about them.

- Plans for home care visits so that the parents know when to expect the visit and what it entails (see information in Chapter 32∞).

Use this final opportunity before discharge to reassure the couple of their ability to be successful parents. Stress the infant's need to feel loved and secure, and urge parents to talk to each other and work together to solve any problems that arise. A sample postpartal teaching checklist is found on the Companion Website.

EVALUATION

Anticipated outcomes of nursing care of the postpartum family include the following:

- The mother is reasonably comfortable and has learned pain relief measures.

- The mother is rested and understands how to add activity over the next few days and weeks.

- The mother's physiologic and psychologic well-being have been supported.

- The mother verbalizes her understanding of self-care measures.

- The new parents demonstrate how to care for their baby.

- The new parents have had opportunities to form attachment with their baby.

- The cesarean birth mother has been supported and has received safe care.

Critical Concept Review

LEARNING OBJECTIVES

CONCEPTS

Relate the use of nursing diagnoses to the findings of the "normal" postpartum assessment and analysis.	1. Nursing diagnoses focus on the normal and expected postpartal course. 2. Nursing diagnoses allow the nurse to identify expected outcomes and select nursing interventions that will help the family meet the expected outcomes.
Delineate strategies for promoting family learning during the early postpartum period.	The nurse should: 1. Discuss desired outcomes and goals with the mother and family members. 2. Design interventions to achieve optimal health promotion.
Discuss appropriate nursing interventions to promote maternal comfort and well-being.	1. The nurse can promote and restore maternal physical well-being by monitoring uterine status, vital signs, cardiovascular status, elimination patterns, nutritional needs, sleep and rest, and support and educational needs. 2. In addition, the postpartum woman may need medications to promote comfort, treat anemia, provide immunity to rubella, and prevent development of antigens (in the nonsensitized Rh-negative woman).

LEARNING OBJECTIVES

CONCEPTS

Describe the nurse's role in promoting maternal rest and helping the mother to gradually resume an appropriate level of activity.

→

1. The nurse should:
   - Encourage the new mother to rest when the infant rests.
   - Counsel the new mother to resume activities gradually.
   - Recommend exercise to provide health benefits to the new mother.

Identify client teaching topics for promoting postpartal family wellness.

→

1. Possible reactions of siblings.
2. Resumption of sexual activity:
   - Discuss possible temporary problems such as sleep deprivation, vaginal dryness, and lack of time together
3. Contraception.
4. Parent-infant attachment:
   - Help parents realize there will be both positive and negative feelings about parenthood.
   - New parents need to understand that the infant is unique with a distinctive personality.

Compare the postpartal nursing needs of the woman who experienced a cesarean birth with the needs of a woman who gave birth vaginally.

→

1. Woman who experienced a cesarean birth has all the needs of the woman who had a vaginal birth:
   - Assessment of the fundus.
   - Assessment of breasts.
   - Perineal evaluation (may have varicose veins or hemorrhoids from pregnancy).
   - Assessment of lochia flow.
   - Assessment of bowel and bladder.
2. After a cesarean birth the woman needs assessment of the abdomen:
   - Incision.
   - Turn, cough, and deep breathe.
   - Bowel sounds.
3. After a cesarean birth the mother will have a greater need for pain medication. She will also have increased fatigue because of the surgical intervention. The mother may need encouragement to interact with the infant.

Summarize the nursing needs of the childbearing adolescent during the postpartal period.

→

1. The nurse should evaluate the adolescent mother in terms of her level of maturity, available support systems, cultural background, and existing knowledge, and then plan care accordingly.

Describe possible approaches to sensitive, holistic nursing care for the woman who relinquishes her newborn.

→

1. The mother who decides to relinquish her baby needs emotional support. She should be able to decide whether to see and hold her baby, and any special requests regarding the birth should be honored.

Delineate criteria and teaching topics related to postpartum discharge.

→

1. Prior to discharge the couple should be given any information necessary for the woman to provide appropriate self-care.
2. Parents should have a beginning skill in caring for their newborn and should be familiar with warning signs of possible complications for mother or baby.
3. Printed information is valuable in helping couples deal with questions that may arise at home.

CRITICAL THINKING IN ACTION

*View the **Critical Thinking in Action** video in Chapter 24 of the CD-ROM. Then, answer the questions that follow.*

Wendy Calahan, a 31-year-old G3, P2, gave birth to a 8.5 pound baby boy by primary cesarean birth for failure to progress. The baby's Apgar scores were 9 and 9 at 1 and 5 minutes. The baby was admitted to the newborn nursery for transitional observation. Wendy was transferred to the postpartum unit where you assume her care. You introduce yourself and orient her to the room, call bell, and safety measures. You perform an initial assessment, with all findings within normal limits. Wendy tells you she is very tired and would like to rest while her baby is in the nursery. Her husband and family have left the hospital after spending time with her in the recovery room but will return later. She admits she is disappointed that she could not give birth vaginally even though she pushed for 2 hours. She says, "This baby was just too big."

1. How would you discuss with Wendy the need for frequent assessments after birth?
2. Explain "maternity or baby blues."
3. Explore activities to minimize maternity blues.
4. Discuss concerns of a woman experiencing her second pregnancy.
5. Discuss behaviors that inhibit paternal attachment.

MEDIALINK

www.prenhall.com/london

- NCLEX-RN® Review, case studies, and other interactive resources for this chapter can be found on the Companion Website at http://www.prenhall.com/london. Click on "Chapter 24" to select the activities for this chapter.

MediaLink Applications

This activity contains 2 questions.

1. **Design a booklet for the postpartum client that focuses on maternal rest and activity. Include various postpartum exercises. Identify signs and symptoms that are abnormal during the postpartum period.**

To create paragraphs in your essay response, type <p> at the beginning of the paragraph, and </p> at the end.

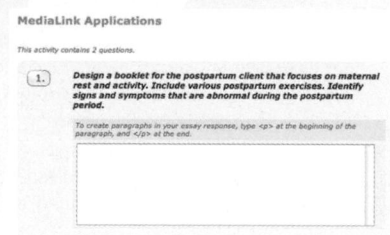

- For animations, more NCLEX-RN® Review questions, and an audio glossary, access the accompanying CD-ROM in this textbook.

REFERENCES

Arms, S. (1990). *Adoption: A handbook of hope.* Berkeley, CA: Celestial Arts.

deMontigny, F., & Lacharité, C. (2004). Fathers' perceptions of the immediate postpartal period. *Journal of Obstetric, Gynecologic, and Neonatal Nursing, 33*(3), 328–338.

Davis, R. E. (2001). The postpartum experience for Southeast Asian women in the United States. *American Journal of Maternal-Child Nursing, 26*(4), 208–213.

Gabbe, S. G., Niebyl, J. R., & Simpson, J. L. (2002). *Obstetrics: Normal and problem pregnancies* (4th ed.). Philadelphia: Churchill Livingstone.

Hughes, S. C., Levinson, G., & Rosen, M. A. (2002). *Shnider and Levinson's anesthesia for obstetrics* (4th ed.). Philadelphia: Lippincott Williams & Wilkins.

Kim-Godwin, Y. S. (2003). Postpartum beliefs and practices among non-Western cultures. *MCN. American Journal of Maternal Child Nursing, 28*(2), 74–78.

Larson-Meyer, D. E. (2002). Effect of postpartum exercise on mothers and their offspring: A review of the literature. *Obesity Research, 10*(8), 841–853.

Martell, L. K. (2003). Postpartum women's perceptions of the hospital environment. *Journal of Obstetric, Gynecologic, and Neonatal Nursing, 32*(4), 478–485.

Montgomery, K. S. (2001). Maternal-newborn nursing: Thirteen challenges that influence excellence in practice. *Journal of Perinatal Education, 10*(1), 31–40.

Spector, R. E. (2004). *Cultural diversity in health and illness* (6th ed.). Upper Saddle River, NJ: Prentice Hall Health.

Varney, H., Kriebs, J. M., & Gegor, C. L. (2004). *Varney's midwifery* (4th ed.). Sudbury, MA: Jones & Bartlett.

Wilson, B. A., Shannon, M. T., & Stang, C. L. (2006). *Nurse's drug guide 2006.* Upper Saddle River, NJ: Prentice-Hall.

The Postpartal Family at Risk

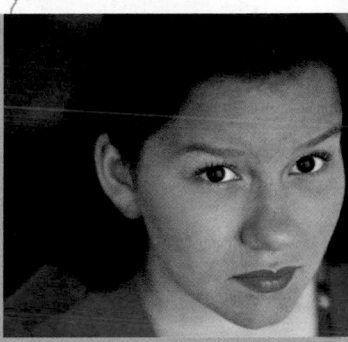

We are surviving. Maybe just. I was told that babies ate at six-ten-two-six-ten-two, but no one said that he would eat at five-seven-nine-eleven or so it seems. I am either getting ready to feed him or just finished feeding and changing him. But I love him without bounds. I feel a need to protect him from ever being hurt or wounded. During that first week, when I was tired and recovering from the emergency cesarean, I was afraid that I would not be able to shelter and help this young son grow up.

—*Kate, 34*

LEARNING OBJECTIVES

- Describe assessment of the postpartum woman for predisposing factors, onset, signs, and symptoms of various postpartum complications.

- Summarize the preventive measures for various complications of the postpartum period that should be incorporated into nursing care of the postpartum woman.

- List the causes of and appropriate nursing interventions for hemorrhage during the postpartal period.

- Develop nursing care plans that reflect a knowledge of etiology, pathophysiology, and current medical management for the woman experiencing postpartum hemorrhage, reproductive tract infection, urinary tract infection, mastitis, thromboembolic disease, or a postpartal psychiatric disorder.

- Evaluate the woman's knowledge of self-care measures, signs of complications to be reported to the primary care provider, and measures to prevent recurrence of complications.

MEDIALINK

www.prenhall.com/london

CD-ROM
NCLEX-RN® Review
Audio Glossary

Companion Website
NCLEX-RN® Review
MediaLink Applications:
    Case Study: Postpartal Client
    Care Plan Activity: Postpartal Care Following
        Vaginal Birth
    Care Plan Activity: Postpartal Care Following
        Cesarean Birth
Thinking Critically
Nursing Care Plan: The Woman with a Puerperal
    Infection

The postpartal period is typically viewed as a smooth, uneventful transition time—and it usually is. However, the nurse must be aware of problems that may develop in order to teach the family the signs of postpartal complications, findings to report to the physician or certified nurse-midwife, and preventive measures if available.

Written instructions to supplement any discussion will be of great value in the early weeks at home with a newborn, when life can be chaotic and instructions may be forgotten. The family should have telephone numbers for postpartum follow-up services and other resources to answer questions. By communicating an attitude of willingness to answer questions and listen to concerns, the nurse enhances the parents' comfort in making calls later for what they might otherwise perceive as issues "too trivial to bother someone about."

When a telephone follow-up or an examination at the home visit provides evidence of a developing complication, the nurse shares these findings or impressions with the woman, and they mutually plan an appropriate next step. In the case of telephone follow-up, the nurse usually counsels the woman to notify her physician or certified nurse-midwife, being prepared to schedule an appointment immediately if risk assessment indicates. The nurse who identifies a complication at the home visit will need to communicate the clinical findings to the certified nurse-midwife or physician and document them and any interventions for the permanent record. (See Chapter 31 for a more detailed discussion of home care for the postpartal family. ∞)

Complications suggest the need for immediate collaborative management. The most common complications of the postpartal period are hemorrhage, infection, thromboembolic disease, and postpartal psychiatric disorders. These are the focus of this chapter.

CARE OF THE WOMAN WITH POSTPARTAL HEMORRHAGE

Hemorrhage in the postpartal period is described as either early (immediate) or late (delayed) postpartal hemorrhage. **Early postpartal hemorrhage** occurs in the first 24 hours after childbirth. **Late postpartal hemorrhage** occurs from 24 hours to 6 weeks after birth. Postpartal hemorrhage continues to be a cause of significant maternal mortality and morbidity and accounts for 11% of maternal deaths attributed to pregnancy-related hemorrhage in the United States (Shevell & Malone, 2003).

The traditional definition of postpartal hemorrhage has been a loss of more than 500 mL of blood following childbirth. That definition is currently being questioned, however, because careful quantification indicates that the average blood loss in a vaginal birth is actually greater than 500 mL, and the average blood loss after cesarean childbirth exceeds 1000 mL (Shevell & Malone, 2003). Some clinicians think postpartal hemorrhage can be objectively and reliably defined as either a decrease in the hematocrit of 10 points between the time of admission and the time postbirth or the need for fluid replacement following childbirth. Clinical estimation of blood loss at childbirth is difficult because blood mixes with amniotic fluid and is obscured as it oozes onto sterile drapes or is sponged away. Without vigilance it may be difficult over the next hours to appreciate the significance of slow, steady blood loss. As the amount of blood loss increases, as in the case of hemorrhage, estimates are likely to be even less accurate. Given the increased blood volume of pregnancy, the clinical signs of hemorrhage—such as decreasing blood pressure, increasing pulse, and decreasing urinary output—do not appear until as much as 1800 to 2100 mL has been lost, shortly before the woman becomes hemodynamically unstable (Gilbert & Harmon, 2003).

EARLY POSTPARTAL HEMORRHAGE

At term, blood volume and cardiac output have increased so that 20% of cardiac output perfuses the pregnant uterus, supporting the developing fetus. When the placenta separates, the many uterine vessels that carried blood to and from the placenta are severed abruptly. The normal mechanism for hemostasis after expulsion of the placenta is contraction of the interlacing uterine muscles to occlude the open sinuses that previously brought blood into the placenta. Uterine atony, the absence of prompt and sustained uterine contractions, can result in significant blood loss. Other causes of postpartal hemorrhage include laceration of the genital tract; episiotomy; retained placental fragments; vulvar, vaginal, or subperitoneal hematomas; uterine inversion; and coagulation disorders.

UTERINE ATONY

Uterine atony (relaxation of the uterus) is a common cause of early postpartal hemorrhage (Shevell & Malone, 2003). Although uterine atony can occur after any childbirth, its contributing factors include the following:

- Overdistention of the uterus due to multiple gestation, hydramnios, or a large infant (macrosomia)
- Rapid or prolonged labor, which indicates that the uterus is contracting abnormally
- Oxytocin augmentation or induction of labor
- Grand multiparity, because stretched uterine musculature contracts less vigorously
- Use of anesthesia or other drugs, such as magnesium sulfate and terbutaline (Brethine), that cause the uterus to relax
- Intra-amniotic infection
- Preeclampsia
- Operative birth
- Retained placental fragments
- Placenta previa
- Asian or Hispanic heritage

Hemorrhage from uterine atony may be slow and steady rather than sudden and massive. The blood may escape the vagina or collect in the uterus, evident as large clots. The uterine cavity may distend with up to 1000 mL or more blood while the perineal pad and linen protectors remain suspiciously dry. Because of the increased blood volume associated with pregnancy, changes in maternal blood pressure and pulse may not occur until blood loss has been significant. The woman with preeclampsia is an exception because she does not have the normal hypervolemia of pregnancy and cannot tolerate even normal post-childbirth blood loss.

Ideally, postpartal hemorrhage is prevented, beginning with adequate prenatal care, good nutrition, avoidance of traumatic procedures, risk assessment, early recognition, and management of complications as they arise. Any woman at risk should be typed and crossmatched for blood and have intravenous lines in place with needles suitable for blood transfusion (18-gauge minimum).

After expulsion of the placenta, the fundus is palpated to ensure that it is firmly contracted. If it is not firm (if it is boggy), fundal massage is performed until the uterus contracts. Fundal massage is painful for the woman who has not received regional anesthesia; consequently she will need explanation for why this uncomfortable procedure is necessary and support as massage is initiated. If bleeding is excessive, the clinician will likely order intravenous oxytocin at a rapid infusion rate and may elect to do a bimanual massage (Figure 25–1A ●). Other uterine stimulants may be necessary to manage postpartal uterine atony. Table 25–1 summarizes critical nursing information about the use of uterine stimulants. The clinician uses hemoglobin and hematocrit results to determine the need for intravenous fluid replacement and blood transfusion.

In addition to the previously described measures, severe uncontrolled hemorrhage may require radio-guided embolization of the pelvic vessels (Poggi & Kapernick, 2003). Vessel ligation may be used to slow blood loss and allow normal clotting mechanisms to occur. Uterine packing, commonly used in postpartal hemorrhage in the past, is no longer advocated because it dilates the uterine cavity and may actually increase bleeding. Hysterectomy is done as a last resort for women of high parity when other measures have failed and excessive bleeding has been life threatening regardless of parity.

● **FIGURE 25–1**

A, Manual compression of the uterus and massage with the abdominal hand will usually control hemorrhage from uterine atony. **B,** Manual removal of placenta. The fingers are alternately abducted, adducted, and advanced until the placenta is completely detached. Both procedures are performed only by the medical clinician.

Adapted from Cunningham, F. G., MacDonald, P. C., & Gant, N. F. (Eds.). (1989). Williams obstetrics (18th ed., pp. 417–418). Norwalk, CT: Appleton & Lange.

LACERATIONS OF THE REPRODUCTIVE TRACT

Early postpartum hemorrhage is associated with lacerations of the perineum, vagina, or cervix. Several factors predispose women to higher risk of reproductive tract lacerations:

- Nulliparity
- Epidural anesthesia
- Precipitous childbirth
- Forceps- or vacuum-assisted birth
- Macrosomia

Thorough inspection of the reproductive tract by the birth attendant facilitates recognition and timely repair of most lacerations. Genital tract lacerations should be suspected when vaginal bleeding persists in the presence of a firmly contracted uterus. The nurse who suspects a laceration should notify the clinician so that the laceration can be immediately sutured to control the hemorrhage and restore the integrity of the reproductive tract. Episiotomies can be a source of postpartal blood loss.

Episiotomy is an often underappreciated source of blood loss because of slow, steady bleeding. The risk for bleeding is increased with mediolateral episiotomies. (See Care of the Woman During an Episiotomy in Chapter 22. ∞) Most deaths from postpartal hemorrhage are not due to gross bleeding but to ineffective management of slow, steady blood loss.

RETAINED PLACENTAL FRAGMENTS

Retained placental fragments and a retained placental lobe may both cause early postpartal hemorrhage and are the most common causes of late hemorrhage. The most common cause of partial separation of the placenta with retention of fragments is massage of the fundus prior to spontaneous placental separation, so this practice should be avoided.

Following birth the placenta should always be inspected for intactness and for evidence of missing fragments or cotyledons on the maternal side and for vessels that transverse to the edge of the placenta outward along the membranes of the fetal side, which may indicate succenturiate placenta and a retained lobe. Uterine exploration may be required to remove missing fragments. This cause should be immediately suspected if bleeding persists and no lacerations are noted (Figure 25–1B ●). Sonography may be used to diagnose retained placental fragments. Curettage, formerly standard treatment, is now thought by some to traumatize the implantation site, thereby increasing bleeding and the potential for uterine adhesions. It may be necessitated by the degree of hemorrhage, however (Shevell & Malone, 2003).

VULVAR, VAGINAL, AND PELVIC HEMATOMAS

Hematomas occur as a result of injury to a blood vessel from birth trauma, often without noticeable trauma to the superficial tissue, or from inadequate hemostasis at the site of incision or laceration repair. The soft tissue in the area offers no resistance, and hematomas containing 250 to 500 mL of blood may develop rapidly. Signs and symptoms vary somewhat with the type of hematoma. Hematomas may be vulvar, vaginal (especially in the area of the ischial spines), or subperitoneal. The latter are rare but the most dangerous because of the large amount of blood loss that can occur without clinical symptoms until the woman becomes hemodynamically

TABLE 25–1 ✤ **Uterine Stimulants Used to Prevent and Manage Uterine Atony**

Drug	Dosing Information	Contraindications	Expected Effects	Side Effects
Oxytocin (Pitocin, Syntocinon)	IV use: 10–40 units in 500–1000 mL crystalloid fluid @ 50 milliunits/min administration rate. Onset: immediate. Duration: 1 h. **IV bolus administration not recommended.** IM use: 10–20 units. Onset: 3–5 min. Duration: 2–3 h.		Rhythmic uterine contractions that help to prevent or reverse postpartal hemorrhage caused by uterine atony.	Uterine hyperstimulation, mild transient hypertension, water intoxication rare in postpartum use.
Methylergonovine maleate (Methergine)	IM use: 0.2 mg q2–4h. Onset: 2–5 min. Duration: 3 h (× 5 dose maximum). PO use: 0.2 mg q6–12h. Onset: 7–15 min. Duration: 3 h (× 1 week). **IV administration not recommended.**	Women with labile or high blood pressure or known sensitivity to drug.	Sustained uterine contractions that help to prevent or reverse postpartal hemorrhage caused by uterine atony; management of postpartal subinvolution.	Hypertension, dizziness, headache, flushing/hot flashes, tinnitus, nausea and vomiting, palpitations, chest pain. Overdose or hypersensitivity is recognized by seizures; tingling and numbness of fingers and toes from vasoconstrictive effect, leading rarely to gangrene; hypertension; weak pulse; chest pain.
Ergonovine maleate (Ergotrate Maleate)	IM use: 0.2 mg q2–4h. Onset: 7 min. Duration: 3 h (5 dose maximum). PO use: 0.2 mg q6–12h. Onset: 15 min. Duration: 3 h (× 2–7 days). **IV administration not recommended.**	Women with labile or high blood pressure or known sensitivity to drug.	Sustained uterine contractions that help to prevent or reverse postpartal hemorrhage caused by uterine atony; management of postpartal subinvolution.	Hypertension, dizziness, headache, nausea and vomiting, chest pain. Hypersensitivity is noted on systemic vasoconstrictive effects: seizure, chest pain, and tingling and numbness of fingers and toes that lead rarely to gangrene.
Prostaglandin (PGF$_{2\alpha}$, Hemabate, Prostin/15M)	IM use: 0.25 mg repeated up to maximum 5 doses; may be repeated q15–90 min. Physician may elect to administer by direct intramyometrial injection.	Women with active cardiovascular, renal, liver disease, or asthma or with known hypersensitivity to drug.	Control of refractory cases of postpartal hemorrhage caused by uterine atony; generally used after failed attempts at control of hemorrhage with oxytoxic agents.	Nausea, vomiting, diarrhea, headache, flushing, bradycardia, bronchospasm, wheezing, cough, chills, fever.

Implications for Nursing Management of the Postpartal Woman Receiving Uterine Stimulants

- Assess fundus for evidence of contraction and amount of uterine bleeding at least q10–15min × 1–2 h after administration, then q30–60min until stable. **More frequent assessments are determined by the woman's condition or by orders of the physician or certified nurse-midwife.**
- Weigh pads to estimate blood loss.
- Monitor blood pressure and pulse q15 min for at least 1 h after administration, then q30–60 min until stable.
- Note expected duration of action of drug being administered and take care to recheck fundus at that time.
- When the drug is ineffective, the fundus remains atonic (boggy or uncontracted), and bleeding continues, massage the fundus. If massage fails to cause sustained contraction, notify the physician or certified nurse-midwife immediately.
- Monitor woman for signs of known side effects of the drug; report to physician or certified nurse-midwife if side effects occur.

- Remind the woman and her support person that uterine cramping is an expected result of these drugs and that medication is available for discomfort. Administer analgesic medications as needed for pain relief. Provide nonpharmacologic comfort measures. If analgesic medication ordered is insufficient for pain relief, notify the physician or certified nurse-midwife.

When Prostaglandin Is Used

- Check temperature q1–2h and/or after chill. Administer antipyretic medication as ordered for prostaglandin-induced fever.
- Auscultate breath sounds frequently for signs of adverse respiratory effects.
- Assess for nausea, vomiting, and diarrhea. Administer antiemetic and antidiarrheal medications as ordered. (In some settings, women are premedicated with these drugs.)

unstable. The most common hematomas are of the vagina and vulva.

Risk factors for hematomas include preeclampsia, pudendal anesthesia, first full-term birth, precipitous labor, prolonged second stage of labor, macrosomia, forceps- or vacuum-assisted birth, and history of vulvar varicosities.

Nonexpanding hematomas less than 5 cm in size are managed with ice packs and analgesia. They usually resolve over several days. For larger hematomas and those that expand, surgical management is usually required; the hematoma is evacuated, the bleeding vessel ligated, and the wound closed, with or without vaginal packing. An indwelling urinary catheter may be necessary for 24 to 36 hours because voiding may be difficult with a vaginal pack in place.

The hematoma site is an ideal medium for the growth of flora normally present in the genital tract. Consequently, broad-spectrum antibiotics are usually ordered to prevent infection or abscess. The nurse can decrease the risk of vulvar or vaginal hematoma by applying an ice pack to the woman's perineum during the first hour after birth and intermittently for up to 24 hours thereafter. If a hematoma develops despite preventive measures, a sitz bath (four to six times a day) after the first 24 hours can aid fluid absorption once bleeding has stopped and will promote comfort, as will the judicious use of analgesic agents.

UTERINE INVERSION

Puerperal uterine inversion is the prolapse of the fundus to or through the cervix so that the uterus is turned inside out. Most cases of uterine inversion occur after birth and may be worsened by excess traction on the cord before placental separation (Poggi & Kapernick, 2003). Today nearly all cases of uterine inversion are recognized, and the potential complications of postpartum hemorrhage are treated immediately after birth.

LATE POSTPARTAL HEMORRHAGE

Although early postpartal hemorrhage usually occurs within hours after birth, delayed hemorrhage generally occurs within 1 to 2 weeks after childbirth, most frequently as a result of **subinvolution** (failure to return to normal size) of the placental site due to retained placental fragments. Blood loss may be excessive but rarely poses the same risk as immediate postpartal hemorrhage.

The site of placental implantation is always the last area of the uterus to regenerate after childbirth. Faulty implantation in the less vascular lower uterine segment (placenta previa), retention of placental tissue, or infection may contribute. With subinvolution the postpartum fundal height is greater than expected, and lochial flow often fails to progress normally from rubra to serosa to alba. Lochia rubra that persists longer than 2 weeks postpartum is highly suggestive of subinvolution. Some women report scant brown lochia or irregular heavy bleeding. Leukorrhea, backache, and foul lochia may occur if infection is a cause. There may be a history of heavy early postpartal bleeding or difficulty in expulsion of the placenta.

Subinvolution is most commonly diagnosed during the routine postpartal examination at 4 to 6 weeks. The woman may relate a history of irregular or excessive bleeding or describe the symptoms listed previously. An enlarged, softer-than-normal uterus palpated bimanually is an objective indication of subinvolution. Treatment includes administration of methylergonovine maleate 0.2 mg orally every 6 hours for at least 48 hours. See "Drug Guide: Methylergonovine Maleate (Methergine)" in Chapter 24. ∞ With uterine infection, antibiotics are also administered and the uterus is reevaluated in 2 weeks. If retained placenta is suspected or other treatment is ineffective, curettage may be indicated (Poggi & Kapernick, 2003).

NURSING MANAGEMENT

NURSING ASSESSMENT AND DIAGNOSIS

Carefully evaluate the woman's prenatal history and the results of ongoing assessment during labor and birth to identify factors that put the woman at risk for postpartal hemorrhage. Following birth, periodic assessment for evidence of vaginal bleeding is a major nursing responsibility. Rely on regular and frequent assessment of fundal height and evidence of uterine tone or contractility to indicate the possible development or recurrence of hemorrhage. Observe and document vaginal bleeding to determine whether further medical intervention is needed. Perform this assessment visually, by pad counts, or by weighing the perineal pads.

When regional anesthesia is used, frequent assessment of the woman's perineum is especially significant. Once the effects of anesthesia have subsided, vaginal and vulvar hematomas generally cause perineal pain. The pain is often intense, out of proportion, or excessive, and usually from the woman's "stitches." If the hematoma is in the posterior vaginal area, rectal pressure may also be a presenting complaint. Hematomas in the upper vagina may cause difficulty voiding because of pressure against the urinary meatus or urethra. Rather than automatically attributing complaints of perineal pain to an episiotomy, examine the perineal area for signs of hematomas: ecchymosis; edema; tenseness of tissue overlying the hematomas; fluctuant, bulging mass at the introitus; and extreme tenderness to palpation. Estimate the size of the hematoma on first assessment of the perineum so that it is easier to identify increases in size and the potential blood loss. Notify the physician or certified nurse-midwife if a hematoma is suspected.

Nursing diagnoses that may apply to a woman experiencing postpartal hemorrhage include the following:

- *Deficient Knowledge* related to lack of information about signs of delayed postpartal hemorrhage
- *Fluid Volume Deficit* related to blood loss secondary to uterine atony, lacerations, or retained placental fragments

PLANNING AND IMPLEMENTATION

If the uterus is soft and boggy, massage it until firm. If the uterus is not contracting firmly and appears larger than anticipated, clots may be expressed during fundal massage. Once clots are removed, the uterus tends to contract more effectively.

If the woman seems to have a slow, steady, free flow of blood, begin to weigh the perineal pads (1 mL = 1 g) and monitor the woman's vital signs every 15 minutes or more frequently if indicated. If the fundus is displaced upward or to one side because of a full bladder, encourage the woman to empty her bladder—or catheterize her if she is unable to void—to allow for sustained uterine contractions.

During the initial postpartum period, maintain the vascular access (IV) started during labor in case additional fluid or blood is necessary. When physicians and certified nurse-midwives write orders that specify "discontinue IV after present bottle," the astute postpartum nurse assesses the consistency of the fundus and the presence of normal versus excessive lochia before discontinuing the infusion. If the assessments are not reassuring, the nurse continues the intravenous (IV) infusion and notifies the physician or certified nurse-midwife.

Assess the woman for signs of anemia, such as fatigue, pallor, headache, thirst, and orthostatic changes in pulse or blood pressure and review the results of all hematocrit determinations. Monitor all medical interventions, IV infusions, blood transfusions, oxygen therapy, and medications such as uterine stimulants as necessary and evaluate them for effectiveness. Also monitor urinary output to determine adequacy of fluid replacement and renal perfusion and report amounts less than 30 mL/hr to the physician. Help the woman plan activities so that she can rest adequately.

The woman experiencing anemia and fatigue related to hemorrhage may need assistance with self-care and progressive ambulation for several days. When she is able to be out of bed to shower, a shower chair permits independence while providing a measure of safety in case the woman feels weak or dizzy. The emergency call light should be easily accessible.

The mother may find it difficult to care for her baby because of the fatigue associated with blood loss. It is often possible to find ways to promote maternal-infant attachment while accommodating the health needs of the mother. The mother may need extra help caring for her infant. If she has IV lines in place, even carrying the newborn may be awkward. For the mother who feels compelled to do as much as possible, the nurse may also need to "give permission" to the mother to return her infant to the nursery so she can have adequate periods of uninterrupted rest. Work with the woman's partner and family to find ways to help the mother cope and assist her if the nursery is an uncomfortable alternative.

The woman and her family or other support persons should receive clear, preferably written, explanations of the normal postpartum course, including changes in the lochia and fundus and signs of abnormal bleeding. Instructions for managing bleeding should include fundal massage, ways to assess the fundal height and consistency, and inspection of any episiotomy and lacerations, if possible. Advise the woman and her family to contact her caregiver if any signs of postpartal hemorrhage occur (Table 25–2). If iron supplementation is ordered, provide instructions for proper dosage to enhance absorption and avoid constipation and nausea.

Nursing Care in the Community

For most postpartal women, routine discharge instructions include advice such as: "You care for your baby, and let someone else care for you, the family, and the household." Because of her fatigue and weakened condition, the woman who experienced postpartal hemorrhage may be unable even to care for her newborn unassisted.

Advise her to rise slowly to minimize the likelihood of orthostatic hypotension. Until she regains strength, she should be seated when holding the newborn.

The support person who assumes responsibility for grocery shopping and meal preparation needs advice about the importance of including foods high in iron in the daily menus. Having the woman indicate her preferences from a list of such foods will promote cooperation with the diet. Explain the rationale for continuing medications containing iron.

TABLE 25–2 ✤ Signs of Postpartal Hemorrhage
Excessive or bright-red bleeding
A boggy fundus that does not respond to massage
Abnormal clots
Any unusual pelvic discomfort or backache
Persistent bleeding in the presence of a firmly contracted uterus
Rise in the level of the fundus of the uterus
Increased pulse or decreased BP
Hematoma formation or bulging/shiny skin in the perineal area
Decreased level of consciousness

The woman should continue to count perineal pads for several days so that she can recognize any recurring problems with excessive blood loss. The debilitated condition and anemia associated with hemorrhage increase the woman's risk of puerperal infection. She and her caregivers should use good handwashing and minimize exposure to infection in the home. Give the woman's caregiver a list of the signs of infection and ensure that he or she understands the importance of alerting the physician immediately if signs occur.

A sense of emergency often accompanies late postpartal hemorrhage. Because it commonly occurs 1 to 2 weeks after birth, the couple is generally at home, involved in the day-to-day activities demanded by their new roles, when the unexpected, excessive bleeding begins. Quick decisions about childcare arrangements must often be made so that the mother can return to the hospital. Both mother and father are likely to be alarmed by the excessive bleeding and concerned about her prognosis. There may be additional worries about separation from the newborn, especially when the mother is breastfeeding. The father may find himself torn between the needs of the mother and those of the newborn. Ideally, arrangements can be made to minimize separation of the family members.

EVALUATION

Expected outcomes of nursing care include the following:

- Signs of postpartal hemorrhage are detected quickly and managed effectively.
- Maternal-infant attachment is maintained successfully.
- The woman can identify abnormal changes that might occur following discharge and understands the importance of notifying her caregiver if they develop.

CARE OF THE WOMAN WITH A REPRODUCTIVE TRACT INFECTION OR WOUND INFECTION

Puerperal infection affects the reproductive tract; it is associated with childbirth and occurs any time up to 6 weeks postpartum. The most common infection is metritis (endometritis), which is limited to the uterus. Indeed the cause of postpartal fever is presumed to be metritis until proven otherwise. However, infection can spread by way of the lymphatic system to become a progressive disease resulting in parametrial cellulitis and peritonitis. The women's prognosis is directly related to the stage of the disease at the time of diagnosis, the causative organism, and the state of her health and immune system.

The standard definition of **puerperal morbidity**, established in the 1930s by the Joint Committee on Maternal Welfare, is a temperature of 38°C (100.4°F) or higher, with the temperature occurring on any 2 of the first 10 postpartum days, exclusive of the first 24 hours, and when taken by mouth by standard technique at least four times a day. However, serious infections can occur in the first 24 hours or may cause only persistent low-grade temperatures. Therefore, careful assessment of all postpartum women with elevated temperatures is essential. The vagina and cervix of approximately 70% of all healthy pregnant women contain pathogenic bacteria that, alone or in combination, are sufficiently virulent to cause excessive infection. However, other factors must be present for infection to occur, such as the change to an alkaline pH of the vagina postpartally that favors growth of aerobes. Uterine infections are relatively uncommon following uncomplicated vaginal births, but they continue to be a major source of morbidity for women who give birth by cesarean. See "Nursing Care Plan: The Woman with a Puerperal Infection."

POSTPARTAL UTERINE INFECTION

Postpartal uterine infection is known variously as *metritis, endometritis, endomyometritis,* and *endoparametritis.* Risk factors for postpartal uterine infection include the following:

- Cesarean birth, which is the single most significant risk (20 times greater than in vaginal births) (Gibbs, Sweet, & Duff, 2004)
- Prolonged premature rupture of the amniotic membranes (PPROM)
- Prolonged labor preceding cesarean birth
- Multiple vaginal examinations during labor
- Compromised health status (due to low socioeconomic status, anemia, obesity, cigarette smoking, use of illicit drugs or alcohol)
- Use of fetal scalp electrode or intrauterine pressure catheter for internal monitoring during labor
- Obstetric trauma (including episiotomy and lacerations of perineum, vagina, or cervix)
- Chorioamnionitis
- Diabetes (4 times more common than in nondiabetic mothers) (Minkoff & Gibbs, 2003)
- Preexisting bacterial vaginosis or *Chlamydia trachomatis* infection.
- Instrument-assisted childbirth (vacuum or forceps)
- Manual removal of the placenta
- Lapses in aseptic technique by surgical staff

ENDOMETRITIS (METRITIS)

Endometritis or metritis, an inflammation of the endometrium, occurs postpartally in 1% to 3% of women who give birth vaginally and up to 27% of women who give

(text continues on page 623)

NURSING CARE PLAN

THE WOMAN WITH A PUERPERAL INFECTION

Intervention	Rationale	Expected Outcome
1. Nursing Diagnosis: Risk for Spread of Infection related to traumatized tissues		
NIC Intervention: **Infection control:** *Minimizing the acquisition and transmission of infectious agents*		**NOC Outcome:** **Risk control:** *Actions to eliminate or reduce actual, personal, and modifiable health threats*

Goal: The patient will be free of complications associated with infection.

■ Encourage patient, staff, and family members to adhere to a strict handwashing policy. ■ Review the patient's prenatal, intrapartal, and postpartal records for underlying problems that could contribute to poor wound healing or increase risk for spread of infection. ■ Monitor blood pressure, pulse, respiration, and temperature. ■ Instruct patient on proper perineal care, including wiping perineum front to back after voiding, perineal washes after voiding and defecating, and changing peri-pads frequently. ■ Encourage patient to consume 2000 mL of fluid a day. ■ Encourage use of the sitz bath, surgigator, or the perineal light two to four times a day for at least 10–15 minutes. ■ Encourage early ambulation. ■ Assess and report signs and symptoms of infection in perineum, including erythema, edema, discharge, pain, and approximation of wound edges (REEDA). **Collaborative:** Obtain lab work as ordered by physician, including culture and sensitivity, CBC with differential, and WBC count. ■ Administer antibiotic therapy as ordered by the physician. ■ Promote wound drainage by assisting physician in opening wound if necessary. If wound is greater than 2–3 cm, pack with iodoform gauze. ■ Report signs and symptoms of severe infections: foul-smelling lochia, uterine subinvolution, uterine tenderness, severe lower abdominal pain, elevated temperature, elevated WBC count, general malaise, chills, lethargy, tachycardia, nausea and vomiting, and abdominal rigidity.	■ Handwashing kills bacteria and prevents cross-contamination. ■ Identifying underlying problems gives the caregiver an opportunity to initiate preventive measures that will promote healthy wound healing and stop the spread of infection. ■ Obtain baseline data; signs and symptoms of septic shock produce a ↓ in blood pressure and an ↑ in respirations. ■ Proper perineal care techniques enhance good hygiene and assist in removing urine and fecal contaminants from perineum. Changing peri-pads frequently decreases skin contact with a moist medium that favors bacteria growth. ■ Maintains hydration and increases circulating volume. ■ Moist or dry heat to the perineum increases blood flow and promotes healing. ■ Enhances circulation and drainage of lochia. ■ Identifying signs and symptoms of infection early allows for prompt treatment and healing. ■ Identifies abnormal lab values for early intervention. In addition, identifies infection and its causative organism for appropriate antibiotic treatment. ■ Fights present infection and helps prevent the spread of further infection. ■ Iodoform gauze is used to maintain patency of wound opening. This promotes drainage and prevents abscesses from developing. ■ Reporting signs and symptoms of severe infections early allows for initiation of appropriate therapy by physician and prevents further spread of the invading pathogen.	■ The patient will be remain free of complications associated with infection as evidenced by practicing behaviors that prevent the spread of infection and promote timely wound healing.

(continued)

NURSING CARE PLAN—continued

THE WOMAN WITH A PUERPERAL INFECTION

Intervention	Rationale	Expected Outcome
2. Nursing Diagnosis: Pain related to the infection process		
NIC Intervention: **Pain management:** *Alleviation of pain or a reduction in pain to a level of comfort that is acceptable to the patient*		**NOC Outcome:** **Pain level:** *Amount of reported or demonstrated pain.*
Goal: The patient will be free of pain.		
■ Assess pain location and intensity, have patient describe on a scale from 1 (mild) to 10 (severe). Assess nonverbal signs of pain, including facial grimacing and agitation. ■ Encourage patient to discuss anxiety and fears. ■ Encourage frequent rest periods and decrease disturbing environmental stimuli. ■ Promote relaxation by encouraging the use of exercises and diversional activities, including radio/television, reading, guided imagery, deep breathing techniques, massage, visualization, and meditation. **Collaborative:** Administer analgesics as ordered by the physician.	■ Assesses the need for pain management and evaluates interventions already implemented. ■ Reduces anxiety and fear and may decrease the patient's perception of pain. ■ Uses frequent rest periods to conserve patient's energy. Increasing environmental stimuli may increase patient's pain perception. ■ Promotes relaxation and refocuses patient's attention away from the intensity of pain. ■ Relieves pain and reduces anxiety.	■ Patient is free of pain as evidenced by verbalization of pain relief and the exhibition of a relaxed demeanor.
3. Nursing Diagnosis: Risk for Impaired Parent-Infant Attachment related to pain secondary to maternal infection		
NIC Intervention: **Attachment promotion:** Facilitation of the development of the parent-infant relationship		**NOC Outcome:** **Parent-infant attachment:** Behaviors that demonstrate an enduring affectionate bond between a parent and infant
Goal: Mother will have no problems bonding with infant and assuming responsibility for the care of the infant.		
■ Provide quality time for mother and infant contact. ■ Encourage partner or family members to give patient videos and pictures of the infant if the mother's condition requires separation from the infant. ■ Encourage partner and family members to become involved with the care of the infant and verbalize interaction to the mother. ■ Encourage mother to feed (breast or bottle) infant if her condition is stable. If mother is unable to breastfeed, encourage and assist her in pumping her breasts to maintain milk production. ■ Assess maternal support systems. **Collaborative:** Offer referrals to home health services, doula services, and support groups.	■ Aids in the bonding process. ■ Promotes bonding and gives the mother reassurance that the infant is being cared for. ■ Allows mother to feel as though she is involved in the care of the infant. ■ Gives mother a positive outlook through hands-on participation in the infant's care. ■ As mother is recovering, she will need assistance in household organization and personal care. ■ Ensures patient's well-being, and identifies problems that may require intervention.	■ Mother will bond with infant as evidenced by exhibiting appropriate attachment behaviors when interacting with infant, providing care to self and infant, and verbalization of understanding of the parenting role.

birth by cesarean (Minkoff & Gibbs, 2003). After expulsion of the placenta, the placental site provides an excellent culture medium for bacterial growth. The remaining portion of the decidua is also susceptible to pathogenic bacteria because of its thinness (approximately 2 mm) and its large blood supply. The cervix may also be a bacterial breeding ground because of the multiple small lacerations attending normal labor and spontaneous birth.

Both aerobic and anaerobic organisms cause metritis that is often polymicrobial (Minkoff & Gibbs, 2003). Clinical findings of metritis in the initial 24 to 36 hours postpartally tend to be related to group B streptococcus (GBS). Late-onset postpartum metritis is most commonly associated with genital mycoplasmas and *Chlamydia trachomatis*. These microbes have a longer replication time and latency period than other bacteria and are not consistently eradicated by antibiotics used for early postpartal infections.

In mild cases of metritis, the woman generally has discharge that is bloody, foul smelling, and either scant or profuse. In more severe cases, she also has uterine tenderness, sawtooth temperature spikes that are usually between 38.3°C and 40°C (101°F and 104°F), tachycardia, and chills. Foul-smelling lochia is cited as a classic sign of metritis, but in the case of infection with β-hemolytic streptococcus, the lochia may be scant, serosanguineous, and odorless (Gibbs et al., 2004).

PELVIC CELLULITIS (PARAMETRITIS) AND PERITONITIS

Pelvic cellulitis (parametritis) is infection involving the connective tissue of the broad ligament or, in more severe forms, the connective tissue of all the pelvic structures. The infection generally ascends upward in the pelvis by way of the lymphatics in the uterine wall, but this may also occur if pathogenic organisms invade a cervical laceration that extends upward into the connective tissue of the broad ligament—a direct pathway into the pelvis.

A pelvic abscess may form in postpartal **peritonitis** (infection involving the peritoneal cavity) and is most commonly found in the uterine ligaments, the cul-de-sac of Douglas, and the subdiaphragmatic space. Parametritis may be a secondary result of pelvic vein thrombophlebitis. This condition occurs when the clot, usually in the right ovarian vein, becomes infected and the wall of the vein breaks down from necrosis, spilling the infection into the connective tissues of the pelvis.

A woman with parametritis may have a variety of symptoms, including marked high temperature (38.9°C to 40°C [102°F to 104°F]) chills, malaise, lethargy, abdominal pain, subinvolution of the uterus, tachycardia, and local and referred rebound tenderness. If peritonitis develops, the woman becomes acutely ill, with severe pain, marked anxiety, high fever, rapid and shallow respirations, pronounced tachycardia, excessive thirst, abdominal distention, nausea, and vomiting.

PERINEAL WOUND INFECTIONS

Given the degree of bacterial contamination that occurs with normal vaginal birth, it is surprising that more women do not have infections of the episiotomy or repaired lacerations of the perineum, vagina, or vulva. When perineal wound infection occurs, it is recognized by the classic signs: redness, warmth, edema, purulent drainage, and, later, gaping of the previously approximated wound. Local pain may be severe. Infected perineal wounds, like other infected wounds, are treated by draining purulent material. Sutures are removed, and the wound is left open. A regimen of broad-spectrum antibiotics is used. When the surface of the wound is free of infectious exudate and tissue granulation is evident, the mother returns for secondary closure of the wound under regional anesthesia.

CESAREAN WOUND INFECTION

The infection rate following cesarean births is 3% to 5%, with the highest rate occurring after emergency cesarean because there is more traumatization of the tissue (Gibbs et al., 2004). Predisposing factors include obesity, diabetes mellitus, prolonged postpartal hospitalization, PROM, metritis, prolonged labor, anemia, steroid therapy, and immunosuppression (Gibbs et al., 2004). Signs of an abdominal wound infection, which may not be evident until after discharge, include erythema, warmth, skin discoloration, edema, tenderness, purulent drainage that is sometimes mixed with sanguineous liquid, and gaping of the wound edges. Fever, pain, malodorous lochia, and other systemic signs are also common. Abdominal distention and decreased bowel sounds may be noted. Culture of the wound drainage commonly reveals mixed pathogens.

CLINICAL THERAPY

The infection site and causative organism are diagnosed by careful history and complete physical examination, blood tests, aerobic and anaerobic endometrial cultures (which may be of limited value because multiple organisms are usually present), and urinalysis to rule out urinary tract infection. When a localized infection develops, it is treated with antibiotics, sitz baths, and analgesics as necessary for pain relief. If an abscess has developed or a stitch site is infected, the suture is removed and the area is allowed to drain. Packing the wound with saline gauze twice to three times daily, using aseptic technique, allows removal of necrotic debris when packing is removed. Broad-spectrum antibiotic coverage treats postpartal wound infections. Cephalosporins, penicillinase-resistant penicillin, and vancomycin are commonly used with anaerobic coverage by clindamycin or ampicillin/sulbactam (Newton, 2003).

The incidence of metritis has been reduced by prophylactic administration of antibiotics to women undergoing cesarean birth. Metritis, once diagnosed, is treated aggressively with antibiotics (Minkoff & Gibbs, 2003). With appropriate antibiotic coverage, improvement should occur within a few days. Antibiotics are generally continued until the woman is afebrile for 24 to 48 hours. The severity of the infection determines the route and dosage. Careful monitoring is also necessary to prevent the development of a more serious infection.

Parametritis and peritonitis are treated with intravenous antibiotics. Treatment begins with broad-spectrum antibiotics effective against the most commonly occurring causative organisms, until the results of culture and sensitivity reports are available. If multiple organisms are present, the approach to antibiotic therapy is continued unless no improvement is observed; then the antibiotic is changed. Antibiotics are generally continued until the woman has been afebrile for 48 hours. Oral antibiotics are rarely needed on discharge.

An abscess is frequently manifested by the development of a palpable mass and may be confirmed with ultrasound. It usually requires incision and drainage to prevent rupture into the peritoneal cavity and the possible development of peritonitis. After drainage the cavity may be packed with iodoform gauze to promote drainage and facilitate healing.

The woman with a severe systemic infection is acutely ill and may require care in an intensive care unit. Supportive therapy includes maintenance of adequate hydration with intravenous fluids, analgesic medications, ongoing assessment of the infection, and possibly continuous nasogastric suctioning if paralytic ileus develops.

NURSING MANAGEMENT

NURSING ASSESSMENT AND DIAGNOSIS

Inspect the woman's perineum every 8 to 12 hours for signs of early infection. The REEDA scale is a reminder to consider redness, edema, ecchymosis, discharge, and approximation. Immediately report any degree of induration (hardening) to the clinician. Note and report fever, malaise, abdominal pain, foul-smelling lochia, tachycardia, and other signs of infection so that treatment can begin. The white blood cell (WBC) count, a usual objective measure of infection, cannot be used reliably because of the normal increase in WBCs during the postpartum period. A WBC count of 14,000 to 16,000 mm^3 is not an unusual finding. An increase in WBC level of more than 30% in a 6-hour period, however, is indicative of infection.

Nursing diagnoses that may apply to the woman with a puerperal infection include the following:

- *Risk for Injury* related to the spread of infection
- *Pain* related to the presence of infection
- *Risk for Altered Parenting* related to delayed parent-infant attachment secondary to woman's pain and other symptoms of infection

PLANNING AND IMPLEMENTATION

Hospital-Based Nursing Care

The nurse caring for a woman during the postpartal period is responsible for teaching the woman self-care measures that are helpful in preventing infection. The woman should understand the importance of perineal care, good hygiene practices to prevent contamination of the perineum (including wiping from front to back, changing perineal pads after voiding), and thorough handwashing. Once edema and perineal pain are under control, encourage sitz baths, which are cleansing and promote healing. Adequate fluid intake and a diet high in protein and vitamin C, which are necessary for wound healing, also help prevent infection.

If the woman has a draining wound or purulent lochia, it is especially important that those in contact with soiled items and linens practice good handwashing. Clear, concise instructions about wound care and how to discard soiled dressings appropriately must be provided to safeguard the woman and her caregivers. If the woman is seriously ill, ongoing assessment of urine specific gravity and intake and output is necessary. Carefully administer antibiotics as ordered and regulate the intravenous fluid rate. Ongoing assessment of the woman's condition is vital to detect subtle changes in her health status. Keep the woman comfortable by providing hygiene, positioning, oral care, and pain relief.

Promoting maternal-infant attachment can be difficult with the acutely ill woman. It may help to provide pictures of the infant and keep the mother informed of the infant's well-being. The partner of a seriously ill woman will be concerned about her condition and torn about spending time with her and with their newborn. Because maternal-infant bonding may be compromised, father-newborn bonding can be especially important. See "Nursing Care Plan: The Woman with a Puerperal Infection," earlier in this chapter.

Nursing Care in the Community

The woman with a puerperal infection needs assistance when she is discharged from the hospital. If the family cannot provide it, a referral to home care services is needed. Home care services should be contacted as soon as puerperal infection is diagnosed so that the nurse can meet with the woman for a family and home assessment and development of a home care plan.

The family needs instruction in the care of a newborn, including feeding, bathing, cord care, immunizations, and significant observations that should be reported. A well-baby appointment should be scheduled. The woman who wishes to breastfeed when her condition allows can maintain lactation by pumping her breasts regularly. Understanding that the opportunity to breastfeed is simply delayed, not eliminated, by the infectious process may improve the woman's morale. Breastfeeding mothers receiving antibiotics should be instructed to inspect the infant's mouth for signs of thrush and to report the finding to their physician.

Teach the mother about activity, rest, medications, diet, and signs and symptoms of complications, and schedule a return medical visit. She needs to know the importance of taking the entire course of prescribed antibiotics even though she may begin to feel better before the bottle is empty. She also needs to know the importance of pelvic rest; that is, she should not use tampons or douches or have intercourse until she has been examined by the physician and told it is safe to resume those activities.

EVALUATION

Expected outcomes of nursing care include the following:

- The infection is quickly identified and treated successfully, without further complications.
- The woman understands the infection and the purpose of therapy; she cooperates with ongoing antibiotic therapy after discharge.
- Maternal-infant attachment is maintained.

CARE OF THE WOMAN WITH A URINARY TRACT INFECTION

The postpartal woman is at increased risk for urinary tract problems due to the normal postpartal diuresis, increased bladder capacity, decreased bladder sensitivity from stretching or trauma, and possible inhibited neural control of the bladder after general or regional anesthesia and contamination from catheterization.

Emptying the bladder completely with each voiding is vital.

OVERDISTENTION OF THE BLADDER

Overdistention occurs postpartally when the woman is unable to empty her bladder, usually because of trauma or the effects of anesthesia. Women who have not sufficiently recovered from the effects of anesthesia cannot void spontaneously, and catheterization is necessary. After the effects of regional anesthesia have worn off, postpartal urinary retention is highly indicative of urinary tract infection (UTI).

CLINICAL THERAPY

Overdistention in the early postpartal period is often managed by draining the bladder with a straight catheter as a onetime measure. If the overdistention recurs or is diagnosed later in the postpartal period, an indwelling catheter is generally ordered for 24 hours.

NURSING MANAGEMENT

NURSING ASSESSMENT AND DIAGNOSIS

The overdistended bladder appears as a large mass, reaching sometimes to the umbilicus and displacing the uterine fundus upward. Increased vaginal bleeding occurs, the fundus is boggy, and the woman may complain of cramping as the uterus attempts to contract. Some women also experience backache and restlessness.

Nursing diagnoses that may apply when a woman has difficulties with overdistention of the bladder include the following:

- *Risk for Infection* related to urinary stasis secondary to overdistention
- *Urinary Retention* related to decreased bladder sensitivity and normal postpartal diuresis

PLANNING AND IMPLEMENTATION

Diligent monitoring of the bladder during the recovery period and preventive health measures greatly reduce the chances for overdistention of the bladder. Encouraging the mother to void spontaneously and helping her use the toilet, if possible, or the bedpan, if she has received conductive anesthesia, prevents overdistention in most cases. Help the woman to a normal position for voiding (i.e., sitting with the legs and feet lower than the trunk) and provide privacy to encourage voiding. The woman should receive medication for whatever pain she may be having before she attempts to void because pain may cause a reflex spasm of the urethra. Applying perineal ice packs after childbirth helps minimize edema, which may interfere with voiding. Pouring warm water over the perineum or having the woman void in the sitz bath may also be effective.

If catheterization becomes necessary, use careful, meticulous aseptic technique. The vagina and vulva are traumatized to some degree by vaginal birth, and edema is common. Because this edema may obscure the urinary meatus, be extremely careful cleansing the vulva and inserting the catheter. It is imperative to discard a catheter that has inadvertently been introduced into the vagina and thus contaminated. Because postpartal trauma and edema make catheterization uncomfortable, be careful and gentle not only in inserting the catheter but also in handling and cleaning the perineal area.

If the amount of urine drained from the bladder reaches 900 to 1000 mL, the catheter is clamped and taped firmly to the woman's leg. Take the woman's vital signs before and after the procedure and note the woman's responses. Then carefully document the procedure and assessment findings. After an hour the catheter may be unclamped and placed on gravity drainage. This technique protects the bladder and prevents rapid intra-abdominal decompression. When the indwelling catheter is removed, a urine specimen is often sent to the laboratory. The tip of the catheter may also be removed and sent for culture.

EVALUATION

Expected outcomes of nursing care include the following:

- The woman voids adequately.
- The woman does not develop infection due to stasis of urine.
- The woman uses self-care measures to decrease bladder overdistention.

CYSTITIS (LOWER URINARY TRACT INFECTION)

Retention of residual urine, bacteria introduced at the time of catheterization, and a bladder traumatized by birth combine to provide an excellent environment for the development of cystitis. *Escherichia coli* has been demonstrated to be the causative agent in most cases of postpartal cystitis and pyelonephritis (in both lower and upper UTI). Generally the infection ascends the urinary tract from the urethra to the bladder and then to the kidneys because vesiculoureteral reflux (backward flow of urine) forces contaminated urine into the renal pelvis.

CLINICAL THERAPY

When cystitis is suspected, a clean-catch midstream urine sample is obtained for microscopic examination, culture, and sensitivity tests. The specimen may require collection by the nurse with the woman on a bedpan because few postpartal women can collect a true midstream clean-catch specimen without contaminating the specimen with lochia. A catheterized specimen is avoided when possible because of the increased risk of infection. When the bacterial concentration is greater than 100,000 colonies of the same organism per milliliter of fresh urine, infection is generally present. Counts between 10,000 and 100,000 suggest infection, particularly if clinical symptoms are noted.

In the clinical setting, antibiotic therapy is often begun before culture and sensitivity reports are available. Frequently used antibiotics include a preparation of trimethoprim-

sulfamethoxazole-double strength (Bactrim DS, Septra DS), one of the short-acting sulfonamides, nitrofurantoin (Macrodantin), and, in the case of sulfa allergy, ampicillin or amoxicillin-clavulanic acid. The antibiotic is changed later if indicated by the results of the sensitivity report (Poggi & Kapernick, 2003). Antispasmodics or urinary analgesic agents, such as phenazopyridine hydrochloride (Pyridium), may be given to relieve discomfort.

NURSING MANAGEMENT

NURSING ASSESSMENT AND DIAGNOSIS

Symptoms of cystitis often appear 2 to 3 days after childbirth. The initial symptoms of cystitis may include frequency, urgency, dysuria, and nocturia. Hematuria and suprapubic pain may also be present. A slightly elevated temperature may occur, but systemic symptoms are often absent. When a UTI progresses to pyelonephritis, systemic symptoms usually occur, and the woman becomes acutely ill. Symptoms include chills, high fever, flank pain (unilateral or bilateral), nausea, and vomiting, in addition to all the signs of lower UTI. Costovertebral angle tenderness on palpation and pain may or may not be present. Obtain a urine culture so that sensitivity can identify the causative organism.

Nursing diagnoses that may apply if a woman develops a UTI postpartally include the following:

- *Pain with Voiding* related to dysuria secondary to infection
- *Health-Seeking Behaviors* related to self-care measures to prevent UTI

PLANNING AND IMPLEMENTATION

Screening for asymptomatic bacteriuria in pregnancy should be routine. Encourage frequent emptying of the bladder during labor and postpartum to prevent overdistention and trauma to the bladder. Catheterization technique and nursing actions to prevent overdistention (previously discussed) also apply. Be sure the woman with pyelonephritis understands the importance of follow-up care after discharge to prevent recurrence or further complications.

Advise the postpartal woman to continue good perineal hygiene after discharge, to maintain a good fluid intake (at least 8 to 10 8-oz glasses daily), especially of water, and to empty her bladder whenever she feels the urge to void, but at least every 2 to 4 hours while awake. Once sexual intercourse is resumed, the new mother should void before (to prevent bladder trauma) and after intercourse (to wash contaminants from the vicinity of the urinary meatus). Wearing underwear with a cotton crotch to facilitate air circulation also reduces the risk of UTI.

Acidification of the urine is thought to aid in preventing and managing UTI. Therefore, advise the woman to avoid carbonated beverages, which increase the alkalinity of urine, and to drink unsweetened cranberry, plum, apricot, and prune juices and take vitamin C, which increases the acidity of urine (Gilbert & Harmon, 2003).

EVALUATION

Expected outcomes of nursing care include the following:

- The woman identifies the signs of UTI, and her condition is treated successfully.

- The woman uses self-care measures to prevent the recurrence of UTI as part of her personal hygiene routine.

- The woman cooperates with any long-term therapy or follow-up.

- Maternal-infant attachment is maintained and the woman is able to care for her newborn effectively.

CARE OF THE WOMAN WITH MASTITIS

Mastitis is an infection of the breast connective tissue that occurs primarily in lactating women. The usual causative organisms are *Staphylococcus aureus*, *Haemophilus parainfluenzae*, *H. influenzae*, *Escherichia coli*, and *Streptococcus* species. Infectious mastitis is a more serious infection, with fever, headache, flulike symptoms, and a warm, reddened, painful area of the breast, often wedge shaped because of the connective tissue septal divisions of the breast (Figure 25–2 ●). Because symptoms of mastitis seldom occur before the second to fourth week postpartum, birthing unit nurses often are not fully aware of how uncomfortable and acutely ill the woman can be; they must ensure that all breastfeeding women are taught preventive techniques, ways of recognizing it, and the appropriate response of immediate notification of their physician or certified nurse-midwife.

The infection usually begins when bacteria invade the breast tissue after it has been traumatized in some way (see the factors commonly associated with mastitis in Table 25–3). Milk serves as a favorable medium for the invasive bacteria; thus, milk is another risk factor. The most common sources of pathogenic organisms are the infant's nose and throat, although other sources include the hands of the mother or birthing unit personnel and the woman's circulating blood. Infants of women with mastitis generally remain well.

In some cases *Candida albicans* is the causative organism of mastitis, entering the breast through a small fissure or abrasion on the nipple; the baby will often have thrush,

● **FIGURE 25–2**

Mastitis. Erythema and swelling are present in the upper outer quadrant of the breast. Axillary lymph nodes are often enlarged and tender. The segmental anatomy of the breast accounts for the demarcated, often V-shaped wedge of inflammation.

a candidal infection of the mouth. There may be a history of a recent course of antibiotics in the woman. Signs include late-onset nipple pain, followed by shooting pain during and between feedings. Eventually the skin of the affected breast becomes pink, flaking, and pruritic. Women may notice a yeasty odor.

COMPLEMENTARY CARE

PROBIOTICS

Probiotics are a category of dietary supplements consisting of beneficial microorganisms (*pro* means "for" and *biotic* means "life" versus *antibiotics*, which literally means "against life"). Probiotics compete with disease-causing microorganisms in the gastrointestinal tract. When antibiotics are taken, they kill many of the beneficial bacteria that exist naturally in the digestive tract. Supplementing with probiotics after a course of antibiotics is frequently prescribed by nutritionists and complementary practitioners. Commonly used probiotics include *Lactobacillus acidophilus* and *Bifidobacterium bifidum;* other species of *Lactobacillus* and *Bifidobacterium* have been shown to be effective in such conditions as diarrhea and vaginal infections (Reid & Bocking, 2003). *Bifidobacterium* also competes against *Candida albicans*. Probiotics can be taken in the form of powder, capsules, and suppositories, or in fermented milk products such as yogurt or kefir.

TABLE 25–3 ❖ Factors Associated with Development of Mastitis

Milk stasis

Failure to change infant position to allow emptying all lobes
Failure to alternate breasts at feedings
Poor suck
Poor letdown

Actions that promote access/multiplication of bacteria

Poor handwashing technique
Improper breast hygiene
Failure to air dry breasts after breastfeeding
Use of plastic-lined breast pads that trap moisture against nipple

Breast/nipple trauma

Incorrect positioning for breastfeeding
Poor latch-on
Failure to rotate position on nipple
Incorrect or aggressive pumping technique

Obstruction of ducts

Restrictive clothing
Constricting bra
Underwire bra

Change in number of feedings/failure to empty breasts

Attempted weaning
Missed feeding
Prolonged sleeping, including sleeping through night
Favoring side of nipple soreness

Lowered maternal defenses

Fatigue
Stress

CLINICAL THERAPY

Diagnosis is usually based on history and physical examination; a culture and sensitivity testing of breast milk obtained by a midstream-type collection process may be done. The nipple is washed first; then the first 3 mL of breast milk are manually expressed and discarded, after which the actual specimen is collected. A leukocyte count of 1 million/mL and bacterial colony count of greater than 10,000/mL is diagnostic (Gibbs et al., 2004). Treatment involves bed rest for at least 24 hours, increased fluid intake (at least 2 to 3 L/day), a supportive bra, frequent breastfeeding, local application of warm moist-heat compresses, and analgesics that are compatible with breastfeeding. Nonsteroidal anti-inflammatory agents are recommended to treat both fever and inflammation. Also a course of 7 to 10 days of antibiotics is appropriate, usually a penicillinase-resistant penicillin or cephalosporin (Poggi & Kapernick, 2003).

Candidal infections can be especially stubborn. Initial treatment generally involves antifungal creams or ointments once or twice daily. Oral Diflucan is excreted in breast milk but it is not considered toxic to the infant and can be used if other agents fail. Women should be instructed to cleanse their nipples with warm water and allow air-drying before application of the antifungal medication. For women who prefer to avoid medication, an alternative treatment is cleansing of the nipples with a solution of 1 tablespoon of vinegar in 1 cup of water, or 1 teaspoon of baking soda in 1 cup of water, followed by air-drying.

Improved outcome, decreased duration of symptoms, and decreased incidence of breast abscess result if the breasts continue to be emptied by nursing or pumping. Thus, continued breastfeeding is recommended in the presence of mastitis. The woman should be contacted within 24 hours of initiation of treatment to ensure that symptoms are subsiding.

Early treatment may prevent the progression of milk stasis and noninfectious inflammation to mastitis; 10% of all cases will progress to abscess formation if mastitis remains untreated, treatment fails, or the infant is abruptly weaned. Breast abscess may require incision and drainage, and intravenous antistaphylococcic antibiotics (Gibbs et al., 2004).

NURSING MANAGEMENT

NURSING ASSESSMENT AND DIAGNOSIS

Each day, assess breast consistency, skin color, surface temperature, nipple condition, and presence of pain to detect early signs of problems that may predispose a woman to mastitis. Watch the mother breastfeeding her baby to ensure proper technique.

If an infection develops, assess for contributing factors such as cracked nipples, poor hygiene, engorgement, supplemental feedings, change in routine or infant feeding pattern, abrupt weaning, and lack of proper breast support so that these factors can be corrected as part of the treatment plan.

Nursing diagnoses that may apply to the woman with mastitis include the following:

■ *Health-Seeking Behaviors* related to lack of information about appropriate breastfeeding practices
■ *Ineffective Breastfeeding* related to pain secondary to development of mastitis

PLANNING AND IMPLEMENTATION

Preventing mastitis is far simpler than treating it. Ideally, mothers learn proper breastfeeding technique prenatally. The nurse helps the mother breastfeed soon after childbirth and reviews correct technique. Comanagement of breastfeeding between the nurse and a certified lactation specialist is often possible. Encourage new mothers, even those not breastfeeding, to wear a good supportive bra at all times to prevent milk stasis, especially in the lower lobes.

Meticulous handwashing by the breastfeeding mother and all personnel is the primary measure in preventing epidemic nursery infections and subsequent maternal mastitis. Prompt attention to mothers who have blocked milk ducts eliminates stagnant milk as a growth medium for bacteria. If the mother finds that one area of her breast feels distended, she can rotate the position of her infant for breastfeeding, manually express milk remaining in the breast after feeding (usually necessary only if the infant is not sucking well), or massage the caked area toward the nipple as the infant nurses. Mothers who develop mastitis can apply warm, moist compresses to the affected area before and during breastfeeding. Encourage the mother to breastfeed frequently, starting with the unaffected breast until letdown occurs in the affected breast and then feeding from the affected breast until it is emptied completely. After breastfeeding, the mother can leave a small amount of milk on each nipple to prevent cracking and allow nipples to air-dry. Early identification of and intervention for sore nipples is also essential, as is prompt assessment of the breastfeeding mother's breast when thrush is discovered in her newborn's mouth.

Discharge Planning and Home Care Teaching

Stress to the breastfeeding woman the importance of adequate breast and nipple care to prevent the development of cracks and fissures, a common portal for bacterial entry. (For a detailed discussion of breastfeeding, see Breastfeeding Concerns Following Discharge in Chapter 32. ∞)

The woman should be aware of the importance of regular, complete emptying of the breasts to prevent engorgement and stasis. She should also understand the role of letdown in successful breastfeeding, correct positioning of the infant on the nipple, proper latch-on, and the principle of supply and demand. If the mother is taking antibiotics, she needs to understand the importance of completing the full course of antibiotics, even if the infection seems to clear quickly. Infants tolerate the small amount of antibiotics in breast milk without difficulty. The infant should also be checked for possible colonization with the same bacteria present in the mother's breast (Poggi & Kapernick, 2003). Breastfeeding mothers returning to work outside the home need information on how to do so successfully. Because mastitis tends to develop after discharge, it is important to include information about signs and symptoms in the discharge teaching and printed materials (Table 25–4). All flulike symptoms should be considered a sign of

mastitis until proven otherwise. If symptoms develop, the woman should contact her caregiver immediately because prompt treatment helps to prevent abscess formation.

Nursing Care in the Community

The home care nurse who suspects mastitis on the basis of assessment findings refers the woman to the physician. The nurse may be asked to obtain a sample of breast milk to be cultured for the causative organism.

If the mother feels too ill to breastfeed or develops an abscess that prevents breastfeeding, the home care nurse can help the mother obtain a breast pump to help her maintain lactation and can provide opportunities for demonstration and return demonstration of pumping. Referral to a lactation consultant or to La Leche League can be invaluable to the woman's physical and emotional adjustment to mastitis.

EVALUATION

Expected outcomes of nursing care include the following:

- The woman is aware of the signs and symptoms of mastitis.
- The woman reports the mastitis signs and symptoms early and is treated successfully.
- The woman can continue breastfeeding if she chooses.
- The woman understands self-care measures she can employ to prevent the recurrence of the mastitis.

CARE OF THE WOMAN WITH POSTPARTAL THROMBOEMBOLIC DISEASE

Thromboembolic disease may occur antepartally, but it is generally considered a postpartal complication. *Venous thrombosis* refers to thrombus formation in a superficial or deep vein, usually in the legs. When the thrombus is formed in response to inflammation in the vein wall, it is termed **thrombophlebitis**. Pulmonary embolism, a rare, life-threatening condition, occurs when thrombi formed in the deep leg veins are carried to the pulmonary artery, obstructing pulmonary blood flow to one or both lungs. These vascular occlusive processes—venous thrombosis, thrombophlebitis, septic pelvic thrombophlebitis, and pulmonary embolism—are known as thromboembolic diseases (Laros, 2004).

Changes in the woman's coagulation system in pregnancy contribute to hypercoagulability. At the same time, compression of the common iliac vein by the gravid uterus leads to venous stasis. These factors increase the risk of thromboembolic disease in pregnant and postpartal women approximately fivefold (Laros, 2004). Thrombosis

TABLE 25–4 ✤ Comparison of Findings of Engorgement, Plugged Duct, and Mastitis

Characteristics	Engorgement	Plugged Duct	Mastitis
Onset	Gradual, immediately postpartum	Gradual, after feedings	Sudden, after 10 days
Site	Bilateral	Unilateral	Usually unilateral
Swelling and heat	Generalized	May shift, little or no heat	Localized, red, hot, and swollen
Pain	Generalized	Mild but localized	Intense but localized
Body temperature	<38.4°C (101.1°F)	<38.4°C (101.1°F)	>38.4°C (101.1°F)
Systemic symptoms	Feels well	Feels well	Flulike symptoms

Used with permission from Lawrence, R. A. (1994). *Breastfeeding: A guide for the medical profession* (p. 261). St. Louis, MO: Mosby.

of the superficial veins complicates the general childbearing period for 1 in 500 to 750 women. Deep vein thrombosis (DVT), which is more serious, occurs most commonly in postpartum women between postpartum days 10 and 20 (Matteson, 2001). These types are discussed shortly.

Factors associated with increased risk of thromboembolic disease are identified in Table 25–5. Factors contributing directly to the development of thromboembolic disease postpartally include (1) increased amounts of certain blood-clotting factors; (2) postpartal thrombocytosis (increased quantity of circulating platelets and their increased adhesiveness); (3) release of thromboplastin substances from the tissue of the decidua, placenta, and fetal membranes; and (4) increased amounts of fibrinolysis inhibitors. Because all women are at risk for thromboembolic disease during the childbearing period, attention should be given to measures that might prevent this complication (Table 25–6).

TABLE 25–5 ✤ Factors Associated with Increased Risk of Thromboembolic Disease

- Cesarean birth
- Inactivity
- Obesity
- Cigarette smoking
- Previous thromboembolic disease
- Trauma to extremity (can include injury from incorrect positioning or prolonged interval in stirrups during labor)
- Varicose veins
- Diabetes mellitus
- Advanced maternal age
- Inherited coagulation disorders
- Multiparity
- Anemia

SUPERFICIAL VEIN LEG DISEASE

Superficial thrombophlebitis is far more common postpartally than during pregnancy. Often the clot involves one of the saphenous veins. This disorder is more common in women with preexisting varices (enlarged veins), although it is not limited to these women. Symptoms—including tenderness in a portion of the vein, some local heat and redness, normal temperature or low-grade fever, and occasionally slight elevation of the pulse—usually become apparent about the third or fourth postpartal day. A tender palpable cord may be noted along a portion of the veins. Treatment involves application of local heat, elevation of the affected limb, bed rest, analgesics, and the use of elastic support hose. Anticoagulants are usually not necessary unless complications develop. Pulmonary embolism is extremely rare.

DEEP VEIN THROMBOSIS

Deep vein thrombosis (DVT) is more frequently seen in women with a history of thrombosis. Certain obstetric complications, such as hydramnios, preeclampsia, and operative birth, are associated with an increased incidence.

Clinical manifestations may include edema of the ankle and leg and an initial low-grade fever often followed by high temperature and chills. Depending on the vein involved, the woman may complain of pain in the popliteal and lateral tibial areas (popliteal vein), pain in the entire lower leg and foot (anterior and posterior tibial veins), inguinal tenderness (femoral vein), or pain in the lower abdomen (iliofemoral vein). The Homans' sign (refer to Figure 23–9 in Chapter 23 ∞) may or may not be positive, but pain often results from calf pressure. Although a positive Homans' sign is specific, the test is not very sensitive (about 25%) (Aronson, Chelmow, & Lee, 2003). Because of reflex arterial spasm, sometimes the limb is pale and cool to the touch—the so-called *milk leg* or *phlegmasia alba dolens*—and peripheral pulses may be decreased.

TABLE 25–6 ✣ Measures to Decrease Risk of Thromboembolic Disease in Childbearing Women

Antepartum Measures	Intrapartum Measures	Postpartum Measures
Advise woman to avoid sedentary lifestyle and to exercise as possible (walking is ideal).	Encourage ambulation unless contraindicated in early labor. Later, encourage leg exercises.	Encourage early ambulation.
Recommend plenty of fluids to avoid dehydration.	Do not gatch bed or use pillows under knees.	For clients on bed rest, advise or assist with turning and leg exercises every 2 hours (woman may be encouraged to rotate ankles and to "write baby's name in the air with her toes").
Advise to quit smoking.	Pad stirrups.	
Teach to avoid prolonged standing or sitting in one position or sitting with legs crossed.	Ensure correct positioning in stirrups that minimizes pressure on the popliteal area.	Encourage fluids to avoid dehydration.
Encourage elevation of legs when sitting.	Limit time in stirrups as possible.	Advise no smoking.
Teach to avoid tight knee-high hose or other constrictive garments.	After cesarean birth, initiate leg/foot exercises as soon as possible (in recovery).	Use antiembolism stockings with those at risk, including after cesarean birth.
Encourage to take frequent breaks during long car trips to walk around, thereby preventing prolonged venous stasis.	Use antiembolism stockings for women at risk for DVT.	Advise against prolonged sitting and crossing legs.
		Encourage elevation of legs while sitting.

SEPTIC PELVIC THROMBOPHLEBITIS

Septic pelvic thrombophlebitis is a complication that develops in conjunction with infections of the reproductive tract and is more common in women who have had a cesarean birth. Infection ascends upward along the venous system, and thrombophlebitis develops in the uterine, ovarian, or hypogastric veins. The diagnosis is suspected with clinical findings resembling metritis that fails to respond to being treated with only antibiotics. Abdominal pain, flank pain, or both, sometimes accompanied by guarding, occur on the second or third day postpartum, along with fever and tachycardia. Bimanual examination may reveal a parametrial mass. On occasion, paralytic ileus develops. Treatment consists of anticoagulation and broad-spectrum antibiotic therapy. Within 48 to 72 hours of initiation of heparin therapy, fever should resolve (Laros, 2004). Resolution of the fever with heparin anticoagulation will help in the presumptive diagnosis (Laros, 2004).

CLINICAL THERAPY

Because cases of thromboembolic disease are seldom clear-cut, diagnosis involves a variety of approaches, such as client history and physical examination, occlusive cuff impedance plethysmography (IPG), Doppler ultrasonography, and contrast venography (increased circumference of affected extremity). In questionable cases, venography provides the most accurate diagnosis of DVT; unfortunately, it is not practical for multiple examinations or prospective screening and may itself induce phlebitis.

Treatment involves the administration of intravenous heparin, using an infusion pump to permit continuous, accurate infusion of medication. Strict bed rest and elevation

THINKING CRITICALLY

ASSESSING POSTPARTUM LEG PAIN

Lei Chang, G1P1, had a cesarean birth after a prolonged labor and failure to progress. As she is walking in the hallway with her husband, you notice that Lei is limping slightly, and you comment on that observation. Lei responds that she is having pain in her right lower leg. She says, "Maybe I pulled a muscle during labor." What would you do?

of the leg are required; analgesics are given as necessary to relieve discomfort. If fever is present, deep thrombophlebitis is suspected, and the woman is also given antibiotics. In most cases, thrombectomy (surgical removal of the clot) is not necessary.

Once the symptoms have subsided (usually in several days), the woman may begin ambulation while wearing elastic support stockings. Intravenous heparin is continued until prothrombin time reaches 1.5 to 2, and treatment with sodium warfarin (Coumadin) is begun. The woman continues taking Coumadin for 2 to 6 months at home. While taking warfarin, prothrombin times are assessed periodically to maintain correct dosage levels.

NURSING MANAGEMENT

NURSING ASSESSMENT AND DIAGNOSIS

Carefully assess the woman's history for factors predisposing her to development of thrombosis or thrombophlebitis. Be alert to any complaints of pain in the legs, inguinal area, or lower abdomen because such pain may indicate DVT.

Also assess the woman's legs for edema, temperature change, or pain with palpation.

Nursing diagnoses that may apply to a postpartal woman with a thrombolic disease include the following:

- *Altered Tissue Perfusion in Periphery* related to obstructed venous return
- *Pain* related to tissue hypoxia and edema secondary to vascular obstruction
- *Risk for Altered Parenting* related to decreased maternal-infant interaction secondary to bed rest and intravenous lines

PLANNING AND IMPLEMENTATION

Evaluate the need for support hose for women with varicosities during labor and the postpartum period. Adequate fluid intake is necessary during labor to prevent dehydration. Because trauma is often a factor in the development of thrombophlebitis, avoid keeping the woman's legs elevated in stirrups for prolonged periods. If stirrups are used, they should be comfortably padded and adjusted to provide correct support and prevent pressure on popliteal vessels. Encourage early ambulation after birth; the knee gatch on the bed should be avoided. Encourage women confined to bed after a cesarean birth to perform regular leg exercises to promote venous return.

Once DVT is diagnosed, maintain the heparin therapy, provide appropriate comfort measures, and monitor the woman closely for signs of pulmonary embolism. Also assess for evidence of bleeding related to heparin and keep the antagonist for heparin, protamine sulfate, readily available.

Tell the woman to avoid prolonged standing or sitting because these positions contribute to venous stasis. Advise the woman to avoid crossing her legs because of the pressure it causes. Recommend that the woman take frequent breaks during car trips and while working if she sits most of the day. Walking is acceptable because it promotes venous return. Remind the woman to mention her history of thrombosis or thrombophlebitis to her physician during subsequent pregnancies so that preventive measures can be instituted early.

Women discharged while taking warfarin must understand the purpose of the medication and be alert for signs of bleeding such as bleeding gums, epistaxis, petechiae or ecchymosis, and evidence of blood in the urine or stool. While taking anticoagulants the woman will be asked to undergo frequent tests to guide dosing. Point-of-care testing is now available to decrease the inconvenience of going to the laboratory. Home self-testing involves a single capillary finger stick (Coaguchek, ProTime, Aocet) to test thromboplastin-mediated clotting expressed as prothrombin (PT) or international normalized ratio (INR). The risk of bleeding increases significantly when the INR is greater than 4 (Zajac, 2004). Bleeding should be reported if it fails to stop within 10

minutes. Encourage the woman to carry a MedicAlert card in case of emergency, to inform all healthcare providers (including dentists) that she is taking anticoagulants, and to have vitamin K available in case of bleeding.

Certain medications such as aspirin and other non-steroidal anti-inflammatory drugs increase anticoagulant activity and should be avoided; when she is taking warfarin, the woman should check for possible medication interaction before taking *any* other medication. Binge alcohol use inhibits warfarin metabolism; an occasional alcoholic beverage does not affect coagulation adversely. Many multivitamins contain vitamin K; clients on warfarin may take them but should do so consistently. Many herbals affect the efficacy of warfarin; for example, garlic, ginger, and ginkgo prolong prothrombin and should be avoided. (See "Nursing Care Plan: The Woman with Thromboembolic Disease" for specific nursing care measures.)

Nursing Care in the Community

Because the mother with postpartal thromboembolic disease will depend on others for much of her initial home care, it is helpful for the father of the newborn to be involved in preparations for discharge. Allow ample time to answer questions and clarify instructions, verbally and in writing. Evaluate how well both mother and father have understood instructions about the plan of care. It is especially important to assess the couple's plans to ensure complete bed rest for the mother. They might explore ways for her to maintain bed rest and still spend quality time with her newborn and any other children. For example, young children can sit on the bed for storytelling or play quiet games, and the newborn's crib can be placed next to the mother's bed.

Many concerns will not surface until the couple returns home and fully comprehends the reality of their situation. For that reason it is valuable to provide them with an accessible resource person and to plan telephone or home visit follow-up care.

Signs of postpartum thrombophlebitis may not occur until after discharge from the birthing unit. Therefore, teach all couples to recognize its signs and symptoms and appreciate the importance of reporting them immediately and of not massaging the affected leg. If signs and symptoms occur after discharge, a short readmission may be required. In that case every effort is made to allow mother, father, and newborn to remain together.

EVALUATION

Expected outcomes of nursing care include the following:

- The woman seeks treatment for her thrombophlebitis early and is managed successfully, without further complications.

NURSING CARE PLAN

THE WOMAN WITH THROMBOEMBOLIC DISEASE

Intervention	Rationale	Expected Outcome

1. Nursing Diagnosis: Ineffective Tissue Perfusion: Peripheral related to interruption of venous blood flow secondary to complications of labor and birth

NIC Intervention: **Embolus care: Peripheral:** Limitation of complications for a patient experiencing, or at risk for, occlusion of peripheral circulation		**NOC Outcome:** **Tissue perfusion: Peripheral:** Extent to which blood flows through the small vessels of the extremities and maintains tissue function

Goal: The patient's presenting signs and symptoms are relieved.

■ Assess, record, and report signs of thrombophlebitis.	■ Early detection of developing thrombophlebitis permits prompt treatment. As the thrombus increases in size, signs of obstruction also increase.	■ Patient will have increased venous return from lower leg as evidenced by decreased edema in lower leg, negative Homans' sign, and no pain or tenderness in lower leg.
■ Assess leg for edema, peripheral pulse, temperature, color, and tenderness every 8 hours.	■ Assessment provides baseline data that may be used to monitor success of treatment. Edema/swelling, diminished or absent peripheral pulse, pallor, cool skin temperature, and tenderness are symptoms of DVT and indicate dysfunction of peripheral circulation in the lower extremities. Measure circumference of lower leg to monitor for swelling. Peripheral pulses in both legs should be palpated for pulse rate and pulse strength to allow for comparison. Lower extremities that are cool to the touch may be due to reflex arterial spasm.	
■ Assess Homans' sign every 8 hours.	■ Normally there is no pain or discomfort associated with this procedure. Pain is caused by inflammation of the vessel. If pain is elicited, the nurse documents the response as a positive Homans' sign and reports findings to the physician.	
■ Maintain bed rest during the acute phase.	■ Bed rest is ordered to decrease possibility that portion of clot will dislodge and result in pulmonary embolism.	
■ Provide warm, moist soaks as ordered.	■ Warmth promotes blood flow to affected area.	
■ Maintain limb in elevated position.	■ Elevation of affected limb promotes venous return and helps decrease edema.	
■ Initiate progressive ambulation following the acute phase and provide properly fitting elastic stockings prior to ambulation.	■ Elastic stockings or "Teds" help prevent pooling of venous blood in lower extremities. Patient may begin to ambulate within a few days when symptoms subside.	
■ Collaborative Activities Administer intravenous heparin as ordered, by continuous intravenous drip, heparin lock, or subcutaneously, including: 1. Monitor IV or heparin lock site for signs of infiltration. 2. Obtain international normalized ratio (INR) and partial thromboplastin time (PTT) per physician order and review prior to administering heparin.	■ Heparin does not dissolve blood clot but is administered to prevent further clotting and improve tissue perfusion. It is safe for breastfeeding mothers because heparin is not excreted in mother's milk.	

(continued)

NURSING CARE PLAN—continued

THE WOMAN WITH THROMBOEMBOLIC DISEASE

Intervention	Rationale	Expected Outcome

3. Observe for signs of anticoagulant overdose with resultant bleeding, including:
  a. Hematuria
  b. Epistaxis
  c. Ecchymosis
  d. Bleeding gums
4. Provide protamine sulfate, per physician order, to combat bleeding problems related to heparin overdose.
 	
5. Monitor and report any signs of pulmonary embolism.
6. Initiate or support any emergency treatment.
 	
7. Obtain prothrombin time (PT) and review prior to beginning warfarin. Repeat periodically per physician order.
	■ Protamine sulfate is heparin antagonist, given intravenously, which is almost immediately effective in counteracting bleeding complications caused by heparin overdose.
	■ Pulmonary embolism is a major complication of DVT/thrombophlebitis. Signs and symptoms may occur suddenly and require immediate emergency treatment; prognosis is related to size and location of embolism.
	■ PT is the test most commonly used to monitor the blood of clients receiving warfarin.	

2. Nursing Diagnosis: Pain related to tissue hypoxia and edema secondary to vascular obstruction

NIC Intervention:		NOC Outcome:
Pain Management: Alleviation of pain or a reduction in pain to a level of comfort that is acceptable to the patient		**Pain: Disruptive effects:** Observed or reported disruptive effects of pain on emotions and behavior

Goal: Patient will obtain relief of pain.

■ Administer analgesics per physician order. Notify physician if pain is not relieved. ■ Provide supportive nursing comfort measures such as back rubs, quiet time for sleep, and diversional activities.	■ Analgesics act to relieve pain and enable the woman to rest. Aspirin or ibuprofen products are contraindicated because they inhibit platelet adhesiveness. Acetaminophen may be ordered by the physician. ■ Once pain decreases, client is more likely to ambulate which will help increase venous return and decrease edema.	■ Patient will have reduction in pain as evidenced by a pain level < 5 at all times.

3. Nursing Diagnosis: Risk for Impaired Parenting related to decreased maternal-infant interaction secondary to bed rest and IVs

NIC Intervention:		NOC Outcome:
Attachment promotion: Facilitation of the development of the parent-infant relationship		**Parent-infant attachment:** Behavior that demonstrates an enduring affectionate bond between a parent and infant

Goal: Patient will demonstrate evidence of positive physical and social interaction with newborn.

■ Maintain mother-infant attachment when mother is on bed rest:
  1. Provide frequent contacts for mother and infant; modified rooming-in if possible by having the crib placed close to the mother's bed and nurse check often to help mother lift or move infant.
  2. Encourage mother to continue feeding infant.
	■ Maternal-infant attachment is enhanced by frequent contact and opportunities to interact.	■ Patient will develop attachment bonds as evidenced by physical interactions (good eye contact, touching the baby, holding baby close, attempting to comfort baby, kissing baby) and social interactions (calling baby by name, making positive comments about baby, asking questions about baby, asking questions about baby care, and talking to baby).

NURSING CARE PLAN—continued

THE WOMAN WITH THROMBOEMBOLIC DISEASE

Intervention	Rationale	Expected Outcome
4. Nursing Diagnosis: Interrupted Family Processes related to illness of family member		
NIC Intervention: **Family integrity promotion:** Promotion of family cohesion and unity		**NOC Outcome:** **Family functioning:** Ability of the family to meet the needs of its members through developmental transitions
Goal: Patient and her family will cope effectively with her illness.		
■ Encourage woman to express her concerns to her partner. Assist couple in planning ways to manage while woman is hospitalized and after her discharge. ■ Encourage partner or support person to bring other children to hospital to visit mother and meet new sibling. ■ Encourage partner or support person to bring in family pictures and notes from other children. Encourage phone calls. ■ Contact social services if indicated to obtain additional assistance for family if needed.	■ Illness of any family member affects the entire family. This is especially true when the family situation is such that the mother is the primary nurturer and she is absent. Family members attempt to continue their own roles while also assuming the tasks of the missing mother. This can result in crisis.	■ Patient expresses assurance that her family misses her but is coping effectively as evidenced by: Family visits woman frequently. Woman and family verbalize plan for division of family tasks while the woman is hospitalized, and understanding of potential needs of woman once released from hospital.
5. Nursing Diagnosis: Health-Seeking Behaviors related to lack of information about DVT/thrombophlebitis, its treatment, preventive measures, and the medication warfarin		
NIC Intervention: **Health education:** Development and provision of instruction and learning experiences to facilitate voluntary adaptation of behavior conducive to health in individuals, families, groups, or communities		**NOC Outcome:** **Knowledge: Health promotion:** Extent of understanding conveyed about the promotion and protection of health
Goal: Patient will understand her condition, its treatment, and long-term implications.		
■ Discuss ways of avoiding circulatory stasis such as avoiding prolonged standing, sitting, and crossing legs. ■ Review need to wear support stockings and to plan for rest periods with legs elevated. ■ In the presence of DVT, discuss the following: 1. The use of warfarin, its side effects, possible interactions with other medications, and the need to have dosage assessed through periodic checks of the prothrombin time.	■ Such discussion is essential to help the woman understand the condition, her medication, and its implications. She must have a clear understanding to be able to provide effective self-care. ■ Prolonged sitting, standing, and crossing legs should be avoided as these activities decrease venous return. ■ Patient placed on warfarin (Coumadin) therapy for 2-6 months at home.	■ Patient has health promotion knowledge as evidenced by: Woman verbalizes understanding of ways to avoid circulatory stasis, need to wear supportive stockings, medication's dosage and side effects, and the importance of a balanced diet which includes vitamin K foods. Woman verbalizes understanding of signs and symptoms of bleeding that need to be reported to healthcare provider.

(continued)

NURSING CARE PLAN—continued

THE WOMAN WITH THROMBOEMBOLIC DISEASE

Intervention	Rationale	Expected Outcome

2. Signs of bleeding, which may be associated with warfarin sodium and need to be reported immediately, include the following: hematuria, epistaxis, ecchymosis, bleeding gums, and rectal bleeding.
3. Monitor menstrual flow: bleeding may be heavier.
4. Review need for woman to eat a *consistent* amount of leafy green vegetables (lettuce, cabbage, brussels sprouts, broccoli) every day.
5. Instruct the woman to report *any* bleeding that continues more than 10 minutes.
6. Instruct the woman to do the following:
  ■ Routinely inspect the body for bruising.
  ■ Carry MedicAlert card indicating she is on anticoagulant therapy.
  ■ Use electric razor to avoid scratching skin.
  ■ Use soft bristle toothbrush.
  ■ Avoid alcohol intake or keep at minimum.
  ■ Avoid taking certain herbs such as ginger, garlic, and ginkgo and any other drugs without checking with the physician.
  ■ Note that stools may change color to pink, red, or black as a result of anticoagulant use.
  ■ Advise all health providers, including dentists, that she is taking anticoagulants.
	■ These foods are high in vitamin K and will affect balance between dose of warfarin and prothrombin time.	

■ At discharge the woman can explain the purpose, dosage regimen, and necessary precautions of any prescribed medications such as anticoagulants.

■ The woman can discuss the self-care measures and ongoing therapies (such as the use of elastic stockings) indicated.

■ The woman has bonded successfully with her newborn and is able to care for her baby effectively.

CARE OF THE WOMAN WITH A POSTPARTUM PSYCHIATRIC DISORDER

The relationship of affective disorders to childbirth is reflected in the fact that the rate of admission to a psychiatric hospital is greater during the year after childbirth than at any other time in a woman's life.

TYPES OF POSTPARTUM PSYCHIATRIC DISORDERS

The classification of postpartum psychiatric disorders is a subject of some controversy. The *Diagnostic and Statistical Manual of Mental Disorders* (American Psychiatric Association, 2000) has an added postpartum onset specifier to the mood disorder diagnostic category of psychiatric disorders. It is proposed that postpartum psychiatric disorders be considered one diagnosable syndrome with three subclasses: (1) adjustment reaction with depressed mood, (2) postpartum psychosis, and (3) postpartum major mood disorder. The incidence, etiology, symptoms, treatment, and prognosis vary with each subclass.

ADJUSTMENT REACTION WITH DEPRESSED MOOD

Adjustment reaction with depressed mood is also known as postpartum blues, *maternal blues,* or *"baby blues."* It occurs in as many as 50% to 80% of mothers and is characterized by mild depression interspersed with happier feelings (Parry, 2004). Postpartum blues typically occur within a few days after the baby's birth and are self-limiting, lasting from a few hours to 10 days or longer. The depression is more severe in primiparas than in multiparas and seems related to the rapid alteration of estrogen, progesterone, and prolactin levels after birth. New mothers experiencing postpartum blues commonly report feeling overwhelmed, unable to cope, fatigued, anxious, irritable, and oversensitive. A key feature is episodic tearfulness, often without an identifiable reason.

Validating the existence of this phenomenon, labeling it as a real but normal adjustment reaction, and providing reassurance can offer a measure of relief. Assistance with self- and infant care, information, and family support aids recovery. The partner should be encouraged to watch for and report signs that the new mother is not returning to a more normal mood but slipping into a deeper depression.

POSTPARTUM PSYCHOSIS

Postpartum psychosis, which has an incidence of 1 to 2 per 1000, usually becomes evident within the first 3 months postpartum (Haessler & Rosenthal, 2003). Symptoms include agitation, hyperactivity, insomnia, mood lability, confusion, irrationality, difficulty remembering or concentrating, poor judgment, delusions, and hallucinations. With appropriate treatment, improvement is seen in 95% of women in 2 to 3 months. There is an increased recurrence rate in subsequent pregnancies (Parry, 2004).

POSTPARTUM MAJOR MOOD DISORDER

Postpartum major mood disorder, also known as postpartum depression, develops in about 7% to 30% of all postpartum women in North America (Haessler & Rosenthal, 2003; Parry, 2004). Although it may occur at any time during the first postpartum year, the periods of greatest risk occur around the fourth week, just before the initiation of menses, and upon weaning. Surprisingly, it is not associated with depression during pregnancy.

Risk factors for postpartum depression include the following:

- Primiparity
- Ambivalence about maintaining the pregnancy
- History of postpartum depression or bipolar illness
- Lack of social support
- Lack of a stable and supportive relationship with parents or partner
- Lack of a supportive relationship with her parents, especially her father, as a child
- The woman's dissatisfaction with herself, including body image problems and eating disorders

CLINICAL THERAPY

Women with a history of postpartum psychosis or depression or other risk factors should be referred to a mental health professional for counseling and biweekly visits between the second and sixth week postpartum for evaluation. Medication, individual or group psychotherapy, and practical assistance with child care and other demands of daily life are common treatment measures for both disorders; however, specific therapies used may vary.

Treatment of postpartum psychosis is directed at the specific type of psychotic symptoms displayed and may include lithium, antipsychotics, or electroconvulsive therapy in combination with psychotherapy, removal of the infant, and social support.

Treatment of postpartum depression is not unlike treatment of any significant depression: psychotherapy and antidepression medications, usually the selective serotonin reuptake inhibitors. Support groups have proved to be successful adjuncts to such treatment. Within a support group of postpartal women and their partners, a couple may feel consolation that they are not alone in their experience. Moreover the group provides a forum for exchanging information about postpartum depression, learning stress reduction measures, and experiencing renewed self-esteem and support. If a support group is not available locally, the woman and her family may be encouraged to contact Depression after Delivery (DAD), a national support network that provides literature and volunteers (P.O. Box 1282, Morrisville, PA 19067, or 800–944–4773).

It is important to realize that many of the drugs used in treating postpartum psychiatric conditions may be contraindicated in breastfeeding women.

NURSING MANAGEMENT

NURSING ASSESSMENT AND DIAGNOSIS

Assessment for factors predisposing a client to postpartal depression or psychosis should begin prenatally (Beck, 2002). Questions designed to detect problems can be included as part of the routine prenatal history interview or questionnaire. Ideally a depression assessment should be completed each trimester to update a pregnant woman's risk status (Beck, 2002). If the assessment has not been done previously, the nurse assesses the woman for predisposing factors during labor and the postpartum stay. Several depression scales are available for assessing postpartum depression. The Edinburgh Postnatal Depression Scale (Table 25–7) is the most widely used screening tool for postpartum depression in large populations of women. Mothers who score above 12 on the Edinburgh Postpartum Depression Scale are likely to be suffering

EVIDENCE-BASED NURSING

TREATMENT OF POSTPARTUM DEPRESSION

Clinical Question

What nursing interventions will provide support for the new mother with postpartum depression?

Evidence

Estimates of the incidence of postpartum depression range from 7% to 30%. Controversy exists as to the causes of postpartum depression; current theories include biochemical changes of pregnancy and various psychoanalytic explanations. Experts at Brigham and Women's Hospital evaluated pharmacologic treatment of postpartum depression and developed a practice guideline. Noting that little has focused on the effects of social factors, two experts for the Cochrane Library analyzed randomized controlled trials to determine the effect of social support interventions for the treatment of postpartum depression. Taken together the evidence indicates that a combination of pharmacologic management and social support interventions are effective in treating postpartum depression.

Pharmacologic management remains the treatment of choice for moderate or severe depression, particularly in mothers who are not breastfeeding. However, the social isolation experienced by many mothers may be a contributing factor in postpartum depression. These reviewers found indication that professional or social support may help the treatment of postpartum depression. Professional or social support included emotional support, individual or group counseling, home or clinic visits, or telephone support networks. Although medication is the standard treatment for postpartum depression, compliance is often poor. Social support may provide an alternative or complementary approach to medication for some women.

Only a few studies have examined the transfer of antidepressants in breast milk. Those that were reviewed indicate that concentrations of antidepressants in either the breast milk or serum of breastfed infants are very low or undetectable. The majority of reports suggest minimal risk of toxicity in infants, but more study is needed to ensure long-term safety.

Implications

Mothers who are moderately or severely depressed in the postpartum period should seek professional evaluation and will likely be prescribed an antidepressant regimen. You can reassure the mother that it is unlikely that antidepressants have a negative effect on the baby, even when the mother is breastfeeding. Encourage compliance with the treatment plan. Because social isolation may contribute to depression, the provision of formal professional or social support interventions may complement the medical management of postpartum depression.

Critical Thinking

What signs and symptoms indicate that your patient may be experiencing postpartum depression? What resources are available for your patients to get professional or social support in the postpartum period?

References

Brigham and Women's Hospital. (2001). *Depression: A guide to diagnosis and treatment.* Boston, MA: Author.

Ray, K. L., & Hodnett, E. D. (2003). Caregiver support for postpartum depression (Cochrane Review). In: *The Cochrane Library,* Issue 4. Chichester, UK: John Wiley & Sons.

---

from postpartum depression. Another tool is Beck's (2002) revised Postpartum Depression Predictors Inventory (PDPI-Revised). This tool is also a practical and simple screening checklist to use during routine care with all postpartum women to identify those who might be experiencing postpartum depression so that early management might be initiated (Table 25–8).

No matter which approach the nurse uses to assess for postpartum depression, enabling the woman's voice to be heard about her feelings of maternal role transition and how she is adjusting in this vulnerable time is of inestimable value (Hanna, Jarman, Savage et al., 2004). Listening to her story provides a critical emie (insider's) view of her circumstances as opposed to an etic (outsider's) view.

In providing daily care, observe the woman for objective signs of depression—anxiety, irritability, poor concentration, forgetfulness, sleep difficulties, appetite change, fatigue, and tearfulness—and listen for statements indicating feelings of failure and self-accusation. Note severity and duration of symptoms. Behavior and verbalizations that

are bizarre or seem to indicate a potential for violence against herself or others, including the infant, are reported as soon as possible for further evaluation.

Be aware that many normal physiologic changes of the puerperium are similar to symptoms of depression (lack of sexual interest, appetite change, fatigue). It is essential that observations be as specific and as objective as possible and that they be carefully documented.

Possible nursing diagnoses that may apply to a woman with a postpartum psychiatric disorder include the following:

- *Ineffective Individual Coping* related to postpartum depression
- *Risk for Altered Parenting* related to postpartal mental illness

PLANNING AND IMPLEMENTATION

Nurses working in antepartal settings or teaching childbirth classes play indispensable roles in helping prospective

TABLE 25–7 ❖ Edinburgh Postnatal Depression Scale

In the past 7 days:

1. I have been able to laugh and see the funny side of things
   - As much as I always could
   - Not quite so much now
   - Definitely not so much now
   - Not at all

2. I have looked forward with enjoyment of things
   - As much as I ever did
   - Rather less than I used to
   - Definitely less than I used to
   - Hardly at all

*3. I have blamed myself unnecessarily when things went wrong
   - Yes, most of the time
   - Yes, some of the time
   - Not very often
   - No, never

4. I have been anxious or worried for no good reason
   - No, not at all
   - Hardly ever
   - Yes, sometimes
   - Yes, very often

*5. I have felt scared or panicky for no very good reason
   - Yes, quite a lot
   - Yes, sometimes
   - No, not much
   - No, not at all

*6. Things have been getting on top of me
   - Yes, most of the time I haven't been able to cope at all
   - Yes, sometimes I haven't been coping as well as usual
   - No, I have been coping quite well
   - No, I have been coping as well as ever

*7. I have been so unhappy that I have had difficulty sleeping
   - Yes, most of the time
   - Yes, sometimes
   - Not very often
   - No, not at all

*8. I have felt sad or miserable
   - Yes, most of the time
   - Yes, quite often
   - Not very often
   - No, not at all

*9. I have been so unhappy that I have been crying
   - Yes, most of the time
   - Yes, quite often
   - Only occasionally
   - No, never

*10. The thought of harming myself has occurred to me
   - Yes, quite often
   - Sometimes
   - Hardly ever
   - Never

Note: Response categories are scored 0, 1, 2, and 3 according to increased severity of the symptoms. Items marked with an asterisk are reverse scored (3, 2, 1, 0). The total score is calculated by adding together the scores for each of the 10 items. A score above the threshold of 12–13 out of 30 indicates, with 86% sensitivity, that the woman is suffering from postpartum depression.

Cox, J. L., Holden, J. M., & Sagovsky, R. (1987). Detection of postnatal depression: Development of the 10-item Edinburgh Postnatal Depression Scale. *British Journal of Psychiatry,* 150, 782–786. Users may reproduce the scale without further permission provided they respect copyright by quoting the names of the authors, the title, and the source of the paper in all reproduced copies.

parents appreciate the lifestyle changes and role demands of parenthood. Offering realistic information and anticipatory guidance and debunking myths about the perfect mother or perfect newborn may help prevent postpartum depression. Social support teaching guides are available for nurses to help postpartum women explore their needs for postpartum support. Alert the mother, spouse, and other family members to the possibility of postpartum blues in the early days after birth, and reassure them of the short-term nature of the condition. Describe symptoms of postpartum depression and encourage the mother to call her healthcare provider if symptoms become severe, if they fail to subside quickly, or if at any time she feels she is unable to function. Encouraging the mother to plan how she will manage at home and providing concrete suggestions on how to cope aid in her adjustment to motherhood. Table 25–9 provides suggestions that serve as primary prevention measures for postpartum depression.

Nursing Care in the Community

Home visits, especially for early-discharge families, are essential to fostering positive adjustments for the new family constellation. Telephone follow-up at 3 weeks postpartum to ask whether the mother is experiencing difficulties is also helpful.

If a woman presents with either three symptoms or one symptom that is present for 3 days, it may signal serious depression and requires immediate referral to a mental health professional. Also make an immediate referral if the mother has rejected the infant or threatened or been aggressive against the infant. In such cases the newborn is never left unattended with the mother. Depression does appear to interfere with optimal mothering; there is less interaction between mother and child, an increased incidence of mood and cognitive development problems, and more visits to the doctor in these children (Beck, 2002).

TABLE 25–8 ✢ **Postpartum Depression Predictors Inventory (PDPI)—Revised and Guide Questions for Its Use**

During Pregnancy

Marital Status	Check One	
1. Single	0	
2. Married/cohabitating	0	
3. Separated	0	
4. Divorced	0	
5. Widowed	0	
6. Partnered	0	

Socioeconomic status		
Low	0	
Middle	0	
High	0	

Self-esteem	Yes	No
Do you feel good about yourself as a person?	0	0
Do you feel worthwhile?	0	0
Do you feel you have a number of good qualities as a person?	0	0

Prenatal depression		
1. Have you felt depressed during your pregnancy?	0	0
If yes, when and how long have you been feeling this way?		
If yes, how mild or severe would you consider your depression?		

Prenatal anxiety		
Have you been feeling anxious during your pregnancy?	0	0
If yes, how long have you been feeling this way?		

Unplanned/unwanted pregnancy		
Was the pregnancy planned?	0	0
Is the pregnancy unwanted?	0	0

History of previous depression		
1. Before this pregnancy, have you ever been depressed?	0	0
If yes, when did you experience this depression?		
If yes, have you been under a physician's care for this past depression?	0	0
If yes, did the physician prescribe any medication for your depression?	0	0

Social support		
1. Do you feel you receive adequate emotional support from your partner?	0	0
2. Do you feel you receive adequate instrumental support from your partner (e.g., help with household chores or baby-sitting)?	0	0
3. Do you feel you can rely on your partner when you need help?	0	0
4. Do you feel you can confide in your partner? (repeat same questions for family and again for friends)	0	0

Marital satisfaction		
1. Are you satisfied with your marriage (or living arrangement)?	0	0
2. Are you currently experiencing any marital problems?	0	0
3. Are things going well between you and your partner?	0	0

Life stress		
1. Are you currently experiencing any stressful events in your life such as:		
financial problems	0	0
marital problems	0	0
death in the family	0	0
serious illness in the family	0	0
moving	0	0
unemployment	0	0
job change	0	0

TABLE 25–8 ❖ **Postpartum Depression Predictors Inventory (PDPI)—Revised and Guide Questions for Its Use—continued**

After delivery, add the following items

	Yes	No
Child care stress		
1. Is your infant experiencing any health problems?	O	O
2. Are you having problems with your baby feeding?	O	O
3. Are you having problems with your baby sleeping?	O	O
Infant temperament		
1. Would you consider your baby irritable or fussy?	O	O
2. Does your baby cry a lot?	O	O
3. Is your baby difficult to console or soothe?	O	O
Maternity blues		
1. Did you experience a brief period of tearfulness and mood swings during the first week after delivery?	O	O

Comments:

_____

_____

_____

A diagnosis of postpartum depression or other psychiatric disorder poses major problems for the family, especially the father. The symptoms of these disorders are difficult to witness and may be harder to understand than physical problems such as hemorrhage and infection. The father may feel hurt by his partner's hostility, worry that she is becoming insane, or be baffled by her mood swings and lack of concern about herself, the newborn, or household responsibilities. Very real practical matters—running the household, managing the children, caring for the totally dependent newborn,

---

TABLE 25–9 ❖ **Primary Prevention Strategies for Postpartum Depression**

1. Celebrate childbirth but appreciate that it is a life-changing transition that can be stressful—at times it can seem overwhelming. Share your feelings with each other and/or others.

2. Consider keeping a journal where you write down feelings. Not only is it emotionally cathartic, but it provides a great memory book.

3. Appreciate that you do not have to know everything to be a good parent—it is okay to seek advice during this transition.

4. Connect to others who are parents—use them as a support and information network.

5. Set a daily schedule and follow it even if you do not feel like it. Structuring activity helps counteract inertia that comes with feeling sad or unsettled.

6. Prioritize daily tasks. Decide what must be done and what can wait. Try to get one major thing done every day. Remember, you do not always have to look like a magazine fashion model.

7. Remember that you do not have to entertain or care for everyone who drops by. Doing something for someone else, however, often tends to make you feel better.

8. If someone volunteers to help you with tasks or baby care, take them up on it. While your volunteer is in action, do something pleasurable or get some rest.

9. Maintain outside interests. Plan some time every day—even if it's just 15 minutes—to do something exclusively for "you" that is pleasurable.

10. Eat a healthful diet. Limit alcohol. Quit smoking. Get some exercise. (All of these can positively affect the immune system.)

11. Get as much sleep as possible. Rest whenever you can, such as when the baby is napping. If you have other young children, bring them onto your bed to read or play quietly while you lie down.

12. Limit major changes (moves, job changes, etc.) the first year insofar as possible.

13. Spend time with others.

14. If things get overwhelming, and you feel yourself slipping into depression, reach out to someone for help.

15. Attend a postpartum support group if one is available. Consider also an international program:

Postpartum Support International
927 North Kellogg Avenue
Santa Barbara, CA 93111
1-805-967-7636 or online at http://www.postpartum.net

and caring for the mother—may be added to his usual routines and work responsibilities. It is not surprising that, even in the most supportive families, relationships may suffer in response to these circumstances. It is often the father or another close family member who in desperation makes contact with the healthcare agency. This is especially difficult when the mother is reluctant to admit she is suffering emotional difficulty or is too ill to recognize her own needs.

Information, emotional support, and assistance in providing or obtaining care for the infant may be needed. Help family members by identifying community resources and making referrals to public health nursing services and social services. Postpartum follow-up and visits from a psy-

chiatric home health nurse are especially important.

EVALUATION

Expected outcomes of nursing care include the following:

- The woman's signs of depression are identified and she receives therapy quickly.

- The newborn is cared for effectively by the father or another support person until the mother is able to participate more fully.

Critical Concept Review

LEARNING OBJECTIVES

CONCEPTS

Describe assessment of the postpartum woman for predisposing factors, onset, signs, and symptoms of various postpartum complications.

1. Predisposing factors for complications:
   - Overdistention of uterus due to a large baby, multiple gestation, or multiparity.
   - Rapid or prolonged labor.
   - Oxytocin induction of labor.
   - Precipitous delivery.
   - C-section.
   - PROM.
   - Urinary catheterization.
2. Nursing assessments include:
   - Frequent fundal checks and massage of fundus if bogginess is detected.
   - Frequent perineal pad checks.
   - Prevention of overdistention of the bladder.
   - Frequent vital sign assesments.
   - Assessment for Homans' sign each shift.
   - Inspection of the perineum and breasts each shift.
   - Assessment for signs of postpartum "blues" or depression.
3. Signs and symptoms:
   - Postpartum hemorrhage: excessive vaginal bleeding.
   - Infection: fever, purulent discharge from vagina or incision, burning during urination, redness and pain in the breast about fourth postpartum week.
   - Thrombophlebitis: pain and swelling in the lower extremities.
   - Postpartum depression: feelings of overwhelming sadness and lack of desire to care for infant.

Summarize the preventive measures for various complications of the postpartum period that should be incorporated into nursing care of the postpartum woman.

1. To prevent complications the nurse will:
   - Assess fundus for signs of bogginess.
   - Assess perineal pads for excessive bleeding.
   - Assess incisions for signs of infection.
   - Assess bladder for signs of distention and encourage woman to void frequently.
   - Use good handwashing techniques to prevent transmission of infective material.
   - Assess breasts for cracking, plugged ducts, and signs of mastitis. Teach mother proper latching-on techniques and breast care.
   - Assess lower extremities for signs of thrombophlebitis, encourage early ambulation, and assess for pulmonary embolus.
   - Assess woman for signs of depression.

LEARNING OBJECTIVES

CONCEPTS

List the causes of and appropriate nursing interventions for hemorrhage during the postpartal period.

1. The main causes of postpartum hemorrhage and the appropriate nursing interventions include:
   - Uterine atony: perform fundal massage and check for clots.
   - Laceration of vagina and cervix (suspect if mother is bleeding heavily in presence of firmly contracted fundus): contact physician to suture the laceration.
   - Retained placental fragments (suspect if client is bleeding, fundus is firm and no lacerations are present): thoroughly inspect placenta.
   - Subinvolution (usually occurs 1–2 weeks after birth): provide mother with discharge instructions, including information about possible complications.

Develop a nursing care plan that reflects a knowledge of etiology, pathophysiology, and current medical management for the woman experiencing postpartum hemorrhage, reproductive tract infection, urinary tract infection, mastitis, thromboembolic disease, or a postpartal psychiatric disorder.

1. Nursing care for the postpartal woman experiencing postpartum complications includes:
   - Thorough nursing history for any predisposing factors.
   - Frequent assessments of all body systems to detect signs and symptoms of complications. These assessments include:
     - Vital signs.
     - Fundal checks.
     - Lochial flow.
     - Perineum.
     - All incisions.
     - Homans' sign.
     - Breasts and nipples.
     - Emotional status.
     - Discharge teaching that includes ongoing medical management and self-care measures, signs and symptoms of further complications.

Evaluate the woman's knowledge of self-care measures, signs of complications to be reported to the primary care provider, and measures to prevent recurrence of complications.

1. Teaching for self care includes:
   - Knowledge of progress of involution.
   - Care of the breasts.
   - Prevention of infection.
   - Expected emotional changes.
   - Need for extra rest.
   - Nutritional needs.
   - Knowledge of dosage regimens and side effects of prescribed medication.
   - Signs and symptoms of complications:
     - Increased vaginal bleeding.
     - Fever.
     - Foul smelling vaginal discharge.
     - Pain and/or redness in an incision.
     - Pain, redness, or swelling in the breasts and/or legs.
     - Overwhelming feelings of sadness or inability to care for infant.

CRITICAL THINKING IN ACTION

*View the **Critical Thinking in Action** video in Chapter 25 of the CD-ROM. Then, answer the questions that follow.*

Betty Jones, a 32-year-old G4 P2012, is admitted to the postpartum unit after a precipitous birth of a preterm (35 weeks' gestation) 4 pound baby girl followed by a postpartum tubal ligation. Betty's vital signs and postpartum assessment are within normal limits. She has an abdominal dressing which is dry and intact and she is able to void. Her IV with 10 units of Pitocin is infusing well in her lower left arm. She admits to 3 on a pain scale of 10. Betty admits to active use of crack cocaine throughout her pregnancy, and smoked it most recently 5 hours before she gave birth. She is HIV positive with a CD_4 count of 726 cells/mm^3 and was treated with zidovudine during the pregnancy, labor, and birth. She also has a history of genital herpes and had been treated for chlamydia during the pregnancy. Her infant has been admitted to the special care nursery because of her preterm status. Betty anticipates her baby will be taken into foster care when discharged from the nursery. Wishing to establish as much of a relationship with her infant as possible before that happens, she asks if she can breastfeed the baby while she is in the hospital.

1. What is your response to Betty's request to breastfeed her infant?
2. Over the course of the first postpartum day, Betty appears lethargic and spends most of her time sleeping. After her evening visitors leave, you observe that she is highly energetic and excitable. Would urine testing be useful to help determine if Betty has used cocaine this evening?
3. Discuss supportive nursing care for infants born of HIV-positive mothers.
4. Betty wishes for an early discharge from the hospital. What physical criteria must be met before leaving the hospital?
5. Discuss when she should contact her physician/CNM after her discharge.

MEDIALINK

www.prenhall.com/london

- NCLEX-RN® Review, case studies, and other interactive resources for this chapter can be found on the Companion Website at http://www.prenhall.com/london. Click on "Chapter 25" to select the activities for this chapter.

- For animations, more NCLEX-RN® Review questions, and an audio glossary, access the accompanying CD-ROM in this textbook.

REFERENCES

American Psychiatric Association. (2000). *Diagnostic and statistical manual of mental disorders: DSM-IV-TR* (4th ed., text rev.). Washington, DC: Author.

Aronson, M. P., Chelmow, D., & Lee, S. B. (2003). Intraoperative and postoperative complications of gynecologic surgery. In A. H. DeCherney & L. Nathan (Eds.), *Current obstetrics & gynecologic: Diagnosis & treatment* (9th ed., pp. 838–855). New York: Lange Medical Books/McGraw-Hill.

Beck, C. T. (2001). Predictors of postpartum depression: An update. *Nursing Research, 50,* 275–285.

Beck, C. T. (2002). Revision of the postpartum depression predictors inventory. *Journal of Obstetric, Gynecologic, and Neonatal Nursing, 31*(4), 394–402.

Gibbs, R. S., Sweet, R. L., & Duff, W. P. (2004). Maternal and fetal infectious disorders. In R. K. Creasy & R. Resnik (Eds.), *Maternal-fetal medicine: Principles and practice* (5th ed., pp. 741–800). Philadelphia: Saunders.

Gilbert, E. S., & Harmon, J. S. (2003). *Manual of high risk pregnancy and delivery* (3rd ed.). St. Louis, MO: Mosby.

Haessler, A., & Rosenthal, M. B. (2003). Psychological aspects of obstetrics & gynecology. In

A. H. DeCherney & L. Nathan (Eds.), *Current obstetrics & gynecologic: Diagnosis & treatment* (9th ed., pp. 1066–1086). New York: Lange Medical Books/McGraw-Hill.

Hanna, B., Jarman, H., Savage, S., & Layton, K. (2004). The early detection of postpartum depression: Midwives and nurses trial a checklist. *Journal of Obstetric, Gynecologic, and Neonatal Nursing, 33*(2), 191–208.

Laros, R. K. (2004). Thromboembolic disease. In R. K. Creasy & R. Resnik (Eds.), *Maternal-fetal medicine: Principles and practice* (5th ed., pp. 845–857). Philadelphia: Saunders.

Matteson, P. S. (2001). *Women's health during the childbearing years: A community-based approach.* St. Louis, MO: C.V. Mosby.

Minkoff, H. L., & Gibbs, R. S. (2003). Obstetric and perinatal infections. In J. R. Scott, R. S. Gibbs, B. Y. Karlan, & A. F. Haney (Eds.), *Danforth's obstetrics and gynecology* (9th ed., pp. 339–364). Philadelphia: Lippincott Williams & Wilkins.

Newton, E. R. (2003). Antibiotics in maternal-fetal medicine. In J. J. Sciarri (Ed.), *Gynecology and obstetrics* (Vol. 3, pp. 1–34). Philadelphia: Lippincott Williams & Wilkins.

Parry, B. L. (2004). Management of depression and psychoses during pregnancy and the puerperium. In R. K. Creasy & R. Resnik (Eds.), *Maternal-fetal medicine: Principles and practice* (5th ed., pp. 1193–1200). Philadelphia: Saunders.

Poggi, S. B. H., & Kapernick, P. S. (2003). Postpartum hemorrhage & the abnormal puerperium. In A. H. DeCherney & L. Nathan (Eds.), *Current obstetrics & gynecologic: Diagnosis & treatment* (9th ed., pp. 531–552). New York: Lange Medical Books/McGraw-Hill.

Reid, G., & Bocking, A. (2003). The potential for probiotics to prevent bacterial vaginosis and preterm labor. *American Journal of Obstetrics and Gynecology, 189*(4), 1202–1208.

Shevell, T., & Malone, F. D. (2003). Management of obstetric hemorrhage. *Seminars in Perinatology, 27*(1), 86–104.

Zajac, P. M. (2004). Going with the flow: Warfarin. *Nursing Made Incredibly Easy, 2*(4), 52–57.

The Physiologic Responses of the Newborn to Birth

I remember clearly when they held him up for us to see and my husband and I cried and laughed and it was so amazing. He was 9 1/2 pounds and was so beautiful. Even though my labor was long, his Apgars were high, and he didn't even cry—not until we dressed him, anyway.

—Crystal, 26

LEARNING OBJECTIVES

- Summarize the respiratory and cardiovascular changes that occur during the transition to extrauterine life and during stabilization.

- Describe how various factors affect the newborn's blood values.

- Correlate the major mechanisms of heat loss in the newborn to the process of thermogenesis in the newborn.

- Explain the steps involved in the conjugation and excretion of bilirubin in the newborn.

- Discuss the reasons a newborn may develop jaundice.

- Describe the functional abilities of the newborn's gastrointestinal tract and liver.

- Identify three reasons a newborn's kidneys have difficulty in maintaining fluid and electrolyte balance.

- List the immunologic responses available to the newborn.

- Explain the physiologic and behavioral responses of newborns during the periods of reactivity and identify possible interventions.

- Describe the normal sensory-perceptual abilities and behavioral states seen in the newborn period.

MEDIALINK

www.prenhall.com/london

CD-ROM

NCLEX-RN® Review
Skill 5-1: Performing Nasal Pharyngeal Suctioning
Audio Glossary

Companion Website

NCLEX-RN® Review
Case Study: Newborn Responses to Birth

The newborn period includes the time from birth through the 28th day of life. During this period the newborn adjusts from intrauterine to extrauterine life. The nurse needs to be knowledgeable about a newborn's normal physiologic and behavioral adaptations and to recognize alterations from normal.

The first few hours of life, in which the newborn stabilizes respiratory and circulatory functions, are called **neonatal transition**. All other newborn body systems change their level of functioning and become established over a longer period of time during the neonatal period.

RESPIRATORY ADAPTATIONS

To begin life as a separate being, the baby must begin to breathe immediately, establishing respiratory gas exchange in conjunction with marked circulatory changes. These radical and rapid changes are crucial to extrauterine life.

INTRAUTERINE FACTORS SUPPORTING RESPIRATORY FUNCTION

Even before the significant respiratory events that occur at birth, certain intrauterine factors also enhance the newborn's ability to breathe. Adequate fetal lung development allows the newborn to expand its lungs and exchange oxygen and carbon dioxide gases. Even before birth the fetus practices breathing movements, which allow it to breathe immediately after birth.

Fetal Lung Development

The respiratory system is in an ongoing state of development during fetal life, and lung development continues into early childhood. During the first 20 weeks' gestation, development is limited to the differentiation of pulmonary, vascular, and lymphatic structures.

At 20 to 24 weeks, alveolar ducts begin to appear, followed by primitive alveoli at 24 to 28 weeks. During this time the alveolar epithelial cells begin to differentiate into type I cells (structures necessary for gas exchange) and type II cells (structures that provide for the synthesis and storage of surfactant). **Surfactant** is a mixture of surface-active phospholipids (lecithin and sphingomyelin), which are critical for alveolar stability. At 28 to 32 weeks' gestation, the number of type II cells increases further, and surfactant is produced by a choline pathway within them. Surfactant production by this pathway peaks at about 35 weeks' gestation and remains high until term, paralleling late fetal lung development. At this time the lungs are structurally developed enough to permit maintenance of lung expansion and adequate exchange of gases.

Clinically the peak production of lecithin corresponds closely with a marked decrease in the incidence of respiratory distress syndrome for babies born after 35 weeks' gestation. Production of sphingomyelin (another component of surfactant) remains constant throughout gestation. The newborn born before the lecithin/sphingomyelin (L/S) ratio is 2:1 will have varying degrees of respiratory distress. (See discussion of L/S ratio, "Respiratory Distress Syndrome," in Chapter 31. ∞)

Fetal Breathing Movements

The newborn's ability to breathe air immediately after its birth appears to result from weeks of intrauterine practice. In this respect, breathing can be seen as a continuation of an intrauterine process; the lungs convert from a fluid-filled organ to an air-filled organ capable of gas exchange.

Fetal breathing movements (FBMs) occur as early as 11 weeks' gestation (see "Biophysical Profile" in Chapter 16 for discussion ∞). These breathing movements are essential for developing the chest wall muscles and the diaphragm. To a lesser extent, they regulate lung fluid volume and resulting lung growth.

INITIATION OF BREATHING

To maintain life the newborn's lungs must function immediately after birth. Two radical changes must take place for the lungs to function:

1. Pulmonary ventilation must be established through lung expansion following birth.

2. A marked increase in the pulmonary circulation must occur.

The first breath of life—the gasp in response to mechanical and reabsorptive, chemical, thermal, and sensory changes associated with birth—starts the serial opening of the alveoli.

So begins the transition from a fluid-filled environment to an air-breathing, independent, extrauterine life. Figure 26–1 ● summarizes the initiation of respiration.

During the latter half of gestation, the fetal lungs continuously produce fluid. This fluid expands the lungs almost completely, filling the air spaces. Some of the lung fluid moves up into the trachea and out into the amniotic fluid.

Production of lung fluid diminishes 2 to 4 days before labor, and fetal breathing movements decrease 24 to 36 hours before the onset of labor (Laughlin & Knuppel, 2003). However, approximately 80 to 100 mL of fluid remains in the respiratory passages of a normal full-term newborn at birth. It must be removed from the lungs to permit adequate movement of air (Polin, Fox, & Abman, 2004).

As the fetus experiences labor, there is a fetal gasp and active exhalation that initiates the removal of fluid from the lungs (Polin et al., 2004). During birth the fetal chest is compressed, increasing intrathoracic pressure and squeezing a small amount of fluid out of the lungs. After the birth of the newborn's trunk, the chest wall recoils.

● **FIGURE 26–1**

Initiation of respiration in the newborn.

This chest recoil creates an empty space in the chest, causing negative intrathoracic pressure. The negative pressure in the chest is thought to produce a small, passive inspiration of air that replaces the fluid that is squeezed out. The significance of the "thoracic squeeze" is controversial, and it is now thought that the process of labor is primarily responsible for the initial movement of lung fluid out of the lungs (Polin et al., 2004).

After this first inspiration, the newborn exhales, with crying, against a partially closed glottis, creating positive intrathoracic pressure. The high positive intrathoracic pressure distributes the inspired air throughout the alveoli and begins to establish *functional residual capacity (FRC),* the air left in the lungs at the end of a normal expiration. The higher intrathoracic pressure also increases absorption of fluid via the capillaries and lymphatic system. The negative intrathoracic pressure created when the diaphragm moves down with inspiration causes lung fluid to flow from the alveoli across the alveolar membranes into the pulmonary interstitial tissue.

At birth the alveolar epithelium is temporarily more permeable. This, combined with decreased cellular resistance at the onset of breathing, may facilitate passive liquid absorption. With each succeeding breath, the lungs continue to expand. Protein molecules are too large to pass through capillary walls. The presence of more protein molecules in the pulmonary capillaries than in the interstitial tissue creates oncotic pressure. This pressure draws the interstitial fluid into the capillaries and lymphatic tissue to balance the concentration of protein. Lung expansion helps the remaining lung fluid move into the interstitial tissue. Pulmonary blood flow increases as pulmonary vascular resistance decreases, and more interstitial tissue fluid is absorbed into the bloodstream. In the healthy term newborn, lung fluid moves rapidly into the interstitial tissue but may take several hours to move into the lymph and blood vessels. Most of the lung fluid is reabsorbed within 2 hours after birth, and it is completely absorbed within 12 to 24 hours after birth (Polin et al., 2004).

Although the initial chest recoil assists in clearing fluid from the airways and permits further inspiration, most clinicians believe mucus and fluid should be suctioned from the newborn's mouth, nose, and throat. They may use a bulb syringe or mucus trap attached to suction as soon as the newborn's head and shoulders are born and again as the newborn adapts to extrauterine life and stabilizes (see Skill 5–1). **SKILLS**

Newborns may have problems clearing the fluid in lungs and beginning respiration for a variety of reasons:

- The lymphatic system may be underdeveloped, decreasing the rate at which the fluid is absorbed from the lungs.
- Complications that occur before or during labor and birth can interfere with adequate lung expansion and cause failure to decrease pulmonary vascular resistance,

resulting in decreased pulmonary blood flow. These complications include inadequate compression of the chest wall in a very small newborn, the absence of chest wall compression in a newborn born by cesarean birth, respiratory depression due to maternal anesthesia, or aspiration of amniotic fluid or meconium.

Chemical Stimuli

An important chemical stimulator that contributes to the onset of breathing is temporary asphyxia of the fetus and newborn. The first breath is an inspiratory gasp triggered by elevation in PCO_2 and decrease in pH and PO_2, the natural result of a normal vaginal birth with cessation of placental gas exchange when the cord is clamped.

These changes, present in all newborns to some degree, stimulate the aortic and carotid chemoreceptors, initiating impulses that trigger the brain's respiratory center. Although this brief period of asphyxia is a significant stimulator, prolonged asphyxia is abnormal and depresses respiration.

Thermal Stimuli

A significant decrease in environmental temperature after birth, 37°C to 21°C–23.9°C (98.6°F to 70°F–75°F), results in sudden chilling of the moist newborn (Cheffer, 2004). The cold stimulates skin nerve endings, and the newborn responds with rhythmic respirations. Normal temperature changes at birth are apparently within acceptable physiologic limits. However, excessive cooling may cause profound depression and evidence of cold stress (see "Care of the Newborn with Cold Stress" in Chapter 31 for discussion of cold stress ∞).

Sensory Stimuli

During intrauterine life the fetus is in a dark, sound-dampened, fluid-filled environment and is nearly weightless. After birth the newborn experiences light, sounds, and the effects of gravity for the first time. As the fetus moves from a familiar, comfortable, quiet environment to one of sensory abundance, a number of physical and sensory influences help respiration begin. They include the numerous tactile, auditory, and visual stimuli of birth.

NURSING PRACTICE

Historically, slapping the buttocks or heels of the newborn was a common way to stimulate breathing, but today the emphasis is on gentle physical contact. Thoroughly dry the newborn and place the baby in skin-to-skin contact with the mother's chest and abdomen. This will provide ample stimulation in a far more comforting way and also decrease heat loss.

FACTORS OPPOSING THE FIRST BREATH

Three major factors may oppose the initiation of respiratory activity: (1) the contracting force between alveoli—called *alveolar surface tension;* (2) the viscosity of lung fluid within the respiratory tract, which is influenced by surfactant levels; and (3) how easily the lung is able to fill with air—called *lung compliance.*

Alveolar surface tension is the contracting force between the moist surfaces of the alveoli. This tension is necessary for healthy respiratory function but would cause the small airways and alveoli to collapse between each inspiration if surfactant were not present.

Surfactant is important because it reduces the attracting force between alveoli. This prevents the alveoli from completely collapsing with each expiration and thus promotes lung expansion. Similarly, surfactant promotes lung compliance, the ability of the lung to fill with air easily. When surfactant decreases, compliance also decreases, and the pressure needed to expand the alveoli with air increases.

Resistive forces of the fluid-filled lung, combined with the small radii of the airways, mean that 30 to 40 cm of water pressure are needed to open the lung initially (Thureen, Deacon, Hernandez et al., 2005). The first breath usually establishes functional residual capacity (FRC) that is 30% to 40% of the fully expanded lung volume. This FRC allows alveolar sacs to remain partially expanded on expiration, decreasing the need for continuous high pressures for each of the following breaths. Subsequent breaths require only 6 to 8 cm of water pressure to open alveoli during inspiration. Therefore, the first breath of life is usually the most difficult.

CARDIOPULMONARY PHYSIOLOGY

The onset of respiration stimulates cardiovascular system changes necessary for successful transition to extrauterine life, hence the term **cardiopulmonary adaptation.** As air enters the lungs, Po_2 rises in the alveoli, relaxing the pulmonary arteries and triggering a decrease in pulmonary vascular resistance. As pulmonary vascular resistance decreases, the vascular flow in the lung increases rapidly and achieves 100% normal flow at 24 hours of life. The delivery of greater blood volume to the lungs contributes to the conversion from fetal circulation to newborn circulation.

After pulmonary circulation is established, blood is distributed throughout the lung, although the alveoli may or may not be fully open. For adequate oxygenation to occur, the heart must deliver sufficient blood to functional, open alveoli. Shunting of blood is common in the early newborn period. Bidirectional blood flow, or right-to-left shunting through the ductus arteriosus, may divert a sig-

nificant amount of blood away from the lungs, depending on the pressure changes of respiration, crying, and the cardiac cycle. This shunting in the newborn period is also responsible for the unstable transitional period in cardiopulmonary function.

OXYGEN TRANSPORT

The transportation of oxygen to the peripheral tissues depends on the type of hemoglobin in the red blood cells. In the fetus and newborn, a variety of hemoglobins exist, the most significant being fetal hemoglobin (Hb F) and adult hemoglobin (Hb A). Approximately 70% to 90% of the hemoglobin in the fetus and newborn is of the fetal variety. The greatest difference between Hb F and Hb A is related to the transport of oxygen.

Since Hb F has a greater affinity for oxygen than does Hb A, the oxygen saturation in the newborn's blood is greater than in the adult's, but the amount of oxygen available to the tissues is less. This situation is beneficial prenatally, because the fetus must maintain adequate oxygen uptake in the presence of very low oxygen tension (umbilical venous Po_2 cannot exceed the uterine venous Po_2). This high concentration of oxygen in the blood makes hypoxia and signs of cyanosis in the newborn particularly difficult to recognize. In addition, alkalosis (increased pH) and hypothermia can result in less oxygen being available to the body tissues, whereas acidosis, hypercarbia, and hyperthermia can result in less oxygen being bound to hemoglobin and more oxygen being released to the body tissues.

MAINTAINING RESPIRATORY FUNCTION

The lung's ability to maintain oxygenation and ventilation (the exchange of oxygen and carbon dioxide) is influenced by such factors as lung compliance and airway resistance. Lung compliance is influenced by the elastic recoil of the lung tissue and anatomic differences in the newborn. The newborn has a relatively large heart and mediastinal structures that reduce available lung space. Also the newborn chest is equipped with weak intercostal muscles and a rigid rib cage with horizontal ribs and a high diaphragm, which restricts the space available for lung expansion. The large abdomen further encroaches on the high diaphragm to decrease lung space. Another factor that limits ventilation is airway resistance, which depends on the radii, length, and number of airways. Airway resistance is increased in the newborn when compared to the adult.

CHARACTERISTICS OF NEWBORN RESPIRATION

The normal newborn respiratory rate is 30 to 60 breaths per minute. Initial respirations may be largely diaphragmatic and shallow and irregular in depth and rhythm. The abdomen's movements are synchronous with the chest movements. When the breathing pattern includes pauses lasting 5 to 15 seconds, **periodic breathing** is occurring. Periodic breathing is rarely associated with differences in skin color or heart rate changes, and it has no prognostic significance. Tactile or other sensory stimulation increases the inspired oxygen and converts periodic breathing patterns to normal breathing patterns during neonatal transition. With deep sleep, the pattern is reasonably regular. Periodic breathing occurs with rapid-eye-movement (REM) sleep, and grossly irregular breathing is evident with motor activity, sucking, and crying. Cessation of breathing lasting more than 20 seconds is defined as *apnea* and is abnormal in term newborns. Apnea may or may not be associated with changes in skin color or heart rate (drop below 100 beats per minute). Apnea always needs to be further evaluated.

The newborn must breathe through the nose. Any obstruction will cause respiratory distress, so it is important to keep the nose and throat clear. Immediately after birth and for about the next 2 hours, respiratory rates of 60 to 70 breaths per minute are normal. Some cyanosis and acrocyanosis are normal for several hours; after that the infant's color improves steadily. If respirations drop below 30 or exceed 60 per minute when the infant is at rest, or if retractions, cyanosis, or nasal flaring and expiratory grunting occur, the clinician should be notified. Any increased use of the intercostal muscles (retractions) may indicate respiratory distress. (See "Respiratory Distress Syndrome" in Chapter 31 and Table 31–1 for signs of respiratory distress. ∞)

CARDIOVASCULAR ADAPTATIONS

As described earlier, the onset of respiration triggers increased blood flow to the lungs after birth. This greater blood volume contributes to the conversion from fetal circulation to neonatal circulation.

FETAL-NEWBORN TRANSITIONAL PHYSIOLOGY

During fetal life, blood with the higher oxygen content is diverted to the heart and brain. Blood in the descending aorta is less oxygenated and supplies the kidney and intestinal tract before it is returned to the placenta. Limited amounts of blood, pumped from the right ventricle toward the lungs, enter the pulmonary vessels. In the fetus, increased pulmonary resistance forces most of this blood through the ductus arteriosus into the descending aorta (Table 26–1). See the fetal heart animation on the CD-ROM ⊙.

Marked cardiovascular system changes occur at birth. Expansion of the lungs with the first breath decreases pulmonary vascular resistance and increases pulmonary blood flow. Pressure in the left atrium increases as blood returns

TABLE 26–1 ✤ Fetal and Neonatal Circulation

System	Fetal	Neonatal
Pulmonary blood vessels	Constricted, with very little blood flow; lungs not expanded	Vasodilation and increased blood flow; lungs expanded; increased oxygen stimulates vasodilation.
Systemic blood vessels	Dilated, with low resistance; blood mostly in placenta	Arterial pressure rises due to loss of placenta; increased systemic blood volume and resistance.
Ductus arteriosus	Large, with no tone; blood flow from pulmonary artery to aorta	Reversal of blood flow; now from aorta to pulmonary artery because of increased left atrial pressure. Ductus is sensitive to increased oxygen and body chemicals and begins to constrict.
Foramen ovale	Patent, with increased blood flow from right atrium to left atrium	Increased pressure in left atrium attempts to reverse blood flow and shuts one-way valve.

from the pulmonary veins. Pressure in the right atrium drops, and systematic vascular resistance increases as umbilical venous blood flow is halted when the cord is clamped. These physiologic mechanisms mark the transition from fetal to neonatal circulation and show the interplay of cardiovascular and respiratory systems (Figure 26–2 ⊙).

Five major areas of change occur in cardiopulmonary adaptation (Figure 26–3 ⊙):

1. **Increased aortic pressure and decreased venous pressure.** Clamping of the umbilical cord eliminates the placental vascular bed and reduces the intravascular space. Consequently, aortic (systemic) blood pressure increases. At the same time, blood return via the inferior vena cava decreases, resulting in a decreased right atrial pressure and a small decrease in pressure in the venous circulation.

2. **Increased systemic pressure and decreased pulmonary artery pressure.** With the loss of the low-resistance placenta, systemic resistance pressure increases, resulting in greater systemic pressure. At the same time, lung expansion increases pulmonary blood flow, and the increased blood PO_2 associated with initiation of respirations dilates pulmonary blood vessels. The combination of vasodilation and

● **FIGURE 26–2**

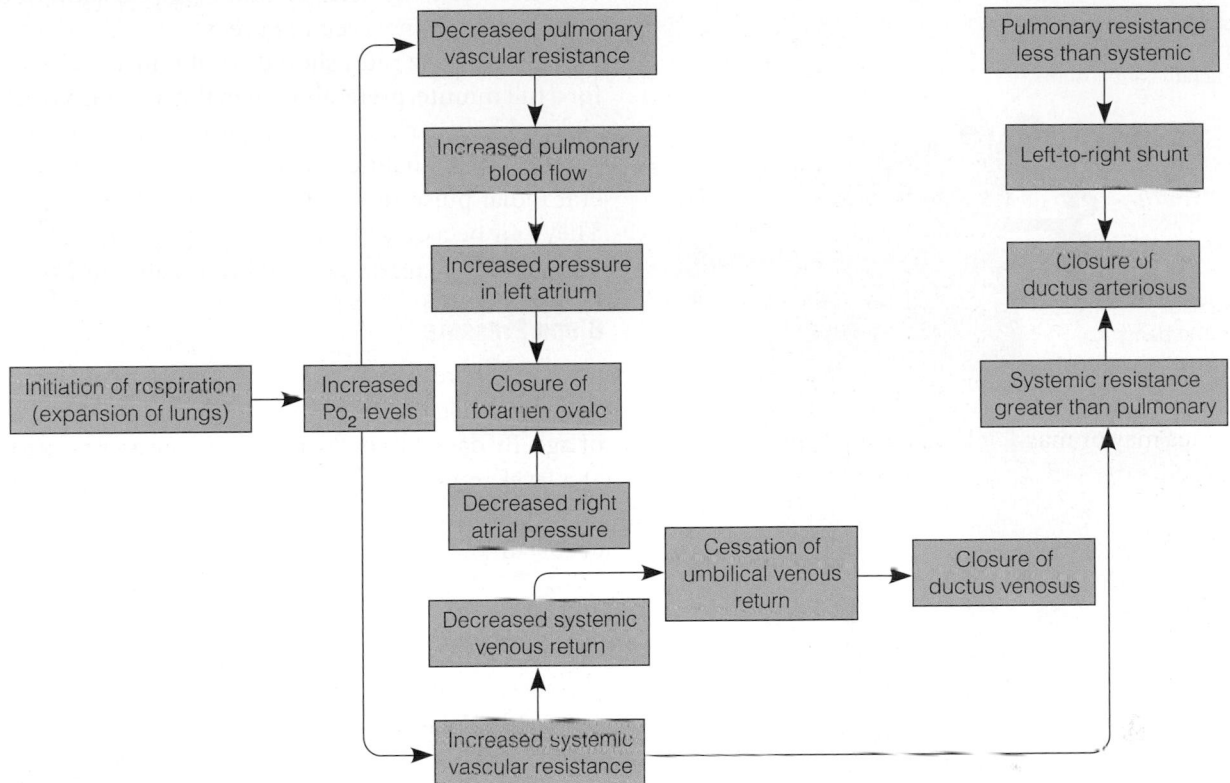

Transitional circulation: conversion from fetal to neonatal circulation.

increased pulmonary blood flow decreases pulmonary artery resistance. As the pulmonary vascular beds open, the systemic vascular pressure increases, enhancing perfusion of the other body systems.

3. **Closure of the foramen ovale.** Closure of the foramen ovale is a function of changing atrial pressures. In utero, pressure is greater in the right atrium, and the foramen ovale is open after birth. Decreased pulmonary resistance and increased pulmonary blood flow increase the pulmonary venous return into the left atrium, raising left atrial pressure slightly. The decreased pulmonary vascular resistance and the decreased umbilical venous return to the right atrium also lower right atrial pressure. The pressure gradients across the atria are now reversed, left atrial pressure is greater, and the foramen ovale is functionally closed 1 to 2 hours after birth. However, a slight right-to-left shunting may occur in the early newborn period. Any increase in pulmonary resistance or right atrial pressure, such as occurs with crying, acidosis, or cold stress, may cause the foramen ovale to reopen, resulting in a temporary right-to-left shunt. Permanent closure occurs within 6 months.

4. **Closure of the ductus arteriosus.** Initial elevation of the systemic vascular pressure above the pulmonary vascular pressure increases pulmonary blood flow by reversing the flow through the ductus arteriosus. Blood now flows from the aorta into the pulmonary artery. Furthermore, although oxygen causes the pulmonary arterioles to dilate, an increase in blood PO_2 triggers the opposite response in the ductus arteriosus—it constricts.

   In utero the placenta provides prostaglandin E_2 (PGE_2), which causes ductus vasodilation. With the loss of the placenta and increased pulmonary blood flow, PGE_2 levels drop, leaving the active constriction by PO_2 unopposed. If the lungs fail to expand or if PO_2 levels drop, the ductus remains patent. Fibrosis of the ductus occurs within 3 weeks after birth, but functional closure happens within 15 hours after birth (Blackburn, 2003).

5. **Closure of the ductus venosus.** Although the mechanism initiating closure of the ductus venosus is not known, it appears to be related to mechanical pressure changes after severing of the cord, redistribution of blood, and cardiac output. Closure

● FIGURE 26–3

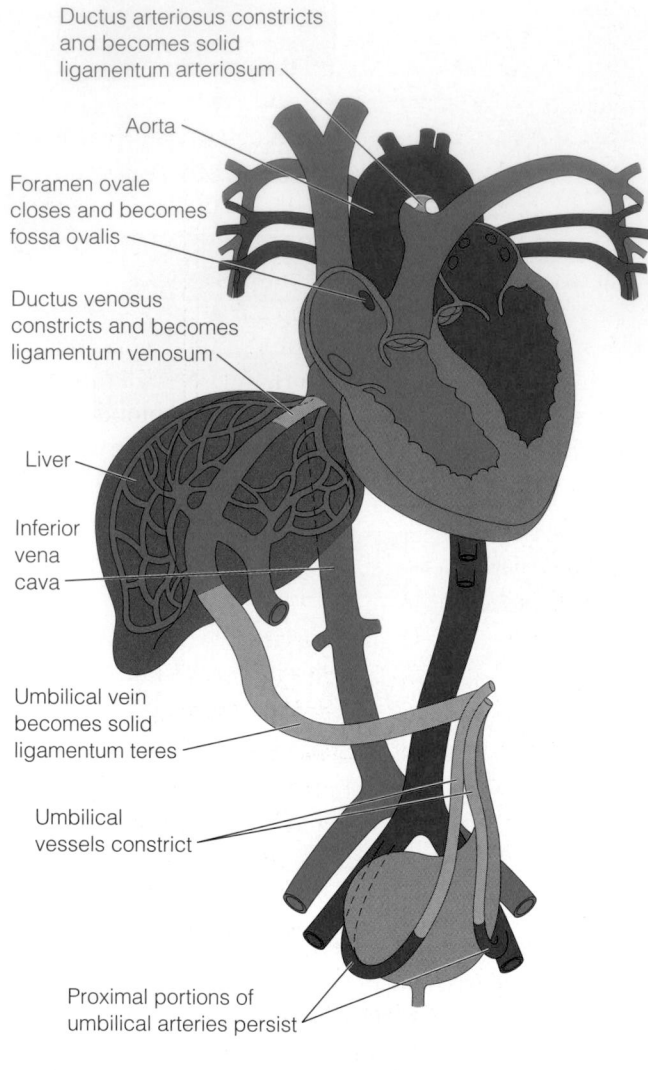

Ductus arteriosus constricts and becomes solid ligamentum arteriosum

Aorta

Foramen ovale closes and becomes fossa ovalis

Ductus venosus constricts and becomes ligamentum venosum

Liver

Inferior vena cava

Umbilical vein becomes solid ligamentum teres

Umbilical vessels constrict

Proximal portions of umbilical arteries persist

■ Blood high in oxygen

■ Blood low in oxygen

Major changes that occur in the newborn's circulatory system.

Used with permission from Hole, J. W. (1993). Human anatomy and physiology (6th ed.). Dubuque, IA: W. C. Brown. All rights reserved.

of the bypass forces perfusion of the liver. Fibrosis of the ductus venosus occurs within 2 months.

CHARACTERISTICS OF CARDIAC FUNCTION

Heart Rate

Shortly after the first cry and the start of changes in cardiopulmonary circulation, the newborn heart rate can accelerate to 180 beats per minute. The average resting heart rate in the first week of life is 120 to 160 beats per minute in a healthy full-term newborn, but it may vary signifi-

cantly during deep sleep or active awake states. In the full-term newborn, the heart rate may drop to a low of 80 beats per minute during sleep (Thureen et al., 2005).

Apical pulse rates should be obtained by auscultation for a full minute, preferably when the newborn is asleep. Peripheral pulses of all extremities should also be evaluated to detect any inequalities or unusual characteristics. Peripheral radial pulses are difficult to palpate in the newborn. They can be assessed when blood pressure is measured if blood pressure readings are taken on all four extremities.

Blood Pressure

The blood pressure tends to be highest immediately after birth and then descends to its lowest level at about 3 hours of age. By days 4 to 6, the blood pressure rises and plateaus at a level approximately the same as the initial level. Blood pressure is sensitive to the changes in blood volume that occur in the transition to newborn circulation (Figure 26–4 ●). Peripheral perfusion pressure is a particularly sensitive indicator of the newborn's ability to compensate for alterations in blood volume prior to changes in blood pressure. Capillary refill should be less than 2 to 3 seconds when the skin is blanched.

Blood pressure during the first 12 hours of life varies with the birth weight. The average mean blood pressure is 50 to 55 mm Hg in newborns over 3 kg during the first 12 hours of life (Thureen et al., 2005). Crying may cause an elevation of 20 mm Hg in both the systolic and diastolic blood pressure; thus, accuracy is more likely in the quiet newborn. The measurement of blood pressure is best obtained with the Doppler technique or a 1- to 2-inch cuff and a stethoscope over the brachial artery.

● FIGURE 26–4

Response of blood pressure (BP) to neonatal changes in blood volume.

Heart Murmurs

Murmurs are produced by turbulent blood flow. They may be heard when blood flows across an abnormal valve or across a stenosed valve, when there is an atrial or ventricular septal defect, or when there is increased flow across a normal valve. In newborns, 90% of all murmurs are transient and not associated with anomalies. Because of the current practice of early discharge, murmurs associated with ventricular septal defect and patent ductus arteriosus are not often picked up until the first well-baby checkup at 4 to 6 weeks of age. Murmurs are sometimes absent even in seriously malformed hearts.

Cardiac Workload

Before birth the right ventricle does approximately two thirds of the cardiac work, resulting in increased size and thickness of the right ventricle at birth. After birth the left ventricle must assume a larger share of the cardiac workload, and it progressively increases in size and thickness.

HEMATOPOIETIC SYSTEM

The hematopoietic system is responsible for the physiologic process of creating new blood cells. This process is called hematopoiesis. After birth the red blood cell (RBC) count gradually increases as cell size decreases. In the first days of life, hematocrit may rise 1 to 2 g/dL above fetal levels as a result of placental transfusion, low oral fluid intake, and diminished extracellular fluid volume. By 1 week postnatally, peripheral hemoglobin is comparable to fetal blood counts. The hemoglobin level declines progressively over the first 2 months of life (Polin et al., 2004). This initial decline in hemoglobin creates a phenomenon known as **physiologic anemia of infancy**. Nutritional status in the newborn stage is one factor that influences the degree of physiologic anemia later. Supplies of vitamin E, folic acid, and iron may be inadequate given the amount of growth in the later part of the first year of life. Hemoglobin values fall, mainly from a decrease in red cell mass rather than from the dilutional effect of increasing plasma volume.

The fact that red cell survival is lower in newborns than in adults, and that red cell production is less, also contributes to this anemia. Neonatal RBCs have a life span of 80 to 100 days, approximately two thirds the life span of adult RBCs.

Leukocytosis is a normal finding, because the stress of birth stimulates increased production of neutrophils during the first few days of life. Neutrophils then decrease to 35% of the total leukocyte count by 2 weeks of age. Eventually lymphocytes become the predominant type of leukocyte, and the total white blood cell count falls.

Blood volume of the term infant is estimated to be 80 mL/kg of body weight. For example, an 8-lb (3.6-kg) newborn has a blood volume of 290 mL. Blood volume varies with the amount of placental transfusion during the expulsion of the placenta, as well as other factors, including the following:

1. **Delayed cord clamping and the normal shift of plasma to the extravascular spaces.** Newborn hemoglobin and hematocrit values are higher when a placental transfusion occurs after birth. Placental vessels contain about 75 to 125 mL of blood at term, which can be transfused into the newborn by holding the newborn below the level of the placenta and delaying cord clamping. Blood volume increases by 50% with delayed cord clamping (Polin et al., 2004). The increase is reflected by a rise in hemoglobin level and an increase in the hematocrit. Cord blood provides the most accurate assessment of the newborn's initial hemoglobin and hematocrit.

2. **Gestational age.** There appears to be a positive association between gestational age, RBC numbers, and hemoglobin concentration.

3. **Prenatal or perinatal hemorrhage.** Significant prenatal or perinatal bleeding decreases the hematocrit level and causes hypovolemia.

4. **The site of the blood sample.** Hemoglobin and hematocrit levels are significantly higher in capillary blood than in venous blood. Sluggish peripheral blood flow creates RBC stasis, increasing RBC concentration in the capillaries. Consequently, blood samples from venous blood sites are more accurate than those from capillary sites.

The concentration of serum electrolytes in the blood indicates the fluid and electrolyte status of the newborn. See Table 26–2 for normal term newborn electrolyte and blood values.

TEMPERATURE REGULATION

Temperature regulation is the maintenance of thermal balance by losing heat to the environment at a rate equal to heat production. Newborns are *homeothermic;* they attempt to stabilize their internal (core) body temperatures within a range in spite of significant temperature variations in their environment.

Thermoregulation in the newborn can be closely related to the rate of metabolism and oxygen consumption. Within a specific environmental temperature range, called the **neutral thermal environment (NTE)**, the rates of oxygen consumption and metabolism are minimal, and internal body temperature is maintained because of thermal balance (Thureen et al., 2005). For an unclothed, full-term newborn, the NTE is an ambient environment temperature range of 32°C to 34°C (89.6°F to 93.2°F) within 50% relative

TABLE 26–2 ✤ Normal Term Newborn Cord Blood Values

Laboratory Data	Normal Range
Hemoglobin	14–20 g/dL
Hematocrit	43%–63%
WBC	10,000–30,000/mm^3
Neutrophils	40%–80%
Platelets	150,000–350,000/mm^3
Reticulocytes	3%–7%
Blood volume	82.3 mL/kg (third day after early cord clamping); 92.6 mL/kg (third day after delayed cord clamping)
Sodium	126–166 mEq/L
Potassium	5.6–12.0 mEq/L
Chloride	98–110 mEq/L
Calcium	8.2–11.1 mg/dL
Glucose	45–96 mg/dL

Adapted from Fanaroff, A. A., & Martin, R. J. (Eds.). (2002). *Neonatal-perinatal medicine* (7th ed., pp.1651, 1661). St. Louis, MO: Mosby.

humidity. The limits for an adult are 26°C to 28°C (78.8°F to 82.4°F) (Polin et al., 2004). Thus, the normal newborn requires higher environmental temperatures to maintain a thermoneutral environment. Several newborn characteristics affect the establishment of a thermal stability:

- The newborn has decreased subcutaneous fat and a thin epidermis.
- Blood vessels are closer to the skin than in an adult. Therefore, changes in environmental temperature influence the circulating blood, and in turn influence the hypothalamic temperature-regulating center.
- The flexed posture of the term newborn decreases the surface area exposed to the environment, thereby reducing heat loss.

Size and age may also affect the establishment of an NTE. For example, the preterm or small-for-gestational-age (SGA) newborn has less adipose tissue and is hypoflexed and therefore requires higher environmental temperatures to achieve a thermal neutral environment. Larger, well-insulated newborns may be able to cope with lower environmental temperatures. If the environmental temperature falls below the lower limits of the NTE, the newborn responds with increased oxygen consumption and metabo-

lism, which results in greater heat production. Prolonged exposure to the cold may result in depleted glycogen stores and acidosis. Oxygen consumption also increases if the environmental temperature is above the NTE.

HEAT LOSS

A newborn is at a distinct disadvantage in maintaining a normal temperature. With a large body surface in relation to mass and a limited amount of insulating subcutaneous fat, the full-term newborn loses about four times the heat an adult does. The newborn's poor thermal stability is primarily due to excessive heat loss rather than impaired heat production. Because of the risk of hypothermia and possible cold stress, minimizing heat loss in the newborn after birth is essential (see "Initial Care of the Newborn" in Chapter 19 and "Maintenance of a Neutral Thermal Environment" in Chapter 28 for nursing measures ∞).

Two major routes of heat loss are from the internal core of the body to the body surface and from the external surface to the environment. Usually the core temperature is higher than the skin temperature, resulting in continuous transfer of heat to the surface. The greater the difference in temperature between core and skin, the more rapidly heat transfer occurs. The transfer is accomplished through an increase in oxygen consumption, depletion of glycogen stores, and metabolizing of brown fat. Heat loss from the body surface to the environment takes place in four ways—by convection, radiation, evaporation, and conduction (Figure 26–5 ⊙).

- **Convection** is the loss of heat from the warm body surface to the cooler air currents. Air-conditioned rooms, air currents with a temperature below the infant's skin temperature, oxygen by mask, and removal from an incubator for procedures increase convective heat loss in the newborn.

- **Radiation** losses occur when heat transfers from the heated body surface to cooler surfaces and objects not in direct contact with the body. The walls of a room or of an incubator are potential causes of heat loss by radiation, even if the ambient temperature of the incubator is within the thermal neutral range for that infant. Placing cold objects (such as ice for blood gases) onto the incubator or near the infant in the radiant warmer will increase radiant losses.

- **Evaporation** is the loss of heat incurred when water is converted to a vapor. The newborn is particularly prone to lose heat by evaporation immediately after birth (when wet with amniotic fluid) and during baths; therefore, drying the newborn is critical.

- **Conduction** is the loss of heat to a cooler surface by direct skin contact. Chilled hands, cool scales, cold examination tables, and cold stethoscopes can cause

FIGURE 26–5

A **Convection**

B **Radiation**

C **Evaporation**

D **Conduction**

Methods of heat loss. **A,** Convection. **B,** Radiation. **C,** Evaporation. **D,** Conduction.

loss of heat by conduction. Even if objects are warmed to the incubator temperature, the temperature difference between the infant's core temperature and the ambient temperature may be significant. This difference results in heat transfer.

Once the infant has been dried after birth, the highest losses of heat generally result from radiation and convection, because of the newborn's large body surface compared with weight, and from thermal conduction, because of the marked difference between core temperature and skin temperature. The newborn can respond to the cooler environmental temperature with adequate peripheral vasoconstriction, but this mechanism is not entirely effective because of the minimal amount of fat insulation present, the large body surface, and ongoing thermal conduction. Because of these factors, minimizing the baby's heat loss and preventing hypothermia are imperative. (See "Care of the Newborn with Cold Stress" in Chapter 31 for nursing measures to prevent hypothermia. ∞)

HEAT PRODUCTION (THERMOGENESIS)

When exposed to a cool environment, the newborn requires additional heat. The newborn has several physiologic mechanisms that increase heat production, or *thermogenesis*. They include increased basal metabolic rate, muscular activity, and chemical thermogenesis, also called *nonshivering thermogenesis (NST)* (Polin et al., 2004).

NST, an important mechanism of heat production unique to the newborn, occurs when skin receptors perceive a drop in the environmental temperature and, in response, transmit sensations to stimulate the sympathetic nervous system. NST uses the infant's stores of **brown adipose tissue (BAT)** (also called brown fat) to provide heat. Brown fat receives its name from the dark color caused by its enriched blood supply, dense cellular content, and abundant nerve endings. These characteristics promote rapid metabolism, heat generation, and heat transfer to the peripheral circulation. The large numbers of brown fat cells increase the speed with which triglycerides are metabolized to produce heat.

Thus, nonshivering thermogenesis from BAT is the primary source of heat in the hypothermic newborn. It first appears in the fetus at about 26 to 30 weeks' gestation and continues to increase until 2 to 5 weeks after the birth of a term infant, unless the fat is depleted by cold stress. BAT is deposited in the midscapular area, around the neck, and in the axillas, with deeper placement around the trachea, esophagus, abdominal aorta, kidneys, and adrenal glands (Figure 26–6 ●). BAT constitutes 2% to 6% of the newborn's total body weight.

Shivering is rarely seen in the newborn, although it has been observed at ambient temperatures of 15°C (59°F) or less (Polin et al., 2004). If the newborn shivers, it means the

● FIGURE 26–6

The distribution of brown adipose tissue (brown fat) in the newborn.

Adapted from Davis, V. (1980, November–December). The structure and function of brown adipose tissue in the neonate. Journal of Obstetric, Gynecologic, and Neonatal Nursing, 9, 364.

newborn's metabolic rate has already doubled. The extra muscular activity does little to produce needed heat.

Thermographic studies of newborns exposed to cold show an increase in the skin heat produced over the newborn's brown fat deposits between 1 and 14 days of age (Polin et al., 2004). However, if the brown fat supply has been depleted, the metabolic response to cold is limited or lacking. The resulting hypothermia causes an increase in basal metabolism and an increase in oxygen consumption. A decrease in the environmental temperature of 2°C, from 33°C to 31°C, is sufficient to double the oxygen consumption of a term newborn. Keeping the normal newborn warm promotes normal oxygen requirements, whereas chilling can cause the newborn to show signs of respiratory distress.

When exposed to cold, the normal term newborn is usually able to cope with the increase in oxygen requirements, but the preterm newborn may be unable to increase ventilation to the necessary level of oxygen consumption. Because oxidation of fatty acids depends on the availability of oxygen, glucose, and adenosine triphosphate (ATP), the newborn's ability to generate heat can be altered by pathologic events such as hypoxia, acidosis, and hypoglycemia or by medication that blocks the release of norepinephrine. The effect of certain drugs, such as meperidine (Demerol), may prevent metabolism of brown fat. Meperidine given to the laboring woman leads to a greater fall in the newborn's body temperature during the neonatal period. Newborn hypothermia prolongs as well as potentiates the effects of many analgesic and anesthetic drugs in the newborn.

RESPONSE TO HEAT

Sweating is the usual initial response of the term newborn to hyperthermia. The newborn sweat glands have limited function until after the fourth week of extrauterine life; heat is lost through peripheral vasodilation and evaporation of insensible water loss. The term infant will be flaccid and assume a position of extension to facilitate heat loss (Kenner, 2003). Oxygen consumption and metabolic rate also increase in response to hyperthermia. Severe hyperthermia can lead to death or to gross brain damage if the baby survives.

HEPATIC ADAPTATIONS

The newborn's liver is frequently palpable 2 to 3 cm below the right costal margin. It is relatively large and occupies about 40% of the abdominal cavity. The newborn's liver plays a significant role in iron storage, carbohydrate metabolism, conjugation of bilirubin, and coagulation.

IRON STORAGE AND RBC PRODUCTION

As RBCs are destroyed after birth, the iron is stored in the liver until needed for new RBC production. Newborn iron stores are determined by total body hemoglobin content and length of gestation. The term newborn has about 270 mg of iron at birth, and about 140 to 170 mg of this amount is in the hemoglobin. If the mother's iron intake has been adequate, enough iron will be stored to last until the infant is about 5 months of age. After about 6 months of age, foods containing iron or iron supplements must be given to prevent anemia.

CARBOHYDRATE METABOLISM

At term the newborn's cord blood glucose level is 70% to 80% of the maternal blood glucose level (Cornblath, Hawdon, Williams et al., 2000). Newborn carbohydrate reserves are relatively low. One third of this reserve is in the form of liver glycogen. Newborn glycogen stores are twice those of the adult. The newborn enters an energy crunch at the time of birth, with the removal of the maternal glucose supply and the increased energy expenditure associated with the birth process and extrauterine life. Newborns consume fuel sources at a faster rate because of the work of breathing, loss of heat when exposed to cold, activity, and activation of muscle tone.

Glucose is the main source of energy in the first 4 to 6 hours after birth. During the first 2 hours of life, the serum blood glucose level declines, then rises, and finally reaches a steady state 2 to 3 hours after birth (Cornblath et al., 2000). The nurse may assess the glucose level on admission to the newborn nursery if risk factors are present or per agency protocol. As stores of liver and muscle glycogen and blood glucose decrease, the newborn compensates by changing from a predominantly carbohydrate metabolism to fat metabolism. Energy can be derived from fat and protein, as well as from carbohydrates. The amount and availability of each of these "fuel substrates" depend on the ability of immature metabolic pathways (which lack specific enzymes or hormones) to function in the first few days of life.

CONJUGATION OF BILIRUBIN

Conjugation of bilirubin is the conversion of yellow lipid-soluble pigment into water-soluble pigment. Unconjugated (indirect) bilirubin is a breakdown product derived from hemoglobin released primarily from destroyed RBCs. Unconjugated bilirubin is not in excretable form and is a potential toxin. **Total serum bilirubin** is the sum of conjugated (direct) and unconjugated (indirect) bilirubin.

Fetal unconjugated bilirubin crosses the placenta to be excreted, so the fetus does not need to conjugate bilirubin. Total bilirubin at birth is usually less than 3 mg/dL unless an abnormal hemolytic process has been present in utero. After birth the newborn's liver must begin to conjugate bilirubin by itself. This produces a rise in serum bilirubin levels in the first few days of life.

The bilirubin formed after RBCs are destroyed is transported in the blood bound to albumin. The bilirubin is transferred into the hepatocytes and bound to intracellular binding proteins. These proteins determine the amount of bilirubin held in a liver cell for processing and consequently determine the amount of bilirubin uptake into the liver. The activity of uridine diphosphoglucuronosyl transferase (UDPGT) enzyme results in the attachments of unconjugated bilirubin to glucuronic acid (product of liver glycogen), producing conjugated (direct) bilirubin. Direct bilirubin is excreted into the common duct and duodenum. The conjugated (direct) bilirubin then progresses down the intestines, where bacteria transform it into urobilinogen (urine bilirubin) and stercobilinogen. Stercobilinogen is not reabsorbed but is excreted as a yellow-brown pigment in the stools.

Even after the bilirubin has been conjugated and bound, it can be changed back to unconjugated bilirubin via the enterohepatic circulation. In the intestines, β-glucuronidase enzyme acts to split off (deconjugate) the bilirubin from glucuronic acid if gut bacteria have not first acted on it to produce urobilinogen; the free bilirubin is reabsorbed through the intestinal wall and brought back to the liver via portal vein circulation. This recycling of the bilirubin and decreased ability to clear bilirubin from the system are prevalent in babies with very high β-glucuronidase activity levels and in those with delayed bacterial colonization of the gut (such as those receiving antibiotics) and further increase the newborn's susceptibility to jaundice (Figure 26–7 ●).

The newborn liver has relatively less UDPGT activity in the first few weeks of life than an adult liver. This lower hepatic activity, along with a relatively large bilirubin load, decreases the liver's ability to conjugate bilirubin and increases susceptibility to jaundice.

PHYSIOLOGIC JAUNDICE

Physiologic jaundice is caused by accelerated destruction of fetal RBCs, impaired conjugation of bilirubin, and increased bilirubin reabsorption from the intestinal tract. This condition is not pathologic, but a normal biologic response of the newborn.

Maisels (2005) describes six factors that may interact to create physiologic jaundice:

1. **Increased amounts of bilirubin delivered to the liver.** The increased blood volume due to delayed cord clamping combined with faster RBC destruction in the newborn raises the bilirubin level in the blood. A proportionately larger amount of nonerythrocyte bilirubin forms in the newborn. Therefore, newborns have two to three times greater production or breakdown of bilirubin than do adults. The use of forceps or vacuum extraction, which sometimes cause facial bruising or cephalhematoma (entrapped hemorrhage), can increase the amount of bilirubin to be handled by the liver.

2. **Defective hepatic uptake of bilirubin from the plasma.** If the newborn does not ingest adequate calories, the formation of hepatic binding proteins diminishes, resulting in higher bilirubin levels.

3. **Defective conjugation of the bilirubin.** Decreased uridine diphosphoglucuronosyl activity, as in hypothyroidism, and inadequate caloric intake cause the intracellular binding proteins to remain saturated and result in greater unconjugated bilirubin levels in the blood. The fatty acids in breast milk are thought to compete with bilirubin for albumin-binding sites and therefore impede bilirubin processing.

4. **Defect in bilirubin excretion.** A congenital infection may cause impaired excretion. Delay in introduction of bacterial flora and decreased intestinal motility can also delay excretion and increase enterohepatic circulation of bilirubin.

5. **Inadequate hepatic circulation.** Decreased oxygen supplies to the liver associated with neonatal hypoxia or congenital heart disease increase the bilirubin level.

6. **Increased reabsorption of bilirubin from the intestine.** Reduced bowel motility, intestinal obstruction, or delayed passage of meconium increases the circulation of bilirubin in the enterohepatic pathway, resulting in higher bilirubin values.

FIGURE 26–7

Conjugation of bilirubin in the newborn.

Adapted from Avery, G. B., Fletcher, M. A., & MacDonald, M. G. (1999). Neonatology: Pathophysiology and management of the newborn (5th ed., p. 767, fig. 38-5). Philadelphia: Lippincott Williams & Wilkins.

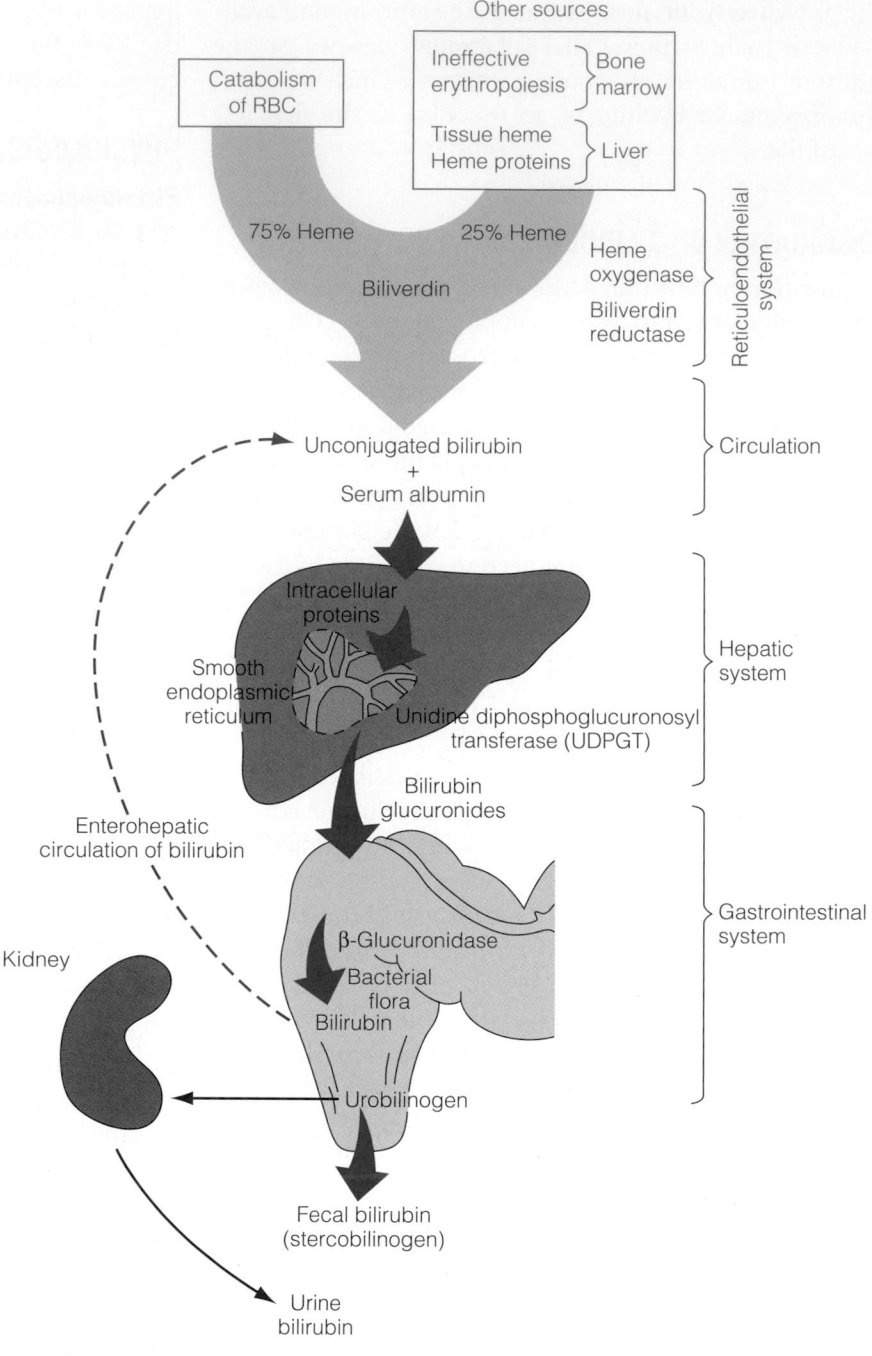

About 50% of term and 80% of preterm newborns exhibit physiologic jaundice on about the second or third day after birth. The characteristic yellow color results from increased levels of unconjugated (indirect) bilirubin, which are a normal product of RBC breakdown and reflect the body's temporary inability to eliminate bilirubin. Serum levels of bilirubin are about 4 to 6 mg/dL before the yellow coloration of the skin and sclera appear. The signs of physiologic jaundice appear after the first 24 hours postnatally. This time frame differentiates physiologic jaundice from pathologic jaundice (see "Physiologic Jaundice" in Chapter 31 ∞), seen at birth or within the first 24 hours of postnatal life.

Peak bilirubin levels are reached between days 3 and 5 in the term infant and between days 5 and 7 in the preterm infant. But these values are established for European and American Caucasian newborns. Chinese, Japanese, Korean, and Native American newborns have considerably higher bilirubin levels that are not as apparent and that persist for longer periods with no apparent ill effects (Maisels, 2005).

The nursery or postpartum room environment, including lighting, may hinder the early detection of the degree and type of jaundice. Pink walls and artificial lights mask the beginning of jaundice in newborns. Daylight assists the observer in early recognition by eliminating distortion caused by artificial light.

If jaundice is suspected, the nurse assesses the newborn's coloring by pressing the skin, generally on the forehead or nose, with a finger. As blanching occurs the nurse observes the icterus (yellow coloring).

Several newborn care procedures will decrease the probability of high bilirubin levels; specifically, the nurse can:

- Maintain the newborn's skin temperature at 36.5°C (97.8°F) or above, because cold stress results in acidosis. Acidosis decreases available serum albumin-binding sites, weakens albumin-binding powers, and causes elevated unconjugated bilirubin levels.

- Monitor stool for frequency and characteristics. Bilirubin is eliminated in the feces; inadequate stooling may result in reabsorption and recycling of bilirubin. Encourage early breastfeeding because the laxative effect of colostrum increases excretion of meconium and transitional stool.

- Encourage early feedings to promote intestinal elimination and bacterial colonization and to provide the calories needed to form hepatic binding proteins.

If jaundice becomes apparent, nursing care is directed toward keeping the newborn well hydrated and promoting intestinal elimination. (For specific nursing management and therapies, see "Nursing Care Plan: The Newborn with Hyperbilirubinemia" in Chapter 31. ∞)

Physiologic jaundice may be very upsetting to parents; they require emotional support and thorough explanation of the condition. If the baby is placed under phototherapy, a few additional days of hospitalization may be required, which may also be disturbing to parents. They can be encouraged to provide for the emotional needs of their newborn by continuing to feed, hold, and caress the infant. If the mother is discharged, the parents are encouraged to return for feedings and to telephone or visit whenever they wish. In many instances the mother, especially if she is breastfeeding, may prefer to remain hospitalized with her newborn; the nurse should support this decision. If insurance limitations make this unrealistic, it may be possible to find an empty room for the discharged mother and her family to use while visiting the newborn. As an alternative to continued hospitalization, the newborn may be treated with home phototherapy. (See "Phototherapy" in Chapter 31 as well as Skill 5–7: Infant Receiving Phototherapy for more information. ∞) **SKILLS**

BREASTFEEDING JAUNDICE AND BREAST MILK JAUNDICE

Breastfeeding is implicated in prolonged jaundice in some newborns. *Breastfeeding jaundice* occurs in the first days of life in breastfed newborns. It appears to be associated with poor feeding practices and not with any change in milk composition. Prevention of early breastfeeding jaundice includes encouraging frequent (every 2 to 3 hours) breastfeeding, avoiding supplementation, and accessing maternal lactation counseling.

In *breast milk jaundice*, the bilirubin begins to rise after the first week of life, when physiologic jaundice is waning after the mother's milk has come in. The level peaks at 5 to 10 mg/dL at 2 to 3 weeks of age and declines over the first several months of life (Maisels, 2005).

In contrast to breastfeeding jaundice, breast milk jaundice is related to milk composition. Some women's breast milk may contain several times the normal concentration of certain free fatty acids. These free fatty acids may compete with bilirubin for binding sites on albumin and inhibit the conjugation of bilirubin or increase lipase activity, disrupting the RBC membrane. Increased lipase activity enhances absorption of bile across the gastrointestinal tract membrane, thereby increasing the enterohepatic circulation of bilirubin. In the past it was thought that the breast milk of women whose newborns have breast milk jaundice contained an enzyme that inhibited glucuronyl transferase, but this hypothesis has not been proven (Thureen et al., 2005).

Newborns with breast milk jaundice appear well, and at present kernicterus (toxic levels of bilirubin in the brain) with this type of jaundice has not been documented. Temporary cessation of breastfeeding may be advised if bilirubin reaches presumed toxic levels of approximately 20 mg/dL or if the interruption is necessary to establish the cause of the hyperbilirubinemia. Most physicians believe that breastfeeding may be resumed once other causes of jaundice have been ruled out and as long as serum bilirubin levels remain below 20 mg/dL. In cases of breast milk jaundice, within 24 to 36 hours after breastfeeding is discontinued, the newborn's serum bilirubin levels begin to fall dramatically. With resumption of breastfeeding, the bilirubin concentration may have a slight rise of 2 to 3 mg/dL with a subsequent decline (Table 26–3).

NURSING PRACTICE

Breastfeeding mothers need encouragement and support in their desire to breastfeed their infants, assistance and instruction about pumping and expressing milk during the interrupted breastfeeding period, and reassurance that nothing is wrong with their milk or mothering abilities.

TABLE 26–3 ✣ Jaundice

Physiologic Jaundice	Breast Milk Jaundice
Physiologic jaundice occurs after the first 24 hours of life.	Bilirubin levels begin to rise after first week of life after mature breast milk comes in.
During the first week of life, bilirubin should not exceed 13 mg/dL. Some pediatricians allow levels up to 15 mg/dL.	Peak of 5–10 mg/dL is reached at 2 to 3 weeks of age.
Bilirubin levels peak at 3 to 5 days in term infants.	It may be necessary to interrupt breastfeeding for a short period when bilirubin reaches 20 mg/dL.

DEVELOPING CULTURAL COMPETENCE

INTERPRETING ILLNESS THROUGH CULTURAL BELIEFS

Cultural Beliefs lead mothers to interpret illness within their cultural framework, especially when left without clear and understood explanations (Hannon, Willis, & Scrimshaw, 2001). For example, some Latina women believe that showing strong maternal emotions during pregnancy and during breastfeeding can be detrimental. They may blame jaundice in their newborn on "bilis" associated with anger. Such maternal reactions can be lessened by careful explanations to the mothers about the diagnosis, prognosis, duration, and management options for jaundice, and possibility for recurrence.

COAGULATION

The liver plays an important part in blood coagulation during fetal life and continues this function to some degree during the first few months after birth. Coagulation factors II, VII, IX, and X (synthesized in the liver) are activated under the influence of vitamin K and therefore are considered vitamin K dependent. The absence of normal flora needed to synthesize vitamin K in the newborn gut results in low levels of vitamin K and creates a transient change in blood coagulation between the second and fifth day of life. From a low point at about 2 to 3 days after birth, these coagulation factors rise slowly, but they do not approach adult levels until 9 months of age or later. Other coagulation factors with low umbilical cord blood levels are XI, XII, and XIII. Fibrinogen and factors V and VII are near adult ranges.

Although newborn bleeding problems are rare, an injection of vitamin K (AquaMEPHYTON) is given prophylactically on the day of birth to combat potential clinical bleeding problems. (Chapter 28 discusses hemorrhagic disease of the newborn in greater depth. ∞)

Platelet counts at birth are in the same range as for older children, but newborns may have mild transient difficulty in platelet aggregation functioning. Phototherapy accentuates this platelet problem.

Prenatal maternal therapy with phenytoin sodium (Dilantin) or phenobarbital also causes abnormal clotting studies and newborn bleeding in the first 24 hours after birth. Infants born to mothers receiving warfarin sodium (Coumadin) may bleed, because these agents cross the placenta and accentuate existing deficiencies in vitamin K-dependent factor. Transient neonatal thrombocytopenia may occur in infants born to mothers with severe hypertension or HELLP syndrome (hemolysis, elevated liver enzymes, and low platelet count) and in infants born to mothers who have idiopathic isoimmune thrombocytopenic purpura.

GASTROINTESTINAL ADAPTATIONS

By 36 to 38 weeks' gestation, the gastrointestinal system is adequately mature, with enzymatic activity and the ability to transport nutrients.

DIGESTION AND ABSORPTION

The full-term newborn has enough intestinal and pancreatic enzymes to digest most simple carbohydrates, proteins, and fats. The carbohydrates newborns must digest are usually disaccharides (lactose, maltose, sucrose), which split into monosaccharides (galactose, fructose, and glucose) by the enzymes of the intestinal mucosa. Lactose is the primary carbohydrate in the breastfeeding newborn and is generally easily digested and well absorbed. The only enzyme lacking is pancreatic amylase, which remains relatively deficient during the first few months of life. Newborns have trouble digesting starches (changing more complex carbohydrates into maltose), so they should not eat them until after the first few months of life.

Although proteins require more digestion than carbohydrates, they are well digested and absorbed from the newborn intestine. The newborn digests and absorbs fats less efficiently because of the minimal activity of the pancreatic enzyme lipase. The newborn excretes about 10% to 20% of the dietary fat intake, compared with 10% for the adult. The newborn absorbs the fat in breast milk more completely than the fat in cows' milk, because breast milk consists of more medium-chain triglycerides and contains lipase. (See "Nutritional Advantages" in Chapter 29 for further discussion of infant nutrition. ∞)

By birth the newborn has experienced swallowing, gastric emptying, and intestinal propulsion. In utero, fetal swallowing is accompanied by gastric emptying and peristalsis of the fetal intestinal tract. By the end of gestation, peristalsis becomes much more active in preparation for extrauterine life. Fetal peristalsis is also stimulated by anoxia, causing the expulsion of meconium into the amniotic fluid in more mature fetuses.

Air enters the stomach immediately after birth. The small intestine is filled with air within 2 to 12 hours and the large bowel within 24 hours. The salivary glands are immature at birth, and the newborn produces little saliva until about age 3 months. The newborn's stomach has a capacity of about 50 to 60 mL. It empties intermittently, starting within a few minutes of the beginning of a feeding and ending 2 to 4 hours after feeding. Bowel sounds are present within the first 30 to 60 minutes of birth, and the newborn can successfully feed during this time. The newborn's gastric pH becomes less acidic about a week after birth and remains less acidic than that of adults for the next 2 to 3 months.

The cardiac sphincter is immature, as is neural control of the stomach, so some regurgitation may happen in the newborn period. Regurgitation of the first few feedings during the first day or two of life can usually be lessened by avoiding overfeeding and by burping the newborn well during and after the feeding.

When no other signs and symptoms are evident, vomiting is limited and ceases within the first few days of life. Continuous vomiting or regurgitation should be observed closely. If the newborn has swallowed bloody or purulent amniotic fluid, lavage of the stomach may be indicated in the term newborn to relieve the problem. Bilious vomiting is abnormal and must be evaluated thoroughly because it might represent a condition that warrants prompt surgical intervention.

Adequate digestion and absorption are essential for newborn growth and development. If optimal nutritional support is available, postnatal growth should parallel intrauterine growth. After 30 weeks' gestation, the fetus gains 30 g/day and adds 1.2 cm to body length daily. To gain weight at the intrauterine rate, the term newborn requires 120 cal/kg/day. After birth, caloric intake is often insufficient for weight gain until the newborn is 5 to 10 days old. During this time, term newborns may lose 5% to 10% of their weight. A shift of intracellular water to extracellular space and insensible water loss account for the 5% to 10% weight loss; thus, failure to lose weight when caloric intake is inadequate may indicate fluid retention.

ELIMINATION

Term newborns usually pass meconium within 8 to 24 hours of life and almost always within 48 hours. **Meconium** is formed in utero from the amniotic fluid and its constituents, intestinal secretions, and shed mucosal cells. It is recognized by its thick, tarry black or dark-green appearance. Transitional (thin brown to green) stools consisting of part meconium and part fecal material are passed for the next day or two, and then the stools become entirely fecal. Generally the stools of a breastfed newborn are pale yellow (but may be pasty green); they are more liquid and more frequent than those of formula-fed newborns, whose stools are paler (Figure 26–8 ○). Frequency of bowel movement varies but ranges from one every 2 to 3 days to as many as 10 daily. Mothers should be counseled that the newborn is not constipated as long as the bowel movement remains soft (Table 26–4).

URINARY ADAPTATIONS

KIDNEY DEVELOPMENT AND FUNCTION

Certain physiologic features of the newborn's kidneys influence the newborn's ability to handle body fluids and excrete urine:

1. The term newborn's kidneys have a full complement of functioning nephrons by 34 to 36 weeks' gestation.

○ **FIGURE 26–8**

Newborn stool samples. **A,** Meconium stool. **B,** Breast milk stool. **C,** Cow's milk stool.

TABLE 26–4 ✤ Physiologic Adaptations to Extrauterine Life

Respiratory, Skin Temperature, and Blood Glucose	Stools (progress from):
Periodic breathing may be present	Meconium (thick, tarry, black)
Desired skin temperature 36–36.5°C (96.8–97.7°F) stabilizes 4 to 6 hours after birth	Transitional stools (thin, brown to green)
Desired blood glucose level reaches 60–70 mg/dL by third postnatal day	Breastfed infants (yellow-gold, soft, or mushy) Formula-fed infants (pale yellow, formed, and pasty)

2. The glomerular filtration rate of the newborn's kidney is low compared with the adult rate. Because of this physiologic inefficiency, the newborn's kidney is unable to dispose of water rapidly when necessary.

The juxtamedullary portion of the nephron has limited capacity to reabsorb HCO_3^- and H^- and concentrate urine. The limitation of tubular reabsorption can lead to inappropriate loss of substances in the glomerular filtrate, such as amino acids, bicarbonate, glucose, and sodium.

Full-term newborns are less able than adults to concentrate urine (reabsorb water back into the blood) because the tubules are short and narrow. They have a greater capacity for glomerular filtration than for tubular reabsorption and secretion. Also, the reduced ability to concentrate urine is due to the limited excretion of solutes (principally sodium, potassium, chloride, bicarbonate, urea, and phosphate) in the growing newborn. Babies gain the ability to concentrate urine fully by 3 months of age. Feeding practices may affect the amount of solutes in urine but have limited effect on concentration of the urine.

Because the newborn has difficulty concentrating urine, the effect of excessive insensible water loss or restricted fluid intake is unpredictable. The newborn kidney is also limited in its dilutional capabilities. Concentrating and dilutional limitations of renal function are important considerations in monitoring fluid therapy to prevent dehydration or overhydration.

CHARACTERISTICS OF NEWBORN URINARY FUNCTION

Many newborns void immediately after birth, and the voiding frequently goes unnoticed. Among normal newborns, 93% void by 24 hours after birth and 100% void by 48 hours after birth (Thureen et al., 2005). A newborn who has not voided by 48 hours should be assessed for adequacy of fluid intake, bladder distention, restlessness, and symptoms of pain. The appropriate clinical personnel should be notified if indicated.

The initial bladder volume is 6 to 44 mL of urine. Unless edema is present, normal urinary output is often limited, and the voidings are scanty until fluid intake increases. The fluid of edema is eliminated by the kidneys, so newborns with edema have a much higher urinary output. The first 2 days postnatally, the newborn voids two to six times daily, with a urine output of 15 mL/day. The newborn subsequently voids 5 to 25 times every 24 hours, with a volume of 25 mL/kg per day.

Following the first voiding, the newborn's urine frequently appears cloudy (due to mucus content) and has a high specific gravity, which decreases as fluid intake increases. Occasionally, pink stains ("brick dust spots") appear on the diaper. These are caused by urates and are innocuous. Blood may occasionally be observed on the diapers of female newborns. This *pseudomenstruation* is related to the withdrawal of maternal hormones. Males may have bloody spotting from a circumcision if performed. In the absence of apparent causes for bleeding, the clinician should be notified. Normal urine during early infancy is straw colored and almost odorless, although odor occurs when certain drugs are given, metabolic disorders exist, or infection is present. Table 26–5 contains urinalysis values for the normal newborn.

IMMUNOLOGIC ADAPTATIONS

The newborn's immune system is not fully activated until sometime after birth. The limitations in the newborn's inflammatory response result in failure to recognize, localize, and destroy invasive bacteria. Thus, the signs and symptoms of infection are often subtle and nonspecific in the newborn. The newborn also has a poor hypothalamic response to pyrogens; therefore, fever is not a reliable indicator of infection. In the neonatal period, hypothermia is a more reliable sign of infection.

Of the three major types of immunoglobulins primarily involved in immunity—IgG, IgA, and IgM—only IgG crosses the placenta. The pregnant woman forms antibodies in response to illness or immunization. This process is called **active acquired immunity**. The transfer of IgG immunoglobulins to

TABLE 26–5 ✤ Newborn Urinalysis Values

Protein < 5–10 mg/dL	Casts 0
WBC < 2–3/hpf	Bacteria 0
RBC 0	Color pale yellow

the fetus in utero results in **passive acquired immunity,** since the fetus does not produce the antibodies itself. IgG immunoglobulins are very active against bacterial toxins.

Because the maternal IgG is transferred primarily during the third trimester, preterm newborns (especially those born prior to 34 weeks' gestation) may be more susceptible to infection. In general, newborns have immunity to tetanus, diphtheria, smallpox, measles, mumps, poliomyelitis, and a variety of other bacterial and viral diseases. The period of resistance varies. Immunity against common viral infections such as measles may last 4 to 8 months, whereas immunity to certain bacteria may disappear within 4 to 8 weeks.

The normal newborn produces antibodies in response to an antigen but not as effectively as an older child does. Immunization usually begins at 2 months of age; then the infant can develop active acquired immunity.

IgM immunoglobulins are produced in response to blood group antigens, gram-negative enteric organisms, and some viruses in the expectant mother. Because IgM does not normally cross the placenta, most or all is produced by the fetus beginning at 10 to 15 weeks' gestation. Elevated levels of IgM at birth may indicate placental leaks or, more commonly, antigenic stimulation in utero. Consequently, elevations suggest that the newborn was exposed to an intrauterine infection such as syphilis or TORCH syndrome (toxoplasmosis, rubella, cytomegalovirus, herpesvirus hominis type 2 infection). (For further discussion, see "Care of the Woman with a Perinatal Infection Affecting the Fetus" in Chapter 15, ∞) The lack of available maternal IgM in the newborn also accounts for the susceptibility to gram-negative enteric organisms such as *Escherichia coli*.

The functions of IgA immunoglobulins are not fully understood. IgA appears to provide protection mainly on secreting surfaces such as the respiratory tract, gastrointestinal tract, and eyes. Serum IgA does not cross the placenta and is not normally produced by the fetus in utero. Unlike the other immunoglobulins, IgA is not affected by gastric action. Colostrum, the forerunner of breast milk, is very high in the secretory form of IgA. It may provide some passive immunity to the infant of a breastfeeding mother. Newborns begin to produce secretory IgA in their intestinal mucosa about 4 weeks after birth.

NEUROLOGIC AND SENSORY-PERCEPTUAL FUNCTIONING

The newborn's brain is about one quarter the size of an adult's, and myelination of nerve fibers is incomplete. Unlike the cardiovascular and respiratory systems, which undergo tremendous changes at birth, the nervous system is minimally influenced by the actual birth process. Because many biochemical and histologic changes have yet to occur in the newborn's brain, the postnatal period is considered a risky time for brain and nervous system development. For neurologic development—including development of intellect—to proceed, the brain and other nervous system structures must mature in an orderly, unhampered fashion.

INTRAUTERINE FACTORS INFLUENCING NEWBORN BEHAVIOR

Newborns respond to and interact with the environment in a predictable pattern of behavior that is somewhat shaped by their intrauterine experience. This intrauterine experience is affected by intrinsic factors such as maternal nutrition and external factors such as the mother's physical environment. Depending on the newborn's intrauterine experience, neonatal behavioral responses to various stresses vary from dealing quietly with the stimulation, to becoming overreactive and tense, to a combination of the two.

Factors such as exposure to intense auditory stimuli in utero can eventually be manifested in the behavior of the newborn. For example, the fetal heart rate (FHR) initially increases when the pregnant woman is exposed to auditory stimuli, but repetition of the stimuli leads to decreased FHR. Thus, the newborn who was exposed to intense noise during fetal life is significantly less reactive to loud sounds postnatally.

CHARACTERISTICS OF NEWBORN NEUROLOGIC FUNCTION

Partially flexed extremities with the legs near the abdomen is the position of the normal newborn. When the newborn is awake, the extremities may exhibit purposeless, uncoordinated bilateral movements. The organization and quality of the newborn's motor activity are influenced by a number of factors, including the following (Brazelton, 1984):

- Sleep-alert states
- Presence of environmental stimuli, such as heat, light, cold, and noise
- Conditions causing a chemical imbalance, such as hypoglycemia
- Hydration status
- State of health
- Recovery from the stress of labor and birth

Eye movements can be seen during the first few days of life. An alert newborn is able to fixate on faces and geometric objects or patterns such as black-and-white stripes. A bright light shining in the newborn's eyes elicits the blinking reflex.

The cry of the newborn should be lusty and vigorous. High-pitched cries, weak cries, and an absence of crying are causes for concern.

The newborn's body grows in a cephalocaudal (head-to-toe), proximal-distal fashion. The newborn is somewhat hypertonic; that is, there is resistance to extending the elbow and knee joints. Muscle tone should be symmetric. Diminished muscle tone and flaccidity may indicate neurologic dysfunction.

Specific symmetric deep tendon reflexes can be elicited in the newborn. Plantar flexion is present. The knee jerk is brisk; a normal ankle clonus may involve three to four beats. Other reflexes, including the Moro, grasping, Babinski, rooting, and sucking reflexes, are characteristic of neurologic integrity (see "Assessment of Neurologic Status" in Chapter 27 ∞).

Complex behavioral patterns reflect the newborn's neurologic maturation and integration. Newborns who can bring a hand to their mouth may be demonstrating motor coordination as well as a **self-quieting ability,** thus increasing the complexity of the behavioral response. Newborns also possess complex, organized defensive motor patterns; for example, they can remove an obstruction such as a cloth across the face.

PERIODS OF REACTIVITY

The baby usually shows a predictable pattern of behavior during the first several hours after birth, characterized by two **periods of reactivity** separated by a sleep phase.

First Period of Reactivity

The first period of reactivity lasts approximately 30 minutes after birth. During this period the newborn is awake and active and may appear hungry and have a strong sucking reflex. This is a natural opportunity to initiate breastfeeding if the mother has chosen it. Bursts of random, diffuse movements alternating with relative immobility may occur. Respirations are rapid, as high as 80 breaths per minute, and there may be retraction of the chest, transient flaring of the nares, and grunting. The heart rate is rapid, and the rhythm may be irregular. Bowel sounds are usually absent.

Period of Inactivity to Sleep Phase

After approximately half an hour, the newborn's activity gradually diminishes. The heart rate and respirations decrease as the newborn enters the sleep phase. The sleep phase may last from a few minutes to 2 to 4 hours. During this period the newborn will be difficult to awaken and will show no interest in sucking. Bowel sounds become audible, and cardiac and respiratory rates return to baseline values.

Second Period of Reactivity

During the second period of reactivity, the newborn is again awake and alert. This period lasts 4 to 6 hours in the normal newborn. Physiologic responses are variable during this stage. The heart and respiratory rates increase; however, it is important to be alert for apneic periods, which may cause a drop in the heart rate. The newborn is stimulated to continue breathing during such times. The newborn may change color rapidly and become mildly cyanotic or mottled during these fluctuations. Production of respiratory and gastric mucus increases, and the newborn responds by gagging, choking, and regurgitating.

Continued close observation and intervention may be required to maintain a clear airway during this period of reactivity. The gastrointestinal tract becomes more active. The newborn often passes the first meconium stool during this second active stage and may also have an initial voiding. The newborn shows he or she is ready to be fed by such behaviors as sucking, rooting, and swallowing. If feeding was not begun in the first period of reactivity, it is done at this time. (See "Initiation of First Feeding" in Chapter 28 and "Initial Feeding" in Chapter 29 for further discussion of this first feeding. ∞)

BEHAVIORAL STATES OF THE NEWBORN

The behavior of the newborn can be divided into two categories, the sleep state and the alert state (Brazelton, 1999). These postnatal behavioral states are similar to those that have been identified during pregnancy. Subcategories are identified under each major category.

Sleep States

The sleep states are as follows:

1. **Deep or quiet sleep.** The baby has closed eyes with no eye movements; regular, even breathing; and jerky motions or startles at regular intervals. Behavioral responses to external stimuli are likely to be delayed. Startles are rapidly suppressed, and changes in state are not likely to occur. Heart rate may range from 100 to 120 beats per minute.

2. **Active rapid eye movement (REM).** The baby has irregular respirations, closed eyes with rapid eye movements visible through the lids, irregular sucking motions, minimal activity, and irregular but smooth movement of the extremities. Environmental and internal stimuli may initiate a startle reaction and a change of state.

Newborn sleep cycles have been recognized and defined according to duration. The length of the cycle depends on the age of the newborn. At term, REM active sleep and quiet sleep occur in intervals of 50 to 60 minutes (Gardner & Goldson, 2002). About 45% to 50% of the total sleep of the newborn is active sleep, 35% to 45% is quiet sleep, and 10% is transitional between these two periods. Growth hormone secretion depends on regular sleep patterns. Any disturbance of the sleep-wake cycle can result in irregular spikes of growth hormone. REM sleep stimulates the highest peaks of growth hormone and the growth of the neural system. Over time the newborn's sleep-wake patterns become diurnal; that is, the newborn sleeps at night and stays awake during the day. (See "Newborn Behavioral Assessment" in Chapter 27 for a short discussion of Brazelton's assessment of newborn states. ∞)

Alert States

In the first 30 to 60 minutes after birth, many newborns display a quiet alert state, characteristic of the first period of reactivity (Figure 26–9 ●). Nurses should use these alert states to encourage bonding and breastfeeding. These periods of alertness tend to be short the first 2 days after birth to allow the baby to recover from the birth process. Subsequent alert states are of choice or of necessity (Brazelton, 1999). The newborn's increasing choice of wakefulness indicates a maturing capacity to achieve and maintain consciousness. Heat, cold, and hunger are but a few of the stimuli that can cause wakefulness by necessity. Once the disturbing stimuli are removed, the baby tends to fall back asleep.

The following are subcategories of the alert state (Brazelton, 1999):

1. **Drowsy or semidozing.** The behaviors common to the drowsy state are open or closed eyes, fluttering eyelids, semidozing appearance, and slow, regular movements of the extremities. Mild startles may be noted from time to time. Although reaction to a sensory stimulus is delayed, it often causes a change of state.

2. **Wide awake.** In the wide-awake state, the newborn is alert and follows and fixates on attractive objects, faces, or auditory stimuli. Motor activity is minimal, and the response to external stimuli is delayed.

● FIGURE 26–9

Mother and newborn gaze at each other. This quiet, alert state is the optimum state for interaction between baby and parents.

3. **Active awake.** In the active-awake state, the newborn's eyes are open and motor activity is quite intense with thrusting movements of the extremities. Environmental stimuli increase startles or motor activity, but individual reactions are difficult to distinguish because of the generally high activity level.

4. **Crying.** Intense crying is accompanied by jerky motor movements. Crying serves several purposes for the newborn. It may be a distraction from disturbing stimuli such as hunger and pain. Fussiness often allows the newborn to discharge energy and reorganize behavior. Most important, crying elicits an appropriate response of help from the parents.

BEHAVIORAL-SENSORY CAPACITIES OF THE NEWBORN

Newborns have several behavioral abilities that assist in their adaptation to extrauterine life. For example, the self quieting ability is their ability to quiet and comfort themselves. They may use hand-to-mouth movements, sucking on a fist or tongue, and attending to external stimuli.

Neurologically impaired newborns cannot use self-quieting activities and require more frequent comforting from caregivers when stimulated. For example, drug-positive newborns often exhibit abnormal sleep and feeding patterns and irritability.

Habituation is the newborn's ability to process and respond to visual and auditory stimulation. For example, when a bright light is flashed into the newborn's eyes, the initial response is blinking, constriction of the pupil, and perhaps a slight startle reaction. However, with repeated stimulation, the newborn's responses gradually diminish and eventually disappear. The capacity to ignore repetitious disturbing stimuli is a newborn defense mechanism readily apparent in the noisy, well-lit nursery.

Visual Capacity

Orientation is the newborn's ability to be alert to, follow, and fixate on complex visual stimuli that are appealing and attractive. The newborn prefers the human face and eyes and bright shiny objects. As the face or object comes into the line of vision, the newborn responds with bright, wide eyes, still limbs, and fixed staring. This intense visual involvement may last several minutes, during which time the newborn can follow the stimulus from side to side. Figure 26–10 ● illustrates this response. The newborn uses this sensory capacity to become familiar with family, friends, and surroundings.

Auditory Capacity

The newborn responds to auditory stimulation with a definite, organized behavior repertoire. The stimulus used to

⊙ **FIGURE 26–10**

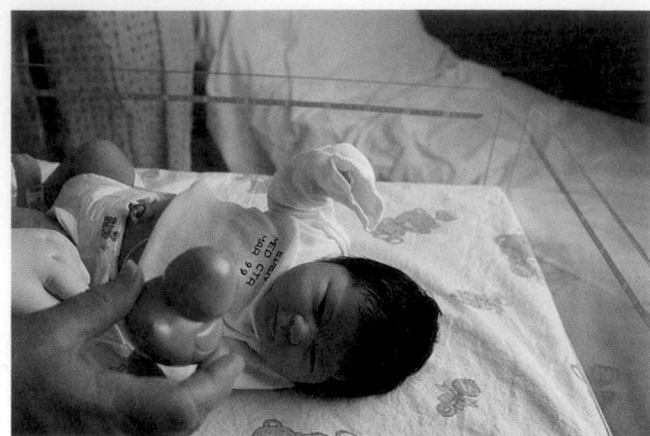

Head turning to follow movement.

assess auditory response should match the state of the newborn. A rattle is appropriate for light sleep, a voice for an awake state, and a clap for deep sleep. As the newborn hears the sound, the cardiac rate rises, and there may be a minimal startle reflex. If the sound is appealing, the newborn will become alert and search for the source of the auditory stimulus.

Olfactory Capacity

Newborns can apparently select people by smell. Newborns were able to distinguish their mothers' breast pads from those of other mothers at just about 1 week postnatally (Gardner & Goldson, 2002).

Taste and Sucking

The newborn responds differently to varying tastes. Sugar, for example, increases sucking. Newborns fed with a rubber nipple versus the breast also show sucking pattern variations. When breastfeeding, the newborn sucks in bursts with frequent regular pauses. The bottle-fed newborn tends to suck at a regular rate with infrequent pauses.

When awake and hungry, the newborn makes rapid searching motions in response to the rooting reflex. Once feeding begins, the newborn establishes a sucking pattern according to the method of feeding. Finger sucking happens not only postnatally but also in utero. The newborn often uses nonnutritive sucking as a self-quieting activity, which helps develop self-regulation. For bottle-fed infants, there is no reason to discourage nonnutritive sucking with a pacifier. For breastfed infants, pacifiers should be offered only after breastfeeding is well established. If the pacifier is offered too soon, the breastfed infant may develop "nipple confusion," may have difficulty learning to suck from the breast, and may nurse less (see "Supplementary Bottle Feeding" in Chapter 29 ∞).

Tactile Capacity

The newborn is very sensitive to being touched, cuddled, and held. Often a mother's first response to an upset or crying newborn is touching or holding. Swaddling, placing a hand on the abdomen, or holding the arms to prevent a startle reflex are other ways to soothe the newborn. The settled newborn can then attend to and interact with the environment.

Critical Concept Review

LEARNING OBJECTIVES

CONCEPTS

| Summarize the respiratory and cardiovascular changes that occur during the transition to extrauterine life and during stabilization. | 1. Newborn respiration is initiated primarily by chemical, mechanical, and reabsorptive processes associated with thermal and sensory stimulation.
2. Onset of respirations stimulates cardiovascular changes:
■ Air enters the lungs, oxygen content rises in alveoli and stimulates relaxation of pulmonary arteries
■ This leads to a decrease in pulmonary vascular resistance, which allows complete vascular flow to lungs
■ With increased oxygenated pulmonary blood flow and loss of the placenta, systemic flood flow increases and the foramen ovale and ductus arteriosus begin to close. |

LEARNING OBJECTIVES

CONCEPTS

| Describe how various factors affect the newborn's blood values. | 1. Newborn blood values are affected by:
■ Site of the blood sample: venous versus capillary
■ Gestational age
■ Prenatal and/or perinatal hemorrhage
■ Timing of the clamping of the umbilical cord |

| Correlate the major mechanisms of heat loss in the newborn to the process of thermogenesis in the newborn. | 1. Thermogenesis is achieved by:
■ Increased basal metabolic rate
■ Muscular activity
■ Nonshivering thermogenesis
■ Metabolizing of brown adipose fat
2. Heat loss is created by:
■ Evaporation (infant is wet from amniotic fluid and/or bath)
■ Convection
■ Radiation
■ Conduction |

| Explain the steps involved in the conjugation and excretion of bilirubin in the newborn. | 1. Unconjugated bilirubin is a byproduct of the destruction of red blood cells.
2. Bilirubin is bound to albumin. It is transferred into liver cells and bound to intracellular proteins. These proteins determine the amount of bilirubin uptake into the liver.
3. UDGPT causes unconjugated bilirubin to attach to glucuronic acid, producing conjugated bilirubin. This is excreted into bile ducts, then into common duct, and into duodenum.
4. In the intestines, bacteria transforms the conjugated bilirubin into urobilinogen (urine bilirubin) and stercobilinogen, and is excreted as a pigment in the stools. |

| Discuss the reasons a newborn may develop jaundice. | 1. Newborn may develop jaundice because of:
■ Accelerated destruction of fetal RBCs
■ Impaired conjugation of bilirubin
■ Increased bilirubin reabsorption from the intestinal tract |

| Describe the functional abilities of the newborn's gastrointestinal tract and liver. | 1. At birth the newborn is able to digest most simple carbohydrates, proteins, and fats. They have trouble digesting starches.
2. The newborn usually passes meconium within 24–48 hours after birth and begins to have normal bowel movements.
3. The newborn liver is slightly less active than the adult liver, which is indicative in the liver's decreased ability to conjugate all of the bilirubin produced by the destruction of fetal RBCs.
4. The liver plays a crucial role in iron storage, carbohydrate metabolism, and coagulation. |

| Identify three reasons a newborn's kidneys have difficulty in maintaining fluid and electrolyte balance. | 1. The following characteristics of a newborn's kidneys cause difficulty in maintaining fluid and electrolyte balance:
■ Decreased rate of glomerular flow and limited excretion of solutes
■ Limited tubular reabsorptions
■ Limited ability to concentrate urine
2. Most newborns void within 48 hours of birth. |

| List the immunologic responses available to the newborn. | 1. The newborn is unable to recognize, localize, and destroy invasive bacteria.
2. The newborn has passive acquired immunity from the mother, lasting from 4 weeks to 8 months.
3. The newborn begins to produce own immunity at about 4 weeks of age. |

(continued)

LEARNING OBJECTIVES

CONCEPTS

Explain the physiologic and behavioral responses of newborns during the periods of reactivity and identify possible interventions.

1. Periods of reactivity
   - First period of reactivity (lasts 30 minutes after birth):
     - The newborn is awake and active, appears hungry, and has a strong suck.
     - The nurse should help mother to initiate breastfeeding.
     - Vital signs are elevated at this time.
   - Period of inactivity to sleep (30 minutes to 4 hours after birth):
     - The newborn is difficult to awaken.
     - Vital signs return to normal.
   - Second period of reactivity (lasts 4–6 hours after period of inactivity):
     - The newborn is awake and alert.
     - Vital signs are variable and the nurse must observe the newborn closely during this time for periods of apnea, gagging, and regurgitation.
     - The newborn often passes meconium stool.
     - The newborn shows a readiness to feed.
2. Behavioral states:
   - Sleep state:
     - Deep or quiet sleep: closed eyes with no eye movement
     - Active rapid eye movements
   - Alert state:
     - Subcategories include: drowsy or semidozing, wide awake, active awake, and crying.
     - The mother and nurse should use this time to facilitate feedings.

Describe the normal sensory-perceptual abilities and behavioral states seen in the newborn period.

1. The normal sensory-perceptual abilities of the newborn are:
   - Visual:
     - The newborn is able to be alert to, follow, and fixate on complex visual stimuli for short periods of time.
   - Auditory:
     - The newborn is able to be alert to and search for an appealing auditory stimulus.
   - Olfactory:
     - The newborn is able to select people by smell.
   - Taste and sucking:
     - The newborn is able to respond selectively to different tastes.
   - Tactile:
     - The newborn is very sensitive to being touched, cuddled, and held.
     - The newborn is able to attend to and interact with the environment.
2. Some of the behavioral capabilities of the newborn that assist in adaptation to extrauterine life include self-quieting ability and habituation.

CRITICAL THINKING IN ACTION

*View the **Critical Thinking in Action** video in Chapter 26 of the CD-ROM. Then, answer the questions that follow.*

Sandra Dee, a 21-year-old, G1, P0000, at 36 weeks' gestation, has been in labor for the last 12 hours and is fully dilated with caput visible on the perineum. The fetal heart rate is 148 to 152 with early deceleration down to 142 with contraction and pushing. Her contractions are 4 to 5 minutes apart of good quality. Sandra's mother and sister are present for the birth. Her prenatal record shows no significant pregnancy problems or complications, and her vital signs have been stable within normal limits. Sandra has received two doses of Stadol for a total of 2 mg IV for pain relief during her labor. The last dose was given 2 hours ago. You assist with the vaginal birth of a live baby without an episiotomy. You observe the sex and time as the midwife places the infant girl on the mother's abdomen, suctions out the baby's mouth and nose, and proceeds to clamp the cord. You dry and stimulate the infant to breathe, remove the wet blanket and replace it with a dry one, and place the infant skin to skin on the mother's chest. You assess the need for infant resuscitation. The baby has a lusty cry spontaneously less than 30 seconds after birth. You palpate the cord obtaining a heart rate of 120, and observe that the baby's chest and face are pink, and the legs and arms are flexed with open fist.

1. Explain the changes that must occur in the infant's cardiopulmonary system at birth.
2. What criteria do you look for when you assess the newborn for adequate cardiopulmonary adaptation at birth?
3. What steps do you take to maintain a neutral thermal environment at birth?
4. Sandra plans to breastfeed. When would you initiate the first feeding?
5. Discuss nursing actions that can decrease the probability of high bilirubin levels in the newborn.

MEDIALINK

www.prenhall.com/london

- NCLEX-RN® Review, case studies, and other interactive resources for this chapter can be found on the Companion Website at http://www.prenhall.com/london. Click on "Chapter 26" to select the activities for this chapter.

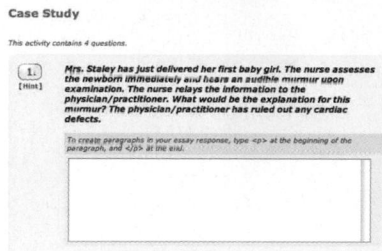

Case Study

This activity contains 4 questions.

1. [Hint]   *Mrs. Staley has just delivered her first baby girl. The nurse assesses the newborn immediately and hears an audible murmur upon examination. The nurse relays the information to the physician/practitioner. What would be the explanation for this murmur? The physician/practitioner has ruled out any cardiac defects.*

To create paragraphs in your essay response, type <p> at the beginning of the paragraph, and </p> at the end.

- For animations, more NCLEX-RN® Review questions, and an audio glossary, access the accompanying CD-ROM in this textbook.

REFERENCES

Blackburn, S. T. (2003). *Maternal, fetal, & neonatal physiology: A clinical perspective* (2nd ed.). St. Louis, MO: Saunders.

Brazelton, T. B. (1984). *Neonatal behavioral assessment scale* (2nd ed.). London: Heineman.

Brazelton, T. B. (1999). Behavioral competence. In G. B. Avery, M. A. Fletcher, & M. G. MacDonald (Eds.), *Neonatology: Pathophysiology and management of the newborn* (5th ed., pp. 321–332). Philadelphia: Lippincott.

Cheffer, N. D. (2004). Adaptation to extrauterine life and immediate nursing care. In S. Mattson & J. E. Smith (Eds.), *Core curriculum for maternal-newborn nursing* (3rd ed., pp. 421–436). St. Louis, MO: Saunders.

Cornblath, M., Hawdon, J. M., Williams, A. F., Aynseley-Green, A., Ward-Platt, M. P., Schwartz, R.,

et al. (2000). Controversies regarding definition of neonatal hypoglycemia: Suggested operational thresholds. *Pediatrics, 105*(5), 1141–1145.

Gardner, S. L., & Goldson, E. (2002). The neonate and the environment: Impact on development. In G. B. Merenstein & S. L. Gardner (Eds.), *Handbook of neonatal intensive care* (5th ed., pp. 219–282). St. Louis, MO: Mosby.

Hannon, P. R., Willis, S. K., & Scrimshaw, S. C. (2001). Persistence of maternal concerns surrounding neonatal jaundice: An exploratory study. *Archives of Pediatrics & Adolescent Medicine, 155*, 1357–1363.

Kenner, C. (2003). Resuscitation and stabilization of the newborn. In C. Kenner & J. W. Lott (Eds.), *Comprehensive neonatal nursing: A physiologic perspective* (3rd ed., pp. 210–228). Philadelphia: Saunders.

Laughlin, D., & Knuppel, R. A. (2003). Maternal-placental-fetal unit: Fetal and early neonatal physiology. In A. H. DeCherney & L. Nathan (Eds.), *Current obstetric & gynecologic diagnosis & treatment* (9th ed., pp. 163–191). New York: Lange Medical Books/McGraw-Hill.

Maisels, M. J. (2005). Jaundice. In M. G. MacDonald, M. D. Mullett, & M. Seshia (Eds.), Avery's Neonatology: *Pathophysiology & management of the newborn*, (6th ed., pp. 768–846). Philadelphia: Lippincott Williams & Wilkins.

Polin, R. A., Fox, W. W., & Abman, S. H. (2004). *Fetal and neonatal physiology* (3rd ed.). Philadelphia: Saunders.

Thureen, P. J., Deacon, J., Hernandez, J., & Hall, D. M. (2005). *Assessment and care of the well newborn* (2nd ed.). Philadelphia: Saunders.

CHAPTER 27

Nursing Assessment of the Newborn

Like most parents, when I held my son for the first time, I checked that all his fingers and toes were present. Then he looked at me with wide, bright, serious eyes and began my introduction to his unique personality.
—Leah, 23

LEARNING OBJECTIVES

- Explain the various components of the gestational age assessment.

- Describe the normal physical and behavioral characteristics of the newborn.

- Summarize the components of a complete newborn assessment and the significance of normal variations and abnormal findings.

- Discuss the neurologic and neuromuscular characteristics of the newborn and the reflexes that may be present at birth.

- Describe the categories of the newborn behavioral assessment.

MEDIALINK

www.prenhall.com/london

CD-ROM

NCLEX-RN® Review
Audio Glossary

Companion Website

NCLEX-RN® Review
MediaLink Applications:
    Case Study: Newborn Maturity Assessment
    Care Plan Activity: Assessment of the Newborn
Thinking Critically

nlike the adult, the newborn communicates needs primarily by behavior. Because the nurse is the most consistent professional observer of the newborn, he or she can translate this behavior into information about the newborn's condition and respond with appropriate nursing interventions. This chapter focuses on the assessment of the newborn and the interpretation of the findings. Newborn assessment is a continuous process designed to evaluate development and adjustments to extrauterine life. In the birth setting, the Apgar scoring procedure (see "Apgar Scoring System" in Chapter 19 for discussion ∞) and careful observation form the basis of assessment and are correlated with information such as the following:

- Maternal prenatal care history
- Birthing history
- Maternal analgesia and anesthesia
- Complications of labor or birth
- Treatment instituted immediately after birth, in conjunction with determination of clinical gestational age
- Consideration of the classification of newborns by weight and gestational age and by neonatal mortality risk
- Physical examination of the newborn

The nurse incorporates data from these sources with the assessment findings during the first 1 to 4 hours after birth to formulate a plan for nursing intervention.

The various newborn assessments and the data obtained from them are only valuable to the degree to which they are shared with the parents. The parents must be included in the assessment process from the moment of their child's birth. The **Apgar score** and its meaning should be explained immediately to the family. As soon as possible, the parents should take part in the physical and behavioral assessments as well.

Encourage the parents to identify their newborn's unique behavioral characteristics. Promote attachment by giving parents a chance to explore their newborn in private and identify individual physical and behavioral characteristics. The nurse's supportive responses to parents' questions and observations are essential throughout the assessment process. The newborn physical examination is the beginning of newborn health surveillance and health education for the newborn's family that continues into the community setting.

TIMING OF NEWBORN ASSESSMENTS

During the first 24 hours of life, the newborn makes the critical transition from intrauterine to extrauterine life. The risk of mortality and morbidity is statistically high during this period. Assessment of the newborn is essential to ensure that the transition proceeds successfully.

There are three major time frames for the assessment of newborns while they are in the birth facility:

- The first assessment is done in the birthing area immediately after birth to determine the need for resuscitation or other interventions. The stable newborn can stay with the family after birth to initiate early attachment. The newborn with complications is usually taken to the nursery for further evaluation and intervention.

- A second assessment is done by the nursery nurse as part of routine admission procedures. During this assessment the nurse carries out a

KEY TERMS

Acrocyanosis, 685

Apgar score, 671

Babinski reflex, 709

Ballard score, 672

Barlow's maneuver, 707

Brazelton Neonatal Behavioral Assessment Scale, 711

Caput succedaneum, 688

Cephalhematoma, 688

Chemical conjunctivitis, 689

Dubowitz tool, 672

Epstein's pearls, 701

Erb-Duchenne paralysis (Erb's palsy), 706

Erythema toxicum, 685

Forceps marks, 686

Gestational age assessment tools, 672

Grasping reflex, 708

Harlequin sign, 685

Jaundice, 685

Lanugo, 674

Milia, 685

Molding, 687

Mongolian blue spots, 686

Moro reflex, 708

Mottling, 685

Nevus flammeus (port-wine stain), 686

Nevus vasculosus (strawberry mark), 687

New Ballard score, 672

Ortolani's maneuver, 707

Pseudomenstruation, 705

Rooting reflex, 709

Skin turgor, 685

Subconjunctival hemorrhage, 689

Sucking reflex, 709

Telangiectatic nevi (stork bites), 686

Thrush, 701

Tonic neck reflex, 708

Trunk incurvation (Galant reflex), 710

Vernix caseosa, 686

brief physical examination to estimate gestational age and evaluate the newborn's adaptation to extrauterine life. No later than 2 hours after birth, the admitting nursery nurse should evaluate the newborn's status and any problems that place the newborn at risk (American Academy of Pediatrics [AAP] & American College of Obstetricians and Gynecologists [ACOG], 2002).

■ Prior to discharge a certified nurse-midwife, physician, or nurse practitioner carries out a behavioral assessment and a complete physical examination to detect any emerging or potential problems.

This chapter presents the procedures for estimating gestational age and performing the complete physical examination and behavioral assessment (Table 27–1). (See "Newborn Physical Assessment by the Nurse" in Chapter 19 for discussion of the immediate postbirth assessment.∞)

ESTIMATION OF GESTATIONAL AGE

Establish the newborn's gestational age in the first 4 hours after birth so that careful attention can be given to age-related problems. Traditionally a newborn's gestational age was determined from the date of the pregnant woman's last menstrual period, but this method was accurate only 75% to 85% of the time. Because of the problems that develop with the preterm newborn or the newborn whose weight is inappropriate for gestational age, a more accurate system was developed to postnatally evaluate the newborn. Once learned, the procedure can be done in a few minutes. *It is essential to wear gloves when assessing the newborn in these early hours after birth and before the first bath until the amniotic fluid, vaginal, and bloody secretions on the skin are removed.*

TABLE 27–1 ✤ Timing and Types of Newborn Assessments

Assess immediately after birth

■ Need for resuscitation
■ If newborn is stable and can be placed with parents to initiate early attachment and bonding

Assessments within 1 to 4 hours after birth

■ Progress of newborn's adaptation to extrauterine life
■ Determination of gestational age
■ Ongoing assessment for high-risk problems

Assessment procedures within first 24 hours or prior to discharge

■ Complete physical examination (Depending on agency protocol, the nurse may complete some components independently, with the certified nurse-midwife, physician, or nurse practitioner completing the exam prior to discharge.)
■ Nutritional status and ability to bottle-feed or breastfeed satisfactorily
■ Behavioral state organization abilities

Clinical **gestational age assessment tools** have two components: external physical characteristics and neurologic or neuromuscular development. Physical characteristics generally include sole creases, amount of breast tissue, amount of lanugo, cartilaginous development of the ear, and testicular descent and scrotal rugae or labial development. These objective clinical criteria are not influenced by labor and birth and do not change significantly within the first 24 hours after birth. Optimal accurate determination of gestational age takes place within 12 hours of birth.

Neurologic examination facilitates assessment of functional or physiologic maturation in addition to physical development. However, the newborn's nervous system is unstable during the first 24 hours of life; neurologic findings based on reflexes or assessments dependent on the higher brain centers may not be reliable. If the neurologic findings drastically deviate from the gestational age derived by evaluation of external characteristics, a second assessment is done in 24 hours.

The neurologic assessment components (excluding reflexes) can aid in assessing the gestational age of newborns of less than 34 weeks' gestation. Between 26 and 34 weeks, neurologic changes are significant, whereas significant physical changes are less evident. One significant neuromuscular change is that muscular tone develops from extension to having the ability to flex the extremity as neurologic maturity develops in a caudocephalad (tail-to-head) progression.

Ballard, Khoury, Wedig et al. (1991) developed the estimation of gestational age by maturity rating, a simplified version of the well-researched **Dubowitz tool**. Ballard's tool gives each physical and neuromuscular finding a value, and the total score is matched to a gestational age (Figure 27–1 ●). The maximum score on Ballard's tool is 50, which corresponds to a gestational age of 44 weeks.

For example, after completing a gestational assessment of a 1-hour-old newborn, the nurse gives a score of 3 to all the physical characteristics, for a total of 18, and gives a score of 3 to all neuromuscular assessments, for a total of 18. The physical characteristics score of 18 is added to the neurologic score of 18 for a total score of 36, which correlates with 38+ weeks' gestation. Because all newborns have slightly varied development of physical characteristics and maturation of neurologic function, scores usually differ instead of all being 3, as in this example.

Postnatal gestational age assessment tools can overestimate preterm gestational age and underestimate postterm gestational age. The tools have been shown to lose accuracy for newborns of less than 28 weeks' or more than 43 weeks' gestation. Ballard et al. (1991) in the **New Ballard score** (NBS) added criteria for more accurate assessment of the gestational age of newborns between 20 and 28 weeks' gestation and less than 1500 g. They suggest that the assessments should be made within 12 hours of birth to

FIGURE 27–1

NEWBORN MATURITY RATING & CLASSIFICATION

ESTIMATION OF GESTATIONAL AGE BY MATURITY RATING
Symbols: X - 1st Exam O - 2nd Exam

NEUROMUSCULAR MATURITY

	−1	0	1	2	3	4	5
Posture							
Square Window (wrist)	>90°	90°	60°	45°	30°	0°	
Arm Recoil		180°	140°–180°	110°–140°	90°–110°	<90°	
Popliteal Angle	180°	160°	140°	120°	100°	90°	<90°
Scarf Sign							
Heel to Ear							

PHYSICAL MATURITY

Skin	sticky friable transparent	gelatinous red, translucent	smooth pink visible veins	superficial peeling &/or rash, few veins	cracking pale areas rare veins	parchment deep cracking no vessels	leathery cracked wrinkled
Lanugo	none	sparse	abundant	thinning	bald areas	mostly bald	
Plantar Surface	heel-toe 40–50mm:−1 <40mm:−2	>50mm no crease	faint red marks	anterior transverse crease only	creases ant. 2/3	creases over entire sole	
Breast	imperceptible	barely perceptible	flat areola no bud	stippled areola 1–2mm bud	raised areola 3–4mm bud	full areola 5–10mm bud	
Eye/Ear	lids fused loosely:−1 tightly:−2	lids open pinna flat stays folded	sl. curved pinna; soft; slow recoil	well curved pinna; soft but ready recoil	formed & firm instant recoil	thick cartilage ear stiff	
Genitals male	scrotum flat, smooth	scrotum empty faint rugae	testes in upper canal rare rugae	testes descending few rugae	testes down good rugae	testes pendulous deep rugae	
Genitals female	clitoris prominent labia flat	prominent clitoris small labia minora	prominent clitoris enlarging minora	majora & minora equally prominent	majora large minora small	majora cover clitoris & minora	

Gestation by Dates _ _ _ _ _ _ _ _ _ _ wks

Birth Date _ _ _ _ _ _ Hour _ _ _ _ _ _ am pm

APGAR _ _ _ _ _ _ 1 min _ _ _ _ _ _ 5 min

MATURITY RATING

score	weeks
−10	20
−5	22
0	24
5	26
10	28
15	30
20	32
25	34
30	36
35	38
40	40
45	42
50	44

SCORING SECTION

	1st Exam = X	2nd Exam = 0
Estimating Gest Age by Maturity Rating	_ _ _ Weeks	_ _ _ Weeks
Time of Exam	Date _ _ _ _ Hour _ _ _ am pm	Date _ _ _ _ Hour _ _ _ am pm
Age at Exam	_ _ _ Hours	_ _ _ Hours
Signature of Examiner	_____ M.D.	_____ M.D.

Newborn maturity rating and classification. If a 1-hour-old newborn is given a score of 3 for each of the physical characteristics and neuromuscular assessments, the newborn's total score would be 36. A total score of 36 correlates with 38+ weeks' gestation.

Used with permission from Ballard, J. L., Khoury, J. C., Wedig, K., Wang, L., Eilers-Walsmann, B. L., & Lipp, R. (1991). New Ballard score, expanded to include extremely premature infants. Journal of Pediatrics, 119, 417.

optimize accuracy, especially in infants of less than 26 weeks' gestational age.

Some maternal conditions, such as preeclampsia, diabetes, and maternal analgesia and anesthesia, may affect certain gestational assessment components and warrant further study. Maternal diabetes, although it appears to accelerate fetal physical growth, seems to retard maturation. Maternal hypertensive states, which retard fetal physical growth, seem to speed maturation.

Newborns of women with preeclampsia have poor muscle tone and edema. Maternal analgesia and anesthesia may cause respiratory depression in the baby. Babies with respiratory distress syndrome (RDS) tend to be flaccid and edematous and assume a "froglike" posture. These characteristics affect the scoring of the neuromuscular components of the assessment tool. The NBS gestational age assessment tool will be used throughout the chapter to demonstrate the assessment of the physical and neuromuscular criteria associated with gestational age.

ASSESSMENT OF PHYSICAL MATURITY CHARACTERISTICS

The first step is to evaluate observable characteristics without disturbing the baby. Selected physical characteristics common to the Dubowitz and Ballard gestational assessment tools are presented here in the order in which they can be evaluated most effectively:

1. *Resting posture,* although a neuromuscular component, should be assessed as the baby lies undisturbed on a flat surface (Figure 27–2 ⊙).

2. *Skin* in the preterm newborn appears thin and transparent, with veins prominent over the abdomen early in gestation. As term approaches, the skin appears opaque because of increased subcutaneous tissue. Disappearance of the protective vernix caseosa promotes skin desquamation and is commonly seen in postmature infants (infants of more than 42 weeks' gestational age and showing signs of placental insufficiency; see "Care of the Postterm Newborn" in Chapter 30 ∞).

3. *Lanugo,* a fine hair covering, decreases as gestational age increases. The amount of **lanugo** is greatest at 28 to 30 weeks and then disappears, first from the face and then from the trunk and extremities.

4. *Sole (plantar) creases* reliably indicate gestational age in the first 12 hours of life. After this the skin of the foot begins drying, and superficial creases appear. Development of sole creases begins at the top (anterior) portion of the sole and, as gestation progresses, proceeds to the heel (Figure 27–3 ⊙). Peeling may also occur. Plantar creases vary with race. In newborns of African descent, sole creases may be less developed at term.

5. Inspect the *areola* and gently palpate the breast bud tissue by applying the forefinger and middle finger to the breast area and measuring the tissue between them

⊙ **FIGURE 27–2**

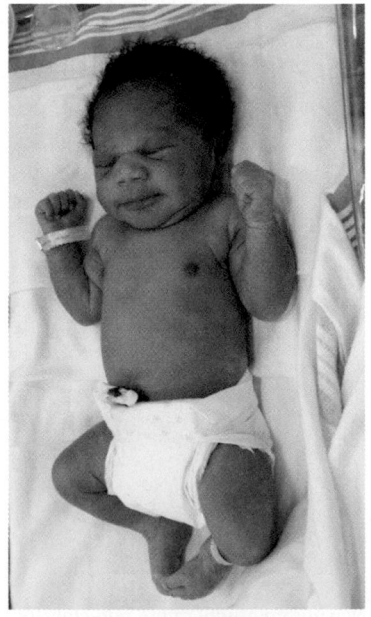

A   B   C

Resting posture. ***A,*** Newborn exhibits beginning of flexion of the thigh. The gestational age is approximately 31 weeks. Note the extension of the upper extremities. Score 1 or 2. ***B,*** Newborn exhibits stronger flexion of the arms, hips, and thighs. Score 3. The gestational age is approximately 35 weeks. ***C,*** The full-term newborn exhibits hypertonic flexion of all extremities. Score 4.

● FIGURE 27–3

  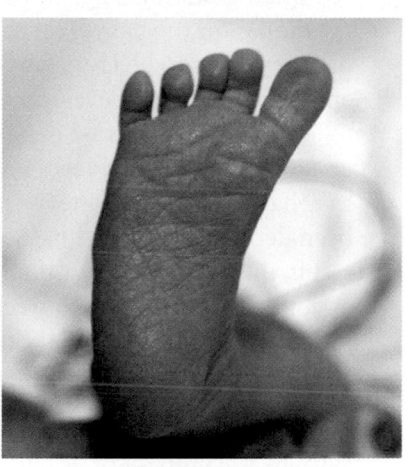

A   B   C

Sole creases. **A,** Newborn has a few sole creases on the anterior portion of the foot. Note the slick heel. Score 2. The gestational age is approximately 35 weeks. **B,** Newborn has a deeper network of sole creases on the anterior two thirds of the sole. Note the slick heel. Score 3. The gestational age is approximately 37 weeks. **C,** The term newborn has deep sole creases down to and including the heel as the skin loses fluid and dries after birth. Score 4. Sole (plantar) creases can be seen even in preterm newborns.

in centimeters or millimeters (Figure 27–4 ●). At term gestation the tissue measures between 0.5 and 1 cm (5 and 10 mm). As gestation progresses the breast tissue mass and areola enlarge. During the assessment the nipple should not be grasped firmly because skin and subcutaneous tissue will prevent accurate estimation of size. Do this procedure gently to avoid causing trauma to the breast tissue.

● FIGURE 27–4

  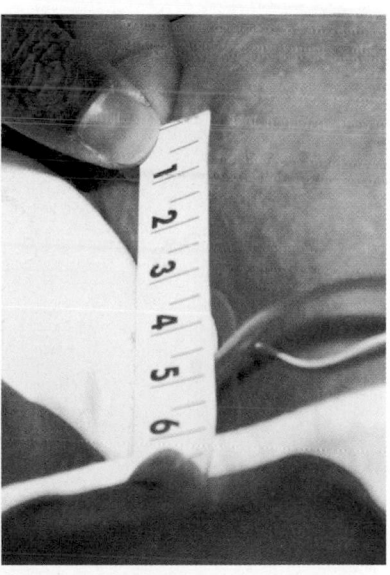

A   B   C

Breast tissue. **A,** Newborn has a visible raised area > 0.75 cm diameter. Score 3. The gestational age is 38 weeks. **B,** Newborn has 10 mm breast tissue area. Score 4. The gestational age is 40 to 44 weeks. **C,** Gently compress the tissue between the middle and index fingers and measure the tissue in centimeters or millimeters. Absence of or decreased breast tissue often indicates premature or small-for-gestational-age newborn.

(B) Used with permission from V. Dubowitz, MD, Hammersmith Hospital, London, England.

As gestation progresses the breast tissue mass and areola enlarge. However, a large breast tissue mass can occur as a result of specific conditions other than advanced gestational age or the effects of maternal hormones on the baby. The newborn of a mother with diabetes tends to be large for gestational age (LGA), and the accelerated development of breast tissue reflects subcutaneous fat deposits. Small-for-gestational-age (SGA) term or postterm newborns may have used subcutaneous fat (which would have been deposited as breast tissue) to survive in utero; as a result, their lack of breast tissue may indicate a gestational age of 34 to 35 weeks, even though other factors indicate a term or postterm newborn.

6. *Ear form* and *cartilage distribution* develop with gestational age. The cartilage gives the ear its shape and substance (Figure 27–5 ●). In a newborn of less than 34 weeks' gestation, the ear is relatively shapeless and flat; it has little cartilage, so the ear folds over on itself and remains folded. (Test this response by holding the top and bottom of the pinna together with the forefinger and thumb and then releasing them or by folding the pinna of the ear forward against the side of the head, releasing it, and observing the response.) By term the newborn's pinna is firm, stands away from the head, and springs back quickly from the folding.

7. *Male genitals* are evaluated for size of the scrotal sac, presence of rugae (wrinkles and ridges in the scrotum), and descent of the testes (Figure 27–6 ●). Prior to 36 weeks, the scrotum has few rugae, and the testes are palpable in the inguinal canal. By 36 to 38 weeks, the testes are in the upper scrotum, and rugae have developed over the anterior portion of the scrotum. By term the testes are generally in the lower scrotum, which is pendulous and covered with rugae.

8. The appearance of the *female genitals* depends in part on subcutaneous fat deposition and therefore relates to fetal nutritional status (Figure 27–7 ●). The clitoris varies in size and occasionally is so swollen that it is difficult to identify the sex of the newborn. This swelling may be due to adrenogenital syndrome, which causes the adrenals to secrete excessive amounts of androgen and other hormones. At 30 to 32 weeks' gestation, the clitoris is prominent, and the labia majora are small and widely separated. As gestational age increases, the labia majora increase in size. At 36 to 40 weeks, they nearly cover the clitoris. At 40 weeks and beyond, the labia majora cover the labia minora and clitoris.

Other physical characteristics assessed by some gestational age scoring tools include the following:

1. *Vernix* covers the preterm newborn. The postterm newborn has little vernix. After noting vernix distribution, the birthing area nurse (wearing gloves) dries the newborn to prevent evaporative heat loss,

● **FIGURE 27–5**

A   B   C

Ear form and cartilage. **A,** The ear of the infant at approximately 36 weeks' gestation shows incurving of the upper two thirds of the pinna. Score 2. **B,** Infant at term shows well-defined incurving of the entire pinna. Score 3. **C,** If the auricle stays in the position in which it is pressed or returns slowly to its original position, it usually means the gestational age is less than 38 weeks.

● FIGURE 27-6

A   B

Male genitals. **A,** Preterm newborn's testes are not within the scrotum. The scrotal surface has few rugae. Score 2. **B,** Term newborn's testes are generally fully descended. The entire surface of the scrotum is covered by rugae. Score 3.

thus disturbing the vernix and potentially altering this gestational age criterion. The birthing area nurse must communicate to the newborn nurse the amount of vernix and the areas of vernix coverage.

2. *Hair* of the preterm newborn has the consistency of matted wool or fur and lies in bunches rather than in the silky, single strands of the term newborn's hair.

3. *Skull firmness* increases as the fetus matures. In a term newborn, the bones are hard and the sutures are not easily displaced. Do not attempt to displace the sutures forcibly.

4. *Nails* appear and cover the nail bed at about 20 weeks' gestation. Nails extending beyond the fingertips may indicate a postterm newborn.

ASSESSMENT OF NEUROMUSCULAR MATURITY CHARACTERISTICS

The central nervous system of the fetus matures at a fairly constant rate. Tests have been designed to evaluate neurologic status as manifested by neuromuscular tone development. In the fetus, neuromuscular tone develops from the lower to the upper extremities.

The neuromuscular evaluation requires more manipulation and disturbances than the physical evaluation of the newborn. The neuromuscular evaluation (see Figure 27-1) is best performed when the baby's condition has stabilized. Evaluate the following characteristics:

1. The *square window sign* is elicited by gently flexing the newborn's hand toward the ventral forearm until

● FIGURE 27-7

A   B   C

Female genitals. **A,** Newborn has a prominent clitoris. The labia majora are widely separated, and the labia minora, viewed laterally, would protrude beyond the labia majora. Score 1. The gestational age is 30 to 35 weeks. **B,** The clitoris is still visible. The labia minora are now covered by the larger labia majora. Score 2. The gestational age is 36 to 40 weeks. **C,** The term newborn has well-developed, large labia majora that cover both clitoris and labia minora. Score 3.

○ **FIGURE 27–8**

A   B   C

Square window sign. **A,** This angle is 90 degrees and suggests an immature newborn of 28 to 32 weeks' gestation. Score 0. **B,** A 30- to 40-degree angle is commonly found from 39 to 40 weeks' gestation. Score 2-3. **C,** A 0-degree angle can occur from 40 to 42 weeks. Score 4.

(C) Used with permission from V. Dubowitz, MD, Hammersmith Hospital, London, England.

resistance is felt. The angle formed at the wrist is measured (Figure 27–8 ○).

2. *Recoil* is a test of flexion development. Because flexion first develops in the lower extremities, test recoil in the legs first. Place the newborn on its back on a flat surface. With a hand on the newborn's knees, place the baby's legs in flexion, then extend them parallel to each other and flat on the surface. The response to this maneuver is recoil of the newborn's legs. According to gestational age, they may not move or they may return slowly or quickly to the flexed position. Preterm infants have less muscle tone than term infants, so preterm infants have less recoil.

Test arm recoil by flexion at the elbow and extension of the arms at the newborn's side. While the baby is in the supine position, completely flex both elbows, hold them in this position for 5 seconds, extend the arms at the baby's side, and release them. On release the elbows of a full-term newborn form an angle of less than 90 degrees and rapidly recoil back to a flexed position. The elbows of a preterm newborn have slower recoil time and form an angle greater than 90 degrees. Arm recoil is also slower in healthy but fatigued newborns after birth; therefore, arm recoil is best elicited after the first hour of birth, when the baby has had time to recover from the stress of the birth. Deep sleep state also decreases the arm recoil response. Assess arm recoil bilaterally to rule out brachial palsy.

3. The *popliteal angle* (degree of knee flexion) is determined with the newborn flat on his or her back. Flex the thigh on the abdomen and chest, place the index finger of the other hand behind the newborn's ankle to extend the lower leg until resistance is met, and measure the angle formed. Results vary from no resistance in the very immature newborn to an 80-degree angle in the term newborn.

4. The *scarf sign* is elicited by placing the newborn supine and drawing an arm across the chest toward the newborn's opposite shoulder until resistance is met. Note the location of the elbow in relation to the midline of the chest (Figure 27–9 ○). A preterm infant's elbow will cross the midline of the chest, whereas a full-term infant's elbow will not cross midline.

5. The *heel-to-ear extension* is performed by placing the newborn in a supine position and then gently drawing the foot toward the ear on the same side until resistance is felt. Allow the knee to bend during the test. It is important to hold the buttocks down to keep from rolling the baby. Assess both the proximity of foot to ear and the degree of knee extension. The leg of a preterm, immature newborn remains straight and the foot goes to the ear or beyond. With advancing gestational age, the newborn demonstrates increasing resistance to this maneuver. Maneuvers involving the

FIGURE 27–9

A

B

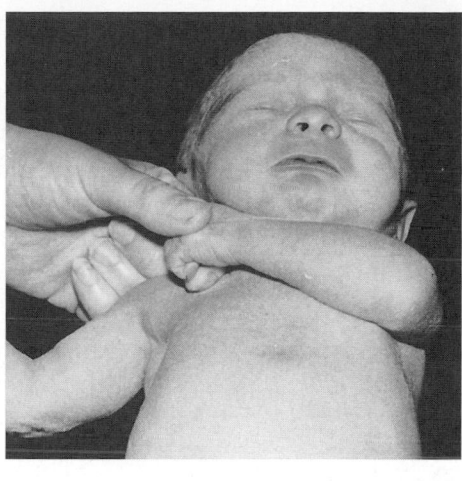
C

Scarf sign. **A,** No resistance is noted until after 30 weeks' gestation. The elbow moves readily past the midline. Score 1. **B,** The elbow is at midline at 36 to 40 weeks' gestation. Score 2. **C,** Beyond 40 weeks' gestation, the elbow will not reach the midline. Score 4.

(C) Used with permission from V. Dubowitz, MD, Hammersmith Hospital, London, England.

FIGURE 27–10

Heel-to-ear. No resistance. Leg fully extended. Score 0.

FIGURE 27–11

A

B

Ankle dorsiflexion. **A,** A 45-degree angle indicates 32 to 36 weeks' gestation. A 20-degree angle indicates 36 to 40 weeks' gestation. Score 2-3. **B,** A 15- to 0-degree angle is common at 40 weeks' or more gestational age. Score 4.

lower extremities of newborns who had frank breech presentation should be delayed to allow for resolution of altered leg positioning (Figure 27–10).

6. *Ankle dorsiflexion* is determined by flexing the ankle on the shin. Use a thumb to push on the sole of the newborn's foot while the fingers support the back of the leg. Then measure the angle formed by the foot and the interior leg (Figure 27–11). Intrauterine position and congenital deformities can influence this sign.

7. *Head lag* (neck flexor) is measured by pulling the newborn to a sitting position and noting the degree of head lag. Total lag is common in newborns up to

34 weeks' gestation, whereas postterm newborns (42+ weeks) hold their heads in front of their body lines. Full-term newborns can support their heads momentarily.

8. *Ventral suspension* (horizontal position) is evaluated by holding the newborn prone on the hand and noting the position of the head and back and the degree of flexion in the arms and legs. Some flexion of arms and legs indicates 36 to 38 weeks' gestation; fully flexed extremities, with head and back even, are characteristic of a term newborn.

9. Major reflexes such as *sucking, rooting, grasping, Moro, tonic neck, Babinski,* and others are evaluated during the newborn examination. (See discussion of reflexes on pages 708-710.)

When the gestational age determination and birth weight are considered together, the newborn can be identified as one whose growth is below the 10th percentile, or small for gestational age (SGA); appropriate for gestational age (AGA); or above the 90th percentile, or large for gestational age (LGA) (Figure 27–12 ●). This determination enables the nurse to anticipate possible physiologic problems and, in conjunction with a complete physical examination, to establish a plan of care appropriate for the individual newborn. For example, an SGA newborn often requires frequent glucose monitoring and early feedings. (See

● **FIGURE 27–12**

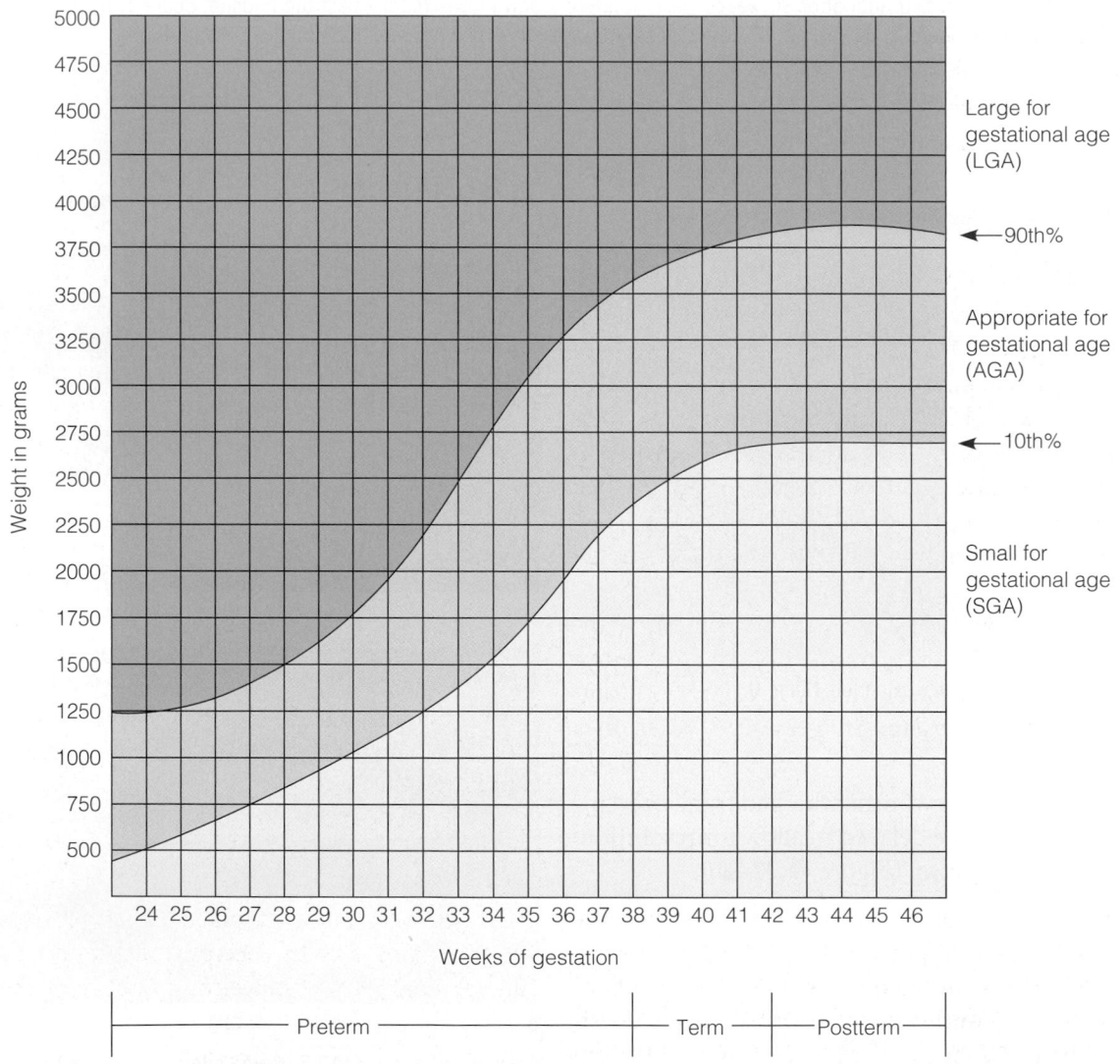

Classification of newborns by birth weight and gestational age. The nurse places the newborn's birth weight and gestational age on the graph and classifies the newborn as large for gestational age (LGA), appropriate for gestational age (AGA), or small for gestational age (SGA).

Used with permission from Battaglia, F. C., & Lubchenco, L. O. (1967). A practical classification of newborn infants by weight and gestational age. Journal of Pediatrics, 71, 161.

"Identification of At-Risk Newborn" in Chapter 30 for a more complete discussion of these categories and the potential problems associated with them. ∞)

NURSING PRACTICE

Measuring weight and height often aggravate newborns and may alter their vital signs. For better accuracy, take the newborn's vital signs before weighing and measuring.

Plot the gestational age against the newborn's length, head circumference, and weight on the appropriate growth chart to determine if these measurements fall within the average range—the 10th to 90th percentile for the corresponding gestational age (Figure 27–13 ●). These correlations further document the level of maturity and appropriate category for the newborn. The comparison of the infant's weight-length ratio further helps identify SGA infants as having symmetric or asymmetric growth restriction. (See Chapter 30 for further discussion. ∞)

PHYSICAL ASSESSMENT

After the initial determination of gestational age and related potential problems, carry out a more extensive physical assessment. Choose a warm, well-lit area that is free of drafts. Completing the physical assessment in the presence of the parents gives a chance to acquaint them with their unique newborn. Perform the examination in a systematic, head-to-toe manner, and record all findings. When assessing the physical and neurologic status of the newborn, first consider general appearance and then proceed to specific areas.

A guide for systematically assessing the newborn appears on pages 690–700. Normal findings, alterations, and related causes are presented and correlated with suggested nursing responses. The findings are typical for a full-term newborn.

GENERAL APPEARANCE

The newborn's head is disproportionately large for its body. The neck looks short because the chin rests on the chest. Newborns have a prominent abdomen, sloping shoulders, narrow hips, and a rounded chest. The center of the baby's body is the umbilicus rather than the symphysis pubis as in the adult. The body appears long and the extremities short.

Newborns tend to stay in a flexed position similar to the one maintained in utero and will offer resistance when the extremities are straightened. The flexed position that the newborn maintains contributes to the short appearance of the extremities. The hands are tightly clenched. After a breech birth, the feet are usually dorsiflexed, and it may take several weeks for the newborn to assume the typical newborn posture.

WEIGHT AND MEASUREMENTS

The normal full-term Caucasian newborn has an average birth weight of 3405 g (7 lb, 8 oz). Newborns of African, Asian, or Mexican descent are usually somewhat smaller at term, whereas Native American infants are often heavier at term (Mandleco, 2004; Wu & Daniel, 2001). Other factors that influence weight are age and size of parents, health of mother (smoking and malnutrition decrease birth weight), and the interval between pregnancies (short intervals, such as every year, result in lower birth weight). After the first week, and for the first 6 months, the newborn's weight increases about 198 g (7 oz) weekly.

Approximately 70% to 75% of the newborn's body weight is water. During the initial newborn period (the first 3 or 4 days), term newborns have a physiologic weight loss of about 5% to 10% because of fluid shifts. This weight loss may reach 15% for preterm newborns. Large babies also tend to lose more weight because of greater fluid loss in proportion to birth weight. If weight loss is greater than 10%, clinical reappraisal is indicated. Factors contributing to weight loss include small fluid intake resulting from delayed breastfeeding or a slow adjustment to the formula, increased volume of meconium excreted, and urination. Weight loss may be marked in the presence of temperature elevation (because of associated dehydration) or consistent chilling (because of nonshivering thermogenesis).

The length of the normal newborn is difficult to measure because the legs are flexed and tensed. To measure length, place babies flat on their backs with their legs extended as much as possible (Figure 27–14 ●). The average length is 50 cm (20 in.), and the range is 48 to 52 cm (18 to 22 in.). The newborn will grow approximately 1 inch a month for the next 6 months. This is the period of most rapid growth.

At birth the newborn's head is one third the size of an adult's head. The circumference (biparietal diameter) of the newborn's head is 32 to 37 cm (12.5 to 14.5 in.). For accurate measurement, place the tape over the most prominent part of the occiput, just above the eyebrows (Figure 27–15A ●). The circumference of the newborn's head is approximately 2 cm greater than the circumference of the newborn's chest at birth, and the two parts remain in this proportion for the next few months. (For factors that alter this measurement, see "Head" later in this chapter.) It is best to take another head circumference on the second day if the newborn experienced significant

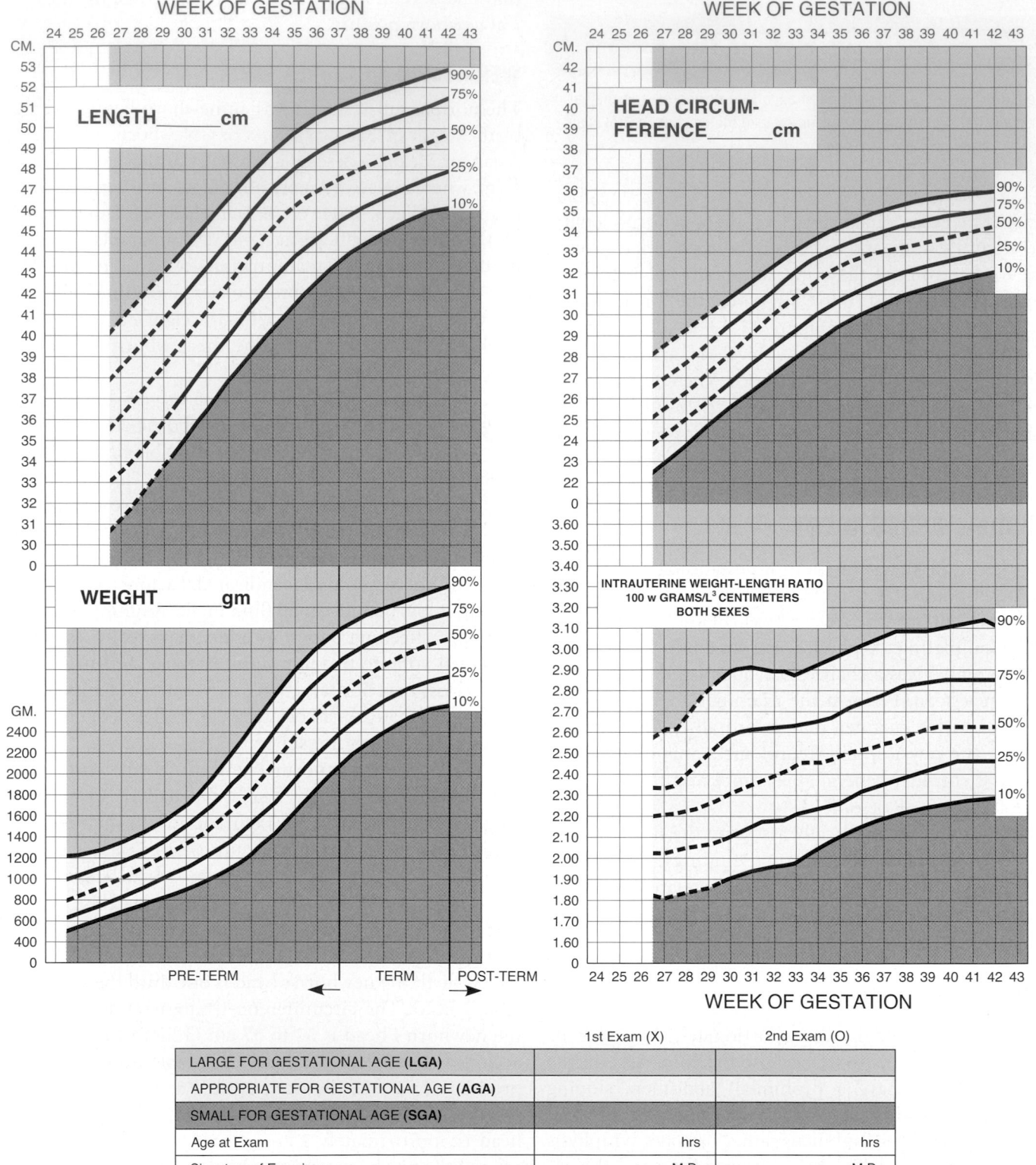

CLASSIFICATION OF NEWBORNS—
BASED ON MATURITY AND INTRAUTERINE GROWTH

Symbols: X-1st Exam O-2nd Exam

	1st Exam (X)	2nd Exam (O)
LARGE FOR GESTATIONAL AGE (**LGA**)		
APPROPRIATE FOR GESTATIONAL AGE (**AGA**)		
SMALL FOR GESTATIONAL AGE (**SGA**)		
Age at Exam	hrs	hrs
Signature of Examiner	M.D.	M.D.

Classification of newborns based on maturity and intrauterine growth.

Used with permission from Lubchenco, L. O., Hansman, C., & Boyd, E. (1966). Intrauterine growth in length and head circumference as estimated from live births at gestational ages from 26 to 42 weeks. Pediatrics, 37, 403–408; and Battaglia, F. C., & Lubchenco, L. O. (1967). A practical classification of newborn infants by weight and gestational age. Journal of Pediatrics, 71, 159.

● **FIGURE 27–14**

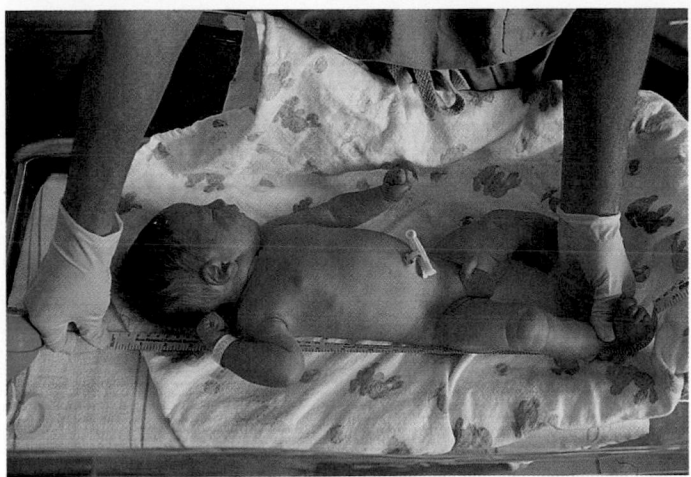

Measuring the length of the newborn.

● **FIGURE 27–15**

A

B

A, Measuring the head circumference of the newborn. **B,** Measuring the chest circumference of the newborn.

head molding or developed a caput from the birth process.

At birth the average circumference of the chest is 32 cm (12.5 in.) and ranges from 30 to 35 cm (12 to 14 in.). Take chest measurements with the tape measure placed at the lower edge of the scapulas and brought around anteriorly, directly over the nipple line (Figure 27–15B). The abdominal circumference, or girth, may also be measured at this time by placing the tape around the newborn's abdomen at the level of the umbilicus, with the bottom edge of the tape at the top edge of the umbilicus (Table 27–2).

TEMPERATURE

Initial assessment of the newborn's temperature is critical. In utero the temperature of the fetus is about the same as, or slightly higher than, the expectant mother's. When babies enter the outside world, their temperature can suddenly drop as a result of exposure to cold drafts and the skin's heat loss mechanisms.

If no heat conservation measures are started, the normal term newborn's deep body temperature falls 0.1°C (0.2°F) per minute; skin temperature drops 0.3°C (0.5°F) per minute. Skin temperature markedly decreases within 10 minutes after exposure to room air. The temperature should stabilize within 8 to 12 hours. Temperature is monitored when the newborn is admitted to the nursery and at least every 30 minutes until the newborn's status has remained stable for 2 hours. After that, assess temperature at least once every 8 hours or according to institutional policy (AAP & ACOG, 2002). (See "Temperature Regulation" in Chapter 26 for a discussion of the physiology of temperature regulation. ∞)

TABLE 27–2 ✥ Newborn Measurements

Weight
- Average: 3405 g (7 lb, 8 oz)
- Range: 2500–4000 g (5 lb, 8 oz–8 lb, 13 oz)
- Weight is influenced by racial origin and maternal age and size
- Physiologic weight loss: 5%–10% for term newborns, up to 15% for preterm newborns
- Growth: 198 g (7 oz) per week for first 6 months

Length
- Average: 50 cm (20 in.)
- Range: 48–52 cm (18–22 in.)
- Growth: 2.5 cm (1 in.) per month for first 6 months

Head Circumference
- 32–37 cm (12.5–14.5 in.)
- Approximately 2 cm larger than chest circumference

Chest Circumference
- Average: 32 cm (12.5 in.)
- Range: 30–35 cm (12–14 in.)

Temperature can be assessed by the axillary skin method, a continuous skin probe, the rectal route, or a tympanic thermometer. Axillary temperature reflects body (core) temperature and the body's compensatory response to the thermal environment. Axillary temperatures are the preferred method and are considered to be a close estimation of the rectal temperature. In preterm and term newborns, there is less than 0.1°C (0.2°F) difference between the two sites. With the axillary method, the thermometer must remain in place at least 3 minutes unless an electronic thermometer is used (Figure 27–16 ●). Axillary temperature ranges from 36.5°C to 37°C (97.7°F to 98.6°F). Axillary temperatures can be misleading, because the friction caused by apposition of the inner arm skin and upper chest wall and the nearness of brown fat to the probe may elevate the temperature.

Skin temperature is measured most accurately by continuous skin probe, especially for small newborns or newborns maintained in incubators or under radiant warmers. Normal skin temperature is 36°C to 36.5°C (96.8°F to 97.7°F). Continuous skin temperature assessment allows time to begin interventions before a more serious fall in core temperature occurs (Figure 27–17 ●).

Rectal temperature is assumed to be the closest approximation to core temperature, but the accuracy of this method depends on the depth to which the thermometer is inserted. Normal rectal temperature is 36.6°C to 37.2°C (97.8°F to 99°F). The rectal route is not recommended as a routine method in the newborn, because it may irritate the rectal mucosa and increase chances of perforation.

Many institutions use tympanic thermometers, portable sensor probes with disposable covers that are placed in the auditory canal. The probe uses infrared technology to measure the temperature of the internal carotid artery blood flow within several seconds. Research suggests that tympanic and digital thermometer axillary tempera-

● **FIGURE 27–17**

Temperature monitoring for the newborn. A skin thermal sensor is placed on the newborn's abdomen, upper thigh, or arm and secured with porous tape or a foil-covered foam pad.

tures are accurate estimations of body temperature in the healthy newborn (Blackburn, 2003). Current research still questions the accuracy of tympanic thermometer readings from sick or potentially ill newborns (Blackburn, 2003).

Temperature instability, a deviation of more than 1°C (2°F) from one reading to the next, or a subnormal temperature may indicate an infection. In contrast to an elevated temperature in older children, an increased temperature in a newborn may indicate reactions to too much covering, too hot a room, or dehydration. Dehydration, which tends to increase body temperature, occurs in newborns whose feedings have been delayed for any reason. Newborns may respond to overheating (a temperature greater than 37.5°C [99.5°F]) by increased restlessness and eventually by perspiration. The perspiration appears initially on the head and face and then on the chest. Many newborns initially cannot perspire, so they increase their respiratory and heart rates, which increase oxygen consumption.

SKIN CHARACTERISTICS

Although the newborn's skin color varies with ethnic background, all healthy newborns have a pink tinge to their skin. The ruddy hue results from increased red blood cell concentrations in the blood vessels and limited subcutaneous fat deposits.

Skin pigmentation is slight in the newborn period, so color changes may be seen even in darker-skinned babies. A newborn who is cyanotic at rest and pink only with crying may have choanal atresia (congenital blockage of the passageway between the nose and pharynx). If crying increases

● **FIGURE 27–16**

Axillary temperature measurement. The thermometer should remain in place for 3 minutes. The nurse presses the newborn's arm tightly but gently against the thermometer and the newborn's side, as illustrated.

● FIGURE 27-18

Acrocyanosis.

the cyanosis, heart or lung problems may be suspected. Very pale newborns may be anemic or have hypovolemia (low blood pressure) and should be evaluated for these problems.

Acrocyanosis (bluish discoloration of the hands and feet) may be present in the first 2 to 6 hours after birth (Figure 27–18 ●). This condition is caused by poor peripheral circulation, which results in vasomotor instability and capillary stasis, especially when the baby is exposed to cold. If the central circulation is adequate, the blood supply should return quickly when the skin is blanched with a finger. Blue hands and nails are a poor indicator of oxygenation in a newborn. The nurse should assess the face and mucous membranes for pinkness reflecting adequate oxygenation.

Mottling (lacy pattern of dilated blood vessels under the skin) occurs as a result of general circulation fluctuations. It may last several hours to several weeks or may come and go periodically. Mottling may be related to chilling or prolonged apnea.

Harlequin sign (clown) color change is occasionally noted: A deep red color develops over one side of the newborn's body while the other side remains pale, so that the skin resembles a clown's suit. This color change results from a vasomotor disturbance in which blood vessels on one side dilate while the vessels on the other side constrict. It usually lasts from 1 to 20 minutes. Affected newborns may have single or multiple episodes, but they are transient and clinically insignificant. Document its occurrence.

Jaundice is first detectable on the face (where skin overlies cartilage) and the mucous membranes of the mouth and has a head-to-toe progression (Varney, Kriebs, & Gegor, 2004). Evaluate it by blanching the tip of the nose, the forehead, the sternum, or the gum line. This procedure must be done in appropriate lighting. If jaundice is present, the area will appear yellowish immediately after blanching.

Another area to assess for jaundice is the sclera. Evaluation and determination of the cause of jaundice must begin immediately to prevent possibly serious sequelae. The jaundice may be related to breastfeeding (in a few cases), hematomas, immature liver function, or bruises from forceps, or it may be caused by blood incompatibility, oxytocin (Pitocin) augmentation or induction, or severe hemolysis process. Report any jaundice noted before a newborn is 24 hours of age to the physician or nurse practitioner. (For detailed discussion of causes and assessment of jaundice, see "Care of Newborn with Jaundice" in Chapter 31. ∞)

Erythema toxicum is an eruption of lesions in the area surrounding a hair follicle that are firm, vary in size from 1 to 3 mm, and consist of a white or pale yellow papule or pustule with an erythematous base. It is often called "newborn rash" or "flea bite" dermatitis. The rash may appear suddenly, usually over the trunk and diaper area, and is frequently widespread (Figure 27–19 ●). The lesions do not appear on the palms of the hands or the soles of the feet. The peak incidence is at 24 to 48 hours of life. The condition rarely presents at birth or after 5 days of life. The cause is unknown, and no treatment is necessary. Some clinicians believe it may be caused by irritation from clothing. The lesions disappear in a few hours or days. If a maculopapular rash appears, a smear of the aspirated papule will show numerous eosinophils on staining; no bacteria will be cultured.

Milia, which are exposed sebaceous glands, appear as raised white spots on the face, especially across the nose (Figure 27–20 ●). No treatment is necessary, because they will clear spontaneously within the first month. Infants of African heritage have a similar condition called transient neonatal pustular melanosis.

Skin turgor is assessed to determine hydration status, the need for early feedings, and the presence of any infectious processes. The usual place to assess skin turgor is over

● FIGURE 27-19

Erythema toxicum on leg.

● **FIGURE 27–20**

Facial milia.

● **FIGURE 27–21**

Stork bites on back of neck.

the abdomen or the thigh. Skin should be elastic and return to its original shape.

Vernix caseosa, a whitish, cheeselike substance, covers the fetus while in utero and lubricates the skin of the newborn. The skin of the term or postterm newborn has less vernix and is frequently dry; peeling is common, especially on the hands and feet.

Forceps marks may be present after a difficult forceps birth. The newborn may have reddened areas over the cheeks and jaws. It is important to reassure the parents that these marks will disappear, usually within 1 or 2 days. Transient facial paralysis resulting from the forceps pressure is a rare complication. Vacuum extractor suction marks on the vertex of the scalp are often seen when vacuum extractors are used to assist with the birth. These marks are benign and do not indicate any underlying brain lesions.

BIRTHMARKS

Telangiectatic nevi (stork bites) appear as pale pink or red spots and are frequently found on the eyelids, nose, lower occipital bone, and nape of the neck (Figure 27–21 ●). These lesions are common in newborns with light complexions and are more noticeable during periods of crying. These areas have no clinical significance and usually fade by the second birthday.

Mongolian blue spots are macular areas of bluish black or gray-blue pigmentation on the dorsal area and the buttocks (Figure 27–22 ●) (Johnston, Flood, & Spinks, 2003). They are common in newborns of Asian and African descent and other dark-skinned races. They gradually fade during the first or second year of life. They may be mistaken for bruises and should be documented in the newborn's chart.

Nevus flammeus (port-wine stain), a capillary angioma directly below the epidermis, is a nonelevated,

sharply demarcated, red-to-purple area of dense capillaries (Figure 27–23 ●). In infants of African descent, it may appear as a purple-black stain. The size and shape vary, but it commonly appears on the face. It does not grow in size, does not fade with time, and does not blanch as a rule. The birthmark may be concealed by using an opaque cosmetic cream. If convulsions and other neurologic problems accompany the nevus flammeus, the clinical picture suggests Sturge-Weber syndrome, with involvement of the fifth cranial nerve (the ophthalmic branch of the trigeminal nerve).

Nevus vasculosus (strawberry mark), a capillary hemangioma, consists of newly formed and enlarged capillaries in the dermal and subdermal layers. It is a raised, clearly delineated, dark-red, rough-surfaced birthmark commonly found in the head region. Such marks usually grow (often rapidly) starting during the second or third

● **FIGURE 27–22**

Mongolian spots.

● **FIGURE 27–23**

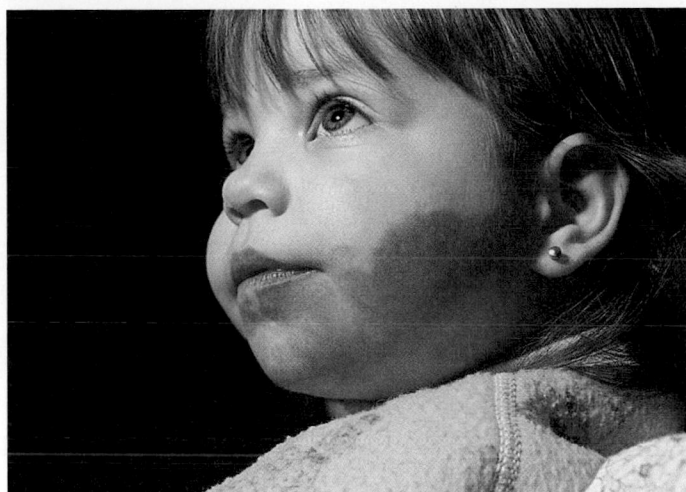

Port-wine stain.

week of life and may not reach their fullest size for 1 to 3 months (Thureen, Deacon, Hernandez et al., 2005). They begin to shrink and start to resolve spontaneously several weeks to months after they reach peak growth. Tell parents that a pale purple or gray spot on the surface of the hemangioma signals the start of resolution. The best cosmetic effect is achieved when the lesions are allowed to resolve spontaneously.

Birthmarks frequently worry parents. The mother may be especially anxious, fearing that she is to blame ("Is my baby 'marked' because of something I did?"). Guilt feelings are common when parents have misconceptions about the cause. Identify and explain them to the parents. Providing appropriate information about the cause and course of birthmarks often relieves the fears and anxieties of the family. Note any bruises, abrasions, or birthmarks seen on admission to the nursery.

HEAD

General Appearance

The newborn's head is large (approximately one fourth of the body size), with soft, pliable skull bones. For most term infants, the occipital-frontal circumference (OFC) is 32 to 37 cm. The head may appear asymmetric in the newborn of a vertex birth. This asymmetry, called **molding**, is caused by overriding of the cranial bones during labor and birth (Figure 27–24 ●). The degree of molding varies with the amount and length of pressure exerted on the head. Within a few days after birth, the overriding usually diminishes and the suture lines become palpable. Because head measurements are affected by molding, a second measurement is indicated a few days after birth. The heads of breech-

born newborns and those born by elective cesarean are characteristically round and well shaped because no pressure was exerted on them during birth. Any extreme differences in head size may indicate microcephaly (an abnormally small head) or hydrocephalus (an abnormal buildup of fluid in the brain). Variations in the shape, size, or appearance of the head may be due to craniostenosis (premature closure of the cranial sutures), which needs to be corrected through surgery to allow brain growth, or plagiocephaly (asymmetry caused by pressure on the fetal head during gestation) (Thureen et al., 2005).

Two fontanelles ("soft spots") may be palpated on the newborn's head. Fontanelles, openings at the juncture of the cranial bones, can be measured with the fingers. Accurate measurement requires the examiner's finger to be measured in centimeters. Carry out the assessment with the newborn in a sitting position and not crying. The diamond-shaped anterior fontanelle is approximately 3 to 4 cm long by 2 to 3 cm wide. It is located at the juncture of the frontal and parietal bones. The posterior fontanelle, smaller and triangular, is formed by the parietal bones and the occipital bone and is 0.5 by 1 cm. The fontanelles are smaller immediately after birth than several days later because of molding. The anterior fontanelle closes within 18 months, whereas the posterior fontanelle closes within 8 to 12 weeks.

The fontanelles are a useful indicator of the newborn's condition. The anterior fontanelle may swell when the newborn cries or passes a stool or may pulsate with the

● **FIGURE 27–24**

Overlapped cranial bones produce a visible ridge in a small, premature newborn. Easily visible overlapping does not occur often in term infants.

Used with permission from Korones, S. B. (1986). High-risk newborn infants (4th ed.). St. Louis, MO: Mosby.

heartbeat, which is normal. A bulging fontanelle usually signifies increased intracranial pressure, and a depressed fontanelle indicates dehydration (Kiesler & Ricer, 2003).

Palpate the sutures between the cranial bones for amount of overlapping. In newborns whose growth has been restricted, the sutures may be wider than normal, and the fontanelles may also be larger due to impaired growth of the cranial bones. In addition to inspecting the newborn's head for degree of molding and size, evaluate it for soft-tissue edema and bruising.

Cephalhematoma

Cephalhematoma is a collection of blood resulting from ruptured blood vessels between the surface of a cranial bone (usually parietal) and the periosteal membrane (Figure 27–25 ⬤). The scalp in these areas feels loose and slightly edematous. These areas emerge as defined hematomas between the first and second day. Although external pressure may cause the mass to fluctuate, it does not increase in size when the newborn cries. Cephalhematomas may be unilateral or bilateral and do not cross suture lines. They are relatively common in vertex births and may disappear within 2 to 3 weeks or very slowly over subsequent months. They may be associated with physiologic jaundice, because extra red blood cells are destroyed within the cephalhematoma.

Caput Succedaneum

Caput succedaneum is a localized, easily identifiable, soft area of the scalp, generally resulting from a long and difficult labor or vacuum extraction. The sustained pressure of the presenting part against the cervix results in compression of local blood vessels, and venous return is slowed. Slowed venous return causes an increase in tissue fluids, an edematous swelling, and occasional bleeding under the periosteum. The caput may vary from a small area to a severely elongated head. The fluid in the caput is reabsorbed within 12 hours to a few days after birth. Caputs resulting from vacuum extractors are sharply outlined, circular areas up to 2 cm thick. They disappear more slowly than naturally occurring edema. It is possible to distinguish between a cephalhematoma and a caput because the caput overrides suture lines (Figure 27–26 ⬤), whereas the cephalhematoma, because of its location, never crosses a suture line (Table 27–3). Caput succedaneum is present at birth, whereas cephalhematoma is not.

HAIR

The term newborn's hair is smooth with texture variations depending on ethnic background. Scalp hair is usually high over the eyebrows. Assessment of the newborn's hair characteristics such as color, quantity, hairlines, direction of growth, and hair whorls can identify genetic, metabolic, and neurologic disorders (Furdon & Clark, 2003). For example, coarse, brittle, and dry hair may indicate hypothyroidism.

⬤ **FIGURE 27–25**

Scalp
Sagittal suture
Periosteum
Blood
Skull bone

Cephalhematoma is a collection of blood between the surface of a cranial bone and the periosteal membrane. This is a cephalhematoma over the left parietal bone.

Used with permission from Potter, E. L., & Craig, J. M. (1975). Pathology of the fetus and infant (3rd ed.). St. Louis, MO: Mosby-Yearbook Medical Publishers.

⊙ FIGURE 27–26

- Sagittal suture
- Serum
- Periosteum
- Skull bone

Caput succedaneum is a collection of fluid (serum) under the scalp.

bral (eyelid) fissure widens (Figure 27–27 ⊙). Paralysis may result from forceps-assisted birth or pressure on the facial nerve from the maternal pelvis during birth. Facial paralysis usually disappears within a few days to 3 weeks, although in some cases it may be permanent.

EYES

The eyes of the newborn of northern European descent are a blue-gray or slate–blue-gray color. Dark-skinned newborns tend to have dark eyes at birth. The sclera tends to be bluish white because of its relative thinness. A blue sclera is

⊙ FIGURE 27–27

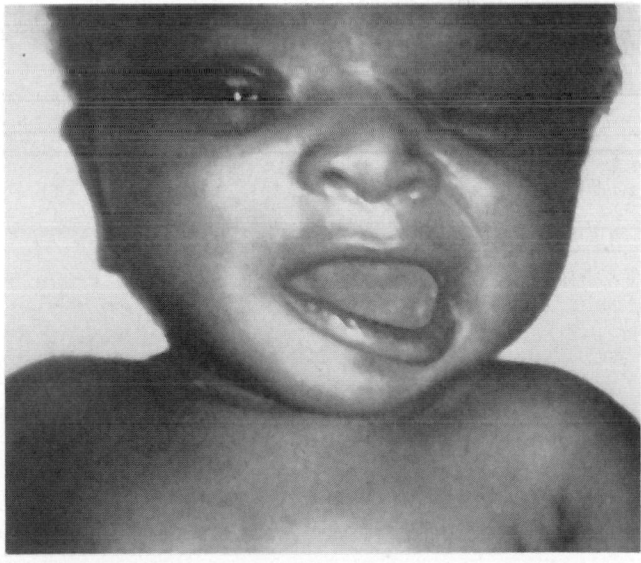

Facial paralysis. Paralysis of the right side of the face from injury to right facial nerve.

Used with permission from Potter, E. L., & Craig, J. M. (1975). Pathology of the fetus and infant (3rd ed.). St. Louis, MO: Mosby-Yearbook Medical Publishers. Courtesy of Dr. Ralph Platow.

FACE

The newborn's face is well designed to help the newborn suckle. Sucking (fat) pads are located in the cheeks, and a labial tubercle (sucking callus) is frequently found in the center of the upper lip. The chin is recessed, and the nose is flattened. The lips are sensitive to touch, and the sucking reflex is easily initiated.

Evaluate symmetry of the eyes, nose, and ears. See "Assessment Guide: Newborn Physical Assessment" on pages 690–700 for deviations in symmetry and variations in size, shape, and spacing of facial features.

Assess facial movement symmetry to determine the presence of facial palsy. Facial paralysis appears when the newborn cries; the affected side is immobile, and the palpe-

(text continues on page 701)

ASSESSMENT GUIDE

NEWBORN PHYSICAL ASSESSMENT

PHYSICAL ASSESSMENT/ NORMAL FINDINGS	ALTERATIONS AND POSSIBLE CAUSES*	NURSING RESPONSES TO DATA†
Vital Signs		
Blood pressure (BP): At birth: 80–60/45–40 mm Hg	Low BP (hypovolemia, shock)	Monitor BP in all cases of distress, prematurity, or suspected anomaly.
Day 10: 100/50 mm Hg (may be unable to measure diastolic pressure with standard sphygmomanometer)		Low BP: Refer to physician immediately so measures to improve circulation are begun.
Pulse: 120–160 bpm (if asleep, as low as 80 bpm; if crying, up to 180 bpm)	Weak pulse (decreased cardiac output) Bradycardia (severe asphyxia, arrhythmia) Tachycardia (over 160 bpm at rest) (infection, CNS problems, arrhythmia)	Assess skin perfusion by blanching (capillary refill test). Correlate finding with BP assessments; refer to physician. Carry out neurologic and thermoregulation assessments.
Respirations: 30–60 breaths/min Synchronization of chest and abdominal movements	Tachypnea (pneumonia, respiratory distress syndrome [RDS])	Identify sleep-wake state; correlate with respiratory pattern.
Diaphragmatic and abdominal breathing	Rapid, shallow breathing (hypermagnesemia due to large doses given to mothers with preeclampsia) Respirations below 30 breaths/min (maternal anesthesia or analgesia)	Evaluate for all signs of respiratory distress; report findings to physician.
Transient tachypnea	Expiratory grunting; subcostal and substernal retractions; flaring of nares (respiratory distress); apnea (cold stress, respiratory disorder)	Evaluate for cold stress. Report findings to physician or neonatal nurse practitioner.
Crying: Strong and lusty Moderate tone and pitch	High pitched, shrill (neurologic disorder, hypoglycemia)	Discuss newborn's use of cry for communication. Assess and record abnormal cries.
Cries vary in length from 3 to 7 min after consoling measures are used	Weak or absent (CNS disorder, laryngeal problem)	Reduce environmental noises.
Temperature: Axilla 36.4–37.2°C (97.5–99°F)	Elevated temperature (room too warm, too much clothing or covers, dehydration, sepsis, brain damage)	Notify physician of elevation or drop.
Rectal 36.6–37.2°C (97.8–99°F); 36.8°C (98.8°F) desired	Subnormal temperature (brain stem involvement, cold, sepsis)	Counsel parents on possible causes of elevated or low temperatures, appropriate home care measures, when to call physician.
Heavier newborns tend to have higher body temperatures	Swings of more than 2°F from one reading to next or subnormal temperature (infection)	Teach parents how to take an axillary temperature; assess parents' knowledge regarding use of thermometer; provide teaching as needed.
Weight: 2500–4000 g (5 lb, 8 oz–8 lb, 13 oz)	<2748 g (<6 lb) = SGA or preterm infant >4050 g (>9 lb) = LGA or infants of diabetic mothers	Plot weight and gestational age on growth chart to identify high-risk infants. Ascertain body build of parents. Counsel parents regarding appropriate caloric intake. Feed the infant early post birth. Check blood glucose according to hospital policy.
Within first 3 to 4 days, normal weight loss of 5%–10% Large babies tend to lose more due to greater fluid loss in proportion to birth weight except infants of diabetic mothers	Loss greater than 15% (small fluid intake, loss of meconium and urine, feeding difficulties)	Notify physician of net losses or gains. Calculate fluid intake and losses from all sources (insensible water loss, radiant warmers, phototherapy lights). Daily weights and before discharge.
Length: 48–52 cm (18–22 in.)	Less than 45 cm (congenital dwarf)	Assess for other signs of dwarfism.
Grows 10 cm (3 in.) during first 3 months	Short/long bones proximally (achondroplasia) Short/long bones distally (Ellis-van Creveld syndrome)	Determine other signs of skeletal system adequacy. Plot progress at subsequent well-baby visits.

*Possible causes of alterations are placed in parentheses.

†This column provides guidelines for further assessment and initial nursing intervention.

ASSESSMENT GUIDE—continued

NEWBORN PHYSICAL ASSESSMENT

PHYSICAL ASSESSMENT/ NORMAL FINDINGS	ALTERATIONS AND POSSIBLE CAUSES*	NURSING RESPONSES TO DATA†
Posture		
Body usually flexed, hands may be tightly clenched, neck appears short because chin rests on chest	Only extension noted, inability to move from midline (trauma, hypoxia, immaturity)	Record spontaneity of motor activity and symmetry of movements.
In breech births, feet are usually dorsiflexed	Constant motion (maternal caffeine intake or drug use)	If parents express concern about newborn's movement patterns, reassure and further evaluate if appropriate.
Skin		
Color: Color consistent with ethnic background	Pallor of face conjunctiva (anemia, hypothermia, anoxia)	Discuss with parents common skin color variations to allay fears. Skin color can vary widely within African-American infants.
Newborns of European descent: pink tinged or ruddy color over face, trunk, extremities	Beefy red (hypoglycemia, immature vasomotor reflexes, polycythemia)	Document extent and time of occurrence of color change.
Newborns of African or Native American descent: pale pink with yellow or red tinge		
Newborns of Asian descent: pink or rosy red to yellow tinge		
Common variations: acrocyanosis, circumoral cyanosis, or harlequin color change	Meconium staining (nonreassuring fetal status) Jaundice (hemolytic reaction from blood incompatibility within first 24 hours, sepsis)	Obtain Hgb and hematocrit values; obtain bilirubin levels. Assess for respiratory difficulty and temperature instability. Differentiate between physiologic and pathologic jaundice.
Mottled when undressed	Cyanosis (choanal atresia, CNS damage or trauma, respiratory or cardiac problem, cold stress)	Assess degree of (central or peripheral) cyanosis and possible causes; refer to physician.
Minor bruising over buttocks in breech presentation and over eyes and forehead in facial presentations		Discuss with parents cause and course of minor bruising related to labor and birth.
Texture: Smooth, soft, flexible; may have dry, peeling hands and feet	Generalized cracked or peeling skin (SGA or postterm; blood incompatibility; metabolic, kidney dysfunction) Seborrheic-dermatitis (cradle cap) Absence of vernix (postmature) Yellow vernix (bilirubin staining)	Report to physician. Instruct parents to shampoo the scalp and anterior fontanelle areas daily with mild soap or baby shampoo; rinse well; avoid use of oil.
Turgor: Elastic, returns to normal shape after pinching	Maintains tent shape (dehydration)	Assess for other signs and symptoms of dehydration.
Pigmentation: Clear; milia across bridge of nose, forehead, or chin will disappear within a few weeks		Advise parents not to pinch or prick these pimplelike areas.
Café-au-lait spots (one or two)	Six or more (neurologic disorder such as von Recklinghausen disease, cutaneous neurofibromatosis)	If there are six or more café-au-lait spots, refer for genetic and neurologic consult.
Mongolian blue spots common over dorsal area and buttocks in dark-skinned infants		Assure parents of normality of this pigmentation; it will fade in first year or two.
Erythema toxicum	Impetigo (group A β-hemolytic streptococcus or *Staphylococcus aureus* infection)	If impetigo occurs, instruct parents about handwashing and linen precautions during home care.
Telangiectatic nevi	Hemangiomas: Nevus flammeus (port-wine stain) Nevus vasculosus (strawberry hemangioma) Cavernous hemangiomas	Collaborate with physician. Counsel parents about birthmark's progression to allay misconceptions. Record size and shape of hemangiomas. Refer for follow-up at well-baby clinic.

*Possible causes of alterations are placed in parentheses.

†This column provides guidelines for further assessment and initial nursing intervention.

ASSESSMENT GUIDE—continued

NEWBORN PHYSICAL ASSESSMENT

PHYSICAL ASSESSMENT/ NORMAL FINDINGS	ALTERATIONS AND POSSIBLE CAUSES*	NURSING RESPONSES TO DATA†
Skin—*continued*		
Rashes	Rashes (infection)	Assess location and type of rash (macular, papular, vesicular). Obtain history of onset, prenatal history, and related signs and symptoms.
Petechiae of head or neck (breech presentation, cord around neck)	Generalized petechiae (clotting abnormalities)	Determine cause; advise parents if further healthcare is needed.
Head		
General appearance, size, movement Round, symmetric, and moves easily from left to right and up and down; soft and pliable	Asymmetric, flattened occiput on either side of the head (plagiocephaly) Head held at angle (torticollis) Unable to move head side to side (neurologic trauma)	Instruct parents to change infant's sleeping positions frequently. When awake, needs to spend "tummy time". Determine adequacy of all neurologic signs.
Circumference: 32–37 cm (12.5-14.5 in.); 2 cm greater than chest circumference Head one fourth of body size	Extreme differences in size may be due to microencephaly (Cornelia de Lange syndrome, cytomegalic inclusion disease [CID]), rubella, toxoplasmosis, chromosome abnormalities, hydrocephalus (meningomyelocele, achondroplasia), anencephaly (neural tube defect) Head is 3 cm or more larger than chest circumference (preterm, hydrocephalus)	Measure circumference from occiput to frontal area using metal or paper tape. Measure chest circumference using metal or paper tape and compare to head circumference. Record measurements on growth chart. Reevaluate at well-baby visits.
Common variations: Molding	Cephalhematoma (trauma during birth, persists up to 3 weeks)	Evaluate neurologic response.
Breech and cesarean newborns' heads are round and well shaped	Caput succedaneum (long labor and birth; disappears in 1 week)	Observe for hyperbilirubinemia. Reassure parents regarding common manifestations due to birth process and when they should disappear.
Fontanelles: Palpation of juncture of cranial bones	Overlapping of anterior fontanelle (malnourished or preterm newborn)	Discuss normal closure times with parents and care of "soft spots" to allay misconceptions.
Anterior fontanelle: 3–4 cm long by 2–3 cm wide, diamond shaped	Premature closure of sutures (craniostenosis)	Refer to physician. Assess fontanelles and sutures daily.
Posterior fontanelle: 1–2 cm at birth, triangle shaped	Late closure (hydrocephalus)	Observe for signs and symptoms of hydrocephalus.
Slight pulsation	Moderate to severe pulsation (vascular problems)	Refer to physician.
Moderate bulging noted with crying, stooling; pulsations with heartbeat	Bulging (increased intracranial pressure, meningitis) Sunken (dehydration)	Report to physician. Evaluate neurologic status. Evaluate hydration status.
Hair		
Texture: Smooth with fine texture variations (*Note:* Variations depend on ethnic background.)	Coarse, brittle, dry hair (hypothyroidism) White forelock (Waardenburg syndrome)	Instruct parents regarding routine care of hair and scalp.
Distribution: Scalp hair high over eyebrows (Spanish-Mexican hairline begins midforehead and extends down back of neck.)	Low forehead and posterior hairlines may indicate chromosomal disorders	Assess for other signs of chromosomal aberrations. Refer to physician.

*Possible causes of alterations are placed in parentheses.

†This column provides guidelines for further assessment and initial nursing intervention.

ASSESSMENT GUIDE—continued

NEWBORN PHYSICAL ASSESSMENT

PHYSICAL ASSESSMENT/ NORMAL FINDINGS	ALTERATIONS AND POSSIBLE CAUSES*	NURSING RESPONSES TO DATA†
Face		
Symmetric movement of all facial features, normal hairline, eyebrows and eyelashes present		Assess and record symmetry of all parts, shape, regularity of features, sameness or differences in features.
Spacing of features: Eyes–ears at same level, nostrils equal size, cheeks full, and sucking pads present	Eyes wide apart—ocular hypertelorism (Apert syndrome, cri-du-chat, Turner syndrome)	Observe for other signs and symptoms indicative of disease states or chromosomal aberrations.
Lips equal on both sides of midline	Atypical face (Down syndrome, cretinism, gargoylism)	
Chin recedes when compared to other bones of face	Atypical small jaw—micrognathia (Pierre Robin syndrome, Treacher Collins syndrome)	Maintain airway; do not position supine. Initiate surgical consultation and referral.
Movement: Makes facial grimaces	Inability to suck, grimace, and close eyelids (cranial nerve injury)	Initiate neurologic assessment and consultation.
Symmetric when resting and crying	Asymmetry (paralysis of facial cranial nerve)	Assess and record symmetry of all parts, shape, regularity of features, and sameness or differences in features.
Eyes		
General placement and appearance: Bright and clear; even placement; slight nystagmus (involuntary cyclic eye movements)	Gross nystagmus (damage to third, fourth, and sixth cranial nerves)	
Concomitant strabismus	Constant and fixed strabismus	Reassure parents that strabismus is considered normal up to 6 months.
Move in all directions Blue-gray or slate–blue-gray	Lack of pigmentation (albinism) Brushfield spots may indicate Down syndrome (a light or white speckling of the outer two thirds of the iris)	Discuss with parents any necessary eye precautions. Assess for other signs of Down syndrome.
Brown color at birth in dark-skinned infants		Discuss with parents that permanent eye color is usually established by 3 months of age.
Eyelids: Position: above pupils but within iris, no drooping	Elevation or retraction of upper lid (hyperthyroidism) "Sunset sign" lid retraction and downward gaze (hydrocephalus), ptosis (congenital or paralysis of oculomotor muscle)	Assess for signs of hydrocephalus and hyperthyroidism. Evaluate interference with vision in subsequent well-baby visits.
Eyes on parallel plane	Upward slant in non-Asians (Down syndrome)	Assess for other signs of Down syndrome.
Epicanthal folds in Asian and 20% of newborns of northern European descent	Epicanthal folds (Down syndrome, cri-du-chat syndrome)	
Movement: Blink reflex in response to light stimulus Eyes open wide in dimly lighted room	Blink absent (CNS injury)	Evaluate neurologic status. Refer to physician.
Inspection: Edematous for first few days of life, resulting from birth and instillation of silver nitrate (chemical conjunctivitis); no lumps or redness	Purulent drainage (infection); infectious conjunctivitis (gonococcus, chlamydia, staphylococcus, or gram-negative organisms) Marginal blepharitis (lid edges red, crusted, scaly)	Initiate good handwashing. Refer to physician. Evaluate infant for seborrheic dermatitis; scales can be removed easily.
Cornea: Clear	Ulceration (herpes infection); large cornea or corneas of unequal size (congenital glaucoma)	Refer to ophthalmologist.
Corneal reflex present	Clouding, opacity of lens (cataract)	Assess for other manifestations of congenital herpes; institute nursing care measures.
Sclera: May appear bluish in newborn, then white; slightly brownish color frequent in newborns of African descent	True blue sclera (osteogenesis imperfecta)	Refer to physician.

*Possible causes of alterations are placed in parentheses.

†This column provides guidelines for further assessment and initial nursing intervention.

(continued)

ASSESSMENT GUIDE—continued

NEWBORN PHYSICAL ASSESSMENT

PHYSICAL ASSESSMENT/ NORMAL FINDINGS	ALTERATIONS AND POSSIBLE CAUSES*	NURSING RESPONSES TO DATA†
Eyes—continued		
Pupils: Pupils equal in size, round, and react to light by accommodation	Anisocoria—unequal pupils (CNS damage) Dilation or constriction (intracranial damage, retinoblastoma, glaucoma) Pupils nonreactive to light or accommodation (brain injury)	Refer for neurologic examination.
Slight nystagmus in newborn who has not learned to focus Pupil light reflex demonstrated at birth or by 3 weeks of age	Nystagmus (labyrinthine disturbance, CNS disorder)	
Conjunctiva: Chemical conjunctivitis Subconjunctival hemorrhage	Pale color (anemia)	Obtain hematocrit and hemoglobin. Reassure parents that chemical conjunctivitis will subside in 1 to 2 days and subconjunctival hemorrhage disappears in a few weeks.
Palpebral conjunctiva (red but not hyperemic)	Inflammation or edema (infection, blocked tear duct)	
Vision: 20/150 Tracks moving object to midline Fixed focus on objects at a distance of about 10–20 inches; may be difficult to evaluate in newborn Prefers faces, geometric designs, and black and white to colors	Cataracts (congenital infection)	Record any questions about visual acuity and initiate follow-up evaluation at first well-baby checkup. May suggest toys for parents to purchase—see Chapter 33. ∞
Lashes and lacrimal glands: Presence of lashes (lashes may be absent in preterm newborns)	No lashes on inner two thirds of lid (Treacher Collins syndrome), bushy lashes (Hurler syndrome), long lashes (Cornelia de Lange syndrome)	
Cry commonly tearless	Excessive tearing (plugged lacrimal duct, natal narcotic withdrawal), glaucoma	Demonstrate to parents how to milk blocked tear duct. Refer to ophthalmologist if tearing is excessive before third month of life.
Nose		
Appearance of external nasal aspects: May appear flattened as a result of birth process	Continued flat or broad bridge of nose (Down syndrome)	Arrange consultation with specialist. May be normal racial variation—Asian or African ancestry.
Small and narrow in midline, even placement in relationship to eyes and mouth	Low bridge of nose, beaklike nose (Apert syndrome, Treacher Collins syndrome) Upturned (Cornelia de Lange syndrome)	Initiate evaluation of chromosomal abnormalities.
Patent nares bilaterally (nose breathers)	Blockage of nares (mucus or secretions), choanal atresia	Inspect for obstruction of nares.
Sneezing common to clear nasal passages	Flaring nares (respiratory distress)	Maintain oral airway until surgical correction is made.
Responds to odors, may smell breast milk	No response to stimulating odors	Inspect for obstruction of nares.
Mouth		
Function of facial, hypoglossal, glossopharyngeal, and vagus nerves: Symmetry of movement and strength	Mouth draws to one side (transient seventh cranial nerve paralysis due to pressure in utero or trauma during birth, congenital paralysis)	Initiate neurologic consultation.
	Fishlike shape (Treacher Collins syndrome)	Administer eye care if eye on affected side of face is unable to close.
Presence of gag, swallowing, coordinated with sucking reflexes	Suppressed or absent reflexes	Evaluate other neurologic functions of these nerves.
Adequate salivation		

*Possible causes of alterations are placed in parentheses.

†This column provides guidelines for further assessment and initial nursing intervention.

ASSESSMENT GUIDE—continued

NEWBORN PHYSICAL ASSESSMENT

PHYSICAL ASSESSMENT/ NORMAL FINDINGS	ALTERATIONS AND POSSIBLE CAUSES*	NURSING RESPONSES TO DATA†
Mouth—*continued*		
Palate (soft and hard): Hard palate dome shaped Uvula midline with symmetric movement of soft palate	High-steepled palate (Treacher Collins syndrome), bifid uvula (congenital anomaly)	Assess for other congenital anomalies.
Palate intact, sucks well when stimulated	Clefts in either hard or soft palate (polygenic disorder)	Initiate a surgical consultation referral. Use special feeding devices.
Epithelial (Epstein's) pearls appear on mucosa		Assure parents that these are normal and will disappear at 2 or 3 months of age.
Esophagus patent, some drooling common in newborn	Excessive drooling or bubbling (esophageal atresia)	Test for patency of esophagus.
Tongue: Free moving in all directions, midline	Lack of movement or asymmetric movement (neurologic damage) Tongue-tied	Further assess neurologic functions. Test reflex elevation of tongue when depressed with tongue blade.
Pink color, smooth to rough texture, noncoated	Deviations from midline (cranial nerve damage) White cheesy coating (thrush) Tongue has deep ridges	Check for signs of weakness or deviation. Differentiate between thrush and milk curds. Reassure parents that tongue pattern may change from day to day.
Tongue proportional to mouth	Large tongue with short frenulum (cretinism, Down syndrome, other syndromes)	Evaluate in well-baby clinic to assess development delays. Initiate referrals.
Ears		
External ear: Without lesions, cysts, or nodules	Nodules, cysts, or sinus tracts in front of ear Adherent earlobes Low set Preauricular skin tags	Evaluate characteristics of lesions. Counsel parents to clean external ear with washcloth only; discourage use of cotton-tip applicators. Refer to physician for ligation.
Hearing: Eustachian tubes are cleared with first cry		
Absence of all risk factors	Presence of one or more risk factors	Assess history of risk factors for hearing loss.
Attends to sounds; sudden or loud noise elicits Moro reflex	No response to sound stimuli (deafness)	Test for Moro reflex.
Neck		
Appearance: Short, straight, creased with skin folds	Abnormally short neck (Turner syndrome) Arching or inability to flex neck (meningitis, congenital anomaly)	Report findings to physician.
Posterior neck lacks loose extra folds of skin	Webbing of neck (Turner syndrome, Down syndrome, trisomy 18)	Assess for other signs of the syndromes.
Clavicles: Straight and intact	Knot or lump on clavicle (fracture during difficult birth)	Obtain detailed labor and birth history; apply figure-eight bandage.
Moro reflex elicitable	Unilateral Moro reflex response on unaffected side (fracture of clavicle, brachial palsy, Erb-Duchenne paralysis)	
Symmetric shoulders	Hypoplasia	

*Possible causes of alterations are placed in parentheses.

†This column provides guidelines for further assessment and initial nursing intervention.

(continued)

ASSESSMENT GUIDE—continued

NEWBORN PHYSICAL ASSESSMENT

PHYSICAL ASSESSMENT/ NORMAL FINDINGS	ALTERATIONS AND POSSIBLE CAUSES*	NURSING RESPONSES TO DATA†
Chest		
Appearance and size: Circumference: 32.5 cm, 1–2 cm less than head		Collaborate with physician.
Wider than it is long		Measure at level of nipples after exhalation.
Normal shape without depressed or prominent sternum	Funnel chest (congenital or associated with Marfan syndrome)	
Lower end of sternum (xiphoid cartilage) may be protruding; less apparent after several weeks	Continued protrusion of xiphoid cartilage (Marfan syndrome, "pigeon chest")	Determine adequacy of other respiratory and circulatory signs.
		Assess for other signs and symptoms of various syndromes.
Sternum 8 cm long	Barrel chest	
Expansion and retraction: Bilateral expansion	Unequal chest expansion (pneumonia, pneumothorax, respiratory distress)	
No intercostal, subcostal, or supraclavicular retractions	Retractions (respiratory distress)	Assess respiratory effort regularity, flaring of nares, difficulty on both inspiration and expiration.
	Seesaw respirations (respiratory distress)	Record and consult physician.
Auscultation: Breath sounds are louder in infants	Decreased breath sounds (decreased respiratory activity, atelectasis, pneumothorax)	
Chest and axilla clear on crying	Increased breath sounds (resolving pneumonia or in cesarean births)	Perform assessment and report to physician any positive findings.
Bronchial breath sounds (heard where trachea and bronchi closest to chest wall, above sternum and between scapulae):		
Bronchial sounds bilaterally	Adventitious or abnormal sounds (respiratory disease or distress)	Evaluate color for pallor or cyanosis.
Air entry clear		Monitor every shift or more frequently.
Rales may indicate normal newborn atelectasis		Report to physician.
Cough reflex absent at birth, appears in 2 or more days		
Breasts: Flat with symmetric nipples	Lack of breast tissue (preterm or SGA)	
Breast tissue diameter 5 cm or more at term	Discharge	Evaluate for infection.
Average distance between nipples 8 cm	Breast abscesses	
Breast engorgement occurs on third day of life; liquid discharge may be expressed in term newborns	Enlargement	Reassure parents of normality of breast engorgement.
Nipples	Supernumerary nipples	No intervention is necessary.
	Dark-colored nipples	
Heart		
Auscultation: Location: lies horizontally, with left border extending to left of midclavicle		
Regular rhythm and rate	Arrhythmia (anoxia), tachycardia, bradycardia	Refer all arrhythmia and gallop rhythms.
Determination of point of maximal impulse (PMI) Usually lateral to midclavicular line at third or fourth intercostal space	Malpositioning (enlargement, abnormal placement, pneumothorax, dextrocardia, diaphragmatic hernia)	Initiate cardiac evaluation.
Functional murmurs	Location of murmurs (possible congenital cardiac anomaly)	Evaluate murmur: location, timing, and duration; observe for accompanying cardiac pathology symptoms; ascertain family history.
No thrills		
Horizontal groove at diaphragm shows flaring of rib cage to mild degree	Marked rib flaring (vitamin D deficiency) Inadequacy of respiratory movement	Initiate cardiopulmonary evaluation; assess pulses and blood pressures in all four extremities for equality and quality.

*Possible causes of alterations are placed in parentheses.

†This column provides guidelines for further assessment and initial nursing intervention.

ASSESSMENT GUIDE—continued

NEWBORN PHYSICAL ASSESSMENT

PHYSICAL ASSESSMENT/ NORMAL FINDINGS	ALTERATIONS AND POSSIBLE CAUSES*	NURSING RESPONSES TO DATA†
Abdomen		
Appearance: Cylindric, with some protrusion; appears large in relation to pelvis; some laxness of abdominal muscles	Distention, shiny abdomen with engorged vessels (gastrointestinal abnormalities, infection, congenital megacolon)	Examine abdomen thoroughly for mass or organomegaly. Measure abdominal girth.
No cyanosis, few vessels seen	Scaphoid abdominal appearance (diaphragmatic hernia)	Report deviations of abdominal size.
Diastasis recti—common in infants of African descent		
	Increased or decreased peristalsis (duodenal stenosis, small bowel obstruction)	Assess other signs and symptoms of obstruction.
	Localized flank bulging (enlarged kidneys, ascites, absent abdominal muscles)	Refer to physician.
Umbilicus: No protrusion of umbilicus (protrusion of umbilicus common in infants of African descent)	Umbilical hernia Patent urachus (congenital malformation)	Measure umbilical hernia by palpating the opening and record; it should close by 1–2 years of age; if not, refer to physician. Be aware of cultural practices. Taping or belly bands do not enhance closure.
Bluish white color	Omphalocele Gastroschisis	Cover omphalocele with sterile, moist dressing.
Cutis navel (umbilical cord projects), granulation tissue present in navel	Redness or exudate around cord (infection) Yellow discoloration (hemolytic disease, meconium staining)	Instruct parents on cord care and hygiene.
Two arteries and one vein apparent	Single umbilical artery (congenital anomalies)	Refer anomalies to physician.
Begins drying 1 to 2 hours after birth	Discharge or oozing of blood from the cord	
No bleeding		
Auscultation and percussion	Bowel sounds in chest (diaphragmatic hernia)	Collaborate with physician.
Soft bowel sounds heard shortly after birth every 10–30 seconds	Absence of bowel sounds Hyperperistalsis (intestinal obstruction)	Assess for other signs of dehydration or infection.
Femoral pulses: Palpable, equal, bilateral	Absent or diminished femoral pulses (coarctation of aorta)	Monitor blood pressure in upper and lower extremities.
Inguinal area: No bulges along inguinal area	Inguinal hernia	Initiate referral.
No inguinal lymph nodes felt		Continue follow-up in well baby clinic.
Bladder: Percusses 1–4 cm above symphysis	Failure to void within 24–48 hours after birth	Determine whether baby voided at birth.
Emptied about 3 hours after birth; if not, at time of birth	Exposure of bladder mucosa (exstrophy of bladder)	Consult with clinician. Cover exstrophy with sterile moist gauze.
Urine—inoffensive, mild odor	Foul odor (infection)	Obtain urine specimen if infection is suspected.
Genitals		
Gender clearly delineated	Ambiguous genitals	Refer for genetic consultation.
Male		
Penis: Slender in appearance, about 2.5 cm long, 1 cm wide at birth	Micropenis (congenital anomaly) Meatal atresia	Observe and record first voiding.
Normal urinary orifice, urethral meatus at tip of penis	Hypospadias, epispadias	Collaborate with physician in presence of abnormality. Delay circumcision.

*Possible causes of alterations are placed in parentheses.

†This column provides guidelines for further assessment and initial nursing intervention.

(continued)

ASSESSMENT GUIDE—continued

NEWBORN PHYSICAL ASSESSMENT

PHYSICAL ASSESSMENT/ NORMAL FINDINGS	ALTERATIONS AND POSSIBLE CAUSES*	NURSING RESPONSES TO DATA†
Male—continued		
Noninflamed urethral opening	Urethritis (infection)	Palpate for enlarged inguinal lymph nodes and record painful urination.
Foreskin adheres to glans	Ulceration of meatal opening (infection, inflammation)	Evaluate whether ulcer is due to diaper rash; counsel regarding care.
Uncircumcised foreskin tight for 2 to 3 months	Phimosis—if still tight after 3 months	Instruct parents on how to care for uncircumcised penis.
Circumcised		Teach parents how to care for circumcision. Check for voiding after procedure and evaluate for excessive bleeding.
Erectile tissue present		
Scrotum: Skin loose and hanging or tight and small; extensive rugae and normal size	Large scrotum containing fluid (hydrocele) Red, shiny scrotal skin (orchitis)	Shine a light through scrotum (transilluminate) to verify diagnosis.
Normal skin color Scrotal discoloration common in breech	Minimal rugae, small scrotum	Assess for prematurity.
Testes: Descended by birth; not consistently found in scrotum	Undescended testes (cryptorchidism)	If testes cannot be felt in scrotum, gently palpate femoral, inguinal, perineal, and abdominal areas for presence.
Testes size 1.5–2 cm at birth	Enlarged testes (tumor) Small testes (Klinefelter syndrome or adrenal hyperplasia)	Refer to and collaborate with physician for further diagnostic studies.
Female		
Mons: Normal skin color, area pigmented in dark-skinned infants		
Labia majora cover labia minora in term and postterm newborns; symmetric size appropriate for gestational age	Hematoma, lesions (trauma) Labia minora prominent	Evaluate for recent trauma. Assess for prematurity.
Clitoris: Normally large in newborn Edema and bruising in breech birth	Hypertrophy (hermaphroditism)	Refer for genetic workup.
Vagina: Urinary meatus and vaginal orifice visible (0.5 cm circumference)	Inflammation; erythema and discharge (urethritis) Congenital absence of vagina	Collect urine specimen for laboratory examination. Refer to physician.
Vaginal tag or hymenal tag disappears in a few weeks		
Discharge; smegma under labia	Foul-smelling discharge (infection)	Collect data and further evaluate reason for discharge.
Bloody or mucoid discharge	Excessive vaginal bleeding (blood coagulation defect)	
Buttocks and Anus		
Buttocks symmetric	Pilonidal dimple	Examine for possible sinus. Instruct parents about cleansing this area.
Anus patent and passage of meconium within 24–48 hours after birth	Imperforate anus, rectal atresia (congenital gastrointestinal defect)	Evaluate extent of problems. Initiate surgical consultation.
No fissures, tears, or skin tags	Fissures	Perform digital examination to ascertain patency if patency uncertain.
	*Possible causes of alterations are placed in parentheses.	†This column provides guidelines for further assessment and initial nursing intervention.

ASSESSMENT GUIDE—continued

NEWBORN PHYSICAL ASSESSMENT

PHYSICAL ASSESSMENT/ NORMAL FINDINGS	ALTERATIONS AND POSSIBLE CAUSES*	NURSING RESPONSES TO DATA†
Extremities and Trunk		
Short and generally flexed; extremities move symmetrically through range of motion but lack full extension	Unilateral or absence of movement (spinal cord involvement) Fetal position continued or limp (anoxia, CNS problems, hypoglycemia)	Review birth record to assess possible cause.
All joints move spontaneously; good muscle tone, of flexor type, birth to 2 months	Spasticity when infant begins using extensors (cerebral palsy, lack of muscle tone, "floppy baby" syndrome) Hypotonia (Down syndrome)	Collaborate with physician.
Arms: Equal in length	Brachial palsy (difficult birth)	Report to clinician.
Bilateral movement	Erb-Duchenne paralysis	
Flexed when quiet	Muscle weakness, fractured clavicle Absence of limb or change of size (phocomelia, amelia)	
Hands: Normal number of fingers	Polydactyly (Ellis-van Creveld syndrome) Syndactyly—one limb (developmental anomaly) Syndactyly—both limbs (genetic component)	Report to clinician.
Normal palmar crease	Simian line on palm (Down syndrome)	Refer for genetic workup.
Normal-sized hands	Short fingers and broad hand (Hurler syndrome)	Evaluate for history of distress in utero.
Nails present and extend beyond fingertips in term newborn.	Cyanosis and clubbing (cardiac anomalies) Nails long or yellow stained (postterm)	Carry out cardiac respiratory assessments. Check pulseoximetry.
Spine: C-shaped spine	Spina bifida occulta (nevus pilosus)	Evaluate extent of neurologic damage; initiate care of spinal opening.
Flat and straight when prone	Dermal sinus	
Slight lumbar lordosis	Myelomeningocele	
Easily flexed and intact when palpated	Head lag, limp, floppy trunk (neurologic problems)	
At least half of back devoid of lanugo		
Full-term infant in ventral suspension should hold head at 45-degree angle, back straight		Elicit reflex to assess degree of involvement.
Hips: No sign of instability	Sensation of abnormal movement, jerk, or snap of hip dislocation	Examine all newborn infants for dislocated hip prior to discharge from birthing center.
Hips abduct to more than 60 degrees		If this is suspected, refer to orthopedist for further evaluation. Reassess at well-baby visits.
Inguinal and buttock skin creases: Symmetric inguinal and buttock creases	Asymmetry (dislocated hips)	Refer to orthopedist for evaluation. Counsel parents regarding symptoms of concern and discuss therapy.
Legs: Legs equal in length	Shortened leg (dislocated hips)	Refer to orthopedist for evaluation.
Legs shorter than arms at birth	Lack of leg movement (fractures, spinal defects)	Counsel parents regarding symptoms of concern and discuss therapy.
Feet: Foot is in straight line	Talipes equinovarus (true clubfoot)	Discuss differences between positional and true clubfoot with parents.
Positional clubfoot—based on position in utero		Teach parents passive manipulation of foot.
Fat pads and creases on soles of feet	Incomplete sole creases in first 24 hours of life (premature)	
Talipes planus (flat feet) normal under 3 years of age		Refer to orthopedist if not corrected by 3 months of age. Reassure parents that flat feet are normal in infants.

*Possible causes of alterations are placed in parentheses.

†This column provides guidelines for further assessment and initial nursing intervention.

(continued)

NEWBORN PHYSICAL ASSESSMENT

PHYSICAL ASSESSMENT/ NORMAL FINDINGS	ALTERATIONS AND POSSIBLE CAUSES*	NURSING RESPONSES TO DATA†
Neuromuscular		
Motor function: Symmetric movement and strength in all extremities	Limp, flaccid, or hypertonic (CNS disorders, infection, dehydration, fracture)	Appraise newborn's posture and motor functions by observing activities and motor characteristics.
May be jerky or have brief twitchings	Tremors (hypoglycemia, hypocalcemia, infection, neurologic damage)	Evaluate electrolyte imbalance, hypoglycemia, and neurologic functioning.
Head lag not over 45 degrees	Delayed or abnormal development (preterm, neurologic involvement)	
Neck control adequate to maintain head erect briefly	Asymmetry of tone or strength (neurologic damage)	Refer for genetic evaluation.
Reflexes		
Blink: Stimulated by flash of light; response is closure of eyelids	Lack of blink response (damage to cranial nerve, CNS injury)	Assess neurologic status.
Pupillary reflex: Stimulated by flash of light; response is constriction of pupil	Lack of reflex (damage to cranial nerve, CNS injury)	
Moro: Response to sudden movement or loud noise should be one of symmetric extension and abduction of arms with fingers extended; then return to normal relaxed flexion	Asymmetry of body response (fractured clavicle, injury to brachial plexus)	Discuss normality of this reflex in response to loud noises or sudden movements.
Infant lying on back: slightly raised head suddenly released; infant held horizontally, lowered quickly about 6 inches, and stopped abruptly Fingers form a C Present at birth; disappears by 6 months of age	Consistent absence (brain damage)	Absence of reflex requires neurologic evaluation.
Rooting and sucking: Turns in direction of stimulus to cheek or mouth; opens mouth and begins to suck rhythmically when finger or nipple is inserted into mouth; difficult to elicit after feeding; disappears by 4 to 7 months of age	Poor sucking or easily fatigable (preterm, breastfed infants of barbiturate-addicted mothers, possible cardiac problem) Absence of response (preterm, neurologic involvement, depressed newborns)	Evaluate strength and coordination of sucking. Observe newborn during feeding, and counsel parents about mutuality of feeding experience and newborn's responses.
Sucking is adequate for nutritional intake and meeting oral stimulation needs; disappears by 12 months		
Palmar grasp: Fingers grasp adult finger when palm is stimulated and held momentarily; lessens at 3 to 4 months of age	Asymmetry of response (neurologic problems)	Evaluate other reflexes and general neurologic functioning.
Plantar grasp: Toes curl downward when sole of foot is stimulated; lessens by 8 months	Absent (defects of lower spinal column)	Assess for other lower extremity neurologic problems.
Stepping: When held upright and one foot touching a flat surface, will step alternately; disappears at 4 to 8 weeks of age	Asymmetry of stepping (neurologic abnormality)	Evaluate muscle tone and function on each side of body. Refer to specialist.
Babinski: Fanning and extension of all toes when one side of sole is stroked from heel upward across ball of foot; disappears at about 12 months	Absence of response (low spinal cord defects)	Refer for further neurologic evaluation.
Tonic neck: Fencer position—when head is turned to one side, extremities on same side extend and on opposite side flex; this reflex may not be evident during early neonatal period; disappears at 3 to 4 months of age Response often more dominant in leg than in arm	Absent after 1 month of age or persistent asymmetry (cerebral lesion)	Assess neurologic functioning.
Prone crawl: While on abdomen, newborn pushes up and tries to crawl	Absence or variance of response (preterm, weak, or depressed newborns)	Evaluate motor functioning. Refer to specialist.
Trunk incurvation (Galant): In prone position, stroking of spine causes pelvis to turn to stimulated side	Failure to rotate to stimulated side (neurologic damage)	

*Possible causes of alterations are placed in parentheses.

†This column provides guidelines for further assessment and initial nursing interventions.

associated with osteogenesis imperfecta. The infant's eye color is established at approximately 3 months, although it may change any time up to 1 year.

Check the eyes for size, equality of pupil size, reaction of pupils to light, blink reflex to light, and edema and inflammation of the eyelids. The eyelids are usually edematous during the first few days of life because of the pressure associated with birth.

Erythromycin and tetracycline are frequently used prophylactically instead of silver nitrate and usually do not cause chemical irritation of the eye. The instillation of silver nitrate drops in the newborn's eyes may cause edema; **chemical conjunctivitis** may appear a few hours after instillation, but it disappears in 1 to 2 days. If infectious conjunctivitis exists, the newborn has the same purulent (greenish yellow) discharge exudate as in chemical conjunctivitis, but it is caused by gonococcus, *Chlamydia,* staphylococci, or a variety of gram-negative bacteria and requires treatment with ophthalmic antibiotics. Onset is usually after the second day. Edema of the orbits or eyelids may persist for several days, until the newborn's kidneys can eliminate the fluid.

Small **subconjunctival hemorrhages** appear in about 10% of newborns and are commonly found on the sclera. These hemorrhages are caused by the changes in vascular tension or ocular pressure during birth. They will remain for a few weeks and are of no pathologic significance. Parents need reassurance that the newborn is not bleeding from within the eye and that vision will not be impaired.

The newborn may demonstrate transient strabismus caused by poor neuromuscular control of eye muscles (Figure 27–28 ●). It gradually regresses in 3 to 4 months. The "doll's eye" phenomenon is also present for about 10

● **FIGURE 27–28**

Transient strabismus may be present in the newborn due to poor neuromuscular control.

Used with permission from Mead Johnson Nutritionals, Evansville, IN.

days after birth. As the newborn's head position is changed to the left and then to the right, the eyes move to the opposite direction. This results from underdeveloped integration of head-eye coordination.

Observe the newborn's pupils for opacities or whiteness and for the absence of a normal red retinal reflex. Red retinal reflex is a red-orange flash of color observed when an ophthalmoscope light reflects off the retina. In a newborn with dark skin color, the retina may appear paler or more grayish. Absence of red reflex occurs with cataracts. Congenital cataracts should be suspected in newborns of mothers with a history of rubella, cytomegalic inclusion disease, or syphilis.

The newborn's cry is commonly tearless because the lacrimal structures are immature at birth and are not usually fully functional until the second month of life. However, some newborns produce tears.

Poor oculomotor coordination and absence of accommodation limit visual abilities, but newborns have peripheral vision, can fixate on objects near (8 to 10 in.) their face for short periods, can accommodate to large objects (3 in. tall by 3 in. wide), and can seek out high-contrast geometric shapes. Newborns can perceive faces, shapes, and colors and begin to show visual preferences early. Newborns generally blink in response to bright lights, to a tap on the bridge of the nose (glabellar reflex), or to a light touch on the eyelids. Pupillary light reflex is also present. Examination of the eye is best accomplished by rocking the newborn from an upright position to the horizontal a few times or by other methods such as diminishing overhead lights, which elicits an opened-eye response.

NOSE

The newborn's nose is small and narrow. Infants are characteristically obligatory nose breathers for the first few months of life and generally remove obstructions by sneezing. The nose is patent if the newborn breathes easily with the mouth closed. If respiratory difficulty occurs, check for choanal atresia (congenital blockage of the passageway between nose and pharynx). Historically, choanal atresia can be checked by attempting to gently pass a soft # 5 French catheter into both nostrils. Because of possible trauma, a cold, flat metal object may also be held under the nose to observe for fogging (Thureen et al., 2005).

The newborn can smell after the nasal passages are cleared of amniotic fluid and mucus. They demonstrate this ability by searching for milk. Newborns turn their heads toward a milk source, whether bottle or breast. Newborns react to strong odors, such as alcohol, by turning their heads away or blinking.

MOUTH

The lips of the newborn should be pink, and a touch on the lips should produce sucking motions. Saliva is normally

● FIGURE 27–29

The nurse inserts a gloved index (or "pinky") finger into the newborn's mouth and feels for any openings along the hard and soft palates. *Note:* Gloves or a finger cot are always worn to examine the palate.

© Stella Johnson (www.stellajohnson.com)

scant. The taste buds develop before birth, and the newborn can easily discriminate between sweet and bitter flavors.

The easiest way to examine the mouth completely is to stimulate infants gently to cry by depressing their tongue, thereby causing them to open the mouth fully. It is extremely important to examine the entire mouth to check for a cleft palate, which can be present even in the absence of a cleft lip (Figure 27–29 ●).

Occasionally an examination of the gums will reveal precocious teeth over the area where the lower central incisor will erupt. If they appear loose, they should be removed to prevent aspiration. Gray-white lesions (inclusion cysts) on the gums may be confused with teeth. On the hard palate and gum margins, **Epstein's pearls**, small glistening white specks (keratin-containing cysts) that feel hard to the touch, are often present. They usually disappear in a few weeks and are of no significance. Thrush may appear as white patches that look like milk curds adhering to the mucous membranes and cause bleeding when removed. **Thrush** is caused by *Candida albicans,* often acquired from an infected vaginal tract during birth or if the mother uses poor handwashing when handling her newborn. Thrush is treated with a preparation of nystatin (Mycostatin).

A newborn who is tongue-tied has a ridge of frenulum tissue attached to the underside of the tongue at varying lengths from its base, causing a heart shape at the tip of the tongue. "Clipping the tongue," or cutting the ridge of tissue, is not recommended. This ridge does not affect speech or eating, but cutting creates an entry for infection.

Transient nerve paralysis resulting from birth trauma may be manifested by asymmetric mouth movements when the newborn cries or by difficulty with sucking and feeding.

EARS

The ears of the newborn should be soft and pliable and should recoil readily when folded and released. In the nor-

mal newborn, the insertion site of the ear (pinna) should be parallel to the inner canthus of the eye. Inspect the ears for shape, size, position, and firmness of cartilage. Low-set ears are characteristic of many syndromes and may indicate chromosomal abnormalities (especially trisomy 13 and 18), mental retardation, and internal organ abnormalities, especially bilateral renal agenesis as a result of embryologic developmental deviations (Figure 27–30 ●). Preauricular skin tags may be present just in front of the ear.

After the first cry, the newborn's hearing becomes acute as mucus from the middle ear is absorbed, the eustachian tube becomes aerated, and the tympanic membrane becomes visible. Evaluate the newborn's hearing by noting the baby's response to loud or moderately loud noises unaccompanied by vibrations. The sleeping newborn should stir or awaken in response to nearby sounds. (This is not a very accurate test, but it may alert the examiner to a possible problem.) The newborn can discriminate the individual characteristics of the human voice and is especially sensitive to sound levels within the normal conversational range. The newborn in a noisy nursery may habituate to the sounds and not stir unless the sound is sudden or much louder than usual.

The AAP has endorsed universal newborn hearing screening (UNHS) in birthing units as the standard of care (Thureen et al., 2005). The current goal is to screen all infants by 1 month of age, confirm hearing loss with audiologic examination by 3 months of age, and treat with comprehensive early intervention services before 6 months of age (AAP & ACOG, 2002). Families need to be educated about appropriate interpretation of screening test results and the appropriate steps for follow-up.

NECK

A short neck, creased with skin folds, is characteristic of the normal newborn. Because muscle tone is not well developed,

● FIGURE 27–30

A   B

The position of the external ear may be assessed by drawing a line across the inner and outer canthus of the eye to the insertion of the ear. *A,* Normal position. *B,* True low-set position.

Used with permission from Mead Johnson Nutritionals, Evansville, IN.

the neck cannot support the full weight of the head, which rotates freely. The head lags considerably when the newborn is pulled from a supine to a sitting position, but the prone newborn is able to raise the head slightly. Palpate the neck for masses and lymph nodes, inspect it for webbing, and determine adequacy of range of motion and neck muscle function by fully extending the head in all directions. It is important to consider injury to the sternocleidomastoid muscle (congenital torticollis) if the neck is rigid.

Evaluate the clavicles for evidence of fractures, which occasionally occur during difficult births or in newborns with broad shoulders. The normal clavicle is straight. If fractured, a lump and a grating sensation (crepitus) during movements may be palpated along the course of the side of the break. Elicit the Moro reflex (see page 708 to evaluate bilateral equal movement of the arms). If the clavicle is fractured, the response will be demonstrated only on the unaffected side.

CHEST

The thorax is cylindric at birth, and the ribs are flexible. Assess the general appearance of the chest. A protrusion at the lower end of the sternum, called the xiphoid cartilage, is frequently seen. It is under the skin and will become less apparent after several weeks as adipose tissue accumulates.

Engorged breasts occur frequently in both male and female newborns. This condition, which occurs by the third day, is a result of maternal hormonal influences and may last up to 2 weeks (Figure 27–31 ●). A whitish secretion from the nipples may also be noted. The newborn's breast should not be massaged or squeezed, because this may cause a breast abscess. Extra nipples, or supernumerary nipples, are occasionally noted below and medial to the true nipples. These harmless pink or brown (in dark-skinned newborns) spots vary in size and do not contain glandular tissue. Differentiate accessory nipples from a pigmented nevi (mole) by placing the fingertips alongside the accessory nipple and pulling the adjacent tissue laterally. The accessory nipple will appear dimpled. At puberty the accessory nipple may darken.

CRY

The newborn's cry should be strong, lusty, and of medium pitch. A high-pitched, shrill cry is abnormal and may indicate neurologic disorders or hypoglycemia. Periods of crying usually vary in length after consoling measures are used. Babies' cries are an important method of communication and alert caregivers to changes in their baby's condition and needs.

RESPIRATION

Normal breathing for a term newborn is 30 to 60 respirations per minute and is predominantly diaphragmatic, with

● **FIGURE 27–31**

Breast hypertrophy.

Used with permission from Korones, S. B. (1986). High-risk newborn infants (4th ed.). St. Louis, MO: Mosby.

associated rising and falling of the abdomen during inspiration and expiration. Note any signs of respiratory distress, nasal flaring, intercostal or xiphoid retraction, expiratory grunt or sigh, seesaw respirations, tachypnea (greater than 60 breaths per minute), hyperexpansion (chest appears high), or hypoexpansion (chest appears low) of the anteroposterior diameter of the chest. Both the anterior and posterior chest are auscultated. Some breath sounds are heard better when the newborn is crying, but localizing and identifying breath sounds are difficult in the newborn. Upper airway noises and bowel sounds may also be heard over the chest wall and make auscultation difficult. Because sounds may be transmitted from the unaffected lung to the affected lung, the absence of breath sounds may not be diagnosed. Air entry may be noisy in the first couple of hours until lung fluid resolves, especially after cesarean births. Brief periods of apnea (episodic breathing) occur, but no color or heart rate changes occur in healthy term newborns.

NURSING PRACTICE

Vital sign assessments are most accurate if the newborn is at rest, so measure pulse and respirations first if the baby is quiet. To soothe a crying baby, try placing your moistened gloved finger in the baby's mouth and then complete your assessment while the baby suckles.

● FIGURE 27–32

A

B

A, Bilaterally palpate the femoral arteries for rate and intensity of the pulses. Press fingertip gently at the groin as shown. *B,* Compare the femoral pulses to the brachial pulses by palpating the pulses simultaneously for comparison of rate and intensity.

HEART

Heart rates can be as rapid as 180 beats per minute in newborns and fluctuate a great deal, especially if the baby moves or is startled. The normal range is 120 to 160 beats per minute. The heart is examined for rate and rhythm, position of the apical impulse, and heart sound intensity. The physician should reassess dysrhythmias.

The pulse rate is variable and is influenced by physical activity, crying, state of wakefulness, and body temperature. The examiner auscultates over the entire heart region (precordium), below the left axilla, and below the scapula. Apical pulse rates are obtained by auscultation for a full minute, preferably when the newborn is asleep.

The placement of the heart in the chest should be determined when the newborn is in a quiet state. The heart is relatively large at birth and is located high in the chest, with its apex somewhere between the fourth and fifth intercostal space.

A shift of heart tones in the mediastinal area to either side may indicate pneumothorax, dextrocardia (heart placement on the right side of the chest), or a diaphragmatic hernia. The experienced nurse can diagnose these and many other problems early with a stethoscope.

Normally the heartbeat has a "toc tic" sound. A slur or slushing sound (usually after the first sound) may indicate a murmur. Although 90% of all murmurs are transient and are considered normal, a physician should monitor them closely. Many murmurs are related to a patent ductus arteriosus, which closes in about 1 to 2 days. Occasionally, significant murmurs are heard, including the murmur of a patent ductus arteriosus, aortic or pulmonary stenosis, or small ventricular septal defect. (See Chapter 30 for a discussion of congenital heart defects. ∞)

Peripheral pulses (brachial, femoral, pedal) are also evaluated to detect any lags or unusual characteristics. Palpate brachial pulses bilaterally for equality and compare them with the femoral pulses. Palpate femoral pulses by applying gentle pressure with the middle finger over the femoral canal (Figure 27–32 ●). Decreased or absent femoral pulses indicate coarctation of the aorta and require additional investigation. A wide difference in blood pressure between the upper and lower extremities also indicates coarctation.

The measurement of blood pressure is best accomplished by using the Doppler technique or a 1- to 2-inch cuff and a stethoscope over the brachial artery (Figure 27–33 ●). When assessing the newborn's blood pressure, the extremity should be immobilized and the cuff should cover two thirds of the upper arm or upper leg. Movement, crying, and inap-

● FIGURE 27–33

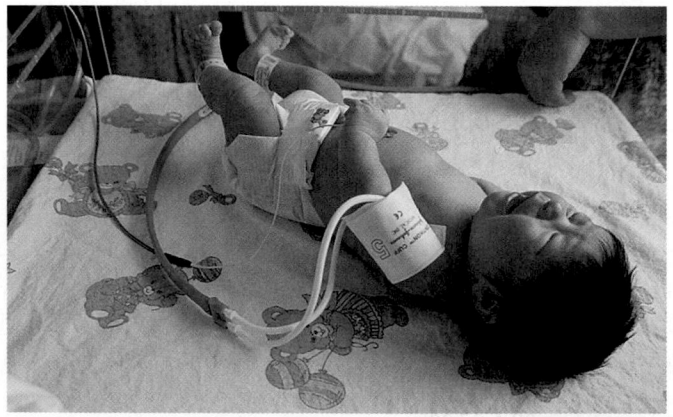

Blood pressure measurement using a Doppler device. The cuff can be applied to the upper arm or thigh.

propriate cuff size can give inaccurate measurements of the blood pressure.

Blood pressure may not be measured routinely on healthy newborns, but it is essential for newborns who are having distress, are premature, or are suspected of cardiac anomaly (Thureen et al., 2005). Infants who have birth asphyxia and are on ventilators have significantly lower systolic and diastolic blood pressures than healthy infants. If cardiac anomaly is suspected, blood pressure is measured in all four extremities (Table 27–4). At birth, systolic values usually range from 80 to 45 mm Hg and diastolic values from 60 to 40 mm Hg. By the tenth day of life, blood pressure rises to 100/50 mm Hg.

ABDOMEN

The nurse can learn a great deal about the newborn's abdomen without disturbing the infant. The abdomen should be cylindric and protrude slightly. A certain amount of laxness of the abdominal muscles is normal. A scaphoid (hollow-shaped) appearance suggests the absence of abdominal contents. No cyanosis should be present, and few if any blood vessels should be apparent to the eye. There should be no gross distention or bulging. The more distended the abdomen, the tighter the skin becomes, with engorged vessels appearing. Distention is the first sign of many of the abnormalities found in the gastrointestinal tract.

Before palpating the abdomen, auscultate for bowel sounds in all four quadrants. Bowel sounds may be present by 1 hour after birth. Palpation can cause a transient decrease in intensity of the bowel sounds.

Abdominal palpation should be done systematically. Palpate each of the four abdominal quadrants and move in a clockwise direction until all four quadrants have been palpated for softness, tenderness, and the presence of masses. Place one hand under the back for support during palpation.

UMBILICAL CORD

Initially the umbilical cord is white and gelatinous in appearance, with the two umbilical arteries and one umbilical vein readily apparent. Because a single umbilical artery is frequently associated with congenital anomalies, it is important to count the vessels during the newborn assessment. The cord begins drying within 1 or 2 hours of birth and is shriveled and blackened by the second or third day. Within 7 to 10 days it sloughs off, although a granulating area may remain for a few days longer.

Cord bleeding is abnormal and may result because the cord was inadvertently pulled or the cord clamp was loosened. Foul-smelling drainage is also abnormal and is generally caused by infection, which requires immediate treatment to prevent septicemia. If the newborn has a patent urachus (abnormal connection between the umbilicus and bladder), moistness or draining urine may be apparent at the base of the cord. Another umbilical cord anomaly that must be assessed for is umbilical cord hernia, which is more common in African-American infants than Caucasian infants (Thureen et al., 2005) (Figure 27–34 ●).

Serous or serosanguineous drainage that continues after the cord falls off may indicate a granuloma. It appears as a small red button deep in the umbilicus. A physician may cauterize it with a silver nitrate stick (Thureen et al., 2005).

GENITALS

Female Infants

Examine the labia majora, labia minora, and clitoris and note the size of each as appropriate for gestational age. A vaginal tag or hymenal tag is often evident and usually disappears in

TABLE 27–4 ✤ Newborn Vital Signs

Pulse
- 120–160 bpm
- During sleep as low as 80 bpm; if crying, up to 180 bpm
- Apical pulse counted for 1 full minute

Respirations
- 30–60 respirations/minute
- Predominantly diaphragmatic but synchronous with abdominal movements
- Respirations are counted for 1 full minute

Blood Pressure
- 80–60/45–40 mm Hg at birth
- 100/50 mm Hg at day 10

Temperature
- Normal range: 36.5–37.5°C (97.7–99.4°F)
- Axillary: 36.4–37.2°C (97.5–99°F)
- Skin: 36–36.5°C (96.8–97.7°F)
- Rectal: 36.6–37.2°C (97.8–99°F)

● **FIGURE 27–34**

Umbilical hernia.

a few weeks. During the first week of life, the female newborn may have a vaginal discharge composed of thick, whitish mucus. This discharge, which can become tinged with blood, is called **pseudomenstruation** and is caused by the withdrawal of maternal hormones. Smegma, a white cheeselike substance, is often present between the labia. Removing it may traumatize tender tissue.

Male Infants

Inspect the penis to determine whether the urinary meatus is correctly positioned. Hypospadias occurs when the urinary meatus is located on the ventral surface of the penis. It occurs most commonly among people of western European descent. Phimosis is a condition in which the opening of the foreskin (prepuce) is small and the foreskin cannot be pulled back over the glans at all. This condition may interfere with urination, so the adequacy of the urinary stream should be evaluated.

Hands should be warm when inspecting the scrotum for size and symmetry, and when palpating to verify the presence of both testes and to rule out cryptorchidism (failure of testes to descend). Palpate the testes separately between the thumb and forefinger, with the thumb and forefinger of the other hand placed together over the inguinal canal. Scrotal edema and discoloration are common in breech births. Hydrocele (a collection of fluid surrounding the testes in the scrotum) is common in newborns and should be identified. It usually resolves without intervention. A discolored or dusky scrotum and solid testis should raise the suspicion of testicular torsion.

ANUS

Inspect the anal area to verify that it is patent and has no fissure. Imperforate anus and rectal atresia may be ruled out by observation. Digital examination, if necessary, is done by a physician or nurse practitioner. The nurse also notes the passage of the first meconium stool. Atresia of the gastrointestinal tract or meconium ileus with resultant obstruction must be considered if the newborn does not pass meconium in the first 24 hours of life.

EXTREMITIES

Examine extremities for gross deformities, extra digits or webbing, clubfoot, and range of motion. Normal newborn extremities appear short, are generally flexible, and move symmetrically.

Arms and Hands

Nails extend beyond the fingertips in term newborns. Count fingers and toes. Polydactyly is the presence of extra digits on either the hands or the feet. Syndactyly refers to fusion (webbing) of fingers or toes. Inspect the hands for normal palmar creases. A single palmar crease, called a simian line (see Figure 6–15 in Chapter 6 ∞), is frequently present in children with Down syndrome.

Brachial palsy, paralysis of portions of the arm, results from trauma to the brachial plexus during a difficult birth. It occurs commonly when strong traction is exerted on the head of the newborn in an attempt to free a shoulder lodged behind the symphysis pubis in the presence of shoulder dystocia. Brachial palsy may also occur during a breech birth if an arm becomes trapped over the head and traction is exerted.

The portion of the arm affected is determined by the nerves damaged. **Erb-Duchenne paralysis (Erb's palsy)** involves damage to the upper arm (fifth and sixth cervical nerves) and is the most common type. Injury to the eighth cervical and first thoracic nerve roots and the lower portion of the plexus produces the relatively rare lower arm injury. The whole-arm type results from damage to the entire plexus.

With Erb-Duchenne paralysis the newborn's arm lies limply at the side. The elbow is held in extension with the forearm pronated. The newborn is unable to elevate the arm, and the Moro reflex cannot be elicited on the affected side (Figure 27–35 ⊙). Lower arm injury causes paralysis of the hand and wrist; complete paralysis of the limb occurs with the whole-arm type.

Carefully instruct the parents in the correct method of performing passive range of motion exercises (to prevent muscle contractures and restore function) and arrange su-

⊙ **FIGURE 27–35**

Right Erb's palsy resulting from injury to the fifth and sixth cervical roots of the brachial plexus.

Used with permission from Potter, E. L., & Craig, J. M. (1975). Pathology of the fetus and infant (3rd ed.). St. Louis, MO: Mosby–Yearbook Medical Publishers.

pervised practice sessions. In more severe cases, splinting of the arm is indicated until the edema decreases. The arm is held in a position of abduction and external rotation with the elbow flexed 90 degrees, often called the "Statue of Liberty" position. The "Statue of Liberty" splint is commonly used, although similar results are obtained by attaching a strip of muslin to the head of the crib and tying the other end around the wrist, thereby holding the arm up.

Prognosis is related to the amount of nerve damage resulting from trauma and hemorrhage within the nerve sheath. Complete recovery occurs within a few months with minimal trauma. Moderate trauma may result in partial paralysis. Recovery is unlikely with severe trauma, and muscle wasting may develop.

NURSING PRACTICE

Always examine more closely any infant who is reluctant to move an extremity. Fractures are often asymptomatic in the newborn; paralytic injuries are characterized by immobility of an extremity.

Legs and Feet

The newborn's legs should be of equal length, with symmetric skin folds. However, they may assume a "fetal posture" secondary to position in utero, and it may take several days for the legs to relax into a normal position. Perform **Ortolani's maneuver** to rule out the possibility of congenital hip dysplasia (hip dislocation). With the newborn relaxed and quiet on a firm surface, with hips and knees flexed at a 90-degree angle, grasp the infant's thigh with the middle finger over the greater trochanter and lift the thigh to bring the femoral head from its posterior position toward the acetabulum. With gentle abduction of the thigh, the femoral head is returned to the acetabulum. Simultaneously the examiner feels a sense of reduction or a "clunk" as the femoral head returns. This reduction is audible. To perform **Barlow's maneuver**, grasp and adduct the infant's thigh and apply gentle downward pressure. Dislocation is felt as the femoral head is then returned to the acetabulum using Ortolani's maneuver, confirming the diagnosis of an unstable or dislocated hip (Figure 27–36 ⊙).

Examine the feet for evidence of a talipes deformity (clubfoot). Intrauterine position frequently causes the feet to appear to turn inward (Figure 27–37 ⊙). This finding is termed a "positional" clubfoot. If the feet can easily be returned to the midline by manipulation, no treatment is indicated; it is important to teach range of motion exercises to the family. Further investigation is indicated when the foot will not turn to a midline position or align readily. The most severe type of "true clubfoot" is called talipes equinovarus. For detailed discussion of various types of foot deformity and management, see Chapter 54. ∞

BACK

With the newborn prone, examine the back. The spine should appear straight and flat, since the lumbar and sacral curves do not develop until the newborn begins to sit. Examine the base of the spine for a dermal sinus. A nevus pilosus ("hairy nerve") is only occasionally found at the base of the spine in newborns, but it is significant because it is often associated with spina bifida and spina bifida occulta. A pilonidal dimple should be examined to ascertain that there is no connection to the spinal canal.

ASSESSMENT OF NEUROLOGIC STATUS

The neurologic examination should begin with a period of observation, noting the general physical characteristics and behaviors of the newborn. Important behaviors to assess are the state of alertness, resting posture, cry, and quality of muscle tone and motor activity.

The usual position of the newborn is with partially flexed extremities, with the legs abducted to the abdomen. When awake, the newborn may exhibit purposeless, uncoordinated bilateral movements of the extremities. If these movements are absent, minimal, or obviously asymmetric, neurologic dysfunction should be suspected. Eye movements are observable during the first few days of life. An alert newborn is able to fixate on faces and brightly colored objects. A bright light shining in the newborn's eyes elicits the blinking response.

Evaluate muscle tone by moving various parts of the body while the head of the newborn is in a neutral position. The newborn is somewhat hypertonic; that is, there should be resistance to extending the elbow and knee joints. Muscle tone should be symmetric. Diminished muscle tone and flaccidity require further evaluation.

Jitteriness (tremorlike movements) is common in the full-term newborn and must be evaluated to differentiate the tremors from convulsions. Tremors may also be related to hypoglycemia, hypocalcemia, or substance withdrawal. Environmental stimuli may initiate tremors. Jitteriness may be distinguished from tonic-clonic seizure activity because it can usually be stopped by the infant sucking on the extremity or by the nurse holding or passively flexing the involved extremity. A fine jumping of the muscle is likely to be a central nervous system (CNS) disorder and requires further evaluation. Newborn seizures may consist of no more than smacking of lips, chewing or swallowing movements, deviations of the eyes, rigidity, or flaccidity because of CNS immaturity. In contrast to tremors, seizures are not usually initiated by stimuli and cannot be stopped by holding.

It is possible to elicit specific deep tendon reflexes, but they have limited value unless they are obviously asymmetric. The knee jerk is typically brisk; a normal ankle clonus may involve three or four beats. Plantar flexion is present.

● FIGURE 27–36

A

B

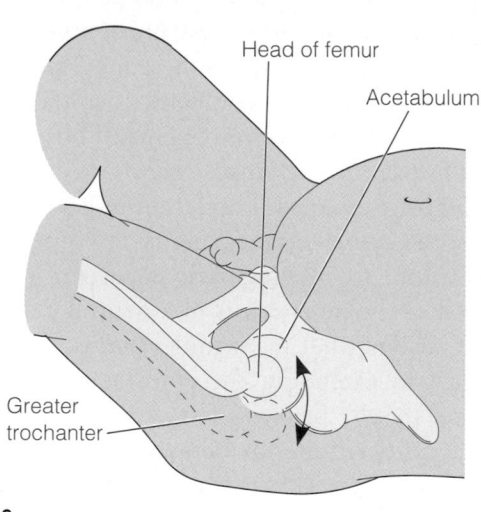

Head of femur

Acetabulum

Greater
trochanter

C

D

A, The asymmetry of gluteal and thigh fat folds seen in infant with left developmental dysplasia of the hip. **B,** Barlow's (dislocation) maneuver. Baby's thigh is grasped and adducted (placed together) with gentle downward pressure. **C,** Dislocation is palpable as femoral head slips out of acetabulum. **D,** Ortolani's maneuver puts downward pressure on the hip and then inward rotation. If the hip is dislocated, this maneuver forces the femoral head over the acetabular rim with a noticeable "clunk."

The immature CNS of the newborn is characterized by a variety of reflexes. Because the newborn's movements are uncoordinated, methods of communication are limited, and control of body functions is drastically limited, the reflexes serve a variety of purposes. Some are protective (blink, gag, sneeze), some aid in feeding (rooting, sucking) and may not be very active if the infant has eaten recently, and some stimulate human interaction (grasping).

The most common reflexes found in the normal newborn are the following:

- The **tonic neck reflex** (fencer position) is elicited when the newborn is supine and the head is turned to one side. In response, the extremities on the same side straighten, whereas on the opposite side they flex (Figure 27–38 ●). This reflex may not be seen during the early newborn period, but once it appears it persists until about the third month.

- The **Moro reflex** is elicited when the newborn is startled by a loud noise or lifted slightly above the crib and then suddenly lowered. In response, the newborn straightens arms and hands outward while the knees flex. Slowly the arms return to the chest, as in an embrace. The fingers spread, forming a C, and the newborn may cry (Figure 27–39 ●). This reflex may persist until about 6 months of age.

FIGURE 27–37

A

B

A, Unilateral talipes equinovarus (clubfoot). **B,** To determine the presence of clubfoot, the nurse moves the foot to the midline. Resistance indicates true clubfoot.

(A) Used with permission from Mead Johnson Nutritionals.

FIGURE 27–38

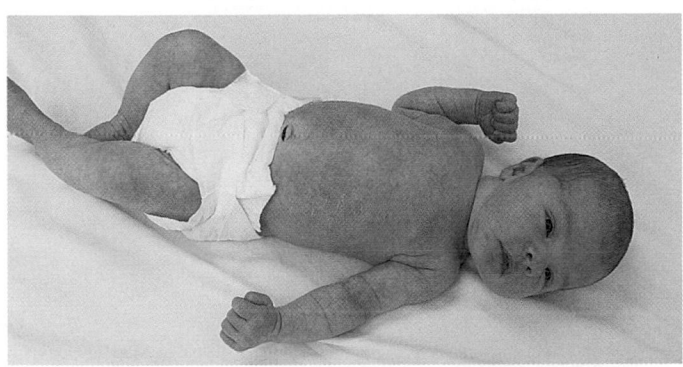

Tonic neck reflex.

© Stella Johnson (www.stellajohnson.com)

FIGURE 27–39

Moro reflex.

FIGURE 27–40

Palmar grasping reflex.

- The **grasping reflex** is elicited by stimulating the newborn's palm with a finger or object; the newborn grasps and holds the object or finger firmly enough to be lifted momentarily from the crib (Figure 27–40 ●). This reflex lessens at 3 to 4 months of age.

- The **rooting reflex** is elicited when the side of the newborn's mouth or cheek is touched. In response, the newborn turns toward that side and opens the lips to suck (if not fed recently) (Figure 27–41 ●).

- The **sucking reflex** is elicited when an object is placed in the newborn's mouth or anything touches the lips. Newborns suck even while sleeping; this is called nonnutritive sucking, and it can have a quieting effect on the baby.

● **FIGURE 27–41**

Rooting reflex.

- The **Babinski reflex** response, or fanning and hyperextension of all toes and dorsiflexion of the big toe, occurs when the lateral aspect of the sole is stroked from the heel upward across the ball of the foot (Mandleco, 2004). In children older than 24 months, it is considered an abnormal response if there is extension or fanning of the toes; this Babinski response indicates upper motor neuron abnormalities (Figure 27–42 ●).

- **Trunk incurvation (Galant reflex)** is seen when the newborn is prone. Stroking the spine causes the pelvis to turn to the stimulated side.

● **FIGURE 27–42**

The Babinski reflex.

In addition to these reflexes, newborns can blink, yawn, cough, sneeze, and draw back from pain (protective reflexes). They can even move a little on their own. When placed on their stomachs, they push up and try to crawl (prone crawl). When held upright with one foot touching a flat surface, the newborn puts one foot in front of the other and "walks" (stepping reflex) (Figure 27–43 ●). This reflex is more pronounced at birth and is lost in 4 to 8 weeks.

Use the following steps to assess CNS integration:

1. Insert a gloved finger into the newborn's mouth to elicit a sucking reflex.

2. As soon as the newborn is sucking vigorously, assess hearing and vision responses by noting changes in sucking in the presence of a light, a rattle, and a voice.

3. The newborn should respond to such stimuli with a brief cessation of sucking, followed by continuous sucking with repetitious stimulation.

This examination demonstrates auditory and visual integrity as well as the capability of complex behavioral interactions. Refer to "Newborn Physical Assessment Guide" in this chapter for a summary of the stimulus for, and response of, the common newborn reflexes. As healthcare providers carry out the newborn physical and neurologic assessment, they are always on the alert to recognize possible alterations and possible injuries related to the birth

● **FIGURE 27–43**

The stepping reflex disappears between 4 and 8 weeks of age.

process that require further investigation and intervention. (See Table 27–5 for potential birth injuries.)

NEWBORN PHYSICAL ASSESSMENT GUIDE

Refer to the guide for systematically assessing the newborn earlier in the chapter. Normal findings, alterations, and related causes are presented and correlated with suggested nursing responses. The findings are typical for a full-term newborn.

NEWBORN BEHAVIORAL ASSESSMENT

Two conflicting forces influence parents' perceptions of their newborn. One is their preconceptions, based on hopes and fears, of what their newborn will be like. The other is their initial reaction to the baby's temperament, behaviors, and physical appearance. Nurses can help parents identify their baby's specific behaviors.

The **Brazelton Neonatal Behavioral Assessment Scale** provides valuable guidelines for assessing the newborn's state changes, temperament, and individual behavior patterns. It provides a way for the healthcare provider, in conjunction with the parents (primary caregivers), to

THINKING CRITICALLY

ASSESSING NEWBORN BEHAVIOR

Maria Reyes, a 19-year-old G2 now P2 mother, gave birth to a 40-week-old female newborn 24 hours ago. The newborn examination was normal. Mrs. Reyes asks about the newborn's exam. She says she has noticed that the baby cries more than her first child did and seems to require holding for longer periods of time after feeding before "quieting down." She is concerned that she is doing something wrong and wants to know when her newborn will start to act like her first baby. What should you discuss with her about newborn behavior?

identify and understand the individual newborn's states and capabilities. Families learn which responses, interventions, or activities best meet the special needs of their newborn, and this understanding fosters positive attachment experiences.

The assessment tool identifies the newborn's repertoire of behavioral responses to the environment and also documents the newborn's neurologic adequacy and capabilities. The examination usually takes 20 to 30 minutes and involves about 30 tests. Some items are scored according to the newborn's response to specific stimuli. Others, such as consolability and alertness, are scored as a result of continuous behavioral observations throughout the assessment. (For a complete discussion of all test items and maneuvers, see Brazelton & Nugent, 1995.)

Because the first few days after birth are a period of behavioral disorganization, the nurse should make every effort to elicit the best response. The best response may be obtained when the parents are holding, cuddling, rocking, or singing to their baby.

It is best to assess the newborn initially in a quiet, softly lit room. The nurse first determines the newborn's state of consciousness, because scoring and introduction of the test items are correlated with the sleep or waking state. The newborn's state depends on physiologic variables, such as the amount of time from the last feeding, positioning, environmental temperature, and health status; presence of such external stimuli as noises and bright lights; and the wake-sleep cycle of the newborn. An important characteristic of the newborn period is the pattern of states, as well as the transitions from one state to another. The pattern of states predicts the newborn's receptivity and ability to respond to stimuli in a cognitive manner. Babies learn best in a quiet, alert state and in a supportive, protective environment that provides appropriate stimuli.

Observe the newborn's sleep-wake patterns (as discussed in Chapter 26 ∞), including the rapidity with which the newborn moves from one state to another, ability to be consoled, and ability to diminish the impact of

TABLE 27–5 ✣ **Potential Birth Injuries**	
Classification	**Examples***
Soft-tissue injuries	Lacerations, abrasions, bruising, fat necrosis
Skull injuries	Cephalhematoma,* fractures
Scalp laceration	Fetal scalp electrode
Scalp abscess	Fetal scalp electrode
Intracranial hemorrhage	Subdural, subarachnoid
Eye injuries	Subconjunctival* and retinal hemorrhages
Fractures	Clavicle,* facial bones, humerus, femur
Dislocations	
Torticollis	Sternocleidomastoid muscle
Nerve injuries	Facial nerve,* brachial plexus,* phrenic nerve, recurrent laryngeal nerve (vocal cord paralysis), Horner syndrome
Spinal cord injuries	
Visceral rupture	Liver, spleen

*Most common birth injuries seen in newborns.

disturbing stimuli. The following questions may provide a framework for assessment:

- Does the newborn's response style and ability to adapt to stimuli indicate a need for parental interventions that will alert the newborn to the environment so that he or she can grow socially and cognitively?

- Are parental interventions necessary to lessen the outside stimuli, as in the case of the baby who responds to sensory input with intensity?

- Can the baby control the amount of sensory input that he or she must deal with?

The behaviors, and the sleep-wake states in which they are assessed, are categorized as follows:

1. **Habituation.** Assess the newborn's ability to diminish or shut down innate responses to specific repeated stimuli, such as a rattle, bell, light, or pinprick to heel.

2. **Orientation to inanimate and animate visual and auditory assessment stimuli.** Observe how often and where the newborn attends to auditory and visual stimuli. Orientation to the environment is determined by an ability to respond to clues given by others and by a natural ability to fix on and follow a visual object horizontally and vertically. This capacity and parental appreciation of it are important for positive communication between infant and parents; the parents' visual (en face) and auditory (soft, continuous voice) presence stimulates their newborn to orient to them. Inability or lack of response may indicate visual or auditory problems. It is important for parents to know that their newborn can turn to voices soon after birth or by 3 days of age and can become alert at different times with a varying degree of intensity in response to sounds.

3. **Motor activity.** Evaluate several components. Assess motor tone of the newborn in the most characteristic state of responsiveness. This summary assessment includes overall use of tone as the newborn responds to being handled—whether during spontaneous activity, prone placement, or horizontal holding—and overall assessment of body tone as the newborn reacts to all stimuli.

4. **Variations.** Assess frequency of alert states, state changes, color changes (throughout all states as examination progresses), activity, and peaks of excitement.

● FIGURE 27–44

The newborn can bring hand to mouth as a self-soothing activity.

5. **Self-quieting activity.** This assessment is based on how often, how quickly, and how effectively newborns can use their resources to quiet and console themselves when upset or distressed. Considered in this assessment are such self-consoling activities as putting hand to mouth, sucking on a fist or the tongue, and attuning to an object or sound (Figure 27–44 ●). Also consider the newborn's need for outside consolation (e.g., seeing a face; being rocked, held, or dressed; using a pacifier; being swaddled).

6. **Cuddliness or social behaviors.** This area encompasses the newborn's need for, and response to, being held. Also consider how often the newborn smiles. These behaviors influence the parents' self-esteem and feelings of acceptance or rejection. Cuddling also appears to be an indicator of personality. Cuddlers appear to enjoy, accept, and seek physical contact; they are easier to placate, sleep more, and form earlier and more intense attachments. Noncuddlers are active and restless, have accelerated motor development, and are intolerant of physical restraint. Smiling, even as a grimace reflex, greatly influences parent-newborn feedback. Parents identify this response as positive.

Critical Concept Review

LEARNING OBJECTIVES

CONCEPTS

Explain the various components of the gestational age assessment.

1. The common physical characteristics included in the gestational age assessment are:
   - Skin
   - Lanugo
   - Sole (plantar) creases
   - Breast tissue and size
   - Ear form and cartilage
   - Genitalia
2. The neuromuscular components of gestational age scoring tools are:
   - Posture
   - Square window sign
   - Popliteal angle
   - Arm recoil
   - Heel-to-toe extension
   - Scarf sign
3. By assessing the physical and neuromuscular components specified in a gestational age tool, the nurse determines the gestational age of the newborn and identifies the newborn as SGA, AGA, or LGA and prioritizes individual needs.

Describe the normal physical and behavioral characteristics of the newborn.

1. Normal ranges for newborn vital signs include:
   - heart rate, 120 to 160 beats per minute
   - respirations, 30 to 60 respirations per minute
   - axillary temperature, 36.1 to 37.2°C (97.5 to 99°F); skin temperature, 36 to 36.5°C (96.8 to 97.7°F); rectal temperature, 36.6 to 37.2°C (97.8 to 99°F);
   - blood pressure at birth, 80-60/45-40 mm Hg.
2. Normal newborn measurements include:
   - weight range, 2500 to 4000 g (5 lb, 8 oz to 8 lb, 13 oz), with weight dependent on maternal size and age
   - length range, 46 to 56 cm (18 to 22 in.);
   - head circumference range, 32 to 37 cm (12.5 to 14.5 in.)—approximately 2 cm larger than the chest circumference.
3. The newborn infant should have a head that appears large for its body.
4. The normal newborn has a prominent abdomen, sloping shoulders, narrow hips, and rounded chest. The body appears long and the extremities short.
5. Newborns tend to stay in a flexed position and will resist straightening of the extremities. Hands remain clenched.
6. Behaviorally, the infant will sleep the majority of the time and wake for feeding. The infant should be easily consoled when upset.

Summarize the components of a complete newborn assessment and the significance of normal variations and abnormal findings.

1. Basis for complete newborn assessment include:
   - Perinatal history
   - Determination of gestational age
   - Physical assessment
   - Behavioral assessment
2. Components of a complete newborn physical assessment include:
   - Vital signs
   - Weight length, and head circumference
   - Skin appearance and presence of birthmarks
   - Examination of the head for size, appearance, symmetry, presence, and status of fontanels
   - Hair appearance
   - Appearance, condition, and symmetry of face, eyes, and ears
   - Appearance and condition of nose and mouth
   - Appearance of chest and auscultation of lungs and heart
   - Appearance of abdomen and presence of bowel sounds
   - Inspection of umbilical stump for 2 arteries and 1 vein

(continued)

LEARNING OBJECTIVES	CONCEPTS
Summarize the components of a complete newborn assessment and the significance of normal variations and abnormal findings.—continued	■ Appearance of appropriate genitalia ■ Condition and patency of anus ■ Position and condition of extremities, trunk, and spine 3. The nurse should be knowledgeable about variations that are indicative of normal newborn responses as well as those that indicate a need for further investigation. 4. An important role of the nurse during the physical and behavioral assessments of the newborn is to teach about their newborn and involve them in their baby's care. This involvement facilitates the parents' identification of their newborn's uniqueness and allays their concerns.
Discuss the neurologic and neuromuscular characteristics of the newborn and the reflexes that may be present at birth.	1. Neurologic assessment characteristics are: ■ State of alertness ■ Resting position ■ Muscle tone ■ Cry ■ Motor activity 2. Neuromuscular assessment characteristics are: ■ Symmetric movements and strength of all extremities ■ Head lag less than 45 degrees ■ Ability to hold head erect briefly 3. Normal reflexes ■ Blink ■ Pupillary reflex ■ Moro ■ Rooting and sucking ■ Palmar grasp ■ Plantar grasp ■ Stepping ■ Babinski ■ Tonic neck ■ Prone crawl ■ Trunk incurvation
Describe the categories of the newborn behavioral assessment.	1. The categories of the newborn behavioral assessment are: ■ Habitation ■ Orientation to inanimate and animate visual and auditory assessment stimuli ■ Motor activity ■ Frequency of alert states, state changes, color changes, activity, and peaks of activity ■ Self-quieting activity ■ Cuddliness

CRITICAL THINKING IN ACTION

*View the **Critical Thinking in Action** video in Chapter 27 of the CD-ROM. Then, answer the questions that follow.*

Susan Pine, a 21-year-old G2, now P1011, delivers a 39 2/7-weeks gestation female newborn. The vaginal birth is assisted with a vacuum extractor. The prenatal record is significant for an increase of maternal blood pressure to 140/90 on the day of birth. Susan is treated with magnesium sulfate during her labor and has an epidural analgesia for the pain of labor. The baby's Apgar is 8 and 9 at 1 and 5 minutes, and she has been admitted to the newborn nursery. The newborn's admission exam is normal except for a 2-cm round caput succedaneum. Now, 8 hours later, the baby's condition is stable and she needs to be bottle-fed. You take her to her mother's room where you observe that Susan does not reach out to take her from you. She seems unsure when handling her baby. Susan asks you about the swelling on her baby's head and wonders if it will ever go away.

1. How would you explain the cause of Susan's baby's caput succedaneum?
2. Compare the difference between a cephalhematoma and caput succedaneum.
3. Explore with Susan her baby's reflexes and state of alertness.
4. Susan asks you how she will know what her baby needs. How would you respond?

MEDIALINK

www.prenhall.com/london

■ NCLEX-RN® Review, case studies, and other interactive resources for this chapter can be found on the Companion Website at http://www.prenhall.com/london. Click on "Chapter 27" to select the activities for this chapter.

Case Study
A nurse has completed the gestational assessment on a newborn who weighs 3000 g, is 48 cm long, with a head circumference of 33 cm. His Apgar scores were 8 at one minute and 9 at five minutes. Other assessment data include skin dry and cracking, no lanugo, sole creases covering the whole heel, areola 3 mm, pinna soft with slow recoil, testes descended with moderate rugae. Reflex data include square window at 0°; arm recoil 100°; popliteal angle 100°; scarf sign yield elbow at midline; heel to ear 90°; and posture fully flexed. The parents express concerns over his small size.

This activity contains 5 questions.

1. *What is the newborn's neuromuscular maturity score?*
[Hint]

To create paragraphs in your essay response, type <p> at the beginning of the paragraph, and </p> at the end.

■ For animations, more NCLEX-RN® Review questions, and an audio glossary, access the accompanying CD-ROM in this textbook.

REFERENCES

American Academy of Pediatrics (AAP), Committee on Fetus and Newborn, & American College of Obstetricians and Gynecologists (ACOG), Committee on Obstetrics. (2002). *Guidelines for perinatal care* (5th ed.). Evanston, IL: Author.

Ballard, J. L., Khoury, J. C., Wedig, K., Wang, L., Eilers-Walsmann, B. L., & Lipp, R. (1991). New Ballard score, expanded to include extremely premature infants. *Journal of Pediatrics, 119*(3), 417–423.

Blackburn, S. T. (2003). *Maternal-fetal, neonatal physiology: A clinical perspective*. St. Louis, MO: Saunders.

Brazelton, T. B., & Nugent, J. K. (1995), *The neonatal behavioral assessment scale* (3rd ed.). London: MacKeith.

Donovan, E. F., Tyson, J. E., Ehrenkranz, R. A., Verter, J., Wright, L. L., Korones, S. B., et al. (1999, August). Inaccuracy of Ballard scores before 28 weeks' gestation. *Journal of Pediatrics, 135,* 147–152.

Furdon, S. A., & Clark, D. A. (2003). Scalp hair characteristics in the newborn infant. *Advances in Neonatal Care, 3*(6), 286–296.

Johnston, P., Flood, K., & Spinks, K. (2003). *The newborn child* (9th ed.). Edinburgh: Churchill Livingstone.

Kiesler, J., & Ricer, R. (2003). The abnormal fontanel. *American Family Physician, 67*(12), 2547–2552.

Mandleco, B. L. (2004). *Growth and development handbook: Newborn through adolescence.* Clifton Park, NY: Thomson/Delmar Learning.

Thureen, P. J., Deacon, J., Hernandez, J. A., & Hall, D. M. (2005). *Assessment and care of the well newborn* (2nd ed.). St. Louis, MO: Elsevier.

Varney, H., Kriebs, J. M., & Gegor, C. L. (2004). *Varney's midwifery* (4th ed.). Sudbury, MA: Jones & Bartlett.

Wu, T. Y., & Daniel, L. (2001). Growth of immigrant Chinese infants in the first year of life. *MCN. American Journal of Maternal Child Nursing, 26*(4), 202–207.

Normal Newborn: Needs and Care

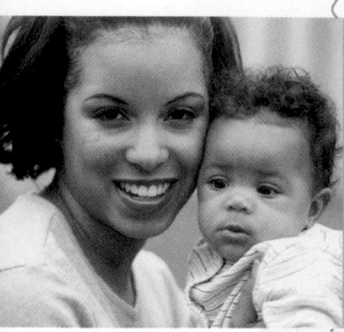

When our daughter was laid in my arms right after birth she was so delicate. I had not dared to hope that we would be blessed with a girl because there were so few girls in my husband's family. Our 2-year-old niece was the first girl in 107 years, so I had pretty much decided that another boy would be just fine. But here she was, right here in my arms.

—*Catherine, 32*

LEARNING OBJECTIVES

- Summarize the essential areas of information to be obtained about a newborn's birth experience and immediate postnatal period.

- Relate the physiologic and behavioral responses of the newborn to possible interventions needed.

- Discuss the major nursing considerations and activities to be carried out during the first 4 hours after birth (admission and transitional period) and subsequent daily care.

- Identify the activities that should be included in a daily care plan for a normal newborn.

- Determine common concerns of families regarding their newborns.

- Describe topics and related content to be included in parent teaching on newborn and infant care.

- Identify opportunities to individualize parent teaching and enhance each parent's abilities and confidence while providing infant care in the birthing unit.

- Delineate the information to be included in discharge planning with the newborn's family.

MEDIALINK www.prenhall.com/london

CD-ROM

NCLEX-RN® Review
Video: Newborn Care
Skill 4-4: Assisting with Breastfeeding after
  Childbirth
Skill 5-1: Performing Nasal Pharyngeal Suctioning
Skill 5-3: Thermoregulation of the Newborn
Skill 10-1: Performing a Capillary Puncture
Audio Glossary

Companion Website

NCLEX-RN® Review
Case Study: Newborn Care
Care Plan Activity: Initial Newborn Care
Care Plan Activity: Infant Care During Transition
Thinking Critically

At the moment of birth, numerous physiologic adaptations begin to take place in the newborn's body. Because of these dramatic changes, newborns require close observation to determine how smoothly they are making the transition to extrauterine life. Newborns also require specific care that enhances their chances of making the transition successfully.

The two broad goals of nursing care during this period are to promote the physical well-being of the newborn and to enhance the establishment of a well-functioning family unit. The nurse meets the first goal by providing comprehensive care to the newborn in the mother-baby unit. The nurse meets the second goal by teaching family members how to care for their new baby and by supporting their efforts so that they feel confident and competent. Thus, the nurse must be knowledgeable about family adjustments that need to be made as well as the healthcare needs of the newborn. It is important that the family return home with the positive feeling that they have the support, information, and skills to care for their newborn. Equally important is the need for each member of the family to begin a unique relationship with the newborn. The cultural and social expectations of individual families and communities affect the way normal newborn care is carried out. The previous two chapters presented an informational database of the physiologic and behavioral changes occurring in the newborn and the pertinent nursing assessments that are needed. This chapter discusses the nursing care management while the newborn is in the birthing unit. The "Clinical Pathway for Newborn Care" starts on page 719.

NURSING MANAGEMENT DURING ADMISSION AND THE FIRST FOUR HOURS OF LIFE

Immediately after birth the baby is formally admitted to the healthcare facility.

NURSING ASSESSMENT AND DIAGNOSIS

During the first 4 hours after birth, carry out a preliminary physical examination, including an assessment of the newborn's physiologic adaptations. In many birthing units, the nurse performs and documents the initial head-to-toe physical assessment during the first hour of transition. Notify the physician or nurse practitioner of any deviation from normal. A complete physical examination is also performed later by the physician or nurse practitioner, within 24 hours after birth and within 24 hours before discharge. This can be accomplished with one physical examination (American Academy of Pediatrics [AAP] & American College of Obstetricians and Gynecologists [ACOG], 2002) (see Table 27–1 ∞).

Nursing diagnoses are based on an analysis of the assessment findings. Physiologic alterations of the newborn form the basis of many nursing diagnoses, as does the family members' incorporation of them in caring for their new baby. Nursing diagnoses that may apply to a newborn include the following:

- *Ineffective Airway Clearance* related to presence of mucus and retained lung fluid
- *Risk for Imbalanced Body Temperature* related to evaporative, radiant, conductive, and convective heat losses
- *Acute Pain* related to heel sticks for glucose or hematocrit tests or vitamin K injection

MEDIALINK

Video: Newborn Care

717

TABLE 28–1 ✣ Signs of Newborn Transition

Normal findings for the newborn during the first few days of life include the following:

Pulse: 120-160 beats/minute

> During sleep as low as 80 beats/minute
>
> If crying, up to 180 beats/minute
>
> Apical pulse is counted for 1 full minute because rate may fluctuate

Respirations: 30-60 respirations/minute

> Predominantly diaphragmatic but synchronous with abdominal movements
>
> Brief periods of apnea (less than 15 seconds) with no color or heart rate changes

Temperature

> Axillary: 36.5-37°C (97.5-98.6°F)
>
> Skin: 36-36.5°C (96.8-97.7°F)

Blood pressure: 80-60/45-40 mm Hg at birth; 100/50 mm Hg at day 10

Blood glucose: greater than or equal to 40 mg%

Hematocrit: < 65%-70% central venous sample

As discussed in Chapter 27, the newborn's physiologic adaptation to extrauterine life occurs rapidly. All body systems are affected. Therefore, many of these nursing diagnoses and associated interventions must be identified and implemented in a very short period (Table 28–1). The newborn requires close monitoring during the first few hours of life to immediately identify any deviation from normal and begin appropriate interventions.

PLANNING AND IMPLEMENTATION

Initiate newborn admission procedures and evaluate the newborn's need to remain under observation. This monitoring may take place in a special transition area or at the mother's bedside. It includes the following:

- Maternal and birth history
- Airway clearance
- Vital signs
- Body temperature
- Neurologic status
- Ability to feed
- Evidence of complications

If the evaluation is normal, the baby is successfully making the transition to extrauterine life and may need less frequent observations. In some settings this may also be a time for moving the mother and baby to another care unit.

Initiation of Admission Procedures

After birth the baby is formally admitted to the healthcare facility. The admission procedures include a review of prenatal and birth information for possible risk factors, a gestational age assessment, and an assessment to ensure that the newborn's adaptation to extrauterine life is proceeding normally. This evaluation of the newborn's status and risk factors must be done no later than 2 hours after birth (AAP & ACOG, 2002).

If the initial assessment indicates that the newborn is not at risk physiologically, perform many of the routine admission procedures in the presence of the parents in the birthing area. Some care measures indicated by the assessment findings may be performed by the nurse or by the parents under the guidance of the nurse in an effort to educate and support the family. Other interventions may be delayed until the newborn has been transferred to an observational nursery. Check and confirm the newborn's identification with the mother's identification and then obtain and record all significant information. The essential data to be recorded on the newborn's chart include the following:

1. **Condition of the newborn.** Pertinent information includes the newborn's Apgar scores at 1 and 5 minutes, resuscitative measures required in the birthing area, physical examination, vital signs, voidings, and passing of meconium. Complications to be noted are excessive mucus, delayed spontaneous respirations or responsiveness, abnormal number of cord vessels, and obvious physical abnormalities.

2. **Labor and birth record.** A copy of the labor and birth record should be placed in the newborn's chart or be accessible on computer. The record contains the significant data about the birth, including duration, course, and status of mother and fetus throughout labor and birth and any analgesia or anesthesia administered to the mother. Take particular care to note any variation or difficulties, such as prolonged rupture of membranes, abnormal fetal position, meconium-stained amniotic fluid, signs of nonreassuring fetal status during labor, nuchal cord (cord around the newborn's neck at birth), precipitous birth, use of forceps or vacuum-assisted device, maternal analgesics and anesthesia received within 1 hour before birth, and administration of antibiotics during labor.

3. **Antepartum history.** Any maternal problems that may have compromised the fetus in utero, such as preeclampsia, spotting, illness, recent infections, rubella status, serology results, hepatitis B screen results, exposure to group B streptococci, or a history of maternal substance abuse, are of immediate concern in newborn assessment. The

CLINICAL PATHWAY

FOR NEWBORN CARE

CATEGORY	FIRST 4 HOURS	4–8 HOURS PAST BIRTH	8–24 HOURS PAST BIRTH
Referral	Review labor/birth record Review transitional nursing record Check ID bands and security alarm if present Consult prn: orthopedics, genetics, infectious disease	Check ID bands and security alarm if present Transfer to mother-baby care at 4-6 hours of age if stable As parents desire, obtain circumcision permit after their discussion with physician Check ID bands and crib cards to ensure infant is in the correct crib Lactation consult prn	Check ID bands and security alarm q shift **EXPECTED OUTCOMES** Mother/baby ID bands correlate at time of discharge and security alarms in place at all times; consults completed prn
Assessments	Continue assessments begun first hour after birth Vital signs: TPR, BP prn, q1h × 4 (skin temp 97.7–98.6°F (36.5°C–37°C), resp may be irregular but within 30–60 per min) **Newborn Assessments** ■ Respiratory status with resp distress scale × 1 then prn. If resp distress, assess q 5–15 min ■ Cord: bluish white color, clamp in place and free of skin ■ Color: skin, mucous membranes, extremities, trunk pink with slight acrocyanosis of hands and feet ■ Wt (5 lb, 8 oz–8 lb, 13 oz) 2500–4000 g, length (18–22 in.) 46–56 cm, HC (12.5–14.5 in.) 32–37 cm, CC (32.5 cm, 1–2 in. less than head) ■ Extremity movement may be jerky or brief twitches ■ Gestational age classification—term AGA ■ Anomalies (cong. anomalies can interfere with normal extrauterine adaptation)	Assess newborn's progress through periods of reactivity Vital signs: TPR q8h and prn or per agency protocol, BP prn **Newborn Assessments** ■ Skin color q4h prn (circulatory system stabilizing, acrocyanosis decreased) ■ Eyes for drainage, redness, hemorrhage ■ Auscultate lungs q4h (noisy, wet resp. normal) ■ Increased mucus production (normal in 2nd period of reactivity) ■ Check apical pulse q4h ■ Umbilical cord base for redness, drainage, foul odor, drying, clamp in place ■ Extremity movement q4h ■ Check for expected reflexes (suck, rooting, Moro, grasp, blink, yawn, sneeze, tonic neck, Babinski) ■ Note common normal variations ■ Assess suck and swallow during feeding ■ Note behavioral characteristics ■ Temp before and after admission bath	VS q8h; normal ranges: T, 97.5-99°F (36.3–37.2°C); P, 120–160; R, 30–60; BP, 60-80/45–40 mm Hg **Continue Newborn Assessments** ■ Skin color q4h ■ Signs of drying or infection in cord area ■ Check that clamp is in place until removed before discharge ■ Check circ for bleeding after procedure, then q30min × 2, then q4h and prn **EXPECTED OUTCOMES** Vital signs medically acceptable, color pink, or appropriate for racial group, assessments WNL, circ site without s/s infection, cord site without s/s infection and clamp removed; newborn behavior WNL
Teaching/ psychosocial	Admission activities performed at mother's bedside if possible, orient to nursery prn, handwashing, assess teaching needs Teach parents use of bulb syringe, signs of choking, positioning, and when to call for assistance Teach reasons for use of radiant warmer, infant hat, and warmed blankets when out of warmer Discuss/teach infant security, identification	Reinforce teaching about choking, bulb syringe use, positioning, temperature maintenance with clothing and blankets Teach infant positioning to facilitate breathing and digestion Teach new parents holding and feeding skills Teach parents soothing and calming techniques Teach parents about introducing newborn to sibling	Final discharge teaching: diapering, normal void and stool patterns, bathing, nail and cord care, circumcision/uncircumcised penis/genital care and normal characteristics, rashes, jaundice, sleep-wake cycles, soothing activities, taking temperatures, thermometer reading Explain s/s of illness and when to call healthcare provider Infant safety: car seats, immunizations, metabolic screening **EXPECTED OUTCOMES** Mother/family verbalize comprehension of teaching; demonstrate care capabilities

AGA, average for gestational age; Appt, appointment; CC, chest circumference; cong, congenital; esp, especially; Circ, circumcision; HC, head circumference; Hct, hematocrit; Hx, history; ID, identification; OU, both eyes; PKU, phenylketonuria; s/s, signs and symptoms; temp, temperature; TPR, temperature, pulse, respirations; VS, vital signs; WNL, within normal limits.

(continued)

MEDIALINK ● Skill 4-4: Assisting with Breastfeeding after Childbirth

CLINICAL PATHWAY—continued

FOR NEWBORN CARE

CATEGORY	FIRST 4 HOURS	4–8 HOURS PAST BIRTH	8–24 HOURS PAST BIRTH
Nursing care management and reports	Place under radiant warmer Place hat on newborn (decreases convection heat loss) Suction nares/mouth with bulb syringe prn Keep bulb syringe with infant Attach security alarm sensor Obtain lab tests: blood glucose; as needed Obtain blood type, Rh, Coombs on cord blood, HSV culture if parental hx Notify physician's office of infant's birth and any change in status Maintain Universal Precautions	Wean from radiant warmer [T 98°F (37°C) axillary] Chemstrips prn; BP prn Oxygen saturation prn Bathe infant if temp > 97.7°F (36.5°C) Position on side Suction nares prn (esp during 2nd period of reactivity) Obtain peripheral Hct per protocol Cord assessment per protocol Fold diaper below cord (for plastic diapers, turn plastic layer away from skin)	Check for hearing test results Weigh before discharge Cord assessment q shift DC cord clamp before discharge Perform newborn metabolic/genetic and hearing screening tests before discharge Circumcision if indicated; circumcision care: change diaper prn, noting ability to void; follow policy for circumcision clamp or Plastibell care **EXPECTED OUTCOMES** Newborn maintains temp, lab test WNL, cord dry without s/s infection and clamp removed, screening tests accomplished, circ site without s/s infection or bleeding
Activity and comfort	Immediately after birth, place under radiant warmer or maintain skin-to-skin contact with mother until stable Soothe baby as needed with voice, touch, cuddling, nesting in warmer	Leave in warmer or with mother until stable, then swaddle Position on back after each feeding	Place in open crib Swaddle to allow movement of extremities in blanket, including hands to face **EXPECTED OUTCOMES** Infant maintains temp WNL in open crib; infant attempts self-calming
Nutrition	Assist newborn to breastfeed as soon as mother/baby condition allows Supplement breast only when medically indicated or per agency policy Initiate glucose or formula-feeding within first hour Gavage feed if necessary to prevent hypoglycemia	Breastfeed on demand, at least q2–3h Teach positions, observe/assist with feeding, breast/nipple care, establishing milk supply, breaking suction, feeding cues, latching-on techniques, nutritive suck, burping Formula-feed on demand, at least q3-4h Determine readiness to feed and feeding tolerance	Continue breastfeeding or formula-feeding pattern Assess feeding tolerance q4h Discuss normal feeding requirements, signs of hunger and satiation, handling feeding problems, and when to seek help **EXPECTED OUTCOMES** Mother verbalizes knowledge of feeding information; breastfeeds on demand without supplement; bottle—tolerates formula-feeding, nipples without problems
Elimination	Note first void and stool if not noted at birth	Note all voids, amount, and color of stools q4h	Evaluate all voids and stool color q8h **EXPECTED OUTCOMES** Voids qs; stools qs without difficulty; stool character WNL; diaper area without s/s skin breakdown or rashes
Medication	Prophylactic ophthalmic ointment OU after baby makes eye contact with parents within 1 hr after birth Administer AquaMEPHYTON IM, dosage according to infant weight per MD/NP order and within 1 hr of birth	Hepatitis B injection as ordered by physician after consent signed by parents	Hepatitis B vaccine within 2 hr of birth or before discharge **EXPECTED OUTCOMES** Baby has received ophthalmic ointment and vitamin K injection; baby has received first Hep B vaccine if ordered and parental permission received

CLINICAL PATHWAY—continued

FOR NEWBORN CARE

CATEGORY	FIRST 4 HOURS	4–8 HOURS PAST BIRTH	8–24 HOURS PAST BIRTH
Discharge planning/ home care	Hepatitis B consent signed Hearing screen consent signed Plan discharge call with parent or guardian in 24 hr to 2 days Assess parents' discharge plans, needs, and support systems	Review/reinforce teaching with mother and significant other Review home preparedness Present birth certificate instructions	Initial newborn screening tests (hearing, blood tests, metabolic screen; i.e., PKU) before discharge Bath and feeding classes, videos, or written information given Give written copy of discharge instructions Newborn photographs Set up appointment for follow-up PKU test Have car seat available before discharge All discharge referrals made, follow-up appt. scheduled **EXPECTED OUTCOMES** Infant discharged home with family; mother verbalizes follow-up appt. time/date
Family involvement	Facilitate early investigation of baby's physical characteristics (maintain temp during unwrapping), hold infant *en face* Dim lights to help infant keep eyes open	Assess parents' knowledge of newborn behaviors, such as alertness, suck and rooting, attention to human voice, response to calming techniques	Assess mother baby bonding/interaction Incorporate father and siblings in care Enhance parent-infant interaction by sharing characteristics and behavioral assessment Support positive parenting behaviors Identify community referral needs and refer to community agencies **EXPECTED OUTCOME** Demonstrates caring and family incorporation of infant
Date			

chart should also include information about maternal age, estimated date of birth (EDB), previous pregnancies, and presence of any congenital anomalies. An HIV test result, if obtained, is also relevant. Be aware of your state's statutes regarding who is allowed access to this information (AAP & ACOG, 2002).

4. **Parent-newborn interaction information.** Note parents' interactions with their newborn and their desires regarding care, such as rooming-in, circumcision, and the type of feeding. Information about other children in the home, available support systems, and interactional patterns within each family unit helps in providing comprehensive care.

As part of the admission procedure, weigh the newborn in both grams and pounds. In the United States, parents understand weight best when it is stated in pounds and ounces (Figure 28–1 ●). Clean and cover the scales each time a newborn is weighed to prevent cross-infection and heat loss from conduction.

Then measure the newborn, recording the measurements in both centimeters and inches. The three routine

● **FIGURE 28-1**

Weighing of newborns. The scale is cleaned and balanced before each weighing, with the protective pad in place. The caregiver should be near the newborn as a safety measure.

measurements are length, circumference of the head, and circumference of the chest. In some facilities, abdominal girth may also be measured. Rapidly assess the baby's color, muscle tone, alertness, and general state. It is important to remember that the first period of reactivity may have concluded, and the baby may be in the sleep-inactive phase, which makes the infant hard to arouse. Do basic assessments for estimating gestational age and finish the physical assessment (see "Newborn Physical Assessment Guide" in Chapter 27 ∞).

In addition to obtaining vital signs, perform a hematocrit and blood glucose evaluation on at-risk newborns or as clinically indicated (such as for small-for-gestational-age [SGA] or large-for-gestational-age [LGA] infants, or if the newborn is jittery). These procedures may be done on admission or within the first 2 hours after birth (AAP & ACOG, 2002) (see Skill 10–1). **SKILLS**

Maintenance of a Clear Airway and Stable Vital Signs

Free flow oxygen should be readily available. Position the newborn on his or her back (or side, if infant has copious secretions). If necessary, use a bulb syringe or DeLee wall suction (see "Initial Care of the Newborn" in Chapter 19 ∞ and Skill 5–1), **SKILLS** to remove mucus from the newborn's nasal passages and oral cavity. A DeLee catheter attached to suction may be used to remove mucus from the stomach to help prevent possible aspiration. When possible, this procedure should be delayed for 10 to 15 minutes after birth, reducing the potential for severe vasovagal reflex apnea.

In the absence of any newborn distress, continue with the admission by taking the newborn's vital signs. The initial temperature is taken by the axillary method; a normal axillary temperature range is 36.5°C to 37°C (97.7°F to 98.6°F).

Once the initial temperature is taken, monitor the core temperature either by obtaining axillary temperatures at intervals or by placing a skin sensor on the newborn for continuous reading. The usual skin sensor placement site is the newborn's abdomen, but placement on the upper thigh or arm can give a reading closely correlated with the mean body temperature. Monitor the vital signs for a healthy term newborn at least every 30 minutes until the newborn's condition has remained stable for 2 hours (AAP & ACOG, 2002). The newborn's respirations may be irregular yet still be normal. Brief periods of apnea, lasting only 5 to 10 seconds with no color or heart rate changes, are considered normal. The normal pulse range is 120 to 160 beats per minute (bpm), and the normal respiratory range is 30 to 60 respirations per minute.

Maintenance of a Neutral Thermal Environment

A neutral thermal environment is essential to minimize the newborn's need for increased oxygen consumption and use of calories to maintain body heat in the optimal range of 36.4°C to 37.2°C (97.5°F to 99°F). If the newborn becomes

THINKING CRITICALLY

"CUTE LITTLE NOISES?"

You overhear Mr. Johannson speaking to his mother on the phone. He is telling her about the "cute little noises" his 30-minute-old baby makes. The infant is in the room with the mother. What is your best course of action?

hypothermic, the body's response can lead to metabolic acidosis, hypoxia, and shock.

A neutral thermal environment is best achieved by performing the newborn assessment and interventions with the newborn unclothed and under a radiant warmer. The radiant warmer thermostat is controlled by a thermal skin sensor taped to the newborn's abdomen, upper thigh, or arm (Figure 28–2 ●). The sensor indicates when the newborn's temperature exceeds or falls below the acceptable temperature range. Be aware that leaning over the newborn may block the radiant heat waves from reaching the newborn.

It is common practice in some institutions to cover the newborn's head with a cap made of wool lined with gauze and cotton, Thinsulate, or cotton and polyester fill terry cloth to prevent further heat loss, in addition to placing the baby under a radiant warmer (Blackburn, 2003).

When the newborn's temperature is normal and vital signs are stable (about 2 to 4 hours after birth), the baby may be given a sponge bath. However, this admission bath may be postponed for some hours if the newborn's condition dictates or the parents wish to give the first bath. In light of early discharge practices (12 to 48 hours), healthy term infants can be safely bathed immediately after the admission assessment is completed (Behring, Vezeau, & Fink, 2003). The baby is bathed while still under the radiant

● **FIGURE 28–2**

Temperature monitoring of the newborn. A skin thermal sensor is placed on the newborn's abdomen, upper thigh, or arm and secured with porous tape or a foil-covered foam pad.

EVIDENCE-BASED NURSING

NEONATAL SKIN CARE

Clinical Question (Problem)

Bathing the newborn is not an innocuous procedure. Newborns have immature thermoregulation mechanisms and so are prone to hypothermia. The skin of the newborn is sensitive and easily damaged. The benefits of daily bathing have not been clearly justified relative to the risks. Decisions about the frequency of bathing should be based on assessment of the individual newborn's needs and the family's beliefs and values. When and how should a newborn be bathed?

Evidence

The Association of Women's Health, Obstetric and Neonatal Nurses (AWHONN) assembled an expert team to evaluate research on neonatal skin care and develop a practice guideline. The group evaluated clinical trials as well as public health studies, and solicited the opinions of respected authorities in the field. They developed detailed guidelines for comprehensive neonatal skin care that include guidelines for bathing newborns.

Implications

Bathe the newborn only when necessary for hygiene; routine bathing is not recommended. During the procedure, focus on protecting the infant's skin and maintaining an adequate body temperature.

The first bath should be given only once the neonatal temperature has stabilized and is in the normal range for 2 to 4 hours. Wear gloves to handle the baby until after the first bath. After the first bath, bathe only

to remove debris. Daily soap bathing is discouraged during the neonatal period, and water-only baths can be alternated with cleansing baths. When you do use soap, use a mild cleansing bar or solution with a neutral pH. Avoid rubbing the skin, and use soft materials (such as cotton balls) to wash; rinse by squeezing water over the skin.

Consider immersion bathing once the umbilical cord clamp is in place (or after umbilical lines have been discontinued for preterm infants). After the bath, immediately dry the infant, diaper the infant, and place a cap on the head; double wrap in blankets. Dress the infant 10 minutes later, and wrap in dry, warm blankets.

It is often the mother's preference that vernix be removed in the initial bath, but removal is unnecessary for hygienic purposes. Vigorous attempts to remove all vernix may result in skin damage. Generally, excessive vernix can be removed in the initial bath, but there are no studies about the benefits or drawbacks of removing all vernix during the first bath.

Critical Thinking

What neonatal assessments would tell you that a bath should be postponed? What will you teach the parents about bathing their new baby?

Reference

Association of Women's Health, Obstetric and Neonatal Nurses (AWHONN). (2001, January). Neonatal skin care. *Evidence-based clinical practice guideline.* Washington, DC: Author.

---

warmer; the bathing may be done in the parents' room and by the parents (Medves & O'Brien, 2004). Bathing the newborn offers an excellent opportunity for teaching and welcoming parents' involvement in the care of their baby.

Recheck the baby's temperature after the bath. If it is stable, dress the newborn in a shirt, diaper, and cap; wrap the baby; and place the newborn in an open crib at room temperature. If the baby's axillary temperature is below 36.4°C (97.5°F), the baby returns to the radiant warmer for gradual rewarming and to prevent hypothermia. Once the newborn is rewarmed, take steps to prevent further heat loss, such as keeping the newborn away from cool surfaces or instruments. Protect the newborn from drafts, open windows or doors, and air conditioners. Blankets and clothing are stored in a warm place. (See "Temperature Regulation" in Chapter 26. ∞) Newborns are often "double-wrapped" in two or more blankets for temperature maintenance.

NURSING PRACTICE

A cap can be fashioned from a piece of stockinette to help reduce heat loss from the head.

Prevention of Complication of Hemorrhagic Disease of Newborn

A prophylactic injection of vitamin K_1 (AquaMEPHYTON) is given to prevent hemorrhage, which can occur due to low prothrombin levels in the first few days of life. See "Drug Guide: Vitamin K_1 Phytonadione (AquaMEPHYTON)." The potential for hemorrhage is thought to result from the absence of gut bacterial flora, which influences the production of vitamin K_1 in the newborn (see Chapter 31 for further discussion ∞). Newborns receive a single dose of 0.5 to 1 mg of natural vitamin K_1 (phytonadione) within the birthing area or within 1 hour of birth (AAP & ACOG, 2002; Wilson, Shannon, & Stang, 2005). Some researchers have questioned the need to give vitamin K to newborns who have had a nontraumatic birth.

The vitamin K_1 injection is given intramuscularly in the middle third of the vastus lateralis muscle, in the lateral aspect of the thigh (Figure 28–3 ●). Before injecting, thoroughly clean the newborn's skin site for the injection with a small alcohol swab. Use a 25-gauge, 5/8-inch needle for the injection. An alternative site is the rectus femoris muscle in the anterior aspect of the thigh. However, this site is near the sciatic nerve and femoral artery and should be used with caution (Figure 28–4 ●).

MEDIALINK Skill 5–3: Thermoregulation of the Newborn

DRUG GUIDE

VITAMIN K₁ PHYTONADIONE (AQUAMEPHYTON)

Overview of Neonatal Action

Phytonadione is used in prophylaxis and treatment of hemorrhagic disease of the newborn. It promotes liver formation of the clotting factors, II, VII, IX, and X. At birth the newborn does not have the bacteria in the colon that are necessary for synthesizing fat-soluble vitamin K₁. Therefore, the newborn may have decreased levels of prothrombin during the first 5 to 8 days of life, reflected by a prolongation of prothrombin time.

Route, Dosage, Frequency

Intramuscular injection is given in the vastus lateralis thigh muscle. A one-time-only prophylactic dose of 0.5 to 1 mg is given intramuscularly in the birthing area or within 1 hour of birth (Wilson, Shannon, & Stang, 2005).

If the mother received anticoagulants during pregnancy, an additional dose may be ordered by the physician and is given at 6 to 8 hours after the first injection. IM concentration: 1 mg/0.5 mL

(neonatal strength); can use 10 mg/mL concentration to minimize volume injected.

Neonatal Side Effects

Pain and edema may occur at injection site. Allergic reactions, such as rash and urticaria, may also occur.

Nursing Considerations

- Protect drug from light.
- Give vitamin K₁ before circumcision procedure.
- Observe for signs of local inflammation.
- Observe for jaundice and severe hemolytic anemia, especially in preterm infants.
- Observe for bleeding (usually occurs on second or third day). Bleeding may be seen as generalized ecchymoses or bleeding from umbilical cord, circumcision site, nose, or gastrointestinal tract. Results of serial prothrombin time (PT) and international normalized ratio (INR) should be assessed.

Prevention of Eye Infection

The nurse is also responsible for giving the legally required prophylactic eye treatment for *Neisseria gonorrhoeae*, which may have infected the newborn of an infected mother during the birth process. A variety of topical agents appear to be equally effective. Ophthalmic ointments that are used include 1% silver nitrate, 0.5% erythromycin (Ilotycin Ophthalmic) (see "Drug Guide: Erythromycin Ophthalmic Ointment [Ilotycin Ophthalmic]"), 1% tetracycline, and ophthalmic solution of povidone-iodine (2.5%). All are also effective against chlamydia, which has a higher incidence rate than gonorrhea.

● FIGURE 28–3

Procedure for vitamin K injection. Cleanse area thoroughly with alcohol swab and allow skin to dry. Bunch the tissue of the upper outer thigh (vastus lateralis muscle) and quickly insert a 25-gauge 5/8-inch needle at a 90-degree angle to the thigh. Aspirate, then slowly inject the solution to distribute the medication evenly and minimize the baby's discomfort. Remove the needle and gently massage the site with an alcohol swab.

● FIGURE 28–4

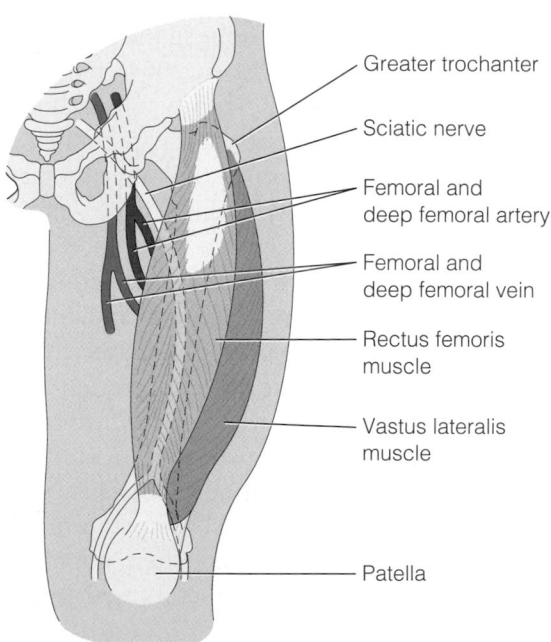

Greater trochanter
Sciatic nerve
Femoral and deep femoral artery
Femoral and deep femoral vein
Rectus femoris muscle
Vastus lateralis muscle
Patella

Injection sites. The middle third of the vastus lateralis muscle is the preferred site for intramuscular injection in the newborn. The middle third of the rectus femoris is an alternative site, but its proximity to major vessels and the sciatic nerve requires caution in using this site for injection.

DRUG GUIDE

ERYTHROMYCIN OPHTHALMIC OINTMENT (ILOTYCIN OPHTHALMIC)

Overview of Neonatal Action

Erythromycin (Ilotycin Ophthalmic) is used as prophylactic treatment of ophthalmia neonatorum, which is caused by the bacteria *Neisseria gonorrhoeae*. Preventive treatment of gonorrhea in the newborn is required by law. Erythromycin is also effective treatment against ophthalmic chlamydial infections. It is either bacteriostatic or bactericidal, depending on the organisms involved and the concentration of drug.

Pregnancy risk category: C

Route, Dosage, Frequency

Ophthalmic ointment (0.5%) is instilled as a narrow ribbon or strand, 1/4 inch long, along the lower conjunctival surface of each eye, starting at the inner canthus. It is instilled only once in each eye. The ointment may be administered in the birthing area or, alternatively, later in the nursery so that eye contact between infant and parent Is facilitated and the bonding process immediately after birth is not interrupted. After administration, gently close eye and gently manipulate to ensure spread of ointment (Wilson, Shannon, & Stang, 2005).

Neonatal Side Effects

Sensitivity reaction, such as edema, inflammation, or drainage, may interfere with ability to focus and may cause edema and inflammation. Side effects usually disappear in 24 to 48 hours.

Nursing Considerations

- Wash hands immediately prior to instillation to prevent introduction of bacteria.
- Do not irrigate the eyes after instillation. Use new tube or single-use container for ophthalmic ointment administration shortly after birth. May wipe away excess after 1 minute.
- Observe for hypersensitivity.
- Teach parents about need for eye prophylaxis. Educate them regarding side effects and signs that need to be reported to the healthcare provider.

Successful eye prophylaxis requires that the medication be instilled into the lower conjunctival sac of each eye (Figure 28–5 ●). Massage the eyelid gently to distribute the ointment. Instillation may be delayed up to 1 hour after birth to allow eye contact during parent-newborn bonding.

Eye prophylaxis medications can cause chemical conjunctivitis, which gives the newborn some discomfort and may interfere with the ability to focus on the parents' faces. The resulting edema, inflammation, and discharge may cause concern if the parents have not been told that the side effects will clear in 24 to 48 hours and that this prophylactic eye treatment is necessary for the newborn's well-being.

Early Assessment of Neonatal Distress

During the first 24 hours of life, be constantly alert for signs of distress in the newborn. If the newborn is with the parents during this period, take extra care to teach them how to maintain their newborn's temperature, recognize the hallmarks of newborn distress, and respond immediately to signs of respiratory problems. Teach the parents to observe the newborn for changes in color or activity, rapid breathing with chest retractions, or facial grimacing. Their interventions include nasal and oral suctioning with a bulb syringe, positioning, and vigorous fingertip stroking of the newborn's spine to stimulate respiratory activity if necessary. Be immediately available in case the newborn develops distress (Table 28–2).

A common cause of neonatal distress is early-onset group B streptococcal (GBS) disease. Infected mothers transmit

● **FIGURE 28–5**

Ophthalmic ointment. Retract lower eyelid outward to instill 1/4-inch-long strand of ointment from a single-dose tube along the lower conjunctival surface.

TABLE 28–2 ❖ Signs of Newborn Distress

Increased respiratory rate (more than 60/min) or difficult respirations

Sternal retractions

Nasal flaring

Grunting

Excessive mucus

Facial grimacing

Cyanosis (central: skin, lips, tongue)

Abdominal distention or mass

Vomiting of bile-stained material

Absence of meconium elimination within 24 hours of birth

Absence of urine elimination within 24 hours of birth

Jaundice of the skin within 24 hours of birth or due to hemolytic process

Temperature instability (hypothermia or hyperthermia)

Jitteriness or blood glucose < 40 mg%

GBS infection to their infants during labor and birth; thus, it is recommended that at-risk mothers receive intrapartum antimicrobial prophylaxis (IAP) for GBS disease. Assess and observe all infants of mothers identified as at risk for signs and symptoms of sepsis (see "Group B Streptococcal Infection" in Chapter 15 for discussion of maternal care ∞).

Initiation of First Feeding

The timing of the first feeding varies depending on whether the newborn is to be breastfed or formula-fed and whether there were any complications during pregnancy or birth, such as maternal diabetes or intrauterine growth restriction (IUGR).

Mothers who choose to breastfeed their newborns may seek to put their baby to the breast during the first period of reactivity. Encourage this practice because successful, long-term breastfeeding during infancy appears to be related to beginning breastfeedings in the first few hours of life. Sleep-wake states affect feeding behavior and need to be considered when evaluating the newborn's sucking ability (Karl, 2004).

Formula-fed newborns usually begin the first feedings by 5 hours of age, during the second period of reactivity when they awaken and appear hungry. Signs indicating newborn readiness for the first feeding are active bowel sounds, absence of abdominal distention, and a lusty cry that quiets with rooting and sucking behaviors when a stimulus is placed near the lips.

Facilitation of Parent-Newborn Attachment

Eye-to-eye contact between the parents and their newborn is extremely important during the early hours after birth, when the newborn is in the first period of reactivity. The newborn is alert during this time, the eyes are wide open, and the baby often makes direct eye contact with human faces within optimal range for visual acuity (7 to 8 inches). It is theorized that this eye contact is an important foundation in establishing attachment in human relationships (Klaus & Klaus, 1985). Consequently, administration of the prophylactic eye medication is often delayed, but no more than 1 hour, to provide an opportunity for a period of eye contact between parents and their newborn, thus facilitating the attachment process (AAP & ACOG, 2002). Parents who cannot be with their newborns in this first period due to maternal or infant distress may need reassurance that the bonding process can proceed normally as soon as both mother and baby are stable.

Another situation that can facilitate attachment is the interactive bath. While bathing their newborn for the first time, parents attend closely to their baby's behavior. In this way the newborn becomes an active participant, and parents are drawn into an interaction with their newborn. The nurse can interpret the infant's behavior, model ways to respond to the behavior, and support parental strategies for doing so (Karl, 2004).

EVALUATION

When evaluating the nursing care provided during the period immediately after birth, the nurse may anticipate the following outcomes:

■ The newborn's adaptation to extrauterine life is supported and complete.

■ The baby's physiologic and psychologic integrity is supported.

NURSING MANAGEMENT OF THE NEWBORN FOLLOWING TRANSITION

Once healthy newborns have demonstrated successful adaptation to extrauterine life, they need appropriate observations for the first 6 to 12 hours after birth and the remainder of their stay in the birthing facility.

NURSING DIAGNOSIS

Examples of nursing diagnoses that may apply during daily care of the newborn include the following:

■ *Risk for Ineffective Breathing Pattern* related to periodic breathing

- *Imbalanced Nutrition: Less than Body Requirements* related to limited nutritional and fluid intake and increased caloric expenditure

- *Impaired Urinary Elimination* related to meatal edema secondary to circumcision

- *Risk for Infection* related to umbilical cord healing, circumcision site, immature immune system, or potential birth trauma (forceps or vacuum extraction birth)

- *Health-Seeking Behaviors* related to lack of information about basic baby care, male circumcision, and breastfeeding or formula-feeding

PLANNING AND IMPLEMENTATION

Maintenance of Cardiopulmonary Function

Assess vital signs every 6 to 8 hours or more, depending on the newborn's status. The newborn should be placed on the back (supine) for sleeping. Keep a bulb syringe within easy reach, and teach parents to do so, in case the baby needs oral-nasal suctioning. If the newborn has respiratory difficulty, clear the airway. Vigorous fingertip stroking of the baby's spine will frequently stimulate respiratory activity. A cardiorespiratory monitor can be used on newborns who are not being observed at all times and are at risk for decreased respiratory or cardiac function. Indicators of risk are pallor, cyanosis, ruddy color, apnea, and other signs of instability. Changes in skin color may indicate the need for closer assessment of temperature, cardiopulmonary status, and hematocrit, and bilirubin levels.

Maintenance of a Neutral Thermal Environment

Make every effort to maintain the newborn's temperature within the normal range. Make certain the newborn is dried completely after the bath, dressed and exposed to the air as little as possible. Use a head covering for the small newborn, who has less subcutaneous fat to act as insulation in maintaining body heat. Ambient temperature of the room where the newborn is kept should be monitored to prevent excessive cooling. Parents may be advised to dress the newborn in one more layer of clothing than is necessary for an adult to maintain thermal comfort. The use of

THINKING CRITICALLY

A NEWBORN WITH RESPIRATORY DIFFICULTY

Aisha Khan gave birth to a healthy girl 2 hours ago. Now she calls you to her room. She sounds frightened and says her baby cannot breathe. You find Aisha cradling her infant in her arms. The infant is mildly cyanotic, waving her arms, and has mucus coming from her nose and mouth. What would you do?

clothes layering allows for flexibility as the infant is moved from one area to another.

A newborn whose temperature falls below optimal levels uses calories to maintain body heat rather than for growth. Chilling also decreases the affinity of serum albumin for bilirubin, thereby increasing the likelihood of newborn jaundice. In addition it increases oxygen use and may cause respiratory distress.

An overheated newborn will increase activity and respiratory rate in an attempt to cool the body. Both measures deplete caloric reserves, and the increased respiratory rate leads to increased insensible fluid loss (Blackburn, 2003).

Promotion of Adequate Hydration and Nutrition

Newborn nutrition is addressed in depth in Chapter 29. ∞ Record caloric and fluid intake and enhance adequate hydration by maintaining a neutral thermal environment and offering early and frequent feedings. Early feedings promote gastric emptying and increase peristalsis, thereby decreasing the potential for hyperbilirubinemia by decreasing the amount of time fecal material is in contact with beta glucuronidase in the small intestine. This enzyme frees the bilirubin from the feces, allowing it to be reabsorbed into the vascular system. Record voiding and stooling patterns. The first voiding should occur within 24 hours and the first passage of stool within 48 hours. When they do not occur, continue the normal observation routine while assessing for abdominal distention, bowel sounds, hydration, fluid intake, and temperature stability.

Weigh the newborn at the same time each day for accurate comparisons. A weight loss of up to 10% for term newborns is considered normal during the first week of life. This weight loss is the result of limited intake, loss of excess extracellular fluid, and passage of meconium. Tell parents about the expected weight loss, the reason for it, and the expectations for regaining the birth weight. Birth weight is usually regained by 2 weeks if feedings are adequate.

Excessive handling can cause an increase in the newborn's metabolic rate and caloric use and cause fatigue. Be alert to the newborn's subtle cues of fatigue, including a decrease in muscle tension and activity in the extremities and neck, as well as loss of eye contact, which may be manifested by fluttering or closure of the eyelids. Quickly cease stimulation when signs of fatigue appear and demonstrate to parents the need to be aware of newborn cues and to wait for periods of alertness for contact and stimulation. Assess the woman's comfort and latching-on techniques, if breastfeeding, or bottle-feeding techniques.

Promotion of Skin Integrity

Newborn skin care, including bathing, is important for the health and appearance of the individual newborn and for infection control within the nursery. Ongoing skin care involves cleansing the buttock and perianal areas with fresh water and cotton or a mild soap and water with diaper changes. If commercial baby wipes are used, those without alcohol should be selected. Wipes that are perfume- and latex-free are also available.

Assess the umbilical cord for signs of bleeding or infection. Removal of the cord clamp within 24-48 hours reduces the chance of tension injury to the area. Keeping the umbilical stump clean and dry can reduce the chance of infection (Figure 28–6 ●). Many types of routine cord care are practiced, including the use of triple dye, an antimicrobial agent such as bacitracin, or application of 70% alcohol to the cord stump. The skin absorption and toxicity of triple-dye agents in newborns have not been carefully studied (AAP & ACOG, 2002). Recent studies have shown that alcohol may not be helpful in promoting drying or preventing infection. Folding the diaper down to avoid covering the cord stump can prevent contamination of the area and promote drying (AWHONN, 2001). The nurse is responsible for cord care per agency policy. It is also the nurse's responsibility to instruct parents in caring for the cord and observing for signs and symptoms of infection after discharge, such as foul smell, redness and drainage, localized heat and tenderness, or bleeding.

Promotion of Safety

Safety of the newborn is paramount. It is essential that the nurse and other caregivers verify the identity of the newborn by comparing the numbers and names on the identification bracelets of mother and newborn before giving a baby to a parent. Another form of identification band or sensor attached to the umbilical cord has a built-in sensor unit that sounds an alarm if the baby is transported beyond

● **FIGURE 28–6**

The umbilical cord base is carefully cleansed.

set birthing unit boundaries. Individual birthing units should practice safety measures to prevent infant abduction and provide information to parents regarding their role in this area (Carroll, 2000). Parental measures to prevent abduction include the following:

- Checking that identification bands are in place as they care for their infant and, if not, having them replaced immediately
- Allowing only people with proper birthing unit identification to remove their baby from the parent's room
- Returning baby to nursery or having baby accompany the parent when leaving the room
- Reporting presence of any suspicious people on the birthing unit

Prevention of Complications

Newborns are at continued risk for the complications of hemorrhage, late-onset cardiac symptoms, and infection. Pallor may be an early sign of hemorrhage and must be reported to the physician. The newborn is placed on a cardiorespiratory monitor to permit continuous assessment. Several newborn conditions put newborns at risk for hemorrhage. Cyanosis that is not relieved by oxygen administration requires emergency intervention, may indicate a congenital cardiac condition or shock, and requires ongoing assessment.

Infection in the nursery is best prevented by requiring that all personnel who have direct contact with newborns scrub for 2 to 3 minutes from the fingertips to and including the elbows at the beginning of each shift. The hands must also be washed with soap and rubbed vigorously for 15 seconds before and after contact with every newborn and after touching any soiled surface such as the floor or one's hair or face. Parents are often instructed to use an antiseptic hand cleaner before touching the baby. They are also instructed that anyone holding the baby should practice good handwashing even after the family returns home. In some clinical settings, family members are asked to wear gowns (preferably disposable) over their street clothes. These are good opportunities to reinforce the efficacy of handwashing in preventing the spread of infection.

Circumcision

Circumcision is a surgical procedure in which the prepuce, an epithelial layer covering the penis, is separated from the glans penis and excised. This procedure supposedly permits exposure of the glans for easier cleaning.

Circumcision was originally a religious rite practiced by Jews and Muslims. The practice gained widespread cultural acceptance in the United States but is much less common in Europe. Many parents choose circumcision because they want their male child to have a physical appearance similar to that of his father or the majority of other children. Other parents feel that it is expected by society. Another commonly cited reason for circumcising newborn males is to prevent the need for anesthesia, hospitalization, pain, and trauma if the procedure is needed later in life (AAP & ACOG, 2002). During the prenatal period, ensure that parents have clear and current information regarding the risks and benefits of circumcision.

The parents make the decision about circumcision for their newborn male child. In most cases the choice is based on cultural, social, and family tradition. To ensure informed consent, parents should be informed during the prenatal period about possible long-term medical effects of circumcision and noncircumcision.

Current Recommendations. As in the past, recommendations regarding circumcision vary. The 1999 AAP policy statement does not recommend routine circumcision but acknowledges that medical indications for circumcision still exist. The organization recommends that analgesia (e.g., EMLA cream, dorsal penile nerve block [DPNB], subcutaneous ring block) be used during circumcision to decrease procedural pain (AAP & ACOG, 2002). The DPNB and subcutaneous ring block are the most effective options. If a circumcision is to be performed, it should be done using the least painful method.

Circumcision should not be performed if the newborn is premature or compromised, has a known bleeding problem, or is born with a genitourinary defect such as hypospadias or epispadias, because the foreskin may be needed in future surgical repairs.

Nurse's Role. The nurse plays an essential role in providing parents with current information regarding the medical, social, and psychologic aspects of newborn circumcision. A well-informed nurse can allay parents' anxiety by sharing information and allowing them to express their concerns. Parents must be informed about potential risks and benefits of circumcision. Hemorrhage, infection, difficulty in voiding, separation of the edges of the circumcision, discomfort, and restlessness are early potential problems. Later there is a risk that the glans and urethral meatus may become irritated and inflamed from contact with the ammonia in urine. Ulcerations and progressive stenosis may develop. Adhesions, progressive stenosis, entrapment of the penis, and damage to the urethra are all potential complications that could require surgical correction (AAP & ACOG, 2002).

Be sure the parents of an uncircumcised male infant have information about hygienic practices. Tell them that the foreskin and glans are two similar layers of cells that separate from each other. The separation process begins prenatally and is normally completed between 3 to 5 years of age. In the process of separation, sterile sloughed cells build up between the layers. This buildup looks similar to the smegma secreted after puberty, and it is harmless. Occasionally during the daily bath, the parent can gently test for retraction. If retraction has occurred, daily gentle washing of the glans with soap and water is sufficient to maintain adequate cleanliness. The parents should teach the child to incorporate this practice into his daily self-care activities. Most uncircumcised males have no difficulty doing so.

If circumcision is desired, the procedure is performed when the newborn is well stabilized and has received his initial physical examination by a healthcare provider. The parents may also choose to have the circumcision done after discharge. However, they need to be advised that if the baby is older than 1 month, the current practice is to hospitalize him for the procedure.

Prior to a circumcision, ensure that the physician has explained the procedure. Determine whether anesthesia is to be used and whether the parents have any further questions about the procedure. Ensure that the circumcision permit is signed. Gather the equipment and prepare the newborn by removing the diaper and placing him on a circumcision board or some other type of restraint, but restraining only the legs. In Jewish circumcision ceremonies, the infant is held by the father or godfather and given wine before the procedure.

A variety of techniques may be used for circumcision (Figures 28–7 ⬤ and 28–8 ⬤), and all produce minimal bleeding. Therefore, make special note of infants with a family history of bleeding disorders or with mothers who took anticoagulants, including aspirin, prenatally. During

⬤ **FIGURE 28–7**

Circumcision using a circumcision clamp. **A,** The prepuce is drawn over the cone, and **B,** the clamp is applied. Pressure is maintained for 3 to 4 minutes, and then excess prepuce is cut away.

◉ FIGURE 28-8

Circumcision using the Plastibell. The bell is fitted over the glans. A suture is tied around the bell's rim and the excess prepuce is cut away. The plastic rim remains in place for 3 to 4 days until healing occurs. The bell may be allowed to fall off; it is removed if still in place after 8 days.

the procedure, assess the newborn's response. One consideration is pain being experienced by the newborn. A DPNB using 1% lidocaine without epinephrine significantly minimizes the pain and the shifts in behavioral patterns associated with circumcision, such as crying, irritability, and erratic sleep cycles. Other studies are investigating the use of topical anesthetic applied 60 to 90 minutes before prepuce removal, acetaminophen, and cryoanalgesia.

Provide comfort measures such as lightly stroking the baby's head, providing a pacifier, and talking to him. Following the circumcision the infant should be held and comforted by a family member or the nurse. Be alert to any cues that these measures are overstimulating the newborn instead of comforting him. Such cues include turning away of the head, increased generalized body movement, skin color changes, hyperalertness, and hiccuping.

Ideally the circumcision should be assessed every 30 minutes for at least 2 hours following the procedure. It is important to observe the first voiding after a circumcision to evaluate for urinary obstruction related to penile injury or edema. Petroleum ointment and gauze may be applied to the site immediately following the procedure to help prevent bleeding and can be used to protect the healing tissue afterward.

Teach family members how to assess for unusual bleeding, how to respond if it is present, and how to care for the newly circumcised penis. Parents of babies circumcised with a method other than the Plastibell should receive the following information:

- Apply petroleum ointment for the next few diaper changes to help prevent further bleeding (Figure 28-9 ◉).

- If bleeding does occur, apply light pressure with a sterile gauze pad to stop the bleeding within a short time. If this is not effective, contact the physician immediately, or take the baby to the healthcare provider's office.

- The glans normally has granulation tissue (yellowish film) on it during healing. Continued application of petroleum ointment (or ointment suggested by the healthcare provider) can help protect the granulation tissue that forms as the glans heals.

- Report to the care provider any signs or symptoms of infection, such as increasing swelling, pus drainage, and cessation of urination.

- Ensure that diapers are not loose enough to cause rubbing with movement or tight enough to cause pain.

- If the infant's care provider recommends oral analgesics, follow instructions for proper measuring and administration.

If the Plastibell is used, parents should receive information on its appearance and how to observe for infection. Inform the parents that the Plastibell should fall off within 8 days. If it is still in place after 8 days, parents should consult with their physician. Though no ointment or creams should be used while the bell remains, application of petroleum ointment may protect granulation tissue afterward.

Enhancement of Parent-Newborn Attachment

Encourage **parent-newborn attachment** by involving both parents with the new family member. (For specific inter-

◉ FIGURE 28-9

Following circumcision, petroleum ointment may be applied to the site for the next few diaper changes.

TEACHING HIGHLIGHTS

WHAT PARENTS NEED TO KNOW ABOUT ENHANCING ATTACHMENT

- Information on the periods of reactivity, expected newborn responses, and normal newborn physical characteristics (see Chapters 26 and 27 ∞).
- The gradual developmental nature of the bonding process and the reciprocal interactive nature of the process.
- The infant's capabilities for interaction such as nonverbal communication abilities. Nonverbal communications include movement, gaze, touch, facial expressions, and vocalizations—including crying. Eye contact is considered one of the cardinal factors in developing infant-parent attachment and will be integrated with touching and vocal behaviors.
- Touching, including stroking, patting, massaging, and kissing, will progress to interactive touch between parent and infant; parents need to assimilate these behaviors into daily routines with their baby.
- Parents need to incorporate comforting techniques, including use of sound, swaddling, rocking, stroking, and massage, into their daily baby care routines.
- The infant's behaviors will change as the infant matures, and it is important for parents to be consistent in response to their infant's cues and needs.
- Information about available pamphlets, videos, and support groups in the community.

ventions, see "Enhancing Attachment" in Chapter 19, "Newborn Behavioral Assessment" in Chapter 24, and "Teaching Highlights: What Parents Need to Know About Enhancing Attachment." ∞)

Infant massage is a common childcare practice in many parts of the world, especially Africa and Asia, and has recently gained attention in the United States (see "Complementary Care" on infant massage in Chapter 30 ∞). Parents can be taught to use infant massage as a method to facilitate the bonding process and to reduce the stress and pain associated with colic, constipation, inoculations, and teething. Infant massage not only induces relaxation for the infant but also provides a calming and feel-good interaction for the parents, which fosters the development of warm, positive relationships.

Discuss waking activities such as talking with the baby while making eye contact, holding the baby in an upright position (sitting or standing), gently bending the baby back and forth while grasping under the knees and supporting the head and back with the other hand, and gently rubbing the baby's hands and feet. Quieting activities may include swaddling or bundling the baby to increase a sense of security; using slow, calming movements; and talking softly, singing, or humming to the baby. Also be aware of cultural

variations in newborn care such as timing of naming the newborn, giving compliments about the baby, and needing good luck charms. As a nurse, you play a vital role in fostering parent-infant attachment.

EVALUATION

When evaluating the nursing care provided during the newborn period, the nurse may anticipate the following outcome:

- The baby's physiologic and psychologic integrity is supported.
- The parents express understanding of the bonding process and display attachment behaviors.

NURSING MANAGEMENT IN PREPARATION FOR DISCHARGE

While the adjustment to parenting is a normal process, going home presents a critical transition for the family. The parents become the primary caregivers for the newborn and must provide a nurturing environment in which the emotional and physical needs of the newborn can be met. Nursing interventions focus on promoting health and preventing possible problems.

NURSING ASSESSMENT AND DIAGNOSIS

When preparing for discharge, assess whether parents have realistic expectations of the newborn's behavior and the depth of their knowledge in caring for their newborn.

Nursing diagnoses that may apply to the newborn's family include the following:

- *Readiness for Enhanced Parenting* related to appropriate behavioral expectations of the newborn
- *Readiness for Enhanced Family Processes* related to integration of newborn into family unit or demands of newborn care and feeding

PLANNING AND IMPLEMENTATION

Parent Teaching

To meet the parent's need for information, the nurse who is responsible for the care of the mother and newborn should assume the primary responsibility for parent education. Nearly every contact with the parents presents an opportunity for sharing information that can facilitate their sense of competence in newborn care. Recognize and respect the many ways of providing safe care. Unless harmful to the newborn, the parents' methods of giving care should be reinforced rather than contradicted. In addition, be sensitive to the cultural beliefs and values of the family (see "Developing Cultural Competence").

DEVELOPING CULTURAL COMPETENCE

CULTURAL BELIEFS AND PRACTICES REGARDING BABY CARE*

Umbilical Cord

- People of Latin American or Filipino cultural backgrounds may use an abdominal binder or bellyband to protect against dirt, injury, and umbilical hernia. They may also apply oils to the stump of the cord or tape metal to the umbilicus to ward off evil spirits.
- People of northern European ancestry may expect a sterile cutting of the cord at birth. They may allow the stump to air-dry and discard the cord once it falls off.
- Some Latin American cultures cauterize the stump with a hot flame, hot coal, or the like (World Health Organization [WHO], 1999).
- In Kenya, women may express colostrum to the cord stump (WHO, 1999).
- In Ecuador, the cord is left long in girls to prevent a small uterus and problems with childbirth (WHO, 1999).

Parent-Infant Contact

- People of Asian ancestry may pick up the baby as soon as it cries, or they may carry the baby at all times.
- Some Native Americans, notably the Navajos, may use cradle boards so the infant can be with the family even during work (Andrews, 2003).
- Korean mothers may be reluctant to pick up or touch their infant, deferring infant care to the paternal grandmother (Schneiderman, 1996).
- The Muslim father traditionally calls praise to Allah in the newborn's right ear and cleans the infant after birth (Hedayat, 2001).

Feeding

- Some women of Asian heritage may breastfeed their babies for the first 1 to 2 years of life. Many Cambodian refugees practice breastfeeding on demand without restriction or, if bottle-feeding, provide a "comfort bottle" in between feedings (Rasbridge & Kulig, 1995).
- People of Iranian heritage may breastfeed female babies longer than male babies. Some people of African ancestry may wean their babies after they begin to walk.

- Muslim women would not breastfeed in public (Hedayat, 2001; Ott, Al-Khadhuri, & Al-Junaibi, 2003).
- Most Korean mothers resist breastfeeding in the hospital, contending that they do not have "milk," and state that they will begin breastfeeding at home (Schneiderman, 1996).
- Some Asians, Hispanics, Eastern Europeans, and Native Americans may delay breastfeeding because they believe colostrum is "bad" (D'Avanzo & Geissler, 2003).

Circumcision

- People of Muslim and Jewish ancestry practice circumcision as a religious ritual (Ott et al., 2003).
- Many natives of Africa and Australia practice circumcision as a puberty rite.
- Native Americans and people of Asian and Latin American cultures rarely perform circumcision.
- Only 15% of the world's male population is circumcised.

Health and Illness

- Some people from Latin American cultural backgrounds may believe that touching the face or head of an infant when admiring it will ward off the "evil eye." They may also neglect to cut the baby's nails to avoid nearsightedness and instead put mittens on the baby's hands to prevent scratching. They also may believe that fat babies are healthy (Andrews, 2003).
- Some people of Asian heritage may not allow anyone to touch the baby's head without asking permission.
- Some Orthodox Jews believe that saying the baby's name before the formal naming ceremony will harm the baby.
- Some Asians and Haitians delay naming their infants (D'Avanzo & Geissler, 2003).
- Some people of Vietnamese ancestry believe that cutting a baby's hair or nails will cause illness.

The information is meant only to provide examples of some of the behaviors that may be found within certain cultures. Not all members of a culture practice the behaviors described.

The information that follows is provided to increase the nurse's knowledge of newborn care and can also be used to meet parents' needs for information (Figure 28–10 ⬤). Parents may be familiar with handling and caring for infants, or this may be their first time to interact with a newborn. If they are new parents, the sensitive nurse gently teaches them by example and provides instructions geared to their needs and previous knowledge about the various aspects of newborn care.

The length of stay in the birthing unit for mother and baby after birth is often 48 hours or less. The challenge for the nurse is to use every opportunity to teach, guide, and support individual parents, fostering their capabilities and confidence in caring for their newborn. Including mother-

baby care and home care instruction on the night shift assists with education needs for early-discharge parents.

Observe how parents interact with their newborn during feeding and caregiving activities. Even during a short stay, there are opportunities to provide information and observe whether the parents are comfortable with changing diapers and wrapping, handling, and feeding their newborn (Figure 28–11 ⬤). Do both parents get involved in the newborn's care? Is the mother depending on someone else to help her at home? Does the mother give reasons (e.g., "I'm too tired," "My stitches hurt," or "I'll learn later") for not wanting to be involved in her newborn's care? As the family provides care, enhance parental confidence by giving them positive feedback. If the par-

● FIGURE 28-10

A Letter From Your Baby

Dear Parents:

I come to you a small, immature being with my own style and personality. I am yours for only a short time; enjoy me.

1. Please take time to find out who I am, how I differ from you, and how much I can bring you joy.

2. Please feed me when I am hungry. I never knew hunger in the womb, and clocks and time mean little to me.

3. Please hold, cuddle, kiss, touch, stroke, and croon to me. I was always held closely in the womb and was never alone before.

4. Please don't be disappointed when I am not the perfect baby that you expected, nor disappointed with yourselves that you are not the perfect parents.

5. Please don't expect too much from me as your newborn baby, or too much from yourself as a parent. Give us both six weeks as a birthday present—six weeks for me to grow, develop, mature, and become more stable and predictable, and six weeks for you to rest and relax and allow your body to get back to normal.

6. Please forgive me if I cry a lot. Bear with me and in a short time, as I mature, I will spend less and less time crying and more time socializing.

7. Please watch me carefully and I can tell you the things that soothe, console, and please me. I am not a tyrant who was sent to make your life miserable, but the only way I can tell you that I am not happy is with my cry.

8. Please remember that I am resilient and can withstand the many natural mistakes you will make with me. As long as you make them with love, you cannot ruin me.

9. Please take care of yourself and eat a balanced diet, rest, and exercise so that when we are together, you have the health and strength to take care of me.

10. Please take care of your relationship with others. Relationships that are good for you support both you and me.

Although I may have turned your life upside down, please realize that things will be back to normal before long.

Thank you,

Your Loving Child

A letter from your baby.

● FIGURE 28-11

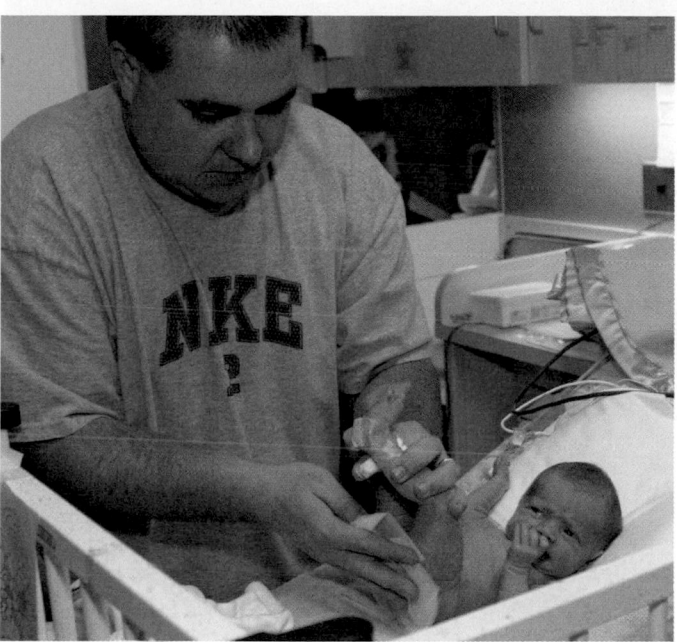

A father demonstrates competence and confidence in diapering his newborn daughter.

ents encounter problems, express confidence in their abilities to master the new skill or information, suggest alternatives, and serve as a role model. All these factors need to be considered when evaluating the educational needs of the parents (Ruchala, 2000).

Several methods may be used to teach families about newborn care. Daily newborn care videos or classes are a nonthreatening way to convey general information. Individual instruction is helpful to answer specific questions or to clarify something that may have been confusing in class. Many birthing centers have 24-hour educational video channels or videos to be viewed in the mother's room on a variety of postpartum and newborn care issues.

One-to-one teaching in the mother's room is the most effective educational method. Both first-time and experienced postpartum mothers rate individual teaching as the most effective method of instruction. Individual instruction is helpful both to answer specific questions and to clarify something that the parents may have found confusing in the educational video. With shorter stays, most teaching unfortunately tends to focus on infant feeding and immediate physical care needs of the mothers, with limited anticipatory guidance provided in other areas. (See "Teaching Highlights: What Parents Need to Know about Newborn Care," which includes a broad range of information important to share with new parents. These topics are discussed in more detail next.)

NURSING PRACTICE

For clients who are hearing impaired, videotapes with the information in both spoken and signed formats will be most helpful. Also birthing centers should have handouts available for families who do not speak English and either birthing center interpreters (not family members) or language interpreter phones.

General Instructions for Newborn Care

Picking up a newborn is one of the first concerns of both student nurses and parents who have not had the experience. The newborn is easily picked up by sliding one hand under the neck and shoulders and the other hand under the buttocks or between the legs and then gently lifting the newborn. This technique provides security and support for the head (which the newborn is unable to support until 3 or 4 months of age).

TEACHING HIGHLIGHTS

WHAT PARENTS NEED TO KNOW ABOUT NEWBORN CARE

Immediate Safety Measures for the Newborn
- Watch for excessive mucus: use bulb syringe to remove mucus.
- Have baby sleep on his or her back in crib or in someone's arms.

Voiding and Stool Characteristics and Patterns
- Urine is straw to amber color without foul smell.
- At least 6 to 10 wet diapers a day after first few days of life.
- Normal progression of stool changes: (1) meconium (thick, tarry, dark green); (2) transitional stools (thin, brown to green); (3a) breastfed infant: yellow-gold, soft or mushy stools; (3b) formula-fed infant: pale yellow, formed and pasty stools.
- Only 1 to 2 stools a day for formula-fed baby.
- Six to 10 small, loose yellow stools per day or only one stool every few days after breastfeeding is well established (after about 1 month).

Cord Care
- Wash hands with clean water and soap before and after care. Keep the cord dry and exposed to air or loosely covered with clean clothes. (If cultural custom demands binding of the abdomen, a sanitary method such as the use of a clean piece of gauze can be recommended.)
- Clean cord and skin around base with a cotton swab or cotton ball. Clean two to three times a day or with each diaper change. Touching the cord, applying unclean substances to it, and applying bandages should be avoided. Do not give tub baths until cord falls off in 7 to 14 days.
- Fold diapers below umbilical cord to air-dry the cord (contact with wet or soiled diapers slows the drying process and increases the possibility of infection).
- Check cord each day for any odor, oozing of greenish yellow material, or reddened areas around the cord. Expect tenderness around the cord and darkening and shriveling of cord. Report to healthcare provider any signs of infection.
- Normal changes in cord: Cord should look dark and dry up before falling off. A small drop of blood may present when cord falls off.
- Never pull the cord or attempt to loosen it.

Care Required for Circumcision and Uncircumcised Infants
Circumcision Care:
- Squeeze water over circumcision site once a day.
- Rinse area off with warm water and pat dry.

- Apply small amount of petroleum jelly (unless a Plastibell is in place) with each diaper change.
- Fasten diaper loosely over penis.
- Since the glans is sensitive, avoid placing baby on his stomach.
- Check for any foul-smelling drainage or bleeding at least once a day.
- Let Plastibell fall off by itself (about 8 days after circumcision).
- Plastibell should not be pulled off.
- Light, sticky, yellow drainage (part of healing process) may form over head of penis.

Uncircumcised Care:
- Clean uncircumcised penis with water during diaper changes and with bath.
- Do not force foreskin back over the penis; foreskin will retract normally over time (may take 3 to 5 years).

Techniques for Waking and Quieting Newborns
Techniques for Waking Baby:
- Loosen clothing, change diaper.
- Hand-express milk onto baby's lips.
- Talk with baby while making eye contact.
- Hold baby in upright position (sitting or standing).
- Have baby do sit-ups (gently and rhythmically bend baby back and forth while grasping the baby under his or her knees and supporting baby's head and back with your other hand).
- Play patty-cake with baby.
- Stimulate rooting reflex (brush one cheek with hand or nipple).
- Increase skin contact (gently rub hands and feet).

Techniques for Quieting Baby:
- Check for soiled diaper.
- Swaddle or bundle baby (bring arms and legs into midline, which increases sense of security).
- Use slow, calming movements with baby.
- Softly talk, sing, or hum to baby.

Signs of Illness
See Table 28–3, see page 739.

● FIGURE 28–12

THINKING CRITICALLY

SIGNS OF ILLNESS?

You are caring for Sarah Feldstein, who had her first child, a daughter, about 4 hours ago. She appears visibly upset when changing her infant's diaper and says she thinks something is wrong because her daughter has tissue protruding from her vagina and some blood in her diaper. What would you do?

Nasal and oral suctioning. The bulb is compressed, the tip is placed in either the mouth or the nose, and the bulb is released.

The nurse can be an excellent role model for families in the area of safety. Safety topics include proper positioning of the newborn on the back to sleep and correct use of the bulb syringe (discussed shortly). The baby should never be left alone anywhere but in the crib. Remind the mother that while she and the newborn are together in the birthing unit, she should never leave the baby alone for security reasons and because newborns spit up frequently the first day or two after birth. Other newborn safety measures are discussed in detail in "Safety Considerations" in Chapter 32. ∞

Demonstrating a bath (see "Bathing" in Chapter 32 ∞), cord care, and temperature assessment is the best way for the nurse to provide information on these topics to parents. Tell parents to call their healthcare provider if redness, foul odor, bright-red bleeding, or greenish yellow drainage occurs at the cord site or if the area remains unhealed 2 to 3 days after the cord stump has sloughed off.

Review with the family how to take axillary or tympanic temperatures and discourage the use of mercury thermometers. It is important that families understand the differences and know how to select a thermometer. The newborn's temperature needs to be taken only when signs of illness are present. Advise parents to call their physician or pediatric nurse practitioner immediately if they observe any signs of illness.

Nasal and Oral Suctioning

Most newborns are obligatory nose breathers for the first months of life. They generally maintain air passage patency by coughing or sneezing. During the first few days of life, however, the newborn has increased mucus, and gentle suctioning with a bulb syringe may be indicated. Demonstrate the use of the bulb syringe in the mouth and nose and have the parents do a return demonstration. The parents should repeat this demonstration of suctioning and cleansing the bulb before discharge so they feel confident in performing the procedure. Care should be taken to apply only gentle suction to prevent nasal bleeding.

To suction the newborn, compress the bulb syringe before placing the tip in the nostril. Take care not to occlude the passageway. Let the bulb reexpand slowly by releasing the compression on the bulb (Figure 28–12 ●). Remove the bulb syringe from the nostril, and compress the drainage

out of the bulb and onto a tissue. The bulb syringe may also be used in the mouth if the newborn is spitting up and unable to handle the excess secretions. Once the bulb is compressed, place the tip of the bulb syringe about 1 inch to one side of the newborn's mouth, and release the compression. The resulting suction draws up the excess secretions. Repeat the procedure on the other side of the mouth. Avoid the roof of the mouth and back of the throat because suction in these areas might stimulate the gag reflex. The bulb syringe should be washed in warm, soapy water and rinsed in warm water daily and as needed after use. Rinsing with a half-strength white vinegar solution followed by clear water may help to extend the useful life of the bulb syringe by inhibiting bacterial growth. A bulb syringe should always be kept near the newborn. New parents and nurses who are inexperienced with newborns may fear that the baby will choke and are relieved to know how to take action if such an event occurs. They should be advised to turn the newborn's head to the side or down as soon as there is any indication of gagging or vomiting and to use the bulb syringe as needed.

Swaddling the Newborn

Swaddling (wrapping) helps the newborn maintain body temperature, provides a feeling of closeness and security, and may be effective in quieting a crying baby by having the newborn's hands near their mouth to allow for sucking (Roach, 2004). Place a blanket on the crib (or secure surface) in the shape of a diamond. Fold down the top corner of the blanket slightly, and place the newborn with the head at the upper edge of the blanket. Wrap the right corner of the blanket around the newborn and tuck it under the left side (not too tightly—the newborn needs a little room to

FIGURE 28–13

Steps in wrapping a baby.

move and to allow for hands to get to the mouth). Pull the bottom corner up to the chest, and wrap the left corner around the newborn's right side (Figure 28–13 ●). Show this wrapping technique to a new mother so she will feel more skilled in handling her baby.

NURSING PRACTICE

Remember that left-handed people tend to hold the baby over their right shoulder, and right-handed people do the opposite. This keeps the dominant hand free. However, most health personnel wear their name tags on the left side. To avoid scratching the baby's face, wear your name tag on the same side as your dominant hand.

Sleep and Activity

The National Institute of Child Health and Human Development and the American Academy of Pediatrics recommend that healthy term infants be placed on their back to sleep. Parents are taught the importance of following "Back to Sleep Guidelines" to reduce the incidence of sudden infant death syndrome (SIDS). Though infants may need to be placed on their sides initially because of copious or thick secretions, placing them on their backs in the newborn period serves to educate parents regarding infant positioning. Studies indicate that parents position their babies in the same positions they observe in the hospital setting, so nurses must demonstrate this behavior to reduce the risk of SIDS. If exceptions are warranted, these should be explained to families so they do not misinterpret what they observe. The placement of babies in a prone position during wakeful play sessions should be encouraged

as well (National Institute of Child Health and Human Development, 2002).

Perhaps nothing is more individual to each newborn than the sleep-activity cycle. It is important to recognize the individual variations of each newborn and to assist parents as they develop sensitivity to their newborn's communication signals and rhythms of activity and sleep (Roach, 2004). (See "Behavioral States of the Newborn" in Chapter 26 for a more detailed discussion of sleep-wake activity. ∞)

Car Safety Considerations

Half the children killed or injured in automobile accidents could have been protected by federally approved car seats. Newborns should go home from the birthing unit in a car seat adapted to fit newborns (Figure 28–14 ●). Ensure that all parents understand the benefits of child safety seat use and proper installation (AAP Committee on Injury and Poison Prevention, 2002). For more detail, see "Injury Prevention" in Chapter 33. ∞

Newborn Screening and Immunization Programs

Before the newborn and mother are discharged from the birthing unit, inform the parents about the normal **newborn screening tests** and tell them when to return to the birthing center or clinic if further tests are needed. Some of the genetic and metabolic disorders that can be identified from a drop of blood obtained by a heel stick are cystic fibrosis, galactosemia, congenital adrenal hyperplasia, congenital hypothyroidism, biotinidase deficiency, maple syrup urine disease, phenylke-

FIGURE 28–14

Infant car restraint for use from birth to about 12 months of age.

tonuria (PKU), medium-chain acyl-CoA dehydrogenase deficiency, and hemoglobinopathies. See "Sickle Cell Anemia" in Chapter 49 and "Endocrine Disorders" in Chapter 56 for detailed discussion of management. ∞

The Expanded Newborn Screening Program allows parents to have their babies screened for over 20 disorders. Early discharge puts infants at risk for delayed or even missed diagnosis of PKU and congenital hypothyroidism because of decreased sensitivity of screening; infants should be retested by 2 weeks of age if the first test was done prior to 24 hours after birth.

Hearing loss is found in 1 to 3 per 1000 infants in the normal newborn population (Thureen, Deacon, Hernandez et al., 2005). The AAP Task Force on Newborn and Infant Hearing endorses the Joint Committee on Infant Hearing recommendation of implementing universal newborn screening in all hospitals providing obstetric services prior to discharge (AAP, 1999).

Immunization programs against the hepatitis B virus during the newborn period and infancy are in place in many states, at least 20 countries, and high-incidence areas such as American Samoa. Universal vaccination of infants is recommended. Infants should receive the first dose of hepatitis B (Hep B) vaccine at birth to 2 months of age. The second dose should be administered at least 1 month after the first dose

The third dose should be administered at least 4 months after the first dose and at least 2 months after the second dose, but not before 6 months of age (Centers for Disease Control, 2004) (see "Drug Guide: Hepatitis B Vaccine"). Parents need to be advised if the birthing center provides newborn hepatitis vaccinations so that an appropriate follow-up program can be set in motion.

Early discharge has affected both the timing of newborn metabolic screening tests and the acquisition of subsequent immunization.

Teach the family all necessary caregiving methods before discharge. A checklist may be helpful to determine whether the teaching has been completed and to verify the parents' knowledge on leaving the birthing unit (Figure 28–15 ●). Review all areas with the mother and father, without rushing, and take time to answer all queries. Note any concerns of the parents.

Nursing Care In the Community

Discuss with parents ways to meet their newborn's needs, ensure safety, and appreciate the newborn's unique characteristics and behaviors. Assist parents in establishing links with their community-based healthcare provider. Parents need to know the signs of illness, how to reach the pediatrician or after-hours clinic, and the importance of follow-up

DRUG GUIDE

HEPATITIS B VACCINE (ENGERIX-B, RECOMBIVAX HB)

Overview of Neonatal Action

Hepatitis B vaccine is used as a prophylactic treatment against all subtypes of hepatitis B virus. It provides passive immunization for newborns of HBsAg-negative and HBsAg-positive mothers. Hepatitis B can be transmitted across the placenta, but most newborns are infected during birth.

The vaccine is produced from baker's yeast and plasmid containing HBsAg gene.

Hepatitis B (thimerosal-free) vaccine contains more than 95% HBsAg protein and is an inactivated (noninfective) product. Universal immunization is recommended.

Infants of HBsAg-positive mothers should concurrently receive 0.5 mL of HBIG prophylaxis at separate injection sites (Centers for Disease Control, 2004).

Route, Dosage, Frequency

First dose of 0.5 mL (10 mcg) is given intramuscularly into the anterolateral thigh within 12 hours of birth for infants born to HBsAg-positive mothers. The second dose of vaccine is given at 1 month of age and is followed by a final dose at 6 months of age.

Infants born to HBsAg-negative mothers receive their first dose of vaccine at birth, the second dose at 1 to 2 months of age, and the third dose at 6 to 18 months (Thureen et al., 2005).

Infants whose mother's HBsAg status is unknown receive the same doses of vaccine as infants born to HBsAg-positive mothers.

Neonatal Side Effects

The only common side effect is soreness at the injection site. Occasional side effects include erythema, swelling, warmth and induration at the injection site, irritability, or low-grade fever (37.7°C [99.8°F]).

Nursing Considerations

Delay administration during active infection; the vaccine will not prevent infection during the incubation period.

- The vaccine should be used as supplied. Do not dilute. Shake well.
- Store in refrigerator at 2°C to 8°C. Do not freeze.
- Do not inject intravenously or interdermally.
- Monitor for adverse reactions. Monitor temperature closely.
- Have epinephrine available to treat possible allergic reactions.
- Responsiveness to the vaccine is age dependent. Preterm infants weighing less than 1000 g have lower seroconversion rates. Consider delaying the first dose until infant is term PCA (postconceptual age) or use a 4-dose schedule.

● **FIGURE 28–15**

NURSERY TEACHING CHECKLIST

Please read the *Mother/Baby* information booklet given to you after birth. After reading it, please go through the following list and check whether you understand each topic or need to know more.

FOR NURSES ONLY

		I know this already	Doesn't apply to me	I need to know more	Taught/ reviewed/ demonstrated
Baby Care	What to do if baby is choking or gagging				
	Safety				
	How to do skin care/cord care				
	How to take care of the circumcision or genital area				
	How to know if my baby is sick and what to do				
	What is jaundice and how to detect it				
	Use of thermometer				
	Use of bulb syringe				
	How and when to burp baby				
	Newborn behavior: crying/comforting				
	How to position baby after feeding				
	What does demand scheduling mean?				
Breastfeeding	I attended breastfeeding class/watched breastfeeding video	YES ☐ NO ☐			
	How to position baby for feeding				
	How to get baby to latch on to my nipple properly				
	When and how long to breastfeed				
	Removal of baby from my nipple				
	What is the supply and demand concept?				
	What is the let-down reflex?				
	When does breast milk come in?				
	Supplementing				
	Proper diet for breastfeeding mothers				
	Prevention and comfort measures for sore nipples				
	Prevention and comfort measures for engorgement				
	When and how to use a breast pump				
	How to express milk by hand				
	How to go back to work and continue to breastfeed				
Bottle-Feeding	How to feed my baby a bottle				
	Reasons for NOT propping bottles				
	How to clean nipple/bottle				
	How to prepare formula				
	What formula should my baby drink				
Safety	**Use of infant car seat**				
	Back to Sleep				
	Shaken Baby Syndrome				

Other information:
_____
_____
_____
_____
_____

I have received and understand the instructions given on the above topics.

_____   _____
MOTHER'S SIGNATURE   DATE

Videos viewed/ Literature given:
_____

Language Spoken by Mother:
☐ English ☐ Spanish ☐ Other _____
Interpreter Used? ☐ Yes ☐ No ☐ Family Interprets
Nurse's Signature(s):
_____
_____
_____

The infant teaching checklist is completed by the time of discharge.

Adapted from Presbyterian/St. Luke's Medical Center, Denver, CO.

TABLE 28–3 �֍ When Parents Should Call Their Healthcare Provider

Temperature above 38°C (100.4°F) axillary or below 36.6°C (97.8°F) axillary

Continual rise in temperature

More than one episode of forceful vomiting or frequent vomiting (over 6 hours)

Refusal of two feedings in a row

Lethargy (listlessness), difficulty in awakening baby

Inconsolable infant (quieting techniques are not effective) or continuous high-pitched cry

Cyanosis (bluish discoloration of skin) with or without a feeding

Absence of breathing longer than 20 seconds

Discharge or bleeding from umbilical cord, circumcision, or any opening (except vaginal mucus or pseudomenstruation)

Two consecutive green watery or black stools or increased frequency of stools

No wet diapers for 18 to 24 hours or fewer than six wet diapers per day after 4 days of age

Pustules, rashes, or blisters other than normal newborn rash

Development of eye drainage

after discharge (Table 28–3). Parents should also check with their clinician for advice about over-the-counter medications to be kept in the medicine cabinet.

Give the family the care provider's phone number and address and any specific instructions. Having the birthing unit or nursery phone number is also reassuring to a newborn's family. Encourage them to call with questions. Follow-up calls lend added support by providing another opportunity for parents to have their questions answered.

Some institutions have initiated postpartum and newborn follow-up home visits 48 to 72 hours after birth when the family is unable to visit their primary healthcare provider within that time period (Lieu, Braverman, Escobar et al., 2000). The home visit focuses on normal newborn care, assessments for hyperbilirubinemia (jaundice), extreme weight loss, feeding problems, and knowledge related to newborn care and feeding within the family unit.

Routine well-baby appointments should be scheduled with the clinic, pediatric nurse practitioner, or physician. Regardless of the type of follow-up services available in the community, the nurse contributes to the newborn's health by stressing the importance of routine care and by helping families who have no follow-up plans to connect to local resources for care.

EVALUATION

When evaluating the nursing care provided in preparation for discharge, the expected outcomes of nursing care include the following:

- The parents demonstrate safe techniques in caring for their newborn.
- The parents verbalize developmentally appropriate behavioral expectations of their newborn and knowledge of community-based newborn follow-up care.

Critical Concept Review

LEARNING OBJECTIVES

CONCEPTS

Summarize the essential areas of information to be obtained about a newborn's birth experience and immediate postnatal period.	Information is gathered from these sources:
	1. Condition of the newborn:
	  ■ Apgar scores.
	  ■ Any resuscitation effort.
	  ■ Vital signs.
	  ■ Voiding.
	  ■ Passage of meconium.

(continued)

LEARNING OBJECTIVES   CONCEPTS

Summarize the essential areas of information to be obtained about a newborn's birth experience and immediate postnatal period.—*continued*

2. Labor and birth record:
   - Length and course of labor.
   - Type of delivery.
   - Conditions at delivery.
   - Medications given during labor.
3. Antepartal record:
   - Infections during pregnancy.
   - EDB.
   - Previous pregnancies.
   - Any congenital anomalies.
   - HIV test result.
4. Parent-newborn interaction information:
   - Type of infant feeding desired.
   - Desire for circumcision if infant is male.
   - Support system available.
   - Whether rooming-in is desired.

Relate the physiologic and behavioral responses of the newborn to possible interventions needed.

1. Maintenance of a clear airway and stable vital signs:
   - The infant's cardiovascular and respiratory systems are changing rapidly.
   - The infant is dried and stimulated to breathe.
   - Free flow oxygen is available if needed, to assist the infant's transition.
   - Apgar score and vital signs are used to assess the infant's transition.
2. Maintenance of a neutral thermal environment:
   - The infant is stressed by the change from the warm, moist environment of the uterus to the dry, drafty environment of the birthing room and nursery.
   - A neutral thermal environment is needed to prevent the need for increased oxygen and calories.
   - The newborn is dried and placed under a radiant warmer.
   - A cap is placed on the infant's head to prevent heat loss.
   - Temperature is checked frequently and the infant is kept from drafts and open windows.
3. Prevention of hemorrhagic disease in the newborn:
   - Newborn lacks intestinal bacterial flora, which is necessary for the production of Vitamin K.
   - Prothrombin levels are low during the first few days of life.
   - Vitamin K injection is given IM quickly after birth.
4. Prevention of eye infection:
   - Infant may come in contact with infected material during birth.
   - Eye prophylaxis is given to all newborns to prevent serious eye infection.
5. Assessment of neonatal distress:
   - The nurse assesses and teaches parents signs and symptoms of respiratory distress such as tachypnea, grunting, retractions, or change in color.
   - Parents are taught to use the bulb syringe and proper positioning to prevent respiratory problems.
6. Expected periods of reactivity:
   - The infant is usually alert for the first hour after birth.
   - The nurse should encourage eye-to-eye contact between the infant and parents.
   - The nurse should initiate first feedings if the infant is stable.

Discuss the major nursing considerations and activities to be carried out during the first 4 hours after birth (admission and transitional period) and subsequent daily care.

1. Nursing interventions during the first 4 hours after birth include:
   - Monitor vital signs: every hour, four times daily.
   - Assess and monitor skin color, including acrocyanosis.
   - Assess condition of cord (note number and type of vessels).
   - Assess weight, length, and head circumference.
   - Determine gestational age classification.
   - Assess for the presence of any anomalies.
   - Identify infant and initiate security system.
   - Check for expected reflexes.
   - Assess ability to suck and swallow.
   - Bathe infant when temperature is stable.
   - Assist mother to feed as soon as infant is stable.
   - Administer necessary medications.

LEARNING OBJECTIVES   ## CONCEPTS

2. Subsequent daily care includes:
   - Monitor vital signs every 6 to 8 hours.
   - Assess condition of umbilical cord and circumcision, if performed.
   - Initiate hearing screening, if applicable.
   - Assess infant's ability to void and stool.
   - Determine if infant is feeding adequately.
   - Swaddle infant to provide for warmth.
   - Initiate necessary immunizations.
   - Initiate newborn screening tests.
   - Provide teaching to parents concerning newborn care.

Identify the activities that should be included in a daily care plan for a normal newborn.

Essential daily care includes:
1. Assessing vital signs.
2. Assessing weight.
3. Assessing overall color.
4. Assessing intake and output.
5. Assessing and caring for umbilical cord and circumcision, if performed.
6. Assessing nutritional status.
7. Assessing parent attachment.
8. Educating parents.

Determine common concerns of families regarding their newborns.

Most parents are concerned about:
1. Immediate health of the newborn.
2. Measures taken to ensure infant safety.
3. How to provide general infant care.
4. How to properly feed infant.

Describe topics and related content to be included in parent teaching on newborn and infant care.

Parent teaching of newborn and infant care include:
1. Safety measures:
   - How to properly use bulb syringe.
   - How to safely position infant in crib.
2. Voiding and stool characteristics and patterns:
   - Normal color of urine and appropriate number of voidings.
   - Color, type, and number of expected stools.
3. Cord care:
   - How to keep cord clean and dry.
   - How to keep diapers from irritating cord.
   - Normal changes of cord.
   - Possible cord complications.
4. Male genitalia care:
   - Care of circumcision site.
   - Signs and symptoms of complications from circumcision.
   - Care and cleaning of uncircumcised infant.
5. How to awaken infant:
   - Dress, undress, or bathe hands and feet of infant.
   - Change diaper.
   - Talk to infant, place in upright position.
   - Increase skin contact.
6. How to quiet infant:
   - Move infant slowly and calmly.
   - Burp infant or change soiled diaper.
   - Swaddle infant.
   - Talk to or coo to infant.
7. Signs of illness:
   - How to take temperature.
   - Know when to call the physician.

(continued)

LEARNING OBJECTIVES

CONCEPTS

Identify opportunities to individualize parent teaching and enhance each parent's abilities and confidence while providing infant care in the birthing unit.

→

Individualized parent teaching is best accomplished by:
1. Observation and demonstration of common infant activities such as:
   - Feeding.
   - Bathing.
   - Diaper changing.
   - Cord care.
   - Circumcision care.
2. Video tapes of selected infant care activities.
3. Written handouts of selected infant care activities.
4. Return demonstration of parents completing selected infant care activities.

Delineate the information to be included in discharge planning with the newborn's family.

→

Prior to discharge the parents are instructed in:
1. General baby care:
   - Safety measures.
   - Skin and cord care.
   - How to detect jaundice.
   - Normal newborn behavior.
   - How to know if infant is sick and phone number of infant's healthcare provider.
   - How to burp and position baby.
   - Circumcision care of male infant.
2. Breastfeeding, if applicable:
   - Position of baby.
   - Supply and demand.
   - Latching on and breaking suction.
   - Supplementing.
   - Care of sore nipples and engorgement.
   - How to express milk by hand and the use of a breast pump.
3. Bottle-feeding, if applicable:
   - Position for feeding.
   - How to prepare formula and how to clean bottles and nipples.
   - Determination of proper formula.
4. Place baby on back to sleep.
5. The proper use of car seats.
6. Remaining newborn screenings.
7. Schedule for newborn immunizations.
8. Appointment for infant's next visit with healthcare provider.

CRITICAL THINKING IN ACTION

*View the **Critical Thinking in Action** video in Chapter 28 of the CD-ROM. Then, answer the questions that follow.*

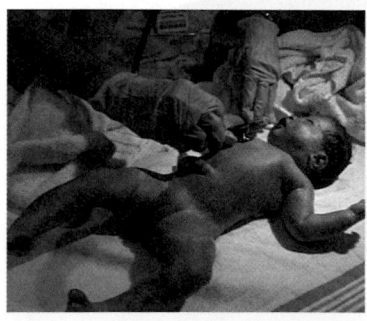

Alice Fine, age 32, G1, now P1001, spontaneously delivers a 7.25 pound baby girl over a median episiotomy. The baby's Apgars are 7 and 9 at 1 and 5 minutes. The baby is suctioned, stimulated, and given free flow oxygen at birth. As the nurse on duty, you admit baby Fine to the newborn nursery, place her under a radiant heater, and perform a newborn assessment. You obtain the vital signs of temperature 97°F, heart rate 128, respiration 55. A physical exam demonstrates no abnormalities, and you note that there were no significant problems with the pregnancy, the mother's blood type is A+, and she plans to bottle-feed. You monitor the baby until her vital signs are stable and then take her to the mother's room for her first bottle-feeding at 60 minutes old.

1. How would you review measures to promote the safety of the newborn from abduction?
2. How would you explain the technique to suction the newborn with a bulb syringe?
3. Describe the care of the newborn's cord.
4. How would you review bottle-feeding with the mother?

MediaLink   www.prenhall.com/london

- NCLEX-RN® Review, case studies, and other interactive resources for this chapter can be found on the Companion Website at http://www.prenhall.com/london. Click on "Chapter 28" to select the activities for this chapter.

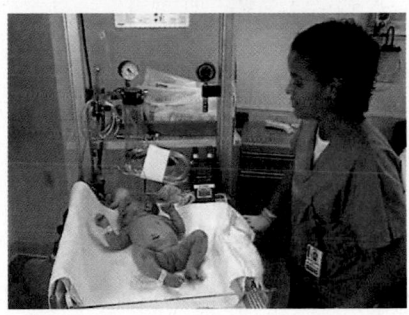

- For animations, more NCLEX-RN® Review questions, and an audio glossary, access the accompanying CD-ROM in this textbook.

REFERENCES

American Academy of Pediatrics (AAP). (1999). Newborn and infant hearing loss: Detection and intervention. *Pediatrics, 103,* 527–530.

American Academy of Pediatrics (AAP), Committee on Fetus and Newborn & American College of Obstetricians and Gynecologists (ACOG). (2002). *Guidelines for perinatal care* (5th ed.). Evanston, IL: Author.

American Academy of Pediatrics (AAP), Committee on Injury and Poison Prevention. (2002). Selecting and using the most appropriate car safety seats for growing children: Guidelines for counseling parents. *Pediatrics, 109*(3), 550–553.

American College of Obstetricians and Gynecologists (ACOG), Committee on Genetics. (2003). Newborn screening (ACOG Committee Opinion No. 287). *Obstetrics and Gynecology, 102,* 887–889.

Andrews, M. M. (2003). Transcultural perspectives in the nursing care of children and adolescents. In M. M. Andrews & J. S. Boyle (Eds.), *Transcultural concepts in nursing care* (4th ed., pp. 132–180). Philadelphia: Lippincott.

Association of Women's Health, Obstetric and Neonatal Nurses (AWHONN). (2001). *Evidence-based clinical practice guideline: Neonatal skin care.* Washington, DC: Author.

Behring, A., Vezeau, T. M., & Fink, R. (2003). Timing of the newborn first bath: A replication. *Neonatal Network, 22*(1), 39–46.

Blackburn, S. T. (2003). *Maternal, fetal, & neonatal physiology: A clinical perspective.* St. Louis, MO: Saunders.

Carroll, V. (2000). Infant abduction: Lowering the risk. *AWHONN Lifelines, 3*(6), 25–27.

Centers for Disease Control, Advisory Committee on Immunization Practices. (2004).

Recommended childhood and adolescent immunization schedule, United States July–December 2004. Retrieved September 20, 2004, from http://www.cdc.gov/nip/acip

D'Avanzo, C. E., & Geissler, E. M. (2003). *Pocket guide to cultural assessment* (3rd ed.). St. Louis, MO: Mosby.

Hedayat, K. M. (2001). Issues in Islamic biomedical ethics: A primer for the pediatrician. *Pediatrics, 108*(4), 965–971.

Karl, D. J. (2004). Using principles of newborn behavioral state organization to facilitate breastfeeding. *MCN. American Journal of Maternal Child Nursing, 29*(5), 292–298.

Karl Klaus, M., & Klaus, P. (1985). *The amazing newborn.* Menlo Park, CA: Addison-Wesley.

Lieu, T. A., Braverman, P. A., Escobar, G. J., Fischer, A. F., Jensvold, N. G., & Capra, A. M. (2000). A randomized comparison of home and clinic follow-up visits after early postpartum hospital discharge. *Pediatrics, 105*(5), 1058–1065.

MacMullen, N. J., & Dulski, L. A. (2000). Factors related to sucking ability in healthy newborns. *Journal of Obstetric, Gynecologic, and Neonatal Nursing, 29*(4), 390–396.

Medves, J. M., & O'Brien, B. (2004). The effect of bather and location of first bath on maintaining thermal stability in newborns. *Journal of Obstetric, Gynecologic, and Neonatal Nursing, 33*(2), 175–182.

Murray, G., Ormson, M. C., Loh, M. H., Ninan, B., Ninan, D., Dockery, L., & Fanaroff, A. A. (2004). Evaluation of Natus ALGO 3 newborn hearing screener. *Journal of Obstetric, Gynecologic, and Neonatal Nursing, 33*(2), 183–190.

National Institute of Child Health and Human Development. (2002). *Babies sleep best on*

their backs: Reduce the risk of sudden infant death syndrome. Retrieved January 10, 2003, from http://www.NIH.gov

Ott, B., Al-Khadhuri, J., & Al-Junaibi, S. (2003). Preventing ethical dilemmas: Understanding Islamic health care practices. *Pediatrics, 29*(3), 227–230.

Rasbridge, L. A., & Kulig, J. C. (1995). Infant feeding among Cambodian refugees. *MCN. American Journal of Maternal Child Nursing, 20*(4), 213–218.

Reynolds, R. D. (1996). Use of the Mogen clamp for neonatal circumcision. *American Family Physician, 54*(1), 177–182.

Roach, J. A. (2004). Newborn stimulation: Preventing over-stimulation is key for optimal growth and well-being. *AWHONN Lifelines, 7*(6), 531–535.

Ruchala, P. L. (2000). Teaching new mothers: Priorities of nurses and postpartum women. *Journal of Obstetric, Gynecologic, and Neonatal Nursing, 29*(3), 265–273.

Schneiderman, J. U. (1996). Postpartum nursing for Korean mothers. *MCN. American Journal of Maternal Child Nursing, 21*(3), 155–158.

Thureen, P. J., Deacon, J., Hernandez, J. A., & Hall, D. M. (2005). *Assessment and care of the well newborn* (2nd ed.). St. Louis, MO: Elsevier Saunders.

Wilson, B. A., Shannon, M. T., & Stang, C. L. (2005). *Prentice Hall nurse's drug guide 2005.* Upper Saddle River, NJ: Pearson Education.

World Health Organization. (1999). *Care of the umbilical cord: A review of the evidence.* [On-line] available www.who.int/rht/documents/MSM98-4

CHAPTER 29

Newborn Nutrition

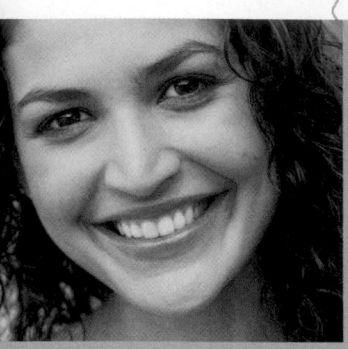

I had been told that most babies ate every 3 to 4 hours and slept the rest of the time. But not my son! He wanted to nurse every 2 hours, and sometimes more often than that. I wanted to meet his needs but felt consumed by them. It was hard to adjust to the fact that I could not get done what I usually accomplished. Once I accepted this fact, I felt free to enjoy the time I was spending with my son.

—*Ryan's mother, 30*

LEARNING OBJECTIVES

- Compare the nutritional value and composition of breast milk and formula preparations.

- Discuss the advantages and disadvantages of breastfeeding and formula-feeding for both mother and newborn.

- Develop guidelines for helping both breast- and formula-feeding mothers to feed their newborns successfully.

- Recognize the influence of cultural values on infant care, especially feeding practices.

- Delineate nursing responsibilities for client education about problems the breastfeeding mother may encounter at home.

- Incorporate knowledge of newborn nutrition and normal growth patterns into parent education and infant assessment.

MEDIALINK www.prenhall.com/london

CD-ROM

NCLEX-RN® Review
Nursing in Action: Breastfeeding
Audio Glossary

Companion Website

NCLEX-RN® Review
Thinking Critically
Case Study: Breastfeeding Client
Care Plan Activity: Breastfeeding Concerns
Actions and Effects of Selected Drugs During
    Breastfeeding

Feeding their newborn is an exciting, satisfying, but often worrisome task for parents. Meeting this essential need of their new child helps parents strengthen their attachment to their child and fosters their self-images as nurturers and providers, yet carries great responsibility. Whether a woman chooses to breastfeed or formula-feed, she can be reassured that she can adequately meet her infant's needs. As questions about feeding arise, the nurse works with the woman to help her develop skill in her chosen method. In every interaction it is the nurse's responsibility to support the parents and promote the family's sense of confidence.

NUTRITIONAL NEEDS OF THE NEWBORN

The newborn's diet must supply nutrients to meet the rapid rate of physical growth and development. A neonatal diet should include protein, carbohydrate, fat, water, vitamins, and minerals. The recommended dietary allowances (RDAs) for birth through the first 6 months have been established. The calories (105 to 108 kcal/kg/day or 50 to 55 kcal/lb/day) in the newborn's diet are divided among protein, carbohydrate, and fat. Protein is needed for rapid cellular growth and maintenance. Carbohydrates provide energy. Fat provides calories, regulates fluid and electrolyte balance, and develops the newborn brain and neurologic system.

Fluid requirements are high (140 to 160 mL/kg/day or 64 to 73 mL/lb/day) because the newborn cannot concentrate urine. Fluid needs increase further during illness or hot weather.

NURSING PRACTICE

Following are newborn caloric and fluid needs:

- Caloric intake: 50 to 55 kcal/lb/day or 105 to 108 kcal/kg/day
- Fluid requirements: 64 to 73 mL/lb/day or 140 to 160 mL/kg/day
- First 6 months weight gain: Formula fed—1 oz/day, Breastfed—0.5 oz/day

The infant's iron needs are affected by accumulation of iron stores during fetal life and the mother's iron and other food intake if she is breastfeeding. Ascorbic acid (usually in the form of fruit juices) and meat, poultry, and fish enhance iron absorption in the mother, just as they do later in the infant. The newborn needs adequate minerals and vitamins to prevent deficiency states such as scurvy, cheilosis, and pellagra.

Formula-fed babies gain weight faster than breastfed babies because of the higher protein in commercially prepared formula and the larger volumes of formula needed to obtain the necessary nutrients. (Because breast milk is digested more easily than formula, the nutrients are more readily available.) Formula-fed infants tend to regain their birth weight by 10 days after birth and may gain 30 g (1 oz) or more per day, up to 6 months of age. Healthy breastfed babies tend to regain their birth weight about 14 days after birth and gain approximately 15 g (0.5 oz) per day in the first 6 months of life. Formula-fed infants generally double their weight within 3.5 to 4 months, whereas breastfeeding infants double their weight at about 5 months of age.

BREAST MILK FEEDING

The composition of human milk varies with the stage of lactation, the time of day, the time during the feeding, maternal nutrition, and gestational age of the newborn at birth. Prolactin and oxytocin work in concert to establish and maintain milk supply (see discussion on the physiology of the breasts later in this chapter). During the establishment of lactation, there are three stages of human milk: colostrum, transitional milk, and mature milk.

Colostrum is a yellowish or creamy-appearing fluid that is thicker than the mature milk and contains more protein, fat-soluble vitamins, and minerals (Orr, 2004). It also contains high levels of immunoglobulins (antibodies such as IgA) and can be a source of passive immunity for the newborn. Colostrum production begins early in pregnancy and may last for several days after birth. In most cases colostrum is replaced by transitional milk within 2 to 4 days after birth.

Transitional milk is produced from the end of colostrum production until approximately 2 weeks postpartum. This milk contains lactose, water-soluble vitamins, elevated levels of fat, and more calories than colostrum.

The final milk produced, **mature milk**, contains about 10% solids (carbohydrates, proteins, fats) for energy and growth; the rest is water, which is vital for maintaining hydration. The composition of mature milk varies according to the time during the feeding. **Foremilk** is obtained at the beginning of the feeding. It is high in water content and contains vitamins and protein. **Hindmilk** is released after the initial letdown, or release of milk, and has a higher fat concentration.

Although mature milk appears similar to skim milk (watery and somewhat bluish in color) and may cause mothers to question whether their milk is "rich enough," mature breast milk provides 20 kcal/oz, as do most prepared formulas. However, the percentage of calories derived from protein is lower in breast milk than in formulas, and a greater percentage of calories is derived from fat. In breastfed babies, protein metabolism produces less nitrogen waste, which has a positive effect on the infant's immature renal system.

The American Academy of Pediatrics (AAP) recommends breast milk exclusively as the optimal food for the first 6 months of life, and breastfeeding in combination with solid foods through at least 12 months of life (Meeks & Tippins, 2002). It is believed that breastfeeding provides newborns and infants with immunologic, nutritional, and psychosocial advantages.

Immunologic Advantages

Immunologic advantages of breastfeeding include varying degrees of protection from respiratory and gastrointestinal infections, otitis media, meningitis, sepsis, and allergies (Thureen, Deacon, Hernandez et al., 2005). This protection of the breastfed baby extends from the neonatal period through age 18 months, when the baby's own immunoglobulins become active.

Secretory IgA, an immunoglobulin in colostrum and breast milk, has antiviral, antibacterial, and antigenic-inhibiting properties. Secretory IgA plays a role in decreasing the permeability of the small intestine to antigenic macromolecules. Other properties in colostrum and breast milk that inhibit the growth of bacteria and viruses are *Lactobacillus bifidus*, lysozymes, lactoperoxidase, lactoferrin, transferrin, and various immunoglobulins (Biancuzzo, 2003). In addition to its immunologic properties, breast milk is known to be nonallergenic.

Nutritional Advantages

Breast milk is composed of lactose, lipids, polyunsaturated fatty acids, and amino acids, especially taurine, and has a whey-to-casein protein ratio that facilitates its digestion, absorption, and full use compared to formulas (Biancuzzo, 2003). Some researchers believe that the high concentration of cholesterol, long-chain polyunsaturated fatty acids (LC-PUFA), and the balance of amino acids in breast milk make it the best food for myelination and neurologic development (Biancuzzo, 2003; Blackburn, 2003). High cholesterol levels in breast milk may stimulate the production of enzymes that lead to efficient metabolism of cholesterol, thereby reducing its harmful long-term effects on the cardiovascular system.

Breast milk provides newborns with minerals in more appropriate doses than do formulas (Riordan, 2005). Although the concentration of iron in breast milk is much lower than that in prepared formulas, it is much more readily and fully absorbed and appears sufficient to meet the infant's iron needs for the first 6 months. The AAP and ACOG (2002) state that breastfed newborns generally do not need supplemental iron before the age of 6 months. Furthermore, supplemental iron may decrease the ability of breast milk to protect the newborn by interfering with lactoferrin, an iron-binding protein that enhances the absorption of iron and has anti-infective properties.

Another advantage of breast milk is that all its components are delivered to the infant in an unchanged form, and vitamins are not lost through processing and heating. If the breastfeeding mother is taking daily multivitamins, if her diet is adequate, and if the baby is exposed to sunlight for 30 minutes a week wearing a diaper or 2 hours a week fully clothed, vitamin D supplements are not necessary for the exclusively breastfed infant (Shinskie & Lauwers, 2002). If the mother's diet or vitamin intake is inadequate or questionable, healthcare providers may choose to prescribe additional vitamins for the infant.

Psychosocial Advantages

The psychosocial advantages of breastfeeding are primarily those associated with maternal-infant attachment. The mother's level of oxytocin generally increases with breastfeeding, and studies indicate that this hormonal change coincides with more even mood responses and increased feelings of maternal well-being. Breastfeeding enhances attachment by providing the opportunity for frequent, direct skin contact between the newborn and the mother. The newborn's sense of touch is highly developed at birth and is a primary means of communication. The tactile stimulation associated with breastfeeding can communicate warmth, closeness, and comfort. The increased closeness lets both newborn and mother learn each other's behavioral cues and needs. The mother's sense of accomplishment in being able to satisfy her baby's needs for nourishment and comfort is enhanced when the newborn sucks vigorously and is satiated and calmed by the breastfeeding. Some mothers prefer breastfeeding as a way to extend the close, unique, nourishing relationship between mother and baby that existed before the baby's birth. Breastfeeding strengthens attachment, and attachment facilitates breastfeeding success (Karl, 2004).

Breastfeeding twins not only is possible but can enhance the mother's individualization and attachment to each newborn. The fantasy of a single baby is replaced more readily with the reality of two individual babies when the mother has close and frequent contact with each. Fathers are encouraged to be a part of the feeding experience by offering fresh or thawed (frozen), pumped breast milk to the baby at one or more feedings daily.

Contraindications and Disadvantages

There are some potential medical contraindications to breastfeeding. A mother with a diagnosis of breast cancer should not breastfeed so that she can begin treatment immediately. Women with HIV or AIDS are counseled against breastfeeding except in countries where the risk of neonatal death from diarrhea and other disease (excluding AIDS) is high (Riordan, 2005).

Maternal medications may preclude breastfeeding, as discussed in Chapters 14 and 30.∞ Management of newborn jaundice may include a brief suspension of breastfeeding (see further information in Chapter 31 ∞).

In the dominant Western culture, in which women actively pursue activities outside the home, being "tied down" to an infant for 9 to 12 feedings every day may be considered inconvenient and stressful. Another often-cited disadvantage of breastfeeding is the exclusion of the father from the nurturing involved in feeding the infant. However, nurturing encompasses more than just feeding, and the father can comfort and attend to the baby in many other ways (Figure 29–1 ◉).

Opinions vary on the advisability of continuing breastfeeding in the event of another pregnancy. Some believe the nutritional demands on the pregnant mother are too great and advocate gradual weaning. Others suggest that with adequate rest, a proper diet, and strong emotional support, continued breastfeeding during pregnancy is a valid choice. The practice of breastfeeding one infant throughout preg-

◉ **FIGURE 29–1**

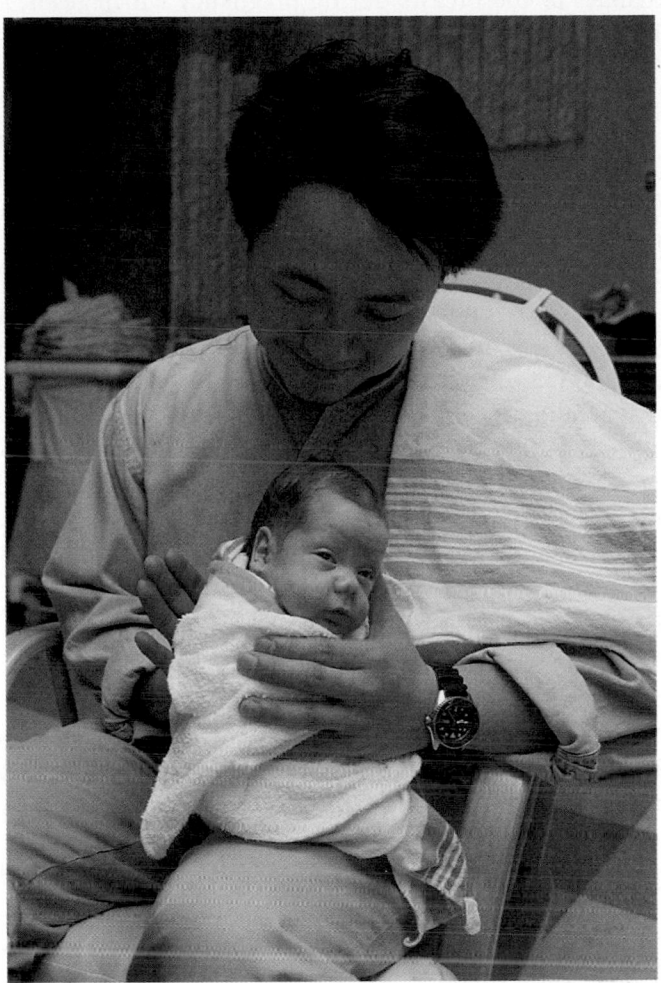

A father can participate in the breastfeeding experience by assisting with burping of his infant.

© Stella Johnson (www.stellajohnson.com).

nancy and then breastfeeding both infants after birth is called tandem nursing. When pregnancy occurs, the decision is best made individually after considering maternal health and motivation and the age of the first child.

Maternal smoking can result in breast milk concentrations of nicotine of 1.5 to 3 times the maternal plasma concentration. Although there is no documented infant health risk related to breastfeeding and smoking, smoking cessation is urged for maternal health reasons (Thureen et al., 2005).

There is some concern about whether women with breast implants should breastfeed or are able to breastfeed. Some research on breast augmentation using the periareolar approach suggests an increased incidence of lactation insufficiency (inadequate expressed milk volume, infant growth, or both). Factors that may influence a mother's ability to breastfeed after breast augmentation include the surgical approach used, alterations in nipple sensation, amount of breast tissue present, and the lack of or limited changes to the breasts during pregnancy which result in little or no postpartum engorgement (Hill, Wilhelm, Aldag et al., 2004).

Another concern is related to the possible toxicity of the silicone in some breast implants. The silicone concentrations in formula and cow milk are higher than that found in the milk of mothers with implants; therefore, the silicone in breast implants is not a contraindication to breastfeeding (Thureen et al., 2005).

Although many mothers learn about breastfeeding from written sources, family and friends, and **La Leche League** (an international lay support and information group), the nurse needs to be a ready source of information, encouragement, and support as well. The nurse can be helpful when parents are deciding whether to breastfeed, after the birth process when breastfeeding is just being established, and after the family returns home.

FORMULA-FEEDING

Although breastfeeding is increasing in popularity, formula-feeding is a viable and nurturing choice, particularly in developed countries, and meets the goal of successful growth of the baby. The closeness and warmth that can occur during breastfeeding is also an integral part of formula-feeding. An advantage of formula-feeding is that parents can share equally in this nurturing, caring experience with their baby.

Types of Infant Formulas

Numerous types of commercially prepared lactose formulas meet the nutritional needs of the infant. There are three categories: formula based on cow's milk proteins, soy protein-based formulas, and specialized or therapeutic formulas.

Commercial formulas that use a cow's milk base tend to have a high renal solute load, high protein and casein content, high proportion of saturated fats, low amounts of linoleic acid, poor mineral bioavailability, and increased risk for allergies to cow's milk proteins.

Companies are developing cow's milk–based formulas that minimize the harmful components. Many formulas are enriched with macronutrients, iron, and LC-PUFA. All of them are enriched with vitamins, particularly vitamin D. Long-term use of low-iron formulas puts infants at risk for anemia. LC-PUFA supplementation to term newborn formulas is thought to benefit the infant's visual function, growth, and neurodevelopment, but its use is still controversial (Morin, 2004).

Soy protein–based formulas (e.g., Isomil, Prosobee, Gerber Soy) substitute soy protein supplemented with methionine for cow's milk protein and are used for primary lactase deficiency or galactosemia conditions, as well as infants of formula-feeding vegan parents. Low-fat or nonfat soymilk should not be used for infants less than 2 years of age; this is the same as restrictions on low-fat or nonfat cow's milk for infants of nonvegan mothers (Morin, 2004). Soy–based infant formulas should not be confused with soy milk, which is not appropriate for infant feeding.

Specialized formulas such as casein-hydrolysated formulas or whey-hydrolysated formulas are used when an infant has an allergy or intolerance to cow's milk protein. The AAP recommends hydrolysated formulas (e.g., Nutramigen, Pregestimil, Alimentum) for infants with allergy or intolerance to cow's milk protein to avoid risk of concomitant allergy to soy protein (AAP Committee on Nutrition, 2000). Casein-hydrolysate is essentially a "predigested" protein that presents protein fragments too small to be recognized by the infant's immune system as an antigen, thereby decreasing the baby's allergic response. Whey-hydrolysated formulas, such as Carnation Good Start, can also be used for infants with cow's milk allergy, but not if the child has an IgE-mediated allergy to cow's milk.

Potential Contraindications

If formula is prepared improperly (such as by adding too much powder), the excess salts (i.e., sodium) may harm the newborn's kidneys and may lead to thirst in the formula-fed infant, causing overfeeding. If formula is overdiluted, the infant will not receive adequate nutrients.

Another potential problem with formulas is an allergic reaction in the newborn. The infant's small intestine is permeable to macromolecules such as those found in cow's milk–based formulas and soy-based formulas. The introduction of a formula's foreign protein can cause an allergic reaction, with signs such as vomiting, colic, diarrhea, colitis, reluctance to feed, and eczema (Table 29–1).

Clinicians recommend that parents who formula-feed use iron-fortified formulas or supplements because iron deficiency anemia can still occur (AAP & ACOG, 2002). However, parents must be aware that too much iron in the form of iron-fortified cereal may interfere with the infant's natural ability to defend against disease. Parents also need to be informed about the constipation that sometimes results from iron-enriched formula and about various methods of alleviating it (Morin, 2004). Many companies make enriched formulas that are similar to breast milk. These formulas have sufficient levels of carbohydrate, protein, fat, vitamins, and minerals to meet the newborn's nutritional needs.

The AAP and ACOG (2002) recommended that infants be given breast milk or iron-fortified formula rather than whole milk until 1 year of age. Neither unmodified cow's milk (i.e., whole milk) nor skim milk is an acceptable alternative for infant feeding. The level of protein in unmodified cow's milk is much higher (50% to 75% greater) than in human milk, is poorly digested, and may cause bleeding of the gastrointestinal tract. It also has higher levels of calcium, phosphorus, sodium, and potassium, which increase renal solute load and result in greater obligatory water loss. Skim milk lacks adequate calories, fat content, and essential fatty acids necessary for proper development of the infant's neurologic system. Nutritionists advise against giving cow's milk with decreased fat content (2% milk) or skim milk to children under 1 year of age.

TABLE 29–1 ✤ Comparison of Breastfeeding and Formula-Feeding

Breastfeeding	Formula-Feeding (Iron-Fortified Formula)
Nutrition	
Breast milk is species specific (i.e., perfect balance of proteins, carbohydrates, fats, vitamins, and minerals for human infants).	Formula is as close to human milk as possible, but nutrients are not as efficiently utilized.
Breast milk contains higher levels of lactose, cystine, and cholesterol, which are necessary for brain and nerve growth.	Nutritional adequacy depends on proper preparation (overdilution results in decreased nutrients delivered to infant).
Proteins are easily digested and fats are well absorbed.	Some babies cannot tolerate the fats or carbohydrates found in regular formula. Companies offer alternative formulas.
Composition varies according to gestational age and stage of lactation, thereby meeting the changing nutritional requirements of individual infants as they grow.	
Infants determine the volume of milk consumed.	Pediatrician or caregiver determines the volume consumed. Overfeeding may occur if caregiver is determined that baby empty bottle.
Frequency of feeding is determined by infant cues.	Feeding is determined by infant's cues.
Anti-infective and Antiallergic Properties	
Breast milk contains immunoglobulins, enzymes, and leukocytes that protect against pathogens.	Formula is linked to an increased number of GI and respiratory infections.
Bacteriostatic properties permit storage at room temperature up to 6 hours, in refrigerator for 24 hours, and freezing for 6 months.	Potential for bacterial contamination exists during preparation and storage.
Breast milk decreases the incidence of allergy by eliminating exposure to potential antigens (cow and soy protein).	Some babies are allergic to cow or soy protein. Formula companies are offering alternative formulas suitable for babies who develop allergies.
Psychosocial Aspects	
Skin-to-skin contact enhances closeness.	Formula feeding provides an opportunity for positive parent-infant interaction.
Hormones of lactation promote maternal feelings and sense of well-being.	
The value system of an industrial society can create barriers to successful breastfeeding: Mother may feel ashamed or embarrassed. Breastfeeding after return to work may be difficult.	
Father is not able to breastfeed, but he can feed expressed breast milk from a bottle and nurture the infant in ways other than feeding.	Father can feed the baby.
Cost	
Healthy diet for mother.	Formula is an expense.
Optional, but recommended, items include nursing pads, nursing bras.	Bottles or disposable nursers with plastic liners, nipples, and nipple caps must be purchased.
A breast pump may be needed.	
Refrigeration is necessary for storing expressed milk.	
Convenience	
The milk is always the perfect temperature.	A refrigeration system is necessary if mixing formula for more than one feeding at a time or using large containers or ready-to-feed formula.
No preparation time is needed.	Varying amounts of time are involved in formula preparation.
The mother must be available to feed or provide expressed milk to be given in her absence.	Anyone can feed the baby.
If she misses a feeding, the mother must express milk to maintain lactation.	
The mother may experience slight discomfort in the early days of lactation.	
Maternal medication may interrupt breastfeeding.	

TIMING OF NEWBORN FEEDINGS

The timing of newborn feedings is determined by physiologic and behavioral cues rather than a set schedule.

INITIAL FEEDING

The nurse should assess for active bowel sounds, absence of abdominal distention, and a lusty cry that quiets and is replaced with rooting and sucking behaviors when a stimulus is placed near the lips. These signs indicate that the newborn is hungry and physically ready to tolerate the initial feeding. Contraindications to immediate breastfeeding include heavy sedation of the mother and physical compromise of either mother or baby.

Because colostrum is not irritating if aspirated (which may occur because of the newborn's initial uncoordinated sucking and swallowing abilities) and is readily absorbed by the respiratory system, breastfeeding can usually begin immediately after birth. The mother who plans to breastfeed may be encouraged to do so immediately after birth and to allow the baby to breastfeed to satiety. Early breastfeeding benefits both mother and newborn because oxytocin helps expel the placenta and prevent excessive maternal blood loss, lactation is accelerated, and the infant receives the immunologic protection of colostrum.

Throughout the first 2 hours after birth, especially during the first 20 to 30 minutes, the infant is usually alert and ready to breastfeed. However, newborn suckling patterns vary, and although many babies are eager to suckle at this time, some simply lick or nuzzle the nipple. This behavior is beneficial because the licking stimulates the release of oxytocin, which aids uterine involution and lactation (letdown). This is a positive breastfeeding interaction (Riordan, 2005). Within minutes after birth, the newborn shows early odor-based recognition of the mother's breasts. Maternal breast odors elicit preferential head orientation, which helps guide the newborn to the nipple.

Formula-feeding newborns are offered formula as soon as they show an interest. For both breastfed and formula-fed infants, early feeding stimulates peristalsis, helping to eliminate the by-products of bilirubin conjugation (which decreases the risk of jaundice), and enhances maternal-infant attachment.

Assessment of the newborn's physiologic status is of primary and ongoing concern to the nurse throughout the first feeding. Extreme fatigue coupled with rapid respiration, circumoral cyanosis, and diaphoresis of the head and face may indicate cardiovascular complications and should be assessed further.

The first feeding also provides an opportunity for the nurse to assess the effectiveness of the newborn's suck, swallow, and gag reflexes. The initial feeding also requires assessment of the infant for the rare congenital anomalies such as tracheoesophageal fistula and esophageal atresia (see information in Chapter 30 ∞). Findings associated with esophageal anomalies include maternal polyhydramnios and increased oral mucus in the infant. In cases of esophageal atresia, the newborn takes the feeding well initially, but as the esophageal pouch fills, the feeding is quickly regurgitated unchanged. If a fistula is present, the infant gags, chokes, regurgitates mucus, and may become cyanotic as fluid passes through the fistula and into the lungs.

It is not unusual for the newborn to regurgitate some mucus and feeding, even if the feeding was taken without difficulty, because of initial uncoordinated suck and swallow abilities. It is important to observe the newborn closely and position the baby on the side after the first feeding to aid drainage and facilitate gastric emptying. Once the infant is tolerating feeding, the normal position after feeding is on his or her back.

ESTABLISHING A FEEDING PATTERN

An on-demand feeding program facilitates each baby's own rhythm and helps a new mother establish lactation. The newborn rapidly digests breast milk and may want to feed 8 to 10 times in a 24-hour period. After the initial period of alertness and eagerness to suckle, the infant progresses to light sleep, then deep sleep, followed by increased wakefulness and interest in breastfeeding. As wakefulness and interest in breastfeeding increase, the infant will often cluster 5 to 10 feeding episodes over 2 to 3 hours, followed by a 4- to 5-hour deep sleep. After this cluster of minifeeds and deep sleep, the infant will feed frequently but at more regular intervals. Maternal medications received during labor may affect newborn feeding behavior by delaying early cluster feedings. Delays in the normal feeding patterns depend on the specific drug and its half-life.

Some newborns whose mothers received epidural analgesia have been noted to be irritable and demonstrate reduced motor organization, poor self-quieting skills, and decreased visual skills and alertness (Biancuzzo, 2003).

Couplet care (mother and baby remain in the same room and are cared for by the same nurse) permits the mother to learn about and respond to her infant's early feeding cues. Early cues that indicate a newborn is interested in feeding include hand-to-mouth or hand-passing-mouth motion, whimpering, sucking, and rooting (Mulford, 1992). Crying is a late sign of hunger. Satiety behaviors can include withdrawal of head from nipple, falling asleep, relaxation of hands, and relief of body tension. When couplet care is not available, a supportive nursing staff and flexible nursery policies allow the mother to feed her infant on cue. It is very frustrating to a new mother to attempt to feed a newborn who is sound asleep because he or she is either not hungry or exhausted from crying. Although people often accept crying as normal and healthy behavior for newborns, it may actually delay the transition to extrauterine life. Crying involves a Valsalva maneuver that increases pulmonary vascular pressure, which may cause unoxygenated blood to be shunted into systemic circulation through the foramen ovale and ductus arteriosus. Therefore, it may be advantageous for the baby to be in the room with the mother; she will respond to the baby's needs more quickly than the nursery staff may be able to, resulting in less infant crying.

Formula-fed newborns may awaken for feedings every 2 to 5 hours but are frequently satisfied with feedings every 3 to 4 hours. Because formula is digested more slowly, the formula-fed infant may go longer between feedings but should not go longer than 4 hours. Babies may begin skipping the night feeding about 8 to 12 weeks after birth. The need for a night feeding is individual and depends on the size and development of the infant.

Both breastfed and formula-fed infants experience growth spurts at certain times and require increased feeding. The breastfeeding mother may meet these increased demands by feeding the baby more frequently to increase her milk supply. It takes about 72 hours for the milk supply to increase adequately to meet the new demand (Biancuzzo, 2003). A slight increase in feedings meets the formula-fed infant's needs.

Nourishing her newborn is a major concern of the new mother. Her feelings of success or failure may influence her self-concept as she assumes her maternal role. With proper instruction, support, and encouragement from professionals, feeding becomes a source of pleasure and satisfaction to both the parents and infant.

DEVELOPING CULTURAL COMPETENCE

BREASTFEEDING IN OTHER CULTURES

Some people of Asian heritage may breastfeed their babies for the first 1 to 2 years of life. Many Cambodian refugees practice breastfeeding on demand without restriction or, if bottle-feeding, provide a "comfort bottle" in between feedings (Rasbridge & Kulig, 1995).

People of Iranian heritage may breastfeed female babies longer than male babies. Some people of African ancestry may wean their babies after they begin to walk.

Most Muslim women do not breastfeed in public (Hedayat, 2001; Ott, Al-Khadhuri, & Al-Junaibi, 2003).

Most Korean mothers resist breastfeeding in the hospital, contending that they do not have "milk," and state that they will begin breastfeeding at home (Schneiderman, 1996). Some Asians, Hispanics, Eastern Europeans, and Native Americans may delay breastfeeding because they believe colostrum is "bad" (Riordan, 2005).

CULTURAL CONSIDERATIONS IN INFANT FEEDING

It is important to understand how culture and society influence infant feeding. Motherhood itself changes the woman's lifestyle. Perceptions of the mother's role and of breastfeeding as a biologic act also influence the mother's comfort with breastfeeding. In one study, some mothers identified shame, modesty, and embarrassment as reasons they chose not to breastfeed. The amount of body contact considered acceptable also influences parental behaviors. North American and European societies sometimes consider it indecent to expose the breast, believe that too much handling spoils children, and regard weaning as a sign of infant development (Biancuzzo, 2003).

The nurse needs to understand the impact of culture on the idiosyncrasies of specific feeding practices. How soon women want to begin breastfeeding after birth is culturally determined. For example, in many cultures (Mexican-American, Navajo, Filipino, and Vietnamese) and in some countries (Guinea, Pakistan, Bangladesh) colostrum is not offered to the newborn (Riordan, 2005). Breastfeeding begins only after the milk flow is established. In many Asian cultures, the newborn is given boiled water until the mother's milk flows. The newborn is fed on demand, and cries are responded to immediately. If the crying continues, evil spirits may be blamed and a priest's blessing may be sought. Although many of the Hmong women of Laos combine breastfeeding with some formula-feeding, they usually find expressing their milk or pumping their breasts unacceptable. Thus, other methods of providing relief should be suggested if breast engorgement develops. Most Muslim mothers breastfeed because the Qur'an (Koran) encourages it until the child is 2 years old (Ott, Al-Khadhuri, & Al-Junaibi, 2003). Japanese women are returning to breastfeeding as the method of feeding for the baby's first year.

The African-American culture tends to emphasize plentiful feeding. Solid foods are introduced early and may even be added to the infant's formula. African-American mothers view frequent feeding as an expression of hardiness and a positive behavioral characteristic for their children for the future (Biancuzzo, 2003). For the traditional Mexican, a fat baby is considered healthy and infants are fed on demand. "Spoiling" is encouraged.

These are but a few of the cultural practices related to feeding. (See "Developing Cultural Competence.") When faced with an infant care practice different from the ones to which they are accustomed, nurses need to evaluate the effect of the practice. Different practices are not necessarily inferior. The nurse should intervene only if the practice is actually harmful to the mother or baby.

PROMOTION OF SUCCESSFUL INFANT FEEDING

Parents may see feeding their baby as the center of their relationship with this new family member. Whether the mother has chosen to formula-feed or breastfeed, the nurse can be instrumental in the mother's success while in the birthing unit and in the early days at home. Feeding and caring for newborns may be routine tasks for the nurse, but the mother's success or failure during the first few times may determine whether she sees herself as an adequate mother.

The newborn's response to caring is an expression of personality but often has great significance for parents. A parent may interpret the newborn's behavior as rejection, which may alter the progress of parent-child relationships. A parent may also interpret the sleepy infant's refusal to suck or inability to retain formula as evidence of parental incompetence. The breastfeeding mother may deduce that the newborn does not like her if he or she fails to take her nipple readily. Conversely, infants pick up messages from the muscular tension of those holding them.

A nurse who is sensitive to the needs of the mother can form a relationship with her that permits teaching about techniques and emotions connected with the feeding. Breastfeeding women frequently express disappointment in the help birthing unit nurses give them; they say they would like more encouragement, support, and practical information about feeding their newborn, especially with early discharge. Nonbreastfeeding mothers express similar concerns. Consistency in teaching by nurses is essential. A new mother becomes very frustrated if she is shown a number of different methods of feeding her newborn. With the technologic advances in formula production and the availability of knowledge about breastfeeding techniques, the mother should be confident that the choice she makes will promote normal growth and development of her newborn.

Supporting the Parents' Feeding Choice

The mother usually decides to breastfeed or formula-feed by the sixth month of pregnancy and often even before conception. However, she may not make her final decision until admission to the birth center. The decision is often influenced by relatives, especially the baby's father and maternal grandmother (Chezem, Friesen, & Boettcher, 2003), by friends, and by social customs rather than being based on knowledge about the nutritional and psychologic needs of the mother and her newborn.

The goals of *Healthy People 2010* continue to be 75% of infants breastfeeding in the early postpartum period and 50% taking in at least some human milk until age 6 months (Riordan, 2005). A recent survey of breastfeeding in the United States showed that the continuation of breastfeeding until 6 to 12 months of age still falls short of the desired goal (Thureen et al., 2005). It is the healthcare provider's respon-

sibility to provide the parents with accurate information about the distinct advantages of breastfeeding to the mother and infant. In these times of short stays, the Baby-Friendly Hospital Initiative program promotes breastfeeding by designating hospitals as centers for breastfeeding education. Unfortunately, only a few hospitals in the United States have implemented the program. Parents have a right to hear about the data so they can make their own informed choices.

Once the parents have made an informed choice of feeding method, the nurse's primary responsibilities are to support the family's decision and to help the family achieve a positive result. No woman should be made to feel either inadequate or superior because of her choice in feeding. There are advantages and disadvantages to breastfeeding and formula-feeding, but positive bonds in parent-child relationships can be developed with either method.

Preparing for Infant Feeding

Before a feeding, the mother should be as comfortable as possible. Preparations may include voiding, washing her hands, and assuming a comfortable position. See Figure 29–2 ● for a variety of breastfeeding positions. These positions can also be used for formula-feeding the newborn in situations such as post-cesarean birth.

The woman who has had a cesarean birth needs support so that the infant does not rest on her abdomen for long periods. When breastfeeding, she may be more comfortable lying on her side with a pillow behind her back and one between her legs. The nurse should position the newborn next to the woman's breast and place a rolled towel or small pillow behind the infant for support. Initially the mother will need assistance in turning from side to side and burping the newborn. She may prefer to breastfeed sitting up with a pillow on her lap and the infant resting on the pillow rather than directly on her abdomen. It may be helpful to place a rolled pillow under the arm supporting the infant's head. The football hold, an alternative position, prevents pressure on the incision while allowing the mother a clear view of the infant's face. Mothers who have undergone cesarean birth frequently use the sitting position to formula-feed. If incisional pain makes this position difficult, she may want to assume the lying-down position. The infant can be moved to a semisitting position against a pillow close to the mother.

Depending on the newborn's level of hunger, the parents may want to use the time before feeding to get acquainted with their infant. The presence of the nurse during part of this time to answer questions and provide reinforcement of parenting skills will be helpful for the family.

Mothers of newborns should not expect alertness as a condition for latching their babies. The mother is more likely to discover that her hungry baby is drowsy, fussy, or crying when her baby comes to breast. She may have to

EVIDENCE-BASED NURSING

SUPPORT FOR THE BREASTFEEDING MOTHER

Clinical Question (Problem)

It is universally accepted that breast milk is the most desirable source of nutrition for newborns, yet mothers need support to successfully initiate and maintain breastfeeding. Nursing assessments can identify conditions that may hinder a mother's desire or ability to breastfeed. A recent survey of breastfeeding prevalence in the United States shows initiation of breastfeeding nears the national goal of 75%; however, continuation of breastfeeding to 6 and 12 months falls far short of the desired goals (Li, Zhao, Mokdad et al., 2003). What nursing actions can best encourage successful breastfeeding?

Evidence

The Association of Women's Health, Obstetric and Neonatal Nurses (AWHONN) assembled a team of nurse experts to evaluate both quantitative and qualitative research and develop a practice guideline. The guideline encompasses a continuum of breastfeeding education that extends from the prenatal period through the first year of life. Factors affecting the breasts and nipples that may impede breastfeeding can include flat or inverted nipples, scarring from breast surgery, significantly asymmetric breasts, or lack of normal pregnancy breast changes. While the experts who developed this guideline noted that these conditions may make breastfeeding more difficult, there is no clinical evidence that breastfeeding is always precluded in these cases. Mothers with these conditions may need additional support during the postpartum period.

Implications

Education should start early in the pregnancy and continue through the postpartum period. The mother's motivation, the attitude of significant others, and cultural variables may affect commitment to breastfeeding. Ideally, offer breastfeeding information early during pregnancy, and help women identify their personal breastfeeding goals. The prenatal period is not too early to develop a breastfeeding plan. Educate family members and other providers to relay consistent, supportive messages about the breastfeeding choice. You can provide valuable support to the mother in planning and successfully maintaining breastfeeding.

After the birth the woman should be assisted to breastfeed as soon as possible, once she is comfortable. Ideally, this should occur within the first hour. While mother and baby are inpatients, observe an entire infant feeding episode to determine if breastfeeding is successful and to provide verbal validation for the mother. Assess the infant's position at the breast and his or her ability to latch, suck, and transfer milk. Avoid the use of pacifiers until the infant is able to latch on and successfully breastfeed.

If the mother needs pain medication, administer it immediately prior to breastfeeding to minimize effects on the newborn. Monitor the success of breastfeeding by tracking the newborn's weight; no more than 7% of birth weight should be lost, and the baby should return to birth weight by 1 to 2 weeks of age. Consider incorporating lay counselors into the breastfeeding plan to provide support and resources for the mother.

Critical Thinking

What will be your teaching plan for the prenatal period through postpartum discharge? How might you encourage a mother's commitment to breastfeeding when initial feedings are difficult? What assessments indicate that the infant is not breastfeeding adequately?

References

Association of Women's Health, Obstetric and Neonatal Nurses (AWHONN). (2000, January). *Breastfeeding support: Prenatal care through the first year. Evidence-based clinical practice guideline* (pp. 1-33). Washington, DC: Author.

Li, R., Zhao, Z., Mokdad, A., et al. (2003). Prevalence of breast-feeding in the United States: The 2001 national immunization survey. *Pediatrics, 111*(5), 1198-1201.

---

wake her infant for morning feeds when newborns like to sleep, and calm the infant at night during expected periods of irritable crying (Karl, 2004). For the sleepy baby, a period of playful activity—such as gently rubbing the feet and hands or adjusting clothing and loosening coverings to expose the infant to room air—may increase alertness so that, when the feeding is initiated, the infant is ready and sucks eagerly. If an infant is overly hungry and upset, talking quietly and rocking gently may help the baby calm down so that he or she can find and grasp the nipple effectively (Karl, 2004).

Routines must be flexible enough to allow this time for the family. Couplet care offers spontaneous, frequent encounters for the family and provides opportunities to practice handling skills, thereby increasing confidence in care after discharge. It also encourages feeding in response to the baby's cues rather than feeding by a fixed schedule. Women who continue to breastfeed tend to be more aware of and responsive to their infant's cues and behavioral state (e.g., quiet alert) than are mothers who wean earlier than planned (Biancuzzo, 2003).

However, the nurse should understand and support the mother's choice to have her newborn cared for in the nursery so she can rest. This rest time is especially important if she must care for herself, the newborn, and other children without adult help at home.

NURSING PRACTICE

As you help new mothers with breastfeeding, it is important to create a relaxed environment and approach to breastfeeding. Encourage the mom to get into a comfortable position, well supported with pillows. Remind her to bring the baby to her breast rather than leaning forward to the baby.

⬤ **FIGURE 29–2**

A

B

Football hold

- Hold the baby's back and shoulders in the palm of your hand.
- Tuck the baby up under the arm, keeping the baby's ear, shoulder, and hip in a straight line.
- Support the breast to touch baby's lips. Once the baby's mouth is open wide, pull the baby quickly to you.
- Hold your breast until the baby nurses easily.

Lying Down

- Lie on your side with a pillow at your back and lay the baby so you are facing each other.
- To start, prop yourself up on your elbow and support your breast with that hand.
- Pull the baby close to you, lining up the baby's mouth with your nipple.
- Hold your breast with the opposite hand. Once the baby is nursing well, lie back down.

C

D

Cradling

- Cradle the baby in the arm closest to the breast, with the baby's head in the crook of the arm.
- Have the baby's body facing you, tummy-to-tummy.
- Use your opposite hand to support the breast.

Across the lap

- Lay your baby on pillows across your lap.
- Turn the baby to face you.
- Reach across your lap to support the baby's back and shoulders with the palm of your hand.
- Support your breast from underneath. Once the baby's mouth is open wide, pull your baby quickly onto your breast.

Four common breastfeeding positions. **A,** Football hold. **B,** Lying down. **C,** Cradling. **D,** Across the lap.

Used with permission from Breastfeeding: A special relationship. *Breastfeeding Education Resources, 1-800-869-7892, Raleigh, NC. Copyright Lactation Consultants of NC.*

CLIENT EDUCATION FOR BREASTFEEDING

The nurse caring for the breastfeeding mother should help the woman achieve independence and success in her feeding efforts (Figure 29–3 ⬤). Prepared with a knowledge of the anatomy and physiology of the breast and lactation, the components and positive effects of breast milk, and techniques of breastfeeding, the nurse can help the woman and her family use their own resources to achieve a successful experience.

PHYSIOLOGY OF THE BREASTS AND LACTATION

The female breast is divided into 15 to 24 lobes separated from one another by fat and connective tissue. These lobes

For many mothers, the nurse's support and knowledge are instrumental in establishing successful breastfeeding.

Used with permission from Jenny Thomas.

TEACHING HIGHLIGHTS

BREASTFEEDING

Following is information that is helpful to breastfeeding mothers:

Basics of Milk Production

Milk produced according to demand

Milk stored in sinuses under areola

Adequate maternal fluid intake required

Milk supply established by frequent breastfeeding (every 1½ to 3 hours)

Letdown reflex: flow of milk initiated by newborn's sucking, presence, or cry; by mother's thoughts; or during maternal orgasm

Positioning Baby at the Breast

Turn baby's entire body toward mother with mouth adjacent to nipple and the ear; shoulder and hip are in direct alignment

Mother should assume a comfortable position with arms supported

Direct nipple straight into baby's mouth so that during sucking, jaw compresses ducts directly beneath areola

Lightly brush infant's mouth with breast to stimulate rooting reflex (but avoid touching both cheeks)

Procedure for Feeding

Avoid arbitrary time limits (since letdown reflex may take up to 3 minutes)

Allow baby to nurse at first breast until breast is emptied

Insert finger in baby's mouth near nipple to break suction

Burp baby before changing breast

Burp baby again at end of feeding

To prevent skin breakdown, wash nipple with warm water and dry thoroughly

Helpful Hints

Be certain baby is well awake before attempting feeding

Alternate breast at which baby begins feeding (use safety pin as reminder)

Lift breast slightly or press lightly on breast above nose if mother's breast occludes infant's nares

Rotate baby's position at breast to avoid undue trauma to nipples and improve emptying of ducts

Avoid supplementary formula feedings until lactation is established

Check with healthcare provider before taking any medication while breastfeeding (because medications may cross into breast milk)

are subdivided into lobules, composed of small units called alveoli, where milk is synthesized by the alveolar secretory epithelium. The lobules have a system of lactiferous ductules that join larger ducts and eventually open onto the nipple surface. During pregnancy, increased levels of estrogen stimulate breast development in preparation for lactation.

Birth results in a rapid drop in estrogen and progesterone with a concomitant increase in the secretion of **prolactin**. This hormone promotes milk production by stimulating the alveolar cells of the breast. Prolactin levels rise in response to the infant suckling. The newborn's suckling also stimulates the release of **oxytocin** from the posterior pituitary. This hormone increases the contractility of the myoepithelial cells lining the walls of the mammary ducts, and a flow of milk results. This is called the **letdown reflex**, or milk ejection reflex. Mothers have described the letdown reflex as a prickling or tingling sensation during

which they feel the milk coming down. Other signs of letdown include increased uterine cramps and increased lochia (during the early postpartum period), milk leaking from the other breast, and a feeling of relaxation. It is not unusual for the breasts to leak some milk before feeding.

The letdown reflex can be stimulated by the newborn's sucking, presence, or cry, or even by maternal thoughts about her baby. It may also occur during sexual orgasm because oxytocin is released. Conversely the mother's lack of self-confidence, fear of embarrassment, or pain connected with breastfeeding may prevent the milk from being ejected into the duct system.

Milk production decreases with repeated inhibition of the milk ejection reflex. Failure to empty the breasts frequently and completely also decreases production. As milk accumulates and is not withdrawn, the buildup of pressure in the alveoli suppresses secretion. Once lactation is established, prolactin production decreases. Oxytocin and sucking continue to facilitate milk production.

Breastfeeding Process

The objectives involved in breastfeeding are (1) to provide adequate nutrition by ensuring proper maternal nutrition to include appropriate fluid intake (see Chapter 12 ∞), (2) to facilitate maternal-infant attachment, and (3) to prevent trauma to the nipples. Information and support are aimed toward these goals. When assisting the mother with breastfeeding, the nurse must use disposable gloves because breast milk and newborn saliva are body substances that call for standard precautions. To facilitate successful breastfeeding, the nurse should arrange for privacy, help the mother find a comfortable position, and position the baby comfortably close to the mother. The mother should support her breast with her hand, using the C-hold. In the C-hold the mother places her thumb well above the areola and the rest of her fingers below the areola and under the breast (Figure 29–4A ●). The mother may also use the scissors hold, placing her index finger above the areola and her other three fingers below the areola and under the

breast. It is important when presenting the breast to the infant that the mother's hand is well away from the nipple so the baby can "latch on" to the breast (Figure 29–4B ●).

The mother positions the baby so that the infant's nose is at the level of the nipple. She lightly tickles the baby's lower lip with her nipple until the baby opens her or his mouth wide and then brings the baby to the breast (Figure 29–5 ●). The baby needs to take the whole nipple into the mouth so that the gums are on the areola. This allows the jaws to compress the milk ducts directly beneath the areola when the baby suckles. The baby's nose and chin should touch the breast. If the breast occludes the baby's airway, simply lifting up on the breast will usually clear the nares. The baby's lips should be relaxed and flanged outward, with the tongue over the lower gum. At this point the baby should be facing the mother (tummy to tummy or chest to chest), with the ear, shoulder, and hip aligned (Figure 29–6 ●).

During early feedings the infant should be offered both breasts at each feeding to stimulate the supply-demand response. In some cases the newborn will suckle only one breast well before falling asleep. As long as each breast is offered frequently (at least every 2 hours), single-breast feeds of whatever duration the baby wishes are appropriate until the baby shows a desire for both breasts. The mother should breastfeed until she becomes relaxed to the point of sleepiness—a delightful side effect of oxytocin secretion—or until she notes cues from the infant suggesting satiety (suckling activity ceases or the baby falls asleep). The length of the feedings is up to the mother; she need not watch a clock. Literature suggests that imposing time limits for

● **FIGURE 29–4**

Nipple

Areola

A

B

A, C-hold. *B,* Mother using C-hold.

Used with permission from Childbirth Graphics Ltd., Rochester, NY.

● FIGURE 29–5

A mother helps her newborn to latch on by tickling the baby's lower lip with her nipple until the baby opens her mouth.

breastfeeding does not prevent nipple soreness and in fact interferes with successful feeding. For example, the length of feeding time necessary to stimulate the milk ejection reflex varies with the individual. If the mother feeds according to the clock and disengages the baby before letdown, the baby will not get the hindmilk. Because the hindmilk is higher in fat and calories than the foremilk, the baby will be less satisfied, will need to feed again sooner, and will gain less weight. The mother should learn to feed in response to her baby's cues and her body, not an arbitrary time sched-

● FIGURE 29–6

Infant in good breastfeeding position: tummy-to-tummy, with ear, shoulder, and hip aligned.

Adapted with permission from Riordan, J., & Auerbach, K. (1993). Breastfeeding and lactation (p. 248). Boston: Jones & Bartlett.

ule. If the mother wishes to end the feeding before the infant falls asleep or detaches from the breast, she should break the suction by gently inserting her finger into the corner of the baby's mouth, pulling down on the baby's chin, or pressing down on the breast near the baby's mouth. Burping between feedings on each breast and at the end of the feeding continues to be necessary. If the infant has been crying, it is also advisable to burp before beginning feeding.

NURSING PRACTICE

To encourage a sleepy baby to breastfeed, unwrap the baby and provide for lots of skin-to-skin contact between the mother and baby. Have the mother rest with the baby near her breast so the baby can feel and smell the breast. Encourage the mother to watch for feeding cues, such as hand-to-mouth activity, fluttering eyelids, vocalization but not necessarily crying, and mouthing activities.

Leaking

Initially more milk is produced than the infant requires. During the first few weeks, infant needs and maternal responses are not yet well attuned, daily variabilities of feeding frequency and duration are greatest, and most women experience breast leaking. Stimuli that result in letdown or leaking breast milk include hearing a baby cry and even thinking about the baby. The nurse should forewarn the mother about this possibility, recommend that she place breast pads in her bra to absorb the secretions, and caution the woman to remove wet pads frequently to prevent irritation to the nipples and infection. (Breast pads with plastic liners interfere with air circulation; the plastic should be removed before using them.) Once breastfeeding is well established (usually after the first month) the mother may also be taught to apply direct pressure to the breast with her hand or forearm when leaking occurs.

NURSING PRACTICE

If the baby is pulling the tongue back, humping the tongue, or thrusting the tongue, you can use digital suck training to bring the tongue down and forward. Place a finger in the baby's mouth, pad side up. When the baby starts sucking well, turn your finger so that the pad is down. If the baby is sucking correctly, the tongue will come forward and cup the finger, and the baby will continue to suckle. Performing this technique before feedings encourages the baby to use the tongue correctly.

Supplementary Bottle-Feeding

Supplementary bottle feedings for the breastfeeding infant may weaken or confuse the sucking reflex or decrease the infant's interest in breastfeeding. The newborn has to open her or his mouth wider to grasp the mother's nipple than to grasp a bottle nipple. The shape of the mouth and lips and the sucking mechanism are also different for sucking the breast and the bottle nipple. While suckling at the breast, the infant's tongue moves front to back, squeezing the milk from the nipple. While sucking on a rubber nipple, the tongue pushes forward against the nipple to control the milk flow. Some breastfeeding babies who are given supplementary bottles cannot adjust to these different techniques and push the mother's nipple out of their mouth in subsequent breastfeeding attempts. This can be frustrating for both mother and baby. Breastfeeding mothers should avoid introducing bottles until breastfeeding is well established.

Parents are often concerned because they have no visual assurance about the amount of breast milk consumed. It is helpful to teach the mother the signs of milk transfer to the infant (i.e., audible swallowing, milk appearing in the baby's mouth, her breast feeling soft after feeding, milk leaking from the opposite breast) (Mulford, 1992). If the infant gains weight and has six or more wet diapers per day without supplementary feedings of water or formula after the first week of life, he or she is receiving adequate amounts of milk. Parents should know that because breast milk is more easily digested than formula, the breastfed infant becomes hungry sooner. Thus, the frequency of breastfeeding is greater than that of bottle-feeding. The parents may also expect the infant to demand more frequent breastfeeding during growth spurts, such as ages 10 days to 2 weeks, 5 to 6 weeks, and 2.5 to 3 months.

Expression of Milk

If the mother who wants to breastfeed is unable to do so for medical or workplace reasons, she needs information about other means of stimulating milk production and storing the breast milk. The choice of method (manual or with breast pump) may depend on the mother's physiologic capabilities to produce the desired amount of milk and her personal preference. During the early postpartum period, if the baby cannot feed at the breast (as in the case of some preterm or sick infants), the mother needs frequent breast stimulation to establish and increase her milk supply to prepare for later breastfeeding. She should use an electric breast pump at least eight times in each 24-hour period (Riordan, 2005). Research has shown that a pulsatile electric pump and double setup (allowing both breasts to be stimulated simultaneously) results in higher prolactin levels and a greater volume of milk than does manual expression (Riordan, 2005). After lactation is established, the mother may express the breast milk by the method that she finds most effective and convenient.

NURSING PRACTICE

Babies are probably getting enough milk if:

- They are breastfeeding at least eight times in 24 hours.
- In a quiet room, their mothers can hear them swallow while feeding.
- Their mothers' breasts appear to soften after feeding.
- The number of wet diapers increases by the fourth or fifth day after birth, or there are at least six to eight wet diapers every 24 hours after day 5.
- The baby's stools are yellow or are beginning to lighten in color by the fourth or fifth day after birth.

Offering a supplemental bottle is not a reliable indicator; most babies will take a few ounces even if they are getting enough breast milk.

To express her milk manually, the woman washes her hands, then massages her breast to stimulate letdown. To massage her breast, the woman grasps the breast with both hands at the base of the breast near the chest wall. Using her palms, she firmly slides her hands toward her nipple. She repeats this process several times. Then she is ready to begin hand expression. The woman generally uses her left hand for her right breast and her right hand for her left breast. However, some women prefer to use the hand on the same side as the breast. The woman should use the method she finds most effective. The woman grasps the areola with her thumb on the top and her first two fingers on the lower portion (Figure 29–7 ●). Without allowing her fingers to slide on her skin, she pushes inward toward the chest and then squeezes her fingers together while pulling forward on the areola. She can use a container to catch any fluid that is squeezed out. She rotates her hand slightly so that she can repeat the process. She continues to reposition her hand and repeat the process to empty all the milk sinuses. The nurse should encourage the mother to drink fluids while pumping. Having a picture of her baby or other momentos of her baby with the mother during pumping will assist with letdown.

Breast pumps use suction to express milk. Some have collection systems to conveniently store the milk. Hand pumps are portable and inexpensive. Battery-operated pumps are more efficient than hand pumps but are also more expensive. Electric pumps are more efficient but are bulky and expensive; however, they can be rented in many areas. Many agencies have a variety of pumps available and provide instruction on correct use (Table 29–2). Videotapes and photographs are also useful in demonstrating the process to new mothers.

Storing Breast Milk

Breast milk has bacteriostatic qualities because of its IgA and IgG antibodies, which retard bacterial growth. It is recommended that refrigerated milk be used within 3 days

FIGURE 29-7

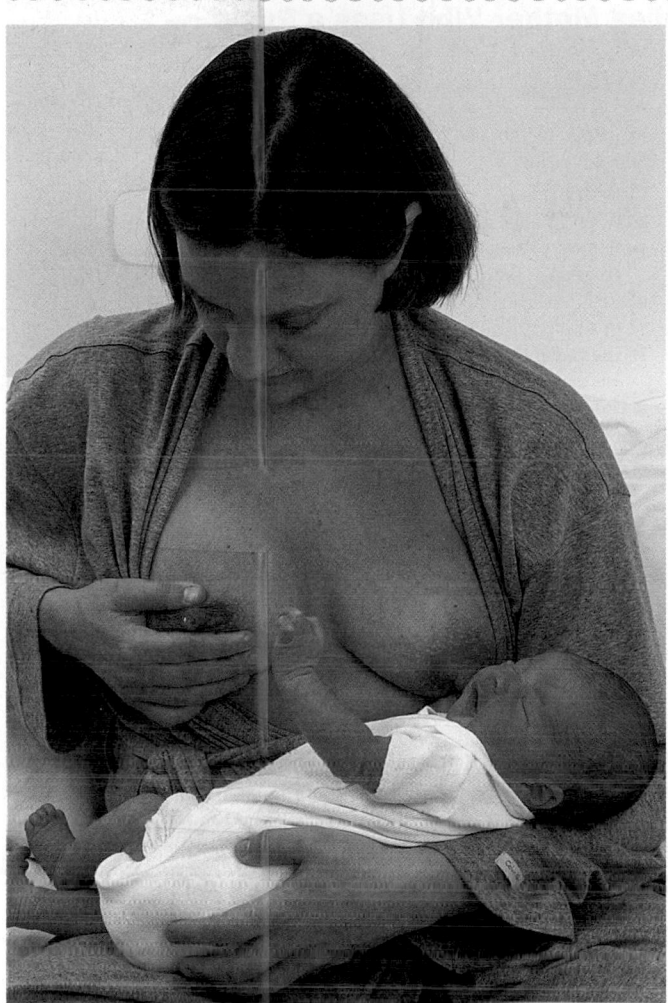

Hand position for manual expression of milk.

© Stella Johnson (www.stellajohnson.com).

(Shinskie & Lauwers, 2002). If breast milk is to be refrigerated and then fed to the infant, it should be stored in clean plastic containers; the white blood cells will adhere to glass, and their protective effect will be lost. Breast milk can be frozen in either glass or plastic; freezing destroys the white blood cells anyway. Breast milk can be stored in a freezer compartment inside the refrigerator for up to 2 weeks, in a self-contained freezer unit of a refrigerator for up to 3 to 4 months, and in a separate deep freeze unit at 0°F or less for up to 6 months. Frozen breast milk can be thawed by initially running cool water over the container, then gradually adding warm water until the milk is thawed. The container should then be gently shaken to return to suspension the fat molecules that separate during freezing. Breast milk should not be defrosted under hot running water or in boiling water. Breast milk must *never* be microwaved. Uneven heating patterns may alter the composition of the milk and can create hot spots that can burn the baby's mouth.

External Supports

Childbirth and the beginning of motherhood are critical times in a woman's life, so physical, psychologic, and social supports are of paramount importance. The father or other partner is the most important support person for her, although the baby can also provide some support in the form of positive feedback. However, extensive family support systems may not be available. The woman's mother, mother-in-law, sisters, and other female relatives who could mentor and care for the new mother may live at a distance or work full-time. As evidenced by the frequent discontinuing of breastfeeding in the early postpartum weeks, there is a need for assistance and follow-up in this area. Nurses, dietitians, childbirth educators, certified nurse-midwives, lactation consultants, mother-to-mother support groups, and physicians must collaborate to provide consistent, timely information and support and to attend to the new mother's special needs.

Breastfeeding mothers who work outside the home and are supported in their decision tend to breastfeed their infants for longer periods than mothers who work but do not receive support. A baby-friendly workplace needs to be seen as another item in a benefit package offered by a company. Families and nurses who believe in breastfeeding need to be part of the solution to breastfeeding and workplace issues by educating employers in their communities (Rojjanasrirat, 2004).

La Leche League International is an organized group of volunteers who provide education about breastfeeding and assistance to women who are breastfeeding infants. Through its small, neighborhood-based groups, it sponsors activities, provides printed materials, rents electric breast pumps, offers one-to-one counseling to mothers with questions or problems, and provides group support to breastfeeding mothers.

Certified lactation consultants are specially trained to offer a variety of services through private practice and healthcare facilities. A variety of lactation education programs are offered with differing prerequisites and objectives. Numerous books, pamphlets, and educational videos are also available to help the breastfeeding mother. The mother needs the support of all family members, her physician or certified nurse-midwife, the pediatrician or certified nurse practitioner, and all nursing personnel. Often the attitudes of these people ultimately lead the woman to success or failure.

Drugs and Breastfeeding

It has long been recognized that certain medications taken by the mother may affect her infant. It should be noted that (1) most drugs pass into breast milk, (2) almost all medications appear in only small amounts in human milk (usually less than 1% of the maternal dosage), and (3) very few drugs are contraindicated for breastfeeding women.

TABLE 29–2 ✤ Recommendations for Breastfeeding Mother Who Uses a Pump

General Pumping Recommendations	Recommendations for Specific Types of Pumps
1. Read the instructions on the use and cleaning of a pump before expressing milk.	1. Avoid pumps that use rubber bulbs to generate vacuum; they can cause bruising.
2. Wash hands before each pumping session.	2. Cylinder pumps:
3. Frequency: For occasional pumping, pump during, after, or between feedings, whichever gives the best results. Most mothers tend to express more milk in the morning. Working mothers should use the pump on a regular basis for the number of feedings that are missed. For premature or ill babies who are not at breast, the number of pumpings should total eight or more in 24 hours. Initiation of pumping should be delayed no longer than 6 hours following birth unless medically indicated. This ensures appropriate development and sensitivity of prolactin receptors. More frequent pumping will avoid the buildup of excessive back pressure of milk during engorgement.	■ When "O" rings are used, they must be in place for proper suction. ■ Remove gaskets after each use for cleaning to avoid harboring bacteria in the pump. ■ Roll the gasket on the inner cylinder back and forth to restore it to its original shape. ■ The pump stroke may need to be shortened as the outer cylinder fills with milk. ■ The user may need to empty the outer cylinder once or twice during pumping. ■ Hand position should be palm up with the elbow held close to the body.
4. Duration: With single-sided pumping, optimal duration is 10 to 15 minutes with an electric pump and 10 to 20 minutes with a manual pump. If double pumping with an electric or two battery-operated pumps, 8 to 10 minutes is optimal. Encourage mothers to tailor these times to their own situation.	3. Battery-operated pumps: ■ Use alkaline batteries. ■ Replace batteries when cycles per minute decrease. ■ Interrupt vacuum frequently to avoid nipple pain and damage. ■ Use an AC adapter when possible, especially if the pump generates fewer than six cycles per minute. ■ Consider renting an electric pump for pumping that will continue for longer than 1 or 2 months. ■ Use two pumps simultaneously if pumping time is limited or to increase the quantity of milk obtained. ■ Choose a pump in which the vacuum can be regulated. ■ Massage the breast by quadrants during pumping.
5. Technique: ■ Elicit the milk ejection reflex before using any pump. ■ Use only as much suction as is needed to maintain milk flow. ■ Massage the breast in quadrants during pumping to increase intramammary pressure. ■ Allow enough time for pumping to avoid anxiety. ■ Use inserts or different flanges if needed to obtain the best fit between pump and breast. ■ Avoid long periods of uninterrupted vacuum. ■ Stop pumping when the milk flow is minimal or has ceased.	4. Semiautomatic pumps: ■ Vacuum may be easier to control if the mother does not lift her finger completely off the hole but rolls it back and forth rhythmically so that the vacuum is efficient but not painful. 5. Automatic electric pumps: ■ Use the lowest pressure setting that is efficient. ■ Use a double setup (simultaneous pumping) when time is limited to increase the milk supply and for prematurity, maternal or infant illness, or other special situations.

Adapted with permission from Riordan, J., & Auerbach, K. (1999). *Breastfeeding and human lactation* (2nd ed., p. 397). Boston: Jones & Bartlett Publishers, Sudbury, MA. www.jbpub.com.

MEDIALINK Actions and Effects of Selected Drugs During Breastfeeding

The properties of a drug influence its passage into breast milk, as does the amount of the drug taken, the frequency and route of administration, and the timing of the dose in relationship to infant feeding. The drug's effects are influenced by the infant's age, the feeding frequency, the volume of milk taken, and the degree of absorption through the gastrointestinal tract.

Five adjustments should be made when administering drugs to a breastfeeding mother to decrease the effects on the infant (Blackburn, 2003):

1. Long-acting forms of drugs should be avoided. The infant may have difficulty metabolizing and excreting them, and accumulation may be a problem.

2. Absorption rates and peak blood levels should be considered in scheduling the administration of the drugs. Less of the drug crosses into the milk if the medication can be given immediately after the woman has breastfed her baby.

3. The infant should be closely observed for any signs of drug reaction, including rash, fussiness, lethargy, or changes in sleeping habits or feeding pattern.

4. Whenever alternatives are available, the drug that shows the least tendency to pass into breast milk should be selected.

5. Single-symptom drugs should be used versus multisymptom drugs.

The mother should be informed about the potential of most drugs to cross into breast milk. She should also be advised to tell any physician who prescribes medications for her that she is breastfeeding.

In counseling the breastfeeding mother, the healthcare provider needs to weigh the benefits of the medication against the possible risk to the infant and its possible effect on breastfeeding. The potential risk to the infant must also be weighed against the effect of interrupting breastfeeding.

Potential Problems in Breastfeeding

Because mothers are discharged from the birthing unit before breastfeeding is well established, they are frequently alone when they encounter changes in the process. Many women stop breastfeeding if the situations they encounter seem problematic. The nurse should offer anticipatory guidance regarding common breastfeeding phenomena and give the woman resources to use after discharge. See "Breastfeeding Concerns Following Discharge" in Chapter 32 for a detailed discussion of self-care measures the nurse can suggest to a woman with a breastfeeding problem (such as cracked nipples) after discharge from the birthing unit. ∞

COMPLEMENTARY CARE

HERBS, HOMEOPATHY, AND ESSENTIAL OILS FOR BREASTFEEDING

Herbs: Herbs thought to increase milk supply include alfalfa, dandelion, fennel, horsetail, red raspberry, caraway, and anise. The mother may drink caraway tea to reduce colic in the breastfeeding infant. Caraway tea also may be given directly to infants to treat colic (Skidmore-Roth, 2004). The following herbs may decrease milk supply, so they should be avoided until a woman is no longer breastfeeding: black walnut, sage, parsley, and yarrow (Balch & Balch, 2001). Black cohosh, blessed thistle, cascara sagrada, horseradish, garlic, cinnamon bark, kava kava, and senna are also contraindicated during lactation (Blumenthal, 2000).

Homeopathy: Pulsatilla, a homeopathic remedy, is used to improve a deficient flow of milk or dry up the milk if the mother is weaning the child.

Essential Oils: Cracked nipples often respond to calendula cream or ointment, found in health food stores. The breastfeeding mother should wash her nipples off very well before feeding her child. Oil of peppermint, as a cold compress, may relieve breast engorgement or assist in the process of weaning. Place four to five drops of peppermint oil in ice cold water. Although essential oils feel like water, chemically they are oils and as such do not mix with the water. Dip a piece of clean fabric into the water so that the cloth picks up the essential oil on the surface. Wring out the fabric and place it on the breasts. Again, the breast should be washed completely before feeding. Women who are allergic to ragweed may find they are also allergic to calendula.

Breastfeeding Evaluation

During the birthing unit stay, the nurse should carefully monitor the progress of the breastfeeding mother and child. A systematic assessment of several breastfeeding episodes gives a chance to teach the new mother about lactation and the breastfeeding process, to provide anticipatory guidance, and to evaluate the need for follow-up care after discharge. Criteria for evaluating a breastfeeding session include maternal and infant cues, latch-on, position, letdown, nipple condition, infant response, and maternal response. The literature provides various tools to guide the assessment and documentation of the breastfeeding efforts. The LATCH scoring table is one example (Figure 29–8 ⚫).

CLIENT EDUCATION FOR FORMULA-FEEDING

With the great emphasis placed on successful breastfeeding, the teaching needs of the formula-feeding new mother may be overlooked. The nurse should encourage the mother who has chosen to formula-feed her infant to assume a comfortable position with adequate arm support so that she can easily hold her infant. Most women cradle their infants in the crook of the arm close to the body, which provides the intimacy and cuddling so essential to an infant and offers the same benefits of closeness as breastfeeding. If the mother has had only limited experience in feeding infants, she may need some guidelines to feed her newborn successfully. The following information helps parents facilitate adequate nutrition and foster attachment:

1. Always hold bottles; never prop them. Positional otitis media may develop if the infant is fed horizontally, because milk and nasal mucus may block the eustachian tube. Holding the infant provides social and close physical contact for the baby and an opportunity for parent-child interaction and bonding (Figure 29–9 ⚫).

2. The nipple should have a hole big enough to allow milk to flow in drops when the bottle is inverted. Too large an opening may cause overfeeding or regurgitation because of rapid feeding. If feeding is too fast, change the nipple and help the infant eat more slowly by stopping the feeding frequently for burping and cuddling.

3. Point the nipple directly into the mouth, not toward the palate or tongue, and place it on top of the tongue. The nipple should be full of liquid at all times to prevent ingestion of extra air, which decreases the amount of feeding and increases discomfort. Nipples vary in shape, amount of energy needed to obtain the formula, and rate of formula flow through the nipple unit.

4. Burp the infant at intervals, preferably at the middle and end of the feeding. An infant who seems to swallow a great deal of air while sucking may need more frequent burping. If the infant has cried before being fed, he or she may have swallowed air; in such cases, burp the infant before beginning to feed or after taking just enough to calm down. Burp the

● FIGURE 29-8

	0	1	2
L Latch	Too sleepy or reluctant No latch achieved	Repeated attempts Hold nipple in mouth Stimulate to suck	Grasps breast Tongue down Lips flanged Rhythmic sucking
A Audible swallowing	None	A few with stimulation	Spontaneous and intermittent <24 hours old Spontaneous and frequent >24 hours old
T Type of nipple	Inverted	Flat	Everted (after stimulation)
C Comfort (breast/ nipple)	Engorged Cracked, bleeding, large blisters or bruises Severe discomfort	Filling Reddened/small blisters or bruises Mild/moderate discomfort	Soft Nontender
H Hold (positioning)	Full assist (staff holds infant at breast)	Minimal assist (i.e., elevate head of bed, place pillows for support) Teach one side; mother does other Staff holds and then mother takes over	No assist from staff Mother able to position and hold infant

LATCH: a breastfeeding charting and documentation tool. LATCH was created to provide a systematic method for breastfeeding assessment and charting. It can be used to assist the mother in establishing breastfeeding and to define areas of needed intervention.

Used with permission from AWHONN. (1994). Jensen, D., Wallace, S., & Kelsay, P. A breastfeeding charting system and documentation tool. Journal of Obstetric, Gynecologic, and Neonatal Nursing, 23(1), 27–32 (Table 1 Latch Scoring Table, p. 29). Washington, DC: Author. © by the Association of Women's Health, Obstetric and Neonatal Nurses. All rights reserved.

infant by holding him or her upright on the shoulder or in a sitting position on the lap with the infant's chin and chest supported on one hand. Then gently pat or stroke the infant's back with the other hand. Too frequent burping may confuse a newborn attempting to coordinate sucking, swallowing, and breathing simultaneously.

5. Newborns frequently regurgitate small amounts of feedings. The amount may look large to the inexperienced parent, but it is normal. Initially it may be due to excessive mucus and gastric irritation from foreign substances such as aspirated blood in the stomach from birth. Later, regurgitation may result when the infant feeds too rapidly and swallows air. It may also happen when the infant is overfed and the cardiac sphincter allows the excess to be regurgitated. Because this is common, experienced mothers and nurses generally keep a "burp cloth" available. Although regurgitation is normal, vomiting or a forceful expulsion of fluid is not. When forceful expulsion occurs, further evaluation may be indicated, especially if other symptoms are present.

6. A fat baby is not necessarily a healthy one. Avoid overfeeding or feeding infants every time they cry.

Encourage but do not force the infant to feed, and allow the infant to set the pace once feedings are established. Parents sometimes set artificial goals—"the baby must take all 5 oz"—and keep feeding the child until those goals are met, even though the infant may not be hungry. Overfeeding results in infant obesity. During early feedings, however, the infant may need simple tactile stimulation—such as gently rubbing feet and hands, adjusting clothing, and loosening coverings—to maintain adequate sucking long enough to complete a full feeding. The desirable amount and frequency of formula-feeding vary with the infant's postnatal age. From birth to 2 months of age, the baby takes six to eight feedings of approximately 2 to 4 oz of formula at each feeding within a 24-hour period.

The three forms of formula are ready-to-feed, liquid concentrate, and powdered (Table 29–3).

The nurse is responsible for discussing formula preparation and sterilization techniques with families. Cleanliness is essential, but sterilization is necessary only if the water source is questionable. Bottles may be effectively prepared in the dishwasher or washed thoroughly in warm, soapy water and rinsed well. The temperature of dishwash-

● **FIGURE 29–9**

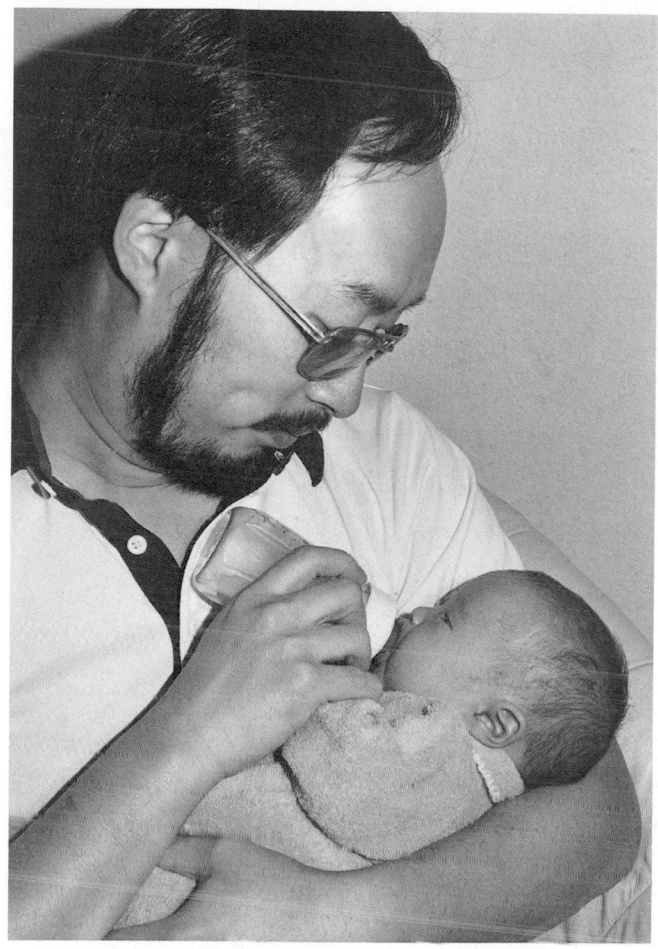

An infant is supported comfortably during bottle-feeding.

formulas, which are less expensive than the concentrated or ready-to-use formulas. Honey should not be used as a "sugar source" because of the danger of infant botulism.

NURSING PRACTICE

When you help a mother bottle-feed her baby for the first time, you can help her avoid many potential frustrations. The first is often "flying arms" as the baby waves his or her arms in the air. The second is the "chin plunge" as the baby's head falls forward in the mother's tentative hold. To avoid the latter, help the mother with positioning. A third frustration may arise when she tries to correctly place the nipple in the mouth. To ensure correct placement, put your index finger on the baby's chin and gently pull downward while quickly sliding the nipple in over the tongue.

Bottles may be prepared individually, or up to one day's supply of formula may be prepared at one time. Extra bottles can be stored in the refrigerator and warmed slightly before feeding by placing them in a container of warm water until at room temperature. Ready-to-use disposable bottles of formula are convenient but expensive. Formula left in bottles after a feeding should be discarded.

The Special Supplemental Food Program for Women, Infants, and Children (WIC) provides 8 lb of powdered formula or 403 oz of concentrated liquid formula (when mixed as directed on the can or container) per month. Individual states make provisions about when WIC nutritionists may distribute soy formulas and whether prescriptions are needed for special or therapeutic formulas.

NUTRITIONAL ASSESSMENT OF THE INFANT

During the early months of life, the food offered to and consumed by infants will be instrumental in their proper

ers may weaken nipples, so they should be washed thoroughly by hand and rinsed well. Tap water, if from an uncontaminated source, may be used to mix powdered

TABLE 29–3 ✤ **Formula Preparation**

Ready-to-Feed	Formula Concentrate	Powdered Formula
(20 kcal/oz; available in 32-oz cans or 4-oz bottles)	(available in 13-oz cans)	(52 scoops per can) Mix one unpacked level scoop of powdered formula with each 60 mL (2 oz) of warm water.
Use within 30 minutes to 1 hour once opened.	Mix equal amounts of concentrate and water from uncontaminated source. This provides a 20 kcal/30 mL (1 oz) dilution.	Always pour water into bottle first; then add powder and stir well.
Do not dilute. Use directly from can, no mixing required.	For example, for a 4-oz feeding, mix 2 oz of formula concentrate with 2 oz water.	Make sure the powder and water are well mixed to ensure the formula composition is 20 kcal/30 mL (1 oz).
Just add clean nipple to bottle.	Wash punch-type can opener and top of formula can before opening.	After opening, keep can tightly covered and use contents within 1 month to ensure freshness.
Most expensive type of formula preparation.	Prepare a single feeding by measuring water and liquid directly into nursing bottle.	Least expensive type.
	Cover opened concentrate formula cans with foil or plastic wrap and refrigerate until next bottle is made up.	

growth and development. The infant's nutritional status is assessed at each well-baby visit.

Nutritional assessment of the infant includes nutritional history from the parents, weight gain, growth chart percentiles, and physical examination. See "Nutritional Assessment" in Chapter 34 for more in-depth discussion of infant nutrition. ∞

TEACHING HIGHLIGHTS

NEWBORN FORMULA-FEEDING

Following is information that is helpful for formula-feeding families:

Types of Formula

Ready-to-feed: use directly from the can.

Concentrate: dilute with water before feeding.

Powder: add water and mix well for proper concentration.

Amount of Formula

Start with 3 oz in each bottle (since a newborn usually takes 1 to 3 oz every 2½ to 4 hours).

Expect increases in baby's appetite with demand feeding (as baby needs more he or she will start finishing each bottle).

Don't feed the baby a partially used bottle after 1 hour at room temperature.

Don't feed the baby a partially used bottle after 4 hours in refrigerator.

Prepare a fresh bottle for each feeding; don't add new formula to old.

Refrigerate bottles made in advance.

Don't feed the baby an opened, refrigerated can of concentrated or ready-to-feed formula after 48 hours.

Temperature of Formula

Mother or family member can try a bottle directly from the refrigerator, but most babies prefer warm formula, close in temperature to breast milk.

Warm bottle under hot tap water, in bottle warmer, or in pan of heated water.

Always test temperature of formula by sprinkling a few drops on wrist.

BE VERY CAREFUL if using a microwave oven to warm formula, as milk is superheated and plastic bottle bags may burst; use "defrost" setting on microwave oven and carefully check temperature of formula before feeding.

Positioning the Baby for Feeding

Hold baby close, establishing eye contact as in breastfeeding.

Hold baby's bottom or foot firmly, keeping his or her back straight to aid digestion and provide a sense of security.

Quiet baby before feeding.

Alternate the side baby is fed from to give baby two-sided stimulation.

Avoid feeding while baby is on his or her back.

Don't prop the bottle.

Procedure for Feeding

Nipple hole should allow only drops of milk to flow.

Keep nipple full with milk to decrease air ingestion.

How to Burp a Baby

Position baby so his or her head rests on mother's shoulder or face down on lap, or sit baby on lap with baby's chin and chest supported.

Gently pat or stroke baby's back.

Burp baby halfway through feeding and at end of feeding.

Learn baby's preferred burping position and whether baby is a slow or quick burper.

Regurgitation of small amounts of formula is common.

Have "burp cloth" available.

Critical Concept Review

LEARNING OBJECTIVES

CONCEPTS

Compare the nutritional value and composition of breast milk and formula preparations.

1. Composition of breast milk:
   - 10% solids consisting of carbohydrates, proteins, and fats
   - 90% is water
2. Breast milk has immunologic and nutritional (biodegradable) properties that make it the optimal food for first year of life.
3. Most common cow milk protein-based formulas attempt to duplicate the same concentration of carbohydrates, proteins, and fats as 20 kcal/oz breast milk.

LEARNING OBJECTIVES

CONCEPTS

Discuss the advantages and disadvantages of breastfeeding and formula-feeding for both mother and newborn.	1. Advantages of breastfeeding:
	  ■ Provides immunologic protection.
	  ■ Infant digests and absorbs components of breast milk easier.
	  ■ Provides most vitamins to infant if mother's diet is adequate.
	  ■ Strengthens the mother-infant attachment.
	  ■ No additional cost.
	  ■ Breast milk requires no preparation.
	2. Disadvantages of breastfeeding:
	  ■ Many medications pass through to breast milk.
	  ■ Father is unable to participate equally in actual feeding of infant.
	  ■ Mother may have difficulty being separated from infant.
	3. Advantages of bottle-feeding:
	  ■ Provides good nutrition to infant.
	  ■ Father can participate in infant feeding activities.
	4. Disadvantages of bottle-feeding:
	  ■ May need to try different formulas before finding one that is well-tolerated by the infant.
	  ■ Formula must be purchased and prepared.
	  ■ Proper preparation is necessary for nutritional adequacy.

Develop guidelines for helping both breast- and formula-feeding mothers to feed their newborns successfully.	1. The breastfeeding mother needs to know:
	  ■ How breast milk is produced.
	  ■ How to correctly position the infant for feeding.
	  ■ The procedure for feeding the infant.
	  ■ How to express leaking of milk.
	  ■ How to express and store breast milk.
	  ■ How and when to supplement with formula.
	  ■ How to care for the breasts
	  ■ Medications that pass through breast milk.
	  ■ Support groups for breastfeeding.
	2. The bottle-feeding mother needs to know:
	  ■ Types of formula available and how to prepare each type.
	  ■ The procedure for feeding the infant
	  ■ How to correctly position the infant for bottle-feeding.
	  ■ How to safely store the formula.
	  ■ How to safely care for bottles and nipples.

Recognize the influence of cultural values on infant care, especially feeding practices.	Nurses must: 1. Recognize that cultural values influence infant feeding practice. 2. Be sensitive to ethnic backgrounds of minority populations. 3. Understand that the dominant culture in any society defines normal maternal infant feeding interactions.
Delineate nursing responsibilities for client education about problems the breastfeeding mother may encounter at home.	Nursing responsibilities include: 1. Teaching signs and symptoms of mastitis, cracked nipples, and other breastfeeding concerns—see Chapter 32. ∞ 2. Reinforcing parents' understanding of the supply-demand nature of breastfeeding. 3. Helping mother to find ways to get adequate rest while breastfeeding. 4. Providing information about who to contact for problems encountered at home.
Incorporate knowledge of newborn nutrition and normal growth patterns into parent education and infant assessment.	Parents need to know: 1. Amount of formula to feed infant at each feeding and how often to feed infant. 2. Number of times per day the breastfed infant should be put to the breast. 3. The expected weight gain of both formula and breastfed infants. 4. The proper diet for the breastfeeding mother.

CRITICAL THINKING IN ACTION

*View the **Critical Thinking in Action** video in Chapter 29 of the CD-ROM. Then, answer the questions that follow.*

Patty Kline, age 28, G1, now P1, delivers a 7.3 pound baby girl by spontaneous vaginal birth over a median episiotomy. The newborn's Apgar scores are 8 and 9 at 1 and 5 minutes. The infant is suctioned in the nose and mouth and given free flow oxygen on the mother's abdomen. Patty received an epidural during her labor and birth. Patty initiated breastfeeding within the first hour after the birth, but at that time the newborn did not latch on. The infant was held to the mother's breast, rooted, and licked the nipple. You are the nurse caring for the infant at 2 hours of age. The admission assessment is significant for asymmetric head with a 3-cm caput succedaneum. The infant's temperature is stable. You bring the infant to the mother's room to assist her with breastfeeding.

1. Describe clues that indicate the infant is ready to breastfeed with the mother.
2. How would you explain how to position the infant at the breast?
3. Explain what to observe for the infant's proper latch-on.
4. Explain the basics of milk production.
5. Explore helpful measures the mother can attempt in support of breastfeeding.

MEDIALINK

www.prenhall.com/london

■ NCLEX-RN® Review, case studies, and other interactive resources for this chapter can be found on the Companion Website at http://www.prenhall.com/london. Click on "Chapter 29" to select the activities for this chapter.

■ For animations, more NCLEX-RN® Review questions, and an audio glossary, access the accompanying CD-ROM in this textbook.

REFERENCES

American Academy of Pediatrics, Committee on Nutrition. (2000). Hypoallergenic infant formulas. *Pediatrics, 106*(2), 346–349.

American Academy of Pediatrics (AAP) & American College of Obstetricians and Gynecologists (ACOG). (2002). *Guidelines for perinatal care* (5th ed.). Washington, DC: Author.

Balch, J. F., & Balch, P. A. (2001). *Prescription for nutritional healing* (3rd ed.). Garden City, NY: Avery Publishing Group.

Biancuzzo, M. (2003). *Breastfeeding the newborn: Clinical strategies for nurses* (2nd ed.). St. Louis, MO: Mosby.

Blackburn, S. T. (2003). *Maternal-fetal, & neonatal physiology: Clinical perspective* (2nd ed.). St. Louis, MO: Saunders.

Blumenthal, M. (2000). *Herbal medicine: Expanded Commission E Monographs.* Austin, TX: American Botanical Council.

Chezem, J., Friesen, C., & Boettcher, J. (2003). Breastfeeding knowledge, breastfeeding confidence, and infant feeding plans: Effects on actual feeding practices. *Journal of Obstetric, Gynecologic, & Neonatal Nursing, 32*(1), 40–47.

Hedayat, K. M. (2001). Issues in Islamic biomedical ethics: A primer for the pediatrician. *Pediatrics, 108*(4), 965–91.

Hill, P. D., Wilhelm, P. A., Aldag, J. C., & Chatterton, R. T. (2004). Breast augmentation and lactation outcome: A case report. *MCN. American Journal of Maternal Child Nursing, 29*(4), 238–242.

Karl, D. J. (2004). Using principles of newborn behavioral state organization to facilitate breastfeeding. *MCN. American Journal of Maternal Child Nursing, 29*(5), 292–298.

Meeks, J. Y., & Tippins, S. (2002). *American Academy of Pediatrics new mother's guide to breastfeeding.* New York: Bantam Books.

Morin, K. H. (2004). Current thoughts on healthy term infant nutrition: The first twelve months. *MCN. American Journal of Maternal Child Nursing, 29*(5), 312–319.

Mulford, C. (1992). The mother-baby assessment (MBA): An "Apgar score" for breastfeeding. *Journal of Human Lactation, 8*(2), 79–82.

Orr, S. S. (2004). Breastfeeding. In S. Mattson & J. E. Smith (Eds.), *Core curriculum for maternalnewborn nursing* (3rd ed.). St. Louis, MO: ElsevierSaunders.

Ott, B. B., Al-Khadhuri, J., & Al-Junaibi, S. (2003). Preventing ethical dilemmas: Understanding Islamic health care practices. *Pediatric Nursing, 29*(3), 227–230.

Rasbridge, L. A., & Kulig, J. C. (1995). Infant feeding among Cambodian refugees. *MCN. American Journal of Maternal Child Nursing, 20*(4), 213–218.

Riordan, J. (2005). *Breastfeeding and human lactation.* Sudbury, MA: Jones & Bartlett.

Rojjanasrirat, W. (2004). Working women's breastfeeding experience. *MCN. American Journal of Maternal Child Nursing, 29*(4), 222–228.

Schneiderman, J. U. (1996). Postpartum nursing for Korean mothers. *MCN. American Journal of Maternal Child Nursing, 21*(3), 155–158.

Shinskie, D., & Lauwers, J. (2002). *Pocket guide for counseling the nursing mother: A lactation consultant's guide.* Sudbury, MA: Jones & Bartlett.

Skidmore-Roth, L. (2004). *Mosby's handbook of herbs and natural supplements.* St. Louis, MO: Mosby.

Thureen, P. J., Deacon, J., Hernandez, J. A., & Hall, D. M. (2005). *Assessment and care of the well newborn* (2nd ed.). St. Louis, MO: ElsevierSaunders.

The Newborn at Risk: Conditions Present at Birth

There is an initial flurry of activity when my baby is taken into the NICU. Now my entire universe, everything that I am, constricts down to focus on our little one. She hardly dents this world, a withery face that shows a kind of infinitely pained acceptance, breath and heartbeat almost nothing, and a pose that moves to rest, resisting nothing. I look at my small daughter with eyes naked with amazement and unsure joy.

—Jontelle, 42

LEARNING OBJECTIVES

- Identify factors present at birth that indicate an at-risk newborn.

- Compare the underlying etiologies of the physiologic complications of small-for-gestational age (SGA) newborns and preterm appropriate for-gestational-age (Pr AGA) newborns.

- Describe the impact of maternal diabetes mellitus on the newborn.

- Compare the characteristics and potential complications of the postterm newborn and the newborn with postmaturity syndrome.

- Discuss the physiologic characteristics of the preterm newborn that predispose each body system to various complications and are used in development of plan of care.

- Summarize the nursing assessments of and initial interventions for a newborn born with selected congenital anomalies.

- Explain the special care needed by an alcohol- or drug-exposed newborn.

- Relate the consequences of maternal HIV/AIDS to management of the newborn in the neonatal period.

- Identify the physical examination findings during the early newborn period that would make the nurse suspect a congenital cardiac defect.

- Explain the special care needed by newborns with an inborn error of metabolism.

MEDIALINK   www.prenhall.com/london

CD-ROM

NCLEX-RN® Review
Skill 15-3: Administering a Gavage Feeding
Audio Glossary

Companion Website

NCLEX-RN® Review
Case Study: Postterm Newborn
Care Plan Activity: Infant of a Diabetic Mother
Complementary Care: Infant Massage
Thinking Critically

The field of neonatology has expanded greatly. Many levels of nursery care have evolved in response to increasing knowledge about at-risk newborns: special care, intensive care, and convalescent or transitional care. As a professional member of the multidisciplinary healthcare team, the nurse provides the holistic care necessary in the often high-tech perinatal environment.

Other factors influencing the outcome of these at-risk infants include the following:

- Birth weight
- Gestational age
- Type and length of newborn illness
- Environmental factors
- Maternal factors
- Maternal-infant separation

IDENTIFICATION OF AT-RISK NEWBORNS

An at-risk newborn is one susceptible to illness (morbidity) or even death because of dysmaturity, immaturity, physical disorders, or complications during or after birth. In most cases the infant is the product of a pregnancy involving one or more predictable risk factors, such as the following:

- Low socioeconomic level of the mother and limited access to healthcare
- Exposure to environmental dangers such as toxic chemicals and illicit drugs
- Preexisting maternal conditions such as heart disease, diabetes, hypertension, and renal disease
- Maternal factors such as age and parity
- Medical conditions related to pregnancy and their associated complications
- Pregnancy complications such as abruptio placentae

Various risk factors and their specific effects on the pregnancy outcome are listed in Table 10–1 in Chapter 10. ∞ Because these factors and the perinatal risks associated with them are known, the birth of at-risk newborns can often be anticipated. The pregnancy can be closely monitored, treatment can be started as necessary, and arrangements can be made for birth to occur at a facility with appropriate resources to care for both mother and baby.

Whether or not prenatal assessment indicates that the fetus is at risk, the course of labor and birth and the infant's ability to withstand the stress of labor cannot be predicted. Thus, the nurse's use of electronic fetal heart monitoring or fetal heart rate auscultation by Doppler plays a significant role in detecting stress or distress in the fetus. Immediately after birth the Apgar score helps identify the at-risk newborn, but it is not the only indicator of possible long-term outcome.

The newborn classification and neonatal mortality risk chart is another useful tool for identifying newborns at risk. Before this classification tool was developed, birth weight of less than 2500 g was the sole criterion for determining immaturity. Clinicians then recognized that a newborn could weigh more than 2500 g and still be immature. Conversely, an infant weighing less than 2500 g might be functionally at term or beyond. Birth weight and gestational age together are now the criteria used to assess neonatal maturity and mortality risk.

Newborn classification and neonatal mortality risk chart. Infants are classified according to weight as small for gestational age (SGA), appropriate for gestational age (AGA), or large for gestational age (LGA) and by weeks of newborn gestation as preterm (Pr), term (F), or postterm (Po). Corresponding neonatal mortality risks are indicated by the percentage in the various colored regions.

Used with permission from Koops, B. L., Morgan, L. P., & Battaglia, F. C. (1982). Neonatal mortality risk in relationship to birth weight and gestational age. Journal of Pediatrics, 101(6), 969.

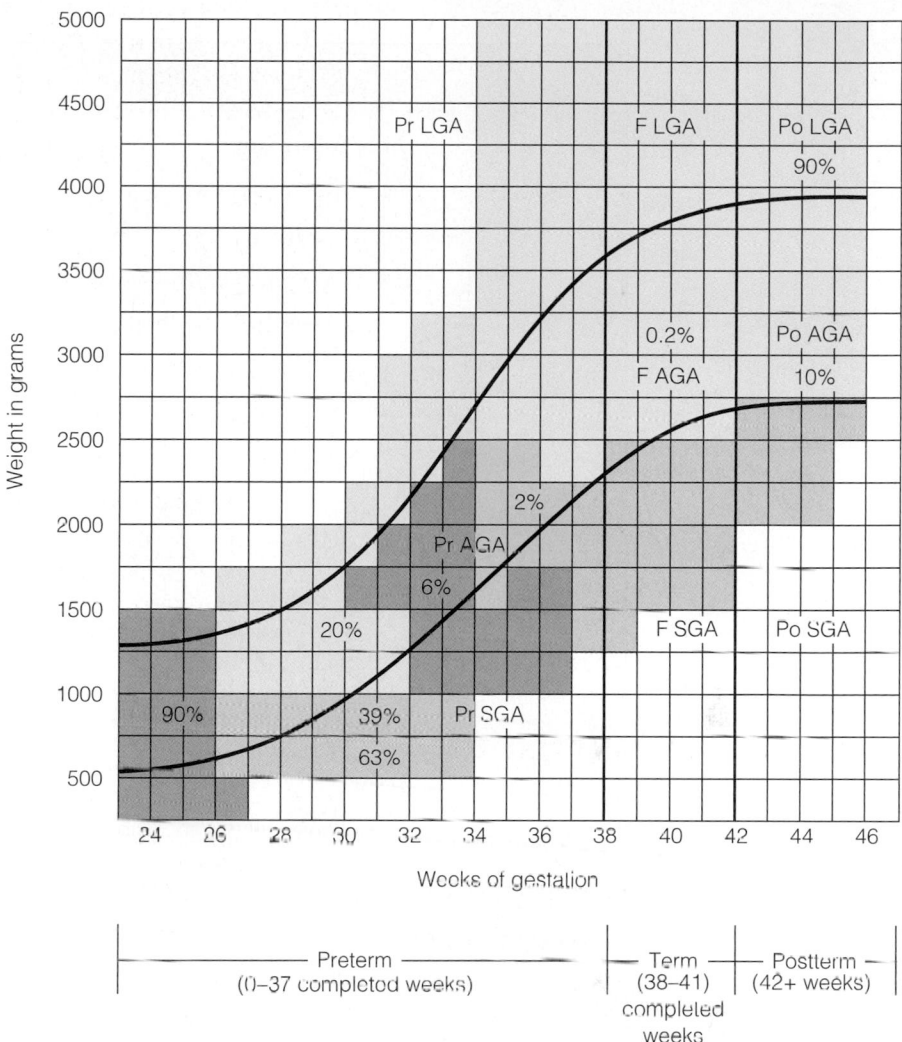

According to the newborn classification and neonatal mortality risk chart, gestation is divided as follows:

- Preterm: less than 37 (completed) weeks
- Term: 38 to 41 (completed) weeks
- Postterm: greater than 42 weeks

As shown in Figure 30–1 ●, large-for-gestational-age (LGA) newborns are those above the 90th percentile curve. Appropriate-for-gestational-age (AGA) newborns are those between the 10th percentile and 90th percentile curves. Small-for-gestational-age (SGA) newborns are those below the 10th percentile curve. A newborn is assigned to a category depending on birth weight and gestational age. For example, a newborn classified as Pr SGA is preterm and small for gestational age. The full-term newborn whose weight is appropriate for gestational age is classified F AGA. It is important to remember that intrauterine growth curve charts are influenced by altitude and the ethnicity of the newborn population used to create the chart. Also the assigned newborn classification may vary according to the intrauterine growth curve chart used; therefore, the chart used should correlate with the characteristics of the client population.

Neonatal mortality risk is the chance of death during the newborn period—that is, the first 28 days of life. As indicated in Figure 30–1, the neonatal mortality risk decreases as both gestational age and birth weight increase. Infants who are preterm and SGA have the highest neonatal mortality risk. The previously high mortality rates for LGA newborns have decreased at most perinatal centers because of improved management of diabetes in pregnancy and increased recognition of potential problems of LGA newborns.

Neonatal morbidity can be anticipated based on birth weight and gestational age. In Figure 30–2 ● the infant's birth weight is located on the vertical axis, and the gestational age

⊙ FIGURE 30-2

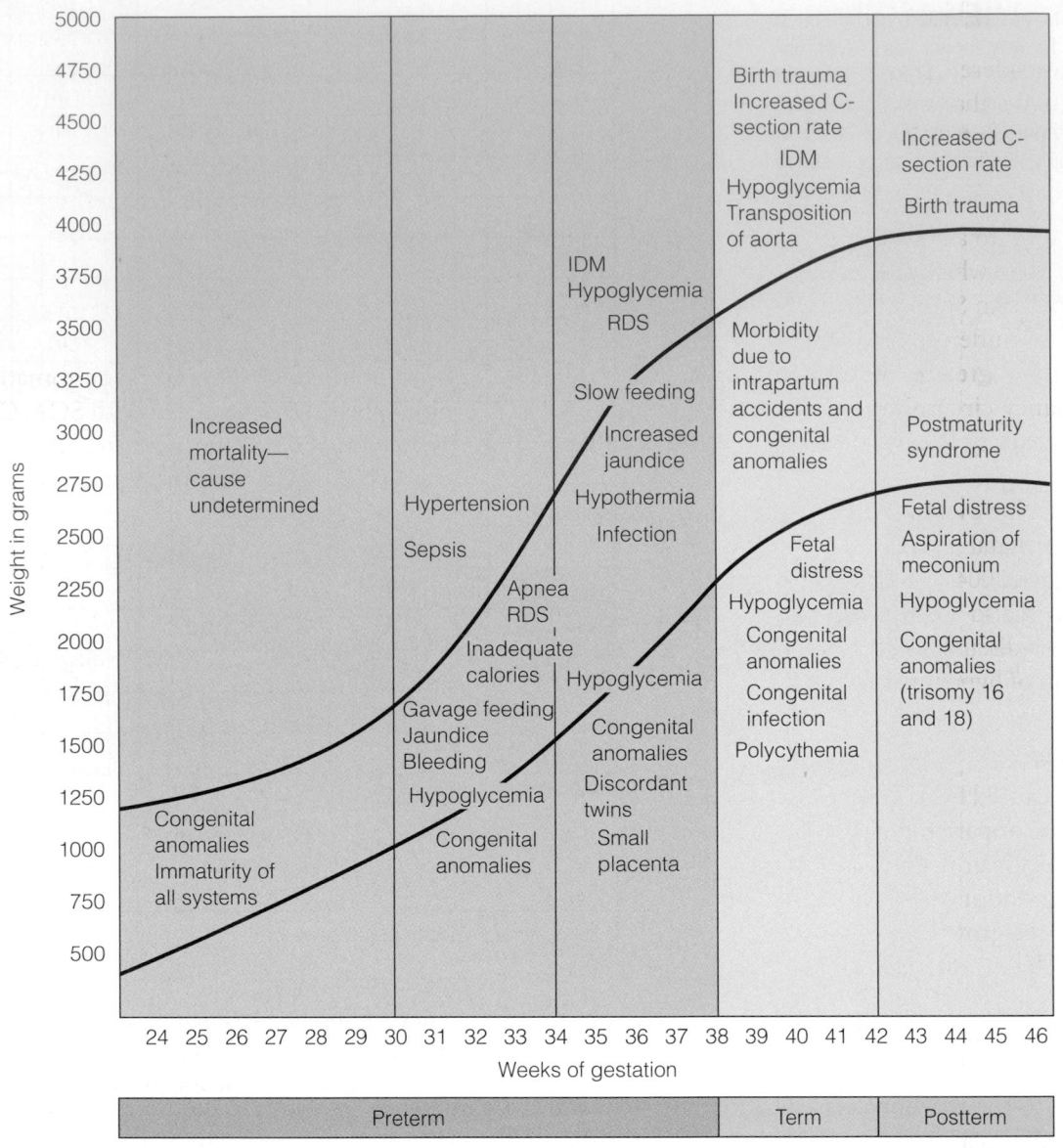

Neonatal morbidity by birth weight and gestational age.

From Lubchenco, L. O. (1976). The high-risk infant *(p. 122). Philadelphia: Saunders.*

in weeks is found along the horizontal axis. The area where the two meet on the graph identifies common problems. This tool helps determine the needs of particular infants for special observation and care. For example, an infant of 2000 g at 40 weeks' gestation should be carefully assessed for evidence of neonatal distress, hypoglycemia, congenital anomalies, congenital infection, and polycythemia.

Identifying the nursing care needs of the at-risk newborn depends on minute-to-minute observations of the changes in the newborn's physiologic status. Nursing care should be directed toward the following:

- Decreasing physiologically stressful situations
- Constantly observing for subtle signs of change in clinical condition
- Interpreting laboratory data and coordinating interventions
- Conserving the infant's energy for healing and growth
- Providing for developmental stimulation and maintenance of sleep cycle
- Helping the family develop attachment behaviors
- Involving the family in planning and providing care

CARE OF THE SMALL-FOR-GESTATIONAL-AGE/INTRAUTERINE GROWTH RESTRICTION NEWBORN

Infants are considered **small for gestational age (SGA)** when they are less than two standard deviations or at less than the third percentile (10th for Denver curves because of the lower birth weight at higher altitudes) (Figure 30–3 ●). When possible, the birth weight charts used to assign the SGA classification to a newborn should be based on the local population into which the newborn is born (Martinez & Simmons, 2005). An SGA newborn may be preterm, term, or postterm. An undergrown newborn may also be said to have **intrauterine growth restriction (IUGR)**, which describes pregnancy circumstances resulting in limited fetal growth. The terms SGA and IUGR are not necessarily interchangeable.

SGA infants have an increased incidence of perinatal asphyxia and perinatal mortality compared to AGA infants (Resnik & Creasy, 2004). The incidence of polycythemia and hypoglycemia is also higher in this group of infants. See Chapter 48 for a discussion of polycythemia and Chapter 31 for a discussion of hypoglycemia. ∞

FACTORS CONTRIBUTING TO IUGR

IUGR may be caused by maternal, placental, or fetal factors and may not be apparent antenatally. In the normal pregnancy, intrauterine growth is linear from approximately 28 to 38 weeks' gestation. After 38 weeks, growth is variable, depending on the growth potential of the fetus and placental function. The most common causes of growth restriction are as follows:

● **FIGURE 30–3**

Thirty-five-week gestational age twins. Twin B (on left) is SGA and weighs 1260 g. Twin A (on right) is AGA and weighs 2605 g.

Courtesy of Carol Harrigan, RNC, MSN, NNP.

- **Maternal factors.** Primiparity, grand multiparity, multiple-gestation pregnancy (twins and higher order multiples), smoking, lack of prenatal care, age extremes (< 16 years or > 40 years), and low socioeconomic status (which can result in inadequate healthcare, inadequate education, and inadequate living conditions) affect IUGR (Martinez & Simmons, 2005). Before the third trimester, the nutritional supply to the fetus far exceeds its needs. Only in the third trimester does maternal malnutrition limit fetal growth.

- **Maternal disease.** Maternal heart disease, substance abuse (drugs, alcohol, smoking), sickle cell anemia, **phenylketonuria (PKU)**, and asymptomatic pyelonephritis are associated with SGA. Complications associated with preeclampsia, chronic hypertensive vascular disease, and advanced diabetes mellitus cause diminished blood flow to the uterus.

- **Environmental factors.** High altitude, exposure to x-rays, excessive exercise, work-related exposure to toxins, hyperthermia, and maternal use of teratogenic drugs (such as nicotine, alcohol, antimetabolites, anticonvulsants, narcotics, and cocaine) affect fetal growth (Resnik & Creasy, 2004).

- **Placental factors.** Placental conditions such as small placenta, infarcted areas, abnormal cord insertions, placenta previa, and thrombosis may affect circulation to the fetus; the circulation becomes more deficient with increasing gestational age.

- **Fetal factors.** Congenital infections (rubella, toxoplasmosis, syphilis, cytomegalic inclusion disease), congenital malformations, discordant twins (see "Twins" in Chapter 7 ∞), sex of the fetus (females tend to be smaller), chromosomal syndromes, and inborn errors of metabolism can predispose a fetus to fetal growth disturbances.

Identifying fetuses with IUGR is the first step in detecting common disorders associated with affected newborns. The perinatal history of maternal conditions, early dating of pregnancy by first-trimester ultrasound measurements, antepartum testing (nonstress test, contraction stress test, biophysical profile [see Chapter 16 ∞]), Doppler velocimetry, gestational age assessment, and the physical and neurologic assessment of the newborn are also important (Resnik & Creasy, 2004).

PATTERNS OF IUGR

Intrauterine growth occurs by an increase in both cell number and cell size. If insult occurs early during the critical period of organ development in the fetus, fewer new cells are formed, organs are small, and organ weight is subnormal. In contrast, growth failure that begins later in pregnancy does not affect the total number of cells, only their size. The organs are normal, but their size is diminished. There are two clinical pictures of newborns:

- **Symmetric (proportional) IUGR** is caused by long-term maternal conditions (such as chronic hypertension, severe malnutrition, chronic intrauterine infection, substance abuse, anemia) or fetal genetic abnormalities (Martinez & Simmons, 2005). Symmetric IUGR can be noted by ultrasound in the first half of the second trimester. In symmetric IUGR there is chronic, prolonged retardation of growth in the size of organs, weight, length, and, in severe cases, head circumference.

- **Asymmetric (disproportional) IUGR** is associated with an acute compromise of uteroplacental blood flow. Some causes are placental infarcts, preeclampsia, and poor weight gain in pregnancy. The growth restriction may not be evident before the third trimester because, although weight is decreased, length and head circumference remain appropriate for that gestational age. Birth weight is below the 10th percentile, whereas head circumference, length, or both may be between the 10th and 90th percentiles. Asymmetric IUGR newborns are particularly at risk for perinatal asphyxia, pulmonary hemorrhage, hypocalcemia, and hypoglycemia in the newborn period.

Despite growth restriction, physiologic maturity develops according to gestational age. Therefore, the SGA newborn may be more physiologically mature than the preterm AGA newborn and less predisposed to complications of prematurity such as respiratory distress syndrome and hyperbilirubinemia. The SGA newborn's chances for survival are better than those of the preterm AGA newborn because of organ maturity, although this newborn still faces many other potential difficulties.

COMMON COMPLICATIONS OF THE SGA NEWBORN

The complications occurring most frequently in the SGA newborn include:

- **Asphyxia.** The SGA newborn suffers chronic hypoxia in utero, which leaves little reserve to withstand the demands of normal labor and birth. Thus, fetal hypoxia and its potential systemic problems can occur. Cesarean birth may be necessary.

- **Aspiration syndrome.** In utero, hypoxia can cause the fetus to gasp during birth, aspirating amniotic fluid into the lower airways. It can also lead to relaxation of the anal sphincter and passage of meconium. This can result in aspiration of the meconium with the first breaths after birth.

- **Hypothermia.** Diminished subcutaneous fat (used for survival in utero), depletion of brown fat in utero, and a large surface area decrease the IUGR newborn's ability to conserve heat. The flexed position assumed by the term SGA newborn diminishes the effect of surface area somewhat.

- **Hypoglycemia.** An increase in metabolic rate in response to heat loss and poor hepatic glycogen stores causes hypoglycemia. In addition the newborn is compromised by inadequate supplies of enzymes to activate gluconeogenesis (conversion of nonglucogen sources such as fatty acids and proteins to glucose).

- **Polycythemia.** The increased number of red blood cells in the SGA newborn is considered a physiologic response to in utero chronic hypoxic stress.

Newborns with significant IUGR tend to have a poor prognosis, especially when born before 37 weeks' gestation. Factors contributing to poor outcome include the following:

- **Congenital malformations.** Congenital malformations occur in 8% of SGA infants (Martinez & Simmons, 2005); the more severe the IUGR, the greater the chance for malformation as a result of impaired mitotic activity and cellular hypoplasia.

- **Intrauterine infections.** Fetuses exposed to intrauterine infections such as rubella and cytomegalovirus are profoundly affected by the offending virus's direct invasion of the brain and other vital organs, resulting in IUGR.

- **Continued growth difficulties.** SGA newborns tend to be shorter than newborns of the same gestational age. Asymmetric IUGR infants can be expected to catch up in weight and approach their inherited growth potential when given an optimal environment. Symmetric SGA infants reportedly have varied growth potential but tend not to catch up to their peers (Martinez & Simmons, 2005).

- **Cognitive difficulties.** Often, SGA newborns can exhibit subsequent learning disabilities. The disabilities are characterized by hyperactivity, short attention span, and poor fine motor coordination (writing and drawing). Some hearing loss and speech defects also occur.

CLINICAL THERAPY

The goal of clinical therapy is early recognition and implementation of the medical management of potential problems.

NURSING MANAGEMENT

NURSING ASSESSMENT AND DIAGNOSIS

The nurse assesses gestational age and identifies signs of potential complications associated with SGA infants. All body parts of the symmetric IUGR infant are in proportion, but they are below normal size for the baby's gestational age. Therefore, the head does not appear overly large or the length excessive in relation to the other body parts. These newborns are generally vigorous.

The asymmetric IUGR infant appears long, thin, and emaciated, with loss of subcutaneous fat and muscle mass. The baby may have loose skin folds; dry, desquamating skin; and a thin and often meconium-stained cord. The head appears relatively large (although it approaches normal size) because the chest size and abdominal girth are decreased. The baby may have a vigorous cry and appear alert and wide eyed.

Nursing diagnoses that may apply to the SGA newborn include the following:

- *Risk for Impaired Gas Exchange* related to aspiration of meconium
- *Risk for Ineffective Thermoregulation and Cold Stress* secondary to decreased subcutaneous fat
- *Risk for Injury to Tissues* related to decreased glycogen stores and impaired gluconeogenesis
- *Altered Nutrition: Less than Body Requirements* related to increased metabolic needs in the infant
- *Risk for Altered Parenting* related to lack of knowledge of infant care and prolonged separation of infant and parents secondary to illness

PLANNING AND IMPLEMENTATION

Hospital-Based Nursing Care

Hypoglycemia, the most common metabolic complication of IUGR, produces such sequelae as central nervous system (CNS) abnormalities and mental retardation. Conditions such as asphyxia, hyperviscosity, and cold stress may also affect the baby's outcome. Pay meticulous attention to physiologic parameters for immediate nursing management and reduction of long-term disorders. (See "Nursing Care Plan: The Small-for-Gestational-Age Newborn," pages 774–777.)

Nursing Care in the Community

The long-term needs of the SGA newborn include careful follow-up evaluation of patterns of growth and possible disabilities that may later interfere with learning or motor functioning. Long-term follow-up care is essential for infants with congenital malformations, congenital infections, and obvious sequelae from physiologic problems. Parents of the IUGR newborn need support, because a positive environment can enhance the baby's growth and the child's ultimate outcome.

EVALUATION

Anticipated outcomes of nursing care include the following:

- The SGA newborn is free from respiratory compromise.
- The SGA newborn maintains a stable temperature and glucose homeostasis.
- The SGA newborn gains weight and takes breast- or formula-feedings without developing physiologic distress or fatigue.
- The parents verbalize their concerns about their baby's health problems and understand the rationale behind management of their newborn.

CARE OF THE LARGE-FOR-GESTATIONAL-AGE (LGA) NEWBORN

A newborn whose birth weight is at or above the 90th percentile on the intrauterine growth curve (at any week of gestation) is considered **large for gestational age (LGA)**. Some AGA newborns have been incorrectly categorized as LGA because of miscalculation of the date of conception due to postconceptual bleeding. Careful gestational age assessment is essential to identify the potential needs and problems of such infants.

The most well-known condition associated with excessive fetal growth is maternal diabetes (White's classes A–C; see Table 14–3 in Chapter 14 ∞); however, only a minority of large newborns are born to mothers with diabetes. The cause of the majority of cases of LGA newborns is unclear, but certain factors or situations have been found to correlate with their birth (Martinez & Simmons, 2005):

- Genetic predisposition is correlated proportionately to the mother's prepregnancy weight and to weight gain during pregnancy. Large parents tend to have large infants.
- Multiparous women have two to three times the number of LGA infants as primigravidas.
- Male infants are typically larger than female infants.
- Infants with erythroblastosis fetalis, Beckwith-Wiedemann syndrome (a genetic condition associated with omphalocele and neonatal hypoglycemia and hyperinsulinemia), or transposition of the great vessels are usually large.

(Text continued on page 777)

NURSING CARE PLAN

THE SMALL-FOR-GESTATIONAL-AGE NEWBORN

Intervention	Rationale	Expected Outcome

1. Nursing Diagnosis: Risk for Impaired Gas Exchange related to meconium aspiration

Intervention	Rationale	Expected Outcome
NIC Intervention: **Respiratory monitoring:** Collection and analysis of patient data to ensure airway patency and adequate gas exchange		**NOC Outcome:** **Respiratory status:** Gas exchange: Alveolar exchange of CO_2 or O_2 to maintain arterial blood gas concentrations

Goal: The newborn's respirations will be stable and maintained with normal limits.

Intervention	Rationale	Expected Outcome
Obtain maternal prenatal, labor, and birth records.	Provides information of fetal stress that may have occurred during the prenatal or intrapartum period. In addition, the birth record will provide information concerning infant's respiratory status at birth; for example, the Apgar score.	■ The infant will maintain adequate respiratory gas exchange as evidenced by respirations of 30–60 /min with no periods of apnea or evidence of worsening distress.
■ Maintain airway patency through judicious suctioning.	■ Respiratory distress in SGA newborns is due to in utero hypoxia and aspiration of meconium.	
■ Observe for worsening signs of respiratory distress such as generalized cyanosis; worsening retractions, grunting, and nasal flaring, as evidenced by Silverman respiratory index; sustained tachypnea; apnea episodes; inequality of breath sounds; presence of rales and rhonchi.		
■ Monitor and maintain adequate body temperature ($36°C+/-0.2°C$ [$97.7°F+/-0.5°F$]) to avoid increased oxygen consumption.	■ Temperature elevation may cause metabolic rate and oxygen needs to increase when associated with meconium aspiration.	
■ Administer oxygen per order for relief of respiratory distress signs (see "Care of the Newborn with Respiratory Distress" in Chapter 31 for nursing care and treatment of meconium aspiration, infant resuscitation).	■ Provides healthcare personnel with cardiac and pulmonary status.	
■ Implement treatment plan for respiratory distress.		
■ Monitor glucose levels.	■ Respiratory distress increases consumption of glucose.	
■ Collaborative: Obtain arterial blood gases per physician's orders.		
■ Monitor infant's cardiac status and pulmonary status pulse oximetry and arterial blood gases (ABGs).	■ Oxygen demands increase with meconium aspiration. Obtaining ABGs will provide medical personnel baseline information of infant's respiratory status, and effective medical interventions can be initiated.	

2. Nursing Diagnosis: Risk for Ineffective Thermoregulation and Cold Stress secondary to decreased subcutaneous fat

Intervention	Rationale	Expected Outcome
NIC Intervention: **Temperature regulation:** Attaining and/or maintaining body temperature within a normal range		**NOC Outcome:** **Thermoregulation:** Newborn: Balance among heat production, heat gain, and heat loss during the neonatal period

Goal: The infant's temperature will be stable and maintained within normal limits.

Intervention	Rationale	Expected Outcome
■ Provide neutral thermal zone (NTZ) range for infant based on postnatal weight.	■ Neutral thermal environment charts used for preterm infant are not reliable for weight of SGA infant.	■ The infant will not exhibit signs and symptoms of hypothermia as evidenced by temperature maintenance of 97.7–99.1°F and no signs and symptoms of respiratory distress.

THE SMALL-FOR-GESTATIONAL-AGE NEWBORN

Intervention	Rationale	Expected Outcome

■ Use a skin probe to maintain infant's skin temperature at 36–36.5°C.
 	
■ Obtain axillary temps and compare to registered skin probe temp. If discrepancy exists evaluate potential cause.
 	
■ Adjust and monitor incubator or radiant warmer to maintain skin temp.
■ Minimize heat losses and prevent cold stress by:
  ■ Warming and humidifying oxygen without blowing over face in order to avoid increasing oxygen consumption.
  ■ Keeping skin dry.
  ■ Keeping isolettes, radiant warmers, and cribs away from windows and cold external walls and out of drafts.
  ■ Avoiding placing infant on cold surfaces such as metal treatment tables, cold x-ray plates.
  ■ Padding cold surfaces with diapers and using radiant warmers during procedures.
  ■ Warming blood for exchange transfusions.
■ Observe for signs and symptoms of cold stress: decreased temperature, lethargy, pallor (for further discussion see Chapter 31 ∞).
	■ A neutral thermal environment requires minimal oxygen consumption to maintain a normal core temp.
	■ Discrepancies between axillary and skin probe monitor temp may be due to mechanical causes or the burning of brown fat.
	
	■ Physical principles of heat loss effects include:
	  ■ Evaporation—lungs and skin when cooling occurs as a result of water evaporation.
	  ■ Convection—air currents.
	  ■ Conduction—skin contact with cooler object.
	  ■ Radiation—loss of warmth to cooler surrounding objects.
	
	■ Hypothermia is a potential problem for SGA infant because:
	  ■ SGA infant has decreased stores of brown fat available for thermogenesis, because SGA infant has used these stores in utero for survival.
	  ■ SGA infant has poor insulation due to use of subcutaneous tissues in utero for survival.	

3. Nursing Diagnosis: Risk for Injury to Tissues related to decreased glycogen stores and impaired gluconeogenesis

NIC Intervention:		NOC Outcome:
High-risk infant care: Identification and management of a high-risk infant to promote healthy outcomes for the baby		**Risk control:** Actions to eliminate or reduce actual, personal, and modifiable health threats

Goal: Newborn will have a normal blood glucose level.

■ Monitor chemstrip per SGA protocol and report values <45 mg/dL. ■ Observe, record, and report signs of hypoglycemia: cyanosis, lethargy, jitteriness, seizure activity, and apnea. ■ Initiate feeding schedule for SGA newborns per agency protocol.	■ Combined with depletion of glycogen stores, impaired gluconeogenesis predisposes SGA infants to profound hypoglycemia within first 2 days of life. ■ Hypoglycemia in SGA infant is indicated by whole blood sugar less than 20 mg/dL. ■ Frequent monitoring of Dextrostix assists in identifying decreasing glucose levels.	■ The fetus will not exhibit signs and symptoms of hypoglycemia as evidenced by a euglycemic state and blood glucose greater than 20 mg/dL.

(continued)

NURSING CARE PLAN—continued

THE SMALL-FOR-GESTATIONAL-AGE NEWBORN

Intervention	Rationale	Expected Outcome
■ Provide glucose intake either through early enteral feeding (before 4 hr) or by IV per physician's order. See further discussion of hypoglycemia in Chapter 31	■ Provision of glucose through early feedings (begin before 4 hr of age) assists in maintaining glucose levels.	

4. Nursing Diagnosis: Altered Nutrition: Less than Body Requirements related to increased metabolic needs in the infant

NIC Intervention: **Newborn monitoring:** Measurement and interpretation of physiologic status of the newborn for the first 24 hours		NOC Outcome: **Nutritional status:** Food and fluid intake: Amount of food and fluid taken into the body over a 24-hr period

Goal: Infant will gain weight and tolerate nipple-feedings without tiring.

■ Assess suck, swallow, gag, and cough reflexes. ■ Initiate test water feeding at 1 hour of age, then proceed to 5% glucose/water. Move early to formula-feeding q2–3 hr. ■ Supplement oral feedings with intravenous intake per orders. ■ Use concentrated formulas that supply more calories in less volume, such as Similac 24. ■ Promote growth by providing caloric intake of 120–150 cal/kg/day in small amounts. ■ Observe, record, and report signs of respiratory distress or fatigue occurring during feedings. ■ Supplement gavage or nipple-feedings with intravenous therapy per physician order until oral intake is sufficient to support growth. ■ Establish a nipple-feeding program that is begun slowly and progresses slowly, such as nipple-feed once per day, nipple-feed once per shift, and then nipple-feed every other feeding. ■ Monitor daily weight with anticipation of small amount of weight loss when nipple-feedings start.	■ Prevents feeding problems and assists in determining the best method of feeding for infant. ■ Sterile water is desirable for first feedings because it causes fewer pulmonary complications in the presence of gastrointestinal tract abnormalities or aspiration of feeding. ■ SGA newborns require more calories/kg for growth than AGA newborns because of increased metabolic activity and oxygen consumption secondary to increased percentage of body weight made up by visceral organs. ■ Small, frequent feedings of high-caloric formula are used because of limited gastric capacity and decreased gastric emptying. ■ Growth is evaluated by increase in weight, length, and body measurements. ■ Decrease in exhaustion is an important consideration in feeding SGA infant. ■ Adequate nutritional intake promotes growth and prevents such complications as metabolic catabolism and hypoglycemia. ■ Gavage feedings require less energy expenditure on the part of the newborn. ■ Nipple-feeding, an active rather than passive intake of nutrition, requires energy expenditure and burning of calories by infant.	■ The infant will maintain steady weight gain as evidenced by <2%/day weight loss, tolerates oral feedings, and urine output is 1–3 mL/kg/hr.

NURSING CARE PLAN—continued

THE SMALL-FOR-GESTATIONAL-AGE NEWBORN

Intervention	Rationale	Expected Outcome

5. Nursing Diagnosis: Risk for Altered Parenting related to lack of knowledge of infant care and prolonged separation of infant and parents secondary to illness

NIC Intervention: **Teaching:** Infant care: Instruction on nurturing and physical care needed during the first year of life		**NOC Outcome:** **Parenting:** Provision of an environment that promotes optimum growth and development of dependent children.

Goal: Parents will bond with infant and have realistic expectations about infant. Parents are comfortable taking infant home. They are able to demonstrate normal infant care and assessments of possible complications, and know when to return for follow-up.

■ Support emotionally the psychologic well-being of family, including positive parent-infant bonding and sensory stimulation of infant. ■ Include parents in determining infant's plan of care and encourage their participation. Encourage parents to visit frequently. Provide opportunities for parents to touch, hold, talk to, and care for infant. Determine the type and amount of appropriate sensory stimulation and implement sensory stimulation program. ■ Prepare for discharge by instructing parents in such areas as feeding techniques, formula preparation, and breastfeeding; bathing, diapering, and hygiene; temperature monitoring; administration of vitamins, care of complications, and preventing exposure to infections; normal elimination patterns, normal reflexes and activity, and how to promote normal growth and development without being overprotective; returning for continued medical care; and availability of community resources if indicated.	■ Parent-infant bonding begins in first few hours or days following birth. SGA infants may experience prolonged periods of separation from their parents, which necessitates intervention to ensure parent-infant bonding. ■ Parents should receive the same postpartum teaching as any parent taking a new infant home. ■ Parents need to understand the changes to expect in color of the infant's stool and number of bowel movements plus odor from formula or breastfeeding in order to avoid unnecessary concern. SGA infants usually do not require referral to community agencies such as visiting nurse associations unless there is a specific problem requiring assistance.	■ The parent will demonstrate ability to perform basic infant care tasks as evidenced by exhibiting appropriate attachment behaviors (i.e., talking and holding infant), feeding infant, and bathing infant.

The increase in the LGA infant's body size is characteristically proportional, although head circumference and body length are in the upper limits of intrauterine growth. The exception to this rule is the infant of the diabetic mother, whose body weight increases while length and head circumference may remain in the normal range. Macrosomic infants have poor motor skills and have difficulty in regulating behavioral states. LGA infants tend to be more difficult to arouse to a quiet alert state and may have feeding difficulties.

COMMON COMPLICATIONS OF THE LGA NEWBORN

Disorders of the LGA newborn can include the following:

■ **Birth trauma due to cephalopelvic disproportion (CPD).** Often, LGA newborns have a biparietal diameter greater than 10 cm (4 in.) or are associated with a maternal fundal height measurement greater than 42 cm (16 in.) without hydramnios. Because of their excessive size, there are more breech presentations and shoulder dystocias. These complications may result in asphyxia, fractured clavicles, brachial palsy, facial paralysis, phrenic nerve palsy, depressed skull fractures, hematomas, and bleeding due to birth trauma.

- **Increased incidence of cesarean births due to fetal size.** Mothers and infants have all the risk factors associated with cesarean births (Martinez & Simmons, 2005).

- **Hypoglycemia, polycythemia, and hyperviscosity.** These disorders are most often seen in infants with diabetic mothers, erythroblastosis fetalis, and Beckwith-Wiedemann syndrome.

Nursing Management

The perinatal history, in conjunction with ultrasonic measurement of fetal skull and gestational age testing, is important in identifying an at-risk LGA newborn. Direct essential nursing care toward monitoring vital signs, screening for hypoglycemia and polycythemia, and observing for signs and symptoms related to birth trauma. Address parental concerns about the visual signs of birth trauma and the potential for continuation of the overweight pattern. Help parents learn to arouse and console their newborn and facilitate attachment behaviors. Mothers of LGA infants with facial or head bruising may be reluctant to interact with their newborns because they fear hurting their infant. The nursing care provided for complications associated with LGA newborns is similar to the care needed by the infant of a diabetic mother and will be discussed in the next section.

CARE OF THE INFANT OF A DIABETIC MOTHER (IDM)

The infant of a diabetic mother (IDM) is considered at risk and requires close observation the first few hours to the first few days of life. Mothers with severe diabetes or diabetes of long duration, associated with vascular complications, may give birth to SGA infants. The typical IDM (type 1 or 2 when the diabetes is poorly controlled, or gestational diabetes), however, is LGA. The infant is macrosomic, ruddy in color, and has excessive adipose tissue (Figure 30–4 ◉). The umbilical cord and placenta are large. There is a higher incidence of macrosomic infants born to certain ethnic groups (Native Americans, Mexican Americans, African Americans, Pacific Islanders) (Chmait & Moore, 2005).

IDMs have decreased total body water, particularly in the extracellular spaces, and are therefore not edematous. Their excessive weight is due to increased weight of the visceral organs, cardiomegaly (hypertrophy), and increased body fat. The only organ not affected is the brain.

The excessive fetal growth of the IDM is caused by exposure to high levels of maternal glucose, which readily crosses the placenta. The fetus responds to these high glu-

● FIGURE 30–4

Macrosomic infant of diabetic mother.

cose levels with increased insulin production and hyperplasia of the pancreatic beta cells. The insulin's main action is to help glucose enter muscle and fat cells. Once in the cells, glucose is converted to glycogen and stored. Insulin also inhibits the breakdown of fat to free fatty acids, thereby maintaining lipid synthesis, increasing the uptake of amino acids, and promoting protein synthesis. Insulin is an important regulator of fetal metabolism and has a "growth hormone" effect that increases linear growth. IDMs may be obese as children.

COMMON COMPLICATIONS OF THE IDM

Although IDMs are usually large, they are immature in physiologic functions and exhibit many of the problems of the preterm (premature) infant. The complications most often seen in an IDM are as follows:

- **Hypoglycemia.** Even without the high-glucose maternal blood supply, this newborn continues to produce high levels of insulin, which deplete the blood glucose within hours after birth. IDMs also have less ability to release glucagon and catecholamines, which normally stimulate glucagon breakdown and glucose release. The incidence of hypoglycemia in IDMs varies from 30% to 50% (Moore, 2004), according to the degree of success in controlling the maternal diabetes, the maternal blood sugar level at birth, the length of labor, the class of maternal diabetes, and early versus late feedings of the newborn. Signs and symptoms of hypoglycemia include tremors, cyanosis, apnea, temperature instability, poor feeding, and hypotonia. Seizures may occur in severe cases.

- **Hypocalcemia.** Tremors are the obvious clinical sign of hypocalcemia. They may be due to the IDM's prematurity and to the stresses of difficult pregnancy, labor, and birth, which predispose any infant to hypocalcemia. Women who have diabetes tend to have decreased serum magnesium levels at term because of increased urinary calcium excretion, which causes secondary hypoparathyroidism in their infants.

NURSING PRACTICE

When beginning fluids on an IDM, it is sometimes best to start at a higher concentration of dextrose to avoid hypoglycemia episodes.

- **Hyperbilirubinemia.** This condition may be seen at 48 to 72 hours after birth. It may be caused by slightly decreased extracellular fluid volume, which increases the hematocrit level. This in turn causes an increase in red blood cell breakdown that increases bilirubin. The presence of hepatic immaturity may impair bilirubin conjugation. Enclosed hemorrhages resulting from complicated vaginal birth may also cause hyperbilirubinemia.

- **Birth trauma.** Since most IDMs are LGA, trauma may occur during labor and birth from shoulder dystocia.

- **Polycythemia.** An IDM's decreased extracellular volume may cause this condition. Fetal hyperglycemia and hyperinsulinism result in increased oxygen consumption, leading to fetal hypoxia (Moore, 2004). Hemoglobin A_{lc} binds oxygen, decreasing the oxygen available to the fetal tissues. This tissue hypoxia stimulates increased erythropoietin production, which increases both the hematocrit level and the potential for hyperbilirubinemia. See "Influence of Diabetes on Pregnancy Outcome" in Chapter 14 for discussion of hemoglobin A_{lc}. ∞

- **Respiratory distress syndrome (RDS).** This complication occurs especially in newborns of diabetic mothers in White's classes A–C who are not well controlled. Insulin antagonizes the cortisol-induced stimulation of lecithin synthesis that is necessary for lung maturation. Therefore, IDMs may have less mature lungs than expected for their gestational age. There is also a decrease in the phospholipid phosphatidylglycerol (PG), which stabilizes surfactant. The insufficiency of PG increases the incidence of RDS. Therefore, it is important to test for the presence of PG in the amniotic fluid.

  RDS does not appear to be a problem for infants born of diabetic mothers in White's classes D–F; instead, the stresses of poor uterine blood supply may lead to increased production of steroids, which accelerates lung maturation. IDMs may also have a delay in closure of the ductus arteriosus and decreases in postnatal pulmonary artery pressure (Moore, 2004).

- **Congenital birth defects.** These may include transposition of the great vessels, ventricular septal defect, patent ductus arteriosus, small left colon syndrome, and sacral agenesis (caudal regression) (Moore, 2004). Early close control of maternal glucose levels before and during pregnancy decreases the risk of birth defects.

CLINICAL THERAPY

Prenatal management is directed toward controlling maternal glucose levels, which minimizes the common complications of IDMs. Because the onset of hypoglycemia occurs between 1 and 3 hours after birth in IDMs (with a spontaneous rise to normal levels by 4 to 6 hours), blood glucose determinations should be done initially on cord blood, hourly during the first 4 hours after birth, and at 4-hour intervals until the risk period (about 24 hours) has passed or per agency protocol.

IDMs whose serum glucose level falls below 40 mg/dL should have early feedings with formula or breast milk (colostrum). If normal glucose levels cannot be maintained with oral feedings, an intravenous infusion of D10W at a rate of 4 to 6 mg/kg/min usually maintains normoglycemia in the IDM. If higher glucose concentrations are needed to maintain normal serum glucose levels, a central line will be placed to minimize tissue extravasation. Newborns with refractory hypoglycemia may benefit from the administration of intravenous corticosteroids. Once the blood glucose level has been stable for 24 hours, the infusion rate can be decreased as oral feedings are increased. The newborn's blood glucose levels must be carefully monitored. Repeat dextrose as bolus infusion is contraindicated because it may lead to severe rebound hypoglycemia after an initial brief increase in glucose level.

NURSING MANAGEMENT

NURSING ASSESSMENT AND DIAGNOSIS

Do not be lulled into thinking that a big baby is a mature baby. In almost every case, because of the infant's large size, the IDM will appear older than gestational age scoring indicates. Consider both the gestational age and whether the baby is AGA or LGA in planning and providing safe care. In caring for the IDM, assess for signs of respiratory distress, hyperbilirubinemia, birth trauma, and congenital anomalies. Nursing diagnoses that may apply to IDMs include the following:

- *Altered Nutrition: Less than Body Requirements* related to increased glucose metabolism secondary to hyperinsulinemia

- *Impaired Gas Exchange* related to respiratory distress secondary to impaired production of surfactant
- *Ineffective Family Coping: Compromise* related to the illness of the baby

PLANNING AND IMPLEMENTATION

Nursing care of the IDM is directed toward early detection and ongoing monitoring of hypoglycemia (with glucose tests) and polycythemia (with central hematocrits), RDS, and hyperbilirubinemia. (These conditions are presented in Chapter 31. ∞) Also assess for signs of birth trauma and congenital anomalies.

Parent teaching is directed toward preventing macrosomia and the resulting fetal-neonatal problems with early and ongoing diabetic control. Advise parents that with early identification and care, most IDMs' neonatal problems have no significant sequelae.

EVALUATION

Expected outcomes of nursing care include the following:

- The IDM's respiratory distress and metabolic problems are minimized.
- The parents understand the effects of maternal diabetes on the baby and the preventive steps they can initiate to decrease its impact on subsequent fetuses.
- The parents verbalize their concerns about their baby's health problems and understand the rationale behind management of their newborn.

CARE OF THE POSTTERM NEWBORN

The **postterm newborn** is any newborn born after 42 weeks' gestation.

Postterm, or prolonged, pregnancy occurs in approximately 4% to 14% of all pregnancies (Resnik & Resnik, 2004). The cause of postterm pregnancy is not completely understood, but there are several associated factors. (See Chapter 21 for discussion of maternal factors. ∞) Many pregnancies classified as prolonged are thought to be a result of inaccurate estimates of date of birth (EDB). Postterm pregnancy is more common in Australian, Greek, and Italian ethnic groups.

Most babies born after prolonged pregnancy are of normal size and health; some continue growing and are over 4000 g at birth, which supports the contention that the postterm fetus can remain well nourished. Potential intrapartal problems for these healthy but large fetuses are cephalopelvic (CPD) and shoulder dystocia. See "Care of the Woman and Fetus at Risk for Macrosomia" in Chapter 21 for discussion of the necessary assessments and interventions for CPD and shoulder dystocia. ∞

COMMON COMPLICATIONS OF THE NEWBORN WITH POSTMATURITY SYNDROME

The term **postmaturity** applies only to the infant who is born after 42 completed weeks of gestation and also demonstrates characteristics of *postmaturity syndrome.* Only about 5% of postterm newborns show signs of postmaturity syndrome.

The truly postmature newborn is at high risk for morbidity and has a mortality rate two to three times greater than that of term infants. Although today the percentages are extremely low, most postmature fetal deaths occur during labor because the fetus uses up necessary body reserves.

Decreased placental function impairs oxygenation and nutrition transport, leaving the fetus prone to hypoglycemia and asphyxia when the stresses of labor begin. The following are common disorders of the postmature newborn:

- *Hypoglycemia,* from nutritional deprivation and depleted glycogen stores.
- *Meconium aspiration* in response to in utero hypoxia. Oligohydramnios increases the danger of aspirating thick meconium. Severe meconium aspiration syndrome increases the baby's chance of developing persistent pulmonary hypertension, pneumothorax, and pneumonia.
- *Polycythemia* due to increased production of red blood cells (RBCs) in response to hypoxia.
- *Congenital anomalies* of unknown cause.
- *Seizure* activity because of hypoxic insult.
- *Cold stress* because of loss or poor development of subcutaneous fat.

The long-term effects of postmaturity syndrome are unclear. At present, studies do not agree on how postmaturity syndrome affects weight gain and IQ scores (Resnik & Resnik, 2004).

Prolonged pregnancy itself is not solely responsible for the postmaturity syndrome. The characteristics of postmature newborns are primarily caused by a combination of advanced gestational age, placental aging and subsequent insufficiency, and continued exposure to amniotic fluid.

CLINICAL THERAPY

The aim of antenatal management is to differentiate the fetus who has postmaturity syndrome from the fetus who is large, well nourished, alert, and tolerating the prolonged (postterm) pregnancy. (Antenatal and intrapartal tests to evaluate fetal status and determine obstetric management are discussed in more depth in Chapter 16 and in Chapter 21. ∞) If the amniotic fluid is meconium stained, an amnioinfusion may be done during labor. This procedure dilutes the meconium, decreasing the risk of meconium aspiration syndrome. (For detailed discussion of clinical management and care of the newborn at risk for meconium aspiration, see "Meconium Aspiration Syndrome" in Chapter 31. ∞)

Hypoglycemia is monitored by serial glucose determinations per agency protocols. If not in respiratory distress, the baby may be given glucose infusions or early feedings, but these measures must be instituted with caution because of the possibility of asphyxia in the first 24 hours. Postmature newborns are often voracious eaters.

As with SGA infants, peripheral and central hematocrits are tested to determine the presence of polycythemia. Fluid resuscitation can be initiated. In extreme cases a partial exchange transfusion may be necessary to prevent polycythemia and adverse sequelae such as hyperviscosity. Oxygen is provided for respiratory distress. In addition, decreased liver glycogen stores can cause temperature instability and excessive loss of heat. (See "Care of the Newborn with Cold Stress" in Chapter 31 for thermoregulation techniques. ∞)

NURSING MANAGEMENT

NURSING ASSESSMENT AND DIAGNOSIS

The newborn with postmaturity syndrome appears alert; this wide-eyed, alert appearance is not necessarily a positive sign because it may indicate chronic intrauterine hypoxia.

The infant typically has dry, cracking, parchmentlike skin without vernix or lanugo (Figure 30–5 ●). Fingernails are long, and scalp hair is profuse. The infant's body appears long and thin. The wasting involves depletion of previously stored subcutaneous tissue, causing the skin to be loose. Fat layers are almost nonexistent.

Postmature newborns frequently have meconium staining, which colors the nails, skin, and umbilical cord. The varying shades (yellow to green) of meconium staining can give some clue as to whether the expulsion of meconium in utero was a recent or chronic problem. Green coloring indicates a more recent event.

Nursing diagnoses that may apply to the postmature newborn include the following:

- *Hypothermia* related to decreased liver glycogen and brown fat stores
- *Altered Nutrition: Less than Body Requirements* related to increased use of glucose secondary to in utero stress and decreased placenta perfusion
- *Impaired Gas Exchange in the Lungs and at the Cellular Level* related to airway obstruction from meconium aspiration

● FIGURE 30–5

Postterm infant demonstrates deep cracking and peeling of skin.
Reprinted by permission of V. Dubowitz, MD, Hammersmith Hospital, London, England.

MEDIALINK Case Study: Postterm Newborn

PLANNING AND IMPLEMENTATION

Hospital-Based Nursing Care

Nursing interventions are primarily supportive. The nurse needs to do the following:

- Monitor cardiopulmonary status, because the stresses of labor are poorly tolerated and can result in hypoxemia in utero and possible asphyxia at birth.
- Provide warmth to counterbalance the infant's poor response to cold stress and decreased liver glycogen and brown fat stores.
- Frequently monitor blood glucose per agency protocol and initiate early feeding (at 1 or 2 hours of age) or intravenous glucose per physician order.
- Obtain a central line hematocrit to determine accurately the presence of polycythemia.

Encourage parents to express their feelings and fears about the newborn's condition and potential long-term problems. Give careful explanations of procedures, include the parents in the development of care plans for their baby, and encourage follow-up care as needed.

EVALUATION

Expected outcomes of nursing care include the following:

- The postterm newborn establishes effective respiratory function.
- The postmature baby is free of metabolic alterations (hypoglycemia) and maintains a stable temperature.

CARE OF THE PRETERM (PREMATURE) NEWBORN

A **preterm infant** is any infant born before the completion of 37 weeks' gestation (Figure 30–6 ◉). With the help of modern technology, infants are surviving at younger gestational ages, but not without significant morbidity. The incidence of all preterm births in the United States is approximately 12%, and 18% of African-American newborns are preterm (Als & Lawhon, 2004). The rise in multiple birth rates has markedly influenced overall rates of low-birth-weight (LBW) infants. Prematurity and low birth weight are common in single and young mothers. (See "Care of Woman at Risk due to Preterm Labor" in Chapter 15 or a discussion of preterm labor. ∞)

The major problem of the preterm newborn is the variable immaturity of all systems, which depends on the length of gestation. The preterm newborn must traverse the same complex, interconnected pathways from intrauterine to extrauterine life as the term newborn. Immaturity means the premature newborn is ill equipped to make this transition smoothly. Maintenance of the preterm newborn falls within narrow physiologic parameters.

ALTERATION IN RESPIRATORY AND CARDIAC PHYSIOLOGY

The preterm newborn is at risk for respiratory problems because the lungs are not fully mature and not fully ready to take over the process of oxygen and carbon dioxide exchange without assistance until 37 to 38 weeks' gestation. Critical factors in the development of respiratory distress include the following:

1. The preterm infant is unable to produce adequate amounts of surfactant. (See "Fetal Lung

Development" in Chapter 26 ∞ for discussion of respiratory adaptation and development.) Inadequate surfactant lessens compliance (ability of the lung to fill with air easily), so the inspiratory pressure needed to expand the lungs with air is higher. The collapsed (or atelectatic) alveoli will not exchange oxygen and carbon dioxide. As a result, the infant becomes hypoxic, pulmonary blood flow is inefficient, and the preterm newborn's available energy is depleted.

2. The muscular coat of pulmonary blood vessels is incompletely developed. Consequently the pulmonary arterioles do not constrict as well in response to decreased oxygen levels. Lower pulmonary vascular resistance leads to left-to-right shunting of blood through the ductus arteriosus back into the lungs.

The ductus arteriosus usually responds to increasing oxygen levels and prostaglandin E levels by vasoconstriction; in the preterm infant, who is more susceptible to hypoxia, the ductus may remain open. A patent ductus increases the blood volume to the lungs, causing pulmonary congestion, increased respiratory effort, carbon dioxide retention, and bounding femoral pulses.

The common complications of the cardiopulmonary system in preterm infants are discussed later in this chapter and in Chapter 31. ∞

ALTERATION IN THERMOREGULATION

Heat loss is a major problem in preterm newborns, but the nurse can do much to prevent it. Two factors limiting heat production, however, are the availability of glycogen in the liver and the amount of brown fat available for metabolism. Both of these limiting factors appear in the third trimester. In the cold-stressed baby, norepinephrine is released, which stimulates the metabolism of brown fat for heat production. As a complicating factor, the hypoxic newborn cannot increase oxygen consumption in response to cold stress because of the already limited reserves and thereby becomes progressively colder. Since the muscle mass is small in preterm infants, and muscular activity is diminished (they are unable to shiver), little heat is produced.

Five physiologic and anatomic factors cause heat loss in the preterm infant:

1. The preterm baby has a higher ratio of body surface to body weight. This means that the baby's ability to produce heat (based on body weight) is much less than the potential for losing heat (based on surface area). Heat loss in a preterm infant weighing 1500 g is five times greater per unit of body weight than in an adult.

2. The preterm baby has very little subcutaneous fat, which is the human body's insulation. Without

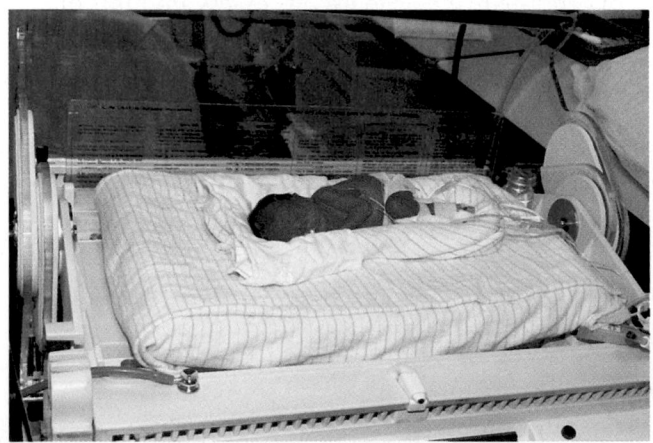

◉ **FIGURE 30–6**

A 6-day-old, 28-week gestational age, 960-g preterm infant.
Courtesy of Carol Harrigan, RNC, MSN, NNP.

adequate insulation, heat is easily conducted from the core of the body (warmer temperature) to the surface of the body (cooler temperature). The body loses heat as the blood vessels, which lie close to the skin surface in the preterm infant, transport blood from the body core to the subcutaneous tissues.

3. The preterm baby has thinner, more permeable skin than the term infant, contributing to a greater insensible water loss as well as to heat loss.

4. The posture of the preterm baby is another important factor influencing heat loss. Flexion of the extremities decreases the amount of surface area exposed to the environment. Extension increases the surface area exposed to the environment and thus increases heat loss. The gestational age of the infant influences the amount of flexion, from completely hypotonic and extended at 28 weeks to strong flexion displayed by 36 weeks.

5. The preterm baby has a decreased ability to vasoconstrict superficial blood vessels and conserve heat in the body core.

In summary, gestational age is directly proportional to the ability to maintain thermoregulation; thus, the more preterm the newborn, the less able the infant is to maintain heat balance. Preventing heat loss with a neutral thermal environment is one of the most important considerations in nursing management of the preterm infant. Cold stress, with its accompanying severe complications, can be prevented (see "Care of the Newborn with Cold Stress" in Chapter 31 ∞).

ALTERATION IN GASTROINTESTINAL PHYSIOLOGY

The basic structure of the gastrointestinal (GI) tract is formed early in gestation. Maturation of the digestive and absorptive process is more variable, however, and occurs later in gestation. As a result of GI immaturity, the preterm newborn has the following ingestion, digestive, and absorption problems:

■ A marked danger of aspiration and its complications due to the infant's poorly developed gag reflex, incompetent esophageal cardiac sphincter, and poor sucking and swallowing reflex.

■ Difficulty in meeting high caloric and fluid needs for growth due to small stomach capacity.

■ Limited ability to convert certain essential amino acids to nonessential amino acids. Certain amino acids, such as histidine, taurine, and cysteine, are essential to the preterm infant but not to the term infant.

■ Inability to handle the increased osmolarity of formula protein due to kidney immaturity. The preterm infant requires a higher concentration of whey protein than of casein.

■ Difficulty absorbing saturated fats because of decreased bile salts and pancreatic lipase. Severe illness may also prevent intake of adequate nutrients.

■ Difficulty with lactose digestion initially because processes may not be fully functional during the first few days of a preterm infant's life. The preterm newborn can digest and absorb most simple sugars.

■ Rickets and significant bone demineralization due to deficiency of calcium and phosphorus, which are deposited primarily in the last trimester.

■ Increased basal metabolic rate and increased oxygen requirements due to fatigue associated with sucking.

■ Feeding intolerance and necrotizing enterocolitis (NEC) as a result of diminished blood flow and tissue perfusion to the intestinal tract due to prolonged hypoxia and hypoxemia at birth.

ALTERATION IN RENAL PHYSIOLOGY

The kidneys of the preterm infant are immature compared with those of the term infant. This situation poses clinical problems in the management of fluid and electrolyte balance. Specific characteristics of the preterm infant include the following:

■ The glomerular filtration rate (GFR) is lower because of decreased renal blood flow. The GFR is directly related to lower gestational age, so the more preterm the newborn, the lower the GFR. The GFR is also decreased in the presence of diseases or conditions that decrease the renal blood flow and perfusion, such as severe respiratory distress, hypotension, and asphyxia. Anuria and oliguria may also be observed.

■ The preterm infant's kidneys have a limited ability to concentrate urine or to excrete excess amounts of fluid. This means that if excess fluid is administered, the infant is at risk for fluid retention and overhydration. If too little is administered, the infant will become dehydrated because of the inability to retain adequate fluid.

■ The kidneys of the preterm infant begin excreting glucose (glycosuria) at a lower serum glucose level than those of the term infant. Therefore, glycosuria with hyperglycemia is common.

■ The kidney's buffering capacity is reduced, predisposing the infant to metabolic acidosis. Bicarbonate is excreted at a lower serum level, and acid is excreted more slowly. Therefore, after periods of hypoxia or insult, the preterm infant's kidneys need a longer time to excrete the lactic acid that accumulates.

Sodium bicarbonate is frequently required to treat the metabolic acidosis.

■ The immaturity of the renal system affects the preterm infant's ability to excrete drugs. Because excretion time is longer, many drugs are given over longer intervals in the preterm infant (i.e., every 24 hours instead of every 12 hours). Urine output must be carefully monitored when the infant is receiving nephrotoxic drugs such as gentamicin, nafcillin, and vancomycin. If urine output is poor, drugs can become toxic in the infant much more quickly than in the adult.

ALTERATION IN REACTIVITY PERIODS AND BEHAVIORAL STATES

The newborn infant's response to extrauterine life is characterized by two periods of reactivity (see "Periods of Reactivity" in Chapter 26 ∞). The preterm infant's periods of reactivity are delayed. In the very ill infant, these periods of reactivity may not be observed at all because the infant may be hypotonic and unreactive for several days after birth.

As the preterm newborn grows and the condition stabilizes, identifying behavioral states and traits unique to each infant becomes increasingly possible. In general, stable preterm infants do not demonstrate the same behavioral states as term infants. Preterm infants tend to be more disorganized in their sleep-wake cycles and are unable to attend as well to the human face and objects in the environment. Neurologically, their responses (sucking, muscle tone, states of arousal) are weaker than full-term infants' responses.

By observing each infant's patterns of behavior and responses, especially the sleep-wake states, the parent and nurse can plan nursing care around the times when the infant is alert and best able to attend. The more knowledge parents have about the meaning of their infant's responses and behaviors, the better prepared they will be to meet their newborn's needs and to form a positive attachment with their child. See discussion of developmental care for the preterm newborn later in this section.

TEACHING HIGHLIGHTS

OPTIMAL TIMING FOR TEACHING

After observing an infant's pattern of behavior and responses, especially the sleep-wake states, use the time when the infant is alert and best able to attend to help parents learn about and provide newborn care.

MANAGEMENT OF NUTRITION AND FLUID REQUIREMENTS

Early feedings are extremely valuable in maintaining normal metabolism and lowering the possibility of such complications as hypoglycemia, hyperbilirubinemia, hyperkalemia, and azotemia. However, the preterm infant is at risk for complications that may develop because of immaturity of the digestive system.

Nutritional Requirements

The oral (enteral) caloric intake necessary for growth in a healthy preterm newborn is 95 to 130 kcal/kg/day (Blackburn, 2003). In addition to these relatively high caloric needs, the preterm newborn requires more protein than the full-term infant. To meet these needs, many institutions use breast milk or special preterm formulas.

Whether breast milk or formula is used, feeding regimens are established based on the infant's weight and estimated stomach capacity (Table 30–1). Initial formula feedings are gradually increased as the infant tolerates them. It may be necessary to supplement oral feedings with parenteral fluids to maintain adequate hydration and caloric intake until the baby is on full oral feedings. Preterm infants who cannot tolerate any oral (enteral) feedings are given nutrition by total parenteral nutrition (TPN).

In addition to a higher calorie and protein formula, preterm infants should receive supplemental multivitamins, including vitamin E and trace minerals. A diet high in polyunsaturated fats (which preterm infants tolerate best) increases the requirement for vitamin E. Preterm infants fed iron-fortified formulas have higher red cell hemolysis and lower vitamin E concentrations and thus require additional vitamin E. Preterm formulas also need to contain medium-chain triglycerides (MCTs) and additional amino acids such as cysteine, as well as calcium, phosphorus, and vitamin D supplements to increase mineralization of bones. Rickets and significant bone demineralization have been documented in very-low-birth-weight infants and otherwise healthy preterm infants.

Nutritional intake is considered adequate when there is consistent weight gain 20 to 30 g/day. Initially, no weight gain may be noted for several days, but total weight loss should not exceed 15% of the total birth weight or more than 1% to 2% per day. Some institutions add the criteria of head circumference growth and increase in body length of 1 cm per week, once the newborn is stable.

Methods of Feeding

The preterm infant is fed by various methods depending on the infant's gestational age, health and physical condition, and neurologic status. The three most common oral feeding methods are bottle, breast, and gavage.

Bottle-Feeding. Preterm infants who have a coordinated, as well as rhythmic, suck-swallow-breathing pattern between 35 and 36 weeks' postconceptual age may be fed by bottle. Nutritive sucking is a multifaceted process involving the

TABLE 30–1 ✣ Suggested Feeding Guidelines for the Preterm Infant

Weight (g)	Feeding Interval	Beginning Volume (mL/kg/d)	Feeding Increments (mL/kg/d)	Days to Full Feedings[†]
< 1000	q 3 hour	10–20	10–20	16–13
1000–1500	q 3 hour	10–20	15–20	10–7
1501–1800 sick[‡]	q 3 hour	10–20	20–30	7–5
1501–1800 healthy[‡]	q 3 hour	20–40	30–50	5–3
> 1800 sick[‡]	q 3 hour	20–40	30–75	5–2

[†]Full feedings are defined as 120 kcal/kg/day of a 24 kcal/oz formula or human milk.

[‡] *Sick* refers to infants who have had symptoms of any medical or surgical condition, other than uncomplicated prematurity.

Healthy refers to term or preterm infants who have had no symptomatic medical or surgical conditions.

1. Advancement of feedings should occur only as the infant demonstrates tolerance of enteral feedings. Clinical signs of feeding intolerance or illness dictate discontinuing or holding the advancement of feedings.

2. Infants are started on either full-strength human milk or 24 kcal/oz premature infant formula.

3. At 100–120 mL/kg, fortifier is added to human milk.

4. Iron supplements are added at 2–4 mg/kg/day for the human milk fed infant at full feeds.

central nervous system and the musculoskeletal system of the mouth, pharynx, esophagus, and face (McGrath, 2004). To avoid excessive expenditure of energy, a soft, yellow, single-hole nipple may be used (milk flow is less rapid). The infant is fed in a semisitting position and burped gently after each 1/2 to 1 oz. The feeding should take no longer than 15 to 20 minutes (nippling requires more energy than other methods). Babies who are progressing from gavage feedings to bottle-feeding should start with one session of bottle-feeding a day and slowly increase the number of times per day a bottle is given until the baby tolerates all feedings from a bottle.

The nurse also assesses the infant's ability to suck. Sucking may be affected by age, asphyxia, sepsis, intraventricular hemorrhage, or other neurologic insult. Before initiating bottle-feeding, the nurse should observe for signs of stress, such as tachypnea (more than 60 respirations per minute), respiratory distress, or hypothermia, which may increase the risk of aspiration. During the feeding, the nurse should observe the infant for signs of feeding difficulty (tachypnea, cyanosis, bradycardia, lethargy, uncoordinated suck and swallow). Difficulty in bottle-feeding is often associated with a milk bolus that is too large for the infant's oral cavity, which can lead to aspiration.

Breastfeeding. Mothers who wish to breastfeed their preterm infants are given the opportunity to put the infant to the breast as soon as the infant has demonstrated a coordinated suck and swallow reflex, is showing consistent weight gain, and can control body temperature

outside of the incubator, regardless of weight. Preterm infants tolerate breastfeeding with higher transcutaneous oxygen pressures and better maintenance of body temperature than during bottle-feeding. In addition to breast milk's many benefits for the infant, breastfeeding allows the mother to contribute actively to the infant's well-being (Figure 30–7 ◉). Mothers should be encouraged to breastfeed because of the numerous benefits if they choose to do so. It is important to be aware of the advantages of breastfeeding, as well as the possible disadvantages of breast milk as the sole source of food for the preterm infant (see "Breast Milk Feeding" in Chapter 29 ∞). Even if the infant cannot be put to the breast, mothers can pump their breasts, and the breast milk can be given via gavage. A double pumping system produces higher levels of prolactin than sequential pumping of the breasts.

By initiating skin-to-skin holding of preterm infants in the early intensive care phase, mothers can significantly increase milk volume and thereby overcome lactation problems (Turnage-Carrier, 2004). Preterm infants tolerate breastfeeding with higher transcutaneous oxygen saturation and better maintenance of body temperature than during bottle feedings.

The football hold is suggested as a convenient position for breastfeeding preterm babies. Feeding may take up to 45 minutes, and babies should be burped as they alternate breasts. It is important to monitor the length of feeding time so that the preterm infant does not burn too many calories.

○ **FIGURE 30-7**

Mother breastfeeding her premature infant.

A flexible feeding schedule should be coordinated so babies can breastfeed during alert times and be allowed to set their own pace. Feedings should be on demand, but a maximum number of hours between feedings should be set. A similar regimen should be used for the baby who is progressing from gavage to breastfeeding. The mother begins with one feeding at the breast and then gradually increases the number of times during the day that the baby breastfeeds. When breastfeeding is not possible because the infant is too small or too weak to suck at the breast, the mother may express her breast milk into a cup. The milk touches the infant's lips and is lapped by the protruding motions of the tongue.

NURSING PRACTICE

For an otherwise healthy, growing premature infant who is receiving total enteral intake and has started to experience apnea and bradycardia, one differential diagnosis to think about is reflux rather than sepsis, although sepsis may need to be ruled out.

Gavage Feeding. The gavage feeding method is used with preterm infants (less than 34 weeks' gestation) who lack or have a poorly coordinated suck and swallow reflex or are ill and ventilator dependent. Gavage feeding may be used as an adjunct to nipple-feeding if the infant tires easily or as an al-

ternative if an infant is losing weight because of the energy expenditure required for nippling, which increases the chance of aspiration (see Skill 15-3 ∞).

Gavage feedings are administered by either the nasogastric or orogastric route and by intermittent bolus or continuous drip method (see Figures 30-8 ● and 30-9 ●).

NURSING PRACTICE

Orogastric gavage catheter placement is preferable to nasogastric because most infants are obligatory nose breathers. If nasogastric is used, a 5 French catheter is often used to minimize airway obstruction.

Total Parenteral Nutrition. TPN is used in situations that do not allow feeding the infant through the GI tract. The TPN method provides complete nutrition to the infant intravenously. TPN uses hyperalimentation to provide calories, vitamins, minerals, protein, and glucose, and intralipids to provide essential fatty acids.

Fluid Requirements

Fluid requirement calculations take into account the infant's weight and postnatal age. Recommendations for fluid therapy in the preterm infant are approximately 80 to 100 mL/kg/day for day 1, 100 to 120 mL/kg/day for day 2, and 120 to 150 mL/kg/day by day 3 of life. These amounts may be increased up to 200 mL/kg/day if the infant is very small, receiving phototherapy, or under a radiant warmer because of increased insensible water losses. Fluid losses can be minimized through the use of heat shields and humidity, or "swamping."

○ **FIGURE 30-8**

Measuring gavage tube length. (See Clinical Skill 15-3. **SKILLS**)

FIGURE 30–9

Auscultation for placement of gavage tube. (See Clinical Skill 15-3. **SKILLS**)

COMMON COMPLICATIONS OF PRETERM NEWBORNS

The goals of medical and nursing care are to anticipate and manage the complications associated with prematurity and to meet the preterm infant's growth and development needs. The most common of these complications are as follows:

1. **Apnea of prematurity.** Apnea of prematurity refers to cessation of breathing for 20 seconds or longer or for less than 20 seconds when associated with cyanosis and bradycardia. Apnea is a common problem in the preterm infant (less than 37 weeks' gestation), presenting between day 2 and day 7 of life. The etiology of apnea is multifactorial but is thought to be primarily a result of neuronal immaturity, which contributes to the preterm infant's irregular breathing patterns (central apnea). Obstructive apnea can occur when there is cessation of airflow associated with blockage of the upper airway (small airway diameter, increased pharyngeal secretions, altered body alignment and positioning). Gastroesophageal reflux (GER) has been implicated in apnea. GER is defined as a movement of gastric contents into the lower esophagus due to poor esophageal sphincter tone, causing laryngospasm, which leads to bradycardia and apnea. As such, apnea of prematurity is a diagnosis of exclusion.

2. **Patent ductus arteriosus (PDA).** The ductus arteriosus fails to close because of decreased pulmonary arteriole musculature and hypoxemia. Symptomatic PDA is often seen when premature infants are recovering from RDS. Patent ductus arteriosus often prolongs the course of illness in a preterm newborn and leads to chronic pulmonary dysfunction.

3. **Respiratory distress syndrome.** Respiratory distress results from inadequate surfactant production (see Chapter 31 ∞).

4. **Intraventricular hemorrhage (IVH).** Intraventricular hemorrhage is the most common type of intracranial hemorrhage in small preterm infants, especially those weighing less than 1500 g or of less than 34 weeks' gestation. Up to 34 weeks' gestation, the preterm's brain ventricles are lined by the germinal matrix, which is highly susceptible to hypoxic events such as respiratory distress, birth trauma, and birth asphyxia. The germinal matrix is very vascular, and its blood vessels rupture in the presence of hypoxia.

5. **Anemia of prematurity.** The preterm infant is at risk for anemia because of the rapid rate of growth required, shorter RBC life, excessive blood sampling, decreased iron stores, and deficiency of vitamin E. The hemoglobin usually reaches its lowest level by 3 to 12 weeks and remains low for 3 to 6 months.

Other common problems of preterm infants such as feeding difficulties are briefly discussed earlier in the physiologic sections. (For an in-depth discussion of RDS, hyperbilirubinemia, hypoglycemia, and sepsis, see Chapter 31. ∞)

LONG-TERM NEEDS AND OUTCOME

The care of preterm infants and their families continues after they leave the nursery. Follow-up care is extremely important because many developmental problems are not noted until an infant is older and begins to demonstrate motor delays or sensory disability.

Within the first year of life, low-birth-weight preterm infants face higher mortality rates than term infants. Causes of death include sudden infant death syndrome (SIDS)—which occurs about five times more frequently in the preterm infant—respiratory infections, and neurologic defects. Morbidity is also much higher among preterm infants, with those weighing less than 1500 g at highest risk for long-term complications. The most common long-term needs observed in preterm infants include the following:

■ **Retinopathy of prematurity (ROP).** Premature newborns are particularly susceptible to characteristic retinal changes, known as ROP, which can impair vision. The disease is now viewed as multifactorial in origin with hyperoxemia (increased oxygen levels) as one factor. Increased survival of very-low-birth-weight (VLBW) infants may be the most important factor in the increased incidence of ROP.

- **Bronchopulmonary dysplasia (BPD).** Long-term lung disease results when positive pressure respirator therapy and high oxygen concentration damage the alveolar epithelium. Infants with BPD have long-term dependence on oxygen therapy and an increased incidence of respiratory infection during their first few years of life. For further discussion see "Bronchopulmonary Dysplasia" in Chapter 46. ∞

- **Speech defects.** The most common speech defects involve delayed development of receptive and expressive ability that may persist into the school-age years.

- **Neurologic defects.** The most common neurologic defects include cerebral palsy, hydrocephalus, seizure disorders, lower IQ, and learning disabilities. However, the socioeconomic climate and family support systems are extremely important influences on the child's ultimate school performance when there are no major neurologic defects. Families can be reminded that risk does not equal injury, injury does not equal damage, and description of damage does not allow a precise prediction about recovery or outcome.

- **Auditory defects.** Preterm infants have a 1% to 4% incidence of moderate to profound hearing loss and should have a formal audiologic examination before discharge and at 3 to 6 months (corrected age). Tests currently used to measure newborn hearing functions are the evoked otoacoustic emissions (EOAE) or the automated auditory brain response (AABR) test. Any infant with repeated abnormal results should be referred to speech-and-language specialists.

When evaluating the infant's abilities and disabilities, it is important for parents to understand that developmental progress must be evaluated based on chronological age from the expected date of birth, not from the actual date of birth (corrected age). Parents need consistent support from healthcare professionals in the long-term management of their infant to promote the highest quality of life possible.

NURSING MANAGEMENT

NURSING ASSESSMENT AND DIAGNOSIS

Assess the physical characteristics and gestational age of the preterm newborn accurately to anticipate the special needs and problems of the baby. Physical characteristics vary greatly depending on gestational age, but these characteristics are common:

- *Color* is usually pink or ruddy but may be acrocyanotic. (Cyanosis, jaundice, and pallor are abnormal and should be noted.)

- *Skin* is reddened and translucent, blood vessels are readily apparent, and there is little subcutaneous fat.

- *Vernix caseosa* is abundant.

- *Lanugo* is plentiful and widely distributed.

- *Head size* appears large in relation to body.

- *Skull bones* are pliable; fontanelle is smooth and flat.

- *Ears* have minimal cartilage and are pliable, folded over.

- *Nails* are soft and short.

- *Genitals* are small; testes may not be descended.

- *Resting position* is flaccid, froglike.

- *Cry* is weak and feeble.

- *Reflexes* (sucking, swallowing, gag) are poor.

- *Activity* consists of jerky, generalized movements. (Seizure activity is abnormal.)

Determination of gestational age in preterm newborns requires knowledge and experience in administering gestational assessment tools. The tool used should be specific, reliable, and valid. (For a discussion of gestational age assessment tools, see Chapter 27. ∞)

Nursing diagnoses that may apply to the preterm newborn include the following:

- *Impaired Gas Exchange* related to immature pulmonary vasculature and inadequate surfactant production

- *Altered Nutrition: Less than Body Requirements* related to weak suck and swallow reflexes and decreased ability to absorb nutrients

- *Ineffective Thermoregulation* related to hypothermia secondary to decreased glycogen and brown fat stores

- *Fluid Volume Deficit* related to high insensible water losses and inability of kidneys to concentrate urine

- *Ineffective Family Coping* related to anger or guilt at having given birth to a premature baby

PLANNING AND IMPLEMENTATION

Maintenance of Respiratory Function

Preterm newborns have increased danger of respiratory obstruction. Their bronchi and trachea are so narrow that mucus can obstruct the airway. Maintain patency through judicious suctioning, but only suction as needed.

Positioning can also affect respiratory function, especially in the preterm newborn. If the baby is in the supine position, slightly elevate the infant's head to maintain the airway, being careful to avoid hyperextension of the neck because the trachea will collapse. Also, because the newborn has weak neck muscles and cannot control head movement, maintain this head position by placing a small roll under the shoulders. Because the prone position splints the chest wall and decreases the amount of respiratory effort used to move the chest wall, it facilitates chest expansion and improves air entry and oxygenation. Weak or absent cough or gag reflexes increase the premature newborn's chance of aspiration. Ensure that the infant's position facilitates drainage of mucus or regurgitated formula.

Monitor heart and respiratory rates with cardiorespiratory monitors and observe the newborn for alterations in cardiopulmonary status. Signs of respiratory distress include the following:

- Cyanosis (serious sign when generalized)
- Tachypnea (sustained respiratory rate greater than 60/minute after first 4 hours of life)
- Retractions
- Expiratory grunting
- Nasal flaring
- Apneic episodes
- Presence of rales or rhonchi on auscultation
- Diminished air entry

If respiratory distress occurs, administer oxygen per physician or nurse practitioner order to relieve hypoxemia. If hypoxemia is not treated immediately, it may result in patent ductus arteriosus or metabolic acidosis. When administering oxygen to the newborn, monitor the oxygen concentration with devices such as the transcutaneous oxygen monitor ($tcPO_2$) or the pulse oximeter. Periodic arterial blood gas sampling to monitor oxygen concentration in the baby's blood is essential since hyperoxemia may lead to ROP.

Consider respiratory function during feeding. To prevent aspiration and increased energy expenditure and oxygen consumption, ensure that the infant's gag and suck reflexes are intact before starting oral feedings.

Maintenance of Neutral Thermal Environment

Providing a neutral thermal environment minimizes the oxygen consumption required to maintain a normal core temperature; it also prevents cold stress and facilitates growth by decreasing the calories needed to maintain body temperature. The preterm infant's immature central nervous system provides poor temperature control, and stores of brown fat are decreased. A small infant (< 1200 g) can lose 80 kcal/kg/day through radiation of body heat.

Use all the usual thermoregulation measures discussed in Chapter 28. ∞ In addition, to minimize heat loss and temperature instability effects:

1. Allow skin-to-skin contact between mother and newborn to maintain warmth and foster security (see "kangaroo care" discussion later in this chapter).

2. Warm and humidify oxygen to minimize evaporative heat loss and decrease oxygen consumption.

3. Place the baby in a double-walled incubator or use a Plexiglas heat shield over small preterm infants in single-walled incubators to avoid radiative heat losses. Some institutions use radiant warmers and plastic wrap over the baby and pipe in humidity (swamping). Do not use Plexiglas shields on radiant warmer beds because they block the infrared heat.

4. Avoid placing the baby on cold surfaces such as metal treatment tables and cold x-ray plates (conductive heat loss). Pad cold surfaces with diapers and use radiant warmers during procedures, place infant on prewarmed mattresses, and warm hands before handling the baby to prevent heat transfer via conduction.

5. Use warmed ambient humidity. The use of humidity and its role in decreasing insensible water loss remains controversial (Blackburn, 2003).

6. Keep the skin dry and place a cap on the baby's head to prevent heat loss via evaporation. (The head makes up 25% of the total body size.)

7. Keep radiant warmers, incubators, and cribs away from windows and cold external walls and out of drafts to prevent heat loss by radiation.

8. Open incubator portholes and doors only when necessary, and use plastic sleeves on portholes to decrease convective heat loss.

9. Use a skin probe to monitor the baby's skin temperature. Correlate ambient temperatures with the skin probe in the incubator using the servocontrol rather than the manual mode. The temperature should be 36°C to 37°C (96.8°F to 97.7°F). Temperature fluctuations indicate hypothermia or hyperthermia. Be careful not to place skin temperature probes over bony prominences, areas of brown fat, poorly vasoreactive areas such as extremities, or excoriated areas.

10. Warm formula or stored breast milk before feeding.

11. Use reflector patch over the skin temperature probe when using a radiant warmer bed so that the probe does not sense the higher infrared temperature as the baby's skin temperature and therefore decrease the heater output.

Once preterm infants are medically stable, they can be clothed with a double-thickness cap, cotton shirt, and diaper and, if possible, swaddled in a blanket. Begin the process of weaning to a crib when the premature infant is medically stable, does not require assisted ventilation, weighs approximately 1500 g, has 5 days of consistent weight gain, and is taking oral feedings and when apnea and bradycardia episodes have stabilized. Be familiar with the institution's protocol for weaning to a crib.

Maintenance of Fluid and Electrolyte Status

Keep the newborn hydrated by providing adequate intake based on weight, gestational age, chronologic age, and volume of sensible and insensible water losses. Adequate fluid intake should compensate for increased insensible losses and the amount needed for renal excretion of metabolic products. Minimize insensible water losses by providing high ambient humidity, humidifying oxygen, using heat shields, covering the skin with plastic wrap, and placing the infant in a double-walled incubator.

Evaluate the hydration status of the baby by assessing and recording the following signs of dehydration:

- Sunken fontanelle, loss of weight
- Poor skin turgor (skin returns to position slowly when squeezed gently)
- Dry oral mucous membranes
- Decreased urine output
- Increased specific gravity (>1.013)

Also identify signs of overhydration by observing the newborn for edema or excessive weight gain and by comparing urine output with fluid intake.

Weigh the preterm infant at least once daily at the same time each day. *Weight change is one of the most sensitive indicators of fluid balance.* Weighing diapers is also important for accurate input and output measurement (1 mL = 1 g). A comparison of intake and output measurements over an 8- or 24-hour period provides important information about renal function and fluid balance. Assessment of patterns and whether they show a net gain or loss over several days is also essential to fluid management. In addition, monitor blood serum levels and pH to evaluate for electrolyte imbalances.

Accurate hourly intake calculations when administering intravenous fluids are essential to prevent overload. Accuracy can be ensured by using neonatal or pediatric infusion pumps. To prevent electrolyte imbalance and dehydration, take care to give the correct intravenous (IV) solutions and volumes and concentrations of formulas. Periodically obtain urine specific gravity and pH. Urine osmolality provides an indication of hydration, although this factor must be correlated with other assessments (e.g., serum sodium). Hydration is considered adequate when the urine output is 1 to 3 mL/kg/hr.

Provision of Adequate Nutrition and Prevention of Fatigue During Feeding

The feeding method depends on the preterm newborn's feeding abilities and health status. Both nipple and gavage methods are initially supplemented with IV therapy until oral intake is sufficient to support growth (110 to 130 kcal/kg/day). Early, small-volume enteral feedings called *minimal enteral nutrition* via gavage have proved to be of benefit to the very-low-birth-weight infant (see "Methods of Feeding" earlier in the chapter). Formula or breast milk (with or without fortifiers to increase caloric content) is incorporated into the feedings slowly. Gastrointestinal priming with these small-volume enteral feedings is not intended to contribute to the total nutritional intake but rather to enhance gut metabolism. Trophic feedings may also help encourage earlier advancement to full feedings, thereby decreasing the development of NEC and the complications of parenteral nutrition.

Before each feeding, measure abdominal girth and auscultate the abdomen to determine the presence and quality of bowel sounds. Such assessments permit early detection of abdominal distention, visible bowel loops, and decreased peristaltic activity, which may indicate NEC or paralytic ileus. Also check for residual formula in the stomach before feeding when the newborn is fed by gavage. This procedure also can be performed when the nipple-fed newborn presents with abdominal distention. Carefully watch for other signs of feeding intolerance including guaiac-positive stools (occult blood in stools), lactose in the stools (reducing substance in the stools), vomiting, and diarrhea.

Preterm newborns who are ill or who fatigue easily with nipple-feedings are usually fed by gavage. The infant is essentially passive with these methods, thus conserving energy and calories. As the baby matures, gavage feedings are replaced with breast- or bottle-feedings to help strengthen the sucking reflex and meet oral and emotional needs. Signs that indicate readiness for oral feedings are a strong gag reflex, nonnutritive sucking, and rooting behavior. Both low-birth-weight and preterm infants nipple-feed more effectively in a quiet state. Establish a gradual nipple-feeding program, such as one nipple-feeding per day, then one nipple-feeding per shift, and then a nipple-feeding every other feeding. Monitor daily weights because often there is a small weight loss when nipple-feedings are started. After feedings, place the baby on the left side (with support to maintain this position) or on the abdomen to enhance gastric emptying and decrease the chance of aspiration if regurgitation occurs. Gastroesophageal reflux is not uncommon in preterm newborns. Long-term gavage feeding may create nipple aversion that will require developmental occupational therapy interventions.

Involve the parents in feeding their preterm baby (Figure 30–10 ⦿). This involvement is essential to the development of attachment between parents and infant. In addition it teaches parents about the care of their infant and helps them cope with the situation.

● FIGURE 30–10

Father participates in feeding experience with his premature infant.

Prevention of Infection

The nurse is responsible for minimizing the preterm newborn's exposure to pathogenic organisms. The preterm newborn is susceptible to infection because of an immature immune system and thin and permeable skin. Invasive procedures, techniques such as umbilical catheterization and mechanical ventilation, and prolonged hospitalization place the infant at greater risk for infection.

Strict handwashing, reverse isolation, and use of equipment for only one infant help minimize the preterm newborn's exposure to infectious agents. Most nurseries have adopted the standard precautions recommended by the Centers for Disease Control and Prevention (CDC) of isolating every baby, and the Joint Commission on Accreditation of Healthcare Organizations (JCAHO) requirement that staff have short trimmed nails and no artificial nails. Staff members are required to complete a 2- to 3-minute scrub using antibacterial solutions, which inhibit growth of gram-positive cocci and gram-negative rod organisms. Other specific nursing interventions include limiting visitors and requiring visitors to wash their hands. Maintain strict aseptic practices when changing IV tubing and solutions (IV solutions and tubing should be changed every 24 hours or per agency protocols), administering parenteral fluids, and assisting with sterile procedures. Incubators and radiant warmers should be changed weekly. Prevent pressure-area breakdown by changing the baby's position regularly, doing range of motion exercises, and using a sheepskin (covered with a blanket or diaper beneath the infant's head), a water bed, or an air mattress. To avoid skin tears, a protective trans-

parent covering can be applied over vulnerable joints but is used sparingly (Association of Women's Health, Obstetric and Neonatal Nurses [AWHONN], 2001). Chemical skin preps and tape may cause skin trauma and should be avoided as much as possible.

If infection (sepsis) occurs in the preterm newborn, the nurse may be the first to identify its subtle clinical signs. Inform the clinician of the findings immediately and implement the treatment plan per clinician orders. (For specific nursing care required for the newborn with an infection, see "Care of the Newborn with Infection" in Chapter 31. ∞)

Promotion of Parent-Infant Attachment

Preterm newborns can be separated from their parents for prolonged periods after illness or complications that are detected in the first few hours or days following birth. The resultant interruption in parent-newborn bonding necessitates intervention to ensure successful attachment.

Nurses need to take measures to promote positive parental feelings toward the preterm newborn. For example, give photographs of the baby to parents to take home or to the mother if she is in a different hospital or too ill to come to the nursery and visit. Place the infant's first name on the incubator as soon as it is known to help the parents feel that their infant is a unique and special person. Provide a weekly card with the baby's footprint, weight, and length to promote bonding. Give parents the telephone number of the nursery or intensive care unit and the names of staff members so that they have access to information about their baby at any time of the day or night. Encourage visits from siblings and grandparents to foster attachment.

Early parental involvement in the care of and decisions about their baby gives the parents more realistic expectations for their baby. The unique combination of personality characteristics of the infant and of the parents influences the bonding and interactive process for the family. By observing each infant's patterns of behavior and responses, especially sleep-wake states, the nurse can teach parents optimal times for interacting with their infant. Parents need education to develop caregiving skills and to understand the premature infant's behavioral characteristics. Their daily participation (if possible) is encouraged, as are early and frequent visits. Provide opportunities for parents to touch, hold, talk to, and care for the baby. Skin-to-skin (kangaroo care) helps parents feel close to their small infant (Figure 30–11 ●). Kangaroo care has been shown to improve sleep periods and parents' perception of their caregiving ability (Turnage-Carrier, 2004).

The parents and nurse can plan nursing care around the times when the infant is alert and best able to attend. The more knowledge parents have about the meaning of their infant's responses, behaviors, and cues for interaction, the better prepared they will be to meet their newborn's needs and form a positive attachment with their child.

● **FIGURE 30–11**

Kangaroo (skin-to-skin) care facilitates closeness and attachment between parents and their premature infant.

Courtesy of Carol Harrigan, RNC, MSN, NNP.

Parental involvement in difficult care decisions is essential and discussed in greater detail in Chapter 31. ∞

Some parents progress easily to touching and cuddling their infant; others do not. Parents need to know that their feelings are normal and that the progression of acquaintanceship is slow. Rooming-in can provide another opportunity for the stable preterm infant and family to get acquainted; it offers both privacy and readily available help (Figure 30–12 ●).

Promotion of Developmentally Supportive Care

Prolonged separation and the neonatal intensive care unit (NICU) environment necessitate individualized baby sensory stimulation programs. The nurse plays a key role in determining the appropriate type and amount of visual, tactile, and auditory stimulation.

Some preterm infants are not developmentally able to deal with more than one sensory input at a time. The Assessment of Preterm Infant Behavior (APIB) scale (Als, Lester, Tronick et al., 1982) identifies individual preterm newborn behaviors according to five areas of development. The preterm baby's behavioral reactions to stimulation are observed, and developmental interventions are then based on reducing detrimental environmental stimuli to the lowest possible level and providing appropriate opportunities for development (Blackburn, 2003).

The NICU environment contains many detrimental stimuli that the nurse can help reduce. Noise levels can be lowered by replacing alarms with lights or silencing them quickly and keeping conversations away from the baby's bedside. Dimmer switches should be used to shield the baby's eyes from bright lights, and blankets may be placed over the top portion of the incubator. Dimming the lights may encourage infants to open their eyes and be more responsive to their parents. Plan nursing care to decrease the number of times the baby is disturbed. Place signs (e.g., "Quiet Please") near the bedside to allow the baby some periods of uninterrupted sleep (Blackburn, 2003). Some other suggested developmentally supportive interventions include the following:

- Use containment measures when turning or moving the infant or doing procedures such as suctioning. Use the hands to hold the infant's arms and legs, flexed, close to the midline of the body. Containment measures help stabilize the infant's motor and physiologic subsystems during stressful activities.
- Touch the infant gently and avoid sudden postural changes.

● **FIGURE 30–12**

Family bonding occurs when parents have opportunities to spend time with their infant.

Courtesy of Carol Harrigan, RNC, MSN, NNP.

COMPLEMENTARY CARE

COMPLEMENTARY AND ALTERNATIVE MEDICINE (CAM) IN THE NICU

As NICUs are becoming more and more "developmentally" friendly, complementary and alternative medicine (CAM) has now become an adjunct to that nurturing environment. This holistic approach in caring for the low-birth-weight infant attempts not only to mimic the intrauterine environment, but also to foster parent-infant bonding by simultaneously caring for the body, spirit, and mind.

Aromatherapy is the use of scent to alter mood or behavior to produce a calming and sedating effect. There is an enhanced bonding process between mothers and newborns associated with the natural body odor emitted from the mother (Jones, Kassity, & Duncan, 2001). Aromatherapy is utilized in the NICU by placing an article of clothing belonging to the mother next to the infant to produce a soothing and consoling effect on the infant in her absence. Researchers are also investigating other aromatherapies, including peppermint as a respiratory stimulant, chamomile as a method to regulate sleep-wake cycles, Brazilian guava for its analgesic effects, and lavendar sitz baths for management of diaper rash.

Skin-to-skin (kangaroo) care is becoming more prevalent in NICUs across the United States. It was first practiced in Bogota, Colombia, in the early 1980s because of the fear of the spread of infection from sharing incubators (Turnage-Carrier, 2004). Skin-to-skin care is defined as the practice of holding infants skin-to-skin next to their parents. The infant is usually naked, except for a diaper, and placed on his/her parent's bare chest. They are then both covered with a blanket. Benefits of skin-to-skin care as a developmental intervention include the following: improved oxygenation as evidenced by an increase in transcutaneous oxygen levels, enhanced temperature regulation, a decline in the episodes of apnea and bradycardia, increased periods of quiet sleep, stabilization of vital signs, positive interaction between parent and infant which enhances attachment and bonding, increased growth parameters, and early discharge

(McGrath, 2004). Limitations to skin-to-skin care may be due to staff uneasiness when moving the infant while attached to multiple IV lines, monitor leads, and a ventilator. The limited confines of the nursery may be another limiting factor.

Music therapy as a noninvasive auditory stimulus has been shown to be advantageous for the premature infant (Standley, 2001). The music used in NICUs includes primarily lullabies and soft acoustical pieces which are pleasant, soothing, and calming. Such music has been shown to effect newborn physiologic responses, improving oxygenation and increasing weight gain. It also has behavioral effects, leading to enhanced parental bonding and increased intervals of nonnutritive sucking periods. Language development is also enhanced if the music is live and sung by the mother or another female, which is preferential to the infant (Standley, 2001). The overall noise level in the NICU needs to be considered before including any extra auditory stimulation, including music therapy.

Infant massage and gentle touch have been practiced for many centuries. The types of stimulation include massage with stroking, gentle touch without stroking, and therapeutic touch or "hands on" containment. Practitioners report such physiologic benefits as stimulating blood and lymphatic flow, promoting weight gain in premature infants, and regulating sleep patterns. Many emotional and behavioral benefits are also cited by practitioners. Classes are available to teach parents how to perform massage on their infants. Massage demonstrates compassion while increasing the parent's empathy and understanding of the baby. It helps parents learn to interpret their baby's behavioral cues such as facial expression, various crying patterns, and other body language. At the same time it helps infants learn about their various body parts and boundaries and feel how they integrate into the whole. Therapeutic touch reduces motor activity and energy expenditure by the infant and promotes comfort (Harrison, 2001).

- Promote self-consoling and soothing activities, such as placing blanket rolls or approved manufactured devices next to the infant's sides and against the feet to provide "nesting." Swaddle the infant with the extremities in a flexed position and ensure that the hands can reach the face for hand-to-mouth activities, which can be consoling (Figure 30–13 ●).
- Simulate the kinesthetic advantages (decreased motor activity, improved sleep, fewer behavior state changes) of the intrauterine environment by using sheepskin or approved water beds.
- Provide opportunities for nonnutritive sucking with a pacifier. Nonnutritive sucking improves oxygen saturation; decreases body movements; improves sleep, especially after feedings; and increases weight gain.

- Provide objects for the infant to grasp (e.g., a piece of blanket, oxygen tubing, a finger) during caregiving. Grasping may comfort the baby.

Teaching the parents to read behavioral cues will help them move at their infant's own pace when providing stimulation. Parents are ideally equipped to meet the baby's need for stimulation. Stroking, rocking, cuddling, quiet singing, and talking to the baby can all be integral parts of the baby's care. Visual stimulation in the form of *en face* interaction with caregivers and mobiles is also important.

Preparation for Home Care

Parents are often anxious when their premature infant is transferred out of the NICU or is discharged home. Parents of preterm babies should receive the same postpartal teaching as any parent taking a new infant home. In preparing

⊙ FIGURE 30–13

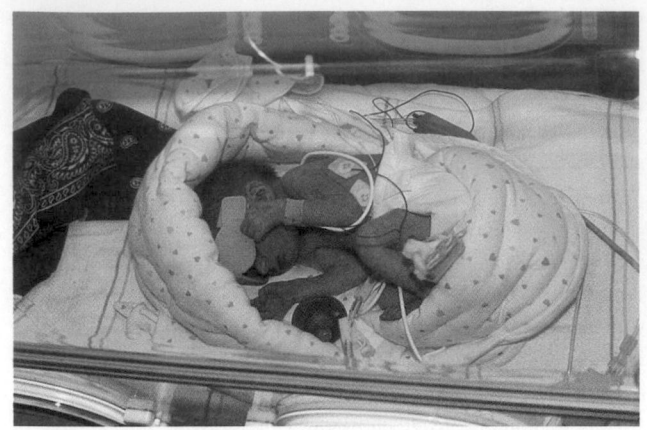

Infant is "nested." Hand-to-mouth behavior facilitates self-consoling and soothing activities.

Courtesy of Theresa Kledzik, RN, Developmental Nurse, Memorial Hospital, Colorado Springs, Colorado.

for discharge, encourage the parents to spend time caring directly for their baby. Direct caregiving familiarizes them with their baby's behavior patterns and helps them establish realistic expectations about the infant. Some NICUs have a special room near the nursery where parents can spend the night with their baby before discharge.

Discharge instruction includes breast- and bottle-feeding techniques, formula preparation, and vitamin administration. If the mother wishes to breastfeed, teach her to pump her breasts to keep the milk flowing and provide milk even before discharge. Give information on bathing, diapering, hygiene, and normal elimination patterns and prepare the parents to expect changes in the color of the baby's stool, number of bowel movements, and timing of elimination when the infant is switched from bottle- to breastfeeding. This information can prevent unnecessary concern by the parents. Also discuss normal growth and development patterns, reflexes, and activity for preterm infants. In these discussions, emphasize ways to promote bonding behaviors and deal with newborn crying. Care of the preterm infant with complications, preventing infections, recognizing signs of a sick baby, and the need for continued medical follow-up are other key issues.

Families with preterm infants usually do not need to be referred to community agencies, such as visiting nurse assistance. However, referral may be necessary if the infant has severe congenital abnormalities, feeding problems, or complications with infections or respiratory problems or if the parents seem unable to cope with an at-risk baby.

Preterm and low-birth-weight infants are at greater risk of increased morbidity from vaccine preventable diseases (Saari & Committee on Infectious Diseases, 2003). The medically stable preterm infant and low-birth-weight infant should receive full doses of diphtheria, tetanus, acellular pertussis, *Haemophilus influenzae* type b, hepatitis B, poliovirus, and pneumococcal conjugate vaccines at a chronologic age consistent with the schedule recommended for full-term infants (Saari & Committee on Infectious Diseases, 2003). The influenza vaccine should be administered at 6 months of age before the beginning of and during the influenza season.

Parents of preterm infants can benefit from meeting with others in a similar situation to share common experiences and concerns. Refer parents to support groups and make connections for parents with early education intervention centers.

EVALUATION

Expected outcomes of nursing care include the following:

■ The preterm newborn is free of respiratory distress and establishes effective respiratory function.

■ The preterm newborn gains weight and shows no signs of fatigue or aspiration during feedings.

■ The parents verbalize their anger and guilt feelings about the birth of a preterm baby and show attachment behavior such as frequent visits and growing confidence in their caregiving activities.

CARE OF THE NEWBORN WITH CONGENITAL ANOMALIES

The birth of a baby with a congenital defect places both newborn and family at risk. Many congenital anomalies can be life threatening if not corrected within hours after birth; others are very visible and cause the families emotional distress. When one congenital anomaly is found, healthcare providers should look for others, particularly in body systems that develop at the same time during gestation. Table 30–2 identifies some common anomalies and their early management and nursing care in the neonatal period. More detailed discussions of these congenital anomalies are found in the appropriate system alterations chapters later in the text.

CARE OF THE NEWBORN OF A SUBSTANCE-ABUSING MOTHER

An **infant of a substance-abusing mother (ISAM)** may also be alcohol or drug dependent. After birth, when an infant's connection with the maternal blood supply is severed, the newborn may suffer withdrawal. In addition the drugs ingested by the mother may be teratogenic, resulting in congenital anomalies or in developmental problems.

ALCOHOL DEPENDENCE

The **fetal alcohol syndrome (FAS)** includes a series of malformations frequently found in infants exposed to alcohol in utero. It has been estimated that complete FAS occurs in up to 5 live births per 1000 (Martinez, Partridge, & Taeusch, 2005). FAS rates are higher among Native Americans, Alaska Natives, African Americans, and women of low socioeconomic status. Fetal alcohol effects (FAE), or **alcohol-related birth defects (ARBD)**, are usually determined only by a positive maternal drinking history and

TABLE 30–2 ✤ Congenital Anomalies: Identification and Care in Newborn Period

Congenital Anomaly	Nursing Assessments	Nursing Goals and Interventions
Congenital hydrocephalus (*Enlarged head*)	Enlarged or full fontanelles Split or widened sutures "Setting sun" eyes Head circumference > 90% on growth chart	Assess presence of hydrocephalus: Measure and plot occipital–frontal baseline measurements; then measure head circumference once a day. Check fontanelle for bulging and sutures for widening. Assist with head ultrasound and transillumination. Maintain skin integrity. Change position frequently. Clean skin creases after feeding or vomiting. Use sheepskin pillow under head. Postoperatively, position head off operative site. Watch for signs of infection.
Choanal atresia (*Occlusion of posterior nares*)	Cyanosis and retractions at rest Snorting respirations Difficulty breathing during feeding Obstruction by thick mucus	Assess patency of nares: Listen for breath sounds while holding baby's mouth closed and alternately compressing each nostril. Assist with passing feeding tube to confirm diagnosis. Maintain respiratory function: Assist with taping airway in mouth to prevent respiratory distress. Position with head elevated to improve air exchange.
Cleft lip (*Unilateral or bilateral visible defect*)	May involve external nares, nasal cartilage, nasal septum, and alveolar process Flattening or depression of midfacial contour (At left) Unilateral cleft lip with cleft abnormality involving both hard and soft palates. (*Courtesy Marcia London RNC, APRN, NNP*)	Provide nutrition: Feed with special nipple. Burp frequently (increased tendency to swallow air and reflex vomiting). Clean cleft with sterile water (to prevent crusting on cleft prior to repair). Support parental coping: Assist parents with grief over loss of idealized baby. Encourage verbalization of their feelings about visible defect. Provide role model in interacting with infant: Parents internalize others' responses to their newborn.
Cleft palate (*Fissure connecting oral and nasal cavity*)	May involve uvula and soft palate May extend forward to nostril involving hard palate and maxillary aveolar ridge Difficulty in sucking Expulsion of formula through nose	Prevent aspiration/infection: Place prone or in side-lying position to facilitate drainage. Suction nasopharyngeal cavity (to prevent aspiration or airway obstruction). During newborn period, feed in upright position with head and chest tilted slightly backward (to aid swallowing and discourage aspiration). Provide nutrition: Feed with special nipple that fills cleft and allows sucking. Also decreases chance of aspiration through nasal cavity. Clean mouth with water after feedings. Burp after each ounce (tend to swallow large amounts of air). Thicken formula to provide extra calories. Plot weight gain patterns to assess adequacy of diet. Provide parental support: Refer parents to community agencies and support groups. Encourage verbalization of frustrations because feeding process is long and frustrating. Praise all parental efforts. Encourage parents to seek prompt treatment for upper respiratory infection (URI) and teach them ways to decrease URI.

(continued)

TABLE 30–2 ✤ Congenital Anomalies: Identification and Care in Newborn Period—continued

Congenital Anomaly	Nursing Assessments	Nursing Goals and Interventions
Tracheoesophageal fistula (type 3) (*Connection between trachea and esophagus*)	History of maternal hydramnios Excessive mucous secretions Constant drooling Abdominal distention beginning soon after birth Periodic choking and cyanotic episodes Immediate regurgitation of feeding Clinical symptoms of aspiration pneumonia (tachypnea, retractions, rhonchi, decreased breath sounds, cyanotic spells) Failure to pass nasogastric tube	Maintain respiratory status and prevent aspiration. Withhold feeding until esophageal patency is determined. Quickly assess patency before putting to breast in birth area. Place on low intermittent suction to control saliva and mucus (to prevent aspiration pneumonia). Place in warmed, humidified incubator (liquefies secretions, facilitating removal). Elevate head of bed 20–40 degrees (to prevent reflux of gastric juices). Keep quiet (crying causes air to pass through fistula and to distend intestines, causing respiratory embarrassment). Maintain fluid and electrolyte balance. Give fluids to replace esophageal drainage and maintain hydration. Provide parent education: Explain staged repair—provision of gastrostomy and ligation of fistula, then repair of atresia. Keep parents informed; clarify and reinforce physician's explanations regarding malformation, surgical repair, pre- and postoperative care, and prognosis (knowledge is ego strengthening). Involve parents in care of infant and in planning for future; facilitate touch and eye contact (to dispel feelings of inadequacy, increase self-esteem and self-worth, and promote incorporation of infant into family).

Esophagus

Trachea

(At left) The most frequently seen type of congenital tracheoesophageal fistula and esophageal atresia.

Diaphragmatic hernia (*Portion of intestines in the thoracic cavity through abnormal opening in diaphragm*)	Difficulty initiating respirations Gasping respirations with nasal flaring and chest retraction Barrel chest and scaphoid abdomen Asymmetric chest expansion Breath sounds may be absent, usually on left side Heart sounds displaced to right Spasmodic attacks of cyanosis and difficulty in feeding Bowel sounds may be heard in thoracic cavity	Never ventilate with bag and mask O$_2$ because the stomach will inflate, further compressing the lungs. Maintain respiratory status: Immediately administer oxygen. Initiate gastric decompression. Place in high semi-Fowler's position (to use gravity to keep abdominal organs' pressure off diaphragm). Turn to affected side to allow unaffected lung expansion. Carry out interventions to alleviate respiratory and metabolic acidosis. Assess for increased secretions around suction tube (denotes possible obstruction). Aspirate and irrigate tube with air or sterile water.

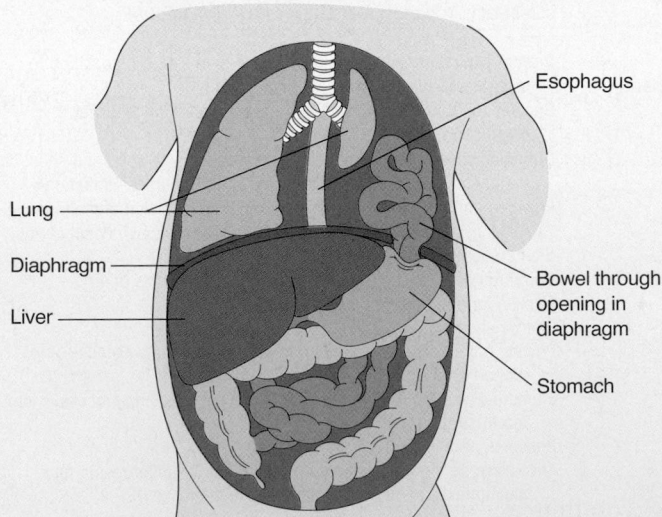

Esophagus

Lung

Diaphragm

Liver

Bowel through opening in diaphragm

Stomach

(At left) Diaphragmatic hernia. Note compression of the lung by the intestine on the affected side. (*Used with permission from Nancy Houck, RNC, BSN, NNP*)

TABLE 30-2 ✤ Congenital Anomalies: Identification and Care in Newborn Period—continued

Congenital Anomaly	Nursing Assessments	Nursing Goals and Interventions
Myelomeningocele (Saclike cyst containing meninges, spinal cord, and nerve roots in thoracic and/or lumbar area)	Myelomeningocele directly connects to subarachnoid space, so hydrocephalus is often associated No response or varying response to sensation below level of sac May have constant dribbling of urine Incontinence or retention of stool Anal opening may be flaccid 	Prevent trauma and infection. Position on abdomen or on side and restrain (to prevent pressure and trauma to sac). Meticulously clean buttocks and genitals after each voiding and defecation (to prevent contamination of sac and decrease possibility of infection). May put protective covering over sac (to prevent rupture and drying). Observe sac for oozing of fluid or pus. Credé bladder (apply downward pressure on bladder with thumbs, moving urine toward the urethra) as ordered to prevent urinary stasis. Assess amount of sensation and movement below defect. Observe for complications. Obtain occipital frontal circumference baseline measurements; then measure head circumference once a day (to detect hydrocephalus). Check fontanelle for bulging. (At left) Newborn with lumbar myelomeningocele. (Used with permission from Dr. Paul Winchester)
Omphalocele (Herniation of abdominal contents into base of umbilical cord)	May have an enclosed transparent sac covering	Maintain hydration and temperature. Provide D₅LR and albumin for hypovolemia. Place infant in sterile bag up to and covering defect. Cover sac with moistened sterile gauze, and place plastic wrap over dressing (to prevent rupture of sac and infection). Initiate gastric decompression by insertion of nasogastric tube attached to low suction (to prevent distention of lower bowel and impairment of blood flow). Prevent infection and trauma to defect. Position to prevent trauma to defect. Administer broad-spectrum antibiotics.
Imperforate anus, congenital dislocated hip, and clubfoot	See discussion starting in Chapter 27, "Anus and Extremities" ∞	Identify defect and initiate appropriate referral early.

cognitive difficulties. These infants usually do not exhibit the classic facial dysmorphology (Moran, 2004). Another term applied to these children is alcohol-related neurodevelopmental disorder (ARND). These children have CNS, behavior, and cognitive abnormalities (Moran, 2004). The new diagnostic categories for FAS take into consideration the various clinical manifestations of FAS, the social and family environment, and, if available, the maternal alcohol history.

Although it is known that ethanol freely crosses the placenta to the fetus, it is still not known whether the alcohol alone or the breakdown products of alcohol cause the damage. ("Care of the Woman with Substance Abuse Problems" in Chapter 14 discusses alcohol abuse in pregnancy. ∞) The effects of other substances often com-bined with alcohol, such as nicotine, diazepam (Valium), marijuana, and caffeine, as well as poor diet, enhance the likelihood of FAS.

Long-Term Complications for the Infant with FAS

The long-term prognosis for the FAS newborn is less than favorable. Many FAS infants are evaluated for organic and inorganic failure to thrive. These infants have a delay in oral feeding development but have a normal progression of oral motor function. Many FAS infants feed poorly and have persistent vomiting until 6 to 7 months of age. They have difficulty adjusting to solid foods and show little spontaneous interest in food.

Central nervous system dysfunctions are the most common and serious problem associated with FAS. Hypotonicity and increased placidity are seen in these infants. They also have a decreased ability to block out repetitive stimuli. Children exhibiting FAS can be severely mentally retarded or have normal intelligence. Generally the more abnormal the facial features, the lower the IQ scores. Often there is little improvement in intelligence (as measured by IQ) despite positive environmental and educational factors (Moran, 2004). These children show impulsivity, cognitive impairment, and speech and language abnormalities indicative of CNS involvement (Moran, 2004).

NURSING MANAGEMENT

NURSING ASSESSMENT AND DIAGNOSIS

The nurse assesses the newborn for the following characteristics typical of FAS:

- **Abnormal structural development and CNS dysfunction.** Examples include mental retardation, microcephaly, and hyperactivity.

- **Growth deficiencies.** Infants with FAS are often growth retarded; weight, length, and head circumference are affected. These infants show a persistent postnatal growth deficiency, with head circumference and linear growth most affected.

- **Distinctive facial abnormalities.** These include short palpebral fissures; epicanthal folds; broad nasal bridge; flattened midfacies; short, upturned, or beaklike nose; micrognathia (abnormally small lower jaw); hypoplastic maxilla; thin upper lip or vermilion border; and smooth philtrum (groove on upper lip) (Martinez et al., 2005).

- **Associated anomalies.** Abnormalities affecting cardiac (primarily septal and valvular defects), ocular, renal, and skeletal (especially involving joints, such as congenital dislocated hips) systems are often noted.

In the first week of life, an alcohol-exposed newborn may show symptoms that include sleeplessness, excessive arousal states, unconsolable crying, abnormal reflexes, hyperactivity with little ability to maintain alertness and attentiveness to environment, jitteriness, abdominal distention, and exaggerated mouthing behaviors such as hyperactive rooting and increased nonnutritive sucking. These symptoms commonly persist throughout the first month of life but may continue longer. The infant's alcohol dependence is physiologic, not psychologic. Signs and symptoms of withdrawal often appear within 6 to 12 hours and at least within the first 3 days of life. Seizures after the neonatal period are rare.

NURSING DIAGNOSIS

Nursing diagnoses that may apply to the FAS newborn include the following:

- *Altered Nutrition: Less than Body Requirement* related to decreased food intake and hyperirritability

- *Alteration in Neurodevelopment Status* related to central nervous system involvement secondary to maternal alcohol use

- *Ineffective Coping* related to dysfunctional family dynamics and substance-dependent mother

PLANNING AND IMPLEMENTATION

Hospital-Based Nursing Care

Nursing care of the FAS newborn is aimed at avoiding heat loss, providing adequate nutrition, and reducing environmental stimuli. The FAS baby is most comfortable in a quiet, dimly lit environment. Because of their feeding problems, these infants require extra time and patience during feedings. It is important to provide consistency in the staff working with the baby and parents and to keep personnel and visitors to a minimum at any one time.

Tell the alcohol-dependent mother that breastfeeding is not contraindicated but that excessive alcohol consumption may intoxicate the newborn and inhibit the letdown reflex. Monitor the newborn's vital signs closely and observe for evidence of seizure activity and respiratory distress.

Nursing Care in the Community

Infants affected by maternal alcohol abuse are also at risk psychologically. Restlessness, sleeplessness, agitation, resistance to cuddling or holding, and frequent crying can be frustrating to parents because their efforts to relieve the distress are unrewarded. Feeding difficulties can also result in frustrations for the caregiver and digestive upsets for the infant. Frustration may cause the parents to punish the baby or result in the unconscious desire to stay away from the infant. Either outcome may create an unstable family environment and result in failure to thrive.

Focus on providing support for the parents and reinforcing positive parenting activity. Prior to discharge, give parents opportunities to provide baby care so that they can feel confident about interpreting their baby's cues and meeting the baby's needs. Referring the family to social services and visiting nurse or public health nurse associations is essential for the well-being of the infant. Follow-up care and teaching can strengthen the parents' skills and coping abilities and help them create a stable, healthy environment for their family. The infant with FAS or ARBD should be involved in intervention programs that monitor the child's developmental progress, health, and home environment.

EVALUATION

Expected outcomes of nursing care include the following:

- The FAS newborn is able to tolerate feedings and gain weight.

- The FAS infant's hyperirritability or seizures are controlled, and the baby has suffered no physical injuries.

- The parents are able to identify the special needs of their newborn and accept outside assistance as needed.

DRUG DEPENDENCY

Drugs abused by the pregnant woman can include the following legal and illegal substances, used alone or in combination: tobacco, cocaine, phencyclidine (PCP), methamphetamines, inhalants, marijuana, heroin, and methadone. Patterns of abuse of alcohol, marijuana, and heroin in childbearing women have changed very little in the past few years. The incidence of cocaine (especially "crack") use may have stabilized but oxycodone (OxyContin) use has risen dramatically (see "Substances Commonly Abused During Pregnancy" in Chapter 14 for more discussion of maternal substance abuse ∞). Marijuana, alcohol, and nicotine are sometimes used in conjunction with cocaine.

Drug-dependent infants are predisposed to a number of problems. Since almost all drugs cross the placenta and enter the fetal circulation, the fetus can develop problems in utero or soon after birth. The effects of polydrug use on the newborn must always be taken into consideration.

The greatest risks to the fetus of the drug-abusing mother are as follows:

- **Intrauterine asphyxia.** Asphyxia is often a direct result of fetal withdrawal secondary to maternal withdrawal. Fetal withdrawal is accompanied by hyperactivity, with increased oxygen consumption. Insufficiency of oxygen can lead to fetal asphyxia. Moreover, women addicted to narcotics tend to have a higher incidence of preeclampsia, abruptio placentae, and placenta previa, resulting in placental insufficiency and fetal asphyxia.

- **Intrauterine infection.** Sexually transmitted infection, HIV infection, and hepatitis are often connected with the pregnant addict's lifestyle. Such infections can involve the fetus.

- **Alterations in birth weight.** These alterations may depend on the type of drug the mother uses. Women who smoke or use heroin have infants of lower birth weight who are SGA. Women maintained on methadone have infants of higher birth weight, some of whom are LGA.

- **Low Apgar scores.** Low scores may be related to the intrauterine asphyxia or the medication the woman received during labor. The use of a narcotic antagonist (nalorphine or naloxone) to reverse respiratory depression is contraindicated because it may precipitate acute withdrawal in the infant.

Common Complications of the Drug-Dependent Newborn

The newborn of a woman who abused drugs during her pregnancy is predisposed to the following problems:

- **Respiratory distress.** The heroin-addicted newborn frequently suffers respiratory stress, mainly meconium-aspiration pneumonia and transient tachypnea. Meconium aspiration is usually secondary to increased oxygen consumption and activity experienced by the fetus during intrauterine withdrawal. Transient tachypnea may develop because narcotics inhibit the reflex responsible for clearing the lungs. Respiratory distress syndrome, however, occurs less often in heroin-addicted newborns, even in those who are premature, because they have tissue-oxygen-unloading capabilities comparable to those of a 6-week-old term infant. In addition, heroin stimulates production of glucocorticoids via the anterior pituitary gland.

- **Jaundice.** Newborns of methadone-addicted women may develop jaundice due to prematurity. By contrast, infants of mothers addicted to heroin or cocaine have a lower incidence of hyperbilirubinemia because these substances contribute to early maturity of the liver.

- **Congenital anomalies and growth retardation.** Anomalies of the genitourinary and cardiovascular systems are slightly more common in infants of heroin- and cocaine-addicted mothers. Infants of cocaine-addicted mothers exhibit congenital malformations involving bony skull defects, such as microencephaly, and symmetric intrauterine growth restriction, cardiac defects, and genitourinary defects.

- **Behavioral abnormalities.** Babies exposed to cocaine have poor state organization. They exhibit decreased interactive behaviors when tested with the Brazelton Neonatal Behavioral Assessment Scale. These infants also have difficulty moving through the various sleep and awake states and have problems attending to and actively engaging in auditory and visual stimuli.

- **Withdrawal.** The most significant postnatal problem of the drug-exposed newborn is opiate withdrawal (usually from heroin or methadone). Withdrawal manifestations often begin after discharge, especially with short birthing unit stays. See "Clinical Manifestations" for a discussion of withdrawal symptoms.

CLINICAL MANIFESTATIONS

NEWBORN WITHDRAWAL

Central Nervous System Signs

- Hyperactivity
- Hyperirritability (persistent shrill cry)
- Increased muscle tone
- Exaggerated reflexes
- Tremors and myoclonic jerks
- Sneezing, hiccups, yawning
- Short, unquiet sleep
- Fever (accompanies the increased neuromuscular activities)

Respiratory Signs

- Tachypnea (> 60 breaths per minute when quiet)
- Excessive secretions

Gastrointestinal Signs

- Disorganized, vigorous suck
- Vomiting
- Drooling
- Sensitive gag reflex
- Hyperphagia
- Diarrhea
- Abdominal cramping
- Poor feeding (< 15 mL on first day of life; takes longer than 30 minutes per feeding)

Vasomotor Signs

- Stuffy nose, yawning, sneezing
- Flushing
- Sweating
- Sudden, circumoral pallor

Cutaneous signs

- Excoriated buttocks, knees, elbows
- Facial scratches
- Pressure-point abrasions

Long-Term Effects

During the first 2 years of life, many cocaine-exposed infants demonstrate behavior lability and are unable to express strong feelings such as pleasure, anger, or distress, or even a strong reaction to being separated from their parents. Cocaine-exposed infants may be at higher risk for motor development problems, delays in expressive language skills, and feeding difficulties because of swallowing problems (Martinez et al., 2005).

Infants of drug-addicted mothers often have a higher incidence of gastrointestinal and respiratory illnesses. These illnesses can be related not to drug exposure but to the mother's lack of education regarding proper infant care, feeding, and hygiene.

Another important long-term complication is the high rate of SIDS in heroin- or methadone-exposed infants and for infants who have a high neonatal abstinence score (Moran, 2004). The infant born to a drug-dependent mother may also be neglected, abused, or both.

Clinical Therapy

For optimal fetal and neonatal outcome, the opiate-addicted woman should receive complete prenatal care as early as possible (see Chapter 14 ∞) and pharmacologic management of neonatal withdrawal. She should be started on a methadone program (Martinez et al., 2005) that prevents heroin use during pregnancy. It is not recommended that the woman be withdrawn completely from narcotics while pregnant because it induces fetal withdrawal with poor newborn outcomes. Unfortunately, pregnant women may be denied access to programs for substance abusers.

Newborn treatment may include management of newborn complications; serologic tests for syphilis, HIV, and hepatitis B; urine drug screen and meconium analysis; and social service referral. Drugs used to control withdrawal symptoms vary and may be regionally based. They include phenobarbital, paregoric, oral morphine sulfate solution, and diazepam (Blackburn, 2003). Nutritional support is important in light of the increase in energy expenditure that withdrawal may entail.

NURSING MANAGEMENT

NURSING ASSESSMENT AND DIAGNOSIS

Early identification of the newborn needing medical or pharmacologic interventions because of maternal substance abuse decreases the incidence of neonatal mortality and morbidity. During the newborn period, nursing assessment focuses on:

- Discovering the mother's last drug intake and dosage level through the perinatal history and laboratory tests. Women may be reluctant to disclose this information; therefore, a nonjudgmental interview technique is essential (Andres, 2004).

- Assessing for congenital malformations and the complications related to intrauterine withdrawal such as SGA, intrauterine asphyxia, meconium aspiration, and prematurity.

- Identifying the signs and symptoms of newborn withdrawal or neonatal abstinence syndrome.

Although many signs and symptoms of drug withdrawal are similar to those seen with hypoglycemia and hypocalcemia, drug-addicted babies have normal glucose, and calcium values are reported to be within normal limits for these infants.

Neonatal abstinence syndrome includes both physiologic and behavioral responses. Assess the severity of withdrawal with a scoring system such as the Finnegan scale that is based on observations and measurement of the responses to neonatal abstinence. The system evaluates the infant on potentially life-threatening signs such as vomiting, diarrhea, weight loss, irritability, tremors, and tachypnea (Table 30–3).

Nursing diagnoses that may apply to drug-dependent newborns include the following:

- *High Risk for Infant CNS Injury* related to perinatal substance abuse
- *Risk for Ineffective Airway Clearance* related to suppression of respiratory system
- *Altered Nutrition: Less than Body Requirements* related to vomiting and diarrhea, uncoordinated suck and swallow reflex, and hypertonia secondary to withdrawal
- *Impaired Skin Integrity* related to constant activity

TABLE 30–3 ✤ Neonatal Abstinence Score Sheet

NEONATAL ABSTINENCE SCORING SYSTEM

System	Signs and Symptoms	Score	am	pm	Comments
Central Nervous System Disturbances	Excessive high-pitched (or other) cry	2			Daily weight:
	Continuous high-pitched (or other) cry	3			
	Sleeps < 1 hour after feeding	3			
	Sleeps < 2 hours after feeding	2			
	Sleeps < 3 hours after feeding	1			
	Hyperactive Moro reflex	2			
	Markedly hyperactive Moro reflex	3			
	Mild tremors disturbed	1			
	Moderate-severe tremors disturbed	2			
	Mild tremors undisturbed	3			
	Moderate-severe tremors undisturbed	4			
	Increased muscle tone	2			
	Excoriation (specific area)	1			
	Myoclonic jerks	3			
	Generalized convulsions	5			
Metabolic/Vasomotor/ Respiratory Disturbances	Sweating	1			
	Fever < 101 (99–100.8°F/37.2–38.2°C)	1			
	Fever > 101 (38.4°C and higher)	2			
	Frequent yawning (> 3–4 times/interval)	1			
	Mottling	1			
	Nasal stuffiness	1			
	Sneezing (> 3–4 times/interval)	1			
	Nasal flaring	2			
	Respiratory rate > 60/min	1			
	Respiratory rate > 60/min with retractions	2			
Gastrointestinal Disturbances	Excessive sucking	1			
	Poor feeding	2			
	Regurgitation	2			
	Projectile vomiting	3			
	Loose stools	2			
	Watery stools	3			
	Total Score				
	Initials of Scorer				

Used with permission from Finnegan, L. P. (1990). Neonatal abstinence syndrome. In Nelson, N. (Ed.), *Current therapy in neonatal-perinatal medicine* (2nd ed.). Ontario: BC Decker.

- *Sleep Pattern Disturbance* related to CNS excitation secondary to drug withdrawal
- *Risk for Altered Parenting* related to lack of knowledge of infant care
- *Ineffective Family Coping: Disabling* related to drug-dependent parent

PLANNING AND IMPLEMENTATION

Hospital-Based Nursing Care

Care of the drug-dependent newborn is based on reducing withdrawal symptoms and promoting adequate respiration, temperature, and nutrition. See "Nursing Care Plan: The Newborn of a Substance-Abusing Mother" for specific nursing measures.

General nursery care measures include:

- Monitoring temperature for hypothermia.
- Careful monitoring of pulse and respirations every 15 minutes until stable; stimulation if apnea occurs.
- Small, frequent feedings, especially if the infant has vomiting, regurgitation, and diarrhea.
- Intravenous therapy as needed.
- Medications as ordered, such as oral morphine, phenobarbital, tincture of opium, and paregoric. Use of paregoric is controversial because it contains alcohol and camphor (Thureen, Deacon, Hernandez et al., 2005).
- Proper positioning on the right side-lying or semi-Fowler's to avoid possible aspiration of vomitus or secretions.
- Monitoring frequency of diarrhea and vomiting and weighing infant every 8 hours during withdrawal.
- Observing for problems of SGA or LGA newborns.
- Swaddling with hands near mouth to minimize injury and help achieve more organized behavioral state. (Offer a pacifier for nonnutritive, excessive sucking. Gentle, vertical rocking can be successful in calming an infant who is out of control.) (See Figure 30–14 ⊙ .)
- Placing newborn in quiet, dimly lit area of nursery.
- Protecting face and extremities from excoriation by using mittens and soft sheets or sheepskin.

Nursing Care in the Community

Parents need assistance to prepare for what they can expect in the first few months at home. At the time of discharge, tell the mother to anticipate mild jitteriness and irritability in the newborn, which may persist from 6 days to 8 weeks, depending on the initial severity of the withdrawal (Blackburn, 2003). Infants with neonatal abstinence syndrome are at a significantly higher risk for SIDS when the mother

⊙ **FIGURE 30–14**

Nonnutritive suckling on a pacifier has a calming effect on a newborn.

used heroin or cocaine. The infant should sleep supine, and home apnea monitoring should be implemented. Help the mother learn feeding techniques, comforting measures, how to recognize newborn cues, and appropriate parenting responses. Counsel parents about available resources, such as support groups, and when to seek further care. Ongoing evaluation is necessary because of the potential for long-term problems. Follow-up on missed appointments can bring parents back into the healthcare system, thereby improving parent and infant outcomes and promoting a positive, interactive environment after birth.

EVALUATION

Expected outcomes of nursing care include the following:

- The newborn tolerates feedings, gains weight, and has a decreased number of stools.
- The parents learn ways to comfort their newborn.
- The parents cope with their frustrations and begin to use outside resources as needed.

INFANTS OF MOTHERS WHO ARE TOBACCO DEPENDENT

Despite increased knowledge about the dangers of smoking to the fetus and newborn, 15–25% of women continue to smoke during pregnancy (Martinez et al., 2005). The common consequence of tobacco use is addiction to nicotine. Most smokers report true enjoyment, associated with a sense

NURSING CARE PLAN

THE NEWBORN OF A SUBSTANCE-ABUSING MOTHER

Intervention	Rationale	Expected Outcome

1. Nursing Diagnosis: High Risk for Infant CNS Injury related to perinatal substance abuse

NIC Intervention: **Newborn monitoring:** Measurement and interpretation of physiologic status of the newborn the first 24 hours after birth		**NOC Outcome:** **Neurologic status:** Extent to which the peripheral and central nervous systems receive, process, and respond to internal and external stimuli

Goal: The newborn will be free of signs and symptoms of CNS injury.

■ Obtain prenatal records and question patient about history of drug addiction. Include duration, type of drug or drugs used, and time and amount of last dose taken prior to birth. ■ Assess newborn for signs and symptoms of withdrawal (i.e., high-pitched shrill cry, sneezing, vomiting, diarrhea, hypertonicity, restlessness, and wakefulness). ■ Provide a quiet and calm environment. Swaddle infant tightly and place in a side-lying or prone position. ■ Carefully plan tests and treatments to avoid excessive stimuli. ■ Use soothing techniques such as rocking, cuddling, soft music, and soft tones when speaking. ■ Administer appropriate medications as ordered by physician. Monitor efficacy and side effects of these medications, which may include paregoric and phenobarbital.	■ Noting the mother's last drug ingestion will provide the medical staff with an approximate time frame to expect the infant to exhibit withdrawal symptoms. ■ The average symptoms of withdrawal occur 72 hours after birth; however, symptoms may appear as early as 6-24 hours after birth. ■ Providing a quiet environment decreases stimuli, therefore reducing CNS symptoms. ■ Planning care promotes rest and reduces external stimuli. ■ These activities promote comfort, security, and infant bonding. ■ These medications aid patient in alleviating symptoms related to withdrawal.	■ Infant will have no signs and symptoms of CNS injury as evidenced by reduced hyperactivity and irritability, normal sleep-wake pattern, no jitteriness, and no seizure activity.

2. Nursing Diagnosis: Risk for Ineffective Airway Clearance related to suppression of respiratory system

NIC Intervention: **Respiratory monitoring:** Collection and analysis of patient data to ensure airway patency and adequate gas exchange		**NOC Outcome:** **Respiratory status:** Gas exchange: Alveolar exchange of CO_2 or O_2 to maintain arterial blood gas concentrations

Goal: Infant will be free of signs and symptoms of respiratory distress after birth.

■ Obtain maternal prenatal, labor, and birth records. ■ Assess infant's respiratory rate and effort, skin color, heart rate, presence or absence of cough reflex, and symptoms of respiratory distress. ■ Position infant in a side-lying or semi-Fowler's position. ■ Monitor infant for temperature elevation.	■ Provides information of fetal stress that may have occurred during the prenatal or intrapartum period. In addition the birth record will provide information concerning infant's respiratory status at birth; for example, the Apgar score. ■ Maternal narcotic consumption may depress the cough reflex and respiratory center of the infant after birth. Symptoms such as cyanosis, tachycardia, grunting, retractions, and nasal flaring may indicate hypoxia. ■ Prevents aspiration. ■ Temperature elevation may cause metabolic rate and oxygen needs to increase when associated with CNS stimulation.	■ The infant will maintain adequate respiratory gas exchange as evidenced by: respirations are 30–60 breaths/min and arterial blood gases are within normal range.

(continued)

THE NEWBORN OF A SUBSTANCE-ABUSING MOTHER

Intervention	Rationale	Expected Outcome
Collaboration: Obtain arterial blood gases (ABGs) as ordered by physician. ■ Monitor infant's cardiac status and pulmonary status using ECG and pulse oximetry.	■ Oxygen demands increase with drug withdrawal. Obtaining ABGs will provide medical personnel baseline information of infant's respiratory status, and effective medical interventions can be initiated. ■ Provides medical personnel with cardiac and pulmonary status.	

3. Nursing Diagnosis: Altered Nutrition: Less than Body Requirements related to vomiting and diarrhea, uncoordinated suck and swallow reflex, and hypertonia secondary to withdrawal

NIC Intervention: **Nutrition therapy:** Administration of food and fluids to support metabolic processes of a patient who is malnourished or at high risk for becoming malnourished		**NOC Outcome:** **Nutritional status:** Extent to which nutrients are available to meet metabolic needs

Goal: The infant will gain or maintain weight.

■ Review gestational age assessment. ■ Assess infant's sucking and swallowing reflexes. ■ Monitor regurgitation, vomiting, and diarrhea. ■ Use bulb syringe before feedings if having problems with nasal stuffiness and congestion. ■ Initiate appropriate feedings per physician's orders (i.e., oral, gavage, or IV feedings). ■ Provide small frequent feedings of a high-calorie formula. ■ Position infant on right side after feedings. ■ Monitor infant's weight and document on graph.	■ Oral feeding may be difficult due to CNS hyperactivity and GI hypermobility. ■ GI hypermobility, irritation, and CNS stimulation can increase nutritional needs. ■ Allows infant to breathe easier by ridding the nasal passages of excessive mucus. ■ Facilitates nutritional intake because SGA infants require 110-120 kcal/kg/day for adequate nutrition. ■ Prevents regurgitation and promotes gastric emptying. ■ Identifies abnormalities in weight gain or loss and allows for early intervention when necessary.	■ The infant will tolerate feedings, maintain weight, or gain weight as evidenced by no regurgitation or aspiration of feedings, and adequate weight gain according to weight graph.

4. Nursing Diagnosis: Risk for Altered Parenting related to lack of knowledge of infant care

NIC Intervention: **Teaching:** Infant care: Instruction on nurturing and physical care needed during the first year of life		**NOC Outcome:** **Parenting:** Provision of an environment that promotes optimum growth and development of dependent children

Goal: The parent will demonstrate ability to independently provide infant care.

■ Assess mother's desire to learn infant care tasks. Evaluate her present physical and emotional stability. ■ Instruct mother on coping strategies (i.e., exercise, listening to music, and discussing concerns openly) to manage stressful situations. ■ Assess mother's insight into her own chemical dependency. ■ Instruct mother on signs and symptoms of withdrawal and treatment interventions. ■ Encourage mother and family members to perform basic infant care tasks.	■ Will provide knowledge of mother's ability to care for infant. ■ Will give mother the tools to handle stress, thereby decreasing the chances of exhibiting abusive behavior. ■ Assistance in enrollment into a chemical dependency program may be necessary before mother can independently care for infant. ■ Assists the mother in understanding infant's behaviors and gives her the tools to intervene without feeling anxious. ■ Facilitates attachment and increases parenting competence.	■ The parent will demonstrate ability to perform basic infant care tasks as evidenced by exhibiting appropriate attachment behaviors (i.e., talking and holding infant), feeding infant, and bathing infant.

of relaxation during stress, especially with the first cigarette of the day (CDC, 2005). The tobacco-induced hazards on the pregnant woman and her developing fetus may be one of the most underrated health issues, at least in public opinion.

Preconceptual cigarette smoking has been found to increase infertility. Fortunately the reduction in fertility is reversible if the woman stops smoking. Smoking during pregnancy has been associated with spontaneous abortion, placenta previa, and abruptio placentae. See "Tobacco" in Chapter 11 for discussion of maternal care. ∞

Risks of Tobacco to the Fetus and Newborn

The most studied compound found in cigarette smoke that can adversely affect the intrauterine environment is carbon monoxide. Carbon monoxide binds hemoglobin to form carboxyhemoglobin, which reduces the oxygen-carrying capacity of the blood. It also increases the binding of hemoglobin to oxygen, which impairs the release of oxygen to the tissues. Therefore, the fetus can experience intrauterine hypoxia (Martinez et al., 2005). Mothers who smoke during pregnancy are nearly twice as likely to have a LBW infant, and smoking during pregnancy is responsible for 20% to 30% of all LBW infants (Law, Stroud, LaGasse et al., 2003). The nicotine in cigarettes acts as a neuroteratogen that interferes with fetal development, specifically the developing nervous system. The greatest risks to the fetus and newborn of the mother who smokes include the following (Law et al., 2003):

- *Intrauterine growth restriction or prematurity* secondary to cigarette metabolites crossing the placenta, which cause vasoconstriction and decreased uterine blood flow
- *Intrauterine distress* presenting as meconium staining and low Apgar scores
- *Neonatal neurobehavioral abnormalities* such as impaired habituation, orientation, consolability, orientation to sound
- *Hypertonia or hypotonia, tremors, hyperactive Moro reflex*
- *Signs of nicotine toxicity* (tachycardia, irritability, poor feeding)

Clinical Therapy

Prevention is always the best intervention. Inquiry into tobacco and smoke exposure should be a routine part of the prenatal history. Preconception and prenatal counseling about the effects of cigarette smoking on pregnancy and the fetus should occur. It is estimated that there would be a 10% reduction in perinatal mortality and an 11% reduction in the incidence of low birth weight if smoking during pregnancy were eliminated (AAP & ACOG, 2002).

Cotinine, a metabolite of nicotine, has been found in fetal body fluids. There is also a positive correlation between the number of cigarettes smoked per day and concentration of cotinine in maternal urine. Other factors that influence fetal and maternal serum cotinine concentrations are nicotine content of the cigarette and the time elapsed between the last cigarette smoked and the sampling. These findings indicate that cotinine may be used as a marker of maternal-fetal tobacco exposure during pregnancy (Martinez et al., 2005).

NURSING CARE MANAGEMENT

Mothers should be counseled that eliminating or reducing smoking even late in pregnancy can improve fetal growth. The use of nicotine patches (instead of smoking) reduces the absorption of nicotine and thereby may result in increased birth weight of the fetus. See "Tobacco" in Chapter 11 for further discussion of prenatal smoking cessation and other intervention programs. ∞ Newborns of mothers who are tobacco dependent may be screened with the NICU Network Neurobehavioral Scale (NNNS) to assess their neurologic, behavioral, and stress/abstinence neurobehavioral function (Law et al., 2003).

The potential for long-term respiratory problems such as asthma, as well as cognitive and receptive language delays that may persist into school age, should be evaluated.

CARE OF THE NEWBORN AT RISK FOR HIV/AIDS

An increasing number of newborns are born infected with HIV or at risk for acquiring it in the newborn period or early infancy. Perinatal and neonatal transmission can occur across the placenta or through breast milk or contaminated blood. Maternal-to-newborn vertical transmission rates are about 13% to 40% in the United States (Thureen et al., 2005). The risk of vertical transmission can be decreased in mothers taking zidovudine during gestation. (For discussion of maternal and fetal HIV/AIDS, see "Care of the Woman with HIV Infection" in Chapter 14. ∞ For the infant with HIV/AIDS, see "Acquired Immune Deficiency Syndrome" in Chapter 44. ∞)

CARE OF THE NEWBORN WITH CONGENITAL HEART DEFECTS

Congenital heart defects occur in 1% of live births. Because accurate diagnosis and surgical treatment are now available, many deaths that could result from congenital heart defects can be prevented (American Heart Association, 2005). Corrective cardiac surgery is being done at earlier ages; for example, more than half the children undergoing surgery are less than 1 year of age, and one fourth are less than 1 month old. It is crucial for the nurse to have comprehensive knowledge of congenital heart disease to detect deviations from normal and initiate interventions.

OVERVIEW OF CONGENITAL HEART DEFECTS

The majority of congenital heart malformations are multifactorial with no specific trigger or cause. Factors that can contribute to congenital heart malformation can be classified as environmental or genetic. For example, infections of the pregnant woman, such as rubella, cytomegalovirus, coxsackie B, and influenza, have been implicated. Steroids, alcohol, lithium, and some anticonvulsants have been shown to cause malformations of the heart. Seasonal spraying of pesticides has also been linked to an increase in congenital heart defects.

Clinicians are also beginning to see cardiac defects in infants of mothers with PKU who do not follow their diets. Chromosomal factors may include Down syndrome, Turner syndrome, and Holt-Oram syndrome. Trisomy 13/15 and 16/18 infants frequently have heart lesions. Increased incidence and risk of recurrence of specific defects occur in families.

The most common cardiac defects seen in the first 6 days of life are left ventricular outflow obstructions (mitral stenosis, aortic stenosis or atresia), hypoplastic left heart, coarctation of the aorta, patent ductus arteriosus (the most common defect, especially in premature infants), transposition of the great vessels, tetralogy of Fallot, and large ventricular septal defect or atrial septal defects. Many cardiac defects may not manifest themselves until after discharge from the birthing unit.

NURSING MANAGEMENT

The neonatal nurse's primary goal is to identify cardiac defects early and notify the physician. The three most common manifestations of cardiac defect are cyanosis, detectable heart murmur, and congestive heart failure signs (tachycardia, tachypnea, diaphoresis, hepatomegaly, cardiomegaly). "Pathophysiology Illustrated: Cardiac Defects of the Early Newborn Period" shows the pathophysiology as well as the clinical manifestations and medical-surgical management of selected cardiac defects.

PATHOPHYSIOLOGY ILLUSTRATED

Cardiac Defects of the Early Newborn Period

CONGENITAL HEART DEFECT	CLINICAL FINDINGS	MEDICAL-SURGICAL MANAGEMENT
Increased Pulmonary Blood Flow		
Patent ductus arteriosus (PDA) ↑ in females, maternal rubella, RDS, < 1500 g preterm newborns, high-altitude births 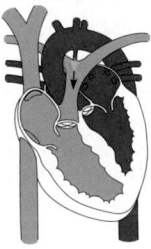	Harsh grade 2–3 machinery murmur upper left sternal border (LSB) just beneath clavicle ↑ difference between systolic and diastolic pulse pressure Can lead to right heart failure and pulmonary congestion ↑ left atrial (LA) and left ventricular (LV) enlargement, dilated ascending aorta ↑ pulmonary vascularity	Indomethacin—0.2 mg/kg orally (prostaglandin inhibitor) 3 doses q 12–24 hours Surgical ligation, occlusion coil Use of O$_2$ therapy and blood transfusion to improve tissue oxygenation and perfusion Fluid restriction and diuretics
	The patent ductus arteriosus is a vascular connection that, during fetal life, short-circuits the pulmonary vascular bed and directs blood from the pulmonary artery to the aorta. Postnatally, blood shunts through the ductus from the aorta to the pulmonary artery.	
Atrial septal defect (ASD) ↑ in females and Down syndrome	Initially frequently asymptomatic Systolic murmur second left intercostal space (LICS) With large ASD, diastolic rumbling murmur lower left sternal (LLS) border Failure to thrive, upper respiratory infection (URI), poor exercise tolerance	Umbrella occluder Surgical closure with patch or suture
Ventricular septal defect (VSD) ↑ in males	Initially asymptomatic until end of first month or if large enough to cause pulmonary edema Loud, blowing systolic murmur at third to fourth intercostal space (ICS) Increased pulmonary blood flow Right ventricular hypertrophy Rapid respirations, growth failure, feeding difficulties CHF at 6 weeks to 2 months of age	Follow medically—some spontaneously close Use of Lanoxin and diuretics in right congestive heart failure (CHF) Surgical closure with Dacron patch or umbrella occluder

PATHOPHYSIOLOGY ILLUSTRATED

Cardiac Defects of the Early Newborn Period—continued

CONGENITAL HEART DEFECT	CLINICAL FINDINGS	MEDICAL-SURGICAL MANAGEMENT

Obstruction to Systemic Blood Flow

Coarctation of aorta

Can be preductal or postductal

Absent or diminished femoral pulses

Increased brachial pulses

Late systolic murmur left intrascapular area

Systolic BP in lower extremities

Enlarged left ventricle

Can present in CHF at 7–21 days of life

   Coarctation of the aorta is characterized by a narrowed aortic lumen. The lesion produces an obstruction to the flow of blood through the aorta, causing an increased left ventricular pressure and workload.

Surgical resection of narrowed portion of aorta

Prostaglandin E_1 to maintain peripheral perfusion

No afterload reducer drugs

Hypoplastic left heart syndrome

Normal at birth—cyanosis and shocklike CHF develop within a few hours to days

Soft systolic murmur just left of the sternum

Diminished pulses

Aortic and/or mitral atresia

Tiny, thick-walled left ventricle

Large, dilated, hypertrophied right ventricle

X ray, cardiac enlargement and pulmonary venous congestion

PGE_1 until decision made

Norwood procedure

Transplant

Decreased Pulmonary Blood Flow

Tetralogy of Fallot

(Most common cyanotic heart defect)

Pulmonary stenosis

Overriding aorta

Right ventricular hypertrophy

Ventricular septal defect (VSD)

May be cyanotic at birth or within first few months of life

Harsh systolic murmur LSB

Crying or feeding increases cyanosis and respiratory distress

X-ray boot-shaped appearance secondary to small pulmonary artery

Right ventricular enlargement

   In tetralogy of Fallot, the severity of symptoms depends on the degree of pulmonary stenosis, the size of the ventricular septal defect, and the degree to which the aorta overrides the septal defect.

Prevention of dehydration, intercurrent infections

Alleviation of paroxysmal dyspneic attacks

Palliative surgery to increase blood flow to the lungs

Corrective surgery—resection of pulmonic stenosis, closure of VSD with Dacron patch

---

Mixed Defects*

Transposition of great vessels (TGA)

(↑ females, IDMs, LGAs)

Cyanosis at birth or within 3 days

Possible pulmonic stenosis murmur

Right ventricular hypertrophy

Polycythemia

"Egg on its side" x-ray

   Complete transposition of great vessels is an embryonic defect caused by a straight division of the bulbar trunk without normal spiraling. As a result the aorta originates from the right ventricle, and the pulmonary artery from the left ventricle. An abnormal communication between the two circulations must be present to sustain life.

Prostaglandin E to vasodilate ductus to keep it open

Inotropic support

Initial surgery to create opening between right and left side of heart if none exists

Total surgical repair—usually the arterial switch procedure—done within first few days of life

---

Mixed defects—postnatal survival is dependent upon mixing of systemic and pulmonary blood flow.

Initial repair of heart defects in the newborn period is becoming more commonplace. The NICU staff is involved in both the preoperative and postoperative care of newborns. The benefits for the infant include the NICU staff's knowledge of neonatal anatomy and physiology, experience in supporting the family, and an awareness of the developmental needs of the newborn.

After the baby is stabilized, decisions are made about ongoing care. The parents need careful and complete explanations and the chance to take part in decision making. They also require ongoing emotional support. Families with any baby born with a congenital anomaly also need genetic counseling about future conception. Parents need opportunities to verbalize their concerns about their baby's health. Be sure they understand the rationale for follow-up care.

CARE OF THE NEWBORN WITH INBORN ERRORS OF METABOLISM

Inborn errors of metabolism are a group of hereditary disorders transmitted by mutant genes. Most are transmitted by an autosomal recessive gene, requiring two heterozygous parents to produce a homozygous infant with the disorder. Carriers of some disorders can be identified by special tests, and some inborn errors of metabolism can be detected in utero. Some of the inborn errors of metabolism (especially those associated with mental retardation) are now detected neonatally through newborn screening programs (see "Care of the Newborn with an Inborn Error of Metabolism" in Chapter 28 ∞). For more extensive discussion of inborn errors of metabolism, see "Inborn Errors of Metabolism" in Chapter 56. ∞

Critical Concept Review

LEARNING OBJECTIVES

CONCEPTS

| Identify factors present at birth that indicate an at-risk newborn. | Factors present at birth that may place an infant at risk include:
1. Maternal low socioeconomic level:
   ■ Decreased access to healthcare.
2. Exposure to environmental dangers:
   ■ Toxic chemicals.
   ■ Illicit drugs.
3. Preexisting maternal conditions:
   ■ Heart disease.
   ■ Diabetes.
   ■ Hypertension.
   ■ Renal disease.
4. Maternal age and parity.
5. Pregnancy complications:
   ■ Abruptio placenta.
   ■ Placenta previa.
   ■ Preeclampsia. |
| Compare the underlying etiologies of the physiologic complications of small-for-gestational age (SGA) newborns and preterm appropriate-for-gestational-age (Pr AGA) newborns. | Many of the same factors contribute to the common complications of the SGA newborn and the Pr AGA newborn:
1. Maternal factors:
   ■ Grand multiparity.
   ■ Multiple gestation pregnancy.
   ■ Low socioeconomic status.
   ■ Poor maternal nutrition.
2. Maternal disease:
   ■ Heart disease.
   ■ Hypertension.
   ■ Preeclampsia.
3. Environmental factors:
   ■ Maternal use of drugs.
   ■ Exposure to toxins.
   ■ High altitude. |

LEARNING OBJECTIVES   **CONCEPTS**

4. Placental factors:
   - Small placenta.
   - Placenta previa.
   - Abnormal cord insertions.
5. Fetal factors:
   - Congenital infections.
   - Chromosomal syndromes.

Describe the impact of maternal diabetes mellitus on the newborn.

The most common complications of maternal diabetes mellitus are:
1. Hypoglycemia.
2. Hypocalcemia.
3. Hyperbilirubiemia.
4. Birth trauma.
5. Polycythemia.
6. Respiratory distress syndrome.
7. Congenital birth defects:
   - Cardiac anomalies.
   - Gastrointestinal anomalies.
   - Sacral agenesis.

Compare the characteristics and potential complications of the postterm newborn and the newborn with postmaturity syndrome.

1. Postmaturity:
   - Applies to any newborn born after 42 weeks gestation.
   - Most are of normal size and health.
   - Large fetus may have difficult time passing through birth passage.
2. Postmaturity syndrome, in which the fetus is exposed to poor placental function, which impairs nutrition and oxygenation and has the following characteristics:
   - Hypoglycemia.
   - Meconium aspiration.
   - Polycythemia.
   - Congenital anomalies.
   - Seizure activity.
   - Cold stress.

Discuss the physiologic characteristics of the preterm newborn that predispose each body system to various complications and are used in developing a plan of care.

1. Respiratory difficulties:
   - Lack of surfactant causes the alveoli to collapse and infant becomes hypoxic.
   - Incomplete development of the muscular coat of the pulmonary blood vessels, which leads to left to right shunting of blood through the ductus arteriosus back into lungs.
2. Cardiac difficulties:
   - Ductus arteriosus remains open due to low oxygen levels and low prostaglandin E levels.
   - Patent ductus remains open, causing more blood to flow to lungs, increased respiratory effort, carbon dioxide retention, and bounding femoral pulses.
3. Temperature control difficulties:
   - Less able to produce heat because of the higher ratio of body surface to body weight.
   - Lack of brown fat.
   - Thin skin, which causes greater insensible water loss.
   - Lack of flexion increases heat loss.
4. Gastrointestinal difficulties:
   - Poor suck effort.
   - High caloric needs and limited ability to take in nutrition.
   - Increased basal metabolic rate and oxygen needs related to increased effort at sucking.
   - Increased chance of aspiration.
   - Decreased ability of convert amino acids.
   - Decreased ability to handle increased osmolarity of formula protein.
   - Difficulty absorbing saturated fats.
   - Difficulty digesting lactose.
   - Diminished blood flow to the intestines resulting in necrotizing enterocolitis.

(continued)

LEARNING OBJECTIVES

CONCEPTS

Discuss the physiologic characteristics of the preterm newborn that predispose each body system to various complications and are used in developing a plan of care.—continued

→

5. Renal difficulties:
   - Decreased glomerular filtration rate due to decreased renal blood flow.
   - Inability to concentrate urine.
   - Decreased ability of kidney to buffer.
   - Delayed drug excretion time.
   - Spilling of glucose at a lower serum glucose rate.
6. Reactivity and behavioral state difficulties:
   - Delayed or lack of periods of reactivity due to poor condition of newborn.
   - More disorganized in sleep–wake cycle.

Summarize the nursing assessments of and initial interventions for a newborn born with selected congenital anomalies.

→

Nursing assessments and initial interventions focus on:
1. Respiratory:
   - Ability of infant to breathe.
   - Maintain respiratory function.
2. Nutritional:
   - Is infant able to suck and swallow?
   - Does feeding cause respiratory distress?
   - Provide calories by breast, nipple, gastrointestinal tube, or IV.
3. Neurological:
   - Is infant able to move all extremities?
   - Is there a visible defect present on the spine?
   - Is head circumference normal size and does it maintain normal size?
   - Keep infant in prone position if necessary.
   - Keep defect covered with sterile saline soaks until surgery.
   - Keep HOB elevated if head circumference is larger than normal.
4. Parental involvement:
   - Assess parents' knowledge of infant's anomaly.
   - Keep parents informed about infant's condition.
   - Teach parents appropriate home care of infant.

Explain the special care needed by an alcohol- or drug-exposed newborn.

→

Special care of the infant who was exposed to drugs or alcohol focuses on:
1. Assessment of the mother's last drug intake and dosage.
2. Assessment for congenital anomalies and complications.
3. Assessment for signs and symptoms of withdrawal.

Relate the consequences of maternal HIV/AIDS to the management of the newborn in the neonatal period.

→

Infant of the mother who has HIV/AIDS receives the same care as all newborn infants. The nurse also includes the following aspects of care:
1. Uses standard precautions when drawing blood samples.
2. Uses disposable gloves when changing diapers.
3. Protects infant from opportunistic diseases.
4. Keeps newborn well-nourished to prevent failure to thrive.

Identify the physical examination findings during the early newborn period that would make the nurse suspect a congenital cardiac defect.

→

The three most common manifestations of cardiac defects are:
1. Cyanosis.
2. Detectable heart murmur.
3. Signs of congestive heart failure:
   - Tachycardia.
   - Tachypnea.
   - Diaphoresis.
   - Hepatomegaly.
   - Cardiomegaly.

Explain the special care needed by newborns with an inborn error of metabolism.

→

Most infants with inborn errors of metabolism need care that centers around:
1. Specially prepared formulas.
2. Dietary modifications.
3. Replacement hormones.
4. Continual assessment for physical abnormalities and cognitive delays.

CRITICAL THINKING IN ACTION

View the **Critical Thinking in Action** *video in Chapter 30 of the CD-ROM. Then, answer the questions that follow.*

As the nurse on duty, you are caring for baby Erin, a 38-week IDM female born by repeat cesarean birth to a 32-year-old G3 now P3 mother. Erin's Apgar scores are 7 and 9 at 1 and 5 minutes. At 2 hours of age, the baby has an elevated respiratory rate of 100 to 110, heart rate of 165 with Grade II/VI intermittent machinery murmur, and mild cyanosis. She is now receiving 30% oxygen and has a respiratory rate of 70 to 80. The baby's clinical course, chest x-ray, and lab results are all consistent with transient tachypnea of the newborn

and patent ductus arteriosus. The mother calls you to ask about how her baby is doing. She tells you that her last child was born at 30 weeks and had to be hospitalized for 6 weeks. She says, "I really tried to do it right this time," and asks you if this baby will have the same respiratory problem.

1. What should you tell the mother?
2. What can you do to facilitate mother–infant attachment?
3. Discuss the emotional response of parents to the birth of an ill or at-risk infant. (See Chapter 31 for additional information. ∞)
4. Discuss the four psychologic tasks essential for coping with the stress of an at-risk newborn and providing a basis for the maternal-infant relationship. (See Chapter 31. ∞)
5. Baby Erin is being discharged tomorrow. Review the elements of discharge and home care instructions.

MEDIALINK   www.prenhall.com/london

REFERENCES

Als, H., & Lawhon, G. (2004). Theoretic perspective for developmentally supportive care. In C. Kenner & J. M. McGrath (Eds.), *Developmental care of newborns and infants: A guide for health professionals.* St. Louis, MO: Elsevier Mosby.

Als, H., Lester, B. M., Tronick, E., & Brazelton, T. B. (1982). Assessment of preterm infant behavior (APIB). In B. M. Fitzgerald Lester & M. W. Yogman (Eds.), *Theory and research in behavioral pediatrics* (Vol. 1, pp. 35–82). New York: Plenum.

American Academy of Pediatrics (AAP) & American College of Obstetricians and Gynecologists (ACOG). (2002). *Guidelines for perinatal care* (5th ed.). Elk Grove Village, IL: Author.

American College of Obstetricians and Gynecologists (ACOG), Committee on Genetics. (2003). Newborn screening (ACOG Committee Opinion No. 287). *Obstetrics and Gynecology, 102,* 887–889.

American Heart Association. (2005). *Congenital cardiovascular disease statistics.* Retrieved October 21, 2005, from http://www.americanheart.org/ children

Andres, R. L. (2004). Effects of therapeutic, diagnostics and environmental agents and exposure to social and illicit drugs. In R. K. Creasy & R. Resnik (Eds.), *Maternal-fetal medicine: Principles and practice* (5th ed., pp. 281–305). Philadelphia: Saunders.

Association of Women's Health, Obstetric and Neonatal Nurses (AWHONN). (2001). *Evidence based clinical practice guidelines: Neonatal skin care.* Washington, DC: Author.

Blackburn, S. (2003). *Maternal-fetal-neonatal physiology: A clinical perspective* (2nd ed.). Philadelphia: Saunders.

Centers for Disease Control and Prevention (CDC), National Center for Chronic Disease Prevention and Health Promotion. (2005). *Pattern of tobacco use among women and girls: Fact sheet.* Retrieved January 31, 2005, from http:// www.cdc.gov/tobacco/sgr_forwomen/factsheet_ tobaccouse.htm

Chmait, R., & Moore, T. R. (2005). *Endocrine disorders in pregnancy.* In H. W. Taeusch, R. A. Ballard,

& C. A. Gleason (Eds.), *Avery's diseases of the newborn* (8th ed., pp. 71–86). Philadelphia: Saunders.

Harrison, L. (2001). The use of comforting touch and massage to reduce stress for preterm infants in the neonatal intensive care unit. *Newborn and Infant Nursing Review, 1*(4), 235–241.

Horns, K. M. (2004). Immunology and infectious disease. In M. T. Verklan & M. Walden (Eds.), *Core curriculum for neonatal care nursing* (3rd ed., pp. 759–793). St. Louis, MO: Elsevier Saunders.

Jones, J., Kassity, N., & Duncan, K. (2001). Complementary care: Alternatives for the neonatal intensive care unit. *Newborn and Infant Nursing Reviews, 1*(4), 207–210.

Law, K. L., Stroud, L. R., LaGasse, L. L., Niaura, R., Liu, J., & Lester, B. M. (2003). Smoking during pregnancy and newborn neurobehavior. *Pediatrics, 111*(6), 1318–1332.

Martinez, A., & Simmons, R. (2005). Abnormalities of fetal growth. In H. W. Taeusch, R. A. Ballard, & C. A. Gleason (Eds.), *Avery's diseases of the newborn* (8th ed., pp. 32–45). Philadelphia: Saunders.

Martinez, A., Partridge, J. C., & Taeusch, H. W. (2005). Perinatal substance abuse. In H. W. Taeusch, R. A. Ballard, & C. A. Gleason (Eds.), *Avery's diseases of the newborn* (8th ed., pp. 106–126). Philadelphia: Saunders.

McGrath, J. M. (2004). Feeding. In C. Kenner & J. M. McGrath (Eds.), *Developmental care of newborns & infants: A guide for health professionals*. St. Louis, MO: Elsevier Mosby.

Moore, T. R. (2004). Diabetes in pregnancy. In R. K. Creasy & R. Resnik (Eds.), *Maternal-fetal medicine: Principles and practice* (5th ed., pp. 1023–1061). Philadelphia: Saunders.

Moran, B. A. (2004). Substance abuse in pregnancy. In S. Mattson & J. E. Smith (Eds.), *Core curriculum for maternal-newborn nursing* (3rd ed., pp. 750–770). St. Louis, MO: Elsevier Saunders.

Resnik, J. L., & Resnik, R. (2004). Post-term pregnancy. In R. K. Creasy & R. Resnik (Eds.), *Maternal-fetal medicine: Principles and practice* (5th ed., pp. 663–669). Philadelphia: Saunders.

Resnik, R., & Creasy, R. K. (2004). Intrauterine growth restriction. In R. K. Creasy & R. Resnik (Eds.), *Maternal-fetal medicine: Principles and practice* (5th ed., pp. 495–512). Philadelphia: Saunders.

Saari, T. N., & Committee on Infectious Diseases. (2003). Immunization of preterm and low birth weight infants. *Pediatrics, 112*(1), 193–198.

Standley, J. M. (2001). Music therapy for the neonate. *Newborn and Infant Nursing Reviews, 1*(4), 211–216.

Sterk, L. (2004). Congenital anomalies. In M. T. Verklan & M. Walden (Eds.), *Core curriculum for neonatal care nursing* (3rd ed., pp. 858–892). St. Louis, MO: Elsevier Saunders.

Thureen, P. J., Deacon, J., Hernandez, J., & Hall, D. M. (2005). *Assessment and care of the well newborn*. St. Louis, MO: Elsevier Saunders.

Turnage-Carrier, C. S. (2004). Caregiving and the environment. In C. Kenner & J. M. McGrath (Eds.), *Developmental care of newborns and infants: A guide for health professionals*. St. Louis, MO: Elsevier Mosby.

The Newborn at Risk: Birth-Related Stressors

We watched him breathe every precious breath. He was covered with wires and tubes. The rhythmic tides of his sleeping and feeding spaciously measured his days and nights. We kept watch. He was special to us and we would say over and over, "Daddy and mommy are here and we love you."
—*Alan and Claudia, parents of a baby with RDS*

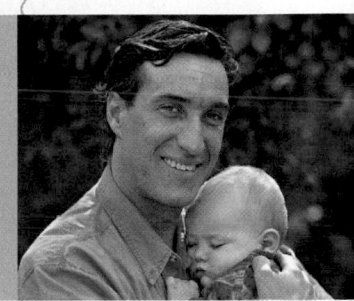

LEARNING OBJECTIVES

- Discuss how to identify infants in need of resuscitation and the appropriate method of resuscitation based on the labor record and observable physiologic indicators.

- Based on clinical manifestations, differentiate between the various types of respiratory distress (respiratory distress syndrome, transient tachypnea of the newborn, and meconium aspiration syndrome) in the newborn and their related nursing care.

- Discuss selected metabolic abnormalities (including cold stress and hypoglycemia), their effects on the newborn, and the nursing implications.

- Differentiate between physiologic and pathologic jaundice based on onset, cause, possible sequelae, and specific management.

- Explain how Rh incompatibility or ABO incompatibility can lead to the development of hyperbilirubinemia.

- Identify nursing responsibilities in caring for the newborn receiving phototherapy.

- Discuss selected hematologic problems such as anemia and polycythemia and the nursing implications associated with each one.

- Describe the nursing assessments that would lead the nurse to suspect newborn sepsis.

- Relate the consequences of selected maternally transmitted infections, such as maternal syphilis, gonorrhea, herpesvirus, and chlamydia, to the management of the infant in the neonatal period.

- Describe the interventions to facilitate parental attachment with the at-risk newborn.

- Identify the special initial and long-term needs of parents of at-risk infants.

MEDIALINK

www.prenhall.com/london

CD-ROM

NCLEX-RN® Review
Skill 10-1: Performing a Capillary Puncture
Nursing in Action: Infant Receiving Phototherapy
Audio Glossary

Companion Website

NCLEX RN® Review
Case Study: Newborn with Jaundice
Care Plan Activity: Infection in a Newborn
MediaLink Application:
   Infant Respiratory Distress Syndrome
Thinking Critically

arked homeostatic changes happen during the transition from fetal to neonatal life. The most rapid anatomic and physiologic changes of this period occur in the cardiopulmonary system, so the newborn's major problems are usually related to this system. These problems include asphyxia, respiratory distress, cold stress, jaundice, hemolytic disease, and anemia. Ideally, problems are anticipated and identified prenatally, and appropriate intervention measures are begun at or immediately after birth.

CARE OF THE NEWBORN AT RISK DUE TO ASPHYXIA

Neonatal asphyxia results in circulatory, respiratory, and biochemical changes. Circulatory patterns that accompany asphyxia indicate the newborn's inability to make the transition to extrauterine circulation—in effect, a return to fetal circulatory patterns. Failure of lung expansion and establishment of respiration rapidly produces serious biochemical changes, including hypoxia (decreased oxygen concentration available to tissues), acidosis (increased acidity of blood reflected by low pH), and hypercarbia (excess levels of carbon dioxide in the blood).

These biochemical changes cause abnormal changes in pulmonary circulation. Arterioles constrict, resulting in vascular resistance and diminished pulmonary blood flow to the organs and the lungs, and a large right-to-left shunt through the ductus arteriosus. The foramen ovale reopens as right atrial pressure exceeds left atrial pressure, and blood flows from right to left. (See Chapter 26 for a review of normal newborn cardiopulmonary adaptation. ∞)

However, the most serious biochemical abnormality caused by hypoxia is a change from aerobic to anaerobic metabolism. This change results in the buildup of lactate and development of metabolic acidosis. Simultaneous respiratory acidosis may also occur due to a rapid increase in carbon dioxide (PCO_2) during asphyxia. In response to hypoxia and anaerobic metabolism, glycogen stores are mobilized to provide a continuous glucose source for the brain, and the amounts of free fatty acids (FFAs) and glycerol in the blood increase.

The newborn has several protective mechanisms against hypoxic insults. These include a relatively immature brain and a resting metabolic rate lower than that of adults, an ability to mobilize substances within the body for anaerobic metabolism and to use energy more efficiently, and an intact circulatory system able to redistribute lactate and hydrogen ions in tissues still being perfused. Unfortunately, the body's stores of glycogen may be used up rapidly during an asphyxial attack. Severe, prolonged hypoxia overcomes the body's protective mechanisms, resulting in brain damage or death of the newborn.

The newborn suffering apnea requires immediate resuscitative efforts. The need for resuscitation can be anticipated if specific risk factors are present during the pregnancy or labor and birth.

RISK FACTORS PREDISPOSING TO ASPHYXIA

The need for resuscitation may be anticipated if the mother demonstrates the antepartal and intrapartum risk factors described in Table 10–1 in Chapter 10 and Table 18–1 in Chapter 18. ∞ Neonatal risk factors for resuscitation are as follows (Thureen, Deacon, Hernandez et al., 2005):

- Nonreassuring fetal heart rate pattern
- Difficult birth
- Fetal scalp/capillary blood sample-acidosis

- Apneic episode unresponsive to tactile stimulation
- Inadequate ventilation
- Male infant
- Prematurity
- Small for gestational age
- Multiple births
- Structural lung abnormality (congenital diaphragmatic hernia, lung hypoplasia)
- Congenital heart disease
- Sepsis with cardiovascular collapse

Risk factors are not always apparent prenatally. Particular attention must be paid to all at-risk pregnancies during the intrapartal period. Certain aspects of labor and birth challenge the oxygen supply to the fetus, and often the at-risk fetus has less tolerance for the stress of labor and birth.

CLINICAL THERAPY

The initial goal of medical management is to identify the fetus at risk for asphyxia, so that resuscitative efforts can begin at birth. Fetal biophysical assessment (see Chapter 16 ∞), combined with monitoring of fetal pH, fetal heart rates, and fetal oximetry if available, may help identify the presence of nonreassuring fetal status. If nonreassuring fetal status is present, appropriate measures can be taken to deliver the fetus immediately, before major damage occurs, and to treat the asphyxiated newborn.

The fetal biophysical profile enhances the ability to predict an abnormal perinatal outcome. In addition to the fetal biophysical profile, fetal scalp blood sampling may indicate asphyxic insult and the degree of fetal acidosis, when considered in relation to the stage of labor, uterine contractions, and the presence of nonreassuring fetal heart rate (FHR) patterns. The stress of labor causes an intermittent decrease in exchange of gases in the placental intervillous space, which causes the fall in pH and fetal acidosis. The acidosis is primarily metabolic.

During labor a fetal pH of 7.25 or higher is considered normal (nonacidemia). A pH value of 7.2 or less is considered an ominous sign of intrauterine asphyxia (acidemia). However, low fetal pH without associated hypoxia can be caused by maternal acidosis secondary to prolonged labor, dehydration, and maternal lactate production.

Assessment of the newborn's need for resuscitation begins at the time of birth. The nurse should note the time of the first gasp, first cry, and onset of sustained respirations in order of occurrence. The Apgar score (see information in Chapter 19 ∞) may be helpful in determining the severity of the neonatal depression and may be predictive of neonatal survival (de Ungria & Steinhorn, 2003; Fanaroff, Martin, & Rodriguez, 2004).

The treatment of fetal or newborn asphyxia is resuscitation. The goals of resuscitation are to provide an adequate airway with expansion of the lungs, to decrease the P_{CO_2} and increase the P_{O_2}, to support adequate cardiac output, and to minimize oxygen consumption by reducing heat loss.

RESUSCITATION MANAGEMENT

Initial resuscitative management of the newborn is extremely important. Suctioning is always performed before resuscitation so that mucus, blood, or meconium is not aspirated into the lungs. Caregivers should keep the infant in a head-down position before the first gasp to avoid aspiration of the oropharyngeal secretions and must suction the oropharynx and nasopharynx immediately. Clearing the nasal and oral passages of obstructive fluid establishes a patent airway.

Breathing is established with the simplest form of resuscitative measures initially, with progression to more complicated methods as required. For example:

1. Simple stimulation is provided by rubbing the newborn's back.

2. If respirations have not been initiated or are inadequate (gasping or occasional respirations), the lungs must be inflated with positive pressure. The mask is positioned securely on the face (over nose and mouth, avoiding the eyes), with the infant's head in a "sniffing" or neutral position (Figure 31–1 ●).

● FIGURE 31–1

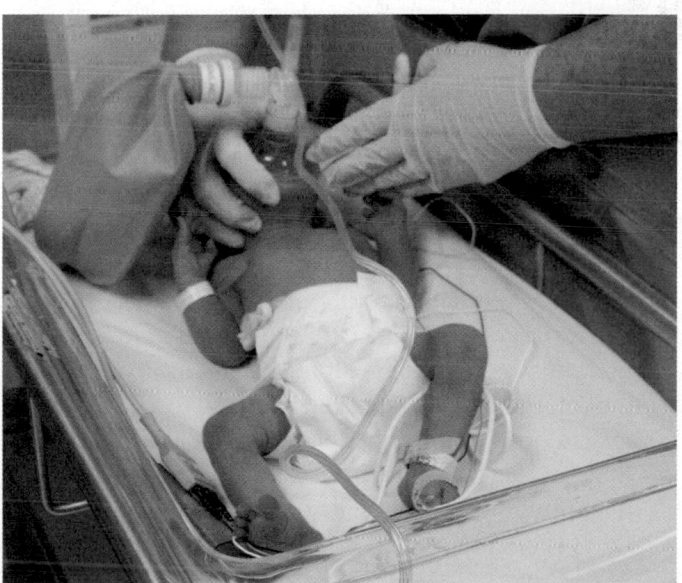

Demonstration of resuscitation of an infant with bag and mask. Note that the mask covers the nose and mouth, and the head is in a neutral position. The resuscitating bag is placed to the side of the baby so that chest movement can be seen.

Hyperextension of the infant's neck obstructs the trachea and must be avoided. An airtight connection is made between the baby's face and the mask (thus allowing the bag to inflate). The lungs are inflated rhythmically by squeezing the bag. Oxygen can be delivered at 100% with an anesthesia bag with manometer or modified self-inflating bag and adequate liter flow of at least 5 L/min. The self-inflating (Ambu or Hope) bag delivers only 40% oxygen unless it has been adapted with an attached oxygen reservoir (American Academy of Pediatrics [AAP] Committee on Fetus and Newborn & American College of Obstetricians and Gynecologists [ACOG] Committee on Obstetrics, 2002). It may not be possible to maintain adequate inspiratory pressure with Ambu or Hope bags. In a crisis situation, it is crucial that 100% oxygen be delivered with adequate pressure.

3. The rise and fall of the chest are observed for proper ventilation. Air entry and heart rate are checked by auscultation. Manual resuscitation is coordinated with any voluntary efforts. The rate of ventilation should be between 40 and 60 breaths per minute. Pressure should be adequate to move the chest wall. The pressure gauge (manometer) must be in place to avoid overdistention of the newborn's lungs and other problems such as pneumothorax or abdominal distention. In newborns with normal lungs, 15 to 25 cm H_2O may be adequate. If the newborn has lung disease, 20 to 40 cm H_2O may be necessary. If the newborn has not taken a first breath after birth, pressures of > 30 cm H_2O may be transiently required to expand collapsed alveoli. If ventilation is adequate, the chest moves with each inspiration, bilateral breath sounds are audible, and the lips and mucous membranes become pink. Distention of the stomach is controlled by inserting a nasogastric tube for decompression.

4. Endotracheal intubation may be needed. However, most newborns, except for very-low-birth-weight (VLBW) infants (< 1500 g), can be resuscitated by bag and mask ventilation. With preterm newborns, positive end expiratory pressure (PEEP) is required to help prevent alveolar collapse. If the baby is intubated and the color and heart rate fail to respond to ventilatory efforts, poor or improper placement of an endotracheal tube may be the cause. If the baby is intubated properly, pneumothorax, diaphragmatic hernia, or hypoplastic lungs (Potter's association) may exist.

Once breathing is established, the heart rate should increase to over 100 beats per minute. If the heart rate is absent or if it remains less than 60 beats per minute after 30 seconds of adequate assisted ventilation with 100% oxygen, external cardiac massage (chest compression) is be-

gun. Chest compressions are started immediately if there is no detectable heartbeat. The procedure for performing chest compressions is as follows:

1. The infant is positioned on a firm surface.
2. The resuscitator stands at the foot of the infant and places both thumbs over the lower third of the sternum (just below an imaginary line drawn between the nipples), with the fingers wrapped around and supporting the back (Figure 31–2A ⊙).

⊙ **FIGURE 31–2**

A

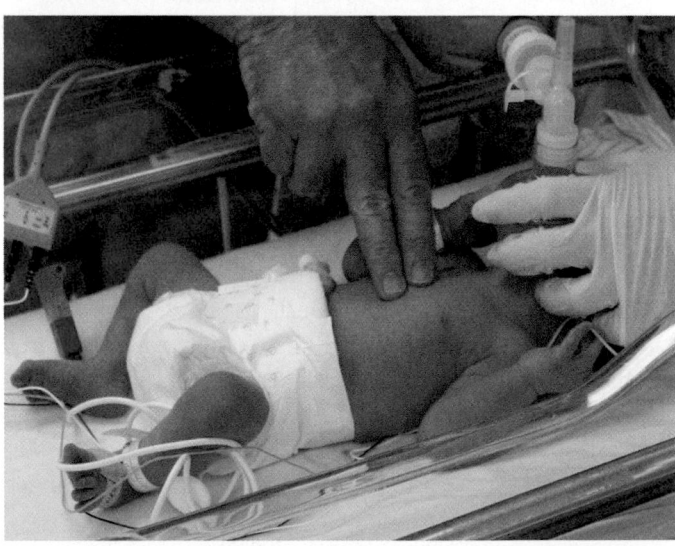

B

External cardiac massage. The lower third of the sternum is compressed with two fingertips or thumbs at a rate of 90 compressions per minute. **A,** The thumb method uses the fingers to support the infant's back and uses both thumbs to compress the sternum. **B,** The two-fingers method uses the tips of two fingers of one hand to compress the sternum and the other hand or a firm surface to support the infant's back.

Alternatively, the resuscitator may use two fingers instead of thumbs (Figure 31–2B). The two-thumb method is preferred because it may provide better coronary perfusion pressure; however, it makes access to the umbilical cord for medication administration more difficult (de Ungria & Steinhorn, 2003).

3. The sternum is depressed to sufficient depth to generate a palpable pulse or approximately one third of the anterior-posterior depth of the chest at a rate of 90 compressions per minute (AAP & ACOG, 2002). Use a 3:1 ratio of heartbeat to assisted ventilation.

Drugs needed in the treatment of shock, cardiac arrest, and narcosis should be available in the birthing area. Oxygen is the drug most often used because of its effectiveness in ventilation.

After 30 seconds of ventilation and cardiac compression, the newborn's cardiopulmonary status is reassessed by palpating the umbilical cord for a pulse. If the newborn has not responded with spontaneous respirations and a heart rate above 60 beats per minute, resuscitative medications are necessary (AAP & ACOG, 2002). The most accessible route for administering medications is the umbilical vein. If bradycardia is present, epinephrine (0.1 to 0.3 mL/kg of a 1:10,000 solution or 0.01 to 0.03 mg/kg) is given through the umbilical vein catheter or the peripheral intravenous (IV) setup. When epinephrine is administered by endotracheal tube, the IV dose of epinephrine should be diluted with 1 mL of normal saline (Glomella, 2004). *Sodium bicarbonate is rarely given in the birthing room* and only to correct metabolic acidosis after effective ventilation is established. Dextrose is given to prevent progression of hypoglycemia. A 10% dextrose in water IV solution is usually sufficient to prevent or treat hypoglycemia in the birthing area. Naloxone hydrochloride (0.1 mg/kg), a narcotic antagonist, is used to reverse narcotic depression. See "Drug Guide: Naloxone Hydrochloride (Narcan)."

If shock develops (low blood pressure or poor peripheral perfusion), the baby may be given a volume expander such as normal saline, or lactated Ringer's solution in a dose of 10 mL/kg given over 5 to 10 minutes. Whole blood (O negative crossmatched against the mother), fresh frozen plasma, and packed red blood cells can also be used for volume expansion and treatment of shock. In some instances of prolonged resuscitation associated with shock and poor response to resuscitation, dopamine (5 mg/kg/min) may be necessary.

DRUG GUIDE

NALOXONE HYDROCHLORIDE (NARCAN)

Overview of Neonatal Action
Naloxone hydrochloride (Narcan) is used to reverse respiratory depression due to acute narcotic toxicity. It displaces morphinelike drugs from receptor sites on the neurons; therefore, the narcotics can no longer exert their depressive effects. Naloxone reverses narcotic-induced respiratory depression, analgesia, sedation, hypotension, and pupillary constriction.

Route, Dosage, Frequency
Intravenous dose is 0.1 mg/kg (0.25 mL/kg of 0.4 mg/mL preparation 0.1 mL/kg of 1 mg/mL) concentration at birth, including premature infants. This drug is usually given through endotracheal tube (ET) or IV, although naloxone can be given intramuscularly (IM) if adequate perfusion exists. For IV push, infuse over at least 1 minute; for ET administration, dilute in 1 to 2 millimeters of (NS) normal saline.

Reversal of drug depression occurs within 1 to 2 minutes after IV administration and within 15 minutes of IM administration. The duration of action is variable (minutes to hours) and depends on the amount of the drug present and the rate of excretion. Dose may be repeated in 3 to 5 minutes. If there is no improvement after two or three doses, discontinue naloxone administration. If initial reversal occurs, repeat dose as needed (Young & Mangum, 2005).

Neonatal Contraindications
Naloxone should not be administered to infants of narcotic-addicted mothers because it may precipitate acute withdrawal syndrome (increased heart rate and blood pressure, vomiting, tremors).

Respiratory depression may result from nonmorphine drugs, such as sedatives, hypnotics, anesthetics, or other nonnarcotic CNS depressants.

Neonatal Side Effects
Excessive doses may result in irritability, increased crying, and possible prolongation of partial thromboplastin time (PTT). Tachycardia may occur.

Nursing Considerations
■ Monitor respirations closely—rate and depth for improved respiratory effort.

■ Assess for return of respiratory depression when naloxone effects wear off and effects of longer acting narcotics reappear.

■ Have resuscitative equipment, O₂, and ventilatory equipment available.

■ Monitor bleeding studies.

■ Note that naloxone is incompatible with alkaline solutions such as sodium bicarbonate.

■ Store at room temperature and protect from light.

■ Compatible with heparin.

NURSING MANAGEMENT

NURSING ASSESSMENT AND DIAGNOSIS

Communication between the obstetric office or clinic and the birthing area helps the birthing area nurse identify newborns who may need resuscitation. When the woman arrives in the birthing area, have the antepartal record ready. Note any contributory perinatal history factors and assess present fetal status. As labor progresses, continue ongoing monitoring of fetal heartbeat and its response to contractions, assist with fetal scalp blood sampling, and observe for the presence of meconium in the amniotic fluid to assess for fetal asphyxia. Alert the resuscitation team and the practitioner responsible for the newborn's care of any potential high-risk laboring women.

Nursing diagnoses that may apply to the newborn with asphyxia and the newborn's parents include the following:

- *Ineffective Breathing Pattern* related to lack of spontaneous respirations at birth secondary to in utero asphyxia
- *Decreased Cardiac Output* related to impaired oxygenation
- *Ineffective Family Coping: Compromised* related to baby's lack of spontaneous respirations at birth and fear of losing their newborn

PLANNING AND IMPLEMENTATION

Hospital-Based Nursing Care

In the high-risk nursery, resuscitation may be needed at any time. Check and maintain equipment to ensure its reliability at all times. Inspect all equipment—bag and mask, oxygen and flow meter, laryngoscope, and suction machine—for damaged or nonfunctioning parts before a birth or when setting up an admission bed. Sterilize resuscitative equipment in the birthing room after each use. A systematic check of the emergency cart and equipment is a routine responsibility of each shift. It is a good idea to be prepared by assembling equipment for pH and blood gas determination.

During resuscitation it is essential to keep the newborn warm. Dry the newborn quickly with warmed towels or blankets to prevent evaporative heat loss, remove the wet blankets, and place him or her under the radiant warmer. This device provides an overhead radiant heat source (a thermostatic mechanism taped to the infant's abdomen triggers the radiant warmer to turn on or off to maintain consistent temperature). Set the servocontrol at 36.5°C (97.7°F). Cover the newborn's head with a hat as the head is a major source of heat loss (de Ungria & Steinhorn, 2003). An open bed is necessary for easy access to the newborn.

Training and knowledge about resuscitation are vital to personnel in the birth setting for both normal and at-risk births. Since resuscitation must be a two-person effort for high-risk newborns, call for additional support as needed. One member must have the skill to perform airway management and ventilation. Record resuscitative efforts on the newborn's chart so that all members of the healthcare team have access to the information.

Parent Teaching

The new CPR guidelines favor family members being present during resuscitation in the birthing room and in the neonatal intensive care unit (NICU), but the procedure is particularly distressing for parents. Advise parents that a support person will be available for them if resuscitation is necessary. As soon as the infant's condition has stabilized, a member of the interdisciplinary team needs to discuss the newborn's condition with the parents. The parents may have many fears about the reasons for resuscitation and the condition of their baby after resuscitation.

EVALUATION

Expected outcomes of nursing care include the following:

- The newborn requiring resuscitation is promptly identified, and intervention is started early.
- The newborn's metabolic and physiologic processes are stabilized, and recovery is proceeding without complications.
- The parents can verbalize the reason for resuscitation and what was done to resuscitate their newborn.
- The parents can verbalize their fears about the resuscitation process and potential implications for their baby's future.

CARE OF THE NEWBORN WITH RESPIRATORY DISTRESS

Respiratory distress is an inappropriate respiratory adaptation to extrauterine life. It is one of the most severe conditions that may affect the newborn. The nurse caring for a baby with respiratory distress needs to understand the normal pulmonary and circulatory physiology (see "Respiratory Adaptation" in Chapter 26 ∞), the pathophysiology of the disease process, clinical manifestations, and supportive and corrective therapies. Only with this knowledge can the nurse make appropriate observations about responses to therapy and development of complications. Unlike the verbalizing adult client, the newborn communicates needs only by behavior or physiologic parameters that must be interpreted by the NICU nurse. The neonatal nurse interprets this behavior as clues about the baby's condition. In this section, we discuss respiratory distress syndrome, transient tachypnea of the newborn, and meconium aspiration syndrome.

RESPIRATORY DISTRESS SYNDROME

Respiratory distress syndrome (RDS), also called *hyaline membrane disease (HMD)*, is the result of a primary absence, deficiency, or alteration in the production of pulmonary surfactant. It is a complex disease that affects approximately 20,000 to 30,000 infants a year in the United States, most of whom are preterm infants. RDS is a complication in about 1% of pregnancies. The syndrome occurs more frequently in premature Causasian infants than in infants of African descent and almost twice as often in males as in females.

Not all the factors precipitating the pathologic changes of RDS have been determined, but two main factors associated with its development include:

1. **Prematurity.** All preterm newborns—whether AGA, SGA, or LGA—and especially infants of diabetic mothers are at risk for RDS. The incidence of RDS increases with the degree of prematurity, and most deaths occur in newborns weighing less than 1500 g. The maternal and fetal factors resulting in preterm labor and birth, complications of pregnancy, cesarean birth (and its indications), and familial tendency are all associated with RDS.

2. **Surfactant deficiency disease.** Normal pulmonary adaptation requires adequate surfactant, a lipoprotein that coats the inner surfaces of the alveoli. Surfactant provides alveolar stability by decreasing the alveoli's surface tension and tendency to collapse. Surfactant is produced by type II alveolar cells starting at about 24 weeks' gestation. In the normal or mature newborn lung, it is continuously synthesized, oxidized during breathing, and replenished. Adequate surfactant levels lead to better lung compliance and permit breathing with less work. RDS is due to alterations in surfactant quantity, composition, function, or production.

TEACHING HIGHLIGHTS

RESPIRATORY DISTRESS

You can help parents understand their baby's respiratory distress by having them think of the air sacs (alveoli) of the lungs as tiny balloons filled with water and no air. When the tiny balloon (alveolus) is emptied (as in expiration), water droplets can remain inside the balloon. The sides of the balloon stick together, increasing the surface tension, making the next inspiration breath very difficult.

Development of RDS indicates a failure to synthesize surfactant, which is required to maintain alveolar stability (see "Factors Opposing the First Breath" in Chapter 26 ∞). On expiration this instability increases atelectasis (lung collapse), which causes hypoxia and acidosis because of the lack of gas exchange. These conditions further inhibit surfactant production and cause pulmonary vasoconstriction. The resulting lung instability causes the biochemical problems of hypoxemia (decreased Po_2), hypercarbia (increased Pco_2), and acidemia (decreased pH), which further increases pulmonary vasoconstriction and hypoperfusion. The cycle of events of RDS leading to eventual respiratory failure is diagrammed in "Pathophysiology Illustrated: Respiratory Distress Syndrome (RDS)."

Because of these pathophysiologic conditions, the newborn must expend increasing amounts of energy to reopen the collapsed alveoli with every breath, so that each breath becomes as difficult as the first. The progressive expiratory atelectasis upsets the physiologic homeostasis of the pulmonary and cardiovascular systems and prevents adequate gas exchange. Breathing becomes progressively harder as lung compliance decreases, which makes it more difficult for the newborn to inflate the lungs and breathe.

The physiologic alterations of RDS produce the following complications:

1. **Hypoxia.** As a result of hypoxia, pulmonary blood vessels constrict and their resistance increases, which reduces pulmonary blood flow. The increase in pulmonary blood vessel resistance may cause a return to fetal circulation as the ductus opens and blood flow is shunted around the lungs. This shunting increases the hypoxia and further decreases pulmonary perfusion. Hypoxia also causes impairment or absence of metabolic response to cold; reversion to anaerobic metabolism, resulting in lactate accumulation (acidosis); and impaired cardiac output, which decreases perfusion to vital organs.

2. **Respiratory acidosis.** Persistently rising Pco_2 and decreases in pH are poor prognostic signs of pulmonary function and adequacy because increased Pco_2 and decreased pH are results of alveolar hypoventilation.

3. **Metabolic acidosis.** Because the cells lack oxygen, the newborn begins an anaerobic pathway of metabolism, with an increase in lactate levels and a resulting base deficit (loss of bicarbonate). As the lactate levels increase, the pH decreases in an attempt to maintain acid-balance homeostasis.

The classic radiologic picture of RDS is diffuse bilateral reticulogranular density, with portions of the air-filled tracheobronchial tree (air bronchogram) outlined by the

PATHOPHYSIOLOGY ILLUSTRATED

Respiratory Distress Syndrome (RDS)

↓ Surfactant

↓ Lung compliance

Atelectasis → ↑ Work of breathing

↓ Ventilation

↓ Po₂ → Anaerobic metabolism —Metabolic→ Acidosis ←Respiratory— ↑ CO₂

Pulmonary and peripheral vasoconstriction

↑ R → L Shunting   ↑ Pulmonary artery pressure   ↓ Pulmonary blood flow   Poor peripheral perfusion

↓ Surfactant   ↓ Arterial blood pressure

A

A, Cycle of events of RDS leading to eventual respiratory failure.
Used with permission from Gluck, L., & Kulovich, M. V. (1973). Fetal lung development. Pediatric Clinics of North America, 20, 375. Modified.
B, RDS chest x-ray. Chest radiograph of respiratory distress syndrome characterized by a reticulogranular pattern with areas of microatelectasis of uniform opacity and air bronchograms.
Courtesy of Carol Harrigan, RNC, MSN, NNP

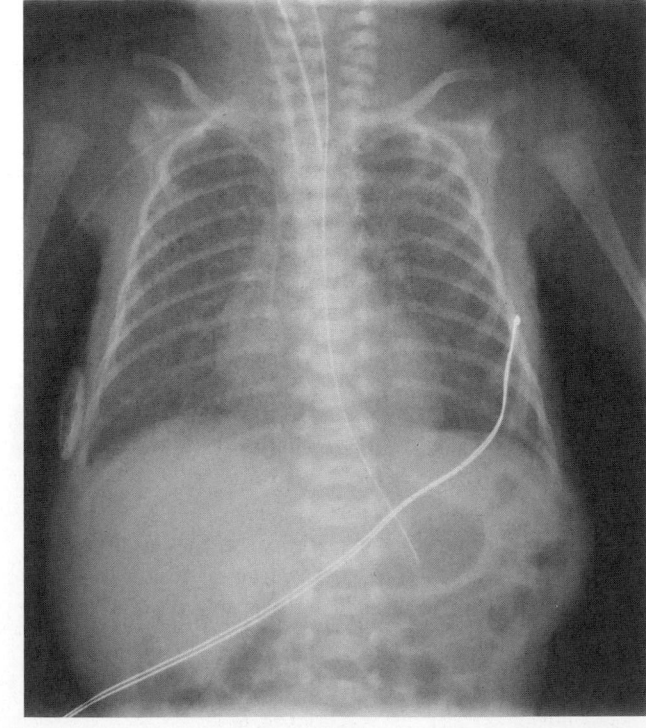

B

opaque ("white-out") lungs and widespread atelectasis (Thureen et al., 2005). See "Pathophysiology Illustrated." The progression of x-ray findings parallels the pattern of resolution, which usually occurs in 7 to 10 days, and the time of surfactant reappearance, unless surfactant replacement therapy and mechanical ventilation have been used (Blackburn, 2003). Echocardiography is a valuable tool in diagnosing vascular shunts that move blood either away from or toward the lungs.

CLINICAL THERAPY

Antenatally, respiratory distress due to preterm labor is treated with therapies to enhance fetal lung development (see "Care of the Woman at Risk Due to Preterm Labor" in Chapter 15 ∞). The goals of postnatal therapy are to maintain adequate oxygenation and ventilation, correct acid-base imbalance, and provide the supportive care required to maintain homeostasis.

Surfactant replacement therapy decreases the severity of RDS in low-birth-weight newborns. Surfactant replacement therapy is delivered through an endotracheal tube and may be given in either the birthing room or the nursery, as indicated by the severity of RDS. Repeat doses are often required. The most frequently reported response to treatment is rapidly improved oxygenation and decreased need for ventilatory support.

Supportive medical management consists of ventilation therapy, transcutaneous oxygen and carbon dioxide

monitoring, blood gas monitoring, correction of acid-base imbalance, environmental temperature regulation, adequate nutrition, and protection from infection. Ventilation therapy is directed toward preventing hypoventilation and hypoxia. Mild cases of RDS may require only increased humidified oxygen concentrations. Moderately afflicted infants may need continuous positive airway pressure (CPAP). Babies with severe RDS require mechanical ventilatory assistance from a respirator (Figure 31–3 ●).

● FIGURE 31–3

One-day-old, 29 weeks' gestational age, 1450-g baby on respirator and in isolette.

Courtesy of Carol Harrigan, RNC, MSN, NNP.

EVIDENCE-BASED NURSING

CONTINUOUS POSITIVE AIRWAY PRESSURE FOR RESPIRATORY DISTRESS SYNDROME

Clinical Question

Can continuous positive airway pressure (CPAP) reduce the use of intermittent positive pressure ventilation (IPPV) in preterm infants, without an increase in adverse effects?

Evidence

The standard treatment for many newborns with RDS is intermittent positive pressure ventilation. IPPV has been demonstrated effective, but it is invasive and may result in airway and lung injury. In order to determine if CPAP was a viable alternative for spontaneously breathing infants with RDS, four neonatal specialists conducted a systematic review for the Cochrane Library. CPAP by mask, nasal prong, nasopharyngeal tube, or endotracheal tube was included. In these trials, CPAP was associated with benefits in terms of reduced respiratory failure and mortality. The studies had varying levels of pressure and delivery mode, so no final conclusions can be drawn about optimal administration methods. Babies on CPAP were reported to have a high rate of pneumothorax.

Implications

CPAP can be effective in reducing respiratory failure in spontaneously breathing preterm infants. It is less invasive, results in fewer complica-

tions, and costs less than IPPV. The infants in these trials tended to have a greater birth weight, but very small preterm infants may still require IPPV, even if spontaneously breathing. You can assure parents that CPAP is an effective treatment for RDS in preterm infants who are breathing spontaneously, particularly if they are of greater birth weight. It is a less invasive procedure resulting in fewer injuries, and it is as effective as IPPV when used correctly and judiciously. More research is needed to identify specific characteristics of those preterm infants who can safely forgo IPPV for CPAP.

Critical Thinking

What assessments will you plan for the preterm infant on CPAP to help you identify early signs of pneumothorax?

Reference

Ho, J. J., Subramaniam, P., Henderon-Smart, D. J., & Davis, P. G. (2003). Continuous distending pressure for respiratory distress syndrome in preterm infants (Cochrane Review). In: *The Cochrane Library*, Issue 4. Chichester, UK: John Wiley & Sons.

High-frequency and extracorporeal membrane oxygenation (ECMO), a form of heart-lung bypass, has been tried when conventional ventilator therapy has not been successful. Both of these have specific protocols for eligibility for use and require specially trained nurses and respiratory therapists. Nitric oxide inhalation therapy may also be a useful adjunctive therapy for infants with RDS (Glomella, 2004). In some institutions, morphine or fentanyl is used for its analgesic and sedative effects. Sedation may be indicated for infants who have air leak respiratory problems. Use of pancuronium (Pavulon) for muscle relaxation in infants with RDS is controversial.

NURSING MANAGEMENT

NURSING ASSESSMENT AND DIAGNOSIS

Look for characteristics of RDS such as increasing cyanosis, tachypnea (> 60 respirations/min), grunting respirations, nasal flaring, significant retractions, and apnea. Table 31–1 reviews clinical findings associated with respiratory distress in general. The Silverman-Andersen index (Figure 31–4 ●) may be helpful in evaluating the signs of respiratory distress in the birthing area.

Nursing diagnoses that may apply to the newborn with RDS include the following:

- *Risk for Ineffective Breathing Pattern* related to immature lung development
- *Ineffective Thermoregulation* related to increased respiratory effort
- *Altered Nutrition: Less than Body Requirements* related to increased metabolic needs in the infant
- *Risk for Fluid Volume Deficit* related to increased insensible water losses

PLANNING AND IMPLEMENTATION

Hospital-Based Nursing Care

Based on clinical parameters, the neonatal nurse implements therapeutic approaches to maintain physiologic homeostasis and provides supportive care to the newborn with RDS. (See "Nursing Care Plan: The Newborn with Respiratory Distress Syndrome.")

Nursing interventions and criteria for instituting mechanical ventilation depend on institutional protocol. Methods of oxygen monitoring and nursing interventions are included in Table 31–2. The nursing care of infants on ventilators or with umbilical artery catheters is not discussed here. These infants have severe respiratory distress and are cared for in NICUs by nurses with advanced knowledge and training. Ventilatory assistance with high-frequency ventilators has shown positive results.

The parents of a baby with respiratory distress will need a very supportive environment.

EVALUATION

Expected outcomes of nursing care include the following:

- The newborn at risk of RDS is promptly identified and early intervention is initiated.

TABLE 31–1 ✤ Clinical Assessments Associated with Respiratory Distress

Clinical Picture	Significance
Skin Color	
Pallor or mottling	These represent poor peripheral circulation due to systemic hypotension and vasoconstriction and pooling of independent areas (usually in conjunction with severe hypoxia).
Cyanosis (bluish tint)	Depending on hemoglobin concentration, peripheral circulation, intensity and quality of viewing light, and acuity of observer's color vision, this is frankly visible in advanced hypoxia. Central cyanosis is most easily detected by examination of mucous membranes and tongue.
Jaundice (yellow discoloration of skin and mucous membranes due to presence of unconjugated [indirect] bilirubin)	Metabolic alterations (acidosis, hypercarbia, asphyxia) of respiratory distress mean the newborn is predisposed to having bilirubin dissociate from albumin-binding sites and be deposited in the skin and central nervous system.
Edema (presents as slick, shiny skin)	This is characteristic of preterm infants because their total protein concentration is low, with a decrease in colloidal osmotic pressure and transudation of fluid. Edema of hands and feet is frequently seen within first 24 hours and resolved by fifth day in infants with severe RDS.

TABLE 31–1 ❖ Clinical Assessments Associated with Respiratory Distress—continued

Clinical Picture	Significance
Respiratory System	
Tachypnea (normal respiratory rate 30–60/minute, elevated respiratory rate 60+/minute)	Increased respiratory rate is the most frequent and easily detectable sign of respiratory distress after birth. This compensatory mechanism attempts to increase respiratory dead space to maintain alveolar ventilation and gas exchange in the face of an increase in mechanical resistance. As a decompensatory mechanism, it increases workload and energy output by increasing respiratory rate, which causes increased metabolic demand for oxygen and thus increases alveolar ventilation on an already overstressed system. Shallow, rapid respirations increase dead space ventilation, thus decreasing alveolar ventilation.
Apnea (episode of nonbreathing for more than 20 seconds; periodic breathing, a common "normal" occurrence in preterm infants, is defined as apnea of 5–10 seconds alternating with 10–15 seconds of ventilation)	This poor prognostic sign indicates cardiorespiratory disease, CNS disease, metabolic alterations, intracranial hemorrhage, sepsis, or immaturity. Physiologic alterations include decreased oxygen saturation, respiratory acidosis, and bradycardia.
Chest	Inspection of the thoracic cage includes shape, size, and symmetry of movement. Respiratory movements should be symmetric and diaphragmatic; asymmetry reflects pathology (pneumothorax, diaphragmatic hernia). Increased anteroposterior diameter indicates air trapping (meconium aspiration syndrome).
Labored respirations (Silverman-Andersen index in Figure 31–4 indicates severity of retractions, grunting, and nasal flaring, which are signs of labored respirations)	Indicates marked increase in the work of breathing.
Retractions (inward pulling of soft parts of the chest cage—suprasternal, substernal, intercostal, subcostal—at inspiration)	These reflect the significant increase in negative intrathoracic pressure necessary to inflate stiff, noncompliant lungs. Infants try to increase lung compliance by using accessory muscles. Lung expansion markedly decreases. Seesaw respirations are seen when the chest flattens with inspiration and the abdomen bulges. Retractions increase the work of breathing and oxygen need so that assisted ventilation may be necessary due to exhaustion.
Flaring nares (inspiratory dilation of nostrils)	This compensatory mechanism attempts to lessen the resistance of the narrow nasal passage.
Expiratory grunt (Valsalva maneuver in which the infant exhales against a closed glottis, thus producing an audible moan)	This increases transpulmonary pressure, which decreases or prevents atelectasis, thus improving oxygenation and alveolar ventilation. Intubation should not be tried unless the infant's condition is rapidly deteriorating, because it prevents this maneuver and allows the alveoli to collapse.
Rhythmic body movement with labored respirations (chin tug, head bobbing, retractions of anal area)	This is a result of using abdominal and other respiratory accessory muscles during prolonged forced respirations.
Auscultation of chest reveals decreased air exchange, with harsh breath sounds or fine inspiratory rales; rhonchi may be present	Decrease in breath sounds and distant quality may indicate interstitial or intrapleural air or fluid.
Cardiovascular System	
Continuous systolic murmur may be audible	Patent ductus arteriosus is common with hypoxia, pulmonary vasoconstriction, right-to-left shunting, and congestive heart failure.
Heart rate usually within normal limits (fixed heart rate may occur with a rate of 110–120/minute)	A fixed heart rate indicates a decrease in vagal control.
Point of maximal impulse usually located at fourth to fifth intercostal space, left sternal border	Displacement may reflect dextrocardia, pneumothorax, or diaphragmatic hernia.
Hypothermia	This is inadequate functioning of metabolic processes that require oxygen to produce necessary body heat.
Muscle Tone	
Flaccid, hypotonic, unresponsive to stimuli Hypertonia and/or seizure activity	These may indicate deterioration in the newborn's condition and possible CNS damage due to hypoxia, acidemia, or hemorrhage.

● **FIGURE 31–4**

Evaluation of respiratory status using the Silverman-Andersen index. The baby's respiratory status is assessed. A grade of 0, 1, or 2 is determined for each area, and a total score is charted in the baby's record or on a copy of this tool and placed in the chart.

Used with permission from Ross Laboratories, Nursing Aid No. 2. Columbus, OH; Silverman, W. A., & Andersen, D. H. (1956). Pediatrics, 17, 1–10. Copyright 1956, American Academy of Pediatrics.

■ The newborn is free of respiratory distress and metabolic alterations.

■ The parents verbalize their concerns about their baby's health problem and survival and understand the rationale behind the management of their newborn.

TRANSIENT TACHYPNEA OF THE NEWBORN

Some AGA preterm and near-term infants may develop progressive respiratory distress that can resemble classic RDS. They may have had intrauterine or intrapartal asphyxia due to maternal oversedation, maternal bleeding, prolapsed cord, breech birth, or maternal diabetes. The newborn then fails to clear the airway of lung fluid, mucus, and other debris or has an excess of fluid in the lungs due to aspiration of amniotic or tracheal fluid. Transient tachypnea occurs in 11 per 1000 live births. It is also more prevalent in cesarean birth newborns who have not had the thoracic squeeze that occurs during vaginal birth and removes some of the lung fluid (Glomella, 2004).

Usually the newborn experiences little or no difficulty at the onset of breathing. However, shortly after birth, expiratory grunting, flaring of the nares, and mild cyanosis may be noted in the newborn breathing room air. Tachypnea is usually present by 6 hours of age, with respiratory rates as high as 100 to 140 breaths per minute. Mild respiratory and metabolic acidosis may be present at 2 to 6 hours.

Clinical Therapy

Initial x-ray findings may be identical to those showing RDS within the first 3 hours. However, radiographs of infants with transient tachypnea usually reveal a generalized overexpansion of the lungs (hyperaeration of alveoli), which is identified principally by flattened contours of the diaphragm. Dense streaks (increased vascularity) radiate from the hilar region and represent engorgement of the lymphatic vessels, which clear alveolar fluid when air breathing begins. Within 48–72 hours the chest x-ray examination is normal (Glomella, 2004).

NURSING PRACTICE

In babies with RDS who are on ventilators, increased urination (determined by weighing diapers) may be an early clue that the baby's condition is improving. As fluid moves out of the lungs and into the bloodstream, alveoli open and kidney perfusion increases, which results in increased voiding. At this point, monitor chest expansion closely. If chest expansion is increasing, ventilator settings may have to be decreased. Too high a ventilator setting may "blow the lung," resulting in pneumothorax.

Ambient oxygen concentrations of 30% to 50%, usually under an oxygen hood, may be required to correct

(continues on page 826)

TABLE 31–2 ✛ Oxygen Monitors

Type	Function and Rationale	Nursing Interventions
Pulse Oximetry—SPo$_2$		
Estimates beat-to-beat arterial oxygen saturation.	Calibration is automatic.	Understand and use oxyhemoglobin dissociation curve.
Microprocessor measures saturation by the absorption of red and infrared light as it passes through tissue.	Less dependent on perfusion than TcPo$_2$ and TcPCo$_2$; however, functions poorly if peripheral perfusion is decreased due to low cardiac output.	Monitor trends over time and correlate with arterial blood gases. Check disposable sensor at least q8h.
Changes in absorption related to blood pulsation through vessel determine saturation and pulse rate.	Much more rapid response time than TcPo$_2$— offers real-time readings.	Use disposable cuffs (reusable cuffs allow too much ambient light to enter, and readings may be inaccurate).
	Can be located on extremity, digit, or palm of hand, leaving chest free; not affected by skin characteristics.	
	Requires understanding of oxyhemoglobin dissociation curve.	
	Pulse oximeter reading of 87% to 95% reflects clinically safe range of saturation.	
	Extreme sensitivity to movement; decreases if average of 7th or 14th beat is selected rather than beat to beat.	
	Poor correlation with extreme hyperoxia.	
Transcutaneous Oxygen Monitor—TcPo$_2$		
Measures oxygen diffusion across the skin.	When transcutaneous monitors are properly calibrated and electrodes are appropriately positioned, they provide reliable, continuous, noninvasive measurements of Po$_2$, PCo$_2$, and oxygen saturation.	Use TcPo$_2$ to monitor trends of oxygenation with routine nursing care procedures.
Clark electrode is heated to 43°C (preterm) or 44°C (term) to warm the skin beneath the electrode and promote diffusion of oxygen across the skin surface. Po$_2$ is measured when oxygen diffuses across the capillary membrane, skin, and electrode membrane (Askin & Diehl Jones, 2004).	Readings vary when skin perfusion is decreased. Reliable as trend monitor. Frequent calibration necessary to overcome mechanical drift. Following membrane change, machine must "warm up" 1 hour prior to initial calibration; otherwise, after turning it on, it must equilibrate for 30 minutes prior to calibration. When placed on infant, values will be low until skin is heated; approximately 15 minutes required to stabilize.	Clean electrode surface to remove electrolyte deposits; change solution and membrane once a week. Allow machine to stabilize before drawing arterial gases; note reading when gases are drawn and use values to correlate. Ensure airtight seal between skin surface and electrode; place electrodes on clean, dry skin on upper chest, abdomen, or inner aspect of thigh; avoid bony prominences.
	Second-degree burns are rare but possible if electrodes remain in place too long. Decreased correlations noted with older infants (related to skin thickness), with infants with low cardiac output (decreased skin perfusion), and with hyperoxic infants.	Change skin site and recalibrate at least every 4 hours; inspect skin for burns; if burns occur, use lowest temperature setting and change position of electrode more frequently.
	The adhesive that attaches the electrode may abrade the fragile skin of the preterm infant. May be used for both preductal and postductal monitoring of oxygenation for observations of shunting.	Adhesive disks may be cut to a smaller size, or skin prep may be used under the adhesive circle only; allow membrane to touch skin surface at center.

NURSING CARE PLAN

THE NEWBORN WITH RESPIRATORY DISTRESS SYNDROME

Intervention	Rationale	Expected Outcome
1. Nursing Diagnosis: Risk for Ineffective Breathing Pattern related to immature lung development		
NIC Intervention: **Respiratory monitoring:** Collection and analysis of patient data to ensure airway patency and adequate gas exchange		**NOC Outcome:** **Respiratory status:** Ventilation: Movement of air in and out of the lungs

Goal: The infant will maintain an effective breathing pattern.

■ Review maternal birth records noting medications given to mother prior to birth and the infant's condition at birth such as Apgar scores and resuscitative measures. ■ Initiate cardiac and respiratory monitoring and calibrate these monitors every 8 hours. ■ Monitor infant's respiratory rate and rhythm, pulse, blood pressure, and activity. ■ Assess skin color; note signs of cyanosis, duskiness, and pallor. ■ Clear infant's airway by suctioning prn with bulb syringe. ■ Administer warmed, humidified oxygen by oxygen hood and monitor the oxygen concentrations every 30 minutes. ■ Do not allow oxyhood to touch infant's face; maintain a stable oxygen concentration by increasing and decreasing oxygen by 5%–10% increments.	■ Several drugs suppress respiratory function in the newborn. ■ Close monitoring detects periodic apneic spells and allows for medical intervention if necessary. ■ Increases in respiratory rate and pulse, alteration in rhythm, and blood pressure may indicate respiratory distress. ■ Any changes in the normal skin color may indicate a physiologic change occurring. ■ Opens airway by clearing mucus and allows maximum respiratory effort. ■ Prevents mucosal dryness and maintains an even level of oxygen administration. ■ Allowing oxyhood to touch infant's face may cause apnea by stimulating the facial nerve.	■ The infant will maintain an effective breathing pattern as evidenced by: respirations are 30–60 breaths/min, arterial blood gases are within a normal range, infant is free of signs of retractions or nasal flaring, and blood pH is 7.35–7.45.
Collaborative: Obtain arterial blood gases (ABGs) per physician orders. 1. Maintain constant O_2 concentration for 15–30 minutes before sample is obtained. 2. Avoid stimulating infant 15 minutes prior to obtaining sample. 3. Avoid suctioning infant prior to obtaining sample. 4. Obtain sample in heparinized tuberculin syringe and maintain the temperature of the sample. 5. Assess the patency of the IV line to prevent clot formation, then replace blood used to clear line. 6. Flush line with 2 mL heparinized solution before restarting flow of IV fluids. 7. Monitor transcutaneous pulse oximeter continuously or hourly and record. Rotate sensor site every 3–4 hours.	■ Obtaining arterial blood gases is essential in managing an infant receiving oxygen. Suctioning may cause a discrepancy in ABG readings and should be avoided.	
■ Assess infant's need for mechanical ventilation: apnea present, hypoxia (PaO_2 < 50 mm Hg), hypercapnia ($PaCO_2$ > 60 mm Hg), respiratory acidosis (pH < 7.2). ■ Administer mechanical ventilation per hospital protocol.	■ Mechanical ventilation improves oxygenation and ventilation, resulting in rise in PaO_2 and decrease in $PaCO_2$. ■ CPAP or PEEP can be administered by nasal prongs or by nasopharyngeal or oral intubation.	

NURSING CARE PLAN—continued

THE NEWBORN WITH RESPIRATORY DISTRESS SYNDROME

Intervention	Rationale	Expected Outcome
2. Nursing Diagnosis: Ineffective Thermoregulation related to increased respiratory effort		
NIC Intervention: **Temperature regulation:** Attaining or maintaining body temperature within a normal range		**NOC Outcome:** **Thermoregulation: Newborn:** Balance among heat production, heat gain, and heat loss during the neonatal period
Goal: The infant will exhibit no signs of hypothermia.		
■ Review maternal prenatal and intrapartum records. Note any medications mother received during these times. ■ Assess infant's temperature frequently. ■ Observe for signs of increased oxygen consumption and metabolic acidosis. ■ Warm all inspired gases and record temperature of delivered gases. ■ Use radiant warmers or isolettes with servocontrols, incubators, and open cribs with appropriate clothing. ■ Note signs and symptoms of respiratory distress, including tachypnea, apnea, cyanosis, acrocyanosis, bradycardia, lethargy, weak cry, and hypotonia.	■ Medications such as Demerol and magnesium sulfate used by the mother during the prenatal or intrapartum periods significantly interfere with the infant's ability to retain heat. ■ Hypothermia leads to pulmonary vasoconstriction because of the increase in oxygen consumption. ■ Cold stress leads to increased oxygen needs; thereby, brown fat is used to maintain body temperature. ■ Hypoxia and acidosis further depresses surfactant production. ■ Maintains neutral thermal environment. ■ These signs can predispose the infant to metabolic acidosis.	■ The infant will not exhibit signs and symptoms of hypothermia as evidenced by temperature maintenance of 97.7–99.1°F and no signs and symptoms of respiratory distress. ■ Cold air/oxygen blown in face of newborn is stimulus for consumption of oxygen and glucose and increased metabolic rate.
3. Nursing Diagnosis: Altered Nutrition: Less than Body Requirements related to increased metabolic needs in the Infant		
NIC Intervention: **Newborn monitoring:** Measurement and interpretation of physiologic status of the newborn the first 24 hours		**NOC Outcome:** **Nutritional status: Food and fluid intake:** Amount of food and fluid taken into the body over a 24-hour period
Goal: Infant will gain weight in a normal curve.		
■ Assess suck, swallow, gag, and cough reflexes. ■ Assess respiratory status of infant. If problems are noted, notify physician. ■ Monitor IV rates per infusion pump (starting at 60 mL/kg/day) or as ordered by physician. ■ Record hourly intake and output (I&O) and daily weights. ■ Provide total parenteral nutrition (TPN) when indicated.	■ Prevents feeding problems and assists in determining the best method of feeding for infant. ■ In the presence of respiratory distress, avoid oral fluids and initiate parenteral nutrition per physician's orders. ■ Allows for close monitoring of fluid intake. ■ IV fluids are administered to replace sensible and insensible water loss, as well as evaporative water loss secondary to infant respiratory distress. Monitoring I&O will prevent circulatory system overload that can lead to pulmonary edema and cardiac problems. ■ TPN is used as nutritional alternative if bowel sounds are not present and/or infant remains in acute distress.	■ The infant will maintain steady weight gain as evidenced by < 2%/day weight loss, tolerates oral feedings, and urine output is 1–3 mL/kg/hour.

(continued)

NURSING CARE PLAN—continued

THE NEWBORN WITH RESPIRATORY DISTRESS SYNDROME

Intervention	Rationale	Expected Outcome
■ Advance, based on tolerance, from intravenous to gastrointestinal (GI) feedings. Gavage or nipple-feedings are used, and IV is used as supplement (discontinued when oral intake is sufficient). ■ Provide adequate caloric intake: consider amount of intake, type of formula, route of administration, and need for supplementation of intake by other routes. ■ Assess infusion site for signs and symptoms of infection, including erythema, edema, and drainage with a foul odor.	■ If IV is discontinued before oral intake is established, baby will not receive adequate calories. ■ Formula or breast milk stimulate GI hormones necessary for a functional absorptive GI tract. ■ Avoid complications associated with nutrition by IV route only. ■ Calories are essential to prevent catabolism of body proteins, and metabolic acidosis due to starvation or inadequate caloric intake. ■ Appropriate intervention can be initiated when signs and symptoms of infection are detected early. Treatment may avoid infection and sepsis in the infant.	

4. Nursing Diagnosis: Risk for Fluid Volume Deficit related to increased insensible water losses

NIC Intervention:		NOC Outcome:
Fluid monitoring: Collection and analysis of patient data to regulate fluid balance		**Fluid balance:** Balance of water in the intracellular and extracellular compartments of the body

Goal: The infant will not exhibit signs of dehydration and will display appropriate weight gain.

■ Observe for weight fluctuations by obtaining daily weights. ■ Document cumulative balances of intake (IV fluid administration and feedings) and output (urine collection bags, weighing or counting diapers) hourly. ■ Obtain urinalysis, monitor closely specific gravity and nitrites. ■ Monitor vital signs, including blood pressure, pulse, temperature, and mean arterial pressure (MAP). ■ Assess client for signs of dehydration (i.e., poor skin turgor, pale mucous membranes, and sunken anterior fontanelle). ■ Assess IV site for signs of infection (erythema and edema) and infiltration. **Collaborative:** Obtain labs for Hct, serum calcium, serum magnesium, serum potassium, blood urea nitrogen (BUN), creatinine, and uric acid levels. ■ Administer fluids, blood products, and electrolytes as ordered by physician.	■ Fluctuations in weight may indicate water imbalance or inadequate caloric intake. ■ Balanced fluid intake and output suggest homeostasis. ■ Specific gravity > 1.013 and nitrites present in the urine are indicative of not enough fluid intake. ■ A MAP of less than 20 mm Hg may indicate hypotension. ■ Detecting signs and symptoms of dehydration early in the infant is important because early intervention is vital to prevent further damage. ■ If signs and symptoms of infection are noted, intervention is necessary and IV site should be changed. ■ Determines necessity for TPN administration. ■ Replaces low nutrient stores and treats anemia if present.	■ The infant will be free of signs and symptoms of dehydration as evidenced by intake equaling output, urine specific gravity in normal range, and a weight gain of at least 20–30 grams/day.

Premature infant under an oxygen hood. Infant is nested and has a non-nutritive sucking pacifier.

Courtesy of Lisa Smith-Pedersen, RNC, MSN, NNP.

the hypoxemia (Figure 31–5 ●). Fluid and electrolyte requirements should be met with IV fluids during the acute phase of the disease. Oral feedings are contraindicated because of rapid respiratory rates. The infant should be improving by 8 to 24 hours. The clinical course of transient tachypnea lasts approximately 72 hours (Glomella, 2004).

When hypoxemia is severe and tachypnea continues, persistent pulmonary hypertension must be considered and treatment measures initiated. If pneumonia is suspected initially, antibiotics may be administered prophylactically.

Nursing Management

For nursing actions, see "Nursing Care Plan: The Newborn with Respiratory Distress Syndrome."

THINKING CRITICALLY

TRANSIENT TACHYPNEA OF THE NEWBORN

You are caring for baby girl Linn, who is a 39-week, AGA female born by repeat cesarean birth to a 34-year-old G3, now P3, mother. Baby Linn's Apgar scores were 7 and 9 at 1 and 5 minutes. At 2 hours of age, an elevated respiratory rate of 100 to 120 and mild cyanosis were noted. She is now receiving 30% oxygen and has a respiratory rate of 70 to 80. The baby's clinical course, chest x-ray examination, and lab work are all consistent with transient tachypnea of the newborn. Her mother calls you to ask about her baby. She tells you that her last child was born at 30 weeks' gestation, has respiratory distress syndrome requiring ventilator support, and was hospitalized for 6 weeks. She asks you, "Is this the same respiratory distress?" What will you tell her?

CARE OF THE NEWBORN WITH MECONIUM ASPIRATION SYNDROME

Because the body's response to asphyxia is increased peristalsis (movement) within the bowels and relaxation of the anal sphincter, the presence of meconium in the amniotic fluid indicates that the fetus may be suffering asphyxia. However, if the fetus is in a breech position, the presence of meconium in the amniotic fluid does not necessarily indicate asphyxia.

Approximately 13% of live-born infants are born through meconium-stained amniotic fluid (MSAF). Of the newborns born through MSAF, an average of 5% develop **meconium aspiration syndrome (MAS)** (Gelfand, Fanaroff, & Walsh, 2004). This fluid may be aspirated into the tracheobronchial tree in utero or during the first few breaths taken by the newborn. This syndrome primarily affects term, SGA, and postterm newborns and those who have experienced a long labor.

Meconium in the lungs produces a ball-valve action (air is allowed in but not exhaled), so that alveoli overdistend and rupture, resulting in pulmonary air leaks such as pneumomediastinum or pneumothorax. The meconium also triggers a chemical pneumonitis in the lung, causing oxygen and carbon dioxide to be trapped there and the lungs to hyperinflate. Secondary bacterial pneumonia can occur.

CLINICAL MANIFESTATIONS OF MAS

Clinical manifestations of MAS include (1) fetal hypoxia in utero a few days or a few minutes before birth, indicated by a sudden increase in fetal activity followed by diminished activity, slowing of FHR or weak and irregular heartbeat, loss of beat-to-beat variability, and meconium staining of amniotic fluid; and (2) signs of distress at birth, such as pallor, cyanosis, apnea, slow heartbeat, and low Apgar scores (below 6) at 1 and 5 minutes. Newborns with intrauterine asphyxia, meconium-stained newborns, or newborns that have aspirated meconium are depressed at birth and require resuscitation to establish adequate respiratory effort.

After the initial resuscitation, the severity of clinical symptoms depends on the extent of aspiration. Many infants need mechanical ventilation at birth because of immediate signs of distress (generalized cyanosis, tachypnea, and severe retractions). An overdistended, barrel-shaped chest with increased anteroposterior diameter is common. Auscultation reveals diminished air movement, with prominent rales and rhonchi. Abdominal palpation may reveal a displaced liver caused by diaphragmatic depression resulting from the overexpansion of the lungs. The skin, nails, and umbilical cord usually have yellowish staining.

The chest x-ray film reveals nonuniform, coarse, patchy densities and hyperinflation (9 to 11 rib expansion)

(Glomella, 2004). Evidence of pulmonary air leak is frequently present. Extreme hypoxia is also caused by the cardiopulmonary shunting and resultant failure to oxygenate and can lead to persistent pulmonary hypertension of the newborn (PPHN).

CLINICAL THERAPY

The maternity and pediatric teams must work together to prevent MAS. The most effective form of preventive management is as follows:

1. After the head is born and while the shoulders and chest are still in the birth canal, the baby's oropharynx and then nasopharynx are suctioned by the birth attendant with the use of a bulb syringe or DeLee attached to wall suction. (This is also done with a cesarean birth.) To decrease the possibility of HIV transmission, low-pressure wall suction is used.

2. If the infant is vigorous even if there is thick or thin meconium in the amniotic fluid, no subsequent special resuscitation is indicated (de Ungria & Steinhorn, 2003).

3. If the infant has absent or depressed respirations, heart rate less than 100 beats per minute, or poor muscle tone, direct tracheal suctioning by specially trained personnel such as a neonatal nurse practitioner, an experienced NICU nurse trained in those skills, a respiratory therapist, or a nurse anesthetist is recommended. The glottis is visualized with a laryngoscope and the trachea suctioned (Gelfand et al., 2004).

If the newborn's head is not adequately suctioned at the time the head is born but the shoulder and chest are still in the vagina, respiratory or resuscitative efforts will push meconium into the airway and into the lungs. Stimulation of the newborn should be avoided to minimize respiratory movements. Further resuscitative efforts are undertaken as indicated, following the same principles of clinical therapy used for asphyxia (discussed earlier in this chapter). Resuscitated newborns should be transferred immediately to the NICU for closer observation. An umbilical arterial line may be used for direct monitoring of arterial blood pressures; blood sampling for pH and blood gases; and infusion of intravenous fluids, blood, or medications.

Treatment usually involves delivering high levels of oxygen and high-pressure ventilation. Ventilation with low PEEP is preferred to avoid pulmonary air leaks such as pneumothorax. Unfortunately, high pressures may be needed to cause sufficient expiratory expansion of obstructed airways or to stabilize airways weakened by inflammation so that the most distal atelectatic alveoli are ventilated.

Surfactant replacement therapy is most effective when used prophylactically. It improves oxygenation and de-creases the incidence of air leaks. Systemic blood pressure and pulmonary blood flow must be maintained. Dopamine or dobutamine, volume expanders, or both may be used to maintain systemic blood pressure.

Newborns over 2 kg (7 lb) with respiratory failure who are not responding to conventional ventilator therapy may need treatment with high-frequency ventilation and/or nitric oxide therapy or ECMO (Zukowsky, 2004). ECMO treatment has proved successful for newborns with meconium aspiration, pneumonia, and PPHN who are not responding to traditional treatments.

Treatment includes chest physiotherapy (chest percussion, vibration, and drainage) to remove debris. Frequently, prophylactic intravenous antibiotics are given. Bicarbonate (to correct metabolic acidosis) may be necessary for several days for severely ill newborns. Mortality in term or postterm infants is very high, because the cycle of hypoxemia and acidemia is difficult to break.

NURSING MANAGEMENT

NURSING ASSESSMENT AND DIAGNOSIS

During the intrapartum period, observe for signs of fetal hypoxia and meconium staining of amniotic fluid. At birth assess the newborn for signs of distress. Carefully observe for complications such as pulmonary air leaks; anoxic cerebral injury manifested by convulsions; myocardial injury evidenced by congestive heart failure or cardiomegaly; disseminated intravascular coagulation (DIC) resulting from hypoxic hepatic damage that depresses liver-dependent clotting factors; anoxic renal damage demonstrated by hematuria, oliguria, or anuria; fluid overload; sepsis secondary to bacterial pneumonia; and any signs of intestinal necrosis from ischemia, including gastrointestinal obstruction or hemorrhage.

Nursing diagnoses that may apply to the newborn with MAS and the infant's parents include the following:

- *Impaired Gas Exchange* related to aspiration of meconium and amniotic fluid during birth

- *Altered Nutrition: Less than Body Requirements* related to respiratory distress and increased energy requirements

- *Ineffective Family Coping: Compromised* related to life-threatening illness in term newborn

PLANNING AND IMPLEMENTATION

Hospital-Based Nursing Care

Initial interventions are aimed at preventing aspiration by helping remove the meconium from the infant's oropharynx and nasopharynx before the first extrauterine breath. When significant aspiration occurs, the primary goals of therapy are to maintain appropriate gas exchange and minimize complications. Nursing interventions after resuscitation should include maintaining adequate oxygenation and ventilation, regulating temperature, performing glucose testing by glucometer at 2 hours of age to check for hypoglycemia, observing intravenous fluids administration, calculating necessary fluids (which may be restricted in the first 48 to 72 hours due to cerebral edema), providing caloric requirements, and monitoring intravenous antibiotic therapy.

EVALUATION

Expected outcomes of nursing care include the following:

- The newborn at risk of MAS is promptly identified, and early intervention is initiated.
- The newborn is free of respiratory distress and metabolic alterations.
- The parents verbalize their concerns about their baby's health problem and survival and understand the rationale behind the management of their newborn.

CARE OF THE NEWBORN WITH COLD STRESS

Cold stress is excessive heat loss that requires a newborn to use compensatory mechanisms (such as increased respirations and nonshivering thermogenesis) to maintain core body temperature. Newborns experience heat loss that results in cold stress through the mechanisms of evaporation, convection, conduction, and radiation. (See "Heat Loss" in Chapter 26 for types of thermoregulation. ∞)

Heat loss at birth that leads to cold stress can play a significant role in the severity of RDS and the ultimate outcome for the infant. Both preterm and SGA newborns are at risk for cold stress because they have decreased adipose tissue, brown fat stores, and glycogen available for metabolism. As discussed in Chapter 26, the newborn infant's major source of heat production in nonshivering thermogenesis (NST) is brown fat metabolism. ∞ The infant's ability to respond to cold stress by NST is impaired in the presence of several conditions:

- Hypoxemia (Po_2 less than 50 torr)
- Intracranial hemorrhage or any CNS abnormality
- Hypoglycemia (blood glucose level < 40 mg/dL)

When these conditions occur, the infant's temperature should be monitored closely and the neutral thermal environment conscientiously maintained. The nurse must recognize these conditions and treat them as soon as possible. The metabolic consequences of cold stress can be devastating and potentially fatal to an infant. Oxygen requirements rise, glucose use increases, acids are released into the bloodstream, and surfactant production decreases. The effects are graphically depicted in Figure 31–6 ⦿.

NURSING MANAGEMENT

The amount of heat an infant loses depends largely on the actions of the nurse or caregiver. For example, following the transfer of a NICU newborn from one bed to another, a transient, although not significant, decrease in temperature for up to 1 hour may be noted. Prevention of heat loss is especially critical in the VLBW infant. Placing the VLBW

⦿ **FIGURE 31–6**

Cold stress chain of events. The hypothermic, or cold-stressed, newborn attempts to compensate by conserving heat and increasing heat production. These physiologic compensatory mechanisms initiate a series of metabolic events that result in hypoxemia and altered surfactant production, metabolic acidosis, hypoglycemia, and hyperbilirubinemia.

newborn in a polyethylene wrapping immediately following birth can decrease the postnatal fall in temperature that normally occurs. Both convective and evaporative heat loss can be reduced (Blackburn, 2003).

Observe the baby for signs of cold stress, including increased movement and respirations, decreased skin temperature and peripheral perfusion, development of hypoglycemia, and possibly development of metabolic acidosis.

Vasoconstriction is the initial response to cold stress. Because it initially decreases skin temperature, monitor and assess skin temperature instead of rectal temperature. A decrease in rectal temperature means that the core temperature of the infant has decreased and the infant has long-standing cold stress. By monitoring skin temperature, possible decrease will become apparent before the infant's core temperature is affected.

If skin temperature decreases, determine whether hypoglycemia is present. Hypoglycemia is a result of the metabolic effects of cold stress and is suggested by glucometer values below 45 mg/dL, tremors, irritability or lethargy, apnea, or seizure activity.

If the baby becomes hypothermic, initiate the following care plan (Blackburn, 2003):

- Keep the ambient air temperature 1°C to 1.5°C higher than the infant's temperature.

- Warm the newborn slowly because rapid temperature elevation may cause hypotension and apnea.

- Increase the air temperature in hourly increments of 1°C until the infant's temperature is stable.

- Monitor skin temperature every 15 to 30 minutes to determine if the newborn's temperature is increasing.

- Remove plastic wrap, caps, and heat shields while rewarming the infant so that cool air is not trapped along with the warm air.

- Warm intravenous fluids prior to infusion.

- Block heat loss by evaporation, radiation, convection, and conduction and maintain the newborn in a neutral thermal environment.

Assess for anaerobic metabolism and treat the resulting metabolic acidosis. Burning brown fat increases oxygen consumption, lactic acid levels, and metabolic acidosis. Hypoglycemia may be reversed by adequate glucose intake, as described in the following section.

CARE OF THE NEWBORN WITH HYPOGLYCEMIA

A widely used cutoff point or threshold for intervention in newborn hypoglycemia is a *plasma glucose concentration at or below* 40 mg/dL (Armentrout, 2004). *Plasma glucose*

values less than 20 to 25 mg/dL should be treated with parenteral glucose, regardless of the age or gestation. **Hypoglycemia** is the most common metabolic disorder in IDMs, SGA infants, and preterm AGA infants. The pathophysiology of hypoglycemia differs for each classification.

AGA preterm infants have not been in utero long enough to store glycogen and fat. As a result they have decreased ability to carry out gluconeogenesis. This situation is further aggravated by the tissues' increased use of glucose (especially in the brain and heart) during stress and illness (chilling, asphyxia, sepsis, RDS).

Infants of White's classes A–C or type 1 diabetic mothers have increased stores of glycogen and fat (see "Common Complication of the IDM" in Chapter 30 ∞) and higher circulating insulin and insulin responsiveness levels than other newborns. Because the high in utero glucose loads stop at birth, the newborn experiences rapid, profound hypoglycemia (Armentrout, 2004).

The SGA infant has used up glycogen and fat stores because of intrauterine malnutrition and has a blunted hepatic enzymatic response with which to produce and use glucose. Any newborn stressed at birth (from asphyxia or hypothermia) also quickly uses up available glucose stores and becomes hypoglycemic. Epidural anesthesia may alter maternal-fetal glucose homeostasis, resulting in hypoglycemia.

CLINICAL THERAPY

The goal of management includes early identification of hypoglycemia through observation and screening of newborns at risk (Sperling & Menon, 2004). The newborn may be asymptomatic, or any of the following may occur:

- Lethargy, jitteriness
- Poor feeding
- Vomiting
- Pallor
- Apnea, irregular respirations, respiratory distress, cyanosis
- Hypotonia, possible loss of swallowing reflex
- Tremors, jerkiness, seizure activity
- High-pitched cry
- Exaggerated Moro reflex

Aggressive treatment is recommended after a single low blood glucose value if the infant shows any of these symptoms. In at-risk infants, routine screening should be done frequently during the first 4 hours of life and then whenever any of the noted clinical manifestations appear or at 4-hour intervals until the risk period has passed.

Differential diagnosis of a newborn with nonspecific hypoglycemic symptoms includes determining if the newborn has any of the following:

- CNS disease
- Sepsis
- Metabolic aberrations
- Polycythemia
- Congenital heart disease
- Drug withdrawal
- Temperature instability
- Hypocalcemia

Hypoglycemia may also be defined as a *glucose oxidase reagent strip* below 45 mg/dL, but only when corroborated with laboratory plasma glucose testing (see Skill 10–1 **SKILLS**). Common bedside methods use whole blood, an enzymatic reagent strip, and a reflectance meter or color chart. Bedside glucose oxidase strip tests can screen for hypoglycemia, but laboratory determinations must confirm the results before a diagnosis of hypoglycemia can be made. Glucose reagent strips should not be used by themselves to screen for and diagnose hypoglycemia, because their results depend on the baby's hematocrit and there is a wide variance (5 to 15 mg/dL) between their results and laboratory plasma determinations.

NURSING PRACTICE

Wrapping the foot in a warm washcloth or disposable diaper is a simple way to create adequate vasodilation for taking a blood specimen.

Blood glucose sampling techniques can significantly affect the accuracy of the blood glucose value. Whole blood glucose concentrations are 10% to 15% lower than plasma glucose concentrations—the higher the hematocrit, the greater the difference between whole blood and plasma values. Also, venous blood glucose concentrations are approximately 15% to 19% lower than arterial blood glucose concentrations because the tissues extract some glucose before the blood enters the venous system ("Neonatal Hypoglycemia," 2000). Newer techniques, such as using a glucose oxidase analyzer or an optical bedside glucose analyzer, are more reliable for bedside screening but must also be validated with laboratory chemical analysis.

NURSING PRACTICE

Blood samples for the laboratory should be placed on ice and analyzed within 30 minutes of drawing to prevent the red blood cells from continuing to metabolize glucose and giving a falsely low reading.

Adequate caloric intake is important. Early formula-feeding or breastfeeding is a major preventive approach. If early feeding meets the infant's fluid and caloric needs, the blood glucose concentration is likely to remain above the hypoglycemic level. During the first hours after birth, asymptomatic newborns may also be given oral glucose. Another plasma glucose measurement is then obtained 30 to 60 minutes after feeding.

Intravenous infusions of a dextrose solution (5% to 10%) begun immediately after birth also should prevent hypoglycemia. Plasma glucose levels are obtained when the parenteral infusion is started. However, in the very small AGA infant, infusions of 10% dextrose solution may cause hyperglycemia to develop, requiring an alteration in the glucose concentration. Infants require 6 to 8 mg/kg/min of glucose to maintain normal glucose concentrations. Therefore, an intravenous glucose solution should be calculated based on the infant's body weight, with blood glucose tests to determine adequacy of the infusion treatment.

A rapid infusion of 25% to 50% dextrose is contraindicated because it may lead to profound rebound hypoglycemia following an initial brief increase. In more severe hypoglycemic periods, corticosteroids may be administered. It is thought that steroids enhance gluconeogenesis from noncarbohydrate protein sources (Armentrout, 2004). The untreated hypoglycemia may result in permanent, untreatable CNS damage or death.

NURSING MANAGEMENT

NURSING ASSESSMENT AND DIAGNOSIS

The objectives of nursing assessment are to identify newborns at risk and to screen symptomatic infants. For

---

COMPLEMENTARY CARE

PAIN RELIEF IN THE NICU

Oral administration of sucrose for pain management from procedural pain (heel sticks, venipuncture, IM injections, oral suctioning, etc.) has been introduced in the NICU. The sweetness of the sucrose, a disaccharide, elevates the infant's pain threshold through endogenous opioid release in the central nervous system. A range of 0.05 to 2 mL of 24% sucrose is administered on the anterior part of the baby's tongue via a syringe or nipple approximately 2 minutes prior to the procedure (Walden & Jorgensen, 2004). But it is important to be careful because with repeated doses of sucrose, hyperglycemia may arise in the infant. Also, repeated use of sucrose analgesia in preterm infants may impact their neurologic development and behavioral outcomes. Until further research is done, repeated doses of sucrose are not recommended (Mitchell & Waltman, 2003).

newborns diagnosed with hypoglycemia, assessment is ongoing and includes careful monitoring of glucose values. In addition, urine dipstick and urine volume tests (monitor only if above 1 to 3 mL/kg/hr) may be evaluated frequently for osmotic diuresis and glycosuria.

Nursing diagnoses that may apply to the newborn with hypoglycemia include the following:

- *Altered Nutrition: Less than Body Requirements* related to increased glucose use secondary to physiologic stress
- *Ineffective Breathing Pattern* related to tachypnea and apnea
- *Acute Pain* related to frequent heel sticks secondary to glucose monitoring

PLANNING AND IMPLEMENTATION

Monitor infants in at-risk groups no later than 2 hours after birth and before feedings or whenever there are abnormal signs (Armentrout, 2004). Monitor the IDM within 30 minutes of birth. Once an at-risk infant's blood sugar level is stable, glucose testing every 2 to 4 hours (or per agency protocol), or prior to feedings, adequately monitors glucose levels. The infant's lateral heel is the preferred site for the glucose sample, so that the posterior tibial nerve and artery and the important longitudinally oriented fat pad of the heel will not be damaged (Figures 31–7 ⦿ and 31–8 ⦿).

Calculate glucose requirements and maintain intravenous glucose levels for any symptomatic infant with low serum glucose levels. The method of feeding greatly influences glucose and energy requirements; thus, pay careful attention to glucose monitoring during the transition

⦿ **FIGURE 31–7**

Heel stick. With a quick, piercing motion, puncture the lateral heel with a microlance. Be careful not to puncture too deeply.

⦿ **FIGURE 31–8**

Puncture sites

Potential sites for heel sticks. Avoid shaded areas to prevent injury to arteries and nerves in the foot and the important longitudinally oriented fat pad of the heel, which in later years could impede walking.

from intravenous to oral feedings. Titration of intravenous glucose may be required until the infant can take adequate amounts of formula or breast milk to maintain a normal blood sugar level. Titrate by decreasing the concentration of parenteral glucose gradually to 5%, then reducing the rate of infusion to 6 mg/kg/min, then to 4 mg/kg/min, and slowly discontinuing it over 4 to 6 hours. Enteral feedings are increased to maintain an adequate glucose and caloric intake.

Identify any discrepancies between the baby's caloric requirements and received calories. Weigh the newborn daily at consistent times, preferably before feeding. Only then can findings of unusual losses or gains, as well as the pattern of weight gain, be considered reliable.

The therapeutic nursing measure of nonnutritive sucking during gavage feedings has been reported to increase the baby's daily weight gain and lead to earlier bottle-feeding or breastfeeding and discharge. Nonnutritive sucking may also lower activity levels, which allows newborns to conserve their energy stores. Activity can increase energy requirements; crying alone can double the baby's metabolic rate.

Establishing and maintaining a neutral thermal environment has a potent influence on the newborn's metabolism. Pay careful attention to environmental conditions, physical activity, and organization of care, and integrate these factors into nursing care.

EVALUATION

Expected outcomes of nursing care include the following:

- The newborn at risk for hypoglycemia is promptly identified, and intervention is started early.
- The newborn's glucose level is stabilized, and recovery is proceeding without sequelae.

CARE OF THE NEWBORN WITH JAUNDICE

The most common abnormal physical finding in newborns is jaundice. **Jaundice** is a yellowish coloration of the skin and sclera of the eyes that develops from deposits of the yellow pigment bilirubin in lipid tissues. Normally the placenta clears fetal unconjugated (indirect) bilirubin in utero, so total bilirubin at birth is usually less than 3 mg/dL unless an abnormal hemolytic process has been present. Postnatally the infant must conjugate bilirubin (convert a lipid-soluble pigment into a water-soluble pigment) in the liver.

The rate and amount of conjugation of bilirubin depend on the rate of hemolysis, the bilirubin load, the maturity of the liver, and the presence of albumin-binding sites. (See Chapter 26 for discussion of conjugation of bilirubin. ∞) The liver of a normal, healthy term infant is usually mature enough and producing enough glucuronyl transferase that the total serum bilirubin does not reach a pathologic level.

PHYSIOLOGIC JAUNDICE

Physiologic or neonatal jaundice is a normal process that occurs during transition from intrauterine to extrauterine life and appears after 24 hours of life. Some degree of jaundice occurs in about half of all healthy term newborns and in 80% of preterm newborns (Madan, MacMahon, & Stevenson, 2005). It is due to the newborn's shortened cell life span, slower uptake by the liver, lack of intestinal bacteria, and poorly established hydration.

Lab tests reveal a predominance of unconjugated bilirubin. The average level of unconjugated bilirubin in cord blood is approximately 2 mg/dL at birth. This level rises to an average of 5 to 6 mg/dL between the third and fifth days of life. The jaundice is usually not visible after 10 days. The pattern of physiologic jaundice differs between breastfed and formula-fed newborns (for further discussion of physiologic jaundice, see "Physiologic Jaundice" in Chapter 26 ∞). Physiologic jaundice remains a common problem for the term newborn and may require treatment with phototherapy.

PATHOPHYSIOLOGY OF HYPERBILIRUBINEMIA

Serum albumin-binding sites are usually able to conjugate enough bilirubin to meet the demands of the normal newborn. However, certain conditions tend to decrease the number of sites available. Fetal or neonatal asphyxia and neonatal drugs such as indomethacin decrease the binding affinity of bilirubin to albumin, because acidosis impairs albumin's capacity to hold bilirubin. Hypothermia and hypoglycemia release free fatty acids that dislocate bilirubin from albumin. Maternal use of sulfa drugs or salicylates interferes with conjugation or with serum albumin-binding sites by competing with bilirubin for these sites. Finally, premature infants have less albumin available for binding with bilirubin. Neurotoxicity is possible because unconjugated bilirubin has a high affinity for extravascular tissue, such as fatty tissue (subcutaneous tissue) and cerebral tissue.

Bilirubin not bound to albumin can cross the blood-brain barrier, damage cells of the CNS, and produce kernicterus or bilirubin encephalopathy (Watson, 2004). **Kernicterus** (meaning "yellow nucleus") refers to deposits of indirect or unconjugated bilirubin in the basal ganglia of the brain and to the permanent neurologic sequelae of untreated **hyperbilirubinemia** (elevation of bilirubin level).

The classic bilirubin encephalopathy of kernicterus most commonly found with Rh and ABO blood group incompatibility is less common today due to aggressive treatment with phototherapy and exchange transfusions. But cases of kernicterus are reappearing as a result of early discharge and the increased incidence of dehydration (as a result of discharge before the mother's milk is established). Current therapy can reduce the incidence of kernicterus encephalopathy but cannot distinguish all infants who are at risk.

CAUSES OF HYPERBILIRUBINEMIA

A primary cause of pathologic hyperbilirubinemia is hemolytic disease of the newborn secondary to Rh incompatibility. All pregnant women who are Rh negative or who have blood type O (possible ABO blood incompatibility) should be asked about outcomes of any previous pregnancies and history of blood transfusion. Prenatal amniocentesis with spectrophotographic examination may be indicated. Cord blood from newborns is evaluated for bilirubin level, which should not exceed 5 mg/dL. Newborns of Rh-negative and O blood type mothers are carefully assessed for jaundice and levels of serum bilirubin.

Alloimmune hemolytic disease, also known as **erythroblastosis fetalis**, occurs when an Rh-negative mother is pregnant with an Rh-positive fetus and maternal antibodies cross the placenta. Maternal antibodies enter the fetal circulation, then attach to and destroy the fetal red blood cells (RBCs). The fetal system responds by increasing RBC production. Jaundice, anemia, and compensatory erythropoiesis result. A marked increase in immature RBCs (erythroblasts) also occurs, hence the designation erythroblastosis fetalis. Because of the use of Rh immune globulin (RhoGAM), the incidence of erythroblastosis fetalis has dropped dramatically.

Hydrops fetalis, the most severe form of erythroblastosis fetalis, occurs when maternal antibodies attach to the Rh site on the fetal RBCs, making them susceptible to destruction; severe anemia and multiorgan system failure result. Cardiomegaly with severe cardiac decompensation and hepatosplenomegaly occurs. Severe generalized massive edema (anasarca) and generalized fluid effusion into the pleural cavity (hydrothorax), pericardial sac, and peritoneal cavity (ascites) develop. Jaundice is not present initially because the bilirubin pigments are excreted through the placenta into the maternal circulation. The hydropic hemolytic disease process is also characterized by hyperplasia of the pancreatic islets, which predisposes the infant to neonatal hypoglycemia similar to that of IDMs. In addition the associated thrombocytopenia and hypoxic damage to the capillaries means these infants have increased bleeding tendencies. Hydrops is a frequent cause of intrauterine death among infants with Rh disease.

ABO incompatibility (the mother is blood type O and the baby is blood type A or B) may result in jaundice, although it rarely results in hemolytic disease severe enough to be clinically diagnosed and treated. Hepatosplenomegaly may be found occasionally in newborns with ABO incompatibility, but hydrops fetalis and stillbirth are rare.

Other prenatal and perinatal factors predispose the newborn to hyperbilirubinemia. During pregnancy, predisposing maternal conditions include hereditary spherocytosis, diabetes, intrauterine infections, and gram-negative bacilli infections that stimulate production of maternal alloimmune antibodies, drug ingestion (such as sulfas, salicylates, novobiocin, diazepam), and oxytocin administration.

In addition to Rh or ABO incompatibility, other conditions predispose the newborn to hyperbilirubinemia: polycythemia (central hematocrit 65% or more), pyloric stenosis, obstruction or atresia of the biliary duct or of the lower bowel, low-grade urinary tract infection, sepsis, hypothyroidism, enclosed hemorrhage (cephalhematoma, large bruises), asphyxia neonatorum, hypothermia, acidemia, and hypoglycemia. Neonatal hepatitis, atresia of the bile ducts, and gastrointestinal atresia all can alter bilirubin metabolism and excretion.

The prognosis for a newborn with hyperbilirubinemia depends on the extent of the hemolytic process and the underlying cause. Severe hemolytic disease results in fetal and early neonatal death from the effects of severe anemia—cardiac decompensation, edema, ascites, and hydrothorax. Hyperbilirubinemia may lead to kernicterus if not aggressively treated. The resulting neurologic damage may cause death, cerebral palsy, possible mental retardation, or hearing loss or, to a lesser degree, perceptual impairment, delayed speech development, hyperactivity, muscle incoordination, or learning difficulties.

DEVELOPING CULTURAL COMPETENCE

ETHNIC VARIATIONS AND JAUNDICE

East Asian infants (Japanese, Chinese, and Filipino ethnic groups) have a higher occurrence of hyperbilirubinemia than Caucasian infants. Infants with Asian fathers and Caucasian mothers have a higher incidence of jaundice than if both parents are Caucasian. Other ethnic groups at risk for increased bilirubinemia are Navajo, Eskimo, and Sioux Native American newborns; Greek newborns; Sephardic-Jewish (oriental ancestry) newborns; and some Hispanic newborns.

CLINICAL THERAPY

Neonatal hyperbilirubinemia can be considered pathologic and requires further investigation if any of the following criteria are met (American Academy of Pediatrics Subcommittee on Hyperbilirubinemia, 2004; Madan et al., 2005):

1. Clinically evident jaundice before first 24 hours of life
2. Serum bilirubin concentration rising more than 0.2 mg/dL/hour or 5 mg/dL/per day
3. Total serum bilirubin (TSB) exceeding the 95th percentile on the nomogram
4. Signs of underlying illness in any infant (vomiting, lethargy, poor feeding, excessive weight loss, apnea, tachypnea, or temperature instability)
5. Clinical jaundice persisting for more than two weeks in a term newborn
6. Conjugated bilirubin concentrations greater than 2 mg/dL or more than 20% of the total serum bilirubin concentration

Initial diagnostic procedures are aimed at differentiating jaundice resulting from increased bilirubin production, impaired conjugation or excretion, or a combination of these factors. When one or more predisposing factors for jaundice are present, the maternal and neonatal blood types should be tested in the laboratory for Rh or ABO incompatibility. Early prenatal identification of the fetus at risk for Rh or ABO incompatibility allows prompt treatment. (See Chapter 15 for discussion of in utero management of this condition. ∞)

Because of the shorter life span of red blood cells in the newborn, a significant bilirubin load is produced. When bilirubin breaks down, carbon monoxide (CO) is released. This production of carbon monoxide is being investigated as a marker in the study of bilirubin production. Measuring end-tidal CO (ETCO) has been shown to provide results similar to laboratory measures of bilirubin (Madan et al., 2005).

Other needed laboratory evaluations are Coombs' test, serum bilirubin levels (direct and total), hemoglobin, reticulocyte percentage, white cell count, and positive smear for cellular morphology.

The Coombs' test determines whether jaundice is due to Rh or ABO incompatibility. The indirect Coombs' test measures the amount of Rh-positive antibodies in the mother's blood. Rh-positive RBCs are added to the maternal blood sample. If the mother's serum contains antibodies, the Rh-positive RBCs agglutinate (clump) when rabbit immune antiglobulin is added, which is a positive test result.

The direct Coombs' test reveals antibody-coated (sensitized) Rh-positive RBCs in the newborn. Rabbit immune antiglobulin is added to the specimen of neonatal blood cells. If the neonatal RBCs agglutinate, they have been coated with maternal antibodies, a positive result.

If the hemolytic process is due to Rh sensitization, laboratory findings will reveal the following: (1) an Rh-positive newborn with a positive Coombs' test; (2) increased erythropoiesis with many immature circulating red blood cells (nucleated blastocysts); (3) anemia, in most cases; (4) elevated levels of bilirubin in cord blood (5 mg/dL or more); and (5) a reduction in albumin-binding capacity. Maternal data may include an elevated anti-Rh titer and spectrophotometric evidence of a fetal hemolytic process.

Laboratory findings reveal an increase in immature blood cells (reticulocytes) when the hemolytic process is due to ABO incompatibility. The resulting anemia is usually not significant during the newborn period and is rare later on. The direct Coombs' test may be negative or mildly positive, whereas the indirect Coombs' test may be strongly positive. Infants with a positive direct Coombs' test have increased incidence of jaundice, with bilirubin levels above 10 mg/dL. Increased numbers of spherocytes (spherical, plump, mature erythrocytes) are seen on a peripheral blood smear. Increased numbers of spherocytes are not seen on blood smears from infants with Rh disease.

THERAPEUTIC MANAGEMENT

Whatever the cause of hyperbilirubinemia, management of these infants is directed toward alleviating anemia, removing maternal antibodies and sensitized erythrocytes, increasing serum albumin levels, reducing serum bilirubin levels, and minimizing the consequences of hyperbilirubinemia. Early discharge of newborns from birthing centers has significantly affected the diagnosis and management of neonatal jaundice in that setting and increased the emphasis on outpatient and home care management.

Hemolytic disease may be treated with phototherapy, exchange transfusion, and drug therapy. When determining the appropriate management of hyperbilirubinemia due to hemolytic disease, the three relevant variables are the newborn's (1) serum bilirubin level, (2) birth weight, and (3) age in hours. If a newborn has hemolysis with an unconjugated bilirubin level of 14 mg/dL, weighs less than 2500 g (birth weight), and is 24 hours old or less, an exchange transfusion may be the best management. However, if that same newborn is over 24 hours of age, which is past the time when an increase in bilirubin would be due to pathologic causes, phototherapy may be the treatment of choice to prevent the possible complication of kernicterus.

Phototherapy is the exposure of the newborn to high-intensity light. It may be used alone or in conjunction with exchange transfusion to reduce serum bilirubin levels. Exposure of the newborn to high-intensity light (fluorescent light bulbs or bulbs in the blue-light spectrum) decreases serum bilirubin levels in the skin by facilitating biliary excretion of unconjugated bilirubin. Phototherapy decreases serum bilirubin levels by changing bilirubin from the non-water soluble (lipophilic) form to water-soluble by-products that can then be excreted. When bilirubin absorbs light, three forms of photochemical reaction occur: photo-oxidation, photoisomerization, and structural isomerization. Photo-oxidation is a minor contributor to bilirubin elimination. Structural isomerization is the most important pathway for decreasing serum bilirubin levels. Bilirubin is converted to lumirubin which is bound to albumin and transported to the liver. It is a stable water-soluble molecule so it is excreted into the urine and bile for excretion. Photoisomerization occurs when the natural form of bilirubin is exposed to light at a certain wavelength and the bilirubin is converted to a less toxic form. The new isomer, photobilirubin, is created rapidly, but is quite unstable. Photobilirubin is bound to albumin, transported to the liver, and is incorporated into bile. If it is not quickly eliminated from the bowel it can convert back to its original form and return to the bloodstream.

Phototherapy is an intervention that is used more for the prevention of hyperbilirubinemia in order to halt bilirubin levels from climbing dangerously high. The decision to start phototherapy is based on 2 factors: gestational age and age in hours. Phototherapy is the most effective in the first 24 to 48 hours of usage; frequently the light can be discontinued during or immediately after this time frame.

Phototherapy plays an important role in preventing a rise in bilirubin levels but does not alter the underlying cause of jaundice, and hemolysis may continue to produce anemia. Many authors have recommended initiating phototherapy "prophylactically" in the first 24 hours of life in high-risk, very-low-birth-weight or severely bruised infants.

Phototherapy can be provided through halogen spotlights, (although this is less often used due to the risk of thermal burns), conventional banks of phototherapy lights or by a fiberoptic blanket attached to a halogen light source around the trunk of the newborn or a combination of both delivery methods. The banks of bilirubin lights utilize light in the blue spectrum. This is the most effective source available, but can mask cyanosis, and causes dizziness and nausea in the staff. With the fiberoptic blanket, the light stays on at all times, and the newborn is accessible for care, feeding, and diaper changes; greater surface area is exposed and there are no thermoregulation issues. The eyes are not covered. Fluid and weight loss are not complications of this system. Furthermore, it makes the infant accessible to the parents and is less alarming to parents than standard phototherapy. A combination of a fiberoptic light source in the mattress under the baby and a standard light source above may also be used. This is termed intensive phototherapy. Intensive phototherapy should reduce the TSB by 1–2 mg/dL within 4–6 hours and should continue to decline. If this goal is not reached then an exchange transfusion should be considered. Many institutions and pediatricians use fiberoptic blankets for home care (see Figure 31–9 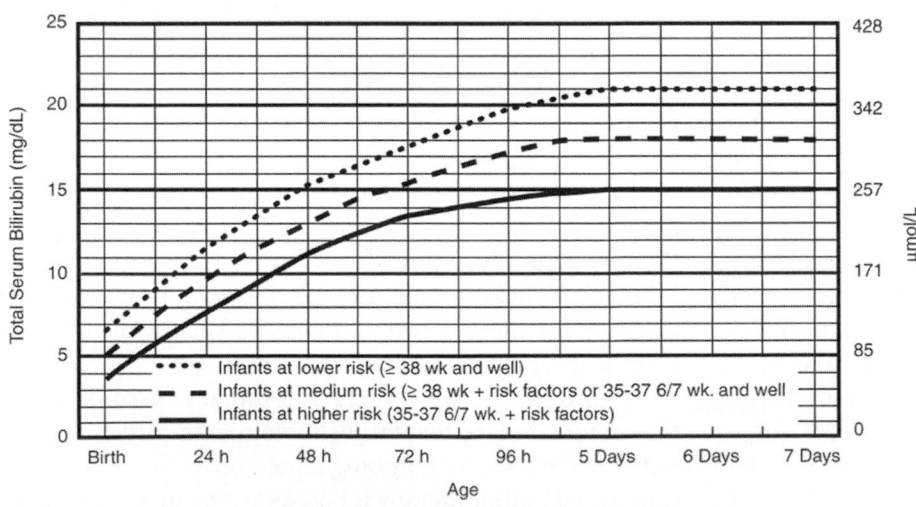).

Exchange Transfusion

Exchange transfusion is the withdrawal and replacement of the newborn's blood with donor blood. It is used to treat anemia with RBCs that are susceptible to maternal antibodies, remove sensitized RBCs that would be lysed soon, remove serum bilirubin, and provide bilirubin-free albumin to increase the binding sites for bilirubin. Concerns about exchange transfusion are related to the use of blood products, which include the potential for HIV infection and hepatitis.

If the TSB is at or approaching the exchange level, send blood for immediate type and crossmatch. Blood for exchange transfusion is modified whole blood (red cells and plasma) crossmatched against the mother and compatible with the infant.

NURSING MANAGEMENT

NURSING ASSESSMENT AND DIAGNOSIS

Assessment is aimed at identifying prenatal and perinatal factors that predispose the newborn to the development of jaundice and at recognizing the jaundice as soon as it is apparent. (See "Nursing Care Plan: The Newborn with Hyperbilirubinemia.") Clinically, ABO incompatibility presents as jaundice and occasionally as hepatosplenomegaly. Fetal hydrops or erythroblastosis is rare. Suspect **hemolytic disease of the newborn** if the placenta is enlarged, if the newborn is edematous with pleural and pericardial effusion plus ascites, if pallor or jaundice is noted during the first 24 to 36 hours, if hemolytic anemia is diagnosed, or if the spleen and

(continues on page 842)

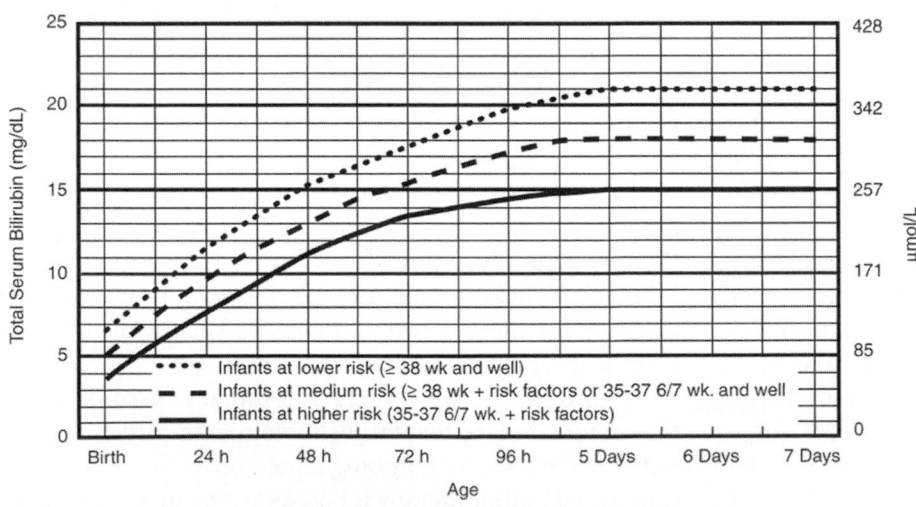

◉ FIGURE 31–9

- Use total bilirubin. Do not subtract direct reacting or conjugated bilirubin.
- Risk factors = isoimmune hemolytic disease, G6PD deficiency, asphyxia, significant lethargy, temperature instability, sepsis, acidosis, or albumin < 3.0g/dL (if measured)
- For well infants 35-37 6/7 wk can adjust TSB levels for intervention around the medium risk line. It is an option to intervene at lower TSB levels for infants closer to 35 wks and at higher TSB levels for those closer to 37 6/7 wk.
- It is an option to provide conventional phototherapy in hospital or at home at TSB levels 2-3 mg/dL (35-50mmol/L) below those shown but home phototherapy should not be used in any infant with risk factors.

Guidelines for phototherapy in hospitalized infants of 35 or more weeks' gestation.
American Academy of Pediatrics Subcommittee on Hyperbilirubinemia (2004). Management of hyperbilirubinemia in the newborn infant 35 or more weeks of gestation. Pediatrics, 114(1), 297–316. Used with permission.

NURSING CARE PLAN

THE NEWBORN WITH HYPERBILIRUBINEMIA

Intervention	Rationale	Expected Outcome

1. Nursing Diagnosis: Impaired Tissue Integrity related to predisposing factors associated with hyperbilirubinemia

Intervention	Rationale	Expected Outcome
NIC Intervention: **High–risk newborn care:** Identification and management of a high-risk newborn to promote healthy outcomes for baby		**NOC Outcome:** **Risk control:** Actions to eliminate or reduce actual, personal, and modifiable health threats

Goal: Babies at risk for jaundice and early signs of jaundice will be identified.

Intervention	Rationale	Expected Outcome

■ Evaluate baby's history for predisposing factors for hyperbilirubinemia.
 	
■ Observe color of amniotic fluid at time of rupture of membranes.
■ Assess baby for developing jaundice in daylight if possible.
 	
  1. Observe sclera.
 	
  2. Observe skin color and assess by blanching.
 	
  3. Check oral mucosa, posterior portion of hard palate, and conjunctival sacs for yellow pigmentation in dark-skinned newborns.
Report jaundice occurring within 24 hours of birth.
	Early identification of risk factors enables the nurse to monitor babies for early signs of hyperbilirubinemia. Acidosis, hypoxia, and hypothermia increase the risk of hyperbilirubinemia at lower bilirubin levels.
	■ Amber-colored amniotic fluid indicates hyperbilirubinemia.
	■ Early detection is affected by nursery environment. Artificial lights (with pink tint) may mask beginning of jaundice.
	1. Most visible sign of hyperbilirubinemia is jaundice noted in skin, sclera, or oral mucosa. Onset is first seen on face and then progresses down trunk.
	2. Blanching the skin leaves a yellow color to the skin immediately after pressure is released.
	3. Underlying pigment of dark-skinned people may normally appear yellow.
		■ Baby's jaundice is identified early.

2. Nursing Diagnosis: Risk for Fluid Volume Deficit related to phototherapy

Intervention	Rationale	Expected Outcome
NIC Intervention: **Fluid monitoring:** Collection and analysis of patient data to regulate fluid balance		**NOC Outcome:** **Fluid balance:** Balance of water in the intracellular and extracellular compartments of the body

Goal: The infant will not exhibit signs of dehydration and will display appropriate weight gain.

Intervention	Rationale	Expected Outcome

■ Offer feedings every 2 to 3 hr. Breastfeed on demand with no supplementation unless excessive weight loss or increasing TSB with adequate feeding.
■ Provide 25% extra fluid intake.
 	
■ Assess for dehydration:
  1. Poor skin turgor
  2. Depressed fontanelles
  3. Sunken eyes
  4. Decreased urine output
  5. Weight loss
  6. Changes in electrolytes
	■ Adequate hydration increases peristalsis and excretion of bilirubin.
	
	■ Replace fluid losses due to watery stools, if under phototherapy.
	
	■ Phototherapy treatment may cause liquid stools and increased insensible water loss, which increases risk of dehydration.
		■ Baby will have good skin turgor, clear amber urine output of 1-3 mL/kg/hr, six to eight wet diapers/day, and will maintain weight.

(continued)

NURSING CARE PLAN—continued

THE NEWBORN WITH HYPERBILIRUBINEMIA

Intervention	Rationale	Expected Outcome

Monitor intake and output (I & O). Weigh daily. Report signs of dehydration.
■ Administer IV fluids:
  1. Monitor flow rates.
  2. Assess insertion sites for signs of infection.
	■ Prevents fluid overload. IV fluids may be used if baby is dehydrated or in presence of other complications. IV may be started if exchange transfusion is to be done.	

3. Nursing Diagnosis: Potential for Injury related to use of phototherapy lights

NIC Intervention:		NOC Outcome:
Newborn monitoring: Measurement and interpretation of physiologic status of the newborn the first 24 hr after birth		**Risk Control:** Actions to eliminate or reduce actual, personal, and modifiable health threats

Goal: Baby will not have any corneal irritation or drainage, skin breakdown, or major fluctuations in temperature.

■ Cover baby's eyes with eye patches while under phototherapy lights. Cover testes/penis in male infants. ■ Make certain that eyelids are closed prior to applying eye patches. ■ Remove baby from under phototherapy and remove eye patches during feedings. ■ Inspect eyes each shift for conjunctivitis, drainage, and corneal abrasions due to irritation from eye patches. ■ Administer thorough perianal cleansing with each stool or change of perianal protective covering. ■ Provide minimal coverage—only of diaper area. ■ Avoid the use of oily applications on the skin. ■ Reposition baby q 2 hours. ■ Observe for bronzing of skin. ■ Place Plexiglas shield between baby and light. Monitor baby's skin and core temperature frequently until temperature is stable. ■ Check axillary temperature with readings on servo-controlled unit on incubator. Regulate incubator temperature as needed.	■ Protects retina from damage due to high-intensity light and testes from damage from heat. ■ Prevents corneal abrasions. ■ Provides visual stimulation and facilitates attachment behaviors. ■ Prevents or facilitates prompt treatment of purulent conjunctivitis. ■ Frequent stooling increases risk of skin breakdown. Prevents infection. ■ Provides maximal exposure. Shielded areas become more jaundiced, so maximum exposure is essential. ■ Prevents superficial burns to skin. ■ Provides equal exposure of all skin areas and prevents pressure areas. ■ Bronzing is related to use of phototherapy with increased direct bilirubin levels or liver damage; may last for 2 to 4 months. ■ Hypothermia and hyperthermia are common complications of phototherapy. Hypothermia results from exposure to lights, subsequent radiation, and convection losses. ■ Hyperthermia may result from the increased environmental heat. Additional heat from phototherapy lights frequently causes a rise in the baby's and incubator's temperatures. Fluctuations in temperature may occur in response to radiation and convection.	■ Baby's eyes are protected, skin is intact, and baby maintains a stable temperature.

NURSING CARE PLAN—continued

THE NEWBORN WITH HYPERBILIRUBINEMIA

Intervention	Rationale	Expected Outcome

4. Nursing Diagnosis: Risk for Impaired Parenting related to deficient knowledge of infant care and prolonged separation of infant and parents secondary to illness

NIC Intervention: **Teaching:** Infant care: Instruction on nurturing and physical care needed during the first year of life		**NOC Outcome:** **Parenting:** Provision of an environment that promotes optimum growth and development of dependent children

Goal: Parents will bond with infant and have realistic expectations about their infant. Parents are comfortable taking their infant home. They are able to demonstrate normal infant care and assessments of possible complications, and they know when to return for follow-up.

■ Encourage parents to provide tactile stimulation during feeding and diaper changes.
■ Encourage cuddling and eye contact during feedings.
■ Offer suggestions to comfort restless infant:
  1. Nesting when beneath bili lights
  2. Talking softly and singing quietly to infant
  3. Taped music or tape recording of evening activities from home
  4. Rhythmic patting of buttocks
  5. Firm, nonstroking touch, assisting with control of extremities
  6. Pacifier for nonnutritive sucking
■ Encourage family/friend support of mother/parents (i.e., meals, rest, child care for siblings, allow expressions of concerns/feelings).
■ Evaluate additional psychosocial needs.
 	
■ Discuss rationale for treatment and possible side effects of phototherapy with family (stool changes, increased fluid loss, possible temp instability, slight lethargy, rash, altered sleep-wake patterns).
Instruct family on infant's care while undergoing phototherapy:
  1. Safety precautions—bili mask, incubator door closed and latched, covering genitalia per policy.
  2. Skin care, cord care, circumcision care as appropriate.
  3. Lab draws, rationale for intake and output.
■ Encourage parent/significant other/sibling involvement in infant care as possible.
■ Evaluate family's understanding of information.
■ Give explanation of equipment being used and changes in bilirubin levels. Allow parents an opportunity to ask questions; reinforce or clarify information as needed.
	■ Newborn has normal needs for tactile stimulation.
	
	■ Provides opportunity for parents to bond with their newborn.
	■ Provides comfort and decreases sensory deprivation. Presence of equipment may discourage parents from interacting with newborn.
	
	■ Decreases strain on mother/parents by assisting with other responsibilities and allows for additional time with newborn for bonding, care, etc.
	■ Parents may not understand what is happening or why.
	■ Physician preference of treatment modalities may vary. Parents may not understand why their newborn is not receiving a treatment that another with the same condition is receiving.
		■ The parent will demonstrate ability to perform basic infant care tasks as evidenced by exhibiting appropriate attachment behaviors (i.e., talking to and holding infant), feeding infant, and caring for infant under home bili therapy.
		
		■ Parents verbalize understanding of rationale and possible side effects from phototherapy; parents/family demonstrate safety precautions when caring for infant; parents getting meals and rest; parents verbalize support given.

(continued)

NURSING CARE PLAN—continued

THE NEWBORN WITH HYPERBILIRUBINEMIA

Intervention	Rationale	Expected Outcome
■ As necessary, review role of pumping breasts and offering formula for limited time. ■ Assist mother to pump her breasts to maintain milk supply.	■ The etiology of breast milk jaundice remains uncertain. The serum bilirubin levels begin to fall within 48 hr after discontinuation of breastfeeding. Opinion of physicians varies regarding the need for discontinuing breastfeeding. ■ If breastfeeding is temporarily discontinued, assess mother's knowledge of pumping her breasts and provide information and support as needed.	

liver are enlarged. Carefully note changes in behavior and observe for evidence of bleeding. If laboratory tests indicate elevated bilirubin levels, check the newborn for jaundice about every 2 hours and record observations.

To check for jaundice in lighter-skinned babies, blanch the skin over a bony prominence (forehead, nose, sternum) by pressing firmly with the thumb. After pressure is released, if jaundice is present, the area appears yellow before normal color returns. In darker-skinned babies, check oral mucosa and the posterior portion of the hard palate and conjunctival sacs for yellow pigmentation. Because birthing units are often decorated with pink walls and surroundings, which may mask yellowish tints, and because yellow light makes differentiation of jaundice difficult, perform the assessment in daylight for the best results.

In addition to visually inspecting the newborn, use reflectance photometers that measure transcutaneous bilirubin (TcB) to screen and monitor neonatal jaundice. Analysis for end-tidal carbon monoxide is another portable screening tool. This analysis allows quick identification of those newborns with significant hemolytic disease who may be at risk for further complications of unconjugated hyperbilirubinemia (American Academy of Pediatrics Subcommittee on Hyperbilirubinemia, 2004).

If jaundice appears, record and report the time of onset and carefully observe for any increase in depth of color or changes in the newborn's behavior. Assess the newborn's behavior for neurologic signs associated with hyperbilirubinemia, which are rare but may include hypotonia, diminished reflexes, lethargy, or seizures.

Some hospitals have developed a mandatory screening policy of all newborns prior to discharge utilizing the TcB monitor. If the level comes back as high as earlier levels then a follow-up TSB will be performed.

Nursing diagnoses that may apply to care of a newborn with jaundice include the following:

■ *Risk for Fluid Volume Deficit* related to phototherapy, increased insensible water loss, and frequent loose stools

■ *Potential for Injury* related to use of phototherapy

■ *Sensory-Perceptual Alterations* related to neurologic damage secondary to kernicterus

■ *Risk for Altered Parenting* related to deficient knowledge of infant care and prolonged separation of infant and parents secondary to illness

PLANNING AND IMPLEMENTATION

Hospital-Based Nursing Care

Hospital-based care is described in "Nursing Care Plan: The Newborn with Hyperbilirubinemia." If phototherapy lights are used, expose the newborn's entire skin surface to the light. Minimal covering may be applied over the genitals and buttocks to expose maximum skin surface while still protecting the bedding from soiling. Measure phototherapy success every 12 hours or with daily serum bilirubin levels (more frequently if there is hemolysis or a higher level prior to initiation of phototherapy). Turn lights off while blood is drawn to ensure accurate serum bilirubin levels. Because it is not known if phototherapy injures the delicate eye structures, particularly the retina, apply eye patches over the newborn's closed eyes during exposure to banks of phototherapy lights (Figure 31–10 ●). Stop phototherapy and remove the eye patches at least once per shift to assess the eyes for conjunctivitis. Also remove patches to allow eye contact during feeding (social stimulation) or when parents are visiting (to promote parental attachment).

O FIGURE 31–10

Infant receiving phototherapy via overhead bilirubin lights. The phototherapy light is positioned over the isolette. Bilateral eye patches are always used to protect the baby's eyes during phototherapy.

Courtesy of Lisa Smith-Pederson, RNC, MSN, NNP.

NURSING PRACTICE

If the area of jaundice around the eyes begins to disappear, then the eye patches are allowing light to enter and better eye protection is needed.

Most phototherapy units provide the desired level of irradiance when the infant is 45 to 50 cm below the lamps. Use a photometer to measure and maintain desired irradiance levels. Disadvantages of lights are that they create a difficult work environment and can distort an infant's color. A harmless, temporary bronze discoloration of the skin may occur with phototherapy when the infant has elevated direct serum bilirubin levels or liver disease. As a side effect of phototherapy, some newborns develop a maculopapular rash.

Monitor the newborn's temperature to prevent hyperthermia and hypothermia. The newborn needs additional fluids to compensate for the increased loss of water through the skin and loose stools. Loose stools and increased urine output result from increased bilirubin excretion. Observe the infant for signs of dehydration and perianal excoriation (see Skill 5–7 **SKILLS**).

When assessing the newborn's skin color for jaundice and bronzing, also examine the skin for developing pressure areas. Reposition the newborn at least every 2 hours to permit the light to reach all skin surfaces, to prevent pressure areas, and to vary the stimulation to the infant. Keep track of the number of hours each lamp is used so that it

can be replaced before its effectiveness is lost. Be careful about using ointment under bilirubin lights because this combination may cause burns.

To parents, the terms *jaundice, hyperbilirubinemia, exchange transfusion,* and *phototherapy* may sound frightening and threatening. Some parents may feel guilty about their baby's condition and think they have caused the problem. Under stress, parents may not be able to understand the physician's first explanations. Anticipate that the parents will need explanations repeated and clarified and that they may need help voicing their questions and fears. Coach parents when they visit with the baby and encourage eye and tactile contact with the newborn. After the mother's discharge, keep parents informed of their infant's condition and encourage them to return to the hospital or call at any time so that they can be fully involved in the care of their infant. Advise parents that they can expect a rebound of 1 to 2 mg/dL after discontinuation of phototherapy and that a follow-up bilirubin test may be done (Watson, 2004).

While the mother is still hospitalized, phototherapy can also be carried out in the parents' room if the only problem is hyperbilirubinemia. The parents must be willing to keep the baby in the room for 24 hours a day, be able to take emergency action (e.g., for choking) if necessary, and complete instruction checklists. Some institutions require that parents sign a consent form. Instruct the parents but also continue to monitor the infant's temperature, activity, intake and output, and positioning of eye patches (if conventional light banks are used) at regular intervals (Table 31–3).

Nursing Care in the Community

Some studies have shown that with early discharge of newborns and their mothers comes an increase in hospital readmission and elevated risk of pathologic hyperbilirubinemia. Home phototherapy use is only recommended if

---

TABLE 31–3 ✤ **Instructional Checklist for In-Room Phototherapy**

Explain and demonstrate the placement of eye patches and explain that they must be in place when the infant is under the lights.

Explain the clothing to be worn (diaper under lights, dress and wrap when away from the lights).

Explain the importance of taking the infant's temperature regularly.

Explain the importance of adequate fluid intake.

Explain the charting flow sheet (intake, output, eyes covered).

Explain how to position the lights at a proper distance.

Explain the need to keep the infant under phototherapy except during feeding and diaper changes.

the bilirubin level is plotted on the nomogram and found to be in the "optional phototherapy" range. Any neonate with a level in the higher range should be hospitalized for continual phototherapy and serum bilirubin levels closely monitored on a regular schedule (American Academy of Pediatrics Subcommittee on Hyperbilirubinemia, 2004).

Jaundice and its treatment can be very disturbing to parents and may generate feelings of guilt and fear. Reassurance and support are vital especially for the breastfeeding mother, who may question her ability to adequately nourish her newborn. The parents' perception of and/or misconceptions about jaundice can affect parent-infant interactions. The nurse should explain the causes of jaundice and emphasize that is is usually a transient problem and one to which all infants must adapt after birth. It is essential that the impact of cultural beliefs be considered. Some Latina women believe that showing strong maternal emotions during pregnancy and during breastfeeding can be detrimental. "Bilis" associated with anger may be blamed by some Latina women for jaundice. Cultural beliefs lead mothers to interpret illness within their cultural framework, especially when left without clear and understood explanations. Maternal reactions can be lessened by careful explanations to the mothers about the diagnosis, prognosis, duration, management options for jaundice, and possibility of recurrence.

If the baby is to receive phototherapy at home, teach the parents to record the infant's temperature, weight, fluid intake and output, stools, and feedings and to use the phototherapy equipment. If phototherapy lights are being used, parents must agree that the baby will be exposed to the lights for long periods of time; that they will hold the baby for only short periods for feeding, comforting, and diaper changing; and that the room temperature will be regulated to minimize heat loss. A combination of phototherapy lights and fiberoptic mattress may be used (Figure 31–11). Fiberoptic phototherapy blankets eliminate the need for eye patches, decrease heat loss because the baby is covered, and provide more chances for baby-parent interaction. The best method of home phototherapy depends on the cause of the hyperbilirubinemia and the rate of progression of the jaundice. Ongoing monitoring of bilirubin levels is essential with home phototherapy and can be carried out in the home, in the follow-up clinic, or in the clinician's office.

EVALUATION

Expected outcomes of nursing care include the following:

■ The newborn at risk for development of hyperbilirubinemia is identified, and care is provided to minimize the potential impact of hyperbilirubinemia.

● FIGURE 31–11

Newborn on fiberoptic "bili" mattress and under phototherapy lights. A combination of fiberoptic light source and standard phototherapy light source above baby may also be used.

■ The baby does not have any corneal irritation or drainage, skin breakdown, or major fluctuations in temperature.

■ Parents understand the rationale for, goal of, and expected outcome of therapy.

■ Parents verbalize their concerns about their baby's condition and identify how they can facilitate their baby's improvement.

CARE OF THE NEWBORN WITH ANEMIA

Neonatal anemia is often difficult to recognize by clinical evaluation alone. The hemoglobin concentration in a term newborn is 15 to 20 g/dL, slightly higher than that in premature newborns, in whom the mean hemoglobin is 14 to 18 g/dL. Infants with hemoglobin values of less than 14 g/dL (term) and 13 g/dL (preterm) are usually considered anemic. The most common causes of neonatal anemia are blood loss, hemolysis, and impaired RBC production.

Blood loss (hypovolemia) occurs in utero from placental bleeding (placenta previa or abruptio placentae). Intrapartal blood loss may be fetomaternal, fetofetal, or the result of umbilical cord bleeding. Birth trauma to abdominal organs or the cranium may produce significant blood loss, and cerebral bleeding may occur because of hypoxia.

Excessive hemolysis of RBCs is usually a result of blood group incompatibilities but may be caused by infection. The most common cause of impaired RBC production is a genetically transmitted deficiency in glucose-6-phosphate dehydrogenase (G6PD) deficiency. Anemia and jaundice are the presenting signs.

A condition known as **physiologic anemia** results from the normal gradual drop in hemoglobin for the first 6 to 12 weeks of life or corresponds with the decline in fetal hemoglobin. Theoretically the bone marrow stops production of RBCs in response to higher oxygen levels that result from breathing changes after birth. When the amount of hemoglobin decreases to levels of 10 to 11 g/dL at about 6 to 12 weeks of age in term newborns, the bone marrow begins production of RBCs again, and the anemia disappears.

Anemia in preterm newborns is seen earlier than in term newborns, and increased production of RBCs does not start until hemoglobin is 7 to 9 g/dL. The preterm baby's hemoglobin reaches a low sooner (by 4 to 8 weeks after birth) than does a term newborn's (6 to 12 weeks) because a preterm infant's RBC survival time is shorter than that of a term newborn (Diehl-Jones & Askin, 2004). This difference is due to several factors: the preterm infant's rapid growth rate, decreased iron stores, and an inadequate production of erythropoietin (EPO).

CLINICAL THERAPY

Hematologic problems can be anticipated based on the pregnancy history and clinical manifestations. The age at which anemia is first noted is also of diagnostic value. Clinically, light-skinned anemic infants are very pale when they do not have other symptoms of shock and usually have abnormally low RBC counts. In acute blood loss, symptoms of shock (such as pallor, low arterial blood pressure, and a decreasing hematocrit value) may be present.

The initial laboratory workup should include hemoglobin and hematocrit measurements, reticulocyte count, ferritin concentrations, examination of peripheral blood smear, bilirubin determinations, direct Coombs' test of infant's blood, and examination of maternal blood smear for fetal erythrocytes (Kleihauer-Betke test). Clinical management depends on the severity of the anemia and whether blood loss is acute or chronic. The baby should be placed on constant cardiac and respiratory monitoring. Mild or slow chronic anemia may be treated adequately with iron supplements alone or with iron-fortified formulas. Frequent determinations of hemoglobin, hematocrit, and bilirubin levels (in hemolytic disease) are essential. In severe cases of anemia, transfusions are the treatment of choice. Management of anemia due to prematurity includes recombinant human erythropoietin (rEPO) and supplemental iron. Blood transfusions (dedicated units of blood) are kept to a minimum.

NURSING MANAGEMENT

Assess the newborn for symptoms of anemia (pallor). If the blood loss is acute, the baby may show signs of shock (a capillary filling time greater than 3 seconds, decreased pulses, tachycardia, and low blood pressure). Continued observation identifies physiologic anemia as the preterm newborn

grows. Signs of compromise include poor weight gain, tachycardia, tachypnea, and apneic episodes. Promptly report any symptoms indicating anemia or shock. Record the amount of blood drawn for all laboratory tests so that total blood removed can be assessed and replaced by transfusion when necessary. For long-term management, see "Normocytic Anemia" in Chapter 49. ∞

CARE OF THE NEWBORN WITH POLYCYTHEMIA

Polycythemia, a condition in which blood volume and hematocrit values are increased, is more common in SGA and full-term infants with delayed cord clamping, maternal-fetal and twin-to-twin transfusions, or chronic intrauterine hypoxia than in other newborns (Diehl-Jones & Askin, 2004). An infant is considered polycythemic when the central venous hematocrit value is greater than 65% to 70% or the venous hemoglobin level is greater than 22 g/dL during the first week of life. Other conditions that present with polycythemia are chromosomal anomalies such as trisomy 21, 18, and 13; endocrine disorders such as hypoglycemia and hypocalcemia; and births at altitudes over 5000 feet.

CLINICAL THERAPY

The goal of therapy is to reduce the central venous hematocrit value to a range of 55% to 60% in symptomatic infants. To decrease the RBC mass, the symptomatic infant receives a partial exchange transfusion in which blood is removed from the infant and replaced milliliter for milliliter with fresh frozen plasma or 5% albumin. The infant needs supportive treatment of presenting symptoms until the condition is resolved; this usually happens spontaneously after the partial exchange transfusion.

NURSING MANAGEMENT

Assess for, record, and report symptoms of polycythemia. Also do an initial screening of the newborn's hematocrit value on admission to the nursery. If a capillary hematocrit is done, warming the heel prior to obtaining the blood helps to decrease falsely high values. Peripheral venous hematocrit samples are usually obtained from the antecubital fossa.

Many infants are asymptomatic, but as symptoms develop, they are related to the increased blood volume, hyperviscosity (thickness) of the blood, and decreased deformability of RBCs, all of which result in poor perfusion of tissues. The infants have a characteristic plethoric (ruddy) appearance. The most common symptoms include:

- Tachycardia and congestive heart failure due to the increased blood volume.

- Respiratory distress with grunting, tachypnea, and cyanosis; increased oxygen need; or respiratory hemorrhage due to pulmonary venous congestion, edema, and hypoxemia.

- Hyperbilirubinemia due to increased numbers of RBCs breaking down.

- Decrease in peripheral pulses, discoloration of extremities, alteration in activity or neurologic depression, renal vein thrombosis with decreased urine output, hematuria, or proteinuria due to thromboembolism.

- Jitteriness, decreased activity and tone, and seizures due to decreased perfusion of the brain and increased vascular resistance secondary to sluggish blood flow, which can result in neurologic or developmental problems.

Observe closely for the signs of distress or change in vital signs during the partial exchange. Assess carefully for partial exchange transfusion complications such as transfusion overload (which may result in congestive heart failure), irregular cardiac rhythm, bacterial infection, hypovolemia, and anemia. Reunite the newborn with the parents as soon as the baby's status permits.

CARE OF THE NEWBORN WITH INFECTION

Newborns up to 1 month of age are particularly susceptible to an infection, referred to as **sepsis neonatorum**, caused by organisms that do not cause significant disease in older children. Once any infection occurs in the newborn, it can spread rapidly through the bloodstream, regardless of its primary site. The incidence of primary neonatal sepsis is 0.1 to 0.8 per 1000 live births (1% to 8%) (Glomella, 2004). The frequency of nosocomial infection is less in normal newborn infants and increases for infants in the NICU.

Prematurity and low birth weight are associated with nosocomial infection rates up to 15 times higher than average. The general debilitation and underlying illnesses often associated with prematurity necessitate invasive procedures such as umbilical catheterization, intubation, resuscitation, ventilator support, monitoring, parenteral alimentation (especially lipid emulsions), and prior broad-spectrum antibiotic therapy.

However, even full-term infants are susceptible, because their immunologic systems are immature. They lack the complex factors involved in effective phagocytosis and the ability to localize infection or to respond with a well-defined, recognizable inflammatory response. In addition, newborns lack the IgM immunoglobulin necessary to protect against bacteria, because it does not cross the placenta (refer to "Immunologic Adaptations" in Chapter 26 for immunologic adaptations in the newborn period ∞).

Most nosocomial infections in the NICU present as bacteremia or sepsis, urinary tract infections, meningitis, or pneumonia. Maternal antepartal infections such as rubella, toxoplasmosis, cytomegalic inclusion disease, and herpes may cause congenital infections and resulting disorders in the newborn. Intrapartum maternal infections, such as amnionitis and those resulting from premature rupture of membranes (PROM) and precipitous birth, are sources of neonatal infection (see "Care of the Woman with a Perinatal Infection" in Chapter 15 for more detailed information ∞). Passage through the birth canal and contact with the vaginal flora (β-hemolytic streptococci, herpes, *Listeria*, gonococci) expose the infant to infection (Table 31–4). When the fetus or newborn has an infection anywhere, the adjacent tissues or organs are easily penetrated. The blood-brain barrier is ineffective. Septicemia is more common in males, except for infections caused by group B β-hemolytic streptococcus.

Gram-negative organisms (especially *Escherichia coli, Enterobacter, Proteus,* and *Klebsiella*) and the gram-positive organism β-hemolytic streptococcus are the most common causative agents. *Pseudomonas* is a common fomite contaminant of ventilator support and oxygen therapy equipment. Gram-positive bacteria, especially coagulase-negative staphylococci, are common pathogens in nosocomial bacteremias, pneumonias, and urinary tract infections. Other gram-positive bacteria that commonly cause infection are enterococci and *Staphylococcus aureus* (Glomella, 2004).

Protection of the newborn from infections starts prenatally and continues throughout pregnancy and birth. Prenatal prevention should include maternal screening for sexually transmitted infections and monitoring of rubella titers in women who test negative. Intrapartum sterile technique is essential. Smears from genital lesions are taken, and placental and amniotic fluid cultures are obtained if amnionitis is suspected. If genital herpes is present toward term, cesarean birth may be indicated. All newborns' eyes should be treated with an antibiotic ophthalmic ointment to prevent damage from gonococcal infection. Prophylactic antibiotic therapy for asymptomatic women who test positive for group B streptococcus (GBS) during the intrapartum period helps prevent early-onset sepsis.

CLINICAL THERAPY

Cultures should be taken as soon after birth as possible for infants with a history of possible exposure to infection in utero (e.g., PROM more than 24 hours before birth or questionable maternal history of infection). They should be obtained before antibiotic therapy is begun.

1. One blood culture is obtained from different peripheral sites. They are taken from a peripheral rather than an umbilical vessel, because catheters may

TABLE 31–4 ✤ Maternally Transmitted Newborn Infections

Infection	Nursing Assessment	Nursing Plan and Implementation
Group B Streptococcus 1%–2% colonized, with 1 in 10 developing disease Early onset—usually within hours of birth or within first week Late onset—1 week to 3 months	Severe respiratory distress (grunting and cyanosis) May become apneic or demonstrate symptoms of shock Meconium-stained amniotic fluid seen at birth	Early assessment of clinical signs necessary. Assist with x-ray examination—shows aspiration pneumonia or hyaline membrane disease. Immediately obtain blood, gastric aspirate, external ear canal, and nasopharynx cultures. Administer antibiotics, usually aqueous penicillin or ampicillin combined with gentamicin, as soon as cultures are obtained. Early assessment and intervention are essential to survival.
Syphilis Spirochetes cross placenta after 16th–18th week of gestation	Check perinatal history for positive maternal serology Assess infant for Elevated cord serum IgM and FTA-ABS IgM Rhinitis (snuffles) Fissures on mouth corners and excoriated upper lip Red rash around mouth and anus Copper-colored rash over face, palms, and soles Irritability Generalized edema, particularly over joints, bone lesions; painful extremities Hepatosplenomegaly, jaundice Congenital cataracts SGA and failure to thrive	Refer to evaluate for blindness, deafness, learning or behavioral problems. Use isolation techniques until infants have been on antibiotics for 48 hours. Administer penicillin. Provide emotional support for parents because of their feelings about mode of transmission and potential long-term sequelae.
Gonorrhea Approximately 30%–35% of newborns born vaginally to infected mothers acquire the infection	Assess for Ophthalmia neonatorum (conjunctivitis) Purulent discharge and corneal ulcerations Neonatal sepsis with temperature instability, poor feeding response, and/or hypotonia, jaundice	Administer 1% silver nitrate solution or ophthalmic antibiotic ointment (see "Drug Guide: Erythromycin [Ilotycin] Ophthalmic Ointment" in Chapter 28 ∞) or penicillin. Make a follow-up referral to evaluate any loss of vision.
Herpes Type 2 1 in 7500 births Usually transmitted during vaginal birth; a few cases of in utero transmission have been reported	Small cluster vesicular skin lesions over all the body Check perinatal history for active herpes genital lesions Disseminated form—DIC, pneumonia, hepatitis with jaundice, hepatosplenomegaly, and neurologic abnormalities. Without skin lesions, assess for fever or subnormal temperature, respiratory congestion, tachypnea, and tachycardia	Carry out careful handwashing and gown and glove isolation with linen precautions. Administer intravenous vidarabine (Vira A) or acyclovir (Zovirax). Make a follow-up referral to evaluate potential sequelae of microcephaly, spasticity, seizures, deafness, or blindness. Encourage parental rooming-in and touching of their newborn. Show parents appropriate handwashing procedures and precautions to be used at home if mother's lesions are active. Obtain throat, conjunctiva, cerebral spinal fluid (CSF), blood, urine, and lesion cultures to identify herpesvirus type 2 antibiotics in serum IgM fraction. Cultures positive in 24–48 hours.
Oral Candidal Infection (Thrush) Acquired during passage through birth canal	Assess newborn's buccal mucosa, tongue, gums, and inside the cheeks for white plaques (seen 5 to 7 days of age) Check diaper area for bright-red, well-demarcated eruptions Assess for thrush periodically when newborn is on long-term antibiotic therapy	Differentiate white plaque areas from milk curds by using cotton tip applicator (if it is thrush, removal of white areas causes raw, bleeding areas). Maintain cleanliness of hands, linen, clothing, diapers, and feeding apparatus. Instruct breastfeeding mothers on treating their nipples with nystatin. Administer gentian violet (1%–2%) swabbed on oral lesions 1 hour after feeding or nystatin instilled in baby's oral cavity and on mucosa. Swab skin lesions with topical nystatin. Discuss with parents that gentian violet stains mouth and clothing. Avoid placing gentian violet on normal mucosa; it causes irritation.
Chlamydia Trachomatis Acquired during passage through birth canal	Assess for perinatal history of preterm birth Symptomatic newborns present with pneumonia—conjunctivitis after 3–4 days Chronic follicular conjunctivitis (corneal neovascularization and conjunctival scarring)	Instill ophthalmic erythromycin (see "Drug Guide: Erythromycin [Ilotycin] Ophthalmic Ointment" in Chapter 28 ∞). Make a follow-up referral for eye complications and late development of pneumonia at 4–11 weeks postnatally.

yield false-positive results due to contamination. The skin is prepared by cleaning with an unit-specific antiseptic solution and allowed to dry; the specimen is obtained with a sterile needle and syringe.

2. Spinal fluid culture is done following a spinal tap/lumbar puncture if there is concern of CNS symptoms/pathology.

3. The specimen for urine culture is best obtained by sterile catheterization or suprapubic bladder aspiration.

4. Skin cultures are taken of any lesions or drainage from lesions or reddened areas.

5. Nasopharyngeal, rectal, ear canal, conjunctival, and gastric aspirate cultures may be obtained.

Other laboratory investigations include a complete blood count, C-reactive protein (CRP), chest x-ray examination, serology, and Gram stains of cerebrospinal fluid, urine, skin exudate, and umbilicus. White blood cell (WBC) count with differential may indicate the presence or absence of sepsis. A level of 30,000–40,000 mm^3 WBCs may be normal in the first 24 hours of life, and a low WBC count (< 5000–7500/mm^3) may indicate sepsis. A low neutrophil count and a high band (immature WBCs) count indicate an infection. Stomach aspirate should be sent for culture and smear if a gonococcal infection or amnionitis is suspected. The C-reactive protein level may or may not be elevated. Serum IgM levels are elevated (normal level less than 20 mg/dL) in response to transplacental infections. If available, counterimmunoelectrophoresis tests for specific bacterial antigens are performed.

Evidence of congenital infections may be seen on skull x-ray films (cerebral calcifications such as in cytomegalovirus or toxoplasmosis), on bone x-ray films (syphilis or cytomegalovirus), and in serum-specific IgM levels (rubella). Cytomegalovirus infection is best diagnosed by urine culture.

Because neonatal infection causes high mortality, therapy begins before results of the septic workup are obtained. A combination of two broad-spectrum antibiotics, such as ampicillin and gentamicin, is given in large doses until a culture with sensitivities is obtained.

After the pathogen and its sensitivities are determined, appropriate specific antibiotic therapy is begun. Combinations of penicillin and gentamicin are increasingly being used because of kanamycin-resistant enterobacteria and penicillin-resistant staphylococcus. Rotating aminoglycosides has been suggested to prevent development of resistance. Use of cephalosporins and, in particular, cefotaxime has emerged as an alternative to aminoglycoside therapy in the treatment of neonatal infections. Duration of therapy varies from 7 to 14 days (Table 31–5). If cultures are nega-

tive and symptoms subside, antibiotics may be discontinued after 3 days. Supportive physiologic care may be required to maintain respiratory, hemodynamic, nutritional, and metabolic homeostasis.

NURSING MANAGEMENT

NURSING ASSESSMENT AND DIAGNOSIS

The nurse most often notices symptoms of infection during daily care of the newborn (Short, 2004). The infant may deteriorate rapidly in the first 12 to 24 hours after birth if β-hemolytic streptococcal infection is present, with signs and symptoms mimicking RDS. In other cases the onset of sepsis may be gradual, with more subtle signs and symptoms. The most common signs include the following:

1. Subtle behavioral changes; the infant "is not doing well" and is often lethargic or irritable (especially after the first 24 hours) and hypotonic; color changes may include pallor, duskiness, cyanosis, or a "shocky" appearance; skin is cool and clammy

2. Temperature instability, manifested by either hypothermia (recognized by a decrease in skin temperature) or, rarely in newborns, hyperthermia (elevation of skin temperature) necessitating a corresponding increase or decrease in isolette temperature to maintain a neutral thermal environment

3. Feeding intolerance, as evidenced by a decrease in total intake, abdominal distention, vomiting, poor sucking, lack of interest in feeding, and diarrhea

4. Hyperbilirubinemia

5. Tachycardia initially, followed by spells of apnea or bradycardia

Signs and symptoms may suggest CNS disease (jitteriness, tremors, seizure activity), respiratory system disease (tachypnea, labored respirations, apnea, cyanosis), hematologic disease (jaundice, petechial hemorrhages, hepatosplenomegaly), or gastrointestinal disease (diarrhea, vomiting, bile-stained aspirate, hepatomegaly). A differential diagnosis is necessary because symptoms are similar to those of other more specific conditions.

Nursing diagnoses that may apply to the infant with sepsis neonatorum and the family include the following:

- *Risk for Infection* related to newborn's immature immunologic system

- *Fluid Volume Deficit* related to feeding intolerance

- *Ineffective Family Coping* related to present illness resulting in prolonged hospital stay for the newborn

TABLE 31-5 ❖ Neonatal Sepsis Antibiotic Therapy

Drug	Dose (mg/kg) Total Daily Dose	Schedule for Divided Doses	Route	Comments
Ampicillin	50–100 mg/kg	Every 12 hours* Every 8 hours†	IM or IV	Effective against gram-positive microorganisms, *Haemophilus influenzae*, and most *Escherichia coli* strains. Higher doses indicated for meningitis. Used with aminoglycoside for synergy.
Cefotaxime	50 mg/kg 100–150 mg/kg/day	Every 12 hours* Every 8 hours	IM or IV	Active against most major pathogens in infants; effective against aminoglycoside-resistant organisms; achieves CSF bactericidal activity; lack of ototoxicity and nephrotoxicity; wide therapeutic index (levels not required); resistant organisms can develop rapidly if used extensively; ineffective against *Pseudomonas*, *Listeria*.
Gentamicin	2.5–3 mg/kg 5–7.5 mg/kg/day	Every 12–24 hours*‡ Every 8–24 hours†	IM or IV	Effective against gram-negative rods and staphylococci; may be used instead of kanamycin against penicillin-resistant staphylococci and *E. coli* strains and *Pseudomonas aeruginosa*. May cause ototoxicity and nephrotoxicity. Need to follow serum levels. Must never be given as IV push. Must be given over at least 30–60 minutes. In presence of oliguria or anuria, dose must be decreased or discontinued. In infants less than 1000 g or 29 weeks, lower dosage 2.5–3 mg/kg/day. Monitor serum levels before administration of second dose.
	4–5 mg/kg/dose (first week of life)	Every 24–48 hours		Peak 5–10 mcg/mL Trough 1–2 mcg/mL
Methicillin	25–50 mg/dose 50–100 mg/kg/day	Every 12 hours* Every 6–8 hours†	IM or IV	Effective against penicillinase-resistant staphylococci. Monitor CBC and UA. Slow IV push.
Nafcillin	25–50 mg/kg 50–100 mg/kg/day	Every 8–12 hours* Every 6–8 hours†	IM or IV	Effective against penicillinase-resistant staphylococci. Caution in presence of jaundice.
Penicillin G (aqueous crystalline)	25,000–50,000 units/kg 50,000–125,000 units/kg/day	Every 12 hours* Every 8 hours†	IM or IV	Initial sepsis therapy effective against most gram-positive microorganisms except resistant staphylococci; can cause heart block in infants.
Vancomycin	10–20 mg/kg 30 mg/kg/day	Every 12–24 hours*‡ Every 8 hours†	IV	Effective for methicillin-resistant strains (*Staphylococcus epidermidis*); must be administered by slow intravenous infusion to avoid prolonged cutaneous eruption. For smaller infants, < 1200 g, < 29 weeks, smaller dosages and longer intervals between doses. Nephrotoxic, especially in combination with aminoglycosides. Slow IV infusion over at least 60 minutes. Peak 25–40 mcg/mL Trough 5–10 mcg/mL

*Up to 7 days of age.
†Greater than 7 days of age.
‡Dependent on gestational age.

PLANNING AND IMPLEMENTATION

In the nursery, environmental control and prevention of acquired infection are the responsibilities of the neonatal nurse. An infected newborn can be effectively isolated in an isolette and receive close observation. Promote strict hand-washing technique for all who enter the nursery, including nursing colleagues; physicians; laboratory, x-ray, and respiratory therapists; and parents. Discourage visits to the nursery area by unnecessary personnel. Be prepared to assist in the aseptic collection of specimens for laboratory investigations. Scrupulous equipment care (per agency protocol)—changing and cleaning of isolettes, removing and sterilizing wet equipment, preventing cross use of linen and equipment, cleaning sink-side equipment such as soap containers periodically, and taking special care with the open radiant warmers (access without prior handwashing is much more likely than with the closed isolette)—prevents contamination.

Provision of Antibiotic Therapy

Administer antibiotics as ordered by the nurse practitioner or physician. In addition to the five rights of drug administration, be knowledgeable about the following:

- The proper dose to be administered, based on the weight of the newborn and desired peak and trough levels

- The appropriate route of administration, because some antibiotics cannot be given intravenously

- Admixture incompatibilities, because some antibiotics are precipitated by intravenous solutions or by other antibiotics

- Side effects and toxicity

In term infants being treated for infections, neonatal home infusion of antibiotics should be considered as a viable alternative to continued hospitalization. The infusion of antibiotics at home by skilled RNs facilitates parent-infant bonding while meeting the infant's ongoing healthcare needs.

Provision of Supportive Care

In addition to antibiotic therapy, physiologic supportive care is essential in caring for a septic infant. Responsibilities of the nurse include the following:

- Observe for resolution of symptoms or development of other symptoms of sepsis.

- Maintain neutral thermal environment with accurate regulation of humidity and oxygen administration.

- Provide respiratory support: administer oxygen and observe and monitor respiratory effort.

- Provide cardiovascular support: observe and monitor pulse and blood pressure; observe for hyperbilirubinemia, anemia, and hemorrhagic symptoms.

- Provide adequate calories; oral feedings may be discontinued due to increased mucus, abdominal distention, vomiting, and aspiration.

- Provide fluids and electrolytes to maintain homeostasis; monitor weight changes, urine output, and urine specific gravity.

- Observe for the development of hypoglycemia, hyperglycemia, acidosis, hyponatremia, and hypocalcemia.

Restricting parents' visits to the nursery has not been shown to have any effect on the rate of infection and may be harmful for the newborn's psychologic development. With instruction and guidance, both parents should be allowed to handle the baby and participate in daily care. Support of the parents is crucial. They need to be informed of the newborn's prognosis as treatment continues and to be involved in care as much as possible. They also need to understand how infection is transmitted.

EVALUATION

Expected outcomes of nursing care include the following:

- The risks for development of sepsis are identified early, and immediate action is taken to minimize the development of the illness.

- Appropriate use of aseptic technique protects the newborn from further exposure to illness.

- The baby's symptoms are relieved, and the infection is treated.

- The parents verbalize their concerns about their baby's illness and understand the rationale behind the management of their newborn.

CARE OF THE FAMILY OF AN AT-RISK NEWBORN

The birth of a preterm or ill infant or an infant with a congenital anomaly is a serious crisis for a family. Throughout the pregnancy, the parents have felt excitement, experienced thoughts of acceptance, and pictured what their baby would look like. Both parents have wished for a perfect baby and feared an unhealthy one. Each parent and family member must accept and adjust when the fantasized fears become reality.

PARENTAL RESPONSES

Family members have acute grief reactions to the loss of the idealized baby they have envisioned. In a preterm birth, the mother is denied the last few weeks of pregnancy that seem to prepare her psychologically for the stress of birth and the attachment process. Attachment at this time is fragile, and interruption of the process by separation can affect the future mother-child relationship. Parents express grief as shock and disbelief, denial of reality, anger toward self and others, guilt, blame, and concern for the future. Self-esteem and feelings of self-worth are jeopardized.

Feelings of guilt and failure often plague mothers of preterm newborns. They may question themselves: "Why did labor start?" or "What did I do [or not do]?" A woman may have guilt fantasies and wonder: "Was it because I had sex with my husband [a week, 3 days, a day] ago?" "Was it because I carried three loads of wash up from the basement?" or "Am I being punished for something done in the past—even in childhood?"

The period of waiting between suspicion and confirmation of abnormality or dysfunction is a very anxious one for parents because it is difficult, if not impossible, to begin attachment to the infant if the newborn's future is questionable. During the waiting period, parents need support and acknowledgment that this is an anxious time. They must be kept informed about tests and efforts to gather additional data, as well as efforts to improve their baby's outcome. It is helpful to tell both parents about the problem at the same time, with the baby present. An honest discussion of the problem and anticipatory management at the earliest possible time by health professionals help the parents (1) maintain trust in the physician and nurse, (2) appreciate the reality of the situation by dispelling fantasy and misconception, (3) begin the grieving process, and (4) mobilize internal and external support.

Although reactions and steps of attachment are altered by the birth of these infants, a healthy parent-child relationship can occur. Kaplan and Mason (1974) identified four psychologic tasks as essential for coping with the stress of an at-risk newborn and for providing a basis for the maternal-infant relationship:

1. Anticipatory grief as a psychologic preparation for possible loss of the child while still hoping for his or her survival
2. Acknowledgment of maternal failure to produce a term or perfect newborn expressed as anticipatory grief and depression and lasting until the chances of survival seem secure
3. Resumption of the process of relating to the infant, which was interrupted by the threat of nonsurvival; continuous threat of death or abnormality may impair this task, and the mother may be slow in her response of hope for the infant's survival
4. Understanding of the special needs and growth patterns of the at-risk newborn, which are temporary and yield to normal patterns

Solnit and Stark (1961) postulated that grief and mourning over the loss of the loved object—the idealized child—mark parental reactions to a child with abnormalities. *Grief work,* the emotional reaction to a significant loss, must occur before adequate attachment to the actual child is possible. Parental detachment precedes parental attachment. The parents must first grieve the loss of the wished-for perfect child and then must adopt the imperfect child as the new love object.

Parental responses to a child with health problems may be viewed as a five-stage process (Klaus & Kennell, 1982):

1. *Shock* is felt at the reality of the birth of this child. This stage may be characterized by forgetfulness, amnesia about the situation, and a feeling of desperation.
2. There is disbelief *(denial)* of the reality of the situation, characterized by a refusal to believe the child has a problem. This stage is exemplified by assertions that "It didn't really happen!" or "There has been a mistake; it's someone else's baby."
3. *Depression* over the reality of the situation and a corresponding grief reaction follows acceptance of the situation. This stage is characterized by much crying and sadness. Anger may also emerge at this stage. A projection of blame on others or on self and feelings of "not me" are characteristic of this stage.
4. *Equilibrium and acceptance* are characteristic of a decrease in the emotional reactions of the parents. This stage is variable and may be prolonged by a continuing threat to the infant's survival. Some parents feel chronic sorrow in relation to their child.
5. *Reorganization* of the family is necessary to deal with the child's problems. Mutual support of the parents facilitates this process, but the crisis of the situation may precipitate alienation between the mother and father.

DEVELOPMENTAL CONSEQUENCES

The baby who is born prematurely, is ill, or has a malformation or disorder is at risk for emotional, intellectual, and cognitive developmental delays. The risk is directly proportional to the seriousness of the problem and the length of treatment. The necessary physical separation of family and infant and the tremendous emotional and financial burdens may adversely affect the parent-child relationship. The recent trend to involve the parents with their newborn early, repeatedly, and over protracted periods of time has done much to facilitate positive parent-child relationships.

Parents must have a clear picture of the reality of the disability and the types of developmental hurdles ahead. Unexpected behaviors and responses from the baby due to his or her problem or disorder can be upsetting and frightening.

The demands of care for the child and disputes regarding management or behavior stress family relationships. The entire multidisciplinary team may need to pool their resources and expertise to help parents of children born with problems or disorders so that both parents and children can thrive.

NURSING MANAGEMENT

NURSING ASSESSMENT AND DIAGNOSIS

A positive nurse-family relationship helps information gathering in areas of concern. A concurrent illness of the mother or other family members or other concurrent stress (lack of hospitalization insurance, loss of job, age of parents) may change the family response to the baby. Feelings of apprehension, guilt, failure, and grief expressed verbally or nonverbally are important aspects of the nursing history. These observations enable all professionals to be aware of the parental state, coping behaviors, and readiness for attachment, bonding, and caretaking. Appropriate nursing assessments during interviewing and relating to the family include the following:

1. **Level of understanding:** observations concerning the ability to assimilate the information given and to ask appropriate questions; the need for constant repetition of information

2. **Behavioral responses:** appropriateness of behavior in relation to information given; lack of response; flat affect

3. **Difficulties with communication:** deafness (reads lips only); blindness; dysphagia; understanding only of foreign language

4. **Paternal and maternal education level:** parents unable to read or write; parents with eighth-grade-level education; parents with a graduate-level degree or healthcare background

Documenting such information, gathered through continuing contact and development of a therapeutic relationship with the family, lets all professionals understand and use the nursing history to provide continuous individual care.

Visiting and caregiving patterns indicate the level or lack of parental attachment. A record of visits, caretaking procedures, affect (in relating to the newborn), and telephone calls is essential. It is important to note serial observations rather than just isolated observations that cause concern. Grant (1978) developed a conceptual framework depicting adaptive and maladaptive responses to parenting an infant with an actual or potential problem (Figure 31–12 ●).

If a pattern of distancing behaviors evolves, intervene appropriately. Follow-up studies have found that a statistically significant number of preterm, sick, and congenitally defective infants suffer from failure to thrive, battering, or other parenting disorders. Early detection and intervention prevents these aberrations in parenting behaviors from leading to irreparable damage or death.

Nursing diagnoses that may apply to the family of a newborn at risk include the following:

■ *Dysfunctional Grieving* related to loss of idealized newborn

■ *Fear* related to emotional involvement with an at-risk newborn

■ *Altered Parenting* related to impaired bonding secondary to feelings of inadequacy about caretaking activities

PLANNING AND IMPLEMENTATION

Hospital-Based Nursing Care

In their sensitive and vulnerable state, parents are acutely perceptive of others' responses and reactions (particularly nonverbal) to the child. Parents can be expected to identify with the responses of others. Therefore, it is imperative that medical and nursing staff be fully aware of and come to terms with their own feelings so they are comfortable and at ease with the baby and grieving family.

Nurses may feel uncomfortable, may not know what to say to parents, or may fear confronting their own feelings as well as those of the parents. Each nurse must work out personal reactions with instructors, peers, clergy, parents, or significant others. It is helpful to have a stockpile of therapeutic questions and statements to initiate meaningful dialogue with parents. Opening statements might include the following: "You must be wondering what could have caused this," "Are you thinking that you (or someone else) may have done something?" "How can I help?" and "Are you wondering how you are going to manage?" Avoid statements such as "It could have been worse," "It's God's will," "You have other children," "You are still young and can have more," and "I understand how you feel." This child is important now.

Support of Parents for Initial Visit to the Newborn.   Before parents see their child, prepare them for the visit. Maintain a positive, realistic attitude about the infant. An overly negative, fatalistic attitude further alienates the parents from their infant and retards attachment behaviors. Instead of beginning to bond with their child, the parents will anticipate their loss and begin the process of grieving. Once started, the grieving process is difficult to reverse.

Before preparing parents for the first view of their infant, observe the baby. All infants exhibit strengths as well

○ FIGURE 31-12

Parental Tasks				
Realistically perceive infant's medical condition and needs	Adapt to infant's hospital environment	Assume primary caretaking role	Assume total responsibility for infant upon discharge	Cope with death of infant

Maladaptive Responses

Failure to visit infant or call

Emotional withdrawal from infant

Difficulty interacting comfortably with infant during hospitalization

Resistance to providing minimal caretaking during hospitalization

Failure to achieve sense of parental competence

Failure to achieve sense of attachment to infant

Distortion of medical information received

Debilitating preoccupation with infant's condition

Ascribing blame for infant's condition

Fear of taking infant home

Distorted view of infant and potential needs at time of discharge

Failure to verbalize needs and concerns to staff and family

Hostility toward and distrust of staff

Adaptive Responses

Frequent visits and calls

Emotional involvement with infant

Development of comfortable interaction with infant during hospitalization

Interest in assuming maximum amount of caretaking during hospitalization

Growing sense of parental competence

Growing sense of attachment to infant

Objective interpretation of medical information received

Acceptance of and constructive adaptation to infant's condition

Objective understanding of the causes of infant's condition

Confidence in assuming total responsibility for infant

Realistic view of infant and potential needs at time of discharge

Free verbalization of needs and concerns to staff and family

Realistic view of expectations of staff

Unhealthy Outcome

Disturbed parent-child relationship

Failure to thrive

Vulnerable child syndrome

Deterioration of marital and family equilibrium

Healthy Outcome

Positive parent-child relationship

Maintenance of marital and family equilibrium

Maladaptive and adaptive parental responses during crisis period, showing unhealthy and healthy outcomes.

Used with permission from Grant, P. (1978). Psychological needs of families of high-risk infants. Family and Community Health, 11(3), 93; with permission of Aspen Publishers, Inc., © 1978. 11, 93, Fig. 1, Philadelphia: Lippincott Williams & Wilkins.

as deficiencies; prepare the parents to see both the deviations and the normal aspects of their infant. The nurse may say, "Your baby is small, about the length of my two hands. She weighs 2 lb, 3 oz, but is very active and cries when we disturb her. She is having some difficulty breathing but is breathing without assistance and in only 35% oxygen."

Describe the equipment being used for the at-risk newborn and its purpose before the parents enter the intensive care unit. Many NICUs have booklets for parents to read before entering the units. Explanations and pictures make the parents better prepared to deal with the feelings they may experience when they see their infant for the first time (Figure 31–13 ○).

Upon entering the unit, parents may be overwhelmed by the sounds of monitors, alarms, and respirators, as well as by the unfamiliar language and "foreign" atmosphere. Preparing the parents by having the same healthcare professionals accompany them to the unit can be reassuring. The primary nurse and physician caring for the newborn need to be with the parents when they first visit their baby. Parental reactions vary, but initially there is usually an element of shock. Help them by providing chairs and time to regain composure. Slow, complete, and simple explanations—first about the infant and then about the equipment—allay fear and anxiety.

As parents attempt to deal with the initial stages of shock and grief, they may fail to grasp new information.

● **FIGURE 31–13**

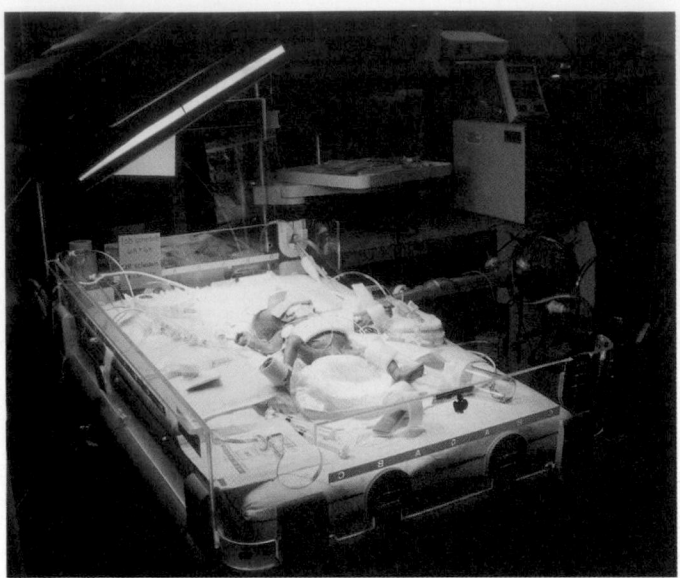

This 25 weeks' gestational age infant with respiratory distress syndrome may be frightening for her parents to see for the first time due to the technology that is attached to her.

Courtesy of Lisa Smith-Pedersen, RNC, MSN, NNP.

They may need repeated explanations to accept the reality of the situation, procedures, equipment, and the infant's condition on subsequent visits.

Concern about the infant's physical appearance is common yet may remain unvoiced. Parents may express such concerns as, "He looks so small and red—like a drowned rat," "Why do her genitals look so abnormal?" and "Will that awful-looking mouth [cleft lip and palate] ever be normal?" Anticipate and address such questions. Use of pictures, such as of an infant after cleft lip repair, may be reassuring to doubting parents. Knowledge of the development of a "normal" preterm infant allows the nurse to make reassuring statements such as, "The baby's skin may look very red and transparent with lots of visible veins, but it is normal for her maturity. As she grows, subcutaneous fat will be laid down, and these superficial veins will begin to disappear."

The nursing staff set the tone of the NICU. Nurses foster the development of a safe, trusting environment by viewing the parents as essential caregivers, not as visitors or nuisances in the unit. Providing privacy when needed and offering easy access to staff and facilities are important in developing an open, comfortable environment. An uncrowded and welcoming atmosphere lets parents know they are welcome there. However, even in crowded physical surroundings, the nurses can convey an attitude of openness and trust.

A trusting relationship is essential for collaborative efforts in caring for the infant. Therapeutically use personal responses to relate to the parents on a one-to-one basis. Each person has different needs, different ways of adapting to crisis, and different means of support. Use techniques that feel real and spontaneous, and avoid words or actions that feel foreign. Gauge interventions so that they match the parents' pace and needs.

Facilitation of Attachment if Neonatal Transport Occurs. Transport to a regional referral center that may be some distance from the parents' community may be necessary. It is essential that the mother see and touch her infant before the infant is transported. Bring the mother to the nursery or take the infant in a warmed transport isolette to the mother's bedside to let her see the infant before transportation to the center. When the infant reaches the referral center, a staff member should call the parents with information about the infant's condition during transport, safe arrival at the center, and present condition.

Support of parents with explanations from the professional staff is crucial. Occasionally the mother may be unable to see the infant before transport (e.g., if she is still under general anesthesia or experiencing complications such as shock, hemorrhage, or seizures). In these cases, take a photograph of the infant to give to the mother, and provide an explanation of the infant's condition and problems and a detailed description of the infant's characteristics. An additional photograph is also helpful for the father to share with siblings or extended family. With the increased attention on improved fetal outcome, prenatal maternal transports, rather than neonatal transports, are occurring more frequently. This practice gives the mother of an at-risk infant the opportunity to visit and care for her infant during the early postpartal period.

Promotion of Touching and Parental Caretaking. Parents visiting a small or sick infant may need several visits to become comfortable and confident in their ability to touch the infant without injuring him or her. Barriers such as isolettes, incisions, monitor electrodes, and tubes may delay the mother's development of comfort in touching the newborn. Knowledge of this normal delay in touching behavior will help the nurse understand parental behavior.

Klaus and Kennell (1982) demonstrated a significant difference in the amount of eye contact and touching behaviors of mothers of normal newborns and mothers of preterm infants. Whereas mothers of normal newborns progress within minutes to palm contact of the infant's trunk, mothers of preterm infants are slower to progress from fingertip to palm contact and from the extremities to the trunk. The progression to palm contact with the infant's trunk may take several visits to the nursery.

Use support, reassurance, and encouragement to help the mother develop positive feelings about her parenting abilities and her importance to her infant. Touching facilitates familiarity with the infant and thus establishes a bond between mother and infant. Touching and seeing the infant help the mother realize the "normal" aspects and potential of her baby (Figure 31–14 ◉).

Encourage parents to meet their newborn's need for stimulation. Stroking, rocking, cuddling, singing, and talking should be an integral part of the parents' caretaking responsibilities. Promote bonding by encouraging parents to visit and become involved in their baby's care (Figure 31–15 ◉). When visiting is impossible, the parents should feel free to phone whenever they wish to receive information about their baby. A warm, receptive attitude provides support. Facilitate parenting by personalizing a baby to the parents, by referring to the infant by name, or by relating personal behavioral characteristics. Remarks such as "Jenny loves her pacifier" help make the infant seem individual and unique.

The variety of equipment needed for life support is hardly conducive to anxiety-free caretaking by the parents. However, parents may care for even the sickest infant, if only in a small way. Promote the parents' success by facilitating parental caretaking. Demonstration and explanation, followed by support of the parents in initial caretaking behaviors, positively reinforce this behavior. Changing their infant's diaper, providing skin or oral care, or helping turn the infant may at first provoke anxiety, but the parents will become more comfortable and confident in caretaking and feel satisfied by the baby's reactions and their ability "to do something." Complimenting the parents' competence in

◉ FIGURE 31–15

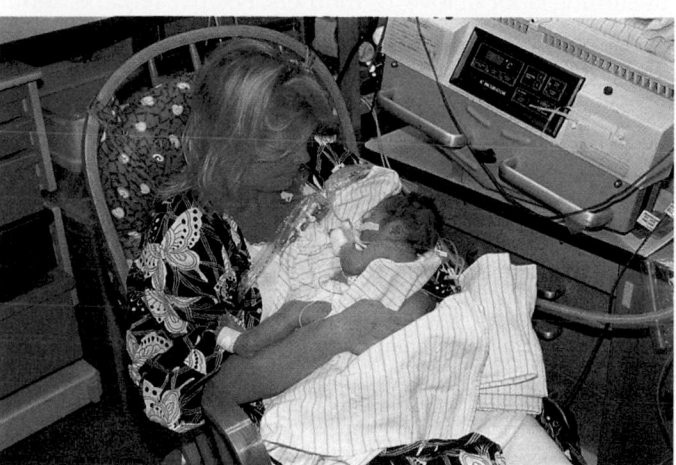

This mother of a 35 weeks' gestational age infant with respiratory distress syndrome is spending time with her newborn and meeting the baby's need for cuddling.

Courtesy of Carol Harrigan, RNC, MSN, NNP.

caretaking also increases their self-esteem, which may have been damaged by feelings of guilt and failure. *Never give the parents a task that they might not be able to accomplish.* Cues that the parents are ready to become involved with the child's care include their reference to the baby by name and their questioning as to amount of feeding taken, sleeping patterns, appearance today, and the like (Loo, Espinosa, Tyler et al., 2003).

Often parents of high-risk infants have ambivalent feelings toward the nurse. As they watch the nurse competently perform caretaking tasks, they may feel both grateful for the nurse's abilities and expertise and jealous of the nurse's ability to care for their infant (Bruns & McCollum, 2002). These feelings may take the form of criticism of the care of the infant, manipulation of staff, or personal guilt. Instead of fostering (by silence) these inferiority feelings of parents, recognize that such feelings are needed to intervene appropriately to enhance parent-infant attachment. For example, avoid making unfavorable comparisons between the baby's responses to parental and nursing caretaking. During a quiet time it may help to encourage the parents to talk about their hopes and fears and to facilitate their involvement in parent groups. Parents are also often anxious when their baby is transferred from the NICU to the "regular nursery." They may feel that their infant is not being cared for as proficiently because the nurses are not at the infant's bedside as often as they were in the NICU.

Verbalizations that improve parental self-esteem are essential and easily shared. For example, point out that, in addition to physiologic use, breast milk is important because of the emotional investment of the mother. Pumping, storing,

◉ FIGURE 31–14

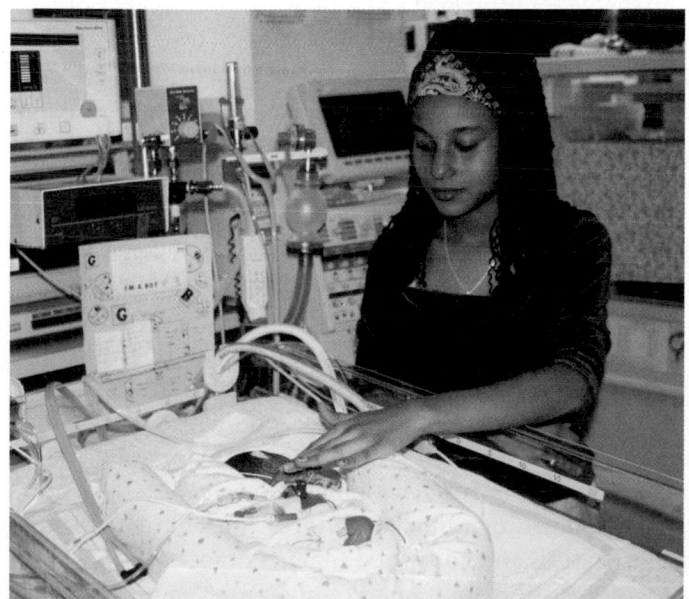

Mother of this 26 weeks' gestational age, 600-g baby begins attachment through fingertip touch.

Courtesy of Lisa Smith-Pedersen, RNC, MSN, NNP.

labeling, and delivering quantities of breast milk is a time-consuming labor of love for mothers. Positive remarks about breast milk reinforce the maternal behavior of caretaking and providing for her infant: "Breast milk is something that only you can give your baby," "You really have brought a lot of milk today," "Look how rich this breast milk is," or "Even small amounts of milk are important, and look how rich it is."

If the infant begins to gain weight while being fed breast milk, it is important to point this correlation out to the mother. Advise the parents that initial weight loss with beginning nipple-feedings is common because of the increased energy expended when the infant begins active rather than passive nutritional intake.

Encourage parents to provide care for their infant even if the baby is very sick and likely to die. Detachment is easier after attachment, because the parents are comforted by the knowledge that they did all they could for their child while he or she was alive.

Facilitation of Family Adjustment. During crisis it is difficult to maintain interpersonal relationships. Yet in a newborn intensive care area, the parents are expected to relate to many different care providers. It is important that parents have as few professionals as possible relaying information to them. A primary nurse should coordinate care and provide continuity for parents. Care providers are individuals and thus will use different terms, inflections, and attitudes. These subtle differences are monumental to parents and may confuse, confound, and produce anxiety. The transfer of the baby from NICU to a step-down unit or transport back to the home hospital provokes parental anxiety because they must now deal with new healthcare professionals. The nurse not only functions as a liaison between the parents and the various professionals interacting with the infant and parents but also offers clarification, explanation, interpretation of information, and support to the parents.

Encourage parents to deal with the crisis with help from their support system. The support system attempts to meet the emotional needs and to provide support for the family members in crisis and stress situations. Biologic kinship is not the only valid criterion for a support system; an emotional kinship is the most important factor. In our mobile society of isolated nuclear families, the support system may be a next-door neighbor, a best friend, or perhaps a schoolmate. Search out the significant others in the lives of the parents and help them understand the problems so that they can support the parents.

The impact of the crisis on the family is individual and varied. Interact with the family to find out about the family's ability to adapt to the situation. To begin appropriate interventions, view the birth of the infant (normal newborn, preterm infant, or infant with congenital anomaly) as it is defined by the family.

It is important to encourage open communication within the family. Discourage family members from keeping secrets from one another, especially between spouses, because secrets undermine the trust of relationships. Well-meaning rationales such as "I want to protect her," "I don't want him to worry about it," and so on can be destructive to open communication and to the basic element of a relationship—trust.

Open communication is especially important when the mother is hospitalized apart from the infant. The first person to visit the infant relays information regarding the infant's care and condition to the mother and family. In this situation the mother has had minimal contact, if any, with her infant. Because of her anxiety and isolation, she may mistrust all those who provide information (the father, nurse, physician, or extended family) until she sees the infant for herself. This can put tremendous stress on the relationship between spouses. The parents (and family) should be given information together. This practice helps overcome misunderstandings and misinterpretations and promotes cooperative "working through" of problems.

Encourage the entire family—siblings as well as other relatives—to visit and obtain information about the baby. Interventions that help the family cope with the situation include providing support, confronting the crisis, and understanding the reality. Support, explanations, and the helping role must include the extended family, as well as the nuclear family, to aid the extended family in communication and to support ties with the nuclear family.

Do not overlook the needs of siblings. Siblings have been looking forward to the new baby, and they too suffer a degree of loss. Young children may react with hostility and older ones with shame at the birth of an infant with an anomaly. Both reactions may make them feel guilty. Parents, who may be preoccupied with working through their own feelings, often cannot give the other children the attention and support they need. Sometimes another child becomes the focus of family tension. Anxiety can take the form of finding fault or of overconcern. This is a form of denial; the parents cannot face the real worry—the infant at risk. After assessing the situation, the observant nurse can ensure that another family member or friend steps in to support the siblings of the affected baby.

Respect and seek to meet the desires and needs of the people involved and understand that differences can exist side by side. It is often possible to elicit the parents' feelings about the experience by asking "How are you doing?" The emphasis is on the word *you*, and the interest must be sincere.

Parents from minority cultures must deal with language barriers and cultural differences that can make feelings of isolation and uncertainty more acute (Shah & Campbell, 2004). Feelings of isolation and uncertainty influence not only the parents' emotional responses to the ill newborn, but also their ability to access and use services as well as their interaction with health professionals. Hospital cultural interpreter programs can assist families with interactions with staff, and provide translation during family meetings and multidisciplinary family conferences.

Families with children in the NICU may become friends and support one another. To encourage the development of these friendships and to provide support, many units have established parent groups. The core of the groups consists of parents whose infants were once in the intensive care unit. Most groups make contact with families within a day or two of the infant's admission to the unit, through either phone calls or visits to the hospital. Early one-on-one parent contacts are more effective than discussion groups in helping families work through their feelings. This personalized method gives the grieving parents a chance to express personal feelings about the pregnancy, labor, and birth and their different-than-expected infant with others who have experienced the same feelings and with whom they can identify.

Nursing Care in the Community

Predischarge planning begins once the infant's condition becomes stable and it seems likely the newborn will survive (AAP & ACOG, 2002). Discharge preparation and care conferences should involve a multidisciplinary team approach. NICU nursing staff is the fulcrum for aiding in the transition of high-risk infants from the intensive care unit to the home. Effective open communication with families during the entire discharge-planning phase of care empowers them to assume the role of primary caregiver for their children (Allen, Donohue, & Porter, 2002).

Adequate predischarge teaching helps parents transform any feelings of inadequacy they may have into feelings of self-assurance and attachment. From the beginning, teach the parents about their infant's special needs and growth patterns. This teaching and involvement are best facilitated by a nurse who is familiar with the infant and his or her family and who has developed a comfortable and supportive relationship with them. When twins are being discharged, inform parents that cobedding of twins allows for clustering of care and facilitates the parents' ability to spend time with both of their children (Figure 31–16 ●).

Provide home care instructions in an optimal environment for parental learning. Learning should take place over time, to avoid bombarding the parents with instructions in the day or hour before discharge. Parents often enjoy performing minimal caretaking tasks, with gradual expansion of their role.

Many NICUs provide facilities for parents to room-in with their infants for a few days before discharge. This

COMPLEMENTARY CARE

COBEDDING OF TWINS

As NICUs have become more and more "developmentally" friendly, complementary and alternative therapies have become an adjunct to that nurturing environment.

Cobedding of stable twins and higher order multiples replicates the closeness of the in utero environment whereby the siblings are placed together in the same incubator or crib to maintain physical contact. Clustering of care provided by the bedside nurse is a true advantage to cobedding. This in turn proves beneficial to the parents because they have interactions with fewer nurses and other members of the healthcare team. In addition the parents can care for and visit with all the infants at one time (Lutes & Altimier, 2001). Discharge teaching, therefore, is easily facilitated. Cobedding is also a strategy to maximize the synchronization of sleep-wake cycles (Hayward, 2003; Lutes & Altimier, 2001).

● **FIGURE 31–16**

Cobedding of twins facilitates delivery of care and parent interaction with healthcare members.

Courtesy of Carol Harrigan, RNC, MSN, NNP.

practice allows parents a degree of independence in the care of their infant with the security of nursing help nearby. It is particularly helpful for anxious parents, parents who have not had the opportunity to spend extended time with their infant, or parents who will be giving complex physical care at home, such as tracheostomy care.

Transitional care centers (TCCs) also allow parents to master caring for the at-risk newborn prior to discharge. The TCCs shorten the length of hospitalization and decrease readmission rates (Allen et al., 2002). Families are able to interact with the staff while gradually transitioning to the role of sole caretakers of their medically complex, high-risk infant. When discharging a medically fragile infant to home, schedule a predischarge home visit by a public health nurse or home health agency. This predischarge visit evaluates the home for any possible issues that may complicate the parents' ability to care for their at-risk infant, especially if there are multiple monitoring-equipment needs.

The basic elements of discharge and home care instruction are as follows:

1. Teach the parents routine well-baby care, such as bathing, taking a temperature, preparing formula, and breastfeeding.

2. Help parents learn to do special procedures as needed by the newborn, such as gavage or gastrostomy feedings, tracheostomy or enterostomy care, medication administration, cardiopulmonary resuscitation (CPR), and operation of the apnea monitor. Before discharge, the parents should be as comfortable as possible with these tasks and should demonstrate independence. Written instructions are useful for parents to refer to once they are home with the infant, but they should not replace actual participation in the infant's care.

3. Make sure that all applicable screening (metabolic, vision, hearing) tests, immunization, and respiratory syncytial virus (RSV) prophylaxis are done prior to discharge and that all records are given to the primary care provider and parents.

4. Refer parents to community health and support organizations. The Visiting Nurses' Association, public health nurses, or social services can assist the parents in the stressful transition from hospital to home by providing predischarge home visits and then the necessary home teaching and support. Some NICUs have their own parent support groups to help bridge the gap between hospital and home care. Parents can also find support from a variety of community organizations, such as mothers-of-twins groups, trisomy 13 clubs, the March of Dimes Birth Defects Foundation, handicapped children services, and teen mother and child programs. Each community has numerous agencies capable of assisting the family in adapting emotionally, physically, and financially to the chronically ill infant. Be familiar with community resources and help the parents identify which agencies may benefit them.

5. Help parents recognize the growth and development needs of their infant. A development program begun in the hospital can be continued at home, or refer parents to an infant development program in the community.

6. Arrange medical follow-up care before discharge. A family pediatrician, a well-baby clinic, or a specialty clinic may provide follow-up care for the infant. The first appointment should be made before the infant is discharged from the hospital.

7. Evaluate the need for special equipment for infant care (such as a respirator, oxygen, apnea monitor) in the home. Any equipment or supplies should be in the home before the infant's discharge.

8. Arrange for neonatal hospice for parents of the medically fragile infant as needed.

Further evaluation after the infant has gone home is useful in determining whether the crisis has been resolved satisfactorily. The parents are usually given the intensive care nursery's telephone number to call for support and advice. It is a good idea for staff to follow up with each family with visits or telephone calls at intervals for several weeks to assess and evaluate the infant's (and parents') progress.

EVALUATION

Expected outcomes of nursing care include the following:

- The parents are able to verbalize their feelings of grief and loss.
- The parents verbalize their concerns about their baby's health problems, care needs, and potential outcome.
- The parents participate in their infant's care and show attachment behaviors.

CONSIDERATIONS FOR THE NURSE WHO WORKS WITH AT-RISK NEWBORNS

The birth of a baby with a problem is a traumatic event with the potential for either disruption or growth of the involved family. The staff NICU nurses may never see the long-term results of the specialized, sensitive care they give to parents and their newborns. Their only immediate evidence of effective care may be the beginning of resolution of parental grief; discharge of a recovered, thriving infant to the care of happy parents; and the beginning of reintegration of family life.

Nurses cannot provide support unless they themselves are supported. Working in an emotional environment of life-and-death situations takes its toll on staff. NICUs are among the most stressful areas in healthcare for patients, families, and nurses. Nurses bear most of the stress and largely determine the atmosphere of the NICU. The nurse's ability to cope with stress is the key to creating an emotionally healthy environment and a positive working atmosphere. The emotional needs and feelings of the staff must be recognized and dealt with so that staff can support the parents. An environment of openness to feelings and support in dealing with their human needs and emotions is essential for personnel.

As caregivers, nurses may be unaware of their need to grieve for their own losses in the NICU. Nurses must also go through the grief work that parents experience. Techniques such as group meetings, individual support, and primary care nursing may help maintain staff mental health.

Critical Concept Review

LEARNING OBJECTIVES

CONCEPTS

Discuss how to identify infants in need of resuscitation and the appropriate method of resuscitation based on the labor record and observable physiologic indicators.

1. Infants at risk for resuscitation include:
   - Nonreassuring fetal heart pattern, meconium-stained amniotic fluid and/or acidosis detected by fetal scalp sample.
   - Cardiac disease diagnosed prenatally.
   - Other congenital abnormality diagnosed prenatally.
   - Premature birth.
   - Infant of multiple pregnancy.
   - Prolonged or difficult delivery.
2. Infants needing resuscitation:
   - Weak cry at birth.
   - Poor respiratory effort at birth.
   - Retractions at birth.
3. Resuscitation methods:
   - Stimulation by rubbing the newborn's back. (Done initially to all infants.)
   - Use of positive pressure to inflate the lungs. (Used if respirations are inadequate or have not been initiated.)
   - Endotracheal intubation. (Used immediately for severely premature infants, infants with known congenital anomalies, and infants who do not respond to stimulation or bag and mask.)
   - Medications: Naloxone (Narcan) may be used to reverse effects of narcotics given to mother prior to birth.

Based on clinical manifestations, differentiate between the various types of respiratory distress (respiratory distress syndrome, transient tachypnea of the newborn, and meconium aspiration syndrome) in the newborn and their related nursing care.

1. Respiratory distress syndrome:
   - Lack of sufficient surfactant causes labored respirations and increased work at breathing.
   - Seen most frequently in premature newborns.
   - Nursing care involves administration of surfactant, close assessment, and supportive care if mechanical ventilation is needed.
2. Transient tachypnea of the newborn (TTNB):
   - Usually results from excess fluid in the lungs.
   - Infant breathes normally at birth, but develops symptoms of respiratory distress by 4-6 hours of age.
   - Nursing care involves initiating oxygen therapy and restricting oral feedings until respiratory status improves.
3. Meconium aspiration syndrome:
   - Signs and symptoms of respiratory distress beginning at birth.
   - May depend upon the amount of meconium that is aspirated.
   - Nursing care involves suctioning of oropharynx and nasopharynx prior to infant's first breath.
   - After initial suctioning and resuscitation efforts, nursing care involves ongoing assessment for signs and symptoms of respiratory distress and supportive care of the infant requiring mechanical ventilation or ECMO.

(continued)

LEARNING OBJECTIVES

CONCEPTS

Discuss selected metabolic abnormalities (including cold stress and hypoglycemia), their effects on the newborn, and the nursing implications.	1. Cold stress sets up the chain of physiologic events of hypoglycemia, pulmonary vasconstriction, hyperbilirubinemia, respiratory distress, and metabolic acidosis.
	2. Nursing interventions include:
	  ■ Keep infant warmed during any transport.
	  ■ Observe for any signs of hypoglycemia.
	  ■ Have infant go to breast or feed early in neonatal period.
	  ■ Assess blood glucose frequently.

Differentiate between physiologic and pathologic jaundice based on onset, cause, possible sequelae, and specific management.	1. Physiologic jaundice:
	  ■ Occurs in 50% of all newborns.
	  ■ Appears after 24 hours of age.
	  ■ Not visible after 10 days of age.
	  ■ May require phototherapy.
	2. Pathologic jaundice:
	  ■ Usually caused by ABO or Rh incompatibility.
	  ■ Jaundice may be present within 24 hours of birth.
	  ■ Treatment begins with phototherapy, but may progress to exchange transfusions.
	3. Untreated hyperbilirubinemia (due to either type of jaundice) may result in neurotoxicity.

Explain how Rh incompatibility or ABO incompatibility can lead to the development of hyperbilirubinemia.	1. Rh incompatibility:
	  ■ Maternal antibodies enter the fetal circulation, then attach to and destroy fetal red blood cells.
	  ■ Fetal system produces more RBCs.
	  ■ Hyperbilirubinemia, anemia, and jaundice result.
	2. ABO incompatibility:
	  ■ Mother is type O and infant is type A or B.
	  ■ Less severe than Rh incompatibility.

Identify nursing responsibilities in caring for the newborn receiving phototherapy.	Nursing responsibilities for the newborn receiving phototherapy include: 1. Expose maximum amount of skin surface for optimal therapeutic results. 2. Apply eye patches while phototherapy is in progress. 3. Assess eyes for signs/symptoms of conjunctivitis per agency protocol. 4. Frequently monitor temperature. 5. Offer infant water and formula frequently to assist in excretion of bilirubin. 6. Keep parents informed of need for phototherapy and encourage parents to hold and care for infant while undergoing phototherapy.

Discuss selected hematologic problems such as anemia and polycythemia and the nursing implications associated with each one.	1. Anemia in newborns results from prenatal blood loss, birth trauma, infection, or blood group incompatibility:
	  ■ Nursing assessments for signs and symptoms of anemia.
	  ■ Record all amounts of blood taken during laboratory testing.
	2. Polycythemia may result from delayed cord clamping, twin-to-twin transfusion, or chronic intrauterine hypoxia:
	  ■ Nursing assessments for signs and symptoms of polycythemia.

Describe the nursing assessments that would lead the nurse to suspect newborn sepsis.	The most common signs of newborn sepsis include: 1. Lethargy or irritability. 2. Pallor or duskiness. 3. Hypothermia. 4. Feeding intolerance. 5. Hyperbilirubinemia. 6. Tachycardia, bradycardia, or apneic spells.
Relate the consequences of selected maternally transmitted infections, such as maternal syphilis, gonorrhea, herpesvirus, and chlamydia, to the care of the infant in the neonatal period.	1. All infants receive eye prophylaxis with opthalmic antibiotic due to possibility of transmission of gonorrhea or chlamydia during the birth process. 2. Maternal syphilis requires that the infant be isolated from other newborns and receive antibiotics at birth. 3. Maternal herpes virus infection requires administration of IV antiviral medications in the immediate newborn period as well as multiple cultures (skin, spinal fluid) for presence of herpesvirus.

LEARNING OBJECTIVES

CONCEPTS

Describe the interventions to facilitate parental attachment with the at-risk newborn.

1. Assess the parent's level of understanding of the infant's problem.
2. Prepare and facilitate the parents' viewing of the infant.
3. Promote touching and facilitate parental participation in care of the infant.
4. Facilitate parental adjustment to the infant's special needs.

Identify the special initial and long-term needs of parents of at-risk infants.

1. Initially, the parents need to understand the infant's problem, including expected treatments.
2. Need to understand routine well-baby care.
3. Need to understand how to perform any special procedures needed to care for the infant.
4. Need referral for normal infant screening procedures.
5. Need to understand normal growth and development of infants.
6. Need to have medical follow-up arranged.
7. Need referral for any special equipment required at home.

CRITICAL THINKING IN ACTION

*View the **Critical Thinking in Action** video in Chapter 31 of the CD-ROM. Then, answer the questions that follow.*

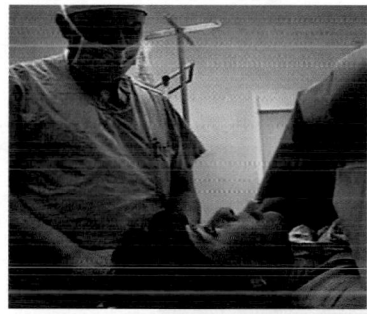

Rebecca Prince, age 21, G2 now P2, gives birth to a 5 pound baby at 38 weeks' gestation by primary cesarean birth for fetal distress. The infant's Apgars are 7 and 9 at 1 and 5 minutes. The infant is suctioned and given free flow oxygen at birth, then is admitted to the newborn nursery for transitional care and does well. You are the nurse caring for baby Prince at 36 hours old. You review the newborn's record and note that the baby's blood type is A+ and his mother is O+. Rebecca wants to breastfeed. You are performing a shift assessment on baby Prince when you observe the infant has a unilateral cephalhematoma and is lethargic. You blanch the skin over the sternum and observe a yellow discoloration of the skin. Lab tests reveal a serum bilirubin level of 12 mg/dL, hematocrit 55%, a mildly positive direct Coombs' test, and a positive indirect Coombs' test. Baby Prince is diagnosed with hyperbilirubinemia secondary to ABO incompatibility and cephalhematoma. You provide phototherapy by fiberoptic blanket around the trunk of the infant and take the baby to his mother's room.

1. How would you explain the purpose of phototherapy with the mother?
2. Describe the care the mother can give to the newborn.
3. Discuss the advantage of the fiberoptic blanket phototherapy for the newborn.
4. Newborns up to 1 month of age are susceptible to organisms that do not cause significant disease in older children. Explore the circumstances that cause susceptibility to infection.
5. Describe how to distinguish between oral thrush and milk curds.

MEDIALINK

www.prenhall.com/london

■ NCLEX-RN® Review, case studies, and other interactive resources for this chapter can be found on the Companion Website at http://www.prenhall.com/london. Click on "Chapter 31" to select the activities for this chapter.

■ For animations, more NCLEX-RN® Review questions, and an audio glossary, access the accompanying CD-ROM in this textbook.

REFERENCES

Abbasi, S., Hirsch, D., Davis, J., Tolosa, J., Stouffer, N., Debbs, R., et al. (2000). Effect of single versus multiple courses of antenatal corticosteroids on maternal and neonatal outcome. *American Journal of Obstetrics and Gynecology, 182*(5), 1243–1249.

Allen, M. C., Donohue, P. K., & Porter, M. (2002). Follow-up of the NICU infant. In G. B. Merenstein & S. L. Gardner, *Handbook of intensive care* (5th ed., pp. 787–800). St Louis, MO: Mosby.

American Academy of Pediatrics (AAP) Committee on Fetus and Newborn & American College of Obstetricians and Gynecologists (ACOG) Committee on Obstetrics. (2002). *Guidelines for perinatal care* (5th ed.). Evanston, IL: Author.

American Academy of Pediatrics Subcommittee on Hyperbilirubinemia. (2004). Management of hyperbilirubinemia in the newborn infant 35 or more weeks of gestation. *Pediatrics, 114*(1), 297–316.

Armentrout, D. (2004). Glucose management. In M. T. Verklan & M. Walden (Eds.), *Core curriculum for neonatal intensive care nursing* (3rd ed., pp. 192–204). St. Louis, MO: Elsevier Saunders.

Askin, D. F., & Diehl-Jones, W. (2004). Assisted ventilation. In M. T. Verklan & M. Walden (Eds.), *Core curriculum for neonatal intensive care nursing* (3rd ed., pp. 536–568). St. Louis, MO: Elsevier Saunders.

Blackburn, S. T. (2003). *Maternal, fetal, & neonatal physiology: A clinical perspective* (2nd ed.). St. Louis, MO: Saunders.

Bruns, D. A., & McCollum, J. A. (2002). Partnerships between mothers and professionals in the NICU: Caregiving, information exchange, and relationships. *Neonatal Network, 21*(7), 15–23.

Cloherty, J. P., Eichenwald, E. C., & Stark, A. R. (2004). *Manual of neonatal care* (5th ed.). Philadelphia: Lippincott Williams & Wilkins.

Dargaville, P. A., South, M., & McDougall, P. N. (2001). Surfactant and surfactant inhibitors in meconium aspiration syndrome. *Journal of Pediatrics, 138*(1), 113–115.

de Ungria, M., & Steinhorn, R. H. (2003). Neonatal resuscitation. In J. J. Sciarra (Eds.), *Gynecology and obstetrics* (Vol. 3, chap. 68, pp. 1–15). Philadelphia: Lippincott Williams & Wilkins.

Diehl-Jones, W., & Askin, D. F. (2004). Hematologic disorders. In M. T. Verklan & M. Walden (Eds.), *Core curriculum for neonatal intensive care nursing* (3rd ed., pp. 728–758). St. Louis, MO: Elsevier Saunders.

Fanaroff, A. A., Martin, R. J., & Rodriguez, R. J. (2004). Identification and management of problems in the high-risk neonate. In R. K. Creasy & R. Resnik (Eds.), *Maternal-fetal medicine: Principles and practice* (5th ed., pp. 1263–1301). Philadelphia: Saunders.

Gelfand, S. L., Fanaroff, J. M., & Walsh, M. C. (2004). Meconium stained fluid: Approach to the mother and the baby. *Pediatric Clinics of North America, 51*(3), 655–667.

Glomella, T. L. (2004). *Neonatology: Management, procedures, on-call problems, diseases, and drugs* (5th ed.). New York: Lange Medical Books/McGraw-Hill.

Grant, P. (1978). Psychological needs of families of high-risk infants. *Family and Community Health, 1*(3), 93–97.

Hayward, K. (2003). Cobedding of twins: A natural extension of the socialization process? *MCN. American Journal of Maternal Child Nursing, 28*(6), 260–263.

Kaplan, D. M., & Mason, E. A. (1974). Maternal reactions to premature birth viewed as an acute emotional disorder. In H. J. Parad (Ed.), *Crisis intervention* (pp. 118–128). New York: Family Services Association of America.

Klaus, M. H., & Kennell, J. H. (1982). *Maternal-infant bonding* (2nd ed.). St. Louis, MO: Mosby.

Loo, K. K., Espinosa, M., Tyler, R., & Howard, J. (2003). Using knowledge to cope with stress in the NICU: How parents integrate learning to read the physiologic and behavioral cues of the infant. *Neonatal Network, 22*(1), 31–37.

Lutes, L. M., & Altimier, L. (2001). Co-bedding multiples. *Newborn and Infant Nursing Reviews, 1,* 242–246.

Madan, A., MacMahon, J. R., & Stevenson, D. K. (2005). Neonatal hyperbilirubinemia. In H. W. Taeusch, R. A. Ballard, & C. A. Gleason (Eds.), *Avery's diseases of the newborn* (8th ed., pp. 1226–1257). Philadelphia, PA: Elsevier Saunders.

Mitchell, A., & Waltman, P. A. (2003). *Oral sucrose and pain relief for preterm infants. Pain Management Nursing, 4*(2), 62–69. 2003 W. B. Saunders. Retrieved July 28, 2003, from http://www.medscape.com/viewarticle/458592

Neonatal hypoglycemia. (2000). *NANN guidelines for practice* (pp. 1–16). Des Plaines, IL: National Association of Neonatal Nurses.

Shah, M. A. & Campbell, D. (2004). *Transcultural aspects of perinatal health: A resource guide. American Academy of Pediatrics: National Perinatal Association.* Elk Grove Village, IL: American Academy of Pediatrics.

Short, M. A. (2004). Guide to a systematic physical assessment in the infant with suspected infection and/or sepsis. *Advances in Neonatal Care, 4*(3), 141–153.

Solnit, A., & Stark, M. (1961). Mourning and the birth of a defective child. *Psychoanalytic Study of the Child, 16,* 505.

Sperling, M. A. & Menon, R. K. (2004). *Differential diagnosis and management of neonatal hypoglycemia. Pediatric Clinics of North America, 51*(3), 703–723.

Thureen, P. J., Deacon, J., Hernandez, J. A., & Hall, D. M. (2005). *Assessment and care of the well newborn* (2nd ed.). St. Louis, MO: Elsevier Saunders.

Walden, M., & Jorgensen, K. M. (2004). Pain management. In C. Kenner & J. M. McGrath (Eds.), *Developmental care of newborn & infants: A guide for health professionals* (pp. 197–222). St. Louis, MO: Mosby.

Watson, R. L. (2004). Gastrointestinal disorders. In M. T. Verklan & M. Walden (Eds.), *Core curriculum for neonatal intensive care nursing* (3rd ed., pp. 643–702). St. Louis, MO: Elsevier Saunders.

Young, T. E., & Mangum, O. B. (2005). *Neofax*®: *A manual of drugs used in neonatal care* (18th ed.). Raleigh, NC: Acorn.

Zukowsky, K. (2004). Respiratory distress. In M. T. Verklan & M. Walden (Eds.), *Core curriculum for neonatal intensive care nursing* (3rd ed., pp. 487–523). St. Louis, MO: Elsevier Saunders.

Home Care of the Postpartum Family

I remember how frightened I was when we brought our first child home from the hospital. Neither of our mothers could come to stay and I was absolutely terrified. I survived, but it was hard. My daughter is expecting her first child next month and she wants me to come out to help her. Thank God. I don't want to be a "buttinski" mother, but I really want to be there for her . . . and I guess for me, too!

—Lois, 53

LEARNING OBJECTIVES

- Discuss the components of postpartal home care.
- Identify the main purposes of home visits during the postpartum period.
- Summarize actions a nurse should take to ensure personal safety during a home visit.
- Delineate aspects of fostering a caring relationship in the home.
- Describe assessment and care of the newborn and reinforcement of parent teaching in the home.
- Discuss maternal and family assessment and anticipated progress after birth.
- Delineate interventions to address the common concerns of breastfeeding mothers following discharge.
- In addition to home visits, identify other types of follow-up care available to postpartum families.

MEDIALINK

www.prenhall.com/london

CD-ROM
Audio Glossary
NCLEX-RN® Review

Companion Website
Thinking Critically
NCLEX-RN® Review
Case Study: Follow-Up with the Client at Home
Care Plan Activity: Breastfeeding Care Plan

In the 1990s, in an effort to contain costs, discharge within 48 hours of birth became the norm and, indeed, discharge within 24 hours of vaginal birth was not uncommon. In 1998 the U.S. federal government passed legislation that guaranteed a minimum stay of up to 48 hours following vaginal birth and up to 96 hours following cesarean birth at the discretion of the mother and her care provider. Research has demonstrated that extending the length of stay does not increase costs when death rates and readmission costs are considered (Malkin, Keeler, Broder et al., 2003).

Discharge prior to 48 hours now occurs only at the family's request. These early discharges present a challenge to nurses because the time available for nursing assessments and client teaching is greatly reduced. In addition, many conditions in the newborn, such as jaundice, ductal-dependent cardiac lesions, and gastrointestinal obstructions, may take longer than 2 days to develop, and identification of these problems depends on a skilled, experienced professional. Other experts contend that breastfeeding may not be well established prior to 48 hours and discharge before this time can lead to increased rates of dehydration and poor breastfeeding outcomes (Heck, Schoendorf, Gilberto et al., 2003).

Early discharge also has implications for the mother. Opportunities to become comfortable with her new baby may be compromised. In addition, extended family members who live at a distance and have agreed to assist the new family in the first few weeks after birth may not have arrived yet. Furthermore, in the first 24 hours after childbirth, the mother may be too tired or may not be ready emotionally to participate in learning activities.

In all cases of early discharge, a home visit by an experienced postpartal nurse can be invaluable. However, home visits are not the norm universally. In many areas, support for low-risk women and newborns is provided through telephone follow-up and clinic or office visits. Nevertheless, home care is becoming an essential component of perinatal nursing care, particularly as caregivers struggle to find an appropriate balance between providing quality client care and managing escalating healthcare costs.

THE HOME VISIT

Home care for the postpartum family is focused more on assessment, teaching, and counseling than on physical care. Postpartum home care gives nurses a chance to enhance information and self- and infant care techniques initially presented in the birth setting. Moreover the home setting lets the nurse and family interact in a more relaxed environment in which the family has control of the setting. In some instances, the challenges of assessing and enhancing self-care and infant care may be unique in the home, and the nurse has many opportunities to exercise critical thinking to develop creative options with the family.

In planning a home visit, the nurse should clearly understand the purpose of the visit and the content to be addressed. Other important considerations include ways of creating and fostering relationships with families, techniques for preplanning and executing the visit while maintaining safety, documentation of the visit, and telephone follow-up.

The postpartum home visit differs from community health visits in that only one or two home visits are typically planned, and long-term follow-up by the postpartum nurse is not anticipated. Although the postpartum home visit is comprehensive, it focuses specifically on the postpartum family's needs and care.

The established guidelines for discharge of the mother and baby mean the nurse can expect certain levels of health and wellness. However, because the status of the mother and newborn can change, the nurse should stay alert for deviations from the norm.

PURPOSES OF THE HOME VISIT

The postpartum home visit usually occurs within 24 to 48 hours of discharge and is conducted by a registered nurse who is experienced in postpartum maternal and newborn care. Before the home visit, the nurse prepares by identifying the purpose of the home visit and gathering anticipated materials and equipment. A personal contact while the woman is still in the birth setting or a previsit telephone call is used to arrange the appointment with the woman and her family. During the previsit contact, it is important for the nurse to identify clearly the purpose and goals of the visit and to begin establishing rapport.

The postpartum home visit has many purposes. It provides an opportunity to assess the status of the mother and infant after birth for signs of any complications, to complete follow-up blood work if needed, and to ascertain current informational needs. The home visit also provides time to cover additional information in a more relaxed setting. In addition the nurse assesses adaptation of the family to the new baby and adjustment of any siblings and addresses the need for referrals to clinics, classes, community agencies, or postpartum support groups.

FOSTERING A CARING RELATIONSHIP WITH THE FAMILY

The dynamics of the home visit are different from those of the hospital or birthing center. In the home, the family members have control of their environment and the nurse is an invited visitor. The nurse can rely on the same characteristics of a caring relationship that have been integral to hospital-based practice—regard, genuineness, empathy, trust, and rapport—but the relationship may take on new elements as the nurse moves into the home setting for the first time.

MAINTAINING SAFETY

In the past, nurses were perceived as a mainstay of communities and could move in most settings without fear or concern for safety. However, today some communities are not safe for visiting nurses. It is important to follow some basic safety rules when making a home visit. Specifically, know the address and ask for directions during the previsit contact. If the area is not familiar, trace out the route on a map before leaving for the visit and take the map along. It is also wise to wear a name tag and sensible shoes. Avoid wearing expensive jewelry or pins of a religious or political nature that might be seen as offensive. A cellular phone or pager is advisable for any community visitor, as is a working flashlight, especially for night visits. In addition, carry sufficient change to call from a pay phone if necessary. Notify a supervisor when leaving for a visit and check in as soon as the visit is done.

Many agencies that provide home care services have established violence prevention programs to help ensure safety. Nurses in the community need to be aware of their environment and alert to environmental cues, whether overt or subtle. In addition the following recommendations are important (Aisenstein, 2003):

- Drive around a neighborhood before making a visit to identify potential cues to violence. Avoid walking through a crowd or staying in an elevator with others if it makes you uneasy.

- In high-risk areas, visit the family during daylight hours. Inform the family as to when you plan to arrive and advise them to call your supervisor if you do not arrive within 15 minutes of the arranged time. Provide them with a contact name and phone number.

- Do not park in deserted or unlit areas. Make sure your car is in good working order and has gas. Keep doors locked and windows closed.

- Lock personal belongings in the trunk of the car, out of sight. Do not carry a purse, medications, or other items.

- In accordance with agency policy, wear scrubs or a lab coat or other uniform that identifies you as a nurse.

- Pay attention to the body language of anyone present, not just the client. Be alert for signs that a person is becoming angry (reddened neck and face, clenched fists, pacing).

- Be aware of personal body language and how it might be interpreted. (For example, avoid crossing arms or shoving hands in pockets, which may suggest hostility; remain calm and convey a sense of respect at all times.)

- Leave the home immediately if a gun is visible and the client or family member refuses to put it away.

- If a situation arises that feels unsafe, end the visit.

If the visit is in an area that seems very unsafe, it may be wise for two nurses to go together. Avoid entering areas where violence is in progress. In such cases, return to the car and call 911.

It is always important to be aware of one's surroundings and the people who are nearby. First home visits may feel uncomfortable because they are unfamiliar, but experience increases comfort (Figure 32–1 ●).

CARRYING OUT THE HOME VISIT

When the client or family answers the door, the nurse introduces himself or herself and confirms that the location

○ **FIGURE 32-1**

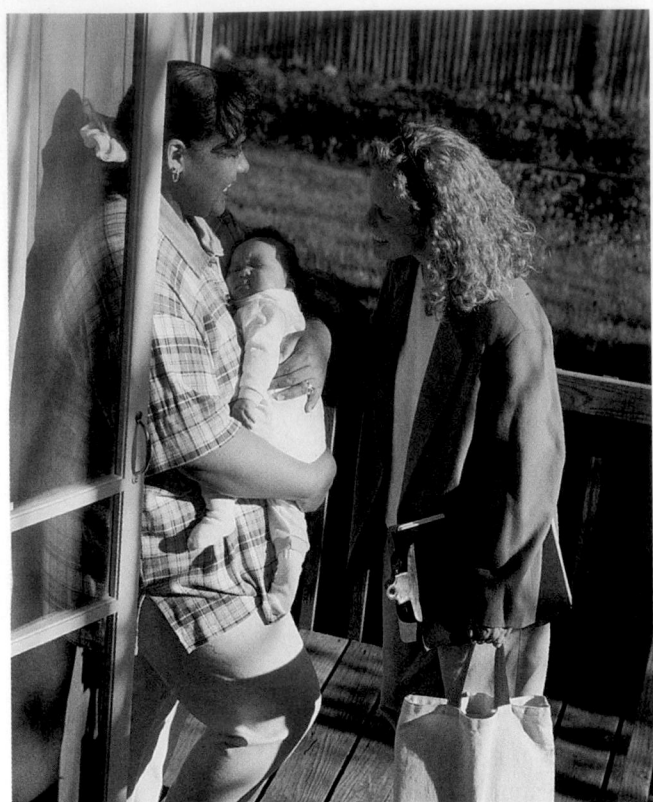

Nurse arriving for a home visit.

is correct. If a place to sit is not indicated, ask "Where is the best place to sit so that we can talk for a while?" In some homes the mother or family may offer refreshments, and this may be an important aspect of welcoming a visitor. In this case it is helpful to accept the refreshment graciously.

DEVELOPING CULTURAL COMPETENCE

CULTURAL CUES IN A HOME VISIT

During a home visit, be sensitive to cultural cues. In most cultures there is a designated family caretaker—possibly a mother, aunt, or grandmother. Seek her cooperation and support for any interventions. Your client is more likely to agree to your suggestion if the designated caregiver approves.

Complete planned assessments, provide direct care as necessary, carry out family and client teaching, make necessary referrals to community agencies, and schedule additional home visits or telephone contact. Report significant medical concerns to the certified nurse-midwife or physician immediately and plan for appropriate follow-up. The aspects assessed and addressed during the home visit are discussed in the following sections.

HOME CARE: THE NEWBORN

POSITIONING AND HANDLING

If the mother or other family members seem unsure about handling or positioning the baby, show them how to position and handle the newborn as needed. As the family members provide care, instill confidence by giving them positive feedback. If a family member encounters problems, suggest alternatives and serve as a role model.

When the newborn is out of the crib, one of the following holds can be used (Figure 32–2 ○). The *cradle hold* is frequently used during feeding. It provides a sense of warmth and closeness, permits eye contact, frees one of the adult's hands, and provides security because the cradling protects the newborn's body. Gripping the baby's thigh with the hand while the arm supports the newborn's body provides extra security. The *upright position* provides security and a sense of closeness and is ideal for burping. One hand should support the neck and shoulders, while the other hand holds the buttocks or is placed between the newborn's legs. The newborn may also be held upright in a cloth sling carrier that gently holds the baby against the parent's chest and frees the hands for other tasks. The *football hold* frees one of the caregiver's hands and permits eye contact. This hold is ideal for shampooing, carrying, or breastfeeding. It frees the caregiver to talk on the telephone or do the myriad tasks that await attention at this busy time.

The infant's position should be changed periodically throughout the early months of life, because skull bones are soft, and permanently flattened areas may develop if the newborn consistently lies in one position. The awake newborn is frequently positioned on her or his side with the dependent arm forward to provide support and to prevent rolling. The side-lying position aids drainage of mucus and allows air to circulate around the cord. It is also comfortable for the newly circumcised male. After feeding, the newborn may be placed on the right side to aid digestion and to prevent aspiration of regurgitated feedings; this position also makes it easier to expel air bubbles from the stomach.

Although the side-lying position is appropriate when the infant is awake and under observation, infants should sleep on their backs (Figure 32–3 ○). The American Academy of Pediatrics has recommended sleeping in nonprone positions since 1992 to reduce the risk of sudden infant death syndrome (SIDS). The phrase "back to sleep" is used to convey this important concept to families.

NEWBORN FEEDING

Newborn feeding is discussed in detail in Chapter 29. ∞ Problems a breastfeeding mother may face at home are discussed later in this chapter.

● **FIGURE 32–2**

Various positions for holding an infant. **A,** Cradle hold. **B,** Upright position. **C,** Football hold.

● **FIGURE 32–3**

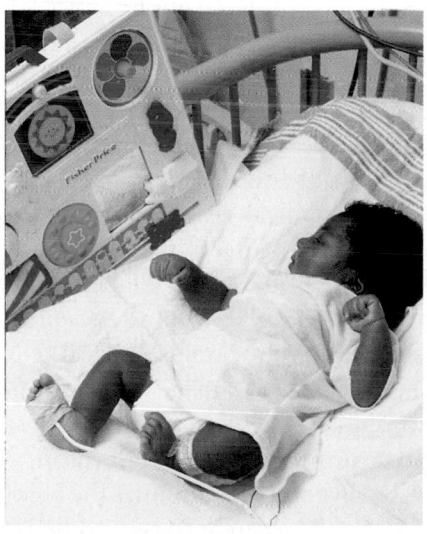

Babies should be placed on their backs to sleep.

BATHING

If the parents are not comfortable about bathing their newborn, a bath demonstration is a straightforward way to provide information to them. Because excess bathing and the use of soap remove natural skin oils and dry out the newborn's sensitive skin, bathing should be done every other day or twice a week. Sponge baths are recommended for the first 2 weeks or until the umbilical cord completely falls off and the umbilicus has healed. Some agencies use a tub bath for the bath demonstration.

At home the family may want to use a small plastic tub, a clean kitchen or bathroom sink, or a large bowl as the baby's tub. Expensive baby tubs are not necessary, but some prefer to purchase them. Before starting, if no one else is at home, the parent may want to take the phone off the hook and put a sign on the door to prevent being disturbed. Having someone home during the first few baths will be helpful, because that person can get forgotten items, attend to interruptions, and provide moral support. The room should be warm and free of drafts.

Sponge Baths

After the supplies are gathered, the tub is filled with water that is warm to the touch. Even though the newborn will not be placed in the tub, the bath giver carefully tests the water temperature with an elbow or forearm. An unperfumed, mild soap such as Castile or Neutrogena should be used and kept on a soap dish or paper towel, not added to the water. Liquid soap products are also available for infant bathing. The newborn should be wrapped in a blanket, with a T-shirt and diaper on, to keep her or him warm and secure. It is important to keep the baby warm and to avoid chilling. Thus, parents are encouraged to keep the baby partially covered during the sponge bath, uncovering areas as they are bathed.

To start the bath, the adult wraps a washcloth once around the index finger and wets it with water. Soap is not used on the face. The bath giver gently wipes each eye from inner to outer corner. This direction prevents the potential for clogging the tear duct at the inner corner, where the eye naturally drains. A different portion of the washcloth is used for each eye to prevent cross-contamination. Cotton balls can also be used for this purpose, a new one for each eye. Some swelling and drainage may be present the first few days after birth because of eye prophylaxis. The bath giver washes the ears next by wrapping the washcloth once around an index finger and gently cleaning the external ear and behind the ear. Cotton swabs are never used in the ear canal because it is possible to put the swab too far into the ear and damage the ear drum. In addition the swab may push any discharge farther down into the ear canal. The caregiver then wipes the remainder of the baby's face. Many babies start to cry at this point. The face should be washed every day and the mouth and chin wiped off after each feeding.

The neck is washed thoroughly with the washcloth. Soap may now be used. Formula or breast milk and lint collect in the skin folds of the neck, so it may be helpful to sit the newborn up, supporting the neck and shoulders with one hand while washing the neck with the other hand.

Next the bath giver unwraps the blanket, removes the T-shirt, and wets the chest, back, and arms with the washcloth. The bath giver may then lather the hands with a small amount of soap and wash the baby's chest, back, and arms. Wetting the cord is avoided, if possible, because it delays drying. Soap is rinsed off with the wet washcloth, and the upper part of the body is dried with a towel or blanket. The newborn's upper body is then wrapped with a clean, dry blanket to prevent a chill. The bath giver then unwraps the newborn's legs, wets them with the washcloth, and lathers, rinses, and dries them well. If the newborn has dry skin, a small amount of unscented lotion or ointment (petroleum jelly or A + D ointment) may be used. Ointments are thought to be better than lotions for dry, cracked feet and hands. Baby oil is not recommended, because it clogs skin pores. Powders are not currently recommended. Families should be warned that baby powder can cause serious respiratory problems if inhaled. If parents want to use powder, they should be advised to use one that is talc-free. They should also shake the powder into the hand and then pat it on the newborn rather than shaking it directly onto the baby.

The genital area should be cleansed with soap and water daily and with water or commercially available wipes after each wet or dirty diaper. Females should be washed from the front of the genitalia toward the rectum to prevent fecal contamination of the urethra and thus the bladder. Newborn girls often have a thick, white mucus discharge or a slight bloody discharge from the vaginal area. This discharge is normal for the first 1 to 2 weeks after birth and should be wiped off with a damp cloth during diaper changes.

Parents of uncircumcised males should cleanse the penis daily. Even minimal retraction of the foreskin is not advised (see in-depth discussion of care of uncircumcised male babies in Chapter 26 ∞). Males who have been circumcised also need daily gentle cleansing. The bath giver rubs a very wet washcloth over a bar of soap, then squeezes the washcloth above the baby's penis, letting the soapy water run over the circumcision site. The area is rinsed off with plain warm water and lightly patted dry. A small amount of petroleum jelly, A + D ointment, or bactericidal ointment may be put on the circumcised area, but excessive amounts may block the meatus and should be avoided. It is important to avoid using ointments if a Plastibell is in place because use of ointments may cause the Plastibell ring to slip off the penis too early. The Plastibell usually falls off within 5 to 8 days. If it does not, the family needs to call the healthcare provider.

The diaper area is cleansed with each diaper change to prevent diaper rash. Despite routine cleansing, a diaper rash may still occur. Baby powder or cornstarch is not recommended for diaper rash. Baby powder may cake with urine and irritate the perineal area; cornstarch may promote fungal infection. Ointments that provide a barrier, such as zinc oxide, A + D ointment, and petroleum jelly, are more effective. If the ointment does not help the rash, families using disposable diapers should try another brand. If they use cloth diapers, a different detergent or fabric softener, more thorough rinsing, and hanging them in the sun to dry may solve the problem. If the rash persists, parents should discuss the problem with their nurse practitioner or physician, because it may be due to a yeast or fungal infection.

The umbilical cord should be kept clean and dry. The presence of the umbilical vessels in the cord makes it a common entry area for infection. The cord stump generally falls off in 7 to 14 days. The diaper should be folded down to allow air to circulate around the cord. The parents should consult their healthcare provider if redness, bright-red bleeding, or puslike drainage with foul odor appears around the umbilicus or if the area remains unhealed 2 to 3 days after the cord stump has sloughed off.

The last step in bathing is washing the hair (a step some suggest doing first). The newborn is swaddled in a dry blanket, leaving only the head exposed, and held in the football hold with the head tilted slightly downward to prevent water from running in the eyes. Water should be brought to the head by a cupped hand. The hair is moistened and lathered with a small amount of mild shampoo. A very soft brush may be used to massage the shampoo over the entire head, including the soft spots. The hair is then rinsed and toweled dry. Oils or lotions are not used on the newborn's head unless there is evidence of cradle cap. Moistening the scaly area with lotion or mineral oil half an hour or more before shampooing softens the crusts or scales and makes it easier to remove them with a soft brush during the shampoo.

Tub Baths

The baby may be put in a small tub after the cord has fallen off and the circumcision site is healed (approximately 2 weeks) (Figure 32–4 ●). Newborns usually enjoy a tub bath more than a sponge bath, although some cry during either type.

Only 3 or 4 inches of water are needed in the tub. To prevent slipping, a washcloth is placed in the bottom of the tub or sink. Some parents choose to bring the newborn into the tub with them. The baby's face is washed in the same manner as for a sponge bath. The parent then places the newborn in the tub using the cradle hold and grasping the distal thigh. The neck is supported by the parent's elbow in the cradle position. An alternative hold is to support the newborn's head and neck with the forearm while grasping the distal shoulder and arm.

Because wet newborns are slippery, some parents pull a cotton sock (with holes cut out for the fingers) over the supporting arm to provide a "nonskid" surface. The newborn's body may be washed with a soapy washcloth or hand. To wash the back, the bath giver places his or her noncradling hand on the newborn's chest with the thumb under the newborn's arm closest to the adult. Gently tipping the newborn forward onto the supporting hand frees the cradling arm to wash the back. After the bath the newborn is lifted out of the tub in the cradle position, dried well, and wrapped in a dry blanket. The hair is then washed in the same way as for a sponge bath.

NAIL CARE

The nails of the newborn are seldom cut in the birthing center. During the first days of life, the nails may adhere to the skin of the fingers, and cutting is contraindicated. Within a week the nails separate from the skin and frequently break off. If the nails are long or if the baby is scratching his or her face, the nails may be trimmed. Trimming is most easily done while the infant is asleep. Nails should be cut straight across using blunt-ended cuticle scissors.

DRESSING THE NEWBORN

Newborns need to wear a T-shirt, diaper (with a diaper cover or plastic pants if using cloth diapers), and a sleeper. On a fairly cool day, they should be wrapped in a light blanket while being fed. Newborns should be covered with a blanket in air-conditioned buildings. The blanket should be unwrapped or removed when inside a warm building. At home the temperature determines the amount of clothing the newborn wears. Families who keep their home at 60°F to 65°F should dress the infant more warmly than those who maintain a temperature of 70°F to 75°F.

Newborns should wear head coverings outdoors to protect their sensitive ears from drafts. A blanket can be wrapped around the baby, leaving one corner free to place over the head while outdoors or in crowds for added protection. Advise families about how easily a newborn's skin can burn in the sun. To prevent sunburn the newborn should remain shaded and wear a light layer of clothing with a tight weave. The American Academy of Pediatrics does not recommend sunscreen for infants under 6 months of age, although sunscreen may be applied to small areas of skin such as the tops of feet or lower arms.

Diaper shapes vary (Figure 32–5 ●). Prefolded and disposable diapers are usually rectangular. Cloth diapers may also be triangular or kite folded. Extra material is placed in front for males and toward the back for females to increase absorbency.

Baby clothing should be laundered separately with a mild soap or detergent. Diapers may be presoaked before washing. If the infant develops a rash, it may be necessary for his or her clothing to be rinsed twice to remove soap and residue. Some newborns may not tolerate clothing treated with fabric softeners added to the washer or dryer.

TEMPERATURE ASSESSMENT

When teaching parents about taking their baby's temperature, provide opportunities for discussion and demonstration. Clarify the times when the family should call their

● **FIGURE 32–4**

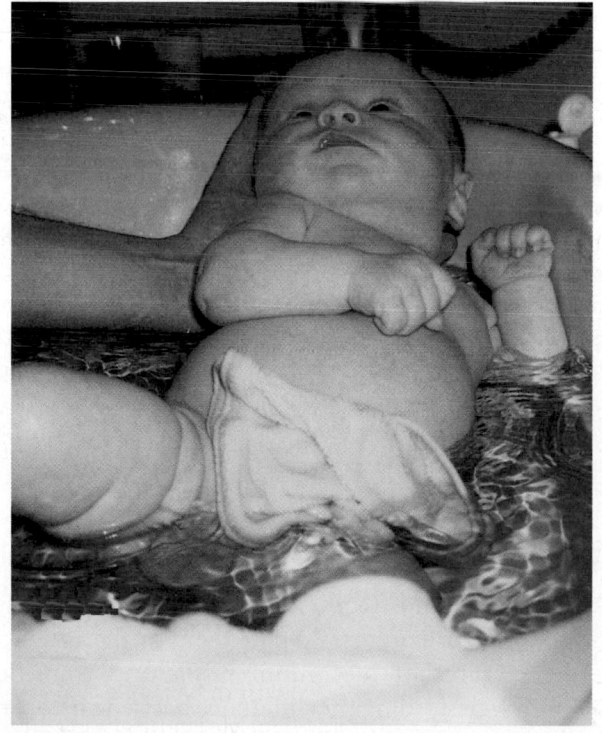

When bathing the newborn, it is important to support the head. Wet babies are very slippery.

● **FIGURE 32-5**

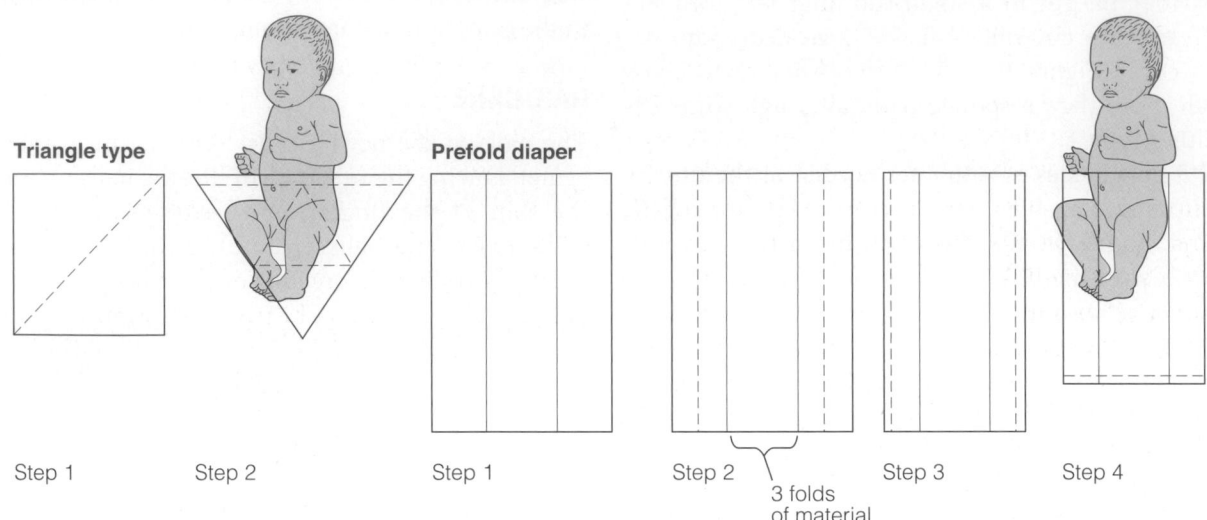

Triangle type   Prefold diaper

Step 1   Step 2   Step 1   Step 2   Step 3   Step 4

3 folds
of material

Two basic cloth diaper shapes. Dotted lines indicate folds.

primary healthcare provider. Discuss the different types of thermometers available for home use. It is important that parents understand the differences and how to select the appropriate one. Although tympanic (ear) thermometers are more expensive, many parents choose them because they are fast and easy to use. Other parents use a digital thermometer. Review the correct procedure for using the chosen thermometer.

Parents need to take the newborn's temperature only if he or she seems ill. They should call their physician or pediatric nurse practitioner immediately if any signs of illness are present. They should call their pediatrican or nurse practitioner if the temperature exceeds 38°C (100.4°F) axillary. Parents should also check with their clinician about over-the-counter medications to be kept in the medicine cabinet.

When parents find their newborn has a fever, they may expect to give an antipyretic such as acetaminophen (Tylenol). They should not give any form of aspirin for an illness that may be viral; use of aspirin in viral illnesses has been linked to Reye syndrome in children. Parents should discuss management of flu, colds, teething, constipation, diarrhea, and other common ailments with their clinician before they occur. When analgesic or antipyretic medication is needed, clinicians generally recommend acetaminophen drops. Ibuprofen (children's Motrin) may also be used in children 6 months of age or older.

STOOLS AND URINE

The appearance and frequency of a newborn's stools can cause concern for parents. Prepare them by discussing and showing pictures of meconium stools and transitional stools and by describing the difference between breast milk and formula stools. Although each baby develops his or her own stooling patterns, parents can get an idea of what to expect (see Figure 26–8 in Chapter 26 ∞).

- Breastfed newborns may have 6 to 10 small, semiliquid, yellow stools per day by the third or fourth day, when milk production is established, unless the mother is having problems with her milk supply. Once breastfeeding is well established, usually by 1 month, the newborn may have only 1 stool every few days because of the increased digestibility of breast milk, or still may have several daily. Constipation is unlikely in newborns receiving only breast milk. Infrequent stooling in the first few weeks may indicate inadequate milk intake.

- Formula-fed babies may have only one or two stools a day; they are more formed and yellow or yellow-brown.

The parents may also be shown pictures of a constipated stool (small, pelletlike) and diarrhea (loose, green, or perhaps blood tinged). Families need to understand that a green color is common in transitional stools, so that transitional stools are not confused with diarrhea during the first week of a newborn's life. Constipation may indicate that the newborn needs additional fluid. Parents may try offering additional water in an attempt to reverse the constipation.

Babies normally void five to eight times per day. Fewer than six to eight wet diapers a day may indicate that the newborn needs more fluids. Voiding is easy to assess with cloth diapers. Parents who use superabsorbent disposable diapers may have difficulty determining voiding because the surface of the diaper feels dry. The liquid pools inside the filling of the diaper.

SLEEP AND ACTIVITY

The newborn demonstrates several sleep-wake states after the initial periods of reactivity described in Chapter 26. ∞ It is not uncommon for a newborn to sleep almost continuously for the first 2 to 3 days following birth, awakening only for feedings every 3 to 4 hours. Some newborns bypass this stage of deep sleep and require only 12 to 16 hours of sleep. The parents need to know that this pattern is normal.

Deep sleep is characterized by regular breathing and no movement except for sudden body jerks. During this sleep state, normal household noise will not awaken the infant. In **light sleep** the baby has irregular breathing and fine muscular twitching. The baby may cry out during sleep, but this does not mean he or she is uncomfortable or awake. Unusual noise may awaken the newborn more easily in this state; however, he or she will quickly go back to sleep. In the **drowsy** state, newborns open and close their eyes, but the eyes appear glazed and the face is often still. Newborns return to sleep easily from this state, or awaken in response to stimuli.

Quiet alert state is a state in which newborns are quietly involved with the environment. They watch a moving mobile, smile, and, as they age, discover and play with their hands and feet. When newborns become uncomfortable due to wet diapers, hunger, or cold, they enter the **active alert state** and **crying state**. In these states, parents should identify and eliminate the cause of the crying. Sometimes families are frustrated as they try to identify the external or internal stimuli that are causing the angry, hurt crying. Tell parents that the state may be changed from crying to quiet alert by moving the newborn to a more upright position where he or she can scan and explore. (See Table 32–1.)

CRYING

For the newborn, crying is the only way to express needs vocally. Families learn to distinguish different tones and qualities of the newborn's cry. The amount of crying is highly individual. Some cry as little as 15 to 30 minutes in 24 hours, and others cry as long as 2 hours every 24 hours. When crying continues after causes such as discomfort and hunger are eliminated, the newborn may be comforted by swaddling or by rocking and other reassuring activities. There is some indication that newborns who are held more tend to be calmer and cry less when not being held. Some parents are afraid that holding may "spoil" the newborn and need reassurance that this is not the case. Picking babies up when they cry teaches them that adults try to meet their needs and are responsive to them. This helps build a sense of trust in humankind. Excessive crying should be noted and assessed, taking other factors into consideration. After the first 2 or 3 days, newborns settle into individual patterns.

To increase parents' coping abilities, suggest that they initially respond to the baby's crying by checking for hunger, a wet or soiled diaper, excessive cold or heat, restrictive or chafing clothing or blankets, or other comfort concerns. If these are not present, suggest holding or rocking the infant as discussed above. Other calming measures include burping the infant (which provides repetitive tactile stimulation and disperses air bubbles), placing the infant in a mechanized infant swing, or taking the infant for a ride in a stroller or car. Some infants are soothed by white noise such as the sound of a dryer or the static on an untuned radio, whereas others are soothed when bound "papoose style" on the mother's or father's chest, swaddled, bathed, or massaged.

SAFETY CONSIDERATIONS

Newborns should not have pillows or stuffed animals in the crib while they sleep; these items could cause suffocation. Mattresses should fit snugly in a crib to prevent entrapment and suffocation, and the crib should be inspected regularly to determine whether it is in safe working order. Crib slats should be no more than 2 3/8 inches apart. Encourage parents to attend infant cardiopulmonary resuscitation (CPR) classes, especially if there is a family history of SIDS or the infant requires special care.

TABLE 32–1 ✤ Infant State* Chart (Sleep and Awake States)

CHARACTERISTICS OF STATE

Sleep States	Body Activity	Eye Movement	Facial Movement	Breathing Pattern	Level of Response	Implications for Caregiving
Deep sleep	Nearly still except for occasional startle or twitch	None	Without facial movements except for occasional sucking movement at regular intervals	Smooth and regular	Only very intense and disturbing stimuli will arouse infants.	Caregivers trying to feed infants in deep sleep will probably find the experience frustrating. Infants will be unresponsive, even if caregivers use disturbing stimuli (flicking feet) to arouse infants. Infants may arouse only briefly and then become unresponsive as they return to deep sleep. If caregivers wait until infants move to a higher, more responsive state, feeding or caregiving will be much more pleasant.
Light sleep	Some body movements	Rapid eye movement (REM): fluttering of eyes beneath closed eyelids	May smile and make brief fussy or crying sounds	Irregular	Infants are more responsive to internal and external stimuli. When these stimuli occur, infants may remain in light sleep or move to drowsy state.	Light sleep makes up the highest proportion of newborn sleep and usually precedes awakening. Caregivers who are not aware that the brief fussy or crying sounds made during this state occur normally may think it is time for feeding and may try to feed infants before they are ready to eat.
Awake States						
Drowsy	Activity level variable, with mild startles interspersed from time to time; movements usually smooth	Eyes open and close occasionally; are heavy lidded, with dull glazed appearance	May have some facial movements; often there are none and the face appears still	Irregular	Infants react to sensory stimuli, although responses are delayed. State change after stimulation is frequently noted.	From the drowsy state infants may return to sleep or awaken further. To wake them, caregivers can provide something for infants to see, hear, or suck. This may arouse them to a quiet alert state, a more responsive state. Infants left alone without stimuli may return to a sleep state.
Quiet alert	Minimal	Brightening and widening of eyes	Faces have bright, shining, sparkling looks	Regular	Infants attend most to environment, focusing attention on any stimuli that are present.	Infants in this state provide much pleasure and positive feedback for caregivers. Providing something for infants to see, hear, or suck will often maintain a quiet alert state in the first few hours after birth. Most newborns commonly experience a period of intense alertness before going into a long sleeping period.
Active alert	Much body activity; may have periods of fussiness	Eyes open, with less brightening	Much facial movement; faces not as bright as in alert state	Irregular	Infants are increasingly sensitive to disturbing stimuli (hunger, fatigue, noise, excessive handling).	Caregivers may intervene at this stage to console and to bring infants to a lower state.
Crying	Increased motor activity, with color changes	Eyes may be tightly closed or open	Grimaces	More irregular	Infants are extremely responsive to unpleasant external or internal stimuli.	Crying is the infant's communication signal. It is a response to unpleasant stimuli from the environment or from within infants (fatigue, hunger, discomfort). Crying tells us infants have been reached. Sometimes infants can console themselves and return to lower states. At other times they need help from caregivers.

*State is a group of characteristics that regularly occur together: body activity, eye movements, facial movements, breathing pattern, and level of response to external stimuli (e.g., handling) and internal stimuli (e.g., hunger).

Used with permission from Blackburn, S., & Kang, R. (1991). Early parent-infant relationships (2nd ed., module 3, series 1). In The first six hours after birth. White Plains, NY: March of Dimes Birth Defects Foundation. Reprinted with permission of the copyright holder.

Many families, especially breastfeeding families, practice **cosleeping**, in which the infant sleeps with the mother or both parents during the night. Cosleeping families should be counseled to observe the following safety guidelines:

- Place the infant on a firm mattress, never on comforters, pillows, or a water bed.
- Never sleep with your infant if you have been using drugs or have become intoxicated.
- Ensure that the infant is protected from rolling off the bed or becoming entrapped in bed rails or in a space between the frame and mattress.
- As with crib sleeping, remove all decorative pillows, stuffed animals, toys, or blankets that could impair the baby's breathing. Do not cover the baby with blankets, sheets, or down comforters.
- Make sure the baby is sleeping on his or her back.
- Ensure plenty of ventilation to the infant.
- Avoid overdressing the infant since the parent's body heat will reduce the need for excess clothing.
- Never smoke in bed with an infant because of the risk of falling asleep with a lit cigarette. (*Note:* Family members who smoke should smoke outdoors and not in the household with the infant because of the risks associated with secondhand smoke.)

NEWBORN SCREENING AND IMMUNIZATION PROGRAM

Before the newborn and mother are discharged from the hospital, inform the parents about the normal screening tests for newborns and tell them when to return for further tests if needed. Newborn screening tests detect disorders that cause mental retardation, physical disabilities, or death if left undiscovered. Inborn errors of metabolism that can usually be detected from a drop of blood obtained by a heel stick on the second or third day include phenylketonuria (PKU) and congenital hypothyroidism (mandatory screening in all states in the United States), as well as sickle cell disease, galactosemia, and homocystinuria. Some states are now requiring or offering as optional several additional screening tests. Inform parents that a second blood specimen will be required from the newborn after 7 to 14 days; in some states the second blood specimen is not recommended if the first specimen is obtained 48 hours or longer after birth. Stress that an abnormal test result is not diagnostic. More specific tests must be performed to verify the results.

If additional tests are positive, treatment is begun. Explain to parents that these conditions may be treated by diet or by administration of missing hormones. The inborn conditions cannot be cured, but they can be treated. They are not contagious, but they may be inherited.

Many states now require hearing screenings prior to discharge. Sometimes infants fail to pass these tests for reasons other than hearing loss. Amniotic fluid in the ear canals is a frequent cause of suboptimal test results. In these cases, infants are retested in a week or two. Parents should be informed of the need for retesting and the importance of follow-up.

HOME CARE: THE MOTHER AND FAMILY

During the first home visit, the nurse completes a physical assessment of the mother and a psychosocial assessment of the family. Teaching for self-care is commonly required for new mothers, especially breastfeeding mothers with nipple soreness, engorgement, and other concerns. Family teaching related to resumption of sexual activity and contraception may also be required.

ASSESSMENT OF THE MOTHER AND FAMILY

During the first home visit, complete a physical and psychologic assessment. Before doing so, ensure privacy. The physical assessment focuses on the mother's physical adaptation, determined by evaluating vital signs, breasts, abdominal musculature, elimination patterns, reproductive tract, and laboratory values. Talk with the mother about her diet, level of fatigue, ability to rest and sleep, pain management, and signs of postpartum complications. For breastfeeding mothers, assess the woman's feeding technique and give her information about possible problems that may occur.

The psychologic assessment focuses on attachment, adjustment to the parental role, emotional response to childbirth and parenting, sibling adjustment, and educational needs. Ask specifically about feelings of depression, anger, and the like (see the discussion of postpartum depression in Chapter 25 ∞). When appropriate, mention available community resources, including public health department follow-up visits. If not already discussed, teaching about family planning is appropriate at this time, coupled with information about birth control methods.

In ideal situations a family-centered approach with the father or partner and any siblings present provides an opportunity to observe family interactions and gives all family members a chance to ask questions and express concerns. In addition any questionable family interaction pattern such as one suggestive of abuse or neglect may be evident and further referral could be considered if needed.

If the partner or any siblings of the newborn are not present, it is important to ask the new mother how she believes the family members are adjusting and to seek her perceptions of family dynamics. It is also useful to ask about the role the grandparents play in the family and the support and assistance that they are able and willing to provide. (See "Assessment Guide: Postpartal—First Home Visit and Anticipated Progress at 6 Weeks.")

ASSESSMENT GUIDE

POSTPARTAL—FIRST HOME VISIT AND ANTICIPATED PROGRESS AT 6 WEEKS

PHYSICAL ASSESSMENT/ NORMAL FINDINGS	ALTERATIONS AND POSSIBLE CAUSES*	NURSING RESPONSES TO DATA†
Vital Signs		
Blood pressure: Return to normal prepregnant level.	Elevated blood pressure (anxiety, essential hypertension, renal disease).	Review history, evaluate normal baseline; refer to physician or CNM if necessary.
Pulse: 60–90 beats/minute (or prepregnant normal rate).	Increased pulse rate (excitement, anxiety, cardiac disorders).	Count pulse for full minute and note irregularities; marked tachycardia or beat irregularities require additional assessment and possible physician or CNM referral.
Respirations: 16–24/minute.	Marked tachypnea or abnormal patterns (respiratory disorders).	Evaluate for respiratory disease, refer to physician or CNM if necessary.
Temperature: 36.2–37.6°C (98–99.6°F)	Increased temperature (infection).	Assess for signs and symptoms of infection or disease state.
Weight		
2 days: Possible weight loss of 12–20+ lb.	Minimal weight loss (fluid retention, preeclampsia).	Evaluate for fluid retention, edema, deep tendon reflexes, and blood pressure elevation.
6 weeks: Returning to normal prepregnant weight.	Retained weight (excessive caloric intake).	Determine amount of daily exercise. Provide dietary teaching. Refer to dietitian if necessary for additional dietary counseling.
	Extreme weight loss (excessive dieting, inadequate caloric intake).	Discuss appropriate diets; refer to dietitian for additional counseling if necessary.
Breasts		
Nonbreastfeeding 2 days: May have mild tenderness; small amount of milk may be expressed. 6 weeks: Soft with no tenderness; return to prepregnant size.	Some engorgement (incomplete suppression of lactation). Redness; marked tenderness (mastitis). Palpable mass (tumor).	Engorgement may be seen in nonbreastfeeding mothers. Advise client to wear a supportive, well-fitted bra, avoid very warm showers, use ice packs for comfort; evaluate for signs and symptoms of mastitis (rare in nonbreastfeeding mothers).
Breastfeeding Full with prominent nipples, lactation established.	Cracked, fissured nipples (feeding problems). Redness, marked tenderness, or even abscess formation (mastitis). Palpable mass (full milk duct tumor).	Counsel about nipple care. Evaluate woman's condition, evidence of fever; refer to physician, or certified nurse midwife for initiation of antibiotic therapy, if indicated. Opinion varies as to value of breast examination for lactating mothers; some feel a lactating mother should examine her breasts monthly, after feeding, when breasts are empty; if palpable mass is felt, refer to physician for further evaluation. For breast inflammation instruct the mother to 1. Keep breast empty by frequent feeding. 2. Rest when possible. 3. Take prescribed pain relief med. 4. Force fluids. If symptoms persist for more than 24 hours, instruct her to call her physician or CNM.

*Possible causes of alterations are placed in parentheses.

†This column provides guidelines for further assessment and initial nursing interventions.

ASSESSMENT GUIDE—continued

POSTPARTAL—FIRST HOME VISIT AND ANTICIPATED PROGRESS AT 6 WEEKS

PHYSICAL ASSESSMENT/ NORMAL FINDINGS	ALTERATIONS AND POSSIBLE CAUSES*	NURSING RESPONSES TO DATA[†]
Abdominal Musculature		
2 days: Improved firmness, although "bread dough" consistency is not unusual, especially in multipara.	Marked relaxation of muscles.	Evaluate exercise level; provide information on appropriate exercise program.
Striae pink and obvious. Cesarean incision healing.	Drainage, redness, tenderness, pain, edema (infection).	Evaluate for infection; refer to physician or CNM if necessary.
6 weeks: Muscle tone continues to improve; striae may be beginning to fade, may not achieve a silvery appearance for several more weeks, linea nigra fading.		
Elimination Pattern		
Urinary Tract		
Return to prepregrant urinary elimination routine.	Urinary incontinence, especially with lifting, coughing, laughing, and so on (urethral trauma, cystocele).	Assess for cystocele; instruct in appropriate muscle tightening exercises; refer to physician or CNM.
	Pain or burning when voiding urgency and/or frequency, pus or white blood cells (WBC) in urine, pathogenic organisms in culture (urinary tract infection).	Evaluate for urinary tract infection; obtain clean-catch urine sample; refer to physician or CNM for treatment if indicated.
Routine urinalysis within normal limits (proteinuria disappeared).	Sugar or ketone in urine—may be some lactose present in urine of breastfeeding mothers (diabetes).	Evaluate diet; assess for signs and symptoms of diabetes; refer to physician or CNM.
Bowel Habits		
2 days: May be some discomfort with defecation, especially if client had severe hemorrhoids or third- or fourth-degree extension.	Severe constipation or pain when defecating (trauma or hemorrhoids).	Discuss dietary patterns; encourage fluid, adequate roughage.
		Continue use of stool softener if necessary to prevent pain associated with straining; continue sitz baths, periods of rest for severe hemorrhoids; assess healing of episiotomy or lacerations; severe constipation may require administration of laxatives, stool softeners, and an enema.
6 weeks: Return to normal prepregnancy bowel elimination patterns.	Marked constipation.	See previous discussion.
	Fecal incontinence or constipation (rectocele).	Assess for evidence of rectocele; instruct in muscle-tightening exercises; refer to physician or CNM.
Reproductive Tract		
Lochia		
2 days: Lochia rubra or lochia serosa, scant amounts, fleshy odor.	Excessive amounts (nonfirm uterus), foul odor (infection).	Assess for evidence of infection or failure of the uterus to decrease in size; refer to physician or CNM.
6 weeks: No lochia, or return to normal menstruation pattern.	See above.	See above.
Fundus and Perineum		
2 days: Fundus is at least two finger-breadths below the umbilicus; uterine muscles still somewhat lax; introitus of vagina lacks tone—gapes when intra-abdominal pressure is increased by coughing or straining.	Uterus not decreasing in size appropriately (infection).	Assess fundus for firmness and/or signs of infection, refer to physician or CNM if indicated.

*Possible causes of alterations are placed in parentheses.

[†]This column provides guidelines for further assessment and initial nursing interventions.

(continued)

ASSESSMENT GUIDE—continued

POSTPARTAL—FIRST HOME VISIT AND ANTICIPATED PROGRESS AT 6 WEEKS

PHYSICAL ASSESSMENT/ NORMAL FINDINGS	ALTERATIONS AND POSSIBLE CAUSES*	NURSING RESPONSES TO DATA†
Reproductive Tract *(continued)*		
Episiotomy and/or lacerations healing; no signs of infection. 6 weeks: Uterus almost returned to prepregnant size, with almost completely restored muscle tone.	Evidence of redness, tenderness, poor tissue approximation in eplsiotomy and/or laceration (wound infection). Continued flow of lochia, failure to decrease appropriately in size (subinvolution).	Assess for evidence of subinvolution or infection; refer to physician for further evaluation and for dilation and curettage if necessary.
Hemoglobin and Hematocrit Levels		
6 weeks: Hb 12 g/dL. Hct 37% plus or minus 5%.	Hb less than 12 g/dL. Hct 32% (anemia).	Assess nutritional status, begin (or continue) supplemental iron for marked anemia (Hb less than or equal to 9 g/dL). Additional assessment and physician or CNM referral may be necessary.
Attachment		
Bonding process demonstrated by soothing, cuddling, and talking to infant; appropriate feeding techniques; eye-to-eye contact; calling infant by name.	Failure to bond demonstrated by lack of behaviors associated with bonding process, calling infant by nickname that promotes ridicule; inadequate infant weight gain, infant is dirty, hygienic measures are not being maintained, severe diaper rash, failure to obtain adequate supplies to provide infant care (malattachment).	Provide counseling, talk with the woman about her feelings regarding the infant; provide support for the caretaking activities that are being performed; refer to public health nurse for continued home visits.
Parent interacts with infant and provides soothing, caretaking activities.	Parent is unable to respond to infant needs (inability to recognize needs; inadequate education and support, fear, family stress).	Provide support for caretaking activities observed; provide information about caretaking activities, such as responding to infant cry; methods of wrapping infant; methods of soothing the infant such as swaddling, rocking, increasing stimuli by singing to the infant or decreasing stimuli by putting infant to rest in quiet room; methods of holding the infant; differences in the cry. Identify support system such as friends, neighbors; provide information regarding community resources and support groups.
Parents express feelings of comfort and success with the parent role.	Evidence of stress and anxiety (difficulty moving into or dealing with the parent role).	Provide support and encouragement; provide information regarding progression into parent role and assist parents in talking through their feelings; refer to community resources and support groups.
Woman is in the informal or personal stage of maternal role attainment.	Woman is still greatly influenced by others, has not developed an image or style of her own (woman remains in the anticipatory stage).	Provide role modeling for the woman in working through problem solving with the infant; provide encouragement as she thinks through decisions and develops her sense of problem solving; encourage her to make decisions regarding infant care.
Adjustment to Parental Role		
Parents are coping with new roles in terms of division of labor, financial status, communication, readjustment of sexual relations, and adjusting to new daily tasks.	Inability to adjust to new roles (immaturity, inadequate education and preparation, ineffective communication patterns, inadequate support, current family crisis).	Provide counseling; refer to parent groups.

*Possible causes of alterations are placed in parentheses.

†This column provides guidelines for further assessment and initial nursing intervention.

ASSESSMENT GUIDE—continued

POSTPARTAL—FIRST HOME VISIT AND ANTICIPATED PROGRESS AT 6 WEEKS

PHYSICAL ASSESSMENT/ NORMAL FINDINGS	ALTERATIONS AND POSSIBLE CAUSES*	NURSING RESPONSES TO DATA[†]
Education		
Mother understands self-care measures.	Inadequate knowledge of self-care (inadequate education).	Provide education and counseling.
Parents are knowledgeable regarding infant care.	Inadequate knowledge of infant care (inadequate education).	
Siblings are adjusting to new baby.	Excessive sibling rivalry.	
Parents have a method of contraception.	Birth control method not chosen.	
	*Possible causes of alterations are placed in parentheses.	[†]This column provides guidelines for further assessment and initial nursing intervention

Continue to teach the mother and her family as needed, including descriptions of relevant self-care measures. Discuss infant care and answer questions the family may have. Generally the new mother has a final postpartum examination with her caregiver about 6 weeks after childbirth. However, if the assessment indicates a need, refer the woman to her healthcare provider for further care before the 6-week check.

BREASTFEEDING CONCERNS FOLLOWING DISCHARGE

The mother-baby nurse in the birthing area can offer anticipatory guidance about common breastfeeding issues and provide resources for the woman's use after discharge. Nursing support for breastfeeding mothers can take many forms. Informational support includes written materials, verbal information, demonstration, answering questions, offering tips, providing feedback, and giving nonverbal assistance (such as moving a baby closer to the mother's breast).

Encouragement and interpersonal support (such as staying with a breastfeeding woman and supporting the mother's decisions) are also helpful. The nurse can also tell the family about various Web sites that might be helpful. This should include the site for the La Leche League, an international organization designed to help women breastfeed successfully.

Chapter 29 provides in-depth discussion of breastfeeding, including the physiology of breastfeeding, cultural aspects of the process, hints for getting started, and so forth. ∞ Because mothers are discharged from the birthing unit before breastfeeding is well established, they are frequently alone when they encounter changes in the breastfeeding process. Many women stop breastfeeding if the situations they encounter seem too hard to handle. Risk factors for suboptimal breastfeeding include maternal obesity, primiparity, use of formula supplementation, use of pacifiers, cesarean birth, second stage greater than 1 hour, low birth weight, and flat or inverted nipples (Dewey, Nommsen-Rivers, Heinig et al., 2003).

Table 32–2 summarizes self-care measures to suggest to a woman with a breastfeeding problem.

Nipple Soreness

Some discomfort often occurs initially with breastfeeding; it usually peaks between the third and sixth days and then lessens (Heck et al., 2003). However, the mother should not switch to bottle-feeding or delay feedings at this point because these measures cause engorgement and more soreness. Discomfort that lasts throughout the feeding or past the first week demands attention.

The baby's position at the breast is a critical factor in nipple soreness. The mother's hand should be off the areola, and the baby should be facing the mother's chest, with ear, shoulder, and hip aligned (see Figure 29–5). To help decrease nipple soreness, encourage the mother to rotate positions when feeding her infant. Changing positions alters the focus of greatest stress and promotes more complete breast emptying.

Nipple soreness may also develop if the infant has faulty sucking habits. Nipples may have injured tips that are bruised, scabbed, or blistered from the nipple entering the baby's mouth at an upward angle and rubbing against the roof of the mouth or from poor latch-on (Page, Lockwood, & Guest, 2003). Soreness may also result from continuous negative pressure if the infant falls asleep with the breast in his or her mouth.

Chewed nipples, which result from improper positioning, are cracked or tender at or near the base. In these cases the baby's jaws close only on the nipple instead of on the areola, the baby's mouth is not opened wide enough, or the infant's mouth has slipped down to the nipple from the areola

TABLE 32–2 ✤ Breastfeeding Problems and Remedies

Nipples Not Graspable

Flat or inverted nipples

- Use Hoffman technique to break adhesions.
- Wear milk cups to encourage nipples to protrude.
- Use nipple tug and roll to increase protractility.
- Form the nipple prior to breastfeeding by hand shaping, ice, wearing milk cups a half-hour before feeding.
- As a last resort, use nipple shield for first few minutes of feeding to draw out nipple; then place baby on breast.

Engorged breasts

Treat engorgement by relieving fullness with hand expression of milk prior to breastfeeding and instituting frequent feeding so nipple is more prominent.

Large breasts

- Support breast with opposite hand or use rolled towel under breast to bring nipple to the level of baby's mouth.
- Use C-hold to make nipple accessible to baby.

Engorgement

Missed or infrequent feedings

- Breastfeed frequently (every 1 1/2 hours).
- Massage and hand express or pump to empty breasts completely when feedings are missed or when a full feeling develops in breasts and baby is not available or willing to nurse.

Breasts not emptied at feedings

- Breastfeed long enough to empty breasts (10–15 minutes on each side at each feeding).
- If baby will not nurse long enough to empty breasts, hand express or pump after feeding.

Inadequate letdown

- Use relaxation techniques, massage, and warm or cool compresses before breastfeeding.
- Relax in warm shower with water running from back over shoulders and breasts, hand expressing to relieve fullness.
- If due to anxiety, try to eliminate the source of tension.

Baby sleepy or not eager to nurse

- Use rousing techniques (e.g., hold baby upright, unwrap blanket, change diaper).
- Preexpress milk onto nipple or baby's lips to entice baby.
- Avoid use of bottles of water or formula; these will decrease baby's willingness to suckle.

Inadequate Letdown

Letdown not well established

- Give the baby ample time at the breast (at least 15 minutes per side) to allow for letdown and complete emptying.
- Breastfeed in a quiet spot away from distractions.
- Massage breasts before breastfeeding.
- Drink juice, water, tea (no caffeine) before and during feeding.
- Condition letdown by setting up a routine for beginning feedings.
- Use relaxation and breathing techniques.
- Stimulate the nipple manually before breastfeeding.
- Concentrate thought on the baby and milk flow; turn on a faucet so that the sound of running water helps stimulate letdown.
- Use synthetic oxytocin nasal spray several times during a feeding. This should condition letdown within 24 hours. Then it is no longer needed. Spray must be prescribed by a doctor.

Mother overtired or overextended

- Nap or rest when the baby rests.
- Lie down to breastfeed.
- Breastfeed the baby in bed at night.
- Simplify daily chores; set priorities.

Mother tense, pressured

- Identify the causes of tensions and eliminate or minimize them.
- Decrease fatigue.

Mother caught in cycle of little milk, worry, less milk

- Try all the actions mentioned earlier.
- Develop confidence in mothering skills. (A home visit by a counselor may help.)

Cracked Nipples

All causes of sore nipples carried to extreme

- Refer to all actions for sore nipples.
- Consult doctor about using aspirin, acetaminophen (Tylenol), or other painkiller.
- Improve nutritional status, increasing protein, vitamin C, zinc.

Local infection (baby with staph or other organism may have infected mother's nipples)

Refer to physician.

Plugged Ducts

Poor positioning

- Try a variety of positions for complete emptying.

Incomplete emptying of breast

- Breastfeed at least 10 minutes per side after letdown.
- Alternate breastfeeding positions.
- If baby does not empty breasts, pump or express milk after feedings.

External pressure on breast

- Use larger size bras, insert bra extender, or go braless.
- Use nursing bra instead of pulling up conventional bra to breastfeed to avoid pressure on ducts.
- Avoid bunching up sweater or nightgown under arm during feeding.

Sore Nipples

Poor positioning

- Alternate breastfeeding positions throughout the day.
- Bring the baby close to feed so the baby does not pull on the breast.
- Place the nipple and some of the areola in the baby's mouth.
- Check to ensure the baby is put on and off the breast properly.
- Check to ensure the nipple is back far enough in the baby's mouth.
- Hold the baby closely during feeding so the nipple is not constantly being pulled.

Baby chewing or nuzzling onto nipple

- Form the nipple for the baby.
- Set up a pattern of getting the baby onto the breast using the rooting reflex.

Baby nursing on end of nipple

- Ensure the nipple is way back in the baby's mouth by getting the baby properly onto the breast.
- Check for an inverted nipple.
- Check for engorgement.

TABLE 32–2 ✤ Breastfeeding Problems and Remedies—continued

Baby chewing his or her way off the nipple (nipple being pulled out of baby's mouth at end of feeding)
- Remove the baby from the breast by placing a finger between the baby's gums to ensure suction is broken.
- End feeding when the baby's suckling slows, before he or she has a chance to chew on the nipple.

Baby overly eager to breastfeed
- Breastfeed more often.
- Preexpress milk to hasten letdown, avoiding vigorous suckling.

Dry colostrum or milk causing nipple to stick to bra or breast pads
Moisten bra or pads before taking off so as not to remove keratin.

Nipples not allowed to dry
- Remove plastic liners from milk pads.
- Air-dry breasts completely after feeding.
- Change milk pads frequently.

Improper use of breast shield
- Use shield only to draw out nipple; then have the baby suckle on the breast.
- Cut tip of shield back bit by bit and eventually discard.

Nipple skin not resistant to stress
- Improve diet, especially adding fresh fruits and vegetables and vitamin supplements.
- Eliminate or decrease use of sugary foods, alcohol, caffeine, cigarettes.
- Check use of cleansing or drying agents.

Natural oils removed or keratin layers broken down by drying agents (soap, alcohol, shampoo, deodorant)
- Eliminate irritants.
- Wash breasts with water only.

Adapted with permission from "Breastfeeding Problems and Remedies," copyright © 2005 by Judith Lauwers and Anna Swisher, from *Counseling the Nursing Mother*, 4th edition by Judith Lauwers and Anna Swisher. Used by permission of Jones and Bartlett.

---

as a result of engorgement. Soreness on the underside of the nipple is caused by the infant nursing with his or her bottom lip tucked in rather than out, causing a friction burn. In such cases, even vigorous sucking produces little milk because the milk sinuses under the areola are not compressed. This situation results in a frustrated infant and marked soreness for the mother. The problem is overcome by positioning the infant with as much areola as possible in his or her mouth and rotating the baby's positions at the breast.

Nipple soreness is especially pronounced during the first few minutes of a feeding. If the mother is not expecting this discomfort, she may become discouraged and quickly stop. The letdown reflex may take a few minutes to activate, and it may not occur if the mother stops breastfeeding too quickly. The infant is unsatisfied, and the possibility of breast engorgement increases.

Nipple soreness can also result from the vigorous feeding of an overeager infant. In this case the mother may find it helpful to breastfeed more frequently. The woman can also apply ice to her nipples and areola for a few minutes before feeding to promote nipple erectness and numb the tissue initially. To prevent skin breakdown, after feeding the mother can wash her nipples and areolae with water and allow them to air dry well. To promote dryness the mother may leave her bra flaps down for a few minutes after feeding (Figure 32–6 ⬤) or expose her nipples to sunlight or ultraviolet light for 30 seconds at first, gradually increasing to 3 minutes. Drying the nipples with a hair dryer on a low heat setting also facilitates drying and promotes healing (Page et al., 2003).

⬤ **FIGURE 32–6**

Mothers with sore nipples can leave bra flaps down after feedings to promote air drying and prevent chapping.

The use of petroleum-based products such as Vaseline, A + D ointment, cocoa butter, and baby oil to lubricate the nipples is discouraged because petroleum interferes with skin respiration and may prolong soreness. Because of the risk of allergic reactions, products such as Massé cream (risk of peanut allergy) and lubricants containing lanolin (risk of wool allergy) are also discouraged. In addition, products that are washed off before breastfeeding should be avoided because washing irritates the nipples (Page et al., 2003).

Many lactation experts recommend that the mother's own milk be applied to the nipples and allowed to air dry. Breast milk is high in fat, fights infection, and will not irritate the nipples. Moreover, it is readily available at no cost to the mother. In cases of very dry or sore nipples, hypoallergenic medical-grade anhydrous lanolin may be helpful. This product poses a low risk of allergy because the alcohols that contribute to the allergic response have been removed (Page et al., 2003).

If the woman finds that her bra or clothing rubs against her nipples and adds to her discomfort, she may put shields in her bra. Both Medela Shells and Woolrich Shields relieve friction and promote air circulation. If a woman uses breast pads inside her bra to keep milk from leaking onto her clothes, she should change the pads frequently so the nipples remain dry.

NURSING PRACTICE

If the mother continually has soreness due to a delay in letdown, encourage her to massage the breast in a circular pattern and apply warm compresses just before each breastfeeding session. These activities encourage letdown, increasing the chance that it will occur at the same time that the infant is placed on the breast.

Nipple dermatitis, which causes swollen, reddened, burning nipples, is most commonly caused by thrush or by allergic response to breast cream preparations. If the nipple soreness has a sudden onset and is accompanied by burning or itching, shooting pains through the breast, and a deep pink coloration of the nipple, it may be caused by a thrush infection spread from the infant to the mother. White patches or streaks in the infant's mouth indicate a need for treatment of the mouth and nipple infection. The disease can be treated with a variety of antifungal preparations and does not prevent breastfeeding.

Cracked Nipples

Nipple soreness is often coupled with cracked nipples. When a breastfeeding mother complains of soreness, carefully examine the nipples for fissures or cracks and observe the mother during breastfeeding to see whether the infant is correctly positioned at the breast. If the positioning is correct and cracks exist, interventions are necessary. All the interventions described for sore nipples may be used. It may also help the mother to begin nursing on the breast that is less sore. This approach allows the letdown reflex to occur in the affected breast and permits the infant to more vigorously suck the less tender breast, which decreases trauma to the cracked nipple. With severe cases the temporary use of a nipple shield for breastfeeding may be appropriate. For the mother's comfort, analgesics may be taken after breastfeeding.

Breast Engorgement

Breast fullness and breast engorgement are not the same. All lactating women experience a transitional fullness at first, initially due to venous congestion and later due to accumulating milk. However, this fullness generally lasts only 24 hours, the breasts remain soft enough for the newborn to suckle, and there is no pain. Engorged breasts are hard, painful, and warm and appear taut and shiny.

The infant should nurse for an average of 15 minutes per feeding and should feed at least 8 to 12 times in 24 hours (Varney, Kriebs, & Gegor, 2004). If the baby is unable to nurse more frequently, the mother may express some milk manually or with a pump, taking care to avoid traumatizing the breast tissue. Warm or cool compresses before breastfeeding stimulate letdown and soften the breast so that the infant can grasp the areola more easily. Wearing a well-fitting nursing bra 24 hours a day supports the breasts and prevents discomfort.

The use of fresh green cabbage leaves placed inside the bra to treat engorgement is a long-recognized home remedy that has sparked renewed interest. Although the exact action of the cabbage is not understood, it appears to reduce the edema of engorgement. The amount of relief women experience varies. Some women report relief in as little as 30 minutes, whereas other women require more continuous use to perceive an effect. Prolonged use of cabbage can cause the milk to dry up, which may be helpful if sudden weaning is necessary (Lauwers & Swisher, 2005). Analgesics such as acetaminophen and ibuprofen, alone or in combination with codeine, are appropriate, especially if taken just before breastfeeding. The pain will be relieved, but the medication will not reach the milk for some time.

Plugged Ducts

Some mothers experience plugging of one or more ducts, especially in conjunction with or following engorgement. When breast milk pools within a duct and then dries, it forms a white, hardened plug that is typically visible at the outlet of the duct at the nipple surface. Because milk accumulates behind a plugged duct, women also experience an area of fullness, tenderness, or lumpiness in the associated area of the breast.

Plugging may be relieved by heat and massage. Encourage the mother to massage her breasts from her chest wall forward to the nipple while standing in a warm shower or after applying moist heat to the breast. The mother should then breastfeed her infant, starting on the unaffected breast if the plugged breast is tender. Some lactation consultants advocate starting on the affected side since the more vigorous sucking may help dislodge the plug. A breast pump may be effective in unplugging the duct. Frequent breastfeeding and varying positions to ensure complete emptying helps prevent the problem.

Effect of Alcohol and Medications

Mothers may ask the home care nurse about the use of alcohol and medications when breastfeeding. Although moderate alcohol consumption was considered acceptable in the past, it is no longer recommended for breastfeeding women. Alcohol levels in breast milk parallel those found in the maternal plasma, peaking 30 to 60 minutes after consumption. Mothers who do occasionally drink while lactating should be advised to consume the alcohol after breastfeeding rather than shortly before a feeding in order to minimize the amount the infant receives.

As discussed in Chapter 28, most medications do pass into the breast milk. ∞ Women should consult their primary care provider or other practitioner prior to taking over-the-counter medications, prescription medications, or herbal supplements.

Breastfeeding and the Working Mother

The best preparation for maintaining lactation after return to work is frequent, unlimited breastfeeding. Even when well planned, the first day back to work may be filled with emotional and physical distress. Anticipatory guidance may ease the transition from maternity leave to work. The earlier the breastfeeding mother returns to work, the more often she will need to pump her breasts to express the breast milk. Because milk production follows the principle of supply and demand, if breasts are not pumped, the milk supply will decrease.

An electric breast pump and double collection system are the best way of expressing milk. However, it is not the only method. Sometimes a mother has a flexible schedule and can return home or have the baby brought to her to nurse at lunch. If this is not possible, the infant may be fed expressed milk via bottle or spoon. (For proper storage of breast milk, see "Storing Breast Milk" in Chapter 28 ∞.) If the baby is 3 months or older, cup feeding is an option. The mother should wait until lactation is well established before introducing the bottle. Most babies adjust to the bottle within 7 to 10 days.

To maintain a milk supply, the working mother must pay special attention to her fluid intake. She can ensure adequate intake by drinking extra fluid at each break and whenever possible during the day. It is also helpful to breastfeed more on weekends and during the night, to eat a nutritionally sound diet, and to continue manual expression or pumping when not breastfeeding.

Night breastfeeding presents a dilemma: it may help a working mother maintain her milk supply, but it may also contribute to fatigue. Some women choose to have the infant sleep with them so that breastfeeding is more easily accomplished; other women find it difficult to sleep soundly when the infant is in the same bed. For the mother who works long hours or has a rigid work schedule, the best alternative may be to limit breastfeeding to morning and evening feedings, with supplemental feedings at other times. This choice allows her to maintain a close relationship with the infant and provides some of the unique benefits of breast milk. Her milk production will adjust to this feeding schedule within a few days to a week.

Weaning

The decision to wean the baby from the breast may be made for a variety of reasons, including family or cultural pressures, changes in the home situation, or a personal opinion about when weaning should occur. For the woman who is comfortable with breastfeeding and well informed about the process, the appropriate time to wean her infant will become evident if she is sensitive to the child's cues. Often weaning falls between periods of great developmental activity for the child. Thus, weaning commonly occurs at 8 to 9 months, 12 to 14 months, 18 months, 2 years, and 3 years of age. The infant weaned before 12 months should be given iron-fortified infant formula, not cows' milk (American College of Obstetricians and Gynecologists, 2000).

If weaning is timed to respond to the child's cues, and if the mother is comfortable with the timing, it can be accomplished with less difficulty than if the process begins before mother and child are ready emotionally. Nevertheless, weaning is a time of emotional separation for mother and baby; it may be difficult for them to give up the closeness of their breastfeeding sessions. The nurse who is understanding about this possibility can help the mother see that her infant is growing up and plan other comforting, consoling, and play activities to replace breastfeeding. A gradual approach is the easiest and most comforting way to wean the child from breastfeedings.

During weaning the mother should substitute one cup feeding or bottle-feeding for one breastfeeding session over a few days to a week so that her breasts gradually produce less milk. Eliminating the breastfeedings associated with meals first helps the mother wean the infant more easily. Over a period of several weeks, she can substitute more cup feedings or bottle-feedings for breastfeedings. The slow method of weaning prevents breast engorgement, allows infants to alter their eating methods at their own rates, and provides time for psychologic adjustment.

RESUMPTION OF SEXUAL ACTIVITY

Typically, postpartum couples resume sexual intercourse once the episiotomy is healed and the lochial flow has stopped. Because this usually occurs by the end of the third week, prior to the 6-week check, it is important that the woman and her partner have information about what to expect. Inform the couple that, because the vaginal vault is "dry" (hormone poor), some form of lubrication such as K-Y jelly or Astroglide may be necessary during intercourse. The female-superior and side-lying coital positions may be preferable because they allow the woman to control the depth of penile penetration.

Forewarn breastfeeding couples that, during orgasm, milk may spurt from the nipples due to the release of oxytocin. Some couples find this spurt pleasurable or amusing, but others feel more comfortable if the woman wears a bra during sexual activity. Breastfeeding the baby before lovemaking may reduce the chance of milk release.

Other factors may interfere with satisfactory sexual experiences: the baby's crying may "spoil the mood," the woman's changed body may seem unattractive to her or her partner, maternal sleep deprivation may interfere with desire, and the woman's physiologic response to sexual stimulation may be altered due to hormonal changes. By 3 months postpartum, sexual interest and activity are generally regular in frequency. However, a return to prepregnant levels of sexual activity varies by couple and may take from a few weeks to a year after childbirth.

With anticipatory guidance during the prenatal and postpartum periods, the couple can be forewarned of potential temporary problems. Anticipatory guidance is enhanced if the couple can discuss their feelings and reactions as they are experienced. See "Teaching Highlights: Resumption of Sexual Activity After Childbirth."

Contraception

Information on contraception is often provided as part of discharge teaching. However, the nurse can also be an im-

TEACHING HIGHLIGHTS

RESUMPTION OF SEXUAL ACTIVITY AFTER CHILDBIRTH

- Delay intercourse until no lochia is present because lochia indicates that healing is not yet complete.
- Tenderness of the vagina and perineum may cause discomfort. The partner may test the woman's level of comfort by slipping a lubricated finger inside her vagina. The female-superior and side-lying positions may be preferable because they let the woman control the depth of penetration of the penis.
- Vaginal dryness may occur because the vagina is "hormone poor." It can be avoided by using a water-soluble lubricant.
- Based on the amount of breast engorgement and tenderness present, the partner may need to avoid breast stimulation during foreplay or use a very gentle approach.
- Escape of milk during sexual activity can be minimized by breastfeeding immediately beforehand.
- Fatigue and the new baby's schedule may have a negative impact on the woman's feelings of desire. Napping when the baby sleeps helps decrease fatigue. However, fatigue may be a reality couples need to accept during the early postpartum months.
- Contraception is important even during the early postpartum period. The woman's body needs adequate time to heal and recover from the stress of pregnancy and childbirth. Couples opposed to contraception may choose abstinence at this time.

portant resource for the woman and her partner during postpartum follow-up. Couples typically choose to use contraception to control the number of children they will have or to determine the spacing of future children. Whatever the method, consistency of use is essential. Identify the advantages, disadvantages, risks, and contraindications of the various methods to help the couple, or the single mother, make an informed choice. (For a more detailed discussion of contraceptive methods, see Chapter 4. ∞)

ADDITIONAL TYPES OF FOLLOW-UP CARE

Other types of follow-up care may include return home visits, telephone follow-up, and postpartum classes and support groups.

RETURN VISITS

If the mother, family, and physician or certified nurse-midwife have chosen discharge earlier than 48 hours after vaginal birth, in some states the mother may request a total of three home visits. In such cases the nurse would schedule the first visit about 24 hours after discharge and then space out the other two visits over the next week. In other instances the nurse may schedule additional home visits based on the findings of the first home visit and the follow-up phone call.

TELEPHONE FOLLOW-UP

Telephone follow-up is offered to families prior to discharge, and a mutually agreed upon time is set for the call. Typically the call is made within 3 days after discharge or earlier if desired, lasts about 20 minutes, and is goal directed. To perform effective telephone assessment, the nurse must be able to listen skillfully, ask open-ended questions, and project an attitude of caring. Care provided during a telephone conversation is limited to supportive counseling, teaching, and referral. It is also fairly common for a home care nurse to make a telephone follow-up call to a family a few days after a home visit to provide additional information, address questions or areas of confusion, and make referrals if indicated.

In addition to these scheduled follow-up telephone calls, nurses in birthing, newborn, and postpartum units, and clinic nurses often receive phone calls from postpartal families seeking advice or care. These calls must be triaged immediately. Calls with urgent or life-threatening implications should be referred appropriately, either by initiating an immediate call to the practitioner or, in rare circumstances, calling 911.

Finally, many communities have established 24-hour help lines for new parents to call when they have questions or need support. In areas where help lines are not available, parents may be directed to call the birthing center. In either case the nurse provides the number so that it is readily accessible for the family.

POSTPARTUM CLASSES AND SUPPORT GROUPS

Postpartum classes are available in many areas to help meet the continuing needs of the childbearing family. Classes may focus on topics such as parenting, postpartum exercise, or nutrition, or there may be loosely structured group sessions that address mothers' concerns as they arise. Such classes offer chances for the new mother to socialize, share her concerns, and receive encouragement. Because babysitting arrangements may be difficult or expensive, it is desirable to provide child care for newborns and siblings; in some classes infants may remain with mothers.

Many parents today look to the Internet for information and advice. Help them learn criteria that suggest that Internet information is reliable and of high quality, including affiliation with a university medical or nursing school; inclusion of authors' credentials, education, board certification, and affiliations; referencing of information; currency of information; similarity of information when compared with other sources; and easy accessibility.

Critical Concept Review

LEARNING OBJECTIVES

CONCEPTS

Discuss the components of postpartal home care.	→	The components of the postpartal home visit include: 1. Establish contact with the mother prior to the visit. 2. Identify the purpose and goals of the visit. 3. Establish rapport with the mother. 4. Maintain safety during the visit. 5. Assess the status of the mother, newborn, and family. 6. Reinforce teaching concerning maternal and newborn care.
Identify the main purposes of home visits during the postpartum period.	→	The main purposes of the home visit: 1. Assess the status of the mother and infant. 2. Assess adaptation and adjustment of the family to the new baby. 3. Determine current informational needs. 4. Provide teaching as needed. 5. Use as an opportunity to answer additional questions related to infant care and feeding, and to provide emotional support to the mother and family.
Summarize actions a nurse should take to ensure personal safety during a home visit.	→	Nurses need to act proactively to maintain their safety when making home visits by exercising reasonable caution and remaining alert to environmental cues.

(continued)

LEARNING OBJECTIVES

CONCEPTS

Delineate aspects of fostering a caring relationship in the home.

→

Fostering a caring relationship in the home involves:
1. Evidence of genuineness and empathy.
2. Establishment of trust and rapport.
3. Positive regard for the mother and family.

Describe assessment and care of the newborn and reinforcement of parent teaching in the home.

→

1. Assess the infant's weight, length, heart rate, head circumference, and any signs of jaundice.
2. Watch the mother feed the baby and discuss any concerns she has about feeding.
3. Reinforce teaching in the following areas:
   - Position and handling.
   - Bathing.
   - Dressing.
   - Temperature assessment.
   - Stool and urine.
   - Sleep and activity.
   - Crying.
   - Safety considerations.
   - Newborn screening and necessary immunizations.

Discuss maternal and family assessment and anticipated progress after birth.

→

1. Expected maternal assessments:
   - Vital signs. (Should be at prepregnancy level.)
   - Weight. (Expect weight to be near prepregnancy level at 6 weeks postpartum.)
   - Condition of the breasts.
   - Condition of the abdomen, including a healing cesarean incision, if applicable.
   - Elimination pattern. (Should return to normal by 4 to 6 weeks postpartum.)
   - Lochia. (Should progress from lochia rubra to lochia serosa to lochia alba. If not breastfeeding, menstrual pattern should return at 6 weeks postpartum.)
   - Fundus. (Fundus should decrease in size one finger-breadth per day after the birth of the baby. Uterus should return to normal size by 6 weeks postpartum.)
   - Perineum. (Episiotomy and lacerations should show signs of healing.)
2. Family assessment:
   - Bonding. (Appropriate demonstration of bonding should be apparent.)
   - Level of comfort. (Parents should display appropriate levels of comfort with the infant.)
   - Siblings are adjusting to new baby.
   - Parental role adjustment. (Parents should be working on division of labor, changes in financial status, communication changes, readjustment of sexual relations, and adjustment to new daily tasks.)
   - Contraception. (Parents understand need to choose and use a method of contraception.)

Delineate interventions to address the common concerns of breastfeeding mothers following discharge.

→

Common concerns of the breastfeeding mother include:
1. Nipple soreness.
2. Cracked nipples.
3. Engorgement.
4. Plugged ducts.

Breastfeeding mothers are encouraged to:
1. Nurse frequently.
2. Change the infant's position regularly.
3. Allow nipples to air dry after breastfeeding.

In addition to home visits, identify other types of follow-up care available to postpartum families.

→

Other types of follow-up care:
1. Telephone calls.
2. Return visits.
3. Baby care/postpartum classes.
4. New mother support groups.

CRITICAL THINKING IN ACTION

*View the **Critical Thinking in Action** video in Chapter 32 of the CD-ROM. Then, answer the questions that follow.*

Jane Benne, age 23, G1, P1 gave birth by cesarean for cephalopelvic disproportion to a healthy 7 pound 1 ounce baby boy 5 days ago. You are making a home visit 2 days after Jane was discharged from the hospital to her two-story home. When you arrive the baby is sleeping in a bassinet in Jane's bedroom on the second level. Jane has been trying to breastfeed and complains to you of sore nipples and swollen breasts. She is also having problems getting the baby to latch on and says that she has been supplementing her baby's feedings with a bottle because she is afraid her baby is not getting enough milk from her breasts alone. She also mentions that the baby seems more satisfied after she gives the bottle and seems to sleep longer. You ask her how she has been feeling, and she tells you that she is very tired and upset about her body not making enough milk to feed her child. You assess Jane's breasts and find them to be full and firm, but the nipples are cracked and blistered.

1. What is your focus in the home postpartum visit?
2. What counseling can you give Jane regarding her sore nipples?
3. What suggestion do you give Jane regarding supplemental bottle-feedings?
4. Explain your assessment of Jane's abdominal incision and provide suggestions for healing.
5. How would you discuss the baby's voiding patterns to ensure adequate hydration?

MEDIALINK

www.prenhall.com/london

- NCLEX-RN® Review, case studies, and other interactive resources for this chapter can be found on the Companion Website at http://www.prenhall.com/london. Click on "Chapter 32" to select the activities for this chapter.

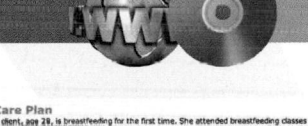

- For animations, more NCLEX-RN® Review questions, and an audio glossary, access the accompanying CD-ROM in this textbook.

REFERENCES

Aisenstein, T. (2003). For nurses new to home care. *Nursing Spectrum.* Retrieved on December 5, 2003, from http://nsweb.nursingspectrum.com/ce/ce109.htm

American Academy of Pediatrics, Committee on Fetus and Newborn. (1995). Hospital stay for healthy term newborns. *Pediatrics, 96*(4, Pt. 1), 788–790.

American College of Obstetricians and Gynecologists. (2000). *Breastfeeding: Maternal and infant aspects* (ACOG Educational Bulletin No. 258). Washington, DC: Author.

Association of Women's Health, Obstetric and Neonatal Nurses (AWHONN). (1999). *Breastfeeding: Clinical position statement.* Washington, DC: Author.

Center for Medicaid and Medicare Services. (2002). *Newborn and Mother's Health Protection Act statutory text.* Retrieved December 5, 2003, from http://www.cms.hhs.gov/hipaa/hipaa1/content/nmhpastat.asp

Dewey, K. G., Nommsen-Rivers, L. A., Heinig, M. J., & Cohen, R. J. (2003). Risk factors for suboptimal infant breastfeeding behavior, delayed onset of lactation, and excess neonatal weight loss. *Pediatrics, 112*(3 Pt 1), 607–619.

Heck, K. E., Schoendorf, K. C., Gilberto, F. C., & Braveman, P. (2003). Does postpartum length of stay affect breastfeeding duration? A population-based study. *Birth, 30*(3), 153–158.

Lauwers, J., & Swisher, A. (2005). *Counseling the nursing mother.* Boston: Jones & Bartlett.

Madlon-Kay, D., DeFor, D. A., & Egerter, S. (2003). Newborn length of stay, health care utiliza-tion, and the effect of Minnesota legislation. *Archives of Pediatric & Adolescent Medicine, 157,* 579–583.

Malkin, J. D., Keeler, E., Broder, M. S., & Garber, S. (2003). Postpartum length of stay and newborn health: A cost-effectiveness analysis. *Pediatrics, 3*(4), e316–e322. Retrieved December 5, 2003, from http://www.pediatrics.aappublications.org/cgi/content/abstract/111/4/e316

Page, T., Lockwood, C., & Guest, K. (2003). Management of nipple pain and/or trauma associated with breastfeeding. *Joanna Briggs Institute (JBI) Reports, 1*(4), 127–134.

Varney, H., Kriebs, J. M., & Gegor, C. L. (2004). *Varney's midwifery* (4th ed.). Boston: Jones & Bartlett.

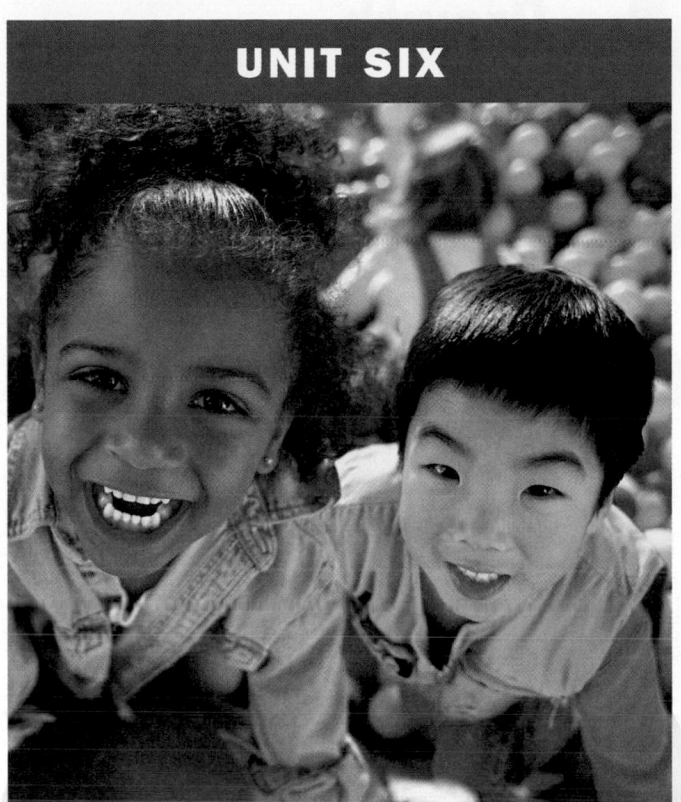

UNIT SIX

Care and Needs of Children

Growth and Development

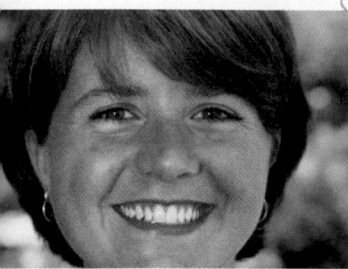

We want to help our adopted daughter Irena grow into a normal and special child. She had challenges in her short life in Romania that we can only imagine. We worry about how we can help her grow and develop.

Mother of Irena, 2

LEARNING OBJECTIVES

- Describe major theories of development as formulated by Freud, Erikson, Piaget, Kohlberg, social learning theorists, and behaviorists.

- Plan nursing interventions for children that are appropriate for the child's developmental state, based on theoretical frameworks.

- Explain contemporary developmental approaches such as temperament theory, ecologic theory, and the resilience framework.

- Recognize major developmental milestones for infants, toddlers, preschoolers, school-age children, and adolescents.

- Synthesize information from several theoretical approaches to plan assessments of the child's physical growth and developmental milestones.

- Describe the role of play in the growth and development of children.

- Use data collected during developmental assessments to implement activities that promote development of children and adolescents.

MEDIALINK www.prenhall.com/london

Video: Growth and Development
NCLEX–RN® Review
Audio Glossary

Objectives
NCLEX–RN® Review
Thinking Critically
Critical Thinking: Linking Theory and Research
MediaLink Applications:
    Preparing a Preschooler for Surgery
    Developing Values in Adolescence

Children develop as they interact with their surroundings. They learn skills at different ages, but the order in which they learn them is universal. Development is affected by factors such as nutrition and cultural practices, as well as the social situation in the country or neighborhood. While each child will develop in a unique manner influenced by genetic makeup, life experiences, and the interaction between these factors, certain principles of development assist parents and the nurse in fostering positive adaptations for the child.

This chapter will cover general principles of growth and development and will explore several theories related to childhood development, as well as their nursing applications. Each age group, from infancy through adolescence, is described in detail. Developmental milestones, physical and cognitive characteristics, play patterns, and communication strategies are presented. This basic information helps guide developmentally appropriate care for children in each age group. These concepts can be applied when caring for all children, including those in special situations.

PRINCIPLES OF GROWTH AND DEVELOPMENT

It is essential to understand the concepts of growth and development when learning to care for children. A skilled pediatric nurse integrates knowledge of physical growth and psychosocial development into each child healthcare encounter. **Growth** refers to an increase in physical size. Growth represents quantitative changes such as height, weight, blood pressure, and number of words in the child's vocabulary. **Development** refers to a qualitative increase in capability or function. Developmental skills unfold in a complex manner influenced by the relationship between the child's innate, unfolding capabilities and the stimuli and support provided in the environment. Examples include the ability to sit without support or to throw a ball overhand. These quantitative and qualitative changes in body organ functioning, ability to communicate, and performance of motor skills unfold over time and are key components in the process of planning pediatric healthcare.

Each child displays a unique maturational pattern during the process of development. Although the exact age at which skills emerge differs, the sequence or order of skill performance is uniform among children. Skill development proceeds according to two processes: from the head down and from the center of the body out to the extremities. Development that proceeds from the head downward through the body and toward the feet is called **cephalocaudal development** (Figure 33–1 ◉). For example, at birth an infant's head is much larger proportionately than the trunk or extremities. Similarly, infants learn to hold up their heads before sitting and to sit before standing. Skills such as walking that involve the legs and feet develop last in infancy. Development that proceeds from the center of the body outward to the extremities is called **proximodistal development** (see Figure 33–1). For example, infants are first able to control the trunk, then the arms; only later are fine motor movements of the fingers possible. As the child grows, both physical and cognitive skills differentiate from general to more specific skills. Pediatric nurses use these concepts of predictable and sequential developmental direction to analyze the infant's and child's present state and to partner with parents to plan ways to encourage and support the next emerging developmental abilities.

During the childhood years, extraordinary changes occur in all aspects of development. Physical size, motor skills, cognitive ability, language, sensory ability, and psychosocial patterns all undergo major transformations. Nurses

KEY TERMS

accommodation, 892

adaptation phase, 901

adjustment phase, 901

anticipatory guidance, 890

assimilation, 892

associative play, 914

autosomal chromosomes, 902

cephalocaudal development, 889

conservation, 917

cooperative play, 918

defense mechanisms, 891

development, 889

dramatic play, 915

ecologic theory, 897

expressive jargon, 911

growth, 889

nature, 897

nurture, 897

object permanence, 895

parallel play, 910

protective factors, 900

proximodistal development, 889

puberty, 920

resilience, 900

risk factors, 900

sex chromosomes, 907

solitary play, 907

● FIGURE 33–1

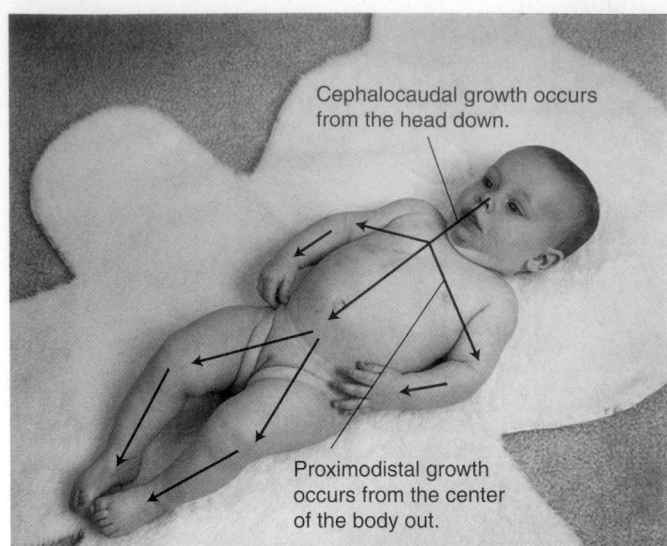

Cephalocaudal growth occurs from the head down.

Proximodistal growth occurs from the center of the body out.

In normal cephalocaudal growth, the child gains control of the head and neck before the trunk and limbs. In normal proximodistal growth, the child controls arm movements before hand movements. For example, the child reaches for objects before being able to grasp them. Children gain control of their hands before their fingers; that is, they can hold things with the entire hand before they can pick something up with just their fingers.

study normal patterns of development so they can perform thorough pediatric assessments and identify children who demonstrate unexpected developmental findings. These assessments can guide the nurse in planning interventions for the child and family, such as referring the child for a diagnostic evaluation or rehabilitation, or teaching the parents how to provide adequate stimulation for the child. Nurses

use **anticipatory guidance** to predict upcoming developmental tasks or needs of a child and performing appropriate teaching related to them. When development is proceeding normally, the nurse uses his or her knowledge of these normal patterns to provide approaches based on the child's cognitive and language ability, to offer appropriate toys and activities during illness, and to respond therapeutically during interactions with the child. For situations with special challenges, such as in adoptions, additional interventions may be needed (see "Growth and Development").

MAJOR THEORIES OF DEVELOPMENT

Child development is a complex process. Many theorists have attempted to organize their observations of behavior into a description of principles or a set of stages. Each theory focuses on a particular facet of development. Most developmental theorists separate children into age groups by common characteristics (Table 33–1).

FREUD'S THEORY OF PSYCHOSEXUAL DEVELOPMENT

Theoretical Framework

Sigmund Freud (1856–1939) was a physician in Vienna, Austria. His work with adults experiencing a variety of nervous disorders led him to develop the approach called psychoanalysis, which explored the driving forces of the unconscious mind. These psychoanalytic techniques led Freud to believe that early childhood experiences form the unconscious motivation for actions in later life. He believed that sexual energy is centered in specific parts of the body at certain ages. Unresolved conflict and unmet needs

GROWTH AND DEVELOPMENT

Over 20,000 international adoptions occurred in 2001 in the United States, up from less than half that number one decade before. China, Russia, Guatemala, South Korea, Ukraine, Kazakhstan, and Vietnam are presently the most frequent countries of origin for orphans being adopted in the United States (Chamberlain, 2003). Average age of adoptees is 2 years (Jenista, 2000). Although these children may have an array of medical conditions such as infectious diseases, inadequate immunizations, and nutritional disorders, the effects of their early life experiences on development can also be profound. Institutionalization and multiple foster care placements can result in emotional neglect, growth and developmental delays, and behavior problems (Aronson, 2000; Chamberlain, 2001; Chen, Barnett, & Wilson, 2003; Faber, 2000; Johnson, 2000; Miller, 2000).

Many international adoptees are small in size, due to poor nutrition of the mother during pregnancy and of the infant after birth, and to growth delay related to emotional issues. The child should be

examined closely at the time of adoption for length, weight, and head circumference. Within 6 months of arrival, most children show improvement in growth patterns. If growth does not improve by this time, the child is further assessed for problems such as intestinal parasites, chronic diseases, or other medical problems (Chen et al., 2003; Miller, 2000). The psychosocially based problem of eating disorder of infancy and childhood should also be considered (see Chapter 34 for a thorough discussion of this condition ∞).

Although it is expected that international adoptees may have some developmental delays and often improve dramatically after adoption, testing of development, including verbal skills, upon arrival with their adoptive family is important. It provides a baseline upon which to measure future developmental test results and provides information needed to help parents encourage and stimulate the child appropriately (Miller, 2000). Nurses perform careful developmental monitoring and assist adoptive parents in fostering normal growth and development.

THINKING CRITICALLY

INTERNATIONAL ADOPTION COUNSELING

Michael and Alyssa had tried for several years to have a biologic child. After an unsuccessful in vitro fertilization, they decided to try to adopt a child. They explored opportunities with adoption agencies and learned that international adoption would be possible for them. They adopted 2-year-old Irena from Romania several months ago.

Despite thorough investigation of Michael and Alyssa by the adoption agency, they received only scant information about Irena's history. She was given to an orphanage by her mother when she was about 7 months old; the mother stated that the pregnancy and birth were normal. She was giving the child up because she had two older children to care for and her husband had left home nearly a year before and had not been heard from since. Irena appears small for her age, but she is thriving in her new environment. She is learning to say a few English words and is responding appropriately to care and interactions.

How can you work with Michael and Alyssa to ensure special attention to Irena's growth and healthcare needs? What challenges in her early life may have influenced Irena's physical growth, her ability to interact with others, the timing of developmental milestones, and speech?

What will Irena's cultural needs be as she grows older? How can Michael and Alyssa prepare to tell her about her adoption and background someday? How can they learn about Irena's country of origin?

TABLE 33–1 ✤ Developmental Age Groups

Infancy—Birth to 12 months. Includes infants or babies up to 1 year of age who require a high level of care in daily activities.

Toddlerhood—1–3 years. Characterized by increased motor ability and independent behavior.

Preschool—3–6 years. The preschooler refines gross and fine motor ability and language skills and often participates in a preschool learning program.

School age—6–12 years. Begins with entry into a school system and is characterized by growing intellectual skills, physical ability, and independence.

Adolescence—12–18 years. Begins with entry into the teen years. Mature cognitive thought, formation of identity, and influence of peers are important characteristics of adolescence.

TABLE 33–2 ✤ Common Defense Mechanisms Used by Children

Defense Mechanism	Definition	Example
Regression	Return to an earlier behavior	A previously toilet-trained child becomes incontinent when separated from parents during a hospitalization.
Repression	Involuntary forgetting of uncomfortable situations	An abused child cannot consciously recall episodes of abuse.
Rationalization	An attempt to make unacceptable feelings acceptable	A child explains hitting another because "he took my toy."
Fantasy	A creation of the mind to help deal with unacceptable fear	A hospitalized child who is weak pretends to be Superman.

---

at a certain stage lead to a fixation of development at that stage (Lerner, 2002).

Freud viewed the personality as a structure with three parts: the id is the basic sexual energy that is present at birth and drives the individual to seek pleasure; the ego is the realistic part of the person, which develops during infancy and searches for acceptable methods of meeting impulses; and the superego is the moral/ethical system, which develops in childhood and contains a set of values and conscience (Craig & Baucum, 2001). The ego diverts impulses and protects itself from excess anxiety by use of **defense mechanisms**, including regression to earlier stages and repression or forgetting of painful experiences such as child abuse (Table 33–2).

Stages

Oral (Birth to 1 Year). The infant derives pleasure largely from the mouth, with sucking and eating as primary desires.

Anal (1 to 3 Years). The young child's pleasure is centered in the anal area, with control over body secretions as a prime force in behavior.

Phallic (3 to 6 Years). Sexual energy becomes centered in the genitalia as the child works out relationships with parents of the same and opposite sexes.

Latency (6 to 12 Years). Sexual energy is at rest in the passage between earlier stages and adolescence.

Genital (12 Years to Adulthood). Mature sexuality is achieved as physical growth is completed and relationships with others occur.

Nursing Application

Freud emphasized the importance of meeting the needs of each stage in order to move successfully into future developmental stages. The crisis of illness can interfere with normal developmental processes and add challenges for the nurse striving to meet an ill child's needs. For example, the importance of sucking in infancy guides the nurse to provide a pacifier for the infant who cannot have oral fluids. The preschool child's concern about sexuality guides the nurse to provide privacy and clear explanations during any procedures involving the genital area. It may be necessary to teach parents that masturbation by the young child is normal and to help parents deal with it. The adolescent's focus on relationships suggests that the nurse should include questions about significant friends during history taking. Table 33–3 summarizes ways to apply these theoretical concepts to the care of children.

ERIKSON'S THEORY OF PSYCHOSOCIAL DEVELOPMENT

Theoretical Framework

Erik Erikson (1902–1994) studied Freud's theory of psychoanalysis under Freud's daughter, Anna. He later established his own developmental theory which describes psychosocial stages during eight periods of human life. For each stage, Erikson identified a crisis, that is, a particular challenge that exists for healthy personality development to occur (Erikson, 1963, 1968). The word "crisis" in this context refers to normal maturational social needs rather than to a single critical event. Each developmental crisis has two possible outcomes. When needs are met, the consequence is healthy and the individual moves on to future stages with particular strengths. When needs are not met, an unhealthy outcome occurs that will influence future social relationships.

Stages

Trust Versus Mistrust (Birth to 1 Year). The task of the first year of life is to establish trust in the people providing care. Trust is fostered by provision of food, clean clothing, touch, and comfort. If basic needs are not met, the infant will eventually learn to mistrust others.

Autonomy Versus Shame and Doubt (1 to 3 Years). The toddler's sense of autonomy or independence is shown by controlling body excretions, saying no when asked to do something, and directing motor activity and play. Children who are consistently criticized for expressions of autonomy or for lack of control—for example, during toilet training—will develop a sense of shame about themselves and doubt in their abilities.

Initiative Versus Guilt (3 to 6 Years). The young child initiates new activities and considers new ideas. This interest in exploring the world creates a child who is involved and busy. Constant criticism, on the other hand, leads to feelings of guilt and a lack of purpose.

Industry Versus Inferiority (6 to 12 Years). The middle years of childhood are characterized by development of new interests and by involvement in activities. The child takes pride in accomplishments in sports, school, home, and community. If the child cannot accomplish what is expected, however, the result will be a sense of inferiority.

Identity Versus Role Confusion (12 to 18 Years). In adolescence, as the body matures and thought processes become more complex, a new sense of identity or self is established. The self, family, peer group, and community are all examined and redefined. The adolescent who is unable to establish a meaningful definition of self will experience confusion in one or more roles of life.

Nursing Application

Erikson's theory is directly applicable to the nursing care of children. Health promotion and health maintenance visits in the community provide opportunities for helping caregivers meet children's needs. Parents benefit from learning what the child's developmental tasks are at each stage and from discussing ideas about how to encourage healthy psychosocial development. Such discussions also may highlight parental concerns and provide a forum for reassurance about normal developmental characteristics, such as a child who does not follow through on each activity as a preschooler or tries different hairstyles each month as an adolescent. The child's usual support from family, peers, and others is interrupted by hospitalization. The challenge of hospitalization also adds a situational crisis to the normal developmental crisis a child is experiencing. Although the nurse may meet many of the hospitalized child's needs, continued parental involvement is necessary both during and after hospitalization to ensure progression through expected developmental stages (see Table 33–3).

PIAGET'S THEORY OF COGNITIVE DEVELOPMENT

Theoretical Framework

Jean Piaget (1896–1980) was a Swiss scientist who wrote detailed observations of the behavior of his own and other children. Based on these observations, Piaget formulated a theory of cognitive (or intellectual) development. He believed that the child's view of the world is influenced largely by age and maturational ability. Given nurturing experiences, the child's ability to think matures naturally (Ginsberg & Opper, 1988; Piaget, 1972). The child incorporates new experiences via **assimilation** and changes to deal with these experiences by the process of **accommodation**. An example of assimilation occurs when the infant uses reflexes to suck on objects that touch the lips. With more experience the infant accommodates to learn that not all objects are pleasant to suck and cognitive structures change to integrate and learn from the experiences.

TABLE 33–3 ✤ Nursing Applications of Theories of Freud, Erikson, Piaget

Age Group	Developmental Stages	Nursing Applications
Infant (birth to 1 year)	Oral stage (Freud): The baby obtains pleasure and comfort through the mouth.	When a baby is not able to take foods or fluids, offer a pacifier if not contraindicated. After painful procedures, offer a baby a bottle or pacifier or have the mother breastfeed.
	Trust versus mistrust stage (Erikson): The baby establishes a sense of trust when basic needs are met.	Hold the hospitalized baby often. (**A**) Offer comfort after painful procedures. Meet the baby's needs for food and hygiene. Encourage parents to room in. Manage pain effectively with use of pain medications and other measures.
	Sensorimotor stage (Piaget): The baby learns from movement and sensory input.	Use crib mobiles, manipulative toys, wall murals, and bright colors to provide interesting stimuli and comfort. Use toys to distract the baby during procedures and assessments.
Toddler (1–3 years)	Anal stage (Freud): The child derives gratification from control over body excretions.	Ask about toilet training and the child's rituals and words for elimination during admission history. Continue child's normal patterns of elimination in the hospital. Do not begin toilet training during illness or hospitalization. Accept regression in toileting during illness or hospitalization. Have potty chairs available in hospital and childcare centers.
	Autonomy versus shame and doubt stage (Erikson): The child is increasingly independent in many spheres of life.	Allow self-feeding opportunities. Encourage child to remove and put on own clothes, brush teeth, or assist with hygiene. (**B**) If immobilization for a procedure is necessary, proceed quickly, providing explanations and comfort.
	Sensorimotor stage (end); preoperational stage (beginning) (Piaget): The child shows increasing curiosity and explorative behavior. Language skills improve.	Ensure safe surroundings to allow opportunities to manipulate objects. Name objects and give simple explanations.
Preschooler (3–6 years)	Phallic stage (Freud): The child initially identifies with the parent of the opposite sex but by the end of this stage identifies with the same-sex parent.	Be alert for children who appear more comfortable with male or female nurses, and attempt to accommodate them. Encourage parental involvement in care. Plan for playtime and offer a variety of materials from which to choose.
	Initiative versus guilt stage (Erikson): The child likes to initiate play activities.	Offer medical equipment for play to lessen anxiety about strange objects. (**C**) Assess children's concerns as expressed through their drawings. Accept the child's choices and expressions of feelings.
	Preoperational stage (Piaget): The child is increasingly verbal but has some limitations in thought processes. Causality is often confused, so the child may feel responsible for causing an illness.	Offer explanations about all procedures and treatments. Clearly explain that the child is not responsible for causing the illness.

A

B

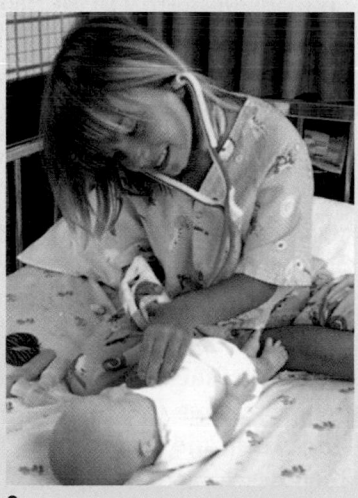

C

(continued)

TABLE 33–3 ✤ Nursing Applications of Theories of Freud, Erikson, Piaget—continued

Age Group	Developmental Stages	Nursing Applications
School age (6–12 years)	Latency stage (Freud): The child places importance on privacy and understanding the baby.	Provide gowns, covers, and underwear. Knock on door before entering. Explain treatments and procedures.
	Industry versus inferiority stage (Erikson): The child gains a sense of self-worth from involvement in activities.	Encourage the child to continue school work while hospitalized. Encourage child to bring favorite pastimes to the hospital. (**D**) Help child adjust to limitations on favorite activities.
	Concrete operational stage (Piaget): The child is capable of mature thought when allowed to manipulate and see objects.	Give clear instructions about details of treatment. Show the child equipment that will be used in treatment.
Adolescent (12–18 years)	Genital stage (Freud): The adolescent's focus is on genital function and relationships.	Ensure access to gynecologic care for adolescent girls. Provide information on sexuality. Ensure privacy during healthcare. Have brochures and videos available for teaching about sexuality.
	Identity versus role confusion stage (Erikson): The adolescent's search for self-identity leads to independence from parents and reliance on peers.	Provide a separate recreation room for teens who are hospitalized. (**E**) Take health history and perform examinations without parents present. Introduce adolescent to other teens with same health problem.
	Formal operational stage (Piaget): The adolescent is capable of mature, abstract thought.	Give clear and complete information about healthcare and treatments. Offer both written and verbal instructions. Continue to provide education about the disease to the adolescent with a chronic illness, as mature thought now leads to greater understanding.

D

E

Stages

Sensorimotor (Birth to 2 Years). Infants learn about the world by input obtained through the senses and by their motor activity. Six substages are characteristic of this stage.

Use of Reflexes (Birth to 1 Month). The infant begins life with a set of reflexes such as sucking, rooting, and grasping. By using these reflexes, the infant receives stimulation via touch, sound, smell, and vision. The reflexes thus pave the way for the first learning to occur.

Primary Circular Reactions (1 to 4 Months). Once the infant responds reflexively, the pleasure gained from that response causes repetition of the behavior. For example, if a toy grasped reflexively makes noise and is interesting to look at, the infant will grasp it again.

Secondary Circular Reactions (4 to 8 Months). Awareness of the environment grows as the infant begins to connect cause and effect. The sounds of bottle preparation will lead to excited behavior. If an object is partially hidden, the infant will attempt to uncover and retrieve it.

Coordination of Secondary Schemes (8 to 12 Months). Intentional behavior is observed as the infant uses learned behavior to obtain objects, create sounds, or engage in other pleasurable activity. **Object permanence** (the knowledge that something continues to exist even when out of sight) begins when the infant remembers where a hidden object is likely to be found; it is no longer "out of sight, out of mind." The concept of object permanence is not fully developed however. The infant knows the parent well, objects to new people, and seems very worried when the parent leaves. Other caretakers may be rejected as the infant does not understand that the parent will return. This phase of "stranger anxiety" is quite common and heralds the infant's growing recognition of and desire to be cared for by the parent.

Tertiary Circular Reactions (12 to 18 Months). Curiosity, experimentation, and exploration predominate as the toddler tries out actions to learn results. The child turns objects in every direction, places them in the mouth, uses them for banging, and inserts them in containers as he or she explores their qualities and uses.

Mental Combinations (18 to 24 Months). Language provides a new tool for the toddler to use in understanding the world. Language enables the child to think about events and objects before or after they occur. Object permanence is now fully developed as the child actively searches for objects in various locations and out of view. The child who has had successful separations from the parents followed by return, such as hours spent in another's home or childcare center, begins to understand that the missing parent will return.

Preoperational (2 to 7 Years). The young child thinks by using words as symbols, but logic is not well developed. During the preconceptual substage (2 to 4 years), vocabulary and comprehension increase greatly but the child is egocentric (that is, unable to see things from the perspective of another). In the intuitive substage (4 to 7 years), the child relies on transductive reasoning (that is, drawing conclusions from one general fact to another). For example, when a child disobeys a parent and then falls and breaks an arm that day, the child may ascribe the broken arm to bad behavior. Cause-and-effect relationships are often unrealistic or a result of "magical thinking" (the belief that events occur because of thoughts or wishes). Additional characteristics noted in the thought of preschoolers include centration, or the ability to consider only one aspect of a situation at a time, and animism, or giving life to inanimate objects because they move, make noise, or have certain other qualities.

Concrete Operational (7 to 11 Years). Transductive reasoning has given way to a more accurate understanding of cause and effect. The child can reason quite well if concrete objects are used in teaching or experimentation. The concept of conservation (that matter does not change when its form is altered) is learned at this age.

Formal Operational (11 Years to Adulthood). Fully mature intellectual thought has now been attained. The adolescent can think abstractly about objects or concepts and consider different alternatives or outcomes.

Nursing Application

Piaget's theory is essential to pediatric nursing. The nurse must understand a child's thought processes in order to design stimulating activities and meaningful, appropriate teaching plans. What activities could be planned for a hospitalized child based on his or her expected cognitive level? How can cognitive development be encouraged in a school-age child receiving home health services? Understanding a child's concept of time suggests how far in advance to prepare that child for procedures. Similarly, decisions about offering manipulative toys, reading stories, drawing pictures, or giving the child reading matter to explain healthcare measures depend on the child's cognitive stage of development (see Table 33–3).

KOHLBERG'S THEORY OF MORAL DEVELOPMENT

Theoretical Framework

Lawrence Kohlberg (1927–1987) was a German theorist who used Piaget's cognitive theory as a basis for his theory of moral development. He presented stories involving moral dilemmas to children and adults and asked them to solve the dilemmas. Kohlberg then analyzed the motives they expressed when making decisions about the best course to take. Based on the explanations given, Kohlberg established three levels of moral reasoning. Although he provided age guidelines, he stated that they are approximate and that many people never reach the highest (postconventional) stage of development (Santrock, 2004).

Stages

Preconventional (4 to 7 Years). Decisions are based on the desire to please others and to avoid punishment.

Conventional (7 to 12 Years). Conscience or an internal set of standards becomes important. Rules are important and must be followed to please other people and "be good."

Postconventional (12 Years and Older). The individual has internalized ethical standards on which to base decisions. Social responsibility is recognized. The value in each of two differing moral approaches can be considered and a decision made.

Nursing Application

Decision making is required in many areas of healthcare. Children can be assisted to make decisions about healthcare and to consider alternatives when available. Keep in mind that young children may agree to participate in research simply because they want to comply with adults and appear cooperative. Guidelines for child participation in research are available (see Chapter 1 ∞).

Parents can be provided with information so that they can assist their children in moral judgments. Encourage talking with a child or adolescent about how a given decision was made. Parents can then add information and help the child learn to integrate more factors into decision making. Talking about the process is important in helping children progress to higher moral development stages. Focusing on the feelings of others, using positive discipline techniques, and clearly identifying positive and negative behaviors are important.

SOCIAL LEARNING THEORY

Theoretical Framework

Originally from Canada, psychologist Albert Bandura (1925–) has conducted research at Stanford University for many years. He believes that children learn attitudes, beliefs, customs, and values through their social contacts with adults and other children. Children imitate (or model) the behavior they see; if the behavior is positively reinforced, they tend to repeat it. The external environment and the child's internal processes are key elements in social learning theory (Bandura, 1986, 1997a).

Bandura believes that an important determinant of behavior is self-efficacy, or the expectation that someone can produce a desired outcome. For example, if adolescents believe they can avoid use of drugs or alcohol, they are more likely to do so. A child who has confidence in his or her ability to exercise regularly or lose weight has a greater chance of success with these behavior changes. Parents who have confidence in their ability to care adequately for their infants are more likely to do so (Bandura, 1997b). See "Evidence-Based Nursing" for further examples of application of the concept of self-efficacy.

Nursing Application

The importance of modeling behavior can readily be applied in healthcare. Children are more likely to cooperate if they see adults or other children performing a task willingly. A frightened child may watch another child perform vision screening or have blood drawn and then decide to allow the procedure to take place. Contact with positive

EVIDENCE-BASED NURSING

CONCEPT OF SELF-EFFICACY

Clinical Question
How can nurses use the concept of self-efficacy when planning interventions for children and families?

Evidence
Nurses often provide information for parents and children that will encourage them to adopt healthy lifestyles. Providing information may not be enough; many of us know about health behaviors but do not consistently apply them. The concept of self-efficacy helps to explain why some people take on healthy behaviors while others do not. People who are convinced they can make a positive change are more likely to do so. A number of research projects test and apply self-efficacy in teaching about health. Two examples follow:

- Few effective interventions have been found that prevent or lower obesity rates in early adolescents. Nurses tested a health promotion program designed to increase self-efficacy and provide information in a group of 60 middle-school youth, matched with 57 youth who did not receive the teaching. Children who had low self-efficacy scores tended to have greater consumption of high-fat foods. The intervention was associated with significantly lowered fat in the diet. Approaches that address diet choices, consciousness, efficacy, and other behavioral factors are more likely to contribute to dietary change than simple presentation of facts about dietary intake (Frenn, Malin, & Bansal, 2003).
- Violence among youth is a complex problem that presents challenges to nurses in many settings. The authors examined factors that influence extent and likelihood of youth violence among 318 middle-school students. Self-efficacy was identified as

a key concept for testing and was defined as the confidence of students to avoid engaging in physically violent behaviors. Lower self-efficacy was associated with, and a strong predictor of, more frequent violent behaviors. Interventions can be targeted at increasing students' self-efficacy so that violent behaviors will decrease (Riner & Saywell, 2002).

Implications
When planning interventions to encourage health behaviors in children and adolescents, assess the youth's belief that the new behaviors are important and that they can be adopted. Include interventions that demonstrate that others have adopted the health behaviors and plan approaches to enhance the child's belief in ability to change.

Critical Thinking
Plan a teaching project about the importance of physical activity for presentation to a group of 12-year-olds. What approaches will enhance the self-efficacy of the children? How would interventions to enhance self-efficacy differ for young elementary-school children from those in middle or high school? What theoretical approaches discussed earlier in this chapter help you to understand the cognitive abilities of children at various ages and suggest ways to influence their self-efficacy?

References
Frenn, M., Malin, S., & Bansal, N. K. (2003). Stage-based interventions for low-fat diet with middle school students. *Journal of Pediatric Nursing, 18*, 36–45.

Riner, M. E., & Saywell, R. M. (2002). Development of the Social Ecology Model of Adolescent Interpersonal Violence Prevention (SEMAIVP). *Journal of School Health, 72*, 65–70.

role models is useful when teaching children and adolescents self-care for chronic diseases such as diabetes. Give positive reinforcement for desired performance.

Nurses can use the concept of self-efficacy to increase the chance of success with lifestyle behavior changes. For example, encouraging youth who are trying to quit smoking, providing them with role models, and pointing out parental successes with their children all demonstrate methods of fostering self-efficacy.

BEHAVIORISM

Theoretical Framework

John Watson (1878–1958) was an American scientist who applied the research of animal behaviorists like Pavlov and Skinner to children. Pavlov and, later, Skinner worked with animals, presenting a stimulus such as food and pairing it with another stimulus such as a ringing bell. Eventually the animal being fed began to salivate when the bell rang. As Skinner and then Watson began to apply these concepts to children, they showed that behaviors can be elicited by positive reinforcement, such as a food treat, or extinguished by negative reinforcement, such as scolding or withdrawal of attention. Watson believed that he could make of a child anyone he desired—from a professional to a thief or beggar—simply by reinforcing behavior in certain ways (Santrock, 2004).

Nursing Application

Behaviorism has been criticized for its simplicity and its denial of the inherent capability of persons to respond willfully to events in the environment. This theory does, however, have some use in healthcare. When particular behaviors are desired, positive reinforcement can be established to encourage these behaviors. Behavioral techniques are also used to alter behavior of misbehaving children or to teach skills to children with disabilities. Parents often use reinforcement in toilet training and other skills learned in childhood.

ECOLOGIC THEORY

Theoretical Framework

There is controversy among theorists concerning the relative importance of heredity versus environment—or nature versus nurture—in human development. **Nature** refers to the genetic or hereditary capability of an individual. **Nurture** refers to the effects of the environment on a person's performance (Figure 33–2 ●). Piaget believed in the importance of internal cognitive structures that unfold at their appointed times, given any environment that provides basic opportunities. He emphasized the strength of nature. The behaviorist John Watson, on the other hand,

● **FIGURE 33–2**

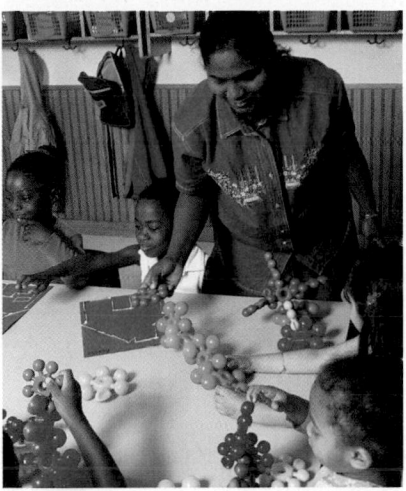

Children exposed to pleasant stimulation and who are supported by an adult will develop and refine their skills faster. Group activities such as these provide an opportunity for both motor skill and psychosocial development. Can you identify which skills are being developed?

believed that behaviors are primarily shaped by environmental responses; he thus stressed the predominance of nurture. Contemporary developmental theories increasingly recognize the interaction of nature and nurture in determining the child's development.

Urie Bronfenbrenner (1917–2005), a professor at Cornell University, formulated the ecologic theory of development to explain the unique relationship of the child in all of life's settings, from close to remote (Bronfenbrenner, 1986, 2005; Bronfenbrenner, McClelland, Ceci et al., 1996). **Ecologic theory** emphasizes the presence of mutual interactions between the child and these various settings. Neither nature nor nurture is considered of more importance. Bronfenbrenner believes each child brings a unique set of genes—as well as specific attributes such as age, gender, health, and other characteristics—to his or her interactions with the environment. The child then interacts in many settings at different levels or systems (Figure 33–3 ●).

Levels/Systems. *Microsystem.* This level is defined as the daily, consistent, close relationships such as home, child care, school, friends, and neighbors. For the child with a chronic illness requiring regular care, the healthcare providers may even be part of the microsystem. In the ecologic model, the child influences each of these settings in addition to being influenced by them, with reciprocal interactions.

Mesosystem. This level includes relationships of microsystems with one another. For example, two microsystems for most children are the home and the school. The relationships between these microsystems are shown by parents' involvement in their children's school. This involvement, in

● **FIGURE 33–3**

Chronosystem
Patterning of environmental events and transitions over the life course of the individual and the historical events of a particular time

Macrosystem
Attitudes and ideologies of the culture

Exosystem

Mesosystem

Microsystem

The individual

1929

Depression

Mass media

Parents' workplace

School

Family

Community centers

Famine

Values

War

Extended family

Religious group

Peers

Legal services

Medical advances

Social welfare services

Friends of family

Laws

Health services

The information age

Bronfenbrenner's ecologic theory of development views the individual as interacting within five levels or systems.

Data from Santrock, J. W. (2004). Life span development. Madison, WI: Brown & Benchmark. Based on Bronfenbrenner's (1979, 1986) works in Contexts of child rearing: Problems and prospects. American Psychologist, 34, 844–850; Ecology of the family as a context for human development: Research perspectives. Developmental Psychology, 22, 723–742.

turn, influences the effects of the home and school settings on the children.

Exosystem. This level is composed of those settings that influence the child even though the child is not in close daily contact with the system. Examples include the parents' jobs and the governing board of the local school district. Al-

though the child may not go to the parents' workplaces, he or she can be influenced by policies related to healthcare, sick leave, inflexible work hours, overtime, or travel, or even by the mood of the boss (through its impact on the parent). The child's needs may influence a parent to give up a certain job, or to work harder to obtain money for the child's education. Likewise, when a local school board votes

TABLE 33-4 ❖ Assessment of Ecologic Systems in Childhood—Bronfenbrenner

Microsystems	Mesosystems	Exosystems	Macrosystems	Chronosystems
Parents	Parents' involvement in childcare or school	Community centers	Cultural group membership	Child's age
Significant others in close contact	Parents' involvement in community	Local political influences	Beliefs and values of group	Parents' ages
Childcare arrangements	Parents' relationships with significant others (e.g., grandparents, care providers)	Parents' work	Political structure	
School		Parents' friends and activities		
Neighborhood contacts	Influences of religious community (e.g., church, synagogue, mosque) or parents and school	Social services		
Clubs		Healthcare		
Friends, peers		Libraries		
Religious community (e.g., churches, synagogues, mosques)				

to ban certain books or to finance a field trip, the child is influenced by these decisions; the child, in turn, can help establish an atmosphere that will guide future school board decisions.

Macrosystem. This level includes the beliefs, values, and behaviors expressed in the child's environment. Culture is a powerful influence in the macrosystem, as is the political system. For instance, a democratic system creates different beliefs, values, and even eating practices than an anarchic system.

Chronosystem. This final level brings the perspective of time to the previous settings. The time period during which the child grows up influences views of health and illness. For example, the experiences of children with influenza in the 19th versus 20th centuries were quite different.

Nursing Application

Nurses use ecologic theory when they assess the child's settings to identify influences on development. Table 33–4 provides an assessment tool based on this theory. Interventions are planned to enhance the strengths of the child's settings and to improve on areas that are not supportive.

TEMPERAMENT THEORY

Theoretical Framework

In contrast to behaviorists such as Watson or maturational theorists such as Piaget, Stella Chess and Alexander Thomas recognize the innate qualities of personality that each individual brings to the events of daily life. They, like Bronfenbrenner, believe the child is an individual who both influences and is influenced by the environment. However, Chess and Thomas focus on one specific aspect of development—the wide spectrum of behaviors possible in children, identifying nine parameters of response to

daily events (Table 33–5). Their theory is based on a research study entitled the New York Longitudinal Study, which began with infants in 1956 and has continued into the adulthood of these participating individuals. By careful observations of responses to life events, Chess and Thomas identified characteristics of personality that provide the

TABLE 33-5 ❖ Nine Parameters of Personality

1. **Activity level.** The degree of motion during eating, playing, sleeping, bathing. Scored as high, medium, or low.
2. **Rhythmicity.** The regularity of schedule maintained for sleep, hunger, elimination. Scored as regular, variable, or irregular.
3. **Approach or withdrawal.** The response to a new stimulus such as a food, activity, or person. Scored as approachable, variable, or withdrawn.
4. **Adaptability.** The degree of adaptation to new situations. Scored as adaptive, variable, or nonadaptive.
5. **Threshold of responsiveness.** The intensity of stimulation needed to elicit a response to sensory input, objects in the environment, or people. Scored as high, medium, or low.
6. **Intensity of reaction.** The degree of response to situations. Scored as positive, variable, or negative.
7. **Quality of mood.** The predominant mood during daily activity and in response to stimuli. Scored as positive, variable, or negative.
8. **Distractibility.** The ability of environmental stimuli to interfere with the child's activity. Scored as distractible, variable, or nondistractible.
9. **Attention span and persistence.** The amount of time devoted to activities (compared with other children of the same age) and the degree of ability to stick with an activity in spite of obstacles. Scored as persistent, variable, or nonpersistent.

Data from Chess, S., & Thomas, A. (1996). *Temperament: Theory and practice.* Philadelphia: Brunner/Mazel, div. of Taylor & Francis.

 MediaLink Developing Values in Adolescence

TABLE 33–6 ✤ Patterns of Temperament

The "easy" child is generally moderate in activity; shows regularity in patterns of eating, sleeping, and elimination; and is usually positive in mood and when subjected to new stimuli. The easy child adapts to new situations and is able to accept rules and work well with others. About 40% of children in the New York Longitudinal Study displayed this personality type.

The "difficult" child displays irregular schedules for eating, sleeping, and elimination; adapts slowly to new situations and persons; and displays a predominantly negative mood. Intense reactions to the environment are common. About 10% of children in the New York Longitudinal Study displayed this personality type.

The "slow-to-warm-up" child has reactions of mild intensity and slow adaptability to new situations. The child displays initial withdrawal followed by gradual, quiet, and slow interaction with the environment. About 15% of children in the New York Longitudinal Study displayed this personality type.

The remaining 35% of children studied showed some characteristics of each personality type (Chess & Thomas, 1995).

basis for the study on temperament. Infants generally display clusters of responses, which are classified into three major personality types (Table 33–6). Although most children do not demonstrate all behaviors described for a particular type, they usually show a grouping indicative of one personality type (Chess & Thomas, 1995, 1996).

Recent research demonstrates that personality characteristics displayed during infancy are often consistent with those seen later in life. Predicting future characteristics is not possible, however, because of the complex and dynamic interaction of personality traits and environmental reactions.

Many other researchers have expanded the work of Chess and Thomas, developing assessment tools for temperament types. The concept of "goodness of fit" is an outgrowth of this theory. Goodness of fit refers to whether parents' expectations of their child's behavior are consistent with the child's temperament type. There is a "good fit" when the properties of the environment are in accord with the child's capabilities, characteristics, and style of behavior (Chess & Thomas, 1999; Turecki, 2003). For example, an infant who is very active and reacts strongly to verbal stimuli may be unable to sleep well when placed in a room with older siblings. A child who is slow to warm up may not perform well in the first few months at a new school, much to the parents' disappointment. When parents understand a child's temperament characteristics, they are better able to shape the environment to meet the child's needs.

Nursing Application

The concept of personality type or temperament is a useful one for nurses (Melvin, 1995). Nurses can assess the tem-

perament of young children and alter the environment to meet their needs. This may involve moving a hospitalized child to a single room to ensure adequate rest if the child is easily stimulated, or allowing a shy child time to become accustomed to new surroundings and equipment before beginning procedures or treatments.

Parents are often relieved to learn about temperament characteristics. They learn to appreciate their children's qualities and to adapt the environment to meet the children's needs. A burden of guilt can also be lifted from parents who feel that they are responsible for their child's actions. Teach parents ways of enhancing goodness of fit between the child's personality and the environment (Table 33–7).

RESILIENCY THEORY

Theoretical Framework

Why do some children coming from similar backgrounds have such different behavioral outcomes? The resiliency theory examines both the individual's characteristics as well as the interaction of these characteristics with the environment. **Resilience** is the ability to function with healthy responses, even when faced with significant stress and adversity (Stewart, Reid, & Mangham, 1997). In this model the individual or family members experience a crisis that provides a source of stress, and the family interprets or deals with the crisis based on resources available. Families and individuals have **protective factors**, which are characteristics that provide strength and assistance in dealing with crises, and **risk factors**, which are characteristics that promote or contribute to their challenges. Risk and protective factors can be identified in children, in their families, and in their communities (see Chapter 36 for fur-

TABLE 33–7 ✤ Ways to Improve Goodness of Fit Between Parents and Child

Child's Behavior	Parent's Activity
Extremely active	Plan periods of active play several times a day. Have restful periods before bedtime to foster sleep.
Shy	Allow time to adapt at own pace to new people and situations.
Easily stimulated	Have quiet room for sleeping for an infant. Have quiet room for homework for a school-age child.
Short attention span	Provide projects that can be completed in a short period. Gradually encourage longer periods at activities.

TABLE 33–8 ✤ Components of Resiliency Model

Component	Meaning	Example
A = Crisis event or health challenge	Nature of healthcare challenge	Parent leaving home
V = Vulnerability; risk factors	Stresses and risks related to dealing with the health challenge	Prior abandonment; financial instability; child's developmental understanding of abandonment
T = Typology	Family methods of functioning	Reliance on extended family; parent alcoholism
B = Protective factors	Strengths for dealing with challenge	Child's desire to succeed in school; positive role modeling of maternal grandparents
C = Appraisal	Family's interpretation of crisis event	Abandonment by loved one; inability to trust others
PS = Problem solving or coping techniques	Skills that help family work toward solution	Use of community resources; acceptance of school and community counselors; child's involvement in classroom activities
X = Response	Positive or negative response to tension created by the health challenge	Remaining parent using counseling available; child identifying with a teacher in school; establishment of sense of mutual interdependence among remaining family members

Data from Malone, J. A. (1998). The resiliency model of family stress, adjustment, and adaptation. In B. Vaughn-Cole, M. A. Johnson, J. A. Malone, & B. L. Walker, *Family nursing practice*. Philadelphia: W. B. Saunders, p. 52. Adapted.

ther description of the interplay of social and environmental factors with individual characteristics ∞). A crisis for a young child might be a transfer to a new childcare provider. Protective factors could involve past positive experiences with new people, an "easy" temperament, and awareness of the new childcare provider about adaptation needs of young children to new experiences. Risk factors for a similar child might be repeated moves to new care providers, limited close relationships with adults, and a "slow-to-warm-up" temperament.

Once confronted by a crisis, the child and family first experience the **adjustment phase**, characterized by disorganization and unsuccessful attempts at meeting the crisis. In the **adaptation phase**, the child and family meet the challenge and use resources to deal with the crisis (Malone, 1998). Adaptation may lead to increasing resilience as well when the child and family learn about new resources and inner strengths and develop the ability to deal more effectively with future crises. The model and examples are described in Table 33–8.

Nursing Application

Nurses gather information about the individual characteristics, prior life experiences, and environmental factors that act as protective and risk factors for children. Table 33–9 lists questions that can be helpful as the nurse gathers information from a child or family members. Nurses then use concepts of resiliency theory in planning interventions for children and families. Nursing strategies can target risk factors, such as encouraging gun

safety by teaching about use of gun trigger locks and locked gun cabinets in families with firearms. In addition, protective factors can be emphasized, such as encouraging holding and verbalization to parents of infants to provide an environment that meets needs for trust establishment and speech development.

TABLE 33–9 ✤ Assessment Questions to Determine Resilience Capability

Questions to determine risk factors:

- Describe the event that occurred and what it has been like for your family.
- What other stressors do you have in your family right now?
- Are there financial worries?
- Are there things you think and worry about late at night?
- Describe your job, your friends.
- What is a typical day like?
- Describe your neighborhood.
- Do you have friends, people to call in emergencies?

Questions to determine protective factors:

- What gives you strength?
- How do you deal with this stress?
- What do you think you do well in your family?
- Who do you call when you need help?
- Do you have a computer? Internet access?
- Are you religious? Spiritual?
- Do you exercise regularly?
- How do you spend free time?

INFLUENCES ON DEVELOPMENT

Both nature and nurture are important in determining individual patterns of development. The interaction of these two forces can explain differences in time frames for acquisition of developmental skills, personality variations between identical twins, and other unique characteristics of individuals. Genetic and environmental factors interact and contribute to individual differences in rates and outcomes of child development. Several of these influences are discussed in this section.

Genetic inheritance plays an important part in the child's potential and the unfolding of developmental milestones. Each child inherits 23 chromosomes from the mother's egg and 23 from the father's sperm, resulting in a unique individual with 46 chromosomes. Two of these are **sex chromosomes**, and determine the child's gender; the rest are called **autosomal chromosomes**, and govern all remaining characteristics.

Every chromosome carries many genes that determine physical characteristics, intellectual potential, personality type, and other traits. Children are born with the potential for certain features; however, their interaction with the environment influences how and to what extent particular traits are manifested. See Chapter 7 for further discussion of genetic transmission and health-related conditions. ∞

Some Asian cultures calculate age from the time of conception. This practice acknowledges the profound influence of the prenatal period. The mother's nutrition and general state of health play a part in pregnancy outcome. Poor nutrition can lead to small infants and infants with compromised neurologic performance, slow development, or impaired immune status with resultant high disease rates. Low maternal stores of iron can result in anemia in the infant (American Academy of Pediatrics, 2004). Maternal smoking is associated with low-birth-weight infants. Ingestion of alcoholic beverages, including beer and wine, during pregnancy may lead to fetal alcohol syndrome (Figure 33–4 ◉). Illicit drug use by the mother may result in neonatal addiction, convulsions, hyperirritability, poor social responsiveness, and other neurologic disturbances.

Even prescription or over-the-counter drugs may adversely affect the fetus. This was brought to general attention with the drug thalidomide, commonly used in Europe to treat nausea during the 1950s. This drug resulted in the birth of infants with limb abnormalities to women who used the drug during pregnancy. Differences in physiology related to gastric emptying, renal clearance, drug distribution, and other factors contribute to variations in pharmacokinetics during pregnancy. Drugs can cause teratogenesis (abnormal development of the fetus) or mutagenesis (permanent changes in the fetus' genetic material) (McCarter-Spaulding, 2005). The U.S. Food

◉ FIGURE 33–4

Fetal alcohol syndrome.

Used with permission from Dr. Sterling Clarren, Seattle, WA. Clarren, S. K., & Smith, D. W. (1978). The fetal alcohol syndrome. New England Journal of Medicine, 298, 1063–1067. Copyright 1978, Massachusetts Medical Society. All rights reserved.

and Drug Administration (FDA) has established risk categories for drugs in pregnancy (Table 33–10).

Some maternal illnesses are harmful to the developing fetus. An example is rubella (German measles), which is rarely a serious disease for adults but which can cause deafness, vision defects, heart defects, and mental retardation in the fetus if it is acquired by a pregnant woman. A fetus can also acquire diseases such as acquired immunodeficiency syndrome (AIDS)/human immunodeficiency virus (HIV) infection or hepatitis B from the mother.

Radiation, chemicals, and other environmental hazards may adversely affect a fetus when the mother is exposed to these influences during her pregnancy. The best outcomes for infants occur when mothers eat well; exercise regularly; seek early prenatal care; refrain from use of drugs, alcohol, tobacco, and excessive caffeine; and follow general principles of good health.

As we have seen, both nature and nurture are important in determining individual patterns of development. These two forces interact in unique ways in each individual, explaining differences in time frames for acquisition of developmental skills among children, personality variations between identical twins, and other unique characteristics of individuals. An environmental factor that is extremely important in the development of children is the profile of family characteristics. The family is an important

TABLE 33–10 ✤ FDA Pregnancy Categories for Drugs

Category A—controlled studies with humans have not demonstrated a risk of the drug to the fetus

Category B—controlled studies with animals have not demonstrated a risk of the drug to the fetus

Category C—animal studies have found adverse effects of the drug on the fetus and there are no controlled studies with humans, or no animal or human studies are available; drug is used only if benefit justifies the potential risk

Category D—there is evidence of risk to the fetus in humans; drug may be used in life-threatening situations or to treat a serious disease

Category X—animal and/or human studies have shown harm to the fetus from the drug that outweighs any potential benefit; drug is contraindicated in pregnancy

component in the lives of all children and plays an essential role in fostering the development of youth. A significant concept in families is that of parenting. How children are parented interacts with their individual characteristics to influence risk and protective factors, personality characteristics, and developmental outcomes. Chapter 38 discusses types of families, frameworks used to understand families, the roles of families in fostering the development of children, and types of parenting styles. ∞

The families into which children are born influence them profoundly. Children are supported in different ways and acquire different world views depending on such factors as whether one or both parents work, how many siblings are present, and whether an extended family is close by. Note should be made of variations in family structure such as single parent, homosexual parents, extended family, and stepparents. How might a nontraditional "family" setting, such as an adoptive home with many children, influence a child's development?

Another factor that influences child development is that of culture. The traditional customs of the many cultural groups represented in North American society influence the development of the children in these groups. Foods commonly eaten vary among people with different cultural backgrounds and influence the incidence of health problems such as cardiovascular disease in these groups. The Native American practice of carrying infants on boards often delays walking when measured against the norm for walking on some developmental tests. Children who are carried by straddling the mother's hips or back for extended periods have a low incidence of developmental

dysplasia of the hip since this keeps their hips in an abducted position. It is important for nurses to take cultural practices into account when performing developmental screening; some tests may not be culturally sensitive and can inaccurately label a child as delayed when the pattern of development is simply different in the group, perhaps due to childrearing practices in the family. In addition, certain groups are more prone to develop certain diseases due to genetic variations (Table 33–11).

All cultural groups have rules regarding patterns of social interaction. Schedules of language acquisition are determined by the number of languages spoken and the amount of speech in the home. The particular social roles assumed by men and women in the culture affect school activities and ultimately career choices. Attitudes toward touching and other methods of encouraging developmental skills vary among cultures. Beginning on page 1029, Chapter 36 includes further description of other factors that influence child development such as school and child care, community services, and additional community and family factors. ∞

TABLE 33–11 ✤ Diseases and Conditions More Common among Cultural Groups

African Americans
Sickle cell disease
Hypertension
Stomach and esophageal cancer
Lactose intolerance

Asians/Pacific Islanders
Hypertension
Stomach and liver cancer
Lactose intolerance
Thalassemia

American Indians/ Aleuts/Eskimos
Diabetes
Ear infections
Accidents and suicides
Cirrhosis of the liver
Overweight

Hispanic Americans
Diabetes
Overweight
Lactose intolerance

Jews
Tay-Sachs disease
Niemann-Pick disease
Werdnig-Hoffman disease

Mediterraneans
G6PD deficiency
β-Thalassemia
Familial Mediterranean fever

United Kingdom
Cystic fibrosis
Phenylketonuria
Hereditary amyloidosis
Hyperhomocystinemia

Used with permission from Jarvis, C. (2000). *Physical examination and health assessment* (3rd ed.). Philadelphia: WB Saunders; and Spector, R. (2000). *Guides to heritage assessment and health traditions.* Upper Saddle River, NJ: Prentice Hall Health. Adapted.

INFANT (BIRTH TO 1 YEAR)

Imagine the experience of tripling body weight in 1 year, or becoming proficient in understanding fundamental words in a new language and even speaking a few. These and many more accomplishments take place in the first year of life. Starting the year as a mainly reflexive creature, the infant can walk and communicate by the year's end. Never again in life is development so swift.

PHYSICAL GROWTH AND DEVELOPMENT

The first year of life is one of rapid change for the infant. The birth weight usually doubles by about 5 months and triples by the end of the first year (Figure 33–5 ●). Height increases by about a foot during this year. Teeth begin to erupt at about 6 months, and by the end of the first year the infant has six to eight deciduous teeth (see Chapter 35 ∞). Physical growth is closely associated with type and quality of feeding (see Chapter 34 for a discussion of nutrition in infancy ∞).

Body organs and systems, although not fully mature at 1 year, function differently than they did at birth. Kidney and liver maturation helps the 1-year-old excrete drugs or other toxic substances more readily than in the first weeks of life. The changing body proportions mirror changes in developing internal organs. Maturation of the nervous system is demonstrated by increased control over body movements with growing differentiation from general to specific skills, thus enabling the infant to sit, stand, and walk. Sensory function also increases as the infant begins to discriminate visual images, sounds, and tastes (Table 33–12).

COGNITIVE DEVELOPMENT

The brain continues to increase in complexity during the first year. Most of the growth involves maturation of cells, with only a small increase in number of cells. This growth of the brain is accompanied by development of its functions. One has only to compare the behavior of an infant shortly after birth with that of a 1-year-old to understand the incredible maturation of brain function. The newborn's eyes widen in response to sound; the 1-year-old turns to the sound and recognizes its significance. The 2-month-old cries and coos; the 1-year-old says a few words and understands many more. The 6-week-old grasps a rattle for the first time; the 1-year-old reaches for toys and feeds himself or herself.

The infant's behaviors provide clues about thought processes. Piaget's work outlines the infant's actions in a set of rapidly progressing changes in the first year of life. The infant receives stimulation through sight, sound, and feeling, which the maturing brain interprets. This input from the environment interacts with internal cognitive abilities to enhance cognitive functioning.

COMPLEMENTARY CARE

INFANT MASSAGE

Infant massage is a technique for communicating with and soothing infants. This technique has been used in many cultures throughout history, but it is not traditional within most families in the United States and Canada. It has many benefits for both infants and parents and can be taught to families who are interested. Some of the benefits for babies include improved sleep, soothability, and decreased stress hormones. Premature infants have been shown to have enhanced growth and motor ability (Field, 2002; Mainous, 2003). Massage periods of 10 to 15 minutes daily can be encouraged and facilitated. Such episodes will enhance bonding and attachment between parents and infant.

● **FIGURE 33–5**

Body proportions at various ages.

| 3 mo. fetus | Newborn | 2 yr | 5 yr | 13 yr | Adult |

TABLE 33–12 ❖ Physical Growth and Development Milestones During Infancy

Age	Physical Growth	Fine Motor Ability	Gross Motor Ability	Sensory Ability
Birth to 1 month	Gains 140–200 g (5–7 oz)/week Grows 1.5 cm (1/2 in.) in first month Head circumference increases 1.5 cm (1/2 in.)/month	Holds hand in fist (**A**) Draws arms and legs to body when crying	Inborn reflexes such as startle and rooting are predominant activity May lift head briefly if prone (**B**) Alerts to high-pitched voices Comforts with touch (**C**)	Prefers to look at faces and black-and-white geometric designs Follows objects in line of vision (**D**)
2–4 months	Gains 140–200 g (5–7 oz)/week Grows 1.5 cm (1/2 in.)/month Head circumference increases 1.5 cm (1/2 in.)/month Posterior fontanelle closes Eats 120 mL/kg/24 hr (2 oz/lb/24 hr)	Holds rattle when placed in hand (**E**) Looks at and plays with own fingers Readily brings objects from hand to mouth	Moro reflex fading in strength Can turn from side to back and then return (**F**) Decrease in head lag when pulled to sitting; sits with head held in midline with some bobbing When prone, holds head and supports weight on forearms (**G**)	Follows objects 180 degrees Turns head to look for voices and sounds

A Holds hand in fist

B May lift head

C Comforts with touch

D Follows objects

E Holds rattle

F Can turn from side to back

G Holds head up and supports weight with arms

(continued)

TABLE 33–12 ✣ **Physical Growth and Development Milestones During Infancy—continued**

Age	Physical Growth	Fine Motor Ability	Gross Motor Ability	Sensory Ability
4–6 months	Gains 140-200 g (5-7 oz)/week Doubles birth weight 5-6 months Grows 1.5 cm (1/2 in.)/month Head circumference increases 1.5 cm (1/2 in.)/month Teeth may begin erupting by 6 months Eats 100 mL/kg/24 hr (1 1/2 oz/lb/24 hr)	Grasps rattles and other objects at will; drops them to pick up another offered object (*H*) Mouths objects Holds feet and pulls to mouth Holds bottle Grasps with whole hand (palmar grasp) Manipulates objects (*I*)	Head held steady when sitting No head lag when pulled to sitting Turns from abdomen to back by 4 months and then back to abdomen by 6 months When held standing supports much of own weight (*J*)	Examines complex visual images Watches the course of a falling object Responds readily to sounds

H Grasps objects at will

I Manipulates objects

J Supports most of weight when held standing

Age	Physical Growth	Fine Motor Ability	Gross Motor Ability	Sensory Ability
6–8 months	Gains 85-140 g (3-5 oz)/week Grows 1 cm (3/8 in.)/month Growth rate slower than first 6 months	Bangs objects held in hands Transfers objects from one hand to the other Beginning pincer grasp at times	Most inborn reflexes extinguished Sits alone steadily without support by 8 months (*K*) Likes to bounce on legs when held in standing position	Recognizes own name and responds by looking and smiling Enjoys small and complex objects at play

K Sits alone without support

TABLE 33–12 ✤ Physical Growth and Development Milestones During Infancy—continued

Age	Physical Growth	Fine Motor Ability	Gross Motor Ability	Sensory Ability
8–10 months	Gains 85–140 g (3–5 oz)/week Grows 1 cm (3/8 in.)/month	Picks up small objects (**L**) Uses pincer grasp well (**M**)	Crawls or pulls whole body along floor by arms (**N**) Creeps by using hands and knees to keep trunk off floor Pulls self to standing and sitting by 10 months Recovers balance when sitting	Understands words such as "no" and "cracker" May say one word in addition to "mama" and "dada" Recognizes sound without difficulty

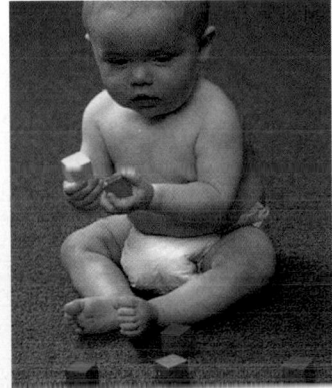

L Picks up small objects

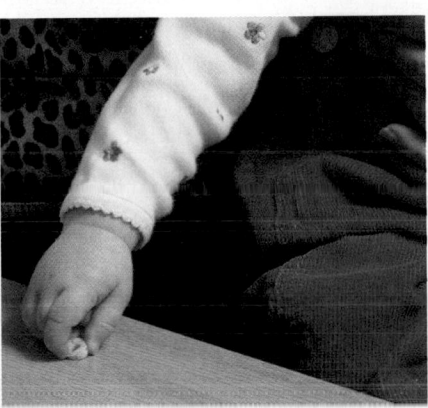

M Uses pincer grasp well

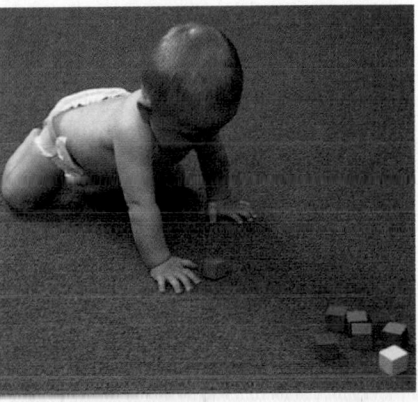

N Crawls or pulls body by arms

Age	Physical Growth	Fine Motor Ability	Gross Motor Ability	Sensory Ability
10–12 months	Gains 85–140 g (3–5 oz)/week Grows 1 cm (3/8 in.)/month Head circumference equals chest circumference Triples birth weight by 1 year	May hold crayon or pencil and make mark on paper Places objects into containers through holes (**P**)	Stands alone (**Q**) Walks holding onto furniture Sits down from standing (**R**)	Plays peek-a-boo and patty cake

P Places objects in container through holes

Q Stands alone

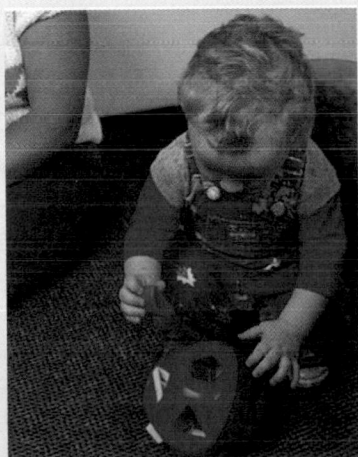

R Sits down from standing

PLAY

An 8-month-old infant is sitting on the floor, grasping blocks and banging them on the floor. Infants spend much of their time engaging in **solitary play**, or playing by themselves. When a parent walks by, the infant laughs and waves hands and feet wildly. Physical capabilities enable the infant to move toward and reach out for objects of interest. Cognitive ability is reflected in manipulation of the blocks to create different sounds. Social interaction enhances play. The presence of a parent or other person increases interest in surroundings and teaches the infant different ways to play.

The play of infants begins in a reflexive manner. When an infant moves extremities or grasps objects, the foundations of play are established. The feel and sound of these activities give pleasure to the infant, who gradually performs them purposefully. For example, when a parent places a rattle in the hand of a 6-week-old infant, the infant grasps it reflexively. As the hands move randomly, the rattle makes an enjoyable sound. The infant learns to move the rattle to create the sound and then finally to grasp the rattle at will to play with it.

The next phase of infant play focuses on manipulative behavior. The infant examines toys closely, looking at them, touching them, and placing them in the mouth. The infant learns a great deal about texture, qualities of objects, and all aspects of the surroundings. At the same time, interaction with others becomes an important part of play. The social nature of play is obvious as the infant plays with other children and adults.

Toward the end of the first year, the infant's ability to move in space enlarges the sphere of play (Table 33–12). Once the infant is crawling or walking, he or she can get to new places, find new toys, discover forgotten objects, or seek out other people for interaction. Play is a reflection of every aspect of development, as well as a method for enhancing learning and maturation.

PERSONALITY AND TEMPERAMENT

Why does one infant frequently awaken at night crying while another sleeps for 8 to 10 hours undisturbed? Why does one infant smile much of the time and react positively to interactions while another is withdrawn with unfamiliar people and frequently frowns and cries? Such differences in responses to the environment are believed to be inborn characteristics of temperament. Infants are born with a tendency to react in certain ways to noise and to interact differently with people. They may display varying degrees of regularity in activities of eating and sleeping, and manifest a capacity for concentrating on tasks for different amounts of time.

Nursing assessment identifies personality characteristics of the infant that the nurse can share with the parents. With this information the parents can appreciate more fully the uniqueness of their infant and design experiences to meet the infant's needs. Parents can learn to modify the environment to promote adaptation. For example, an infant who does not adapt easily to new situations may cry, withdraw, or develop another way of coping when adjusting to new people or places. Parents might be advised to use one or two babysitters rather than engaging new sitters frequently. If the infant is easily distracted when eating, parents can feed the infant in a quiet setting to encourage a focus on eating. Although the infant's temperament is unchanged, the ability to fit with the environment is enhanced. See Chapter 37 for further application of this information to health promotion of the infant. ∞

COMMUNICATION

Even at a few weeks of age, infants communicate and engage in two-way interaction. Comfort is expressed by soft sounds, cuddling, and eye contact. The infant displays discomfort by thrashing the extremities, arching the back, and crying vigorously. From these rudimentary skills, communication ability continues to develop until the infant speaks several words at the end of the first year of life (Table 33–13).

Nurses assess communication to identify possible abnormalities or developmental delays. Language ability may be assessed with the Denver II Developmental Test and other specialized language screening tools (see Chapters 37 and 38 ∞). Normal infants understand (receptive speech) more words than they can speak (expressive speech). Abnormalities may be caused by a hearing deficit, developmental delay, or lack of verbal stimulation from caretakers. Further assessment may be required to pinpoint the cause of the abnormality.

Nursing interventions focus on providing a stimulating environment. Encourage parents to speak to infants and teach words. Hospital nurses should include the infant's known words when providing care.

GROWTH AND DEVELOPMENT

Following are strategies for communicating with the infant:

Hold for feedings.

Hold, rock, and talk to infant often.

Talk and sing frequently during care.

Tell names of objects.

Use high-pitched voice with newborns.

When the infant is upset, swaddle and hold securely.

TODDLER (1 TO 3 YEARS)

Toddlerhood is sometimes called the first adolescence. An infant only months before, the child from 1 to 3 years is now displaying independence and negativism. Pride in newfound accomplishments emerges.

PHYSICAL GROWTH AND DEVELOPMENT

The rate of growth slows during the second year of life. Parents may become concerned because the child has a limited food intake, and need reassurance that this is normal (see Chapter 34 for further discussion of nutrition in toddlerhood ∞). By age 2 years, the birth weight has usually quadrupled and the child is about one half of the adult height. Body proportions begin to change, with the legs longer and the head smaller in proportion to body size than during infancy (see Figure 33–5). The toddler has a pot-bellied appearance and stands with feet apart to provide a

TABLE 33–13 ✣ Psychosocial Development During Infancy

Age	Play and Toys	Communication
Birth–3 months	Prefers visual stimuli of mobiles, black-and-white patterns, mirrors Auditory stimuli are music boxes, tape players, soft voices Responds to rocking and cuddling Moves legs and arms while adult sings and talks Likes varying stimuli—different rooms, sounds, visual images	Coos Babbles Cries
3–6 months	Prefers noise-making objects that are easily grasped like rattles Enjoys stuffed animals and soft toys with contrasting colors	Vocalizes during play and with familiar people Laughs Cries less Squeals and makes pleasure sounds Babbles multisyllabically (mamamamama)
6–9 months	Likes teething toys Increasingly desires social interaction with adults and other children Soft toys that can be manipulated and mouthed are favorites	Increases vowel and consonant sounds Links syllables together Uses speechlike rhythm when vocalizing with others
9–12 months	Enjoys large blocks, toys that pop apart and go back together, nesting cups and other objects Laughs at surprise toys like jack-in-the-box Plays interactive games like peek-a-boo Uses push-and-pull toys	Understands "no" and other simple commands Says "dada" and "mama" to identify parents Learns one or two other words Receptive speech surpasses expressive speech

wide base of support. By approximately 33 months, eruption of deciduous teeth is complete, with 20 teeth present.

Gross motor activity develops rapidly (Table 33–14), as the toddler progresses from walking to running, kicking, and riding a Big Wheel tricycle (Figure 33–6 ◉). As physical maturation occurs, the toddler develops the ability to control elimination patterns (Table 33–15 and "Developing Cultural Competence").

DEVELOPING CULTURAL COMPETENCE

CHILDREARING PRACTICES

In traditional Native American families, children are allowed to unfold and develop naturally at their own pace. Children thus wean and toilet train themselves with little interference or pressure from parents. The nurse should be sensitive to the childrearing practices of the family and support them in these culturally accepted practices, rather than imposing a more structured approach to toilet training.

COGNITIVE DEVELOPMENT

During the toddler years, the child moves from the sensorimotor to the preoperational stage of development. The early use of language awakens in the 1-year-old the ability to think about objects or people when they are absent. Object permanence is well developed.

At about 2 years of age, the increasing use of words as symbols enables the toddler to use preoperational thought. Rudimentary problem solving, creative thought, and an understanding of cause-and-effect relationships are now possible.

TABLE 33–14 ✣ Growth and Development Milestones During Toddlerhood

Age	Physical Growth	Fine Motor Ability	Gross Motor Ability	Sensory Ability
1–2 years	Gains 227 g (8 oz) or more per month Grows 9–12 cm (3.5–5 in.) during this year Anterior fontanelle closes	By end of 2nd year, builds a tower of four blocks (**A**) Scribbles on paper (**B**) Can undress self (**C**) Throws a ball	Runs Walks up and down stairs (**E**) Likes push and pull toys (**F**)	Visual acuity 20/50
2–3 years	Gains 1.4–2.3 kg (3–5 lb)/year Grows 5–6.5 cm (2–2.5 in.)/year	Draws a circle and other rudimentary forms Learns to pour Learning to dress self (**D**)	Jumps Kicks ball Throws ball overhand	

A Second year tower of four blocks

B Scribbles on paper

C Can undress self

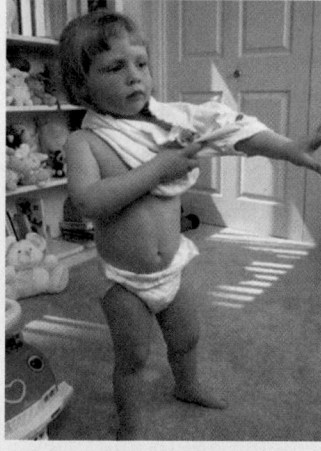

D Learning to dress self

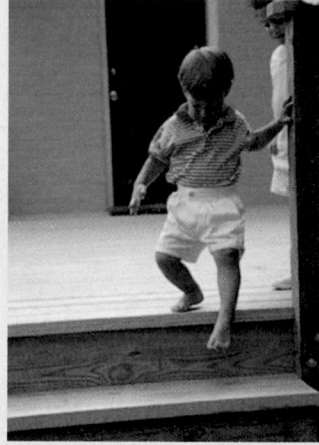

E Walks up and down stairs

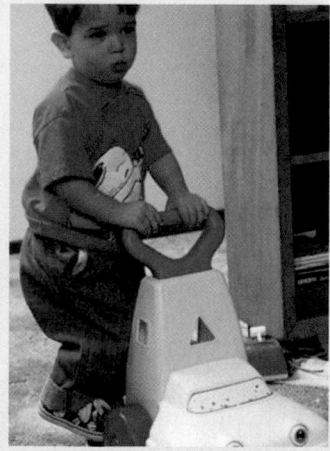

F Likes push and pull toys

PLAY

Many changes in play patterns occur between infancy and toddlerhood. The toddler's motor skills enable him or her to bang pegs into a pounding board with a hammer, for example. The social nature of toddler play is also readily seen. Toddlers find the company of other children pleasurable, even though socially interactive play may not occur. Two toddlers tend to play with similar objects side by side, occasionally trading toys and words. This is called **parallel play**. This playtime with other children helps toddlers develop social skills. Toddlers engage in play activities they have seen at home, such as pounding with a hammer and talking on the phone. This imitative behavior teaches them new actions and skills.

Physical skills are manifested in play as toddlers push and pull objects, climb in and out and up and down, run, ride a Big Wheel, turn the pages of books, and scribble with a pen. Both gross motor and fine motor abilities are enhanced during this age period.

Cognitive understanding enables the toddler to manipulate objects and learn about their qualities. Stacking blocks and placing rings on a building tower teach spatial

● **FIGURE 33–6**

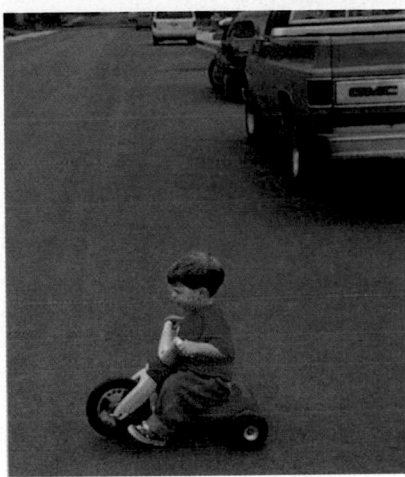

This toddler has learned to ride a Big Wheel, which he is doing right into the street. Toddlers must be closely watched to prevent injury.

relationships and other lessons that provide a foundation for future learning. Various kinds of play objects should be provided for the toddler to meet play needs. These play needs can easily be met whether the child is hospitalized or at home (Table 33–16).

PERSONALITY AND TEMPERAMENT

The toddler retains most of the temperamental characteristics identified during infancy but may demonstrate some changes. The normal developmental progression of toddlerhood also plays a part in responses. For example, the infant who previously responded positively to stimuli, such as a new babysitter, may appear more negative in toddlerhood. The increasing independence characteristic of this age is shown by the toddler's use of the word "no." The parent and child constantly adapt their responses to each other and learn anew how to communicate with each other.

COMMUNICATION

Because of the phenomenal growth of language skills during the toddler period, adults should communicate frequently with children in this age group. Toddlers imitate words and speech intonations, as well as the social interactions they observe.

At the beginning of toddlerhood, the child may use four to six words in addition to "mama" and "dada." Receptive speech (the ability to understand words) far outpaces expressive speech. By the end of toddlerhood, however, the 3-year-old has a vocabulary of almost 1000 words and uses short sentences.

Communication occurs in many ways, some of which are nonverbal. Toddler communication includes pointing, pulling an adult over to a room or object, and speaking in expressive jargon. **Expressive jargon** is using unintelligible words with normal speech intonations as if truly communicating in words. Another communication method occurs when the toddler cries, pounds feet, displays a temper tantrum, or uses other means to illustrate dismay. These powerful communication methods can upset parents, who often need suggestions for handling them. It is best to verbalize the feelings shown by the toddler, for example, by saying, "You must be very upset that you cannot have that

TABLE 33–15 ❖ Toilet Training

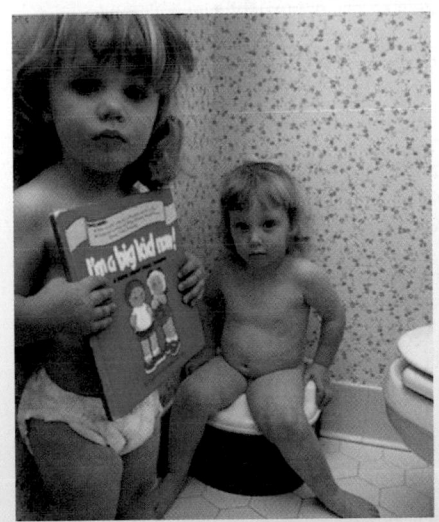

When are children ready to learn toileting? Are parents responsible for the differences in ages at which toilet training is accomplished? Does toilet training provide clues to a child's intellectual ability?

We know that children are not ready for toilet training until several developmental capabilities exist: to stand and walk well, to pull pants up and down, to recognize the need to eliminate and then to be able to wait until in the bathroom. Once this readiness is apparent, the child can be given a small potty chair and the procedure explained.

Children often prefer their own chair on the floor to using the large toilet. The child should be placed on the chair at regular intervals for a few moments and can be given reward or praise for successes. If the child seems not to understand or does not wish to cooperate, it is best to wait a few weeks and then try again. Just as all of development is subject to individual timetables, toilet training occurs with considerable variability from one child to another. Identify for parents the developmental characteristics of their child and encourage them to appreciate without anxiety the unfolding of skills. These timetables are not predictive of future development.

The child who is ill or hospitalized or has other stress often regresses in toilet-training activities. It is best to quietly reinstitute attempts at training after the trauma. Potty chairs should be available on pediatric units and toileting habits identified during initial assessment so that regular routines can be followed and the child's usual words for elimination can be used.

TABLE 33–16 ✧ Psychosocial Development During Toddlerhood

Age	Play and Toys	Communication
1–3 years 	Refines fine motor skills by use of cloth books, large pencil and paper, wooden puzzles Facilitates imitative behavior by playing kitchen, grocery shopping, toy telephone Learns gross motor activities by riding Big Wheel tricycle, playing with soft ball and bat, molding water and sand, tossing ball or bean bag Cognitive skills develop by educational television shows, music, stories, and books	Increasingly enjoys talking Exponential growth of vocabulary especially when spoken and read to Needs to release stress by pounding board, frequent gross motor activities, and occasional temper tantrums Likes contact with other children and learns interpersonal skills

candy. When you stop crying you can come out of your room," and then to ignore further negative behavior. The toddler's search for autonomy and independence creates a need for such behavior. Sometimes an upset toddler responds well to holding, rocking, and stroking.

GROWTH AND DEVELOPMENT

Following are strategies for communicating with the toddler:

Give short, clear instructions.

Do not give choices if none exist.

Offer a choice of two alternatives when possible.

Approach positively and slowly, allowing time for the toddler to adjust.

Tell toddler what you are doing, and say the names of objects.

Parents and nurses can promote a toddler's communication by speaking frequently, naming objects, explaining procedures in simple terms, expressing feelings that the toddler seems to be displaying, and encouraging speech. The toddler from a bilingual home is at an optimal age to learn two languages. If the parents do not speak English, the toddler will benefit from a daycare experience in which the providers do, so that he or she can learn both languages.

The nurse who understands the communication skills of toddlers is able to assess expressive and receptive language and communicate effectively, thereby promoting positive healthcare experiences for these children (Table 33–17).

PRESCHOOL CHILD (3 TO 6 YEARS)

The preschool years are a time of new initiative and independence. Most children are in a daycare center or school for part of the day and learn a great deal from this social contact. Language skills are well developed, and the child is able to understand and speak clearly. Endless projects characterize the world of busy preschoolers. They may work with play dough to form animals, then cut out and paste paper, then draw and color.

PHYSICAL GROWTH AND DEVELOPMENT

Preschoolers grow slowly and steadily, with most growth taking place in long bones of the arms and legs. The short, chubby toddler gradually gives way to a slender, long-legged preschooler (Table 33–18).

TABLE 33–17 ✧ Communicating with a Toddler

Procedures such as drawing blood can be frightening for a toddler. Effective communication minimizes the trauma caused by such procedures:

- Avoid telling toddlers about the procedure too far in advance. They do not have an understanding of time and can become quite anxious.
- Use simple terminology. "We need to get a little blood from your arm. It will help us to find out if you are getting better." If the parent is willing, say, "Your mom will hold your arm still so we can do it quickly."
- Allow the toddler to cry. Acknowledge that it must be frightening and that you understand.
- Perform the procedure in a treatment room so that the toddler's bed and room are a safe haven.
- Be sure the toddler is restrained, with the joints above and below the procedure immobilized.
- Use a Band-Aid to cover up the site. This can reassure the toddler that the body is still intact.
- Allow the toddler to choose a reward such as a sticker after the procedure.
- Praise the toddler for cooperation and acknowledge that you know this was difficult.
- Comfort the toddler by rocking, offering a favorite drink, playing music, and holding. If parents are present, they can offer the comfort needed.

TABLE 33–18 ✤ Physical Growth and Development Milestones During the Preschool Years

Physical Growth		Fine Motor Ability
Gains 1.5–2.5 kg (3–5 lb)/year	Grows 4–6 cm (1 1/2–2 1/2 in.)/year	Uses scissors (**A**) Draws circle, square, cross (**B**) Draws at least a six-part person Enjoys art projects such as pasting, stringing beads, using clay Learns to tie shoes at end of preschool years (**C**) Buttons (**D**) Brushes teeth (**E**)

A Uses scissors

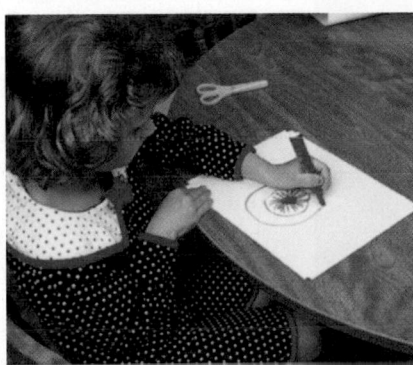

B Draws circle, square, cross

C Ties shoes

D Buttons clothes

E Brushes teeth

Gross Motor Ability	Sensory Ability	Fine Motor Ability
Throws a ball overhand Climbs well (**F**) Rides bicycle (**G**)	Visual acuity continues to improve Can focus on and learn letters and numbers (**H**)	Eats three meals with snacks Uses spoon, fork, and knife

F Climbs well

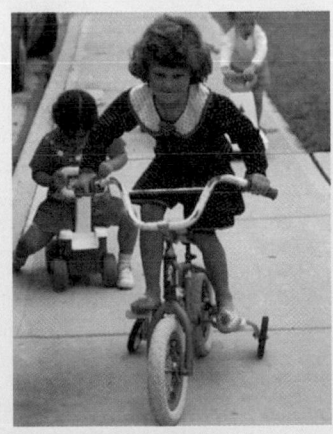

G Rides bicycle or bicycle with training wheels

H Learns letters and numbers

● **FIGURE 33–7**

Preschoolers continue to develop more advanced skills such as kicking a ball without falling down.

Physical skills continue to develop (Figure 33–7 ●). The preschooler runs with ease, holds a bat, and throws balls of various types. Writing ability increases, and the preschooler enjoys drawing and learning to write a few letters.

The preschool period is a good time to encourage good dental habits. Children can begin to brush their own teeth with parental supervision and help to reach all tooth surfaces. Parents should floss children's teeth, give fluoride as prescribed if the water supply is not fluoridated, and schedule the first dental visit so the child can become accustomed to the routine of periodic dental care.

COGNITIVE DEVELOPMENT

The preschooler exhibits characteristics of preoperational thought. Symbols or words are used to represent objects and people, enabling the young child to think about them. This is a milestone in intellectual development; however, the preschooler still has some limitations in thought (Table 33–19).

PLAY

The preschooler has begun playing in a new way. Toddlers simply play side by side with friends, each engaging in his or her own activities, but preschoolers interact with others during play. One child cuts out colored paper, for example, while her friend glues it on paper in a design. This new type of interaction is called **associative play** (Figure 33–8 ●).

In addition to this social dimension of play, other aspects of play also differ. The preschooler enjoys large motor activities such as swinging, riding a tricycle, and throwing a ball. Increasing manual dexterity is demonstrated in greater complexity of drawings and manipulation of blocks and modeling. These changes necessitate planning of playtime to include appropriate activities. Preschool programs and child life departments in hospitals help meet this important need.

Materials provided for play can be simple but should guide activities in which the child engages. Since fine motor activities are popular, paper, pens, scissors, glue, and a

TABLE 33–19 ✤ Characteristics of Preoperational Thought

Characteristic	Definition	Example
Egocentrism	Ability to see things only from one's own point of view	The child who cannot understand why parents may need to leave the hospital for work when the child wishes them to be present
Transductive reasoning	Connecting two events in a cause-effect relationship simply because they occur together in time	A child who, awakening after surgery and feeling pain, notices the intravenous infusion and believes that it is causing the pain
Centration	Focusing on only one particular aspect of a situation	The child who is concerned about breathing through an anesthesia mask and will not listen to any other aspects of preoperative teaching
Animism	Giving lifelike qualities to nonliving things	The child who views a monitoring machine as alive because it beeps

variety of other such objects should be available. The child can use them to create important images such as pictures of people, hospital beds, or friends. A collection of dolls, furniture, and clothing can be manipulated to represent parents and children, nurses and physicians, teachers, or other significant people. Because fantasy life is so powerful at this age, the preschooler readily uses props to engage in **dramatic play**, that is, the living out of the drama of human life (Figure 33–9 ⊙).

The nurse can use playtime to assess the preschool child's developmental level, knowledge about healthcare, and emotions related to healthcare experiences. Observations about objects chosen for play, content of dramatic

⊙ **FIGURE 33–8**

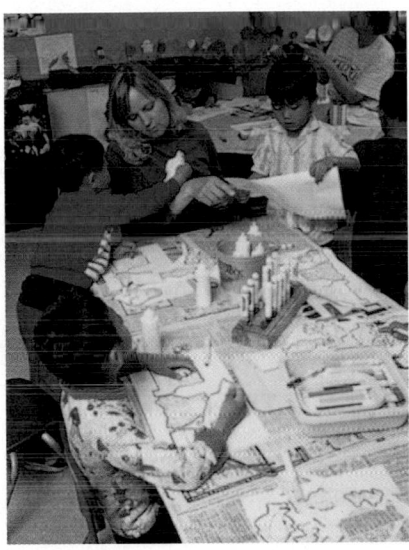

These preschoolers are participating in associative play, which means they can interact. One child is cutting out shapes, and the other is gluing them in place.

⊙ **FIGURE 33–9**

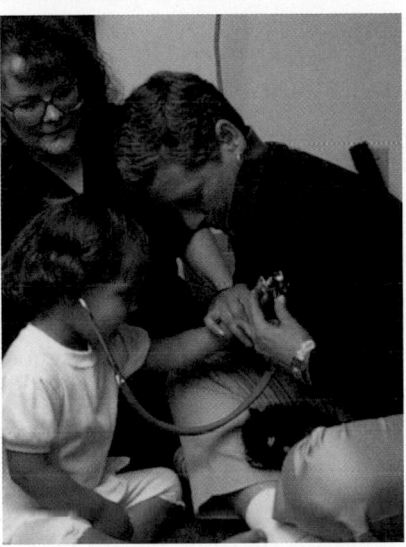

Jasmine is participating in dramatic play with a nurse while her mother looks on. In dramatic play the child uses props to play out the drama of human life. It can be an excellent way for a nurse to assess the developmental level of children while talking to them. Notice that the child and the nurse are on the floor at the same level and the atmosphere is informal. Why is it important to be at the same level as the child?

play, and pictures drawn can provide important assessment data. The nurse can also use play periods to teach the child about healthcare procedures and offer an outlet for expression of emotions (Table 33–20).

PERSONALITY AND TEMPERAMENT

Characteristics of personality observed in infancy tend to persist over time. The preschooler may need assistance as these characteristics are expressed in the new situations of preschool or nursery school. An excessively active child, for

---

TABLE 33–20 ✣ Psychosocial Development During the Preschool Years

Age	Play and Toys	Communication
3–6 years	Associative play is facilitated by simple games, puzzles, nursery rhymes, songs Dramatic play is fostered by dolls and doll clothes, play houses and hospitals, dress-up clothes, puppets Stress is relieved by pens, paper, glue, scissors Cognitive growth is fostered by educational television shows, music, stories, and books	All parts of speech are developed and used, occasionally incorrectly Communicates with a widening array of people Play with other children is a favorite activity Health professionals can ■ Verbalize and explain procedures to children ■ Use drawings and stories to explain care ■ Use accurate names for body functions ■ Allow the child to talk, ask questions, and make choices

example, will need gentle, consistent handling to adjust to the structure of a classroom. Encourage parents to visit preschool programs to choose the one that would best foster growth in their child. Some preschoolers enjoy the structured learning of a program that focuses on cognitive skills, whereas others are happier and more open to learning in a small group that provides much time for free play. Nurses can help parents to identify their child's personality or temperament characteristics and to find the best environment for growth.

COMMUNICATION

Language skills blossom during the preschool years. The vocabulary grows to over 2000 words, and children speak in complete sentences of several words and use all parts of speech. They practice these newfound language skills by endlessly talking and asking questions.

The sophisticated speech of preschoolers mirrors the development occurring in their minds and helps them to learn about the world around them. However, this speech can be quite deceptive. Although preschoolers use many words, their grasp of meaning is usually literal and may not match that of adults. These literal interpretations have important implications for healthcare providers. For example, the preschooler who is told she will be "put to sleep" for surgery may think of a pet recently euthanized; the child who is told that a dye will be injected for a diagnostic test may think he is going to die; mention of "a little stick" in the arm can cause images of tree branches rather than of a simple immunization.

The child may also have difficulty focusing on the content of a conversation. The preschooler is egocentric and may be unable to move from individual thoughts to those the nurse is proposing in a teaching situation.

GROWTH AND DEVELOPMENT

Following are strategies for communicating with the preschooler:

Allow time for child to integrate explanations.

Verbalize frequently to the child.

Use drawings and stories to explain care.

Use accurate names for body functions.

Allow choices.

Concrete visual aids such as pictures of a child undergoing the same procedure or a book to read together enhance teaching by meeting the child's developmental needs. Handling medical equipment such as intravenous bags and stethoscopes increases interest and helps the child to focus. Teaching may have to be done in several short sessions rather than one long session.

SCHOOL–AGE CHILD (6 TO 12 YEARS)

Errol, 10 years old, arrives home from school shortly after 3 p.m. each day. He immediately calls his friends and goes to visit one of them. They are building models of cars and collecting baseball cards. Endless hours are spent on these projects and on discussions of events at school that day (Figure 33–10 ●).

Nine-year-old Karen practices soccer two afternoons a week and plays in games each weekend. She also is learning to play the flute and spends her free time at home practicing. Although practice time is not her favorite part of music, Karen enjoys the performances and wants to play well in front of her friends and teacher. Her parents now allow

● FIGURE 33–10

A, School–age children may take part in activities that require practice. This is a consideration when children are hospitalized and unable to practice or perform. Why? *B,* School–age children enjoy spending time with others the same age on projects and discussing the activities of the day. This is an important consideration when they are in an acute care setting. When you are in the clinical setting, look for examples of this type of interaction taking place.

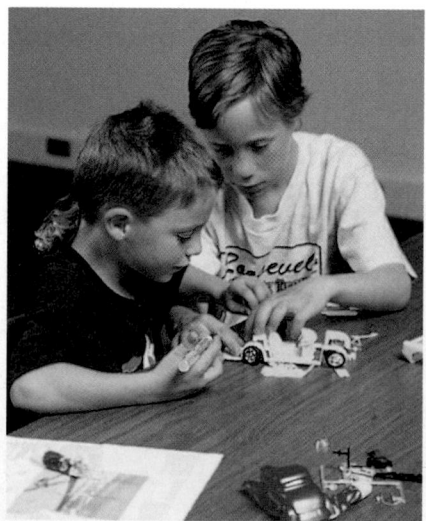

A

B

her to ride her bike unaccompanied to the store or to a friend's house.

These two school-age children demonstrate common characteristics of their age group. They are in a stage of industry in which it is important to the child to perform useful work. Meaningful activities take on great importance and are usually carried out in the company of peers. A sense of achievement in these activities is important to develop self-esteem and to prevent a sense of inferiority or poor self-worth.

PHYSICAL GROWTH AND DEVELOPMENT

School age is the last period in which girls and boys are close in size and body proportions. As the long bones continue to grow, leg length increases (see Figure 33–5). Fat gives way to muscle, and the child appears leaner. Jaw proportions change as the first deciduous tooth is lost at 6 years and permanent teeth begin to erupt. Body organs and the immune system mature, resulting in fewer illnesses among school-age children. Medications are less likely to cause serious side effects, since they can be metabolized more easily. The urinary system can adjust to changes in fluid status. Physical skills are also refined as children begin to play sports, and fine motor skills are well developed through school activities (Table 33–21 and Figure 33–11 ◉).

Although it is commonly believed that the start of adolescence (age 12 years) heralds a growth spurt, the rapid increases in size commonly occur during school age. Girls may begin a growth spurt by 9 or 10 years and boys a year or so later. Nutritional needs increase dramatically with this spurt.

The loss of the first deciduous teeth and the eruption of permanent teeth usually occur at about age 6, or at the beginning of the school-age period. Of the 30 permanent teeth, 22 to 26 erupt by age 12 and the remaining molars follow during the teenage years. The school-age child should be closely monitored to ensure that brushing and flossing are adequate, that fluoride is taken if the water supply is not fluoridated, that dental care is obtained to provide for examination of teeth and alignment, and that loose teeth are identified before surgery or other events that may lead to loss of a tooth.

COGNITIVE DEVELOPMENT

The child enters the stage of concrete operational thought at about 7 years. This stage enables school-age children to consider alternative solutions and solve problems. However, school-age children continue to rely on concrete experiences and materials to form their thought content.

During the school-age years, the child learns the concept of **conservation** (that matter is not changed when its form is altered). At earlier ages a child believes that when water is poured from a short, wide glass into a tall, thin glass, there is more water in the taller glass. The school-age

---

TABLE 33–21 ✤ Physical Growth and Development Milestones During the School-Age Years

Physical Growth	Fine Motor Ability	Gross Motor Ability	Sensory Ability
Gains 1.4–2.2 kg (3–5 lb)/year	Enjoys craft projects	Rides two-wheeler (**A**)	Can read
Grows 4–6 cm (1 1/2–2 1/2 in.)/year	Plays card and board games	Jumps rope (**B**)	Able to concentrate for longer periods on activities by filtering out surrounding sounds (**C**)
		Roller skates or ice skates	

A Rides two-wheeler   **B** Jumps rope   **C** Concentrates an activities for longer periods

● **FIGURE 33–11**

School-age girls and boys enjoy participating in sports. They begin to lose fat while developing their muscles, so they appear leaner than at earlier ages. *Left,* Front teeth are lost around age 6 years. The family may have rituals associated with the loss of teeth that could affect the child's behavior if he loses a tooth while in the hospital.

child recognizes that although it may look like the taller glass holds more water, the quantity is the same. The concept of conservation is helpful when the nurse explains medical treatments. The school-age child understands that an incision will heal, that a cast will be removed, and that an arm will look the same as before once the intravenous infusion is removed.

PLAY

When the preschool teacher tries to organize a game of baseball, both the teacher and the children become frustrated. Not only are the children physically unable to hold a bat and hit a ball, but they seem to have no understanding of the rules of the game and do not want to wait for their turn at bat. By 6 years of age, however, children have acquired the physical ability to hold the bat properly and may occasionally hit the ball. School-age children also understand that everyone has a role—the pitcher, the catcher, the batter, the outfielders. They cooperate with one another to form a team, are eager to learn the rules of the game, and want to ensure that these rules are followed exactly (Table 33–22).

The characteristics of play exhibited by the school-age child are cooperation with others and the ability to play a part in order to contribute to a unified whole. This type of play is called **cooperative play**. The concrete nature of cognitive thought leads to a reliance on rules to provide structure and security. Children have an increasing desire to spend much of playtime with friends, which demonstrates the social component of play. Play is an extremely important method of learning and living for the school-age child. Active physical play has decreased in recent years as televi-

---

TABLE 33–22 ✣ Psychosocial Development During the School-Age Years

Age	Activities	Communication
6–12 years 	Gross motor development is fostered by ball sports, skating, dance lessons, water and snow skiing/boarding, biking A sense of industry is fostered by playing a musical instrument, gathering collections, starting hobbies, playing board and video games Cognitive growth is facilitated by reading, crafts, word puzzles, school work	Mature use of language Ability to converse and discuss topics for increasing lengths of time Spends many hours at school and with friends in sports or other activities Health professionals can: ■ Assess child's knowledge before teaching ■ Allow the child to select rewards following procedures ■ Teach techniques such as counting or visualization to manage difficult situations ■ Include both parent and child in healthcare decisions

sion viewing and playing of computer games have increased, leading to poor nutritional status and a high rate of overweight among children. See Chapter 34 for further discussion of nutrition and physical activity in children. ∞

When a child is hospitalized, the separation from playmates can lead to feelings of sadness and purposelessness. School-age children often feel better when placed in multibed units with other children. Games can be devised even when children are wheelchair bound (Figure 33–12). Normal, rewarding parts of play should be integrated into care. Friends should be encouraged to visit or call a hospitalized child. Discharge planning for the child who has had a cast or brace applied should address the activities the child can engage in and those the child must avoid. Reinforce the importance of playing games with friends.

PERSONALITY AND TEMPERAMENT

The enduring aspects of temperament continue to be manifested during the school years. The child classified as "difficult" at an earlier age may now have trouble in the classroom. Advise parents to provide a quiet setting for homework and to reward the child for concentration. For example, after homework is completed, the child can watch a television show. Creative efforts and alternative methods of learning should be valued. Encourage parents to see their children as individuals who may not all learn in the same way. The "slow-to-warm-up" child may need encouragement to try new activities and to share experiences with

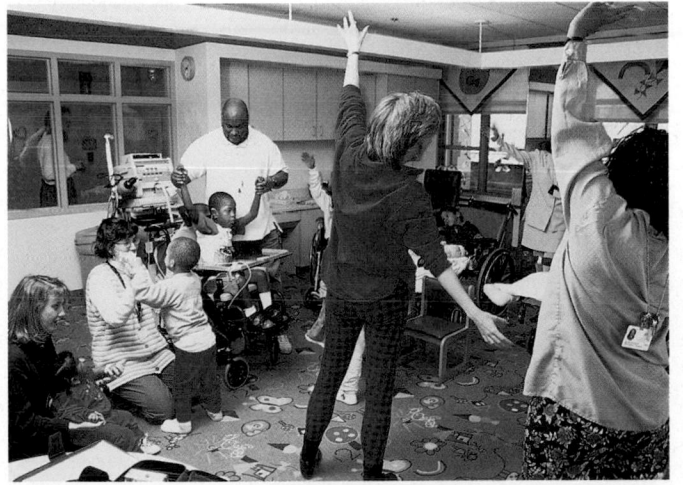

● FIGURE 33–12

The nurse can help the child and family accept and adjust to new circumstances. Encouraging the child in a wheelchair to participate in group activities can help build confidence in physical skills. Good self-esteem, goal attainment, personal satisfaction, and general health are the continued benefits.

others, while the "easy" child will readily adapt to new schools, people, and experiences.

COMMUNICATION

During the school-age years, the child should learn how to correct any lingering pronunciation or grammatical errors. Vocabulary increases, and the child is taught about parts of speech in school. School-age children enjoy writing and can be encouraged to keep a journal of their experiences while in the hospital as a method of dealing with anxiety. It is uncommon for school-age children to understand words as literally as preschoolers.

> ### GROWTH AND DEVELOPMENT
>
> Following are strategies for communicating with the school-age child:
>
> Provide concrete examples of pictures or materials to accompany verbal descriptions.
>
> Assess knowledge before planning teaching.
>
> Allow child to select rewards following procedures.
>
> Teach techniques such as counting or visualization to manage difficult situations.
>
> Include child in discussions and history with parent.
>
> Be honest in explanations and all communications.

SEXUALITY

While children become aware of sexual differences between genders during preschool years, they deal much more consciously with sexuality during school age. As children mature physically, they need information about their body changes so that they can develop a healthy self-image, and an understanding of the relationships between their bodies and sexuality. Children become interested in sexual issues and are often exposed to erroneous information on television shows, in magazines, or from friends and siblings. Schools and families need to use opportunities to teach school-age children factual information about sex, as well as fostering healthy concepts of self and others. It is advisable to ask occasional questions about sexual issues to learn how much the child knows and to provide correct information when answers demonstrate confusion. Both friends and the media are common sources of erroneous ideas. Appropriate and inappropriate touch should be discussed, with lists of trusted people who can be approached (teachers, clergy, school counselors, family members, neighbors) to discuss any episodes with which the child feels uncomfortable. Even these trusted people can be implicated in inappropriate episodes, so encourage the child to go to more than one person, an important approach if the child is uncomfortable about a relationship with any individual.

ADOLESCENT (12 TO 18 YEARS)

Adolescence is a time of passage signaling the end of childhood and the beginning of adulthood. Although adolescents differ in behaviors and accomplishments, they are in a period of identity formation. If a healthy identity and sense of self-worth are not developed in this period, role confusion and purposeless struggling will ensue. The adolescents encountered in nursing practice represent various degrees of identity formation, and each will offer unique challenges.

PHYSICAL GROWTH AND DEVELOPMENT

The physical changes ending in **puberty**, or sexual maturity, begin near the end of the school-age period. The prepubescent period is marked by a growth spurt at an average age of 10 years for girls and 13 years for boys. The increase in height and weight is generally remarkable and is completed in 2 to 3 years (Table 33–23). The growth spurt in girls is accompanied by an increase in breast size and growth of pubic hair. Menstruation occurs last and signals achievement of puberty. In boys the growth spurt is accompanied by growth in size of the penis and testes and by growth of pubic hair. Deepening of the voice and growth of facial hair occur later, at the time of puberty. See Chapter 33 for a description of the pubertal stages. ∞

During adolescence children grow stronger and more muscular and establish characteristic male and female patterns of fat distribution. The apocrine and eccrine glands mature, leading to increased sweating and a distinct odor to perspiration. All body organs are now fully mature, enabling the adolescent to take adult doses of medications.

The adolescent must adapt to a rapidly changing body for several years. These physical changes and hormonal variations offer challenges to identity formation.

COGNITIVE DEVELOPMENT

Adolescence marks the beginning of Piaget's last stage of cognitive development, the stage of formal operational thought. The adolescent no longer depends on concrete experiences as the basis of thought but develops the ability to reason abstractly. Such concepts as justice, truth, beauty, and power can be understood. The adolescent revels in this newfound ability and spends a great deal of time thinking, reading, and talking about abstract concepts.

The ability to think and act independently leads many adolescents to rebel against parental authority. Through these actions, adolescents seek to establish their own identity and values.

ACTIVITIES

Maturity leads to new activities. Adolescents may drive, ride buses, or bike independently. They are less dependent on parents for transportation and spend more time with

---

TABLE 33–23 ✛ **Physical Growth and Development Milestones During Adolescence**

Physical Growth	Fine Motor Ability	Gross Motor Ability	Sensory Ability
Variation in age of growth spurt During growth spurt, girls gain 7–25 kg (15–55 lb) and grow 2.5–20 cm (2–8 in.); boys gain approximately 7–29.5 kg (15–65 lb) and grow 11–30 cm (4 1/2–12 in.)	Skills are well developed (**A**)	New sports activities attempted and muscle development continues (**B**) Some lack of coordination common during growth spurt	Fully developed

A Skills are well developed

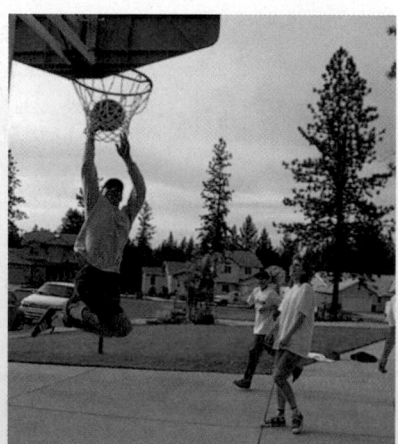

B New sports activities attempted

TABLE 33–24 ✤ **Psychosocial Development During Adolescence**

Age	Activities	Communication
12–18 years 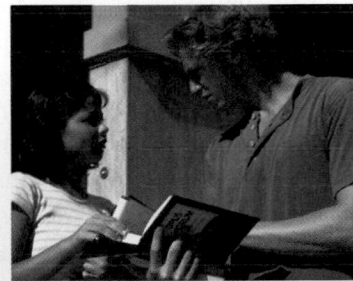	Sports—ball games, gymnastics, water and snow skiing/boarding, swimming, school sports School activities—drama, yearbook, class office, club participation Quiet activities—reading, school work, television, computer, video games, music	Increasing communication and time with peer group—movies, dances, driving, eating out, attending sports events Applying abstract thought and analysis in conversations at home and school

friends. Activities include participation in sports and extracurricular school activities, as well as "hanging out" and attending movies or concerts with friends (Table 33–24). The peer group becomes the focus of activities (Figure 33–13 ◉), regardless of the teen's interests. Peers are important in establishing identity and providing meaning. Although same-sex interactions predominate, boy-girl relationships are more common than at earlier stages. Adolescents thus participate in and learn from social interactions fundamental to adult relationships.

PERSONALITY AND TEMPERAMENT

Characteristics of temperament manifested during childhood usually remain stable in the teenage years. For instance, the adolescent who was a calm, scheduled infant and child often demonstrates initiative to regulate study times and other routines. Similarly the adolescent who was an easily stimulated infant may now have a messy room, a harried schedule with assignments always completed late,

and an interest in many activities. It is also common for an adolescent who was an easy child to become more difficult because of the psychologic changes of adolescence and the need to assert independence.

As during the child's earlier ages, the nurse's role may be to inform parents of different personality types and to help them support the teen's uniqueness while providing necessary structure and feedback. Nurses can help parents understand their teen's personality type and work with the adolescent to meet expectations set by teachers and others in authority.

COMMUNICATION

The adolescent uses and understands all parts of speech. Colloquialisms and slang are commonly used with the peer group. The adolescent often studies a foreign language in school, having the ability to understand and analyze grammar and sentence structure.

The adolescent increasingly leaves the home base and establishes close ties with peers. These relationships become

◉ **FIGURE 33–13**

Social interaction between children of same and opposite sex is as important inside the acute care setting as it is outside. **A,** Teenagers enjoy playing together. **B,** Emotional relationships form during adolescence.

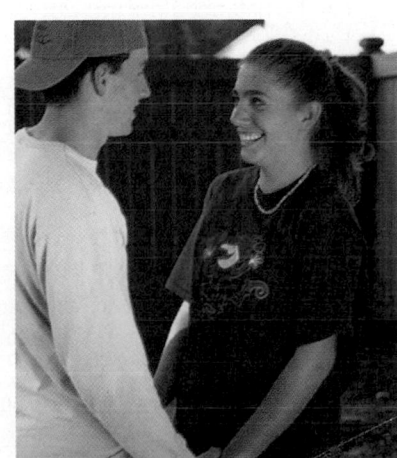

A   B

the basis for identity formation. There is generally a period of stress or crisis before a strong identity can emerge. The adolescent may try out new roles by learning a new sport or other skills, experimenting with drugs or alcohol, wearing different styles of clothing, or trying other activities. It is important to provide positive role models and a variety of experiences to help the adolescent make wise choices.

The adolescent also has a need to leave the past, to be different, and to change from former patterns to establish his or her own identity. Rules that are repeated constantly and dogmatically will probably be broken in the adolescent's quest for self-identity. This poses difficulties when the adolescent has a health problem, such as diabetes, or a heart problem that requires ongoing care. Introducing the adolescent to other teens who manage the same problem appropriately is usually more successful than telling the adolescent what to do.

Ensure privacy during the taking of health histories or interventions with teens. Even if a parent is present for part of a history or examination, the adolescent should be given the opportunity to relay information or ask questions alone with the healthcare provider. The adolescent should be given a choice of whether to have a parent present during an examination or while care is provided. Most information shared by an adolescent is confidential. Some states mandate disclosure of certain information to parents, such as an adolescent's desire for an abortion. In these cases the adolescent should be informed of what will be disclosed to the parent.

Setting up teen rooms (recreation rooms for use only by adolescents) or separate adolescent units in hospitals can provide necessary peer support during hospitalization. Most adolescents are not pleased when placed on a unit or in a room with young children. Choices should be allowed whenever possible. These might include preference for evening or morning bathing, the type of clothes to wear while hospitalized, timing of treatments, and who should be allowed to visit and for how long. Use of contracts with adolescents may increase compliance. Firmness, gentleness, choices, and respect must all be balanced during care of adolescent patients.

 GROWTH AND DEVELOPMENT

Following are strategies for communicating with the adolescent:

Provide written as well as verbal explanations.

Direct history and explanations to teen alone; then include parent.

Allow for safe exploration of topics by suggesting that teen is similar to other teens. ("Many teens with diabetes have questions about.... How about you?")

Arrange meetings for discussions with other teens.

SEXUALITY

With maturation of the body and increased secretion of hormones, the adolescent achieves sexual maturity. This is a complex process involving growing interactions with members of the opposite sex, an interplay of the forces of society and family, and identity formation. The early adolescent progresses from dances and other social events with members of the opposite sex; the late adolescent is mature sexually and may have regular sexual encounters. About 47% of all high-school students in the United States have had intercourse, and 34% are currently sexually active. Only 63% used a condom at their last sexual encounter, putting this age group at high risk of acquiring sexually transmitted infections (Grunbaum et al., 2004).

Teenagers need information about their bodies and emerging sexuality. Developmental changes vary among teens and these differences should be explained. They should understand the interests and forces they experience. Including sex education in school classes and healthcare encounters is important. Information on how to prevent sexually transmitted diseases is given, with most school districts now providing some teaching on AIDS. Far more common risks to teens, however, are diseases such as gonorrhea and herpes. Health histories should include questions on sexual activity, sexually transmitted diseases, and birth control use and understanding. Most hospitals routinely perform pregnancy screening on adolescent girls before elective procedures.

Adolescents benefit from clear information about sexuality, an opportunity to develop relationships with adolescents in various settings, an open atmosphere at home and school where problems and issues can be discussed, and previous experience in problem solving and self-decision making. Sexual issues should be among topics that adolescents can discuss openly in a variety of settings. Alternatives and support for their decisions should be available.

Some adolescents identify with a sexual minority group such as lesbian, gay, bisexual, or transgender. They are at particular risk of being stigmatized and harassed by other youth or adults. They are more likely to suffer a variety of problems such as isolation, rejection by significant others, violence, suicide, and taking sexual risks (Stevens & Morgan, 1999, 2001). Nurses are instrumental in helping these youth by providing information for them and their parents, integrating sexual minority content into school sexual curricula, and providing referrals for healthcare and social care when needed. See Chapter 36 for further information about the health issues related to homosexuality and other sexual minority practices. ∞

Critical Concept Review

LEARNING OBJECTIVES

CONCEPTS

Describe major theories of development as formulated by Freud, Erikson, Piaget, Kohlberg, social learning theorists, and behaviorists.

1. Freud:
   - Early childhood experiences form the unconscious motivation for action in later life.
2. Erikson:
   - There are eight periods that determine an individual's future social relationships.
3. Piaget:
   - Child's view of the world is influenced largely by age, experience, and maturational ability.
4. Kohlberg:
   - Developed a framework for understanding moral decision making.
5. Social learning theorists:
   - Children learn attitudes, beliefs, and customs through social contact with adults and other children.
6. Behaviorists:
   - Behavior can be elicited by positive reinforcement and extinguished by negative reinforcement.

Plan nursing interventions for children that are appropriate for the child's developmental state, based on theoretical frameworks.

1. Infant:
   - Encourage parents to hold and stay with infant.
   - Provide opportunities for sucking.
   - Provide infant with toys that give comfort or stimulate interest.
2. Toddler:
   - Maintain toilet-training procedures.
   - Encourage appropriate independent behavior.
   - Give short explanations.
   - Provide rewards for appropriate behaviors.
3. Preschooler:
   - Encourage parents to be involved in care of child.
   - Provide safe versions of medical equipment for playtime.
   - Give clear explanations about procedures and illnesses.
4. School-age:
   - Provide for privacy and modesty.
   - Explain treatments and procedures clearly.
   - Encourage continuation of school work.
5. Adolescent:
   - Provide privacy.
   - Interview and examine adolescent without parents present, if possible.
   - Encourage adolescent participation in treatment and decision making.
   - Encourage visitation of peers.

Explain contemporary developmental approaches such as temperament theory, ecologic theory, and the resilience framework.

1. Ecologic theory:
   - Emphasizes the presence of mutual interactions between the child (who is unique) and various settings.
2. Temperament theory:
   - All children can be categorized into three patterns of temperament, which can be used to assist in adaptation of the child's environment and for a better understanding of the child.
3. Resiliency theory:
   - All individuals experience crises that lead to adaptation and development of inner strengths and the ability to handle future crises.

(continued)

LEARNING OBJECTIVES

CONCEPTS

Recognize major developmental milestones for infants, toddlers, preschoolers, school-age children, and adolescents.

1. Infant:
   - Rolls over.
   - Sits up.
   - Stands.
   - Able to say one to two words.
   - Uses pincer grasp well.
2. Toddler:
   - Walks up and down stairs.
   - Undresses self.
   - Scribbles on paper.
   - Kicks a ball.
   - Has a vocabulary of 1000 words and uses short sentences.
3. Preschooler:
   - Uses scissors.
   - Rides bicycle with training wheels.
   - Throws a ball.
   - Writes a few letters.
   - All parts of speech well-developed.
4. School-age:
   - Possesses reading ability.
   - Rides a two-wheeled bike.
   - Jumps rope.
   - Plays organized sports.
   - Mature use of language.
5. Adolescent:
   - Fine motor skills well-developed.
   - Gross motor skills improve due to growth spurts.
   - Able to apply abstract thought and analysis.

Synthesize information from several theoretical approaches to plan assessments of the child's physical growth and developmental milestones.

The nurse plans assessments of the child's:
1. Physical growth and development and prenatal influences.
2. Cognitive development.
3. Psychosocial development.
4. Personality and temperament.
5. Communication.
6. Sexuality.

Describe the role of play in the growth and development of children.

1. Infant:
   - Engages primarily in solitary play, although social interaction enhances play.
   - Learns and matures through feel and sound of activities and objects.
   - As the infant begins to crawl and walk, the sphere of play enlarges and the effect of play on growth and development increases.
2. Toddler:
   - Increased motor skills enable the toddler to engage in new ways of playing.
   - Play becomes more social, and often includes parallel play with other toddlers.
   - Engages in imitative behavior, which teaches them new actions and skills.
   - Increased cognitive abilities enable the toddler to manipulate objects and learn about their qualities.
3. Preschooler:
   - Interacts with others in associative play.
   - Enjoys large motor activities.
   - Increased manual dexterity is demonstrated in greater complexity of play activities.
   - Fantasy play enhances growth and development.
4. School-age:
   - Increased physical abilities allow greater range and complexity of activities.
   - Engages in cooperative play, which increases social and cognitive skills.
5. Adolescent:
   - Increased maturity leads to new activities and ways to play.
   - The peer group—as the focus of activities—plays an important role in establishing the adolescent's identity.
   - Participate in and learn from social interactions fundamental to adult relationships.

LEARNING OBJECTIVES

CONCEPTS

Use data collected during developmental assessments to implement activities that promote development of children and adolescents.

1. Discuss proper nutrition and feeding techniques.
2. Conduct health teachings and screenings that are appropriate for child's age.
3. Encourage family to discover child's personality characteristics and temperament.
4. Instruct parents in expected language skills and refer to appropriate providers for assistance.
5. Give parents information regarding appropriate and normal sexual behavior in young children.
6. Instruct school-age children concerning the expected body changes of puberty.
7. Give adolescent information concerning birth control and sexually transmitted diseases.

CRITICAL THINKING IN ACTION

View the **Critical Thinking in Action** video in Chapter 33 of the CD-ROM. Then, answer the questions that follow.

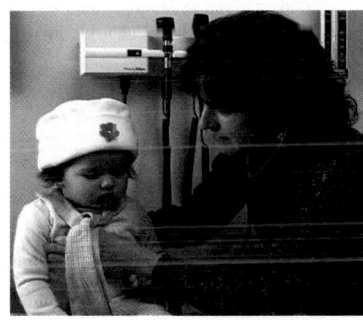

You encounter a 12 month old child, Julia, while working in the developmental clinic. Her mother tells you that their family practice physician had concerns that Julia might have a developmental delay. She was a full-term baby and there were no complications throughout her mother's pregnancy or delivery. Julia's mother tells you that she has a generally shy and slow-to-warm-up temperament. She makes little eye contact with you and prefers to sit on her mother's lap and cling to her arms if a stranger gets close. The baby in the video is demonstrating some of the skills Julia is able to accomplish. She is able to pick up small objects, babble, crawl, and use her pincer grasp. She is not able to walk, hold a crayon, or speak any words. Julia clearly has a developmental delay.

1. What are some examples of toys you can suggest to Julia's parents based on her developmental level (not based on her age)?
2. What are some examples of hazards you can advise Julia's parents about avoiding based on her developmental level?
3. What is a suggestion you can give the parents about dealing with a child like Julia who has a shy or slow-to-warm-up temperament?

MEDIALINK **www.prenhall.com/london**

- NCLEX-RN® Review questions, case studies, and other interactive resources for this chapter can be found on the Companion Website at http://www.prenhall.com/London. Click on "Chapter 33" to select the activities for this chapter.

- For tutorials including animations and videos, more NCLEX-RN® Review questions, and an audio glossary, access the accompanying CD-ROM in this book.

REFERENCES

American Academy of Pediatrics. (2004). *Pediatric nutrition handbook* (5th ed.). Elk Grove Village, IL: Author.

Aronson, J. (2000). Medical evaluation and infectious considerations on arrival. *Pediatric Annals, 29,* 218–223.

Bandura, A. (1986). *Social foundations of thought and actions: A social cognitive theory.* Englewood Cliffs, NJ: Prentice Hall.

Bandura, A. (1997a). *Self efficacy in changing societies.* New York: Cambridge University Press.

Bandura, A. (1997b). *Self efficacy: The exercise of control.* New York: WH Freeman.

Bronfenbrenner, U. (1986). Ecology of the family as a context for human development: Research perspectives. *Developmental Psychology, 22,* 723–742.

Bronfenbrenner, U. (Ed.). (2005). *Making human beings human: Bioecological perspectives on human development.* Thousand Oaks, CA: Sage Publications.

Bronfenbrenner, U., McClelland, P. D., Ceci, S. J., Moen, P., & Wethington, E. (1996). *The state of Americans.* New York: Free Press.

Chamberlain, L. J. (2001). Children adopted abroad could face life–long psychological problems. *Infectious Diseases in Children, 14*(1), 20.

Chamberlain, L. J. (2003). Initial medical examination important for international adoptees. *Infectious Diseases in Children, 16*(3), 52, 59.

Centers for Disease Control and Prevention (CDC). (2000). *Advance Data, 314,* 1–28.

Chen, L. H., Barnett, E. D., & Wilson, M. E. (2003). Preventing infectious diseases during and after international adoption. *Annals of Internal Medicine, 139,* 371–378.

Chess, S., & Thomas, A. (1995). *Temperament in clinical practice.* New York: Guilford Press.

Chess, S., & Thomas, A. (1996). *Temperament: Theory and practice.* Philadelphia: Brunner/Mazel.

Chess, S., & Thomas, A. (1999). *Goodness of fit: Clinical applications from infancy through adult life.* Philadelphia: Brunner/Mazel.

Craig, G. J., & Baucum, D. (2001). *Human development.* Upper Saddle River, NJ: Pearson Education.

Erikson, E. (1963). *Childhood and society.* New York: W.W. Norton.

Erikson, E. (1968). *Identity: Youth and crisis.* New York: W.W. Norton.

Faber, S. (2000). Behavioral sequelae of orphanage life. *Pediatric Annals, 29,* 242–248.

Federal Interagency Forum on Child and Family Statistics. (2000). *America's children: Key national indicators of well-being.* Washington, DC: U.S. Government Printing Office.

Field, T. (2002). Preterm infant massage therapy studies: An American approach. *Seminars in Neonatology, 7,* 487–494.

Fields, J., Smith, K., Bass, L. E., & Lugaila, T. (2001). *A child's day: Home, school, and play (selected indicators of child well-being).* Washington, DC: U.S. Department of Commerce.

Frenn, M., Malin, S., & Bansal, N. K. (2003). Stage-based interventions for low-fat diet with middle school students. *Journal of Pediatric Nursing, 18,* 36–45.

Ginsberg, H., & Opper, S. (1988). *Piaget's theory of intellectual development* (3rd ed.). Paramus, NJ: Prentice Hall.

Grunbaum, J. A., Kann, L., Kinchen, S., Ross, J., Hawkins, J., Lowry, R., et al. (2004). *Youth Risk Behavior Surveillance—United States, 2003, Morbidity and Mortality Weekly Report, 53* (SS02), 1–96.

Jarvis, C. (2000). *Physical examination and health assessment* (3rd ed.). Philadelphia: WB Saunders.

Jenista, J. A. (2000). Preadoption review of medical records. *Pediatric Annals, 29,* 212–217.

Johnson, D. E. (2000). Long-term medical issues in international adoptees. *Pediatric Annals, 29,* 234–241.

Lerner, R. M. (2002). *Adolescence.* Upper Saddle River, NJ: Pearson Education.

Mainous, R. O. (2003). Infant massage as a component of developmental care: Past, present, and future. *Holistic Nursing Practice, 17,* 1–7.

Malone, J. A. (1998). The resiliency model of family stress, adjustment, and adaptation. In B. Vaughan-Cole, M. A. Johnson, J. A. Malone, & B. L. Walker, *Family nursing practice* (pp. 49–60). Philadelphia: WB Saunders.

McCarter-Spaulding, D. E. (2005). Medications in pregnancy and lactation. *MCN. American Journal of Maternal Child Nursing, 30,* 10–17.

Melvin, N. (1995). Children's temperament: Intervention for parents. *Journal of Pediatric Nursing, 10,* 152–159.

Miller, L. C. (2000). Initial assessment of growth, development, and the effects of institutionalization in internationally adopted children. *Pediatric Annals, 29,* 224–233.

Piaget, J. (1972). *The child's conception of the world.* Totowa, NJ: Littlefield, Adams.

Riner, M. E., & Saywell, R. M. (2002). Development of the social ecology model of adolescent interpersonal violence prevention (SEMAIVP). *Journal of School Health, 72,* 65-70.

Santrock, J. (2004). *Life-span development* (9th ed.). Boston: McGraw-Hill.

Spector, R. (2000). *Guides to heritage assessment and health traditions.* Upper Saddle River, NJ: Prentice Hall Health.

Stevens, P., & Morgan, S. (1999). Health of lesbian, gay, bisexual, and transgender youth. *Journal of Child and Family Nursing, 2,* 237–249.

Stevens, P., & Morgan, S. (2001). Health of lesbian, gay, bisexual, and transgender youth. *Journal of Pediatric Health Care, 15,* 24–34.

Stewart, M., Reid, G., & Mangham, C. (1997). Fostering children's resilience. *Journal of Pediatric Nursing, 12,* 21–31.

Turecki, S. (2003). The behavioral complaint: Symptom of a psychiatric disorder or a matter of temperament? *Contemporary Pediatrics, 20,* 111–119.

Infant, Child, and Adolescent Nutrition

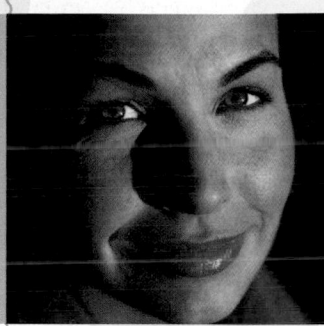

It is exciting to see Joey progressing into the school setting. Being with children his age will really help him develop in many ways. We're just worried because he needs to get only foods he can chew and swallow so he does not choke. He also needs his tube feedings during school to be sure he gets enough energy to do well.

Mother of Joey, 11 years old

LEARNING OBJECTIVES

- Discuss major nutritional concepts pertaining to the growth and development of children.

- Describe and plan nursing interventions to meet nutritional needs for all age groups from infancy through adolescence.

- Integrate methods of nutritional assessment into nursing care of infants, children, and adolescents.

- Discuss common nutritional problems of children in developed countries.

- Apply the nursing process to care for children with eating disorders.

MEDIALINK

www.prenhall.com/london

CD-ROM

Videos:
  Anorexia Nervosa
  Breastfeeding and First Foods
  Children and Overweight
  Nutritional Status
Nursing in Action: Administering a Gavage/Tube
  Feeding
Skills 9-1 to 9-7: Growth Measurements
Skill 15-3: Administering a Gavage Feeding
NCLEX-RN® Review
Audio Glossary

Companion Website

Objectives
NCLEX-RN® Review
Thinking Critically
Case Study: Manage a Child's Peanut Allergy at School
Dietary Reference Intakes
Typical Daily Intake at Various Ages
MediaLink Applications:
  Growth Chart Analysis
  Diet and Culture
  Analyze Your Diet
  Fast Food Analysis
  Plan a Nutrition Teaching Session
  Vegetarian Teens: Plan a 2-Day Menu
  Youth Adolescent Questionnaire
Audio Glossary

Adequate nutrition is an essential component of growth and development. The child's nutritional status begins before birth and is related to the mother's nutritional state. All children must be assessed for nutritional status, followed by teaching or other interventions to enhance health. Nurses are instrumental in giving parents information about normal nutritional needs of infants and young children. Common techniques to assess nutrition, such as measuring growth and monitoring hematocrit, provide needed information about whether intake of nutrients is adequate.

While all children and parents can benefit from information about nutritional needs, some children have additional issues that must be considered. The nurse recognizes the special requirements of children with conditions such as feeding disorder, food allergies, cystic fibrosis, cerebral palsy, or diabetes. Nutrition monitoring is provided throughout childhood so that dietary counseling can be integrated with other teaching to promote development. How can the nurse bridge the various settings in which children's nutritional needs are met? These might include the home, childcare settings, schools, and hospitals. How can the nurse help the family prepare for meeting the nutritional needs of a child who has special needs during car or plane travel?

Some children have unique nutritional needs due to their social environments. Parents may not be knowledgeable about child nutritional requirements. Perhaps the family is vegetarian and needs extra help to ensure intake of essential nutrients. If finances are limited, the family may need resources such as food stamps, food banks, or budget planning. The nurse considers the high rate of childhood obesity and common nutritional deficits when applying concepts of health promotion with families. Whatever the nurse's setting, knowledge of nutrition must be integrated within nursing care.

GENERAL CONCEPTS IN NUTRITION

Nutrition refers to taking in food and assimilating it metabolically for use by the body. It is an essential component of life and therefore an important body of knowledge to consider in discussions of child growth and development. The body requires a wide array of intake products. **Macronutrients**, or the major building blocks of the body, are carbohydrates, protein, and fat. Vitamins and minerals are **micronutrients**, or substances needed in small quantities for healthy body functioning. The need for nutrients is dependent on activity level, state of health, and presence of disease or other stress- and age-related requirements.

The **Dietary Reference Intakes (DRIs)** are a set of values established by the Food and Nutrition Board of the Institute of Medicine and the National Academy of Science that can be used to assess and plan intake for individuals of different ages. They commonly include four different values that can be considered by nursing, nutrition, and other health personnel. While the DRIs are the approach used in the United States, other countries have developed their own approaches to dietary standards. For example, Canada uses Adequate Intake and Reference Nutrient Intake, while the United Kingdom uses Recommended Daily Nutrient Intakes. The aims of these standards are to provide a method to evaluate individual and population diets and to plan nutrition programs and education. DRIs are generally specific to males and females in several age categories. See Appendix J ∞ for a list of DRIs for children and adolescents.

While the DRIs provide useful information when evaluating diets, their use can be time consuming. What "quick check" can provide feedback about the daily diets of children? The nurse should learn the Food Guide Pyramid and hang it in schools, clinics, and hospitals. It is a fast way to look at children's intakes for one day and see if they meet most requirements. Instead of calculating amounts of nutrients ingested, the pyramid focuses on categories of foods, which readily reflects the actual intake. The numbers of servings from various categories stay constant throughout childhood, while the serving sizes increase as the child gets older. See Figure 34–1 ● for the Food Guide Pyramid, and consult Web sites for alternative pyramids for vegetarians and those from various ethnic groups, such as Hispanic and Native American.

NUTRITIONAL NEEDS

Nutritional needs evolve during all of infancy and childhood. They support growth and development, and influence the progression of the child along the developmental path. Nutritional intake helps to maintain the health of the child and fosters a state of maximal potential or health promotion. Specific needs during each developmental stage are discussed in this section.

INFANCY

Breast Milk and Formula-Feeding

From the first feeding of a few ounces of breast milk to a meal of soft table foods with the family at 1 year of age, the infant demonstrates an amazing growth in ability to ingest and digest a wide variety of foods. Never again will the individual have such a high metabolic rate or high intake requirements in relation to size, or such a change in the types of foods eaten. Infants have an extremely fast rate of growth, since birth weight is usually doubled by about 5 months of age, and tripled by 1 year. Meeting nutritional needs is made difficult by the small size of the infant's stomach and the immaturity of the digestive system. Their great physical activity also necessitates high caloric intake. Nutrient demands for protein and vitamins must be met for the cells of the nervous system and body organs to develop properly.

The natural first food is breast milk and its intake should be encouraged for all infants. See Chapter 29 for a discussion of newborn nutrition. ∞ The American Academy of Pediatrics believes that breastfeeding is the best source of nutrition for babies through the first birthday and should be encouraged by health professionals (Committee on Nutrition, 2004). The American Diabetes Association states that broad-based efforts are needed to break barriers to breastfeeding, citing that exclusive breastfeeding for 6 months, and

● FIGURE 34–1

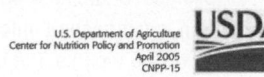

The Food Guide Pyramid is used to provide teaching about amounts of foods recommended for daily intake.

Courtesy of the U.S. Department of Agriculture and U.S. Department of Health and Human Services (2005).

breastfeeding with supplementary foods for at least 12 months, is the ideal feeding pattern for infants. The U.S. Preventive Services Task Force recommends breastfeeding education and behavioral counseling in 30- to 90-minute individual or group sessions with specially trained nurses or lactation specialists (*http://www.preventiveservices.arhq.gov*). The Canadian Task Force on Preventive Health Care also recommends counseling for women to encourage breastfeeding. Breast milk can be the only food for the first 6 months and should continue through 12 months of age, with addition of solid foods from 6 to 12 months. Many advantages to breastfeeding are known, including excellent nutritional balance, promotion of gastrointestinal function, fostering immune defense, psychologic benefits, and economic advantage. While breast milk is the best nutritional source for infants, babies may need some limited supplements.

Providing breastfeeding information and instruction positively influences the number of women who decide to breastfeed and increases the number of months they choose to continue breastfeeding (Kramer, 2001). The most effective programs for encouraging breastfeeding are those that involve education and skill/problem-solving information given in at least one session by a health professional (U.S. Preventive Services Task Force, 2003). Some hospitals have lactation specialists who assist breastfeeding mothers; in others, nurses provide this service. Home visits, phone calls from hospital nursing staff, early visits after the birth to obstetric and pediatric offices, and resources such as LaLeche League can provide mothers with needed breastfeeding information and problem-solving suggestions. Information is needed so that the mother gets adequate nutritional intake and sufficient rest. Support programs are especially helpful to mothers who have difficulty breastfeeding, feel unsure how it will fit into family and work life, are very young, or have an infant with problems related to feeding. The mother of a hospitalized infant needs special support to continue breastfeeding. The mother should be encouraged to come to the hospital to feed her baby on the same schedule as at home. If the infant cannot breastfeed, the hospital can provide an electric pump so the mother can maintain lactation. Often hospitals provide meals for the mother of a hospitalized baby so that she can maintain good nutrition and quality breast milk while she stays in the hospital with the baby.

Some women decide not to breastfeed or are unable to do so. After several months of breastfeeding, some mothers begin to use supplemental bottles when the infant is away from them. Nurses give these mothers information about formula preparation and feeding. Three types of formula are available—ready to feed, concentrate, and powder. All are nutritionally adequate for infants. Nurses can help parents decide which preparation of formula is best suited for their infants (see Table 34–1) and teach methods of preparation (see "Nursing Practice"). Some infants, such as those with phenylketonuria or other metabolic disorders, or babies with cow milk allergies, require specialized formulas. Breast- or bottle-feeding is discussed at each contact with health professionals to identify potential teaching needs.

NURSING PRACTICE

Formula can be mixed with tap water but must be refrigerated once mixed. Formula that the infant does not drink should be discarded after use and not kept for future feedings. This minimizes the chance for bacteria to grow and to cause illness in the baby. When the family lives in older housing, caution them to run tap water for about 2 minutes before using it and to use only cold water for formula preparation. These practices minimize the chance that lead will be leached from the older pipes in the house (see Chapter 51 for further discussion of lead poisoning ∞).

TEACHING HIGHLIGHTS

SUPPLEMENTS FOR BREASTFED BABIES

1. Each baby receives a vitamin K injection after birth to promote adequate blood clotting. After that, no further vitamin K is needed since the child manufactures this vitamin in the gut once he or she begins eating.
2. The need for vitamin D is not fully established, but 400 IU/day is recommended for infants who are breastfed, live in northern climates and urban settings (especially in winter), are dark skinned, or are kept well covered when outside.
3. Iron is not needed unless the infant is not eating food with iron by 4 to 6 months. The baby may need an iron source earlier if the mother was anemic during pregnancy or while breastfeeding.
4. Fluoride 0.25 mg is given after 6 months of age if water is not fluoridated to a level of 0.3 parts per million (ppm), or if the baby is not drinking any water.

NURSING PRACTICE

Advise parents to use caution when providing finger foods to the infant. Hard foods and some soft and malleable ones slip easily into the throat and may cause choking. Avoid hot dogs, hard vegetables, candy, and chunks of peanut butter. Infants and other young children should always be supervised while eating. Be sure parents are familiar with techniques for airway obstruction removal and have emergency numbers clearly listed on their phones.

During infancy and toddlerhood, nurses should carefully examine the patterns of breast- and bottle-feeding. **Early childhood caries** can occur when a young child is allowed to breastfeed or drink from a bottle for long periods, especially

TABLE 34-1 ❖ Advantages and Disadvantages of Formula Preparations

Formula Preparation	How Packaged	Advantages	Disadvantages
Ready to feed	Bottles or cans	No preparation needed	Most expensive type of formula
Concentrate	Cans of concentrated liquid	Easy to add equal amounts of formula concentrate and water directly into bottle and shake	Can be incorrectly measured, leading to inadequate or unsafe nutrition for infant; requires access to clean water supply such as city tap water or bottled water; well water may have too high a mineral concentration
Powder	Cans	Least expensive type of formula	Can be incorrectly measured, leading to inadequate or unsafe nutrition for infant; requires shaking to mix thoroughly; requires access to clean water supply such as city tap water or bottled water; well water may have too high a mineral concentration

when sleeping (Figure 34–2 ◉). The milk, juice, or other fluid pools around the upper anterior teeth, salivary flow decreases, and acid buffering is decreased, resulting in tooth decay. Nurses should teach parents to avoid putting the child to bed with a bottle and encourage pacifier use or a bottle of water instead. The child should not walk around with a bottle during the day. Mothers who breastfeed should also be cautioned to limit feeding to specific times so that milk will not pool in the mouth during sleep.

Parents can be taught beginning dental care for the infant, which includes wiping the teeth off daily once they erupt with a piece of moist gauze or a small infant toothbrush. Some pediatric dentists like to see the child for a first dental visit at about 1 year of age, while others wait until the child is older. The nurse should encourage the parents to select and establish contact with a dental provider when the child is nearing the end of infancy.

◉ FIGURE 34-2

Early childhood caries. This child has had major tooth decay related to sleeping as an infant and toddler while sucking bottles of juice and milk.

Courtesy of Dr. Lezley McIlveen, Department of Dentistry, Children's National Medical Center, Washington, DC.

Introduction of Supplemental Foods

When should other foods be added to the infant's diet? Although some parents add other foods when the infant is only days or weeks old, it is best to take cues from the infant's developmental milestones. The American Academy of Pediatrics recommends introducing semisolid food at 4 to 6 months (Committee on Nutrition, 2004). At this age the extrusion reflex (or tongue thrust) decreases and the infant can sit well with support. The infant is also developing the ability to appreciate texture and swallow nonliquid foods and can indicate desire for food or turn away when full.

The first food added to the infant's diet is usually rice cereal. The advantages of introducing cereal first is that it provides iron at an age when the infant's prenatal iron stores begin to decrease, it seldom causes allergy, and it is easy to digest. A tablespoon or two is fed to the infant once or twice daily just before formula or breastfeeding. The infant may appear to spit out food at first because of normal back-and-forth tongue movement. Parents should not interpret this early feeding behavior as indicating dislike for the food. With a little practice the infant becomes adept at spoon feeding.

Once the infant eats 1/4 cup of cereal twice daily, usually at 6 to 8 months of age, vegetables or fruits can be introduced (Table 34–2). By 8 to 10 months of age, most fruits and vegetables have been introduced and strained meats or other protein (e.g., tofu, cheese, mashed cooked beans) can be added to the infant's diet. Finger foods are introduced during the second half of the first year as the infant's palmar and then finger grasp develops and as teeth begin to erupt (Figure 34–3 ◉). Infants enjoy toast, O-shaped cereal, finely sliced meats, cheese and tofu, and small pieces of cooked, softened vegetables. Certain foods are more commonly associated with development of food allergies, and avoiding them in infancy may decrease allergy incidence. One new food should be added no more than every several days in order to identify any allergies. Recommendations

TABLE 34–2 ✤ Introduction of Solid Foods in Infancy

Recommendation	Rationale
Introduce rice cereal at 4–6 months.	Rice cereal is easy to digest, has low allergenic potential, and contains iron.
Introduce fruits or vegetables at 6–8 months. Some healthcare providers recommend vegetable introduction before fruits.	Fruits and vegetables provide needed vitamins. Vegetables are not as sweet as fruits; introducing them first may enhance acceptability to the infant.
Introduce meats at 8–10 months.	Meats are harder to digest, have high protein load, and should not be fed until close to 1 year of age.
Use single-food prepared baby foods rather than combination meals.	Combination meals usually contain more sugar, salt, and fillers.
Introduce one new food at a time, waiting at least 3 days to introduce another. Delay feeding eggs, strawberries, wheat, corn, fish, and nut products until close to 1 year of age.	If a food allergy or intolerance develops, it will be easy to identify. The foods listed are those most commonly associated with food allergy.
Avoid carrots, beets, and spinach before 4 months of age. Have well water evaluated for nitrates.	Nitrates in these foods and in water near agricultural runoff can be converted to nitrite by young infants, causing methemoglobinemia.
Infants can be fed mashed portions of table foods such as carrots, rice, and potatoes.	This is a less expensive alternative to jars of commercially prepared baby food; it allows parents of various cultural groups to feed ethnic foods to infants.
Avoid adding sugar, salt, and spices when mixing own baby foods.	Infants need not become accustomed to these flavors; they may get too much sodium from salt or develop gastric distress from some spices.
Avoid honey until at least 1 year of age.	Infants cannot detoxify *Clostridium botulinum* spores sometimes present in honey and can develop botulism.

● FIGURE 34–3

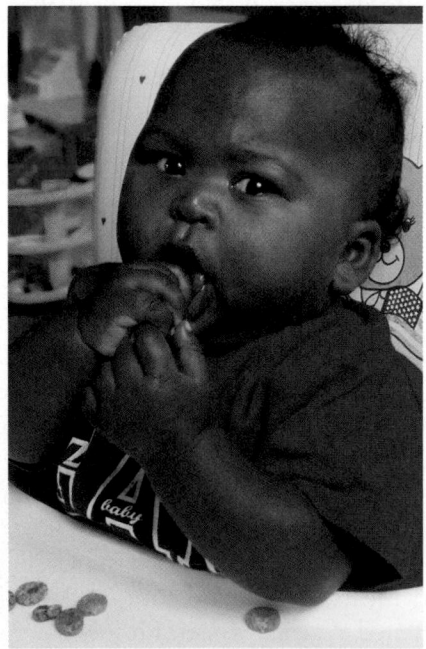

The baby who has developed the ability to grasp with thumb and forefinger should receive some foods that can be held in the hand.

for infants at risk due to family history of allergy are to delay feeding of cow milk until 1 year, eggs until 2 years, and peanuts, nuts, fish, and shellfish until 3 years (Committee on Nutrition, 2004). As food and juice intake increase, formula- or breastfeedings decrease in amount and frequency (Table 34–3).

If breastfeeding is not chosen, or if supplemental feedings are given, only iron-fortified infant formula should be used during the first year of life. Cow milk (including evaporated milk) can lead to bleeding and anemia (see content on iron and anemia on p. 945 in this chapter), can interfere with absorption of some nutrients, and has a high solute load which immature kidneys can have difficulty excreting. ∞ Iron-fortified formula should always be used when the infant under 12 months drinks formula. When breastfed babies are not eating foods with iron by 4 to 6 months, supplemental iron may need to be added. Careful dietary assessment and discussion of intake by the nurse at health visits helps the practitioner decide if supplemental iron is needed. Weaning is the term used when babies give up breastfeeding or a bottle and obtain most fluids by cup. At about 8 to 9 months, a cup should be offered to the baby with assistance provided so that learning about drinking from a cup can begin. By about 1 year of age, babies are

TABLE 34–3 ✤ Infant Nutritional Pattern

Birth–1 month
- Eats every 2–3 hours, breast or bottle
- 2–3 ounces (60–90 mL) per feeding

2–4 months
- Has coordinated suck-swallow
- Eats every 3–4 hours
- 3–4 ounces (90–120 mL) per feeding

4–6 months
- Begins baby food, usually rice cereal
- Eats 4 or more times daily
- 4–5 ounces (100–150 mL) per feeding

6–8 months
- Eats baby food such as rice cereal, fruits, and vegetables
- Eats 4 times daily
- 6–8 ounces (160–225 mL) per feeding

8–10 months
- Enjoys soft finger foods
- Eats 4 times daily
- 6 ounces (160 mL) per feeding
- Uses cup with lid

10–12 months
- Eats most soft table foods with family
- Uses cup with or without lid
- Attempts to feed self with spoon though spills often
- Eats 4 times daily
- 6–8 ounces (160–225 mL) per feeding

usually able to drink most liquids from a cup with a lid so bottles can be slowly withdrawn and replaced by cups. Breastfeeding may continue if the parent and infant desire, but introduction of other foods and a cup for drinking water or juice are still required. Babies should only be offered cups at meal and snack times so they become accustomed to drinking when thirsty rather than carrying a bottle or cup for much of the day, in order to decrease the chance for dental caries and increased calorie intake.

Parents who want to make baby foods at home can be encouraged and instructed to do so. Some commercially prepared foods have unnecessary additives such as salt, sugar, and food starch, and they may be costly for some families. Parents can easily blend fruits and vegetables the family is eating before adding salt, sugar, or seasoning. Prepared foods should be used promptly and stored in the refrigerator between feedings. Foods can also be placed into ice cube trays and frozen; a cube or two can be defrosted at mealtime. Nurses should caution parents not to use honey in foods for infants as it can lead to infant botulism. If foods or fluids are microwaved, they should be shaken,

stirred, and checked for temperature so that hot areas in the food do not burn the infant.

TODDLERHOOD

Why do parents of toddlers frequently become concerned about the small amount of food their children eat? Why do toddlers seem to survive and even thrive with minimal food intake? The toddler often displays the phenomenon of **physiologic anorexia**, caused when the extremely high metabolic demands of infancy slow to keep pace with the more moderate growth rate of toddlerhood. Although it can appear that the toddler eats nothing at times, intake over days or a week is generally sufficient and balanced enough to meet the body's demands for nutrients and energy.

Parents often need knowledge about the types of foods that constitute a healthy diet. Some easy to prepare foods are high in salt and other additives and can lead to exceeding the recommendation of *Healthy People 2010* for sodium intake. The nurse can offer alternatives to hot dogs, microwave meals, or fast foods by providing information about easy preparation of sliced meats, cheese, tofu, fruits, and vegetables. Healthy snacks for young children include yogurt, cheese, milk, slices of bread with peanut butter, thinly sliced fruits, and soft vegetables.

Parents should be advised to offer a variety of nutritious foods several times daily (three meals and two snacks) and let the toddler make choices from the foods offered. They should offer foods only at mealtimes and have the child sit in a high chair or on a special seat at the table to eat (Figure 34–4 ◉). Small portions are most appealing to

◉ FIGURE 34–4

Toddlers should sit at a table or in a high chair to eat, to minimize the chance of choking and to foster positive eating patterns.

the toddler. A general guideline for food quantity at a meal is one tablespoon of each food per year of age. The toddler should drink 16 to 24 oz (1/2 to 3/4 L) of milk daily. Parents should be cautioned against giving the toddler more than a quart (one liter) of milk daily, since this interferes with the desire to eat other foods, leading to dietary deficiencies. Recall that the child should not be put to bed with a bottle or allowed to carry a bottle of milk or juice around during the day, due to the risk of early childhood caries (see earlier discussion). In addition, parents should be advised to limit fruit juice to 4 to 6 ounces daily for children ages 1 to 6 years to decrease the opportunity for overweight, early childhood dental caries, and abdominal discomfort (American Academy of Pediatrics Committee on Nutrition, 2001). Unpasteurized juice should never be used since it may contain pathogens particularly harmful to young children. Drinking water and eating whole fruits, which provide fiber, are healthier alternatives. Avoid more than one meal weekly from a fast food restaurant due to the generally high fat and low fiber content of such meals.

GROWTH AND DEVELOPMENT

Toddlers generally eat three meals and two to three snacks daily. Toddlers can drink 2% milk starting at 2 years of age, or "follow-up" formula. Cups are recommended, with bottle use discontinued. Drinks should be consumed at mealtimes and for snacks while sitting at a table; carrying cups during the day while playing or at other activities is not recommended. The child is learning to use utensils but may prefer fingers and still needs small serving sizes.

Learning how to eat with others is an important task of toddlerhood. The toddler displays characteristic autonomy or independence during mealtime. Advise parents to provide opportunities for self-feeding of food with fingers and utensils, and to allow some simple choices, such as type of liquid or cup to use. Young children should eat at a table with others, not be allowed to run and play while eating, and eat at specified meal and snack times. Because social skills are developing, the hospitalized toddler may eat better if allowed to have meals with parents or other hospitalized children. See Chapter 40 for further suggestions about management of nutrition in hospitalized children. ∞

PRESCHOOL

The diet of the preschooler is similar to that of the toddler, but mealtime is now a more social event. Preschoolers like the company of others while they eat, and they enjoy helping with food preparation and table setting (Figure 34–5 ●). Involving them in these tasks can provide a forum for teaching about nutritious foods and principles of preparation, such as the need for refrigeration, safety around stoves, and cleanliness. Visits to fast food restaurants should be limited to about once weekly and the opportunity used to assist the child in making wise choices of nutritionally adequate foods in that setting.

Although the rate of growth is slow and steady during the preschool years, the child may have periods of **food jags** (eating only a few foods for several days or weeks) and greater or lesser intake. Parents should be advised to assess food intake over a 1- or 2-week period rather than at each meal to obtain a more accurate impression of total intake. Food jags can be handled by providing the desired food along with other foods to foster choice. The child who chooses not to eat at snacktime or mealtime should not be given other foods in between. The child will become hungry and get accustomed to eating when food is provided.

● **FIGURE 34–5**

Preschoolers learn food habits by eating with others. Engaging them in food preparation enhances knowledge of food and promotes intake at meals.

Three meals and two or three snacks daily are the norm. Fruit juice should be limited to 8 to 12 ounces daily.

The preschool period is a good time to continue encouraging good dental habits. Children can begin to brush their own teeth with parental supervision and help to reach all tooth surfaces. See Chapter 37 for recommended doses of fluoride when the water supply is not fluoridated. ∞ If the child has not yet visited a dentist, the first dental visit should be scheduled so the child can become accustomed to the routine of dental care.

SCHOOL-AGE

The school-age years are a period of gradual growth when energy requirements remain at a steady level, although at some point during these years, most children experience a preadolescent growth spurt. Girls may begin a growth spurt by 10 or 11 years, and boys a year or so later. Nutritional needs increase dramatically with this spurt, with large numbers of calories and increased amounts of other nutrients required (see Appendix J for RDAs ∞).

School-age children are increasingly responsible for preparing snacks, lunches, and even some other meals. These years are a good time to teach children how to choose nutritious foods and plan a well-balanced meal. Because school-age children operate at the concrete level of cognitive thought, nutrition teaching is best presented by using pictures, samples of foods, videotapes, handouts, and hands-on experience.

School-age children often prefer the types of food eaten at home and may be resistant to new food items. A hospitalized child may refuse to eat, slowing the recuperative process. Nurses should encourage family members to bring favorite foods from home that meet nutritional requirements. This can be especially helpful when the hospital serves food only from the dominant cultural group. A child accustomed to a diet of rice, tofu, and vegetables may not enjoy a hospital meal of hamburger and fries. By school-age, food has become strongly associated with social interaction, so it is beneficial to have children eat together or to invite family members to take the child off the unit to eat or to bring in food from home and eat with the child. Many hospitals allow children to plan a pizza night or sponsor other events to encourage eating in a social atmosphere.

Most children consume at least one meal daily in school. While children may bring lunches to school, most participate in school lunch programs, and perhaps school breakfast programs. Nurses should become familiar with the policies of school districts in their areas for providing foods, snacks, and reduced price food to students in need. Over the past decade, many school systems in the United States have allowed vending machines for carbonated sweetened beverages and snacks to be installed in public schools. Part of the profits from these machines has enabled revenue-strapped school districts to enhance their incomes. However, schools are increasingly challenged about the presence of the machines, especially in light of the growing problem of overweight among youth. Some school districts have now limited the number of machines or the hours during which they can be used by students. Nurses are able to provide information for districts about the problems of obesity and the need for healthy foods for youth.

The opening quote in this chapter is from the mother of Joey, a young boy with cerebral palsy who has a gastrostomy feeding tube to assist him in ingestion of adequate nutrients. Joey is attending school and the teacher has been taught to administer his tube feedings. Nurses often assist families who have children with special needs to integrate them into the school environment. How might the nurse plan for Joey to participate in school lunchtime with peers? Since he can eat some soft foods by mouth, what types of foods are commonly available at school that he might be able to enjoy?

The loss of the first deciduous teeth and the eruption of permanent teeth usually occur at about 6 years, or at the beginning of the school-age period. Of the 32 permanent teeth, 22 to 26 erupt by age 12 years, and the remaining molars follow in the teenage years. See Chapter 35 for the typical sequence of tooth eruption and Chapter 37 for dental care needs during childhood. ∞ The school-age child should be closely monitored to ensure that brushing and flossing are adequate, that fluoride is taken if the water supply is not fluoridated, that dental care is obtained to provide for examination of teeth and alignment, and that loose teeth are identified before surgery or sports participation.

ADOLESCENCE

Most adolescents need well over 2000 calories daily to support the growth spurt, and some adolescent boys require nearly 3000 calories daily. When teenagers are active in a variety of sports, these requirements increase further. Because adolescents prepare much of their own food and often eat with friends, they need to be taught about good nutrition. Developing a diet that includes a large number of calories, meets vitamin and mineral requirements, and is acceptable to the teen may be a challenge. The pregnant adolescent has even more challenging nutrient requirements. See Chapter 12 for details about needs during pregnancy. ∞ An adolescent who is hospitalized and does not like the hospital lunch sometimes has a friend who visits bring a soft drink and chips; however, the teen may be receptive to offers of juice and pizza, a more nutritious meal. Small improvements should be viewed positively as they may lead to further changes.

Fast food represents a significant intake for many adolescents. It is commonly high in fat, calories, and sodium while being low in essential nutrients such as calcium, folic acid, riboflavin, vitamins A and C, and fiber. Many schools are redesigning cafeterias and food programs to entice more teens to eat at school rather than nearby fast food restaurants. Adding fruits and salads and allowing choice can enhance quality of food intake (Calderon, 2002). School nurses play a vital role in helping to tailor a healthy school nutrition program and teaching teens about the most healthy choices at their favorite fast food restaurants.

Peer group influence is important, so group sessions in which adolescents eat lunch together can provide a forum for influencing food habits. What other methods might encourage positive nutritional habits among teens?

NUTRITIONAL ASSESSMENT

What is the best indication that the child's nutrition is adequate? Which data-collection methods provide the most accurate information about a child's dietary intake? The nurse plays an important role in assessing the diets of children and in seeking additional evaluation from dietitians and nutritionists in complex situations.

PHYSICAL AND BEHAVIORAL MEASUREMENT

Growth Measurement

A common method of evaluating the adequacy of diet is measurement of growth. **Anthropometric measurement** is the term used to refer to assessment of various parts of the body. Anthropometry of young children commonly includes weight, length, and head circumference. Standing height is substituted for length once the child can stand. Head circumference, also known as occipital-frontal circumference (OFC), is measured during infancy, and into early years when there are growth concerns. Additional measurements that may be included in special circumstances include chest circumference, mid-upper arm circumference, and skinfold measurement at sites such as triceps, abdomen, and subscapular regions. Skills 9–1 through 9–7 in the accompanying CD-ROM and the Clinical Skills Manual present techniques for accurate measurement of weight, length, height, chest circumference, and head circumference. SKILLS

After collecting the measurements, the nurse plots them on the appropriate standardized growth curves for weight, length to height, head circumference, and body mass index (Figure 34–6 ●). **Body mass index** (BMI) is a calculation based on the child's weight and height, or length, and is calculated as kilograms of weight/m² of height. This is a useful calculation for determining if the child's height and weight are in proportion and identifies which percentile the child falls in for each measurement.

Children normally fall between the 10th and 90th percentiles. A measurement below the 10th percentile, especially for BMI, may indicate undernutrition, while one over the 90th percentile can indicate overnutrition. However, it is important to look at the differences between measurements. An infant in the 90th percentile for length, weight, and head circumference is proportional and may be a naturally large baby. On the other hand, a child who is consistently in the 10th percentile for all measurements, but is growing steadily and is at a normal development level, may simply be a small child. Much cultural and individual variation exists in size. See Appendix C for standardized growth curves by gender and age for infants, children, and adolescents. ∞ Visit the Companion Website at *http://www.prenhall.com/london* to find out more about the growth curves and a course in accurate assessment techniques.

DEVELOPING CULTURAL COMPETENCE

GROWTH PATTERNS AMONG IMMIGRANT CHILDREN

The revised growth grids now in use were standardized using a cross section of the U.S. population and generally reflect most children. However, children from some other countries or cultures may fall outside of these curves. For example, new immigrants or adoptees may be in lower percentiles, and "catch up" over several months or years. Children of immigrants from developing countries tend to be larger than their parents. Even when small, children should follow normal growth patterns. For example, a child may remain at the 10th or 25th percentile for height but continues to slowly grow and does not fall to a lower percentile.

The nurse should plot measurements on the same growth curve with earlier percentiles for the child. When measurements follow the same percentile over time, growth is generally normal for the child and nutrition is likely adequate. However, a sudden or sustained change in percentile may indicate a chronic disorder, emotional difficulty, or a nutritional intake problem. Further assessment of physical status and dietary intake will be needed.

Additional Physical Measurement

Many observations from the physical assessment provide clues to nutritional status. Dietary intake can affect every body system, and a combination of certain symptoms may suggest specific nutritional problems. Some common physical manifestations of nutritional status are outlined in Table 34–4.

Laboratory measurements can provide useful information when nutritional status is questionable. Some common studies include hematocrit and hemoglobin, serum glucose

● FIGURE 34–6

The nurse accurately measures the child and then places height and weight on appropriate growth grids for the child's age and gender.

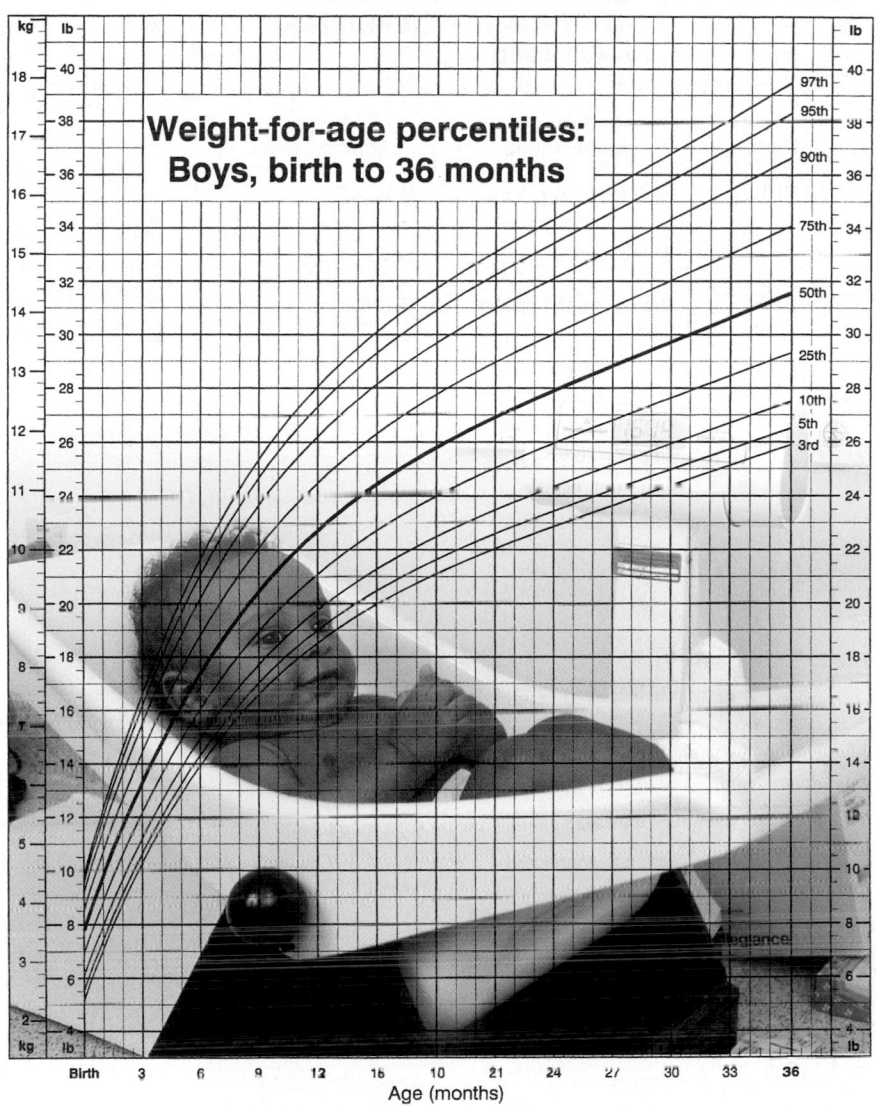

Weight-for-age percentiles: Boys, birth to 36 months

and fasting insulin, lipids and lipoproteins, and liver and renal function studies. Adding some further measurements such as chest circumference and skinfolds (measurement of fat at certain body sites such as triceps, scapular, and abdominal areas) may also be useful (Bessler, 1999).

DIETARY INTAKE

The mother's dietary intake during pregnancy may provide information about the child's nutritional state and it can be assessed for pertinent information. The nurse should obtain detailed information about the child's dietary intake when there is a potential for nutritional deficiency due to disease, knowledge deficit, or socioeconomic status. After the information is collected, the dietary intake should be compared to the recommended levels for a

child of that age and gender (see Figure 34–1 for Food Guide Pyramid; see Appendix J for Recommended Dietary Allowances ∞). The 24-hour recall of intake, a food frequency questionnaire, and a dietary screening history (Tables 34–5 and 34–6) provide a good overview of the infant's or child's intake and eating patterns. A food diary provides precise information about the child's food intake.

Twenty-Four-Hour Recall of Food Intake

The 24-hour diet recall is frequently used to assess the adequacy of the diet. People can generally remember their intake in the past day so results are fairly accurate, it is easy to gather the data and analyze results, and only a few minutes are needed. The nurse should ask the parent or child to list all

MediaLink Youth Adolescent Questionnaire

TABLE 34–4 ✤ Clinical Manifestations of Dietary Deficiencies/Excesses

Nutrient	Deficiency Manifestation	Excess Manifestation
Vitamin A	Night blindness Skin dryness and scaling	Headache Drowsiness Hepatomegaly
Vitamin C	Abnormal hair (coiled shape) Skin abnormalities (dermatitis and lesions) Purpura Bleeding gums Joint tenderness Sudden heart failure	Usually none—excess is excreted in urine
Vitamin D	Rib abnormalities Bowed legs	Drowsiness
B vitamins	Weakness Decreased deep tendon reflexes Dermatitis	Usually none—excess is excreted in urine
Protein	Hepatomegaly Edema Scant, depigmented hair	Kidney failure
Carbohydrate	Emaciation Decreased energy Retarded growth and development	Overweight
Iron	Lethargy Slowed growth and developmental progression Pallor	Vomiting, diarrhea, abdominal pain Pallor Cyanosis Drowsiness Shock

plates so accurate amounts can be indicated is helpful)

- Types of specific foods used, such as whole milk vs. nonfat or 2%, brand names of cereals, specific types of margarine or butter
- Additives used, such as condiments, table salt, spices, milk to mix formula
- Food preparation methods, including adding fats to cook, removal or retention of fats on meats
- Vitamins and supplements, types and doses
- Whether the intake is typical (in situations such as illness or vacation, intake may be different than usual)

TABLE 34–5 ✤ Dietary Screening History for Infants

Overview Questions

What was the infant's birth weight?

At what age did the birth weight double and triple?

Was the infant premature?

Does the infant have any feeding problems such as difficulty sucking and swallowing, spitting up, fatigue, or fussiness?

If Infant Is Breastfed

How long does the baby nurse at each breast?

What is the usual schedule for breastfeeding?

Does the baby also take any milk or formula? Amount and frequency? What type?

If Infant Is Fed Other Foods

What formula is used? Is it iron fortified?

How is it prepared?

Do you hold or prop the bottle for feedings?

How much formula is taken at each feeding?

How many bottles are taken each day?

Does the baby take a bottle to bed for naps or nighttime? What is in the bottle?

If Infant Is Formula-Fed

At what age did the baby start eating other foods?

Cereal	Finger foods
Fruit/juices	Meats
Vegetables	Other protein sources

Do you use commercial baby food or make your own?

Does the baby eat any table foods?

How often does the baby take solid foods?

How is the baby's appetite?

Do you have any concerns about the baby's feeding habits?

Does the baby take a vitamin supplement? Fluoride?

Have there been any allergic reactions to foods? Which ones?

    Does the baby spit up frequently?

    Have there been any rashes?

What types of stools does the baby have? Frequency? Consistency?

foods eaten during the past 24 hours (Figure 34–7 ⊙). It is usually helpful to ask for a description of activities in the last day, then start with the most recent event and move backwards, integrating food intake into the daily schedule. For example, the nurse might begin by saying, "You mentioned you got up early to come to the clinic today. What did Sam eat at home before you left? Did he have a snack as you traveled here or after you arrived?" While asking about the foods eaten, the nurse should inquire specifically about the following:

- All meals and snacks
- Amounts of each food item consumed (having various size measuring cups, bowls, and

NURSING CARE PLAN

THE CHILD WHO IS OVERWEIGHT

Intervention	Rationale	Expected Outcome

1. Nursing Diagnosis: Imbalanced Nutrition: More than Body Requirements related to excessive intake in comparison to metabolic needs

Intervention	Rationale	Expected Outcome
NIC Priority Intervention: **Weight reduction assistance:** Facilitating loss of weight and body fat		**NOC Suggested Outcome:** **Respiratory status: weight control:** Personal actions resulting in achievement and maintenance of optimum body weight for health

Goal: The child will demonstrate adequate intake of all nutrients without excessive energy intake.

Intervention	Rationale	Expected Outcome
■ Perform thorough nutritional assessment of child. ■ Share results of assessment with child and family by showing weight, height, and body mass index grids. ■ Identify with the child and family 2–3 target areas to begin weight management. Examples might include: 　■ Having fast food only once weekly 　■ Switching to low-fat dairy products 　■ Keeping two more fresh fruits and vegetables in the house and two less snack foods ■ Integrate nutrition information into each visit. Examples of topics include: 　■ Dietary requirements for age group 　■ Effects of simple sugar and fat intake on weight 　■ Beneficial effects of fruits, vegetables, whole grains, and nonfat dairy 　■ Reading food labels 　■ Healthy choices in fast food restaurants 　■ Calculation of fat content of foods ■ Use growth grids to help child and family establish a weight reduction or maintenance goal.	■ Assessment assists in identification of dietary risks and strengths as well as health conditions related to nutrition. ■ Many families do not consider their child overweight. Concrete information about the child's size in comparison with recommendations assists in establishing the importance of weight management. ■ Changing dietary patterns drastically is difficult and may lead to giving up the attempt at weight management. Partnering with the family to set goals enhances chances of success. ■ Nutrition information is best learned in an ongoing program. ■ Goals motivate families to achieve desired health behaviors. The goal for a young child may be weight maintenance so that as the child grows in height, the correct proportion is reached, while weight reduction may be needed for older children or youth who are very obese.	■ Child meets all dietary requirements while achieving weight and body mass index goal.

2. Nursing Diagnosis: Readiness for Enhanced Family Coping related to need to foster health of family member

Intervention	Rationale	Expected Outcome
NIC Priority Intervention: **Health system guidance:** Facilitating child's use of appropriate nutrition and health services to foster weight control		**NOC Suggested Outcome:** **Health-promoting behavior:** Actions to promote, sustain, and increase wellness

Goal: The family will assist child to manage stressors and to develop new strategies to support weight control goals.

Intervention	Rationale	Expected Outcome
■ Include key family members in some of the counseling sessions with the overweight child.	■ Key members of the family are those who purchase foods, provide support for the child, and participate in decisions about health.	■ Child expresses satisfaction with family understanding and support of weight.

(continued)

NURSING CARE PLAN—continued

THE CHILD WHO IS OVERWEIGHT

Intervention	Rationale	Expected Outcome
■ Encourage the family to eat together at least once daily if possible or to increase number of meals eaten together weekly. ■ Seek a resource for the child to be monitored about twice monthly; this may be a healthcare provider office, nutritionist, school nurse, or other person.	■ The family is an important support system in weight loss programs. Eating as a family or in a social situation can provide a chance to promote healthy foods; intake is generally lower fat and calorie than when eating alone. ■ Provides opportunity to monitor the child's progress and to offer support, additional information, and problem-solving techniques.	

3. Nursing Diagnosis: Activity Intolerance related to sedentary lifestyle

NIC Priority Intervention:		NOC Suggested Outcome:
Exercise promotion: Facilitating regular exercise to maintain and increase endurance and energy use		**Endurance:** Extent that energy enables the child to sustain activity

Goal: The child will demonstrate activity tolerance by adequate oxygenation, respiratory effort, and ability to speak during brisk walking, biking, or other activity.

■ Establish daily exercise routine beginning with 15–30 minutes daily of walking. ■ Gradually increase activity over 1–2 months until 60 minutes of daily exercise is maintained. ■ Use activities enjoyed by the child and suggest options as necessary; refer the family to community resources such as swimming pools, organized sports, and biking groups. ■ Have families plan at least 1–2 activities they can do together weekly. ■ Limit screen activities to a maximum of 2 hours daily. 　Have child keep a log of hours of television, video games, computer, and other similar activities. 　Tell child never to snack while doing screen activities. ■ Ask about use of tobacco in children in 5th grade or higher. 　Inquire about exposure to environmental tobacco smoke at all ages. 　Perform teaching to discourage tobacco use or offer cessation programs as needed.	■ Starting with brief amounts of exercise makes the child feel comfortable and enhances potential for success. ■ Gradual increase as the cardiovascular and respiratory systems adapt is generally comfortable for children; 60 minutes of moderate activity daily is recommended for children. ■ Activities the child enjoys will be more likely to remain in usual activity patterns; exercising with others in groups increases motivation. ■ This fosters family relationships and provides support and motivation for the child. ■ Increased use of screen activities is related to poor dietary habits and increased sedentary behaviors and excess weight. ■ Most adults who smoke began the habit in childhood; middle school years are the most common age for smoking initiation. 　Smoking by others in the household can be harmful to children. 　Smoking decreases respiratory reserves and worsens several cardiovascular disease risks.	■ Child demonstrates ability to engage in moderate activity for 60 minutes with minimal respiratory discomfort.

4. Nursing Diagnosis: Chronic Low Self-Esteem related to weight

NIC Priority Intervention:		NOC Suggested Outcome:
Self-esteem enhancement: Assisting the child to increase personal judgment of self-worth		**Quality of life and self-esteem:** Expressed satisfaction with life circumstances and positive judgment of self-worth

NURSING CARE PLAN—continued

THE CHILD WHO IS OVERWEIGHT

Intervention	Rationale	Expected Outcome
Goal: The child expresses positive perception of self-worth and confidence in ability to deal with issues related to weight.		
■ Facilitate development of a positive outlook by exposing child to others who have been successful with weight loss. ■ Praise child for weight loss, weight maintenance, increased physical activity, and other achievements. Help the child establish rewards for meeting goals, such as purchase of new clothing. ■ Partner with parents so that they understand the value of praise and never label the child by derogatory words such as "fat."	■ Increases motivation and feelings of self-efficacy. ■ Enhances judgment of self-worth and pride in accomplishments. ■ Family members are usually the most intimate support system for the child.	■ Child speaks positively about accomplishments in weight control management.

TABLE 34–6 ✢ **Dietary Screening History for Children**

What types of food or beverage does the child especially like?

What foods or beverages does the child dislike?

What is the child's typical eating schedule? Meals and snacks?

Does the child eat with the family or at separate times?
 Where does the child eat each meal?

Who prepares the food for the family?
 What methods of cooking are used? Baking? Frying? Broiling?
 What ethnic foods are commonly eaten?

Does the family eat in a restaurant frequently? What type?
 What type of food does the child usually order?

Is the child on a special diet?

Does the child need to be fed, feed himself or herself, need assistance eating, or need any adaptive devices for eating?

What is the child's appetite like?

Does the child take any vitamin supplements (iron, fluoride)?

Does the child have any allergies? What types of symptoms?

What types of regular exercise does the child get?

Are there any concerns about the child's eating habits?

Once the 24-hour recall is obtained, the nurse needs to analyze the intake by first doing a quick check to compare servings of various food types with the Food Guide Pyramid, as described earlier. Next the nurse should do a detailed analysis to compute calories, carbohydrate, protein, and fat intake and compare them to recommended amounts. All major vitamins and minerals are also computed and comparisons made to the DRIs. This computation may be done by hand, using a book of nutrients in common foods, or may be done on the computer. Several

computer programs are available, and the federal government has a Web site that provides intake levels and comparisons to the RDAs. It may be useful to compute a personal 24-hour recall or that of a child in the clinical setting with the Healthy Eating Index.

Food Frequency Questionnaire

Food frequency questionnaires are available that can be easily administered to parents or children. Usually they ask about how often certain types of foods are eaten in a specified period such as a week. Questionnaires can be long and evaluate a total diet, or short and focus on specific

◉ **FIGURE 34–7**

The nurse is interviewing a child about foods eaten in the last day. Note the models of food and dishes for accurate assessment of serving sizes.

items such as fruit and vegetable intake. A short questionnaire about milk intake or fruit and vegetable intake may be helpful before planning a teaching project on nutrition to a class of school-age children. Knowing their usual intake of a food item can provide helpful information for planning the project. See the Companion Website for one example of questions from a food frequency questionnaire.

Dietary Screening History

The nurse should ask the parent about the infant's or child's eating habits using questions in Tables 34–5 and 34–6. Responses provide information about the family's eating habits and food beliefs beyond that collected on a 24-hour dietary recall or food frequency questionnaire.

DEVELOPING CULTURAL COMPETENCE

DIETARY INTAKE VARIES AMONG CULTURES

Each culture has eating practices that influence dietary intake. It is important to understand the foods commonly eaten by each cultural group and their contribution to the total nutrition of the child. Depending on the populations nurses work with, they may need to ask about intake of freshly caught fish or wild game such as pheasants and elk. Home-prepared sausages and cheese may be part of diets. Berries and garden produce might be eaten. Foods from ethnic markets may include spices, dried mushrooms, and other products. Using open-ended questions in gathering data will increase the likelihood of obtaining an accurate evaluation of diet.

Food Diary

Parents are asked to keep a food diary when the child has a nutrition problem or disorder that requires dietary management, such as malnutrition, obesity, or type 1 diabetes. All meals and snacks, with food preparation method and quantities eaten over a 1- to 7-day period, are recorded. Eating patterns change significantly for holidays or family gatherings, so parents should be asked to select typical days for the food diary or to record specific events affecting food intake. Including one weekday and one weekend day may be helpful. Parents need to be reminded of all the places children might have eaten, such as the childcare center, school, friends' houses, or neighbors. Food diaries can provide a great deal of helpful information, but they take time and motivation to complete well (Lee & Nieman, 2003). The nurse should be sure instructions are complete and that the form has a place to record amounts, preparation, events occurring, and where food was eaten. The nurse or parent may need to obtain the school lunch menu and talk with the school lunch personnel to add accurate school intake.

The nurse completes the nutritional assessment indicated for a child and may consult with or refer the family to a dietitian or nutritionist for additional assessment and teaching.

COMMON NUTRITIONAL CONCERNS

CHILDHOOD HUNGER

While most Americans live in a land of plenty, significant numbers of children periodically experience hunger. **Food security** is access at all times to enough nourishment for an active, healthy life (Federal Interagency Forum on Child and Family Statistics, 2000). In contrast, **food insecurity** indicates an inability to acquire or consume adequate quality or quantity of foods in socially acceptable ways, or the uncertainty that one will be able to do so (Boyle & Morris, 1999).

The major cause of hunger in children is poverty, and since one in five children is poor, their families may be unable to provide sustainable nutrition at all times (Children's Defense Fund, 2004). Many single-income families have a head of household moving into the workforce, so incomes are often not sufficient to provide for family food needs (see Chapter 1 for a description of Temporary Assistance for Needy Families [TANF] ∞). Families may be ineligible for food assistance programs even though they cannot afford enough food for all their members. Children with special nutritional needs are at particular risk since it may be more costly to buy and prepare formula or foods for a child with allergies, diabetes, or an immune disorder.

Children with insufficient dietary intake are at risk for a wide array of health problems. They may become anemic; have a high rate of infectious disease due to lowered immune response; have slowed developmental maturation, delayed or stunted physical growth, and learning disorders; and be at greater risk of overweight, cardiovascular disease, and diabetes in adulthood (Committee on Nutrition, 2004; Hanson, Dahlman-Hoglund, Lundin et al., 1997; Walter, Olivares, Pizarro et al., 1997). Subsequently, the national and individual cost of childhood hunger is great.

Nurses are well positioned to evaluate families for food insecurity in a variety of hospital, clinic, school, and home settings. In addition to the assessment of the individual child's nutritional status, further questions can determine families with potential problems. Nurses should administer the screening tool to identify risk in families (Table 34–7). Most parents go without food themselves in order to feed their children, so food insecurity may not have directly affected all children. However, anxiety over providing food can be very stressful for families, and diet quality deteriorates as insecurity increases. If families have experienced food insecurity or may be likely to at some time, nurses should be sure to provide them with access to community agencies and programs that can help. What resources are available locally to help families with food insecurity?

TABLE 34–7 ✣ Food Insecurity Screening

1. Does your household ever run out of money to buy food to make a meal?
2. Do you or members of your household ever eat less than you feel you should because there is not enough money for food?
3. Do you or members of your household ever cut the size of meals or skip meals because there is not enough money for food?
4. Do your children ever eat less than you feel they should because there is not enough money for food?
5. Do you ever cut the size of your children's meals or do they skip meals because there is not enough money for food?
6. Do your children ever say they are hungry because there is not enough food in the house?
7. Do you ever rely on a limited number of foods to feed your children because you are running out of money to buy foods for a meal?
8. Do any of your children ever go to bed hungry because there is not enough money to buy food?

Scoring: 5–8 yes responses = hungry; 1–4 yes responses = risk of hunger. From Washington State Department of Health.

TEACHING HIGHLIGHTS

COMMUNITY RESOURCES FOR FOOD

Food Stamp Program Eligibility based on household size and income; refer students and those with low incomes, especially when they have young children; education services often available

Child Nutrition Programs—School lunch, breakfast, and milk programs; free and lowered cost meals in schools; assist parents to apply

Special Child Programs—Summer programs, Head Start, child care centers and homeless children programs may provide nutritional support in some communities

Women, Infants, and Children (WIC)—Supplemental foods and nutrition education to pregnant, breastfeeding, and postpartum women and to their young children; assessment of child growth often included

Nutrition Education and Training Program—Nutrition education for teachers and school food service personnel

Community Services—May include food banks, field gleaning, and other programs

Find out what services are available to provide food and nutrition education in your community. Make a list to use in clinical settings with families.

OVERWEIGHT AND OBESITY

After several decades of similar statistics regarding overweight in children, the numbers are now skyrocketing. The current incidence of overweight in the United States has been called an epidemic and is associated with a wide array of health problems, such as the appearance of type 2 diabetes in youth (Ludwig & Ebbeling, 2001). See Chapter 56 for a discussion of diabetes. ∞ Overweight can also influence self-image, dietary quality, and amount of physical activity. The National Health and Nutrition Examination Survey has found that 16% of child and adolescent groups are now overweight (Hedley, Ogden, Johnson, Carroll, Curtin, & Flegal, 2004). When using the 85th percentile of BMI as an indicator of risk overweight, from 20% to 33% of youth are affected (Ogden, Flegal, Carroll et al., 2002). Since overweight in childhood and adolescence frequently tracks into adulthood, the implications for healthcare are obvious.

GROWTH AND DEVELOPMENT

When a child has one obese parent, chances of the child being overweight are increased. In families with two overweight parents, the incidence of obesity in children increases even more. The child who has obese parents and is overweight as an adolescent is at very high risk of becoming an obese adult (Whitaker, Wright, Pepe et al., 1997). Be alert for families with overweight adults and begin prevention early with the children in these families.

DEVELOPING CULTURAL COMPETENCE

OVERWEIGHT CAUSES HEALTH DISPARITIES AMONG CERTAIN GROUPS

Overweight is more common among some ethnic and socioeconomic groups. Lack of knowledge about foods and physical activity, limited access to fresh produce and safe places to exercise, and easy access to increasing numbers of fast foods may all constitute risk factors. Lower income, and Hispanic, black, or Native-American ethnic identity are all associated with higher incidence of overweight, especially among women. National goals to eliminate health disparities in income and ethnic groups have been set (*Healthy People 2010,* 2000).

Many reasons are cited for the increase in overweight children. The number of calories consumed is not increasing. However, children tend to exercise less, particularly in daily life. They infrequently walk or ride bikes, either because of the convenience of driving or due to unsafe neighborhoods. Television viewing is very high among youth and contributes to overweight both from the inactivity associated with it and the pattern of snacking during commercial time. As many as 60% of obese children view television excessively, defined as more than 4 hours daily; over 25% of all children watch 4 or more hours of television daily and 67% watch at least 2 hours daily (Crespo, Smit, Troiano et al., 2001). Children may spend additional time with computer activities and playing video games.

The percentage of calories from fat consumed in the United States is among the highest in the world. Although no more than 30% of calories should come from total dietary fat, and no more than 10% from saturated fat, about 35% of calories consumed in the United States are supplied by fat and 12% by saturated fat (Krauss, Eckel, Howard et al., 2001; National Cholesterol Education Program, 1991). High levels of dietary fat are associated with higher cholesterol levels and decreased activity. The high rate of dietary fat is related to the large amount of fast food consumed, as fast food restaurants are convenient and fit well into today's lifestyles. Another factor that contributes to overweight is a pattern of snacking, and there has been an increase in this activity in the last decade. Snacks are often nutrient-poor and calorie-dense (Zizza, Siega-Riz, & Popkin, 2001).

Nurses can help parents and children build good nutritional and exercise habits throughout life, thus decreasing the incidence of overweight and its attendant health risks. Beginning with an assessment of growth patterns starting early in life, nurses can address patterns of eating fast foods, meals on the run, and while watching television in early health promotion and health maintenance visits. Parents should be advised that television viewing should be limited to a maximum of 2 hours daily, and that television and video games should not be placed in children's bedrooms. Daily exercise routines of at least 30 minutes can be included in most families. Also, nurses should teach about the Food Guide Pyramid and its integration into a healthy life. Healthy snacks include fruits, vegetables, grains, and nuts. "Super sizing" fast foods and eating out often should be avoided.

Risks for poor health often cluster together in individuals and families. Nurses need to be alert for situations in which parents are overweight and children have elevated blood pressure, exercise infrequently, or are in upper percentiles for weight, BMI, or skinfold. Girls who have menarche before 11 years of age are more often overweight. Being alert for early menarche can help identify overweight girls who need intervention for obesity prevention (Adair & Gordon-Larsen, 2001). The presence of risk factors necessitates further dietary and risk assessment so that a management plan can be implemented. Visit the Companion Website for information that will be helpful to families in the clinical setting. See resources such as "Helping Your Overweight Child" and "Take Charge of Your Health: A Teenager's Guide to Better Health."

Consult the "Nursing Care Plan" in this chapter for further interventions appropriate for the overweight child.

FOOD SAFETY

Every year in the United States, about 76 million people contract foodborne illnesses. Some are quite mild, while others can be very severe. Children are at greater risk of severe illness and death from food and water due to their immature gastrointestinal and immune systems. The most common pathogens are *Campylobacter, Salmonella, Shigella,* and *Escherichia coli;* infants are at extremely high risk of *Campylobacter, Rotavirus,* and *Salmonella* illness (MMWR, 2001a). A former common cause of food-related illness was hepatitis A. Although hepatitis A is still prevalent in some parts of the country, effective management and prevention through immunization has decreased its incidence (see Chapter 51 ∞). Worldwide over 3 million people die of illness related to unsafe drinking water each year, and most of those deaths are among children.

Foodborne illness is relayed by food preparation and storage practices, lack of adequate training of retail employees about foods and hygiene, and increasing amounts and types of foods being imported from other countries. Some examples of contaminated foods in the last few years include undercooked hamburger meat, cross-contamination of salad bar items from meats, unpasteurized apple cider, green onions, prepackaged salad and delicatessen meat, and sprouts. While most infected persons experience acute diarrhea, some can develop complications such as hemolytic uremic syndrome or thrombocytic purpura. Health personnel should integrate teaching regularly so that families can decrease risks of foodborne illness.

TEACHING HIGHLIGHTS

FOODBORNE SAFETY GUIDELINES

Four Key Food Safety Practices:

1. *Clean:* Wash hands and surfaces often.
2. *Separate:* Don't cross-contaminate.
3. *Cook:* Cook to proper temperatures.
4. *Chill:* Refrigerate promptly.

(U.S. Department of Health and Human Services, 2000)

Food may carry products other than microorganisms that can be harmful. An example is mercury, which may be concentrated in certain types of fish. This metal can cause harm to the developing nervous system of fetuses, infants, and young children when consumed regularly. The U.S. Food and Drug Administration (FDA) and Environmental Protection Agency (EPA) note that fish are an important part of a healthy diet, but that certain recommendations should be followed to lower risk of mercury's detrimental effects. Women who may become pregnant, are pregnant or breastfeeding, and young children should:

■ Eliminate shellfish, shark, swordfish, king mackerel, and tilefish from the diet.

- Eat up to 12 ounces (two average meals) a week of a variety of low-mercury fish and shellfish, such as shrimp, canned light tuna, salmon, pollock, and catfish. Albacore or white tuna has more mercury than light tuna, so limit white tuna to one meal weekly.

Check for local advisories about the safety of fish caught in local waters. In the absence of advice, up to 6 ounces (one meal) weekly may be eaten from local waters. Do not eat other fish during that week (FDA, 2004).

COMMON DIETARY DEFICIENCIES

Dietary deficiencies can occur in individual children, and some are common in populations. While children can have deficits in nearly any nutrient, a number of nutrient deficits are more common in childhood. Limitations in the food supply or patterns of dietary intake cause most deficiencies, while children with certain disease processes, such as metabolic diseases, may have difficulty absorbing or using nutrients ingested (see Chapter 56 for a discussion of inborn errors of metabolism ∞). The nutrient deficiencies of a population are a result of genetic factors, characteristics of the food supply, and intake patterns of particular groups.

DEVELOPING CULTURAL COMPETENCE

VITAMIN A DEFICIENCY

Vitamin A deficiency is common in developing countries. The vitamin is found in liver, dairy products, and fish. Provitamin A sources are yellow and dark green vegetables. The vitamin is fat soluble and stored in the liver. When deficient, children develop night blindness, vision loss, and high rates of infection. Public health efforts have been directed at identifying children with low vitamin A status and providing the vitamin in capsule form or in commonly ingested foods.

Iron

Newborns have a store of iron obtained from their mothers in the uterus, if the maternal nutritional state was satisfactory and the baby is normal gestational age. Breast milk contains little iron, but the iron it does contain has high bioavailability. However, by 4 to 6 months of age, the baby's iron stores begin to decrease and a dietary source of iron must be added. Enriched rice cereal is commonly used to meet these initial iron needs. In babies who do not have adequate stores or do not take in enough iron, **anemia**, or a reduction in the number of red blood cells, can result (Figure 34–8 ●). Feeding cow milk during infancy can also cause anemia by irritating the gut and leading to small but consistent loss of blood from the gastrointestinal tract; cow's milk should not be fed in the first year of life. When

● FIGURE 34–8

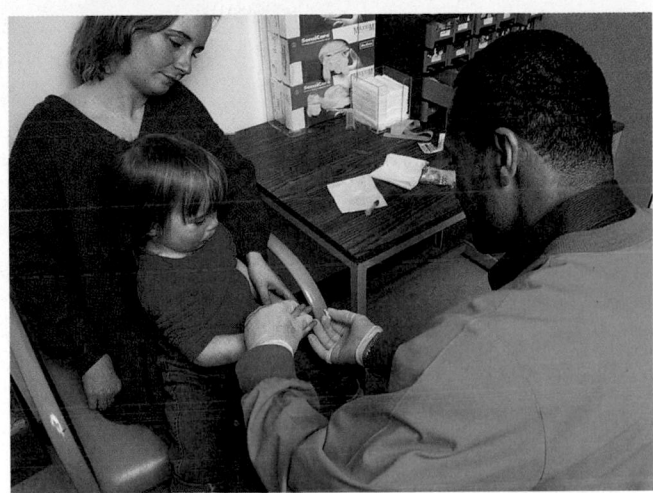

Most Head Start centers participate in screening programs to identify children at risk for anemia.

formulas are used, they should be iron fortified to help avoid iron deficiency anemia.

The other group most commonly deficient in iron is adolescent females, related to loss of blood in menses, metabolic need of the growth spurt, and poor dietary balance due to sporadic dieting. Further discussion of the symptoms and treatment of iron deficiency anemia can be found in Chapter 49. ∞ Encourage intake of good iron sources such as meats, eggs, dried fruits, iron-fortified cereal, and iron-fortified baby cereal for infants.

Calcium

Calcium is an essential nutrient for bone development during childhood and adolescence. An increased intake of soda pop and fruit juices is related to a decrease in calcium intake, especially among adolescents. During the adolescent growth spurt, almost 40% of the adult bone mass is accumulated (Trahms, 2000). Inadequate intake puts the person at risk for osteoporosis later in life since it is not possible to make up for earlier deficits. Although genetic variables account for some of the influence on adult bone mass, increasing calcium intake has been shown to promote bone formation. While the recommended daily intake for adolescents is 1500 mg, the average intake for adolescent males is 1169 mg and for females is only 753 mg (only half of the recommended level) (Food & Nutrition Board, 2001). Nurses should encourage foods such as milk and milk products, egg yolks, grains, legumes, nuts, and fruit juice with added calcium.

Adolescents at highest risk for impaired bone development include female athletes and others who diet to a great degree to maintain slimness. Teens who exercise excessively may manifest the "female athlete triad" of excessive thinness,

DRUG GUIDE

IRON

Overview of Action

Iron is a necessary component of hemoglobin and is therefore essential in the oxygen transfer carried out by red blood cells. It is used in microcytic and hypochromic anemia, which result from iron deficiency. Supplements are frequently used during pregnancy when intake often does not meet iron needs, and in infants with decreased iron stores, such as with small-for-gestational-age and premature infants.

Route, Dosage, Frequency

Ferrous Fumarate: 3 mg/kg/day po

Ferrous Gluconate: 8 mg/kg/day po—over 2 years

Ferrous Sulfate: 5 mg/kg/day po

Ferrous Sulfate Dried: 160 mg/day po

Iron Dextran: up to 25 mg/day (under 5 kg weight); up to 50 mg/day (5–10 kg weight); up to 100 mg/day (over 10 kg)—IM, IV

RDAs for Iron:

7–12 months: 11 mg

1–3 years: 7 mg

4–8 years: 10 mg

9–13 years: 8 mg

14–18 years: males 11 mg; females 15 mg

Pregnancy: 27 mg

Lactation: 9–10 mg

Nursing Considerations

Administer PO: The mg doses of various forms of iron are not equivalent; rather, the amount of elemental iron in various preparations is important.

Administration with a snack decreases absorption but is often recommended, as GI irritation will be lessened. Accompanying iron with vitamin C may enhance iron absorption.

Liquid preparations should be given with fluid, such as juice, and by a dropper or straw because they can stain teeth. **IM:** Do not mix with other medications. Given to the upper outer buttock; therefore, this form is used only in older children and adults. Change needle after drawing up iron. Use long needle and **Z–track** injection technique. Permanent tissue staining can occur if not deep IM. Aspirate after inserting needle and inject slowly. **IV:** Given undiluted. Do not mix with other medications (known to be incompatible with some other medicines) and do not use the multidose bottle (latter only for IM injection). Give at rate slower than 1 mL/minute. Test dose of 25 mg or less given over 5 minutes. If no reaction, remaining dose can be given over 1–6 hours. Flush vein after infusion with normal saline.

Assess: Obtain a diet history. Be alert for elements that can decrease iron absorption, such as low-calcium or high-phosphate diet, infection, or decreased GI acid. Watch for signs of deficiency in infants after 4–6 months of age when maternal iron stores are depleted (earlier in premature infants). A CBC including hematocrit, hemoglobin, and reticulocytes is done to establish iron deficiency anemia. Before administering parenteral iron, a test dose of 0.5 mL is given.

Monitor: Epinephrine 1:1000 available for parenteral administration. Watch for hypersensitivity. Hemoglobin, hematocrit, other lab studies regularly.

Teaching: Take oral preparation between meals unless GI distress occurs. Teach food sources of iron. Take liquid forms with straw and water to decrease chance of teeth staining. Dairy products, eggs, whole grains, tea, and coffee decrease iron absorption.

Data from information in Bindler, R. M., & Howry, L. B. (2005). Pediatric drug guide. Upper Saddle River, NJ: Prentice Hall-Health.

---

excessive exercise, and amenorrhea. A high rate of fractures and osteomalacia can result, in addition to an extreme risk of osteoporosis in adulthood. Asking about menstrual patterns as well as exercise and diet can be combined with physical measurements of height and weight to obtain pertinent information about the teen athlete. See the discussion of the eating disorders anorexia nervosa and bulimia nervosa later in this chapter.

Vitamin D

Vitamin D deficiencies are rare since the vitamin can be synthesized in the skin upon exposure to sunlight. However, an increase in cases of vitamin D-deficient rickets has recently been observed. This vitamin is needed to enhance absorption of calcium, so a lack of vitamin D can contribute to calcium deficiency as well. Human milk contains little vitamin D, and if infants are kept wrapped when outside, live in northern climates and rarely get outside in win-

GROWTH AND DEVELOPMENT

Vitamin D rickets had virtually disappeared from the United States, but several cases have recently been identified. Suggested reasons for the resurgence include failure to provide vitamin D supplementation when breastfeeding is the sole source of intake for over 6 months, use of nonfortified products such as soy milk, and use of sunscreens or covers when infants are outside. Be alert for infants and toddlers with neurologic conditions such as seizures, low height for age, slowness in learning to walk, and malformations (bowing) of spine, legs, and arms. Encourage sunscreen use, but be aware that children who are dark skinned or are kept covered due to religious beliefs may be at higher risk. Be certain that breastfed babies receive vitamin D supplements until other vitamin D sources are added to the diet (MMWR, 2001b). When rickets is suspected, laboratory studies should include serum calcium, phosphorus, 25–OH vitamin D, alkaline phosphatase, parathyroid hormone, and hematocrit (Oken & Lightdale, 2001).

ter months, have extensive sunscreens applied, or are dark in skin color, vitamin D deficiency can result. This has led to a recommendation by the American Academy of Pediatrics that all breastfed infants receive a 400 international units supplement of vitamin D daily. Formula-fed babies receive adequate amounts in commercial formulas.

Folic Acid

Epidemiologic evidence has linked increasing maternal folic acid (the most common form of folate in the human body) intake with decreased incidence of neural tube defects such as spina bifida in offspring. More recently, cleft lip and palate incidence has also been found to decrease when folate intake increases, and research is examining the role of folate and B vitamins in prevention of depression. Folate levels are low among adolescents, putting them at particular risk of birth defects when they have babies. The FDA approved fortification of cereals and breads with folate to decrease the population risk of related congenital anomalies. Other good sources of folate include spinach, avocado, green leafy vegetables, beans and peas, liver, and many fruits.

Protein-Energy Malnutrition

Although the micronutrient deficiencies described above are the most common problems in developed countries, macronutrient deficiencies are the most common nutritional problems worldwide. While kwashiorkor indicates protein deficiency, and marasmus is a lack of energy-producing calories, both deficiencies often occur together and are referred to as protein-energy malnutrition (PEM). Protein deficiency manifests with edema, leading to the large abdomens and rounded faces seen in severely malnourished children. Other symptoms include scant, depigmented hair, skin changes, and decreased serum proteins. It can occur following severe diarrhea or other infection in susceptible children. Caloric deficiency results in emaciation, decreased energy levels, and retarded development (see Table 34–4). PEM may occur when a child is weaned in order for the mother to provide breast milk to a new baby. Adoptees and immigrants to developed countries sometimes manifest with at least mild PEM, so careful nutritional assessment is needed to provide adequate nutrition.

FEEDING AND EATING DISORDERS

Deficiencies in food intake related to available nutrients and safety of the food supply were discussed in the previous section. In addition to these issues of availability, nutrient intake is affected by psychologic issues of individuals as well. Disorders of food intake span the entire developmental spectrum and can affect pregnant women, young children, and adolescents. Some of the most common feeding and eating disorders are discussed below.

Pica

Pica is an eating disorder characterized by ingestion of nonfood items or food items consumed in abnormal quantities or forms. Examples of ingested items include starch, peeling paint, paper, soil components, flour, and coffee grounds. Clinical manifestations include zinc and iron deficiencies as well as symptoms of lead or other poisoning (see Chapter 51 ∞) if these substances are contained in peeling paint or other ingested material. The disorder most commonly manifests in pregnancy when women have abnormal cravings for nonfood products, and it can seriously impair the developing fetus (see Chapter 12 for more information ∞). Some children also ingest abnormal amounts of nonfood items and fail to take in adequate nutrients from food. Treatment for children involves removing them from the substances, ensuring an adequate and nutritious diet, and treating any dietary deficiencies noted.

Feeding Disorder of Infancy and Early Childhood (Failure to Thrive)

Feeding disorder of infancy and early childhood, or failure to thrive (FTT), describes a syndrome in which infants or young children fail to eat enough food to be adequately nourished. This disorder accounts for 5% to 10% of pediatric hospitalizations in children under 1 year of age, and many more children are managed in community settings (Behrman, Kliegman, & Jenson, 2004).

Etiology and Pathophysiology. The cause of feeding disorder can be organic, as in congenital acquired immunodeficiency syndrome (AIDS) (see Chapter 43 ∞), inborn errors of metabolism (see Chapter 56 ∞), congenital heart defect (see Chapter 47 ∞), neurologic disease (see Chapter 53 ∞), and esophageal reflux (see Chapter 51 ∞). However, most cases are nonorganic in origin. When the cause is nonorganic, the condition is called feeding disorder of infancy or early childhood.

Infants and children whose parents or caretakers suffer from depression, substance abuse, mental retardation, or psychosis are at risk for this disorder. Parents may be socially and emotionally isolated, or may lack knowledge of infant nutritional and nurturing needs. A reciprocal interaction pattern may exist in which the parent does not offer enough food or is not responsive to the infant's hunger cues, and the infant is irritable, not soothed, and does not give clear cues about hunger (Corrales & Utter, 1999). Premature and small-for-gestational-age babies more commonly have eating disorders.

Clinical Manifestations. The characteristics of this feeding disorder are persistent failure to eat adequately with no

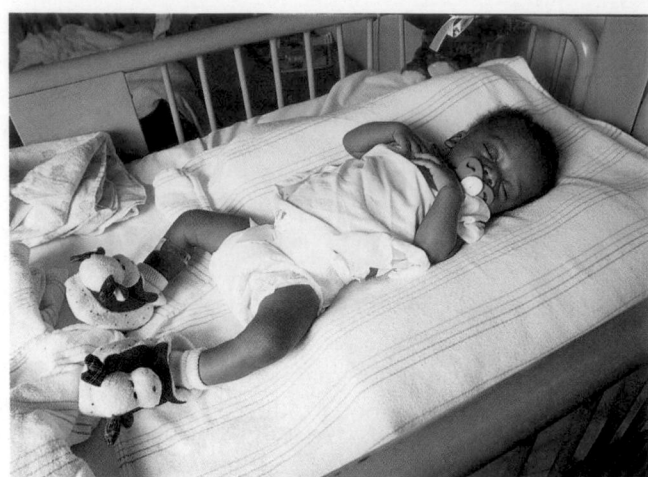

Infants with failure to thrive may not look severely malnourished, but they fall well below the expected weight and height norms for their age. This infant, who appears to be about 4 months old, is actually 8 months old. He has been hospitalized for feeding disorder of infancy.

weight gain or with weight loss in a child under 6 years of age, which is not associated with other medical conditions or mental disorders, and is not caused by lack of or unavailability of food (American Psychiatric Association Working Group on Eating Disorders, 2000). Infants with feeding disorder refuse food, may have erratic sleep patterns, are irritable and difficult to soothe, and are often developmentally delayed (Figure 34–9 ●).

Clinical Therapy. A thorough history and physical examination are needed to rule out any chronic physical illness. The infant or child may be hospitalized so that healthcare providers can establish a routine for feeding and sleeping. The goals of treatment are to provide adequate caloric and nutritional intake, promote normal growth and development, and assist parents in developing feeding routines and responding to the infant's cues of physical and psychologic hunger.

DEVELOPING CULTURAL COMPETENCE

HEIGHT AND WEIGHT GROWTH STANDARDS

Each child should maintain a height and weight growth pattern similar to the population standard. Asian-American children may normally be below the fifth percentile on growth charts and not have an eating disorder. Suspect an eating disorder when the infant or child falls one standard deviation below his or her own curve and either fails to gain weight or loses weight over several months.

NURSING MANAGEMENT

NURSING ASSESSMENT AND DIAGNOSIS

Nursing assessment of the child is essential for establishing the best intervention plan. Accurate weight and height each time any child is seen for healthcare provides an important record of growth patterns over time. This helps identify the child with an eating disorder. The child's activity level, developmental milestones, and interaction patterns provide important information. When feeding the child, observe how the child indicates hunger or satiety, the ability of the child to be soothed, and general interaction patterns such as eye contact, touch, and "cuddliness."

Ask parents about stresses in their lives; these may prevent appropriate interaction with the child. Asking about the pregnancy and birth can elicit information about early disturbances in the child-parent relationship. Are there other children in the family and have eating problems occurred with them? Observe the child and parent behaviors while they feed the child; cues given by each person and interactional modes such as rocking, singing, talking, and body postures are important.

Some of the nursing diagnoses pertinent for the young child with an eating disorder include the following:

- *Imbalanced Nutrition: Less than Body Requirements* related to inability to ingest proper amounts of food

- *Delayed Growth and Development* related to inadequate intake

- *Risk for Impaired Parenting* related to lack of knowledge about nutritional needs

- *Fatigue* related to malnutrition

PLANNING AND IMPLEMENTATION

Nursing care centers on performing a thorough history and physical assessment, observing parent-child interactions during feeding times, and providing necessary teaching to enable parents to respond appropriately to their child's needs. The child is often hospitalized initially and evaluated for physical growth while staff members feed the child. Accurate weights, nutritional assessments, and developmental evaluation should be done to see if the child grows more normally. Additional diagnostic tests may be carried out at this time to rule out organic causes of poor growth.

Once a diagnosis of nonorganic failure to thrive is confirmed, parents become involved in feeding the child. Observations of feeding and continued careful physical assessments are needed. Carefully record the child's intake at each meal or feeding. Teach parents how to understand and respond to the child's cues of hunger and satiety. Teach them to hold, rock, and touch the infant during feedings and establish eye contact with infants and older children.

Upon discharge, referral to an agency that can continue monitoring of the home situation is needed. This provides an opportunity to observe feeding during a home visit and evaluate stresses and behavior patterns among family members. Frequent growth measurement and development must be ensured so the child is adequately nourished. Parents may need referral to community resources to help them manage stressful situations in their lives and to enhance their parenting skills.

EVALUATION

Expected outcomes of nursing care include the following:

- Adequate growth and normal development of the infant is achieved.
- An improved parent-child relationship is established.

Anorexia Nervosa

Anorexia nervosa is a potentially life-threatening eating disorder that occurs primarily in teenage girls and young women, affecting an estimated 5% of young women and 1% of young men in the United States (American Dietetic Association, 2001). The typical patient is white and from a middle- to upper-middle-class family. Age at onset varies, and incidence peaks at 12 to 13 years and again at 17 to 18 years.

Etiology and Pathophysiology. Many causes are now thought to contribute to the onset of anorexia. Cultural overemphasis on thinness may contribute to the excessive concern with dieting, body image, and fear of becoming fat that is experienced by many adolescents. Chemical changes have been found in the brain and blood of individuals with anorexia, leading to theories about a biologic cause. Often a significant life stress, loss, or change precedes the onset of anorexia. Stress hormones are commonly elevated in anorectics, and immune system function may be disturbed (Brambilla, 2001; White, 2000).

Many authorities view family issues as contributory to anorexia. Intrafamilial conflicts and dysfunctional family patterns may occur when parents are overly controlling and perfectionistic. The adolescent's eating behaviors may be an attempt to exercise independence and resolve internal psychologic conflicts.

The adolescent may engage in lengthy and vigorous exercise (up to 4 hours daily) to prevent weight gain. Laxatives or diuretics may be used to induce weight loss. As the disorder progresses, the adolescent perceives the ever-thinner body as becoming more beautiful. Youths may share weight loss techniques with anorectic friends and search out Internet sites that are positive about anorexia. The body responds to the abnormal eating behaviors as if starvation

were occurring. Leukopenia, electrolyte imbalance, and hypoglycemia develop as a result of PEM. Once the body mass decreases below a critical level, menstruation ceases.

Clinical Manifestations. Anorectic adolescents are characterized by extreme weight loss accompanied by a preoccupation with weight and food, excessive compulsive exercising, peculiar patterns of eating and handling food, and distorted body image. They may prepare elaborate meals for others but eat only low-calorie foods. Characteristically, the fear of becoming fat does not decrease with continued weight loss. Accompanying signs and symptoms of depression, crying spells, feelings of isolation and loneliness, and suicidal thoughts and feelings are common. The disorder is often associated with mental illness such as obsessive-compulsive disorder, anxiety disorders (see Chapter 54 ∞), and history of abuse (Herpertz-Dahlmann, Muller, Herpertz et al., 2001).

Physical findings include cold intolerance, dizziness, constipation, abdominal discomfort, bloating, irregular menses, and malnutrition (Figure 34–10 ●). Hypothalamic suppression can lead to disturbances of gynecologic function, osteoporosis, decreased bone density, and fractures (Seidenfeld & Rickert, 2001). Lanugo (fine, downy body hair) may be present. Fluid and electrolyte imbalances, especially potassium imbalances, are common. The child or adolescent is usually energetic despite significant weight loss. Extreme weight loss often leads to cardiac arrhythmias (bradycardia).

● **FIGURE 34–10**

This young lady began to have symptoms of anorexia at age 12 years. Her parents obtained ongoing counseling for her and the family. She died of the disorder in her early 20s.

TABLE 34–8 ✣ *DSM-IV* Diagnostic Criteria for Anorexia Nervosa

A. Refusal to maintain body weight at or above a minimally normal weight for age and height (e.g., weight loss leading to maintenance of body weight less than 85% of that expected; or failure to make expected weight gain during period of growth, leading to body weight less than 85% of that expected).

B. Intense fear of gaining weight or becoming fat, even though underweight.

C. Disturbance in the way in which one's weight or shape is experienced, undue influence of body weight or shape on self-evaluation, or denial of the seriousness of the current body weight.

D. In postmenarcheal females, amenorrhea, i.e., the absence of at least three consecutive menstrual cycles. (A woman is considered to have amenorrhea if her periods occur only following hormone, e.g., estrogen, administration).

Used with permission from the Diagnostic and Statistical Manual of Mental Disorders, 4th ed., © 2000. American Psychiatric Association.

Clinical Therapy. Diagnosis is based on a comprehensive history, physical examination revealing characteristic clinical manifestations, and the *DSM-IV* criteria included in Table 34–8. Diagnostic tests commonly include hematocrit and hemoglobin, serum electrolytes, and serum vitamins and vitamin-precursors.

The goal of treatment is to address the physiologic problems associated with malnutrition, as well as the behavioral and cognitive components of the disorder. A firm focus is placed on reaching a targeted weight with a gradual weight gain of 0.1 to 0.2 kg/day (0.25 to 0.5 lb/day). Enteral feedings or total parenteral nutrition (TPN) may be necessary to replace lost fluid, protein, and nutrients, although the adolescent often perceives these feedings as a punitive measure.

Individual treatment and family therapy are used to address dysfunctional family patterns and assist the family to accept and deal with the adolescent as an independent and less than perfect individual. Family involvement is crucial to effect a lasting change in the adolescent. Nurses, psychologists, family therapists, and dietitians commonly partner to plan and implement therapy.

Long-term outpatient treatment, in either an individual or a group setting, is frequently necessary. Counseling may be continued for 2 to 3 years to ensure that weight gain and self-image are maintained. Antidepressant drugs such as imipramine (Tofranil) or desipramine (Norpramin) may be prescribed for coexisting conditions such as depression, anxiety, or obsessive-compulsive disorders.

Indications for hospitalization include loss of 25% to 30% of body weight, fluid and electrolyte imbalances or arrhythmias, or the need to provide a more intense period of therapy if outpatient treatment fails to produce improvement. Behavior modification techniques are used extensively in combination with counseling and other methods in the care of the hospitalized anorectic adolescent.

NURSING MANAGEMENT

NURSING ASSESSMENT AND DIAGNOSIS

Obtain a thorough individual and family history. Ask about usual eating patterns, daily caloric intake, exercise patterns, and menstrual history. Ask about medication use; include prescription, nonprescription, and herbal products. Is there a family history of eating disorders? Assess for signs of malnutrition. Obtain height and weight measurements and compare with norms for the general population. Because the anorectic patient often wears layers of clothes when being weighed, strive to obtain an accurate measurement.

Nursing diagnoses for the adolescent with anorexia nervosa include the following:

- *Imbalanced Nutrition: Less than Body Requirements* related to inadequate intake
- *Risk for Deficient Fluid Volume* related to inadequate fluid intake or fluid volume loss from overuse of laxatives and diuretics
- *Risk for Imbalanced Body Temperature* related to excessive weight loss and absence of subcutaneous fat
- *Constipation* related to inadequate food intake and overuse of laxatives
- *Disturbed Body Image* related to distorted perception of body size and shape
- *Chronic Low Self-Esteem* related to dysfunctional family dynamics
- *Compromised Family Coping* related to parental tendency to be overly controlling and perfectionistic

PLANNING AND IMPLEMENTATION

Nursing care centers on meeting nutritional and fluid needs, preventing complications, administering medications, and providing referral to appropriate resources. Specific treatment measures vary depending on physical complications, length and degree of illness, emotional symptoms accompanying the disorder, and family dynamics. Resistance to treatment is common, and nurses who care for anorectic adolescents must deal with their own feelings of frustration and anger.

Meet Nutritional and Fluid Needs

Monitor nutritional and fluid intake, encourage consumption of food, and observe eating behaviors at mealtime. Elimination patterns may be altered as a result of increased intake during hospitalization. Monitor for possible problems, including abdominal distention, constipation, or diarrhea. Daily monitoring of serum electrolytes is necessary.

If TPN is administered, watch for complications such as circulatory overload, hyperglycemia, or hypoglycemia. Use strict aseptic technique when changing tubing or dressings.

Administer Medications

Monitor vital signs if the adolescent is receiving antidepressants. Watch for signs of hypertension and tachycardia. Administer medications after meals because it helps to prevent gastric irritation. Be alert for substance abuse. Anorectics often use products such as excess laxatives or ephedra (also known as ma huang) to induce weight loss. Changes in the central nervous system, vital signs, and other findings may indicate over-the-counter or herbal drug use.

Provide Referral to Appropriate Resources

Refer parents and other family members to the American Anorexia and Bulimia Association, National Anorectic Aid Society, and National Association of Anorexia Nervosa & Associated Disorders for further information about the disorder and a list of support groups in their area.

EVALUATION

Expected outcomes for nursing care include weight gain, maintenance of adequate fluid volume, beginning of positive sense of self-esteem, intake of nutritionally balanced diet, and use of psychologic counseling to understand the disorder.

Bulimia Nervosa

Bulimia nervosa is an eating disorder characterized by binge eating (a compulsion to consume large quantities of food in a short period of time). Usually the episodes of bingeing are followed by various methods of weight control (purging), such as self-induced vomiting, large doses of laxatives or diuretics, or a combination of methods. Bulimia affects 5% or more of young women. Like anorexia, it affects mainly adolescent girls and young women who are white and in the higher socioeconomic classes (Orbanic, 2001). The disorder usually begins in middle to late adolescence, frequently emerging during college.

Etiology and Pathophysiology. Causes of bulimia nervosa are similar to those of anorexia nervosa: sensitivity to social pressure for thinness, body image difficulties, and long-standing dysfunctional family patterns. Families may be chaotic and distant from the girl, rather than overinvolved as with the anorectic. Many bulimic individuals experience depression. It is not clear whether the depression is a cause or a result of the bulimic individual's inability to control the bingeing and purging cycles. A bulimic adolescent often binges after any stressful event.

Bingeing usually occurs in secret for several hours until the individual is stopped by abdominal discomfort, by an-

other person, or by vomiting. At first the episodes of binge eating are pleasurable. Immediately following the binge episode, however, feelings of guilt, shame, anger, depression, and fear of loss of control and weight gain arise. As these feelings intensify, the bulimic adolescent becomes increasingly anxious. This usually initiates the purge behaviors.

Purging eliminates the discomfort from bloating and also prevents weight gain. This relieves the feelings of depression and guilt, but only temporarily. Adolescents with bulimia commonly practice the binge-purge cycle many times a day, losing their ability to respond to normal cues of hunger and satiety.

Clinical Manifestations. Bulimic adolescents, like anorectics, are preoccupied with body shape, size, and weight. They may appear overweight or thin and usually report a wide range of average body weight over the years. Physical findings depend on the degree of purging, starvation, dehydration, and electrolyte disturbance. Erosion of tooth enamel, increased dental caries, and gum recession, which result from vomiting of gastric acids, are common findings. The back of a hand can have calluses from inducing vomiting. Abdominal distention is often seen. Esophageal tears and esophagitis may also occur.

Clinical Therapy. A comprehensive history is necessary because most bulimic adolescents appear normal in weight or only slightly underweight. Diagnostic tests include hematocrit, hemoglobin, and serum electrolytes; they may identify signs of altered electrolyte and hematologic status. The diagnosis is confirmed by the presence of specific *DSM-IV* criteria (Table 34–9).

TABLE 34–9 ✢ *DSM-IV* Criteria for Bulimia Nervosa

A. Recurrent episodes of binge eating. An episode of binge eating is characterized by both of the following:
   1. Eating, in a discrete period of time (e.g., within any 2-hour period), an amount of food that is definitely larger than most people would eat during a similar period of time and under similar circumstances
   2. A sense of lack of control over eating during the episode (e.g., a feeling that one cannot stop eating or control what or how much one is eating)
B. Recurrent inappropriate compensatory behavior in order to prevent weight gain, such as self-induced vomiting; misuse of laxatives, diuretics, enemas, or other medications; fasting; or excessive exercise.
C. The binge eating and inappropriate compensatory behaviors both occur, on average, at least twice a week for 3 months.
D. Self-evaluation is unduly influenced by body weight and shape.
E. The disturbance does not occur exclusively during episodes of anorexia nervosa.

Used with permission from the Diagnostic and Statistical Manual of Mental Disorders, 4th ed., © 2000. American Psychiatric Association.

[Right margin: MediaLink — Video: Anorexia Nervosa]

Treatment includes management of physiologic problems, behavior modification, and psychotherapy. Such management involves a variety of healthcare providers such as physicians, nurses, and therapists. Behavior modification focuses on modifying the dysfunctional eating patterns and restoring a normal pattern. Until the episodes of bingeing and purging are under control, feelings of discouragement and hopelessness prevail. Thus, the focus early in treatment is on initiating an immediate behavioral change. Once initial interventions have been successful, group therapy sessions work well for persons with anorexia or bulimia. Specific treatment measures may include the following:

- Educating the adolescent about good nutrition (including food choice and caloric content)
- Encouraging the adolescent to keep a log or food journal and assisting the adolescent to make connections between emotional states, stress, and the impulse to binge or purge
- Setting up a daily dietary routine of three meals and three snacks a day (using the same foods for each meal and snack every day to change misconceptions about the weight-gaining potential of certain foods and to decrease anxiety about what food must be eaten at the next meal)

Once these initial measures have been taken, the underlying psychosocial issues are explored. The goals of therapy are to provide the bulimic adolescent with adaptive coping skills and to improve self-esteem.

Most bulimic adolescents do not require hospitalization. Serious abnormalities in fluid and electrolyte levels caused by uncontrollable cycles of bingeing and vomiting, accompanied by depression or suicidal activity, are indications of the need for hospitalization. The prognosis is good with long-term therapy.

NURSING MANAGEMENT

NURSING ASSESSMENT AND DIAGNOSIS

Obtain a thorough individual and family history, including daily dietary intake and weight fluctuations. Inquire about problems such as abdominal pain or distention, which may indicate an abnormal eating or elimination pattern. Assess the oral mucosa for signs of damage to tooth enamel caused by purging; examine hands for evidence of vomiting-induced calluses.

Following are nursing diagnoses that may be appropriate for the adolescent with bulimia nervosa:

- *Imbalanced Nutrition: Less than or More than Body Requirements* related to inadequate intake

- *Risk for Deficient Fluid Volume* related to fluid volume loss
- *Impaired Oral Mucous Membrane* related to chemical effects of vomited gastric acids
- *Deficient Knowledge (child)* related to health risks of excessive use of laxatives and diuretics
- *Anxiety* related to discomfort with weight and eating patterns
- *Chronic Low Self-Esteem* related to dysfunctional family dynamics
- *Ineffective Individual Coping* related to life stressors

PLANNING AND IMPLEMENTATION

Nursing care includes monitoring nutritional intake and elimination patterns, preventing complications, and providing appropriate referrals.

During hospitalization the patient should keep a food diary. Be alert to the adolescent who hides, gives away, or discards food from the tray or who exits to use the bathroom after meals. The adolescent should be monitored for at least 30 minutes after meals by remaining in a central area in the company of the nurse or other responsible individuals. Withdrawal from laxatives and diuretics is managed with careful observation for alterations in fluid and electrolyte status. Cardiac monitoring may be necessary if potassium levels are seriously altered. Esophageal tearing or esophagitis is treated to promote mucosal healing. Medications such as antidepressants may be administered. Encourage continuation of group and other therapy sessions.

Bulimic adolescents and their families can be referred to organizations such as those listed earlier in the section on anorexia for assistance and information about the disorder.

EVALUATION

Expected outcomes for nursing care for the adolescent with bulimia include healthy mucous membranes and skin, adequate intake of fluids and food, balanced food intake, maintenance of normal weight, and absence of bingeing and purging.

FOOD REACTIONS

Food reaction encompasses any adverse reaction to foods or substances ingested in foods. Allergies are the most serious type of reaction. The foods that most commonly cause allergy are fish, shellfish, nuts, eggs, soy, wheat, corn, strawberries, and cow's milk products. Allergies are IgE-mediated reactions that are potentially systemic and are characteristically rapid in onset. They may be manifested as swelling of the lips, mouth, uvula, or glottis; generalized urticaria; and, in severe reactions, anaphylaxis. Food allergies are the most common cause of anaphylaxis and are more prevalent in children with a family history of allergic reactions to various substances and foods (**atopy**). Children with allergies may experience reddened cheeks and urticaria of the lips, mouth, and throat when they eat certain foods (Pongracic, 2000). Allergic individuals need to be aware of hidden substances in prepared foods. For example, the child allergic to nuts will experience a reaction to a food if nut extracts are used in its preparation.

Delayed hypersensitivity reactions are attributed to digestive products of food and require a thorough diet history over several days to identify the offending food. These reactions are more difficult to diagnose, since the reaction can occur up to 24 hours after ingestion of the food. There may also be biphasic reactions that occur 1 to 30 hours after an initial anaphylaxis. Such reactions can be severe and life threatening.

Food intolerance refers to an abnormal physiologic response to a food and is not IgE-mediated. Examples might include indigestion or flatulence upon eating certain foods, or a sweating reaction to some spices (Burks, 2000).

Cow milk may cause an allergy or food intolerance. In allergy an IgE-mediated systemic reaction occurs. In intolerance there is a gastrointestinal response to milk proteins (diarrhea, vomiting, abdominal pain) as a result of the lack of the enzyme lactase in the gastrointestinal tract. Infants have difficulty absorbing cow's milk; when ingesting it, they may have vomiting and watery, blood-streaked, mucoid diarrhea. Even without such overt signs, they may have anemia induced by blood loss not noted by care providers.

DEVELOPING CULTURAL COMPETENCE

LACTOSE INTOLERANCE

Some ethnic groups have a high incidence of lactose intolerance due to low amounts of the enzyme lactase in the gut. While most members of the group have adequate amounts of lactase in childhood to drink milk products, by adulthood 70% to 100% of some groups are lactose intolerant. Blacks, Native Americans, and Asians often have lactase deficiency which may begin to emerge during childhood. When a child develops intolerance to milk products, suggest alternative sources of calcium and other nutrients found in milk.

Diagnostic tests to identify suspected food allergies include measurement of serum IgE levels, scratch tests, and the **radioallergosorbent test (RAST)**, in which radioimmunoassay measures IgE antibodies to specific allergens (see Chapter 44 ∞). A diet diary is kept, noting date, type of foods eaten, and reaction, if any. Foods should be eaten singly for several days to determine whether they cause a reaction.

Treatment consists of eliminating the offending foods from the child's diet.

Nursing Management

Prevention is the first step. Instruct parents of infants to introduce new foods at a rate of not more than one new food every 3 to 5 days. If a sensitivity is noted, the causative food can be easily identified. Discuss any changes in diet or preparation of formula. Reassure parents that the child's symptoms will disappear when the offending foods are removed from the diet.

Be alert for skin, respiratory, and other characteristic manifestations of sensitivity or allergy. Many nurses are involved in administering and measuring skin prick tests for possible allergies.

Nursing care of a child with food allergies is primarily supportive. Help the family identify the offending foods. Explain to parents all tests, use of a food diary, and care of the child should a reaction occur. The child and school may need an EpiPen or other emergency treatment for the allergic child. Emphasize the importance of reading food labels for hidden foods that can trigger an allergic reaction (Bock, Munoz-Furlong, & Sampson, 2001). The child with a food allergy should wear a medical alert bracelet. Be sure that school personnel know about the allergy and know to avoid giving the child the food product. Some allergies can create expense for the family as they search for special foods; ask if this is an issue for them. Refer the family to the Food Allergy Network (see our Companion Website). Recognize that food allergies can be life threatening and plan carefully with the family, childcare facilities, schools, and other community contacts to ensure avoidance of the offending food and fast treatment if needed.

NURSING PRACTICE

Children with food allergies should wear an alert bracelet and carry an emergency medication such as EpiPen. Nurses in schools and offices must instruct families, schoolteachers, and others about the child's allergy and what to do in case of accidental ingestion of the food product. Assist them to set up prevention and emergency treatment plans.

NUTRITIONAL SUPPORT

SPORTS NUTRITION

Regular physical activity should be encouraged for all children, with at least 30 to 60 minutes of activity recommended daily. However, during vigorous or prolonged exercise, or during hot weather, child and adolescent athletes may have special nutritional needs. A well-balanced diet, reflective of the Food Guide Pyramid, is needed. A wide variety of fresh fruits and vegetables, grains, and complex carbohydrates usually provides for adequate caloric intake. When the child is hungry, extra calories should come from the food groups listed here, rather than from increased intake of fat. When the child or teen is very active, sports bars or drinks can provide the additional needed calories in a nutritionally balanced manner. As always, the height, weight, and BMI percentiles are the best assurance that the child is growing adequately over time. Adequate energy to perform the sport as well as be attentive and productive at school and for other activities should also be considered.

Water should be increased during activity both to minimize chance of dehydration and also to maximize performance. About 1 hour before vigorous exercise, the child should drink 1 to 2 glasses (8 to 16 ounces) of water and should repeat the same amount of fluid just before the exercise begins. Young children may not feel thirsty and should be encouraged to drink 4 to 6 ounces of fluid every 15 minutes during exercise (Trahms, 2000). Water is usually the best replacement, but during extended exercise, sports drinks may be a good alternative for some of the fluid intake. More water is needed after activity. Weight loss of 1 pound indicates a loss of about ½ quart of fluid. The nurse should be sure the child takes in fluid to replace all losses.

Some common nutrients that may be deficient in all teens, but even more often in the athlete, are calcium and iron. The increased blood volume common in the well-conditioned person necessitates greater intake. Calcium-rich foods such as milk products and dark green vegetables, and iron-rich foods such as meats and grains can guard against deficiencies. While many adolescents believe that they need extra protein during athletic season, most Americans eat adequate protein to meet even the increased needs of sports. On the other hand, the vegetarian child or adolescent may need help to plan a diet with adequate protein.

Many teens take a wide variety of dietary supplements, believing that they enhance performance during sports. Most of the claims of these products are unproven, and their safety has not usually been investigated, especially in the young. The nurse should offer guidance and help the family and teen investigate claims before choosing to use a product. They should be instructed in doses, desired effects, and potential side effects of supplements. Some sports and coaches may encourage small size and dieting. Children and adolescents in activities such as ballet, wrestling, track or running, and horse racing may have health risks associated with inconsistent or poor intake.

Some common amino acid nutritional supplements include creatine, carnitine, and glutamine. Although the side effects of these substances are minimal, their possible enhancement of performance is temporary and outcomes of long-term use are unknown. Increasing protein intake

to meet needs during high activity is a better alternative. Creatine has been studied more than most supplements; it is made by the body and is present in many protein sources. Supplemental creatine increases the creatine level in muscle and may help to increase performance in short bursts of activity, while not affecting endurance sports. The increase in muscle mass that can occur is actually due to water and is lost quickly when the supplement is discontinued (Johnson, 2001). Some athletes obtain steroids, which can cause serious side effects and can lead to endocrine disturbance and interfere with growth; their use is

COMPLEMENTARY CARE

USE OF DIETARY SUPPLEMENTS IN CHILDREN

The use of complementary and alternative therapies has continued to increase over the last 10 years, and this includes the use of dietary supplements in children. Approximately one in two infants or preschoolers and one in three school-age children use at least one vitamin and mineral supplement, typically a multivitamin. Adolescents are most likely to use two or more supplements, often a vitamin/mineral or multiple vitamin supplement plus single vitamins (Briefel, 2002). Dietary supplements—which include herbs or botanicals, vitamins, minerals, and homeopathic remedies—have been promoted to improve health, prevent illness, and be a "safer" alternative to conventional medications such as antibiotics.

Dietary supplements come in many forms and are marketed as capsules, tablets, tinctures, extracts, and tea. Many parents have learned about the use of dietary supplements from magazine and newspaper articles that often claim cures for common childhood conditions. There have been few well-controlled studies using dietary supplements in children. Although dietary supplements and pharmaceuticals have similarities such as similar appearance (pills, capsules, etc.) and biochemical remedies, they have significant differences as well. Dietary supplements do not have similar regulation in regard to processing, purity, and potency, as does the pharmaceutical industry.

Some dietary supplements—specifically, herbs—are considered safe and effective for children and adolescents, such as echinacea (see Chapter 42 ∞), and chamomile (see Chapter 51 ∞). There are many more dietary supplements used in children and adolescents, some with studies to support their use. Since dietary supplements are not controlled well for quality or purity, the healthcare provider is the best advisor to parents and adolescents as to which products to use. Though advertised as "natural," dietary supplements are not always safe to use and may have druglike effects. Parents and children should be told that if a product claims to be a "miracle cure" to treat multiple different conditions, and the medical and scientific communities are trying to suppress its use, then that dietary supplement is one to avoid. Until federal regulations improve (including good manufacturing practices) and studies including children are done, the widespread use of dietary supplements in children should be minimal and cautious.

also illegal in sports. Minerals such as chromium, iron, and calcium are used by some youths. The nurse should ask careful and sensitive questions such as "Many athletes take supplements to aid in performance in sports. What supplements do you take or are you considering?" Information should be provided to enhance the youth's understanding of nutrition and sports performance. Generally, a balanced diet with adequate carbohydrate, protein, and fat will meet the needs of most athletes and lead to maximal sport performance.

HEALTH-RELATED CONDITIONS

Many health conditions influence the child's nutritional state. Conversely, the child's nutritional state can influence the state of health. See "Pathophysiology Illustrated" for examples of some common conditions that influence nutritional needs. These conditions are discussed in various chapters throughout the text. When reading about them, discuss with classmates how to adjust normal nutritional assessment and teaching due to the presence of a healthcare

PATHOPHYSIOLOGY ILLUSTRATED
Conditions That Influence Nutritional Needs

Cerebral palsy or other brain damage can influence the child's ability to chew and swallow food.

Lack of sufficient vitamin A intake causes blindness or impaired vision in many children in developing countries.

Child with renal disease may have trouble regulating fluids and proteins in the body.

Cystic fibrosis influences the child's ability to absorb nutrients.

Liver disease alters the child's ability to break down metabolic waste products.

Child with diabetes needs close monitoring and regulation of dietary intake.

concern. Which conditions influence absorption of nutrients? Which cause changes in nutritional intake requirements? Some children benefit from special dietary aids, such as eating utensils and cups that are easy to grasp. Therapists can evaluate and make recommendations about devices that can assist the child at meals.

VEGETARIANISM

Some families choose to eat vegetarian diets and can be helped and encouraged in their endeavors. Several variations in intake occur. **Vegetarians** eat no poultry, meat, or fish. Lacto-ovovegetarians eat eggs and dairy products, while lacto-vegetarians eat dairy products. In contrast, **vegans** are strict vegetarians and eat no animal products. When someone says they are vegetarian, it is best if the nurse asks specific questions about what the individual will and will not eat.

GROWTH AND DEVELOPMENT

When a pregnant teen follows a vegetarian diet, she needs additional help to encourage adequate nutrition (Rudys-Shapard, 2001). A 24-hour or 2-day diet record helps identify nutritional needs. Consider additional pregnancy needs for protein, iron, and calcium, and note that Vitamin B$_{12}$ is recommended as a supplement. Use the vegetarian Food Guide Pyramid available through the American Dietetic Association.

The vegetarian can be very healthy, but may need some additional help to ensure nutritional adequacy. Some common deficiencies include vitamins D and B$_{12}$, zinc, iron, calories, protein, and fat. Completing a 24-hour diet recall for pregnant or lactating women and vegetarian children, with analysis for RDAs, can be helpful. The nurse should be sure to routinely assess growth and other nutritional measures, as well as provide ideas of various foods to meet nutritional needs and perform other general nutritional teaching. When a vegetarian child is hospitalized, the nurse should plan with the nutrition department and the child's family to meet intake needs.

ENTERAL THERAPY

Enteral therapy is a form of nutritional support provided when a child cannot take in enough food orally to sustain health. Since it is the closest form of nutritional support to the natural method of eating, it has the least untoward effects and greatest rate of success. Some children who use enteral therapy are those with cerebral palsy or other neurologic conditions which lead to weakness of the throat and mouth, those with neoplasm or immune dysfunction, and those in acute states of recovery from accidents or illness (Figure 34–11 ⊙). Although a tube can be inserted into the nasal opening and

FIGURE 34–11

This child has returned to school following surgery. Due to cerebral palsy, he has difficulty chewing and swallowing food. The school nurse has taught his teacher to safely administer some enteral feedings during school hours.

placed through the esophagus into the stomach, a tube surgically placed into the stomach through an abdominal opening, a jejunal or gastric tube, is preferred for long-term use. As long as the child can absorb and use nutrients, enteral therapy can be successful in providing calories and essential nutrients. Commercially prepared formulas are available, and specially formulated solutions can be adapted for children with specific dietary needs. The tube and entry site are cared for to prevent infection and skin breakdown. See Chapter 51 for suggestions on management of nursing care during tube feedings. ∞ See also Skill 15–3 on the accompanying CD-ROM, and the Clinical Skills Manual. **SKILLS**

Some of the concerns with enteral feedings relate to the inability to adequately develop hunger/satiety cues in the child, the potential for infection or skin breakdown at the tube site related to action of gastric juice and feedings on the skin, and the need for ongoing care several times daily. Ideally, enteral feedings are temporary and children can begin to take in more foods orally as they grow and develop.

TOTAL PARENTERAL NUTRITION (TPN)

Parenteral nutrition makes it possible to provide intravenous nutritional support for people who cannot eat or are unable to absorb nutrients from the intestinal tract in a normal manner and are at risk of severe malnutrition (Matarese & Gottschlich, 2002). Examples of children who benefit from this method of nutrition are those with congenital malformation of the gastrointestinal tract,

THINKING CRITICALLY

THE CHILD WITH SPECIAL NUTRITIONAL NEEDS

Joey was diagnosed with cerebral palsy early in life. He is now 11 years old and has recently been enrolled in school. Part of the healthcare plan being implemented in the school involves fostering a positive nutritional state. Joey has limited ability to swallow, related to muscle weakness of cerebral palsy, and is therefore unable to ingest enough calories by mouth to ensure his optimal growth and development. Joey had a feeding tube inserted into his stomach at an early age and receives some of his nutrition by this method.

The school nurse has met with Joey's parents and his home health nurse to learn about the amount and type of tube feedings he receives, as well as the texture of oral feedings he can manage. The nurse will plan the feeding schedule at school to facilitate adequate nutrition in that setting. In addition, careful ongoing nutritional assessment will be needed to evaluate if Joey is getting the calories and other nutrients he needs for growth and development. The school nurse is also educating the classroom teachers and other school personnel about Joey's unique nutritional requirements.

- What do the teachers need to know about Joey's nutritional needs during school?
- How will you organize Joey's care if you are the case manager for his integration within the school system?
- How can the nurse help the family prepare for meeting nutritional needs of a child who has special needs like Joey's during travel by car or plane?
- If Joey's family plans to visit another state on a car trip this summer, what will they need to bring with them? (His feeding solution, tubing, and other supplies, and they may need refrigeration to maintain enteral solutions.)

head injury, or severe burns; it may also be used for support after bone marrow transplant, sepsis, or other critical conditions. A catheter is inserted so that a sterile nutrition solution is infused directly into the bloodstream. A central venous catheter is used to promote safe infusion. Fluids usually contain glucose; electrolytes like sodium, potassium, calcium, magnesium, phosphate, and chloride; vitamins; and proteins. Lipid emulsions are another type of TPN used in some children. Meticulous care is needed, whether in the hospital or at home, to ensure safe TPN infusion and treatment. The nurse performs initial assessment, ongoing evaluation, and monitoring of treatment, and administers the solutions in the hospital or other settings (Skipper, 1998). See Skill 12–7 for the protocols for TPN management in the Clinical Skills Manual. **SKILLS**

Critical Concept Review

LEARNING OBJECTIVES

CONCEPTS

Discuss major nutritional concepts pertaining to the growth and development of children.

Infancy:
1. Increased need for calories because of:
   - Rapid physical growth.
   - Increased physical activity.
2. Proper nutrition is needed for development of the nervous system and organs.
3. Should receive only breast milk or formula until tongue thrust has decreased and infant can sit well.
4. No cow milk until 1 year of age.
5. Food introduction principles are needed by parents.

Toddlerhood:
1. Development of physiologic anorexia.
2. Amount of milk and fruit juice should be limited so child will eat nutritious solid food.
3. Should begin to learn to eat in social situations.

Preschool:
1. Should begin to help with simple food preparation.
2. May exhibit extreme food preferences (food jag).
3. Emphasize brushing of teeth and first dental visit.

School-age:
1. Time of gradual growth with preadolescent growth spurt.
2. Increased need for calories during growth spurt.
3. May be resistant to trying new foods.
4. Expect loss of first deciduous teeth and eruption of permanent teeth.

Adolescence:
1. Need for increased calories during growth spurt.
2. Increased physical activity (such as sports) will increase caloric needs.
3. Encourage balanced intake and minimize fast foods.

Describe and plan nursing interventions to meet nutritional needs for all age groups from infancy through adolescence.

Infancy:
1. Encourage breastfeeding, if possible.
2. Assist mother to continue to breastfeed the hospitalized infant.
3. Discuss feeding during each contact with the mother.
4. To decrease occurrence of dental caries, teach parents that infant should not be given a bottle at bedtime.
5. Teach beginning dental care.
6. Supplemental foods begin with rice cereal and progress to vegetables and then fruit.
7. Begin use of cup for liquids at 8-9 months of age.

Toddlerhood:
1. Encourage parents to provide health foods that are easily eaten:
   - Small portions.
   - Place 1 tablespoon of food per year of age on child's plate.
2. Limit milk to 1 quart per day.
3. Limit fruit juice to 6 ounces per day.
4. Parents should establish meal time rules.

Preschool:
1. Encourage parents to use meal preparation as time for teaching about proper nutrition and kitchen safety.
2. Limit fruit juice to 12 ounces per day.
3. Encourage parents to limit fast food to once per week.

School-age:
1. Present nutritional teaching to child by using pictures and providing hands-on experiences.
2. Encourage families to bring food from home for the hospitalized child.
3. Allow hospitalized children to eat together.
4. Become knowledgeable concerning nutritional assistance available to the child and family.

Adolescence:
1. Encourage teen to drink fruit juice in place of soft drinks.
2. Provide healthy choices of food for teen.
3. Allow peer interaction during meals, if possible.

(continued)

LEARNING OBJECTIVES

CONCEPTS

Integrate methods of nutritional assessment into nursing care of infants, children, and adolescents.

→

Nutritional assessments include:
1. Growth measurements:
   - Height (length).
   - Weight.
   - Head circumference.
   - Skinfold measurement.
2. Body mass index.
3. Laboratory tests:
   - Hemoglobin and hematocrit.
   - Lipid profile.
   - Liver function.
   - Renal function.
   - Serum glucose.
4. Mother's dietary intake during pregnancy.
5. 24-hour food recall.
6. Food frequency questionnaire.
7. Food diary.

Discuss common nutritional problems of children in developed countries.

→

Common nutritional problems include:
1. Hunger due to poverty.
2. Obesity.
3. Foodborne illness.
4. Dietary deficiencies.

Apply the nursing process to care for children with eating disorders.

→

1. Assessment:
   - Obtain individual and family history.
   - Obtain accurate height and weight.
   - Observe eating behaviors.
   - Investigate use of prescription and OTC medications.
2. Planning and implementation:
   - Monitor nutritional and fluid intake.
   - Encourage nutritious food consumption.
   - Monitor elimination pattern.
   - Administer medications as needed.
3. Evaluation:
   - Promote adequate food and fluid to establish healthy nutritional lifestyle.
   - Encourage positive self-esteem.

CRITICAL THINKING IN ACTION

*View the **Critical Thinking in Action** video in Chapter 34 of the CD-ROM. Then, answer the questions that follow.*

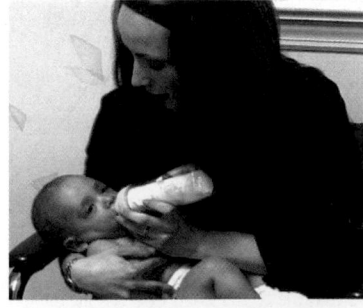

A mother is seeing the Pediatric Nurse Practitioner you are working with for her son Jonathan's 3-month, well-baby checkup at the local community health clinic. The baby is in the 90th percentile for weight and in the 50th percentile for height and is fed Similac formula with Iron. According to the medical history, Jonathan had RSV when he was 1 month old and there are smokers in the house. The nurse practitioner has asked you to educate the mother about feeding her 3-month-old baby. The mother has raised concerns that the baby is not sleeping through the night and the baby's grandmother has suggested adding cereal to his bottle at night to help him sleep. Jonathan has met all developmental milestones and has not yet developed teeth.

1. What type of advice can you give the mother about adding cereal to the bottle?
2. Why is rice cereal recommended as the first food to introduce when Jonathan is able to start solid foods?
3. What is the reason only iron-fortified formula or breast milk is recommended the entire first year of life for Jonathan, rather than cow milk?
4. Based on Jonathan's height and weight percentiles on the growth chart, his mother wonders if he should be put on a "diet." What would be the appropriate response to her concern?

MEDIALINK   www.prenhall.com/london

- NCLEX RN® Review, case studies, and other interactive resources for this chapter can be found on the Companion Website at http://www.prenhall.com/london. Click on "Chapter 34" to select the activities for this chapter.

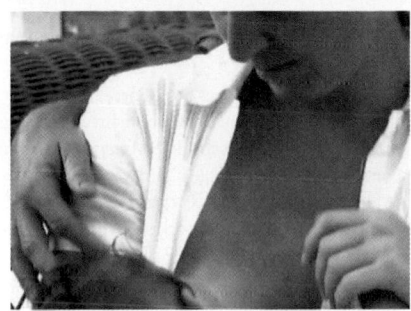

- For animations, more NCLEX-RN® Review questions, and an audio glossary, access the accompanying CD-ROM in this book.

REFERENCES

Adair, L. S., & Gordon–Larsen, P. (2001). Maturational timing and overweight prevalence in US adolescent girls. *American Journal of Public Health, 91,* 642–644.

American Academy of Pediatrics Committee on Nutrition. (2001). The use and misuse of fruit juice in pediatrics. *Pediatrics, 107,* 1210–1213.

American Dietetic Association. (2001). Position of the American Dietetic Association: Breaking the barriers to breastfeeding. *Journal of the American Dietetic Association, 101,* 1213–1220.

American Psychiatric Association Working Group on Eating Disorders. (2000). Practice guidelines for the treatment of patients with eating disorders. *American Journal of Psychiatry, 157,* 1–39.

Behrman, R. E., Kliegman, R. M. & Jenson, H. B. (2004). *Nelson textbook of pediatrics* (17th ed.) Philadelphia: Saunders.

Bessler, S. (1999). Nutritional assessment. In P. Q. Samour, K. K. Helm, & C. E. Lang, *Handbook of pediatric nutrition* (2nd ed., pp. 17–42). Gaithersburg, MD: Aspen.

Bock, S. A., Munoz–Furlong, A., & Sampson, H. A. (2001). Fatalities due to anaphylactic reactions to foods. *Journal of Allergy and Clinical Immunology, 107,* 191–193.

Boyle, M. A., & Morris, D. H. (1999). *Community nutrition in action* (2nd ed.). Belmont, CA: West/Wadsworth.

Brambilla, F. (2001). Social stress in anorexia nervosa: A review of immuno–endocrine relationships. *Physiology and Behavior, 73,* 365–369.

Breier, S. J. (2000). Ethics and total parenteral nutrition. *Journal of Intravenous Nursing, 23,* 52–57.

Briefel, R. R. (2002). National nutrition data: Contributions and challenges. *Nutrition Today, 37(3),* 126–127.

Burks, W. (2000). Diagnosis of allergic reactions to food. *Pediatric Annals, 29,* 744–752.

Calderon, L. (2002). Promoting a healthful lifestyle and encouraging advocacy among university and high school students. *Journal of American Dietetic Association 102(3 Suppl),* S71–S72.

Children's Defense Fund. (2004). *The state of America's children.* Washington, DC: Author.

Committee on Nutrition. (2004). *Pediatric nutrition handbook* (5th ed.). Elk Grove Village, IL: American Academy of Pediatrics.

Corrales, K. M., & Utter, S. L. (1999). Failure to thrive. In P. Q. Samour, K.K. Helm, & C. E. Lang, *Handbook of pediatric nutrition* (2nd ed., pp. 395–412). Gaithersburg, MD: Aspen.

Crespo, C. J., Smit, E., Troiano, R. P., Bartlett, S. J., Macera, C. A., & Anderson, R. E. (2001). Television watching, energy intake, and obesity in US children: Results from the third National Health and Nutrition Examination Survey. *Archives of Pediatric and Adolescent Medicine, 155,* 360–365.

Falciglia, G. A., Troyer, A. G., & Couch, S. C. (2004). Dietary variety increases as a function of time and influences dietary quality in children. *Journal of Nutrition Education and Behavior, 36,* 77–83.

Federal Interagency Forum on Child and Family Statistics. (2000). *America's children: Key national indicators of well–being, 2000.* Washington, DC: Author.

Food and Drug Administration. (2004). *Backgrounder for the 2004 FDA/EPA consumer advisory: What you need to know about mercury in fish and shellfish.* Washington, DC: Department of Health and Human Services. Retrieved June 8, 2004, from http:www.fda.gov/oc/opacom/hottopics/ mercury/backgrounder.html

Food and Nutrition Board. (2001). *Dietary reference intakes.* Washington, DC: National Academy Press.

Hanson, L. A., Dahlman–Hoglund, A., Lundin, S., Karllson, M., Dahlgren, U., Ahlstedt, S., & Telemo, E. (1997). Early determinants of immunocompetence. *Nutrition Reviews, 55,* S12–S17.

Hedley, A. A., Ogden, C. L., Johnson, C. L., Carroll, M. D., Curtin, L. R., & Flegal, K. M (2004). Overweight and obesity among US children, adolescents, and adults, 1999–2002. *JAMA 291,* 2847–2850.

Hensrud, D. D. (1999). Nutrition screening and assessment. *Medical Clinics of North America, 83,* 1525–1546.

Herpertz–Dahlmann, B., Muller, B., Herpertz, S., Heussen, N., Hedebrand, J., & Remschmidt, H. (2001). Prospective 10–year follow–up in adolescent anorexia nervosa—course, outcome, psychiatric co morbidity, and psychosocial adaptation. *Journal of Child Psychology and Psychiatry, 42,* 603–612.

Johnson, W. A. (2001). Nutritional supplements: What you need to know. *Contemporary Pediatrics, 18(7),* 63–74.

Kramer, M. S. (2001). Promotion of breastfeeding intervention trial (PROBIT). *Journal of the American Medical Association, 285,* 413–420.

Krauss, R. M., Eckel, R. H., Howard, G., Appel, L. J., Daniels, S. R., Deckelbaum, R. J., et al. (2001). AHA scientific statement: AHA dietary guideline. *Journal of Nutrition, 131,* 132–146.

Lee, R. D., & Nieman, D. C. (2003). *Nutrition assessment* (3rd ed.). Boston: McGraw–Hill.

Ludwig, D. S., & Ebbeling, C. B. (2001). Type 2 diabetes in children. *Journal of the American Medical Association, 286,* 1427–1430.

Matarese, L. E., & Gottschlich, M. M. (2002). *Contemporary nutrition support practice.* St. Louis, MO: Elsevier.

McDonough, A. B. (1999). Eating disorders. In P.Q. Samour, K. K. Helm, & C. E. Lang, *Handbook of pediatric nutrition* (2nd ed., pp. 191–204). Gaithersburg, MD: Aspen.

MMWR. (2001a). Preliminary FoodNet data on the incidence of foodborne illnesses. *Morbidity and Mortality Weekly Report, 50,* 241–246.

MMWR. (2001b). Severe malnutrition among young children—Georgia, January 1997–June 1999. *Morbidity and Mortality Weekly Report, 50,* 224–227.

National Cholesterol Education Program. (1991). *Report of the expert panel on blood cholesterol levels in children and adolescents.* Washington, DC: U.S. Department of Health and Human Services.

Neumark–Sztainer, D. (2000). Primary prevention of disordered eating among preadolescent girls. *Journal of the American Dietetic Association, 100,* 1466–1473.

Ogden, C. L., Flegal, K. M., Carroll, M. D., & Johnson, C. L. (2002). Prevalence and trends in overweight among US children and adolescents, 1999–2000. *Journal of the American Medical Association, 288,* 1728–1732.

Oken, E., & Lightdale, J. R. (2001). Updates in pediatric nutrition. *Current Opinions in Pediatrics, 13,* 280–288.

Orbanic, S. (2001). Understanding bulimia. *American Journal of Nursing, 101*(3), 35–41.

Pongracic, J. A. (2000). Is it food allergy? *Contemporary Pediatrics, 17,* 101–112, 117–121.

Rudys–Shapard, R. (2001). Adolescent, pregnant, and vegetarian: A turbulent time for a teen. *Journal of Pediatric Health Care, 15,* 35–40.

Seidenfeld, M. E., & Rickert, V. I. (2001). Impact of anorexia, bulimia and obesity on the gynecologic health of adolescents. *American Family Physician, 64,* 445–450.

Skipper, A. (1998). *Dietitian's handbook of enteral and parenteral nutrition* (2nd ed.). Gaithersburg, MD: Aspen.

Trahms, C. M. (2000). *Nutrition in infancy and childhood* (7th ed.). New York: WCB/McGraw–Hill.

U.S. Department of Health and Human Services. (2000). *Healthy People 2010.* Washington, DC Author.

U.S. Preventive Services Task Force. (2003). Behavioral interventions to promote breastfeeding: Recommendations and rationale. *American Journal for Nurse Practitioners, 7*(11), 23–32.

Walter, T., Olivares, M., Pizarro, F., & Munoz, C. (1997). Iron, anemia, and infection. *Nutrition Reviews, 55,* 111–124.

Whitaker, R., Wright, J. A., Pepe, M. S., Seidel, K. D., & Dietz, W. H. (1997). Predicting obesity in young adulthood from childhood and parental obesity. *New England Journal of Medicine, 337,* 869–873.

White, J. H. (2000). The prevention of eating disorder: A review of the research on risk factors with implications for practice. *Journal of Child and Adolescent Psychiatric Nursing, 123,* 76–88.

Willett, W. (2001). *Eat, drink, and be healthy.* New York: Simon & Schuster.

Zizza, C., Siega–Riz, A. M., & Popkin, B. M. (2001). Significant increase in young children's snacking between 1977–1978 and 1994–1996 represents a cause for concern! *Preventive Medicine, 32,* 303–310.

Pediatric Assessment

I was scared when we brought Latoya to the hospital. She looked helpless, afraid, and sick. The nurses and doctors took over when we got to the hospital, and I felt better because they seemed to know what to do.
—Father of Latoya, 6 months old

LEARNING OBJECTIVES

- Describe the elements of a health history for an infant or child of different ages.

- Identify communication strategies to improve the quality of historical data collected.

- Describe the strategies to gain cooperation of a young child for assessment.

- Describe the differences in sequence of the physical assessment for infants, children, and adolescents.

- Modify physical assessment techniques according to the age and developmental stage of the child.

- Determine the sexual maturity rating of males and females based upon physical signs of secondary sexual characteristics present.

- Recognize at least five important signs of a serious alteration in health condition that require urgent nursing intervention.

MEDIALINK

www.prenhall.com/london

CD-ROM

Audio Glossary
Animations:
   Otoscope Examination
   Mouth and Throat Examination
   3D Eye
   Movement of Joints
Skills 9-1–9-7: Growth Measurements
Skill 9-10: Blood Pressure
Skills 9-11–9-14: Body Temperature Measurements
Skills 9-18 and 9-19: Visual Acuity Screening
NCLEX-RN® Review

Companion Website

New Pediatric Blood Pressure Tables
Techniques for Assessing Selected Primitive Reflexes,
   with Normal Findings and Their
   Expected Age of Occurrence
Thinking Critically
NCLEX-RN® Review
Case Study

How do examination techniques vary by the age of the child? How does the nurse encourage infants and toddlers to cooperate with the examination? This chapter provides an overview of pediatric assessment, including history taking and examination techniques geared to the unique needs of pediatric patients. Strategies for obtaining the child's history are presented first. The remainder of the chapter then outlines a systematic process for physical examination of the child.

ANATOMIC AND PHYSIOLOGIC CHARACTERISTICS OF INFANTS AND CHILDREN

Children and infants are not only smaller than adults, but also significantly different physiologically. Knowledge of pediatric anatomic and physiologic differences will aid in recognizing normal variations found during the physical examination. It also assists with understanding the different physiologic responses children have to illness and injury. The illustration in "As Children Grow" provides an overview of important anatomic and physiologic differences between children and adults.

OBTAINING THE CHILD'S HISTORY

COMMUNICATION STRATEGIES

The health history interview is a very personal conversation with a parent, caretaker, or adolescent during which private concerns and feelings are shared. Try to ensure that this exchange of information with the parent or the child is clearly understood by both parties and that it is an effective communication. Effective communication is difficult to accomplish because parents and children often do not correctly interpret what the nurse says, just as the nurse may not understand completely what the parent or child says. People's interpretation of information is based on their life experiences, culture, and education.

Strategies to Build a Rapport with the Family

When beginning the history, make sure the parents understand the purpose of the interview and that the information will be used appropriately. To develop rapport, demonstrate interest in and concern for the child and family during the interview. This rapport forms the foundation for the collaborative relationship between the nurse and parent that will provide the best nursing care for the child. The following strategies help to establish rapport with the child's family during the nursing history:

- Make a self-introduction (name, title or position, and role in caring for the child). To demonstrate respect, ask all family members present what name they prefer you to use when talking with them.
- Explain the purpose of the interview and why the nursing history is different from the information collected by other health professionals. For example, "The nurses will use this information to plan nursing care best suited for your child."
- Provide privacy and remove as many distractions as possible during the interview. If the patient's room does not offer privacy, attempt to find a vacant patient room or lounge. Assure the parents and the child that the information provided during the assessment is protected under the Health Insurance Portability and Accountability Act (HIPAA), a federal law that requires written consent to be provided before health information can be shared with healthcare providers outside the facility.

AS CHILDREN GROW

Children Are Not Just Small Adults

Body surface area large for weight, making infants susceptible to hypothermia.

Anterior fontanelle and open sutures palpable up to about 18 months. Posterior fontanelle closes between 2 and 3 months.

Tongue large relative to small nasal and oral airway passages.

Short, narrow trachea in children under 5 years makes them susceptible to foreign body obstruction.

Until late school age and adolescence, cardiac output is rate dependent not stroke volume dependent, making heart rate more rapid.

Abdomen offers poor protection for the liver and spleen, making them susceptible to trauma.

Until 12 to 18 months of age, kidneys do not concentrate urine effectively and do not exert optimal control over electrolyte secretion and absorption.

Until later school age, proportion of body weight in water is larger, with more water in extracellular spaces. Daily water exchange rate is much higher.

All brain cells present at birth; myelinization and further development of nerve fibers occur during first year.

Head proportionately larger, making child susceptible to head injury.

Higher metabolic rate, higher oxygen needs, higher caloric needs.

Until puberty, percentage of cartilage in ribs is higher, making them more flexible and compliant.

Until about 10 years, there is a faster respiratory rate, fewer and smaller alveoli, and less lung volume. Tidal volume is proportional to weight (7 to 10 mL/kg).

Up to about 4 or 5 years, diaphragm is primary breathing muscle. CO_2 is not effectively expired when child is distressed, making child susceptible to metabolic acidosis.

Until puberty, bones are soft and more easily bent and fractured.

Muscles lack tone, power, and coordination during infancy. Muscles are 25% of weight in infants versus 40% in adults.

Blood volume is weight dependent: 80 mL/kg.

Children are not just small adults. There are important anatomic and physiologic differences between children and adults that will change based on a child's growth and development.

■ Direct the focus of the interview with open-ended questions. Use close-ended questions or directing statements to clarify information. Open-ended questions are useful to initiate the interview, develop a rapport, and understand the parent's perceptions of the child's problem. For example: "Tell me what problems led to Roberto's admission to the hospital." Close-ended questions are used to obtain detailed information. For example: "How high was Tommy's fever this morning?"

■ Ask one question at a time so that the parent or child understands what piece of information is desired and so that it is clear which question the parent is answering. "Does any member of your family have diabetes, heart disease, or sickle cell anemia?" is a multiple question. Ask about each disease separately to ensure the most accurate response.

DEVELOPING CULTURAL COMPETENCE

PHRASING YOUR QUESTIONS

Some cultural groups, particularly Asians, try to anticipate the answers you want to hear, or say yes even if they do not understand the question. This is done in an effort to please you or as an expression of politeness. Remember to phrase your questions in a neutral manner.

- Involve the child in the interview by asking age-appropriate questions. Young children can be asked, "What is your doll's name?" or "Where does it hurt?" Demonstrating an interest in the child initiates development of rapport with both child and parents. Ask older children and teens questions about their illness or injury. Offer them an opportunity to privately discuss their major concerns when their parents are not present.

- Be honest with the child when answering questions or when giving information about what will happen. Children need to learn that they can trust their nurse.

- Choose the language style best understood by the parent and child. Commonly used phrases can have different meanings to persons in various regions of the country or to different ethnic groups. To improve communication, request frequent feedback from the parents or child to ensure that their interpretation of phrases is accurate.

- Use an interpreter to improve communication when not fluent in the family's primary language. To ensure confidentiality of information for parents, avoid using a family member for history taking.

Careful Listening

Complete attention is necessary to "hear" and accurately interpret information the parents and child give during the nursing history. Carefully listen to the information provided by the parent, as well as how it is expressed, and observe behavior during the interaction.

- Does the parent hesitate or avoid answering certain questions?

- Pay attention to the parent's attitude or tone of voice when the child's problems are discussed. Determine if it is consistent with the seriousness of the child's problem. The tone of voice can reveal anxiety, anger, or lack of concern.

- Be alert to any underlying themes. For example, the parent who talks about the child's diagnosis, but repeatedly refers to the impact of the illness on the family's finances or on meeting the needs of other family members, is requesting that these issues be addressed.

- Observe the parent's nonverbal behavior (posture, gestures, body movements, eye contact, and facial expression) for consistency with the words and tone of voice used. Is the parent interested in and appropriately concerned about the child's condition? Behaviors such as sitting up straight, making eye contact, and appearing apprehensive reflect appropriate concern for the child. Physical withdrawal, failure to make eye contact, or a happy expression could be inconsistent with the child's serious condition.

DEVELOPING CULTURAL COMPETENCE

EYE CONTACT

Eye contact with the interviewer may be avoided by many cultural groups (Asian, Native American, and Middle Eastern patients) because it is considered impolite, aggressive, or a sign of disrespect (Spector, 2000). Europeans, such as the French and Spanish, use firm eye contact and look for a response or impact regarding what has been said. Some Americans may make brief eye contact and then let the eyes wander (Seidel, Ball, Dains et al., 2003).

Subtle nonverbal and verbal cues often indicate that the parent has not provided complete information about the child's problem. Observe for behaviors such as avoiding eye contact, change in voice pitch, or hesitation when responding to a question. Being supportive and asking clarifying questions encourage further description or the expression of information that is difficult for the parent or child to share. For example: "It sounds like that was a very difficult experience. How did Latasha react?"

Encourage parents to share information, even if it is private or sensitive, especially when it influences nursing care planning. Often parents avoid sharing some information because they want to make a good impression, or they do not understand the value of the missing information. If parents hesitate to share information, briefly explain why the question was asked—for example, to make their child's hospital experience more pleasant or to begin planning for the child's discharge and home care.

In some cases the parent becomes too agitated, upset, or angry to continue responding to questions. When the information is not needed immediately, move on to another portion of the history to determine whether the parent is able to respond to other questions. Depending on the emotional status of the parent, it may be more appropriate to collect the remaining historical data later.

DATA TO BE COLLECTED

Collect and organize the child's health, medical, and personal-social history to plan the child's nursing care. This text uses a modification of the Burns Classification System as the data-collection framework selected (Burns, 1992; Byrnes, 1996). Physiologic, psychosocial, and developmental data are organized to help develop the nursing diagnoses and the nursing care plan. Be alert for nonverbal cues.

Patient Information

Obtain the child's name and nickname, age, sex, and ethnic origin. The child's birth date, race, religion, address, and phone number can be obtained from the admission form. Ask the parent for an emergency contact address and phone number, as well as a work phone number. Record the person providing the patient history and that person's relationship to the patient.

Physiologic Data

Collect information about the child's health problems and diseases chronologically in a format similar to the traditional medical history.

- The chief complaint is the child's primary problem or reason for hospital admission or visit to a healthcare setting, stated in the parent's or child's exact words.
- The history of the present illness or injury is a detailed description of the current health problem. This includes the onset and sequence of events, characteristics of and changes in symptoms over time, influencing factors, and the current status of the problem. Each problem is described separately. Table 35–1 lists the specific data to be collected about each illness and injury.
- The past history is a more detailed description of the child's prior health problems. It includes the birth history and all major past illnesses and injuries. A detailed and complete birth history is obtained when the child's present problem may be related to the birth history (Table 35–2).

TABLE 35–1 ✛ History of Present Illness or Injury

Characteristic	Defining Variables
Onset	Sudden or gradual, previous episodes, date and time began
Type of symptom	Pain, itching, cough, vomiting, runny nose, diarrhea, rash, etc.
Location	Generalized or localized—anatomically precise
Duration	Continuous or episodic, length of episodes
Severity	Effect on daily activities, e.g., interrupted sleep, decreased appetite, incapacitation
Influencing factors	What relieves or aggravates symptoms, what precipitated the problem, recent exposure to infection or allergen
Past evaluation for the problem	Laboratory studies, physician's office or hospital where done, results of past examinations
Previous and current treatment	Prescribed and over-the-counter drugs used, complementary and alternative therapies, other treatments tried (heat, ice, rest), response to treatments

TABLE 35–2 ✛ Birth History

Prenatal	■ Mother's age, health during pregnancy, prenatal care, weight gained, special diet, expected date of birth ■ Details of illnesses, x-ray findings, hospitalizations, medications, complications, and timing during pregnancy ■ Prior obstetric history
Antenatal—description of birth	■ Site of birth (hospital, home, birthing center) ■ Labor induced or spontaneous, length of labor, time/duration or rupture of membranes ■ Vaginal or cesarean birth, forceps or suction used, vertex or breech position ■ Gestation at birth, single or multiple birth
Condition of baby at birth	■ Weight, Apgar score, cried immediately ■ Need for incubator, oxygen, suctioning, ventilator ■ Any abnormalities detected, meconium staining
Postnatal	■ Difficulties in the nursery—feeding, respiratory difficulties, jaundice, cyanosis, rashes ■ Length of hospital stay, special nursery, home with mother ■ Breast- or bottle-fed, weight lost/gained in hospital ■ Medical care needed in first week—readmission to hospital

Identify all major illnesses, including common communicable diseases. Identify major injuries, their cause or mechanism, and their severity. For past surgeries obtain information about the specific type and if the surgery was performed as day surgery or required at least a night of hospitalization. For all hospitalizations, record the reason and length of hospitalization. If any transfusions (blood or blood products) have been given in the past, identify the circumstances, type of transfusion, and reaction. Obtain information about each specific diagnosis, treatment, outcome, complication or residual problem, and the child's reaction to the event.

- The current health status is a detailed description of the child's typical health status:

    Health maintenance—child's primary care provider, dentist, and other healthcare providers, timing of last visit to each.

    Medications—prescribed and over-the-counter medications taken daily, frequently, or for home management of fever, colds, coughs, cuts, and rashes.

Ask about the use of plants, herbs, teas, or other complementary therapies.

Allergies—to food, medication, animals, insect bites, or environmental exposure, and the type of reaction (e.g., respiratory difficulty, rash, hives, itching).

Immunizations—review child's record for immunization status, vaccines and dates received, any unexpected reactions.

Safety measures used—car restraint system, window guards, medication storage, sports protective gear, smoke detectors, bicycle helmet, firearm storage, and others.

Activities and exercise—physical mobility and limitations, adaptive equipment used; play and/or sports activities.

Nutrition—formula-fed or breastfed, if breastfed, for how long, type and amount of daily formula intake; when solid foods were introduced, enrollment in the WIC (Women, Infants, and Children) Program; eating and snacking habits, variety of foods consumed, "junk foods" eaten, appetite.

Sleep—length and timing of naps and nighttime sleep; nightmares or night terrors, other sleep disturbances; where the child sleeps, and bedtime rituals.

- The familial and hereditary diseases summarize the major familial and hereditary diseases in three generations of family members, including the parents, grandparents, aunts, uncles, cousins, child, and siblings. Collect information about the health status of each parent. Record information in either a pedigree or a narrative format. Specific diseases to ask about are listed in Table 35–3.

- The review of systems provides a comprehensive overview of the child's health. This is an opportunity to identify additional signs and symptoms associated with the child's condition. Other problems may also be revealed that have no direct relationship to the child's significant health problem but could be factors complicating nursing care or home care. For example, asking about any urinary problems may reveal that a child still wets the bed at 7 years of age, although the admission is for a femur fracture. The nurse would then need to consider how bed-wetting might cause problems with the spica cast. For each problem, obtain the treatment, outcomes, residual problems, and age at time of onset. Data-collection guidelines are given in Table 35–4.

Psychosocial Data

Obtain information about family composition to establish a socioeconomic and sociologic context for planning the child's care in the hospital, community, and at home.

TABLE 35–3 ❖ Familial or Hereditary Diseases

Infectious diseases	Tuberculosis, HIV, hepatitis, varicella
Heart disease	Heart defects, myocardial infarctions, hypertension, hyperlipidemia, sudden childhood deaths
Allergic disorders	Eczema, hay fever, or asthma
Eye disorders	Glaucoma, cataracts, vision loss
Ear disorders	Hearing loss
Hematologic disorders	Sickle cell anemia, thalassemia, G6PD deficiency, leukemia
Lung disorders	Cystic fibrosis
Cancer	Type, early age of onset
Endocrine disorders	Diabetes mellitus, hypothyroidism, hyperthyroidism
Mental disorders	Mental retardation, epilepsy, Huntington chorea, psychiatric disorders
Musculoskeletal disorders	Arthritis, muscular dystrophy
Gastrointestinal disorders	Ulcers, colitis, kidney disease
Problem pregnancies	Repeated miscarriages, stillbirths
Learning problems	Attention deficit disorder, Down syndrome

- Family composition, including family members living in the home, their relationship to the child, marital status of parents or other family structure, and people helping to care for the child

- Household members employed, family income, and financial resources or agencies used such as health insurance, food stamps, or Temporary Assistance for Needy Families (TANF)

- Description of the housing and home environment (atmosphere, emotional stresses, family activities); safe play area; use of city or well water; and availability of electricity, heat, and refrigeration

- School or childcare arrangements; description of the neighborhood, including playgrounds, transportation, and proximity to stores

- Changes in family or lifestyle since last seen; number of times the family has moved; how the child and family members have coped with the changes

TABLE 35–4 ✣ Review of Systems

Body Systems	Examples of Problems to Identify
General	General growth pattern, overall health status, ability to keep up with other children or tires easily with feeding or activity, fever, sleep patterns
	Allergies, type of reaction (hives, rash, respiratory difficulty, swelling, nausea), seasonal or with each exposure
Skin and lymph	Rashes, dry skin, itching, changes in skin color or texture, tendency for bruising, swollen or tender lymph glands
Hair and nails	Hair loss, changes in color or texture, use of dye or chemicals on hair
	Abnormalities of nail growth or color
Head	Headaches
Eyes	Vision problems, squinting, crossed eyes, lazy eye, wears glasses, eye infections, redness, tearing, burning, rubbing, swelling eyelids
Ears	Ear infections, frequent discharge from ears, or tubes in ears
	Hearing loss (no response to loud noises or questions, inattentiveness, was hearing test ever done?), hearing aids or cochlear implant
Nose and sinuses	Nosebleeds, nasal congestion, colds with runny nose, sinus pain or infections
	Nasal obstruction, difficulty breathing, snoring at night
Mouth and throat	Mouth breathing, difficulty swallowing, sore throats, strep infections, mouth odor
	Tooth eruption, cavities, braces
	Voice change, hoarseness, speech problems
Cardiac and hematologic	Heart murmur, anemia, hypertension, cyanosis, edema, rheumatic fever, chest pain
Chest and respiratory	Trouble breathing, choking episodes, cough, wheezing, cyanosis, exposure to tuberculosis, other infections
Gastrointestinal	Bowel movements, frequency, color, regularity, consistency, discomfort, constipation or diarrhea, abdominal pain, bleeding from rectum, flatulence
	Nausea or vomiting, appetite
Urinary	Frequency, urgency, dysuria, dribbling, strength of urinary stream
	Toilet trained—age when day and night dryness attained, enuresis
Reproductive	For pubescent children
Female	Menses onset, amount, duration, frequency, discomfort, problems; vaginal discharge, breast development
Male	Puberty onset, emissions, erections, pain or discharge from penis, swelling or pain in testicles
Both	Sexual activity, use of contraception, sexually transmitted diseases
Musculoskeletal	Weakness, clumsiness, poor coordination, balance, tremors, abnormal gait, painful muscles or joints, swelling or redness of joints, fractures
Neurologic	Brain or head injuries
	Seizures, fainting spells, dizziness, numbness
	Learning problems, attention span, hyperactivity, memory problems

Information about daily routines, psychosocial data, and other living patterns forms the basis for many nursing diagnoses as well as the nursing care plan. Collection of information should focus on issues that have an impact on the quality of daily living, even if some data seem to overlap with disease data (Table 35–5).

The psychosocial history for adolescents should focus on critical areas in their lives that may contribute to a less than optimal environment for normal growth and development (Goldenring & Rosen, 2004). Possible screening questions are found in Table 35–6.

~~~~~~

TABLE 35–5 ✤ Daily Living Patterns

Role relationships	■ Family relationships/alterations in family process ■ Peer relationships ■ Social interactions: e.g., child care, preschool, school, neighborhood
Self-perception/ self-concept	■ Personal identity and role identity ■ Self-esteem, body image/nonvisible disorder
Coping/stress tolerance	■ Temperament ■ Coping behaviors ■ Discipline ■ Any substance abuse
Values and beliefs	■ Religion, belong to any spiritual group or community ■ Any foods or drinks not allowed according to spiritual beliefs, special food preparation ■ Any medical interventions prohibited ■ Personal values/beliefs
Home care provided for child's condition	■ Resources needed/available, respite care available ■ Knowledge and skills of parents, other family members
Sensory/perceptual problems	■ Adaptations to daily living for any sensory loss (vision, hearing, cognitive, or motor)

Adapted with permission from Burns, C. (1992). A new assessment model and tool for pediatric nurse practitioners. *Journal of Pediatric Health Care, 6,* 73–81.

Developmental Data

Information about the child's motor, cognitive, language, and social development will help to plan nursing care. Ask the parent about the child's milestones and current fine and gross motor skills. Obtain the age at which the child first used words appropriately and the current words used or language ability. For children in school, ask about academic performance to assess cognitive development. Ask the parent about the child's manner of interaction with other children, family members, and strangers. Guidelines for a nursing assessment of development can be found in Chapter 33. ∞

DEVELOPMENTAL APPROACH TO THE EXAMINATION

The sequence and approach to the examination varies by age. Provide a comfortable atmosphere for the examination with privacy so that modesty is respected. Explain the procedures as you begin to perform them. In young children, a foot-to-head sequence is often used so that the least distressing parts of the examination are completed first. In older cooperative children, the head-to-toe approach is generally used.

Newborns and Infants under 6 Months of Age

Infants are among the easiest children to examine, as they do not resist the examination procedure. Keep the parent present to provide security to the infant. Provide physical comfort during the examination by feeding, using a pacifier, cuddling, or changing the diaper to keep the infant calm and quiet. Distraction such as rocking or clicking noises may help when the infant begins to get distressed. Observe the infant for general level of activity, overall mood, and responsiveness to handling.

Keep the sequence of the examination flexible to take advantage of times the infant is quiet or asleep to auscultate the lungs, heart, and abdomen. If the infant continues to be quiet or can be quieted with a pacifier, palpate the abdomen while the muscles are relaxed. The remainder of the examination can proceed in a head-to-toe sequence. Portions of the examination that will disturb the infant, such as the examination of the hips, should be performed at the end.

Infants over 6 Months of Age

Because of developing separation and stranger anxiety, it is often best to keep the older infant with the parent. The infant and toddler can be examined on the parent's lap and then held against the parent's chest for some steps, such as the ear examination. The infant will not object to having clothing removed, but make sure the room is warm for the infant's comfort. Observe the infant's general level of activity, mood, and responsiveness to handling by the parent.

Smile and talk soothingly to the infant during the procedure. Use toys to distract the older infant. Use a pacifier or bottle to quiet the child when necessary. Because the infant may be fearful of being touched by a stranger, begin with the feet and hands before moving to the trunk. However, take advantage of opportunities presented when the infant is sleeping or quiet to auscultate the heart and lungs.

Toddlers

Toddlers may be active, curious, shy, cautious, or slow to warm up. Because of stranger anxiety, keep toddlers with their parents, often examining them on the parent's lap. It is possible to create a flat surface for the abdominal and genital examination by sitting close to the parent with knees together. For invasive procedures (ear, eye, and mouth exam) the parent can hold the child closely to the chest with legs between the parent's legs. The cranial nerve assessment or developmental assessment can be used as a method to gain cooperation for other procedures. Much of the neurologic and musculoskeletal assessment can be conducted by observing the child play and walk around in the examining room.

Tell the child what you will do at each step of the examination, using a confident voice that expects cooperation rather than asking. When a choice is possible, let the

TABLE 35–6 ✣ Adolescent Psychosocial Assessment Using the HEEADSSS Screening Tool

	Screening Questions
Home environment	Who lives with you? Where do you live? Do you have your own room? What are relationships like at home? To whom are you closest at home? To whom can you talk at home? Is there anyone new at home? Has someone left recently? Have you ever had to live away from home? (Why?)
Employment and education	Are you currently in school? What are your favorite subjects at school? Your least favorite subjects? How are your grades? Any recent changes? Any dramatic changes in the past? Have you changed schools in the past few years? What are your future education/employment plans/goals? Are you working? Where? How much? Tell me about your friends at school.
Eating	What do you like and not like about your body? Have there been any recent changes in your weight? Have you dieted in the last year? How? How often? Have you done anything else to try to manage your weight? How much exercise do you get in an average day? Week? What do you think would be a healthy diet? How does that compare with your current eating patterns?
Activities	What do you and your friends do for fun? (with whom, where, and when?) What do you and your family do for fun? (with whom, where, and when?) Do you participate in any sports or other activities? Do you regularly attend a church group, club, or other organized activity?
Drugs (substance use)	Do any of your friends use tobacco? Alcohol? Other drugs? Does anyone in your family use tobacco? Alcohol? Other drugs? Do you use tobacco? Alcohol? Other drugs? Is there any history of alcohol or drug problems in your family? Does anyone at home use tobacco?
Sexuality	Have you ever been in a romantic relationship? Tell me about the people that you've dated. OR Tell me about your sex life. Have any of your relationships ever been sexual relationships? Are your sexual activities enjoyable? What does the term "safer sex" mean to you? Are you interested in boys? Girls? Both?
Suicide/depression	Do you feel sad or down more than usual? Do you find yourself crying more than usual? Are you "bored" all the time? Have you thought a lot about hurting yourself or someone else?
Safety (savagery)	Have you ever been seriously injured? (How?) How about anyone else you know? Do you always wear a seat belt in the car? Have you ever ridden with a driver who was drunk or high? When? How often? Do you use safety equipment for sports or other physical activities (for example, helmets for biking or skateboarding)? Is there any violence in your home? Does the violence ever get physical? Is there a lot of violence at your school? In your neighborhood? Among your friends? Have you ever been physically or sexually abused? Have you ever been raped, on a date or at any other time? (If not asked previously)

Adapted with permission from Goldenring, J. M., & Rosen, D. S. (2004). Getting into adolescent heads: An essential update. *Contemporary Pediatrics, 21*(1), 64–90.

child have some control. For example, let the toddler choose which ear to examine first or to stand or sit for a certain part of the examination. Let the child hold a security object if it helps. Attempt to reduce the child's anxiety by demonstrating the use of instruments on the parent or security object. Begin the examination by touching the feet and then moving gradually toward the body and head. Instruments to examine the ears, eyes, and mouth are usually viewed as the most fearful and should be used at the end of the examination.

Preschoolers

Assess the willingness of the child to be separated from the parent. Younger children will often prefer to be examined on the parent's lap, while older children will be comfortable on the examining table. Most children are willing to undress, but leave the underpants on until conducting the genital examination. Most children in this age group are cooperative during the physical examination. Some children will prefer to have the head, eyes, ears, and mouth examined first while others will prefer to postpone them to the end.

Allow the child to touch and play with the equipment. Give simple explanations about the assessment procedures, and offer choice where there is one during the examination. Use distraction to gain the child's cooperation during the examination, such as asking the child to count, name colors, or talk about a favorite activity. Give positive feedback when the child cooperates.

School-age Children

School-age children willingly cooperate during the examination and sit on the examining table. Anticipate the development of modesty in school-age children and offer a patient gown to cover the underwear. Let the older school age child determine if the examination will be conducted in privacy or with the parent or siblings present.

A head-to-toe sequence can be used in this age group. Demonstrate how the instruments are used and let the child handle them if they wish. During the examination, tell the child what you are doing and why. Offer as many choices as possible to help the child feel empowered. The examination is a good opportunity to teach the child about how the body works, such as letting the child listen to heart and breath sounds.

Adolescents

Protect the adolescent's modesty by providing a private place to undress and put on the patient gown, and then during the examination by covering the parts of the body not being assessed. Use the head-to-toe sequence and the same procedures used for adults. Perform the examination in private without parent or siblings unless the adolescent specifically requests the parent's presence. Provide a chaperone when the parent or accompanying adult is not present during the examination.

Adolescents often have a lot of concerns regarding their developing bodies. When appropriate, provide reassurance about the normal progression of secondary sexual characteristic development and what further changes to expect.

GENERAL APPRAISAL

The examination begins upon first meeting the child (Figure 35–1 ○). Measure the infant's weight, length, and head circumference (see Skills 9–1 through 9–7 in the accompanying CD-ROM, as well as the Clinical Skills Manual). **SKILLS**

If the child can stand, substitute a standing height measurement for length. Plot the measurements on the appropriate growth curves. Take the child's temperature, heart rate, respiratory rate, and blood pressure (see Skills 9–8 through 9–14). **SKILLS**

NURSING PRACTICE

Following are the specific examination techniques:

Inspection. Purposeful observation of the child's physical features and behaviors. Physical feature characteristics include size, shape, color, movement, position, and location. Detection of odors is also a part of inspection.

Palpation. Use of touch to identify characteristics of the skin, internal organs, and masses. Characteristics include texture, moistness, tenderness, temperature, position, shape, consistency, and mobility of masses and organs. The palmar surface of the fingers and finger pads helps determine position, size, consistency, and masses. The ulnar surface of the hand is best to detect vibrations.

Auscultation. Listening to sounds produced by the airway, lungs, stomach, heart, and blood vessels to identify their characteristics. Auscultation is usually performed with a stethoscope to enhance the sounds heard.

Percussion. Striking the surface of the body, either directly or indirectly, to set up vibrations that reveal the density of underlying tissues and borders of internal organs.

Observe the child's general appearance and behavior. The child should appear well nourished and well developed. Infants and young children are often fearful and seek reassurance from their parents. The child may resist interacting with the nurse until rapport is established.

Observe the behavior and tone of voice used by the parent when he or she is talking to the child. Is the child encouraged to speak? Is the child appropriately reassured or supported by the parent? The child should feel secure with the parent and perceive permission to interact with the nurse.

FIGURE 35-1

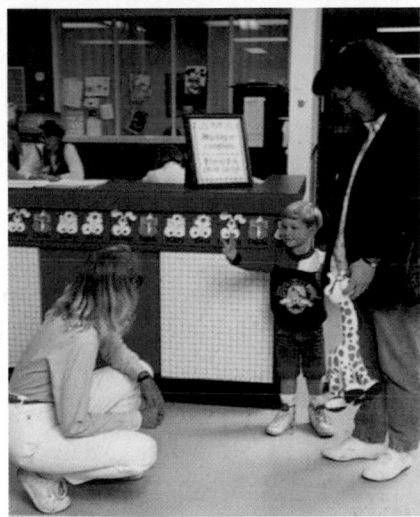

Examination of the child begins from the first contact. You should be observing the behavior of the child and parent by using visual cues to make a proper assessment. Does the child appear well nourished? Does the child appear secure with the parent?

ASSESSING SKIN AND HAIR CHARACTERISTICS

Examination of the skin requires good lighting to detect variations in skin color and to identify lesions. Daylight is preferred when available. Rather than inspecting the entire skin surface of the child at one time, examine the skin simultaneously with other body systems as each region of the body is exposed.

DEVELOPING CULTURAL COMPETENCE

SKIN TONE DIFFERENCES

The palms of the hands and soles of the feet are often lighter than the rest of the skin surface in darker-skinned children. In addition, their lips may appear slightly bluish.

INSPECTION OF THE SKIN

Use gloves to inspect the child's skin for color and the presence of imperfections, elevations, or other lesions.

Skin Color

The color of the child's skin usually has an even distribution. Check for color variations—such as increased or decreased pigmentation, pallor, mottling, bruises, erythema, cyanosis, or jaundice—that may be associated with local or generalized conditions. Some variations in skin color are common and normal, such as freckles found in the white population and Mongolian spots found on dark-skinned

infants. See "Newborn Skin" in Chapter 27 for more information. ∞ Bruises are common on the knees, shins, and lower arms as children stumble and fall. Bruises on other parts of the body, especially in various stages of healing, should raise a suspicion of child abuse. Bruises often go through various color changes as the body reabsorbs blood over several days. The transition of color often progresses through reddish blue, brownish blue, brownish green, greenish yellow, and yellow-brown before returning to normal skin color. Note any tattoos or body piercings.

When a skin color abnormality is suspected, inspect the buccal mucosa and tongue to confirm the color change. This is especially important in darker-skinned children because the mucous membranes are usually pink, regardless of skin color. Press the gums lightly for 1 to 2 seconds. Any residual color, such as that seen in jaundice or cyanosis, is more easily detected in blanched skin. Jaundice may also be noticed in the sclerae of the eyes. Generalized cyanosis is associated with respiratory and cardiac disorders. Jaundice is associated with liver disorders.

PALPATION OF THE SKIN

Palpation of the skin provides a sense of its characteristics: temperature, texture, moistness, and resilience or turgor. To evaluate these characteristics, lightly touch or stroke the skin surface. Follow standard precautions by wearing gloves when palpating mucous membranes, open wounds, and lesions. The following list provides details on each of the characteristics of skin palpation.

Temperature

The child's skin normally feels cool to the touch when placing the wrist or dorsum of the hand against the child's skin. Excessively warm skin may indicate the presence of fever or inflammation, whereas abnormally cool skin may be a sign of shock or cold exposure.

Texture

Children have soft, smooth skin over the entire body. Identify any areas of roughness, thickening, or *induration* (area of extra firmness with a distinct border). Abnormalities in texture are associated with endocrine disorders, chronic irritation, and inflammation.

Moistness

The child's skin is normally dry to the touch. The skin may feel slightly damp when the child has been exercising or crying. Excessive sweating without exertion is associated with a fever or with an uncorrected congenital heart defect.

Resilience

The child's skin is taut, elastic, and mobile because of the balanced distribution of intracellular and extracellular fluids.

◉ FIGURE 35–2

Tenting of the skin associated with poor skin turgor. Assess skin turgor on the abdomen, forearm, or thigh. Skin with normal turgor will return to a flat position quickly.

To evaluate skin turgor, pinch a small amount of skin on the abdomen between the thumb and forefinger, release the skin, and watch the speed of recoil (Figure 35–2 ◉). Skin with good turgor rapidly returns to its previous contour. Skin with poor turgor tents or stands up rather than resuming its previous contour. Poor skin turgor is commonly associated with dehydration.

If *edema,* an accumulation of excess fluid in the interstitial spaces, is present, the skin feels doughy or boggy. To test for the degree of edema present, press for 5 seconds against a bone beneath the area of puffy skin, release the pressure, and observe how rapidly the indentation disappears. If the indentation disappears rapidly, the edema is "nonpitting." Slow disappearance of the indentation indicates "pitting" edema, which is commonly associated with kidney or heart disorders.

NURSING PRACTICE

The degree of dehydration, or weight loss caused by dehydration, can be estimated from the time it takes tented skin to return to its natural contour (Seidel, Ball, Dains et al., 2003).

Weight Loss from Dehydration	Time to Return to Normal
< 5%	< 2 sec
5% to 8%	2 to 3 sec
9% to 10%	3 to 4 sec
> 10%	> 4 sec

CAPILLARY REFILL AND SMALL-VEIN FILLING TIMES

Two techniques can determine the adequacy of tissue *perfusion* (oxygen circulating to the tissues). When capil-

lary refill time or small-vein filling times suggest that tissue perfusion is inadequate, immediately assess the child for shock or a physical constriction such as a cast or bandage that is too tight. The capillary refill time is normally less than 2 seconds (Figure 35–3A and B ◉). The small-vein filling time is normally less than 4 seconds (Figure 35–3C and D).

SKIN LESIONS

Skin lesions usually indicate an abnormal skin condition. Characteristics such as location, size, type of lesion, pattern, and discharge, if present, provide clues about the cause of the condition. Inspect and palpate the isolated or generalized skin color abnormalities, elevations, lesions, or injuries to describe all characteristics present.

Primary lesions (such as macules, papules, and vesicles) are often the skin's initial response to injury or infection. Mongolian spots and freckles are normal findings also classified as primary lesions. Secondary lesions (such as scars, ulcers, and fissures) are the result of irritation, infection, and delayed healing of primary lesions (see "Pathophysiology Illustrated—Skin Lesions" in Chapter 57 ∞). The illustrations in "Pathophysiology Illustrated" on page 974 describe common primary lesions.

NURSING PRACTICE

Following are common patterns of skin lesions:

Annular:	Circular, begins in center and spreads to periphery
Polycyclic:	Annular lesions running together
Linear:	In a row or stripe
Herpetiform:	Grouped or clustered
Gyrate:	Twisted, spiral, coiled

INSPECTION OF THE HAIR

Inspect the scalp hair for color, distribution, and cleanliness. The hair shafts should be evenly colored, shiny, and either curly or straight. Variation in hair color not caused by bleaching can be associated with a nutritional deficiency. Normally, hair is distributed evenly over the scalp. Investigate areas of hair loss. Hair loss in a child may result from tight braids or skin lesions such as ringworm (see "Fungal Infections" in Chapter 57 ∞). Notice any unusual hair growth patterns. An unusually low hairline on the neck or forehead may be associated with a congenital disorder such as hypothyroidism.

Children are frequently exposed to head lice. Inspect the individual hair shafts for small nits (lice eggs) that adhere to the hair (Figure 35–4 ◉). None should be present.

○ FIGURE 35-3

A

B

C

D

Capillary refill technique: **A,** Pinch the end of a finger until the skin is blanched. **B,** Quickly release the finger and watch the blood return to the veins. Count the seconds it takes for the color to return or veins to fill. Slow color return or vein filling time could be related to shock or constriction due to a tight bandage or cast. Small-vein filling time technique: **C,** Using the index finger, milk a vein on the dorsum of the hand or foot from proximal to distal. **D,** Release your pressure and color should return promptly.

Observe the distribution of body hair as other skin surfaces are exposed during examination. Fine hair covers most areas of the body. Body hair in unexpected places should be noted. For example, a tuft of hair at the base of the spine often indicates a spinal defect.

It is important to note the age at which pubic and axillary hair develops in the child. Development at an unusually young age is associated with precocious puberty.

GROWTH AND DEVELOPMENT

Pubic hair begins to develop in children between 8 and 12 years of age, and axillary hair develops about 6 months later. Facial hair is noted in boys shortly after axillary hair develops.

PALPATION OF THE HAIR

Palpate the hair shafts for texture. Hair should feel soft or silky with fine or thick shafts. Endocrine conditions such as hypothyroidism may result in coarse, brittle hair. Part the hair in various spots over the head to inspect and palpate the scalp for crusting or other lesions. If lesions are present, describe them using the characteristics in "Pathophysiology Illustrated."

ASSESSING THE HEAD FOR SKULL CHARACTERISTICS AND FACIAL FEATURES

What can cause a child's head or face to be asymmetric? How does a normal fontanelle feel?

INSPECTION OF THE HEAD AND FACE

During early childhood the skull's sutures permit expansion for brain growth. Infants and young children normally have a rounded skull with a prominent occipital area. The shape of the head changes during childhood, and the occipital area becomes less prominent. An abnormal skull shape can result from premature closure of the sutures. Children who were

PATHOPHYSIOLOGY ILLUSTRATED
Common Primary Skin Lesions and Associated Conditions

Lesion Name: Macule
Description:
Flat, nonpalpable, diameter <1 cm (½ in.)
Example: Freckle, rubella, rubeola, petechiae

Lesion Name: Patch
Description:
Macule, diameter >1 cm (½ in.)
Example: Vitiligo, Mongolian spot

Lesion Name: Papule
Description:
Elevated, firm, diameter <1 cm (½ in.)
Example: Warts, pigmented nevi

Lesion Name: Nodule
Description:
Elevated, firm, deeper in dermis than papule, diameter 1–2 cm (½ in.-1 in.)
Example: Erythema nodosum

Lesion Name: Tumor
Description:
Elevated, solid, diameter >2 cm (1 in.)
Example: Neoplasm, hemangioma

Lesion Name: Vesicle
Description:
Elevated, filled with fluid, diameter <1 cm (½ in.)
Example: Early chicken pox, herpes simplex

Lesion Name: Pustule
Description:
Vesicle filled with purulent fluid
Example: Impetigo, acne

Lesion Name: Bulla
Description:
Vesicle diameter >1 cm (½ in.)
Example: Burn blister

Lesion Name: Wheal
Description:
Irregular elevated solid area of edematous skin
Example: Urticaria, insect bite

● FIGURE 35-4

A

Nit

B

A, Inspecting for head lice with a fine-tooth comb. **B,** Nits on hair.
(B) Courtesy of Centers for Disease Control.

low-birth-weight infants often have a flat, elongated skull because the soft skull bones were flattened by the weight of the head early in infancy. Head flattening is also associated with the back-lying sleep positions in infants.

The head circumference of infants and young children is routinely measured until 3 years of age to ensure that adequate growth for brain development has occurred. The Clinical Skills Manual **SKILLS** as well as the CD-ROM describes the proper technique for use of the tape measure. A larger-than-normal head is associated with hydrocephalus, and a smaller-than-normal head suggests microcephaly.

Inspect the child's face for symmetry during several facial expressions such as resting, smiling, talking, and crying (Figure 35–5 ●). Significant asymmetry may result from paralysis of trigeminal or facial nerves (cranial nerves V or VII), in utero positioning, and swelling from infection, allergy, or trauma.

Next inspect the face for unusual facial features such as coarseness, wide eye spacing, or disproportionate size. Tremors, tics, and twitching of facial muscles are often associated with seizures.

PALPATION OF THE SKULL

Palpate the skull in infants and young children to assess the sutures and fontanelles and to detect soft bones (see "As Children Grow").

Sutures

Use your fingerpads to palpate each suture line. The edge of each bone in the suture line can be felt, but normally there is no separation of the two bones. If additional bone edges are felt, it may indicate a skull fracture. The suture lines of the skull are seldom palpated after 2 years of age. After that time the sutures rarely split.

Fontanelles

At the intersection of the sutures, palpate the anterior and posterior fontanelles. The fontanelle should feel flat and

● FIGURE 35-5

Draw an imaginary line down the middle of the face over the nose and compare the features on each side. Significant asymmetry may be caused by paralysis of cranial nerve V or VII, in utero positioning, or swelling from infection, allergy, or trauma.

AS CHILDREN GROW

Sutures

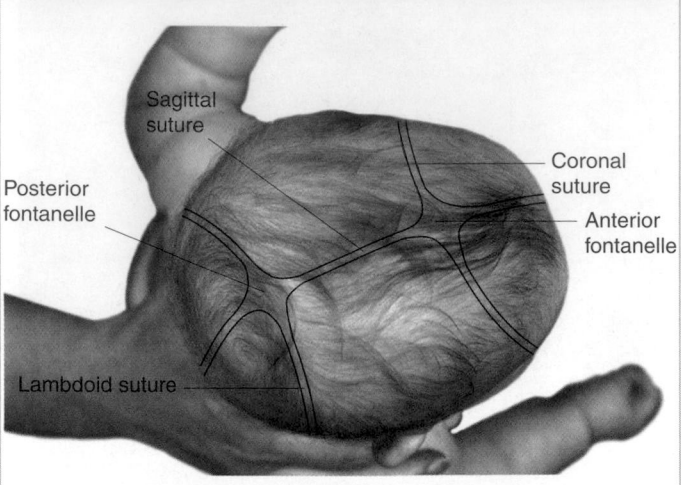

Sagittal suture

Coronal suture

Posterior fontanelle

Anterior fontanelle

Lambdoid suture

The sutures are separations between the bones of the skull that have not yet joined. The fontanelles are formed at the intersection of these sutures where bone has not yet formed. Fontanelles are covered by tough membranous tissue that protects the brain. The posterior fontanelle closes between 2 and 3 months. The anterior fontanelle and sutures are palpable up to the age of 18 months.

firm inside the bony edges. The anterior fontanelle is normally smaller than 5 cm (2 in.) in diameter at 6 months of age and then becomes progressively smaller. It closes between 12 and 18 months of age. The posterior fontanelle closes between 2 and 3 months of age.

A tense fontanelle, bulging above the margin of the skull, is an indication of increased intracranial pressure. A soft fontanelle, sunken below the margin of the skull, is associated with dehydration.

DEVELOPING CULTURAL COMPETENCE

TOUCHING THE CHILD'S HEAD

The head is a sacred part of the body to Southeast Asians. Ask for permission before touching the infant's head to palpate the sutures and fontanelles (Spector, 2000). When a Hispanic child is examined, however, not touching the head is considered bad luck.

ASSESSING EYE STRUCTURES, FUNCTION, AND VISION

INSPECTION OF THE EXTERNAL EYE STRUCTURES

The function of the external and internal eye structures and related cranial nerves makes vision possible. Inspect the ex-

ternal eye structures, including the eyeballs, eyelids, and eye muscles. Test the function of cranial nerves II, III, IV, and VI, which innervate the eye structures. Equipment needed for this examination includes an ophthalmoscope, vision chart, penlight, small toy, and an index card or paper cup.

Eye Size and Spacing

Inspect the eyes and surrounding tissues simultaneously when examining facial features (Figure 35–6 ●). The eyes should be the same size but not unusually large or small. Observe for eye bulging, which can be identified by retracted eyelids or a sunken appearance. Bulging may be associated with a tumor, and a sunken appearance may reflect dehydration.

Next inspect the eyes to see if they are appropriately distanced from each other. **Hypertelorism**, or widely spaced eyes, can be a normal variation in children.

Eyelids and Eyelashes

Inspect the eyelids for color, size, position, mobility, and condition of the eyelashes. Eyelids should be the same color as surrounding facial skin and free of swelling or inflammation along the edges. Sebaceous glands that look like yellow striations are often present near the hair follicles. Eyelashes curl away from the eye to prevent irritation of the conjunctivae.

Inspect the conjunctivae lining the eyelids by pulling down the lower lid and then everting the upper lid. The conjunctivae should be pink and glossy. The lacrimal punctum, the opening for the lacrimal gland on each lid, is located near the medial canthus. No redness or excess tearing should be present.

When the eyes are open, inspect the level at which the upper and lower lids cross the eye. Each lid normally covers part of the iris but not any portion of the pupil. The lids

● FIGURE 35–6

Lacrimal gland

Inner canthus

Lacrimal caruncle

Lacrimal punctum

Iris Pupil

Sclera Conjunctiva

Outer canthus

External structures of the eye. Notice that the light reflex is at the same location on each eye.

should also close completely over the iris and cornea. Ptosis, drooping of the lid over the pupil, is often associated with injury to the oculomotor nerve, cranial nerve III. Sunset sign, in which the sclera is seen between the upper lid and the iris, may indicate retracted eyelids or hydrocephalus.

Inspect the eyes for the palpebral slant (Figure 35–7 ●). The eyelids of most people open horizontally. Children of Asian descent often have an extra fold of skin, known as the epicanthal fold, covering all or part of the medial canthus of the eye. An upward or Mongolian slant is a normal finding in Asian children; however, children with Down syndrome also often have a Mongolian slant (Figure 35–8 ●). A downward or anti-Mongolian slant is seen in some children as a normal variation.

Eye Color

Inspect the color of each sclera, iris, and bulbar conjunctiva. The sclera is normally white or ivory in darker-skinned children. Sclerae of another color suggest the presence of an underlying disease. For example, yellow sclerae indicate jaundice. Typically the iris is blue or light colored at birth and becomes pigmented within 6 months. Inspect the iris for the presence of Brushfield spots, white specks in a linear pattern around the iris circumference, which are often

● **FIGURE 35–8**

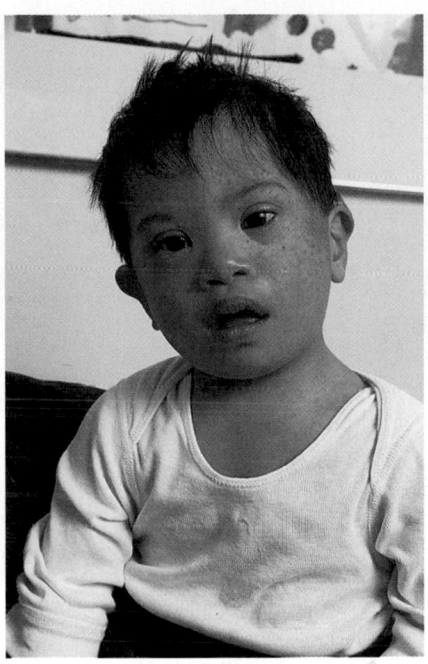

The eyes of this boy with Down syndrome show a Mongolian slant.

● **FIGURE 35–7**

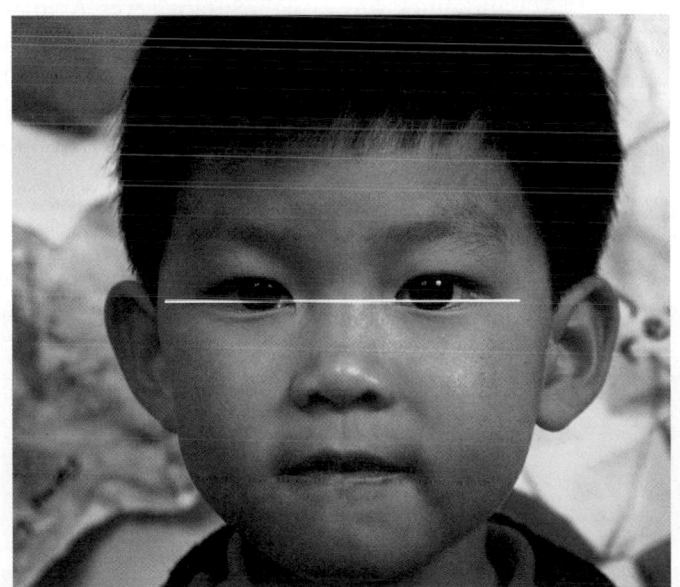

Draw an imaginary line across the medial canthi and extend it to each side of the face to identify the slant of the palpebral fissures. When the line crosses the lateral canthi, the palpebral fissures are horizontal and no slant is present. When the lateral canthi fall above the imaginary line, the eyes have an upward or Mongolian slant. A downward or anti-Mongolian slant is present when the lateral canthi fall below the imaginary line. Epicanthal folds are present when an extra fold of skin partially or completely covers the caruncles in the medial canthi. Which type of slant does this child have?

associated with Down syndrome. The bulbar conjunctivae, which cover the sclera to the edge of the cornea, are normally clear. Redness can indicate eyestrain, allergies, or irritation.

Pupils

Inspect the pupils for size and shape. Normally the pupils are round, clear, and equal in size. Some children have a **coloboma**, a keyhole-shaped pupil caused by a notch in the iris. This sign can indicate that the child has other congenital anomalies.

To test the pupillary response to light, shine a bright light into one eye. A brisk constriction of both the pupil exposed to direct light and the other pupil is a normal finding.

To test pupillary response to accommodation, ask the child to look first at a near object (for example, a toy) and then at a distant object (for example, a picture on the wall). The expected response is pupil constriction with near objects and pupil dilation with distant objects. This procedure tests the optic nerve, cranial nerve II.

INSPECTION OF THE EYE MUSCLES

It is important to detect strabismus, or crossed eyes, because if uncorrected it can cause vision impairment. The evaluation of extraocular movements, the corneal light reflex, and the cover-uncover test are used to detect a muscle imbalance.

⊙ **FIGURE 35–9**

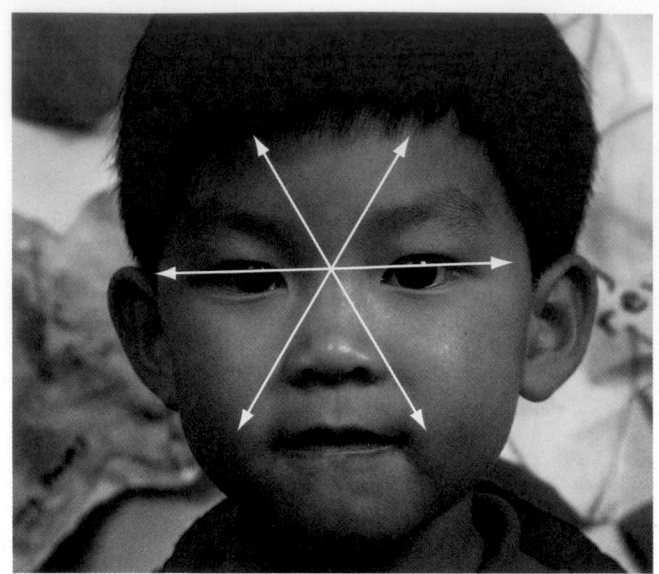

Begin the eye muscle examination with inspection of the extraocular movements. Have the child sit at your eye level. Hold a toy or penlight about 30 cm (12 in.) from the child's eyes and move it through the six cardinal fields of gaze. Both eyes should move together, tracking the object. This procedure tests cranial nerves III, IV, and VI.

Extraocular Movements

Seat the child at eye level to evaluate the extraocular movements. Hold a toy or penlight 30 cm (12 in.) from the child's eyes and move it through the six cardinal fields of gaze. The child's head may need to be held still until fine motor eye movement develops. Both eyes should move together, tracking the object. This procedure tests the oculomotor, trochlear, and abducens nerves (cranial nerves III, IV, and VI) (Figure 35–9 ⊙).

Corneal Light Reflex

To test the corneal light reflex, shine a light on the child's nose, midway between the eyes. Identify the location where the light is reflected on each eye. The light reflection is normally symmetric, at the same spot on each cornea (see Figure 35–6). An asymmetric corneal light reflex indicates strabismus.

Cover-Uncover Test

The cover-uncover test can be used to test for eye muscle weakness for older, cooperative children, usually at about 4 or 5 years. See Figure 35–10 ⊙ for the technique. Because the eyes work together, no obvious movement of either eye is expected. Eye movement indicates a muscle imbalance.

VISION ASSESSMENT

Because vision is such an important sense for learning, assessment is essential to detect any serious problems. Vision is evaluated using an age-appropriate vision test, but no simple method exists. It is possible to assess vision in infants and children by observing their behavior in response to certain maneuvers and during play.

Infants and Toddlers

When the infant's eyes are open, test the blink reflex by moving your hand quickly toward the infant's eyes. A quick blink is the normal response. Absence of the blink reflex can indicate that the infant is blind.

To test an infant's ability to visually track an object, hold a light or toy about 15 cm (6 in.) from the infant's

⊙ **FIGURE 35–10**

The cover–uncover test. With the child at your eye level, ask the child to look at a picture on the wall. *A,* As you cover one eye with an index card or paper cup, simultaneously observe for any movement of the uncovered eye. If it jumps to fixate on the picture, the uncovered eye has a muscle weakness. *B,* As you remove the cover from the eye, simultaneously observe the covered eye for any movement to fixate on the picture. If the eye has a muscle weakness, it drifts to a relaxed position once covered.

A Right, uncovered eye is weaker. **B** Left, covered eye is weaker.

GROWTH AND DEVELOPMENT

Research has discovered that newborns have vision good enough at birth to prefer faces to other patterns and to follow a moving object. The child's visual acuity develops during early childhood (Seidel et al., 2003).

Age	Visual Acuity
3 years	20/40
4 years	20/40
5 years	20/30
6 years	20/20

● FIGURE 35–11

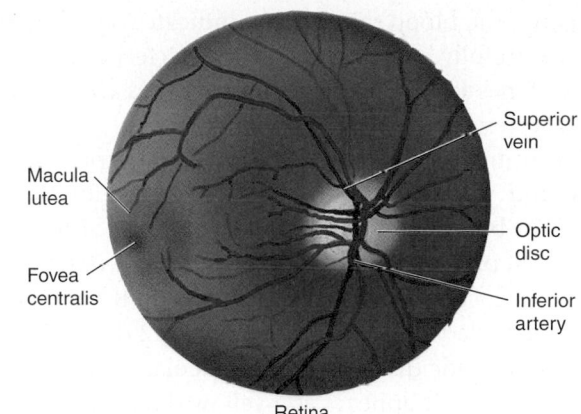

Normal fundus.

eyes. When the infant has fixated on or is staring at the object, move it slowly to each side. The infant should follow the object with the eyes and by moving the head.

Once an infant has developed skills to reach for and then pick up objects, observe play behavior to evaluate vision. The ability to easily find and pick up small toys is a good indicator of vision in children under 3 years of age.

Standardized Vision Charts

Standardized vision charts cannot be used to test vision until the child can understand directions and can cooperate, usually at about 3 or 4 years of age. The Snellen E chart, HOTV chart, and the Picture chart are used to test visual acuity of preschool-age children just as the Snellen Letter chart is used for school-age children and adolescents. Skills 9–18 through 9–19 in the Clinical Skills Manual, as well as the accompanying CD-ROM, describes the use of these charts.

NURSING PRACTICE

Indications for further evaluation include visual acuity of 20/40 or less in either eye by 3 to 5 years of age, visual acuity of 20/30 or less in either eye by 6 years of age, or a difference in vision of 2 lines or more on the Snellen eye chart between the eyes, even within the passing range (American Academy of Pediatrics, 2003).

INSPECTION OF THE INTERNAL EYE STRUCTURES

The funduscopic examination allows inspection of the internal eye structures—the retina, optic disc, arteries and veins, and macula (Figure 35–11 ●). The ophthalmoscope is a complex instrument and requires practice to master. The examination is difficult to perform on uncooperative children, and most often it is performed by experienced examiners.

Darken the room so the child's pupils dilate. Explain the procedure to the child to gain his or her cooperation. Have a picture on the wall or have the parent or assistant

hold a toy for the child to stare at so that the child's eye will not have to be held open forcibly.

Using the Ophthalmoscope

The ophthalmoscope has a lens-and-mirror system and a bright light for inspecting the structures of the internal eye. Turn the ophthalmoscope on and set the lens power at 0. Keep a forefinger on the disk to change the lens power as needed. Look through the lens of the ophthalmoscope, stabilizing it by resting the top against an eyebrow and the handle against a cheek. Use your right eye to examine the child's right eye and your left eye to examine the child's left eye. This position is best for visualizing the eye, and it reduces direct exposure to infection. Place a hand on the child's head for stabilization.

Red Reflex. Shine the ophthalmoscope light at the child's eye from a distance of 30 cm (12 in.). The first image seen is the red reflex, the red glow of the vascular retina. When the red reflex is seen, the ophthalmoscope is being used correctly and the child's lens is clear. The red reflexes should be equal in color, intensity, and clarity (American Academy of Pediatrics Section on Opthalmology, 2002). Black spots or opacities within the red reflex are abnormal and may indicate congenital cataracts. If a white reflex is seen rather than a red reflex, a retinoblastoma may be present. The red reflex can also be tested by shining a small flashlight into the eye.

Visualizing the Internal Eye Structures. Slowly move closer to the child. Deeper levels of the vitreous humor are inspected before the pink retina comes into view. The retina is a deeper pink in dark-skinned children. A blood vessel is the first retinal structure usually seen. Continue moving closer to the child's eye and adjust the plus or minus lenses to focus on this blood vessel. Retinal arteries appear smaller and brighter red than veins. The blood vessels branch to spread and cover the retina.

MEDIALINK ● Skills 9-18 and 9-19: Visual Acuity Screening

Inspect and follow the branching of the blood vessels toward the nose until they merge into the optic disc. Dark areas along the blood vessels may indicate retinal hemorrhages. Carefully inspect sites where arteries and veins cross. Notches and indentations at these sites are associated with hypertension.

The optic disc margin is normally sharply defined, round, and yellow to creamy pink. Blurring of the disc margins or bulging of the optic disc is a sign of increased intracranial pressure. Use the diameter of the optic disc to identify the location of other landmarks on the retina.

The macula is located approximately 2 disc diameters lateral to the optic disc. To see the macula, ask the child to look at the light. It appears as a yellow dot surrounded by deep pink. The macula is inspected last because the bright light causes the child to blink and look away.

NURSING PRACTICE

Keep the red reflex in view to make sure your head and the ophthalmoscope move as one unit. If you lose the red reflex when moving closer to the child, move back, find the red reflex, and start again.

ASSESSING THE EAR STRUCTURES AND HEARING

Equipment needed for this examination includes an otoscope, noisemakers (bell, rattle, tissue paper), and a tuning fork 500 to 1000 Hz.

INSPECTION OF THE EXTERNAL EAR STRUCTURES

The position and characteristics of the pinna, the external ear, are inspected as a continuation of the head and eye examination. The pinna is considered "low set" when the top lies completely below an imaginary line drawn through the medial and lateral canthi of the eye toward the ear. Low-set ears are often associated with congenital renal disorders (Figure 35–12 ◉).

Inspect the pinna for any malformation. The pinna should be completely formed, with an open auditory canal. Next, inspect the tissue around the pinna for abnormalities. A pit or hole in front of the auditory canal may indicate the presence of a sinus. If the pinna protrudes outward, there may be swelling behind the ear, a sign of mastoiditis.

Inspect the external auditory canal for any discharge. A foul-smelling, purulent discharge may indicate the presence of a foreign body or an infection in the external canal. Clear fluid or a blood-tinged discharge may indicate a cerebrospinal fluid leak caused by a basilar skull fracture.

◉ **FIGURE 35–12**

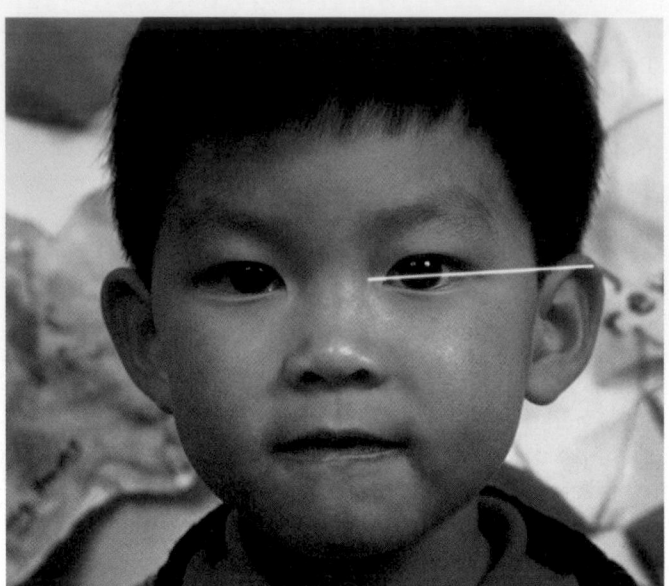

To detect the correct placement of the external ears, draw an imaginary line through the medial and lateral canthi of the eye toward the ear. This line normally passes through the upper portion of the pinna. The pinna is considered "low set" when the top lies completely below the imaginary line. Low-set ears are often associated with renal disorders. Is this a normal ear placement? Yes, it is.

INSPECTION OF THE TYMPANIC MEMBRANE

Examination of the tympanic membrane is important in infants and young children because they are prone to otitis media, a middle ear infection. The eustachian tubes are shorter, wider, and more horizontally positioned in infants and young children than in older children and adults. This positioning enables bacteria to move up the eustachian tube from the pharynx, causing an infection. See As Children Grow: Eustachian Tube in Chapter 45. ∞

The otoscope, an instrument with a magnifying lens, bright light, and speculum, is used to examine the internal auditory canal and tympanic membrane. Infants and young children often resist having their ears inspected with the otoscope because of past painful experiences. For that reason it may be wise to delay the otoscopic examination until portions of the assessment requiring cooperation are completed. Use simple explanations to prepare the child. Let the child play with the otoscope or demonstrate how it is used on the parent or a doll. Figure 35–13 ◉ illustrates one method for restraining an uncooperative child. See also Skill 7–3 in the Clinical Skills Manual. **SKILLS**

Using the Otoscope

To begin the otoscopic examination, hold the handle of the otoscope in the palm with the thumb pointed toward the base of the handle. If using a pneumatic squeeze bulb, hold

⊙ **FIGURE 35–13**

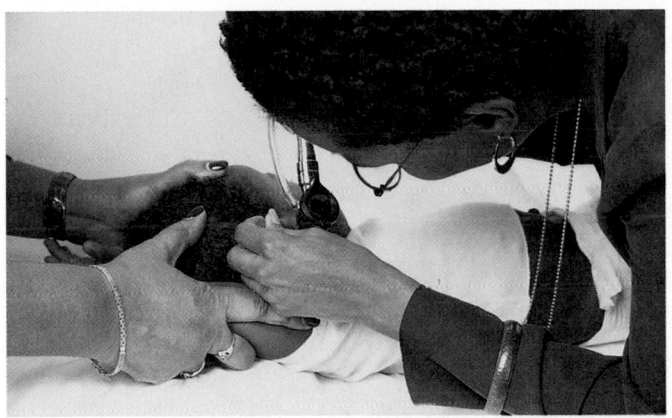

To restrain an uncooperative child, place the child prone on the examining table. Have an assistant hold the child's arms next to the head to restrain the child's head movements. Restrain the child's body movements by lying across the child's body. Keep your hands free to hold the otoscope and position the external ear.

it between the index finger and the handle. Choose the largest ear speculum that fits into the auditory canal to form a seal for testing the movement of the tympanic membrane. A large speculum is also less likely to injure the auditory canal if the child moves suddenly.

Hold the otoscope in the hand closest to the child's face. When the child is cooperative, rest the back of that hand against the child's head to stabilize it. Use the other hand to pull the pinna toward the back of the head and either up or down. Pulling the pinna straightens the auditory canal and improves inspection of the tympanic membrane (Figure 35–14 ⊙).

⊙ **FIGURE 35–14**

To straighten the auditory canal, pull the pinna back and up for children over 3 years of age. Pull the pinna down and back for children under 3 years of age.

Slowly insert the speculum into the auditory canal, inspecting the walls for signs of irritation, discharge, or a foreign body. The walls of the auditory canal are normally pink, and some cerumen is present. Children often put beads, peas, or other small objects into their ears. If the auditory canal is obstructed by cerumen or a foreign body, warm water irrigation can be used to clean the canal.

NURSING PRACTICE

Never irrigate the ear canal if any discharge is present, the tympanic membrane may be ruptured. Water could enter the middle ear and potentially worsen the infection.

The tympanic membrane, which separates the outer ear from the middle ear, is usually pearly gray and translucent. It reflects light, and the bones (ossicles) in the middle ear are normally visible (Figure 35–15 ⊙). When the pneumatic attachment is squeezed, the tympanic membrane normally moves in and out in response to the positive and negative pressure applied. Table 35–7 lists the abnormal findings of a tympanic membrane examination and their associated conditions.

HEARING ASSESSMENT

Hearing evaluation is important in children of all ages because hearing is essential for normal speech development and learning. Often hearing must be evaluated by inspection of the child's responses to various auditory stimuli. Hearing loss may occur at any time during early childhood as the result of birth trauma, frequent otitis media, meningitis, or antibiotics that damage cranial nerve VIII. Hearing loss may also be associated with congenital anomalies and genetic syndromes.

Use hearing and speech articulation milestones as an initial hearing screen. Select an age-appropriate method to screen hearing. When a hearing deficiency is suspected as a result of screening, refer the child for audiometry, tympanometry, or evoked response to obtain the most accurate evaluation of hearing. See Skills 9–20 and 9–21 in the Clinical Skills Manual. **SKILLS**

GROWTH AND DEVELOPMENT

Indicators of hearing loss in an infant:
- No startle reaction to loud noises
- Does not turn toward sounds by 4 months of age
- Babbles as a young infant but does not keep babbling or develop speech sounds after 6 months of age

Indicators of hearing loss in a young child:
- No speech by 2 years of age
- Speech sounds are not distinct at appropriate ages

● **FIGURE 35-15**

Cross-section of the ear. The tympanic membrane normally has a triangular light reflex with the base on the nasal side pointing toward the center. The bony landmarks, the umbo and handle of malleus, are seen through the tympanic membrane.

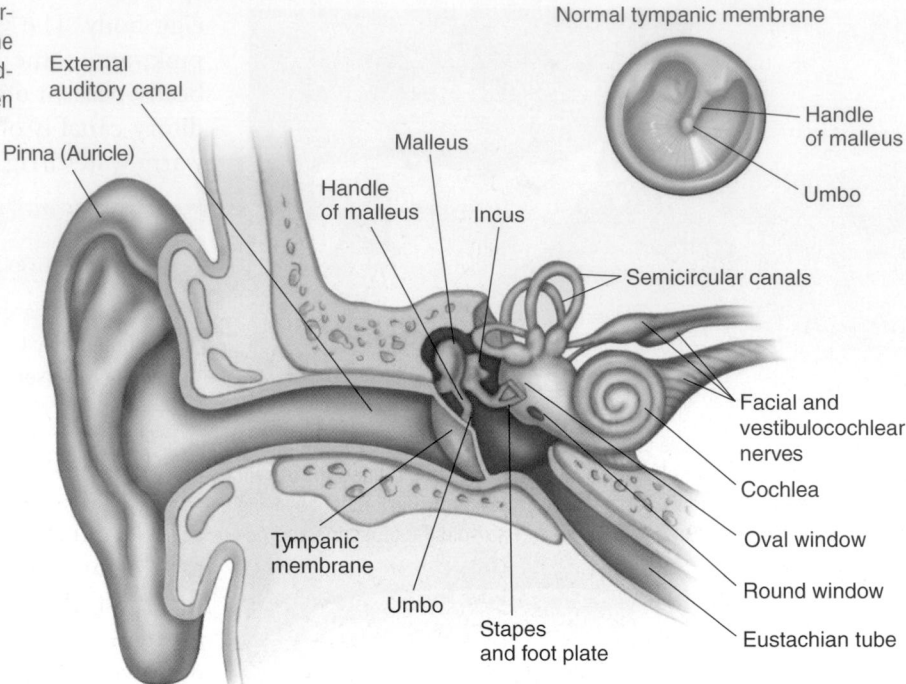

Infants and Toddlers

Select noisemakers with different frequencies, such as a rattle, bell, and tissue paper, that will attract the young child's attention. Ask the parent or an assistant to entertain the infant with a quiet toy, such as a teddy bear. Stand behind the infant, about 2 feet (60 cm) away from the infant's ear but outside the infant's field of vision, and make a soft sound with the noisemaker. Have the parent or assistant observe the child for any of the following responses when the noisemaker is used: widening the eyes, briefly stopping all activity to listen, or turning the head toward the sound. Repeat the test in the other ear and with the other noisemakers.

Preschool and Older Children

Use whispered words to evaluate the hearing of children over 3 years of age. Position your head about 12 inches (30 cm) away from the child's ear, but out of the range of vision so the child cannot read your lips. Use words easily recognized by the child, such as Mickey Mouse, hot dog, and Popsicle, and ask the child to repeat the words. Repeat the

TABLE 35-7 ❖ Unexpected Findings on Examination of the Tympanic Membrane and Their Associated Conditions

Characteristics of Tympanic Membrane	Unexpected Findings	Associated Conditions
Color	Redness	Infection in middle ear
	Slight redness	Prolonged crying
	Amber	Serous fluid in middle ear
	Deep red or blue	Blood in middle ear
Light reflex	Absent	Bulging tympanic membrane, infection in middle ear
	Distorted, loss of triangular shape	Retracted tympanic membrane, serous fluid in middle ear
Bony landmarks	Extra prominent	Retracted tympanic membrane, serous fluid in middle ear
Movement	No motility	Infection or fluid in middle ear
	Excess motility	Healed perforation

test with different words in the opposite ear. The child should correctly repeat the whispered words.

NURSING PRACTICE

An alternative procedure is used to assess hearing when the child will not cooperate by repeating whispered words. In a whisper, direct the child to point to different parts of the body or objects, for example, "Show me your eyes" and "Point to your mouth." Children should point to the correct body part each time.

Bone and Air Conduction of Sound

Use a tuning fork to evaluate the hearing of school-age children who can follow directions. Stroke the tines of the tuning fork to begin the vibration. Avoid touching the vibrating tines, which will dampen the sound. Test bone conduction by placing the handle of the tuning fork on the child's skull. Test air conduction by holding the vibrating tines close to the child's ear (Figure 35–16 ⊙).

To perform the *Weber test*, place the vibrating tuning fork on top of the child's skull in the midline. Ask the child to say where the sound is heard best, either in both ears equally or in one ear. The sound should be heard equally in both ears.

To perform the *Rinne test*, place the vibrating tuning fork handle on the mastoid process behind an ear. Ask the child to say when the sound is no longer heard. Immediately move the tuning fork, holding the vibrating tines about 2.5 to 5 cm (1 to 2 in.) from the same ear. Again, ask the child to indicate when the sound is no longer heard. The child normally hears the air-conducted sound twice as long as the bone-conducted sound. Repeat the Rinne test on the other ear. Table 35–8 provides an interpretation of the Weber and Rinne tests.

TABLE 35–8 ✤ Interpretation of the Weber and Rinne Tests of Hearing

Test and Result	Associated Condition
Weber Test	
Sound heard equally in both ears	No hearing loss
Sound heard better in one ear (lateralized)	Conductive hearing loss if sound lateralized to deaf ear
Rinne Test	
Sound heard by air conduction twice as long as bone conduction	No hearing loss
Sound heard longer by bone conduction than air conduction	Conductive hearing loss in affected ear
Sound heard longer by air conduction than bone conduction, but less than twice as long	Sensorineural hearing loss in affected ear

ASSESSING THE NOSE AND SINUSES FOR AIRWAY PATENCY AND DISCHARGE

An otoscope with a nasal speculum or a penlight is needed for this examination.

INSPECTION OF THE EXTERNAL NOSE

Examine the external nose characteristics and placement on the face simultaneously with the facial features. Inspect the external nose for size, shape, symmetry, and midline placement on the face. The nose should be proportional in

⊙ **FIGURE 35–16**

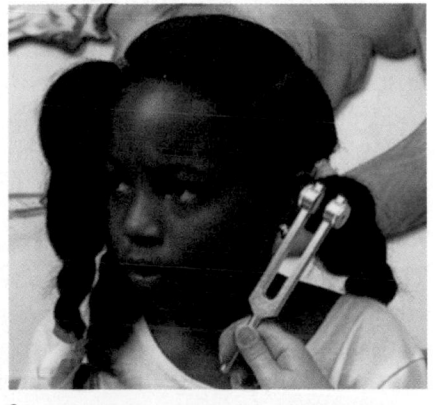

A   B   C

A, Weber test. Place vibrating tuning fork on midline of the child's head. **B,** Rinne test, step 1. Place vibrating tuning fork on mastoid process. **C,** Rinne test, step 2. Reposition still vibrating tines between 2.5 and 5 cm (1 and 2 in.) from ear.

size to other facial features and positioned in the middle of the face. A flattened nasal bridge is the expected finding in Asian and black children.

The nasolabial folds are normally symmetric. Asymmetry of the nasolabial folds may be associated with injury to the facial nerve (cranial nerve VII). A saddle-shaped nose is associated with congenital defects such as cleft palate.

Inspect the external nose for unusual characteristics. For example, a crease across the nose between the cartilage and bone is often caused by the allergic child's wiping an itchy nose upward with a hand.

PALPATION OF THE EXTERNAL NOSE

When a deformity is noted, gently palpate the nose to detect any pain or break in contour. No tenderness or masses are expected. Pain and a contour deviation are usually the result of trauma.

Nasal Patency

The child's airway must be patent to ensure adequate oxygenation. To test for nasal patency, occlude one nostril and observe the child's effort to breathe through the open nostril with the mouth closed. Repeat the procedure with the other nostril. Breathing should be noiseless and effortless. **Nasal flaring**, an effort the child makes to widen the airway, is a sign of respiratory distress and should not be present.

GROWTH AND DEVELOPMENT

Infants under 6 months of age will not automatically open their mouths to breathe when their nose is occluded, such as by mucus.

If the child struggles to breathe, a nasal obstruction may be present. Nasal obstruction may be caused by a foreign body, congenital defect, dry mucus, discharge, polyp, or trauma. Newborns may have respiratory distress because of choanal atresia, a congenital membranous or bony obstruction between the nose and the nasopharynx. Young children commonly place objects up their nose, and unilateral nasal flaring is a sign of such an obstruction.

ASSESSMENT OF SMELL

The olfactory nerve (cranial nerve I) can be tested in school-age children and adolescents. When testing smell, choose scents the child will easily recognize such as orange, chocolate, and mint. When the child's eyes are closed, occlude one nostril and hold the scent under the nose. Ask the child to take a deep sniff and identify the scent. Alternate odors between the nares. The child can normally identify common scents.

INSPECTION OF THE INTERNAL NOSE

Inspect the internal nose for color of the mucous membranes and the presence of any discharge, swelling, lesions, or other abnormalities. Use a bright light, such as an otoscope light or penlight. For infants and young children, push the tip of the nose upward and shine the light at the end of the nose. The nasal speculum of the otoscope can be used in older children (Figure 35–17 ●). Avoid touching the septum of the nose with the speculum. Injury to the septum can cause a nosebleed.

Mucous Membranes and Nasal Septum

The mucous membranes should be dark pink and glistening. A film of clear discharge may also be present. Turbinates, if visible, should be the same color as the mucous membranes and have a firm consistency. When the turbinates are pale or bluish gray, the child may have allergies. A polyp, a rounded mass projecting from the turbinate, is also associated with allergies. The nasal septum should be straight without perforations, bleeding, or crusting. Crusting will be noted over the site of a nosebleed.

Discharge

Observe for the presence of nasal discharge, noting if the drainage is from one or both nares. Nasal discharge is not a normal finding unless the child is crying. Discharge may be watery, mucoid, purulent, or bloody, depending on the condition present. A foul-smelling discharge in only one nostril is often associated with a foreign body. Table 35–9 lists conditions associated with nasal discharge.

● **FIGURE 35–17**

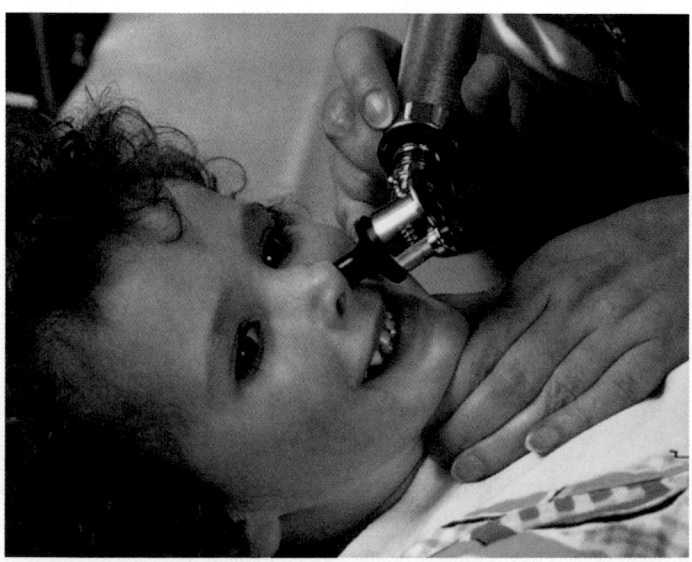

Technique for examining nose.

<table>
<tr><td colspan="2">TABLE 35–9 ✢ Nasal Discharge Characteristics and Associated Conditions</td></tr>
</table>

Discharge Description	Associated Condition
Watery	
Clear, bilateral	Allergy
Serous, unilateral	Spinal fluid from fracture of cribriform plate
Mucoid or purulent	
Bilateral	Upper respiratory infection
Unilateral	Foreign body
Bloody	Nose bleed, trauma

INSPECTION OF THE SINUSES

The illustration in "As Children Grow" shows how the maxillary and ethmoid sinuses develop during early childhood. Sinus infections can occasionally occur in young children. Suspect a sinus problem when the child has a headache or pain and swelling around one or both eyes.

Inspect the face for any puffiness and swelling around one or both eyes. Puffiness and swelling are not normally present. To palpate over the maxillary sinuses, press up under both zygomatic arches with the thumbs. To palpate the ethmoid sinuses, press up against the bone above both eyes with the thumbs. No swelling or tenderness is expected. Tenderness may indicate sinusitis.

ASSESSING THE MOUTH AND THROAT FOR COLOR, FUNCTION, AND SIGNS OF ABNORMAL CONDITIONS

Equipment needed to examine the mouth and throat includes a tongue blade and penlight.

INSPECTION OF THE MOUTH

Young children often need coaxing and simple explanations before they will cooperate with the mouth and throat examination. Most children readily show their teeth. If the child resists by clenching the teeth, they can be gently separated with a tongue blade. Wear gloves when examining the mouth (Figure 35–18 ⊙).

AS CHILDREN GROW

Growth and Development of Sinuses

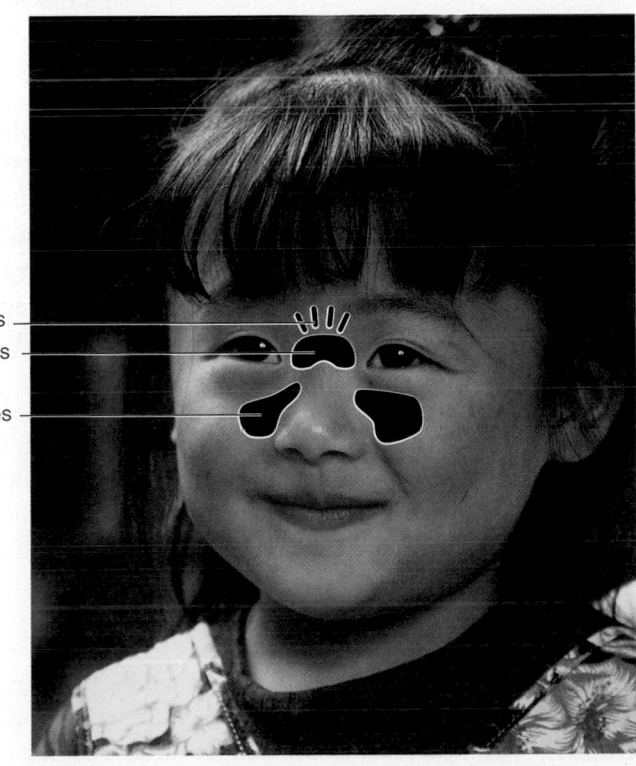

Ethmoid sinuses
Sphenoid sinus
Maxillary sinuses

Sinuses grow and develop during childhood. Maxillary sinuses can be identified in 1-year-old children. Ethmoid sinuses have developed in children by 6 years of age. Sinus problems under 7 years occur infrequently.

○ FIGURE 35-18

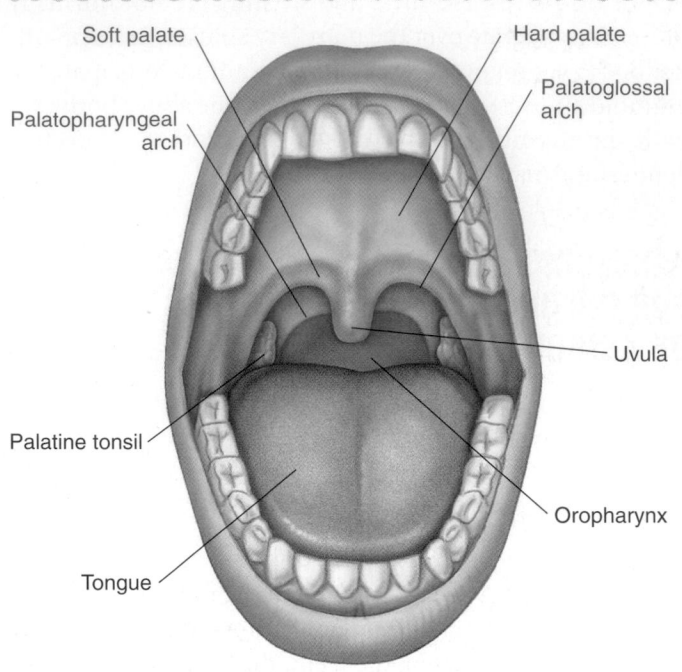

Soft palate

Hard palate

Palatoglossal arch

Palatopharyngeal arch

Uvula

Palatine tonsil

Oropharynx

Tongue

The structures of the mouth.

NURSING PRACTICE

Avoid examining the mouth if there are signs of respiratory distress, high fever, drooling, and intense apprehension. These may be signs of epiglottitis. Inspecting the mouth may trigger a total airway obstruction. See "Laryngotracheobronchitis" in Chapter 47 for more information. ∞

Lips

Inspect the lips for color, shape, symmetry, moisture, and lesions. The lips are normally symmetric without drying, cracking, or other lesions. Lip color is normally pink in white children and more bluish in darker-skinned children. Pale, cyanotic, or cherry-red lips indicate poor tissue perfusion caused by various conditions. Note any clefts or edema.

Teeth

Inspect and count the child's teeth. The timing of tooth eruption is often genetically determined, but there is a regular sequence of tooth eruption. Figure 35–19 ○ presents the typical sequence of tooth eruption for both deciduous and permanent teeth.

Inspect the condition of the teeth, look for loose teeth, and note any spaces where teeth are missing. Compare empty tooth spaces with the child's developmental stage of tooth eruption. Once the permanent teeth have erupted, none should be missing. Teeth are normally white, without

a flattened, mottled, or pitted appearance. Discolorations on the crown of a tooth may indicate caries. Discolorations on the tooth surface may be associated with some medications and fluorosis. See Chapter 46. ∞

Mouth Odors

During inspection of the teeth, be alert to any abnormal odors that may indicate problems such as diabetic ketoacidosis, infection, or poor hygiene. Be alert for alcohol odors in older children that could signal substance abuse.

Gums

Inspect the gums for color and adherence to the teeth. The gums are normally pink, with a stippled or dotted appearance. Use a tongue blade to help visualize the gums around the upper and lower molars. No raised or receding gum areas should be apparent around the teeth. When inflammation, swelling, or bleeding is observed, palpate the gums to detect tenderness. Inflammation and tenderness are associated with infection and poor nutrition.

Buccal Mucosa

Inspect the mucous membrane lining the cheeks for color and moisture. The mucous membrane is usually pink, but patches of hyperpigmentation are commonly seen in darker-skinned children. The Stensen duct, the parotid gland opening, is opposite the upper second molar bilaterally. Normally pink, the duct opening becomes red when the child is infected with mumps. Small pink sucking pads can be present in infants. No areas of redness, swelling, or ulcerative lesions should be present.

Tongue

Inspect the tongue for color, moistness, size, tremors, and lesions. The child's tongue is normally pink and moist, without a coating, and it fits easily into the mouth. A pattern of gray, irregular borders that form a design (geographic tongue) is often normal, but it may be associated with fever, allergies, or drug reactions. Tremors are abnormal. A white adherent coating on an infant's tongue may be caused by thrush, a *Candida* infection.

Observe the mobility of the tongue. Ask the child to touch the gums above the upper teeth with the tongue. This tongue movement is adequate to enunciate all speech sounds clearly. Ask the child to stick out the tongue and lift it so the underside of the tongue and the floor of the mouth can be inspected for distended veins.

Palate

Inspect the hard and soft palate to detect any clefts or masses or an unusually high arch. The palate is normally pink, with a dome-shaped arch and no cleft. The uvula hangs freely from the soft palate. Newborns often have Ep-

● **FIGURE 35–19**

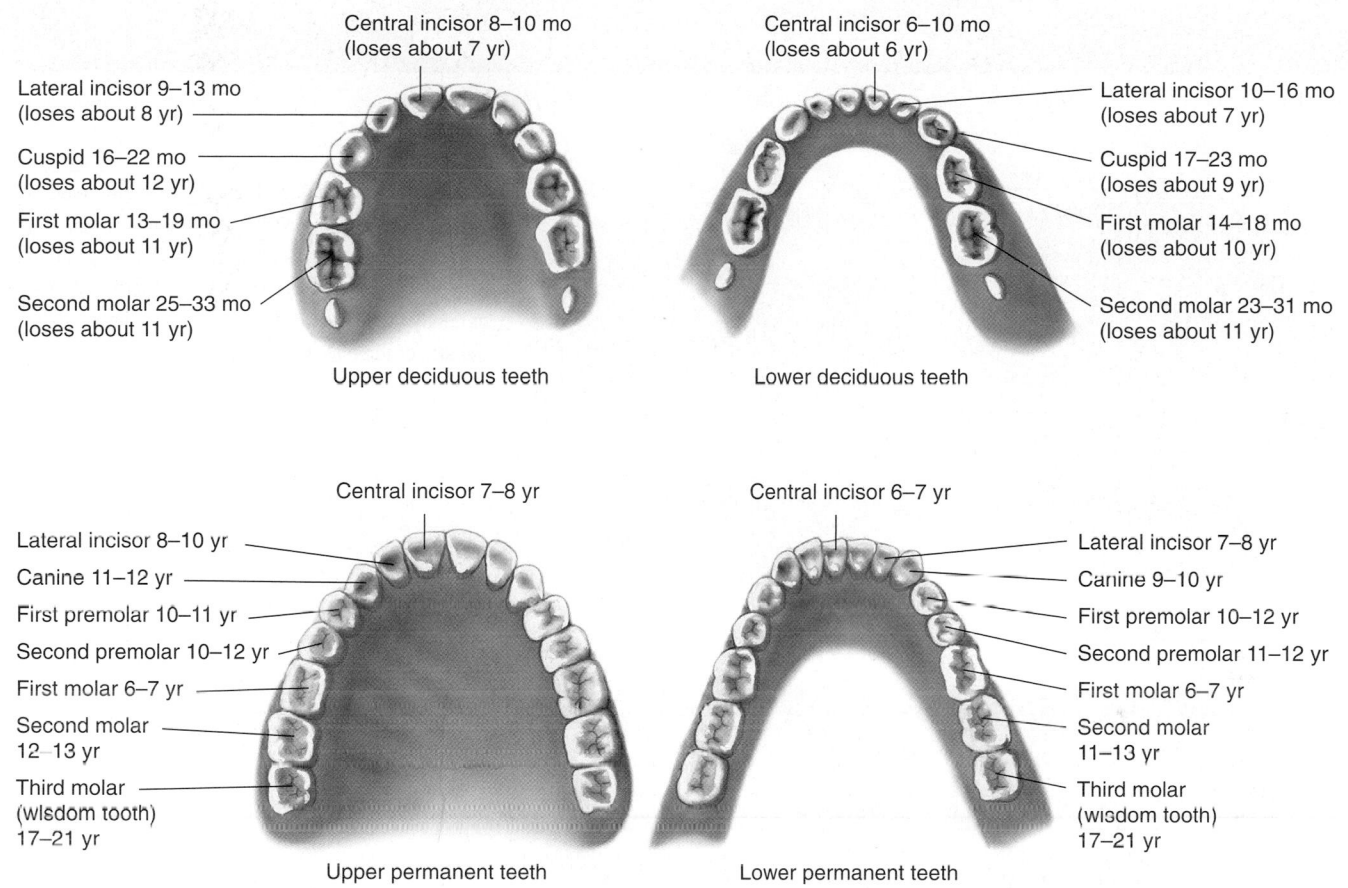

Central incisor 8–10 mo (loses about 7 yr)

Lateral incisor 9–13 mo (loses about 8 yr)

Cuspid 16–22 mo (loses about 12 yr)

First molar 13–19 mo (loses about 11 yr)

Second molar 25–33 mo (loses about 11 yr)

Upper deciduous teeth

Central incisor 6–10 mo (loses about 6 yr)

Lateral incisor 10–16 mo (loses about 7 yr)

Cuspid 17–23 mo (loses about 9 yr)

First molar 14–18 mo (loses about 10 yr)

Second molar 23–31 mo (loses about 11 yr)

Lower deciduous teeth

Central incisor 7–8 yr

Lateral incisor 8–10 yr
Canine 11–12 yr
First premolar 10–11 yr
Second premolar 10–12 yr
First molar 6–7 yr
Second molar 12–13 yr
Third molar (wisdom tooth) 17–21 yr

Upper permanent teeth

Central incisor 6–7 yr

Lateral incisor 7–8 yr
Canine 9–10 yr
First premolar 10–12 yr
Second premolar 11–12 yr
First molar 6–7 yr
Second molar 11–13 yr
Third molar (wisdom tooth) 17–21 yr

Lower permanent teeth

Typical sequence of tooth eruption for both deciduous and permanent teeth. Notice that bottom deciduous teeth are shed first and bottom permanent teeth erupt first.

stein pearls, white papules in the midline of the palate that disappear in a few weeks. A high-arched palate can be associated with sucking difficulties in young infants.

PALPATION OF THE MOUTH STRUCTURES

Palpate any masses seen in the mouth to determine their characteristics, such as size, shape, firmness, and tenderness. No masses should be found.

Tongue

To assess the tongue's strength, while simultaneously testing the hypoglossal nerve (cranial nerve XII), place the index finger against the child's cheek and ask the child to push against your finger with the tongue. Some pressure against the finger is normally felt.

Palate

To palpate the palate, insert the little finger, with the fingerpad upward, into the mouth. While the infant sucks against your finger, palpate the entire palate. This procedure also tests the strength of the sucking reflex, innervated

by the hypoglossal nerve (cranial nerve XII). No clefts should be palpated.

INSPECTION OF THE THROAT

Inspect the throat for color, swelling, lesions, and the condition of the tonsils. Ask the child to open the mouth wide and stick out the tongue. Illuminate the throat with a flashlight. Use a tongue blade, if needed, to visualize the posterior pharynx. Moistening the tongue blade may decrease the child's tendency to gag. The throat is normally pink without lesions, drainage, or swelling. Swelling or bulging in the posterior pharynx may be associated with a peritonsillar abscess.

Tonsils

During childhood the tonsils are large in proportion to the size of the pharynx because lymphoid tissue grows fastest in early childhood. The tonsils should be pink without exudate, but crypts (fissures) may be present as a result of prior infections. The size of the tonsils can be graded as indicated in the "Pathophysiology Illustrated" diagram.

PATHOPHYSIOLOGY ILLUSTRATED
Tonsil Size with Infection

Tonsil size can be graded from 1+ to 4+ in relation to how much of the airway is obstructed. Tonsil size of 1+ and 2+ is normal. Tonsil size of 3+ is common with infections such as strep throat. Tonsils that "kiss" or nearly touch each other (4+) significantly reduce the size of the airway.

A

B

C

D

Gag Reflex

Use a tongue blade when you are unable to see the posterior pharynx or need to test the gag reflex. Do this at the end of the examination because children dislike the gagging sensation. Prepare the child for what will happen. Ask the child to say "Ah." A symmetric rising movement of the uvula is observed. If the uvula does not rise or rises to one side, cranial nerves IX and X may be paralyzed. The epiglottis lies behind the tongue and is normally pink like the rest of the buccal mucosa.

ASSESSING THE NECK FOR CHARACTERISTICS, RANGE OF MOTION, AND LYMPH NODES

INSPECTION OF THE NECK

Inspect the neck for size, symmetry, swelling, and any abnormalities. A short neck with skin folds is normal for infants. The neck is normally symmetric. No swelling should be present. Swelling may be caused by local infections such as mumps or a congenital defect. The neck lengthens between 3 and 4 years of age.

Inspect the child's neck for webbing, an extra skin fold on each side of the neck. Webbing is commonly associated with Turner syndrome. See "Turner Syndrome" in Chapter 56. ∞

Infants develop head control by 2 months of age. By this age an infant can lift the head up and look around when lying on the stomach. A lack of head control can result from neurologic injury, such as an anoxic episode.

PALPATION OF THE NECK

Face the child and use your fingerpads to simultaneously palpate both sides of the neck for lymph nodes, as well as the trachea and thyroid.

Lymph Nodes

To palpate the lymph nodes, slide your fingerpads gently over the lymph node chains in the head and neck. The sequence for lymph node palpation is as follows: around the ears, under the jaw, the occipital area, and the cervical chain in the neck (Figure 35–20 ●). Firm, clearly defined, non tender, movable lymph nodes up to 1 cm (1/2 in.) in diameter are common in young children. Enlarged, firm, warm, tender lymph nodes indicate a local infection.

Trachea

Palpate the trachea to determine its position and to detect the presence of any masses. The trachea is normally in the midline of the neck. It is difficult to palpate in children less than 3 years of age because of their short necks. To palpate the trachea, place your thumb and forefinger on each side of the child's trachea near the chin and slowly slide them down the trachea. Any shift to the right or left of midline may indicate a tumor or a collapsed lung.

Thyroid

As the fingers slide over the trachea in the lower neck, attempt to feel the isthmus of the thyroid, a band of glandular tissue crossing over the trachea. The lobes of the thyroid wrap behind the trachea and are normally covered by the sternocleidomastoid muscle. Because of the anatomic position of the thyroid, its lobes are not usually palpable in the child unless they are enlarged.

RANGE OF MOTION ASSESSMENT

To test the neck's range of motion, ask the child to touch the chin to each shoulder and to the chest and then to look at the ceiling. Move a light or toy in all four directions when assessing infants. Children should freely move the neck and head in all four directions without pain.

When the child is unable to move the head voluntarily in all directions, passively move the child's neck through the expected range of motion. Limited horizontal range of motion may be a sign of torticollis, persistent head tilting. Torticollis results from a birth injury to the sternocleidomastoid muscle or from unilateral vision or hearing impairment. Pain with flexion of the neck toward the chest (Brudzinski's sign) may indicate meningitis. See "meningitis" in Chapter 53. ∞

ASSESSING THE CHEST FOR SHAPE, MOVEMENT, RESPIRATORY EFFORT, AND LUNG FUNCTION

What terms describe the location of specific sounds heard when auscultating the chest? What are retractions and what do they indicate? How can normal and adventitious breath sounds be distinguished when auscultating the lungs?

Examination of the chest includes the following procedures: inspecting the size and shape of the chest, palpating chest movement that occurs during respiration, observing

● **FIGURE 35–20**

The neck is palpated for enlarged lymph nodes around the ears, under the jaw, in the occipital area, and in the cervical chain of the neck.

Maxillary
Buccal
Sublingual
Submandibular
Supraclavicular
Anterior auricular
Posterior auricular
Occipital
Superficial cervical
Tonsillar
Posterior cervical
Superior deep cervical

the effort of breathing, and auscultating breath sounds. A stethoscope is needed.

TOPOGRAPHIC LANDMARKS OF THE CHEST

The chest skeleton provides most of the landmarks used to describe the location of findings during examination of the chest, lungs, and heart. The intercostal spaces are the horizontal markers. The sternum and spine are the vertical landmarks. When both a horizontal and a vertical landmark are used, the location of findings can be precisely described on the right or left side of the patient's chest (Figures 35–21 ● and 35–22 ●).

INSPECTION OF THE CHEST

Position the child on the parent's lap or on the examining table with all clothing above the waist removed to inspect the chest. The thoracic muscles and subcutaneous tissue are less developed in children than in adults, so the chest wall is thinner. As a result the rib cage is more prominent.

Size and Shape of the Chest

Inspect the chest for any irregularities in shape. A chest is considered rounded when the anteroposterior diameter is approximately equal to the lateral diameter. If a child over 2 years of age has a rounded chest, a chronic obstructive lung condition such as asthma or cystic fibrosis may be present.

GROWTH AND DEVELOPMENT

In infants the chest is rounded with the anteroposterior diameter approximately equal to the lateral diameter. The chest becomes more oval with growth. By 2 years of age the lateral diameter is greater than the anteroposterior diameter.

An abnormal chest shape results from two different structural deformities (Figure 35–23 ●). If the sternum protrudes, increasing the anteroposterior diameter, pigeon chest (pectus carinatum) may be present. If the

● **FIGURE 35–21**

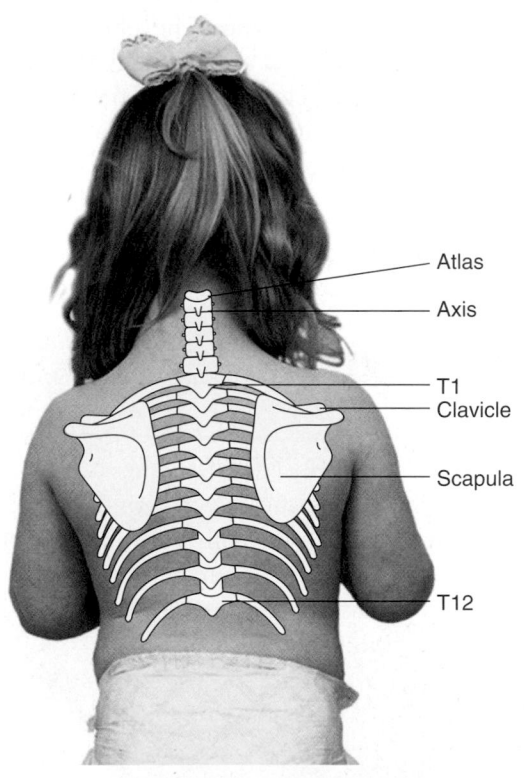

A   **B**

Intercostal spaces and ribs are numbered to describe the location of findings. **A,** To determine the rib number on the anterior chest, palpate down from the top of the sternum until a horizontal ridge, the angle of Louis, is felt. Directly to the right and left of that ridge is the second rib. The second intercostal space is immediately below the second rib. Ribs 3–12 and the corresponding intercostal spaces can be counted as the fingers move toward the abdomen. **B,** To determine the rib number on the posterior chest, find the protruding spinal process of the seventh cervical vertebra at the shoulder level. The next spinal process belongs to the first thoracic vertebra, which attaches to the first rib.

● **FIGURE 35-22**

Right midclavicular line

Sternal line

Right upper lobe

Left upper lobe

Right middle lobe

Right lower lobe

Left lower lobe

Right anterior axillary line

Vertebral line

Right scapular line

Right posterior axillary line

A

B

The sternum and spine are the vertical landmarks used to describe the anatomic location of findings. The distance between the finding and the center of the sternum (midsternal line) or the spinal line can be measured with a ruler. Imaginary vertical lines, parallel to the midsternal and spinal lines, are used to further describe the location of findings. **A,** anterior vertical landmarks, **B,** posterior vertical landmarks.

lower portion of the sternum is depressed, decreasing the anteroposterior diameter, funnel chest (pectus excavatum) may be present. Scoliosis, curvature of the spine, causes a lateral deviation of the chest. See "Scoliosis" in Chapter 55. ∞

Chest Movement and Respiratory Effort

Inspect for simultaneous chest expansion and abdominal rise. Chest movement is normally symmetric bilaterally, rising with inspiration and falling with expiration. The chest movement of infants and young children is less pronounced than the abdominal movement. The diaphragm is the primary breathing muscle in infants and children under 6 years old. The thoracic muscles are less developed and serve as accessory muscles in cases of respiratory distress. As the thoracic muscles develop, they become primarily responsible for ventilation. On inspiration the chest and abdomen should rise simultaneously. Asymmetric chest rise is associated with a collapsed lung. **Retractions**, depression of sections of the chest wall with each inspiration, are seen when the accessory muscles are used for breathing in cases of respiratory distress.

● **FIGURE 35-23**

A

B

Two types of abnormal chest shape. **A,** Funnel chest (pectus excavatum). **B,** Pigeon chest (pectus carinatum).

GROWTH AND DEVELOPMENT

Infants and children have a faster respiratory rate than adults because of a higher metabolic rate and need for oxygen. Young children are also unable to increase the depth of respirations because not all the alveoli are developed (Hazinski, 1999).

Respiratory Rate

Because young children use the diaphragm as the primary breathing muscle, observe or feel the rise and fall of the abdomen to count the respiratory rate in children under age 6 years (see Skill 9–9 in the Clinical Skills Manual **SKILLS**). Table 35–10 gives the normal respiratory rates for each age group. Make every effort to count the respiratory rate when the child is quiet. The respiratory rate rises in response to excitement, fear, respiratory distress, fever, and other conditions that increase oxygen needs.

NURSING PRACTICE

To get the most accurate reading of a newborn's and young infant's respiratory rate, wait until the baby is sleeping or resting quietly. Use the stethoscope to auscultate the rate or place your hand on the abdomen. Count the number of breaths for an entire minute, because newborns and young infants can have irregular respirations.

A sustained respiratory rate greater than 60 breaths per minute is an important sign in respiratory distress. At that rate, children develop hypoxemia if treatment is not started. The child's airway is very narrow, resulting in higher airway resistance than occurs in adults. When the respiratory rate exceeds 60 breaths per minute, inspired oxygen does not reach the alveoli for gas exchange because air moves no farther than the upper airway (Eichelberger, Ball, Pratsch et al., 1998).

PALPATION OF THE CHEST

Use palpation to evaluate chest movement, respiratory effort, deformities of the chest wall, and tactile fremitus.

Chest Wall

To palpate the chest motion with respiration, place your palms and outspread fingers on each side of the child's chest. Confirm the bilateral symmetry of chest motion. Use your fingerpads to palpate any depressions, bulges, or unusual chest wall shape that might indicate abnormal findings such as tenderness, cysts, other growths, crepitus, or fractures. None should be found. **Crepitus**, a crinkly sensation palpated on the chest surface, is caused by air escaping into the subcutaneous tissues. It often indicates a serious injury to the upper or lower airway. Crepitus may also be felt near a fracture.

Tactile Fremitus

Crying and talking produce vibrations, known as **tactile fremitus**, that can be palpated on the chest. Place the palms of your hands on each side of the chest to evaluate the quality and distribution of these vibrations. Ask the child to repeat a series of words or numbers, such as Mickey Mouse or ice cream. As the child repeats the words, move your hands systematically over the anterior and posterior chest, comparing the quality of findings side to side. The vibration or tingling sensation is normally palpated over the entire chest. Decreased sensations indicate that air is trapped in the lungs, as occurs with asthma. Increased sensations indicate lung consolidation, as occurs with pneumonia.

AUSCULTATION OF THE CHEST

Auscultate the chest with a stethoscope to assess the quality and characteristics of breath sounds, to identify abnormal breath sounds, and to evaluate vocal resonance. Use an infant or pediatric stethoscope when available to help localize any unexpected breath sounds. Use the stethoscope diaphragm because it transmits the high-pitched breath sounds better.

Breath Sounds

Evaluate the quality and characteristics of breath sounds over the entire chest, comparing sounds between the sides. Select a routine sequence for auscultating the entire chest so assessment of all lobes of the lungs will be consistently performed. Figure 35–24 ● shows one suggested chest auscultation sequence. Listen to an entire inspiratory and expiratory phase at each spot on the chest before moving to the next site.

TABLE 35–10 ✤ **Normal Respiratory Rate Ranges for Each Age Group**

Age	Respiratory Rate per Minute
Newborn	30–60
1 year	20–40
3 years	20–30
6 years	16–22
10 years	16–20
17 years	12–20

NURSING PRACTICE

Auscultation of breath sounds is difficult when an infant is crying. First, try to quiet the infant with a pacifier, bottle, or toy. If the infant continues to cry, all is not lost. At the end of each cry the infant takes a deep breath, which you can use to assess breath sounds, vocal resonance, and tactile fremitus. Encourage toddlers and preschoolers to take deep breaths by providing a pinwheel or mobile to blow.

GROWTH AND DEVELOPMENT

Infants and young children have a thin chest wall because of immature muscle development. The breath sounds of one lung are heard over the entire chest. It takes practice to accurately identify absent or diminished breath sounds in infants and young children. Because the distance between the lungs is greatest at the apices and midaxillary areas in young children, these sites are best for identifying absent or diminished breath sounds. Carefully auscultate, comparing the quality of breath sounds heard bilaterally.

Three types of normal breath sounds are usually heard when the chest is auscultated. *Vesicular breath sounds* are low-pitched, swishing, soft, short expiratory sounds. They are usually heard in older children but not in infants and young children. *Bronchovesicular breath sounds* are medium-pitched, hollow, blowing sounds heard equally on inspiration and expiration in all age groups. The location of these sounds on the chest is related to the child's developmental status. *Bronchial/tracheal breath sounds* are hollow and higher pitched than vesicular breath sounds.

Breath sounds normally have equal intensity, pitch, and rhythm bilaterally. Absent or diminished breath sounds generally indicate a partial or total obstruction, such as from a foreign body or mucus, that does not permit airflow.

Vocal Resonance

Auscultate the chest to evaluate how well voice sounds are transmitted. Have the child repeat a series of words, either the same as or different from those used for evaluating tactile fremitus. Use the stethoscope to auscultate the chest, comparing the quality of sounds from side to side and over the entire chest. Voice sounds, with words and syllables muffled and indistinct, are normally heard throughout the chest.

If voice sounds are absent or more muffled than usual, an airway obstruction condition such as asthma may be present. When a lung consolidation condition such as pneumonia is

● FIGURE 35-21

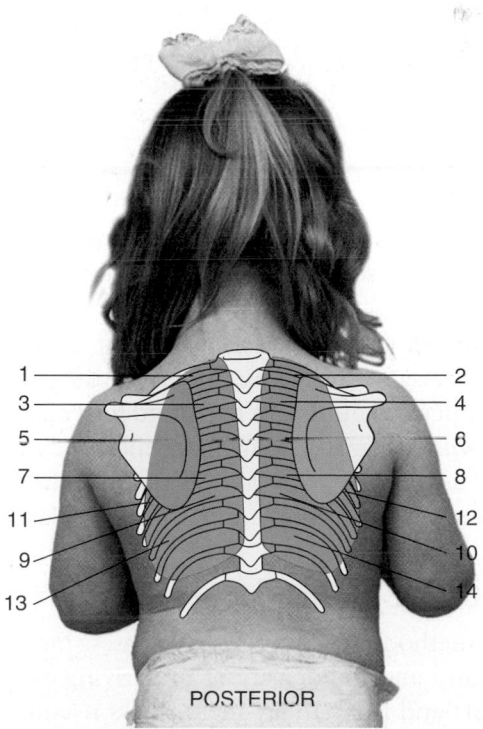

One example of a sequence for auscultation of the chest.

TABLE 35–11 ✤ **Description of Selected Adventitious Sounds and Their Cause**

Type	Description	Cause
Fine crackles	High-pitched, discrete, noncontinuous sound heard at end of inspiration *(Rub pieces of hair together beside your ear to duplicate the sound.)*	Air passing through watery secretions in the smaller airways (alveoli and bronchioles)
Sibilant rhonchi	Musical, squeaking, or hissing noise heard during inspiration or expiration, but generally louder on expiration	Bronchospasm or an anatomic narrowing of the trachea, bronchi, or bronchioles
Sonorous rhonchi	Coarse, low-pitched sound like a snore, heard during inspiration or expiration; may clear with coughing	Air passing through thick secretions that partially obstruct the larger bronchi and trachea

present, the vocal resonance quality changes in characteristic ways. These abnormal characteristics are called whispered pectoriloquy, bronchophony, and egophony. **Whispered pectoriloquy** is present when syllables are heard distinctly in a whisper. **Bronchophony** is the increased intensity and clarity of sounds while the words remain indistinct. **Egophony** is the transmission of the "eee" sound as a nasal "ay" sound.

Abnormal Breath Sounds

Abnormal breath sounds, also called adventitious sounds, generally indicate disease. Examples of abnormal breath sounds are crackles, rhonchi, and friction rubs. To further assess abnormal breath sounds, the examiner determines their location, the respiratory phase in which they are present, and whether they change or disappear when the child coughs or shifts position. To routinely identify these adventitious sounds takes practice. Table 35–11 describes adventitious sounds.

Abnormal Voice Sounds

Observing the quality of the voice and other audible sounds is also important during an examination of the lungs. Examples of these sounds are hoarseness, stridor, and cough. *Stridor* is a noise resulting from air moving through a narrowed trachea and larynx; it is associated with croup. *Wheezing* is a noise resulting from the passage of air through mucus or fluids in a narrowed lower airway; it is associated with asthma. A cough is a reflexive clearing of the airway associated with a respiratory infection. Hoarseness is associated with inflammation of the larynx.

PERCUSSION OF THE CHEST

Percussion is a method sometimes used to assess the resonance of the lungs and the density of underlying organs, such as the heart and liver. Today there is less reliance on percussion to evaluate the lungs because of the frequent use of radiologic examination.

When percussing the anterior and posterior chest, choose a sequence that covers the entire chest and permits comparison bilaterally. The same sequence as that used for auscultation is effective. To perform *indirect percussion,* lay your middle finger of the nondominant hand on the child's chest at an intercostal space. Keep your other fingers off the chest. With a springlike motion, use the fingertip of the other hand to tap the finger in contact with the chest (Figure 35–25A ⦿). Direct percussion is a technique effective for infants. Tap the chest at an intercostal space with a fingertip to elicit the quality of resonance (Figure 35–25B).

⦿ **FIGURE 35–25**

A   B

A, Indirect percussion. Place the middle finger on the child's chest at an intercostal space with the other fingers off the chest. Tap the finger with a springlike motion with the fingertip of the other hand. **B,** Direct percussion. Tap the infant's chest with the fingertip directly at an intercostal space.

● **FIGURE 35–26**

Normal resonance patterns expected over the chest. Tympany is a loud, high-pitched sound, like a drum. It is usually heard over an air-filled stomach. Flatness is a soft, dull sound, like the sound made when percussing your thigh. It is heard over dense muscle and bone. Dullness is a moderately loud, thudlike sound. It is heard when percussing over the liver and heart, and at the base of the lungs (at the level of the diaphragm). Resonance is a loud, low-pitched, hollow sound, like the sound made when percussing a table. It is heard over the lungs. Hyperresonance is a loud, very low-pitched, booming sound. It is usually heard over superinflated lungs. However, because of the thin chest wall in young children, hyperresonance may be a normal finding.

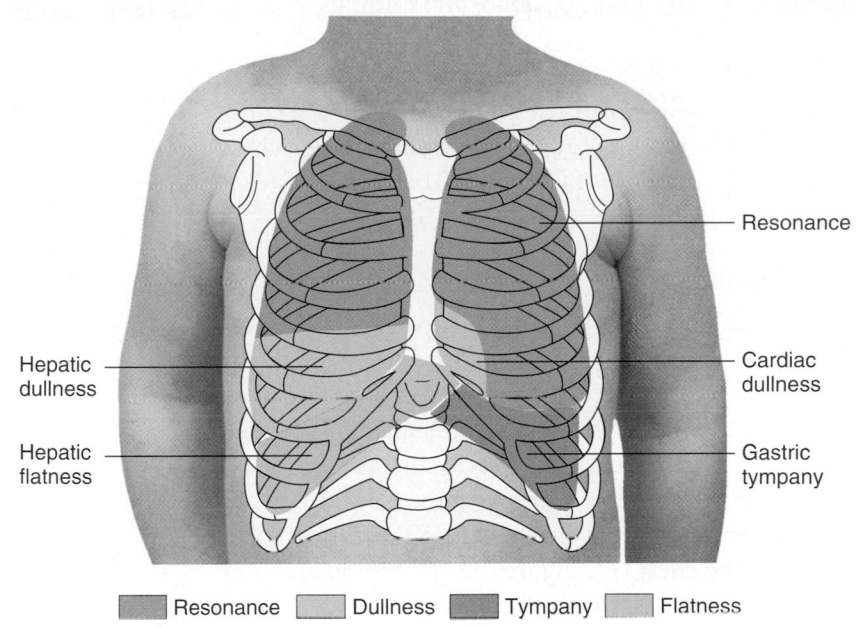

Resonance

Hepatic dullness

Hepatic flatness

Cardiac dullness

Gastric tympany

☐ Resonance ☐ Dullness ☐ Tympany ☐ Flatness

Characteristic patterns of percussion resonance are expected (Figure 35–26 ●). Characteristic descriptions of sounds heard with percussion of the chest include tympany, flatness, dullness, resonance, and hyperresonance.

ASSESSING THE BREASTS

INSPECTION OF THE BREASTS

The nipples of prepubertal boys and girls are symmetrically located near the midclavicular line at the fourth to sixth ribs. The areola is normally round and more darkly pigmented than the surrounding skin. Inspect the anterior chest for other dark spots that may indicate supernumerary nipples, which are small, undeveloped nipples and areola that may be mistaken for moles. Their presence may be associated with congenital renal or cardiac anomalies.

See page 1008 for pubertal development.

PALPATION OF THE BREASTS

Palpate the developing breasts of adolescent females for abnormal masses or hard nodules while the child is supine. Use a concentric pattern covering all quadrants of each breast, including the axilla, all around the areola, and then around the nipple. Breast tissue normally feels dense, firm, and elastic.

The majority of boys have unilateral or bilateral breast enlargement during adolescence called gynecomastia. It is often most noticeable around 14 years of age and commonly disappears by the time of full sexual maturity. Palpate the tissue to differentiate actual breast tissue from fatty tissue in the pectoral area, and to detect any masses.

ASSESSING THE HEART FOR HEART SOUNDS AND FUNCTION

A stethoscope and sphygmomanometer is needed to assess the heart.

INSPECTION OF THE PRECORDIUM

Begin the heart examination by inspecting the precordium, or anterior chest. Place the child in a reclining or semi-Fowler's position, either on the parent's lap or on the examining table. Inspect the shape and symmetry of the anterior chest from the front and side views. The rib cage is normally symmetric. Bulging of the left side of the chest wall may indicate an enlarged heart.

Observe for any chest movement associated with the heart's contraction. The **apical impulse**, sometimes called the point of maximum intensity, is located where the left ventricle taps the chest wall during contraction. The apical impulse can normally be seen in thin children. A heave, an obvious lifting of the chest wall during contraction, may indicate an enlarged heart.

PALPATION OF THE PRECORDIUM

Place the entire palmar surface of your fingers together on the chest wall to palpate the precordium. Systematically palpate the entire precordium to detect any pulsations, heaves, or vibrations. Palpating with minimal pressure increases the chance of detecting abnormal findings.

Apical Impulse

The apical impulse is normally felt as a slight tap against one fingertip. Use the topographic landmarks of the chest to describe its location (see Figures 35–21 and 35–22). Any other sensation palpated is usually abnormal.

Abnormal Sensations

A *lift* is the sensation of the heart lifting up against the chest wall. It may be associated with an enlarged heart or a heart contracting with extra force. A *thrill* is a rushing vibration that feels like a cat's purr. It is caused by turbulent blood flow from a defective heart valve and a heart murmur. If present, the thrill is palpated in the right or left second intercostal space. To describe a thrill's location, use the topographic landmarks of the chest (see Figures 35–21 and 35–22) and estimate the diameter of the thrill palpated.

GROWTH AND DEVELOPMENT

The location of the apical impulse changes as the child's rib cage grows. In children under 7 years old, it is located in the fourth intercostal space just medial to the left midclavicular line. In children over 7 years old, it is located in the fifth intercostal space at the left midclavicular line.

PERCUSSION OF THE HEART BORDERS

Percussion of the heart borders is rarely performed during physical examination. The borders of the heart are better identified by radiologic examination.

AUSCULTATION OF THE HEART

Auscultation is used to count the apical pulse, to assess the characteristics of the heart sounds, and to detect abnormal heart sounds. Use the bell of the stethoscope to detect these lower pitched sounds.

To assess heart sounds completely, auscultate the heart with the child in both sitting and reclining positions. Differences in heart sounds caused by a change in the child's position or by a change in the position of the heart near the chest wall can then be detected. If differences in heart sounds are detected with a position change, place the child in the left lateral recumbent position and auscultate again.

Heart Rate and Rhythm

The apical heart rate can be counted at the site of the apical impulse (Skill 9–8) **SKILLS** either by palpation or by auscultation. Count the apical rate for 1 minute in infants and in children who have an irregular rhythm. The brachial or

TABLE 35–12 ✤ Normal Heart Rates for Children of Different Ages

Age	Heart Rate Range (beats/min)	Average Heart Rate (beats/min)
Newborns	100–170	120
Infants to 2 years	80–130	110
2–6 years	70–120	100
6–10 years	70–110	90
10–16 years	60–100	85

radial pulse rate should be the same as the auscultated apical heart rate. Table 35–12 gives normal heart rates in children of different ages.

GROWTH AND DEVELOPMENT

The child's heart rate varies with age, decreasing as the child grows older. The heart rate also increases in response to exercise, excitement, anxiety, and fever. Such stresses increase the child's metabolic rate, creating a simultaneous need for more oxygen. Children respond to the need for more oxygen by increasing their heart rate, a response called sinus tachycardia. They cannot increase their cardiac stroke volume to deliver more oxygen to the tissues as adults do.

Listen carefully to the heart rate rhythm. Children often have a normal cycle of irregular rhythm associated with respiration called sinus arrhythmia. With *sinus arrhythmia* the child's heart rate is faster on inspiration and slower on expiration. When any rhythm irregularity is detected, ask the child to take a breath and hold it while you listen to the heart rate. The rhythm should become regular during inspiration and expiration. Other rhythm irregularities are abnormal.

Differentiation of Heart Sounds

Heart sounds are due to the closure of the valves and vibration or turbulence of blood produced by that valve closure. Two primary sounds, S_1 and S_2, are heard when the chest is auscultated.

S_1, the first heart sound, is produced by closure of the tricuspid and mitral valves when the ventricular contraction begins. The two valves close almost simultaneously, so only one sound is normally heard.

S_2, the second heart sound, is produced by the closure of the aortic and pulmonic valves. Once blood has reached the pulmonic and aortic arteries, the valves close to prevent leakage back into the ventricles during diastole. The timing

● FIGURE 35–27

Sound travels in the direction of blood flow. Rather than listen for heart sounds over each heart valve, auscultate heart sounds at specific areas on the chest wall away from the valve itself. These areas are named for the valve producing the sound. Aortic: Second right intercostal space near the sternum. Pulmonic: Second left intercostal space near the sternum. Tricuspid: Fifth right or left intercostal space near the sternum. Mitral (apical): In infants—third or fourth intercostal space, just left of the left midclavicular line. In children—fifth intercostal space at the left midclavicular line.

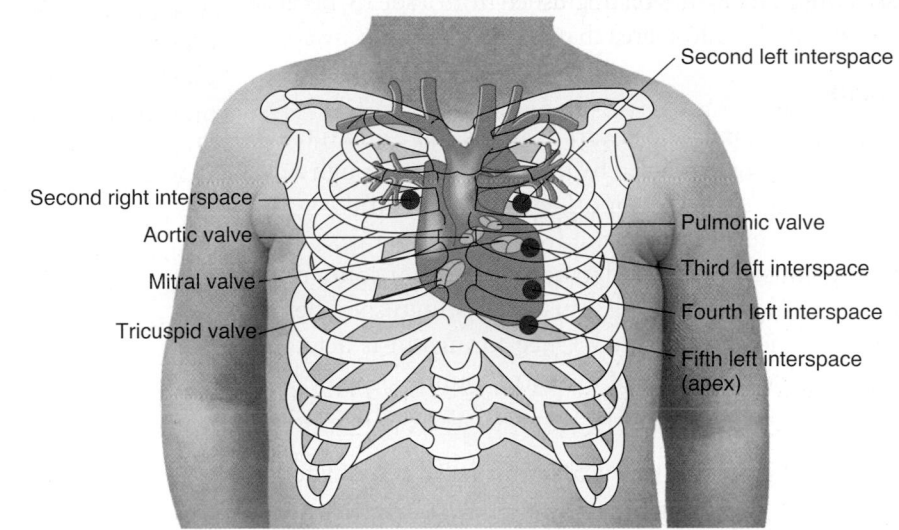

of the valve closure varies with respirations. Sometimes S_2 is heard as a single sound and at other times as a split sound, that is, two sounds heard a fraction of a second apart.

Sound is easily transmitted in liquid, and it travels best in the direction of blood flow. Auscultate heart sounds at specific areas on the chest wall in the direction of blood flow, just beyond the valve (Figure 35–27 ●). The sounds produced by the heart valves or blood turbulence are heard throughout the chest in thin infants and children. Both S_1 and S_2 can be heard in all listening areas.

Auscultate heart sounds for quality (distinct versus muffled) and intensity (loud versus weak). First, distinguish between S_1 and S_2 in each listening area. Heart sounds are usually distinct and crisp in children because of their thin chest wall. Muffling or indistinct sounds may indicate a heart defect or congestive heart failure. Document the area where heart sounds are heard the best. Table 35–13 and Figure 35–27 review the location where each sound is normally best heard for assessment of quality and intensity. If the child has a potential murmur, auscultate the heart in the sitting, reclining, and standing positions to see if differences are noted by position change.

NURSING PRACTICE

Palpate the carotid pulse when auscultating the heart to distinguish between the two heart sounds. The heart sound heard simultaneously with the pulsation is S_1.

Splitting of the Heart Sounds

After distinguishing the first and second heart sounds, try to detect physiologic splitting. A split S_2 is more apparent dur-

ing inspiration when the child takes a deep breath. More blood returns to the right ventricle, causing the pulmonic valve to close a fraction of a second later than the aortic valve. To detect physiologic splitting, auscultate over the pulmonic area while the child breathes normally and then while the child takes a deep breath. Splitting is normally more easily detected after a deep breath. The splitting returns to a single sound with regular breathing. If splitting does not vary with respiration, it is called fixed splitting. This is an abnormal finding associated with an atrial septal defect.

Third Heart Sound

A third heart sound, S_3, is occasionally heard in children as a normal finding. S_3 is caused when blood rushes through the

TABLE 35–13 ❖ Identification of the Listening Sites for Auscultation of the Quality and Intensity of Heart Sounds

Heart Sound	Locations Best Heard	Where Heard Softly
S_1	Apex of the heart Tricuspid area Mitral area	Base of the heart Aortic area Pulmonic area
S_2	Base of the heart Aortic area Pulmonic area	Apex of the heart Tricuspid area Mitral area
Physiologic splitting	Pulmonic area	
S_3	Mitral area	

mitral valve and splashes into the left ventricle. It is heard in diastole, just after S_2. It is distinguished from a split S_2 because it is louder in the mitral area than in the pulmonic area.

Murmurs

Occasionally abnormal heart sounds are auscultated. These sounds are produced by blood passing through a defective valve, great vessel, or other heart structure.

To hear murmurs in children takes practice. Often, murmurs must be very loud to be detected. For softer murmurs, normal heart sounds must be distinguished before an extra sound is recognized. Once a murmur is detected, define the characteristics of the extra sound.

Murmurs are classified by the following characteristics:

- *Intensity.* How loud is it? Can a thrill also be palpated?
- *Location.* Where is the murmur the loudest? Identify the listening area and precise topographic landmarks. Is the child sitting or lying down?
- *Radiation.* Is the sound transmitted over a larger area of the chest, to the axilla, or to the back?
- *Timing.* Is the murmur heard best after S_1 or S_2? Is it heard during the entire phase between S_1 and S_2?
- *Quality.* Describe what the murmur sounds like—for example, machinelike, musical, or blowing.

NURSING PRACTICE

Following are guidelines for grading the intensity of a murmur:

Intensity	Description
Grade I	Barely heard in a quiet room
Grade II	Quiet, but clearly heard
Grade III	Moderately loud, no thrill palpated
Grade IV	Loud, a thrill is usually palpated
Grade V	Very loud, a thrill is easily palpated
Grade VI	Heard without the stethoscope in direct contact with the chest wall

Auscultate for a venous hum over the supraclavicular fossa above the middle of the clavicle or over the upper anterior chest with the bell of the stethoscope. A venous hum is heard as a continuous low-pitched hum throughout the cardiac cycle. It may be loudest during diastole or when the child stands, and it does not change with respirations. It may be quieted by having the child turn the neck. A venous hum may be associated with anemia, but it has no pathologic significance.

COMPLETING THE HEART EXAMINATION

A complete assessment of cardiac function also includes measuring the blood pressure, palpating the pulses, and evaluating signs from other systems.

Blood Pressure

Assessment of blood pressure is important to detect conditions of hypertension or hypovolemic shock. The child should be seated and quiet for 3 to 5 minutes before the blood pressure is taken. See Skill 9–10 **SKILLS** for the technique for obtaining the blood pressure in children in the Clinical Skills Manual, as well as the CD-ROM accompanying this text.

Compare the systolic and diastolic readings with the standard blood pressure values by age, sex, and height in Table 35–14a & b. Use the child's height percentile for age and sex from the standard growth curves. A blood pressure value at the 50th percentile for the child's age, sex, and height percentile is considered the midpoint of the normal range. A reading above the 95th percentile indicates hypertension.

NURSING PRACTICE

In any child in which there is a concern about a heart condition, obtain a blood pressure reading in both an arm and a leg and compare the readings. The blood pressure in the leg should be the same or up to 10 mm Hg higher than the arm reading. If the reading in the leg is lower than the arm, coarctation of the aorta may be present.

Palpation of the Pulses

Palpate the characteristics of the pulses in the extremities to assess the circulation. The technique and sites for palpating the pulse are the same as those used for adults. Evaluate the pulsation for rate, regularity of rhythm, and strength in each extremity and compare your findings bilaterally. The femoral and brachial pulses are the most important pulses to evaluate.

Palpate the femoral arteries and compare their strength with the strength of the brachial pulse. The femoral pulsations are usually stronger than or as strong as the brachial pulsations. A weaker femoral pulse is associated with coarctation of the aorta.

GROWTH AND DEVELOPMENT

Infants have a low systolic blood pressure, and detecting the distal pulses is often difficult. Use the brachial artery in the arms and the popliteal or femoral artery in the legs to evaluate the pulses. The radial and distal tibial pulses are normally palpated easily in older children.

Other Signs

To assess the heart and tissue perfusion, consider other signs, including skin color, capillary refill, and respiratory distress. The mucous membranes are usually pink. Cyanosis is most commonly associated with a congenital heart defect in children. Capillary refill is normally less than 2 seconds, indicating good circulation and perfusion of the tissues. Signs of

TABLE 35–14(a) �֍ Systolic and Diastolic Blood Pressure Values for Children of Different Ages by Sex and Selected Height Percentiles

Blood Pressure Levels for Girls by Age and Height Percentile

Age (Year)	BP Percentile ↓	Systolic BP (mm Hg) ← Percentile of Height →							Diastolic BP (mm Hg) ← Percentile of Height →						
		5th	10th	25th	50th	75th	90th	95th	5th	10th	25th	50th	75th	90th	95th
1	50th	83	84	85	86	88	89	90	38	39	39	40	41	41	42
	90th	97	97	98	100	101	102	103	52	53	53	54	55	55	56
	95th	100	101	102	104	105	106	107	56	57	57	58	59	59	60
	99th	108	108	109	111	112	113	114	64	64	65	65	66	67	67
2	50th	85	85	87	88	89	91	91	43	44	44	45	46	46	47
	90th	98	99	100	101	103	104	105	57	58	58	59	60	61	61
	95th	102	103	104	105	107	108	109	61	62	62	63	64	65	65
	99th	109	110	111	112	114	115	117	69	69	70	70	71	72	72
3	50th	86	87	88	89	91	92	93	47	48	48	49	50	50	51
	90th	100	100	102	103	104	106	106	61	62	62	63	64	64	65
	95th	104	104	105	107	108	109	110	65	66	66	67	68	68	69
	99th	111	111	113	114	115	116	117	73	73	74	74	75	76	76
4	50th	88	88	90	91	92	94	94	50	50	51	52	52	53	54
	90th	101	102	103	104	106	107	108	64	64	65	66	67	67	68
	95th	105	106	107	108	110	111	112	68	68	69	70	71	71	72
	99th	112	113	114	115	117	118	119	76	76	76	77	78	79	79
5	50th	89	90	91	93	94	95	96	52	53	53	54	55	55	56
	90th	103	103	105	106	107	109	109	66	67	67	68	69	69	70
	95th	107	107	108	110	111	112	113	70	71	71	72	73	73	74
	99th	114	114	116	117	118	120	120	78	78	79	79	80	81	81
6	50th	91	92	93	94	96	97	98	54	54	55	56	56	57	58
	90th	104	105	106	108	109	110	111	68	68	69	70	70	71	72
	95th	108	109	110	111	113	114	115	72	72	73	74	74	75	76
	99th	115	116	117	119	120	121	122	80	80	80	81	82	83	83
7	50th	93	93	95	96	97	99	99	55	56	56	57	58	58	59
	90th	106	107	108	109	111	112	113	69	70	70	71	72	72	73
	95th	110	111	112	113	115	116	116	73	74	74	75	76	76	77
	99th	117	118	119	120	122	123	124	81	81	82	82	83	84	84
8	50th	95	95	96	98	99	100	101	57	57	57	58	59	60	60
	90th	108	109	110	111	113	114	114	71	71	71	72	73	74	74
	95th	112	112	114	115	116	118	118	75	75	75	76	77	78	78
	99th	119	120	121	122	123	125	125	82	82	83	83	84	85	86
9	50th	96	97	98	100	101	102	103	58	58	58	59	60	61	61
	90th	110	110	112	113	114	116	116	72	72	72	73	74	75	75
	95th	114	114	115	117	118	119	120	76	76	76	77	78	79	79
	99th	121	121	123	124	125	127	127	83	83	84	84	85	86	87
10	50th	98	99	100	102	103	104	105	59	59	59	60	61	62	62
	90th	112	112	114	115	116	118	118	73	73	73	74	75	76	76
	95th	116	116	117	119	120	121	122	77	77	77	78	79	80	80
	99th	123	123	125	126	127	129	129	84	84	85	86	86	87	88
11	50th	100	101	102	103	105	106	107	60	60	60	61	62	63	63
	90th	114	114	116	117	118	119	120	74	74	74	75	76	77	77
	95th	118	118	119	121	122	123	124	78	78	78	79	80	81	81
	99th	125	125	126	128	129	130	131	85	85	86	87	87	88	89
12	50th	102	103	104	105	107	108	109	61	61	61	62	63	64	64
	90th	116	116	117	119	120	121	122	75	75	75	76	77	78	78
	95th	119	120	121	123	124	125	126	79	79	79	80	81	82	82
	99th	127	127	128	130	131	132	133	86	86	87	88	88	89	90

(continued)

TABLE 35–14(a) ✥ Systolic and Diastolic Blood Pressure Values for Children of Different Ages by Sex and Selected Height Percentiles—continued

Blood Pressure Levels for Girls by Age and Height Percentile

Age (Year)	BP Percentile ↓	Systolic BP (mm Hg) ← Percentile of Height →							Diastolic BP (mm Hg) ← Percentile of Height →						
		5th	10th	25th	50th	75th	90th	95th	5th	10th	25th	50th	75th	90th	95th
13	50th	104	105	106	107	109	110	110	62	62	62	63	64	65	65
	90th	117	118	119	121	122	123	124	76	76	76	77	78	79	79
	95th	121	122	123	124	126	127	128	80	80	80	81	82	83	83
	99th	128	129	130	132	133	134	135	87	87	88	89	89	90	91
14	50th	106	106	107	109	110	111	112	63	63	63	64	65	66	66
	90th	119	120	121	122	124	125	125	77	77	77	78	79	80	80
	95th	123	123	125	126	127	129	129	81	81	81	82	83	84	84
	99th	130	131	132	133	135	136	136	88	88	89	90	90	91	92
15	50th	107	108	109	110	111	113	113	64	64	64	65	66	67	67
	90th	120	121	122	123	125	126	127	78	78	78	79	80	81	81
	95th	124	125	126	127	129	130	131	82	82	82	83	84	85	85
	99th	131	132	133	134	136	137	138	89	89	90	91	91	92	93
16	50th	108	108	110	111	112	114	114	64	64	65	66	66	67	68
	90th	121	122	123	124	126	127	128	78	78	79	80	81	81	82
	95th	125	126	127	128	130	131	132	82	82	83	84	85	85	86
	99th	132	133	134	135	137	138	139	90	90	90	91	92	93	93
17	50th	108	109	110	111	113	114	115	64	65	65	66	67	67	68
	90th	122	122	123	125	126	127	128	78	79	79	80	81	81	82
	95th	125	126	127	129	130	131	132	82	83	83	84	85	85	86
	99th	133	133	134	136	137	138	139	90	90	91	91	92	93	93

BP, blood pressure

*The 90th percentile is 1.28 SD, 95th percentile is 1.645 SD, and the 99th percentile is 2.326 SD over the mean.

National Heart, Lung, and Blood Institute. (2004). Blood pressure tables for children and adolescents from the fourth report on the diagnosis, evaluation, and treatment of high blood pressure in children and adolescents.

Retrieved June 11, 2004, from http://www.nhlbi.nih.gov/guidelines/hypertension/child_tble.htm

respiratory distress, such as tachypnea, flaring, and retractions, may be associated with the child's attempts to compensate for hypoxemia caused by a congenital heart defect.

ASSESSING THE ABDOMEN FOR SHAPE, BOWEL SOUNDS, AND UNDERLYING ORGANS

TOPOGRAPHIC LANDMARKS OF THE ABDOMEN

The location of underlying organs and structures of the abdomen must be considered when the abdomen is examined. The abdomen is commonly divided by imaginary lines into quadrants for the purpose of identifying underlying structures (Figure 35–28 ⬤ on page 1003).

INSPECTION OF THE ABDOMEN

Begin the examination of the abdomen by inspecting the shape and contour, condition of the umbilicus and rectus muscle, and abdominal movement. Inspect the child's abdomen from the front and side with good lighting. Perform

---

THINKING CRITICALLY

ASSESSING A CHILD WITH BRONCHIOLITIS

Latoya, 6 months old, is brought by her mother and father to the emergency room. She is an emergency admission from the local pediatrician's office with a diagnosis of bronchiolitis. As Latoya's nurse, you are responsible for assessing her condition after she arrives on the pediatric nursing unit.

What historical information do you collect, and what approach do you take to examine Latoya? What procedures are used to perform a physical examination on a 6-month-old? Identify all the components of the physical assessment used to detect signs of respiratory difficulty and inadequate tissue perfusion. How do you organize your findings to make sense of them to plan nursing care?

---

inspection and auscultation before palpation and percussion because touching the abdomen may change the characteristics of bowel sounds.

TABLE 35–14(b) ✤ Systolic and Diastolic Blood Pressure Values for Children of Different Ages by Sex and Selected Height Percentiles

Blood Pressure Levels for Boys by Age and Height Percentile

Age (Year)	BP Percentile ↓	Systolic BP (mm Hg) ← Percentile of Height →							Diastolic BP (mm Hg) ← Percentile of Height →						
		5th	10th	25th	50th	75th	90th	95th	5th	10th	25th	50th	75th	90th	95th
1	50th	80	81	83	85	87	88	89	34	35	36	37	38	39	39
	90th	94	95	97	99	100	102	103	49	50	51	52	53	53	54
	95th	98	99	101	103	104	106	106	54	54	55	56	57	58	58
	99th	105	106	108	110	112	113	114	61	62	63	64	65	66	66
2	50th	84	85	87	88	90	92	92	39	40	41	42	43	44	44
	90th	97	99	100	102	104	105	106	54	55	56	57	58	58	59
	95th	101	102	104	106	108	109	110	59	59	60	61	62	63	63
	99th	109	110	111	113	115	117	117	66	67	68	69	70	71	71
3	50th	86	87	89	91	93	94	95	44	44	45	46	47	48	48
	90th	100	101	103	105	107	108	109	59	59	60	61	62	63	63
	95th	104	105	107	109	110	112	113	63	63	64	65	66	67	67
	99th	111	112	114	116	118	119	120	71	71	72	73	74	75	75
4	50th	88	89	91	93	95	96	97	47	48	49	50	51	51	52
	90th	102	103	105	107	109	110	111	62	63	64	65	66	66	67
	95th	106	107	109	111	112	114	115	66	67	68	69	70	71	71
	99th	113	114	116	118	120	121	122	74	75	76	77	78	78	79
5	50th	90	91	93	95	96	98	98	50	51	52	53	54	55	55
	90th	104	105	106	108	110	111	112	65	66	67	68	69	69	70
	95th	108	109	110	112	114	115	116	69	70	71	72	73	74	74
	99th	115	116	118	120	121	123	123	77	78	79	80	81	81	82
6	50th	91	92	94	96	98	99	100	53	53	54	55	56	57	57
	90th	105	106	108	110	111	113	113	68	68	69	70	71	72	72
	95th	109	110	112	114	115	117	117	72	72	73	74	75	76	76
	99th	116	117	119	121	123	124	125	80	80	81	82	83	84	84
7	50th	92	94	95	97	99	100	101	55	55	56	57	58	59	59
	90th	106	107	109	111	113	114	115	70	70	71	72	73	74	74
	95th	110	111	113	115	117	118	119	74	74	75	76	77	78	78
	99th	117	118	120	122	124	125	126	82	82	83	84	85	86	86
8	50th	94	95	97	99	100	102	102	56	57	58	59	60	60	61
	90th	107	109	110	112	114	115	116	71	72	72	73	74	75	76
	95th	111	112	114	116	118	119	120	75	76	77	78	79	79	80
	99th	119	120	122	123	125	127	127	83	84	85	86	87	87	88
9	50th	95	96	98	100	102	103	104	57	58	59	60	61	61	62
	90th	109	110	112	114	115	117	118	72	73	74	75	76	76	77
	95th	113	114	116	118	119	121	121	76	77	78	79	80	81	81
	99th	120	121	123	125	127	128	129	84	85	86	87	88	88	89
10	50th	97	98	100	102	103	105	106	58	59	60	61	61	62	63
	90th	111	112	114	115	117	119	119	73	73	74	75	76	77	78
	95th	115	116	117	119	121	122	123	77	78	79	80	81	81	82
	99th	122	123	125	127	128	130	130	85	86	86	88	88	89	90
11	50th	99	100	102	104	105	107	107	59	59	60	61	62	63	63
	90th	113	114	115	117	119	120	121	74	74	75	76	77	78	78
	95th	117	118	119	121	123	124	125	78	78	79	80	81	82	82
	99th	124	125	127	129	130	132	132	86	86	87	88	89	90	90
12	50th	101	102	104	106	108	109	110	59	60	61	62	63	63	64
	90th	115	116	118	120	121	123	123	74	75	75	76	77	78	79
	95th	119	120	122	123	125	127	127	78	79	80	81	82	82	83
	99th	126	127	129	131	133	134	135	86	87	88	89	90	90	91

(continued)

TABLE 35–14(b) ✤ Systolic and Diastolic Blood Pressure Values for Children of Different Ages by Sex and Selected Height Percentiles—continued

Blood Pressure Levels for Girls by Age and Height Percentile

Age (Year)	BP Percentile ↓	Systolic BP (mm Hg) ← Percentile of Height →							Diastolic BP (mm Hg) ← Percentile of Height →						
		5th	10th	25th	50th	75th	90th	95th	5th	10th	25th	50th	75th	90th	95th
13	50th	104	105	106	108	110	111	112	60	60	61	62	63	64	64
	90th	117	118	120	122	124	125	126	75	75	76	77	78	79	79
	95th	121	122	124	126	128	129	130	79	79	80	81	82	83	83
	99th	128	130	131	133	135	136	137	87	87	88	89	90	91	91
14	50th	106	107	109	111	113	114	115	60	61	62	63	64	65	65
	90th	120	121	123	125	126	128	128	75	76	77	78	79	79	80
	95th	124	125	127	128	130	132	132	80	80	81	82	83	84	84
	99th	131	132	134	136	138	139	140	87	88	89	90	91	92	92
15	50th	109	110	112	113	115	117	117	61	62	63	64	65	66	66
	90th	122	124	125	127	129	130	131	76	77	78	79	80	80	81
	95th	126	127	129	131	133	134	135	81	81	82	83	84	85	85
	99th	134	135	136	138	140	142	142	88	89	90	91	92	93	93
16	50th	111	112	114	116	118	119	120	63	63	64	65	66	67	67
	90th	125	126	128	130	131	133	134	78	78	79	80	81	82	82
	95th	129	130	132	134	135	137	137	82	83	83	84	85	86	87
	99th	136	137	139	141	143	144	145	90	90	91	92	93	94	94
17	50th	114	115	116	118	120	121	122	65	66	66	67	68	69	70
	90th	127	128	130	132	134	135	136	80	80	81	82	83	84	84
	95th	131	132	134	136	138	139	140	84	85	86	87	87	88	89
	99th	139	140	141	143	145	146	147	92	93	93	94	95	96	97

BP, blood pressure

*The 90th percentile is 1.28 SD, 95th percentile is 1.645 SD, and the 99th percentile is 2.326 SD over the mean.

National Heart, Lung, and Blood Institute. (2004). Blood pressure tables for children and adolescents from the fourth report on the diagnosis, evaluation, and treatment of high blood pressure in children and adolescents.

Retrieved June 11, 2004, from http://www.nhlbi.nih.gov/guidelines/hypertension/child_tble.htm

Shape

Inspect the shape of the abdomen to identify an abnormal contour. The child's abdomen is normally symmetric and rounded or flat when the child is supine. A scaphoid or sunken abdomen is abnormal and may indicate dehydration.

Umbilicus

Observe the newborn's umbilical stump for color, bleeding, odor, and drainage. See Chapter 27 for more information. ∞ After the stump falls off, inspect the umbilicus for continued drainage which may indicate an infection or a granuloma.

Inspect the umbilicus in older infants and toddlers. Children in these age groups often have an umbilical hernia, a protrusion of abdominal contents through an open umbilical muscle ring.

Rectus Muscle

Inspect the abdominal wall for any depression or bulging at midline above or below the umbilicus, indicating sepa-
ration of the rectus abdominis muscles. The depression may be up to 5 cm (2 in.) wide. Measure the width of the separation to monitor change over time. As abdominal muscle strength develops, the separation usually becomes less prominent. However, the splitting may persist if congenital muscle weakness is present.

Abdominal Movement

Infants and children up to 6 years of age breathe with the diaphragm. The abdomen rises with inspiration and falls with expiration, simultaneously with the chest rise and fall. When the abdomen does not rise as expected, peritonitis may be present.

Other abdominal movements such as peristaltic waves are abnormal. Peristaltic waves are visible rhythmic contractions of the intestinal wall smooth muscle, which move food through the digestive tract. Their presence generally indicates an intestinal obstruction, such as pyloric stenosis.

● FIGURE 35–28

Topographic landmarks of the abdomen. The abdomen is commonly divided by imaginary lines into quadrants for the purpose of identifying underlying structures.

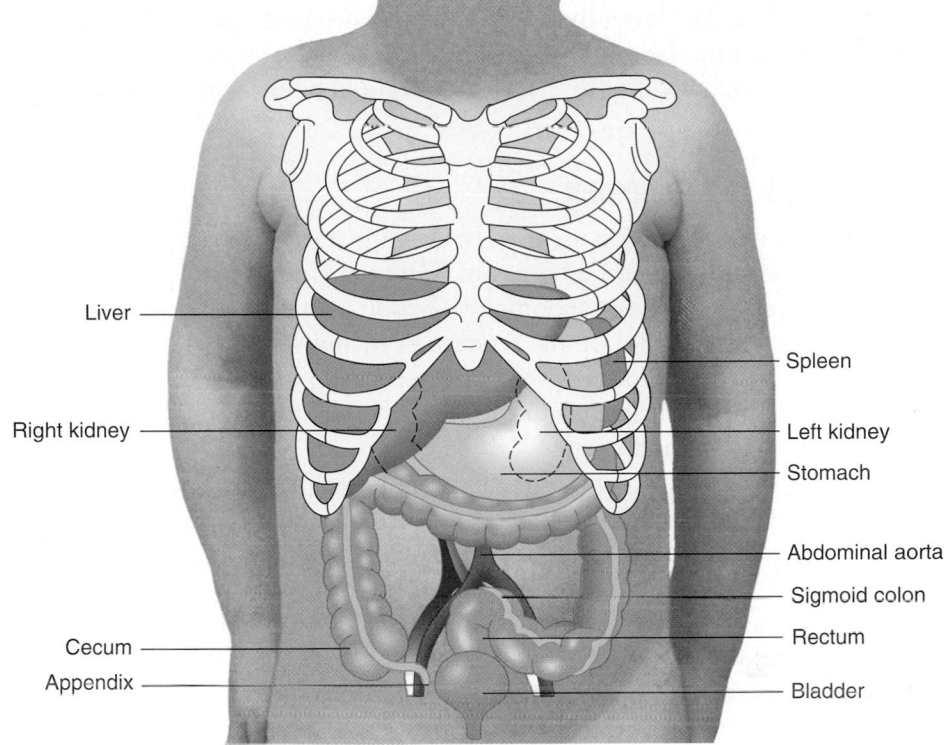

AUSCULTATION OF THE ABDOMEN

To evaluate bowel sounds, auscultate the abdomen with the diaphragm of the stethoscope. Bowel sounds normally occur every 10 to 30 seconds. They have a high-pitched, tinkling, metallic quality. Loud gurgling (borborygmi) is heard when the child is hungry. Listen in each quadrant long enough to hear at least one bowel sound. Before determining that bowel sounds are absent, auscultate at least 5 minutes in each quadrant. Absence of bowel sounds may indicate peritonitis or a paralytic ileus. Hyperactive bowel sounds may indicate gastroenteritis or a bowel obstruction.

Next auscultate over the abdominal aorta and the renal arteries for a vascular hum or murmur. No murmur should be heard. A murmur may indicate a narrowed or defective artery.

PERCUSSION OF THE ABDOMEN

Use indirect percussion to evaluate borders and sizes of abdominal organs and masses. Percussion is performed with the child supine. Choose a sequence to systematically percuss the entire abdomen (Figure 35–29 ●).

Different tones are expected when the abdomen is percussed, depending on the underlying structures. Dullness is found over the liver, spleen, and full bladder. Tympany is found over the stomach or the intestines when an obstruction is present. Tympany may be found over areas beyond

the stomach in infants because of air swallowing. A resonant tone may be heard over other areas.

Organ size can be identified by listening for a percussion tone change at the border of an organ. For example, when the examiner percusses down the chest, the upper

● FIGURE 35–29

Sequence for indirect percussion of the abdomen.

edge of the liver is usually detected by a tone change from resonant to dull near the fifth intercostal space at the right midclavicular line. The lower liver edge is usually detected 2 to 3 cm (about 1 in.) below the right costal margin in infants and toddlers, but closer to the costal margin in older children.

PALPATION OF THE ABDOMEN

Both light and deep palpation are used to examine the abdomen's organs and to detect any masses. Light palpation evaluates the tenseness of the abdomen (how soft or hard it is), the liver, the presence of any tenderness or masses, and any defects in the abdominal wall. Deep palpation detects masses, defines their shape and consistency, and identifies tenderness in the abdomen.

To make the most accurate interpretation, perform the abdominal examination when the child is calm and cooperative. Organs and other masses are more easily palpated when the abdominal wall is relaxed. Infants and toddlers often feel more secure lying supine across both the parent's and the examiner's laps. A bottle, pacifier, or toy may distract the child and improve cooperation for the examination.

To begin palpation, position the child supine with knees flexed. Stand beside the child and place warmed fingertips across the child's abdomen. Palpate with the edge of your fingers, not just your fingerpads, and palpate in a sequence to examine the entire abdomen. Watch the child's face during palpation for a grimace or constriction of the pupils, which indicates pain.

NURSING PRACTICE

Use suggestive words to help the child relax so you can palpate the abdomen. "How soft will your tummy get when my hand feels it? Does it get softer than this? Yes. See, it softens as you breathe out. Will it also be softer here?" In this way, the child learns to relax the abdomen and is challenged to do it better.

When children are ticklish, some special approaches are needed to gain their cooperation. Use a firm touch and do not pretend to tickle the child at any point in the examination. Alternatively, put the child's hand on the abdomen and place your hand over the child's. Let your fingertips slide over to touch the abdomen. The child has a sense of being in control, and you may be able to palpate directly.

Older children often need distraction, especially when there is a question of abdominal tenderness and guarding or when the child is ticklish. Have the child perform a task that requires some concentration, such as pressing the hands together or pulling locked hands apart.

Light Palpation

For light palpation, use a superficial, gentle touch that slightly depresses the abdomen. Usually the abdomen feels soft and no tenderness is detected. Palpate any bulging along the abdominal wall, especially along the rectus muscle and umbilical ring, which could indicate a hernia. Measure the diameter of the muscle ring, rather than the protrusion, to monitor change over time. The muscle ring normally becomes smaller and closes by 4 years of age. An umbilical hernia that persists beyond this age may need surgical repair.

Liver. Locate and lightly palpate the lower liver edge. Place the fingers in the right midclavicular line at the level of the umbilicus and gently move them toward the costal margin during expiration. As the liver edge descends with inspiration, a flat, narrow ridge is usually felt. Measure the distance of the liver edge from the right costal margin at the right midclavicular line. The liver edge is normally palpated 2 to 3 cm (1 in.) below the right costal margin in infants and toddlers. It may not be palpable in older children. The liver is enlarged when the edge is more than 3 cm (1 in.) below the right costal margin. An enlarged liver may be associated with congestive heart failure or hepatic disease.

Deep Palpation

To perform deep palpation, press the fingers of one hand (for small children) or two hands (for older children) more deeply into the abdomen. Because the abdominal muscles are most relaxed when the child takes a deep breath, ask the child to take regular deep breaths when palpating each area of the abdomen.

Spleen. Palpate for the spleen at the left costal margin in the midclavicular line. The spleen tip may be felt when the child takes a deep breath. The spleen is enlarged when it can be easily palpated below the left costal margin.

Kidneys. Palpate for the kidneys deep in the abdomen along each side of the spinal column. The kidneys are difficult to palpate in all children, except newborns, because of the deep layer of abdominal muscles and intestines. If a kidney is actually palpated, an abnormal mass may be present.

NURSING PRACTICE

If an enlarged kidney or mass is detected, do not continue to palpate the kidney. Pressure on the mass may release cancerous cells.

Other Masses. Occasionally other masses, both normal and abnormal, can be palpated in the abdomen. A tubular mass commonly palpated in the lower left or right quadrant is often an intestine filled with feces. A distended bladder is often palpated as a firm, central, dome-shaped mass above the symphysis pubis in young children. Any fixed mass that moves laterally, pulsates, or is located along the vertebral column may be a neoplasm.

ASSESSMENT OF THE INGUINAL AREA

The inguinal area is inspected and palpated during the abdominal examination to detect enlarged lymph nodes or masses. The femoral pulse, a part of the heart examination, may be assessed simultaneously with the abdominal examination.

Inspection

Inspect the inguinal area for any change in contour, comparing sides. A small bulging noted over the femoral canal in girls may be associated with a femoral hernia. A bulging in the inguinal area in boys may be associated with an inguinal hernia.

Palpation

Palpate the inguinal area for lymph nodes and other masses. Small lymph nodes, less than 1 cm (1/2 in.) in diameter, are often present in the inguinal area because of minor injuries on the legs. Any tenderness, heat, or inflammation in these palpated lymph nodes could be associated with a local infection.

ASSESSING THE GENITAL AND PERINEAL AREAS FOR EXTERNAL STRUCTURAL ABNORMALITIES

What can a vaginal discharge indicate in a preadolescent girl? Is swelling in a newborn's scrotum normal? Where is the proper location of the urethral meatus on the penis?

PREPARATION OF CHILDREN FOR THE EXAMINATION

Examination of the genitalia and perineal area can cause stress in children because they sense their privacy has been invaded. To make young children feel more secure, position them on the parent's lap with their legs spread apart. Children can also be positioned on the examining table with their knees flexed and the legs spread apart like a frog.

In younger children the genital and perineal examination is performed immediately after assessment of the abdomen. The genitals and perineum may be examined last in older children and adolescents. Equipment needed for this examination includes gloves, lubricant, and a penlight.

✿ GROWTH AND DEVELOPMENT

Preschool-age children are often taught that strangers are not permitted to touch their "private parts." When a child this age actively resists examination of the genital area, ask the parent to tell the child you have permission to look at and touch these parts of the body. Some children develop modesty during the preschool period. Briefly explain what you need to examine and why. Then calmly and efficiently examine the child.

INSPECTION OF THE FEMALE GENITALIA

Inspect the external genitalia of girls for color, size, and symmetry of the mons pubis, labia, urethra, and vaginal opening (Figure 35–30 ◉). At that time, determine the stage of pubertal maturation. Simultaneously look for any abnormal findings such as swelling, inflammation, masses, lacerations, or discharge.

Mons Pubis

Inspect the mons pubis for pubic hair and its characteristics. See page 1008 for guidelines to assess the stage of pubic hair development.

Labia

The labia minora are usually thin and pale in preadolescent girls but become dark pink and moist after puberty. In young infants the labia minora may be fused and cover the structures in the vestibule. These adhesions may need to be separated. See Chapter 27 ∞ for more information.

Hymen

Use the thumb and forefinger of one gloved hand to separate the labia minora for viewing structures in the vestibule. The hymen is just inside the vaginal opening. In preadolescents it is usually a thin membrane with a crescent-shaped opening. The vaginal opening is usually about 1 cm (1/2 in.) in adolescents when the hymen is intact. Sexually active adolescents may have a vaginal opening with irregular edges.

◉ **FIGURE 35–30**

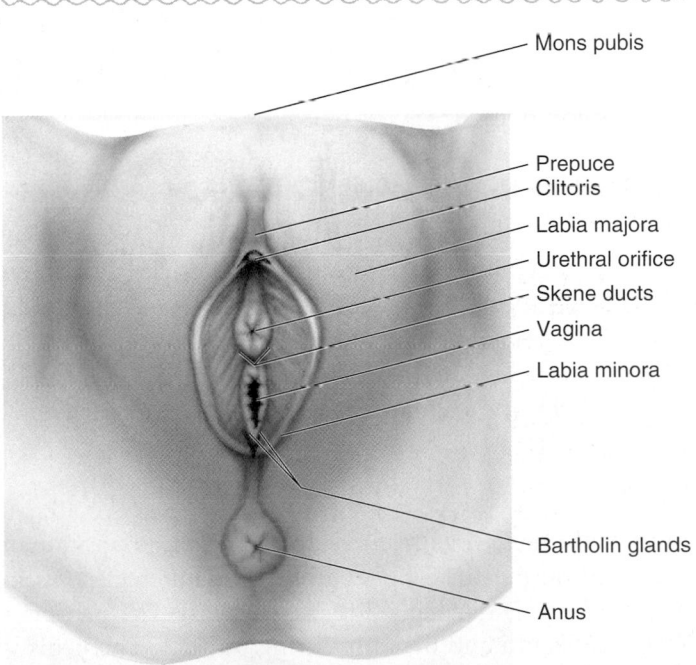

Mons pubis

Prepuce
Clitoris
Labia majora
Urethral orifice
Skene ducts
Vagina
Labia minora

Bartholin glands

Anus

Anatomic structures of the female genital and perineal area.

Urethral and Vaginal Openings

Inspect the vestibule for lesions. No lesions or signs of inflammation are expected around the urethral or vaginal opening. Redness and excoriation are often associated with an irritant such as bubble bath.

Vaginal Discharge

Preadolescent girls do not normally have a vaginal discharge. Adolescents often have a clear discharge without a foul odor. Menses generally begin approximately 2 years after breast bud development. A foul-smelling discharge in preschool-age children may be associated with a foreign body. Various organisms may cause a vaginal infection in older children.

NURSING PRACTICE

Signs of sexual abuse in young children include bruising or swelling of the vulva, foul-smelling vaginal discharge, enlarged opening of the vagina, and rash or sores in the perineal area.

An internal vaginal examination is indicated when abnormal findings such as a vaginal discharge or trauma to the external structures is noted. Only an experienced examiner should perform the vaginal examination of the child.

PALPATION OF THE FEMALE GENITALIA

Palpate the vaginal opening with a finger of your free, gloved hand. The Bartholin and Skene glands are not usually palpable. Palpation of these glands in preadolescent children indicates enlargement because of an infection such as gonorrhea.

INSPECTION OF THE MALE GENITALIA

Inspect the male genitalia for the structural and pubertal development of the penis, scrotum, and testicles. Place boys in tailor position, seated with their legs crossed in front of them. This position puts pressure on the abdominal wall to push the testicles into the scrotum. See page 1009 for guidelines to assess the staging of pubic hair and external genital development.

Penis

Inspect the penis for size, foreskin, hygiene, and position of the urethral meatus. The length of the nonerect penis in the newborn is normally 2 to 3 cm (1 in.). The penis enlarges in length and breadth during puberty. The penis is normally straight. A downward bowing of the penis may be caused by a chordee, a fibrous band of tissue associated with hypospadias.

GROWTH AND DEVELOPMENT

The foreskin is usually not completely separated from the glans at birth. Separation is normally completed by 3 to 6 years of age. A foreskin opening large enough for a good urinary stream is normal, even when the foreskin does not fully retract.

When the penis is circumcised, the glans penis is exposed. To inspect the glans penis of an uncircumcised boy, ask the child or parent to pull the foreskin back. Alternatively, the examiner may retract the foreskin. The foreskin of children over 6 years of age normally retracts past the corona easily. If the foreskin is tight and cannot be retracted, phimosis is present.

NURSING PRACTICE

When the boy's foreskin does not easily retract, do not forcefully pull it back. Force may result in torn tissues that heal with adhesions between the foreskin and the glans. Preputial adhesions are normal in infants and young boys, and usually resolve on their own.

The glans penis is normally clean and smooth without inflammation or ulceration. The urethral meatus is a slit-shaped opening near the tip of the glans. No discharge should be present. A round, pinpoint urethral meatus may indicate meatal stenosis. Location of the urethral meatus at another site on the penis is abnormal, indicating hypospadias or epispadias. Inspect the urinary stream. The stream is normally strong without dribbling. Erythema and edema of the glans (balanitis) may result from infection or trauma. In the uncircumcised penis, purulent discharge and an edematous foreskin may be seen.

Scrotum

Inspect the scrotum for size, symmetry, presence of the testicles, and any abnormalities. The scrotum is normally loose and pendulous with rugae, or wrinkles. The scrotum of infants often appears large in comparison to the penis. A small, undeveloped scrotum that has no rugae indicates that the testicles are undescended. Enlargement or swelling of the scrotum is abnormal. It may indicate an inguinal hernia, hydrocele, torsion of the spermatic cord, or testicular inflammation. A deep cleft in the scrotum may indicate ambiguous genitalia.

PALPATION OF THE MALE GENITALIA

Penis

Palpate the shaft of the penis for nodules and masses. None should be present.

Testicles

Palpate the scrotum for the presence of the testicles. Make sure your hands are warm to avoid stimulating the cremasteric reflex that causes the testicles to retract. Place your index finger and thumb over both inguinal canals on each side of the penis. This keeps the testicles from retracting into the abdomen (Figure 35–31 ●).

Gently palpate each testicle with only enough pressure to identify the shape and size. The testicles are normally smooth and equal in size. They are approximately 1 to 1.5 cm (1/2 in) in diameter until puberty, when they increase in size. A hard, enlarged, painless testicle may indicate a tumor.

If a testicle is not palpated in the scrotum, the examiner palpates the inguinal canal for a soft mass. When the testicle is found in the inguinal canal, try to move it to the scrotum to palpate the size and shape. The testicle is descendable when it can be moved into the scrotum. An undescended testicle is one that does not descend into the scrotum or cannot be palpated in the inguinal canal.

Spermatic Cord

Palpate the length of the spermatic cord between the thumb and forefinger from the testicle to the inguinal canal. It normally feels solid and smooth. No tenderness is expected.

Enlarged Scrotum

When bulging or swelling of the scrotum is present, palpate the scrotum to identify the characteristics of the mass. Try to determine whether the mass is unilateral or bilateral

● FIGURE 35–31

Palpating the scrotum for descended testicles and spermatic cords.

and attempt to reduce the mass by pushing it back through the external inguinal ring. A mass that decreases may indicate an inguinal hernia. A mass that does not decrease may indicate a hydrocele or an incarcerated hernia. To distinguish between a hydrocele and an incarcerated hernia, place a bright penlight under the scrotum and look for a red glow or transillumination through the scrotum. A hydrocele transilluminates; a hernia does not.

Inguinal Canal

Attempt to insert the little finger into the external inguinal canal to determine whether the external inguinal ring is dilated. The inguinal ring is normally too small for the finger to pass into the canal. If the finger passes into the inguinal canal, ask the child to cough. A sensation of abdominal contents coming down to touch the fingertip may indicate an inguinal hernia.

Cremasteric Reflex

Stroke the inner thigh of each leg to stimulate the cremasteric reflex. The testicle and scrotum normally rise on the stroked side. This response indicates intact function of the spinal cord at the T12, L1, and L2 levels.

INSPECTION OF THE ANUS AND RECTUM

Inspect the anus for sphincter control and any abnormal findings such as inflammation, fissures, or lesions. The external sphincter is usually closed. Inflammation and scratch marks around the anus may be associated with pinworms. A protrusion from the rectum may be associated with a rectal wall prolapse or a hemorrhoid.

PALPATION OF THE ANUS AND RECTUM

Lightly touching the anal opening should stimulate an anal contraction or "wink." Absence of a contraction may indicate the presence of a lower spinal cord lesion.

Patency of the Anus

Passage of meconium by newborns indicates a patent anus. When passage of meconium is delayed, a lubricated catheter can be inserted 1 cm (1/2 in.) into the anus. Resistance in passage of the catheter may indicate an obstruction.

Rectal Examination

A rectal examination is not routinely performed on children. It is indicated for symptoms of intra-abdominal, rectal, bowel, or stool abnormalities. Only an experienced examiner should perform a rectal examination.

ASSESSMENT OF PUBERTAL DEVELOPMENT AND SEXUAL MATURATION

The age of onset of secondary sexual characteristics can vary with race and ethnicity, environmental conditions, geographic location, and nutrition. For example, sexual maturity begins earlier in taller and heavier girls. Black girls have an earlier onset of breast and pubic hair development than whites (Herman-Giddens, Slora, Wasserman et al., 1997).

◉ FIGURE 35–32

Normal stages of breast development.

Used with permission from Van Wieringen et al. (1971). Growth diagrams 1965 Netherlands, Groningen: Wolters-Noordhof.

FEMALES

Inspect the child's breasts while the child is sitting. Breast development in girls usually precedes other pubertal changes. Figure 35–32 ◉ shows the Tanner stages of breast development. Breast budding, the first stage of pubertal development in girls, normally occurs between 9 and 14 years of age. The mean age for breast development in African-American girls is 8.87 years, and for Caucasian girls it is 9.96 years (Herman-Giddens et al., 1997). Breast development before 6 years of age in African Americans and 7 years of age in Caucasians is abnormal (Herman-Giddens et al., 1997; Kaplowitz, Oberfield, and the Drug and Therapeutics and Executive Committees of the Lawson Wilkins Pediatric Endocrine Society, 1999). A girl's breasts may develop at different rates and appear asymmetric.

The presence, amount, and distribution of pubic hair indicates the sexual maturation stage in the girl. Preadolescent girls have no pubic hair. Initial pubic hair is lightly pigmented, sparse, and straight. Pubic hair develops in consistent stages for all girls, but the timing of pubic hair stages is individually determined (Tanner, 1962). Figure 35–33 ◉ illustrates the normal stages of female pubic hair development. Breast development usually precedes pubic hair development. The presence of pubic hair before 8 years of age is unusual.

◉ FIGURE 35–33

The stages of female pubic hair development with sexual maturation. Soft downy hair along the labia majora is an indication that sexual maturation is beginning. Hair grows progressively coarse and curly as development proceeds.

Used with permission from Van Wieringen et al. (1971). Growth diagrams 1965 Netherlands, Groningen: Wolters-Noordhof.

● FIGURE 35–34

The stages of male pubic hair and external genital development with sexual maturation.

Used with permission from Van Wieringen et al. (1971). Growth diagrams 1965 Netherlands, Groningen: Wolters-Noordhof.

MALES

Initial signs of pubertal development in males are enlargement of the testicles and thinning of the scrotum. Straight, downy pubic hair first appears at the base of the penis 6 months later. The hair becomes darker, dense, and curly, extending over the pubic area in a diamond pattern by the com-

pletion of puberty. The presence of pubic hair before 9 years of age is uncommon, and delayed onset of testicular enlargement after 14 years of age needs evaluation. Penile enlargement generally follows testicular enlargement about one year later in genitalia Tanner stage 3. Stages of pubic hair development follow a standard pattern, as seen in Figure 35–34 ●.

SEXUAL MATURITY RATING

The sexual maturity rating (SMR) is an average of the breast and pubic hair Tanner stages in females and of the genital and pubic hair Tanner stages in males. The rating is a number between 2 and 5, as stage 1 is prepubertal. The SMR is then related to other physiologic events that happen during puberty. Compare the stage of the child's secondary sexual characteristics with information in Figure 35–35 ●.

In females, menarche generally occurs in SMR 4 or breast stage 3 to 4. The peak height velocity usually occurs before menarche at a mean age of 11.5 years. In males, ejaculation usually occurs at SMR 3, with semen noted between SMR 3 and 4. The peak height velocity usually occurs in SMR 4 or genital stage 4 to 5, at about 13.5 years of age.

ASSESSING THE MUSCULOSKELETAL SYSTEM FOR BONE AND JOINT STRUCTURE, MOVEMENT, AND MUSCLE STRENGTH

INSPECTION OF THE BONES, MUSCLES, AND JOINTS

Inspect and compare the arms and then the legs for differences in alignment, contour, skin folds, length, and

● FIGURE 35–35

A

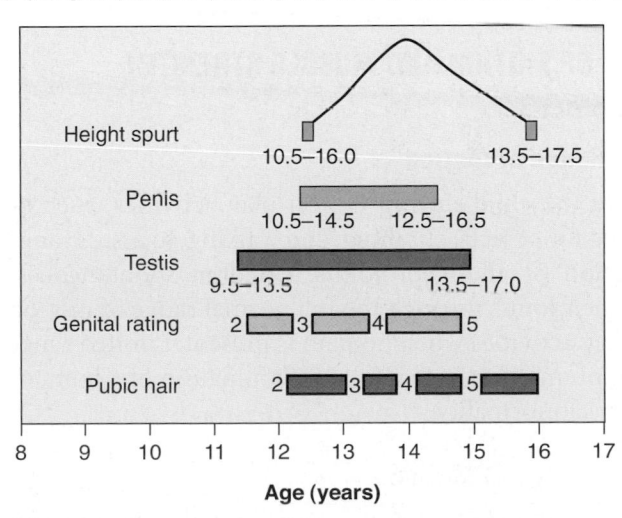

B

Sexual maturity rating—approximate timing of developmental changes. The numbers indicate stages of development. Range of ages during which some changes occur is indicated by the inclusive numbers below them. **A,** Females. **B,** Males.

Used with permission from Marshall, W. A., & Tanner, J. M. (1969). Archives of Disease in Childhood, 44, 291.

deformities. The extremities normally have equal length, circumference, and numbers of skin folds bilaterally. Extra skin folds and a larger circumference may indicate a shorter extremity.

Inspect and compare the joints bilaterally for size, discoloration, and ease of voluntary movement. Joints are normally the same color as surrounding skin, with no sign of swelling. Children should voluntarily flex and extend joints during normal activities without pain. Redness, swelling, and pain with movement may indicate injury or infection.

PALPATION OF THE BONES, MUSCLES, AND JOINTS

Palpate the bones and muscles in each extremity for muscle tone, masses, or tenderness. Muscles normally feel firm, and bony masses are not normally present. Doughy muscles may indicate poor muscle tone. Rigid muscles, or hypertonia, may be associated with an active seizure or cerebral palsy. A mass over a long bone may indicate a recent fracture or a bone tumor.

Palpate each joint and surrounding muscles to detect any swelling, masses, heat, or tenderness. None is expected when the joint is palpated. Tenderness, heat, swelling, and redness can result from injury or a chronic joint inflammation such as juvenile rheumatoid arthritis.

GROWTH AND DEVELOPMENT

Palpate the clavicles of the newborn from the sternum to the shoulder. These bones are often fractured during the birth process. A mass and crepitus may indicate a fracture.

RANGE OF MOTION AND MUSCLE STRENGTH ASSESSMENT

Active Range of Motion

Observe the child during typical play activities, such as reaching for objects, climbing, and walking, to assess range of motion of all major joints. Children spontaneously move their joints through the full normal range of motion with play activities when no pain is present. Limited range of motion may indicate injury, inflammation of a joint, or a muscle abnormality.

Passive Range of Motion

When a joint is suspected of having limited active range of motion, perform passive range of motion. Flex and extend, abduct and adduct, or rotate the affected joint cautiously to avoid causing extra pain. Full range of motion without pain is normal. Limitations in movement may indicate in-

jury, inflammation, or malformation. Increased passive range of motion may indicate muscle weakness.

Muscle Strength

Observe the child's ability to climb onto an examining table, throw a ball, clap the hands, or move around on the bed. The child's ability to perform age-appropriate play activities indicates good muscle tone and strength. Attainment of age-appropriate motor development is another indicator of good muscle strength (Table 35–15).

To assess the strength of specific muscles in the extremities, engage the child in some games. Compare muscle strength bilaterally to identify muscle weakness. For example, the child squeezes the examiner's fingers tightly with each hand; pushes against and pulls the examiner's hands with his or her hands, lower legs, and feet; and resists extension of a flexed elbow or knee. Children normally have good muscle strength bilaterally. Unilateral muscle weakness may be associated with a nerve injury. Bilateral muscle weakness may result from hypoxemia or a congenital disorder such as Down syndrome. Asymmetric weakness may be associated with conditions such as cerebral palsy.

When generalized muscle weakness is suspected in a preschool- or school-age child, ask the child to stand up from the supine position. Children are normally able to rise to a standing position without using their arms as levers. Children who push their body upright using the arms and hands may have generalized muscle weakness, known as a positive Gowers' sign. This may indicate muscular dystrophy (see Chapter 55 ∞).

TABLE 35–15 ❖ Selected Gross Motor Milestones for Age

Gross Motor Milestones	Age Attained
Rolls over from prone to supine position	4 months
Sits without support	8 months
Pulls self to standing position	10 months
Walks around room holding onto objects	11 months
Walks alone well	15 months
Kicks ball	24 months
Jumps in place	30 months
Throws ball overhand	36 months

Note: From Frankenburg, W. K., Dodds, J., Archer, P., Shapiro, H., & Bresnick, B. (1992). The Denver II: A major revision and restandardization of the Denver Developmental Screening Test. *Pediatrics, 89,* 91-97. Reproduced with permission from *Pediatrics,* Figure 2, © 1992.

TABLE 35–16 ✣	Normal Development of Posture and Spinal Curves
Age	**Posture and Spinal Curves**
2–3 months	Holds head erect when held upright; thoracic kyphosis when sitting.
6–8 months	Sits without support; spine is straight.
10–15 months	Walks independently; straight spine.
Toddler	Protruding abdomen; lumbar lordosis.
School-age child	Height of shoulders and hips is level; balanced thoracic convex and lumbar concave curves.

POSTURE AND SPINAL ALIGNMENT

Posture

Inspect the child's posture when standing from a front, side, and back view. The shoulders and hips are normally level. The head is held erect without a tilt, and the shoulder contour is symmetric. After beginning to walk, young children often have a pot-bellied stance because of lumbar lordosis. The spine has normal thoracic convex and lumbar concave curves after 6 years of age. Table 35–16 shows normal posture and spinal curvature development.

Spinal Alignment

Assess the school-age child and adolescent for scoliosis, a lateral spine curvature. Stand behind the child, observing the height of the shoulders and hips (Figure 35–36 ●). Ask the child to bend forward slowly at the waist, with arms extended toward the floor. No lateral curve should be present in either position. The ribs normally stay flat bilaterally. The lumbar concave curve should flatten with forward flexion (Figure 35–37 ●). A lateral curve to the spine or a one-sided rib hump is an indication of scoliosis (see Chapter 55 ∞).

INSPECTION OF THE UPPER EXTREMITIES

Arms

The alignment of the arms is normally straight, with a minimal angle at the elbows, where the bones articulate.

Hands

Count the fingers. Extra finger digits (polydactyly) or webbed fingers (syndactyly) are abnormal. Inspect the creases on the palmar surface of each hand. Multiple creases across the palm are normal. A single crease that crosses the entire palm of the hand, a simian crease, is associated with Down syndrome (Figure 35–38 ●).

● **FIGURE 35–36**

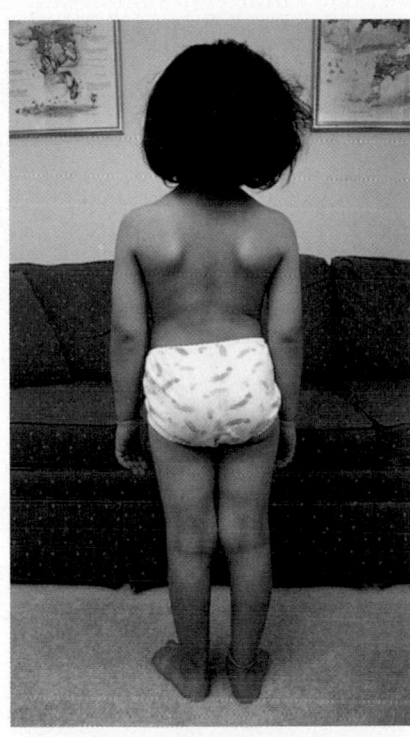

Does this child have legs of different lengths or scoliosis? Look at the level of the iliac crests and shoulders to see if they are level. See the more prominent crease at the waist on the right side? This child could have scoliosis.

Nails

Inspect the nails for size, shape, and color. Nails are normally convex, smooth, and pink. Clubbing, widening of the nailbed with an increased angle between the proximal nail fold and nail, is abnormal (see Figure 48–46 in Chapter 48 ∞).

● **FIGURE 35–37**

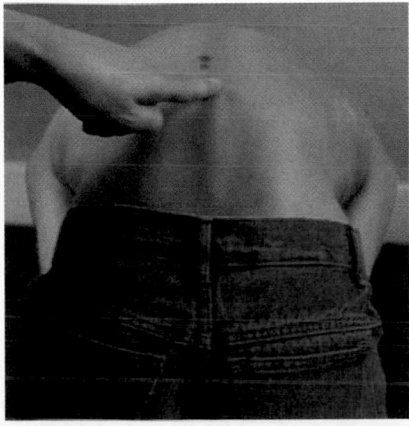

Inspection of the spine for scoliosis. Ask the child to slowly bend forward at the waist, with arms extended toward the floor. Run your forefinger down the spinal processes, palpating each vertebra for a change in alignment. A lateral curve to the spine or a one-sided rib hump is an indication of scoliosis.

● FIGURE 35-38

A

B

A, Normal palmar creases. **B,** Simian crease associated with Down syndrome.

Used with permission from Zitelli, B. J., & Davis, H. W. (Eds.). (1997). Atlas of pediatric physical diagnosis (3rd ed.). St. Louis, MO: Mosby–Year Book.

Clubbing is associated with chronic respiratory and cardiac conditions.

INSPECTION OF THE LOWER EXTREMITIES

Hips

Assess the hips of newborns and young infants for dislocation or subluxation. First inspect the skin folds on the upper legs. The same number of skin folds should be present on each leg. Uneven skin folds may indicate a hip dislocation or difference in leg length (Allis' sign). Then check for a difference in knee height symmetry (Figure 35–39 ●). The Ortolani-Barlow maneuver is used to as-

sess an infant's hips for dislocation or subluxation. See Chapter 27. ∞

Ask the child to stand on one leg and then the other. The iliac crests should stay level. If the iliac crest opposite the weight-bearing leg appears lower, the hip bearing weight may be dislocated.

Legs

Inspect the alignment of the legs. After a child is 4 years of age, the alignment of the long bones is straight, with minimal angle at the knees and feet where the bones articulate. Assess alignment of the lower extremities in infants and toddlers to ensure that normal changes are occurring. To evaluate the toddler with bowlegs, have the child stand on a firm surface. Measure the distance between the knees when the child's ankles are together. No more than 1.5 in (3.5 cm) between the knees is normal. See Figure 35–40 ● for assessment of knock-knees.

GROWTH AND DEVELOPMENT

Infants are often born with a twisting of the tibia caused by positioning in utero (tibial torsion). The infant's toes turn in as a result of the tibial torsion. Toddlers go through a skeletal alignment sequence of bowlegs (genu varum) and knock-knees (genu valgum) before the legs assume a straight alignment.

Feet

Inspect the feet for alignment, the presence of all toes, and any deformities. The weight-bearing line of the feet is usually in alignment with the legs. Many newborns

● FIGURE 35-39

Flex the infant's hips and knees so the heels are as close to the buttocks as possible. Place the feet flat on the examining table. The knees are usually the same height. A difference in knee height (Allis sign) is an indicator of hip dislocation (see also "Barlow-Ortolani Maneuver" in Chapter 27 ∞).

Courtesy of Dee Corbett, RN, Children's National Medical Center, Washington, DC.

● FIGURE 35–40

To evaluate the child with knock-knees, have the child stand on a firm surface. Measure the distance between the ankles when the child stands with the knees together. The normal distance is not more than 2 in. (5 cm) between the ankles.

have a flexible forefoot inversion (metatarsus adductus) that results from uterine positioning. Any fixed deformity is abnormal.

Inspect the feet for the presence of an arch when the child is standing. Children up to 3 years of age normally have a fat pad over the arch, giving the appearance of flat feet. Older children normally have a longitudinal arch. The arch is usually seen when the child stands on tiptoe or is sitting. Inspect the nails of the feet as for the hands.

ASSESSING THE NERVOUS SYSTEM FOR COGNITIVE FUNCTION, BALANCE, COORDINATION, CRANIAL NERVE FUNCTION, SENSATION, AND REFLEXES

Equipment needed for this examination includes a reflex hammer, cotton balls, a penlight, and tongue blades.

COGNITIVE FUNCTION

Observe the child's behavior, facial expressions, gestures, communication skills, activity level, and level of consciousness to assess cognitive functioning. Match the neurologic examination to the child's stage of development. For example, cognitive function is evaluated much differently in infants than in older children because infants cannot use words to communicate.

Behavior

The behavior of infants and children during the assessment indicates their alertness. Infants and toddlers are curious but seek the security of the parent, either by clinging or by making frequent eye contact. Older children are often anxious and watch all of the examiner's actions. Lack of interest in assessment or treatment procedures may indicate a serious illness. Excessive activity or an unusually short attention span may be associated with an attention deficit hyperactivity disorder.

Communication Skills

Speech, language development, and social skills provide good clues to cognitive functioning. Listen to speech articulation and words used, comparing the child's performance with standards of social development and speech articulation for the child's age (Table 35–17). Toddlers can normally follow simple directions such as "Show me your mouth." By 3 years of age, the child's speech should be easily understood. Delay in language and social skill development may be associated with mental retardation.

TABLE 35–17 ❖ Expected Language Development for Age

Language Milestones	Age Attained
Understands Mama and Dada	10 months
Says Mama, Dada, 2 other words; imitates animal sounds	12 months
4–6 word vocabulary, points to desired objects	13–15 months
7–20 word vocabulary, points to 5 body parts	18 months
2-word combinations	20 months
3-word sentences, plurals	36 months

Note: From Capute, A. J., Shapiro, B. K., & Palmer, R. B. (1987). Marking the milestones of language development. Contemporary Pediatrics, 4, 24–41.

Memory

Immediate, recent, and remote memory can be tested in children starting at approximately 4 years of age. To evaluate recent memory, ask the child to remember a special name or object. Then 5 to 10 minutes later during the examination, have the child recall the name or object. To evaluate remote memory, ask the child to repeat his or her address or birth date or a nursery rhyme. By 5 or 6 years of age, children are normally able to recall this information without difficulty.

GROWTH AND DEVELOPMENT

Test immediate memory by asking the child to repeat a series of words or numbers, such as the names of Disney or Sesame Street characters. Children can remember more words or numbers with age.

Age	Recall Ability
4 years	3 words or numbers
5 years	4 words or numbers
6 years	5 words or numbers

Level of Consciousness

When approaching the infant or child, observe his or her level of consciousness and activity, including facial expressions, gestures, and interaction. Children are normally alert, and sleeping children arouse easily. The child who cannot be awakened is unconscious. A lowered level of consciousness may be associated with a number of neurologic conditions such as a head injury, seizure, infection, or brain tumor.

CEREBELLAR FUNCTION

Observe the young child at play to assess coordination and balance. Development of fine motor skills in infants and preschool children provides clues to cerebellar function.

Balance

Observe the child's balance during play activities such as walking, standing on one foot, and hopping (Table 35–18). The Romberg procedure can also be used to test balance in children over 3 years of age (Figure 35–41 ◉). Once balance and other motor skills are attained, children do not normally stumble or fall when tested. Poor balance may indicate cerebellar dysfunction or an inner ear disturbance.

Coordination

Tests of coordination assess the smoothness and accuracy of movement. Development of fine motor skills can be used to assess coordination in young children (Table 35–19). After 6 years of age, the tests for adults (finger-to-nose, finger-to-finger, heel-to-shin, and alternating motion) can be used (Figure 35–42 ◉). The child usually

TABLE 35–18 ✣ Expected Balance Development for Age

Balance Milestones	Age Attained
Stands without support briefly	12 months
Walks alone well	15 months
Walks backwards	2 years
Balances on 1 foot for 5 seconds	4 years
Hops on 1 foot, heel-toe walking	5 years
Heel-toe walking backwards	6 years

responds enthusiastically when these tests are presented as games. Jerky movements or inaccurate pointing (past pointing) indicate poor coordination, which can be associated with delayed development or a cerebellar lesion.

Gait

A normal gait requires intact bones and joints, muscle strength, coordination, and balance. Inspect the child when

◉ **FIGURE 35–41**

Romberg procedure. Ask the child to stand with feet together and eyes closed. Protect the child from falling by standing close. Preschool–age children may extend their arms to maintain balance, but older children can normally stand with their arms at their sides. Leaning or falling to one side is abnormal and indicates poor balance.

TABLE 35–19 Expected Fine Motor Development for Age

Fine Motor Milestones	Age Attained
Transfers objects between hands	7 months
Picks up small objects	10 months
Feeds self with cup and spoon	12 months
Scribbles with crayon or pencil	18 months
Builds 2-block tower	24 months
Builds 4-block tower	30 months
Unfastens front buttons	36 months

Note: From Frankenburg, W. K., Dodds, J., Archer, P., Shapiro, H., & Bresnick, B. (1992). The Denver II: A major revision and restandardization of the Denver Developmental Screening Test. *Pediatrics, 89,* 91–97. Reproduced with permission from *Pediatrics,* Table 2, © 1992.

walking from both a front and a rear view. The iliac crests are normally level during walking, and no limp is expected. A limp may indicate injury or joint disease. Staggering or falling may indicate cerebellar ataxia. Scissoring, in which the thighs tend to cross forward over each other with each step, may be associated with cerebral palsy or other spastic conditions.

GROWTH AND DEVELOPMENT

Gait is related to the motor development of the child. Toddlers beginning to walk have a wide-based gait and limited balance. With practice the toddler's balance improves and the gait develops a narrower base.

CRANIAL NERVE FUNCTION

To assess the cranial nerves in infants and young children, modify the procedures used to assess school-age children and adults (Table 35–20). Abnormalities of cranial nerves

● FIGURE 35–42

Tests of coordination. **A,** Finger-to-nose test. Ask the child to close the eyes and touch his or her nose, alternating the index fingers of the hands. **B,** Finger-to-finger test. Ask the child to alternately touch his or her nose and your index finger with his or her index finger. Move your hand to several positions within the child's reach to test pointing accuracy. Repeat the test with the child's other hand. **C,** Heel-to-shin test. Ask the child to rub his or her leg from the knee to the ankle with the heel of the other foot. Repeat the test with the other foot. This test is normally performed without hesitation or inappropriate placement of the foot. **D,** Rapid alternating motion test. Ask the child to rapidly rotate his or her wrist so the palm and dorsum of the hand alternately pat the thigh. Repeat the test with the other hand. Hesitating movements are abnormal. Mirroring movements of the hand not being tested indicate a delay in coordination skill refinement.

TABLE 35–20 ✣ **Age-Specific Procedures for Assessment of Cranial Nerves in Infants and Children**

Cranial Nerve[a]	Assessment Procedure and Normal Findings[b]
I Olfactory	Infant: Not tested.
	Child: Not routinely tested. Give familiar odors to child to smell, one naris at a time. *Identifies odors such as orange, peanut butter, and chocolate.*
II Optic	Infant: Shine a bright light in eyes. *A quick blink reflex and dorsal head flexion indicates light perception.*
	Child: Test vision and visual fields if cooperative. *Visual acuity appropriate for age.*
III Oculomotor IV Trochlear VI Abducens	Infant: Shine a penlight at the eyes and move it side to side. *Focuses on and tracks the light to each side.* Child: Move an object through the six cardinal points of gaze. *Tracks object through all fields of gaze.* All ages: Inspect eyelids for drooping. Inspect pupillary response to light. *Eyelids do not droop and pupils are equal size and briskly respond to light.*
V Trigeminal	Infant: Stimulate the rooting and sucking reflex. *Turns head toward stimulation at side of mouth and sucking has good strength and pattern.*
	Child: Observe the child chewing a cracker. Touch forehead and cheeks with cotton ball when eyes are closed. *Bilateral jaw strength is good. Child pushes cotton ball away.*
VII Facial	All ages: Observe facial expressions when crying, smiling, frowning, etc. *Facial features stay symmetric bilaterally.*
VIII Acoustic	Infant: Produce a loud sound near the head. *Blinks in response to sound, moves head toward sound or freezes position.*
	Child: Use a noisemaker near each ear or whisper words to be repeated. *Turns head toward sound and repeats words correctly.*
IX Glossopharyngeal X Vagus	Infant: Observe swallowing during feeding. *Good swallowing pattern.* All ages: Elicit gag reflex. *Gags with stimulation.*
XI Spinal accessory	Infant: Not tested.
	Child: Ask child to raise the shoulders and turn the head side to side against resistance. *Good strength in neck and shoulders.*
XII Hypoglossal	Infant: Observe feeding. *Sucking and swallowing are coordinated.*
	Child: Tell the child to stick out the tongue. Listen to speech. *Tongue is midline with no tremors. Words are clearly articulated.*

[a]Bracketed nerves are tested together.
[b]Italic indicates normal findings.

---

may be associated with compression of an individual nerve, head injury, or infections.

SENSORY FUNCTION

To assess sensory function, compare the responses of the body to various types of stimulation. Bilateral equal responses are normal. Loss of sensation may indicate a brain or spinal cord lesion. Withdrawal responses to painful procedures indicate normal sensory function in an infant.

Superficial Tactile Sensation

Stroke the skin on the lower leg or arm with a cotton ball or a finger while the child's eyes are closed. Cooperative children over 2 years of age can normally point to the location touched.

Superficial Pain Sensation

Break a tongue blade to get a sharp point. After asking the child to close the eyes, touch the child in various places on each arm and leg, alternating the sharp and dull ends of the tongue blade. A paper clip may also be used. Children over 4 years of age can normally distinguish between a sharp and dull sensation each time. To improve the child's accuracy with the test, let the child practice describing the difference between the sharp and dull stimulation.

An inability to identify superficial touch and pain sensation may indicate sensory loss. Identify the extent of sensory loss, such as all areas below the knee. Other sensory function tests (temperature, vibratory, deep pressure pain, and position sense) are performed when sensory loss is found. Refer to other texts for a description of these procedures.

INFANT PRIMITIVE REFLEXES

Evaluate the movement and posture of newborns and young infants by the Moro, palmar grasp, plantar grasp, placing, stepping, and tonic neck primitive reflexes. These reflexes appear and disappear at expected intervals in the first few months of life as the central nervous system develops. Movements are normally equal bilaterally. An asymmetric response may indicate a serious neurologic problem on the less responsive side. See "Newborn Primitive Reflexes" in Chapter 27 for more information. ∞

SUPERFICIAL AND DEEP TENDON REFLEXES

Evaluate the superficial and deep tendon reflexes to assess the function of specific segments of the spine.

Superficial Reflexes

Assess superficial reflexes by stroking a specific area of the body. The plantar reflex, testing spine levels L4 to S2, is routinely evaluated in children (Figure 35–43 ◉). Assess the cremasteric reflex in boys (see page 1007).

◉ **FIGURE 35–43**

To assess the plantar reflex, stroke the bottom of the infant's or child's foot in the direction of the arrow. Watch the toes for plantar flexion or the Babinski response, fanning and dorsiflexion of the big toe. The Babinski response is normal in children under 2 years of age. Plantar flexion of the toes is the normal response in older children. A Babinski response in children over 2 years of age can indicate neurologic disease.

Deep Tendon Reflexes

To assess the deep tendon reflexes, tap a tendon near specific joints with a reflex hammer (or with the index finger for infants), comparing responses bilaterally. The biceps, triceps, brachioradialis, patellar, and Achilles tendons are usually evaluated in children. Inspect for movement in the associated joint and palpate the strength of the expected muscle contraction (Table 35–21). The numeric scoring of deep tendon reflexes is as follows:

Grade	Response Interpretation
0	No response
1+	Slow, minimal response
2+	Expected response, active
3+	More active or pronounced than expected
4+	Hyperactive, clonus may be present

Responses are normally symmetric bilaterally. The absence of a response is associated with decreased muscle tone and strength. Hyperactive responses are associated with muscle spasticity.

NURSING PRACTICE

The best response to deep tendon reflex testing is achieved when the child is relaxed or distracted. Children often anticipate the knee jerk and either tighten up or exaggerate the response. Making the child focus on another set of muscles may provide a more accurate response. When testing the reflexes on the lower legs, have the child press his or her hands together or try to pull them apart when gripped together.

ANALYZING DATA FROM THE PHYSICAL EXAMINATION

Once the physical examination has been completed, group any abnormal findings for each system with those of other systems. Use clinical judgment to identify common patterns of physiologic responses associated with health conditions. Individual abnormal physiologic responses are also the basis of many nursing diagnoses. Be sure to record all findings from the physical assessment legibly, in detail, and in the format approved by your institution.

TABLE 35–21 ❖ **Assessment of Deep Tendon Reflexes and the Spinal Segment Tested with Each**

Deep Tendon Reflex	Technique and Normal Findings[a]	Spine Segment Tested
Biceps 	Flex the child's arm at the elbow, and place your thumb over the biceps tendon in the antecubital fossa. Tap your thumb. *Elbow flexes as the biceps muscle contracts.*	C5 and C6
Triceps 	With the child's arm flexed, tap the triceps tendon above the elbow. *Elbow extends as the triceps muscle contracts.*	C6, C7, and C8
Brachioradialis 	Lay the child's arm with the thumb upright over your arm. Tap the brachioradial tendon 2.5 cm (1 in) above the wrist. *Forearm pronates (palm facing downward) and elbow flexes.*	C5 and C6

TABLE 35-21 ✣ Assessment of Deep Tendon Reflexes and the Spinal Segment Tested with Each—continued

Deep Tendon Reflex	Technique and Normal Findings[a]	Spine Segment Tested
Patellar 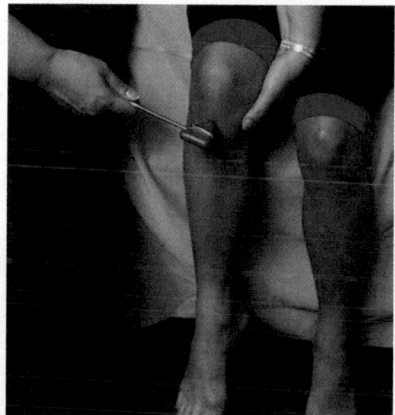	Flex the child's knees, and when the legs are relaxed, tap the patellar tendon just below the knee. *Knee extends (knee jerk) as the quadriceps muscle contracts.*	L2, L3, and L4
Achilles 	While the child's legs are flexed, support the foot and tap the Achilles' tendon. *Plantar flexion (ankle jerk) as the gastrocnemius muscle contracts.*	S1 and S2

[a]*Italics indicate normal findings.*

Critical Concept Review

LEARNING OBJECTIVES

Describe the elements of a health history for an infant or child of different ages.

CONCEPTS

Historical data to collect includes:
1. Chief complaint.
2. History of the present illness or injury.
3. Past history.
4. Current health status.
5. Review of systems.
6. Family history.
7. Psychosocial data.
8. Developmental data.

(continued)

LEARNING OBJECTIVES

CONCEPTS

Identify communication strategies to improve the quality of historical data collected.	1. Introduce self, including purpose of interview. 2. Provide privacy, including confirmation confidentiality. 3. Use open-ended questions. 4. Ask one question at a time. 5. Direct question to the child when appropriate. 6. Be honest with the child and family. 7. Obtain feedback from parents to confirm understanding.
Describe strategies to gain cooperation of a young child for assessment.	1. Allow the young child to stay in caretaker's lap for most of the examination. 2. Allow the young child to hold and examine any equipment before it is used on the child. 3. Avoid the use of any quick, jerky movements when performing assessments.
Describe the differences in sequence of the physical assessment for infants, children, and adolescents.	1. Any painful or frightening procedures (examination of throat and ears) should be delayed until the end of the physical assessment of the infant and young child. 2. Physical examination of the school-age child should proceed in a head-to-toe fashion, with the exception of the genitalia examination (should be done last). 3. The physical examination of the adolescent may be completed without the presence of the parent, especially the examination of the genitalia.
Modify physical assessment techniques according to the age and developmental stage of the child.	Infants and toddlers: 1. Head circumference is required until age 3. 2. Palpate fontanels until closure. 3. Assess vision and hearing response with the use of toys and familiar objects. 4. Perform the abdominal examination with the infant and toddler on the lap of the caregiver and use distraction. 5. Use direct percussion of the chest to evaluate resonance. Preschooler: 1. Ask young child to show teeth to begin assessment of the mouth and throat. 2. Gently pry teeth apart with a tongue depressor if teeth remain clenched. 3. Use familiar objects and words easily recognized to assess vision and hearing. 4. Males should sit "tailor fashion" to assess genitalia. Adolescent: 1. Assess breast development in both males and females.
Determine the sexual maturity rating of males and females based upon physical signs of secondary sexual characteristics present.	The sexual maturity rating (SMR) for: 1. Females: Average of breast development and pubic hair (Tanner stages). 2. Males: Average of genital development and pubic hair (Tanner stages).
Recognize at least five important signs of a serious alteration in health condition that require urgent nursing intervention.	1. Altered level of consciousness. 2. Bradycardia. 3. Tachypnea (greater than 60 breaths per minute). 4. Pain. 5. Signs of dehydration (no tears, dry mucous membranes, doughy skin turgor, sunken fontancile, increased urine concentration). 6. Stridor. 7. Retractions. 8. Cyanosis.

CRITICAL THINKING IN ACTION

*View the **Critical Thinking in Action** video in Chapter 35 of the CD-ROM. Then, answer the questions that follow.*

It is a relatively calm night in the Children's hospital emergency room when a 6-month-old infant named Colby is brought in by emergency personnel from an automobile accident. Colby was in his infant, rear-facing, car seat, riding with his parents when another car rear-ended them. The parents were not hurt and did not need to go to the hospital. The father immediately called 911 on his cell phone after the accident. When the ambulance arrived at the emergency room, you were given the report from the EMT. He stated that Colby was alert and quiet in his father's arms when they arrived on the scene and he did not have any obvious signs of trauma. He is being brought to the hospital to make sure he did not sustain any injuries from the accident. His vital signs are as follows: temperature—98.9 degrees fahrenheit, respirations—40, pulse—110 and blood pressure is 95/55.

Colby is alert with no apparent distress. His pupils are equal, round, and reactive to light. His anterior fontanelle is flat and he has equal movements of extremities. His breath sounds are clear and equal bilaterally. His heart sounds have a regular rate and rhythm without murmur. He voided around 2 hours ago, before the accident.

1. The fontanelles are an extremely important body part to examine in children. In the scenario with Colby, it can give an indication if there is increased intracranial pressure related to a head injury. How can you describe the placement of the fontanelles, and when should they close and become unpalpable? Also, describe why the head would be more likely to sustain injury in an infant like Colby versus an adult.

2. After reviewing the scenario, what can you tell the parents about Colby's vital signs and stability at this time? What is the difference between adult vital signs and Colby's vital signs?

3. Describe what structures in the chest and abdominal area of Colby's body would be of concern with the type of accident he sustained.

4. If a heart murmur were to be found on examination of Colby, what would be the five ways to describe it?

MEDIALINK   www.prenhall.com/london

- NCLEX-RN® Review, case studies, and other interactive resources for this chapter can be found on the Companion Website at http://www.prenhall.com/london. Click on "Chapter 35" to select the activities for this chapter.

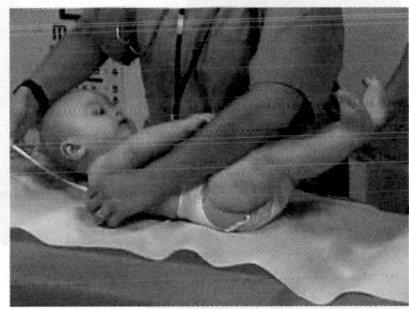

- For animations, more NCLEX-RN® Review questions, and an audio glossary, access the accompanying CD-ROM in this textbook.

REFERENCES

American Academy of Pediatrics. (2003). Eye examination in infants, children, and young adults by pediatricians. *Pediatrics, 111*(4), 902–907.

American Academy of Pediatrics Section on Ophthalmology. (2002). Red reflex examination in infants. *Pediatrics, 109*(5), 980–981.

Burns, C. (1992). A new assessment model and tool for pediatric nurse practitioners. *Journal of Pediatric Health Care, 6*, 73–81.

Byrnes, K. (1996). Conducting the pediatric health history: A guide. *Pediatric Nursing, 22*, 135–137.

Eichelberger, M. R., Ball, J. W., Pratsch, G. S., & Clark, J. R. (1998). *Pediatric emergencies: A manual for prehospital care providers* (2nd ed.). Upper Saddle River, NJ: Brady, Prentice Hall.

Ganel, A., Dudkiewicz, I., & Grogan, D. P. (2003). Pediatric orthopedic physical examination of the infant: A 5 minute assessment. *Journal of Pediatric Health Care, 17*(1), 39–41.

Goldenring, J. M., & Rosen, D. S. (2004). Getting into adolescent heads: An essential update. *Contemporary Pediatrics, 21*(1), 64–90.

Green, M., Sullivan, P., & Eichberg, C. (2002). Avoid a "Swiss cheese" history when psychosocial complaints are on the menu. *Contemporary Pediatrics, 19*(10), 115–125.

Hazinski, M. F. (1999). *Manual of pediatric critical care* (pp. 289–293). St. Louis, MO: Mosby.

Herman–Giddens, M. E., Slora, E. J., Wasserman, R. C., Bourdony, C. J., Bhapkar, M. V., Koch, G. G., et al. (1997). Secondary sexual characteristics and menses in young girls seen in office practice: A study from the pediatric research in office setting network. *Pediatrics, 99*(4), 505–512.

Instone, S. L. (2002). Developmental strategies for interviewing children. *Journal of Pediatric Health Care, 16*(6), 304–305.

Kaplowitz, P. B., Oberfield, S. E., and the Drug and Therapeutics and Executive Committees of the Lawson Wilkins Pediatric Endocrine Society. (1999). Reexamination of the age limit for defining when puberty is precocious in girls in the United States: Implications for evaluation and treatment. *Pediatrics, 104*(4), 936–941.

McEvoy, M. (2000). An added dimension to the pediatric health maintenance visit: The spiritual history. *Journal of Pediatric Health Care, 14*(5), 216–220.

Muntner, P., He, J., Cutler, J. A., Wildman, R. P., & Whelton, P. K. (2004). Trends in blood pressure among children and adolescents. *Journal of the American Medical Association, 291*(17), 2107–2113.

National Heart, Lung, and Blood Institute. (2004). Blood pressure tables for children and adolescents from the fourth report on the diagnosis, evaluation, and treatment of high blood pressure in children and adolescents. Retrieved June 11, 2004, from *http://www.nhlbi.nih.gov/guidelines/ hypertension/child_tbl.htm*

Seidel, H. M., Ball, J. W., Dains, J., & Benedict, G. W. (2003). *Mosby's guide to physical examination* (5th ed.). St. Louis, MO: Mosby.

Spector, R. E. (2000). *Cultural diversity in health and illness* (5th ed.). Upper Saddle River, NJ: Prentice Hall Health.

Tanner, J. M. (1962). *Growth at adolescence* (2nd ed.). Oxford, England: Blackwell Scientific Publications.

Social and Environmental Influences on the Child

Amy has always been a challenge. She has already left home a couple of times and lived on the streets. Lately she has been more interested in school and is at home and trying to do well. We want her to succeed and learn the skills she needs in her life. I wish she would not have all of these body piercings, but we don't want to make too big an issue of it as long as she is doing well in school.

Mother of Amy, 15 years old

LEARNING OBJECTIVES

- Identify major social and environmental factors that influence the health of children and adolescents.

- List external influences that influence child and adolescent health.

- Apply the ecologic model and resiliency theory to assessment of the social and environmental factors in children's lives.

- Examine the effects of substance use, physical activity, and other lifestyle patterns on health.

- Plan nursing interventions for children who experience violence.

- Explore the nursing role in prevention and treatment of child abuse and neglect.

MEDIALINK www.prenhall.com/london

CD-ROM

Videos:
   Extreme Sports
   Violence in the Media
   Identifying Child Abuse
   Smoking and Smoking Cessation
   Identifying Youth Who Abuse Drugs and Alcohol
Audio Glossary
NCLEX-RN® Review
Objectives
Critical Thinking

Companion Website

MediaLink Applications:
   Develop a Teaching Plan: Individualized Sport
   Music and Violence

M any of the major causes of mortality and morbidity in children are closely linked with social influences in the child's environment. The social contexts for young children growing up today are different from those of even a decade ago. Examining the social contexts in which children live and grow can provide insights into behavior, and present opportunities for nursing interventions. All nurses must examine the social influences and apply the knowledge gained to plan healthcare that will benefit youth as they grow into adulthood.

What are the settings where nurses might work with youth in the community? What are the challenges of today's society that children must often face at very young ages? How can nurses help children face these challenges, and emerge healthy and contributing members of society? What roles do nurses play in identifying and using the protective factors and in minimizing the risk factors of youth? This chapter will examine and apply these concepts in a variety of nursing settings.

Examine again the major causes of death for children from 1 year of age through adolescence that are presented on the Companion Website 🌐. See Chapter 1 for more discussion. ∞ Notice that most morbidity is related to preventable causes linked to present-day lifestyles. Car crashes, fires, drowning, and homicides are a few examples of common causes of death in children.

Now examine the major reasons for hospitalization on the Website 🌐. By the time children are 5 years of age, injuries rank as the second cause, and by 10 years, mental disorders are the major cause of hospitalization. By the teen years, pregnancy and mental disorders are the most common admitting diagnoses to hospitals. All of these conditions are related, at least in part, to the social and environmental settings in which children live. These settings and their influences must be examined to understand how best to intervene with children.

BASIC CONCEPTS

In this chapter, two main theories will provide a framework for examining societal influences on children. The ecologic model and resiliency theory are discussed in Chapter 33, ∞ and should be reviewed now to assist in evaluating the environmental settings that influence children.

The ecologic theory views the child and the environment as interacting forces, with children influencing systems around them, even while they are influenced by these systems (Bronfenbrenner, 2005; Lackey & Walker, 1998). Close systems providing daily contact are microsystems, but other systems such as parental work and political or cultural environments are also important. Understanding these systems, or the forces in which children function, can provide information that guides care providers. For example, if the parents' employers do not provide healthcare insurance, their children may not get needed healthcare such as immunizations, treatment for diseases, and growth monitoring.

Resiliency theory examines risk and protective factors in the child's environment as they influence the child's adaptation to stressful events, and can be modified to lead to more productive and healthy outcomes. For example, if a young child is hospitalized for treatment of an acute infectious illness, some **protective factors** might include the ability of one parent to stay with the child at all times, the ability of a grandmother to care for siblings at home during this time, and the child's ability to adapt to new situations and communicate readily with staff members. On the other hand, **risk factors** might include lack of comprehensive health insurance to pay for the hospitalization, lack of an identified healthcare "home" (consistent care provider) for the child, and missing some immunizations. The concepts of resiliency theory can be applied to Amy's family as described in the opening quotation. She experienced disruption in family stability. The risk and protective factors interacted with her own personality in ways that resulted in her desire to appear as an independent person, establishing her identity through body art, and finally, a desire to return to school.

The National Longitudinal Study of Adolescent Health (ADD) was conducted with over 100,000 adolescents in the United States, and found that parent-family connectedness, school connectedness, a belief in a higher being, and academic success were predictive of youth having lower health risks (Franke, 2003). Nurses can assist adolescents and their families in establishing a sense of attachment to each other. Encourage families to include adolescents in activities, attend their sports and other school events, have meals together regularly, and attend faith-based activities or other community events as a family.

Theoretical frameworks are discussed in Chapter 33 ∞ and are useful when examining social and environmental influences on children because they guide us to examine certain factors that can be altered or understood. They suggest the assessment data to collect and pertinent nursing interventions to use. They also foster partnerships with other care providers who use these and similar theories to plan social, psychologic, and other care for children and their families.

EXTERNAL INFLUENCES ON CHILD HEALTH

POVERTY

An important risk factor that influences the health of children is poverty. Conversely, basic financial stability is a protective factor that contributes to the general health and well-being of children. Children who are poor are overrepresented in nearly every health indicator. One in six children is poor, or in a family earning less than $14,128 annually for a family of three or $18,104 for a U.S. family of four (Children's Defense Fund, 2004). Children who are poor are more likely to have unmet health needs, to have difficulty in school, to become teen parents, and to experience multiple health problems. Children are the poorest group in this country, and more children are poor now than at any time in the past (Board on Children, Youth, and Families, 2001). Inadequate or unsafe housing, food insecurity, and poor dietary quality are more common. What is the face of poverty? Some statistics that may prove surprising include the following:

- The children most likely to be living in poor households are those below 6 years of age.

- About 39% of children living in a single-headed household are poor, while only 8% in married-couple households are poor.

- Ethnic variations are startling; 10% of white, 30% of Hispanic, and 34% of black children live in poverty.

- Poverty rates are higher in suburban and rural areas than in central cities.

- Nearly 80% of poor children have at least one parent working full time.

(Federal Interagency Forum on Child and Family Statistics, 2004)

DEVELOPING CULTURAL COMPETENCE

ETHNIC DISPARITY IN POVERTY RATES

Ethnic disparities occur with 10% of white children classified as poor, 30% of Hispanic children, and 34% of black children (Federal Interagency Forum on Child and Family Statistics, 2004).

Poverty leads to homelessness for some children. Children comprise one third of the homeless, women represent 20%, and families comprise 39% of the homeless population. Families are the fastest growing group of homeless people. On any night, about 100,000 children are homeless in the United States (DeForge, Zehnder, Minick et al., 2001). The reasons for homelessness are also common risks for a number of the other challenges to health discussed in this chapter. Homeless people often have poor finances, may have been abused or victims of other violence, and may have mental instability. Children who experience homelessness often have multiple physical and mental

---

THINKING CRITICALLY

DEMOGRAPHICS AND NURSING CARE

Nurses should understand the demographics in the areas where they work. What is the poverty rate in your community? What ethnic groups are overrepresented among the poor? Locate the resources such as food services, healthcare for the underserved, and enhanced school programs in order to refer poor families. Recognize that health promotion services may not be high priority when a family does not have adequate housing or food. When children are seen in any setting, such as in school or in an emergency room or hospital for acute care, perform needed assessments and intervention. Measure growth, assess vision and hearing, evaluate dietary intake, and check immunization status. Find out the stresses the family experiences and what resources they need to meet basic necessities. Construct a nursing care plan for a family living in poverty with two young children.

health problems, and lack health insurance to provide care for these problems. Some of the common problems faced by homeless children and families include trauma, alcoholism, respiratory and skin infections, tuberculosis and HIV, and nutritional disorders (Stratigos & Katsambas, 2003). Teens who have been homeless are more likely to engage in other risky behavior, such as unprotected sex, sex with multiple partners, and substance abuse. They are more likely to need emergency care, to be depressed, and to become pregnant than other teens (Steele, Ramgoolam, & Evans, 2003).

Health problems related to homelessness, and other family characteristics, continue even after finding a place to live. Even after families leave homeless shelters, children frequently become separated from their mothers due to parent stress, lack of access to resources, and inability of parents to provide adequate settings for the children (Cowal, Shinn, Weitzman et al., 2002). Complex, ongoing care is needed. This may begin in a shelter for the homeless, but should continue while the family obtains a place to live, accesses other community services, gets the children safely enrolled in school, and has financial and mental stability. Nursing management for families with children that are poor or homeless focuses on identification of poverty, careful assessment of health risks, and linking the family to resources that can assist with stability and health. There is often no way to identify a poor child from appearance, and they may hide their status when they are in school or come to a healthcare facility. Addresses given may not be accurate, or the address of a shelter might be used. Children living at shelters or in cars and on the street usually do not take the school bus but prefer to walk to avoid stigma. Be alert for children who have multiple health problems and repeated infectious diseases. They are often hungry at times. Degrees of personal hygiene may vary depending on access to laundry and bathing facilities. See Table 36–1 for examples of nursing care needs for homeless children and families.

STRESS

The adverse effect of stress on adults is well documented. More recently the impact of stress on children has been recognized. Children manifest stress in a variety of ways, including regressive behavior, interrupted sleep, hyperactive behavior, gastrointestinal symptoms, crying, and withdrawal from normal events. Common stressful events for children include moving to a new home or school, marital difficulties in the family, abuse, a parent deployed in the military, and being expected to achieve at an extremely high level in school or sports (Figure 36–1 ●). The busy pace of today's lifestyles and the media's encouragement of early development in children may put undue stress upon some children and preteens (Elkind, 2001).

Adolescents may be stressed by fulfilling many roles, such as student, part-time worker, and active member of a family. They may be in school all day, be in sport or music practice for 2 to 3 hours after school, and then have a job for several additional hours. Lack of adequate sleep is common and adds further to stress, in addition to putting the teen at risk for car crashes and poor school performance. For poor families, commonly reported stressors are related to food, shelter, transportation, medical care, and personal-time needs.

The child experiencing stress has more frequent respiratory and gastrointestinal illnesses and is more likely to be the victim of an injury. The negative long-term effects of stress on body organs and systems suggest that children under stress are more likely to develop illnesses such as strokes, hypertension, and heart attacks later in life.

Nurses help children manage stress by encouraging good coping strategies. With all children, emphasize healthy lifestyles including good nutrition, exercise, and plenty of sleep. The National Heart, Lung, and Blood Institute has launched a program to encourage children to get at least 9 hours of sleep nightly and offers tips for sleep for children and teens. Encourage parents to provide youth with activities that foster self-esteem, and to avoid unrealistic expectations about performance in sports and other activities. Provide resources to help with food acquisition, shelter, transportation, and medical care for families needing them. Adolescents may benefit from various approaches for stress management such as massage, rest, physical activity, and yoga.

COMPLEMENTARY CARE

YOUTH AND COMPLEMENTARY THERAPY

Many healthcare providers assume that youth use few complementary and alternative medicine (CAM) approaches. A study at a Texas university suggests that this may not be accurate. Researchers received a total of 913 questionnaires from college students who answered questions related to use of CAM; 66% of the students reported use of such therapy in the past year. The most common types were high-dose vitamin/nutritional supplements, herbal medicine, relaxation/meditation, and massage. Less common were chiropractic medicine, yoga, and acupuncture. Most students had positive attitudes about CAM. Those engaging in the practices were more commonly female and holistic in approach to health, and expressed a sense of control over their own health. The researchers suggest that healthcare providers working with youth assess their use of CAM and provide written and other materials to provide information. Those who are self-directed and take control of their own health may benefit most from resources provided on CAM approaches (Chng, Neill, & Fogle, 2003).

TABLE 36–1 ❖ Common Health Problems and Nursing Management of Poor and Homeless Children

Common Health Problems	Nursing Management
Lack of immunizations	Check immunization records Provide immunizations at schools and in homeless shelters
Common infectious diseases	Facilitate free clinics in shelters, schools, community settings Teach hygiene measures Provide resources for disease management Arrange for medications when needed Provide information about resources for bathing, hygiene
Sleep deficits	Inform parents about respite facilities Arrange for children to have quiet sleep time in school if possible
Vision and hearing deficits	Perform screening for deficits Provide resources for eye glasses, hearing aids, care for ear infections (Service organizations such as Lion's Club are good options)
Nutritional deficits	Perform height and weight checks and nutritional assessment Evaluate family for food security (see Chapter 31 ∞) Be sure child is registered for school breakfast and lunch programs if available Ensure that children are linked to summer food programs at end of academic year Link to Women, Infants, and Children (WIC) Nutrition Program Inform about resources for meals and field gleaning in the community
Dental care problems	Teach oral hygiene Provide toothbrushes and toothpaste Provide bottled water if child lives in a car or on the street Perform oral assessment Refer to dental programs for people with low incomes
Injuries	Teach basic safety precautions Visit the living situation if possible to assess for safety hazards Teach "street safe" skills Provide helmets, car seats, or other gear needed
Adolescent pregnancy and sexually transmitted diseases	Provide sexuality teaching Inform about access to family planning services Assess for child abuse and prostitution
Mental illness	Assess for depression Evaluate for suicide potential Provide links to services Plan programs to foster self-esteem Arrange for a "Big Brother" or "Big Sister" Refer to extracurricular activities in the school and community Arrange for a school bus stop away from a shelter so other students do not stigmatize the homeless child

Partner with military families to assist them as one or both parents are deployed for duty in a remote location. Connect parents with resources for child care, psychologic support, and arrangements that need to be made to prepare for the absence. Because of frequent moves, the family may not be strongly connected to resources in the community. Help families explain to children why and where the parents are going, and how they will keep in touch during absence. They need to know who they will stay with, whether they will attend the same school, and how food and other needs will be provided (Stafford & Grady, 2003).

EVIDENCE-BASED NURSING

HOMELESSNESS FROM THE VIEWPOINT OF CHILDREN

Problem

Children are the age group showing the fastest growth in homelessness, accounting for about 39% of the homeless population. Due to their ages, children are vulnerable to developmental delays, mental health problems, and effects of violence. Most nurses have not been homeless and do not understand the experience of homelessness for children.

Evidence

A study by four nurses sought to describe the homeless experience from the perspective of children. They interviewed 14 children with an average age of 10 years who were located in shelters in a metropolitan area. The children had been in the shelters from 2 weeks to 6 months, and most had prior periods living in shelters, in hotels, or with relatives. The researchers identified five themes common to the children:

- "I'm not homeless." The children viewed homelessness as having no resources and having to live outside. They felt that they had resources and felt they might be ridiculed if people thought they were homeless.
- "I like living in a shelter sometimes." While the children had mixed feelings about living in shelters, most were glad to have food, a place to sleep, and a feeling of safety. They described friends in the shelter and were glad to have those relationships.
- "Living in a shelter is hard." The children complained about rules and rigid schedules in the shelters. They missed freedom of movement, play space, and privacy.
- "Stop the violence." All children described living in violent neighborhoods and the wish that violence would stop. Fighting back was perceived as important to protecting oneself.

- "I need approval." Children frequently described how important it was to be noticed and praised by teachers and other adults.

Implications

While this study was small, there were important findings for nurses. The stigma of being homeless should be considered when interacting with children. The researchers suggest reading stories and describing families that lose a home to all children in schools so that the topic is addressed. Nurses can partner with teachers to plan collaborative approaches. The privacy of children should be considered, and school buses should not stop directly in front of shelters to pick up children. Integrating positive reinforcement for children into shelter routines, school classrooms, and other settings is important for the child's sense of self-esteem (DeForge et al., 2001).

Critical Thinking

Find at least two shelters in your community. Are nurses involved in planning healthcare? How long do families usually remain? Do the schools know that children are homeless? Do they strive to preserve the privacy of homeless children while supporting their needs for growth, health, and education? What is the nursing role in the shelter, in the school, and in the community?

Reference

DeForge, V., Zehnder, S., Minick, P., & Carmon, M. (2001). Children's perspectives of homelessness. *Pediatric Nursing, 27,* 377–383.

FAMILY STRUCTURE

The families into which children are born influence them greatly. Children are supported in different ways and acquire different world views depending on such factors as whether one or both parents work, how many siblings are present, and whether an extended family is close by. Note variations in family structure such as single parent, adolescent parent, homosexual parents, extended family, grandparents raising grandchildren, and stepparents. Societal changes have impacted family life and the needs of children in profound ways. Working parents often raise children with little time for quality relationships and without the financial resources needed for optimum development (Board on Children, Youth, and Families, 2001). All of these factors influence the physical and mental health of children, and can determine their needs for nursing intervention.

About 45% of all marriages in the United States end in divorce (Hetherington, 2005). Divorce has a profound effect on children, varying with the child's age and cognitive stage. Young children who have limited ability to under-

stand divorce may show such behavioral manifestations as crying, sleep disturbance, regression, and aggressive behavior (Wallerstein, Corbin, & Lewis, 1988; Wallerstein, Lewis, & Blakeslee, 2000) (see Table 36–2). Older children and adolescents more commonly show inadequate social skills related to cooperation and negotiation, increased aggression, and substance abuse (Thompson, 1998). After divorce, children most often live (about 80% of the time) in a single-parent household with the mother (Friedman, 2003). This can lead to financial strain, decreased health insurance coverage, parental role strain, and other stresses that affect the children. Remarriage, stepparenting, and joint custody arrangements all create additional challenges for families. Children with additional risk factors are more challenged by divorce than those with many protective factors. Nurses can help families recognize the challenges the children are experiencing, evaluate the child's risk and protective factors, help them cope with their particular needs, and provide resources such as mediation sessions, parenting skills sessions, financial assistance, and support groups (Hetherington, 2005).

○ FIGURE 36–1

 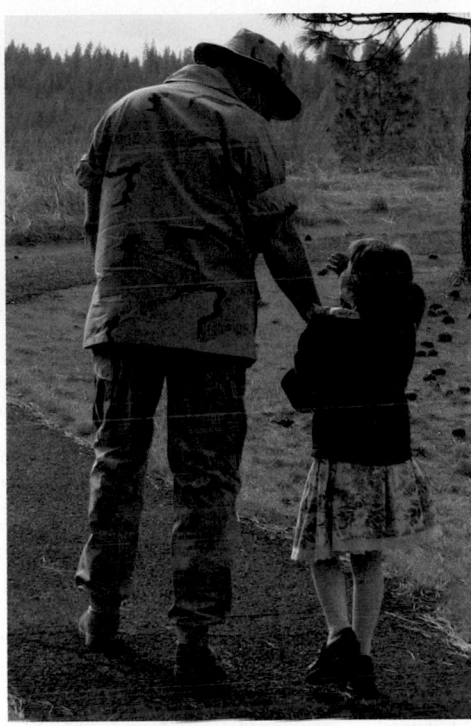

The special relationship between a father about to be deployed in the military and his young daughter is clear. This father has two other children and is spending time with each of them, as well as with the family together, before leaving. The cycle of leaving and returning home can be stressful for families. Nurses can assist military families in making plans for healthcare, finances, and communication while gone and providing resources for emotional support for the entire family.

TABLE 36–2 ✤ **Effects of Divorce**

Age (years)	Behavior
3–5	Fear, anxiety, and dread in daily life events Regression Searching and questioning Self-blame Increased aggression
6–8	Extreme sadness Fantasies and panic Worries about lack of food, money, caretaking
9–12	Intense anger Somatic complaints Confused self-identity
13–18	Withdrawal from family Concern about sex and marriage Sense of loss Anger

Adapted from Wallerstein, J., & Kelly, J. (2000). *Surviving the breakup*. New York: Harper Collins.

SCHOOL AND CHILD CARE

Once a child is 5 or 6 years of age, several hours daily are spent in a school setting. Children develop physical skills through participation in education and sports. Psychosocial stages are met as the child interacts with children and adults and achieves social interaction patterns and pride in accomplishments. The presentation of concepts that challenge thought processes enhances cognitive development.

Although the primary role of schools is educational, they also perform several health-related functions. School health screening programs play an important role in identifying children with such health problems as hearing loss, visual impairment, and scoliosis. Nurses provide assessment, teaching, and clinical management related to some health problems. Some schools have clinics that examine and provide even more complete healthcare for children. Many schools teach good nutrition, healthful living, safe sexual practices, and other health-related subjects. A school nurse may be present, at least part time, to plan these classes or to work with teachers. Nurses assist school districts in providing plans for emergency healthcare when needed. With the increase in mainstreaming, school staff now have the responsibility for administering medications, maintaining urinary catheters,

● FIGURE 36–2

Most children will spend time in childcare settings. It is important to explore options and find the best fit for the child's needs.

and providing respiratory care and other treatments to ensure the child's proper growth and development. See Chapter 35 for further discussion of school nurse activities. ∞

Some children spend part or nearly all of their days in childcare settings (Figure 36–2 ●). Nearly half of all children are in regular child care by their first birthday (Fields, Smith, Bass et al., 2001). While there has been debate about whether child care has a positive or negative impact on children, it appears now that the closeness of the parent-child relationship, the quality of care, and the length of the child-care day are important in determining daycare effects on children (National Institute of Child Health and Human Development, 1997).

Nursing management involves helping parents to explore types of daycare options available and to evaluate programs in their communities (Table 36–3). Care options for young school-age children, either before or after school, can also be shared with parents. When available, recommend early intervention programs with at-risk children, such as the Zero to Three Project and Head Start, which contribute to children's health and welfare. Nurses frequently manage the health programs in early intervention, providing screening, doing health evaluations, and establishing early intervention education plans. Nurses and parents can consult the National Association for the Education of Young Children for recommendations about evaluation of childcare experiences (National Association, 2004).

TEACHING HIGHLIGHTS

EVALUATION OF CHILD CARE

The nurse can help parents to evaluate childcare options and make decisions about placement for their children. Parents should always be welcomed to visit an agency or home child care—this is essential so they can see the routines in action. Some questions they can ask are suggested as follows.

Administration
Is the facility licensed?
Who are the administrators? What is their training and experience?
How many staff are employed? What is their training?
Is there a parent board? What part do they play in administering the center?

Physical Environment, Health, and Safety
What is the neighborhood like? Is transportation to the center convenient?
What is the condition of lighting, heat, cooling, ventilation system, play spaces (inside and out), and the building's general condition?
Is playground equipment safe?
Is there a soft material such as bark, sand, or rubber tiles under climbing equipment?
Is there always supervision for the children?
Are there emergency medical forms and signed forms for field trips?
Who may pick up children? How are they signed in and out?

What is the immunization policy and how are records examined and maintained?
Are criminal background checks of staff done for potential child abuse and other problems?
What is the policy for children with infectious diseases and other illness?
How are foods prepared? Are staff licensed in food handling?
What is the state of general cleanliness?
Who changes diapers? Are recommendations for standard precautions to prevent pathogen transfer followed?
What arrangements and routines are made for naps and quiet times?

Developmental Approaches
Is the curriculum appropriate for different age groups?
Are there materials and plans for gross motor, fine motor, language, and social development?
How much time do children spend in structured time? Free time?
How is discipline handled?
Do the children appear occupied and happy?
What reading materials are available?
What type and quantity of field trips are planned?
What is the educational level and longevity of the childcare workers?
Is there a diversity among the children's backgrounds and experiences?

TABLE 36–3 ✤ Types of Child Care

Type of Care	Description	Advantage/Disadvantage
In home	Caretaker comes to home of the child	Child can remain at home Little exposure to infectious diseases No need for alternative care when child is ill Limited contact with other children to encourage development Most costly
Family child care	Parent brings child to home of a caretaker	Limited number of children Some exposure to other children and encouragement of development Family type atmosphere Little governmental regulation or examination
Center care a. Private, nonprofit (i.e., church, YMCA) b. Public (i.e., Head Start) c. Private proprietary	Parent brings child to a center where many children receive care	A learning curriculum plan is in place Contact with other children can enhance development Exposure to multiple children increases infectious disease risk

COMMUNITY

The community in which a child lives may support the child's development or, conversely, expose the child to hazards. Social programs such as Head Start preschools, sports activities, after-school programs, and child abuse treatment centers offer valuable services that improve the experience of growing children. On the other hand, an economically depressed community with scant services and a high homicide rate is unsupportive and hazardous for growing children.

The physical environment is supportive when the child has sidewalks on which to walk to school, open spaces in which to learn and play, and clean air to breathe. Children who must walk to school on unsafe roads, have access to contaminated drinking supplies, or live near polluting manufacturing companies or in crowded housing or old structures are at risk for injuries and health problems such as lead poisoning (see Chapter 51 ∞).

The following developmental variations place children at high risk for environmental contaminant exposure:

■ Children are smaller than adults and thus are closer to the ground. They are more likely to be exposed to contaminants in soil and on floors, including lead-based paint dust, chemicals, and other pollutants.

■ During infancy and toddlerhood, hand-to-mouth behaviors are common, so young children are more likely to ingest toxic substances.

■ Higher metabolic rates and fluid turnover expose children to air, food, and water contaminants.

■ The nervous system and growth/development of children are vulnerable to toxic insults during early developmental periods (Sattler, Afzal, Condon et al., 2003).

See Table 36–4 for some common contaminants in children's environments and nursing implications.

Nurses should be aware of the types of neighborhoods in the community. Learn about local resources and hazards. Assessment of every child involves getting information about the community and the healthcare that the family needs help to obtain. Refer children when appropriate for lead testing and for safe programs after school. Teach them about injury prevention specific to their communities.

CULTURE

The child's cultural group may influence the use of traditional and contemporary healthcare practices. If the parents or children are recent immigrants, they may still be learning the English language and finding out about healthcare resources. Children and adolescents of immigrants may feel stress as they combine their family's traditional culture with the new culture in which the family now lives. They may also have a great deal of responsibility to interpret for the family since they often can speak two languages and understand practices in the new culture.

Recent immigrants may experience culture shock, a state of crisis related to the difference in values and lifestyle. This can lead to stress-related symptoms, and create a need for healthcare intervention. Children whose parents emigrated from another country may feel different from peers and develop conflict with their parents, particularly during adolescence. Even in families that have been in this country for some time, challenges to mental and physical health can occur.

All cultural groups have rules about patterns of social interaction. Schedules of language acquisition are determined by the number of languages spoken and the amount

TABLE 36–4 ✣ Examples of Environmental Contaminants

Contaminant	Effects	Nursing Implications
Radon	Lung cancer	Radon is a radioactive gas that can seep into homes undetected. Homes should be tested for radon presence. Ask if testing has been done and recommend home test kit or local contractor.
Carbon monoxide	Tissue anoxia from CO combination with hemoglobin, leading to its inability to transport oxygen.	CO is formed during combustion. Newborns and infants are especially vulnerable. Check chimneys for proper burning and ventilation. Do not leave children in or around running cars or place them near the exhaust of motor boats or other vehicles. Do not use charcoal grills inside.
Pesticides	Cancer, neurologic damage	Avoid infestations by storing food and pet supplies correctly. Teach families to follow directions on pesticides and avoid use around children. Wash clothes and skin after use before coming in contact with children. Store pesticides locked out of reach of children.
Food and water contaminants	Gastrointestinal distress, neurologic damage	Common contaminants are mercury (in household batteries and thermometers and in fish), lead (in older homes with peeling lead-based paint), and water (bacterial growth, especially in untreated well water). Assess the home environment for ingestible contaminants. Instruct in safe removal. Be alert for signs of gastrointestinal distress, neurologic changes, or slow development in young children. Newborns and infants are at greatest risk.

Adapted from Sattler, Afzal, Condon et al., 2003.

of speech in the home. The particular social roles assumed by men and women in the culture affect school activities and ultimately career choices. Attitudes toward touching and other methods of encouraging developmental skills vary among cultures. Nurses must become aware of common characteristics of the cultural groups they serve so that they can provide culturally competent nursing care. Arrange for translators when needed. Be aware that families often accept and use both traditional and westernized healthcare, and remain nonjudgmental about traditional healing practices. Provide ethnic foods in healthcare facilities. Evaluate youth in immigrant families for conflict between family and societal expectations.

LIFESTYLE ACTIVITIES AND THEIR INFLUENCE ON CHILD HEALTH

Many patterns of daily life play a part in determining the length and quality of one's life. The child's use of tobacco products and controlled substances influences both physical and mental health. Patterns of exercise and use of protective gear protect against early disabilities. The use of decorative patterns that affect the skin and can introduce pathogens is an example of a lifestyle pattern that influences mental health, body image, and the body's physical health.

TOBACCO USE

Tobacco use is the most preventable cause of adult death in the United States. It leads to 430,000 deaths annually, and will be responsible for the premature death of 5 million of today's youth as they reach adult years (U.S. Department of Health & Human Services, 2000). Major health problems linked to tobacco use include cardiovascular disease, cancer, chronic lung disease, low birth weight, and other maternal problems. Even passive smoking or environmental tobacco smoke (ETS) is linked to increased heart disease, blood pressure, and respiratory problems (Leone, 2003). While cigarettes are most common, chewing tobacco, snuff, cigars, and bidis (small, brown, hand-rolled cigarettes) also pose significant health hazards.

Many nurses view tobacco use as an adult issue. Although sale of tobacco products to children and advertisements aimed at this age group are forbidden by federal law, many youths obtain and use tobacco. After steadily increasing rates of youth smoking for many years, rates began to decrease in 1997. However, a significant number of youth still continue to use tobacco, making this an important health topic. About 30% of high schoolers and 13% of middle schoolers in the United States have smoked within the last 30 days (MMWR, 2003); about 14% of students are frequent smokers (MMWR, 2002). When including children who have ever smoked, the numbers are even larger. About 64% have tried smoking by the time they enter high school (MMWR, 2002). Significant numbers of youth also report using chewing tobacco and cigars in the month prior to being surveyed (U.S. Department of Health & Human Services, 2000). Approximately 3000 youths per day try their first cigarette; the major ages for trying tobacco are 9 to 14 years, between sixth and ninth grade. Early initiation of smoking becomes an extremely risky behavior when it is recognized that 80% of current adult smokers began smoking before 18 years of age (MMWR, 2001). Nicotine is highly addictive, and most people become addicted to the substance in adolescent years.

Certain characteristics contribute to the likelihood of tobacco use. They include increasing age, male gender, ethnic group, ease of obtaining tobacco products, and smoking among family members. Low socioeconomic group membership, access to tobacco products, low price of products, advertising, and lack of parental involvement in the youths' lives are associated with tobacco use (U.S. Department of Health & Human Services, 2000). Girls commonly cite reasons for smoking such as a desire to be slim and to appear mature, while boys more often view smoking as a way to be tough and rebellious. Both genders admit that smoking helps them to feel part of a group (Hanson, 1999) (Figure 36–3 ●).

DEVELOPING CULTURAL COMPETENCE

SMOKING RATES AMONG YOUTH

Among youth in the United States, white youth are significantly more likely to smoke than either Hispanic or black peers. About 32% of white students reported smoking in the previous month, while 27% of Hispanic and 15% of black students report this behavior (MMWR, 2002). American Indian and Alaska Natives also have high smoking rates, while Asian Americans have low rates (U.S. Department of Health & Human Services, 2000).

Several programs have been developed to encourage youth to avoid tobacco use. In addition, smoking cessation programs are available to assist youth who are already regular smokers, and successfully achieve the goals of cessation or decrease in tobacco use (Coleman-Wallace, Lee, Montgomery et al., 1999). Smoking cessation efforts are more successful in teens who smoke occasionally rather than daily, so keeping occasional smokers from becoming regular smokers is important. Smoking cessation may involve use of peer leadership and support, counseling, and computer instruction. When teens have become regular smokers, nicotine replacement therapy may be needed since they are likely addicted to nicotine (Donovan, 2000). Once a teen is identified as a smoker, using a biologic marker such as urine cotinine (a by-product of tobacco)

● FIGURE 36–3

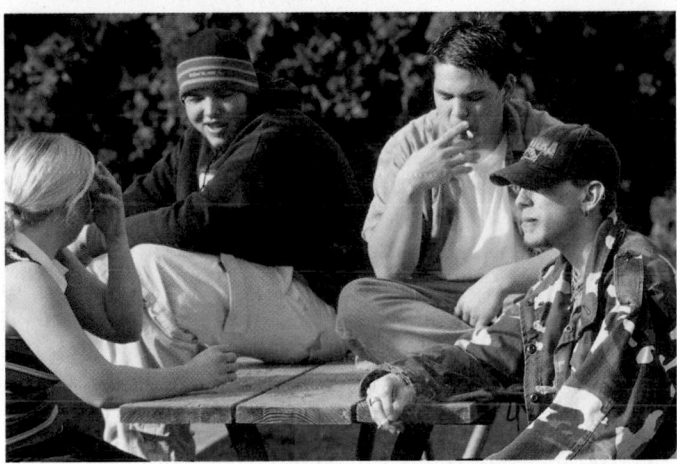

Approximately 70% of children have tried smoking by their high school years. Early intervention can begin with discussions about smoking starting at 9 or 10 years of age.

levels can help to identify the frequency of smoking. This information can be used to make suggestions to the teen about the potential outcomes of the behavior and the cessation program which is most likely to be helpful.

NURSING MANAGEMENT

NURSING ASSESSMENT AND DIAGNOSIS

Nurses are in a unique position to inquire about the incidence of smoking and other tobacco use among youth. Insert questions into all well-child visits, beginning at about 9 to 10 years of age. Inquire about whether family members (especially parents and siblings) smoke or chew, and ask if some of the child's friends have tried smoking. Try to find out the child's knowledge and beliefs about the benefits and risks of tobacco use. As the child gets older, ask more direct and detailed questions. A nonjudgmental approach will be best to obtain a truthful response. School nurses can make observations about numbers of teens smoking and general attitudes about tobacco use. When children come to hospitals and other health facilities for care, use of tobacco should be part of general admission questions.

Some nursing diagnoses that may apply to youth who smoke or show potential for this behavior include the following:

- *Activity Intolerance* related to lowered oxygen supply
- *Impaired Gas Exchange* related to ventilation-perfusion imbalance
- *Chronic Low Self-Esteem* related to negative self-appraisal

- *Health-Seeking Behaviors of Dangers of Tobacco Use* related to developmental focus on present
- *Imbalanced Nutrition, Less than Body Requirements* related to effects of chemical dependence

PLANNING AND IMPLEMENTATION

The roles of nurses in preventing and intervening in youth smoking are to inform youth, identify smokers, and implement programs (Table 36–5). Provide developmentally appropriate information about the hazards of tobacco use in all settings where youth are present. Posters, flyers, and speakers are particularly useful. Addicted teens who share their stories of difficult withdrawal from tobacco, and adults who have had cancer of the lungs or larynx may be effective speakers. Find out where teens obtain tobacco products in the community and where they use the products in order to target these places. Offer information on prevention and cessation programs to youths and families in clinics, outpatient surgery centers, community activities, and hospitals. Use opportunities such as adolescent pregnancy and illness to reinforce the hazardous effects of tobacco on the individual and on those around. Speak to young athletes about the effects of tobacco on athletic performance. Show youth the ways this product can interfere with meeting life goals. Role-play how to tell other youth "no" when tobacco is offered. Establish programs that increase the sense of self-esteem without tobacco use. Be sure to include parents in the programs so that they see and acknowledge their role in setting an example about tobacco use, and in providing guidelines for the child. Provide information on the influence of environmental tobacco (secondhand smoke).

Adopt a nonjudgmental attitude when asking questions about smoking so that youth using tobacco can be identified. Ask questions without parents present and assure youth that the information will not be shared. Encourage youth to cut back and to quit use of tobacco products. Offer assistance to them in these efforts.

Work with the schools and school districts to help establish preventive and cessation programs. There should be clear guidelines about school policies regarding smoking on school grounds. Keeping occasional youth smokers from becoming regular users should be a goal in order to avoid nicotine addiction. Find out what positive incentives can be offered to youth who are successful in quitting smoking. Contract with them to achieve their goals.

EVALUATION

Expected outcomes of nursing interventions regarding tobacco use are lowered rates of regular use, delayed initiation of use, and success of cessation programs. Use the *Healthy People 2010* (U.S. Department of Health and Human Services, 2000) objectives as guidelines:

- Reduce the proportion of children who are regularly exposed to tobacco smoke at home to 10%.
- Increase smoke-free and tobacco-free environments in schools, including all school facilities, property, vehicles, and school events, to 100%.
- Eliminate tobacco advertising and promotions that influence adolescents and young adults.
- Increase adolescents' disapproval of smoking to 95%.
- Reduce tobacco use by adolescents to 21%.
- Increase the average age of first use of tobacco products from 12 years to 14 years.

TABLE 36–5 ✣ Nursing Role in Youth Smoking Prevention

Inform

- Hang posters, provide brochures, and facilitate presentations about smoking risks in all settings where youth are present.
- Target smokers with special information about the effects of nicotine on their bodies.

Identify

- Ask questions about smoking and other tobacco use at every health encounter beginning at about 9 to 10 years of age.
- For users, ask amount and type of tobacco.
- Find resources where youth obtain tobacco in the community and become proactive in stopping sales.

Implement

- Encourage youth tobacco users to quit.
- Facilitate referral to cessation programs.
- Arrange positive rewards for youth successful in cessation.

SUBSTANCE USE

Substance abuse occurs in children and adolescents of all socioeconomic levels and is a growing health problem. The use of any drug can pose a serious psychologic and physical risk to children and adolescents.

Although a decline in the daily use of marijuana by adolescents has been reported, abuse of other substances, particularly alcohol, cocaine, crack, and heroin, remains high. The Youth Risk Behavior Surveillance of high school seniors reported the following alarming statistics: 75% have had alcohol to drink, 45% had an alcoholic drink in the last month, 28% engaged in binge drinking of alcohol, and the average age for beginning alcohol and cigarette use was 12 years (MMWR, 2004). Prevalence increases with advancing age and grade in school, and 47% of children have had their first drink by 9 years of age (Fetro, Coyle, & Pham, 2001). About 40% of students have used marijuana; 9% have used cocaine;

● **FIGURE 36–4**

 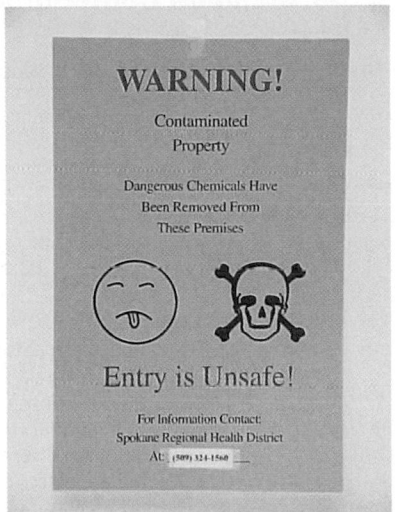

Methamphetamine is a popular drug because it can be manufactured with items that are available to the lay public. Manufacture of the substance in homes has become a concern of health departments and communities at large. Children can be harmed by the chemicals produced and may experience neglect and abuse. They may suffer even after the home is found and adults are apprehended as they must be placed in foster homes.

Courtesy of Spokane Regional Health District, Spokane, WA

12% report inhalant use of glue, paints, or other substances; 8% report methamphetamine use (Figure 36–4 ●); 11% report ecstasy use; and 3% have used heroin (MMWR, 2004). Synthetic drugs such as phencyclidine (PCP) (commonly called "designer" drugs) mimic other narcotics, stimulants, and hallucinogens and are also dangerous.

Over-the-counter medications are legal, but frequently abused. Easily obtainable at grocery stores and drugstores, these drugs include antihistamines, atropine, bromides, caffeine, ephedrine, pseudoephedrine, phenylpropanolamine, and amphetamine-like substitutes. Volatile inhalants, such as glues, are dangerous substances of abuse, and their use appears to be rising among school-age children and adolescents. Anabolic steroids are the drugs of abuse most commonly used by athletes. Some common contemporary drugs and street names are listed in Table 36–6.

Etiology and Pathophysiology

In most cases substance abuse represents a maladaptive coping response to the stressors of childhood and adoles-

NURSING PRACTICE

Following are common inhalant agents:

Aerosols	**Solvents**
Cooking spray	Nail polish remover
Whipped cream	Paint thinner or cleaner
Spray paint	Lighter fluid
Cosmetic sprays	Degreaser
Adhesives	**Other**
Model glues	Gasoline
Rubber cements	Helium

Note: From Cook (1999). Adapted.

cence. A child may begin using drugs or alcohol to deal with stress because family members or peers do so. Children in families with a history of substance abuse are at higher risk of abusing drugs and alcohol. Other risk factors include rebelliousness, aggressiveness, low self-esteem, dysfunctional parental relationships, lack of adequate support systems, academic underachievement, poor judgment, and poor impulse control. Adolescents and young adults most commonly use "club drugs" to achieve greater satisfaction during nights of dancing, drinking, and attending clubs. Use of these drugs with alcohol can lead to deadly consequences. See Table 36–6 for common club drugs.

Initial experimentation with alcohol or drugs may be unpleasant. With continued use, however, the adolescent learns to "achieve the high," an illusion of power and well-being. The adolescent wants the high more frequently and

TABLE 36–6 ✤ Common Contemporary Club Drugs, Street Names, and Drug Information

Drug	Action	Street Names	Route	Time of Action
Methylenedioxymethamphetamine (MDMA)	Stimulant; appetite suppressant; increased pulse, BP, temperature, overhydration, hyponatremia, memory loss	Ecstasy, XTC, X, Adam, Clarity, Lover's speed	PO (tablets, capsules)	3–6 hours
Gamma-hydroxybutyrate (GHB)	CNS depressant, euphoria, growth hormone release	Grievous Bodily Harm, G., Liquid Ecstasy, Georgia Home Boy	PO (liquid, powder, tablets, capsules)	4 hours
Ketamine	Anesthetic; decreased memory, attention, learning; increased BP; respiratory collapse	Special K, K, Vitamin K, Cat Valiums	IV, respiratory (injected, snorted or smoked; liquid or powder)	1–2 hours
Rohypnol (benzodiazepine)	Amnesia, sedative; decreased BP, urinary retention; given prior to sexual assault	Roffies, Rophies, Roche, Forget-me Pill	PO, respiratory (snorted; tablets)	8–12 hours
Methamphetamine	Stimulant; highly addictive; memory loss, violence, psychosis; cardiac and neurologic damage	Speed, Ice, Chalk, Meth, Crystal, Crank, Fire, Glass	PO, respiratory, IV (smoked, snorted, injected)	Several hours; long-term permanent effects
Lysergic acid diethylamide (LSD)	Hallucinogen; increased pulse, BP, temperature; psychosis, flashbacks	Acid, Boomers, Yellow Sunshines	PO (liquid, tablets, capsules)	1–2 hours; possible flashbacks later

Data from National Institute on Drug Abuse. 2004. *NIDA Community Drug Alert Bulletin—Club Drugs.* Bethesda, MD: U.S. Department of Health and Human Services.

actively seeks alcohol or drugs. Tolerance to the substance occurs with continued use, and ever-increasing amounts are required to achieve a pleasurable high. Physical and psychologic dependence ensues as the body's tissues require the substance to function properly. Withdrawal symptoms occur when the child or adolescent is deprived of the substance.

Clinical Manifestations

Substance abuse in children and adolescents is commonly overlooked and underdiagnosed by healthcare providers (Pagliaro & Pagliaro, 1996). This is due in part to the wide range of clinical presentations, which vary according to type of drug abused, amount, frequency, time of last use, and severity of drug dependence.

Common physical manifestations include alterations in vital signs, weight loss, chronic fatigue, chronic cough, respiratory congestion, red eyes, and general apathy and malaise. Withdrawal may be shown by anxiety, headache, tremors, nausea and vomiting, malaise, weakness, insomnia, depressed mood or irritability, and hallucinations. The mental status examination (refer to Chapter 35 ∞) may reveal alterations in level of consciousness, impaired attention and concentration, impaired thought processes, delusions, and hallucinations. Low self-esteem, feelings of guilt or worthlessness, and suicidal or homicidal thoughts are also common.

Poor school performance and changes in mood, sleep habits, appetite, dress, and social relationships are nonspecific characteristics of the substance-abusing child.

Clinical Therapy

Multiple psychiatric diagnostic criteria exist for each drug class. Children and adolescents who have other psychosocial disorders commonly use or abuse drugs or alcohol. Treatment should therefore focus not only on the substance use or abuse, but also on the issues underlying the problem. Intervention includes the family as well as the substance-abusing child or adolescent.

The primary goal of treatment is to teach the child and other family members to develop and sustain positive coping patterns, and to support them during this process. Most treatment programs offer inpatient and outpatient services, as well as after-care programs. These programs usually consist of peer support that focuses on developing a drug- and alcohol-free lifestyle, healthy family relationships, and positive coping skills. Family involvement is strongly encouraged. Hospitalization is required if the physical dependence is significant and withdrawal places the child at risk for complications such as seizures, depression, or suicidal behavior.

CLINICAL MANIFESTATIONS

COMMONLY ABUSED DRUGS

DRUG	POTENTIAL FOR DEPENDENCE	CLINICAL MANIFESTATIONS
Depressants Alcohol, barbiturates (amobarbital, pentobarbital, secobarbital)	*Physical and psychologic:* High; varies somewhat among drugs	*Physical:* Decreased muscle tone and coordination, tremors *Psychologic:* Impaired speech, memory, and judgment, confusion; decreased attention span; emotional lability
Stimulants Amphetamines (e.g., Benzedrine), caffeine, cocaine	*Physical:* Low to moderate *Psychologic:* High; withdrawal from amphetamines and cocaine can lead to severe depression	*Physical:* Dilated pupils, increased pulse and blood pressure, flushing, nausea, loss of appetite, tremors *Psychologic:* Euphoria; increased alertness, agitation, or irritability; hallucinations; insomnia
Opiates Codeine, heroin, meperidine (Demerol), methadone, morphine, opium, oxycodone (Percodan)	*Physical and psychologic:* High; varies somewhat among drugs; withdrawal effects are uncomfortable but rarely life threatening	*Physical:* Analgesia, depressed respirations and muscle tone (may lead to coma or death), nausea, constricted pupils *Psychologic:* Changes in mood (usually euphoria), drowsiness, impaired attention or memory, sense of tranquility
Hallucinogens Lysergic acid diethylamide (LSD), mescaline, phencyclidine (PCP)	*Physical:* None *Psychologic:* Unknown	*Physical:* Lack of coordination, dilated pupils, hypertension, elevated temperature; severe PCP intoxication can result in seizures, respiratory depression, coma, and death *Psychologic:* Visual illusions and hallucinations, altered perceptions of time and space, emotional lability, psychosis
Volatile Inhalants Glues, typing correction fluid, acrylic paints, spot removers, lighter fluid, gasoline, butane	*Physical and psychologic:* Varies with drug used	*Physical:* Impaired coordination, liver damage (in some cases) *Psychologic:* Impaired judgment, delirium
Marijuana	*Physical:* Low *Psychologic:* Usually low; occasionally moderate to high	*Physical:* Tachycardia, reddened conjunctiva, dry mouth, increased appetite *Psychologic:* Initial anxiety followed by euphoria; giddiness; impaired attention, judgment, and memory

NURSING MANAGEMENT

NURSING ASSESSMENT AND DIAGNOSIS

Nurses may encounter the substance-abusing child or adolescent in the emergency department or outpatient clinic, in schools and other community settings, or during hospitalization for an injury or other acute problem.

Nursing assessment includes taking a thorough history from the parents and child, observing the child's behavior, and performing a physical examination. The history should include the age at which drug use began, pattern of use, length of time the drug has been used, amount of drug used, and psychologic state while on drugs. A history of parental drug use and noninvolvement in parenting the child puts the child at higher risk for substance abuse, reflecting the combined effects of genetic and environmental influences. Assessment tools provide useful information. One tool known as PACES collects information about parents and peers, accidents and alcohol or other drug use, cigarette use, emotional problems, and school and sexuality issues (Knight, 1997). Another useful assessment tool, called HEEADSS, is described in Table 35–6 in Chapter 35.∞ It is used to evaluate the home, education, alcohol, drugs, smoking, and sex practices of the teen.

Physiologic Assessment

Look for physical signs and symptoms of substance abuse, including bloodshot eyes, dilated pupils, slurred speech, and weight loss. The adolescent may appear sleepy or restless, or may show signs of clumsiness or inconsistent behavior. Consider all types of substance abuse, including model glue, gasoline, and other sources. Consider signs of withdrawal as well as current intoxication.

Psychologic Assessment

Changes in social habits may indicate substance abuse. Parents may report a drop in the school-age child's or adolescent's grades or decreased interest in school activities. The adolescent does not introduce new friends to parents, and has less contact with parents, teachers, and other adults who were previously important. Note the child's current drug use, potential for violence, and motivation to make changes. Assess the degree of family support available.

Nursing diagnoses for children and adolescents who abuse drugs or alcohol might include the following:

- *Impaired Social Interaction* related to altered thought processes
- *Chronic Low Self-Esteem* related to dysfunctional family and social relationships
- *Risk for Injury* related to altered perceptions and sensorium
- *Risk for Violence: Self-Directed or Other-Directed* related to physiologic dependence on drugs, alcohol, and other substances

PLANNING AND IMPLEMENTATION

Care of children and adolescents who abuse drugs, alcohol, and other substances is challenging and often frustrating. Long-term mental health counseling may be necessary to resolve underlying issues and foster lifestyle and behavioral changes.

Prevention is the most desirable intervention. The nurse can play a major role in teaching children and their families about substance abuse. Education should begin in primary school, and continue with intensification during

TEACHING HIGHLIGHTS

IDENTIFYING THE YOUTH WHO IS ABUSING SUBSTANCES

Families are often confused about the behavior of adolescents and unsure whether it represents normal development or abuse of substances. Some characteristics of normal development that help to differentiate these occurrences are listed as follows. When concerned about possible substance use, the parent can confront the child or talk with school nurses or counselors.

- Many youth are periodically distant with parents but remain involved with peers in school sports and other activities. Withdrawal from all activities and friends may indicate substance abuse.
- Adolescents often complain about school, but when teachers report the student meets expectations and is consistently performing in the classroom, this is normal behavior.
- Teens may be weepy on occasion when having a difficult time with friends or not performing as desired. Continued, consistent weepiness is more likely to indicate depression or substance abuse.
- Teens like to stay up late and are frequently tired in the morning, whereas abusing teens may "nod off" frequently during the day.
- Many adolescents like to achieve a disheveled look in clothing, but the teen who frequently neglects basic hygiene or does not seem to have the energy to wash and dress may be depressed or be abusing substances.
- All teens get some infections, but abusing teens may have reddened eyes, oral sores, and constant respiratory discomfort from "snorting" substances.

middle school and high school. Nurses also can play a major role in community education. Various prevention programs have been developed by federal and private organizations. Referral to support organizations may be beneficial for the child, parents, and other family members. Self-help groups, available in most communities, include Alcoholics Anonymous, Narcotics Anonymous, Al-Anon, Nar-Anon, and Ala-Teen. Parents may receive support from a group such as Parents Anonymous.

The youth's protective factors can be identified and used in planning appropriate interventions. For example, a child with goals for a future career can be helped to see how substance use will interfere with goal attainment. Identifying a strong role model through a program like Big Brothers or Big Sisters can assist children who lack that strength in their families.

Expected outcomes of nursing interventions include abstention from alcohol and street drugs, successful participation in substance abuse programs, and developmentally appropriate social and cognitive skills.

PHYSICAL INACTIVITY

In the past few decades, children have become increasingly sedentary. This change is a reflection of lifestyles in which car travel is valued, computers and televisions are part of daily life, neighborhoods are sometimes unsafe places for play, and schools do not routinely require daily physical education classes (Figure 36–5 ●). Children and adolescents spend an average of almost 3 hours per day watching television; when video games and computers are included, the total average is 6 1/2 hours daily (Committee on Public Education, American Academy of Pediatrics, 2001). Children who watch 4 or more hours of television daily get significantly less physical activity and have poorer sports performance than those who watch 1 hour or less (Crespo, Smit, Troiano et al., 2001). There is often a high intake of fatty snacks during television viewing. Even at very young ages, children are immersed in various types of media. A nationally representative survey of 1065 parents of children from 6 months to 6 years found that 25% of children under 2 years of age and 36% of those under 6 years have a television in their bedrooms (Rideout, Vandewater, & Wartella, 2003).

Physical inactivity leads to many health concerns. A primary outcome is overweight or obesity (see Chapter 34 ∞). Other outcomes can be an increased rate of type 2 diabetes (see Chapter 56 ∞), increased exposure to television/computer game violence and sexual activity at early ages, and early progression of cardiovascular disease (see Chapter 48 ∞).

On the other hand, patterns of physical activity established in childhood can increase exercise behaviors in adulthood; contribute to lower rates of low back pain, overweight, osteoporosis, heart disease, diabetes, colon cancer, and high blood pressure; and lead to a more positive self-image.

Although many children demonstrate low levels of physical activity, a profound decrease in vigorous activity is common in grades 9 through 12. Boys who do remain active generally engage in team sports and weight training, while girls more commonly enjoy aerobics and dance classes (*U.S. Department of Health and Human Services,* 2000).

Health professionals can integrate assessment of physical activity into all healthcare, and make recommendations to children and families that will help to increase opportunities for physical activity. Nurses can assess height, weight, and body mass index to look for signs of overweight (see Chapter 34 ∞). Children should be asked about how they like to spend free time. Community and school activities should be encouraged and rewarded. Examples include fun runs, walks of benefit causes, aerobics classes, team sports, roadside cleanups, fairs, and carnivals. Help parents and children learn what they can do for physical fitness. Work with school physical education personnel to plan activities both in and out of physical education class that promote lifelong exercise routines.

INJURY AND PROTECTIVE EQUIPMENT

In the discussion of causes of childhood and adolescent morbidities and mortalities in Chapter 1, unintentional injuries are listed as a common problem. In fact, 71% of all deaths from age 10 years onward result from four causes—motor-vehicle crashes, other unintentional injury, homicide, and suicide (MMWR, 2004). Chapter 37 and Chapter 38

● **FIGURE 36–5**

Physical inactivity is a growing problem among children and can contribute to poor health. It is important to balance sedentary activities, such as playing computer games, with physical and social activities. Sports are an excellent way for children to develop their psychosocial, cognitive, and motor skills.

Soccer photo courtesy of Rebecca Scheirer, Kensington, Maryland.

MediaLink ● Extreme Sports Video

TEACHING HIGHLIGHTS

PHYSICAL ACTIVITY GUIDELINES FOR YOUTH

- Engage in moderate physical activity (bike-riding, walking, baseball, rollerblading) at least 30 minutes 5 times weekly.
- Engage in vigorous physical activity that causes sweating and hard breathing (soccer, running, ice hockey) at least 20 minutes 3 times weekly.
- Encourage schools to offer physical education to all students, and have students sign up when this is an elective.
- Encourage walking and bike-riding to friends' homes and stores whenever safe.
- Plan physical activities together as a family.
- Get a pet and plan to walk the pet together daily.
- Limit television and other similar sedentary activities to no more than 2 hours daily.
- On days home, allow the child to watch television for up to 1 hour, and then insist that 1 hour of reading, 1 hour of physical activity, and 1 hour of socializing with others take place before returning to more television.

● **FIGURE 36–6**

What protective gear should children use for skateboarding? How would you convince them to use the protection?

discuss the frequent injuries seen in children at different developmental ages, and safety precautions to avoid injuries from car crashes, falls, poisonings, and other developmentally related injuries. ∞ Many common injuries are preventable with simple use of protective gear and following of safety guidelines (Figure 36–6 ●). Some sports and activities that require safety gear include rollerblading, skateboarding, roller hockey, ice hockey, football, soccer, baseball, scooters, and skiing or snowboarding fast or using jumps.

It is important to consider that 18% of youths rarely or never wear seat belts in automobiles and 38% of those who ride motorcycles do not wear helmets (MMWR, 2004). Emphasize safe automobile and motorcycle behaviors in adolescence, with the recognition that risks increase if driving is combined with use of alcohol and controlled substances. Adolescents sometimes engage in practices that put them at particular risk, and nurses should be alert for such activities in their communities. Examples include car surfing (standing on the trunk, hood, or roof of a moving vehicle) (Geiger, Drongowski, & Lenni, 2001) or street racing (racing cars down a street at extremely high speed).

Many children ride bicycles, but only about 14% are protected by helmet use, contributing to 23,000 bicycle-related head injuries annually. Bike helmets could prevent up to 88% of serious brain injuries from bicycle crashes (Committee on Injury and Poison Prevention, American Academy of Pediatrics, 2001). Strategies to make helmet use more attractive to children and adolescents are needed. Nurses can play a major role in programs to educate and reward children for helmet use, and can assist families to find affordable helmets. Nurses can be active in identifying behaviors in youths in specific communities and working with schools and other community groups to establish educational programs. Efforts should also include adequate conditioning for sports, proper treatment of injuries, and prevention of overuse injuries (Committee on Sports Medicine and Fitness, 2001).

DEVELOPING CULTURAL COMPETENCE

ETHNIC DISPARITY IN UNINTENTIONAL CHILDHOOD INJURIES

Striking ethnic disparity rates exist in the rates of unintentional injury among children. These differences are due mainly to living in impoverished communities rather than any innate biologic variations. Although the unintentional injury rate in children under 14 years declined 39% from 1987 to 2000, the smallest reductions were among American Indian/Alaskan Natives (20% decline) and African-American children (36% decline), while higher reductions were seen in Asian/Pacific Islanders (52% decline) and white children (39% decline) (National Safe Kids Campaign, 2003). What are the major causes of unintentional injury in your community and state? What ethnic and age groups are at greatest risk? How can you integrate teaching in your practice that is specific to the findings in your community?

A growing number of children engage in "extreme" sports, those that carry a high degree of risk and have not traditionally been common. Some examples are mountain biking, three-wheeling, ski racing, snowboarding through trees and on courses with pikes and other challenges, ice climbing, rock climbing, and wake boarding. While the nurse is probably unable to dissuade youth from engaging in these activities, safety measures should be emphasized. Find out what protective gear the youth wears and what is recommended. Provide examples of stories of youth who have been saved by use of such gear. Encourage the youth to engage in sports activities only when others are present and to have a plan for emergencies, including a working cell phone, leaving information with an adult about plans and expected return, and planning for harsh weather with items such as emergency blankets, gear, and food. Encourage the youth to talk with parents and other adults about the risks and benefits of the activities.

BODY ART

Body art in the form of painting, tattooing, and piercing has been used by humans throughout history. In recent years, there has been a resurgence of interest in this decorative art among teens. Many adolescents have multiple body piercings and tattoos and may even resort to performing these decorations on themselves or friends.

From 10% to 25% of adolescents have tattoos, and even more have at least one body piercing (Armstrong & Kelly, 2001). In some states, teens must be 18 years of age or have parental permission to obtain body art, but students often report that it is easy to have an adult present who signs and claims to be a parent. Amy, described at the opening of this chapter, had her piercing done by a friend. In some states, tattoo and body piercing businesses must be licensed and comply with certain regulations, while in others there are no regulations. Amy demonstrates some common characteristics of teens that choose to use body art. It may be seen as a way to establish individualism and independence, and helps some teens to feel part of a peer group. Multiple tattoos and piercings are common, as is the case with Amy (Figure 36–7 ●).

Body art is a common source of infections with skin pathogens, as well as hepatitis B and C. Body piercing is a major method of transmission of hepatitis C, a disease that may not even become manifested until years later. It can be a source of HIV if proper techniques are not followed. Piercings in parts of the body such as the mouth or navel are most prone to bacterial infection and continued redness and irritation. Serious systemic infections such as endocarditis have occurred after some piercings. The pierced site may not appear infected, but transfer of organisms causes serious infection and heart damage. Com-

Talk openly with adolescents about their health and teach them to avoid health risks connected with tattoos and piercing.

mon infective agents include *Neisseria* and *Staphylococcus*. When noting signs of systemic infection such as fever, weakness, malaise, and arthralgia (see Chapter 48 for full discussion of endocarditis ∞), gather history about body piercings and refer for care to the primary healthcare provider (Goldrick, 2003). Pierced tongues can lead to chipped teeth or even be the cause of choking if dislodged from the site.

Another issue that the teen should consider is the relationship of the tattoos to future lifestyle changes. Advise teens to avoid tattooing the name of a person or musical group since relationships change and tastes in music evolve. Be sure they know the meaning of phrases, foreign words, or Asian symbols. Consider the visibility of the tattoo and its effect on future employment. Tattoos on the face, neck, or other readily visible places may be a detriment during employment interviews. Tattoos should always be considered permanent. Methods for removal may be costly, painful, and unsuccessful (Selekman, 2003).

Another form of body art that is regarded as disfigurement is *branding* or scarification. In this process, the skin is burned to result in a scar. Commonly a desired sign, symbol, or word is inscribed. Results are usually not precise and do not adhere to expected designs. This procedure is done on the self or friend, using common household metal implements heated in fires or stoves. Others cut themselves in the form of a desired design, a process called *cutting*. These practices can result in infection, often do not yield the desired result, and may indicate underlying problems. They should be discouraged, and the youth involved should be referred for further assessment by primary care providers or counselors.

Since teens may choose to obtain body art even if parents object and if there are state laws to prohibit or make it difficult, nursing care must focus on providing information for the teen, assessing sites, identifying infections, and referring if needed. Care is almost always provided in community settings such as clinics or schools. Consider asking teens if they are thinking about body art since they often do not seek advice before obtaining the art and may not get adequate teaching (Montgomery & Parks, 2001).

SEXUAL ORIENTATION

Adolescence is a time of identifying emerging sexuality. Most teens establish relationships with members of the opposite sex and learn how to interact in ways guided by their peer group, family, and culture. For some youth, the transition into adult sexuality is more challenging, as they feel emotional and sexual attraction to people of the same sex (**homosexuality**). The term **gay** is often used for homosexual males and **lesbian** for homosexual females. Other youth are **bisexual**, or attracted to both men and women, and some are **transgendered**, or are attracted to dress and act like members of the opposite sex. The abbreviation LGBT is sometimes used to refer collectively to these minority sexuality choices. From 1% to 10% of youth identify as homosexual (Benton, 2003).

THINKING CRITICALLY

THE ADOLESCENT WITH BODY PIERCINGS

Amy is 15 years old and attends an alternative high school. She recently had an ear piercing and it is sore. She comes to the health room to ask the advice of the school nurse. The area around the piercing is inflamed and mildly edematous. After asking some questions, the nurse learns that Amy's ear was pierced by a friend, using a needle that had been "sterilized" by passing it through a match flame. She has had a slight fever, but otherwise feels fine.

In her home state, adolescents under 18 years of age must have the signature of a parent for body piercings and tattoos, so Amy chose to have the procedure done by a friend. She believes this is safe since her friend has done many piercings on others. She admits that her parents are not very pleased with her body art, but that they allow her to do it as long as she agrees to stay in high school. She had previously run away and spent several weeks living on the streets.

- What healthcare and social needs does Amy have?
- How can you support both Amy and her parents?
- What physical care does Amy need to treat potential infection at her piercing site?
- What systemic infectious diseases is Amy at risk of acquiring due to repeated body piercings with unsterile technique?

TEACHING HIGHLIGHTS

CARE FOR TATTOOS AND BODY PIERCINGS

Before the Procedure
- Does the studio look clean?
- Visit several studios to make comparisons of techniques, quality, and cleanliness.
- Ask to watch a tattoo or piercing done on someone else.
- What are the artist's sterilization and hygiene practices?
- Is the artist licensed? Trained?
- Look at pictures of completed art and talk with former clients.
- Insist that new, sterile equipment be opened in front of the person to be decorated.
- Consider if this permanent body decoration is desired for a lifetime.
- Consider what the tattoo or piercing will look like in several years.
- Consider the possible side effects of infection, dislike for the art, and allergy to dyes or metals.
- Be sure that hepatitis B vaccination is completed before the procedure.
- Be aware that no immunization is available to protect against the health risks of hepatitis C and HIV.

Care after the Procedure
- Touch the area only after carefully washing your hands.
- Keep the area elevated and use ice for the first 2 days to minimize swelling.

- Avoid contact with another person's body fluids until well healed.
- Turn the piercing jewelry gently several times daily using washed hands.
- Use antibacterial mouthwash or cleaner or ointment as recommended.
- Avoid pressure and rubbing on the site (such as belts on navel piercings).
- Watch carefully for signs of infection and report them to a healthcare provider:
  - Increased redness
  - Swelling
  - Pain
  - Hot feeling
  - Discharge
- Ask the artist how long healing will take. It varies from 2 months in the mouth or up to 6 or 8 months for a navel.
- Metal is dangerous during some medical procedures such as magnetic resonance imaging (MRI) or during surgery. Be sure to tell doctors and nurses about your piercings when you are hospitalized or receiving medical care, especially if they are in a part of the body not readily visible.
- If you decide to remove a piece of jewelry soon after it is placed, the skin may heal with only a slight scar.

Sexual attractions and practices different than the mainstream are not deviant nor symptoms of a mental disorder but should be viewed as part of a continuum of sexual expression. Although there are psychodynamic, genetic, and biologic theories about homosexuality, the reasons why some individuals become homosexual are not clear. For some teens the process of "coming out" or telling others they are homosexual can be a difficult experience (Sadock & Sadock, 2003).

LGBT youth are at risk for a variety of problems related to emotional and physical health. These include rejection by family members and peers, verbal harassment, sexual abuse and physical assault, a high rate of suicide, substance abuse, high rate of homelessness, and sexual risks of HIV and other sexually transmitted diseases (Stevens & Morgan, 2001). Their health risks need to be identified and appropriate care provided.

Nurses can provide healthcare for LGBT youth in a variety of settings. School nurses and clinics can display a sign to demonstrate that they are accepting of persons with minority sexual preferences. These signs are rainbows or triangles with several colors shown and can be obtained from local "gay pride" or other groups. Terminology in assessment should be gender-free. Ask "Do you have one or more sexual partners?" rather than "Do you have a boyfriend?" When youth identify as LGBT, provide usual care of all kinds. This includes preventive care such as immunizations, sports assessments, and injury prevention teaching. Be alert that the youth may have additional health challenges. Ask about peer and parental support; refer to support groups if needed. Provide resources for homelessness and when the teen is depressed or suicidal (see Chapter 54 ∞). Perform testing for sexually transmitted diseases if the teen is having sexual contact, and teach preventive measures. Foster a positive sense of self-esteem through encouraging positive activities such as sports, music, and friendships with peers.

EFFECTS OF VIOLENCE

Violence is a threatened or actual use of physical force that leads to actual or potential physical or emotional trauma. In the past several years, adults and children alike have been shocked by the violent episodes in schools. Although these incidents had much media coverage, they are just one type of violence to which children may be regularly exposed. Children can be the recipients of violence during child abuse and homicides, and they themselves can perform acts of violence on others. They may be touched by violence when parents, siblings, or other family members are killed in gang conflicts, in terrorist attacks, or in wars. The effects of violence are far-reaching and ongoing; they permeate the victim's entire lifetime. This section explores some types of violence affecting children.

SCHOOLS AND COMMUNITIES

At a time when firearm deaths are decreasing overall, unintentional deaths and suicides have increased among children. About 75% of these deaths are committed with firearms found in the home. Forty percent of households with children have guns, and in 25% of those homes the firearms are stored loaded or are not secured under lock (Society for Pediatric Nurses, 2000).

Homicide in children has gained attention in the last several years due to several shootings at schools. While homicide is an extreme example, there are other types of violence. Children report being threatened verbally and with guns or knives at home, in schools, and in their neighborhoods. They may be beaten up or bullied or harassed. They may view domestic violence in their own homes. They may be subjected to dangerous situations in their neighborhoods or during times of homelessness. About half of youths report experiencing serious threats to their well-being (Pratt & Greydanus, 2000). Date rape or other sexual violence is reported by up to 15% of teens (Spencer & Bryant, 2000).

MediaLink Video: Violence in the Media

NURSING PRACTICE

When a group of children is attacked or killed in a school shooting, this tragic occurrence has the attention of the media. Little do many realize that this tragedy is really part of daily life. About 9 children are killed by a firearm every day in the United States, or about 60 per week. An additional 200 to 300 children suffer from nonfatal firearm injuries (Children's Defense Fund, 2004). Nurses must intervene in this national tragedy. Become familiar with firearm injury statistics in your community. Teach families about the dangers of firearms. Urge safe storage. Teach children and youth about the danger of firearms. Help schools establish programs to ensure safety for students.

Risk factors more commonly seen in situations where violence has been committed against children have been identified (see Table 36–7). In addition, children who commit violence more commonly have ready access to firearms, are exposed to violence in the home or community, watch violent media, and have poor self-esteem or depression.

Another type of violence is terrorism. The events of September 11, 2001, in the United States, and other examples in various countries take a large toll on the mental health of children and adolescents. Likewise, children who live through wars or have a parent or sibling die in war can be permanently affected by these events. The response of children to terrorism is not well studied. Disasters such as the World Trade Center attack can lead to sleep and eating problems, fears of entering tall buildings, regression in school performance and other behaviors, and post-traumatic stress disorder (see Chapter 54 ∞). Most children and adolescents

TABLE 36–7 ✣ Risk Factors Common in Families with Child Victims of Violence

- History of mental illness, domestic violence, incarceration, or substance abuse in the home
- Family stresses
- Inadequate child care or supervision
- Inadequate family social support
- Use of corporal punishment for the child
- Child abuse
- Access to firearms
- Gang membership in family or neighborhood
- High exposure to media violence
- Child hyperactivity and other developmental behavioral disorders

Adapted from Task Force on Violence, American Academy of Pediatrics. (1999). The role of the pediatrician in youth violence prevention in clinical practice and at the community level. *Pediatrics, 103,* 173-181.

experience profound sadness, cling to adults who provide security, and have a variety of somatic complaints (Murray, 2002). Several resources have been developed to help families and health professionals help children deal with war and violence. See the resources on the National Center for Children Exposed to Violence, Society of Pediatric Nurses, and American Academy of Child and Adolescent Psychiatry.

BULLYING

One type of violence that frequently occurs in schools is **bullying**, or aggressive behavior that is intended to cause harm, exists in a relationship with imbalance of power, and occurs repeatedly (Limber, 2003). Bullying behaviors include verbal abuse (taunting, teasing), name calling, threats, spreading rumors, social exclusion, and physical abuse (hitting, shoving, kicking, tripping). About 16% of children in a large national survey had suffered bullying, most commonly in grades 6 through 8, and more frequently among males. Almost 30% of 11- to 15-year-olds have been either a victim or a perpetrator of bullying. Up to 160,000 U.S. children may miss school every day in efforts to avoid bullying (Limber, 2003; Nansel, Overpeck, Pilla et al., 2001). Although bullying is most commonly reported in schools, it can occur in neighborhoods as children go to and from school, on school buses, on sports teams, and in other settings.

Bullies are more likely to smoke, drink alcohol, and perform poorly in school, and one in four bullies has a criminal record by age 30 years (Health Resources and Services Administration, 2003). Bullies are more likely to bring weapons to school, putting other children at risk (Fox, Elliot, Kerlikowske et al., 2003), and bullying is associated with future delinquent behavior (Van der Wal, de Wit, & Hirasing, 2003). They are aggressive, impulsive, and need to dominate others.

On the other hand, children who are bullied are more commonly socially isolated and anxious (Nansel et al., 2001). This social isolation has many negative outcomes. This includes feelings of depression, low self-esteem, loneliness, and suicidal ideation among those bullied. Health problems such as migraines, stomach pains, suicidal thoughts, and other problems can result. Academic performance commonly deteriorates and rates of school absenteeism increase (Children's Safety Network, National Injury and Violence Prevention Resource Center, 2003; Limber, 2003). Realizing the serious effects of such behaviors, a number of states have now passed legislation that reiterates the rights of all children to attend school in a safe and peaceful manner. Some state education departments mandate school district programs for students about bullying, and clear school policies about dealing with the behavior.

Nurses can be active in setting up school policies about bullying and integrating assessment and interventions related to bullying into health promotion visits. School programs should:

- Inform all students that bullying is not tolerated.
- Train teachers and other personnel about signs of bullying.
- Ensure adult supervision in hallways and on playgrounds, sites where bullying is most common.
- Teach children to promptly report bullying that is experienced or observed.
- Set up peer support for those who are bullied.
- Arrange therapeutic treatment through school counselors and other resources for those who bully; involve parents in the treatment plan.
- Measure incidence of bullying, monitor outcomes of policies, and use data to evaluate policies in schools.

Nurses who are in clinics, offices, and other health promotion settings can:

- Be alert for children with behavior changes (irritability, anxiety, poor self-concept).
- Consider bullying as a potential cause when fear or refusal to attend school is reported by child or parents.
- Ask questions during visits, such as "Have you ever been afraid to go to school?" or "What are the best and worst things about going to your school?" "What are the other kids in your neighborhood like?"

- Ask parents what they have done about any situations identified. Partner with the parent to act as liaison to the school or other agency.
- Refer identified bullies and victims of bullying to mental health specialists.

A campaign is being developed by the Health Resources and Services Administration's (HRSA) Maternal and Child Health Bureau, which will target 9- to 13-year-old youths, to prevent bullying. Access their Web site for information about dealing with this issue in schools in your state.

INCARCERATION

A growing number of children are entering the judicial system, and many are admitted at young ages. Juveniles were responsible for 12% of arrests for violent crimes in 2001 (Snyder, 2003). Girls represent an increasing number of children in juvenile justice. Children in detention, courts, and other facilities have frequently been victims as well as perpetrators of violence. They often have multiple risks such as substance abuse, early sexual activity, multiple sexual partners, lack of a healthcare home, and mental health issues (Guthrie, Hoey, Ravoira et al., 2002). Nurses may work within the juvenile justice system to provide episodic care for children or to partner with others to establish health-related programs within facilities. Youth need the following:

- Basic physical care such as immunizations, vision and hearing screening
- Nutrition assessment and teaching
- Skin assessment and hygiene practice teaching
- Information about sexuality, sexual practices, and sexually transmitted diseases
- Assessment for substance abuse
- Teaching about hazards of substance use and assistance with quitting
- Mental health services
- Developmental assessment
- Individualized education plans to meet cognitive needs

NURSING MANAGEMENT

NURSING ASSESSMENT AND DIAGNOSIS

Nurses are in key positions to identify children at risk of being recipients and victims of violence. The ecologic framework can be used to assess children. Some questions that can be asked are listed in Table 36–8. It is important to detect both the risks that lead to vulnerability and the protective factors that can promote resilience and safety. Adapt

---

TABLE 36–8 ❖ Assessment Questions to Identify Violence Risk and Protective Factors

Microsystem
- Have you been hurt by your parents or anyone else at home?
- When was the last time you were made fun of or bullied at school? What did you do?
- Have you ever brought a gun or knife or other weapon to school?
- Do you have access to guns and knives at home? At friends' houses?
- What stresses are there in your family now?
- Tell me about school—what you like and don't like.

Mesosystem
- Do your parents attend school meetings? Talk with your teachers?
- Do you participate in any church, synagogue, or mosque services?
- Do you participate in any community activities?

Exosystem
- What stresses do your parents have at work, in their families, with their health or finances?
- Do you feel like your school helps to keep you safe?
- Are there plans for handling violent episodes at your school if they were to occur?
- Do you feel safe in your neighborhood?
- Where would you go or who would you call if you felt unsafe or were hurt and no one was at home?

---

questions to each age group and insert them in every healthcare encounter.

Nursing care for violence is discussed in the nursing care plan on pages 1046–1048. The following nursing diagnoses may be appropriate:

- *Risk for Violence: Self-Directed* related to history of violence
- *Chronic Low Self-Esteem* related to history of abuse
- *Dysfunctional Family Processes* related to situational crises
- *Delayed Growth and Development* related to environmental deficiencies

PLANNING AND INTERVENTION

Nurses intervene with individual children, with families, and in schools and communities to increase safety and decrease violence. Help children and families meet basic needs and access resources to assist with finances, respite care, domestic violence, and other issues. Education is a key element of intervention.

Providing Information

Teach the family the dangers of firearms and the necessity for using gun locks and locked cabinets, storing guns unloaded, and storing guns and ammunition in separate places. Suggest alternative activities to minimize child exposure to violence

MEDIALINK Music and Violence

NURSING CARE PLAN

THE CHILD AND VIOLENT BEHAVIOR

Intervention	Rationale	Expected Outcome
1. Nursing Diagnosis: Risk for Violence: Other-Directed related to history of family violence		
NIC Priority Intervention: **Environmental management:** Violence prevention: Monitoring and manipulation of the environment to decrease the potential for violent behavior directed toward self, others, or the environment		**NOC Suggested Outcome:** **Impulse control:** Ability to restrain compulsive or impulsive behavior in child and others
Goal: The child demonstrates impulse control.		
■ Identify violent behaviors in the child. ■ Provide a safe place for exploration of feelings by referral to school or other counseling, support groups, and other resources. ■ Provide strategies for managing anger and alternative ways for coping with problems.	■ Violence in the child usually develops over time. ■ The child needs an opportunity to explore feelings and vulnerability. ■ Coping strategies can be learned from others and can help in dealing with a stressful home situation.	The child expresses the ability to manage problems in acceptable ways.
Goal: The child is secure in a safe environment.		
■ Perform a thorough assessment of hazards to the physical and emotional state in the child's home, neighborhood, and school. ■ Institute actions that will result in removal of child from unsafe situations. ■ Use community resources to provide respite care, teaching for families, and safety instructions for the child.	■ Hazards to physical and emotional health promote violence to and from the child. ■ Removal from family, community, or school may be needed to ensure child safety. ■ Stress reduction measures may help to decrease violent behaviors.	The child expresses a sense of physical and emotional safety in daily life.
2. Nursing Diagnosis: Impaired Home Maintenance related to insufficient family organization		
NIC Priority Intervention: **Home maintenance assistance:** Helping the family to maintain the home as a safe place to live		**NOC Suggested Outcome:** **Role performance:** Congruence of an individual's role behavior with role expectations
Goal: Family members are able to meet role expectations.		
■ Provide information on child's developmental needs. ■ Provide ongoing assessment in the home via home healthcare visits. ■ Assist the family in identifying hazards in the environment that can impair the child's growth and development. ■ Evaluate ability of adults to provide a safe, secure, nurturing environment.	■ Parents need to understand the developmental progression of their children. ■ Early identification of hazards can lead to proper interventions to protect against harm to the child. ■ Families may need respite care, information about child needs, financial assistance, or other resources to meet the needs of the child.	Family members meet role expectations, contributing to making the home a safe and secure place for the child.

NURSING CARE PLAN—continued

THE CHILD AND VIOLENT BEHAVIOR

Intervention	Rationale	Expected Outcome
3. Nursing Diagnosis: Hopelessness related to long-term family stress		
NIC Priority Intervention: **Hope instillation:** Facilitation of the development of a positive outlook in the given situation		**NOC Suggested Outcome:** **Hope:** Presence of internal state of optimism that is personally satisfying and life supporting
Goal: The child will have adequate food and sleep, and will express satisfaction with life.		
■ Monitor child's nutritional state and growth and daily patterns. ■ Monitor child's developmental status. ■ Determine adequacy of relationships and support systems.	■ The child's nutrition, sleep, and other patterns provide clues to the family's ability to perceive hope and provide care for the child. ■ The child needs close personal relationships in order to grow and learn.	The child demonstrates normal growth patterns and meets expected developmental outcomes.
Goal: The family will identify resources to achieve life goals.		
■ Monitor the family's decision-making ability. ■ Provide information on community resources. ■ Refer for psychiatric and other services if needed. ■ Assist in goal setting.	■ Feeling overwhelmed by daily life events leads to an inability to set goals and make decisions to meet the goals. ■ Resources can assist the family members in setting and achieving realistic goals.	The family establishes realistic goals for growth and development of its members, and takes steps to meet the goals.
4. Nursing Diagnosis: Risk for Injury related to physical or psychological conditions in the environment		
NIC Priority Intervention: **Safety behavior:** Family actions to minimize risk of physical or emotional trauma		**NOC Suggested Outcome:** **Parenting:** Social safety: Parental actions to avoid social relationships that might cause harm or injury **Risk control:** Actions to eliminate or reduce actual, personal, and modifiable health risks
Goal: Risk for physical and emotional injury to the child is decreased.		
■ Identify physical and psychologic factors that affect the child's safety. ■ Assist family to deal with issues such as mental status challenges, fatigue, financial concern, substance abuse, lack of adequate childcare resources, and other factors. ■ Instruct family on methods of keeping the child safe.	■ Multiple factors in the family can contribute to risk of violence and lack of safety for the child. ■ Families need information about the impact of unsafe settings on the child and methods that can decrease risk of injury.	The child is not injured in physical or emotional ways in the home or other immediate settings.
5. Nursing Diagnosis: Post-Trauma Syndrome related to physical or psychosocial abuse		
NIC Priority Intervention: **Counseling:** Use of an interactive helping process focusing on the needs, problems, and feelings of the child who is a victim of abuse or other violence		**NOC Suggested Outcome:** **Abuse/violence recovery:** Healing of psychologic and physical wounds of abuse or violence

(continued)

NURSING CARE PLAN—continued

THE CHILD AND VIOLENT BEHAVIOR

Intervention	Rationale	Expected Outcome
Goal: The child demonstrates abuse or violence recovery		
■ Assess the child's affect and behaviors. ■ Evaluate social interactions and sense of trust in others. ■ Assist the child in identifying feelings and coping strategies by providing counseling, art therapy, and other strategies.	■ Disturbed child behaviors can demonstrate a sense of mistrust and insecurity. ■ Establishment of close interactions with others demonstrates reestablishment of a sense of trust. ■ A child who has experienced abuse or other violence needs a therapeutic relationship with a counselor to deal with the trauma and begin to rebuild trust and respect, and to learn coping mechanisms.	The child identifies feelings related to violent episode(s) and expresses healing of the self.

in the media. Inform parents about rating systems for television and other media, and about lockout mechanisms for televisions and computers. Discuss the harmful effects of verbal and physical abuse to the child or other family members and explore alternatives.

Present the school-age child and adolescent with information about bullying and strategies for dealing with it. Provide school and community resources where the child can go if there are threats of any kind. Discuss date rape and violence with all teens and encourage them to report it.

NURSING CARE IN THE COMMUNITY

Both in schools and in community settings, nurses can plan peer mentoring to provide assistance to children at high risk of experiencing violence. Nurses can link and co-

ordinate school and community programs for children to provide for parent involvement and child support. Discuss safety issues, both risks and protective actions, in schools and community groups. Report children who are at risk. Work to establish extended programs for children so that they are safe after school. Help children learn behaviors that will help them to be safe in their communities and at home. Teach positive problem solving and conflict management techniques to children and parents.

Youth with special needs are a special concern of nurses. Jails and detention centers often have a nurse who visits youth on a regular basis or when health problems occur. Health teaching may be provided in some facilities. Halfway houses and homeless shelters are examples of settings where violence prevention and intervention can occur with youth. Mental health centers and other programs

TEACHING HIGHLIGHTS

RATING SYSTEMS FOR MEDIA

TELEVISION RATING	TELEVISION MA CATEGORIES	VIDEO & COMPUTER	MOVIES
TV-Y: for all	FV: fantasy violence	E: for everyone	G: general audience
TV-Y7: for older children	L: language	T: for teen	PG: parental guidance suggested
G: general audience	V: violence	M: mature user	PG13: parents strongly cautioned
TV-PG: parental guidance suggested	S: sexual situation	AO: adults only	R: restricted to above 18 years without adult
TV-14: parents strongly cautioned	D: sexual dialogue		NC17: no one under 18 years admitted
TV-MA: mature audience			

have nurses that work with children who are victims of violence (for example, have witnessed domestic violence, have witnessed or had a family member murdered, have been abused at home or school) or perpetrators of violence. See Chapter 54 for a discussion of post-traumatic stress disorder and its effects on the child and adolescent. ∞

Partner with families to assist them in dealing with children about war and terrorism. Recognize that youth who have experienced such events themselves are more at risk for mental health disruptions with future events. Answer questions from children honestly but reassure them that many people are trying to make the situation safe. Other suggestions for parents include the following:

- Limit television viewing and other media exposure because of its constant replaying of the events of terrorism or war. Preschoolers may think the events continue to happen, rather than being a onetime occurrence. Watch with children and talk with them about what is happening.

- Continue with structured family events such as meals, recreation, and faith-based activities. Spend time with your child.

- Take cues from the child about how much to discuss. Use words the child or adolescent can understand.

- Partner with the school so teachers know what parents have discussed and parents are aware of how events are discussed at school.

- If youth decide to become active by writing letters or joining campaigns, allow them to participate in this way.

- Be alert for regression in behavior, sleep and eating problems, or other indications of stress. Consider talking with the healthcare provider or a counselor in such situations.

- Expect that even after the child has adjusted, there may be delayed reactions. Anniversaries of events, holidays, and birthdays often bring renewed pain and sadness.

- Realize that adults must care for themselves, obtain stress relief, and talk with others in order to have strength and resources available for children.

EVALUATION

The expected outcomes of nursing care for violence prevention include a decrease in incidents of homicides, firearm injuries, abuse, date rape, and other violence among children. Additional outcomes are establishment of programs to decrease violence, and verbalization by all children of what to do if violence occurs and how to solve problems without becoming violent.

CHILD ABUSE

One of the most common types of violence against children is child abuse. This type of violence can have implications for both the physical and mental health of children, and can influence their health status even long after the abuse has occurred. Awareness of the problem of child abuse is increasing. More cases are being reported; however, these are probably only a small percentage of the total. Approximately 10% to 20% of children between the ages of 3 and 17 years—about 2.8 million children—are physically abused each year (Murry, Baker, & Lewin, 2000).

Physical abuse is only one part of a larger problem. The definition of child abuse has expanded over the past 10 years to include physical neglect, emotional abuse and neglect, verbal abuse, and sexual abuse, as well as physical abuse. Many sexually abused children are under the age of 5 years, with some as young as 3 months of age. The average age for sexual molestation is 4 years. The perpetrator is the parent or another person legally responsible who:

- Inflicts or allows another to inflict physical or emotional pain or injury,

- Creates or allows another to create a significant risk of serious physical or emotional pain or injury, or

- Commits or allows another to commit an act of sexual abuse, as defined by law, against the child.

Abuse generally involves an act of commission, that is, actively doing something to a child physically, emotionally, or sexually, such as hitting, belittling, or molesting. Neglect more often involves an act of omission, such as not providing adequate nutrition, emotional contact, or necessary physical care. Because the evidence is often not visible, emotional abuse and neglect are more difficult to identify and prove than physical abuse or neglect. Risk factors for abuse and neglect are listed in Table 36–9.

PHYSICAL ABUSE

Physical abuse is the deliberate maltreatment of another individual that inflicts pain or injury and may result in permanent or temporary disfigurement or even death. Common methods of physical abuse in children are listed in Table 36–10.

PHYSICAL NEGLECT

Physical neglect is the deliberate withholding of or failure to provide the necessary and available resources to the child. Behaviors constituting physical neglect include failure to provide for the following basic needs: adequate nutrition and hydration, hygiene (e.g., clean diapers and clothes, bathing and toileting facilities), shelter (e.g., warmth in winter), and appropriate healthcare (e.g., immunizations, dental care, medications, eyeglasses).

TABLE 36–9 ✣ Risk Factors for Child Abuse and Neglect

Factors Increasing Risk for Physical Abuse

Poverty

Violence in the family

Prematurity

Unrelated male primary caretaker

Parents who were abused as children

Age less than 3 years

Handicap or condition that requires a great deal of care (e.g., mental retardation, attention deficit hyperactivity disorder)

Parental substance abuse or social isolation

Factors Increasing Risk for Sexual Abuse

Absence of natural father or having a stepfather

Being female

Mother's employment outside the home

Poor relationship with parent

Parental relationship characterized by conflict

Parental substance abuse or social isolation

EMOTIONAL ABUSE

Emotional abuse usually involves shaming, ridiculing, embarrassing, or insulting the child. It can also include the destruction of a child's personal property, such as tearing up the child's favorite family photographs or letters or harming, killing, or giving away the child's pet. These actions are frequently used as a means of frightening or controlling the child.

Verbal abuse is a common method of emotional abuse. Words can be a violent and volatile weapon against a child, eroding the child's fragile sense of self and destroying self-esteem. Common examples of verbal abuse include yelling obscenities at the child, calling the child names, threatening to "put the child away" or to give away or kill the child's pet, telling the child "I wish you were never born" or "You're worthless," and using words to humiliate, shame, or degrade the child.

EMOTIONAL NEGLECT

Emotional neglect is characterized by the caretaker's emotional unavailability to the child. The usual style of interaction is cold and lacking in sensitive personal attention. The child suffers from a lack of nurturance and failure of the parent or caretaker to meet basic dependency needs.

SEXUAL ABUSE

Child sexual abuse is the exploitation of a child for the sexual gratification of an adult. Between 100,000 and 500,000 children in the United States are sexually abused each year.

Approximately 75% to 80% of child sexual abusers are immediate family members, other relatives, friends, or neighbors. The word "child" in sexual abuse and molestation refers to anyone who has not reached the age of consent, even if a teenager. **Incest** is sexual activity between close

TABLE 36–10 ✣ Methods of Physical Abuse in Children

A

B

Hitting, slapping, kicking, or punching

Whipping with belts, shoes, or electrical cords (**A**)

Inflicting burns with a lit cigarette or lighter (**B**)

Immersing child or body part in scalding water (commonly legs, perineal area, hands, or feet; see Figure 57-14A)

Shaking the child violently ("shaken child" syndrome)

Tying the child to a fence, bed, tree, or other object

Throwing the child against a wall, down stairs, or against a window

Choking or gagging the child

Fracturing the legs, arms, ribs, or skull

Deliberately administering excessive doses of prescribed or nonprescribed drugs

Deliberately withholding prescribed medication

Photographs used with permission. Copyright © AAP/Kempe.

family members, so that marriage would be legally or culturally prohibited. Male perpetrators make up 92% to 98% of all abusers (Frederickson, 1999; Murry et al., 2000). Abusers often threaten to harm or kill the child or another family member if the child discloses the abuse. Some abusers are pedophiles, people who have sexual impulses toward preadolescent children. The pedophile is at least 16 years of age and is at least 5 years older than the victim, and the victim is 13 years of age or younger. Another form of sexual abuse is exhibitionism, or obtaining sexual arousal by exposing one's genitals to a stranger.

NURSING PRACTICE

Following are common forms of sexual abuse:
- Oral-genital contact
- Fondling and caressing the genitals
- Anal intercourse
- Sexual intercourse
- Rape
- Sodomy
- Prostitution
- Forcing viewing of or participation in pornography

Etiology and Pathophysiology

Regardless of the type of abuse, the most common abuser is the child's parent or guardian or the boyfriend of the child's mother. Risk factors associated with abusive behavior in adults include the following:

- Psychopathology, such as drug addiction or alcoholism, low self-esteem, poor impulse control, and other personality disorders

- Poor parenting experiences, such as abuse in the abuser's own childhood, rejection by the abuser's own parent(s), lack of knowledge of alternative methods of discipline, strong belief in or family tradition of harsh discipline, and lack of parental affection

- Marital stressors and problems with partners, such as hostile-dependent, abusive, or nonsupportive relationships, and one-sided decision making

- Environmental stressors, such as legal, financial, medical, or housing problems

- Social isolation, such as few friends and limited use of sitters, family, or other resources

- Inappropriate expectations for the developmental level of the child

Clinical Manifestations

Clinical manifestations of physical abuse are listed on this page. Behaviors inconsistent with developmental stage may

be apparent. For example, the toddler or preschool child may be indiscriminately friendly with unfamiliar adults, including healthcare providers, rather than demonstrating shyness or anxiety. For the infant or young child with "shaken baby syndrome" or "shaken child syndrome," the symptoms are those of central nervous system injury from repeated coup and contrecoup injury (see Chapter 53 ∞). These may include vomiting, irritability, fatigue, poor feeding, bradycardia, apnea, enlarged fontanelle, and seizures. Bruises are usually not present (Castiglia, 2001).

Manifestations of physical neglect include undernourishment (evidenced by constantly feeling hungry, hoarding or stealing food, and being underweight), unclean clothes and body, poor dental health (extensive cavities or generally poor condition of teeth), and inappropriate clothing for the season.

Manifestations of emotional abuse, verbal abuse, and emotional neglect include fear, poor physical growth, and failure to meet appropriate developmental milestones. The child may have difficulty relating to adults, impaired communication skills, and developmental delays. Behavioral manifestations include anxiety, fear, shame, aggression, delinquency, and depression (Frederickson, 1999).

Children who have been sexually abused may exhibit a variety of physical and behavioral signs and symptoms. However, sexual abuse does not always result in apparent injury. Among the many long-term consequences of child sexual abuse are ongoing feelings of shame, guilt, anger, and hostility; decreased self-esteem, which leads to increased self-destructive behavior and risk of suicide; recurrence of victimization experiences; substance abuse; and eating disorders. The results can be long-lasting, with children experiencing post-traumatic stress disorder (PTSD) or substance abuse in adulthood (Walker, Scott, & Koppersmith, 1998). Factors associated with greater psychologic harm to the child include (1) a long period of abuse, (2) use of violent force or threat of

CLINICAL MANIFESTATIONS

CHILD ABUSE

- Multiple bruises in various stages of healing
- Scald burns with clear lines of demarcation and in a glove or stocking distribution (see Figure 57–14 in Chapter 57 ∞)
- Rope, belt, or cord marks, usually seen on the mouth, buttocks, back, legs, and arms (see Figure A in Table 36–10)
- Burn scars in various stages of healing
- Multiple fractures in various stages of healing
- Shortness of breath and distress upon being moved, indicating chest contusions and possible rib fractures
- Sedation from overmedication
- Exacerbation of chronic illness (such as diabetes or asthma) because of withholding of medication

CLINICAL MANIFESTATIONS

SEXUAL ABUSE IN CHILDREN AND ADOLESCENTS

- Vaginal discharge
- Blood-stained underpants or diaper
- Genital redness, pain, itching, or bruising
- Difficulty walking or sitting
- Urinary tract infection
- Sexually transmitted disease
- Somatic complaints, such as headaches or stomachaches
- Sleeping problems, such as nightmares or night terrors
- Bed-wetting
- Unwillingness to go to babysitter, family member, neighbor, or other person

- Fear of strangers
- New or excessive sexual curiosity or play
- Constant masturbation
- Curling into fetal position
- Excessively seductive behavior
- Phobias about particular places, people, or things
- Abrupt changes in school performance and attendance
- Changes in eating habits
- Abrupt changes in behavior (especially withdrawal)
- Child or adolescent female acts like a wife or mother

violence, (3) abuse involving penetration (intercourse or oral–genital sex), and (4) abuse involving family members, especially the father or stepfather.

Clinical Therapy

Diagnosis of abuse is made on the basis of a careful history and thorough physical examination. X-ray, CT, and MRI studies may be ordered to identify signs of recurrent abuse (e.g., healed fractures). Laboratory studies may involve urine culture for signs of infection or screening for sexually transmitted diseases. Genitourinary examination may be performed if sexual abuse is suspected. Some children are admitted directly to the hospital with the diagnosis of suspected abuse or neglect. Less obvious as a victim of abuse is the child admitted with a skull fracture who "fell off a chair."

Neglect, which is more difficult to define and identify, frequently requires hospitalization with a comprehensive medical, social, and psychiatric evaluation. Five basic categories must be considered when attempting to diagnose neglect: (1) medical care neglect (lack of necessary medical care), (2) gross safety neglect (lack of appropriate supervision), (3) physical neglect (lack of food and shelter), (4) emotional neglect, and (5) educational neglect.

All 50 states have extensive, complex statutes about reporting child abuse and neglect. A specialist must be consulted, especially if the child's testimony will be used in court.

Children do not routinely make false allegations of abuse. If indeed there is reason to believe the allegations are false, a child and adolescent therapist (psychiatrist, psychologist, psychiatric clinical nurse specialist, or social worker) with special expertise should be consulted to determine the truth. Keep in mind that children who withdraw their accusations have often been threatened or coerced into doing so. Because children who have been physically, emotionally, or sexually abused are at risk for major depression, they require skilled care by mental health professionals who are specially trained in this area. Initially the treatment goals include prevention of self-destructive or other dangerous acts. Children must be encouraged to express their fears and feelings in a safe and supportive environment. Equally important is the child's need to build coping skills and self-esteem. The child must be reassured and convinced that he or she is in no way responsible or to blame for what happened.

Individual treatment with art therapy is used initially because it is the least threatening method in the early stages of treatment, it can easily be tailored to meet the child's individual needs, and it prepares the child for other forms of treatment such as family and group therapy (Figure 36–8 ⬤). Family or group therapy may be of benefit in exploring the child's concerns and feelings. Anger is common, especially in children who were abused by a trusted adult such as the father or stepfather.

NURSING MANAGEMENT

NURSING ASSESSMENT AND DIAGNOSIS

Nursing assessment in instances of suspected child abuse or neglect requires a comprehensive history and physical examination, with documentation of findings. Consultation with social service agencies in the community is important if the family is receiving services.

NURSING PRACTICE

Every state has a child abuse law specifying the particular behaviors that define every type of abuse. Any professional who works with children and reasonably suspects that a child has been abused is required to report his or her suspicions to the local agency for child protective services. Reports made in good faith are not liable to countersuits. However, professionals who suspect abuse and do not report it may be held responsible by the judicial system.

● FIGURE 36-8

Therapeutic strategies with young children involve various methods of communication, such as dramatic play and art.

Obtaining the history can be stressful for both the nurse and the parent. Use of therapeutic communication techniques and a quiet, unhurried environment are helpful. Be open, nonjudgmental, and calm. A statement such as "Hello, Mr. S. My name is Joan T. I'm Jonathan's nurse, and I will be asking you some questions about his overall health" may be a good start. It is important to differentiate true child abuse from cultural variations that might inaccurately be assumed to indicate abuse (Figure 36–9A and B ●). Obtaining information about abusive and neglectful behaviors requires a trusting relationship with parents, who are often afraid to trust any professional.

> ## DEVELOPING CULTURAL COMPETENCE
>
> ### CUPPING AND CAO GIO
>
> Traditional treatment practices are sometimes mistaken for signs of physical abuse. The Chinese practice of cupping, which involves heating a bamboo cup and placing it on the skin, is a traditional treatment for headaches or abdominal pain. The Vietnamese practice of cao gio (rubbing out the wind), in which a coin or the fingers are forcefully rubbed on the chest, back, or neck, is used to treat minor ailments.

The health history sequence should include (1) parental concerns, (2) general family history, and (3) specific child history. This sequence begins with nonthreatening topics and allows the nurse to demonstrate concern before asking about abuse-related concerns. Obtain details about how injuries occurred. Document the parents' and child's own words verbatim using quotation marks. Compare reports obtained from each family member for lack of consistency and details that change over time.

It is desirable to interview the parent and child separately as well as together. Parent-child interaction during an intensive history-taking session provides an opportunity to

● FIGURE 36-9

It is important to differentiate cultural practices, such as **A**, cupping, and **B**, coining, from signs of child abuse.

Used with permission of the American Academy of Pediatrics, Visual Diagnosis of Child Physical Abuse Slide Kit. Photographs copyright © AAP/Kempe.

A

B

observe the child's behavior and the parent's method of handling and responding to the child.

Data gathered during history taking are particularly important in light of physical findings. Are there discrepancies between the history and physical assessment data? Do the parents give a history of an uncontrollable, inattentive toddler when the nurse observes a child who is attentive throughout a 15-minute examination? Assess the child's general appearance, including dress and behavior during the assessment. How do the child's affect, behavior, and development compare with those of other children the same age? Be alert for the signs of shaken child syndrome; this most often appears as a subtle neurologic condition. Measure head circumference and perform a neurologic examination (see Chapter 53 ∞).

Documentation of findings is important in all situations but is essential in cases of suspected child abuse and neglect. Each person who handles a laboratory specimen or other item (e.g., clothing soiled with semen) in cases of suspected child abuse must be identified in the patient's record, and the specimen must never be left unattended. Record physical findings as observed. Use figure diagrams to document skin injuries. Take photographs to document the location, nature, and extent of injuries.

Among the nursing diagnoses that might be appropriate for the physically abused or neglected child are the following:

- *Pain* related to inflicted injuries
- *Impaired Skin Integrity* related to inflicted injuries
- *Delayed Growth and Development* related to lack of supportive parenting and environment
- *Imbalanced Nutrition: Less than Body Requirements* related to inadequate caloric intake
- *Impaired Health Maintenance* related to lack of parental provision of child's essential needs
- *Fear* related to actual physical harm or repeated risk of injury
- *Risk for Injury* related to physical abuse
- *Risk for Other-Directed Violence (Parent)* related to inability to manage anger

Additional diagnoses that might apply to the emotionally abused or neglected child include the following:

- *Defensive Coping* related to psychologic impairment
- *Chronic Low Self-Esteem* related to lack of appropriate emotional support from parents
- *Disabled Family Coping* related to dysfunctional family dynamics and pattern of physical abuse

Diagnoses that might apply to the sexually abused child include the following:

- *Anxiety* related to potential separation from parent
- *Rape-Trauma Syndrome* related to sexual exploitation
- *Ineffective Role Performance* related to domestic violence
- *Disturbed Personal Identity* related to disturbance of usual activities of childhood

PLANNING AND IMPLEMENTATION

Nursing care focuses on helping to remove the child from an abusive environment, preventing further injury, providing supportive care, and reinforcing the importance of follow-up care and counseling.

Prevent Further Injury

Work with social services and community agencies to assess the child's home environment, individuals living in the home, and the actions surrounding the abuse. Assist in removing the child from the home to temporary custody of the court or foster care of another relative, if indicated. Counsel family members about abuse and refer them for appropriate therapy.

Provide Supportive Care

Protect and treat the child's injuries (e.g., fractures, burns). Include parents in the child's treatment plan, and keep them informed about the child's progress. Even if suspected of inflicting injuries to the child, the parent is still the child's primary caretaker. Talk with the parent as you would with any parent. Be supportive of any guilt expressed. Encourage the parent to assist with the child's care. Observe parent–child interactions and document supportive behaviors and the child's response to the parent versus other care providers.

Interacting nonjudgmentally with a parent suspected of abusing his or her child can be difficult. Nurses should talk with a colleague about any anger they feel toward the parents or about the child's injuries or specific actions surrounding the abuse. Use team meetings to develop strategies that enable healthcare professionals to work with the parents and child.

Home Care Teaching

If there is any question about the child returning to a potentially dangerous situation, support the child's removal from the situation. The child may receive supervised care in the home by court order. Day care, home nursing, and social worker visits may be arranged. Parents should be referred to parent effectiveness classes, family therapy, and support groups as necessary. When a neighbor or friend is the abuser, the family may need support and legal advice when a term of incarceration is finished and the perpetrator returns to the community. Some states and communities have sexual offender laws that publicize the presence of an offender on parole within neighborhoods.

Encourage the family to inform other care providers when the child's abuse history may affect a response to care. They should be alert to signs of PTSD so they can seek assistance if the child has continuing problems (see Chapter 53 ∞).

NURSING PRACTICE

When children have been abused, they are often frightened in new situations. Sexually abused children may resist removing clothes for a physical examination or medical test. They may want to wear undergarments to the surgical suite. They may distrust members of the gender that abused. When aware of a history of abuse, ask the parents or guardians how to best facilitate the child's healthcare. Be sensitive to fears and allow the child to wear clothing, have a support person present, or whatever may provide a sense of security.

EVALUATION

Expected outcomes of nursing care for the child who has been abused or neglected include the following:

- Maintenance of normal growth and development
- Establishment of a positive sense of self-esteem
- Provision of parenting information and stress relief for parents
- Provision of a nurturing environment for the child
- Absence of episodes of abuse

ADDITIONAL ABUSIVE AND VIOLENT SITUATIONS

ABANDONED BABIES

There are no accurate statistics on numbers of babies that are abandoned in dumpsters, on doorsteps, and in other locations. This tragedy has been addressed by "Safe Haven" laws in some states that allow women to drop unwanted babies at certain locations such as hospitals and fire stations without legal recrimination. In spite of these laws, babies continue to be abandoned, perhaps because mothers do not know about the laws or because they do not believe they will not be found guilty. Young teen mothers may not want others to know they had a baby. In addition, placement of these babies in adoptive homes is difficult because of paternity suits. Nurses should know their state's "Safe Haven" law details. Inform adolescents and young women about the law and post information in community sites frequented by women. Partner with young pregnant women to link them to resources such as adoption agencies when they might not want to keep a baby.

HAZING

Hazing is an activity that is forced upon an individual, which causes humiliation and is required for membership in an organization or group. It can sometimes be potentially harmful. In the past 30 years, about 60 college students have died of events linked to hazing, and even middle and high school athletes commonly engage in hazing activities (Gershel, Katz-Sidlow, Small et al., 2003). Activities might include removing clothes, drinking large amounts of alcohol, using snuff or other substances, being locked in small places, being beaten, and many other behaviors. In spite of its common practice, many coaches are not aware of it, and many students do not know what to do about hazing practices. Ask during health visits if the student has ever had to do something to belong to the group or team. Ask about "scary" things others have had them do. Assist schools and colleges in setting up antihazing policies. Encourage students to report hazing. Be aware of the possibility of hazing when seeing children with traumatic injuries.

DOMESTIC VIOLENCE

Domestic violence or intimate partner abuse is that which occurs between adult partners in a family. It may involve the parents of a child, or one parent and the significant other. Even teens who are in a sexual relationship with another person can be direct victims of domestic violence. This type of abuse then injures the child or adolescent either by witnessing a loved one being abused, or by being the victim. About 3.3 million children annually in the United States are exposed to violence against their mothers or other female care providers. Children who live in homes where intimate partner abuse occurs are 10 times more likely to be abused themselves, so the behavior is often a precursor to child abuse (Regan, 2003).

DATING VIOLENCE

Dating violence is another type of intimate partner abuse; this type occurs in relationships among youth. Most dating violence is directed at females, and studies have focused largely on girls. In one questionnaire, over 9% of adolescent girls reported being victims of dating violence. African-American girls more commonly report dating violence than Hispanic or white girls (Howard & Wang, 2003). In another study, about 20% of high school females reported dating violence (Silverman, Raj, Mucci et al., 2001). Girls who report dating violence were also more likely to report other risk behaviors, such as feeling sad, having attempted suicide, or having used substances such as tobacco and drugs. Early sexual activity, having a higher number of sex partners, and being less likely to use birth control are also associated with higher incidence of dating violence. A cluster risk profile may therefore put adolescents more at risk for dating violence.

Date rape is a term used when dating violence takes the form of rape. This can be particularly harmful to females who often do not want to share the event or press charges against the attacker.

Nurses should screen for violence at each health promotion visit, including gynecologic visits and prenatal care. Ask what is going well and not going well in intimate relationships, and whether the person ever feels unsafe or is forced to do things she does not wish to do. Recognize that while not as common, males may even be victims of violence in close relationships. Recognize that alcohol and other drugs are often connected with violence in relationships so ask about their use. Organize peer discussion groups about intimacy in order to help youth develop a sense of self-confidence and self-efficacy that will empower them to refuse activities in relationships in which they do not wish to engage (Rickert, Vaughan, & Wiemann, 2002).

MUNCHAUSEN SYNDROME BY PROXY

Munchausen syndrome by proxy is a potentially deadly form of child abuse that involves the fabrication of signs and symptoms of a health condition in a child. Usually it is the mother who creates these fictitious signs in her child (the proxy). The victim is usually under 6 years of age, and commonly under 1 year of age (Hettler, 2002; Paulk, 2001). Frequently the child's symptoms of illness are used to gain entry into the medical system to meet the abuser's own needs.

The issues of abuse are multidimensional. The child is a victim of the feigned illness, repeated hospitalizations, and invasive procedures. Equally disruptive is the deprivation of the child's daily routine caused by the periodic medical crises.

Munchausen syndrome by proxy should be suspected when unexplained, recurrent, or extremely rare conditions occur; illness is unresponsive to treatment; and the history and clinical findings are inconsistent. The most commonly reported signs and symptoms are central nervous system dysfunction, apnea, diarrhea, vomiting, fever, seizures, signs of bleeding (in urine or stool), and rashes. The parent may overdose the child on medications, such as nonprescription drugs and even syrup of ipecac, causing a variety of side effects. The symptoms occur in the presence of the same caretaker and disappear when the child is separated from that caretaker.

The child often appears uncooperative, extremely anxious, fearful, and negative. The caretaker, who in contrast appears very cooperative, competent, and loving, often expresses a desire for the child to recover. The caretaker may even suggest diagnostic procedures to try to determine "what's wrong." Characteristically the caretaker thrives in the healthcare environment.

The cause of Munchausen syndrome by proxy is often complex and rooted in the caretaker's own abusive or neglectful childhood. The disorder occurs in all socioeconomic classes. Often the perpetrator has some type of healthcare background, such as nursing or another allied health profession. The abuser is often young, married, and middle socioeconomic class (Paulk, 2001).

A suspicion of Munchausen syndrome by proxy requires a coordinated evaluation by an interdisciplinary team. Members of the team must organize and communicate a strategic plan regarding collection of evidence, confrontation of the abuser, and management of the hospitalized child. The child's safety is the ultimate concern. The case must also be reported to the appropriate child protective services.

Nursing Management

Take special care to maintain a trusting relationship with the caretaker so that he or she does not become suspicious and leave the hospital. Often the best person on the team to function in the role of "trusted other" is a member of the psychiatric consultation team.

Careful documentation of parent-child interactions, presence or absence of symptoms, and other pertinent observations is essential. The child must be closely monitored. If blood is present in the child's urine, stool, or vomitus, carefully document whether the nurse was present or whether the sample was provided by the parent. Covert video surveillance may be ordered by the hospital when the syndrome is highly suspected in a particular situation. Expert consultants may be needed to ensure legal requirements for investigation are met. When enough evidence is collected to prove Munchausen syndrome by proxy, the physician or another member of the psychiatric team confronts the caretaker.

Critical Concept Review

LEARNING OBJECTIVES

CONCEPTS

Identify major social and environmental factors that influence the health of children and adolescents.

1. Present-day lifestyles:
   - Availability of firearms.
   - Availability of alcohol.
2. Importance of "fitting in" with a group.
3. Need for two incomes in the household.
4. Early sexual involvement.

List external influences that influence child and adolescent health.

1. Poverty.
2. Homelessness.
3. Stress.
4. Family structure.
5. School and child care.
6. Community.
7. Culture.

Apply the ecological model and resiliency theory to assessment of the social and environmental factors in children's lives.

1. The theory of ecologic development provides a framework to use in assessing the interactions of children with the environment.
2. The theory of resilience examines risk and protective factors of children in order to formulate interventions to assist the child dealing with health problems.

Examine the effects of substance use, physical activity, and other lifestyle patterns on health.

1. Children and adolescents are more vulnerable to addiction and negative effects due to developing cognition, organ, and body systems.
2. Increased use of computers, televisions, and video games have led to decreased physical activity, which may contribute to obesity.
3. Body art and piercing may lead to a variety of health concerns.
4. Concerns over sexual orientation are normal during adolescence. Homosexual orientation may sometimes be associated with higher rates of rejection by family, abuse and harassment, suicide, and sexually transmitted diseases.

Plan nursing interventions for children who experience violence.

1. Assist family in dealing with issues such as mental status challenges, fatigue, financial concerns, and substance abuse.
2. Instruct family in methods to help child feel safe.
3. Assess child's behaviors.
4. Evaluate social interactions and trust in others.
5. Assist child in identifying feelings and coping strategies by providing counseling and other therapies.

Explore the nursing role in prevention and treatment of child abuse and neglect.

1. All nurses have the responsibility to report suspected abuse and neglect.
2. Teach children that no one has the right to touch and feel certain places in the body.
3. Teach children the importance of reporting any incidence of abuse.
4. Assist in the interview and examination of the abused child.
5. Help to remove the child from the abusive environment, prevent further injury, and ensure supportive care and counseling are provided.

CRITICAL THINKING IN ACTION

*View the **Critical Thinking in Action** video in Chapter 36 of the CD-ROM. Then, answer the questions that follow.*

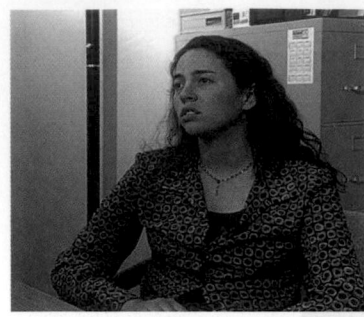

You are working at the inpatient adolescent psychiatric unit where there are approximately 20 teens between the ages of 12 and 17 years old. The teens are admitted for several different diagnoses, including: depression, suicide attempts, bipolar disorders, and eating disorders. The nurses are in charge of medication administration, vital signs, unit safety issues, physical assessments, and basic therapeutic interventions. You are working with a client named Cindy, 15 years old, who was admitted due to a suicide attempt and has been given a dual diagnosis of bulimia nervosa and depression. She has had extreme weight loss and gain over the past year and is currently 67 inches tall and weighs 140 pounds. She has stated she tried to commit suicide with a knife due to being upset with the loss of a boyfriend. She

thought she was fat and was trying to lose weight by laxative use and vomiting after meals. There is a family history of depression and substance abuse, but Cindy denies any substance use. She lives with her mother and has no contact with her father. She does not feel she has anyone to discuss her feelings with and states her mother is gone from the house frequently. Cindy admits to often eating fast food and snacking on other junk food and soda. She has been in the hospital for 2 weeks and was resistant to treatment at first, but seems to be improving with therapy and medication. She has lost 3 pounds while she has been hospitalized and her vital signs are usually: temperature—98.7°F, pulse—70, respirations—12, and blood pressure—110/70. (Review the content on bulimia in Chapter 34 to answer the following questions. ∞)

1. What are some of the signs of bulimia Cindy may exhibit?
2. What can you tell the mother about Cindy's vital signs and stability at this time? How can you explain the weight loss?
3. What behavioral signs of bulimia should be part of your nursing assessment of Cindy while she was hospitalized?
4. What are the treatment recommendations for Cindy?

MEDIALINK

www.prenhall.com/london

- NCLEX–RN® Review questions, case studies, and other interactive resources for this chapter can be found on the Companion Website at http://www.prenhall.com/london. Click on "Chapter 36" to select the activities for this chapter.

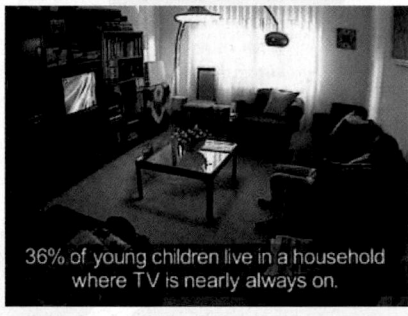

36% of young children live in a household where TV is nearly always on.

- For tutorials including animations, more NCLEX–RN® Review questions, and an audio glossary, access the accompanying CD-ROM in this book.

REFERENCES

Anderson, R. E., Crespo, C. J., Bartlett, S. J., Cheskin, L. J., & Pratt, M. (1998). Relationship of physical activity and television watching with body weight and level of fatness among children: Results from the third National Health and Nutrition Examination Survey. *Journal of the American Medical Association, 279,* 938–942.

Armstrong, M. L. & Kelly, L. (2001). Tattooing, body piercing, and branding are on the rise: Perspectives for school nurses. *Journal of School Nursing, 17,* 12–23

Behrman, R. E. (Ed.). (2000). *The future of children: Unintentional injuries in childhood.* Los Altos, CA: The David and Lucille Packard Foundation.

Benton, J. (2003). Making schools safer and healthier for lesbian gay bisexual and questioning students. *Journal of School Nursing, 19,* 257–259.

Board on Children, Youth, and Families. National Research Council and Institute of Medicine (2001). *From neurons to neighborhoods.* Washington, DC: National Academy Press.

Bronfenbrenner, U. (2005). *Making human beings human: Bioecological perspectives.* Thousand Oaks, CA: Sage Publications.

Castiglia, P. T. (2001). Shaken baby syndrome. *Journal of Pediatric Health Care, 15,* 78–80.

Children's Defense Fund. (2004). *Basic facts on poverty.* Washington, DC: Author. Retrieved January

26, 2004, from http://www.childrensdefense.org/fs_cpfaq_facts.php

Children's Safety Network, National Injury and Violence Prevention Resource Center. (2003). *Preventing bulleying: The role of the public health professional.* Retrieved January 23, 2004, from http://www.childrenssafetynetwork.org

Chng, C. L., Neill, K., & Fogle, P. (2003). Predictors of college students' use of complementary and alternative medicine. *American Journal of Health Education, 39,* 269–271.

Coleman-Wallace, D., Lee, J. W., Montgomery, S., Blix, G., & Wang, D. T. (1999). Evaluation of developmentally appropriate programs for adolescent tobacco cessation. *Journal of School Health, 69,* 314–319.

Committee on Injury and Poison Prevention, American Academy of Pediatrics. (2001). Bicycle helmets. *Pediatrics, 108,* 1030–1032.

Committee on Public Education, American Academy of Pediatrics. (2001). Children, adolescents and television. *Pediatrics, 107,* 423–426.

Committee on Sports Medicine and Fitness, American Academy of Pediatrics. (2001). Risk of injury from baseball and softball in children. *Pediatrics, 107,* 782–784.

Cook, K. R. (1999). Assessment of potential inhalant use by students. *Journal of School Nursing, 15*(20), 20–23.

Cowal, K., Shinn, M., Weitzman, B. C., Stojanovic, D., & Labay, L. (2002). Mother-child separations among homeless and housed families receiving public assistance in New York City. *American Journal of Community Psychology, 30,* 711–730.

Crespo, C., Smit, E., Troiano, R., Bartlett, S. J., Macera, C. A., & Anderson, R. E. (2001). Television watching energy intake and obesity in United States children. *Archives of Pediatric and Adolescent Medicine, 155,* 360–363.

DeForge, V., Zehnder, S., Minick, P., & Carmon, M. (2001). Children's perspectives of homelessness. *Pediatric Nursing, 27,* 377–383.

Donovan, K. A. (2000). Smoking cessation programs for adolescents. *Journal of School Nursing, 16*(4), 36–43.

Elders, J. (2003). *The role of the pediatrician in violence in the school.* Retrieved January 30, 2004, from http://www.schoolhealth.org/reduviol.html

Elkind, D. (2001). *The hurried child: Growing up too fast too soon.* Reading, MA: Perseus Books.

Federal Interagency Forum on Child and Family Statistics. (2004). *America's children: Key national indicators of well-being 2004.* Washington, DC: U.S. Government Printing Office.

Fetro, J. V., Coyle, K. K., & Pham, P. (2001). Health-risk behaviors among middle school students in a large majority-minority school district. *Journal of School Health, 71,* 30–37.

Fields, J., Smith, K., Bass, L. E., & Lugaila, T. (2001). *A child's day: Home, school, and play (selected indicators of child well-being).* Washington, DC: U.S. Department of Commerce.

Fox, J. A., Elliot, D. S., Kerlikowske, R. G., Newman, S. A., & Christeson, W. (2003). *Bullying prevention is crime prevention.* Washington, DC: Fight Crime: Invest in Kids.

Franke, T. M. (2003). The effect of attachment on adolescent violence. *The Prevention Researcher, 10,* 14–16.

Frederickson, D. (1999). Maltreatment of children. *Journal of Child and Family Nursing, 2,* 393–401.

Friedman, M. M. (2003). *Family nursing* (5th ed.). Upper Saddle River, NJ: Prentice Hall.

Geiger, J. D., Drongowski, R. A., & Lenni, J. L. (2001). Car surfing: An underreported mechanism of serious injury in children and adolescents. *Journal of Pediatric Surgery, 36,* 232–234.

Gershel, J. C., Katz-Sidlow, R. J., Small, E., & Zandieh, S. (2003). Hazing of suburban middle school and high school athletes. *Journal of Adolescent Health, 32,* 333–335.

Goldrick, B. A. (2003). Endocarditis associated with body piercing. *American Journal of Nursing, 103,* 26–27.

Guthrie, B. J., Hoey, E., Ravoira, L. W., & Kintner, E. (2002). Girls in the juvenile justice system: Leave no girl's health un-addressed. *Journal of Pediatric Nursing, 17,* 414–423.

Hanson, M. (1999). Which straw will break the camel's back? *American Journal of Nursing, 99,* 63–69.

Health Resources and Services Administration. (2003). *The National Bullying Prevention Campaign.* Washington, DC: Author.

Herrenkohl, T. I., Maguin, E., Hill, K. G., Hawkins, J. D., Abbott, R. D., & Catalano, R. F. (2000). Developmental risk factors for youth violence. *Journal of Adolescent Health, 26,* 176–186.

Hetherington, E. M. (2005). Divorce and the adjustment of children. *Pediatrics in Review, 26,* 163–169.

Hettler, J. (2002). Munchausen syndrome by proxy. *Pediatric Emergency Care, 18,* 371–374.

Howard, D. E., & Wang, M. Q. (2003). Risk profiles of adolescent girls who were victims of dating violence. *Adolescence, 38,* 1–14.

Knight, J. R. (1997). Adolescent substance use: Screening, assessment, and intervention. *Contemporary Pediatrics, 14,* 45, 51–56, 61–72.

Lackey, N., & Walker, B. L. (1998). An ecological framework for family nursing practice and research. In B. Vaughan-Cole, M. A. Johnson, J. A. Malone, & B. L. Walker, *Family nursing practice* (pp. 38–48). Philadelphia: WB Saunders.

Leone, A. (2003). Relationship between cigarette smoking and other coronary risk factors in atherosclerosis: Risk of cardiovascular disease and preventive measures. *Current Pharmacological Design, 9,* 2117–2123.

Limber, S. (2003). *Youth development program: Olweus bullying prevention.* Retrieved January 20, 2004, from http://www.clemson.edu.scg/youth/IFNLbully.htm

Malone, J. A. (1998). The resiliency model of family stress, adjustment, and adaptation. In B. Vaughan-Cole, M. A. Johnson, J. A. Malone, & B. L. Walker, *Family nursing practice* (pp. 49–60). Philadelphia: WB Saunders.

MMWR. (2001). Youth tobacco surveillance—United States, 2000. *Morbidity and Mortality Weekly Report, 50* (SS4), 1–84.

MMWR. (2002). Trends in cigarette smoking among high school students. *Morbidity and Mortality Weekly Report, 51,* 409–412.

MMWR. (2003). Tobacco use among middle and high school students—United States, 2002. *Morbidity and Mortality Weekly Report, 52,* 1096–1098.

MMWR. (2004). Youth risk behavior surveillance—United States, 2003. *Morbidity and Mortality Weekly Report, 53* (SS-2), 1–95.

Montgomery, D. F., & Parks, D. (2001). Tattoos: Counseling the adolescent. *Journal of Pediatric Health Care, 15,* 14–19.

Murray, J. S. (2002). Helping children cope with separation during war. *Journal of Specialists in Pediatric Nursing, 7,* 127–130.

Murry, S. K., Baker, A. W., & Lewin, L. (2000). Screening families with young children for child maltreatment potential. *Pediatric Nursing, 26,* 47–54.

Nansel, T. R., Overpeck, M., Pilla, R. S., Ruan, W. J., Simons-Morton, B., & Scheidt, P. (2001). Bullying behaviors among US youth: Prevalence and association with psychosocial adjustment. *Journal of the American Medical Association, 285,* 2094–2100, 2131–2132.

National Association for Education of Young Children. (2004). *NAEYC early childhood programs standards.* Retrieved August 10, 2004, from http://www.naeyc.org/accreditation

National Institute of Child Health and Human Development. (1997). The effects of infant child care on infant-mother attachment security. *Child Development, 68,* 860–879.

National Institute on Drug Abuse. (1999). *Some facts about club drugs.* Bethesda, MD: U.S. Department of Health and Human Services.

National Safe Kids Campaign. (2003). *Report to the nation: Trends in international childhood injury mortality 1987–2000.* Washington, DC: Author.

Pagliaro, A. M., & Pagliaro, L. A. (1996). *Substance abuse among children and adolescents.* New York: John Wiley & Sons.

Paulk, D. (2001). Munchausen syndrome by proxy. *Clinician Reviews, 11*(8), 51–56.

Piper, F. M. (1988). *Stress management techniques for young children.* Nova University. (ERIC Document Reproduction Service No. ED299052)

Pratt, H. D., & Greydanus, D. E. (2000). Adolescent violence: Concepts for a new millennium. *Adolescent Medicine, 11,* 103–125.

Regan, K. (2003, October). When daddy hits mommy. *Advance for Nurses,* 27–28.

Rickert, V. I., Vaughan, R. D., & Wiemann, C. M. (2002). Adolescent dating violence and date rape. *Current Opinions in Obstetrics and Gynecology, 14,* 495–500.

Rideout, V. J., Vandewater, E. A., & Wartella, E. A. (2003). *Electronic media in the lives of infants, toddlers, and preschoolers.* Menlo Park, CA: Kaiser Family Foundation, Pub # 3378.

Sadock, B. J., & Sadock, V. A. (2003). *Kaplan & Sadock's Synopsis of Psychiatry* (9th ed.). Philadelphia: Lippincott Williams & Wilkins.

Santrock, J. (2004). *Life-span development* (9th ed.). Boston: McGraw-Hill.

Sattler, B., Afzal, B. M., Condon, M. E., Belka, E. K., & McKee, B. A. (2003). *Children's health and the environment: Environmentally healthy homes and communities.* American Nurses Association. http://www.medscape.com/viewprogram/2660_pnt

Selekman, J. (2003). A new era of body decorations: What are kids doing to their bodies? *Pediatric Nursing 29,* 77–79.

Silverman, J. G., Raj, A., Mucci, L. A., & Hathaway, J. E. (2001). Dating violence in adolescent girls and associated substance use, unhealthy weight control, sexual risk behavior, pregnancy and suicidiality. *Journal of the American Medical Association, 286,* 572–579.

Snyder, H. (2003, December). Juvenile arrests. *Juvenile Justice Bulletin,* 1–12.

Society for Pediatric Nurses, SPN Public Policy Committee. (2000). Gun accidents, suicides increase among children. *SPN News, 9,* 6.

Spencer, G. A., & Bryant, S. A. (2000). Dating violence: A comparison of rural, suburban, and urban teens. *Journal of Adolescent Health, 27,* 302–305.

Stafford, E. M., & Grady, B. A. (2003). Military family support. *Pediatric Annals, 32,* 111–115.

Steele, R. W., Ramgoolam, A., & Evans, J. (2003). Health services for homeless adolescents. *Seminars in Pediatric Infectious Diseases, 14,* 38–42.

Stevens, P. E., & Morgan, S. (2001). Health of lesbian, gay, bisexual, and transgender youth. *Journal of Pediatric Health Care, 15,* 24–34.

Stewart, M., Reid, G., & Mangham, C. (1997). Fostering children's resilience. *Journal of Pediatric Nursing, 12,* 21–31.

Stratigos, A. J., & Katsambas, A. D. (2003). Medical and cutaneous disorders associated with homelessness. *Skinmed, 2,* 168–172.

Swerdlow, J. L. (2000). *Nature's medicine: Plants that heal.* Washington, DC: National Geographic Society.

Task Force on Violence, American Academy of Pediatrics. (1999). The role of the pediatrician in youth violence prevention in clinical practice and at the community level. *Pediatrics, 103,* 173–181.

Telles, S., Narendran, S., Raghuraj, P., Nagarathna, R., & Nagendra, H. R. (1997). Comparisons of changes in autonomic and respiratory parameters of girls after yoga and games at a community home. *Perceptual and Motor Skills, 84*(1), 251–257.

Telles, S., & Srinivas, R. B. (1998). Autonomic and respiratory measures in children with impaired vision following yoga and physical activity programs. *International Journal of Rehabilitation and Health, 4*(2), 117–122.

Thompson, P. (1998). Adolescents from families of divorce: Vulnerability to physiological and psychological disturbances. *Journal of Psychosocial Nursing, 36,* 34–39.

U.S. Department of Health and Human Services. (2000). Healthy People 2010. Washington, DC: Author.

Van der Wal, M. F., de Wit, C. A. M., & Hirasing, R.A. (2003). Psychosocial health among young victims and offenders of direct and indirect bullying. *Pediatrics, 111,* 1312–1317.

Walker, G. C., Scott, P. S., & Koppersmith, G. (1998). The impact of child sexual abuse on addiction severity and analysis of trauma processing. *Journal of Psychosocial Nursing, 36*(3), 10–18.

Wallerstein, J. S., Corbin, S. B., & Lewis, J. M. (1988). Children of divorce: A ten year study. In E. M. Hetherington & J. B. Arasteh (Eds.), *Impact of divorce, single parenting, and stepparenting on children.* Hillsdale, NJ: Erlbaum.

Wallerstein, J., Lewis, J., & Blakeslee, S. (2000). *The unexpected legacy of divorce: A 25 year landmark study.* New York: Hyperion.

Health Promotion and Health Maintenance for the Infant and Young Child

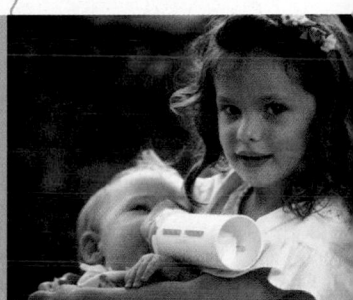

Mommy was really glad to go see the nurse today. She took our baby and me. Grandma said that they would give us a card that would help us buy food. I'm glad because I'm tired of eating peanut butter. Mommy said we could get some milk and juice, and even some chicken.

Melody, age 4, sister of 7-month-old Amanda

LEARNING OBJECTIVES

- Define health promotion and health maintenance.

- Describe how health promotion and health maintenance are addressed by partnering with families during health supervision visits.

- Describe the components of a health supervision visit.

- Explore the nurse's role in providing health promotion and health maintenance for the infant and young child.

- Describe the general observations made of infants and their families as they come to the pediatric healthcare home for health supervision visits.

- Describe the areas of assessment and intervention for health supervision visits of infants and young children—growth and developmental surveillance,

nutrition, physical activity, oral health, mental and spiritual health, family and social relations, disease prevention strategies, and injury prevention strategies.

- Plan health promotion and health maintenance strategies employed during health supervision visits of infants and young children.

- Recognize the importance of family in infant and child healthcare, and include family assessment in each health supervision visit.

- Integrate pertinent mental healthcare into health supervision visits for young children.

- Synthesize data about the family and other social relationships to promote and maintain health of infants, toddlers and preschoolers.

MEDIALINK

www.prenhall.com/london

CD-ROM

Videos:
  Temper Tantrums
  Making the Pacifier Decision
NCLEX-RN® Review
Audio Glossary

Companion Website

NCLEX-RN® Review
MediaLink Applications:
  Case Study: Domestic Violence

One of the two major goals of *Healthy People 2010* is to help individuals of all ages to increase life expectancy and improve their quality of life. The concepts of health promotion and health maintenance provide for nursing interventions that contribute to meeting this goal. Many students in health professions begin their studies with a strong interest in care of ill individuals. However, as time progresses, they learn that "well" people need care also. They need teaching to improve diet, reduce stress, and obtain immunizations. They may seek information about how to exercise properly or ensure a safe environment for their children. These examples of care and teaching are components of health promotion and health maintenance.

Nursing is a holistic profession that examines and works with all aspects of the lives of individuals, and has a strong focus on family and community as well. Nurses are uniquely positioned to provide health promotion and health maintenance activities, and indeed these activities should be a part of each encounter with families. What is the difference between health promotion and health maintenance? When should nurses engage in activities that focus on health? How are these activities integrated into health supervision visits for the infant and young child? How do nurses partner with other healthcare professionals to offer comprehensive health services in settings accessible to parents and young children? How can nurses help children and their families to maximize length and quality of life? These are some of the questions that will be explored in this chapter, with specific activities that target families with infants and young children.

GENERAL CONCEPTS

In order to understand health promotion and health maintenance it is important to develop a definition of health. The World Health Organization defines **health** as a state of complete physical, mental, and social well-being and not merely the absence of disease and infirmity (World Health Organization, 2001). Even individuals with chronic disease can be viewed as healthy if they are successfully adapting to their conditions. Health is viewed as dynamic, changing, and unfolding; it is the realization of a state of actualization or potential (Pender, Murdaugh, & Parsons, 2002). It is a basic human right and is necessary for development of societies.

Health promotion refers to activities that increase well-being and enhance wellness or health (Pender et al., 2002). These activities lead to actualization of positive health potential for all individuals, even those with chronic or acute conditions. Examples include providing information and resources in order to:

■ Enhance good nutrition at each developmental stage.

■ Integrate physical activity into the child's daily events.

■ Provide adequate housing.

■ Promote oral health.

■ Foster positive personality development.

Health promotion is concerned with development of strategies that seek to foster conditions that allow populations to be healthy and to make healthy choices (World Health Organization, 2001). Nurses engage in health promotion by partnering with children and families to promote family strengths in the areas of lifestyles, social development, coping, and family interactions. They also provide **anticipatory guidance** for families because they understand the child's upcoming developmental stages and teach families how to provide an environment to assist in meeting the milestones of the stages. This concept is explored more fully later in this chapter.

Health maintenance (or health protection) refers to activities that preserve an individual's present state of health and that prevent disease or injury occurrence. Examples of these activities include developmental screening or surveillance to identify early deviations from normal development, providing immunizations to prevent illnesses, and teaching about common childhood safety hazards. Health maintenance activities are commonly preventive in nature, and terminology common to community or public health nursing explains the levels and aims of preventive actions. Prevention levels are identified as primary prevention, secondary prevention, and tertiary prevention (Table 37–1).

While it is clear that health promotion and health maintenance activities are closely linked and often overlap, there are some differences. Health maintenance focuses on known potential health risks and seeks to prevent them or to identify them early so that intervention can occur. Health promotion looks at the strengths and goals of individuals, families, and populations, and seeks to use them to assist in reaching higher levels of wellness. It involves partnerships with the family as health goals are set, and with other health professionals and resources to provide for meeting the goals. Nurses apply both health promotion and health maintenance concepts when providing healthcare, recognizing that the concepts overlap. Health promotion and health maintenance are integrated into healthcare visits for children, with the care provider applying both knowledge of health maintenance concepts and adding information the family has identified that will assist in increasing health or wellness (health promotion). These activities commonly take place at "well child" or health supervision visits.

Health supervision is the provision of services that focus on disease and injury prevention (health mainte-

nance), growth and developmental surveillance, and health promotion at key intervals during the child's life. What health promotion and health maintenance activities are parts of health supervision visits? How can these activities be integrated into all settings where care is provided for children? What are the recommended times for health visits to occur and what care is provided at certain times? How can health supervision visits be organized to accomplish the goals of the family and health professionals? These and other questions will be answered in this section and the following section focused on nursing management.

All children need a medical home, where ongoing health supervision is provided during the developmental years. A medical home or **pediatric healthcare home** is the site of comprehensive healthcare by a pediatric healthcare professional in order to ensure optimal health (National Association of Pediatric Nurse Associates and Practitioners [NAPNAP], 2002). When a family has an established partnership with a care provider, comprehensive, family-centered health services can be provided based on the family's risks and protective factors. These services may be provided in physicians' offices, community health clinics, the home, schools, childcare centers, shelters, or mobile vans (Figure 37–1 ⦿). National guidelines for preventive health services have been developed for infants, children, and adolescents by the U.S. Department of Health and Human Services (DHHS), the American Academy of Pediatrics (AAP), and the American Medical Association. NAPNAP supports the list of comprehensive services of a pediatric healthcare home identified by the AAP (see "Nursing Practice").

TABLE 37–1 ❖ Levels of Preventive Health Maintenance Activities

Level	Description	Example of Nursing Actions
Primary Prevention	Activities that decrease opportunity for illness or injury	Giving immunizations Teaching about car safety seats
Secondary Prevention	Early diagnosis and treatment of a condition to lessen its severity	Developmental screening Vision and hearing screening
Tertiary Prevention	Restoration to optimum function	Rehabilitation activities for child after a car crash

Data from Murray & Zentner, 2001, p. 53.

NURSING PRACTICE

The American Academy of Pediatrics and the National Association of Pediatric Nurse Associates and Practitioners concur that a pediatric healthcare home should offer the following:

- Family-centered care and trusting partnership
- Sharing of unbiased and clear information
- Provision of primary care to include acute and chronic care, breastfeeding promotion, immunizations, growth and development, screenings, healthcare supervision, and counseling about health, nutrition, safety, parenting, and psychosocial issues
- Continuous available care
- Continuity of care
- Referral to specialists as needed
- Referral to early intervention and child care
- Coordination of services
- Maintenance of a comprehensive central record
- Provision of developmentally appropriate and culturally competent care

(AAP, 2002; NAPNAP, 2002)

FIGURE 37-1

A
B

A, The nurse is providing a health supervision visit in the child's home after discharge from the hospital for an acute illness. *B,* A nurse is providing information to a child visiting a mobile healthcare van.

The health supervision visit is individualized to the family and child. Standardized screenings and examinations are included, and time is provided for the family's specific concerns and questions about the child's health. Nurses play an integral part in these comprehensive visits, and they partner with other healthcare providers to accomplish health supervision.

A tracking system in the pediatric healthcare home site helps to identify appropriate health supervision activities for each child at every visit. Most often computers are used to list appropriate topics for visits at specific ages. If a child misses a visit, the family can be contacted by phone and encouraged to come in for the recommended care. A family may be called if their young child is lacking some immunizations. Recognizing that not all families get into the healthcare home for each recommended visit, every health encounter, including an episodic illness visit or care for a chronic illness, is a potential time to complete health promotion and health maintenance activities. For example, immunizations may sometimes be given during a visit for an acute condition such as otitis media (ear infection) if the child has missed a prior health supervision visit. Even when children are seen in hospitals, emergency rooms, or other settings, it is important to ask about their pediatric healthcare home and when the last visit occurred. Identify children who need basic health supervision services and provide them or refer to other settings for meeting these needs at another time.

Nurses play an important role in managing health supervision visits. Depending on the setting, the nurse may provide all services or support other care providers by obtaining an updated health history, screening for diseases and other conditions, conducting a developmental assessment, and providing immunizations, anticipatory guidance, and health education. Nurses in all settings are instrumental in identifying children who need health supervision and are not obtaining recommended care (Figure 37–2 ⦿).

While health supervision visits can address many health-related topics, there is generally a limited time in which to engage a child or family. The nurse needs to direct the encounters and have some ideas for pertinent agendas. *Bright Futures* booklets provide guidance about how the nurse can manage health supervision visits. Six concepts should be integrated into care:

1. The care provider *builds effective partnerships* with the family. A **partnership** is a relationship in which participants join together to ensure healthcare delivery in a way that recognizes the critical roles and contributions of each partner in promoting health and preventing illness. The partners in child health include the child, family, health professionals, and the community.

2. The nurse *fosters family-centered communication* by showing interest in the child and family, and effectively conveying information and understanding.

3. The nurse *focuses on health promotion and health maintenance topics during visits,* recognizing that families may not initiate these discussions.

● FIGURE 37-2

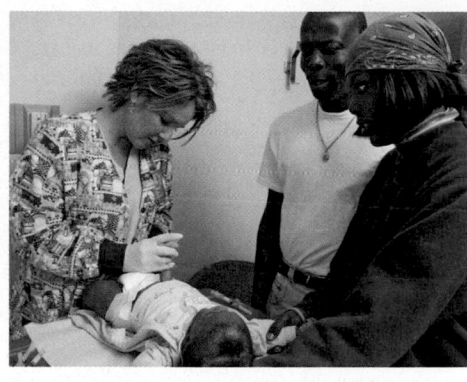

A   B   C

The nurse plays many roles in providing health promotion and health maintenance for children. **A,** Data are collected from the time a nurse calls the child and family to the examination room and during the history-taking phase. The nurse asks questions while observing the child's behaviors and the relationship between parent and child. The nurse also performs screening tests, including blood pressure, tuberculosis, vision and hearing, and developmental screening. **B,** Interventions that include teaching may take place. **C,** A nurse may administer immunizations as parents watch and assist by holding the child. Nurses also play important roles in teaching families information to enhance health.

4. The nurse *manages time well* to enable health promotion topics to be addressed during visits. This includes reviewing the child's health record and selecting topics pertinent for the child's age and the family's situation.

5. The nurse *educates the family during "teachable moments."* Large teaching plans are not always needed; children and families often learn best when presented with small bits of information based on the parent's questions or the nurse's observations.

6. The nurse *becomes an advocate for child health issues.* When an issue arises while caring for a child, seek additional data from various sources, talk with others, and strategize how the problem could be solved.

(Green & Palfrey, 2002)

COMPONENTS OF HEALTH PROMOTION/HEALTH MAINTENANCE VISITS

The nurse identifies and isolates pertinent topics for health promotion and health maintenance during health supervision visits. Nurses also apply their knowledge of areas that need to be addressed with an infant or child of a particular age, and then make general observations of the child and family to identify additional topics for discussion. While categories to consider vary depending on the age of the child, the family's particular needs, and community resources, there are some common topics that generally require attention. Often, nurses start with the topics described as follows, integrating general observations as they progress with a visit, and further identifying assessment areas needed in particular situations.

Pediatric nurses make *general observations* of infants and their families whenever they encounter them. Nurses who are observant during the health supervision visit have many opportunities for assessing the family. These general observations begin when the family is called in and welcomed by the nurse to the facility. They continue as the infant or child is weighed and measured, and throughout the visit. Nurses observe the physical contact between the child and other family members, the developmental tasks displayed by the child, and parental level of stress or ease in conducting childcare activities.

Growth and developmental surveillance provide important clues about the child's condition and environment. The child's height, weight, and body mass index are calculated at each health supervision visit, and results are placed on percentile charts (see Chapter 34 and Chapter 35 for more information ∞). Parents are given the information in written form and it is interpreted for them. Physical assessment is performed to be sure the child is growing as expected and has no abnormal or unexplained physical findings (see Chapter 35 ∞). Developmental surveillance is a flexible, continuous process of skilled observations that also provides data about the child's capabilities, allows for early identification of any neurologic problems, and helps to verify that the home environment is stimulating. Information may be collected from several sources, for instance, a questionnaire that the parent completes, questions asked during the interview, or observation of the child during the visit. Parents can also be interviewed to identify any developmental concerns they may have about the child or adolescent. When talking with parents, review physical, social, and communication milestones for infants, young children, older children, or adolescents. Detailed milestones for each age group are found in Chapter 33. ∞

⊙ **FIGURE 37–3**

Follow all directions for performing the Denver II assessment and for interpreting responses. Develop rapport with the child and approach the assessment as fun. This often helps the child participate more actively during the entire Denver II assessment. This 9-month-old boy is able to perform the following age-appropriate behaviors: **A,** Banging two cubes; **B,** playing ball with the examiner; **C,** using a thumb-finger grasp; **D,** pulling to stand.

 A
 B
 C
 D

Standardized developmental questionnaires are effective for developmental surveillance of most children, especially when time for health supervision visits is limited. A commonly used test is the Denver II, which can be applied as a developmental chart, like a growth curve, to monitor the child's developmental progress (Figure 37–3 ⊙ and Figure 37–4 ⊙). When performing developmental screening with the Denver II or any other standardized screening tools, nurses make sure all directions are followed by:

- Choosing the proper test for the child's age and desired information.

- Reading directions thoroughly or using specific training tools available.

- Practicing as needed until proficient with the test.

- Calculating the infant's or child's age correctly, especially if premature.

- Attempting to develop rapport with the infant or child to get the best performance.

- Following directions for administration of items; in some cases, parents can be asked if a child demonstrates specific skills at home, especially if the child is not willing to perform an item during testing.

- Noting the behavior and cooperativeness of the child during the screening process.

- Analyzing the findings using the test instructions to make the correct interpretation.

Failure to perform an item in a single domain does not mean the child has failed the test (see "Developing Cultural Competence"). The child should be reevaluated at a future visit. Schedule the appointment at a time of day when the child is awake and rested. Provide parents with guidance on specific methods for stimulating the child. Failure of multiple items within one domain or across multiple domains is of greatest concern. When poor development patterns in one or more domains are revealed, referral for diagnostic developmental assessment is needed.

DEVELOPING CULTURAL COMPETENCE

ENGLISH AS A SECOND LANGUAGE AND DEVELOPMENTAL TESTING

Children who have recently come from other countries and even some born in this country who live in families from minority ethnic groups may have difficulty with some items on developmental tests. For example, children who are not skilled in the English language may not understand some instructions or be able to answer questions about definitions of words. When parents do not have English as a primary language and the examiner uses English, common terms might be misinterpreted. Parents might not understand what is meant if you ask, "Does your baby have a mobile over the crib at home?" or "Is she starting to be afraid of strangers?" How can you be alert for language differences and become sensitive to miscommunication?

Nutrition is a vital part of each health supervision visit. It makes important contributions to general health and fosters growth and development. Include observations and screening relevant to nutritional intake at each health supervision visit. Eating proper foods for age and activity ensures that children have the energy for proper growth, physical activity, cognition, and immune function. Nutrition is closely linked to both health promotion and health maintenance. See Chapter 34 for detailed nutritional assessment recommendations. ∞ For specific nutritional questions to ask for each age group, see Chapter 38. ∞ Find out what questions parents have about feeding their children. Use the information gathered to provide both health promotion and health maintenance interventions.

Physical activity provides many physical and psychologic health benefits. However, there is growing disparity between recommendations and reality among most children (Patrick, Spear, Holt et al., 2001). Research by the Centers for Disease Control and Prevention (CDC) using the Youth Media Campaign Longitudinal Survey (YMCLS) of parents and children found that 61.5% of 9- to 13-year-old children report that they do not participate in any organized physical activity during hours outside of school. Although organized activities are important and consistent forms of exercise, not all children can participate or desire to do so. However, 22.6% of these children reported that they do not engage in ANY physical activity outside of school. Parents noted that barriers to physical activities included transportation problems, lack of opportunities in area, expense, lack of parental time, and lack of neighborhood safety (MMWR, 2003). Inquire about activities the child prefers and amount of time for activity during the day. As the child grows older, include questions about sedentary activities such as number of hours spent watching television or playing computer games. See if the child plays sports at school or in the community. Ask about activities in a typical day to measure amount of activity. Once the nurse gathers data about physical activity, interventions are implemented to enhance activity patterns.

While *oral health* may seem to require the knowledge of a specialist, there are many implications that relate to general healthcare. Oral health is important because teeth assist in language development, impacted or infected teeth lead to systemic illness, and teeth are related to positive self-image formation. Between 4 and 5 million children in the United States are affected by tooth decay and pain that interfere with activities of daily living such as eating, sleeping, attending school, and speaking (Ryan, 2003). The nurse applies health promotion to dental health by teaching about oral care and access to dental visits. Health maintenance activities relate to prevention of caries and illness related to dental disease.

NURSING PRACTICE

Children from homes with low income are especially prone to poor dental health, so efforts are being extended to help families receive care. Many of the State Children's Health Insurance Programs (SCHIP) offer dental services (VanLandeghen, Bronstein, & Brach, 2003). All children in the Medicaid program are eligible for dental coverage in the Early and Periodic Screening, Diagnostic, and Treatment Services (EPSDT). Private and public clinics in many communities provide low-cost or free care for families with limited financial resources (Ryan, 2003). Many families do not realize their children could receive these services. Find out what resources are available in your state and community, and refer as needed. See Chapter 1 for further description of programs mentioned here. ∞

Mental and spiritual health are important concepts to address in health promotion and health maintenance visits. Parents can be encouraged to keep a record of mental health issues to bring to health supervision visits. This helps them understand that the healthcare professional is willing to partner with them to assist in dealing with mental health. Suggest topics such as child and parental mood, child temperament, stresses and ways that family members manage stress, or sleep patterns. Make notes in the record as a reminder of questions to ask at the next visit (Jellinek, Patel, & Froehle, 2002). The child and family are both observed for appropriateness of affect and mood. Be alert for signs of depression, stress, anxiety, and child abuse or neglect. The nurse establishes both health promotion and health maintenance goals related to child and family mental health. Health promotion goals relate to adequate resources to meet family challenges, and protective factors such as involvement in extended family and the community. Teaching stress reduction techniques such as meditation, relaxation, and imagery, as well as providing resources for yoga or other techniques, is helpful. Health maintenance goals relate to prevention of mental health problems. Examples include providing resources when domestic violence occurs, or referring cases of suspected child abuse or neglect. The **spiritual dimension** is a connection with a greater power than that in the self, and guides a person to strive for inspiration, respect, meaning, and purpose in life (Murray & Zentner, 2001). Spiritual health is seen in the large context as those entities that provide meaning in life. For some, this may be membership in a faith-based group; for others it may be feeling part of a society with a purpose of greater good, or setting goals for the future. Ask about the family's meaningful activities. Provide links to faith-based groups as needed.

The *relationships* that a child establishes with others begin at birth. The first and most important set of relationships

FIGURE 37-4

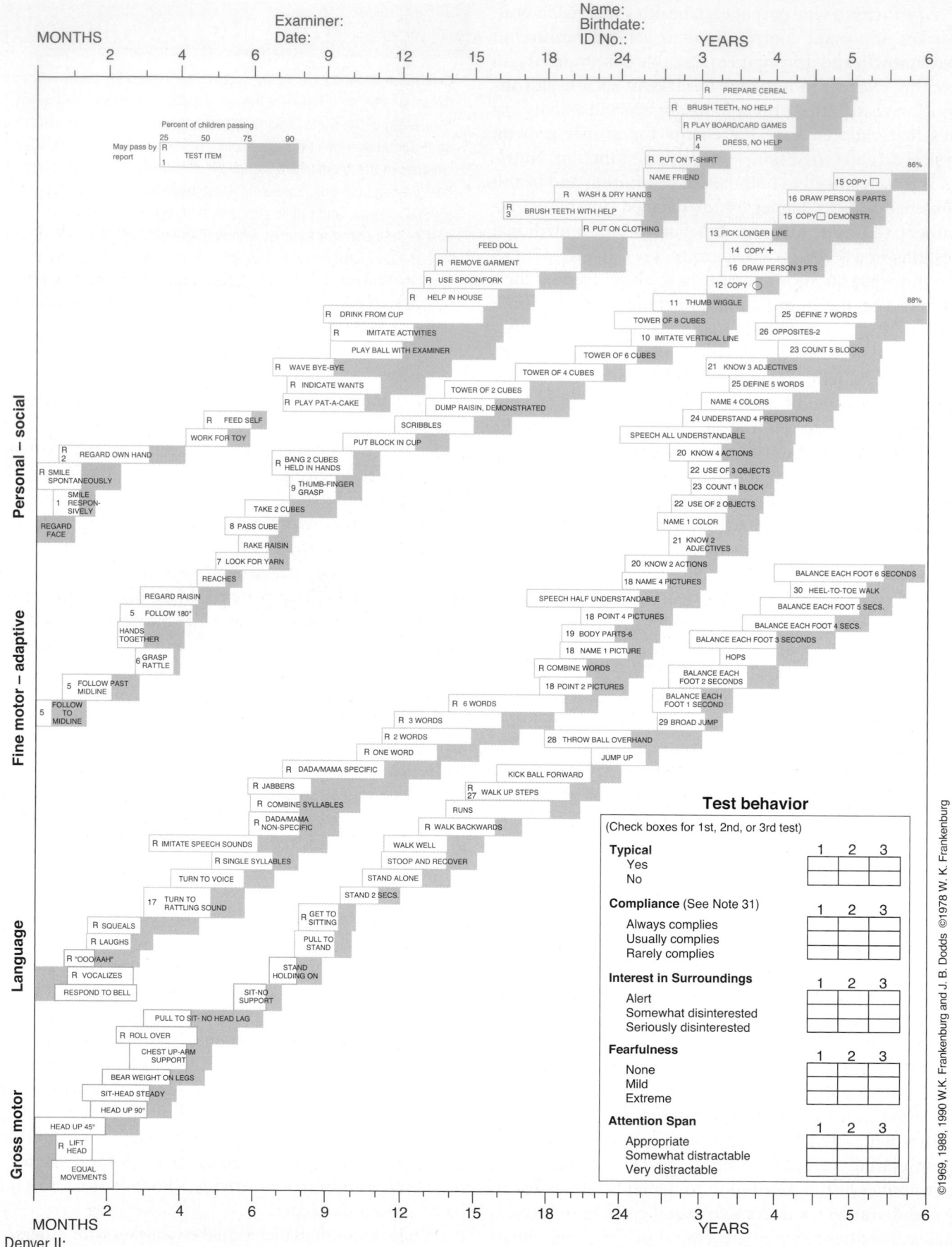

A, Denver II;

DIRECTIONS FOR ADMINISTRATION

1. Try to get child to smile by smiling, talking, or waving. Do not touch him/her.
2. Child must stare at hand several seconds.
3. Parent may help guide toothbrush and put toothpaste on brush.
4. Child does not have to be able to tie shoes or button/zip in the back.
5. Move yarn slowly in an arc from one side to the other, about 8" above child's face.
6. Pass if child grasps rattle when it is touched to the backs or tips of fingers.
7. Pass if child tries to see where yarn went. Yarn should be dropped quickly from sight from tester's hand without arm movement.
8. Child must transfer cube from hand to hand without help of body, mouth, or table.
9. Pass if child picks up raisin with any part of thumb and finger.
10. Line can vary only 30 degrees or less from tester's line.
11. Make a fist with thumb pointing upward and wiggle only the thumb. Pass if child imitates and does not move any fingers other than the thumb.

12. Pass any enclosed form. Fail continuous round motions.
13. Which line is longer? (Not bigger.) Turn paper upside down and repeat. (pass 3 of 3 or 5 of 6).
14. Pass any lines crossing near midpoint.
15. Have child copy first. If failed, demonstrate.

When giving items 12, 14, and 15, do not name the forms. Do not demonstrate 12 and 14.

16. When scoring, each pair (2 arms, 2 legs, etc.) counts as one part.
17. Place one cube in cup and shake gently near child's ear, but out of sight. Repeat for other ear.
18. Point to picture and have child name it. (No credit is given for sounds only.)
    If less than 4 pictures are named correctly, have child point to picture as each is named by tester.

19. Using doll, tell child: Show me the nose, eyes, ears, mouth, hands, feet, tummy, hair. Pass 6 of 8.
20. Using pictures, ask child: Which one flies?... says meow?... talks?... barks?... gallops? Pass 2 of 5, 4 of 5.
21. Ask child: What do you do when you are cold?... tired?... hungry? Pass 2 of 3, 3 of 3.
22. Ask child: What do you do with a cup? What is a chair used for? What is a pencil used for? Action words must be included in answers.
23. Pass if child correctly places <u>and</u> says how many blocks are on paper. (1, 5).
24. Tell child: Put block **on** table; **under** table: **in front of** me, **behind** me. Pass 4 of 4. (Do not help child by pointing, moving head or eyes.)
25. Ask child: What is a ball?... lake?... desk?... house?... banana?... curtain?... fence?... ceiling? Pass if defined in terms of use, shape, what it is made of, or general category (such as banana is fruit, not just yellow). Pass 5 of 8, 7 of 8.
26. Ask child: If a horse is big, a mouse is_____? If fire is hot, ice is_____? If sun shines during the day, the moon shines during the _____? Pass 2 of 3.
27. Child may use wall or rail only, not person. May not crawl.
28. Child must throw ball overhand 3 feet to within arm's reach of tester.
29. Child must perform standing broad jump over width of test sheet (8 1/2 inches).
30. Tell child to walk forward, ⊂⊃⊂⊃⊂⊃⊂⊃ → heel within 1 inch of toe. Tester may demonstrate. Child must walk 4 consecutive steps.
31. In the second year, half of normal children are non-compliant.

OBSERVATIONS:

B, Directions for administration of Denver II.

develops with the family. The mother, father, siblings, and perhaps extended family are the contexts in which the baby learns to relate with others. With growth the world widens to encompass other children, friends of the family, peers, school, and the larger community network. Analyzing the child's relationships at all ages provides important clues to social interactions. From the moment the family is called in from a waiting area, be alert for clues to family interactions. Likewise, other social interactions are important to evaluate. Does the young infant interact in an age-appropriate manner with the healthcare provider or other children in the area? Ask the parents questions about family and social interactions. Once assessment has taken place, establish goals and interventions related to family and social relationships.

Disease prevention strategies focus mainly on health maintenance, or prevention of disease. Some health disruptions can be detected early and treatment for the condition can begin. **Screening** is a procedure used to detect the possible presence of a health condition before symptoms are apparent. It is usually conducted on large groups of individuals at risk for a condition and represents the secondary level of prevention (Figure 37–5 ●). Most screening tests are not diagnostic by themselves but are followed by further diagnostic tests if the screening result is positive. Once a screening test identifies the existence of a health condition, early intervention can begin, with the goal of reducing the severity or complications of the condition. Another way to prevent diseases is to immunize children against common communicable diseases. See Chapter 45 for the complete list of childhood immunizations and schedules for administration. ∞

Most childhood mortality and hospitalization is related to injury (see Chapter 1 for more information ∞). Therefore, it is important for the nurse to integrate *injury prevention* strategies in all health supervision visits. The family is constantly challenged to maintain a safe environment as the child grows older, reaches more advanced developmental levels, is exposed to a widening world outside of the family, and has less supervision. Safety teaching should be integrated with developmental progression. Asking parents to bring their questions about safety to each visit can be a good starting point for discussion. The nurse considers knowledge about the age of the child and information from the health supervision visit to plan health maintenance interventions related to injury. Teaching is performed, resources are made available, and parents and children who have experienced injury are invited to present their experiences.

Many other topics might be discussed during health supervision visits. They may relate to either health maintenance activities designed to preserve health, or health promotion activities designed to enhance or improve the state of wellness. They include topics such as extended family members and their role in the child's life, cultural variations or inclusion, or development of moral values and ethical behaviors.

● **FIGURE 37–5**

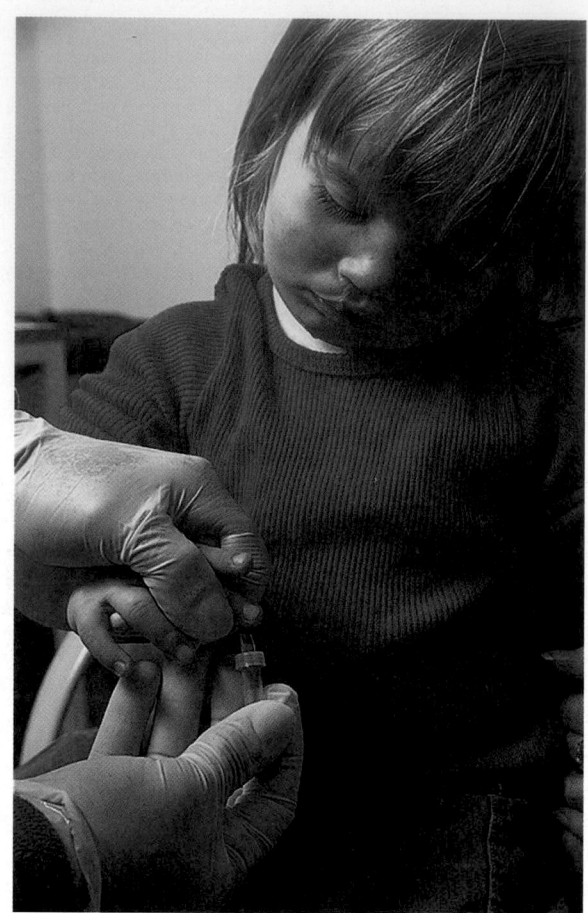

This 18-month-old toddler is having a blood screening test to detect iron deficiency anemia. Children are often screened for adequate levels of iron in later infancy and during toddlerhood.

HEALTH PROMOTION AND HEALTH MAINTENANCE OF THE INFANT

Infancy is a major life transition for the baby and parents. The infant accomplishes phenomenal physical growth and many developmental milestones while the family adapts to the addition of a new member and establishes new goals for each of its existing members. Infant health supervision visits are very important to support the health of the baby and the family unit. These visits begin after the newborn period, at about 1 month of age. This is the time when parents establish an ongoing partnership with a healthcare provider. A "medical home" or "pediatric healthcare home" is identified to serve the baby's health needs. The goals of health supervision visits are to identify and address the health promotion and health maintenance needs of the infant.

Facilitating breastfeeding, helping parents to understand their infant's temperament, and employing strategies to ensure adequate sleep by the baby and parents are examples of health promotion activities. Health maintenance activities focus on disease and injury prevention. Some examples of these interventions include administering immunizations and teaching about infant car seats.

An established relationship with a healthcare provider and agency is important so that trust develops and the family will feel comfortable about turning to the professionals for information and guidance as the baby grows. Nurses play a vital role in welcoming new families into office and clinic settings, establishing rapport, and applying principles of communication so that trust and positive partnerships develop between providers and families. Infancy is a time when the child grows in physical, psychologic, and cognitive ways; health supervision visits play a key role in fostering healthy growth and development. When should the infant be seen for health supervision visits? What are key components of these visits? How can the nurse best assess and intervene to ensure the infant's health and safety? These are some of the questions that will be answered in this section of the chapter.

EARLY CONTACTS WITH THE FAMILY

Health promotion and health maintenance occur in a series of health supervision visits during the first year of life. Schedules vary among facilities, but a common pattern includes visits at about 1 month, 2 months, 4 months, 6 months, 9 months, and 1 year of age. In addition, most children have some episodic illnesses such as gastrointestinal illness or otitis media and visit the facility at other times for treatment of these illnesses. A few children have chronic or serious healthcare problems during the first year, and have extensive contact with the healthcare home and other services.

During these first visits, assess the family for protective factors and risks. Protective factors might include knowledge level of infant needs, support from family and friends, and the mother's good health and nutritional state during pregnancy. Risk factors could include limited financial resources, lack of preparation for the baby, and illness or other stress among family members. Knowledge of these factors will shape the nursing interventions in the first health supervision in infancy. The nurse applies health promotion principles by building on strengths and fosters health maintenance by intervening to minimize risks.

GENERAL OBSERVATIONS

When the family comes to the clinic or office for care with an infant, general observations should begin at first contact (Figure 37–6 ●). Welcome the family warmly to the facility and comment on the baby. Ask how the family is doing with the baby and how the adjustment is going. Be alert for signs of fatigue or depression in the parents, as these can occur when caring for an infant and can interfere with bonding and positive transition. Upon entering the

● **FIGURE 37–6**

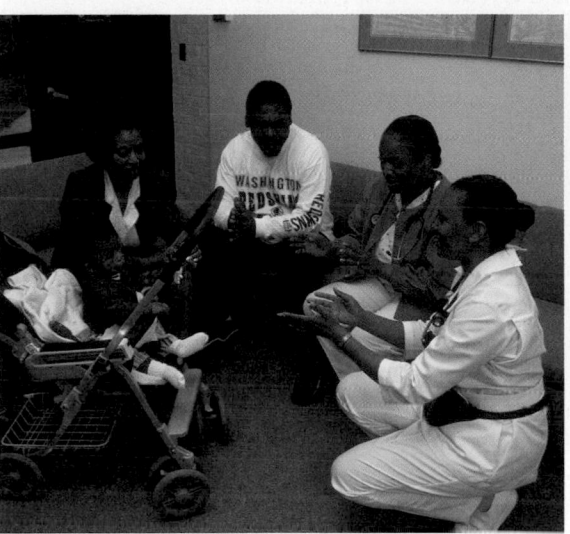

The nurse begins assessment of the infant's family when they are seen in the waiting room and called in for care. What observations can you make of the infant's general appearance? Developmental accomplishments? Interaction of parents with the baby?

examination room, it is helpful to explain the plans for the visit, such as "I will weigh and measure Sarah now and show you how she is growing. Then I'll ask a few questions about her eating, sleeping, and other things. Then the nurse practitioner will be in to do Sarah's physical examination. Do you have any questions as we start? Will you undress Sarah now so we can weigh her accurately?"

GROWTH AND DEVELOPMENTAL SURVEILLANCE

Physical growth and meeting of developmental milestones provide important information about infants. The baby is measured for accurate length, weight, and head circumference. (See the Skills Manual SKILLS and Chapter 35 ∞ for more information; also see Figure 37–7 ●.) The measurements should be placed on growth grids and interpreted. Parents enjoy seeing how the baby is progressing and are usually eager to learn about the child's weight gain and growth percentiles. Be alert for an infant who demonstrates a change in percentile range. For example, if the baby was in the 75th percentile for length and weight at birth, but has fallen to below the 50th percentile for weight, additional assessment of the baby's feedings is needed. Likewise, if the head circumference is much lower or higher than the length and weight percentiles, further neurologic and developmental assessment should be done.

Growth measurement is followed by a physical assessment. The nurse may complete parts of the assessment, with the remainder performed by the physician, nurse practitioner, or other primary care provider. The

● FIGURE 37-7

Weighing and measuring length during health supervision visits provides important information about the child's nutrition and general development. This young infant was measured and then while the parents dressed the child the nurse placed the findings on the growth grid.

assessment evaluates each body system, with particular attention paid to the heart, skin, musculoskeletal system, abdomen, and neurologic status. See Chapter 35 for a thorough discussion of physical assessment. ∞

Developmental surveillance is integrated into each infant healthcare visit by observing developmental milestones in the infant (see Chapter 33 for a summary of milestones expected at different ages ∞). When there is no opportunity to observe a skill directly, ask parents about whether the infant performs the skill (see "Developing Cultural Competence"). In addition to direct observation, parents are usually requested to fill in a form that asks questions about common developmental tasks. Review the results and determine if additional questions should be asked. When some milestones have not been met, make an appointment for the infant to have a developmental test by a certified examiner.

DEVELOPING CULTURAL COMPETENCE

CULTURAL INFLUENCES ON DEVELOPMENTAL TESTS

Be alert for differences in cultural practices and beliefs that may influence developmental milestones. For example, if a child is kept on a cradleboard for much of the time, the baby may be slow in learning to crawl. This baby may progress directly to standing by furniture without demonstrating as much creeping or crawling as other infants. If an item such as "waves good-bye" or "plays patty-cake" represents a practice not common in another culture, the child may not have had exposure to the skill. Be alert for cultural variations, allow the child time to learn a developmental skill, and retest on other occasions.

The nurse establishes health promotion and health maintenance interventions related to growth and development assessment data. Anticipatory guidance related to development is a major component of health promotion. The nurse anticipates the next milestones the infant will be meeting, and recommends ways for the parents to support the infant in progression. Some health promotion activities include:

- Teaching about food introduction that will foster growth.
- Encouraging toys and activities that will assist in meeting the next developmental milestones.
- Demonstrating gross and fine motor skills that the infant has achieved.
- Demonstrating to parents how the child will focus on their faces and mimic their vocal sounds.

Other interventions are focused on health maintenance or disease and injury prevention. Safety hazards and ways to avoid them are discussed, and parents are given brochures, Web sites, or videotapes to enhance injury prevention information. Can you outline additional health promotion and health maintenance interventions that relate to the infant's growth and development?

NUTRITION

The importance of nutrition during the first year of life cannot be overestimated. The baby will triple his or her birth weight by 1 year of age and has a great need for nutritional balance. From the first sips of breast milk or formula as a newborn, to eating the family meal at 1 year of age, the fast progression of nutritional intake patterns is obvious. See Chapter 34 for a thorough description of nutritional needs during infancy. ∞

During each visit the nurse seeks to learn what the baby is eating, and whether the family has any questions or concerns related to intake (Story, Holt, & Sofka, 2002). Open-ended questions are a good way to begin, with more specific questions inserted after the parent's perceptions are known. Once the baby is in the second half of the first year, food patterns of the family become more important. Consider childcare settings as well.

Observations from other portions of the visit can provide clues about additional questions to ask. If an infant has not gained weight as expected and has fallen into a lower channel of weight percentile, more specific analysis of intake is needed. Ask for a recall of the baby's intake in the previous day. When the baby does not meet developmental milestones on schedule or is lethargic, intake may be inadequate for age. In these cases support may be needed to ensure adequate intake; a thorough description of feeding may be the first step in analyzing the problem and planning interventions. When the child's ability to take in nutrients or the parent's ability to feed the baby is questioned, an observation of a feeding might take place, either at the health-care setting or during a home visit.

Additional nutritional assessment measures are used at certain points in the first year. A hematocrit or hemoglobin is generally performed between 9 and 12 months of age. Lead screening may be needed in certain population groups (see Chapter 51 for more information ∞). Food security screening can be used when appropriate (see Chapter 34 ∞). Each visit includes nutritional teaching about important items. The topics for discussion vary according to age group. See Table 37–2 for suggested teaching topics at specific ages. Desired outcomes for nutrition in infancy include adequate growth, normal nutritional assessment findings, and knowledge by parents of the nutritional needs of the infant.

PHYSICAL ACTIVITY

Physical activity is needed for adequate development of fine and gross motor skills in infancy. Unlike other times of life, the focus is on providing only the opportunities for activity, without a need to focus on motivation. As long as infants are meeting developmental milestones and have a stimulating environment that provides opportunity for fine and gross motor activity, they will use their motor skills, thus enhancing their performance. Time should be provided each day for the infant to reach for objects, freely exercise legs and arms, and increasingly use head control.

Playing with parents or others and being surrounded by toys and other stimulating items will encourage motor behavior in all body parts. Ask the parents for a description of the baby's typical day and listen for these types of play periods. While babies should sleep on their backs, they need supervised play periods when they are awake that are spent on the stomach. This encourages developmental skills and lessens flattening of the back of the head from excessive positioning on back. Observe the physical skills of the infant (see Chapter 33 ∞) for motor developmental

---

TABLE 37–2 ✤ Nutrition Teaching for Health Promotion and Health Maintenance Visits

Age	Nutrition Teaching	
1 month	Support breastfeeding efforts. Teach correct formula types and preparation if used. Teach burping and rate of feeding information. Suggest water during hot weather or if family wants to use a bottle at baby's bedtime.	Encourage families to view feedings as social interactions; emphasize importance of holding the infant and not propping bottles.
2 months	Continue above. Review fluid needs of infants. Reinforce food safety for partially used bottles of breast milk or formula. Use warm water for heating bottles rather than microwave to avoid burning.	Warn against feeding honey in the first year of life due to risk of botulism. Begin daily cleaning of infant gums. Provide information about any supplements needed (for example, iron for premature infant, vitamin D for babies not exposed to adequate sunlight).
4 months	Continue above. Discuss introduction of first foods between 4 and 6 months, and surveillance for symptoms of allergy or intolerance.	Discuss changing food patterns such as increasing amounts and decreasing numbers of daily milk feedings.
6 months	Continue above. Reinforce proper introduction of new foods, to include rice cereal, vegetables, and fruits. Discuss any unusual food reactions observed. Introduce cup for drinking. Introduce soft finger foods.	Serve juice only in a cup and limit to no more than 6 ounces daily. Caution about common choking foods and items. Provide information about fluoride supplement if water supply is not fluoridated.
9 months	Continue above. If mother does not continue to breastfeed, teach family to use iron-fortified formula for the first year of life. Encourage self-feeding of finger foods, integrating common foods for the family.	Introduce source of protein such as tofu, cheese, mashed beans, and slivers of meats.
12 months	Continue above. Support mother who wishes to continue breastfeeding beyond 1 year of age.	Encourage cups for all feedings other than breast.

TABLE 37–3 ✣ Risk and Protective Factors Regarding Physical Activity in Infancy

Risk Factors	Protective Factors
■ Premature birth ■ Delayed developmental milestones ■ Limited stimulation by family or other care providers ■ Lack of knowledge by family about infant's physical activity needs ■ Limited community resources for families with infants	■ Meets developmental milestones at expected ages ■ Has contact with parents, siblings, and others for significant time each day ■ A supportive environment with room to play safely, stimulating surroundings ■ Physically active family ■ Family knowledge about infant's physical activity needs ■ Community programs that promote physical activity in infants and information for families

Data from Patrick, K., Spear, B., Holt, K., & Sofka, D. (Eds.). (2001). *Bright futures in practice: Physical activity.* Arlington, VA: National Center for Education in Maternal and Child Health.

norms, ask questions about play periods provided, and compose a list of the family protective factors and risk factors in this area. Table 37–3 lists some risk and protective factors related to physical activity during infancy.

Based on the results of assessment and using the concept of anticipatory guidance, the nurse plans appropriate teaching for the family. Health maintenance deals with prevention of physical development delays. The nurse evaluates success of interventions by the child's progression in physical activity milestones at the next health supervision visit. Adequate parental understanding of the importance of physical activity and the means of supporting the child's activities is an important outcome of care.

ORAL HEALTH

The first teeth begin to erupt about midway during infancy. Two front teeth are common at about 6 months of age. However, even before this, parents lay the foundation for good oral health. The mother's intake during pregnancy and breastfeeding are essential to ensuring adequate availability of calcium and other nutrients that will be used as the infant's teeth develop. The nurse in child health supervision settings ensures that the baby has adequate intake of these nutrients via breastfeeding and other foods. A dietary recall of the mother's intake, as well as the infant's, is one way of assessing for nutrients. When the water supply is not fluoridated, inquire about use of fluoride drops.

Help the family establish healthy dental habits. The parents should wipe the infant's gums with soft moist gauze once or twice daily. This helps to clean residues of food from the gums and gets the baby accustomed to having something wiping the gums, a practice that may assist when toothbrushing begins. Families are also cautioned to avoid having the baby breastfeed when sleeping, to avoid use of bottles in bed, and not to allow the baby to drink at will from a bottle during the day. These practices are linked to early childhood caries (see Chapter 34 ∞) and can lead to tooth decay. Nurses assess for the presence of teeth and whether patterns are similar to those expected (see Chapter 35 for additional information ∞). It is wise to ask if the baby has had any difficulty with teeth eruption. Many babies have increased crying and parents have disrupted sleeping during these periods. Suggest comfort measures such as offering cool beverages and safe "teething toys" for the baby.

MENTAL AND SPIRITUAL HEALTH

The baby's mental health is related to early experiences, inborn characteristics such as temperament and resilience, and relationships with caregivers. The first year of life provides many opportunities for the infant to develop positive mental health; interventions during this important period can enhance the child's future mental status.

One way to evaluate mental health is to look carefully at the growth and development surveillance data that were described earlier. Children who feel secure and have nurturing environments usually grow as expected and perform milestones at usual times. Slow growth and delayed development are sometimes related to feeding disorder of infancy and early childhood (see Chapter 34 for more details ∞). In these cases a disturbed relationship with the primary caregiver influences the psychologic state of the infant and results in decreased food intake. Another way to assess mental health is to observe the child and parent interacting. Does the parent hold the baby securely and does the child cuddle and settle in to the parent's arms? (See Figure 37–8 ◉.) Is there eye contact between parent and child? Does the parent appear comfortable in holding and comforting the baby? These interactions indicate bonding or positive attachment.

During the first year, the baby learns to identify parents; beginning at about 6 months of age, infants may cry or protest when another person holds them. This is called **stranger anxiety** and indicates expected attachment to parents. Similarly, infants in the second half of the first year of life may exhibit **separation anxiety** by inconsolable crying and other signs of distress when parents are not present. These behaviors are normal, demonstrate healthy attachment to primary caregivers, and indicate mental health. Help parents to recognize them as expected occurrences. Provide them ideas of how to deal with this behavior. They can remain in sight and talk to the baby during

FIGURE 37-8

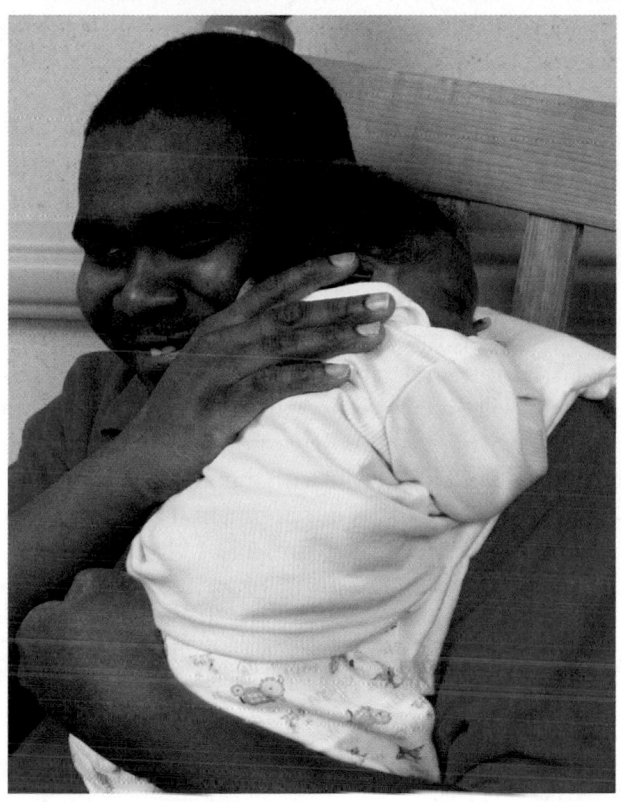

Interactions between the parent and infant provide clues to mental health. Do the adult and child appear comfortable with each other? Is eye contact and vocalization present? Are their bodies soft and relaxed or tense?

health supervision examinations. They should be encouraged to hold and comfort the baby after painful procedures like immunizations. Once the baby has experienced that the parent leaves and returns, security in the care of others can emerge.

Another important indication of infant mental health is the ability to comfort oneself. **Self-regulation** is the process of dealing with feelings, learning to soothe self, and focusing on activities for increasing periods of time. Infants learn early how to comfort and calm themselves. Ask parents if the child sucks a finger, softly rocks, or otherwise comforts self when distressed. Some babies prefer to be alone and quiet when tired or distressed; others calm better when held, rocked, or placed in an infant swing. Help the parents to identify and reinforce the baby's methods of self-soothing, and teach swaddling and rocking techniques. Self-regulation is needed by the baby when learning to go to sleep while tired and agitated. Nurses use health promotion principles to teach about sleep patterns in infants, and implement health maintenance when partnering with families to deal with problem sleep behaviors that lead to infant and parent fatigue (see "As Children Grow" and "Evidence-Based Nursing").

The baby is born into a family with spiritual strengths and limitations. The nurse assesses the family and provides additional resources when needed. Although the infant is not mature enough to understand the family's spiritual framework, the atmosphere in the family that relates to nurturing, valuing children, providing a safe and secure

EVIDENCE-BASED NURSING

INFANT SLEEP

Problem

Many babies have limited sleeping periods during the night, and their night awakenings disturb parents' sleep. Parents may have busy days and be unable to nap for adequate sleep to perform at a safe and productive level during the day. In an effort to increase sleep, some parents may feed the infant frequently during the day, believing that if the baby has fed well, longer night sleep periods may occur.

Evidence

It had been noted that infants with more than 11 feeds in 24 hours at 1 week of age were nearly 3 times more likely to have night wakenings than infants who had fewer feedings. A group of 316 newborns with more than 11 feedings daily and their families participated in a study and were randomly assigned to receive one of three interventions:

- Three-step behavioral program
- Educational booklet
- Helpline for sleeping problems

After 12 weeks, 82% of the babies in the behavioral program slept through the night, compared with 61% for the other two interventions. The behavioral program taught parents to minimize light and social interaction at night, avoid feeding or cuddling at night, and beginning at 3 weeks of age, delay feeding when the baby awoke at night.

Implications

This evidence-based practice provides implications for nursing practice. Ask parents of young newborns to keep track of the number of daily feedings and nighttime awakenings of the infant. For infants with 11 or more daily feedings, teach parents how to minimize stimulation and interaction at night, as previously described. Provide opportunities to review results at future health supervision visits.

Critical Thinking

What reasons might working parents have for responding eagerly and interacting with an infant who awakens at night?

Do you think there are other reasons why babies awake at night? What clues help you to decide if an infant sleep problem exists?

Reference

Nikolopoulou, M., & St. James-Roberts, I. (2003). Preventing sleeping problems in infants who are at risk of developing them. *Archives of Disease in Childhood, 88*, 108-111.

AS CHILDREN GROW

Infant Sleep Patterns

Birth—3 months

10–16 hours of sleep daily in about five sleep periods of 30 minutes to 3 hours

3–6 months

14 hours of sleep daily with a longer sleep at night plus two to three naps daily

By 4–6 weeks, a consistent sleep pattern should emerge

6–12 months

12–14 hours of sleep daily with a longer sleep at night plus one to two naps daily

(Green & Palfrey, 2002, p. 24)

environment, and recognizing mental balance is conveyed readily to the infant. The infant's social and psychologic health are closely related to these factors. Assess the family's meaningful activities and practices and engagement in faith-based practices. Ask if they have needs or desires for referrals in the community such as to an organized religious body or other meaningful activities.

Many of the nurse's interventions are aimed at healthy mental health development in the baby. Health promotion activities focus on teaching parents the needs of infants for security and interaction. Suggest healthy sleep patterns and how they can be achieved. Teach self-regulation skills so that the parents can help the child become quiet and calm. Health maintenance seeks to identify babies with disruptions in mental health status, often manifested by growth or interaction abnormalities. When the infant has disturbed sleep patterns or difficulty calming self when upset, or the parents do not interpret infant cues related to hunger or discomfort, the nurse plans interventions to help prevent further problems. An expected outcome for these activities is the reestablishment of expected growth and development, and age-appropriate interactions of the infant with others.

RELATIONSHIPS

The family is the primary site where the infant learns to interact with other people. Therefore, family dynamics must be examined during health supervision visits. Some factors in the mental health of the parents directly affect the atmosphere in the home, and the resulting health of the baby. Depression in parents or other family members is an important condition that has the potential to influence the infant's health. Interactions with parents who are depressed will be altered; caretaking, both physical and emotional,

can be impaired. Another challenge to the mental health of families and the infants in these families is that of domestic violence, a situation in which parents or adult care providers commit violent acts toward one another. Another risk that occurs in some families with infants is child abuse or maltreatment. This problem is a serious issue that causes disturbed mental status in the baby. See Chapter 36 for a detailed description of child abuse and its effect on infants and older children. ∞ Suspected child abuse must be reported to legal authorities in order to protect children.

The infant's social interactions both within and outside the family display unbelievable growth in the first year. The role of the nurse related to infant social interactions in health supervision visits is to evaluate the social skills of the infant, learn what parents have noticed about the baby's temperament and how it fits with their lives, and make suggestions for positive social development. Desired outcomes for the infant include establishment of close relationships with parents and other family members, a stimulating home environment that is responsive to the baby's temperament, and developmental progression in social interactions.

DISEASE PREVENTION STRATEGIES

Infants are prone to many infectious diseases, especially once passive immunity from the mother wanes at about 6 months of age (see Chapter 44 and Chapter 45 ∞). Recommended immunizations are administered on schedule to provide protection from some diseases. Recommended immunizations for infancy are listed in Table 37–4. Further details on immunizations can be found in Chapter 19. ∞ Instruct parents about coming immunizations and when

TABLE 37–4 ✣ Routine Immunizations Recommended During Infancy

Immunization	Age Recommended
Hepatitis B	After birth up to 2 months (1st dose) 1–4 months (2nd dose) 6–18 months (3rd dose)
Diphtheria, tetanus, pertussis	2, 4, and 6 months (3 doses)
Haemophilus influenzae type b	2, 4, and 6 months (3 doses; 3rd dose is not needed if PRP-OMP [Pedvax HIB or Comvax] are used for primary series)
Inactivated poliovirus	2, 4, and 6–18 months (3 doses)
Pneumococcal	2, 4, and 6 months (3 doses)
Influenza	6–23 months (1 dose annually)

the baby should be seen again. Be sure the parent understands the risks and benefits of each immunization. Answer their questions truthfully, and have resources on hand such as brochures and videotapes for interested parents.

During each health supervision visit, the nurse performs recommended screenings and counsels the parents about why such screening is important. Vision and hearing screenings are consistently performed. Screenings for anemia and lead poisoning are added at particular times or with certain groups. Families with certain genetic diseases such as sickle cell disease or cystic fibrosis may choose to have screening for the infant so that supportive care could begin early if the child has the disease. Parents benefit from teaching about common diseases and conditions of young children and measures for their prevention. Ask about environmental tobacco smoke (ETS) and encourage smoking parents to quit. Teach parents to put babies to sleep on their backs to assist in lowering the chance of sudden infant death syndrome. Be sure parents have a phone number to call when they have questions about conditions or whether the baby should be seen by the healthcare provider (see "Teaching Highlights: When to Contact the Healthcare Provider"). Desired outcomes for disease prevention strategies include adequate management of health problems, integration of immunization and other preventive measures into care of the infant, and family understanding of preventive measures recommended for infants.

TEACHING HIGHLIGHTS

WHEN TO CONTACT THE HEALTHCARE PROVIDER

Instruct parents to contact a provider if the child has:

- Rectal temperature ≥ 100.4°F (38.0°C)
- Seizure
- Skin rash, purplish spots, petechiae
- Change in activity or behavior that makes the parent uncomfortable
- Unusual irritability, lethargy
- Failure to eat
- Vomiting
- Diarrhea
- Dehydration
- Cough

Data from Green, M., & Palfrey, J. S. (Eds.). (2002). Bright futures: Guidelines for health supervision of infants, children, and adolescents (2nd ed.). Arlington, VA: National Center for Education in Maternal and Child Health.

INJURY PREVENTION STRATEGIES

During the first year of life, injury becomes an increasingly common cause of mortality. Strategies must be included in each health supervision visit to lower the risk of injury. Nurses should never assume that parents understand how

to insert an infant car seat correctly or what types of toys and foods can lead to choking. Know the most common hazards at each age and teach parents methods of avoiding them (Tables 37–5 and 37–6).

Begin the conversation by asking parents what safety hazards they are aware of in the child's environment. Use this information as the starting point for discussion. Give positive feedback for their awareness of hazards and measures they have taken to prevent them. Consider using a home assessment survey that assists parents in identifying hazards that may be present in their homes. When infants visit friends, relatives, or neighbors, they may be exposed to other hazardous situations. Grandparents may not have a home that is "baby-proofed" and the infant could have access to electrical cords, machinery, medicines, or other hazards. Help the parents to evaluate the childcare home or center. Focus on car safety since this is a frequent cause of injury for infants. Provide brochures and other types of information about recommendations. Refer every family for a car seat examination at a certified examination center. Provide resources for car seats if the family is not able to afford one. Discuss other possible safety hazards such as extensions on the parent's bicycle and use of baby strollers in areas where cars are present.

NURSING MANAGEMENT

NURSING ASSESSMENT AND DIAGNOSIS

The nurse working in clinics, offices, and other settings that offer primary care for infants should be skillful in assessing health promotion and health maintenance. The infant's growth, developmental level, general physical health, and mental/social health are assessed. Family interactions and other settings where the infant spends time are evaluated for risks and protective factors that influence the child's development. Assess the health of siblings and patterns of integrating the infant into the rest of the family. Particular attention is directed at assessment of risk for diseases and injuries. The data-gathering phase always provides parents with the opportunity to ask questions and relay concerns. Further assessment may need to be directed at these areas.

Based on the assessment data, the nurse establishes nursing diagnoses that become the basis for nursing interventions. Both areas of strength and need are included; often the family's strengths can be used to further promote health. Nursing diagnoses established during a health supervision visit of an infant might include the following:

- *Effective Breastfeeding* related to the mother's confidence and knowledge
- *Interrupted Breastfeeding* related to the mother's resumption of employment outside the home

TABLE 37–5 ❖ Injury Prevention in Infancy

Hazard	Development Characteristics	Preventive Measures
Falls	Mobility increases in first year of life, progressing from squirming movements to crawling, rolling, and standing.	Do not leave infant unsecured in infant seat, even in newborn period. Do not place on high surfaces such as tables or beds unless holding child. **(A)** Once mobile by crawling, keep doors to stairways closed or use gates. Standing walkers have led to many injuries and are not recommended.
Burns	Infant is dependent on caretakers for environmental control. The second half of the first year is marked by crawling and increased mobility. Objects are explored by touching and placing in mouth.	Check temperature of bath water and food/liquids for drinking. Cover electrical outlets. Supervise infant so that play with electrical cords cannot occur.
Motor vehicle crashes	Infant is dependent on caretakers for placement in car. On impact with another motor vehicle, an infant held on a lap acts as a torpedo.	Use only approved restraint systems (according to federal Motor Vehicle Safety Standards). The seat must be used for every trip, even if very short. The seat must be properly buckled to the car's lap belt system. **(B)**
Drowning	Infant cannot swim and is unable to lift head.	Never leave infant alone in a bath of even 2.5 cm (1 in.) of water. Supervise when in water even when a life preserver is worn. Flotation devices such as arm inflatables are not certified life preservers.
Poisoning	Infant is dependent on caretakers to keep harmful substances out of reach.	Keep medicines out of reach. Teach proper dosage and administration of medicines to parents. Cleaning products and other harmful substances should not be stored where the infant can reach them. Remove plants from play areas. Have poison control center number by telephone.
Choking	The second half of infancy is marked by exploratory reaching and mouthing objects. Infant explores objects by placing them in the mouth. **(C)**	Avoid foods that commonly cause choking. Keep small toys away from infants, especially toys labeled "not intended for use by those under 3 years."
Suffocation	Young infant has minimal head control and may be unable to move if vomiting or having difficulty breathing.	Position infant on back for sleep. **(D)** Do not place pillows, stuffed toys, or other objects near head. Do not use plastic in crib. Avoid latex balloons.
Strangulation	Infant is able to get head into railings or crib slats but cannot remove it.	Be sure older cribs have slats spaced 6 cm (2 3/8 in.) or less apart. The mattress must fit tightly against the crib rails.

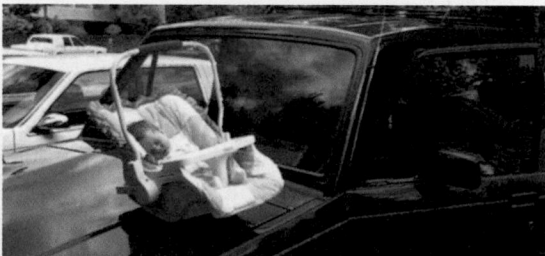

(A) Never leave infant unsecured or on high surface.

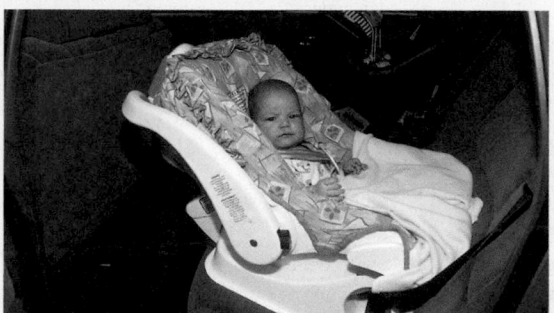

(B) Always use approved restraint system. Place infant in rear-facing seat in backseat of car

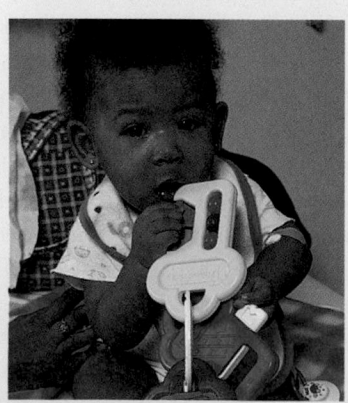

(C) Explores objects with mouth.

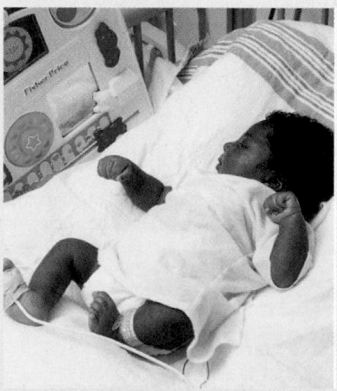

(D) Place infant on back for sleeping, keep toys clear.

TABLE 37–6 ✜ Injury Prevention Topics by Age

Age	Injury Prevention Teaching Topics	
1 month	Use infant car safety seat. Put baby to sleep on back. Avoid loose bedding and toys in crib; avoid clothes and blankets with loose strings and do not tie a pacifier around the neck or with a string. Avoid tobacco use in the environment. Provide adult supervision of the baby at all times by trusted individuals. Test bath water temperature and never leave baby alone in bath.	Never place baby on high object such as counter, table, or bed; always keep one hand on the baby during activities like diaper changes to prevent falling. Wash hands correctly and often. Avoid contact with persons with communicable diseases. Have smoke alarms and avoid fire hazards. Learn infant CPR and airway obstruction removal. Never shake the baby. Have plans for emergency care.
2 months	Follow the above. Use only recommended playpens or cribs and keep sides up. Avoid moldy environments. Keep baby toys cleaned.	Avoid direct sunlight for the baby. Keep sharp and small objects out of baby's environment. Keep hot water heater lower than 120°F. Review emergency plan with all care providers.
4 months	Follow the above. Get all poisonous substances out of baby's view and reach; install locks to keep them inaccessible.	Do not use latex balloons or plastic bags near the baby.
6 months	Follow the above. If an infant-only car seat was used, switch to rear-facing convertible safety seat (intended for babies up to 40 lb) when baby is 20 to 30 lb or 26 inches. Empty containers of water immediately after use; be sure pools or other bodies of water are locked and not accessible to baby. Use sunscreen, hat, and long sleeves when baby is in the sun. Keep heavy and sharp objects out of reach; check that all poisons are locked away including in homes visited; keep pet food and cosmetics out of reach.	Do not drink hot liquids or eat soup while holding the baby. Have poison control number by phones and programmed into cell phones. Be alert for dangers of hot curling irons and other appliances. Have electrical cords out of reach and not hanging down. Have home and environment checked for lead hazards. Lower infant crib mattress if still in upper position. Install gates and guards on stairs and windows. Never use an infant walker.
9 months	Follow the above. Crawl on the floor and look for hazards at baby's eye level. Pad sharp corners on tables and other furniture.	Watch for tables, chairs, and other devices the baby may use for climbing to unsafe places.
12 months	Follow the above. Change to forward-facing car safety seat if baby is at least 20 lb; install correctly and have installation checked; place in back seat and never in front seat with a passenger air bag. Start teaching the child to wash hands frequently, showing how. Provide own personal items such as clothing and blankets to childcare providers; wash often. Change batteries in home smoke alarms and check system.	Turn handles to back of stove; use back rather than front burners; watch for hot liquids. Check care provider setting for safety hazards. Remember that responsible adults should always supervise your infant, not other children. Peruse home once again for hazards now that the child is more active, climbing, and walking. Check playgrounds for hazards and always supervise the child in a playground.

Data from Green, M., & Palfrey, J. S. (Eds.).(2002). *Bright futures: Guidelines for health supervision of infants, children, and adolescents* (2nd ed.). Arlington, VA: National Center for Education in Maternal and Child Health.

- *Compromised Family Coping* related to recent role changes
- *Risk for Altered Parent/Child Attachment* related to anxiety associated with parenting role
- *Sleep Pattern Disturbance (infant)* related to frequently changing sleep routines and cycles
- *Impaired Skin Integrity (infant)* related to developmental factors
- *Risk for Infection (infant)* related to inadequate acquired immunity
- *Risk for Injury (infant)* related to design of environment

■ *Risk for Altered Growth and Development* related to parental substance abuse

PLANNING AND IMPLEMENTATION

The nurse plays a vital role in successful health promotion and health maintenance activities. Explain to the parents what procedures are being performed and their purpose. Encourage them to ask questions and share their perceptions of the infant's personality, development, and other traits. This will enhance their understanding that healthcare involves a partnership between them and the care providers. It will lead to trust that promotes their ability to share concerns honestly. The first year of the baby's life is a key time for establishing a trusting relationship with health professionals.

Recognize the importance of data provided by simple assessments such as length and weight. Analyze all findings to learn if the child is developing as expected. Much of the visit is spent in teaching parents about topics such as safety measures, providing anticipatory guidance related to development, assisting with integration of the new baby into the family, and relaying resources for support of the family in the community, on the Internet, or in other areas. Parenting classes, childcare facilities, and family planning resources are examples of common parental needs. Perform recommended physical and developmental assessment, administer screening tests, and give immunizations. Be sure parents understand the need for tests and treatments, and relay the results of tests to them.

Nurses who work in hospitals, emergency services, and other facilities are an important link in health supervision. Ask where and how often the child is seen for care. Check immunization schedules to be sure they are up-to-date. When the child is not being seen regularly, find out if the family does not know the importance of these visits or lacks resources to obtain the necessary care. Refer them to resources as needed so that they can identify a pediatric healthcare home. Some agencies that provide health supervision are equipped to perform home visits on a regular basis or in case of special need. When nurses make regular home visits to families with many risk factors, health outcomes are improved. Seeing the family in the natural setting enables the nurse to tailor interventions to the specific situation. Nutrition, safety, and other teaching is more effective when it matches the family's needs. For example, showing how to set up a stimulating environment with safe materials, even if toys are limited, is an effective nursing strategy. Ensure that home visits are performed whenever appropriate and available, either through the pediatric healthcare home or other community agency.

Before the family leaves the facility, be sure they have the next appointment scheduled. Summarize content of the present visit, emphasizing the family's strengths and the baby's newly acquired developmental skills. Sensitively list any areas that require work in the coming weeks, such as "baby-proofing" the home or encouraging the infant to reach for objects. Provide a journal or notebook in which the parents can record the infant's development and write down questions to ask in future visits. Suggest possible topics for the parents to think about, and provide books, brochures, and other printed material.

EVALUATION

Expected outcomes of nursing care for the infant and family in health promotion and health maintenance include the following:

■ Parents state common safety hazards at the child's present and upcoming ages.

■ The infant demonstrates normal patterns of growth and progression in developmental milestones.

■ The infant remains free of disease and injury.

■ The infant is well adjusted, showing positive response to the environment and interactions with significant others.

HEALTH PROMOTION AND HEALTH MAINTENANCE OF THE YOUNG CHILD

The years following infancy are challenging for parents as the child grows and acquires new developmental skills. The child progresses from the first tentative steps and words at a year of age through the "terrible twos" of toddlerhood and into preschool age when most children attend some type of education program, have well-developed verbal communication, and acquire many gross and fine motor skills. Toddler and preschool ages are often grouped as "young childhood" since the family remains the primary system within which the child interacts, and there are many common health concerns such as nutrition, sleep, and growing independence. Facing consistent changes in development, parents rely on the pediatric healthcare home (medical home) for advice and information. Regular visits are recommended for 12, 15, and 18 months, and at about 2, 3, 4, and 5 years of age. Nurses apply concepts of anticipatory guidance during visits for health promotion and health maintenance to assist parents in the transitions they face.

Recommendations for developmental health supervision of young children include four main categories. Use this framework to plan these health supervision visits:

1. *Assessment* is performed, using screening tests, evaluations, and observations.

2. *Education* provides information about parent-child interactions, sleep, discipline, and other developmental tasks.

3. *Intervention* includes counseling the parent, making home visits, and ensuring ongoing contacts with health professionals.

4. *Care coordination* between the office setting and community resources ensures that proper referrals occur.

(Halfon, Regalado, McLearn et al., 2003)

GENERAL OBSERVATIONS

The relationship with the family should be established as a partnership in care of the child. If, however, the family is new to this care provider, reach out to welcome them warmly and express interest in them as individuals and parents. Families often feel uncomfortable in healthcare settings, and it is important to establish positive rapport so they will be able to ask questions and bring up concerns about the child.

While calling the toddler in from the waiting room, it is wise to recall the child just 1 year before. It is amazing that this young child is now able to walk in, even if with a bit of help. Watch for the child's desire for independence or signs of continuing reliance on the parent. By preschool age, the child is totally independent in walking and usually engages in conversations easily. Welcoming the preschool child warmly, assess the child's social skills and motor activities. Direct greetings or questions to the child to evaluate stranger anxiety and ability to understand simple commands or questions. What verbal skills are observed? Observe the child's general appearance, nutrition, and state of health.

Health supervision visits are adapted for older toddlers and preschoolers to include observations of parental discipline and interaction style. Does the parent respond to the child's questions? Were age-appropriate toys or activities brought to the visit to help occupy the child while waiting? Is the child observant of the environment and alert?

GROWTH AND DEVELOPMENTAL SURVEILLANCE

The first assessment skill integrated into the visit is generally measurement of growth. Weight and length are measured and compared to expected patterns of growth. Once the child can stand to be measured, sometime between 2 and 3 years of age, charts for standing height rather than recumbent length are used. Body mass index (BMI) is first calculated at 2 years of age and provides information about the relationship of height and weight (see Chapter 34 for additional information ∞). Head circumference is usually measured until 1 to 2 years of age. (Consult growth grids in Appendix C. ∞)

Growth continues to be a primary way of evaluating the child's nutritional status. It may also provide clues about conditions that have not yet been evaluated such as endocrine, cardiac, or other disorders. Depending on the results of growth measurement, additional data may be gathered. For a child under the 5th percentile for weight or BMI, detailed nutritional intake records should begin. Laboratory studies such as hematocrit and hemoglobin can be performed. Patterns of family growth can be examined. What size are the parents and siblings? Ask if the child has had any illness or hospitalization. For children above the 85th percentile for BMI, detailed dietary intake and physical activity history should be taken.

The physical assessment is performed, with some parts conducted by the nurse and others by the primary care provider such as a physician or nurse practitioner. See Chapter 35 for a thorough discussion of physical examination. ∞ The order of the examination and the approaches to the child are particularly important at this age. Leave intrusive procedures such as ear and eye examinations, and visualization of genitalia until the end of the examination. Integrate techniques such as allowing the child to play with the stethoscope, asking the child to "blow out" the light from the otoscope, or having the child make a game of pushing the legs against the examiner to measure symmetry of strength (Figure 37–9 ●). Preschoolers are generally interested in their bodies, and teaching about parts of the examination is helpful. During the physical examination, ask the parents pertinent questions. Consider the young child's expected developmental milestones (see information in Chapter 33 ∞) and ask questions related to these milestones. Developmental surveillance is integrated throughout the visit and developmental screening or testing is performed. Ask if the child has had developmental testing done at a childcare agency or another site.

Nurses generally have in-depth knowledge of child development, through growth and development courses and pediatric nursing curricula, and are thus well positioned to address parental concerns related to child development. Topics pertinent at health supervision visits of young children include sleep patterns, discipline techniques, toilet training, learning and reading practices, communication, and parental issues and questions. Many children, especially by preschool age, are attending a childcare center. Ask about the experience and whether developmental skills are a focus of activity. Ask if the parent is pleased with childcare experience or needs further resources.

Health promotion growth and development issues for toddlers and preschoolers are addressed at each visit. Some common examples include:

- Explaining growth patterns and what is expected in the months ahead.

- Providing toys that encourage development of the coming developmental milestones.

- Showing parents the child's developmental progression on a screening tool.

● **FIGURE 37–9**

A

B

The approach to examination of the toddler or preschooler is important in order to elicit cooperation. **A,** The toddler may accept parts of the examination best when seated on the parent's lap such as shown in this photo of a boy with his father. **B,** The preschooler likes the opportunity to touch and become comfortable with equipment used, or in this case, holds a doll that receives the same examinations as the child.

Likewise, health maintenance activities are included in health supervision visits, with the primary purpose being prevention of disease and injury. Specific examples are included throughout the chapter, but some general areas addressed are:

- Connecting developmental skills with risks for injury such as drowning and car crashes.
- Recognizing the possibility of infectious diseases as the child begins a childcare experience and addressing recognition of and treatments for common diseases.

Expected outcomes for the child include normal growth and development patterns for motor, language, and social skills; parental knowledge of stimulating activities for the child; awareness of the family about risks to growth and development; and healthy body systems for the child.

NUTRITION

The child's nutritional status continues to play an important part in promoting health and preventing health disruptions during toddler and preschooler years. Good nutrition fosters normal growth patterns, promotes developmental progression, and helps prevent disorders such as anemia, tooth decay, and immune dysfunction. Intake of food takes on an increasingly social dimension during early childhood as children interact more with adults and other children at mealtimes.

For toddlers, questions for the family focus on introduction of foods, the child's eating patterns, and transition from breast or bottle to other liquids. The toddler often consumes small amounts of foods, and parents consequently worry about the change in appetite. Showing them that the child is growing normally can help allay their anxiety about this common developmental variation. Preschoolers increasingly interact with others during food preparation and meal consumption. Questions focus on the child's likes and dislikes for particular foods, behavior at the table, and establishment of healthy family eating patterns. Ask how often the family eats out, especially at fast food restaurants. When parents are busy and older siblings are in activities, both toddlers and preschoolers may be eating foods such as french fries or milk shakes several times weekly. Suggest alternative approaches to the busy lifestyle, such as bringing fresh fruit slices along when an older sibling is at a sporting event, keeping a cooler in the car to maintain cool items, and limiting fast food meals to no more than one or two weekly. Encourage the family to set times when they all eat together, even if only a few times weekly. If children help with preparations for this family meal, and then eat together, nutritional knowledge and intake can be positively enhanced. When the child is in a childcare center or home, encourage the parents to find out what food is provided for the child in that setting.

During the toddler and preschool years, children are gaining much more independence about food choices and patterns of eating. At the same time, their eating patterns depend mainly on the family and so assessment should involve the entire family unit (see "Developing Cultural Competence: Family Nutrition"). Parents can benefit from receiving information about nutrition in young children (Table 37–7).

DEVELOPING CULTURAL COMPETENCE

FAMILY NUTRITION

Each family integrates their own cultural backgrounds and past experiences into food preparation and choices. Ask what foods are common in the child's cultural group and help the family learn when to introduce each food. For example, rice may be a first food for an Asian baby, rather than rice cereal. Be sure the child also takes in adequate iron sources in the first foods offered. Tofu or bean paste may be a common protein source in some diets. A Native American child may eat fish or wild game, along with berries and roots. Ask and learn about each family's cultural patterns. Learn what you can about cultural groups in your community. Encourage the family to offer the young child their usual foods, as long as they meet needs for requirements, are prepared with minimal salt and seasoning, and are soft enough to avoid choking. Perform diet recalls and analyses to check for any specific teaching needs in all families.

Health promotion interventions include actions such as supporting breastfeeding for young toddlers and being sure preschoolers have a role in selecting foods for healthy snacks. Important health promotion teaching to include with every family is the importance of including "5 a day," or 5 servings of fruits and vegetables into the daily diet. Nurses and parents partner together to ensure that the young child establishes healthy eating habits at home and in other daily settings. Health maintenance activities focus primarily on disease and injury prevention, with examples of feeding practices that do not include common choking foods, and limiting daily fruit juice intake to prevent dental caries and excessive caloric intake. Desired outcomes related to nutrition include meeting normal growth and development milestones, maintenance of recommended weight, increasing understanding of healthy food patterns, and prevention of nutrition-related disorders.

PHYSICAL ACTIVITY

The toddler and preschooler consistently show gains in fine and gross motor abilities. They move around independently and have more physical activity away from the home base. They commonly visit parks, swim, attend childcare centers, and help with some household tasks. These activities are important, both because they assist the child to continue to develop motor skills and because they limit the amount of time spent in sedentary behavior. The toddler and preschool years are an important time for setting the habits for physical activity during all of childhood.

TABLE 37–7 ❖ Nutrition Teaching for Health Promotion and Health Maintenance Visits

Age	Nutrition Teaching	
1 year	Support mother who continues to breastfeed. Wean child from bottle by substituting cup. If beginning to use cow milk, use whole milk. Limit juice to 4–6 ounces daily; offer water several times daily. Encourage safety measures—use high chair with strap, secure child and use caution in grocery carts, do not allow foods to be eaten in car. Provide information on choking and airway obstruction removal training.	Provide food and water safety guidelines (see Chapter 34). Be sure all major food groups have been introduced. Limit high-fat and high-sugar foods. Review amounts of food commonly consumed and frequency of feedings. Review use of fluoride if water supply is not fluoridated.
2 years	Encourage total removal of bottle if still in use. Ensure that all foods common to family have been offered. Offer child-sized eating utensils. Child can change to low-fat or skim milk if family desires. Limit milk to 2 servings daily.	Teach parents methods for dealing with temper tantrums over food—make food available at meal and snack times only, do not force intake, offer a variety of foods. Teach that child may have days of very low intake due to slowing growth rate.
3 years	Teach normal intake and decreasing number of snacks. Engage child in food preparation and pouring liquids from small pitcher. Recognize that food jags (periods when only 1 or 2 foods are eaten) are common.	Recognize importance of social nature of eating; expect child to sit for a short period at meals with family. Meals and snacks should not be eaten while watching television.
4 years	Encourage involving child in snack selection and preparation. Start to teach food groups and importance of nutrition for the body.	Alter intake as appropriate depending on weight and BMI. Dairy products consumed should all be low or reduced fat.

During toddler years the main emphasis is on providing experiences that encourage further motor development. The child needs to walk, run, hop, push and pull objects, and throw balls. Motor activity is a major component in all play times, and activities should engage the child's large and small muscle groups (Figure 37–10 ⦿). By the preschool years, coordination becomes increasingly important. Physical activity is important for all children, including those with developmental disabilities. The preschooler learns to balance, walk on one foot, skip, and throw and catch with greater accuracy. Kinesthesia, or the sense of one's body position and movement, develops during these years. Eye-hand coordination improves at the same time that visual acuity matures (Patrick et al., 2001). The social component plays an important role as children learn to engage in games and activities cooperatively with others.

The nurse applies the concept of resilience by identifying both risk and protective factors related to physical activity (Table 37–8). The assessment becomes the basis for nursing interventions, both to reinforce positive physical activity and to make recommendations for changes where needed.

Since both children and adults are commonly overweight and sedentary in today's society, emphasis on phys-

⦿ FIGURE 37–10

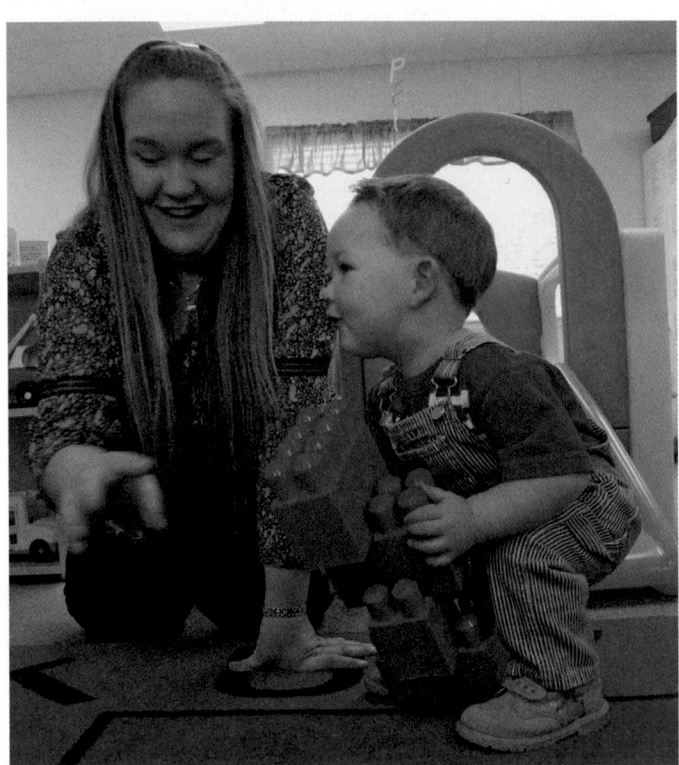

This toddler enjoys motor activity that uses large muscle groups. The preschooler begins to spend increasing amounts of time in coordination of both small and large muscle mass. List several physical activities that you can suggest for the parents of children in each of these age groups.

TABLE 37–8 ✣ **Risk and Protective Factors Regarding Physical Activity in Toddlerhood and Preschool**

Risk Factors	Protective Factors
▪ Limited stimulation by family or other care providers	▪ Expected developmental progression
▪ Long work hours by parents	▪ Daily contact with other young children
▪ Parents who have little physical activity on a daily basis	▪ Easily engaged socially with others
▪ Limited social time with other children	▪ Eagerness to try new physical activity
▪ Limited access to balls, slides, balance beams, tricycles, and other materials that foster physical activity	▪ Access to balls, slides, balance beams, tricycles, and other materials that foster physical activity
▪ Adequate safety gear for activities is not available	▪ Adequate safety gear that properly fits child is available
▪ Reluctance to try new physical activity	▪ Family members engage in daily physical activity
▪ Television or other screen activities are engaged in for more than 2 hours daily	▪ Family members spend time daily in physical activity with child
▪ Developmental delay	▪ Family understands motor developmental milestones and importance of physical activity in childhood
▪ Slow development of social skills	
▪ Lack of knowledge by family about child physical activity needs	▪ Television and other screen activities are limited to no more than 2 hours daily
▪ Limited community resources for child care and physical activity	▪ Neighborhood contains access to child care which integrates physical activity
▪ Unsafe neighborhood and lack of lawns, parks, and other facilities	▪ Neighborhood is safe, and contains lawns, parks, and other facilities

Data from Patrick, K., Spear, B., Holt, K., & Sofka, D. (Eds.). (2001). *Bright futures in practice: Physical activity*. Arlington, VA: National Center for Education in Maternal and Child Health.

ical activity should be a part of each health supervision visit. Nurses and parents are partners in planning activities for the young child; patterns set in motion at this early age will continue into the rest of childhood and into adulthood. Suggestions for the family may include setting guidelines to limit television and other screen activities to a maximum of 2 hours daily in order to facilitate adequate physical activity time. Children should not have television and computers in their bedrooms. Health promotion teaching imparts to parents the benefits of activity, such as a healthy immune and cardiovascular system, positive self-concept of the child, and the child's learning of important motor skills. Health maintenance teaching focuses on disease prevention, such as avoidance of overweight, and injury prevention, with use of protective gear for sports.

Expected outcomes of health promotion and health supervision related to physical activity are daily inclusion of at least 60 minutes of activity into life patterns, normal developmental progression of the musculoskeletal system, growth in coordination, and appropriate balance between dietary intake and physical activity so that normal weight is maintained.

ORAL HEALTH

The early childhood years play an important part in the child's future oral health, and yet dental care remains one of the most preventable and common unmet healthcare needs for children in developed countries (VanLandeghen et al., 2003). **Early childhood caries (ECC)** is defined as one or more decayed, missing, or filled tooth surfaces in a child 71 months of age or younger (American Academy of Pediatric Dentistry, 2003). This condition is caused by inadequate preventive care, which can include diet, brushing, and feeding habits. ECC is serious because young children with the condition are more likely to have continuing dental problems that can influence speech, cause pain, and delay development. Teaching prevention at an early age is key to preventing the problem.

The nurse assists the family to ensure oral health for the young child. At about 1 year of age, the child should have made a first visit to the dentist. By about 2 years of age, the toddler has a full set of 20 primary teeth, called **deciduous teeth**, that will be lost during childhood, beginning at about 6 years. Evaluate these teeth for condition and number. They help to maintain space for the permanent teeth, foster positive eating habits, and are needed for language development. Inquire about how the family cleans the teeth and ask them to demonstrate if the child has any dental decay. At the end of preschool, the first of these deciduous teeth are lost, an important developmental event for most children.

Based on the results of the assessment of the child's teeth, observation of language skills, and answers to questions directed at parents, plan interventions that will foster maintenance of oral health, thus preventing dental disease. (See Chapter 46 for emergency treatment of dental injury. ∞) These may include referral to low-cost dental clinics, provision of toothbrush and toothpaste, demonstration to the parents and young child about proper brushing technique, and teaching about limiting sweet snacks and drinks. Remember to positively reinforce health promotion practices such as good oral hygiene for toddlers and preschoolers who brush, visit the dentist, and are careful to limit intake of sweets. Desired outcomes for oral health are eruption of a normal set of deciduous teeth, regular dental care, nutrition and hygiene practices that foster dental health, and knowledge of child and parent about oral health.

MENTAL AND SPIRITUAL HEALTH

The family is key in fostering a positive self-image and setting the stage for the young child's mental health. As the family is called in for the visit, begin an assessment of the family's methods of influencing mental health. Observe communication and interactions in the family and the child's ability to interact with healthcare providers. Ask for a description of a typical day or what the child has recently begun to do. The child's sense of self and mental status are related to new accomplishments. Inquire about toilet training, toothbrushing, choosing clothes and getting dressed, using crayons, or other developmental tasks.

Self-regulation by the infant was described as the ability to soothe and comfort the self. By toddler and preschool periods, the young child self-regulates other activities to control anger, desires for objects or foods, and other behaviors. In order to assist the child in developing the ability to control and regulate self, parents often use discipline techniques. Ask about how the parent deals with the child who is having a temper tantrum or showing other undesirable behaviors. Reinforce positive ways of helping the child set limits for self and make suggestions when parents need assistance (see "Teaching Highlights: Positive Discipline"). The goal of discipline is to help the child develop a sense of right and wrong, and to learn acceptable ways of dealing with other people.

Adequate sleep and rest are needed for children to master self-regulation. Most toddlers have established regular sleeping patterns with occasional night awakenings. They sleep about 10 to 12 hours at night with one or two daytime naps (Murray & Zentner, 2001). Parents have usually learned to establish clear routines such as reading a story, rubbing a back, and then leaving the child alone. Occasionally parents who work during the day may feel guilty about putting the child to sleep. Help them to spend quality time with the child after arriving home, and then to establish clear sleeping expectations. Transitional objects such as blankets or toys are important for the toddler and can be used during childcare experiences to provide comfort and help maintain normal routines. Some families prefer to have children sleep in the bed with parents. If this is the parents' decision, be sure they are aware of safety hazards such as excessive bedding, falling between headboard and frame, parental smoking that could lead to a fire, or parental alcohol and drug use which can lead to not being alert to the child.

The preschooler sleeps about 9 to 11 hours and may have one or no naps each day (Murray & Zentner, 2001). Some quiet playtime can be beneficial even for the preschooler who does not nap. At this age, some children develop awakenings at night and may need some assistance in falling back to sleep. **Nightmares** are frightening dreams that awaken the child who is often crying and upset. Parents

TEACHING HIGHLIGHTS

POSITIVE DISCIPLINE

First, provide structure that enhances the possibility of desirable behaviors:

- Limit rules to those that are essential. It will be easier to enforce a few important rules than many that are nonessential.
- Provide an environment where the child is mainly free to explore safely in order to avoid constant cautions. For example, have adequate play space for toddlers with limited fragile glassware in the usual daily environment. It is easier for the toddler to learn not to touch a few objects when adequate objects are provided for play.
- Spend time interacting with the child several times each day. Praise positive behaviors frequently. Preschoolers often like to have charts with stars to record picking up toys, helping a parent, and other positive behaviors. Once a certain number of stars is reached, a reward, such as stickers or an outing with the parent, is earned.

When the child shows undesirable behaviors:

- Use distraction as the first approach and praise the child for selecting the new activity suggested by the parent.
- Tell the child one time that the behavior is unsatisfactory and what will happen if the behavior persists.

- Separate the child from a setting in which behavior is undesirable. Place the child in "time out," a separate place that is safe. Toddlers can be placed in a playpen or crib, while preschoolers are told to sit on a chair. One minute of time out per year of age is a good length of time. Once time out is over, provide a positive activity and move the child directly toward the activity.

When undesirable behaviors include other people, such as biting or hitting:

- Tell the child clearly that it is not okay to hurt another person.
- Separate the child immediately from the situation and use time out.
- If there are repeated episodes, be sure the child is getting adequate sleep and food, has opportunities for active play that releases energy, and has positive attention from many people in the environment. Be sensitive to stresses such as a recent trauma or a new sibling.
- Encourage the child to "use words" instead of hitting or biting. Until able to do so on their own, parents can model this behavior. "You feel like saying 'I am really upset that you took my toy away.' Let's use words instead of hitting so your sister knows that."

---

can reassure the child, rub the child's back, provide some repeat of a bedtime routine such as reading a story, and then allow the child to settle into sleep again. It is not advisable to bring children to the parental bed since they may start to awaken at night in order to continue this practice. **Night terrors** are characterized by a child who cries out and appears frightened. However, in contrast to nightmares, the child having a night terror is not fully awake and may appear disoriented (Edelman & Mandle, 2002). Parents should quietly talk to and comfort the child, allowing the child to return to sleep. There is no recollection of these events the next morning.

The toddler gains more independence in many aspects of life such as mobility and speech. The control over toileting is another milestone that signals greater independence and can lead to a sense of self-control. Ask parents if the toddler has shown interest in toilet training and how they intend to work with the child to attain control over bowel and bladder (see Chapter 33 for further discussion about toilet training ∞). Preschoolers are generally well trained for bowel and bladder with only occasional accidents. These should be treated with understanding rather than blame in order for healthy self-concept to develop.

Preschoolers are increasingly aware of gender and sexuality issues. They may ask questions about kissing, love, or their genitals. These questions should be truthfully an-

swered, leaving the child with a positive sense of sexuality. Some exploration of genitals can occur, and children should be told simply that it is something that should occur in private, and then offered other activities to engage them when with other people.

The family's spiritual orientation takes on additional meaning for the toddler and preschooler. They can participate in the family's faith-based practices, which enlarge their microsystem influences to include that of the religious group, thus reinforcing the child's learning about right and wrong. The nurse assesses the family's faith-based or spiritual beliefs and provides support for the family's approach, whether it is in established religious organizations or in the family's other meaningful activities.

Health promotion activities focus on development of a healthy self-concept in the toddler and young child by helping parents to set up successful play experiences, to praise the child for successes, to use effective limit-setting techniques, and to realize and appreciate the child's unique characteristics. Health maintenance seeks to avoid poor self-image that can occur with constant criticism or expectations not in alignment with the toddler or preschooler developmental capabilities. Further examples of the family interactions that can influence the child's self-concept are provided in the following section on relationships.

Desired outcomes for the child related to mental and spiritual health include emergence of a positive self-esteem, ability to self-regulate behaviors, emergence of methods to handle daily stressors, and normal developmental progression in tasks such as toilet training and sleep.

RELATIONSHIPS

Family members are part of the microsystem for the toddler and preschooler, and as such, form a vital part of the child's environment. Families with members who handle stress well and have healthy lifestyle patterns offer security for the young child. When parents are stressed or depressed, the mental status of all family members can be affected. Ask how things are going for the family in general. Inquire about siblings and whether there are any issues of concern that might influence the toddler or preschooler. Illness or behavior problems in a sibling can decrease the parent's ability to deal with other children. The focus on a sibling in need can be confusing to a toddler or preschooler. Be alert for signs of child abuse and for substance abuse in family members. Have the parents become separated or divorced? Is there a new stepparent?

During questions and observations, the nurse identifies family risk and protective factors. Reinforce strengths and provide services and referrals to deal with risks. Some strengths include the following:

- The family spends time together each day.
- Parents are proud of the child's accomplishments and knowledgeable about developmental progression.
- Childcare center personnel and family members interact regularly to plan consistent approaches for the toddler and preschooler.
- The teen mother of a toddler is enrolled in a high school continuation program with a childcare component.

Examples of risks to mental health include the following:

- Mother has been diagnosed with depression.
- Uncle in home uses street drugs.
- Child awakens with night terrors.
- Child was recently in a serious car accident.
- Teen mother is estranged from own family and has few goals and resources.

Toddlers continue to grow in social abilities, while preschoolers demonstrate large strides in socializing with others. Expect that most toddlers will enjoy playing with other children, although they play "side by side" and not cooperatively. They also engage in play with adults for short periods, such as throwing a ball. However, preschoolers begin to engage in activities that involve other children directly. They play "house" where one child plays the mother, and another the child. They engage in simple games where each plays a separate role. Their interactions with adults display similar maturity as they take on tasks such as setting the table for dinner or picking up books from the floor. Social skills involve getting along with others. Young children exhibit increasing skill in language development, a primary medium for social exchange. From just a few words at 1 year, the child has progressed to stating three-word sentences by 3 years of age. While all parts of speech are not in place, young children certainly have the ability to make needs and thoughts known. Assessment of language skills provides a mirror into this important means of socializing.

Successful social skills involve separating from the parent at times. During toddlerhood, most children spend some time away from parents. Initially they may be fearful and display crying, but gradually they learn to adapt to the new person and place. Preschoolers need to begin developing relationships with other adults and children in order to adapt to the school setting at about 5 years of age. Ask how many people the child has contact with each week and how they manage separation from the parent. Encourage parents to see separation as a skill the child is learning rather than something that is guilt-producing for them. When they leave the child in a secure setting, they should hug, provide a favorite object, and leave. Short periods initially will teach the child that the parent can be trusted to return.

Expected outcomes of health promotion and health maintenance activities with young children include increasing social skills with parents, siblings, and other children and adults; successful management of temperament characteristics; adjustment to time away from the home; and improving language/communication skills.

DISEASE PREVENTION STRATEGIES

Toddlers remain prone to many infectious diseases due to immature immune systems. By the preschool age, immune defenses are more mature and communicable diseases are less common. Some immunizations are given during this age period in order to complete a basic series. For the child who has not had all immunizations, extra visits to catch them up to recommended levels may be needed. At the end of the preschool period, the child has a complete review of the immunization record so any needed injections are given before school entry. See Table 37–9 for immunizations recommended during toddlerhood and preschool. Toddlers and preschoolers also need screening for several health conditions. Earlier visits may have failed to identify a problem due to the child's young age, so areas such as vision, hearing, and developmental milestones are always included.

Recognize that the environment is a powerful influence on the health of children. Ask if parents or others in the home smoke. Discourage this practice and describe the

TABLE 37–9 ❖ Routine Immunizations Recommended During Toddlerhood and Preschool Age

Immunization	Age Recommended
Hepatitis B	6-18 months: Administer #3 if series not completed during infancy
Diphtheria, tetanus, pertussis	15-18 months (#4) 4-6 years (#5)
Haemophilus influenzae type b	12-15 months (#4 or will be #3 for PRP-OMP type that requires only 3 doses for whole series)
Inactivated poliovirus	4-6 years (#4)
Measles, mumps, rubella	12-15 months (#1)
Varicella	12-18 months (only 1 dose needed at this age)
Pneumococcal	12-15 months (#4)

Note: Schedule may need to be adapted if child did not receive all recommended immunizations during infancy. See the CDC and AAP Web sites for recommended catch-up schedules.

health implications for the child. Is the neighborhood generally safe? Are there air, water, or other toxic exposures? Ask about lead exposure in the home (see Chapter 51 for more information ∞). How much television and other screen time is common in the home? Older siblings who allow the preschooler to play violent video games or watch many hours of inappropriate television can be affecting the mental health of the young child. Do parents watch the evening news, even when it involves violence, in front of young children? Do they discuss television shows with the child?

Ask if the child has had any diseases, whether common ones such as middle ear infection, or less common ones such as a serious respiratory infection. Has the child been diagnosed with a chronic disorder like cystic fibrosis or hemophilia? How has that affected their general health and family functioning?

Desired outcomes for disease prevention include integration of prevention methods into the family's daily life, prompt treatment of acute diseases, and individualization of all health supervision topics for the child with a chronic condition or special healthcare need.

INJURY PREVENTION STRATEGIES

Injuries remain a common healthcare problem for children during the toddler and preschooler years. The child's mobility, physical skills, and lack of understanding of the presence of hazards put them at particular risk. In addition, children are generally left to play alone for short periods, and toddlers and preschoolers can quickly get into dangerous situations. Every healthcare visit needs to include an assessment of risks and teaching to prevent injuries. Tables 37–10 and 37–11 list injury hazards during these age periods.

Ask parents what they think the most common hazards are for the age of the child, and add other hazards to their awareness. Car safety always needs reinforcing as the types of seats change when the child reaches 20 and then 40 lb. Be certain that children from 20 to 40 lb:

- Use a convertible forward-facing seat that has been placed in the back seat.
- Have harness straps at or above the shoulders.

Children over 40 lb should be placed in a belt-positioning booster seat:

- In the back seat.
- That uses both lap and shoulder belts.
- With the lap belt low and tight across the lap/upper thigh area and shoulder belt snug across the chest and shoulder.

Recommend that parents have their car seat checked by a childcare inspector. Give them the addresses of the closest inspection stations. These can be located by going through the National Highway Traffic Safety Administration (http://www.nhtsa.dot.gov) .

Some additional common and serious safety hazards are falls and drowning. In addition to providing general guidelines about safety, these most common injuries should be directly addressed. Children often fall down stairs, from counters where they have been placed or crawled, and from grocery carts. Drowning episodes occur when toddlers and preschoolers are not watched every moment while at a lake or ocean, fall from boats without personal flotation devices on, fall into a backyard pool, or drown in a bathtub or other body of water. While all young children should begin to take swimming lessons, this does not guarantee their safety around water. Nursing interventions concentrate on relaying to parents the severity of the risk of falls and drowning for children. Teach them to be aware of the dangers and to avoid them, both at home and in other settings. Refer them to classes on first aid and cardiopulmonary resuscitation.

The child spends increasing time away from the parent. Childcare situations should provide the same supervision the child receives at home. Help parents to ask questions and feel confident in safety at other settings. For example, while parents may be cautious about gun safety at home, few of them inquire if a home the child is visiting has guns and how they are stored.

TABLE 37–10 ✢ Injury Prevention in Toddlerhood

	Hazard	Developmental Characteristics	Preventive Measures
	Falls	Gross motor skills improve: Toddler is able to move chairs to counters and can climb up ladders.	Supervise toddler closely. Provide safe climbing toys. Begin to teach acceptable places for climbing.
	Poisoning	Gross motor skills enable toddler to climb onto chairs and then cabinets. Medicines, cosmetics, and other poisonous substances are easily reached.	Keep medicines and other poisonous material locked away. Use child-resistant containers and cupboard closures. Have Poison Control Center number (1–800–222–1222) by telephone.
	Burns	Toddler is tall enough to reach stove top. Toddler can walk to fireplace and may reach into fire.	Keep pot handles turned inward on stove. Do not burn fires without close supervision. Use a fire screen.
	Drowning	Toddler can walk onto docks or pool decks. Toddler may stand on or climb seats on boat. Toddler may fall into buckets, toilets, and fish tanks and be unable to get top of body out.	Supervise any child near water. Swimming classes do not protect a toddler from drowning. Use child-resistant pool covers. Use approved child life jackets near water and on boats. Empty buckets when not in use.
	Motor vehicle crashes	Toddler may be able to undo seat belt, may resist using car seat, demonstrating characteristic negativism and autonomy.	Insist on safety seat use for all trips. Use approved safety only, such as forward-facing convertible seat. Toddler is not large enough to use car seat belts.

TABLE 37–11 ✤ Injury Prevention in the Preschool Years

	Hazard	Developmental Characteristics	Preventive Measures
	Motor vehicle crashes	Older preschooler independently gets into car and puts on seat belt. Child may forget to belt up or may do so incorrectly.	Verify that child is belted in properly before starting car. Child restraint systems must be used until child weighs 18 kg (40 lb) and is 100 cm (40 in.) tall.
	Motor vehicle and pedestrian accidents	Preschooler increasingly plays outside alone or with friends. Preschooler is unable to judge speed of moving car and assumes driver knows that he or she is present.	Teach child never to go into road. A safe, preferably enclosed, play yard is recommended.
	Drowning	Preschooler who has had swimming lessons may choose to go into a lake or pool.	Teach child never to go into water without an adult. Provide supervision whenever child is near water.
	Burns	Preschooler can understand the hazards of fire.	Teach child to stop, drop, and roll if clothes are on fire. Practice escapes from home are useful. A visit to a fire station can reinforce learning. Teach child how to call 911.
	Needle sticks in hospital	Preschooler can ambulate and is interested in new objects.	Keep needles out of reach. Remove from unit immediately after use.
	Electrical injury in hospital	Preschooler is mobile and may trip over cords and equipment or may choose to examine them.	Avoid use of electrical cords if possible. Keep equipment out of major traffic areas. Keep beds away from electrical outlets. Monitor child closely.

Preschoolers are generally interested in health and their bodies. This is a time when teaching can become directed both to the parents and to their children. Preschoolers are receptive to practicing street crossing and tricycle/bicycle riding skills. It may be helpful to have a place in the clinic or office where they can be taught basic skills such as handwashing or street crossing. Consider the time of year and geographic location and teach appropriately. Spring is often a good time to teach bicycle and water safety, while winter hazards may include wood stoves or other heating devices. See Table 37–12 for further information about toddler and preschooler hazards and safety teaching needed.

Desired outcomes for the child are integration of safe practices into car restraints and other daily activities, progression through toddlerhood and preschool with no serious injuries, prompt care for minor injuries, and increasing understanding by child, parent, and other care providers of the common safety hazards at this age.

TABLE 37–12 ✤ Disease and Injury Prevention Topics by Age

Age	Injury Prevention Teaching Topics	
15 months	Wash adult and toddler hands frequently.	Have poison control number by phones and programmed into cell phones.
	Clean toys with soap and water regularly.	Be alert for dangers of hot curling irons and other appliances.
	Provide child's own bedding for childcare setting and wash weekly.	Have electrical cords out of reach and not hanging down.
	Use forward-facing car safety seat if child is 20 lb; install correctly and have installation checked; place in back seat and never in front seat with a passenger air bag.	Keep water temperature from being too hot to touch.
		Have home environment checked for lead hazards.
	Empty containers of water immediately after use; be sure pools or other bodies of water are locked and not accessible.	Secure the child in shopping carts.
		Do not let child have access to alcoholic drinks.
	Use sunscreen, hat, and long sleeves in the sun.	Remember that responsible adults should always supervise your child, not other children.
	Keep heavy and sharp objects out of reach; check that all poisons are locked away including in homes visited; keep pet food and cosmetics out of reach.	Know CPR, airway obstruction removal, and other first aid.
18 months	Follow the above.	Use a helmet on the child when taking the child on the back of a bicycle.
	Bolt heavy objects that might be pulled down securely to the wall.	Check batteries in home smoke alarms and check system.
	Be cautious of the toddler near machinery in the yard like lawn mowers and farm equipment.	Ask care providers about discipline methods; do not allow corporal punishment.
2–3 years	Follow the above.	Teach how to cross streets.
	When the child is 40 lb, switch to a belt-positioning booster seat, using vehicle lap and shoulder belt; place in rear seat.	Provide a helmet for riding tricycles.
	Teach handwashing after toileting and other activities.	Check playgrounds for safety hazards and hard surfaces under equipment.
	Clean potty chair thoroughly.	
	Keep guns unloaded and locked away in a different locked place than ammunition; have trigger locks installed.	
3–4 years	Follow the above.	Know CPR, airway obstruction removal, and other first aid for the child who has become a preschooler.
	Do not let child play unsupervised.	
4–5 years	Follow the above.	Teach safety around strangers (never go with a stranger; find a trusted person like parent or police).
	Continue teaching safety skills to the child.	
	Continue supervising when near streets or water sources.	

Data from Green, M., & Palfrey, J. S. (Eds.). (2002). *Bright futures: Guidelines for health supervision of infants, children and adolescents* (2nd ed.). Arlington, VA: National Center for Education in Maternal and Child Health.

NURSING MANAGEMENT ∎

NURSING ASSESSMENT AND DIAGNOSIS

Nurses partner with other healthcare professionals such as physicians, nurse practitioners, and speech therapists to assess health promotion and health maintenance status of young children. The toddler and preschool years are characterized by much developmental progression, and strategies need to be constantly adapted to meet the particular needs of the child and family. It is important to realize that the parents are partners in the care of the child and that every health supervision visit should address their questions and concerns. Their observations of the child are an invaluable part of the process. As the preschooler becomes more verbal, another partner is added to the healthcare team. Ask preschoolers what they want to learn, what questions they have about staying well, and other pertinent questions.

Toddlers and preschoolers are examined for growth, physical health status, and mental/social characteristics. Development is an area that many pediatricians feel ill-prepared to address but which parents commonly want addressed (Halfon et al., 2003). Nurses are adept at describing normal developmental milestones, evaluating the progression of children, and using anticipatory guidance to address parental developmental concerns.

Based on a thorough assessment, you will establish nursing diagnoses that are appropriate for the young child and family. Potential nursing diagnoses established during a health supervision of a toddler or preschooler might include the following:

- *Anxiety* related to change of environment (new care provider)
- *Parental Role Conflict* related to lack of support from significant others
- *Risk for Delayed Growth and Development* related to lead exposure
- *Health-Seeking Behaviors* related to parental desire for safety information
- *Impaired Skin Integrity* related to hyperthermia (sunburn)

PLANNING AND IMPLEMENTATION

Based on the nursing diagnoses established, the nurse works with other partners to plan strategies to meet the needs of the family. Explain that assessment questions are asked to provide a picture of the child that can be helpful in partnering with parents to plan healthcare. Reinforce the importance of the family coming to health supervision visits with their own list of issues. Work with other healthcare professionals to be sure all needs of a particular child and family are addressed.

Some teaching takes place as the examination occurs. Explain the height and weight measurements and what they mean. Relate them to questions about dietary intake and family food patterns. During the physical examination, insert information about common infections such as otitis media (middle ear infection) and share immunization information.

If the family has been reluctant to ask questions, reflect on the child's development. "Many children have trouble sleeping through the night; is that the case for Cassandra? What helps her to sleep? What is it like at her bed time?" Developmental areas such as sleep, discipline, toilet training, and expected developmental milestones should be addressed. If the parents were provided in an earlier visit with a journal to record observations and questions, ask if they have brought it with them.

A key part of the visit involves health promotion activities. It is essential to apply concepts of anticipatory guidance as you address the child's coming developmental progression. If the child will soon be toilet trained, provide information about possible approaches. If the child is learning to swim or has access to water, reinforce safety precautions near water. For the child going to a new childcare center, provide the parents with a list of questions they can ask the care provider, and tips to assist in the transition to a new setting.

Health maintenance activities are added to the visit as you give immunizations and screen for tuberculosis, lead screening, or problems with language, vision, or hearing. The focus of these activities is to prevent disease or to find it early before there are serious consequences. Whenever you find information that may indicate a problem, be sure to refer the child to the primary care provider, such as the physician or nurse practitioner. You may even recommend that the child be seen by another specialist such as a speech pathologist or dentist. Other health maintenance activities that must be part of each visit with a toddler or preschooler involve teaching about common hazards and how to avoid them. Emergency care in case of injury is also helpful information for parents, so first aid classes can be recommended.

Conclude the visit with some words of praise about the parent and child accomplishments. Provide the date for the next visit. List any resources helpful to the family, including the clinic/office contact information and emergency services.

EVALUATION

Parents should be asked occasionally to evaluate the care they are receiving at the health promotion and health maintenance site. Use these comments to monitor and adjust procedures as needed. The expected outcomes for nursing care of the toddler and preschooler include the following:

- The child demonstrates normal patterns of growth and progression in developmental milestones.
- The child remains free of disease and injury.
- Parents relay satisfaction with the pediatric healthcare home.
- The child manifests positive physical, social, and emotional adjustment.

Critical Concept Review

LEARNING OBJECTIVES

CONCEPTS

Define health promotion and health maintenance.	1. Health promotion:
	  ■ Activities that increase well-being and enhance wellness or health.
	2. Health maintenance:
	  ■ Activities that preserve an individual's present state of health and prevent disease or injury occurrence.

Describe how health promotion and health maintenance are addressed by partnering with families during health supervision visits.	1. Health promotion and health maintenance are integrated into healthcare visits. 2. Care provider adds identified information gathered at the visit which the nurse can then use to direct the activities.

Describe the components of a health supervision visit.	1. Assessment of:
	  ■ Growth and development.
	  ■ Amount and type of physical activity.
	  ■ Oral health.
	  ■ Mental and spiritual health.
	  ■ Relationships.
	2. Conduct disease and injury prevention screenings.

Explore the nurse's role in providing health promotion and health maintenance for the infant and young child.	1. Build effective partnerships with families. 2. Foster family-centered communication. 3. Address health promotion and health maintenance needs. 4. Manage time to provide for health promotion during routine healthcare visits. 5. Educate in family's teachable moments. 6. Advocate for children and their families.
Describe the general observations made of infants and their families as they come to the pediatric healthcare home for health supervision visits.	1. Do child and parent have close physical contact, eye contact, and vocalization during visit? 2. Do parents appear relaxed or stressed? 3. Does child behave as expected for age and situation? 4. Is parent able to effectively handle child being seen as well as any siblings present? 5. Does the baby respond to eye contact, movements, and vocalizations by the nurse?

Describe the areas of assessment and intervention for health supervision visits of infants and young children—growth and developmental surveillance, nutrition, physical activity, oral health, mental and spiritual health, family and social relations, disease prevention strategies, and injury prevention strategies.	1. Growth and development:
	  ■ Obtain length, weight, and head circumference.
	  ■ Observe and interview family to determine if infant is reaching appropriate developmental milestones.
	2. Nutrition:
	  ■ Determine type of infant feeding family is using.
	  ■ Instruct family concerning appropriate nutrition for infant's age.
	3. Physical activity:
	  ■ Assess daily routines and infant's ability to participate.
	  ■ Provide instruction concerning appropriate toys.
	4. Oral health:
	  ■ Inspect infant's mouth.
	  ■ Instruct parents concerning importance of toothbrushing.
	5. Mental and spiritual health:
	  ■ Instruct family concerning expected stranger anxiety and separation anxiety.
	  ■ Explain need for infant to develop self-regulating (self-comforting) behaviors.

(continued)

LEARNING OBJECTIVES

CONCEPTS

Describe the areas of assessment and intervention for health supervision visits of infants and young children—growth and developmental surveillance, nutrition, physical activity, oral health, mental and spiritual health, family and social relations, disease prevention strategies, and injury prevention strategies.—continued	6. Family and social relations:
	  ■ Encourage parents to play daily with infant and take a break when infant care becomes frustrating.
	7. Disease prevention strategies:
	  ■ Administer necessary immunizations.
	  ■ Instruct parents concerning when to call the physician.
	8. Injury prevention strategies:
	  ■ Instruct parents in proper use of car seats and prevention of falls.

Plan health promotion and health maintenance strategies employed during health supervision visits of infants and young children.	1. Explain procedures and the purpose of these procedures. 2. Encourage parents to ask questions and share general perceptions of the child.

Recognize the importance of family in infant and child healthcare, and include family assessment in each health supervision visit.	1. Health supervision visits begin with collaborative planning with the family.
	2. Each visit should include:
	  ■ Interview with family concerning developmental status of the child.
	  ■ Observation of family interaction.
	  ■ Discussion of parental concerns.

Integrate pertinent mental healthcare into health supervision visits for young children.	1. Mental health issues to be addressed include:
	  ■ Assessment of occurrence of common problems such as nightmares and temper tantrums.
	  ■ Explanation of the promotion of a positive self-esteem.
	  ■ Guidance in assisting child in self-regulating behaviors.
	  ■ Explanation of emergence of methods to assist child in handling daily stressors.
	  ■ Instruction in normal developmental tasks such as toilet training.

Synthesize data about the family and other social relationships to promote and maintain health of infants, toddlers and preschoolers.	1. Health promotion and maintenance activities related to social relationships focus on:
	  ■ Increasing social skills with the people in the child's environment.
	  ■ Successful management of temperament characteristics.
	  ■ Adjusting to time away from home.
	  ■ Improving language and communication skills.

CRITICAL THINKING IN ACTION

*View the **Critical Thinking in Action** video in Chapter 37 of the CD-ROM. Then, answer the questions that follow.*

Quinton and his mother have come into the office for his 2-year-old well-child check-up. During the visit you learn that his mother stays home with him during the day and his father often works overtime. His only significant medical history incident was when he had stitches placed in his forehead for falling on the edge of a table when he was 15 months old. There is a family history of attention deficit disorder and Crohn's disease. His height is in the 75th percentile, weight is in the 50th percentile, and body mass index is between the 25th and 50th percentiles. His temperature is 98.9°F and his pulse is 80. He is described by his parents as a picky eater and tends to eat the same foods frequently. They also say he tends to eat well on some days and other days will hardly eat anything. On the days he is not eating well, his mother will often resort to giving him soda or a sugary snack just so he is "getting something." Quinton sleeps about 7 hours per night and his mother usually ends up sleeping with him because he continues to fight going to sleep after being put to bed. He does not have a regular bedtime or rest routine and he usually naps in the car during the day. His mother tells you that her only break during the day when she is at home with Quinton is when he is watching television in his bedroom, so he often watches 2-4 hours per day. Quinton has a soft stool every day and has not showed any interest in potty training at this time. He is developmentally able to go up and down stairs, kick a ball, scribble on paper, and is able to speak in 3-4 word sentences. During the visit at the office, it is obvious his parents have difficulty controlling him and frequently make threats and offer bribes to get him to behave properly. He starts screaming and kicking when his parents set limits on his behavior in the office and his parents say they are frequently exhausted and do not know what to do about his high energy level. They also are concerned because they feel like the discipline methods they have been using are not working, and he is getting into so many things in the home that they are concerned he may hurt himself. They have used spanking and time-outs, but they do not seem to improve his behavior. They think he may have some type of medical condition like attention deficit disorder considering it does run in their family.

1. At 2 years of age, a consistent routine will help a toddler behave more appropriately. What are some of the things you can tell Quinton's parents regarding his sleep and nutrition habits to help establish a better routine?

2. How can you advise Quinton's parents about positive approaches to disciplining him?

3. How can you advise Quinton's parents about disciplining him when it is needed?

4. What are some suggestions you can give Quinton's parents about handling his temper tantrums?

MEDIALINK   www.prenhall.com/london

REFERENCES

American Academy of Pediatric Dentistry. (2003). *Policy on early childhood caries (ECC): Unique challenges and treatment options.* Retrieved August 25, 2005, from http://www.aapd.org

American Academy of Pediatrics. (2002). The medical home. Policy statement. *Pediatrics, 110,* 184–186.

Borghese-Lang, R., Morrison, L., Ogle, A., & Wright, A. (2003). Successful bottle feeding of the young infant. *Journal of Pediatric Health Care, 17,* 94–101.

Brenner, R. A., and the Committee on Injury, Violence, and Poison Prevention. (2003). Prevention of drowning in infants, children, and adolescents. *Pediatrics, 112,* 440–445.

Colyar, M. R. (2003). *Well-child assessment for primary care providers.* Philadelphia: F. A. Davis.

Denehy, J. (1999). Health promotion: A golden opportunity for school nurses. *Journal of School Nursing, 15,* 4–5.

Edelman, C. L., & Mandle, C. L. (2002). *Health promotion throughout the life span* (5th ed.). St. Louis, MO: Mosby.

Gafney, K. F., & Altieri, L. B. (2001). Mothers' ranking of clinical intervention strategies used to promote infant health. *Pediatric Nursing, 27,* 510–515.

Glascoe, F. P. (2003). How you can implement the AAP's new policy on developmental and behavioral screening? *Contemporary Pediatrics, 20,* 85–95.

Green, M., & Palfrey, J. S. (Eds.).(2002). *Bright futures: Guidelines for health supervision of infants, children, and adolescents* (2nd ed.). Arlington, VA: National Center for Education in Maternal and Child Health.

Halfon, N., McLearn, K. T., & Schuster, M. A. (Eds.). (2002). *Child rearing in America.* Cambridge, U. K.: Cambridge Press.

Halfon, N., Regalado, M., McLearn, K. T., Kuo, A. A., & Wright, K. (2003). *Building a bridge from birth to school: Improving developmental and behavioral health services for young children.* New York: Commonwealth Fund.

Hammermeister, J., & Peterson, M. (2001). Does spirituality make a difference? Psychosocial and health-related characteristics of spiritual well-being. *American Journal of Healthy Education, 32,* 293–297.

Harrell, W. A. (2003). Effect of two warning signs on adult supervision and risky activities by children in grocery shopping carts. *Psychological Reports, 92,* 889–898.

Jellinek, M., Patel, B. P., & Froehle, M. C. (Eds.).(2002). *Bright futures in practice: Mental health* (Vol. I & II). Arlington, VA: National Center for Education in Maternal and Child Health.

Lipman, T. H., & Hayman, L. L. (2000). Celebrating 25 years of pediatric nursing research: Progress and prospects. *MCN. American Journal of Maternal Child Nursing, 25,* 331–335.

Mindell, J. (2003). *Sleep, infants, and parents.* National Sleep Foundation. Retrieved August 28, 2003, from http://www.sleepfoundation.org/ask/ infantsandparents. *html*

MMWR. (2003). Physical activity levels among children aged 9–13 years—United States, 2002. *Morbidity and Mortality Weekly Report, 52,* 785–788.

Murray, R. B., & Zentner, J. P. (2001). *Health promotion strategies through the life span* (7th ed.). Upper Saddle River, NJ: Prentice Hall.

National Association of Pediatric Nurse Associates and Practitioners (NAPNAP). (2002). *NAPNAP position statement on the pediatric health care home.* Retrieved August 25, 2003, from http:// www.napnap.org/practice/positions/ healthcarehome.html

Nikolopoulou, M., & St. James-Roberts, I. (2003). Preventing sleeping problems in infants who are at risk of developing them. *Archives of Disease in Childhood, 88,* 108–111.

Patrick, K., Spear, B., Holt, K., & Sofka, D. (Eds.).(2001). *Bright futures in practice: Physical activity.* Arlington, VA: National Center for Education in Maternal and Child Health.

Pender, N. J., Murdaugh, C. L., & Parsons, M. A. (2002). *Health promotion in nursing practice* (4th ed.). Upper Saddle River, NJ: Prentice Hall.

Ryan, J. (2003). Improving oral health: Promise and prospects. *National Health Policy Forum Background Paper.* Washington, DC: George Washington University.

Schuster, M. A. (2000). Anticipatory guidance: What information do parents receive: What information do they want? *Archives of Pediatric and Adolescent Medicine, 154,* 1191–1198.

Sessanna, L. (2003). Teaching holistic child health promotion using Watson's theory of human science and human care. *Journal of Pediatric Nursing, 18,* 64–68.

Squires, J., & Nickel, R. (2003). Never too soon: Identifying social-emotional problems in infants and toddlers. *Contemporary Pediatrics, 20,* 117–125.

Story, M., Holt, K., & Sofka, D. (Eds.).(2002). *Bright futures in practice: Nutrition.* Arlington, VA: National Center for Education in Maternal and Child Health.

Thompson, K. M. (2003). The role of bath seats in unintentional infant bathtub drowning deaths. *Medscape General Medicine 5.* Retrieved April 2, 2003, from http://www.medscape.com/viewarticle/ 450989

VanLandeghen, L., Bronstein, J., & Brach, C. (2003). *Children's dental care access in Medicaid. The role of medical care use and dentist participation* (CHIRI Issue Brief 2. AHRQ Publication No. 03–0032). Rockville, MD: Agency for Healthcare Research and Quality. Retrieved June 30, 2003, from http://www.ahrq.gov/about/cods/chirident.htm

World Health Organization. (2001). *Background information about health promotion.* Retrieved June 6, 2003, from http://www.who.int/hpr/backgroundhp/

Young, L. E., & Hayes, V. (2002). *Transforming health promotion practice: Concepts, issues, and applications.* Philadelphia: F. A. Davis.

Health Promotion and Health Maintenance for the Older Child and Adolescent

Our school nurse is really great. She answers our questions about diabetes without making us feel like we're different than other kids. We can keep equipment like syringes in her office and she helps us to program our insulin pumps.

Jessalyn, age 12, child with diabetes

LEARNING OBJECTIVES

- Apply knowledge of school-age growth and development to identify needed assessment of nutrition and physical activity.

- State components of self-concept for school-age children.

- Describe the growing importance of peers in planning teaching strategies with school-age children.

- Use knowledge of the major injury risks of school-age children to plan nursing interventions that contribute to their prevention.

- Identify the major health concerns of the adolescent years.

- Apply communication skills to interactions with adolescents and their families.

- Apply assessment skills to plan data-gathering methods for nutrition, physical activity, and mental health status of youth.

- Intervene with adolescents by integrating activities to promote health and to prevent disease and injury.

MEDIALINK

www.prenhall.com/london

CD-ROM

Video: Teen Mental and Spiritual Health
NCLEX-RN® Review
Audio Glossary

Companion Website

NCLEX-RN® Review
MediaLink Applications:
   Develop a Teaching Plan: Smoking Education
   Case Study: Immunization Update

HEALTH PROMOTION AND HEALTH MAINTENANCE OF THE OLDER CHILD

The older childhood years span the time when most children enter kindergarten at about 5 years of age, and progress until about 12 to 13 years of age when adolescence begins. Even though health promotion and health maintenance needs continue during this time, less frequent visits to the pediatric healthcare home are recommended. In addition, most children are relatively healthy and need few immunizations, which may lead to only sporadic visits for care. Whenever older school-age children are seen in healthcare, even for illness or emergency care, it is wise to ask when the last "well-child" or health supervision visit was scheduled. Encourage the parents to make an appointment if the child is due for a visit. Visits are generally recommended at about 5 years of age, when most children are going to kindergarten, and then at 6 to 8 years, at 8 to 10 years, and at 10 to 12 years. The visits during this time will focus on establishing good health habits related to important issues such as nutrition, physical activity, and mental health; learning the importance of avoiding tobacco and drugs; ensuring success in school, family, and extracurricular activities; and fostering good decision-making and problem-solving skills.

GENERAL OBSERVATIONS

The first school-age visit usually occurs just before entry into kindergarten. During this visit the child has a thorough examination to be certain that physical development is normal, developmental milestones have been met for fine and gross motor skills, school readiness is displayed in social skills and language, and final sets of basic immunizations are completed. The child is often excited about the visit because it is associated with beginning school; some anxiety is often felt as it may be the first time the child is aware of getting "shots." As with earlier visits, the nurse's observations begin as the child is called in for the visit. It is wise to speak to the child first, introducing yourself and welcoming the child and parents to the office or clinic. Many children of this age actively participate in conversations, making teaching and gathering data easy. For children who are quiet or look to the parents, allow more time for them to get to know the personnel, directing most initial questions to parents. This may be the first visit where the child is old enough to be a partner in the healthcare visit. Establishing positive rapport with the child will be more likely to enhance efforts designed to teach about health.

Observe if the child brought a book, toy, or some other object to the visit. How are the parents interacting with the child? What types of speech tones are used? Is there mutual respect or are parents and child ignoring each other or having disagreements? The child should walk showing symmetry and ease of movement, follow instructions about where to go and taking off shoes for weighing, and demonstrate clear language skills with parent or healthcare personnel.

By the time children come for the 6- to 8-year visit and 8- to 10-year visit, they are expected to be increasingly active in sports, school activities, music, or other interests. Look for clues about their interests as they arrive. Did they bring books or a CD player? What are the book topics or favorite types of music? Ask what they are doing during the summer, or what their two favorite after-school activities entail. Have them describe a typical day to obtain clues about their life.

Some children do not commonly come to clinics, offices, or other settings for health supervision visits. School nurses or nurse practitioners in school-based clinics sometimes offer health promotion/health maintenance activities in the school setting. A major focus of school nurses is making the environment conducive to health for groups of children. School nurses may offer some parts of examination to individual children, such as growth and developmental surveillance; may conduct health screening, such as vision, hearing, or scoliosis; may work with food service personnel and administration to improve meal and snack quality and minimize unhealthy choices in vending machines; and may work with teachers to integrate concepts such as physical activity and self-esteem into classroom activities (Wainwright, Thomas, & Jones, 2000). The nurse often links children with healthcare needs to other community services.

During health supervision visits, watch the parents' responses as children answer questions. Be alert for the parent who interrupts the child or constantly "corrects" what is said. Some comments by the parent should involve praise of the child or looking to the child for opinions on certain topics. This indicates that a partnership is developing in the family and that family members work together and value each other. Direct some questions to the parents also. Ask if they came with specific questions or concerns that should be addressed. If the child has an individualized education or health plan (see Chapter 39 ∞), ask if the parent brought a copy, if the plan is still appropriate, or if it needs updating. Allow the parent an opportunity to meet with the physician, nurse practitioner, or other professional in a private place and without the child present if desired. Be alert for family dynamics that can influence mental health status. Ask if there have been any important changes in the family and how they have influenced the child. During conversations, be alert for reports of separation, divorce, remarriages, ill siblings or grandparents, recent or upcoming moves, parent job changes, substance abuse, incarceration of family members in jail, custody disputes, or other issues. Such topics can be followed up with further questions, as described later in the mental health section, to learn how they influence the child.

GROWTH AND DEVELOPMENTAL SURVEILLANCE

As the child comes into the health supervision site, height and weight are measured. Be sure to have the child remove shoes and coats. Ask the child and parents if they know the child's current height and weight, and if they have any questions. Plot the percentiles for these measurements, calculate body mass index (BMI) and its percentile, and explain the meaning of these findings later in the visit. Recognize that children do not grow uniformly; they have periods of slow growth followed by fast spurts. Similar to earlier ages, watch for children who have changed channels on a growth grid, and for those above the 85th percentile or below the 3rd

percentile for body mass index, and gather additional nutritional data in these cases (see Chapter 34 ∞).

School-age children have logical thought processes and are learning about their bodies. They should be active participants in the physical examination. Explain what you are doing and why. A head-to-toe examination is carried out, with particular attention to systems and skills that influence success in school. Vision, hearing, muscular strength, and coordination are examples of areas that affect school performance. See Chapter 35 for detailed information about the physical examination. ∞ Remember to provide feedback about the findings; families appreciate knowing that the child's vision is normal and strength is well developed. They should be told what is normal as well as areas that may need more assessment or intervention. Inquire about the child's sleep patterns. During the examination, ask for a description of any illnesses the child has had. Children of school age are generally healthy, with only a few upper respiratory infections or other minor illnesses annually. Unusual complaints may indicate a need for further testing; examples will be discussed in the disease prevention section later in this chapter.

School-age children frequently have minor injuries. These might include falls from bicycles, skin rashes from exposure to plants on a hiking trip, bruises from a ball sport, and other minor mishaps. Be alert for more serious problems that may indicate a need for additional detailed data gathering and teaching. Examples will be discussed in the injury prevention section.

Developmental surveillance continues to be an important part of the examination for school-age children. Some milestones can be observed during the visit while other information is obtained by report of parent and child. This information is combined with reports about school and other activities in order to establish that the child is developing as desired.

Desired outcomes for growth and developmental surveillance include normal progression with developmental tasks, absence of physical and psychosocial abnormalities or trauma, and integration of safe practices into daily life.

NUTRITION

Key concepts related to nutrition in school-age children are independence and formation of habits that influence the future. First, children are increasingly independent in food choices. They usually have strong likes and dislikes for certain foods. They may come home alone and prepare snacks. During school, they choose what to eat from the school lunch or the sack lunch sent by family. They may even have access to vending machines or sales of snacks during school hours. While independence in food choices is growing, the child is greatly influenced in those choices by friends and the media. Foods that may be rejected often include fresh vegetables and fruits, since they get little media attention, and friends may not prefer them.

At a time when the child chooses many of the foods in the daily diet, habits are being formed that will affect nutrition and health in general in the years to come. Good choices will help to promote health—to maintain weight at a recommended level, provide nutrients for adequate growth and activity, and prevent onset of some chronic diseases. Conversely, poor choices can lead to overweight and its accompanying problems, lack of adequate calcium and resultant osteoporosis, eating disorders, or lack of energy for brain growth and optimal performance in school. The patterns established during this period are often influential in later nutritional status. Knowledge about foods, family participation in good nutritional practices, and access to healthy foods can all be enhanced by nursing intervention during this critical formative period.

The first nutritional status assessment includes height and weight measurement, body mass index calculation, and examination of percentiles for each measurement on growth grids. Slow, steady growth is the norm during the early school-age years; it will be followed by a growth spurt when the child nears puberty.

During the visit, observations provide information about nutritional status. What is the condition of the nails, skin, and hair? What is the energy level and reported physical activity? Does the child look lean or overweight? As the child nears puberty, there may be an increase in fat stores as a preparation for the pubertal growth spurt (Story, Holt, & Sofka, 2002). Integrate some questions for the parent and child into the visit that provide clues about diet. While observing the child and family and asking dietary questions, list risks and protective factors related to nutrition. Perhaps protective factors relate to adequate access to nutritious foods, a family garden, and weight and height within normal limits. Reinforce the positive practices of the family and inform the child of how food choices relate to energy level, school performance, and general health. Risk factors become the basis for teaching and planning with the family for necessary change. It is difficult to tackle several nutritional changes at one time, so concentrate on those most needing attention, and on those the family agrees are important. Provide information about healthy snacks to keep at home, ways to improve calcium intake, the importance of getting at least five fruit/vegetable servings daily, limitation of soda pop to one can daily, and the importance of family meals (Figure 38–1 ●). Desired outcomes for health maintenance include absence of overweight and future chronic disease, adequate intake of all nutrients, and increasing child and family knowledge about nutrition.

● **FIGURE 38–1**

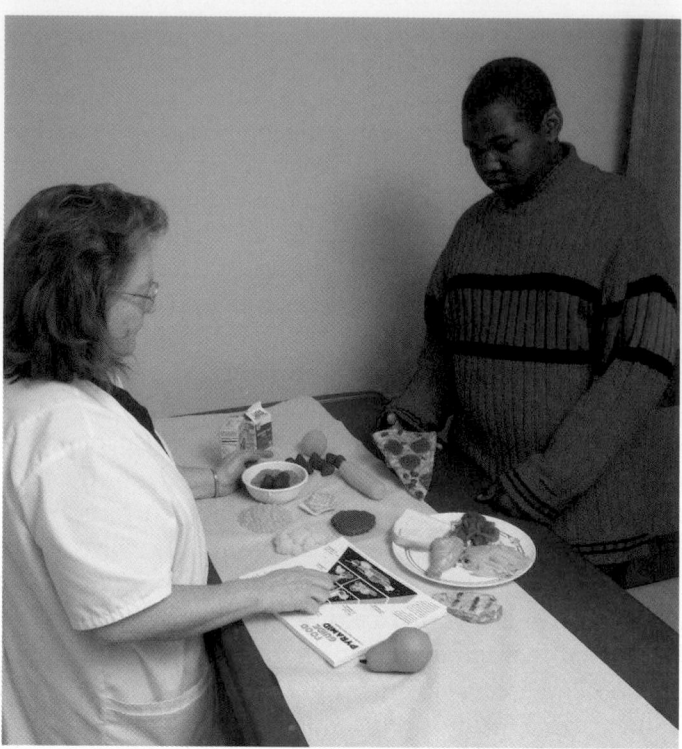

This school-age child is receiving teaching from the nurse about food choices. What benefit do the food models provide in this situation? What other teaching techniques can you suggest?

PHYSICAL ACTIVITY

Just as food choices during the school-age years are likely to influence the child's future nutrition, physical activity during these years is often crucial to development of lifelong exercise. During these years, the child who is physically active continues to refine skills such as eye-hand coordination, muscular strength, agility, and speed. Some children become skilled at ball sports such as basketball, football, soccer, or baseball. Others focus on gymnastics, wrestling, horseback riding, or hockey (Figure 38–2 ●). Some do not like team or organized sports but choose skateboarding, skiing, or biking. Whatever the interest, it is important that children identify some physical activity and continue to develop motor skills. The benefits include socialization, positive sense of accomplishment and self-esteem, weight control, and increasing physical ability (Figure 38–3 ●). Children who do not have an activity of importance often fall behind their peers in agility and skill, making future attempts at an activity very difficult and less likely to be successful.

Similar to earlier periods in life, the nurse lists risk and protective factors related to school-age physical activity (Table 38–1). Families are often significant in promoting physical activity for children. Find out what the parents do for physical activity and how often. Do they attend a sports

● FIGURE 38-2

Everyone needs to be physically active. Some children participate in school sports. Others, such as these boys playing hockey, choose a sport that is available in the community. Other children prefer to walk, ride a bike, or engage in other more solitary activities. Determine what is enjoyable for a particular child and provide assistance in integrating desired activity into daily routines.

● FIGURE 38-3

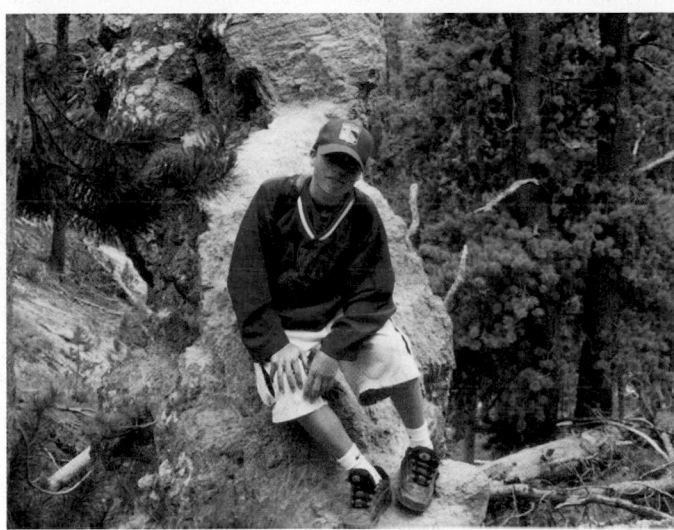

School-age children often enjoy hikes with family, clubs, or other groups. What are the physical and mental health benefits from this activity?

club after work or does the child see them engaging in exercise? Most families can include some walking, yard work, or other activity that is done together in order to engage the child. Do they walk to a neighbor's house or a nearby store rather than driving? Do they always take elevators, or choose the stairs in buildings? What is the activity level of siblings? When older siblings are involved in sports, the

---

TABLE 38-1 ✤ Risk and Protective Factors Regarding Physical Activity in School-Age Children

Risk Factors	Protective Factors
■ Limited role modeling of daily physical activity by parents and other family members ■ Limited facilities in the neighborhood to encourage activity, such as parks, skateboard facilities, rinks, ball courts ■ Inadequate financial resources to join clubs or pay for organized sports ■ School cuts to physical education programs and recess ■ School tryouts for sports that eliminate all but the best players in certain sports ■ Reluctance to try new activity ■ Worry about competence and physical appearance ■ Television viewing or other screen activities for more than 2 hours daily ■ Developmental delay and special needs	■ Expected developmental skill level ■ Feels self-confident in ability and physical appearance ■ Willing to try new activities ■ Sets goals for learning physical skills ■ Parents exercise daily and exercise with the child some of this time in a setting the child can see ■ Parents set expectation that everyone in family will choose a physical activity and engage in it regularly ■ Schools provide physical education each day with a variety of offerings; student gets to choose and set goals for some activities ■ Schools schedule recess or physical activity breaks twice daily ■ Sports teams are leveled so that all students desiring to play a particular sport, such as soccer, are able to do so ■ Adequate safety gear that properly fits child is available ■ Neighborhood provides access to parks, skateboard facilities, rinks, ball courts, and other facilities ■ Family has adequate financial resources to pay for health club or organized sports ■ Television viewing and other screen activities limited to no more than 2 hours daily

Data from Patrick, K., Spear, B., Holt, K., & Sofka, D. (Eds.). (2001). *Bright futures in practice: Physical activity.* Arlington, VA: National Center for Education in Maternal and Child Health.

younger child often is encouraged to develop skills in the same sport.

The child spends much of the day in school, and so this setting is important to consider. In an effort to conserve financial resources, some schools have decreased physical education (PE) programs. Children may not have regular PE classes, and there may be few standards of performance. In addition, many states and provinces have established tests and standards for performance in certain cognitive areas. In an attempt to increase teaching time to meet standards, some schools have cut out recess and other breaks. Some schools are located in unsafe areas and outside recreation is not advisable. It is unrealistic to expect children to sit for long periods without physical activity, and such practice reinforces the poor habits of inadequate exercise among children. Nurses are influential members of school committees and can encourage the integration of activity in the school day. They may be able to serve on a school or community committee, informing other committee members of the benefits of exercise to enhance cognitive performance and general health. Teachers and school administrators can be supplied with models of successful school activity programs. Nurses can often be influential in finding community volunteers to work with teams of students. Student nurses, physical education students, senior citizens, and others in the community may be able to help young children play baseball, tennis, or soccer. Other volunteers may teach stretching or warmup activities. Community partners such as businesses may provide protective gear or uniforms for school sports, especially if the business name can be displayed. In addition, schools can offer alternative activities that some children might prefer to traditional organized sports.

It is essential to consider physical activity for the child who has special healthcare needs. It may be difficult for schools to plan an activity for the child with cerebral palsy, visual impairment, or developmental delay. Search for other community resources and help the family to access them. There may be programs for children to ride horses, swim, ski, and engage in other physical activities. Imagine the thrill that waits a child who has rarely moved quickly when riding a sled or sliding on skis. In summary, the nurse plays an important role in meeting desired outcomes of health promotion by suggesting activities that parents can do together, becoming active in physical education programs in schools, acting as a positive role model, and helping interested children to partner with community resources for activity. Health maintenance outcomes include use of safety gear and correct techniques to prevent injury from sport participation.

ORAL HEALTH

Many changes occur in the mouth during the school-age years, necessitating periodic examination. About 6 years of age, most children lose a tooth, usually in the front. Following that, all 20 of the deciduous or primary teeth will be lost, and the permanent teeth will simultaneously begin to erupt. See Chapter 35 ∞ for the schedule of tooth loss and tooth eruption. In addition the jaw line elongates and teeth move into new positions. Periodic dental visits focus on both the placement of teeth and oral hygiene.

During the health promotion visit, examine the teeth. Look to see how many deciduous and permanent teeth are present. Describe the child's oral hygiene. Ask how often the child brushes, flosses, and visits the dentist. The child should have learned how to brush and floss during preschool years but is now performing the skills independently. If there are caries or poor oral hygiene is apparent, ask the child to demonstrate brushing and flossing. Reinforce the need for brushing twice daily and flossing once daily. Provide toothpaste and toothbrushes as gifts during health supervision visits. Local dentists will often provide these supplies to encourage oral hygiene.

Dental visits are recommended every 6 months. If the child is not visiting on that schedule, ask if finances or transportation is an issue, if the family needs a referral to a dentist, or if there is some other reason. If caries or malocclusion is present, stress the need for a dental appointment soon. Inquire about use of fluoride if the water supply is not fluoridated. Ask if the child has had sealants applied to the permanent teeth; these will help to prevent future caries.

Many children have a high intake of sugared foods and snacks. If this is apparent from the nutritional assessment, discuss the importance of limiting these foods and brushing after their consumption. Frequent brushing is needed when the child has braces. Ask how they are caring for them and what the orthodontist has recommended.

The nurse's health promotion activities include positive reinforcement of good hygiene habits, and health maintenance involves teaching about the need for improved care and limiting food that furthers the formation of caries. Desired outcomes include good oral hygiene, attendance at recommended dental visits, and absence of dental caries.

MENTAL AND SPIRITUAL HEALTH

The school-age years are marked by the emergence of new cognitive skills, ability to interact cooperatively with others, and a feeling of accomplishment in achievements. The child's self-concept and mental health are linked to these important developmental tasks. **Self-concept** is the mental idea that one has of the self. School age is an important period in the development of one's self-concept. **Self-esteem** reflects a positive self-concept; it includes the feelings and beliefs of children about their competence and worth as individuals, ability to meet challenges, and ability to learn lessons from success and failure (Jellinek, Patel, & Froehle,

2002). The aim is to establish a positive sense of self-esteem, even in the face of adversity and challenge. The child who believes in his or her ability to face good times and bad has a lowered chance of mental illness such as depression, eating disorder, and anxiety. Parents are encouraged to evaluate and help to build the child's sense of self-esteem (see "Teaching Highlights: Evaluating and Fostering Self-Esteem").

Many of the areas discussed already in this chapter provide clues to the child's self-concept. Are there sports or other physical activities? They may reflect a positive self-concept and body image. However, if the child is forced to do these sports by parents and feels inadequate in their performance, they may promote a negative self-concept and body image. Ask about children's activities and how they feel about them. Do they enjoy them? How do they rate their performance?

Inquire about school performance and best friends. Is there an increasing independence and responsibility for self? Success in achieving developmental milestones leads to a positive sense of self-esteem in the child. Parents are encouraged to evaluate and help to build the child's sense of self-esteem. A low sense of self-esteem is noted when the child states a disinterest in exercise, school clubs, and family activities. This can lead to loneliness, depression, and mental health problems such as eating disorders (Jellinek et al., 2002). When these feelings are noted during a health supervision visit, the nurse should recommend that the child see a counselor at school or another setting, and should recommend that parents be included in the sessions so that they can best help the child.

It is obvious that the family plays a critical part in the child's developing self-esteem and mental health. In order to understand the child, it is necessary to ask questions about and explore dynamics in the family. Several protective factors have been identified for families:

- Communication is open and clear, and parents use problem-solving skills.
- Members are encouraged and appreciated.
- Family is committed to each other, including spending time together.
- Religious or spiritual orientation is present.
- Social connectedness or support is available.
- Resilience or the ability to adapt to new situations is present (Wertlieb, 2003).

Ask about and observe the family's relationships. Evaluate the effect of family interactions on the child. Model respectful interchanges by listening carefully to the child, as well as the parent. Gently recognize the child if parents answer for the child or seem to put him or her down. Provide brochures and examples of ways to show children their importance. Encourage both parents to come to child healthcare visits and support the involvement of both parents in childrearing (Task Force on the Family, 2003). Ask about family stressors such as job changes, financial concerns, illness, substance abuse, and domestic violence. About one half of marriages end in divorce, so be prepared to offer suggestions to deal with this situation (see Chapter 36 ∞ for further discussion of effects of divorce on children). Ask about and identify risk factors and protective factors. The child's strengths are used to assist the family functioning and will, in turn, give the child a sense of accomplishment. Some examples include the following:

- A child who is able to act independently can be given responsibility for parts of the home or family function,

---

TEACHING HIGHLIGHTS

EVALUATING AND FOSTERING SELF-ESTEEM

Parents play an important part in fostering the child's self-esteem. The nurse can ask them to evaluate the child and provide suggestions about positive actions.

EVALUATION QUESTIONS	POSITIVE ACTIONS
What does your child do well?	Build on the child's strengths and talents; point out the child's abilities.
How does your child respond to failure?	Assist the child to assess performance; help the child see that mistakes are expected and have lessons to teach.
Does your child have close friends?	Arrange structured play times such as going to a movie or cooking with a friend.
How does your child respond to new challenges?	Give the child responsibilities at home; encourage your child to try new experiences; help the child feel a sense of control over outcomes.
How does your own personality compare to your child's?	Recognize differences in style; appreciate the unique qualities of the child; tailor expectations to the child and not to self or other children.
Are you setting reasonable and attainable expectations for your child?	Ask the child what is attainable; establish goals for behaviors together.

Data from Spratt, E. (2002). Assessing and reinforcing your child's self-esteem. In M. Jellinek, B. P. Patel, & M.C. Froehle (Eds.), Bright futures in practice: Mental health—Volume II. Tool kit (p. 94). Arlington, VA: National Center for Education in Maternal and Child Health.

such as planning the menu for dinner two evenings weekly.

- A creative child can be given the task of planning books and other activities for a younger sibling.
- A child with a talent for design can be asked to set the table for dinner guests.

Self-concept and self-esteem include all parts of the person such as cognitive, spiritual, sexual, and physical. **Body image** refers to a specific part of the self-concept—to the idea that one forms about one's body. **Sexuality** is another part of the self-concept and refers to the person's view of self as a sexual being, and what that means for one's life. The school-age child is developing a sense of body image and sexuality. Look at the child's appearance and dress. Some children may have poor posture, display a sense of insecurity, and seem uncomfortable with themselves. Others may dress as if they were much older, seem sophisticated, and are clearly assuming the role identification with their gender group. Ask the parents in a private setting what observations they have about the child's body image and sexuality. Inquire about friends of the opposite sex and whether the parent has concerns. Questions related to sexuality will emerge during school years. They should be answered truthfully and fully. Even children who do not ask questions usually need information related to sexuality education. They may get information in school beginning in about fourth grade, but often still have misconceptions about the bodies of men and women, sexual intercourse, how babies are born, and other topics. Suggest that parents read books with their children that deal with these issues at a level children understand. If books are available at home, children will be likely to look at them and ask questions. They should be in the home from third grade on since many young girls have body changes as early as 9 or 10 years of age (see Chapter 33 ∞). This can often put both parent and child at ease and open the door to discussion. Parents should be advised to talk with teachers to learn what is presented in school and be able to supplement and clarify this information. Having discussions at a young age will help lead to further discussion as the child gets older.

Suggest to parents that computer and other media provide information that can confuse children. Encourage them to watch movies with children, encourage frank discussions related to sexuality observed, and answer questions truthfully. Children generally learn about topics such as sexual intercourse, homosexuality, and childbirth from school discussions and the media. It is better to learn from parents than from friends or the media. A few moments alone with parents and child at healthcare visits may help to identify the concerns of each related to sexuality.

By about fourth to sixth grades, most girls have started to have prepubertal body changes and may have begun to menstruate. This is another opening to discussions about mature bodies of men and women and the transformation from childhood to greater maturity. Boys mature about 2 years later than girls. Without an event such as menstruation, parents may be less likely to start discussions with male children. Suggest that parents consciously begin conversations with boys periodically to explain changes they see in themselves and their peers. See Chapter 33 ∞ for further discussion of the body changes seen in the prepubertal period and during puberty.

School-age children continue to develop an ability to self-regulate activities and responses to situations. At this age the abilities to solve problems and assume more responsibility for self are important. Encourage parents to discuss issues with the child and to seek solutions together when appropriate. The child assumes more responsibility for assisting with meal preparation and home chores, coming home alone after school, and caring for younger siblings. Encourage the parents to praise the child for assuming more family responsibilities and recognize that the child will need some guidance when taking on new tasks.

Sleep is still important for children in order to have the energy to perform well in school and other activities. They generally take charge of bedtime routines with reminders about the time to go to sleep, and they sleep through the night. Sleep time varies from 8 to 12 hours, depending on child and activity level. Busy schedules may interrupt this pattern, leading to irritability, lack of concentration, or even hyperactive behavior (Colyar, 2003). Help children and families plan what the bedtime should be.

Sleepwalking and sleep talking sometimes occur at this age, but usually decrease as the child nears adolescence. Children who have stress at home, such as parental fighting, ill family members, or inadequate food or shelter, may not get enough sleep and fall asleep at school. Ask the child if falling asleep in class is occurring, and seek additional information about family stressors. This can lead to interventions such as recommending family counseling or referring to resources to obtain better housing or more stable food sources.

School is a major microsystem influence in the lives of children, and it plays a role in self-concept and mental health formation. Ask the child to describe a best friend; if unable to do so, isolation may be occurring. Inquire about what the three best and three worst things are about school. Children with low self-concepts often have trouble talking about and evaluating school. Find out where the child attends school, if the area is generally safe, and how the child gets to school. Encourage the parents to meet the child's teachers, to become active in school activities, and to be available to solve problems with school personnel when needed. Partner with the parents and child when interventions are needed. An office nurse may contact a school nurse when the child needs support in the school environment. This may occur if the child has become ill and missed school, has family stressors, does not get along well with a teacher, or has a condition such as attention deficit disorder. Identify the risk and protective factors in the school environment and plan interventions to support the child when risks are present. Certain mental health disorders are commonly seen during the school years. One example includes anxiety problems that result in worries, fears, physical symptoms, stress, and sleep disorder, without significantly impairing daily functioning. However, some anxiety disorders affect functioning and have more striking characteristics such as clinging, abdominal pain and headache, and refusal to attend school (American Psychiatric Association, 2000). Post-traumatic stress syndrome and depression may also be seen. See Chapter 54 for further description of these disorders. ∞ Anxiety disorder, post-traumatic stress, and depression should be referred to a mental health specialist for treatment. However, all children worry at times and this type of anxiety can be helped by learning coping skills and relaxation techniques.

Spiritual health is the ability to develop a spiritual nature, including awareness of a life purpose and fulfillment (Pender et al., 2002). School age is a time when children learn more about the people and the world around them, and begin to find their place in that world. Connection with faith-based groups assists some children and families in defining the purpose of life, while others may do so through social activity or a strong moral sense of responsibility. Ask children what brings happiness, how they help other people, or if they are members of a church, synagogue, or mosque. If families seem to have little purpose, parents are withdrawn or depressed, or the child has difficulty answering questions about meaningful activities, suggest methods of engagement in the community. These might include providing contacts at local religious events, posting flyers about community events designed to bring unity to various cultural groups, or suggesting services needing volunteers in the community. Families who spend time together and find meaning in supporting each other nurture the spiritual health of their members. Suggest that every family plan a "family night" weekly when they play games, talk, eat, or engage in other activities together.

The nurse has an important role in fostering the mental and spiritual health of school-age children. Health promotion fosters strengths of families and children, leading to healthy self-concept and positive self-esteem. Health maintenance seeks to prevent mental health disruptions. Be alert for risk factors in families since they represent the need for intervention. Expected outcomes for health promotion and health maintenance activities with school-age children include formation of a positive sense of self-esteem and healthy body image, use of coping skills to deal with stress, sleep patterns that meet needs for rest, and a growing purpose and meaning in life.

RELATIONSHIPS

While the school-age child is gradually moving away from the family as the center of life, the family remains an important anchor. The preceding section discusses several issues where the parents foster development. Ask also about siblings, grandparents, and other extended family members. Sometimes these persons assist in the child's formation of a self-concept. Peers are increasingly important to the school-age child's self-identity. School age is a time of cooperative engagement with others. All children need to learn how to make and maintain friendships and work with others on projects and in recreation.

Inquire about the child's best friends at school. In private, ask parents if they are comfortable with the child's selection of friends. Find out if the parents facilitate friendships by allowing other children to come to the home and providing transportation as needed. When the child experiences a risk factor such as a move to a new town or school, role-play how to meet new children and how to make friends. If the child feels like an outcast or outsider among peers at school, explore how the family can create a safe and secure place for the child in extracurricular activities with children who have similar interests. When children are home schooled, the family may need to plan social events and contacts after usual school hours.

Since peers are important to the school-age child, pressure begins to appear like others, to fit in, and to do what others encourage. Although such pressures are often associated with teen years, they usually begin earlier, at least by 8 or 9 years of age. Ask children what things friends try to get them to do that they know they should not do, or if friends have tried to get them to smoke. Middle school years are the most common age for beginning to smoke, so always ask if the child has tried smoking, being careful to do this when the parent is not present and the child is more likely to be honest. They may tell you about activities when parents are not in the room, such as playing with guns, trying alcohol or other substances, or other risky behavior. It is best to ask children what they do in these situations, what they want to do, and who they can talk to about these events. Offer information about the risks connected with behaviors that are described, and suggest people such as parents, teachers, counselors, or clergy who are possible resources. If the child's health is at risk, be sure to report the activity to the physician or other healthcare provider so that it can be pursued and the child's safety can be assured. Activities such as playing with firearms or visiting a friend whose parents are making methamphetamine, for example, place children in extreme danger.

School age is often a time when children first experience violence in relationships with others. Some children are bullied, while others are the bullies. Anger and aggression can occur, and children get in fights with each other. Ask children to describe when they last had a disagreement with someone and how the problem was solved. Suggest people like school nurses, teachers, and counselors who can help, and be sure that children feel safe in schools, neighborhoods, and homes. Ask parents how they resolve arguments between children at home and what help they need to help children learn problem-solving skills. Find out what policies the local schools have to assist in decreasing harassment of and by children. Become active on school committees that help children learn how to solve problems peacefully and how to respond to episodes of violence. See Chapter 36 for further discussion of violence in children and a detailed discussion of bullying. ∞

The child's temperament still plays a part in response to situations and the ability to self-regulate. The "difficult" child may have trouble getting to sleep or being quiet in the classroom. Have parents plan more physical activity for this child. Teach the child that bedtime routines are helpful and that sitting near the front of the class can help with concentration. The "slow to warm up" child may need ideas about what to say when meeting new people. Parents can help the child prepare for a new school by visiting with the child, talking about it, and meeting with the teacher so that a warm welcome can occur. The "easy" child is usually adaptable in most situations and is regular in activities. However, this child may object when other children interrupt, fail to take turns, or otherwise "break the rules" of behavior. They might need help to understand differences in temperament in order to be more tolerant of classmates and their behaviors. Often nurses in schools address the issue of individual differences by speaking with classes or small groups of children.

The nurse takes an active role in promoting the child's health by anticipating developmental issues and preparing parents and child to deal with them. Health maintenance outcomes include preventing problems in interactions.

DISEASE PREVENTION STRATEGIES

School-age children are generally healthy. The immune system is mature (see Chapter 44 ∞), personal hygiene practices are more mature than at earlier ages, and immunizations are usually complete. Engage school-age children in active pursuit of their own health. Teach strategies that can enhance the prevention of diseases. Nurses in offices and schools can teach children how to wash hands effectively, how respiratory infections are transmitted, what can cause gastrointestinal illness, and how to best manage their own health problems (Figure 38–4 ⊙). Ask children in your settings what topics are of most interest to them and

⊙ FIGURE 38–4

A student with diabetes is showing the school nurse how she programs her insulin pump. The nurse has partnered with nurses in the endocrinology office to learn about the type of pump the student is using. Such collaboration contributes to the monitoring and management of diabetes.

be prepared to suggest common areas of concern such as safety, skin care, athletics, and illnesses. Children are interested in their bodies and can understand the connection between eating well and avoiding illness, maintaining normal weight and preventing type 2 diabetes, avoiding smoking to prevent cancer and other respiratory diseases, and exercising to prevent hypertension.

School-age children are in the concrete stage of intellectual development (see Chapter 33 ∞). This means that teaching is most effective when opportunities are provided to touch, feel, and otherwise become actively engaged in learning. When teaching about smoking, provide models of lungs and have the students breathe through a straw to demonstrate the effects of airway narrowing. These concrete activities will teach them concepts better than simple lecture or reading (Figure 38–5 ⊙). Concepts of health promotion tend to be abstract since they deal with supporting one's highest potential for wellness. Thus, it becomes even more important to provide concrete methods of learning.

Immunizations are generally up-to-date for school-age children. However, some children may have missed earlier doses due to illness or missed healthcare visits. Evaluate the immunization record to be sure it meets all recommendations. The most common immunization needs at this time include the following:

- Hepatitis B (whole series or a missed third shot)
- Hepatitis A (if in state with recommendation for immunization)
- Tetanus-diphtheria, polio, or measles-mumps-rubella (if booster dose was not given prior to school entry)

● FIGURE 38-5

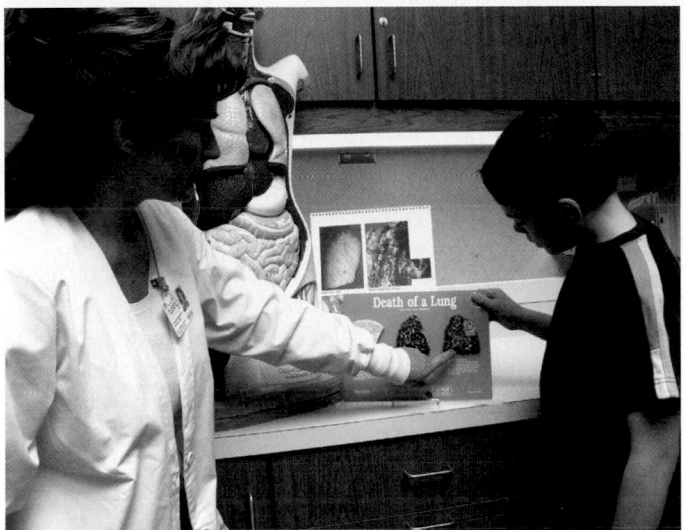

This boy is learning about the effects of smoking on the body through the concrete experience of examining a model of the lungs. Why does this type of hands-on technique help school-age children to learn concepts?

- Varicella if not given earlier and the child has not had the disease
- Meningococcal vaccine
- Certain vaccines for children at high risk, such as pneumococcal and influenza (see Chapter 15 for further information on immunizations ∞)

Screening for health risks should occur during the visit. These include hearing and vision screening, blood pressure monitoring, tuberculin skin test, and in some cases screening for hyperlipidemia and lead exposure. Unusual complaints may indicate a need for further testing; examples include the following:

- Pain other than brief discomfort after an injury
- Headaches
- Bruising
- Lack of coordination
- Repeated infections
- Decreasing vision or hearing
- Problems or changes in school performance or behavior

Children who have an identified health problem or developmental disability may have additional needs for screening and for interventions to assist with health maintenance. For example, the child with cystic fibrosis will need information to lessen risk of respiratory infection, and the child with diabetes may need additional blood studies. The child who has difficulty reading will need al-ternative approaches to teaching correct handwashing; demonstration with explanation may be the best approach. A family history of some diseases increases the child's risk and necessitates testing. For example, if a parent has had early cardiovascular disease (before age 55 years), a lipid profile should be performed on the child.

Parents should receive explanations about the screening tests performed and the results obtained. Inform them about vision and hearing results. Send home or call about results of blood tests when available. Be sure they understand the findings and have resources to assist in preventing or treating the specific disease in their children. Have them call with questions about health problems the child develops, and provide information about lowering risks of diseases. Be sure that families know when to keep children home from school (elevated temperature, active vomiting or diarrhea, coughing up brown or green mucus). Assist schools in setting guidelines for management of infectious diseases in that setting. Contact the local county and state health department for infectious disease guidelines for schools. Desired outcomes for the school-age child include prevention of infectious diseases, prompt treatment for acute infections, and careful management of existing health conditions in order to maximize health potential.

INJURY PREVENTION STRATEGIES

Injuries are a common cause of morbidity and mortality among school-age children, and each health maintenance encounter should include injury prevention strategies. Children have more independence and may be harmed by activities they engage in without adults, such as playing with fire or firearms. They participate in many sports and other physical activities and may suffer related injuries. Some children unfortunately suffer harm due to physical abuse or other forms of violence (see Chapter 36 ∞).

Many common injuries are preventable with simple use of protective gear and following safety guidelines. Eighteen percent of youth rarely or never wear seat belts in automobiles (MMWR, 2004). Many children ride bicycles, but only about 14% are protected by helmet use, contributing to 23,000 bicycle-related head injuries annually. Bike helmets could prevent up to 88% of serious brain injuries from bicycle crashes (Committee on Injury and Poison Prevention, American Academy of Pediatrics, 2001). Strategies to make helmet use more attractive and to ensure correct wearing of helmets are needed (see "Evidence-Based Nursing").

Identify youth engaging in risky activities and teach them safe practices. Join with schools and community groups to establish education programs. Provide information about adequate conditioning for sports in order to decrease chance of overuse injury (Committee on Sports Medicine and Fitness, American Academy of Pediatrics,

BICYCLE HELMET EFFECTIVENESS AND USE

Problem

About 900 children die of bicycle-related injuries annually in the United States. Although helmets can reduce injury, many times they are not worn correctly.

Evidence

Nearly 500 children visiting a pediatric office were asked to bring their helmet to their health supervision visit, or were supplied with one when they came. Although about 73% of the children claimed to wear a helmet when bicycling, only 4% were able to demonstrate correct fitting and wearing of the helmet. Commonly the helmets were worn too high on the head, were not properly strapped on, or were secured so that they moved around the head excessively. The researchers suggest that helmet assessment be integrated into health supervision visits.

Implications

Nurses should not assume that reports of safety precautions such as wearing helmets or seat belts mean that children use these measures correctly. Ask for demonstrations and provide suggestions to improve technique as needed. Common injury causes such as car and bicycle crashes necessitate including at least these evaluations as part of health maintenance activities (Parkinson & Hike, 2003).

Critical Thinking

What are the reasons that children might not wear protective gear during sports? Are there laws in your community about wearing helmets for biking? How can nurses work with parents and schools to increase helmet use? To what incentives would school-age children be most likely to respond?

References

Lohse, J. L. (2003). A bicycle safety education program for parents of young children. *Journal of School Nursing, 19,* 100–110.

Parkinson, G. W., & Hike, K. E. (2003). Bicycle helmet assessment during well visits reveals severe shortcomings in condition and fit. *Pediatrics, 112,* 320–323.

2001). Each visit should contain basic history questions related to injury prevention. Pursue topics that appear to indicate problems. Once information is collected during the visit, plan two or three health maintenance topics that seem most important for injury prevention in this family. When there is a history of injury in the child, partner with the family to plan ways to avoid repeated harm. See Table 38–2 for some common injury hazards during the school years. See Table 38–3 for injury prevention teaching.

NURSING MANAGEMENT

NURSING ASSESSMENT AND DIAGNOSIS

Assessment of health promotion and health maintenance topics occurs in many settings with school-age children. They may be seen in offices, clinics, or other settings designed to provide such care. They may come for episodic care for a fracture or infection when health promotion and health maintenance can be easily integrated. They may be seen in the home or neighborhood center, and are frequently encountered by nurses in schools. Opportunities for assessment and intervention should be used whenever they occur. The individual child is examined, and the family, friends, school, and community are addressed. In addition these visits provide an opportunity to identify early and intervene for health-related problems that emerge or become apparent in school age.

Assessment can be considered on two levels with school-age children. Individual children may be assessed for height and weight, for immunization status, and for use of protective gear during sports. Populations of children may also be assessed since school age is the first time that large numbers of children are together in certain settings. The findings from such assessments will become the basis of an **individualized approach** or a **population-based approach** to health promotion and health maintenance. For example, nurses commonly measure height and weight, and calculate body mass index for *individual* children seen in a clinic. The results are shared with the family, and appropriate teaching about weight control and nutritious intake can be addressed. In other settings, nurses may measure a *classroom* of children and use the collective data to plan appropriate interventions. If 40% of children in a school are classified as overweight by BMI percentile, much emphasis should be placed on teaching about dietary intake, physical activity, and the relationship of recommended weight levels to chronic disease risk. However, if only a small number of children are overweight, interventions may not be as extensive about this topic.

Nurses perform assessment of growth in school-age children, look for achievement of developmental tasks, assess physical and mental health, and assess social characteristics. Based on the assessment of the individual child or populations of children, nursing diagnoses for children and families are established. Possible nursing diagnoses include the following:

- *Delayed Growth and Development* related to abuse

- *Impaired Parenting* related to lack of knowledge about child health maintenance

- *Sleep Deprivation* related to sleep terrors

TABLE 38–2 ✣ Injury Hazards in the School-Age Years

	Hazard	Developmental Characteristics	Preventive Measures
	Motor vehicle/ pedestrian/ biking crashes	Child plays outside; may follow ball into road; rides two-wheeler.	Teach child safe outside play, especially near streets. Reinforce use of bike helmet. Teach biking safety rules and provide safe places for riding.
	Firearms	Child may have been shown location of guns; is interested in showing them to friends.	Teach child never to touch guns without parent present. Guns should be kept unloaded and locked away. Guns and ammunition should be stored in different locations. Be sure guns have trigger locks.
	Burns	Child may perform experiments with flames or toxic substances.	Teach child what to do in case of fire or if toxic substances touch skin or eyes. Reinforce teaching about 911.
	Assault	Child may be left alone after school and may walk, bike, or take public transportation alone.	Provide telephone numbers of people to contact in case of an emergency or if child feels lonely. Leave child alone for brief periods initially, and evaluate child's success in managing time. Teach child not to accept rides from or talk to or open doors to strangers. Teach child how to answer the phone.

- *Risk for Violence Directed at Others* related to history of witnessing family violence
- *Risk for Loneliness* related to long periods alone after school
- *Health-Seeking Behaviors* related to locating swimming classes

PLANNING AND IMPLEMENTATION

The nurse is instrumental in planning interventions to promote and maintain health in school-age children. These interventions may take place in offices, homes, or clinics with an individual child, or in schools and other community settings with groups of children.

When working with individuals, summarize the strengths and needs that you have identified during the visit, and ask the child and family if they concur. Plan together with them to provide the needed information for topics you all have developed. Be sure to emphasize those areas where the family excels. For example, positively reinforce use of car seat belts (see "Teaching Highlights: Car Safety for the School-Age Child"), use of protective sports

TABLE 38–3 ✿ Injury Prevention Topics by Age

Age	Injury Prevention Teaching	
5–8 years	Use a booster seat, properly positioned in the back seat of the car; use lap and shoulder belts.	Teach safety with strangers.
	Never place the child in a front car seat with a passenger air bag.	Provide a list of people a child can approach if feeling threatened by touch or other experience.
	Be sure the child knows how to swim and works on these skills regularly.	Choose care providers carefully; occasionally pick up child earlier than expected; ask about policies regarding discipline and do not leave child with someone who uses corporal punishment.
	Protect the child with sunscreen when outside.	Be sure the child knows emergency numbers, names, and plans.
	Check smoke alarms and keep them in proper function.	
	Have an escape plan in case of fire in the home.	Review carefully any hazardous event that has occurred with the child and summarize what was done correctly and how response could be improved.
	Keep poisons, electrical appliances, and fire starters locked.	
	Keep firearms unloaded and locked; store ammunition in a separate locked location; have trigger locks installed on guns; keep dangerous knives locked.	Limit screen time to 2 hours daily; do not allow violent games or viewing.
	Provide protective gear for bicycling and other activities and insist that it be worn.	Review behavior with strangers regularly such as not getting in cars, and not engaging in phone or Internet conversations.
	Teach safety precautions for bicycling and other activities.	
8–10 years	Use car booster seat until child sits upright against back seat with bent knees over edge of seat; insist on use of lap and shoulder belts.	Do not allow child to operate power tools or machinery.
		Continue to reinforce other teaching described above, include child more fully, and enlarge responsibility to the child with increasing age.
	Do not place child in front seat of car with a passenger air bag.	
10–12 years	Continue to reinforce teaching described above.	Avoid high noise levels such as when listening to music through earphones.
	Parents and child should attend class on cardiopulmonary resuscitation and airway obstruction removal.	

Data from Green, M., & Palfrey, J.S. (Eds.). (2002). *Bright futures: Guidelines for health supervision of infants, children, and adolescents* (2nd ed.). Arlington, VA: National Center for Education in Maternal and Child Health.

gear, and being current with immunizations. Summarize the next expected developmental tasks, such as increasing independence and growing self-responsibility for choosing snacks and television shows. Then provide anticipatory guidance to assist with the child's growing independence. As peers are becoming more important, always focus some discussion on maintaining healthy social relationships through school peers, religious or community events, and sibling contacts. A combination of discussion and reading material or pertinent Web sites for later exploration is welcomed by most families. Provide telephone numbers of resources for questions and community contacts. Tell the parents when the next health promotion/maintenance visit is recommended. If you come in contact with school children for episodic care, ask when the last health maintenance visit occurred. If a child is seen for healthcare after a bicycling accident, the family may be receptive to teaching about safety precautions. When exposed to injuries to the skin, a review of the last tetanus booster may review health maintenance needs. Use every opportunity to work with individual children and insert appropriate health promotion/health maintenance topics.

When you are working with groups of children, health promotion focuses on known needs, interests, and risk areas. Nurses in school settings have used a variety of creative approaches to promote the health of youth. Nurses in

TEACHING HIGHLIGHTS

CAR SAFETY FOR THE SCHOOL-AGE CHILD

Recommendations include the following:

- For children over 40 lb (generally 4 to 8 years of age), use a belt positioning, forward-facing booster seat located in the back seat. Always use both lap and shoulder belt. Make sure the lap belt fits low and tight across the lap/upper thigh area, and the shoulder belt is snug across the chest and shoulder to avoid abdominal injuries.
- Children 4′9″ and taller can sit in a regular car seat restrained with lap and shoulder belt that are snug and correctly located across the lap and chest. The back seat is preferred for all children and necessary for children 12 years and younger.

Note: ALL children 12 years and younger should ride in the back seat.

schools can set up a program to train students in health topics; these students then become peer coaches or health advocates in working with other students (Streng, 2000). Another activity is evaluating the components of school health programs and making recommendations for additions as needed. The Centers for Disease Control and Prevention (CDC) has identified several areas for health policies in schools; they include health education, physical education, health services, mental health and social services, food service, environment, faculty and staff health promotion, and family and community involvement (Kolbe, Kann, & Brener, 2001). Bulletin boards, community newspapers, television, and community group membership may all be as effective as teaching in school classrooms. Stress reduction teaching should be provided on group and individual levels. Nurses can teach or assist in development of progressive relaxation, deep breathing, biofeedback, yoga, or meditation (Dombrowski, 1999). Interventions will be most effective if they begin with an understanding of the population served.

EVALUATION

Seek evaluation from parents during visits for care. Were their questions answered? Do they know where to turn for advice? Do they know when the child should be seen again for health promotion/maintenance?

The expected outcomes for nursing care of individual school-age children include the following:

- The child demonstrates normal patterns of growth and development.
- The child, family, and community provide a supportive and nurturing environment for the child.
- The child shows growing independence in directing own health promotion activities.

Expected outcomes of nursing care for groups of children include the following:

- The children identify lifestyle decisions that influence their health status.
- The school and community offer resources that help to lessen risk factors related to health, and disease/injury prevention.

HEALTH PROMOTION AND HEALTH MAINTENANCE OF THE ADOLESCENT

Adolescents are often seen only sporadically for healthcare, even though visits are recommended annually. They are usually healthy, may not need immunizations, and consequently do not often come for healthcare. If they have a minor illness,

come in for birth control, or need a sports examination, the visit should be viewed as a health supervision opportunity. While all components of the usual visit may not be performed, at least those parts most important are inserted into care. If time is limited, the nurse has to decide which topics to address during a healthcare visit. It is advisable to start with the topic of most interest to the teen and then to insert some injury prevention teaching, since injury is the greatest risk to teens. Health promotion topics such as dietary and exercise habits could be discussed if there is time. Mental health assessment and teaching are other areas of prime importance. Of course, if the teen is at immediate risk, such as considering suicide in response to depression, this must be dealt with immediately by collaborating with a mental health specialist.

What general principles can guide programs to promote health in adolescents? Some researchers have analyzed theory application and approaches of programs, and others have suggested key elements of programs (see "Thinking Critically"). Programs that assist adolescents in taking on health promotion behaviors foster a sense of competence, confidence in the youth's own abilities, building of a sense of character and responsibility, connection to other youth and beneficial programs, and the qualities of caring and compassion (Lerner & Thompson, 2002). When establishing youth programs, whether with individual adolescents or with groups, the nurse includes evaluation of effectiveness, and plans methods to enlarge and sustain successful approaches.

GENERAL OBSERVATIONS

The beginning of the visit with an adolescent can be an important source of information, just as it is with younger children. However, the adolescent is at a more advanced stage of development, and the observations the nurse makes will relate to this developmental stage.

Ideally the facility has a waiting area that is designed for teens. Teens often dislike waiting for healthcare with either young children or older adults. Teen waiting areas are popular because they provide a special place, thereby relaying that the teen is important, and they use video and other popular methods to impart health information while the teen waits (Figure 38–6 ●). When calling the adolescent back for care, observe if parents or friends are present, or if the teen is alone. Young adolescents often come with parents to the facility, and parents often then wait in the waiting room during the examination. Sometimes, if the teen comes in for a special problem, such as a skin lesion or other health concern, the parent follows the adolescent into the examination room. Watch to see if a parent or friend is present, and if that person comes with the teen when called. If someone comes with the teen, it may be necessary to provide some private time by asking the other person to wait outside for a moment. Reassure the parents that there

THINKING CRITICALLY

APPLYING THEORY TO PLAN FOR ADOLESCENT HEALTH

A review that analyzed articles describing adolescent health promotion identified the most common theories used by healthcare providers (Montgomery, 2002). A major theory is *social cognitive theory.* This theory was developed by Walter Bandura, who is described in Chapter 33 (Bandura, 1977). ∞ The key components of his theory involve **self-efficacy** (the person's belief in the ability to perform a behavior) and **outcome expectancy** (what the person expects to get from performing a certain behavior). Learning a new behavior occurs through **modeling**, or imitation of the behavior of someone else. Bandura believes that individuals make decisions about health behaviors based on thought about the consequences and outcomes of those behaviors. The *person's characteristics,* such as self-efficacy and outcome expectancy, interact with the external *environment* and the *behavioral choices* available. All of these components together determine health behaviors, and all can be influenced to promote health.

When seeking to promote physical activity behaviors in youth, some essential components are:

■ Encouraging the youth to believe they could perform the activity (self-efficacy).

■ Pointing out the positive aspects of the behavior (outcome expectancy).

■ Showing the youth how to do the activity (modeling).

■ Providing a physical setting and opportunity for performing the behavior (environment).

■ Allowing trial and error, choice in time and extent of activity (behavioral choices).

Compose a teaching plan to encourage increased physical activity for a teen, using all components of the social cognitive theory. List the outcome measures or goals for the teaching, the interventions, and methods of evaluation.

● FIGURE 38–6

Parents often accompany teens with a healthcare problem in for the examination. Provide an opportunity to see both the teen and parent privately and integrate general health promotion and health maintenance into the visit. What questions can you ask this teen? What teaching might be needed?

will be time to talk with them about any of their concerns and questions. Provide them with an opportunity to ask questions and get information also.

Some teens are comfortable in healthcare settings and actively engage in conversation, while others are nervous and will need more explanations and reassurance during the first steps of measurement and blood pressure. By adolescence, boys and girls should be assuming more of a partnership role in their own healthcare. As the visit begins, greet adolescents warmly, ask what concerns and questions they have, and ask for their opinions and reactions throughout the visit. This will show that their thoughts are important and that they play an important role in guiding the healthcare visits. When adolescents are visiting the same office or clinic that they came to during childhood, they usually know and feel comfortable with the care providers. If the setting is new to them, explain procedures and introduce personnel so they feel more at ease.

GROWTH AND DEVELOPMENTAL SURVEILLANCE

Adolescence spans several years, and growth and developmental issues vary throughout the period. For young adolescents, or those from about 12 to 13 years of age, growth measurement remains important. Many youth are still growing, and use of percentile grids continues to be an important part of care. Growth should remain in the same percentile channel as during childhood, with girls reaching nearly adult height at this age, and boys still continuing to grow. Be alert as always for youth who have either increased or decreased channels, or are above the 85th percentile or below the 5th percentile for body mass index. They will need additional assessment of nutritional intake and physical activity.

By middle and late adolescence, adult growth is nearly achieved, earlier for girls than boys. While measurement continues to be performed, nurses assess the BMI more carefully to be sure the height and weight indicate appropriate intake and exercise. Overweight at this age is likely to continue into adulthood, particularly if parents are overweight, so early intervention will be needed to decrease this potential. Other youth may have eating disorders and should be referred to a specialist for care. Children from homes without sufficient financial resources may be hungry and lack food. Parents who were eligible for Women, Infants, and Children (WIC) Nutrition Program services when children were younger may not receive them once the child is an adolescent, so the increasing dietary intake needs of their teens cannot be met. If an adolescent is thin and has little energy, consider this possibility; administer the food security questionnaire found in Chapter 34. ∞

There are few options for measuring the developmental competence of adolescents, but observations and questions during care provide information about the meeting of developmental milestones. Key tasks for adolescents involve separating from the parents and establishing positive relationships with peers. The young teen may come to an appointment with a parent and still rely on that parent to answer some questions during the examination. However, the middle and late teen should be increasingly able to come alone, answer questions, and assume responsibility for healthcare decisions. Offer older teens the option of coming into the room alone, stating, "Your mom can wait here and we can come and get her later. Does that sound all right?" During time with the adolescent, ask questions to learn about peer interactions and activities.

The adolescent receives a physical examination, often by the nurse practitioner or physician. See Chapter 35 for components of the examination. ∞ Some particular parts of the examination to include for teens are scoliosis screening, sexual maturity rating (Tanner stages), breast exam, testing for sexually transmitted diseases (among those sexually active), pelvic exam and pap smear (for sexually active females), hematocrit for anemia annually in menstruating adolescents, hearing screening (at 12, 15, and 18 years), blood pressure annually, lipid screening for those with family history of early heart disease or other risk factors, and tuberculosis screening for those in high-risk areas. Most adolescents do not want their parents present during the examination, but occasionally will want a parent for something like a first pelvic examination or a blood draw. Ask them their wishes in a confidential setting so they can freely make the choice. They also may choose to have a healthcare provider of the same gender as them complete the genitourinary examination. Expected outcomes of care include screening and early identification for common health problems, normal patterns of growth, and meeting of developmental milestones.

NUTRITION

The young adolescent needs a well-balanced diet to support the growth of this period, and the late adolescent requires intake that supports physical activity and provides nutrients for metabolism and to promote the immune system. While nutritional intake is important, teens often do not eat well. They may be busy and do not want to plan meals, they like to eat foods that are popular with other teens so high fat and sugar intake can be common, they may be dieting to achieve weight loss, and some do not have enough financial resources to access proper foods.

Combine the information from measurement of the adolescent with the answers to questions about diet to identify possible areas for intervention. Find out what questions the teen has about foods, diet, maintaining desired weight, and topics like vegetarianism or supplements to enhance athletic performance. See Chapter 34 for further detail about these special nutritional topics. ∞ Health promotion plans focus on practices that lead to healthy growth and development. They may include teaching about:

- Getting five fruits and vegetables daily.
- Including whole grain products to replace refined products whenever possible.
- The importance of eating three meals each day, including breakfast and lunch.
- Eating together as a family several times weekly, which enhances quality food intake.
- How to plan menus and prepare foods for balanced intake.

Health maintenance plans center on those practices that prevent disease, including:

- Limiting refined sugar and high-fat intake (such as soft drinks and fried foods) to maintain weight at recommended level.
- Including two to three servings of dairy products daily to enhance bone formation and decrease chance of osteoporosis as an adult.
- Using resources for treatment of eating disorders if they are identified.

While much of nutrition teaching should be aimed directly at the adolescent, parents are also included. They can be effective contributors to healthy intake by providing plenty of fruits and vegetables for snacks, having foods attractively prepared and ready for consumption when the teen is hungry, planning several meals together as a family each week, encouraging milk or other forms of calcium intake, and setting a good example for food intake. Help them to identify the youth with an eating disorder and provide resources for intervention in these cases. Consider as well the teen with a baby. The adolescent who is pregnant or breastfeeding has even more need for nutritional teaching and may need financial resources to access sufficient food. How can the nurse combine the growth and developmental needs of an adolescent with those of her new baby when planning teaching?

PHYSICAL ACTIVITY

Many adolescents suffer from the effects of inadequate physical activity. As children get older and enter the teenage years, physical activity decreases, particularly in girls. Only about 30% to 60% of adolescents report daily vigorous activity, and the percentage is lower among some groups (Epstein, Paluch, Kalanus et al., 2001). The recommendation of *Healthy People 2010* (U. S. Department of Health & Human Services, 2000) is quite moderate, stating that adolescents should get at least 20 minutes of vigorous activity 3 days weekly. At a time when teens are not very active as a group, physical education requirements in school are also decreasing, with only 19% of 12th-grade students regularly attending a PE class (Lowry, Wechsler, Kann et al., 2001). Physical activity levels must therefore be assessed at each health supervision visit or in other contacts with adolescents. Apply resilience theory and assess youth, family, and community for risk and protective factors regarding physical activity (Table 38–4).

Some youth have established regular physical activity programs, and their behaviors should be encouraged (Figure 38–7 ●). Be alert for those who exercise but have other health problems. Some athletes try to eat very little to remain a certain weight for wrestling, running, or other sports. Integrate nutritional teaching that includes the importance of adequate intake for sports performance. Other athletes use nutritional supplements to enhance performance. While most are not harmful, few have proven benefits and their cost is not warranted; some may actually be harmful to adolescents.

Other youth have very little physical activity and feel incompetent in performing many sports. Work with them to find at least one thing they can do on a daily basis—walking their dog in the neighborhood, riding a bike to the store, using stairs instead of elevators when possible, parking on the far side of the school lot and walking further, swimming at a club their parents belong to or at a local YMCA or YWCA, or saving money to take lessons for something they have always dreamed of doing such as horseback riding or golf. Form interest groups at schools and community centers that provide an outlet for adolescents who cannot "make the team" for school sports. Encourage parents and adolescents to set goals together to integrate some physical activity daily.

The nurse's activities for health promotion concentrate on teaching the health and mental benefits of physical ac-

tivity such as increased energy, weight control, and a feeling of control and success. Health maintenance focuses on viewing physical activity as a method to prevent disease such as cardiovascular disease and diabetes. Youth who have family members with these diseases or meet adults who have them are more likely to understand the importance of their own activity. Desired outcomes include maintenance of weight within recommended level, daily exercise of 20 to 60 minutes, and establishment of lifetime routines for exercise.

TABLE 38–4 ✦ Risk and Protective Factors Regarding Physical Activity in Adolescence

Risk Factors	Protective Factors
■ Lives in isolated setting with little opportunity for contact with other teens	■ Has opportunities for participation in physical activity at home, at school, and in the community
■ Has a developmental disability that impairs physical movement	■ Likes physical activity
■ Does not like physical activity	■ Has exercised during all of childhood, often with parents
■ Has a pattern and history of low activity levels	■ Knowledgeable about benefits of activity; committed to maintaining exercise patterns
■ Is overweight	
■ Does not feel competent in most sports	
■ Limited financial resources to pay registration fees or buy protective gear for sports	■ Has many friends living close who participate in physical activity
■ Family members who have little physical activity	■ Youth and parents agree to a limit of 2 hours daily of screen time
■ Parents who are not active in school sports and committees	■ Availability of financial and other resources for sports gear and protective equipment
■ Parents who do not like physical activity and have had low levels while their teen was growing up	■ Parents participate in regular physical activity and encourage the adolescent to do so also
■ Parents who have little time or facilities for exercise, or always exercise at a club out of view of their family	■ Neighborhood and community provide physical activity options
■ Lack of youth and parent knowledge about physical activity needs and benefits	■ Public policies maintain parks, green spaces, biking trails, playgrounds
■ Lack of neighborhood programs for physical activity promotion	■ Programs are available for adolescents with developmental disabilities or other healthcare needs
■ Presence of neighborhood hazards and unsafe areas	

Data from Green & Palfrey, 2002.

What risk and protective factors for physical activity are present in your community? Go to http://www.activelivingbydesign.org to examine the positive effect community planning can have on its members' exercise levels.

● FIGURE 38–7

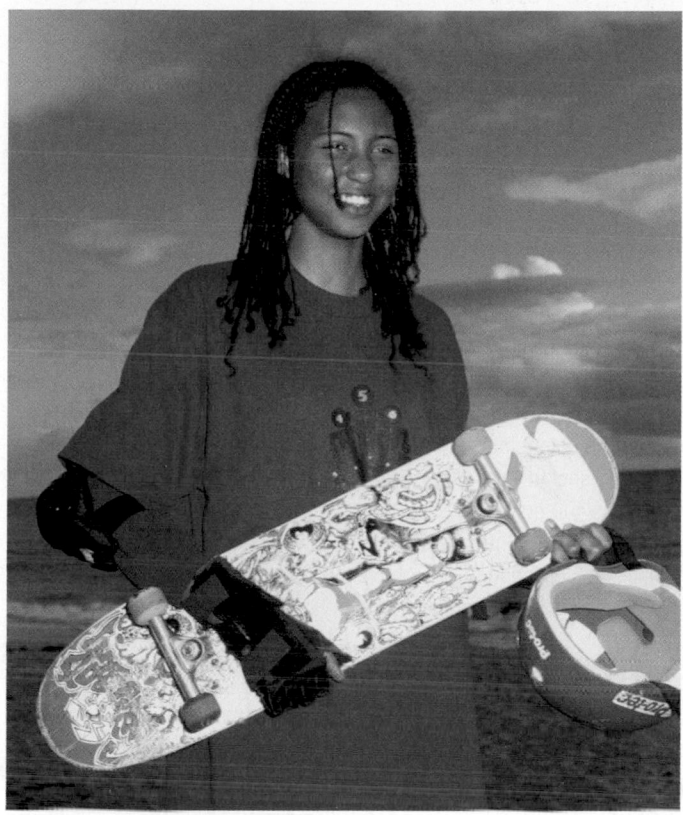

This teen girl is an avid "boarder." How can you encourage and praise her for this activity? What clues do you have that she is using adequate safety measures?

ORAL HEALTH

Continued dental care during the adolescent years can ensure oral health. The recommendations remain the same as those for young children. The adolescent should floss daily, brush twice daily with a small amount of fluoridated toothpaste, and visit a dental provider every 6 months. By about 14 years of age, those adolescents who do not have fluoridated water and have been taking fluoride can stop this supplement. Even the molars have been formed by that age so fluoride tablets are no longer needed. Continue to examine the condition of the teeth and the number of erupted permanent teeth present. Be alert for any unusual growths and ulcers in the mouth and refer for care as needed.

One potential concern that should be addressed includes the availability of dental insurance for the adolescent. The teen whose family does not have dental insurance needs referrals for care to affordable resources. Dental specialists clean off plaque that has formed, apply sealants to erupting molars, examine the teeth for caries, and perform restorative care. There are particular groups more at risk

for inadequate dental care (see "Developing Cultural Competence"). When working with these populations, nurses can question access to care, and make recommendations that foster regular checkups. Some teens may wish to whiten the teeth or get orthodontia to improve appearance. The nurse helps the youth and parents to find resources for needed care. Expected outcomes are dental visits twice annually with recommended follow-up care for problems, and good oral health.

DEVELOPING CULTURAL COMPETENCE

DENTAL CARE

Several ethnic groups are more likely to have inadequate dental care than other groups. When you work with these populations, be certain to include dental assessment in health supervision visits, and have resources for care readily available.

An analysis of several national surveys such as the National Health and Nutrition Examination Survey (NHANES) reported that rural children were more likely (41%) to be uninsured for dental care than urban children (35%). They were also less likely to have visited a dentist in the last year (70%) than urban children (74%). More rural children (8%) had unmet dental needs than did urban children (6%) (Vargas, Ronzio, & Hayes, 2003). When children live in rural areas, be sure to ask about their access to dental care.

Another analysis of NHANES data examined African-American respondents. Sixty-two percent reported that they only visit a dentist when needed rather than regularly. Those who were poor, unemployed, uninsured, or living in the South had poorer dental health. If you work with African-American youth, be conscious of the need to integrate oral assessment into care, and to encourage utilization of services (Green, Person, Crowther et al., 2003).

National Health Interview Surveys (NHISs) data were analyzed for dental care utilization by Asians and Native Hawaiians and other Pacific Islanders. Native Hawaiian and other Pacific Islander children were most likely (82%) to have had a dental visit in the last year, while Asian Indians were least likely to have a visit (60%). Once again, children with no insurance and who were poor were more likely to have less care. Children living with a single parent or someone other than a parent, and those whose parents had under 12 years of education, were more likely to have unmet dental needs (Qui & Ni, 2003).

All children need oral assessment and questions about dental care, but rural and poor groups, particularly African Americans and Asian groups, may need teaching about the importance of dental care and referral to appropriate resources.

MENTAL AND SPIRITUAL HEALTH

Adolescents have many challenges to their mental health and need support to emerge from adolescence with mental and spiritual strengths. Mental health topics must be addressed at each health supervision opportunity to promote mental health among teens. Mental health is closely linked to developmental tasks such as growing independence, formation of close relationships with peers, becoming confident in accomplishments, and setting goals for the future. Some chronic mental health disorders such as schizophrenia can emerge during adolescence, so mental health screening is important to perform with this age group.

As during other ages, the self-concept continues to develop and tailors reactions to the environment. Self-regulation in the form of making decisions to govern oneself is important. Self-esteem, or a positive feeling about the self, is key to meeting life's challenges. Ask what the teen is proud of and has accomplished and what disappointments have occurred as well. Provide resources to deal with disappointments and give praise for the teen's accomplishments. Another part of the self-concept that continues to develop is that of body image. Factors such as early or late maturation, overweight or underweight, or the role of the media can influence the teen's body image. A healthy image includes the realization that the body has positive and less positive attributes and that the individual can influence the body by healthy eating and physical activity. Be alert for the teen whose wish for a different body leads to eating disorders and excessive exercise or intake of nutritional supplements.

Sexuality involves both body changes that signal mature sexual development, and the mental concept of oneself as a sexual being. Body changes and mental concepts do not necessarily mature at the same time, and adolescents may not be ready for sexual maturity and the decisions about sexual behavior simply due to achieving sexual maturation. Most young adolescent girls have begun menstruating, and by early to middle adolescence, boys are having nocturnal emissions and ejaculations. Ask teens if they have received information about puberty, body changes, and sexuality. Tell young adolescents that most teens have questions and that they may ask about any areas of interest, including contraception, and sexually transmitted diseases. Ask older adolescents directly if they have had sexual intercourse and if so, what they are doing to protect against pregnancy and sexually transmitted diseases. Provide support for adolescents who have decided not to have sexual intercourse, encouraging them to continue this plan, telling them that sexual feelings are normal, but that decisions about sexual intercourse are their right and privilege. Ask if teens have confusion about their sexuality. If teens have identified as homosexual, let them know they are welcome and ask about decisions regarding sexual practices, reinforcing the need for protection against sexually transmitted diseases. Provide community resources to support gay or lesbian teens so that they can develop a social group in which they feel comfortable. Some adolescents are seen for healthcare at the time they become sexually active. Use this opportunity to reinforce and correct prior knowledge about the body and protection against pregnancy and sexually transmitted diseases (see "Nursing Practice").

NURSING PRACTICE

The nurse who works with adolescents dealing with sexuality issues may find that the values of some teens are very different from one's personal values. How do you react when a teen decides to have sexual intercourse or has become pregnant? Can you help teens to make wise decisions without telling them what they should do?

It is important for adolescents to learn the significance of sexual intercourse and the meaning of close relationships. Teaching them early about this will enable them to respect others at the time they do have intimate relations. Respect is also the key to working with teens. Nurses should treat them with respect, expecting them to consider options and make wise decisions. Nurses who cannot work with certain groups of teens because of moral values differing from their own have the obligation to refer the teens for care to resources where they can receive the information and services they are requesting.

Most adolescents still need discipline or guidance from parents at certain times. Rather than a constant battle over daily events, it is best if there are just a few important rules that parents have to enforce only rarely. When working with parents, nurses can assist them to set useful boundaries for teens and offer resources such as parenting groups and Web sites for assistance.

Sleep is necessary for anyone to function safely and at a level of one's potential. Unfortunately, many youth do not get the sleep needed for healthy functioning. Teens have an increased need for sleep due to their growth rates and activity levels. At the same time, their internal clocks change, making it more difficult to get to sleep at the usual time. It is thought that a decrease in secretion of melatonin occurs, so the teen does not feel tired in the late evening. However, they often do not have the number of hours of sleep needed by the time they wake up for school or work. The problem may be worsened if the student participates in sports or other activities. They may need to get to school before normal starting hours for music, sports, or other activities, or perhaps stay late into the evening for practices. Some adolescents then work weekends or evenings as well. And of course social activities usually fill much of their time. While about 9 hours of sleep is needed, most adolescents get about 6 hours (Mayo Clinic, 2005). The effects of sleep deprivation can be serious. Teens cannot perform to their potential in school or at work. Many parents state that adolescents are moody and difficult to communicate with when they are tired. There may be a connection between lack of sleep and substance abuse, and teens commonly use caffeinated beverages to stay awake. Some people tend to eat more when they are tired, and get less physical activity. Perhaps one of the most serious consequences deals with the danger of driving while sleepy; this is a common cause of accidents. Ask adolescents about what time they go to bed, when they awaken, and whether they are frequently tired. Provide suggestions for regular sleep schedules, avoiding caffeine products in the evening, and planning a day of relaxation into every week.

Temperament or personality type characteristics continue into adolescence, but they generally do not change from earlier years. For example, the active infant and young child is usually an active teenager. The slow-to-warm-up baby may be the adolescent who needs more time to adjust to a new school or teachers. If the adolescent or parent has trouble with personality characteristics, it may be helpful to talk about these traits, help them to establish a positive sense about the attributes, and discuss ways to adapt the environment as needed. For example, parents should not expect a slow-to-warm-up teen to be interested in running for a class office. Someone with irregular sleep and eating habits will find it difficult to have a job at a set time and will need to set alarms and other reminders.

Spirituality offers comfort and support for the adolescent. Being a member of a teen group in a faith-based home can offer a peer group with similar values and bring meaning to life. Some adolescents reject the faith of their parents and seek a different group; others seek to leave religious practices totally while others become more committed to them. Ask them if they have the resources they need to bring meaning to their lives; provide them if needed. Realize that participation in community food kitchens, raising money for causes, and other activities also provide meaning for many adolescents (Figure 38–8 ◉).

The nurse actively promotes the mental health of youth by understanding their developmental needs and providing information and resources. Gentle guidance and active partnership with youth help to provide the resources to ensure healthy self-concept, sexuality, and personality development. While most teenagers have many protective factors that can be identified and fostered, a few have risks that can harm mental health. It is important to identify the risks also, and to use health maintenance techniques to lessen the risk factors. Depression and substance use are two common risks to mental health. Depression is discussed in Chapter 54 ∞ and substance abuse is discussed in Chapter 36. ∞ See the quick checklists in Table 38–5 to help in identification of these problems during health supervision visits.

Although health promotion and health maintenance activities commonly occur in office or clinic settings, there are many other settings where nurses work with adolescents,

◉ **FIGURE 38–8**

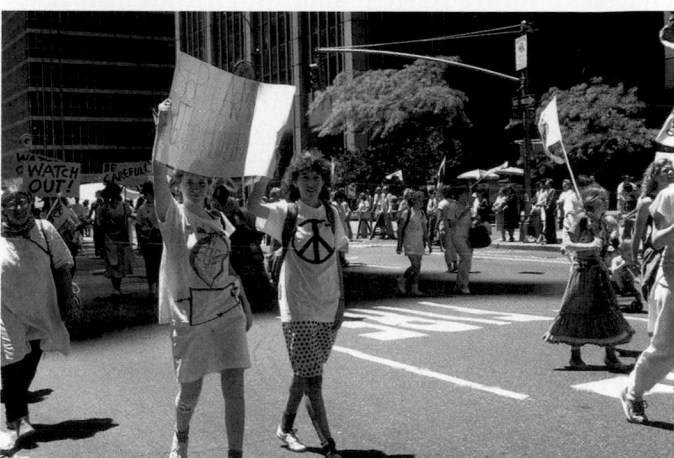

Teens often become associated with causes. This helps them to feel part of a social group and also provides the opportunities to examine belief systems and to make decisions about meaningful activities.

and mental health activities are often integrated into these settings. Consider offering health promotion/maintenance wherever students might be found. Some nontraditional settings include correctional facilities, school-based health centers, and programs for pregnant teens. Adolescents in these facilities can benefit from services to improve diet, physical activity, and lifestyle behaviors that influence mental health.

The desired outcomes for mental and spiritual health promotion and maintenance include meaningful activities in the adolescent's life, emerging independence, good choices about lifestyle behaviors, and development of successful coping skills.

TABLE 38–5 ✢ Signs of Depression and Substance Abuse	
Depression	**Substance Use**
Changes in behavior, school performance, sleep, and appetite	Changes in behavior, school performance, sleep, and appetite
Physical complaints	Accidents and other unexplained events
Loss of interest in usual activities	Lack of responsibility
Difficulty in motivating self and setting goals	Labile mood and attitude
Change in friends	Hopelessness
Feelings of worthlessness	Depression
Consideration of death or suicide	Feelings of ambivalence
	A variety of physical changes depending on the substance

Data from Jellinek, Patel, & Froehle, 2002.

RELATIONSHIPS

Adolescents form stronger bonds with friends than at any time earlier in development; at the same time they need their parents for guidance and reassurance as they become more independent. As teenagers strive for independence, they frequently strike out at parents, test limits, and have conflicts with parents. Interactions in the family provide consistent and important ties at the same time that social interactions become a central part of life. Health promotion helps teens to form strong friendships with peers and to continue to value and participate in the family. It helps parents to understand the developmental needs and their role in establishing a new type of relationship with the emerging young adult in the family. Partnerships with care providers are important to help families work together to achieve these outcomes.

When adolescents are seen for healthcare visits, assess relationships with others. Provide time alone with both the adolescent and the parents (if they are present) so that everyone has time to talk freely and to ask questions. Some areas already discussed, such as school performance and activities, provide information about the adolescent's friends and how time is spent. Ask teens to describe their best friends and what they do together. Ask parents their opinions of the youth's friends. Inquire about the youth's roles in the family. Does the teen have jobs and responsibilities? What freedom is allowed? What are relationships like with siblings and extended family members such as grandparents and cousins? What activities are done together as a family? Are there differences in the teen's and the parents' answers to these questions? What are the teen's and parents' desires for how the family unit functions together?

Provide an opportunity alone with the teen to talk about issues such as domestic violence. Is the youth abused or is there violence between adults in the family? Are there stressors such as lack of sufficient finances, an ill parent, or a lost job? How have these occurrences affected the adolescent? Minor adjustments can be helped by discussion, whereas some major problems will need referral to mental health specialists.

In their relationships with peers, adolescents often have many of the same issues that emerge with parents. They may have disagreements with friends or feel hurt by things that are said or done. Ask teens about how things are going with friends and what problems they have. Talk about negotiating, joining groups to form new friendships, and the importance of respecting and not making fun of others. Give them strategies for living up to their own standards even when friends are enticing them to do other things. Suggest that having friends one can trust and who have the same ideals can be very sup-portive and fun in adolescent years. Expected outcomes are the formation of strong relationships both within and outside of the family, along with independence in decision making.

DISEASE PREVENTION STRATEGIES

Teenagers typically do not have many diseases and most are minor illnesses like respiratory and gastrointestinal illness. However, there are some diseases that occur and nurses must always be aware of signs of potential disease. Some common health issues that are described throughout this book include the following:

- Acne and skin infections
- Body piercing and tattooing
- Sports overuse injuries
- Constipation and diarrhea
- Dental problems

Other observations may signal more serious health concerns and need to be referred for further evaluation. Some examples include the following:

- Scoliosis
- Anemia
- Excessive tiredness
- Bruising
- Sexually transmitted diseases
- Eating disorder
- Abuse or severe bullying

Several screening tests should be performed during health supervision visits with adolescents, including vision, hearing, smoking, depression, stress, alcohol or other substance use, blood pressure, urinalysis, sexually transmitted infection risk, and in some cases pap smears and breast examinations. Screening tests with abnormal results require follow-up and intervention. For example, if the adolescent is anemic, iron tablets may be needed and teaching about high-iron foods should be done. Vision impairment requires referral to an eye specialist. Presence of sexually transmitted diseases requires teaching and medication treatment. History of sexual activity will guide the nurse to tests that should be included in the examination (see "Nursing Practice").

The adolescent should receive extensive information about ways to protect health and prevent disease. The hazardous outcomes of smoking are discussed, and smoking cessation programs are encouraged for smokers. Unprotected sexual activity is presented as a serious health threat. Use of sunscreens to prevent burns and future skin cancer

MediaLink

Immunization Update

NURSING PRACTICE

Sexually active teens should be screened annually for the following:

- Chlamydia
- Gonorrhea
- Trichomoniasis
- Human papillomavirus
- Herpes simplex virus
- Bacterial vaginosis

Teens should be screened for syphilis and HIV/AIDS if requesting testing or meeting any of these criteria:

- History of sexually transmitted infection
- More than one sexual partner in past 6 months
- Intravenous drug use
- Sexual intercourse with a partner at risk
- Sex in exchange for drugs or money
- Homelessness
- Males—sex with other males
- Syphilis—residence in areas where disease is prevalent
- HIV/AIDS—blood or blood product transfusion before 1985

See Chapter 52 for further information on screening procedures. ∞

Data from Green, M., & Palfrey, J. S. (2002). Bright futures: Guidelines for health supervision of infants, children, and adolescents (2nd ed., p. 268). Arlington, VA: National Center for Education in Maternal and Child Health.

is encouraged. Females are taught breast self-exam, and males are taught testicular exam. For youth who are overweight and sedentary, the possible outcomes such as type 2 diabetes and cardiovascular disease are mentioned. While it would not be advisable to threaten or frighten an adolescent with descriptions of diseases, an understanding of the potential serious outcomes can be motivators for behavior change.

In addition to teaching to prevent disease, the nurse also administers any needed immunizations. Many adolescents have not had immunizations since about school entry time, so their record should be carefully reviewed. Some common immunizations needed by adolescents include the following:

- When was the last tetanus-diphtheria booster? It is recommended every 10 years if no wounds have required an update in the interim. If the child received it at age 5 years, a booster is needed at 15 years.

- Was a second measles-mumps-rubella administered? A second dose may not have been routine when teens were younger so they may need it now.

- Is hepatitis A common in your state? If so, the teen needs to get that vaccine.

- Has the youth had hepatitis B vaccine? This is important for all youth, and some may not have received it as infants.

- Did the youth have a clear history of varicella disease? If not, the vaccine is needed.

- Meningococcal vaccine is now recommended for all youth.

The results of health screening are shared with the teen and with the parent as appropriate. Teaching and other interventions for disease prevention are examples of health maintenance activities. Expected outcomes are increasing knowledge of common diseases and methods of prevention among teen and parent, use of screening tests by the healthcare provider, and use of the healthcare home by the adolescent for treatment of diseases.

INJURY PREVENTION STRATEGIES

Injury is the greatest health hazard for adolescents, so injury prevention must be integrated into every health contact with youth. The major hazard is automobile crashes (see Chapter 1 ∞). Many teens learn to drive and have a license by 16 years of age. They often transport friends, get distracted by social interactions in the car, have little experience about what to do if a car slides or has mechanical problems, may drink and drive, talk on cell phones while driving, and are often tired when driving (Figure 38-9). Several states have instituted graduated driving licensing to help decrease some risks. Commonly, the youth cannot drive other youth for the first few months, cannot drive from about 1 a.m. to 6 a.m., and has serious consequences for speeding or other infractions.

◉ FIGURE 38-9

Adolescents often drive motorized vehicles and may be at risk for injury if not properly prepared or protected. What teaching and experience do these youth need for safe enjoyment of the experience of driving and riding with friends? Do schools in your area offer driver education classes? What are the state requirements for youth driver licensure?

Parents in states without these laws may wish to establish them for their own adolescents. Driving should always be presented as a privilege and a responsibility. Serious consequences such as losing the ability to drive for a time after any infraction can be suggested to parents. Because of the great risk of injury and death from car crashes, ask at each health visit if the teen drives, rides with other teens, what rules parents have established about driving, and whether the teen ever drinks and drives or rides with someone who does. Reinforce the need to wear a lap and shoulder belt at all times and to never drink and drive.

Youth are at risk for injury with other motorized vehicles. Motorcycles, four-wheelers, boats, jet skis, farm machinery, and tools are other sources of injury. Ask about the youth's exposure to various machines and teach about avoiding alcohol and drug use, and safety gear and precautions to be used. Every health visit should include other questions that help to identify a wide variety of injury hazards. Be sure to discuss and provide written material to perform injury prevention teaching. Such measures are important health maintenance activities (Table 38–6 and Table 38–7). Desired outcomes for nursing care include absence of serious injury, the ability to state sources of risk for injury, and emergency plans for assistance when engaging in any risky activities.

NURSING MANAGEMENT

NURSING ASSESSMENT AND DIAGNOSIS

Nurses assess adolescents in a variety of settings, including offices, clinics, schools, home, correctional facilities, extended care facilities, sports-related endeavors, and family planning clinics. A wide array of health concerns should be included in these assessments. They include measurement of growth; presence of any unusual findings on physical examination; lifestyle choices related to dietary intake, physical activity, and oral hygiene; assessment of mental status, family interactions, and social connections with peers; and

TABLE 38–6 ✣ Injury Prevention in Adolescence

	Hazard	Developmental Characteristics	Preventive Measures
	Motor vehicle crashes	Adolescents learn to drive, enjoy new independence, and often feel invulnerable.	Insist on driver's education classes. Enforce rules about safe driving. Seat belts should be used for every trip. Discourage drug and alcohol use. Get treatment for teenagers who are known substance abusers.
	Sporting injuries	Adolescents may participate in physically challenging sports such as soccer, gymnastics, or football. They may be allowed to drive motorboats.	Encourage use of protective sporting gear. Teach safe boating practices. Perform teaching related to hazards of drug and alcohol use, especially when using motorized equipment.
	Drowning	Adolescents overestimate endurance when swimming. They take risks diving.	Encourage swimming only with friends. Reinforce rules and teach them about risks.

TABLE 38–7 ❖ Injury Prevention Topics for Adolescence

Topic	Teaching
Driving	Always wear seat and shoulder belt.
	Do not drink and drive or ride with others who do.
	Do not talk on a cell phone as you drive.
	Do not drive when you are tired.
	Drive with parents or other adults for several months in winter driving conditions if you live where there is snow, ice, or heavy rains.
	Keep your car in good repair.
Sun	Wear sunscreen.
	Limit time outside especially early in summer.
Machinery	Learn how to use power tools correctly.
	Always have someone near when you use tools or machinery.
Emergency care	Learn first aid, CPR, and airway obstruction removal.
Water safety	Learn to swim well.
	If you supervise younger children near water, never leave them alone, even for a minute.
Fires	Do not play with fire.
	Follow guidelines to avoid igniting gasoline.
	Test smoke alarms in your house every 6 months and change batteries annually.
Firearms	Know and follow rules to keep firearms locked, with ammunition locked in a separate place.
	Never take out a gun to show a friend unless your parent is also present.
	Take firearm safety classes if you hunt or target shoot.
Hearing	Avoid loud music especially for long periods and through ear phones.
Sports	Wear protective gear recommended for your sport.
Abuse	Report any abuse to an adult you trust.
	Date with other couples whenever possible and report date rape.
	Do not drink or take drugs.

Data from Green & Palfrey (2002).

protective factors. The protective factors can be used during implementation to enhance the youth's resilience.

Based on a thorough assessment, you will establish nursing diagnoses that are appropriate for the adolescent and family. Some possible nursing diagnoses might include the following:

■ *Rape-Trauma Syndrome* related to date rape

■ *Impaired Dentition* related to ineffective oral hygiene

■ *Imbalanced Nutrition: More than Body Requirements* related to lack of basic nutritional knowledge and obesity in both parents

■ *Disturbed Sleep Pattern* related to frequently changing sleep/wake schedule

■ *Low Self-Esteem* related to situational crisis of friends making fun of adolescent

PLANNING AND IMPLEMENTATION

Whatever the setting, the nurse partners with the adolescent, the parents, and other persons such as teachers or school counselors to plan appropriate goals and related interventions. Nurses work with individual adolescents in offices, schools, and other settings, and often work with groups of adolescents to perform teaching. Apply communication skills that are effective with teens, such as listening to concerns, allowing for discussion, and bringing peers who have had experiences related to the topic being discussed.

Many of your interventions will involve teaching, so it is wise to develop a number of resources for working with teens. Consult the Web resources on the CD with this book, and visit agencies in your community to gather appropriate materials. Teaching topics will be directed both at health promotion (providing information to enhance the adolescent's state of health) and at health maintenance (sharing tips about how to avoid disease and injury). A good starting point is to have the adolescent identify a personal health goal and begin teaching there. In addition to teaching, you will provide direct care when you administer immunizations, perform vision screening, and examine the spine and posture for scoliosis.

One of the challenges during health supervision for adolescents is including the right mix of teen and parent decision making and involvement. You will again apply communication skills by tactfully allowing time for both parent and adolescent to be seen alone. Realize that you are supporting and providing information for parents, like useful discipline techniques, recognition of common parental feelings about teens, and the need for growing independence by their youth. When you provide teaching to groups of teens in schools, there may be policies about what needs to be sent home to parents. Some schools require an outline of topics such as sexually transmitted diseases or substance

any risky behaviors the adolescent engages in such as smoking, unprotected sexual relations, alcohol or drug use, or unsafe driving practices. The people and organizations around the adolescent such as family, school, and neighborhood are all assessed. Remember to list both risks and use be sent home for parents to read. Parents may call you with questions about content and approach, or some may choose to attend and sit in on your presentation. This obviously requires that you partner with the school administration, teachers, parents, and others to be effective in your presentation. Collaboration with many individuals and agencies are important skills.

Whether you see adolescents in offices or other private settings, or in schools, correction facilities, or other places with groups present, leave information about how you or another nurse or care provider can be contacted. Provide brochures, referral numbers, names, and emails related to the topics discussed. Encourage annual visits for health supervision visits and suggest a variety of places to obtain this care. For example, if a youth will soon graduate from high school, find out if he or she will be working or attending college and provide links to health insurance or care providers in the new location.

EVALUATION

Expected outcomes for care of adolescents and their families during health promotion and health maintenance include the following:

- Evidence that a rape victim is no longer abused
- Absence of debris and plaque on dental surfaces
- Approaching ideal weight
- Demonstration of amount and pattern of sleep for mental and physical rejuvenation
- Positive personal judgment of self-worth

Critical Concept Review

LEARNING OBJECTIVES

CONCEPTS

LEARNING OBJECTIVES	CONCEPTS

Apply knowledge of school-age growth and development to identify needed assessment of nutrition and physical activity.	Nutrition:
	1. Height, weight, and BMI.
	2. Assessment of nutritional status.
	3. Educate child and family about healthy nutritious practices:
	   ■ Healthy snacks at home.
	   ■ Need for increased calcium intake.
	Physical activity:
	1. Educate child and family in risk and protective factors related to physical activity.
	2. Assess physical activity of the family:
	   ■ Suggest activities that child and parent can do together.
	3. Encourage child to become active in physical education activities at school.

State components of self-concept for school-age children.	1. Self-esteem:
	   ■ Does child believe he/she is able to handle challenges?
	2. Body image:
	   ■ Does child's appearance and dress reflect a positive self-esteem?
	3. Sexuality:
	   ■ Does child ask appropriate questions about his or her own sexuality and opposite sex?

Describe the growing importance of peers in planning teaching strategies with school-age children.	1. School-age children feel pressure to appear like others, to fit in, and to do what others encourage. 2. Teaching strategies must appeal to the group as a whole. 3. Educational methods must be interesting and varied.
Use knowledge of the major injury risks of school-age children to plan nursing interventions that contribute to their prevention.	Injury prevention efforts should focus on the common causes of mortality and morbidity in school-age children, including: 1. Firearms. 2. Abuse. 3. Motor vehicle crashes. 4. Sports-related injuries.

LEARNING OBJECTIVES	CONCEPTS
Identify the major health concerns of the adolescent years.	1. School performance. 2. Sexual issues. 3. Body image Issues. 4. The need for independence.
Apply communication skills to interactions with adolescents and their families.	1. Assist parents to understand that the adolescent is striving to be independent. 2. Reassure adolescent that the parent is trying to provide guidance during a confusing time of life. 3. Encourage parents to reward positive behaviors. 4. Encourage adolescent to discuss specific issues rather than global subjects.
Apply assessment skills to plan data-gathering methods for nutrition, physical activity, and mental health status of youth.	Nutrition: 1. Discuss weight changes since last healthcare visit. 2. Discuss usual meal routines and favorite foods. Physical activity: 1. Question adolescent regarding participation in sports, including amount of practice. 2. Discuss other forms of physical activity engaged in daily or weekly. Mental health status: 1. Assess adolescent's perception of accomplishments and disappointments in life. 2. Ask adolescent about sexual activity.

Intervene with adolescents by integrating activities to promote health and to prevent disease and injury.	1. Screening tests:
	  ■ Scoliosis.
	  ■ Mental health status.
	  ■ Anemia.
	  ■ Sexually transmitted diseases.
	2. Review immunization status.
	3. Review information concerning need for sun protection
	4. Discussion of birth control and prevention of sexually transmitted diseases.
	5. Discussion of safe driving practices:
	  ■ Seat belts.
	  ■ Do not drink and drive.
	6. Discussion of prevention of common sports injuries.

CRITICAL THINKING IN ACTION

View the **Critical Thinking in Action** video in Chapter 38 of the CD-ROM. Then, answer the questions that follow.

Tammy is a 13-year-old coming into the office for her yearly check-up and she has never been in the hospital or had surgery. She is a good student and is excited to start 7th grade next year. She has not had any immunizations since going into kindergarten. Tammy arrives with her mother, with whom she lives; she has no contact with her biological father. Her mother decides to stay in the waiting room, but did note on the written history form that there is a family history of high cholesterol and heart disease in family members under 50 years old. Tammy's mother is a single parent working full time with 2 other children at home. Tammy's body mass index is in the 85th percentile and she passed her hearing and vision tests. Her blood pressure is 115/70 and her urinalysis shows blood, but Tammy has her menses today. Tammy has a period every month and menarche started at 10 years old. Her menses lasts 5-7 days and she denies experiencing cramping or excessively heavy menses. Tammy enjoys being a member of the volleyball team and is involved in a church youth group. She does not get to spend much time with her friends because she watches her 2 younger siblings in the afternoons while her mother is at work. When her mother is away, she admits to sitting and playing video games or watching TV most of the day. Tammy says she has had a boyfriend, but denies sexual activity. She also denies any experimentation with substance use.

1. What vaccines is Tammy due for at this age if she has not already had them?
2. Based on the information you collected about Tammy, what are some of the areas of recommended health teaching?
3. A dietary assessment demonstrates that Tammy frequently skips meals and eats fast food almost daily. What are some of the suggestions you can give Tammy to improve her nutritional status?
4. What are some of the injury prevention topics you can discuss with Tammy?

MEDIALINK

www.prenhall.com/london

- NCLEX-RN® Review, case studies, and other interactive resources for this chapter can be found on the Companion Website at http://www.prenhall.com/london. Click on "Chapter 38" to select the activities for this chapter.

What are some of your disappointments? How have you dealt with them?

- For animations, more NCLEX-RN® Review questions, and an audio glossary, access the accompanying CD-ROM in this textbook.

REFERENCES

Adderly-Kelly, B., & Green, P. M. (2000). Health promotion for urban middle school students: A survey of learning needs. *Journal of National Black Nurses Association, 22,* 34–38.

American Psychiatric Association. (2000). *Diagnostic and statistical manual of mental disorders: DSM-IV-TR.* Washington, DC: Author.

Bandura, A. (1977). *Self-efficacy in changing societies.* New York: Cambridge University.

Colyar, M. R. (2003). *Well-child assessment for primary care providers.* Philadelphia: FA Davis.

Committee on Injury and Poison Prevention, American Academy of Pediatrics. (2001). Bicycle helmets. *Pediatrics, 108,* 1030–1032.

Committee on Sports Medicine and Fitness, American Academy of Pediatrics. (2001). Risk of injury from baseball and softball in children. *Pediatrics, 107,* 782–784.

Dickey, S. B., & Deatrick, J. (2000). Autonomy and decision making for health promotion in adolescence. *Pediatric Nursing, 26,* 461–467.

Dombrowski, M. A. (1999). Preventing disease with stress management in elementary schools. *Journal of School Health, 69,* 136–127.

Edelman, C. L., & Mandle, C. L. (2002). *Health promotion throughout the life span* (5th ed.). St. Louis, MO: Mosby.

Eisenberg, M. E., Neumark-Sztainer, D., & Story, M. (2003). Associations of weight-based teasing and emotional well-being among adolescents. *Archives of Pediatric and Adolescent Medicine, 157,* 733–738.

Epstein, L. H., Paluch, R. A., Kalanus, L. E., Goldfield, G. S., Cerny, F. J., & Roemmich, J. N. (2001). How much physical activity do youth get: A quantitative review of heart-rate measured activity. *Pediatrics, 108,* e44 (electronic article). Retrieved October 16, 2005, from http://pediatrics.aappublications. org/cgi/content/full/108/3/e44

Green, B. L., Person, S., Crowther, M., Frison, S., Shipp, M., Lee, P., & Martin, M. (2003). Demographic and geographic variations of oral health among African Americans based on NHANES III. *Community Dental Health, 20,* 117–122.

Green, M., & Palfrey, J. S. (Eds.). (2002). *Bright futures: Guidelines for health supervision of infants, children, and adolescents* (2nd ed.). Arlington, VA: National Center for Education in Maternal and Child Health.

Halfon, N. (2002). *Child rearing in America: Challenges facing parents with young children.* New York: Cambridge University Press.

Halfon, N., Regalado, M., McLearn, K. T., Kuo, A. A., & Wright, K. (2003). *Building a bridge from birth to school: Improving developmental and behavioral health services for young children.* New York: Commonwealth Fund.

Jellinek, M., Patel, B. P., & Froehle, M. C. (Eds.). (2002). *Bright futures in practice: Mental health* (Vol. I & II). Arlington, VA: National Center for Education in Maternal and Child Health.

Kerker, B. D., Horwitz, S.M., Leventhal, J. M., Plichta, S., & Leaf, P. J. (2000). Identification of violence in the home: Pediatric and parental reports. *Archives of Pediatric and Adolescent Medicine, 154,* 457–462.

Kolbe, L. J., Kann, L., & Brener, N. D. (2001). Overview and summary of findings: School health policies and programs study 2000. *Journal of School Health, 71,* 253–259.

Lerner, R. M., & Thompson, L. S. (2002). Promoting healthy adolescent behavior and development: Issues in the design and evaluation of effective youth programs. *Journal of Pediatric Nursing, 17,* 338–344.

Little, D. C., Vermillion, J.M., Dikis, E. J., Little, R. J., Custer, M. D., & Cooney, D. R. (2003). Life on the farm—children at risk. *Journal of Pediatric Surgery, 38,* 804–807.

Lohse, J. L. (2003). A bicycle safety education program for parents of young children. *Journal of School Nursing, 19,* 100–110.

Lowry, R., Wechsler, H., Kann, L., & Collins, J. S. (2001). Recent trends in participation in physical education among US high school students. *Journal of School Health, 71,* 145–152.

Mayo Clinic. (2005). *Adolescent sleep problems.* Retrieved October 16, 2005, from http:www. mayoclinic.com

MMWR. (2004). Youth risk behavior surveillance—United States, 2003. *Morbidity and Mortality Weekly Report, 53* (SS02), 1–96.

Montgomery, K. S. (2002). Health promotion with adolescent: Examining theoretical perspectives to guide research. *Research and Theory for Nursing Practice: An International Journal, 16,* 119–134.

Murray, R. B., & Zentner, J. P. (2001). *Health promotion strategies through the life span* (7th ed.). Upper Saddle River, NJ: Prentice Hall.

Nygard, P., Waiters, E. D., Grube, J. W., & Keege, D. (2003). Why do they do it? A qualitative study of adolescent drinking and driving. *Substance Abuse and Misuse, 38,* 835–863.

O'Donnell, G. W., & Mickalide, A. D. (1998). *SAFE KIDS at home, at play and on the way: A report to the nation on unintentional childhood injury.* Washington, DC: National SAFE KIDS Campaign.

Parkinson, G. W., & Hike, K. E. (2003). Bicycle helmet assessment during well visits reveals severe shortcomings in condition and fit. *Pediatrics, 112,* 320–323.

Pate, R. R., Freedson, P.S., Sallis, J. F., Taylor, W. C., Sirard, J., Trost, S. G., & Dowda, M. (2002). Compliance with physical activity guidelines: Prevalence in a population of children and youth. *Annals of Epidemiology, 12,* 303–308.

Patrick, K., Spear, B., Holt, K., & Sofka, D. (Eds.). (2001). *Bright futures in practice: Physical activity.* Arlington, VA: National Center for Education in Maternal and Child Health.

Pender, N. J., Murdaugh, C.L., & Parsons, M. A. (2002). *Health promotion in nursing practice* (4th ed.). Upper Saddle River, NJ: Prentice Hall.

Qui, Y., & Ni, H. (2003). Utilization of dental care services by Asians and native Hawaiian or other Pacific Islanders: United States, 1997–2000. *Advances in Data, 336,* 1–11.

Simons-Morton, B. G., Hartos, J. L., & Beck, K. H. (2003). Persistence of effects of a brief intervention on parental restrictions of teen driving privileges. *Injury Prevention, 9,* 142–146.

Story, M., Holt, K., & Sofka, D. (Eds.). (2002). *Bright futures in practice: Nutrition.* Arlington, VA:

National Center for Education in Maternal and Child Health.

Streng, N. (2000). A student health advocate program. *Journal of School Nursing, 16,* 50–53.

Task Force on the Family. (2003). Family pediatrics: Report of the Task Force on the Family. *Pediatrics, 111,* 1541–1571.

U. S. Department of Health and Human Services (2000). *Healthy People 2010.* Washington, D.C.: Author.

VanLandeghen, K., Bronstein, J., & Brach, C. (2003). *Children's dental access in Medicaid. The role of medical care use and dentist participation* (CHIRI Issue Brief 2. AHRQ Publication No. 03–0032).

Rockville, MD: Agency for Healthcare Research and Quality. Retrieved June 30, 2003, from http://www.ahrq.gov/about/chirident.htm

Vargas, C. M., Ronzio, C. R., & Hayes, K. L. (2003). Oral health status of children and adolescents by rural residence, United States. *Journal of Rural Health, 19,* 260–268.

Wainwright, P., Thomas, J., & Jones, M. (2000). Health promotion and the role of the school nurse: A systematic review. *Journal of Advanced Nursing, 32,* 1083–1091.

Weist, M. D., Goldstein, A., Morris, L., & Bryant, T. (2003). Integrating expanded school

mental health programs and school-based health centers. *Psychology in the Schools, 40,* 297–308.

Young, K. T. (1998). Listening to parents: A national survey of parents with young children. *Archives of Pediatric and Adolescent Medicine, 152,* 255–262.

Young, L. E., & Hayes, V. (2002). *Transforming health promotion practice: Concepts, issues, and applications.* Philadelphia: F.A. Davis.

Wertlieb, D. (2003). Converging trends in family research and pediatrics: Recent findings for the American Academy of Pediatrics Task Force on the Family. *Pediatrics, 111* (Supp.), 1572–1587.

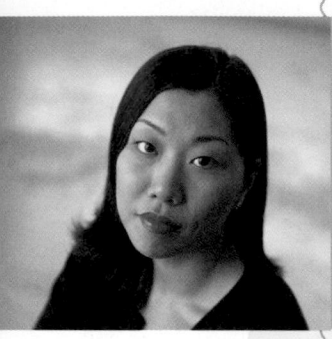

Nursing Considerations for the Child and Family in the Community

Sometimes Jessica's asthma attacks really frighten me because she struggles so hard to breathe. She has a lot of trouble with asthma in the summertime with all the heat. I am afraid to let her play outside with her friends for fear that she will have another attack. I would really like to know how to keep Jessica's asthma under control.

—Mother of Jessica, 8

LEARNING OBJECTIVES

- List the categories of family strengths that help families cope with stressors.

- Describe the advantages of using a family assessment tool.

- List the variety of community healthcare settings where nurses provide health services to children.

- Describe the role of the nurse in each identified healthcare setting.

- Describe the responses of children to disasters by developmental stage.

- Define the child with a chronic condition by categories of impairments.

- List the skills and knowledge needed by the nurse to effectively care for the child with a chronic condition in the community.

- Describe nursing interventions to support the transition of a child with a chronic condition to school and adult living.

- Discuss the family's role in care coordination.

MEDIALINK www.prenhall.com/london

CD-ROM

Videos:
    Disaster Preparedness
    EMS for Children
Audio Glossary
NCLEX-RN® Review

Companion Website

MediaLink Applications:
    Identify Health Issues in Childcare Settings
    Develop an Individualized Health Plan (IHP)
    Complete an Emergency Information Form (EIF)
School Policy Review
Teaching Plans:
    Disasters and the Family with an Infant
    Disasters and the Family with a Child
    Disasters and the Child Assisted by Technology
Thinking Critically
NCLEX-RN® Review
Case Study

Children receive most of their healthcare in community settings. Depending upon the community, healthcare resources, and age of the child, this care may be provided in a variety of settings. When providing care to the child and family in the community, it is important for the nurse to assess the family's strengths, be aware of community resources, and help families manage the complex healthcare that is often provided in the home.

FAMILY ASSESSMENT

The **family** is an interdependent network of individuals that mutually influence each other. Families must be understood in their own context. It is important to understand each family's strengths and uniqueness and how the family and its members respond to the complex and often conflicting demands for time and attention. Nurses need to be able to assess family strengths and support mechanisms, to identify coping strategies, and to determine when families have overextended their resources and need additional support. In some cases nurses can provide the additional support needed, and at other times referral to other health professionals is appropriate to address the family's needs.

Children and families live within a variety of settings and interact with those settings in ways that directly or indirectly influence behaviors and learning. Because of these environmental influences on the family, it is important to consider the relationship of the family with the social networks within the community.

FAMILY STRESSORS

Families experience many stressors as an inevitable part of life. Some stressors are positive, such as the birth of a child that leads to transitions within the family. Other stressors are unexpected and not considered positive, such as learning that a child has a serious health condition. A child's illness or injury affects the entire family. Such a stressor demands a response from the family members that can lead to change within the family's interactions among its members and with the environment. Identifying how families respond to the stress of illness or injury of a child or other family member is important because of the potential hardships it causes the entire family.

Many families live in a stressed state due to inadequate finances, healthcare concerns, relationship challenges, and other pressures. Stressors are also cumulative and can come from many sources (work demands, school issues, extended family demands, achieving quality family time, and community roles). Most families have developed coping strategies to deal with daily routine stressors. Unexpected events are often more stressful as the family has not had time to consider available resources and prepare a response.

FAMILY STRENGTHS

Family strengths are the relationships and processes that support and protect families and family members during times of adversity and change. These strengths help maintain family cohesion while supporting the development and well-being of individual family members (Moore, Chalk, Scarpa et al., 2002). There are four types of strengths that enable families to develop, adapt to change, and cope with challenges (Feeley & Gottlieb, 2000):

- Individual or family traits, such as optimism or resilience
- Individual or family assets, such as finances

- Individual or family capabilities, skills, and competencies, such as problem solving
- Another quality less permanent than a trait or asset, such as motivation

Identifying the family's **resilience**—the family's capacity to develop their strengths and abilities, to "bounce back" from the stresses and challenges faced, and to eliminate or minimize negative outcomes—is an important focus for family assessment prior to planning nursing interventions. Resilience of children is discussed in Chapter 36. ∞

When a family can control and deal with events satisfactorily, they gain a sense of competence, making them more resilient, in contrast to families who are overwhelmed by traumatic experiences. Characteristics of a resilient family include the following (Patterson, 1991):

- Balancing the child's illness with other family needs
- Forming collaborative relationships with healthcare professionals
- Maintaining a professional relationship rather than a friendship relationship with providers
- Developing competence in communication skills
- Maintaining family flexibility and adapting to changing circumstances
- Maintaining a commitment to the family as a unit
- Attributing positive meaning to the situation
- Maintaining supportive relationships outside the family
- Engaging in active coping efforts with effective and efficient problem-solving abilities

Most families do not naturally develop resilience. Often nursing support is needed to help family members learn new skills, make adaptations, and gain confidence in their abilities to manage the challenges they face. Potential resources include religious faith, finances, social support, physical health, family flexibility, and family coping mechanisms. If resources are diminished and the family defines the stressor as significant enough to cause a crisis, then the family will be susceptible to more serious disruption by the event. Nurses need to help families identify their strengths and areas for improvement that will lead to increased resiliency.

Functional families use a variety of coping strategies for stress management and they successfully reduce stress. Coping strategies of dysfunctional families are defensive and do not effectively manage the stress. See Table 39–1 for coping strategies used by functional and dysfunctional families.

Recognition of family strengths can be used to develop a rapport and relationship with the family. Focus on family competence, and acknowledge and validate family members' emotions. Once the family recognizes the strengths it brings to the management of their child's healthcare prob-

lem, the more likely the family will become an effective partner in the process. The nurse can often help families recognize that the strengths used in prior life experiences may transfer to the current healthcare experience.

COLLECTING DATA FOR FAMILY ASSESSMENT

To obtain an accurate and concise family assessment, the nurse needs to establish a trusting relationship with the child and family. Identify the parent's and the child's greatest concern, and expect these concerns to be different. It is important

---

TABLE 39–1 ❖ Coping Strategies Used by Functional Families and Dysfunctional Families

Functional Family Coping Strategies	Dysfunctional Family Coping Strategies
■ Family relationships—increased structure and organization within the home and family, strengthening family cohesion, and increased role flexibility of family members.	■ Denial of family problems.
■ Gathering information and knowledge, family joint problem solving.	■ Exploiting a family member such as by scapegoating (negatively labeling and stigmatizing a family member) to avoid examining the real problem in the family.
■ **Normalization**—the process of family management that involves acknowledging a life-changing situation, such as the child has a chronic health problem, but family makes an effort to lead a normal life. Family life is perceived to be normal because the impact of the condition on the family functioning is minimized, as demonstrated by behaviors, rituals, and routines that show others that the family is normal.	■ Use of threat or withdrawal of affection and support to keep family members together at the expense of the emotional health of its members.
■ Passive acceptance about an event or situation about which little or nothing can be done and determining that it will take care of itself over time.	■ Myths or images the family has of itself that obscure reality and enable the family to deny some of its problems.
■ Direct, open, honest, and clear communication.	■ Extreme dominance and submission patterns.
■ Use of humor and laughter.	■ Family addictions (drug or alcohol).
■ Maintaining active linkages with the community and using social support networks.	■ Domestic violence (partner, child, sibling to sibling, and elder abuse).
■ Spiritual supports.	

Data from Friedman, M. M., Bowden, V. R., & Jones, E. G. (2003). *Family nursing: Research, theory, and practice* (5th ed., pp. 476–494). Upper Saddle River, NJ: Prentice Hall.

to acknowledge these multiple concerns and demonstrate respect for the diversity of the family. The goal is to obtain family information that will be helpful in planning nursing interventions that will help the family care for the child and improve the child's outcomes while valuing each person within the family.

Information about the family is collected continuously during the healthcare process, through interviews, observations of the family interactions, reports from other healthcare providers or agencies working with the family, and with a family assessment tool. Family assessment data that are important to collect include the following:

- Name, age, sex, and family relationship of all people residing in the household
- Family type, structure, roles, and values
- Cultural associations, including cultural norms and customs related to childrearing and infant feeding
- Faith-based affiliations
- Support systems network, including extended family, friends, and faith-based and community associations
- Communication patterns, including language barriers
- Environmental data—place of residence, condition of housing, number of persons living in the residence, sleeping arrangements, play areas, neighborhood characteristics

See Chapter 35 for suggested data to collect about the psychosocial history and daily living patterns. ∞ Observation of the home and family members is recommended in some cases to obtain valuable information about family functioning.

FAMILY ASSESSMENT TOOLS

Family assessment tools can be used to gather additional information about the family's functioning and can place particular focus on family stresses, coping strategies, and family strengths. Information about the way the family functions in nurturing its members, problem solving, and communicating may help identify strategies that are potentially more effective for management of the child's healthcare. They enable the nurse to work more effectively with the family, such as collaborating with the family in planning for health maintenance and health promotion strategies.

Family APGAR

The Family APGAR is a quick five-item questionnaire that may be used as an initial screening tool for family assessment. The five family concepts measured include family adaptability, partnership, growth, affection, and resolve (Table 39–2). The five-item questionnaire can be administered quickly to family members over 10 years of age. Ask all family members to complete a separate copy of the questionnaire to gain a picture of the family's perspective on family functioning. Be more concerned if the majority of responses fall in the "hardly ever" category or responses vary a lot among family members. This may indicate a family that needs much more support to cope with the demands of daily life and management of the child's condition.

Home Observation for Measurement of the Environment (HOME)

The HOME Inventory is an assessment tool developed to measure the quality and quantity of stimulation and support available to the child in the home environment (Caldwell & Bradley, 1984). Four age-specific scales are available (birth to 3 years, 3 to 6 years, 6 to 10 years, and 10 to 15 years). Examples of subscales within each age-specific scale include parental responsivity, acceptance of child, the physical environment, learning materials, variety in experience, and parental involvement. Data are collected during an informal, low-stress interview and observation over 45 to 90 minutes in the home setting (Figure 39–1 ●). The child's primary caregiver and the child must be present and awake during the interview. Observation of the parent-child interaction is an essential part of the assessment. The intent is to allow family members to act normally. Assessment of the home environment will help to identify factors that promote the child's growth and development. Examples of nursing interventions that could result from the HOME assessment include items that can be used in the home for toys and strategies for interacting with the child to promote learning.

Nursing Family Assessment Tools

The Friedman Family Assessment Tool (FFAM), developed by Marilyn Friedman, and the Calgary Family Assessment Model, developed by Lorraine Wright and Maureen Leahy, have been developed to assist nurses with family assessment (see Appendix H). ∞ Each contains information to collect data about a family's relationships, functioning, strengths, and problems. Refer to family nursing texts to obtain copies of these tools.

FAMILY SUPPORT SERVICES IN THE COMMUNITY

Services exist in all communities with a purpose of supporting families to promote the health and development of children as well as family positive relationships. Examples of these family support services include the following:

- Head Start and Early Head Start
- Before- and after-school programs for children of working parents
- School-based health and counseling services
- Play groups for preschool children
- Peer support groups
- Social service programs offered by the faith community

TABLE 39–2 ❖ The Family APGAR Questionnaire

Directions:

The following questions have been designed to help us better understand you and your family. You should feel free to ask questions about any item in the questionnaire.

The space for comments should be used when you wish to give additional information or if you wish to discuss the way the question is applied to your family. Please try to answer all questions.

Family is defined as the individual(s) with whom you usually live. If you live alone, your "family" consists of persons with whom you now have the strongest emotional ties.[a]

For each question, check only one box

	Almost always 2	Some of the time 1	Hardly ever 0
I am satisfied that I can turn to my family for help when something is troubling me. Comments: _____			
I am satisfied with the way my family talks over things with me and shares problems with me. Comments: _____			
I am satisfied that my family accepts and supports my wishes to take on new activities or directions. Comments: _____			
I am satisfied with the way my family expresses affection and responds to my emotions, such as anger, sorrow, and love. Comments: _____			
I am satisfied with the way my family and I share time together. Comments: _____			

[a]According to which member of the family is being interviewed, the interviewer may substitute for the word *family* either *spouse, significant other, parents,* or *children.*

Responses are scored (either 2, 1, 0) and summed. The total score ranges from 0 to 10. The larger the score, the greater amount of satisfaction with family functioning.

Adapted with permission from Smilkstein, G. (1978). The family APGAR: A proposal for a family function test and its use by physicians. *Journal of Family Practice, 6*(6), 1231–1239.

- Home visiting programs for high-risk children and parents
- Job skills training, adult education, and literacy programs
- Crisis care and respite care programs

Many of these family support services work to promote positive family relationships, parental competencies, and behaviors that contribute to the health and development of the children and family. Most programs are designed with the premise that no family is entirely self-sufficient and most can benefit from some external support.

Think about the formal and informal family support services in your community. Nurses play an important role in helping to link families to the types of community support services they need after performing a family assessment and collaborating with families to identify and seek assistance most beneficial to their needs.

SETTINGS FOR COMMUNITY HEALTHCARE

Nurses care for children in a wide variety of community settings. Some of these settings include childcare centers,

● FIGURE 39–1

A visit to the home when all family members are present provides the best information for completion of an assessment tool such as the Home Observation for Measurement of the Environment (HOME).

schools, camps, physician offices, hospital or public health clinics, homeless shelters, and the home. The range of nursing care varies from monitoring the health and safety of children in childcare centers and schools to the provision of acute care to a child at home. Falling within this range are the provision of health supervision or well-child care, care for episodic illnesses and injuries, and assisting families to learn optimal management of their child's chronic conditions. Each of these nursing roles is important in promoting the health of children in the community.

Children receive most of their healthcare (health promotion and episodic healthcare for acute illnesses and injuries) in community settings. Depending on the community, healthcare resources, and age of the child, this care may be provided in any of the settings previously listed. Patterns of healthcare delivery have changed over the past decade due to technology developments and efforts to reduce healthcare costs. Day surgery in ambulatory surgical centers, newborn discharge after 24 to 48 hours, home care for long-term intravenous antibiotics, and short stay units associated with emergency departments are common. Options to provide safe, high-quality care with fewer hospitalizations or shorter stays when hospitalization is needed are explored. Home care services have developed to support families who care for more acutely ill children in their homes.

Care of children continues to shift rapidly from the hospital to community settings. This trend in out-of-hospital care is seen among children with chronic health conditions and advanced disease states. Technologic advances, such as portable medical equipment, now make it possible to provide complex healthcare services in the home and other community settings. Strategies to support families who pro-

vide care to their children in the home have developed. Additionally, federal law mandates that education be provided to all children with disabilities, and there are no exceptions based on healthcare status. As a result, schools are now obligated to provide complex healthcare to children.

The nurse working with families in a community setting must use the knowledge of how the larger environment influences the child's health and development and the family's activities. Nurses have a variety of positions within these settings, such as community health nurse, home health nurse, school nurse, pediatric nurse in an office setting, and nurse practitioner or advanced practice nurse. The nurse may assume the role of direct care provider, educator, advocate, or planner in any of these positions. To work effectively in the community, the nurse needs to gain experience and skills in:

- Conducting child and family assessments and working with families to plan individualized healthcare strategies, as well as implementing and evaluating nursing care strategies to match family economic, cultural, and social situation, and available resources.

- Working with community agencies (schools, churches, and other community-based resources) to assess, plan strategies, and implement and evaluate approaches addressed to the healthcare needs of the community's children.

OFFICE OR HEALTHCARE CENTER SETTING

Every child should have a **healthcare home** or **medical home**, a consistent, continuous, comprehensive, family-centered, and compassionate source of primary health care. The healthcare providers in the healthcare home or medical home assume responsibility for coordinating the healthcare needed by the child between all healthcare settings. Important elements of a healthcare home or medical home include the following (American Academy of Pediatrics, 2002):

- Family-centered care that involves a trusting relationship, respecting the diversity and importance of the family in the child's life

- Continuity of care from infancy through adolescence, and transition of adolescents with chronic conditions to adult healthcare

- Family-centered health promotion and health maintenance care

- Interaction with child care, school, and community agencies as needed, coordinating care with all health providers

A physician office or health center is often the site of the healthcare home. Health promotion and health maintenance services are provided to the child and family, as well as episodic acute illness and injury care at this location. See Chapter 37 and Chapter 38 for the specific health promotion services provided in the community setting. ∞

Role of the Pediatric Nurse in an Office or Health Center

The nursing process is used when providing care for children in the health center. The range of assessment responsibilities may vary by setting as well as the preparation and experience of the nurse (Figure 39–2 ◉). Specific functions of the pediatric nurse in this setting include the following:

- Identifying children in need of urgent care or isolation
- Performing nursing assessments, including the health history, vital signs, growth and development, nutritional status, immunization status, family strengths and challenges, and physical examination
- Performing screening tests to detect health problems such as vision, hearing, anemia, and lead poisoning (see Chapter 37 ∞)
- Assisting with physician examinations and performing diagnostic tests as well as providing information about procedures and offering reassurance
- Developing nursing diagnoses and implementing a plan of care, including immunizations, patient education for health promotion, or management of a health condition
- Linking families with community resources

◉ FIGURE 39–2

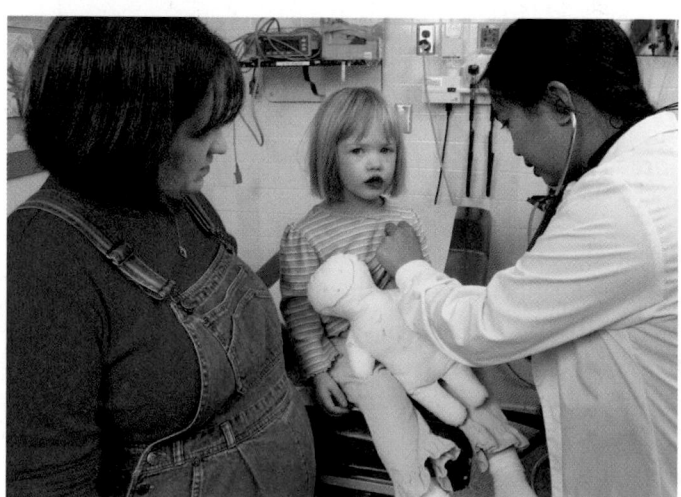

Nurses carefully assess children in the office setting who present with an acute care illness. It is important to identify how serious the child's illness is and to monitor the child for progression of symptoms during the visit. This is also a time to gather information about the child's illness and to identify health information that will be needed for the family to care for the child at home.

- Ensuring a safe environment and that infection control guidelines are followed

An important goal is to develop a positive relationship with the child and family so that optimal healthcare is provided. This relationship is strengthened over the months and years of providing care to the child and family.

Identifying Severely Ill and Injured Children. Assessment of the child with an episodic illness or injury upon arrival in the health center is important to determine the urgency of care needed. A rapid assessment for changes in mental status, airway patency, breathing, and circulation is used to identify the child that needs immediate medical attention. The child with an urgent condition must be monitored frequently to detect any worsening of condition and need for emergency care.

The nurse collaborates with the physician to develop an emergency response plan for the health center. The nurse is often responsible for teaching the office receptionist to recognize a child that needs immediate assessment by the nurse. The nurse is also often responsible for ensuring that all emergency care equipment, supplies, and medications are organized and readily available in the central treatment room. See "Nursing Practice" for equipment needed for office emergency preparedness. The nurse takes a leadership role in coordinating mock drills with all staff in the healthcare setting so that all employees know and perform their designated role when a true emergency occurs.

NURSING PRACTICE

Essential equipment needed for managing an emergency in an office setting includes the following: oxygen and an oxygen delivery system, bag-valve-mask resuscitator in a pediatric and adult size, clear oxygen masks in various pediatric sizes (both simple face masks and non-rebreather masks with a reservoir), oral airways in various sizes, suction devices, peak flow meter, and a nebulizer or metered dose inhaler with a spacer/mask. Essential medications are epinephrine 1:1000 and albuterol (American Academy of Pediatrics Committee on Pediatric Emergency Medicine, 2000). Locate the emergency equipment in every clinical setting where you have assignments.

Educating the Child and Family. Child and family education regarding injury prevention, growth and development, nutrition, healthy lifestyles, and the home care of episodic illnesses and injuries are important nursing roles in primary care. The nurse also may be responsible for selecting patient education materials for the waiting area and those specifically used to teach families about various conditions. Knowledge of the community and population served by the health center enables the nurse to select appropriate education materials.

Nurses teach families to provide the condition-specific care for the child at home. Examples of information provided include:

- Signs that the condition is not improving as expected and when to return to the physician.
- How and when to administer prescribed medications and their potential side effects.
- Modifications in diet and activity.
- Other supportive care for the child's condition.
- Education to help the child and family recognize the need to initiate care for a new episode of a chronic condition (i.e., asthma, sickle cell anemia, or hemophilia) that may prevent the need for a healthcare visit or reduce the severity of the episode.

Identifying Community Resources. Nurses in primary care settings are often involved in identifying community resources that are needed by the child and family to help promote the child's health. Compiling a manual of community resources and regularly updating names and phone numbers of contacts will make it easier to provide information efficiently. Examples of community resources that might be included are early intervention programs, support groups, language and translation services, food banks, lead paint abatement services, social services, and mental health services.

Ensuring a Safe Environment for Children. The health center has many potential hazards such as equipment, cleaning supplies, sharps, medications, and laboratory materials from which the child needs to be protected. The nurse should ensure a safe environment for the child. Guidelines for infection control must be developed and implemented to reduce the transmission of infectious diseases between child patients and between the healthcare providers and children.

SPECIALTY HEALTHCARE SETTINGS

Pediatric nurses also provide care for children with acute and chronic conditions within hospital outpatient or specialty care ambulatory settings. Children may be referred to physician specialists for diagnostic workups or the long-term management of their chronic conditions. In some cases health promotion, health maintenance, and episodic illness care are provided to children with chronic conditions in these settings. With experience, pediatric nurses working in a hospital ambulatory setting develop specialized knowledge and skill to meet the specific needs of the population of children cared for in that setting. The roles for nurses in these settings are similar to those described for the health center.

SCHOOL SETTINGS

School nurses practice independently as the only licensed healthcare provider in the educational setting and, depending on the community, serve up to 3000 children in one or more schools. School nursing is a specialized practice of professional nursing that advances the well-being, academic success, and lifelong achievement of children. School nurses facilitate positive student responses to normal development; facilitate health promotion, health maintenance, and safety; intervene in actual and potential health problems; provide case management services; and actively collaborate with others to build student and family capacity for adaptation, self-management, self-advocacy, and learning (National Association of School Nurses and American Nurses Association, 2001). See "Nursing Practice" for the Standards of Professional School Nursing Practice.

NURSING PRACTICE

Standards of professional school nursing practice include the following:

1. The school nurse collects client data.
2. The school nurse analyzes the assessment data in determining nursing diagnoses.
3. The school nurse identifies expected outcomes individualized to the client.
4. The school nurse develops a plan of care/action that specifies interventions to attain expected outcomes.
5. The school nurse implements the interventions identified in the plan of care/action.
6. The school nurse evaluates the client's progress toward attainment of outcomes.
7. The school nurse systematically evaluates the quality and effectiveness of school nursing practice.
8. The school nurse evaluates one's own nursing practice in relation to professional practice standards and relevant statutes, regulations, and policies.
9. The school nurse acquires and maintains current knowledge and competency in school nursing practice.
10. The school nurse interacts with and contributes to the professional development of peers and school personnel as colleagues.
11. The school nurse's decisions and actions on behalf of clients are determined in an ethical manner.
12. The school nurse collaborates with the student, family, school staff, community, and other providers in providing student care.
13. The school nurse promotes use of research findings in school nursing practice.
14. The school nurse considers factors related to safety, effectiveness, and cost when planning and delivering care.
15. The school nurse uses effective written, verbal, and nonverbal communication skills.
16. The school nurse manages school health services.
17. The school nurse assists students, families, school staff, and community to achieve optimal levels of wellness through appropriately designed and delivered health education.

Used with permission from the National Association of School Nurses and American Nurses Association. (2001). Scope and standards of professional school nursing practice. Silver Spring, MD: American Nurses Publishing.

School nurses work to remove or minimize the health barriers to learning so students can improve school performance. School health services include preventive services, health promotion and health maintenance, health education, emergency care, and the referral and management of acute and chronic health problems. The traditional tasks of screening, first aid, and monitoring immunization status are still performed. The following "Nursing Practice" lists the *Healthy People 2010* national health objectives that illustrate the breadth of school nursing.

NURSING PRACTICE

The *Healthy People 2010* objectives that relate to school health issues include the following:

- Increase high school completion rate.
- Increase the percentage of middle, junior high, and senior high schools that provide health education to prevent health problems in the following areas: unintentional injury, violence, suicide, tobacco use and addiction, alcohol and other drug use, unintended pregnancy, HIV/AIDS and STD infection, unhealthy dietary patterns, inadequate physical activity, and environmental health.
- Increase the percentage of the nation's elementary, middle, junior high, and senior high schools that have a nurse-to-student ratio of at least 1 to 750.
- Increase the percentage of the nation's primary and secondary schools that have official school policies ensuring the safety of students and staff from environmental hazards, such as chemicals in special classrooms, poor indoor air quality, asbestos, and exposure to pesticides.
- Increase the percentage of public and private schools that require use of appropriate head, face, eye, and mouth protection for students participating in school-sponsored physical activities.
- Reduce weapon-carrying on school property.
- Increase the percentage of children and adolescents age 6 to 19 years whose intake of meals and snacks at school contributes to good overall dietary quality.
- Increase the percentage of school-based health centers with an oral health component.
- Increase the percentage of the nation's public and private schools that require daily physical education for all students.
- Increase the percentage of adolescents who participate in daily school physical education.
- Increase the percentage of adolescents who spend 50% of school physical education time being physically active.
- Increase the percentage of the nation's public and private schools that provide access to their physical activity spaces and facilities for all persons outside of normal school hours.
- Reduce the number of school or workdays missed by persons due to asthma.

Data from U.S. Department of Health and Human Services. (2000). Healthy People 2010 (2nd ed.). Washington, DC: U.S. Government Printing Office. http://www.healthypeople.gov

Role of the Nurse in the School Setting

Nursing roles in the school setting focus on promoting the health and safety of the population of children enrolled (including faculty and staff) and providing direct care to ill and injured children (Figure 39–3 ⊙). Specific activities include infection control, health education, assessment for conditions that affect health and learning, administering medications, participating on teams to develop individualized education plans (IEPs) and individualized health plans (IHPs), advocating for better nutrition and physical activity to improve overall health, investigating environmental safety hazards, and planning for crisis intervention and support services (Robinson, 2002). The nurse is an important liaison in planning for the access of emergency medical services personnel when a child becomes acutely ill or injured.

Collaboration with the other health professionals in the community is becoming increasingly important to promote health in the school setting. Working with the school's physician consultant to discuss and update standing orders for the care of children is important so that the nurse can provide care for urgent and emergency health threats that students may potentially experience. Communicating with the child's

⊙ **FIGURE 39–3**

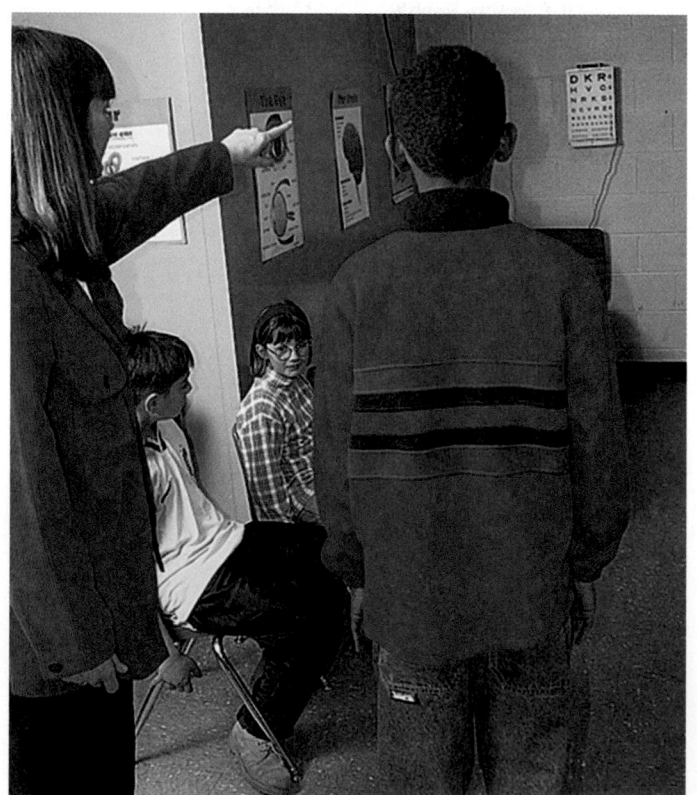

The school is often the setting for screening tests of large groups of students to identify those that may have a problem that interferes with learning. Screening tests are often organized so all children in a particular grade are assessed, as in this vision screening test.

healthcare provider about the child's specific health conditions makes it possible for the nurse to plan for management of the child's condition in the school setting. The school nurse often has valuable information to help the child's healthcare providers with their ongoing management.

Facilitating a Child's Return to School. The school nurse also helps the child return to the classroom following an acute illness or injury, especially when environmental adaptation is required or when a change in health status has occurred. The transition back to school is assisted when the pediatric nurse in the hospital or community setting or the child's healthcare provider contacts the school nurse to coordinate the child's return to school rather than having the parent take full responsibility for informing the school. Educational materials about the child's condition can be recommended to educate students, faculty, and staff. The school nurse then begins to work with the family to prepare teachers and school administrators for the child's special needs. The child's teacher and classmates can be prepared for the child's physical changes if appropriate. Sometimes the teacher's expectations of the child need to be modified, such as a child with a mild brain injury who may have decreased ability to concentrate for several weeks during recovery. Often an IHP must be developed or modified. See page 1146.

Children with Complex Healthcare Conditions. Previously homebound children, who are **medically fragile**, needing skilled nursing care with or without medical equipment to support vital functions, now attend school. See page 1147 for a discussion of these children and their care in the community.

THINKING CRITICALLY

ASTHMA ATTACKS AT SCHOOL

Carrie, 8 years old, is anxious because her asthma attack is getting worse. Her teacher sees that she is having trouble breathing, so she sends her to the school health office for treatment. Carrie has such severe asthma that a nebulizer is kept at school for her to use. This treatment often relieves Carrie's symptoms and permits her to return to classes. However, in this case, the asthma attack does not respond to the treatment, and the school contacts her mother to come pick her up from school. This means another visit to the emergency department for treatment.

Carrie does not like to miss school or to worry her mother. Her mother wishes there were some way to reduce the number and severity of her asthma attacks.

What are some possible triggers of Carrie's asthma attacks at school? What measures can be taken to control her asthma on a daily basis and reduce the number of attacks? What special arrangements are needed to permit a child to receive care for asthma or another chronic condition while at school? What education does the teacher need to make an assessment and decision for Carrie to go to get her treatment?

CHILDCARE SETTINGS

Many young children are cared for in childcare settings while parents are at work. Many types of childcare arrangements exist, such as in-home care by a family member or nanny, a licensed childcare family home setting for up to five children, or a licensed childcare center for six or more children. States establish minimum licensure requirements and guidelines for the safe operation of childcare settings that address the staff qualifications, staff-child ratio, staff training requirements, safe food handling, safe health practices, and environmental safety. Guidelines for the safe operation of childcare centers are available through the National Resource Center for Health and Safety in Child Care.

Role of the Nurse in Childcare Settings

Nurses can assume an important consultant role in the establishment of the childcare center's policies for health practices, teaching staff about safe health practices, and monitoring and promoting health practices in the setting. The nurse consultant can also teach staff to identify children with illnesses and to provide first aid for injured children. In some cases, especially in childcare centers for ill children, nurses provide health screening and direct care to children (Evers, 2002).

Reducing Disease Transmission. Children are close together in large numbers, put things in their mouths, may be contagious before symptoms occur, and are susceptible to most infectious agents. The nurse can educate and work with the childcare center manager and staff to reduce disease transmission in the following ways:

- Developing guidelines for review of immunizations and plans for exclusion of unimmunized children when a vaccine-preventable disease occurs in the facility (see "Immunization Information" in Chapter 45 for further information ∞)
- Checking each child daily for signs and symptoms of illness (e.g., behavior changes, rashes, fever, vomiting, diarrhea, and eye drainage) and developing guidelines for the exclusion and return of children with different infectious conditions
- Teaching staff when and how to handwash, manage secretions, sanitize toys and surfaces, and manage cuts and scrapes
- Developing guidelines for diapering infants and toddlers
- Caring for the sick child and reducing exposure to others until the child is picked up by the parents

Health Promotion and Health Maintenance. Health promotion activities are those that further the child's highest level of functioning and development, such as having activities that stimulate physical development, nutrition that fosters growth

MediaLink ► National Resource Center for Health and Safety in Child Care

EVIDENCE-BASED NURSING

INJURY PREVENTION IN CHILDCARE SETTINGS

Clinical Question

What are the most common injuries that occur in childcare settings and how do the types of injuries vary by the age of the child?

Evidence

Injury data were collected for a full year from incident reports about the types of injuries occurring to children in two urban childcare centers. A total of 131 children between 6 weeks and 7 years of age (mean age of 24 months) were enrolled full- or part-time in the centers. During the year, a total of 897 incident reports identified 1023 injuries. The distribution of injuries was as follows: bites (39%), falls (23%), bumps and bruises (22%), and scratches, cuts, blisters, and fracture (16%). Only two children required medical attention. The remainder received first aid on site. Infants and toddlers (0 to 36 months of age) had the highest frequency of injury, reflecting in large part the high frequency of biting reported in this age group. Approximately 60% of all injuries occurred in the morning hours (Waibel & Misra, 2003).

Implications

Understanding the type of injuries that happen in childcare centers, the age group most affected, and other information, such as time of day,

provides the nurse with important information to help the childcare center to promote the health of enrolled children and make efforts to reduce injuries. Injury prevention strategies can potentially be developed based upon collected data. The number of minor injuries in childcare centers illustrates the importance of having childcare center staff who are trained in first aid. It is also important to have guidelines for management of injuries and notification of parents when injuries happen.

Critical Thinking

Consider the distribution of injuries and identify potential strategies that could be used to reduce the number of biting and fall incidents. What actions could the childcare center workers take to reduce the number of incidents that occur during morning hours? Outline the first aid guidelines that a childcare center should have in place to manage each of the most common injuries reported. What guidelines should exist for notifying parents about injuries that occur?

Reference

Waibel, R., & Misra, R. (2003). Injuries to preschool children and infection control practices in childcare programs. *Journal of School Health, 73*(4), 167–172.

and ability to perform at maximum level, and a well-rounded program that considers all types of development, from fine and gross motor, to language, emotional growth, cognition, and social skills. Nurses can design and offer health education programs for the children (toothbrushing, handwashing, and blowing the nose into a tissue) to promote healthy habits. Health maintenance activities are those that prevent injury or disease, such as immunization monitoring, infection control, and practices like putting infants on their back to sleep. See "Sudden Infant Death Syndrome" in Chapter 47 for additional information. ∞

Environmental Safety. The nurse should inspect the childcare environment to identify hazards that could cause injury to the children. Cleaning supplies and other toxins must be stored in a locked cabinet to prevent children from exposure. Inspect toys used by children to ensure that there are no sharp edges or points, small parts, or pinching parts. Playground equipment should also be checked for safety (Figure 39–4 ●).

Emergency Care Planning. The nurse can help the childcare administrator develop a guideline to assess and identify the child with an emergency health condition and to develop an emergency care plan for instances when a child becomes acutely ill or injured. This plan should include the following elements: giving first aid, calling emergency medical services to transport the child to the emergency department, notifying the parent about the child's condition, and accompanying the child to the emergency department until the parent arrives.

HOME HEALTHCARE SETTING

Home healthcare is a component of the continuum of comprehensive healthcare provided to children and families in their home. Children with episodic or long-term health conditions can benefit from home health services. Only a small number of these children have conditions serious enough to need continuous (daily, up to 24 hours a day) private duty care in the home. Most children receive intermittent skilled nursing visits to assess the child to see how family members are managing the child's healthcare needs. Intermittent home healthcare services (one to several visits a week) may be provided to help families during the child's acute recovery, such as a child receiving home antibiotic infusion therapy.

Many children needing home healthcare are medically fragile, dependent upon a medical device for survival or prevention of further disability. Parents and other care providers without backgrounds in healthcare are given tremendous responsibilities to provide technology-assisted healthcare to their child. Technology-assisted care in the home may include any of the following: ventilators; tracheostomies; suctioning; nasogastric, gastrostomy, or parenteral feeding with feeding pumps; and intravenous fluids and medications with intravenous pumps. In some cases, families have created mini-intensive care units in their home. Examples of some serious chronic conditions cared for by families in the home include children with congenital heart defects before corrective surgery, bronchopulmonary dysplasia, and cancer in its terminal stage. The home envi-

● **FIGURE 39-4**

Assess the childcare center's environment for safety hazards. Check the area around playground equipment, making sure there are wood chips or cushioned tiles under the equipment. Inspect the playground equipment for protruding screws, loose nuts and bolts, and instability at least monthly.

- Knowledge and experience in acute care practice with various medical technologies used with children. These skills enable nurses to provide direct care, teach the family and child self-care practices, and monitor the child's progress.

- Community assessment skills; an understanding of community resources, financing mechanisms, and multiagency collaboration; and good communication skills.

- An understanding of the community's health resources to better assist families to find the most supportive services to match the child's and family's needs.

- An understanding of the community's cultural diversity and the cultural values of the families served.

- Skill in educating family members to assume care of the child.

Nurses in the home care setting use the nursing process to assess child, family, and home environment. Then the nurse assists the family to manage care of a child with a chronic condition more independently while promoting the child's growth and development. A major goal of working with families in the home care setting includes promoting or restoring the child's health while attempting to minimize the effects of the disability and illness, including terminal illness (Figure 39–5 ●).

Assessment of the Home Care Environment. Assessment of the home is focused on the safety of the environment for the

● **FIGURE 39-5**

ronment is believed to be optimal for the long-term care of these children so they can participate as part of the family and have their growth and development promoted. The family gains some control over their lives by having the child in the home versus coordinating visits to the child and trying to maintain family (Balinsky & Marié, 2001).

Health insurers pay many of the costs associated with home care; however, the family pays some costs out-of-pocket, such as medications, supplies, and transportation, causing a financial burden. In some cases a parent must give up employment to provide care to the child. Healthcare systems (healthcare providers and insurers) are challenged to simultaneously address the child's illness and developmental needs while providing the support needed by these families so that children do well in their home environments. The family also needs help to support the growing child in the school and other peer settings.

Role of the Nurse in Home Healthcare

Nurses need a variety of skills and knowledge to work in the home care setting, including the following:

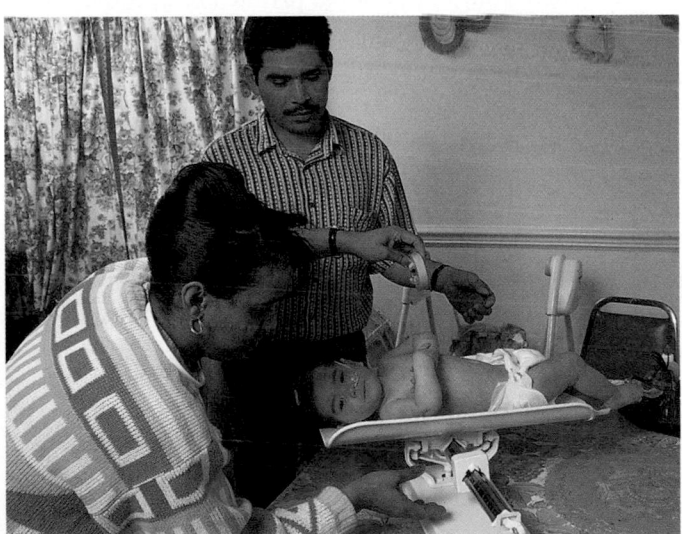

Nurses provide both short-term and long-term services to families in the home setting. In some cases, families need support for a short time after the child is discharged from the hospital following an acute illness. In other cases, families need assistance with complex nursing care for the child dependent on technology for survival.

child and the resources needed for the child's care such as the following:

- Home readiness (safe sleeping arrangements, adequate supplies, ability to meet nutritional and fluid needs, telephone access, heat, electricity, refrigeration, and lack of any communicable diseases in the home).

- Potential hazards related to the child's age, condition, and requirements for technology-assisted care (extension cords that are needed to reach electrical outlets could trip and injure family members).

- Features in the home environment that could cause an acute illness, such as use of a woodstove or fireplace for heating that could cause respiratory distress, or renovation of a house built before 1960 that could expose the child to lead dust. Additionally the nurse may identify family members who smoke.

Assessment of Family Abilities to Provide Needed Care. The parents and other family members in the home are assessed for parenting skills and the ability to provide care needed by the child and to monitor the child's health status. Family strengths and coping abilities are evaluated using the family assessment guidelines on page 1129. The presence of siblings, their developmental and physical status, and their needs should also be assessed.

Partnership with the Family. Control belongs to the family in the home care setting. The parents are the nurse's employer, so every interaction is negotiated with the family, or between the family and child if there are differences in what they want. The nurse must be flexible and able to set aside power. House rules for such things as parking, private areas in the home, routines, and discipline of the child must all be followed. Role expectations of the nurse must be clearly understood to reduce stress in the family. The success of home care is also based upon effective cultural communication as described in "Developing Cultural Competence."

DEVELOPING CULTURAL COMPETENCE

FAMILY PERSPECTIVE OF HEALTH AND DISEASE

When providing care in the home, recognize potential conflicts between "mainstream" medical care and the family's cultural preferences after carefully listening to the parents' perspectives. Learn and use the family's perspectives of health and disease in discussions and in development of the plan of care (Ahmann, 1996).

Informed consent is needed for invasive treatments and decisions for provision of emergency care to avoid serious risk for life and limb. When the family caregiver is not present and the home care nurse provides such care, the

home health agency and the nurse are at significant liability risk (Hogue, 1993).

Nursing Management Focus. Nurses help families in the home setting in the following ways:

- Assuring competent care to the child

- Educating them about the child's condition and physical signs and symptoms that may indicate a change in health status

- Educating them and demonstrating methods to promote the child's development

- Linking them to community resources, including support groups, respite care, and therapeutic recreation

- Assisting families in time management skills and patient care management

- Advocating for increased insurance coverage or locating other sources of financial assistance

The range of nursing care activities that may be included in a child's care plan in the home setting include sensory stimulation, routines of daily living, positioning and skin care with gentle handling, respiratory care, nutrition and elimination, medications, and other supportive therapies. Other providers, such as physical therapists, speech-language therapists, occupational therapists, and social workers, may provide other healthcare services in collaboration with the home health nurse. See "Teaching Highlights" for information to help families develop a plan for safe evacuation of the home in case of fire.

Emergency Preparedness. The nurse should work with the family to develop an emergency care plan for any child whose condition could worsen rapidly and become life threatening, such as serious congenital heart defects, tracheostomies, and apnea. Elements of the plan should include the following:

- When to call 911 or the local emergency number.

- Notifying the local electricity service providers when a child requires technology assistance so the home is given high priority for resources during power outages.

- Notifying the local emergency medical services unit that a child with special needs is in the community, allowing the emergency medical technicians to visit before an emergency and become knowledgeable of the child's potential emergency care needs.

- Preparing a written emergency medical history that gives emergency healthcare providers enough basic information to understand the child's health condition, to prevent delays in disease-specific treatment, and to minimize unnecessary interventions until the child's personal physician can be consulted. A recommended Emergency Information Form is available through the American Academy of Pediatrics.

TEACHING HIGHLIGHTS

HAVING A FIRE ESCAPE PLAN

Developing a fire escape plan is important when the family has one or more children with special healthcare needs. Important steps to have families take in developing the plan include:

- Have working smoke detectors in the home and teach children what the alarm means.
- Draw a diagram of your house. Mark all windows and doors.
- Plan two routes out of every room.
- Think about an escape plan if the fire starts in the kitchen, bedroom, or basement.
- Figure out the best way to get infants and young children out of the house. Will you carry them? Is there more than one small child, and if so, how will you get them out if you are the only adult?
- Teach preschool and school-age children to follow the escape plan by crawling, touching doors, and going to the window if the door is hot. Show children how to cover their nose and mouth to reduce smoke inhalation.
- Prepare an alternate fire escape plan in case you are alone with the child when the fire begins.
- Keep home exits clear of toys and debris.
- Select a safe meeting place outside the home. Teach children not to go back inside the burning home.

DISASTER PREPAREDNESS

Many types of disasters occur each year in the United States. Natural disasters include floods, ice storms, hurricanes, earthquakes, tornados, and fires. Other types of disasters can occur when trains or trucks carrying toxic chemicals and nuclear waste crash or explode. Concerns of terrorism with infectious organisms, toxic chemicals, or radioactive agents have elevated the need for disaster and emergency preparedness. (See Chapter 45 for information about infectious agents used for bioterrorism. ∞) State agencies, hospitals, and emergency medical services systems collaborate in **disaster preparedness**, the development of community plans for mass casualty events involving natural disasters and man-made disasters. Efforts to ensure appropriate planning and availability of resources for children during disasters in all communities are ongoing through the funding and coordination of several federal agencies.

Children have special vulnerabilities during a disaster. Their developmental ability and cognitive levels may interfere with their ability to escape danger. They have unique psychologic vulnerabilities and need special plans for management. The impact of other disasters on the mental health of children is significant, such as the following:

- Fewer coping skills to help deal with the impact of witnessing injuries.

- Limited understanding due to cognitive level/abilities.
- Fear and anxiety is heightened with hoaxes, actual incidents, and the associated media coverage. Fear increases after a disaster has occurred, with the worry that it will happen again, that someone will be injured or killed, that they will be separated from their family, or that they will be left alone. Children may believe that repeated television broadcasts of mass casualty events are additional events.
- The disruption of normal life patterns (reliability, cohesion, and predictability) may be prolonged and causes stress.

See Table 39–3 for the developmental responses to disasters. See Chapter 36, "Societal and Environmental Influences on the Child," for more information about promoting coping skills and resilience in children to promote healthier responses in the times of disasters. ∞

Children are likely to have emergency needs different from adults due to their size and earlier stages of development. Because of their anatomy and physiology (thinner skin, increased body surface area, faster respiratory rate, and closer to the ground where heavier aerosol agents fall), they have different vulnerabilities in response to various terrorism agents (Cieslak & Henretig, 2003). Special developmental considerations with young children include the following:

- They are unable to flee or take evasive action to escape danger.
- Caregivers or parents may become incapacitated, and child care with mental health support will be needed.
- They are unable to follow the instructions given to adults regarding evacuation or safe actions.
- They cannot distinguish between reality and fantasy.
- Young children may fear emergency responders in protective suits and hoods.

Role of the Nurse in Disaster Preparedness

Pediatric nurses in schools and other community settings have a significant role in working with families in preparing for a disaster. They can help families use developmentally appropriate information to talk with their children about disaster planning and information about disasters when they occur. They can help the family develop a disaster plan. Families must prepare to manage on their own for at least 72 hours following a major disaster (unless the child needs special technology for life support) because it will take this long for nationally coordinated help and relief to arrive.

Nurses will be actively involved in caring for children injured during the disaster. Nurses can also help after the

TABLE 39–3 ❖ **Responses to Disasters by Children of Different Age Groups**

Age Group	Responses
Toddlers and preschoolers	Reaction reflects that of parents
	Regressive behaviors
	Decreased appetite
	Vomiting, constipation, diarrhea
	Sleep disorders (insomnia, nightmares)
	Tics, stuttering, muteness
	Clinging
	Re-enactment by play
	Irritability
	Post-traumatic stress disorder
School age	Fear, anxiety
	Increased hostility with siblings
	Somatic complaints
	Sleep disorders
	School problems
	Social withdrawal, apathy, decreased interest in peers, hobbies, school
	Re-enactment by play
	Post-traumatic stress disorder
Preadolescents	Increased hostility with siblings
	Somatic complaints
	Eating disorders
	Decreased interest in peers, hobbies, school
	Rebellion
	Refusal to do chores
	Interpersonal difficulties
	Post-traumatic stress disorder
Adolescents	Decreased interest in social activities, peers, hobbies, school
	Inability to experience pleasure
	Decline in responsible behaviors
	Rebellion, behavior problems, risk-taking behaviors
	Somatic complaints
	Sleep disorders
	Eating disorders
	Change in physical activity
	Confusion
	Lack of concentration

Adapted with permission from Aghababian, R. V. (1999). *Pediatric Disaster Life Support—PDLS.* Boston: University of Massachusetts Medical School.

disaster by assessing children for distress or post-traumatic stress disorder, and promoting security and stability (Ferguson, 2002).

THE CHILD WITH A CHRONIC CONDITION

Children with a **chronic condition**, a condition that at the time of diagnosis is expected to last 3 months or more, receive most of their healthcare in the community. Chronic conditions are often defined by diagnostic categories or by functional or social limitations. Examples of these categories include the following (Allen, 2004):

- Limitations in function that would typically be expected for the child's age and development
- Disfigurement
- Dependency on medications or a special diet for control of the condition
- Dependency on medical technology for functioning
- Need for more medical care and related services than typically used by a healthy child of the same age
- Special ongoing treatments at home or school

Some of these children have a **handicap** or **disability**, a limitation that interferes with the child's ability to fully participate in society which can be related to one of the following (Msall, Avery, Tremont et al., 2003):

- Medical impairment (chronic condition)
- Functional limitation (mobility, self-care, communication, or learning-behavior impairment)
- Difficulty maintaining a social role in school or play

See Figure 39–6 ● for children with visible and invisible disabilities. Some children who are medically fragile are **technology-assisted**, depending on a medical device that is required to sustain life (mechanical ventilators, intravenous nutrition or drugs, tracheostomy, suctioning, oxygen, or tube feedings). Other children depend on medical devices that compensate for vital body functions and require nursing care management such as renal dialysis, urinary catheters, and colostomies.

Many of these children require specialized healthcare. The term **children with special healthcare needs (CSHCN)** is applied to "those who have or are at risk for a chronic physical, developmental, behavioral, or emotional condition and who also require health and related services of a type or amount beyond that required by children generally" (McPherson, Arango, Fox et al., 1998). A national survey revealed that 12.8% (9.3 million) of children in the United States under the age of 18 years have special healthcare needs (Van Dyke, Kogan, McPherson et al., 2004). With improved healthcare and technology, approximately

● FIGURE 39–6

Children with chronic conditions may have a visible or nonvisible health condition, or nonvisible until an acute episode of their condition makes the condition visible. **A,** The child in a wheelchair has a visible disability. **B,** The child with a seizure may have no visible signs of the condition unless a seizure is witnessed.

A

B

90% of children with chronic conditions will reach their 20th birthday, and most of these survivors will live on into adulthood (Lindeke, Leonard, Presler et al., 2002).

The 12.8% of children with special healthcare needs consume an estimated 45% of all pediatric healthcare costs, demonstrating their need for increased health services (Allen, 2004). Efforts to reduce health costs have resulted in fewer hospitalizations and more care in the community. Families need considerable assistance for care coordination to ensure that their children have access to the needed care. See "Nursing Practice" for national health objectives in *Healthy People 2010* that are focused on the health status and healthcare delivery to these children.

NURSING PRACTICE

The *Healthy People 2010* objectives for children with special health-care needs include the following:

■ All CSHCN will receive regular ongoing comprehensive care within a medical home.
■ All families with CSHCN will have adequate private and/or public insurance to pay for the services they need.
■ Services for CSHCN and their families will be organized in ways that families can use them easily.
■ Families of CSHCN will participate in decision making at all levels and will be satisfied with the services they receive.

Courtesy of the U.S. Department of Health and Human Services. (2000). Healthy People 2010 *(2nd ed.). Washington, DC: U.S. Government Printing Office.* http://www.healthypeople.gov

---

ROLE OF THE NURSE

Nurses providing care to children with specific chronic conditions need the following knowledge and skills (Allen, 2004):

■ Knowledge of the pathophysiology of the chronic condition and anticipated disease trajectory
■ Knowledge of child and family reactions to the stress of the chronic condition
■ The ability to work with the family in their efforts to manage the child's normal growth and development
■ The ability to provide culturally sensitive care to the child and family experiencing a chronic health condition
■ Assessment skills to identify any changes in the child's condition requiring referral or consultation
■ The ability to communicate effectively with appropriate health professionals regarding any changes in the child's physical or psychosocial health
■ The ability to work collaboratively with other health professionals
■ Knowledge of resources (community agencies, tertiary care centers, specialty professionals) appropriate for the child and family with a chronic condition
■ The ability to identify a dysfunctional family needing intervention

This knowledge and these skills make it possible for the nurse to provide the health promotion and health maintenance care as well as condition-specific care needed by the child and family. Family assessment provides information about the family's strengths, resilence, and coping mechanisms to help plan the nursing care provided. Nurses play a significant role in teaching the parents to manage the child's condition and provide care at home, providing guidelines to promote the child's growth and development, monitoring the child's health status, supporting families during crisis episodes, and referring the family to appropriate community services. For example, the recommended care of children with asthma has changed from episodic care for acute asthma attacks with minimal daily management to guidelines for aggressive daily management by the child and family. Recognition of early warning signs of an asthma attack can lead to the initiation of extra medications in an effort to avert a severe attack. (See Chapter 47 for a discussion of asthma management. ∞) Refer to "Nursing Care Plan: The Child with Asthma in the Community Setting" for strategies that can be used when working with the child and family to improve asthma management.

Care Coordination

Care coordination involves promoting timely access to services, providing continuity of care, and enhancing the family's well-being (Lindeke et al., 2002). The nurse partners with the family and healthcare team to coordinate care and services to meet the individualized needs of the child and family. It also involves matching the family's needs for services based upon assessment findings. The goals of care coordination include (American Academy of Pediatrics, 1999):

- Gaining access to and integrating services and resources on behalf of the child.
- Linking service systems with the family.
- Preventing duplication of services and unnecessary cost.
- Advocating for improved individual outcomes.

Because numerous healthcare providers and healthcare agencies are often involved in the care of the child with a chronic illness or an injury requiring long-term care, coordination of health services is important to prevent gaps and overlaps. The nurse may work as a **case manager** to help the family with care coordination. The role includes coordinating the healthcare team, determining family needs, identifying resources, and arranging for healthcare needs.

Once management goals are set by the multidisciplinary team, the case manager collaborates with the family to assist in decision making about which healthcare provider or agency is responsible for assisting the child to meet each goal. An important role is helping the family to determine cost-effective strategies to meet healthcare goals in order to prevent the child from reaching the cap on health insurance benefits for as long as possible. The case manager sup-

ports the parents in taking an active role in the treatment planning and decision-making process in preparation for becoming the child's care coordinator.

COMMUNITY SITES OF CARE

Most children with chronic conditions are cared for in the home without home nursing or other health services. The healthcare provider for children with chronic conditions varies by the type of condition, type of health insurance coverage, preferences of the family, and availability of pediatric specialty resources.

Office or Health Center

A healthcare home or medical home for these children is especially important as children with chronic conditions need regular preventive healthcare just as healthy children do. Health promotion, disease prevention, and anticipatory guidance have greater significance for the child with special healthcare needs. This child already has a condition that places him or her at higher risk for additional problems, such as infectious diseases, injury, or developmental delay. Information about community resources that may help the child and family is usually more extensive when the child's healthcare home is in the local community. The goal is for the child to have as normal a childhood as possible.

Specialty Referral Centers

The child with a chronic condition is often referred to pediatric specialists, as needed, for a review of the management of the child's health condition, and to make new recommendations according to the child's health status. These specialists are often based in hospital outpatient or specialty health centers. The pediatric specialist and advanced practice nurses may collaborate with the child's primary care provider to coordinate care for the child with chronic conditions such as spina bifida, cystic fibrosis, or diabetes mellitus. In this manner, the child benefits from the most current healthcare guidelines and expertise in care for the specific condition (Figure 39–7 ●).

The child and family usually retain a primary care provider, who provides health supervision care and episodic illness care while serving as the child's advocate in the larger healthcare system. Sometimes a pediatric specialist serves as the child's primary care provider, but it is important to make sure regular health supervision services are not forgotten during the care of acute exacerbations of the chronic condition. Some children with chronic conditions may even require additional health supervision visits for added immunizations, such as meningococcal and influenza vaccines.

Nurses working in hospital specialty clinics and other community settings can help ensure that these children re-

NURSING CARE PLAN

THE CHILD WITH ASTHMA IN THE COMMUNITY SETTING

Intervention	Rationale	Expected Outcome

1. Nursing Diagnosis: Family Coping: Readiness for Enhanced related to increased control of asthma with daily therapeutic care

Intervention	Rationale	Expected Outcome
NIC Priority Intervention: **Normalization promotion:** Assisting parents and other family members of children with chronic illnesses or disabilities in providing normal life experiences for their children and families		**NOC Suggested Outcome:** **Information processing:** Family gains the ability to acquire, organize, and use information to manage stressors and provide more normal life experiences

Goal: The child and parents will work in partnership with the nurse to improve the child's asthma management.

Intervention	Rationale	Expected Outcome
■ Listen to the family's concerns about asthma management and respond with information to correct any misconceptions. ■ Teach the family skills (assessment, use of equipment, and giving medications) for managing the child's asthma episodes. ■ Provide telephone consultation to the parents during management of the first few asthma episodes. ■ Educate the parents about when to call for future medical advice or to seek emergency treatment.	■ The parents' concerns may not be the same as the nurse's. If the parents' concerns are not addressed, the parents may not comply with recommended care. ■ Proper use of equipment and appropriate medication dosage will help alleviate asthma symptoms. ■ Support and reinforcement of learning during an asthma episode will increase the parents' confidence in managing future episodes. ■ Parents need guidelines for judging the severity of asthma episodes.	The parents express greater confidence in averting and managing their child's asthma episodes.

2. Nursing Diagnosis: Knowledge Deficit (asthma management) related to lack of exposure to new treatment regimen

Intervention	Rationale	Expected Outcome
NIC Priority Intervention: **Teaching, procedure/treatment:** Preparing a patient to understand and mentally prepare for a prescribed procedure and treatment		**NOC Suggested Outcome:** **Knowledge:** Extent of understanding conveyed about daily asthma treatment regimen

Goal: The child and family will begin daily medication management of asthma.

Intervention	Rationale	Expected Outcome
■ Teach the child and parents the importance of daily medications for asthma management.	■ Daily controller medications reduce the inflammation that is the underlying cause of asthma episodes.	The number of asthma episodes is reduced.

Goal: The child and parents will recognize early signs of an asthma episode and begin taking medications.

Intervention	Rationale	Expected Outcome
■ Teach the child and parents to use a peak flow meter. ■ Help the child recognize his or her personal best peak flow and range indicating development of asthma symptoms. ■ Teach the family and child to give medications when the peak flow falls to the yellow range. ■ Teach the child and family to monitor the child's response to medications with the peak flow meter.	■ The peak flow meter helps quantify changes in respiratory status before symptoms are detected. ■ Identifying a personal best peak flow helps establish the ranges to be used for future symptom identification. ■ Giving medications before an asthma episode becomes established may help avert the actual episode. ■ Monitoring the response gives the family information to determine when home care is inadequate and medical intervention is needed.	The number of asthma episodes requiring emergency department intervention is reduced.

(continued)

NURSING CARE PLAN—continued

THE CHILD WITH ASTHMA IN THE COMMUNITY SETTING

Intervention	Rationale	Expected Outcome
3. Nursing Diagnosis: Ineffective Health Maintenance related to lack of school asthma management plan		
NIC Priority Intervention: **Health system guidance:** Facilitating a patient's location and use of appropriate health services		**NOC Suggested Outcome:** **Health-promoting behavior:** Actions to sustain or promote optimal wellness
Goal: An individualized health plan (IHP) will be developed to help control and manage the child's asthma symptoms.		
■ Ensure that the family has the physician order for the child's asthma management at school. ■ Provide the family with educational materials to give to the school nurse and school administrators. ■ Advocate for all children to have an asthma management plan developed. ■ Support the family to have a customized IHP that matches the physician's written orders. Provide support for the child with beginning asthma symptoms to get medications early. ■ Include in the IHP participation in regular school/class activities such as field trips and physical education, and what to do if asthma symptoms occur at school. ■ Help the family to obtain extra equipment and medications that can be provided to the school. ■ Work with the parents and school nurse to teach the specific asthma interventions to a designated person in the school nurse's absence.	■ School personnel need the child's physician orders to provide medications during the school day. ■ School personnel need the latest information about effective asthma management in school settings. ■ Establishing a school policy will help all children with asthma receive appropriate care. ■ The child with severe asthma needs a personalized care plan to be most successful in controlling asthma episodes. ■ Participation, even with modification or premedication prior to activities, promotes self-esteem and peer relationships. ■ Schools will provide care, but the families must provide all supplies, equipment, and medications. ■ School nurses often travel between several schools. The school administrator or secretary often serves as the backup care provider.	Implementation of the IHP reduces the number of school absences for asthma episodes that occur during school hours and increases participation in school activities.
4. Nursing Diagnosis: Situational Low Self-Esteem (Child) related to need to seek special care during school hours		
NIC Priority Intervention: **Self-esteem enhancement:** Assisting a patient to increase his/her personal judgment of self-worth		**NOC Suggested Outcome:** **Self-esteem:** Personal judgment of self-worth
Goal: The child's improved control over asthma will increase his or her self-esteem and peer relationships.		
■ Assess the child's peer relationships and opportunities for age-appropriate interactions. ■ Motivate the child and family to gain increased control of asthma so the child can participate in normal childhood activities. ■ Identify types of conflict and teasing the child experiences with peers, and teach the child defense tactics to deal with them.	■ Assessment is important to identify the best strategies to support the child and family. ■ Motivation may increase compliance with recommended daily asthma control interventions. ■ If the child is able to gain some control over these situations, his or her self-esteem will be improved.	The child establishes friendships and engages in activities with peers.

● FIGURE 39–7

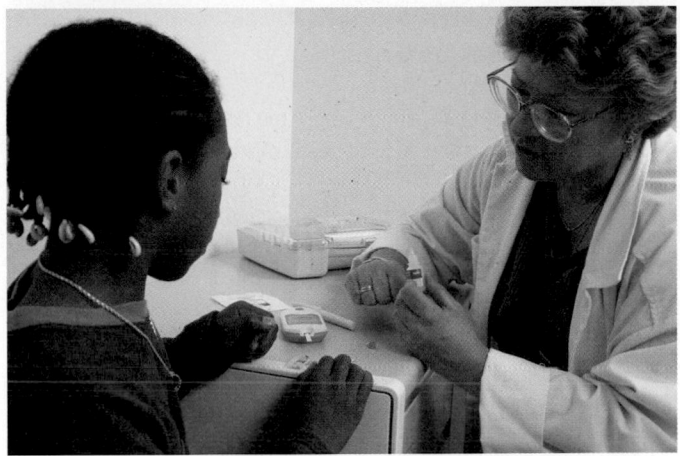

Nurses often assume a larger role in working with children and families with a chronic health condition in the hospital ambulatory setting. Developing a care plan and educating the family to manage diabetes type 1 is an important role of this pediatric nurse, who is also a certified diabetes educator.

ceive the appropriate health promotion services. The nurse in a tertiary care facility needs to identify appropriate resources and to help the family connect with local community resources. This is a greater challenge if the child and family have traveled a distance to obtain the specialty services. It is often best to make sure the child has a primary care provider in the home community to provide regular care and to help coordinate local community resources.

Schools

Many children with chronic conditions have school activity limitations that can range from inability to attend school, to receiving or needing special education services, to limited school attendance. The majority of children with a functional disability need special education services (Msall et al., 2003). Chronic health impairments by themselves or in combination with other functional disabilities also cause school activity limitations.

All children, including those with chronic conditions and special healthcare needs, are entitled to a free education that is matched to their developmental and functional capabilities by federal law. The age range for educational services includes infants and toddlers, with the hope that early intervention in provision of educational services will lower the total cost of educational services for these children. Provisions for transitional planning for adult living, including vocational training and independent living, are also included in the Individuals with Disabilities Education Act. See "Nursing Practice" for federal laws that provide assurances for educational services.

Attending school is an important transition for children with special healthcare needs and their families. Send-

NURSING PRACTICE

FEDERAL LAWS FOR PROVIDING EDUCATION SERVICES FOR CHILDREN WITH SPECIAL HEALTHCARE NEEDS

- Rehabilitation Act, Public Law (PL) 93–112 of 1973 prohibited discrimination against people with a disability. Section 504 specifies that each student who has a disability is entitled to accommodations needed to attend school and participate as fully as possible in school activities (Betz, 2001).
- The Education for All Handicapped Children Act, Public Law (PL) 94–142 of 1975, mandated that all children, even those with handicaps, be provided with public education and related services.
- Education for All Handicapped Children Amendments, PL 99–457 of 1986, expanded the scope of PL 94–142 to include appropriate services for infants and toddlers with disabilities and their families.
- Individuals with Disabilities Education Act (IDEA), PL 105–17 of 1997, ensures that all children with disabilities have available to them a free appropriate public education that emphasizes special education and related services designed to meet their unique needs and prepare them for employment and independent living. Every child with a disability must have a written individualized education plan, and parents have the right to question placement decisions and to due process when settling differences.

ing the child to school has several benefits for the child and family. Children have an opportunity for socialization with children and adults beyond the immediate family. Parents gain a sense of normalization as the child attends school like all other children. Parents also benefit by some respite from the child's care during the school day (Rehm & Rohr, 2002).

Educational System Planning. Careful planning is needed when a child with special needs attends school or receives other education services. Many children have chronic medical conditions that require management during the day in the school environment, such as asthma, diabetes, and attention deficit disorder. Some children just need medications administered regularly or episodically. Other children need more extensive interventions integrated into the school day, such as blood glucose monitoring or intermittent self-catheterization. The education system is obligated to provide reasonable accommodations to ensure that the child's medical needs are met during the school day. The education system's obligation is negotiated with the family in formalized plans.

- An **individualized family service plan (IFSP)** is developed for the early intervention process for infants with special healthcare needs and/or developmental delays and their families. The IFSP contains information about the services required to support a child's development and enhance the family's capacity to facilitate the child's development. The family and education service providers work as a team to plan, implement, and evaluate services specific to the family's unique concerns, priorities, and resources.

- An **individualized education plan (IEP)** is developed for a child with cognitive, motor, social, and communication impairments who needs special education services. The IEP is jointly planned with the school administrator, teacher, parents, and other special support professionals as appropriate for the child's condition. The child is also included in the process when possible. The plan is developed after an assessment of the child's abilities and specific functional limitations.

- An **individualized health plan (IHP)** is developed for the child with medical conditions that need to be managed within the school setting. An IHP may be developed simultaneously with the IEP for the child with a health problem and a coexisting functional impairment. Some children need only an IHP for management of their chronic medical condition at school, such as daily medication administration or for glucose monitoring and insulin injection. A physician order is required for medication administration and special treatments. Learning may be challenged when the child has frequent acute illness episodes that result in missed days of school, and the IHP often integrates methods to prevent the child from being penalized for those absences.

- An **individualized transition plan (ITP)** is included in the development of an IEP for each child with a chronic disability who is 14 years or older. The ITP focuses on assisting the individual to receive vocational training and in moving successfully from the home into other community living settings as they grow older.

Parents have an important role in advocating for their child to ensure that the child receives the most appropriate educational services. School systems must provide a full range of educational services for the children with special healthcare needs, including services that support cognitive development, self-care skills, mobility, improved communication, and social skills (Figure 39–8 ●). Because each child's severity and combination of impairments is unique, identifying and matching the specific services for each child requires discussion and negotiation. Parents should make an effort to learn about the different types of educational services that address a child's specific disability in preparation for the IEP meeting. In this way, the parents are better prepared to participate in the educational planning and development of their child's IEP. (See "Nursing Practice" for the elements of an IEP.)

NURSING PRACTICE

The elements of an IEP are the following:
- Student's name
- Date of meeting to develop or review the IEP
- Statement of transition service needs of student beginning at age 14 years
- Present level of assessments and education performance, including how the child's disability affects the child's involvement and progress in a general curriculum or participation in appropriate activities
- Measurable annual goals that include benchmarks or short-term objectives in meeting the child's needs that enable the child to be involved in or progress in the general curriculum or participate in appropriate activities
- Special education and related services, supplementary aids and services, and program modifications or supports for school personnel needed to enable the child to make advancements toward attaining annual goals
- Explanation to the extent that the child will or will not participate with nondisabled children
- Any specific modification in the administration of state or districtwide assessments of achievement that are needed for the child to participate in the assessment, or reasons for excluding the child from assessment of achievement
- How the child's progress toward annual goals will be measured
- How the child's parents will be regularly informed of the child's progress toward annual goals and the extent to which the child's progress is sufficient to meet goals by the end of the year

Data from the U.S. Department of Education. (2004). A guide to the individualized education program. Retrieved October 14, 2004, from http://www.ed.gov/parents/needs/speced/iepguide/index.htm

● **FIGURE 39–8**

Because some children need medications or other therapies during school hours, the parents and child, school nurse, teacher, and school administrators develop a plan to manage the child's condition during school hours. This document is the child's individual school health plan.

The Child's Response to Entering School. Children with chronic conditions, whether they cause minimal interference in the child's daily life or are dependent upon technology, face certain challenges in the school setting. School-age children with special healthcare needs may for the first time recognize differences between themselves and other children, such as appearance, abilities, social skills, or special treatment needs. They also may experience social stigma for the first time, experience teasing, or have difficulties forming friendships (Melnyk, Feinstein, Moldenhouer et al., 2001). Some children, particularly adolescents, may attempt to hide their condition or fail to adhere to necessary recommendations, such as dietary restrictions, in order to appear like their peers.

Education for Children Who Are Medically Fragile. Children who are medically fragile or technology-assisted are also entitled to education services in the school setting. The child's need for skilled supportive nursing care must be carefully considered by the parents and the school system. Parents are often anxious about how well the child will be cared for by others during the school day. Risks for the child in the school setting include safety issues related to ventilators, tracheostomy, and medication therapy, as well as exposure to infectious diseases.

The school administration must provide the personnel resources and equipment needed to ensure that care is consistently available. Modifications to the school setting for the child, such as wheelchair ramps or an elevator, may be needed. Sometimes the child is placed in a classroom with healthy children, and the teacher is expected to monitor and provide care as needed. Health aides may be assigned to provide care for one or more children with school nurse supervision. Some children are placed in classes composed of children with special healthcare needs where health aides are more available to provide needed care.

Nurses play a key role in assisting the family to understand that a teacher's primary responsibility is to teach, not to provide healthcare. The teacher is responsible for the health and safety of all children in the classroom. Parents need to have realistic expectations about the level of skilled support services that can be provided in a classroom. Teachers and education leaders are often challenged to meet the obligations for the child's special education services in balance with the needs of all other children in the classroom.

Home schooling is an option for these children with resources provided through the school system. Home schooling may be used full time or for periods when the child is too ill to attend school. Home schooling provides education continuity when the child cannot attend school, and it reduces the child's stress and fatigue. However, the child loses the opportunity for peer and social interaction.

Transition to Adulthood. Adolescents with chronic conditions that may affect the future ability to work and live independently should have customized transition planning in preparation for adulthood and self-determination. An ITP is developed through the IEP process, using a multidisciplinary approach in collaboration with the family to assist in identifying appropriate support programs, living arrangements, and employment (Beckman, 2002). Transition planning needs to focus on the following areas (American Academy of Pediatrics, 2000):

- Identifying and transitioning the adolescent or young adult to adult-oriented healthcare services
- Identifying and selecting an alternative living arrangement so the child can leave home and live in the community
- Helping the adolescent learn work skills and apply them in the workplace in preparation for leaving the school environment

Healthy Ready to Work services may be particularly helpful to adolescents and families in planning for the transition to adulthood.

Home

Many families become the primary caregiver for the child that is medically fragile, taking responsibility in spite of the level of skill and complexity involved in that care. The family faces numerous challenges for home care, including modification of the home. Management of the condition involves technologic support, medications, and treatment regimens, all potential necessities to maintain the child in the home. Family members must decide who has responsibility for different aspects of the child's care.

While health plans claim that home care of these children costs less, families assume responsibility for many out-of-pocket expenses, such as supplies and frequent visits to healthcare providers. Many question the true financial savings since many families of children who are medically fragile report limited access to healthcare services and limited insurance to meet their child's needs (Newacheck, McManus, Fox et al., 2000). Many families give up employment income when one parent stays home to care for the child. Home health nursing care may be needed if both parents continue to work or to cover the night shift so parents can sleep. Because of the burden of care, parent caregivers may experience depression, social isolation, poor physical health, and high degrees of stress associated with caring for the medically fragile child.

Moving the child who is chronically ill or the technology-assisted child to the home setting is a life-changing decision for the family, and it must be done with collaboration between the family and the healthcare team. Preparation for the transition of the child with a chronic condition or technology assistance to the home requires that the family receive extensive training and instructions on the care of the child. This transition is often challenging and intimidating for the family who now must assume the role of independent caregiver. Family members often feel unprepared to handle the complex situation of the chronic condition and technologic supports. The family may be assuming care of a child who has been hospitalized for months or even years before being discharged home (Harrigan, Ratliffe, Patrinos et al., 2002). The family needs to be highly motivated and possess the strength and resiliency factors to overcome the obstacles that will arise in order to be successful in assuming management responsibility for the child's care (Figure 39–9 ⬤).

Respite care is an important support service to help families keep the child with a chronic condition in the home. Respite care and other support services (home health services and parent support groups) may also reduce the risk of abuse. Many states have passed legislation for in-home family support services that include respite care. Because many respite services charge for their assistance, the family may require help in identifying respite waiver subsidies available to them. Reliable child care and enrollment in school are other mechanisms for families to obtain respite care.

Emergency Preparedness

Emergency preparedness, or advance planning, is needed to ensure that medically fragile children who need technology for survival or have the potential for a life-threatening episode have the resources needed in the event of a disaster. The designated shelter—with health professionals and elec-

⬤ **FIGURE 39–9**

Daily caregiving demands of the child who is medically fragile continue 24 hours a day, 7 days a week. Parents need to identify ways to share the care of the child and other family care management. When the child lives with a single parent, additional healthcare resources are needed so the parent can sleep.

trical power for the needed equipment—for such children should be identified and known to the family. In the meantime, battery packs for power backup should be available at all times. Additionally, parents need to arrange for durable power of attorney so that consent for emergency medical care can be available as needed. The child and parents may become separated during the disaster, or the parents may become injured and unable to care for the child.

Critical Concept Review

LEARNING OBJECTIVES

CONCEPTS

List the categories of family strengths that help families cope with stressors.

1. Individual or family traits:
   - Optimism or resilience.
2. Individual or family assets:
   - Finances.
3. Individual or family capabilities, skills, or competencies:
   - Problem solving.

Describe the advantages of using a family assessment tool.

Family assessment tools can be used to collect information about:
1. The family's functioning.
2. The way it nurtures its members.
3. Problem solving and communication.
4. Strategies that are potentially more effective for management of the child's healthcare.

LEARNING OBJECTIVES

CONCEPTS

List the variety of community healthcare settings where nurses provide health services to children.	1. Childcare centers. 2. Schools. 3. Camps. 4. Physician's office. 5. Hospital out patient clinic. 6. Public health clinic. 7. Homeless shelters. 8. The home.
Describe the role of the nurse in each identified healthcare setting.	1. Nurses in childcare centers, schools, and camps triage emergent problems, maintain immunization records of each child, perform regular vision and hearing screenings, and refer children for other therapies. 2. Nurses in a physician's office perform routine growth and development screenings and administer immunizations. 3. Nurses in hospital out-patient clinics care for children with acute illnesses and arrange referrals for other community services. 4. Nurses in public health clinics administer growth and development assessments as well as necessary immunizations. 5. Nurses in homeless shelters assess children for developmental level, determine immunization status, and assist in arranging community services. 6. Nurses in the home assess the environment and coordinate and assist families to plan care for chronically ill children.
Describe the responses of children to disasters by developmental stage.	1. Toddler and preschooler: Regressive behaviors. Difficulty separating from parents. Eating and sleeping difficulties. 2. School-age: Generalized fear and anxiety. Difficulties with school, play, and sleep. 3. Preadolescents and adolescents: Interpersonal difficulties. Rebellious attitudes. Lack of concentration. Risk-taking behaviors.
Define the child with a chronic condition by categories of impairments.	1. Limitations in function that would typically be expected for the child's age and development. 2. Disfigurement. 3. Dependency on medications or a special diet for control of the condition. 4. Dependency on medical technology for functioning. 5. Need for more medical care and related services than typically used by a healthy child of the same age. 6. Special ongoing treatments at home or school.
List the skills and knowledge needed by the nurse to effectively care for the child with a chronic condition in the community.	1. Knowledge of the pathophysiology of the chronic condition and anticipated disease trajectory. 2. Knowledge of child and family reactions to the stress of the chronic condition. 3. The ability to work with the family in their efforts to manage the child's normal growth and development. 4. The ability to provide culturally sensitive care to the child and family experiencing a chronic health condition. 5. Assessment skills to identify any changes in the child's condition requiring referral or consultation. 6. The ability to communicate effectively with appropriate health professionals regarding any changes in the child's physical or psychosocial health. 7. The ability to work collaboratively with other health professionals. 8. Knowledge of resources (community agencies, tertiary care centers, specialty professionals) appropriate for the child and family with a chronic condition. 9. The ability to identify a dysfunctional family needing intervention.

(continued)

LEARNING OBJECTIVES

CONCEPTS

Describe nursing interventions to support the transition of a child with a chronic condition to school and adult living.

→

1. Assist family to understand the educational role of the teacher.
2. Educate teachers and staff about the unique needs of the child.
3. Provide instruction concerning medical equipment needed by the child.
4. Supervise the healthcare aides attending the child at school.
5. Identify adult-oriented healthcare services for the adolescent or young adult.
6. Assist the family to identify and select alternative living arrangements.
7. Provide referrals to agencies that can assist in the acquisition of workplace skills.

Discuss the family's role in care coordination.

→

1. Family decides who has responsibility for different aspects of the child's care.
2. Family assumes responsibility for many expenses of the child.
3. Family becomes the primary caregiver of the child.
4. Family may become the child's case manager.

CRITICAL THINKING IN ACTION

*View the **Critical Thinking in Action** video in Chapter 39 of the CD-ROM. Then, answer the questions that follow.*

Gavin is a 1-year-old coming into the clinic for his well-child check. The clinic is set up to see teen mothers and their babies for well-child visits and immunizations. Diane, his mother, has been bringing him there since he was born. Gavin qualifies for healthcare coverage through the Medicaid system in their state. He was born full term and has never been in the hospital or had surgery. Diane is still attending high school and plans to graduate this year. She and Gavin are living with her boyfriend's (Gavin's father) parents until they can raise enough money to live on their own. Gavin's father does not come to the well-baby visits. Gavin attends daycare while his mother is at school. He is up-to-date on immunizations so far and there is no significant family medical history, but there is smoking in the home. Gavin has been walking since he was 9 months old. He is able to point, wave, clap, and has 2 words. He is able to drink from a cup and put objects into a cup. He has been growing and thriving at an appropriate pace. Diane describes him as a good eater and tells you that he is currently on whole milk. He has soft stools daily and 5-6 wet diapers per day. He sleeps through the night and takes 2 naps per day. Diane describes him as an extremely active child and has worked on childproofing everything in the house.

1. What is the role of the nurse in caring for Gavin and his parents in the clinic?
2. What data does the nurse collect to perform a family assessment?
3. What strengths and stressors are likely to be present in this family?
4. What are the elements of a healthcare or medical home?

MEDIALINK   www.prenhall.com/london

■ NCLEX-RN® Review, case studies, and other interactive resources for this chapter can be found on the Companion Website at http://www.prenhall.com/london. Click on "Chapter 39" to select the activities for this chapter.

■ For animations, more NCLEX-RN® Review questions, and an audio glossary, access the accompanying CD-ROM in this textbook.

REFERENCES

Ahmann, E. (1996). *Home care for the high risk infant: A family centered approach* (2nd ed.). Gaithersburg, MD: Aspen.

Allen, P. J. (2004). The primary care provider and children with chronic conditions. In P. J. Allen & J. A. Vessey, *Primary care of the child with a chronic condition* (4th ed., pp. 3–22). St. Louis, MO: Mosby.

American Academy of Pediatrics. (2000). The role of the pediatrician in transitioning children and adolescents with developmental disabilities and chronic illness from school to work or college. *Pediatrics, 106*(4), 854–856.

American Academy of Pediatrics. (2002). The medical home. *Pediatrics, 110*(1), 184–186.

American Academy of Pediatrics Committee on Children with Disabilities. (1999). Care coordination: Integrating health and related systems of care for children with special health care needs. *Pediatrics, 104*, 978–981.

American Academy of Pediatrics Committee on Pediatric Emergency Medicine, Seidel, J. S., & Knapp, J. F. (Eds.). (2000). *Childhood emergencies in the office, hospital, and community: Organizing systems of care.* Elk Grove Village, IL: American Academy of Pediatrics.

Balinsky, W., & Marié, J. (2001, June). Pediatric home care: A cost benefit and cost effectiveness update. *Caring Magazine,* pp. 16–19.

Beckman, P. J. (2002). Providing family-centered services. In M. L. Batshaw (Ed.), *Children with disabilities* (5th ed., pp. 683–691). Baltimore: Paul H. Brookes.

Betz, C. L. (2001). Use of 504 plans for children and youth with disabilities: Nursing application. *Pediatric Nursing, 27*(4), 347–352.

Caldwell, B. M., & Bradley, R. H. (1984). *The Home Observation for Measurement of the Environment.* Little Rock: University of Arkansas.

Cieslak, T. J., & Henretig, F. M. (2003). Ring-a-ring a roses: Bioterrorism and its peculiar relevance to pediatrics. *Current Opinion in Pediatrics, 19,* 107–111.

Evers, D. B. (2002). The pediatric nurse's role as health consultant to a child care center. *Pediatric Nursing, 22*(3), 231–235.

Feeley, N., & Gottlieb, L. N. (2000). Nursing approaches to working with family strengths and resources. *Journal of Family Nursing, 6*(1), 9–24.

Ferguson, S. L. (2002). Preparing for disasters: Enhancing the role of pediatric nurses in wartime. *Journal of Pediatric Nurses, 17*(4), 307–308.

Harrigan, R. C., Ratliffe, C., Patrinos, M. E., & Alice, T. (2002). Medically fragile children: An integrative review of the literature and recommendations for future research. *Issues in Comprehensive Pediatric Nursing, 25*, 1–20.

Hogue, E. (1993). Care in the absence of primary caregivers. *Pediatric Nursing, 19*(1), 49–50.

Lindeke, L. L., Leonard, B. J., Presler, B., & Garwick, A. (2002). Family-centered care coordination for children with special needs across multiple settings. *Journal of Pediatric Health Care, 16*(6), 290–297.

McPherson, M., Arango, P., Fox, H., Lauver, C., McManus, M., Newacheck, P. W., et al. (1998). A new definition of children with special health care needs. *Pediatrics, 102*(1), 137–140.

Melnyk, B. M., Feinstein, N. F., Moldenhouer, Z., & Small, L. (2001). Coping in parents of children who are chronically ill: Strategies for assessment and intervention. *Pediatric Nursing, 27*(6), 548–558.

Moore, K. A., Chalk, R., Scarpa, J., & Vandivere, S. (2002). Family strengths: Often overlooked, but real. *Child Trends Research Brief.* Retrieved December 5, 2003, from http://www.childtrends.org

Msall, M. E., Avery, R. C., Tremont, M. R., Lima, J. C., Rogers, M. L., & Hogan, D. P. (2003). Functional disability and school activity limitations in 41,300 school children: Relationship to medical impairments. *Pediatrics, 111*(3), 548–553.

National Association of School Nurses and American Nurses Association. (2001). *Scope and standards of professional school nursing practice.* Silver Spring, MD: American Nurses Publishing.

Newacheck, P. A., McManus, M., Fox, H. B., Hung, Y. Y., & Halfon, N. (2000). Access to health care for children with special health care needs. *Pediatrics, 105*(4), 760–766.

Office of Technology Assessment. (1987). *Technology-dependent children: Hospital vs. home care. A technical memorandum.* Washington, DC: Congress of the United States.

Patterson, J. M. (1991). Family resilience to the challenge of a child's disability. *Pediatric Annals, 20*(9), 491–499.

Rehm, R. S., & Rohr, J. A. (2002). Parents', nurses', and educators' perceptions of risks and benefits of school attendance by children who are medically fragile/technology dependent. *Journal of Pediatric Nursing, 17*(5), 345–354.

Robinson, J. (2002). The changing role of the school nurse: A partner in infection control and disease prevention. *Journal of School Nursing, 18* (Suppl., October), 12–14.

U.S. Department of Health and Human Services. (2000). *Healthy People 2010* (2nd ed.). Washington, DC: U.S. Government Printing Office Retrieved December 28, 2004, from http://www.healthypeople.gov

Van Dyke, P. C., Kogan, M. D., McPherson, M., Weissman, G. R., & Newacheck, P. W. (2004). Prevalence and characteristics of children with special health care needs. *Archives of Pediatric and Adolescent Medicine, 158*(9), 884–890.

Waibel, R., & Misra, R. (2003) Injuries to preschool children and infection control practices in childcare programs. *Journal of School Health, 73*(4), 167–172.

40

Nursing Considerations for the Hospitalized Child

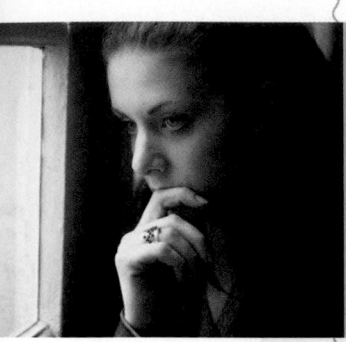

We live 50 miles from the hospital, and have three other children. We were worried about how we were going to be able to stay with Sabrina. She's only 4, and it's her first time in the hospital. Fortunately, they have beds for parents, so one of us can always be by her side throughout her procedure and recuperation.

—*Mother of Sabrina, age 4*

LEARNING OBJECTIVES

- Discuss the child's understanding of health and illness according to the child's psychosocial and developmental levels.

- Recognize the effect of hospitalization on the child and family.

- Assess the family's risk and protective factors that will influence adaptation to hospitalization.

- Identify several types of hospital units and the needs that children and families have in each unit.

- Identify methods that the child and family use to adapt to hospitalization.

- Describe types of therapeutic play and recreation used with hospitalized children.

- Use knowledge of child and family response to hospitalization to plan nursing interventions to facilitate coping with hospitalization.

MEDIALINK www.prenhall.com/london

CD-ROM

Video: Treatment Room
Skill 10-4: Performing a Venipuncture
Skill 11-1: Administering an Oral Medication
Skill 11-2: Administering an Intramuscular Injection
Skill 11-4: Administering an Intravenous Medication
Skill 11-12: Using a Metered Dose Inhaler (MDI)
NCLEX-RN® Review
Audio Glossary

Companion Website

NCLEX-RN® Review
MediaLink Applications:
    Communication Strategy: Preparing a Toddler for
      Venipuncture
    Case Study: Preparing an Adolescent for Surgery
    Care Plan: Preparing a School-Age Child for Surgery
Audio Glossary

Hospitalization, whether it is elective, planned in advance, or the result of an emergency or trauma, is stressful for children of all ages and their families. Today, children are infrequently hospitalized, because most pediatric conditions can be managed within the community. Hospitalized children are usually very ill. They find themselves in an unknown environment, surrounded by strange people and equipment and frightening sights and sounds. They are subjected to unfamiliar procedures, some of which are invasive, and may even have surgery or be in an intensive care unit. For both children and families, routines are disrupted and normal coping strategies are tested.

To minimize the stress of hospitalization, nurses need to provide support to children and their families before, during, and after hospitalization. Through preadmission preparation, children and their families are introduced to the acute care setting. During hospitalization, nurses work collaboratively with parents to use various strategies that promote coping and adaptation, or prepare children for procedures and surgery. Nurses are instrumental in ensuring that the developmental and educational needs of children are met, especially when hospitalization is prolonged. Nurses also work with families to help prepare for discharge or transfer to a long-term care or rehabilitation facility.

EFFECTS OF ILLNESS AND HOSPITALIZATION ON CHILDREN AND FAMILIES

CHILDREN'S UNDERSTANDING OF HEALTH AND ILLNESS

Children have limited knowledge about the body and its relation to health and illness. A young child is likely to think that misbehavior toward his or her mother caused an illness to occur if the two events occur close in time. Older children sometimes feel responsible or guilty about an illness. Adolescents often feel invulnerable and may believe that they will never become ill or have an accident. However, if an adolescent has had a close friend who experienced a life changing event like a car crash, the adolescent may fear being in a car crash like that of the friend. The nurse realizes that the understanding of the child or adolescent about an illness and hospitalization is based primarily on their cognitive ability at various developmental stages and on previous experiences with healthcare professionals. The nurse uses this knowledge to plan care that will help children use coping strategies appropriate to assist the child (Vessey, 2003).

Infant

By about 6 months of age, infants have developed an awareness of themselves as separate from their mothers or fathers. They are able to identify primary caretakers and to feel anxious when in contact with strangers. Hospitalization can be a traumatic time for an infant, particularly if the parents are not staying with the child. They can sense the anxiety their parents are experiencing during a hospitalization.

Three phases of **separation anxiety** were first identified in young children who were separated from their parents for long periods or permanently and lacked a close relationship with one caretaker after separation (Bowlby, 1960). Characteristic behaviors of children in the three phases of separation anxiety are listed in Table 40–1. Hospitalized infants and young children often display some of these behaviors, particularly if parents are unable to remain with the child.

TABLE 40–1 ✛ **Stages of Separation Anxiety in Young Children**

Protest
Screaming, crying
Clinging to parents
Withdrawal from other adults

Despair
Sadness, depression
Withdrawal or compliant behavior
Crying when parents appear

Denial
Lack of protest when parents leave
Appearance of being happy and content with everyone
Close relationships not established
Developmental delay possible

Data from Bowlby, J. (1960). Separation anxiety. *International Journal of Psychoanalysis, 41,* 89–113.

Before the 1970s, healthcare professionals assumed that the despair and denial manifested by infants and young children after prolonged separation were signs of positive adaptation, since the child in these stages seemed calm and quiet. Infants sometimes protested when their parents visited, and parents were therefore advised not to visit often. However, the protest phase is now viewed as a healthy response to separation from loved ones and as an indication that the infant has meaningful, close relationships. Parents should be encouraged to remain with and provide care to the hospitalized infant, and to visit as often as possible if they cannot remain with the young child.

Toddler and Preschooler

Toddlers and preschoolers are beginning to understand illness but not its cause. Two unrelated events may appear to have a cause-and-effect relationship for young children, who may consider the sun, an animal, bad behavior, or even magic to be the cause of their illnesses. These children may blame other people, events, or themselves for an illness (Bibace & Walsh, 1981). This is especially true if the other event occurs shortly before the illness.

The child's concept of the body usually is limited to names and locations of some body parts. Although toddlers and preschoolers are not likely to understand how the lungs, heart, bones, or other body parts function, they are learning concepts of safety, hygiene, and other health-related issues.

Separation from parents remains the major stressor for the child. When a parent cannot be present, reminders can

be left with the child. These might include a piece of cloth saturated with the mother's favorite perfume or father's cologne, an object belonging to the parent, or an audiotape with messages from the parents. Toddlers and preschoolers fear body mutilation and change. If the child is undergoing an operation, the nurse should explain to the child that surgery will "fix" the body, and take the child on a tour of the unit and operating room if possible. A picture book of the hospital unit, equipment, and personnel can be used to prepare the child. Having a doll on which the same procedures are done can be helpful. The nurse should encourage the parents to be present as much as possible for important rituals such as toileting, carrying out bedtime routines, and singing favorite nursery rhymes.

School-Age Child

Older children have a more realistic understanding of the reasons for illness and are able to comprehend explanations. They benefit from use of models and pictures to understand explanations. The child's concept of body parts and function is maturing. However, understanding should be evaluated so that teaching can be geared to the child's level of understanding. Concepts of time are well formed, and parents should be encouraged to tell the child when they will return. Parents should also be available for telephone calls to provide support and comfort. The child may feel lonely because of separation from parents, family, and friends. The child may worry about pain, stitches, and bandages, and wonder if his or her body will return to normal. Stressful procedures can lead to regression or other behavioral changes. The child relies on parents and others for support and understanding during these events.

Adolescent

After 11 years of age, adolescents become increasingly aware of the physiologic, psychologic, and behavioral causes of illness and injury. Adolescents are concerned with appearance and perceive an illness or injury in terms of its effect on their body image. Allowing choices in clothing worn in the hospital, hair style and care, and music played on CDs or other devices acknowledges the importance of their self-identity. Privacy and modesty are major concerns of adolescents because their physical characteristics are rapidly changing. Nurses should respect their feelings. Adolescents are in the process of becoming independent of their parents' influence, so control over aspects of their care is important. The peer group is a major influence in their lives, and having recreation and teen lounge facilities available are among their major recommendations. Separation from peers, home, and school are cited as major stressors of hospitalization by adolescents (Gusella, Ward, & Butler, 1998).

GROWTH AND DEVELOPMENT

School-age children between the ages of 5 and 8 years believe that the internal body consists mainly of a heart and bones. They view the digestive system as having two parts, the mouth and the stomach. Showing them how parts of the body are related can be helpful to enhance their understanding. However, young adolescents, ages 11 to 13 years, can describe the location and function of major organs such as the brain, nose, eyes, heart, and stomach. They usually have gaps in understanding and may have misconceptions, however, so evaluating their knowledge is a part of the nursing plan in order to plan teaching to meet their knowledge needs.

DEVELOPING CULTURAL COMPETENCE

RESPECTING THE WISHES OF FAMILIES OF HOSPITALIZED CHILDREN

There are many cultural influences on health beliefs and practices. For example, Mexican Americans view family as a strong support. Extended family and godparents (compadres) may want to be with a hospitalized child. Although the father of the child is often the spokesperson, mothers commonly are influential in decisions regarding child healthcare. As another example, Hawaiian families also often wish to have many family members present with a hospitalized child, and may value playing native music and use of aromatherapy (Lassetter & Baldwin, 2005). The nurse should be inclusive of all people the family wishes to have present in the hospital and for explanations about healthcare.

FAMILY RESPONSES TO HOSPITALIZATION

The illness and hospitalization of a child disrupt a family's usual routines. Sometimes roles are altered as one parent stays at the hospital while the other parent or siblings take on additional tasks at home. Family members may be anxious and fearful, especially when the outcome is unknown or potentially serious. Watching a child in pain is difficult for a parent. A serious emergency, lengthy illness, chronic condition, poor prognosis, lack of family support, and lack of financial or community services make adjustment more difficult. (See Chapter 41 for a description of nursing support for the child with life-threatening illness or injury. ∞)

Parents report greater satisfaction with their children's care when nurses tailor actions to the family needs and preferences. Positive communication with medical personnel and viewing care as a partnership between parents (as well as other key family members) and clinicians are viewed as predictive of parental satisfaction with their child's hospital care (Marino & Marino, 2000). Nurses need to see the parents as the ones who know and understand the child best, ask for their participation and partnership in care, and carefully explain all aspects of treatment. Parents need support to lessen their anxiety since those with many fears may not be able to parent children effectively and perform protective, nurturing, and decision-making roles (Melnyk, 2000). Nurses are alert to cultural patterns in the family that can influence the response to hospitalization and the family's management of the experience. The cultural background influences such areas as views of health, illness, and causation of illness; may determine who the decision maker is in the family regarding healthcare practices; and provides guidance for acceptable treatments (Spector, 2004).

The siblings of an ill child often receive little attention from the parents. Parents are preoccupied and may not think to take the siblings to visit the child in the hospital. The siblings may fantasize about the illness or injury and the appearance of their brother or sister. Siblings who are not adequately informed about the hospitalized child's condition may fear that the child will be disabled or die, even when this is unlikely. They may feel guilty about fighting with or being mean to their brother or sister in the past and believe that they played a role in causing the illness. They may believe that they will also become ill and hospitalized.

As family roles and routines change, siblings may feel insecure and anxious. Behavioral problems may develop, or school performance may deteriorate. Siblings may feel jealous because the ill brother or sister seems to monopolize the parents' attention. Given support, however, the siblings of an ill child manage well. See Chapter 41 for a description of additional strategies for working with the siblings of a hospitalized child. ∞

Nurses encourage the family to consider the siblings' experiences and needs when a child in the family is hospitalized. Encourage the family to bring the siblings to the hospital for a visit if possible. They may need preparation so that they understand what is happening in the hospital and with the child's condition (see "Teaching Highlights: Strategies for Assisting the Sibling of a Hospitalized Child" for teaching needed prior to the visit).

PREPARATION FOR HOSPITALIZATION

Hospitalization may be planned or unexpected. A child may be hospitalized for one of the following reasons:

- The child who has been ill at home gradually or suddenly becomes worse.

- The child needs diagnostic or treatment procedures or requires elective surgery.

- The child who was previously healthy suffers an injury, necessitating unexpected hospitalization.

TEACHING HIGHLIGHTS

STRATEGIES FOR ASSISTING THE SIBLING OF A HOSPITALIZED CHILD

1. Be truthful. Explain why the child is hospitalized, what the treatment involves, and how long the hospitalization is expected to last.
2. Assure siblings that neither they nor the hospitalized child is the cause of the need for treatment. If the sibling was involved in a situation in which the hospitalized child was injured, mental health counseling should be recommended.
3. Allow time for questions and expression of fears and other feelings during the preparation period.
4. Prepare the sibling for the child's appearance. This may include presence of tubes, bandages, or other treatments. It may be appropriate to cover some wounds, remove or cover some drainage tubes or bags, or otherwise prepare the environment. Be present to explain what the sibling is seeing and answer questions.
5. Prepare the sibling for the child's communication status. If the child cannot speak, tell the sibling what to expect. Suggest things to say and help the child to touch the hospitalized child.
6. Be present following the visit and encourage the sibling to share feelings about the visit. Provide opportunity for the sibling to express the effects of the treatment on the family.

When hospitalization is planned, both children and their parents have time to prepare for the experience. Assess the family's knowledge and expectations and then provide information about what is likely to happen. A variety of approaches can be used to provide information and allay fears.

- Tours of the hospital unit or surgical area are helpful. During tours, allow preschoolers and school-age children to see and touch items with which they will come in contact. The surgical team's attire is less frightening if the child has had a chance to try it on (Figure 40–1 ⊙). Medical equipment is not as scary when the child learns what it does and sees how it is used, for example, through demonstration on a doll (Figure 40–2 ⊙).

- If a tour is not possible, photographs or a videotape can show the medical setting and procedures. Tailor preparation time to age of child. For example, very young children may be told a day or two in advance with stories read to explain procedures. Older children can be told several days or a week ahead to allow time for explanations and questions.

- Many hospitals offer health fairs to explain health procedures to children. During a tour, while hospitalized, or at home, the child can be exposed to books or films that explain in age-appropriate terms

⊙ **FIGURE 40–1**

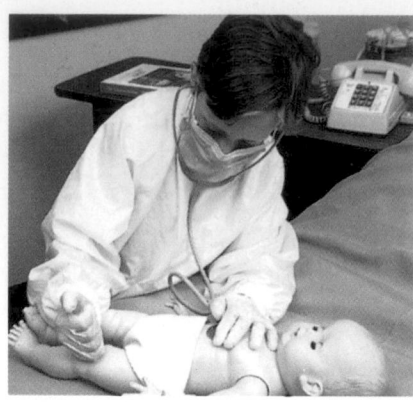

Allowing the child to dress up as a doctor or a nurse helps prepare the child for hospitalization. This helps the child adjust to treatment care and the recovery process. Why? What might the child's concerns be? Can you think of any concerns that could be related to cultural background?

what to expect during various procedures (Table 40–2). Use coloring books and other concrete methods for teaching, as they can help children to cope emotionally with hospitalization (LaMontagne, 2000).

Parents can be instrumental in preparing a child for hospitalization by reviewing material presented, being available to answer questions, and being truthful and supportive (Table 40–3, Figure 40–3 ⊙).

Different approaches are useful when adolescents are being prepared for hospitalization. They learn not only from written materials, models, and videotapes, but also

⊙ **FIGURE 40–2**

The child's anxiety and fear often will be reduced if the nurse explains what is going to happen and demonstrates how the procedure will be done by using a doll. Based on your experience, can you list five things you can do to prepare a school-age child for hospitalization?

TABLE 40–2 ✤ Sample Teaching Materials for Children Regarding Hospitalization and Healthcare

Videotapes

Clean Intermittent Catheterization.	Learner Managed Designs, Inc.
I Have Epilepsy Too.	Epilepsy Foundation
What Do I Tell My Children? How to Help a Child Cope with the Death of a Loved One.	Life Cycle Productions

Books

Barney Is Best. Carlstrom, N. W.	HarperCollins
Barney and Baby Bop Go to the Doctor. Larsen, M.	Lyrick Publishers
The Berenstain Bears Go to the Doctor. Berenstain, S., & Berenstain, J.	Random House
Chris Gets Ear Tubes. Pace, B., & Hutton, K.	Kendall Green Publishers
Curious George Goes to the Hospital. Rey, M., & Rey, H. A.	Houghton Mifflin Company
Cut. McCormick, P., & McCormick, P.	Front Street Publishers
(Mental health hospitalization of a teen)	
David's Story: A Book about Surgery. Drink, B.	Lerner Publications
Doctors and Nurses: What Do They Do? Green, C.	HarperCollins
The Fall of Freddie the Leaf. Buscaglia, L.	Henry Holt & Co.
Going to the Hospital. Rogers, F., & Judkis, J.	Penguin Putnam Books
The Hospital Book. Howe, J.	Crown Publishers
Let's Talk about Going to the Hospital. Johnston, M.	Rosen Publisher
A Night Without Stars. Howe, J.	Avon
No Measles, No Mumps for Me. Showers, P.	Thomas Y. Crowell
Corduroy Goes to the Doctor. Freeman, D., & McCue, L.	A Golden Book
Rita Goes to the Hospital. Davison, M.	Random Books
Tubes in My Ears: My Trip to the Hospital. Dooley, V., & Katon, M.	Mondo Publishers
A Visit to the Sesame Street Hospital. Hautzig, D.	Random Books
When Molly Was in the Hospital: A Book for Brothers and Sisters of Hospitalized Children. Duncan, D.	Rayve Productions
Why Am I Going to the Hospital? Cilliota, C., & Livingston, C.	Lyle Stuart

TABLE 40–3 ✤ Parental Preparation of Children for Hospitalization

- Read stories to the child about the experience.
- Talk about going to the hospital, what it will be like. Talk about coming home.
- Encourage the child to ask questions.
- Encourage the child to draw pictures of what the hospital will be like.
- Visit the hospital unit if possible.
- Let the child touch or see equipment if possible.
- Plan for support via parents' presence, telephone calls, special items of the parents that child can keep during the stay.
- Be honest. Tell about expected pain and management of this experience.

ADAPTATION TO HOSPITALIZATION

SPECIAL UNITS AND TYPES OF CARE

Children who are admitted to a hospital may be cared for in one or more of the following units: emergency department, intensive care unit, or short-stay unit. They may require surgical treatment involving preoperative and postoperative care. Children with infectious diseases may require isolation precautions. Other children may need rehabilitative care to achieve or restore maximum potential.

Emergency Care

When a child is brought to an emergency department, the parents are usually frightened and insecure and may even

● FIGURE 40–3

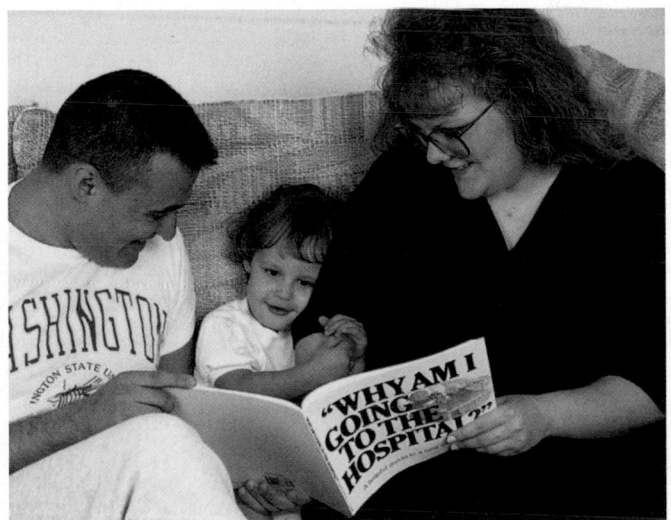

Jasmine's parents are taking the time to prepare her for hospitalization by reading a book recommended by the nurse. Such material should be appropriate to the child's age and culture. Why do you think that having parents read this material to the child is valuable?

from talking with peers who have had similar experiences. A few weeks of preparation may be helpful to provide time for these exchanges of information and support. Provide a forum for asking questions without parents present.

be in a state of shock. They may demonstrate panic behaviors and need clear directions and frequent repetitions of material. The fast pace and critical nature of the unit create an atmosphere in which parents are hesitant to ask questions and are anxious about the outcome. Keep both the child and the family informed about what is being done and when more news may be available. The parents and child should remain together as much as possible. Help parents identify support systems that can help them during this stressful time. It is recommended that parents who wish to remain with a child during even invasive procedures or resuscitation efforts should be allowed to do so (Emergency Nurses Association, 2001). Nurses ask family members about whether they want to be present in critical situations, provide support, and keep them informed about the healthcare provided whatever their desired level of participation.

Intensive Care

Parents of a child in an intensive care unit are also likely to be anxious, particularly since the child's illness may be severe and the prognosis may be guarded. The unfamiliar equipment may create an atmosphere of fear. Numerous healthcare professionals come and go, and parents may not know whom to turn to or even what questions to ask. Nurses should provide emotional support, explain the purpose of treatments and machines, help parents to hold or touch their child, and provide support and referral to other services if appropriate. (See Table 41–1 in Chapter 41 for a discussion of stressors in parents and children in an intensive care unit and the nursing strategies intended to address these stressors. ∞)

Preoperative and Postoperative Areas

Many hospitals now allow parents to be with their child until anesthesia induction and again in the postanesthesia recovery area. Parents often want to support their child before and immediately after a surgical procedure, and their presence may offer reassurance and comfort to the child.

Prepare family members for what will happen and what is expected of them. In some hospitals, only one or two close family members are allowed to see the child. They may need to wear special gowns, shoes, or hats, and they may be restricted to certain areas. Explain special equipment such as intravenous setups and monitoring devices.

Short-Stay Units

Hospitalizations have generally become short, with minor surgery, diagnostic tests such as radiology studies or cardiac catheterizations, and treatments such as chemotherapy performed within a day. The child may be admitted in the morning and go home in the afternoon. In addition, children who have potentially serious illnesses may be

● FIGURE 40–4

The nurse is monitoring a young child who is in a short-stay unit for treatment of dehydration and fever. What support does the mother need?

placed on a short-stay or 23-hour unit for monitoring or limited treatment, after which a decision is made to either hospitalize the child for additional treatment or send the child home if improvement occurs (Figure 40–4 ●). These short stays are beneficial because they cause minimal disruption of family patterns and are cost effective. Nurses can help parents prepare the child properly for planned admissions, monitor the child during the procedures, encourage family participation in care, and keep families well informed (Table 40–4).

TABLE 40–4 ✣ **Nursing Considerations in Preparing Parents and Child for Planned Short-Stay Admission**

- Are there special requirements, such as not being permitted food or drink or needing extra fluid intake?
- What time and where must the child appear?
- Are any special forms, insurance numbers, or previous records needed?
- How long will the child stay in the hospital?
- Are parents expected or encouraged to be with the child or stay in the health facility?
- Is there a chance the child may need to remain longer than expected?
- What will the child's condition be for transfer home?
- Will special equipment or care be needed?
- What symptoms can indicate problems?
- Where can the family go or whom can they call in case of problems or questions?

THINKING CRITICALLY

PREPARING CHILDREN FOR HOSPITALIZATION OR SHORT-STAY SURGERY

Six-year-old Kate has had several nosebleeds and fainting spells recently. After examination by her physician and a number of diagnostic studies such as chest x-ray examination, echocardiography, and electrocardiography, coarctation of the aorta is diagnosed. Kate will come in this week for a cardiac catheterization. In 2 weeks, she is scheduled to have open heart surgery.

Kate has had few health problems, and her experiences with healthcare professionals are limited. Her parents, who are anxious about the heart surgery, are concerned about how their daughter will adapt to hospitalization.

How should you prepare Kate for the cardiac catheterization and later for the surgery? Include knowledge of her developmental stages and cognitive understanding in your planned intervention approaches. How far in advance should teaching take place? What teaching aids are helpful? How can Kate's parents be involved in and reinforce the teaching? What kind of support do her parents, siblings, and friends need during hospitalization? See Table 40-4 for nursing considerations in preparing children for short hospitalizations; these guidelines will be useful for your plan of preparation for the cardiac catheterization.

● **FIGURE 40–5**

Rehabilitation units provide an opportunity for the child to relearn tasks like walking and climbing stairs. They provide an important transition from hospital to home community.

Isolation

Children who are placed in isolation may suffer lack of stimulation due to limited contact with other children. Frequent family visits are important and should be encouraged. Family members may be reluctant to wear protective garments either out of fear of using them incorrectly or a belief that they are unnecessary. Be sure the family understands the reason for isolation and any special procedures. Having contact with and holding the child should be encouraged whenever possible. (Standard precautions are described in the Quick Reference to Maternal-Child Procedures, as well as the CD-ROM accompanying this text.) **SKILLS**

Rehabilitation

Rehabilitation units provide children with ongoing care and support to continue recovery beyond the initial period of illness or injury. These may be separate units within a hospital or independent centers. The objective of **rehabilitation** is to help the child with physical or mental challenges reach his or her fullest potential and to promote achievement of developmentally appropriate skills. Parental involvement is essential (Figure 40–5 ●).

FAMILY ASSESSMENT

To develop a plan of care that involves all family members, assess the impact of the child's illness or hospitalization on the family (Table 40–5). Teaching the child and family, providing support, and referring them to community resources are key elements of the plan.

Assess the family's resources frequently. These resources include the coping strategies of family members, financial resources, access to healthcare, and availability of community services. One family may manage quite well with limited financial support because they have good coping strategies, while another family with greater financial resources may have difficulty caring for an ill child. Staying with a hospitalized child can be a financial drain for parents if they must miss work and perhaps travel to another location and stay away from home.

It is important to assess the family dynamics. Evaluate the quality of communication, methods of handling problems, and sources of strength. Examine how the family has been dealing with the health needs of their child if the child has been hospitalized or required home care in the past. Ask about the roles they want to play in the child's treatment and the roles they would like the nurse to fulfill. Referrals to the hospital social service department, family service agencies, or other community organizations may be needed. Support groups in the community or agencies that provide medical equipment can also be helpful. Assess the cultural characteristics of the family and how they might influence the care response as well as alternative treatments. Integrate the family's desired types of approaches into care whenever possible.

TABLE 40–5 ✣ Family Assessment

Family Roles
- What changes will the child's illness create in the family?
- Will household tasks need to be reallocated?
- Will a burden be placed on certain family members?
- Will one parent room in or spend a great deal of time in the hospital?

Knowledge
- What knowledge does the family have about the child's condition and treatment? Do they need further information?
- At what time should discharge planning and teaching begin?

Support Systems
- Does the family have medical insurance? What percentage of costs will it cover? Will other financial support be needed?
- Are close friends or family available to provide child care for other children, assist with family tasks, or help in other ways?
- Are there community services such as support groups, camps for children with disabilities, education sessions, or equipment and financial resources to which the nurse can refer the family?

Siblings
- Have they been informed of the ill child's condition and the expected outcome?
- Have they been reassured that they did not cause the illness?
- Do they understand the change in roles and family routines?
- Are they able to visit the ill child?
- Have their teachers been informed of the family stress?
- If the hospitalized child's life is threatened, are the siblings involved in a therapy plan to assist them in dealing with that stress?

DEVELOPING CULTURAL COMPETENCE

INTEGRATING CULTURAL PRACTICES

Many ethnic groups such as Chinese Americans and Mexican Americans use a combination of Western medicine and traditional therapies such as home treatments or a traditional healer (curandismo for Mexican Americans). This information may not be shared with nurses or physicians, both out of respect and in fear that they will be told not to use these methods. Recognizing and supporting use of both Western and traditional practices can promote health and provide comfort for children and families. Ask about care practices in an inviting and accepting manner so that all forms of treatment can be integrated into the plan of care.

CHILD AND FAMILY TEACHING

Teaching is an essential part of the nurse's role in care of hospitalized children and their parents. Teaching may be informal, as when the nurse provides an explanation during routine care, or structured, as when the nurse plans and implements a formal teaching program. Be sure that explanations or reading materials are at a level the parent can understand. If translators are needed to facilitate understanding, be sure they are available for teaching sessions. Teaching about the behaviors seen in hospitalized children and strategies to deal with these behaviors are helpful for parents. For instance, nurses can provide information for parents of hospitalized toddlers about the possibility of regression in behavior, and for parents of teens the fact that loss of independence is a difficult transition. Then strategies can be suggested to assist the family in dealing with the behaviors observed. How can nurses plan to provide such developmental information for parents? When and where should the nurse address these issues?

NURSING PRACTICE

When children are hospitalized for illness or injury, they are in a vulnerable position. Whereas adults are able to refuse or question treatment, children are often not given those rights. This may be in conflict with the United Nations Convention on the Rights of the Child, which gives children the right to be heard in all matters affecting them. Nurses can carefully examine each situation, being careful not to take for granted that hospitalized children will be unhappy and in pain. We can seek to allow them to speak their wishes and to provide strategies that will best help them during healthcare (Bricher, 2000).

Teaching directed at children must take into account their developmental levels and cognitive abilities. Learning is easier when teaching involves more than one sense (such as hearing, vision, and touch). Teaching directed at parents must also be geared to their level of understanding. If English is the parents' second language, a translator may be necessary.

Timing is a critical factor in teaching. Parents and children are less receptive to teaching when they are preoccupied with other thoughts or activities. Scheduling specific times for teaching sessions may be helpful.

Depending on the information to be presented, teaching may use the cognitive, psychomotor, or affective domains of learning. Teaching that includes all three of these domains is more effective.

GROWTH AND DEVELOPMENT

For children who can hear, touch, see a model or equipment, read, look at pictures, or even smell things like alcohol swabs, learning is more complete. This is particularly important for the school-age child in the stage of concrete operational thought, who must be able to manipulate materials in order to learn.

Teaching Plans

A teaching plan is a written plan that includes goals and expected outcomes, interventions needed to achieve the specified goals, and a method and time for evaluation of the expected outcomes. The teaching plan may also specify teaching methods and types of materials to be used. Developing a teaching plan helps ensure that all the necessary information is included and makes teaching more efficient.

The child's primary caretaker should participate in the teaching. The primary caretaker is most often a parent but may be a close family member (uncle, aunt, grandparent). The first step in establishing a teaching plan is to assess the child's or parent's knowledge, skills, and feelings by finding the answers to the following questions:

- What does the parent or child know about the health issue?
- What is the cognitive level or ability to learn?
- Is there a desire to learn?
- What previous experiences affect the learning experience, either positively or negatively?
- What resources are available to the parents, child, and nurse to enhance understanding of the health condition?
- Are there feelings or beliefs that might interfere with the learning process?

The second step involves deciding what knowledge, skill, or change in attitude is desired. Outcome criteria or objectives are established for the parent and child:

- A learning objective for a parent might be: The parent states the importance of checking the child's toes in the casted leg twice daily for temperature, movement, sensations, color, and edema (cognitive domain).
- An objective for a child might be: The child self-catheterizes using correct technique and records the amount of urine in a log (psychomotor domain).
- An objective for an adolescent might be: The adolescent explores methods of managing feelings of loss of control related to diabetes management (affective domain).

Explore possible teaching methods and approaches. A variety of sources, including written materials (books, pamphlets, handouts, and stories), computer software, audiovisual presentations, and others, are available (see Table 40–2). In some settings, audiovisual and computer resources may be limited. Small-group teaching sessions (e.g., for children with recently diagnosed diabetes or cystic fibrosis) may be another option. Gathering two or three parents or children together on a unit to learn and share experiences may be helpful.

For some conditions, standardized teaching plans are available in books and from healthcare agencies. These plans can serve as a guide in developing an individualized teaching plan.

Children with Special Needs

Children with disabilities may have special learning needs (Allen & Vessey, 2004). If they have visual impairment or visual perceptual difficulty, material must be presented in auditory and tactile ways. Children with hearing deficits need visual and tactile presentations. Children with learning disabilities may need more frequent reinforcement and shorter teaching sessions. Evaluate them for comprehension often and adjust teaching as necessary. When psychomotor skill performance is needed, special aids may be necessary so the child can hold a syringe, draw up a liquid, or perform other tasks. Adequate assessment of the child's strengths and disabilities, along with consultation with parents and the child's teachers, can help the nurse plan teaching methods.

Children who have chronic illnesses may have been hospitalized numerous times and have received other healthcare at home and in the community. They usually have adapted coping mechanisms that help them deal with the chronic illness. Talk to them to see what has helped in the past, provide information about what to expect during current hospitalizations, assign staff members familiar to the children when possible, and follow the children's lead in helping them cope. Their frequent hospitalizations may serve as a strength if they adapt quickly and understand what to expect, or may contribute to a depressing situation if the hospitalization reflects a worsening of condition.

STRATEGIES TO PROMOTE COPING AND NORMAL DEVELOPMENT

During hospitalization, care of the child focuses not only on meeting physiologic needs, but also on meeting psychosocial and developmental needs. Several strategies may help children adapt to the hospital environment, promote effective coping, and provide developmentally appropriate activities. These strategies include child life programs, rooming-in, therapeutic play, and therapeutic recreation.

Child Life Programs

Many hospitals have child life programs that focus on the psychosocial needs of hospitalized children. Professional child life specialists, paraprofessionals, and volunteers staff these departments. Due to changes in the healthcare system, more children today are receiving care in outpatient centers, day surgery units, and other community agencies. Pediatric inpatient units are consequently small, and play therapy programs are sometimes curtailed. Nurses need to plan to provide play, whatever the size or services of the unit (DePasquale, 1999). A **child life specialist** plans activities to provide age-appropriate playtime for children either in the child's room or in a playroom. Some activities are designed to assist children in working through feelings about illness. Examples include playing with medical equipment or drawing pictures about hospital treatments. A trusted child life specialist may stay with a child during a particularly frightening procedure such as a venipuncture or bone marrow aspiration.

Both the child life department and the nursing staff focus on the emotional needs of hospitalized children, plan play experiences that promote optimal development, and support the family in providing the child's care and support (American Academy of Pediatrics, 2000). Child life specialists and nurses collaborate to meet the child's desired outcomes related to coping with and adjusting to hospitalization.

Rooming-In

Rooming-in is the practice of having a parent stay in the child's hospital room and care for the hospitalized child. Some hospitals provide cots, others have special built-in beds on pediatric wards, and in some institutions a parent stays in a separate room on the unit. A parent who is rooming-in may want to perform all of the child's basic care or help with some of the medical care. Communication between nurse and parent is important so that the parent's desire for involvement is supported. The nurse also facilitates the parent's comfort by providing towels and privacy for showering, offering information about where to obtain

food, and in all ways assisting the parent in the ability to be present to support the child.

Therapeutic Play

Play is an important part of childhood. The stress of illness and hospitalization increases the value of play. Not only does play facilitate normal development, but play sessions can help the child learn about healthcare, express anxieties, work through feelings, and achieve a sense of mastery or control over frightening or little-understood situations. In the present era of cost containment, play programs may be minimized in hospitals, so nurses should document the need for and benefits of play. Play that presents an opportunity to deal with the fears and concerns of health experiences is called **therapeutic play** (Figure 40–6 ⊙).

Through therapeutic play the child's knowledge of his or her illness or injury can be assessed. A common technique involves using an outline drawing of the body (Figure 40–7 ⊙) or stories and asking the child to draw in or talk about what the illness or injury means to him or her (Ramsey, 2000). Alternatively, the child may be asked to draw a picture or make up a story, enabling the nurse to assess fears and other emotions. The Goodenough Draw-A-Person test helps to assess the cognitive level of children between 3 and 13 years of age (Table 40–6). The Gellert Index is another tool that helps to assess the child's knowledge of the body (Table 40–7). In addition to assessment, drawing can be used as a nursing intervention. Show the child on a drawing what will happen during surgery or a

⊙ FIGURE 40–6

A, Volunteers such as this foster grandmother can provide stimulation and nurturing to help young children adapt to lengthy hospitalizations. **B,** Child life specialists plan activities for young children in the hospital to facilitate play and stress reduction.

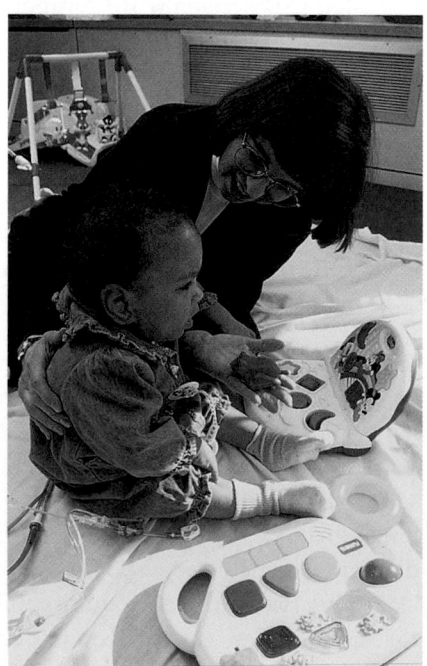

A   B

● **FIGURE 40–7**

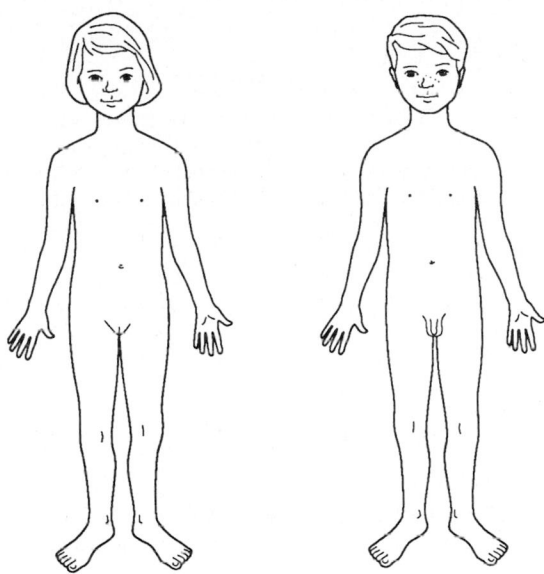

The nurse can use a simple gender-specific outline drawing of a child's body to encourage children to draw what they think about their medical problem. Such drawings reveal a child's interpretation, which the nurse can work with to provide appropriate care.

treatment. The child's drawings of healthcare experiences allow him or her to express fears and gain mastery over the situation.

Dramatic play, or acting out the experiences of healthcare encounters, is an effective form of play that enables young children to relive and feel control over the events that have occurred to them. A variety of techniques that may be used to promote therapeutic play are described in Table 40–8. Specific techniques are chosen to reflect the child's developmental stage.

TABLE 40–6 ✢ Goodenough Draw-A-Person Test

- The child is asked to draw a picture of a person and to do so carefully and completely, taking his or her time. It is preferable to have the child take the test alone, away from parents.
- Points are assigned for specific details included in the drawing, for example, 1 point each for the presence of head, legs, arms, trunk, and eyes. Additional points are assigned depending on the complexity of details.
- For every 4 points assigned, another year is added to a baseline age of 3 years. For example, a child who scores 24 points (by including 24 details) would have a total score of 9 years (6 plus 3 baseline years). This number is compared to the child's chronologic age to determine his or her cognitive level.

The Goodenough Test may be obtained from the Psychological Corporation, 555 Academic Court, San Antonio, TX 78204; 1-800-872-1726.

TABLE 40–7 ✢ Gellert Index of Body Knowledge

Part A

What do you have inside you? Tell me as many things as you can think of that are inside you.

Part B

1. Show me the head. What is in the head? (Tell me all the things that are in the head.)
2. Make a circle showing where and about how big the heart is. What does the heart do? (What is it for?) What would happen if we didn't have a heart?
3. Show me some places where you have bones. (Try for a minimum of five locations.) What do we have bones for? What would happen if we didn't have bones?
4. Make a circle showing where and about how big the stomach is. What does the stomach do? Show me where the food goes after you swallow it. (Sketch in diagram.) And then? (If excretion is not mentioned spontaneously, ask: Does it ever come out anywhere? If the answer is affirmative, ask: Show me where it comes out.)
5. Make a circle showing about where and about how big the ribs are. Why do we have ribs? (What for?) What would happen if we didn't have ribs?
6. Make a circle showing about where and about how big the liver is. What does the liver do? What would happen if we didn't have a liver?
7. What do you think we have a skin for? What would happen if we didn't have a skin?
8. Make a circle showing where and about how big the lungs are. How many lungs are there? What do we have lungs for? What would happen if we didn't have lungs?
9. Do you have any nerves? (If no, ask: Does anybody else? If so, who?) What would happen if we didn't have any nerves?
10. Make a circle showing where and about how big the bladder is. What do we have a bladder for? What would happen if we didn't have a bladder?
11. How come we have bowel movements? (What for?) Where do bowel movements come from? (Probe for derivation from food, stomach, intestines.) Show me on the diagram. What would happen if we didn't have bowel movements? About how often (how many times) should people have bowel movements? About how often do you have bowel movements?

Part C

1. What do you think is the most important part of you? (If you picked one part of you as the most important, which one would you pick?)
2. Are there any parts of you that you could live (get along) without? Which ones?

From Gellert, E. (1962). Children's conceptions of the content and functions of the human body. *Genetic Psychology Monographs, 65,* 293–405. Used with permission of the Helen Dwight Reid Education Foundation. Published by Heidref Publications, 1319 18th St. NW, Washington, DC 20036-1802.

Infant and Toddler. Infants engage in play readily. Crib mobiles, soft toys, music, and familiar toys from home facilitate development and help the infant to relax. Play is important for toddlers. Through play they explore the environment and

TABLE 40–8 ✤ Therapeutic Play Techniques

Technique	Assessment	Intervention
Stories	Have the child make up a story about a picture. Analyze content and emotional clues in the story. Have children tell a story about an important experience in a group of other children.	Read or make up stories to explain illness, hospitalization, or other specific aspects of healthcare. Emotions such as fear can be included. Make a picture book of the hospital unit and use it to talk with the child about the experience.
Drawings	Administer Goodenough Draw-A-Person test (see Table 40–6) to evaluate cognitive level. Consider subject matter, size and placement of items in drawings, colors used, presence or absence of physical barriers, and general emotional feeling. Administer Gellert Index (Table 40–7) to learn about the child's knowledge of the body and its functioning before planning teaching.	Use the child's drawings or outlines of the body to explain care, procedures, or conditions. Provide an opportunity for the child to draw pictures of his or her choice or directed topics such as a picture of the child's family or healthcare encounter. Ask the child: "Tell me about your picture." Be alert to the child's emotions: "This child must be frightened by the big x-ray machine."
Music	Observe types of music chosen and effects of played music on behavior.	Encourage parents and children to bring favorite tapes to the hospital for stress relief. Have tapes playing during tests and procedures. Parents can tape their voices to play for infants and young children during separations. During longer hospitalizations, children can tape messages for siblings or classmates, who are then encouraged to retape their responses. Playtime can include the opportunity to play instruments and sing.
Puppets	The puppets can ask questions of young children, who are often more likely to answer the puppet than a person.	Perform short skits to teach children necessary healthcare information. Include emotional content when appropriate.
Dramatic play	Provide dolls and medical equipment, and analyze the roles assigned to dolls by the child, the behavior demonstrated by the dolls in the child's play, and the apparent emotions. Dolls with disabilities like those of the child are especially helpful (see Figure 40–10).	Provide dolls and equipment for play sessions. To ensure safety, supervise closely when actual equipment is used. Respond to emotions and behavior shown. Use dolls and equipment such as casts, nebulizer, intravenous apparatus, and stethoscope to explain care. Use dolls with problems or disabilities similar to those of the child, when available. Provide toys that foster expression of emotion, such as a pounding board and indoor darts.
Pets	Provide pet therapy. Watch the interaction between child and animal (see Figure 40-9).	Respond to emotions the child shows. Facilitate touch and contact with animals.

Additional techniques, such as sand or water play, may be appropriate in specific situations.

learn to identify with significant people in their lives. Play is also an acceptable way for toddlers to release tensions caused by stress or aggressive impulses.

Toddlers should be approached slowly, and the initial approach should be made in their parents' presence, if possible, to decrease feelings of stranger anxiety (wariness of strangers). Playing a variation of peek-a-boo or hide-and-seek using the curtain surrounding the toddler's crib or bed helps promote the realization that objects out of sight, such as parents, do return. Transitional objects, such as a familiar blanket or stuffed animal, can temporarily substitute for the security of parents. The toddler who is restrained can be read familiar stories. Repetition of stories promotes a sense of stability in the unfamiliar hospital environment.

A doll is a familiar toy that can be used to recreate a stressful environment, thereby providing an opportunity for the child to express and work through feelings. Other developmentally appropriate toys for toddlers include familiar objects from home such as measuring cups or spoons, wooden puzzles, building blocks, and push-and-pull toys. Playing with safe hospital equipment (bandages, syringes without needles, and stethoscopes) helps toddlers overcome the anxiety associated with these items. Supervise these play sessions and remove hospital equipment when you leave.

Preschooler. The nurse can intervene to reduce the stress produced by preschoolers' fears through the use of some kinds of play. A simple outline of the body or a doll can be used to address the child's fantasies and fears of bodily harm (see Figure 40–7). Playing with safe hospital equipment may help preschoolers to work through feelings such as aggression (Figure 40–8 ⬤).

● **FIGURE 40-8**

A child life specialist works with children being treated for cancer. Special dolls are used to familiarize children with the procedures that they will undergo.

● **FIGURE 40-9**

Hospitals may have pet therapy from specially trained animals to provide comfort and distraction during healthcare. Both the child and the dog seem to be smiling.

Preschoolers like crayons and coloring books, puppets, felt and magnetic boards, play dough, books, and recorded stories. Preschoolers and older children often enjoy pet therapy. Children's hospitals and units can have visits from pets, most commonly dogs, that provide diversion and physical contact (Figure 40-9 ●). Both preschool and school-age children may enjoy playing with a toy hospital.

School-Age Child. Although play begins to lose its importance in the school-age years, the nurse can still use some techniques of therapeutic play to help the hospitalized child deal with stress. School-age children often regress developmentally during hospitalization, demonstrating behaviors characteristic of an earlier state, such as separation anxiety and fear of body injury. Outlines of the body and, occasionally, dolls can be used to illustrate the cause and treatment of the child's illness (Figure 40-10 ●). Use terms for body parts that

● **FIGURE 40-10**

A

B

A, Age-appropriate play will help the child adjust to hospitalization and care. **B,** Having the child play with dolls that have "disabilities" similar to his or her own will help the child adjust. Such play helps the child realize what activities are possible.

are suitable for older children. Drawings provide an outlet for expression of fears and anger.

School-age children enjoy collecting and organizing objects and often ask to keep disposable equipment that has been used in their care. They may use these items later to relive the experience with their friends. Games, books, schoolwork, crafts, tape recordings, and computers provide an outlet for aggression and increase self-esteem in the school-age child. The type of play used should promote a sense of mastery and achievement.

NURSING PRACTICE

Technology can be used as a therapeutic tool with hospitalized children. In one creative project, children with chronic illness made their own videos about living with illness, thereby gaining control over the experience. Another example of technology application is Starbright World, a computer network where seriously ill children can interact in a "virtual community" (Rode, Capitulo, Fishman et al., 1998). For more information, visit our Web site.

Therapeutic Recreation

Many of the special play techniques used with younger children are not suitable for adolescents. However, adolescents do need a planned recreation program to help them meet developmental needs during hospitalization. Peers are important, and the isolation of hospitalization can be difficult. Telephone contact with other teenagers and visits from friends should be encouraged. Interactions with other teenagers at a pizza party, video game, or movie night or during other activities can help adolescents feel normal (Figure 40–11 ●). Physical activities that provide an outlet for stress are recommended. Even adolescents on bed rest or in wheelchairs can play a modified form of basketball.

The independence of adolescence is interrupted by illness. Give teenagers choices to assist them in regaining control. Giving them options and letting them choose an evening recreational activity can promote their feelings of independence. Passes to leave the hospital for special activities may be possible.

STRATEGIES TO MEET EDUCATIONAL NEEDS

Some hospitalizations are so short that the absence of the child or adolescent from school and peers is of minimal concern. However, if hospitalization is expected to last longer than a few days or if the child's condition will change so that he or she needs special school arrangements, the nurse should assess the effects of hospitalization on the child's education. Parents, teachers, school nurse, and other care providers may need to plan together to meet the child's educational needs and to establish an Individualized Education Plan (IEP).

● **FIGURE 40–11**

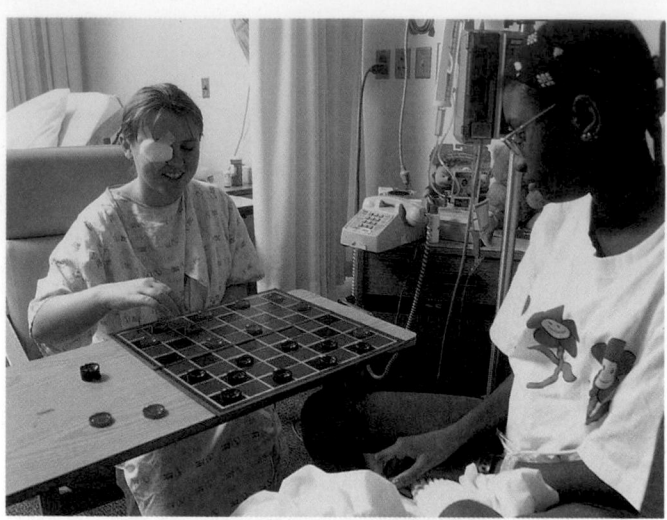

Having interaction with other hospitalized adolescents and maintaining contact with friends outside the hospital are very important so that the teenager does not feel isolated and alone. A friendly yet competitive checkers game helps to stimulate these teenagers and allows for self-expression. What are the other benefits?

When an elective procedure occurs, encourage families to arrange the extended school absence with teachers. The child can then be provided with schoolwork to do in the hospital or at home when well enough. This minimizes educational deficits and future problems for the child. Pencils, paper, comfortable work areas, computers, and quiet work times should be provided. Telephone calls or Internet connections with teachers can be arranged as needed. Tutors can provide teaching and facilitate the return to school. The nurse assesses the school environment and helps to plan for the child's return if special arrangements such as wheelchairs, medications during school hours, or shortened school days will be needed.

The social aspects of school and peers should also be considered. Peers can be encouraged to visit a hospitalized classmate, send cards and letters, call on the phone, or communicate via the Internet. Classmates can videotape a class or messages to the hospitalized child. When the child returns to school, information may be shared about the child's special needs. Maintain the child's and family's privacy by discussing with them the information needed by others, and obtaining written permission before disclosing any information. The hospital and school nurse often collaborate with each other, as well as the child and family, to plan for the child's needs. The child with chronic health problems or requiring long-term hospitalization has other school-related needs. Hospitals or rehabilitation units may have classrooms, teachers, and facilities to promote learning (Figure 40–12 ●). Many school districts provide tutors or computer connections for students who are hospitalized or receiving home care for long periods. Teachers can visit

FIGURE 40-12

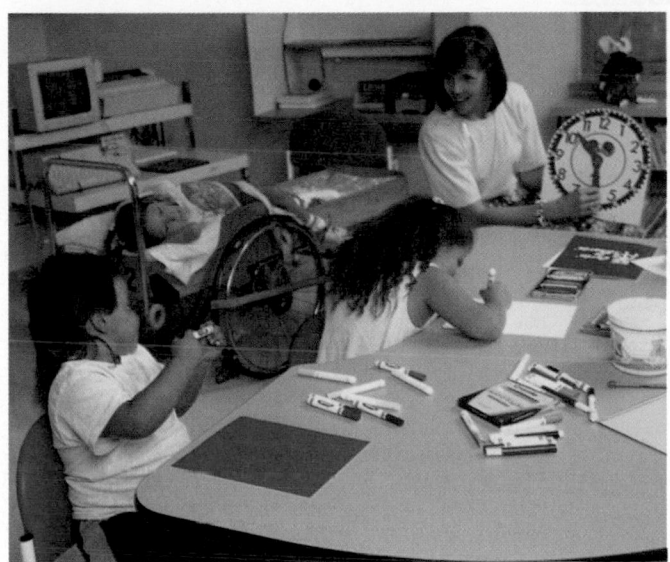

Shriners Hospital in Spokane, Washington, has a special classroom and teacher for children undergoing a lengthy hospital stay, enabling them to remain current with their schoolwork. The child who falls behind other students might not fit in when he or she returns to school or might be required to repeat a grade. What are the potential consequences of these situations?

children at the hospital or at home. Parents are often pivotal in making arrangements to meet the child's educational needs, since they interact with the child, the school, and the healthcare team.

PREPARATION FOR PROCEDURES

A number of procedures take place during hospitalization, from collection of urine or blood specimens to spinal taps and surgery. Special techniques can help the child to understand and cope with feelings about these procedures. Never assume that a procedure will not be traumatic for the child. Even providing urine in a specimen cup or undergoing x-ray examination can be frightening if the child does not understand the reason for the procedure or what to expect. Administration of medication can also be frustrating for the child. Prepare the child for medication administration and adapt techniques from those used with adults, so the correct medication is safely given (Table 40–11). See Skills 11–1 through 11–13 in the *Clinical Skills Manual*; Skills 11–1, 11–2, 11–4, and 11–11 can also be found on the CD-ROM that accompanies this text. **SKILLS**

To assess the child's feelings about the procedure, ask the following questions:

- Does the child know the purpose of the procedure?

- Has the child experienced this procedure before? Was the experience painful, frightening, or reassuring?

- What does the child think will happen? Are the child's beliefs accurate?

- Is the procedure painful?

- What techniques does the child use to gain control in challenging situations?

- Will the parents or adult friends be present to provide support?

Preparation may begin a few moments to several days before the procedure, depending on the child's age. Use words that the child understands to describe the procedure and its purpose (see Chapter 33 ∞). Older children need explanations geared to their cognitive level and previous experiences. They will want to know what is happening, why, and what they can do to cope during the procedure (Table 40–9).

Provide written information for adolescents, and schedule time for questions and discussions. Adolescents can make many choices about their own healthcare. They can be asked such questions as, "Do you want a local or general anesthetic?" or "Do you want your hand numbed for the intravenous start?" Some adolescents want their parents involved in their care, while others prefer to minimize the parents' role.

NURSING PRACTICE

When a potentially painful procedure will be occurring, an anesthetic cream or disk, such as EMLA, should be applied from 1 to 2 hours before the planned procedure. This can lessen discomfort and, therefore, fear in the child. Obtain a medical order and apply the cream as ordered or instruct parents if the child will be coming from home for a procedure.

The procedure should be performed as quickly and efficiently as possible. Parents may wish to be involved or may prefer to be available afterward to comfort the child. The parents or nurse can be designated to support the child. This may involve gentle touch, talking, singing, reassurance, praying, or a stress reduction technique. Ask the child and family what stress reduction practice may be helpful to them. Personal preference and cultural practices may differ among individuals.

DEVELOPING CULTURAL COMPETENCE

NATIVE AMERICAN TECHNIQUES FOR HEALING AND PROTECTING

Many American Indian tribes use "smudging," or burning of native plants, as a blessing and purifying of the spirit. This is thought to enhance healing and protect the child. The nurse can provide a safe and facilitative environment for this important ceremony in the hospital.

MediaLink Case Study: Preparing an Adolescent for Surgery

MediaLink Skills 11-1, 11-2, 11-4, and 11-12

TABLE 40–9 ✤ Assisting Children Through Procedures

Development Stage	Before Procedure	During Procedure
Infant	None for infant. Explain to parents the procedure, the reason for it, and their role.	Restrain infant securely and gently. Perform procedure quickly. Use touch, voice, pacifier, and bottle as distractions. Have parent hold, rock, and sing to infant after procedure.
Toddler	Give explanation just before procedure, since toddler's concept of time is limited. Explain that child did nothing wrong; the procedure is simply necessary.	Perform in treatment room. Give short explanations and directions in a positive manner. Avoid giving choices when none are available. For example, "We are going to do this now" is better than "Is it okay to do this now?" Allow child to cry or scream. Comfort child after procedure. Give child a choice of favorite drink or special sticker.
Preschool child	Give simple explanations of procedure. Basic drawings may be useful. While providing supervision, allow the child to touch and play with equipment to be used if possible. Since any entry into the body is viewed as a threat, state that the child's body will remain the same, and use adhesive bandages to reassure the child that the body is intact and parts will not "fall out."	Perform in treatment room. Restrain securely. Give short explanations and directions in a positive manner. Encourage control by having the child count to 10 or spell name. Allow child to cry. Give positive feedback for cooperation and getting through procedure. Encourage the child to draw afterward to explore the experience.
School-age child	Clear, thorough explanations are helpful. Use drawings, pictures, books, and contact with equipment. Teach stress reduction techniques such as deep breathing and visualization. Offer a choice of reward after procedure is completed.	Be ready to restrain child if needed. Allow child to remain in position by self if child is able to be still. Explain throughout procedure what is happening. Facilitate use of stress control techniques. Praise cooperative efforts.
Adolescent	Give clear explanations orally and in writing. Teach stress reduction techniques. Explore fear of certain procedures, such as staple removal or venipuncture.	Assist adolescent in self-control. Avoid using restraints. Assist with use of stress control techniques. Explain expected outcome and tell when results of test will be completed.

Procedures on young children are generally performed in a treatment room so the child's own room is viewed as a "safe" and relatively pain-free site. After the procedure the child can be taken back to his or her room for comfort and reassurance. A choice of reward often soothes the young child. An example of a common procedure which children need assistance with during hospitalization is venipuncture (see Table 40–9 and Skill 10–4). **SKILLS**

Preparation for Surgery

A child's surgical experience can be elective, planned in advance, or a result of an emergency or trauma. How a child responds to the experience depends on the psychologic and physical preparation he or she receives. See "Nursing Care Plan: The Child Undergoing Surgery" for a summary of the key elements of preoperative and postoperative care.

Preoperative Care

Preoperative care of the child includes both psychosocial and physical preparation for surgery.

Psychosocial Preparation. The goal of preoperative teaching is to reduce the fear associated with the unknown and decrease stress and anxiety associated with surgery. Teaching should be geared to the child's developmental level. If child life specialists are available, they can play an important role in preparing the child for surgery.

If the child will be in an intensive care unit or recovery room after surgery, a visit there before surgery can reduce the fear and anxiety associated with waking up in a strange environment filled with frightening sights, sounds, and smells. The use of tapes, anatomically correct puppets and dolls, drawings, and models is encouraged to teach the child about the surgical procedure. For example, a doll was used as a teaching aid in preparing Sabrina, the preschooler described in the opening quote, for surgery. Playing with stethoscopes, gowns, masks, and syringes without needles also helps the child feel more in control. Reassure children that their parents can accompany them to the operating room floor and will be waiting when they awaken from surgery.

Physical Preparation. Preoperative procedures and guidelines vary among hospitals and outpatient surgical centers. In ambulatory and acute care settings, preoperative checklists

NURSING CARE PLAN

THE CHILD UNDERGOING SURGERY

Intervention	Rationale	Expected Outcome
Preoperative Care		
1. Nursing Diagnosis: Deficient Knowledge related to preoperative and postoperative events		
NIC Priority Intervention: **Teaching, preoperative:** Assisting a patient to understand and mentally prepare for surgery and postoperative recovery		**NOC Suggested Outcome:** **Knowledge:** Extent of understanding conveyed about treatment regimen
Goal: The child and family will acquire knowledge related to the operation.		
■ Ask questions of the parent and child about surgery. ■ Teach about preoperative and postoperative events using appropriate developmental methods such as dolls, drawings, stories, and tours. ■ Reinforce information the family has received about the purpose of surgery. ■ Have the child demonstrate postoperative events that pertain to his or her care such as deep breathing, putting bandage on doll, taping intravenous line on doll, and pressing patient-controlled analgesia button. ■ Allow the parents and child to ask questions.	■ Prior knowledge and understanding can be reinforced and used to guide your presentation. ■ Developmental level determines the cognitive approach that works best for teaching. ■ The physician may have explained operation. ■ Concrete experience promotes learning. ■ Learners must have opportunity to ask questions.	The child and family are able to verbalize details about expected preoperative and postoperative events. They ask questions that demonstrate understanding. The child demonstrates skills needed in the postoperative period.
2. Nursing Diagnosis: Anxiety related to change in health status		
NIC Priority Intervention: **Anxiety reduction:** Minimizing apprehension, dread, foreboding, or uneasiness related to an unidentified source of anticipated danger		**NOC Suggested Outcome:** **Coping:** Actions to manage stressors that tax an individual's resources
Goal: The child and family will show decreased behavior indicating anxiety.		
■ Question the child about expectations of hospitalization and previous experiences. ■ Orient the child to the hospital setting, routines, staff, and other patients. ■ Institute age-appropriate play and interactions with the child. ■ Explain procedures and prepare for those that might cause trauma. ■ Allow the parents and child to ask questions.	■ Previous experiences can influence present anxiety level. ■ Familiarity with the setting and people can decrease anxiety by removing unknown factors. ■ Play can increase trust level and decrease anxiety. ■ The child is more likely to trust caregivers if they are truthful and if parents are present. ■ Questioning provides an opportunity to explain the unknown, which decreases anxiety.	The child and family demonstrate less anxiety. They verbalize understanding and comfort in hospital routines. Parents support the child for traumatic procedures.
3. Nursing Diagnosis: Risk for Infection and Injury related to exposure to nosocomial infection and use of preoperative medication		
NIC Priority Intervention: **Infection control and fall prevention:** Minimizing the acquisition and transmission of infectious agents, and instituting special precautions with patient at risk of falling		**NOC Suggested Outcome:** Actions to eliminate or reduce actual, personal, and modifiable health risks

(continued)

NURSING CARE PLAN—continued

THE CHILD UNDERGOING SURGERY

Intervention	Rationale	Expected Outcome
Goal: The child will show no signs of infection. The child will remain free of injury.		
■ Monitor vital signs at least every 4 hours. Inspect skin and respiratory status each shift. ■ Report any variation from expected vital signs. ■ Keep side rails up after preoperative medication is given. Maintain NPO status when ordered. Transport the child to the operating room safely secured.	■ Increase in vital sign levels, skin lesions, nasal drainage, or adventitious breath sounds can indicate signs of infection in the child. ■ Symptoms are reported so surgery can be canceled if necessary. ■ Preoperative medication can alter level of consciousness. NPO status prevents aspiration.	The child's vital signs and assessments are within normal limits. The child is transported safely to the operating room.

Postoperative Care

4. Nursing Diagnosis: Impaired Skin Integrity related to disruption of skin surface

NIC Priority Intervention:		NOC Suggested Outcome:
Wound care: Prevention of wound complications and promotion of wound healing		**Wound healing:** The extent to which cells and tissue have regenerated following intentional closure
Goal: The child will be free of infection.		
■ Monitor vital signs per hospital routine. Record and report changes from baseline. ■ Monitor surgical dressing and drains every hour. ■ Change or reinforce dressings when wet. ■ Check the intravenous site every hour for redness, swelling, pain, or pallor. ■ Teach parents signs of infection before discharge. Teach parents aseptic technique for dressing change and wound care.	■ Changes in vital signs, especially increased temperature and pulse, can indicate infection. ■ Excess drainage may indicate infection. ■ Wet dressing can allow organisms to come into contact with surgical wound. ■ Intravenous lines may become infiltrated or cause thrombophlebitis. ■ Parents report signs of infection and perform home care as needed.	The surgical wound heals without infection. The intravenous line remains patent without signs of infection. The child continues to demonstrate no signs of infection at home.

5. Nursing Diagnosis: Risk for Constipation related to surgical procedure and anesthetics

NIC Priority Intervention:		NOC Suggested Outcome:
Constipation management: Establishment and maintenance of regular bowel elimination		**Bowel elimination:** Ability of the gastrointestinal tract to form and evacuate stool effectively
Goal: The child will achieve and maintain normal bowel functioning by the fourth postoperative day.		
■ Auscultate bowel signs every 4 hours. Offer liquids only when bowel sounds are present. Assess the abdomen for distention. ■ Document the character and frequency of bowel movements. ■ Advance the diet as tolerated. ■ Increase activity as ordered and tolerated.	■ Restricting fluids avoids distention if peristalsis is not normal. ■ Knowledge of bowel status ensures early identification of constipation. ■ Fluids and roughage promote a normal bowel functioning. ■ Physical activity promotes peristalsis.	The child has bowel movement within 2 to 3 days after surgery with normal pattern by the fourth postoperative day.

NURSING CARE PLAN—continued

THE CHILD UNDERGOING SURGERY

Intervention	Rationale	Expected Outcome
6. Nursing Diagnosis: Risk for Fluid Volume Imbalance related to intravenous infusion and NPO status		
NIC Priority Intervention: Fluid management		**NOC Suggested Outcome:** **Fluid balance:** The child remains in fluid balance with no vomiting in postoperative period
Goal: The child will achieve and maintain proper circulating volume. The child will tolerate oral intake when started, with no nausea, vomiting, or dehydration present.		
■ Monitor vital signs per hospital routines. ■ Record intake and output. Be alert for fluid loss via dressings or watery stools. Evaluate hydration status by skin turgor and mucous membranes. ■ Monitor laboratory values of hematocrit and hemoglobin. ■ Begin oral intake after assessment of bowel sounds. Record vomiting. Administer antiemetics if indicated.	■ Changes in vital signs, especially pulse and blood pressure, can indicate fluid imbalance. ■ Intake and output are roughly equivalent. Urinary retention sometimes occurs postoperatively as a result of anesthesia. Fluid status can be assessed by skin and mucous membrane hydration. ■ Increased hematocrit and hemoglobin can indicate hemoconcentration and underhydration. Decreased serum values can indicate hemodilution of overhydration. ■ Vomiting can cause fluid loss.	
7. Nursing Diagnosis: Impaired Gas Exchange related to anesthetics and pain		
NIC Priority Intervention: **Airway management:** Facilitation of patency of air passages		**NOC Suggested Outcome:** **Respiratory status:** Ventilation: Movement of air in and out of lungs
Goal: The child will maintain adequate ventilation with no respiratory impairment.		
■ Auscultate lungs every 2 hours. Record rate, rhythm, and quality of respiration. Evaluate respiratory rate after analgesics. ■ Administer oxygen if ordered. ■ Reposition the child every 2 hours. ■ Encourage deep breathing and coughing every 2 hours. Use incentive spirometer, pinwheels, or other blow toys appropriate for the developmental level of the child. ■ Ensure proper intake and output.	■ Early identification of respiratory difficulty aids early treatment. Analgesics, especially morphine, may slow respiratory rate. ■ Oxygen may facilitate breathing status postoperatively. ■ Repositioning ensures expansion of all lung fields. ■ All areas of the lungs must be expanded. Mucus is expectorated. ■ Balanced fluid status ensures liquefication of secretions and prevents excess fluid accumulation.	The child moves adequate air in and out of lungs.
8. Nursing Diagnosis: Pain related to surgical procedure		
NIC Priority Intervention: **Pain management:** Alleviation of pain or a reduction in pain to a level of comfort that is acceptable to the patient		**NOC Suggested Outcome:** **Pain control behavior:** Personal actions to control pain

(continued)

NURSING CARE PLAN—continued

THE CHILD UNDERGOING SURGERY

Intervention	Rationale	Expected Outcome
Goal: The child will maintain an adequate comfort level.		
■ Assess behavioral cues (e.g., crying, movement, guarding ability to participate in activities of daily living). ■ Use an appropriate pain scale with verbal children. ■ Administer prescribed pain medications on a regular basis. ■ Use age-appropriate methods of pain control (e.g., distraction, repositioning).	■ Behavior of preverbal children provides clues to pain experience. ■ Pain scales allow children to quantify the amount of pain (see Chapter 42). ■ Narcotics and nonnarcotic analgesics alter pain perception. ■ Nonpharmacologic interventions interfere with pain perception and may decrease the child's anxiety.	The child's pain is controlled as demonstrated by a low number on the pain scale (behavioral or verbal).

9. Nursing Diagnosis: Risk for Impaired Skin Integrity related to limited mobility after surgery

NIC Priority Intervention: **Skin surveillance and pressure management:** Collection and analysis of patient data to maintain skin integrity and minimize pressure to body part		**NOC Suggested Outcome:** **Risk control:** Actions to eliminate or reduce actual personal and modifiable health threats
Goal: The child's skin will remain intact.		
■ Turn and reposition the child every 2 hours. ■ Keep linens clean and dry. ■ Check pressure areas when turning and rub erythematous areas with lotion. ■ Get the child up and ambulating when ordered. ■ Check the incision for drainage, redness, and intactness of staples or stitches every 4 to 8 hours.	■ Repositioning takes pressure off the skin and allows increased circulation. ■ Clean linen decreases the chance of skin breakdown. ■ Rubbing increases circulation. ■ Movement decreases pressure on skin. ■ Early identification of infection or problems with wound healing can ensure fast treatment.	The child develops no pressure areas. The wound heals without complication.

10. Nursing Diagnosis: Anxiety (Child and Family) related to change in health status and environment

NIC Priority Intervention: **Anxiety reduction:** Minimizing apprehension, dread, foreboding, or uneasiness related to an identified source of danger		**NOC Suggested Outcome:** **Coping:** Actions to manage stressors that tax an individual's resources
Goal: The child and family will verbalize comfort with postoperative care and outcome.		
■ Explain monitors, drains, dressings, intravenous lines, and procedures. ■ Reassure the child and family that anxiety is a normal response to the stressful event of surgery. ■ Encourage parental presence and care of the child. ■ Use touch and other nonverbal and verbal communication with the child and family.	■ Knowledge of purpose decreases anxiety. ■ Knowledge of what is expected decreases anxiety. ■ The child's anxiety decreases with parental presence. ■ Effective communication reassures child and family.	The child and family demonstrate coping skills to deal with hospitalization.

NURSING CARE PLAN—continued

THE CHILD UNDERGOING SURGERY

Intervention	Rationale	Expected Outcome
11. Nursing Diagnosis: Deficient Knowledge (Child and Family) related to lack of exposure to needed home care		
NIC Priority Intervention: **Teaching postoperative:** Health system guidance: Facilitating a patient's location and use of appropriate health services		**NOC Suggested Outcome:** **Knowledge:** Home care: Extent of understanding conveyed about home care
Goal: The child and family will verbalize self-care required at home.		
■ Provide oral and written home care instructions regarding surgical wound care, medications, activities, and diet. ■ Provide a number to call for questions or concerns. Instruct on follow-up visits.	■ Teaching regarding home care is necessary early in hospitalization. ■ Parents need to know emergency information and that follow up care is required.	The child and family demonstrate skills needed for home care following discharge. They verbalize plans for future care.

ensure proper physical preparation of patients for surgery. A sample checklist appears in Table 40–10.

Postoperative Care

Postoperative care of the child includes both physical and psychologic care. Evaluate the child's level of consciousness, and take vital signs frequently. Observe the surgical site for drainage, and check dressings. Monitor the child's intake and output and provide comfort and pain relief. (See Chapter 42 for details concerning pain management. ∞) Administer medications in a developmentally appropriate manner (Table 40–11). Ensure safety by taking measures to prevent infections, administering accurate medication doses, and performing all needed monitoring and reporting of assessment results (Miller & Zhan, 2004). Allow parents to visit with the child as soon after surgery as possible and provide culturally competent care (Figure 40–13 ☻). Provide information and support for families that choose to use

☻ FIGURE 40–13

This child has just undergone surgery and is in the PICU. Although the child's physical care is immediate and important, remember that both the child and the family have strong psychosocial needs that must be addressed concurrently. It is important to reunite the family as soon as possible after surgery.

TABLE 40–10 ✛ Preoperative Checklist

_____ Check that consent forms are witnessed and signed and in the patient's chart.

_____ Be sure the child's name band is in place.

_____ Be sure any allergies are prominently noted in the child's chart and on a special name band.

_____ Remove any prosthetic devices, including orthodontic appliances and body piercings.

_____ Check the child's mouth for loose teeth and tongue piercings.

_____ Remove eyeglasses and jewelry.

_____ Bathe and cleanse the operative site if ordered.

_____ Put the child in an operating room gown, allowing the child to wear underwear.

_____ Check that all special tests have been completed and the results are in the child's chart.

_____ Have the child void before surgery.

_____ Keep the child NPO (with nothing by mouth) before surgery.

_____ Give the child prescribed medications.

_____ Transport the child safely to the operating room.

TABLE 40–11 ❖ Variations in Medication Administration to Children

Route	Developmental Consideration	Techniques
Oral	Children under 5 years cannot generally swallow pills and capsules.	■ Medications are usually given in liquid form (elixir, syrup, or suspension). ■ Sometimes tablets are crushed or capsules are opened and mixed with one spoon of food. Check with pharmacy to be sure this does not inactivate the drug. Never crush enteric-coated or timed-release medicine. ■ When choosing a vehicle for crushed tablets, use only one spoonful of applesauce, pudding, jelly, or similar food. ■ Medication cups, nipples, and oral syringes can be used to administer liquid medication. Use TB syringe for amounts less than 1 mL to increase accuracy.
	Children may not want to take medicine.	■ Position young children upright to avoid choking and aspiration. ■ Give liquid medicines slowly by oral syringe (for infants) aimed at the inside of the cheek or by medicine cup (for toddler and preschooler) for drinking. ■ Have the expectation that the medicine will be taken. Let children choose the type of fluid to drink after but do not ask if they will take their medicine now.
Rectal	Colon is small in size.	■ For children under 3 years, the nurse's gloved fifth finger is used for insertion. After this age the index finger can usually be used. ■ Lubricate the tip of the suppository.
Ophthalmic and otic	Young children may be fearful of medicines placed in the eyes or ears.	■ Adequate restraint is needed to avoid injury. ■ The nurse's hand can be stabilized by resting the wrist on the child's head. ■ Explanations and therapeutic play can be used with children old enough to explain the process of administration. ■ Have medication at room temperature.
Topical	Skin of infants is thin and fragile.	■ Only prescribed doses and medicines appropriate for young children should be used on the skin. ■ Covering the area or keeping the child's hands occupied may be necessary to ensure adequate contact of medication with the skin.
Intramuscular	Anatomy and physiology of children differs from that of adults.	■ Gluteus maximus muscle (dorsal gluteal site) must not be used until the child has been walking for at least 1 year. ■ Vastus lateralis site is preferred for young children. ■ Amounts to be administered should be limited to no more than 1 to 2 mL for ventrogluteal site depending on muscle size. ■ The deltoid muscle is rarely used in young children except for the small amounts injected in some vaccines.
Intravenous	Veins are small and fragile.	■ Careful maintenance of sites is needed. ■ Common infusion sites include hands and feet, although scalp veins are sometimes used in infants.
	Fluid balance is critical.	■ Infusion pumps require frequent monitoring. ■ Syringe pumps are often used when minimal fluid is to be given over an extended period of time. ■ Central lines are commonly used for long-term intravenous medication therapy.

complementary care (see "Complementary Care: Reiki"). Refer to "Nursing Care Plan: The Child Undergoing Surgery."

PREPARATION FOR LONG-TERM CARE

When ill or injured children require long-term care, they are often transferred from an acute care hospital to a rehabilitation center or other long-term care facility. The rehabilitation phase of the treatment does not begin at the time of discharge from the acute care hospital but, instead, early in the hospitalization phase. The plan of care is instituted in the hospital, interventions and therapies are begun, and plans are made for continued care.

When it becomes apparent that a child will need long-term care, the healthcare team explores with the family the options and resources available to provide such care:

■ Home care with support services such as visiting nurses and physical therapists

■ A long-term care facility

■ A specialized rehabilitation center that can provide care for an extended period

COMPLEMENTARY CARE

REIKI

Reiki therapy is becoming an increasingly popular complementary modality throughout the United States. Reiki is a treatment modality classified as an energetic healing therapy and shares its foundational principles with other energy-based modalities such as therapeutic touch, polarity therapy, healing touch, and some forms of massage. Therapeutic touch and healing touch both have origins in the nursing profession (Kemper & Kelly, 2004). See our Companion Website at http://www.prenhall.com/london for more information regarding the origins of Reiki, and the training and licensing of Reiki practitioners.

Practitioners of Reiki use "laying on of hands" techniques to confer universal life energy to the client for the purpose of healing a wide variety of physical and psycho-spiritual problems. Hand positions during the Reiki treatment session correspond with the body's endocrine and lymphatic systems, major body organs, and the *chakra* system known to yoga and other Eastern healing practices. Although there is great need for further empiric research regarding the efficacy of Reiki, preliminary studies have documented relaxation response during a Reiki treatment. The relaxation response components measured after a Reiki treatment include a decrease in systolic blood pressure, decrease in pain, decrease in anxiety, and an overall feeling of well-being (Nield-Anderson & Ameling, 2001; Wardell & Engebretson, 2001). One small study also documented an increase in IgA measurements, which might suggest a biochemical reaction as well (Wardell & Engebretson, 2001). This direction of research may help identify the exact mechanism involved in Reiki healing.

Because Reiki is a noninvasive treatment modality fostering relaxation, it may help children undergoing painful or anxiety-producing procedures. Children often describe the Reiki practitioner's hands as "really warm" and seem to settle during a treatment.

The family should make the decision about which option will work best, considering the needs of the child, the financial implications, the roles and supports available to the family unit, and the resources available in the community. Guidelines to assist parents in evaluating rehabilitation centers are available from the Brain Injury Association. See the Companion Website for links to such resources. Nurses in acute care hospitals frequently coordinate services when transfer to another facility occurs. This involves giving information about the child's history, plan of care, and treatment to the new facility. Forms are available to assist the person responsible for coordinating the transfer. Families will need support and assistance in dealing with the transfer from the acute care setting to another facility.

PREPARATION FOR HOME CARE

Nurses play an important role in preparing the child and family for discharge home; this preparation starts early during the hospitalization. The nurse works with the social service department, home care agencies, and the family to plan for equipment, procedures, and other home care needs. Parents of newborns who have been hospitalized will need assistance to bond with and learn interaction skills with the baby in addition to assistance with physical care (Whitfield, 2003). Home care nurses collaborate with the hospital nurse and assist families to meet the child's healthcare needs.

ASSESSING THE CHILD IN PREPARATION FOR DISCHARGE

Discharge plans should begin early in the child's hospitalization. A healthcare team, including the physician, nurse, social worker, discharge planner, and family, works together to ensure a smooth transition home. An assessment of the family's ability to manage the child's care and of the appropriateness of the home for providing care should be made.

Children with multisystem problems may require home care involving specialized equipment and personnel. Early planning gives the family time to investigate health insurance benefits, support services in the community, and other needs before discharge.

When a child is to be discharged home, the school district should be contacted and plans for education made. This involves an assessment of the child by the school district and formulation of an **individualized education plan** (IEP). The IEP may include home tutors, specialized services from persons such as physical or speech therapists, or arrangements for transport of the child with a disability to the school and provisions for special medical care as needed. For each child with a chronic disability who is 14 years or older, an **individualized transition plan** focuses on assisting the individual in moving successfully from school into the community (Allen & Vessey, 2004).

Some common problems that interfere with successful discharge planning include financial concerns, the family's unavailability for teaching and planning, long distance between home and hospital, and poor communication and lack of teamwork among involved healthcare disciplines. Nurses should be alert to these potential problems from the initial contact with the child and family and should implement measures to deal with them.

PREPARING THE FAMILY FOR HOME CARE

The family may need to learn physical and rehabilitative procedures for the child's care. Short-term care may be necessary until the child regains full function. In other situations, care may be required throughout the child's life. This may involve measuring vital signs or determining blood glucose levels. For the child requiring complex long-term care, parents may need to learn about intra-

EVIDENCE-BASED NURSING

PREPARING FAMILIES TO PROVIDE HEALTHCARE FOR CHILDREN AT HOME

Problem

Children are often discharged from hospitals while still requiring complicated healthcare procedures, so parents need to learn how to perform these procedures safely. Parents may not be able to be in the hospital consistently during the hospitalization or they may not be as involved in the child's care as would be helpful for learning the needed skills.

Evidence

Using a qualitative approach, researchers interviewed families of 14 children hospitalized for a variety of chronic illnesses. Parents identified a lack of support by personnel when they were present in the hospital; they often felt in the way and did not want to disturb the routines of the unit. Parents reported that they were frequently not included in decision making about the child, and yet felt responsibility for managing the multiple needs of the child's condition once they returned home (Ygge & Arnetz, 2004). Other authors have noted that teaching families is often viewed as a short-term task, but that instead it is ongoing and needs to be integrated into all interactions to adequately prepare the family for discharge (London, 2004).

Implications

Preparing families for care of their children is a complex task, and the situation in the hospital is sometimes not conducive to teaching and learning. Nurses can support parents during rooming-in by making them comfortable and integrating them into discussions and decisions about the child's care; they are collaborators in all of the care involved. Nurses can also view every interaction as a teachable moment and constantly include teaching whenever a parent is present. Explain medications,

what assessments are being performed, and how this will all be adapted in the home situation. Provide resources for the responsibility the parent takes on as the child returns home, including phone numbers, parent support groups, reading material, and Internet sources. Ask parents what care they feel comfortable with and what they need more assistance to perform. Involve them in the decision about referral to home healthcare or a school nurse.

Critical Thinking

What conditions in the hospital will assist parents to feel welcome and part of the hospital routine? Is there a comfortable and relatively quiet place to sleep, a place to eat, and other needed comforts? How can parents become a part of rounds to their own child? What questions can they be asked? How can the nurse help to explain to parents the meaning of conversations that take place near the child by healthcare personnel? How can you adapt your teaching plan to include integration into every interaction with the parents? How can you record the teaching needs of parents so that other nurses can continue with needed information, demonstrations, and assessments? What techniques need to be part of discharge care so that parents leave with resources to get future questions answered as they take over total care of the child?

References

London, F. (2004). How to prepare families for discharge in the limited time available. *Pediatric Nursing, 30,* 212–214, 227.

Ygge, B. M., & Arnetz, J. E. (2004). A study of parental involvement in pediatric hospital care: Implications for clinical practice. *Journal of Pediatric Nursing, 19,* 217–223.

---

venous lines, medications, oxygen administration, or ventilators (Figure 40–14 ⊙).

Parents need to be taught how to use the equipment needed for the child's care and must show that they can use it correctly. They must be able to identify symptoms of distress and report them immediately to the healthcare provider. The education provided and the parents' ability to perform care are discussed with a visiting nurse or individual who manages the home care program. Parents should be encouraged to learn cardiopulmonary resuscitation. (Refer to "Nursing Considerations for the Child and Family in the Community" in Chapter 39. ∞)

Help parents explore options for respite. If they cannot provide daily care or need a break, they should be able to rely on others for a short period. Some agencies are available to provide respite care. Ongoing assistance may be needed to help families deal with financial, time, and other challenges. If parents must take a leave of absence from work to provide care for the child, inform them about the coverage provided by the Family Medical Leave Act (U.S. Department of Labor, 2004).

⊙ **FIGURE 40–14**

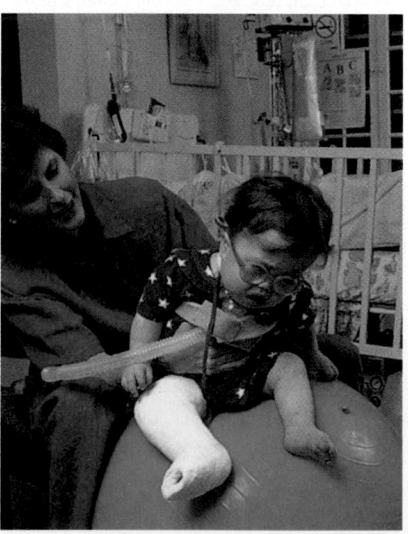

This child with chronic medical problems is being cared for at home. Are there any legal implications for the hospital and the nurse associated with the preparation of the child and family for home care?

PREPARING PARENTS TO ACT AS CASE MANAGERS

The family is an integral part of the plan of care for an ill or hospitalized child. The child with a chronic illness or an injury requiring long-term care will probably require the services of numerous healthcare personnel or healthcare agencies. One person needs to be identified as a **case manager** to coordinate healthcare and to prevent gaps and overlaps. In some hospitals nurses act as case managers. They may organize a patient care conference while the child with a chronic condition is hospitalized. Management goals are set and decisions are made about which healthcare provider or agency is responsible for helping the child meet each goal.

Parents can also be case managers. The parent as case manager coordinates medical care, hospital stays, and visits to specialists; meets with school district representatives to plan the individualized education program for the child; finds equipment, personnel, and other services for home care; and manages the child's overall care.

Nurses should strongly encourage parents who want to take over case management to do so. Help them learn the management skills required. Many community agencies such as social service or home health agencies hold workshops for parents managing the complex care of their children.

Critical Concept Review

LEARNING OBJECTIVES

CONCEPTS

Discuss the child's understanding of health and illness according to the child's psychosocial and developmental levels.

1. Infant:
   - Has no concept of illness. Distressed by separation from parent.
2. Toddler and preschooler:
   - Blames other people, events, or themselves for an illness. Distressed by parental separation and fear of body mutilation and change.
3. School-age child:
   - Understands basic reason for illness. Also understands body parts and functions. Fear their body will not return to normal after an illness.
4. Adolescent:
   - Understands cause of illness. Concerned with the effect of illness on body image. Concerned about modesty and privacy.

Recognize the effect of hospitalization on the child and family.

1. Disruption of usual routines.
2. Anxiety and fear:
   - Unknown or serious outcome.
   - Pain.
   - Financial difficulties.
   - Lack of family support.
   - Lack of community support.
3. Parents report increased satisfaction when family needs and preferences are considered.
4. Sibling difficulties:
   - Lack of parental attention.
   - Jealousy over attention given to sick child.
   - Lack of information about child who is ill.
   - Guilt over role in illness.
   - Anxiety and insecurity over changing roles.

Assess the family's risk and protective factors that will influence adaptation to hospitalization.

1. Alteration in family roles.
2. Additional, unplanned expenses.
3. Care of children left at home.
4. Knowledge of child's condition.
5. Community services needed at discharge.
6. Support groups available.
7. Persons available to support family.

(continued)

LEARNING OBJECTIVES	CONCEPTS

Identify several types of hospital units and the needs that children and families have in each unit.

1. Emergency units:
   - Family needs information about procedures and outcomes.
   - Have parents and child remain together as much as possible.
   - Identify the support system that family has available.
2. Intensive care:
   - Provide emotional support.
   - Explain purpose of treatments and machines.
   - Help parents hold and touch child.
   - Provide support and referral for services.
3. Pre-and postoperative areas:
   - Allow parents to be with child.
   - Prepare parents for what they will see.
4. Short-stay units:
   - Prepare child for admission.
   - Encourage family participation.
   - Keep family well-informed.
5. Isolation:
   - Encourage frequent family visits.
   - Help parents understand need for protective equipment.
6. Rehabilitation units:
   - Encourage parental involvement.
   - Explain relation to home care.

Identify methods that the child and family use to adapt to hospitalization.

1. Child life programs.
2. Rooming-in.
3. Therapeutic play.
4. Therapeutic recreation.

Describe types of therapeutic play and recreation used with hospitalized children.

1. Activities designed to help children work through feelings about illness:
   - Child will play with equipment and draw pictures about treatments.
2. Dramatic play:
   - Acting out experiences of healthcare encounters.
3. Pet therapy:
   - Time with pets helps to reduce anxiety in children.
4. Movie night or pizza party:
   - Provides socialization for adolescent.

Use knowledge of child and family response to hospitalization to plan nursing interventions to facilitate coping with hospitalization.

1. Provide tour of hospital unit, if possible.
2. Provide written materials explaining hospital policies and procedures.
3. Provide age-appropriate material to the child.
4. Allow child to play with examples of medical equipment.
5. Include parents and child in the establishment of a plan of care for the child.

CRITICAL THINKING IN ACTION

*View the **Critical Thinking in Action** video in Chapter 40 of the CD-ROM. Then, answer the questions that follow.*

Today the hospital is sponsoring an orientation day for a group of children preparing to have surgery. Each child is given a time to tour the surgery suite. One 8-year-old girl, Lauren, is extremely nervous about having a tonsillectomy. Both her parents are with her today and she clings to them. You decide to ask Lauren to draw a picture of a person. Lauren seems excited to do this and draws a person with a lot of detail, which, you analyze afterwards, demonstrates that she has a cognitive level of a 9-year-old. You next ask Lauren to describe what all the parts are in the human body. You ask her to describe what is inside them to see what she understands about the body. When she is asked about the head, she says, "There are gooey brains in there." When asked about the heart and what would happen if she didn't have a heart, she says, "A person would die in the hospital like grandpa." After hearing this comment you see it as a good opportunity to discuss her fears of the hospital. She is afraid she is going to die like her grandpa did when his heart stopped beating. You explain that her procedure is different than that of her grandpa. You read a book to Lauren entitled, "Why Am I Going to the Hospital?" by Lyle Stuart. Lauren appears to relax and asks to see the place for surgery. You let Lauren dress up like a surgeon, touch the instruments, and give the family the tour. You offer more suggestions about books they could read before coming back for surgery and suggest getting a doll to practice procedures on at home. You provide phone numbers for the parents if they have additional questions.

1. Describe the role of a child life specialist.
2. Besides the types of techniques used with Lauren to help her deal with her feelings based on her age, what are examples of other techniques that can be used?
3. Describe the concept of rooming in.
4. After surgery, what assessments are needed to monitor Lauren for signs of infection?

MEDIALINK   www.prenhall.com/london

- NCLEX-RN® Review, case studies, and other interactive resources for this chapter can be found on the Companion Website at http://www.prenhall.com/london. Click on "Chapter 40" to select the activities for this chapter.

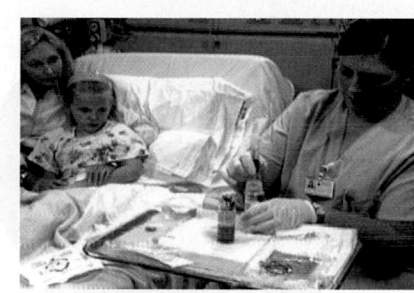

- For animations, more NCLEX-RN® Review questions, and an audio glossary, access the accompanying CD-ROM in this textbook.

REFERENCES

Allen, P. J., & Vessey, J. A. (2004). *Primary care of the child with a chronic condition* (4th ed.). St. Louis, MO. Mosby.

American Academy of Pediatrics, Committee on Hospital Care. (2000). Child life services. *Pediatrics, 106,* 1156–1159.

Ball, J. W. (1998). *Pediatric patient teaching guides.* St. Louis, MO: Mosby-Yearbook.

Bibace, R., & Walsh, M. (1981). Children's conception of illness. In R. Bibace & M. Walsh (Eds.), *Children's conceptions of health, illness and bodily function.* San Francisco: Jossey-Bass.

Bowlby, J. (1960). Separation anxiety. *International Journal of Psychoanalysis, 41*(2/3), 89–113.

Bricher, G. (2000). Children in the hospital: Issues of power and vulnerability. *Pediatric Nursing, 26,* 277–282.

De Pasquale, S. (1999, November). Serious play. *Johns Hopkins Magazine,* 30–36.

Emergency Nurses Association. (2001). *Family presence at the bedside during invasive procedures and resuscitation.* Retrieved June 13, 2005, from http://www.ena.org/about/position/PDFs/FamilyPresence.PDF

Gellert, E. (1962). Children's conception of the content and functions of the human body. *Genetic Psychology Monographs, 65,* 293–405.

Gusella, J. L., Ward, A. M., & Butler, G. S. (1998). The experience of hospitalized adolescents:

How well do we meet their developmental needs? *Children's Health Care, 27,* 131–145.

Kemper, K. J., & Kelly, E. A. (2004). Treating children with therapeutic and healing touch. *Pediatric Annals, 33*(4), 248–252.

LaMontagne, L. L. (2000). Effects of surgery type and attention focus on children's coping. *Nursing Research, 49,* 245–252.

Lassetter, J. H., & Baldwin, J. H. (2005). Improving the experience of hospitalization for Hawaiian children on the mainland through cultural sensitivity to Hawaiian ways of healing. *Journal of Pediatric Nursing, 20,* 170–176.

London, F. (2004). How to prepare families for discharge in the limited time available. *Pediatric Nursing, 30,* 212–214, 227.

Marino, B. L., & Marino, E. K. (2000). Practice applications of research. Parents' report of children's hospital care: What it means for your practice. *Pediatric Nursing, 26,* 195–198.

Melnyk, B. M. (2000). Intervention studies involving parents of hospitalized young children: An analysis of the past and future recommendations. *Journal of Pediatric Nursing, 15,* 4–13.

Miller, M. R., & Zhan, C. (2004). Pediatric patient safety in hospitals: A national picture in 2000. *Pediatrics, 113,* 1741–1746.

Nield-Anderson, L., & Ameling, A. (2001). Reiki. A complementary therapy for nursing prac-

tice. *Journal of Psychosocial Nursing Mental Health Services, 39*(4), 42–49.

Proctor, E. K., Morrow-Howell, N., Kitchen, A., & Wang, Y. T. (1995). Pediatric discharge planning: Complications, efficiency, and adequacy. *Social Work in Health Care, 22,* 1–18.

Ramsey, C. A. (2000). Storytelling can be a valuable teaching aid. *Association of Operating Room Nurses Journal, 72,* 497–499.

Rode, D., Capitulo, K. L., Fishman, M., & Holden, G. (1998). The therapeutic use of technology. *American Journal of Nursing, 98*(12), 32–35.

U.S. Department of Labor. (2004). *Family and Medical Leave Act.* http://www.dol.gov/esa/shd/ fmla/ Retrieved 1/25/05.

Vessey, J. A. (2003). Children's psychological responses to hospitalization. *Annual Review of Nursing Research, 21,* 173–201.

Wardell, D. W., & Engebretson, J. (2001). Biological correlates of Reiki touch healing. *Journal of Advanced Nursing, 33*(4), 439–445.

Whitfield, M. F. (2003). Psychosocial effects of intensive care on infants and families after discharge. *Seminars in Neonatology 8,* 185–193.

Ygge, B. M., & Arnetz, J. E. (2004). A study of parental involvement in pediatric hospital care: Implications for clinical practice. *Journal of Pediatric Nursing, 19,* 217–223.

The Child with a Life-Threatening Condition and End-of-Life Care

It all happened so fast. We didn't even see the car coming. Next thing I knew, we were in the emergency room talking about abdominal and head injuries. Now we are in the intensive care unit, and I'm worried because Alexa is still unconscious and on a ventilator. It was helpful for the nurse to tell me that even though Alexa couldn't respond it was good to talk to her, because she will probably hear me and be comforted.

—*Mother of Alexa, 6*

LEARNING OBJECTIVES

- Describe the child's responses to having a life-threatening illness or injury by developmental level.

- Discuss the responses of parents and siblings when the child has a life-threatening illness or injury.

- Describe the coping mechanisms used by the child and family in response to stress.

- Develop a nursing care plan for the child with a life-threatening illness or injury.

- Identify the physiologic and psychologic changes that occur in the dying child.

- Develop a nursing care plan to provide family-centered care for the dying child and family.

- Describe the development of the child's concept of death.

- Describe the responses of nurses caring for children who die.

MEDIALINK www.prenhall.com/london

CD-ROM

Videos:
 Involving Family in NICU Setting
 Presenting Bad News to Families
 Parental Reactions to Death of a Child
Audio Glossary
NCLEX-RN® Review

Companion Website

MediaLink Applications:
 Case Study: Newborn in NICU with
  Bronchopulmonary Dysplasia
 Care Plan: Adolescent in PICU for a Brain Injury
 Case Study: Loss of a Schoolmate
 Family-Centered Care Plan: Death of a Child
 Helping Families Grieve
 Preparing the Family for Hospice
 Complementary Care: Use of Music Therapy in Grief
 Grief Resources for Nurses
Thinking Critically
NCLEX-RN® Review

W hat do children like Alexa face after admission to the pediatric intensive care unit (PICU)? What nursing strategies can help a critically ill or injured child cope with the experience? What stressors will families face during the child's hospitalization? What interventions could help them in this crisis? What interventions are needed when the child is dying? This chapter will give guidance about providing supportive care to critically ill and injured or dying children like Alexa and to their families.

The intense emotional and physical demands placed on the critically ill or injured child present a challenge to nurses' attempts to provide developmentally appropriate care. The child's parents and siblings are confronted with a stressful situation. A family-centered model of nursing practice offers a framework for performing interventions that help to minimize stress and enhance coping by parents, siblings, and the ill or injured child.

LIFE-THREATENING ILLNESS OR INJURY

A threat to a child's life may be expected, as in a chronic illness or progressive disabling disease, or unexpected, as in an unintentional injury. How children, parents, and siblings cope with the threat will depend on the anticipated or unanticipated nature of the event and the conditions surrounding the child's admission to the hospital.

When death results from a chronic disease or terminal illness, the child and family have time to adjust to the impending death. Parents can become involved in the child's therapy as integral members of the treatment team. Emergency admission for an acute illness or unintentional injury, however, brings with it sudden stressors as the child and family are thrust into an unfamiliar environment, confronted with frightening or invasive procedures, and faced with an uncertain outcome.

Nursing care of children and families coping with specific chronic diseases or terminal illnesses such as cancer, cystic fibrosis, or muscular dystrophy is discussed elsewhere in this book. The following discussion focuses on care of children with life-threatening illnesses or injuries and care of the dying child.

CHILD'S EXPERIENCE

Admission to the hospital, emergency department, or PICU is one of the most frightening experiences a child can have. The critically ill child may appear extremely anxious and fearful, or withdrawn, solemn, and preoccupied with his or her physical condition. The illness or injury often brings pain, decreases energy, and changes the child's level of consciousness. Younger children may be unable to understand what is happening to them. The PICU environment appears overwhelming, fast paced, and frightening. The child's normal sleep patterns can be disrupted because of the lack of day–night patterns in many intensive care units (Figure 41–1 ●). Being cared for by strangers produces anxiety in the child. The child's limited ability to move intensifies feelings of powerlessness and vulnerability. Children admitted to a PICU are at risk for post-traumatic stress disorder (Melnyk, Small, & Carno, 2004). See Chapter 54. ∞

NURSING PRACTICE

Seriously injured children requiring hospitalization for injury are at risk for post-traumatic stress disorder (PTSD). Variables predictive of PTSD include child acute stress, parental stress, and the degree of the psychologic trauma exposure. One study reported 12.5% of injured children met diagnostic criteria for PTSD at one month after the injury (Daviss, Mooney, Racusin et al., 2000).

FIGURE 41–1

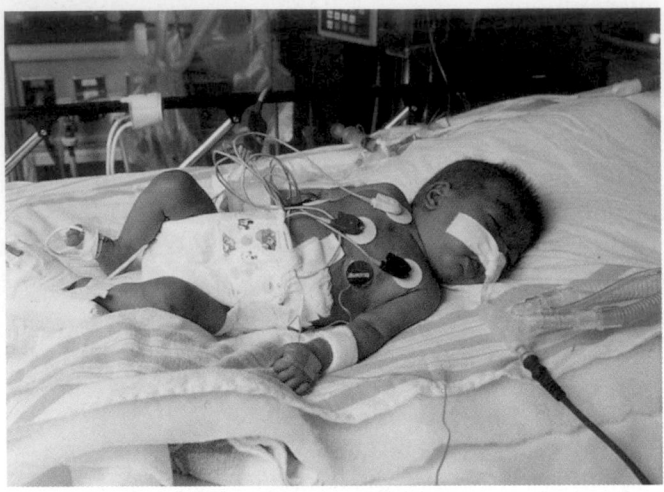

Jooti feels pain, hears noises, has her sleep disrupted, and has limited mobility because of all the equipment attached to her.

Children's responses to stress are influenced by their developmental levels, past experiences, types of illness, coping mechanisms, and available emotional support. Nurses need to take into consideration how the child's developmental level and coping skills will influence his or her ability to deal with the PICU experience. Successful coping can provide the child with the skills to handle difficult situations in the future.

STRESSORS TO THE CHILD

The four most significant stressors for hospitalized children of all ages are (1) separation from parents or the primary caretaker; (2) loss of self-control, autonomy, and privacy; (3) being subjected to multiple painful and invasive procedures; and (4) fear of body injury and disfigurement. Table 41–1 highlights key stressors of hospitalization for children at each developmental stage.

In addition to dealing with these stressors, the critically ill child experiences an intense emotional and physical threat to his or her well-being.

An unanticipated admission places the child at emotional risk for several reasons, including the lack of preparation for the experience, the uncertainty and unpredictability of events that follow, the unfamiliarity of the environment, and the heightened anxiety of parents. An admission for exacerbation of a disease such as cystic fibrosis or leukemia can provoke feelings of depression or hopelessness. See Chapter 40 for responses to hospitalization by age group. ∞

COPING MECHANISMS

Coping is cognitive and behavioral responses to manage specific internal and external demands that exceed a per-

GROWTH AND DEVELOPMENT

Coping behavior is influenced by maturation, cognitive development (increased attention span, problem-solving ability, and understanding of cause and effect), and increased impulse control. Young children use more behavioral strategies and ventilate feelings (Ryan-Wenger, 1996).

son's resources, enabling the person to solve problems and to respond emotionally. The child may mirror the parents' behaviors and responses, which may help or hinder the child's response to stress. The child's temperament, previous coping experiences, and availability of **support systems** all combine to influence his or her ability to cope with the current experience.

The nature and severity of the illness and an emergency admission to the hospital stress a child's coping capabilities. Defense mechanisms displayed by children in these situations include regression, or return to an earlier behavior (a common reaction to stress), denial, repression (involuntary forgetting), postponement, and bargaining.

THINKING CRITICALLY

PICU STRESSORS

The PICU receives a call from a community hospital requesting transport for an unstable 12-year-old boy who is in status epilepticus. Jeremiah has a seizure disorder controlled with medications, but several days ago he decided to stop taking his medications. So many seizure medications have been given in the community hospital emergency department to stop Jeremiah's seizures that he is now unconscious and must be intubated to maintain his airway until the medications wear off.

The transport team is in the air within minutes and arrives at the rural community hospital 25 minutes later. They stabilize Jeremiah and receive reports from the medical and nursing teams, meet briefly with his parents, answer a few questions, and are back in the air.

Jeremiah is admitted directly to the PICU, where the unit team has been preparing for his arrival. He is connected to cardiorespiratory and noninvasive blood pressure monitors, while his existing intravenous lines and endotracheal tube are evaluated for patency. Team members quickly complete a head-to-toe assessment. The unit clerk enters Jeremiah's room to say that his parents have arrived in the emergency department and are being escorted to the PICU.

What stressors do children like Jeremiah face after sudden admission to the PICU? What age-specific strategies can you use to help him cope with the experience? What stressors will parents face during the initial period when you work with them? How can you intervene to help them in this crisis?

TABLE 41–1 ✤ Stressors of Hospitalization for Children at Various Developmental Stages

Developmental Stages	Responses	Nursing Implications
Infant		
Separation anxiety Stranger anxiety Painful, invasive procedures Immobilization Sleep deprivation, sensory overload	Sleep–awake cycle disrupted Feeding routines disrupted Displays excessive irritability	Encourage parental presence Adhere to infant's home routine as much as possible Utilize topical anesthetics or preprocedural sedation as prescribed Promote a quiet environment and reduce excess stimuli
Toddler		
Separation anxiety Loss of self-control Immobilization Painful, invasive procedures Bodily injury or mutilation Fear of the dark	Is frightened if forced to lie supine Associates pain with punishment Wonders why parents don't come to the rescue	Encourage parental presence Allow choices when possible Utilize topical anesthetics or preprocedural sedation as prescribed Explain all procedures and equipment used Provide a night-light or flashlight
Preschooler		
Separation anxiety and fear of abandonment Loss of self-control Bodily injury or mutilation Painful, invasive procedures Fear of the dark, ghosts, and monsters	Displays difficulty separating reality from fantasy Demonstrates withdrawal, projection, aggression, regression Fears body parts will leak out when skin is not intact Fears that tubes are permanent Fears ghosts and monsters	Encourage parental presence Allow choices when possible Utilize topical anesthetics or preprocedural sedation as prescribed Explain all procedures Provide a night-light or flashlight
School-Age Child		
Loss of control Loss of privacy and control over bodily functions Bodily injury Painful, invasive procedures Fear of death	Displays increased sensitivity to the environment Demonstrates detailed recall of events to self and other patients	Encourage parental participation Allow the child choices when possible Explain all procedures and offer reassurance Utilize topical anesthetics or preprocedural sedation as prescribed Encourage peer interaction
Adolescent		
Loss of control Fear of altered body image, disfigurement, disability, and death Separation from peer group Loss of privacy and identity	Displays denial, regression, withdrawal, intellectualization, projection, displacement	Include the adolescent in the plan of care Encourage discussion of fears and anxieties Explain all procedures Ask the adolescent his or her desire for parental involvement Encourage peer interaction

NURSING MANAGEMENT

NURSING ASSESSMENT AND DIAGNOSIS

Nursing assessment involves, in addition to physiologic parameters, skilled observation of the child's psychosocial and emotional needs. It is important for the nurse to understand normal psychosocial and cognitive development in order to plan developmentally appropriate interventions. Assessment should include the child's response to illness, the environment, coping strategies, and the need for information and support.

The accompanying "Nursing Care Plan" includes common nursing diagnoses for the child coping with a critical illness or injury. The following nursing diagnoses may also be appropriate:

- *Impaired Verbal Communication* related to the effects of endotracheal intubation and mechanical ventilation
- *Spiritual Distress* related to the crisis of illness or suffering
- *Disturbed Sleep Pattern* related to circadian asynchrony, excessive stimulation, pain, and anxiety caused by the critical care unit environment

NURSING CARE PLAN

THE CHILD COPING WITH A LIFE-THREATENING ILLNESS OR INJURY

Intervention	Rationale	Expected Outcome
1. Nursing Diagnosis: Anxiety (Child) related to separation from parents, foreign environment, strangers as caretakers, invasive procedures		

NIC Priority Intervention:		**NOC Suggested Outcome:**
Anxiety reduction: Minimizing apprehension, dread, foreboding, or uneasiness related to an unidentified source of anticipated danger		**Anxiety control:** Ability to eliminate or reduce feelings of apprehension and tension from unidentified source

Goal: The child will exhibit or express an increased sense of security.

■ Encourage parents to remain at the bedside (open visitation) and to participate in the child's care by touching, talking to, reading to, and singing to the child.	■ Presence of parents is comforting to the child.	The child appears more relaxed and acknowledges parents' presence. Behavioral manifestations of anxiety are absent.
■ Talk with the child. Avoid discussions at bedside that the child should not overhear.	■ The child may overhear and remember, even if unconscious.	
■ Offer to arrange a visit from the chaplain or other spiritual support.	■ Spiritual support often provides comfort and sustenance in a time of crisis.	
■ Provide the child with developmentally appropriate explanations when possible. Encourage the child to ask questions and express concerns.	■ Information reduces anxiety and builds trust.	
■ Prepare child in advance for procedures using developmentally appropriate techniques.	■ Preparation decreases anxiety related to the unknown.	
■ Make the child's bedside more personal and familiar by encouraging parents to bring in security objects, family photos, and favorite toys from home.	■ Security objects decrease foreignness of hospital environment. The child derives comfort from presence of personal items.	
■ Involve the child in play appropriate to developmental age (see Chapter 33 ∞).	■ Play provides familiarity, decreases fantasy, and provides motor activity.	
■ Provide care using a primary nursing care model.	■ Consistency in caregivers helps to build the child's trust.	

2. Nursing Diagnosis: Powerlessness (Moderate) related to inability to communicate, and control relinquished to the healthcare team		

NIC Priority Intervention:		**NOC Suggested Outcome:**
Mutual goal setting: Collaborating with patient to identify and prioritize care goals, then developing a plan for achieving those goals		**Participation: Healthcare decisions:** Personal involvement in selecting and evaluating healthcare options

Goal: The child or adolescent will have an increased sense of control over the situation.

■ Provide opportunities for choices when possible. Encourage participation in self-care.	■ Such opportunities provide sense of control and autonomy through decision making.	The child or adolescent expresses satisfaction over ability to control some elements of situation.
■ Prepare the child or adolescent in advance (timing dependent on developmental level) for procedures. Describe the sensations that will be experienced. Allow some choice in timing or method of pain relief.	■ Information reduces anxiety and fear associated with the unknown and helps the child maintain self-control.	

NURSING CARE PLAN—continued

THE CHILD COPING WITH A LIFE-THREATENING ILLNESS OR INJURY

Intervention	Rationale	Expected Outcome
2. Nursing Diagnosis: Powerlessness (Moderate) related to inability to communicate, and control relinquished to the healthcare team (continued)		
■ Provide routines for the child both within a 24-hour period and for scheduled care. Tell the child before (timing dependent upon developmental level), repeat explanation of why procedure is necessary, complete procedure in a consistent manner, and offer praise or a special story when completed. When possible, incorporate rituals from home.	■ Self-control is maintained through rituals.	
■ Encourage play as a means of expressing feelings.	■ Play is a normal activity for children and provides freedom of expression.	
■ Provide other means of communication to the intubated child (e.g., a word board or finger board).	■ Maintaining communication provides autonomy and independence for the child.	
■ For the child requiring restraints, use as seldom as possible, provide appropriate explanations, and release at regular intervals. Wrapping IV lines well and using armboards can help maintain lines and avoid restraints.	■ Release from restraints helps diminish the sense of powerlessness that accompanies their use.	
3. Nursing Diagnosis: Acute Pain related to injuries, invasive procedures, surgery		
NIC Priority Intervention: **Pain management:** Alleviation of pain or a reduction in pain to a level of comfort that is acceptable to the patient		**NOC Suggested Outcome:** **Comfort level:** Feelings of physical and psychologic ease
Goal: The child will experience reduced pain and improved comfort.		
■ Assess the child's pain: location, intensity, what makes it better or worse.	■ Assessment provides baseline information from which a plan of care can be developed.	The child experiences a perceived or actual improvement in comfort level.
■ If appropriate, use pain assessment scale (see Chapter 42 ∞).	■ Use of scale provides continuity and consistency in monitoring of the child's pain.	
■ Provide optimal pain relief with prescribed analgesics. Provide comfort measures—position changes, back rubs, etc. Provide diversional activities as appropriate or possible. Incorporate the family in pain relief modality.	■ Physiologic and psychologic methods of pain control can be used in combination to maximally improve outcomes.	

■ *Deficient Diversional Activity* related to forced inactivity

■ *Hopelessness* related to critical illness, deteriorating physical condition, or prolonged activity restrictions creating isolation

■ *Anticipatory Grieving* related to potential loss of body function or impending death of self

PLANNING AND IMPLEMENTATION

Nursing care focuses on promoting a sense of trust, providing education about the illness or injury, preparing the child for procedures, facilitating the use of play, and promoting a sense of control. General care for the child in the PICU may include the following: frequent physiologic assessment, pain and sedation management, nutritional support, medication administration, managing multiple IV lines and pumps, maintaining ventilatory and hemodynamic monitoring equipment, and wound care.

Provide Psychosocial Care for the Child

Children admitted to a PICU need support for the stressful experience. Children often feel and hear even when unconscious, so touch and verbal interchanges are important. Nurses play a key role in providing developmentally appropriate support to the child. Nursing interventions are directed at building a trusting relationship, minimizing the stressors experienced by the child, and promoting coping. Ongoing reassessment of progress in meeting the child's needs is critical. The accompanying "Nursing Care Plan" summarizes care for the child coping with a life-threatening illness or injury.

Promote a Sense of Security

For children of all ages, feeling secure depends on a sense of physical and psychologic safety. A sense of physical security is difficult to attain within the PICU because of the constant barrage of procedures that are part of the child's treatment plan. The presence of the parents provides the best sense of psychologic safety. An open visitation policy that enables parents to be at the bedside is optimal. Including parents as partners in the child's care provides comfort and reassurance to the child. Children whose parents have high anxiety levels pick up their parents' emotional cues and become more anxious. Consistency of staff is invaluable in developing familiarity and a trusting relationship with the child.

Personalizing the child's bedside can promote comfort and a sense of security. Pictures from home, a favorite blanket or toy, music tapes, or posters can make the environment friendlier and more familiar to the child (Figure 41–2 ●). Religious or spiritual icons may also provide psychologic support.

Provide Education About the Illness or Injury and Prepare the Child for Procedures

A child's ability to understand the cause of the illness and its therapy depends on his or her cognitive abilities. Help younger children to understand that illness and hospitalization are not a punishment.

Preparation for procedures is important at all ages, even for the unconscious or sedated child. Toddlers will benefit from being talked to, soothed, and touched during and after the procedure. Provide preschoolers, school-age children, and adolescents with an explanation of the sensations they can expect to experience (temperature, vibrations, sounds, smells, tastes, sight). (See Chapter 40. ∞)

● **FIGURE 41–2**

By their very nature, PICUs are ominous and sterile. To lessen this effect, it can help to personalize the child's space. Being there with the child and parent, answering questions, or just talking can be a comfort to both.

Facilitate the Use of Play

The use of play is important in alleviating stress and helping children to prepare for procedures. It is also another way for the nurse to assess the child's developmental level. Therapeutic play adds familiarity, diminishes fantasies, provides motor activity, and helps the child develop a sense of mastery (see Chapter 40 ∞). Children who are immobilized by tubes and restraints can still feel a sense of accomplishment, for example, by completing a puzzle, even if the nurse points to each piece and responds when the child, through nods and gestures, indicates where it should be placed. Play can help children work through a painful situation, making it more tolerable.

Promote a Sense of Control

Children between toddlerhood and adolescence experience a loss of control during a life-threatening illness. This loss of control may be related to the body, emotions, normal routines, or privacy. Nursing interventions should promote a sense of control over these areas.

Give the child choices whenever possible. Even the simple choice of which color gown to wear can help the child feel in control. Scheduling routine activities and treatments at the same time each day adds predictability and lessens anxiety. Limited mobility and the use of restraints, although sometimes necessary, contribute to the child's sense of powerlessness.

Physical immobilizers are sometimes used in children with altered consciousness to prevent the unintentional removal of technologic devices or equipment. The Joint Commission on Accreditation of Healthcare Organizations requires that hospitals have policies and procedures for the use of restraints or immobilizers. If immobilizers must be used, plan to release them regularly for short periods. Restrain all children as little as possible, and explain the rationale for immobilizers, emphasizing that they are not a punishment (see Skills 7–1 to 7–6 **SKILLS**). Provide diversional activities for the child, for example, by reading stories, playing music, or watching videotapes (see Chapter 40 ∞).

Enhance the child's coping skills by teaching the child and family a combination of relaxation, visual imagery, or distraction techniques, and comforting self-talk phrases, such as "This will be over soon. If I stay calm, it will be all right. It will be over faster and then I can do something fun." Help the parents become the child's coping coaches.

EVALUATION

Expected outcomes of nursing care include the following:

- A trusting relationship is developed with the child and family.
- The child's social interactions, coping, and growth and development are promoted through diversional activities.
- The child's and family's coping is promoted through education and preparation for procedures.

PARENTS' EXPERIENCE

The uncertainty and unpredictability of a child's life-threatening illness or injury challenge a family's coping and stability. Families will display many different reactions and coping strategies. Children who are hospitalized for a critical illness cannot be adequately cared for if their families' needs are not met. Not only will parents find it difficult to support the child if their own needs are not met, but they also can transmit their anxiety to the child, who then becomes even more anxious.

WHAT MAKES A PROBLEM A CRISIS?

A **family crisis** occurs when a family encounters a problem that seems insurmountable and with which the family cannot cope in its usual ways. The critical care environment and the implications of a life-threatening illness or injury are far removed from the everyday experiences of most families. The unfamiliarity of the environment and the uncertainty and seriousness of the illness or injury create a crisis for the family.

Unexpected illness or injury adds another dimension of stress, since families have little time to prepare for the experience. A sudden admission threatens family integrity, causing enormous stress and separation from loved ones. The interruption of the unique parent-child relationship can be more stressful to parents than the physical PICU environment. Stresses are intensified when divorce, separation, and stepparenting are involved. Other current family stresses such as financial problems, long distance from home to hospital, or another family member with an illness can add to the state of crisis. See Chapter 39 for a discussion on family assessment and family resiliency. ∞

REACTIONS TO LIFE-THREATENING ILLNESS OR INJURY

Parents typically progress through stages that might include shock and disbelief; anger and guilt; deprivation and loss; anticipatory waiting; and readjustment or mourning.

Shock and Disbelief

The universal reaction of parents is shock and disbelief. As the familiar is disrupted, parents experience a loss of control, an inability to regain their bearings, and feelings of immobility. The hospital environment, emergency department, or PICU may seem unreal. The emotions parents experience initially are intensified by the physical appearance of their child (particularly after a major injury); the presence of monitors, tubing, and equipment; and the actual injury or illness. As the mother of a 5-year-old trauma patient said, "I felt distanced, in a daze, in and out of it that first day after the accident."

Shock and disbelief begin in the first few moments after hearing the "news" and can last for days. The shock helps postpone the full impact of the crisis. For most parents, however, the overwhelming sense of shock passes during the first 24 hours. During this period, parents grope for answers and explanations about the illness or injury. Information must be repeated many times to parents, since in this stage they are often unable to assimilate information easily.

Anger and Guilt

Anger and guilt surface as parents become more aware of their child's illness or injury. Their anger may be directed toward themselves, each other, healthcare providers, or other children or parents, as in the case of a motor vehicle crash involving a group of teenagers. Parents may also be angry with their child. This anger may be a result of injuries the child sustained when breaking known rules such as drinking and driving, playing with matches, or riding a bike without a helmet. Lastly, the anger may not be directed at anyone specifically. Injuries caused by natural disasters such as an earthquake, flood, or hurricane provoke just as much anger as those that result from the actions of people. This may create a challenge to the parents' spiritual beliefs.

Parents typically react to their child's illness or injury with some degree of guilt. This reaction may be magnified in the PICU environment. The fact that the guilt usually has no basis in real events does not lessen the feeling. A question parents frequently ask at this stage is, "Why not me instead of my child?" Parents' feelings of guilt may have one of two causes:

1. *They may feel responsible for causing the illness or injury.* Statements such as, "If only I hadn't sent him to the store on his bike, this wouldn't have happened," or, from the father of a 2-year-old who nearly drowned, "Maybe if I hadn't been working, he would have been in my care and this wouldn't have happened," reflect feelings of guilt for causing or failing to prevent the injury.

2. *They may feel guilty about not noticing the onset of an illness or disregarding earlier symptoms of an illness.* The mother of a 1-year-old with meningitis repeatedly said, "I shouldn't have waited so long to take her to the doctor!"

Deprivation and Loss

As the shock slowly recedes, parents enter a stage of deprivation and loss related to their parental role. Within minutes or hours, parents have gone from the familiar role of being a parent of a healthy child to the unexpected and unfamiliar role of being a parent of a critically ill child. Parents have compared this deprivation and loss to that experienced when a family member dies.

Parents' difficulties and ambivalence in releasing to strangers a part of their responsibility as the child's primary caretakers can threaten their self-esteem and self-control. Moreover, if parents cannot participate in the child's care, they may feel helpless or worthless.

Anticipatory Waiting

Once the child's condition is stabilized and survival seems likely, parents often move into a period of anticipatory waiting. This stage is characterized as "life suspended in time." Parents spend a great deal of time waiting: for test results, for explanations, for their child to become conscious, or for surgery to be over. Parents may fear leaving the area because they may miss an important procedure, physician visit, or decisions or changes in treatment. Lack of mobility decreases the parents' use of typical coping mechanisms, so anxiety and the sense of powerlessness may increase. Pagers provided to family members of critically ill children allow them to take breaks away from the child's bedside but know they can be quickly reached when needed (Gavaghan & Carroll, 2002). The use of pagers and cellular phones can decrease feelings of frustration and anger associated with arriving at the bedside to find that there has been a change in the child's condition (Griffin, 2003).

Parents may have a preoccupation with medical details. During this period, parents may ask questions about the long-term effects of the illness or injury on the child, about the potential for brain damage, or about the need for additional surgeries. Parents may place demands on staff and be frustrated when the child's progress is slow.

Readjustment or Mourning

The last stage that parents experience is readjustment or mourning. Readjustment is experienced as the child recovers, improves steadily, and prepares for transfer and discharge. In contrast, parents of the child who dies reenter the cycle of emotions characteristic of grief. Parents also mourn when the child remains seriously ill or unresponsive, when the outcome remains uncertain for an extended period, or when long-term care is required.

Table 41–2 lists the most important needs of parents during a child's critical illness or injury.

NURSING MANAGEMENT

NURSING ASSESSMENT AND DIAGNOSIS

Nurses who work with families of critically ill children have a unique opportunity to help them adapt and to promote family functioning. Begin by assessing the family's reaction to the illness, coping skills, stressors, and needs. See Chapter 39. ∞ This initial assessment provides a baseline of information for developing a care plan and strategies to meet the psychosocial as well as physiologic needs of families.

Several nursing diagnoses may apply to parents who are dealing with their child's critical illness or injury. Examples include the following:

- *Interrupted Family Processes* related to the impact of a critically ill child on the family system
- *Spiritual Distress* related to the child's critical illness, suffering, or death
- *Disabled Family Coping* related to the child's severe or fatal illness
- *Fatigue* related to extreme stress, sleep deprivation, and crisis
- *Anticipatory Grieving* related to potential death of the child or loss of body functions
- *Readiness for Enhanced Family Coping* related to constructive crisis management

PLANNING AND IMPLEMENTATION

Nursing care focuses on providing information and building trust, promoting parental involvement, providing for

TABLE 41–2 ❖ Parental Needs During Hospitalization of a Critically Ill or Injured Child

Information (the most important identified need)
- Information and frequent updates about the child's condition. Repeat the information and provide other materials frequently as parents forget or cannot concentrate on details due to stress.
- Explanations they can understand about the child's condition, equipment being used, and procedures of care.
- Discussion with a physician or care coordinator daily.
- General information about unit policies, team members, phone numbers, etc.

Proximity
- Permission to remain at the bedside.
- Permission to touch and speak with the child.
- Open, flexible visiting hours.

Reestablishment of the parental control
- Recognition as important to the child's recovery.
- Recognition as the decision maker of the child's treatment options.

Participation in the child's care
- Performance of care (bathing, diaper changes, feeding, range of motion exercises, massages, hair care).
- Provision of comfort measures (reading, singing, telling stories, touching, talking).
- Explanation of equipment and procedures to the child to decrease the child's fears.

Confidence in the treatment plan and caregivers
- Continuity in staffing and healthcare contacts.
- Evidence that staff care about the child.
- Assurance that the child is receiving appropriate treatment and pain management.

Psychologic support
- Acknowledgment that the situation is difficult.
- Help to focus on the positive or unchanged aspects of the child's appearance.
- Rest and nutrition to maintain physical resources necessary for coping.
- Space and privacy as needed.
- Hope—an essential component of coping.
- Choice of other family members to be present.
- Preparation for responses of siblings and the long-term emotional responses of the pediatric patient.

---

parents' physical and emotional needs, facilitating positive staff–parent relationships and communication, and maintaining or strengthening family support systems. A family-centered approach will help meet the needs of families, minimize stress, and enhance family coping. See Table 1–1 in Chapter 1. ∞ The challenge to nurses is to blend and balance technology with caring.

Provide Information and Build Trust

The information given to parents must be provided frequently and accurately. Deliver information on the child's illness, condition, and plan of care in a manner and language readily understandable to parents. Upon admission, parents need to be given an idea of what to expect in the days ahead and prepared for special procedures or major changes in therapy that may become necessary. Parents and siblings also need to be prepared before they see the child the first time. Tell them what tubes and monitors are present and how the child will look and react.

Honesty in discussions with parents is extremely important. If parents feel misled or that information is being withheld, a trusting relationship will be impossible. Informed parents, however, will feel that they are active participants in decision making and care planning for their child. Trust is facilitated when parents believe that the staff truly cares about the child and sees him or her as an individual, special child.

NURSING PRACTICE

Explain to the child and parents, in easy-to-understand terms, the purpose of equipment that is being used. Answer alarms quickly. Follow with an explanation of why alarms sound.

Parents also need a sense of hope regarding their child's illness to help them cope. Focus on the positives as the child progresses through the different phases of the critical illness.

Promote Parental Involvement

An important role of nurses is to encourage and support parents in their parenting role. The parents' place when possible is at the bedside—their very presence can comfort the child, minimize fears, and reduce the child's distress during invasive procedures. They provide continuity and may notice subtle condition changes that a newly assigned nurse may miss. Throughout the child's hospitalization, parents will continue to need reassurance and encouragement. Open visitation by parents is important to maintain their parenting role.

Participation in care of the child helps parents cope with the child's life-threatening illness or injury (Katz, 2002). Encourage family member involvement in the care of the infant or child. The parents gain a sense of control over the situation and a sense of empowerment (Sydnor-Greenberg & Dokken, 2000). Parents who do not remain with their child at the bedside may feel undervalued (Griffin, 2003). Giving parents a role at the bedside, such as providing personal care, is one way to promote involvement.

Family Presence During Resuscitation and Invasive Procedures

Many hospitals are implementing policies that permit families to be present during resuscitation and invasive procedures. Some parents who choose to witness a child's resuscitation express that it was important to know that everything possible was done to help the child. When parents are permitted to be present, a support person is with them and these steps are usually followed (Levetown, 2004):

1. Prior to entering the room, the parents are informed about the environment, equipment near to and on the child and its purpose, and who is in the room and caring for the child.

2. The parents are told that if they feel uncomfortable or get in the way of the resuscitation team, they will be escorted out.

3. Position the parents so they can see the child's face and hold his or her hand. Encourage the parents to tell the child how much he or she is loved.

4. If the parents are looking around, explain what is being done for the child and why.

5. If the child is declared dead, reassure the parents that they were present at the child's last moment and that the child (use child's name) felt loved.

NURSING PRACTICE

If parents choose not to witness the resuscitation, regular updates (5- to 10-minute intervals) should be provided to the parents as they wait in a private area. A designated support person (chaplain or family support team member) should be present with the parents as they wait.

Provide for Physical and Emotional Needs

The experience of having a child with a critical illness drains parents' physical and emotional reserves. Parents often need encouragement to take care of themselves and to take a break periodically. A statement such as "It is important for you to eat and rest because Alexa is really going to need you when she wakes up" helps parents to realize that becoming exhausted benefits neither them

nor the child. Provision of a beeper may help reduce the parents' anxiety.

Orienting parents to the hospital, as well as to the unit routines, helps them to adapt to their surroundings. Many communities now have a Ronald McDonald house—an inexpensive but warm and supportive environment for parents of ill children. Computer resources at the Ronald McDonald house may make it possible for parents to stay in contact with concerned family and friends. When financial burdens are a consideration, parents may need family support and social service referrals.

Parents are often at different levels of coping during a crisis. The child's critical illness may foster cohesion between the couple and build a stronger relationship. Unfortunately, the reverse may also be true—differences in styles or levels of coping may foster a sense of isolation, placing a strain on the couple's relationship. Be alert to family dynamics and refer the family for counseling or therapy, if indicated.

Facilitate Positive Staff–Parent Relationships and Communication

Given the intensity of the parents' experience when their child is critically ill, it is easy to see how problems can arise between staff and parents. Each healthcare team member must be aware of the child's current status so that parents receive the same information from all staff. Consistency in the message can instill confidence. Provide explanations geared to the parents' level of understanding, using language the parents can understand.

Parents need to know who has the overall responsibility for the care of their child. They should be introduced to the nurse and physician responsible for the child's care. This is especially important in teaching hospitals that have rotating staff. The staff physician with the overall responsibility should meet with parents as often as necessary to talk about changes in the child's condition or treatment plan and to allow time for parents to ask questions (Figure 41–3 ●). Encourage parents to keep a daily log or notebook to record information on the child's care, progress, and needs. Family care conferences can be helpful when a large number of team members provide care.

Maintain or Strengthen Family Support Systems

Support systems are the extended network of family, friends, and religious and community contacts that provide nurturance, emotional support, and direct assistance to parents, enabling them to cope with overwhelming problems and crises. Most parents indicate that having family or friends nearby is crucial as a support system.

Parents may need to be reassured that it is all right to ask for help from family, friends, or community services. They may be uncomfortable asking for help, instead attempting to handle multiple responsibilities themselves,

FIGURE 41-3

In times of crisis, everyone likes to know that someone is in charge and who that person is. The parents should meet and talk with the staff physician in charge and the nurses as often as possible. Parents need to know that someone is responsible, even if different people are providing care.

often to the point of exhaustion. Some parents are unable to respond to offers of help because it requires too great a mental effort on their part.

Nurses may need to intervene on parents' behalf when they have inappropriate support. Parents may be frustrated by people who come to visit unannounced, stay too long, or visit too often, and may find it difficult to tell well-meaning but insensitive friends that they cannot deal with visitors right now. In these situations, offering to serve as a gatekeeper may be helpful. Suggest that parents inform family and friends about specific times for visits or phone calls to allow for rest periods. An extended family member may be given the responsibility of relaying information to others.

Families of critically ill or dying children often have emotional needs beyond the support capabilities of the nurse caring for the child. Referrals to family and support services or pastoral care may be beneficial in these instances.

EVALUATION

Expected outcomes of nursing care include the following:

- The nurse establishes a trusting relationship and effective communication with the family.
- Parents participate in their child's care as much as desired.
- Family members receive emotional support and nurturance needed to sustain them through their child's illness.

SIBLINGS' EXPERIENCE

As the parents' focus shifts to the critically ill child, they may need support in dealing with the healthy siblings. Siblings also need care and may feel left out when everyone's attention is focused on the ill child. Siblings of critically ill children may demonstrate behaviors ranging from jealousy or envy to resentment, guilt, hostility, anger, insecurity, regression, and fear. Nurses should recognize that siblings may fear becoming ill themselves or believe that they played a role in the child's illness. Siblings often have nightmares about the illness or injury their brother or sister has sustained and about the ill child dying.

The nurse should tell siblings about their brother or sister using language and concepts appropriate to their ages and developmental levels. As appropriate, siblings should be allowed to visit. Such a visit should be encouraged if the child could potentially die, to allow the sibling to say goodbye. These visits often help to lift the spirits of the ill child. Because children's fantasies are often worse than reality, unfounded fears may be relieved by a visit.

Preparation for the visit is important. Before the visit, the nurse should talk with the siblings about what to expect and describe how their brother or sister will look. If the ill child acts, moves, talks, or looks different than usual, provide an explanation beforehand. Describe the hospital environment, including equipment, sounds, and smells. Using a doll, drawing pictures, or showing an actual picture of the child can help prepare the siblings. Table 41-3 summarizes strategies for working with siblings of an ill or injured child.

During the visit the nurse should demonstrate how to talk to and touch the ill child and encourage the siblings to do the same (Figure 41-4 ●). After the visit the nurse should discuss with siblings what they saw and felt, and answer any

---

TABLE 41-3 ✤ **Strategies for Working with Siblings of an Ill or Injured Child**

- Be truthful. Tell why the child is hospitalized, what the treatment involves, and how long the hospitalization is expected to last.
- Assure siblings that they did not cause the illness and that the ill child did nothing wrong. If a sibling had some involvement in or responsibility for the health crisis, referral for psychologic counseling is needed.
- Allow siblings to ask questions and state fears and other feelings.
- Allow siblings to visit if possible. Cover tubes and wires with a sheet. Wash off blood or cover bloody bandages if possible. Prepare them for any equipment, dressing, and procedures they might see.
- Warn them if the ill child is not speaking. Say something like, "John can't talk now. He seems to be sleeping deeply. He may be able to hear, though, so you can touch him and talk to him."
- Encourage siblings to express their feelings related to the disruptive effect of the child's hospitalization on family life.

FIGURE 41–4

During the sibling's visit to the ill child, it is important to talk with the sibling and answer any questions in an honest manner at a level the child can understand.

questions they may have. When a sibling cannot visit, contact with the ill child can be maintained by sending pictures, drawings, cards, and messages recorded on audiotapes or videotapes (Figure 41–5 ●).

FIGURE 41–5

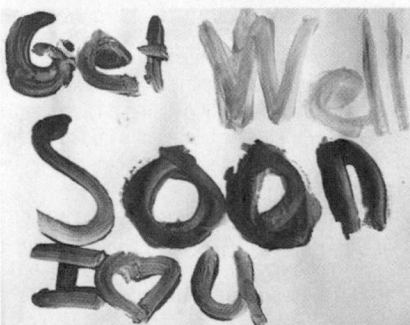

It is important that parents and siblings feel comfortable communicating with the seriously ill child. If siblings cannot visit, they should be encouraged to paint or record messages. They need to be able to express themselves and to feel that they are helping.

If parents are staying at the hospital with the ill child, encourage them to call the siblings at home at a regular time each night. Allowing the siblings at home the opportunity to share their day as well as to receive an update on the ill child provides a feeling of connectedness. The phone call offers siblings a consistent link to the parents as well as the reassurance that they are important and loved.

END-OF-LIFE CARE

When the family is faced with end-of-life decision making and care because of a child's chronic condition or multiple acute care episodes, the family relies on the nurse and other members of the healthcare team to provide honest information about various treatment options and potential outcomes (Table 41–4). Depending on cognitive abilities, developmental stage, physical and mental status, and prior experiences with healthcare, the child may also participate in the decision-making process (Haddad, 2000). The family may need to consider issues such as **palliative care**, **hospice care**, do-not-resuscitate requests, continuation of schooling, organ/tissue donation, and autopsy.

PALLIATIVE CARE

The World Health Organization defines palliative care as the total care of patients whose disease is not responsive to

---

TABLE 41–4 ✛ **Nursing Roles in Improving Pediatric Palliative, End-of-Life, and Bereavement Care**

The nurse and other members of the healthcare team work collaboratively to improve end-of-life care for children and their families through the following actions:

1. Plan nursing care for children with life-threatening medical conditions and their families that matches the child's physical, cognitive, emotional, and spiritual level of development.
2. Implement family-centered care, ensuring that families are part of the care team and their beliefs, feelings, and desires are respected.
3. Plan and provide compassionate care for children with life-threatening conditions and for their families beginning at the time of diagnosis through death and bereavement.
4. Seek information, education, and mentoring to gain proficiency and skill in working effectively with children who are dying and their families.
5. Work within the healthcare facility to promote needed changes that will improve the palliative, end-of-life, and bereavement care for children and their families.
6. Participate in research designed to increase healthcare professional understanding of clinical, cultural, organizational, and other practices or perspectives that can improve palliative, end-of-life, and bereavement care for children and their families.

Data from Institute of Medicine. (2003). *When children die: Improving palliative and end-of-life care for children and their families.* Washington, DC: National Academies Press, p. 7.

curative treatment (Ferrell & Coyle, 2002). It combines active and compassionate therapies intended to soothe, comfort, and relieve persons with life-limiting conditions (Institute of Medicine [IOM], 2003). These therapies may be combined with other therapies aimed at reducing or curing the illness and treating symptoms more aggressively than hospice care. It is estimated that approximately 5000 children die each year from conditions such as cancer, congenital defects, cystic fibrosis, and HIV infection who could benefit from palliative care (Chaffee, 2001). A significant barrier to palliative care for children is the cultural denial of the fact that children actually die, often resulting in poor access to healthcare supports and services that could improve the quality of life (Rushton & Catlin, 2002).

HOSPICE CARE

Hospice care helps patients with short life expectancies to live their remaining time to the fullest—alert, without pain, and with choices and dignity. Families and children receive emotional, spiritual, and medical support. It is estimated that less than 1% of dying children receive hospice services (American Academy of Pediatrics, 2000b). Some families do not see hospice as an acceptable alternative because it requires them to accept the child's impending death and may imply that they are giving up hope (Klopfenstein & Young-Saleme, 2002). Families may need assistance to see that hospice is an opportunity to focus on the time left with the child. Home hospice care allows the family to spend time with the terminally ill infant or child without technical equipment and the presence of strangers. The hospice nurse provides anticipatory guidance to the child and family so they are not alarmed by the signs and symptoms of impending death, such as nausea and respiratory difficulty. Appropriate pain management is also provided. Grief counseling and support is also provided to families for a year following the death of the child.

When a child receives palliative or hospice care, the family and healthcare providers collaborate to determine which treatments are appropriate to continue with the child's end-of-life care, such as total parenteral nutrition, intravenous fluids, gastric or nasogastric feedings, and certain medications. Nurses participate on the multidisciplinary team to ensure comprehensive care to the dying child and family. Health plan coverage for pediatric palliative/hospice care services or alternative financial assistance is investigated.

ETHICAL ISSUES SURROUNDING A CHILD'S DEATH

Because the death of a child is so emotionally charged, many potential misunderstandings and conflicts can develop between families and healthcare providers. The more common ethical issues that need to be addressed include withdrawing or withholding treatment, parental treatment refusal, and do-not-resuscitate orders.

WITHDRAWAL OF OR WITHHOLDING TREATMENT

The decision to withdraw or withhold life-sustaining treatments from the dying child is very difficult and emotional for parents. Withholding nutrition and hydration may be especially difficult because parents often associate food with nurturing and love, or the fear that death will be hastened. Other treatments such as medications, mechanical ventilation, and dialysis may be withdrawn if the outcome for the child is inevitable death and continuing treatment causes more suffering than benefit.

The nurse may feel conflicted when parents are unable to discontinue aggressive therapies that the nurse feels are extending the child's suffering. Consultation with a member of the hospital ethics committee can help clarify the issues involved and reduce the emotions associated with the conflict. During the consultation an unbiased professional collects facts about the child's condition, clarifies the beliefs and values of parents and health professionals, and improves communication while investigating options for compromise (Rushton, 2004).

CONFLICTS REGARDING PARENTAL TREATMENT REFUSAL

Parents and healthcare providers sometimes disagree over what, if any, medical interventions should be provided when the child is dying. Parents may refuse treatments based on religious convictions or because they wish to avoid prolonging the child's life in order to provide a peaceful death (IOM, 2003). Initiating highly technical, but possibly futile, interventions may cause emotional and financial stress that overwhelms young parents.

Court intervention may be initiated by the healthcare team to have a surrogate legal guardian appointed in certain situations when recommended care is refused. Intervention is based on the legal principle that failure to obtain adequate medical care for a child violates the state child neglect laws (IOM, 2003). Consultation with the hospital's ethics committee should also be obtained to help resolve the conflict. The nurse is sometimes in the uncomfortable position of trying to provide care to the infant or child while an adversarial rather than a supportive relationship exists with the parents.

DO-NOT-RESUSCITATE ORDERS

Parents faced with a child's inevitable death may be asked to consider a do-not-resuscitate or do-not-intubate

EVIDENCE-BASED NURSING

IMPROVING THE QUALITY OF PEDIATRIC END-OF-LIFE CARE IN THE PICU

Clinical Question (Problem)

The majority of children who die because of life-limiting conditions die in the hospital setting, and many times in the pediatric intensive care unit (PICU). What are the parents' perspectives with regard to improving their child's quality of care?

Evidence

A study involving parents of 56 children who had died in the pediatric intensive care unit focused on care provided to the child and parental end-of-life decision making. Parents struggled with issues such as how adequate information was about particular aspects of the child's care and loss of control. The study results indicated that when parents considered withdrawal of life support, they placed the highest priorities on quality of life, likelihood of improvement, and their perception of their child's pain and discomfort (Meyer, Burns, Griffith et al., 2002). Another study was conducted by interviewing parents of 44 children who had died at one children's hospital. Themes emerging from the interviews included the following: parents appreciated being highly involved in decision making, difficult news should be delivered by a familiar person, one caregiver should be in charge throughout all phases of treatment, improved services for siblings are needed, and pain management is critical. Effective caregivers were described as those who were honest, clinically accurate, compassionate, and available. Language barriers

with Spanish-speaking families compromised the ability of these families to fully understand the child's care and caused them to feel isolated (Contro, Larson, Scofield et al., 2002).

Implications

Identifying the specific care valued by parents when a child is dying in the PICU is important for planning nursing care and multidisciplinary palliative care. Nurses can assist the family through the decision-making process by providing honest, factual responses to the family's questions. Communication and nursing care planning should ensure that family-centered care is provided by integrating values important to the family.

Critical Thinking

Consider the special needs of parents of a newborn with a cardiac congenital anomaly that cannot be corrected by surgery. Identify a family-centered palliative care plan for the infant who is expected to die within the next few days.

References

Meyer, E. C., Burns, J. P., Griffith, J. L., & Truog, R. D. (2002). Parental perspectives on end-of-life care in the pediatric intensive care unit. *Critical Care Medicine, 30*(1), 226–231; Contro, N., Larson, J., Scofield, S., Sourkes, B., & Cohen, H. (2002). Family perspectives on quality of pediatric palliative care. *Archives of Pediatric and Adolescent Medicine, 156*(1), 14–19.

MediaLink Case Study: Loss of a Schoolmate

(DNR or DNI) order. The family and healthcare providers must decide if a resuscitation attempt would be in the best interest of a child with an end-stage condition. Factors such as allowing the child to die with dignity and the possibility of causing more harm and suffering if resuscitative measures are implemented are considered. Parents need ongoing support as they may feel they are "giving up" on their child. Provide honest information and make sure that the family understands that compliance with a DNR or DNI order does not mean the child will not receive further care or interventions. Oxygen, suctioning, and control of pain, as well as other comfort measures and supportive nursing care, continue in the presence of a DNR order.

NURSING PRACTICE

Some healthcare facilities are replacing the do-not-resuscitate (DNR) order with the phrase "allow natural death" (AND). This phrase may be more acceptable to families, as they are allowing the child to die peacefully rather than requesting that intervention be withheld. This helps them consider the option as being in the child's best interest, rather than "giving up" (Ramer-Chrastek, Brunnquell, & Hasse, 2002).

SCHOOL CONSIDERATIONS

The Americans with Disabilities Act of 1990 and the Education for All Handicapped Children Act mandate that all children with disabilities—including those with terminal illnesses—are entitled to the same education as other students. Children with a chronic or terminal illness may be at high risk of dying while at school. School officials have many concerns about accepting a DNR order, including the effect of the death of a student on a classmate, liability issues, and the potential misinterpretation of the DNR order for an emergency such as choking (American Academy of Pediatrics, 2000a). Some school districts will not honor DNR orders (Ramer-Chrastek, 2000).

CARE OF THE DYING CHILD

Care of the dying child presents one of the greatest challenges to the nurse, requiring the utmost sensitivity and compassion. Children as young as 5 years of age can sense when they are seriously ill. A child's awareness of death develops more rapidly when he or she is experiencing the progression of a disease and related medical treatment. Children with life-limiting illnesses often learn about death and their own illness from exposure to other seriously ill and dying children during hospitalization or clinic visits.

AWARENESS OF DYING BY DEVELOPMENTAL AGE

Infants and toddlers are not actually aware of death, but they are aware of and react to changes in normal routines and the behavior of parents. Toddlers may know they feel bad, but they do not understand that their physical symptoms are associated with impending death. See Figure 41–6 ◉.

Preschool children can see their bodies deteriorate and feel the effects of medications used during disease progression and treatment. Changes in self-concept occur as they perceive these body changes. They often describe their illness in terms of mutilation to their body. They may realize that they are dying because of these physical changes.

School-age children also have subtle fears about body integrity and anxieties about the seriousness of their illness. This greater preoccupation with illness is considered by many professionals as the child's version of **death anxiety**, a feeling of apprehension or fear of death. Children may express death anxiety as a concern with treatments that invade the body or interfere with normal body functions.

◉ **FIGURE 41–6**

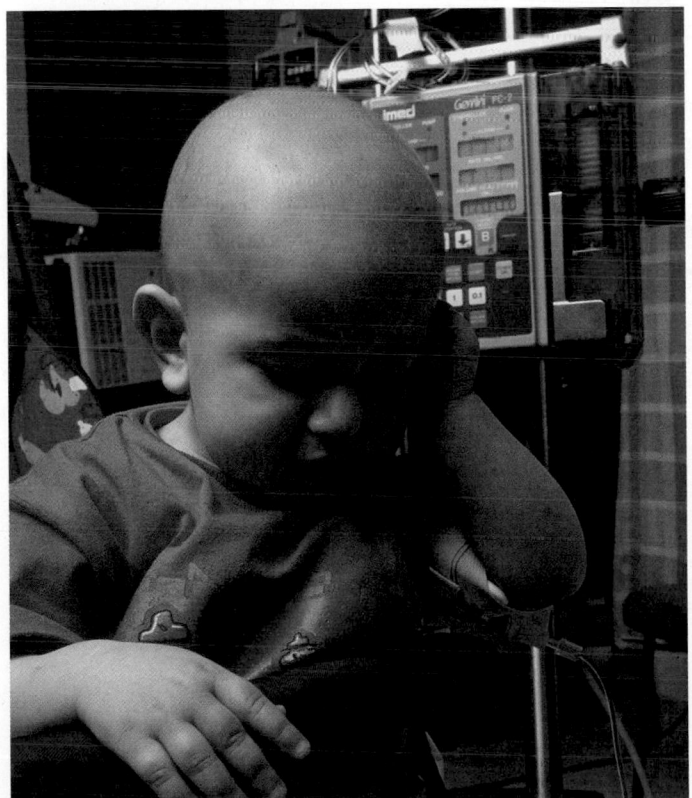

The toddler with a life-limiting condition recognizes that he feels bad and that routines are different. His anxiety may increase due to the concern and feelings of sadness exhibited by his parents.

Adolescents have a mature understanding of death, but the normal developmental milestones of adolescence add to their problems in facing a terminal illness. They are struggling to establish their own identity and plans for the future. At a time when body image is extremely important, they may be faced with the possibility of mutilation and disfigurement. Dying adolescents are often isolated from their peers during a period when peers are the most essential social group. Adolescents with terminal illnesses may be angry because they recognize their loss when the whole world is opening up to them.

Do not expect adolescents to handle feelings in the same way that adults do. Adolescents often avoid expressing anger, an expected stage of grieving, against the family, seeking to control and direct these feelings elsewhere. They often become angry at changes in treatment procedures, lack of explanations, and threats to their independence. As death nears, the adolescent may permit comforting and support and may accept care from warm and loving family members, as long as he or she is not treated condescendingly.

NURSING MANAGEMENT

Nursing care of the dying child and family focuses on providing family-centered support for their physical and psychosocial needs.

NURSING ASSESSMENT AND DIAGNOSIS

Assess the child's physiologic status and comfort level. Physiologic changes in the dying child may be directly related to the child's disease process or injury. Signs and symptoms of approaching death are provided in "Clinical Manifestations: The Dying Child."

Assess the child's awareness of impending death. Examples of questions the child may ask include: "What will death be like? What happens after I die? When will I be with [person closest to child] again? Will my parents be all right? Will you remember me?" Assess the ability of the parents to talk with the child about dying.

Assess the family for coping skills and need for social supports. Identify any cultural or spiritual traditions, rituals, and beliefs related to loss and grieving.

Examples of nursing diagnoses that apply to the dying child and family include the following:

- *Fear (Child)* related to unanswered questions and concerns of abandonment
- *Death Anxiety (Child)* related to impending death
- *Anticipatory Grieving (Parents)* related to imminent death of child
- *Hopelessness (Parents)* related to failure of therapies to prolong life

CLINICAL MANIFESTATIONS

THE DYING CHILD

SYSTEM	CLINICAL MANIFESTATIONS
Cardiovascular System	■ The heart rate may initially increase as hypoxia develops, then the heart rate and blood pressure decrease, resulting in decreased cardiac output. ■ A change in pulse pressure and a decrease in the volume of Korotkoff's sounds indicate imminent death. ■ Peripheral circulation decreases, leading to diaphoresis, clammy cool skin, and changes in skin coloring (mottled to cyanotic). Mottling is a sign of imminent death.
Respiratory System	■ Impaired cardiac function leads to pulmonary congestion, tachypnea, diminished breath sounds, and hypoxia. ■ Dyspnea; **air hunger**, the most severe form of dyspnea, may cause the child to look panicked, gasp for breath, and sit upright. ■ Cheyne-Stokes breathing (periods of shallow breathing alternating with apnea) is a sign of imminent death. ■ As muscles relax, secretions accumulate in the oropharynx and bronchi. The "death rattle" is caused by air passing through these secretions. ■ Moaning or grunting with breathing is not uncommon.
Neurologic System	■ Decreased cerebral perfusion, hypoxemia, metabolic acidosis, the influences of disease-related factors, and an accumulation of toxins from renal and liver failure lead to neurologic dysfunction. ■ Agitation or restlessness, withdrawal, increasing drowsiness, confusion; may be unconscious during final hours. ■ The child may speak of visions (persons or objects) not visible to others. ■ Hearing and vision acuity may deteriorate, but remember that hearing is considered to be the last of the senses to diminish before death.
Musculoskeletal System	■ Extreme muscle weakness and fatigue, difficulty with swallowing. ■ May be unable to reposition self, toilet self, or effectively cough and clear secretions.
Renal System	■ Decreased kidney function and urine production. ■ Sphincters relax and incontinence can occur.
Gastrointestinal System	■ Decreased oral fluid intake and anorexia are common. ■ Parenteral fluids may cause edema and increased respiratory secretions leading to shortness of breath and cough. ■ Sphincters relax and bowel incontinence can occur.

PLANNING AND IMPLEMENTATION

Nursing care for the dying child and the family includes providing comfort, assisting the child in a peaceful death, assisting the child and family with coping strategies, and facilitating grief.

Physiologic Care

A major goal in care of the dying child is to promote comfort and keep the child pain-free. Provide analgesia to promote optimal pain relief. Oral or rectal analgesia is available for families who choose to withhold intravenous fluids. Complementary care for comfort and pain management as described in Chapter 42 can be used by the nurse and family members. ∞

If air hunger occurs, elevate the head of the bed, open a window, or use a circulating fan. An opioid may be prescribed for air hunger or tachypnea as its action dilates the pulmonary vessels, reduces oxygen consumption, and decreases pulmonary congestion.

Other physiologic care includes keeping the airway clear of secretions, bathing and keeping the skin dry and intact, changing the child's position frequently, and encouraging favorite foods and liquids as tolerated. Involve the parents in physical care and encourage them to hold and comfort the child.

DEVELOPING CULTURAL COMPETENCE

ASSESSING CULTURAL DIFFERENCES IN DEALING WITH DEATH

Consider the customs and attitudes that might reflect the family's cultural heritage and affect their response to death. Information about these customs will help plan nursing care to families. For example, try to learn about the following:

- How much to reveal to a child about the diagnosis and prognosis
- How much the child and family want to participate in medical decision making
- The degree of trust in the medical system
- The amount of emotional display that is appropriate
- The role of children, women, and the elderly
- The concept of an afterlife and how it is prepared for (e.g., special ceremonies)
- Whether death should take place alone, with the family, or with an extended group
- Whether death should take place in the home or in the hospital
- Funeral and burial customs
- The length of the mourning period

Used with permission from Lewis, L., Brecher, M., Reaman, G. H., & Sahler, O. J. (2002). How can you help meet the needs of dying children? Contemporary Pediatrics, 19(4), 147–159.

Psychologic Care

Parents may prefer not to talk with the child about the seriousness of the illness and potential for death out of a desire to protect the child from bad news, and a fear that the child will lose hope (Mazanec & Tyler, 2003). Even when children are not told they are dying, they know their condition is worsening. They are undergoing treatments, not feeling well, and picking up cues from their parents. They usually do not have the same fears about dying that adults do. Kübler-Ross (1983) noted that children are more fearful of abandonment than death. A recent study that investigated whether parents had talked about death with their child who had advanced cancer revealed that a third had done so, and none of the parents regretted having the discussion. Parents were more likely to talk with their child if they sensed the child was aware of his or her imminent death, if they were religious, or if the child was older at the time of diagnosis (Kreicbergs, Valdimarsdóttir, Onelöv et al., 2004).

Some children keep most of their thoughts about death to themselves. If they have not been told that they are dying, they may feel isolated and get the message not to discuss their condition. They may fear that the family members will abandon them emotionally. Children often avoid displaying anger, since they fear desertion more than death. They may also believe that expressing their awareness of death and their fears will place added emotional burdens on family members that could be unbearable to the family.

TABLE 41–5 ❖ Strategies for Talking with a Dying Child

- Be flexible.
- Recognize that some children communicate best through nonverbal means (i.e., art or music). The child may be willing to talk through a puppet or a stuffed animal.
- Respect the child's need to be alone and the desire to share. Allow communication, but do not force it.
- Be receptive when children initiate a conversation.
- Be specific and literal in explanation of death.
- Acknowledge that a child's life can be complete, even if it is brief. Let dying children know they will always be loved and remembered. Help children find a sense of accomplishment and purpose in the lives they have led.
- Empower children as much as possible in circumstances concerning their deaths. Reassure them of continued love and physical closeness.

Used with permission from Faulkner, K. W. (1997). Talking about death with a dying child. American Journal of Nursing, 97(6), 64–69.

Provide the child with opportunities for fantasy play, drawing, and storytelling, without emphasizing or reinforcing death themes. Listen to what children tell you about themselves and their lives. **Death imagery**, references to death or death-related topics (going away, separation, funerals) may be themes of their stories. Strategies for talking with a dying child are described in Table 41–5.

When caring for adolescents, remember that outbursts of anger are common but not personally directed at the nurse. Provide activities to help adolescents channel their feelings. Continue providing support in spite of their behavior. This approach may encourage adolescents to accept comforting without losing face. Be available to listen when the adolescent wants to talk and express feelings and frustrations. Promote friendships with other adolescents who have similar interests or problems.

Parents may not recognize the child's death anxiety because of their own fears, concerns, and feelings of helplessness. Depending on the family's cultural and religious beliefs, a chaplain or other healthcare professional who specializes in working with terminally ill children and families may help reduce a child's spiritual fears and promote peace and comfort among family members.

DEVELOPING CULTURAL COMPETENCE

CULTURAL INFLUENCES AND DEATH

Many culturally influenced rules and customs surround dying. For instance, the Hmong belief system holds that children will live in eternity in the same state in which they existed at the time of death. Therefore, it is important that the child's body be intact at death.

NURSING PRACTICE

Some parents ask that their child not be told he or she is dying. Do you abide by their wishes when the child asks you if he or she is dying? Tell the parents that the child asked the question. Offer to set up a meeting with the healthcare team to discuss their fears and concerns about telling their child the truth. Offer words and phrases parents can use to talk with their child about his or her death at a developmentally appropriate level. Some parents may prefer that the child's questions be answered honestly by another professional. A professional who has special bereavement counseling training can assist children and families with discussions.

Family Support

Work closely with the family when the child's death is imminent, because they will remember the experience and words spoken for the rest of their lives. Prepare the family for changes in the child's appearance and behavior. Providing the parents with a room to be alone with the child ensures privacy at this extremely personal time. Ask the family in a nonjudgmental, supportive manner what is important to them in the final moments and hours of their child's life and what will be important to them in the grief process. Certain religious or cultural practices may need to be planned and should be accommodated when possible. Holding the child is a universal request and should be permitted, along with touching, stroking, kissing, and talking soothingly. Many families find that saying good-bye as a group is helpful. Families need to cry together and to tell each other how much they will miss each other. They need to be assured that the vigil with the child is important so the child does not feel isolated or abandoned as death approaches. See Table 41–6 for more common mourning and after-death rituals.

Tissue and Organ Donation

Families may be asked about making an anatomic gift. Information about organ and tissue donation is usually shared with families by specially trained personnel who identify the appropriate time to talk with families. Nurses can become better prepared to serve the family of the dying child and potential organ recipients by becoming familiar with the healthcare facility's criteria for organ and tissue procurement. Generally an organ procurement organization coordinator will collaborate with the nurses and healthcare team to support the process.

Need for Autopsy

When the exact cause of death is not clear, an autopsy may be suggested. In the event of an unnatural or unexpected death (suicide, homicide, sudden infant death syndrome), an autopsy may be required by state law. Parents may be hesitant to consent to autopsy when they have a choice because they are uneasy about the child's body being further invaded. Support the family during decision making by explaining that the autopsy will likely reveal the cause of death. This information may be especially important if the death is potentially due to a genetic disorder, affecting future childbearing decisions.

Postmortem Care and Family Support

Offer ongoing support after the child dies. Questions like the following may help begin the conversation: "I am sorry for your loss. How can I help?" "What are your traditions when an infant or child dies?" "Is there someone I can call for you?"

Identify the family's wishes for postmortem care before performing any care. Ask before removing any jewelry or other item from the child because cultural and spiritual practices may specify that the article remain on the child after death. Follow the healthcare facility's guidelines for postmortem care. The child should be positioned according to guidelines or cultural/religious practices, the room should be cleaned, and medical equipment should be removed.

After the child's death, allow the family to spend as much time as they need with the child's body. Never rush family members who are saying good-bye to the child. Save all of the child's personal items—especially in the case of an infant, whose parents may have few mementos. A lock of hair, hand- or footprints, the infant's identification band, the child's weight and height, the last clothes or patient gown worn by the child sealed in a plastic bag to retain the child's scent, or a picture of the infant can be sources of comfort and remembrance for families. It may be traumatic to receive the child's possessions, so when possible, use a special remembrance box or container for this purpose.

When a newborn or young infant has died, wrap the baby in a blanket and offer the mother and other family members the opportunity to hold the baby. Parents may want to bathe and dress the infant. The family experiencing the death of a newborn may appreciate an offer to take pictures of the baby and family together, if picture taking is not prohibited by religious or cultural traditions. Some families may feel uncomfortable taking pictures with their dead baby and refuse the offer. Ask for permission before cutting a lock of hair as some cultural and religious groups prohibit it, such as Native Americans. Handprints and footprints may be captured using ink pads or clay and given to the parents. Some parents may initially refuse to take any of the baby's personal items or pictures. These items should be stored to allow the parents the opportunity to obtain them later.

Parents may need direction about resources available to help with a memorial service or funeral. Information about organ and tissue donation, as well as the need for an au-

TABLE 41–6 ❖ Cultural Traditions in Mourning and After-Death Rites

Religious Group	Rituals You Might Observe	Organ Donation or Autopsy Beliefs
American Indians	■ Beliefs and practices vary widely ■ Navajo do not touch the deceased or their belongings	Varies among tribes
Buddhism	■ Last-rite chanting at bedside ■ Cremation common	Organ donation considered act of mercy, autopsy individual choice
Catholicism	■ Sacrament of the sick ■ Obligated to take ordinary but not extraordinary means to prolong life ■ Burial is common	Autopsy, organ donation acceptable
Christian Science	■ Unlikely to seek medical help to prolong life ■ Disposal of body and parts decided by family	Individual decides about organ donation
Hinduism	■ No restrictions to right-to-die issue ■ Religious prayers chanted before and after death ■ Cremation common ■ Men and women display outward grief ■ Thread tied around wrist signifies a blessing, do not remove	Autopsy, organ donation acceptable
Islam	■ Attempts to shorten life prohibited ■ Body is washed only by Muslim of same gender	Organ donation acceptable Autopsy only for medical or legal reasons
Jehovah's Witness	■ Use of extraordinary means to prolong life is individual choice ■ Burial determined by family preference	Autopsy if required by law Organ donation forbidden
Judaism	■ If death is inevitable, no new procedures needed, but must continue those ongoing ■ Body ritually washed ■ Burial as soon as possible, all body parts must be buried together ■ Seven-day mourning period	Autopsy permitted in certain circumstances, organ donation is complex issue
Mennonite	■ Do not believe life must be continued at all cost	Autopsy and organ donation acceptable
Mormonism	■ If death inevitable, promote a peaceful and dignified death ■ Burial in "temple clothes"	Autopsy permitted with permission of next of kin, organ donation is permitted
Protestantism	■ Burial or cremation is individual decision	Organ donation, autopsy are individual decisions
Seventh Day Adventist	■ Follow ethic of prolonging life ■ Disposal of body and burial are individual decisions	Autopsy, organ donation acceptable

Adapted from Spector, R. E. (2000). *Cultural diversity in health and illness* (5th ed., pp. 137–138, 144–149). Upper Saddle River, NJ: Prentice Hall Health.

topsy, if required, needs to be discussed. Acknowledge with parents that certain dates—such as the day of the week the child died, the child's birthday, or family holidays—will be difficult and may trigger intense sadness again. Parents may benefit from keeping a journal of their thoughts and memories, or writing letters or poems to or about their child.

EVALUATION

Expected outcomes of caring for the dying child and family may include the following:

■ The child is pain-free and comfortable, and the child's physiologic needs are met.

■ The cultural and spiritual needs of the dying child and family are met.

■ The dying child and family receive support during the dying process.

■ The family receives continued support after the child's death.

BEREAVEMENT

PARENTS' REACTIONS

The death of one's child is probably the most painful experience for a parent. Grief, an individual's feelings and behaviors in response to death, is painful, individualized, and exhausting. Many factors influence the parents' grief responses, including their perception of the preventability of the illness or injury, the suddenness and other circumstances of the death, the nature of their attachment to the child, previous losses, spiritual or religious orientation, and culture.

SUDDEN DEATH OF A CHILD

Although many children die because of chronic illness or terminal condition, more than 40% of child deaths between 1 and 19 years of age are caused by unexpected injuries (Health Resources and Services Administration, 2002). The sudden and unexpected death that results from sudden infant death syndrome, injury, illness, suicide, or violence can lead to more intense grief that takes longer to resolve than grief experienced after an expected death (Menke, 2002). Parents have not had time to prepare for the child's death. Parents need support to deal with the death of the child and to deal with their surviving children. See Table 41–7 for nursing care strategies to provide comfort and support for parents whose child dies suddenly.

DEATH OF A NEWBORN OR YOUNG INFANT

Approximately 15,000 infants are born each year who are dying at birth or have conditions that are incompatible with prolonged life beyond the first year (Catlin & Carter, 2002). The death of a newborn forces parents to experience their child's entire life in a short period of time, and they are faced with overwhelming grief at the time when they anticipated the experience of joy. Unique experiences may

occur with multiple birth, such as the death of one or more of the infants, leading to conflicting emotions for the parents. While they mourn the death of one child, they must parent and bond with the survivor. Concerns arise as the parents fear losing the other infant (Lundqvist, Nilstun, & Dykes, 2002). Refer parents to a perinatal bereavement program or support group.

Although parents progress through distinct stages of grief, as described on page 1187, the time line and nature of the grief process differ for each individual. The intense pain and shock initially felt by parents gradually give way to feelings of anger, guilt, depression, and loneliness. Very slowly, and with much support, energy returns and parents again begin to enjoy life experiences. Spouses may need additional support when they are at different levels of grieving to prevent a sense of loneliness and isolation.

The nurse should emphasize to parents that although the period surrounding their child's death is difficult, caring for themselves physically and mentally is important. Parents may experience friction due to differing rates and intensity of grief. The nurse can give a list of appropriate support groups, books, and articles to parents for later use. Parents can be referred to national organizations, such as the Candlelighters Foundation or Compassionate Friends, and to local support groups for bereaved parents or siblings. (See the Companion Website for links to such resources.) Some institutions have formal follow-up programs for bereaved parents to encourage a healthy progression through the grieving process.

SIBLINGS' REACTIONS

Siblings experiencing the death of a brother or sister require supportive and compassionate care. In the course of the child's illness, the siblings probably will have received less attention from parents. They may fear that they caused their brother or sister to be injured or become ill, or worry that bad thoughts on their part brought on the illness. Nurses and other support personnel can assist the surviving children to adapt to their parents' distraction, grief, and increased protectiveness of them. The siblings need to hear that the parents' grief in no way diminishes the love felt for them. Table 41–8 highlights children's understanding of death at different developmental stages, some of the possible behavioral responses, and nursing considerations for family education.

When talking to the siblings of a child who has died, honesty is most important and questions should be answered truthfully. The nurse should provide explanations in language that is developmentally appropriate and reassure siblings that they did not cause their brother or sister to die and that death was not a punishment for wrongdoing. The nurse should allow the siblings to ask questions

---

TABLE 41–7 ✤ **Strategies for Working With Parents Whose Child Dies Suddenly**

- Identify a spokesperson for the medical team to keep the family informed during resuscitation efforts. Have both parents present if possible.
- Provide private space with telephone access.
- Create time for families to assimilate the child's worsening status by providing several updates during the resuscitation. Prepare them for what is to come.
- Offer to telephone clergy, family, and friends.
- After the death, prepare the body for viewing.
- Provide time and a place for the family to say good-bye.
- Sit close and make eye contact. Share your emotions with the family. Accept whatever emotions family members express.
- Convey information to the family about the cause of death, autopsy, funeral preparations, and the normal grief process.
- Arrange for family follow-up to see how they are responding to the child's loss and to review autopsy findings.

Data from Anderson, J. E. (1996). Helping parents cope with sudden death. *Contemporary Pediatrics, 13*(12), 42–57. © 1996 Thomson Medical Economics. All rights reserved.

TABLE 41–8 ❖ Children's Understanding of Death and Possible Behavioral Responses

Understanding of Death	Possible Behaviors	Nursing Considerations
Infant ■ Lacks understanding of concept of death ■ May sense caregivers are tense, routines are altered	■ May show sadness by turning away from your gaze ■ Resists cuddling and eats less ■ Excessive crying, clingy ■ Sleeping more than usual	■ Encourage parents to hold and cuddle the infant to help reduce the fear of separation. ■ Use a soft and comforting voice. ■ Follow familiar routines.
Toddler ■ Unable to distinguish fact from fantasy ■ No understanding of true concept of death ■ Aware someone is missing—separation anxiety ■ Unable to distinguish death from temporary separation or abandonment	■ Clingy, refuses to let parent out of sight ■ Stops walking and talking, regression from previously achieved milestones ■ Shows distress by biting, hitting, tears ■ Fearfulness ■ Problems eating and sleeping ■ Sleep disturbances	■ Encourage parents to hold and cuddle the toddler to help reduce the fear of separation. ■ Follow familiar routines. ■ Be tolerant of regressive behaviors. ■ Talk and answer questions in terms that the child will understand.
Preschooler ■ Believes death is temporary ■ Magical thinking—believes dead person can be brought back to life ■ Believes bad thoughts cause death ■ Has beginning experience with death of animals and plants	■ May fear going to sleep, has nightmares, afraid of dark ■ Out-of-control behavior, hyperactivity, tantrums, regression ■ Problems with bowel and bladder control ■ Crying spells ■ Seems morbidly fascinated with death ■ Asks lots of questions ■ Displays anger at failure to keep person "alive," breaks toys, aggressive to friends ■ Regression to baby talk or thumb-sucking ■ Complaints of abdominal pain	■ Listen to the child and answer questions honestly. ■ Try to follow usual routines. ■ Be tolerant of regressive behaviors, provide play activities. ■ Reassure the child that his thoughts or actions did not contribute to the death. ■ Keep memories alive with pictures and other things that remind the child of the loved one. ■ Participate in rituals such as going to cemetery, releasing helium balloons, and planting flowers.
School-Age Child ■ Acquires more realistic understanding of death ■ By 8–10 years, understands that death is permanent and irreversible, and that people die from internal and external causes ■ Believes that death is universal and will happen to him or her ■ May have exaggerated concerns about death	■ May deny sadness by hiding tears and acting more like adults ■ Difficulty concentrating on school work ■ Psychosomatic complaints—stomachache or headache ■ Acting-out behavior, aggression, anger at being abandoned ■ May try to comfort parents by taking over tasks ■ May fear someone else they love will die	■ Listen to the child and answer questions honestly. The school-age child copes by gathering as much information as possible. ■ Return to usual routines and activities. ■ Keep memories alive through activities such as art, music, creating a memory book, sewing a quilt, and planting a garden. ■ Share Internet resources. ■ Use coping support groups.
Adolescent ■ Intellectually capable of understanding death ■ Has a better grasp of association between illness and death ■ Sense of invincibility conflicts with fear of death ■ Able to recognize effect of death on others	■ Same as school-age child ■ May have severe depression ■ Acting-out behavior, risk-taking behavior, delinquency, suicide attempts, promiscuity, pseudo-indifference	■ Be available and foster open communication. ■ Share grief and feelings with the adolescent. ■ Keep memories alive with pictures and other things that remind the child of the loved one. ■ Access counseling and support groups. ■ Share Internet resources.

Adapted with permission from Menke, E. M. (2002). Handling children's grief at the first anniversary. *Journal of Pediatric Health Care, 16*(5), 267–270.

GROWTH AND DEVELOPMENT

Children need to understand the finality of death—that all body functions have stopped. Simple statements that can be told to children include, "Adam's heart will never beat again," "He will never get cold or hungry," and "He will never come home again." These simple statements may need to be repeated several times since young children will test to see if the same answers are given each time.

and acknowledge the emotions they are feeling by emphasizing that it is all right for them to be sad, angry, frightened, or tearful. The nurse should use the same amount of energy and concern in acknowledging their grief as acknowledging that of adults. Siblings should be asked how they feel about saying good-bye to the dying child, and provided with physical and emotional support. Preparation of the siblings before seeing the dying child involves a brief explanation of what they will see, feel, hear, and smell. Siblings may have to hear information several times.

As appropriate and comfortable, siblings should be permitted to participate in planning the child's memorial or funeral service. Being able to grieve as a family provides siblings with a sense of connectedness to parents and provides security at a vulnerable time. If siblings attend the funeral, the nurse should prepare them for what to expect, such as an open casket or behaviors of mourners. The nurse can suggest designating a support person, such as a family member or close friend, who can monitor the siblings' needs while the parents attend to other matters. It is important to keep the family together as much as possible.

As with parental bereavement, sibling bereavement is a lifelong process. The nurse should encourage parents to make sure other caregivers and teachers know about the sibling's loss. The child should be allowed to express feelings other than sadness (e.g., guilt and anger) and encouraged to express grief through art, stories, and writing. Children can be encouraged to celebrate their sibling's life by preparing collages of photographs, collecting the child's favorite toys, and making a keepsake box.

STAFF REACTIONS TO THE DEATH OF A CHILD

Children are highly valued by society because of their potential future contributions. Children are expected to have a normal life span, and the death of a child is often viewed as a tragedy. Caring for dying children is especially stressful and demanding for healthcare professionals. Nurses involved in long-term relationships with children experience grief when these children die. Some nurses

cope by distancing themselves socially from the dying child and family to maintain composure and a professional demeanor.

Caring for the dying child may be especially difficult for nurses with young children of their own. They tend to identify with the child, making it more likely that they will have difficulty dealing with the death in a professional manner. Nurses may not be able to recognize the dying child's anxiety and fears because of their own personal defenses against their sense of helplessness to alter the course of the child's disease.

Nurses who work with terminally ill children and their families need special preparation to meet the needs of these individuals and to manage personal stress simultaneously. Mentorship with experienced hospice nurses, as well as additional educational experiences, may help promote professional nursing care. Nurses who work with dying children and their families must learn to cope effectively with grief and develop empathy, competence, and confidence in their ability to provide more humane and effective nursing care. Although crying with families was once considered unprofessional to some, it is now recognized as an expression of caring and empathy. Nurses should feel

● FIGURE 41–7

Nurses need to express grief in a supportive environment after a child's death. Sharing the sadness and grief or futility of resuscitation efforts with colleagues can often help nurses continue to provide supportive care to the next families who need compassionate care.

free to express their sorrow and grief for the child and family. Some nurses attend funeral and memorial services when invited by the patient's family.

Nurses working in emergency departments caring for children who die suddenly or in hospice settings and hospital units that care for terminally ill children need support systems to help balance the stresses of working with dying children. The workplace should acknowledge the stress nurses experience when working with terminally ill children. Support systems may include discussions with peers or debriefing group sessions with mental health professionals that provide an opportunity for nurses to discuss their feelings and concerns (Figure 41–7 ◉). Participating in team decisions regarding the dying child's plan of care (palliative rather than curative) helps many nurses manage their distress.

Critical Concept Review

LEARNING OBJECTIVES

CONCEPTS

Describe the child's responses to having a life-threatening illness or injury by developmental level.

1. Infant:
   - Sleep-wake cycle and feeding routine are disrupted.
   - Excessive irritability.
2. Toddler:
   - Frightened by immobilizers
   - Associates pain with punishment
3. Preschooler:
   - Fears mutilation of genitals.
   - Easily regresses to earlier stages.
4. School-age child:
   - Fears body injury and death.
   - Fears loss of control.
5. Adolescent:
   - Displays anger, rebellion, and withdrawal.

Discuss the responses of parents and siblings when the child has a life-threatening illness or injury.

1. Parents go through different stages:
   - Shock and disbelief.
   - Anger and guilt.
   - Deprivation and loss.
   - Anticipatory waiting.
   - Readjustment or mourning.
2. Siblings:
   - Insecurity and anxiety.
   - Jealousy or envy of attention given to sick child.
   - Resentment, fear, and anger.

Describe the coping mechanisms used by the child and family in response to stress.

Child:
1. Regression.
2. Denial.
3. Repression.
4. Postponement.
5. Bargaining.

Family:
1. Participation in care.
2. Participation in decision making.
3. Family support.
4. Anger and hostility.

(continued)

LEARNING OBJECTIVES	CONCEPTS

Develop a nursing care plan for the child with a life-threatening illness or injury.

1. Encourage parents to stay at bedside.
2. Provide developmentally appropriate explanations about all procedures and equipment.
3. Provide opportunities for play where possible.
4. Use the primary nurse model.
5. Provide opportunities for choice where appropriate.
6. Provide routines for scheduled care.
7. Treat the child's pain and fear.

Identify the physiologic and psychologic changes that occur in the dying child.

1. Physiologic changes:
   - Decrease in peripheral circulation, skin appears cool and mottled.
   - Cheyne-Stokes respirations.
   - Increase of secretions in the back of the throat.
   - Decreased perfusion to the brain leads to restlessness, agitation, increased lack of awareness of surroundings, leading to coma.
   - Kidney function decreases, leading to decreased urine output.
   - Child usually incontinent as death approaches.
2. Psychologic changes:
   - Aware of impending death with or without being told about terminal condition.
   - Fear of separation from parents, or abandonment.
   - Death anxiety.

Develop a nursing care plan to provide family-centered care for the dying child and family.

1. Provide physical comfort for the child.
   - Treat pain effectively.
   - Instruct parents in nonpharmacologic pain relief.
2. Provide emotional comfort.
   - Encourage family to stay with child.
3. Establish homelike routines for child and family.
   - Allow child to take part in decision making.
   - Refer parents to support groups.
4. Maintain family functioning.
   - Encourage parents to take breaks.
   - Provide time for sibling interaction.
5. Promote cultural and spiritual values.
   - Incorporate family rituals in care of child.
6. Prepare family and child for impending death.

Describe the development of the child's concept of death.

1. Infant:
   - No understanding of death.
   - Senses caregivers' anxiety and tension.
2. Toddler:
   - Equates death with separation.
3. Preschooler:
   - Believes death is temporary.
   - Believes bad thoughts cause death.
4. School-age child:
   - By age 8–10, believes death is permanent.
   - Understands all persons will die.
5. Adolescent:
   - Understands connection between illness and death.
   - Recognizes effect of death on others.
   - Sense of invincibility conflicts with fear of death.

Describe the responses of nurses caring for children who die.

1. Development of severe grief when caring for child over a long period of time.
2. Feelings of helplessness to change the end results.
3. Reluctance to form connections with other terminally ill children.
4. Identification with terminally ill child if own child is near same age.

CRITICAL THINKING IN ACTION

*View the **Critical Thinking in Action** video in Chapter 41 of the CD-ROM. Then, answer the questions that follow.*

Kelly is a 24-week-old premature baby born to her parents, Shawn and Lori, who are of Navajo Indian descent. The mother had a premature rupture of membranes and Kelly was kept alive by life support. Kelly's condition is extremely critical with her weight at 500 grams. You know that when infants are this small and their condition is critical, any amount of touch can be extremely stressful to their bodies. The mother has been pumping and freezing breast milk for future use. The parents are encouraged to assist the nurse in any way they can, but they are not able to touch Kelly. The parents have been educated about how critical Kelly's condition is and the machines and medications being used. They still have confusion and uncertainty about the situation. The grandparents have been helping care for Roseanne, Kelly's 7-year-old sister and she has visited her sister once. The parents have not left the hospital at all. On the third day of life, Kelly gained weight and started to show an increase in activity. The parents thought this could be a positive sign, but the nurse explained that the weight gain was from swelling and the increased activity was from agitation as Kelly's struggled to breathe. When the parents were at the bedside, Kelly started to become cyanotic and her oxygen saturation level dropped to the 60s. Several nurses, doctors, and respiratory therapists tried to save her, but were unsuccessful. This was an extremely devastating loss to all the medical personnel and family involved.

1. What are some of the stressors Kelly experienced while in the hospital?
2. What are the stages of grief a family is likely to experience with Kelly's situation?
3. What are some of the strategies that can be used when helping Kelly's sibling deal with the loss of her sister?
4. What are some of the strategies for helping Kelly's parents deal with losing her?

MEDIALINK

www.prenhall.com/london

- NCLEX-RN® Review, case studies, and other interactive resources for this chapter can be found on the Companion Website at http://www.prenhall.com/london. Click on "Chapter 41" and select the activities for this chapter.

- For animations, more NCLEX-RN® Review questions, and an audio glossary, access the accompanying CD-ROM in this textbook.

REFERENCES

American Academy of Pediatrics. (2000a). Policy statement: Do not resuscitate orders in schools. *Pediatrics, 105*(4), 878–879.

American Academy of Pediatrics Committee on Bioethics and Committee on Hospital Care. (2000b). Palliative care for children. *Pediatrics, 106*(2), 351–357.

Anderson, J. E. (1996). Helping parents cope with sudden death. *Contemporary Pediatrics, 13*(12), 42–57.

Catlin, A., & Carter, B. (2002). Creation of a neonatal end-of-life palliative care protocol. *Neonatal Network, 21*(4), 37–49.

Chaffee, S. (2001). Pediatric palliative care. *Primary Care Clinics in Office Practice, 28*(2), 365–390.

Contro, N., Larson, J., Scofield, S., Sourkes, B., & Cohen, H. (2002). Family perspectives on quality of pediatric palliative care. *Archives of Pediatric and Adolescent Medicine, 156*(1), 14–19.

Daviss, W. B., Mooney, D., Racusin, R., Ford, J. D., Fleischer, A., & McHugo, G. J. (2000). Predicting posttraumatic stress after hospitalization for pediatric injury. *Journal of American Academy of Child and Adolescent Psychiatry, 39*(5), 576–583.

Faulkner, K. W. (1997). Talking about death with a dying child. *American Journal of Nursing, 97*(6), 64–69.

Ferrell, B. R., & Coyle, N. (2002). An overview of palliative care. *American Journal of Nursing, 102*(10), 18.

Gavaghan, S. R., & Carroll, D. L. (2002). Families of critically ill patients and the effect of nursing interventions. *Dimensions of Critical Care Nursing, 21*(2), 64–71.

Griffin, T. (2003). Facing challenges to family-centered care II: Anger in the clinical setting. *Pediatric Nursing, 29*(3), 212–214.

Haddad, A. (2000). Ethics in action. *RN, 63*(11), 21–23.

Health Resources and Services Administration, Maternal and Child Health Bureau. (2002). *Child health USA, 2002.* Rockville, MD: U.S. Department of Health and Human Services.

Institute of Medicine. (2003). Patterns of child-hood death in America. In *When children die:*

Improving palliative and end-of-life care for children and their families (pp. 41–71). Washington, DC: National Academy Press.

Katz, S. (2002). When the child's illness is life-threatening: Impact on parents. *Pediatric Nursing, 28*(5), 453–464.

Klopfenstein, K. J., & Young-Saleme, T. (2002). Your role in the spectrum of adolescent cancer: Diagnosis through the treatment to care at life's end. *Contemporary Pediatrics, 19*(8), 105–127.

Kreicbergs, U., Valdimarsdóttir, U., Onelöv, E., Henter, J. I., & Steineck, G. (2004). Talking about death with children who have severe malignant disease. *New England Journal of Medicine, 351*(12), 1251–1253.

Kübler-Ross, E. (1983). *On children and death.* New York: Macmillan.

Levetown, M. (2004). Breaking bad news in the emergency department: When seconds count. *Topics in Emergency Medicine, 26*(1), 35–43.

Lewis, L., Brecher, M., Reaman, G. H., & Sahler, O. J. (2002). How can you help meet the needs of dying children. *Contemporary Pediatrics, 19*(4), 147–159.

Lundqvist, A., Nilstun, T., & Dykes, A. (2002). Experiencing neonatal death: An ambivalent transition into motherhood. *Pediatric Nursing, 28*(6), 621–626.

Mazanec, P., & Tyler, M. K. (2003). Cultural considerations in end-of-life care. *American Journal of Nursing, 103*(3), 50–58.

Melnyk, B. M., Small, L., & Carno, M. (2004). The effectiveness of parent-focused interventions in improving coping/mental health outcomes in critically ill children and their parents: An evidence base to guide clinical practice. *Pediatric Nursing, 30*(2), 143–148.

Menke, E. M. (2002). Handling children's grief at the first anniversary. *Journal of Pediatric Health Care, 16*(5), 267–270.

Meyer, E. C., Burns, J. P., Griffith, J. L., & Truog, R. D. (2002). Parental perspectives on end-of-life care in the pediatric intensive care unit. *Critical Care Medicine, 30*(1), 226–231.

Ramer-Chrastek, J. (2000). Hospice care for a terminally ill child in the school setting. *Journal of School Nursing, 16*(2), 52–56.

Ramer-Chrastek, J., Brunnquell, D., & Hasse, S. (2002). Letting nature take its course. *American Journal of Nursing, 102*(10), 24CC–24JJ.

Rushton, C. H. (2004). Ethics and palliative care in pediatrics. *American Journal of Nursing, 104*(4), 54–63.

Rushton, C. H., & Catlin, A. (2002). Pediatric palliative care: The time is now? *Pediatric Nursing, 28*(1), 57–70.

Ryan-Wenger, N. A. (1996). Children, coping, and the stress of illness: A synthesis of research. *Journal of the Society of Pediatric Nurses, 1*(3), 126–138.

Sydnor-Greenberg, N., & Dokken, D. (2000). Coping and caring in different ways: Understanding and meaningful involvement. *Pediatric Nursing, 26*(2), 185–190.

Pain Assessment and Management in Children

Felicia must be in pain so soon after her surgery. I know I would have pain if it were me. Can she get pain medicine without getting another needle?
—*Mother of Felicia, 5*

LEARNING OBJECTIVES

- Describe the physiologic and behavioral consequences of pain in children.

- Select an appropriate tool to assess the pain of infants and children in each age group.

- Describe the nursing assessment and management for a child receiving an opioid analgesic.

- Explain the rationale for the effectiveness of nonpharmacologic (complementary) methods of pain control.

- Assess children of different ages with acute pain and develop a nursing care plan that integrates pharmacologic interventions and developmentally appropriate nonpharmacologic (complementary) therapies.

- Develop a nursing care plan for assessing and monitoring the child having sedation and analgesia for a medical procedure.

MEDIALINK

www.prenhall.com/london

CD-ROM

NCLEX-RN® Review
Animation: Morphine
Videos:
    Pain Management Kit
    Pain Perception
Nursing in Action: Administering Patient-Controlled
    Analgesia
Nursing in Action: Sedation Monitoring
Postoperative Pain Flow Chart
Audio Glossary
Skill 13-1 Selected Pediatric Pain Scales
Skill 13-2 Patient-Controlled Analgesia
Skill 13-3 Monitoring Sedation
Skill 13-4 Local Pain Blocks

Companion Website

NCLEX-RN® Review
Case Study
Thinking Critically
MediaLink Applications:
    Managing Light Sedation
    Calculating Opioid Dosage
    Postoperative Pain Assessment
Complementary Care: Hypnotherapy for Children

Everyone has his or her own perception of pain. A neurologic response to tissue injury, **pain** is an unpleasant sensory and emotional experience associated with actual or potential tissue damage (see "Pathophysiology Illustrated"). Effective pain management is every child's right.

ACUTE AND CHRONIC PAIN

Pain exists when the patient says it does (McCaffrey & Pasero, 1999). Pain may be either acute or chronic. **Acute pain** is sudden and of short duration; it may be associated with a single event, such as surgery, or an acute exacerbation of a condition such as a sickle cell crisis. The inflammatory response that follows the initial tissue injury causes a sustained pain response (Fuller, 2001). **Chronic pain** is a persistent pattern of pain, lasting longer than 6 months; it is generally associated with a prolonged disease process such as juvenile rheumatoid arthritis.

In 2001 the Joint Commission on Accreditation of Healthcare Organizations introduced standards for the assessment and management of pain in patients. All patients are assessed for pain, and they have the right to appropriate pain management. Patient education includes managing pain as a part of treatment.

MISCONCEPTIONS ABOUT PAIN IN CHILDREN

Healthcare professionals once believed that children feel less pain than adults. Undertreatment of pain was based on these attitudes about pain, the difficulty and complexity of pain assessment in children, and inadequate research. Some nurses still undertreat pain, either not giving pain medication on a fixed schedule around the clock as ordered by the physician or giving less than 40% of the pain medication ordered (Vincent, 2001). For a review of past myths and the contrasting reality, see Table 42–1.

Research has shown that past beliefs about children's perception of pain were incorrect. Even newborns feel pain. All the necessary peripheral and central nervous system anatomic structures and functional ability to process pain are present by 20 weeks' gestation (Pasero, 2002). Pain impulses are transmitted along the nonmyelinated C fibers, and the pain signal is less precise. Pain conduction may be slower in newborns, but the distance the pain stimuli must travel is much shorter than in adults. Because the descending neurotransmitters are less developed, newborns are less able to reduce the pain impulses. Premature and newborn infants may be even more sensitive to pain than older children. Newborns and infants also remember pain. By 6 months of age, children demonstrate anticipatory fear of pain when taken to a location where they once experienced pain (McGrath & Craig, 1989).

DEVELOPING CULTURAL COMPETENCE

HEALTH PROFESSIONAL'S ATTITUDES ABOUT CHILDREN'S PAIN

Think about your personal pain experiences during childhood and how your family members encouraged you to be stoic or to express pain. These types of experiences often contribute to a health professional's attitudes about pain experienced by children. For example, healthcare workers may believe that being in pain for a little while is not so bad or that pain helps build character.

PATHOPHYSIOLOGY ILLUSTRATED

Pain Perception

Nociceptors (free nerve endings at the site of tissue damage) transmit information by specialized nerve fibers to the spinal cord. Unmyelinated C fibers slowly transmit dull, burning, diffuse pain as well as chronic pain. Large, myelinated A-delta fibers quickly transmit sharp, well-localized pain. Nociceptors are stimulated by mechanical, thermal, and chemical injury. Biochemical mediators (bradykinin, prostaglandin, leukotrienes, serotonin, histamine, catecholamines, and substance P) are produced in response to tissue damage. These substances help move the pain impulse from the nerve endings to the spinal cord. After the sensory information reaches the substantia gelatinosa in the dorsal horn of the spinal cord, the pain signal may be modified depending on the presence of other stimuli, from either the brain or the periphery. The pain signal is then transmitted to the brain through the spinothalamic, reticulospinal, and spinomesoencephalic nerve pathways, where perception occurs. Once the sensation reaches the brain, emotional responses may increase or decrease the intensity of the pain perceived.

The gate control theory of pain helps explain how the pain impulses are allowed to proceed to the brain. The substantia gelatinosa serves as a gate and regulates the transmission of pain and other impulses to the brain (Huether & Leo, 2002). Since pain and nonpain impulses are sent along the same pathways, nonpain impulses can compete with pain impulses for transmission.

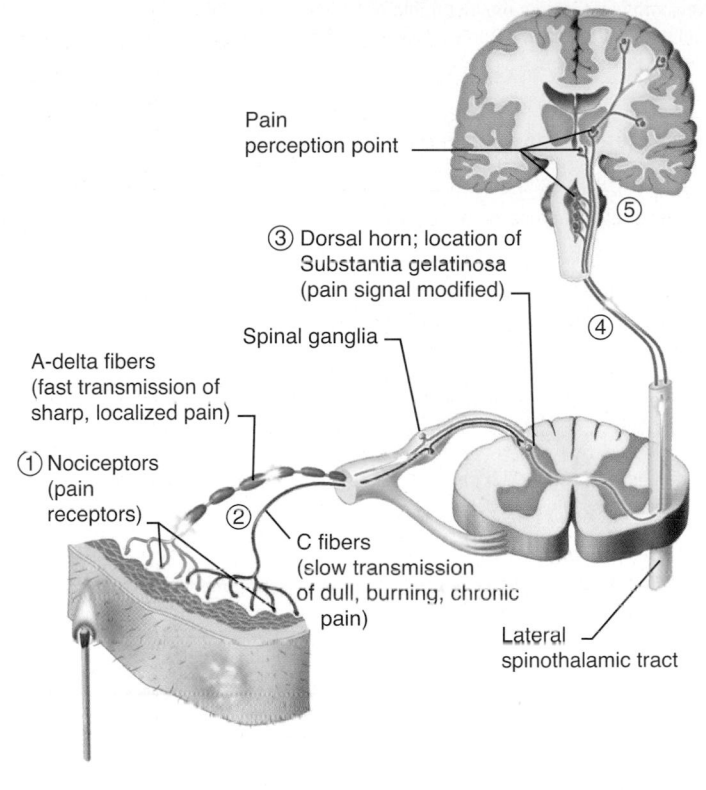

CLINICAL MANIFESTATIONS

Physiologic Indicators

Acute pain stimulates the adrenergic nervous system and results in physiologic changes, including tachycardia, tachypnea, hypertension, pupil dilation, pallor, increased perspiration, and increased secretion of catecholamines and adrenocorticoid hormones. Changes in these signs demonstrate a complex stress response. These signs are not specific to pain, so they cannot be used for monitoring pain.

Chronic pain of long duration permits physiologic adaptation, so normal heart rate, respiratory rate, and blood pressure levels are often seen (Huether & Leo, 2002).

Behavioral Indicators

Children in acute pain behave in many of the same ways as children who show signs of fear and anxiety (Hazinski, 1999; Tesler, Holzemer, & Spreker, 1999). These behaviors include the following:

- Short attention span (child is difficult to distract)
- Irritability (child is difficult to comfort)
- Facial grimacing, biting or pursing lips; see Figure 42–1 ● on p. 1211 for facial expression of newborns and infants
- Posturing (guarding a painful joint by avoiding movement), remaining immobile, or protecting the painful area
- Drawing up knees, flexing limbs, massaging affected area
- Lethargy, remaining quiet, or withdrawal
- Sleep disturbances

Preverbal children may show conflicting signs of pain (restlessness, agitation or withdrawal, hyperalert or vigilant, grimacing, crying, or anger), making pain assessment and management more challenging.

Children often suffer additional emotional distress and fear that the discomfort will worsen. Depression and aggressive behavior are frequently overlooked as indicators of pain.

CONSEQUENCES OF PAIN

Unrelieved pain is stressful and has many undesirable physiologic consequences (Table 42–2). For example, the

TABLE 42–1 ❖ Misconceptions about Pain in Infants and Children

Myth	Reality
Newborns and infants are incapable of feeling pain. Children do not feel pain with the same intensity as adults because a child's nervous system is immature.	By 20 weeks' gestation, a fetus has most of the anatomic and functional requirements for pain processing. Term infants have the same level of sensitivity to pain as older infants and children. Preterm infants may actually have greater sensitivity.
Infants are incapable of expressing pain.	Infants express pain with both behavioral and physiologic cues that can be assessed.
Infants and children have no memory of pain.	Preterm infants have been noticed to associate the smell of alcohol with heel sticks and to try to pull the foot away to avoid the pain. Infants cry in anticipation of immunizations.
Parents exaggerate or aggravate their child's pain.	Parents know their child and are able to identify when the child is in pain.
Children are not in pain if they can be distracted or if they are sleeping.	Children use distraction to cope with pain, but they soon become exhausted when coping with pain and fall asleep.
Repeated experience with pain teaches the child to be more tolerant of pain and cope with it better.	Children who have more experience with pain respond more vigorously to pain. Experience with pain teaches how severe the pain can become.
Children tolerate discomfort well. They become accustomed to pain after having it for a while.	Children do not tolerate pain any better than adults, and may have less tolerance with prior painful experiences. They do not become accustomed to pain or cope with it better than adults.
Children recover more quickly than adults from painful experiences such as surgery.	Children heal quickly from surgery, but they have the same amount of pain from surgery as an adult.
Children tell you if they are in pain. They do not need medication unless they appear to be in pain.	Children may be too young to express pain or afraid to tell anyone other than a parent about the pain. The child fears the treatment for pain may be worse than the pain itself.
Children without obvious physical reasons for pain are not likely to have pain.	The cause of pain cannot always be determined. The feeling of pain is subjective and should be accepted by nurses.
Children run the risk of becoming addicted to pain medication when used for pain management.	Addiction is extremely rare when the child is treated for an acute condition.

child with acute postoperative pain takes shallow breaths and suppresses coughing to avoid more pain. These self-protective actions increase the potential for respiratory complications. Unrelieved pain may also delay the return of normal gastric and bowel functions and cause a stress ulcer. Anorexia associated with pain may delay the healing process. The long-term effects of pain on the child's physical or psychologic condition are unknown.

PAIN ASSESSMENT

The goal of pain assessment is to provide accurate information about the location and intensity of pain and its effects on the child's functioning. No laboratory tests are routinely used to assess pain. Prolonged, severe pain produces a physiologic stress response that includes the chemical release of catecholamines, cortisol, aldosterone, and other corticosteroids.

Insulin secretion also decreases, leading to increased amounts of glucose and severe hyperglycemia (Hazinski, 1999).

PAIN HISTORY

Parents can provide a great deal of information about the child's response to pain, such as the following:

- How the child typically expresses pain, both verbally and behaviorally. Children and parents use similar terms to describe pain. Some examples of words used are a *hurt, owie, boo-boo, stinging, sore, cutting, burning, itching, hot,* and *tight.* Knowing the appropriate word to use makes communicating with the child easier. The parent can often provide signs used to recognize the child's pain.

- The child's previous experiences with painful situations and reactions.

● FIGURE 42–1

Bulged brows

Brows lowered,
drawn together

Eyes squeezed shut

Furrowed nasolabial
creases

Taut tongue

Open, angular, squarish
lips and mouth

Quivering chin

Neonatal characteristic facial responses to pain include bulged brow, eyes squeezed shut, furrowed nasolabial creases, open lips, pursed lips, stretched mouth, taut tongue, and a quivering chin.

Adapted from Carlson, K. L., Clement, B. A., & Nash, P. (1996). Neonatal pain: From concept to research questions and the role of the advanced practice nurse. Journal of Perinatal Neonatal Nursing, 10 (1), 64–71.

- How the child copes with and manages pain. The child with several past pain experiences may not exhibit the same types of stressful behaviors as the child with few pain experiences.

 THINKING CRITICALLY

DETERMINING WHEN A CHILD IS IN PAIN

Felicia, who is 5 years old, was struck by a car. Six hours ago, she had surgery to repair a liver laceration, but she also has numerous bruises and abrasions on her body. After spending 3 hours in the postanesthesia unit, she was moved to the pediatric inpatient unit. She has an intravenous line in place, as well as a nasogastric tube attached to low suction. Her abdominal dressing is clean and dry. Felicia has orders for morphine IV every 3 hours around the clock for the first 24 hours.

Felicia's mother is rooming in with her during her hospital stay. Twelve hours after surgery, Felicia is dozing but is responsive to verbal stimuli. Her most recent IV morphine was given 2 hours ago. The nurse attempts to determine how well Felicia's pain is managed. Her facial expression indicates that she is not in pain. Felicia's mother feels that she is resting fairly comfortably.

How do you know whether Felicia is in pain? Can you expect her to tell you if she feels pain? Is any additional assessment needed to justify giving Felicia more pain medication? What other pain relief measures could reduce or help to control her pain in the first 24 hours?

What is the appropriate dose of IV morphine for Felicia, who weighs 25 kg? What is the timing of assessments of response to pain and potential side effects? What signs of respiratory distress indicate a need for naloxone administration?

- What works best to reduce the child's pain?
- The parent's and child's preferences for analgesic use and other pain interventions.

TABLE 42–2 ✤ Physiologic Consequences of Unrelieved Pain in Children

Responses to Pain	Potential Physiologic Consequences
Respiratory Changes	
Rapid shallow breathing	Alkalosis
Inadequate lung expansion	Decreased oxygen saturation, atelectasis
Inadequate cough	Retention of secretions
Neurologic Changes	
Increased sympathetic nervous system activity	Tachycardia, change in sleep patterns, increased blood glucose and cortisol levels
Metabolic Changes	
Increased metabolic rate with increased perspiration	Increased fluid and electrolyte losses
Immune System Changes	
Depression of immune response	Increased risk of infection
Gastrointestinal Changes	
Increased intestinal secretions and smooth muscle sphincter tone	Impaired gastrointestinal functioning, ileus

Data from Eland, J. M. (1990). Pain in children. *Nursing Clinics of North America, 25,* 871–884; Altimier, L., Norwood, S., Dick, M. J., et al. (1994). Postoperative pain management in preverbal children: The prescription and administration of analgesia with and without caudal analgesia. *Journal of Pediatric Nursing, 9*(4), 226–232; McCaffrey, M., & Pasero, C. (1999). *Pain: Clinical manual* (2nd ed., p. 24, 27). St. Louis, MO: Mosby; and Mitchell, A., & Boss, B. J. (2002). Adverse effects of pain on the central nervous systems of newborns and young children: A review of the literature. *Journal of Neuroscience Nursing, 34*(5), 228–236.

DEVELOPING CULTURAL COMPETENCE

TERMS THAT DESCRIBE PAIN INTENSITY

The terms *pain, hurt,* and *ache* have been found to describe pain intensity across cultures. Pain is most intense, hurt is less severe, and ache is least severe (Gaston-Johansson, Albert, Fagan et al., 1990). Similarly, pain and hurt mean greater pain than ache in school-age children and adolescents (LaFleur & Raway, 1999). The term *tender* or *tenderness* may be confusing for some families in which English is a second language. Tender or tenderness is more commonly associated with caring or romance or with meat rather than soreness or pain.

Older children may be able to give a history of painful procedures. When attempting to obtain information about the child's pain experiences and present level of pain, keep in mind that many children modify their pain descriptions depending on the type of questions asked and what they expect will happen as a result of their response. Examples of questions to ask include the following:

■ What kinds of things caused hurt in the past and what made it feel better?

■ Does the child tell others about being in pain and what does the child want others to do for the pain?

■ What does the child not want done when he or she is hurting? What would the child like the nurse to do for the hurt?

■ Where is the hurt, and what does it feel like? What could be causing the hurting?

CULTURAL INFLUENCES ON PAIN

Children's culture and social learning have a tremendous influence on their expression of pain. Cultural traditions often guide children about self-control, coping, and enlisting the assistance of others (Huether & Leo, 2002). Children learn directly and indirectly from their parents about how to respond to pain. By showing approval and disapproval, parents teach their children how to behave when in pain. This instruction includes the following:

■ How much discomfort justifies a complaint

■ How to express the complaint

■ How and when to stop complaining

■ Whom to approach for pain relief

For example, boys in the United States are usually encouraged to hide their pain by acting brave and not crying. Girls are often encouraged to express their pain openly. Children also observe other family members in pain and imitate their responses (Abu-Saad, 1984).

DEVELOPING CULTURAL COMPETENCE

EXPRESSION OF PAIN

Some ethnic groups, such as Asian, Anglo-Saxon–Germanic, and Irish, do not openly express pain. People of Italian and Jewish descent are more likely to use both verbal and nonverbal methods to express pain freely. However, children have individualized responses, and younger children have had less time to acquire culturally learned behaviors.

DEVELOPMENTAL RESPONSES TO PAIN

A child's responses to and understanding of pain depend on the child's age and stage of development. See Tables 42–3 and 42–4 to learn more about the child's responses at each age. A child's responses to pain also depend upon situational factors that influence pain responses (McGrath, 1995):

■ Cognitive—understanding of the pain source, ability to control what will happen, focus of attention is on the pain or a distraction

■ Behavioral—use of a pain control strategy, ability to continue usual activities, response of parents and healthcare providers

■ Emotional—presence of fear, anxiety, frustration, anger, depression

Young children are unable to give a detailed description of their pain because of their limited vocabulary and pain experiences. Depending on their developmental stage, children use different coping strategies, such as escape, postponement or avoidance, diversion, and imagery, to deal with pain. Healthcare providers now recognize that children do not complain of pain for several reasons:

■ Some children believe they need to be brave.

■ Preschoolers and adolescents may assume the nurse knows they have pain.

■ Some children are afraid that an injection to relieve pain will hurt more than the pain they have.

GROWTH AND DEVELOPMENT

School-age children and adolescents may not exhibit distress in direct proportion to their pain intensity. Thus, behavioral measures may not match the child's self-report of pain intensity. Older children often appear calm, are expressionless, and limit movement following surgery, but report pain of moderate to severe levels (Tesler et al., 1999). Because children in these age groups can accurately report pain intensity, use the self-report of pain as a valid pain assessment.

TABLE 42–3 ❖ Behavioral Responses and Verbal Descriptions of Pain by Children of Different Developmental Stages

Age Group	Behavioral Response	Verbal Description
Infants		
<6 months	Generalized body movements, chin quivering, facial grimacing, poor feeding	Cries
6–12 months	Reflex withdrawal to stimulus, facial grimacing, disturbed sleep, irritability, restlessness	Cries
Toddlers		
1–3 years	Localized withdrawal, resistance of entire body, aggressive behavior, disturbed sleep	Cries and screams, cannot describe intensity or type of pain
Preschoolers		
3–6 years (preoperational)	Active physical resistance, directed aggressive behavior, strikes out physically and verbally when hurt, low frustration level	Can identify location and intensity of pain, denies pain, may believe his or her pain is obvious to others
School-Age Children		
7–9 years (concrete operations)	Passive resistance, clenches fists, holds body rigidly still, suffers emotional withdrawal, engages in plea bargaining	Can specify location and intensity of pain and describe its physical characteristics in relation to body parts
10–12 years (transitional)	May pretend comfort to project bravery, may regress with stress and anxiety	Able to describe intensity and location with more characteristics, able to describe psychologic pain
Adolescents		
13–18 years (formal operations)	Want to behave in a socially acceptable manner (like adults), show a controlled behavioral response	More sophisticated descriptions as experience is gained; may think nurses are in tune with their thoughts, so they don't need to tell the nurse about their pain

PAIN ASSESSMENT SCALES

Various pain scales are used to assess pain in children.

Nonverbal Children

Physical and behavioral indicators are used to quantify pain in nonverbal children. For example, the Neonatal Infant Pain Scale (NIPS) and the FLACC Behavioral Pain Assessment Scale rely on the nurse's observation of the child's behavior.

The NIPS is designed to measure procedural pain in preterm and full-term newborns up to 6 weeks after birth. The newborn facial expression, cry quality, breathing patterns, arm and leg position, and state of arousal are observed. This tool has high inter-rater reliability and validity. See Table 42–5 on p. 1215.

The FLACC is designed to measure acute pain in infants and young children following surgery, and it can be used until the child is able to self-report pain with another pain scale. FLACC is an acronym for the five categories that are assessed: Face, Legs, Activity, Cry, and Consolability. To use FLACC the nurse observes the child during routine care for 1 to 5 minutes, and then selects the score that most closely matches each behavior noted. The scores for the five categories are added together for the total score. The tool has validity and reliability for evaluation of postoperative pain (Manworren & Hynan, 2003; Willis, Merkel, Voepel-Lewis, et al., 2003). See Table 42–6 on p. 1215.

Young children (3 years and older) can localize pain if given an outline of the front and back of the body. The child can mark where the pain is located or color the area of pain with crayons. The child should use one color for the place where it hurts the most, and another color for areas with less pain.

Self-Report Pain Scales

Other scales depend on the child's self-report of pain intensity (see Skill 13–1). **SKILLS** To use pain scales, the child must be developmentally ready and understand the concept of a little or a lot of pain well enough to tell the nurse. Children 2 to 3 years of age are usually able to understand the concept of "more or less." This child cannot be given more than three choices on a pain scale (none, some, a lot) when assessing pain. When the child can understand rank order and is able to classify, match, and estimate, a numeric scale can be used. A child who correctly responds to either of the following items is developmentally ready for a numeric scale (Merkel, 2002):

■ Which number is larger, 5 or 9? Which number is smaller, 7 or 4?

TABLE 42–4 ✤ Children's Understanding of Pain by Developmental Stage

Developmental Stage	Understanding of Pain
Infants	
< 6 months	No apparent understanding of pain; newborns exposed to repeated painful experiences in ICU demonstrate memory of pain by holding their breath when approached by care providers
6–12 months	Anticipate a painful event such as an immunization with fear; responsive to parental anxiety
Toddlers	
1–3 years	Do not understand what causes pain and why they might have pain; demonstrate fear of painful situations; use common words for pain such as *owie* and *boo-boo*
Preschoolers	
3–6 years (preoperational)	Pain is a hurt; have language skills to express pain, and skills increase with age; do not relate pain to illness but may relate pain to an injury; often believe pain is punishment; do not understand why a painful procedure will make them feel better or why an injection takes pain away
School-Age Children	
7–9 years (concrete operations)	Can understand simple relationships between pain and disease but have no clear understanding of the cause of pain; can understand the need for painful procedures to monitor or treat disease; may associate pain with feeling bad or angry; may recognize psychologic pain related to grief and hurt feelings
10–12 years (transitional)	Better able to understand the relationship between an event and pain; have a more complex awareness of physical and psychologic pain, such as moral dilemmas and mental pain
Adolescents	
13–18 years (formal operations)	Have a sophisticated understanding of the causes of physical and mental pain; relate to the pain experienced by others; pain has both qualitative and quantitative characteristics

■ Ask the child to place several blocks or pieces of paper of different sizes in a row from biggest to smallest.

Examples of self-report pain scales include the Faces Pain Scale and the Oucher Scale. The Oucher Scale presents a series of six photographs of a child expressing increased intensity of pain in combination with a vertical Visual Analog Scale (Figure 42–2 ◉ on p. 1216). The child selects a face that best fits his or her level of pain; an older child can select a number between 0 and 10. The nurse should *not* compare the photos with the child's facial expression to determine pain level. The tool has been developed for three cultural groups with validity and reliability for children between 3 and 12 years of age.

The Faces Pain Rating Scale has a series of six cartoonlike faces with expressions from smiling to tearful that can be used by children starting at 3 years of age (Figure 42–3 ◉). The nurse explains the meaning of each face and asks the child to select the face that is the closest match to the pain felt. As with the Oucher Scale, the nurse should not compare the faces with the child's facial expression to determine pain level. Comparison of faces pain scales has revealed that those scales with a smiling face as the indicator of no pain resulted in significantly higher pain ratings by children and parents than scales using a neutral expression face as an indicator of no pain (Chambers, Gresbrecht, Craig et al., 1999).

School-age children and adolescents have better number concepts and language skills, so additional tools can be used to assess their pain. The nurse should ask the child to describe the pain and give its location. At about 8 years of age, children can give a separate rating for the intensity of pain and describe how unpleasant it is (Jedlinksy, McCarthy, & Michel, 1999). Providing some words such as sharp, dull, aching, pounding, cold, hot, burning, throbbing, stinging, tingling, or cutting can help children describe their pain.

The Numeric Pain Scale or Visual Analog Scale is a single 10-cm horizontal or vertical line that has descriptors of pain at each end (no pain, worst possible pain). Marks and numbers are placed at each cm on the line.

The Poker Chip Tool uses four checkers or poker chips to quantify pain. The child is asked to pick the number of chips that best match the pain felt, with one chip being a little pain and four being the most pain he or she could have.

The Word-Graphic-Rating Scale has words describing increasing pain intensity across a horizontal line. The child marks the line that is closest to the level of pain felt. A millimeter ruler can be used to quantify the pain and record the pain score (Figure 42–4 ◉ on p. 1217).

The Adolescent Pediatric Pain Tool includes a human figure drawing, the Word-Graphic Rating Scale, and a choice of descriptive words. Adolescents indicate pain sites on the human figure outline, use the Word-Graphic-Rating Scale as described, and use the word choices to characterize the pain felt.

TABLE 42–5 ❖ Neonatal Infant Pain Scale (NIPS)

Characteristic	Scoring Criteria	Characteristic	Scoring Criteria
Facial Expression 0 = Relaxed muscles 1 = Grimace	■ Restful face with neutral expression ■ Tight facial muscles; furrowed brow, chin, and jaw (Note: At low gestational ages, infants may have no facial expression)	**Arm Movements** 0 = Relaxed/restrained (with soft restraints) 1 = Flexed/extended	■ Relaxed, no muscle rigidity, random movements of arms ■ Tense, straight arms; rigid; or rapid extension and flexion
Cry 0 = No cry 1 = Whimper 2 = Vigorous cry	■ Quiet, not crying ■ Mild moaning, intermittent cry ■ Loud screaming, rising, shrill, and continuous (Note: silent cry may be scored if infant is intubated, as indicated by obvious facial movements)	**Leg Movements** 0 = Relaxed/restrained (with soft restraints) 1 = Flexed/extended	■ Relaxed, no muscle rigidity, occasional random movements of legs ■ Tense, straight legs; rigid; or rapid extension and flexion
Breathing Patterns 0 = Relaxed 1 = Change in breathing	■ Relaxed, usual breathing pattern maintained ■ Change in drawing breath; irregular, faster than usual, gagging, or holding breath	**State of Arousal** 0 = Sleeping/awake 1 = Fussy	■ Quiet, peaceful, sleeping; or alert and settled ■ Alert and restless or thrashing; fussy

Used with permission from Lawrence, J., Alcock, D., McGrath, D. P., et al. (1993). The development of a tool to assess neonatal pain. *Neonatal Network, 12*(6), 61.

CLINICAL THERAPY FOR PAIN

Pain management includes both drug and nondrug measures. Children need adequate pain medication, but nondrug measures can enhance pain management and ultimately reduce the amount of pain medication needed.

PAIN MEDICATIONS

Drug interventions include the use of **opioids, nonsteroidal anti-inflammatory drugs (NSAIDs)**, and nonnarcotic analgesics (acetaminophen).

TABLE 42–6 ❖ FLACC Behavioral Pain Assessment Scale

Categories	SCORING		
	0	**1**	**2**
Face	No particular expression or smile	Occasional grimace or frown; withdrawn, disinterested	Frequent to constant frown, clenched jaw, quivering chin
Legs	Normal position or relaxed	Uneasy, restless, tense	Kicking or legs drawn up
Activity	Lying quietly, normal position, moves easily	Squirming, shifting back and forth, tense	Arched, rigid, or jerking
Cry	No cry (awake or asleep)	Moans or whimpers, occasional complaint	Crying steadily, screams or sobs; frequent complaints
Consolability	Content, relaxed	Reassured by occasional touching, hugging, or being talked to; distractable	Difficult to console or comfort

Observe the child for 5 minutes or longer. Observe the legs and body uncovered. Reposition the patient or observe activity. Assess body for tenseness and tone. Initiate consoling interventions if needed. Each of the five categories is scored from 0 to 2, resulting in a total score between 0 and 10. A total score of 0 = relaxed and comfortable; 1–3 = mild discomfort; 4–6 = moderate pain; 7–10 = severe discomfort or pain.

Used with permission from Merkel, S. I., Voepel-Lewis, T., Shayevitz, J. R., & Malviya, S. (1997). The FLACC: A behavioral scale for scoring post-operative pain in young children. *Pediatric Nursing, 23*(3), 293–297.

● **FIGURE 42–2**

Use the Oucher Scale that is the best match for the ethnicity of the child. After determining that the child has an understanding of number concepts, teach the child to use the scale. Point to each photo and explain that the bottom picture is "no hurt," the second picture is a "little hurt," the third picture is "a little more hurt," the fourth picture is "even more hurt," the fifth picture is "a lot of hurt," and the sixth picture is the "biggest or most hurt you could ever have." The numbers beside the photos can be used to score the amount of pain the child reports.

The Caucasian version of the Oucher used with permission from Judith E. Beyer, RN, PhD, 1983. The African-American version of the Oucher used with permission from Mary J. Denyes, RN, PhD, and Antonia M. Villarruel, RN, PhD, 1990. The Hispanic version of the Oucher used with permission from Antonia M. Villarruel, RN, PhD, 1990.

Opioids

Opioids are commonly given for severe pain, such as after surgery or a severe injury. Opioids (e.g., morphine and codeine) may be administered by oral, subcutaneous, intramuscular, and intravenous routes. Administration of opioids by an oral route is as effective as by intramuscular and intravenous routes when the drug is given in an **equianalgesic dose** (the amount of drug, whether given by oral or parenteral routes, needed to produce the same analgesic effect) (Table 42–7). Oral and intravenous routes

● **FIGURE 42–3**

| 0 | 1 | 2 | 3 | 4 | 5 |
| No Hurt | Hurts Little Bit | Hurts Little More | Hurts Even More | Hurts Whole Lot | Hurts Worst |

The Faces Pain Rating Scale is valid and reliable in helping children to report their level of pain. Make sure the child has an understanding of number concepts and then teach the child to use the scale. Point to each face and use the words under the picture to describe the amount of pain the child feels. Then ask the child to select the face that comes closest to the amount of pain felt.

Used with permission from Wong, D. L., & Baker, C. M. (1988). Pain in children: Comparison of assessment scales. Pediatric Nursing, 14, 9–16.

FIGURE 42–4

No	Little	Moderate	Large	Worst
Pain	Pain	Pain	Pain	Possible
				Pain

Word-Graphic Rating Scale has words rather than numbers under the line. It may be used by itself or with the Adolescent Pediatric Pain tool. Teach the child to use the tool by pointing to the side of the line that is no pain. Then run your finger along the line and tell the child that this location is the worst possible pain. If the child has some pain, ask the child to make a mark along the line that is the best match for the amount of pain felt. Use a millimeter ruler to measure from the "no pain" end of the line to the marked location to identify the pain score. Make sure the line is the same length each time pain is assessed so comparisons can be made.

Used with permission from Sinkin-Feldman, L., Tesler, M., & Savedra, M. (1997). Word placement on the Word-Graphic Rating Scale by pediatric patients. Pediatric Nursing, 23, 31–34.

are preferred for children. Rectal preparations of some opioids are also available. The optimal analgesic dose varies widely among patients in all age groups (American Pain Society, 1999).

Common side effects include sedation, nausea, vomiting, constipation, and itching. Potential complications of opioids include respiratory depression, cardiovascular collapse, and addiction. When the child's condition is unstable, as in trauma or critical illness, the dosage of opioids must be carefully calculated to match the child's cardiorespiratory status, although infants and children are no more likely than adults to develop respiratory depression following administration of a weight-specific dose of narcotics (Holder & Patt, 1995). Addiction is a rare complication in adults and children treated for painful conditions.

When giving opioids over an extended period of time, children may experience **withdrawal**, the physical signs and symptoms that occur when a sedative or pain drug is stopped suddenly in a patient with physical dependence. An example would be a child in an intensive care setting who experienced

TABLE 42–7 ❖ Opioid Analgesics and Recommended Doses for Children and Adolescents[*]

Drug	Approximate Equianalgesic Oral Dose	Approximate Equianalgesic Parenteral Dose	Recommended Starting Dose (Adults >50 kg) Oral	Parenteral	Recommended Starting Dose (Children & Adults <50 kg) Oral	Parenteral
Morphine	30 mg	10 mg	15–30 mg every 3–4 hr	10 mg every 3–4 hr	0.3 mg/kg every 3–4 hr	0.1 mg/kg every 3–4 hr
Codeine	130 mg	75 mg IM or Subcutaneous	30–60 mg every 3–4 hr	60 mg every 2 hr	0.5–1 mg every 3–4 hr[a]	NR
Hydromorphone (Dilaudid)	7.5 mg	1.5 mg	4–8 mg every 3–4 hr	1.5 mg every 3–4 hr	0.06 mg/kg every 3–4 hr	0.015 mg/kg every 3–4 hr
Levorphanol (Levo-Dromoran)	4 mg (acute) 1 mg (chronic)	2 mg (acute) 1 mg (chronic)	2–4 mg every 6–8 hr	2 mg every 6–8 hr	0.04 mg/kg every 6–8 hr	0.02 mg/kg every 6–8 hr
Meperidine (Demerol)	300 mg	100 mg	NR	100 mg every 3 hr	NR	0.05–1.5 mg/kg every 2–4 hr
Methadone (Dolophine, others)	20 mg (acute) 2–4 mg (chronic)	10 mg (acute) 2–4 mg (chronic)	5–10 mg every 6–8 hr	10 mg every 6–8 hr	0.2 mg/kg every 6–8 hr	0.1 mg/kg every 6–8 hr
Oxycodone (Roxicodone)	30 mg	NA	5–10 mg every 3–4 hr	NA	0.1–0.2 mg/kg every 3–4 hr[a]	NA
Fentanyl	NA	0.01 mg	5 mcg/kg Lozenge	50–100 mcg every 1–2 hr	5–15 mcg/kg Oralet[b]	1 mcg/kg

NR = Not recommended; NA = Not available

*For all parenteral opioids, start with the low dose and titrate to effective pain control.

[a] Caution: Doses of aspirin and acetaminophen in combination with opioid/NSAID preparation must also be adjusted to the patient's body weight.

[b] The Oralet is not widely used because of nausea and vomiting side effects.

Data from American Pain Society. (1999). *Principles of analgesic use in the treatment of acute pain and cancer pain* (4th ed., pp. 6–8, 14–15, 20). Glenview, IL: Author; Hazinski, M. F. (1999). Analgesia, sedation, and neuromuscular blockade in pediatric critical care. In M. F. Hazinski, *Manual of pediatric critical care* (pp. 44–72). St. Louis, MO: Mosby; and Acute Pain Management Guideline Panel. (1992). *Acute pain management in infants, children, and adolescents: Operative and medical procedures. Quick reference guide for clinicians* (AHCPR Pub. No. 92-0020). Rockville, MD: Agency for Healthcare Policy and Research, U.S. Public Health Service, Department of Health and Human Services.

NURSING PRACTICE

Respiratory depression (unresponsiveness and a respiratory rate less than 12 breaths/min in children less than 2 years of age) may progress to respiratory arrest and is the major life-threatening complication of opioid administration. Clinical signs that predict the development of respiratory depression include sleepiness, small pupils, and shallow breathing. Children at particular risk for respiratory depression induced by an opioid are those with an altered level of consciousness, an unstable circulatory status, a history of apnea, or a known airway problem. Some hospitals use continuous pulse oximetry when children at risk for respiratory depression receive opioids.

Respiratory depression is most likely to occur when the child is sleeping. This augments the depressant effect on the respiratory center and potential airway obstruction by the tongue (American Pain Society, 1999). Identify the time interval before drug-specific peak respiratory depression occurs, and then carefully monitor the child's vital signs during that period to detect respiratory depression. Naloxone is the drug used for reversal of opioids' adverse effects.

TABLE 42–8 ✜ Signs and Symptoms of Opioid or Sedative Withdrawal

System	Signs and Symptoms
Central nervous system	Irritability, increased wakefulness, tremulousness, hyperactive deep tendon reflexes, clonus, inability to concentrate, frequent yawning, sneezing, delirium, hypertonicity, visual or auditory hallucinations
Gastrointestinal system	Feeding intolerance with vomiting, diarrhea, uncoordinated suck and swallow
Sympathetic nervous system	Tachycardia, tachypnea, increased blood pressure, nasal stuffiness, sweating, fever

Data from Tobias, J. D. (2000). Tolerance, withdrawal, and physical dependency after long term sedation and analgesia of children in the pediatric intensive care unit. *Critical Care Medicine, 28*(6), 2122–2132. Adapted.

life-threatening injuries, multiple surgeries, and invasive procedures for long-term treatment. Slowly weaning the child off the opioid over 2 to 4 weeks will prevent withdrawal symptoms. See Table 42–8 for signs and symptoms of withdrawal.

Acetaminophen and Nonsteroidal Anti-inflammatory Drugs

NSAIDs such as aspirin, primarily given orally, are effective for the relief of mild to moderate pain and chronic pain. Table 42–9 presents recommended dosages of these drugs. They are most commonly used for bone, inflammatory, and connective tissue conditions. An NSAID may be prescribed in combination with an opioid to increase the effectiveness of the narcotic drug, which may ultimately reduce the amount of opioids needed.

Acetaminophen is a nonnarcotic analgesic that is used like an NSAID. It works by raising the pain threshold and is equal to aspirin in analgesic properties.

DRUG ADMINISTRATION

Pain from surgery, major trauma, or cancer is present for predictable periods because of the effects of tissue damage.

TABLE 42–9 ✜ Acetaminophen, NSAIDs and Recommended Doses for Children and Adolescents

Oral NSAID Peak Action Time	Usual Adult Dose	Usual Pediatric Dose	Comments
Acetaminophen 0.5–2 hr	500–1000 mg every 4–6 hr	10–15 mg/kg every 4–6 hr	Lacks the peripheral anti-inflammatory activity of other NSAIDs; rectal suppository available
Aspirin 1–2 hr	650–975 mg every 4–6 hr	10–15 mg/kg every 4 hr	Do not use in children under 12 years with possible viral illness; may cause gastric upset and bleeding; rectal suppository available
Choline magnesium trisalicylate (Trilisate) 2 hr	1000–1500 mg every 12 hr	25 mg/kg every 12 hr	Does not increase bleeding time like other NSAIDs; also available as oral liquid
Ibuprofen (Motrin, others) 0.5 hr	200–400 mg every 4–6 hr	10 mg/kg every 6–8 hr	Available as oral suspension
Naproxen (Naprosyn) 2–4 hr	500 mg initial dose followed by 250 mg every 6–8 hr	5 mg/kg every 12 hr	Available as oral liquid

Data from American Pain Society. (1999). *Principles of analgesic use in the treatment of acute pain and cancer pain* (4th ed., pp. 6–8, 14–15, 20). Glenview, IL: Author; Hazinski, M. F. (1999). Analgesia, sedation, and neuromuscular blockade in pediatric critical care. In M. F. Hazinski, *Manual of pediatric critical care* (pp. 44–72). St. Louis, MO: Mosby; and Acute Pain Management Guideline Panel. (1992). *Acute pain management in infants, children, and adolescents: Operative and medical procedures. Quick reference guide for clinicians* (AHCPR Pub. No. 92-0020). Rockville, MD: Agency for Healthcare Policy and Research, U.S. Public Health Service, Department of Health and Human Services.

DRUG GUIDE

ACETAMINOPHEN

Overview of Action

Produces analgesia by unknown mechanism. Acts in the hypothalamus to cause antipyresis. Used in treatment of mild to moderate pain and of fever. Does not have anti-inflammatory effects. Does not affect bleeding time.

Routes, Dosage, Frequency

Oral or rectal: 10 to 15 mg/kg/dose every 4 to 6 hours, as needed. Do not exceed 5 doses/day. If not prescribed by healthcare provider, seek medical advice after 5 doses for either fever or pain. Children 12 years and older should not exceed 4 g per day.

Contraindications: Previous allergy to the drug and G6PD deficiency. Do not give preparations with aspartame to children with phenylketonuria. Use cautiously in children with hepatic dysfunction, anemia, renal dysfunction, or rheumatoid arthritis.

Drug interactions: Chronic coadministration with carbamazepine, phenytoin, barbiturates, and rifampin may increase potential for chronic hepatotoxicity.

Side effects: Liver damage with overdose.

Nursing Implications

- Assess: Note hepatic and renal function. Assess pain level or actual temperature prior to administration.
- Administer: Follow dosage directions carefully for different liquid preparations. Concentration differs between drops and elixir. Plain or chewable tablets may be crushed and given with fluid; avoid giving with high-carbohydrate meals, which can decrease drug absorption.
- Monitor: Evaluate the response to medication. Periodic renal and hepatic studies may be ordered for patients on long-term therapy.
- Patient teaching: Do not give with other over-the-counter medications unless directed by healthcare provider as they may also contain acetaminophen or aspirin. Consult a physician for dosage in a child younger than 2 to 3 years, if fever or illness persists over 3 days, or if relief is not obtained. Limit child to 5 doses/day. Store out of the child's reach as this medication is a frequent cause of childhood poisoning.

Data from: Wilson, B. A., Shannon, M. T., & Stang, C. L. (2005). Prentice Hall nurse's drug guide. Upper Saddle River, NJ: Prentice Hall; Iaketoma, C. K., Hudding, J. H., & Kraus, D. M. (2002). Pediatric dosage handbook (9th ed.). Hudson, OH: Lexi-Comp.

Pain relief should be provided around the clock. Every effort should be made to give the child analgesics without causing more pain. The preferred routes of administration are intravenous, local nerve block, and oral.

Continuous infusion analgesia is recommended for children with continuous or persistent severe pain because constant drug levels eliminate peaks and valleys in pain control. Analgesics may also be given intravenously on a scheduled basis (e.g., every 3 to 4 hours). Delays in giving analgesics increase the chances of breakthrough pain and the subsequent anticipation of pain. Giving analgesics on an as-needed basis for acute pain also results in the loss of pain control. More medications are often needed to restore pain control than would have been required for continuous infusion analgesia.

Patient-Controlled Analgesia

Patient-controlled analgesia (PCA) is a method of administering an intravenous analgesic, such as morphine, using a computerized pump programmed by the healthcare professional and controlled by the child (Skill 13–2). **SKILLS** A continuous infusion of opioid prevents a recurrence of pain during long sleeping periods. This method of pain management is especially useful for pain control in the first 48 hours after surgery when oral pain management is not possible. PCA is prescribed mostly for children 5 years of age and older. Children selected for PCA should be able to push the injection button and understand that pushing the

button will give them medication to relieve pain. Parents are sometimes given responsibility for pushing the injection button for younger children or those with disabilities.

After initial pain control has been achieved with an IV infusion by the nurse, the child presses a button to receive a smaller analgesic dose for episodic pain relief. Safety features that include the ability to set the maximum number of infusions per hour and the maximum amount of drug received in a given time period prevent overdoses. Additional pain medication is often ordered as needed to supplement the continuous and patient-administered infusion when pain control is not maintained.

Children and adolescents benefit from PCA by receiving continuous pain control and having the ability to control their comfort level with no trauma from injections. Once children can take oral analgesics, PCA is discontinued.

REGIONAL PAIN MANAGEMENT

Epidural pain control provides selective analgesia and has become more common for postoperative pain management. A catheter is inserted into either the lumbar or the caudal space. Only minute doses of drugs are needed because of the high concentration achieved at the opioid receptors in the spinal cord's dorsal horn (Pasero, 2003).

Local nerve blocks, such as a popliteal block for anesthesia and analgesia of an extremity, are used more frequently for pain control after surgery. A subcutaneous catheter is inserted into the local area for infusion of the

MEDIALINK Skill 13-2: Patient Controlled Analgesia

analgesia. Pain control is achieved without systemic side effects from the medication. Tingling felt in the fingers or toes of the affected extremity is the first sign that the nerve block is receding.

NURSING MANAGEMENT

NURSING ASSESSMENT AND DIAGNOSIS

Nurses have an ethical obligation to relieve a child's suffering not only because of the consequences of unrelieved pain but also because appropriate pain management may have benefits such as earlier mobilization, shortened hospital stays, and reduced costs. To provide effective nursing management of children in pain, anticipate the presence of pain and recognize the child's right to pain control.

When assessing pain in children, keep the following questions in mind:

- What is happening in tissues that might cause pain? Assume that children who have had surgery, injury, vaso-occlusive episode, or illness are experiencing pain, since these events also cause pain in adults.
- What external factors could be causing pain? For example, is the cast too tight or is the child poorly positioned in bed?
- Are there any indicators of pain, either physiologic or behavioral?
- How is the child responding emotionally?
- How does the child or parent rate the pain?

Physiologic symptoms such as nausea, fatigue, dyspnea, bladder and bowel distention, and fever may influence the intensity of pain felt by a child. Fear, anxiety, separation from parents, anger, culture, age, or a previous pain experience may also affect the child's behavior or responses to pain stimuli.

When working with an infant or child, determine which pain scale is the most appropriate for the circumstance and developmental stage. When using a self-report pain assessment tool, *use the same tool each time* you assess for pain or for the evaluation of pain management. This makes comparison of assessment results possible. A chronologic record of the child's pain assessments must be documented along with actions taken to relieve pain, in addition to the follow-up assessments to determine the effectiveness of those actions.

Remember that surgery and trauma can result in multiple sites of pain (incision or laceration, cut or bruised muscles, interrupted blood supply, nasogastric tube placement, insertion sites of intravenous lines). When using pain scales in the assessment of a verbal child, attempt to identify all sites of pain. Then evaluate the intensity of pain at each site.

Examples of nursing diagnoses for children in pain include the following:

- *Acute Pain (abdominal)* related to injury and surgery
- *Anxiety* related to anticipation of pain from an invasive procedure
- *Sleep Pattern Disturbed* related to inadequate pain control
- *Ineffective Individual Therapeutic Regimen Management* related to self-management of pain control, and use of nonpharmacologic pain-control measures
- *Ineffective Breathing Pattern: Potential for,* related to opioid overdose
- *Risk for Constipation* related to opioid pain medication and limited activity

PLANNING AND IMPLEMENTATION

Nursing management involves the following actions to increase and maintain patient comfort once the assessment is completed and nursing diagnoses are developed: pharmacologic intervention; nonpharmacologic intervention; monitoring, evaluating, and documenting the effectiveness of pain-control measures to provide optimal comfort; and patient education.

The accompanying "Nursing Care Plan" summarizes nursing care for the child with postoperative pain.

NURSING CARE PLAN

THE CHILD WITH POSTOPERATIVE PAIN

Intervention	Rationale	Expected Outcome
1. Nursing Diagnosis: Severe Abdominal Pain related to surgery and injury		
NIC Priority Intervention: **Pain management:** Alleviation of pain or a reduction in pain to a level of comfort that is acceptable to the patient		**NOC Suggested Outcome:** **Comfort level:** Feelings of physical and psychologic ease
Goal: The child will report relief (to a level acceptable to the child on a pain scale).		
■ Give analgesic by a pain-free method. ■ Have the child select a pain scale and rate the amount of pain perceived before and 30–60 minutes after analgesia is given to ensure pain relief. ■ Assess pain control each hour to ensure that the child's pain is relieved. ■ Reposition the child every 2 hr to maintain good body alignment. ■ Provide therapeutic touch or massage. Encourage the parents to read a story or play favorite music.	■ The child may deny pain to avoid analgesia by painful route. ■ The child's pain rating is the best indicator of pain. Maintenance of pain control requires less analgesia than treating each acute pain episode. ■ Frequent monitoring identifies inadequate pain control before it becomes significant. ■ New positions decrease muscle cramping and skin pressure. ■ Complementary therapy reduces stress and enhances the analgesic action.	The child reports pain relief after administration of analgesia.
2. Nursing Diagnosis: Disturbed Sleep Pattern related to inadequate pain control		
NIC Priority Intervention: **Sleep enhancement:** Facilitation of regular sleep/awake cycles		**NOC Suggested Outcome:** **Sleep:** Extent and pattern of sleep for mental and physical rejuvenation
Goal: The child will experience fewer disruptions of sleep by pain.		
■ Give analgesia by continuous infusion or every 3–4 hr around the clock.	■ Pain breakthrough occurs even during sleep and disturbs the healing effects of sleep.	The child's sleep is undisturbed by pain. Child sleeps for age-appropriate number of hours per day.
3. Nursing Diagnosis: Ineffective Individual Therapeutic Regimen Management related to self-management of pain control and use of nondrug pain-control measures		
NIC Priority Intervention: **Self-modification assistance:** Reinforcement of self-directed change initiated by the patient to achieve personally important goals		**NOC Suggested Outcome:** **Treatment behavior pain control:** Personal actions to palliate or eliminate pain
Goal: The child and family will effectively use patient-controlled analgesia (PCA) and complementary therapy pain-control measures.		
■ Teach the child how the PCA works and when to push the button. ■ Teach the family and the child how to use age-appropriate imagery, distraction, relaxation techniques, and other complementary therapy pain-control measures.	■ The child must know that pushing the PCA button will keep pain under control. ■ Complementary therapy pain-control measures reduce the amount of analgesia needed.	The child's pain rating stays low. The child and family independently use complementary therapies for pain control.
Goal: The child and family will use appropriate analgesia after discharge.		
■ Discuss appropriate pain control to use at home after discharge.	■ The family and child may be anxious about pain management at home.	The family understands pain-relief measures for use at home and knows where to call if help is needed.

(continued)

NURSING CARE PLAN—continued

THE CHILD WITH POSTOPERATIVE PAIN

Intervention	Rationale	Expected Outcome
4. Nursing Diagnosis: Risk for Ineffective Breathing Pattern related to opioid overdose		
NIC Priority Intervention: **Respiratory monitoring:** Collection and analysis of patient data to ensure airway patency and adequate gas exchange		**NOC Suggested Outcome:** **Vital signs status:** Temperature, pulse, respirations, and blood pressure within expected range for the individual
Goal: The child will maintain adequate ventilations.		
■ Verify that correct dose of opioid analgesia is given for the child's weight. ■ Monitor vital signs and depth of inspirations before analgesic is administered and at time of peak drug action. ■ Calculate agonist dose ordered by physician to be sure it will reverse respiratory depression, but not counteract effect of analgesia.	■ Respiratory depression is a significant complication of opioid analgesia when too much analgesia is given. ■ Respiratory depression episode must not progress to respiratory arrest. All opioids act on brainstem center, which decreases responsiveness to CO_2 tension. ■ Valuable time will be saved if agonist is needed for episode of respiratory depression. Complete reversal of analgesia will cause the child to have significant pain.	There is no episode of respiratory depression associated with analgesia.
5. Nursing Diagnosis: Constipation related to opioid administration and decreased motility of gastrointestinal tract		
NIC Priority Intervention: **Constipation management:** Prevention and alleviation of constipation		**NOC Suggested Outcome:** **Bowel elimination:** Ability of gastrointestinal tract to form and evacuate stool effectively.
Goal: The child will have minimal constipation.		
■ Palpate the abdomen, and assess bowel sounds and abdominal distention. ■ Request physician order for stimulating laxative and stool softener. ■ Provide fluids of choice to increase fluid intake when IV fluids are decreased. ■ Inform family and child that constipation is a side effect of pain medication.	■ Signs of constipation must be anticipated and identified. ■ Opioids increase the transit time of feces and interfere with bile enzymes needed for evacuation. ■ Extra fluids will counteract opioid action of increasing the absorption of water from the large intestine. ■ Parents can become partners in managing fluid intake and monitoring bowel movements.	The child has bowel movements at least every 2 days while on opioid pain control.

Pharmacologic Intervention

Give analgesics as ordered by the physician, ensuring that the dose is appropriate for the child's weight. When administering an opioid by intravenous infusion or PCA, monitor the flow rate and the site for infiltration. Monitor the child's vital signs for complications related to opioids, such as respiratory depression. Vital signs (heart rate and blood pressure) may not change in response to effective analgesia when infection, trauma, or other stressors keep them elevated. Check for the presence of other side effects of analgesics, such as sedation, nausea, vomiting, itching, urinary retention, and constipation. Make sure analgesic antagonists such as naloxone are available should complications develop.

NURSING PRACTICE

Naloxone may be used to treat respiratory depression caused by an opioid drug at a dose and slow infusion rate that does not reverse the pain-control effects of the narcotic. A continuous infusion or repeated doses may be needed for severe overdoses.

When a regional nerve block is used, the analgesic effect does not recede for several hours after the catheter is removed. Be careful when ambulating a child with a regional nerve block in an extremity. Protect the extremity from injury because the child has reduced feeling in the limb. Monitor the child for tingling of fingers or toes, an indication that the analgesic effect is receding. Begin oral analgesia to maintain pain control.

Oral NSAIDs are generally ordered for less severe pain or chronic pain. These drugs may mask fever. Be alert to the potential complication of gastrointestinal hemorrhage in critically ill children who have increased gastric acids as a physiologic stress response to pain.

Assess the child for pain 15 to 30 minutes following intravenous pain medication and 1 hour after oral pain medication to determine if adequate pain control was achieved. Evaluate the child's level of pain frequently to identify any increase in pain intensity. Use information collected from the child and parent, as well as from an appropriate pain scale. Dramatic reductions in pain should occur, although not all pain may disappear. Be certain to record results of pain-control measures to guide future nursing actions. Use a flowsheet to document assessments and medication administration during the postoperative period.

Many children sleep after receiving an analgesic. This sleep is not a side effect of the drug or a sign of an overdose, but the result of pain relief. Pain interrupts sleep, and once pain is relieved, the child can sleep comfortably. However, sleep does not always indicate pain control. A child in pain may fall asleep in exhaustion. Look for other symptoms of pain, such as excess movement or moaning.

Become an advocate for children when the dose or type of analgesic ordered is inadequate. **Tolerance** is a decrease in a drug's effect over time or the need for increasing amounts of the drug to produce or maintain the same level of pain relief or sedation effect. This may occur when children with severe pain have been taking opioids or sedatives for several days. Breakthrough pain occurs, and an increase in dosage is needed to achieve the previous level of pain relief. Tolerance can be delayed with effective use of pain scales to allow appropriate drug dosing, and often less analgesia is needed. Magnesium may also slow the development of tolerance (Tobias, 2000).

Before asking the physician to change the analgesia, review the child's record for documentation that the prescribed drug has been given at the appropriate dose and frequency and that the child's pain relief is ineffective despite the drug administration. After verifying the record, provide the physician with information about the characteristics of the child's pain and ask that the medication be changed.

Nonpharmacologic Intervention

Complementary therapies are the nonpharmacologic methods of pain control that can be used with or without analgesics. The gate control theory helps explain why complementary pain management techniques are effective in helping to control pain. Stimulation of the larger A-delta

---

EVIDENCE-BASED NURSING

GIVING CHILDREN ADEQUATE PAIN MEDICATION

Clinical Question

Why does adequate management of children with acute pain continue to be a problem?

Evidence

In several recent studies, researchers found that some children continue to be undermedicated for moderate and severe pain despite continuing efforts to promote effective pain management for children (Higgins, Turley, Harr et al., 1999; Vincent, 2001; Vincent & Denyes, 2004). A study by Vincent and Denyes in 2004 explored factors related to the actions 67 nurses took to relieve children's pain in actual clinical situations in a children's hospital. The 132 children were experiencing pain from surgery, burns, vaso-occlusive episodes, and trauma. Nurses studied had a moderately high level of knowledge and attitudes about relieving children's pain. Behavioral manifestations of pain led more nurses to believe a child's self-report of pain. Nurses did tend to give more analgesia to children reporting higher pain levels, meaning that the child's pain level is what triggered the nurses to administer analgesia.

Implications

Surprisingly, 26% of children reporting pain received no analgesia, and the 51% of children with moderate to high levels of reported pain received markedly less than the recommended and ordered amounts of

analgesia. Pediatric nurses have an obligation to ask children to report their pain levels and then to accept that this pain rating is accurate. Behavioral cues that pain exists should not be necessary to evaluate pain in children who can self-report pain. Crying and grimacing in pain are not the only pain behaviors to look for. Pain behaviors vary among children. For example, children use play as a distraction to self-manage pain, and they sleep after becoming fatigued from dealing with pain. Children are entitled to comfort and pain relief, so all information that informs the nurse that the child is experiencing pain should be used in making decisions to relieve pain.

Critical Thinking

What could be some reasons for undermedication of children by nurses? What is your role in improving the pain management of children in all settings?

References

Vincent, C. V., & Denyes, M. J. (2004). Relieving children's pain: Nurses' abilities and analgesic practices. *Journal of Pediatric Nursing, 19*(1), 40–50.

Vincent, C. V. (2001). Nurses' analgesic practices with hospitalized children. *Journal of Child and Family Nursing, 4*(2), 79–89.

Higgins, S. S., Turley, K. M., Harr, J., & Turley, K. (1999). Prescription and administration of around the clock analgesics in postoperative pediatric cardiovascular surgery patients. *Progress in Cardiovascular Nursing, 14*(1), 19–24.

TEACHING HIGHLIGHTS

HELPING A CHILD COPE WITH PAIN

Parents are the single most powerful nonpharmacologic method of pain relief available to children. A parent's presence greatly reduces the anxiety associated with pain and hospitalization (Broome, 2000). Children often feel more secure telling their parents about their pain and anxiety. When parents are actively participating in the child's care during hospitalization, teach them about how complementary therapies can be used to enhance the child's pain management. Help the parent select the age-appropriate complementary therapy for the child:

- Infants: holding, cuddling, sucking a pacifier, massage
- Toddlers: massage, stories, bubbles, touch, holding and rocking, music (Figure 42–5)
- Preschoolers: engaging in play, stories, music, imagining being a superhero, watching television or a video
- School-age children: rhythmic breathing, muscle relaxation, guided imagery, talking about pleasant experiences, playing games, listening to radio, watching television or a video
- Adolescents: rhythmic breathing, muscle relaxation, guided imagery, having visitors, playing games, watching television, listening to radio or CD player

fibers by nonpainful touch and pressure such as massage causes the substantia gelatinosa in the dorsal horn of the spinal cord to "close the gate" and decrease the transmission of pain impulses to the brain (Franck, Greenberg, & Stevens, 2000; Huether & Leo, 2002). See "Pathophysiology Illustrated" on page 1209."

One or more of these methods may provide adequate relief of low levels of pain. When used with analgesics, nonpharmacologic techniques often increase the effectiveness of the analgesic or reduce the dosage required. When used in association with a medical procedure, remember to use an intervention before, during, and after the procedure. This gives the child a chance to recover, feel mastery, and remember coping (Fanurik, Koh, Schitz et al., 1997).

Assemble a pain management kit to promote distraction, imagery, and relaxation in children. Items that might be included are magic wands, pinwheels, bubble liquid, a slinky spring toy, a foam ball, party noisemakers, and pop-up books. It may also be helpful to include items for therapeutic play such as syringes, adhesive bandages, alcohol swabs, and other supplies from a medical kit. The pain management kit may be especially helpful for distracting children who are being prepared for surgery or for painful procedures.

Distraction. **Distraction** involves engaging a child in a wide variety of activities to help him or her focus attention on something other than pain and the anxiety associated with the procedure. Examples of distracting activities are listening to music, singing a song, playing a game, watching tele-

vision or a video, and focusing on a picture while counting. Select activities that are developmentally appropriate for the child. Children in severe pain cannot be distracted, but do not assume the pain is gone if a child can be distracted.

Cutaneous Stimulation. Cutaneous stimulation involves gently rubbing the painful area, massaging the skin gently, and holding or rocking the child. Touching provides a stimulus to compete with the pain stimuli transmitted from the peripheral nerves to the spinal cord. These actions may reduce the pain felt by the child. Swaddling and blanket rolls may calm a distressed newborn by decreasing tactile stimulation and containing gross motor behaviors (Lynn, Ulma, & Spreker, 1999).

Sucrose Solution. Concentrated sucrose solutions (12% or 24%) with a pacifier may be used as a pain relief measure in newborns. Sucrose may provide a natural pain relief by activating endogenous opioid systems in the body. The analgesic effect of sucrose lasts approximately 3 to 5 minutes, with a peak action in 2 minutes (Mitchell & Waltman, 2003). A moistened pacifier dipped in a packet of sugar given to the infant during a painful procedure reduced pain behaviors such as duration of crying and vagal tone during a heel stick (Greenberg, 2002).

● FIGURE 42–5

The presence of the parent is an important part of pain management. Children often feel more secure telling their parents about their pain and anxiety.

Electroanalgesia. Also known as transcutaneous electrical nerve stimulation (TENS), **electroanalgesia** delivers small amounts of electrical stimulation to the skin by electrodes. This electrical stimulation is stronger than the pain impulses, and because of the gate control theory, is thought to interfere with the transmission of pain from the peripheral nerves to the spinal cord. TENS may be used for both acute and chronic pain management. The only known side effect is skin irritation at the electrode site.

Guided Imagery. Imagery is a cognitive process that encourages the child to focus concentration on an event or place unrelated to the pain process. The focus can be on exploring a favorite place, doing a favorite activity, remembering a funny story, or being a superhero. This method is most effective in children over 6 years of age. Ask the child to think about all the sights, sounds, smells, tastes, and feelings that will help him or her to experience the favorite place, activity, or story. Guided imagery is a form of self-hypnosis, and it is most effective when preceded by a relaxation exercise.

Relaxation Techniques. Relaxation techniques are used to reduce muscle tension, which aggravates pain. Relaxation methods include rhythmic breathing and alternately tensing and relaxing selected muscle groups for 10 seconds each. Progressively move from specific muscle groups to more central muscles. Enhance relaxation by focusing the child's attention on something pleasant.

Hypnosis. An altered state of consciousness occurs when appropriate suggestions distort perception, memory, and mood. Children who respond to hypnotic suggestions are often more relaxed and experience less pain. The precise physiologic mechanism for the success of hypnosis in pain control is not known; however, the gate control theory may be a factor.

Application of Heat and Cold. Heat application promotes dilation of blood vessels. The increased blood circulation permits the removal of debris of cell breakdown from the site. Heat also promotes muscle relaxation, breaking the pain–spasm–pain cycle. To reduce edema, do not apply heat in the first 24 hours after an injury.

The application of cold is believed to slow the ability of pain fibers to transmit pain impulses. Cold also controls pain by decreasing edema and inflammation and by causing partial or complete anesthesia or numbness of the skin. When cold is applied, assess the skin for redness or signs of irritation. Take care to avoid causing thermal injury. Discontinue cold applications immediately if the skin alternately blanches and reddens afterwards or if blisters or redness do not subside between applications.

Discharge Planning and Home Care Teaching

Children are frequently discharged from the hospital with oral analgesics following surgery, injury, or treatment of acute medical conditions. Parents have the responsibility

COMPLEMENTARY CARE

HYPNOTHERAPY FOR CHILDREN

The most widely studied of the complementary/alternative therapies, hypnotherapy is often successfully prescribed as the primary treatment for a variety of childhood problems, including pain, bed-wetting, asthma, stool-withholding, habit disorders, anxiety and fears, migraine headaches, nausea from chemotherapy, needle phobias, warts, insomnia, tics, and other problems (Anbar, 2003; Thompson, 2004).

Children have a great capacity to use their imaginations and fantasy worlds for therapeutic gain and are actually more successful than adults in attaining a hypnotic state. Children entering a healthcare environment are often fearful. As the nurse, you can induce a more relaxed state in children by speaking quietly, focusing them on their breathing, and suggesting they imagine something pleasant—the ingredients of hypnotic induction.

Hypnosis is an altered state of awareness facilitating heightened concentration, decreased awareness of external stimuli, increased relaxation, and increased suggestibility. Hypnotherapy can be as simple as teaching a child to blow on a pinwheel while getting an injection. This diminishes the pain and fear of the needle by focusing the child's heightened attention elsewhere. More formal hypnotherapy is done by a therapist trained in pediatric hypnotherapeutic techniques that use the images and language of the child to induce relaxation and give posthypnotic suggestions. Language such as, "You are the boss of your body and can help make this headache not bother you anymore" is used to help children gain mastery over their physical symptoms.

to provide adequate pain control for their child after day surgery. The child usually leaves the surgical center pain-free, and the parents may not anticipate pain. Take the time to discuss the importance of pain management and its benefits in promoting the child's healing. Make sure parents know that a sudden increase in pain intensity indicates the development of a complication requiring medical attention.

Provide guidance to help parents assess their child's pain, and for school-age children and adolescents to assess their own pain. Teach parents and children about the dosage and frequency of administration and the side effects of the analgesic ordered. Review nonpharmacologic methods of pain control with parents and children. Encourage children and parents to use the techniques that work best for them.

Remember that many common health problems (otitis media, pharyngitis, and urinary tract infection) have pain as one of the presenting symptoms. Often the only medication prescribed is an antibiotic to clear the infection. This may leave the child in pain for 48 to 72 hours until the antibiotic brings the infection under control. Give parents recommendations for pain control and comfort measures during this period. Review the dose, dosing device, and formulation of acetaminophen used by parents to identify any risk for overdose.

EVALUATION

Expected outcomes of nursing care include the following:

- The child's pain level is assessed frequently and pain management is effective in improving the child's comfort.
- The child successfully uses a PCA pump to control acute pain.
- Age-appropriate nonpharmacologic methods of pain management enhance the comfort provided by medications.

NURSING MANAGEMENT OF CHRONIC PAIN

Some children have medical conditions that cause chronic pain and episodic acute pain, such as rheumatoid arthritis, cancer, headaches, recurrent abdominal pain, and HIV infection. Chronic pain does not arouse the sympathetic nervous system in the same way that acute pain does. Therefore the child may perceive pain but not appear to be in pain.

Physical and psychologic signs and symptoms should be viewed together. No tools have been developed to assess chronic pain for any child age group. Assessment and evaluation of chronic pain in children should include the following aspects (American Pain Society, 2003):

- Approach pain as the present problem and obtain the history of pain onset, its development over time, intensity, duration, location, what makes it worse or relieves it, and its impact on daily life (sleeping, appetite, school, and social interactions).
- Determine the amount of distress the child and family experience with pain, including anxiety, depression, and hopelessness.
- Clarify what the family and child believe causes the pain and their response to it.
- Identify past pain problems in the family and the current methods of treatment.
- Observe the child's appearance, posture, gait, and emotional and cognitive state.
- Assess muscle spasms, trigger points, areas sensitive to light touch, and a complete neurologic examination.

Older children with recurrent episodes of pain can be encouraged to keep a diary or log to describe the characteristics, timing, activities, and potential triggers of their pain, as well as their response to pain treatment measures. A pain assessment scale should be used to rate the pain intensity before and after medications and other pain-control measures are used. This record can help improve pain management.

Examples of nursing diagnoses for children with chronic pain include the following:

- *Chronic Pain* related to arthritic joint inflammation and degeneration
- *Disturbed Sleep Pattern* related to ineffective management of chronic pain
- *Impaired Physical Mobility* related to ineffective management of chronic pain

Children with chronic conditions (arthritis, sickle cell disease, hemophilia, cancer, recurrent headaches, etc.) often need long-term pain management. NSAIDs and acetaminophen are often ordered for pain management. Strategies for chronic pain management include the following:

- Explain and validate pain and its causes.
- Encourage the use of a pain diary.
- Discuss treatment goals with the child and family and jointly develop a care plan that integrates pharmacologic and nonpharmacologic (complementary) methods.
- Develop a care plan for sudden painful episodes associated with acute flare-ups of their condition.
- Provide effective preventive pain management for procedural pain, as many of these children have numerous medical procedures.

Parents should be actively engaged in pain control for their child. Teach parents the importance of pain control and how to use a variety of complementary therapies with their child to supplement the pain medications administered. Refer children with long-term pain to a pediatric pain program to be evaluated for customized strategies to manage pain.

SEDATION AND PAIN MANAGEMENT FOR MEDICAL PROCEDURES

Children undergo a wide variety of painful diagnostic and treatment procedures in the hospital and in outpatient settings. Procedures such as chest tube insertion, arterial puncture, lumbar puncture, bone marrow aspiration, fracture reduction, laceration repair, insertion of a central or peripheral intravenous line, and burn debridement cause significant pain in children. The anticipation of these procedures causes anxiety and emotional distress that can lead to greater intensity of pain. Children who have experienced severe pain in the past may be unwilling to cooperate with healthcare personnel.

CLINICAL THERAPY

Minor Medical Procedures

Topical anesthetics can be used to reduce the pain associated with the first needle stick. Vapocoolant sprays can be used for injections. Eutectic mixture of local anesthetics (EMLA) cream, a mixture of 2.5% lidocaine and 2.5% prilocaine in an emulsion, is effective if applied 60 minutes before a needle stick procedure on intact skin (Rogers & Ostrow, 2004). See Figure 42–6 ⊙. A new preparation (ELA-MAX, 4% liposomal lidocaine) is effective if applied 30 minutes before a needle stick (Eichenfield, Funk, Fallon-Friedlander et al., 2002).

A local anesthetic such as lidocaine buffered by sodium bicarbonate is often injected to provide analgesia for emergency invasive procedures. Lidocaine can also be injected subcutaneously in a small area to reduce the pain of deeper needle insertion.

Sedation

Sedation is a medically controlled state of depressed consciousness (light to deep) used for painful diagnostic and therapeutic procedures. Procedures such as burn debridement, laceration repair, bone marrow aspiration, and fracture reduction are associated with so much pain and anxiety

⊙ **FIGURE 42–6**

A

B

When painful procedures are planned, use EMLA cream to anesthetize the skin where the painful stick will be made. **A,** Apply a thick layer of cream over intact skin (one half of a 5-g tube). **B,** Cover the cream with a transparent adhesive dressing, sealing all the sides. The cream anesthetizes the dermal surface in 45 to 60 minutes.

that children need premedication with analgesia and **anxiolysis**, mild sedation. Sedation is often used to gain the cooperation of the child for the medical procedure. Drugs for sedation include the following (Proudfoot, 2002):

- Benzodiazepines: diazepam (Valium), midazolam (Versed), and lorazepam (Ativan)
- Hypnotics or barbiturates: thiopental, pentobarbital
- Ketamine
- Propofol (Diprivan)
- Analgesics: Fentanyl, Alfentanil

When sedatives are given in lower doses, **light sedation** occurs during which the child maintains protective reflexes, maintains a patent airway, and appropriately responds to verbal stimuli. **Deep sedation** is a controlled state of depressed consciousness or unconsciousness in which the protective reflexes are lost. See Table 42–10. Analgesia must be given in association with sedation because the sedated child can still feel pain but not communicate its presence.

Guidelines should exist in every healthcare facility where pediatric sedation is performed to ensure safe healthcare practices. These guidelines often require that the health professionals monitoring the child have specific qualifications, such as pediatric advanced life support training. With the combined effects of analgesia and sedatives, the child must be carefully monitored for respiratory depression and signs of deep sedation. Antagonist agents are available for opioids and benzodiazepines when the effects of sedation and respiratory depression need to be reversed. (See Skills 13–3 and 13–4 for more information. **SKILLS**)

NURSING MANAGEMENT

Increase Comfort During Painful Procedures

Help the child cope with a painful procedure by telling the child what sensations to expect and what will happen during the procedure. This reduces stress more effectively than just providing information about the procedure. See Chapter 39 for methods of preparing children of different developmental ages for procedures.

MediaLink Skills 13-3 and 13-4

NURSING PRACTICE

Whenever sedation is given, be sure to have the resources available to monitor the child's vital signs and to provide advanced life support if the child should progress to deep sedation. In case complications occur, the following equipment should be immediately available: suction apparatus, a bag-valve mask for assisted ventilation with capability of 90% to 100% oxygen delivery, and an oxygen supply (5 L/min for more than 60 minutes). Antagonists to sedative medication must be premeasured and ready to administer.

TABLE 42–10 ✤ Characteristics of Light and Deep Sedation

Assessment Factors	Light Sedation	Deep Sedation
Airway	Able to maintain airway independently and continuously	Unable to maintain airway independently or continuously
Cough and gag reflexes	Reflexes intact	Partial or complete loss of reflexes
Level of consciousness	Easily aroused with verbal or gentle physical stimulation	Not easily aroused, may not respond purposefully to verbal or gentle physical stimulation

Data from Proudfoot, J. (2002). Pediatric procedural sedation and analgesia (PSA): Keeping it simple and safe. *Pediatric Emergency Medicine Reports, 7*(2), 1–2.

Drug therapy is not always used for quick procedures, such as a dressing change, or an unexpected intravenous insertion, injection, or venipuncture. Complementary therapies, especially guided imagery, relaxation techniques, and distraction, may reduce the anxiety associated with the anticipation of the procedure. Teach parents and children to use these interventions before procedures. Help children control their anxiety through therapeutic play.

When pharmacologic pain management is used for a procedure, the nurse's responsibilities include the following:

■ Treat anticipated procedure-related pain prophylactically. For example, give an analgesic before a bone marrow aspiration or fracture reduction. Permit time for the drug to become effective.

■ Manage preexisting pain before beginning a procedure such as scrubbing a burn.

■ Whenever possible, administer drugs by a nonpainful route (oral, transmucosal, intravenous). Avoid intramuscular or subcutaneous injections.

■ When procedures must be repeated (for example, bone marrow aspirations for children with leukemia), give optimal analgesia for the first procedure to reduce anxiety about future procedures.

■ To prevent increased anxiety, avoid delays in performing procedures.

■ Document the results of pain management.

When the child receives sedation, monitoring the child's status is important. Nursing assessments include visual confirmation of respiratory effort, color, and vital signs. Pulse oximetry and other technology may be used for monitoring, but the equipment must not replace visual assessment. Vital signs must be checked every 15 minutes until the child regains full consciousness and level of functioning. If light sedation progresses to deep sedation, airway management is essential; check vital signs every 5 minutes.

Criteria for discharge after sedation include the following (Bindler & Ball, 2003):

■ Satisfactory and stable cardiovascular function and airway patency.

■ Easily arousable, protective reflexes intact.

■ Adequate hydration.

■ Infant is able to hold the head up and sit up unassisted if old enough to do so, or the child can stand and walk without assistance.

■ Discharge status is the same as admission status.

Critical Concept Review

LEARNING OBJECTIVES

CONCEPTS

Describe the physiologic and behavioral consequences of pain in children.

1. Physiologic consequences of acute pain:
   ■ Tachycardia and rapid shallow breathing.
   ■ Inadequate cough.
   ■ Inadequate lung expansion.
   ■ Depressed immune response.
   ■ Increased perspiration and loss of electrolytes and fluids.
   ■ Increased intestinal secretions.

LEARNING OBJECTIVES

CONCEPTS

Describe the physiologic and behavioral consequences of pain in children.—continued

2. Behavioral consequences of acute pain:
   - Short attention span.
   - Irritability.
   - Facial grimacing.
   - Posturing, protecting painful area, immobility.
   - Lethargy or withdrawal.
   - Sleep disturbance.

Select an appropriate tool to assess the pain of infants and children in each age group.

1. Infants and nonverbal children:
   - Neonatal infant pain scale.
   - FLACC Behavioral Pain Assessment Scale.
2. Young children:
   - Color area of pain on outline of body.
   - Faces pain scale.
   - Oucher scale.
3. Older children and adolescents:
   - Visual analog scale.
   - Poker chip scale.
   - Word graphic scale.
   - Adolescent pediatric pain tool.

Describe the nursing assessment and management for a child receiving an opioid analgesic.

1. Use oral and intravenous route, if possible.
2. Titrate dose to match child's cardiorespiratory status.
3. Identify line of peak drug effect and monitor child's vital signs to detect respiratory depression.
4. Observe for nausea, constipation and itching.
5. Have naloxone (Narcan) available for treatment of respiratory distress.

Explain the rationale for the effectiveness for nonpharmacologic (complementary) methods of pain control.

Nonpharmacologic methods of pain control are effective in children due to the Gate Control Theory. The use of methods such as nonpainful touch and massage stimulate the larger A-delta fibers and decrease the transmission of pain impulses to the brain.

Assess children of different ages with acute pain and develop a nursing care plan that integrates pharmacologic interventions and developmentally appropriate nonpharmacologic (complementary) therapies.

Interventions common to all ages:
1. Assess pain frequently.
2. Anticipate need for pain medication.
3. Monitor vital signs.

Pharmacologic and nonpharmacologic interventions by age group:
1. Infants and toddlers:
   - Administer oral or intravenous medications around the clock.
   - Hold, swaddle, rock, or provide nonnutritive sucking.
   - Allow infant to suck sucrose solution.
   - Have toddler blow bubbles.
2. Preschooler:
   - Use distraction techniques with the use of a magic wand, pinwheel, or noise maker.
   - Allow child to watch appropriate TV shows or videos.
3. School-age child and adolescent:
   - Instruct in use of PCA or epidural until able to take oral medications.
   - Use hypnotherapy if child is able to cooperate.
   - Engage child in breathing techniques for relaxation.
   - Use guided imagery, visitors, TV, radio, tapes, or CDs for distraction.

Develop a nursing care plan for assessing and monitoring the child having sedation and analgesia for a medical procedure.

1. Explain procedure to the child and parents.
2. Administer medications by oral or intravenous route, if possible.
3. Employ nonpharmacologic methods such as distraction and guided imagery to decrease anxiety.
4. Use pulse oximetry and a cardiorespiratory monitor during procedure.
5. After procedure is completed, check vital signs and level of consciousness frequently until child is stable and awake.

CRITICAL THINKING IN ACTION

*View the **Critical Thinking in Action** video in Chapter 42 of the CD-ROM. Then, answer the questions that follow.*

A 12-year-old boy, Kevin, is recovering from a 4-wheeler accident on the medical surgical unit at a local children's hospital. He was riding the 4-wheeler unsupervised and without permission while his parents were at work. He suffered an abdominal injury requiring surgery, three broken bones and several lacerations that needed stitches. His parents are very worried about his injuries and at the same time angry with him for not following the rules. Kevin appears expressionless in his hospital bed, but cries and grimaces at any slight movement. When asked on a scale of 1–10 (10 being the most pain) how much pain he is feeling, he says a 10. His parents are reluctant to let him have any pain medications because they fear he may become dependent on the medication. His father states that

Kevin should be a man and tolerate the pain, and he thinks enduring the pain will teach him a lesson about responsibility. The nurse explains that pain management is necessary to improve Kevin's healing, help him mobilize sooner, and potentially shorten his hospital stay. She explains the physiological consequences of ineffective pain management and discusses how the medication will help him sleep and rest. She explains that some of pain medications can be addicting, but the chances of Kevin becoming addicted to pain medications for this injury are extremely rare. She also reviews the nonpharmacological methods of relieving pain. The parents are still reluctant to the medications, but agree to conform to the doctor's orders.

1. What are some of the potential physiological consequences to letting Kevin suffer pain?
2. What are some examples of opioid analgesics available to Kevin?
3. What are some examples of NSAIDs available to Kevin?
4. What are the signs and symptoms of opioid withdrawal and how long should it take for Kevin to be weaned off an opioid?

MEDIALINK   www.prenhall.com/london

- NCLEX-RN® Review, case studies, and other interactive resources for this chapter can be found on the Companion Website at http://www.prenhall.com/london. Click on "Chapter 42" and select the activities for this chapter.

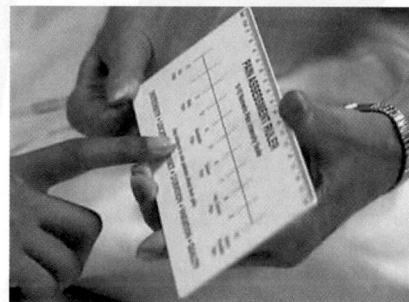

- For animations, more NCLEX-RN® Review questions, and an audio glossary, access the accompanying CD-ROM in this textbook.

REFERENCES

Abu-Saad, H. (1984). Cultural components of pain: The Asian-American child. *Children's Health Care, 13,* 11–14.

American Pain Society. (1999). *Principles of analgesic use in the treatment of acute pain and cancer pain* (4th ed.). Glenview, IL: Author.

American Pain Society. (2003). Pediatric chronic pain: A position statement from the American Pain Society. Retrieved October 22, 2003 from www.ampainsoc.org/cgi-bin/print/print/pl.

Anbar, R. (2001). Self-hypnosis for management of chronic dyspnea in pediatric patients. *Pediatrics, 2,* 21.

Anbar, R. D. (2003). Self-hypnosis for anxiety associated with severe asthma: A case report. *BMC Pediatrics, 3*(1), 3 7.

Bindler, R. C., & Ball, J. W. (2003). *Clinical skills manual for pediatric nursing: Caring for children.* (3rd ed.). Upper Saddle River, NJ: Prentice Hall.

Broome, M. E. (2000). Helping parents support their child in pain. *Pediatric Nursing, 26*(3), 315–317.

Chambers, C. T., Gresbrecht, K., Craig, K. D., Bennett, S. M., & Huntsman, E. (1999). A comparison of faces scales for the measurement of pediatric pain: Children's and parent's ratings. *Pain, 83,* 25–35.

Eichenfield, L. F., Funk, A., Fallon-Friedlander, S., & Cunningham, B. B. (2002). A clinical study to evaluate ELA-MAX (4% liposomal lidocaine) as compared with eutectic mixture of local anesthetics cream for pain reduction of venipuncture in children. *Pediatrics, 109*(5), 1093–1099.

Fanurik, D., Koh, J., Schitz, M., & Brown, R. (1997). Pharmacobehavioral intervention: Integrating pharmacologic and behavioral techniques for pediatric procedures. *Children's Health Care, 26*(1), 1–13.

Franck, L. S., Greenberg, C. S., & Stevens, B. (2000). Pain assessment in infants and children. *Pediatric Clinics of North America, 47*(3), 487–512.

Fuller, B. F. (2001). Infant behaviors as indicators of established pain. *Journal of Society of Pediatric Nurses, 6*(3), 109–115.

Gaston-Johansson, F., Albert, M., Fagan, E., & Zimmerman, L. (1990). Similarities in pain descriptions of four different ethnic-culture groups. *Journal of Pain and Symptom Management, 5*(2), 94–100.

Greenberg, C. S. (2002). A sugar-coated pacifier reduces procedural pain in newborns. *Pediatric Nursing, 22*(3), 271–277.

Hazinski, M. F. (1999). Analgesia, sedation, and neuromuscular blockage in pediatric critical care. In M. F. Hazinski, *Manual of pediatric critical care* (pp. 44–72). St. Louis, MO: Mosby.

Higgins, S. S., Turley, K. M., Harr, J. & Turley, K. (1999). Prescription and administration of around the clock analgesics in postoperative pediatric cardiovascular surgery patients. *Progress in Cardiovascular Nursing, 14*(1), 19–24.

Holder, K. A., & Patt, R. B. (1995). Taming the pain monster: Pediatric postoperative pain management. *Pediatric Annals, 24*(3), 164–168.

Huether, S. E., & Leo, J. (2002). Pain, temperature regulation, sleep, and sensory function. In K. L. McCance & S. E. Huether (Eds.), *Pathophysiology: The biologic basis for disease in adults and children* (4th ed., pp. 401–410). St. Louis, MO: Mosby–Year Book.

Jedlinsky, B. P., McCarthy, C. F., & Michel, T. H. (1999). Validating pediatric pain measurement: Sensory and affective components. *Pediatric Physical Therapy, 11*, 368–374.

Joint Commission on Accreditation of Healthcare Organizations. (2001). *Pain standards for 2001.* Oakbrook Terrace, IL: Author.

LaFleur, C. J., & Raway, B. (1999). School-age child and adolescent perception of the pain intensity associated with three word descriptors. *Pediatric Nursing, 25*(1), 45–55.

Lynn, A. M., Ulma, G. A., & Spreker, M. (1999). Pain control in very young infants: An update. *Contemporary Pediatrics, 16*(11), 39–66.

Manworren, R. C. B., & Hynan, L. S. (2003). Clinical validation of FLACC: Preverbal patient pain scale. *Pediatric Nursing, 29*(2), 140–146.

McCaffrey, M., & Pasero, C. (1999). *Pain: Clinical manual* (2nd ed.). St. Louis, MO: Mosby.

McGrath, P. A. (1995). Pain in the pediatric patient: Practical aspects of assessment. *Pediatric Annals, 24*(3), 126–138.

McGrath, P. J., & Craig, K. D. (1989). Developmental and psychological factors in children's pain. *Pediatric Clinics of North America, 36*(4), 823–836.

Merkel, S. (2002). Pain assessment in infants and children: The finger span scale. *American Journal of Nursing, 102*(11), 55–56.

Merkel, S. I., Voepel-Lewis, T., Shayevitz, J. R., & Malviya, S. (1997). The FLACC: A behavioral scale for scoring post-operative pain in young children. *Pediatric Nursing, 23*(3), 293–297.

Mitchell, A., & Waltman, P. A. (2003). Oral sucrose and pain relief in preterm infants. *Pain Management Nursing, 4*(2), 62–69.

Pasero, C. (2002). Pain assessment in infants and young children: Neonates. *American Journal of Nursing, 102*(8), 61–65.

Pasero, C. (2003). Epidural analgesia for postoperative pain. *American Journal of Nursing, 103*(10), 62–64.

Proudfoot, J. (2002). Pediatric procedural sedation and analgesia (PSA): Keeping it simple and safe. *Pediatric Emergency Medicine Reports, 7*(2), 1–2.

Rogers, T. L., & Ostrow, C. L. (2004). The use of EMLA cream to decrease venipuncture pain in children. *Journal of Pediatric Nursing, 19*(1), 33–39.

Shapiro, B. S. (1995). Treatment of chronic pain in children and adolescents. *Pediatric Annals, 24*(3), 148–156.

Sinkin-Feldman, L., Tesler, M., & Savedra, M. (1997). Word placement on the Word-Graphic Rating Scale by pediatric patients. *Pediatric Nursing, 23*, 31–34.

Tesler, M. D., Holzemer, W. L., & Spreker, M. (1999). Pain behaviors: Postsurgical responses of children and adolescents. *Journal of Pediatric Nursing, 13*(1), 41–47.

Thompson, N. L. (2004). *Hypnotherapy for children.* Frederick, MD: Publish America.

Tobias, J. D. (2000). Tolerance, withdrawal, and physical dependency after long term sedation and analgesia of children in the pediatric intensive care unit. *Critical Care Medicine, 28*(6), 2122–2132.

Vincent, C. V. (2001). Nurses' analgesic practices with hospitalized children. *Journal of Child and Family Nursing, 4*(2), 79–89.

Vincent, C. V., & Denyes, M. J. (2004). Relieving children's pain: Nurses' abilities and analgesic practices. *Journal of Pediatric Nursing, 19*(1), 40–50.

Willis, M. H. W., Merkel, S. I., Voepel-Lewis, T., & Malviya, S. (2003). FLACC behavioral pain assessment scale: A comparison with the child's self-report. *Pediatric Nursing, 29*(3), 195–198.

Wong, D. L., & Baker, C. M. (1988). Pain in children: Comparison of assessment scales. *Pediatric Nursing, 14*, 9–16.

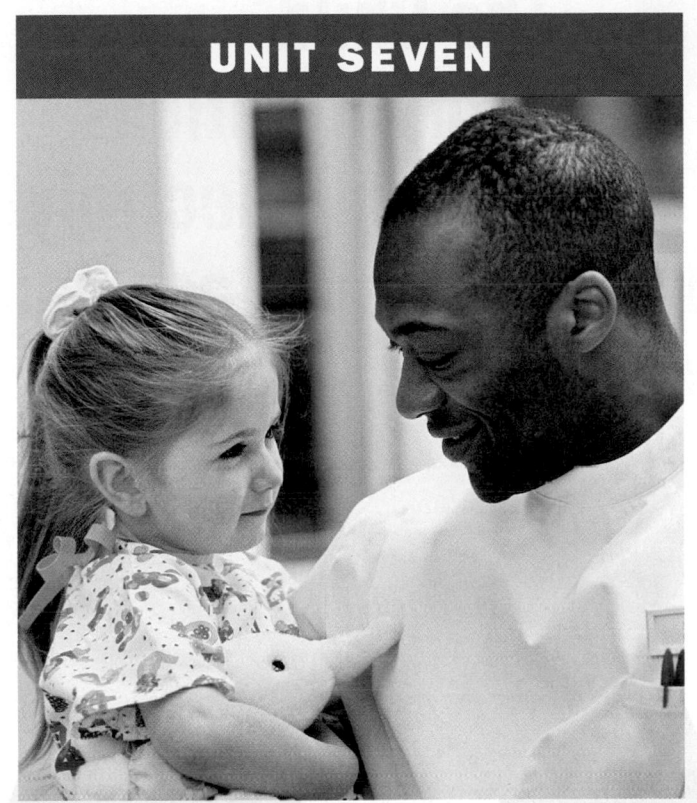

UNIT SEVEN

Caring for Children with Alterations in Health Status

CHAPTER 43

The Child with Alterations in Fluid, Electrolyte, and Acid-Base Balance

LeShan always likes to eat, so when he won't even drink I know he is sick. We just didn't know how sick he was or that he had gotten dehydrated. I wonder if we should have done something else for him at home.

—*Mother of LeShan, 18 months*

LEARNING OBJECTIVES

- Describe normal fluid and electrolyte status for children at various ages.

- Identify regulatory mechanisms for fluid and electrolyte balance.

- Recognize threats to fluid and electrolyte balance in children.

- Describe acid-base balance and recognize disruptions common in children.

- Analyze assessment findings to recognize fluid-electrolyte problems and acid-base imbalance in children.

- Describe appropriate nursing interventions for children experiencing fluid-electrolyte problems and acid-base imbalance.

MEDIALINK www.prenhall.com/london

CD-ROM

Acid-Base Balance Animation
Audio Glossary
NCLEX-RN® Review

Companion Website

Case Study: Dehydration and Fluid Calculation
Care Plan: Hyponatremic Dehydration in
  Breastfeeding
MediaLink Applications:
  Care Plan: Infant Feeding
  Formula Preparation at a Home Visit
  Identifying Intravenous Fluids
  Interpreting Blood Gases
  Understanding School-Age Athletes and Fluid
    Needs
Audio Glossary
NCLEX-RN® Review

A thorough understanding of fluid, electrolyte, and acid-base homeostasis and imbalances is essential when providing nursing care to children like LeShan. This chapter presents information about the processes that maintain fluid and electrolyte balance, and describes the common imbalances that may occur in children. It also describes how the body regulates acid-base status and explains the management of acid-base imbalances.

Many health conditions cause changes in body fluids that must be regulated and managed. Sometimes management of fluid status in the home or in a short-term ambulatory facility can prevent more serious illness or hospitalization.

ANATOMY AND PHYSIOLOGY OF PEDIATRIC DIFFERENCES

Infants and young children differ physiologically from adults in ways that make them vulnerable to fluid, electrolyte, and acid-base imbalances.

Fluid in the body is in a dynamic state. Much of the human body is composed of water. **Body fluid** is body water that has solutes dissolved in it. Some of the solutes are **electrolytes**, or charged particles (ions). Electrolytes such as sodium (Na^+), potassium (K^+), calcium (Ca^{++}), magnesium (Mg^{++}), chloride (Cl^-), and inorganic phosphorus (Pi) ions must be present in the proper concentrations for cells to function effectively. In persons of all ages, fluid continuously leaves the body through the skin, in feces and urine, and during respiration. **Sensible water loss** is that which is measurable and observable, such as in urine through drainage tubes. **Insensible water loss** cannot be directly measured or observed, such as that lost through the skin and respirations. For adults and children, intake of oral fluid is approximately equivalent to urinary output in normal circumstances. Likewise, water provided in food and by the body's metabolic processes is approximately the same as insensible loss from feces, skin, and respirations. In people of all ages, body fluid is located in several compartments. The two major fluid compartments contain the **intracellular fluid** (fluid inside the cells) and the **extracellular fluid** (outside the cells). The extracellular fluid is made up of **intravascular fluid** (within the blood vessels) and **interstitial fluid** (between the cells and outside the blood and lymphatic vessels) (Figure 43–1 ●). Extracellular fluid accounts for about one third of total body water, and intracellular fluid for about two thirds. The concentrations of electrolytes in the fluid differ depending on the fluid compartment. For example, extracellular fluid is rich in sodium ions; intracellular fluid, by contrast, is low in sodium ions but rich in potassium ions (Table 43–1).

Fluid moves between the intravascular and interstitial compartments by a process called filtration. Water moves into and out of the cells by the process of osmosis. These processes are discussed later in the chapter.

The percentage of body weight composed of water varies with age. The percentage of total body water is highest at birth (and higher in premature than in full-term infants) and decreases with age (See "As Children Grow: Fluid and Electrolyte Differences"). Newborns and young infants also have a proportionately larger extracellular fluid volume than older children and adults because their brain and skin (both rich in interstitial fluid) occupy a greater proportion of their body weight. Much of the body's extracellular fluid is exchanged each day. Infants have a high daily fluid requirement with little fluid volume reserve; this makes the infant vulnerable to dehydration. As an infant grows, the proportion of water inside the cells increases (Bindler & Howry, 2005).

FIGURE 43–1

The major body fluid compartments. Extracellular fluid is composed mainly of *vascular fluid* (fluid in blood vessels) and *interstitial fluid* (fluid between cells and outside the blood and lymphatic vessels). Intracellular fluid is that within cells.

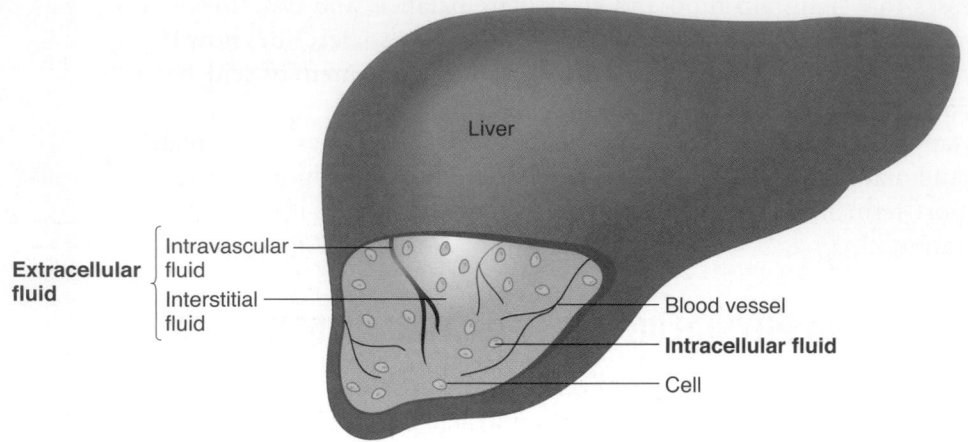

Infants and children under 2 years of age lose a greater proportion of fluid each day than older children and adults and are thus more dependent on adequate intake. They have a greater amount of skin surface or body surface area (BSA) and thus have greater insensible water losses through the skin. Because of this relatively large BSA, they are also at greater risk when skin is affected such as in burns. In addition, respiratory and metabolic rates are high during early childhood, so children have greater water loss from the lungs and greater water demand to fuel the body's metabolic processes (Figure 43–2 ●). Due to these factors, the exercising child dehydrates easily and must consume more fluid during physical activity, particularly during hot weather (Committee on Sports Medicine and Fitness, 2000).

When fluid status is compromised, a number of body mechanisms are activated to help restore balance. Several of these mechanisms occur in the kidney. The kidneys conserve water and needed electrolytes while excreting waste products and drug metabolites. In children under 2 years of age, however, the glomeruli, tubules, and nephrons of the kidneys are immature. They are thus unable to conserve or excrete water and solutes effectively (see Chapter 52 ∞). Because more water is generally excreted, the infant and young child can become dehydrated quickly or develop electrolyte imbalances. In addition, infants have a weaker transport system for ions and bicarbonate, placing them at greater risk for acidosis and acid-base imbalances. Children under 2 years of age also have difficulty regulating electrolytes such as sodium

TABLE 43–1 ❖ **Electrolyte Concentrations in Body Fluid Compartments**

Components	EXTRACELLULAR FLUID (ECF)		Intracellular Fluid
	Vascular	Interstitial	
Na+	High	High	Low
K+	Low	Low	High
Ca++	Low	Low	Low (higher than ECF)
Mg++	Low	Low	High
Pi	Low	Low	High
Cl−	High	High	Low
Proteins	High	Low	High

FIGURE 43–2

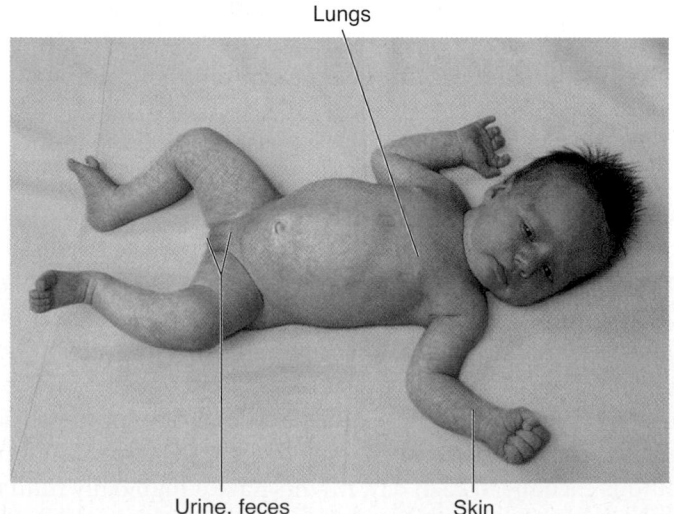

Normal routes of fluid excretion from infants and children.

AS CHILDREN GROW

Fluid and Electrolyte Differences

Newborn

75% Total
body water
• ECF 45%
• ICF 30%

Brain and skin occupy
a greater proportion of
body weight and are
high in interstitial fluid

Infant

65% Total
body water
• ECF 25%
• ICF 30–40%

High BSA
promotes fluid loss

Little fluid reserve
in intracellular fluid

5–6x greater fluid
exchange daily

High metabolic rate requires
generous fluid intake

Child/Adolescent

50% Total
body water
• ECF 10–15%
• ICF 40%

Kidneys are immature
until 2 years and unable
to conserve water and
electrolytes or fully assist
in acid–base balance

The newborn and infant have a high percentage of body weight composed of water, especially extracellular fluid, which is lost from the body easily. Note the small stomach size which limits ability to rehydrate quickly.

and calcium. Renal response to high solute loads is slower and less developed, with function improving gradually during the first year of life (Hewitt-Taylor, 1999).

Finally, in addition to the immaturity of physiologic processes, many health conditions make young children more vulnerable to fluid deficit. Examples include water loss due to phototherapy used to treat newborns with hyperbilirubinemia; water loss with increased respiratory rate during illness, fever, vomiting, and diarrhea; and drainage from blood loss or drainage tubes.

✿ FLUID VOLUME IMBALANCES

When fluid excretion and losses are balanced by the proper volume and type of fluid intake, fluid balance will be maintained. If, however, fluid output and intake are not matched, fluid imbalance may occur rapidly. The major types of fluid imbalances are extracellular fluid volume deficit (dehydration), extracellular fluid volume excess, and interstitial fluid volume excess (edema).

EXTRACELLULAR FLUID VOLUME IMBALANCES

EXTRACELLULAR FLUID VOLUME DEFICIT (DEHYDRATION)

Extracellular fluid volume deficit occurs when there is not enough fluid in the extracellular compartment (vascular and interstitial). Depending on the cause of dehydration, sodium may be at normal, low, or elevated levels. (Hyponatremia and hypernatremia are described later in the chapter, on pages 1252 and 1250.) The state of body water deficit is called **dehydration**. There are three major types of dehydration:

■ **Isotonic dehydration (or isonatremic dehydration)** occurs when fluid loss is not balanced by intake, and the loss of water and sodium are in proportion. The serum sodium is therefore within normal limits or slighty low, even though the circulating blood volume is lowered. Most of the fluid lost is from the extracellular component. This type of dehydration is commonly manifested in the illnesses of young children such as vomiting and diarrhea.

- **Hypotonic dehydration (or hyponatremic dehydration)** occurs when fluid loss is characterized by a proportionately greater loss of sodium than water. Serum sodium is below normal levels. Compensatory fluid shifts occur from the extracellular to intracellular components in an attempt to establish normal proportions, thus leading to even greater extracellular dehydration. Severe and prolonged vomiting and diarrhea, burns, and renal disease can lead to this condition, as well as administration of intravenous fluid without electrolytes in treatment of dehydration.

- **Hypertonic dehydration (or hypernatremic dehydration)** occurs when fluid loss is characterized by a proportionately greater loss of water than sodium. Serum sodium is above normal levels. Compensatory fluid shifts occur from the intracellular to extracellular components in an attempt to establish normal proportions. The extracellular component therefore remains fairly normal, delaying the onset of signs and symptoms of dehydration until the condition is quite serious. Neurologic symptoms reflecting intracellular imbalance may occur simultaneously with more common symptoms of dehydration. The condition may be caused by health problems such as diabetes insipidus or administration of intravenous fluid or tube feedings with high electrolyte levels.

The body continuously attempts to compensate for fluid and electrolyte imbalance by shifting fluid and electrolytes from one component to another. Therefore, it is rare for only one type of dehydration to occur; the child's fluid and electrolyte status and symptoms are constantly changing. Ongoing assessment and management are needed.

Etiology and Pathophysiology

Extracellular fluid volume deficit is usually caused by the loss of sodium-containing fluid from the body. Vomiting, diarrhea, nasogastric suction, hemorrhage, and burns most often cause loss of fluid containing sodium. Vomiting and diarrhea are common manifestations of disease in children throughout the world, and each year up to 5 million children die from dehydration related to diarrhea. In the United States, about 300 to 500 die annually from this problem, about 220,000 are hospitalized, and many more receive outpatient care (Nager & Wang, 2002; Shamir, Zahavi, Abramowich et al., 1998).

Another cause of extracellular fluid volume deficit in infants is increased water loss in low-birth-weight in-

FIGURE 43–3

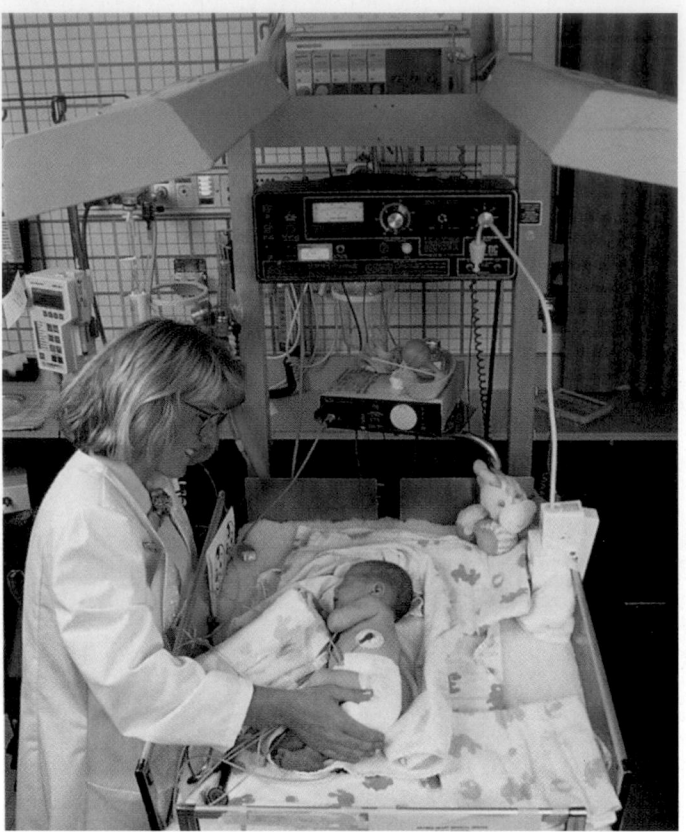

Use of an overhead warmer or phototherapy increases insensible fluid excretion through the skin, thus increasing the fluid intake needed.

fants kept under radiant warmers to maintain heat (Figure 43–3). Less frequently, adrenal insufficiency, accumulation of extracellular fluid in a "third space" such as the peritoneal cavity, and overuse of diuretics may be the cause. The latter etiology is most often seen in bulimic adolescents who are trying to control their weights (see Chapter 34 ∞).

Excessive exercise during very hot weather without sufficient fluid replacement can lead to fluid and electrolyte imbalance. Children are more prone than adults to imbalance from exercise, for several of the physiologic differences described in the pediatric variations section earlier. Since children have a greater BSA, they can gain more heat from the environment when it is hot and lose more when it is cold (Binkley, Beckett, Casa et al., 2002). The high metabolic rate of children is further increased during exercise so that fluid lost in metabolism is significant. Young children do not sweat effectively and may be unable to eliminate heat by this method. Children may not feel thirsty and so fail to drink even when dehydrated (Committee on Sports Medicine and Fitness, 2000).

For burns, gastroenteritis, and other illness, initial dehydration in the first 3 days reflects a high loss of extracel-

TABLE 43–2 ✤ Severity of Clinical Dehydration

	Mild	Moderate	Severe
Percent of body weight lost	Up to 5% (40–50 mL/kg)	6%–9% (60–90 mL/kg)	10% or more (100+mL/kg)
Level of consciousness	Alert, restless, thirsty	Irritable or lethargic (infants and very young children); alert, thirsty, restless (older children and adolescents)	Lethargic to comatose (infants and young children); often conscious, apprehensive (older children and adolescents)
Blood pressure	Normal	Normal or low; postural hypotension (older children and adolescents)	Low to undetectable
Pulse	Normal	Rapid	Rapid, weak to nonpalpable
Skin turgor	Normal	Poor	Very poor
Mucous membranes	Moist	Dry	Parched
Urine	May appear normal	Decreased output (<1 mL/kg/hr); dark color; increased specific gravity	Very decreased or absent output
Thirst	Slightly increased	Moderately increased	Greatly increased unless lethargic
Fontanelle	Normal	Sunken	Sunken
Extremities	Warm; normal capillary refill	Delayed capillary refill (>2 sec)	Cool, discolored; delayed capillary refill (>3–4 sec)
Respirations	Normal	Normal or rapid	Changing rate and pattern

lular fluid. About 80% of the fluid loss is extracellular, and only about 20% intracellular. However, with time the relationship begins to change, so that in illnesses over 3 days, about 60% of fluid loss is extracellular while 40% is intracellular (Johns Hopkins, 2005). Since the electrolyte composition of extracellular and intracellular fluids differs (see Table 43–1), electrolyte management will need to change for long-term conditions.

Clinical Manifestations

The signs of dehydration relate to the severity or degree of the body water deficit (Table 43–2). They are a result of both the decreased fluid (e.g., diminished turgor and mucous membrane moisture) and the body's response to the fluid deficit (e.g., pulse and blood pressure changes).

Mild dehydration is hard to detect, because children appear alert and have moist mucous membranes. Infants

CLINICAL MANIFESTATIONS

EXTRACELLULAR FLUID VOLUME DEFICIT

SIGNS AND SYMPTOMS	PHYSIOLOGIC BASIS
Weight loss	Decreased fluid volume; 1 L of fluid weighs 1 kg
Postural blood pressure drop (older children)	Inadequate circulating blood volume to offset the force of gravity when in upright position
Increased small vein filling time	Decreased vascular volume
Delayed capillary refill time	Decreased vascular volume
Flat neck veins when supine (older children)	Decreased vascular volume
Dizziness, syncope	Inadequate circulation to brain
Oliguria	Inadequate circulation to kidneys
Thready, rapid pulse	Cardiac reflex response to decreased vascular volume
Sunken fontanelle (infants)	Decreased fluid volume
Decreased skin turgor	Decreased interstitial fluid volume

GROWTH AND DEVELOPMENT

Urine specific gravity may increase in older children who are dehydrated, but children under 2 years of age are not able to concentrate urine effectively. A rising specific gravity may not be seen in the younger dehydrated child.

may be irritable and older children are thirsty. In moderate dehydration the child is often lethargic and sleepy, but there may be periods of restlessness and irritability, especially in infants. Skin turgor is diminished, mucous membranes appear dry, and urine is dark in color and diminished in amount. Pulse rate is usually increased, and blood pressure can be normal or low. Severe dehydration is manifested by increasing lethargy or nonresponsiveness, markedly decreased blood pressure, rapid pulse, nonelastic skin turgor, dry mucous membranes, sunken and dry eyes, and markedly decreased or absent urinary output.

Clinical Therapy

Medical management depends on accurate identification of the degree of dehydration. In addition to physical signs and symptoms (see Table 43–2), elevated blood urea nitrogen (BUN) (>25 mg/dL) and serum bicarbonate (>17 mEq/L) are useful to identify moderate and severe diarrhea (Eliason

& Lewan, 1998; Vega & Avner, 1997). The treatment of extracellular fluid volume deficit is administration of fluid containing sodium, by oral rehydration therapy or by intravenous fluids.

Oral rehydration therapy has been used for years in developing countries without an accessible supply of intravenous fluids. More recently, experts have recognized the benefits of its early use to prevent severe dehydration and to treat mild and moderate dehydration in children in developed countries. The therapy successfully treats the dehydration caused by many gastrointestinal illnesses and prevents hospitalization for many infants and young children (Armon, Stephenson, MacFaul et al., 2001). It is the treatment of choice for children with diarrhea who have mild to moderate dehydration. Commercially available solutions contain water, carbohydrate (sugar), sodium, potassium, chloride, and lactate. Examples include Pedialyte, Infalyte, Rehydralate, Ricelyte, Resol, Nutralyte, Hydralyte, and Lytren. Some clinicians allow lactose-free milk, breast milk, or half-strength milk to be given in addition to oral rehydration therapy solution.

When the child is severely dehydrated, electrolytes are measured by laboratory analysis, and intravenous fluid is given, often accompanied by oral rehydration. The intravenous fluid is commonly Ringer's lactate or dilute saline, such as one half or one quarter normal saline (see Table 43–3

TABLE 43–3 ✤ Common Intravenous Solutions, Uses, and Components

IV Solution	Uses	CHO (g/100 mL)	Protein (g/100 mL)	Cal/L	NA+ (mEq/L)	K+ (mEq/L)	Cl− (mEq/L)	HCO₃ (mEq/L)	Ca++ (mEq/L)
D₅W	Restores water loss, plasma volume, and calories; lowers sodium levels	5	–	170	–	–	–	–	–
Normal saline (0.9% NaCl)	Restores water and sodium loss; maintains sodium and chloride at present levels	–	–	–	154	–	154	–	–
Ringer's solution	Expands intracellular fluid; replaces extracellular losses	0–10	–	0–340	147	4	155.5	–	4
Lactated Ringer's solution	Replaces fluid loss from burns, bleeding, and severe diarrhea	0–10	–	0–340	130	4	109	28	3
Albumin 25% (salt poor albumin)	Restores major plasma protein in blood loss that has been treated with NS (plasma expander)	–	25	1000	100–160	–	< 120	–	–

Note: Variations and combinations are available to tailor intake to needs of the child. For example, ½ NS (0.45% NaCl) or ¼ NS (0.225% NaCl) are often used in young children; the lower sodium content helps to avoid inadvertent hypernatremia. D₅W ½ NS and D₅W ¼ NS are combinations of D₅W and NS; they provide both carbohydrate and sodium. Amino acid 8.5% is an additional plasma expander to restore loss of plasma proteins.

Adapted with permission from Johns Hopkins Hospital (2005). *The Harriet Lane handbook* (17th ed.). Johns Hopkins University Press; and LeMone, P., & Burke, K. M. (2004). *Medical surgical nursing* (3rd ed.). Upper Saddle River, NJ: Prentice Hall Health.

THINKING CRITICALLY

THE DEHYDRATED CHILD

LeShan is 18 months old. Several days ago he developed vomiting and diarrhea. His parents tried to get him to eat, but he had little appetite. He drank a little water and a few sips of juice, but the next morning he was listless and would not drink anything. The diarrhea continued.

His mother has brought him to the urgent care center. LeShan is irritable on arrival, and his mother reports that he has been alternately irritable and lethargic. His mucous membranes and tongue appear dry, and skin turgor over the abdomen is slightly decreased. His mother notes that LeShan has had only two wet diapers today and says the urine in his diaper was dark in color. She also reports that he weighed 12 kg (26 lb) at the clinic last week. However, when the nurse weighs him, the scale reads only 11 kg (24½ lb). What do LeShan's symptoms suggest about his degree of dehydration? What nursing interventions should be planned?

for types of intravenous fluids and their uses). The fluid combination replenishes the extracellular fluid volume and adds solutes to return the body fluid back to normal. The child may be hospitalized or treated with intravenous fluids in a short-stay unit until the dehydration is controlled. Once hydrated, the child resumes an age appropriate diet (Burkhart, 1999).

NURSING MANAGEMENT

NURSING ASSESSMENT AND DIAGNOSIS

Weigh the child daily with the same scale and without clothing. Compare to past weights and calculate weight loss. Carefully measure intake and output, urine specific gravity, level of consciousness, pulse rate and quality, skin turgor, mucous membrane moisture, quality and rate of respirations, and blood pressure. Compare the blood pressure when the child is supine with the pressure when the child is sitting with legs hanging down or standing. If the child is dehydrated, the sitting or standing blood pressure will be lower than the supine blood pressure, because blood accumulates in the dependent legs. Obtain samples of urine and blood as needed for dehydration evaluation.

NURSING PRACTICE

To obtain urine from an infant for testing specific gravity, place two cotton balls in the diaper. When they are wet, push them into a 10-mL syringe and squeeze out the urine with the plunger. Remember to use gloves for this procedure.

The nursing diagnosis *Deficient Fluid Volume* applies to all children who have an extracellular fluid volume deficit. Other diagnoses depend on the severity of the condition and the age of the child. Several nursing diagnoses that might be appropriate for the mildly to severely dehydrated child are included in the accompanying "Nursing Care Plans." Additional care of the child with dehydration from gastroenteritis can be found in Chapter 51. ∞ Nursing diagnoses might include the following:

- *Deficient Fluid Volume* related to active fluid volume loss or failure of regulatory mechanisms
- *Risk for Ineffective Peripheral Tissue Perfusion* related to hypovolemia
- *Risk for Injury* related to postural hypotension

PLANNING AND IMPLEMENTATION

Nursing care of the dehydrated child focuses first on prevention of the problem, and then on providing oral rehydration fluids, teaching parents oral rehydration methods, and, if necessary, administering intravenous fluids to restore fluid balance. The accompanying "Nursing Care Plans" summarize care of the child with mild to severe dehydration.

Prevent Dehydration

Nursing care can often prevent dehydration. Carefully monitor temperature probes in radiant warmers and isolettes for newborns to prevent overheating and resulting dehydration. Teach parents proper clothing for infants to prevent overheating. Nurses play an important role in educating parents, youth, school personnel, and coaches about the dangers of heat-related illness. Prevention is key, so that children can exercise safely. Prior to a new exercise regimen, assessment for risk factors is performed. This includes medical conditions that put the child at high risk, such as cystic fibrosis, diabetes, obesity, or mental retardation. Prior history of heat-related illness or recent change from a cooler to hotter environment increase risk. Long exercise periods increase the stress upon the body. The major nursing interventions are partnering with families and athletic coaches to prevent problems and to recognize and treat them promptly.

Provide Oral Rehydration Fluids

In mild or moderate dehydration, oral rehydration fluid is the first intervention. It is given in frequent small amounts; for example, 1 to 3 teaspoons of fluid every 10 to 15 minutes is a useful guideline for starting oral rehydration. For the first 2 to 4 hours of treatment, 50 mL of fluid for each kg of the child's weight should be the target intake (Endsley & Galbraith, 1998; Larson, 2000). Instruct parents to continue to administer 1 teaspoon every 2 to 3 minutes even if the child vomits, as small amounts

MEDIALINK Case Study: Dehydration and Fluid Calculation

NURSING CARE PLAN

THE CHILD WITH MILD OR MODERATE DEHYDRATION

Intervention	Rationale	Expected Outcome
1. Nursing Diagnosis: Ineffective Management of Therapeutic Regimen related to knowledge deficit about diarrhea and vomiting		
NIC Priority Intervention: **Family involvement:** Facilitate family participation in care of the child		**NOC Suggested Outcome:** Effective therapeutic regimen management
Goal: Parents will describe appropriate home management of fluid replacement for diarrhea and vomiting.		
■ Explain how to replace body fluid with an oral rehydration solution. Encourage parents to keep the solution at home and begin use with the first sign of diarrhea. ■ Teach parents to continue the child's normal diet in addition to providing replacement fluids for diarrhea. ■ Provide verbal and written instructions to parents at each well-child visit.	■ Use of an oral rehydration solution can enable successful treatment of vomiting and diarrhea at home. ■ Diet plus fluid supplementation leads to faster recovery. ■ Parents are provided with a reference for later use.	Parents are successfully able to treat the child's diarrhea and vomiting at home.
2. Nursing Diagnosis: Deficient Knowledge (Parent) related to causes of dehydration		
NIC Priority Intervention: **Teaching:** Teach causes of dehydration		**NOC Suggested Outcome:** **Knowledge:** Treatment regimen
Goal: Parents will state common causes of childhood dehydration.		
■ Teach parents childhood conditions that commonly lead to dehydration.	■ If parents recognize situations that can lead to dehydration, they will be more alert to its appearance.	Parents recognize conditions of risk for dehydration in children.
3. Nursing Diagnosis: Risk for Deficient Fluid Volume related to worsening of child's condition		
NIC Priority Intervention: **Fluid management:** Promote fluid balance		**NOC Suggested Outcome:** **Fluid balance:** Balance of water in extra- and intracellular compartments of body
Goal: Parents will seek healthcare for the child's worsening condition.		
■ Teach parents to seek care when the child's vomiting or diarrhea worsens, or the child's mental alertness changes.	■ Severe dehydration may occur if milder forms are not successfully treated.	Parents seek prompt attention for the child's worsening condition, preventing the development of severe dehydration.

of the fluid may still be absorbed. Table 43–4 outlines guidelines for oral rehydration therapy.

Teach Parents Oral Rehydration Methods

Instruct parents about the types of fluids and amounts to be given. Begin teaching with parents of all newborns and reinforce teaching at each well-child visit. Advise parents to continue the child's normal diet in addition to providing the rehydration solution. Cereal, starches, soup, fruits, and vegetables are all allowed. Tell parents to avoid simple sugars, which can worsen diarrhea because of osmotic effects. This includes soft drinks (if used, they should be diluted with equal parts of water), undiluted juice, Jell-O, and sweetened cereal.

NURSING PRACTICE

Encourage parents to keep an oral rehydration solution in liquid or powder form on hand at all times and to use these solutions rather than juice, soda, or other drinks when the child first develops diarrhea.

If an oral rehydration solution is too concentrated, it can make diarrhea worse. Juice and cola are very concentrated and should be diluted to half strength if they are the only fluids available to be given to a child who has diarrhea. Sugar facilitates the absorption of sodium in oral rehydration fluids. In addition, tell parents not to give diet beverages for oral rehydration because they contain no sugar and will not be effectively absorbed.

NURSING CARE PLAN

THE CHILD WITH SEVERE DEHYDRATION

Intervention	Rationale	Expected Outcome
1. Nursing Diagnosis: Deficient Fluid Volume related to excess losses and inadequate intake		
NIC Priority Intervention: **Fluid management:** Promote fluid balance		**NOC Suggested Outcome:** **Fluid balance:** Balance of water in extra- and intracellular components of the body
Goal: The child will return to normal hydration status and will not develop hypovolemic shock.		
■ Monitor weight daily. Assess intake and output every shift. Assess heart rate, postural blood pressure, skin turgor, small vein filling time, capillary refill time, fontanelle (infant), and urine specific gravity every 4 hours or more frequently as indicated. ■ Administer intravenous fluid as ordered. Monitor for crackles in dependent portions of the lungs.	■ Frequent assessment of hydration status facilitates rapid intervention and evaluation of the effectiveness of fluid replacement. ■ Replace fluid lost from the body. Excessive replacement of sodium-containing fluids could cause extracellular fluid volume excess.	The child has signs of normal hydration.
2. Nursing Diagnosis: Risk for Injury related to decreased level of consciousness		
NIC Priority Intervention: **Fall prevention:** Institute special precautions		**NOC Suggested Outcome:** **Fall prevention:** Minimize risk factors that precipitate falls
Goal: The child will not experience injury.		
■ Raise the side rails of the bed. Ensure that a small child does not become tangled in bed covers. ■ Monitor level of consciousness every 2–4 hours or more often as indicated. ■ Monitor serum sodium concentration daily or more often. ■ Have the child sit before rising from bed and assist to stand slowly.	■ Safety measures protect the child. ■ Frequent assessment provides evidence of the need for safety interventions and of the effectiveness of therapy. ■ Elevated serum sodium concentration causes brain cell shrinkage and decreased level of consciousness. ■ Slow adjustment to upright posture reduces light-headedness from decreased blood volume.	The child does not fall or suffer other injuries.
3. Nursing Diagnosis: Activity Intolerance related to bedrest immobility		
NIC Priority Intervention: **Activity therapy:** Plan activities to meet child's developmental needs		**NOC Suggested Outcome:** **Energy conservation:** Manage energy to sustain activity
Goal: The child will engage in normal activity for age.		
■ Plan activities appropriate for the age of the child that can be done in bed. ■ Group nursing interventions to provide time for the child to rest. ■ Provide asistance during meals and other activities as needed.	■ Activities will provide distraction and promote recovery. ■ The child will require more rest than usual. ■ Prevention of overexertion will conserve body fluid and promote healing.	The child engages in normal developmental activities and receives adequate rest.

TABLE 43–4 ✣ Oral Rehydration Therapy Guidelines

- Children with diarrhea and no dehydration should be continued on age-appropriate diets.
- For mild dehydration, give 50 mL/kg oral rehydration therapy in 4 hours in addition to replacing fluids lost in stool and emesis. (Measure emesis and give 10 mL/kg of fluid for each diarrheal stool.)
- For moderate dehydration, give 100 mL/kg oral rehydration therapy in 4 hours in addition to replacing fluids lost as described above.
- For severe dehydration, the child is hospitalized and treated with intravenous fluids. When hydrated adequately or concurrently with intravenous rehydration, begin oral rehydration therapy with 50 to 100 mL/kg of fluid in 4 hours and stool replacement as described above.
- When rehydration is complete, resume normal diet.

Adapted from Provisional Committee on Quality Improvement, Subcommittee on Acute Gastroenteritis. (1996). Practice parameter: The management of acute gastroenteritis in young children. *Pediatrics, 97,* 424–436.

Repeated vomiting of large volumes of fluid, increasing diarrhea, or a worsening of the child's condition can indicate the need for intravenous therapy. Teach parents when to seek further medical care. If the child's condition worsens or does not improve after 4 hours of oral rehydration therapy, parents should contact a healthcare professional. Dizziness or lethargy are symptoms that can be manifestations of dehydration and indicate need for further healthcare.

Monitor Intravenous Fluid Administration

The hospitalized child usually requires intravenous fluids. Use volume control devices for measuring and monitoring intake. Be sure that the amount of fluid administered corresponds with the diagnosed dehydration state of the child (Table 43–5). Usually, about one half of the 24-hour total maintenance and replacement needs are given in the first 6

TABLE 43–5 ✣ Calculation of Intravenous Fluid Needs

1. First, calculate the maintenance fluid needs of the child, according to the following guideline:

   Usual Weight Maintenance Amount
Usual Weight	Maintenance Amount
Up to 10 kg	100 mL/kg/24 hr
11–20 kg	1000 mL + (50 mL/kg for weight above 10 kg)/24 hr
>20 kg	1500 mL + (20 mL/kg for weight above 20 kg)/24 hr

2. Next, calculate replacement fluid for that loss: Multiply the percentage of body weight loss × 10 × normal weight to obtain the mL/kg/24 hr required.
3. Finally, calculate continued losses and add them to the total of maintenance and replacement needs.

---

to 8 hours, with a slower rate infused for the remainder of the 24 hours. During the first 1 to 3 hours, the infusion rate may be highest to rapidly expand the vascular space. Electrolytes, such as potassium, are not added until the child has voided a sufficient quantity of urine, in order to avoid hyperkalemia. Rapid infusion of 20 to 30 mL/kg over 1 to 2 hours is sometimes used in outpatient settings, followed by oral fluids. Careful monitoring of intake and output is needed to ensure that the intravenous line remains in place until the child is tolerating oral fluids and taking in enough to maintain hydration. When oral fluids are maintained, the child may be discharged and hospitalization avoided.

Maintain the intravenous line carefully so fluid infusion can be kept on schedule (refer to the *Clinical Skills Manual* as well as the CD-ROM that accompanies this text). **SKILLS** See "Evidence-Based Nursing: Intravenous Starts." Use a pump to prevent inadvertent, rapid infusion, which can lead to fluid overload and electrolyte imbalance (Figure 43–4 ●). Play with the toddler and preschool child frequently and use diversionary methods, as necessary, to distract the child from the intravenous line. Monitor the child carefully and implement safety precautions as necessary. Once the child begins to tolerate some oral fluids, substitute oral rehydration therapy for intravenous fluids; frequent administration of appropriate fluids is needed.

Discharge Planning and Home Care Teaching

Prior to discharge, parents need instructions about types of fluids and amounts to encourage. Teach the signs of dehydration (see Table 43–2) so that if the child does not take in adequate fluids, parents can seek help immediately. Instruct

● **FIGURE 43–4**

The use of a volume control device with an intravenous saline solution is important to prevent a sudden extracellular fluid volume overload.

EVIDENCE-BASED NURSING

INTRAVENOUS STARTS

Problem

Parents often voice dissatisfaction with the number of intravenous starts to which their young hospitalized children are subjected, as children experience pain and anxiety when intravenous lines are inserted.

Evidence

The Children's Hospital of Denver created a task force to address problems of venous access. Co-chairs in this collaborative project included a nurse from the neonatal intensive care unit, a general surgeon, and a radiologist. Additional nurses from units using peripheral intravenous lines served as committee members. A tracking tool was developed to collect information on intravenous placements for a 1-month period. Other children's hospitals were also surveyed for their practices regarding venous access policies and procedures.

Implications

Based on the analysis of internal and external data, the task force developed recommendations to (1) develop a group of specially trained nurses to act as resources for other staff nurses, (2) create an algorithm

to provide guidelines for decisions about peripheral vs. peripherally inserted central venous catheters vs. central venous catheter insertion, (3) use the specially trained nurses to educate staff members about the new algorithm, and (4) develop a tracking/evaluation mechanism for the new algorithm and trained nurse group.

Critical Thinking

This clinical situation is an example of partnership among healthcare specialists in order to improve care for hospitalized children. What were the benefits of having an interdisciplinary group examine the topic of intravenous starts? How would you suggest that parent satisfaction before and after a program like this be measured? What could be the benefits of having a nursing resource group and an intravenous start guideline to positively influence the hospitalization of young children requiring intravenous infusion for dehydration?

Reference

The Venous Access Task Force. (2002). Using evidence-based practice to create a venous access team. *Journal of Pediatric Nursing, 17,* 450-454.

---

them to begin the child's normal diet once hydration is completed, determined by adequate urinary output and normal behaviors. Review methods of minimizing the child's chance of acquiring gastrointestinal infections (e.g., avoiding contact with other children who are infected; using careful handwashing and dishwashing procedures when another child in the home is sick). During well-child visits, encourage all parents to keep oral rehydration fluids at home in case they are needed; they are available in most grocery stores and pharmacies. Address the needs for increasing fluids in hot weather and when the child is exercising.

EVALUATION

Expected outcomes of nursing care include the following:

- Balance of water and electrolytes in intracellular and extracellular compartments
- Normal urinary output
- Adequate fluid intake for maintenance needs
- Vital signs within normal limits

EXTRACELLULAR FLUID VOLUME EXCESS

Extracellular fluid volume excess occurs when there is too much fluid in the vascular and interstitial compartment. This imbalance may also be called saline excess or extracellular volume overload. If this disorder occurs by itself (without saline disturbance), the serum sodium concentration is normal. There is simply too much extracellular fluid, even though it has a normal concentration.

Infants and children who develop an extracellular fluid volume excess have a condition that causes them to retain **saline** (sodium and water) or have been given an overload of sodium-containing isotonic intravenous fluid (Figure 43–5 ●). What conditions cause retention of saline? The hormone aldosterone is secreted by the adrenal cortex. One of its normal functions is to cause the

● **FIGURE 43–5**

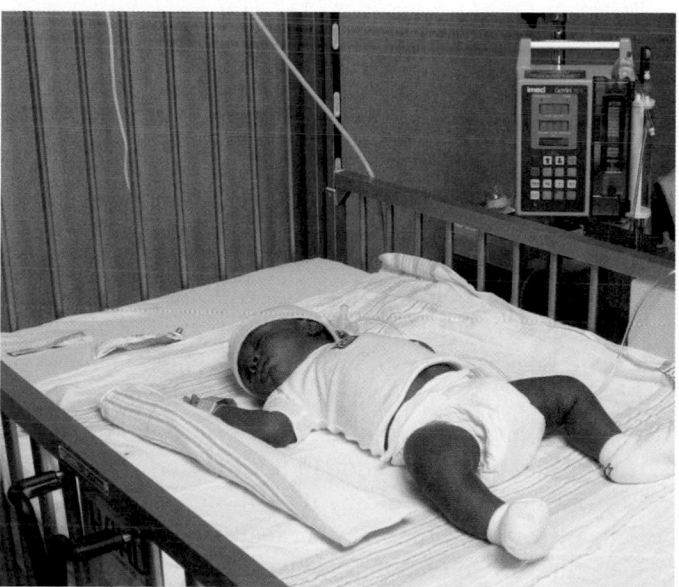

If isotonic fluid containing sodium is given too rapidly or in too great an amount, an extracellular fluid volume excess will develop. Carefully monitor fluid intake, excretion, and retention in infants and children.

PATHOPHYSIOLOGY ILLUSTRATED

Aldosterone Effects

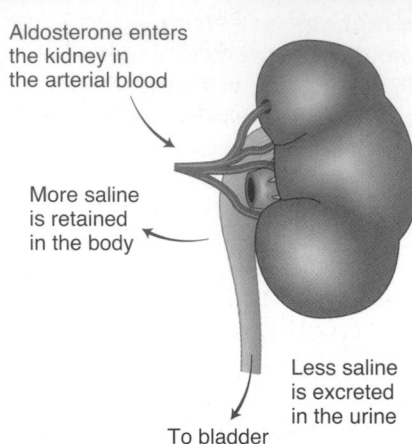

Aldosterone enters the kidney in the arterial blood

More saline is retained in the body

Less saline is excreted in the urine

To bladder

Aldosterone has a saline-retaining effect. Increased aldosterone secretion can be caused by adrenal tumors or congestive heart failure.

● FIGURE 43–6

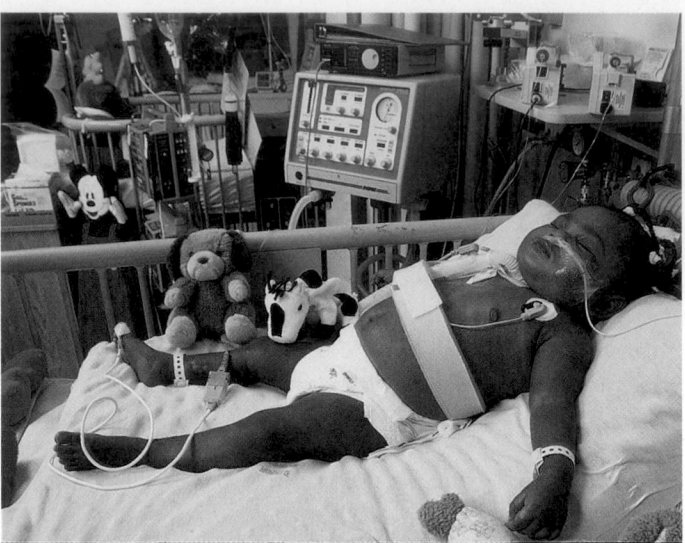

This infant with congenital heart disease has signs of generalized edema. Note the fluid retention in the face and abdomen.

kidneys to retain saline in the body (see "Pathophysiology Illustrated: Aldosterone Effects"). Saline excess can be caused by any condition that results in excessive aldosterone secretion, such as adrenal tumors that secrete aldosterone, congestive heart failure, liver cirrhosis, and chronic renal failure. Most glucocorticoid medications (such as prednisone) have a mild saline-retaining effect when taken on a long-term basis.

Extracellular fluid volume excess is characterized by sudden weight gain. A gain of 0.5 kg (1 lb) in a day is related to fluid, and represents 500 mL of saline. An overload of fluid in the blood vessels and interstitial spaces can cause clinical manifestations such as bounding pulse, distended neck veins in children (not usually evident in infants), periorbital edema, hepatomegaly, dyspnea, orthopnea, and lung crackles. Edema is the sign of overload of the interstitial fluid compartment. In an infant, edema is often generalized (Figure 43–6 ●). Edema in children with extracellular fluid volume excess occurs in the dependent parts of the body, that is, in the parts closest to the ground. Thus, edema is evident in sacral areas in a child supine in bed. Scrotum or labia may be edematous. (Edema that develops from other causes is described in the next section of this chapter.)

Intravenous fluid volume regulation is important, especially in young children. Either inaccurate calculation of needed fluid or inadvertent infusion of excess fluids can cause overload.

The clinical therapy for extracellular fluid volume excess focuses on treating the underlying cause of the disor-

der. For example, a child who has congestive heart failure is given medications to strengthen the heart's ability to contract. Managing the cause also helps to reduce the extracellular fluid volume excess. Diuretics may be given to remove fluid from the body, thus reducing the extracellular fluid volume directly.

Nursing Management

Rapid weight gain is the most sensitive index of extracellular fluid volume excess. Therefore, daily weighing with the same scale and articles of clothing is an important nursing assessment. Measure the child's intake and output. For babies in diapers, a diaper is weighed dry and then wet, with grams of weight increase equal to urine volume in milliliters. When treatment is successful, output is greater than intake. Assess the character of the pulse and observe for neck vein distention when the child is sitting (usually visible only in older children). Monitor for signs of pulmonary edema (an indication of severe imbalance) by listening to lung sounds in the dependent lung fields (crackles) and assessing for respiratory distress (rapid respiratory rate, use of accessory muscles of respiration). Observe for edema.

A child may develop a fluid overload whenever an isotonic intravenous solution containing sodium, such as normal saline or Ringer's solution, is administered. Therefore, monitor the infusion rate frequently and carefully and use a volume control device and pump whenever possible to aid in accurate administration. Use only small bags (e.g., 250 or 500 mL) for infants and young children, and check pumps frequently. If an excess of fluid has already developed, administer the medical therapy as prescribed and monitor for any complications of the medical therapy. For example, many diuretics increase potassium excretion in the urine, which may lead to an abnormally low plasma potassium concentration unless potassium intake is increased. (Refer to the discussion of hypokalemia later in this chapter.) It is also important to monitor for the development of extracellular fluid volume deficit as a result of diuretic therapy.

If edema is present, provide careful skin care and protection for edematous areas. Teach parents how to provide skin care and perform position changes at home. See the following section for additional interventions related to edema.

If a child has a long-term condition such as chronic renal failure that predisposes to extracellular fluid volume excess, a dietary sodium restriction may be prescribed (see Chapter 52 for further detail ∞). Teach parents how to manage sodium restriction. Plan low-sodium meals that fit the family's cultural practices. If the child is old enough to participate, incorporate games into the teaching. If a scale is available, teach parents to take and record an accurate daily weight.

Desired outcomes include electrolyte balance, maintenance of intact skin, and dietary intake as prescribed.

INTERSTITIAL FLUID VOLUME EXCESS (EDEMA)

Edema is an abnormal increase in the volume of the interstitial fluid. It may be caused by an extracellular fluid volume excess or it may be due to other causes.

The causes of edema are best understood in the context of normal capillary dynamics. Fluid moves between the vascular and interstitial compartment by the process of **filtration**. Filtration is the net result of forces that tend to move fluid in opposing directions. The strongest forces determine the direction of fluid movement.

At the capillary level, two forces (blood hydrostatic pressure and interstitial osmotic pressure) tend to move fluid from the capillaries into the interstitial fluid, while two other forces (blood colloid osmotic pressure and interstitial fluid hydrostatic pressure) tend to move fluid in the opposite direction (from the interstitial fluid into the capillaries). The net result of these forces usually moves fluid from the capillaries into the interstitial compartment at the arterial end of the capillaries and fluid from the interstitial compartment back into the capillaries at the venous end of the capillaries. This process brings oxygen and nutrients to the cells and removes carbon dioxide and other waste products.

Edema occurs if the balance of these four forces is altered so that excess fluid either enters or leaves the interstitial compartment (see "Pathophysiology Illustrated:

Capillary Dynamics and Edema"). This may occur through (1) increased blood hydrostatic pressure, (2) decreased blood colloid osmotic pressure, (3) increased interstitial fluid osmotic pressure, or (4) blocked lymphatic drainage. Many clinical conditions are associated with these altered forces (Table 43–6), described in the following list:

1. **Increased blood hydrostatic pressure.** When extracellular fluid volume excess occurs, the increased fluid volume in the vascular compartment congests the veins. The pressure against the sides of the capillary is increased and more fluid then enters the interstitial compartment.

2. **Decreased blood colloid osmotic pressure.** Much of the osmotic pressure that pulls fluid into the capillaries is due to the presence of albumin and other plasma proteins made by the liver. The part of the blood osmotic pressure that is due to plasma proteins is often called **oncotic pressure** or blood colloid osmotic pressure. Any condition that decreases plasma proteins will decrease blood colloid osmotic pressure and cause edema. For example, if a clinical condition causes large amounts of albumin to leak into the urine, the liver will not be able to make albumin fast enough to replace it. As a result the plasma protein level will fall, decreasing the blood osmotic pressure. Without this pulling force to return fluid to the capillaries, edema will occur. This is the cause of edema in children who have nephrotic syndrome (see Chapter 52 ∞).

3. **Increased interstitial fluid osmotic pressure.** Ordinarily, only a few small proteins enter the interstitial fluid, and the interstitial fluid osmotic

PATHOPHYSIOLOGY ILLUSTRATED
Capillary Dynamics and Edema

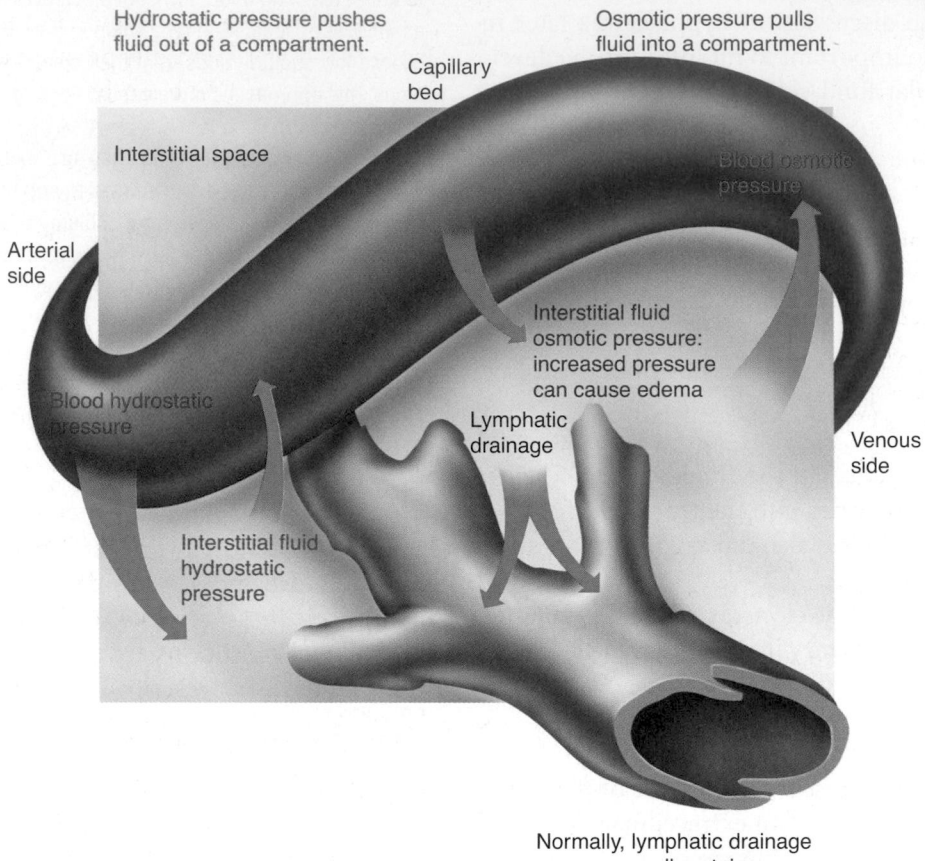

Hydrostatic pressure pushes fluid out of a compartment.

Osmotic pressure pulls fluid into a compartment.

Capillary bed

Interstitial space

Blood osmotic pressure

Arterial side

Blood hydrostatic pressure

Interstitial fluid osmotic pressure: increased pressure can cause edema

Lymphatic drainage

Venous side

Interstitial fluid hydrostatic pressure

Normally, lymphatic drainage removes small proteins and excess interstitial fluid. Blocked lymphatic drainage can cause edema.

With normal capillary dynamics, fluid moves out of the compartment by the force of hydrostatic pressure in the blood vessel and is pulled out by interstitial osmotic pressure. Fluid is forced into the compartment by interstitial hydrostatic pressure and pulled in by compartment osmotic pressure. Abnormal capillary dynamics can cause edema.

pressure is small. If the capillary becomes abnormally permeable to proteins, however, the influx of large amounts of proteins into the interstitial fluid causes a dramatic increase in interstitial fluid osmotic pressure. The increased pulling force keeps an abnormal amount of fluid in the interstitial compartment. This mechanism plays an important part in the edema caused by a bee sting or a sprained ankle. It occurs to a greater extent in burns, leading to swelling at the same time that there is a great loss of fluid volume through the burned skin (see Chapter 57 ∞).

4. **Blocked lymphatic drainage.** The lymph vessels normally drain small proteins and excess fluid from the interstitial compartment and return them to the blood vessels. If lymph vessels are blocked, fluid accumulates in the interstitial compartment. This may occur when a tumor blocks lymphatic drainage.

Edema causes localized or generalized swelling, which may cause pain and restrict motion. Edema due to extracellular fluid volume excess or right-sided heart failure usually occurs in the dependent portion of the body. In a child who is walking, dependent edema is observed in the ankles; in a bedfast, supine child, it is seen in the sacral area. The skin over an edematous area often appears thin and shiny.

The main focus of clinical therapy for edema is to treat the underlying condition that caused the edema. Such conditions are discussed throughout this book. The edema

TABLE 43–6 ✤ **Clinical Conditions That Cause Edema**

Edema Due to Increased Blood Hydrostatic Pressure

Increased Capillary Blood Flow
Inflammation
Local infection

Venous Congestion
Extracellular fluid volume excess
Right heart failure
Venous thrombosis
External pressure on vein
Muscle paralysis

Edema Due to Decreased Blood Osmotic Pressure

Increased Albumin Excretion
Nephrotic syndrome (albumin leaks into urine)
Protein-losing enteropathies (excess albumin in feces)

Decreased Albumin Synthesis
Kwashiorkor (low-protein, high-carbohydrate starvation diet provides too few amino acids for liver to make albumin)
Liver cirrhosis (diseased liver unable to make enough albumin)

Edema Due to Increased Interstitial Fluid Osmotic Pressure

Increased Capillary Permeability
Inflammation
Toxins
Hypersensitivity reactions
Burns

Edema Due to Blocked Lymphatic Drainage

Tumors
Goiter
Parasites that obstruct lymph nodes
Surgery that removes lymph nodes

from inflammation of an injury is initially treated with cold to reduce capillary blood flow and thus reduce blood hydrostatic pressure.

Nursing Management

A child or parent may make comments that alert the nurse to the development of edema. Shoes may become tight by the end of the day (dependent edema); the waistband of pants or a skirt may be "outgrown" suddenly (generalized edema or ascites [accumulation of fluid in the peritoneal cavity]); the eyes may be puffy (periorbital edema); a ring may be too tight; fingers may "feel like sausages." In many cases visual inspection is sufficient to recognize edema. Observe for pitting edema. To detect changes in the amount of swelling, measure around the edematous part. If the edema is caused by extracellular fluid volume excess, daily measurements of weight and intake and output are a necessary part of the daily assessment. Nursing assessment

should also focus on the integrity of the skin, presence of pain, restricted motion, and alterations in the child's body image.

Elevation of an area of localized edema helps to reduce the swelling. The skin over an edematous area needs extra care because it is fragile and prone to breakdown (Figure 43–7 ◉). Carefully position an infant or child on bed rest and turn frequently to prevent pressure sores. Perform turning carefully to avoid skin abrasion by rubbing against the sheets. Pat the skin dry after cleansing rather than rubbing it. Trim the child's fingernails smooth to prevent scratching. Teach parents skin care for the child at home. Teach older children to inspect their skin carefully to identify areas needing special care.

If restricted mobility is a problem, make specific plans to help the child manage activities. For example, if an edematous finger restricts the motion of a hand, food can be cut into bite-sized portions before the meal is served, so that the child can still eat independently.

Discomfort from edema may require creative nursing interventions. Distraction with toys or activities appropriate to the child's developmental level can be useful. Interventions to treat the underlying problem can also reduce the edema and its accompanying discomfort. Interventions for edema should be added to the nursing management of the underlying condition that causes the edema. Administration of the prescribed medical therapy and observation for the complications of therapy are nursing responsibilities.

Discuss with school-age children and adolescents feelings of embarrassment about the edematous appearance. They need to understand the reason for edema and be able

◉ **FIGURE 43–7**

Edematous tissue is easily damaged. It must be kept clean and dry and free of pressure.

to explain it to peers. Arrange for the child to meet other children with similar concerns.

Desired outcomes of care include maintenance of intact skin, normal respiratory sounds and effort, and normal weight patterns.

ELECTROLYTE IMBALANCES

All body fluids contain electrolytes, although the concentration of those electrolytes varies, depending on the type and location of the fluid. When a serum electrolyte value is reported from the laboratory, it provides information about the concentration of that electrolyte in the blood. It may not necessarily reflect the concentration of the electrolyte in other body compartments. Refer to Table 43–1 to see which electrolytes have the highest and lowest concentrations in the blood and other fluid compartments.

Electrolytes are normally gained and lost in relatively equal amounts so the body remains in balance. However, when a child has an abnormal route of loss, such as vomiting, wound drainage, or nasogastric suction, electrolyte balance can be disturbed. In addition, supplementation with electrolytes via intravenous fluids in proportions different than body fluids can also cause electrolyte imbalance. Children with disease states that interfere with normal mechanisms of electrolyte regulation, such as renal disease, also have disturbance in electrolyte levels. Monitoring for signs of imbalance becomes important in all of these situations.

SODIUM IMBALANCES

The serum sodium concentration reflects the **osmolality** of body fluids; that is, their degree of concentration or dilution. It refers to the number of moles of the substance per kilogram of water in the solution. Serum sodium concentration reflects the proportion of water and sodium in the extracellular compartment. When the osmolality of body fluids becomes abnormal, the cells swell or shrink. These cell size changes are due to **osmosis**, the movement of water across a semipermeable membrane into an area of higher particle concentration. Sodium levels are maintained at high extracellular and low intracellular levels by the sodium-potassium pump, which moves these electrolytes against their expected concentration gradients (Figure 43–8 ●).

HYPERNATREMIA

Hypernatremia is a condition of increased osmolality of the blood. The body fluids are too concentrated, containing excess sodium relative to water. A serum sodium level above 148 mmol/L in children (146 mmol/L in newborns) is diagnostic of hypernatremia (Table 43–7).

Hypernatremia is caused by conditions that cause the body to lose relatively more water than sodium or to gain relatively more sodium than water (Table 43–8). Special circumstances in which a high solute intake may occur without adequate water include an infant formula that is too concentrated or one that is prepared with salt instead

● **FIGURE 43-8**

A, Water balance is maintained by the simple passage of molecules from greater to lesser concentration across cell membranes. **B,** Sodium levels are maintained by an active transport system, the sodium-potassium pump, which moves these electrolytes across cell membranes in spite of their concentration.

TABLE 43–7 ✣ Normal Serum Values

Blood Component	Values
Sodium	Newborn: 131–144 mmol/L
	Children: 132–141 mmol/L
Potassium	Premature infants: 4.5–7.2 mmol/L
	Full-term infants: 3.2–5.7 mmol/L
	Children: 3.3–4.7 mmol/L
Calcium	Premature infants: 3.5–4.5 mEq/L (1.7–2.3 mmol/L)
	Full-term infants: 4–5 mEq/L (2–2.5 mmol/L)
	Children: 4.4–5.3 mEq/L (2.2–2.7 mmol/L)
Magnesium	Children: 1.3–2.7 mg/dL (0.5–1.1 mmol/L)
Arterial pH	Infants: 7.18–7.5
	Children: 7.27–7.49
	Adolescents: 7.35–7.41
Arterial Po_2	Infants: 60–70 mm Hg (8–9.3 pKa)
	Children: 80–108 mm Hg (10.7–14.4 pKa)
	Adolescents: 80–100 mm Hg (4.3–6.4 pKa)
Arterial Pco_2	Infants: 27–41 mm Hg (3.6–5.5 pKa)
	Children and adolescents: 32–48 mm Hg (4.3–6.4 pKa)
Arterial bicarbonate	Infants: 19–24 mmol/L
	Children: 18–25 mmol/L
	Adolescents: 20–29 mmol/L

TABLE 43–8 ✣ Causes of Hypernatremia

Loss of Relatively More Water than Sodium	Gain of Relatively More Sodium than Water
Inadequate breastfeeding intake with normal output	Inability to communicate thirst
Diabetes insipidus (not enough antidiuretic hormone)	Limited or no access to water
Diarrhea or vomiting without fluid replacement	High solute intake without adequate water (e.g., tube feedings)
Excessive sweating without fluid replacement	Intravenous hypertonic saline
High solute intake without adequate water (causes kidneys to excrete water)	Improper formula preparation leading to excessive concentration
Increased aldosterone	

NURSING MANAGEMENT

Monitor serum sodium level and measure intake and output and urine specific gravity. Normal specific gravity under 2 years is 1.001 to 1.015, while in children over 2 years 1.010 to 1.030 is the normal range. Specific gravity changes toward normal levels as therapy progresses. Frequently assess responsiveness to monitor the effect of hypernatremia on brain cells. As the concentration of body fluids returns to normal, the child will become more alert and responsive. Watch for rebound hyponatremia while monitoring the fluid replacement. Implement safety interventions such as raised bed rails for protection. Ensure adequate rest and introduce developmentally appropriate activities when the child is alert.

Water deprivation is a form of child neglect or abuse. In neglect, the parents simply do not provide adequate water for the child. A form of child abuse that sometimes includes water deprivation is Munchausen syndrome by proxy (see Chapter 36 ∞). A small child who is hospitalized with hypernatremia that does not have a detectable cause may be subject to water deprivation. Assess the child's general condition, developmental tasks, the family dynamics, and the parents' understanding of formula preparation and the child's fluid intake needs.

Teaching can prevent many cases of hypernatremia. Be sure the breastfeeding mother has instruction and resources about lactation before discharge after birth. If discharged soon after birth, be sure the infant has an appointment to have weight checked within the first few days, and alert the parents to expected output of at least six wet diapers daily. By about 10 days, infants should have regained the birth weight.

When an infant is sick or developing slowly, parents sometimes want to feed the infant more concentrated formula to make him or her stronger. Parents and caregivers of

of sugar. A breastfed baby not receiving adequate breast milk who has normal water loss may develop hypernatremic dehydration (Livingstone, Willis, Abdel-Wareth et al., 2000)

An infant or child who has hypernatremia is generally thirsty. The urine output is small unless the hypernatremia is caused by diabetes insipidus. A decreased level of consciousness manifested by confusion, lethargy, or coma results from shrinking of the brain cells. Seizures can occur when hypernatremia occurs rapidly or is severe. Severe hypernatremia can be fatal.

Hypernatremia is treated by intravenous administration of **hypotonic fluid**, or fluid that is more dilute than normal body fluid. This therapy dilutes the body fluids back to normal concentration. If a child is dehydrated, **isotonic fluids** (those with the osmolality of body fluids) may be administered first to replenish the volume, followed by hypotonic fluid to correct the osmolality. The underlying cause of the disorder is also treated.

TABLE 43–9 ✤ **Causes of Hyponatremia**

Gain of Relatively More Water than Sodium	Loss of Relatively More Sodium than Water
Excessive intravenous D_5W (5% dextrose in water)	Diarrhea or vomiting with replacement by tap water only instead of fluid containing sodium
Excessive tap water enemas	
Irrigation of body cavities with distilled water	Excessive sweating
Excessive antidiuretic hormone	Diuretics, especially thiazides
Forced excessive oral intake of tap water	
Congestive heart failure	

bottle-fed babies should be taught never to give undiluted formula concentrate or evaporated milk. Parents should be cautioned to keep salt out of reach, since eating handfuls of salt has caused hypernatremia. Teach parents to offer extra fluids during hot weather. Teach oral rehydration therapy for use at home during mild vomiting and diarrhea (see page 1244).

Nurses can prevent hypernatremia in hospitalized infants and children by administering water between tube feedings, keeping water available, and offering it frequently. Offering frequent small amounts and using Popsicles and other creative interventions can increase children's intake.

Desired outcomes of treatment for hypernatremia include balance of electrolytes and fluid in the intracellular and extracellular compartments, and alert level of consciousness.

HYPONATREMIA

In hyponatremia the osmolality of the blood is decreased. The body fluids are too dilute, containing excess water relative to sodium. Hyponatremia is the most common sodium imbalance in children (Behrman, Kliegman, & Jenson, 2004). A serum sodium level below 132 mmol/L in children (131 mmol/L in newborns) is diagnostic of hyponatremia.

ETIOLOGY AND PATHOPHYSIOLOGY

Hyponatremia is caused by conditions that cause gain of relatively more water than sodium or loss of relatively more sodium than water (Table 43–9). Oral intake of water causes hyponatremia in unusual conditions such as forced fluid intake. More commonly, parents feed an infant only water or dilute formula to save money instead of regular-strength formula or breast milk. Excessive swallowing of swimming pool water by an infant can have the same effect.

Infants are vulnerable to the type of hyponatremia caused by water intoxication since they have a poorly developed thirst mechanism and may continue to drink, and then are unable to excrete excess water quickly due to immature kidney function (Behrman et al., 2004). Forced water intake is another cause and a form of child abuse.

CLINICAL MANIFESTATIONS

The child with hyponatremia has a decreased level of consciousness, which results from swelling of brain cells. This can be manifested as anorexia, headache, muscle weakness, decreased deep tendon reflexes, lethargy, confusion, or coma. If hyponatremia arises rapidly or is extreme, seizures may occur. Hyponatremia is a frequent cause of seizures in infants under 6 months of age who also have a low body temperature. Nausea and vomiting also occur in some children. Severe hyponatremia can be fatal.

CLINICAL THERAPY

In most cases, hyponatremia is treated by restricting the intake of water. This therapy allows the kidneys to correct the imbalance by excreting excess water from the body. If a child is having seizures from hyponatremia, intravenous **hypertonic saline** (more concentrated than body fluid) may be administered. Use of this concentrated fluid is a way to rapidly increase body fluid concentration, but it must be monitored carefully because it can easily cause rebound hypernatremia.

NURSING MANAGEMENT

NURSING ASSESSMENT AND DIAGNOSIS

Monitor serum sodium level and measure intake and output. If an infant with hyponatremia has normal antidiuretic hormone (ADH) levels, and other causes have been ruled out, carefully question parents about proper preparation of formula and feeding practices. A toddler or school-age child may be subjected to forced fluid intake as a form of child abuse. Sensitive interviewing and a caring manner can help identify such problems in a family.

Since hyponatremia is characterized by decreased level of consciousness, frequently assess responsiveness to monitor the response to therapy. The child will become more alert and responsive as the concentration of body fluids returns to normal.

The highest priority nursing diagnosis for hyponatremia addresses the *Risk for Injury* related to the child's decreased level of consciousness. The following diagnoses might also apply:

- *Self-Care Deficit* related to weakness and tiredness
- *Ineffective Health Maintenance* related to parental misinterpretation about infant formula preparation
- *Ineffective Breastfeeding* related to inadequate sucking by infant or inadequate milk production

PLANNING AND IMPLEMENTATION

Nurses can prevent hyponatremia in hospitalized children by using normal saline instead of distilled water for irrigations and by avoiding tap water enemas. It is important to help the child comply with any prescribed fluid restrictions. Allow the child to choose favorite fluids to drink. Teach parents to replace body fluids lost through diarrhea or vomiting with oral electrolyte solutions (see pp. 1242 and 1244).

Expected outcomes are avoidance of injury, balance of fluid and electrolytes, and establishment of adequate formula or breastfeeding intake.

POTASSIUM IMBALANCES

Potassium, an essential electrolyte, performs many necessary functions in the body such as muscle contraction and enzymatic reactions. Potassium intake in healthy children comes from potassium-rich foods such as fruits and vegetables. Potassium is absorbed easily from the intestine. A normal potassium distribution is important for proper function.

A potassium imbalance arises when the serum potassium concentration rises or falls outside the normal range. Potassium imbalances are caused by alterations in potassium intake, distribution, or excretion; or by loss of potassium through an abnormal route such as burns, emesis, or renal failure.

Most potassium ions in the body are found inside the cells. The sodium-potassium pump in cell membranes moves potassium ions into cells to maintain the high in-

PATHOPHYSIOLOGY ILLUSTRATED
Potassium Ions

Factors that shift potassium ions into or out of cells.

tracellular potassium concentration. Potassium ions can be shifted into or out of cells by various physiologic factors (see "Pathophysiology Illustrated: Potassium Ions"). Potassium is excreted from the body through urine, feces, and sweat. The hormone aldosterone increases potassium excretion in the urine.

HYPERKALEMIA

Hyperkalemia is an excess of potassium in the blood. It is reflected by a level above 5.8 mmol/L in children or above 5.2 mmol/L in newborns (see Table 13-7).

ETIOLOGY AND PATHOPHYSIOLOGY

Hyperkalemia is caused by conditions that include increased potassium intake, shift of potassium from cells into the extracellular fluid, and decreased potassium excretion. Renal insufficiency is a primary cause of hyperkalemia (Blonshine, 2000). Premature infants commonly have low systemic blood flow and resultant poor renal function, leading to hyperkalemia (Kluckow & Evans, 2001). Increased potassium intake is frequently due to intravenous potassium overload. Excessive or too rapid intravenous administration of potassium-containing solutions can occur if the potassium requirement is overestimated or if the intravenous infusion runs in too fast.

Blood transfusion is another source of potassium intake that may cause hyperkalemia. Potassium ions leak out of red blood cells that are stored in a blood bank. The longer the blood is stored, the more potassium leaks out of cells and accumulates in the fluid portion of the transfusion. Hyperkalemia from administration of stored blood arises when multiple units are transfused, as when infants receive exchange transfusions or children receive multiple blood transfusions after a serious injury or in surgery.

Shift of potassium from cells into the extracellular fluid occurs when there is massive cell death, as with a crush injury, in sickle cell anemia (hemolytic crisis), or when chemotherapy for a malignancy is rapidly effective (tumor lysis syndrome). In these situations the dead cells release their high-potassium contents into the extracellular fluid. Potassium ions also shift out of cells in metabolic acidosis caused by diarrhea and in diabetes mellitus when insulin levels are low.

Decreased potassium excretion occurs with acute or chronic oliguria during renal failure, severe hypovolemia, and conditions that decrease the secretion of aldosterone by the adrenal cortex (lead poisoning, Addison's disease, hypoaldosteronism). Several medications can cause hyperkalemia, including some cancer chemotherapy, potassium-sparing diuretics, angiotensin-converting enzyme inhibitors, and nonsteroidal anti-inflammatory analgesics.

CLINICAL MANIFESTATIONS

The clinical manifestations of hyperkalemia are all related to muscle dysfunction since potassium plays a vital role in muscle activity. Hyperactivity of gastrointestinal smooth muscle causes intestinal cramping and diarrhea in some children. The skeletal muscles become weak, beginning typically with leg weakness and ascending. Weakness can progress to flaccid paralysis. The child is often lethargic. Dysfunction of cardiac muscle causes cardiac arrhythmias such as tachycardia and may result in heart failure and cardiac arrest. Abnormalities in the electrocardiogram include a prolonged QRS complex, a peak in T waves, atrioventricular block, and ventricular dysrhythmia (Johns Hopkins Hospital, 2005).

CLINICAL THERAPY

Hyperkalemia is treated by management of the underlying condition that caused the imbalance. If the serum potassium concentration is very high or is causing dangerous cardiac arrhythmias, treatment to decrease the serum potassium level may be ordered. These treatments may remove potassium from the body or drive it from the extracellular fluid into the cells. Potassium is removed from the body by peritoneal dialysis or hemodialysis, by potassium-wasting diuretics, or with a cation exchange resin (Kayexalate) administered orally or rectally. Medical treatments that drive potassium ions into cells are intravenous bicarbonate, intravenous insulin, and glucose.

NURSING MANAGEMENT

NURSING ASSESSMENT AND DIAGNOSIS

Monitor serum potassium levels with prescribed laboratory analysis. Ongoing assessment of muscle strength is important because the muscle weakness may progress to flaccid paralysis. (This paralysis is reversible on correction of the potassium imbalance.) Diarrhea can occur in infants and children. An older child may complain of intestinal cramping. Monitor the pulse rate carefully.

GROWTH AND DEVELOPMENT

The nursing diagnoses for hyperkalemic children will prompt a nurse to provide safety measures appropriate to the child's developmental level and to assist the child with activities that muscle weakness makes difficult. It is important to provide play and diversional activities that take into account the child's degree of muscle strength as well as the appropriate developmental level.

Nursing diagnoses for a child who has hyperkalemia depend on the severity of the clinical manifestations. The cause of the imbalance may also lead to useful diagnoses that guide teaching for the child and the parents. The following nursing diagnoses may apply:

- *Activity Intolerance* related to decreased cardiac output secondary to cardiac arrhythmias
- *Risk for Injury* related to muscle weakness
- *Self-Care Deficit: Hygiene and Dressing* related to neuromuscular impairment
- *Anxiety* related to change in health status
- *Ineffective Health Maintenance* related to parental lack of exposure about potassium intake in chronic renal failure
- *Ineffective Management of Therapeutic Regimen by Family* related to complexity of therapy

PLANNING AND IMPLEMENTATION

Nursing care includes measures to prevent hyperkalemia from developing in hospitalized children. If hyperkalemia does develop, care shifts to administering intravenous solutions, monitoring cardiopulmonary status, ensuring safety, promoting adequate nutrition, and preparing the child and family for discharge.

Prevent Hyperkalemia

Any child receiving an intravenous infusion that contains potassium is at risk for hyperkalemia. Check that urine output is normal (1–2 mL/kg/hr) before administering intravenous potassium solutions. Turn over intravenous solutions to which potassium has been added several times to mix the contents thoroughly before connecting them to the infusion tubing. Double-check the potassium order and intravenous dosage with another nurse.

Be sure blood or packed red blood cells are fresh, especially for the child receiving multiple transfusions, and for all newborns. Use a cardiac monitor during infusion of these products to watch for arrhythmias.

Administer Intravenous Solutions

Once a child is diagnosed as hyperkalemic, ensure that any infusions with added potassium are stopped. Several infusions may need to be managed, including glucose, bicarbonate, and calcium gluconate. Maintain the infusion at the prescribed rate and monitor the child's condition frequently.

Monitor Cardiopulmonary Status

Upon diagnosis of hyperkalemia, an electrocardiogram is performed and a cardiac monitor applied. Monitor for any changes in cardiac status and for cardiac arrhythmias. Report abnormal rate and character of pulse as well as shortness of breath.

Ensure Safety

Since the child is weak, raise side rails. Position the child carefully. Assist the child with activities requiring leg muscle strength, such as climbing into bed or pushing up in bed. Encourage quiet activities with frequent rest periods. Document and report any change in muscle weakness.

Promote Adequate Nutritional Intake

Adequate caloric intake is necessary to prevent tissue breakdown and the resultant potassium release from cells. Offer the child nourishing snacks if his or her appetite is decreased. Restrict potassium-rich foods.

Discharge Planning and Home Care Teaching

If the child has chronic renal failure or another condition that decreases aldosterone secretion, teach parents and children to restrict foods high in potassium. Most oral rehydration solutions, including Pedialyte, contain potassium and should not be used to provide fluid for the child. Instruct the family not to use salt substitutes, which commonly contain potassium. Parents should check with the care provider and pharmacist before giving even over-the-counter products to the child, as some of these medications contain potassium. Management of renal failure at home with frequent visits for dialysis and other treatments can be challenging. Refer to Chapter 52 for further suggestions to help parents handle this condition. ∞

EVALUATION

Expected outcomes for the child with hyperkalemia include the following:

- Return to a state of fluid and electrolyte balance
- Maintenance of safety
- Adequate nutritional intake to provide essential potassium
- Normal cardiac rate and rhythm

HYPOKALEMIA

Hypokalemia occurs when the serum potassium concentration is too low. Total body potassium may be decreased, normal, or even increased when the serum level is low, depending on the cause of the imbalance. Serum potassium levels below 3.5 mmol/L in children (3.7 mmol/L for newborns) are diagnostic of hypokalemia.

ETIOLOGY AND PATHOPHYSIOLOGY

Hypokalemia is caused by conditions that include increased potassium excretion, decreased potassium intake, shift of potassium from the extracellular fluid into cells, and loss of potassium by an abnormal route.

Increased potassium excretion is a major cause of hypokalemia in children. In addition to diuretics and other medications, causes of increased urinary potassium excretion are osmotic diuresis (glucose present in urine), hypomagnesemia, increased aldosterone (hyperaldosteronism, congestive heart failure, nephrotic syndrome, cirrhosis), and increased cortisol (Cushing's disease and syndrome). Eating large amounts of black licorice increases renal excretion of potassium. Diarrhea causes potassium to be excreted in the feces.

Decreased potassium intake will lead to hypokalemia slowly, or more rapidly if combined with increased excretion or loss of potassium. Hospitalized children that are placed on NPO status and receive prolonged intravenous therapy should have added potassium. Adolescents concerned about weight loss or those with anorexia nervosa may embark on fad diets low in potassium.

Shift of potassium from the extracellular fluid into cells occurs in alkalosis and hypothermia (unintentional or induced for surgery). Hyperalimentation often causes hypersecretion of insulin, which also shifts potassium into cells.

Vomiting is a route for the loss of potassium; self-induced vomiting in bulimia, for example, can cause hypokalemia. Nasogastric suctioning (Figure 43–9 ⦿) and intestinal decompression can cause potassium loss. Hypokalemia can also be caused by several medications (Table 43–10).

CLINICAL MANIFESTATIONS

Since the ratio of intracellular to extracellular potassium determines the responsiveness of muscle cells to neural stimuli, it is not surprising that the clinical manifestations of hypokalemia involve muscle dysfunction. Gastrointestinal smooth muscle activity is slowed, leading to abdominal distention, constipation, or paralytic ileus. Skeletal muscles are weak and unresponsive to stimuli, and weakness may progress to flaccid paralysis. The respiratory muscles may be impaired. Cardiac arrhythmias can occur. Polyuria results from changes

● FIGURE 43–9

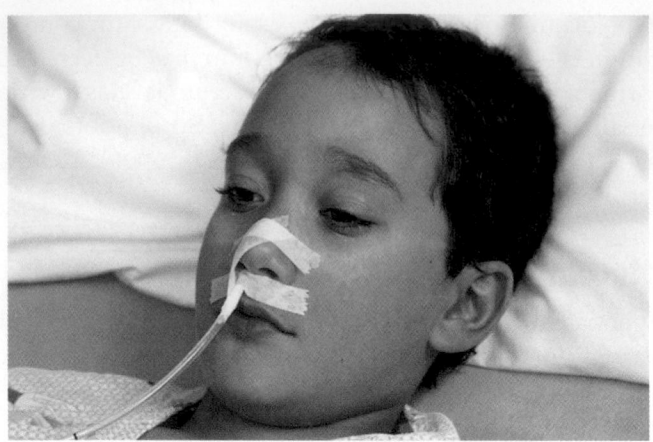

Because this child has a nasogastric tube in place, it is important to monitor his potassium levels.

in the kidney caused by hypokalemia. Symptoms may range from mild fatigue with potassium levels < 3.5 mmol/L, to muscle necrosis at < 2.5 mmol/L, and flaccidity and respiratory problems at < 2 mmol/L (English, 2002).

CLINICAL THERAPY

Medical management of hypokalemia focuses on replacement of potassium while treating the cause of the imbalance. Potassium replacement may be given intravenously or orally.

NURSING MANAGEMENT

NURSING ASSESSMENT AND DIAGNOSIS

Monitor serum potassium levels. Observe for muscle weakness, which is frequently detected first in the legs. Parents may report that muscle weakness restricts the child's activities and impairs interactions with peers. Skeletal muscle strength can be difficult to assess if the child is lethargic.

Muscle weakness may affect the respiratory muscles. Assess the child frequently to determine the need for assisted ventilation. Cardiac monitoring is important for continued assessment of hypokalemia-associated arrhythmias. Apical pulse rate should be monitored.

Assess for diminished bowel sounds. Ask the parents if the child has recently been awakening to use the toilet at night or has begun bed-wetting after previously being dry at night. These may be symptoms of polyuria associated with chronic hypokalemia.

The most important nursing diagnoses in the child with severe hypokalemia relate to cardiac arrhythmias and respiratory muscle weakness. The following nursing diagnoses may apply:

- *Risk for Activity Intolerance* related to decreased cardiac output secondary to cardiac arrhythmia
- *Ineffective Breathing Pattern* related to respiratory musculoskeletal impairment
- *Risk for Injury* related to muscle weakness
- *Self-Care Deficit: Hygiene and Dressing* related to neuromuscular impairment
- *Constipation* related to decreased motility
- *Anxiety* related to change in health status
- *Ineffective Health Maintenance* related to management of potassium supplements or high-potassium diet
- *Ineffective Management of Therapeutic Regimen* related to complexity of potassium therapy
- *Imbalanced Nutrition: Less than Body Requirements* related to lack of basic nutritional knowledge regarding safe weight-loss diet

TABLE 43–10 ✤ Drugs That May Cause Electrolyte Disturbance

Hyperkalemia	Hypokalemia	Hypocalcemia	Hypermagnesemia	Hypomagnesemia
Potassium-containing medications	Beta-adrenergic agonists	Antacids (if overused)	Magnesium-containing cathartics	Magnesium-wasting diuretics
Potassium-sparing diuretics	Insulin	Laxatives (if overused)	Magnesium antacids	Antineoplastics
Angiotensin-converting enzyme inhibitors	Potassium-wasting diuretics	Oil-based bowel lubricants		Systemic antifungals
Cytotoxic agents	Parenteral penicillins	Anticonvulsants		Aminoglycoside antimicrobials
	Glucocorticoids	Phosphate-containing preparations		Laxatives
	Aminoglycoside antimicrobials	Protein-type plasma expanders during rapid infusion		
	Systemic antifungals	Antineoplastics		
	Antineoplastics			
	Laxatives			

TABLE 43–11 ✤ Food Sources of Electrolytes

Potassium-Rich Foods		Calcium-Rich Foods		Magnesium-Rich Foods
Apricots	Orange juice	Milk	Legumes	Whole-grain cereal
Bananas	Peaches	Cheese	Nuts	Dark green vegetables
Cantaloupe	Potatoes	Yogurt	Figs	Soy
Cherries	Prunes	Pudding	Chicken	Almonds
Dates	Raisins	Egg yolks	Salmon (canned with bones)	Peanut butter
Figs	Strawberries	Grains (cream of wheat,	Tofu	Bananas
Molasses	Tomato juice	farina, bran muffins)	Fruit drinks with added calcium	Egg yolk
		Sardines (canned)		

PLANNING AND IMPLEMENTATION

Nursing care of the child with hypokalemia focuses on ensuring adequate potassium intake, monitoring cardiopulmonary status, promoting normal bowel function, ensuring safety, providing dietary counseling, and preparing the child and family for discharge.

Ensure Adequate Potassium Intake

Since potassium is excreted from the body every day, daily potassium intake is necessary to prevent hypokalemia. A hypokalemic child who is able to eat should be given a high-potassium diet. Teach parents (and the child if old enough) which foods are high in potassium and how to incorporate them into the daily diet (Table 43–11).

Children who have no oral intake for a period of time should receive intravenous fluids that contain potassium. Calculate the dosage to be sure it is accurate. Ensure that the infusion runs on schedule. Sometimes the child will complain of burning along the vein when potassium is infused. The infusion may need to be slowed temporarily to allow it to continue. Check serum potassium to watch for high or low potassium levels. Monitor urine output. An oliguric child can develop hyperkalemia when receiving supplements.

Monitor Cardiopulmonary Status

Hypokalemia potentiates digitalis toxicity. A hypokalemic child receiving digitalis needs careful surveillance for digitalis toxicity, which is manifested as anorexia, nausea, vomiting, and bradycardia. Observe for these effects. Take the pulse rate and rhythm regularly. Monitor respirations and ease of breathing to watch for decreased respiratory muscle activity.

Promote Normal Bowel Function

Ensure adequate fluids and fiber in the diet. Monitor and record the number of stools and report inadequate stools.

Ensure Safety

Keep bed side rails up. Assist the child as needed to move into and out of bed. Reposition the child frequently to preserve skin integrity of limbs that are not moved regularly. Perform passive range of motion if the child is not moving. Use supportive pillows to position the child properly.

Provide Dietary Counseling

The adolescent trying to lose weight and not consuming a nutritious diet needs dietary teaching. More intensive treatment will be needed for teens who are anorexic or bulimic (see Chapter 36 for interventions ∞).

Discharge Planning and Home Care Teaching

Teach parents how to give potassium supplements, if prescribed. Liquid or powdered potassium supplements can be mixed with juice or sherbet to improve the bitter taste. The parent should call the mixture "medicine" so that the child does not learn to dislike all juices. Teach the parents signs of hypokalemia and hyperkalemia and whom to call to report these symptoms. These signs must be reported promptly so medications can be adjusted.

EVALUATION

Expected outcomes for the child with potassium imbalance include normal rate and rhythm of heart and respiratory system, regular bowel movements, maintenance of safety, and knowledge of child and family regarding food sources of potassium.

GROWTH AND DEVELOPMENT

Bradycardia occurs at a different level for children of various ages. For infants, a pulse rate below 100 is considered bradycardia. For young children, 80 may be the identified number, whereas for adolescents, a pulse below 60 is bradycardia. Look at the child's age and normal pulse range to find changes that indicate bradycardia.

CALCIUM IMBALANCES

A normal serum calcium concentration is important for many physiologic functions, including muscle and nerve function, secretion of hormones, bone formation and strength, and clotting of the blood. Calcium is the most abundant mineral in the body, with about 98% of it being present in bones (Umpaichitra, Bastian, & Castells, 2001). A discussion of dietary calcium intake and its importance in bone formation can be found in Chapter 34 (also see "Developing Cultural Competence: Calcium Intake and Osteoporosis").

DEVELOPING CULTURAL COMPETENCE

CALCIUM INTAKE AND OSTEOPOROSIS

Ingestion and absorption of calcium is important in the growing child to ensure formation of strong bones. Adolescents who ingest more calcium have less risk of osteoporosis later in life. It has been noted that black women have less bone loss and fewer fractures than white women. A study with black and white adolescent girls showed that the blacks absorbed more calcium from the diet, and lost less in their urine, leading to increased bone density (Bryant et al., 2003). Nurses should recognize this difference and monitor intake of all adolescents. Recognize the high risk of developing osteoporosis in those who are white and consuming little calcium. Interventions should focus on ways of increasing intake.

Calcium imbalances are caused by alterations in calcium intake, absorption, distribution, or excretion. Calcium absorption requires vitamin D for maximum efficiency and is greatest in the duodenum. Calcium distribution involves calcium entry into and exit from bones and the distribution of different forms of calcium in the plasma. Ionized calcium is the only physiologically active form; additional calcium is bound to protein or ions. Calcium is excreted in urine, feces, and sweat (see "Pathophysiology Illustrated: Calcium Imbalances").

Parathyroid hormone is the major regulator of the plasma calcium concentration. It increases the plasma calcium concentration by increasing calcium absorption, increasing calcium withdrawal from bones, and decreasing calcium excretion in the urine. The plasma calcium concentration has an important influence on cell membrane permeability and influences the threshold potential of excitable cells. For this reason, calcium imbalances alter neuromuscular irritability.

HYPERCALCEMIA

Hypercalcemia refers to a plasma excess of calcium (above 5.3 mEq/L [2.7 mmol/L] in children or 5 mEq/L [2.5 mmol/L] in newborns) (see Table 43–7). Because so much calcium is stored in the bones, however, the serum levels of calcium may not reflect body stores.

PATHOPHYSIOLOGY ILLUSTRATED

Calcium Imbalances

Some causes of excess calcium in the blood (hypercalcemia)

Ca²⁺
Ca²⁺
Ca²⁺

- Vitamin D overdose
- Hyperparathyroidism
- Bone tumors and other cancers
- Thiazide diuretics
- Familial hypercalcemia

Some causes of decreased calcium in the blood (hypocalcemia)

Ca²⁺
Ca²⁺
Ca²⁺

- Insufficient dietary calcium and vitamin D intake
- Chronic diarrhea
- Laxative abuse
- Malabsorption
- Chronic renal insufficiency
- Hypoparathyroidism
- Alkalosis
- Large transfusion of citrated blood
- Rapid infusion of plasma expanders

A variety of conditions can lead to hypercalcemia and hypocalcemia.

ETIOLOGY AND PATHOPHYSIOLOGY

Hypercalcemia is caused by conditions that include increased calcium intake or absorption, shift of calcium from bones into the extracellular fluid, and decreased calcium excretion. Hypercalcemia due to increased calcium intake or absorption may occur if an infant is fed large amounts of chicken liver (source of vitamin A) or is given megadoses of vitamin D or vitamin A, or if a child or adolescent consumes large amounts of calcium-rich foods concurrently with antacids (milk-alkali syndrome). Infants with very low birth weight can develop hypercalcemia if they have inadequate phosphorus intake, as bone phosphorus and calcium will be resorbed. Hypercalcemia may also occur when children receiving total parenteral nutrition are given excessive doses of calcium.

Most cases of hypercalcemia in children are due to a shift of calcium from bones into the extracellular fluid. The excessive amounts of parathyroid hormone produced in hyperparathyroidism cause calcium withdrawal from bones. Prolonged immobilization also causes withdrawal of calcium from bones. Often, the excess calcium ions are excreted in the urine. However, if calcium is withdrawn from bones faster than the kidneys can excrete it, hypercalcemia results. Hypercalcemia also occurs with many types of malignancies such as leukemias. The malignant cells produce substances that circulate in the blood to the bones and cause bone resorption. The calcium from the bones then enters the extracellular fluid, causing hypercalcemia. Bone tumors destroy bone directly, leading to the release of calcium. Familial hypercalcemia and infantile hypercalcemia are rare congenital disorders.

Thiazide diuretics (e.g., thiazide and hydrochlorthiazide) decrease calcium excretion in the urine and may contribute to development of hypercalcemia.

CLINICAL MANIFESTATIONS

Hypercalcemia may have nonspecific symptoms, making diagnosis difficult. Many signs and symptoms of hypercalcemia are manifestations of decreased neuromuscular excitability. Constipation, anorexia, nausea, and vomiting can occur. Fatigue and skeletal muscle weakness predominate. Confusion, lethargy, and decreased attention span are common. Polyuria develops. Severe hypercalcemia may cause cardiac arrhythmias and arrest. Newborns with hypercalcemia have flaccid muscles and exhibit failure to thrive. Hypercalcemia increases sodium and potassium excretion by the kidneys and can lead to polyuria and polydipsia.

CLINICAL THERAPY

Hypercalcemia is treated by increasing fluids and administering the diuretic furosemide (Lasix) to increase excretion of calcium in the urine. Treatment to decrease intestinal absorption of calcium involves effective use of glucocorticoids. Bone resorption can be decreased by administration of glucocorticoids and calcitonin. Phosphate is sometimes given to treat hypercalcemia, but it may cause dangerous precipitation of calcium phosphate salts in body tissues. Dialysis may be used, if necessary.

NURSING MANAGEMENT

NURSING ASSESSMENT AND DIAGNOSIS

Nursing assessment of a child with hypercalcemia includes monitoring serum calcium levels, level of consciousness, gastrointestinal function, urine volume, specific gravity, cardiac rhythm, and pH. With chronic hypercalcemia, assessment of activity tolerance and developmental level becomes important.

Many nursing diagnoses are appropriate for children who have hypercalcemia. Diagnoses that address cardiac and neuromuscular manifestation are especially important. The following nursing diagnoses may apply:

- *Risk for Activity Intolerance* related to decreased cardiac output secondary to cardiac arrhythmia
- *Risk for Injury* related to decreased level of consciousness
- *Risk for Injury* related to neuromuscular impairment
- *Risk for Injury* related to possibility of spontaneous fractures
- *Self-Care Deficit: Hygiene and Dressing* related to neuromuscular impairment
- *Anxiety* related to change in health status
- *Constipation* related to decreased motility
- *Risk for Imbalanced Nutrition: Less than Body Requirements* related to anorexia and nausea
- *Risk for Impaired Urinary Elimination* related to renal calculi

PLANNING AND INTERVENTION

Carefully calculate calcium in total parenteral nutrition and other solutions, administer these solutions with caution, and use cardiac monitoring to prevent hypercalcemia in hospitalized children.

Interventions to increase fluid intake are important for children with hypercalcemia or those who are immobilized. An increased fluid intake, appropriate to the child's age, is necessary to keep the urine dilute and to help reduce constipation (a common symptom of hypercalcemia). An acidic urine helps to keep calcium from forming stones. Because urinary tract infections may cause the urine to be alkaline, institute nursing interventions to prevent urinary tract infection. Thiazide diuretics, which decrease calcium excretion, should not be given to the hypercalcemic child. Provide a high-fiber diet to help reduce constipation.

Increasing mobility through assisted weight bearing helps decrease the withdrawal of calcium from bones that is caused by immobility. If the hypercalcemia is caused by withdrawal of calcium from bones, the child is at risk for fractures with minor trauma and must be handled with special care. See Chapter 55 for further discussion of care following fractures and prolonged casting. ∞

Teach parents to avoid giving calcium-rich foods (such as dairy products) and calcium antacids (e.g., Tums) to children with hypercalcemia. Vitamin D supplements should be avoided as they increase calcium absorption from the gastrointestinal tract.

Expected outcomes include cardiac pump effectiveness, safety, normal bowel excretion, and adequate nutritional status.

HYPOCALCEMIA

Hypocalcemia is a serum deficit of calcium (below 4.4 mEq/L [2.2 mmol/L] in children, 4 mEq/L [2 mmol/L] in newborns, or 3.4 mEq/L [1.7 mmol/L] in premature infants) (Umpaichitra et al., 2001). Remember that serum calcium levels may not reflect body stores of this mineral, as most of the body's calcium is stored in bone.

ETIOLOGY AND PATHOPHYSIOLOGY

Hypocalcemia is caused by conditions that include decreased calcium intake or absorption, shift of calcium to a physiologically unavailable form, increased calcium excretion, and loss of calcium by an abnormal route.

Decreased calcium intake or absorption causes hypocalcemia in children with chronic generalized malnutrition, or with a diet low in vitamin D and calcium. Female adolescents trying to lose weight or maintain a low weight often decrease foods that contain calcium and may develop chronic hypocalcemia. They may have premature bone loss and inadequate bone. (See Chapter 34 for further discussion of calcium intake during adolescence ∞). This deficit cannot be made up later in life, increasing the risk of osteoporosis.

Even with a normal calcium intake, hypocalcemia occurs if the mineral is not absorbed. If a child does not have enough vitamin D, calcium is not absorbed efficiently from the duodenum. Sunlight speeds formation of vitamin D in the skin. Children institutionalized without access to sunlight (e.g., severely developmentally delayed children, those with very dark skin, or children kept well covered when outside) may become hypocalcemic because of the lack of vitamin D (see Chapter 34 ∞). Uremic syndrome is another cause of vitamin D deficiency. It interferes with the kidney's ability to activate vitamin D. High phosphate in-

take can cause hypocalcemia. Chronic diarrhea and steatorrhea (fatty stools) also reduce calcium absorption from the gastrointestinal tract.

Calcium becomes physiologically unavailable when calcium shifts into bone or free ionized calcium in plasma binds to proteins or small organic ions in the plasma. Too much calcium shifts into bones in various types of hypoparathyroidism, including DiGeorge syndrome (congenital absence of the parathyroid glands). Hypomagnesemia impairs parathyroid hormone function and may cause hypocalcemia. Some types of neonatal hypocalcemia are associated with delayed parathyroid hormone function or hypomagnesemia. Calcium shifts rapidly into bone when rickets is treated. A high plasma phosphate concentration causes plasma calcium to decrease. Ionized hypocalcemia, due to an increased binding of plasma ionized calcium, occurs very rapidly. The ionized hypocalcemia persists until the alkalosis resolves or the citrate is metabolized by the liver. Children who receive liver transplants are hypocalcemic for several days because of impaired citrate metabolism.

NURSING PRACTICE

Following are causes of ionized hypocalcemia:
- Alkalosis, which causes more calcium to bind to plasma proteins
- Citrate in transfused blood products, which binds calcium

Increased calcium excretion occurs in steatorrhea, when calcium secreted into the gastrointestinal fluid binds to the fecal fat in addition to the dietary calcium that is bound in the feces. A similar situation occurs in acute pancreatitis.

Loss of calcium by an abnormal route may contribute to hypocalcemia; calcium is lost through burn or wound drainage or sequestered in acute pancreatitis. Many medications can cause hypocalcemia (see Table 43–10).

CLINICAL MANIFESTATIONS

The signs and symptoms of hypocalcemia are manifestations of increased muscular excitability (tetany). In children they include twitching and cramping, tingling around the mouth or in the fingers, carpal spasm, and pedal spasm. Laryngospasm, seizures, and cardiac arrhythmias are more severe manifestations of hypocalcemia and may be fatal. Hypocalcemia may cause congestive heart failure, especially in newborns.

GROWTH AND DEVELOPMENT

Hypocalcemia in infants is more often seen as tremors, muscle twitches, and brief tonic-clonic seizures. Perform careful neurologic assessments on infants at risk of electrolyte imbalance.

DRUG GUIDE

CALCIUM GLUCONATE

Overview of Action

Calcium is a normal body electrolyte and may need to be infused in infants or young children with health problems leading to low calcium. It is also used during exchange transfusion in newborns since citrate in the blood transfusion can bind body calcium. In the form of CaCl, calcium may be used during resuscitation. Calcium regulates excitability of muscles and nerves, and therefore affects cardiac function (inotropic effect); is necessary for blood clotting; plays a role in storage and release of neurotransmitters, in renal function, and in maintaining cell membranes; and is an antidote to excessive magnesium infusion.

Routes, Dosage, Frequency

Hypocalcemia

    Neonate: IV 200-800 mg/kg/day divided into doses given q6hrs

    Infant: PO 400-800 mg/kg/day divided into doses given q6hrs

        IV: 200-500 mg/kg/day divided into doses given q6hrs

    Child: PO or IV 200-500 mg/kg/day divided into doses given q6hrs

    Adolescent: PO or IV 5-15 g/day divided into doses given q6hrs

Cardiac Arrest

    Infant/Child: IV 100 mg/kg/dose (or 1 ml/kg/dose) q 10 minutes as needed for resuscitation

Adolescent: IV 500-800 mg/dose (or 5-8 mL/dose) q 10 minutes as needed for resuscitation (maximum of 3g/dose)

Contraindications

Ventricular fibrillation, metastatic bone disease, renal calculi, hypercalcemia, pregnancy (category B); not to be injected into myocardium or given by SC or IM routes

Side Effects

Tingling, heat sensation, fainting, hypotension, bradycardia, cardiac arrhythmias, cardiac arrest, pain at IV infusion site, venous thrombosis; with PO administration, constipation, increased gastric acid secretion

Nursing Implications

- Verify dose carefully with the prescriber and another nurse.
- Monitor heart rate and rhythm—hypotension and bradycardia can occur.
- Use extreme caution if given in cardiac or renal disease.
- Maintain IV carefully to avoid extravasation; do **not** administer by peripheral infusion, scalp vein, IM, or SC.
- Precipitates when given in infusion with bicarbonate.

Data from Bindler, R. & Howry, L. (2005). Pediatric Drug Guide. Upper Saddle River, NJ: Prentice Hall Health, pp. 223–226.

Although these symptoms are diagnostic of acute calcium deficiency, a more common state in children and adolescents is chronic low intake of calcium. This may be manifested by spontaneous fractures in infants and in adolescents who exercise excessively.

CLINICAL THERAPY

Hypocalcemia is treated by oral or intravenous administration of calcium (see "Drug Guide: Calcium Gluconate"). The original cause of the imbalance is also treated. If the hypocalcemia is due to hypomagnesemia, the magnesium must be replenished before the calcium replacement can be successful. When the cause is chronic low dietary intake, counseling is needed about high-calcium foods, and perhaps the necessity for vitamin D intake or supplements.

NURSING MANAGEMENT

NURSING ASSESSMENT AND DIAGNOSIS

Carefully assess growth in the young female who is trying to diet. Whenever an adolescent female is very thin, be sure to ask about excessive sports and other activities, and about regularity of menstrual periods. If periods are irregular or not occurring, collect additional dietary information to help determine whether the girl is lacking in intake of calcium, calories, and other nutrients. These assessments are needed even if serum calcium values are normal. Look for signs of inadequate nutrition such as fat and muscle wasting, dry hair, and cold hands and feet. Assess for muscle cramps, stiffness, and clumsiness; grimacing caused by spasms of facial muscles and twitching of arm muscles; and laryngospasm. Increased neuromuscular excitability may be detected by testing for Trousseau's sign or Chvostek's sign. Many healthy newborns have a positive Chvostek's sign; however, this assessment should be reserved for children over several months of age. Monitor serum calcium levels and perform cardiac monitoring to observe for cardiac arrhythmias.

The effects of increased neuromuscular excitability in the child with hypocalcemia are the basis for several nursing diagnoses. These include the following:

- *Risk for Injury* related to potential for fractures
- *Risk for Injury* related to increased neuromuscular excitability
- *Risk for Ineffective Breathing Pattern* related to laryngospasm
- *Activity Intolerance* related to decreased cardiac output secondary to cardiac arrhythmias

MediaLink   Understanding School-Age Athletes and Fluid Needs

- *Disturbed Sensory Perception* related to electrolyte imbalance
- *Anxiety* related to change in health status
- *Imbalanced Nutrition: Less than Body Requirement* related to lack of basic nutritional knowledge of sources and recommended amounts of calcium intake

PLANNING AND IMPLEMENTATION

To correct calcium deficiency in the hospitalized child, give oral or intravenous calcium as prescribed. Monitor for complications of calcium supplementation. Monitor for the side effect of constipation to oral supplements, or for tissue sloughing, elevated serum calcium, or decreased serum phosphate with intravenous supplementation. Calcium is never given intramuscularly because it causes tissue necrosis. A 10% calcium gluconate intravenous solution should be readily available for emergency use in severe hypocalcemia.

Take measures to ensure safety for the child who is hospitalized with hypocalcemia. Seizure precautions may be necessary. Explain the cause of muscle cramps to parents and older children.

Counsel the family about dairy products and nondairy foods rich in calcium (see Table 43–11). For the adolescent female whose weight and menstrual patterns show irregularities, total calories and calcium intake should be increased. Teaching may also be needed about proper calcium intake and its importance both to athletic performance and to prevention of osteoporosis. Encourage three glasses of nonfat milk per day. Teach ways to use milk in the diet. For example, sprinkle nonfat dry milk on cereal and other foods. If the child is lactose-intolerant, emphasize nondairy sources of calcium and advise parents to purchase special milk treated with lactase. This milk is more costly, and inadequate family finances may prevent its use. If a child has a health condition leading to chronic diarrhea, encourage increased intake of calcium-rich foods. Calcium supplements in the form of calcium carbonate tablets may be used.

EVALUATION

Expected outcomes of nursing care include ingestion of recommended dietary allowances for calcium, absence of discomfort related to calcium imbalance, and freedom from injury.

MAGNESIUM IMBALANCES

Magnesium is necessary for enzyme function in cells, acetylcholine release, glycolysis, stimulation of ATPases, and bone formation. Since magnesium is a component of chlorophyll, dark green leafy vegetables are a good dietary source of magnesium. Nuts and grains are also good sources of magnesium. Magnesium is absorbed primarily from the terminal ileum. Magnesium is distributed among the extracellular fluid (small amounts), the cells (larger amounts), and the bones (large amounts). Magnesium excretion occurs in urine, feces, and sweat.

Magnesium imbalances are caused by alterations in magnesium intake, distribution, or excretion; by loss of magnesium through an abnormal route; or by a combination of these factors. The plasma magnesium concentration influences the release of acetylcholine at neuromuscular junctions. Thus, magnesium imbalances are characterized by alterations in neuromuscular irritability.

HYPERMAGNESEMIA

Hypermagnesemia occurs when the plasma magnesium concentration is too high (above 2.4 mg/dL [0.99 mmol/L]) (see Table 43–7). Keep in mind that the serum levels measured in the laboratory may not reflect body magnesium stores, because most magnesium in the body is located in the bones and inside the cells.

Hypermagnesemia is caused by conditions that involve increased magnesium intake and decreased magnesium excretion. Impaired renal function leading to decreased magnesium excretion is the most common cause of hypermagnesemia in children. In both oliguric renal failure and adrenal insufficiency, magnesium ions that cannot be excreted in the urine accumulate in the extracellular fluid.

Less frequently, increased magnesium intake may cause hypermagnesemia. Magnesium sulfate given to treat eclampsia in the mother before birth causes hypermagnesemia in the newborn. Abnormally high amounts may also be taken in magnesium-containing enemas, laxatives, antacids, and intravenous fluids (see Table 43–10). Aspiration of seawater, as in near-drowning, is an uncommon but potentially serious source of excessive magnesium intake. Children with Addison's disease can have abnormally high magnesium levels.

Clinical manifestations of hypermagnesemia include decreased muscle irritability, hypotension, bradycardia, drowsiness, lethargy, and weak or absent deep tendon reflexes. In severe hypermagnesemia, flaccid muscle paralysis, fatal respiratory depression, cardiac arrhythmias, and cardiac arrest occur.

Hypermagnesemia is managed primarily by increasing the urinary excretion of magnesium. This is usually accomplished by increasing fluid intake (except in oliguric renal failure) and by the administration of diuretics. Dialysis may sometimes be necessary.

NURSING MANAGEMENT

Monitor serum magnesium levels. Take the child's blood pressure (to watch for hypotension), heart rate and rhythm (to monitor for bradycardia and cardiac arrhythmias), respiratory rate and depth (to watch for respiratory depression), and deep tendon reflexes (to check muscle tone and paralysis or movement). Keep the side rails of the bed raised. Children with hypermagnesemia or oliguria should not be given magnesium-containing medications or sea salt.

Teach parents of children with chronic renal failure that these children should never be given milk of magnesia, antacids that contain magnesium, or other sources of magnesium. When hypermagnesemia is treated with diuretics, monitor potassium levels to watch for hypokalemia.

Expected outcomes of nursing care include maintenance of electrolyte balance, normal neuromuscular tone, safety, and regular heart rate and rhythm.

NURSING PRACTICE

Instruct parents of a child with chronic renal failure to read labels to detect magnesium in antacids and cathartics. Encourage them to check with their pharmacist and other healthcare providers before administering any over-the-counter medication to the child.

HYPOMAGNESEMIA

Hypomagnesemia refers to a plasma magnesium concentration that is too low (below 1.5 to 1.7 mg/dL [0.62 to 0.70 mmol/L]). Remember that the serum levels of magnesium may not reflect body stores, since most of the magnesium in the body is found in cells and bones.

Hypomagnesemia is caused by conditions that include decreased magnesium intake or absorption, shift of magnesium to a physiologically unavailable form, increased magnesium excretion, and loss of magnesium by an abnormal route.

Decreased magnesium intake or absorption can occur if a child who is not eating has prolonged intravenous therapy without magnesium. Chronic malnutrition is another cause of decreased magnesium intake. Magnesium absorption is decreased in chronic diarrhea, short bowel syndrome, malabsorption syndromes, and steatorrhea.

Magnesium may shift to a physiologically unavailable form after transfusion of many units of citrated blood products; magnesium bound to the citrate is not physiologically active. Such transfusions cause prolonged hypomagnesemia in liver transplant patients, who have impaired citrate metabolism. Magnesium shifts rapidly into bones that have been deprived of adequate stores.

Increased magnesium excretion in the urine occurs with diuretic therapy, the diuretic phase of acute renal failure, diabetic ketoacidosis, and hyperaldosteronism. Chronic alcoholism, occasionally seen in adolescents, increases urinary magnesium excretion. Magnesium contained in gastrointestinal secretions is bound to fat and excreted in the stool.

Loss of magnesium by an abnormal route occurs with prolonged nasogastric suction and through sequestration of magnesium in acute pancreatitis. Several medications may cause hypomagnesemia (see Table 43–10).

Hypomagnesemia is characterized by increased neuromuscular excitability (tetany). The clinical manifestations are hyperactive reflexes, skeletal muscle cramps, twitching, tremors, and cardiac arrhythmias. Seizures can occur with severe hypomagnesemia.

Hypomagnesemia is managed by administering magnesium and treating the underlying cause of the imbalance.

NURSING MANAGEMENT

In addition to monitoring serum magnesium levels, nursing assessment of hypomagnesemia includes monitoring deep tendon reflexes, testing for Trousseau's and Chvostek's signs, monitoring cardiac function, and observing for muscle twitching. Children able to talk report muscle cramping. Because magnesium levels are not routinely measured in many settings, request the test for any child who has risk factors and early manifestations of hypomagnesemia. When intramuscular or intravenous magnesium is ordered, administer carefully as directed and monitor vital signs. Electrocardiogram and renal studies may precede drug administration. Have resuscitative drugs and equipment readily available during drug administration.

Teach parents of a child with hypomagnesemia or continuing risk factors such as chronic diarrhea to include magnesium-rich foods in the diet (see Table 43–11). Before administering magnesium supplements, verify that the child's urine output is adequate. Monitor deep tendon reflexes if intravenous magnesium is given, and observe for complications of magnesium supplementation. Oral magnesium may lead to diarrhea, and intravenous magnesium can cause flushing, elevated serum magnesium, cardiac arrhythmias, or decreased deep tendon reflexes.

Expected outcomes of nursing care for the child with an imbalance in magnesium are restoration and maintenance of electrolyte balance.

CLINICAL ASSESSMENT OF FLUID AND ELECTROLYTE IMBALANCE

How can a nurse assess children appropriately for fluid and electrolyte imbalance without thinking through the clinical

TABLE 43–12 ✤ Risk Factor Assessment for Fluid Imbalances

Isotonic Fluid (Extracellular Fluid Volume Imbalances)
- Source of increased intake?
- Aldosterone secretion increased or decreased?
- Source of loss from the body?

Water
- Source of increased intake?
- Antidiuretic hormone secretion increased or decreased?
- Source of unusual loss from the body?

manifestations of every possible disorder one after the other? First, perform a rapid risk factor assessment on each child to see which factors are present (Tables 43–12 and 43–13).

A risk factor assessment may be performed mentally while providing care. Look for factors that alter the intake, retention, and loss of isotonic fluid and water. Use this information to evaluate which fluid imbalance is most likely to occur in a particular child. Next, look for factors that alter electrolyte intake and absorption, distribution between plasma and other electrolyte pools, excretion, and abnormal routes of electrolyte loss. Use this information to evaluate which electrolyte imbalances are most likely to occur in the child. A review of pathophysiology is important to understand the role of the other electrolytes and substances, such as phosphorus, in the body.

After evaluating possible imbalances for the child, perform a clinical assessment. Assess for fluid imbalances by assessing weight changes, vascular volume, interstitial vol-

TABLE 43–13 ✤ Risk Factor Assessment for Electrolyte Imbalances

Electrolyte Intake and Absorption
- Increased?
- Decreased?

Electrolyte Shifts
- From electrolyte pool to plasma?
- From plasma to electrolyte pool?

Electrolyte Excretion
- Increased?
- Decreased?

Electrolyte Loss by Abnormal Route
- Vomiting?
- Diarrhea?
- Nasogastric suction?
- Wound?
- Burn?
- Excessive sweating?

ume, and cerebral function (Table 43–14). Assess for electrolyte imbalances by assessing serum electrolyte levels, skeletal muscle strength, neuromuscular excitability, gastrointestinal tract function, and cardiac rhythm (Table 43–15). Next, check for other manifestations specific to a particular high-risk imbalance (e.g., polyuria in hypokalemia). Evaluate any serum laboratory values available. This method of risk factor assessment followed by clinical assessment provides a rapid yet thorough approach to assessment for fluid and electrolyte imbalances.

✤ PHYSIOLOGY OF ACID-BASE BALANCE

Normal acid-base balance is necessary for proper function of the cells and the body. The number of hydrogen ions (H^+) present in a fluid determines how acidic it is. Increasing the hydrogen ion concentration makes a solution more acidic. Because the hydrogen ion concentration in body fluids is very small, acidity is expressed as **pH** (the negative logarithm of the hydrogen ion concentration) rather than as the hydrogen ion concentration itself. The range of possible pH values is 1 to 14. A pH of 7 is neutral. The lower the pH, the more acidic the solution. A pH above 7 is basic. The higher the pH, the more basic the solution. Body fluids are normally slightly basic (see Table 43–7).

The pH of body fluids is regulated carefully to provide a suitable environment for cell function. The pH of the blood influences the pH inside the cells. **Acidemia** refers to a decreased blood pH below normal levels, while **alkalemia** is an increased blood pH. Normal arterial blood pH ranges are 7.36 to 7.42 for infants, 7.37 to 7.43 for children, and 7.35 to 7.41 for adolescents. For the enzymes outside the cells to function optimally, the pH must be in the normal range. If the pH inside the cells becomes too high or too low, then the speed of chemical reactions becomes inappropriate for proper cell function. Cell protein function relies on the correct level of hydrogen ions. Thus, acid-base imbalances result in clinical signs and symptoms, and, in severe cases, they may cause death.

In the course of their normal function, all cells in the body produce acids. Cells produce two kinds of acids: carbonic acid (H_2CO_3) and metabolic (noncarbonic) acids. Carbonic acid is formed from carbon dioxide and water, while common metabolic acids are pyruvic, sulfuric, lactic, and hydrochloric acids. These acids are released into the extracellular fluid and must be neutralized or excreted from the body to prevent dangerous accumulation. They can be neutralized to some degree by the buffers in body fluids. The lungs excrete carbonic acid in the form of carbon dioxide and water. Metabolic acids are excreted by the kidneys.

~~~
TABLE 43–14  ✣  **Summary of Clinical Assessment of Fluid Imbalances**
~~~

Assessment Category	Specific Assessments	Changes with Fluid Imbalances
Rapid changes in weight	Daily weights	Weight gain—extracellular volume excess
		Weight loss—extracellular volume deficit; clinical dehydration
Vascular volume	Small vein filling time	Increased—extracellular volume deficit; clinical dehydration
	Capillary refill time	Increased—extracellular volume deficit; clinical dehydration
	Character of pulse	Bounding—extracellular volume excess
		Thready—extracellular volume deficit; clinical dehydration
	Postural blood pressure measurements	Postural drop—extracellular volume deficit; clinical dehydration
	Lung sounds in dependent portions	Crackles—extracellular volume excess
	Central venous pressure	Increased—extracellular volume excess
		Decreased—extracellular volume deficit; clinical dehydration
	Tenseness of fontanelle (infants)	Bulging—extracellular volume excess
		Sunken—extracellular volume deficit; clinical dehydration
	Neck vein filling (older children)	Full with upright—extracellular volume excess
		Flat when supine—extracellular volume deficit; clinical dehydration
Interstitial volume	Skin turgor	Skin tents—extracellular volume deficit; clinical dehydration
	Presence or absence of edema	Edema—extracellular volume excess
Cerebral function	Level of consciousness	Decreased—clinical dehydration

BUFFERS

The maintenance of hydrogen ions within normal range relies heavily on buffers. A **buffer** is a compound that binds hydrogen ions when their concentration rises and releases them when the concentration falls (see "Pathophysiology Illustrated: Buffer Responses to Acid and Base"). Several kinds of buffers are present in the body, such as bicarbonate, protein, hemoglobin, and phosphate. Various body fluids have buffers to meet their special needs. The bicarbonate buffer system neutralizes metabolic acids (see "Pathophysiology Illustrated: The Bicarbonate Buffer System"); however, it cannot neutralize carbonic acid.

~~~
TABLE 43–15  ✣  **Summary of Clinical Assessment of Electrolyte Imbalances**
~~~

Assessment Category	Specific Assessments	Changes with Electrolyte Imbalances
Skeletal muscle function	Muscle strength	Weakness, flaccid paralysis—hyperkalemia; hypokalemia
Neuromuscular excitability	Deep tendon reflexes	Depressed—hypercalcemia; hypermagnesemia
		Hyperactive—hypocalcemia; hypomagnesemia
	Chvostek's sign (not infants)	Positive—hypocalcemia; hypomagnesemia
	Trousseau's sign	Positive—hypocalcemia; hypomagnesemia
	Paresthesias	Digital or perioral—hypocalcemia
	Muscle cramping or twitching	Present—hypocalcemia; hypomagnesemia
Gastrointestinal tract function	Bowel sounds	Decreased or absent—hypokalemia
	Elimination pattern	Constipation—hypokalemia; hypercalcemia
		Diarrhea—hyperkalemia
Cardiac rhythm	Arrhythmia	Irregular—hyperkalemia; hypokalemia; hypercalcemia; hypocalcemia; hypermagnesemia; hypomagnesemia
	Electrocardiogram	Abnormal—hyperkalemia; hypokalemia; hypercalcemia; hypocalcemia; hypermagnesemia; hypomagnesemia
Cerebral function	Level of consciousness	Decreased—hyponatremia; hypernatremia

PATHOPHYSIOLOGY ILLUSTRATED

Buffer Responses to Acid and Base

A, How buffers respond to an excess of base. If the blood has too much base, the acid portion of a buffer pair (e.g., H_2CO_3 of the bicarbonate buffer system) releases hydrogen ions (H^+) to help return the pH to normal. **B,** How buffers respond to an excess of acid. If the blood has too much acid, the base portion of a buffer pair (e.g., HCO_3^- of the bicarbonate buffer system) takes up hydrogen ions (H^+) to help return the pH to normal.

All buffer systems have limits. For example, if there are too many metabolic acids, the bicarbonate buffers become depleted. The acids then accumulate in the body until they are excreted by the kidneys. Clinically, this is seen as a decreased serum bicarbonate concentration and decreased blood pH.

ROLE OF THE LUNGS

The lungs are responsible for excreting excess carbonic acid from the body. A child breathes out carbon dioxide and water, the components of carbonic acid, with each breath. With faster and deeper breaths, more carbonic acid is excreted. Since carbonic acid is converted in the body to carbon dioxide and water by the enzyme carbonic anhydrase, an indirect laboratory measurement of carbonic acid is PCO_2 (see Table 43–7).

Although a child can voluntarily increase or decrease the rate and depth of respirations, they are usually involuntarily controlled. Chemoreceptors in the hypothalamus

PATHOPHYSIOLOGY ILLUSTRATED

The Bicarbonate Buffer System

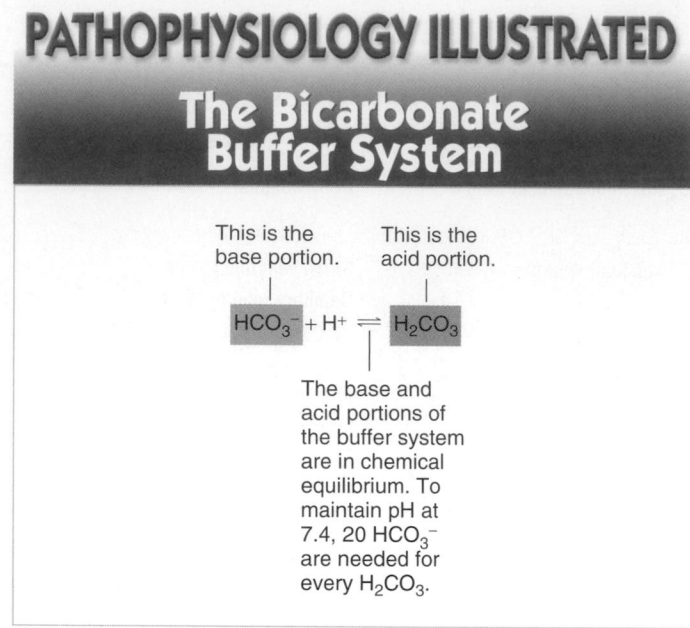

of the brain and in the aorta and carotid arteries monitor the PCO_2 and pH of the blood. These arteries also monitor the PO_2 of the blood. The input from the chemoreceptors is combined with other neural input to change breathing according to needs. Rate and depth increase or decrease according to the amount of carbonic acid that needs to be excreted.

If a child has a condition that decreases the excretion of carbonic acid or causes breathing to be too slow or shallow (such as overmedication following surgery), carbonic acid accumulates in the blood. Clinically, this is seen as an increased blood PCO_2. The reverse will also be true.

ROLE OF THE KIDNEYS

The kidneys excrete metabolic acids from the body in two ways. They reabsorb filtered bicarbonate and form bicarbonate when needed to restore balance. Bicarbonate is formed when acids and ammonium combine with extra ions. The blood bicarbonate concentration is an indicator of the amount of metabolic acids present, since bicarbonate is used in buffering the acids (see Table 43–7). When the concentration is normal, metabolic acids are present in usual amounts (see "Pathophysiology Illustrated: The Kidneys and Metabolic Acids").

In a healthy child, the result of these renal processes is excretion of metabolic acids and maintenance of blood bicarbonate concentration within normal limits. However, a child whose kidneys are not producing enough urine may be unable to excrete metabolic acids effectively. Accumulation of these acids uses up many of the available bicarbonate buffers, resulting in a decreased serum bicarbonate concentration.

PATHOPHYSIOLOGY ILLUSTRATED

The Kidneys and Metabolic Acids

A

B

A, Recycling of bicarbonate by the kidneys. Bicarbonate ions that are in the blood are filtered into the renal tubules at the glomerulus. In the proximal tubules, bicarbonate ions are reabsorbed into the blood at the same time that hydrogen ions are transported from the blood into the renal tubular fluid. *B,* Secretion and buffering of hydrogen ions in the kidneys. If the urine is too acidic, the cells that line the urinary tract could be damaged. To prevent this problem, hydrogen ions secreted into the distal tubules are neutralized by phosphate buffers or bound to ammonia and excreted in the form of ammonium ions.

ROLE OF THE LIVER

The liver also plays a role in maintaining acid-base balance by metabolizing protein, which produces hydrogen ions. It also synthesizes proteins needed to maintain osmotic pressures in the fluid compartments.

ACID-BASE IMBALANCES

There are four acid-base imbalances. Two are the result of processes that cause too much acid in the body and are referred to as **acidosis**. The other two are the result of processes that cause too little acid in the body and are called **alkalosis** (Noble, 1999). An acid-base disorder caused by too much or too little carbonic acid is called a respiratory acid-base imbalance. A disorder caused by too much or too little metabolic acid is called a metabolic acid-base imbalance.

NURSING PRACTICE

Acidosis: Relatively too much acid in the body
   Respiratory acidosis: Relatively too much carbonic acid
   Metabolic acidosis: Relatively too much metabolic acid

Alkalosis: Relatively too little acid in the body
   Respiratory alkalosis: Relatively too little carbonic acid
   Metabolic alkalosis: Relatively too little metabolic acid

Arterial blood gas measurements (ABGs) provide a laboratory evaluation of a child's current acid-base status. Table 43–16 provides a method that can help interpret the pH, P_{CO_2}, and bicarbonate concentrations, the most important acid-base measures. End-tidal CO_2 can provide a continuous noninvasive measurement. (Remember that P_{CO_2} reflects carbonic acid status, and bicarbonate concentration reflects the metabolic acid status.)

RESPIRATORY ACIDOSIS

Respiratory acidosis is caused by the accumulation of carbon dioxide in the blood. Since carbon dioxide and water can be combined into carbonic acid, respiratory acidosis is sometimes called carbonic acid excess. The condition can be acute or chronic. It is controlled by the lungs.

ETIOLOGY AND PATHOPHYSIOLOGY

Any factor that interferes with the ability of the lungs to excrete carbon dioxide can cause respiratory acidosis. These factors may interfere with the gaseous exchange within the lungs, may impair the neuromuscular pump that moves air in and out of the lungs, or may depress the respiratory rate (Table 43–17; Figure 43–10 ●).

TABLE 43–16 ❖ How to Interpret Arterial Blood Gas Measurements

Ask the following questions to analyze blood gas results.

1. **What is the pH?** If the pH is normal, the child has no imbalance or has compensated for an imbalance. If the pH is below normal, the child has acidosis. If the pH is above normal, the child has alkalosis.

2. **What is the Pco_2?** If the Pco_2 is normal, the child does not have an acid-base imbalance. If the Pco_2 is above normal, the child has respiratory acidosis. This may be the primary disorder or may be a compensatory response to metabolic alkalosis. Looking at the bicarbonate concentration helps you decide. If the Pco_2 is below normal, the child has respiratory alkalosis. Again, this can be the primary disorder or may be a compensatory response to metabolic acidosis.

3. **What is the bicarbonate concentration?** If the bicarbonate concentration is within normal range, the child does not have a metabolic acid-base imbalance. If the bicarbonate is above normal, the child has metabolic alkalosis. This can be a primary disorder or can be compensatory in respiratory acidosis. When bicarbonate is below normal, the child has metabolic acidosis, either as a direct disorder or as a compensatory response to respiratory alkalosis.

4. **What do the results together tell you?** If the pH is abnormal and either the Pco_2 or bicarbonate concentration is normal, there is an uncompensated acid-base disorder. If all three values are abnormal, the child has a partially compensated disorder and the pH will provide the definitive answer. If Pco_2, pH, and bicarbonate are all decreased, then partially compensated metabolic acidosis is most likely. If pH is normal and Pco_2 and bicarbonate are abnormal, there is a fully compensated acid-base disorder.

5. **What are the child's history and clinical signs?** Does your interpretation fit with what you know about the child's medical condition and with assessments you are making? This last step helps you to integrate laboratory data with the clinical picture to strengthen your nursing care of the child with an acid-base imbalance.

● FIGURE 43–10

This child may develop respiratory acidosis or respiratory alkalosis. If the tidal volume is set too low during mechanical ventilation, carbon dioxide (carbonic acid) will accumulate in the body (respiratory acidosis) because it is not being excreted by the lungs. If the tidal volume is set too high, carbon dioxide will be depleted in the body (respiratory alkalosis) because it is being excreted in great quantities.

As the Pco_2 begins to increase, the pH of the blood begins to decrease. Compensatory mechanisms begin to act in the form of nonbicarbonate buffers, additional hydrogen ion excretion by the kidneys, and formation and decreased bicarbonate excretion by the kidneys. These compensatory mechanisms take several days to become active so the child manifests a changing clinical situation, depending on the underlying cause and the amount of compensation occurring (Table 43–18).

TABLE 43–17 ❖ Causes of Respiratory Acidosis

Factors Affecting the Lungs	Factors Affecting the Neuromuscular Pump	Factors Affecting Central Control of Respiration
Aspiration	Flail chest	Sedative overdose
Spasm of the airways	Pneumothorax or hemothorax	General anesthesia
Laryngeal edema	Mechanical underventilation	Head injury
Epiglottitis	Hypokalemic muscle weakness	Brain tumor
Croup	High cervical spinal cord injury	Central sleep apnea
Pulmonary edema	Botulism	
Atelectasis	Tetanus	
Severe pneumonia	Kyphoscoliosis	
Cystic fibrosis	Poliomyelitis	
Bronchopulmonary dysplasia	Muscular dystrophy	
Pulmonary embolism	Congenital diaphragmatic hernia	
	Guillain-Barré syndrome	

TABLE 43–18 ❖ Laboratory Values in Uncompensated and Compensated Respiratory Acidosis

	P_{CO_2}	pH	HCO_3
Uncompensated	Increased	Decreased	Normal
Partially compensated	Increased	Decreasing but moving toward normal	Increasing
Fully compensated	Increased	Normal	Increased

CLINICAL MANIFESTATIONS

Acidosis in the brain cells causes central nervous system depression, manifested by confusion, lethargy, headache, increased intracranial pressure, and even coma. Acute respiratory acidosis can lead to tachycardia and cardiac arrhythmias. The child's arterial blood gases always show an increased P_{CO_2}, the laboratory sign of increased carbonic acid. Serum pH can be decreased or normal.

CLINICAL THERAPY

Treatment of respiratory acidosis requires correction of the underlying cause. For example, treatment may include bronchodilators for bronchospasm, mechanical ventilation for neuromuscular defects, decreasing sedative use, or surgery for kyphoscoliosis.

NURSING MANAGEMENT

NURSING ASSESSMENT AND DIAGNOSIS

Nursing assessment plays a pivotal role in decisions about interventions for respiratory acidosis. This is especially true in chronic conditions such as cystic fibrosis and kyphoscoliosis. Assess respiratory rate, rhythm, and depth carefully. Take the apical pulse and be alert for tachycardia or arrhythmia. A cardiac monitor may be used. Obtain serial arterial blood gas measurements in acute conditions to evaluate changing status. Assess the level of consciousness and energy. Observe for chronic fatigue, headache, or decreased level of consciousness.

Several nursing diagnoses may apply to the child with respiratory acidosis. The most important addresses the child's *Risk for Injury*. Other nursing diagnoses depend on the specific clinical manifestation and the particular cause of the acidosis. Examples include the following:

- *Risk for Injury* related to decreased level of consciousness
- *Activity Intolerance* related to decreased cardiac output secondary to cardiac dysrhythmias
- *Ineffective Breathing Pattern (Hypoventilation)* related to neuromuscular impairment
- *Pain (Headache)* related to cerebral vasodilation
- *Ineffective Family Management of Therapeutic Regimen* related to complexity of bronchodilator therapy

PLANNING AND INTERVENTION

Nursing Care in the Community

Teach children at risk for respiratory acidosis and their parents preventive measures to use at home. For the child with a chronic condition such as cystic fibrosis, muscular dystrophy, or kyphoscoliosis, demonstrate deep breathing and encourage its use several times each day. Teach the family signs of infection—including fever, increased respiratory secretions, and discomfort with breathing—so these problems can be treated promptly, preventing further respiratory involvement. Position the child to facilitate chest expansion. Teach parents about proper administration of any necessary medications. For example, the child with cystic fibrosis may receive antibiotics to prevent respiratory infections. Teach parents and older children about home respirator use (Figure 43–11).

GROWTH AND DEVELOPMENT

It is usually difficult to get a young child to do deep breathing or to use the "blow bottle" that is often given to older children and adults. To make deep breathing fun, use a pinwheel and have the child turn it during play. Alternatively, give a child a straw and have him or her blow bubbles in a glass of water, or have the child use the straw to blow scraps of paper across the bedside table.

Hospital-Based Nursing Care

For the hospitalized child, the focus is on ensuring safety. Keep bed side rails raised, and turn and position the child frequently. Evaluate mental status and document and report any changes in alertness. When laboratory values of blood pH and P_{CO_2} are available, evaluate them promptly

⬢ **FIGURE 43–11**

This child, who has muscular dystrophy, uses a "turtle" respirator at home to assist with breathing. His parents required instructions from the nurse on use of the respirator. The family has a generator to provide electricity for the respirator during power outages.

and report any changes or abnormalities. Administer medications as ordered. Carefully monitor the doses of sedatives to avoid further respiratory depression. Provide suctioning and encourage deep breathing.

EVALUATION

Expected outcomes of nursing care for the child with respiratory acidosis include maintenance of safety, adequate rate and rhythm of respirations, and management of causative disorders. ■

RESPIRATORY ALKALOSIS

Respiratory alkalosis occurs when the blood contains too little carbon dioxide. It is sometimes called carbonic acid deficit.

Excess carbon dioxide loss is caused by hyperventilation, in which more air than normal is moved into and out of the lungs. Some common causes of hyperventilation are hypoxemia, anxiety, pain, fever, salicylate poisoning, meningitis, septicemia, and mechanical overventilation (Foster, Vaziri, & Sassoon, 2001).

In many cases, respiratory alkalosis lasts for several hours only. Renal compensation does not occur, as these compensatory mechanisms take several days to begin action. An example is the hyperventilation that occurs with acute anxiety. If the condition persists, however, the kidneys will begin to retain more acid and excrete more bicarbonate. Hydrogen ions will be released from body buffers to decrease plasma bicarbonate. While the imbalance continues, cellular function is thus protected by returning pH to normal levels (Table 43–19).

Arterial blood gas measurements show a decreased P_{CO_2} in respiratory alkalosis. Blood pH is generally elevated. The lack of carbon dioxide causes neuromuscular irritability and paresthesias in the extremities and around the mouth. Muscle cramping and carpal or pedal spasms can occur. The child may be dizzy or confused.

Medical management focuses on correcting the condition that caused the hyperventilation so that the body's compensatory mechanisms can return carbon dioxide levels to normal.

NURSING MANAGEMENT

Assess the child's level of consciousness and ask if the child feels light-headed or has tingling sensations or numbness in the fingers or toes, or around the mouth. Assess the rate and depth of respirations. Monitor the hospitalized child's P_{O_2} with serial arterial blood gas measurements to evaluate changes in status. Make a careful assessment about the cause of hyperventilation. Did an occurrence cause anxiety for the child? Is the child in pain? (See Chapter 42. ∞) Has the child received salicylates in any form? Is the child mechanically ventilated? Is there a central nervous system infection such as meningitis?

TABLE 43–19 ✤ Laboratory Values in Uncompensated and Compensated Respiratory Alkalosis

	Pco₂	pH	HCO₃
Uncompensated	Decreased	Increased	Normal
Partially compensated	Decreased	Increasing but moving toward normal	Decreasing
Fully compensated	Decreased	Normal	Decreased

PLANNING AND IMPLEMENTATION

Nursing care for the child with respiratory alkalosis centers on preventing injury, teaching stress management techniques, maintaining pain control, promoting respiratory function, ensuring safety, maintaining fluid status, and providing health supervision and home care.

Teach Stress Management Techniques

When anxiety is the cause of respiratory alkalosis, instruct the child to breathe slowly; demonstrate the rhythm. Use a calm voice, stuffed toys, and supportive reassurance. Teach stress-control techniques such as relaxation and imagery for situations that cause anxiety.

Maintain Pain Control

Use medications, imagery, distraction, positioning, massage, and other techniques to decrease pain and maintain pain management. See Chapter 42 for a description of these and other measures to assist with pain control. ∞

Promote Respiratory Function

Have the child cough, or suction as needed. Be certain that mechanical ventilation systems are working properly.

Ensure Safety

Provide a safe environment for the child who has a decreased level of consciousness. Be sure the child is supervised when sitting or standing up. Keep bed rails up.

Regulate Fluid Status

Renal compensation to manage ongoing respiratory alkalosis requires adequate urinary output. Regulate fluid intake to ensure urine output unless fluids are restricted due to medical condition.

Nursing Care in the Community

Teach parents to keep aspirin and other salicylate products out of reach of children, preferably in a locked medicine box. Provide stickers with the number of the Poison Control Center.

EVALUATION

Expected outcomes of nursing care for the child with respiratory alkalosis include normal respiratory rate and rhythm, maintenance of safety, and regulation of fluid status.

METABOLIC ACIDOSIS

Metabolic acidosis is a condition in which there is an excess of any acid other than carbonic acid. For this reason, it is sometimes called noncarbonic acid excess.

ETIOLOGY AND PATHOPHYSIOLOGY

Metabolic acidosis is caused by an imbalance in production and excretion of acid or by excess loss of bicarbonate. Excess accumulation occurs by one of two mechanisms. First, a child can eat or drink acids or substances that are converted to acid in the body. Examples include aspirin, boric acid, and antifreeze. Second, cells can make abnormally high amounts of acid that cannot be excreted. This is the case in ketoacidosis of untreated diabetes mellitus, untreated growth hormone deficiency (Glaser, Shirali, Styne et al., 1998), bladder construction that uses part of the bowel (Mundy, 1999), or the starvation that can occur in anorexia or bulimia. A disorder of excretion occurs in conditions such as oliguric renal failure (Figure 43–12 ●).

The body can lose bicarbonate through the urine or through excessive loss of intestinal fluid. Diarrhea, fistulas, and ileal drainage are all possible sources. Carbonic anhydrase inhibitors can cause loss of excess bicarbonate in the urine.

● **FIGURE 43–12**

With any postoperative or immobilized child, it is important to monitor urine output to detect oliguria. If the kidneys do not produce sufficient urine, the metabolic acids accumulate in the body and cause metabolic acidosis. Inadequate fluid intake in the postoperative or immobilized child can lead to oliguria and, potentially, metabolic acidosis.

TABLE 43–20 ✤ Laboratory Values in Uncompensated and Compensated Metabolic Acidosis

	HCO₃	pH	Pco₂
Uncompensated	Decreased	Decreased	Normal
Partially compensated	Decreased	Decreasing but moving	Decreasing

Below-normal pH of the blood stimulates the chemoreceptors in the brain and arteries and respiratory compensation begins. The child's rate and depth of breathing increase and carbonic acid is removed from the body. The blood pH shifts to a more normal range even though the cause is not corrected. The underlying condition and the degree of compensation alter the clinical laboratory values observed (Table 43–20).

CLINICAL MANIFESTATIONS

Laboratory values show decreased blood pH and decreased HCO₃ and Pco₂. An attempt at respiratory compensation causes one of the most important signs of metabolic acidosis, increased rate and depth of respirations (hyperventilation) or **Kussmaul respirations**. Severe acidosis can cause decreased peripheral vascular resistance and resultant cardiac arrhythmias, hypotension, pulmonary edema, and tissue hypoxia. Confusion or drowsiness may result, as well as headache or abdominal pain.

CLINICAL THERAPY

Treatment of metabolic acidosis depends on identification and treatment of the underlying cause. In severe metabolic acidosis, intravenous sodium bicarbonate may be used to increase the pH and to prevent cardiac arrhythmias. This treatment is difficult to manage, because renal excretion can cause excess retention of bicarbonate; therefore, intravenous sodium bicarbonate is used only in severe situations, such as prolonged cardiac arrest.

NURSING MANAGEMENT

NURSING ASSESSMENT AND DIAGNOSIS

Assess the rate and depth of respirations. Evaluate the child's level of consciousness frequently. Be alert for signs or complaints of headache and abdominal pain. Serial arterial blood gas measurements will usually be obtained to evaluate changes in status.

Several nursing diagnoses can apply to the child with metabolic acidosis, including the following:

- *Risk for Injury* related to confusion/drowsiness or decreased responsiveness
- *Risk for Decreased Cardiac Output* related to cardiac arrhythmias
- *Altered Tissue Perfusion: Cerebral* related to tissue hypoxia
- *Ineffective Family Management of Therapeutic Regimen* related to complexity of management of diabetes mellitus

PLANNING AND IMPLEMENTATION

Ensure safety, taking into account the child's level of consciousness and alertness. Turn the child and change his or her position to prevent pressure on the skin. Limit the child's activities to decrease cardiac workload.

Position the child to facilitate chest expansion. Provide oral care during rapid respirations since the mouth may become dry.

Monitor intravenous solutions and laboratory values indicating acid-base balance. Report changes promptly.

Once the child is stabilized, provide teaching to compensate for knowledge deficits. Teach parents of young children to keep medications and acids locked up and out of reach to prevent poisoning (Figure 43–13 ●). This in-

● FIGURE 43–13

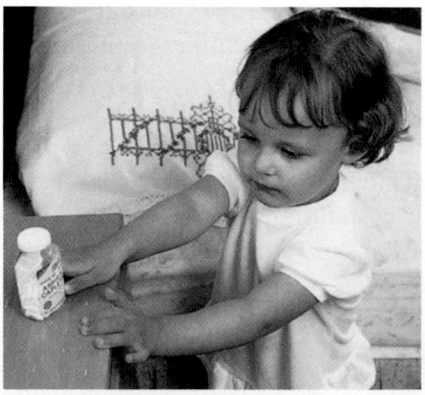

Teaching parents to use safety latches on cabinets to keep aspirin away from small children can help prevent one cause of metabolic acidosis.

cludes medicines with aspirin as well as substances commonly kept in the garage for car maintenance. Teach about home management of diabetes and about early identification and treatment to avoid diabetic ketoacidosis. Expected outcomes of nursing care relate to prevention of acidosis and restoration of normal body balance during disease processes.

METABOLIC ALKALOSIS

Metabolic alkalosis occurs when there are too few metabolic acids. It is sometimes called noncarbonic acid deficit.

A gain in bicarbonate or a loss of metabolic acid can cause metabolic alkalosis. Bicarbonate is gained through excessive intake of bicarbonate antacids or baking soda or through metabolism of bicarbonate precursors such as the citrate contained in blood transfusions. Increased renal absorption of bicarbonate can occur in profound hypokalemia, primary hyperaldosteronism, or extreme deficit in extracellular fluid volume. Acid can be lost through severe vomiting, such as that seen in infants with pyloric stenosis, and through continued removal of gastric contents through suction.

When the chemoreceptors in the brain and arteries detect the rising pH of metabolic alkalosis and respirations decrease, the body retains carbonic acid. This carbonic acid can neutralize the bicarbonate and return pH toward normal.

Blood pH, bicarbonate, and Pco_2 are usually elevated in metabolic alkalosis (Table 43–21). Hypokalemia often occurs simultaneously (refer to pages 1255–1256 to review signs of hypokalemia). Respiratory rate and depth usually decrease. Increased neuromuscular irritability, cramping, paresthesia, tetany, seizures, and excitation can occur. Finally, this state can progress to weakness, confusion, lethargy, and coma.

Clinical therapy is directed at treating the underlying cause of the condition. Increasing the extracellular fluid volume with intravenous normal saline facilitates renal excretion of bicarbonate.

NURSING MANAGEMENT

Assess the child's level of consciousness frequently. Alertness may decrease after an initial period of excitement, so regular assessments are needed. Monitor neuromuscular irritability. Observe for nausea and vomiting. Assess the rate and depth of respirations carefully. Obtain serial arterial blood gas measurements as ordered.

Facilitate ease of respirations. Ensure safety by keeping bed rails elevated and by turning the child frequently. Position the child on the side to avoid aspiration of vomitus.

If antacids were the cause of the alkalosis, teach the child and parents about correct use of these medications.

MIXED ACID-BASE IMBALANCES

It is possible for two acid-base imbalances to occur at the same time. For example, a child with cystic fibrosis can develop respiratory acidosis from lung problems and concurrent metabolic alkalosis from vomiting during an illness. Treatment with diuretics may cause concurrent metabolic alkalosis resulting from extracellular volume depletion and hypokalemia in a child with congestive heart failure and chronic respiratory acidosis. In these cases, all underlying causes must be identified and treated. Care of children with mixed acid-base imbalances is often complicated, requiring hospitalization and careful management. Upon discharge the nurse can teach parents about signs of imbalance that need to be reported and treated to prevent further complications. Evaluation of care is based on outcomes of adequate respiratory ventilation and metabolic balance.

TABLE 43–21 ✤ **Laboratory Values in Uncompensated and Compensated Metabolic Alkalosis**

	HCO$_3$	pH	Pco$_2$
Acute condition; uncompensated	Increased	Increased	Normal
Partially compensated	Increased	Increased but moving toward normal	Increasing
Fully compensated	The need for oxygen drives respirations and limits full compensation for metabolic alkalosis.		

Critical Concept Review

LEARNING OBJECTIVES

CONCEPTS

Describe normal fluid and electrolyte status for children at various ages.

1. Newborn:
   - Basal metabolic rate is double that of children.
   - Approximately four to five times greater water intake needs per kilogram of body weight.
   - Only 10% of ability to excrete sodium.
2. Infants:
   - Larger extracellular fluid volume than older children and adults.
   - High daily fluid requirement with little fluid volume reserve.
3. Child/adolescent:
   - Total body water is 50% of total body weight.
   - Kidneys unable to conserve water and electrolytes until after age 2 years.
   - Children under 2 years have a greater proportion of skin surface.

Identify regulatory mechanisms for fluid and electrolyte balance.

1. Kidneys conserve water and electrolytes while excreting waste products and drug metabolites:
   - Children under 2 years of age have immature glomeruli, tubules, and nephrons.

Recognize threats to fluid and electrolyte balance in children.

1. Higher respiratory and metabolic rates increase water demands and water loss:
   - Allow dehydration to occur more quickly in children.
2. Immature kidneys lead to greater water and electrolyte loss.
3. Higher body surface area (BSA) increases insensible water loss through the skin.
4. Young child unable to communicate thirst.
5. Young child may not cooperate with oral rehydration.

Describe acid-base balance and recognize disruptions common in children.

Acid-base balance:
1. Lungs:
   - Responsible for excreting excess carbonic acid from body.
2. Kidneys:
   - Reabsorb filtered bicarbonate.
   - Form bicarbonate if needed to restore balance.
3. Liver:
   - Metabolizes protein, which produces hydrogen ions.
   - Synthesizes proteins needed to maintain osmotic pressure in the fluid compartments.

Disruptions in acid-base balance:
1. Respiratory acidosis:
   - Associated with chronic diseases that decrease respiratory effort.
2. Respiratory alkalosis:
   - Often seen with severe infections, anxiety, pain, and lowered levels of oxygen.
3. Metabolic acidosis:
   - May be seen in diabetic ketoacidosis or severe anorexia.
4. Metabolic alkalosis:
   - Seen in chronic metabolic conditions and with prolonged vomiting.

Analyze assessment findings to recognize fluid-electrolyte problems and acid-base imbalance in children.

1. Laboratory assessments:
   - Serum electrolyte levels.
   - Serum creatinine.
   - Serum glucose.
   - P_{CO_2}.
   - pH.
   - HCO_3.

LEARNING OBJECTIVES

CONCEPTS

Analyze assessment findings to recognize fluid-electrolyte problems and acid-base imbalance in children.—continued

→

2. Physical assessments:
- Daily weights.
- Vital signs.
- Tenseness of anterior fontanel (infant only).
- Skin turgor.
- Bowel sounds.
- Cardiac rhythm.
- Level of consciousness.
- Respiratory function.
- Intake and output measurement.
- Observation for neck vein distention.

Describe appropriate nursing interventions for children experiencing fluid-electrolyte problems and acid-base imbalance.

→

1. Weigh child daily.
2. Carefully assess skin for any breakdown from diarrhea or edema.
3. Turn and position child carefully to prevent skin breakdown.
4. Administer IV fluids as ordered.
5. Monitor oxygen saturation.
6. Maintain oxygen therapy as ordered.
7. Provide age-appropriate activities.
8. Instruct parents in signs and symptoms of dehydration.
9. Instruct parents in the use of oral rehydration methods.

CRITICAL THINKING IN ACTION

View the **Critical Thinking In Action** video in Chapter 43 of the CD-ROM. Then, answer the questions that follow.

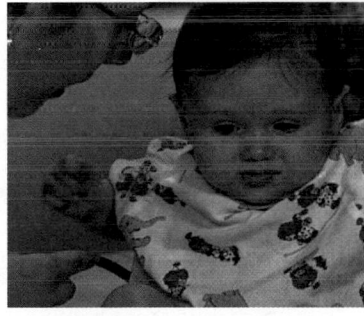

A 10-month-old named Devin comes to the emergency room by ambulance at 3:00 A.M. for respiratory distress. His parents state that he was experiencing a cough for the past week and developed a fever over 103 degrees Fahrenheit tonight. He woke up crying with a frightening cough and could barely catch his breath; the parents called 9-1-1. Devin's respiratory rate is 55 times per minute with moderate retractions, his temperature is 104.2 degrees Fahrenheit, and his heart has a regular rhythm with a rate of 120 beats per minute. His breath sounds demonstrate wheezing and rhonchi throughout all lung fields. At the hospital, he is given a breathing treatment with albuterol 0.5 mL and 2 mL of normal saline per nebulizer. His respiratory rate decreases to 40 and retractions improve. The arterial blood gas measurements show an increased Pco_2, a decreased pH, and a normal HCO_3. A diagnosis of croup syndrome and resultant respiratory acidosis is made. Devin is admitted for monitoring.

1. What are some of the other possible causes of respiratory acidosis in children such as Devin?
2. What are some of the signs and symptoms of respiratory distress and the central nervous system problems associated with Devin's particular acid-base imbalance?
3. Devin's heart rate and rhythm are monitored closely in the hospital. What is the reason for these assessments?
4. What is the treatment for Devin's acid-base imbalance?
5. What are some of the measures taken in the hospital to ensure Devin's safety?

MEDIALINK www.prenhall.com/london

- NCLEX-RN® Review, case studies, and other interactive resources for this chapter can be found on the Companion Website at http://www.prenhall.com/london. Click on "Chapter 43" to select the activities for this chapter.

- For animations, more NCLEX-RN® Review questions, and an audio glossary, access the accompanying CD-ROM in this textbook.

REFERENCES

Aker, J., & O'Sullivan, C. (1998). The selection and administration of perioperative intravenous fluids for the pediatric patient. *Journal of PeriAnesthesia Nursing, 13,* 172–181.

Armon, K., Stephenson, T., MacFaul, R., Eccleston, P., & Werneke, U. (2001). An evidence and consensus based guideline for acute diarrhoea management. *Archives of Disease in Childhood, 85,* 132–142.

Bar-Or, O. (1996). Water and electrolyte replenishment in the exercising child. *International Journal of Sport Nutrition, 6,* 93–99.

Behrman, R. E., Kliegman, R. M., & Jenson, H. B. (Eds.). (2004). *Nelson textbook of pediatrics* (17th ed.). Philadelphia: WB Saunders.

Bindler, R. M., & Howry, L. B. (2005). *Pediatric drug guide.* Upper Saddle River, NJ: Prentice Hall Health.

Binkley, H. M., Beckett, J., Casa, D. J., Kleiner, D. M., & Plummer, P. E. (2002). National Athletic Trainers' Association position statement: Exertional heat illnesses. *Journal of Athletic Training, 37,* 329–343.

Blonshine, S. (2000). Sodium, potassium, and ionized calcium. *AARC Times, 24*(4), 46–48.

Bryant, R. J., Wastney, M. E., Martin, B. R., Wood, O., McCabe, G. P., Morshidi, M., et al., (2003). Racial differences in bone turnover and calcium metabolism in adolescent females. *Journal of Clinical Endocrinology and Metabolism, 88,* 1043–1047.

Burkhart, D. M. (1999). Management of acute gastroenteritis in children. *American Family Physician, 60,* 2555–2563.

Committee on Sports Medicine and Fitness. (2000). Climatic heat stress and the exercising child and adolescent. *Pediatrics, 106,* 158–159.

Davenport, M. (1996). Pediatric fluid balance. *Care of the Chronically Ill Child, 12*(1), 26–28, 30–31.

Eliason, B. C., & Lewan, R. B. (1998). Gastroenteritis in children: Principles of diagnosis

and treatment. *American Family Physician, 58,* 1769–1776.

Endsley, S., & Galbraith, A. (1998). Are you overlooking oral rehydration therapy in childhood diarrhea? *Postgraduate Medicine, 104,* 159–166, 171.

English, M. (2002). Challenges in managing profound hypokalemia. *British Medical Journal, 324,* 269–270.

Foster, G. T., Vaziri, N. D., & Sassoon, C. S. H. (2001). Respiratory alkalosis. *Respiratory Care, 46,* 384–391.

Glaser, N. S., Shirali, A. C., Styne, D. M., & Jones, K. L. (1998). Acid-base homeostasis in children with growth hormone deficiency. *Pediatrics, 102,* 1407–1414.

Hewitt-Taylor, J. (1999). Children in intensive care: Physiological considerations. *Nursing in Critical Care, 4,* 40-45.

Johns Hopkins Hospital. (2005). *The Harriet Lane handbook* (17th ed.). St. Louis, MO: Mosby.

King, C. K., Glass, R., Bresee, J. S., & Duggan, C. (2003). Managing acute gastroenteritis among children. *Morbidity and Mortality Weekly Report, 52*(RR16), 1–16.

Kluckow, M., & Evans, N. (2001). Low systemic blood flow and hyperkalemia in preterm infants. *Journal of Pediatrics, 139,* 227–232.

Larson, C. E. (2000). Safety and efficacy of oral rehydration therapy for the treatment of diarrhea and gastroenteritis in pediatrics. *Pediatric Nursing, 26,* 177–179.

Livingstone, V. H., Willis, C. E., Abdel-Wareth, L. O., Thiessen, P., & Lockitch, G. (2000). Neonatal hypernatremic dehydration associated with breast-feeding malnutrition: A retrospective survey. *Canadian Medical Association Journal, 162,* 647–652.

Mundy, A. R. (1999). Metabolic complications of urinary diversion. *Lancet, 353,* 1813–1814.

Nager, A. L., & Wang, V. J. (2002). Comparison of nasogastric and intravenous methods of rehydration in pediatric patients with acute dehydration. *Pediatrics, 109,* 566–572.

Newman, J. (1996). Decision tree and postpartum management for preventing dehydration in the breastfed baby. *Journal of Human Lactation, 12,* 129–135.

Noble, K. A. (1999, June 28). Putting the puzzle together: Arterial blood gas interpretation. *Advance for Nurses, 19*–22.

Provisional Committee on Quality Improvement, Subcommittee on Acute Gastroenteritis. (1996). Practice parameter: The management of acute gastroenteritis in young children. *Pediatrics, 97,* 424–436.

Rivera-Brown, A. M., Gutierrez, R., Gutierrez, J. C., Frontera, W. R., & Bar-Or, O. (1999). Drink composition, voluntary drinking, and fluid balance in exercising, trained, heat-acclimatized boys. *Journal of Applied Physiology, 86,* 78–84.

Shamir, R., Zahavi, I., Abramowich, T., Poraz, I., Tal, D., Pollak, S., & Dinari, G. (1998). Management of acute gastroenteritis in children in Israel. *Pediatrics, 101,* 892–894.

Straughn, A., & English, B. (1996). Oral rehydration therapy. *MCN. American Journal of Maternal Child Nursing, 21,* 144–147.

Umpaichitra, V., Bastian, W., & Castells, S. (2001). Hypocalcemia in children: Pathogenesis and management. *Clinical Pediatrics, 40,* 305–312.

Venous Access Task Force. (2002). Using evidence-based practice to create a venous access team. *Journal of Pediatric Nursing, 17,* 450–454.

Vega, R., & Avner, J. R. (1997). A prospective study of the usefulness of clinical and laboratory parameters for predicting percentage of dehydration in children. *Pediatric Emergency Care, 13,* 179–182.

The Child with Alterations in Immune Function

We knew that Raymond might have AIDS—my sister was HIV positive. But we have taken him in as our own child and cared for him. Somehow we thought he would be fine. Now, to get the diagnosis is devastating, especially since my sister is also very ill. We need to learn a lot about how to help him. Can we send him to a preschool next year as we had planned? How will we get money to pay for his medicines? What do we tell other people? How do we get him to eat better? We just don't know where to turn right now.
—*Aunt of Raymond, 2 years*

LEARNING OBJECTIVES

- Describe the structure and function of the immune system and apply that knowledge to the care of children with immunologic disorders.

- Explain the differences between active and passive immunity.

- Identify infection control measures to prevent the spread of infection in children with an immunodeficiency.

- Develop a nursing care plan in partnership with the family for a child with human immunodeficiency virus (HIV).

- Describe nursing management for the child with systemic lupus erythematosus or juvenile rheumatoid arthritis.

- Describe exposure prevention measures for the child with latex allergy.

- Apply nursing interventions and prevention measures for the child experiencing other hypersensitivity reactions.

MEDIALINK

www.prenhall.com/london

CD-ROM

Animations:
  HIV Infection/Transmission
  Methotrexate
Video:
  AIDS/HIV
Audio Glossary
NCLEX-RN® Review

Companion Website

MediaLink Applications:
  Case Study: Toddler with HIV
  Case Study: Postexposure Management of
    Needlestick Injuries
Audio Glossary
NCLEX-RN® Review

What are the signs and symptoms of immunologic disorders in children? Often they are nonspecific. The immune system is one of the few body systems that regulates, either directly or indirectly, all other body functions. Thus, a problem with the immune system can have multisystem consequences and may be life threatening. Allergic reactions to food or frequent episodes of otitis media may indicate a disorder of immune function. Immune conditions can be mild to severe and life threatening. Congenital abnormalities sometimes signal a defect in cellular immunity. This chapter will examine some of the more common disorders of immune function and discuss nursing care of children who have these diseases and their families.

ANATOMY AND PHYSIOLOGY OF PEDIATRIC DIFFERENCES

The function of the immune system is to recognize any foreign substances within the body—in simple terms, to distinguish "nonself" from "self"—and to eliminate foreign substances as efficiently as possible. Whenever the body recognizes the presence of a substance that it cannot identify as part of itself, the body protects itself through the immune response. Normally the immune system responds to an invasion of foreign substances, or antigens, in numerous ways. It produces **antibodies**, or proteins that work against **antigens**, the foreign substances that trigger the immune response. There are many types of antibodies, described later in this section. The immune system also produces other types of cells, such as T lymphocytes and natural killer (NK) cells.

Immunity is either natural or acquired. Natural immune defenses are those an infant is born with, such as intact skin, body pH, natural antibodies from the mother, and inflammatory and phagocytic properties. Acquired immunity is composed of humoral (antibody-mediated) and cell-mediated immunity and is not fully developed until a child is about 6 years of age.

Humoral immunity is responsible for destroying bacterial antigens. B lymphocytes, produced in the bone marrow, develop into plasma cells that produce antibodies. Antibodies are a type of protein called **immunoglobulins**. There are five types of immunoglobulins: IgM, IgG, IgA, IgD, and IgE (Table 44–1). IgM, IgG, and IgA act to control a number of body infections, whereas IgE is useful in combating parasitic infections and is part of the allergic response. The role of IgD is not known.

Antibodies are found in serum, body fluids, and certain tissues. When a child is first exposed to an antigen, the B lymphocyte system begins to produce antibodies that react specifically to that antigen (see "Pathophysiology Illustrated: Primary Immune Response"). It takes approximately 3 days for this process, known as **primary immune response**, to occur. Subsequent en-

TABLE 44–1 ✤ Classes of Immunoglobulins

IgM	Present in intravascular spaces
IgG	Present in all body fluids
IgA	Present in secretions of gastrointestinal, respiratory, and genitourinary tracts
IgD	Presence and function not yet described
IgE	Present in internal and external body fluids

PATHOPHYSIOLOGY ILLUSTRATED

Primary Immune Response

Antigen presenting cell

Macrophage ingests antigens and signals helper T cells that antigens are present. B cells also signal T cells.

Message sent

Helper T cells

Helper T cells stimulate rapid cell division in B cells and killer T cells.

Humoral immunity (in body fluids) Stimulates division

Cellular immunity (in body cells) Stimulates division

B cells produce plasma cells.

B cells

Killer T cells

Killer T cells directly attack and destroy body cells infected with antigen.

Plasma cells produce antibodies.

Plasma cells

Memory T cells

Memory B cells and T cells remember how to identify the antigen and will reactivate at future time if same type of antigen is present.

Memory B cells

Antibodies directly attack and destroy antigens either before or after antigens invade body cells.

counters with the antigen trigger memory cells, resulting in a **secondary immune response** within 24 hours.

Infants and children have differing amounts of some immunoglobulins. IgG is the only immunoglobulin that crosses the placenta; as a result, a newborn's levels are similar to those of his or her mother. This maternal IgG disappears by 6 to 8 months of age. The infant's IgG then increases gradually until mature levels are reached at 7 to 8 years. IgM levels are low at birth, rise markedly at 1 week of age, and continue to increase until adult levels are reached at about 1 year. IgA and IgE are not present at birth. Manufacture of these immunoglobulins begins by 2 weeks of age; however, normal values are not achieved until 6 to 7 years. It is thus easy to see why children under 6 years of age become ill so often—they do not have a full complement of immunoglobulins.

In contrast, cell-mediated immunity achieves full function early in life. T lymphocytes, produced in the thymus, provide cellular immunity and protect against most viruses, fungi, slowly developing bacterial infections such as tuberculosis, and tumors. In addition they control the timing of the response in delayed hypersensitivity reactions, such as the purified protein derivative (PPD) test, and they are responsible for the rejection of foreign grafts, such as transplants. For this reason the blood infused into newborns is generally irradiated to prevent **graft-versus-host disease** (a series of immunologic reactions in response to transplanted cells) from transfused lymphocytes. Specialized types of T lymphocytes include killer T cells, suppressor T cells, and helper T cells. Suppressor T cells inhibit B lymphocytes from differentiating into plasma cells. Helper T cells aid in the proliferation and immunologic function of other cells. T lymphocytes have proteins on their surfaces that can be used to measure the immune activity of these cells. For example, some of the common proteins are CD2, CD3, CD4, CD5, CD7, and CD8.

Natural killer cells (also known as non-B/non-T lymphocytes) originate in the bone marrow and thymus and migrate to the blood and spleen. They play a role in control of viral infection, tumors, and autoimmune disease. Newborns have somewhat lower numbers of NK cells than older children and adults, decreasing their ability to respond to certain antigens.

Complement is a component of blood serum consisting of 11 protein compounds. It is an inactive enzyme that activates in response to antigen–antibody functions, resulting in a generalized inflammatory reaction that kills foreign cells. It also plays a role in causing some autoimmune diseases. The levels of some of the complement proteins are lower in newborns than in older children and adults, thus delaying and hampering response to certain infections.

IMMUNODEFICIENCY DISORDERS

Immunodeficiency, a state of decreased responsiveness of the immune system, can occur to varying degrees in response to any number of events. Children with congenital immunodeficiency, or **primary immune deficiency**, are born with a failure of humoral antibody formation (B-cell disorder), a deficient cellular immune system (T-cell disorder), or a combination of both defects. Approximately 50,000 new cases of primary immunodeficiency are diagnosed each year in the United States (Cooper, Pommering, & Koranyi, 2003). In these congenital disorders, the immune deficiency is not caused by another condition. However, immunodeficiency may also be acquired, as in human immunodeficiency virus (HIV) infection. Acquired immunodeficiency is also called **secondary immune deficiency**.

B-CELL AND T-CELL DISORDERS

In B-cell disorders, immunoglobulins may be present in inadequate numbers or nearly absent. X-linked hypogammaglobulinemia, selective IgA deficiency, and common variable immunodeficiency are examples of such disorders. Because newborns are protected from infection by maternal antibodies in the first months after birth, symptoms of B-cell disorders usually become apparent after 3 months of age. Infants with these disorders have frequent recurrent bacterial infections and failure to thrive. With treatment, consisting of intravenous immunoglobulins and antibiotics, most children survive into adulthood. Prognosis depends on the degree of antibody deficiency.

T-cell disorders are characterized by inadequate numbers of T lymphocytes or absence of T-cell functions. Isolated T-cell disorders are rare, usually accompanied by B-cell disorder, and may be associated with congenital abnormalities (as in DiGeorge syndrome) or of unknown cause. DiGeorge syndrome is most often accompanied by

abnormalities in chromosome 22, and is often diagnosed soon after birth. The syndrome is characterized by the absence of parathyroid or thymus glands, resultant hypocalcemia, cardiac defects, low-set ears, hypertelorism (widely set eyes), tetany 48 hours after birth, and viral and fungal infections in the neonatal period. Pneumonia and failure to thrive are common, and T lymphocyte counts are often <1500/mm^3 for CD3 and <1000/mm^3 for CD4 cells (Elder, 2000). Children with the disorder are treated with antibiotics for prophylaxis against pneumonia from *Pneumocystis carinii*, oral calcium, thymus transplantation, and HLA-identical bone marrow transplantation. Without thymus transplantation, few children survive beyond 5 years.

Immunodeficiency with hyper-IgM is a T-cell disorder that affects mainly males and causes decreased T-cell function, variable abnormal levels of immunoglobulins, and high titers of some antibodies. It is usually X-linked but is sometimes autosomal. Pulmonary and sinus bacterial infections generally occur in the first 2 years of life (Koleilat, Williams, & Ryan, 2003). Treatment with Intravenous Immune Globulin (IVIG) therapy is helpful although later malignancies and liver disease can occur (Schwartz, 2000).

Refer to Table 44–2, which compares laboratory values for selected congenital immunodeficiency disorders.

TABLE 44–2 ✣ Selected Congenital Immunodeficiency Disorders

Disorders	Laboratory Findings
B cell	
X-linked hypogammaglobulinemia	Reduced IgA, IgM, IgE, IgG (< 100 mg/dL), absence of B cells in peripheral blood, normal T cells
Selective IgA deficiency	IgA < 10 mg/dL
Common variable immunodeficiency	IgA, IgM reduced; IgG < 250 mg/dL
T cell	
DiGeorge syndrome	Lymphopenia; absent T-cell functions, decreased T cells, normal B cells
X-linked immunodeficiency with hyper-IgM	Reduced IgG, IgA; elevated IgM; mutations in T-cell surface proteins
Combined	
Severe combined immunodeficiency syndrome (SCID)	Complete absence of T- and B-cell and NK immunity
Wiskott–Aldrich syndrome	Thrombocytopenia, low platelet volume, nonfunctional B-cells, normal IgG, decreased IgM, increased IgA, increased IgE; inability to respond to polysaccharide antigens

SEVERE COMBINED IMMUNODEFICIENCY DISEASE

Severe combined immunodeficiency disease (SCID) is a congenital condition characterized by absence of both humoral and cellular immunity. SCID occurs in X-linked recessive, autosomal recessive, and sporadic forms. The disorder is more common in males than females (Cooper et al., 2003). Without appropriate treatment, children born with SCID usually die within the first 2 years of life.

ETIOLOGY AND PATHOPHYSIOLOGY

Severe combined immunodeficiency disease is caused by genetic mutations of cellular receptors to interleukin. The mutations lead to impaired lymphoid development in children with low T and NK cells. The B lymphocytes may appear normal in number but are defective in performance (Candotti, 2000).

CLINICAL MANIFESTATIONS

Symptoms of SCID develop early in life. The newborn often demonstrates a susceptibility to infection by 3 months of age. The disorder is characterized by chronic infection (such as otitis media or pneumonia), failure to completely recover from infection, frequent reinfection, and infection with viruses such as cytomegalovirus and the bacterium *Pneumocystis carinii*. Often the first infection seen is a resistant oral candidiasis. Children are also highly susceptible to serious infections like meningitis, skin or organ infection, osteomyelitis, or sepsis. Failure to thrive is a consequence of persistent illness.

Some infants experience graft-versus-host disease as a result of placental transfer of maternal T lymphocytes. The reaction may be manifested by a perinatal rash that resembles measles or atopic dermatitis (Koleilat et al., 2003). If the child receives foreign tissue (for example, in a blood transfusion), signs such as skin rash, fever, hepatosplenomegaly, and diarrhea may occur.

CLINICAL THERAPY

A marked reduction in lymphocyte counts is indicative of SCID. B and T lymphocytes are generally few in number or absent from the peripheral blood and lymphoid tissues. In some cases the B lymphocyte count may be elevated, although these cells do not function normally. NK cells are few in number. Immunoglobulin levels are significantly reduced. Refer to Table 44–2 for laboratory findings in SCID. Diagnosis is usually made only after extensive laboratory testing. In addition to a complete blood count, erythrocyte sedimentation rate, and B- and T-cell lymphocyte counts, other studies including IgA, IgG, and IgM antibody titers, neutrophil count, and titer levels of immunizations received may be performed (Table 44–3). A chest radiograph is conducted to assess thymus size.

For children with primary immunodeficiencies, prevention of infection is essential. Antibiotic therapy targeting specific infectious agents should be aggressive (Koleilat et al., 2003). Additional management consists of antibiotic prophylaxis and immunizations for encapsulated bacteria (e.g., heptavalent pneumococcal vaccine, *Haemophilus* b conjugate vaccine, meningococcal polysaccharide vaccine). Children with T-cell deficiencies should receive

---

TABLE 44–3 ✤ Cells Evaluated in Laboratory Studies for Immune Conditions

Test and Type of Cell Evaluated	Action	Implication of Increased or Decreased Levels
White Blood Cell (WBC) Count		
Neutrophil (54–62%)	Phagocytic cell that defends against bacteria	Increased in bacterial infection, inflammatory processes, and some malignancies
Eosinophil (1–3%)	Associated with antigen-antibody reaction	Increased in allergic reaction; decreased in children receiving corticosteroids
Basophils (0–3%)	Phagocytic cell; involved in immediate hypersensitivity reaction; stores histamine and has receptor sites for IgE	Increased in leukemia; decreased in allergy, acute infection, collagen and chronic diseases
Monocytes (4–9%)	Phagocytic cell active in chronic infection	Increased in tuberculosis, protozoan infection, monocytic leukemia
Lymphocytes (T, B, non-B/non-T [NK]) (25–33%)	Major components of immune system	Increased in many infections; decreased in children with immune deficiency
Immunoglobulins		
(IgM, IgG, IgA, IgD, IgE) (See appendix for age-specific values.)	Many roles in a number of immunologic reactions	Increased in presence of infection or allergic response; decreased in children with immune deficiency

cytomegalovirus-negative irradiated blood products due to the risk of infection and graft-versus-host disease from lymphocytes in the donor blood (Cooper et al., 2003).

The goal of medical management is to restore immune function. Thymic hormones have been given to some children with limited success. Intravenous immune globulin (IVIG) may be administered. Hematopoietic stem cell and bone marrow transplantation offer hope for children with SCID (see Chapter 50 ∞). The transplantation corrects T-cell function, and new cells appear 3 to 4 months after infusion of the donor or stem cells. Enzyme replacement therapy may be implemented in autosomal recessive SCID caused by adenosine deaminase deficiency. With the identification of the genetic defect for SCID in recent years, gene transfer has been successfully attempted in a small number of children. This experimental therapy will likely be used more often in the future (Champi, 2002).

Prognosis is poor without aggressive therapy. Some children have survived 10 years after a successful bone marrow transplant.

NURSING MANAGEMENT

NURSING ASSESSMENT AND DIAGNOSIS

Obtain a thorough history of infections, including age of onset, type of causal organism, frequency, and severity. Take a family history, and find out if the child has had any unusual reactions to vaccines, medications, or foods. Measure the child's height and weight accurately to identify failure to thrive. Look for any evidence of infections involving the skin, subcutaneous tissues, respiratory system, and mucous membranes. Palpate the abdomen for hepatomegaly and the lymph nodes for lymphadenopathy.

Assess family support systems and coping mechanisms when a child is diagnosed with the disorder.

The primary nursing diagnosis for a child with SCID is *Risk for Infection* related to immunodeficiency. Other nursing diagnoses may include the following:

- *Risk for Imbalanced Nutrition: Less than Body Requirements* related to chronic illness
- *Risk for Impaired Skin Integrity* related to immunologic deficit
- *Risk for Caregiver Role Strain* related to a child with a chronic, life-threatening illness
- *Risk for Delayed Growth and Development* related to physical disability and chronic illness

PLANNING AND IMPLEMENTATION

Nursing care of the immunodeficient child focuses on preventing infection (see "Teaching Highlights: Reducing Risk

TEACHING HIGHLIGHTS

REDUCING RISK OF INFECTION IN THE CHILD WITH IMMUNODEFICIENCY DISEASE

Teach family members the following practices to reduce the risk of transmission of infection to the child with immunodeficiency disease:

- Wash all bottles, nipples, and pacifiers with hot water and soap, or in the dishwasher.
- Change diapers frequently and cleanse skin with mild soap and dry thoroughly.
- Wash hands before handling child, after changing diapers, and before feeding child.
- Do not allow child to share utensils, cups, bottles, or pacifiers with others.
- Maintain clean pets and clean the pet's environment frequently.
- Avoid exposing the child to other family members' illnesses, such as colds.

of Infection in the Child with Immunodeficiency Disease"). However, even with environmental controls, such as keeping children inside special units to maintain a sterile environment, these children are prone to **opportunistic infections** (infections caused by normally nonpathogenic organisms in people who lack normal immunity).

Prevent Systemic Infection

Frequent and thorough handwashing is important. Always use standard precautions, adding transmission-based precautions when needed. **SKILLS** Use sterile aseptic technique when caring for all sites where needles, catheters, central lines, endotracheal tubes, pressure-monitoring lines, and peripheral intravenous lines enter the child's body. Food and other items entering the hospital room may need special treatment. The child should be placed in a negative pressure room, and contact with infectious individuals should be avoided. Refer to the current recommendations for immunizations for the immunocompromised child. (See Chapter 45. ∞)

Promote Skin Integrity

The skin is the only intact defense that many immunodeficient children have. Provide good skin care, and observe all possible pressure areas closely for signs of breakdown or infection. Turn the child frequently. Encourage range of motion exercises. Avoid any skin trauma.

Manage Medication Therapy

Many medications used long term in the treatment of children with SCID have numerous side effects. Monitor closely for side effects of antibiotics, such as overgrowth of resistant organisms (e.g., thrush infections in the mouth, *Clostridium difficile* infections of the gastrointestinal tract) and administer IVIG safely (see "Drug Guide: Immune Globulin").

DRUG GUIDE

IMMUNE GLOBULIN

Overview of Action

Contains globulin protein from large pools of normal human plasma of venous or placental origin. Intramuscular formulation used to provide passive immunity or to modify severity of certain specific infectious diseases, such as measles, varicella-zoster, hepatitis A, and hepatitis B. Intravenous formulation used as maintenance therapy in those unable to manufacture sufficient quantities of IgG antibodies, such as in immunodeficiency diseases, idiopathic thrombocytopenia, and Kawasaki disease.

Routes, Dosage, Frequency

IM: Doses vary with specific products but ranges are generally 0.02 to 0.06 mL/kg after exposure to disease

IV: For immunoglobulin deficiency:

Gammagard or Gamimmune 100 mg/kg/month

Sandoglobulin or Venoglobulin-S 200 mg/kg/month

For idiopathic thrombocytopenia purpura:

400 mg/kg/day for 5 consecutive days or 1 g/day every other day for up to 3 doses

For Kawasaki disease:

2 g/kg given over 10–12 hours or 400 mg/kg/day on 4 consecutive days

Contraindications

Anaphylaxis or severe reaction to human immune globulin or any ingredient in the formulation; hepatitis A

Side Effects

Pain, muscle stiffness, local inflammation at IM injection site; headache, malaise, fever, arthralgia, nephrotic syndrome; hypersensitivity reaction; infusion reactions

Nursing Implications

Monitor vital signs before, during, and after infusion.

Have emergency drugs and equipment readily available; hypersensitivity reactions are most common with large or repeated doses.

Stop infusion immediately and report hypersensitivity reactions.

Consult package insert for IM formulations for specific diseases and inform family of the expected length of time for passive immunity. Active immunization to diseases may be needed following that time period.

Adapted from Bindler, R. M., & Howry, L. B. (2005). Pediatric drug guide. Upper Saddle River, NJ: Prentice Hall Health.

Provide Emotional Support and Referral to Appropriate Support Groups and Services

SCID is a life threatening and devastating disease. Even with aggressive therapy, the prognosis is poor. Evaluate the family's knowledge about the disease. The parents may feel guilt because of the genetic nature of the disease and the difficulties of treatment. Listen closely to their concerns and encourage them to discuss their fears. Refer them to an appropriate support group or counselor if needed. Encourage genetic counseling if the parents plan to have more children.

The family of a child who undergoes hematopoietic or bone marrow transplantation requires additional support and referrals. The transplantation procedure involves surgery for both the ill child and the donor, often another child in the family. (Refer to the discussion on transplantation in Chapter 50. ∞) After the infusion of the donor marrow, the ill child will be hospitalized for several months until T lymphocyte levels are sufficient to provide resistance to infection. During this period, parents may need to rely on social services to help manage the family situation, particularly if the child is hospitalized at a medical center far from the family's home. Assess the family's situation and make appropriate referrals to social services and support groups. Introduce parents to other families undergoing bone marrow transplantation.

EVALUATION

The success of nursing care for the child with SCID is measured by outcomes such as the following:

- Adequate nutritional status as determined by normal growth patterns
- Maintenance of intact skin
- Adaptive coping by family to demands of a chronic illness
- Developmental performance within normal level for age

WISKOTT–ALDRICH SYNDROME

A combined congenital immunodeficiency syndrome, Wiskott–Aldrich syndrome is an X-linked disorder which causes mutation in the WAS gene and changes in WAS protein (Elder, 2000). The gene resides on Xp11.22-23. The incidence is 4 in 1 million live male births (Dibbern & Routes, 2004). It is characterized by thrombocytopenia, eczema, hemorrhagic tendencies, and recurrent infections. Thrombocytopenia with bleeding tendencies appears during the neonatal period. Eczema appears by 1 year of age. Infections involve the middle ear and often lead to chronic otitis media. Children are particularly susceptible to infections from herpes viruses and lymphoreticular malignancies, especially of the lymphatic system.

The diagnosis is made in the early neonatal period on the basis of the thrombocytopenia, which leads to petechiae and bleeding (refer to Table 44–2). How and when Wiskott–Aldrich syndrome manifests itself varies, with some children maintaining normal lymphocyte levels for years. Treatment is symptomatic and includes antibiotic prophylaxis together with platelet infusions and, sometimes, splenectomy. Without bone marrow or stem cell transplantation, most children die within the first 5 years of life. Survival beyond adolescence is unusual. Infection, bleeding, or malignancy (leukemia or lymphoma) may be the cause of death (Elder, 2000).

NURSING MANAGEMENT

Nursing care is similar to that for the child with SCID. Refer the parents for genetic counseling to help them understand the transmission of the disease and the probability of having another child with the same disorder. Arrange for psychologic support for parents overwhelmed with guilt from learning that the illness is inherited.

Help the parents and family cope with the knowledge that the child has a chronic and potentially fatal illness. Referral to family counseling may be appropriate. Expected outcomes are return to normal immunologic function or successful coping with a life-threatening illness.

ACQUIRED IMMUNODEFICIENCY SYNDROME

Soon after acquired immunodeficiency syndrome (AIDS) was recognized in homosexual adults and intravenous drug abusers, cases of AIDS were seen in children. Increasing numbers of children infected with HIV have been diagnosed, making HIV infection a leading cause of immune disease in infants and children and a major cause of death in children 1 to 4 years of age. By December 2003, over 10,300 children in the United States under 14 years were infected. Over 5300 deaths have been reported in children due to AIDS (Centers for Disease Control and Prevention [CDC], 2005).

Most cases of HIV in children—and virtually all new cases—are the result of perinatal transmission. The CDC estimates that approximately 300 infants are born with HIV infection each year in the United States (MMWR, 2003). These numbers have decreased from the previously reported estimates of 1000 to 2000 infants born annually with HIV infection during the 1990s, primarily because of more effective identification and treatment of infected mothers and babies. Because of the high rate of transfer from mother to infant, HIV counseling and voluntary testing are encouraged for all pregnant women. According to the American Academy of Pediatrics (2001), half of all new HIV infections in the United States occur among young

people between the ages of 13 and 24 years. Most cases of HIV during adolescence are acquired through sexual transmission.

The virus affects multiple systems and eventually destroys the child's immune system (see "Pathophysiology Illustrated: Human Immunodeficiency Virus"). An understanding of the natural history of HIV disease is still evolving, and there are several important differences in the disease progression and clinical manifestations of pediatric and adult HIV infection.

ETIOLOGY AND PATHOPHYSIOLOGY

AIDS is caused by HIV-1. Most children acquire HIV in a form of **vertical transmission** from their mothers transplacentally or during birth. Transmission can occur during birth from blood, amniotic fluid, and exposure to genital tract secretions, and after birth through breast milk from HIV-positive mothers. However, risk for perinatal transmission has been significantly reduced since mothers identified as infected receive zidovudine (AZT) during pregnancy, the baby is born by cesarean, and the baby is given drug therapy after birth (Ramstead, 2003).

HIV was also transmitted to children through transfusions of infected blood before mandatory screening of blood and blood products was instituted in 1985. Most of these children were infected during treatment of hemophilia. Although 30% of adolescents with AIDS also have hemophilia, with infected blood the expected etiology, adolescents now most commonly acquire the virus through intravenous drug abuse or through unprotected sexual activities.

HIV selectively targets and destroys T cells, thereby decreasing and eventually eliminating cellular immunity. It also affects humoral immunity. Thus the child is left unprotected against a myriad of bacterial, viral, fungal, and opportunistic infections, which are ultimately fatal. Every organ system can be affected.

CLINICAL MANIFESTATIONS

The interval from HIV infection to the onset of overt AIDS is shorter in children than in adults, and shorter in children infected perinatally than in those infected through transfusion. Most children with AIDS have nonspecific findings, including lymphadenopathy, hepatosplenomegaly, nephropathy, oral candidiasis, failure to thrive and weight loss, diarrhea, chronic eczema and dermatitis, and fever. Raymond, described at the beginning of this chapter, had several of these findings, as well as a history of recurrent, acute infections (bronchitis, otitis media, and colds).

Bacterial and opportunistic infections, such as *Streptococcus, Haemophilus influenzae, Salmonella,* and *Pneumocystis carinii* pneumonia (PCP), as well as malignancies such as lymphomas, frequently occur as the disease

PATHOPHYSIOLOGY ILLUSTRATED
Human Immunodeficiency Virus

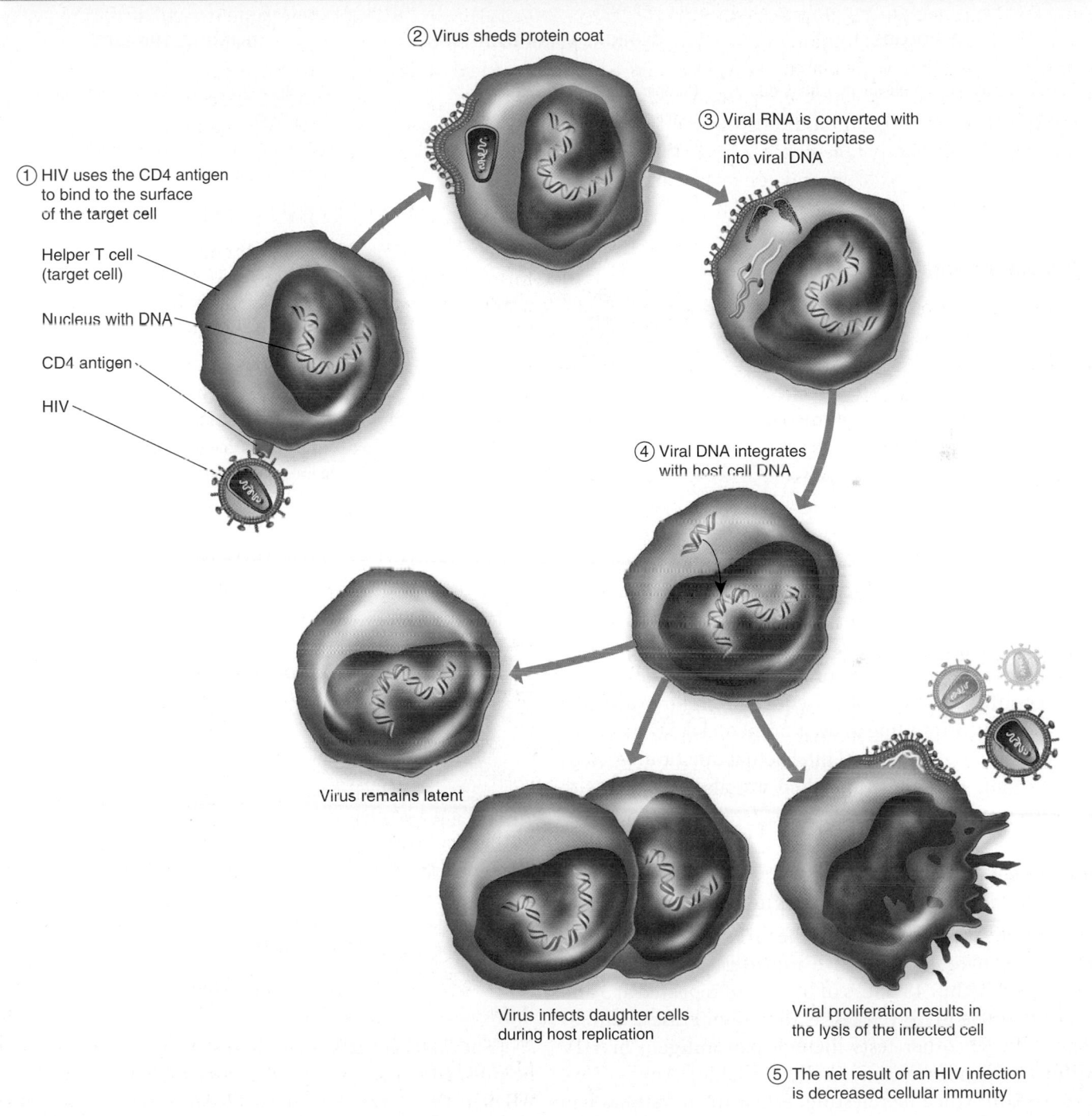

② Virus sheds protein coat

③ Viral RNA is converted with reverse transcriptase into viral DNA

① HIV uses the CD4 antigen to bind to the surface of the target cell

Helper T cell (target cell)

Nucleus with DNA

CD4 antigen

HIV

④ Viral DNA integrates with host cell DNA

Virus remains latent

Virus infects daughter cells during host replication

Viral proliferation results in the lysis of the infected cell

⑤ The net result of an HIV infection is decreased cellular immunity

progresses. Laboratory tests are used to determine the severity of disease. The viral load is the number of circulating HIV particles per millimeter:

- Viral loads of less than 10,000 are low risk.
- Viral loads of 10,000 to 100,000 are moderate risk.
- Viral loads greater than 100,000 are high risk.

- A T4 (CD4) count of 650 to 1200 cells/mm^3 represents a competent immune system.
- A T4 count of 500 to 200 cells/mm^3 indicates a suppressed immune system.
- A T4 count of less than 200 cells/mm^3 is an AIDS indicator value.

CLINICAL MANIFESTATIONS

HUMAN IMMUNODEFICIENCY VIRUS IN CHILDREN

ETIOLOGY	CLINICAL MANIFESTATIONS	CLINICAL THERAPY
Frequent, chronic, or unusual infections due to poor immune response	Chronic bilateral otitis media Oral candidiasis *Pneumocystis carinii* pneumonia (PCP) Skin disorders Fever	Vigorous antimicrobial therapy for treatment of infections Limit exposure to groups of people Obtain recommended immunizations
Poor nutritional intake due to lack of appetite caused by disease and medications	Failure to thrive (eating disorder of childhood) Weight and body mass index below 10th percentile Chronic diarrhea Skin irritation	Monitor growth Supplemental intake such as enteral feedings at night, and TPN if needed Meticulous skin care to prevent breakdown
Immune system overgrowth to compensate for lack of proper immune response	Hepatosplenomegaly and lymphadenopathy	Assess abdomen frequently Teach about safe transport to avoid injury to liver and spleen

Note: Be alert for the possibility of HIV infection in infants with combinations of listed clinical manifestations, especially in infants known to be at risk.

Children infected with HIV around the time of birth have a higher cancer risk than other children, with the average age of cancer diagnosis at 5 to 6 years (Caselli, 2000). Lymphocytic interstitial pneumonitis is a common manifestation of pediatric AIDS. Frequently children develop encephalopathy resulting in developmental delay or a deterioration of motor skills and intellectual functioning. Adolescents with HIV infection often are also infected with hepatitis B virus (Rogers, 2000).

CLINICAL THERAPY

Most children with AIDS are diagnosed early in life. Serologic tests for detection of the virus are monitored in infants born to HIV-positive mothers. These tests are performed within 48 hours of birth and repeated at 3 and 6 months. The preferred test is the polymerase chain reaction (PCR); other tests include p24 antigen, or HIV culture (which is not universally available). Any positive result is confirmed by retesting. When the infant has had two negative tests, testing with enzyme-linked immunosorbent assay (ELISA; HIV antibody) should be done at 12, 15, and 18 months. After two consecutive negative results with ELISA, the child is considered free of HIV. In addition a complete blood count (CBC) and CD4+ T-cell subset is performed at 3 to 6 months. Rapid serologic tests are under study and results are showing promise. Their future use may shorten the diagnosis time

and promote better follow-up of potential cases (Nielsen & Bryson, 2000).

NURSING PRACTICE

Two types of tests are commonly used to test for HIV infection. One is enzyme-linked immunosorbent assay (ELISA), and the other is polymerase chain reaction (PCR). Although the PCR has the greatest sensitivity, it is costly (about $175) and identifies some false-positive results. ELISA is less expensive (about $50) but not as sensitive, especially for children under 18 months. For this reason, repeated tests are recommended, especially in the infant who may become HIV positive after birth to an infected mother. In developing countries where expense prohibits repeated tests, the ELISA is often used with astute clinical observations of the child at risk.

The CDC considers children under 13 years of age to be infected if their symptoms meet the CDC criteria for AIDS, if they have HIV in the blood or tissues, or if they have antibodies to HIV. The CDC criteria address two issues: first, the diagnosis of HIV, and second, the clinical classification of children infected with HIV (Table 44–4).

Because of the rapidity of disease progression in perinatally transmitted HIV infection, early identification of infected infants is important to ensure the most effective treatment. HIV-infected mothers should be identified during pregnancy, and their infants should undergo periodic

TABLE 44–4 ✤ Clinical Staging of Pediatric HIV Infection

Diagnosis of HIV infection in children

- HIV infected (two or more positive tests for HIV or demonstrates AIDS)
- Perinatally exposed (born to a mother known to be infected with HIV)
- Seroconverter (born to a mother known to be infected with HIV but has had two negative HIV tests)

When infected, the child with HIV is classified as

- Category N (not symptomatic)
- Category A (mildly symptomatic)
- Category B (moderately symptomatic)
- Category C (severely symptomatic; multiple, recurrent infection)

Data from Guidelines for the use of antiretroviral agents in pediatric HIV infection. (1998). *Morbidity and Mortality Weekly Report, 47* (RR-4), 1–43.

laboratory testing, as previously described. Regardless of the results of these tests, all infants of infected mothers should start prophylaxis against PCP (a commonly serious or fatal outcome in infants) by the age of 4 to 6 weeks and continue to 12 months, or until two negative HIV tests have been documented (at 1 and 4 months of age). Drugs used for PCP prophylaxis include trimethoprim-sulfamethoxazole (Bactrim or Septra), dapsone, or aerosolized pentamidine. In addition, all infected mothers should receive oral zidovudine (AZT) after the first trimester of pregnancy and intravenous AZT during labor and birth; the newborn should receive 6 weeks of oral AZT after birth. A CBC with differential is performed at birth, 4 to 6 weeks, and 12 weeks to monitor for drug side effects.

Medical management is supportive, as there is no cure for AIDS. Intravenous immune globulin (see "Drug Guide: Immune Globulin") has been used to prevent bacterial infections in children under the age of 2 years. Prompt therapy for bacterial and opportunistic infections is needed. Treatment with highly active antiretroviral therapy (HAART) has had a dramatic impact on the health of HIV-infected children (Table 44–5). Combination therapy is recommended for all infants, children, and adolescents who are treated with antiretroviral agents including nucleoside reverse transcriptase inhibitors such as zidovudine (AZT), didanosine (DDI), zalcitabine (DDC), lamivudine (3TC), and stavudine (D4T) (Edmunds & Mayhew, 2004).

The protease inhibitors (PIs) ritonavir and nelfinavir have been approved for use in children over 2 years, and other PIs are under investigation (Temple, Koranyi, & Nahata, 2001). The protease inhibitors are most effective in combination with nucleoside reverse transcriptase inhibitors, which slow replication of the virus. Drug trials

have demonstrated reduction of serum HIV load in perinatally infected infants who were treated with a combination of several antiviral drugs. The antineoplastic drug hydroxyurea can be used in combination with nucleoside reverse transcriptase inhibitors (Kline et al., 2000).

The earlier the child develops AIDS, the poorer the prognosis. However, as treatment improves, more children are living longer with the disease. Younger children are more likely to die of pulmonary diseases or infection, while those who survive past 10 years of age are more likely to die of cardiac disease, wasting syndrome, encephalopathy, and infection with *Mycobacterium avium* complex. The average age for survival of a child after diagnosis of HIV infection is 8 years (Langston, Cooper, Goldfarb et al., 2001).

NURSING MANAGEMENT

NURSING ASSESSMENT AND DIAGNOSIS

For infants at risk of HIV infection, obtain the HIV test results of the mother if available. When these are positive, the infant will need to be screened numerous times during infancy for HIV infection, as described in the previous section. Facilitate the screening and explain its necessity to the family.

Physiologic Assessment

Assessment centers on observation and evaluation of potential sites of infection. Assess breath sounds, respiratory status, arterial blood gases, level of consciousness, and mental status. Report any evidence of lymphocytic interstitial pneumonitis or neurologic abnormalities. Assess the child's height and weight frequently. Observe for signs of failure to thrive and assess for anemia. Look for *Candida* infections in the mouth and the diaper area. Note any developmental delays in motor skills or intellectual functioning, which could result from encephalopathy and poor nutrition, and can signal the progression from HIV infection into AIDS (Pearson, McGrath, Nozyce et al., 2000). Report them so that the child can receive further medical evaluation.

Psychosocial Assessment

Assess family support systems and coping mechanisms, as the stress of caring for a child with AIDS may overwhelm parents. Assess the family's ability to care for the child. If the mother is infected, ask about the extended family's ability to provide daily care and emotional support. Support the family when they decide to inform a school-age child or adolescent of the diagnosis. When assessing an adolescent with AIDS, evaluate the teen's understanding of how AIDS is transmitted and the response to the diagnosis.

MEDIALINK Animation: HIV Infection/Transmission

MEDIALINK Case Study: Toddler with HIV

TABLE 44-5 ✣ Medications Used to Treat Human Immunodeficiency Virus

Medication	Action	Nursing Implications
Nucleoside Analogs or Nucleoside Reverse Transcriptase Inhibitors (NRTIs)		
Examples: Zidovudine (AZT) Didanosine Zalcitabine Stavudine Lamivudine	Inhibits action of viral reverse transcriptase, an enzyme in the conversion of RNA to DNA	Baseline data include physical assessment, laboratory studies (especially measurement of white and red blood cell counts); monitored at least monthly for changes. Common side effects include fever, headache, insomnia, myalgia, nausea, vomiting, diarrhea, anorexia, bone marrow suppression with resulting granulocytopenia and anemia, dyspnea, cough, skin rash. Teach signs and symptoms of infection. Be sure family realizes that the drug neither cures HIV nor prevents transfer from the person infected to others.
Protease Inhibitors		
Examples: Saquinavir Ritonavir Indinavir Nelfinavir Kaletra (lopinavir/ritonavir combination) Fosamprenavir	Blocks the function of the enzyme protease needed for viral formation and growth	Baseline data include physical assessment and laboratory studies (such as serum electrolytes, CBC, liver function studies, blood glucose, hemoglobin A_{1c}, serum amylase, CPK); monitored at least monthly for changes. Side effects include CNS, CV changes, life-threatening hematologic changes, respiratory distress, and allergy; monitor for specific side effects of the particular drug administered. Oral forms taken within 2 hours of a full meal. Be sure family realizes that the drug neither cures HIV nor prevents transfer from the person infected to others.
Nonnucleoside Reverse Transcriptase Inhibitors		
Examples: nevirapine, delavirdine	Bind to viral reverse transcriptase and disrupt the conversion of RNA to DNA	Baseline data include physical assessment and laboratory studies (such as liver and kidney function tests, CBC and differential); monitored at least monthly for changes. Side effects include fever, headache, nausea, diarrhea, hepatitis, altered liver function, anemia, neutropenia, drowsiness and fatigue, rash, Stevens-Johnson syndrome. Be sure family realizes that the drug neither cures HIV nor prevents transfer from the person infected to others. Teach the family to: Notify healthcare provider immediately if rash appears. Use caution in driving or other hazardous activity due to fatigue. Avoid St. John's wort which may decrease the medication's activity.

Note: The average cost of annual therapy with a combination of drugs as recommended is about $10,000 (Burpo, 2000). What special financial needs will families have when someone is treated for HIV?

The accompanying "Nursing Care Plan" includes common nursing diagnoses that may apply to a child hospitalized with AIDS. Other nursing diagnoses may include the following:

- *Diarrhea* related to gastrointestinal infection, malignancy, or drug reactions
- *Impaired Gas Exchange* related to pulmonary disease
- *Delayed Growth and Development* related to chronic infection and poor nutrition
- *Risk for Compromised Family Coping* related to life-threatening illness

PLANNING AND IMPLEMENTATION

The first step in dealing with HIV infection is prevention. Nurses must be active in evaluating test results and instituting measures to prevent vertical transmission of HIV to the infants of infected mothers. Adequate testing, prophylaxis for HIV and PCP, and follow-up visits for evaluation

NURSING PRACTICE

The American Academy of Pediatrics Committee on Pediatric AIDS recommends that school children and adolescents with HIV be informed of their diagnosis. Telling the child is difficult for parents and they often avoid doing so. Since parents usually want to be the ones to tell the child, they need help planning how to discuss the issue and ongoing support in the process of communication (Instone, 2000). Nurses can help parents understand the need to discuss the diagnosis with the child, provide information about how to tell the child, and emotionally support them with this difficult task. Provide hope about the success of treatment and ability to maintain an active life. Assist the family in identifying support groups, Web sites and other information, and respite care.

of general health and development for all infants at risk of the disease is advised. Guidelines from the American Academy of Pediatrics recommend that pediatricians offer HIV testing and counseling to adolescents who are sexually active or involved in substance abuse (Committee on Pediatric AIDS, 2001). There are also recommendations for including HIV and AIDS education in comprehensive health education for students from kindergarten through 12th grade (Committee on Pediatric AIDS, 1998). Nurses can implement these policies and counsel teens about the dangers and prevention measures for HIV (Committee on Pediatric AIDS, 1998).

NURSING PRACTICE

The American Academy of Pediatrics recommends that HIV and AIDS education be part of health education in grades kindergarten through 12. School nurses should be educated about HIV/AIDS, ethics, testing, and counseling. The particular roles defined for nurses in school settings include:

1. Participate in education programs for teachers
2. Assist schools and other organizations to develop education programs
3. Review, adapt, and develop educational materials
4. Participate in public discussions about HIV/AIDS
5. Take part in meetings with school administrators, staff, and parents
6. Facilitate networking among parents and AIDS community groups

(Committee on Pediatric AIDS, 1998)

If the child is diagnosed with HIV, close health supervision is needed to ensure medications are taken and examinations are carried out. When HIV progresses to AIDS, nursing care is similar to that of a child with any serious, chronic, life-threatening disease. It centers on preventing infection, managing pain, promoting respiratory and other

organ function, promoting adequate nutritional intake, and providing emotional support to the parents and child, while promoting the child's growth and development. The accompanying "Nursing Care Plan" summarizes nursing care for the child hospitalized with AIDS.

Prevent Infection

Protection of the newborn from HIV-infected maternal secretions is essential. Measures to implement include avoidance of the use of fetal scalp electrodes and other invasive devices during labor. Bathe the newborn as soon as possible after birth and wash the eyes and face before administration of prophylactic eyedrops or ointment. Heel sticks and newborn injections should be delayed until after the newborn has been bathed. In order to avoid transmission of HIV through breast milk, encourage the mother to formula-feed the baby instead of breastfeeding (Luxner, 2003).

Proper disposal of needles and contaminated materials or equipment is essential to reduce the transmission of HIV (Figure 44–1 ●). Standard precautions (see Skills Manual) are implemented to prevent exposure to HIV. **SKILLS**

Immunosuppressed children become infected with bacteria as well as other common organisms. Frequent handwashing and limiting the child's exposure to people

● **FIGURE 44–1**

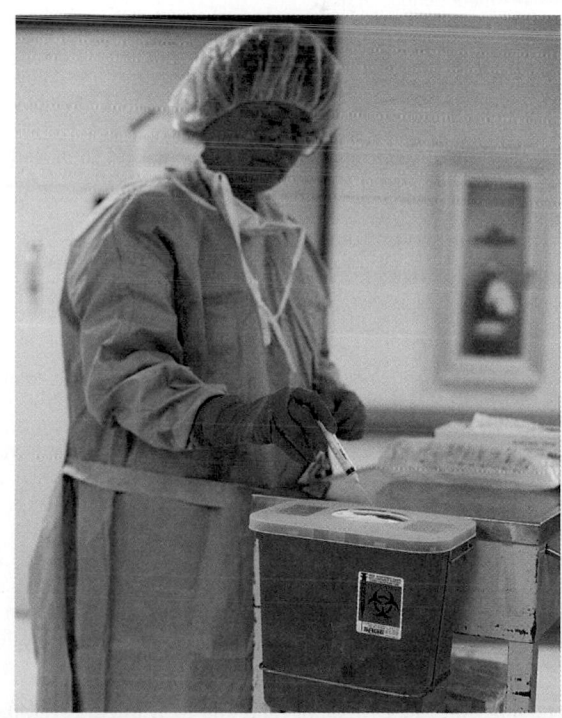

This nurse is disposing of a needle and syringe in a biohazard container, a necessary practice to avoid the transmission of HIV through needle sticks with contaminated needles. This universal precaution provides protection even when the immune status of the patient is not known.

NURSING CARE PLAN

THE CHILD WITH ACQUIRED IMMUNODEFICIENCY SYNDROME

Intervention	Rationale	Expected Outcome
1. Nursing Diagnosis: Risk for Infection related to immunosuppression		
NIC Priority Intervention: **Infection control:** Minimizing the acquisition and transmission of infectious agents		**NOC Suggested Outcome:** **Risk control:** Answers to eliminate or reduce actual, personal, and modifiable health threats
Goal: Risk Factors for Infection will be eliminated as evidenced by infection control.		
■ Assess the child every 2–4 hours for fever; lesions in the mouth; and redness, inflammation, soreness, and lesions on the skin or around intravenous lines. ■ Auscultate for changes in breath sounds every 2 hours. Perform pulmonary toilet (coughing, deep breathing, incentive spirometry) every 2–4 hours. ■ Enforce strict handwashing. Allow no fresh flowers, fruits, or vegetables in child's room. Screen visitors for colds or recent exposure to varicella. Use blood and body fluid precautions (refer to *Clinical Skills Manual*). **SKILLS** Practice strict asepsis for dressing changes and suctioning. ■ Coordinate patient care assignments to avoid exposing the child to individuals with recent infections or immunizations. ■ Organize patient care activities to allow for adequate periods of rest. ■ Follow recommendations of CDC and AAP for immunizing immunosuppressed children. Avoid varicella vaccine. Perform annual TB testing.	■ Fever is one of the few signs of infection in the immunosuppressed child who does not have a sufficient number of white blood cells. ■ Pneumonia is a likely infection in the child with AIDS. ■ Control of environmental factors helps prevent infection. ■ Planning minimizes chances for infection. ■ Rest periods allow the child to regain energy. ■ Special recommendations consider the child's decreased immune response and the danger of acquiring disease from certain live virus vaccines.	The child has no fever and shows no other signs of infection.
2. Nursing Diagnosis: Imbalanced Nutrition: Less than Body Requirements related to loss of appetite and decreased absorption of nutrients		
NIC Priority Intervention: **Nutrition management:** Assistance with or provision of a balanced dietary intake of food and fluids		**NOC Suggested Outcome:** **Nutritional status:** Nutrient value: adequacy of nutrients taken into the body
Goal: The child will demonstrate adequate nutritional status to meet metabolic needs.		
■ Encourage frequent small meals to promote nutritional and fluid intake. ■ Maintain nasogastric tube feeding, if ordered. Total parenteral nutrition may be necessary to ensure adequate nutrition. ■ Eliminate unpleasant stimuli and odors from the environment during meals. ■ Monitor skin turgor every shift. ■ Involve a nutritionist in planning a diet for the child that includes favorite foods.	■ Additional nutrition is required to rebuild the immune system. ■ Unpleasant stimuli decrease the desire for food. ■ Skin turgor reflects hydration status. ■ Including favorite food encourages intake.	The child eats frequent meals of adequate nutritional content.
3. Nursing Diagnosis: Risk for Impaired Skin Integrity related to skin infection, immobility, or diarrhea		
NIC Priority Intervention: **Skin surveillance:** Collection and analysis of patient data to maintain skin integrity		**NOC Suggested Outcome:** **Risk control:** Actions to eliminate or reduce actual, personal, and modifiable health threats

NURSING CARE PLAN—continued

THE CHILD WITH ACQUIRED IMMUNODEFICIENCY SYNDROME

Intervention	Rationale	Expected Outcome
Goal: The child will have structural intactness and normal physiologic function of skin.		
■ Observe all pressure areas closely for signs of infection or breakdown. ■ Keep skin clean and dry. Provide perineal care to minimize irritation from diarrhea.	■ Skin care is important in the immunocompromised child. The skin may be the only intact defense the child has. ■ Prevents breaking or cracking of skin.	The child is free of preventable skin breakdown.

4. Nursing Diagnosis: Risk for Impaired Oral Mucous Membrane related to infection

NIC Priority Intervention: **Oral health restoration:** Promotion of healing for a patient who has an oral mucosa lesion		**NOC Suggested Outcome:** **Tissue integrity:** Structural intactness and normal physiologic function of mucous membranes
Goal: The child will have intact oral mucous membranes.		
■ Inspect mouth for signs of blistering or lesions. ■ Provide mouth care with normal saline solution or lemon-glycerine swabs every 2–4 hours.	■ Candidal infection is frequently associated with immunodeficiency. ■ Provides comfort and promotes healing.	The child has intact oral mucous membranes.

5. Nursing Diagnosis: Pain related to Infections

NIC Priority Intervention: **Pain management:** Alleviation of pain or a reduction in pain to level of comfort that is acceptable to the patient		**NOC Suggested Outcome:** **Comfort level:** Feelings of physical and psychologic ease
Goal: The child will be free of pain or experience only mild pain/discomfort.		
■ Observe for signs of pain and discomfort. ■ Medicate for pain as ordered and document results. ■ Implement general comfort measures (holding, rocking, etc.).	■ Pain relief adds to the comfort of the child and family.	The child shows evidence of pain relief.

6. Nursing Diagnosis: Deficient Knowledge (Parent) related to home care of child with AIDS

NIC Priority Intervention: **Teaching, treatment:** Preparing a patient and family to understand and mentally prepare for a treatment		**NOC Suggested Outcome:** **Knowledge, treatment regimen:** Extent of understanding conveyed about AIDS treatment
Goal: The parent(s) will demonstrate knowledge about home care, measures to prevent infection, and signs and symptoms to report to healthcare providers.		
■ Explain the importance of optimizing the child's health status and reducing risk of complications through diet, rest, and meticulous personal hygiene. Be sure that parents and other family members understand how AIDS is spread and appropriate precautions. ■ Discuss with the parents and the child reasons for protective measures.	■ Knowledge about the disorder and preventive measures is necessary to provide safe and effective home care for the child. ■ Knowledge of rationale increases compliance.	The parent describes appropriate home care and preventive measures for a child with AIDS.

(continued)

NURSING CARE PLAN—continued

THE CHILD WITH ACQUIRED IMMUNODEFICIENCY SYNDROME

Intervention	Rationale	Expected Outcome
6. Nursing Diagnosis: Deficient Knowledge (Parent) related to home care of child with AIDS—Continued		
■ Inform the family about signs and symptoms of infection that should be reported promptly to the physician or nurse (fever, chills, cough, mild erythema).	■ Prompt treatment increases outcome.	
7. Nursing Diagnosis: Caregiver Role Strain related to anxiety about child's condition and demands of providing care		
NIC Priority Intervention: **Caregiver support:** Provision of the necessary information, advocacy, and support to facilitate primary patient care by someone other than a health professional		**NOC Suggested Outcome:** **Caregiver emotional health:** Feelings, attitudes, and emotions of a family care provider while caring for the child over an extended period of time
Goal: The parent(s) will demonstrate emotional health as evidenced by decreased anxiety related to the child's condition and care.		
■ Encourage family members to express fears and concerns regarding the child's prognosis. ■ Advise families about support services or other resources available in the community.	■ Expression of fears helps to decrease anxiety. ■ Provides additional support to help the family cope with the child's illness and the dying process, when needed.	The parent states decreased anxiety.

with upper respiratory or other infections are the best interventions to protect the child with HIV from acquiring other infections. The child should follow a modified immunization schedule that avoids exposure to live varicella vaccine. Live measles-mumps-rubella vaccine is used unless the child is severely affected with AIDS, since the risk of serious outcomes for measles disease is great (see Chapter 45 for further information about immunization schedules ∞). Tuberculosis is more common in children with AIDS so they should have annual skin tests read by health professionals (Cohen, Chen, Sunkle et al., 2000). Teach sexually active adolescents the importance of practicing safe sex and the ramifications of high-risk sexual behaviors and intravenous drug abuse.

Promote Medication Regimen Adherence

The treatment regimen with the use of antiretroviral therapies for the child with HIV or AIDS may be complex and time consuming, presenting an overwhelming challenge to the child and the family. Nonadherence to the prescribed antiretroviral treatment regimen will likely result in increased morbidity and mortality. Some common reasons for nonadherence include frequent dosing, child's displeasure with medication (large pills, gritty powders, bitter taste), and associated side effects including nausea and rashes (Brackis-Cott, Mellins, Abrams et al., 2003).

Strategies for achieving optimal management of the treatment regimen include educating the parent or care provider, and the child when old enough to understand, regarding the purpose of the medication, the benefits of adhering to the regimen, and the potential consequences of failure to adhere to the regimen. Behavior modification techniques, using positive reinforcement, can be very effective in promoting the child's adherence. Support should be provided to the family, and the medication regimen should be tailored to the family's routine. Praise should be offered to the child and parent for adhering to the regimen. If problems exist in the management of the treatment regimen, carefully listen to the family to help determine the cause. Collaborate with the family in establishing goals to help meet the prescribed treatment regimen. Consider the effect of cultural beliefs on medication adherence (see "Developing Cultural Competence: HIV/AIDS and Hispanics" and "Evidence-Based Nursing: Adolescents with HIV Infection and Medication Regimen Adherence"). If further intervention is required, other options include direct observational therapy or home visits.

Promote Respiratory Function

Because many children with AIDS develop pneumonia, encourage the child to cough and deep breathe every 2 to 4 hours. Blowing cotton balls with a straw, blowing bubbles,

DEVELOPING CULTURAL COMPETENCE

HIV/AIDS AND HISPANICS

Hispanics account for approximately 14% of the total U.S. population; however, they account for a disproportionate 18% of the total AIDS cases diagnosed due primarily to poverty and inadequate access to quality healthcare. Additionally, women may be reluctant to ask male partners to wear a condom due to machismo behavior displayed by some Hispanic males; this can increase the risk of heterosexual spread of disease. Nurses need to be aware of these cultural concerns in the Hispanic population and provide them an opportunity to discuss concerns about HIV/AIDS. CDC funded programs are now providing community-based free health clinics and other bilingual services (CDC, 2004a).

or other games may engage the interest of a younger child. Reposition infants frequently so all areas of the lungs can aerate. Rest periods to conserve energy and lower the body's demand for oxygen are important.

Promote Adequate Nutritional Intake

Because many children with AIDS have failure to thrive, nutrition is an important part of their care. (See Chapter 34 for information to include in a detailed nutritional assessment. ∞) A nutritionist should be involved in planning an appropriate diet for the child that provides necessary calories, protein, and other nutrients. Vitamins may be especially lacking in the diets of infected children. Antioxidants (vitamin A, vitamin E, zinc, and selenium) enhance general immune system function; children should get recommended levels. Periodic dietary analysis and teaching are needed. Adequate nutrition is sometimes provided by hyperalimentation.

Diarrhea resulting from gastrointestinal infection and lactose intolerance is common in these children and complicates other nutritional disturbances. Antidiarrheal medications may be prescribed or alternative formulas tried. Keep the child's lips and mouth moist and pay close attention to hydration status. Monitor the skin turgor and urine output, and provide careful perineal skin care to prevent infection.

Frequent *Candida* infections lead to blisters, cracking, and discharge involving the oral mucous membranes. Mouth care with a non-alcohol-based solution such as normal saline or lemon-glycerine swabs should be done every 2 to 4 hours.

Provide Emotional Support

The family of the child with AIDS is under great strain. The mother and others in the family may also be infected. Integrate social services and support groups into the care of the child as soon as the diagnosis is made.

EVIDENCE-BASED NURSING

ADOLESCENTS WITH HIV INFECTION AND MEDICATION REGIMEN ADHERENCE

Problem
Medication adherence is a major problem in the HIV-infected adolescent.

Evidence
An increase in incidence of human immunodeficiency virus has been seen in the United States, particularly among young people ages 13 to 19 years. Adherence to highly active antiretroviral therapy (HAART) has been shown to decrease morbidity and mortality. However, medication adherence in this age group is often poor. The REACH (Reaching for Excellence in Adolescent Care) project has conducted studies evaluating medication adherence in the HIV-positive adolescent.

In face-to-face interviews of HIV-infected adolescents enrolled in REACH from several U.S. cities, only 41% ($n = 161$) reported consistently taking their medication as prescribed. Depressed mood was a major factor in nonadherence.

In another REACH study, 114 HIV-positive adolescents prescribed HAART were interviewed regarding barriers associated with medication adherence. Participants reported simply forgetting to take their medication, not having medication available to take (e.g., left medication at home), and variations in their daily routine as key reasons for not taking the prescribed medications as directed.

Nursing Implications
In these studies adherence to medication regimens was noted to be closely tied to depressed mood, to lack of understanding of the importance of strictly following medication directions, as well as to daily routine. This suggests that improving organizational skills, better education, and treatment for depression could have a positive impact on medication adherence.

Critical Thinking
1. What are some barriers that may lead to medication nonadherence in the HIV-positive adolescent?
2. What support does the adolescent need to improve medication adherence?
3. What measures can the nurse take to improve medication adherence in the adolescent?

Reference
Murphy, D. A., Wilson, C. M., Durako, S. J., Muenz, L. R., & Belzer, M. (2001). Antiretroviral medication adherence among the REACH HIV-infected adolescent cohort in the USA. *AIDS Care, 13*(1), 27–41.

THINKING CRITICALLY

THE TODDLER WITH AIDS

Raymond, a 2-year-old child, has had recurrent infections since he was born. After a recent illness with fever, vomiting, and diarrhea, blood tests were done to evaluate his immune function. He was diagnosed with AIDS and admitted to a special unit of the hospital for children with AIDS.

- What physical needs does Raymond have at this time?
- He manifests failure to thrive, a frequent occurrence with AIDS. How can the nurse and dietitian work together to plan a diet for him to enable him to grow?
- What information does Raymond's family need?
- What can you do to provide emotional support for them?
- What community and Internet resources could be helpful?

Spend time talking with the family about their fears and feelings. In many parts of the United States, AIDS still carries a tremendous stigma, and the family may not be able to discuss their feelings outside the healthcare environment. Safeguard the family's wishes about the privacy of the diagnosis.

Clarify any misconceptions the older child with AIDS may have about transmission of the disease. Clearly discuss routes of transmission and the need for safe sexual practices with adolescents. Providing support for adolescents is particularly important, as the dependence which this chronic and terminal disease brings can make it difficult to meet the developmental task of independence. Adolescents may benefit from contact with other infected peers.

NURSING PRACTICE

Disclosure of patient information is a breach of confidentiality that may subject you to legal action. Disclosure of confidential information occurs whenever a patient's condition—for example, a diagnosis of AIDS—is discussed inappropriately with any third party.

Discharge Planning

The diagnosis of AIDS is surrounded by strong emotions and fears. Be honest and direct. Education is essential. Explain that there is no evidence that casual contact among family members can spread the infection. For the child hospitalized, identify home care needs well in advance of discharge.

Discuss the family's finances as well as health insurance coverage for the child's care. Assess the family's ability to provide nutritious food, required medications, and a supportive environment. Refer to services as needed to ensure that the child gets quality care after discharge.

Support groups, home healthcare nursing services, financial assistance, and psychologic counseling are usually needed at some point during the child's illness, and the family should be aware of the availability of such services. Help the family deal with guilt feelings about the child's condition.

Nursing Care in the Community

Much of the care of the child with HIV infection or AIDS takes place in the community. Evaluate the family and community support systems and provide resources and referrals as needed. Many children with HIV infection are placed in foster homes, and these families need careful instruction to manage this multifaceted illness.

School attendance guidelines for children with AIDS by the American Academy of Pediatrics (AAP) and the CDC recommend unrestricted school attendance for children with AIDS or AIDS-related complex as long as their physician approves. Contraindications to school attendance include lack of control of body secretions, biting, and open wounds that cannot be covered. The nurse often prepares the school personnel with training related to care for children with known and unknown cases of HIV. The nurse also may be responsible for providing medicines or other care for the HIV-infected child at school.

NURSING PRACTICE

Because children with HIV or other bloodborne infections may be enrolled in childcare centers, staff in these centers should use standard precautions in handling blood and body fluids. Instruct daycare center personnel in use of these precautions. Help childcare centers establish procedures to notify all parents when a child with an infectious disease has been at the center. Parents of immunocompromised children can then take any necessary precautions to minimize the chances of their children becoming ill. Parents of HIV-infected children must be very cautious to limit the exposure of their children to infectious diseases.

Help the family alter the home environment to provide standard precautions during care. Make sure the child and family understand that HIV is transmitted through blood, urine, stool, and other body secretions. Teach family members the importance of careful hygiene. Encourage careful handwashing and tell parents to use precautions when handling body fluids. Explain that they should wear gloves when changing diapers; disposing of urine, stool, and emesis; or treating the child's cuts and scrapes. Instruct parents to use a bleach solution for disinfection of objects when necessary and to avoid contact with people with infectious illnesses. Precautions to guard against foodborne illness are particularly important for the HIV-infected child. Parents also need instruction on correct administration and side effects of any medications the child is taking. Giving a child a complicated combination of drugs can be challenging for all families, so use teaching tailored to the particular family and repeatedly evaluate the family's success with medication administration.

Emphasize the importance of promoting the child's development. Perform frequent developmental screenings. Teach the parents how to support the child in achieving developmental milestones. Encourage contact with other children and adults, provide for appropriate toys, teach parents how to encourage the child's communication, and praise the family for what the child has already accomplished. Children who manifest decreasing developmental milestones or other neurologic symptoms should be assessed for HIV-induced encephalopathy by the primary care provider. The nurse's record of development will be of great importance in this situation.

The child needs regular health maintenance care, such as child health supervision visits, immunizations, and care for any other health conditions. (See "Health Promotion: The Child with HIV or AIDS.")

EVALUATION

There are many desired outcomes of care for the child with HIV infection or AIDS. These include the following:

- Decreased numbers of cases of pediatric HIV due to vertical transmission from known infected mothers
- Prevention of infectious diseases in children with the virus
- Adequate respiratory function and perfusion
- Nutritional intake to support normal growth patterns and prevent malnutrition
- Adequate family coping with the stress of chronic disease
- School attendance and support in the educational process

AUTOIMMUNE DISORDERS

An immune system damaged by pathologic changes may react to some of the body's own proteins, resulting in the production of autoantibodies. These pathologic conditions in which the body directs the immune response against itself—identifying "self" as "nonself"—are called autoimmune disorders.

The primary feature of autoimmune disorders is tissue injury caused by a probable immunologic reaction of the host with its own tissues. Structural or functional changes occur as immune cells attack other cells in the body.

The autoimmune disorders are grouped into systemic and organ-specific diseases. Systemic diseases, which largely involve more than one organ, include systemic lupus erythematosus and juvenile rheumatoid arthritis. Organ-specific diseases, which primarily affect a single organ, include type 1 diabetes mellitus (see Chapter 56 ∞) and thyroiditis. Idiopathic (or immune) thrombocytic purpura is an immune disease affecting blood platelets and clotting and is discussed in Chapter 49. ∞

SYSTEMIC LUPUS ERYTHEMATOSUS

Systemic lupus erythematosus (SLE) is a chronic inflammatory disease of unknown origin that involves many organ systems. SLE affects 7 per 100,000 individuals and is more common in African Americans, Hispanics, and Asians than in Caucasians. Females are affected more than males with a 9:1 ratio (Mulvihill, 2003). The majority of cases are diagnosed during the teenage and early adult years.

The three classifications of systemic lupus erythematosus are as follows:

- **Systemic lupus**—involves one or more of the following systems: cardiovascular, central nervous system, hematologic, kidneys, lungs, musculoskeletal.
- **Drug-induced lupus**—associated with some antineoplastic drugs, isoniazid (INH), hydralazine

(Apresoline), and others. The symptoms generally subside after the drugs are discontinued.

- **Discoid lupus**—involvement of the disorder is limited to the skin.

ETIOLOGY AND PATHOPHYSIOLOGY

The exact etiology of SLE is unknown. It is believed that an outside environmental agent causes the body to initiate an abnormal immune system response to its own tissues. A genetic component is suspected as the disease is often more prevalent in members of the same family. Specific medications, diet, hormones, sunlight, stress, and viruses have been linked to systemic lupus erythematosus (Mulvihill, 2003). Approximately 5% of the children born to individuals with lupus will develop the illness (Lupus Foundation of America, 2004).

The body produces autoantibodies and combines with antigens to form immune complexes. These antigen–antibody complexes are deposited in the connective tissue, triggering an inflammatory response. The chronic inflammation then destroys connective tissue. The tissue damage varies according to the organ involvement, though the tissues most likely to be affected are the small blood vessels, glomeruli, joints, spleen, and heart valves. Because many systems can be affected simultaneously, organ damage with subsequent multisystem failure may occur.

CLINICAL MANIFESTATIONS

Manifestations of SLE may be acute, with onset of nephritis, arthritis, or vasculitis, or may be noted as a gradual onset with nonspecific symptoms. Symptoms depend on the organ involved and the amount of tissue damage that has occurred. Initial nonspecific symptoms include fever, chills, fatigue, malaise, and weight loss. The most common symptoms are arthritis and skin rash. A butterfly rash on the face, consisting of a pink or red rash over the bridge of the nose extending to the cheeks, is a characteristic finding. Children with SLE may have hemolytic anemia, with a low white blood cell and platelet count; bleeding disorders; hypergammaglobulinemia; and vasculitis. See "Clinical Manifestations: Systemic Lupus Erythematosus" for a comprehensive list of the clinical manifestations of SLE.

Systemic lupus erythematosus is characterized by periods of remission and exacerbation (flares). Flares are triggered by a variety of causes, including sun exposure, a cold or other infection, and stress. The child or family may be able to identify other triggers to flares, such as particular events, activities, or situations.

CLINICAL THERAPY

Blood tests reveal anemia, an elevated blood urea nitrogen (BUN), abnormal plasma proteins, abnormal erythrocyte sedimentation rate (ESR), presence of antinuclear antibodies, and a positive LE (lupus erythematosus) cell reaction, which indicates nonspecific inflammation. The Coombs' test is positive. Radiologic examinations include chest radiographs and CT scans, as well as MRI of affected joints. A 24-hour urine collection and imaging studies, as well as renal biopsies, may be performed to evaluate lupus nephritis. Urinalysis may reveal proteinuria.

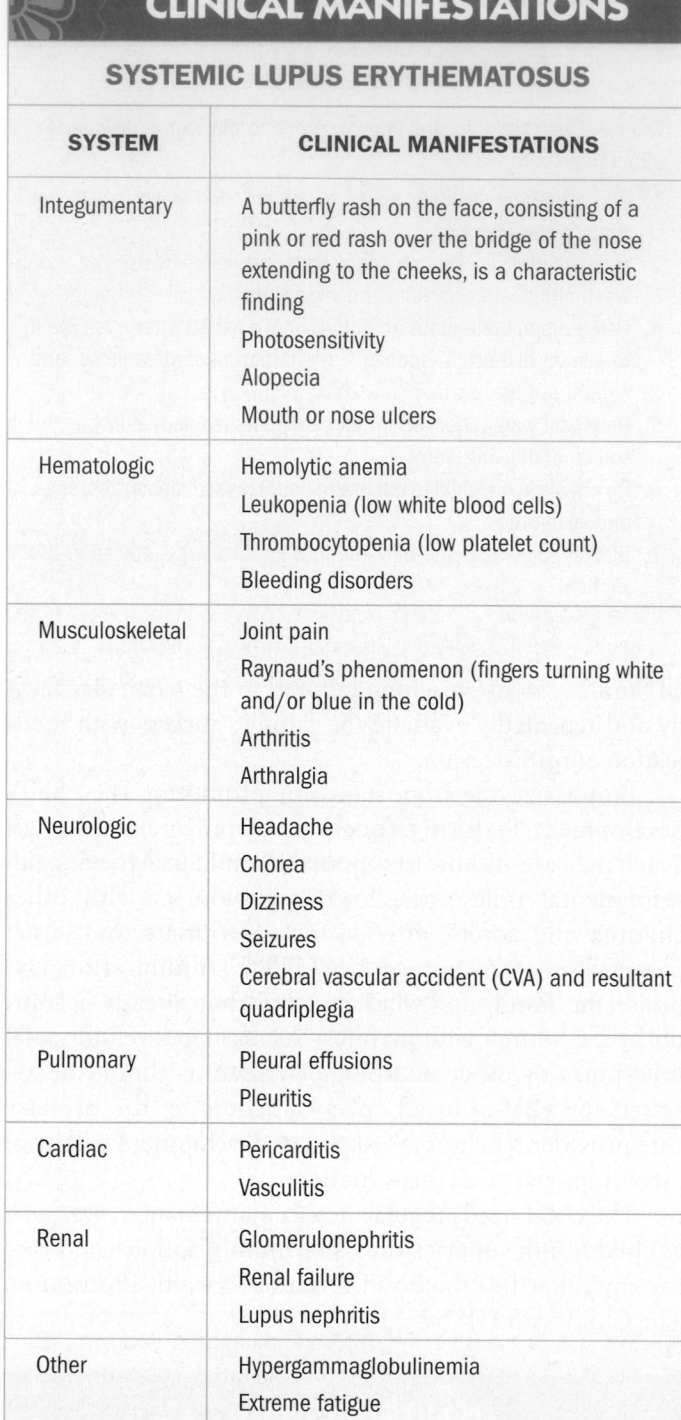

CLINICAL MANIFESTATIONS

SYSTEMIC LUPUS ERYTHEMATOSUS

SYSTEM	CLINICAL MANIFESTATIONS
Integumentary	A butterfly rash on the face, consisting of a pink or red rash over the bridge of the nose extending to the cheeks, is a characteristic finding Photosensitivity Alopecia Mouth or nose ulcers
Hematologic	Hemolytic anemia Leukopenia (low white blood cells) Thrombocytopenia (low platelet count) Bleeding disorders
Musculoskeletal	Joint pain Raynaud's phenomenon (fingers turning white and/or blue in the cold) Arthritis Arthralgia
Neurologic	Headache Chorea Dizziness Seizures Cerebral vascular accident (CVA) and resultant quadriplegia
Pulmonary	Pleural effusions Pleuritis
Cardiac	Pericarditis Vasculitis
Renal	Glomerulonephritis Renal failure Lupus nephritis
Other	Hypergammaglobulinemia Extreme fatigue

The goals of medical management are to create a remission of symptoms and to prevent complications. Corticosteroids, such as prednisone, are prescribed to control inflammation. Antimalarial preparations, such as hydroxychloroquine and chloroquine, are used to treat symptoms associated with skin lesions and renal and arthritic problems. Although the exact action of these drugs on SLE is not known, they often permit continued remission with a lowered dose of steroids. Nonsteroidal anti-inflammatory drugs (aspirin, ibuprofen, naproxen) are used to relieve muscle and joint pain. Immunosuppressant drugs, such as cyclosporin and methotrexate, have been used to help control SLE. Diet may be restricted if the child has excessive weight gain or fluid retention from steroids and renal damage.

NURSING PRACTICE

The side effects of the corticosteroids, immunosuppressants, and antimalarial drugs used in the treatment of children with SLE are significant and include hair loss, susceptibility to infection, "moon face," retinal damage, and bone loss. These are significant side effects for the adolescent who is commonly concerned about appearance. Teens with SLE may need special teaching, guidance, and support. Support groups or Internet chat rooms may be helpful.

Prognosis depends on the severity of the internal organ involvement; however, while SLE was once considered a fatal disease, the survival rate is now more than 97% (American College of Rheumatology, 2003). Kidney failure is managed by hemodialysis or peritoneal dialysis. Renal transplantation has been very successful for treatment of renal failure secondary to lupus nephritis.

NURSING MANAGEMENT

NURSING ASSESSMENT AND DIAGNOSIS

Physiologic Assessment

A thorough assessment is needed, as symptoms are widespread. Assess the child's nutritional status, including baseline weight and history of recent weight loss or weight gain. The skin is assessed for rashes, ulcers, photosensitivity, ecchymosis, petechiae, cyanosis, and hair loss. Respiratory assessment includes breath sounds and respiratory rate and assessing for pleural effusion or pleuritis. Cardiovascular assessment includes vital signs and assessing heart sounds and for symptoms of pericarditis or friction rub. Musculoskeletal assessment includes joint pain, joint deformity, pain, weakness, and ability to perform activities of daily living. Neurologic assessment includes changes in affect or cognitive abilities and seizure activity. Gastrointestinal assessment includes splenomegaly.

Psychosocial Assessment

Because SLE is a chronic disease that affects primarily adolescents, psychosocial assessment is indicated. Assess family interactions, exploring stressful situations such as divorce or trauma. Treatment-related restrictions and changes in appearance can lead to withdrawal, depression, and suicidal tendencies. Perform psychosocial assessments periodically as the child grows and adapts to the disorder or faces new developmental challenges with a chronic disease.

Several nursing diagnoses may apply to the child with SLE. These include the following:

- *Risk for Ineffective Management of Therapeutic Regimen, Family,* related to complexity of therapeutic regimen
- *Risk for Ineffective Tissue Perfusion (Renal)* related to interrupted blood flow in kidneys
- *Risk for Impaired Skin Integrity* related to immunologic deficit
- *Risk for Activity Intolerance* related to chronic disease
- *Risk for Disturbed Body Image* related to side effects of medications and skin alterations
- *Risk for Infection* related to immunosuppressive medications
- *Pain* related to joint inflammation and injury

PLANNING AND IMPLEMENTATION

The goals of nursing care are to help the child manage and cope with a chronic disease, prevent infection, promote nutrition, facilitate a remission, and recognize and avoid triggers for flares.

Maintain Fluid Balance

Because most children with SLE have renal involvement, monitor intake and output and frequently evaluate the child's fluid and electrolyte status. Renal dysfunction can manifest itself by edema, muscle cramps, diarrhea, tetany, and convulsions.

Promote Adequate Nutrition

Currently, there are no specific dietary plans for the child with SLE; however, the diet may be restricted according to renal involvement, weight gain, weight loss, or other complications. The child is at risk for weight gain associated with treatment with steroids and a decreased activity level during exacerbations of this disease. A well-balanced, nutritious diet as well as appropriate fluid intake for age should be encouraged.

Promote Skin Integrity

The rash on mucous membranes can cause weakening of the tissues, placing the child at increased risk for infection. Encourage good hygienic measures and a mild soap.

Recommend that adolescents limit their use of cosmetics. Reinforce the importance of avoiding sunlight as much as possible and the use of sun protection factor (SPF) of 15 or higher at all times when in the sun. Encourage the child to wear protective clothing to limit exposure to sunlight (see Chapter 57 for discussion of sun exposure ∞). Avoidance of unprotected fluorescent lighting is recommended since exacerbations of systemic lupus erythematosus have been reported following this exposure (Mulvihill, 2003). Encourage the adolescent to avoid the use of tanning beds. Provide instructions on oral care to maintain intact oral mucosa. Provide instructions on the care of the head if alopecia occurs.

Promote Rest and Comfort

Because of fatigue and joint pain, the child has little energy reserve during acute episodes of the disease. Encourage frequent rest periods and a nutritious diet to maximize energy stores. A physical therapist can plan a program to encourage mobility and increase muscle strength.

Manage Side Effects of Medications

Observe for side effects of medications used for treatment, and teach the child and family about these effects. For example, immunosuppressant drugs can promote infection anywhere in the body, and nonsteroidal anti-inflammatory drugs commonly cause gastric distress and bleeding of the gastrointestinal tract. The antimalarial drug hydroxychloroquine can cause serious vision changes; thus, frequent eye examinations are needed.

Avoid Triggers for Disease Flares

Many children and their parents can recognize the signs of an impending flare and the triggers that precede them. Partner with the parents and child to implement measures to avoid these triggers. Discuss preventive behaviors such as avoiding sun exposure and avoiding stressors. Adolescents should be warned that alcohol, smoking, and drugs also pose an increased risk due to the potential to stimulate flares. Female adolescents who are sexually active should avoid birth control pills which contain the hormone estrogen since the extra estrogen may exacerbate symptoms. Alternative birth control methods should be discussed with the adolescent. See "Complementary Care: SLE and Stress" for application of stress reduction.

Prevent Infection

Infections are a leading cause of death for patients with systemic lupus erythematosus. Prophylactic antibiotics may be required for dental work and surgical procedures. Instruct the patient and family to inform all healthcare providers of the disease to plan for prophylactic measures. Educate the patient and family on the importance of ad-

---

COMPLEMENTARY CARE

SLE AND STRESS

Systemic lupus erythematosus exacerbations have been linked to stress. Stress-reducing techniques such as guided imagery, reading, and quiet games can benefit the child or adolescent and reduce exacerbations of SLE. A study by Greco, Rudy, and Manzi (2004) showed that a stress management program can provide improvement in pain and psychological and physical function. Since SLE is most common in adolescents, what stress reduction might be possible? Consider a busy teen who plays sports, has many social activities, and excels in school; how can you assist this teen to see the importance of stress reduction? How can stress reduction techniques be integrated into the daily life of an active teen?

---

hering to the immunization schedule, and to obtain a yearly influenza vaccine to prevent infection. Instruct the family on handwashing and infection control measures in the home. Warn adolescents about the dangers of tattooing and body piercing because of the risk of infection.

Provide Emotional Support

Adolescents may have an altered body image as a result of rash, alopecia, arthritic changes in the joints, and chronic disease. Referral to a lupus support group, social services, or counseling may be helpful. The American Lupus Society and the Lupus Foundation of America can provide information to help parents and children adjust to the disease The Arthritis Foundation also publishes a useful pamphlet, *Meeting the Challenge: A Young Person's Guide to Living with Lupus.*

EVALUATION

Successful outcomes of nursing care involve management of this chronic disease. Expected outcomes of nursing care include the following:

- Normal intake and output levels, with demonstrated fluid and electrolyte balance
- Maintenance of intact skin
- A balance of rest and activity to promote development
- Medication management
- Positive body image

JUVENILE RHEUMATOID ARTHRITIS

Juvenile rheumatoid arthritis (JRA) is a chronic autoimmune inflammatory disease characterized by joint inflammation resulting in decreased mobility, swelling, and pain that occurs slightly more often in girls than in boys. Juvenile rheumatoid arthritis is the most common type of arthritis in children and adolescents, and usually occurs in children between 2 and 5 or between 9 and 12 years of age. It may enter remission or occasionally continue as a chronic disease. Approximately 5 to 18 of every 100,000 children develop juvenile rheumatoid arthritis each year (Ilowite, 2002).

Remission may last for months, years, or a lifetime. Juvenile rheumatoid arthritis affects joints and surrounding tissues in addition to possibly affecting other organs such as the heart, lungs, liver, and eyes. During its course, the child may experience pain, impaired mobility, and interference with normal growth and development. Seventy percent of children with juvenile rheumatoid arthritis experience permanent remission of the disease by adulthood. Rarely the disease is unresponsive to treatment or the child may suffer lasting impairment such as bone and joint changes. Children with early onset have a better prognosis for complete recovery.

ETIOLOGY AND PATHOPHYSIOLOGY

The cause of JRA is unknown, but it is thought to have an autoimmune basis. Inflammation begins in the joint and leads to pain and swelling. Scar tissue eventually develops, resulting in limited range of motion. There are three types of JRA: pauciarticular, systemic, and polyarticular. *Pauciarticular arthritis* primarily affects the knees, ankles, and elbows, and occurs more frequently in females. *Systemic arthritis* affects males and females equally and characteristically is manifested by high fever, polyarthritis, and rheumatoid rash. Systemic arthritis affects internal organs and joints. *Polyarticular arthritis* involves many joints (five or more), particularly the small joints of the hands and fingers. It may also affect the hips, knees, feet, ankles, and neck.

CLINICAL MANIFESTATIONS

JRA may be restricted to a few joints or be systemic with involvement of multiple joints. Symptoms can include fever, rash, lymphadenopathy, splenomegaly, and hepatomegaly. The child may develop a limp or obviously favor one extremity over the other. A slow rate of growth or uneven growth of extremities may also be noted. Pain, stiffness, loss of motion, and swelling occur in the large joints such as the knees. Older children may develop symmetric involvement of the small joints of the hand. The disease is frequently chronic, extending over several years after an initial manifestation with pain and other symptoms. Remissions and exacerbations are characteristic.

CLINICAL THERAPY

Diagnosis is made primarily on the basis of the history and assessment findings, in particular, arthritis having an onset before 16 years of age and persisting for at least 6 weeks, with no other identifiable cause (Gottlieb & Ilowite, 2000). There are no specific laboratory tests for the disease. In some children, rheumatoid factor, human leukocyte anti-

gen (HLA) B27, and antinuclear antibody (ANA) tests are positive, and the ESR may be elevated.

Medical management involves drug therapy, physical therapy, and, when necessary, surgery. The goals of treatment are to relieve pain and prevent contractures. Salicylates (aspirin) or nonsteroidal anti-inflammatory drugs (tolmetin sodium, naproxen, diclofenac, ibuprofen) are prescribed to reduce inflammation. Steroids may be used with children who have moderately active disease. Children who do not respond to aspirin or nonsteroidal anti-inflammatory drugs may be treated with sulfasalazine and methotrexate. Physical therapy increases strength and mobility of joints while protecting them from injury. Surgery is occasionally performed to relieve pain and maintain or improve joint function in children with joint contractures.

> ### NURSING PRACTICE
>
> Infants and children with juvenile rheumatoid arthritis who are receiving aspirin therapy are at risk of developing Reye syndrome if they contract influenza or chickenpox. These children should be immunized with varicella vaccine and should receive influenza vaccine in the fall of each year. See Chapter 53 for further information about Reye syndrome. ∞

Complications such as eye chronic uveitis, which results from chronic inflammation, may occur in children with juvenile rheumatoid arthritis, especially those with pauciarticular arthritis. Children with polyarticular and systemic juvenile rheumatoid arthritis should be examined by an ophthalmologist for eye inflammation every 6 months, and children with pauciarticular arthritis should be examined every 3 months.

Growth interference for the child with juvenile rheumatoid arthritis is a potential complication. The specific disorder may result in bone growth disturbance such as contractures or effusions, and the administration of corticosteroids can also inhibit growth.

NURSING MANAGEMENT

NURSING ASSESSMENT AND DIAGNOSIS

A careful history is important, as it is sometimes the primary mode of diagnosis. Assess for joint swelling and deformities, fever, nodules under the skin, growth delays, and enlarged lymph nodes. Several nursing diagnoses may apply to the child with JRA. They include the following:

- *Activity Intolerance* related to chronic pain
- *Impaired Physical Mobility* related to joint stiffness
- *Anxiety* related to stress of chronic illness
- *Pain* related to joint inflammation
- *Disturbed Body Image* related to illness

MEDIALINK Animation: Methotrexate

PLANNING AND IMPLEMENTATION

Nursing care focuses on preventing pain, planning measures to enhance development in spite of illness, promoting mobility, encouraging adequate nutrition, and teaching the parents and child about the disease and its management. Most care occurs in the community, including physical therapy, with only occasional hospitalizations during an exacerbation of the disease.

Promote Improved Mobility

Physical therapists play an essential role in the child's treatment. The goals of physical therapy are to maintain joint function, strengthen muscles, increase tone, maintain body alignment, and prevent permanent deformities such as contractures. Range of motion exercises, stretching, hydrotherapy, and swimming exercises help to prevent deformities (Figure 44–2 ●). Encourage the child to perform activities of daily living. Medications may be given to reduce joint swelling and inflammation. Warm compresses to the involved joints are soothing.

Encourage Adequate Nutrition

Promote general health by encouraging a well-balanced diet. Children with decreased mobility may have reduced metabolic needs, and excess weight causes additional muscle strain. Periodically perform diet recalls and nutritional assessments. Plot growth carefully and watch for changes in growth percentiles (see Chapter 34 for additional information regarding nutrition assessment ∞).

Nursing Care in the Community

The child with JRA may never, or rarely, be hospitalized. Most care takes place during visits to healthcare offices, clin-ics, and physical therapy. Teach parents about the child's condition and prognosis, and answer their questions about the child's treatment. The child may need support to adjust to the diagnosis of a chronic illness. Encourage the child to maintain contact with peers and to attend school whenever possible. Explain to the child and parents that overexertion may exacerbate the disease. Inform parents about possible complications of JRA, such as altered growth related to early closure of epiphyseal plates, small joint contractures, and synovitis. Refer parents and children to the Arthritis Foundation and the American Juvenile Arthritis Foundation for further information and support.

Partner with the family and school officials to meet the child's needs. Accommodations at school may include providing a set of books for the home so that the child is not required to carry the books home daily. Additional time may be required for the child to move from class to class. Adaptive computers and tutors during exacerbations may be helpful. School nurses work with the child, family, and school personnel to establish the child's Individualized Education Plan (IEP).

EVALUATION

Desired outcomes for the child with JRA include the following:

- Maintenance of joint mobility
- Comfort and freedom from pain
- Positive body image
- Avoidance of infection
- Parental understanding and support of the therapeutic process

● FIGURE 44–2

The physical therapist uses hydrotherapy to help maintain joint function in a child who has juvenile rheumatoid arthritis.

ALLERGIC REACTIONS

Allergy is one of the major chronic illnesses of children today. Why are some children allergic to cats, for instance, while no one else in the family has allergies? In order to answer this question, the nurse needs a basic understanding of the mechanisms of allergy.

Allergy is an abnormal or altered reaction to an antigen. Antigens responsible for clinical manifestations of allergy are called **allergens**. Allergens can be ingested in food or drugs or injected or absorbed through contact with unbroken skin. Common allergens in children include medications (such as penicillin); animal dander; dust, mites, and mold; plant pollens; and foods (such as nuts, seafood, or egg white). An allergic reaction is an antigen–antibody reaction and can manifest itself as anaphylaxis, atopic disease, serum sickness, or contact dermatitis. Therefore, the symptoms can be mild to severe or life threatening, and they can be localized or systemic. Characteristic findings in children with allergies are summarized in Table 44–6.

TABLE 44–6 ✣ Characteristic Findings in Children with Allergies

Respiratory system: Asthma, rhinitis (seasonal and perennial), serous otitis media, cough, pneumonia, croup, edema of glottis

Gastrointestinal system: Abdominal pain and colic, stomatitis, constipation, diarrhea, bloody stools, geographical tongue, vomiting

Skin: Angioedema, urticaria, eczema, atopic dermatitis, erythema multiforme, purpura, drug and food rashes, contact dermatitis

Nervous system: Headache, tension, fatigue, convulsions, Ménière syndrome, tremor

Eye: Conjunctivitis, cataract, ciliary spasm, iritis

Blood: Thrombocytopenic purpura, hemolytic anemia, leukopenia, agranulocytosis

Musculoskeletal system: Arthralgia, myalgia, rheumatoid arthritis, torticollis

Genitourinary system: Dysuria, vulvovaginitis, enuresis

Miscellaneous: Anaphylactic shock, serum sickness, autoimmune diseases

The **hypersensitivity response**, an overreaction of the immune system, is responsible for allergic reactions. Hypersensitivity reactions have been classified into four types. Type I hypersensitivity reactions are immediate; they occur within seconds or minutes of exposure to the antigen. Symptoms can include a wheal and flare in the skin, edema, spasm of smooth muscle, wheezing, vomiting, diarrhea, or anaphylaxis. The release of chemical substances such as histamine is responsible for the signs and symptoms. The first time a child is exposed to the allergen, there is no reaction. With every exposure thereafter, however, the allergic child may have a reaction to the allergen.

NURSING PRACTICE

Anaphylaxis is an exaggerated hypersensitivity reaction that may manifest with itching; localized or generalized hives on the hands, feet, or mucosa; soft tissue swelling; cough; dyspnea; pallor; sweating; and tachycardia. Severe reactions may lead to respiratory distress or death. Nursing roles involve preventing anaphylactic reactions by teaching families how to minimize exposure and by alerting all healthcare personnel in hospitals and clinics to the child's allergy. In addition, it is important to know emergency procedures in all facilities such as schools, homes, and hospitals.

CLINICAL MANIFESTATIONS

TYPES OF HYPERSENSITIVITY REACTIONS

TYPE	ETIOLOGY	CLINICAL MANIFESTATIONS	EXAMPLES
Type I Localized or systemic reactions (anaphylaxis)	Antibodies bind to certain cells, causing release of chemical substances that produce an inflammatory reaction.	Hypotension, wheezing, gastrointestinal spasm, uterine spasm; stridor, urticaria	Extrinsic asthma Hay fever
Type II Tissue-specific reactions	Antibodies cause activation of complement system, which leads to tissue damage.	Variable; may include dyspnea or fever	Transfusion reaction ABO incompatibility Hemolytic disease of the newborn
Type III Immune-complex reactions	Immune complexes are deposited in tissues, where they activate complement, which results in a generalized inflammatory reaction.	Urticaria, fever, joint pain	Acute glomerulonephritis Serum sickness
Type IV Delayed reactions	Antigens stimulate T cells that release lymphokines, which cause inflammation and tissue damage.	Variable; may include fever, erythema, pruritus	Contact dermatitis Tuberculin skin test Graft-versus-host disease Allograft rejection

Type IV reactions are delayed responses that do not appear until several hours after exposure and require 24 to 72 hours to develop fully. A type IV reaction, which is not confined to any specific tissue, is elicited by relatively complex antigens such as those of bacteria and viruses and by simple antigens such as drugs and metals. Symptoms include contact dermatitis, itching, and blistering.

Assessment of the child with an allergy includes a complete physical examination; laboratory, x-ray, and pulmonary function studies; tests of nasal function; and skin testing. Treatment generally involves avoidance of the allergen, such as substitution of a different drug when the child has a drug allergy. Desensitization may sometimes be used with increasing doses of the allergen administered intradermally in an office where resuscitation is readily available. This treatment is useful for allergy to bees or some pollens. For skin allergies, the allergen is avoided, skin is kept well lubricated, and topical steroids may be used. Oral antihistamines are sometimes used to treat allergy. When exposure to an allergen occurs, medical care may include treatment of anaphylaxis.

NURSING MANAGEMENT

The child with allergies requires a thorough assessment, including a complete past medical history, family history, personal and social history, and review of symptoms. The history focuses on the following areas:

- What symptoms does the child experience? Encourage the child to describe the difficulty in his or her own words.

- Are the symptoms continuous or intermittent? What are the frequency and duration of episodes?

- When did the child first begin to experience symptoms? Did the child have eczema or a feeding problem in infancy or childhood? Did the infant have frequent bouts of colic or skin problems when new foods were introduced? Was there a change in symptoms at puberty? Are the symptoms becoming worse or spontaneously improving?

- What known agents in the environment cause difficulties?

- Are there seasonal variations in symptoms? At what time of the day or night do symptoms usually occur?

The nurse may be responsible for performing intradermal skin tests for allergies (Figure 44–3 ●). Nursing care focuses on treating the symptoms, alleviating the anxiety of the child and parents, and identifying the allergens. Teaching the child and family how to minimize or avoid exposure to allergens is important. Teach parents of children who have had severe reactions to bee or wasp stings how to take precautions and how to provide emergency treatment if the child is stung.

● **FIGURE 44–3**

Results of intradermal skin testing on the forearm. Injections are given on each side of the markings. Note the positive results marked by induration and erythema in response to certain antigens.

Used with permission from VU/Southern Illinois University/Visuals Unlimited.

Families may need instructions on allergy-proofing the home. Pets, dust, carpets, fabrics, feather pillows and bedding, and cigarette smoke can all cause allergic reactions. If families are reluctant to give up pets, frequent baths can reduce dander, which is the usual allergen. Instruct the family on proper use of epinephrine (Figure 44–4 ●).

When the child has type I reactions to an environmental substance, avoidance of the allergen is most critical. In addition, care providers, families, and school personnel must be able to treat anaphylaxis if exposure to the allergen occurs. Be sure to label the child's chart and bed and apply a red armband to alert others to allergies when the child is hospitalized. School nurses keep records about children's allergies and inform school personnel about the allergies and cautions that need to be followed. See Chapter 34 for more information about serious reactions to food, such as

● **FIGURE 44–4**

The school nurse is teaching a parent and a teacher about the correct use of the EpiPen, which is being maintained at home and at school in case of allergic reaction in a child who has a peanut allergy.

peanut allergy. ∞ Nurses must be aware of the resuscitation procedures and equipment in all facilities such as hospital units, offices, childcare centers, and schools. See Chapter 47 for airway maintenance. ∞

LATEX ALLERGY

Latex allergy is common among healthcare workers, those in other occupations, and patients. About 10% of healthcare workers, 50% of children with spina bifida, and 34% of children with three or more surgeries are sensitive to latex (Brehler & Kutting, 2001). Many healthcare products, such as gloves, drains, catheters, and intravenous ports, contain latex, a sap from the rubber tree. Latex allergy is caused by an IgE-mediated response that develops after repeated exposure to latex. In some cases, intraoperative deaths have occurred when allergic individuals were exposed to latex products during surgery. A reaction to latex products can be manifested as irritant reaction of the skin, type IV of delayed hypersensitivity with redness, inflam-

mation, and blisters on the skin, or type I hypersensitivity, which is immediate and often has systemic manifestations (itchy eyes, asthma, or anaphylaxis).

Children most at risk for latex allergy include those with myelodysplasia and congenital urinary tract anomalies. Up to 70% of children with spina bifida have immunoglobulin E (IgE) antibodies to latex, and other at-risk groups include children with bladder exstrophy (Houribane, Allard, Wade et al., 2002). People who have had repeated surgeries are also at higher risk due to high exposure to latex during surgery. Healthcare personnel are also at risk for latex allergy because of exposure in the workplace (Table 44–7).

Children and adolescents at high risk should receive allergy testing for latex; the radioallergosorbent test (RAST) is most often used. This test measures circulating IgE antibodies to many allergens, and correlates well with results of allergy skin testing. Healthcare personnel should use alternative products when caring for people at risk.

When a positive skin test has occurred or when the person has had a reaction to latex, all latex products

TABLE 44–7 ✣ Measures to Protect Latex Allergy

Healthcare personnel are at high risk of developing latex allergy because of intense exposure to products containing latex. An estimated 8–12% of healthcare workers are latex sensitive. You can protect yourself by using the following measures:

- Decrease exposure by using alternative products whenever available (use synthetic rubbers, polyethylene, nitrile, neoprene, vinyl gloves).
- Use powder-free gloves if using latex gloves (the powder has high amounts of latex, which are inhaled).
- Avoid oil-based hand creams and lotions before putting on latex gloves, as these preparations break down the latex.
- When you have symptoms of sensitivity to latex on exposure (rash, hives, nasal congestion, conjunctivitis, cough, or wheeze), contact the Employee Health Department of your facility.
- If severely allergic, avoid all contact and wear a medical identification bracelet.
- Contact the National Institute of Occupational Safety and Health (NIOSH) at 800-346-4647 or the American Nurses Association at 800-637-0323 for more information.

TABLE 44–8 ❖ **Sources of Latex in Hospital, Home, and Community with Recommended Alternatives**

Frequently Contain Latex	Examples of LATEX-SAFE Alternatives/Barriers
Latex in the Hospital	
Adhesives, skin (Smith+Nephew)	Mastisol (Ferndale)
Anesthesia circuits, bags, oxygen masks	Neoprene (Anesthesia Associates, Ohmeda adult), some Vital Signs
Bandaids	Active Strip (3M), CURAD Neon, Readi-Bandages, NHP, some Airstrip
Blood pressure cuff, tubing (J&J)	Cleen Cuff (Vital Signs), nylon (some Trimline)
Bulb syringe	selected Davol, Medline, Rusch, Premium, Baxter
Casts: Delta-Lite Podiatry, Orthoflex (J&J)	Scotchcast soft, Delta-Lites, recent Conformable (J&J), Caraglas Ultra, liners (Gore)
Catheters, condom	Clear Advantage, ProSys NL, selected Coloplast, Rochester, PolyTech (Hollister)
Catheters, indwelling & systems, UDS	some Am BioMed, Argyle, Bard, Cook, Dale, Kendall, Lifetech, Mentor, Rochester, Rusch, Vitaid. Adapters & plug (Addto)
Catheters, cardiac, vascular, pulmonary	some World Medical, Am BioMed
Catheters, straight, coude	Mentor, RobNel (Sherwood), Coloplast, selected Bard, Rusch catheters
Catheters, feeding	Accumark feeding catheter (Sims Portex)
CPR manikins & Medical training aids	most Laerdal products
Dressings: Dyna-flex, butterfly closures (J&J) BDF Elastoplast, Action Wrap, Coban (3M) Lyofoam (Acme), Spandage (Medi-tech), Telfa	Duoderm, Reston foam (3M), Opsite, Venigard, Comfeel, Sorbaview, Telfa (some) Xeroform, PinCare, Bioclusive, Montg'ry strap (J&J), Webril, Metalline, Selopor, Opraflex, Centurion brief, some Airstrips, Rainbow Net (Surgilast), VAC

Note: latex in package only: Steri-strip wound closure system, Tegaderm, Tegasorb, Active Strips (3M), Nu-Derm (J&J), CURAD

Ear Plugs	Grainger (5F767)
Elastic wrap: ACE, Esmarch, Zimmer Dyna-flex, Elastikon (J&J)	E-Cotton, CEB elastic (coNco), Champ (Carolon), Adban Adhesive, X-Mark (Avcor) Co-Flex, PowerFlex (Andover), Comprilan (Jobst), Esmark (DeRoyal), NHP)
Electrode bulbs, pads, grounding	some Baxter, Dantec EMG, Conmed, ValleyLab, Vermont Med, Staodyn, Neotrode
Endotracheal tubes, airways	selected Berman, Mallinckrodt, Polamedco, Portex, Rusch, Sheridan, Shiley
Enemas	BabyLax, Theravac, Bowel Man't Tube (MIC), Pharmaseal set, all Fleet Ready-to-use, cone irrigation set (Convatec), silicone retention cuff tip (Lafayette)
G-tubes, buttons	Silicone (Bard, Flexiflo, MIC, Rusch, Stomate)
Gloves: sterile, clean, surgical, orthodontic	Allergard (J&J), dermaprene (Ansell), N-DEX (Best), Safeskin Nitrile, Neolon, SensiCare, Tru-touch (Maxxim), Nitrex, Tactyl 1,2 (SmartPractice), Duraprene (Allegiance Healthcare), Elastyren (Hermal, Center Labs), Boston Medical, Masel, Neotech
Incentive deep breathing exerciser	Voldyne 5000 (Sherwood David & Geck), Triflo II
IV access: injection ports, Y-sites, bags, pumps, buretrol ports, PRN adapters, needleless systems	**Cover Y-sites and bag ports – do not puncture. Use stopcocks for meds.** Polymer injection caps + burettes + Safsite (Braun), Abbot systems, Walrus, Gemini (IMED), selected Baxter (InterLink), Statlock, Ready Med, ConMed, Clave, Alaris, Hudson, select Sims, IV boards (Avcor), Terumo Pumps: Mach II, ADS 100; Clic-Open (vial top remover – Sepha Pharm.)
OR/Infection Control masks, hats, shoe covers	some by Kimberly Clark, TECNOL; OR & sterile packs (CML, DeRoyal) twill ties
Medication vial stoppers	some AmRegent, Astra, Bedford Labs, Fujisawa, Gensia, Glaxo, Lilly, Roche
Miscellaneous items	Soft-Grip fabric clamp covers (Scanlan), Precision Dynamics I.D. bracelets
Penrose drains	Jackson-Pratt, Zimmer Hemovac
Pulse oximeters, thermometer probes	Nonin oximeters, **selected** Nellcor sensors, Diatec probe covers
Reflex hammers	Cover with plastic bag
Respirators	Advantage (MSA), HEPA-Tech (Uvex), PFR 95 (Tecnol), 3M 1860
Resuscitators, manual	certain Ambu, Armstrong, Laerdal, Puriton Bennett, Vital Blue, Respironics, Rusch
Spacer (for metered dose inhalers)	ACE spacer (Center Labs), OptiHaler (HealthScan)
Stethoscope tubing	PVC (some Littman) cover with ScopeCoat or latex-free stockinette (Albahealth)
Suction tubing	PVC (Davol, Laerdal, Mallinckrodt, Superior, Yankauer) Medline, Ballard
Syringes, disposable	Terumo Medical, Abbott PCA Abboject, Norm-Ject (Air-Tite), EpiPen, selected BD syringes, AdvantaJet (Activa)

Used with permission from the Spina Bifida Association of America. www.sbaa.org.4590 MacArthur Blvd NW Suite 250 Washington DC: 20001-4226.

Frequently Contain Latex	Examples of LATEX-SAFE Alternatives/Barriers
Tapes: pink, Waterproof (3M), Zonas, Moleskin, cloth, Waterproof (J&J), adhesive felt (Acme)	Dermicel (J&J), Durapore, Microfoam, Micropore, Transpore (3M) Cath-Strip (Genetic Labs), Ice Tape (P.O.Pak), All-Felt (Universal Foot Care)
Tonopen disposable covers (glaucoma tester)	
Tourniquets	Children's Medical, Grafco, VelcroPedic, X-Tourn straps (Avcor), Free-Band (Kent)
Theraband (also strip, tube), Other OT supplies	REP Bands & Cords (OPTP), Exercise putty (Rolyan), new Thera-Band Exercisers plastic tubing-Tygon LR-40
Tubing, sheeting	(Norton), elastic thread, sheets (JPS Elastomerics)
Vascular stockings (Jobst)	Compriform Custom (Jobst)
Latex in the Home and Community	
Art supplies: paints, glue, erasers, fabric paints	Elmers (School Glue, Glue-All, GluColors, Carpenters Wood Glue, Sno-Drift paste) FaberCastel erasers, Crayola (**except** stamps, erasers), Liquitex paints, DickBlick Tempera & acrylic paints & soap erasers, Play-Doh
Balloons	Mylar balloons, self-sealing *Myloons*
Balls: Koosh balls, tennis balls, bowling balls	PVC (Hedstrom Sports Ball), Nerf Foam Balls
Carpet backing, gym floor, basement sealant	Provide barrier–cloth or mat
Chewing gum	Bubblicious, Trident (Warner-Lambert), Wrigley gums (check new products)
Clothes: applique on Tees, elastic on socks, underwear, sneakers, sandals	Cloth-covered elastic, neoprene (Decent Exposures, NOLATEX Industries) Buster Brown elastic-free socks (Vermont Country Store)
Condoms, contraceptive sponges, diaphragm	Polyurethane (Avanti), female condom (Reality), Wideseal Silicone Diaphragms (Milex), Trojan Supra Condom
Crutches: tips, axillary pads, hand grips	Cover with cloth, tape
Dental dams, cups, bands, root canal material orthodontic rubber bands	PURO/M27 intraoral elastics (Midwest Orthodontic), wire springs, sealant (Delton) dams (Meer Dental, Hygenic Corp), John O Butler, Earloop masks (Richmond)
Diapers, Incontinence pads, rubber pants	Huggies, First Quality, Gold Seal, Tranquility, Always, some Attends, Drypers Diapers (not training pants), Confidence (Paper-Pak), Pampers, Luvs
Feeding nipples	Silicone, vinyl (**selected** Gerber, Evenflo, MAM, Ross, Mead Johnson)
Food handled with latex gloves	Synthetic gloves for food handling
Note: associated allergies are reported to banana, avocado, chestnut, kiwi, and other fruits	
Handles on racquets, tools, bicycles	Vinyl, leather handles, or cover with cloth or tape
Infant toothbrush-massager	Soft bristle brush or cloth, Gerber/NUK
Kitchen cleaning gloves	PVC MYPLEX (Magla), cotton liners (Allerderm)
Miscellaneous items	*some* medical stickers by MediBadge, UAL, Cushie Tushie Potty Seat
Newsprint, ads, coupons, lottery scratch tickets	
Pacifiers	Soothies (Children's Med Ventures), **selected** Binky, Gerber, Infa, Kip, MAM
Rubber bands, bungee cords	Plasti bands
Toys–Stretch Armstrong, old Barbies	Jurassic Park figures (Kenner), 1993 Barbie, Disney dolls (Mattel), many toys by Fisher Price, Little Tikes, Playskool, Discovery, Trolls (Norfin), Silly-putty
Water toys & equipment: beach thongs, masks, bathing suits, caps, scuba gear, goggles	PVC, plastic, nylon, Suits Me Swimwear
Wheelchair cushions, tires	Jay, ROHO cushions, Use leather gloves, Sof Care bed/chair cushions (Gaymar)
Zippered plastic storage bags	Waxed paper, plain plastic bags, Ziploc bags

must be removed from the allergic individual's environment. Alternative products, such as nonlatex gloves and catheters, must be used when providing healthcare. People allergic to latex should also wear a medical identification bracelet at all times and should have an epinephrine kit readily available at home and school. Nurses should be alert for any signs of hypersensitivity when the child is receiving healthcare, and be prepared with drugs and equipment to treat anaphylaxis. This is especially important in operative settings when acute anaphylaxis is often life threatening. Nurses should emphasize to parents and children that many everyday products contain latex, including latex balloons and condoms (Table 44–8).

GRAFT-VERSUS-HOST DISEASE

Graft-versus-host disease can occur when bone marrow or stem cells are transfused into a recipient, typically as treatment for leukemia or severe combined immunodeficiency disease. The donated cells attach to the recipient child's bone marrow and begin production. The child's lymphocyte production increases and immune response develops. However, despite prior blood and tissue typing, sometimes the donor cells are incompatible with the recipient cells and the new cells begin to mount a type IV hypersensitivity/immunologic response in the child who has received the transplant (Behrman, Kliegman, & Jenson, 2004; Vogelsang, Lee, & Bensen-Kennedy, 2003).

Graft-versus-host disease may be either acute or chronic. Acute disease occurs in the first 100 days after transplant. The skin manifests a pruritic and macular-papular rash that begins on the extremities and progresses to the trunk. Gastrointestinal effects include nausea, vom-

iting, anorexia, diarrhea, cramping, and abdominal pain. Impaired liver function tests and jaundice often occur. On the other hand, chronic graft-versus-host disease occurs after the first 100 days. Recurrent infections, skin reactions, and thrombocytopenia are evidenced, with mouth, throat, and esophageal ulcers, gastrointestinal disorders, cholestasis, and eye irritation (Higman & Vogelsang, 2004).

Careful physical examination and laboratory tests are used to diagnose and stage the disease. Early identification is key to beginning therapy and stopping progression of the life-threatening condition. Several immunosuppressant drugs are used in treatment. Nursing care focuses on careful assessments of all children who have received transplants and partnering with other health professionals for treatment. Skin, gastrointestinal system, nutrition and growth, and eye examinations are commonly stressed during the therapeutic phase. Children and their families need information and support about this immune system complication of transplantation of bone marrow or stem cells.

Critical Concept Review

LEARNING OBJECTIVES

CONCEPTS

LEARNING OBJECTIVES	CONCEPTS
Describe the structure and function of the immune system and apply that knowledge to the care of children with immunological disorders.	1. Structure: ■ The immune system is composed of antibodies, leukocytes (white blood cells), and lymphoid tissue. ■ A child's immune system is not fully developed until age 6. 2. Function: ■ Recognizes any foreign substances within the body and eliminates them as efficiently as possible. 3. Immune system disorders may result in multisystem consequences because the immune system is involved in the regulation of all body functions.
Explain the differences between active and passive immunity.	1. Active immunity: ■ An antigen (in the form of a vaccine) is given to a child. This stimulates the body to produce antibodies without causing clinical disease. 2. Passive immunity: ■ Antibodies that are produced in another human or animal host are given to a child in order to confer immediate immunity.
Identify infection control measures to prevent the spread of infection in children with an immunodeficiency.	1. Perform frequent handwashing, standard precautions, and strict asepsis for invasive procedures. 2. Place the child in a negative-pressure room. 3. Avoid contact with persons with infectious disorders. 4. Avoid immunizations with live vaccines for child, siblings, and family members. 5. Food and items entering the child's room should receive special treatment.

LEARNING OBJECTIVES

CONCEPTS

Develop a nursing care plan in partnership with the family for a child with human immunodeficiency virus (HIV).

1. Prevent infection:
   - Perform frequent handwashing.
   - Prevent child's exposure to people with infections of any kind.
   - Instruct parents to follow modified immunization schedule.
2. Promote medication regimen adherence:
   - Instruct parents concerning the importance of compliance with medication regimen.
3. Promote respiratory function:
   - Inform parents of importance of deep breathing exercises for the prevention of pneumonia.
   - Instruct parents to include rest periods in the child's daily activities.
4. Promote adequate nutritional intake:
   - Encourage parents to provide nutritious meals.
   - Instruct parents concerning the importance of administering necessary vitamins to the child.
5. Provide emotional support:
   - Allow family to discuss fears and feelings about diagnosis.
   - Assist the family and child with the child's integration into the school environment.

Describe nursing management for the child with systemic lupus erythematosus or juvenile rheumatoid arthritis.

1. Nursing interventions common to both disorders include:
   - Promote adequate nutrition.
   - Assist in avoidance of flare-ups.
   - Manage side effects of medication.
   - Promote rest and comfort.
   - Provide emotional support.
2. Nursing interventions specific to SLE include:
   - Promote skin integrity.
   - Prevent infection.
   - Maintain fluid balance.
3. Nursing interventions specific to JRA include:
   - Promote improved mobility.

Describe exposure prevention measures for the child with latex allergy.

1. Products that come in contact with child must be free of latex.
2. Encourage parents to place a medical alert identification bracelet on the child.
3. Instruct parents to keep an epinephrine kit available at home and at school.
4. Instruct parents concerning everyday products that contain latex.

Apply nursing interventions and prevention measures for the child experiencing other hypersensitivity reactions.

1. Careful physical assessment:
   - Monitor for early signs and symptoms of hypersensitivity reactions.
   - Careful attention must be given to assessment of the skin and GI system.
2. Instruct the family in proper immunization schedule for the child.
3. Instruct the family concerning signs and symptoms of infection.
4. Teach the family the importance of protecting the child from contact with individuals with infections:
   - Child should avoid all crowded areas.
5. Assist families to follow proper medication schedule:
   - Inform parents of possible side effects of medication.

CRITICAL THINKING IN ACTION

*View the **Critical Thinking in Action** video in Chapter 44 of the CD-ROM. Then, answer the questions that follow.*

You are working at a pediatrician's office when 11-year-old Nirah and his parents come in. The husband, wife, and Nirah are all human immunodeficiency virus (HIV) positive. Nirah does not know he is HIV positive, but he has been very compliant with taking his antiretroviral medications. However, he has recently developed a cough and his parents decided to visit the pediatrician's office.

The pediatrician finds that Nirah has a fever of 102°F, respiratory rate of 60 breaths per minute, no visible retractions during respiration, and a pulse of 120 beats per minute. The physician decides to admit him to the hospital.

After the laboratory tests and radiographs are completed in the hospital, the physician tells the family that Nirah has pneumonia and strep throat. Nirah is started on IV antibiotics and shows improvement after three days of treatment. You monitor Nirah frequently and have him deep breathe. You also teach the parents how to encourage deep-breathing exercises.

1. How does HIV interfere with normal function of the child's immune system?
2. What are some of the measures of infection control for Nirah while he is hospitalized with HIV?
3. How can you promote Nirah's respiratory function?
4. When children, especially those with an immune system problem, are on antibiotics, they can develop thrush (Candida in the mouth). What is the treatment to prevent this side effect?

MEDIALINK

www.prenhall.com/london

- NCLEX-RN® Review, case studies, and other interactive resources for this chapter can be found on the Companion Website at http://www.prenhall.com/london. Click on "Chapter 44" to select the activities for this chapter.

How HIV destroys a T-Cell

- For animations, more NCLEX-RN® Review questions, and an audio glossary, access the accompanying CD-ROM in this textbook.

REFERENCES

American Academy of Pediatrics, Committee on Pediatric AIDS and Committee on Adolescence. (2001). Adolescents and human immunodeficiency virus infection: The role of the pediatrician in prevention and intervention. *Pediatrics, 107,* 188–190.

American College of Rheumatology. (2003). Retrieved December 22, 2003, from http://rarediseases.about.com/gi/dynamic/offsite. htm?site=http%3A%2F%2Fwww.rheumatology. org%2Fpatients%2Ffactsheet%2Fsle.html

Behrman, R. E., Kliegman, R. M., & Jenson, H. B. (2004). *Nelson textbook of pediatrics* (17th ed., pp. 738–741). Philadelphia: Saunders.

Bindler, R. M., & Howry, L. B. (2005). *Pediatric drug guide.* Upper Saddle River, NJ: Prentice Hall Health.

Brackis-Cott, E., Mellins, C. A., Abrams, E., Reval, T., & Dolezal, C. (2003). Pediatric HIV medication adherence: The views of medical providers from two primary care programs. *Journal of Pediatric Health Care, 17,* 252–260.

Brehler, R., & Kutting, B. (2001). Natural rubber latex allergy. *Archives of Internal Medicine, 161,* 1057–1064.

Burpo, R. H. (2000). Common antiviral agents used in women's and children's care. *Journal of Obstetric, Gynecologic and Neonatal Nursing, 29,* 181–200.

Candotti, F. (2000). The potential for therapy of immune disorders with gene therapy. *Pediatric Clinics of North America, 47,* 1389–1408.

Caselli, D. (2000). Human immunodeficiency virus-related cancer in children: Incidence and

treatment outcome—report of the Italian Register. *Journal of Clinical Oncology, 18,* 3854–3861.

Centers for Disease Control and Prevention. (2004a). *HIV/AIDS among Hispanics.* Retrieved December 5, 2004, from http://www.cdc.gov/hiv/pubs/facts/hispanic.htm

Centers for Disease Control and Prevention. (2004b). *OraQuick rapid HIV test for oral fluid. Frequently asked questions.* Retrieved December 4, 2004, from http://www.cdc.gov

Centers for Disease Control and Prevention. (2005). Retrieved March 16, 2005 from AIDS statics. www.cdc.gov/hiv/stats/htm.

Champi, C. (2002). Primary immunodeficiency disorders in children: Prompt diagnosis can lead to lifesaving treatment. *Journal of Pediatric Health, 16,* 16–21.

Chapman, E. H., Weintraub, R. J., Milburn, M. A., Pirozzi, T. O., & Woo, E. (1999). Homeopathic treatment of mild traumatic brain injury: A randomized, double-blind, placebo-controlled clinical trial. *Journal of Head Trauma Rehabilitation, 14,* 521–542.

Cohen, H., Chen, X. C., Sunkle, S., Davis, L., Geromanos, K., Xanthos, G., & Shearer, W. (2000). Ability of caregivers to read delayed hypersensitivity skin tests in children exposed to and infected by HIV. *Journal of Pediatric Health Care, 14,* 50–55.

Committee on Pediatric AIDS. (1998). Human immunodeficiency virus/acquired immunodeficiency syndrome education in schools. *Pediatrics, 101,* 933–935.

Committee on Pediatric AIDS and Committee on Adolescence. (2001). Adolescents and human immunodeficiency virus infections: The role of the pediatrician in prevention and intervention. *Pediatrics, 107,* 188–190.

Cooper, M. A., Pommering, T. L., & Koranyi, K. (2003). Primary immunodeficiencies. *American Family Physician, 68,* 2001.

Davenas, E., Beauvais, J., Oberbaum, M., Robinson, B., Miadonna, A., Tedeschi, A., et al. (1988). Human basophil degranulation triggered by very dilute antiserum against IgE. *Nature, 333,* 816–818.

Dibbern, D. A., & Routes, J. M. (2004). *Wiscott-Aldrich syndrome.* Retrieved June 20, 2004, from http://www.emedicine.com/med/topic1162.htm

Elder, M. E. (2000). T cell immunodeficiencies. *Pediatric Clinics of North America, 47,* 1253–1274.

Edmunds, M. W., & Mayhew, M. S. (2004). *Pharmacology for the Health Care Provider* (2nd ed.). St. Louis: Elsevier Mosby.

Gottlieb, B. S., & Ilowite, N. T. (2000). Meeting the challenge of rheumatologic diseases in teens. *Contemporary Pediatrics, 17,* 61–98.

Greco, C. M., Rudy, T. E., & Manzi, S. (2004). Effects of a stress-reduction program on psycho-logical function, pain, and physical function of systemic lupus erythematosus patients: A randomized controlled trial. *Arthritis and Rheumatology, 51*(4), 625–634.

Higman, M. A., & Vogelsang, G. B. (2004). Chronic graft-versus-host disease. *British Journal of Haematology, 125,* 435–454.

Houribane, J. O., Allard, J. M., Wade, A. M., & McEwan, A. I. (2002). Impact of repeated surgical procedures on the incidence and prevalence of latex allergy: A prospective study of 1263 children. *Journal of Pediatrics, 140,* 479–482.

Ilowite, N. T. (2002). Current treatment of juvenile rheumatoid arthritis. *Pediatrics, 109,* 109–115.

Instone, S. L. (2000). Perception of children with HIV infection when not told for so long: Implications for diagnosis disclosure. *Journal of Pediatric Health Care, 14,* 235–243.

Kline, M. W., Calles, N. R., Simon, C., & Schwarzwald, H. (2000). Pilot study of hydroxyurea in human immunodeficiency virus infected children receiving didanasine and/or stavudine. *Pediatric Infectious Disease Journal, 19,* 1083–1086.

Koleilat, M. A., Williams, L. W., & Ryan, M. E. (2003). Read the warning signs of primary immunodeficiency. *Contemporary Pediatrics, 20,* 65–81.

Langston, C., Cooper, E. R., Goldfarb, J., Easley, K. A., Husak, S., Sunkle, S., et al. (2001). Human immunodeficiency virus-related mortality in infants and children: Data from the pediatric pulmonary and cardiovascular complications of vertically transmitted HIV study. *Pediatrics, 107,* 328–338.

Lindegren, M. L., Steinberg, S., & Byers, R. H. (2000). Epidemiology of HIV/AIDS in children. *Pediatric Clinics of North America, 47,* 1–20.

Lupus Foundation of America. (2004) Retrieved December 4, 2004, from http://www.lupus.org/education/types/html system Lupus Erythematosus.

Luxner, K. L. (2003). The complicated prenatal experience. In M. H. Hogan & R. S. Glazebrook (Eds.), *Maternal-newborn nursing.* Upper Saddle River, NJ: Prentice-Hall.

MMWR. (2003). Advancing HIV prevention: New strategies for a changing epidemic—United States. *Morbidity and Mortality Weekly Report, 52,* 329–332.

Mulvihill, K. (2003). Systemic lupus erythematosus: Early identification, co-management are key KP contributions. *Advances for Nurse Practitioners, 11,* 32–36.

Nielsen, K., & Bryson, Y. J. (2000). Diagnosis of HIV infection in children. *Pediatric Clinics of North America, 47,* 39–64.

Pearson, D. A., McGrath, N. M., Nozyce, M., Nichols, S. L., Raskino, C., Brouwers, P., et al. (2000). Predicting HIV progression in children using measures of neuropsychological and neurological functioning. *Pediatrics, 106*(6), E76. Retrieved October 20, 2005, from http://www.pediatrics.org/cgi/content/full/ 106/6/376

Ramstead, C. (2003). HIV counseling, testing, and referral: Putting revised guidelines to use. *Clinician Reviews, 13,* 58–64.

Rogers, A. S. (2000). Serologic examination of hepatitis B infection and immunization in HIV-positive youth and associated risks. *AIDS Patient Care and STDs, 14,* 651–657.

Schwartz, S. A. (2000). Intravenous immunoglobulin treatment of immunodeficiency disorders. *Pediatric Clinics of North America, 47,* 1355–1370.

Temple, M. E., Koranyi, K., & Nahata, M. C. (2001). The safety and antiviral effect of protease inhibitors in children. *Pharmacotherapy, 21,* 287–294.

Vickers, A. J. (2000). Clinical trials of homeopathy and placebo: Analysis of a scientific debate. *Journal of Complementary and Alternative Medicine, 6,* 49–56.

Vogelsang, G. B., Lee, L., & Bensen-Kennedy, D. M. (2003). Pathogenesis and treatment of graft-versus-host disease after bone marrow transplant. *Annual Review of Medicine, 54,* 29–54.

CHAPTER

45

The Child with Infectious and Communicable Diseases

We came in today because Chang has a fever. I know Lian and Chang need immunizations. Lian will be going to kindergarten in the fall, so it is very important for her to get all of the immunizations she needs now.
—Mother of Lian, 5 years old, and Chang, 2 years old

LEARNING OBJECTIVES

- Describe the reasons why children are more vulnerable than adults to infectious and communicable diseases.

- Describe the process of infection and modes of transmission.

- Explain the role that vaccines play in reduction and elimination of infectious and communicable diseases.

- Develop a nursing care plan for children of all ages needing immunizations.

- Recognize common infectious and communicable diseases.

- Develop a nursing care plan for a child with a common infectious disease.

MEDIALINK www.prenhall.com/london

CD-ROM

Skill 9–11: Oral Route (Body Temperature)
Skill 9–12: Axillary Route (Body Temperature)
Skill 9–13: Rectal Route (Body Temperature)
Skill 9–14: Tympanic Route (Body Temperature)
NCLEX-RN® Review
Audio Glossary

Companion Website

NCLEX-RN® Review
MediaLink Applications:
  Care Plan: Develop an Immunizations Schedule:
    Infant with HIV, Healthy Infant, Preschooler
  Immunizations and Older Children
  Vaccine Administration Record
  Immunization FAQ
  Case Study: Reporting an Adverse Vaccine Event
  Bioterrorism Preparedness
Thinking Critically
Vaccine Safety Information
Immunization Safety Research
Catch-Up Schedule for Immunizations
Audio Glossary

An **infectious disease** is any communicable disease caused by microorganisms that are commonly transmitted from one person to another or from an animal to a person. A **communicable disease** is an illness directly or indirectly transmitted from one person or animal to another by contact with body fluids, by contact with contaminated items, or by vectors (ticks, mosquitoes, other insects). Infectious and communicable diseases are a major cause of morbidity in infants and children in the United States, and can sometimes result in death.

For a communicable disease to occur, the following three links need to be present (see "Pathophysiology Illustrated: The Chain of Infection"): an infectious agent or pathogen, an effective means of transmission, and a susceptible host. An effective chain of transmission for infection requires a suitable habitat, or reservoir, for the pathogen. A reservoir may be living or nonliving, and transmission may be direct or indirect. **Direct transmission** involves physical contact between the source of the infection and the new host. **Indirect transmission** occurs when pathogens survive outside humans before causing infection and disease.

Infants and young children are often susceptible hosts because their immune systems are immature and they have not yet developed antibodies to many agents (see Chapter 44 ∞). Immunodeficiency and poor health may also increase a child's risk of contracting an infectious disease.

Control of infectious diseases is usually directed at interrupting the chain of transmission or eliminating one or more of the habitats or reservoirs (e.g., spraying insecticide to kill mosquitoes that carry malaria). Isolating an infected individual interferes with disease transmission, and killing the pathogen eliminates the causal agent. Public health authorities monitor patterns of disease occurrence, and healthcare workers are required to report cases of many infectious diseases to state health officials.

PATHOPHYSIOLOGY ILLUSTRATED
The Chain of Infection

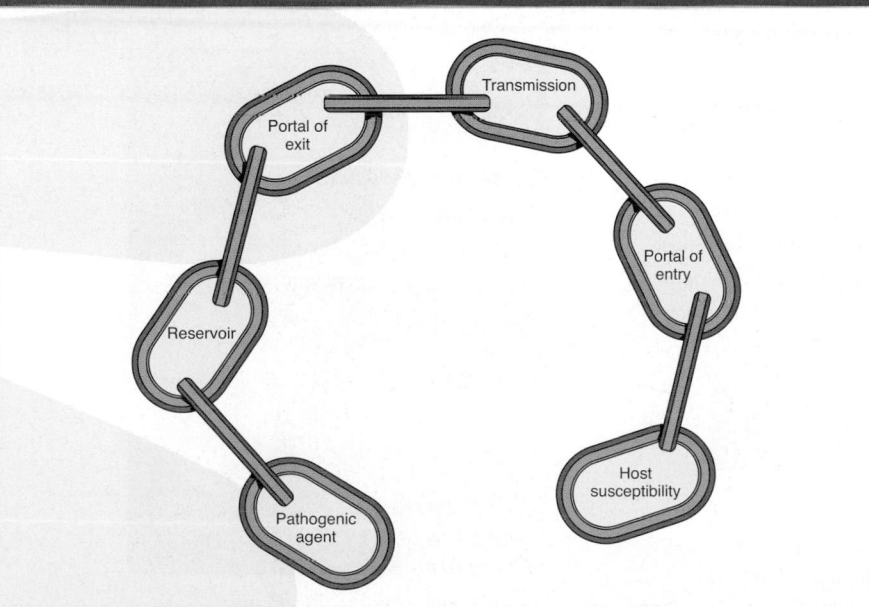

To achieve infection control, one of the links in the chain must be broken.

Major public health programs and scientific advances such as safer drinking water, better sanitation, improved standards of living, immunizations, and advanced medical treatment have decreased the occurrence of infectious and communicable diseases. Reducing the number of preventable childhood illnesses is a major national goal in *Healthy People 2010,* and nurses are important partners in this effort. Specific objectives are targeted at the reduction or elimination of the following infectious diseases (Department of Health and Human Services, 1999):

■ Elimination—rubella and congenital rubella syndrome, diphtheria, *Haemophilus influenza* type b, measles, mumps, polio, and tetanus

■ Reduction—pertussis, hepatitis B, varicella, foodborne pathogens, and HIV infections

SPECIAL VULNERABILITY OF CHILDREN

The capability and function of the immune system, especially of infants, is becoming better understood. Infants are particularly vulnerable to infectious diseases for the following reasons:

■ Their immune system is not fully mature at birth.

■ Passively acquired maternal antibodies provide limited protection, and this protection decreases over several months after birth.

■ Disease protection through immunization is as yet incomplete.

As children grow, they develop immunity through immunization or exposure to the natural disease. As children mature and become more active, they interact more frequently with other children and adults, which increases their exposure to infectious agents (Figure 45–1 ◉). As healthy children are exposed to more infections, they develop antibodies naturally. Thus, subsequent infections with the same type of organism may be less severe or avoided. (Refer to "Anatomy and Physiology of Pediatric Differences" in Chapter 44. ∞)

DEVELOPING CULTURAL COMPETENCE

ORIGINS OF INFECTIOUS DISEASE

In some cultures, infectious diseases are seen as punishment or the result of curses or evil spirits. For example, Native Americans traditionally view illnesses as the result of disharmony or displeasing the spirits. They may not believe in the germ theory of disease causation.

◉ **FIGURE 45–1**

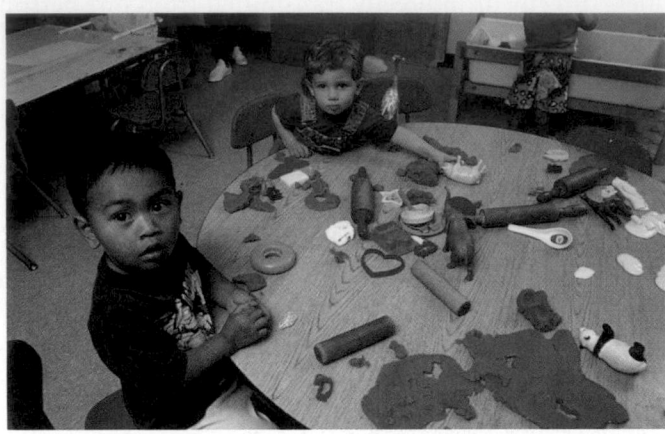

Infectious diseases are easily transmitted in settings such as childcare centers where children handle common objects.

The poor hygiene behaviors of young children facilitate transmission of infectious diseases in child care and other close environments. The fecal-oral and respiratory routes are the most common sources of transmission in children. Children usually do not wash their hands after toileting unless they are closely supervised. They put toys and their hands in their mouths, and then rub their nose and eyes. They often are unable to care for a runny nose without help. Diapers may leak stool and provide the fecal exposure to organisms. In addition, the staff in childcare centers or other people caring for children may not use proper handwashing techniques (Figure 45–2 ◉). All

◉ **FIGURE 45–2**

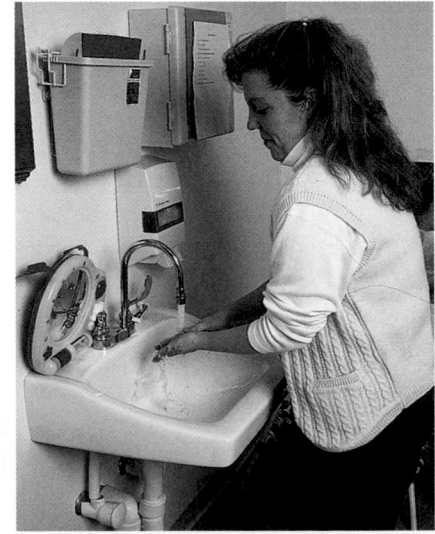

Proper handwashing is one of the most effective measures in preventing transmission of microorganisms.

of these behaviors promote the transmission of infection. (See "Teaching Highlights: Reducing the Transmission of Infection.")

IMMUNIZATION

The development and widespread use of immunizations has been one of the great breakthroughs of modern medicine. Immunization introduces an **antigen** (a foreign substance that triggers an immune system response) into the body, allowing immunity against a disease to develop naturally. The person produces **antibodies**, proteins capable of responding to specific antigens.

In **active immunity** (in which antibody production is stimulated without causing clinical disease) an antigen is given in the form of a vaccine. When a child may need antibodies faster than the body can develop them, **passive immunity** may be induced with antibodies produced in another human or animal host and given to the child. This approach is also used with at-risk children after a single exposure to a disease to prevent the disease from occurring or to reduce its severity. For example, if a child who has never had a tetanus immunization steps on a rusty nail, the child

needs immediate protection (passive immunity) from tetanus. Tetanus immune globulin injection is given to combat the tetanus toxin produced by the bacterial spores introduced by the nail. Because passive immunity does not confer lasting immunity, the process of antibody development (active immunity) is then begun by administering a tetanus toxoid vaccine.

Since the first vaccines were developed in the late 1800s, many diseases have decreased dramatically in incidence. The introduction of vaccines against childhood diseases such as measles, mumps, rubella, polio, whooping cough, diphtheria, smallpox, *Haemophilus influenzae* type b, hepatitis B, and chickenpox has greatly improved the quality of life for children and adults. Since the introduction of the pneumococcal conjugate vaccine in 2000, there has been a 35% reduction in invasive disease (meningitis and pneumonia) caused by pneumococcal strains resistant to penicillin, and a 78% reduction in disease caused by strains targeted in the vaccine among children less than 2 years of age (Peters & Edwards, 2002; Whitney, Farley, & Hadler, 2003).

Types of vaccines against childhood illnesses used in the United States include the following:

- **Killed virus vaccine.** A vaccine that contains a microorganism that has been killed but is still capable of inducing the human body to produce antibodies. Example: inactivated poliovirus vaccine.
- **Toxoid.** A toxin that has been treated (by heat or chemical) to weaken its toxic effects but retain its antigenicity. Example: tetanus toxoid.
- **Live virus vaccine.** A vaccine that contains a microorganism in live but attenuated, or weakened, form. Example: measles and varicella vaccines.
- **Recombinant forms.** An organism that has been genetically altered for use in vaccines. Examples: hepatitis B and **acellular pertussis vaccine** (a vaccine that uses proteins from pertussis rather than the whole cell to stimulate the process of active immunity).
- **Conjugated forms.** An altered organism joined with another substance to increase the immune response. Example: The *Haemophilus influenzae* type b (Hib) vaccine is conjugated with a protein-carrier like tetanus toxoid (PRP-T); however, this specific vaccine brand confers no immunity to tetanus.

Improvements in vaccine technology continue to improve the safety and efficacy of immunization against an increasing number of diseases. Today's vaccines are often produced synthetically with recombinant DNA technology or genetic engineering to reduce side effects.

NURSING PRACTICE

Thimerosal, a bacteriostatic agent that contains ethyl mercury, was used to sterilize vaccines in multidose vials. Because of the possible association between mercury poisoning and nerve and brain damage, vaccine manufacturers are working to eliminate thimerosal from vaccines. The cumulative mercury exposure in vaccines continues to fall. The Immunization Safety Review Committee reported that there is no causal relationship between thimerosal exposures in vaccines and subsequent development of autism, attention deficit hyperactivity disorder, and speech and language delay (Institute of Medicine, 2001).

Vaccines should be administered at specific ages and intervals. Timing for first immunizations is determined by the age at which **transplacental immunity** (passive immunity transferred from mother to infant) decreases or disappears, and the infant or child develops the ability to make antibodies in response to the vaccine. Scientists continue to study the duration of protection from vaccines. Some vaccines do not confer lifelong immunity.

The recommended schedule for immunization is updated at least annually to reflect new vaccines and the need for repeat immunization. The Advisory Committee on Immunization Practices (ACIP) of the Centers for Disease Control (CDC), the American Academy of Pediatrics (AAP), and the American Academy of Family Practitioners (AAFP) collaborate on the recommended schedule. The 2005 recommendations are given in Table 45–1. This schedule applies to immunizations all children should receive, and schedules and recommendations vary for children who begin immunizations later in childhood or need catch-up doses. Other immunization recommendations are made for children who recently received blood products or immunosuppressive agents. Supplemental immunizations for meningococcal and pneumococcal infections are recommended for certain children, as noted in Table 45–2. Visit the CDC Web site for the most current vaccine schedules and recommendations for catch-up doses.

The effectiveness of vaccines depends on their proper storage and on the immunization of all susceptible individuals. Lower immunization rates of children are often associated with economic factors, limited access to healthcare, the lack of primary care at hours convenient for working parents, inadequate education about the importance of immunization, and religious prohibitions. Efforts to administer vaccines and monitor immunization status in children are increasing. For example, managed care organizations require that contracted healthcare providers comply with the pediatric immunization standards, and patient records are audited to ensure compliance. The federal Vaccines for Children program provides free vaccines for qualified children and adolescents up to 19 years of age, and it has resolved some of the economic factors associated with vaccine coverage.

However, an increasing number of parents are choosing not to immunize their children for philosophic reasons, such as the following (Coyer, 2002; Mera & Hackley, 2003):

- Concerns that vaccines are dangerous (such as mercury in thimerosol) and can cause harm to their child, such as autism and sudden infant death syndrome.

- The belief that vaccines do not work—even some vaccinated children get the infectious disease, so the vaccines are not all that protective.

- Disagreement with government regulation and monitoring of immunizations.

- The belief that the threat of the disease has diminished with vaccine success and improved sanitary conditions and the need for immunization of their child is less important.

- The number of adverse events to vaccines now exceeds the number of cases of vaccine-preventable diseases, and the public has increased access to this information.

- The belief that they can control their child's susceptibility to disease and the outcome if they become infected.

All healthcare providers need to be consistent in the message about the value of vaccines and to clear up any misconceptions parents may have.

NURSING PRACTICE

Special care must be taken to ensure the potency of vaccines by storing them properly in the refrigerator or freezer. Read the package inserts of vaccines to determine proper storage conditions. Store vaccines in a refrigerator with separate doors for the refrigerator and freezer units. Check the temperature of each unit twice daily and record the temperatures on a log. The refrigerator should have a consistent temperature range of 35° to 46°F (2°C to 8°C), and the freezer should have a consistent temperature of 5°F (−15°C) or lower. Keep jugs of water in the refrigerator and trays of ice in the freezer to help keep the temperature in the units consistent. Store the vaccines in the middle of the units, placing the older vaccines in the front. Make sure the facility has an emergency plan for safe storage of vaccines in case of a power outage or natural disaster.

Check the expiration of vaccines prior to use. When reconstituting vaccines, it is important to use the solution provided and follow the manufacturer's directions. Write the date and time on the bottle if it is a multidose vial. Some reconstituted vaccines (varicella and MMR) have a short shelf life and are available only in single-dose vials.

TABLE 45–1 ✛ Recommended Immunization Schedule for United States Children and Adolescents, United States, 2006

Vaccine ▼ / Age ▶	Birth	1 month	2 months	4 months	6 months	12 months	15 months	18 months	24 months	4–6 years	11–12 years	13–14 years	15 years	16–18 years
Hepatitis B¹	HepB	HepB		HepB¹		HepB					HepB Series			
Diphtheria, Tetanus, Pertussis²			DTaP	DTaP	DTaP		DTaP			DTaP	Tdap		Tdap	
Haemophilus influenzae type b³			Hib	Hib	Hib³	Hib								
Inactivated Poliovirus			IPV	IPV		IPV				IPV				
Measles, Mumps, Rubella⁴						MMR				MMR		MMR		
Varicella⁵						Varicella				Varicella				
Meningococcal⁶									MPSV4		MCV4		MCV4 / MCV4	
Pneumococcal⁷			PCV	PCV	PCV	PCV			PCV		PPV			
Influenza⁸					Influenza (Yearly)					Influenza (Yearly)				
Hepatitis A⁹									HepA Series					

Vaccines within broken line are for selected populations

■ Range of recommended ages ■ Catch-up immunization ■ 11–12 year old assessment

This schedule indicates the recommended ages for routine administration of currently licensed childhood vaccines, as of December 1, 2005, for children through age 18 years. Any dose not administered at the recommended age should be administered at any subsequent visit when indicated and feasible. ■ Indicates age groups that warrant special effort to administer those vaccines not previously administered. Additional vaccines may be licensed and recommended during the year. Licensed combination vaccines may be used whenever any components of the combination are indicated and other components of the vaccine are not contraindicated and if approved by the Food and Drug Administration for that dose of the series. Providers should consult the respective ACIP statement for detailed recommendations. Clinically significant adverse events that follow immunization should be reported to the Vaccine Adverse Event Reporting System (VAERS). Guidance about how to obtain and complete a VAERS form is available at www.vaers.hhs.gov or by telephone, 800-822-7967.

1. **Hepatitis B vaccine (HepB).** *AT BIRTH:* All newborns should receive monovalent HepB soon after birth and before hospital discharge. **Infants born to mothers who are HBsAg-positive** should receive HepB and 0.5 mL of hepatitis B immune globulin (HBIG) within 12 hours of birth. **Infants born to mothers whose HBsAg status is unknown** should receive HepB within 12 hours of birth. The mother should have blood drawn as soon as possible to determine her HBsAg status; if HBsAg-positive, the infant should receive HBIG as soon as possible (no later than age 1 week). **For infants born to HBsAg-negative mothers,** the birth dose can be delayed in rare circumstances but only if a physician's order to withhold the vaccine and a copy of the mother's original HBsAg-negative laboratory report are documented in the infant's medical record. *FOLLOWING THE BIRTHDOSE:* The HepB series should be completed with either monovalent HepB or a combination vaccine containing HepB. The second dose should be administered at age 1–2 months. The final dose should be administered at age ≥24 weeks. It is permissible to administer 4 doses of HepB (e.g., when combination vaccines are given after the birth dose); however, if monovalent HepB is used, a dose at age 4 months is not needed. **Infants born to HBsAg-positive mothers** should be tested for HBsAg and antibody to HBsAg after completion of the HepB series, at age 9–18 months (generally at the next well-child visit after completion of the vaccine series).

2. **Diphtheria and tetanus toxoids and acellular pertussis vaccine (DTaP).** The fourth dose of DTaP may be administered as early as age 12 months, provided 6 months have elapsed since the third dose and the child is unlikely to return at age 15–18 months. The final dose in the series should be given at age ≥4 years.

   Tetanus and diphtheria toxoids and acellular pertussis vaccine (Tdap – adolescent preparation) is recommended at age 11–12 years for those who have completed the recommended childhood DTP/DTaP series and have not received a Td booster dose. Adolescents 13–18 years who missed the 11–12-year Td/Tdap booster dose should also receive a single dose of Tdap if they have completed the recommended childhood DTP/DTaP vaccination series. Subsequent **tetanus and diphtheria toxoids (Td)** are recommended every 10 years.

3. **Haemophilus influenzae type b conjugate vaccine (Hib).** Three Hib conjugate vaccines are licensed for infant use. If PRP-OMP (PedvaxHIB® or ComVax® [Merck]) is administered at ages 2 and 4 months, a dose at age 6 months is not required. DTaP/Hib combination products should not be used for primary immunization in infants at ages 2, 4 or 6 months but can be used as boosters after any Hib vaccine. The final dose in the series should be administered at age ≥12 months.

4. **Measles, mumps, and rubella vaccine (MMR).** The second dose of MMR is recommended routinely at age 4–6 years but may be administered during any visit, provided at least 4 weeks have elapsed since the first dose and both doses are administered beginning at or after age 12 months. Those who have not previously received the second dose should complete the schedule by age 11–12 years.

5. **Varicella vaccine.** Varicella vaccine is recommended at any visit at or after age 12 months for susceptible children (i.e., those who lack a reliable history of chickenpox). Susceptible persons aged ≥13 years should receive 2 doses administered at least 4 weeks apart.

6. **Meningococcal vaccine (MCV4).** Meningococcal conjugate vaccine (MCV4) should be given to all children at the 11–12 year old visit as well as to unvaccinated adolescents at high school entry (15 years of age). Other adolescents who wish to decrease their risk for meningococcal disease may also be vaccinated. All college freshmen living in dormitories should also be vaccinated, preferably with MCV4, although meningococcal polysaccharide vaccine (MPSV4) is an acceptable alternative. Vaccination against invasive meningococcal disease is recommended for children and adolescents aged ≥2 years with terminal complement deficiencies or anatomic or functional asplenia and certain other high risk groups (see *MMWR* 2005;54 [RR-7]:1-21); use MPSV4 for children aged 2–10 years and MCV4 for older children, although MPSV4 is an acceptable alternative.

7. **Pneumococcal vaccine.** The heptavalent **pneumococcal conjugate vaccine (PCV)** is recommended for all children aged 2–23 months and for certain children aged 24–59 months. The final dose in the series should be given at age ≥12 months. **Pneumococcal polysaccharide vaccine (PPV)** is recommended in addition to PCV for certain high-risk groups. See *MMWR* 2000; 49(RR-9):1-35.

8. **Influenza vaccine.** Influenza vaccine is recommended annually for children aged ≥6 months with certain risk factors (including, but not limited to, asthma, cardiac disease, sickle cell disease, human immunodeficiency virus [HIV], diabetes, and conditions that can compromise respiratory function or handling of respiratory secretions or that can increase the risk for aspiration), healthcare workers, and other persons (including household members) in close contact with persons in groups at high risk (see *MMWR* 2005;54[RR-8]:1-55). In addition, healthy children aged 6–23 months and close contacts of healthy children aged 0–5 months are recommended to receive influenza vaccine because children in this age group are at substantially increased risk for influenza-related hospitalizations. For healthy persons aged 5–49 years, the intranasally administered, live, attenuated influenza vaccine (LAIV) is an acceptable alternative to the intramuscular trivalent inactivated influenza vaccine (TIV). See *MMWR* 2005;54(RR-8):1-55. Children receiving TIV should be administered a dosage appropriate for their age (0.25 mL if aged 6–35 months or 0.5 mL if aged ≥3 years). Children aged ≤8 years who are receiving influenza vaccine for the first time should receive 2 doses (separated by at least 4 weeks for TIV and at least 6 weeks for LAIV).

9. **Hepatitis A vaccine (HepA).** HepA is recommended for all children at 1 year of age (i.e., 12–23 months). The 2 doses in the series should be administered at least 6 months apart. States, counties, and communities with existing HepA vaccination programs for children 2–18 years of age are encouraged to maintain these programs. In these areas, new efforts focused on routine vaccination of 1-year-old children should enhance, not replace, ongoing programs directed at a broader population of children. HepA is also recommended for certain high risk groups (see *MMWR* 1999; 48[RR-12]1-37).

The Childhood and Adolescent Immunization Schedule is approved by:
Advisory Committee on Immunization Practices www.cdc.gov/nip/acip • American Academy of Pediatrics www.aap.org • American Academy of Family Physicians www.aafp.org

Source: Department of Health and Human Services, Centers for Disease Control and Prevention.

TABLE 45–2 ✛ Supplemental Immunizations

Vaccine	Recommendation
Meningococcal (MPSV4)	For children older than 2 years of age with asplenia. Vaccine duration is 5 years or longer in children older than 4 years at the time of immunization. The vaccine should be repeated after 1 year if the child is younger than 4 years at the time of initial immunization.
	The vaccine is also recommended for college students residing in dormitories or other group living arrangements as an alternative to the MCV4 vaccine (see Table 45-3).
23-valent Pneumococcal	For children older than 2 years of age with sickle cell disease, asplenia, chronic cardiovascular and pulmonary disorders, nephrotic syndrome, renal failure, HIV infection, cerebrospinal fluid leaks, or those undergoing immunosuppressive therapy.
	Repeat the immunization after 3–5 years if the child is younger than 10 years at the time of first immunization or at severe risk for pneumococcal infection.

NURSING MANAGEMENT

NURSING ASSESSMENT AND DIAGNOSIS

Nurses are responsible for reviewing a child's immunization record and determining whether the child needs immunization. Inquire about the child's health promotion care as well as health problems. Make sure to use the most current guidelines for comparison with the child's record. If the child is behind in appropriate immunizations for age, determine the best combination of vaccines to give at this visit to better protect the child. Also take advantage of opportunities to give needed immunizations to siblings accompanying the family on the visit. A minor illness should not deter immunization.

Healthcare providers miss many opportunities to immunize children. Children (and siblings present) should have their immunization status assessed during all healthcare visits and hospitalizations, and in schools. To reduce the number of missed opportunities for full immunization of children, use the following guidelines (American Academy of Pediatrics, 2003):

- Several vaccines—diphtheria, tetanus, and acellular pertussis (DTaP); measles, mumps, and rubella (MMR); hepatitis B (HBV); *Haemophilus influenzae* type b (Hib); inactivated polio (IPV); varicella; and heptavalent pneumococcal vaccines—can be given at the same visit.

- Combination vaccines such as Pediarix (combining DTaP, HepB, and IPV) can reduce the number of overall injections needed in the first 2 years of life from 20 to 14.

- Two injections can be given in different sites on the same extremity.

- Immunizations can be given when the child has a minor illness with or without a low-grade fever, and with antibiotic treatment. Recent exposure to an infectious disease is not a reason to defer a vaccine.

- Preterm and low-birth-weight infants who are medically stable should receive all routinely recommended vaccines at the same chronologic age and in the same dosage as full-term infants. HepB may be delayed in infants weighing less than 2000 grams whose mother is hepatitis B negative until 30 days of age or upon hospital discharge (Saari & Committee on Infectious Diseases, 2003).

- Immunizations can be given when there was a local reaction to a prior vaccine or a family member had an adverse response.

Assess the child for potential contraindications to vaccines—past reactions and allergies to key vaccine components. True contraindications for a vaccine are an anaphylactic reaction to the vaccine or one of its components and a moderate to severe acute illness. Some additional contraindications for specific vaccines may also exist, such as pregnancy and allergy to some components of the vaccine (e.g., neomycin, gelatin, eggs) (see Table 45–3). Determine if female teens could be pregnant.

The accompanying "Nursing Care Plan" explores three potential nursing diagnoses that may apply to the child

NURSING PRACTICE

Immune globulin inhibits the response to live virus vaccines such as measles, mumps, rubella, and varicella. Ask about recent administration of immune globulin or blood products leading to decreased antibody response to vaccines. Refer to the most current guidelines to identify the appropriate interval (3 or more months) between administration of immune globulin or blood products and live virus vaccine administration.

Similarly, if immune globulin or blood products must be given within 14 days after administration of a live virus vaccine, the vaccine should be administered again after the period specified in the most current guidelines, unless serologic testing determines that the child developed adequate serum antibodies (American Academy of Pediatrics, 2003).

(continues on p. 1323)

TABLE 45–3 ✣ Recommended Pediatric Immunizations

Immunization Type	Side Effects	Contraindications	Nursing Considerations
Diphtheria and Pertussis Vaccines and Tetanus Toxoid (DTaP, Tdap) *Type:* Inactivated *Route:* Intramuscular *Dosage:* 0.5 mL *Age(s) given:* 2, 4, 6, 15–18 months; 4–6 years (5 doses); 11–12 years May give at same time as all other vaccines, in a separate site. *Storage:* Store in body of refrigerator at 2°–8°C (35°–46°F). Do not freeze. Tripedia and Infanrix are licensed for all 5 doses. Daptacel is licensed for the first 4 doses. Pediarix is composed of DTaP, Hep B, and IPV and can be given as the primary series. TriHiBit is composed of DTaP and Hib. A Tdap vaccine for adolescents became part of the 2006 vaccine schedule.	*Common:* Redness, pain, swelling, nodule at injection site; temperature up to 38.3°C (101°F); drowsiness, irritability, fussiness; anorexia within 2 days of injection. Increase in frequency and magnitude of local reactions with 4th and 5th doses, (e.g., entire limb swelling). *Serious:* Allergic reaction, anaphylaxis; shock or collapse (hypotonic-hyperresponsive episode—sudden loss of muscle tone, pallor, fever, and unresponsiveness), fever above 38.8°C (102°F); febrile seizure; persistent inconsolable crying; coma or permanent brain damage.	Gelatin allergy (do not use Tripedia). Occurrence of a serious side effect after previous administration of DTaP, such as anaphylaxis or encephalopathy within 7 days after DTP or DTaP. Precautions in additional doses should be considered in children with the following reactions within 48 hours of the previous dose: —Fever ≥ 40.5°C (105°F) —Continuous inconsolable crying lasting ≥ 3 hours —Pale or limp episode or collapse —Convulsion within 3 days of dose. Administration should be delayed for 1 month after immunosuppressive therapy and until moderate to severe febrile illnesses have resolved. Administration of immune serum globulin within last 90 days.	Use same brand for all doses where feasible. Prior to immunization, ask about previous reactions to immunization. DTaP may coincide with or hasten the recognition of a seizure disorder. In children with a history of seizures with or without fever, give acetaminophen at the time of vaccine and then every 4 hours for 24 hours. Shake vaccine before withdrawing. Solution will be cloudy. If it contains clumps that cannot be resuspended, do not use. Daptacel stopper vial contains latex. Pediarix stopper vial is latex-free. When required, simultaneous administration of tetanus immune globulin or diphtheria antitoxin should be given in separate sites with a new needle and syringe. Inform parents of the chance of increased reaction to the 4th and 5th doses. Defer the vaccine when the child has a progressive neurologic problem until the child is stable. DT is given to children <7 years of age who have had a serious reaction to the pertussis component of the DTP or DTaP vaccine. Td or Tdap is given to children ≥7 years. The series does not need to be restarted, no matter how long since the previous dose was given.
Poliovirus Vaccine (IPV) *Type:* Inactivated *Route:* Subcutaneous or intramuscular depending upon vaccine used *Dosage:* 0.5 mL *Age(s) given:* 2, 4, 12–18 months; 4–6 years (4 doses) May give at same time as all other vaccines in a separate site. *Storage:* Store in body of refrigerator at 2°–8°C (35°–46°F). Do not freeze.	*Common:* Swelling and tenderness, irritability, tiredness. *Serious:* Allergic reaction or anaphylaxis.	Hypersensitivity to vaccine components: neomycin, streptomycin, polymyxin B. Anaphylactic response. Pregnancy.	Prior to immunization, ask if the child has an allergy to neomycin, streptomycin, or polymyxin B (whichever of these antibiotics the specific vaccine to be used contains). Clear, colorless suspension. Do not use if it contains particulate matter, becomes cloudy, or changes color. Recommended for use in all vaccine doses. All doses must be separated by at least 4 weeks.

(continued)

TABLE 45-3 ✤ Recommended Pediatric Immunizations—continued

Immunization Type	Side Effects	Contraindications	Nursing Considerations
Poliovirus Vaccine (IPV)—Cont. Pediarix includes IPV along with DTaP and HepB. IPV may be given as single vaccine preparation.			The series does not need to be restarted, no matter how long since the previous dose was given.
Measles, Mumps, Rubella Vaccines (MMR) *Type:* Live attenuated *Route:* Subcutaneous *Dosage:* 0.5 mL *Age(s) given:* 12-15 months; 4-6 years (2 doses) May give at same time as all other vaccines in a separate site. *Storage:* Store in body of refrigerator at 2°-8°C (35°-46°F). When reconstituted, keep refrigerated and away from light; discard if unused within 8 hours. Diluent is stored at room temperature or in refrigerator. Do not freeze.	*Common:* Elevated temperature 1-2 weeks after immunization; redness or pain at injection site; noncontagious rash; joint pain. *Serious:* Allergic reaction or anaphylaxis; febrile seizure; meningitis (usually mild); encephalopathy; thrombocytopenia purpura; and rare cases of coma and permanent brain damage.	Prior anaphylactic reaction to vaccine. Allergy to neomycin or gelatin. Severely impaired immune system due to malignancy, immune deficiency disease, immunosuppressive therapy. Wait at least 3-11 months after administration of immune serum globulin or blood products (time determined by the type) before giving vaccine. Pregnancy or possibility of pregnancy within 4 weeks. Thrombocytopenia or history of thrombocytopenic purpura. Tuberculosis or positive PPD tuberculin test.	Prior to immunization, ask if child has allergy to neomycin or gelatin. Observe the child with an egg allergy for 90 minutes after injection. Inquire about immunosuppression. MMR vaccine is recommended for those infected with HIV. Instruct adolescent girls of childbearing age to avoid pregnancy for 3 months after immunization. Give tuberculosis (TB) test at same time as MMR or 4-6 weeks later. If MMR and Varivax are not given on the same day, space them ≥28 days apart. Reconstituted vaccine is a clear, yellow solution. Give entire contents of reconstituted vial even if more than 0.5 mL. As college students are at greater risk due to decreasing immunity, make sure they have received a second MMR dose.
Hepatitis B Vaccine (HB) *Type:* Inactivated *Route:* Intramuscular *Dosage:* Engerix-B: 10 mcg or Recombivax HB: 5 mcg *Age(s) given:* Birth-2 months, 1 month after first dose; 6 months after first dose **or** Birth-2 months, 1-4 months, 6-18 months (3 doses) May give at same time as all other vaccines in a separate site. *Storage:* Store in body of refrigerator at 2°-8°C (35°-46°F). Do not freeze. Storage out of recommended temperature range decreases potency.	*Common:* Pain or redness at injection site; headache; photophobia; altered liver enzymes. *Serious:* Allergic reaction or anaphylaxis; fever.	Prior anaphylaxis, liver abnormalities. Serious allergic reaction to past dose. Yeast hypersensitivity.	Prior to immunization, check status of mother's hepatitis B test and presence of other liver disease. *Note:* If mother has HbsAg+ or unknown status, vaccine must be given to infant within 12 hours of birth along with hepatitis B immune globulin at the same time in another site with new needle and syringe. Shake vaccine before withdrawing. Solution will appear cloudy. Various formulations (pediatric, adult, dialysis) are available in different strengths. Read package insert carefully to determine proper dosage for age for the particular formulation used.

TABLE 45–3 ✣ Recommended Pediatric Immunizations—continued

Immunization Type	Side Effects	Contraindications	Nursing Considerations
Hepatitis B Vaccine (HB)—Cont. Engerix-B and Recombivax HB are single vaccine preparations. Comvax is a combination of Hib and HepB. Newborn dose should be monovalent (single vaccine) preparation.			A 3-dose series can be started at any age. Minimum spacing for children and teens is 4 weeks between doses 1 and 2, and 8 weeks between doses 2 and 3. The last dose in an infant series should not be given before 6 months of age. Vaccine brands can be interchanged for 3-dose series. The series does not need to be restarted, no matter how long since the previous dose was given.
***Haemophilus influenzae* Type B (Hib)** *Type:* Inactivated *Route:* Intramuscular *Dosage:* 0.5 mL *Age(s) given:* 2, 4, 6, 12–15 months; (4 doses for HbOC[a] [HibTITER] and PRP-T[a] [ActHib]) **or** 2, 4, 12–15 months (3 doses for PRP-OMP[a] [PedvaxHIB]) May give at same time as all other vaccines in a separate site. *Storage:* Store in body of refrigerator at 2°–8°C (35°–46°F). Do not freeze. Use or discard reconstituted ActHIB and OmniHIB within 30 minutes. Refrigerate reconstituted PedvaxHIB and discard within 24 hours. HibTITER, ActHib, OmniHib, and PedvaxHIB are single vaccine preparations. Comvax is a combination of PRP-OMP plus HepB. TriHiBit is composed of DTaP and Hib.	*Common:* Pain, redness, or swelling at site. *Serious:* Allergic reaction of anaphylaxis (extremely rare); fever.	Prior anaphylactic reaction to this vaccine.	Prior to immunizations, ask if child is immunosuppressed. Solution is clear and colorless. Since schedules for product preparations of different companies vary, it is important to read package inserts carefully. If the first dose is given between 7 and 11 months of age, 3 doses are needed. If the first dose was given at 12 to 14 months of age, give a booster dose in 8 weeks. If the first dose is given when the child is over 15 months or under 5 years, only one dose is needed. Second and third doses can be given 4 to 8 weeks after the first. Use the same vaccine preparation for all doses of the primary series if possible. The series does not need to be restarted, no matter how long since the previous dose was given.
Heptavalent Pneumococcal Conjugate Vaccine (PCV) *Type:* Inactivated *Route:* Intramuscular *Dosage:* 0.5 mL	*Common:* Soreness, swelling, redness at injection site; mild to moderate fever; irritability, drowsiness, restless sleep, decreased appetite, vomiting and diarrhea, rash or hives.	Hypersensitivity to diphtheria toxoid.	Clear, colorless, or slightly opalescent liquid.

(continued)

TABLE 45–3 ✣ Recommended Pediatric Immunizations—continued

Immunization Type	Side Effects	Contraindications	Nursing Considerations
Heptavalent Pneumococcal Conjugate Vaccine (PCV)—Cont. *Age(s) given:* 2, 4, 6, 12-15 months *Storage:* Store in body of refrigerator at 2°–8°C (35°–46°F). Do not freeze. Prevnar is a single vaccine preparation.	*Severe:* Allergic reaction or anaphylaxis.		In addition to infants, this vaccine is a priority for children 2–5 years with sickle cell disease, asplenia, HIV infection, or immunocompromised. The vaccine is also a priority for American Indian and Native Alaskan children 2–5 years because of their increased risk for pneumococcal disease. The series does not need to be restarted, no matter how long since the previous dose was given.
Varicella Virus Vaccine *Type:* Live attenuated *Route:* Subcutaneous *Dosage:* 0.5 mL *Age(s) given:* 12-18 months; or any time up to 12 years of age (1 dose); 13 years or older (2 doses 4–8 weeks apart) *Storage:* Frozen at 5°F or colder. May be stored in refrigerator at 2°–8°C (35°–46°F) up to 72 hours before reconstitution. Once reconstituted, vaccine must be used within 30 minutes or discarded. Do not refreeze. Diluent kept at room temperature. Varivax is a single vaccine preparation.	*Common:* Pain or redness at injection site; fever up to 38.8°C (102°F) in children or up to 37.7°C (100°F) in adults. Less commonly a vaccine-related rash (mild exanthem of 6 to 10 lesions that last for 2 to 3 days) may occur during first month after the injection. *Severe:* Allergic reaction or anaphylaxis; thrombocytopenia; febrile seizure; CNS manifestations.	Prior anaphylactic reaction to vaccine. Allergy to neomycin or gelatin. Immunodeficiency or receiving immunosuppression therapy. Administration of immune serum globulin or blood products in last 3–11 months. Active untreated TB. Pregnancy. Moderate or severe febrile illness.	Prior to immunization, ask if child is immunodeficient or on immunosuppression treatment or has an allergy to neomycin or gelatin. Determine if a family member is immunocompromised. Clear, colorless to pale yellow liquid when reconstituted. Give the entire contents of the vial even if more than 0.5 mL. Instruct adolescent girls of childbearing age to avoid pregnancy for 3 months after immunization. The vaccine is effective. Only very mild cases occurred in children who were immunized, primarily caused by wild type virus (Vazquez, LaRussa, Gershon et al., 2001).
Hepatitis A *Type:* Inactivated *Route:* Intramuscular *Dosage:* 0.5 mL, 1.0 mL over 17 years for Vaqta,[a] 1.0 mL over 18 years for Havrix[a] *Age(s) given:* 12-23 months; 2-18 years, 6-12 months after first dose (2 doses) in areas with increased incidence. May give at same time as all other vaccines in a separate site. *Storage:* Store in body of refrigerator at 2°–8°C (35°–46°F). Do not freeze; do not use if has been frozen. Havrix and Vaqta are single vaccine preparations.	Rare reports of anaphylaxis/anaphylactoid reactions.	Known hypersensitivity to any component of vaccine. Prior hypersensitivity reaction to the vaccine.	Shake well, slightly opaque white suspension. Can be given for post exposure prophylaxis against hepatitis A. Immune globulin and vaccine can be given at the same time in different sites. High incidence areas include the states of Alaska, Arkansas, Arizona, California, Colorado, Idaho, Missouri, Montana, New Mexico, Nevada, Oklahoma, Oregon, South Dakota, Texas, Utah, Washington, and Wyoming. Other high-risk populations to receive this vaccine include incarcerated youth, Native Alaskans, and American Indians.

TABLE 45–3 ✛ Recommended Pediatric Immunizations—continued

Immunization Type	Side Effects	Contraindications	Nursing Considerations
Hepatitis A—Cont.			Do not restart the series, no matter how long since the previous dose. Vaccine brands can be interchanged
Influenza Type: Inactivated (TIV), live attenuated for intranasal use (LAIV) Route: Intramuscular (all ages), intranasal (5 years and older) Dosage: 0.25 mL in infants 6 to 35 months, 0.5 mL beginning at 3 years May give at same time as all other vaccines in a separate site. TIV storage: Store in body of refrigerator at 2°–8°C (35°–46°F). Do not freeze; do not use if has been frozen. LAIV storage: Keep frozen. May be thawed and kept in refrigerator at 2°–8°C (35°–46°F) for no more than 24 hours before use. Flu Shield (Trivalent, inactivated vaccine) Flu Mist (LAIV)	Common after TIV: May have soreness or swelling at injection site, fever, aches. Life-threatening allergic reactions are rare. Common after intranasal vaccine: Runny nose or nasal congestion, fever, headache or muscle aches, abdominal pain and occasional vomiting. No life-threatening problems were detected during clinical trials.	Contraindicated in children with history of anaphylactic reaction to egg or chicken protein, hypersensitivity to thimerosol, known sensitivity to gentamicin or other aminoglycosides. LAIV is contraindicated in children on long-term aspirin therapy; who have known or suspected immune deficiency disorders; who are immunosuppressed; or who have an altered immune status due to various therapies. Should not be given within 3 days of pertussis vaccine (Mosby's Drug Consult, 2004). Postpone vaccine when child has acute febrile illness until symptoms abate, but may be given with minor illness, with or without fever.	Thawed intranasal vaccine is pale yellow, clear to slightly cloudy. Administered annually in autumn. Children with no history of influenza illness or vaccine need 2 doses 1 month apart. Intranasal dose is split (0.25 mL) with a dose divider clip. Administer in each nostril while child is sitting in an upright position. Insert the tip of the sprayer inside the nose and depress the plunger to spray. Children 8 years of age or younger who are receiving the influenza vaccine for the first time should get 2 doses separated by at least 4 weeks (injectable) and 6 weeks (intranasal). Must be reimmunized each year as immunity wanes.
Meningococcal Tetravalent Conjugate Vaccine (MCV4) Type: Inactivated Route: Intramuscular Dosage: 0.5 mL in children Age(s) given: 11–12 years and older May be given at same time as Td vaccine. Storage: Store in body of refrigerator at 2°–8°C (35°–46°F) until use.	Common: Pain at injection site, headache, and fatigue. Less than 5% experienced a severe systemic reaction in vaccine trials (Bilukha & Rosenstein, 2005). A possible association between MCV4 (Menactra) and Guillain Barré syndrome occurring 2 to 4 weeks after vaccination has been reported (Food and Drug Administration, 2005).	Contraindicated in children with known hypersensitivity to any component of vaccine, including diphtheria toxoid. Stopper contains latex. Patients at risk for hemorrhage should not receive vaccine. Pregnant women should receive vaccine only if clearly needed.	May be given to children immunosuppressed by disease or medication. Recommended for control of meningococcal outbreaks caused by serogroups A, C, W-135, and Y. Until adequate supply exists, recommended for preadolescents and adolescents wishing to reduce health risks.

[a]Trade names

Data from American Academy of Pediatrics. (2003). *Red Book: Report of the Committee on Infectious Disease* (26th ed.). Elk Grove Village, IL: Author; Immunization Action Coalition; Mosby. (2004). *Mosby's Drug Consult 2004*. St. Louis, MO: Mosby.; Bindler, R. M., & Howry, L. B. (2005). *Pediatric drugs and nursing implications* (3rd ed.). Upper Saddle River, NJ: Prentice Hall Health; and Buck, M. L. (2005). Meningococcal conjugate vaccine. *Pediatric Pharmacology, 11*(5). Retrieved June 7, 2005, from http://www.medscape.com/viewarticle/505508_print

NURSING CARE PLAN

THE CHILD NEEDING IMMUNIZATIONS

Intervention	Rationale	Expected Outcome
1. Nursing Diagnosis: Risk for Infection related to incomplete immunization series		
NIC Priority Interventions: **Health Screening:** Detecting health risks or problems by means of history, examination, and other procedures.		**NOC Suggested Outcome:** **Immune Status:** Adequacy of natural and acquired appropriately targeted resistance to internal and external antigens
Goal: The child will become adequately protected from disease-preventable illnesses.		
■ Review the child's immunization record for needed vaccines at each healthcare visit. ■ Identify all due vaccines that can be provided simultaneously. ■ Identify potential contraindications to needed vaccines. Review past reactions to vaccines.	■ Assessment identifies the children who have missed needed immunizations. ■ Many vaccines can be given at the same visit to more adequately protect the child. This also saves healthcare trips for families. ■ Reduces the risk for the child and other caretakers to have adverse reactions to vaccines.	The child is adequately protected from vaccine-preventable illnesses.
2. Nursing Diagnosis: Deficient Knowledge (Parent) related to potential side effects of vaccines		
NIC Priority Interventions: **Teaching, prescribed medication:** Preparing a pateint to safely take prescribed medications and monitor their effects.		**NOC Suggested Outcome:** **Knowledge:** Extent of understanding conveyed about vaccine reactions and comfort measures
Goal: Parents will sign consent for vaccines to be given.		
■ Educate the parents about the need for specific vaccines and the risk if not given. Obtain signed consent before giving vaccines.	■ Informed consent is required for all treatments.	The parent(s) complete(s) consent form, which is placed in the child's file.
Goal: Parents will state the side effects of vaccines given.		
■ Review past reactions to vaccines and describe common potential reactions and why they occur. ■ Describe serious side effects that should be reported to the healthcare provider.	■ Parents should expect common reactions and know they indicate the child's body is building protection to the illness. ■ Parents need to be prepared for potential serious side effects so they can obtain care if needed.	Parents report all serious side effects to the healthcare provider.
Goal: Parents will manage common side effects of vaccines.		
■ Teach parents general comfort measures for children's common side effects; for example: 　■ Cool pack to tender leg 　■ Acetaminophen or ibuprofen for fever and discomfort 　■ Rocking and holding the infant 　■ Gentle movement of affected extremity	■ Parents will know how to make the child more comfortable during the 24–48 hours after the vaccine is given.	The child is given comfort measures after vaccine administration.

NURSING CARE PLAN—continued

THE CHILD NEEDING IMMUNIZATIONS

Intervention	Rationale	Expected Outcome
3. Nursing Diagnosis: Risk for Injury related to vaccine reaction		
NIC Priority Interventions: **Surveillance Safety:** Purposeful and ongoing collection and analysis of information about the patient and the environment for use in promoting and maintaining patient saftey.		**NOC Suggested Outcome:** **Risk control:** Actions to eliminate or reduce actual, personal, and modifiable health threats
Goal: The child's potential vaccine reactions will be safely managed.		
■ Prepare for life-threatening reactions by having resuscitation drugs and equipment immediately available. ■ Monitor the child for 15 minutes after the vaccine is given before letting the child go home. ■ Assess the child for extreme anxiety and injection fearfulness. ■ Have the fearful child sit or lie down until symptoms of vasovagal response have disappeared. ■ Report all vaccine-related reactions to the appropriate agency using the standard form.	■ Anaphylactic reactions must be managed quickly and effectively. ■ A life-threatening response will usually become apparent within this time frame. ■ These are potential signs the child may have a vasovagal response to the injection. ■ The child who faints may sustain a head injury. ■ Legal requirements for all healthcare providers.	The child has no reaction, or a severe reaction to a vaccine is managed effectively.

needing immunizations. Additional nursing diagnoses may include the following:

■ *Risk for Impaired Skin Integrity* related to vaccine response

■ *Ineffective Health Maintenance* related to cultural beliefs regarding routine immunization

PLANNING AND IMPLEMENTATION

Nursing management focuses on being a strong advocate for immunization, informing parents about immunizations and possible side effects, addressing their fears about possible reactions, obtaining consent, and reporting adverse reactions. Be well informed about recommended immunization schedules.

Provide written materials (current Vaccine Information Statements [VIS]) about immunizations to the parents or guardian as required by the National Vaccine Injury Act of 1986 and 1993. Written materials do not replace teaching about immunizations that explains the risks and benefits of immunization, risks of disease, how to manage common mild reactions, and how to report serious reactions. Record the child's history carefully, specifying any previous reactions to immunizations, allergies, and immune diseases.

Some parents fear immunization reactions because of stories they have heard. Talk with parents to understand their concerns. Be able to explain the risks and benefits of each immunization. Parents have the right to refuse im-

munizations for their child on the basis of religious beliefs, but they should sign a form documenting informed refusal. If there is a disease outbreak, the nonimmunized child must be kept out of school. Local, city, or state courts decide how to settle any conflicts.

Federal legislation requires consent to be obtained before administering a vaccine. In most institutions it is the nurse's responsibility to inform the parents or the child's legal guardian, supply literature, and obtain written consent before the vaccine is administered. The nurse is required to record the (1) month, day, and year of administration; (2) vaccine given; (3) manufacturer; (4) lot number and expiration date of the immunization given; (5) site and route of administration; and (6) name, title, and address of the person who administers the vaccine. In addition the nurse ensures that any severe immunization reaction is reported to the National Vaccine Injury Compensation Program.

NURSING PRACTICE

Be prepared for potential vaccine anaphylaxis. Keep epinephrine and resuscitation equipment immediately available. The dose for epinephrine (aqueous 1:1000) is 0.01 mL/kg per dose up to 0.5 mL intramuscularly. The dose can be repeated every 10 to 20 minutes for up to a total of 3 doses until symptoms subside or other emergency care interventions are initiated (American Academy of Pediatrics, 2003).

MEDIALINK Develop Immunization Schedules

MEDIALINK Immunization FAQ

● **FIGURE 45–3**

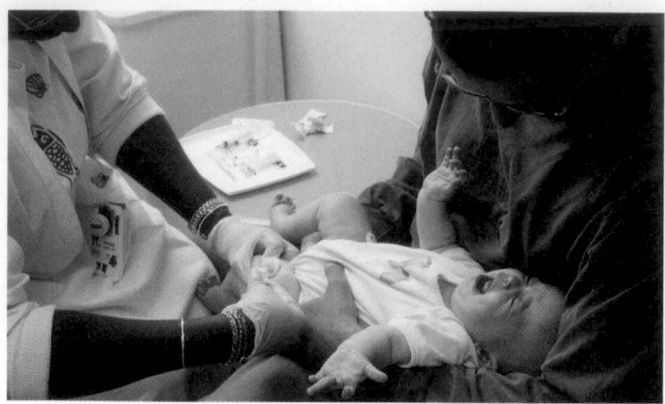

Give immunizations quickly and efficiently. Do not prolong the wait and let fear grow. The child will be anxious, especially if more than one injection must be given.

Give the appropriate immunizations to the child as efficiently as possible, while providing support to the child (Figure 45–3 ●). Longer needles (25 mm rather than 16 mm) reduce the rates of local reactions and tenderness in infant immunizations. This may ensure that the vaccine is given intramuscularly rather than subcutaneously (Diggle & Deek, 2000).

Anticipate ways to reduce pain and anxiety associated with immunizations. Do not prolong the process of giving immunizations, and tell the child honestly that the needles will cause some pain. Let the child select the arm or leg for the injection and forms of distraction to promote coping. When finished giving injections, let the parent comfort the child. Provide guidelines for managing expected mild reactions at home. Schedule the child's next appointment for a health promotion visit to complete needed immunizations. Give parents a record of the child's immunizations, and record the vaccines given in the healthcare agency's official records.

NURSING PRACTICE

Reduce pain and anxiety associated with injections with the following techniques:

- Give young infants 25% sucrose water to drink (mix 1 packet of sugar in 10 mL of tap water) a minute or two before the injection. See pain management of infants in Chapter 42. ∞
- Apply pressure at the site for 10 seconds before the injection.
- Instruct parent how to apply EMLA cream to the site for an hour before the injection.
- Use vapocoolant spray immediately before the injection.
- Give two injections simultaneously in different extremities using two different providers.
- Use age-appropriate distraction techniques. See Chapter 42. ∞

EVIDENCE-BASED NURSING

NURSING CARE DURING IMMUNIZATIONS

Clinical Question

How can nurses reduce the pain and anxiety associated with injections?

Evidence

A study about the use of distraction to reduce the distress of immunizations was conducted with 90 infants age 2 months to 3 years in a rural health department. Nurses performing injections were trained in the use of appropriate behaviors and distraction techniques (age-appropriate toy and a popular cartoon movie) to use with the study children. Infants and children in the control group could be provided with comfort, reassurance, and empathy, but no toy or movie. Interactions were videotaped and scored by researchers. Infants in the distraction group displayed less distress than the control group. In many cases the parents helped supplement the distraction provided by the nurse (Cohen, 2002). Another study explored methods to reduce the pain and stress associated with four immunization injections provided to 116 infants between 6 and 16 weeks of age. The intervention group received a bottle with 10 mL of 25% sucrose 2 minutes before the injections. They were then allowed to suck on a pacifier or bottle of formula throughout the injections and afterwards. Parents were asked to hold the infants on their lap with their upper bodies close to the parent, making the legs available for injection. The control group received immunizations on the examining table with no specific comfort measures provided. Infants in the intervention group cried less and parents expressed the desire for the same procedure to be used in future visits (Reis, Roth, Syphan et al., 2003).

Implications

Infants and young children often receive several injections for immunizations at health promotion visits, and parents are distressed by the number of injections and associated pain. Nurses can use simple comfort measures and distraction to reduce pain and distress associated with immunizations. By assembling a toolkit of distraction devices for infants and children of various ages, the nurse can be quickly prepared to provide age-appropriate distraction. Sucrose solution can be prepared in advance, anticipating the number of young infants that will need immunizations in a morning or afternoon. Nurses can also provide guidance to parents about how they can hold and comfort the infant during the injections.

Critical Thinking

Identify the different methods nurses use for comforting infants receiving immunizations in a busy clinical setting. Compare the effectiveness of those methods with distraction and sucrose solution to help you identify your future nursing care interventions for immunizations.

References

Cohen, L. L. (2002). Reducing infant immunization distress through distraction. *Health Psychology, 21*(2), 207–211.
Reis, E. C., Roth, E. K., Syphan, J. L., Tarbell, S. E., & Holubkov, R. (2003). Effective pain reduction for multiple immunization injections in young infants. *Archives of Pediatrics & Adolescent Medicine, 57*, 1115–1120.

Certain reactions following immunization are reportable by law to the U.S. Department of Health and Human Services (Table 45–4). The National Childhood Vaccine Injury Acts of 1986 and 1993 provide compensation if a link between immunization and a serious adverse effect is found. The first act resulted after serious neurologic adverse reactions from pertussis immunizations were reported, creating significant liability concerns for healthcare professionals. The Vaccine Adverse Event Reporting System was established in 1988 to track serious vaccine reactions (see Table 45–4). Follow guidelines for reporting according to the Vaccine Adverse Event Reporting System. The Vaccine Safety Datalink project continually evaluates vaccine safety on more than 6 million people. See the Companion Website for some of the latest research findings.

EVALUATION

Expected outcomes of nursing care include the following:

- Parents are fully informed and give consent for immunizations.
- All immunizations appropriate for the child's age are given at each health visit.
- The parents are prepared to manage mild reactions to immunizations at home.

INFECTIOUS AND COMMUNICABLE DISEASES IN CHILDREN

Infectious and communicable diseases cause acute illnesses. These diseases are caused by bacterial, viral, protozoan, or fungal organisms. As noted earlier, infants and children develop infectious and communicable diseases

more frequently than adults do. They develop antibodies as they are exposed to infectious organisms, so they frequently become symptomatic after exposure. The epidemiology, clinical manifestations, treatment, prevention, and nursing care of selected infectious and communicable diseases of childhood are described in detail in Table 45–5. Infectious diseases transmitted by animal vectors are detailed in Table 45–6.

CLINICAL MANIFESTATIONS

The child with an infectious or communicable disease has a cluster of symptoms specific to the disease. Initially there may be nonspecific signs such as fatigue, malaise, weakness, and decreased responsiveness or inability to concentrate. Skin rash, poor appetite, malaise, vomiting, diarrhea, and body aches are some common signs and symptoms. Fever is the most common sign of infectious disease in infants and children. Why does fever develop in response to certain illnesses and infections? What methods can be used to manage fever in children?

Physiology of Fever

The hypothalamus is the control center for the regulation of body temperature and is for that reason frequently compared to a thermostat (see "Pathophysiology Illustrated: Fever"). As blood circulates through the hypothalamus, this brain structure directs body systems to conserve or dissipate heat, depending on the temperature of the blood.

- If body temperature is lower than normal, vasoconstriction is initiated to conserve heat. The adrenal glands produce epinephrine and norepinephrine, which cause an increase in metabolism, more vasoconstriction, and more heat production.
- Shivering or chills may occur, which in turn may increase heat production.
- When excess heat is produced, the body's temperature increases. The heart rate and respiratory rate increase.
- Vasodilation occurs and the skin flushes, becoming warm to the touch. As the temperature decreases, the child may start to perspire, and the heart and respiratory rates return to normal.

(continues on p. 1340)

THINKING CRITICALLY

IMMUNIZATIONS

Lian, 5 years old, has accompanied her mother and 2-year-old brother Chang to the pediatric clinic. Her mother is concerned because Chang has had a fever of 38.3°C (101°F) for the past 3 days. Chang has been to this office several times in the past few months for healthcare, but this is the first time Lian has come along.

When the nurse asks about Lian's last visit to the doctor and the status of her immunizations, her mother says Lian has not been seen for about 2 years. She is not sure whether Lian has had all of her shots. In checking Lian's health records, the nurse notes that she needs several immunizations, including DTaP, polio, varicella, and hepatitis B. Chang needs polio, MMR, and Hib vaccines.

Should Lian be given any of these immunizations today, even though her brother is ill? Which immunizations could be given at the same time? Should Chang also receive any immunizations today?

NURSING PRACTICE

One degree of temperature elevation causes an increase in respiratory rate by four breaths per minute and increases the metabolic need for oxygen by 7%.

TABLE 45–4 ✤ National Childhood Vaccine Injury Act—Vaccine Injury Table, July 1, 2005

Vaccine	Adverse Event	Time Interval
I. Tetanus toxoid-containing vaccines (e.g., DTaP, Tdap, DTP-Hib, DT, Td, TT)	A. Anaphylaxis or anaphylactic shock	0–4 hours
	B. Brachial neuritis	2–28 days
	C. Any acute complication or sequela (including death) of above events	Not applicable
II. Pertussis antigen-containing vaccines (e.g., DTaP, Tdap, DTP, P, DTP-Hib)	A. Anaphylaxis or anaphylactic shock	0–4 hours
	B. Encephalopathy (or encephalitis)	0–72 hours
	C. Any acute complication or sequela (including death) of above events	Not applicable
III. Measles, mumps and rubella virus-containing vaccines in any combination (e.g., MMR, MR, M, R)	A. Anaphylaxis or anaphylactic shock	0–4 hours
	B. Encephalopathy (or encephalitis)	5–15 days
	C. Any acute complication or sequela (including death) of above events	Not applicable
IV. Rubella virus-containing vaccines (e.g., MMR, MR, R)	A. Chronic arthritis	7–42 days
	B. Any acute complication or sequela (including death) of above event	Not applicable
V. Measles virus-containing vaccines (e.g., MMR, MR, M)	A. Thrombocytopenic purpura	7–30 days
	B. Vaccine-Strain Measles Viral Infection in an immunodeficient recipient	0–6 months
	C. Any acute complication or sequela (including death) of above events	Not applicable
VI. Polio live virus-containing vaccines (OPV)	A. Paralytic polio	
	—in a non-immunodeficient recipient	0–30 days
	—in an immunodeficient recipient	0–6 months
	—in a vaccine assoc. community case	Not applicable
	B. Vaccine-strain polio viral infection	
	—in a non-immunodeficient recipient	0–30 days
	—in an immunodeficient recipient	0–6 months
	—in a vaccine assoc. community case	Not applicable
	C. Any acute complication or sequela (including death) of above events	Not applicable
VII. Polio inactivated-virus containing vaccines (e.g., IPV)	A. Anaphylaxis or anaphylactic shock	0–4 hours
	B. Any acute complication or sequela (including death) of above event	Not applicable
VIII. Hepatitis B antigen-containing vaccines	A. Anaphylaxis or anaphylactic shock	0–4 hours
	B. Any acute complication or sequela (including death) of above event	Not applicable
IX. Hemophilus influenzae type b polysaccharide conjugate vaccines	A. No condition specified for compensation	Not applicable
X. Varicella vaccine	A. No condition specified for compensation	Not applicable
XI. Rotavirus vaccine	A. No condition specified for compensation	Not applicable
XII. Vaccines containing live, oral, rhesus-based rotavirus	A. Intussusception	0–30 days
	B. Any acute complication or sequela (including death) of above event	Not applicable
XIII. Pneumococcal conjugate vaccines	A. No condition specified for compensation	Not applicable
XIV. Any new vaccine recommended by the Centers for Disease Control and Prevention for routine administration to children, after publication by Secretary, HHS of a notice of coverage[b]	A. No condition specified for compensation	Not applicable

[a]Effective date: July 1, 2005

[b]As of **December 1, 2004,** hepatitis A vaccines have been added to the Vaccine Injury Table (Table) under this category. As of **July 1, 2005,** *trivalent* influenza vaccines have been added to the Table under this category. Trivalent influenza vaccines are given annually during the flu season either by needle and syringe or in a nasal spray. All influenza vaccines routinely administered in the United States are trivalent vaccines covered under this category. See *News* on the VICP Web site for more information (*www.hrsa.gov/osp/vicp*).

Retrieved 10/24/2005

TABLE 45–5 ✣ Selected Infectious and Communicable Diseases in Children

Disease	Clinical Manifestations	Clinical Therapy	Nursing Management
Chickenpox (Varicella)*+ *Causal agent:* Varicella-zoster, human herpesvirus 3. *Epidemiology:* Peak occurrence is in the late fall, winter, and spring. Maternal antibodies disappear 2–3 months after birth. *Transmission:* Direct contact of the virus to the mucous membranes or conjunctiva primarily through airborne spread of secretions and occasionally with lesion contact. When introduced into a susceptible and unvaccinated population, it has an attack rate of nearly 90% (Arvin, 2002). *Incubation period:* 14–21 days *Period of communicability:* As long as 5 days before the onset of the rash to a maximum of 6 days after the appearance of vesicles, when all lesions have crusted over. This period may be prolonged after passive immunization or in immunodeficient children.	Acute onset of mild fever, malaise, anorexia, headache, mild abdominal pain, and irritability occurs before and with eruption. The rash begins as a macule on an erythematous base and progresses to a papule, then to a clear, fluid-filled vesicle. The rash may erupt for 1–5 days and is itchy. Lesions of all stages may be present at any one time. Crusts may remain for 1–3 weeks. The lesions begin on the trunk, scalp, and face, and then spread to the rest of the body. Ulcerative lesions may be seen in the mucous membranes. Lesions in the mouth may lead to decreased fluid intake and dehydration. *Complications:* Complications are rare but can include secondary infection (cellulitis, local abscesses, sepsis, meningitis, encephalitis, pneumonia), thrombocytopenia, and Reye syndrome. Chickenpox can be fatal in immunocompromised children. Children who are undergoing chemotherapy, steroid treatment, or transplant therapy should be carefully monitored after exposure to the disease.	Medical management is supportive. Oral and IV acyclovir is used for immunocompromised patients, children treated with chronic salicylate therapy, and oral or aerosol corticosteroids. Acyclovir is not recommended for healthy children or adolescents with uncomplicated chickenpox (American Academy of Pediatrics, 2003). Varicella-zoster immune globulin is given as soon as possible to newborns of infected mothers and exposed immunocompromised, unimmunized children up to 4 days after exposure. *Prognosis:* Most children recover fully. Children who are immunocompromised must be treated aggressively. The disease is more severe when steroids have been given during the incubation period (Arvin, 2002). *Prevention:* Varicella is vaccine-preventable. See Table 45–3. The vaccine may be given within 72 hours after exposure to prevent or significantly modify the disease. Wild virus cases occur in vaccinated children.	■ Use airborne and contact precautions while children are contagious. ■ Upon admission to the hospital, inquire about varicella immunization or recent exposure. Place all exposed children in isolation to protect newborns and immunocompromised patients. Nurses caring for the exposed or infected child should have documented immunity. ■ When treated at home, isolate the child from all susceptible individuals, especially medically fragile and immuno-compromised children or adults, and women early in pregnancy. Notify the school or childcare facility of the child's illness. ■ Secondary cases are often more severe than the primary case. ■ The child with eczema or sunburn may have a more severe rash. ■ Give nonaspirin antipyretics to control fever. ■ Give oral antihistamines for relief of itching. Oatmeal and Aveeno baths are soothing. Caladryl lotion applied to lesions may also provide relief. ■ Keep the child's fingernails short and clean. Young children may need to wear soft cotton mittens when itching cannot be controlled. ■ Change bed linens frequently. Wash linen in mild soap and rinse well. ■ Reassure the child that the lesions are temporary and will go away. ■ Observe the child closely for symptoms of complications such as drowsiness, meningeal signs, respiratory distress, and dehydration. Disorientation and restlessness may indicate viral encephalitis. ■ Monitor for acyclovir side effects: nausea, vomiting, diarrhea, abdominal pain, as well as allergic skin reactions or headache. Monitor renal function if the child has renal insufficiency.

Chickenpox

Used with permission of the American Academy of Pediatrics, http://www.vaccineinformation.org/photos/varlaap 002.jpg, accessed 6/20/2004.

*Indicates that a vaccine or antitoxin is available for use in high-risk or as-needed situations.
+Indicates that the disease has a safe and effective vaccine.

(continued)

TABLE 45–5 ✢ Selected Infectious and Communicable Diseases in Children—continued

Disease	Clinical Manifestations	Clinical Therapy	Nursing Management
Coxsackievirus *Causal agent:* Coxsackievirus A16 and Enterovirus 71 *Epidemiology:* Occurs worldwide, most commonly in summer and early fall. Sporadic outbreaks are seen, especially among children in out-of-home settings. Immunity probably occurs after clinical or subclinical infection, but duration of the immunity is unknown. *Transmission:* Fecal-oral and respiratory routes. *Incubation period:* 3–6 days. *Period of communicability:* 2 days before rash to 2 days after it disappears.	Each of the coxsackieviruses causes a different set of manifestations. Herpangina is an acute, self-limiting viral disease characterized by the sudden onset of fever, sore throat, and small, discrete grayish papulovesicular ulcerative pharyngeal lesions that gradually increase in size. In hand-foot-and-mouth disease, the lesions are more diffuse and may occur on the buccal surfaces of the cheeks, gums, and sides of the tongue. Papulovesicular lesions occur on the hands and feet and last for 7–10 days. Children may be irritable and have a fever, anorexia, dysphagia, malaise, and a sore throat. *Complications:* Enterovirus 71 caused a fatal epidemic of hand-foot-and-mouth disease in Taiwan in 1998 (Chang, Lin, Hsu et al., 1999).	Diagnostic tests include a cell culture to detect the virus. Medical care is supportive. An antiviral drug, pleconaril, is being evaluated for use in immunodeficient children (American Academy of Pediatrics, 2003). *Prognosis:* Recovery is generally good with supportive care. *Prevention:* Avoid contact with infected persons early in the disease.	■ Isolate the child while contagious. Use standard and contact precautions if the child is hospitalized. ■ Apply topical lotions and give systemic medications as ordered to lessen the pain and relieve the irritation. ■ Offer cool drinks and soft, bland foods (no citrus, salty, or spicy foods). Swallowing may be painful. ■ Offer warm saline mouth rinses. ■ Observe for dehydration. ■ Provide reassurance and support to parents. ■ Give nonaspirin antipyretics for fever. Keep the child out of school or childcare while the child is febrile.
Diphtheria*+ *Causal agent:* Corynebacterium diphtheriae *Epidemiology:* Occurs mostly in colder months in unimmunized, partially immunized, and immunized children with waning immunity. Cases of cutaneous and wound diphtheria occur sporadically in the tropics. Maternal immunity lasts up to 6 months after birth. The disease is endemic in areas where immunization is no longer routine, such as Russia. *Transmission:* Contact with nasal or eye discharge, or skin lesion; or less commonly by indirect contact with contaminated items. Unpasteurized milk has served as a vehicle. *Incubation period:* 2–7 days or longer. *Period of communicability:* Usually 2–4 weeks or until 4 days after antibiotics are started.	Symptoms can be mild or severe with a gradual onset over 1–2 days. Low-grade fever, anorexia, malaise, rhinorrhea with a foul odor, cough, sore throat, hoarseness, stridor or noisy breathing, cervical lymphadenitis, and pharyngitis may be present. In more severe cases the membranes of the tonsils, pharynx, and larynx are affected. The characteristic membranous lesion is a thick, bluish white to grayish black patch that covers the tonsils. It can spread to cover the soft and hard palates and the posterior portion of the pharynx. Attempts to remove the membrane result in bleeding. *Complications:* Produces an endotoxin that causes myocarditis and peripheral neuropathy (diplopia, slurred speech, difficulty swallowing, or paralysis of the palate) or ascending paralysis similar to Guillain-Barré syndrome.	Diagnostic tests include a culture from any mucosal or cutaneous lesion. Administration of IV antitoxin and antibiotics within 3 days of onset of symptoms. The child must be tested for sensitivity to horse serum before giving the antitoxin. When diphtheria is suspected, antibiotic therapy (penicillin G or erythromycin) should be initiated without waiting for laboratory results. Removal of membrane may be needed to treat airway obstruction. *Prognosis:* With treatment, prognosis is good. If untreated, death may occur due to airway obstruction. *Prevention:* Diphtheria is a vaccine-preventable disease. See Table 45–3. This is a reportable disease.	■ Use droplet precautions for pharyngeal disease and contact precautions for cutaneous disease. ■ Monitor closely for signs of increasing respiratory distress, as well as cardiac and neurologic complications. Provide humidified oxygen as necessary. ■ Have emergency airway equipment available. ■ Administer antibiotics. Give no medications containing caffeine or other stimulants. ■ Use oral suction gently as necessary. ■ Allow children to use mouthwash if desired. Gargling is not permitted because it can irritate the pharyngeal surfaces. ■ Encourage liquids as tolerated. Intravenous fluids may be necessary. ■ Provide emotional support to the family. ■ Initiate the search for patient contacts to give antibiotics and immunization boosters.

TABLE 45–5 ✤ Selected Infectious and Communicable Diseases in Children—continued

Disease	Clinical Manifestations	Clinical Therapy	Nursing Management
Erythema Infectiosum (Fifth Disease) *Causal agent:* Human parvovirus B19 *Epidemiology:* Occurs worldwide, most often in winter and spring. The disease also occurs in epidemics, with peak activity every 6 years. The incidence is highest in children between the ages of 5 and 14 years. *Transmission:* Respiratory secretions and blood. *Incubation period:* 6–14 days *Period of communicability:* Believed to be the highest before the onset of the disease.	Stage 1 begins as a flulike illness (headache, chills, malaise, nausea, body ache) lasting 2–3 days. Stage 2 occurs 1 week later with a fiery-red rash on the cheeks giving a "slapped face" appearance. Circumoral pallor is seen. In 1 to 4 days a lacelike symmetric, erythematous, maculopapular rash appears on the truck and limbs, spreading proximal to distal but sparing the palms and soles. During the third stage, lasting 1–3 weeks, the rash fades but can reappear if the skin is irritated or exposed to sunlight. The rash may be mildly pruritic. *Complications:* Children with hemolytic conditions may have transient aplastic crisis.	Diagnosis can be made by a serologic test for immuno-globulin (Ig) M parvovirus B19-specific antibody. Medical treatment is supportive and recovery is usually spontaneous. Children with hemolytic conditions may need blood transfusions if an aplastic crisis occurs. Immunodeficient patients may develop a chronic infection for which IV immune globulin therapy is often effective (American Academy of Pediatrics, 2003). *Prognosis:* Fetal infection may occur resulting in fetal hydrops or spontaneous abortion. *Prevention:* Avoid contact with infected persons.	■ Children with aplastic crisis are often hospitalized. ■ Use standard and droplet precautions. Isolation is needed only for children with aplastic crisis or when immunosuppressed. ■ Nonaspirin antipyretics may be given to control fever. ■ Use soothing oatmeal or Aveeno baths if the rash is pruritic. Antipruritics may also help to relieve itching. ■ Encourage rest and offer frequent fluids. ■ Keep children out of direct sunlight if possible. Provide protective, light, loose clothing if exposure to sunlight cannot be avoided. ■ Provide quiet diversionary activity. There is no reason to keep the immune competent child out of school or day care. ■ Explain the three stages of rash development to parents.

Characteristic facial rash of erythema infectiosum (fifth disease).

Courtesy of Centers for Disease Control and Prevention, Atlanta, GA.

Haemophilus Influenzae, Type B[+] *Causal agent:* Coccobacilli H. influenzae bacteria, which has several serotypes and can be encapsulated or nonencapsulated. *Epidemiology:* Occurs most often in the spring and summer. Most commonly affected are infants and young children in childcare centers. Low-birth-weight children and children with chronic illnesses have an increased susceptibility. *Transmission:* Direct contact or droplet inhalation. The organism is frequently asymptomatically colonized in the respiratory tract.	Begins with a viral upper respiratory infection. The organism passes through the mucosal barrier to directly invade the bloodstream. It can cause several severe invasive illnesses, including meningitis, epiglottitis, pneumonia, septic arthritis, and cellulitis. It is also a cause of sepsis in infants. Other illnesses include sinusitis, otitis media, bronchitis, and pericarditis. Each disease has very specific clinical manifestations. Invasive disease has decreased significantly since introduction of the vaccine.	Treatment consists of antibiotic therapy, but one third of strains are resistant to ampicillin. Rifampin may be given to unprotected household contacts (not pregnant women), if another child has not completed immunizations, within 1 week after diagnosis. In this case, the infected child also gets rifampin to eliminate nasopharyngeal colonization. *Prognosis:* With rapid diagnosis and treatment, recovery is good but highly dependent on the disease the organism has caused. When treatment is delayed, the prognosis for full recovery becomes much more guarded.	■ Use droplet precautions until 24 hours after the initiation of antibiotics. ■ Antibiotic therapy is administered intravenously for severe infections. Infections such as otitis media can be managed with oral antibiotics. ■ Unimmunized children under the age of 4 years are at increased risk for developing disease from H. influenzae. Specific prophylactic measures for susceptible children may be ordered by the physician. ■ Administer antipyretics to help the child feel more comfortable.

*Indicates that a vaccine or antitoxin is available for use in high-risk or as-needed situations.
[+]Indicates that the disease has a safe and effective vaccine.

(continued)

TABLE 45–5 ✛ Selected Infectious and Communicable Diseases in Children—continued

Disease	Clinical Manifestations	Clinical Therapy	Nursing Management
Haemophilus Influenzae, Type B⁺— Cont. *Incubation period:* Unknown. *Period of communicability:* 3 days from onset of symptoms.	*Complications:* Illness caused by *H. influenzae* type B responds to antibiotic therapy. Left untreated, severe sequelae and death, especially in young infants, can occur from conditions such as meningitis, epiglottitis, sinusitis, pneumonitis, and cellulitis.	*Prevention:* Immunization is now available for *H. influenzae* type B. See Table 45–3. Other types of *H. influenzae* are not vaccine-preventable.	■ Closely monitor IV sites for patency and infiltration. ■ Perform nursing care measures specific to the illness. ■ Inform family members that rifampin turns urine and other body fluids orange, and it will cause stains.

Hepatitis A, Hepatitis B, and Hepatitis C, see Chapter 51. ∞

Influenza *Causal agent:* Orthomyxoviridae, types A and B. *Epidemiology:* Prevalent in the United States from October to March, but the virus is active in other parts of the world year-round. During annual epidemics, 10% to 40% of healthy children are infected, and 1% is hospitalized (Cheung & Lieberman, 2002). *Transmission:* Spreads by aerosolized particles and direct contact with respiratory secretions. *Incubation period:* 1 to 4 days. *Period of communicability:* One day before symptoms until 5 days after onset of illness.	Abrupt onset of fever (38°C to 40°C), chills, cough, runny nose, sore throat, malaise, aches, headache, and anorexia. Children may have nausea and vomiting, diarrhea, and abdominal pain. Children may also present with croup, bronchiolitis, conjunctivitis, or other nonspecific febrile illness. *Complications:* Otitis media, exacerbations of chronic lung conditions such as asthma and cystic fibrosis. Pneumonia, croup, bronchiolitis, and wheezing may occur in up to 25% of children. Myositis, myocarditis, encephalitis, transverse myelitis, Reye syndrome, and Guillain-Barré syndrome are all potential complications.	Diagnostic tests may include viral culture, rapid antigen testing from throat or nasopharynx, polymerase chain reaction, and immunofluorescence. Treatment is supportive. Antiviral therapy (amantadine, rimantadine, oseltamivir, and zanamivir) is given to children 1 year of age or older at high risk of complications and those on long-term aspirin therapy (Cheung & Lieberman, 2002). When antiviral medication is initiated within 2 days of symptoms the duration of symptoms may be reduced by 1 to 1½ days. *Prevention:* Influenza vaccine is now recommended for infants and children over 6 months of age. See Table 45–3.	■ Use droplet and contact precautions for hospitalized infants and children. ■ The child is usually cared for at home. Encourage parents to wash hands frequently and to reduce exposure of other family members to the infected child. ■ Provide fluids to keep nasal secretions moist and to prevent dehydration. ■ Provide acetaminophen or ibuprofen for fever management and mild pain. ■ If antiviral medications are given, be alert for nausea and vomiting. Zanamivir can exacerbate asthma. ■ Provide rest and quiet diversional activities. ■ Teach parents to be alert to signs of complications from the viral infection.
Measles (Rubeola)*⁺ *Causal agent:* Morbillivirus, a member of the paramyxovirus group. *Epidemiology:* Occurrence peaks in the late winter and early spring. In developed countries, measles occurs mostly in outbreaks among unimmunized children, or possibly those with declining immunity. Many cases are imported from countries without routine immunization. Maternal immunity is active until the infant is age 12–15 months. In developing countries, measles remains an endemic disease and is a significant cause of infant and child morbidity and mortality. *Transmission:* Airborne, respiratory droplets and contact with infected persons. *Incubation period:* About 8–12 days.	Children are quite ill in the 3–5 day prodromal phase, with symptoms including high fever, conjunctivitis, coryza, cough, anorexia, and malaise. Koplik spots (small, irregular, bluish white spots on a red back-ground) appear on the buccal mucosa about 2 days before and after the rash appears. The characteristic red, blotchy, maculopapular rash that becomes confluent usually appears 2–4 days after onset of prodromal phase. The rash begins on the face and spreads to the trunk and extremities. Symptoms gradually subside in 4–7 days. Other symptoms include anorexia, malaise, fatigue, and generalized lymphadenopathy.	Diagnosis can be made by a serologic test for immunoglobulin (Ig) M measles antibody. Treatment is supportive. Antibiotics are used for secondary bacterial infections. *Prognosis:* Recovery is generally good with supportive care. *Prevention:* Measles is a vaccine-preventable disease. See Table 45–3. Immune globulin, administered up to 6 days after exposure, may be helpful in preventing the disease in susceptible persons (immunocompromised children, infants less than 1 year of age, pregnant women). All healthcare workers should have documented immunity. This is a reportable disease.	■ If the child is hospitalized, maintain airborne precautions during the contagious period. ■ Use a cool-mist vaporizer to help clear respiratory passages. ■ Suction nose and oral cavity very gently as necessary. ■ Give nonaspirin antipyretics for fever and antipruritics for itching. ■ Assess lungs carefully, especially in young children, in whom pneumonias are a common complication. ■ Antitussives may be ordered to control coughing. ■ Keep lights dim, and cover windows if the child has photophobia. ■ Elevate the head of the bed. Keep the room cool with good air circulation. Provide light, nonirritating blankets. ■ Keep skin clean and dry. No soaps should be used.

TABLE 45–5 ✛ Selected Infectious and Communicable Diseases in Children—continued

Disease	Clinical Manifestations	Clinical Therapy	Nursing Management
Measles (Rubeola)[*][+]**—Cont.** *Period of communicability:* Begins during the prodromal phase and ends 2–4 days after the rash appears.	*Complications:* Diarrhea, otitis media, bronchopneumonia, bronchitis, laryngotracheobronchitis, and encephalitis. Complications and sequelae occur most often in children who are malnourished, medically fragile, and immunosuppressed. The younger the child, the greater the risk for complications.		■ Maintain fluid intake. Offer cool liquids frequently in small amounts. Blended, pureed, and mashed foods are most easily tolerated. ■ Maintain bed rest. Visitors should be immune to measles. ■ Provide diversions such as music, stories, and favorite toys.

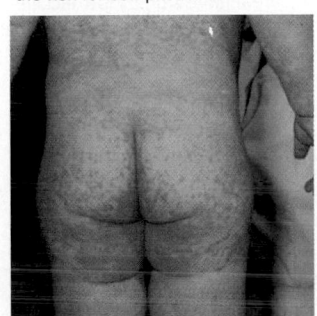

A   **B**

Measles, third day of rash. **A,** Facial rash. **B,** Posterior view.

Courtesy of Centers for Disease Control and Prevention, Atlanta, GA.

Koplik spots on oral mucosa, fifth day of rash.

Courtesy of Centers for Disease Control and Prevention, Atlanta, GA.

Mononucleosis *Causal agent:* Epstein-Barr virus (EBV), a member of the herpesvirus group. *Epidemiology:* Occurs worldwide. In developing countries, the disease occurs in young children and may be asymptomatic or mild. In developed countries, the disease is more common in older children and adolescents. *Transmission:* Direct contact with infected oropharyngeal and genital tract secretions. EBV can survive for several hours outside the body. EBV can also be transmitted by blood transfusion. Approximately 85% of adults have antibody to EBV. *Incubation period:* 10–50 days. *Period of communicability:* Virus is shed for up to 18 months after the clinical course of the disease. The infected individual becomes a lifelong carrier (American Academy of Pediatrics, 2003).	In very young children, mononucleosis may cause irritability, but be otherwise asymptomatic. A maculopapular rash may be seen in a few cases. In other children, the disease is characterized by malaise, headache, anorexia, abdominal pain, fatigue, and fever for 2–3 days, followed by lymphadenopathy and a sore throat. Hepatosplenomegaly may occur. Pain from swelling of the tonsils and lymph nodes may be significant. The syndrome typically lasts 2–3 weeks and is self-limited. Weakness and lethargy may continue for several months. *Complications:* Rare side effects include central nervous system symptoms such as encephalitis, aseptic meningitis, and Guillain-Barré syndrome. Splenic rupture, respiratory failure, and hematologic complications such as thrombocytopenia can also occur. In immunodeficient children, fatal infections or lymphomas can develop.	Diagnostic tests include the serologic monospot test or testing EBV antibodies by immunofluorescence. Abnormal live enzymes may be found. On a blood smear, lymphocytes are enlarged with atypical nuclei (Downey cells). Treatment is supportive. Corticosteroids may be used to control tonsillar swelling and pain when there is impending airway obstruction, massive splenomegaly, myocarditis, or hemolytic anemia. Antibiotics (ampicillin and amoxicillin) should be avoided as a nonallergic rash often develops (American Academy of Pediatrics, 2003). *Prognosis:* After recovery, the virus remains latent in the lymphoid system. It can be reactivated during periods of immunosuppression. *Prevention:* No known prevention.	■ Children are usually treated at home. Standard precautions should be used. ■ Give antipyretics and analgesics for fever and sore throat. Offer warm salt water for gargling. Offer soft foods and encourage fluids. ■ Maintain bed rest during acute phase. ■ Give adolescents a sense of responsibility by involving them in decisions about care whenever possible. Be sure to include parents and adolescents in discussions. ■ Reassure adolescents who may be worried about keeping up with schoolwork that they can return to school when the fever is gone and swallowing is normal. ■ Teens should avoid kissing until the fever has been gone several days. ■ Contact sports should be avoided until the liver and spleen are normal, usually in about 4 weeks. ■ If splenomegaly is present, alcohol should be avoided for 3 months after liver function test results return to normal.

[*]Indicates that a vaccine or antitoxin is available for use in high-risk or as-needed situations.

[+]Indicates that the disease has a safe and effective vaccine.

(continued)

TABLE 45–5 ✿ Selected Infectious and Communicable Diseases in Children—continued

Disease	Clinical Manifestations	Clinical Therapy	Nursing Management
Mumps (Parotitis)[+] *Causal agent: Rubulavirus* in the Paramyxoviridae family. *Epidemiology:* Occurs worldwide in unvaccinated children, most often in winter and spring. Infection and vaccination induce lifelong immunity. Maternal antibodies begin to disappear in infants at the age of 12–15 months. *Transmission:* Contact with respiratory tract secretions. *Incubation period:* 12–25 days. *Period of communicability:* 7 days before parotid swelling until 9 days after swelling subsides.	Malaise; low-grade fever; and earache, headache, pain with chewing, decreased appetite and activity; followed by bilateral or unilateral parotid gland swelling. Swelling peaks around the third day. Meningeal signs (stiff neck, headache, and photophobia) occur in about 15% of patients. *Complications:* Orchitis (inflammation of the epididymis, pain on testicular palpation, and scrotal swelling—most often unilateral) may occur in postpubertal males; sterility is relatively rare (American Academy of Pediatrics, 2003). Oophoritis, pancreatitis, aseptic meningoencephalitis, and unilateral permanent deafness are sometimes seen.	Diagnostic tests include a viral culture from a throat washing, urine, or cerebrospinal fluid. Serum mumps immunoglobulin (Ig) G antibody titer may also be performed. Therapy is supportive, focused on symptom relief. *Prognosis:* Mumps is usually self-limiting. *Prevention:* Mumps is a vaccine-preventable disease. See Table 45–3. This is a reportable disease.	■ Use standard and droplet precautions for hospitalized children while contagious. ■ Children are usually cared for at home. They are generally uncomfortable but are rarely very ill. ■ Avoid exposure to immuno-compromised or susceptible individuals. ■ Give nonaspirin analgesics and antipyretics to control fever and pain. ■ Encourage fluid intake. Swallowing and chewing may be painful. Offer soft and blended foods. Avoid foods and beverages that increase salivary flow (citrus, spices, and candies) because they cause pain. ■ Talking may be painful. Provide a bell or other attention-getting device. ■ Apply warm or cool compresses, whichever is preferred, to the parotid area. ■ Be alert for signs of complications. Headache, stiff neck, vomiting, and photophobia may indicate meningeal irritation. ■ Provide scrotal supports if testicular swelling occurs. ■ Reassure children that the facial swelling will go away. ■ Keep children out of school or childcare until 9 days after parotid swelling occurs. Encourage diversional activities.

A, Side view. **B,** Front view.

This child has mumps with diffuse lymphedema on the neck.

Courtesy of Centers for Disease Control and Prevention, Atlanta, GA.

Disease	Clinical Manifestations	Clinical Therapy	Nursing Management
Pertussis (Whooping Cough)[+] *Causal agent: Bordetella pertussis.* *Epidemiology:* Occurs worldwide. Most common in children under 6 months of age. Epidemic cycles occur every 3–4 years. Pertussis may occur in health-care workers or adults who have incomplete immunity, and these adults can spread the disease to unimmunized children. Approximately 20 to 40 million cases occur annually in the world (World Health Organization, 1999). *Transmission:* Respiratory droplets and direct contact with discharge from the respiratory membranes.	The onset is insidious. *Catarrhal stage:* The disease begins with nasal congestion, a runny nose, low-grade fever, and a mild nonproductive cough, lasting about 2 weeks. *Paroxysmal stage:* The cough becomes more severe at night and changes into spasms of paroxysmal coughing when the child attempts to expel a thick mucoid plug. This is followed by forceful inspiration through a narrowed glottis and stridor, or "whooping." (Young infants do not manifest the "whooping," rather they present with frequent apnea.) Sucking on a bottle may trigger the coughing spell. Coughing may be	Diagnostic tests include culture and polymerase chain reaction (PCR) testing. Treatment consists of antibiotics (erythromycin and other macrolides); corticosteroids, if ordered; and supportive care. *Prognosis:* The disease is most severe in infants under 1 year of age, and most deaths occur in this age group.	■ Use droplet precautions until 5–7 days after antibiotics are initiated. Most hospitalized cases occur in children under the age of 5 years. ■ Closely monitor respirations and oxygen saturation. The smaller the child, the greater the risk for respiratory distress and apnea. ■ Remain with the child during coughing spells, when hypoxic and apneic episodes are most likely. Give oxygen if ordered. Have emergency equipment available. ■ Provide humidification. Gentle suctioning may be necessary. ■ Give nonaspirin antipyretics as needed for fever.

TABLE 45–5 ✣ Selected Infectious and Communicable Diseases in Children—continued

Disease	Clinical Manifestations	Clinical Therapy	Nursing Management
Pertussis (Whooping Cough)[+]— Cont. *Incubation period:* 7–21 days (commonly 7–10 days). *Period of communicability:* Begins about 1 week after exposure. Communicable for 5–7 days after antibiotic therapy is initiated. The disease is most contagious before the paroxysmal cough stage.	accompanied by flushing; cyanosis; vomiting; and profuse drainage from the nose, eyes, and mouth. Paroxysmal coughing may last 1–6 weeks or more. Dehydration may result from decreased oral intake. *Convalescent stage:* Up to 6 weeks when paroxysms gradually subside. *Complications:* Pneumonia, atelectasis, otitis media, encephalopathy, seizures, and death. Highest mortality rate and complication rate is in infants under 1 year. In 2000, 17 infants under 4 months of age died due to pertussis (Centers for Disease Control, 2002a).	*Prevention:* Pertussis is a vaccine-preventable disease. See Table 45–3. Healthcare professionals in close contact with infected children before diagnosis may need antibiotics to prevent transmission. Vaccine protection wanes after 5 to 10 years allowing adolescents and adults to become infected and transmit the infection to susceptible infants. A new vaccine for adolescents and adults (Tdap) is part of the current immunization schedule for children and adolescents. This is a reportable disease.	■ Encourage frequent rest periods. ■ Allow the child to eat desired foods in small frequent feedings. ■ Encourage the child to take fluids. The child may need IV hydration if oral intake is not tolerated. ■ Provide emotional support to parents. ■ Teach parents to watch for signs of respiratory failure and dehydration if the child is managed at home.
Pneumococcal infection[+] *Causative agent:* Streptococcus pneumoniae, a gram-positive diplococcus. *Epidemiology:* The organism is found in the pharynx of healthy people. Outbreaks occur in the winter and spring when people are in more crowded physical settings. In temperate climates, 8 of 90 serotypes account for most of the invasive pediatric infections. The disease is more common in African Americans, American Indians, and Alaskan Natives. It occurs most commonly in the 6-month to 2-year age group, and among children in childcare settings. Of particular concern is the development of penicillin and multiantibiotic-resistant strains. *Transmission:* Respiratory secretions, and droplets. *Incubation period:* 1–3 days. *Period of communicability:* Unknown. Probably less than 24 hours after effective antibiotic therapy is initiated.	The signs and symptoms are related to the focal area of infection. The organism causes otitis media, sinusitis, pharyngitis, laryngotracheobronchitis, pneumonia, meningitis, and bacteremia. In otitis media, upper respiratory infection, fever, ear pain, and decreased appetite are seen. In bacteremia, there is unexplained fever and no localized infection site. In pneumonia, fever, chills, chest pain, dyspnea, malaise, and a productive cough are seen. In meningitis, inconsolable crying, increased irritability, lethargy, refusal to eat, nausea, vomiting, diarrhea, myalgia, photophobia, and seizures are seen. *Complications:* This organism is one of the leading causes of morbidity and mortality. It is the leading cause of acute otitis media, and a major cause of meningitis, bacteremia, and pneumonia (Tan, 2002). Other complications include septic arthritis, osteomyelitis, endo-carditis, and brain abscess.	Symptomatic care is provided. Penicillin is given for penicillin-sensitive strains, but up to 48% of infections are penicillin resistant. Macrolide antibiotics are used for mild disease if the child is allergic to penicillin. Penicillin-resistant strains are treated with third-generation cephalosporins (cefotaxime or ceftriaxone). Vancomycin and rifampin are used in combination when strains are resistant to antibiotics listed above (American Academy of Pediatrics, 2003). *Prevention:* Many serotypes are preventable with immunization. See Table 45–2 and Table 45–3. Significant reduction in pneumonia, meningitis, bacteremia, and otitis media have occurred with the vaccine. No increase of invasive pneumoccal disease with nonvaccine serotypes has been detected (Keyserling, 2002).	■ If the child is hospitalized, maintain standard precautions. ■ Provide nonaspirin antipyretics for control of fever and comfort. ■ Encourage fluids, and monitor intake and output. ■ Monitor vital signs and level of consciousness to identify signs of worsening condition. ■ Educate parents about the need for the vaccine, as the unimmunized child could become infected repeatedly with different serotypes. ■ Many children with mild disease will be treated at home. Educate parents about signs indicating a need to seek additional medical care, the need for proper medication administration, and comfort measures for the child. ■ Individuals with congenital asplenia or traumatic splenectomy, malignancy, sickle cell disease, and nephrotic syndrome are at higher risk for invasive disease with this organism. ■ Additional factors that increase risk of pneumococcal disease include poverty, crowded housing, homelessness, and exposure to tobacco smoke.

*Indicates that a vaccine or antitoxin is available for use in high-risk or as-needed situations.

[+]Indicates that the disease has a safe and effective vaccine.

TABLE 45–5 ✣ Selected Infectious and Communicable Diseases in Children—continued

Disease	Clinical Manifestations	Clinical Therapy	Nursing Management
Poliomyelitis[+] *Causal agent:* Poliovirus is an enterovirus with three serotypes. *Epidemiology:* Occurs worldwide. Polio primarily affects children and immunocompromised or unimmunized adults caring for infants who received live poliovirus vaccine. The vaccine induces lifelong immunity. Since live poliovirus vaccine was discontinued in the United States, no wild poliomyelitis cases have occurred since 2000. *Transmission:* Primarily by the fecal-oral route, but also the respiratory route. *Incubation period:* Usually 7–10 days (range 3–36 days). *Period of communicability:* Greatest shortly before and right after clinical symptoms develop when the virus is in the throat. Excreted in the feces for several weeks.	Affects the central nervous system. Less severe infections may be limited to fever and stiffness in the neck and back, headache, vomiting, and sore throat. In other cases, fever, headache, stiff neck, Kernig or Brudzinski sign, decreased deep tendon reflexes, and progressive weakness occur. With cranial nerve involvement, there may be respiratory difficulties. An increased respiratory rate may interfere with the ability to talk because frequent pauses are needed. Onset of paralysis may be sudden, in hours, or gradual over 3–5 days. Paralysis results from damage to motor neurons. *Complications:* Permanent motor paralysis, respiratory arrest, myocardial failure, aseptic meningitis, and postpolio syndrome.	Diagnosis is made by cell culture from stool or throat swabs. Treatment is supportive. No chemotherapeutic agents that directly kill the poliovirus are available. *Prognosis:* Respiratory complication is life threatening and involves 5–10% of all cases. Respiratory paralysis may lead to death. Motor paralysis may result in long-term disability. *Prevention:* Poliomyelitis is a vaccine-preventable disease. See Table 45–3. This is a reportable disease.	■ Use standard and droplet precautions in the hospital and keep the child on strict bed rest. ■ Observe closely for respiratory paralysis (ineffective cough, talking with frequent pauses, shallow and rapid respiratory rate). Have emergency equipment at bedside. Assist ventilations as needed until mechanical ventilation is set up. ■ Administer sedatives and nonaspirin analgesics as ordered to allow for rest and comfort. Moist hot packs may relieve discomfort. ■ Encourage fluids. ■ Position the child to promote body alignment. ■ Perform range of motion exercises to prevent contractures after the acute phase. ■ Provide emotional support. ■ Patients are alert and aware. Tell them what is happening to them. ■ Long-term orthopedic (physical therapy) support may be needed by some children.
Roseola (Exanthem Subitum, Sixth Disease) *Causal agent:* Herpesvirus type 6. *Epidemiology:* Occurs worldwide, primarily in children 6–24 months of age (after maternal antibodies decline). No seasonal pattern. *Transmission:* Likely to be from respiratory secretions of healthy individuals. *Incubation period:* Appears to be 5–15 days. *Period of communicability:* Lifelong persistent infection and virus shedding in healthy individuals (American Academy of Pediatrics, 2003).	Sudden, high fever up to 40.5°C (105°F) for 3–8 days, during which the child does not appear toxic (normal appetite and behavior). The fever phase is followed by a characteristic pale pink, discrete, maculopapular rash, which starts on the trunk and spreads to the face, neck, and extremities. The rash can last for 1–2 days. The child's appetite is normal. *Complications:* Children may have febrile seizures during high fever stage. Encephalopathy may develop in rare cases.	Roseola is self-limiting, and treatment is supportive. *Prognosis:* Roseola is benign in most cases.	■ Children are rarely hospitalized, but if they are, use standard precautions. ■ Give nonaspirin antipyretics to control fever. ■ Observe closely for any seizure activity, especially during the acute febrile periods. ■ Encourage fluids. ■ Reassure parents that the rash will disappear in a few days.

TABLE 45–5 ❖ Selected Infectious and Communicable Diseases in Children—continued

Disease	Clinical Manifestations	Clinical Therapy	Nursing Management
Rubella (German Measles)[+] *Causal agent:* An RNA virus, member of the family Togaviridae, genus *Rubivirus.* *Epidemiology:* Occurs worldwide and is most prevalent in the winter and spring. Maternal antibodies disappear about 6–9 months after birth. Infection or vaccination induces lifelong immunity. Most cases occur in adults 20–29 years of age. Most U.S. cases occur among foreign-born Hispanic adults from countries that do not have rubella vaccination programs. Congenital rubella syndrome is most likely the result of lack of immunization rather than vaccine failure. Each year an average of 6 infants are born with congenital rubella syndrome (Reef, Frey, Theall, et al., 2002). *Transmission:* Droplet spread, direct contact with infected persons, or contact with articles soiled by nasal secretions. *Incubation period:* 14–21 days (most commonly 16–18 days). *Period of communicability:* 7 days before until 4 days after the rash onset. Infants with congenital rubella may shed the virus for months after birth.	Rubella is generally a mild disease with a characteristic pink, nonconfluent, maculopapular rash. The rash appears on the face, progresses to the neck, trunk, and legs, and disappears in the same order. Prodromal symptoms occur 1–5 days before the rash and include low-grade fever, headache, malaise, coryza, sore throat, and anorexia. Forchheimer spots (discrete, erythematous pinpoint or larger lesions on the soft palate) are seen during the prodromal phase. Generalized lymphadenopathy involving the postauricular, suboccipital, and posterior cervical areas is common up to 7 days before the rash. Many cases are asymptomatic. Signs of congenital rubella syndrome include growth retardation, radiolucent bone disease, hepatosplenomegaly, thrombocytopenia, and purpuric skin lesions (giving a "blueberry muffin" appearance). No obvious signs may be found with mild forms of the disease at birth. *Complications:* Complications are rare, but include arthritis in adolescents, encephalitis, and congenital rubella syndrome.	Diagnostic tests include cell culture from a nasal swab, and detection of IgM or IgG antibodies. Treatment is supportive. Rubella is generally self-limiting in children. *Prognosis:* Disease is usually mild and benign. Major risk is for fetus if the mother is infected in the first trimester. Abortion, stillbirth, or fetal death is common (10% die after birth). Many other anomalies may be present, such as intrauterine growth retardation, cardiac, ear, and eye deficits. *Prevention:* Rubella is a vaccine-preventable disease. See Table 45–3. Females of childbearing age need to be immunized to reduce the risk for congenital rubella syndrome. All healthcare workers should have documented immunity.	■ Maintain standard and droplet precautions for contagious children. ■ Maintain contact precautions for infants with congenital rubella syndrome until 1 year of age unless nasopharyngeal and urine cultures are repeatedly negative after 3 months of age (American Academy of Pediatrics, 2003). ■ Children are usually treated at home. They should be isolated from pregnant women. ■ Give nonaspirin analgesics and antipyretics for any pain and fever. ■ Allow children to choose what they would like to eat and drink. Encourage fluids. ■ Provide quiet activities. ■ Exclude children from childcare or school for 7 days after onset of rash. School and childcare facilities should be notified of the child's illness. Congenital rubella syndrome *Courtesy of Centers for Disease Control and Prevention*
Streptococcus A *Causal agent:* Group A streptococci (GAS). *Epidemiology:* The illness is caused by various M-protein groups of group A alpha- and beta-hemolytic streptococci. In recent years severe infections have appeared, in some cases threatening life and limb. Different strains are associated with pharyngeal and pyodermal infections. Pharyngeal infections tend to occur more in late fall, winter, and spring. Pyodermal infections tend to occur in warmer seasons because of the association with minor skin trauma and insect bites.	*Pharyngeal:* Abrupt onset with a sore throat, dysphagia, malaise, high fever, chills, headache, abdominal pain, anorexia, and vomiting. A beefy red pharynx with exudate (strep throat) and tender cervical nodes are seen. Palatal petechiae may be seen. *GAS respiratory tract infection:* Toddlers may develop serous rhinitis and a respiratory illness with moderate fever, irritability, and anorexia rather than pharyngitis.	Diagnosis can be made by a rapid strep test or a culture of secretions from the pharynx and tonsils. Cultures of skin lesions are not indicated (American Academy of Pediatrics, 2003). Prompt antibiotic treatment is effective. Penicillin V is the drug of choice. Erythromycin is used if the child is allergic to penicillin. The fever decreases after treatment is begun. Uncomplicated impetigo is treated with mupirocin ointment. Invasive strains causing necrotizing fasciitis or myositis need surgical intervention (exploration and debridement of dead tissue).	■ Children with uncomplicated infections are usually cared for at home. ■ Promote bed rest during the febrile stage. ■ Give nonaspirin antipyretics to control fever. Teach parents important signs of a worsening condition. ■ For pharyngeal infections, offer warm salt water for gargling, a soft diet, and nonacidic beverages. Encourage fluids. Provide cool, clear liquids. Swallowing may be difficult. ■ Explain to parents the importance of giving the child the full course of antibiotics. ■ Encourage other family members with sore throats to have throat cultures taken.

*Indicates that a vaccine or antitoxin is available for use in high-risk or as-needed situations.

[+]Indicates that the disease has a safe and effective vaccine.

(continued)

TABLE 45–5 ✢ Selected Infectious and Communicable Diseases in Children—continued

Disease	Clinical Manifestations	Clinical Therapy	Nursing Management
Streptococcus A—Cont. *Transmission:* Contact with respiratory secretions for pharyngitis or skin lesions for pyoderma. *Incubation period:* Pharyngeal: usually 2–5 days. Pyodermal: usually 7–10 days. *Period of communicability:* For weeks in untreated pharyngeal infections. The child is most contagious during the acute stage of the illness.	*Scarlet fever:* A characteristic erythematous, sandpaper rash appears in some cases 12–48 hours after onset of symptoms, starting on the neck and spreading to the trunk and extremities. In 3–4 days, the rash begins to fade and the tips of the toes and fingers begin to peel. The classic strawberry tongue is seen on day 4–5. *Pyodermal:* Lesions (impetigo) are honey-colored crusts at the site of open lesions. *Complications:* If untreated, acute otitis media, sinusitis, peritonsillar or retropharyngeal abscess, cervical lymphadenitis, acute rheumatic fever, acute glomerulonephritis, toxic shock syndrome, bacteremia, and necrotizing fasciitis or myositis can occur.	*Prognosis:* Recovery is usually good with antibiotic therapy; 10% to 20% of school-age children become chronic carriers. *Prevention:* None. Scarlet fever from group A beta-hemolytic streptococcus	■ For impetigo, teach the parents to wash the skin, remove crusts, and apply antibiotic ointment. ■ If the child is hospitalized, maintain droplet precautions for pharyngeal infections and contact precautions for skin lesions for 24 hours after beginning antibiotics. Monitor vital signs, especially temperature. Administer antibiotics as ordered. ■ If the child develops invasive streptococcal infection, use standard precautions. The child with toxic shock syndrome will need intensive care to manage shock and fluid and electrolyte imbalances.
Tetanus *Causal agent: Clostridium tetani* or tetanus bacillus. *Epidemiology:* The bacillus is common and exists as a spore in soil, dust, and animal excretions. The organism produces an endotoxin that affects the central nervous system. *Transmission:* The organism is transmitted to humans through puncture wounds or broken skin. Newborns can acquire tetanus via the umbilical cord if they are born in an unclean area, a contaminated implement is used to cut the cord, or clay is applied to the umbilical cord as a ritual in some Middle Eastern cultures. *Incubation period:* 3 days–3 weeks (average 8 days). *Period of communicability:* Not communicable to other individuals except through skin wounds.	Stiffness of the neck and jaw, with painful facial spasms and difficulty chewing and swallowing over a few days, and headache. Noise or sudden movement may stimulate spasms. Spasms of facial muscles may produce a grinning expression (risus sardonicus). Localized prolonged and painful muscle contraction may occur at the site of the wound. Eventually rigidity of the abdomen and trunk produce **opisthotonos** (rigid hypertextension of the entire body). Spasms and fever occur along with difficulty swallowing the increased oral secretions. Respiratory muscles can be affected and cause airway obstruction and suffocation. Newborns have difficulty with sucking, progressing to an inability to suck, irritability, and nuchal rigidity. *Complications:* Laryngospasm, respiratory distress, death.	Tetanus immune globulin is given to unimmunized persons as soon as possible. Tetanus toxoid is given at the same time in a separate site. Medications are provided to treat muscle spasms. Intensive care is provided with cardiorespiratory monitoring, assisted ventilation, IV metronidazole or penicillin G, nutrition, and supportive care. Wound cleansing and debriding is performed. Survival beyond 4 days indicates an increased chance of recovery. Paroxysms become less frequent and complete recovery may take weeks. *Prognosis:* 30% mortality; much higher in newborns. Intensive care has improved mortality. *Prevention:* Tetanus immunizations are given. See Table 45–3. Tetanus boosters are updated every 10 years, or, if a potentially contaminated wound occurs, in 5 years. Proper surgical debridement of wounds decreases the chance of infection.	■ Prevent disease by checking immunization records and administering immunizations as necessary. ■ Give immune globulin to unimmunized persons. ■ Assist with wound debridement. ■ The child with tetanus is hospitalized. Use standard precautions. ■ Monitor the child's condition. Handle as little as possible. Reduce stimulation by placing child in a quiet, darkened room. ■ Offer skin and respiratory care. The child may need an endotracheal tube, suctioning, and supplemental oxygen for airway support. ■ Provide feedings via total parenteral nutrition or feeding tube. ■ Maintain hydration with IV fluids and electrolytes. ■ Try to reduce the child's anxiety, as mental status may be unaffected. ■ Prepare the family for a possible poor prognosis.

Tuberculosis, see Chapter 47. ∞

TABLE 45–6 ✣ Selected Infectious Diseases Transmitted by Insect or Animal Hosts (Zoonosis)

Disease	Clinical Manifestations	Clinical Therapy	Nursing Management
Lyme Disease* *Causal agent:* Borrelia *burgdorferi,* a spirochete, which is transmitted by ixodid ticks. *Epidemiology:* Distribution in the United States correlates highly with the distribution of various tick carriers (vectors). It occurs in 49 states and the District of Columbia. 80% of cases occur in the Northeastern, Mid-Atlantic, and North Central states (Centers for Disease Control, 2002b). Exposure occurs in any outdoor setting where ticks are endemic. Animals such as dogs and cats can also have the disease. Lyme disease occurs year round, with the highest risk of infection in the summer. Children between 5 and 14 years are at highest risk because of outdoor activities. Infection does not induce immunity. *Transmission:* Tick bite. The tick transmits the infected spirochete when it draws blood. The tick must feed for 30 hours to transmit the disease. Lyme disease is the most common vectorborne illness in North America. *Incubation period:* 3–32 days after an infected tick bite. A rash in 48 hours is an allergic reaction or infection, not Lyme disease. *Period of communicability:* The infection is not contagious from person to person.	The most typical early symptom is a slowly expanding red rash that develops a bull's-eye appearance called erythema migrans at the site of the bite. The bite is often found on the groin, axilla, or thigh. The rash starts as a flat or raised red area and may progress to partial clearing; develop blisters or scabs in the center. It is usually at least 5 cm in diameter. The rash may look like a bruise in dark-skinned patients. It resolves spontaneously within 4 weeks. Only 50%–75% of patients have the rash (Wade, 2000). Stage 1 symptoms, lasting 5–21 days, include malaise, fatigue, headache, stiff neck, mild fever, and muscle and joint aches. Stage 2 (early disseminated) occurs 1–4 months after the bite. The most common symptoms of untreated disease are pain and swelling of the joints, most commonly the knee (Lyme arthritis), facial palsy, meningitis, AV block. Stage 3 (late disseminated) occurs months later and includes problems such as Lyme arthritis and central nervous system changes. These may become chronic problems. *Complications:* Left untreated, Lyme disease can cause significant neurologic deficits, including arm and leg weakness, Bell's palsy, encephalopathy, optic neuropathy, meningitis, severe headaches, and cognitive and behavioral changes as well as chronic arthritis, and disorders of the peripheral nerves. The spirochete can cross the placental barrier and infect the fetus (Wade, 2000).	Diagnostic tests include the enzyme-linked immunosorbent assay (ELISA) plus the Western blot test. Antibiotics are the treatment of choice. Amoxicillin or cefuroxime axetil are most often used in children 8 years of age or younger. Doxycycline or tetracycline is given to children over the age of 8 years. A 2-week course of oral medication is given. If recurrent arthritis, central nervous system difficulty, or carditis occurs, treat for 4 weeks with IV ceftriaxone, cefotaxime, or penicillin G. Relapse can occur. *Prognosis:* Lyme disease does not cause acute life-threatening illness, but it may result in significant morbidity, especially when chronic. *Prevention:* ■ A vaccine, LYMErix, is approved for high-risk patients 15–70 years. Some clinical trials in younger children appear promising. ■ Avoid areas that are heavily tick infested, and wear protective clothing. Check for ticks (especially hidden in hair) after every outing. Check pets because they can carry home ticks that are then transferred to the child. Remove ticks as soon as possible. There is no acquired immunity.	■ Children with early disease are usually treated at home. Children with progressive symptoms may be hospitalized. Use standard precautions. ■ Educate parents about the need for the long course of medications, informing them that the spirochete can go dormant. ■ Tell parents to have the child avoid sun exposure when taking doxycycline. Nonaspirin analgesics and antipyretics may provide relief of mild fevers, headaches, and muscle and joint aches. ■ Children with Lyme disease may tire easily. Promote rest and avoid vigorous activities that may be difficult. ■ Educate parents and children about the disease and early recognition of the symptoms. ■ Teach parents to safely remove ticks. To remove a tick, grasp it gently but firmly with fine-point tweezers where the mouthparts are attached. Pull gently—avoid squeezing of the tick's body—until it releases. Clean the area with soap and water (American Academy of Pediatrics, 2003). ■ Tell parents to mark the date of tick bite on the calendar and monitor the child's health for flulike symptoms over the next 30 days. Encourage them to seek medical attention promptly if symptoms develop. ■ Provide emotional support.

Lyme Disease

---

*Indicates that a vaccine or antitoxin is available for use in high-risk or as-needed situations

(continued)

Disease	Clinical Manifestations	Clinical Therapy	Nursing Management
Malaria *Causal agent: Plasmodium*, four species (*P. falciparum, P. vivax, P. ovale, P. malariae*) *Epidemiology:* Occurs in tropical and subtropical regions on four continents (Africa, Americas, Asia, and Oceana). The highest mortality is in children 6 months to 3 years of age. The disease is acquired during travel to an endemic area. *P. falciparum* causes the most serious disease. *Transmission:* The bite of an infected female Anopheles mosquito during a nocturnal blood meal permits the parasite to enter the human bloodstream. The parasite passes to the liver and infects hepatic cells. During an asymptomatic 5–16 day cycle, the parasite transforms to become a merozoite that can reproduce asexually. The merozoites are released as parasites that infect the red blood cells. Transmission can also occur by blood transfusion. *Incubation period:* Varies by type. *P. falciparum* in 7–10 days, for the other types it can remain dormant for a year or longer. *Period of communicability:* Not communicable except by blood or blood product transfusion, or the transplantation of organs from an infected person.	Nonspecific signs such as myalgia, malaise, headache, abdominal pain, back pain, pallor, diarrhea, nausea, and vomiting are common. Spiking fever >40°C occurs at the time red blood cells rupture, becoming a classical cyclic pattern every 48–72 hours. Periods of symptomatic improvement are sometimes seen between spells. Seizures and altered consciousness indicate the development of cerebral malaria. Hepatosplenomegaly and jaundice from hemolysis are often seen. Attacks may recur over the course of the year after infection, but the parasites die out gradually if reinfection does not occur. Children who live in endemic areas and survive the first 5 years of life develop immunity to the severe effects of the disease as long as they have frequent reexposure to the infection. *Complications:* When more than 5% of red blood cells are infected, severe anemia is seen; cerebral malaria with seizures, increased intracranial pressure, confusion, stupor, coma, and frequently death are most common in children. Pulmonary edema, respiratory failure, renal failure, spontaneous bleeding, and shock are seen in older children and adolescents. Children with asplenia are at high risk for death. Causes 1–2 million deaths worldwide annually. If the fetus becomes infected and survives, intrauterine growth retardation is common (Howell, 2001).	Malaria can be diagnosed by examining blood smears for parasites, or with a plasmodium HRP2 antigen enzyme-linked immunosorbent assay (ELISA). Laboratory tests often reveal anemia (Hgb <12 gm/dl) and thrombocytopenia (<150,000/mm³). The patient is hospitalized to receive fluid replacement, antipyretics, and anemia management. The blood is regularly monitored for parasite density. In severe disease with greater than 5% parasitemia, intensive care and IV treatment is needed. Careful monitoring is needed to detect mental status changes, severe anemia, renal failure, and pulmonary edema. Exchange transfusion may be used in some children with greater than 5% parasitemia (Shingadia & Shulman, 2000). Oral chloroquine is the treatment of choice for all species except *P. faciparum.* Quinine sulfate and tetracycline are used for therapy in children over 8 years for chloroquine-resistant *P. falciparum.* Atovaquone-proguanil was recently approved by the FDA to treat malaria and for prophylaxis. Hypoglycemia may result from quinine treatment. Primaquine (sometimes used along with chloroquine to prevent relapses) will cause severe anemia if given to individuals with G6PD disorder. *Prevention:* Minimize contact with mosquitoes, use DEET insect repellent, screened rooms, DEET-treated mosquito netting, and cover the body with light-colored clothing when traveling in endemic regions.	■ Use standard precautions for the hospitalized patient. ■ Maintain fluid intake. Monitor intake and output. ■ Monitor blood glucose level and be prepared to respond to sudden hypoglycemia. ■ Observe for signs of increasing illness severity such as confusion, seizures, and shock. Be prepared to protect the patient from injury and provide emergency support with airways and oxygen supplementation until the child can be transferred to intensive care. ■ Monitor the hematocrit and hemoglobin levels. ■ Administer antipyretics to control the fever and promote comfort. ■ Provide education and emotional support to parents of children with severe malarial symptoms. ■ Educate families traveling to endemic areas about the importance of antimalarial chemoprophylaxis. Explain the need to take the medication correctly despite the common side effects of nausea and vomiting. Discuss the need to protect children during nocturnal feeding times of mosquitoes with protective clothing, mosquito repellent, and mosquito netting around the bed.
Rabies (Hydrophobia)* *Causal agent: Rhabdoviridae*, two types (urban, in dogs; wild, in wildlife). *Epidemiology:* Occurs worldwide. Urban rabies is generally controlled by vaccination of domestic animals susceptible to the infection, especially dogs and cats. Rabies can occur in many wild animals, particularly bats, foxes, skunks, and raccoons. *Transmission:* Infected saliva from bite of rabid animal. Virus enters the wound and travels along the nerves from point of entry to the brain where it multiplies and migrates along the efferent nerves to the salivary glands.	Children may be free of symptoms during the long incubation period. Initial acute symptoms include pain or paresthesia at the site of exposure along with headache, fever, loss of appetite, and malaise. Painful contractures in the muscles used for swallowing lead to hydrophobia (50% of patients), a reflex contraction at the sight of liquid. Neurologic symptoms such as hallucinations, disorientation, periods of excitability (mania) and quiet, and seizures later occur. Some patients may have confusion with or without agitation with progression to stupor and coma. Symptoms last about 2 weeks.	Diagnosis is made on the basis of history and clinical symptoms. The diagnosis is usually confirmed by fluorescent antibody staining of the dead animal's brain tissue. Diagnostic tests performed on the victim include fluorescent microscopy of skin biopsy from the nape of the neck, from the saliva, from antibody in the cerebrospinal fluid, or by detection of viral nucleic acid in infected tissues (American Academy of Pediatrics, 2003).	■ Work with family members and local animal control to have any animal suspected of having rabies quarantined, if possible. ■ Administer HRIG and HDCV as ordered. Assist family with obtaining help to find and quarantine the animal for observation. ■ Provide emotional support to the family while reinforcing the urgency for the vaccine and the need for a series of injections. ■ Inform parents and the child about the side effects of the vaccine—irritation at the injection site, itching, headache, muscle aches, nausea, and dizziness.

Disease	Clinical Manifestations	Clinical Therapy	Nursing Management
Rabies (Hydrophobia)*—Cont. *Incubation period:* Highly variable (3–7 weeks); average 6 weeks. This period depends on the amount of virus in the saliva, how close to the brain or major nerves the bite occurred, and how deeply the saliva penetrated the skin.	*Complications:* Usually results in death.	Immediately wash animal bites thoroughly with soap and water and irrigate well. Suturing should be avoided if possible. Human rabies immune globulin (HRIG) and human diploid cell rabies vaccine (HDCV) should be given to all persons bitten by animals that may be rabid. Half of the HRIG is infiltrated around the wound and the remainder is given IM. Follow local guidelines for delay in HRIG and HDCV if testing of the animal's brain is done. The vaccine is of no value once rabies symptoms are present. *Prognosis:* If symptoms develop, no drug improves the prognosis. *Prevention:* Postexposure prophylaxis with HRIG and HDCV should be given as soon as possible after exposure. HDCV is repeated on days 3, 7, 14, and 28 after the bite (five doses). The HDCV series may be stopped if the animal is found free of rabies. Expert advice on the administration of these vaccines is available from state and local health officials. Prevention also includes immunizing all domestic animals against rabies.	■ If the child acquires rabies, he or she will be hospitalized. ■ Institute standard and contact precautions. The virus is transmitted primarily in the saliva and cerebrospinal fluid. ■ Make the child as comfortable as possible. ■ Keep liquids out of sight of the hydrophobic child. ■ Use caution in the late stages of the disease when children are usually combative. Various medications, paralyzing agents, and sedatives may be used to provide relief. Coma and death occur after an exhaustive period of excitement and agitation that may last for days. ■ Provide emotional support to the family of the dying child. ■ Participate in local education about rabies and safe interactions with dogs. See Chapter 57. ∞ ■ Teach children to avoid contact with all unknown animals, dead or alive.
Rocky Mountain Spotted Fever (Tickborne Typhus Fever, San Paulo Typhus) *Causal agent:* Rickettsia rickettsii, a bacterium that is transmitted by infected ticks. *Epidemiology:* Rocky Mountain spotted fever (RMSF) occurs in most of the United States, southwestern Canada, and Mexico. Nearly half of all U.S. cases occur in Oklahoma, North Carolina, South Carolina, and Tennessee. Generally occurs between April and September. Most infections occur in children who are less than 15 years of age. Infection induces immunity. *Transmission:* Transmitted by bites of ticks, principally dog and wood ticks. *Incubation period:* 2–12 days (most commonly 7 days) after bite of an infected tick. *Period of communicability:* There is no evidence of person-to-person transmission.	RMSF is a multisystem disease that can be mild, moderate, or severe. Onset may be gradual or rapid. Children may be very ill. Sudden onset is characterized by a moderate to high fever (40°C) that ordinarily lasts for 2–3 weeks, significant malaise, abdominal pain, nausea, vomiting, deep muscle pain, persistent headache, chills, and conjunctival injection. The characteristic rash, which usually appears between the third and fifth days, starts on the extremities, including the palms and soles, and moves to the trunk. Initially the rash is maculopapular and blanches with pressure. It later becomes petechial and more defined; it is rarely pruritic. Up to 25% of children do not develop a rash. The child may have splenomegaly, hepatomegaly, and jaundice. *Complications:* In severe cases bleeding from the gastrointestinal tract and from disseminated intravascular coagulation (DIC) can be significant. Pulmonary complications, especially pneumonitis, pulmonary edema, and respiratory distress syndrome are common and can become life threatening. Central nervous system involvement can cause significant encephalitis and overall severe neurologic dysfunction. Cardiac and renal complications can also occur, leading to shock in severe cases.	Diagnostic tests include the indirect immunofluorescent antibody assay, enzyme immunoassay, or indirect hemagglutination test. Treatment of choice is doxycycline, regardless of the patient's age (Jacobs, Ogborn, & Tunnessen, 2001). *Prognosis:* Without early recognition and treatment, morbidity is significant and mortality in children is 2%–3% in children under 10 years (Centers for Disease Control, 2000). Mortality in untreated cases is 20%–25% (Jacobs et al., 2001). *Prevention:* Avoid areas that are heavily tick infested, and wear protective clothing. Check for ticks and if found remove promptly. Infected ticks must be attached and feeding for 4–6 hours to transmit the disease. Seek medical attention promptly for a child who has been bitten and becomes symptomatic.	■ Use standard precautions. ■ Children may require prolonged hospitalization, including monitoring in the intensive care unit. ■ Have hemodynamic monitoring equipment and emergency supplies readily available. ■ Administer antibiotics as ordered. ■ Observe for any abnormal bleeding. ■ Make the child as comfortable as possible. If the child is unconscious, support the extremities and keep the eyes closed and lubricated. ■ Provide quiet diversion activities. ■ Provide emotional support, and keep parents informed about the child's condition. Rocky Mountain Spotted Fever

*Indicates that a vaccine or antitoxin is available for use in high-risk or as-needed situations

PATHOPHYSIOLOGY ILLUSTRATED
Fever

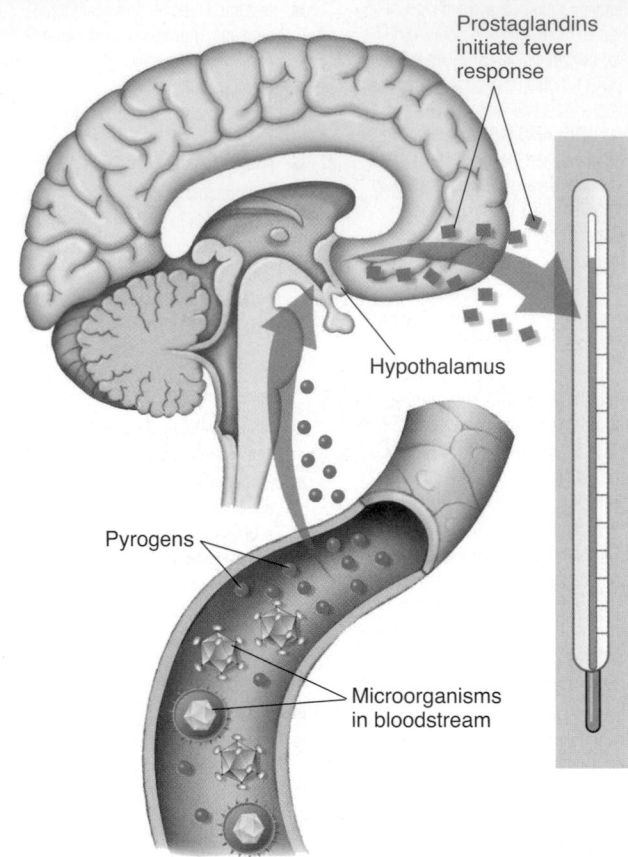

Prostaglandins initiate fever response

Hypothalamus

Pyrogens

Microorganisms in bloodstream

The hypothalamus functions as the body's thermostat, directing the body to conserve or dissipate heat. When microorganisms invade the body, endogenous pyrogens are released into the bloodstream. These substances travel to the hypothalamus, where they trigger the production and release of prostaglandins, which initiate the fever response. Blood is diverted from the extremities to more central vessels. This helps increase the core body temperature by decreasing heat loss. Shivering increases both metabolic action and heat production. The hypothalamus then maintains the temperature at the new set point.

Endogenous pyrogens (interleukins, interferons, and tumor necrosis factor) are released by macrophages in response to an invasive organism. These pyrogens travel through the circulatory system to the hypothalamus, where they trigger the production of prostaglandins. Prostaglandins are believed to raise the body's thermoregulatory set point, causing fever (Cimpella, Goldman, & Khine, 2000).

CLINICAL THERAPY

Diagnostic tests include cultures from sites where the infection may potentially be located (skin, pharynx, blood,

urine, feces, cerebrospinal fluid, etc.). (See Skills 10-4 to 10-18 in the *Clinical Skills Manual* for guidelines for collecting specimens.) **SKILLS** In some cases, x-rays or special imaging may be used to identify localized infection in an organ, such as the lungs.

For many infectious and communicable diseases, management is supportive. (See Skills 9–11 to 9–14 on the accompanying CD-ROM as well as the *Clinical Skills Manual.*) **SKILLS** An elevated temperature can be a beneficial physiologic response, helping to eradicate organisms that thrive at lower body temperatures, and mobilizing the immune response. It may also enhance the effect of antibiotics. In addition, fever decreases the plasma iron concentration, which may limit the growth of microorganisms (Cimpella et al., 2000). Fever is not inherently harmful until it reaches 41°C (105.9°F). For this reason, medical management may include postponing treatment of low-grade fevers under 38.9°C (102°F) to promote the body's natural defenses against an infection. If not managed, elevated temperatures can result in febrile seizures, which usually have no long-term sequelae. Thus, fevers greater than 38.9°C (102°F) should be treated, especially if associated with discomfort. Persistent temperatures of 38.3°C to 38.5°C (101°F to 101.5°F) may also benefit from antipyretic treatment. Acetaminophen and ibuprofen are the preferred antipyretics for children. Aspirin is no longer recommended for children because of its association with Reye syndrome. Antipyretics reduce fever by inhibiting prostaglandin synthesis, thus lowering the body's temperature set point.

Antibiotics are often another component of clinical therapy for infectious diseases. Before the introduction of antibiotics, children were often unable to fight infection and died as the result of overwhelming sepsis; antibiotics have decreased morbidity and mortality from infections among children. However, strains of bacteria have developed resistance to many antibiotics. Children with chronic illnesses such as cystic fibrosis, sickle cell disease, and AIDS are particularly susceptible to infection by drug-resistant pathogens.

 COMPLEMENTARY CARE

HOT AND COLD

Many Latino and Asian cultures subscribe to the hot and cold theory of disease causation. "Hot" and "cold" do not refer to temperature, but to categories. Fever, a hot condition, is treated by giving the patient cold substances (foods or medicines). Cold foods include vegetables, fruits, and fish. Cold medicines include orange flower water, linden, and sage. See Table 2.2 in Chapter 2. ∞

NURSING MANAGEMENT

NURSING ASSESSMENT AND DIAGNOSIS

Assess the child's hydration status and fluid intake, vital signs, comfort level, and appetite. Observe for seizures and for a **toxic appearance** (lethargy, poor perfusion, hypoventilation or hyperventilation, and cyanosis). The child with a fever may be irritable and restless, sleep fitfully, and have nonspecific muscular pain. Identify children who may be at higher risk for a serious illness in association with a fever, in particular:

- Infants and children having a toxic appearance.
- Newborns less than 28 days of age with a temperature over 38°C (100.4°F).
- Children less than 4 years of age with a temperature over 41°C (105.8°F).
- Children with conditions such as a congenital heart disease, ventriculoperitoneal shunt, asplenia, and sickle cell anemia.

Observe the child for other signs of infection, such as a rash, nausea and vomiting, or diarrhea, as well as generalized symptoms of a poor appetite and malaise.

The following nursing diagnoses may be appropriate for children with infectious and communicable diseases:

- *Hyperthermia* related to infectious disease process
- *Risk for Deficient Fluid Volume* related to hypermetabolic state

DRUG GUIDE

CEFTRIAXONE SODIUM (ROCEPHIN)

Overview of Action
Semisynthetic third-generation cephalosporin that acts by binding to one or more of the penicillin-binding proteins located on the bacterial cell wall, inhibiting bacterial cell wall synthesis and killing the bacterium. More active against a wide range of gram-negative bacteria, such as *Neisseria gonorrhoeae, Haemophilus influenzae, Shigella, Enterobacter aerogenes, Escherichia coli, Klebsiella,* and *Pseudomonas aeruginosa.* Also active against some gram-positive strains (e.g., *Staphylococcus aureus, Staphylococcus pyogenes, Streptococcus pneumoniae*). Used to treat infections of acute otitis media, lower respiratory tract, skin, intra-abdominal area, urinary tract, pelvic inflammatory disease, bones, joints, and septicemia and meningitis.

Routes, Dosage, Frequency
IM, IV
- Newborns: 50 mg/kg/day as single dose
- Infants, children: 50 to 75 mg/kg/day in 2 equally divided doses every 12 hours (dosage not to exceed 2 g/day)
- Meningitis: Newborns to 12 years: Loading dose: 75 mg/kg once, then 100 mg/kg/day in 2 equally divided doses every 12 hours (dosage not to exceed 4 g/day)
- Skin and skin structure infections: Less than 12 years: Loading dose: 50 to 75 mg/kg once daily or in equally divided doses twice daily (not to exceed 2 g)
- Prophylaxis for infants of mothers with peripartum gonococcal infections: Single dose 50 mg/kg IM or IV given at birth (125 mg maximum dose)

Contraindications: Hypersensitivity to the drug or cephalosporins, newborns with hyperbilirubinemia. Use with caution if allergic to penicillin and other drugs, or if impaired renal or hepatic function.
Side Effects: Diarrhea, rash, pruritius, hypersensitivity, pain and induration at injection site.

Nursing Implications
- Assess: Determine if previous allergic reaction to ceftriaxone, penicillins, or cephalosporins. Obtain cultures and sensitivity before treatment, but treatment can start before results are obtained.
- Administer: **IM:** Reconstitute with sterile water, normal saline, bacteriostatic water, or 1% lidocaine solution without epinephrine for injection. Solution will be light yellow to amber. Injection is painful. Give into deep muscle appropriate for age and development; adequately restrain child, rotate and record sites. Do not use bacteriostatic water with benzyl alcohol for reconstitution in newborns. **IV:** Reconstitute according to package insert with compatible IV fluid. Intermittent infusion is given over 30 minutes in recommended concentrations of 10 to 40 mg/mL; compatible with D5W, D10W, D5W/0.5% NS, D5W/NS. Do not premix with other aminoglycosides and other bacteriostatic agents. Use of large vein with small-bore needle may reduce local IV reactions. Has 83 mg (3.6 mEq) sodium/1 gram of drug.
- Monitor: Check IM site for induration. Observe IV site for vein irritation and extravasation, and change peripheral site every 48 to 72 hours. Monitor child for hypersensitivity and side effects, especially if renal or hepatic impairment is present, or if on long-term therapy. Monitor CBC, prothrombin time, and hepatic and renal function levels. Watch for symptoms of superinfection or diarrhea (may indicate pseudomembranous colitis), check for fever and report. Yogurt (4 oz) daily may maintain normal intestinal flora. Watch for symptoms of bleeding due to possible prolonged bleeding time especially in malnutrition, children on anticoagulants, and other susceptible patients. If given for group A beta-hemolytic streptococcal infections, a 10-day therapy course is needed to reduce risk of rheumatic fever and glomerulonephritis. Usual therapy course is 4 to 14 days, or 2 days after symptoms subside.
- Patient teaching: Cold compresses for 24 hours after IM injection. Heat to injection site after 24 hours for local pain management.

Data from Wilson, B. A., Shannon, M. T., & Stang, C. L. (2005). Nurse's drug guide 2005. *Upper Saddle River, NJ: Prentice Hall-Health; Mosby. (2004).* Mosby's drug consult 2004. *St. Louis, MO: Author.*

- *Impaired Skin Integrity* related to hyperthermia and scratching skin lesions
- *Impaired Oral Mucous Membranes* related to infectious disease process
- *Deficient Fluid Volume* related to repeated episodes of vomiting and diarrhea
- *Ineffective Therapeutic Regimen Management (Family)* related to complexity of care required by child

PLANNING AND IMPLEMENTATION

Most children with infectious diseases are cared for at home; however, children may be evaluated in various healthcare settings.

Nursing care of children with infectious diseases in healthcare settings focuses on preventing the spread of infection. Isolate children with suspicious rashes from other children. When possible, hard surfaces and toys in the waiting room and examining room where the child was seen should be wiped down with antiseptic solution before another child uses the room. Linens are disposed of in appropriately marked linen bags.

Nursing care for treatment of fever includes administering antipyretics, removing unnecessary clothing, and encouraging increased fluid intake. Tepid baths or sponging has been found to be no more effective than acetaminophen in reducing fevers (Sharber, 1997).

NURSING PRACTICE

Use one medication (acetaminophen or ibuprofen) for fever management as a patient safety initiative. These medications have different durations of action (acetaminophen—4 hours, and ibuprofen—6 hours) and many different preparations, so there is a risk for overdosing the child if the administration schedule is not adhered to strictly (Carson, 2003).

Children are often admitted to the hospital for treatment of severe infections. In addition, countless numbers of **nosocomial** (hospital-acquired) **infections** occur each year. The fecal-oral and respiratory routes are the most common sources of infections in children. All items with which the infected child comes into contact are considered contaminated (linens, toys, medical equipment, etc.). Transmission-based precautions, including isolation, must be implemented to reduce exposure of other children and staff to the infectious agent. Follow the facility's standard precautions and transmission-based precautions to reduce the spread of infectious diseases to staff and other patients. Bring any questions and concerns to the hospital's infection control nurse. (See the Infection Control chapter in the *Clinical Skills Manual* for more detailed information.)
SKILLS

Involve the parents by allowing them to assist with their child's care. Nursing care also includes treating infection, administering antibiotics on schedule, monitoring antibiotic blood levels if indicated to ensure appropriate results, and educating parents.

Nursing Care in the Community

Teach parents to care for their child at home. This includes how and when to give antipyretics and antibiotics if ordered, appropriate foods and beverages to provide, and care of rashes and other topical symptoms. Parents often fear fever, believing it is a disease rather than a symptom of an illness. Provide information and reassurance. Help them to recognize the signs of the child's worsening condition in association with the child's specific disease.

Correct any misconceptions parents and childcare workers may have about the occurrence or cause of the infectious disease in their child. The parents and other providers may feel that they have exposed the child to certain germs or bacteria. Teach them that infection control will reduce exposure of other children and family members to the infectious disease. Specific infection control measures include the following:

- Practice good handwashing; it is one of the best ways to decrease the spread of infection.
- Disinfect hard surfaces such as those touched by the child with a cold, diaper-changing areas, diaper pails, and cribs.
- Tell children not to kiss pets on the mouth.
- Remove toys that the child has mouthed and disinfect them before other children play with them.
- Make sure all children in the house are fully immunized.

EVALUATION

Expected outcomes of nursing care include the following:

- Opportunities for spread of infection between patients and family members are minimized.
- The child's fever is effectively managed with antipyretics.
- The full treatment with antibiotics, if ordered, is completed.

TEACHING HIGHLIGHTS

GUIDELINES FOR EVALUATING AND TREATING FEVER IN CHILDREN

About fevers:

- A fever is not a disease; it is the body's response to an infection. It means the child's body is using natural defenses to fight an infection.
- If the child has a fever and does not look sick, it may be better to let the child use his or her natural defenses to fight off the virus or bacteria causing the fever.

Treating the fever:

- Use a thermometer to check the child's temperature.
- Use either acetaminophen or ibuprofen to lower a fever, giving the correct dose—drops and syrups do not have the same concentration. Do not alternate medications.
- Remove all but a light layer of the child's clothing.
- Monitor the child's behavior and response to fever medication.
- The temperature may rise again 4 hours after giving acetaminophen or 6 hours after ibuprofen. Check the temperature and give another dose of fever medicine. Check for recommendations on the bottle for the maximum number of doses allowed per day.

Call your healthcare provider immediately if:

- The infant is under 2 months old and has a fever over 38.0°C (100.4°F).
- The child has a fever over 40.1°C (104.2°F) and any of the following symptoms are present:

- The child is crying inconsolably or whimpering. The child cries when moved or otherwise touched by the parent or other family members.
- The child is difficult to awaken.
- The child's neck is stiff.
- There are purple spots present on the skin.
- Breathing is difficult and no better after the nose is cleared.
- The child is drooling saliva and is unable to swallow anything.
- The child has a convulsion.
- The child acts or looks very sick.

Call your healthcare provider within 24 hours if:

- The child is 2 to 4 months old (unless fever occurs within 48 hours of a DTaP shot and the infant has no other serious symptoms).
- The fever is higher than 40.1°C (104.2°F) (especially if the child is under 3 years old).
- The child complains of burning or pain with urination.
- The fever has been present more than 24 hours without an obvious cause or location of infection.
- The fever went away for more than 24 hours and then returned.
- The fever has been present for more than 72 hours.

EMERGING INFECTION CONTROL THREATS

Special attention is now directed at disease surveillance associated with infectious agents. Potential weapons of terrorists (anthrax, smallpox, plague, botulism, hemorrhagic fever, or tularemia) or the emergence of rare infectious diseases, such as severe acute respiratory syndrome (SARS), need to be identified as early as possible so that public health measures can be initiated. The state public health system would be activated to identify cases, to control the spread of infection, and to prepare the mass casualty response to care for the potentially large numbers of ill adults and children. See Table 45–7 for the signs and symptoms of biologic agents that could potentially be used for terrorism and appropriate clinical therapy.

NURSING MANAGEMENT

Maintain a high level of suspicion when more than the expected number of individuals with similar signs and symptoms seek care in any healthcare facility. Initiating infection control measures such as airborne and contact precautions may help reduce the transmission of infection. Instituting isolation before a definitive diagnosis is appropriate when the level of suspicion is high. Assess children and provide supportive nursing care for the identified infection.

Nurses should regularly review guidelines posted by the Centers for Disease Control and Prevention about the management of specific health threats.

MEDIALINK   Bioterrorism Preparedness

TABLE 45-7 ✤ Clinical Manifestations of Aerosolized Organisms that Are Potential Biologic Weapons of Terrorists

Organisms	Aerosol Transmission Clinical Manifestations	Clinical Therapy
Anthrax Causal agent: Bacillus anthracis	■ Cutaneous—papule that progresses to a vesicle that develops into a skin ulcer with a depressed black scab area in the center. Not painful. Child may have fever, malaise, headache, and regional lymphadenopathy. ■ Gastrointestinal—nausea, loss of appetite, bloody diarrhea, hematemesis, fever, stomach pain, severe abdominal pain followed by fever and septicemia. ■ Inhalation—brief prodrome with respiratory symptoms like a sore throat, mild fever, malaise, muscle aches followed by development of dyspnea, cough, chest pain, shortness of breath, and systemic symptoms. Shock, pleural effusion, and meningitis may develop without treatment.	■ IV ciprofloxacin or doxycycline for patients over 12 years. For children under 12 years, IV ciprofloxacin plus clindamycin. ■ For postexposure prophylaxis: oral ciprofloxacin or amoxicillin for 60 days.
Botulism Causal agent: Clostridium botulinum	■ Ptosis, diplopia, blurred vision. Sluggishly reactive pupils. ■ Speech and swallowing problems, dysarthria, dysphonia, dysphagia, and loss of gag reflex. ■ Acute, afebrile symmetric descending flaccid paralysis, progressing to loss of head control, hypotonia, generalized weakness, deep tendon reflexes diminish or disappear. Constipation. ■ May be preceded by abdominal cramps, nausea, vomiting, or diarrhea. ■ May become confused or obtunded.	■ Slow IV infusion of equine antitoxin diluted in normal saline. ■ Epinephrine and diphenhydramine for serum sickness or urticaria.
Hemorrhagic Fever Causal agent: Ebola or Marburg virus	■ Abrupt onset of fever, myalgia, headache, nausea, vomiting, abdominal pain, photophobia, diarrhea, chest pain, cough, pharyngitis. ■ Maculopapular rash prominent on trunk soon after fever, bleeding into skin (petechiae, ecchymosis, subconjunctival hemorrhages), shock and circulatory collapse in short period. ■ Ghostlike appearance, looks critically ill.	■ Management of hypotension and shock and maintenance of fluid and electrolyte balance. ■ Replacement of blood, platelets, and plasma for severe hemorrhage.
Plague Causal agent: Yersinia pestis Pneumonic plague with aerosol route of transmission	■ Severe respiratory illness with high fever, chills, headache, cough, breathing difficulty. ■ Rapidly developing pneumonia, bloody or watery sputum. ■ May lead to respiratory failure and shock.	■ Streptomycin IM or gentamicin IV. Alternate antibiotics include IV chloramphenicol or doxycycline.
Smallpox Causal agent: Variola major virus	■ Prodrome 2 to 4 days before rash: abrupt onset with fever (101°F or higher), malaise, headache, muscle pain, prostration, nausea and vomiting, and backache. ■ Rash begins with red spots in mouth and on tongue that develop sores and break open. Then a few macules known as herald spots appear on the forehead, face, and extremities. Over the next few days a generalized rash develops, progressing from macules to papules, to tense vesicles, to tense deep pustules with an umbilicated appearance. Most cases have discrete, semiconfluent to confluent vesicles. Lesions are firm, all in same stage of development, more concentrated on the extremities than the trunk. The temperature usually falls and the patient feels better. ■ The pustules form scabs by the end of the second week, and the scabs fall off after 3–4 weeks.	■ Supportive care. ■ Antibiotics for secondary infection.
Tularemia Causal agent: Francisella tularensis	■ Febrile illness, fatigue, chills, headache, malaise, dyspnea, chest pain. ■ May develop hemorrhagic inflammation of airways that progresses to pneumonia, pleuritis, and hilar lymphadenopathy. ■ May also have pharyngitis, bronchiolitis, and pneumonia with systemic symptoms.	■ Supportive care in the intensive care unit. ■ Streptomycin IM or gentamicin IV, alternate drug is IV ciprofloxacin. For children use gentamicin IV, alternate drugs are doxycycline and chloramphenicol. ■ Postexposure prophylaxis for 14 days with ciprofloxacin, for children use doxycycline.

Source: Data from Yetman, R. J., Parks, D., & Taft, E. (2002). Management of patients exposed to biologic weapons. *Journal of Pediatric Health Care, 16*(5), 256–261; Centers for Disease Control and Prevention. (2003). Retrieved September 24, 2003, from http://www.bt.cdc.gov.

Critical Concept Review

LEARNING OBJECTIVES

CONCEPTS

Describe the reasons why children are more vulnerable than adults to infectious and communicable diseases.

1. Infants and children have immature immune systems.
2. Infants' protection from maternal antibodies decrease with age.
3. Incomplete immunization status.
4. Lack of prior exposure to infectious agents.
5. Poor hygiene practices of infants and children.

Describe the process of infection and modes of transmission.

1. Process of infection requires:
   - An infectious agent.
   - Effective means of transmission.
   - Susceptible host.
2. Modes of transmission:
   - Direct: requires physical contact between source of infection and new host.
   - Indirect: pathogens survive outside host before causing disease.

Explain the role that vaccines play in the reduction and elimination of infectious and communicable diseases.

1. Vaccinations have kept most children from acquiring common childhood diseases.
2. Vaccinations have led to an 80% reduction in pneumonia and meningitis in children under two years of age.

Develop a nursing care plan for children of all ages needing immunizations.

1. Teach the importance of immunization during the prenatal period, including immunizations the infant will receive in the nursery.
2. Review immunization schedule with parents before newborn leaves hospital.
3. Provide written materials about immunizations.
4. Review immunization status of infant and child at every visit with healthcare provider.
5. Assess child for potential contraindications to vaccines prior to administration.
6. Review expected side effects of immunizations with parents.

Recognize common infectious and communicable diseases.

1. Chickenpox (Varicella):
   - Causes fluid-filled vesicles with elevated temperature and itching.
2. Coxsackiviruses:
   - May cause respiratory symptoms or skin and mucous membrane lesions.
3. Diptheria:
   - Seen in countries with low immunization rates.
   - May cause severe respiratory symptoms.
4. Erythema Infectiosum (Fifth disease):
   - Begins with mild, flu-like illness and ends with a red rash on the cheeks.
5. Haemophilus Influenza, Type B:
   - Begins with respiratory symptoms, but may progress to meningitis.
6. Influenza:
   - Very contagious.
   - Sudden onset of respiratory symptoms.
7. Measles (Rubeola):
   - High fever, red rash.
   - Recognized by presence of Koplik spots on buccal mucosa.
8. Mononucleosis:
   - Symptoms begin with high fever, sore throat, and malaise.
   - Child develops severe cervical lymphadenopathy and possibly liver and spleen enlargement.
9. Mumps (Parotitis):
   - Begins with fever and pain while chewing.
   - Child develops swelling of parotid glands.

LEARNING OBJECTIVES

CONCEPTS

Recognize common infectious and communicable diseases.—continued

10. Pertussis (Whooping Cough):
    ■ Begins with vague respiratory symptoms.
    ■ Recognized by paroxysmal cough that sounds like a "whoop."
11. Pneumococcal infection:
    ■ May cause otitis media, sinusitis, and/or pharyngitis.
12. Poliomyelitis:
    ■ Virus affects central nervous system.
    ■ Begins with fever, sore throat, and stiff neck.
    ■ May progress to paralysis.
13. Roseola (Exanthem subitum):
    ■ Sudden high fever in child 6 months to 2 years of age without toxic symptoms.
    ■ Following fever phase, child develops a maculopapular rash over most of body.
14. Rubella:
    ■ Mild disease causing low grade fever and rash.
    ■ Causes birth defects if mother acquires disease during pregnancy.
15. Streptococcus A:
    ■ Rapid onset of severe sore throat with high fever.
    ■ May progress to scarlet fever.
    ■ Pyodermal skin lesions with honey crust.

Develop a nursing care plan for a child with a common infectious disease.

1. Isolate child from others as much as possible.
2. Treat high fever and other symptoms with non-aspirin antipyretic medications.
3. Cut fingernails short to discourage scratching.
4. Encourage use of tepid or colloidal baths to treat itching.
5. Medicate with antihistamines to assist with complaints of itching.

CRITICAL THINKING IN ACTION

*View the **Critical Thinking in Action** video in Chapter 45 of the CD-ROM. Then, answer the questions that follow.*

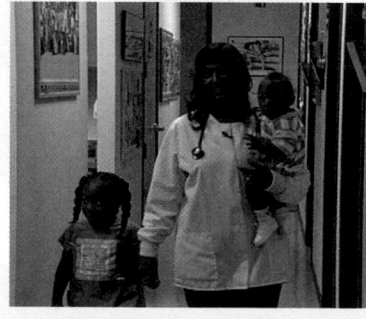

Keisha, 7, and Brandon, 1, are brought to the pediatric clinic, with both needing immunizations. Even though Brandon is sick today, their mother would still like Keisha to have her immunizations, and she would also like both kids to have a complete check-up before their vaccines to make sure they are healthy.

You examine Keisha's vital signs as: 80th percentile in height, 40th percentile in weight, temperature 98.9 degrees, blood pressure 105/62, urinalysis with a trace of leukocytes, and she passes her hearing and vision screening. She seems extremely anxious about having to get a needle. There is evidence of eczema and allergic rhinitis.

You examine Brandon as a sick visit while he clings to his mother. His vital signs are: temperature 102 degrees, respiratory rate of 30 breaths per minute, and heart rate of 90 beats per minute. Brandon's exam exhibits evidence of a coxsackievirus, evidenced by grayish, papulovesicular, ulcerative lesions in his mouth. This type of illness does not respond to antibiotics. You advise the mother to avoid others because it is contagious and to offer cool drinks and bland foods. She is also told warm saline mouth rinses would be helpful, to observe for dehydration, and to give ibuprofen or acetaminophen as needed.

1. Since Brandon has been into the office several times for various infections, what education can be given to his mother to reduce the chances of future infections?
2. Keisha has eczema and allergic rhinitis. Would this be a contraindication to giving vaccines?
3. What are questions the nurse should ask the mother before administering vaccines to Keisha to make sure there are no contraindications to giving them?
4. What should the mother be told about caring for Keisha after her vaccines?
5. How should the mother be told to manage Brandon's fever?

MEDIALINK   www.prenhall.com/london

- NCLEX-RN® Review, case studies, and other interactive resources for this chapter can be found on the Companion Website at http://www.prenhall.com/london. Click on "Chapter 45" to select the activities for this chapter.

MediaLink Applications

Immunization schedules and recommendations for children and adolescents are issued yearly in the United States, and may be revised at six-month intervals. Vaccine shortage notices and guidelines for rationing vaccines may be issued throughout the year. The nurse is responsible for remaining current on immunization recommendations and teaching parents about immunizations. Refer to the www.aap.org, www.aafp.org, www.cdc.gov/nip/acip, and www.medem.com websites to answer the following questions.

This activity contains 11 questions.

1.   **What vaccines are given to special populations, and at what ages?**

To create paragraphs in your essay response, type <p> at the beginning of the paragraph, and </p> at the end.

- For animations, more NCLEX-RN® Review questions, and an audio glossary, access the accompanying CD-ROM in this textbook.

REFERENCES

American Academy of Pediatrics Committee on Infectious Disease. (2003). *Red book: Report of the Committee on Infectious Disease* (26th ed.). Elk Grove Village, IL: American Academy of Pediatrics.

Arvin, A. M. (2002). Antiviral therapy for varicella and herpes zoster. *Seminars in Pediatric Infectious Diseases, 13*(1), 12–21.

Bilukha, O. O., & Rosenstein, N. (2005). Prevention and control of meningococcal disease. *Morbidity and Mortality Weekly Report, 54*(RR07), 1–21.

Buck, M. L. (2005). Meningococcal conjugate vaccine. *Pediatric Pharmacology, 11*(5). Retrieved June 7, 2005, from http://www.medscape.com/viewarticle/505508_print.

Carson, S. M. (2003). Alternating acetaminophen and ibuprofen in the febrile child: Examination of the evidence regarding efficacy and safety. *Pediatric Nursing, 29*(5), 379–382.

Centers for Disease Control and Prevention. (2000). Consequences of delayed diagnosis of Rocky Mountain spotted fever in children—West Virginia, Michigan, Tennessee, and Oklahoma, May–July 2000. *Morbidity and Mortality Weekly Report, 49*(39), 885–888.

Centers for Disease Control and Prevention. (2002a). Pertussis deaths—United States, 2000. *Morbidity and Mortality Weekly Report, 51*(28), 616–618.

Centers for Disease Control and Prevention. (2002b). Lyme disease—United States, 2000. *Morbidity and Mortality Weekly Report, 51*(2), 29–31.

Centers for Disease Control Advisory Committee on Immunization Practices. (2006). *Recommended childhood and adolescent immunization schedule—United States, 2006.* Morbidity and Mortality Weekly Report, 54(52); Q1–Q4. Retrieved January 6, 2006 from http://www.cdc.gov/mmwr/preview/mmwrhtml/mm5451-Immunizational.htm?s_cid-mm5451-Immunizational_e%0d%0a.

Chang, L. Y., Lin, T. Y., Hsu, K. H., Huang, Y. C., Lin, K. L., Hsueh, C., et al. (1999). Clinical features and risk factors of pulmonary edema after enterovirus 71–related hand, foot, and mouth disease. *Lancet, 354*(9191), 1682–1686.

Cheung, M., & Lieberman, J. M. (2002). Influenza: Update on strategies for management. *Contemporary Pediatrics, 19*(10), 82–94.

Cimpella, L. B., Goldman, D. L., & Khine, H. (2000). Fever pathophysiology. *Clinical Pediatric Emergency Medicine, 1*(2), 84–93.

Cohen, L. L. (2002). Reducing infant immunization distress through distraction. *Health Psychology, 21*(2), 207–211.

Coyer, S. M. (2002). Understanding parental concerns about immunizations. *Journal of Pediatric Health Care, 16*(4), 193–196.

Department of Health and Human Services, Office of Disease Prevention and Promotion. (1999). *Healthy People 2010.* Washington, DC: Author.

Diggle, L., & Deek, J. (2000). Effect of needle length on incidence of local reactions to routine immunizations in infants aged 4 months: Randomized control trial. *British Medical Journal, 321*(7266), 931–933.

Food and Drug Administration, (2005). FDA and CDC issue alert on Menactra meningococcal vaccine and Guillain Barre syndrome. Retrieved January 6, 2006 from http://www.fda.gov/bbs/topics/NEWS/2005/NEW01238.htm.

Gottlieb, B. (2000). *Alternative cures.* Emmaus, PA: Rodale Press.

Health Resources and Services Administration Office of Special Programs. (2005). *National Childhood Vaccine Injury Act vaccine injury table.* Retrieved October 24, 2005, from http://www.hrsa.gov/osp/vicp/table.htm.

Howell, K. (2001). Malaria: Part 2. *Practice Nursing, 12*(11), 464–466.

Institute of Medicine Board of Health Promotion and Disease Prevention. (2001). *Immunization safety review: Thimerosol containing vaccines and neurodevelopmental disorders.* Washington, DC: National Academy Press.

Jacobs, E. S., Ogborn, J., & Tunnessen, W. W. (2001). Fever and abdominal pain in a 13 year old: Time for rash decisions. *Contemporary Pediatrics, 18*(10), 20–26.

Keyserling, H. L. (2002). Prevention of pneumococcal disease in children. *Medscape.* Retrieved December 20, 2002, from http://www.medscape.com/viewprogram/1807_pnt.

Mera, K. E., & Hackley, B. (2003). Childhood vaccines: How safe are they? *American Journal of Nursing, 103*(2), 79–88.

Mosby. (2004). *Mosby's drug consult 2004.* St. Louis, MO: Author.

Peters, T. R., & Edwards, K. M. (2002). Pneumococcal vaccines: Present and future. *Pediatric Annals, 31*(4), 261–268.

Reef, S. E., Frey, T. K., Theall, K., Abernathy, E., Burnett, C. L., Icenogle, J., et al. (2002). The changing epidemiology of rubella in the 1990s: On the verge of elimination and new challenges for control and prevention. *Journal of the American Medical Association, 287*(4), 464–472.

Reis, E. C., Roth, E. K., Syphan, J. L., Tarbell, S. E., & Holubkov, R. (2003). Effective pain reduction for multiple immunization injections in young infants. *Archives of Pediatrics & Adolescent Medicine, 57,* 1115–1120.

Saari, T. N., & Committee on Infectious Diseases. (2003). Immunization of preterm and low birth weight infants. *Pediatrics, 112*(1), 193–198.

Sharber, J. (1997). The efficacy of tepid sponge bathing to reduce fever in young children. *American Journal of Emergency Medicine, 15*(2), 211–213.

Shingadia, D., & Shulman, S. T. (2000). Recognition and management of imported malaria in children. *Seminars in Pediatric Infectious Diseases, 11*(3), 172–177.

Tan, T. Q. (2002). Pneumococcal infections in children. *Pediatric Annals, 31*(4), 241–247.

Vazquez, M., LaRussa, P. S., Gershon, A. A., Steinberg, S. P., Freudigman, K., & Shapiro, E. D. (2001). The effectiveness of the varicella vaccine in clinical practice. *New England Journal of Medicine, 344*(13), 955–960.

Wade, C. F. (2000). Keeping Lyme disease at bay: An integrated approach to prevention. *American Journal of Nursing, 100*(7), 26–31.

Whitney, C. G., Farley, M. M., & Hadler, J. (2003). Decline in invasive pneumococcal disease after introduction of protein-polysaccharide conjugate vaccine. *New England Journal of Medicine, 348*(18), 1737–1746.

World Health Organization. (1999). Pertussis vaccines WHO position paper. *Weekly Epidemiological Record, 74,* 137–144.

Yetman, R. J., Parks, D., & Taft, E. (2002). Management of patients exposed to biologic weapons. *Journal of Pediatric Health Care, 16*(5), 256–261.

CHAPTER 46

The Child with Alterations in Eye, Ear, Nose, and Throat Function

The early intervention program that Raeanne attended to help her deal with her visual impairment really helped her to prepare for preschool. We learned a lot too about how to help her. We are still really nervous about her starting at preschool and being with a lot of other children. We want it to go well for her.
—*Mother of Raeanne, 3 years old*

LEARNING OBJECTIVES

- Describe abnormalities of the eyes, ears, nose, throat, and mouth in children.

- Plan for screening programs and identification of children with vision and hearing abnormalities.

- Plan nursing care for children with vision or hearing impairments.

- Use latest recommendations when implementing care and teaching for children with abnormalities of eyes, ears, nose, throat, and mouth.

- Integrate preventive and treatment principles when implementing care for children related to eyes, ears, nose, and throat.

MEDIALINK www.prenhall.com/london

CD-ROM

Animations:
    Ear Abnormalities
    Middle Ear Dynamics
Videos:
    3D Eye/Eye Anatomy
    3D Ear/Ear Anatomy
    Otitis Media
Nursing in Action:
    Eye, Ear, and Nose Medication Administration
    Obtaining a Sample for Throat Culture
Skills 9-18–9-19: Visual Acuity Screening
Skill 10-15: Obtaining a Sample for Throat Culture
Audio Glossary
NCLEX-RN® Review

Companion Website

MediaLink Applications:
    Plan Interventions for Visual Disorders
    Early Identification and Intervention for Hearing
        Loss
    Neonate Screening and the Law
    Plan a Vision Screening Program
    Case Study: Otitis Media
Thinking Critically
NCLEX-RN® Review
Audio Glossary

How are conditions of the eye, ear, nose, and throat related? Which conditions have the potential to affect a child's growth, development, and behavior? In what settings do children with eye, ear, nose, and throat conditions receive care? How can parents be helped to foster development in their children when they have a visual or hearing disorder?

Because the eye, ear, nose, and throat are connected, a malformation, infection, or other condition in one of these structures may affect them all. Intact sensory structures enable children to reach developmental milestones; thus alterations, especially to the eye and ear, may delay a child's development. Most children with eye, ear, nose, and throat disorders are treated at home or in the community rather than in the hospital.

ANATOMY AND PHYSIOLOGY OF PEDIATRIC DIFFERENCES

EYE

How are the eyes of children different from those of adults? Chapter 35 provides a detailed discussion of the assessment of the eyes and **visual acuity**, the ability to discriminate letters or other objects. ∞ The eyes of newborns differ from the eyes of adults in several ways. Visual acuity in newborns ranges between 20/100 and 20/400. The lens is more spherical and cannot accommodate to both near and far objects, which means that the newborn sees best at a distance of about 8 inches (20 cm). Since the optic nerve is not yet completely myelinated, the ability to distinguish color and other details is decreased. If the infant is preterm, especially less than 32 weeks' gestation, retinal vascularization, particularly in the periphery of the retina, may be incomplete. The rectus muscles that control binocular vision may be somewhat uncoordinated at birth. The eyes should be aligned and movement coordinated by the age of 3 months.

The cornea of the infant and young child occupies a larger portion of the orbit than in the adult. Since the eyeball is relatively unprotected laterally, it is more easily injured. The sclera of the newborn is thin and translucent with a bluish tinge, and the iris is blue or gray. Eye color changes during the first 6 months of life. Infants produce tears to nourish and oxygenate the outer layers of the cornea. Parents do not see tears when a young infant cries because the infant's lacrimal system drains them efficiently into the nasal cavity. However, the amount of tears is less in preterm infants, which can lead to dry corneas and concentration of medications administered into the eye (Behrman, Kliegman, & Jenson, 2004).

As infants grow, their eyes mature and their vision improves. By the age of 2 or 3 years, most children have a visual acuity of 20/50, and by the age of 6 or 7 years, it is 20/20. Visual acuity is measured using standardized letter or picture charts. (See Chapter 35. ∞) **Vision** refers to the complex process of acquiring meaning from what is seen, involving the eye, brain, and related neurologic and physiologic structures. Development interacts with a child's maturing physiologic system to bring increasing meaning to objects in sight (Table 46–1).

EAR

Why do infants and young children have more ear problems than adults? The eustachian tube, which connects the nasopharynx to the middle ear, is proportionately shorter, wider, and more horizontal in infants than in older children or adults (see "As Children Grow: Eustachian Tube"). During sucking, yawning, and other movements, the tube opens for milliseconds, allowing free

TABLE 46–1 ✤ Visually Related Developmental Milestones

Age	Milestone
Term neonate	Demonstrates alertness to visual stimulus presented 8-12 in. (20-30 cm) from eyes
1 month	Follows an object 60 degrees horizontally and 30 degrees vertically; blinks at an approaching object
2 months	Follows a person from 6 ft (2 m) away; smiles in response to a face; raises head 30 degrees from prone
3 months	Tracks an object through 180 degrees; regards own hand; begins visual-motor coordination
4–5 months	Social smile; reaches for a cube 12 in (30 cm) away; notices a raisin 12 in (30 cm) away
7–8 months	Picks up a raisin by raking
8–9 months	Pokes at holes in a peg board; neat pincer grasp; crawling
12–14 months	Stacks blocks; places a peg in a round hole; stands and walks

Used with permission from Scheiner, A. P. (1996). Vision problems: Impairment to blindness. In A. M. Rudolph, J. I. E. Hoffman, & C. D. Rudolph (Eds.), *Rudolph's pediatrics* (20th ed., p. 167). Stamford, CT: Appleton & Lange.

The external ear canal is small at birth, although the internal ear and middle ear are relatively large. As a result the tympanic membrane is close to the surface and can be easily injured. Babies can hear at about 20 weeks' gestation, and the auditory nerve function is mature at about 5 months of age in the infant. Before 34 weeks' gestation, the exterior ear is soft with little cartilage apparent. When the ear of a preterm is folded forward and released, its recoil is slow, while with term newborns the recoil is strong and fast.

NOSE AND THROAT

Up to the age of 6 months, infants breathe primarily through the nose and not through the mouth. Edema and nasal discharge may interfere with adequate air intake and feeding. Mucosal swelling and exudate may block the small nasal passages of young children.

The palatine tonsils, visible on oral examination, are located on each side of the oropharynx. The method for examining a child's throat is discussed in Chapter 35. ∞ Although tonsils vary in size considerably during childhood, they are normally large, especially in school-age children. Lymph tissue decreases in size by about 10 years, so its appearance after this age can indicate abnormality. The nasopharyngeal tonsils (adenoids) lie in the posterior wall of the nasopharynx, just above the oropharynx. In children the adenoids may become enlarged, harboring bacteria and interfering with breathing.

The mucosal membranes of the mouth are expected to be intact and without lesions at all ages. The first teeth commonly erupt at about 6 months of age, and the first loss of teeth begins at about 6 years. See Chapter 35 for thor-

passage of air between the nasopharynx and the middle ear. This predisposes young children to development of otitis media or middle ear infection.

AS CHILDREN GROW

Eustachian Tube

Age 2

Age 12

Position of eustachian tube is at less of an angle in the young child, resulting in decreased drainage. (more horizontal)

End of eustachian tube in nasal pharynx opens during sucking.

Eustachian tube equalizes air pressure between the middle ear and the outside environment and allows for drainage of secretions from middle ear mucosa.

Of the three anatomic differences in the eustachian tube between adults and small children (shorter, wider, more horizontal), which do you think could cause more problems for the child and why?

ough descriptions of assessment of the oral cavity in infants and children. ∞

DISORDERS OF THE EYE

INFECTIOUS CONJUNCTIVITIS

Conjunctivitis is an inflammation of the conjunctiva, the clear membrane that lines the inside of the lid and sclera. Bacteria, viruses, allergies, trauma, or irritants cause the conjunctiva to become swollen and red with a yellow or white discharge (Figure 46–1 ●). Some additional less common causes of conjunctivitis include inflammation of eyelash follicle, tumor, or uveitis (Gross, 2002). Parents commonly refer to all conjunctivitis as "pink eye."

Conjunctivitis in an infant under 30 days of age is called ophthalmia neonatorum. These infections are usually acquired from the mother during vaginal birth as a result of contact with infected vaginal discharge containing organisms such as *Chlamydia trachomatis* and *Neisseria gonorrhoeae*. See Chapter 28 for information on prophylactic eye treatment. ∞ Newborns occasionally get chemical conjunctivitis in response to prophylactic eye treatment. This may be a cause when the conjunctivitis develops within 24 to 48 hours after instillation of the medication (Alcorn, 2001).

Another cause of infection in infants is herpesvirus, which requires prompt and vigorous treatment to prevent eye injury or blindness. Infants with herpes virus infections of the eye are treated with intravenous acyclovir as well as topical drops.

● **FIGURE 46–1**

Swollen eyelid

Purulent discharge

Inflamed conjunctiva

Acute conjunctivitis. The major difference between bacterial and viral conjunctivitis is that bacterial conjunctivitis has a purulent discharge that may result in crusting whereas the discharge from viral conjunctivitis is serous (watery). Allergic conjunctivitis produces watery to thick drainage and is characterized by itching.

Used with permission from Newell, F. W. (1996). Ophthalmology: Principles and concepts (8th ed.). St. Louis, MO: Mosby-Year Book.

In infants who have frequent tearing and "mattering" (eyelid discharge that has formed a crust) on awakening, a plugged lacrimal duct may mimic conjunctivitis. Treatment involves massaging the tear duct every 4 hours when the infant is awake. Lacrimal ducts that remain plugged after the age of 1 year may have to be opened surgically.

Bacterial conjunctivitis can occur in older children as well. It is characterized by edema of the eyelid, red conjunctiva, and enlarged preauricular lymph glands. There is usually mucopurulent exudate that causes matting, making the eyes difficult to open upon awakening. Older children with conjunctivitis complain of itching or burning, mild photophobia, and a feeling of scratching under the lids. Parents may notice increased tearing or a mucoid or mucopurulent discharge, redness and swelling of the conjunctiva, a pink sclera, and crusty eyelids, especially in the morning. There is no change in vision. Common infectious organisms in older children include *Haemophilus influenzae, Streptococcus pneumoniae, Moraxella catarrhalis,* and *Escherichia coli*. Most cases are caused by hand to eye contact, and the disease can rapidly spread whenever groups of youth spend time together, such as among young children and adolescents in schools and childcare centers, and even among college students in dormitories, sororities, fraternities, and on sports teams (Gross, 2002; Stephenson, 2003). Although bacterial conjunctivitis can be bilateral, it is more commonly unilateral.

A viral cause is also possible, with adenoviruses the most common organism. Viral conjunctivitis is more often bilateral than unilateral. Herpes simplex virus (HSV) can also cause infection, either by transfer from a herpes-infected mother to her baby during birth or by contact with an infected person in infants or children of any age. Ophthalmic herpes infection is often accompanied by characteristic vesicular lesions on the skin of the face. A culture of the lesions is performed for diagnosis, and any accompanying conjunctivitis is assumed to be caused by herpes virus. For the infection caused by HSV, prompt and vigorous treatment is needed to prevent eye injury or blindness, which can occur in children with recurrent herpes virus infections as a result of antibody reaction to the viral antigen. Herpes virus infections commonly recur so periodic treatment and sometimes prophylaxis may be needed.

When conjunctivitis is caused by an allergy, the child complains of intense itching. Eyes are red with watery discharge, and the conjunctivae have a "cobblestone" appearance.

In most cases a diagnosis of the cause of conjunctivitis is made based on the history and symptoms. Cultures can be taken, especially in infants or in cases suspected of being unusual bacterial illness or herpes viruses. A Gram stain of discharge and conjunctival scraping for potential *Chlamydia* or herpes are performed. Infants and children must be promptly referred to primary care providers or eye specialists for treatment of possible eye infections. When diagnosed in an infant in the neonatal intensive care unit, the infant is isolated to prevent spread to other infants.

Antibiotic eye medication is prescribed in droplet or ointment form if a bacterial infection is suspected. Treatment may be started after a laboratory sample is obtained but before the results are known. Fluoroquinolones are now frequently used to treat bacterial conjunctivitis; drops or ointment can be used. When gonococcal conjunctivitis occurs in newborns, ceftriaxone is recommended; the disease is resistant to penicillin. Chlamydial infections are treated with oral erythromycin or tetracycline. Careful total evaluation of the newborn with any conjunctivitis is also performed to watch for other signs of infection. Instructions for instilling eye medication are provided in the skills manual (see Skill 11–6). **SKILLS**

Viral conjunctivitis may be treated with comfort measures such as cleaning drainage away with a warm clean cloth, and avoiding bright lights and reading. Ophthalmic antibiotics may sometimes be given to prevent bacterial invasion due to frequent rubbing of the eyes. Herpes simplex virus infections of the eye are treated promptly by an ophthalmologist, neonatologist, or others who are trained in this serious disease. Topical drugs are used, and often are combined with a systemic antiviral agent such as acyclovir (Alcorn, 2001; Gross, 2002). Neonatal herpes simplex virus is treated vigorously with parenteral acyclovir for 14 days (or longer if central nervous system involvement is found upon lumbar puncture), and with topical ophthalmic medication (trifluridine, iododeoxyuridine, or vidarabine). Recurrent lesions may necessitate suppressive or prophylactic treatment with oral acyclovir (Committee on Infectious Diseases, 2003).

If an allergen is believed to be the cause, antihistamines administered orally or ophthalmically may be prescribed. Topical steroids and vasoconstrictors may also be used (Alcorn, 2001). Decongestants can be combined with systemic antihistamines for short-term therapy. More current treatment involves use of mast-cell stabilizers to decrease the activation of mast cells that accompanies allergic reactions. Most mast-cell stabilizers have been tested and found to be safe in children 3 years of age and older (Alexander, 2003).

NURSING MANAGEMENT

Nurses routinely instill antibiotics into the eyes of newborns after birth. Perform a careful examination so that any cases of ophthalmia neonatorum can be referred promptly to an ophthalmologist. Women infected with gonococcus or chlamydia should be identified so their babies can receive attention and medication at birth to prevent infection (Brocklehurst & Rooney, 2000). Babies born at home should have ocular examinations soon after birth.

TEACHING HIGHLIGHTS

INSTILLING EYE MEDICATIONS

It can be challenging to safely instill eye medication into young children. Give parents the following suggestions:

- Wash your hands well.
- Be sure the medicine is warmed at least to room temperature.
- Remove any drainage from the eye with a clean or sterile moist, warm cloth or gauze.
- Wash your hands again.
- Have the child lying on the back with eyes closed.
- Gently pull the lower lid down to form a small pocket.
- Apply a thin string (for ointment) or drops of the medicine.
- Allow the eyelid to return to normal position.
- Have the child keep the eye closed for several seconds.
- Help prevent spread of the infection by keeping the child's hands clean.
- Enhance comfort by keeping the head elevated to decrease swelling and avoid exposure to bright light.

In suspected conjunctivitis, gentle pressure for several seconds with a gloved index finger placed next to the inner corner of the eye may cause a discharge of mucopurulent drainage. Refer for care and report the findings. Since infectious conjunctivitis is extremely contagious, tell parents that children should not return to child care or school until they have been taking an antibiotic for 24 hours. Teach parents the importance of careful handwashing and the avoidance of shared towels. Tell parents that children should not rub their eyes. Mittens may help prevent infants from rubbing their eyes. Toddlers may be distracted by activities that keep their hands busy. Teach parents the proper techniques for instilling eye medications. For children with allergies, alert parents to signs of infection so if the child gets an eye infection, they will seek prompt treatment.

PERIORBITAL CELLULITIS

Periorbital cellulitis is an infection of the eyelid and surrounding tissues, usually caused by bacteria. Children present with swollen, tender, red or purple eyelids; restricted, painful movement of the area around the eye; and fever. Periorbital cellulitis should be treated promptly to prevent the spread of the infection to the posterior orbit. Management includes hospitalization for intravenous antibiotics and the application of hot packs. Children usually respond favorably within 48 to 72 hours.

VISUAL DISORDERS

Vision, the complex process of acquiring meaning from what is seen, depends on many factors. The eyes must move quickly and in a coordinated manner. (See Chapter 35 for discussion of eye movement assessment. ∞) They must function together for clear, single vision to occur. If this ability, called **binocularity**, is not present (perhaps due to strabismus or amblyopia), the child cannot make sense of the images the brain receives. Normally, the objects seen are integrated with other senses through eye–hand coordination, and with the brain through visual imagery and discrimination of objects seen. Although visual acuity is essential, the child's movements, mental processes, and other senses all interact to give meaning to objects that are viewed. Vision therefore influences learning and school performance.

Visual disturbances must be diagnosed and treated promptly to prevent impairment or loss of visual acuity. Most children undergo a simple test for visual acuity during healthcare visits as soon as they can cooperate with the examiner. Once in school, children's visual acuity is screened every 2 to 3 years during the elementary years. Nurses often organize vision screening programs for children. Table 46–2 provides a series of questions that can be used to identify visual disturbances in children. A child who does not pass vision screening is referred to an ophthalmologist or optometrist for more detailed examination of near and far vision, eye structure and movement, and color discrimination.

TABLE 46–2 ❖ Assessment Questions for Identifying Visual Disturbances in Children

Young Child

Ask the parents:

Does your child follow you with his or her eyes as you come into a room?

Are other objects followed with ease?

Do both eyes work together or does one seem to wander off?

At what age did your baby sit, stand, walk?

Does your child have any difficulty picking up objects?

School-Age Child

Ask the parents:

Does your child like to look at pictures and read?

Does your child hold toys or books close, or sit very close to the television?

Does your child squint or rub the eyes?

Is he or she at grade level in all subjects?

Has your child demonstrated any learning difficulties?

Does he or she use a computer, watch television, or play computer games?

Does your child play sports and games at the same level of ability as peers?

Some of the common visual disorders in children are:

- *Hyperopia* (farsightedness): Light rays focus posterior to the retina, resulting in an inability to focus on nearby objects. All children have some degree of hyperopia until 9 to 10 years of age. However, their eyes can accommodate sufficiently to enable them to see near objects clearly. Blurring of vision occurs only in children with excessive hyperopia, or a difference in accommodation between the two eyes. Amblyopia, or a weakening of the poorer eye, can occur in these children if treatment is not obtained.

- *Myopia* (nearsightedness): Light rays focus anterior to the retina, resulting in an inability to see far-off objects. Although children of any age can manifest myopia, it most commonly develops at about 8 years of age. The child may complain of headaches and often squints to improve distance vision.

- *Astigmatism*: Light rays are refracted differently depending on their place of entry to the eye. The curvature of the cornea or lens is not uniformly spherical, causing blurred images. The child with astigmatism often holds pages very close to the face to obtain the best visual image (DeRespinis, 2001).

For the description and management of four disorders that can significantly affect vision—strabismus, amblyopia, cataracts, and glaucoma—see "Clinical Manifestations: Visual Disorders."

Compensatory lenses are prescribed for most visual disorders. A significant difference in visual acuity between the eyes is often a result of amblyopia or strabismus, and further treatment may be needed. The visual acuity of a child with compensatory lenses should be reevaluated every 1 to 2 years. More frequent visits to an eye specialist are needed when a child is being treated for amblyopia or strabismus.

NURSING MANAGEMENT

The nurse plays an important role in identifying eye disorders in children and performing careful eye examinations of newborns and children. Observe for symmetry of placement and movement, ability to follow objects with each eye, and any abnormalities in appearance. The light reflex, cover-uncover test, and visual acuity testing are essential tests for every child. See Chapter 35 for a description of eye examination and the Skills Manual for visual acuity tests (Skills 9–18 and 9–19). ∞ **SKILLS**

Nurses in schools plan and carry out visual acuity screening on children. Generally certain grades (such as kindergarten, 2, 5, and 8) are screened annually along with any children new to a district. The nurse performs and records the screening results and informs the school and families of any

PATHOPHYSIOLOGY ILLUSTRATED
Visual Abnormalities

A Hyperopia

B Myopia

C Astigmatism

Vertical
Horizontal
Vertical

In hyperopia light rays focus behind the retina, making it difficult to focus on objects at close range. In myopia light rays focus in front of the retina, making it difficult to focus on objects that are far away. In astigmatism light rays do not uniformly focus on the eye due to abnormal curvature of cornea or lens.

children with abnormal results, who are referred to an eye specialist for care. An important part of the screening process is following up on referrals to be certain that children receive the diagnostic care they need.

When abnormalities are found on screening, nurses refer families to the care of an eye specialist. When prescriptive lenses are used, the nurse instructs the parent and child on correct wear practices and care. If surgery is needed, surgical and postoperative follow-up are needed. This will include pain control, observing for signs of infection (ophthalmic or systemic), and administering needed eye medications. Sterile technique is used postoperatively to provide eye care. Promptly report deviations from normal such as increased pain, redness, discharge, or edema of the eye; increased temperature or pulse, which may indicate infection; increased sensitivity to light; or other abnormalities. Children are usually discharged home with instructions to minimize certain vigorous activities for a certain period of time. Perform postoperative and discharge teaching and emphasize the importance of follow-up visits.

COLOR BLINDNESS

Color blindness is an X-linked recessive disorder found in 8% of white and 4% of black males and almost never in females. The most common form affects the ability to distinguish between the colors red and green, but there are other variations. Preschool boys are tested for color blindness in some clinics to identify those with the disorder. Color blindness is not treatable, and management focuses on issues of safety (e.g., problems in distinguishing between red and green traffic signals) and techniques to improve discrimination of colors in the affected color groups.

RETINOPATHY OF PREMATURITY

Retinopathy of prematurity (ROP) occurs when immature blood vessels in the retina constrict and become necrotic. This condition, which may occur in infants of low birth weight or of short gestation, can heal completely or lead to mild myopia or retinal detachment and blindness.

ETIOLOGY AND PATHOPHYSIOLOGY

Retinopathy of prematurity results from injury to the developing capillaries of the retina. Oxygen therapy is associated with the development of retinopathy of prematurity (Figure 46–2 ●), but other factors such as respiratory distress, artificial ventilation, apnea, bradycardia, heart disease, multiple blood transfusions, infection, hypoxia, hypercarbia, acidosis, shock, and sepsis have also been linked with the disorder. It is most common in infants born before 28 weeks of gestation and weighing under 1600 g (3 lb, 8 oz) at birth. A genetic link may be present as white infants are more commonly affected than those of African heritage, and Alaskan Natives have a high rate of the disorder. In developed countries ROP is the second most

CLINICAL MANIFESTATIONS

VISUAL DISORDERS

ETIOLOGY	CLINICAL MANIFESTATIONS	CLINICAL THERAPY
Strabismus Can be congenital or acquired. Seen in 5% of all children Most common types: **Esotropia:** inward deviation of eyes ("crossed eyes") **Exotropia:** outward deviation of eyes ("wall-eyes") Strabismus *Used with permission from Paediatrics, 2e, Thomas & Harvey, p. 130, 1997, by permission of the publisher Churchill Livingstone.*	Eyes appear misaligned to observer. May occur only when child is tired. Symptoms include squinting and frowning when reading; closing one eye to see; having trouble picking up objects; dizziness and headache. Corneal light reflex and cover–uncover tests confirm diagnosis. Child may have no other abnormalities but certain conditions such as cerebral palsy, hydrocephalus, Down syndrome, and seizure disorder are more commonly accompanied by strabismus.	Occlusion therapy (patching the fixating or good eye to force use of the weak eye) Compensatory lenses Surgery of the rectus muscles to correct muscle imbalance Eye drops to cause blurring of the good eye Prisms Vision therapy (eye exercises) If treatment is begun before 24 months of age, amblyopia (reduced vision in one or both eyes) may be prevented.
Amblyopia ("lazy eye") Reduced vision in one or both eyes; affects 7% of children. Amblyopia can result from anything which causes visual deprivation to one eye. The most common causes are untreated strabismus, with the child "tuning out" the image in deviating eye, congenital cataract, or visual differences between eyes.	Symptoms are the same as for strabismus. Vision testing can be used to diagnose condition.	Compensatory lenses Occlusion therapy for 2–6 hours daily Occasionally vision therapy (eye exercises) is used in an attempt to improve the weaker eye. Atropine 1% 1 gtt/day in unaffected eye. Treatment is discontinued when visual faculty no longer improves; 20/20 acuity rarely attained. Treatment is most successful if received by 5–6 years of age.
Cataracts Occur when all or part of lens of eye becomes opaque, which prevents refraction of light rays onto retina Seen in 1 of every 250 newborns Congenital cataract. *Used with permission from Vaughan, D., Asbury, T., & Riordan-Eva, P. (1992) General ophthalmology (13th ed., p. 172). New York: McGraw-Hill Companies.*	Can affect one or both eyes and may be congenital or acquired. Clouding of lens indicates presence of cataract; however, cataracts are not always visible to naked eye. Symptoms included distorted red reflex, symptoms of vision loss (see strabismus), white pupil. May be present alone but sometimes associated with fetal alcohol syndrome and Down syndrome.	Must be diagnosed at a young age for successful treatment; many cases are missed. Specific treatment depends on whether one or both eyes are affected, extent of clouding and presence of other ocular abnormalities. Surgical removal of lens and corrective lenses; contact lenses frequently used; results of surgery are good; surgery before the age of 2 months is associated with the best results; visual acuity in 55% of children is 20/40 or better. Lens implant may be used. Eye protectors and restraints are used postoperatively to prevent injury; antibiotic or steroid drops may be used for several weeks; treatment for amblyopia may be necessary.

(continued)

CLINICAL MANIFESTATIONS—continued

VISUAL DISORDERS

ETIOLOGY	CLINICAL MANIFESTATIONS	CLINICAL THERAPY
Glaucoma Increased intraocular pressure damages eye and impairs visual function; ciliary body of eye produces aqueous fluid that flows between iris and lens into anterior chamber; if enough fluid accumulates, blindness results; affects 1 in 100,000 newborns. May be congenital (primary) or acquired (secondary) and affect one or both eyes. Congenital glaucoma. *Used with permission from Vaughan, D., Asbury, T. & Riordan-Eva, P. (1992). General ophthalmology (13th ed., p. 172). New York: McGraw-Hill Companies.*	Symptoms of congenital glaucoma include tearing, blinking, corneal clouding, eyelid spasms, and progressive enlargement of eye; photophobia (extreme sensitivity to light). Symptoms of acquired glaucoma include constant bumping into objects in child's periphery (painless visual field loss); seeing halos around objects. Diagnosis is made using tonometer, which measures intraocular pressure.	Surgery to reduce intraocular pressure is treatment of choice, since medications used to combat glaucoma in adults are not as effective in children. Compensatory lenses used following surgery. Treatment is not always successful, especially if the child has congenital glaucoma, so parents' feelings regarding care of a visually impaired child should be explored.

Data from Altemeier, W. A. (2000). Preschool vision screening: The importance of the two-line difference. Pediatric Annals, 29, 264–267; Bacal, D. A., & Wilson, M. C. (2000). Strabismus: Getting it straight. Contemporary Pediatrics, 17, 49–60; Starr, N. B. (2000). Vision therapy for learning disabilities and dyslexia. Journal of Pediatric Health Care, 14, 32–33.

● **FIGURE 46–2**

This premature infant in the neonatal intensive care unit is receiving artificial ventilation—a risk factor for retinopathy of prematurity. The infant will need careful management of oxygen exposure and periodic eye examinations.

common cause of blindness, occurring in 12.5% of infants born from 23 to 26 weeks' gestation (Wheatley, Dickinson, Mackey et al., 2002).

The retina is normally vascularized by about 8 months' gestation. For the premature infant, however, this process must continue after birth, and the environmental and other conditions listed in the preceding paragraph appear to affect its course. Arteriole constriction, followed by vascular proliferation of abnormal vessels, occurs. In most cases the abnormal vessels gradually regress and normal vascularization occurs. Sometimes, however, the abnormal vascularization continues into the vitreous cavity, causing abnormalities of the retina, optic disc, and macula. It is not known why the disease progresses in some cases, but progression is directly linked to lower birth weight, greater prematurity, and duration (not necessarily concentration) of oxygen therapy. Raeanne, the child described in the scenario at the beginning of this chapter, developed retinopathy of prematurity after receiving oxygen therapy to aid her underdeveloped lungs.

Although the developing capillaries are lost, in up to 90% of cases there is some degree of revascularization later. The degree of visual loss, varying from slight to total, is determined by the degree of revascularization.

CLINICAL MANIFESTATIONS

Retinopathy of prematurity is characterized by progressive changes in the retinal blood vessels, and in severe disease, by retinal detachment. Premature and low-birth-weight infants at risk for the disease are given frequent ocular examinations to ensure early detection of these changes. For infants who do not receive ophthalmologic examinations, resulting visual impairment may be detected only later in infancy when the child progresses slowly in meeting developmental milestones, fails to reach for objects, and does not follow objects or faces with the eyes. When visual impairment is present, the child usually manifests myopia. Total loss of vision can occur in the child who suffers a retinal detachment.

CLINICAL THERAPY

Diagnosis is made by ophthalmologic examination. A classification system is used to describe the location, extent, and severity of the disease (American Academy of Pediatrics, 2001). All infants at risk, particularly those under 2000 g (4 lb, 3 oz) at birth or born before 33 weeks of gestation, are assessed frequently by an ophthalmologist experienced with the condition. The disease does not manifest itself before 4 to 6 weeks after birth, so it is important that the infant receive regular eye examinations until the risk is discounted. If the infant shows signs of disease, eye examinations continue every 1 to 2 weeks. Involvement of blood vessels in the periphery of the retina rarely leads to visual impairment. With involvement in other areas of the retina, visual problems are more common.

Treatment of infants with severe retinopathy of prematurity involves using cryotherapy or laser therapy to stop progression of the disease process. Other surgical procedures such as a scleral buckle procedure and vitrectomy have been used in retinal detachments. Prompt treatment of accompanying problems such as strabismus, amblyopia, and myopia can promote maximal development.

NURSING MANAGEMENT

NURSING ASSESSMENT AND DIAGNOSIS

Assessment of the infant at risk for retinopathy of prematurity begins at birth by identifying infants who may require oxygen therapy. Look for risk factors such as prematurity and low birth weight. Assess the infant's breathing efforts and report any changes. Be certain the ventilation equipment is properly set to deliver the correct amount of oxygen (see Skill 14–1). **SKILLS** Note the cumulative risks in a particular case and suggest the need for a referral to an ophthalmologist, as necessary.

"Nursing Care Plan: The Child with a Visual Impairment Secondary to Retinopathy of Prematurity" outlines several nursing diagnoses. Other nursing diagnoses may be appropriate for an infant with the potential to develop retinopathy of prematurity or a child with resulting visual impairment. They include the following:

- *Disturbed Visual Sensory Perception* related to altered transmission of impulses
- *Potential Impaired Gas Exchange* related to ventilation-perfusion imbalance
- *Delayed Growth and Development* related to effects of visual impairment
- *Altered Family Processes* related to a child with a visual impairment

PLANNING AND IMPLEMENTATION

The nurse plays an important role in preventing retinopathy of prematurity. Encourage early and regular prenatal care to prevent unnecessary premature births. Administer oxygen only to newborns who need it, and in the amount specified by the physician. Ensure that the proper ventilatory settings are used. Shield newborns from excessive exposure to light, since that may decrease susceptibility to retinopathy of prematurity. Be alert for infants with multiple risk factors and refer them, when appropriate, for ophthalmologic examination. Parents of infants at risk for retinopathy of prematurity require information about the disorder, as well as support, as the long-term effects on the child's vision are often identified only after subsequent examinations as the child grows.

The accompanying "Nursing Care Plan" summarizes care for the child with a visual impairment resulting from retinopathy of prematurity. The nurse is instrumental in case management for such children. Reinforce to parents the importance of follow-up eye examinations. Teach methods of stimulating development for the visually impaired child (refer to the next section).

EVALUATION

Expected outcomes of nursing care for the child with retinopathy of prematurity include the following:

- Early identification of visual impairment
- Normal developmental milestone achievement
- Positive management of child's visual condition by the family

NURSING CARE PLAN

THE CHILD WITH A VISUAL IMPAIRMENT SECONDARY TO RETINOPATHY OF PREMATURITY

Intervention	Rationale	Expected Outcome
1. Nursing Diagnosis: Disturbed Visual Sensory Perception related to altered reception, transmission, and integration resulting from retinopathy of prematurity		
NIC Priority Intervention: **Visual deficit enhancement:** Assistance in accepting and learning alternate methods for living with diminished vision		**NOC Suggested Outcome:** **Developmental progression:** Compensate for sensory deficits by maximizing use of impaired senses
Goal: The child will receive adequate sensory input.		
■ Provide kinesthetic, tactile, and auditory stimulation during play and in daily care (e.g., talking and playing). Provide music while bathing an infant, using bells and other noises on each side of infant. Verbally describe to a child all actions being carried out by adult.	■ Because visual sensory input is not present, the child needs input from all other senses to compensate and provide adequate sensory stimulation.	The child demonstrates minimal signs of sensory deprivation.
2. Nursing Diagnosis: Risk for injury related to impaired vision		
NIC Priority Intervention: **Fall prevention:** Instituting special precautions with patients at risk for injury		**NOC Suggested Outcome:** **Risk control:** Actions to eliminate or reduce modifiable health threats
Goal: The child will be protected from safety hazards that can lead to injury.		
■ Evaluate environment for potential safety hazards based on age of child and degree of impairment. Be particularly alert to objects that give visual cues to their dangers (e.g., stoves, fireplaces, candles). Eliminate safety hazards and protect the child from exposure. Take the child on a tour of new rooms, explaining safety hazards (e.g., schools, hotel room, hospital room).	■ The child may be at risk for injury related both to developmental stage and to inability to visualize hazards.	The child will experience no injuries.
3. Nursing Diagnosis: Risk for Delayed Growth and Development related to impaired vision		
NIC Priority Intervention: **Developmental enhancement:** Facilitating or teaching parents/caregivers to facilitate optimal growth and development of children		**NOC Suggested Outcome:** **Child growth and development:** Milestones of developmental progression
Goal: The child has experiences necessary to foster normal growth and development.		
■ Help parents plan early, regular social activities with other children. ■ Provide opportunities and encourage self-feeding activities. ■ Provide an environment rich in sensory input. ■ Assess growth and development during regular examinations to identify the child's strengths and needs.	■ The visually impaired child benefits developmentally from contact with other children. ■ To obtain adequate nutrients, the child needs to feel comfortable feeding self. ■ Sensory input is needed for normal development to occur. ■ Regular examinations aid in early identification of growth problems or developmental delays, so that appropriate interventions can be planned.	The child demonstrates normal growth and development milestones.

NURSING CARE PLAN—continued

THE CHILD WITH A VISUAL IMPAIRMENT SECONDARY TO RETINOPATHY OF PREMATURITY

Intervention	Rationale	Expected Outcome
4. Nursing Diagnosis: Risk for Compromised Family Coping related to child's prolonged disability from sensory impairment		
NIC Priority Intervention: **Family mobilization:** Utilization of family strengths to influence child's health positively		**NOC Suggested Outcome:** **Positive coping:** Extent to which family can mobilize resources to deal with the child's needs
Goal: The family identifies methods for coping with their visually impaired child.		
■ Provide explanation of visual impairment as appropriate. ■ Refer parents to organizations, early intervention programs, and other parents of visually impaired children. ■ Assist parents to plan for meeting developmental, educational, and safety needs of their visually impaired child. Offer resources for changing home environment to assist visually impaired child.	■ The parents may feel guilt about the child's visual impairment, which can be allayed by knowledge of the cause. ■ The parents will receive needed information and support from others. ■ The child may require an enhanced environment in order to foster developmental progress.	The family successfully copes with the experience of having a visually impaired child.

THINKING CRITICALLY

THE CHILD WITH ROP

Raeanne, 3 years old, has a severe visual impairment. Born prematurely at 25 weeks of gestation, she received oxygen therapy, which damaged her retinal blood vessels. As a result, Raeanne developed retinopathy of prematurity. While in the hospital, Raeanne was given frequent ophthalmoscopic examinations. She received cryotherapy to the retinal vessels—a treatment designed to prevent detached retinae and the resulting total vision loss. Although this treatment halted progression of the disorder, Raeanne was left severely myopic (near-sighted).

For the first 3 years of life, Raeanne and her mother attended an early-intervention program, which provided stimulation for Raeanne and helped teach her mother techniques for enhancing her developmental progress. Raeanne will soon begin attending preschool. Her speech is well developed for a 3-year-old; she is socially mature, converses readily, and shows no developmental delays. However, she has had little contact with other children.

As the nurse in the preschool Raeanne will be attending, how will you assist both her parents and the preschool staff in helping Raeanne adapt to the preschool experience?

VISUAL IMPAIRMENT

Visual impairment accounts for 11% of chronic medical conditions in children. Legal blindness (defined as visual acuity of 20/200 or worse in the corrected eye or significantly

reduced visual fields) occurs in 1 per 35,000 children. About 1 in 500 children has partial vision. About half of the children who are blind or have partial vision have other disabilities as well. Approximately 5% to 10% of preschoolers and 20% to 30% of school-age children have some type of vision problem (Burns, Brady, Dunn et al., 2000; Halle, 2002).

Many conditions discussed earlier in this chapter lead to temporary or permanent visual impairment. Infants who are premature; whose mothers were infected prenatally with rubella, toxoplasmosis, or other viruses; and who have certain congenital and hereditary conditions have a high risk of visual problems (Table 46–3). Fetal alcohol syndrome (FAS) is a major cause of visual disturbance; 90% of children with FAS have eye abnormalities. See Chapter 54 for further description of FAS. ∞

The signs of visual impairment depend on the cause and degree of the problem and the age of the child (Table 46–4).

GROWTH AND DEVELOPMENT

Infants with visual impairment use kinesthesia, touch, and language to socialize. They appreciate and use touch more than other children and respond to verbal explanations when others use nonverbal communication. Vision affects both fine and gross motor skills, so skills such as hand-to-mouth coordination and walking may be delayed in children who are visually impaired.

TABLE 46–3 ✛ Common Causes of Visual Impairment in Children

Congenital or Hereditary	Acquired
Cataracts	Injury to eye or head
Glaucoma	Infections
Tay–Sachs disease	Rubella
Marfan syndrome	Measles
Down syndrome	Chickenpox
Fetal alcohol syndrome	Brain tumor
Prenatal infections (maternal infection)	Retinopathy of prematurity
Rubella	Cerebral palsy
Toxoplasmosis	
Herpes simplex	
Retinoblastoma	

The child's eyes may appear crossed or watery, and the lids may be crusty. Verbal children may complain of itching, dizziness, headache, or blurred, double, or poor vision.

The American Optometric Association and American Public Health Association recommend comprehensive vision examination starting at 6 months of age, while the American Academy of Ophthalmology and American Academy of Pediatrics recommend screening by 3 years of age (Center for Health and Health Care in Schools, 2004). The U.S. Preventive Services Task Force (USPSTF) recommends screening to detect amblyopia, strabismus, and defects in visual acuity in children younger than 5 years (U.S. Preventive Services Task Force, 2004). In spite of this difference in timing, it is clear that all young children should have vision examinations to identify vision problems early in life. Clinical therapy depends on the child's condition and may include surgery, medication, and supportive aids. In the case of a disorder that results in permanent visual impairment, an interdisciplinary team of specialists works with the child and family. Nurses have an important role in this team to ensure developmental progression for the child and ongoing support for the family.

TABLE 46–4 ✛ Signs of Visual Impairment

Infants	Toddlers and Older Children
May be unable to follow lights or objects	May rub, shut, or cover eyes
Do not make eye contact	Tilt or thrust head forward
Have a dull, vacant stare	Blink frequently
Do not imitate facial expressions	Hold objects close
	Bump into objects
	Squint

NURSING MANAGEMENT

NURSING ASSESSMENT AND DIAGNOSIS

Prevent visual deficits by teaching safety in activities that can injure the eye. For example, be sure that children are not allowed to play with laser pointers since young children are at risk of retinal damage from these pointers due to a slower blink and gaze aversion response.

Vision screening facilitates early detection and treatment of conditions that can lead to vision loss. Visual testing can be done at any age, including immediately after birth. Developmental milestones that require vision, such as following bright lights, reaching for objects, or looking at pictures in a book, can be used to assess vision. For children over the age of 3 years, visual acuity is most frequently measured by means of an age-appropriate acuity test (see Skills 9–18—9–19). **SKILLS** Vision screening should begin at 3 years of age and take place during annual heathcare visits. Most states mandate school screening of vision. (See Chapter 35. ∞) The photo screener, a device that can be used to take a photo of the child's eyes, is useful for infants, toddlers, and preschoolers. The photo can be used to diagnose refraction errors, eye opacities, and misalignment (Gomez & Davis, 2001). Visual fields and the ability to discriminate colors are tested at school age, when children can cooperate.

Children who are visually impaired may lag in development of cognitive and other skills. Sighted children learn the word *cup* using four senses—sight, touch, hearing, and taste—to obtain the information necessary to connect words with the objects they represent. In contrast, children with visual impairments rely on only three senses—touch, hearing, and taste. They learn concepts through differences in sounds, textures, and shapes.

Many visual disorders are linked with conditions that influence development. Thus, a child with cerebral palsy or fetal alcohol syndrome should be assessed frequently to identify a visual disorder, as well as to evaluate normal developmental milestones.

Nursing diagnoses for the child with impaired vision might include the following:

- *Disturbed Sensory/Perceptual Alteration (Visual)* related to altered sensory perception
- *Risk for Injury* related to poor vision
- *Risk for Delayed Growth and Development* related to visual impairment
- *Risk for Ineffective Family Coping* related to demands of a child with a sensory impairment

PLANNING AND IMPLEMENTATION

Nursing care for a child with a visual impairment focuses on encouraging the child's use of all senses, promoting so-

TEACHING HIGHLIGHTS

ENHANCING DEVELOPMENT OF THE VISUALLY IMPAIRED CHILD

- Encourage a toddler or preschooler who is visually impaired to look at pictures in well-lit settings. Have a school-age child read large-print books. Computers designed for the visually impaired are also available. The Optacon (a device that raises print so it can be felt by the child) and View Scan (which magnifies print) improve reading ability.
- Expose the infant and child to everyday sounds.
- Encourage the infant to use the sense of touch to explore people and objects. Have the parents purchase toys with sound and texture in mind. Directional concepts can be taught using games. Responding to the infant's and child's vocalizations encourages the use of speech.
- Teach specific techniques for toileting, dressing, bathing, eating, and safety.
- When the child becomes mobile, furniture and other objects in the environment should be kept in the same positions so the child can safely move around independently. Extra care must be taken to prevent injuries when a child does not see.
- Emphasize the child's abilities. Adolescents can use seeing-eye dogs or a white cane to function independently.
- Encourage the child to function independently within normal developmental parameters.
- If the child goes to a hospital or another strange environment, orient the child to the placement of objects and do not rearrange them.
- Teach those around the child to:
    - Announce their presence to the child when approaching.
    - Walk slightly ahead of the child so he or she can sense their movements.
    - Let the child hold the seeing person's arm rather than the reverse.
    - Identify the contents of meals and encourage the child to feed self.

FIGURE 46–3

This child needs ongoing developmental assessment and a comprehensive individualized education plan. As is true with many children, she has several healthcare needs. Note that she is receiving tube feedings.

- Stroke, rock, and hug infants and children who are visually impaired. Sing and talk to them. These infants do not make eye contact and have rather blank expressions.
- Call the child's name and speak before touching the child. Tell the child when the nurse and others are leaving the room. Describe locations of foods on the plate and tray to orient the child.
- Teach parents to read body language and vocalization as expressions of emotion. Facial expressions give a great deal of information, but infants and children with poor vision do not have the ability to learn by visual imitation. Show parents how to use tactile means to teach appropriate facial expressions. For example, a touch on the arm can be soft and stroking to indicate a smile, but firmer to indicate dismay or frown.
- Describe procedures such as blood pressure, ear examination, or cast application so the child knows what they will feel like. Let the child touch the equipment.
- Explain to parents that discipline and rewards for children with poor vision should be the same as those for other children in the family. The child should be given age-appropriate tasks.
- Encourage contact with peers as the child grows older. Teach the child to look directly at persons who are talking to him or her. Play, sports, and other activities can be modified to give the visually impaired child the same social experiences as a sighted child.

cialization, helping parents to meet the child's developmental and educational needs, and providing emotional support to parents. Refer the parents to an early intervention program as soon as the diagnosis is made. Nearly all care occurs in community and home settings.

Encourage Use of All Senses

Children who are partially sighted or blind use other senses to a great extent. Encouraging the use of the eyes as much as possible is important even if a child has poor vision (Figure 46–3 ◉).

Promote Socialization

The child's interactions and socializations should be as normal as possible (similar to those of sighted children of the same age and development).

Nursing Care in the Community

Public laws require that each state provide educational and related services for children with disabilities (see Chapter 1 ∞). Parents and professionals should develop an individual education plan (as discussed in Chapter 39 ∞) that maximizes the child's learning ability. If possible, the child with a vision problem should attend child care and preschool with children who have normal visual acuity. What nursing actions are needed to help a child with a visual impairment adjust to child care or school?

- Provide parents with information about educational options before their child reaches school age. Education should take place in a setting that allows the child to have contact with other children and to participate in social activities.

- The child may be mainstreamed with a tutor, be partially mainstreamed in a resource room, attend special classes, or be tutored at home. If the child is to attend public school, suggest to parents that they contact the school well before enrollment to ensure that school personnel understand the child's disability.

- Make sure that equipment such as large-print books, braille materials, audio equipment, or an Optacon (described in "Teaching Highlights: Enhancing Development of the Visually Impaired Child" on page 1361) is available. Ensure that frequent eye examinations are performed and assist with proper use and care of prescribed glasses or contact lenses, as necessary. Clean glasses daily with warm water and dry with a clean, soft cloth. Follow family directions for cleaning contact lenses.

- Familiarize the child with the new environment.

Provide Emotional Support

The family often needs help to understand the child's abilities and disabilities. Support them as they learn about their child's visual problems, tell friends and family, and then adjust to supporting the child.

- Encourage habilitation as soon as realistically possible. Make the adjustment easier by providing information about the child's specific type of visual impairment, available community services, and groups or associations for children with similar vision conditions.

- Suggest resources to families of children with visual disorders.

- Be supportive and listen to the family's concerns about the child's visual deficit.

- Make sure the parents meet their own physical and emotional needs so they are better able to care for and provide support to their child.

GROWTH AND DEVELOPMENT

Children with visual impairment may take longer to master self-help skills such as feeding and dressing. Perform regular developmental assessments and suggest adaptive ways that parents can help the child learn these skills.

EVALUATION

Expected outcomes of nursing care for the child with a visual impairment include the following:

- Prevention of injury
- Growth and development to maximum potential
- Establishment of successful individualized education plan

INJURIES OF THE EYE

In the United States, eye injuries are common in boys 11 to 15 years of age and in all children 9 to 11 years of age. Boys from 11 to 15 years have four times more eye injuries than girls. About 42,000 sports injuries occur annually with about half of these in children (Committee on Sports Medicine and Fitness, 2004). Sports, darts, fireworks, air-powered BB guns, blunt and sharp objects, chemical and thermal burns, physical irritants, and abuse may cause eye trauma (Behrman, Kliegman, & Jenson, 2004). Recreational activities such as sports and playing with projectile toys are common causes. Older children may be injured by chemicals in school science laboratories.

Promoting prevention of injury is an important nursing intervention. Protective eyewear should be used by participants in all sports with a risk of eye injury, with extreme caution in those with diminished vision or only one functional eye. The most common injuries occur in baseball, basketball, swimming, bicycling, and football (Center for Health and Health Care in Schools, 2004). Chemicals and objects such as scissors and knives should be placed out of reach.

Some injuries can be treated at home, but many require emergency care or hospitalization. If a tetanus booster has not been given in the last 5 years, the child is reimmunized. A careful history of the injury is taken, assessment of the eye is performed, and visual acuity is mea-

TABLE 46–5 ❖ Emergency Treatment of Eye Injuries

Injury	Treatment
Subconjunctival hemorrhage (caused by coughing, mild trauma, or increased physical activity)	Usually heals spontaneously; child should see ophthalmologist if most of sclera is covered or if condition does not clear up in 1–2 weeks
Periorbital ecchymosis ("black eye")	Apply ice to eye area (both eyes) for 5–15 minutes every hour for the first 1–2 days after injury (even if only one eye is affected, both eyes may discolor); then apply warm compresses
Foreign body on conjunctiva	Do not let child rub eye; remove material on surface of eye by closing upper lid over lower lid, irrigating or everting upper lid, visualizing material, and removing it with slightly damp handkerchief; patch eye and transport child to emergency department if foreign body cannot be removed
Corneal abrasion	Superficial corneal abrasions are diagnosed by touching sterile fluorescein strip to lower conjunctiva; dye remains where corneal epithelial cells are disrupted; most corneal abrasions heal spontaneously or antibiotic ointment may be prescribed and eyes patched in some children
Burns (alkaline burns readily penetrate cornea and are more serious than acid burns)	For child with chemical burn, irrigate eye for 15–30 minutes; transport child to emergency department, where irrigation should continue (see Skills Manual **SKILLS**); pupils are dilated to reduce pain and prevent adhesions; after irrigation is complete, eyes are patched and antibiotics are prescribed
Penetrating & perforating injuries	Obtain medical assistance immediately; never try to remove an object that has penetrated the child's eye; such objects should be removed by an ophthalmologist; prevent the child from rubbing injured eye; cover both eyes with shield before transportation to emergency department
Eye injuries caused by severe blows to head and eye (blunt trauma can seriously injure all eye structures, including orbit, which can be fractured)	Transport immediately to ophthalmologist's office or emergency department for evaluation and treatment

sured. Table 46–5 summarizes emergency treatment of common eye injuries.

DISORDERS OF THE EAR

OTITIS MEDIA

Otitis media, or inflammation of the middle ear, is sometimes accompanied by infection. This condition is one of the most common childhood illnesses. About 70% of infants have at least one case of acute otitis media during the first year of life, and 93% have been diagnosed with the problem by age 7 years. Peak incidence is in the first 2 years of life, particularly from 6 to 12 months of age (Hoberman, Marchant, Kaplan et al., 2002). Otitis media occurs more frequently among boys and in children who attend childcare centers, in those with allergies, in children exposed to tobacco smoke, and in those who use pacifiers several hours daily. It is most common during the winter months. Children with conditions such as cleft lip and palate or Down syndrome more often experience otitis media.

Breastfeeding appears to be protective against otitis media. In the past decade, an increased number of cases have been observed, and recent changes have been made in recommendations for treatment (American Academy of Pediatrics, 2004; Sagraves, 2002).

ETIOLOGY AND PATHOPHYSIOLOGY

The specific cause of otitis media is unknown, but it appears to be related to eustachian tube dysfunction. Often an upper respiratory infection precedes otitis media. This infection causes the mucous membranes of the eustachian tube to become edematous. As a result, air that normally flows to the middle ear is blocked, and the air in the middle ear is reabsorbed into the bloodstream. Fluid is pulled from the mucosal lining into the former air space, providing a medium for the rapid growth of pathogens. The tympanic membrane and fluid behind it become infected. The most common causative organisms are *Streptococcus pneumoniae*, *Haemophilus influenzae*, and *Moraxella catarrhalis* (Hoberman et al., 2002).

GROWTH AND DEVELOPMENT

Fluid accumulation in the middle ear prevents the efficient transmission of sound and can result in hearing loss over time, potentially delaying speech and language development. These delays may manifest as cognitive deficits or behavior problems. Motor development has been found to be impaired in children with chronic ear infections.

Conditions such as enlarged adenoids or edema from allergic rhinitis can also obstruct the eustachian tube and lead to otitis media. Since children with certain facial malformations (cleft palate) and genetic conditions (Down syndrome) usually have compromised eustachian tubes, these children are more vulnerable to otitis media. Children who live in crowded conditions, those exposed to cigarette smoke, and those who attend child care with multiple children are at higher risk. Pacifier use raises the soft palate and thus alters dynamics in the eustacian tube, providing for entry of microorganisms from the nasopharynx (Garrelts & Melnyk, 2001).

CLINICAL MANIFESTATIONS

Otitis media is the general term for inflammation of the middle ear. *Acute otitis media (AOM)* is diagnosed when the child has acute onset of ear pain, marked redness of the tympanic membrane upon otoscopy, and middle ear effusion (Figure 46–4 ◉). Recurrent acute otitis media indicates repeated bouts of AOM, such as three in 6 months, or four in 12 months. *Otitis media with effusion (OME)* is evidence of fluid in the middle ear without inflammation (Figure 46–5 ◉). OME sometimes becomes chronic in nature (continuing more than 3 months) and is more commonly associated with hearing loss.

Infants and young children have characteristic behaviors that indicate otitis media may be present. Pulling at the

DEVELOPING CULTURAL COMPETENCE

OTITIS MEDIA

American Indian and Alaska Native (AI/AN) children have a very high rate of otitis media, perhaps due to culturally related bony structures of the ear, nose, and mouth. A recent study found that AI/AN children are seen about 3 times more frequently in outpatient clinics for otitis media than are other U.S. children (Curns, Holman, Shay et al., 2002). Be alert for the common incidence in these population groups, plan prevention programs, and ensure prompt care and teaching about treatments for families of children affected. *What prevention measures would you emphasize with these families?* See the nursing management section in otitis media for suggestions of preventive approaches.

◉ **FIGURE 46–4**

Acute otitis media is characterized by pain and a red, bulging, nonmobile tympanic membrane.

Courtesy of Kevin Kavanagh, MD, FACS.

◉ **FIGURE 46–5**

Otitis media with effusion is noted on otoscopy by fluid line or air bubbles.

Courtesy of Kevin Kavanagh, MD, FACS.

MEDIALINK Video: Otitis Media

ear is a sign of ear pain (Figure 46–6 ●). Diarrhea, vomiting, and fever are typical of otitis media. Irritability and "acting out" may be signs of a related hearing impairment. The child with otitis media often has night awakenings with crying due to increased pressure when prone or supine. Some children with otitis media are asymptomatic; therefore, an ear examination should be performed at every healthcare visit (see Chapter 35 ∞). A red, bulging, nonmobile tympanic membrane is a sign of otitis media. If fluid lines and air bubbles are visible, the child has otitis media with effusion.

CLINICAL THERAPY

Diagnosis is based on otoscopic examination. Acute otitis media is diagnosed with certainty when there is a history of acute onset, presence of middle ear effusion (bulging or decreased mobility of the tympanic membrane, air fluid behind the membrane or otorrhea or discharge), and signs and symptoms of inflammation (erythema of tympanic membrane or discomfort that makes sleep and other activities difficult for the child) (Subcommittee on Management of Acute Otitis Media, 2004). Otoscopic examination includes visualization and pneumatic otoscopy. The trained clinician can perform pneumatic otoscopy in which positive air pressure in the external canal is used to measure the movement of the tympanic membrane. Special gradient

● **FIGURE 46–6**

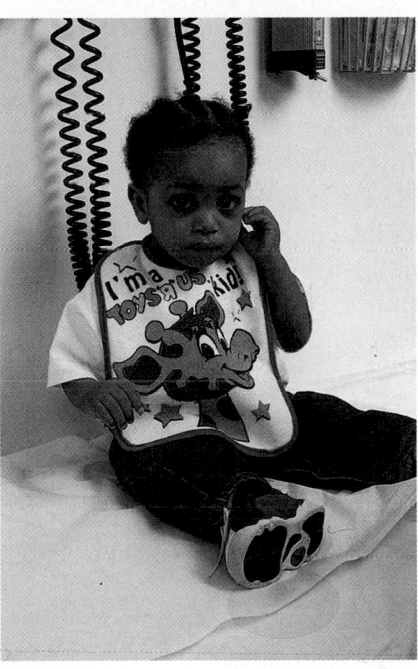

This young child is pulling at the ear and acting fussy, two important signs of otitis media. Ask the parents about presence of fever and night awakenings, additional signs that are often observed in children with this condition.

CLINICAL MANIFESTATIONS

ACUTE OTITIS MEDIA AND OTITIS MEDIA WITH EFFUSION

ETIOLOGY	CLINICAL MANIFESTATIONS	CLINICAL THERAPY
Acute otitis media—bacterial infection in the middle ear from pathogens transferred from the nasopharynx; most common infectious agents are *S. pneumoniae, H. influenzae, M. catarrhalis*	*Behavioral*—ear pain, pulling at ear, rapid onset, irritability, malaise, poor feeding *Examination*—bulging tympanic membrane, air or fluid bubbles present behind tympanic membrane; immobile or poorly mobile tympanic membrane, red (or other color change such as white, gray, or yellow as long as bulging is present) tympanic membrane, reduced visibility of tympanic membrane landmarks with displaced light reflex	Treat ear pain with local anesthetic, local herbal pain products, or systemic acetaminophen or ibuprofen Observe child's condition for 48–72 hours and, if not improved, treat with course of antibiotics
Otitis media with effusion—collection of fluid in the middle ear behind the tympanic membrane which is not infected with bacteria	*Behavioral*—difficulty hearing or responding as expected to sounds *Examination*—signs of acute inflammation are NOT present; tympanic membrane is retracted or neutral; immobile or partly mobile tympanic membrane; yellow or gray tympanic membrane; opaque or thickened tympanic membrane with visibility of landmarks reduced	Symptomatic treatment and pain relief Careful observation of hearing acuity over several months Speech assessment if loss of hearing acuity occurs Developmental assessment

acoustic reflectometry (SGAR) measures the condition of the middle ear by introducing a sound and measuring the tympanic membrane response (Hoberman & Paradise, 2000). A "flat" tympanogram is also suggestive of otitis media. (The tympanogram is described in the next section, on hearing impairment.)

Since otitis media with effusion may only involve fluid in the middle ear, it is best diagnosed by pneumatic otoscopy and tympanometry. Since this type of otitis media is most commonly associated with hearing loss, audiologic testing should be performed in the pediatric healthcare home (medical home) if the effusion persists for 3 months or longer. A referral to an audiologist should be made for children who fail testing in the office or are less than 4 years of age (Otitis Media with Effusion, 2004).

Concern has developed about the increasing appearance of drug-resistant microbials as causative agents in otitis media. These organisms may explain the increase in otitis media observed in the last decade. Based on current knowledge, the American Academy of Pediatrics and the American Academy of Family Physicians joined to establish recommendations in 2004 (Subcommittee on Manage-

ment of Acute Otitis Media, 2004). Acute otitis media is now treated with antibiotic therapy for 10 days in children under 6 years, and 5 to 7 days for children 6 years and over. Consistent with current guidelines, acute otitis media treatment is delayed for 48 to 72 hours after diagnosis in children 6 months to 2 years with nonsevere illness at presentation AND uncertain diagnosis, or in children 2 years and older without severe symptoms OR with uncertain diagnosis.

When prescribed, the choice of antibiotic depends on the probable organism, ease of administration, cost, previous effectiveness, and any history of allergies. First-line therapy is amoxicillin at a dose of 80 to 90 mg/kg/day. Amoxicillin with clavulanate or cefuroxime are second-line drugs. If an intramuscular drug is preferred, cefdinir at 14 mg/kg/day, cefpodoxime at 10 mg/kg/day, or cefuroxime at 30 mg/kg/day can be prescribed (Zacharyczuk, 2004). (See "Drug Guide: Amoxicillin.")

OME is not treated with antibiotics but is evaluated periodically to be sure there is not an additional AOM that needs treatment. Children with OME generally improve within 3 months. Since this type of otitis is more com-

DRUG GUIDE

AMOXICILLIN

Overview of Action

Bactericidal action inhibits cell-wall synthesis, a broader spectrum of activities than penicillin G. Effective on some gram-positive and gram-negative organisms, such as *Haemophilus influenzae, Escherichia coli, Proteus mirabilis, Neisseria gonorrhoeae,* meningococci, enterococci, and *Salmonella.* Used to treat infections of the ear, upper respiratory tract, GU system, skin, and soft tissue and as a prophylaxis against bacterial endocarditis. Topical forms may be used for eye infections.

Routes, Dosage, Frequency

PO

- Under 20 kg: 20 to 40 mg/kg/day in equally divided doses every 6 to 12 hours
- Over 20 kg: 250 to 500 mg every 8 hours (maximum dose 2 to 3 g)

For prophylaxis against bacterial endocarditis in susceptible children who are undergoing procedures:

Child: 25–50 mg/kg/day divided into doses and given q 8–12 hours; commonly for otitis media dose is 80–90 mg/kg/day divided into 2 doses and given q 12 hours (maximum dose 875 mg b.i.d.)

Adolescents: 250–500 mg q 8 hours

Nursing Implications

Assess: Assess previous allergy to this drug, penicillins, cephalosporins, other drugs, asthma, or family history of allergies. Obtain culture and sensitivity before treatment when ordered, but can start treatment before results.

Administer PO: Stable in gastric acid, give without regard to meals. Shake suspension well. Capsules may be taken apart or tablets crushed; mixed in small amount of food or fluid. Chewable tablets should be chewed thoroughly or crushed and followed with fluids.

Side Effects: Nausea, vomiting, diarrhea, pruritus, urticaria, anaphylaxis.

Monitor: Monitor child for hypersensitivity (especially within first 20 minutes following dose), rash (onset and characteristics), and side effects. Monitor blood counts, renal and hepatic function with prolonged or high-dose therapy or with premature infants and newborn. Maintain fluid intake. Watch for signs of superinfection; diarrhea (may indicate pseudomembranous colitis, which can occur while on drug or 4 to 6 weeks after drug is discontinued). If given for β-hemolytic streptococcal infection, 10-day course is needed to prevent risk of acute rheumatic fever or glomerulonephritis. If ampicillin rash occurs, it usually subsides in 6 to 14 days; however, rash can become severe, requiring drug discontinuance. Rash then usually resolves in 1 to 7 days.

Teaching: Child must take the medicine for the recommended time. If a revisit is scheduled, such as one for evaluation of treatment success in otitis media, parents are encouraged to keep this appointment. Report diarrhea, nausea, rash, or other side effects. Report if the child seems to have continued symptoms of infection (fever, irritability, pain, discharge from infected site, fatigue, or lethargy). Encourage generous fluid intake for age. Store medication out of reach of children.

Adapted from Bindler, R. M., & Howry, L. B. (2005). Pediatric Drug Guide. Upper Saddle River, NJ: Prentice Hall-Health.

monly associated with hearing loss and cochlear damage, follow-up with audiology is essential. If hearing is abnormal, speech testing should be performed (Otitis Media with Effusion, 2004).

Neither decongestants nor antihistamines have been shown to be effective in the treatment of otitis media with or without effusion. If infection recurs in spite of antibiotic treatment, **myringotomy** (surgical incision of the tympanic membrane) may be performed and **tympanostomy tubes** (pressure equalizing tubes) inserted to drain fluid from the middle ear. Tube insertion is generally recommended for children with bilateral middle ear effusion and hearing deficiency of greater than 20 decibels (dB) for over 3 months. Enlarged and infected adenoids may be removed at the same time (Paradise, Feldman, Campbell et al., 2001). Alternatively, a tympanostomy may be done to extract middle ear fluid for culture and sensitivity so that antimicrobial therapy can be directed at the cause of infection.

NURSING MANAGEMENT

NURSING ASSESSMENT AND DIAGNOSIS

Assess the tympanic membrane for color, transparency, mobility, presence of landmarks, and light reflex. Ask the parents whether the child has had a fever, been fussy, or been pulling at the ears. Observe for signs of impaired hearing.

Several nursing diagnoses that may apply are included in "Nursing Care Plan: The Child with Otitis Media." Additional nursing diagnoses might include the following:

- *Risk for Imbalanced Body Temperature: Hyperthermia* related to infectious process
- *Fatigue (Child and Parent)* related to sleep deprivation
- *Sensory/Perceptual Alteration Auditory* related to chronic ear infections and altered sensory reception

PLANNING AND IMPLEMENTATION

Most children with otitis media are not hospitalized; therefore, nursing management centers on care of the child in the home. The child having tympanostomy tubes inserted is generally treated in a day surgery setting. Occasionally, children admitted to the hospital for other problems have a concurrent ear infection. The accompanying "Nursing Care Plan" summarizes nursing care for the child with otitis media.

Emphasize preventive measures. Exposure to secondhand smoke in the home increases the incidence of otitis media in children, so encourage parents who smoke to avoid smoking near the child or in the home. If young children are in child care with fewer than 10 children, incidence decreases. Breastfeeding provides some protection from the disease. Placing babies to sleep with a pacifier may increase incidence and should be avoided in the infant with prior infections (Niemela, Pihakari, Pokka et al., 2000). Many cases of otitis media are related to microbials such as *Haemophilus influenzae* and *Pneumococcal pneumoniae,* so immunization against these pathogens (see Chapter 45 ∞) can be effective preventive measures.

Chronic otitis media can create many problems for the family. The child's waking at night with ear pain results in lack of sleep and parental fatigue. Parents often become frustrated and disillusioned by the healthcare system's inability to cure the child and may fear a permanent hearing impairment. Reassure parents that as the child grows older, the recurrent infections eventually cease. Teach them that asking for courses of antibiotics for every infection may not be the best treatment. Provide pain relief techniques such as teaching correct administration of ear drops, oral administration of acetaminophen, and positioning the baby with the head slightly elevated. Provide hearing and language examinations at regular intervals, inform parents of results, and refer to an audiology specialist if hearing problems are identified. Make sure parents of children with tympanostomy tubes know how to care for the child and what symptoms to report. For the child with some hearing loss due to otitis media with effusion, a home environment that fosters math, reading, and verbal skills can overcome the effects of lowered hearing during the time of infection (Roberts, Burchinal, & Zeisel, 2002). Focus interventions on helping parents to read and talk with children frequently who have otitis media with effusion.

EVALUATION

Expected outcomes of nursing care for the child with otitis media include the following:

- Return to normal sleep and feeding patterns
- Maintenance of normal hearing and speech development
- Effective pain and temperature management
- Understanding of treatment regimen by parents

OTITIS EXTERNA

Otitis externa is an inflammation of the skin and surrounding soft tissue of the ear canal. It is sometimes called "swimmer's ear" because it is common in children who swim frequently, especially during hot and muggy weather. The ear canal can also be injured by use of cotton-tipped applicators, foreign objects, or sprays used near the face. If the tympanic membrane is not intact because of tympanostomy tubes or breakage of the membrane, there may be drainage visible in the canal; this drainage may irritate the

NURSING CARE PLAN

THE CHILD WITH OTITIS MEDIA

Intervention	Rationale	Expected Outcome
1. Nursing Diagnosis: Acute Pain related to inflammation and pressure on tympanic membrane		
NIC Priority Intervention: **Pain management:** Alleviation or reduction in pain to a level of comfort acceptable to patient and family		**NOC Suggested Outcome:** **Pain level:** Amount of reported or demonstrated pain
Goal: The child or parent will indicate absence of pain.		
■ Give analgesic such as acetaminophen. Use analgesic eardrops. ■ Have the child sit up, raise head on pillows, or lie on unaffected ear. ■ Apply warmth to the ear. ■ Have the child chew gum or blow on balloon to relieve pressure in ear.	■ Analgesics alter perception or response to pain. ■ Elevation decreases pressure from fluid. ■ Heat increases blood supply and reduces discomfort. ■ Attempts to open the eustachian tube may help aerate the middle ear.	Verbal child states that pain is relieved. Nonverbal child has improved disposition and comfort.
2. Nursing Diagnosis: Infection related to presence of pathogens		
NIC Priority Intervention: **Infection control:** Minimizing the acquisition and transmission of infectious agents		**NOC Suggested Outcome:** **Risk control:** Actions to eliminate or reduce health threats
Goal: The child will be free of infection.		
■ Encourage breastfeeding of infants. ■ Instruct the parents to administer antibiotics exactly as directed and to complete prescribed course of medication. ■ Telephone the parents 2 or 3 days after initial examination. ■ Examine ear 3 or 4 days after completion of antibiotic treatment, or if symptoms worsen in child on symptomatic treatment.	■ Breastfeeding affords natural immunity to infectious agents. ■ Taking antibiotics as prescribed minimizes chance for overgrowth of pathogens. ■ If symptoms have not improved in 36 hours, treatment should be evaluated. ■ Checkup determines whether treatment is effective.	The child's temperature is normal, symptoms have disappeared, and tympanic membrane shows no signs of infection.
3. Nursing Diagnosis: Risk for Caregiver Role Strain related to chronic disease		
NIC Priority Intervention: **Caregiver support:** Provision of necessary support, information, and advocacy to facilitate care by parents		**NOC Suggested Outcome:** **Caregiver performance:** Provision by family care provider of healthcare for child
Goal: The parents will manage the child's condition with minimal stress.		
■ Determine the parents' ability to manage condition. Provide frequent information and feedback. ■ Encourage parental input in managing care. ■ Listen carefully to parental expressions of frustration and fatigue and try to understand parents' feelings.	■ Many parents can treat children at home. Knowledge of condition allows parents to make informed decisions and to manage condition effectively. ■ Active participation increases confidence and ability to manage condition. ■ Reacting empathetically encourages parents to communicate.	The parents express confidence about treating the child and state that stress is reduced.

NURSING CARE PLAN—continued

THE CHILD WITH OTITIS MEDIA

Intervention	Rationale	Expected Outcome
4. Nursing Diagnosis: Risk for Infection related to deficient knowledge about infection in children		
NIC Priority Intervention: **Infection control:** Minimizing the acquisition and transmission of infectious agents		**NOC Suggested Outcome:** **Knowledge:** Extent of understanding conveyed about infectious disease prevention
Goal: The parents will state understanding of preventive measures.		
■ Teach family members to cover mouths and noses when sneezing or coughing and to wash hands frequently. Have parents isolate sick children. ■ Encourage optimal nutrition, rest, and exercise. ■ Position bottle-fed infants upright when feeding. Do not prop bottles. ■ Eliminate allergens and upper respiratory irritants such as tobacco, smoke, and dust.	■ Good hygiene prevents spread of pathogens. ■ Physical well-being helps the body fight disease. ■ Elevated position prevents injection of milk and pathogens into the eustachian tube. ■ Fewer irritants and allergens may decrease susceptibility to respiratory infections. Secondhand smoke contributes to higher incidence of otitis media.	Parents express understanding of measures to lead to fewer infections.
5. Nursing Diagnosis: Risk for Delayed Growth and Development related to hearing loss		
NIC Priority Intervention: **Developmental enhancement:** Facilitating optimal growth and development of the child		**NOC Suggested Outcome:** **Growth and development:** Milestones of developmental progression
Goal: The child will have normal hearing.		
■ Assess hearing ability frequently.	■ Monitoring detects hearing loss early.	The child's general health and hearing improve, and incidence of condition decreases.
Goal: The child will have normal motor and language development.		
■ Assess motor and language development at each healthcare visit.	■ Early detection of developmental delays can lead to appropriate intervention.	The child has language and motor development within norms for age group.

canal and lead to otitis externa. Any irritation of the canal can become infected with bacteria, virus, or fungi; sometimes it represents an allergic reaction. The child usually complains of pain and itching, and may have intense pain when the examiner presses on the tragus, or skin tab in front of the ear. Sometimes the ear appears swollen, and redness or drainage of the canal may be seen upon otoscopic examination.

Treatment of otitis externa requires removing the dried and flaking epithelium and cerumen. Burrows solutions or normal saline are used to irrigate and clean the canal. Steroid eardrops are used to decrease inflammation, and antibiotic drops are also used if a bacterial infection is suspected. Ibuprofen or acetaminophen may be helpful for pain control. The ear canal should then be kept dry by using ear plugs or a swim cap for swimming and gently blow-drying the canal after bathing. The child should not return to swimming for about 5 days. Cotton-tipped applicators or other objects should not be placed in the ear canal so that the skin in the canal can heal. If hair sprays or other solutions are irritating, they should not be used by the child or adolescent.

Nurses should be aware of the signs of otitis externa such as a painful ear, drainage, and irritated canal. Verify that the tympanic membrane is intact during otoscopic examination. Teach families to avoid the irritants identified

EVIDENCE-BASED NURSING

OTITIS MEDIA

Problem

Sometimes rather simple interventions can positively influence a health-care issue. Research can assist in identifying interventions that have an effect on common problems. Acute otitis media is an important pediatric issue since it affects about 70% of all children by their third birthday. Nurses may be able to identify the problem but until recently have had little to offer families to help prevent otitis media.

Evidence

In a type of research that is called a meta-analysis, or summary of studies on a topic, two nurses described the collective results of research that examined relationships between incidence of otitis media and pacifier use. One study enrolled nearly 500 infants and divided them into control and intervention groups (Niemela, Pihakari, Pokka et al., 2000). The control group received usual instructions during healthcare visits, while the intervention group parents were instructed to limit pacifier use after 6 months of age, and to discontinue the pacifier after 10 months when the baby's sucking need was lessened. Incidence of otitis media was recorded and parents reported on pacifier use. Although the intervention group did not show decreased incidence of pacifier use, the babies in that group were using the pacifier significantly less daily than the control group babies. The occurrence of acute otitis media was 29% less in the intervention group than the control group.

In a second study, over 800 children were studied for an average of 10 months (Niemela, Uhari, & Mottonen, 1995). Parents completed questionnaires about their children's health and answered questions about pacifier use. About 29.5% of the children younger than 2 years who used pacifiers had three or more episodes of acute otitis media, while 20.6% of those who did not use pacifiers had the history of otitis media. For children from 2 to 3 years, acute otitis media incidence was 30.6% in pacifier users and 13.2% in nonusers.

In another study of 200 children, charts were reviewed for incidence of otitis media and parents completed questionnaires about

pacifier use (Jackson & Mourino, 1999). Prevalence of otitis media was 36% for pacifier users and 23% for nonusers.

Implications

Many children use pacifiers, and parents are often not aware that this practice can influence incidence of otitis media. The common nature of ear infections makes it important to apply knowledge to decrease its incidence among young children. In addition, some children have hearing loss or need surgery due to the disorder. Parents can be informed that babies over 6 months of age do not have the same need for sucking that younger babies do (Garrelts & Melnyk, 2001). This would be a good age to decrease pacifier use. Perhaps parents will be receptive to offering a pacifier when the baby goes to sleep but not using it during waking hours.

Critical Thinking

How will you phrase questions to ask in a sensitive manner about pacifier use by young children? How can you approach a parent during a well-child visit with a 2-year-old if you notice the child still using a pacifier? If a parent is interested in decreasing pacifier use for a baby, what strategies can you suggest to lessen the number of hours of daily use gradually? Develop an information sheet that can be used in a clinic to teach parents about the connection between pacifier use and acute otitis media.

References

Garrelts, L., & Melnyk, B. M. (2001). Pacifier usage and acute otitis media in infants and young children. *Pediatric Nursing, 27,* 516–518.

Jackson, J. M., & Mourino, A. P. (1999). Pacifier use and otitis media in infants twelve months of age and younger. *Pediatric Dentistry, 21,* 256–260.

Niemela, M., Pihakari, O., Pokka, T., Uhari, M., & Uhari, M. (2000). Pacifier as a risk factor for acute otitis media: A randomized, controlled trial of parental counseling. *Pediatrics, 106,* 483–488.

Niemela, M., Uhari, M., & Mottonen, M. (1995). A pacifier increases the risk of recurrent acute otitis media in children in day-care centers. *Pediatrics, 96,* 884–888.

---

such as cotton-tipped applicators, sprays, and frequent swimming. Demonstrate proper instillation of drops (see Skills Manual) and give instructions for use of acetaminophen for pain relief in the acute period. **SKILLS**

HEARING IMPAIRMENT

Approximately 1 million children in the United States have some form of hearing impairment. Hearing impairment is expressed in terms of **decibels** (dB), which are units of loudness, and rated according to severity (Table 46–6). Children who have only a mild hearing loss (35 to 40 dB) may miss 50% of everyday conversation and are considered at high risk for school failure. Children with a hearing loss of more than 90 dB are considered legally deaf. From 2 to 6 children per 1000 have a hearing loss (Bachman & Arvedson, 1998).

ETIOLOGY AND PATHOPHYSIOLOGY

About 50% of hearing loss is genetically caused, usually with a recessive inheritance pattern. Another 25% is due to environmental causes around the time of birth; the remainder is due to unknown causes. Hearing loss is present in about 1 to 2 infants per 1000 births (Walter et al., 2000). Infants at risk for hearing loss include those with:

- Family history of congenital hearing loss.
- Positive titer for TORCH infections (toxoplasmosis, rubella, cytomegalovirus, syphilis, herpes).
- Craniofacial abnormalities.
- Very low birth weight (<1500 g).
- Bilirubin > 16 mg/dL.
- Aminoglycoside medication administration > 5 days.

TEACHING HIGHLIGHTS

CARE OF THE CHILD WITH TYMPANOTOMY TUBES

After Surgery

Encourage the child to drink generous amounts of fluids.

Reestablish a regular diet as tolerated.

Give pain medication (acetaminophen) as ordered for discomfort and at bedtime.

Place drops in child's ears if instructed.

Restrict the child to quiet activities.

Following Postoperative Period

Follow the physician's instructions regarding swimming and water (some caution against swimming and other activities that might get water in ears; others do not).

Ear plugs can be used to prevent water from getting into ears.

Be alert for tubes becoming dislodged and falling out and alert physician (they usually fall out within 1 year).

Report purulent discharge from the ear, which may indicate a new ear infection. Contact the care provider.

- Low Apgar score at 1 or 5 minutes.
- Bacterial meningitis.
- Mechanical ventilation > 5 days.
- Presence of syndromes associated with hearing loss (Down syndrome, Pierre Robin syndrome, Arnold-Chiari malformation) (Vohr et al., 2000).

COMPLEMENTARY CARE

NATUROPATHIC EXTRACT FOR EAR PAIN IN OTITIS MEDIA

Since many children with otitis media experience ear pain that can disrupt their sleep and that of family members, anesthetic ear drops have been used for their analgesic effect on the tympanic membrane. Since some families might prefer use of natural remedies for ear pain, a study comparing Otikon (a naturopathic herbal extract of *Allium sativum, Verbascum thapsus, Calendula flores,* and *Hypericum peroforatum*) with a local anesthetic of ametocaine and phenazone was conducted. About half of the total 103 children received each of the pain treatments, and parents rated the children after training with a pain tool. Both treatments were effective in decreasing ear pain over the 3 days of the study. There was no significant difference in success rates of local anesthetic and naturopathic agent; in fact, the naturopathic agent was as effective or more effective than anesthetic at each measurement period. It is concluded that herbal pain control may be beneficial for treatment of ear pain, and can help to decrease the need for antibiotic treatment for every case of otitis media (Sarrell, Mandelberg, & Cohen, 2001).

TABLE 46–6 ✣ Severity of Hearing Loss

Type of Loss	Hearing Ability
Slight/mild	Some speech sounds are difficult to perceive, particularly unvoiced consonant sounds
Moderate	Most normal conversational speech sounds are missed
Severe	Speech sounds cannot be heard at a normal conversational level
Profound	No speech sounds can be heard; considered legally deaf
Deaf	No sound at all can be heard

Common causes of conductive hearing loss include impacted cerumen, the most frequent reason for conductive loss; outer ear infection ("swimmer's ear"); trauma; or a foreign body. Conductive loss also occurs if the tympanic membrane does not fully vibrate, as in otitis media. In these cases loss may be restored after the infection clears. Chronic and untreated ear infections may lead to ear structural changes and permanent hearing impairment. The loss of acuity may be gradual or rapid and results in diminished hearing in all ranges.

Conditions leading to sensorineural hearing loss may be congenital (maternal rubella), genetic (Tay-Sachs disease), or acquired (such as from ototoxic drugs, bacterial meningitis, or loud noise). In sensorineural hearing loss, high-frequency sounds are most affected. Such hearing loss may be preceded by **tinnitus** or ringing in the ears. Teenagers who use earphones at high volumes or attend many rock concerts are at risk for hearing loss (Figure 46–7 ●). Other noise hazards include firecrackers, guns, and power and farm equipment.

CLINICAL MANIFESTATIONS

Hearing disorders can be classified according to the location of the deficit. **Conductive hearing loss** occurs when conditions in the external auditory canal or tympanic membrane prevent sound from reaching the middle ear. **Sensorineural hearing loss** occurs when the hair cells in the cochlea or along the auditory nerve (cranial nerve VIII) are damaged. This leads to permanent hearing loss. A **mixed hearing loss** indicates a hearing loss having a combination of conductive and sensorineural causes.

Hearing is both an innate and a learned behavior. Infants and children who are hearing impaired exhibit a range of behaviors, depending on their age and the severity of the deficit. Infants who hear normally respond to sound in both obvious and subtle ways that do not occur

● FIGURE 46–7

Listening to loud music with headphones or at rock concerts is a frequent cause of hearing loss among teenagers and young adults. This adolescent needs to be informed about the possible outcomes of this activity.

in those who are hearing impaired (Table 46–7). As children mature, their hearing impairments affect their language skills. Hearing loss is often manifested as a cognitive deficit, a behavioral problem, or both.

CLINICAL THERAPY

Early identification of hearing loss is a key element in successful treatment. Detection of hearing loss in infants is important to ensure optimal development. Universal screening of all infants is recommended before 1 month of age, with diagnostic audiologic evaluation before 3 months, and beginning of early intervention programs by 6 months of age for those with hearing impairment (Walter et al., 2000). Many state laws now mandate screening of newborns. Observations of response to noise in all newborns should be accompanied by more sophisticated testing such as auditory brain stem response or transient evoked otoacoustic emissions, especially in those at high risk of deficits (Figure 46–8 ●). See Table 46–8.

NURSING PRACTICE

Although it is recommended that infants with significant hearing loss be identified by 3 months of age and receive treatment by 6 months, most children with hearing deficits are not identified until later in childhood. Early intervention is crucial for maximizing the child's ability to use any hearing present and to learn communication methods. Development is profoundly impacted by difficulty in communication. Nurses need to test all newborns and infants for signs of hearing disorders and refer as needed. Parents often are the first to notice a problem with hearing, so ask for their observations of the infant's hearing during each visit (Garganta & Seashore, 2000).

TABLE 46–7 ✣ Behaviors Suggestive of Hearing Impairment

Age	Behavior
Infant	Has a diminished or absent startle reflex to loud sound
	Does not awaken when environment is very noisy
	Awakens only to touch
	Does not turn head to sound at 3–4 months
	Does not localize sound at 6–10 months
	Babbles little or not at all
Toddler and preschooler	Speaks unintelligibly, in a monotone, or not at all
	Communicates needs through gestures
	Appears developmentally delayed
	Appears emotionally immature, yells inappropriately
	Does not respond to doorbell or telephone
	Appears more interested in objects than people and prefers to play alone
	Focuses on facial expressions rather than verbal communications
School-age child and adolescent	Asks to have statements repeated
	Answers questions inappropriately, except when able to view speaker's face
	Daydreams and is inattentive
	Performs poorly at school or is truant
	Has speech abnormalities or speaks in a monotone
	Sits close to or turns television or radio up loudly
	Prefers to play alone

An otoscopic examination with a tympanogram can be performed on an older infant to determine conductive hearing loss. The **tympanogram** is a test that provides a graph of the ability of the middle ear to transmit sound. An airtight probe is inserted into the external ear canal and a tone is emitted. The probe measures the pressure, which is plotted on a graph. A "flat" tympanogram suggests conductive hearing loss. **Audiography** can be used with cooperative children over 3 years of age. Sounds of various frequencies and intensities are presented to the child

GROWTH AND DEVELOPMENT

Infants and young children respond automatically with a blink or the startle reflex to unexpected or loud noises. As they mature, they localize the sound source, then understand speech, and then communicate verbally.

● FIGURE 46–8

Newborn hearing screening is an effective tool in diagnosing some causes of hearing impairment very early in life.

through earphones, and the child is instructed to raise his or her hand when the sound is heard. Audiography cannot detect hearing loss caused by middle ear effusion but can indicate sensorineural loss.

The hearing of preschool and school-age children is tested by asking them to repeat whispered words. Hearing

TABLE 46–8 ✤ Screening Tests for Newborn Hearing

Test	Mechanism of Action
Otoacoustic emission (OAE) (either transient evoked [TEOAE] or distortion-product [DPOAE])	A measure of low-intensity sounds from the cochlear hair cells in response to clicks from a probe placed in the ear canal
	Sensitive in frequency range above 1500 Hz
	May show false negative for loss below 1000–1500 Hz
	Detects inner ear hearing loss by evaluating cochlear and hair cell function
	Does not detect neural damage to 8th cranial nerve
	Can be sensitive to outer ear canal obstruction or middle ear effusion, leading to false positive result
Auditory brainstem response (ABR)	Electrical response to auditory stimuli from three surface scalp electrodes
	Reflects activity of cochlea, cranial nerve 8, and auditory brainstem pathways
	Detects hearing loss from 1000–8000 Hz
	May show false negative results for losses in the 500–2000 Hz levels
	Will give a positive result even if cochlear loss is not present

of school-age children and adolescents also is assessed with the Weber and Rinne tests (see Chapter 35 ∞).

If a hearing loss is uncorrectable, a multidisciplinary team composed of pediatrician, audiologist, otolaryngologist, speech–language pathologist, nurse, teacher, and social worker should help the child and family adapt to the disability (Brookhouse, Beauchaine, & Osberger, 1999). If the deficit is due to recurrent ear infections, tympanostomy tube insertion may improve hearing. Some families choose to have a child treated with a cochlear implant. A cochlear implant is a small electronic device that helps to provide sound for those who are deaf or profoundly hard of hearing. It consists of the following:

1. A microphone to pick up sound that is located outside of the body; it is worn as a headpiece behind the ear

2. A speech processor which organizes sound from the microphone; worn behind the ear or on a belt

3. A transmitter that transfers the sound into electrical impulses; part of the headpiece behind the ear

4. Electrodes which send the signals to the brain; this receiver is implanted in the skin behind the ear with a wire leading to the cochlear fluid in the middle ear

A hearing aid may be prescribed for a conductive loss. A sensorineural loss is more difficult to treat, but cochlear implants and bone conduction hearing aids have been used in some children. Cochlear implants are increasingly being used in children and have restored hearing in some who are profoundly deaf (Cheng, Rubin, Powe et al., 2000).

For children with uncorrectable hearing loss, several approaches are used to enhance communication (Table 46–9). Children with hearing impairment may receive speech therapy and instructions in lipreading, signing, cuing, and fingerspelling.

NURSING MANAGEMENT

NURSING ASSESSMENT AND DIAGNOSIS

Nurses conduct newborn hearing tests soon after birth and make observations of the infant's responses to sound. As the child grows, assess hearing at every well-child visit. The best judges of hearing are parents; ask them if they have any concerns about their child's hearing. An infant's reaction to rattles, bells, or handclapping (about 12 in. [30 cm] from the ear) is an important observation. Evaluate language milestones when examining the older infant and child. Language development is a major area of focus in deaf children. Deaf infants begin to babble at about 5 to 6 months of age, the same age as hearing infants. However, this babbling ceases several months later in the hearing-impaired child.

TABLE 46–9 ✢ Communication Techniques for Children Who Are Hearing Impaired

Technique	Description
Cued speech	Supplement to lipreading; eight hand shapes represent groups of consonant sounds and four positions about the face represent groups of vowel sounds; based on the sounds the letters make, not the letters themselves; child can "see-hear" every spoken syllable a hearing person hears
Oral approach	Uses only spoken language for face-to-face communication; avoids use of formal signs; uses hearing aids and residual hearing
Total communication	Uses speech and sign, fingerspelling, lipreading, and residual hearing simultaneously; child selects communication technique depending on the situation

Used with permission from Schwartz, S. (1996). *Choices in deafness: A parent's guide* (2nd ed.). Rockville, MD: Woodbine House. For publications related to hearing-impaired children, contact Woodbine House.

School nurses use audiometers to evaluate hearing during screening programs in schools, and refer children who do not pass the screening test (see Skills 9–20—9–21) SKILLS. Measures to promote speech and communication development as well as safety are implemented.

Common nursing diagnoses for the child with impaired hearing include the following:

- *Disturbed Sensory/Perception (Auditory)* related to altered sensory perception
- *Risk for Impaired Verbal Communication* related to hearing loss
- *Risk for Delayed Growth and Development* related to communication impairment
- *Readiness for Enhanced Family Coping*, related to caring for a child with a hearing impairment

PLANNING AND IMPLEMENTATION

Nurses can encourage prevention of hearing loss from exposure to loud noises such as loud music and power and farm equipment. Music should be turned down and ear protection worn for other activities. School nurses should be active in hearing conservation education programs in school (Folmer, 2003). Several programs are available to assist the school nurse in teaching children at targeted ages about noise-induced hearing loss. The nurse should develop and deliver hearing conservation curricula to chil-

dren at elementary, middle, and high school levels; inform teachers and other professionals about noise-induced hearing loss; and train volunteers to assist with school programs.

Newborn screening, developmental assessment, and childhood hearing screening facilitate identification of hearing loss in infants and children. Infants should be tested for hearing loss by 3 months of age. In cases of loss, intervention should begin before 6 months of age (Joint Committee on Infant Hearing, 2000).

Nursing care of the child with a hearing impairment focuses on facilitating the child's ability to receive spoken language and to send information, helping parents meet the child's schooling needs, and providing emotional support to parents. Refer the parents to an early intervention program as soon as the diagnosis of hearing impairment is made, in order to foster the child's development. If a cochlear implant is planned, the child needs surgical care and follow-up to monitor results and integrate sound gradually into the child's life (Slattery & Fayad, 1999).

Facilitate Ability to Receive Spoken Language

Be aware of how the child compensates for hearing loss and use these strategies in communication.

- If hearing loss is mild or temporary or if the child reads lips, first obtain the child's visual attention by lightly touching the child or saying the child's name.
- Position your face 3 to 6 ft (1 to 2 m) from the child's face and make sure that the child's eyes are focused on your face and lips. Make sure the room is well lit, with no backlighting. Speak at a normal rate and tone, and use facial expressions that show caring or concern. If the child does not understand, rephrase the information in shorter, simpler sentences. Use specific, concrete explanations, and give the child time to comprehend. Watch for subtle signs of misinterpretations and give consistent and immediate feedback since only 30% of the English language is visible on the lips.
- Be familiar with the different types of hearing aids. Hearing aids, which are microphones that amplify all sounds, can be worn in or behind the ear, in the frame of glasses, or on the body with a wire attached to the ear. Place the hearing aid in the ear with the volume off, then slowly turn up to half volume. Adjust as needed. When talking to a child with a hearing aid, speak slowly within 6 to 18 inches (15 to 45 cm) from the microphone using a normal conversational tone. Talk to the child even if the child is not looking at you. Make sure the batteries are fresh for the best reception. Since all sound is amplified, reduce background noise as much as possible. Clean the hearing aid daily with a damp cloth. Change the batteries as needed, usually

about once a week. The child's growth necessitates a new fitting, usually about once annually.

Acoustic feedback, an audible whistling sound that cannot always be heard by the child, is one of the most common problems with hearing aids. To eliminate this sound, readjust the hearing aid to make sure that it is inserted properly and that no hair or ear wax is caught between the ear mold and canal. Turning down the volume may also help.

A remote microphone system is another type of device designed to improve hearing. This is often used in the classroom situation because it eliminates background noise. The speaker wears a transmitter that picks up the voice and transmits it to a receiver worn by the child.

Facilitate Ability to Send Information

Maintain the child's hearing aid in proper condition. Many children with impaired hearing communicate using speech, which is enhanced through speech therapy. In addition they are taught to sign, fingerspell, or use cued speech (Figure 46–9 ◉). Articulation may be difficult, and understanding what the child is trying to say may be frustrating for both the nurse and the child. Taking time to listen carefully is important.

◉ **FIGURE 46–9**

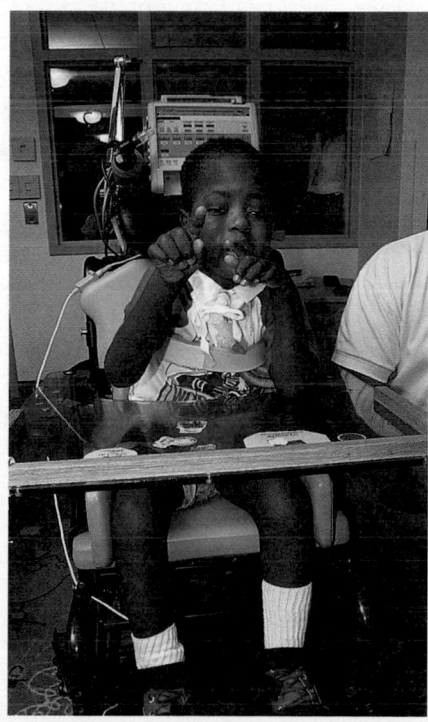

This child with a hearing impairment and tracheostomy is communicating by means of American Sign Language.

Take measures to promote speech and communication development as well as safety. Ask the parents to explain the child's communication techniques and to help interpret words. Have younger children point to pictures. Use assisted technologies such as a computer or picture board as well as drawings or gestures if necessary. This is especially helpful for communicating feelings of pain and hunger during hospitalization. If the child signs or fingerspells, make sure that you understand the signs for important functions. Give older children a pad of paper and pencil to write requests. People other than parents should be able to understand what the child is trying to communicate. Have an interpreter available if the child uses American Sign Language. Learn some common signs to communicate simple words or phrases. Orient the child carefully to new settings such as the hospital room or a new school.

Help Parents to Meet Child's Educational Needs

Public laws apply to the education of children who are hearing impaired (see Chapter 1 ∞). After diagnosis, the parents and professionals together agree on an individualized education plan (see discussion in Chapter 39 ∞). Day care and preschool are recommended for children with hearing problems.

■ Give parents information about adjustments that may have to be made for the hearing-impaired child who attends public school. By sitting at the front of the classroom, the child can hear and see more clearly. The teacher should always face the child when speaking, and background noise should be reduced.

■ Tell parents that children who are hearing impaired have the same intelligence quotient (IQ) distribution as children without hearing impairment. However, communication and learning can be difficult, and extra support is needed.

■ Children with hearing impairment should reach their intellectual potential, although development in certain areas may take place more slowly than it does in non-hearing-impaired children.

Provide Emotional Support

By recognizing the effects of the diagnosis on the family, the nurse can help the family deal with their reaction to the child's hearing loss. Supporting healthy coping is an important intervention to help the parents carry on with their lives.

■ Help the parents understand the child's disability and its effect on speech and language development. Provide accurate information about their concerns. Work jointly with other healthcare professionals and social service workers if necessary.

- Tell the family about the community services available for medical, nursing, psychologic, and financial assistance.

EVALUATION

Expected outcomes of nursing care for a child with hearing impairment include the following:

- Successful establishment of communication method
- Growth and development to maximum potential
- Establishment of successful individualized education plan
- Positive family coping

INJURIES OF THE EAR

Ear injuries of many types commonly occur in children. Lacerations, infections, and hematomas may occur in the external ear structures, especially the pinna. Children may place foreign objects in the ear, and insects may enter the ear canal. Rupture of the tympanic membrane may result from head injuries, blows to the ear, or insertion of objects into the ear canal. Caution children and parents not to place anything into the ear, including cotton swabs for cleaning.

See Table 46–10 for information on the emergency treatment of ear injuries. Any injury resulting in earache, decreased hearing, persistent bleeding, or other discharge should be seen by a physician.

HEALTH PROMOTION

The Child with a Hearing Impairment

Growth and Developmental Surveillance

- Ensure that the child receives all immunizations at scheduled times. All children with cochlear implants should have pneumococcal vaccine (PCV7 for under 5 years or PPV23 for over 5 years). The immunization should be completed 2 weeks before surgery for cochlear implant. Children should be up to date on all immunizations, but rubella, mumps, and measles are especially important since infections with the diseases could cause further hearing loss.
- Complete developmental assessment, including receptive and expressive verbal skills at each visit.
- Teach about safety precautions for those with hearing impairment, such as inability to hear announcements at school, fire alarms at home, or sirens when in travel. Assist the family to install visual stimuli for fire alarms and other safety needs.

Communication

- Review the type of communication used by the child and the family's satisfaction.
- Ask about relationships with other children, both hearing impaired and those with normal hearing.
- Review discipline techniques used by the parents and consistency of limit setting.

Nutrition and Physical Activity

- Complete 24-hour diet recall and be sure the child receives adequate nutrition appropriate in energy for activities.
- Review the child's exercise patterns since some children with hearing impairment may avoid interactions with other children in sports.
- Refer the family to community activity programs as needed.

Mental Health

- Find out stressors parents may feel.
- Locate community resources for early intervention and ongoing programs.
- Assist the youth and family to plan for moves to new schools and communities, and for plans related to transition to young adulthood, including college, trade schools, or work in the community.

Disease Prevention Strategies

- Be sure signs of ear infection such as fever, irritability, disturbed sleep, rubbing ear, or ear drainage are promptly evaluated in the pediatric healthcare home.
- Teach parents to administer antibiotics for ear infections exactly as prescribed.
- Encourage breastfeeding of infants and avoiding smoking to minimize incidence of ear infections.
- Be sure the child has all recommended immunizations.

Injury Prevention Strategies

- Encourage family to preserve any hearing the child may have by avoiding exposure to loud sounds; when children are old enough to understand be sure they safeguard against exposure to loud music, guns, and other risks.
- Teach the child and family to plan for safety when crossing streets, driving cars, escaping house fires, and other situations that normally rely on hearing.

TABLE 46–10 ❖ Emergency Treatment of Ear Injuries

Injury	Treatment
Pinna	
Minor cuts or abrasions	Wash thoroughly with soap and water and rinse well; leave exposed to air if possible or apply adhesive bandage; monitor for infection.
Hematomas	Needle aspiration should be performed and pressure dressing applied; undrained hematomas may become fibrotic; "cauliflower ear" deformity may develop.
Cellulitis or abscesses	Apply moist heat intermittently; make sure that prescribed antibiotic is taken; minor surgery may be performed for an abscess.
Deep lacerations	Apply pressure to stop bleeding; transport to physician's office or emergency department for suturing.
Ear Canal	
Foreign bodies	Have child lie on back and turn head over edge of bed, with affected side down; wiggle earlobe and have child shake head; foreign object may fall out as result of gravity; if object remains in ear, call physician; do not try to remove foreign body with tweezers since this may push the object further into the ear.
Insects	Shine flashlights into ear to try to attract insect; instilling a few drops of mineral oil, olive oil, or alcohol kills insect, and irrigating ear canal gently may remove dead insect. See Skill 11–9. **SKILLS**
Tympanic Membrane	
Ruptures	Call physician if child has persistent ear pain after blow, blast injury, or insertion of foreign object; cover external ear loosely with piece of sterile cotton or gauze; if tympanic membrane has been ruptured, systemic antibiotics are prescribed.

DISORDERS OF THE NOSE, THROAT, AND MOUTH

EPISTAXIS

Epistaxis, or nosebleed, is common in school-age children, especially boys. Kiesselbach's plexus, an area of plentiful veins located in the anterior nares, is the most common source of bleeding. The most common cause is irritation from nosepicking, foreign bodies, or low humidity. Other causes include forceful coughing, allergies, or infections resulting in congestion of the nasal mucosa. Bleeding from the posterior septum is more serious and may be life threatening. Hospitalization may be necessary. Posterior nosebleeds have a variety of causes, some of which may indicate systemic disease (i.e., bleeding disorder) or injury.

NURSING MANAGEMENT

Children with nosebleeds are sometimes brought to the emergency department by a parent who has been unable to stop the flow of blood within a few minutes. Both parent and child may be frightened. Ask the parent briefly about any history of nosebleeds and other contributing factors, including medications. Take the child's pulse and blood pressure to assess for excessive blood loss. Carefully examine the nasal mucosa by asking the child to blow any clots out gently, if possible. Suctioning may be necessary.

Observing the flow may help determine whether the blood is coming from an anterior or a posterior location. A nosebleed confined to one side of the nose is almost always anterior, but posterior bleeding can flow on one or both sides. If blood cannot be seen, the child may be swallowing it and may become nauseated. Suspect posterior bleeding in children who have sustained blunt trauma or in other children at high risk.

The child with anterior bleeding should sit upright quietly. The head should be tilted forward to prevent blood from trickling down the throat, which can lead to vomiting. The nares should be squeezed just below the nasal bone and held for 10 to 15 minutes while the child breathes through the mouth. If the bleeding does not stop, a cotton ball or swab soaked with Neo-Synephrine, epinephrine, thrombin, or lidocaine may be inserted into the affected nostril to promote topical vasoconstriction or anesthesia. Once the bleeding has stopped, the nostril may have to be cauterized with silver nitrate or electrocautery. If the bleeding cannot be stopped, absorbable packing may be used.

Posterior bleeding must also be stopped by packing, and the child must be monitored carefully. Arterial ligation is occasionally needed. Repeated or severe nosebleeds need further evaluation (Newland & Rich, 1998).

Assess the child's hematocrit or hemoglobin if significant bleeding has occurred. Take a complete history and do a physical examination of children with frequent epistaxis to rule out systemic disease.

TEACHING HIGHLIGHTS

PREVENTION AND HOME MANAGEMENT OF EPISTAXIS

Prevention
- Humidify the child's room, especially during the winter.
- Discourage the child from picking or rubbing the nose or inserting foreign objects in the nose.
- Instruct the child to blow the nose gently and release sneezes through the mouth.

Home Management
- Keep the child calm.
- Sit the child upright with head tilted slightly forward so blood does not run down the throat.
- Press a roll of cotton under the upper lip to compress the labial artery.
- Apply steady pressure to both nostrils just below the nasal bone with the thumb and forefinger for 15 to 20 minutes. Time by the clock.
- Apply an ice pack or cold compress to the bridge of the nose or the back of the neck.
- Call healthcare provider if the bleeding does not stop.
- Avoid further bleeds by sleeping with the head elevated on pillows, avoiding hot showers and drinks, and avoiding aspirin or other noncoagulant drugs during the first few days after a nosebleed.

Data from Newland, J. A., & Rich, E. (1998). Epistaxis. American Journal of Nursing, 98, 16HHH.

After the nosebleed has stopped, the child is more vulnerable to recurrent bleeding and should avoid bending over, stooping, strenuous exercise, hot drinks, and hot baths or showers for the next 3 to 4 days. Sleeping with the head elevated on two or three pillows and humidifying the air with a vaporizer may also prevent a recurrence. Give parents suggestions for prevention and home management of epistaxis.

NASOPHARYNGITIS

Nasopharyngitis, also known as the "common cold," causes inflammation and infection of the nose and throat and is probably the most common illness of infancy and childhood. More than 200 viruses and numerous bacteria can cause this condition. The most common viruses include rhinovirus and coronavirus, and the most frequently occurring bacterium is group A *Streptococcus*. The organisms incubate in 1 to 3 days, and the infection is communicable several hours before symptoms develop and for 1 to 2 days after they begin. Symptoms may last 4 to 10 days

or longer. The pathogens are believed to spread when the infected person touches the hand of an uninfected person, who then touches his or her mouth or nose, resulting in self-inoculation.

A red nasal mucosa with clear nasal discharge and an infected throat with enlarged tonsils may be apparent in children with nasopharyngitis. Vesicles may be present on the soft palate and in the pharynx. Accompanying symptoms may vary, depending on the child's age (Table 46–11).

Between episodes of nasopharyngitis, the child should be asymptomatic. If a child continues to have upper respiratory infections, an underlying condition such as allergy, asthma, or polyps should be ruled out.

NURSING MANAGEMENT

For infants who cannot breathe through the mouth, normal saline nose drops can be administered every 3 to 4 hours, especially before feeding (see Skill 11–10). **SKILLS** For infants over 9 months of age, nasal stuffiness can be treated with either normal saline nose drops or a decongestant such as phenylephrine (0.125% to 0.25%, depending on the child's age). Older children can use nasal sprays.

Although nose drops and sprays are more effective than systemic decongestants, they should not be used for more than 4 or 5 days or more often than recommended. Antihistamines may be helpful for children with allergic rhinitis or profuse nasal drainage. Long-acting nasal sprays and medications with several ingredients are not recommended.

TABLE 46–11 ✤ Manifestations of Nasopharyngitis

Infants Younger Than 3 Months of Age

Lethargy	Feeding poorly
Irritability	Fever (may be absent)

Infants 3 Months of Age or Older

Fever	Anorexia
Vomiting	Irritability
Diarrhea	Restlessness
Sneezing	

Older Children

Dry, irritated nose and throat

Chills, fever

Generalized muscle aches

Headache

Malaise

Anorexia

Thin nasal discharge, which may later become thick and purulent

Sneezing

Room humidification may help prevent drying of nasal secretions. Antipyretics such as acetaminophen reduce fever and make the child more comfortable. Aspirin is not recommended because of its association with Reye syndrome (refer to Chapter 53 ∞).

Children should avoid strenuous physical activity and engage in quiet play such as reading, listening to music or stories, or watching television or videotapes. Children should not be forced to eat. Encourage the intake of favorite fluids to liquify secretions. Tell parents that no medicine or vaccine can prevent the common cold, but eliminating contact with infected persons can reduce the spread of infection. Proper handwashing and disposal of tissues helps to decrease the spread of the infection.

SINUSITIS

Sinusitis is an inflammation of one or more of the paranasal sinuses. These sinuses, which have respiratory epithelium and are continuous with the respiratory tract, include the maxillary, ethmoid, frontal, and sphenoid sinuses. The sinuses may become infected with bacteria following a viral upper respiratory infection. In most cases, the child's history reveals a cold for several days, followed by improvement in the cold symptoms but an increase in purulent nasal drainage. There is accompanying facial pain, headache, and fever. Chronic sinusitis may occur in children with uncontrolled allergies and asthma.

Signs and symptoms of sinusitis in children are sometimes nonspecific. A history of recent upper respiratory infection is common, persistent cough from postnasal drip can occur, and nasal discharge or swelling can be apparent. Malodorous breath, fever, mouth breathing, hyponasal speech, and cervical lymphadenopathy may be present (Duchene, 2000; Hayes, 2001; Leung & Kellner, 2004). Young children may be anorexic or have difficulty feeding, and older children may complain of headache.

Diagnosis of sinusitis is usually based on history and physical examination findings. Percussion and illumina-tion of sinuses are not generally useful in children. Computed tomography (CT), magnetic resonance imaging (MRI), and x-rays may be done but they can be costly and require sedation of young children and results may not be conclusive. For the child with repeated sinusitis or who appears toxic, aspiration of sinus aspirate may be performed for culture by an otolaryngologist.

Although most primary care providers treat suspected sinusitis with antibiotics, many cases will clear spontaneously without treatment. Amoxicillin is the first choice for therapy; amoxicillin/clavulanate and cephalosporins are also sometimes used (Kakish, Mahafza, & Batieha et al., 2000; Sinus and Allergy Health Partnership, 2000). Children with recurrent sinusitis should be referred for further care by an otolaryngologist and allergy specialist.

Parents whose child has persistent and purulent nasal drainage should be told to see a healthcare provider, particularly if the drainage is accompanied by facial pain, headache, and fever. Nurses should teach parents to correctly administer antibiotics (e.g., to take medications for the full course) if prescribed, and to use saline nose drops if needed for comfort. Infants may need their noses cleared with nose drops and a bulb syringe prior to feedings. (Refer to the Skills Manual for correct use of a bulb syringe.) SKILLS Antipyretics can be given for fever and to relieve pain.

PHARYNGITIS

Acute pharyngitis is an infection that primarily affects the pharynx, including the tonsils. It is seen most frequently in children 4 to 7 years of age and is rare in children less than 1 year of age. Approximately 80% of these infections are caused by viruses; the rest are caused by bacteria. Bacterial pharyngitis is commonly known as "strep throat," since it is most often caused by group A beta-hemolytic streptococcus (GABHS). Viral pharyngitis is caused by a large number of enteroviruses.

The major complaint is a sore throat. See "Clinical Manifestations: Viral Pharyngitis and Strep Throat." Children with symptoms of strep throat who have minimal throat redness and pain, exudate, mild lymphadenopathy, and a low-grade fever, and who have been exposed to someone who has pharyngitis should have a throat culture. The classic signs of purulent drainage and white patches are not present in all cases of strep throat. A child who finds swallowing difficult or extremely painful, who drools, or who exhibits signs of dehydration or respiratory distress should be seen by a physician immediately. These signs could be indicators of serious conditions such as epiglottitis, peritonsillar or retropharyngeal abscess, or diphtheria.

DEVELOPING CULTURAL COMPETENCE

HOT AND COLD DISEASE THEORY

Many Hispanic and Asian cultural groups believe in the "hot and cold theory" of disease, in which health problems are viewed as the result of imbalance. For example, some Mexican Americans traditionally treat a "cold disease" such as an earache or common cold with "hot" substances. Ask families if they prefer to eat certain foods during an illness. Incorporating such preferences may help the child and increase the confidence of the family in healthcare providers.

CLINICAL MANIFESTATIONS

VIRAL PHARYNGITIS AND STREP THROAT (GROUP A BETA-HEMOLYTIC STREPTOCOCCUS [GABHS])[a]

VIRAL PHARYNGITIS	STREP THROAT
Nasal congestion	Tonsillar exudate[b]
Mild sore throat	Painful cervical lymphadenopathy[b]
Conjunctivitis	Abdominal pain
Cough	Vomiting
Hoarseness	Severe sore throat
Mild pharyngeal redness	Headache
Minimal tonsillar exudate	Fever >38.3°C (101°F)
Mildly tender anterior cervical lymphadenopathy	Petechial mottling of soft palate
Fever <38.3°C (101°F)	

a = Children 6 months to 3 years of age may have streptococcus with symptoms that resemble those of viral pharyngitis. Children with scarlet fever have the symptoms of strep throat plus a sandpaper-textured erythematous generalized rash and pallor of the lips.

b = Classic signs of strep throat

The diagnosis of strep throat is made by throat culture, using the rapid or traditional strep tests (see Skill 10–5). **SKILLS** Results of the rapid strep test may be available within minutes; those for the traditional test are available in 24 to 48 hours. Early signs of strep throat should be treated with oral penicillin for 10 days or with long-acting penicillin given in one injection immediately, even before the result of the culture is available. If the child is allergic to penicillin, erythromycin is given. Acute symptoms should resolve within 24 hours of therapy, at which time the child is no longer contagious. For viral pharyngitis, symptomatic treatment alone is used.

NURSING PRACTICE

Throat cultures must be properly performed for accurate diagnosis. Swab a sterile cotton-tip applicator across the tonsils, posterior edge of the soft palate, and uvula. Ask cooperative children to put their hands under their buttocks, open their mouth, and laugh or pant like a dog. Quickly swab the throat. You can place uncooperative and young children on their backs with their hands next to their heads and have a parent or an assistant hold them. Depress the tongue gently with a tongue blade and swab the throat.

NURSING MANAGEMENT

Nursing care focuses on symptomatic relief. Acetaminophen reduces throat pain and generalized fever. Cool, nonacidic fluids and soft foods, ice chips, or frozen juice pops given frequently in small amounts facilitate swallowing and prevent dehydration. Humidification, chewing gum, and gargling with warm salt water (1 teaspoon [5 g] salt to 8 oz [250 mL] water) soothe an irritated throat. Alternatively, the salt water can be placed in a spray bottle and sprayed gently toward the throat. Commercial throat sprays or throat lozenges are not generally more effective than these home remedies. Encourage the child to rest, to conserve energy and promote recovery.

Teach parents the importance of completing the 10-day course of antibiotics if prescribed for bacterial pharyngitis. Reinforce to parents the importance of treating streptococcal infections, as untreated infections may lead to rheumatic fever, cervical adenitis, sinusitis, glomerulonephritis, or meningitis.

TONSILLITIS

Tonsillitis is an infection or inflammation (hypertrophy) of the palatine tonsils. Although most children with pharyngitis may have infected tonsils, they do not necessarily have tonsillitis.

ETIOLOGY AND PATHOPHYSIOLOGY

Like pharyngitis, tonsillitis may be caused by a virus or bacterium. The primary site of infection is the tonsils.

CLINICAL MANIFESTATIONS

Symptoms suggestive of tonsillitis include frequent throat infections with breathing and swallowing difficulties, persistent redness of the anterior pillars, and enlargement of the cervical lymph nodes. If children breathe through their mouths continuously, the mucous membranes may become dry and irritated.

CLINICAL THERAPY

Diagnosis is made on the basis of visual inspection and clinical manifestations. Symptomatic treatment for tonsillitis is the same as for pharyngitis. Surgical removal of tonsils (tonsillectomy) is often recommended when children have recurrent throat infections (about three per year for 3 years), chronic tonsillitis, obstructive sleep apnea, or malformations causing nasal speech or a facial growth abnormality. If the child is under 3 years of age, the surgery is postponed if possible because it may stimulate growth of other lymphoid tissue in the nasopharynx. If the pharyngeal tonsils (adenoids) are enlarged, as suggested by mouth breathing, cough, impaired taste and smell, a muffled quality to the voice, and chronic otitis media, they may be removed at the same time.

NURSING MANAGEMENT

NURSING ASSESSMENT AND DIAGNOSIS

Assess the throat carefully during each physical examination. Observe for tonsils that are simply large (a common finding in childhood) and those that are inflamed. Look for the degree of redness and presence of any exudate. Ask if the child has pain or difficulty swallowing. Ask about the history of past tonsillar infections and the length of time of the present discomfort.

If surgery is indicated, take a complete history of the child preoperatively. Monitor vital signs and observe for respiratory distress, hemorrhage, and dehydration postoperatively.

Several nursing diagnoses may apply to the child with tonsillitis. They include the following:

- *Pain* related to inflammation of the pharynx
- *Risk for Deficient Fluid Volume* related to inadequate intake
- *Risk for Ineffective Breathing Pattern* related to obstruction by enlarged tonsils
- *Impaired Swallowing* related to inflammation and pain
- *Health-Seeking Behaviors (Parents)* related to home care following discharge

PLANNING AND IMPLEMENTATION

The nurse provides general supportive care and, if medication is prescribed, encourages completion of the full course of treatment. The nursing management of children with tonsillitis is similar to that of children with pharyngitis (see earlier discussion).

If surgery is indicated, help the parents prepare their child for a short-term surgical procedure with a possible overnight stay in the hospital (see Chapter 40 ∞).Children should be free of sore throat, fever, or upper respiratory infection for at least 1 week before surgery. They should not be given aspirin or ibuprofen for 2 weeks before surgery, since these medications can increase bleeding. Check if any herbal medications are taken and report them to the physician and anesthesiologist since some may interfere with anesthetic drugs used in surgery.

Discharge Planning and Home Care Teaching

Discharge planning includes teaching parents about pain management, fluid and nutrition intake, activity restrictions, and possible complications in the postoperative period. Most children have a sore throat for 7 to 10 days after tonsillectomy. Advise parents how to relieve the child's throat pain.

Children may experience ear pain, especially when swallowing, between 4 and 8 days after tonsillectomy. Advise parents that this pain is referred from the tonsillar area and does not indicate an ear infection.

Emphasize to parents the importance of adequate fluid intake. Children should be given any liquid they prefer for the first week, except citrus juices, which may produce a burning sensation in the throat. Soft foods such as gelatin, applesauce, frozen juice pops, and mashed potatoes can be added as tolerated.

TEACHING HIGHLIGHTS

CARE AFTER TONSILLECTOMY

After tonsillectomy the parent can take measures to increase the child's comfort.

- Have the child drink adequate cool fluids or chew gum, as this reduces spasms in the muscles surrounding the throat.
- Give acetaminophen elixir, as ordered.
- Apply an ice collar around the child's neck.
- Have the child gargle with a solution of 1/2 teaspoon (2.5 g) each of baking soda and salt in a glass of water.
- Have the child rinse the mouth well with viscous lidocaine and then swallow the solution.

TEACHING HIGHLIGHTS

COMPLICATIONS OF TONSILLECTOMY AND ADENOIDECTOMY

Bleeding

- To prevent bleeding, aspirin or ibuprofen should not be given for pain for the first postoperative week. Use acetaminophen instead.
- Bleeding is most likely to occur within the first 24 hours or 7 to 10 days after the tonsillectomy, when the scar is forming. Report any trickle of bright red blood to the physician immediately.

Infection

- The back of the throat will look white and have an odor for the first 7 to 8 days after the surgery. The child may also have a low-grade fever. These are not signs of infection.
- For temperatures over 38.3°C (101°F), acetaminophen may be used.
- Call the physician if the child develops a fever above 38.8°C (102°F).

Pain

- Administer acetaminophen as ordered.
- Offer frequent small amounts of cool liquids. Avoid citrus juice.
- Provide for rest and quiet activities for several days.

Children do not need to be confined to bed, but they should avoid vigorous exercise for the first week after surgery. Advise parents that the child may return to school approximately 10 days after tonsillectomy.

Any surgery carries the risk of postoperative complications. Teach parents the normal signs of healing in the postoperative period, as well as signs of complications. See "Clinical Pathway: Tonsillectomy and Adenoidectomy."

CLINICAL PATHWAY

TONSILLECTOMY AND ADENOIDECTOMY

CATEGORY	IMMEDIATE PERIOPERATIVE PERIOD	DISCHARGE TO HOME CARE
Daily outcomes	Parent/client verbalizes understanding of preoperative teaching including IV fluids, antiemetics, ice pack to neck, activity, and pain management Parent/client displays effective coping Validate informed consent	Client has a patent airway and has minimal drainage in the throat Client has stable vital signs and is alert and responsive Client remains free of signs/symptoms of hemorrhage, and hemoglobin and hematocrit remains within normal limits Client manages pain with ordered medications Parent/client verbalizes/demonstrates home care instructions Client tolerates liquids without complaints of severe pain or vomiting
Assessments, tests, and treatments	*Preoperative:* CBC Urinalysis PTT Baseline physical assessment with a focus on respiratory status Anesthesia consult Assess cognitive/developmental level *Postoperative:* Position on side until fully awake; then Fowler's position Level of consciousness Vital signs and O_2 saturation, neurovascular assessment, and bleeding assessment q15min × 4; q30min × 4; q1hr × 4 and then q4hr and prn Assess lung sounds q1–2hr and prn Discourage coughing or clearing of throat Monitor for frequent swallowing Ice pack to neck Monitor intake and output; encourage voiding prior to discharge Offer/administer analgesics on schedule as ordered Assess pain and effectiveness of pain medications	Perform complete discharge assessment
Knowledge deficit	Orient to room and surroundings Include family in teaching Provide simple, brief instructions Review preoperative preparation, including hospital and surgical routines Emphasize probability of the presence of old blood in the nose, between the teeth, and in emesis Reinforce preoperative teaching Evaluate understanding of teaching Provide information at developmental/cognitive level	Review plan of care as well as diet and activity restrictions Complete discharge teaching regarding postoperative assessments, follow-up care, signs and symptoms to report, medications, and diet Explain to client to avoid coughing or clearing throat and to avoid gargling Review the importance of reporting any signs or symptoms of bleeding during the postoperative period up to 10 days following surgery Evaluate understanding of teaching
Psychosocial	Assess anxiety related to pending surgery Assess fears of the unknown related to surgery Encourage verbalization of concerns Provide emotional support to client and family Minimize external stimuli (e.g., noise, movement) Reassure child that he/she will be able to talk	Assess level of anxiety Encourage verbalization of concerns Provide emotional support to client and family Provide information and encouragement to client and family
Diet	*Preoperative:* NPO Baseline nutritional assessment *Postoperative:* Advance to clear liquid to full liquid following surgery; offer cool fluids Encourage large sips of fluids No straws No citrus juices	Advance to regular diet as tolerated

CLINICAL PATHWAY—continued

TONSILLECTOMY AND ADENOIDECTOMY

CATEGORY	IMMEDIATE PERIOPERATIVE PERIOD	DISCHARGE TO HOME CARE
Activity	As desired until premedicated for surgery In bed with rails up once premedicated Progress from bed rest to dangling on side of bed to walking postoperatively as tolerated	Provide safety precautions Encourage bed rest for first 24 hours, then advance as tolerated to normal activity
Medications	Preoperative medications, postoperative analgesics, and antibiotics as ordered	Analgesics as ordered Antibiotics if ordered NO ASPIRIN
Transfer/discharge plans	Assess discharge plans and support system	Probable discharge within 6 hours of surgery Complete discharge home care teaching when fully awake and oriented and before discharge Provide a written copy of discharge instructions Provide telephone number or other resource for questions

Adapted with permission from Beyea, S. C. (1996). Critical pathways for collaborative nursing care. Upper Saddle River, NJ: Prentice Hall–Health.

EVALUATION

Expected outcomes of nursing care for the child with tonsillitis include the following:

- Adequate intake of food and fluids
- Management of pain and fever
- Absence of postoperative complications such as bleeding, hemorrhage, and dehydration
- Healing without impairment following tonsillectomy

MOUTH AND DENTAL EMERGENCIES

Children may have trauma to the mouth and teeth during sporting activities and during other injuries. About 10% of children experience some dental trauma (Diangelis & Bakland, 1998). Nurses inform parents of proper treatment for injuries and may provide emergency treatment in schools and other community settings. Injury prevention includes use of protective gear during sports. See Chapter 50 for a discussion of oral care during treatment for cancer, and see Chapter 36 for a discussion of protective sporting gear and of body piercing which may include the oral cavity.

Since the mouth has a profuse blood supply, bleeding may be extensive for even minor injuries. It is best to use clean cloths to absorb the blood and prevent choking on it, and get the child to an emergency facility to have the lesion carefully examined.

Dental injuries may involve fracture of a tooth, luxation (partial extrusion), or avulsion (complete removal). The child should be transported immediately to an emergency facility. If the child is otherwise stable, an emergency dental visit is the best choice. When avulsion has occurred, fast care can improve chances that a permanent tooth can be reimplanted and kept alive. Chances of tooth survival are best when reimplanted within 30 minutes (Rudy, 2001). Nurses can perform care or teach parents what to do in case of dental emergency. Referral to dental resources may be needed. Families with financial constraints may lack dental care and resources. Seek resources in the local community for families in need of dental assistance.

TEACHING HIGHLIGHTS

CARE OF A TOOTH AVULSION

When a tooth is removed during an injury, prompt treatment may improve the chance that it can be reimplanted. If the child's condition is stable, try to reimplant the tooth and then transfer to an emergency dental facility.

- Handle the tooth only by the crown (its top).
- Gently rinse the tooth in a bowl of tap water. Do NOT place it under running water.
- Insert into the socket.
- Have the child provide gentle pressure by biting a piece of gauze or a tea bag.

If the child is unstable or has other injuries, enlist emergency medical transportation (call 911). In this case the tooth is transported with the child.

- Place the tooth in milk, saline, saliva, or water. If a dental aid kit is available it may contain a transport liquid called Hank's Balanced Salt Solution.

Data from Rudy, C. A. (2001). Dental trauma. School Nurse News, 18(1), 33–35. Adapted.

Critical Concept Review

LEARNING OBJECTIVES

CONCEPTS

Describe abnormalities of the eyes, ears, nose, throat, and mouth in children.

→

Eyes:
1. Conjunctivitis:
   - Inflammation of the conjunctiva.
   - Caused by viruses, bacteria, allergy, trauma, or irritants.
2. Cellulitis:
   - Infection of the eyelid and the surrounding tissues.
3. Visual disorders:
   - Errors of refraction.
   - Abnormal musculature.
   - Malignancies of the eye.
   - Glaucoma and cataracts.
   - Retinopathy of prematurity.
4. Injuries to the eye.

Ears:
1. Otitis media:
   - Inflammation of the middle ear.
2. Otitis externa:
   - Inflammation of the skin and tissue of the ear canal.
3. Hearing impairment:
   - Genetic.
   - Environmental.
   - Unknown causes.

Nose, throat, and mouth:
1. Epistaxis:
   - Caused by low humidity or irritation.
2. Nasopharyangitis:
   - Inflammation or infection of the nose and throat.
3. Sinusitis:
   - Inflammation of one or more of the paranasal sinuses.
4. Pharyngitis:
   - Infection primarily of the tonsils.
5. Tonsillitis:
   - Infection and hypertrophy of the palatine tonsils.
6. Mouth ulcers.
7. Trauma to the mouth and teeth.

Plan for screening programs and identification of children with vision and hearing abnormalities.

→

Vision:
1. Assess for eye symmetry and movement, for ability to follow objects with each eye, and for any abnormalities in appearance of eyes at each well-child visit.
2. Visual acuity screenings should be performed annually beginning at age 5.

Hearing:
1. All newborns should be screened for hearing abnormalities while in the newborn nursery.
2. Hearing and speech development should be assessed at each well-child visit.

Plan nursing care for children with vision or hearing impairments.

→

Vision impairment:
1. Call the child's name and identify self upon entering the room and inform the child before leaving the room.
2. Describe all procedures before they are done.
3. Allow child to touch the equipment if possible.
4. Describe the foods and their location when food trays are delivered.

Hearing impairment:
1. Touch the child to get his or her attention.
2. Stand in front of the child and speak normally.
3. Keep room well-lit.

LEARNING OBJECTIVES

CONCEPTS

Plan nursing care for children with vision or hearing impairments—continued

→

4. Be familiar with the child's hearing amplification system so that it is placed correctly.
5. Provide a picture board to aid in communication.
6. Have an interpreter available if child understands only American Sign Language.

Use latest recommendations when implementing care and teaching for children with abnormalities of eyes, ears, nose, throat, and mouth.

→

1. Prevention of vision and hearing impairment and loss depends on early diagnosis and treatment.
    ■ Screen for visual and hearing acuity at every well-child visit and every 2–3 years during elementary school.
2. Instruct parents in the correct use of a child's adaptive devices (lenses and aides) and use of medication.
3. Inform parents about risks and benefits of cochlear implant surgery.

Integrate preventive and treatment principles when implementing care for children related to eyes, ears, nose, and throat.

→

Eyes:
1. Prevent eye injuries by teaching safety in activities that can injure the eye.
2. Encourage the use of protective eye wear for sports, school projects, and yard work
Ears:
1. Instruct parents and child concerning the dangers of listening to loud music with and without headphones.
2. Encourage the use of ear protection when child is exposed to loud noise.
Nose, throat, and mouth:
1. Instruct parents concerning the importance of completing the entire course of antibiotics when treating a throat infection.
2. Stress the importance of the use of mouth guards when playing sports.

CRITICAL THINKING IN ACTION

*View the **Critical Thinking in Action** video in Chapter 46 of the CD-ROM. Then, answer the questions that follow.*

You are working at a local children's urgent care facility when a couple comes in carrying their screaming 9-month-old child, Becky. The parents are worried as Becky has been crying steadily for the past 2 hours. You ask about recent illnesses or injuries and they tell you that she has had only two colds in her life and the most recent was about a week ago.

You assess Becky's vital signs as follows: weight 19 pounds (8.6 kilograms), temperature 101 degrees F, respirations 60 breaths per minute without retractions, and heart rate 120 beats per minute. She does not have any rashes or evidence of injuries, and upon examination she appears well nourished but clearly in distress. Her heart rate is regular and rhythm and breath sounds are equal bilaterally and clear to auscultation. Both tympanic membranes are red and bulging. Her abdomen is soft and without organomegaly. The doctor diagnoses bilateral acute otitis media and administers analgesic ear drops and ibuprofen in the office. Within 15 minutes, Becky has settled down, stopped crying, and is resting in her father's arms. The family is sent home with instructions to administer analgesics and return with 48 hours for further assessment.

1. What are the three main organisms that may have caused Becky's otitis media?
2. What are some of the guidelines you can give Becky's parents about otitis media treatment?
3. The mother says she has family members who have had tubes placed in their ears because of ear infections and wants to know if this is something that Becky will need to have done.
4. What are some methods parents can use to prevent future otitis media episodes?

MediaLink

www.prenhall.com/london

- NCLEX-RN® Review, case studies, and other interactive resources for this chapter can be found on the Companion Website at http://www.prenhall.com/london. Click on "Chapter 46" to select the activities for this chapter.

- For animations, more NCLEX-RN® Review questions, and an audio glossary, access the accompanying CD-ROM in this textbook.

REFERENCES

Agency for Healthcare Research and Quality. (2001). *Management of acute otitis media* (AHRQ Pub. No. 00-E010). Rockville, MD: Author.

Alcorn, D. M. (2001, March). Red eye: When to treat and when to refer. *Infectious Diseases in Children*, 3–8.

Alexander, M. (2003). Ocular allergy: Treatment options for children. *Contemporary Pediatrics*, Suppl., 3–6.

American Academy of Pediatrics, Section on Ophthalmology. (2001). Screening examination of premature infants for retinopathy of prematurity. *Pediatrics, 108*, 809–811.

American Academy of Pediatrics, Subcommittee on Management of Acute Otitis Media. (2004). Diagnosis and management of acute otitis media. *Pediatrics, 113*, 1451–1465.

Bacal, D. A., & Wilson, M. C. (2000). Strabismus: Getting it straight. *Contemporary Pediatrics, 17*, 49–60.

Bachman, K. R., & Arvedson, J. C. (1998). Early identification and intervention for children who are hearing impaired. *Pediatrics in Review, 19*, 155–165.

Behrman, R. E., Kliegman, R. M., & Jenson, H. B. (2004). *Nelson textbook of pediatrics* (17th ed.). Philadelphia: Saunders.

Brocklehurst, P., & Rooney, G. (2000). Interventions for treating genital *Chlamydia trachomatis* infection in pregnancy. *Cochrane Database Systematic Review 2000, (2)*, CD000054.

Brookhouse, P. E., Beauchaine, K. L., & Osberger, M. J. (1999). Management of the child with sensorineural hearing loss: Medical, surgical, hearing aids, cochlear implants. *Pediatric Clinics of North America, 46*, 121–142.

Burns, C. E., Brady, M. A., Dunn, A. M., & Starr, N. B. (2000). *Pediatric primary care* (2nd ed.). Philadelphia: WB Saunders.

Center for Health and Health Care in Schools. (2004). *Childhood vision: What the research tells us.* Retrieved June 15, 2004, from http://www.healthinschools.org

Cheng, A. K., Rubin, H. R., Powe, N. R., Mellon, N. K., Francis, H. W., & Niparko, J. K.

(2000). Cost-utility of the cochlear implant in children. *Journal of the American Medical Association, 284*, 850–856.

Committee on Infectious Diseases. (2003). *Red book* (26th ed.). Elk Grove Village, IL: American Academy of Pediatrics.

Committee on Sports Medicine and Fitness. (2004). Protective eyewear for young athletes. *Pediatrics, 113*, 619–622.

Coody, D., Banks, J. M., Yetman, R. J., & Musgrove, K. (1997). Eye trauma in children: Epidemiology, management, and prevention. *Journal of Pediatric Health Care, 11*, 182–188.

Curns, A. T., Holman, R. C., Shay, D. K., Cheek, J. E., Kaufman, S. F., Singleton, R. J., & Anderson, L. J. (2002). Outpatient and hospital visits associated with otitis media among American Indian and Alaska Native children younger than 5 years. *Pediatrics, 109*(3). Retrieved October 25, 2005, from www.pediatrics.org/cgi/content/full/109/3/e41.

DeRespinis, P. A. (2001). Eyeglasses: Why and when do children need them? *Pediatric Annals, 30*, 455–461.

Diangelis, A. J., & Bakland, L. K. (1998). Traumatic dental injuries: Current treatment concepts. *Journal of the American Dental Association, 129*, 1401–1414.

Duchene, T. M. (2000). Managing sinusitis in children. *Nurse Practitioner, 25*(9), 42–55.

Folmer, R. L. (2003). The importance of hearing conservation instruction. *Journal of School Nursing, 19*, 140–148.

Garganta, C., & Seashore, M. R. (2000). Universal screening for congenital hearing loss. *Pediatric Annals, 29*, 302–308.

Garrelts, L., & Melnyk, B. M. (2001). Pacifier usage and acute otitis media in infants and young children. *Pediatric Nursing 27*, 516–518.

Gomez, S., & Davis, R. L. (2001). Photoscreening—A viable method for referral. *School Nurse News, 18*(1), 18–20.

Gross, R. D. (2002). Understanding ocular infections and strategies for management. *Contemporary Pediatrics*, Suppl., 4–7, 10–12.

Halle, C. (2002). Achieve new vision screening objectives. *Nurse practitioner, 27*(3), 15–37.

Hayes, D. (1999). State programs for universal newborn hearing screening. *Pediatric Clinics of North America, 46*, 89–94.

Hayes, R. O. (2001). Pediatric sinusitis. *Clinician Reviews, 11*(10). 53–58.

Hoberman, A., Marchant, C. D., Kaplan, S. L., & Feldman, S. (2002). Treatment of acute otitis media consensus recommendations. *Clinical Pediatrics, 41*, 373–390.

Hoberman, A., & Paradise, J. L. (2000). Acute otitis media: Diagnosis and management in the year 2000. *Pediatric Annals, 29*, 609–620.

Jackson, J. M., & Mourino, A. P. (1999). Pacifier use and otitis media in infants twelve months of age and younger. *Pediatric Dentistry, 21*, 256–260.

Joint Committee on Infant Hearing. (2000). Joint committee on infant hearing 2000 position statement: Principles and guidelines for early hearing detection and intervention programs. *Pediatrics, 106*, 798–817.

Kakish, K. S., Mahafza, T., Batieha, A., Ekteish, F., & Daoud, A. (2000). Clinical sinusitis in children attending primary care centers. *Pediatric Infectious Disease Journal, 19*, 1071–1074.

Kemper, K. J. (2001). Complementary and alternative medicine for children: Does it work? *Archives of Disease in Childhood, 84*(1), 6–9.

Kemper, K. J., & Sarah, R. (2000). On pins and needles? Pediatric pain patients' experience with acupuncture. *Pediatrics, 105*, 941–947.

Lee, A. C., Highfield, E. S., Berde, C. B., & Kemper, K. J. (1999). Survey of acupuncturists: Practice characteristics and pediatric care. *Western Journal of Medicine, 171*(3), 153–157.

Leung, A. K. C., & Kellner, J. D. (2004). Acute sinusitis in children: Diagnosis and management. *Journal of Pediatric Health Care, 18*, 72–76.

Little, P., Gould, C., Williamson, I., Moore, M., Warner, G., & Dunleavey, J. (2001). Pragmatic randomized controlled trial of two prescribing strategies for childhood acute otitis media. *British Medical Journal, 322*, 336–342.

Newland, J. A., & Rich, E. (1998). Epistaxis. *American Journal of Nursing, 98,* 16HHH.

Niemela, M., Pihakari, O., Pokka, T., Uhari, M., & Uhari, M. (2000). Pacifier as a risk factor for acute otitis media: A randomized, controlled trial of parental counseling. *Pediatrics, 106,* 483–488.

Niemela, M., Uhari, M., & Mottonen, M. (1995). A pacifier increases the risk of recurrent otitis media in children in day-care centers. *Pediatrics, 96,* 884–888.

Niskar, A. S., Kieszak, S. M., Holmes, A. E., Esteban, E., Rubin, C., & Brody, D. J. (2001). Estimated prevalence of noise-induced hearing threshold shifts among children 6 to 19 years of age: The third national health and nutrition examination survey, 1988–1994, United States. *Pediatrics, 108,* 40–43.

Otitis Media with Effusion, Clinical Practice Guideline. (2004). *Pediatrics, 113,* 1412–1429.

Paradise, J. L., Feldman, H. M., Campbell, T. F., Dollaghan, C. A., Colburn, D. K., Bernard, B. S., et al. (2001). Effect of early or delayed insertion of tympanostomy tubes for persistent otitis media on developmental outcome at the age of 3 years. *New England Journal of Medicine, 344,* 1170–1187.

Roberts, J. E., Burchinal, M. R., & Zeisel, S. A. (2002). Otitis media in early childhood in relation to children's school-age language and academic skills. *Pediatrics, 110,* 696–706.

Rudy, C. A. (2001). Dental trauma. *School Nurse News, 18(1),* 33–35.

Sagraves, R. (2002). Increasing antibiotic resistance: Its effect on the therapy for otitis media. *Journal of Pediatric Health Care, 16,* 79–87.

Sarrell, E. M., Mandelberg, A., & Cohen, H. A. (2001). Efficacy of naturopathic extracts in the management of ear pain associated with acute otitis media. *Archives of Pediatric and Adolescent Medicine, 155,* 796–799.

Scheiner, A. P. (1996). Vision problems: Impairment to blindness. In A. M. Rudolph, J. I. E. Hoffman, & C. D. Rudolph (Eds.), *Rudolph's pediatrics* (20th ed., p. 167). Stamford, CT: Appleton & Lange.

Sinus and Allergy Health Partnership. (2000). Antimicrobial treatment guidelines for acute bacterial rhinosinusitis. *Otolaryngology and Head and Neck Surgery, 123,* 5–31.

Slattery, W. H., & Fayad, J. N. (1999). Cochlear implants in children with sensorineural inner ear hearing loss. *Pediatric Annals, 28,* 359–363.

Starr, N. B. (2000). Vision therapy for learning disabilities and dyslexia. *Journal of Pediatric Health Care, 14,* 32–33.

Stephenson, M. (2003). Mucopurulent discharge is good sign conjunctivitis is bacterial. *Infectious Diseases in Children, 3,* 32–33.

Subcommittee on Management of Acute Otitis Media, American Academy of Pediatrics. (2004). Diagnosis and management of acute otitis media. *Pediatrics, 113,* 1451–1465.

Subcommittee on Management of Sinusitis and Committee on Quality Improvement, American Academy of Pediatrics. (2001). Clinical practice guideline: Management of sinusitis. *Pediatrics, 108,* 798–808.

U.S. Preventive Services Task Force. (2004). *Screening for visual impairment in children younger than age 5 years.* Retrieved June 1, 2004, from http://www.ahrq.gov/clinic/3rduspstf.visionscr/sicshrs.htm

Vohr, B. R., Widen, J. E., Cone-Wesson, B., Sininger, Y. S., Gorga, M. P., Folsom, R. C., & Norton, S.J. (2000). Identification of neonatal hearing impairment: Characteristics of infants in the neonatal intensive care unit and well-baby nursery. *Ear & Hearing, 21,* 373–382.

Walter, W. F., Cunningham, G. C., Davis, J. G., Morton, C. C., Elsas, L. J., Finitzo, T., Fack, R. E. Ing, P. S., Pandya, A., McCube, E. R. B., & Smith, R. J. H. (2000). Statement of the American College of Medical Genetics on universal newborn hearing screening. *Genetics in Medicine, 2,* 149–150.

Wheatley, C. M., Dickinson, J. L., Mackey, D. A., Craing, J. E., & Sale, M. M. (2002). Retinopathy of prematurity: Recent advances in our understanding. *Archives of Disease in Childhood, 87,* F78–F82.

White, K. R., & Maxon, A. B. (1999). *Early identification of hearing loss: Implementing universal newborn hearing screening programs.* Rockville, MD: U.S. Department of Health & Human Services, Maternal & Child Health Bureau.

Zacharyczuk, C. (2004, April). New guidelines outline AOM management options. *Infectious Diseases in Children, 24.*

The Child with Alterations in Respiratory Function

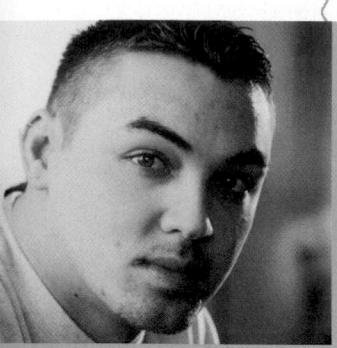

Emily gets sick so much faster than my other children. I guess the bronchopulmonary dysplasia and her tracheostomy make her more susceptible to infections. I really get concerned because she struggles so hard to breathe when she gets all these extra secretions. I have learned to suction and change her tracheostomy, but I am afraid that one day she will completely obstruct her airway. I just hope I remember all the things I have been taught if that happens, and that the emergency medical personnel come quickly.
—Father of Emily, 8 months

LEARNING OBJECTIVES

- Describe unique characteristics of the pediatric respiratory system anatomy and physiology and apply that information to the care of children with respiratory conditions.

- List the different respiratory conditions and injuries that can cause respiratory distress in infants and children.

- Assess the child's respiratory signs and symptoms

to distinguish between respiratory distress and respiratory failure and describe the appropriate nursing care.

- Develop a nursing care plan for a child with common acute respiratory conditions.

- Develop a nursing care plan for the child with a chronic respiratory condition.

MEDIALINK www.prenhall.com/london

CD-ROM

Animations/Videos
   CO_2 and O_2 Transport
   Gas Exchange
   Pediatric Respiratory Emergency Management
   SIDS
Skill 11-12: Using a Metered Dose Inhaler
Skill 14-2: Oxygen Saturation: Pulse Oximetry
Skill 14-5: Peak Expiratory Flow Meter
Skill 14-11: Tracheostomy Care
Skill 14-25: Chest Physiotherapy/Postural Drainage
NCLEX-RN® Review
Audio Glossary

Companion Website

MediaLink Applications
   Teaching Plan: Metered Dose Inhaler
   Nursing Care Plan: The Child with Cystic Fibrosis
   Care Plan: Bronchopulmonary Dysplasia
   Teaching Plan: Dust Mites
   Respiratory Risks in a Childcare Setting
Medication Administration
Bronchial Hygiene Therapy
Asthma Guidelines: For Children Under 5
NCLEX-RN® Review
Audio Glossary

This chapter explores several special factors in the child's respiratory system that create ongoing threats to respiratory function and overall health. Most respiratory problems in children produce mild symptoms, last a short time, and can be managed at home. Nevertheless, acute respiratory problems are the most common cause of illness requiring hospitalization in infants and children under 10 years of age and a leading cause of hospitalization in children between 10 and 15 years of age (Health Resources and Services Administration, 2002).

Pediatric respiratory conditions may occur as a primary problem or as a complication of nonrespiratory conditions and may be life threatening or have long-term implications. Nurses must learn to assess the child's current respiratory status quickly, monitor progress, and anticipate potential complications (Table 47-1).

Respiratory problems may result from structural problems, functional problems, or a combination of both. Structural problems involve alterations in the size and shape of parts of the respiratory tract. Functional problems involve

---

TABLE 47-1 ❖ Assessment Guidelines for a Child in Respiratory Distress[a]

Quality of Respirations

- Inspect the rate, depth, and ease of respirations. See Table 35-8 for expected respiratory rate ranges by age. ∞
- Identify the signs of respiratory distress: **tachypnea** (abnormally rapid rate of respirations), retractions, nasal flaring, inspiratory stridor, expiratory grunting.
- Note lack of simultaneous chest and abdominal rise with inspiration (**paradoxical breathing**).
- Auscultate breath sounds to see if they are bilateral, diminished, or absent, and for presence of **adventitious** sounds (wheezes, crackles, rhonchi).

Quality of Pulse

- Assess the rate and rhythm: *tachycardia may indicate hypoxia.*
- Compare pulse sites (apical to brachial) for strength and rate.

Color

- Observe overall color: with respiratory distress, color progresses from pallor to mottled to cyanosis; *central cyanosis is a late sign of respiratory distress.*
- Compare peripheral and central color: assess capillary refill and nailbed color and inspect mucous membranes; *central cyanosis in mucous membranes is more ominous.*
- Note whether crying improves or worsens color.

Cough

- Quality: note whether it is dry (nonproductive), wet (productive, mucousy), brassy (noisy, musical), or croupy (barking, seal-like).
- Effort: note whether it is forceful or weak; *weak cough may indicate an airway obstruction or fatigue from prolonged respiratory effort (not valid in newborns).*

Behavior Change

- Note level of consciousness: alert or lethargic; *lethargy may indicate hypoxia.*
- Restlessness and irritability are associated with hypoxia.
- Watch for abrupt behavior changes; *restlessness, irritability, and lowered level of consciousness may indicate increasing hypoxia.*

Signs of Dehydration

- Inspect for dry mucous membranes, lack of tears, poor skin turgor, and decreased urine output, which indicate that fluid needs are not being met.

[a]Refer to Chapter 35 for the actual techniques of assessment mentioned in this table.

alterations in gas exchange and threats to this normal process from irritants (such as large particles and chemicals) or invaders (such as viruses or bacteria). Alterations in other organ systems, especially the immune and neurologic systems, may also threaten respiratory function. When reading this chapter, keep the distinction between structural and functional problems in mind to help distinguish between what is normal and what is abnormal about the child's maturing respiratory system. See Chapter 46 for upper respiratory conditions such as colds, otitis, sinusitis, and pharyngitis. ∞

ANATOMY AND PHYSIOLOGY OF PEDIATRIC DIFFERENCES

The child's respiratory tract constantly grows and changes until about 12 years of age. The young child's neck is shorter than an adult's, resulting in airway structures that are closer together.

UPPER AIRWAY DIFFERENCES

The child's airway is shorter and narrower than an adult's. These differences create a greater potential for obstruction (see "As Children Grow: Airway Development"). The infant's airway is approximately 4 mm in diameter, about the width of a drinking straw, in contrast to the adult's airway diameter of 20 mm. The trachea primarily increases in length rather than diameter during the first 5 years of life. The child's little finger is a good estimate for the child's tracheal diameter and can be used for a quick assessment of airway size. The trachea in a child is higher and at a different angle than the adult's (see "As Children Grow: Trachea Position"). The child's narrower airway causes an increase in **airway resistance**, the effort or force needed to move

AS CHILDREN GROW

Airway Development

Smaller nasopharynx, easily occluded during infection.

Lymph tissue (tonsils, adenoids) grows rapidly in early childhood; atrophies after age 12.

Smaller nares, easily occluded.

Small oral cavity and large tongue increase risk of obstruction.

Long, floppy epiglottis vulnerable to swelling with resulting obstruction.

Larynx and glottis are higher in neck, increasing risk of aspiration.

Because thyroid, cricoid, and tracheal cartilages are immature, they may easily collapse when neck is flexed.

Because fewer muscles are functional in airway, it is less able to compensate for edema, spasm, and trauma.

The large amounts of soft tissue and loosely anchored mucous membranes lining the airway increase risk of edema and obstruction.

It is easy to see that a child's airway is smaller and less developed than an adult's airway, but why is this important? An upper respiratory tract infection, allergic reaction, positioning of the head and neck during sleep, and the small objects children play with can have serious consequences in the child.

AS CHILDREN GROW

Trachea Position

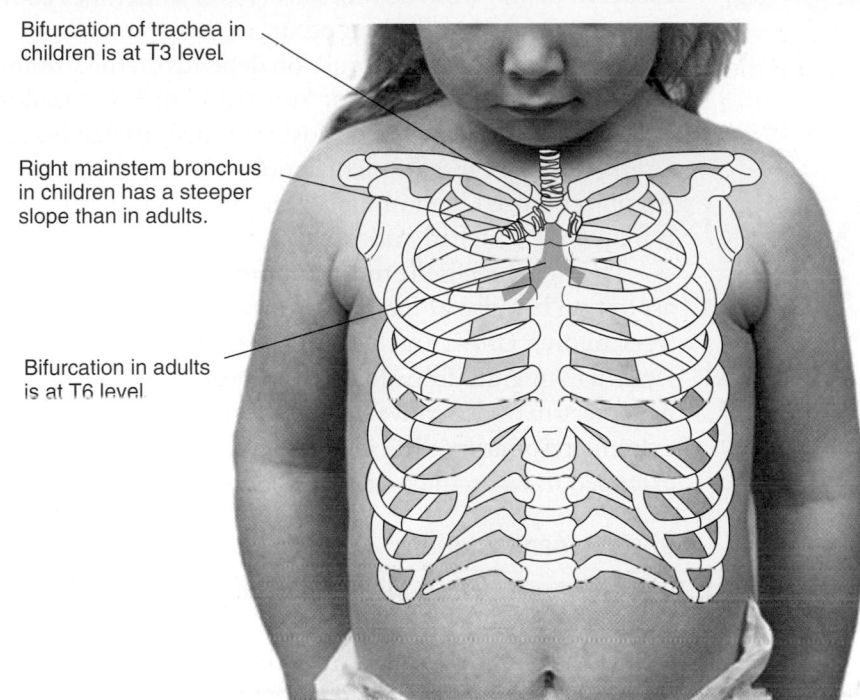

Bifurcation of trachea in children is at T3 level.

Right mainstem bronchus in children has a steeper slope than in adults.

Bifurcation in adults is at T6 level.

In children, the trachea is shorter and the angle of the right bronchus at bifurcation is more acute than in the adult. When you are resuscitating or suctioning, you must allow for the differences. Do you think that this difference is significant in respiratory infection? Why?

oxygen through the trachea to the lungs (see "Pathophysiology Illustrated: Airway Diameter").

Physiologically, the upper airway is the port for inspiration of oxygen and expiration of carbon dioxide. Infants, children, and adults can breathe through either the nose or the mouth. Until 4 weeks of age, newborns are obligatory nose breathers. The coordination of mouth breathing is controlled by maturing neurologic pathways; thus, young infants do not automatically open the mouth to breathe when the nose is obstructed. The only time a newborn breathes through the mouth is when he or she is crying. Nasal patency in newborns is therefore essential for such activities as breathing and eating.

Lower Airway Differences

The developing alveoli change size and shape, and their numbers increase until respiratory maturity is attained at puberty (Froh, 2002). Alveolar growth increases the area available for gas exchange. At birth the distal (peripheral) bronchioles that extend to the alveoli are narrow and fewer in number than in an adult. The child's overall growth can be correlated to the increased branching of the peripheral bronchioles as the alveoli continue to multiply. The taller the child, the greater the lung surface area.

The bronchi and bronchioles are lined with smooth muscle. The newborn does not have enough smooth mus-

GROWTH AND DEVELOPMENT

At birth the lung tissue contains only 25 million alveoli, which are not fully developed. The number of alveoli increases to 300 million by 8 years of age, after which these structures begin increasing in size and complexity until puberty (Froh, 2002).

cle bundles to help trap airway invaders. By 5 months of age, however, a baby has enough muscles to react to irritants by bronchospasm and muscle contraction. Smooth muscle development is complete and comparable to that of an adult by 1 year of age (Webster & Huether, 1998).

Ventilation is the movement of air in and out of the lungs and alveoli. The lungs rely on the diaphragm and intercostal muscles to power respiration. Children under 6 years of age use the diaphragm to breathe as the intercostal muscles are immature. The negative pressure caused by the downward movement of the diaphragm draws in air. By 6 years of age, the child uses the intercostal muscles more effectively. The ribs are primarily cartilage and very flexible, and in cases of respiratory distress, the negative pressure caused by the diaphragm movement causes the chest wall to be drawn inward, causing **retractions** (see "Pathophysiology Illustrated: Retraction Sites").

PATHOPHYSIOLOGY ILLUSTRATED
Airway Diameter

Newborn

1 mm
swelling

4 mm

2 mm

Adult

1 mm
swelling

20 mm
diameter of airway

18 mm
diameter of airway

The diameter of an infant's airway is approximately 4 mm, in contrast to an adult's airway diameter of 20 mm. An inflammatory process in the airway causes swelling that narrows the airway, and airway resistance increases. Note that swelling of 1 mm reduces the infant's airway diameter to 2 mm, but the adult's airway diameter is only narrowed to 18 mm. Air must move more quickly in the infant's narrowed airway to get the same amount of air to the lungs. The friction of the quickly moving air against the side of the airway increases airway resistance. The infant must use more effort to breathe and breathe faster to get adequate oxygen.

RESPIRATORY DISTRESS AND RESPIRATORY FAILURE

Many respiratory conditions associated with difficulty breathing can progress to respiratory distress. If the condition is not managed effectively, it can progress to respiratory failure. Foreign-body aspiration is a common cause of airway obstruction and respiratory distress.

FOREIGN-BODY ASPIRATION

Foreign-body aspiration is the inhalation of any object (solid or liquid, food or nonfood) into the respiratory tract. Aspiration occurs most often during feeding and reaching activities, while crawling, or during playtime in children 6 months to 4 years of age. These young children have a tendency to put small objects in the mouth. However, aspiration may occur in children of any age.

Etiology and Pathophysiology

In infants over 6 months of age and young children, any number of small objects that make their way into the child's mouth may cause aspiration. Foods such as nuts, popcorn, or small pieces of raw vegetables or hot dog; small, loose toy parts such as small wheels and bells; or household objects and substances such as beads, safety pins, coins, buttons, latex balloon pieces, and colorful liquids (mouthwash, perfume) in enticing packages (screw-top bottles) are frequent causes of airway obstruction. Partial and sometimes complete airway obstruction can occur.

The severity of the obstruction depends on the size and composition of the object or substance and its location within the respiratory tract. Most aspirated foreign bodies (AFBs) usually cause bronchial, not tracheal, obstruction. An object lodged high in the airway above the vocal cords is frequently coughed out.

The right lung is the most common site of lower airway aspiration because of the sloped angle of its bronchus (see "As Children Grow: Trachea Position" on page 1391). Objects may migrate from higher to lower airway locations. An object may also move back up to the trachea, creating extreme respiratory difficulty. If oxygen is depleted for an extended time, brain damage may occur.

Clinical Manifestations

Children are usually brought to the hospital after a sudden episode of coughing or gagging. The child may have signs of increased respiratory effort such as **dyspnea** (difficulty breathing), tachypnea (rapid respiratory rate), nasal flaring, and retractions. If the child cannot say the "P" in words like *Pluto* or *Peter Pan,* the foreign body has noticeably diminished expiratory effort. As respiratory distress progresses, the child may have a concentrated focus on breathing, have an anxious expression, and sit in a forward position with the neck extended. As the child becomes increasingly hypoxic, behavior changes such as irritability and decreased responsiveness are seen.

Coughing, choking, gagging, dysphonia, and wheezing may be brief or may persist for several hours if the object drops below the trachea into one of the mainstem bronchi. In some cases the child may become asymptomatic after coughing for 15 to 30 minutes. If the foreign body drops into the lower airway and is not removed, the child may present with a chronic cough, persistent or recurrent pneumonia, or a lung abscess weeks later.

Clinical Therapy

Clinical therapy focuses on taking a careful history to determine whether aspiration has indeed occurred. Coughing, gagging, or choking associated with feeding or crawling on the floor is usually a confirming event for aspiration. The physical examination often reveals decreased breath sounds, stridor, and respiratory distress in the child without a witnessed aspiration. A special radiograph, called a forced expiratory film, may be ordered. This shows local hyperinflation (air trapping) and a mediastinal shift away from the affected side (Hazinski, 1999). Sometimes, when the object aspirated is radiopaque, it

PATHOPHYSIOLOGY ILLUSTRATED

Retraction Sites

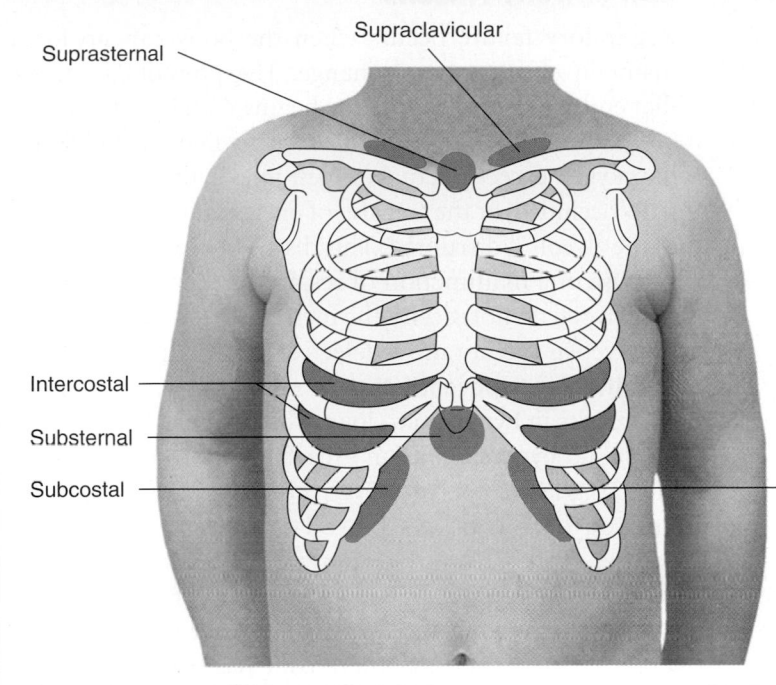

Suprasternal

Supraclavicular

Supraclavicular

Intercostal

Substernal

Subcostal

Subcostal

Retractions may occur in the very young infant in the suprasternal area. In the older infant and child, retractions occur when the airway is severely obstructed, as in croup. The depth and location of retractions is associated with the severity of respiratory distress. Isolated intercostal retractions indicate mild distress. Subcostal, suprasternal, and supraclavicular retractions indicate moderate distress. These retractions accompanied by use of accessory muscles indicate severe distress.

MEDIALINK

Video: Pediatric Respiratory Emergency Management

can be seen on an x-ray film (Figure 47–1 ●). Chest thrusts and back blows or the abdominal thrust are used to remove an object from an obstructed airway. An object lodged in the trachea is a life-threatening situation. (See Skill 14–14.) **SKILLS**

● **FIGURE 47–1**

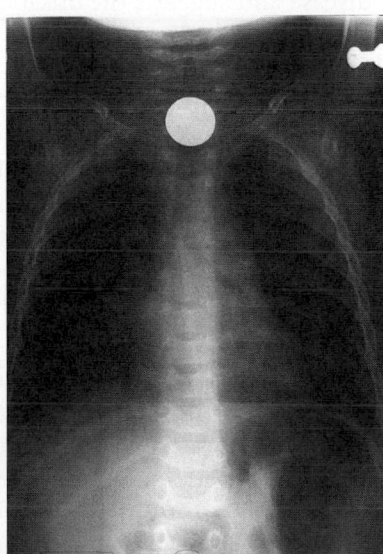

An aspirated foreign body (coin) is clearly visible in the child's trachea on this chest x-ray.

Courtesy of Rockwood Clinic, Spokane, WA.

Fluoroscopy and fiberoptic bronchoscopy may be used to identify, locate, and extract the AFB. See the section on pneumonia, page 1409, for care of the child with complications of aspiration.

NURSING MANAGEMENT

NURSING ASSESSMENT AND DIAGNOSIS

Physiologic Assessment

The child will be in respiratory distress, and constant monitoring is essential. Perform the respiratory assessment following guidelines in Table 47–1. If the object remains lodged, observe the child for increasing signs of respiratory distress, especially vital signs, audible wheezing on auscultation, and retractions. Note changes in breath sounds, from noisy to decreasing to absent, on the affected side. This can indicate that the object is moving and blocking a mainstem bronchus. Attach the child to a cardiorespiratory monitor and pulse oximeter to assess the child for subtle signs of increasing hypoxia.

Psychosocial Assessment

The unexpected and acute nature of the event creates anxiety for both parents and child. The child will be fearful because of difficulty breathing. Assess coping and level of stress.

NURSING PRACTICE

These signs and symptoms signal the body's response to increased metabolic demands for oxygenation as a result of airway stress, obstruction, or impending illness:

- Increasing restlessness, irritability, unexplained sudden confusion
- Rapid heart rate accompanied by rapid respiratory rate

Developmental Assessment

As the child's condition stabilizes, observe how well the child's abilities match the parents' understanding of age-appropriate behaviors. See developmental abilities by age Chapter 33. ∞

Common nursing diagnoses for a child with an AFB include the following:

- *Ineffective Airway Clearance* related to foreign body aspiration
- *Impaired Spontaneous Ventilations* related to foreign body aspiration and respiratory muscle fatigue
- *Fear (Parent or Child)* related to uncertainty of prognosis, unfamiliar surroundings and procedures
- *Risk for Injury* related to developmental age and small objects in environment

PLANNING AND IMPLEMENTATION

The period right after aspiration until AFB removal is critical. Promptly document and report any subtle changes in the child's respiratory status. The nurse must remain with the child who has a significant obstruction, and have resuscitation equipment at the bedside. Permit the child to stay in a position of comfort. Avoid performing procedures that increase the child's anxiety as sudden movements and increased respiratory efforts may cause the obstruction to move and completely obstruct the airway. Be prepared to perform back blows and chest thrusts for an infant or abdominal thrusts for the child with complete obstruction. (See Skill 14–9. **SKILLS**)

After the AFB is removed, the child is stabilized and observed for a few hours in a short-stay unit.

Discharge Planning and Home Care Teaching

Discharge planning centers on anticipatory guidance about childproofing the home (see Chapter 33 ∞). Encourage the parents to learn CPR, choking-prevention techniques, and back blows, chest thrusts, or abdominal thrusts.

EVALUATION

Expected outcomes of nursing care include the following:

- The child regains the ability to ventilate spontaneously after removal of the foreign body.

- Parents complete a safety check of the home to prevent future aspiration incidents.

RESPIRATORY FAILURE

Respiratory failure occurs when the body can no longer maintain effective gas exchange. The physiologic process that ends in respiratory failure begins with hypoventilation of the alveoli. Hypoventilation occurs when the body's need for oxygen exceeds actual oxygen intake, the airway is partially occluded, or the transfer of oxygen and carbon dioxide in the alveoli is disrupted. This disruption may occur either because of a malfunction of respiratory center stimulation (the alveoli do not receive the message to diffuse) or because the alveolar membrane is defective (a structural problem).

Alveolar hypoventilation (poor ventilation of the alveoli) results in **hypoxemia** (lower than normal blood oxygen level) and **hypercapnia** (an excess of carbon dioxide in the blood). Arterial blood gas levels indicative of respiratory failure are a PaO_2 level less than 50 mm Hg and a $PaCO_2$ level greater than 50 mm Hg in a patient breathing room air (Grant & Curley, 2001). See Appendix B for expected laboratory values by age and Skill 10–6. **SKILLS** When the blood levels of oxygen and carbon dioxide reach abnormal levels, **hypoxia** (lower than normal oxygen in the tissues) occurs and respiratory failure begins. *Hypoxemia that persists when supplemental oxygen is given is a sign of respiratory failure.*

Signs of impending respiratory failure include irritability, lethargy, cyanosis, and increased respiratory effort such as dyspnea, tachypnea, nasal flaring, and intercostal retractions. Grunting slows the expiratory flow and increases the lung volume and alveolar pressures. This is a sign of severe disease and suggests the onset of respiratory failure (Margolis & Gadomski, 1998).

Nursing Management

Early recognition of impending respiratory failure is the most important aspect of care for a child with any signs of respiratory compromise. When the child has a chronic respiratory condition, development of respiratory failure may be gradual. Signs will be subtle. Be particularly alert to behavior changes in addition to respiratory signs. Serial blood gases may be needed to monitor the child.

Place a child who has respiratory distress in an upright position (by elevating the head of the bed). Assess respiratory quality and rate, followed by apical pulse rate and temperature. Monitor oxygen saturation with pulse oximetry. Administer oxygen as ordered and keep respiratory emergency equipment at the child's bedside. Monitor the child for changes in vital signs, respiratory status, and level of responsiveness. Be prepared to assist ventilations if respiratory status deteriorates. (See Skills 9–8 to 9–10. **SKILLS**)

CLINICAL MANIFESTATIONS

RESPIRATORY FAILURE AND IMMINENT RESPIRATORY ARREST

PHYSIOLOGIC CAUSE	CLINICAL MANIFESTATIONS
Respiratory failure These signs occur because the child is trying to compensate for oxygen deficit and airway blockage. Oxygen supply is inadequate; behavior and vital signs reflect compensation and beginning hypoxia.	*Initial signs* Restlessness Tachypnea Tachycardia Diaphoresis
The child tries to use accessory muscles to assist oxygen intake; hypoxia persists and efforts now waste more oxygen than is obtained.	*Early decompensation* Nasal flaring Retractions Grunting Wheezing Anxiety and irritability Mood changes Headache Hypertension Confusion
Imminent respiratory arrest These signs occur because oxygen deficit is overwhelming and beyond spontaneous recovery. Cerebral oxygenation is dramatically affected; central nervous system changes are ominous.	*Severe hypoxia* Dyspnea Bradycardia Cyanosis Stupor and coma

Excessive crying and anxiety deplete metabolic reserves. External ventilatory support and vigorous crying may impede diaphragm function if the stomach becomes distended with air. Because the child's metabolic rate is about double that of an adult, the child has a greater need for oxygen. Respiratory distress, anxiety, and even fever can dramatically add to the child's oxygen demand.

Using Artificial Airways

Respiratory problems that do not respond to oxygen therapy, medications, or position changes require the insertion of an artificial airway. As the child's level of responsiveness deteriorates, the ability to keep the airway open decreases. Endotracheal intubation is a short-term, emergency measure to stabilize the airway by placing a tube in the trachea. The tube must be protected and stabilized to prevent its displacement. (See Skills 14–8 and 14–9. SKILLS) A tracheostomy is the creation of a surgical opening into the trachea through the anterior neck at the cricoid cartilage. Surgeons prefer to perform this procedure in the operating room; however, a tracheostomy may also be performed in an emergency department or other setting when immediate intervention is needed. These children usually require admission to the intensive care unit (ICU) for monitoring and ventilatory support. Suction airway secretions as needed and provide tracheostomy care if present. See Skills 14–20—14–24 in the *Clinical Skills Manual.* SKILLS

Because endotracheal and tracheostomy tubes prevent vocal cord vibration, intubated children cannot cry or talk. Infants and young children often express initial frustration when they realize they cannot communicate verbally. When the child is alert, give suggestions for ways to make noise and gain attention, such as striking the mattress. A communication board can be used with older children.

Many children are discharged from the hospital and cared for at home for an extended period with a tracheostomy tube in place. It is essential to teach parents how

THINKING CRITICALLY

OXYGEN DELIVERY DEVICES

Oxygen delivery devices are selected to match the concentration of oxygen needed by the child. In respiratory failure, a higher concentration of oxygen is needed to reverse the hypoxemia. Which oxygen delivery device should be used? Are there any contraindications to oxygen use in a child who is hypoxic?

to maintain the airway, clean the tracheostomy site, and change the tube. A home healthcare nurse can provide follow-up care and support for the child and family. (See Skill 14–11. SKILLS)

APNEA

Infants have **periodic breathing**, an irregular rhythm, and may have pauses of up to 20 seconds between breaths. This breathing pattern is not apnea. **Apnea** is the cessation of respiration lasting longer than 20 seconds, or any pause in respiration associated with cyanosis, marked pallor, hypotonia, or bradycardia. Apnea may be the first major sign of respiratory dysfunction in the newborn (see respiratory distress in Chapter 30 ∞).

APPARENT LIFE-THREATENING EVENT (ALTE)

Apparent life-threatening event (ALTE) is defined as an episode of apnea accompanied by a color change (cyanosis, pallor, or occasionally ruddiness), limp muscle tone, choking, or gagging in a near-term or term infant who is greater than 37 weeks' gestation. The majority of these events occur in infants under 4 months of age, with a peak incidence between 1 week and 2 months (Davies & Gupta, 2002). These episodes may occur during sleep, wakefulness, or

CLINICAL MANIFESTATIONS

CAUSES OF APPARENT LIFE-THREATENING EVENTS

CAUSE	CLINICAL MANIFESTATIONS	DIAGNOSTIC TESTS
Functional or structural airway problem or immaturity	Apnea of 20 sec or longer; accompanied by bradycardia or cyanosis	Cardiorespiratory monitoring, sleep study, pneumogram, sepsis workup
Aspiration as a result of dysfunctional swallowing or gastroesophageal reflux	Choking, coughing, cyanosis, vomiting	Barium swallow, esophageal pH probe
Cardiac problems	Tachycardia, tachypnea, dyspnea	Cardiorespiratory monitoring, electrocardiogram, echocardiogram, arterial blood gases
Drug toxicity or poisoning; maternal history of ingestion	Central nervous system depression, hypotonia	Serum magnesium level, toxicity screen
Environmental, thermoregulation problem	Lethargy, tachypnea, hypothermia or hyperthermia	Cardiorespiratory and temperature monitoring, environmental temperature level (ambient air temperature)
Impaired oxygenation, respiratory disease (pulmonary edema, atelectasis, pneumonia)	Cyanosis, tachypnea, respiratory distress, anemia, choking, coughing	Oximetry, chest radiograph, arterial blood gases, complete blood count, upper airway evaluation, sleep study, serum electrolytes
Acute infection (sepsis, meningitis, necrotizing enterocolitis)	Feeding intolerance, lethargy, temperature instability	Complete blood count, cultures when appropriate, C-reactive protein, chest and abdominal radiographs
Intracranial pathology (intraventricular hemorrhage, ventricular dilation, central nervous system anomalies, meningitis)	Abnormal neurologic examination, seizures	Cranial ultrasound, computed tomography scan, electroencephalogram, magnetic resonance imaging, cerebrospinal fluid evaluation
Metabolic disorders	Jitteriness, poor feeding, lethargy, central nervous system depression or irritability, hypotonia	Serum electrolytes (potassium, sodium, chloride), glucose, calcium, arterial blood gases

Data from Theobald, K., Botwinski, C., Albanna, S., & McWilliam, P. (2000). Apnea of prematurity: Diagnosis, implications for care, and pharmacologic management. Neonatal Network, 19(6), 17–24; and Eichenwald, E., & Stark, A. (1992). Apnea of prematurity: Etiology and management. Tufts University School of Medicine Reports on Neonatal Respiratory Diseases, 2(1), 1–11. Adapted.

feeding. ALTE should not be confused with sudden infant death syndrome (SIDS) (see page 1398).

A variety of identifiable diseases and conditions can cause ALTE, such as infection, gastroesophageal reflux, seizures, cardiac arrhythmias, and metabolic or endocrine problems. In some cases, no cause is identified. ALTE can frighten the parent or observer, who often fears the infant has died. Emergency resuscitation is usually required.

Nursing Management

After ALTE, infants are usually admitted to the hospital for evaluation and cardiorespiratory monitoring. Nursing care includes collecting a detailed history of the event, observing and monitoring cardiorespiratory status, providing supportive care to the infant and family, and anticipating the need for emergency resuscitation and for the diagnostic process.

Monitor Cardiorespiratory Status. Cardiorespiratory monitoring records heart rate and respiratory rate while the infant is awake and asleep. Pulse oximetry provides a noninvasive continuous evaluation of the infant's oxygenation status. A pulse oximetry reading (SpO2) less than 95% indicates hypoxemia. (See Skills 14–2 to 14–4. **SKILLS**)

Provide Emotional Support. Establishing rapport and open communication with the parents is essential for creating a sense of trust. To obtain further information about the episode, use open-ended questions and active listening skills. Parents are fearful and anxious about the infant's prognosis. Explanations of tests and treatment help to decrease their anxiety and increase their understanding of the situation.

During hospitalization the infant should be held and cuddled to provide a sense of security and well-being. Encouraging parents' participation in the infant's care helps to meet these needs and promotes family bonding. Often parents are afraid to touch the infant because they might disconnect the monitoring cable. Wrapping the cable inside the infant's blanket helps secure the wires, increasing parents' feelings of confidence in handling the infant.

Support the mother to continue breastfeeding and maintaining a supply of breast milk by pumping, if necessary. Ensure that the mother gets adequate fluids and nutrition. Provide privacy for breast pumping, and store breast milk for future feedings.

Anticipate Emergency Resuscitation. Because the infant who has had ALTE continues to be at risk for cardiopulmonary arrest, keep emergency resuscitation equipment and drugs readily accessible at all times.

Discharge Planning and Home Care Teaching. Identify and address home care needs well in advance of discharge. Teach parents how to operate an apnea monitor, what to do when the infant has an apneic episode, and how to perform cardiopulmonary resuscitation (CPR) and choking-prevention techniques (see Skill 14–13 **SKILLS**).

OBSTRUCTIVE SLEEP APNEA

Obstructive sleep apnea syndrome (OSA) is a disorder of breathing during sleep that involves prolonged partial upper airway obstruction and/or intermittent complete obstruction that disrupts normal ventilation during sleep and normal sleep patterns (American Academy of Pediatrics, 2002). This results in labored breathing and snoring when the child tries to move air past the obstruction. Its incidence peaks between 2 and 6 years of age when tonsils and adenoids are at their largest in contrast to the airway's size.

The upper airway contains about 30 muscles that permit the pharynx to collapse, enabling the child to talk and swallow, but also maintain airway patency. When the child is awake, muscle tone is maintained and the airway remains patent even when obstructions such as enlarged adenoids and tonsils, craniofacial anomalies, or obesity are present. During sleep, the airway muscles relax and the pharynx becomes obstructed. When the airway muscles are relaxed, the airway resistance is increased. Reduced upper airway tone and obstruction then results in apnea episodes that lead to hypoventilation, hypoxia, hypercapnia, and an elevated blood pressure. Hypertrophy of the adenoids and tonsils is the most common cause of OSA, followed by craniofacial abnormalities. Without treatment, complications develop that can include failure to thrive, pulmonary hypertension, **cor pulmonale** (obstruction of pulmonary blood flow that leads to right ventricular hypertrophy and heart failure), systemic hypertension, and cognitive impairment.

Children with OSA snore and have signs of labored breathing during sleep such as retractions and paradoxical breathing. After pauses in snoring or lack of airflow, the child may be noted to snort, gasp, choke, move, or arouse to take a breath. Sleep is restless and the child may sleep in unusual positions to hyperextend the neck and airway. Daytime sleepiness and other symptoms of sleep deprivation (poor attention, increased activity, aggression, acting-out behavior, poor school performance) may be noted.

Diagnosis is made by **polysomnography**, a sleep study that simultaneously records the brain activity, eye movement, apnea episodes, oxygen desaturation and sleep disturbances. Adenotonsillectomy is the most common treatment for OSA, and resolution of the condition occurs in the majority of children. Weight loss strategies may be implemented for obese children. Continuous positive airway pressure (CPAP) is used for children with surgical contraindications or those with persistent OSA.

Nursing Management

In the community setting, all children should be screened for snoring as part of their routine healthcare. Assess the child for signs of nasal obstruction, mouth breathing, and enlarged tonsils. Determine if the child has symptoms of

TEACHING HIGHLIGHTS

HOME CARE INSTRUCTIONS FOR THE INFANT REQUIRING APNEA MONITORING

Apnea Equipment
- Understand monitor type, lead wires, placement of skin electrodes or chest belt, battery power, manual for troubleshooting.

Emergency Preparation
- Notify telephone company, electric company, local rescue squad, local emergency department (establishes priority status).
- Post phone numbers of rescue squad, physician, equipment company, power company, emergency number, cardiopulmonary resuscitation (CPR) guidelines, other important numbers (neighbor, parents' work numbers) in at least two places in the home; have at least one added extension phone.
- Keep the apnea monitor battery fully charged.

Safety Precautions
- Place monitor on firm surface; keep away from other appliances (television, microwave oven) and water.
- Ensure that alarms are audible from all locations.
- Double-check that monitor is on before going to bed.
- Thread cable and wires through lower end of infant's clothes.
- Ensure integrity of leads, monitor cable, and power cord (replace if frayed).

Routine Care
- Understand reasons for apnea monitor and frequency of use.
- Be able to attach and detach infant chest leads and belt.
- Evaluate skin for irritation or breakdown from electrode placement and give skin care (no oils or lotion; move patches correctly).

Emergency Care
- Develop plan for respiratory failure and power failure.
- Demonstrate CPR and back blows and chest thrusts for airway obstruction.
- Understand how to respond to alarms for apnea, bradycardia, or loose lead.

Apnea Alarm
- Observe infant's respiratory movement.
- If respiration is absent or infant is lethargic, stimulate by calling name and gently touching, proceeding to vigorous touch if needed.
- If no response, proceed with CPR.

Bradycardia Alarm
- Stimulate infant; infant should respond quickly.

Loose Lead
- Check electrode patch. Is it loose? Dirty? Belt loose?
- Check wires from electrode or monitor cable.
- Check power supply. Is battery low? Power failure? Monitor malfunctioning?

---

sleep deprivation or if a condition is present that places the child at high risk for OSA. Coordinate referral to a sleep center for polysomnogram evaluation and explain the purpose of the test. Discuss how to prepare the child for the strange setting and wires that will be attached during the sleep study. Most pediatric centers will allow the parent to stay with the child during the study.

Following adenotonsillectomy, the hospital nurse monitors the child for bleeding and respiratory distress, such as obstructive sleep apnea and pulmonary edema. Continuous pulse oximetry is used to detect oxygen desaturation. See Chapter 46 for care of the child having adenotonsillectomy. ∞

Sleep center nurses provide education and support to families of children who need to use CPAP to treat the OSA. The nurse helps identify the best fitting mask or nasal prong system for CPAP delivery. Parents may need guidance about helping children to go to sleep wearing the mask until they are accustomed to it.

SUDDEN INFANT DEATH SYNDROME (SIDS)

Sudden infant death syndrome (SIDS) has been defined as the sudden unexpected death of an infant under 1 year of age with onset of the fatal episode during sleep that remains unexplained after a thorough investigation, including an autopsy, a review of the circumstances of death, and a review of the clinical history (Krous, 2004). It remains a leading cause of death in infants between 1 month and 1 year of age, with 90% of cases occurring before 6 months of age (American Academy of Pediatrics Committee on Child Abuse and Neglect, 2001). SIDS occurs rarely in infants younger than 2 weeks. It is currently unpredictable and in some cases unpreventable.

SIDS is referred to as a "syndrome" because of the many and varied autopsy and clinical findings that characterize most infants who die of the disorder. The autopsy typically does not identify a disease process that caused the death. Current evidence suggests a genetic susceptibility to SIDS (American Academy of Pediatrics Committee on Fetus and Newborn, 2003). The current thinking is that vulnerable infants have a defect in the arcuate nucleus, a brain structure that plays a role in regulating breathing, heartbeat, body temperature, and arousal (Kato, Franco, Groswasser et al., 2003; Parnigrahy, Filiano, Sleeper et al., 2000). Child abuse and homicide may be associated with 1% to 5% of suspected SIDS cases (American Academy of Pediatrics Committee on Child Abuse and Neglect, 2001). Other proposed causes include *H. pylori* gastrointestinal infection and long QT syndrome, a cardiac arrhythmia. (See cardiac arrhythmias in Chapter 48. ∞) SIDS has not been found to be associated with newborn apnea or immunizations for diphtheria, tetanus, and pertussis (DTaP). See Table 47–2 for infant and maternal factors that place infants at risk for SIDS.

The first symptom is a cardiac arrest. Clinical findings include evidence of a struggle or change in position during sleep and the presence of frothy, blood-tinged secretions from the mouth and nares. Typically parents find the infant dead in the crib in the morning or after a nap and report having heard no cries or disturbances during the night.

Nursing Management

The sudden, unexpected nature of the infant's death is confirmed in the emergency department. The nurse's role is to be empathetic and provide support during one of the greatest crises a family must face. The focus is on supporting the family during the acute grieving period. See Table 47–3.

TABLE 47–2 ❖ Risk Factors for Sudden Infant Death Syndrome (SIDS)

Infant
- Race (in decreasing order of frequency): most common in Native American infants, followed by black, Hispanic, white, and Asian infants
- Gender: more common in males than females
- Age: most common in infants between 2 and 4 months of age
- Time of year: more prevalent in winter months
- Exposure to passive smoke
- Sleeping arrangement: prone or side-lying position and turning to prone, sharing bed with others, use of pillows and quilts with bedding
- Overheating due to excessive blankets, clothing on infant, room temperature

Maternal Risk Factors
- Maternal age less than 20 years at first pregnancy and a short interval between pregnancies
- Prenatal smoking, binge alcohol, and illicit drug use
- Anemia
- Poor prenatal care, low weight gain during pregnancy
- History of sexually transmitted disease or urinary tract infection

TABLE 47–3 ❖ Supportive Care for the Family of an Infant with Sudden Infant Death Syndrome (SIDS)

1. Provide parents with a private area and a support person who reinforces that the infant's death was not their fault. *Parents need to be able to express their grief in their own way and hear that they are not being blamed for the infant's death.*

2. Prepare the family for the viewing of the infant. Describe how the infant will look and feel. *You can say, "Paul's [use the infant's name] skin will feel cool. He will be very still and his eyes will be closed." They probably know this, but a gentle explanation demonstrates empathy. Explain that pooling of blood on the dependent areas will look like bruises.*

3. Allow parents to hold, touch, and rock the infant if desired. *Viewing the infant allows parents a chance to say good-bye. Before bringing the infant to parents, wrap in a clean blanket, comb the hair, wash the face, swab the mouth clean, and apply Vaseline to lips.*

4. Reinforce the physician's explanation about the need for an autopsy. *An autopsy is required for all unexplained deaths. You can say to parents, "It is the only way we can be sure of what caused your baby's death."*

5. Answer parents' questions and provide them with sources for further information. Provide literature and a name of the local contact for a SIDS support group, as well as for the national foundation. *Parents may not be able to take in all of your answers. Many emergency departments and pediatric units have a social worker who provides ongoing contact with the family. Provide names of resource people and phone numbers for SIDS support groups.*

6. Advise parents that surviving siblings may benefit from psychologic support. *Siblings often require emotional support in the weeks and months after the death. Social workers can help the family obtain counseling and support for all members.*

7. Provide parents with a lock of hair, footprints, and handprints, if they desire. *Personal items can be placed in a memory book. This reaffirms the child's existence for many parents.*

NURSING PRACTICE

Guidelines for the support of families experiencing SIDS should include baptism services, religious support, grief counseling, assistance with funeral arrangements, and counseling on cessation of breastfeeding and sibling reactions.

Reassure the parents that they are not responsible for the infant's death and help them contact other family members and mobilize support. Older children may need reassurance that SIDS will not happen to them. They may also believe that bad thoughts or wishes about their baby brother or sister caused the death. Support groups can help parents, siblings, and other family members express these fears and work through their feelings about the infant's death. The SIDS Alliance and SHARE are organizations that can help families locate a support group in their area. See the Companion Website for links.

Nurses can play an important role in educating the public about the link between SIDS and infant positioning during sleep. Educate the parents of all newborns and infants about the recommended sleep position—on the back—for infants, and ask them to make sure this position is used when the infant is cared for by another family member or childcare provider. Parents should also use a firm mattress and avoid the use of loose bedding, toys, and pillows. Place hospitalized infants to sleep in supine position rather than side-lying or prone. See Chapter 53 for issues related to infant skull flattening from sleeping on the back. ∞

CROUP SYNDROMES

Croup is a term applied to a broad classification of upper airway illnesses that result from swelling of the epiglottis and larynx. The swelling usually extends into the trachea and bronchi. Included under the classification of croup syndromes are viral syndromes, such as spasmodic laryngitis (spasmodic croup), laryngotracheitis, and laryngotracheobronchitis (LTB), and bacterial syndromes, such as bacterial tracheitis and epiglottitis (see "Pathophysiology Illustrated: Airway Changes with Croup").

LTB, epiglottitis, and bacterial tracheitis are referred to as the "big three" of pediatric respiratory illness because they affect the greatest number of children across all age groups in both sexes. The initial symptoms of all three conditions include inspiratory **stridor** (a high-pitched, musical sound that is created by narrowing of the airway), a "seal-like" barking cough, and hoarseness. LTB is the most common disorder, but epiglottitis and bacterial tracheitis are more serious.

LARYNGOTRACHEOBRONCHITIS

Although the term *croup* is applied to several viral and bacterial syndromes, it is most often used to refer to LTB, a viral invasion of the upper airway that extends throughout the larynx, trachea, and bronchi. Table 47–4 compares LTB and other croup syndromes.

Etiology and Pathophysiology

Acute viral LTB is most common in children 3 months to 4 years of age but can occur up to 8 years of age. Boys are affected more often than girls. LTB is of greatest concern in infants and children under the age of 6 years, because of potential airway obstruction. The causative organism is usually parainfluenza virus type I, II, or III, that appears during winter months. Other viruses causing LTB include

PATHOPHYSIOLOGY ILLUSTRATED
Airway Changes with Croup

Epiglottis swells occluding airway

Cricoid cartilage

Trachea swells against cricoid cartilage resulting in restriction

There are two important changes in the upper airway in croup: the epiglottis swells, thereby occluding the airway, and the trachea swells against the cricoid cartilage, causing restriction.

influenza A and B, adenovirus, respiratory syncytial virus, and measles (Perkin & Swift, 2002).

Airway tissues respond to the invading virus with inflammation and edema. Copious, tenacious secretions further increase the child's respiratory distress. The laryngeal inflammation causes the airway diameter to narrow in the subglottic area, the narrowest part of the airway. Even small amounts of mucus or edema can quickly obstruct the airway. Both the large and small airways can be affected.

Clinical Manifestations

Most children brought to the emergency department with LTB have been ill for a couple of days with upper respiratory symptoms. These symptoms progress to a cough and hoarseness. Fever may or may not be present. Common presenting signs are tachypnea, inspiratory stridor, and a seal-like barking cough.

Clinical Therapy

Diagnosis is often made by clinical signs. Pulse oximetry is used to detect hypoxemia. If the diagnosis of LTB is in question, anteroposterior (AP) and lateral x-rays of the up-

TABLE 47–4 ✤ Summary of Croup Syndromes

	VIRAL SYNDROMES			BACTERIAL SYNDROMES	
	Acute Spasmodic Laryngitis (Spasmodic Croup)	**Laryngotracheobronchitis**	**Laryngotracheitis**	**Bacterial Tracheitis**	**Epiglottitis (Supraglottitis)**
Severity	Least serious	Most common[a]	Most serious; progresses if untreated	Guarded; requires close observation	Most life threatening (medical emergency)[a]
Age affected	3 months to 3 years	3 months to 8 years	3 months to 8 years	1 month to 13 years[a]	2 years to 8 years
Onset	Abrupt onset; peaks at night, resolves by morning (recurs)[a]	Gradual onset; starts as URI, progresses to moderate respiratory difficulty	Gradual onset; starts as URI, progresses to symptoms of respiratory distress	Progressive from URI (1–2 days)	Progresses rapidly (hours)[a]
Clinical manifestations	Afebrile; mild respiratory distress; barking-seal cough	*Early:* mild fever [<39°C (102.2°F)]; hoarseness; barking-seal, brassy, croupy cough; rhinorrhea; sore throat; stridor (inspiratory); apprehension *Progressing to* labored respirations	*Early:* mild fever [<39°C (102.2°F)]; barking-seal, brassy, croupy cough; rhinorrhea; sore throat; stridor (inspiratory); apprehension; restless/irritable *Progressing to* retractions (progressive); increasing stridor; cyanosis	High fever [>39°C (102.2°F)]; URI appears as viral croupy cough and croup initially; stridor (tracheal); purulent secretions	High fever [>39°C (102.2°F)]; URI; intense sore throat; dysphagia[a]; drooling[a]; increased pulse and respiratory rate; prefers upright position (tripod position with chin thrust)[a]
Etiology	Unknown; suspect viral with allergic/ emotional influences	Parainfluenza, types I and II, RSV, or influenza	Parainfluenza, types I and II, RSV, or influenza	*Staphylococcus*	*Haemophilus influenzae*

[a]Classic parameter or key point (distinguishes condition).

per airway are taken; these may show symmetric subglottic narrowing called a "steeple sign." Throat cultures and visual inspection of the inner mouth and throat are contraindicated in children with LTB and epiglottitis. These procedures can cause **laryngospasms** (spasmodic vibrations that close the larynx) as a result of the child's anxiety or of probing this reactive and already compromised area.

Clinical therapy consists of maintaining and improving respiratory effort with medications, humidification, and supplemental oxygen when the saturated oxygen level is less than 92% (see Table 47–5). Mist tents are rarely used for laryngotracheobronchitis.

Children with a good response to medications are often sent home from the emergency department after an observation period. Children with moderate to severe symptoms after medications are admitted for further observation and treatment. Airway obstruction is a potential complication of LTB. The child may require intubation and transfer to the ICU to maintain airway patency if obstruction is imminent. Most children, however, respond positively to the

TABLE 47–5 ✤ Medications Used for Symptomatic Treatment of Laryngotracheobronchitis

Medication	Action/Indication	Nursing Considerations
Beta-agonists and beta-adrenergics (e.g., albuterol, racemic epinephrine): aerosolized through face mask	Rapid-acting bronchodilator, decreases bronchial and tracheal secretions and mucosal edema, used to decrease symptoms of moderate to severe respiratory distress; and constriction of subglottic mucosa and submucosal capillaries. Used until dexamethasone begins working.	Provides only temporary relief; improvement in 30 minutes which lasts about 2 hours, it gives time for the steroid to work; the child may experience tachycardia (160–200 beats/min) and hypertension; dizziness, headache, and nausea may necessitate stopping medication; reduces the need for artificial airway
Corticosteroids (e.g., dexamethasone): IM, PO, nebulized budesonide	Anti-inflammatory, used to decrease edema; has a long half-life of 36–54 hours	The child may experience cardiovascular symptoms (hypertension): requires close observation for individual response; children less frequently need emergency airways; stridor resolves faster

medications and oxygen therapy and are discharged within 48 to 72 hours.

NURSING MANAGEMENT

NURSING ASSESSMENT AND DIAGNOSIS

The initial and ongoing physical assessment of the child with LTB focuses on adequacy of respiratory functioning. See Tables 47–6 and 47–7. Continuous monitoring is required to identify changes in airway patency. A means of communication (sign language or simple word cues) must be established so the older child can alert nursing staff to respiratory difficulty.

Pay particular attention to the child's respiratory effort, breath sounds, and responsiveness. Physical exhaustion can diminish the intensity of retractions and stridor. As the child uses the remaining energy reserve to maintain ventilation, breath sounds may actually diminish. Noisy breathing (audible airway congestion, coarse breath sounds) in this situation verifies adequate energy stores. Responsiveness decreases as hypoxemia increases.

NURSING PRACTICE

Observe the child continuously for inability to swallow, absence of voice sounds, increasing degree of respiratory distress, and acute onset of drooling (an ominous sign of supraglottic obstruction). If any of these signs occur, get medical assistance immediately. The quieter the child, the greater the cause for concern.

The following nursing diagnoses might be appropriate for the child with acute LTB:

- *Ineffective Breathing Pattern* related to tracheobronchial obstruction, decreased energy, and fatigue
- *Risk for Deficient Fluid Volume* related to inadequate fluid intake prior to admission
- *Fear (Child)* related to unfamiliar surroundings, procedures, and separation from support system

PLANNING AND IMPLEMENTATION

Maintain Airway Patency

Supplemental oxygen with humidity may be needed for hypoxemia. Cool mist is presumed to moisten airway secre-

---

TABLE 47–6 ✣ Clinical Scoring System for Assessing Children with Stridor

Sign	0	1	2	3
Stridor	None	With agitation	Mild at rest	Severe at rest
Retraction	None	Mild	Moderate	Severe
Air entry	Normal	Normal	Decreased	Severe decrease
Color	Normal	Normal	Cyanotic with agitation	Cyanotic with rest
Level of consciousness	Normal	Restless if disturbed	Restless if undisturbed	Lethargic

Scoring: To quantifiy the severity of stridor, add the individual scores for each of the sign categories. A score between 0 and 15 is possible. A rating of severity based on total score is as follows: < 6 is mild, 7–8 is moderate, > 8 is severe.

Source: From Perkin, R. M., & Swift, J. D. (2002). Infectious causes of upper airway obstruction in children. *Pediatric Emergency Medicine Reports, 7*(11), 120.

TABLE 47–7 ✣ Nursing Assessment of Child with Respiratory Difficulty

Nursing Action	Rationale
Assess heart rate and respiratory rate.	Tachypnea and tachycardia indicate increasing respiratory effort.
Check position of the child (sitting, prone, or supine)?	Upright or semi-Fowler's promotes airway patency; the child's own attempt or desire to change to a more upright position may signal increased distress.
Assess overall quality of respiratory effort. Determine inspiratory and expiratory breath sounds, ability to speak, and presence of stridor, cough, retractions, nasal flaring, cyanosis.	Reflects overall adequacy of airway and respiratory function.
Initiate stridor scoring assessment (Table 47-6), continue scoring every 30 minutes or more frequently if distress increases; initiate nursing actions appropriate for stridor score.	Provides consistent and objective assessment data with score for future comparison.
Attach cardiorespiratory monitor and pulse oximeter.	Provides continuous assessment data as part of ongoing physiologic monitoring.

tions and soothe the inflamed mucosa, but research has not documented its benefit (Perkin & Swift, 2002). Allow the child to assume a comfortable position. Be immediately available to attend to the child's respiratory needs, and keep resuscitation equipment at the bedside.

Meet Fluid and Nutritional Needs

The respiratory distress may have interfered with the child's ability and desire to drink fluids and compromised the child's fluid status. Recognizing fluid deficit and monitoring the child's hydration and nutritional status are essential. Fluids promote liquification of secretions and provide calories for energy and metabolism.

Children with LTB usually prefer cool, noncarbonated, nonacidic drinks such as oral rehydration fluids. The parents can be encouraged to give the child oral fluids. An intravenous infusion may be necessary to rehydrate the child, maintain fluid balance, or provide emergency access. Observe the child closely for difficulty in swallowing, which may be an early sign of epiglottitis or bacterial tracheitis.

Discharge Planning and Home Care Teaching

During the child's observation period, take every opportunity to assess the parents' knowledge of symptoms of LTB and discuss actions to take if symptoms recur. For example, instruct parents to call the child's physician if:

- Mild symptoms do not improve after 1 hour of humidity and cool air treatment.
- The child's breathing is rapid and labored.
- The child does not drink adequate fluids and the urine output is reduced.

EVALUATION

Expected outcomes of nursing care include the following:

- The child responds to medications with decreased respiratory distress.
- The child's fear and anxiety is managed with family support and explanations about care.

Epiglottitis (Supraglottitis)

Epiglottitis (also known as supraglottitis) is an inflammation of the epiglottis, the long narrow structure that closes off the glottis during swallowing. Because edema in this area can rapidly (within minutes or hours) obstruct the airway by occluding the trachea, epiglottitis is considered a potentially life-threatening condition. (Table 47–4 compares epiglottitis and other croup syndromes.)

Epiglottitis is caused by bacterial invasion of the soft tissue of the larynx by streptococcus and staphylococcus, and by *Haemophilus influenzae* type B (Hib) in unimmu-

nized children. The resulting inflammation and edema in the tissues and surrounding the epiglottis lead to airway obstruction. Since the widespread use of the Hib vaccination, a tenfold decrease in the incidence of epiglottitis has occurred (Isaacson & Isaacson, 2003).

Characteristically, a previously healthy child suddenly becomes very ill. The child initially develops a high fever (greater than 39°C [102.2°F]), with a sore throat, **dysphonia** (muffled, hoarse, or absent voice sounds), and **dysphagia** (difficulty in swallowing). As the larynx becomes obstructed, inspiratory stridor and respiratory distress develop. The intense throat pain keeps the child from swallowing, resulting in drooling. To fully open the airway and improve air intake, the child sits up and leans forward with the jaw thrust forward in the classic "sniffing" or tripod posture and refuses to lie down. The child's anxiety increases as it becomes more difficult to breathe.

Diagnosis is often based on a lateral neck x-ray (Figure 47–2 ⊙), which reveals a narrowed airway and an enlarged, rounded epiglottis, seen as a mass at the base of the tongue. Laryngospasm and airway obstruction can occur as a result of the severe irritation and hypersensitivity of the airway muscles. For this reason, *visual inspection of the mouth and throat is contraindicated in children with suspected epiglottitis.*

Immediate clinical therapy usually involves insertion of an endotracheal tube to maintain the airway. At the same time, a culture of the epiglottis is taken. Antibiotics effective for gram-positive organisms and *H. influenzae* are given until culture sensitivities are available. Antipyretics (acetaminophen, ibuprofen) may be useful in managing fever and sore throat pain.

⊙ **FIGURE 47–2**

— Enlarged, rounded epiglottis
— Narrow airway

The phrase "thumb sign" has been used to describe this enlargement of the epiglottis. Recall the trachea's usual "little finger" size. Do you see the stiff, enlarged "thumb" above it in this lateral neck x-ray?

Nursing Management. Nursing management consists of airway management, drug therapy, hydration, and emotional and psychosocial support of the child and parents.

Until the child is intubated, the child is usually sedated and needs to be positioned to maintain the airway and breathe more easily. Observe the child's respiratory and airway status closely and often. Note any change in level of consciousness. Anxiety-provoking procedures are postponed until the airway is stabilized. Crying stimulates the airway, increases oxygen consumption, and can precipitate laryngospasm. Supplemental humidified oxygen may be used initially to reverse hypoxemia.

Until the endotracheal tube is removed, the child is usually managed in the ICU to ensure continual observation. (See Skill 14–12. **SKILLS**) Administer antibiotics to treat the infection and IV fluids to provide hydration. Because the child was febrile with a sore throat before admission, fluid intake may have been compromised.

The loss of voice, or even the inability to create sounds, can be frightening to a child. The unfamiliar hospital environment and strange equipment can create stress for child and parent alike. Reassure the parents that the child's voice loss is temporary and explain the need for the various pieces of equipment.

Most children show rapid improvement once oxygen, antibiotics, and fluid therapy are started. The endotracheal tube can usually be removed within 24 to 36 hours (Hazinski, 1999). Home care may involve completing the course of antibiotics. Parents need instructions on proper administration and potential problems of drug therapy.

Bacterial Tracheitis

Bacterial tracheitis is a secondary infection of the upper trachea after viral laryngotracheitis that is most often caused by *Staphylococcus aureus, group A streptococcus, Moraxella catarrhalis,* or *Haemophilus influenzae.* The disorder starts with croupy cough and stridor but progresses to include a high fever (greater than 39°C [102.2°F]), respiratory distress, and a toxic appearance (Stroud & Friedman, 2001). Table 47–4 compares bacterial tracheitis and other croup syndromes.

Because of the similarity of symptoms, bacterial tracheitis is often misdiagnosed initially as LTB. Instead of improving with therapy, however, the child's condition becomes worse. Children generally prefer lying flat to sitting up. This seems to be a position of comfort that allows the child to conserve energy. Diagnosis is often made by blood cultures after the child is found unresponsive to usual LTB management. The subglottis is edematous with ulceration, and thick mucopurulent exudate may obstruct the airway. Antibiotics are given for a full 10- to 14-day course. Most children need a secured artificial airway for 3 to 11 days and ventilatory support.

Nursing Management. The child with bacterial tracheitis is frequently cared for in the PICU after intubation. Mechanical suctioning of the thick tracheal secretions that pool high in the upper airway helps maintain a patent airway. Provide humidified air or oxygen. Antibiotics are administered as ordered. The previous section on epiglottitis discusses other nursing care interventions that may also be appropriate for the child with bacterial tracheitis.

LOWER AIRWAY DISORDERS

The lower airway, or bronchial tree, lies below the trachea and includes the bronchi, bronchioles, and alveoli. Lower airway disorders occur because a structural or functional problem interferes with the lungs' ability to complete the respiratory cycle. Lower airway disorders include bronchopulmonary dysplasia, bronchitis, bronchiolitis, pneumonia, and tuberculosis.

BRONCHITIS

Acute bronchitis, inflammation of the trachea and bronchi, rarely occurs in childhood as an isolated problem. The bronchi can be affected simultaneously with adjacent respiratory structures during a respiratory illness. Bronchitis is caused most often by a virus but may also result from invasion of bacteria or in response to an allergen or irritant.

The classic symptom of bronchitis is a coarse, hacking cough, which increases in severity at night. Children with bronchitis look tired. The chest and ribs may be sore because of the deep and frequent coughing. There is often a deep, rattling quality to breathing. Some children have audible wheezing that can be heard without a stethoscope. Treatment is palliative unless a secondary bacterial infection occurs.

NURSING MANAGEMENT

Nursing management includes supporting respiratory function through rest, humidification, hydration, and symptomatic treatment. Refer to the sections on asthma and pneumonia for detailed information on treatment measures.

Home care should emphasize the self-limiting nature of the disorder. Advise parents who smoke that quitting or refraining from smoking in the child's presence may benefit the child.

BRONCHIOLITIS

Bronchiolitis is a lower respiratory tract illness that occurs when an infecting agent (virus or bacterium) causes inflammation and obstruction of the small airways, the bronchioles. The peak age for bronchiolitis is 2 to 6 months (Cooper, Banasiak, & Allen, 2003). Infection is most severe in infants under 6 months of age and in children with heart and lung disease. Bronchiolitis is responsible for 90,000 hospital admissions and 4500 deaths per year (Agency for Healthcare Research and Quality, 2003).

ETIOLOGY AND PATHOPHYSIOLOGY

Infection with *respiratory syncytial virus* (RSV) is the most common cause, but other viral, bacterial, and mycoplasmal organisms may also be responsible. RSV occurs in annual epidemics from October to March. It is transmitted through direct or close contact with respiratory secretions of infected individuals. Nearly all children have been infected with RSV by 2 years of age, and reinfection (via siblings or close family contacts) throughout life is common (National Respiratory and Enteric Virus Surveillance System, 2000).

Viruses, acting as parasites, are able to invade the mucosal cells that line the small bronchi and bronchioles. The invaded cells die when the virus bursts from inside the cell to invade adjacent cells. The membranes of the infected cells fuse with adjacent cells, creating large masses of cells or "syncytia." The resulting cell debris clogs and obstructs the bronchioles and irritates the airway. In response, the airway lining swells and produces excessive mucus. Despite this protective effort by the bronchioles, the actual effect is partial airway obstruction and bronchospasms.

NURSING PRACTICE

Respiratory syncytial virus (RSV) is the most common cause of lower respiratory tract infections in infants and children. RSV causes severe or fatal illness in infants with conditions such as congenital heart disease, bronchopulmonary dysplasia (BPD), prematurity, and immunosuppression. Healthcare workers should follow principles of good handwashing, as the virus is easily transmitted and can survive on the hands for 30 minutes or more (American Academy of Pediatrics, 2003).

The cycle is repeated throughout both lungs as the airway cells are invaded by the virus. The partially obstructed airways allow air in, but the mucus and airway swelling block expulsion of the air. This creates the wheezing and crackles in the airways. Air trapped below the obstruction also interferes with normal gas exchange, leading to hypoxemia. The child with RSV is therefore at risk for respiratory failure as the oxygen level decreases and the carbon dioxide level increases. Apnea and pulmonary edema may occur.

CLINICAL MANIFESTATIONS

The infant or child with bronchiolitis may have been ill with upper respiratory symptoms such as nasal stuffiness, cough (not usually noted in infants), and fever (less than

39°C [102.2°F]) for a few days. As the illness progresses and the lower respiratory tract becomes involved, symptoms increase and include inspiratory and expiratory wheezing; a deeper, more frequent cough; tachypnea; retractions; and more labored breathing. As severe respiratory distress develops, marked retractions, crackles, cyanosis, and diminished breath sounds are noted. Thus the noisier the lungs, the better, as this indicates that the child is still able to move air in and out of the lungs.

Parents report that the infant or child is acting more ill—appearing sicker, less playful, and less interested in eating. Infants, especially, may refuse to feed or may spit up what they do eat along with thick, clear mucus. Dehydration may be present.

CLINICAL THERAPY

The history and physical examination provide the data needed to diagnose bronchiolitis. Chest radiographs show nonspecific findings of inflammation. Enzyme-linked immunoabsorbent assay (ELISA) or direct fluorescent assay performed on a nasal wash specimen are laboratory tests used to identify the virus causing bronchiolitis (see Skills 10–13 and 10–14 **SKILLS**).

Children who test positive for RSV are isolated, roomed together, or placed on the same ward to minimize the spread of the virus to other hospitalized children. Supportive care is provided, especially when the causative agent is unknown and the condition is mild to moderate in severity. See Table 47–8 for clinical therapies. The child may be intubated and ventilated for apnea or respiratory failure. Ribavirin is the only antiviral drug available for treatment. Studies have not confirmed its effectiveness, so it is reserved for life-threatening cases (Wright, Pomerantz, & Luria, 2002).

The following high-risk infants are recommended to receive 5 monthly injections of palivizumab beginning in October or November to prevent RSV infection (American Academy of Pediatrics Committee on Infectious Diseases and Committee on Fetus and Newborn, 2003):

- Prematurity—born at 32 weeks of gestation or earlier, particularly if less than 6 months of age at the start of the RSV season.
- Chronic lung disease such as BPD who have required supplemental oxygen, bronchodilator, diuretic, or corticosteroid therapy within 6 months of the start of RSV season.
- Complicated congenital heart disease, particularly those on medication to control congestive heart failure, with cyanosis, and with moderate to severe pulmonary hypertension.
- Immunocompromised infants and children may benefit.

TABLE 47–8 ❖ Clinical Therapy for Bronchiolitis

Clinical Therapy	Rationale
Cardiorespiratory monitor and pulse oximetry	Enable provider to follow course and assess need for specific therapies.
Humidified oxygen therapy via hood or face tent, mask, or nasal cannula	Delivery method determined by desired concentration of oxygen, degree of moisture, and child's response.
Intubation and assisted ventilation (PEEP/CPAP)	Used when the child becomes too fatigued to breathe effectively.
Hydration via intravenous or oral fluids	Provider must consider insensible fluid loss, decreased intake, the child's current electrolyte and hydration status, and risk for pulmonary edema.
Systemic medications	Bronchodilators, steroids, and beta-antagonists act directly on inflamed and obstructed airways; bronchodilators help prevent apnea episodes in premature infants; nebulized epinephrine, and corticosteroids are occasionally used.
Postural drainage and chest physiotherapy	Helps to further loosen and mobilize trapped mucus.
High-Risk Infant or Child[a] RespiGam (RSV immune globulin) IV Palivizumab (Synargis) IM	Give for 5 consecutive months during RSV season to high-risk children. May prevent RSV bronchiolitis or reduce severity of disease.

[a]Defined as a child with congenital heart disease, bronchopulmonary dysplasia, chronic lung problems, or cystic fibrosis or who is premature or severely ill and less than 6 months old.

Intravenous RSV immune globulin (RespiGam) may alternatively be used in some children under 2 years of age, and these children should wait 9 months before receiving live virus vaccines (varicella and MMR).

NURSING MANAGEMENT

NURSING ASSESSMENT AND DIAGNOSIS

Physiologic Assessment

Assess airway and respiratory function carefully. Good observation skills are important to ensure timely interventions for worsening respiratory symptoms and prevention of respiratory distress (see Table 47–1 and the clinical manifestations of respiratory failure on page 1392). An oxygen saturation level below 90% is the best indicator of the severity of the disease.

See "Nursing Care Plan: The Child with Bronchiolitis."

Psychosocial Assessment

Observe children and their parents for signs of fear and anxiety (Table 47–9). The unfamiliar hospital environment and procedures can increase stress. Parents' questions, as well as their nonverbal cues, help direct nursing interventions during admission and throughout hospitalization.

Common nursing diagnoses for the child with bronchiolitis include the following:

■ *Ineffective Breathing Pattern* related to increased airway secretions, fatigue from coughing and dyspnea, and air trapping

■ *Activity Intolerance* related to imbalance between oxygen supply and demand

■ *Risk for Deficient Fluid Volume* related to inability to meet fluid needs and increased metabolic demands (insensible loss, fever, thickened or increased respiratory secretions)

TABLE 47–9 ❖ Psychosocial Assessment of the Child with an Acute Respiratory Illness

Child

■ Assess for indications of anxiety or fear that may have an impact on respiratory status.
■ For young children, ask about security objects (such as a blanket or doll), the child's reaction to strangers, and reaction to absence of parents.
■ For older children, ask whether this is the first hospital stay and what previous illness and hospital experiences have meant to the child.

Parents

■ Assess parents' reactions: Are they anxious? Fearful? Verbal or quiet? Asking appropriate questions?
■ Observe for nonverbal cues. Often parents have financial worries (cost of hospital stay, lost work and wages) and personal worries (siblings at home who are ill) that they may not readily share with staff.

NURSING CARE PLAN

THE CHILD WITH BRONCHIOLITIS

Intervention	Rationale	Expected Outcome
1. Nursing Diagnosis: Ineffective Breathing Pattern related to increased work of breathing		
NIC Priority Intervention: **Respiratory monitoring:** Collection and analysis of patient data to ensure airway patency and adequate gas exchange		**NOC Suggested Outcome:** **Vital signs status:** Temperature, pulse, respiration, and blood pressure within expected range for the child's age
Goal: The child will return to respiratory baseline. The child will not experience respiratory failure.		
■ Assess respiratory status (Table 47-1) when child is calm and not crying a minimum of every 2–4 hours, or more often as indicated for an increasing or decreasing respiratory rate and episodes of apnea. Cardiorespiratory monitor and pulse oximeter are attached with alarms set. Record and report changes promptly to physician.	■ Changes in breathing pattern may occur quickly as the child's energy reserves are depleted. Assessment and monitoring baseline reveal rate and quality of air exchange. Frequent assessment and monitoring provides objective evidence of changes in the quality of respiratory effort, enabling prompt and effective intervention.	The child returns to respiratory baseline within 48–72 hours.
Goal: The child's oxygenation status will return to baseline.		
■ Administer humidified oxygen via mask, nasal cannula, hood, or tent. ■ Assess pulse oximetry on room air and compare to reading when child is on oxygen. ■ Note child's response to ordered medications. ■ Position head of bed up or place child in position of comfort on parent's lap, if crying or struggling in crib or bed. ■ Assess tolerance to feeding and activities.	■ Humidified oxygen loosens secretions, helps maintain oxygenation status, and eases respiratory distress. ■ Comparison of pulse oximetry readings provides information about improvement status. ■ Medications act systemically to improve oxygenation and decrease inflammation. ■ Position facilitates improved aeration and promotes decrease in anxiety (especially in toddlers) and energy expenditure. ■ Provides an assessment of condition improvement.	The child's respiratory effort eases. Pulse oximetry reading remains at 95% or higher oxygen saturation during treatment. The child tolerates therapeutic measures with no adverse effects. The child rests quietly in position of comfort.
2. Nursing Diagnosis: Risk for Deficient Fluid Volume related to inability to meet body requirements and increased metabolic demand.		
NIC Priority Intervention: **Fluid management:** Promotion of fluid balance and prevention of complications resulting from abnormal or undesired fluid levels		**NOC Suggested Outcome:** **Hydration:** Amount of water in intracellular and extracellular compartments of body
Goal: Child's immediate fluid deficit is corrected.		
■ Evaluate need for intravenous fluids. Maintain IV, if ordered. ■ Calculate maintenance fluid requirements and give oral fluids, IV fluids, or both.	■ Previous fluid loss may require immediate replacement. ■ Assessment ensures child receives appropriate fluids to maintain hydration while transitioning to oral fluids.	Child's hydration status is maintained during acute phase of illness.
Goal: Child will be adequately hydrated, be able to tolerate oral fluids, and progress to normal diet.		
■ Maintain strict intake and output monitoring and evaluate specific gravity at least every 8 hours. ■ Perform daily weight measurement on the same scale at the same time of day. Evaluate skin turgor.	■ Monitoring provides objective evidence of fluid loss and ongoing hydration status. ■ Further evidence of improvement of hydration status.	Child takes adequate oral fluids after 24–48 hours to maintain hydration. Child's weight stabilizes after 24–48 hours; skin turgor is supple.

(continued)

NURSING CARE PLAN—continued

THE CHILD WITH BRONCHIOLITIS

Intervention	Rationale	Expected Outcome
2. Nursing Diagnosis: Risk for Deficient Fluid Volume related to inability to meet body requirements and increased metabolic demand—Continued		
■ Assess mucous membranes and presence of tears. Report changes promptly to physician. ■ Offer clear fluids and incorporate parent in care. Offer fluid choice when tolerated.	■ Moist mucous membranes and tears provide observable evidence of hydration. ■ Choice of fluid offered by parent gains the child's cooperation.	Child shows evidence of improved hydration. The child accepts beverage of choice from parent or nursing staff.
3. Nursing Diagnosis: Anxiety (Child and Parent) related to acute illness, hospitalization, uncertain course of illness and treatment, and home care needs		
NIC Priority Intervention: **Anxiety reduction:** Minimizing apprehension, dread, foreboding, or uneasiness related to an unidentified source of anticipated danger		**NOC Suggested Outcome:** **Anxiety control:** Ability to eliminate or reduce feelings of apprehension and tension from an unidentifiable source
Goal: Child and parents will demonstrate behaviors that indicate decrease in anxiety.		
■ Encourage parents to express fears and ask questions; provide direct answers and discuss care, procedures, and condition changes. ■ Incorporate parents in the child's care. Encourage parents to bring familiar objects from home. Ask about and incorporate in care plan the home routines for feeding and sleeping.	■ Provides opportunity to vent feelings and receive timely, relevant information. Helps reduce parents' anxiety and increase trust in nursing staff. ■ Familiar people, routines, and objects decrease the child's anxiety and increase parents' sense of control over an unexpected, uncertain situation.	Parents and child show decreasing anxiety and decreasing fear as symptoms improve and as child and parents feel more secure in hospital environment. *Parent* freely asks questions and participates in the child's care. The *child* cries less and allows staff to hold or touch him or her.
Goal: Parents will verbalize knowledge of bronchiolitis symptoms and use of home care methods before the child's discharge from the hospital.		
■ Explain symptoms, treatment, and home care of bronchiolitis. ■ Provide written instructions for follow-up care arrangements, as needed.	■ Anticipate potential for recurrence. Assist family to be prepared should respiratory symptoms recur after discharge. ■ Written, as well as oral, instructions reinforce knowledge. Parents may not "hear" and remember the particulars of home care if presented only orally.	Parent accurately describes respiratory symptoms and initial home care actions.

PLANNING AND IMPLEMENTATION

Nursing management focuses on maintaining respiratory function, supporting overall physiologic function and hydration, reducing the child's and family's anxiety, and preparing the family for home care.

Maintain Respiratory Function

Close monitoring is essential to evaluate the child's improvement or to spot early signs of deterioration. Administer oxygen and pulmonary care therapies. High humidity and supplemental oxygen may be provided with a mist tent if the child requires only moisture and minimal oxygen. If more concentrated oxygen is required, it can be given via nasal cannula, hood, or tent. Use pulse oximetry to evaluate oxygenation.

Patent nares are important to promote oxygen intake. A bulb syringe and saline nose drops can be used to quickly clear the nasal passages. Elevate the head of the bed to ease the work of breathing and drain mucus from the upper airways. Chest physiotherapy is often administered by a respiratory therapist.

Support Physiologic Function

Grouping nursing tasks promotes the child's physiologic function by decreasing stress and promoting rest. Medications may be administered to control temperature and promote comfort as needed. An IV infusion may be ordered to rehydrate and maintain fluid balance until the child is capable of taking sufficient oral fluids. Small frequent feedings will help conserve energy in infants who are formula- or breastfed. Thickened formula may improve swallowing and prevent aspiration in infants with RSV bronchiolitis (Gadomski, 2002).

Reduce Anxiety

The need for hospitalization and assistive therapies creates anxiety and fear in the child and parents. An important part of nursing care is anticipating, recognizing, and acting to decrease the child's and parents' anxiety. The parents may be frightened by the child's continued respiratory difficulty and the assistive equipment at the bedside. Provide parents with thorough explanations and daily updates, and encourage their participation in the child's care. Reassure them that holding or touching the child will not dislodge wires or tubing, and that their presence will calm and support the child.

If the child has been ill for a few days before admission, the parents are likely to be tired. Acknowledging parents' physical and emotional needs creates a spirit of caring and enhances communication between staff and family. Encourage the parents to take turns at the child's bedside and to take breaks for meals and rest.

Discharge Planning and Home Care Teaching

Children are discharged once they show sufficient stability in maintaining adequate oxygenation (as evidenced by easing of respiratory effort, decreased mucus production, and absence of coughing). In most children, symptoms abate within 24 to 72 hours; however, resolution of all symptoms may take weeks. The same supportive therapies implemented in the hospital may be needed at home:

- Use of the bulb syringe to suction the nares of an infant under 1 year of age (see Skill 14–20 **SKILLS**)

- Fluid intake to thin respiratory secretions (making them easier to clear) and provide glucose for energy (since the child's appetite may not return to normal for several days)

- Rest

Children can usually recognize their own activity limits. However, parents should encourage active toddlers to nap and take rest periods. Teach the parents proper administration of medications. Acetaminophen may be prescribed for persistent low-grade fevers and general discomfort. Advise parents that RSV infection can recur; therefore, they need to know how to recognize symptoms and when to call the physician.

TEACHING HIGHLIGHTS

DISCHARGE TEACHING FOR BRONCHIOLITIS

Advise parents to call the physician if:

- Respiratory symptoms interfere with sleep or eating.
- Breathing is rapid or difficult.
- Symptoms persist in a child who is less than 1 year old, has heart or lung disease, or was premature and had lung disease after birth.
- The child acts sicker—appears tired, less playful, and less interested in food (parents just "feel" the child is not improving).

EVALUATION

Expected outcomes of nursing care for the child with bronchiolitis include the following:

- The child returns to respiratory baseline within 48 to 72 hours.

- The child's hydration status is maintained during the acute phase of illness.

- Parents and child show decreasing anxiety and decreasing fear as symptoms improve and as child and parents feel more secure in the hospital environment.

PNEUMONIA

Pneumonia is an inflammation or infection of the bronchioles and alveolar spaces of the lungs. It occurs most often in infants and young children. Pneumonia in children often resolves much sooner than in adults. The key is early recognition, enabling the child to be managed at home rather than in the hospital.

Pneumonia may be viral, mycoplasmal, or bacterial in origin. In children under 5 years, pneumonia is most often caused by viruses such as RSV, influenza, parainfluenza virus, adenovirus, rhinovirus, and enterovirus. In children over 5 years, pneumonia is caused by bacteria, such as *Streptococcus pneumoniae*. Children with a condition such as cystic fibrosis or immunosuppression are susceptible to many other bacterial, parasitic, or fungal infections.

What physiologic process occurs to precipitate the symptoms? Bacterial and viral invaders act differently within the lungs:

- Bacterial invaders circulate through the bloodstream to the lungs, where they damage cells. Cellular debris and mucus cause airway obstruction. Bacteria tend to be distributed evenly throughout one or more lobes of a single lung, a pattern termed *unilateral lobar pneumonia*.

- Viruses frequently enter from the upper respiratory tract, infiltrating the alveoli nearest the bronchi of one or both lungs. There they invade the cells, replicate, and burst out forcefully, killing the cells and sending out cell debris. They rapidly invade adjacent areas, distributing themselves in a scattered, patchy pattern referred to as bronchopneumonia.

- Aspiration of food, emesis, gastric reflux, or hydrocarbons causes a chemical injury and inflammatory response. Materials with a lower pH cause more inflammation which sets the stage for bacterial invasion.

Regardless of the causative agent, symptoms include fever, rhonchi, crackles, wheezes, cough, dyspnea, tachypnea, restlessness, and decreased breath sounds if consolidation exists.

Diagnosis is made by chest radiograph, which shows an abnormal density of tissue, such as a lobar consolidation. There is no clinical way to differentiate bacterial and viral cause. The child's age, severity of symptoms, and presence of an underlying lung, cardiac, or immunodeficiency disease can create varying responses.

Clinical management for all types of pneumonia includes symptomatic therapy (pain and fever control) and supportive care through airway management, fluids, and rest. Mycoplasma and other bacterial pneumonias are treated with organism-sensitive antibiotics; viral pneumonias usually improve without antibiotics. Some children need oxygen and IV fluids to maintain hydration.

NURSING MANAGEMENT

Most children with pneumonia are cared for at home. Nursing care incorporates supportive measures and medical therapies as appropriate. Nursing measures used to manage the child with bronchiolitis are generally applicable to the child with pneumonia.

In addition to ongoing respiratory assessment and supportive therapies (chest physiotherapy, antibiotics, hydration), the child may need relief from pain when coughing and deep breathing. Teach the child and parent how to splint the chest, by hugging a small pillow, teddy bear, or doll, to make coughing less painful. Pain medication (acetaminophen or ibuprofen) can provide the added benefits of temperature control and may aid in sleep.

The goal of nursing care is to restore optimal respiratory function. Medications, especially antibiotics, must be taken at prescribed intervals and for the full course. Teach parents the proper administration of drugs and any side effects. Follow-up may include a chest radiograph to see if the lungs are clear. Symptoms of pneumonia usually disappear long before the lungs are completely healed. Some children continue to have worsening reactive airway problems or abnormal results on pulmonary function tests. Most children, however, recover uneventfully.

Preventive measures against pneumonia are limited. A 23-valent pneumococcal vaccine is recommended for children over 2 years of age who are immunosuppressed or have chronic diseases. (See Immunization information in Chapter 45. ∞)

TUBERCULOSIS

Tuberculosis (TB) is caused by the organism *Mycobacterium tuberculosis,* which is transmitted through the air in infectious particles called droplet nuclei. The overall incidence of TB in the United States is 5.1 cases per 100,000 people. More than 50% of new cases of TB in the United States occur in individuals who are foreign-born (Centers for Disease Control, 2004). The risk of developing TB is greatest during the first 2 years of life and during adolescence (American Thoracic Society, 2000). Adolescents are more likely to develop TB because of hormonal changes and metabolic changes associated with growth spurts (Morisky, Malotte, Ebin et al., 2001). Children with altered immune status are also at risk. In young children, the disease develops as an immediate complication of the primary infection.

Adults with active laryngeal or pulmonary TB may transmit the disease to children. By coughing, sneezing, speaking, or singing, a person with active TB sends out tiny droplets of moisture that remain in the air. If these droplets are inhaled, the bacillus is small enough to travel directly to the alveoli and cause infection. Frequently, however, the organism is trapped in the upper airway, preventing infection.

Once the organism reaches the alveoli, an immune response is initiated and macrophages surround and wall off the bacillus in small hard capsules, called tubercles. There the bacillus can remain dormant (inactive) indefinitely or can progress to active TB. The tubercle bacillus grows slowly, dividing within the macrophage. When the organisms number 1000 to 10,000 after 2 to 12 weeks, cellular immune response to TB can be elicited with the TB skin test. The tubercle bacilli may spread by the lymphatic system to the hilar lymph nodes and then to the bloodstream and other sites, resulting in TB meningitis or miliary (disseminated) TB. This systemic form of TB (meningeal or miliary tuberculosis) may lead to serious illness or death. Miliary tuberculosis is not, however, transmissible; only active pulmonary TB has the potential to infect another individual.

Clinical manifestations of TB in infants include a persistent cough, weight loss or failure to gain weight, and fever. Wheezing and decreased breath sounds may be present. Children with active TB may have fatigue, cough, anorexia, weight loss or growth delay, night sweats, chills, and a low-grade fever. Infants, children, and adolescents with latent TB (exposed and infected) are asymptomatic.

See Table 47–10 for the tests used to confirm the diagnosis. Medical management focuses on diagnosis and treatment of active TB with antitubercular drugs, including isoniazid, rifampicin, pyrazinamide, ethambutol, and streptomycin. Therapy usually involves a 6-month regimen of two or more of these drugs. Children with latent TB receive a single daily dose of isoniazid for 9 months. Challenges to treatment have occurred with the development of multidrug-resistant TB organisms. Tuberculosis is a major public health problem and must be promptly reported to local health departments.

In suspected cases of tuberculosis, the child, immediate family, and supposed carrier should be skin tested for TB. Intradermal testing using purified protein derivative (PPD, the Mantoux test) is considered the most accurate test. For interpretation of PPD tests in children, see the Companion Website. A control skin test verifies the response status of the immune system. Children who should receive a TB skin test include those with a TB contact, with TB-suggestive radiologic or clinical findings, who travel to a TB endemic area, who have contact with adults from TB endemic countries, who are incarcerated adolescents, who have contact with persons at high risk for TB (positive HIV status), who are beginning immunosuppression therapy, or who reside in a high-risk neighborhood (American Academy of Pediatrics, 2003).

NURSING MANAGEMENT

Nursing care centers on administering medications and providing supportive care. Teach parents about the disease process, medications, possible side effects, and the importance of long-term therapy (e.g., that drug therapy may last for 6 to 12 months). Emphasize the importance of taking medications as prescribed on an empty stomach. Children with tuberculosis should receive "directly observed drug therapy" administered by a nurse or other healthcare provider to ensure the drug is being taken. Direct observation should be done daily for at least 2 weeks and then decreased to twice a week if the patient is responding to treatment (Stowe & Jacobs, 1999). Children with latent TB should receive "directly observed drug therapy" twice a week (American Academy of Pediatrics, 2003).

Encourage proper nutrition and rest to promote normal growth and development. The child can return to school or child care when effective therapy has been instituted, adherence to therapy has been documented, and clinical symptoms have diminished substantially (American Academy of Pediatrics, 2003). Most children with TB can lead essentially normal lives. The discussion of pneumonia earlier in this chapter and the discussion of tubercular meningitis in Chapter 53 give other nursing care measures appropriate for the child with TB. ∞

TABLE 47–10 ✤ Diagnostic Tests for Tuberculosis

Test	Indication
Mantoux test (intradermal injection of 5 tuberculin units of purified protein derivative [PPD])	A positive test confirms infection with the TB organism and production of antibodies (3–12 weeks after exposure)
Chest radiograph (anteroposterior and lateral views)	Confirms presence of pulmonary tuberculosis (small, seedlike opacities may be visible)
Blood cultures for *Mycobacterium tuberculosis*	Proves diagnosis; defines specific drug sensitivity
Gastric washings (early morning after overnight fast; 3 consecutive days)	Confirms pulmonary TB. Used in children under 12 years because they do not produce sputum.
Sputum cultures (expectorated or from bronchoscopic examination)	Confirms active pulmonary tuberculosis
Pleural biopsy for culture and tissue examination	Taken when pleural effusion is present
Lumbar puncture	Confirms meningeal TB

CHRONIC LUNG DISEASES

BRONCHOPULMONARY DYSPLASIA

Bronchopulmonary dysplasia (BPD), also called chronic lung disease, is the most serious chronic respiratory disorder that begins during infancy. It results from an acute respiratory disease during the neonatal period. Risk factors for developing BPD include prematurity, lung immaturity, high inspired oxygen concentrations, positive pressure ventilation, patent ductus arteriosus, and vitamin A deficiency. It is estimated that 10% to 35% of very low-birth-weight infants develop BPD (Froh, 2002).

BPD results from positive pressure ventilation and oxygen treatment for respiratory distress syndrome and inflammatory changes to the airways (see newborn respiratory distress information in Chapter 30 ∞). Interruption in alveolar development occurs when preterm infants need mechanical ventilation and supplemental oxygen. Inflammation and persistent hypoxia lead to cellular damage, fibrosis, and edema of the bronchioles. Other disorders that contribute to the development of BPD include neonatal pneumonia, meconium aspiration syndrome, fluid overload, and lung hypoplasia (Capper-Michel, 2004).

The infant with BPD has persistent signs of respiratory distress: tachypnea, wheezing, crackles, irritability, nasal flaring, grunting, retractions, pulmonary edema, and failure to thrive. The infant has intermittent bronchospasms and mucous plugging. Infants may have episodes of sudden respiratory deterioration with tracheobronchial narrowing and associated expiratory airflow limitations that may be caused by a sudden increase in pulmonary vascular resistance. Cyanosis may be seen in severe cases. Normal activities, such as feeding, can create increased oxygen demands that are difficult for the compromised infant to meet.

The chest radiograph often shows hyperexpansion, atelectasis, and interstitial thickening (Capper-Michel, 2004). The air trapping persists and in time causes the chest to assume a barrel shape (see "Pathophysiology Illustrated: Barrel Chest"). Medical management focuses on symptomatic treatment that supports respiratory function and on good nutrition, which helps to accelerate lung maturity. Supplemental oxygen with humidity is used to keep the pulse oximetry between 92% and 97% even during sleep and feeding, but high concentration oxygen is avoided to prevent further lung injury (Grant & Curley, 2001). A tracheostomy may be performed for long-term airway management to prevent narrowing of the trachea. Chest physiotherapy and medications (diuretics, bronchodilators, anti-inflammatories, and inhaled corticosteroids) are also used (Table 47–11). With improvement and adequate weight gain, the child is weaned off oxygen, diuretics, and bronchodilators. Long-

PATHOPHYSIOLOGY ILLUSTRATED

Barrel Chest

A barrel chest may result from chronic respiratory conditions such as asthma or bronchopulmonary dysplasia, in which air trapping or hyperinflation of the alveoli occur.

TABLE 47–11 ❖ Medications Used to Treat Bronchopulmonary Dysplasia

Medication	Action/Indication
Bronchodilators (beta₂-adrenergics, anticholinergics, theophylline, albuterol nebulizer)	Decreases airway resistance; increases expiratory flow in small airways; stimulates mucous clearance; different drugs work together for best response
Anti-inflammatory agents (corticosteroids, inhaled cromolyn, beclomethasone)	Reduces pulmonary edema and inflammation in small airways; enhances effect of bronchodilators; helps decrease the need for other drugs and oxygen; for moderate disease only
Diuretics (furosemide, chlorothiazide, spironolactone)	Helps remove excess fluid from lungs; decreases pulmonary resistance and increases pulmonary compliance; may cause electrolyte imbalances
Potassium chloride	Prevents electrolyte imbalances associated with diuretics
Antibiotics	Low-dose prophylactic therapy to prevent severe illness; specific treatment for identified organisms
Vitamin A	Plays a role in normal lung development
Palivizumab, RSV immune globulin	Prevents respiratory syncytial virus

term sequelae include asthma and respiratory infections with frequent rehospitalization rates. Potential long-term outcomes of BPD include developmental delays, growth retardation, impaired cognitive function, and pulmonary dysfunction in adolescents (Belcastro, 2004).

Nursing Management

Nursing management focuses on promoting respiratory function and preparing the family for home care needs. Infants with BPD do not have the same respiratory reserve as healthy infants, and they may become acutely ill at any time. During hospitalization for acute infections, a cardiorespiratory monitor and pulse oximeter are used. Assess airway and respiratory function, vital signs, color, and behavior changes to identify signs of worsening respiratory symptoms, even when oxygen is provided. Position the infant to facilitate breathing. Observe for airway obstruction when the infant has a tracheostomy and suction as needed. Organize care to reduce unnecessary physical stimulation.

Provide fluids and nutrition to meet energy needs; however, fluid management is important to prevent excess

HEALTH PROMOTION
The Child with Bronchopulmonary Dysplasia

Health Supervision

- Assess blood pressure to detect abnormal findings associated with pulmonary hypertension.
- Perform hematocrit frequently during the first year of life to assess for anemia.
- Perform a chest radiograph and pulmonary function tests annually or as needed for clinical condition.
- Perform routine hearing assessment at each visit.
- Coordinate vision screening by an ophthalmologist every 2–3 months during the first year of life. Myopia and strabismus are common resulting from oxygen therapy as a premie.
- Coordinate pulmonary function tests annually or as needed for clinical condition.
- Perform other screening tests as recommended for age.

Growth and Developmental Surveillance

- Assess growth and plot measurements on a growth chart corrected for gestational age. Even if length and weight are lower than normal, monitor for continued growth following the growth curves.
- Perform the Denver II and record the developmental assessment corrected for gestational age.

Nutrition

- Review caloric intake and ensure that intake is optimal for growth. Assess difficulties with feeding related to oral motor function. Refer to a nutitionist as necessary.

Physical Activity

- Organize care so that child has periods of time to rest during the day.

Relationships

- Identify ways to coordinate care during the night to reduce number of times child and family have sleep disturbed.
- Provide discipline appropriate for developmental age.
- Encourage development. Provide developmentally appropriate toys and activities.

Disease Prevention Strategies

- Reduce exposure to infections. If out-of-home child care is used, select a provider caring for a small number of children. If possible, avoid the use of childcare centers during RSV season.
- Immunize the child with the routine schedule based on chronologic age.
- Give the influenza vaccine annually and 23-valent pneumococcal vaccine at 2 years of age.
- Provide monthly injections of palivizumab throughout the RSV season to protect the child from respiratory syncytial virus.

Condition-Specific Guidance

- Develop an emergency care plan for times when the infant's condition rapidly worsens.

THINKING CRITICALLY

INFANT WITH BPD

Emily, an 8-month-old infant with bronchopulmonary dysplasia, is cared for at home by her mother. She has a tracheostomy and receives humidification. Emily has frequent infections and episodes of respiratory distress that require hospitalization. When she develops a fever, more secretions than usual collect in the trachea. Suctioning is needed to ease Emily's breathing. What signs indicate that Emily needs to be suctioned? How do you select the correctly sized suction catheter? How do you suction Emily without causing hypoxia? When is it necessary to change Emily's tracheostomy tube?

fluids and pulmonary edema. Administer medications as ordered. A formula supplemented with carbohydrates and medium chain triglycerides may be given to promote weight gain. Some children need nasogastric or gastros-tomy tube feedings to get adequate nutrition when cyanosis is noted with feeding.

Once home, many infants need ventilation therapy, oxygen respiratory support, and drug therapy (Figure 47–3 ●). Some families need home nursing assistance. Carefully plan and coordinate referrals for needed respiratory supplies, medications, an early intervention program, and follow-up care well in advance of the infant's discharge. Teach parents to identify the signs of respiratory compromise indicating a need for rapid intervention. Suggest ways to provide for the infant's normal development through rest, nutrition, stimulation, and family support. During regular follow-up visits, ensure that the infant receives RSV prophylaxis as described on page 1405.

ASTHMA

Asthma (also called bronchial asthma) is a chronic inflammatory disorder of the airway with airway obstruction that

○ FIGURE 47–3

Many children with BPD are cared for at home, with the support of a home care program to monitor the family's ability to provide airway management, oxygen, and ventilator support. This premature infant girl, who is now 4 months old but weighs only about 5 pounds, requires respiratory support, which is provided by a portable oxygen tank.

can be partially or completely reversed, and increased airway responsiveness to stimuli (Kieckhefer & Ratcliffe, 2004). It is the most common chronic illness, affecting nearly 9 million children in the United States (National Center for Health Statistics, 2004). Affected children have about 10 days of school absenteeism and 20 days of restricted activity per year (Sydnor-Greenberg & Dokken, 2000). Nearly 53 per 1000 children between 0 and 17 years of age have an asthma attack during a year (Centers for Disease Control and Prevention, National Center for Health Statistics, 2001). Most children with asthma experience their first symptoms before the age of 5 years. See the Companion Website for links.

Passive smoke exposure (secondhand smoke), contaminants in indoor air (pet dander, dust mites, cockroach feces, fungal contamination, chemical gases), and pollutants in outdoor air all contribute significantly to the development of asthma and respiratory problems in children (Solomon, Humphreys, & Miller, 2004). Passive smoke exposure has been linked to an increase in asthma symptoms, emergency department visits, and hospital admissions in children of parents who smoke, as well as to decreased lung function (Gilliland, Yu-Fen, & Peters, 2001; Mannino, Homa, & Redd, 2002).

Asthma is a chronic condition with acute exacerbations or persistent symptoms. Children require continuous coordinated care to control sudden symptoms and minimize long-term airway changes. Although unusual in the past, severe persistent asthma is more common now. Hospitalizations for asthma as well as mortality from asthma in children have increased significantly (Akinbami & Schoendorf, 2002).

ETIOLOGY AND PATHOPHYSIOLOGY

Asthma is a chronic inflammatory disease of the lungs that is caused by multiple factors, including environmental exposures, viral illnesses, allergens, and a genetic predisposition. Several chromosomes are thought to be factors in asthma susceptibility, including chromosomes 5q, 6p, 11q, 12q, and 13q (Foley, 2002). Exposure to environmental factors early in life or in utero is thought to stimulate the onset of asthma. A recent report found strong evidence that house dust mites and environmental tobacco smoke, and suggestive evidence that cockroaches, infections with RSV, and mold from indoor home dampness contributed to the development of asthma (Institute of Medicine, 2000).

Inflammation causes the normal protective mechanisms of the lungs (mucus formation, mucosal swelling, and airway muscle contraction) to react excessively in response to a stimulus and cause airway obstruction. The stimulus, or **trigger**, that initiates an asthmatic episode can be inflammatory or noninflammatory. Triggers increase the frequency and severity of smooth muscle contraction, and airway responsiveness is enhanced through inflammatory mechanisms. Asthmatic triggers include exercise, viral or bacterial agents, allergens (mold, dust, pollen, furry pets, birds), fragrances, food additives, pollutants, weather changes (humidity and temperature), and emotions. Exercise triggers a bronchospasm by the rapid breathing of cooler and drier air than the air in the respiratory tract (Baker, Friedman, & Schmitt, 2002).

The reactive airway responses to stimuli are present before the trigger initiates the asthmatic episode. During the acute allergic reaction, an antigen binds to the specific immunoglobulin E surface on the mucosal mast cells, and histamine is released along with intercellular chemical mediators (leukotrienes, prostaglandins, platelet-activating factor, and certain cytokines) resulting in bronchospasm, mucosal edema, and mucus secretion. The late allergic response starts 6 to 9 hours later when inflammatory cells respond and another wave of mediator release occurs. This stimulates more airway inflammation and bronchospasm (Kieckhefer & Ratcliffe, 2004).

Bronchial constriction, airway swelling, and production of copious amounts of mucus causes airway narrowing. Mucus clogs small airways and traps air (see "Pathophysiology Illustrated: Asthma"). The airways

PATHOPHYSIOLOGY ILLUSTRATED

Asthma

Normal bronchiole and alveoli

Capillaries

Mucous gland

Normal bronchiole

Normal alveoli

Mucous membranes become inflamed and edematous.

Mucus production increases.

Inflammatory reaction such as increased capillary permeability and histamine release

Thickened basement membrane

Mucous glands hypersecrete and proliferate.

Airway narrows, restricting airflow.

Smooth muscles constrict.

Restricted airflow prevents proper filling of alveoli and gas exchange.

Hyperinflated alveoli

Collapsed alveoli

Some asthma triggers are exercise, infection, and allergies. Shown is how asthma obstructs airflow through constriction and narrowing of the airway, along with increased production of mucus.

swell, creating muscle spasms that may become uncontrolled in the large airways. Decreased perfusion of the alveolar capillaries results from hyperinflation of the alveoli. Hypoxemia leads to an increased respiratory rate, but less air is breathed per minute because of airway resistance. Progressive chronic inflammatory changes result in **airway remodeling**, an irreversible thickening of the basement membrane, airway smooth muscle hypertrophy, and mucus gland hypertrophy (Froh, 2002).

Moderate anxiety occurs as the asthma episode begins, and increases as the episode intensifies. Severe anxiety intensifies physical responses and symptoms, and a vicious cycle is established. Recognizing and addressing the child's fear and panic are essential for reestablishing normal respirations.

Clinical Manifestations. Asthma is characterized by airway inflammation, airway obstruction or narrowing, and airway hyperreactivity. The sudden appearance of breathing difficulty (cough, wheeze, or shortness of breath) is often referred to as an asthma episode or "asthma attack." The infant or child who has had episodes of frequent coughing or frequent respiratory infections (especially pneumonia or bronchitis) should also be evaluated for asthma. The coughing, especially at night, is the warning signal that the child's airway is very sensitive to stimuli; it may be the only sign in "silent" asthma.

During an acute episode, respirations are rapid and labored and the child often appears tired because of the ongoing exertion of breathing. Nasal flaring and intercostal retractions may be visible. The child exhibits a productive cough and expiratory wheezing, use of accessory muscles, decreased air movement, and respiratory fatigue. In cases of severe obstruction, wheezing may not be heard because of the lack of airflow. The resulting hypoxia, as well as the cumulative effect of previously administered medications, con-

tributes to behaviors ranging from wide-eyed agitation to lethargic irritability. See "Clinical Manifestations: Asthma in Children by Severity of Acute Exacerbations." In children who have repeated acute exacerbations, a barrel chest and the use of accessory muscles of respiration are common findings.

Clinical Therapy. The diagnosis of asthma has four key elements: symptoms of episodic airflow obstruction, partial reversibility of bronchospasm with bronchodilator treatment, exclusion of alternative diagnosis, and confirmation by spirometry of measurement of forced expiratory flow variability. A spirometer measures the volume of air a child can expel from the lungs after a maximum inspiration. Three readings of the forced vital capacity and forced expiratory volume are taken and compared to predicted normal values to assess the severity of airway obstruction. Because the test requires children to

CLINICAL MANIFESTATIONS

ASTHMA IN CHILDREN BY SEVERITY OF ACUTE EXACERBATIONS

ASSESSMENT CRITERIA	MILD	MODERATE	SEVERE
Peak expiratory flow rate (PEFR)[a]	70%–90% predicted or personal best	50%–70% predicted or personal best	Less than 50% predicted or personal best
Respiratory rate, resting or sleeping	Normal to 30% increase above the mean	30%–50% increase above mean	Increase over 50% above mean
Alertness	Normal	Normal	May be decreased
Dyspnea[b]	Absent or mild; speaks in complete sentences	Moderate; speaks in phrases or partial sentences; infant's cry softer and shorter; has difficulty sucking and feeding	Severe; speaks only in single words or short phrases; infant's cry softer and shorter; stops sucking and feeding
Pulsus paradoxus[c]	Less than 10 mm Hg	10–20 mm Hg	20–40 mm Hg
Accessory muscle use	No intercostal to mild retractions	Moderate intercostal retractions with tracheosternal retractions; use of sternocleidomastoid muscles; chest hyperinflation	Severe intercostal retractions, tracheosternal retractions with nasal flaring during inspiration; chest hyperinflation
Color	Good	Pale	Possibly cyanotic
Auscultation	End-expiratory wheeze only	Wheeze during entire expiration and inspiration	Breath sounds becoming inaudible
Oxygen saturation	Greater than 95%	90%–95%	Less than 90%
Pco_2	Less than 35	Less than 40	Greater than 40

Note: Within each category, the presence of several parameters, but not necessarily all, indicates the general classification of the exacerbation.

[a]For children 5 years of age or older.

[b]Parents' or physicians' impression of degree of children's breathlessness.

[c]Pulsus paradoxus does not correlate with phase of respiration in small children.

Note: From National Asthma Education and Prevention Program. (1994). Acute exacerbations of asthma: Care in a hospital-based emergency department (p. 13). Bethesda, MD: National Heart, Lung, and Blood Institute, National Institutes of Health.

cooperate and follow instructions, it is usually administered to children over 4 or 5 years of age. Skin testing may be used to identify allergens (asthma triggers).

Medical management includes medications, support of parents and child, and education. Pharmacologic treatment is matched to the severity of asthma for long-term control and for management of acute episodes. See Table 47–12 for nationally recommended guidelines for the treatment of children over 5 years of age with acute and chronic asthma. Control of asthma symptoms is the goal, and if control is not achieved with the regimen prescribed, then the regimen should be changed to correspond to the next step in asthma severity. Once control of asthma symptoms is achieved, the treatment plan can be reviewed in 1 to 6 months to determine if a step back in asthma treatment is appropriate (Hogan & Wilson, 2003). See Table 47–13 for medications used to treat asthma.

Some healthcare providers encourage children to use a peak expiratory flow meter to identify when an obstruction is occurring. This device measures the child's ability to push air forcefully out of the lungs, similar to a spirometer. Medication administration can be based on peak expiratory flow rate (PEFR) readings and the effectiveness of treatment confirmed by improved PEFR numbers.

NURSING PRACTICE

Markers of good asthma control include the following:

- Minimal or no chronic symptoms day or night
- Minimal or no exacerbations
- No limitations on activities, no school missed, parents don't miss work
- Minimal use of short-acting beta$_2$-agonists (Less than 1 time a day or less than 1 canister a month)
- Minimal or no adverse effects from medications

Data from National Asthma Education and Prevention Program. (2002). NAEPP Expert Panel Report: Guidelines for the diagnosis and management of asthma. Update on selected topics 2002 (NIH Publication No. 02-5075). Bethesda, MD: National Institutes of Health, NHLBI.

See "Clinical Pathway: Stages of Inpatient Care for Children with Severe Asthma."

Most children with acute exacerbations respond to aggressive management in the emergency department. Children who do not respond or who are already being managed at home on corticosteroids have a greater chance of being admitted. Some children need mechanical ventilation.

DRUG GUIDE

ALBUTEROL

Overview of Action
A synthetic sympathomimetic amine and moderately selective beta$_2$-adrenergic agonist that has effect on bronchial, uterine, and vascular supply to muscles. Produces bronchodilation, decreases airway resistance, facilitates mucus drainage, and increases vital capacity.

Routes, Dosage, Frequency
Oral

- **2 to 6 years:** Initial: 0.1–0.2 mg/kg/day 3 times a day (maximum dosage 4 mg/dose)
- **6 to 12 years:** 2 mg 3 to 4 times per day
- **Over 12 years:** 2 to 4 mg 3 to 4 times per day; extended-release tablets: 4 to 8 mg every 12 hours

Inhalation: Oral inhalation for relief of acute bronchospasms or prevention of asthma symptoms

- **6 to 12 years:** 1 to 2 inhalations every 4 to 6 hours

Contraindications: Hypersensitivity to drug or its ingredients.
Side Effects: Restlessness, nervousness, tremors, dizziness, weakness, headache, hallucination, insomnia, tachycardia, palpitations, hypertension or hypotension, peripheral vasodilation, irritation of nose and throat, blurred vision, dilated pupils, muscle cramps, hoarseness.

Nursing Implications
Assessment: Assess the respiratory status and obtain baseline pulse and peak expiratory flow rate.

Administer: For oral: Plain tablets can be crushed and mixed with small amounts of food or fluids. Do not crush coated tablets. Side effects are more common with oral form. **Inhalation:** Shake container well. If second inhalation is prescribed, manufacturer recommends that 1 minute elapse between doses. **Nebulizer:** Follow agency policy for operation of the nebulizer apparatus. Follow package insert directions for solution dilution. If solution is discolored, do not use. Do not remove nebulization capsules from the original package until just prior to use.

Monitor: Monitor pulse (cardiovascular effects may occur), central nervous system stimulation (hyperactivity, excitement, nervousness, insomnia), therapeutic response to medication. Maintain hydration for weight. Do not use over-the-counter drugs (e.g., cold preparations) without physician approval as many contain drugs that intensify albuterol action. Perform periodic arterial blood gases, pulmonary function tests, and pulse oximetry.

Patient teaching: Review directions for correct use of medication. Teach the proper use and care of the inhaler. Have child demonstrate inhaler use. Emphasize that inhaler should not be used more frequently than prescribed, and to contact physician if albuterol fails to provide relief. Avoid contact of inhalation drug with eyes. Help the family ensure that child has access to medicine during school hours if needed.

Note: From Bindler, R. M., & Howry, L. B. (2005). Pediatric drugs and nursing implications (3rd ed.). Upper Saddle River, NJ: Prentice Hall-Health. Adapted.

TABLE 47-12 ✦ **Asthma Severity Classification and Preferred Clinical Therapy for Children Older than 5 Years of Age**

Classification (Steps)	Description	Medications for Long-Term Control
Step 1: Mild intermittent	Brief exacerbations with symptoms no more often than twice a week. Nighttime symptoms no more than twice a week. Asymptomatic and normal PEFR between exacerbations. No emergent visits and no asthma-related absences from school. PEFR ≥ 80% of predicted with variability < 20%.	No daily medications needed. Severe exacerbation may occur, separated by long periods of normal lung function and no symptoms. A course of systemic corticosteroids is recommended.
Step 2: Mild persistent	Exacerbations more than twice a week, but less than once a day. Nighttime symptoms more than twice a month. Exacerbations may affect activity and cause absences from school. PEFR ≥ 80% of predicted with variability of 20% to 30%.	Preferred treatment ■ Low-dose inhaled steroid. Alternate treatment ■ Cromolyn, leukotriene modifier, or nedocromil. OR ■ Sustained-release theophylline to serum concentration of 5–15 mcg/mL.
Step 3: Moderate persistent	Daily symptoms of coughing and wheezing. Exacerbations at least twice a week that may last for days. Nighttime symptoms more than once per week. Exacerbations affect activity and several school absences occur. PEF or FEV_1 > 60% but < 80% of predicted with variability > 30%	Preferred treatment ■ Low- to medium-dose inhaled corticosteroid. Plus Long-acting β_2-agonists Alternate treatment ■ Increase inhaled corticosteroids to within medium-dose range OR ■ Low-dose inhaled steroid and either leukotriene modifier or theophylline. If needed (particularly in children and adolescents with recurring severe exacerbations) Preferred treatment ■ Increase inhaled corticosteroids within medium-dose range and add long-acting inhaled β_2-agonists. Alternative treatment ■ Increase inhaled corticosteroids within medium-dose range and add either leukotriene modifier or theophylline.
Step 4: Severe persistent	Continuous daytime symptoms, limited physical activity. Frequent exacerbations. Frequent nighttime symptoms. Limited physical activity. Hospitalizations are frequent with PICU admissions for severe exacerbations. PEF or FEV_1 ≤ 60% of predicted, with variability > 30%	Preferred treatment ■ High-dose inhaled corticosteroids. Plus ■ Long-acting inhaled β_2-agonists. And if needed, ■ Oral corticosteroids at 2 mg/kg/day (not to exceed 60 mg per day). Repeated efforts should be made to reduce systemic corticosteroids and maintain control with high-dose inhaled corticosteroids.
Quick relief	Bronchodilator as needed for symptoms. Intensity of treatment will depend on severity of exacerbation. ■ Preferred treatment: Short-acting inhaled β_2-agonists by nebulizer, face mask, and space/holding chamber. ■ Alternative treatment: oral β_2-agonist. With viral respiratory infection ■ Bronchodilator every 4–6 hours up to 24 hours (longer with physician counsel); in general, repeat no more than once every 6 weeks. ■ Consider systemic corticosteroids if exacerbation is severe or patient has a history of previous severe exacerbations. ■ Use of short-acting β_2-agonists > 2 times a week in intermittent asthma (daily or increasing use in persistent asthma) may indicate the need to initiate (increase) long-term control therapy.	

Adapted from National Asthma Education and Prevention Program. (2002). *Expert Panel Report II: Guidelines for the diagnosis and management of asthma. Update on selected topics 2002* (NIH Publication No. 02-5075). Bethesda, MD: National Heart Lung and Blood Institute, National Institutes of Health.

TABLE 47–13 ✤ Medications Used to Treat Asthma

Rescue Medication	Action/Indication	Nursing Considerations
Beta₂-agonists (short-acting) Albuterol, metaproterenol, terbutaline, levalbuterol: inhalation, PO	Relax smooth muscle in airway, increase water content in bronchial mucus to promote muciliary clearance resulting in rapid bronchodilation within 5–10 minutes. Drug of choice for acute therapy (metered-dose inhaler or nebulizer).	■ Use this rescue medication before inhaled steroid, wait 1–2 minutes between puffs, wait 15 minutes to give inhaled steroid. Child should hold breath 10 seconds after inspiring. Then rinse mouth and avoid swallowing medication. Use spacer. ■ Some side effects (tachycardia, nervousness, nausea and vomiting, headaches), but these are usually dose related. ■ Repetitive or excessive use can mask increasing airway inflammation and hyperresponsiveness and increase need for higher dosage to get same effect. ■ Use of more than 1 canister a month indicates inadequate control.
Corticosteroids Methylprednisolone: IV Prednisone Prednisolone: PO	Diminish airway inflammation and obstruction, enhance bronchodilating effect of Beta₂-agonists. Used for moderate to severe acute exacerbations when single Beta₂-agonist dose given in emergency department does not resolve symptoms.	■ Not used as primary treatment. ■ Onset of action is 4–6 hours. ■ Short-term therapy for 3–10 days until symptoms resolve or child achieves 80% peak expiratory flow personal best. ■ Give with food. ■ Give daily oral dose in early morning to mimic normal peak corticosteroid blood level. ■ Assess for potential adverse effects of long-term therapy: decreased growth, unstable blood sugar, immunosuppression.
Anticholinergic Ipratropium: inhalation	Inhibits bronchoconstriction and decreases mucus production. Provides additive effects to short-acting Beta₂-agonists during acute exacerbation.	■ Not for primary treatment. ■ Side effects include increased wheezing, cough, nervousness, dry mouth, tachycardia, dizziness, headache, palpitations. ■ Avoid eye contact.

Controller Medication	Action/Indication	Nursing Considerations
Beta₂-agonists (long acting) Salmeterol Formoterol: inhalation	Relax smooth muscle in airway, used for nocturnal symptoms and prevention of exercise-induced bronchospasm.	■ Should not be used for acute asthma attack. ■ Should not be used in place of inhaled corticosteroids. ■ Caution against overdosage as side effects such as tachycardia, tremor, irritability, insomnia will last 8–12 hours. ■ Report use of more than 4 puffs a day as this may indicate need for stepped-up therapy.
Methylxanthines Theophylline: PO Aminophylline: IV	Relax muscle bundles that constrict airways; dilate airway; provide continuous airway relaxation; sustained release for prevention of nocturnal symptoms. Aminophylline may be used for emergency adjunct therapy in ICU, but use is controversial.	■ Tablet should not be crushed or chewed. ■ Used for long-term control, so continuous administration is needed; works best when a specific amount is maintained in the bloodstream (therapeutic serum level, 10–20 mcg/L). ■ Requires serum level checks and dose adjustment. ■ Side effects include tachycardia, dysrhythmias, restlessness, tremors, seizures, insomnia, hypotension, severe headaches, vomiting, and diarrhea.
Mast-Cell Inhibitors Cromolyn sodium Nedocromil: aerosol	Anti-inflammatory, inhibit early- and late-phase asthma response to allergens and exercise-induced bronchospasm; may be used for unavoidable allergen exposure.	■ Not used at time of symptom development or acute exacerbation. ■ Must be used up to 4 times a day to be effective. ■ Therapeutic response seen in 2 weeks, maximum benefit may not be seen for 4–6 weeks. ■ Adverse reactions include wheezing, bronchospasm, throat irritation, nasal congestion, anaphylaxis.

(continued)

TABLE 47-13 ❖ Medications Used to Treat Asthma—continued

Controller Medication	Action/Indication	Nursing Considerations
Corticosteroids Beclomethasone Budesonide Fluticasone Triamcinolone: inhalation	Anti-inflammatory, controls seasonal, allergic, and exercise-induced asthma. Effectively reduces mucosal edema in airways; usually combined with other asthma medications for control. First-line therapy in asthma management.	■ Administer with spacer or holding chamber. ■ Rinse mouth following treatment to reduce chance of thrush and dysphonia. ■ Monitor growth. ■ Monitor for headache, gastrointestinal upset, dizziness, infection. ■ Use exactly as prescribed.
Leukotriene Modifiers Montelukast: PO Zafirlukast: PO	Reduces inflammation cascade responsible for airway inflammation. Improves lung function and diminishes symptoms and need for rescue medications. Adjunct to inhaled corticosteroids in moderate to severe asthma or substitute for inhaled corticosteroids in mild asthma.	■ Administer montelukast in evening; may be given with or without food. ■ Administer zafirlukast 1 hour before or 2 hours after meal. ■ Family needs to report fever, acute asthma attacks, flulike symptoms, severe headaches, or lethargy. ■ Take as prescribed, do not withdraw abruptly.
Other Hyposensitization (allergy shots), subcutaneous	Series of injections that can reduce sensitivity to unavoidable allergens (e.g., environmental organisms—mold, pollen); gradual dose increase over time (buildup) increases the child's tolerance to allergic substances; has been of help in some children.	■ Use is controversial; some question about actual effect.

Data from Baker, V. O., Friedman, J., & Schmitt, R. (2002). Asthma management, part II: Pharmacologic management. *Journal of School Nursing, 18*(5), 257–269; Belcher, D. (2002, November). Breathing easier with pediatric asthma: Pharmacologic management. *Advance for Nurse Practitioners,* 37–38, 79; Baren, J. M., & Puchalski, A. (2002). Current concepts in the ED treatment of pediatric asthma. *Pediatric Emergency Medicine Reports,* 7(10), 105–115.

COMPLEMENTARY CARE

ALTERNATIVE ASTHMA TREATMENTS

Parents of children from different cultures may have concerns about daily medication regimens. Some prefer to use folk medicines such as rubbing oils or camphor (Vicks VapoRub) preparations on the child's chest. Learn about the family's cultural beliefs and practices (Sydnor-Greenberg & Dokken, 2000). Up to 80% of Hispanic, African-American, and immigrant adolescents attending an inner-city high school reported the use of complementary therapies for the treatment of asthma that included rubs, teas (chamomile, ginger, wild root, and eucalyptus), prayer, and massage. There was no association between complementary therapy use and ethnicity or immigrant status. Nearly all adolescents indicated that they would repeat the use of the complementary therapy. It is important to ask about complementary therapy use by children and adolescents with asthma, and how it is used in conjunction with traditional therapy (Reznik, Ozuah, Franco et al., 2002).

NURSING MANAGEMENT

NURSING ASSESSMENT AND DIAGNOSIS

The nurse usually encounters the child and family in the emergency department or nursing unit. In these settings, acute care has become necessary because the child's level of respiratory compromise cannot be managed at home.

Physiologic Assessment

Identify the child's current respiratory status first by assessing the ABCs—airway, breathing, and circulation—to make sure the child's condition is not life threatening. If the child

DEVELOPING CULTURAL COMPETENCE

ASTHMA MANAGEMENT

The number of asthma attacks among children under 18 years varies greatly by race and ethnicity. Non-Hispanic black children have the highest prevalence followed by non-Hispanic white children and Hispanic children (Centers for Disease Control, 2000). A recent study investigated these disparities and found a difference in preventive medications used for asthma. Findings revealed that differences in health beliefs, fear of steroids, or communication issues rather than financial barriers may play a role in the use of preventive asthma medications (Lieu, Lozano, Finkelstein et al., 2002). Learn about the family's cultural beliefs and practices. Parents of children from different cultures may have concerns about daily medication regimens. Some prefer to use folk medicines such as rubbing oils or Vicks preparations on the child's chest (Sydnor-Greenberg & Dokken, 2000). Individualizing care through education is a key to successful treatment. Education should be based on a "thorough assessment of the child's and family's resources, health care beliefs, access to health care services, and management styles" (Swartz, Cantey-Banasiak, & Meadows-Oliver, 2005, p.78).

CLINICAL PATHWAY

STAGES OF INPATIENT CARE FOR CHILDREN WITH SEVERE ASTHMA

CATEGORY	CONTINUOUS NEBULIZER TREATMENTS	FREQUENT NEBULIZER TREATMENTS	TRANSITION TO DISCHARGE, NEBULIZER TREATMENTS EVERY 4–6 HR
Outcomes	Patient will: ■ Evidence stabilization of vital signs. ■ Exhibit patent airway; experience resolution of acute respiratory distress. ■ Verbalize understanding and demonstrate cooperation with respiratory therapy. ■ Have oral intake equal to fluid maintenance needs. Family verbalizes feelings about illness. Family displays effective coping. Family understands plan of care for hospitalization. Family verbalizes beginning understanding of asthma and ongoing care and treatments.	Patient will: ■ Evidence stable vital signs and be afebrile. ■ Exhibit unlabored respirations and patent airway. ■ Tolerate full diet. ■ Tolerate age-appropriate activity without evidence of respiratory distress, weakness, or exhaustion. ■ Have moist mucous membranes. ■ Verbalize understanding and demonstrate cooperation with respiratory therapy. Family exhibits effective coping mechanisms.	Patient is afebrile with stable vital signs. Patient exhibits a patent airway and unlabored respirations with activity. Patient's respiratory rate and status has returned to baseline. Patient tolerates activity without evidence of respiratory distress, weakness, or exhaustion. Patient's mucous membranes are moist. Family verbalizes/demonstrates home care instructions, including strategies to reduce exposure to infectious illnesses and respiratory irritants. Family exhibits willingness to make lifestyle changes and cope with effects of chronic illness. Family demonstrates/verbalizes ability to cope with ongoing stressors. Family verbalizes beginning understanding of home care instruction including trigger agents, signs and symptoms of impending acute episode, and appropriate actions.
Assessments	Vital signs every 1–2 hr and prn. Continuous pulse oximetry monitoring. Cardiorespiratory monitoring while on continuous nebulizer treatments. Potassium level 12 hr after on continuous nebulizer treatments, then every 12 hr. Assess respiratory status every 1–2 hr and as necessary. Monitor carefully for changes in respiratory rate, skin color, retractions, and/or flaring. Strict intake and output. Urine specific gravity every 8 hr. Humidification as ordered. Position patient in semi-Fowler's or high Fowler's position. Oxygen as ordered to maintain O_2 saturation greater than or equal to 95%. Provide quiet, restful environment. Assess cognitive/developmental level.	Vital signs every 4 hr and prn. Assess respiratory status every 4 hr and prn. Monitor carefully for changes in respiratory rate, skin color, retractions, and/or flaring. Discontinue cardiorespiratory monitor. Strict intake and output. Urine specific gravity every 8 hr. Humidification as ordered. Position patient in semi-Fowler's or high Fowler's position. Continue pulse oximetry monitoring while on oxygen. Wean oxygen, keeping O_2 saturation at greater than or equal to 92%. Provide quiet, restful environment.	Vital signs every 8 hr and prn. Pulse oximetry reading every 4 hr if patient is on oxygen. Continue weaning oxygen if O_2 saturation greater than or equal to 92%. Assess respiratory status every 8 hr and prn. Monitor carefully for changes in respiratory rate, skin color, retractions, and/or flaring. Provide quiet, restful environment.
Knowledge	Initiate teaching regarding ongoing care, including procedures, treatments, and medications. Initiate patient and family teaching about asthma, its treatments, trigger agents, avoidance of respiratory infections and irritants, and early signs and symptoms of infections. Evaluate understanding of teaching. Provide information at developmental/cognitive level.	Reinforce earlier teaching about ongoing care. Reinforce teaching about asthma and treatments. Renew detailed teaching with family and patient about home care including medications, respiratory therapy, activity, trigger agents, avoidance of respiratory infections and irritants, early signs and symptoms of impending acute episode, and follow-up care. Evaluate understanding of teaching.	Reinforce earlier teaching about ongoing care. Complete discharge teaching to include diet, follow-up care, signs and symptoms to report, follow-up physician visit, activity, and medications: name, purpose, dose, frequency, route, dietary interactions, and side effects. Provide family/patient with written discharge instructions. Refer unmet teaching needs to outpatient services. Evaluate understanding of teaching. Refer knowledge deficits to community resources.

(continued)

CLINICAL PATHWAY—continued

STAGES OF INPATIENT CARE FOR CHILDREN WITH SEVERE ASTHMA

CATEGORY	CONTINUOUS NEBULIZER TREATMENTS	FREQUENT NEBULIZER TREATMENTS	TRANSITION TO DISCHARGE, NEBULIZER TREATMENTS EVERY 4–6 HR
Psychosocial	Orient patient to setting. Provide age-appropriate communication and support. Encourage verbalization of concerns. Encourage family to participate in care. Reassure patient and family of ongoing surveillance of patient status and responses to therapy.	Provide age-appropriate communication and support. Encourage verbalization of concerns. Encourage family to participate in care. Reassure patient and family of ongoing surveillance of patient status and responses to therapy.	Provide age-appropriate communication and support. Encourage verbalization of concerns. Provide ongoing support and encouragement to family.
Diet	Clear liquids as tolerated. Avoid cold fluids and foods. Encourage fluid intake.	Age-appropriate diet as tolerated, providing small, frequent, nutritious feedings. Avoid cold fluids and foods. Encourage fluid intake.	Age-appropriate diet as tolerated, providing small, frequent, nutritious feedings. Avoid cold fluids and foods. Encourage fluid intake.
Activity	Assess safety needs and provide adequate precautions. Encourage age- and status-appropriate diversional activities. Balance activity with planned rest periods.	Maintain safety precautions. Balance activity with planned rest periods. Increase activity as tolerated. Encourage age- and status-appropriate diversional activities.	Maintain safety precautions. Balance activity with planned rest periods. Encourage age- and status-appropriate diversional activities. Activity as tolerated.
Medications	IV fluids only if unable to take oral fluids to equal maintenance. Oral steroids as ordered. Ipratropium as ordered. Continuous albuterol nebulizer treatments until respiratory distress decreases. Give oral potassium if K level is less than 3.5. Acetaminophen as ordered for temperature over 38.3°C (101°F).	Oral steroids as ordered. Albuterol nebulizer treatments every 2 hr. Acetaminophen as ordered for temperature over 38.3°C (101°F).	Oral steroids as ordered. Albuterol nebulizer treatment every 4–6 hr. Start or restart home therapy. Observe patient for reaction to new medications, if applicable. Patient sent home with inhaler.
Transfer/ discharge plans	Continue to review progress toward discharge goals. Review discharge plans.	Continue to review progress toward discharge goals. Determine need for home respiratory therapy and outpatient teaching for breathing exercises. Finalize discharge plans. Make appropriate referrals.	Finalize plans for home care if needed. Make appropriate referrals. Complete discharge teaching.

is moving air or talking, assess the quality of breathing. Assess the respiratory rate. Inspect the chest for retractions to assess the severity of respiratory distress. Auscultate the lungs for the quality of breath sounds and for the presence or absence of wheezing. Observe the child's color and assess the heart rate. Note whether a cough or stridor is present. Obtain oxygen saturation via pulse oximeter. Determine the severity of symptoms from the "Clinical Manifestations" table on page 1416. Only move on to other symptoms after finding no life-threatening respiratory distress.

Assess skin turgor, intake and output, and specific gravity. Because asthma can be a symptom of another illness, perform a head-to-toe assessment to identify other associated problems (Tables 47–1 and 47–7). (See Skills 9–1 to 9–22.) **SKILLS**

Psychosocial Assessment

Assess the child's anxiety. (See Table 47–9.) In an older child whose asthma was previously diagnosed, assess whether the child thinks this episode could have been avoided if medication had been taken. Look for clues to hidden stress and self-blaming.

Common nursing diagnoses for the child experiencing an acute asthmatic episode include the following:

- *Ineffective Airway Clearance* related to airway compromise, copious mucus secretions, and coughing
- *Impaired Gas Exchange* related to airway obstruction, possible additional respiratory illness, and poor response to medication
- *Risk for Deficient Fluid Volume* related to difficulty in taking adequate fluids with respiratory distress
- *Anxiety/Fear (Child or Parents)* related to difficulty breathing and change in health status
- *Ineffective Therapeutic Regimen Management (Family)* related to inadequate education on daily management of a chronic disease

PLANNING AND IMPLEMENTATION

Pharmacologic and supportive therapies are used to reverse the airway obstruction and promote respiratory function. Nursing interventions center on maintaining airway patency, meeting fluid needs, promoting rest and stress reduction for the child and parents, supporting the family's participation in care, and giving the family information that lets them manage the child's disease.

Maintain Airway Patency

If the child is exhibiting breathing difficulty, give supplemental oxygen by nasal cannula or face mask. Humidified oxygen should be used to prevent drying and thickening of mucus secretions. Place the child in a sitting (semi-Fowler's) or upright position to promote and ease respiratory effort. Evaluate the effectiveness of positioning and oxygen administration by pulse oximeter and by observing for improved respiratory status. (See Skill 14-1. **SKILLS**)

The respiratory distress and need for supplemental oxygen can be stressful for parents and child alike (Figure 47-4 ●). Encouraging the parents' presence can be reassuring for the child. Keep the parents informed of procedures and results, and get their input when developing the treatment plan.

Many medications are given by the aerosol route (Figure 47-5 ●). The advantages of aerosol are that the medication acts quickly, enabling the pulmonary blood vessels to absorb the inhaled medication, systemic effects are minimized, and the inhaled droplets provide the added benefit of moisture. Continuous aerosol treatments may be used for some children with severe exacerbations. Monitor the child for side effects. The frequency of vital sign assessment is related to the severity of symptoms. (See Skill 11-11. **SKILLS**)

● **FIGURE 47–4**

Acute exacerbations of asthma may require management in the emergency department. The child is placed in a semisitting position to facilitate respiratory effort. Providing support to both the child and parent is an important part of nursing care during these acute episodes. This mother is exhausted after a sleepless night of caring for her son.

NURSING PRACTICE

Spacers with valves are often used with metered dose inhalers (MDIs) for children who cannot coordinate inspiration with medication release. The spacer captures the aerosol released by the MDI in a reservoir for the child to breathe in over a couple of minutes. This provides a benefit similar to nebulizer treatment, but it takes less time and is less expensive (Steinbach, 2000). When teaching the child to use an MDI without a spacer, let the child learn to breathe in slowly with straws.

Meet Fluid Needs

Fluid therapy is often necessary to restore and maintain adequate fluid balance. Adequate hydration is essential to thin and break up trapped mucous plugs in the narrowed airways. An adequate oral intake may not be possible with the child's compromised respiratory status. An intravenous infusion may be needed, and this route also may be used for administering medications and providing glucose. Overhydration must be avoided to prevent pulmonary edema in severe asthma attacks.

As respiratory difficulty diminishes, offer oral fluids slowly. Iced beverages precipitate bronchospasms in some

● **FIGURE 47–5**

Medications given by aerosol therapy allow children the freedom to play and entertain themselves.

children with asthma. It is safest to offer the asthmatic child room-temperature or slightly cooled fluids without ice. Determine the child's fluid preferences and give choices where possible. Monitor intake and output and assess specific gravity frequently to evaluate the child's hydration status. Involving parents in feeding can help gain the child's cooperation in taking oral fluids.

Promote Rest and Stress Reduction

The child who has had an acute asthmatic episode is usually very tired when admitted to the nursing unit. Labored breathing and low oxygen status have left the child exhausted. Put the child in a quiet, private room if possible, but accessible for frequent monitoring to promote relaxation and rest. Avoid repeatedly disturbing the child by grouping tasks.

Support Family Participation

The parents may stay with the child, but may be exhausted after hours of their child's respiratory distress. Give parents the option of assisting with the child's treatments, rather than expecting them to do it in addition to comforting the child. Provide frequent updates about the child's condition and encourage the parents to take breaks as needed.

Length of hospitalization depends on the child's response to therapy. Any underlying or accompanying health problem, such as preexisting lung disease or pneumonia, can complicate and extend the child's hospital stay. Communicate with the family of the hospitalized child at least once a day about the child's condition.

Discharge Planning and Home Care Teaching

Parents need a thorough understanding of asthma—how to prevent attacks and provide treatment to maintain the child's health and avoid unnecessary hospitalization. When possible, educate parents when they are rested but refer the child to a healthcare provider for more extensive education. Support of parents and the child should focus on helping them to understand and cope with the diagnosis and the need for daily management to promote near-normal respiratory function.

Discharge planning for the asthmatic child focuses on increasing the family's knowledge about the disease, medication therapy, and the need for follow-up care according to guidelines of the National Asthma Education and Prevention Program. The required lifestyle changes may be difficult for the child and parents. The need to modify the home by removing a loved pet, for example, may create stress. When a family will not give up a pet, discuss the need to bathe the pet frequently to reduce animal dander. The nurse can facilitate discussion and clarification of ways to prevent asthma episodes. Teach the family how to measure and interpret peak expiratory flow readings (see Skill 11–12 **SKILLS**). Discuss rescue medications to manage asthma episodes, as well as controller medications for daily management. Reassure the family that most children with asthma can lead a normal life with some modifications.

Nursing Care in the Community

Nurses provide care to children with asthma in pediatricians' offices, specialty asthma clinics, schools, and summer camps. Once the stress of the acute episode has passed, the community setting is ideal for ongoing coordinated education about asthma management. Help the parents and child to understand the diagnosis and the need for daily management to promote near-normal respiratory function while the child continues to grow and develop normally.

Key points to cover in asthma education include the following (Hayes, Djaferis, Gattasso et al., 2004):

■ Explain that asthma is a chronic and progressive condition, but parents should expect that it can be controlled.

■ Stress the need to follow the prescribed medication schedule, and discuss strategies to remember daily medications (specific time of day or daily event).

■ Discuss possible adverse drug effects.

■ Review proper use of metered dose inhaler, spacer, and peak flow meter.

EVIDENCE-BASED NURSING

MEDICATION MANAGEMENT IN ASTHMA

Clinical Question (Problem)

Many children with asthma have less than optimal medication management to control symptoms and have increased asthma episodes. What information about the family's knowledge and perceptions about managing the child with asthma could help nurses collaborate more effectively with families to improve asthma management?

Evidence

Recent research on parental beliefs, knowledge, experience of living with a child who has asthma, and attitudes about controller medication was conducted through interviews with 18 mothers of children and adolescents with asthma. Parents indicated that they learned to manage the child's asthma through "trial and error." Even though they learned about medications at one time, they still had gaps in knowledge about medication actions. Parents also wished to have health professionals listen to them regarding their child's healthcare needs. The parents reported that daily medication management was the most difficult aspect of asthma care, but they saw a good response in the child when used (Peterson-Sweeney, McMullen, Yoos et al., 2003). Another study involving the parents of 109 children with asthma explored their attitudes and understanding of asthma. Only 27 of the 78 children with persistent asthma had an appropriate medication regimen, and 17 parents reported using no anti-inflammatory medication even when the child had moderate to severe asthma. Some parents believed inhaled steroids should be a last-resort therapy or if steroids were used for a while they would not work when needed. These parents also anticipated that their children would

have activity limitations and episodic emergency department visits (Yoos, Kitzman, & McMullen, 2003).

Implications

Demonstrating respect for the parent's knowledge of the child's health status and response to asthma management is an essential step in developing an effective partnership with the parent. It is also important to talk with parents about their beliefs about daily medications for asthma management, use of inhaled steroids, and their expectations of how asthma will affect their child. Gaining an understanding of the family's beliefs can help guide nursing education and collaborative development of a plan to manage the child's asthma.

Critical Thinking

Consider the possible perceptions and beliefs of parents and children with asthma in your practice setting. Develop an education program that integrates these beliefs and perceptions to help improve families' understanding of medication actions, the differences between inhaled and oral corticosteroids, and collaboration with health professionals to improve the control of their child's asthma.

References

Peterson-Sweeney, K., McMullen, A., Yoos, H. L., & Kitzman, H. (2003). Parental perceptions of their child's asthma: Management and medication use. *Journal of Pediatric Nursing, 17*(3), 118–125.

Yoos, H. L., Kitzman, H., & McMullen, A. (2003). Barriers to anti-inflammatory medication use in childhood asthma. *Ambulatory Pediatrics, 3*(July), 181–190.

MEDIALINK Medication Administration—Growth and Development

- Explain that exercise is important for health, and asthma induced by exercise can be managed with medication.
- Discuss keeping an asthma symptom diary.

If the child has severe asthma and uses high doses of aerosol or oral glucocorticoids to control asthma attacks, monitor the child's growth every 6 months as the disease and medications may affect overall growth. Review the family's daily plan for monitoring the child's respiratory status and the parent's ability to identify the timing and type of stepped-up care needed to manage worsening symptoms. Review and reinforce the child's technique for use of the metered dose inhaler. The goal is to bring asthma episodes under control with stepped-up care before a significant episode occurs (see Table 47–12).

Make sure the child has a supply of medications at school or child care as well as at home. Help the child learn the signs of early respiratory distress and how to request medications when at school before signs get more serious. Help the parents communicate with school personnel regarding the child's condition, and have an individual health plan developed so that medications are given as needed, even in preparation for ex-

ercise. For a young school-age child, make sure the child's teacher can help recognize respiratory distress and reduce the child's fear of going to the nurse for rescue medications.

Environmental control is an important part of asthma management. When possible, pets should not be kept in the home (and never in the child's bedroom). Active dust mite control should be attempted, but it is challenging as mites live in carpets, bedding, upholstered furniture, and clothes. To help control dust mites in the child's bedroom, encase the pillow and mattress in plastic covers. Initiate cockroach control. Smoke from cigarettes, wood stoves, and fireplaces all have the potential to trigger an asthma attack.

Refer to "Nursing Care Plan: The Child with Asthma in the Community Setting" in Chapter 39 for additional information. ∞

EVALUATION

Expected outcomes of nursing care include the following:

- The child recognizes early asthma symptoms and uses rescue medications, hydration, and relaxation breathing before severe respiratory distress occurs.

TEACHING HIGHLIGHTS

HOME CARE INSTRUCTIONS FOR THE CHILD WITH ASTHMA

Identify parents' knowledge about the condition:

1. Review why asthma occurs and assess parents' understanding of the physiologic process. Ask:
   - What happens in your child's lungs during an asthma attack?
   - What are the early warning signs of an asthma episode in your child?
   - What are your child's symptoms and how does he or she respond to them? Does your child use the peak expiratory flow meter to evaluate symptoms? Is a diary maintained of the child's symptoms?
2. Identify asthma triggers and assess parents' understanding of how to prevent, avoid, or minimize their effect in a timely manner. Ask:
   - Do you know your child's personal asthma triggers? Where do most episodes begin? (Suggest that the parents and child keep a notebook to track episodes so they can learn more about these triggers.)
   - What steps can you take or have you taken to minimize or eliminate your child's exposure to indoor pollutants (quitting smoking, environmental control, etc.)?

Set up a schedule for parents and children to learn asthma management:
- Discuss when and where to seek emergency medical help.
- Discuss actions parents can take before seeking medical assistance.

Review parents' understanding of medication therapy:
- Provide information about medications: name, type of drug, dose, method of administration, expected effect, possible side effects. Make sure they understand when controller and rescue medications should be used.
- Evaluate the child's technique for the type of inhaler used as the techniques vary. Review the technique for use of the peak flow meter. See "Medication Administration—Growth and Development" on the Companion Website for growth and developmental issues regarding the use of inhalers.

Address associated issues:
- Storage and proper transport of medications.
- Financial considerations of medication cost and lifestyle changes.
- Notification of child's school or teacher; arrangements for the child's use of medications at school.
- Medical identification bracelet or medallion to facilitate assistance when the child is away from home.

- The child and family implement a daily treatment plan for asthma and reduce the number of asthma episodes the child has.
- The child with a serious asthma episode responds to oxygen, fluids, and medication therapy, avoiding hospital admission.

STATUS ASTHMATICUS

Status asthmaticus is unrelenting, severe respiratory distress and bronchospasm in an asthmatic child, which persists despite pharmacologic and supportive interventions. Without immediate intervention the child with status asthmaticus may progress to respiratory failure and die. The child is placed in an ICU and may require endotracheal intubation with assisted ventilation. The section on respiratory failure earlier in the chapter gives additional information on the nurse's role in providing emergency respiratory care.

CYSTIC FIBROSIS

Cystic fibrosis (CF) is a common inherited autosomal recessive disorder of the exocrine glands that results in physiologic alterations in the respiratory, gastrointestinal, integumentary, musculoskeletal, and reproductive systems. The incidence of CF varies by race—1:3300 in whites, 1:17,000 in blacks, 1:8000 in Hispanics, and 1:32,000 in Asian Americans (McMullen & Bryson, 2004). Approximately 20,000 children and 10,000 adults have CF in the United States (Cystic Fibrosis Foundation, 2004) (Figure 47–6 ●). The median life span for individuals with cystic fibrosis is 35 years (Cystic Fibrosis Foundation, 2005).

ETIOLOGY AND PATHOPHYSIOLOGY

A gene isolated on the long arm of chromosome 7 directs the function of the CF transmembrane conductance regulator (CFTR). With a defective CFTR, the exocrine and epithelial cells have defective chloride-ion transport and decreased water flows across cell membranes. This results in an abnormal accumulation of viscous, dehydrated mucus that affects the respiratory, gastrointestinal, and genitourinary systems. Inflammation and lung changes are present as early as 4 weeks of age. Ultimately, all body organs with mucous ducts become obstructed and damaged (McMullen & Bryson, 2004).

○ **FIGURE 47–6**

Cystic fibrosis is an inherited autosomal recessive disorder of the exocrine glands, so it is not uncommon to see siblings with it such as this brother and sister.

NURSING PRACTICE

Recent advances in localization of the CF gene have led to successful techniques for prenatal diagnosis and carrier testing. There are nearly 1000 mutations of the CFTR gene that can cause CF (Orenstein, Winnie, & Altman, 2002). Genetic testing to identify the majority of CF gene alterations is available to adults with a positive family history, partners of people with CF, couples planning a pregnancy in a high-risk population, and couples seeking prenatal testing. Rare CF gene alterations are not always detected by genetic testing (Cystic Fibrosis Foundation, 2004).

Because of the blocked pancreatic ducts and resulting pancreatic damage, the natural enzymes necessary to digest fats and proteins are not secreted, and malabsorption results in the majority of children by 1 year of age. In some children, the pancreas may stop producing insulin and the body may fail to use insulin normally, resulting in the development of diabetes mellitus.

The lungs are always filled with mucus, which the respiratory cilia cannot clear. This causes air to become trapped in the small airways, resulting in atelectasis (pulmonary collapse). Secondary respiratory infections occur because secretions provide an environment conducive to bacterial growth. Respiratory failure is the leading cause of mortality.

Nearly all males who have CF are sterile because of blockage or absence of the vas deferens. Females have difficulty conceiving because of chronic illness, and increased mucus secretions in the reproductive tract interfere with the passage of sperm (McMullen & Bryson, 2004).

Metabolic function is altered as a result of the imbalances created by excessive electrolyte loss through perspiration, saliva, and mucus secretion. The children are at risk for dehydration secondary to electrolyte imbalance. The "salty taste" of the skin is the result of sodium chloride that makes its way through skin pores to the skin surface.

CLINICAL MANIFESTATIONS

The primary symptom of CF is the production of thick, sticky mucus. One of the earliest signs is meconium ileus, a small bowel obstruction in the newborn's first 48 hours of life. Stools of the child with cystic fibrosis characteristically are frothy (bulky and large quantity), smell foul, contain fat (are greasy), and float. Constipation is common and intestinal obstruction may occur in older children. Rectal prolapse, resulting from the large, bulky, difficult-to-pass stools, may occur.

Other signs and symptoms include a chronic moist, productive cough and frequent respiratory infections. Frontal headaches, facial tenderness, and purulent nasal discharge are signs of a chronic sinus infection. Nasal polyps are found in 10% of children with CF (McMullen & Bryson, 2004). Most children have difficulty maintaining and gaining weight despite a voracious appetite because of malabsorption and frequent infections. Infants and children may have a delayed bone age, short stature, and delayed onset of puberty. Clubbing of the tips of the fingers and toes occurs as the disease progresses (Figure 47-7 ○).

CLINICAL THERAPY

CF is usually diagnosed in infancy or early childhood with one of three major presentations: newborn meconium ileus, malabsorption or failure to thrive, or chronic recurrent respiratory infections. Some children with a milder form of the disease, however, may reach the teen or young adult years before symptoms appear. The mean age at diagnosis is 4.8 years (Farrell, Kosorok, Rock et al., 2001).

○ **FIGURE 47–7**

Digital clubbing.

Newborn screening using dried blood samples for immunoreactive trypsinogen is mandated in some states, and genetic testing of the child's DNA is performed to confirm a positive test (Parad & Comeau, 2003). A sweat chloride test by pilocarpine iontophoresis is used to test children with classic symptoms or a positive family history (McMullen & Bryson, 2004). A sweat chloride concentration of 50 to 60 mEq/L is suspicious. If the chloride concentration is greater than 60 mEq/L, it is diagnostic with other signs. Two tests are performed to confirm the diagnosis (Figure 47–8 ●). A spirometer is used on children older than 6 years to monitor pulmonary function. Sputum cultures are obtained to identify infectious organisms and antibiotic sensitivities.

Clinical therapy focuses on maintaining respiratory function, managing infection, promoting optimal nutrition and exercise, and preventing gastrointestinal blockage (Table 47–14). See Table 47–15 for medications used to treat CF. Newly diagnosed children will have no or minimal symptoms and near-normal lung function if aggressively treated. Pulmonary function declines 2% to 4% per year even with aggressive treatment (Varlotta, 1998).

Improvements in medical management and optimal nutrition have prolonged the lives of children with CF. However, new complications such as CF-related diabetes must be carefully coordinated along with the progression of the disease. Lung transplantation is occasionally performed,

● **FIGURE 47–8**

This 6-month-old girl is being evaluated for cystic fibrosis using the sweat test.

and approximately 50% of cases survive for the first 5 years (McMullen & Bryson, 2004). CF is ultimately terminal, however, because of the progressive multisystem changes and the difficulty of long-term infection management.

TABLE 47–14 ✤ Clinical Therapy for Cystic Fibrosis

Clinical Therapy	Rationale
Respiratory Therapy	
Exercise and physical fitness	Promotes maintenance of lung function
Chest physiotherapy for all lung segments (bilateral percussion or vibration while the patient is in a position to promote sputum drainage)	In association with coughing and breathing techniques secretions move to bronchi from lung areas
Immunizations	Prevention of viral and some bacterial infections
Chest tube drainage of air leaks	Resolves pneumothorax
Thorocoscopy to sew over ruptured alveoli	Repairs area of recurrent pneumothorax and prevents future episode in same location
Lung transplantation	Reversal of respiratory failure
Gastrointestinal Tract Therapy	
Acid suppression preparation	Gastroesophageal reflux worsens lung function; enteric coating of enzyme supplements is affected by high acid content in duodenum
Hyperosmolar enemas, Isotonic fluid lavage of the intestines orally or by nasogastric tube	Enema relieves meconium ileus in most infants; fluid lavage reduces distal intestinal obstruction
Nutrition	
Well-balanced diet with 120–150% of RDA recommended calories and 200% of RDA recommended protein and moderate fat	Promotes essential nutrient balance for health, growth, and weight maintenance; nutritional counseling to support high-caloric intake; cultural-socioeconomic issues important
Pancreatic enzyme supplements	Assists in digestion of nutrients and decreasing fat and bulk

TABLE 47–15 ✣ Medications Used to Treat Cystic Fibrosis

Medications	Actions
Aerosol bronchodilators	Opens large and small airways; use before chest physiotherapy and with symptoms; few studies exist to demonstrate their effectiveness.
Aerosol DNAse	Loosens, liquefies, and thins pulmonary secretions; decreases risk of developing pulmonary infections requiring parenteral treatment in some patients (McMullen & Bryson, 2004).
Corticosteroids and high-dose ibuprofen on alternate days	Anti-inflammatory agents: reduces inflammatory response to infection; alternate day use to decrease side effects of steroids; decreases progression of lung damage in preadolescents with mild disease.
Antibiotics (oral, IV, and inhalation)	Treats infections. Higher doses than normal and prolonged courses may be needed. Antibiotic selection should be based on culture sensitivities. Intermittent administration of tobramycin by inhalation improves pulmonary function.
Pancreatic enzyme supplements (Cotazym-S, Pancrease, Viokase)	Assists in digestion of nutrients decreasing fat and bulk; given prior to food ingestion, taken with meals and snacks.
Multivitamins and vitamin E in water-soluble form; vitamins A, D, and K given when deficient; iron supplementation	Cystic fibrosis interferes with vitamin production; supplements are required in water-soluble form for better absorption (vitamins A, D, E, and K are naturally fat soluble); iron deficiency results from malabsorption syndrome.
Ursodeoxycholate	May slow progression of hepatic lesion in CF. Given when patient has elevated liver enzymes or evidence of portal hypertension.
Lactulose	May abort early distal intestinal obstruction syndrome and prevent recurrences.

NURSING MANAGEMENT

Care of the child with previously diagnosed CF is the focus of the following discussion.

NURSING ASSESSMENT AND DIAGNOSIS

Physiologic Assessment

Physical assessment of the child focuses on adequacy of respiratory function. The child with CF usually is admitted with symptoms of an upper respiratory infection. Obtain a set of baseline vital signs. Assess the child's respiratory status. Auscultate the chest for breath sounds, crackles, and wheezes. Inquire about the frequency and character of the child's cough and characteristics of sputum as changes may be related to a new infection. Note any cyanosis or clubbing of the extremities.

Evaluate the child's growth, plotting the weight and height on a growth curve. Determine whether the child is maintaining an appropriate growth pattern or is malnourished. Inquire about the child's appetite and dietary intake. How are nutritional supplements, pancreatic enzymes, and vitamins used?

Assess the child's stooling pattern. Identify whether the child has problems with abdominal pain or bloating, and whether these problems can be related to eating, stooling, or other activities. Palpate the abdomen for liver size, fecal masses, and evidence of pain.

Psychosocial Assessment

The emotional stress of this chronic disease may not be readily apparent on admission, particularly if the child's symptoms are mild and not imminently life threatening. Ongoing observation of the child's and parents' behavior helps direct nursing interventions throughout hospitalization (see Table 47–9). Parents may feel guilt as carriers of the disease. Siblings may also show signs of difficulty in dealing with the illness. Link the family to support groups. School-age children and adolescents often are embarrassed at being viewed as different from playmates and peers. Ask how the child and adolescent feel about the need for a special diet, medications, and limitations.

Ask parents how the child's illness has affected day-to-day functioning, any potential conflicts with family activities, and how they have adapted to the child's plan of care. Ask what the parents have told the child and siblings about the disease. What questions have the child and siblings asked about CF, and how have parents answered them? Has the child ever asked about his or her life expectancy? If not, what would parents say if asked?

Developmental Assessment

Growth and development may be altered by the chronic nature of the disease. Children with cystic fibrosis may be growth retarded. Compare the child's height and weight to age norms and observe the adolescent for the appearance of secondary sex characteristics, which are often delayed.

Common nursing diagnoses for the child with cystic fibrosis include the following:

- *Ineffective Airway Clearance* related to thick mucus in lungs
- *Risk for Infection* related to the presence of mucous secretions conducive to bacterial growth
- *Imbalanced Nutrition: Less than Body Requirements* related to inability to digest nutrients
- *Parental Role Conflict* related to interruptions in family life due to the home care regimen and child's frequent exacerbations

PLANNING AND IMPLEMENTATION

Nursing management involves supporting the child and family initially, when the diagnosis is made, during subsequent hospitalizations, and during visits to specialty and primary healthcare providers. The nurse's role begins with implementing specific medical therapies and providing nursing care to meet the child's physiologic and psychosocial needs. Respiratory therapy, medications, and diet must be coordinated to promote optimal body function. Psychosocial support and reinforcement of the child's daily care needs are important in preparation for home care.

Children with cystic fibrosis require periodic hospitalization when a severe infection occurs or for a pulmonary and nutritional "tune-up." The child is usually placed in a single room to reduce the spread of infectious organisms with standard precautions. Children with CF are not co-roomed to reduce the risk for transfer of the infectious organisms *Pseudomonas* and *Burkholderia cepacia* (Cystic Fibrosis Foundation, 2000). Respect the parents' experiences as the child's primary care provider and include them in the child's routine care as much as possible. However, parents may view the hospital stay as a break from the rigorous daily pulmonary routine at home and need support in taking advantage of some "down" time. While the family is often proficient at providing physical care to the child, the nurse should take the opportunity to review basic and new information about respiratory care, medications, and nutrition.

Provide Respiratory Therapy

Chest physiotherapy is usually performed one to three times per day before meals to clear secretions from the lungs, as coughing may stimulate vomiting (Figure 47–9). Parents and other family members can learn to help

⦿ FIGURE 47–9

A   B   C

Postural drainage can be achieved by clapping with a cupped hand on the chest wall over the segment to be drained to create vibrations that are transmitted to the bronchi to dislodge secretions. ***A,*** If the obstruction is in the posterior apical segment of the lung, the nurse can do this with the child sitting up. ***B,*** If the obstruction is in the left posterior segment, the child should be lying on the right side. Several other positions can be used depending on the location of the obstruction. ***C,*** A high-frequency chest wall oscillation vest is another option for chest physiotherapy that the child can independently manage.

with these necessary treatments. Pulmonary care may involve aerosol treatments and antibiotics when indicated (see Table 47–11). (See Skill 14–25.) **SKILLS**

Administer Medications and Meet Nutritional Needs

Antibiotics for acute exacerbation are provided by oral, inhalation, and intravenous routes. Because children with CF have an increased clearance of most antibiotics, they need higher doses and long treatment courses. Renal function needs to be monitored and serum antibiotic levels may be taken to ensure therapeutic dosing.

Digestive problems can be eased with pancreatic enzymes and dietary modification. Pancreatic enzyme supplements come in powder sprinkles and capsule form and are taken orally with all meals and large snacks. The amount needed is individualized based on the child's nutritional needs and digestive response to these supplements. Families need to learn which foods if any to avoid that contribute to a child's gastrointestinal problems. The goal is to achieve near-normal, well-formed stools and adequate weight gain.

Fat-soluble vitamins (A, D, E, and K) are not completely absorbed from food; therefore, they must be taken in water-soluble form. Multivitamins taken twice daily usually are sufficient to prevent deficiency. The diet should be well balanced, with an emphasis on high caloric value. Fats and salt are both necessary in the diet. Balanced with pancreatic enzyme supplements, moderate fat intake adds an important source of extra fuel. Respiratory complications cause additional energy expenditure, and some children require supplemental nasogastric or gastrostomy feedings to gain and maintain weight.

Provide Psychosocial Support

Help the parents and child learn what they must do to maintain health after discharge. Emotional support is essential because the diagnosis of this disorder creates anxiety and fear in both the parents and the child. They need assistance with emotional and psychosocial issues relating to discipline, body image (stooling and odor), frequent rehospitalization, the potential fatal nature of the illness, the child's feeling of being different from friends, and overall financial, social, and family concerns. Because the disorder is inherited, families may have more than one child with cystic fibrosis. Parents may have unspoken feelings of anger and guilt, blaming themselves for their children's condition.

Discharge Planning and Home Care Teaching

Review the family's potential need for financial assistance due to the out-of-pocket costs for medications, supplies, equipment, and medical follow-up. Home care of the child with CF is expensive and can be draining on the family's finances. If the family requires financial assistance, refer them to the appropriate social services.

Review chest physiotherapy techniques with the parents, which should be performed as often as two or three times a day. Alternate bronchial hygiene therapy techniques such as a vest may be more easily accepted by the family. See "Bronchial Hygiene Therapy" on the Companion Website. Encourage the child to exercise and participate in physical activities as this helps improve lung function, endurance, and airway clearance.

Managing the child's nutritional needs is important and takes time and energy. Parents need to learn how to prepare high-calorie foods, provide needed enzymes before meals, what vitamins need to be given daily, and what foods should be avoided or eliminated because of the child's digestive problems. Make a referral to a nutritionist either before or at the time of discharge.

NURSING PRACTICE

Parents often have a difficult time getting the child with cystic fibrosis to eat the extra calories needed for optimal nutrition, setting the stage for a potential mealtime battleground. To be successful, parents need guidance about managing mealtime behaviors in addition to guidelines for preparing nutritional calorie-dense foods. Increase calorie intake by adding fats and high-calorie snacks between meals and before bed. Extra intervention may be needed when the child's weight is 85% to 90% of ideal weight for height. Children with adequate nutrition have a longer life expectancy. See the Companion Website for links.

CF affects all family members and disrupts activities of daily living for everyone. It is important to refer families to family counseling and group therapy with families of other children with CF, if indicated. The Cystic Fibrosis Foundation is a source for family information. See the Companion Website for links.

Nursing Care in the Community

Nurses may encounter the child with cystic fibrosis in any of the following settings: clinics specializing in the disease, pediatricians' offices, and schools. The primary goal is to keep the disease under control by promoting optimal nutrition and assisting the family to reduce the incidence of infection. Nurses may also provide home care to the child with cystic fibrosis following hospitalization for an acute exacerbation or provide hospice care.

Assessment. Perform the physical assessment as described for the hospitalized child. Obtain oxygen saturation and spirometry readings if changes in respiratory status are suspected. Observe the child's physical appearance, noting overall body proportions and any changes characteristic of long-term CF. Assess hearing acuity on a regular basis if the antibiotic tobramycin is used as it has been associated with hearing loss.

MEDIALINK Skill 14–25: Performing Chest Physiotherapy/Postural Drainage

MEDIALINK Bronchial Hygiene Therapy

Inquire about the family's and child's emotional and psychosocial responses to managing the illness. These issues are very important when the child is going through major developmental stages.

Management. Review the child's use of bronchodilators and airway clearance techniques. To prevent a change in pulmonary status from progressing, short-term changes in care may be recommended. These may include intravenous and aerosol medications and antibiotics, an increase in the number of times chest physiotherapy is performed daily, and changes in dietary management. Help the family select the best time to fit the additional treatment into their schedule.

Malnutrition is a major problem for children with CF. Parents often need to plan meals and snacks for the young child to ensure that adequate calories are consumed. Arrange for a consultation with a nutritionist if the family would benefit from new strategies to help meet the child's nutritional needs.

Children with CF lose more than normal amounts of salt in their sweat. This loss can become intensified during hot weather, strenuous exercise, and fever. Parents should allow the child to add extra salt to food and should permit some salty snacks (pretzels with salt, pickles, carbonated soda). During periods of increased sweating, the child should be encouraged to drink more fluids and increase salt intake. Teach parents to recognize early symptoms of salt depletion, including fatigue, weakness, abdominal pain, and vomiting, and to contact the child's healthcare provider if these symptoms occur.

Adolescents with CF need special assistance in coping with their disorder, especially as survival into adulthood is common. Help them identify normal adolescent changes versus those related to CF. Adolescents must learn how to cope with the difference they know exists between themselves and peers. Provide information about potential infertility along with guidelines for safe sexual practices to reduce the risk for sexually transmitted infections. Females with CF may be able to conceive and should be offered contraception.

Gradual assumption of responsibility for daily disease management is necessary. Adherence with the daily disease management may be a problem during adolescence. Individualized planning to achieve their daily care regimen while enabling them to interact with peers and participate in school activities may be most helpful. Link adolescents to services to assist with planning appropriate educational and occupational goals for their future. Palliative care planning should be initiated as the disease progresses to respiratory failure.

EVALUATION

Expected outcomes of nursing care include the following:

- The child and family develop proficiency in providing the daily pulmonary care and reducing the incidence of respiratory infections.

- The child and family develop a schedule and routine for daily pulmonary care that fits into family and school activities.

- The child consumes adequate calories and pancreatic enzymes to support growth and to stay within desirable weight ranges.

INJURIES OF THE RESPIRATORY SYSTEM

Airway compromise after an unintentional injury can cause death if not managed quickly and effectively. Children are vulnerable to changes in respiratory function after injury. A child's airway can become easily obstructed because of its small size. The airway may be obstructed by the tongue, small amounts of blood, mucus, or foreign debris, as well as swelling in the respiratory tract or adjacent neck tissue. If the child's neck is flexed or hyperextended, the soft laryngeal cartilage may also compress and obstruct the airway.

SMOKE-INHALATION INJURY

Exposure to fire conditions sets up dramatic responses in the respiratory tract of children. In every age group, inhalation injury increases the child's chance of death by 20%, and it also increases the likelihood that the child will develop pneumonia (Kim, 2001).

The severity of the smoke-inhalation injury is influenced by the type of material burned and whether the child was found in an open or closed space. The composition of materials determines how easily they ignite, how fast they burn, and how much heat they release. These factors influence the production of smoke and toxic gases. Smoke, a product of the burning process that is composed of gases and particles, is generated in varying volumes and density. The type and concentration of toxic gases, which are usually invisible, affect the severity of pulmonary damage. The duration of exposure to the smoke produced and any toxic gases contribute significantly to the child's prognosis.

Exposure to extreme heat, common in house fires, leads to surface injury and upper airway damage. The upper airway normally removes heat from inhaled gases, sparing the lower airway from thermal damage. However, this action results in marked edema, placing the small child at particular risk for airway obstruction. Edema develops rapidly over a few hours and may lead to acute respiratory distress syndrome.

Carbon monoxide (CO) is a clear, colorless, odorless gas present in all fire conditions as the fire consumes oxygen. The CO molecule binds more firmly to hemoglobin than does oxygen. As a result, it replaces oxygen in circulation and rapidly produces hypoxia in the child. The longer the exposure to CO, the greater the hypoxia. The brain receives inadequate oxygen, resulting in confusion. This accounts for the inability of fire victims to escape as confusion progresses to loss of consciousness. The process can be rapidly reversed, however, by timely administration of 100% oxygen (Schweich & Zempsky, 1999).

Damage to the lower airway most often results from chemicals or toxic gas inhalation. Soot is carried deep into the lungs, where it combines with water in the lungs to deposit acid-producing chemicals on the lung tissue. These acids burn the tissue, causing loss of cilia, loss of surfactant, and edema. Tissue destruction, edema, and disruption of gas exchange produce the initial insult to the lungs and potential airway obstruction. Days later, the damaged tissue sloughs off, obstructing the airways. Because the cilia that normally help remove debris have been destroyed, the lungs become a breeding ground for microorganisms. Pneumonia becomes a major health concern. The damaged alveoli heal by scar tissue formation. This can greatly reduce future lung function.

Burns of the face and neck, singed nasal hairs, soot around the mouth or nose, and hoarseness with stridor or voice change all indicate inhalation injury, even when the child initially has no respiratory distress. Edema develops rapidly over a few hours and may lead to airway obstruction with signs such as tachypnea, stridor, coughing, and wheezing. Respiratory distress develops and can lead to respiratory failure.

NURSING MANAGEMENT

Most children who survive smoke-inhalation injury are admitted for close observation, airway management, and ventilatory support, if indicated. Initial treatment is 100% humidified oxygen administered through a nonrebreather mask. Respiratory assessment and pulmonary therapy are usually required to reestablish adequate oxygenation and respiratory function. If respiratory distress develops, aggressive airway management with an endotracheal tube, mechanical ventilation, and monitoring are usually provided in an intensive care unit. Care is provided as described for the child with respiratory failure.

BLUNT CHEST TRAUMA

Blunt trauma is a common injury in children, especially associated with motor vehicle crashes (Pieper, 2000). Chest injuries may not be obvious and can be extremely difficult to evaluate.

Most children who die after sustaining severe blunt trauma were hypoxic because of poor airway and ventilatory control. A child's elastic, pliable chest wall and thin abdominal muscles provide minimal protection to underlying organs. This elasticity often prevents rib fractures, but the energy from blunt trauma is transferred directly from an external force to the internal organs, often causing a pulmonary contusion or pneumothorax. A rib fracture in children under 12 years old indicates trauma of significant force.

PULMONARY CONTUSION

A pulmonary contusion is defined as bruising damage to the tissues of the lung. This causes bleeding into the alveoli, which may lead to capillary rupture in the air sacs. Pulmonary edema develops in the lower airways as blood and fluid from damaged tissues accumulate. Lower airway obstruction and atelectasis may result in impaired gas exchange, acute respiratory distress, and respiratory failure (Hazinski, 1999).

Pulmonary contusion occurs in the majority of children with nonpenetrating chest trauma. Initially the child may appear asymptomatic. Respiratory distress, along with fever, wheezing, hemoptysis, and crackles, often develops over several hours. Careful observation is required during the first 12 hours after the injury to detect decreased perfusion related to ventilatory impairment.

Nursing Management

Nursing care centers on providing necessary physiologic support, such as oxygen therapy, positioning, positive pressure ventilation, oxygen, and comfort measures. The child's level of consciousness is an excellent indicator of respiratory function. Agitation and lethargy can signal increasing hypoxia. When monitoring the status of a child who has a pulmonary contusion, do not rely on the child's color as an indicator of adequate oxygenation. Cyanosis in children is often a late indicator of respiratory distress. Observe for hemoptysis (fresh blood in the emesis), dyspnea, decreased breath sounds, wheezes, crackles, and a transient temperature elevation.

Inspect the thorax for symmetric chest wall movement and equal presence of breath sounds in both lungs. The child may initially appear well but requires careful and thorough monitoring to detect signs of deterioration. Children with significant injuries are cared for in the ICU. Some children require ventilator support as the pulmonary tissues heal.

PNEUMOTHORAX

A pneumothorax occurs when air enters the pleural space because of tears in the tracheobronchial tree, the esophagus, or the chest wall. If blood collects in the pleural space, it is called a *hemothorax,* and if blood and air collect, it is called a *pneumohemothorax.* A pneumothorax is one of the more common thoracic injuries in pediatric trauma patients.

There are three types of pneumothorax: open, closed, and tension. An open pneumothorax, sometimes referred to as a sucking chest wound, results from any penetrating injury that exposes the pleural space to atmospheric pressure, thereby collapsing the lung. A sucking sound may be heard as the air moves through the opening on the chest wall.

A closed pneumothorax is sometimes caused by blunt chest trauma with no evidence of rib fracture (see "Pathophysiology Illustrated: Pneumothorax"). The chest may be compressed against a closed glottis, causing a sudden increase in pressure within the thoracic cavity. The child spontaneously holds his or her breath when the thorax is struck, accounting for the involuntary closing of the glottis. The pressure increase is transferred to the alveoli, causing them to burst. A single burst alveolus may be able to seal itself off, but with the destruction of many alveoli the lung collapses. Breath sounds are decreased or absent on the injured side, and the child is in respiratory distress. A thoracostomy is performed and a chest tube inserted (see Skill 14–15.) **SKILLS** A closed drainage system is attached to help remove the air and reinflate the lung by reestablishing negative pressure.

A tension pneumothorax is a life-threatening emergency that results when the air leaks into the chest during inspiration but cannot escape during expiration. Internal pressure continues to build, compressing the chest contents and collapsing the lung. Venous return to the heart is impaired as the trachea, heart, vena cava, and esophagus are compressed toward the unaffected lung when the mediastinum shifts, leading to decreased cardiac output. Signs of tension pneumothorax include increasing respiratory distress, decreased breath sounds, and paradoxical breathing.

Nursing Management

Nursing management focuses on airway management and maintaining lung inflation. The child arrives on the nursing unit with a chest tube and drainage system in place. Continued close observation for respiratory distress is essential. Carefully monitor vital signs. Complications include hemothorax (if the thoracostomy and chest tube are improperly placed), lung tissue injury, and scarring from poor tube placement (especially if the tube is placed too near the breast in girls).

PATHOPHYSIOLOGY ILLUSTRATED

Pneumothorax

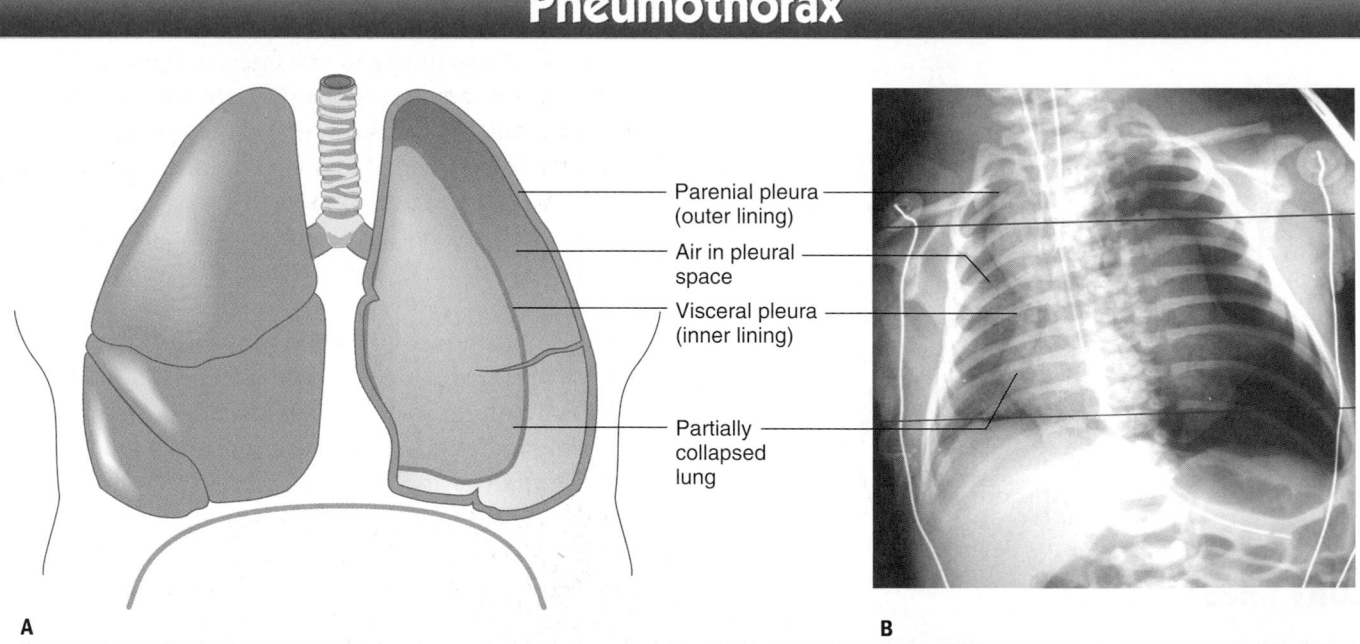

Parenial pleura (outer lining)

Air in pleural space

Visceral pleura (inner lining)

Partially collapsed lung

A, A pneumothorax is air in the pleural space that causes a lung to collapse. Whether the air results from an open injury or from bursting of alveoli due to a blunt injury, it is important to focus on airway management and maintain lung inflation. **B,** Tension pneumothorax, note the collapsed lung on the patient's right side and the deviation of the child's heart and trachea to the right side of the chest. *Courtesy of Dorothy Bulas, M.D., Professor of Radiology and Pediatrics, Children's National Medical Center, Washington, DC.*

Critical Concept Review

LEARNING OBJECTIVES

CONCEPTS

Describe unique characteristics of the pediatric respiratory system anatomy and physiology and apply that information to the care of children with respiratory conditions.

1. A child's airway is shorter and narrower than an adult's:
   - Creates increased potential for obstruction.
2. Trachea is higher and at a different angle:
   - Causes increased risk for right mainstem obstruction.
3. Newborns are obligatory nose breathers:
   - Do not open mouth if nose is obstructed.
4. Newborn doesn't have enough smooth muscle bundles to help trap airway invaders:
   - Increases possibility of upper respiratory infection.
5. Until age 6 the child uses the diaphragm for breathing:
   - Observe the abdomen to count respirations.

List the different respiratory conditions and injuries that can cause respiratory distress in infants and children.

Respiratory conditions and injuries that can cause respiratory distress include:
1. Foreign body aspiration.
2. Obstructive sleep apnea.
3. Croup syndrome.
4. Epiglottitis.
5. Viral and bacterial respiratory infections.
6. Asthma.
7. Smoke inhalation.
8. Blunt chest trauma.
9. Pulmonary contusion.
10. Pneumothorax.

Assess the child's respiratory signs and symptoms to distinguish between respiratory distress and respiratory failure and describe the appropriate nursing care for each level of severity.

Signs of respiratory distress:
- Tachypnea and tachycardia
- Retractions
- Nasal flaring
- Inspiratory stridor
- Pallor or mottled color
- Labored breathing (dyspnea)

Signs of impending respiratory failure include:
- Irritability, anxiety, mood changes
- Lethargy or decreased responsiveness
- Cyanosis
- Wheezing
- Nasal flaring
- Retractions and accessory muscle use
- Grunting

Nursing care includes:
1. Elevate head of the bed.
2. Monitor vital signs and level of responsiveness frequently for any changes.
3. Monitor oxygen saturation.
4. Give oxygen as ordered.
5. Keep emergency equipment at the bedside to assist ventilations if necessary.
6. Keep child from crying, if possible.

(continued)

LEARNING OBJECTIVES

CONCEPTS

Develop a nursing care plan for a child with common acute respiratory conditions. →

1. Maintain airway patency.
2. Frequently assess vital signs.
3. Allow child to assume position of comfort.
4. Meet fluid needs.
5. Promote rest and stress reduction for the child and parents.
6. Support the family's participation in care.
7. Give the family members information that lets them learn to manage the child's disease.

Develop a nursing care plan for the child with a chronic respiratory condition. →

1. Instruct parents in the use of daily medications.
2. Instruct parents in respiratory therapy techniques.
3. Instruct parents about specific nutritional needs of the child.
4. Review the potential need for financial assistance.
5. Encourage child to exercise and to participate in physical activities to the level of child's respiratory condition.
6. Link family to appropriate support groups.
7. Ensure that child gets immunizations and has other health promotion needs addressed.

CRITICAL THINKING IN ACTION

View the **Critical Thinking in Action** video in Chapter 47 of the CD-ROM. Then, answer the questions that follow.

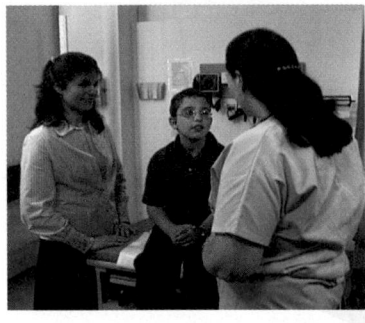

Adam and his mother have come to speak with you to discuss the plan of care for his asthma. Adam, who is 7 years old, has a history of episodic wheezing and nebulizer treatments, but was never was hospitalized for asthma until last week. He was treated in the emergency room and kept 2 days. His parents were educated about how to manage his mild persistent asthma.

His mother has brought a doctor's order along with Adam's Albuterol MDI, his peak flow meter, spacer, and his asthma action plan. She tells you that he is also completing a dose of oral steroids and was placed on Singulair to help prevent the asthma. You discuss the peak flow meter, the guidelines, and what type of action to take as needed. Based on his height of 48 inches, his peak flow meter green zone is 160–128, his yellow zone is 128–80, and his red zone is 80 or below. If he is having problems, he is to take his Albuterol MDI with spacer, two puffs every 4–6 hours as needed.

1. What are some of the side effects associated with Adam's Albuterol MDI?
2. What is the benefit to using a spacer on Adam's Albuterol MDI?
3. What are the signs of respiratory distress to observe for with Adam?
4. Describe the pathophysiology with asthma and why Adam had an asthma attack.

MEDIALINK

www.prenhall.com/london

■ NCLEX-RN® Review, case studies, and other interactive resources for this chapter can be found on the Companion Website at http://www.prenhall.com/london. Click on "Chapter 47" and select the activities for this chapter.

■ For animations, more NCLEX-RN® Review questions, and an audio glossary, access the accompanying CD-ROM in this textbook.

REFERENCES

Agency for Healthcare Research and Quality. (2003). *Management of bronchiolitis in infants and children, summary* (Evidence Report/Technology Assessment: Number 69, AHRQ Publication Number 03-E009). Rockville, MD: Author. Retrieved March 29, 2004, from http://www.ahrq.gov/clinic/epcsums/broncsom.htm

Akinbami, L. J., & Schoendorf, K. C. (2002). Trends in childhood asthma: Prevalence, health care utilization, and mortality. *Pediatrics, 110*(2), 315–322.

American Academies of Pediatrics. (2003). *Red book: 2003 Report of the Committee on Infectious Diseases* (26th ed.). Elk Grove Village, IL: Author.

American Academy of Pediatrics Committee on Child Abuse and Neglect. (2001). Distinguishing sudden infant death syndrome from child abuse fatalities. *Pediatrics, 107*(2), 437–441.

American Academy of Pediatrics Committee on Fetus and Newborn. (2003). Apnea, sudden infant death syndrome, and home monitoring. *Pediatrics, 111*(4), 914–917.

American Academy of Pediatrics Committee on Infectious Diseases and Committee on Fetus and Newborn. (2003). Revised indications for the use of Palivizumab and Respiratory Syncytial Virus Immune Globulin intravenous for the prevention of Respiratory Syncytial Virus infections. *Pediatrics, 112*(6), 1442–1446.

American Academy of Pediatrics Section on Pediatric Pulmonology, Subcommittee on Obstructive Sleep Apnea Syndrome. (2002). Clinical practice guideline: Diagnosis and management of childhood obstructive sleep apnea syndrome. *Pediatrics, 109*(4), 704–712.

American Thoracic Society and Centers for Disease Control and Prevention. (2000). Diagnostic standards and classification of tuberculosis in adults and children. *American Journal of Respiratory and Critical Care Medicine, 161*, 1376–1395.

Anbar, R. D. (2001, February). Self-hypnosis for management of chronic dyspnea in pediatric patients. *Pediatrics, 107*(2), E21.

Baker, V. O., Friedman, J., & Schmitt, R. (2002). Asthma management, part I: An overview of the problem and current trends. *Journal of School Nursing, 18*(3), 128–137.

Baren, J. M., & Puchalski, A. (2002). Current concepts in the ED treatment of pediatric asthma. *Pediatric Emergency Medicine Reports, 7*(10), 105–115.

Belcastro, M. R. (2004). Bronchopulmonary dysplasia: A new look at an old problem. *Newborn and Infant Nursing Reviews, 4*(2), 121–125.

Belcher, D. (2002, November). Breathing easier with pediatric asthma: Pharmacologic management. *Advance for Nurse Practitioners*, 37–38, 79.

Bindler, R. M., & Howry, L. B. (2005). *Pediatric drugs and nursing implications* (3rd ed.). Upper Saddle River, NJ: Prentice Hall-Health.

Capper-Michel, B. (2004). Bronchopulmonary dysplasia. In P. J. Allen & J. A. Vessey, *Primary care of the child with a chronic condition* (4th ed., pp. 282–298). St. Louis, MO: Mosby.

Centers for Disease Control and Prevention. (2000). Measuring childhood asthma prevalence before and after the 1997 redesign of the National

Health Interview Survey. *Morbidity and Mortality Weekly Report, 49*(40), 908–911.

Centers for Disease Control and Prevention. (2004). Trends in tuberculosis—United States, 1998–2003. *Morbidity and Mortality Weekly Report, 53*(10), 209–214.

Centers for Disease Control and Prevention, National Center for Health Statistics. (2001, October). New estimates for asthma tracked. Retrieved January 23, 2003, from www.cdc.gov/nchs/releases/01facts/asthma.htm.

Cooper, A. C., Banasiak, N. C., & Allen, P. J. (2003). Management and prevention strategies for respiratory syncytial virus (RSV) bronchiolitis in infants and young children: A review of evidence-based practice interventions. *Pediatric Nursing, 29*(6), 452–456.

Cote, A., Gerez, T., Brouillette, R. T., & Laplante, S. (2000). Circumstances leading to a change to prone sleeping in sudden infant death syndrome victims. *Pediatrics, 106*(6), 1–5.

Cystic Fibrosis Foundation. (2000). *B. cepacia policy*. Retrieved March 17, 2004, from http://www.cff.org/living_with_cf/B_cepacia_policy.cfm

Cystic Fibrosis Foundation. (2004). *Genetic carrier testing for CF*. Retrieved March 10, 2004, from http://www.cff.org

Cystic Fibrosis Foundation. (2005). *Median age of survival for people with CF increased to 35 years in 2004*. Retrieved July 8, 2005, from http://www.cff.org

Davies, F., & Gupta, R. (2002). Apparent life threatening events in infants presenting to an emergency department. *Emergency Medicine Journal, 19*, 11–16.

Farrell, P. M., Kosorok, M. R., Rock, M. J., Laxova, A., Zeng, L., Lai, H. C., et al. (2001). Early diagnosis of cystic fibrosis through neonatal screening prevents severe malnutrition and improves long term growth. *Pediatrics, 107*(1), 1–13.

Field, T., Henteleff, T., Hernandez-Reif, M., Martinez, E., Mavanda, K., Kuhn, C., et al. (1998). Children with asthma have improved pulmonary functions after massage therapy. *Journal of Pediatrics, 132*(5), 854–858.

Foley, S. M. (2002). Infant asthma: Genetic predisposition and environmental influences. *Newborn and Infant Nursing Reviews, 2*(4), 200–206.

Froh, D. L. (2002). Alterations in pulmonary function in children. In K. L. McCance & S. E. Huether (Eds.), *Pathophysiology: The biologic basis for disease in adults and children* (4th ed., pp. 1145–1169). St. Louis, MO: Mosby.

Gadomski, A. (2002). Bronchiolitis dilemma: A happy wheezer and his unhappy parent. *Contemporary Pediatrics, 19*(11), 40–59.

Gilliland, F. D., Yu-Fen, L., & Peters, J. M. (2001). Effects of maternal smoking during pregnancy and environmental tobacco smoke on asthmatic and wheezing in children. *American Journal of Respiratory and Critical Care Medicine, 163*, 429–436.

Grant, M. J., & Curley, M. A. Q. (2001). Pulmonary critical care problems. In M. A. Q. Curley & P. A. Moloney-Harmon, *Critical care nursing of infants and children* (2nd ed., pp. 655–694). Philadelphia: WB Saunders.

Hayes, E., Djaferis, M., Gattasso, S., Hosmer, T., & Williamson, K. (2004). Documenting to improve pediatric asthma outcomes. *Advance for Nurse Practitioners, 12*(9), 51–56.

Hazinski, M. F. (1999). *Manual of pediatric critical care*. St. Louis, MO: Mosby.

Health Resources and Services Administration, Maternal and Child Health Bureau. (2002). *Child health USA 2002*. Rockville, MD: U.S. Department of Health and Human Services.

Hogan, M. B., & Wilson, N. W. (2003). Asthma in the school-aged child. *Pediatric Annals, 32*(1), 20–25.

Institute of Medicine. (2000). *Clearing the air: Asthma and indoor air exposures*. Washington, DC: National Academy of Sciences.

Isaacson, G., & Isaacson, D. M. (2003). Pediatric epiglottitis caused by group G beta-hemolytic streptococcus. *Pediatric Infectious Disease Journal, 22*(9), 846–847.

Kato, I., Franco, P., Groswasser, J., Scaillet, S., Kelmanson, I., & Kahn, A. (2003). Incomplete arousal processes in infants who were victims of sudden death. *American Journal of Respiratory and Critical Care Medicine, 168*(1), 1298–1303.

Kemper, K. J., & Lester, M. R. (1999). Alternative asthma therapies: An evidence-based review. *Contemporary Pediatrics, 16*, 162–195.

Kieckhefer, G., & Ratcliffe, M. (2004). Asthma. In P. L. Jackson & J. A. Vessey (Eds.), *Primary care of the child with a chronic condition* (4th ed., pp. 174–197). St. Louis, MO: Mosby.

Kim, Y. (2001). Smoke inhalation injury in children. *Office and Emergency Pediatrics, 14*(1), 27–30.

Kohen, D. P., & Wynne, E. (1997). Applying hypnosis in a preschool family asthma education program: Uses of storytelling, imagery and relaxation. *American Journal of Clinical Hypnosis, 39*, 169–181.

Krous, H. F. (2004). Sudden infant death syndrome and unclassified sudden infant deaths: A definitional and diagnostic approach. *Pediatrics, 114*(1), 234–238.

Leung, A. K. C., Kellner, J. D., & Johnson, D. W. (2004). Viral croup: A current perspective. *Journal of Pediatric Health Care, 18*(6), 297–301.

Lieu, T. A., Lozano, P., Finkelstein, J. A., Chi, F. W., Jensvold, N. G., et al. (2002). Racial/ethnic variations in asthma status and management practices among children in managed Medicaid. *Pediatrics, 109*(5), 857–865.

Mannino, D. M., Homa, D. M., & Redd, S. C. (2002). Involuntary smoking and asthma severity in children: Data from the Third National Health and Nutrition Examination Survey. *Chest, 122*(2), 409–415.

Margolis, P., & Gadomski, A. (1998). Does this infant have pneumonia? *Journal of the American Medical Association, 279*(4), 308–313.

Markowitz, G. (2000, April). Don't be sidelined. Managing exercise-induced asthma in children. *Advanced Nurse Practitioner, 8*(4), 77–80.

McMullen, A. H., & Bryson, E. A. (2004). Cystic fibrosis. In P. J. Allen & J. A. Vessey, *Primary care of the child with a chronic condition* (4th ed., pp. 404–425). St. Louis, MO: Mosby.

Milgrom, H., & Taussig, L. M. (1999, September). Keeping children with exercise-induced asthma active. *Pediatrics, 104*(3), e38.

Moon, R. Y., Patel, K. M., & Shaefer, S. J. M. (2000). Sudden infant death syndrome in child care settings. *Pediatrics, 106*(2), 295–300.

Morisky, D. E., Malotte, C. K., Ebin, V., Davidson, P., Cabrera, D., et al. (2001). Behavioral interventions for the control of tuberculosis in adolescents. *Public Health Reports, 116*(6), 568–574.

National Asthma Education and Prevention Program. (2002). *Expert Panel Report II: Guidelines for the diagnosis and management of asthma. Update on selected topics 2002* (NIH Publication No. 02-5075). Bethesda, MD: National Heart Lung and Blood Institute, National Institutes of Health.

National Center for Health Statistics. (2004). *Summary health statistics for U.S. children: National Health Interview Survey, 2002, 10*(221); 87(PHS)-1549. Retrieved February 4, 2005, from www.cdcc.gov/nchs

National Respiratory and Enteric Virus Surveillance System. (2000). Respiratory syncytial virus activity—U.S., 1999–2000 season. *Morbidity and Mortality Weekly Report, 49*(48), 1091–1093.

Orenstein, D. M., Winnie, G. B., & Altman, H. (2002). Cystic fibrosis: A 2002 update. *Journal of Pediatrics, 140*(2), 156–164.

Parad, R. B., & Comeau, A. M. (2003). Newborn screening for cystic fibrosis. *Pediatric Annals, 32*(8), 528–535.

Parnigrahy, A., Filiano, J., Sleeper, L. A., Mandell, F., Valdes-Dapena, M., et al. (2000). Decreased serotonergic receptor binding in rhombic lip-derived regions of the medulla oblongata in the sudden infant death syndrome. *Journal of Neuropathology and Experimental Neurology, 59*(5), 377–384.

Perkin, R. M., & Swift, J. D. (2002). Infectious causes of upper airway obstruction in children. *Pediatric Emergency Medicine Reports, 7*(11), 117–128.

Peterson-Sweeney, K., McMullen, A., Yoos, H. L., & Kitzman, H. (2003). Parental perceptions of their child's asthma: Management and medication use. *Journal of Pediatric Nursing, 17*(3), 118–125.

Pieper, P. (2000). Pediatric trauma. In B. V. Wise, C. McKenna, G. Garvin, & B. J. Harmon (Eds.), *Nursing care of the general pediatric surgical patient* (pp. 459–479). Gaithersburg, MD: Aspen.

Reznik, M., Ozuah, P. O., Franco, K., Cohen, R., & Motlow, F. (2002, October). Use of complementary therapy by adolescents with asthma. *Archives of Pediatric and Adolescent Medicine, 156*, 1042–1044.

Schulte, A., Musolf, J., Meurer, J. R., Cohn, D. H., & Kelly, K. J. (2004). Pediatric asthma case management: A review of evidence and an experimental study design. *Journal of Pediatric Nursing, 19*(4), 304–310.

Schweich, P. J., & Zempsky, W. T. (1999). Emergent issues. In J. A. McMillan, C. D. DeAngelis, R. D. Feigin, & J. B. Warshaw, *Oski's pediatrics: Principles and practice* (3rd ed., pp. 584–585). Philadelphia: Lippincott Williams & Wilkins.

Solomon, G., Humphreys, E. H., & Miller, M. D. (2004). Asthma and the environment: Connecting the dots. *Contemporary Pediatrics, 21*(8), 73–81.

Steinbach, S. F. (2000). Four controversies in pediatric asthma care. *Contemporary Pediatrics, 17*(10), 150–172.

Stowe, C. D., & Jacobs, R. F. (1999). Treatment of tuberculosis infection and disease in children: The North American perspective. *Pediatric Drugs, 1*(4), 299–312.

Stricker, P. R. (2000). Swimming: A case-based approach to exercise-induced asthma and rotator cuff tendonitis. *Pediatric Annals, 29*(3), 166–170.

Stroud, R. H., & Friedman, N. R. (2001). An update on inflammatory disorders of the pediatric airway: Epiglottitis, croup, and tracheitis. *American Journal of Otolaryngology, 22*(4), 268–275.

Swartz, M., Cantey-Banasiak, N., & Meadows-Oliver, N. (2005). Barriers to effective pediatric asthma care. *Journal of Pediatric Health Care, 19*(2), 71–79.

Sydnor-Greenberg, N., & Dokken, D. (2000). Communicating information at diagnosis: Helping families and children manage asthma. *Journal of Child and Family Nursing, 3*(4), 290–295.

Theobald, K., Botwinski, C., Albanna, S., & McWilliam, P. (2000). Apnea of prematurity: Diagnosis, implications for care, and pharmacologic management. *Neonatal Network, 19*(6), 17–24.

van Veldhoven, N. H., Vermeer, A., Bogaard, J. M., Hessels, M. G., Wijnroks, L., Colland, V. T., et al. (2001, August). Children with asthma and physical exercise: Effects of an exercise programme. *Clinical Rehabilitation, 15*(4), 360–370.

Varlotta, L. (1998). Management and care of the newly diagnosed patient with cystic fibrosis. *Current Opinion in Pulmonary Medicine, 4*, 311–318.

Vedanthan, P. K., Kesavalu, L. K., Murthy, K. C., Duvall, K., Hall, M. J., Baker, S., et al. (1998). Clinical study of yoga techniques in university students with asthma: A controlled study. *Allergy and Asthma Proceedings, 19*(1), 3–9.

Webster, H., & Huether, S. E. (1998). Alterations in pulmonary function in children. In K. L. McCance & S. E. Huether (Eds.), *Pathophysiology: The biologic basis for disease in adults and children* (3rd ed., pp. 1201–1220). St. Louis, MO: Mosby.

Wright, R. B., Pomerantz, W. J., & Luria, J. W. (2002). New approaches to respiratory infections in children. *Emergency Medicine Clinics of North America, 20*(1), 93–114.

Yoos, H. L., Kitzman, H., & McMullen, A. (2003, July). Barriers to anti-inflammatory medication use in childhood asthma. *Ambulatory Pediatrics, 3*, 181–190.

The Child with Alterations in Cardiovascular Function

CHAPTER 48

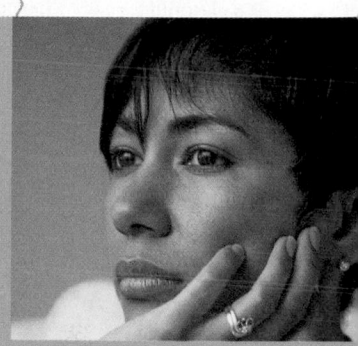

Brandy got sick so fast. Look how hard she is working to breathe. She gets tired before she can finish her formula. We didn't expect her to have to have heart surgery when she was still so small. We were told her chances for successful surgery would improve if she grew some more. I just want her to get stronger and have the chance to grow up to be like other kids.
—*Mother of Brandy, 1 month*

LEARNING OBJECTIVES

- Describe the anatomy and physiology of the cardiovascular system, focusing on the flow of blood and the action of heart valves.

- Recognize the signs of congestive heart failure in an infant and child.

- Develop a nursing care plan for a child with congestive heart failure.

- Describe the pathophysiology associated with congenital heart defects with increased pulmonary circulation, decreased pulmonary circulation, and obstructed systemic blood flow.

- Develop a nursing care plan for the infant with a congenital heart defect cared for at home prior to corrective surgery.

- Develop a nursing care plan for the child undergoing open heart surgery.

- Identify heart diseases acquired during childhood and how they differ from congenital defects.

- Describe the pathophysiology of hypovolemic shock, distributive shock, and cardiogenic shock.

MEDIALINK www.prenhall.com/london

CD-ROM

Animations:
  Blood Pressure
  Congenital Heart Defects
  Digoxin
  Heart Sounds
Skill 9–10: Blood Pressure
Skill 15-2: Inserting and Removing a Nasogastric Tube
Skill 10-6: Blood Gases
Audio Glossary
NCLEX-RN® Review

Companion Website

MediaLink Applications:
  Nursing Care Plan: Pediatric Heart Transplant
  Case Study: Newborn after Heart Surgery
  Teaching Plan: Infective Endocarditis Prophylaxis
  Teaching Plan: Healthy Heart Curricula
Thinking Critically
NCLEX-RN® Review
Audio Glossary

Alterations in cardiovascular function may be a result of a congenital defect, acquired infection, or injury. Congenital heart defects occur in approximately 1 in 170 live births (Neilson & Robin, 2002). Approximately one third of children born with congenital heart disease die as a result of their cardiac disease and about a third of those deaths occur in the first year of life (Connor, 2002). More than 35 types of heart defects have been documented. Rapid advances in the treatment of congenital heart defects allow children to have surgery at younger ages. As a result, nursing care required to identify and manage responses of infants and children with heart disease has become more challenging.

ANATOMY AND PHYSIOLOGY OF PEDIATRIC DIFFERENCES

The transition from fetal to pulmonary circulation is described in Chapter 26. ∞ Systemic vascular resistance increases after the umbilical cord is cut. The increased blood and pressure in the left side of the heart stimulates the closure of the foramen ovale. The ductus arteriosus normally constricts and closes within 10 to 15 hours after birth in response to higher oxygen saturation levels. The ventricles are equal in size at birth, but by 2 months of age the left ventricle is twice as large as the right ventricle. The higher systemic vascular pressures force the left ventricle to develop quickly.

Infants have a greater risk of heart failure than older children because the immature heart is more sensitive to volume or pressure overload. During infancy the muscle fibers of the heart are less developed and less organized, resulting in limited functional capacity. Less **compliance** (amount of distention or expansion the ventricles can achieve to increase stroke volume) of the heart muscle means that the stroke volume (cardiac output) cannot increase substantially. The heart muscle fibers develop during early childhood and by 9 years of age, the weight of the heart has increased by 6 times (Kohr & Sims, 1998). As the child's heart grows and develops, the systolic blood pressure rises, reaching adult levels by puberty.

OXYGENATION

Oxygen bound to hemoglobin is transported to the tissues by the systemic circulation. Hematocrit and hemoglobin concentrations appropriate for the child's age are necessary for adequate oxygen transport (see Chapter 49∞). The oxygen arterial saturation is the amount of oxygen that can potentially be delivered to the tissues. **Desaturated blood** results when oxygenated and unoxygenated blood mix because of a congenital heart defect. Cyanosis, which indicates **hypoxemia** (lower than normal amounts of oxygen in the blood), results from a concentration of 5 or more grams of deoxygenated hemoglobin per 100 mL of blood or from arterial saturations less than 85%. A pulse oximeter provides a noninvasive estimate of arterial oxygen saturation level. A reading of 95% to 98% is normal in children. The following values indicate hypoxemia:

- Mild hypoxemia: 90% to 95%
- Moderate hypoxemia: 85% to 90%
- Severe hypoxemia: < 85%

The child's bone marrow responds to chronic hypoxemia by producing more red blood cells to increase the amount of hemoglobin available for oxygenation. This increase is known as **polycythemia**. A hematocrit value of 50% or higher is common in children with cyanotic heart defects. Extreme polycythemia, a hemoglobin concentration greater than 20 g/dL and a hematocrit greater than 55% to 60%, is dangerous. Blood viscosity is increased, and the child is at risk for a thromboembolism.

CARDIAC FUNCTIONING

The infant's metabolic rate and oxygen requirements double at birth, so the heart rate is high to maintain a high cardiac output and adequate oxygen transport. The infant has little cardiac output reserve capacity until oxygen requirements begin to decrease. **Cardiac output**, the volume of blood ejected from the left ventricle each minute, depends almost completely on heart rate until the heart muscle is fully developed at 5 years of age. Weight-specific cardiac output decreases during childhood. During stress, exercise, fever, or respiratory distress, infants and children have tachycardia, which increases their cardiac output.

Children respond to severe hypoxemia with bradycardia. Cardiac arrest in children generally results from prolonged hypoxemia related to respiratory failure or shock rather than from a primary cardiac insult as in adults. Bradycardia is therefore a significant warning sign of cardiac arrest. Appropriate management of hypoxemia reverses bradycardia and prevents cardiac arrest.

CONGESTIVE HEART FAILURE

Congestive heart failure (CHF) is a disorder of circulation in which cardiac output is inadequate to support the body's circulatory and metabolic needs. It may result from a congenital heart defect that causes increased pulmonary blood flow or obstruction to the systemic blood outflow tract, from problems with heart contractility, or from pathologic conditions that require high cardiac output, such as severe anemia, acidosis, or respiratory disease. CHF also results from acquired heart disease such as cardiomyopathy or Kawasaki disease.

ETIOLOGY AND PATHOPHYSIOLOGY

Blood volume overloads associated with congenital heart defects are the most common cause of congestive heart failure in infants. Up to 90% of infants with uncorrected heart defects develop CHF within the first 6 to 12 months of life (Connor, 2002). Some defects allow blood to flow from the left side of the heart to the right so that extra blood must be pumped to the pulmonary system rather than through the aorta when the left ventricle contracts. This overloads the pulmonary system, and if prolonged can lead to pulmonary artery hypertension, an often irreversible condition leading to life-threatening pulmonary vascular resistance (see p. 1472). Obstructive congenital defects

(i.e., abnormally small pulmonary vessels) restrict the flow of blood, so the heart hypertrophies to work harder to force blood through these structures. This increases cardiac output initially, but eventually the hypertrophied muscle becomes ineffective (Balaguru, Artman, & Auslender, 2000). Initially one side of the heart may fail, but eventually failure is bilateral.

When cardiac output remains insufficient, the body's organs and tissues do not receive adequate oxygen. The kidneys respond to the lowered circulating volume by activating the renin-angiotensin mechanism to retain salt and water. A sympathetic response increases the heart rate, heart muscle contractility, and peripheral vascular resistance. These responses increase cardiac output to the vital organs. Without intervention, the compensatory mechanisms increase their intensity, demanding more effort from the compromised heart. This results in progressive systemic edema and pulmonary congestion.

CLINICAL MANIFESTATIONS

Congestive heart failure often develops subtly, and symptoms may not be recognized at first. The infant tires easily, especially during feeding. Weight loss or lack of normal weight gain, diaphoresis, irritability, and frequent infections may be evident. Older children may have exercise intolerance, dyspnea, abdominal pain or distention, and peripheral edema. See "Clinical Manifestations: Congestive Heart Failure" for clinical manifestations by cause.

As the disease progresses, symptoms such as tachypnea, tachycardia, pallor or cyanosis, nasal flaring, grunting, retractions, cough, or crackles may occur. Generalized fluid

CLINICAL MANIFESTATIONS

CONGESTIVE HEART FAILURE

CAUSE	CLINICAL MANIFESTATIONS
Pulmonary venous congestion	Tachypnea, wheezing, crackles, retractions, cough, grunting, nasal flaring, feeding difficulties, irritability, tiring with play
Systemic venous congestion	Hepatomegaly, ascites, peripheral edema
Impaired cardiac output	Tachycardia, diminished pulses, hypotension, capillary refill time greater than 2 seconds, pallor, cool extremities, oliguria
High metabolic rate	Failure to thrive or slow weight gain

volume overload is seen more commonly in toddlers and older children. Periorbital and facial edema and hepatomegaly are signs of fluid volume excess. Jugular vein distention is seen in older children.

Cardiomegaly, enlargement of the heart by hypertrophy of its walls, occurs as the heart attempts to maintain cardiac output. Cyanosis, weak peripheral pulses, cool extremities, hypotension, and heart murmur are precursors of cardiogenic shock, which can occur if congestive heart failure is not adequately treated. (Cardiogenic shock is discussed on p. 1483.)

CLINICAL THERAPY

Diagnosis is based primarily on clinical manifestations such as tachycardia, respiratory distress, and crackles. A chest x-ray study reveals cardiac enlargement and venous congestion or signs of pulmonary edema. Echocardiography may be performed to diagnose specific cardiac defects or dysfunction. An electrocardiogram may show tachycardia, bradycardia, or ventricular hypertrophy.

The goals of medical management are to make the heart work more efficiently and to remove excess fluid. This decreases the work of the heart and improves systemic circulation without flooding the pulmonary system. Diuretics, such as furosemide, chlorothiazide, and spironolactone, are given to promote fluid excretion. Because most diuretics (except for spironolactone) cause potassium loss, serum potassium levels are monitored and potassium supplements may be ordered.

Inotropic medicines and afterload-reducing agents (angiotensin-converting enzyme inhibitors) are sometimes used to lessen the workload of the heart and help it to work more efficiently. Digoxin is the drug most commonly used to improve the heart's ability to contract and therefore increase its output. A higher than normal dose may be given initially when the child can be monitored, followed by a lower maintenance dose. This process, called **digitalization**, helps the child achieve therapeutic blood levels more quickly. Beta-blockers such as propranolol and carvedilol may be used to treat chronic heart failure (Azeka, Ramires, Valler et al., 2002). See Table 48–1 for medications used to treat CHF.

TABLE 48–1 ✢ Drugs Used to Treat Congestive Heart Failure

Drug	Action
Digoxin	Increases myocardial contractility improving systemic circulation
Furosemide	Rapid diuresis
Thiazides Chlorothiazide (suspension) Hydrochlorthiazide (tablets)	Maintenance diuresis, decreases absorption of sodium, water, potassium, chloride, and bicarbonate in renal tubules
Spironolactone	Maintenance diuresis (potassium-sparing)
ACEi (angiotensin-converting enzyme inhibitor)	Promotes vascular relaxation and reduced peripheral vascular resistance
Propranolol	Increases contractility
Carvedilol	Improves left ventricular function, promotes vasodilation of systemic circulation for chronic heart failure and dilated cardiomyopathy.

Surgery or interventional catheterization to correct a congenital heart defect may become the treatment of choice. Cardiac transplantation may be performed for children with end-stage cardiomyopathy or complex congenital heart defects such as hypoplastic left heart syndrome.

Other medical therapy is supportive. Airway management, ventilatory support, rest, and fluid and dietary management are also part of the treatment plan. Oxygen may be prescribed. Most children improve rapidly after medication is administered.

NURSING MANAGEMENT

NURSING ASSESSMENT AND DIAGNOSIS

Physiologic Assessment

As diagnosis of congestive heart failure depends primarily on physical symptoms, nursing observations are important. Assess the child's vital signs, behavioral patterns (e.g., playfulness, irritability), cardiac function, respiratory function, and fluid status using guidelines in Table 48–2. Use the age-specific heart and respiratory rates in Chapter 35 to identify tachycardia and tachypnea. ∞ Obtain a detailed history of the onset of symptoms from the parents, as congestive heart failure often develops slowly.

NURSING PRACTICE

Digoxin and digitoxin are both digitalis preparations but are not the same drug. Digoxin is the drug of choice in pediatrics. Digitoxin is 10 times more powerful than digoxin, and is rarely used in children. Read labels carefully and double-check doses to ensure that you give the child the right dose of the right drug.

TABLE 48–2 ✛ Guidelines for Assessment of a Child with a Cardiac Condition*

Assessment Focus	Assessment Guidelines
Respirations	■ Inspect the rate, depth, and respiratory effort. ■ Is a cough present? ■ Identify the signs of increased respiratory effort: tachypnea (abnormally rapid rate of respirations), dyspnea, retractions, nasal flaring, and expiratory grunting. ■ Auscultate breath sounds for adventitious sounds (wheezes, crackles).
Pulses	■ Assess the rate, rhythm, and quality. ■ Compare the apical, brachial, and radial pulse rates. ■ Compare the brachial and femoral pulses for strength.
Blood pressure	■ Compare the blood pressure to expected value for age, sex, and height percentiles. (See Table 35-14.) ∞ ■ Compare blood pressure values between upper and lower extremities.
Color	■ Observe overall color: note pallor, dusky color, or cyanosis. ■ Contrast color in peripheral and central locations (e.g., nailbeds to mucous membranes). Note whether crying improves or worsens color.
Heart	■ Inspect the anterior chest for bulging or **heaving** (lifting of the chest wall during contraction). ■ Palpate the chest wall for pulsations, heaves, or vibrations. ■ Locate the point of maximum intensity. ■ Auscultate the heart for the heart sounds and their quality (loud versus weak, distinct versus muffled). Muffled or indistinct sounds are associated with congestive heart failure or a heart defect. ■ Are extra heart sounds or murmurs present? Describe murmurs by intensity, location, radiation, timing, and quality. ■ Auscultate the heart with the child in sitting and reclining positions to detect differences in heart sounds.
Fluid status	■ Observe for signs of periorbital, facial, or peripheral edema. ■ Observe for abdominal distention. ■ Palpate the liver to detect hepatomegaly. ■ Observe for signs of dehydration with acute illnesses.
Activity and behavior	■ Is exercise intolerance present? ■ Does the child tire with feeding? ■ Does the child stop play and squat for rest periods? ■ Identify changes in activity level or behavior (lethargy, decreased responsiveness)
General	■ Assess growth. ■ Note presence of diaphoresis and when it occurs.

*See Chapter 35 for actual techniques of assessment. ∞

Psychosocial Assessment

Take a history of the child's previous hospitalizations and assess the family's knowledge about the child's condition. Families of children with CHF are anxious and fear the potentially serious outcome of the problem and the need to provide ongoing care. Assess the family's anxiety level and coping strategies. Evaluate the family's economic status. Medication is crucial to treatment, and a family's inability to afford or obtain the necessary medications jeopardizes the child's outcome.

Developmental Assessment

Since fatigue limits the activities of the child with congestive heart failure, the child does not have the opportunity to practice the skills needed to attain normal developmental milestones. Assess development with a tool such as the Denver II (see Chapter 33 ∞). In addition, parents can provide information about the attainment of expected developmental milestones such as sitting, manipulating objects, standing, or walking. When CHF is well controlled, the child's energy level increases and developmental skills often improve. In infants and toddlers, assessments every 2 to 3 months are useful to observe development and evaluate disease management.

Parents may limit the child's contact with other children because of frequent infections and exercise intolerance. Ask parents about contact and play with other children and a typical day's activity schedule.

Several nursing diagnoses that may apply to the child with congestive heart failure can be found in the accompanying "Nursing Care Plans." The primary nursing diagnosis is *Decreased Cardiac Output* related to cardiac anomaly.

● **FIGURE 48–1**

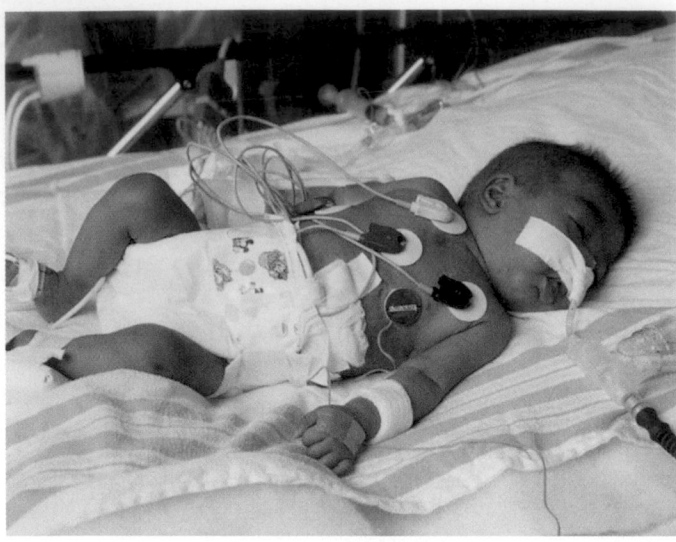

Jooti is receiving intravenous fluids and oxygen. Her condition is being continuously monitored for congestive heart failure.

PLANNING AND IMPLEMENTATION

Nursing care for the child with congestive heart failure focuses on administering and monitoring effects of medications, maintaining adequate oxygenation and myocardial function, promoting rest, fostering development, providing adequate nutrition, and providing emotional support to the child and family (Figure 48–1 ●). (See "Nursing Care Plan: The Child Hospitalized with Congestive Heart Failure.")

Administer and Monitor Prescribed Medications

Children with congestive heart failure usually receive digoxin and furosemide. These medications are potent and must be administered correctly. Measure intake and output carefully (see Skill 9–22). **SKILLS** Weigh the infant's diapers before and after changing (1 g = 1 mL urine). Observe for changes in peripheral edema and circulation. Weigh the child at the same time each day because fluid volume varies throughout the day (see Skill 9–3). **SKILLS** If ascites is present, take serial abdominal measurements to monitor changes (see Skill 9–7). **SKILLS** Turn the child frequently, and provide skin care when edema is present (see Figure 39–8 in Chapter 39 ∞).

Maintain Oxygenation and Myocardial Function

Oxygen therapy may be ordered. Make sure that tubing is patent, the oxygen flow rate is correct, the oxygen delivery device is working properly, and humidification is provided. Keep the child calm and quiet. Position the child in a semi-Fowler's or 45-degree angle position to promote maximum oxygenation.

Promote Rest

Group assessments and interventions together to ensure that the child has some uninterrupted rest each hour. Feedings should last no more than 20 to 30 minutes. Frequent small feedings generally work best, with burping after every half ounce of intake to minimize vomiting. Rocking is restful for infants. Encourage older children to engage in quiet activities such as playing board games or watching television.

Foster Development

Encourage parents to play with the child, using toys to stimulate eye–hand coordination and fine motor movements. Such toys include rattles, blocks, and stuffed animals for infants, and books, paper and pencil, and dolls for older children. Encourage sitting, standing, or walking for short periods with adequate rest afterward to promote the development of large muscles. Singing, talking, and playing music facilitate cognitive and language skills.

Provide Adequate Nutrition

Teach parents about feeding techniques. Encourage the mother who chooses to breastfeed the infant. The antibodies in breast milk reduce infections, and the milk is naturally low in sodium. However, the sucking involved in breast- or bottle-feeding may cause dyspnea that forces the infant to rest frequently during feeding.

Infants should be burped frequently to permit rest and prevent vomiting. They may need small frequent feedings rather than longer feeding periods. Positioning the baby in an infant seat at a 45-degree angle decreases venous return to the heart and decreases its metabolic demand. This is a favorable position for feeding and other activities (Cook & Higgins, 2004). Make sure parents understand that changes in feeding habits (decreased intake, vomiting, sleeping through feedings, increased perspiration with feedings) may indicate deteriorating cardiac status. The infant needs adequate nutrition to support growth. Some infants need a higher caloric formula (24 to 30 calories per ounce) to obtain adequate nutrition. It is not unusual for infants with heart problems to develop failure to thrive as the result of feeding difficulties. (See Chapter 34. ∞) When infants have significant dyspnea with feeding, special feeding techniques are needed such as nutritional supplementation by nasogastric or gastrostomy tube (Figure 48–2 ●). Parents are often advised to give the infant a chance to feed normally for a specific period. The remainder of the formula is then given by nasogastric or gastrostomy tube. (See Skills 15–2 and 15–3. **SKILLS**)

Provide Emotional Support

When a child is hospitalized with CHF, the family is often anxious about his or her condition. Give parents a chance to express concerns about their child's condition. Explain the child's treatment regimen, and make sure family members

NURSING CARE PLAN

THE CHILD HOSPITALIZED WITH CONGESTIVE HEART FAILURE

Intervention	Rationale	Expected Outcome

1. Nursing Diagnosis: Decreased Cardiac Output related to cardiac anomaly (VSD)

NIC Priority Intervention: **Hemodynamic regulation:** Optimization of heart rate, preload, afterload, and contractility		**NOC Suggested Outcome:** **Cardiac pump effectiveness:** Extent to which blood is ejected from the left ventricle per minute to support systemic perfusion pressure

Goal: The child will manifest adequate oxygenation.

■ Evaluate respiratory rate and sounds. Take pulse oximetry readings to determine oxygen saturation. ■ Provide oxygen and humidification if ordered. Observe for diaphoresis, a sign of increased respiratory effort.	■ Absence of tachypnea and adventitious sounds and oxygen saturation above 95% indicate ease of respiration. ■ Supplemental oxygen decreases tachypnea, and humidification moistens secretions to keep airway clear.	The child has normal respiratory rate for age with no evidence of adventitious sounds or diaphoresis.

Goal: The child's cardiac output will be sufficient to meet the body's metabolic demands.

■ Administer digoxin as ordered. ■ Take apical pulse and listen to heart sounds regularly, especially before each dose of digoxin. Record apical pulse with each recorded dose of digoxin. ■ Use cardiac monitor if ordered. ■ Prevent injury by monitoring for digoxin side effects and serum potassium level ■ Provide for rest periods each hour. ■ Place child in semi-Fowler's position.	■ Digoxin increases contractility of the heart and force of contraction. ■ Digoxin may cause bradycardia. Pulse and heart sounds provide information about heart functioning. ■ Monitor notes tachycardia and arrhythmias. ■ Digoxin is a potent drug with serious side effects. Hypokalemia increases risk of digoxin toxicity. ■ Rest decreases need for high cardiac output. ■ Position facilitates lung expansion.	The child's cardiac output is sufficient as indicated by increased energy, adequate feeding intake, and decreased edema. The child maintains normal serum levels of potassium and therapeutic levels of digoxin. The child rests hourly and has adequate energy to eat and play.

2. Nursing Diagnosis: Excess Fluid Volume related to heart failure

NIC Priority Intervention: **Fluid management:** Promotion of fluid balance and prevention of complications resulting from abnormal or undesired fluid levels		**NOC Suggested Outcome:** **Fluid balance:** Balance of water in the intracellular and extracellular compartments of the body

Goal: The child's peripheral and central edema will decrease. Intake and output will be balanced once excess fluid is excreted.

■ Administer diuretics as ordered. ■ Weigh daily. Measure abdominal girth daily. Observe for peripheral edema. ■ Measure intake and output carefully. Weigh diapers to obtain output of young child. ■ Maintain fluid-restricted diet if ordered. ■ Monitor electrolytes.	■ Diuretics mobilize fluids and facilitate excretion. ■ Evaluations demonstrate effectiveness of treatment. ■ Adequate output is a good indicator of renal perfusion. ■ Fluid restriction is sometimes used to decrease cardiac load. ■ Electrolyte imbalance is common when fluids are restricted and diuretics are given.	The child's intake and output are proportional, and electrolyte levels remain within normal ranges.

3. Nursing Diagnosis: Risk for Impaired Skin Integrity related to altered fluid status

NIC Priority Intervention: **Pressure management:** Minimizing pressure to body parts		**NOC Suggested Outcome:** **Tissue integrity: Skin and mucous membranes:** Structural intactness and normal physiologic function of skin and mucous membranes

(continued)

NURSING CARE PLAN—continued

THE CHILD HOSPITALIZED WITH CONGESTIVE HEART FAILURE

Intervention	Rationale	Expected Outcome
Goal: The child's peripheral and central edema will decrease.		
■ Provide skin care for edematous body parts and elevate extremities. ■ Change child's position frequently. ■ Inspect skin frequently for redness and skin breakdown over pressure points.	■ Edematous skin injures easily. Elevation promotes return of fluid from extremities. ■ Position change promotes circulation to skin over pressure points. ■ Inspection identifies earliest stages of skin breakdown.	The child has no skin breakdown after edema resolves.

4. Nursing Diagnosis: Imbalanced Nutrition: Less than Body Requirements related to high metabolic needs and rapid tiring while feeding

NIC Priority Intervention:		**NOC Suggested Outcome:**
Nutrition management: Assistance with or provision of a balanced dietary intake of food and fluids		**Nutrition status:** Extent to which nutrients are available to meet metabolic needs
Goal: The infant or child will demonstrate normal weight gain for age.		
■ Hold infant at 45-degree angle for feeding. ■ Record intake carefully. ■ Weigh child daily. ■ Give frequent small meals with rest periods in between. ■ Use high-calorie formula or give high-calorie snacks. ■ Use soothing approaches such as holding infants for feeding and having parents eat with older child. ■ Transition to supplemental nasogastric feeding if the infant is not able to gain weight.	■ Position facilitates breathing while eating. ■ Evaluation of intake indicates whether caloric and other nutritional needs are met. ■ Weight indicates growth (in absence of edematous symptoms of congestive heart failure). ■ Digesting small meals requires less energy. ■ High-calorie formulas and snacks provide calories efficiently. ■ Restful approach facilitates intake with minimum cardiac work. ■ Nasogastric feeds provide added calories but do not force the infant to use energy to eat.	The infant or child gains recommended weight according to growth grids. All dietary requirements are met, and mealtimes are pleasant.

5. Nursing Diagnosis: Compromised Family Coping related to situational crisis with child's disease

NIC Priority Intervention:		**NOC Suggested Outcome:**
Caregiver support: Provision of necessary information, advocacy, and support to facilitate primary patient care by someone other than healthcare professional		**Family Coping:** Family actions to manage stressors that tax family resources
Goal: Parents will express lessened anxiety as hospitalization proceeds.		
■ Encourage parents to room-in or stay with child. Explain procedures and treatment. Involve parents in care as much as possible. Have parents plan child's play periods. ■ At discharge, provide clear instructions and information about what to do in an emergency, and whom and where to call with questions. ■ Allow parents to verbalize questions, concerns, and feelings. Refer parents to support groups or other resources as needed.	■ Involvement in child's care lessens parental anxiety and fear of unknown. ■ Having resources available provides feelings of security. ■ Emotional support is needed to lessen anxiety.	Parents participate in developing and implementing the treatment plan and providing care to the child.

DRUG GUIDE

DIGOXIN

Action

Digoxin acts on the heart by increasing the force of the myocardial systolic contraction, decreasing the degree of activation of the sympathetic nervous system and renin-angiotensin system, slowing the heart rate, and reducing the conduction velocity through the atrioventricular node. Digoxin is used in the treatment of congestive heart failure and for ventricular rate control in chronic atrial fibrillation.

Routes, Dosage, Frequency

Dosage varies by age and whether giving a digitalizing or maintenance dose.

Digitalizing dose (may be given in divided dosages):

Age	PO dose	IM/IV dose
Premature neonates	20 mcg/kg	15 mcg/kg
Neonate	30 mcg/kg	20 mcg/kg
1 to 24 months	40 to 50 mcg/kg	30 to 40 mcg/kg
2 to 10 years	30 to 40 mcg/kg	20 to 30 mcg/kg
Over 10 years and under 100 kg	10 to 15 mcg/kg	8 to 12 mcg/kg
Adult	10 to 15 mcg/kg (1 mg)	10 to 15 mcg/kg (1 mg)

Maintenance dose:

Age	PO dose	IM/IV dose
Premature neonates	5 mcg/kg	3 to 4 mcg/kg
Neonate	8 to 10 mcg/kg	6 to 8 mcg/kg
1 to 24 months	10 to 12 mcg/kg	7.5 to 9 mcg/kg
2 to 10 years	8 to 10 mcg/kg	6 to 8 mcg/kg
Over 10 years and under 100 kg	2.5 to 5 mcg/kg	2 to 3 mcg/kg
Adult	0.1 to 0.375 mg/day	0.1 to 0.375 mg/day

Doses are reduced in renal dysfunction, especially if creatinine clearance is under 10 mL/minute.

Nursing Management

Assessment: Before giving digitalizing dose, establish baseline vital signs, quality of peripheral pulses, clinical symptoms, and ECG. Check serum electrolytes, and hepatic and renal function. Assess hydration status, and hydrate if hypovolemic.

Administration: Digoxin is given intravenously or orally in extremely small doses. Carefully measure and verify the dose calculation and appropriateness of dose for weight of the child. Verification of the dose and calculation by another nurse is usually required. Digitalizing or loading doses may be divided.

PO: Give at same times daily without regard for food. Food will slow absorption, but it does not decrease total absorption. Use the provided calibrated dropper for the elixir. Be certain to administer digoxin, *not digitoxin,* tablets. Tablet may be crushed and mixed with fluid or food if patient cannot swallow it whole.

IV: Give undiluted or diluted in 4 mL of sterile water, D5W, or saline, and administer over at least 5 minutes. Use immediately after dilution. Do not mix with other medications. Patients are changed from IV to PO form as soon as possible.

Monitor

- *Before giving any dose, take apical pulse for 1 minute.* If bradycardia is detected (< 60 to 100 beats/min in children, dependent upon age, < 60 beats/min in adolescents, or below a guideline noted in the physician's order) or changes in heart rhythm or quality are noted, withhold medication and call for a physician's advice before administering the drug.
- Observe the child carefully for digoxin toxicity. Early signs include cardiac arrhythmias in children. Early indicators in adults (nausea, vomiting, anorexia, diarrhea, visual disturbance) are rarely the initial signs of toxicity in children.
- Serum digoxin levels are taken 6 to 8 hours after a dose. A therapeutic serum level ranges from 0.8 to 2 ng/mL. Levels over 2 ng/mL are toxic.
- Monitor hepatic and renal functions. Dosage will be reduced if creatinine clearance is 50 mL/minute or less. Check serum electrolytes, particularly potassium, calcium, and magnesium; closely monitor those also on diuretics. Careful monitoring of intake and output is required, especially in cases of impaired renal function.
- Monitor serum digoxin levels closely during antibiotic therapy as altered intestinal flora may precipitate toxicity.
- If a child taking digoxin orally is NPO or vomiting, seek a physician's order regarding the course of action; the drug must not be omitted.
- If routes of administration (tablet, elixir, parenteral) are changed, absorption of digoxin may be altered. Generally, tablets and elixir dosages will need to be decreased by 20% to 25% when changing to IV or capsule preparations.

Patient Education

- Take the pulse prior to giving medication. Report to physician when pulse rate falls below or rises above guidelines provided. Administer the medication exactly as prescribed.
- Do not administer over-the-counter medications for colds, coughs, allergies, GI upset, or obesity without approval.
- Keep the medication locked and out of reach of children.

Data from Bindler, R. M., Howry, L. B., Wilson, B. A., Shannon, M. T., & Stang, C. L. (2005). Pediatric drug guide. Upper Saddle River, NJ: Prentice Hall.

● FIGURE 48–2

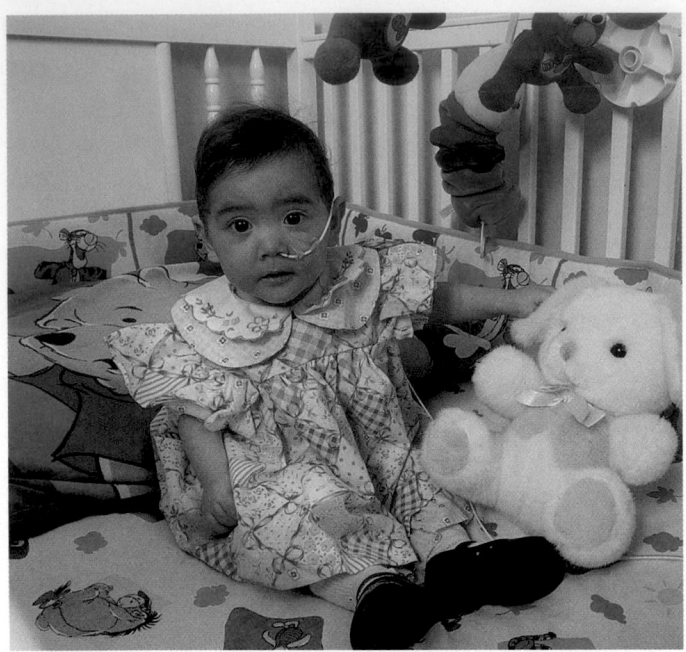

Infants with cardiac conditions often require supplemental feedings to provide sufficient nutrients for growth and development. The parents of this infant girl have been taught how to give her nasogastric feedings at home.

understand the child's need for nutrition and rest. Refer parents to the appropriate support groups as talking with parents of children with cardiac conditions may be a source of emotional support.

Discharge Planning and Home Care Teaching

Identify and address home care needs well in advance of discharge. Show parents how to feed the child to maximize nutritional intake. While the child is hospitalized, teach the family about the administration of medications and signs of a worsening condition. Tell them to watch for symptoms such as increased feeding difficulty, irritability, lethargy, breathing difficulty, and puffiness around the eyes or extremities, which indicate that congestive heart failure is worsening. Parents are frequently taught to take the child's pulse and to report any significant change to the physician. An increase in pulse rate can signal CHF, and a decrease can indicate digoxin toxicity. Teach parents to identify signs of dehydration when the child is managed on diuretics. An acute illness could lead to dehydration more quickly when the child takes these medications.

Demonstrate administration of drugs, and then supervise while the parents measure and administer medications. Teach parents about the toxic effects of digoxin and other drugs. Advise them to notify the physician immediately if any of these side effects occur. Teach parents about the potential interaction between digoxin and certain an-

tibiotics so they can remind the primary care provider to prescribe safe antibiotics when they are needed. Because digoxin is a potential poison, encourage parents to keep it locked up at home and away from children. In case of accidental ingestion, immediate medical care is needed. Be sure parents keep the poison control number on all phones.

Nursing Care in the Community

"Nursing Care Plan: The Child with Congestive Heart Failure Being Cared for at Home" outlines home care. Parents play a critical role in the care of the child with heart disease by facilitating normal development and limiting the incidence of congestive heart failure.

The family is often overprotective and reluctant to leave the child with other caregivers. Find out if a knowledgeable person who can safely administer medications and watch the child is available for respite care. Show the family how to assess the child's energy level, and how to observe for feeding problems and edema. Observe medication administration and correct any errors. Watch the child feeding and make suggestions as necessary.

EVALUATION

Expected outcomes of nursing care can be found in the "Nursing Care Plans."

CONGENITAL HEART DISEASE

Congenital heart disease refers to a defect in the heart or great vessels, or persistence of a fetal structure after birth. Congenital heart defects occur in an estimated 1% of all pregnancies and 1 in every 170 live births (Neilson & Robin, 2002). People with congenital heart disease are living longer. Between 1979 and 1997, deaths from heart defects declined by 39.4% (Boneva, Botto, Moore et al., 2001). This is attributed to diagnostic advances, surgical technique refinements, and intensive care.

ETIOLOGY AND PATHOPHYSIOLOGY

Most congenital heart defects develop during the first 8 weeks of gestation. They are usually the result of a combined or interactive effect of genetic and environmental factors, such as:

■ Fetal exposure to drugs such as phenytoin, lithium, and alcohol.

■ Maternal viral infections such as rubella or coxsackie B5.

■ Maternal metabolic disorders such as phenylketonuria, diabetes mellitus, and hypercalcemia.

■ Maternal complications of pregnancy such as increased age and antepartal bleeding.

NURSING CARE PLAN

THE CHILD WITH CONGESTIVE HEART FAILURE BEING CARED FOR AT HOME

Intervention	Rationale	Expected Outcome

1. Nursing Diagnosis: Delayed Growth and Development related to effects of physical disability

Intervention	Rationale	Expected Outcome
NIC Priority Intervention: **Developmental enhancement:** Teaching parents to facilitate optimal gross motor, fine motor, language, cognitive, social, and emotional growth of preschool children		**NOC Suggested Outcome:** **Child development** (2 years): Milestones of physical, cognitive, and psychosocial progression by 2 years of age

Goal: The child will meet developmental milestones for age group.

Intervention	Rationale	Expected Outcome
■ Perform baseline developmental assessment. ■ Plan for short play periods after rest. ■ Introduce age-appropriate toys and activities such as rattles and blocks for infants and art projects for older children. ■ Plan for interactions with healthy children.	■ Assessment provides comparison for later assessments and basis for planning specific games, toys, and activities. ■ Short play periods maintain energy and facilitate play. ■ Play activities facilitate learning and mastery of developmental tasks. ■ Social skills are learned through contact with others.	The child displays normal language, fine motor, and gross motor activity.

2. Nursing Diagnosis: Ineffective Therapeutic Regimen Management related to complexity of therapeutic regimen

Intervention	Rationale	Expected Outcome
NIC Priority Intervention: **Mutual goal setting:** Collaborating with the family to identify and prioritize care goals, then developing a plan for achieving those goals		**NOC Suggested Outcome:** **Compliance behavior:** Actions taken on the basis of professional advice to promote wellness, recovery, and rehabilitation

Goal: Parents will demonstrate correct administration of medications.

Intervention	Rationale	Expected Outcome
■ Have parents prepare the medication dosages and administer the digoxin, diuretics, and other medications to the child under the supervision of the home health nurse.	■ Demonstrating techniques used to administer medications provides opportunities to identify dosage errors and to suggest methods to help ensure the child gets all needed medications.	Parents report that child continues to demonstrate improvement and adequate cardiac output with absence of congestive heart failure.

Goal: Parents will state side effects of medications and symptoms of congestive heart failure.

Intervention	Rationale	Expected Outcome
■ Describe side effects of medications. Give parents handouts with telephone number to call to ask questions or report side effects. ■ Describe subtle onset of congestive heart failure and its symptoms (increasing weakness, exhaustion, irritability, difficulty feeding, cough or difficult respirations, edema).	■ If side effects are understood, serious complications can be avoided. ■ Parents can evaluate child regularly and note subtle changes requiring medical management.	

3. Nursing Diagnosis: Imbalanced Nutrition: Less than Body Requirements related to chronic illness and tiring while feeding

Intervention	Rationale	Expected Outcome
NIC Priority Intervention: **Weight gain assistance:** Facilitation of body weight gain		**NOC Suggested Outcome:** **Nutritional status: Food and fluid intake:** Amount of food and fluid taken into the body over a 24-hour period

(continued)

NURSING CARE PLAN—continued

THE CHILD WITH CONGESTIVE HEART FAILURE BEING CARED FOR AT HOME

Intervention	Rationale	Expected Outcome
Goal: The infant or child will demonstrate normal weight gain for age.		
■ Teach parents methods to promote food intake related to positioning, size of feedings, food choices. ■ Observe feeding during home visit.	■ Positioning, frequency of feedings, size of feedings, and use of high-caloric foods can enhance nutritional intake. ■ Feedback can assist parents in integrating positive feeding techniques.	The infant or child shows normal weight gain. Parents report and demonstrate successful feedings of child.
4. Nursing Diagnosis: Activity Intolerance (Child) related to poor cardiac output		
NIC Priority Intervention: **Energy management:** Regulating energy use to treat or prevent fatigue and optimize function		**NOC Suggested Outcome:** **Energy conservation:** Extent of active management of energy to initiate or sustain activity
Goal: The child will perform all necessary activities of daily living without undue tiring.		
■ Help parents alternate activities and rest throughout the child's day. ■ Have parents limit child's exposure to persons with contagious disease. ■ Help family plan quiet surroundings to provide for child's rest.	■ Activities to promote development must be alternated with rest due to decreased cardiac output. ■ When the child is ill and tired, the immune system can be compromised. ■ Home setting may need to be altered to promote rest.	The child performs necessary activities and rests frequently each day.
5. Nursing Diagnosis: Caregiver Role Strain (Parent) related to 24-hour responsibility for child's care		
NIC Priority Intervention: **Caregiver support:** Provision of the necessary information, advocacy, and support to facilitate primary patient care by someone other than a healthcare professional		**NOC Suggested Outcome:** **Caregiver endurance potential:** Factors that promote family care provider continuance over an extended period of time
Goal: Parents will express ability to meet own needs.		
■ Assess family and community supports. Provide information related to respite care. ■ Encourage parents to seek activities to meet personal needs.	■ Variable family and community supports are available. ■ Parents need time to meet own personal needs in order to successfully care for child.	Parents report some time away from the child and report renewal in caring for the child.

■ Genetic factors (family recurrence patterns).

■ Chromosomal abnormalities such as Turner syndrome, Noonan syndrome, Marfan syndrome, DiGeorge syndrome, cri du chat syndrome, Down syndrome, and trisomy syndromes 13, 15, 18, and 21 (Kohr & Sims, 1998). The prevalence of heart defects in children with Down syndrome is about 12% to 44%, and in children with trisomy 13 and 18 the incidence increases to 80% or more (Connor, 2002).

Chromosome 22q11 is one of the most frequent genetic sites associated with development of cardiovascular defects such as truncus arteriosus, tetralogy of Fallot, and pulmonary atresia (Lewin, 2000). Knowledge about other chromosome deletions or mutations associated with cardiovascular defects is emerging. Because of this genetic component, the incidence of congenital heart defects is expected to slowly rise as people with some of these defects survive and have children of their own. Depending on the type of defect, signs and symptoms may be present at birth or develop later.

Congenital heart defects are generally categorized by pathophysiology and **hemodynamics**, the pressures generated by blood and the pathways blood takes through the heart and pulmonary system. These categories include the following:

- Increased pulmonary blood flow (see page 1454)
- Decreased pulmonary blood flow (see page 1460)
- Obstructed systemic blood flow (see page 1469)
- Mixed defects in which infant survival is dependent upon mixing of systemic and pulmonary blood (see page 1460)

CLINICAL MANIFESTATIONS

The presence of a heart murmur is often the first indication of a congenital heart defect. A loud murmur indicates blood is flowing with higher pressure than normal to get through a narrowed valve or vessel, or through a **shunt** (movement of blood between the systemic and pulmonary circulation through an abnormal anatomic opening). Other clinical manifestations and the timing of their appearance vary by the pathophysiology and severity of the defect. See "Clinical Manifestations." Some infants and children may be asymptomatic except for a heart murmur, such as with a small atrial septal defect. Signs and symptoms of congenital heart disease in older children include exercise intolerance, chest pain, arrhythmias, syncope, and sudden death.

CLINICAL THERAPY

Multiple tests are used to diagnose cardiac defects. See Table 48–3. Blood tests such as a hematocrit and hemoglobin are taken to assess for anemia or polycythemia.

TABLE 48–3 ❖ Diagnostic Tests Used in Children with Congenital Heart Disease

Diagnostic Test	Purpose
Chest x-ray study	Reveals size and contour of the heart and characteristics of pulmonary vascular markings
Electrocardiogram (ECG)	Records quality of major electrical activity in the heart, identifies arrhythmias
Echocardiogram	Identifies heart's structures, the pattern of movement, hemodynamics, and the presence of defects
Cardiac catheterization	Allows precise measurement of oxygen saturation, cardiac output, and pressures in each chamber and heart vessel; also identifies anatomic alterations
Holter monitor	Allows 24–48 hour ECG recording
Exercise testing	Enables ECG recording with controlled increase in activity to identify significant cardiac compensation or inadequate cardiac output
Hyperoxia test	Measures differences in arterial blood gas level when child is on room air and on 100% oxygen

CLINICAL MANIFESTATIONS

HEART DEFECTS BY PATHOPHYSIOLOGY

PATHOPHYSIOLOGY	CLINICAL MANIFESTATIONS	TYPES OF DEFECTS
Increased pulmonary blood flow	Tachypnea, tachycardia, murmur, congestive heart failure, poor weight gain, diaphoresis, periorbital edema, frequent respiratory infections	Patent ductus arteriosus, atrial septal defect, ventricular septal defect, atrioventricular canal defect (endocardial cushion defect), truncus arteriosus, total anomalous pulmonary venous return
Decreased pulmonary blood flow	Cyanosis, hypercyanotic spells, poor weight gain, polycythemia	Pulmonic stenosis, tetralogy of Fallot, pulmonary atresia, tricuspid atresia, transposition of the great arteries
Obstruction to systemic blood flow	Diminished pulses, poor color, delayed capillary refill time, decreased urine output, congestive heart failure with pulmonary edema	Coarctation of aorta, aortic stenosis, hypoplastic left heart syndrome, mitral stenosis, interrupted aortic arch
Mixed defects—postnatal survival is dependent upon mixing of systemic and pulmonary blood	Cyanosis, poor weight gain, pulmonary congestion, congestive heart failure may occur with increased shunting	Transposition of great arteries, total anomalous pulmonary venous connection, truncus arteriosus, double outlet right ventricle

Arterial blood gases may be obtained, especially when cyanosis or a complex heart defect is suspected.

One third of infants born with congenital heart defects develop life-threatening symptoms in the first few days of life. Treatment for congenital heart defects depends on the severity of symptoms and whether the condition is imminently life threatening. Interventional catheterization or surgical correction is the treatment of choice for many defects. Many heart defects can be completely repaired with restoration of normal hemodynamics and physiology. For complex heart defects, treatment may be *palliative*, a surgical procedure that does not create normal anatomic or hemodynamic results. A **palliative procedure** may be used for children with a potentially fatal or lethal condition or as an initial procedure while the infant is small, with definitive corrective surgery performed at a later time. Table 48–4 lists the types of interventions during cardiac catheterization and surgical procedures performed on children with congenital heart defects.

Children with complex congenital heart defects require long-term care following palliative or corrective heart surgery. Some need multiple stages of surgery, revisions of previous surgeries, valve replacements, or interventional catheterization to reopen valves or vessels that have become stenotic. Some children need an implanted pacemaker for arrhythmias associated with anomalies of the conduction system or unavoidable surgical incisions in areas of the sinoatrial node or sinoventricular node. The Mustard, Senning, and Fontan procedures, as well as repair of tetralogy of Fallot (TOF), are associated with increased risk of arrhythmias. An implantable cardioverter-defibrillator may be used in older children with life-threatening ventricular arrhythmias (LeRoy, 2001).

Infants with complex congenital heart defects with conditions such as CHF, prolonged hypoxemia, profound acidosis, or low cardiac output have an increased risk for long-term neurologic sequelae. Intraventricular hemorrhage has been documented in nearly 25% of newborns with congenital heart defects. Inadequate nutrition during the first year of life may affect brain development. Cardiopulmonary bypass and deep hypothermic circulatory arrest used in most surgery may cause insult to the neurologic system. Seizures have been noted in the immediate postoperative period (Mahle & Wernovsky, 2001).

Most preschool and school-age survivors of congenital heart disease have normal IQ scores. Some children with complex defects such as transposition of the great arteries (TGA) and hypoplastic left heart syndrome (HLHS) are at an increased risk for neurodevelopmental problems due to the severity of their defect, chronic low-normal systemic blood flow, and hypoxemia (Wernovsky & Newburger, 2003). Visuospatial, visual-motor, and speech deficits may be present even when IQ scores are within normal ranges. Children with HLHS are at higher risk for mental retardation than many other children with congenital heart defects (Mahle & Wernovsky, 2001).

NURSING MANAGEMENT OF THE CHILD UNDERGOING A CARDIAC CATHETERIZATION

Cardiac catheterization is often an outpatient procedure, but some children will be admitted for observation. The child is NPO for several hours, except for medications, and arrives at the catheterization laboratory 1 to 2 hours before the procedure. Before entering the laboratory, the child is asked to void and is given an oral sedative.

NURSING ASSESSMENT AND DIAGNOSIS

Before the procedure, assess the child's vital signs, hematocrit and hemoglobin concentrations, and capillary refill time. Collect baseline data on skin temperature, color, and strength of pedal and popliteal pulses for comparison with postcatheterization assessments.

For several hours after the procedure, monitor the child for potential complications such as arrhythmia, bleeding, hematoma development, thrombus formation, and infection. No bleeding should occur at the catheterization site. Assess vital signs, perfusion of the lower extremities (pulses, temperature, color, capillary refill time, and sensation), and the pressure dressing over the catheterization site every 15 minutes for 1 hour and then every 30 minutes for 1 hour. Be sure to check under the buttocks to make sure blood does not ooze out and run under the child. The child's vital signs should remain stable. Monitor intake and output because the contrast medium may cause diuresis. Infants and children treated with diuretics have a greater potential for dehydration. The child's intake and output should be balanced, so additional fluids may be needed.

The following nursing diagnoses may apply to the child who undergoes cardiac catheterization:

- *Fear* related to separation from support system in a stressful situation

- *Risk for Imbalanced Fluid Volume* related to inadequate fluid intake due to NPO status and diuretic effect of contrast medium

- *Impaired Tissue Perfusion (Cardiopulmonary)* related to mechanical reduction of arterial and venous blood flow

- *Decreased Cardiac Output* related to ventricular restriction (obstruction by balloon catheter)

TABLE 48–4 ❖ Clinical Interventions for Congenital Heart Defects

Cardiac Catheterization Interventions	Purpose	Therapeutic Use
Angioplasty	Dilatation of coarctation of aorta or a stenotic vessel during cardiac catheterization.	Palliative or corrective, COA
Balloon valvuloplasty	A deflated balloon is inserted into the opening of a narrowed valve and inflated to stretch the valve open during cardiac catheterization.	Corrective or PS, palliative, AS
Patent ductus arteriosus closure	Closure of ductus arteriosus by surgery or an umbrella or coil device during cardiac catheterization.	Corrective, PDA
Rashkind—Balloon atrial septostomy	Creation of larger defect (at the foramen ovale) between atria to increase blood mixing, performed during cardiac catheterization.	Palliative, TGA
Transcatheter closure	Closure of a septal defect by a septal occluder during cardiac catheterization.	Corrective, ASD, PDA, VSD

Surgical Procedures	Purpose	Therapeutic Use
Aorta end-to-end anastomosis	Resection of the narrowed section of the aorta and connecting the proximal and distal sections.	Corrective, COA
Blalock-Taussig shunt, modified	Creation of aortopulmonary conduit (from the subclavian artery to pulmonary artery) to increase pulmonary blood flow.	Palliative, TOF, other defects of decreased pulmonary blood flow
Brock	Blind incision of pulmonary valve.	Corrective, PS
Damus-Kaye-Stansel	Pulmonary artery is cut in two with the proximal section attached to the ascending aorta and the distal section to the right ventricle.	Corrective, TGA, complex single ventricle defects
Fontan	Creation of conduit between inferior vena cava and pulmonary artery to increase pulmonary blood flow—total right heart bypass. This permits the right ventricle to assume the responsibility for the systemic circulation and eject blood into the aorta.	Palliative, HLHS, single ventricle defects
Glenn, Bi-directional Glenn	Superior vena cava connected to right pulmonary artery along with closure of aortopulmonary shunt. Systemic venous blood from the head is sent to the lungs directly without ventricular pumping.	Palliative, HLHS, single ventricle defects
Jatene (arterial switch)	Aorta and pulmonary arteries are transected and reanastomosed to opposite stumps, coronary arteries are moved to new aorta area.	Corrective, TGA
Mustard or Senning (venous switch or intra-atrial baffle)	Baffling blood in atria to reestablish a proper blood flow in transposition of great vessels.	Palliative, TGA
Norwood	Atrial septectomy, anastomosis of the main pulmonary artery to the aorta, and an arterial-pulmonary shunt.	Palliative, HLHS
Norwood with Sano modification	Creation of a right ventricle to pulmonary artery conduit so that both the direct pulmonary and aorta blood flow originates in the right ventricle.	Palliative, HLHS
Patch aortoplasty	Insertion of a Dacron patch to expand the lumen of the aorta.	Corrective, COA
Pulmonary artery banding	Placement of constricting band around pulmonary artery to reduce pulmonary blood flow.	Palliative, VSD, AV canal, single ventricle defects
Rastelli	Creation of a conduit between the right ventricle to pulmonary artery with closure of the ventricular septal defect. In the case of truncus arteriosus, the pulmonary arteries are removed from the truncus.	Corrective, TGA with pulmonic stenosis, TOF, tricuspid atresia, truncus arteriosus
Ross	The diseased aortic valve is replaced with the patient's pulmonic valve (pulmonary autograft), and a homograft (valve from a human donor) replaces the pulmonic valve.	Corrective, AS
Subclavian flap aortoplasty	Division of the distal subclavian artery and inserting a flap into the aorta through the coarcted segment.	Corrective, COA
Transplant	Replacement of diseased heart with donor heart.	Corrective, HLHS, complex defects, cardiomyopathies

AS—aortic stenosis, ASD—atrial septal defect, AV—atrioventricular, COA—coarctation of aorta, HLHS—hypoplastic left heart syndrome, PDA—patent ductus arteriosus, PS—pulmonic stenosis, TOF—tetralogy of Fallot, TGA—transposition of great arteries, VSD—ventricular septal defect

PLANNING AND IMPLEMENTATION

Prepare the child for cardiac catheterization with age-appropriate information. A tour of the catheterization laboratory may reduce the child's fears about the large equipment. Because the child will be sedated but arousable for the procedure, explain the sensations that he or she will experience.

Nursing care during a cardiac catheterization focuses on monitoring the child's vital signs, reassuring the child, and providing emergency care if necessary. After the catheters and guidewires are removed at the end of the procedure, direct pressure must be applied for 15 minutes. A pressure dressing is then placed over the site for 6 hours.

The child is kept on bed rest for 6 hours with an effort to keep the leg straight for several hours. Avoid elevating the head of the bed as flexion of the hips is not permitted during this period. Activity is then limited for 24 hours. Provide quiet diversional activities to keep the child occupied.

Encourage the child to drink small amounts of clear liquids initially, and then progress to other fluids and food as the child tolerates them. Provide adequate fluids to maintain hydration status.

Discharge Planning and Home Care Teaching

Children are routinely discharged several hours after the cardiac catheterization. Teach the parents to watch the child for signs of complications and make sure they know when to notify the physician.

Children whose heart defect is corrected by cardiac catheterization have the same risks for infective endocarditis as children with surgical correction. Use the information in Table 48–5 to teach parents about infective endocarditis prophylaxis.

TEACHING HIGHLIGHTS

HOME CARE AFTER CARDIAC CATHETERIZATION

Check for signs of complications several times in the first 24 hours after catheterization:

- Bleeding or a bruise increasing in size at the catheterization site
- Foot on side of catheterization site is cooler than other foot
- Loss of feeling in foot on side of catheterization
- Fever

Notify the physician immediately if any of these signs are noted within the first 24 hours after the catheterization.

Encourage fluids to help flush the dye out of the body and to prevent dehydration.

Permit quiet play such as games, puzzles, and videos for the first 24 hours after the procedure.

TABLE 48–5 ✛ Antibiotic Recommendations for Infective Endocarditis Prophylaxis in Children*

Procedure	Antibiotic Recommendations
For dental, oral, or upper respiratory tract procedures	Amoxicillin **For children allergic to penicillin:** Clindamycin, cephalexin, cefadroxil, azithromycin, clarithromycin
For genitourinary and gastrointestinal procedures	Ampicillin, gentamicin, amoxicillin **For children allergic to penicillin:** Vancomycin, gentamicin

*One large dose is given 1 hour before the procedures. In high-risk patients, a smaller dose may be given 6 hours after the procedure.

Used with permission from Dajani, A. S., Taubert, K. A., Wilson, W., Bolger, A. F., Bayer, A., et al. (1997). Prevention of bacterial endocarditis: Recommendations of the American Heart Association. *Journal of the American Medical Association, 277*(22), 1794–1801.

EVALUATION

Expected outcomes of nursing care include the following:

- Any potential complications (thrombosis or hemorrhage) following cardiac catheterization are rapidly identified and cared for.
- The child maintains fluid balance.

CONGENITAL HEART DEFECTS THAT INCREASE PULMONARY BLOOD FLOW

ETIOLOGY AND PATHOPHYSIOLOGY

The most common congenital heart defects result from a connection between the left and right side of the heart (septal defect) or between the great arteries (patent ductus arteriosus) that allows blood to flow between the left and right side of the heart. The pressures on the left side of the heart are higher than on the right side, so blood shunts from the left side of the heart to the right side and increases the amount of blood pumped to the lungs. The size of the connection and how much blood passes through it determine how quickly the child develops signs of CHF. The increased blood flow to the lungs causes increased pulmonary vascular resistance (constriction of the pulmonary vascular bed) in an effort to reduce the blood flow, and pulmonary artery hypertension (see page 1472). Right ventricular hypertrophy (RVH) develops to overcome the increasing pulmonary vascular resistance and deliver the blood to the lungs.

CLINICAL MANIFESTATIONS

The infant's heart rate, respiratory rate, and metabolic rate are increased due to the high pulmonary blood flow. Sucking takes energy and diaphoresis often occurs with feeding. The infant may be unable to take in enough calories to support the metabolic rate and growth, so poor weight gain is noted. If CHF develops, signs include dyspnea, tachypnea, intercostal retractions, and periorbital edema. Frequent respiratory infections occur as the wet environment in the lungs supports bacterial growth. See Table 48–6 for the pathophysiology, clinical manifestations, and clinical therapy for the specific congenital heart defects with increased pulmonary blood flow.

CLINICAL THERAPY

See Table 48–6 for tests used to diagnose the condition. Coagulation studies, platelet counts, and serum electrolytes are often obtained for children having open heart surgery, in addition to a chest x-ray, complete blood count, and urinalysis.

Surgery to correct or manage defects that cause significant increased pulmonary blood flow is performed early in infancy to prevent irreversible pulmonary vascular disease. Unless complications develop before surgery, the child should make a complete recovery without limitations. The major complication of these defects is pulmonary artery hypertension. See Figure 48–3 .

Conservative treatment, such as waiting until the child is symptomatic or older, may be selected for some children with these defects. For example, a small ventricular septal defect may close spontaneously, or repair of an atrial septal defect is postponed until preschool or early school-age years. Indomethacin may be given to preterm infants with a patent ductus arteriosus when immediate closure of the ductus is needed.

Interventional cardiac catheterization may be performed for defects. See Table 48–4.

NURSING MANAGEMENT PRIOR TO SURGERY

NURSING ASSESSMENT AND DIAGNOSIS

Physiologic Assessment

Prior to surgery the infant or child is seen regularly to assess growth and for signs of worsening CHF. Many infants with a small defect will have no problems with growth. Failure to gain weight is an indication of an increased metabolic rate and inability to consume adequate calories for both metabolic function and growth. Assessment of length and head circumference helps to determine the full impact of the condition on growth.

Psychosocial Assessment

Assess the ability of the parents to cope with the infant's diagnosis. Initially parents may be in shock and feel guilty or anxious. Parents need an opportunity to express their feelings and to begin learning to cope with the child's illness. The initial period of diagnosis, hospitalization, and early care of the infant at home are very stressful. Parents need special support if their infant has a life-threatening heart defect.

Examples of nursing diagnoses associated with heart defects having increased pulmonary blood flow and their complications include the following:

- *Excess Fluid Volume* related to heart failure and pulmonary vasculature overload
- *Ineffective Infant Feeding Pattern* related to shortness of breath and fatigue

TABLE 48–6 ❖ Pathophysiology, Clinical Manifestations, and Clinical Therapy for Heart Defects that Increase Pulmonary Blood Flow

Pathophysiology, Clinical Manifestations, and Clinical Therapy	Anatomy

Patent Ductus Arteriosus (PDA)

Pathophysiology

A common congenital defect caused by persistent fetal circulation that accounts for 10% of all congenital heart defects (Rome & Kreutzer, 2004). When pulmonary circulation is established and systemic vascular resistance increases at birth, pressures in the aorta become greater than in the pulmonary arteries. Blood is then shunted from the aorta to the pulmonary arteries, increasing circulation to the pulmonary system. It is a common problem of preterm infants, and is present in nearly all preterm infants less than 27 weeks' gestation (Tran, 2002). The ductus arteriosus in the preterm newborn is not as responsive to the increased oxygen content with the conversion to pulmonary circulation, and it is less likely to close.

Patent ductus arteriosus

Clinical Manifestations

Dyspnea; tachypnea; tachycardia; full, bounding pulses; widened pulse pressure; hypotension may be noted when cardiac output is low.

CHF, intercostal retractions, hepatomegaly, and growth failure when a large PDA exists.

A continuous "machinery" murmur during systole and diastole, and a thrill in the pulmonic area.

High risk for frequent respiratory infections, pneumonia, and infective endocarditis.

Diagnostic Tests

The chest radiograph and ECG show left ventricular hypertrophy.

The PDA can be visualized, and left-to-right shunt can be measured on echocardiogram.

■ Mix of oxygenated and unoxygenated blood

Clinical Therapy

Surgical ligation of PDA is the treatment of choice.

Intravenous indomethacin often stimulates closure of the ductus arteriosus in premature infants.

Transcatheter closure by obstructive device is sometimes attempted in children over 18 months of age. Prophylaxis for infective endocarditis is required until the PDA is closed.

Prognosis: No long-term sequelae occur if treated before pulmonary vascular disease develops. If PDA is not treated, child's life span is shortened because pulmonary artery hypertension and pulmonary vascular obstructive disease develop.

Atrial Septal Defect (ASD)

Pathophysiology

The opening in the atrial septum that permits left-to-right shunting of blood. Three types of ASDs occur: ostium secundum, ostium primum that is an endocardial cushion defect with anomalies of one or both of the tricuspid and mitral valves, and sinus venosus that is associated with partial anomalous pulmonary venous connection. The opening may be small, as when the foramen ovale fails to close, or large, as when the septum may be completely absent. Of children with congenital heart defects, 10% have an ASD (Rome & Kreutzer, 2004).

Atrial septal defect

Clinical Manifestations

Infants and young children usually have no symptoms. Small and moderate-size ASDs may not be diagnosed until preschool years or later.

CHF, easy tiring, and poor growth occur with a large ASD.

A soft systolic ejection murmur in the pulmonic area with wide splitting of S_2. The split second sound is fixed through all phases of respiration.

Diagnostic Procedures

Echocardiogram identifies a dilated right ventricle due to blood overload and the shunt size.

The chest x-ray and ECG reveal little information unless the ASD is large, has excessive shunting, and right ventricular hypertrophy is present.

Clinical Therapy

Spontaneous closure of some ASDs occurs within the first 4 years of life. No activity limitations are needed.

Surgery to close or patch the ASD is performed when significant increased pulmonary blood flow causes CHF, or when spontaneous closure has not occurred by 4 years of age.

Secundum ASDs may be closed by a transcatheter device (septal occluder) during cardiac catheterization.

Prognosis: Many persons with uncorrected small and moderate-size ASDs have lived to middle age without symptoms, but CHF and pulmonary artery hypertension may develop in untreated adults. Atrial arrhythmias may also occur in adults.

TABLE 48–6 ✣ **Pathophysiology, Clinical Manifestations, and Clinical Therapy for Heart Defects that Increase Pulmonary Blood Flow—continued**

Pathophysiology, Clinical Manifestations, and Clinical Therapy	Anatomy

Ventricular Septal Defect (VSD)

Pathophysiology

An opening in the ventricular septum results in increased pulmonary blood flow. Blood is shunted from the left ventricle directly across the open septum into the pulmonary artery. This is the most common congenital heart defect, accounting for 40% of all defects (Rome & Kreutzer, 2004).

Clinical Manifestations

Only 15% of VSDs are large enough to cause CHF, an increased number of pulmonary infections, and pulmonary hypertension.

A systolic murmur is auscultated at the third or fourth left intercostal space at the sternal border.

Diagnostic Procedures

A chest x-ray and ECG reveal little when VSDs are small. An enlarged heart and pulmonary vascular markings on chest x-ray occur in cases of large VSDs with shunting. Right and left ventricular hypertrophy may be seen on ECG.

Echocardiogram establishes the diagnosis if shunting is present.

Cardiac catheterization is used only in preparation for surgery. Findings reveal increased oxygen in the right ventricle and increased systolic pressure in the right ventricle and pulmonary artery.

Clinical Therapy

Most small VSDs close spontaneously within the first 6 months of life. Treatment is conservative when no signs of CHF or pulmonary hypertension are present.

Surgical patching of VSD during infancy is performed when poor growth is evident.

Closure of VSD by transcatheter device (i.e., Rashkind device) during cardiac catheterization may be attempted for some defects.

Prophylaxis for infective endocarditis is required.

Prognosis: Highest risk associated with surgical repair is in the first few months of life. Children respond well to surgery and experience substantial catch-up growth. Tachyarrhythmias and right bundle branch block are possible complications.

Ventricular
septal defect

Atrioventricular Canal (Endocardial Cushion) Defect (AV Canal)

Pathophysiology

Atrioventricular (AV) canal refers to a combination of defects in the atrial and ventricular septa and portions of tricuspid and mitral valves. Up to 4% to 5% of children with congenital heart defects have a total or partial AV canal (Driscoll, 1999). This defect is associated with Down syndrome. Endocardial cushions are fetal growth centers for mitral and tricuspid valves and AV septum. The most complex AV canal defect results in one AV valve and large septal defects between both atria and ventricles.

Clinical Manifestations

Severity of symptoms depends on amount of mitral regurgitation and the left to right shunting of blood across the septum.

Infants have CHF, tachypnea, tachycardia, poor growth, recurrent respiratory infections, and repeated respiratory failure.

A holosystolic murmur is loudest at the left lower sternal border, and the intensity reflects the amount of mitral regurgitation. S_1 is accentuated and S_2 is split.

Diagnostic Procedures

On chest x-ray, cardiomegaly and pulmonary vascular markings are present.

On ECG, atrial enlargement, right ventricular hypertrophy, and an incomplete right bundle branch block are noted.

Echocardiogram reveals dilation of the ventricles, septal defects, and details of valve malformation.

Cardiac catheterization reveals increased oxygen in the right atrium, increased right ventricle and/or pulmonary artery pressure.

Clinical Therapy

Surgery is performed during infancy to prevent pulmonary vascular disease. Palliative pulmonary artery banding may be used to reduce blood flow to the lungs and CHF so the infant can grow before corrective surgery.

Oxygen may be required until surgery, but it may increase pulmonary blood flow and worsen CHF.

Patches are placed over septal defects, and valve tissue is used to form functioning valves. The mitral valve may be replaced.

Prophylaxis for infective endocarditis is required.

Prognosis: Information on long-term survival following successful surgery is lacking. Arrhythmias and mitral valve insufficiency occur postoperatively. There is no difference in short-term survival rates between infants with and without Down syndrome.

Atrioventricular
canal defect

● **FIGURE 48-3**

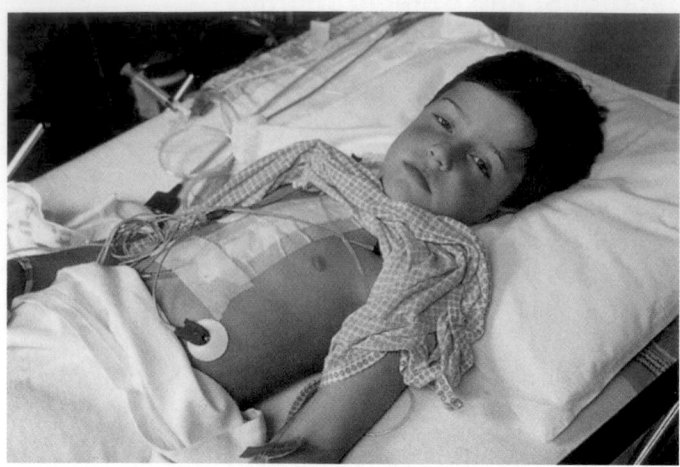

A child with atrial septal defect repair. Surgery is performed with this type of defect to prevent pulmonary artery hypertension.

- *Risk for Infection* related to pulmonary vascular congestion and chronic illness
- *Interrupted Family Processes* related to crisis of child's serious illness

PLANNING AND IMPLEMENTATION

Follow the guidelines for nursing care of the child with CHF. See page 1442.

Family Education

Participate with members of the cardiology team to provide information and educate the family about the child's condition. Information may include the following:

- General information about the congenital heart disease, including a description of the heart's anatomy and physiology and the defect
- Information about genetic and environmental influences associated with congenital heart disease
- Overview of the child's prognosis and timing of medical and surgical interventions

NURSING PRACTICE

Following are some valuable resources for parents of a child with a congenital heart defect:

- *If Your Child Has a Congenital Heart Defect* by the American Heart Association
- *The Parent's Guide to Children's Congenital Heart Defects* by Gerri Freid Kramer and Shari Maurer, Three Rivers Press
- *King of Hearts: The True Story of the Maverick Who Pioneered Open Heart Surgery* by G. Wayne Miller

Psychosocial Support

Parents often need support for anxiety about an uncertain surgical outcome. Determine if parents have a support system as they learn about the infant's diagnosis and make difficult decisions about the child's surgery. Identify some resources for support, such as social services, pastoral services, or a parent of a child with a similar heart defect if the parents do not have adequate support systems. Some parents may be concerned that signing consent for surgery places the child in even more danger of illness or even death.

Parents should be offered genetic counseling if planning a future pregnancy.

Home Care

Children are often managed at home until surgery. Parents should encourage feeding to promote growth, but allow the infant to feed for up to 30 minutes. Breastfeeding is encouraged because of its beneficial effects for the infant. A high-caloric formula may be used if the infant does not gain enough weight. Feedings through a nasogastric or gastrostomy tube may also be given at night or 24 hours a day. Even when nasogastric or gastrostomy feedings are used, encourage the infant to take some formula orally to provide positive oral stimulation. See feeding suggestions for the infant with CHF on page 1443.

Efforts should be made to reduce the infant's exposure to infectious diseases. Wash hands frequently. Respiratory infections make hypoxemia worse in children with cyanosis. Fever increases the metabolic rates and oxygen demands. Vomiting and diarrhea may cause an electrolyte disturbance and digoxin toxicity (Cook & Higgins, 2004). The physician should be notified about fever, poor feeding, vomiting, and diarrhea.

Health promotion visits are important and all immunizations are provided according to the recommended schedule. Monthly prophylaxis for respiratory syncytial virus (RSV) with Palivizumab should be provided during the peak season. See Chapter 47. ∞

Preparation for Surgery

When the child is preschool age or older, prepare the child for the settings, equipment, and experiences to expect before and after surgery. Follow guidelines for preoperative treatment described in Chapter 40. ∞ If an infant or toddler is having surgery, provide parents with information about how the child will look, equipment that will be used, and what care will be provided in the immediate postoperative period.

EVALUATION

- Nutritional intake is adequate with oral feeds and supplemental nasogastric feeding as necessary.

- The child maintains a growth pattern that follows the established growth curve percentile.
- The child receives all immunizations and RSV prophylaxis to reduce the potential for acute illnesses.

NURSING MANAGEMENT AT THE TIME OF SURGERY

The goal of nursing management is to perform assessments, provide supportive care to the family, and meet the child's nursing care needs before and after surgery.

NURSING ASSESSMENT AND DIAGNOSIS

At the time of surgery, the child needs a careful history and physical examination to detect any acute illnesses. Assess the child's behavioral patterns, heart function, respiratory function, weight, and fluid status. Refer to Table 48–2.

In the immediate postoperative period, the child will be cared for in the intensive care unit. When the child returns to the general nursing unit, assessment focuses on signs of surgical complications such as infection, arrhythmias, and impaired tissue perfusion.

- Monitor the child's temperature and inspect the surgical incision site. Fever, excessive incisional pain, spreading erythema around the incision, and wound drainage beginning 3 to 4 days postoperatively may be early signs of infection.
- Assess the respiratory system for breath sounds, respiratory effort, and signs of distress that may indicate pneumonia or fluid in the pleural space.
- Monitor the vital signs, including blood pressure. The child may not be on a cardiac monitor, so auscultation of the apical pulse to detect an irregular heart rate or bradycardia is essential, signs of reduced cardiac output that require immediate intervention.
- Check pulse oximetry, capillary refill, extremity warmth, pedal pulses, level of consciousness, and urine output to assess impaired tissue perfusion. Reduced urine output is a sign of decreased cardiac output.
- Continue to assess the child's pain.

Examples of nursing diagnoses following cardiac surgery include the following:

- *Ineffective Breathing Pattern* related to respiratory muscle fatigue
- *Acute Pain* related to surgical incision and expansion of chest with coughing and deep breathing exercises

- *Risk for Imbalanced Fluid Volume* related to impact of surgery on heart's pumping action
- *Risk for Infection* related to surgery and chronic disease status

PLANNING AND IMPLEMENTATION

Pain Management

Pain management with 24-hour intravenous opioids should be provided for several days postoperatively until the child is taking fluids. Once the child is taking oral fluids and foods, oral analgesics may be given around the clock. Follow the guidelines for pain management provided in Chapter 42.∞ Teach parents and caregivers to lift and move the child so that stress on the incision and potential pain is reduced. Do not lift the child under the arms.

Promote Respiratory Function

Encourage the child to take deep breaths and cough or to perform spirometry exercises regularly to promote full lung expansion (see Skill 14–26). **SKILLS** Provide tips for splinting the chest (a pillow or stuffed animal) to reduce the pain from coughing and deep breathing. Chest physiotherapy may be performed in children under 3 years of age.

Manage Fluids and Nutrition

Encourage the infant or child to begin oral fluids and nutrition when permitted. Although oral fluids are rarely limited following surgery for defects with increased pulmonary blood flow, intake and output should be assessed carefully. Parents may be encouraged to bring in favorite foods for the child when they can be tolerated. Administer antibiotics as prescribed. If intravenous antibiotics are continued after the child's oral intake is normal, the line can be converted to a heparin or saline lock.

Activity

Encourage the child to increase activity gradually with longer periods out of bed every day, but ensure adequate rest periods to promote healing. Provide diversional activities and opportunities for therapeutic play so the child can better manage the stresses associated with pain and frightening procedures.

Discharge Planning and Home Care Teaching

Infants and children may be discharged from the hospital within a few days of surgery. Parents need information spread over several days to prepare for care of the child at home. Encourage a nutritious diet and snacks so the infant or child has an opportunity to catch up for previous growth deficits. Acetaminophen or ibuprofen may be used for pain management after discharge. See "Teaching Highlights: Care of the Child After Cardiac Surgery."

TEACHING HIGHLIGHTS

CARE OF THE CHILD AFTER CARDIAC SURGERY

- Place infants and children in car safety seats for travel home from the hospital. Place a small blanket over the incision to prevent the straps from rubbing.
- Sponge bathe the infant or use a tub bath with a low water level. Avoid soaking the incision until sutures are out and the incision is healed. Clean the incision daily with gentle baby or pH-balanced soap. Do not use oils, creams, lotions, or ointments on the incision. Cover the incision with a clean shirt or bib to keep it clean and dry.
- Pick infants and young children up by placing one hand under the head and the other hand under the hips. Avoid picking the child up under the arms.
- Allow the child to increase activity gradually as tolerated. Report increased fatigue or decreased activity tolerance to the physician. Postpone rough play, bike riding, and climbing for 6 weeks until the sternum incision has healed completely. Allow the child to return to school in about 3 weeks.
- Report any signs of wound infection, fever, flulike symptoms, chest pain, increased respiratory rate or respiratory distress, appetite change, or irritability to the physician.
- Acetaminophen or ibuprofen can be given for pain control. Use the recommended dose for the child's weight.
- Antibiotics should be given for dental and surgical procedures as directed (some children need them for several months and some for the rest of their lives). Report any unexplained fever or illness during the first 2 months following surgery as the child is at higher risk for infective endocarditis during that time.

Children undergoing heart surgery are at risk for post-traumatic stress disorder, especially if the ICU stay is prolonged (Connolly, McClowry, Hayman et al., 2004). See Chapter 54. ∞ Prepare parents for potential behavior problems of young children that may result from the stress of hospitalization, such as nightmares, separation anxiety, and overdependence on parents. Encourage parents to reassure children about their security, and to promote play and other means to deal with their feelings. If the child's symptoms continue for several weeks, a psychologic referral may be needed.

Reassure parents of children with a complete correction of the cardiac defect that there should be no further cardiovascular problems. Provide parents with full information about the child's defect and the surgery performed to share with the child's current and future healthcare providers. Encourage parents to allow the child to live a normal and active life.

Children are at risk for infective endocarditis, especially within the first 6 months after surgery. See Table 48–5 for prophylactic antibiotics needed for procedures. Any unexplained fever or malaise seen in the 2 months following surgical repair or after dental work may be a sign of infection. The child should be examined for petechiae and splenomegaly and evaluated for infective endocarditis. See page 1473.

EVALUATION

Examples of expected outcomes of nursing care include the following:

- The child's pain is effectively managed.
- Full lung expansion is maintained with spirometry exercises or chest physiotherapy.
- The child's incision heals without infection.
- Catch-up growth occurs over the next few months to years.

DEFECTS CAUSING DECREASED PULMONARY BLOOD FLOW AND MIXED DEFECTS

ETIOLOGY AND PATHOPHYSIOLOGY

Defects Causing Decreased Pulmonary Blood Flow

Defects that obstruct the pulmonary blood flow result in little or no blood reaching the lungs to get oxygenated. If an atrial or ventricular septal opening exists between the left and right side of the heart, right-sided pressures exceed those on the left because of the obstructed pulmonary blood flow, resulting in right to left shunting.

The bone marrow is stimulated to produce more red blood cells to increase the hemoglobin available to carry oxygen. Polycythemia, an above-normal increase in the number of red blood cells, may result and place the child at risk for thromboembolism. Over time platelet survival is reduced and clotting factors are impaired, increasing the infant's risk of bleeding with surgery. Brain abscesses are also more common in children with cyanotic heart defects.

When infants and children with cyanosis rise in the morning, they may experience an abrupt decrease in systemic resistance and pulmonary blood flow. This physiologic change can trigger a hypercyanotic (hypoxic or "tet") episode when combined with a sudden increase in cardiac output and venous return associated with crying, feeding, exercise, a warm bath, and straining with defecation. The partial pressure of oxygen (PO_2) is lowered, and the partial pressure of carbon dioxide (PCO_2) rises. Hypoxemia becomes progressively worse as the respiratory center in the brain overreacts, increasing the respiratory effort. The extra respiratory effort further increases the cardiac output and contributes to a life-threatening decline unless rapid intervention is successful.

Mixed Defects

Many complex congenital heart defects involve a combination of defects that make the newborn dependent upon the mixing of the pulmonary and systemic circulations for survival during the postnatal period. This mixing of oxygen-saturated and desaturated blood results in a general desaturated systemic blood flow and cyanosis. Pulmonary congestion occurs because of increased pulmonary blood flow and obstruction of systemic flow.

CLINICAL MANIFESTATIONS

Defects Causing Decreased Pulmonary Blood Flow

Clinical manifestations in infants initially include cyanosis shortly after birth, dyspnea, and a loud murmur. The skin may initially be ruddy or mottled before cyanosis is observed. Cyanosis of mucous membranes may be seen sooner than generalized duskiness. Cyanosis that does not respond as expected to oxygen is a classic sign. Signs and symptoms of chronic hypoxemia include fatigue, clubbing of the fingers and toes, exertional dyspnea, and delayed developmental milestones (Figure 48–4 ●). The infants may need to stop sucking periodically during feedings to breathe, and diaphoresis may be seen with the increased

● **FIGURE 48-4**

A, This infant is cyanotic due to a heart defect that reduces pulmonary blood flow. **B,** Clubbing of the fingers in an older child is one manifestation of a heart defect that reduces pulmonary blood flow.

● **FIGURE 48-5**

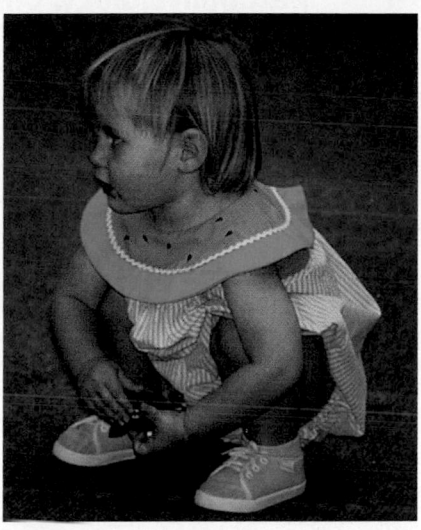

A young child with an uncorrected or partially corrected defect that reduces pulmonary blood flow may squat (assumes a knee–chest position) to reduce systemic blood flow return to the heart.

work of feeding. These infants have a higher metabolic rate, and inadequate calories may be consumed resulting in poor weight gain. See Table 48–7 for the pathophysiology, clinical manifestations, and clinical therapy for these defects.

When the infant or child has severe obstruction to pulmonary blood flow, hypercyanotic episodes can occur suddenly. Toddlers with uncorrected cyanotic heart disease often squat to relieve dyspnea (Figure 48–5 ●). The knee–chest position reduces the cardiac output by decreasing the venous return from the lower extremities and by increasing the systemic vascular resistance. Hypercyanotic episodes usually appear between 2 months and 2 years of age. Signs include increased rate and depth of respirations; increased heart rate; increased cyanosis, pallor, and poor tissue perfusion; diaphoresis; irritability and crying; and seizures and loss of consciousness.

Older children may have additional symptoms such as exercise-induced dizziness and **syncope** (transient loss of consciousness and muscle tone), which are serious signs indicating a need for medical evaluation.

Mixed Defects

These complex congenital heart defects cause varying degrees of cyanosis and CHF. When the pulmonary vascular resistance is lower than the systemic resistance, pulmonary congestion develops, followed by CHF. When the pulmonary blood flow is decreased, the infant will have more severe cyanosis and polycythemia (Suddaby, 2001). See Table 48–8 for the pathophysiology, clinical manifestations, and clinical therapy for these complex mixed defects.

TABLE 48–7 ❖ Pathophysiology, Clinical Manifestations, and Clinical Therapy for Defects with Decreased Pulmonary Blood Flow

Defect Pathophysiology, Clinical Manifestations, and Clinical Therapy	Anatomy

Pulmonic Stenosis (PS)

Pathophysiology

Stenosis (narrowing of valve or valve area) can be above valve, below valve, or at valve. Stenosis obstructs blood flow into the pulmonary artery, which increases preload and results in right ventricular hypertrophy. This is the second most common congenital heart defect, accounting for 8%–12% of all cases (Park, 2002). Stenosis may progress as the heart muscle grows and develops in the subvalvular area.

Clinical Manifestations

Children with mild stenosis may have no symptoms and grow normally.

In moderate stenosis, dyspnea and fatigue occur on exertion. Signs of CHF and hepatosplenomegaly are rare but may result from chronic pressure overload. Heart failure and chest pain on exertion occur in severe cases.

A loud systolic ejection murmur with a widely split S_2 and thrill may be found in the pulmonic listening area.

Diagnostic Tests

The chest x-ray may show an enlarged pulmonary artery with normal heart size and normal pulmonary vascularity.

The ECG may show right atrial enlargement and right ventricular hypertrophy.

An echocardiogram provides information about the pressure gradient across valve and size of valve ring.

Cardiac catheterization findings include increased right ventricular pressure and a normal or slightly lowered pulmonary artery pressure.

Clinical Therapy

Dilation by balloon valvuloplasty, performed during cardiac catheterization, treats simple pulmonic stenosis.

Surgical valvotomy may be used when other defects such as VSD are present.

Surgical resection may be needed for narrowing above the valve area. Pulmonary regurgitation may result, but is not a significant problem.

Prognosis: Pulmonic stenosis does not typically increase in severity. Lifelong infective endocarditis prophylaxis is necessary.

Pulmonic stenosis

☐ Decreased unoxygenated blood flow

Tetralogy of Fallot (TOF)

Pathophysiology

Four defects: pulmonic stenosis, right ventricular hypertrophy, ventricular septal defect (VSD), and overriding of aorta make up the condition. Some children have a fifth defect: open foramen ovale or atrial septal defect (ASD). About 10% of children with congenital heart defects have TOF (Park, 2002). Elevated pressures in the right side of the heart cause a right-to-left shunt.

Clinical Manifestations

The infant becomes hypoxic and cyanotic as the ductus arteriosus closes. The degree of pulmonary stenosis determines severity of symptoms.

A systolic murmur is heard in the pulmonic area and transmitted to the suprasternal notch. A thrill may be palpated in the pulmonic area.

Polycythemia, hypoxic spells, metabolic acidosis, poor growth, clubbing, and exercise intolerance may develop.

Toddlers with uncorrected defects instinctively squat (assume a knee-chest position) to decrease the return of systemic venous blood to the heart. See Figure 48–5.

Diagnostic Tests

A chest x-ray shows the boot-shaped heart due to the large right ventricle, decreased pulmonary vascular markings, and a prominent aorta.

The ECG shows right ventricular hypertrophy.

The echocardiogram shows the VSD, obstruction of pulmonary outflow, an overriding aorta, and the size of the pulmonary arteries.

Cardiac catheterization provides details about the anatomic defects.

Blood tests reveal an elevated hematocrit and hemoglobin and an increased clotting time.

Pulmonic stenosis

Overriding aorta

Ventricular septal defect

Right ventricular hypertrophy

☐ Decreased unoxygenated blood flow

■ Mixed oxygenated and unoxygenated blood

Clinical Therapy

Management of hypercyanotic episodes includes placing the infant in the knee–chest position, calming the child, giving oxygen, and administering morphine and propranolol intravenously. Monitoring the child for metabolic acidosis or prolonged unconsciousness is critical.

A total repair is often performed before 6 months of age when the infant has a hypercyanotic episode. Corrective surgery may be attempted in asymptomatic children by 6 months of age.

Prognosis: Not all children are cured by surgery, but most have improved quality of life and improved longevity. Arrhythmias and right ventricular dysfunction may be residual problems (Waldman & Wernly, 1999). Lifelong infective endocarditis prophylaxis is required.

TABLE 48–7 ✦ Pathophysiology, Clinical Manifestations, and Clinical Therapy for Defects with Decreased Pulmonary Blood Flow—continued

Defect Pathophysiology, Clinical Manifestations, and Clinical Therapy	Anatomy

Pulmonary or Tricuspid Atresia

Pulmonary atresia is the absence of communication between the right ventricle and the pulmonary artery, either at the site of the pulmonary valve or in the main pulmonary artery. In tricuspid atresia, the tricuspid valve is absent. Blood flows to the left side of the heart through the foramen ovale. The PDA provides the only flow of blood to the pulmonary arteries. A ventricular septal defect (VSD) or transposition of the great arteries (TGA) is also often present.

Clinical Manifestations

Cyanosis is present at birth.

Tachypnea, CHF, pulmonary edema, hepatomegaly, acidosis, hypoxic spells, clubbing, polycythemia, and growth delays occur.

A continuous murmur from the PDA is heard in the pulmonic area. A single S_2 is heard in the aortic area, and a harsh systolic murmur may be heard in the tricuspid area.

Diagnostic Tests

The chest x-ray may reveal a normal size or slightly enlarged heart.

The ECG may reveal right atrial hypertrophy.

The echocardiogram shows a small hypoplastic right ventricular cavity and tricuspid valve, an absent right ventricular outflow tract, a dilated right atrium, and right-to-left shunting across the atrial septum.

Clinical Therapy

Prostaglandin E_1 is given immediately to maintain a patent ductus arteriosus. Digoxin and diuretics are also used.

The Rastelli balloon atrial septostomy is performed to increase the atrial opening.

A Rastelli or modified Fontan procedure results in improved survival.

Prognosis: Outcome depends upon the size of the pulmonary outflow tract developed by surgery and the fibrosis in the right ventricle. The child has increased risk for arrhythmia and right ventricular dysfunction.

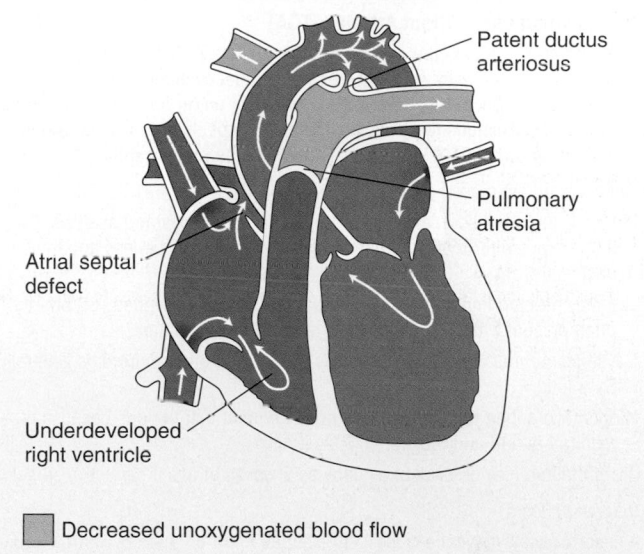

Patent ductus arteriosus

Pulmonary atresia

Atrial septal defect

Underdeveloped right ventricle

▢ Decreased unoxygenated blood flow

CLINICAL THERAPY

Early management of these defects is important to prevent secondary damage to the heart, lungs, and brain, including the adverse effects of hypoxemia on the child's cognitive and psychomotor development. Corrective surgery is often performed in infancy. A palliative procedure may be performed first to preserve life in children with potentially lethal heart defects and complications (see Table 48–4). With some defects, corrective surgery can be postponed with a palliative procedure, giving the infant an opportunity to grow and improve the success of corrective surgery. See Figure 48–6 ◉ for various palliative shunts (surgically created channels for blood flow) that may be performed. See Tables 48–7 and 48–8 for clinical therapy for specific congenital heart defects. Antibiotic prophylaxis for infective endocarditis is needed before and after surgical correction for many of these defects.

If closure of the ductus arteriosus causes life-threatening cyanosis in newborns, prostaglandin E_1 (PGE$_1$) is given to reopen the ductus arteriosus and improve pulmonary or systemic blood flow. Treatment with PGE$_1$ provides time to transfer the newborn to a cardiac center for diagnostic evaluation and surgical intervention. The child's hemoglobin

◉ FIGURE 48–6

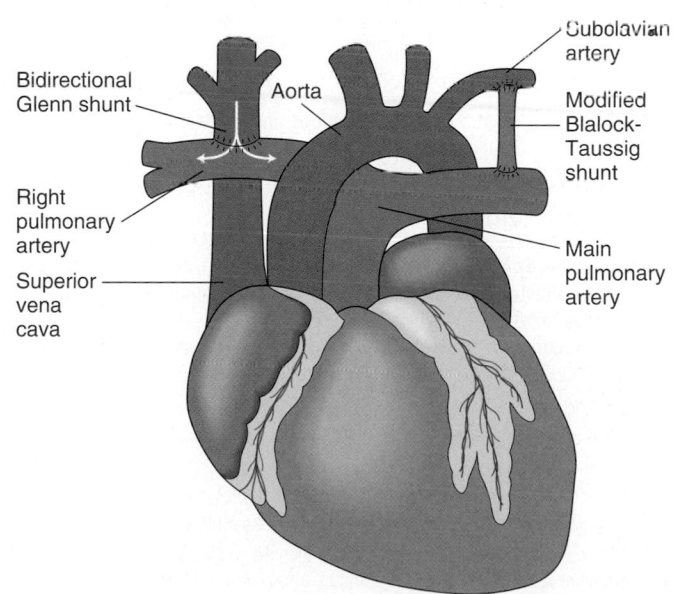

Bidirectional Glenn shunt

Aorta

Subclavian artery

Modified Blalock-Taussig shunt

Right pulmonary artery

Superior vena cava

Main pulmonary artery

Anatomic location of the modified Blalock-Taussig and Glenn shunts for palliative procedures.

TABLE 48–8 ✤ Pathophysiology, Clinical Manifestations, and Clinical Therapy for Mixed Defects

Defect Pathophysiology, Clinical Manifestations, and Clinical Therapy	Anatomy

Transposition of the Great Arteries (TGA)

The pulmonary artery is the outflow tract for the left ventricle, and the aorta is the outflow tract for the right ventricle, creating parallel circulations. The condition is life threatening at birth, and survival initially depends on an open ductus arteriosus and foramen ovale. This condition occurs in about 5% of children with congenital heart disease (Grifka, 1999). An ASD or VSD may also be present with TGA.

Patent ductus arteriosus

Pulmonary artery

Aorta

Clinical Manifestations

Cyanosis, apparent soon after birth, progresses to hypoxia and acidosis. Cyanosis does not improve with oxygen administration. Cyanosis may be less apparent when a large VSD is present.

CHF may develop immediately or over days or weeks. Tachypnea (60 breaths/min) is often present without retractions or other signs of dyspnea.

A systolic murmur is present if a VSD is present; no other murmur is generally heard. S_2 is loud.

Infants take a long time to feed and need frequent rest periods because of rapid respiratory rate and fatigue.

Growth failure may be evident as early as 2 weeks of age if corrective surgery is not performed.

Diagnostic Tests

A chest x-ray may reveal a classic egg-shaped heart on a string (narrow superior mediastinum) with enlarged ventricles and increased pulmonary vascular markings.

The ECG reveals right ventricular hypertrophy.

The echocardiogram often shows the abnormal position of the great arteries rising from the ventricles.

Cardiac catheterization shows increased right ventricular pressure, and the catheter can enter the aorta through the right ventricle.

Blood tests reveal an increased hematocrit and hemoglobin or polycythemia.

Clinical Therapy

Prostaglandin E_1 is ordered to maintain a patent ductus arteriosus until a palliative procedure can be performed.

Corrective surgery (arterial switch) is usually performed before 1 week of age.

Balloon atrial septostomy may be performed during cardiac catheterization in newborns as a first stage. This may also be corrected surgically. Other defects may be repaired in stages as the infant grows.

Prognosis: Survival without surgery is impossible. The 5-year survival following an arterial switch is 82%. Arrhythmias, right ventricular failure, and sudden death are long-term complications (8–15 years) after the Mustard procedure, so the Mustard or Rastelli procedure is performed only when significant pulmonary valve stenosis is present (Grifka, 1999). Other complications of surgical repair include pulmonic or aortic stenosis, coronary artery obstruction, and mitral regurgitation. Infective endocarditis prophylaxis may be necessary.

Truncus Arteriosus

A single large vessel empties both ventricles and provides circulation for the pulmonary, systemic, and coronary circulations. A VSD is usually present. This occurs in less than 1% of congenital heart defects.

Truncus arteriosus Type III

■ Mixed oxygenated and unoxygenated blood

Clinical Manifestations

Cyanosis develops soon after birth; however, this is also a condition of increased pulmonary blood flow. Severe CHF, dyspnea, retractions, fatigue, poor feeding, poor growth, polycythemia, clubbing, increased pulse pressure, bounding peripheral pulses, a widened pulse pressure, frequent respiratory infections, and cardiomegaly occur.

The VSD produces a harsh systolic murmur in the lower sternal border. A systolic click may be heard in the apex and pulmonic area.

Diagnostic Tests

The chest x-ray shows cardiomegaly, a large aorta, and increased pulmonary vascular markings.

The ECG reveals right and left ventricular hypertrophy.

The echocardiogram shows the absence of two semilunar valves.

Cardiac catheterization documents a left-to-right shunt at the level of the ventricle, and equal pressure in the ventricles, the truncus, and pulmonary arteries.

Clinical Therapy

A Rastelli procedure is performed to close the VSD and create a passage to the pulmonary arteries. Repeated surgery is necessary to enlarge the pulmonary artery conduit.

Digoxin and diuretics are given.

Prognosis: Survival is improved, but truncal valve stenosis and regurgitation result. The long-term prognosis is unknown.

TABLE 48–8 ✤ Pathophysiology, Clinical Manifestations, and Clinical Therapy for Mixed Defects—continued

Pathophysiology, Clinical Manifestations, and Clinical Therapy	Anatomy

Total Anomalous Pulmonary Venous Return

The pulmonary veins empty into the right atrium or veins leading to the right atrium rather than into the left atrium. The foramen ovale must remain patent for mixed blood from the right atrium to pass to the systemic circulation. Any obstruction of the pulmonary veins increases the condition's severity.

Clinical Manifestations

Mild cyanosis and frequent respiratory infections occur. Increased cyanosis may occur with feedings as the filled esophagus compresses the common pulmonary vein.

If the pulmonary veins are obstructed in any way, cyanosis will be increased. Increased pulmonary blood flow will result in signs of CHF.

A precordial bulge may be palpated. The S_2 has a wide, fixed split when there is no pulmonary vein obstruction. An ejection murmur and gallop rhythm may be heard in the pulmonic area.

Diagnostic Tests

The chest x-ray shows cardiac enlargement, a large pulmonary artery, and increased pulmonary blood flow.

The ECG reveals hypertrophy of the right atrium and ventricle.

The echocardiogram shows enlargement of the right atrium, a patent foramen ovale, and lack of connection between the pulmonary veins and left atrium.

Cardiac catheterization shows a higher oxygen level in the right atrium and the abnormal circulation.

Clinical Therapy

Prostaglandin E_1 is given to maintain patent ductus arteriosus.

Hypoxemia and CHF are treated.

Balloon atrial septostomy may be performed to promote better mixing of blood so surgery can be delayed until the infant is stabilized.

Surgery to reconnect or baffle the pulmonary veins to the left atrium is performed.

Prognosis: Survivors have lived more than 20 years after correction.

and hematocrit values are monitored for polycythemia or anemia. If the blood viscosity becomes too high, red cell pheresis may be performed. These infants also do not tolerate anemia well with less oxygen-carrying hemoglobin.

Hypercyanotic episodes are treated aggressively. To decrease the pulmonary vascular resistance, the initial treatment involves calming the child, giving oxygen, and administering morphine and propranolol intravenously. Packed red blood cells may be administered to improve oxygen delivery to the tissues when the child is anemic. Postpone all unpleasant procedures. To increase the systemic vascular resistance, the infant is placed in the knee–chest position and given intravenous fluids to expand circulatory volume. Dopamine or phenylephrine (Neo-Synephrine) is also given. Once a hypercyanotic episode has occurred, immediate palliative or corrective surgery is often scheduled.

NURSING MANAGEMENT

Nursing management of the hospitalized child focuses on monitoring PGE$_1$ therapy for newborns, treating hyper-

cyanotic episodes, supporting families to care for the child at home, and providing postsurgical care.

NURSING ASSESSMENT AND DIAGNOSIS

Physiologic Assessment Before Surgery

Infants receiving PGE$_1$ therapy are cared for in an intensive care nursery where their cardiovascular status can be closely monitored until palliative procedures are performed.

Prior to or between stages of surgery, the infant or child is seen regularly to assess growth, and for signs of deterioration in cardiac status. These children are at risk for growth problems that affect height and weight, and potentially the head circumference, so measurements need to be plotted on the same growth curve to monitor the significance of the growth problems.

The child needs careful observation for signs of increased cyanosis in the morning or at other high-risk times. Observe for neurologic signs of thromboembolism due to polycythemia such as headache, dizziness, excessive irritability, and paralysis. Older children with cyanotic defects may have clubbing of the fingers and toes (Figure 48–4).

Assessment Following Surgery

Children are admitted to the ICU following surgery. Refer to the section on nursing assessment of the child with increased pulmonary blood flow on page 1459 for nursing care guidelines. Once the child returns to the general nursing unit, monitor the child's heart functioning. Assess vital signs, pulse oximetry, skin color, and perfusion of the skin by capillary refill and distal pulses. Monitoring fluid intake and output following surgery is critical. A sudden sustained increase in pulse and respirations and a decrease in peripheral perfusion may be early signs of hemorrhage. Signs of respiratory distress may indicate the development of a pneumothorax or CHF.

Psychosocial Assessment

Assess the parents' need for information and emotional support. In many cases, the infant's condition is first identified at birth; however, a defect could have been identified by sonogram prenatally. The parents will be grieving the loss of a perfect newborn and be extremely anxious about the infant's condition and prognosis.

Examples of nursing diagnoses that may apply to a child with decreased pulmonary blood flow include the following:

- *Decreased Cardiac Output* related to ventricular restriction and an obstructed outflow tract
- *Risk for Infection* related to unfiltered bacteria in the blood and sites of blood shunting that promote bacterial growth
- *Caregiver Role Strain* related to care of a child with chronic illness
- *Activity Intolerance* related to cyanosis and dyspnea on exertion
- *Delayed Growth and Development* related to congenital anomaly and hypoxemia

PLANNING AND IMPLEMENTATION

Home Care of the Child Before Surgery

Infants with tetralogy of Fallot and other serious defects are often managed at home to grow and potentially improve surgical outcome. Parents are usually anxious during the wait for surgery. They may fear that the infant will not survive until surgery or that they will be unable to manage any problems the infant may have. Provide information and teach parents how to care for the infant at home. Arrange for home health nursing and other community services that may be required. Many of these children require supplemental nutrition. Oxygen is available only for emergencies as it has no effect on improving the child's usual oxygen saturation level.

Cyanosis with or without CHF often results in delayed gross motor skills. Make referrals to community-based early intervention programs to help parents learn about realistic developmental goals and to promote the child's development. Encourage parents to treat the infant as normally as possible. Children with mild cyanotic lesions do not need to adjust activity. The child with moderate to severe disease should be able to tolerate crying for a few minutes without difficulty. Prolonged crying should not be permitted because it causes fatigue and further hypoxia.

Teach parents to observe for signs of worsening cyanosis, particularly in the morning, that could signal the beginning of a hypercyanotic episode. Provide guidelines for the initial care of the hypercyanotic episode. The parents should call for an ambulance and try to calm and reassure the infant. The infant should be placed in a knee–chest position by holding the infant facing the chest, placing one arm under the knees, and folding the legs upward toward the infant's chest. Use the other arm to support the infant's back. If oxygen is available, provide it in a manner that does not further upset the infant. If none is available in the home, it will be administered in the ambulance during transport to the emergency department.

NURSING PRACTICE

Hypercyanotic episodes become life threatening if not treated immediately. The child becomes progressively more hypoxic and limp, loses consciousness, is likely to have a seizure or cerebrovascular accident, and may die. If they occur when the infant is at home, parents should begin recommended treatment and call 911 or their emergency number.

Teach parents to report signs of illness to the physician. Vomiting and diarrhea may lead to dehydration, which is a particular risk in children with polycythemia because the blood can become even more viscous. Fever increases the metabolic rate and causes further stress on the heart. Aggressive management with antipyretic medication and fluid volume replacement is necessary. Signs of infective endocarditis (low-grade fever, fatigue, and malaise) occurring within 2 months of surgery or a high-risk procedure should be reported. Parents should be taught about the need to request antibiotic prophylaxis for the child.

An emergency plan should be developed for the infant in anticipation of acute problems such as a hypercyanotic episode or respiratory distress, and parents should learn cardiopulmonary resuscitation. The local emergency medical services company should be informed about the presence of a child with special needs in the community. Provide the parents with a card or brief history form with informa-

EVIDENCE-BASED NURSING

PARENTAL STRESS ASSOCIATED WITH HAVING A CHILD WITH A CONGENITAL HEART DEFECT

Clinical Question

Do parents of a child with a congenital heart defect have any more or less stress than parents with children having other chronic conditions?

Evidence

Prior studies identified that parents of infants with congenital heart defects reported higher stress than parents of children with cystic fibrosis or cleft lip and/or cleft palate (Goldberg, Morris, Simmons et al., 1990; Pelchat, Ricard, Bouchard et al., 1999). A 36-item self-report Parenting Stress Index (PSI) was used recently to measure the amount of stress experienced by parents of young children with congenital heart defects. The PSI has three subscales that help interpret the findings: parental distress, parent-child dysfunctional interaction, and difficult child. The 80 parents of children with congenital heart disease reported significantly greater stress than the parent population in whom the PSI had been normalized; 17.5% reported a total stress score at or above the 90th percentile. The parents also had significantly higher stress scores for the difficult child subscale. Parenting stress was not related to the severity of the child's heart disease (Uzark & Jones, 2003). A second study compared the parental stress of 26 children with a complex heart defect requiring multiple surgeries to parental stress of 32 children with a simple defect (ventricular septal defect) requiring a single surgery. No significant differences were found in parental stress (even when scores of mothers and fathers were analyzed separately) by the type of their child's congenital heart defect (Mörelius, Lundh, & Nelson, 2002). These findings were consistent with those of a study that included children with 11 different types of congenital heart defects (Davis, Brown, Bakeman et al., 1998).

Implications

The heart is known to be an organ essential for survival, so it is appropriate for parents to be fearful of their child's survival. However, these studies reveal that most parents of children with congenital heart defects do have significant stress, and the stress is not related to the severity of the heart defect. It is therefore an important nursing role to identify factors that could contribute to the parent's stress and help them find coping mechanisms. Families need information about the child's condition that is reinforced in future visits, especially when the child has a simple heart defect. Allow the parents to tell their stories of living with the child to help understand their stresses and strengths. A family assessment may help identify social supports, strengths, and resources available (see Chapter 39 ∞) . Encourage the parents to raise the child as close to normal as possible. Help them by providing age-appropriate expectations about development and activity and discussing strategies for discipline.

Critical Thinking

Refer back to the statement by Brandy's mother at the beginning of the chapter. What stresses do you believe Brandy's parents are experiencing? What would be important elements of a family assessment for Brandy's parents? Identify two nursing interventions to help this family cope with their stress.

References

Davis, C. C., Brown, R. T., Bakeman, R., & Campbell, R. (1998). Psychological adaptation and adjustment of mothers of children with congenital heart disease: Stress, coping, and family functioning. *Journal of Pediatric Psychology, 23*(4), 219–228.

Goldberg, S., Morris, P., Simmons, R. J., Fowler, R. S., & Levinson, H. (1990). Chronic illness in infancy and parenting stress: A comparison of three groups of parents. *Journal of Pediatric Psychology, 15,* 347–358.

Mörelius, E., Lundh, U., & Nelson, N. (2002). Parental stress in relation to the severity of congenital heart disease in the offspring. *Pediatric Nursing, 28*(1), 28–32.

Pelchat, D., Ricard, N., Bouchard, J. M., Perreault, M., Saucier, J. F., Berrthiaume, M., et al. (1999). Adaptation of parents in relation to their 6-month-old infant's type of disability. *Child: Care, Health, and Development, 25,* 377–397.

Uzark, K. & Jones, K. (2003). Parenting stress and children with heart disease. *Journal of Pediatric Health Care, 17*(4), 163–168.

---

tion about the child's condition, medications, necessary emergency care, and the physician's name so emergency care providers have vital information for medical care.

Although parents may travel with cyanotic children, they should talk with the physician before taking them to areas of high altitude. Supplemental oxygen when traveling on an airplane may be necessary.

Hospital-Based Care of Infant and Child

The newborn receiving continuous infusion of PGE_1 is cared for in the NICU. Side effects of prostaglandin treatment such as cutaneous vasodilation, bradycardia, tachycardia, hypotension, seizure activity, fever, and apnea are monitored and managed.

If a hypercyanotic episode occurs in an infant or toddler prior to surgery, immediately place the child in the knee–chest position and administer oxygen. Administer morphine as ordered. Immediately notify the physician for further instructions if these procedures are ineffective and the episode continues. Avoid any unpleasant or anxiety-provoking procedures.

Following surgery, the child is initially cared for in the intensive care unit until heart function has stabilized. Once the child returns to the general nursing unit, nursing care is the same as described for the child having surgery for increased pulmonary blood flow.

EVALUATION

Examples of expected nursing care outcomes include the following:

■ The parents recognize a hypercyanotic episode and initiate appropriate emergency treatment.

HEALTH PROMOTION

Adolescent with Congenital Heart Disease

Preventive Care

- Encourage regular visits to the primary care provider for general health and illness care. Perform health screening according to recommended schedules (see Chapter 38 ∞). Give all recommended immunizations, including the influenza vaccine.
- Encourage routine dental visits twice a year. Make sure the adolescent knows that regular dental care and antibiotic prophylaxis help reduce endocarditis risk.
- Encourage female adolescents to initiate gynecologic care to ensure that appropriate contraception and other gynecologic care needs are addressed. Ensure that the adolescent understands risks associated with pregnancy and the potential need for special care during pregnancy.
- Provide counseling about health risks associated with tobacco use, alcohol and drug use, and unprotected sex.
- Discuss situations that place the adolescent at risk for endocarditis: body piercing, tattooing, acupuncture, electrolysis, dental care, intrauterine device for contraception, and various diagnostic and surgical procedures (Alderman, 2000).

Exercise and Nutrition

- Inquire about the adolescent's preferred exercise and activity level. An individualized assessment with graded exercise testing on a treadmill or bicycle may be performed to determine specific exercise and activity limitations for the adolescent's condition. Participation in competitive sports and strenuous work may be limited for some adolescents. Those who have had a complete repair can participate in team sports. Adolescents taking anticoagulants may have activity limitations because of the risk for bleeding.
- Encourage adolescents to participate in normal gym activities and other recreational and sports activities to the best of their physical abilities.
- Encourage the adolescent to eat nutritious meals and snacks, and to avoid excess weight gain that could stress the heart function.

Mental and Spiritual Health

- Discuss the adolescent's concerns for the future, as there may be significant uncertainty about the disease course and outcome.
- Identify and refer adolescents as needed for counseling or to a support group of adolescents of similar age with congenital heart disease.

Education for Self-Care

- Begin the process of transitioning the adolescent to adult healthcare. Provide education about the congenital heart defect, surgeries that have been performed, and the types of symptoms resulting. Remember that previous education has been targeted to the parents.
- Provide a written succinct summary of the medical management of the adolescent's condition that can be used when visiting other health professionals that includes the diagnosis, surgeries, medications and their side effects, contraception, exercise prescription, endocarditis prophylaxis, and frequency of medical follow-up (Higgins & Tong, 2003).
- Discuss the medications needed and why, and develop plans for the adolescent to assume responsibility for self-administration.
- Provide education about the need to inform all healthcare providers about the defect and need for prophylaxis. Give the adolescent a copy of the guidelines for antibiotic prophylaxis. See Table 48–5.
- Discuss the future treatment needed for the condition and frequency of cardiac evaluations. Make sure the adolescent understands the need for preventive healthcare and finding a primary care provider.
- Discuss the genetic aspects of the condition and provide resources for genetic counseling if desired.
- Discuss any activity or other limitations, such as strenuous work.
- Discuss the danger signs of the condition (such as arrhythmias, or the potential of dehydration in an adolescent with cyanosis) and how to seek urgent or emergency care.

Vocational Education

- Reassure adolescents who have had complete repairs of the congenital heart defect and have no disabilities that they have no limitations in their career or vocational selection.
- Refer adolescents with cardiac disabilities to career and vocational counseling in an effort to match their interests and physical limitations. These adolescents should be informed about their rights under the Americans with Disabilities Act of 1990.
- Families and patients should be informed to identify health insurance options, and to identify those policies that have fewer restrictions. Educate adolescents about the need to carefully investigate healthcare coverage when considering a job change so that healthcare coverage is not lost (Canobbio, 2001).

- The parents manage fever and medical illnesses to prevent dehydration and thromboembolism.
- The child becomes stable following surgery and has no complications.
- The child attains expected development following surgical repair of the congenital heart defect.

DEFECTS OBSTRUCTING SYSTEMIC BLOOD FLOW

ETIOLOGY AND PATHOPHYSIOLOGY

An anatomic stenosis (narrowing of a valve, of the area around the valve, or in the great artery above the valve) causes obstruction to blood flow and results in a pressure load on the left ventricle and decreased cardiac output. The greater the narrowing, the more obstructed blood flow is to the circulation. This results in higher pressure in the ventricle and decreased cardiac output. Newborns with severe left outflow obstruction or left ventricular dysfunction may develop decreased cardiac output and shock.

CLINICAL MANIFESTATIONS

Low cardiac output is responsible for the clinical manifestations: diminished pulses, poor color, delayed capillary refill time, and decreased urinary output. The blood cannot move past the obstruction, so it backs up into the left atrium and then the lungs, causing CHF and pulmonary edema. The child with mild obstructions may have leg cramps, cooler feet than hands, and stronger pulses in the upper extremities than the lower extremities. The blood pressure may be lower in the legs than the arms rather than the normal expectation of 10 to 15 mm Hg higher in the legs. Decreased blood supply to the gastrointestinal tract may lead to necrotizing enterocolitis. See Chapter 51. ∞ See Table 48–9 for the pathophysiology, clinical manifestations, and clinical therapy for the congenital heart defects that obstruct systemic blood flow.

CLINICAL THERAPY

See Table 48–9 for diagnostic tests and clinical therapy for these defects.

PGE₁ and inotropic medications may be required to support the newborn's systemic circulation until the obstruction is relieved or ventricular function improves.

NURSING MANAGEMENT

Children with aortic stenosis and coarctation of the aorta should have nursing care as described in the nursing management of Defects that Increase Pulmonary Blood Flow on page 1455. Infants with hypoplastic left heart syndrome (HLHS) should have nursing care as described in the nursing management of Defects that Decrease Pulmonary Blood Flow and Mixed Defects on page 1465.

NURSING PRACTICE

Caution parents of children with congenital heart defects to avoid using complementary therapies such as herbal products that may interfere with the medications prescribed to manage the child's heart condition. Products containing ginkgo are known to interact with warfarin, of particular concern for any child on anticoagulant therapy. Full research on many of these herbal remedies has not been conducted, so the potential side effects and interactions with prescribed medications are not known (Cook & Higgins, 2004).

Parents of children with life-threatening defects such as HLHS must make decisions very quickly about the best treatment for their child. There is no cure, and a decision must be made that is best for their individual situation (palliative care, Norwood procedure, or heart transplant). Parents are faced with the potential death of the newborn before having an opportunity to grieve the loss of a normal infant. Parents do not have much time to carefully weigh the information about the various treatment options. However, it is important to try to support parents through this difficult decision-making period. Share the following information with parents so they are fully informed for decision making: information about each of the treatment options and their associated mortality, the intense care that the surviving child will need, potential neurocognitive and neurodevelopmental outcomes, and unknown long-term survival. If parents choose comfort or palliative care, interventions such as PGE₁ are discontinued and the infant is given appropriate pain medication and comfort. Seek the support of clergy, social workers, or other supportive individuals in the family's life to assist them through this period. Reassure parents that they are good parents, no matter what decision they make. See Chapter 41. ∞

CARDIOMYOPATHY

Cardiomyopathy is a serious disorder of the heart's muscle that occurs most often during infancy and adolescence. About 42% of cases (hypertrophic cardiomyopathy) are genetically transmitted as an autosomal dominant trait (Park, 2002). Approximately 36% of young athletes who die suddenly have this form of cardiomyopathy (American Heart Association, 2003). Conditions leading to dilated cardiomyopathy include neuromuscular disorders such as muscular

TABLE 48–9 ❖ Pathophysiology, Clinical Manifestations, and Clinical Therapy for Defects that Obstruct the Systemic Blood Flow

Defect Pathophysiology, Clinical Manifestations, and Clinical Therapy	Anatomy

Aortic Stenosis (AS)

Narrowing of the aortic valve obstructs blood flow to systemic circulation. The valve is often bicuspid rather than tricuspid. The pressure gradient across the valve usually increases as the child grows and cardiac output increases. Aortic stenosis accounts for 3%–6% of all cases of congenital heart defects (Fedderly, 1999).

Clinical Manifestations

Most infants and children are asymptomatic with normal growth and development. Life-threatening aortic stenosis is detected in some newborns. CHF develops in infants with significant stenosis.

The blood pressure is normal, but a narrow pulse pressure may be noted. Peripheral pulses may be weak. The child may complain of chest pain after exercise, but exercise intolerance is uncommon. Fainting and dizziness are serious signs that require intervention.

A systolic heart murmur and thrill may be detected in the aortic or pulmonic areas with transmission to the neck. An ejection click may be heard. Splitting of the S_2 may be noted with severe aortic stenosis.

Diagnostic Tests

The chest x-ray is usually normal, but may reveal a slight prominence of the left ventricle and aorta with increased severity.

The ECG is usually normal in mild cases, but may show mild left ventricular hypertrophy and inverted T waves with increased severity.

An echocardiogram reveals the number of the valve cusps, pressure gradient across valve, and size of the aorta.

Stress testing may be used in asymptomatic children to determine the amount of obstruction present with exercise.

Clinical Therapy

Newborns with life-threatening aortic stenosis need PGE_1 to maintain a patent ductus arteriosus until the aortic valve can be dilated.

The aortic valve may be successfully dilated by balloon valvuloplasty during cardiac catheterization. Surgical valvuloplasty may also be performed. Surgical treatment is palliative rather than curative.

Aortic valve replacement is performed when stenosis is severe or if significant regurgitation results from other interventions.

Prognosis: Chest pain, syncope, and sudden death can occur in symptomatic children, particularly during vigorous exercise. Stenosis is usually progressive during childhood as the valve calcifies. Valve replacement may be necessary once the child reaches adulthood, requiring lifelong anticoagulant therapy. Lifelong infective endocarditis prophylaxis is required.

Aortic stenosis

☐ Decreased oxygenated blood flow

■ Mixed oxygenated and unoxygenated blood

Coarctation of the Aorta (COA)

Narrowing or constriction in the descending aorta, often near the ductus arteriosus or left subclavian artery, obstructs the systemic blood outflow. This defect is common, occurring in 5% of all children with congenital heart disease (Rome & Kreutzer, 2004).

Clinical Manifestations

Many children are asymptomatic and grow normally, but constriction is progressive. 20% to 30% of infants develop CHF by 3 months of age.

Blood pressure in the legs is lower than in the arms. Brachial and radial pulses are typically bounding, but femoral pulses are weak or absent. Older children may complain of weakness and pain in the legs after exercise.

S_2 is loud and single on auscultation. A systolic ejection murmur may be heard at the upper right and middle or lower left sternal border. A thrill may be palpated in the suprasternal notch.

Diagnostic Procedures

The chest x-ray may reveal cardiomegaly, pulmonary venous congestion, and indentation of the descending aorta. Rib notching is rarely seen before 10 years of age. MRI shows the site of coarctation.

ECG shows left ventricular hypertrophy, and right ventricular hypertrophy may be seen in severe cases.

Echocardiogram shows the size of the aorta, the actual coarctation, and functioning of the aortic valve and left ventricle.

Clinical Therapy

Balloon dilation is performed during cardiac catheterization for initial relief and recoarctation. Balloon dilation on infants under 3 months of age may be performed through the umbilical artery to avoid injury to the femoral artery (Rao, Jureidini, Balfour et al., 2003).

Surgical resection with the subclavian artery is used as a patch in the infant. Repair in the first year of life is preferred to decrease exposure to hypertension.

Balloon dilation and surgical resection are palliative, as coarctation may recur.

Prognosis: Post-coarctectomy syndrome (abdominal pain and distention) occurs in 20% of patients (Walters, 2000). Persistent hypertension in adulthood is common. Infective endocarditis prophylaxis is needed.

Coarctation of aorta

TABLE 48–9 ❖ Pathophysiology, Clinical Manifestations, and Clinical Therapy for Defects that Obstruct the Systemic Blood Flow—continued

Defect Pathophysiology, Clinical Manifestations, and Clinical Therapy   **Anatomy**

Hypoplastic Left Heart Syndrome (HLHS)

This is one of the most severe defects with absence or stenosis of mitral and aortic valves, an abnormally small left ventricle, a small aorta, and aortic or mitral stenosis or atresia.

Clinical Manifestations

With closure of the ductus arteriosus, the newborn has progressive cyanosis, tachycardia, tachypnea, dyspnea, retractions, and decreased peripheral pulses.

A systolic murmur may be present or absent.

Poor peripheral perfusion, pulmonary edema, and CHF lead to shock, acidosis, and death.

Diagnostic Procedures

The chest x-ray shows cardiomegaly and increased pulmonary vascularity.

The echocardiogram shows the small left ventricle. This condition may be diagnosed prenatally.

Cardiac catheterization may be performed in preparation of surgical intervention.

Clinical Therapy

Prostaglandin E_1 is given to maintain a patent ductus arteriosus.

Supplemental oxygen is avoided.

Three treatment options include comfort or palliative care, the Norwood procedure, and heart transplantation.

The Norwood procedure is offered to many affected infants in the United States. Surgery is performed in three stages. The Norwood procedure is performed in the first week of life, followed by the Glenn procedure at about 3 to 8 months of age, and the Fontan procedure at between 18 months and 3 years of age.

Up to 63% of infants waiting for a heart transplant die waiting for a donor heart (Jenkins, Flanagan, Jenkins et al., 2000).

In Canada, approximately 50% of parents chose comfort care (Osiovich, Phillips, Byrne et al., 2000).

Prognosis: Without surgery, the median survival time is 3 days. HLHS is the largest contributor of infant deaths due to congenital heart disease. Mortality rates in infants having a first-stage Norwood procedure are approximately 10% to 20% in the first year of life (Cook & Higgins, 2004). Some large centers have achieved a 70% 5-year survival rate with the Norwood procedure (Chang, Chen, & Klitzner, 2002). The child will have some limitations in physical activity because of a single ventricle. Many children have significant neurocognitive and neurodevelopmental impairment (Mahle, Clancy, Moss et al., 2000). Failure of the single ventricle occurs over time, and these children may require a heart transplant during adolescence or adulthood.

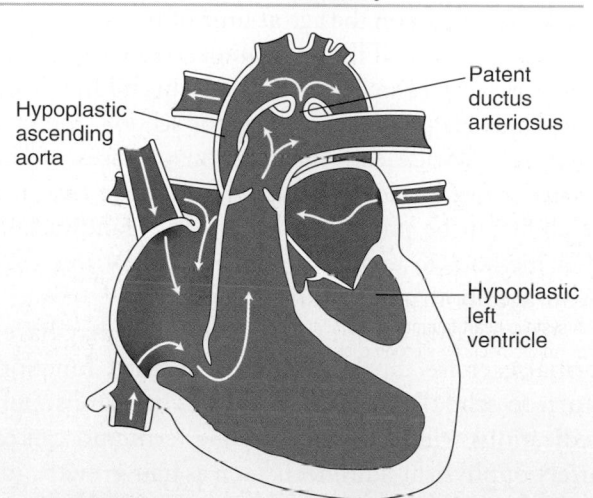

Labels: Hypoplastic ascending aorta; Patent ductus arteriosus; Hypoplastic left ventricle

---

dystrophy and viral myocarditis (Lipshultz, Sleeper, Towbin et al., 2003). Immunosuppression with cyclosporine and prednisone has improved the long-term survival of children with dilated cardiomyopathy (Gagliardi, Bevilacqua, Bassano et al., 2004). Almost 40% of children with symptoms of cardiomyopathy die of the condition within 2 years or receive a heart transplant (Strauss & Lock, 2003).

Nursing management for dilated cardiomyopathy is the same as for children with CHF unless or until a heart transplant is performed. Nursing management for hypertrophic cardiomyopathy involves frequent visits to assess the child's condition and to review progress with antiarrhythmic medications.

❖ HEART TRANSPLANTATION

Approximately 260 heart transplants are performed in children each year (Gabrys, 2005). Conditions associated with transplantation include the following by age group (Odim, Laks, Burch et al., 2000):

- Infants—primarily congenital heart disease, such as hypoplastic left heart syndrome and other complex defects

- Children 1 to 10 years—cardiomyopathy (greater than 50%), congenital heart disease (40%)

- Adolescents—cardiomyopathy (65%), congenital heart disease (25%)

With improved immunosuppressive protocols and surgical techniques, survival rates are increasing (85% at 1 year, 75% at 5 years, and 65% at 10 years) (Gabrys, 2005). The use of ventricular assist devices and extracorporeal membranous oxygenation (ECMO) prior to transplant has been found to improve the child's recovery from end-organ failure and enhance transplantation outcome (Luikart, 2001).

Infection and rejection are the major causes of mortality and morbidity. The immunosuppression regimen usually includes calcineurin inhibitors (cyclosporin or tacrolimus), cell toxins (azathioprine), and corticosteroids. Signs of organ rejection include the following: increasing resting heart rate, arrhythmias, bradycardia; presence of a third heart sound; cool and mottled extremities; inspiratory crackles, diaphoresis, tachypnea, pulmonary edema; hepatosplenomegaly; and oliguria (Duitsman, Suddaby, & Masterson, 1999). As some children may be asymptomatic, endomyocardial biopsy is performed during cardiac catheterization frequently during the first year after transplant to detect rejection, and then annually if no rejection occurs.

Bacterial, fungal, and viral (i.e., cytomegalovirus) infections cause the most problems; however, some common childhood illnesses (acute otitis, colds) may be well tolerated.

Depending upon the age at time of transplant, the child may not have had all immunizations (see Chapter 45 ∞). Live virus vaccines are contraindicated in children with heart transplants. Help parents arrange for schools and childcare centers to provide early notification of cases of measles, mumps, rubella, and chickenpox. Preventive treatment for the child can be provided as necessary. Handwashing and other methods to reduce the spread of infection should be encouraged both at home and at school.

After recovery from surgery, children may have near-normal exercise capabilities, normal heart function, and return to school and other activities. Immunosuppressive medications will be continued long term and can cause a variety of physical side effects such as hair growth, gum hyperplasia, weight gain, moon face, acne, and rashes. Children and adolescents may need support to develop positive self-esteem. Children often develop hypertension and may be treated with calcium channel blockers. Hypercholesterolemia and graft coronary artery disease can become causes of late transplant failure.

Organ rejection is a major concern of families. Provide education for the parents and child to recognize the signs and to seek treatment promptly. Adolescents need special attention to promote adherence to the immunosuppression protocol.

PULMONARY ARTERY HYPERTENSION

Pulmonary artery hypertension is a complication of many congenital heart defects, as well as pulmonary conditions and congenital diaphragmatic hernia. Excessive pulmonary blood flow over time leads to pulmonary vascular vasoconstriction to decrease the blood flow. The smooth muscle in the small pulmonary arteries increases to sustain vasoconstriction if the excess pulmonary blood flow is not controlled. The pulmonary artery pressure must increase to push blood across the vascular bed. Inflammation, hypertrophy of pulmonary vessels, and fibrosis develop. The increased pressure leads to a right-to-left shunt, and right heart function is impaired. The condition may become life threatening (Barst, 1999).

Hypoxemia results from pulmonary hypertension and helps maintain the vasoconstriction. The infant displays tachypnea, cyanosis, retractions, and fatigue. Feeding is difficult, and weight loss with fluid and electrolyte imbal-ance is likely. Older children have exertional dyspnea, chest pain, and syncope.

Clinical therapy involves surgery to correct an obstructive lesion or close a defect. Therapy for pulmonary artery hypertension related to noncardiac conditions involves bronchodilators, antibiotics, corticosteroids, and low-flow oxygen. No cure is available, but these measures can prolong life (Barst, 1999).

Nursing care focuses on promoting rest for oxygen conservation, monitoring fluid intake and output carefully, and administering medications and oxygen. Airplane travel may be possible with supplemental oxygen. Exercise should be tailored to avoid dyspnea. Give parents needed support and information about their child.

ACQUIRED HEART DISEASES

RHEUMATIC FEVER

Rheumatic fever is an inflammatory disorder of connective tissue that follows an initial infection by some strains of group A beta-hemolytic streptococci. This disorder causes changes in the heart, joints, brain, and skin tissues. Although not common, the disorder has occurred more frequently since the 1980s, probably because of a virulent strain of group A streptococcal infections (Steeg, Walsh, & Glickstein, 2000).

The exact cause of the disorder is unknown. Possible causes include an autoimmune response in a genetically predisposed child (Steeg et al., 2000). One to 3 weeks after an untreated streptococcal infection, the hallmark signs of rheumatic fever may occur. Aschoff's bodies (hemorrhagic bullous lesions) develop in the connective tissue of the heart. Endocarditis may lead to permanent mitral or aortic heart valve damage. The child's joints become inflamed and painful (migratory polyarthritis), although this condition improves in several weeks. Subcutaneous nodules may be palpable near joints. A skin rash called erythema marginatum, with pink macules and blanching in the middle of the lesions, is frequently seen on the trunk and proximal extremities. Spiking fever often occurs. A condition known as Sydenham chorea (St. Vitus dance), which is characterized by aimless movements of the extremities and facial grimacing, may be seen if the central nervous system is involved.

Diagnosis is based on clinical signs (Jones criteria; Table 48–10) and laboratory testing for antistreptolysin-O (ASLO). An ASLO titer of 320 Todd units indicates a recent streptococcal infection (Steeg et al., 2000).

Clinical therapy includes antibiotics (penicillin, sulfadiazine, or erythromycin) to eradicate the streptococcal in-

TABLE 48–10 ❖ Guidelines for Diagnosis of Initial Attack of Rheumatic Fever (Jones Criteria, updated 1992)*

Major Manifestations	Minor Manifestations
Carditis	**Clinical findings**
Polyarthritis	Arthralgia
Chorea	Fever
Erythema marginatum	**Laboratory findings**
Subcutaneous nodules	Elevated acute-phase reactants
	Erythrocyte sedimentation rate
	C-reactive protein
	Prolonged PR interval

Supporting evidence of antecedent group A streptococcal infection:
(1) positive throat culture or rapid streptococcal antigen test;
(2) elevated or rising streptococcal antibody titer.

*If supported by evidence of preceding group A streptococcal infection, the presence of two major manifestations or one major and two minor manifestations indicates a high probability of acute rheumatic fever.

Data from Special Writing Group of the Committee on Rheumatic Fever, Endocarditis, and Kawasaki Disease of the Council on Cardiovascular Disease in the Young of the American Heart Association. (1992). Guidelines for the diagnosis of rheumatic fever. Jones criteria, 1992 update. *Journal of the American Medical Association, 268*(15), 2069–2073.

fection. Aspirin is used to treat carditis if present (for 3 to 4 weeks or longer), and to control joint inflammation and reduce fever. Children should be monitored carefully by echocardiogram for potential heart involvement. Steroids may be used for severe carditis with CHF. Most children recover fully. Long-term antibiotic prophylaxis to reduce the risk of recurrent attacks is given well into adulthood. Children with residual valve damage need antibiotic prophylaxis to prevent infectious endocarditis.

NURSING MANAGEMENT

The most important role of the nurse is prevention of rheumatic fever. Nurses in clinics, offices, and schools need to ensure that all children with possible streptococcal infections have a throat culture taken. Even if the sore throat is mild, a culture is needed if family members or other contacts have had a streptococcal infection. Emphasize to the family the importance of giving all doses of the antibiotic prescribed when a culture is positive.

In a case of severe rheumatic fever, the child is hospitalized for a period of time. Nursing care focuses on assessing the child's condition, promoting recovery, and ensuring adherence with the treatment regimen.

During the acute inflammatory phase, take the child's temperature at least every 4 hours and monitor vital signs. The child is on bed rest while monitoring for the onset of carditis, and for 4 weeks if carditis develops. Auscultate the child's heart and note any unusual sounds. Observe the child for changes in skin, joints, or behavior. Be sure family members have throat cultures done to identify possible asymptomatic streptococcal carriers.

Administer antibiotics and aspirin as ordered. The child is usually lethargic and often has joint pain. Aspirin often relieves pain dramatically after a few doses. Position and handle the child's joints carefully. Provide quiet activities, as the child is often confined to bed. Encourage visits or telephone calls from family members and friends. For the child with chorea, provide emotional support; the purposeless involuntary movements that can last for 5 to 15 weeks can be disturbing. Encourage the family to participate in the child's hospital care.

During the recovery phase, the child is generally cared for at home. Activities may be limited, especially if heart damage is suspected. Help parents plan quiet activities, such as playing board games, working with computers, or reading, and arrange rest periods after the child returns to school. Reassure the child and parents that the effects of chorea will eventually subside.

On discharge a daily oral low dose antibiotic is prescribed or a monthly long-acting antibiotic injection is given. Make sure the child and parents understand the importance of taking prescribed medication until adulthood to prevent future infection and possible heart damage from recurrent rheumatic fever. Stress the importance of telling future healthcare providers, including dentists and surgeons, about the child's rheumatic fever history so prophylactic antibiotics can be given to prevent infective endocarditis during invasive procedures.

Make sure the parents understand that the child's future sore throats may be streptococcal and that a throat culture should be taken even when the child is taking daily antibiotics. The child may need additional antibiotics for the infection. Emphasize the importance of follow-up care to prevent new infections and to monitor heart function.

INFECTIVE ENDOCARDITIS

Infective endocarditis is an inflammation of the lining, valves, and arterial vessels of the heart caused by bacterial, enterococci, and fungal infections. Children who have a congenital heart defect, rheumatic heart disease, or a central venous catheter or who have had heart surgery are at risk for infective endocarditis. In children with heart defects, a high velocity or turbulent blood flow can injure the endocardium. Indwelling catheters positioned in the right side of the heart also damage the endocardium or valve endothelium. Infections may occur after the causal organism enters the bloodstream during dental work or surgery and lodges on damaged or abnormal endocardial tissue.

Symptoms can be mild and develop slowly, or they can be severe and develop rapidly. Common symptoms are fever (often with elevations in the afternoon), fatigue, joint and muscle aches, headache, and nausea and vomiting. Signs may include a new or changing murmur, CHF, dyspnea, hematuria, petechia, and splenomegaly (Brook, 1999). Children with indwelling catheters may initially have pulmonary signs related to septic pulmonary embolism.

Infective endocarditis is diagnosed primarily by blood culture; however, urine and cerebrospinal fluid also may be cultured. Elevated erythrocyte sedimentation rate, anemia, elevated C-reactive protein level, increased white blood cell count, alterations in the electrocardiogram, and changes in heart sounds and murmurs are indicators of the condition. Two-dimensional echocardiography is used to identify vegetation or infective lesions in the heart, the extent of valve damage, and cardiac function.

Clinical therapy consists of administering antibiotics such as penicillin G, ampicillin, vancomycin, nafcillin, or gentamicin. Intravenous administration is preferred, with therapy continuing for 2 to 8 weeks until the infective organism is eradicated. Serum levels of antibiotics are monitored to maintain a therapeutic range. Surgery may be necessary to replace a heart valve or because of risk of embolism. If CHF occurs, bed rest and medications such as digoxin and furosemide are prescribed.

NURSING MANAGEMENT

Nursing care focuses on assessing the child's respiratory and cardiovascular status, administering medications, and teaching the parents about the child's care. Take the child's vital signs. Assess oxygen saturation and level of consciousness as CHF and embolism may occur.

Administer medications as ordered and monitor serum antibiotic levels. Monitor for side effects of antibiotics and for infiltration or extravasation at the infusion site. Keep invasive procedures to a minimum. Use careful aseptic technique when managing central lines or venous access devices and when performing venipunctures, urinary catheterizations, and other procedures.

The child is often lethargic and on bed rest. Encourage parents to assist with the child's care and plan quiet age-appropriate activities. At discharge, arrange home health nursing. Home infusion therapy may be ordered. Instruct parents about care needed for the child's recuperation. Reinforce the need for follow-up visits. Home schooling will be needed during the recovery period.

Nursing care also focuses on prevention of endocarditis. Children at high risk for endocarditis should be discouraged from body piercing and tattoos as endocarditis may occur even with prophylaxis. Explain the importance of telling physicians and dentists about the child's history of endocarditis so that they will take care to prevent infection before invasive procedures.

KAWASAKI DISEASE

Kawasaki disease is an acute systemic inflammatory illness. It is the leading cause of acquired heart disease in children in North America and most developed countries. The annual incidence is 18.5 cases per 100,000 children, but incidence is 47.7 cases per 100,000 in Hawaiian children. Children under 5 years of age account for 75% of cases, and nearly half of those cases occurred in children under 2 years. Although this disorder is most common in Asian children, it is seen in all races (Chang, 2002).

The etiology of Kawasaki disease is unknown, but the primary cause is thought to be infectious in genetically predisposed children. It does not appear to be spread by person-to-person contact, but there is often a preceding upper respiratory tract infection. A multisystem inflammatory disease involves the small and medium-sized arteries, including the coronary arteries. Coronary artery damage can lead to aneurysms, ischemic heart disease, and potentially infarcts.

There are three stages of the disease: acute, subacute, and convalescent. The acute stage is characterized by fever, conjunctival hyperemia, red throat, swollen hands and feet, rash on the trunk, enlargement of the cervical lymph nodes, diarrhea, and hepatic dysfunction (Figure 48–7 ●). The subacute stage is characterized by cracking lips and fissures, desquamation of the skin on the tips of the fingers and toes starting at 10 days after the fever begins, joint pain, cardiac disease, and thrombocytosis. In the convalescent stage, 6 to

● **FIGURE 48–7**

This child shows many of the signs of the acute stage of Kawasaki disease: strawberry tongue, dry cracking lips, buccal mucosa erythema.

8 weeks after disease onset, the child appears normal but may have lingering signs of inflammation. Other clinical signs may include abdominal pain, paralytic ileus, diarrhea, vomiting, dysuria, aseptic meningitis, and arthritis.

Diagnosis is based on clinical signs using the criteria given in Table 48–11. Blood studies show some abnormalities such as elevated erythrocyte sedimentation rate, elevated white blood cell count, mild anemia, thrombocytosis, elevated platelet count, and elevated C-reactive protein level. A two-dimensional echocardiogram is used to reveal specific vascular changes in the heart and coronary arteries, including assessment of the internal coronary vessel diameters.

Kawasaki disease is treated with intravenous immunoglobulin (2 g/kg given in a single infusion) and aspirin. High doses of aspirin (80 to 100 mg/kg/day in 4 divided doses) are given while the fever is high. The dose is decreased to 3 to 5 mg/kg/day or less once the fever has dropped for its antiplatelet activity. High doses of immune globulin given before the 10th day of fever reduce the incidence of coronary artery lesions and aneurysms, as well as decrease fever and inflammatory signs (Newburger, Takahashi, Gerber et al., 2004).

Children are usually hospitalized for 3 or more days, depending upon the presence of cardiac lesions and how long the fever persists. Most children recover fully. Careful monitoring for cardiac disease continues for several weeks or months. Coronary aneurysms and coronary artery stenosis with risk of thrombosis are the most serious complications. Children without cardiac complications during the first month of Kawasaki disease generally have no long-term cardiac impairment (Newburger et al., 2004).

NURSING MANAGEMENT

Nursing care focuses on promoting comfort, monitoring for early signs of complications or disease progression, and supporting the family.

Assessment is important in identifying signs of Kawasaki disease, as the acute phase of this disorder is commonly confused with other diseases. The nurse in the community must be alert to early signs and symptoms. When the child is hospitalized, take the temperature every 4 hours and before each dose of aspirin. Carefully assess the extremities for edema, redness, and desquamation every 8 hours. Examine the eyes for conjunctivitis and the mucous membranes for inflammation. Monitor the child's dietary and fluid intake and weigh the child daily. Carefully assess heart sounds and rhythm.

Administer aspirin and immune globulin as ordered. Monitor for side effects of aspirin such as bleeding and gastrointestinal upset. Administer intravenous immune globulin as a blood product, carefully regulating the infusion rate to run slowly according to the physician's orders, and watching for any reactions to the infusion. The infusion rate should not be over 1 mL/min. If symptoms of reaction occur, stop the infusion immediately (see Chapter 49 ∞).

Promote the child's comfort. Keep the child's skin clean and dry, and lubricate the lips. Use cool compresses and tepid sponges to make the feverish child more comfortable. Change the child's clothes and bed linens frequently. Give the child frequent small feedings of soft foods and liquids that are neither too hot nor too cold.

Use passive range of motion exercises to facilitate joint movement. Because the child with Kawasaki disease is often lethargic and irritable, plan rest periods and quiet age-appropriate activities. Encourage the parents to participate in their child's care. This comforts and reassures the child. Give the parents information about the disease and the child's treatment.

Before the child is discharged, teach the parents to administer aspirin as ordered and to watch for side effects. Advise the parents that the child may need to avoid contact sports or other activities that could cause bleeding. Have them take the child's temperature daily and report any fever above 37.8°C (100°F) to the physician. Emphasize the need for follow-up care to monitor for cardiac complications.

Inform the parents of a child with Kawasaki disease to postpone any scheduled immunizations for 5 months after immune globulin administration, as immune response to the vaccine may not be fully effective. Influenza vaccine should be administered, particularly for those children on long-term aspirin therapy because of the risk for Reye syndrome (American Academy of Pediatrics, 2003). See Chapter 53 ∞ for Reye syndrome and its association with aspirin.

TABLE 48–11 ✦ Diagnostic Criteria for Kawasaki Disease

Kawasaki disease is diagnosed when a high spiking fever over 39°C (102.2°F) for 5 days or longer is present along with four of the following five principal features:

- Changes in the extremities: acute changes include erythema of palms and soles and edema of feet, sometimes painful induration of hands and feet; subacute changes include periungual peeling of fingers and toes in weeks 2 and 3.
- Changes in the lips and oral cavity: dry, peeling, cracking lips; strawberry tongue; diffuse erythema of the buccal and pharyngeal mucosae.
- Bilateral bulbar conjunctival redness without exudate, usually painless.
- Polymorphous exanthem (erythematous maculopapular rash) on trunk and extremities, may involve perineal region.
- Cervical lymphadenopathy, > 1.5 cm in diameter, usually unilateral and in anterior cervical triangle.

Adapted with permission from Newburger, J. W., Takahashi, M., Gerber, M. A., et al. (2004). Diagnosis, treatment, and long-term management of Kawasaki disease: A statement for health professionals from the Committee on Rheumatic Fever, Endocarditis, and Kawasaki Disease, Council on Cardiovascular Disease in the Young, American Heart Association. *Circulation, 110* (October 26), 2747-2771.

CARDIAC ARRHYTHMIAS

Cardiac **arrhythmias** (abnormal rhythms or dysrhythmias) occur frequently in children, but less often than in adults. These include tachyarrhythmias (sinus tachycardia) and bradyarrhythmias (sinus bradycardia) that occur with acute conditions such as hypoxia, acidosis, increased intracranial pressure, hypothermia, and hypoglycemia. Most of these arrhythmias resolve once the condition is treated. Less common arrhythmias are often associated with congenital heart disease, including atrial fibrillation, atrial flutter, ventricular fibrillation, and heart block. Arrhythmias must be recognized because they cause decreased cardiac output and CHF, or an even more serious arrhythmia may develop that could result in sudden death.

GROWTH AND DEVELOPMENT

The criteria for bradycardia by age group is as follows (Hanish, 2001):

- Infants to 3 years <100 beats per minute
- Children 3 to 9 years <60 beats per minute
- Children 9 to 16 years <50 beats per minute
- Adolescents over 16 years <40 beats per minute

SUPRAVENTRICULAR TACHYCARDIA

Supraventricular tachycardia (SVT), the most common pathologic tachycardia, is the abrupt onset of a rapid, regular heart rate, often too fast to count. Newborns and young children may be predisposed to the condition because of a congenital heart defect or Wolff-Parkinson-White syndrome. Short periods of arrhythmia (several seconds), which may be caused by paroxysmal atrial tachycardia, are rarely dangerous. However, prolonged episodes of continuous SVT for more than 24 hours may lead to CHF. Cardiac output is affected because diastolic filling cannot occur with such a rapid heart rate. Prolonged episodes of SVT are life threatening and can progress to CHF or cardiogenic shock if untreated.

Early signs in infants include poor feeding, irritability, and pallor. Older children may have episodes of altered consciousness (dizziness or syncope). The presenting heart rate in infants with SVT may be up to 260 beats/min. In older children, a heart rate between 150 and 240 beats/min may be seen.

NURSING PRACTICE

When the heart rate reaches 180 beats/min in a child (220 beats/min in an infant), the time needed for blood to fill the ventricles during diastole is too short. As a result the cardiac output and stroke volume fall. Life-threatening shock may develop if clinical therapy is not initiated to reduce the heart rate (Eichelberger, Ball, Pratsch et al., 1998).

Electrocardiography, including a 24-hour rhythm recording, confirms the diagnosis. Vagal stimulation such as applying ice or iced saline solution to the face may reduce the heart rate. An older child can perform the Valsalva maneuver (holding the breath and straining, or blowing forcefully on the thumb) to increase intrathoracic and venous pressures and thus slow the heart rate. Adenosine or amiodarone are the recommended emergency medications when vagal stimulation does not work. Synchronized cardioversion may be used for life-threatening episodes if other treatments are not effective. Recurrent attacks are common, and digoxin and propranolol may be given to reduce the frequency of episodes (Starr & Freitas-Nichols, 2000). **Radiofrequency ablation** uses energy to destroy a very small section of the myocardium through which an accessory conduction pathway passes that triggers tachycardia. The procedure is performed in a cardiac catheterization laboratory. When successful, medications taken to control SVT can be discontinued.

LONG QT SYNDROME

Long QT syndrome is a rhythm disturbance of autosomal dominant and autosomal recessive inheritance that puts children at risk for ventricular fibrillation and sudden death. It may also result from electrolyte abnormalities, malnutrition associated with anorexia and bulimia, myocarditis, and central nervous system trauma (Berul, 2000). It is thought to be associated with some cases of sudden infant death syndrome.

The arrhythmia commonly occurs without warning and often results in death. It may be triggered by demanding physical exercise, extreme emotional stress, or a loud noise, but some episodes have occurred during rest. Early signs include a fast heart rate (too fast to count), irritability, lethargy, poor feeding, poor perfusion (cool pale skin, increased capillary refill time), decreased responsiveness, decreased blood pressure, and sudden death.

If the child is resuscitated or evaluated because of early signs, the arrhythmia is commonly detected by electrocardiogram. The disorder is treated by beta-adrenergic blockade, antiarrhythmic agents, and often a pacemaker (Lewin, 2000).

NURSING MANAGEMENT

Nursing care of children with SVT or long QT syndrome focuses on assessing the child's condition, administering medications, and providing emotional support to the child and parents. Children are treated in the emergency department or intensive care unit. The child is placed on a cardiac monitor, and frequent assessment is critical. Report continued abnormal rates or rhythms to the physician. Carefully observe and record changes in level of consciousness, color, weakness, irritability, and feeding pattern. Administer medications as ordered. Have emergency drugs and re-suscitation equipment available at the bedside. Provide for rest and adequate nutrition.

Episodes of arrhythmia are frightening for both the child and parents. Carefully explain the treatment plan and home care. Teach parents to take the child's apical pulse. Make sure parents are trained in cardiopulmonary resuscitation. Provide telephone numbers of emergency medical facilities and help parents plan how to seek emergency care. Emphasize that prescribed medications help prevent or reduce the frequency of the episodes. Certain other medications can trigger another episode and should be avoided. The child with SVT should not use cardiac stimulant drugs such as decongestants. The child with long QT syndrome should avoid any medications that prolong the QT interval, such as macrolide antibiotics, tricyclic antidepressants, and antihistamines (Erickson & Jones, 2000).

DYSLIPIDEMIA

Hyperlipidemia is a condition in which one or more lipids (total cholesterol, low-density lipoproteins, triglycerides, high-density lipoproteins) have an abnormal level in the blood. It is important to identify children who have a genetic history or lifestyle that makes them more susceptible to future coronary heart disease and to implement preventive health measures to reduce the child's risk of disease and premature death as an adult. The factors that increase risk for coronary artery calcium are obesity and increased body mass index, elevated blood pressure in childhood, and dyslipidemia (Kavey, Daniels, Lauer et al., 2003).

Some children have primary dyslipidemia due to familial hypercholesterolemia, and may have cholesterol levels as high as 600 to 1000 mg/dL and lipid deposits in their corneas and tendons. As the excessive fat circulates, it causes changes in blood vessels. Children may also have secondary dyslipidemia resulting from a diet rich in saturated fat, too little exercise, diseases such as diabetes, and use of drugs such as anabolic steroids (Kingsbury, 2003). More often children have milder lipid abnormalities that arise from a combination of heredity and lifestyle factors. The fatty streaks that appear in childhood become fibrous plaques in adolescence. These atherosclerotic plaques continue to grow in adulthood and may cause hemorrhage, thrombi, and occlusion of vessels.

A blood test identifies hyperlipidemia. Cholesterol, including total cholesterol (TC) and high-density lipoprotein cholesterol (HDL-C), and triglycerides are measured. See Table 48–12. The low-density lipoprotein cholesterol (LDL-C) level is calculated using an equation based on the triglyceride, HDL, and total cholesterol levels. All children over 2 years of age with the following risk factors should be screened with a fasting lipid panel: a family history of cardiovascular

disease before age 55 years (parents or grandparents) or a parent with elevated total serum cholesterol (240 mg/dL); blood pressure > 90th percentile for age, sex, and height; body mass index > 85th percentile; and diabetes (Kavey et al., 2003).

The primary management of dyslipidemia in most children includes dietary modifications, exercise, and other changes in lifestyle. The child's diet is carefully analyzed and changes are made to satisfy the dietary guidelines given in Table 48–13. It is hoped that careful monitoring and management of lipid levels in childhood will decrease the incidence of cardiovascular disease.

TABLE 48–12 ❖ Laboratory Values for Assessment of Dyslipidemia in Children Between 2 and 19 Years Old

Test	Recommended Level	Levels of Higher Risk
Total Cholesterol	<170 mg/dL	Borderline: 170–199 mg/dL High: ≥200 mg/dL
LDL-C	<110 mg/dL	Borderline: 110–129 mg/dL High: ≥130 mg/dL
Triglyceride	100 mg/dL	Borderline: 100–150 mg/dL High: >150 mg/dL
HDL-C	≥35 mg/dL	<35 mg/dL

Data from National Cholesterol Education Program. (1993). *Expert Panel on Blood Cholesterol in Children and Adolescents, NIH Parent's Guide.* (Publication No. 93-3102) Washington, DC: National Institutes of Health, NHLBI. Retrieved August 4, 2003, from *http://www.americanheart.org/presenter.jhtml?identifier=4499*

TABLE 48–13 ❖ Recommended Nutrient Intake in Children and Adolescents with Hyperlipidemia

Nutrient	Recommended Intake
Saturated fatty acid	Less than 10% of calories
Total fat	No more than 30% of calories
Polyunsaturated fat	Up to 10% of calories
Monounsaturated fat	10–15% of calories
Cholesterol	Less than 300 mg/day

Data from the National Cholesterol Education Program Coordinating Committee. (1991). *Report of the expert panel on blood cholesterol levels in children and adolescents.* Washington, DC: U.S. Department of Health and Human Services; and Kris-Etherton, P., Daniels, S. R., Eckel, R. H., et al. (2001). AHA scientific statement: Summary of the scientific conference on dietary fatty acids and cardiovascular health. Conference summary of the Nutrition Committee of the American Heart Association. *Journal of Nutrition, 131*(4), 1322-1326.

If the child continues to have high serum lipid levels, a lipid specialist should be consulted. Cholestyramine or colestipol, which bind bile acid in the intestine, and niacin are sometimes prescribed in children over 10 years. Lovastatin may be prescribed for adolescents for treatment of familial hypercholesterolemia, and soon may be prescribed for younger children. A recent study of statin therapy in children 8 to 18 years with familial hypercholesterolemia revealed that carotid atherosclerosis regressed without adverse effect on growth, maturation, hormone levels, or liver or muscle tissue (Wiegman, Hutten, de Groot et al., 2004).

NURSING MANAGEMENT

Nursing care focuses on identifying children at risk for dyslipidemia, providing education about diet and exercise, and monitoring eating patterns. Identification and management of dyslipidemia takes place in many community settings. Office and clinic nurses identify children who need to have serum lipid measured. Nurses in schools provide education on ways to reduce risk factors. The child's history of exercise patterns, weight percentile, and dietary intake provides important information. Obtain information on familial heart disease, hypertension, diabetes, and smoking to determine risk factors. Although a screening for total cholesterol level does not require fasting, the child needs to fast for 12 hours before blood is drawn for a complete lipid evaluation.

Work with nutritionists to provide dietary teaching and monitor family eating patterns. Emphasize the importance of teaching and modeling food choices that help lower lipid levels. Help the child select an enjoyable moderate to intense activity such as running, biking, swimming, soccer, hiking, fast walking, aerobic dancing, or rollerblading to participate in for 30 minutes at least 3 to 4 times a week.

Discourage smoking by the child or the parents. Secondhand smoke may affect blood pressure and plaque formation, and thus increase the risk for the development of cardiovascular disease (Giddings, 1999).

Include the entire family in the treatment plan, as changing eating and exercise patterns is difficult for a single family member. The family of a child with dyslipidemia requires continual teaching and reinforcement. Periodically perform nutrition assessments and evaluation of family diet.

HYPERTENSION

Hypertension is present in 350,000 (1% to 5%) children and adolescents (Peters & Flack, 2003). Trends since 1988 have demonstrated a substantially increased systolic and diastolic blood pressure among children and adolescents in the United States. Increasing body mass index accounts for some of the increased blood pressure trends (Muntner, He, Cutler et al., 2004). Secondary hypertension in infants and prepubescent children is often associated with underlying conditions such as kidney disease or heart defects. Primary or essential hypertension may be associated with a genetic or familial predisposition and obesity. Hypertension is defined as a systolic blood pressure and/or diastolic blood pressure that is greater than or equal to the 95th percentile for gender, age, and height, averaged over three readings (National High Blood Pressure Education Program Working Group on High Blood Pressure in Children and Adolescents, 2004).

The child with documented hypertension should have blood chemistry (BUN, creatinine, and electrolytes), complete blood count, urinalysis, and urine culture tests done to detect secondary causes of hypertension. Serum lipid studies and a fasting glucose should be performed to identify dyslipidemia or diabetes. Polysomnography may be performed to identify a sleep disorder as obstructive sleep apnea is associated with hypertension. A drug screen may be appropriate to identify substances that could cause hypertension (National High Blood Pressure Education Program Working Group on High Blood Pressure in Children and Adolescents, 2004).

Nonpharmacologic measures for reduction of blood pressure include dietary counseling for obesity, reduced sedentary activities (television, videos, computer time), increased physical activity, increased fruits and vegetables, and reduced sodium. Medications (ACE inhibitors, angiotensin-receptor blockers, beta-blockers, calcium channel blockers, and diuretics) are used for children with secondary hypertension and poor response to lifestyle modifications.

NURSING MANAGEMENT

A complete history is taken to evaluate the child with persistent high blood pressure, identifying potential risk factors such as family history for hypertension, smoking, or a systemic disease. Is the child obese? How many servings of fruits does the child eat daily? What is the daily number of dairy product servings? What is the child's daily

---

DEVELOPING CULTURAL COMPETENCE

BLOOD PRESSURE AND ETHNICITY

A recent study contrasting the blood pressure of African-American and Caucasian children and adolescents did not find significant differences in blood pressure by ethnicity alone. Differences found were most often attributable to body mass index (BMI). African-American children were more likely to have higher blood pressure and more hypertension at lower levels of BMI. Hypertension in Caucasian children was more likely to occur with higher BMIs (Rosner, Prineas, Daniels et al., 2000).

salt intake? What are the child's daily exercise routines? Take the child's blood pressure regularly to monitor changes (see Skill 9–10 **SKILLS**).Consistently use the right arm for the reading, and compare the blood pressure in the leg to that in the arm (National High Blood Pressure Education Working Group on High Blood Pressure in Children and Adolescents, 2004). Compare readings to the expected blood pressure reading for gender, age, and height (see Table 35–14 in Chapter 35 ∞). Monitor the child's blood pressure every 3 to 6 months. Ensure that the correct sized blood pressure cuff and appropriate technique is used to assess the blood pressure.

Teach both the child and the parents how to improve the diet and develop exercise routines. Provide suggestions about substitute seasonings for salt and a list of salty foods to avoid. Emphasize the importance of avoiding smoking. Teaching that involves the entire family is usually the most

COMPLEMENTARY CARE

TRANSCENDENTAL MEDITATION FOR STRESS MANAGEMENT AND BLOOD PRESSURE CONTROL

The relationship between stress and cardiovascular reactivity and subsequent development of primary hypertension in adults has been documented. African-American adolescents have been found to exhibit greater blood pressure reactivity to stress than Caucasian adolescents. A randomized clinical trial with 35 adolescents 15 to 18 years of age with high normal resting blood pressure (between 85th and 95th percentiles) compared the impact of a 2-month transcendental meditation program with a control group that received lifestyle education sessions. Each group had similar numbers of males and females, but 34 of the participants were African American and 1 was Caucasian. Participants in the transcendental meditation group practiced two 15-minute sessions while sitting comfortably with eyes closed to obtain a deeply restful state of wakefulness. Participants in the control group attended seven weekly 1-hour health education sessions. The study was conducted in collaboration with the public school system. Anthropometric measurements, heart rate, blood pressure, cardiac output, and total peripheral resistance were evaluated at the beginning of the study and during exposure to stressful experiences (a car-driving simulation and a social situation interview). Study results revealed that the transcendental meditation group had greater decreases in resting systolic blood pressure and a trend toward greater decreases in diastolic blood pressure than the control group, particularly with the car-driving simulation. Transcendental meditation shows promise as a potential complementary therapy to help control blood pressure in adolescents. Further study is needed to determine if the blood pressure reductions are sustained long term with this intervention (Barnes, Treiber, & Davis, 2001).

Barnes, V. A., Treiber, F. A., & Davis, H. (2001). Impact of transcendental meditation on cardiovascular function at rest and during acute stress in adolescents with high normal blood pressure. Journal of Psychosomatic Research, 51, *597–605.*

effective. Instruct the family on correct administration of prescribed medications when used.

INJURIES OF THE CARDIOVASCULAR SYSTEM

SHOCK

Shock is an acute, complex state of circulatory dysfunction resulting in failure to deliver sufficient oxygen and other nutrients to meet cell and tissue demands. It can be caused by a variety of conditions such as hemorrhage, dehydration, sepsis, obstruction of blood flow, and cardiac pump failure.

HYPOVOLEMIC SHOCK

Hypovolemic shock is a clinical state of inadequate tissue and organ perfusion resulting from the movement of blood or plasma out of the intravascular compartment leading to inadequate intravascular volume (see "Pathophysiology Illustrated: Hypovolemic Shock"). The blood or plasma in the vascular space may be decreased because of hemorrhage or fluid movement into the interstitial spaces.

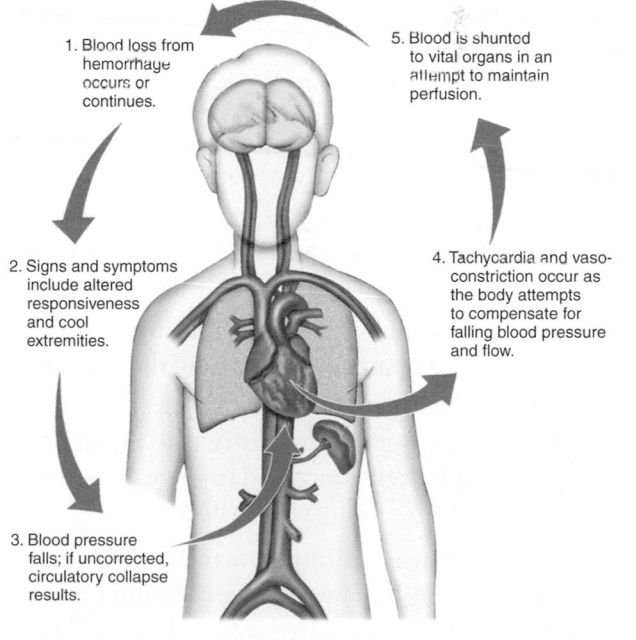

PATHOPHYSIOLOGY ILLUSTRATED
Hypovolemic Shock

1. Blood loss from hemorrhage occurs or continues.

2. Signs and symptoms include altered responsiveness and cool extremities.

3. Blood pressure falls; if uncorrected, circulatory collapse results.

4. Tachycardia and vasoconstriction occur as the body attempts to compensate for falling blood pressure and flow.

5. Blood is shunted to vital organs in an attempt to maintain perfusion.

If hemorrhage reduces the circulating blood volume sufficiently, vasoconstriction occurs, shifting blood to maintain the perfusion of vital organs. When the blood loss exceeds 20% to 25%, the child's body can no longer compensate and hypovolemic shock ensues.

GROWTH AND DEVELOPMENT

The child's total blood volume varies by weight. The child has approximately 80 mL of blood for every kilogram of body weight.

- Newborn: 3 kg × 80 mL = 240 mL (1 cup)
- 5-year-old child: 25 kg × 80 mL = 2000 mL (2 quarts)
- 13-year-old child: 50 kg × 80 mL = 4000 mL (1 gallon)

ETIOLOGY AND PATHOPHYSIOLOGY

Major causes of decreased intravascular blood volume include the following:

- Hemorrhage from significant injury
- Plasma loss from burns, nephrotic syndrome, and sepsis
- Fluid and electrolyte loss associated with dehydration, diabetic ketoacidosis, and diabetes insipidus

Shock results in inadequate delivery of oxygen and nutrients to cells and accumulation of toxic wastes in the capillaries. The reduction in circulating blood volume causes a decrease in cardiac output and mean arterial pressure. Cellular hypoxia and acidosis develop simultaneously. The accumulation of toxins and inadequate tissue oxygenation cause cellular damage.

The child's body attempts to compensate by the following measures:

- The renin-angiotensin-aldosterone system is stimulated to retain sodium and water when perfusion of the kidneys is decreased.
- The antidiuretic hormone is secreted when the atria have reduced blood volume leading to water retention.
- The heart rate and myocardial contractility increase to improve cardiac output.
- The respiratory rate increases to improve oxygenation and decrease waste accumulation in the cells.
- The hydrostatic pressure falls, permitting fluid to shift into the vascular space and increasing the circulating blood volume.
- The peripheral vasculature constricts to maintain the systemic vascular resistance and to increase perfusion to the vital organs as long as possible.

The child can compensate until 20% to 25% of volume loss occurs, and then life-threatening hypotension results.

CLINICAL MANIFESTATIONS

Signs of early hypovolemic shock in children are nonspecific but need to be recognized before hypotension occurs. Signs that the child is compensating for a decreased blood volume are tachycardia, usually sustained at a rate greater than 130 beats per minute; increased respiratory effort; delayed capillary refill (> 2 seconds); weak peripheral pulses; pallor; and cold extremities (signs of decreased perfusion). Urine output decreases (< 0.5 – 1 mL/kg/hr in infants and young children) when renal blood flow drops. In cases of dehydration, dry mucous membranes and poor skin turgor are also present.

If treatment is not begun in the early stages of hypovolemic shock, the condition progresses until the child can no longer compensate. At that time the systolic blood pressure drops and the pulse pressure narrows. Reduced cerebral blood flow ultimately results in a decreased level of consciousness. If shock is not reversed, the condition progresses to cardiopulmonary failure. "Clinical Manifestations: Hypovolemic Shock" compares the signs associated with early, uncompensated, and profound shock.

CLINICAL THERAPY

No laboratory tests can be used to evaluate the volume deficit rapidly enough to diagnose hypovolemic shock. The child is examined for characteristic signs to confirm the diagnosis. Laboratory tests commonly performed after hypovolemic shock is diagnosed include hematocrit and hemoglobin, arterial blood gases, serum electrolytes, glucose, osmolality, blood urea nitrogen, and urinalysis.

Emergency care focuses on improving tissue perfusion. An open airway is established, oxygen is administered, and ventilation is assisted if necessary. Bleeding is controlled, and an intravenous or intraosseous line is started to provide large volumes of crystalloid fluids.

Ringer's lactate solution is the preferred fluid for initial resuscitation. A fluid volume of 20 mL/kg is administered rapidly over 5 minutes. The same amount of fluid is given in 5 minutes if the child's physiologic condition does not improve after fluid is first administered. Signs that a child is responding to fluid resuscitation include improved color, improved responsiveness, lower heart rate, and faster capillary refill time. If no improvement is seen after the second fluid bolus, blood or albumin is usually ordered.

Once the child's physiologic condition is stabilized, the cause of the hypovolemic shock becomes the focus of examination and treatment.

NURSING MANAGEMENT

NURSING ASSESSMENT AND DIAGNOSIS

Ask the parent (or child, if appropriate) about possible injuries or the duration and severity of acute illnesses. If

CLINICAL MANIFESTATIONS

HYPOVOLEMIC SHOCK

SYSTEM	EARLY SHOCK	UNCOMPENSATED SHOCK	PROFOUND SHOCK
Cardiac and respiratory	Tachycardia, weak distal pulses, full central pulses; normal systolic blood pressure; tachypnea	Tachycardia, absent distal pulses, weak central pulses, decreasing systolic blood pressure; tachypnea	Frank hypotension; bradycardia; weak or absent central pulses; bradypnea
Neurologic	Normal, anxious, irritable, or combative behavior	Confusion, lethargy, decreased pain response	Coma
Skin	Mottled appearance; capillary refill time >2 seconds; cool, clammy extremities	Cyanosis; capillary refill time >3 seconds; dusky, cold extremities	Pale, cold skin
Renal	Decreased urine output, increased specific gravity	Markedly decreased urine output; increased specific gravity	No urine output

Data from Waisman, H., & Eichelberger, M. R. (1993). Hypovolemic shock. In M. R. Eichelberger (Ed.), Pediatric trauma: Prevention, acute care, rehabilitation (p. 182). St. Louis, MO: Mosby-Yearbook; Markenson, D. S. (2002). Pediatric prehospital care (p. 174–175). Upper Saddle River, NJ: Brady, Prentice Hall.

no external bleeding is evident, determine whether an injury may be causing internal bleeding. For example, the liver and spleen are highly vascular organs that have little protection from direct blunt forces. Significant bleeding from injury to one of these organs can cause hypovolemic shock without evidence of bleeding. An acute illness such as gastroenteritis with prolonged vomiting and diarrhea can also result in dehydration and hypovolemic shock.

If external bleeding is apparent, determine the amount of blood lost. Although children lose the same amount of blood from a laceration as adults, the total volume of blood lost is proportional to their weight.

Frequently assess the child's heart rate, respiratory rate, blood pressure, capillary refill time, level of consciousness with the Glasgow Coma Scale (see Chapter 53 ∞), color, and skin temperature to identify any changes that indicate improvement or deterioration in the child's condition. Monitor urine output and specific gravity hourly. Signs of the child's improved status include:

- A decrease in heart rate, respiratory rate, and capillary refill time.
- An increase in systolic blood pressure and urine output.
- Improved color, level of consciousness, and skin temperature.
- Regaining of lost weight.

Assess the parents' response and coping mechanisms to the child's potentially life-threatening injury. Families are unprepared for the abrupt change in the child's condition because of the unpredictability of the injury. See Chapter 41. ∞

Several nursing diagnoses may apply to the child with hypovolemic shock. They include the following:

- *Decreased Cardiac Output* related to hypovolemia
- *Deficient Fluid Volume* related to active fluid volume loss
- *Ineffective Tissue Perfusion (Cardiopulmonary, Renal, and Cerebral)* related to impaired transport of oxygen across alveolar and capillary membrane
- *Ineffective Airway Clearance* related to altered level of consciousness
- *Compromised Family Coping* related to life-threatening condition of the child

PLANNING AND IMPLEMENTATION

Nurses in the emergency department operating room and intensive care unit more commonly participate in the resuscitation of the child in hypovolemic shock. Assist with the child's assessment and the establishment of intravenous access. Calculate and prepare the amount of intravenous fluid needed for administration according to the child's weight (20 mL/kg). Ensure rapid fluid administration by intravenous push or pressure bag. Monitor the child's physiologic response to the fluid bolus within 5 minutes. Prepare a second and third fluid bolus.

Use warmed intravenous fluids for resuscitation because hypothermia may interfere with the child's response to treatment. Keep the child covered or use heat lamps to reduce body-heat loss.

When packed red blood cells are administered, verify that the correct blood has been obtained for the child. Change the intravenous fluid to normal saline solution to prevent clotting during blood administration. Assess the child carefully for a transfusion reaction (see Chapter 49 ∞). Monitor the child's physiologic circulatory responses for improvement or deterioration in status. Notify the physician of any deterioration.

Provide support to the child and family during the acute phase of treatment. Parents and children with hypovolemic shock resulting from injury are usually apprehensive. The child may be fearful because of the sudden hospitalization or agitated because of an altered level of consciousness. Determine the causes of the child's anxiety. The parents often fear for the child's life in cases of severe injury. Update the parents about the child's condition frequently. Explain the care being provided and how it helps the child. Listen to their concerns and correct any misconceptions. When hospital policy permits, support the parents who desire to be present during fluid or cardiac resuscitation of the child.

EVALUATION

Examples of expected nursing care outcomes include the following:

- The child receives adequate fluid resuscitation to prevent progression to uncompensated shock.
- The family copes with the stress of the child's injury.

MALDISTRIBUTIVE SHOCK

Maldistributive shock is an abnormal distribution of blood volume, usually resulting from a decrease in systemic vascular resistance. The blood accumulates in the extremities because of vasodilation and capillary permeability. Less blood is returned to the heart, so **preload** (amount of blood in the ventricle at the end of diastole that stretches the heart muscle before contraction) drops and cardiac output falls. Causes of maldistributive shock include anaphylaxis, sepsis, and spinal cord injury.

Immunodeficient children are at high risk for septic shock. Septic shock begins as an infection and progresses to sepsis with a bacterial toxin. Once the toxin enters the circulatory system, the body's inflammatory processes over-

PATHOPHYSIOLOGY ILLUSTRATED
Septic Shock

1. Endotoxin released by microorganisms sets off an out-of-control inflammatory process

2. Macrophage producing cytokines

Red blood cells

4. Neutrophils arrive and multiply occluding capillaries

3. Vasodilation with increased capillary permeability and fluid leak

In septic shock, blood pools in the extremities. Blood flow is sluggish and amounts of oxygen inadequate for cell metabolism are received by the tissues.

respond. White blood cells multiply throughout the body and macrophages produce cytokines, which dilate the blood vessels and increase permeability. Congestion occurs in some tissue beds reducing the delivery of oxygen and nutrients to the cells, and bacteria may be trapped and multiply unchecked. Systemic and pulmonary edema develop as organ ischemia occurs (Hazinski, 1999) (see "Pathophysiology Illustrated: Septic Shock"). As the metabolism is altered, cardiac dysfunction may occur. Toxic shock syndrome is one form of septic shock that may rapidly progress and cause death.

Septic shock has three phases: compensated, uncompensated, and refractory. During the compensated phase, the child has a fever, tachycardia, tachypnea, warm extremities, bounding pulses, and brisk capillary refill. Urine output may be normal. Responsiveness may be decreased. Perfusion appears adequate; however, because of infection and fever, oxygen demand in the tissues is much higher and perfusion is really inadequate.

Cardiac output is high but systemic vascular resistance is low, leading to an uneven flow and pooling in the extremities. Blood moves sluggishly, and anaerobic metabolism and lactic acidosis occur in tissue beds where oxygen no longer circulates. Microvascular thrombi may cause further blood flow obstruction.

In phase two, the child's compensatory mechanisms begin to fail, leading to hypotension and inadeqate oxygen and nutrient delivery to the tissues. Cellular damage from the infection may become so significant that the metabolic processes cannot be supported even when adequate fluids have been given to maintain intravascular volume. Poor tissue perfusion of the vital organs occurs and multiple organ failure begins.

In the refractory phase, the shock becomes irreversible. Cardiac output falls as the myocardium becomes unresponsive. Cardiac arrest soon occurs.

Treatment for septic shock is begun even before the diagnosis is confirmed, with appropriate antibiotics effective for the suspected organism. Fluid resuscitation is used to stabilize the circulation and ensure adequate tissue perfusion. Vasopressors are given during the hypodynamic phase. Metabolic acidosis is treated. Morbidity and mortality are high even when treatment is initiated early. Complications include disseminated intravascular coagulation and adult respiratory distress syndrome.

OBSTRUCTIVE SHOCK

Obstructive shock occurs when a blockage of the main bloodstream interferes with tissue perfusion (see "Pathophysiology Illustrated: Mediastinal Shift"). Causes in children include compression of the vena cava, pericardial tamponade, pulmonary embolism, tension pneumothorax, pleural effusion, and congenital heart defects with outflow obstruction (e.g., coarctation of the aorta). Management is focused on treatment of the underlying condition.

CARDIOGENIC SHOCK

Cardiogenic shock is an abnormality of myocardial function in which the heart fails to maintain adequate cardiac output and tissue perfusion (see "Pathophysiology Illustrated: Cardiogenic Shock"). Causes of cardiogenic

PATHOPHYSIOLOGY ILLUSTRATED
Obstructive Shock Due to Mediastinal Shift

Air

Mediastinal shift

Obstructive shock can occur when a tension pneumothorax obstructs blood flow to and from the heart. Here, the great vessels are compressed during the mediastinal shift.

shock in children may include CHF, cardiovascular surgery, severe obstructive congenital heart disease such as hypoplastic left heart syndrome, cardiomyopathy, and arrhythmias such as bradycardia and supraventricular tachycardia. Cardiogenic shock may also be an end stage for other acute and chronic conditions such as sepsis, prolonged shock, asphyxia, hypoglycemia, and muscular dystrophy.

Clinically, cardiogenic shock resembles hypovolemic shock with low cardiac output. Tachycardia, tachypnea, decreased oxygen saturation, hypotension, diminished peripheral pulses, and cool, pale extremities are common signs. The child becomes disoriented and restless as the compensatory mechanisms fail. Increased systemic vascular resistance puts more stress on the failing heart. Each contraction causes more blood to accumulate in the heart and pulmonary vessels, eventually leading to CHF, metabolic acidosis, and circulatory collapse. Signs of respiratory distress are seen as CHF develops.

The goals of medical treatment are rapid restoration of myocardial function with adequate ventilation, resolution

PATHOPHYSIOLOGY ILLUSTRATED
Cardiogenic Shock

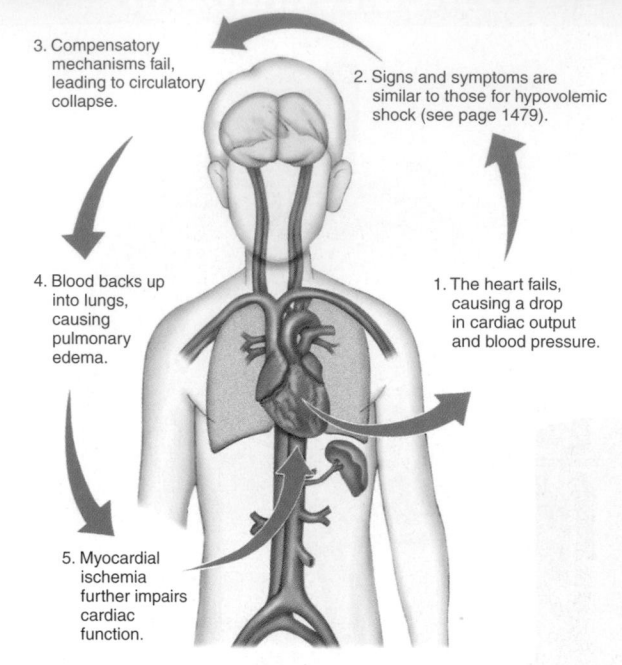

3. Compensatory mechanisms fail, leading to circulatory collapse.

2. Signs and symptoms are similar to those for hypovolemic shock (see page 1479).

4. Blood backs up into lungs, causing pulmonary edema.

1. The heart fails, causing a drop in cardiac output and blood pressure.

5. Myocardial ischemia further impairs cardiac function.

When the heart fails, cardiac output and blood pressure decrease. Blood backs up into the lungs, causing pulmonary edema. Inadequate amounts of oxygen reach the myocardium, further impairing the heart's pumping action. The result is cardiogenic shock.

of the initial metabolic insult, correction of arrhythmias, fluid management, and administration of diuretics and inotropic drugs.

MYOCARDIAL CONTUSION

Myocardial contusion, a rare injury in children, results from a strong, blunt force against the chest wall that injures the heart muscle. Blood flow to areas of the heart muscle is disrupted, or myocardial cells are directly destroyed. This potentially life-threatening condition is often associated with a motor vehicle–related injury. It most often occurs in adolescents who have struck the steering wheel of a motor vehicle during a crash or children who have been struck in the chest with a baseball.

A myocardial contusion should be suspected in cases of injury to the anterior chest. The child has chest discomfort because of fractured ribs or chest wall contusion. An electrocardiogram reveals arrhythmias or signs of myocardial infarct. A two-dimensional echocardiogram may show an abnormality in heart wall movement. Cardiac troponin I levels and cardiac isoenzyme concentrations may be monitored for elevation. Because of the risk of sudden arrhythmias, the child is admitted to the intensive care unit for cardiac monitoring. Long-term problems could potentially include aneurysm, myocardial rupture, and postcontusion pericarditis.

Critical Concept Review

LEARNING OBJECTIVES

CONCEPTS

Describe the anatomy and physiology of the cardiovascular system, focusing on the flow of blood and the action of heart valves.

1. Unoxygenated blood enters the right atrium from the superior and inferior vena cavae.
2. Blood flows through the tricuspid valve into the right ventricle.
3. The blood then moves through the pulmonary valve into the pulmonary artery to the lungs.
4. The blood receives oxygen in the lungs and then enters the left atrium.
5. The blood then travels through the mitral valve and enters the left ventricle.
6. Blood is pumped from the left ventricle through the aortic valve into the aorta and into the rest of the body.

Recognize the signs of congestive heart failure in an infant and child.

1. Infant:
   - Tires easily, especially during feedings.
   - Weight loss or lack of weight gain.
   - Diaphoresis.
   - Irritability.
   - Frequent infections.
   - Tachycardia and tachypnea.

LEARNING OBJECTIVES	CONCEPTS

Recognize the signs of congestive heart failure in an infant and child —*continued*

- Pallor or cyanosis.
- Nasal flaring.
- Grunting.
- Retractions.
2. Child:
   - Exercise intolerance.
   - Abdominal pain.
   - Peripheral edema.
   - Mottling or pallor.
   - Periorbital or facial edema.
   - Jugular vein distention.
   - Hepatomegaly.

Develop a nursing care plan for a child with congestive heart failure

1. Obtain a detailed history of onset of symptoms.
2. Assess vital signs.
3. Assess heart by observation, palpation, and auscultation.
4. Monitor intake and output.
5. Weigh child daily.
6. Turn child frequently and assess skin.
7. Organize nursing actions to provide rest periods.
8. Provide small, frequent feedings.

Describe the pathophysiology associated with congenital heart defects with increased pulmonary circulation, decreased pulmonary circulation, and obstructed systemic blood flow.

1. Defects with increased pulmonary circulation:
   - A connection occurs between the right and left side of the heart, or between the great arteries, which allows blood to flow between the right and left sides of the heart.
   - Blood is shunted to the right side of the heart, which increases blood flow to the lungs.
   - This causes increased pulmonary resistance and pulmonary hypertension.
   - Right ventricular hypertrophy develops.
2. Defects with decreased pulmonary circulation:
   - Structural defects decrease blood flow to the lungs, which decreases systemic oxygen content.
   - If a septal opening is present, increased right-sided pressure causes right-to-left shunting.
   - Decreased oxygen content causes the kidneys to produce a hormonal response, which increases the number of red blood cells leading to polycythemia, increasing the risk for thromboembolism.
   - Abrupt decreases in pulmonary blood flow and systemic vascular resistance combined with activity may cause hypercyanotic episodes.
3. Defects with obstructed blood flow:
   - Decreased cardiac output results from the increased pressure load on the ventricle caused by the obstructed blood flow.

Develop a nursing care plan for the infant with a congenital heart defect cared for at home prior to corrective surgery.

1. Instruct parents in the administration of necessary medications.
2. Instruct parents concerning the need for frequent small feedings.
3. Instruct parents concerning the signs and symptoms of congestive heart failure.
4. Instruct parents concerning the management of hypercyanotic episodes.

Develop a nursing care plan for the child undergoing open heart surgery.

Prior to surgery:
1. Give parents and child a tour of the special care area.
2. Prepare the child for anesthesia and equipment that will be used after surgery.
3. Reassure the child that someone will always be near.
After surgery:
1. Frequent assessment of:
   - Arterial and venous pressures.
   - Vital signs.
   - Oxygen saturation.
   - Core body temperature.
   - Level of consciousness.

(continued)

LEARNING OBJECTIVES

CONCEPTS

Develop a nursing care plan for the child undergoing open heart surgery.—*continued*

→

2. Auscultate heart and lungs:
   - Observe and monitor for arrhythmias.
3. Monitor cardiac output.
4. Monitor intake and output:
   - Urine.
   - Chest tube bleeding and draining.
5. Assess pain level and treat accordingly.
6. Observe for signs and symptoms of infection.

Identify heart diseases acquired during childhood and how they differ from congenital defects.

→

1. Infective endocarditis.
2. Rheumatic fever.
3. Kawasaki syndrome.
All have an infection or inflammatory response cause and may cause serious heart dysfunction. Prompt medical treatment may limit the development of cardiac damage.

Describe the pathophysiology of hypovolemic shock, distributive shock, and cardiogenic shock.

→

1. Hypovolemic shock:
   - Acute, complex state of circulatory dysfunction resulting in failure to deliver sufficient oxygen and other nutrients to meet cell and tissue demands.
   - Caused by severely depleted blood volume or dehydration.
2. Maldistributive shock:
   - Abnormal distribution of the blood volume that results from a decrease in vascular resistance.
   - May be caused by anaphylaxis, sepsis, or spinal cord injury.
3. Cardiogenic shock:
   - Abnormality in myocardial function causes drastically lowered cardiac output.
   - The heart is unable to pump adequate amounts of oxygenated blood to meet cell and tissue demands.

CRITICAL THINKING IN ACTION

View the **Critical Thinking in Action** video in Chapter 48 of the CD-ROM. Then, answer the questions that follow.

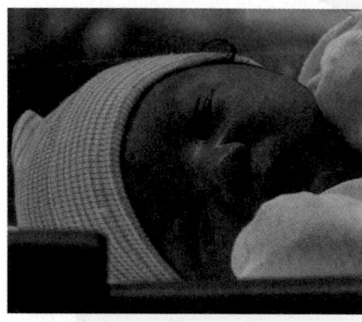

You are working in the hospital when Samantha, a 2-day-old infant, is diagnosed with a continuous, systolic, grade 3, heart murmur in the pulmonic area of the chest. This is the parents' first child and they are extremely worried about their 6-week premature baby. Samantha has full, bounding pulses and weighed 5 pounds 6 ounces at birth, but has lost 3 ounces in the past 2 days. The mother's pregnancy was healthy until her water broke suddenly. The day after Samantha was born, the parents were told about the heart murmur and that an echocardiogram, ECG, and chest x-ray are needed to determine the cause. The tests show that she has a Patent Ductus Arteriosis (PDA). The physician has prescribed 3 doses of a medication to aid in the closure of the duct. You explain that her vital signs and urine output will need to be monitored closely for decreases while she is on this medicine.

Several days later the heart murmur is still heard; the medicine did not work. The parents want to avoid surgery if possible and the doctor explains if the ductus closes by the time she is 9–12 months old, and she is without symptoms, surgery could be avoided. If the PDA is not corrected, her life span will be shortened. She is discharged from the hospital, thriving and breastfeeding well, and the doctor advises about watching for poor weight gain, swelling, intercostal retractions, and breathing more than 60 times per minute. A follow-up appointment is made for 1 week later.

1. How would you explain a PDA to the parents?
2. What was the most likely cause of Samantha's weight loss? Is it the PDA that caused the weight loss?
3. What is the physiological reason Samantha's life span would be shortened if she does not get surgical correction of her PDA?
4. How would you describe congestive heart failure?

MEDIALINK

www.prenhall.com/london

■ NCLEX-RN® Review, case studies, and other interactive resources for this chapter can be found on the Companion Website at http://www.prenhall.com/london. Click on "Chapter 48" and select the activities for this chapter.

■ For animations, more NCLEX-RN® Review questions, and an audio glossary, access the accompanying CD-ROM in this textbook.

REFERENCES

Alderman, L. M. (2000). At risk: Adolescents and adults with congenital heart disease. *Dimension in Critical Care Nursing, 19*(1), 2.

American Academy of Pediatrics Committee on Infectious Disease. (2003). *Red book: Report of the Committee on Infectious Disease* (26th ed.). Elk Grove Village, IL: Author.

American Heart Association (2003). *Youth and cardiovascular diseases—Statistics.* Retrieved August 4, 2003, from http://www.americanheart.org.

Azeka, E., Ramires, J. A. F., Valler, C., & Bocchi, E. A. (2002). Delisting infants and children from the heart transplantation waiting list after carvedilol treatment. *Journal of the American College of Cardiology, 40*(11), 2034–2038.

Balaguru, D., Artman, M., & Auslender, M. (2000). Management of heart failure in children. *Current Problems in Pediatrics, 30*(1), 1–36.

Barnes, V. A., Treiber, F. A., & Davis, H. (2001). Impact of transcendental meditation on cardiovascular function at rest and during acute stress in adolescents with high normal blood pressure. *Journal of Psychosomatic Research, 51*, 597–605.

Barst, R. J. (1999). Recent advances in the treatment of pediatric pulmonary artery hypertension. *Pediatric Clinics of North America, 46*(2), 331–345.

Berul, C. I. (2000). Cardiac evaluation in the young athlete. *Pediatric Annals, 29*(3), 162–165.

Boneva, R. S., Botto, L. D., Moore, C. A., Yang, O., Correa, A., & Erickson, J. D. (2001). Mortality associated with congenital heart defects in the United States: Trends and racial disparities, 1979–1997. *Circulation, 103*(19), 2376–2381.

Brook, M. M. (1999). Pediatric bacterial endocarditis: Treatment and prophylaxis. *Pediatric Clinics of North America, 46*(2), 275–287.

Canobbio, M. M. (2001). Health care issues facing adolescents with congenital heart disease. *Journal of Pediatric Nursing, 16*(5), 363–370.

Chang, R. K. (2002). Hospitalizations for Kawasaki disease among children in the United States, 1988–1997. *Pediatrics, 109*(6), e87–93.

Chang, R. R., Chen, A. Y., & Klitzner, T. S. (2002). Clinical management of infants with hy-

poplastic left heart syndrome in the United States, 1988–1997. *Pediatrics, 110*(2), 292–298.

Connolly, C., McClowry, S., Hayman, L., Mahony, L., & Artman, M. (2004). Posttraumatic stress disorder in children after cardiac surgery. *Journal of Pediatrics, 144*(4), 480–484.

Connor, J. A. (2002). Alterations in cardiovascular function in children. In K. L. McCance & S. E. Huether (Eds.), *Pathophysiology: The biologic basis for disease in adults and children* (4th ed., pp. 1048–1081). St. Louis, MO: Mosby.

Cook, E. H., & Higgins, S. S. (2004). Congenital heart disease. In P. J. Allen & J. A. Vessey, *Primary care of the child with a chronic condition* (4th ed., pp. 382–403). St. Louis, MO: Mosby.

Dajani, A. S., Taubert, K. A., Wilson, W., Bolger, A. F., Bayer, A., Ferrieri, P., et al. (1997). Prevention of bacterial endocarditis: Recommendations of the American Heart Association. *Journal of the American Medical Association, 277*(22), 1794–1801.

Davis, C. C., Brown, R. T., Bakeman, R., & Campbell, R. (1998). Psychological adaptation and adjustment of mothers of children with congenital heart disease: Stress, coping, and family functioning. *Journal of Pediatric Psychology, 23*(4), 219–228.

Driscoll, D. J. (1999). Left-to-right shunt lesions. *Pediatric Clinics of North America, 46*(2), 355–368.

Duitsman, D. M., Suddaby, E. C., & Masterson, G. (1999). Unique considerations for the pediatric heart transplant recipient: The role of the school nurse. *Journal of School Nursing, 15*(3), 10–13.

Eichelberger, M. R., Ball, J. W., Pratsch, G. S., & Clark, J. R. (1998). *Pediatric emergencies* (2nd ed.). Englewood Cliffs, NJ: Brady, Prentice Hall.

Erickson, C. C., & Jones, C. S. (2000). Pediatric sudden cardiac death: What the pediatrician needs to know. *Pediatric Annals, 29*(8), 509–518.

Fedderly, R. T. (1999). Left ventricular outflow obstruction. *Pediatric Clinics of North America, 46*(2), 369–384.

Gabrys, C. A. (2005). Pediatric cardiac transplants: A clinical update. *Journal of Pediatric Nursing, 20*(2), 139–143.

Gagliardi, M. G., Bevilacqua, M., Bassano, C., Leonardi, B., Boldrini, R., et al. (2004). Long term follow up of children with myocarditis treated by immunosuppression and of children with dilated cardiomyopathy. *Heart, 90*, 1167–1171.

Giddings, S. (1999). Preventive pediatric cardiology: Tobacco, cholesterol, obesity, and physical activity. *Pediatric Clinics of North America, 16*(2), 253–262.

Goldberg, S., Morris, P., Simmons, R. J., Fowler, R. S., & Levison, H. (1990). Chronic illness in infancy and parenting stress: A comparison of three groups of parents. *Journal of Pediatric Psychology, 15*, 347–358.

Grifka, R. G. (1999). Cyanotic congenital heart disease with increased blood flow. *Pediatric Clinics of North America, 46*(2), 405–425.

Hanish, D. (2001). Pediatric arrhythmia. *Journal of Pediatric Nursing, 16*(5), 351–362.

Hazinski, M. F. (1999). *Manual of pediatric critical care* (pp. 130–160). St. Louis, MO: Mosby.

Higgins, S. S., & Tong, E. (2003). Transitioning adolescents with congenital heart disease to adult health care. *Progressive Cardiovascular Nursing, 18*(2), 93–98.

Jenkins, P. C., Flanagan, M. F., Jenkins, K. J., Sargent, J. D., Canter, C. E., Chinnock, R. E., et al. (2000). Survival analysis and risk factors for mortality in transplantation and staged surgery in hypoplastic left heart syndrome. *Journal of American College of Cardiology, 36*, 1178–1185.

Kavey, R. E. W., Daniels, S. R., Lauer, R. M., Atkins, D. L., Hayman, L. L., & Taubert, K. (2003). American Heart Association guidelines for primary prevention of atherosclerotic cardiovascular disease beginnings in childhood. *Journal of Pediatrics, 142*(4), 368–372.

Kingsbury, K. J. (2003). Understanding the essentials of blood lipid metabolism. *Progressive Cardiovascular Nursing, 18*(1), 13–18.

Kohr, L. M., & Sims, S. L. (1998). Alterations in cardiovascular function in children. In K. L. McCance & S. E. Huether (Eds.), *Pathophysiology: The biologic basis for disease in adults and children* (3rd ed., pp. 1093–1130). St. Louis, MO: Mosby.

Leroy, S. S. (2001). Clinical dysrhythmias after surgical repair of congenital heart disease. *AACN Clinical Issues, 12*(1), 87–99.

Lewin, M. B. (2000). The genetic basis of congenital heart disease. *Pediatric Annals, 29*(8), 469–480.

Lipshultz, S. E., Sleeper, L. A., Towbin, J. A., Lowe, A. M., Orav, E. J., Cox, G. F., et al. (2003). The incidence of pediatric cardiomyopathy in two regions of the United States. *New England Journal of Medicine, 348* (April 24), 1647–1655.

Luikart, H. (2001). Pediatric cardiac transplantation: Management issues. *Journal of Pediatric Nursing, 16*(5), 320–331.

Mahle, W. T., Clancy, R. R., Moss, E. M., Gerdes, M., Jobes, D. R., & Wernovsky, G. (2000). Neurodevelopmental outcome and lifestyle adjustment in school-aged and adolescent children with hypoplastic left heart syndrome. *Pediatrics, 105* 1082–1089.

Mahle, W. T., & Wernovsky, G. (2001). Long-term developmental outcome of children with complex congenital heart disease. *Clinics in Perinatology, 28*(1), 235–247.

Mörelius, E., Lundh, U., & Nelson, N. (2002). Parental stress in relation to the severity of congenital heart disease in the offspring. *Pediatric Nursing, 28*(1), 28–32.

Muntner, P., He, J., Cutler, J. A., Wildman, R. P., & Whelton, P. K. (2004). Trends in blood pressure among children and adolescents. *Journal of the American Medical Association, 291*(17), 2107–2113.

National Cholesterol Education Program. (1993). *Expert panel on blood cholesterol in children and adolescents, NIH parent's guide* (NIH Publication No. 93-3102). Washington, DC: National Institutes of Health, NHLBI. Retrieved August 4, 2003, from http://www.americanheart.org/ presenter.jhtml?identifier=4499.

National High Blood Pressure Education Program Working Group on High Blood Pressure in Children and Adolescents. (2004). The fourth report on the diagnosis, evaluation, and treatment of high blood pressure in children and adolescents. *Pediatrics, 114*(2), 555–576.

Neilson, D. E., & Robin, N. H. (2002). Advances in the genetics of pediatric heart disease. *Contemporary Pediatrics, 19*(1), 85–100.

Newburger, J. W., Takahashi, M., Gerber, M. A., Gewitz, M. H., Tani, L. Y., Burns, J. C., et al. (2004). Diagnosis, treatment, and long-term management of Kawasaki disease, *Circulation, 110* (Oct 26), 2747–2771.

Odim, J., Laks, H., Burch, C., Komanapalli, C., & Alejos, J. C. (2000). Transplantation for congenital heart disease. *Advances in Cardiac Surgery, 12,* 59–76.

Osiovich, H., Phillips, E., Byrne, P. & Robertson, M. (2000). Transplantation for congenital heart disease. *Advances in Cardiac Surgery, 12,* 59–76.

Park, M. K. (2002). *Pediatric cardiology for practitioners* (4th ed.). St. Louis, MO: Mosby.

Pelchat, D., Ricard, N., Bouchard, J. M., Perreault, M., Saucier, J. F., Berrthiaume, M., et al. (1999). Adaptation of parents in relation to their 6-month-old infant's type of disability. *Child: Care, Health and Development, 25,* 377–397.

Peters, R. M., & Flack, J. M. (2003). Diagnosis and treatment of hypertension in children and adolescents. *Journal of the American Academy of Nurse Practitioners, 15*(2), 56–63.

Rao, P. S., Jureidini, S. B., Balfour, I. C., Singh, G. K., & Chen, S. (2003). Severe aortic coarctation in infants less than three months: Successful palliation by balloon angioplasty. *Journal of Invasive Cardiology, 15*(4), 202–208.

Rome, J. J., & Kreutzer, J. (2004). Pediatric interventional catheterization: Reasonable expectations and outcomes. *Pediatric Clinics of North America, 51,* 1589–1610.

Rosner, B., Prineas, R., Daniels, S. R., & Loggie, J. (2000). Blood pressure differences between Blacks and Whites in relation to body size among US children and adolescents. *American Journal of Epidemiology, 151*(10), 1007–1019.

Starr, N. B., & Freitas-Nichols, J. (2000). Cardiac arrythmias in children. *Journal of Pediatric Health Care, 14*(3), 127–129.

Steeg, C. N., Walsh, C. A., & Glickstein, J. S. (2000). Rheumatic fever: No cause for complaisance. *Contemporary Pediatrics, 17*(1), 128–141.

Strauss, A., & Lock, J. E. (2003). Pediatric cardiomyopathy—A long way to go. *New England Journal of Medicine, 348* (April 24), 1703–1705.

Suddaby, E. C. (2001). Contemporary thinking for congenital heart disease. *Pediatric Nursing, 27*(3), 233–238, 270.

Tran, J. T. (2002). Current treatment strategies of symptomatic patent ductus arteriosus. *Journal of Pediatric Health Care, 16*(6), 306–310.

Uzark, K., & Jones, K. (2003). Parenting stress and children with heart disease. *Journal of Pediatric Health Care, 17*(4), 163–168.

Waldman, J. D., & Wernly, J. A. (1999). Cyanotic congenital heart disease with decreased pulmonary blood flow in children. *Pediatric Clinics of North America, 46*(2), 385–404.

Walters, H. L. (2000). Congenital cardiac surgical strategies and outcomes: HEARTS. *Pediatric Annals, 29*(8), 489–498.

Wernovsky, G., & Newburger, J. (2003). Neurologic and developmental morbidity in children with complex congenital heart disease. *Journal of Pediatrics, 142*(1), 6–8.

Wiegman, A., Hutten, B. A., de Groot, E., Rodenburg, J., Baccker, H. D., et al. (2004). Efficacy and safety of statin therapy in children with familial hypercholesterolemia. *Journal of the American Medical Association, 292*(3), 331–337.

The Child with Alterations in Hematologic Function

Having a child with sickle cell disease is very difficult for us. We know this is a genetic disease, and we feel responsible for Michael's pain. We also never seem to expect the bad times when they come. He'll be doing well and we almost forget . . . then he gets sick or doesn't drink enough and we're in the hospital again. His older sister has started talking about how she worries that sometime she'll have a child with sickle cell disease and we don't know what to tell her.

—Father of Michael, 12 years old

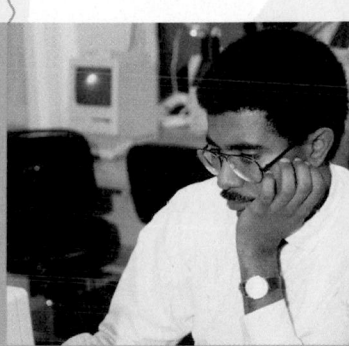

LEARNING OBJECTIVES

- Describe the function of red blood cells, white blood cells, and platelets.

- Discuss the pathophysiology and clinical manifestations of the major disorders of red blood cells affecting the pediatric population.

- Discuss the pathophysiology and clinical manifestations of the major disorders of white blood cells affecting the pediatric population.

- Discuss the pathophysiology and clinical manifestations of the major disorders of platelets affecting the pediatric population.

- Describe the nursing management and collaborative care of a child with a hematologic disorder.

- Discuss nursing implications for a child receiving hematopoietic stem cell transplantation (HSCT).

MEDIALINK

www.prenhall.com/london

CD-ROM

Animations:
  Circulatory System
  Types of Blood Cells
  Sickle Cell Anemia
Nursing in Action: Administering Blood or Blood
  Products
Audio Glossary
NCLEX-RN® Review

Companion Website

MediaLink Applications:
  Ethical Considerations: Hemophilia
  Hematopoietic Stem Cell Transplantation (HSCT)
Care Plan: A School-Age Child with Hemophilia
Case Study: An Adolescent in Sickle Cell Crisis
Thinking Critically
NCLEX-RN® Review
Audio Glossary

MediaLink · Animation: Circulatory System

The hematologic system is one of a few body systems that regulate, directly or indirectly, all other body functions. Because blood is involved in the function of all tissues and organs, changes in the blood may result in altered functioning of many body organs and structures. A tendency toward easy bruising is a characteristic sign of many bleeding disorders. Other signs include nosebleeds, pallor, frequent infections, and lethargy. This chapter discusses the most common disorders of the blood and blood-forming organs in children. (See Chapter 50 for a discussion of leukemia.∞)

ANATOMY AND PHYSIOLOGY OF PEDIATRIC DIFFERENCES

Blood has two components: a fluid portion called plasma and a cellular portion known as the formed elements of the blood. The cellular elements are red blood cells (erythrocytes), white blood cells (leukocytes), and platelets (thrombocytes) (Figure 49–1 ◉). Table 49–1 gives normal values for these blood components in children.

◉ FIGURE 49–1

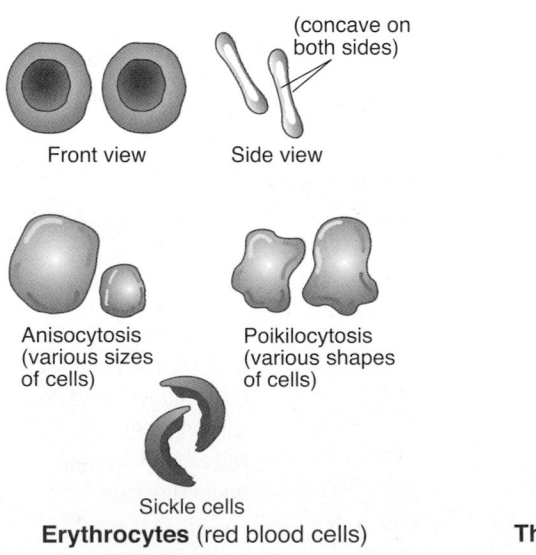

Types of blood cells.

TABLE 49–1 ✣ Normal Blood Values in Children

	Newborn	2 Years	12 Years	18 Years
Red blood cells (RBCs) (values $\times 10^{12}$/L)	4.1–5.74	3.9–5.03	4.93–5.3	3.7–5.5
Hematocrit (Hct) (%)	37.4–56.1	31.7–37.7	34.0–43.9	33.0–46.2
Hemoglobin (Hgb) (g/dL)	12.7–18.6	10.5–12.7	11.2–14.8	10.7–15.7
White blood cells (WBCs) (values $\times 10^3$/µL)	6.8–14.3	5.3–11.5	4.5–10.1	4.4–10.2
Platelets (values $\times 10^9$/L)	164–586	206–459	189–403	175–345

Data from Soldin, S. J., Brugnara, C., & Wong, E. C. (2003). *Pediatric reference ranges* (4th ed.). Washington, DC: AACC Press. Adapted. See additional blood values in Appendix B. ∞

The fetus produces red blood cells by the second week of gestation, with white blood cell and platelet production beginning at 8 weeks. Most of this early production occurs in the liver; however, by 20 to 24 weeks' gestation, liver production decreases as bone marrow production begins to predominate (Ohls & Christensen, 2004).

At birth, **hematopoiesis**, or blood cell production, occurs in the marrow of almost every bone. The flat bones, such as the sternum, ribs, pelvic and shoulder girdles, vertebrae, and hips, retain most of their hematopoietic activity throughout life.

RED BLOOD CELLS

Red blood cells, or erythrocytes, are the most abundant of the cellular elements of blood. They are formed through the process of **erythropoiesis**. The primary function of red blood cells is to transport oxygen from the lungs to the tissues. They also help to carry carbon dioxide back to the lungs. Hemoglobin, a red pigment composed of protein and iron, is essential to this function.

Polycythemia is an above-average increase in the number of red cells in the blood. Any condition that causes the quantity of oxygen transported to the tissues to decrease ordinarily increases the rate of red blood cell production. When a child becomes anemic after a hemorrhage, for instance, the bone marrow immediately begins to produce large quantities of red cells. **Anemia** is a reduction in the number of red blood cells; the various types of anemia will be discussed in the following section.

At birth the newborn has a naturally occurring elevation in red blood cells (RBCs) due to a high level of erythropoietin, which stimulates red cell production (see Table 49–1). Once the newborn begins breathing air and the oxygen level in the blood increases, this production slows. Levels of RBCs fall until about 2 to 3 months of age (to about 9 to 11 g/dL) and then begin increasing. Adult levels are reached during adolescence. Teenage males have RBC levels slightly higher than teenage females (see Appendix B. ∞)

WHITE BLOOD CELLS

White blood cells, or leukocytes, are the mobile units of the body's protective system. They are formed in bone marrow and lymph tissue. The white blood cell count is highest at birth, although levels vary greatly among infants. By 1 week of age, white blood cell values stabilize. Throughout childhood, there is a very slow decrease in white blood cell count (Boxer, 2004).

There are five types of white blood cells, each with a distinct function (Table 49–2). A differential blood count indicates the percentages of the different types of white cells in the blood and is sometimes useful in identifying the cause of an illness. For example, infections cause an increase in neutrophils; and allergies are related to an increase in eosinophils. The role of lymphocytes is discussed with acquired immunodeficiency syndrome in Chapter 44. ∞ A decrease in the number of white blood cells is called **leukopenia**, and can be caused by immune or bone marrow disorders.

TABLE 49–2 ✣ White Blood Cells and Their Functions

Type	Function
Neutrophils	Phagocytosis
Eosinophils	Allergic reactions
Basophils	Inflammatory reactions
Monocytes (macrophages)	Phagocytosis, antigen processing
Lymphocytes	Humoral immunity (B cell), cellular immunity (T cell)

MEDIALINK Animation: Types of Blood Cells

PLATELETS

Platelets, or thrombocytes, are cell fragments that can form hemostatic plugs to stop bleeding. They are synthesized from components in the red bone marrow and are stored in the spleen. Platelet levels in newborns are lower than in older children and adults. Levels of many clotting factors, particularly those requiring vitamin K for activation (factors II, VII, IX, X, and anticoagulant factors—proteins C and S), are also lower in infants. For this reason, all newborns receive a prophylactic injection of vitamin K at birth. Values of platelets and other coagulation products soon reach normal childhood levels (Montgomery & Scott, 2004). A deficiency of platelets can lead to bleeding disorder and is termed **thrombocytopenia**.

✿ ANEMIAS

Anemia is defined as a reduction in the number of RBCs, the quantity of hemoglobin, and the volume of packed red cells to below-normal levels. It can be caused by loss or destruction of existing RBCs or by an impaired or decreased rate of red cell production. Anemia also can be a clinical manifestation of an underlying disorder, such as lead poisoning or hypersplenism (a syndrome characterized by splenomegaly and blood cell deficiencies). The major types of anemia seen in children include iron deficiency anemia, beta-thalassemia, aplastic anemia, normocytic anemia, and sickle cell anemia.

IRON DEFICIENCY ANEMIA

Iron deficiency anemia is the most common type and the most common nutritional deficiency in children. Three percent of children younger than 2 years of age, 9% to 11% of adolescent females, and less than 1% of adolescent males are affected by iron deficiency anemia (Carley, 2003). It can occur because of blood loss, or as a result of increased internal demands (rapid growth) for blood production, or due to poor nutritional intake. See Chapter 34 for a discussion of iron deficiency anemia due to deficits in nutritional intake. ∞

Rapidly growing adolescents whose diets are high in fat and low in vitamins and minerals are particularly susceptible to iron deficiency anemia. Infants who do not take in adequate solid foods after 6 months of age and are fed only breast milk or formula that is not fortified with iron are also at risk because neonatal iron stores have been depleted by this time and their iron needs are not being met. Similarly, if the mother's nutritional status during pregnancy was inadequate, or the infant was born prematurely or as part of a multiple birth, insufficient iron may have been stored in the latter part of pregnancy, placing the infant at higher risk for anemia in the first months of life.

Chronic blood loss is always a potential cause of iron deficiency anemia. The infant who has had bleeding in the neonatal period, the child who loses blood as a result of conditions such as hemophilia or parasitic gastrointestinal illness, and the adolescent girl who has **menorrhagia** (heavy menstrual bleeding) may all be at risk of anemia.

Clinical manifestations depend on the severity of the anemia. Pallor, fatigue, and irritability are characteristic findings. Nailbed deformities, growth retardation, developmental delay, tachycardia, and systolic heart murmur can occur with prolonged anemia. Pica, or consumption of non-food items, is also associated with iron deficiency anemia.

Diagnosis is made on the basis of laboratory studies; findings include low hemoglobin, hematocrit, mean corpuscular volume, serum iron, RBC count, reticulocytes (immature or newly released red blood cells), iron-binding capacity, and serum ferritin <15 ng/mL. Microscopic analysis (Figure 49–2 ⬤) reveals RBCs that are microcytic (small) in size and hypochromic (pale) in appearance (Cook, 2000). A diet history and analysis can provide information about food intake; see Chapter 34 for guidelines about diet history. ∞

Treatment involves correction of the iron deficiency with oral elemental iron preparations and a diet high in

⬤ **FIGURE 49–2**

In iron deficiency anemia, red blood cells appear hypochromic as a result of decreased hemoglobin synthesis.

Courtesy of Dr. Ed Wong, Laboratory Medicine, Children's National Medical Center, Washington, DC.

iron. Ferrous sulfate at a dose of 3 to 6 mg/kg/day for about 4 weeks is a common treatment, followed by evaluation for its effectiveness. If the anemia is improving, treatment usually continues for about 2 months (Carley, 2003; Committee on Nutrition, 2004). Because oral iron preparations cause several side effects such as constipation and gastrointestinal discomfort, the child may receive iron supplements (to restore blood levels of iron) while the iron content of the diet is increased above the recommended dietary allowances (RDAs). Oral supplements can then be tapered off once the child's food intake can supply the needed iron; the child is evaluated in about 6 months for recurring anemia. If the anemia is a result of bleeding, the cause is identified and treated to prevent future excess blood loss.

NURSING MANAGEMENT

The child with iron deficiency anemia is usually identified and treated in the community unless he or she has another serious illness. Nursing care focuses on screening for the disorder and educating the parents and child about the causes of iron deficiency anemia, dietary management, and the importance of complying with the medication regimen.

Screening for anemia is recommended at 9 to 12 months of age, at 15 to 18 months, and again at adolescence (see Chapters 37 and 38 ∞) (Committee on Nutrition, 2004). A hematocrit or hemoglobin level is obtained. More detailed tests are performed if the blood test is abnormal. Children at high risk for nutritional deficiencies, such as those in low-income groups and WIC programs, may require additional tests. Nurses screen most children in Head Start annually. In addition, children showing signs of anemia should be screened. Take height and weight measurements at each healthcare visit, plot them on growth charts, and compare to percentiles obtained at previous visits. Slow downward trends in percentiles are of concern and require further nutritional analysis (see Chapter 34 ∞). Perform developmental screening tests to assess for developmental delays (see Chapter 33 ∞).

DEVELOPING CULTURAL COMPETENCE

BLOOD SAMPLES AND CHINESE AMERICANS

According to traditional Chinese beliefs, a person who does not feel well is lacking in chi (inner energy) and blood. Chinese Americans who follow traditional practices may be hesitant to have blood drawn for laboratory studies for fear of causing body weakness. A person from the same culture may be able to explain the need for analysis of a small sample of blood.

Dietary management is the preferred long-term treatment for iron deficiency anemia. Teach the family and child

about foods rich in iron. The infant over 6 months of age should have a diet that includes breast milk or iron-fortified formula and baby cereals with iron fortification. Avoid cow milk in the first year of life since it can cause bleeding from the gastrointestinal tract, contributing to anemia. Older infants and toddlers can eat finger foods such as thinly sliced meats. Adolescents can be encouraged to eat foods with a high iron content, such as hamburgers and dried fruits.

Oral iron preparations are given to correct anemia (see "Drug Guide," Chapter 34 ∞). Teach the child and family that the liquid iron preparation should be taken through a straw because it stains the teeth. Instruct about side effects such as black stools, constipation, and a foul aftertaste. Emphasize the importance of drinking fluids and eating foods high in dietary fiber to minimize these side effects. The medicine should be stored safely to avoid accidental poisoning. Expected outcomes of care are intake of recommended levels of iron and return to normal hematocrit level.

NORMOCYTIC ANEMIA

In normocytic anemia, the RBCs, although decreased in number, are of normal size with a pale center (Cook, 2000). This type of anemia may occur as a result of hemorrhage, disease-induced inflammation, disseminated intravascular coagulation (DIC; see the discussion later in this chapter), G6PD deficiency, hemolytic uremic syndrome (see Chapter 52 ∞), or several other conditions. When one of these conditions exists in a child diagnosed with anemia, the infectious or inflammatory condition should be suspected as the cause of the identified anemia and treated first. Some infectious and inflammatory causes of anemia are listed in Table 49–3.

Clinical manifestations are similar to those seen in iron deficiency anemia, with the possible occurrence of hepatomegaly and splenomegaly, as well. The etiology of normocytic anemia associated with chronic inflammation or infection is related to increased RBC destruction, de-

---

TABLE 49–3 ✤ **Infectious and Inflammatory Causes of Anemia**

Infections	Inflammations
Haemophilus influenzae type b	Arthritis
HIV/AIDS	Cancers
Orbital cellulitis	Chronic heart or liver disease
Meningitis	
Septic arthritis	

creased iron release from storage sites, and ineffective bone marrow response. In hemorrhage, anemia is a direct result of loss of blood.

Treatment of normocytic anemia depends on the underlying cause. When the anemia is associated with inflammation or infection, the underlying condition is treated. For anemia caused by renal failure, recombinant human erythropoietin is administered. When hemorrhage is the underlying cause, the source of the bleeding is identified and treated. In acute emergencies, blood products are infused to make up for some of the losses.

Nursing management of normocytic anemia depends on the cause of the decreased RBCs. Children with inflammatory or infectious diseases require careful assessment and management of medication and other treatment regimens. Administer blood products and other intravenous fluids as ordered to restore blood volume. Use follow-up and home visits to assess hematocrit, hemoglobin, and dietary intake. (Refer to the discussion later in this chapter for management of DIC, to Chapter 51 for management of intestinal infections, and to Chapter 52 for management of hemolytic uremic syndrome. ∞)

SICKLE CELL ANEMIA

Sickle cell anemia is a hereditary **hemoglobinopathy**, in which normal hemoglobin is partly or completely replaced with abnormal hemoglobin S (Hgb S) (Table 49–4). Sickle cell anemia occurs primarily in blacks, although occasion-

ally it affects people of Mediterranean or Hispanic descent. Sickle cell anemia occurs in about 1 in 375 black infants born in the United States, and 1 in 12 African Americans have sickle cell trait (i.e., they carry one gene for the disease) (Jakubik & Thompson, 2000).

ETIOLOGY AND PATHOPHYSIOLOGY

Sickle cell anemia is an autosomal recessive disorder. If both parents have the trait, with each pregnancy the risk of having a child with the disease is 25%. (See Chapter 3 for a discussion of recessive gene transmission. ∞)

In sickle cell anemia, the hemoglobin in the RBC acquires an elongated crescent or sickle shape (Figure 49–3 ●). The rigid sickled cells obstruct capillary blood flow. Microscopic obstructions lead to engorgement and tissue ischemia. This local tissue hypoxia causes further sickling and ultimately large infarctions. Damaged tissues in organs throughout the body become scarred, resulting in impaired function. For example, children with sickle cell anemia can suffer from splenic sequestration when blood is trapped in the spleen, a life-threatening complication. Many children must undergo splenectomy in early childhood, leading to severely compromised immunity. Frequent infections are common due to impaired immunity, and bacterial infections are the leading cause of death in young children with sickle cell disease. Stroke is a significant risk to children with sickle cell anemia and can lead to developmental delay, mental retardation, and other neurologic problems (National Heart, Lung, and Blood Institute, 2002).

TABLE 49–4 ✤ Sickle Cell Disorders

Sickle Cell Trait (Hgb SA)

Most common form of sickle cell disease in the United States

Heterozygous condition (child has one sickle cell hemoglobin gene and one normal hemoglobin gene)

Child is carrier of sickle cell anemia and rarely has symptoms of the disease

Sickle Cell Anemia (Hgb SS)

Homozygous condition (child has two sickle hemoglobin genes)

Child is subject to sickle cell crises

Sickle Cell Syndromes

Sickle Cell–Hgb C Disease (Hgb SC)

Second most frequent form of sickle cell disease in African Americans

Different from sickle cell anemia only in that the sickle cell assumes a C shape instead of an S shape

Sickle Cell–β–Thalassemia Disease (Hgb SB)

Rarely occurs

Combination of sickle cell trait and thalassemia trait most often seen in people of Mediterranean descent

---

● **FIGURE 49–3**

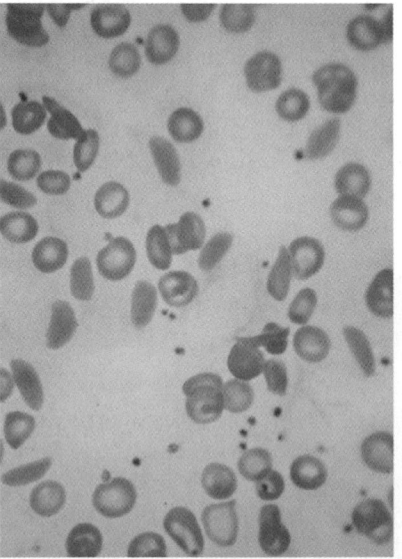

Many of these red blood cells show an elongated crescent shape characteristic of sickle cell anemia.

Courtesy of Dr. Ed Wong, Laboratory Medicine, Children's National Medical Center, Washington, DC.

Precipitating factors for sickle cell crisis include increased blood viscosity (such as from a low fluid intake or fever) and hypoxia or low oxygen tension. Sickling may be triggered by fever and emotional or physical stress. Potential causes of hypoxia or low oxygen tension include high altitudes, poorly pressurized airplanes, hypoventilation, vasoconstriction when cold, or an emotionally stressful event. Any condition that increases the body's need for oxygen or alters the transport of oxygen (such as infection, trauma, or dehydration) may result in sickle cell crisis.

Sickled cells can resume a normal shape when rehydrated and reoxygenated. The membrane of these cells becomes more fragile, however, and cell life is shortened to 10 to 20 days rather than the usual 120 days. In response, bone marrow spaces enlarge to produce more RBCs. Continuous formation and destruction of the child's RBCs contributes to the severe hemolytic anemia that is characteristic of sickle cell anemia (Tanyi, 2003) (see "Pathophysiology Illustrated: Sickle Cell Anemia").

CLINICAL MANIFESTATIONS

Affected children are usually asymptomatic until 4 to 6 months of age because sickling is inhibited by high levels of fetal hemoglobin. Clinical manifestations are directly related to the shortened life span of blood cells (hemolytic anemia) and tissue destruction resulting from **vaso-occlusion** (blockage of a blood vessel). Illness results from recurrent vaso-occlusive events that involve painful crises and chronic organ damage (Odesina, 2001). Pathologic changes happen in most body systems, resulting in multiple signs and symptoms. Examples of common organs affected include the following:

- Brain—cerebrovascular accident, often manifested by headache, aphasia, convulsions, visual changes

- Eyes—retinopathy, retinal detachment, diminished vision

- Bones—chronic ischemia of bones with susceptibility to infection and bone degeneration, manifested by osteoporosis, osteomyelitis, spinal deformities, or aseptic necrosis of the femoral head

- Liver—impaired blood flow from capillary obstruction leads to enlargement and scarring of the liver, manifested by hepatomegaly or cirrhosis

- Spleen—splenic infarct leads to fibrosis and increased rates of infection

- Kidneys—ischemia of kidneys causes enuresis, hematuria, inability to concentrate urine

- Penis—microcirculatory obstruction and engorgement (priapism)

- Extremities—vaso-occlusion and chronic ischemia manifests as peripheral neuropathy, weakness, or arthralgia

- Skin—decreased peripheral circulation causes ulcerations

Sickle cell crises are acute exacerbations of the disease that vary markedly in severity and frequency. Table 49–5 outlines the most common types of crises affecting children with sickle cell disease. These crises may occur individually or in combination.

Children with sickle cell trait rarely have such crises. However, because they have some abnormal hemoglobin, they may develop symptoms of the disease under conditions of abnormally low oxygen such as flying in an unpressurized airplane over 7000 feet, or during anesthesia. The most common symptoms experienced by those with sickle cell trait are splenic infarction and hematuria. However, most persons who carry the trait never have symptoms, even with low oxygen concentrations.

CLINICAL THERAPY

The initial diagnosis of sickle cell anemia in newborns is often made by testing cord blood using hemoglobin electrophoresis. The sickle-turbidity test (Sickledex) may be used for quick screening in children over 6 months of age, once the fetal hemoglobin levels have fallen. Hemoglobin electrophoresis verifies positive Sickledex test results. Newborns are screened for hemoglobinopathies (diseases of the blood) in most states. It is recommended that all newborns be screened, because sickle cell disease can occur in several groups in addition to blacks, such as Mediterranean, South American, Arabian, and East Indian. A child's heritage cannot be predicted from appearance or name alone.

NURSING PRACTICE

Information about genetic testing is confidential and must not be shared with people other than those tested. In the 1970s, when genetic testing for sickle cell disease and trait first became available, many blacks who had the trait for sickle cell disease experienced discrimination in jobs and insurance.

No cure for sickle cell anemia exists. Supportive care is aimed at the prevention and treatment of sickling episodes. Management focuses on pain control, hydration, oxygenation, and prevention of infections and other complications. Penicillin, amoxicillin, Bicillin, or erythromycin are used prophylactically (Wilson, Krishnamurti, & Kamat,

PATHOPHYSIOLOGY ILLUSTRATED

Sickle Cell Anemia

Hemoglobin S and Red Blood Cell Sickling

Sickle cell anemia is caused by an inherited autosomal recessive defect in Hb synthesis. Sickle cell hemoglobin (HbS) differs from normal hemoglobin only in the substitution of the amino acid valine for glutamine in both beta chains of the hemoglobin molecule.

When HbS is oxygenated, it has the same globular shape as normal hemoglobin. However, when HbS loses its oxygen, it becomes insoluble in intra-cellular fluid and crystallizes into rodlike structures. Clusters of rods form polymers (long chains) that bend the erythrocyte into the characteristic crescent shape of the sickle cell.

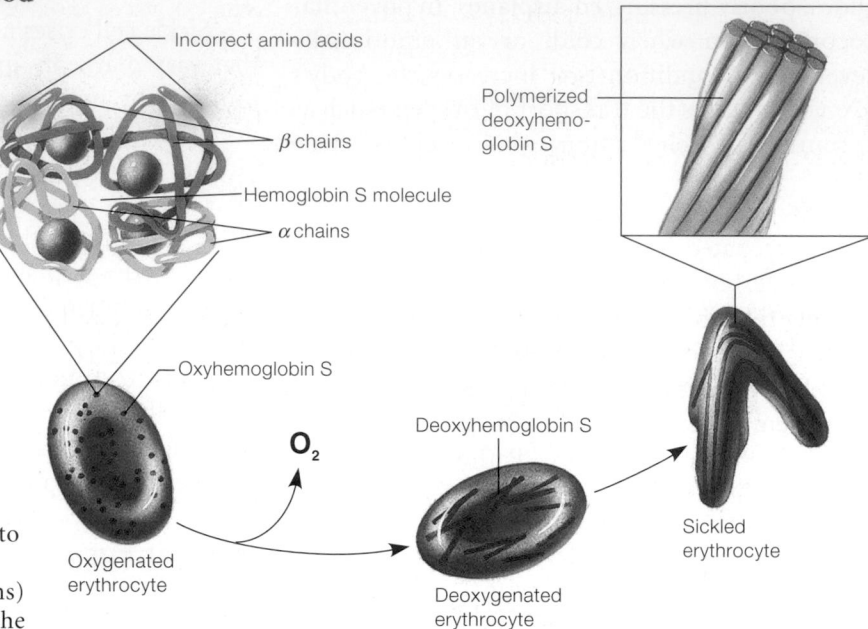

The Sickle Cell Disease Process

Sickle cell disease is characterized by episodes of acute painful crises. Sickling crises are triggered by conditions causing high tissue oxygen demands or that affect cellular pH. As the crisis begins, sickled erythrocytes adhere to capillary walls and to each other, obstructing blood flow and causing cellular hypoxia. The crisis accelerates as tissue hypoxia and acidic metabolic waste products cause further sickling and cell damage.

Sickle cell crises cause microinfarcts in joints and organs, and repeated crises slowly destroy organs and tissues. The spleen and kidneys are especially prone to sickling damage.

The clinical manifestations of sickle cell anemia result from pathologic changes to structures and systems throughout the body.

TABLE 49–5 ✦ Types of Sickle Cell Crises

Vaso–occlusive Crises (Thrombotic)

Most common type of crisis; painful

Caused by stasis of blood with clumping of cells in the microcirculation, ischemia, and infarction

Signs include fever, pain, tissue engorgement

Splenic Sequestration

Life-threatening crisis; death can occur within hours

Caused by pooling of blood in the spleen

Signs include profound anemia, hypovolemia, and shock

Aplastic Crises

Diminished production and increased destruction of red blood cells

Triggered by viral infection or depletion of folic acid

Signs include profound anemia, pallor

2003). All immunizations, particularly pneumococcal vaccine and *Haemophilus influenzae* type b (Hib) vaccine, should be administered on schedule.

Treatment of crises involves hydration, oxygen, pain management, and bed rest to reduce energy expenditure. Cultures (blood, urine, and throat) are taken to identify sources of infection. Other therapeutic measures include blood transfusions to treat the anemia and to make the sickled blood less viscous. Transfusions improve blood and tissue oxygenation, reduce sickling, relieve ischemia in organs affected by the disease, and suppress the production of sickled cells (Ogedegbe, 2002). In children who have had strokes from the disease, periodic transfusions (about every 3 to 4 weeks) can reduce the incidence of future strokes. However, frequent transfusions may result in an overload of iron in the body. The iron is stored in tissues and organs (**hemosiderosis**) because the body has no way of excreting it. For this reason, an iron-chelating drug such as deferoxamine may be given along with vitamin C to promote iron excretion. Treatment with hydroxyurea has been helpful in adults, and is now sometimes used in children. This cytotoxic drug decreases production of abnormal blood cells and leads to less pain (Day & Wynn, 2000). (See Skill 12–6. **SKILLS**)

NURSING PRACTICE

It is important for all health facilities to have current guidelines for transfusion protocols. Become familiar with the policies and procedures where you work. For example, the child's blood type and patient identification needs to be checked by two registered nurses before starting the infusion. See the *Clinical Skills Manual* for further information on blood transfusions. **SKILLS**

Hematopoietic stem cell transplantation (HSCT) may be considered in some cases (refer to later discussion in this chapter about this treatment).

Neonatal screening, early intervention, prophylactic antibiotics, and parent education have allowed children with sickle cell disease to live into adulthood. Prognosis depends on the severity of the child's disease; children with more frequent exacerbations and hospitalization have poorer prognoses.

NURSING MANAGEMENT

NURSING ASSESSMENT AND DIAGNOSIS

The nurse may be involved in sickle cell gene testing to identify carriers and children who have the disease. Once a child is diagnosed with the disease, a comprehensive physical assessment is essential because sickle cell anemia can affect any body system.

THINKING CRITICALLY

SICKLE CELL ANEMIA

Michael is a 12-year-old black child with sickle cell disease who is admitted to the hospital with severe abdominal pain. Which organ is likely filled with sickled cells and causing his pain? Michael is receiving oxygen by nasal cannula; why would he need this? What are the most important nursing assessments and interventions to integrate within Michael's care?

Physiologic Assessment

In children who are known to have sickle cell anemia, take a detailed history from the parents or child about past crises, precipitating events, medical treatment, and home management. Measure the child's height and weight accurately and compare to past measurements, since failure to thrive is common. Ask about chronic or acute pain that the child is experiencing. Pain may occur in nearly any body part, but most commonly manifests as headache, extremity pain, or abdominal discomfort. The ill child with sickle cell disease should receive a careful multisystem assessment. Fever is an emergency necessitating prompt treatment.

When the child is in crisis, assess pain and note the presence of any signs of inflammation or infection. Carefully monitor the child for signs of shock (see Chapter 48 ∞).

Psychosocial Assessment

The family of a child with sickle cell disease requires a thorough psychosocial assessment. Ask if other family members have the diagnosis. If the child is newly diagnosed with the disorder, the family needs assistance to deal with feelings related to the serious, life-threatening nature of the disease. Assess parents' understanding of the disease transmission and ask whether genetic counseling has been obtained. Determine whether the family has adequate healthcare coverage to pay for the child's medical expenses and whether the child qualifies for assistance due to the disease disability. Ask older children about their knowledge of the disease, and explore their feelings related to the management of a chronic condition. When siblings or other family members are carriers, periodic counseling is needed so they can understand implications for dating, marriage, and having children.

Several nursing diagnoses that might apply to the child with sickle cell anemia are presented in the accompanying "Nursing Care Plan." Other nursing diagnoses might include the following:

- *Caregiver Role Strain* related to illness chronicity
- *Risk for Impaired Parenting* related to having a child with a physical illness
- *Delayed Growth and Development* related to effects of physical disability
- *Impaired Physical Mobility* related to pain

PLANNING AND IMPLEMENTATION

The accompanying "Nursing Care Plan" summarizes nursing care for the child with sickle cell anemia. Nursing management for the child in crisis focuses on increasing tissue perfusion, promoting hydration, controlling pain, prevent-ing infection, ensuring adequate nutrition, preventing complications, and providing emotional support to the child and family.

Increase Tissue Perfusion

Administer blood transfusions and oxygen as ordered. To prevent hemolysis, the intravenous fluid used before and after a blood transfusion must be saline rather than D5W. Monitor for transfusion reactions (see "Clinical Manifestations: Blood Transfusion Reactions"). Encourage the child to rest. Work with the child and family to avoid emotional stress. Any activities that increase cellular metabolism also result in tissue hypoxia. Schedule caregiving activities and play to allow for optimal rest.

NURSING PRACTICE

When giving a transfusion, never infuse cold blood since it may increase sickling. Use a blood-warming coil to bring blood to room temperature.

NURSING PRACTICE

Blood reactions can occur as soon as the blood transfusion begins. Administer the first 20 mL of blood slowly and observe the child carefully for a reaction. Repeatedly assess the child according to agency policy and promptly report changes in condition.

CLINICAL MANIFESTATIONS

BLOOD TRANSFUSION REACTIONS

TYPE OF REACTION	ETIOLOGY	CLINICAL MANIFESTATIONS	CLINICAL THERAPY
Allergic reaction	Immune response	Urticaria, itching, respiratory distress	Stop the transfusion; call physician; give antihistamines as ordered; monitor vital signs; maintain intravenous infusion of normal saline; keep intravenous line open; check urine for hematuria
Hemolytic reaction	Mismatched blood, history of multiple transfusions	Fever, chills, hematuria, headache, chest pain; can progress to shock	
Febrile or septic	Usually a result of contamination of blood or idiopathic conditions	Chills, fever, headache, decreased blood pressure, nausea or vomiting, and leg and back pain	Inform primary healthcare provider
Circulatory overload	Results from infusion of excessive amounts of fluid or too rapid administration	Dyspnea, chest or low back pain, productive cough, rales upon auscultation, distended neck veins, increased central venous pressure	Diuretics may be ordered

NURSING CARE PLAN

THE CHILD WITH SICKLE CELL ANEMIA

Intervention	Rationale	Expected Outcome
1. Nursing Diagnosis: Ineffective Tissue Perfusion related to affinity of hemoglobin for oxygen		
NIC Priority Intervention: **Circulatory care:** Promotion of arterial and venous circulation		**NOC Suggested Outcome:** **Tissue perfusion, peripheral:** Extent to which blood flows through the small vessels of the extremities and maintains tissue function
Goal: The child will show few signs and symptoms of tissue hypoxia.		
■ Instruct child to avoid physical exertion, emotional stress, low-oxygen environments (e.g., airplanes, high altitudes), and known sources of infection.	■ Decreased activity and exposure reduce the body's need for oxygen.	The child has no shortness of breath and shows no signs of hypoxia.
Goal: Repeated cerebrovascular accidents will be avoided.		
■ Administer blood transfusions as ordered. ■ Perform several caregiving activities together whenever possible. ■ Give oxygen as ordered. ■ Administer and teach the family to administer prophylactic transfusions for the child who has had a cerebrovascular accident.	■ Packed cells increase number of red blood cells available to carry oxygen to tissue cells. Transfusions promote circulation. ■ Grouping activities allows for optimum rest. ■ High concentration of oxygen in alveoli increases diffusion of gas across membranes. ■ Lowers potential for a future cerebrovascular accident.	The child does not suffer a cerebrovascular accident.
2. Nursing Diagnosis: Risk for Deficient Fluid Volume related to inadequate fluid intake and dehydration		
NIC Priority Intervention: **Fluid management:** Promotion of electrolyte balance and prevention of complications resulting from abnormal or undesired fluid levels		**NOC Suggested Outcome:** **Hydration:** Amount of water in the intracellular and extracellular compartments of the body
Goal: The child will maintain or be restored to adequate hydration.		
■ Calculate the child's daily fluid requirements. Monitor the child's usual fluid consumption and make necessary adjustments. Encourage the child to take fluids. Observe for signs of dehydration. ■ Record intake and output.	■ Optimizing fluid intake ensures that the child gets needed fluid. Dehydration exacerbates crises. ■ Recording enables you to monitor daily fluid intake and spacing throughout the day.	The child shows signs of adequate hydration.
3. Nursing Diagnosis: Pain related to chronic physical disability		
NIC Priority Intervention: **Pain management:** Alleviation of pain or a reduction in pain to a level of comfort acceptable to the patient		**NOC Suggested Outcome:** **Comfort level:** Feelings of physical and psychologic ease

(continued)

NURSING CARE PLAN—continued

THE CHILD WITH SICKLE CELL ANEMIA

Intervention	Rationale	Expected Outcome
Goal: The child will verbalize that pain is controlled.		
■ Administer analgesics, such as morphine or hydromorphone (Dilaudid), as ordered. Continuous intravenous infusion is used for the duration of a painful crisis. ■ Position carefully.	■ Pain of sickle cell crises is excruciating. ■ Joints and extremities can be extremely painful.	The child is pain-free or pain control is significantly improved.

4. Nursing Diagnosis: Risk for Infection related to chronic disease and splenic malfunction

NIC Priority Intervention:		NOC Suggested Outcome:
Infectious control: Minimizing the acquisition and transmission of infectious agents		**Risk control:** Actions to eliminate or reduce actual, personal, and modifiable health threats
Goal: The child will not develop infection.		
■ Ensure adequate nutrition by providing high-calorie, high-protein diet. Make sure that the child's immunizations are up to date. Report any signs of infection to physician immediately. ■ Isolate the child from possible sources of infection. Instruct parents about signs of infection and encourage them to seek prompt healthcare.	■ Chronically ill children are at greater risk of infection. ■ Restriction of persons with infection decreases the child's contact with infectious agents. Prompt care for infection reduces the chance of sickle cell crisis.	The child is free of infection.

5. Nursing Diagnosis: Deficient Knowledge (Child and Parents) related to lack of exposure about cause and treatment of sickle cell anemia

NIC Priority Intervention:		NOC Suggested Outcome:
Teaching disease process: Assisting the patient to understand information related to a specific disease process		**Knowledge:** Extent of understanding conveyed about sickle cell disease
Goal: The child and family will verbalize understanding of risk factors for sickle cell crises and how to minimize them.		
■ Review basics of sickle cell disease. Teach the child and family about signs and symptoms of crises. ■ Arrange for genetic counseling and testing for sickle cell trait for family members if desired.	■ Knowledge of disease helps ensure compliance with treatment regimen and adherence to preventive measures. ■ Questions and concerns regarding future pregnancies can be allayed through knowledge of disease and transmission.	The child and parent can verbalize precipitating events of crises.

Promote Hydration

The child with sickle cell anemia is adversely affected by dehydration. Calculate the child's fluid maintenance requirements (minimum daily fluid intake) (see Chapter 39 ∞) and monitor the child's oral fluid intake. Administer intravenous fluids as ordered. Adjust oral intake as necessary to keep the child well hydrated.

Control Pain

Give prescribed analgesics around the clock during crises. If patient-controlled analgesia is used, be sure that the constant infusions run as ordered and that the parent or child understands the use of bolus infusions, when needed (see Chapter 42 ∞). Help the child assume a comfortable position. Avoid putting stress on painful joints.

GROWTH AND DEVELOPMENT

To encourage fluid intake in a small child:

- Use a favorite cup or glass.
- Use straws.
- Take advantage of times the child is thirsty, such as on awakening or after play.
- Leave a cup within easy reach of the child.
- Offer frozen juice pops, crushed ice drinks, and flavored ice chips.

NURSING PRACTICE

Use neither very hot nor cold compresses for pain management in the child with sickle cell anemia. Ischemic tissue is fragile and has reduced sensation, increasing the risk of burn injury; only mild warmth should be used. Cold compresses promote sickling.

Prevent Infection

Infection makes the child more susceptible to a crisis, and the crisis, in turn, increases susceptibility to infection. Teach the parents how to administer antibiotics for prophylaxis or treatment of infection. Be sure they have the finances and other resources to obtain and give daily antibiotics. Teach food safety practices to prevent food-borne illness (see Chapter 34 ∞). Because infections are particularly virulent in these children, tell parents to get immediate care when the child is ill. Encourage the pneumococcal vaccine in all infants and children with the disease. The *Haemophilus influenzae* type b (Hib) vaccine series should be started by 2 months of age and continued at recommended ages to prevent another common source of infection.

Ensure Adequate Nutrition

Perform regular growth measurements and nutritional assessments. Emphasize the importance of adequate nutri-

EVIDENCE-BASED NURSING

SICKLE CELL ANEMIA AND PAIN MANAGEMENT

Problem

Severe episodes of sickle cell crisis require hospitalization for pain management. Relief of pain is the primary goal for healthcare providers and is most significant to the child experiencing pain. However, different pain management regimens may be used during each hospitalization, and effective regimens are not well documented. Studies are needed to identify effective pain management strategies for children with sickle cell disease. In addition, parents use a variety of pain relief measures at home but these may not be integrated into care when the child becomes hospitalized, leading to poor pain management.

Evidence

Nurse researchers conducted a descriptive longitudinal study with 27 children to evaluate the pain management strategies used in sickle cell disease when they experienced pain during a vaso-occlusive episode. The children ranged in age from 5 to 19 years; there were 40 hospital admissions during the 9-month study. The researchers noted several surprising findings from the study. First, they found that children on average self-administered only 35% of the pain medication that was prescribed. The second finding was that the children did not report significant pain relief. It is assumed that adequate pain relief was not achieved during hospitalization because the dose of analgesics administered was too low. In another study in which 21 female caretakers of children with sickle cell disease were interviewed, a variety of techniques were used to manage pain at home. Oral medications, massage, warmth to painful body parts, and other techniques were considered helpful.

Implications

Hospitalized children who self-administered their medication consistently undermedicated themselves and failed to achieve pain relief. Chil-

dren may not be taught how to use the PCA device properly and may interpret that they should use it as little as possible. Thus, healthcare provider practices influence the child's pain management. In addition, children and families have developed many effective pain relief measures at home that may not be included in hospital care. More information is needed about methods of integrating these techniques into hospital care. Recommendations include the need to evaluate whether increasing analgesic use to the amount prescribed would increase the amount of pain relief. Additional research is needed to determine the effectiveness of different PCA regimens and to evaluate the effectiveness of pain management algorithms. Evaluation tools are needed to measure effectiveness of the child self-medication by PCA. Tools for evaluating home care pain management are needed. Nurses must be willing to integrate the family's measures into care while the child is hospitalized.

Critical Thinking

How will you determine if the child in sickle cell crisis is obtaining adequate pain relief (consult Chapter 42 for ideas ∞)? What personal beliefs of healthcare providers may influence effective pain management? How can these beliefs be addressed? If the primary healthcare provider has prescribed a subtherapeutic dosage of pain medication for a child in sickle cell crisis, what action could you take?

References

Beyer, J. E., & Simmons, L. E. (2004). Home treatment of pain for children and adolescents with sickle cell disease. *Pain Management Nursing, 5,* 126–135.

Jacob, E., Miaskowski, C., Savedra, M., Beyer, J. E., Treadwell, M., & Styles, L. (2003). Management of vaso-occlusive pain in children with sickle cell disease. *Journal of Pediatric Hematology/Oncology, 25,* 307–311.

COMPLEMENTARY CARE

PAIN AND SICKLE CELL ANEMIA

Pain management for children with sickle cell disease is a major challenge, both for healthcare providers and families. A nursing study that determined effectiveness of pain control and types of comfort measures used by families provides information that can be applied in caring for children with sickle cell disease in the hospital and home (Beyer & Simmons, 2004). The mothers in this study described a combination of traditional medicine and complementary approaches. They emphasized the importance of keeping the child healthy, in order to avoid crisis, by avoiding overheating or chilling. Regular medical checkups, adequate hydration, and immunizations were considered important. Being alert to early signs of pain was important so that the families could begin pharmacologic treatment as well as complementary therapies such as applying heat via baths and hot towels to decrease pain and increase relaxation; touching, holding, and massaging the extremities or chest and back; praying together; and distraction and diversionary activities such as playing games and taking drives. Nurses can learn from and apply these approaches with families. Ask them what they do to identify pain early and alleviate it. Add to the list of interventions the family can try and then partner with them to evaluate results. Continue to emphasize medical care while integrating the other comfort measures the family and child find helpful into nursing care plans.

tion to promote growth. Encourage the child to eat a high-protein, high-calorie diet. Emphasize the importance of folic acid and vitamin C supplements as ordered.

Prevent Complications of Crises

Poor growth and delayed maturation are frequently observed, so measure growth and evaluate developmental skills. Watch for signs of increasing anemia, infection, and shock (mental status change, pallor, vital sign changes). Assess the child's neurologic status for evidence of altered cerebral function. If ordered, assess for an enlarged spleen by gentle palpation. Administer blood transfusions and watch the child for any adverse reaction.

Provide Emotional Support

Sickle cell anemia is a chronic disease accompanied by life-threatening episodic crises. Family members often need support to help them deal with their feelings about the diagnosis and its implications. Explore resources in the home and community to see if parents will be able to administer medications and fluids and to provide adequate nutrition. Assess their knowledge of signs of infection and of sickle cell crisis and when to seek medical care for the child. Refer the parents for genetic counseling, particularly if they plan to have more children. Encourage adolescents and young adults in the family to receive genetic counseling

and testing, as well. Referrals to support groups and contact with others with the disease can be helpful.

Discharge Planning and Home Care Teaching

Identify and address home care needs well in advance of discharge. Give parents information about sickle cell disease and the child's treatment. Even parents of a child previously diagnosed with the disorder may benefit from information about the disease process and its management. Explain the basic effect of tissue hypoxia and the effects of sickling on circulation. Refer parents to support groups such as the National Association of Sickle Cell Disease for further information.

Teach parents to look for signs of dehydration, such as dry mucous membranes, weight loss, and sunken fontanelles in infants. Give specific instructions about how many ounces of liquid the child needs to drink each day. Emphasize that increased fluid intake is needed to replace the fluids lost from overheating or exposure to hot weather. Make sure both the child and family understand the triggers and precipitating factors for sickle cell crises. Encourage them to avoid situations that cause crises. Instruct the child and parents about signs and symptoms of crises that should be reported to their healthcare provider (see Table 49–5).

Provide the family with careful instructions about infusion therapy. When regular blood infusions are used, the resulting iron overload is damaging to body organs. These

TEACHING HIGHLIGHTS

HOME CARE CONSIDERATIONS FOR THE CHILD WITH SICKLE CELL ANEMIA

- Follow recommended schedules for well-child care visits.
- Be sure the child is up to date with immunizations, including hepatitis B, annual influenza, pneumococcal vaccine, and tuberculosis skin test.
- Special testing, such as heart and eye examinations, may be needed periodically to check for sequelae of the disease.
- Special medications, such as antibiotics, may be needed; pain relief medicine and blood transfusions may be administered.
- Dehydration is dangerous. Be sure the child gets extra fluids in hot weather, when ill, during physical activity, and during travel.
- As the child develops, provide information about the disease and encourage self-care. Be sure the school personnel understand the child's diagnosis and any care required during school hours.
- Contact your healthcare provider if the child has a high fever, a common illness that lasts more than one day, seizures, change in behavior, severe pain, abnormal skin color or breathing pattern, or any other symptoms that concern you.

children need infusion of deferoxamine (Desferal) for iron overload. The medication is usually given by subcutaneous or intravenous routes over 8 to 10 hours. Prompt recognition of side effects and careful management of the lengthy infusion process are important. The child needs to be monitored for skin reactions and allergic responses. Have parents demonstrate the infusion technique and state what to do in case of reactions. Pain management is needed during infusion as the site may be tender and uncomfortable (Odesina, 2001).

Tell parents that it is important to inform all treating physicians and dentists of the child's medical condition. The child should also wear medical identification (e.g., a medical identification bracelet). Special precautions are necessary when the child undergoes surgery of any kind, as hypoxia resulting from anesthesia is a major surgical risk.

Family members need ongoing support to deal with the stress of having a child with a chronic condition. Provide resources, respite care for parents, and information as needed for siblings.

Encourage older children with sickle cell anemia to participate in activities with other children between crises but to avoid strenuous physical exertion and contact sports. Play and social interactions that promote learning and development are important.

EVALUATION

Expected outcomes of nursing care for the child with sickle cell anemia include the following:

- Management of pain to facilitate comfort level
- Maintenance of adequate hydration state to prevent cell sickling
- Absence of side effects of disease in respiratory system, central nervous system, and body organs
- Maintenance of normal immune status and prevention of infection
- Prompt recognition and treatment of complications of the disease
- Maintenance of normal growth and development for the child
- Provision of necessary services and resources for the parents and other family members
- Knowledge of disease and treatment by family

THALASSEMIAS

The thalassemias are a group of inherited blood disorders of hemoglobin synthesis characterized by anemia that can be mild or severe. β-thalassemia, also known as Cooley anemia, is the most common type. These disorders most often occur in people of Mediterranean descent but are also found among Middle Eastern, Asian, and African populations (Cook, 2000). If both parents carry the abnormal gene, with each pregnancy there is a 25% chance of passing the disorder on to the child.

There are three types of β-thalassemia: thalassemia minor, or thalassemia trait (produces mild anemia); thalassemia intermedia (produces severe anemia); and thalassemia major (produces anemia requiring transfusion). Clinical manifestations of β-thalassemia are caused by the defective synthesis of hemoglobin, structurally impaired RBCs (Figure 49–4 ⊙), and the shortened life span of the RBCs. β-thalassemia can be detected early in infancy. The infant with β-thalassemia manifests pallor, failure to thrive, hepatosplenomegaly, and severe anemia (hemoglobin <6 g/dL). Diagnosis is made by hemoglobin electrophoresis, which shows a decreased production of one of the globin chains in hemoglobin. Characteristic erythrocyte cell changes often can be recognized in infants by 6 weeks of age. Alpha-thalassemia ranges from only having the recessive trait to the fatal disorder alpha-thalassemia major, in which all four alpha-forming genes are defective. Clinical manifestations of this form are similar to those of β-thalassemia minor. Alpha-thalassemia major results in hydrops fetalis, intrauterine congestive heart failure, cardiomegaly, and hepatomegaly.

Diagnosis is made by hemoglobin electrophoresis; decreased hemoglobin, hematocrit, and reticulocyte count are

⊙ **FIGURE 49–4**

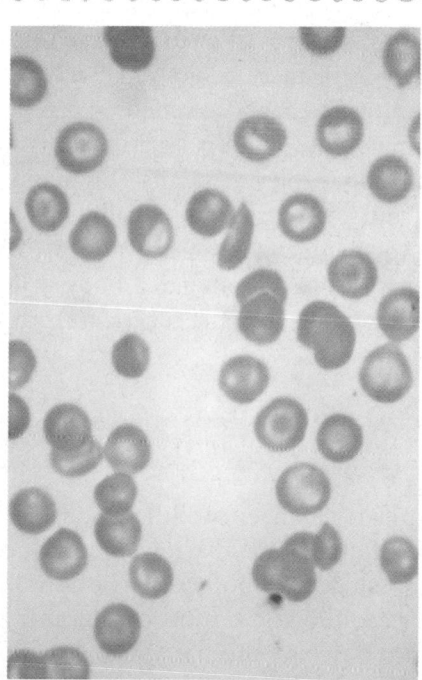

Red blood cell appearance in β-thalassemia. What characteristic abnormalities can be seen on this microscopic view?

Courtesy of Dr. Ed Wong, Laboratory Medicine, Children's National Medical Center, Washington, DC.

seen. Prenatal testing using chorionic villi sampling or amniocentesis can detect the disease in the fetus. Treatment is supportive. The goal of medical management is to maintain normal hemoglobin levels. Blood transfusion is the conventional therapy used to treat children with severe disease. Since iron overload is a side effect of this treatment, children may need to receive an iron-chelating drug such as deferoxamine, which binds excess iron so it can be excreted by the kidneys. Other potential complications of long-term transfusion therapy are transfusion reactions and alloimmunization (antibody formation). Hematopoietic stem cell transplantation is a successful therapy for children newly diagnosed with the disorder (Reed, Walters, & Lubin, 2000).

NURSING MANAGEMENT

Nursing care focuses on observing for complications of transfusion therapy, providing emotional support, and referring the family for genetic counseling. Transfusions of packed cells are often given and careful evaluation for transfusion reactions is needed (see "Clinical Manifestations: Blood Transfusion Reactions" on page 1498). Teach parents the technique for subcutaneous infusion of deferoxamine if that route is to be used for therapy at home. Give parents information about thalassemia and its treatment, and encourage them to obtain genetic counseling. Provide emotional support and encourage parents to take an active role in the child's treatment regimen.

Compliance with transfusion therapy often becomes an issue as children reach adolescence. Offering the adolescent treatment options, such as when to undergo transfusion, can help improve compliance. Adolescents with β-thalassemia and parents of newly diagnosed children can be referred to the Thalassemia Action Group, a national organization for patients, or to the Cooley's Anemia Foundation. Expected outcomes of nursing care include maintenance of normal hemoglobin and hematocrit, safe transfusion of blood products, maintenance of recommended body iron levels, and family understanding about the genetic transmission of the disease.

APLASTIC ANEMIA

Aplastic anemia is a deficiency of the blood cells that results from failure of the bone marrow to produce adequate numbers of circulating blood cells. The condition may be congenital or acquired. It is most common from 15 to 25 years of age, and occurs more often in Asian populations (Derivan & Ferrante, 2000).

Congenital aplastic anemia (Fanconi anemia) is a rare autosomal recessive syndrome consisting of multiple congenital anomalies. Symptoms can include **purpura** (bleeding into the tissues), **petechiae** (pinpoint lesions), bleeding, fa-

CLINICAL MANIFESTATIONS

β-THALASSEMIA

BODY ORGAN	CLINICAL MANIFESTATIONS
Red blood cells (anemia)	Hypochromic and microcytic changes
	Folic acid deficiency
	Frequent epistaxis
Skeletal changes	Osteoporosis
	Delayed growth
	Susceptibility to pathologic fractures
	Facial deformities: enlarged head, prominent forehead due to frontal and parietal bossing, prominent cheek bones, broadened and depressed bridge of nose, enlarged maxilla with protruding front teeth, eyes with mongolian slant and epicanthal fold
Heart	Chronic congestive heart failure
	Myocardial fibrosis
	Murmurs
Liver/gallbladder	Hepatomegaly
	Hepatic insufficiency
Spleen	Splenomegaly
Endocrine system	Delayed sexual maturation
	Fibrotic pancreas, resulting in diabetes mellitus
Skin	Darkening of skin

tigue, and pallor. Laboratory findings include neutropenia or anemia and thrombocytopenia (low platelet count) that progresses to **pancytopenia** (decreased number of blood cell components).

Children with congenital aplastic anemia are at risk for developing malignancies such as acute nonlymphocytic leukemia (D'Andrea & Hord, 2004). The treatment of choice is bone marrow transplantation. However, the prognosis is poor, and death usually results from overwhelming infection, hemorrhage, or malignancy.

Acquired aplastic anemia in children is either idiopathic or occurs from a drug reaction. It can develop after exposure to ionizing radiation or insecticides or after ingestion of drugs such as sulfonamides, chloramphenicol, quinacrine, benzene solvents in model airplane glue, or lead. This type of anemia can also be a result of an infectious process such as viral hepatitis, mononucleosis, cytomegalovirus, tuberculosis, and human immunodeficiency virus.

Symptoms are related to the degree of bone marrow failure and can include petechiae, purpura, bleeding, pallor, weakness, tachycardia, and fatigue. Diagnosis is made by blood studies, which reveal leukopenia (low white blood cell count) with marked neutropenia, thrombocytopenia, and pancytopenia; and by bone marrow aspiration, which reveals yellow, fatty bone marrow instead of red bone marrow.

Supportive treatment includes transfusions of packed cells, platelets, or both. Immunosuppressive drug therapy is effective for many children. The treatment of choice is bone marrow transplantation from a compatible sibling or family member donor.

NURSING MANAGEMENT

Nursing care is similar to that for the child with leukemia (see Chapter 50 ∞). Nursing actions focus on preventing bleeding, administering and monitoring blood transfusions, preventing infection, encouraging mobility as tolerated, educating the parents and child about the disorder, and providing emotional support. Families need support in dealing with a child who has a life-threatening disease. Refer them to support groups for counseling, if indicated, and to social services. Expected outcomes of nursing care include maintenance of normal levels of white and red blood cells and platelets to support body functions.

CLOTTING DISORDERS

HEMOPHILIA

Hemophilia refers to a group of hereditary bleeding disorders that result from a deficiency in specific clotting factors. Hemophilia A, or classic hemophilia, is caused by a deficiency of factor VIII in the blood and accounts for 80% of persons with hemophilia. About 1 in 5000 male babies has hemophilia A. Hemophilia B, known as Christmas disease, is caused by a deficiency of factor IX. Of people with hemophilia, 15% have hemophilia B (Curry, 2004; Nechyba & Gunn, 2002).

ETIOLOGY AND PATHOPHYSIOLOGY

Hemophilia is an X-linked recessive trait, which manifests almost exclusively as affected males and carrier females. Genes for clotting factors VIII and IX are located near the terminal long arm of the X chromosome (Montgomery & Scott, 2004). A daughter who inherits the trait from her father has a 50% chance at each pregnancy of transmitting it to her sons (see Chapter 3 for a description of genetic transmission ∞). However, as many as one third of hemophiliacs have no family members with a history of clotting disorders. In these cases the disorder is caused by a new mutation. The degree of bleeding is related to the amount of clotting factor and the severity of the injury.

CLINICAL MANIFESTATIONS

Hemophilia is manifested in different children by bleeding tendencies that range from mild to moderate or severe. Children with hemophilia often do not manifest symptoms until after 6 months of age as they become more mobile and incur injuries and bleeding from falls or from tooth eruption. Spontaneous bleeding, **hemarthrosis** (bleeding into a joint space), and deep tissue hemorrhage occur. Affected children frequently experience bleeding into the joint spaces of the knees, ankles, and elbows. Bleeding into joint spaces or bursae causes the child to have limited motion because of pain, tenderness, and swelling. Bone changes, contractures, and disabling deformities can result from immobility and from the effects of blood in the joint structures.

Children may have bleeding after circumcision, frequent bruising (**ecchymosis**), epistaxis, hematuria, and bleeding after tooth extraction, minor trauma, or minor surgical procedures. Large subcutaneous and intramuscular hemorrhages sometimes occur. Bleeding into the tissues of the neck, mouth, or chest is particularly serious because of the potential for airway obstruction. Retroperitoneal and intracranial bleeding may also occur and can be life threatening (Stover, 2000).

Females who carry the trait for hemophilia do not usually manifest symptoms of the disease. However, they may have prolonged bleeding during dental work, surgery, or trauma.

CLINICAL THERAPY

Affected people and carriers can be diagnosed before birth through chorionic villus sampling or amniocentesis. Genetic testing of family members is increasingly being used to identify carriers. Diagnosis can also be made on the basis of the history, physical examination, and laboratory data. Laboratory tests show low levels of factor VIII or IX, and prolonged activated partial prothrombin time (APPT). Prothrombin time (PT), thrombin time (TT), fibrinogen, and platelet count are normal.

The goal of medical management is to control bleeding by replacing the missing clotting factor. Replacement therapy is indicated when the child experiences a mild or major hemorrhage or faces a life-threatening situation. Prompt, adequate treatment is needed to prevent serious bleeding episodes and their sequelae (Stover, 2000). A synthetic drug effective against mild hemophilia is desmopressin acetate (DDAVP). An analogue of vasopressin, DDAVP is administered intravenously and causes a two- to fourfold increase in factor VIII activity.

The outlook for children with hemophilia has been greatly improved by the availability of transfusion therapy.

Transfusions started at home and early interventions prevent many disease complications. In the past, many children with factor VIII deficiency died in the first 5 years of life. Today, children with moderate or mild hemophilia can lead normal lives. Gene therapy is being explored for treatment of hemophilia. One approach is to infuse carrier organisms into the body where they would act on target cells to promote manufacture of deficient clotting factor. These research approaches offer the promise of new treatment options in the future (White, 2001).

NURSING MANAGEMENT

NURSING ASSESSMENT AND DIAGNOSIS

Physiologic Assessment

Obtain a complete medical history from the parents or child. In particular, ask about previous episodes of bleeding and the occurrence of hemophilia or any other bleeding disorders in family members. The history of bleeding will vary, depending on the severity of the disease.

Assess the child for any joint pain, swelling, or permanent deformity, particularly around the knees, elbows, ankles, and shoulders. Note the presence of hematuria and mild flank pain. Conduct a neurologic assessment, as the risk for intracranial hemorrhage and bleeding can lead to peripheral neuropathies.

Screen the adolescent with hemophilia for HIV. Present testing methods make transmission of HIV to individuals with hemophilia very unusual. However, before universal testing of the blood supply began in 1985, significant numbers of hemophiliacs acquired HIV from infusions (see Chapter 44 ∞).

Psychosocial Assessment

It is difficult for families to manage care of the child with hemophilia, especially if the disease is severe. Assess the family's coping mechanisms and support systems. Ask whether the family's health insurance covers the child's medical expenses; the factor concentrates and infusion equipment are costly. The child may qualify for financial assistance due to the disease and state of disability. Find out if the parents have respite care that lets them take time for themselves while knowing that the child is cared for safely. Assess older children's understanding of the disease and their adaptation to it.

Developmental Assessment

Because the child with hemophilia may have physical activity restrictions, physical skills may be delayed. Perform frequent developmental assessments, being particularly attentive to fine and gross motor skills.

The most important nursing diagnosis for the child with hemophilia is *Risk for Injury* related to bleeding disorder. Some of the other nursing diagnoses that might apply include the following:

- *Pain* related to bleeding episodes
- *Impaired Physical Mobility* related to joint stiffness or contractures
- *Impaired Home Maintenance Management* related to challenges of hemophilia
- *Interrupted Family Processes* related to family role shift required to care for a child with a chronic illness
- *Delayed Growth and Development* related to effects of physical disability

PLANNING AND IMPLEMENTATION

Nursing care focuses on preventing and controlling bleeding episodes, limiting joint involvement and managing pain, and providing emotional support. Both short-term interventions and long-term management are necessary.

Prevent and Control Bleeding Episodes

Bleeding problems are rare in infants with hemophilia. As children learn to walk and develop other motor skills, however, they often fall and suffer cuts and bruises. The risk of injury can be reduced by emphasizing to parents the need for close supervision and a safe environment. Parents should encourage children to play with safe, age-appropriate toys.

NURSING PRACTICE

Take the following precautions when caring for children with bleeding disorders:

- Avoid taking temperatures rectally or giving suppositories.
- Check blood pressure by cuff as infrequently as possible.
- Avoid intramuscular or subcutaneous injections.
- Use only paper or silk tape for dressings.
- When indicated, perform mouth care every 3 hours with a glycerin swab.
- Except for factor replacement therapy, avoid all venipunctures.
- Use a peripheral finger stick to obtain blood samples.
- Do not give aspirin, ibuprofen, or other drugs that affect bleeding time.

If dental surgery or tooth extraction is necessary, it is performed in a controlled environment by experienced staff. Use of a dental irrigation device is often recommended if the child has excess bleeding from gums. Advise adolescents to shave only with an electric razor.

Control any superficial bleeding by applying pressure to the area for at least 15 minutes. Immobilize and elevate the affected area, and apply ice packs to promote vasoconstriction.

If significant bleeding does occur, offer supportive measures and assist with factor replacement therapy. Carefully monitor the child's condition for any side effects when factor replacement therapy is administered.

Limit Joint Involvement and Manage Pain

During bleeding episodes, hemarthrosis is managed by elevating and immobilizing the joint and applying ice packs. Administer analgesics as ordered. Once bleeding has been controlled, range of motion exercises strengthen muscles and joints and prevent flexion contractures. Physical therapy may be needed. Because excessive weight can place an added stress on joints, encourage the child to maintain an appropriate weight.

Provide Emotional Support

The needs of families with hemophiliac children are best met through a comprehensive team approach. Refer the parents for genetic counseling as soon as possible after diagnosis. It is important to identify family members who carry the trait, as they may suffer excessive bleeding during surgery.

Encourage the parents to verbalize their feelings. Be understanding and sensitive to their needs. Teach the parents about hemophilia and explain how the disorder affects both the child and other family members. Refer the parents and child to organizations such as the National Hemophilia Foundation for further information. (See the Companion Website for links to such resources.)

Discharge Planning and Home Care Teaching

The child may be hospitalized briefly during the first manifestation of bleeding for diagnosis and management. After that, most care takes place in the home. Identify and address home care needs well in advance of discharge. Advise parents to have the child wear a medical identification bracelet. Explain the cause of bleeding so both the child and parents understand the disease process. Teach the child and family how to identify internal bleeding. Signs and symptoms such as joint pain, abdominal pain, and obvious bleeding are indicators for immediate factor infusion. Make sure the child and parents know what situations could cause bleeding to occur. Teach parents to give acetaminophen instead of aspirin to relieve pain.

Instruct the parents and the child, when appropriate, to prepare and administer factor concentrate. If infusion of the missing factor is scheduled regularly, bleeding episodes can be controlled or avoided. Have the parents demonstrate the procedure and make sure they can administer the product correctly. The parents need to be familiar with properties of the factor concentrate to prepare the mixture correctly.

The child will need an individualized school health plan (see Chapter 39 ∞). Members of the school staff should be instructed in management of emergencies, and infusion equipment should be readily available. Identify key school personnel and teach them to provide competent and prompt care for the hemophiliac child.

Help the family and school plan an appropriate schedule of activities without overprotecting the child. Children with hemophilia should not engage in contact sports such as football and soccer, which may result in injury and trauma. Instead, encourage sports such as swimming, hiking, and bicycling.

Explain how the parents can coordinate their child's care with a number of health professionals. Provide ongoing case management, assisting the family to take on this task if able.

Hemophilia is not only a debilitating disorder for the child. It also can be financially draining for the family. Frequent outpatient visits, emergency department visits, hospital admissions, and the cost of factor concentrate can exhaust a family's resources. If indicated, refer families to appropriate social services (e.g., the state's maternal and child health program for children with special healthcare needs) and organizations such as the National Hemophilia Foundation. Sharing experiences with other families of children with hemophilia can provide support.

EVALUATION

Expected outcomes of nursing care include the following:

- Prevention of injury to the child
- Management of pain to promote comfort level
- Promotion of normal growth and development
- Adequate knowledge of child and family for disease management, including recognition of bleeding and prompt initiation of infusions

VON WILLEBRAND DISEASE

Like hemophilia, von Willebrand disease is a hereditary bleeding disorder. There are about 20 different disorders involving a deficiency of von Willebrand factor, a plasma

MediaLink | Ethical Considerations: Hemophilia

protein and the carrier for clotting factor VIII; it plays a necessary role in platelet adhesion (McDaniel, 2000). The most common form of the disorder is transmitted as an autosomal dominant trait, and it can occur in both males and females. The gene for the disease is located on chromosome 12.

The characteristic manifestations are easy bruising and epistaxis. Children with von Willebrand disease frequently have gingival bleeding and increased bleeding with lacerations or during surgery. Affected teenage girls may have menorrhagia (increased menstrual bleeding).

Diagnosis of von Willebrand disease is made after laboratory studies reveal decreased von Willebrand factor levels, von Willebrand factor antigen levels, and factor VIII activity; reduced platelet agglutination; prolonged bleeding time; and prolonged or normal activated partial thromboplastin time (APTT). Treatment is similar to that for the child with hemophilia and involves infusion of von Willebrand protein concentrate. For bleeding episodes or prior to surgery, DDAVP is infused. Locally administered medications such as aminocaproic acid are sometimes used to manage bleeding in the mucous membranes.

NURSING MANAGEMENT

Teach parents about the disorder and instruct them not to give the child any aspirin or other drugs that can cause bleeding or inhibit platelet function. Teach management of bleeding episodes and intravenous infusion techniques, as for hemophilia. The prognosis is good, and children with von Willebrand disease usually have a normal life expectancy. Expected outcomes of nursing care include prompt management of bleeding and prevention of disease complications.

DISSEMINATED INTRAVASCULAR COAGULATION

Disseminated intravascular coagulation (DIC) is a life-threatening, acquired pathologic process in which the clotting system is abnormally activated, resulting in widespread clot formation in the small vessels throughout the body. Excess thrombin is generated, followed by deposition of fibrin strands in body tissues. These changes cause tissue hypoxia, resulting in eventual tissue necrosis. The circulating fibrin fragments later begin to interfere with platelet aggregation and other aspects of the clotting mechanism, resulting in bleeding or hemorrhage.

DIC is a complication of other serious illnesses in infants and children, such as hypoxia, shock, cancer, and viruses. Symptoms can include diffuse bleeding mani-

fested by hematuria, petechiae, or purpura; an injection site that continues to ooze; circulatory collapse; and major vessel thrombosis. The prothrombin time and partial thromboplastin time are prolonged, platelet count and fibrinogen levels are increased, and levels of fibrin–fibrinogen split products are high.

Medical management is supportive and includes identification and treatment of the underlying disorder; replacement of depleted coagulation factors, fibrinogen, and platelets; and anticoagulant therapy (heparin).

NURSING MANAGEMENT

DIC is a complex disorder managed by a critical care team. Nursing care focuses on assessing the bleeding, preventing further injury, and administering prescribed therapies. Observe for petechiae, ecchymoses, and oozing every 1 to 2 hours. Be sure to check dependent areas (those lower than other body parts), as blood pools in these areas. Intravenous sites are particularly prone to oozing and should be assessed every 15 minutes. Examine stool for the presence of blood, and measure blood loss as accurately as possible. Measure intake and output.

Because all body systems can be involved, careful, continuous assessment of all systems is needed. Institute bleeding control precautions, monitor prescribed therapy (transfusion, anticoagulant therapy), and report any signs of complications. Desired outcomes of nursing care are management of bleeding and adequate function of all body systems. Adequate family support in this life-threatening situation is a focus of nursing care.

IDIOPATHIC THROMBOCYTOPENIC PURPURA

Idiopathic thrombocytopenic purpura (ITP), also known as autoimmune thrombocytopenic purpura, is a disorder characterized by increased destruction of platelets, even though platelet production in the bone marrow is normal. When the rate of platelet destruction exceeds the rate of platelet production, the number of circulating platelets decreases and blood clotting slows.

ITP is the most common bleeding disorder in children. It occurs most frequently in children 2 to 10 years of age and usually follows a viral infection such as measles, chickenpox, or rubella, as part of an inappropriate immune response (Bolton-Maggs, 2000). Symptoms include multiple ecchymoses, petechiae, purpura, bleeding from gums or nose, and blood in urine or stools. Diagnosis is made by history and through physical and laboratory findings, which show a decreased platelet count and antiplatelet antibodies in the peripheral blood. Antinuclear antibodies may be present. Treatment includes administering corticosteroids and intravenous immunoglobulins. For children who do not respond to drug therapy over a period of 6 months to 1 year, splenectomy may be the treatment of choice. At least half the children affected have complete remission (Jayabose, Levendoglu-Tugal, Ozkaynkak et al., 2004).

NURSING MANAGEMENT

Nursing care focuses on controlling and reducing the number of bleeding episodes. Preventive measures are similar to those for the child with hemophilia. Teach parents to use acetaminophen, rather than aspirin, to control pain. Provide emotional support to the family. Have the child avoid contact sports. Perform careful assessments of bleeding and take vital signs. Expected outcomes of care are prevention of bleeding and restoration of normal coagulation patterns.

MENINGOCOCCEMIA

Meningococcemia is the most severe disease process that follows infection with *Neisseria meningitidis* or, occasionally, other microorganisms such as *H influenzae* or *Streptococcus pneumoniae*. The disorder is thought to be an immune response to the endotoxins of the organism. Since it seriously affects circulation and is an infection carried by blood it is discussed here although it can have multisystem effects.

Onset is sudden: A respiratory infection is followed by high fever, petechial rash, massive skin and mucosal hemorrhage, hypotension, disseminated intravascular coagulation, and shock. The child, usually under 2 years of age and commonly under 4 months, is critically ill and demonstrates multisystem disease. Symptoms can progress to a critical level within 12 to 48 hours of onset (Smillova & Walker, 2000). Commonly the skin turns pink and then black as the tissues are damaged by reduced oxygen delivery. Limbs may need to be amputated as a result of impaired circulation.

Treatment consists of antibiotics, removal from sources of infection, and multisystem shock management (refer to Chapter 48 for a description of distributive shock ∞). Prompt administration of antibiotics to the child who manifests fever with purpura can decrease the severity of outcome. Depending on the child's condition, total parenteral nutrition, sedation and pain relief, dialysis, or amputation may be required. Close contacts of the child should receive prophylactic antibiotics.

NURSING MANAGEMENT

Nursing care of the child with meningococcemia is complex. Treatment must begin quickly, and the child generally has a lengthy hospitalization in a pediatric intensive care unit (Smillova & Walker, 2000). Perform thorough assessments of all body systems. Administer intravenous infusions when ordered to ensure correct and timely administration of antibiotics and other therapies. Measure urinary output to evaluate kidney function. Meticulous skin care is necessary to preserve the integrity of tissues. Take care to prevent further infections. Nutritional support in the form of total parenteral nutrition is common. The family needs support to deal with the changing critical nature of the child's illness and the possibility that death or permanent, severe deformities will result. When the child improves, continuing comprehensive care in the hospital and then in the community is needed to manage complex issues related to growth, development, nutrition, amputations, and prosthetics. Expected outcomes of nursing care include prevention of further infection, maintenance of body systems during acute phase of illness, and positive adjustment to amputations and deformities resulting from the disease.

HEMATOPOIETIC STEM CELL TRANSPLANTATION (HSCT)

Hematopoietic stem cell transplantation is a treatment used for diseases such as severe combined immunodeficiency disease, severe and unresponsive aplastic anemia, and leukemia. Sources of stem cells include bone marrow, peripheral blood, and cord blood. Hematopoietic stem cells exist primarily in the bone marrow but also circulate in the peripheral blood. These cells can grow into new body cells, and have become useful in treatment of immune and hematologic diseases when restoration of normal cells is needed (Trigg, 2004).

There are three types of transplant: autologous, isogeneic (or syngeneic), and allogeneic. In *autologous* transplantation, the child's own cells are taken, stored, and reinfused after the child has received chemotherapy. In *isogeneic* transplantation, the cells are taken from an identical twin. In *allogeneic* transplantation, the donor, usually a sibling, has a compatible human leukocyte antigen (HLA). When no relative is found to match the child, a histocompatible donor may be sought from the National Marrow Donor Program.

The transplantation procedure begins with chemotherapy and, sometimes, total body irradiation directed at destroying circulating blood cells and the diseased bone

⊙ **FIGURE 49–5**

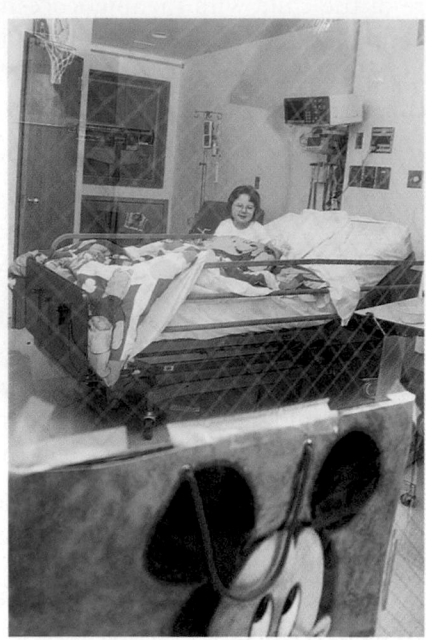

The child undergoing bone marrow transplantation is hospitalized in a special unit while receiving chemotherapy before the transfusion. The child remains in the unit for several weeks afterward until the new marrow produces enough cells to maintain immunity.

marrow in the ill child. Following this treatment, the child is transfused with the donor cells. If the transplantation is successful, the cells implant themselves in the bone and begin to grow. Healthy bone marrow, capable of making blood cells, is the result.

The chemotherapy program for destruction of bone marrow takes 4 to 12 days. During this time, the child is cared for in strict isolation in a special unit that provides a germ-free environment (Figure 49–5 ⊙). Side effects of chemotherapy provide challenges for care in addition to those of preventing infection (see Chapter 50 ∞). The child is without any immunity for a minimum of 10 days after transplantation. It takes 2 to 4 weeks for the donor cells to begin proliferation and maturation. Medications to stimulate the production of red and white blood cells are administered during this period.

Pancytopenia (marked decrease in RBCs, WBCs, and platelets) lasts for several weeks following the transplant. Major risks during this period are anemia, infections, and bleeding. Once the bone marrow begins to produce new cells, graft-versus-host disease (rejection) is the major

threat. Refer to Chapter 44 for a discussion of graft-versus-host disease. ∞

Monitor for this multisystem disorder by assessing the skin, mucous membranes, gastrointestinal function, respiratory function, cardiac function, and hydration status. Because graft-versus-host disease may occur at any time, even after the child returns home, frequent thorough assessments are necessary after discharge.

Supportive care after the transplantation procedure focuses on preventing infection, controlling bleeding, maintaining a nutritious diet and hydration, monitoring for signs of rejection, and providing psychosocial support. The treatment is lengthy, the child is often critically ill, and parents may have traveled to a medical center many miles from home for the procedure. Ask parents about other family members and how they are managing. Provide information about inexpensive housing available near the medical center, such as in a Ronald McDonald house. Encourage parents to discuss their feelings with other parents of children receiving bone marrow transplantation. Organizations such as the Bone Marrow Transplant Family Support Network can serve as resources for families.

When the child is ready for discharge, be sure the family is prepared to administer medications, recognize signs of graft-versus-host disease, provide adequate nutrition for the child, and perform other necessary care. Arrange for follow-up visits and provide the names of local healthcare contact people who can offer support and provide information. The child may need tutors or other educational assistance to promote integration back into the school setting. The major expected outcome of nursing care is the proper activity of bone marrow in the child with resulting normal levels and function of blood cells. Other outcomes are provision of family support, ongoing care and education for the child, adequate nutrition, and prevention of infection. See "Health Promotion: The Child with Hematopoietic Stem Cell Transplantation (HSCT)."

 GROWTH AND DEVELOPMENT

Hospitalizations of children undergoing hematopoietic stem cell transplantation are usually lengthy. Evaluate the child's age and developmental stage and establish developmental goals to be met during the hospitalization. Implement nursing plans to meet the child's developmental needs and encourage further growth. Implement health promotion and health maintenance measures with the family.

HEALTH PROMOTION
The Child with Hematopoietic Stem Cell Transplantation (HSCT)

Growth and Development

- Measure and plot height and weight at each visit using standard growth curve charts.
- Measure onset and progression of puberty using Tanner staging.
- An individualized education plan (IEP) should be performed yearly to identify learning problems.
- Routine hearing screening is advised since hearing loss may occur as a result of ototoxic drug therapy.
- Vision should be screened at each primary care visit since corticosteroid use can cause cataracts, chronic graft versus host disease (GVHD) can result in keratoconjunctivitis, and cytomegalovirus (CMV) can cause retinitis.
- Blood pressure should be monitored each visit since children are commonly placed on medication for hypertension after HSCT because of nephrotoxic medications.
- Instruct parents to record blood pressure at home if necessary.

Nutrition

- Teach family to avoid foods with potential vectors for infection, such as unpasteurized products and undercooked meats.
- A low-sodium diet may be required if the child has hypertension.
- Calcium supplements may be administered to reduce the risk of osteopenia.

Physical Activity

- If the child has thrombocytopenia, physical activity may be restricted.
- The child may experience fatigue. Ask about activity tolerance.

Oral Health

- Dental screening and any required restorative care should be done before transplant to reduce potential sources of infection.

- Routine dental care is resumed once the child's immune system is restored. Ask the family about the child's routine dental care.

Mental and Spiritual Health

- Apply developmental approaches to assess the child's feelings after a HSCT.
- Ask the child about coping with being in the hospital and at home rather than attending school.
- Many physical changes occur with treatment that may interfere with body image. Assess the child's or adolescent's body image in a manner appropriate to age.

Relationships

- In-hospital or in-home schooling is required after HSCT for 6 to 12 months until immune function has been obtained to reduce the risk of infection.
- Encourage peer contact, telephone calls, e-mail, and letters to reduce the child's feelings of isolation.
- On returning to school, the child is encouraged to participate fully in school activities.
- For the adolescent, sex education is important, especially to avoid sexually transmitted infections.

Disease Prevention Strategies

- Teach the family that handwashing is essential to prevent the spread of infection.
- The child should have his or her own eating utensils. Teach safe food preparation techniques.
- In-home childcare is recommended because of the risk of infection in other childcare settings.
- Teach the family that the child should have minimal direct contact with animals to avoid infections.
- Determine the child's immunization schedule and the need for immunizations.
- Encourage the family to obtain an influenza vaccine annually for the child and all household or close contacts.
- Teach signs and symptoms of infection and stress the importance of prompt reporting.

Injury Prevention Strategies

- Ask the family how they store medications.
- Ask the family how they dispose of used needles and syringes.

Critical Concept Review

LEARNING OBJECTIVES	CONCEPTS
Describe the function of red blood cells, white blood cells, and platelets.	1. Red blood cells: ■ Transport oxygen from the lungs to the tissues. ■ Transport carbon dioxide back to the lungs. 2. White blood cells: ■ Protect the body against bacterial invaders. 3. Platelets: ■ Are cells that form hemostatic plugs to stop bleeding.
Discuss the pathophysiology and clinical manifestations of the major disorders of red blood cells affecting the pediatric population.	Iron deficiency anemia: 1. Pathophysiology: ■ Lower than average number of red blood cells caused by blood loss, insufficient oral intake of iron, and increased internal demands due to rapid growth. 2. Clinical manifestations: ■ Pallor. ■ Fatigue. ■ Irritability. Normocytic anemia: 1. Pathophysiology: ■ Increased number of red blood cells that are normal in size with pale centers. ■ Occurs because of hemorrhage, disease-induced inflammation, DIC, G6PD deficiency, and hemolytic uremic syndrome. 2. Clinical manifestations: ■ Same as iron deficiency anemia. ■ Hepatomegaly and splenomegaly. Sickle cell anemia: 1. Pathophysiology: ■ Some or all normal hemoglobin is replaced with sickle-shaped cells. ■ Sickle shape is rigid, fragile, and breaks down faster. ■ Rigidity of cells causes clumping and obstruction of capillary blood flow. 2. Clinical manifestations: ■ Pain. ■ Splenic sequestration. ■ Febrile illnesses. ■ Tissue destruction. ■ Anemia. ■ Vaso-occlusive crisis. Thalassemias: 1. Pathophysiology: ■ Production of beta chain of hemoglobin is impaired. ■ Red blood cells are fragile and have a decreased life span. ■ Increased hemolysis leads to hemosiderin and hemochromatosis. 2. Clinical manifestations: ■ Pallor. ■ Failure to thrive in the infant. ■ Hepatosplenomegaly. ■ Severe anemia.
Discuss the pathophysiology and clinical manifestations of the major disorders of white blood cells affecting the pediatric population.	Aplastic anemia: 1. Pathophysiology: ■ Failure of the bone marrow stem cells to produce all types of blood cells. 2. Clinical manifestations: ■ Anemia. ■ Neutropenia. ■ Infection.

LEARNING OBJECTIVES

CONCEPTS

Discuss the pathophysiology and clinical manifestations of the major disorders of white blood cells affecting the pediatric population.—*continued*

→
- Thrombocytopenia.
- Fever.
- Fatigue.
- Congestive heart failure.
- Tachycardia.

Discuss the pathophysiology and clinical manifestations of the major disorders of platelets affecting the pediatric population.

→
Hemophilia:
1. Pathophysiology:
   - A group of genetic disorders that occurs primarily in males and causes a deficiency of specific clotting factors.
2. Clinical manifestations:
   - Mild to severe bleeding tendencies.
   - Bleeding usually occurs from minor trauma.
   - Hemarthrosis frequently occurs.
Von Willebrand Disease:
1. Pathophysiology:
   - A genetic bleeding disorder that occurs in both men and women, and results in a deficiency of the plasma protein that carries clotting factor VIII.
2. Clinical manifestations:
   - Frequent bruising (ecchymosis).
   - Epistaxis.
   - Increased bleeding with surgery, lacerations, and dental extractions.
   - Teenage girls have increased menstrual bleeding.
Disseminated intravascular coagulation:
1. Pathophysiology:
   - An acquired, abnormal activation of the clotting system resulting in widespread clot formation throughout the body.
   - Results from excessive thrombin formation caused by severe physiologic stress to the body.
2. Clinical manifestations:
   - Diffuse bleeding and oozing.
   - Shock.
   - Hypotension.
   - Impaired tissue perfusion.
Idiopathic thrombocytopenia purpura:
1. Pathophysiology:
   - Increased destruction of platelets in the spleen with normal platelet production.
   - Usually follows a viral illness.
2. Clinical manifestations:
   - Multiple ecchymoses.
   - Petechiae.
   - Bleeding from gums.
   - Epistaxis.
   - Blood in urine and stool.

Describe the nursing management and collaborative care of a child with a hematologic disorder.

→
1. Prepare child for frequent blood tests.
2. Monitor child for transfusion reactions.
3. Prevent infection:
   - Perform frequent handwashing.
   - Limit child's contact with anyone with signs and symptoms of infection.
4. Provide for periods of rest.
5. Encourage intake of foods high in iron content.
6. Limit invasive procedures to prevent bleeding.
7. Teach family and/or child to avoid the use of aspirin products.

Discuss nursing implications for a child receiving hematopoietic stem cell transplantation (HSCT).

→
1. Prevent infection:
   - Child may be placed in protective isolation.
   - Avoid fresh fruit and flowers.

(continued)

LEARNING OBJECTIVES   CONCEPTS

Discuss nursing implications for a child receiving hematopoietic stem cell transplantation (HSCT).—*continued*	2. Control bleeding:
	  ■ Limit invasive procedures.
	  ■ No intramuscular injections or rectal temperature assessment.
	  ■ Maintain pressure on any injection site for at least five minutes.
	  ■ Transfuse with red blood cells or platelets as needed.
	3. Maintain adequate nutrients and hydration:
	  ■ Implement total parenteral nutrition (TPN) as needed.
	  ■ Provide frequent, small meals.
	4. Monitor for signs of rejection:
	  ■ Assess temperature frequently.
	  ■ Assess skin and GI system for signs and symptoms for graft versus host disease (GVHD).
	5. Provide emotional support to the child and family.

CRITICAL THINKING IN ACTION

*View the **Critical Thinking in Action** video in Chapter 49 of the CD-ROM. Then, answer the questions that follow.*

Frederick is admitted to the hospital with severe abdominal pain. He has been hospitalized for his sickle cell anemia several times in the past and now as an 8-year-old, he and his mother are very familiar with the routine. The disease is stable most of the time, but about twice annually he is admitted to the hospital for complications of the disorder. His mother expresses how upsetting it is to watch her son suffering pain from this disease.

In the hospital a priority of nursing intervention is to control Frederick's pain. The doctor diagnoses that the abdominal pain is caused by sickled cells in his spleen. Frederick's hemoglobin is 6 g/dL, so a blood transfusion is ordered. Fluids and oxygen are also administered. Frequent vital signs and other monitoring are performed to identify any infections.

1. Besides correcting the anemia, what is another reason Frederick would be given a transfusion?
2. How would you explain what is happening to Frederick's spleen so that it is causing the abdominal pain?
3. In what way does sickle cell anemia affect the various systems of the body?
4. When giving a blood transfusion to Frederick, should warm or cold blood be given? What is the reason for your answer?

MEDIALINK   www.prenhall.com/london

- NCLEX-RN® Review, case studies, and other interactive resources for this chapter can be found on the Companion Website at http://www.prenhall.com/london. Click on "Chapter 49" and select the activities for this chapter.

Sickled red blood cells

- For animations, more NCLEX-RN® Review questions, and an audio glossary, access the accompanying CD-ROM in this textbook.

REFERENCES

American Academy of Pediatrics. (2000). *Guidelines for health supervision III*. Elk Grove Village, IL: Author.

Beyer, J. E., & Simmons, L. E. (2004). Home treatment of pain for children and adolescents with sickle cell disease. *Pain Management Nursing, 5,* 126–135.

Bolton-Maggs, P. H. B. (2000). Idiopathic thrombocytopenic purpura. *Archives of Disease in Childhood, 83,* 220–223.

Boxer, L. A. (2004). Leukopenia. In R. E. Behrman, R. M. Kliegman, & H. B. Jenson (Eds.), *Nelson textbook of pediatrics* (17th ed., pp. 717–723). Philadelphia: WB Saunders.

Carley, A. (2003). Anemia: When is it iron deficiency? *Pediatric Nursing, 29,* 128–133.

Cook, L. S. (2000). A simple case of anemia: Pathophysiology of a common symptom. *Journal of Intravenous Nursing, 23,* 271–281.

Committee on Nutrition, American Academy of Pediatrics. (2004). *Pediatric nutrition handbook* (5th ed.). Elk Grove Village, IL: American Academy of Pediatrics.

Curry, H. (2004). Bleeding disorder basics. *Pediatric Nursing 30,* 402–429.

D'Andrea, A. D., & Hord, J. D. (2004). The pancytopenias. In R. E. Behrman, R. M. Kliegman, & H. B. Jenson (Eds.), *Nelson textbook of pediatrics* (17th ed., pp. 1642–1646). Philadelphia: WB Saunders.

Day, S. W., & Wynn, L. W. (2000). Sickle cell pain & hydroxyurea. *American Journal of Nursing, 100,* 32–38.

Derivan, M., & Ferrante, C. (2000). Aplastic anemia. *Clinical Journal of Oncology Nursing, 5,* 228–229.

Glader, B. E., & Look, K. A. (1996). Hematologic disorders in children from Southeast Asia. *Pediatric Clinics of North America, 43*(3), 665–682.

Jacob, E., Miaskowski, C., Savedra, M., Beyer, J. E., Treadwell, M., & Styles, L. (2003).

Management of vaso-occlusive pain in children with sickle cell disease. *Journal of Pediatric Hematology/Oncology, 25,* 307–311.

Jakubik, L. D., & Thompson, M. (2000). Care of the child with sickle cell disease: Acute complications. *Pediatric Nursing, 26,* 373–380.

Jarvinen, O., Lehesjoki, A., Lindlof, M., Uutela, A., & Kaariainen, H. (2000). Carrier testing of children for two x-linked diseases: A retrospective study of comprehension of the test results and social and psychological significance of the testing. *Pediatrics, 106,* 1460–1465.

Jayabose, S., Levendoglu-Tugal, O., Ozkaynkak, J. G., Visintainer, P., & Sandor, C. (2004). Long-term outcome of chronic idiopathic thrombocytopenic purpura in children. *Journal of Pediatric Hematology and Oncology, 26,* 724–726.

McDaniel, P. (2000). Focus on factors. *Journal of Intravenous Nursing, 23,* 282–289.

Mentzer, W. C., & Cowan, M. J. (2000). Bone marrow transplantation for beta-thalassemia: The University of California San Francisco experience. *Journal of Pediatric Hematology and Oncology, 22,* 598–601.

Montgomery, R. R., & Scott, J. P. (2004). Hemorrhagic and thrombotic diseases. In R. E. Behrman, R. M. Kliegman, & H. B. Jenson (Eds.), *Nelson textbook of pediatrics* (17th ed., pp. 1651–1674). Philadelphia: WB Saunders.

National Heart, Lung, and Blood Institute. (2002). *The management of sickle cell disease.* Retrieved June 1, 2004, from http://www.nhlbi.nih.gov/health/prof/blood/sickle/sc_mngt.pdf

Nechyba, C., & Gunn, V. L. (Eds.). (2002). *The Harriet Lane handbook* (16th ed., pp. 283–306). Baltimore: Johns Hopkins University Press.

Northington, L. (2000). Chronic sorrow in caregivers of school age children with sickle cell disease:

A grounded theory approach. *Issues in Comprehensive Pediatric Nursing, 23,* 141–154.

Odesina, V. (2001). Intravenous support for the patient in sickle cell crisis. *Journal of Intravenous Nursing, 24,* 32–37.

Ogedegbe, H. O. (2002). Sickle cell disease: An overview. *Laboratory Medicine, 7,* 515–543.

Ohls, R. K., & Christensen, R. D. (2004). The hematopoietic system. In R. E. Behrman, R. M. Kliegman, & H. B. Jenson (Eds.), *Nelson textbook of pediatrics* (17th ed., pp. 1599–1604). Philadelphia: WB Saunders.

Reed, W., Walters, M., & Lubin, B. H. (2000). Collection of sibling donor cord blood for children with thalassemia. *Journal of Pediatric Hematology and Oncology, 22,* 602–604.

Smillova, A., & Walker, E. (2000). Meningococcemia: A critical care emergency. *Critical Care Nurse, 20* (5), 28–38.

Soldin, S. J., Brugnara, C. & Wong, E. C. (2003). *Pediatric reference ranges* (4th ed.) Washington, DC: AACC Press.

Stover, B. (2000). Training the client in self-management of hemophilia. *Journal of Intravenous Nursing, 23,* 304–309.

Tanyi, R. A. (2003). Sickle cell disease: Health promotion and maintenance and the role of primary care nurse practitioners. *Journal of the American Academy of Nurse Practitioners, 15,* 389–397.

Trigg, M. E. (2004). Hematopoietic stem cells. *Pediatrics, 13,* 1051–1057.

White, G. C. (2001). Gene therapy in hemophilia: Clinical trials update. *Thrombosis and Haemostasis, 86,* 172–177.

Wilson, R. E., Krishnamurti, L., & Kamat, D. (2003). Management of sickle cell disease in primary care. *Clinical Pediatrics, 42,* 753–761.

CHAPTER 50

The Child with Alterations in Cellular Growth

Rasheed was just diagnosed with leukemia seven months ago, but already, he has been in the hospital five times. This time he had enterocolitis, an infection of the intestines. But he has now improved and is determined to fight the disease. It is his will and strength that help us all to be strong and to know that he will do well after his treatment is finished.
—Mother of Rasheed, 12 years old

LEARNING OBJECTIVES

- Describe the incidence, known etiologies, and common clinical manifestations of cancer.

- Synthesize information about diagnostic tests and clinical therapy for cancer to plan comprehensive care for children undergoing these procedures.

- Integrate information about oncologic emergencies into plans for monitoring all children with cancer.

- Recognize the most common solid tumors in children, describe their treatment, and plan comprehensive nursing care.

- Plan care for children and adolescents of all ages who have a diagnosis of leukemia.

- Recognize the most common soft-tissue tumors in children, describe their treatment, and plan comprehensive care.

- Describe the impact of cancer survival on children and use this information to plan for ongoing physiologic and psychosocial care in the children's futures.

MEDIALINK

www.prenhall.com/london

CD-ROM

Videos:
    Cancer Overview
    Leukemia
Audio Glossary
NCLEX-RN® Review

Companion Website

Objectives
Drug Guide: Methotrexate
Commonly Used Chemotherapy Drug Combinations
MediaLink Applications:
    Exploring the Controversy: Stem Cell
        Transplantation
    Life with Leukemia: A Teen in Transition
Case Study: Teen with Ewing's Sarcoma
NCLEX-RN® Review

Why do children develop different types of cancers than adults? Cancer in adults is often the result of dietary practices or habits such as smoking. Some adult-onset cancers are the result of oncogenic responses to stimuli—that is, responses that stimulate cancerous changes in cells. Other cancers that occur in adults result from prolonged exposure to toxins such as coal dust and asbestos. Some cancers are known to be related to genetic causes. In adults, prevention through general lifestyle changes is a major focus of interventions. However, in children, cancer is usually embryonic (occurring during development of the fetus) or oncogenic in origin. Thus, lifestyle changes that begin in childhood have little effect on the incidence of childhood cancer, although they may help reduce the incidence of later cancer or other diseases. Occasionally, an environmental exposure is linked to the incidence of cancer in children.

Abnormal cellular growth can occur in any area of the body. Why are some growths called cancer and others not? Changes in cellular growth within the body are called **neoplasms** (meaning new growth). A neoplasm is further classified as benign or malignant. **Benign** means that a growth does not endanger life or health; it tends not to recur after treatment. **Malignant** means that if not treated a tumor will continue to grow, and will spread to other sites in the body (**metastasis**), ending in death. The common term for this type of cellular growth is cancer.

ANATOMY AND PHYSIOLOGY OF PEDIATRIC DIFFERENCES

The major physiologic difference between adults and children that affects cellular growth involves the immune system and how well it defends the body. The rate of cell growth in children also can play a role in the rapid progression of some childhood cancers. The continuing presence of fetal cells in small children is related to some cancers.

The immune system defends the body against foreign organisms and substances through two responses: nonspecific and specific. In a nonspecific response, the components of the immune system attack a variety of targets. Nonspecific components include phagocytic (cell-destroying) cells such as mononuclear leukocytes, polymorphonuclear (PMN) leukocytes, natural killer (NK) cells, and complements (noncellular proteins) that work together to destroy invading cells and substances. During the first month of a child's life, the nonspecific response is immature, so phagocytic cells have little ability to move toward cancer cells and fulfill their function. The nonspecific response is also impaired in premature and small-for-gestational-age (SGA) infants.

In a specific response, T lymphocytes and immunoglobulin (Ig) attack only one type of invader. The specific response capability also is immature in infants. B-cell production of various proteins called immunoglobins (IgM, IgG, and IgA) is below adult levels, so that the infant is vulnerable to bacterial and viral infections. (For a discussion of immune function, see Chapter 44. ∞)

In children, many cells are growing quickly; this fast growth can lead to the proliferation of cancerous as well as normal cells. Cell division that is out of control may normally trigger a mechanism called **apoptosis**, whereby the cell "realizes" something is wrong and destroys itself. The process of apoptosis or physiologic cell death may not be well developed in young children.

CHILDHOOD CANCER

The care of children who have cancer is a challenging specialty in pediatric nursing. For several years the child undergoes aggressive treatments that may

KEY TERMS

Apoptosis, 1517

Benign, 1517

Biotherapy, 1522

Carcinogens, 1518

Chemotherapy, 1522

Complementary therapy, 1527

Extravasation, 1539

Intrathecal, 1522

Leukocytosis, 1550

Leukopenia, 1550

Malignant, 1517

Metastasis, 1517

Myelosuppression, 1539

Nadir, 1530

Neoplasms, 1517

Neutropenia, 1539

Oncogene, 1519

Pancytopenia, 1550

Polypharmacy, 1539

Protocol, 1522

Proto-oncogene, 1519

Radiation, 1525

Secondary cancers, 1532

Thrombocytopenia, 1557

Tumor suppressor genes, 1520

be life threatening and cause serious illness. Sometimes the diagnosis is quite hopeful; at other times, a terminal result may be expected. The child is often cared for at home with outpatient visits for treatment and occasional hospitalization when needed. The periods of hospitalization are times of intense physical vulnerability for the child and intense emotional vulnerability for both the child and the family. To monitor the child closely, nurses need a sound knowledge of physiologic and psychologic responses, medical interventions, and nursing care. Effective communication skills are necessary to support the child and family and promote realistic hope.

INCIDENCE

In 2005, in the United States, new cancer cases are expected to number over 9500 in children under 15 years of age. Cancer causes about 1500–1600 childhood deaths and is the leading cause of disease-related death in children (National Cancer Institute, 2005). However, mortality rates have declined by over 47% since 1975, and have been relatively stable since 1990 (Woodruff, Axelrad, Kyle et al., 2004). Overall survival rate is 80% for childhood cancer (Baggott, Kelly, Fochtman et al., 2002). There is a difference in survival rates for different types of cancer ranging from 69% for neuroblastoma to 94% for Hodgkin disease (American Cancer Society, 2004). Children treated in the 1980s and 1990s have had significantly lower mortality rates than those treated in the 1960s and 1970s due to multimodal therapies including multiagent chemotherapy, surgery, and radiation therapy. Mortality rates are higher for females than males, for those diagnosed before 5 years of age, and for children with central nervous system tumor or leukemia. The cause of death for most children is recurrence of the primary cancer (Moller, Garwicz, Barlow et al., 2001). The most common forms of childhood cancers among children in different age groups are shown in Figure 50–1 (Gurney & Bondy, 2004).

ETIOLOGY AND PATHOPHYSIOLOGY

Alterations in cellular growth occur in response to external and internal stimuli. Neoplasms are caused by one or a combination of three factors: (1) external stimuli that cause genetic mutations, (2) immune system and gene abnormalities, and (3) chromosomal abnormalities.

External Stimuli

External stimuli may affect the child's general health and cause mutations in body cells. **Carcinogens** are chemicals or industrial processes that, when combined with genetic traits and in interaction with one another, result in cancer. Several carcinogens cause cancers that are diagnosed during childhood. Others cause cancers that begin in childhood but are not identified until adulthood. Some chemicals suspected of causing childhood cancer include diethylstilbestrol (maternal use of therapeutic estrogen hormones), anabolic androgenic steroids, alkylating chemotherapy agents, and immunosuppressants used for organ transplantation. Radiation exposure has been known to cause cancers such as leukemia and thyroid tumors in children exposed to nuclear fallout from atomic bombs, other nuclear accidents, and other excessive radiation sources.

External stimuli may also lead to secondary cancers in children, or those occurring after treatment for a primary cancer and of a different cellular type than the primary cancer. Secondary cancers can result when the child is treated for a primary cancer with high doses of radiation. Excessive exposure to ultraviolet radiation from the sun predisposes children to development of skin cancer in adulthood.

Immune System and Gene Abnormalities

One critical function of a normal immune system is immune surveillance, in which phagocytic cells circulate throughout the body, detecting and destroying abnormal and cancerous cells. Children with congenital immune deficiencies, such as Wiskott–Aldrich syndrome, in which immune surveillance may fail, are at high risk for cancer. A form of non-Hodgkin lymphoma develops in some children treated with immune system–suppressing drugs. Children with acquired immunodeficiency syndrome (AIDS) may be at higher risk of certain types of cancer, such as lymphoma, Kaposi sarcoma, and leiomyosarcoma (Biggar, Frisch, & Goedert, 2000).

TEACHING HIGHLIGHTS

WAYS TO DECREASE THE INCIDENCE OF CANCER IN CHILDREN

Many parents ask what they can do to decrease the incidence of cancer in children as they grow into adulthood. The three major teaching areas to address are:

Have children increase intake of fruits and vegetables. Most children do not eat enough of these foods (at least five servings/day are recommended), and increased intake is associated with lower rates of many cancers.

Protect skin with sunscreen. Early excessive exposure to sun and having been sunburned increase the chance of skin cancers in adulthood.

Discourage smoking among children and be sure children are not exposed to environmental tobacco smoke. This will decrease the future chance of developing lung cancer.

○ FIGURE 50-1

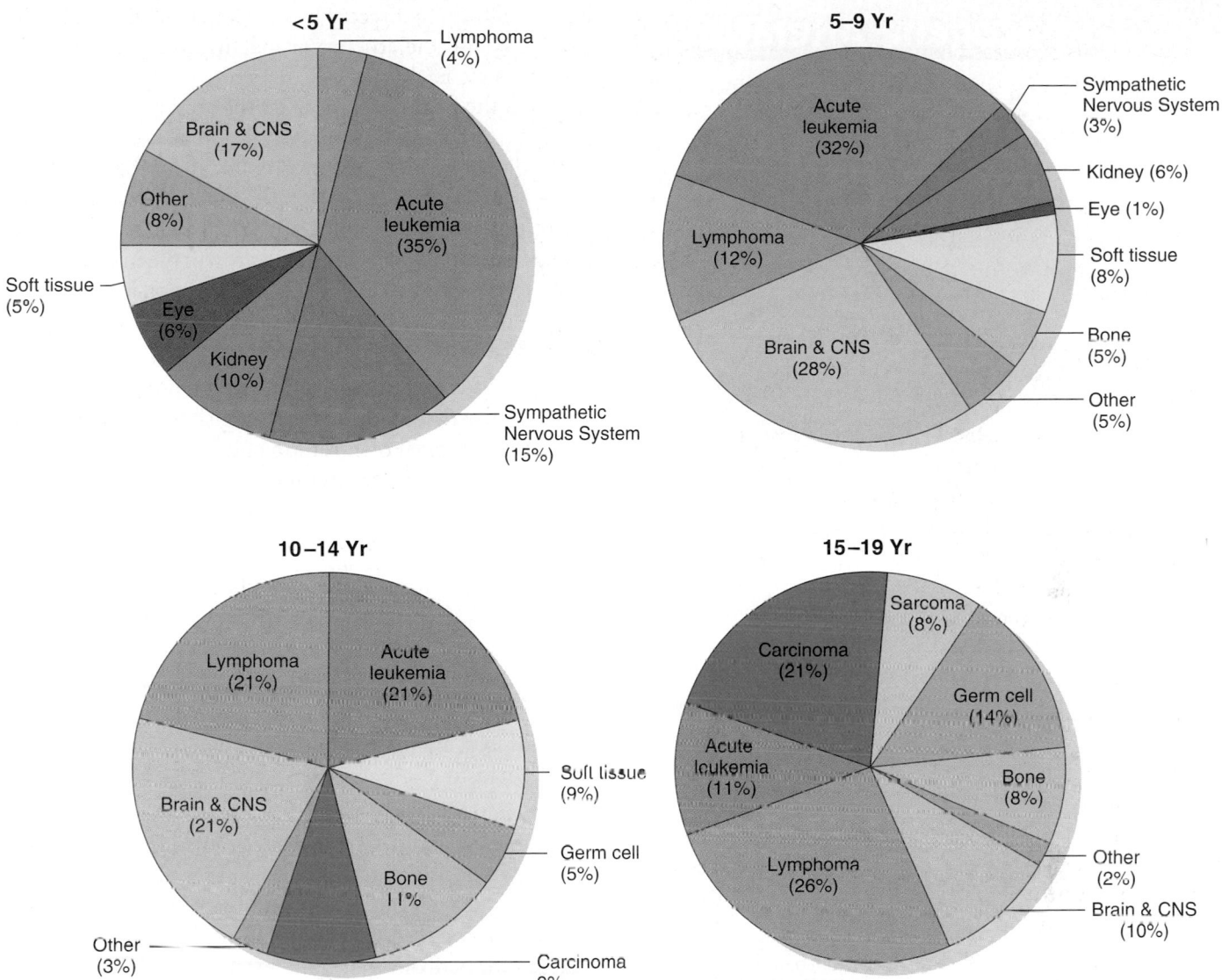

Percentage of primary tumors by site of origin for different age groups.

Data from Gurney, J. G., & Bondy, M. L. (2004). Cancer and benign tumors. In R. E. Behrman & H. B. Jenson (Eds.), Nelson textbook of pediatrics (17th ed., p. 1680). Philadelphia: Saunders.

Viruses and other substances may alter the immune system, thereby allowing cancer to occur (see "Pathophysiology Illustrated: Proto-oncogene Alteration"). Their action is based on changing certain genes that normally regulate cellular growth and development (called **proto-oncogenes**) to related genes that allow unregulated cell division and cancerous growth (called **oncogenes**). Among the cancers thought to be linked to virus action and the change of proto-oncogenes to oncogenes are certain leukemias, rhabdomyosarcoma, Burkitt lymphoma, and some forms of Hodgkin disease.

Sometimes a genetic change that occurs is passed on to future generations of a family. Genetic changes can include autosomal dominant, autosomal recessive, and x-linked transfer. In these cases the resulting cancers often occur rel-

atively early in life. Cancers of these types are typically aggressive since the child has inherited the abnormal gene and it is within each cell, rather than a single mutation of one gene in a specific cell. Due to progress that is being made in the Human Genome Project, there is increasing ability to perform genetic testing for certain familial cancers. Examples of cancers that are sometimes caused by genetic abnormalities within families include retinoblastoma (described later in this chapter), multiple endocrine neoplasia, type 2 (thyroid cancer), and familial adenomatous polyposis (invasive colon cancer). Not all cases of these cancers are familial, but their incidence suggests the need for careful history taking to identify any other cases in the family. Providing recommendations for referral to genetic

PATHOPHYSIOLOGY ILLUSTRATED
Proto-oncogene Alteration

Virus

Proto-oncogene

Oncogene

Tumor-suppressor gene

A proto-oncogene normally regulates cellular growth and development. When altered by a virus or other external cause, it can change to an oncogene, which allows unregulated genetic activity and tumor growth. Tumor-suppressor genes regulate the effects of oncogenes to decrease wildly proliferating cellular growth.

counseling services and following up with further education and psychologic support are important nursing roles (MacDonald & Lessick, 2000).

Tumor suppressor genes counteract the effect of oncogenes, keeping cellular growth within normal limits. When tumor suppressor genes are missing, unstemmed cellular growth can occur. These genes are commonly missing in children with retinoblastoma and Wilms' tumor.

Chromosomal Abnormalities

Normal chromosomes undergo change as a part of the genetic process. Most changes are not harmful. However, some result in chromosomal abnormalities such as hyperploidy (more than the normal number of chromosomes), deletion, translocation, and breakage.

Some chromosomal abnormalities have been linked to an increased incidence of cancer. Children with Down syndrome have a 20 times higher incidence of leukemia than nonaffected children (Ross, Spector, Robison & Olshan, 2005). Children missing a band of genetic material on chromosome 13 often have retinoblastoma. Similarly, a Wilms' tumor often develops in children missing part of the genetic material from chromosome 11.

Regardless of the location of abnormal cellular growth, the pathophysiologic process is similar. The altered cell begins to multiply as directed by the altered genetic structure of its DNA and the absence or inactivation of tumor suppressor genes. Each new cell transmits the new or altered pattern to the next generation. As the abnormal cells replicate, they form a growing neoplastic mass. Normal cells usually die as the increased metabolic rate of the neoplastic cells depletes available nutrition. The altered DNA in the tumor cells may also cause the abnormal cells to invade adjoining tissue. Through continued growth the mass expands until it enters and disrupts a major vessel or a vital organ.

CLINICAL MANIFESTATIONS

Each type of childhood cancer signals its presence differently. Because many of the presenting signs and symptoms of cancer are typical of common childhood illnesses, diagnosis may be delayed. In some cases, no symptoms are noted until the cancer is advanced. Some of the common presenting symptoms of cancer follow.

- *Pain* may be the result of a neoplasm either directly or indirectly affecting nerve receptors through obstruction, inflammation, tissue damage, stretching of visceral tissue, or invasion of susceptible tissue.

- *Cachexia* is a syndrome characterized by anorexia, weight loss, anemia, asthenia (weakness), and early satiety (feeling of being full).

- *Anemia* may be experienced during times of chronic bleeding or iron deficiency. In chronic illness the body uses iron poorly. Anemia is also present in cancers of the bone marrow when the number of red blood cells (RBCs) is reduced, in part because of the presence of large numbers of other bone marrow products. Treatment of cancer often promotes further anemia.

- *Infection* is usually a result of an altered or immature immune system. In addition, infection occurs when bone marrow cancers inhibit maturation of normal immune system cells. Infection may also occur in children treated with corticosteroids. Because their immune response is altered, the normal signs of infection may not appear.

- *Bruising* can occur if the bone marrow cannot produce enough platelets; bleeding after even minor trauma can lead to ecchymosis.

- *Neurologic symptoms* may result from impingement on the brain or nervous system. Signs of increased intracranial pressure, decreased or altered consciousness, eye abnormalities, or other neurologic or behavior changes may be evident.

- *Palpable mass* may be present for certain cancers. This is most commonly abdominal but may be mediastinal, in the neck, or at other sites.

A variety of other symptoms can occur depending on the location of the cancer. Subcutaneous nodules may appear if leukocytosis is present, superior vena cava syndrome or respiratory difficulty can occur with mediastinal tumors (such as neuroblastoma), and enlarged lymph nodes are common with lymphomas (Bleyer, 2004).

COLLABORATIVE CARE

Diagnostic Tests

The most common diagnostic tests performed on children with cancer are complete blood counts with differential, bone marrow aspiration (BMA), bone marrow biopsy (BMBX), lumbar puncture (Table 50–1), peripheral blood studies, radiographic examination, magnetic resonance imaging (MRI), computed tomography (CT; Figure 50–2 ◉), ultrasound, and biopsy of tumor.

NURSING PRACTICE

Any child who has an implanted metallic object in his or her body should not undergo MRI scanning because of the strong magnetic field generated. Metallic objects include orthodontic braces, metal dental bridgework, surgical clips or plates, and orthopedic rods. Remove all jewelry and clothes with metal snaps from the child before the test. Ask about body piercings in places such as the mouth, abdomen, or chest that may not be readily visible. The hardware must be removed for the MRI.

Additional studies helpful for certain cancers are nuclear medicine scans with radioactive isotopes such as gallium or iodine, bone scan with technetium 99m, or positron emission tomography (PET) and single photon emission

FIGURE 50–2

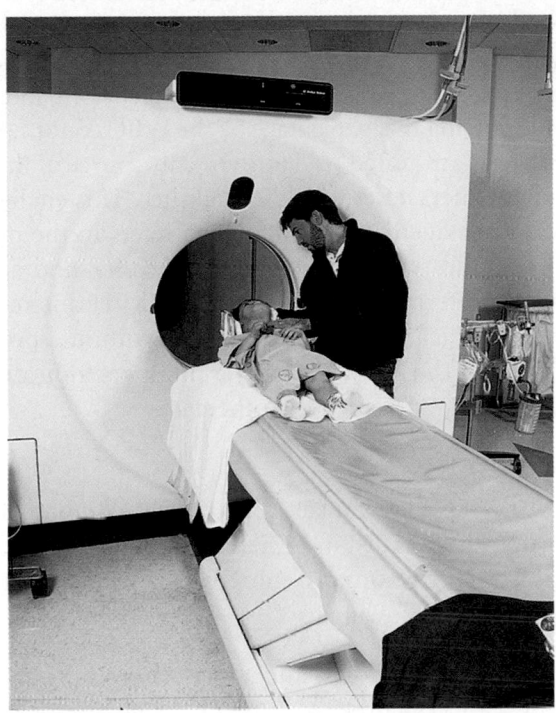

Computed tomography (CT) can be a frightening procedure for children. This 2-year-old boy is comforted by his father before the procedure.

computed tomography (SPECT) that combine nuclear medicine with CT (Leonard, 2002). Specific tests such as pulmonary function tests and echocardiograms may be used in certain situations. Urine analysis is performed.

The blood work is very detailed and includes RBC, WBC, platelets, hematocrit and hemoglobin, serum electrolytes, liver studies, and markers that are elevated in

TABLE 50–1 ✣ Selected Diagnostic Tests for Childhood Cancer

Test	Purpose	Normal Laboratory Values	Diagnostic Values
Bone marrow aspiration	Examines bone marrow	<5% blast cells (immature)	>25% blast cells in acute lymphoblastic leukemia, most with hypercellular marrow
Lumbar puncture	Examines cerebrospinal fluid	Cell count (μL) Polymorphonuclear leukocytes 0 Monocytes 0–5 RBCs 0–5	Presence of malignant cells indicates central nervous system involvement
Complete blood count and differential	Examines cellular components of blood	WBC <10,000/μL Platelets 150,000–400,000/μL Hemoglobin 12–16 g/dL	WBC >10,000/μL Platelets 20,000–100,000/μL Hemoglobin 7–10 g/dL
Absolute Neutrophil Count (ANC)	Blood component ratio: % of segmental neutrophils times % of bands (immature neutrophils) times WBC count	ANC >1000	ANC <500 = risk of infection

specific types of tumors. Absolute neutrophil count (ANC) is important; it uses both the segmented (mature) and bands (immature neutrophils) as a measure of the body's infection-fighting capability. ANC is calculated by adding percent of segmented neutrophils to percent of bands, and then multiplying this percentage by the WBC count.

The tests are aimed at identifying the source of the cancer and any metastases to additional sites. This enables the physician to stage the cancer. Staging refers to the process of labeling the type of cancer cells, severity, and spread, which will determine the recommended treatment. Stage number 1 indicates less severe cancer without spread to other parts of the body, and higher numbers indicate both greater severity and spread to other sites.

Clinical Therapy

Clinical therapy for cancer is extremely complex and is managed by a specialist in pediatric oncology. Recommendations from the National Action Plan for Childhood Cancer include the following:

- Ensure that all children and adolescents suspected of having cancer are referred initially to a pediatric cancer center and have their care coordinated by the center.

- Establish national standards of quality care for children and adolescents with cancer, both medical and psychosocial, as defined by healthcare professionals and patient advocates.

- Quantify current patterns, quality, and outcomes of all phases of childhood and adolescent cancer care.

- Increase participation of children and adolescents in all phases of approved clinical trials (American Cancer Society, 2003).

Cancer itself has many effects on the body, such as altering nutrition and impeding circulation, all of which must be managed carefully. Cancer is treated with one or a combination of therapies: surgery, chemotherapy, radiation, **biotherapy**, and bone marrow transplantation. The choice of treatment is determined by the type of cancer, its location, and the degree of metastasis (spread to other sites in the body). Treatments all have side effects and these will also require clinical management. Many families also choose to use some type of complementary therapy, in addition to traditional medical approaches.

The goal of treatment may be curative, supportive, or palliative. Curative treatment rids the child's body of the cancer. Supportive treatment includes transfusions, pain management, antibiotics, and other interventions to assist the body's defenses and increase the child's comfort. Palliative treatment is designed to make the child as comfortable as possible when no curative treatment is possible (see Chapter 41 for a detailed discussion of palliative care for children ∞). Whatever com-

TEACHING HIGHLIGHTS

CANCER THERAPY

Most parents are not aware of the effects of cancer treatment and how they can help children through this experience. Depending on the stage and type of treatment, there are several ways to help:

- Children in radiation and chemotherapy are fatigued. Provide extra rest periods with shorter activity periods between them.
- Have a bag ready in case the child develops a complication and needs to be taken to stay in the hospital for a few days. Several hospital stays of a few days are normal during treatment.
- When concerned about a symptom in the child, ask the care provider. Parents are often key in identifying problems early.
- Parents are usually concerned about central line care but feel more comfortable after a few days of caring for the line.
- Children may not feel hungry. When they are ready to eat, intake should be nutritious.
- Remember that the child is still at the normal developmental age. Treat them appropriately for their age, not as if they are older or younger.
- Try to maintain contact with the child's peer group and family members.
- Seek information from other parents and resources on cancer care.
- Many families use complementary approaches to deal with the child's cancer. Most of these approaches are not contraindicated. However, be sure to tell the oncologist about what treatments you are choosing to use to be sure none of them will injure your child.
- Take time to get away and relax so that you have enough energy and are better able to deal with your child's therapy.

bination of treatment is used, families have many questions and need resources for information.

Surgery. Surgery is used to remove or debulk (reduce the size of) a solid tumor. An example of a cancer that is commonly treated with surgery is a Wilms' tumor. Surgery may also determine the stage and type of cancer.

Chemotherapy. Chemotherapy is the administration of specific drugs that kill both normal and cancerous cells. The administration of various chemotherapeutic drugs is timed to achieve the greatest cellular destruction. The cell's cycle of replication determines the schedule (see "Pathophysiology Illustrated: Chemotherapy Drug Action"). Several chemotherapeutic drugs are administered simultaneously to maximize their lethal impact on cells at all stages of activity (see Table 50–2). Medications are most commonly oral, intravenous, or **intrathecal** (into spinal canal). Whereas DNA in a normal cell can repair itself after chemotherapy, the DNA in a neoplastic cell cannot. The particular chemotherapy treatment protocol used is based on research into different types of cancer cells. A **protocol** is a plan of action for chemotherapy

PATHOPHYSIOLOGY ILLUSTRATED

Chemotherapy Drug Action

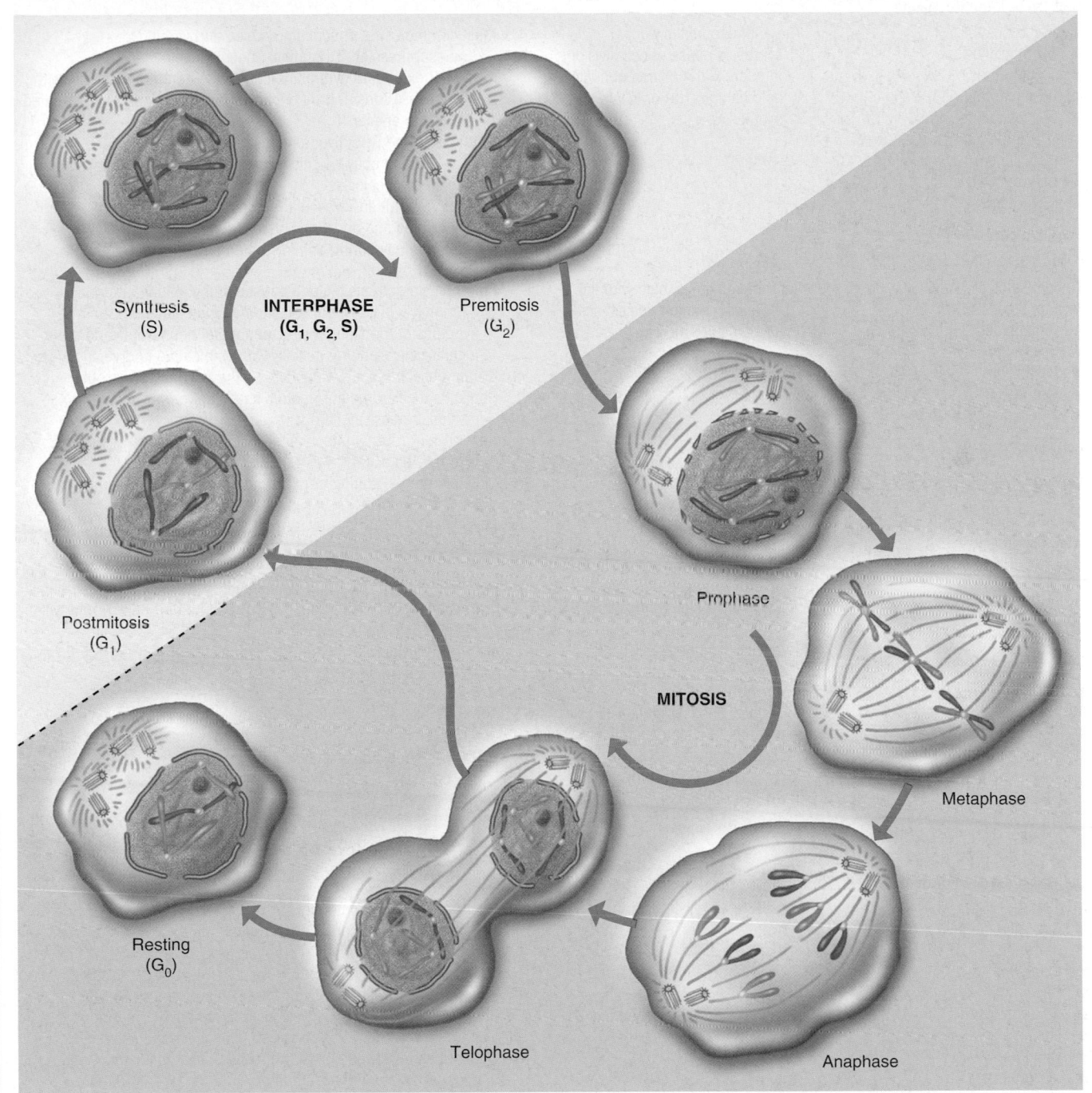

Synthesis
(S)

**INTERPHASE
(G₁, G₂, S)**

Premitosis
(G₂)

Postmitosis
(G₁)

Prophase

MITOSIS

Metaphase

Resting
(G₀)

Telophase

Anaphase

Chemotherapy drugs either act at specific parts of the cell cycle or are nonspecific for action (act throughout all cell phases).

based on the type of cancer, its stage, and the particular cell type (Figure 50–3 ●).

Other drugs used in the treatment of children with cancer include colony-stimulating factors, antiemetics, and nutritional supplements. Colony-stimulating factors are hormonelike glycoproteins that enhance blood cell production and counteract the myelosuppressive effects of chemotherapy drugs. For example, erythropoietin is produced in the kidney, and a recombinant form (epoetin) is available which can be used to treat anemia of cancer,

TABLE 50–2 ✢ Medications Used for Cancer Chemotherapy

Medication	Action/Indication	Nursing Implications
Cell Cycle Specific Agents		
Antimetabolites ■ 5-Azacytidine ■ 5-Fluorouracil ■ 6-Mercaptopurine ■ 6-Thioguanine ■ Cytosine arabinoside (cytarabine) ■ Hydroxyurea ■ Methotrexate	The antimetabolites work at synthesis phase of cell division; interfere with function of nucleic acid; inhibit DNA or RNA synthesis.	Most common side effects are nausea and vomiting, myelosuppression, stomatitis. Specific agents such as methotrexate and cytarabine can cause neurologic toxicity with high doses. Consult drug books and package inserts for detailed list of side effects. Obtain baseline CBC, liver function, renal function. Monitor I&O and body weight. Ensure hydration and output levels ordered by oncologist. Monitor VS and cardiovascular and respiratory function. Watch for bleeding and signs of infection. Monitor carefully during administration for signs of anaphylaxis.
Vinca alkaloids ■ Etoposide ■ Teniposide ■ Irinotecan ■ Paclitaxel ■ Vinblastine ■ Vincristine	Act during mitosis; bind with cell proteins to inhibit nucleic acid and protein synthesis.	Common side effects include nausea and vomiting, abdominal cramping and diarrhea, constipation, paralytic ileus, hair loss, hypotension or hypertension, peripheral neuropathy and neurologic toxicity (latter especially with vinblastine and vincristine). Obtain baseline blood work. Consult specific drug information for period of maximum myelosuppressive effect. Be alert for bruising, infection, and other signs of myelosuppression. Monitor carefully during administration for signs of anaphylaxis.
Miscellaneous—G_1 phase activity ■ L-asparaginase	Causes depletion of asparagine, needed by cancer cells; makes cell in G_1 phase vulnerable to other agents; interferes with prosynthesis. Used in combination with other agents in leukemia and other cancers.	Administered intravenously. Major side effects are severe nausea and vomiting, hypersensitivity, renal failure, myelosuppression, acid–base imbalance. CBC, serum amylase, glucose, coagulation factors, bone marrow function, liver function tests performed before therapy and twice weekly. Monitor I&O, neurologic status, gastrointestinal symptoms, abdominal pain.
Miscellaneous—G_2 phase activity ■ Etoposide	Works at G_2 phase; binds cellular proteins to cause metaphase arrest; also acts on S phase of DNA synthesis. Used with other agents, particularly in recurrent disease.	Administered orally and intravenously. Common side effects are nausea and vomiting, myelosuppression, hair loss, diarrhea. Can cause anaphylaxis; hypotension and IV site pain with rapid infusion. Perform baseline CBC, liver and renal function tests. Check IV site frequently since extravasation can cause necrosis. Monitor VS during infusion and stop drug if hypotension occurs.
Cell Cycle Nonspecific Agents		
Alkylating agents ■ Cyclophosphamide ■ Carboplatin ■ Cisplatin ■ Busulfan ■ Chlorambucil ■ Ifosfamide ■ Thiotepa ■ Mechlorethamine ■ Melphalan ■ Procarbazine ■ Dacarbazine	Substitute an alkyl group for a hydrogen atom, leading to blockage of DNA replication. Used for treatment of many cancers, either alone or in conjunction with other agents.	Most are administered orally and/or intravenously. Array of side effects depending on specific drug. Some common side effects are nausea and vomiting, diarrhea, myelosuppression, hair loss, neuropathies, pulmonary toxicity, renal damage; secondary tumors later in life associated with some agents. Obtain CBC and full blood work before and during treatment. Monitor for side effects of the specific agents administered. Ensure generous hydration and monitor I&O. Teach family the importance of long-term monitoring for secondary tumors.

TABLE 50–2 ✣ Medications Used for Cancer Chemotherapy—continued

Medication	Action/Indication	Nursing Implications
Cell Cycle Nonspecific Agents *(continued)*		
Antibiotics ■ Doxorubicin ■ Mitomycin-C ■ Dactinomycin ■ Bleomycin ■ Daunorubicin ■ Idarubicin ■ Mitoxantrone	Interfere with nucleic acid, inhibiting DNA or RNA synthesis. Used in combination with other agents to treat leukemia and other childhood cancers.	Most are administered intravenously. Common side effects include nausea and vomiting, myelosuppression, oral ulcers, skin and pulmonary toxicity. Several have cumulative dose toxicity, such as cardiac abnormalities (doxorubicin) and skin/pulmonary (bleomycin); total dose the child has received must be monitored. Obtain baseline CBC and other blood studies and monitor throughout therapy. Monitor VS, lung function, cardiac function, neurologic status throughout and following therapy. Be alert for signs of myelosuppression and mucosal ulcers.
Nitrosoureas ■ Carmustine ■ Lomustine	Cross breakage in DNA strands so that DNA and RNA replication cannot occur. Used in lymphomas and other childhood cancers. Can cross blood-brain barrier.	Administered orally (lomustine) or intravenously (carmustine). Major side effect is myelosuppression. Others include pulmonary fibrosis, eye infarction, skin changes, hair loss, nausea, and vomiting. Obtain baseline and periodic CBC and other studies. Monitor pulmonary function, skin, and signs of infection or bleeding.
Hormones ■ Prednisone ■ Prednisolone ■ Dexamethasone	Analog of hydrocortisone; anti-inflammatory; delayed and depressed immune response. Used in conjunction with other agents for many types of childhood cancer.	Often administered orally. Numerous side effects including edema, moon face, mood lability, increased appetite, disturbed sleep, immunosuppression, disturbed glucose control, osteoporosis. Teach child and family the effects of the drug. Minimize exposure to persons with infection. Monitor for infections in all systems. Monitor weight regularly. Take VS. Teach to take as directed. Drug must be tapered slowly at end of therapy.
Topoisomerase I inhibitor ■ Irinotecan ■ Mitoxantrone ■ Topotecan	Inhibit the enzyme topoisomerase I in the cell nucleus, relaxing DNA and preventing its duplication. Used in conjunction with other agents to treat ALL and other childhood cancers.	Administered intravenously; topotecan can be given intrathecally. Common side effects include nausea and vomiting, diarrhea, fever, dehydration, myelosuppression. Can alter liver function and cause skin changes. Obtain baseline and periodic CBC and other studies, including liver function. Monitor for signs of myelosuppression, gastrointestinal distress, change in liver function.

thereby decreasing the number of transfusions needed (Agency for Healthcare Research and Quality, 2001a). Filgrastim (Neupogen) increases production of neutrophils by the bone marrow (see Table 50–3). Antiemetics, such as ondansetron (Zofran), can be used to treat the nausea and vomiting that are common side effects of therapy. Nutritional supplements help maintain nutritional status.

Radiation. **Radiation** therapy involves unstable isotopes that release varying levels of energy to cause breaks in the DNA molecule and thereby destroy cells. Radiation has been used as a treatment method since the early 1900s, shortly after its discovery. It is often used for the local and regional control of cancer, and in combination with surgery and chemotherapy; it may be curative or palliative.

NURSING PRACTICE

Nurses who care for a child receiving implant radiation or who work in a radiation department need to wear a dosimeter film badge at all times to measure their radiation exposure.

The area to be irradiated (treatment field) includes the tumor site and sometimes other involved areas, such as lymph glands. The goal is to irradiate the tumor but not healthy adjacent tissue. The total dose of radiation is divided (or fractionated) and given over several weeks. A common course of radiation treatment might be once daily 4 or 5 days per week for a period of 2 to 6 weeks.

● **FIGURE 50–3**

Protocol = Map or plan of action

Chemotherapy protocol. A protocol is a map or plan of action that directs therapy by identifying the drug and its accompanying treatment.

Tumors highly sensitive to radiation include Hodgkin disease, Wilms' tumor, retinoblastoma, rhabdomyosarcoma, and central nervous system disease in leukemia. Tumors that have a low sensitivity to radiation, such as osteosarcoma and soft-tissue sarcomas, require higher doses of radiation, or other treatments may be preferred.

Biotherapy. Biotherapy is the use of biologic retooling and molecular intervention to produce targeted cancer therapy (Arceci & Cripe, 2002). Biologic retooling uses parts of the human body that are programmed to destroy cells, and applies them to the cancer cells. An example of this technique includes development of antibodies that are tumor-specific to certain cancers. These antibodies promote apoptosis or death of the cancerous cells. Another example is the group of drugs that stimulate the body's own immune response. Cancer vaccines are under development that may work to help the body fight cancers. The actions of many of these agents are not completely understood, and some agents have more than one effect. For example, interferon has both antiviral and antiproliferative effects on some malignant cells. Interferon and tumor necrosis factor (TNF) are undergoing clinical trials to study their effectiveness and to develop protocols

TABLE 50–3 ❖ Medications Used to Treat Cancer: Colony-Stimulating Factors

Medication	Action/Indication	Nursing Implications
Epoetin alfa (human recombinant erythropoietin)	This glycoprotein stimulates the bone marrow in RBC formation; useful when numbers of RBCs are low due to chemotherapy effects	Give subcutaneously or intravenously. Do not shake and do not use if discolored or particles are present. Single-dose vials only so discard any solution that is not used. Obtain blood tests before therapy and periodically after; improvement in hematocrit should be seen in 7–14 days. Monitor blood pressure before and during therapy as hypertension can result. Monitor for change in neurologic response and headache; both seizures and strokes are possible side effects.
Filgrastim (Neupogen) and pegfilgrastim (Neulasta)	This human granulocyte colony-stimulating factor (G-CSF) increases production of neutrophils by the bone marrow	Administered subcutaneously and intravenously; prepare as directed for IV infusion to prevent its absorption by IV tubing. Single-dose vials only so discard any solution that is not used. Incompatible with many medications; check package insert; do not give within 24 hours before or after chemotherapy drugs or their effect may be decreased. Obtain baseline and twice weekly CBC. Monitor for side effects such as bone pain and heart arrhythmias; report fevers and be alert for other signs of infection when neutrophil count is low.
Oprelvekin (Neumega)	A hematopoietic growth factor, interleukin-11, that increases platelet count; useful in low platelet count due to chemotherapy effects on bone marrow	Administered subcutaneously. Single-dose vials only so discard any solution that is not used. Obtain baseline CBC and platelet count; monitor platelets throughout treatment. Monitor for side effects such as edema, fever, CNS changes, tachycardia, respiratory problems, and skin rash. Take daily weights and monitor for fluid retention.

for their safe use against selected cancers. An additional type of biologic therapy is gene therapy or attempting to replace a faulty gene with one that is normal.

Molecular targeting involves interference with metabolic pathways (for example, through enzyme disruption) in the tumor cells. It may also disturb the cell's growth and development and thereby depress proliferation.

Hematopoietic Stem Cell Transplantation. Hematopoietic stem cell transplantation (HSCT) is used to treat leukemia, neuroblastoma, and some noncancerous conditions such as aplastic anemia. The goal of therapy is to administer a lethal dose of chemotherapy and radiation that will kill the cancer, and then to resupply the body with stem cells either from the child's own bone marrow that was previously removed (autologous transplant) and stored or from a compatible donor (allogeneic transplant). Umbilical cord blood is another source of stem cells used for transplant. Peripheral blood stem cells are increasingly being used for transplant. The donor, whether autologous or allogeneic, can be given growth factors prior to donation to stimulate production of stem cells. An advantage of peripheral stem cells is that they can be easily collected rather than by the painful and invasive procedure of a bone marrow aspiration (Reiss & Bolotin, 2002).

HSCT has become the treatment of choice for some cancers when a relapse occurs while the child is receiving another form of cancer therapy and for primary treatment of certain cancers. First, a histocompatible donor must be located. The child then receives intensive chemotherapy, often followed by total body irradiation. Beginning 7 to 10 days before the transplant, this treatment kills all circulating blood cells and bone marrow contents (Alcoser & Burchett, 1999). Following this treatment, the child is intravenously transfused with the donor bone marrow or other source of stem cells. New blood cells usually form within 2 to 6 weeks (Alcoser & Rogers, 2003). (See Chapter 44 for a description of care for the child undergoing transplantation. ∞) Stem cells that become established in the host child's bone marrow can also be obtained from newborn umbilical cord blood. For some children this has become a better option than waiting for a matching bone marrow donor. Cord blood can be easily collected at birth from a sibling of the ill child, as histocompatible matches often occur in siblings, or cord blood banks may offer a match. The umbilical cord blood is then infused into the child undergoing treatment, and the same mechanism occurs as in transplantation of bone marrow—implantation of the stem cells into the child's bone marrow and production of normal blood cells over about 2 to 6 weeks. Advantages of umbilical cord blood are that, unlike bone marrow collection, it is not painful for the donor and does not require anesthesia, there is an opportunity to easily collect samples from many ethnic groups

that are underrepresented in bone marrow donor registries, graft-versus-host disease after treatment is less prevalent, and storage of umbilical cord blood for use later in life is possible. A variety of federally funded and private blood banks are available to store and provide umbilical blood.

Complementary Therapies. Many families use **complementary therapies** in treatment of a child's cancer. These approaches to care are also referred to as alternative or unconventional, and may involve nutritional supplements, oral herbal supplements, touch therapy, and mind/body interventions. Very little research has been done on complementary therapies, although up to 80% of children have used at least one such therapeutic approach (Kelly, Jacobsen, Kennedy et al., 2000). Healthcare providers should be aware of these practices, inquire in a nonjudgmental manner about the therapies, and attempt to learn about specific therapies and practices. Although some herbs and nutritional products such as St. John's wort may decrease serum concentration of chemotherapeutic agents, or some may act as hormones in the body, most are not known to negatively affect contemporary medical treatment, and the families should be assisted in seeking information and supported in use of their chosen therapies (Chase, 2000; Dean, 2000). Eating fruits and vegetables is associated with lower cancer incidence in adults, and some foods such as garlic and oranges may slow cancer growth or enhance medical chemotherapy (Swerdlow, 2000). Some people use some herbal supplements to treat cancer; these include cat's claw (bark of a tree root), mistletoe, and shark cartilage. The U.S. Food and Drug Administration has allowed testing of the efficacy of some herbal treatments for cancer (Kemper & Longwood Herbal Task Force, 1999). Several cancer drugs such as vincristine and paclitaxel are obtained from plant products. Some herbs can decrease nausea and vomiting, and others can boost the immune system's function (Kemper & Longwood Herbal Task Force, 1999).

Palliative Care. In spite of modern medicinal practices and complementary therapies, approximately 25% of children with childhood cancer do not survive (Hurwitz, Duncan, &

DEVELOPING CULTURAL COMPETENCE

CHINESE BLOOD DETOXIFICATION METHODS

Traditional Chinese view cancer as a result of weak or toxic blood, which allows pollutants to accumulate and become toxic. A variety of plant products and acupuncture are used to detoxify the blood, and good nutrition helps it to rebuild. Some common foods used in various cultures to prevent and treat cancer include carrots, garlic, green tea, cabbage, citrus fruits, ginger root, and willow bark (Swerdlow, 2000).

MediaLink — Stem Cell Transplantation

Wolfe, 2004). In these cases the focus of healthcare is to provide comfort and emotional support for the child and family. Too often, healthcare providers feel uncomfortable when a child is expected to die and may withdraw from close contact with the child or family, fail to provide adequate comfort measures, and leave the family without access to needed resources. When recognition of prognosis is delayed, children suffer more and palliative care is less integrated (Wolfe, Klar, Grier et al., 2000). Some symptoms for which children are commonly undertreated include pain, dyspnea, nutrition, elimination, and fatigue (Wolfe, Grier, Klar et al., 2000). However, care for the dying child can be enhanced by a palliative care team; an integrated plan of care; collaboration between families, primary care provider, and other practitioners; and a focus on the child's developmental level and family needs (Chaffee, 2001; Hilden, Emanuel, Fairclogh et al., 2001; Hurwitz, Duncan, & Wolfe, 2005). See Chapter 41 for a detailed description of palliative care for children with terminal disease. ∞

Oncologic Emergencies. Oncologic emergencies can be organized into three groups: metabolic, hematologic, and those involving space-occupying lesions. Overall, the most common oncologic emergencies are tumor lysis syndrome, septic shock, brain herniation, spinal cord compression, and superior vena cava compression from a superior mediastinal mass.

Metabolic Emergencies. Metabolic emergencies result from the lysis (dissolving or decomposing) of tumor cells, a process called tumor lysis syndrome. This cell destruction releases high levels of uric acid, potassium, phosphates, and calcium into the blood and can lower serum sodium levels. It is seen most commonly in children with Burkitt lymphoma and acute lymphocytic leukemia (Baggott et al., 2002). (See "Clinical Manifestations: Management of Tumor Lysis Syndrome.") The nurse collects laboratory studies, including CBC, absolute neutrophil count (ANF), serum electrolytes, bicarbonate, uric acid, blood urea nitrogen (BUN) and creatinine, and urinalysis. The emergency can be life threatening, and the family will need ongoing support and explanations about care.

A second type of metabolic emergency is septic shock. During periods of immune suppression, the child is vulnerable to overwhelming infection, resulting in circulatory failure, inadequate tissue perfusion, and hypotension.

CLINICAL MANIFESTATIONS

MANAGEMENT OF TUMOR LYSIS SYNDROME

ETIOLOGY	CLINICAL MANIFESTATIONS	CLINICAL THERAPY	NURSING IMPLICATIONS
Breakdown of malignant cells releases intracellular components into blood	Hyperuricemia Hyperkalemia Hyperphosphatemia Hypocalcemia	■ Vigorous hydration with 2–4 times maintenance fluid ■ Correction of electrolyte imbalances ■ Administration of allopurinol or urate oxidase (Rasburicase) to reduce conversion of metabolic by-products to uric acid	■ Administration of fluids, beginning before therapy ■ Careful intake and output measures ■ Daily weight ■ Urine specific gravity (should remain <1.010) ■ Monitoring for desired and side effects of drug therapy
Electrolyte imbalance causes metabolic acidosis and serious abnormalities	Cardiac arrhythmias Impaired renal function Tetany, neurologic and mental status changes	■ ECG monitoring ■ Medications such as furosemide to facilitate potassium excretion ■ Dialysis may be needed	■ Administration of electrolytes and medications ■ Urine pH (should remain 7.0 to 7.5) ■ Perform Trousseau's and Chvostek's signs for tetany monitoring and assess neurologic function ■ Perform mental status examination ■ Obtain laboratory specimens as needed

Septic shock can be fatal (see Chapter 48 for a description of septic shock ∞). Factors contributing to massive infection include inadequate neutrophil production, abnormal granulocytes (not able to be actively phagocytic), erosions through normal barriers such as blood vessels and mucous membranes, and altered bone marrow production caused by chemotherapy and some forms of radiation. Such infections may manifest with hyperthermia or hypothermia, tachycardia, tachypnea, hypotension, mental changes, and peripheral cyanosis and coolness, and must be vigorously treated with antimicrobial therapy and hydration management.

A third type of metabolic emergency occurs when treatment destroys large amounts of bone, resulting in hypercalcemia (elevated calcium in the serum). Hypercalcemia is most common in children with acute lymphocytic leukemia and rhabdomyosarcoma. Treatment includes hydration and adequate oral phosphate supplement.

Another emergency occurs when some children develop syndrome of inappropriate antidiuretic hormone (SIADH) and have excessive release of ADH. The resulting decreased urinary output leads to water intoxication. See Chapter 56 for a detailed description of SIADH. ∞

Hematologic Emergencies. Hematologic emergencies result from bone marrow suppression or infiltration of brain and respiratory tissue with high numbers of leukemic blast cells (hyperleukocytosis). Bone marrow suppression results in anemia and thrombocytopenia with resultant hemorrhage. Gastrointestinal and central nervous system bleeding (strokes) are common. Disseminated intravascular coagulation (DIC) occurs in some children and is a life-threatening complication. See Chapter 49 for a thorough description of this condition. ∞ Disruption of normal WBC production and resulting hyperleukocytosis can lead to obstruction of small blood vessels throughout the body.

Treatment involves infusion of packed red blood cells for anemia; and platelet transfusion, vitamin K, and fresh frozen plasma for thrombocytopenia and hemorrhage. Hyperleukocytosis is treated by hydration, bicarbonate infusion, and allopurinol (Baggott et al., 2002).

Space-Occupying Lesions. Extensive tumor growth may result in spinal cord compression, increased intracranial pressure, brain herniation, seizures, massive hepatomegaly, and superior vena cava syndrome (obstruction of the superior vena cava by tumor). These emergencies are often caused by neuroblastoma, medulloblastoma, astrocytoma, Hodgkin disease, or lymphoma. After biopsy of the mass, treatment involves radiation therapy, chemotherapy, and corticosteroids.

Psychosocial Needs. The diagnosis of cancer is devastating for families. They cannot believe that their vibrant, young child or adolescent has a potentially life-threatening disease. Families are in a state of crisis when the diagnosis is made, with the first response one of shock (Hendricks-Ferguson, 2000). At the same time that they are in a state of shock about the diagnosis, parents must gather resources to support the child, make treatment decisions, and adjust family life to integrate the needs of the child with cancer. Some families need to travel a great distance for the child's treatments, and others may have financial constraints that make healthcare costs a major concern. For nearly everyone, parental work schedules as well as arrangements for other children must be adjusted. Most cancer treatment will last for a minimum of several months up to several years, necessitating nearly constant adaptation.

The child reacts to the diagnosis based on age. Infants and toddlers are unaware of the severity of the disease, while preschoolers are beginning to understand illness. However, they may think they caused their illness and are confused about why the parent cannot make the illness go away. School-age children can understand a diagnosis of cancer and benefit from opportunities to talk about the experience. Adolescents find contact with others who have gone through their experience reassuring and supportive. A comprehensive review of studies on communicating with children and adolescents about their cancer did not find clear results and directions (Scott, Entwistle, Sowden et al., 2003). Programs such as group therapy sessions, computer programs about cancer and treatment, and school reintegration all show potential for assisting youth who are adjusting to cancer. Children with cancer may have higher depression scores than healthy children, so they are at risk of disturbed mental health status (Cavusoglu, 2001).

NURSING MANAGEMENT

NURSING ASSESSMENT AND DIAGNOSIS

History

During health promotion visits of all children, nurses are aware of the importance of a history of cancer in the family. Particularly when more than one person has had cancer, and when young children in the extended family have been affected, complete a genogram to isolate cases in the family. (See Chapter 4. ∞) A history of exposure to known carcinogens is also important. Does a parent work in an industry with substances like chemicals or asbestos that might remain on clothing worn home? Was the child treated with radiation or chemotherapy for a previous cancer? Does the child have an identified condition with a high incidence of some type of cancer, such as Down syndrome? Does the child have any recognized congenital anomalies? A number of conditions are more commonly associated with certain types of cancer.

Physiologic Assessment

When performing any physiologic assessment on children, consider the possible signs and symptoms of cancer. These include anemia, frequent infections, bleeding disorders, loss of weight, fatigue, pain, and changes in mental health and neurologic status. Assessment of children with the most significant types of childhood cancers is presented later in the chapter.

Once cancer has been diagnosed, a thorough physical assessment of all systems is needed to help identify the presence and extent of cancer (see Chapter 35 ∞). Systems needing particularly thorough assessments are neurologic, respiratory, cardiac, and gastrointestinal. Assess hydration status and the tumor site if it is visible. Carefully measure height and weight, and compare with prior findings for the child. Observe gait and coordination, as well as any changes in mental status. Evaluate immunization status, pain, nutritional intake, fatigue, infections, bruising, shortness of breath, and elimination problems. Periodic laboratory studies will be performed. Tailor assessments to the side effects of particular treatments. For example, the child on chemotherapy is likely to experience a **nadir** (lowest point) of WBC count about 10 days after drug administration so blood counts are needed then.

Psychosocial Assessment

Assessment of body image, stress and coping abilities, knowledge of the condition and cognitive level, support systems, and developmental level provides data that help determine the appropriate nursing interventions for the child with cancer and the family.

Body Image.   Hair loss, surgical scars, and cushingoid changes are three common treatment-induced threats to body image. Most children being treated for cancer experience hair loss (Figure 50–4 ⊙). Children who have cranial

● FIGURE 50–4

One of the most common threats to a child's body image at any age is hair loss induced by chemotherapy. Use of hats can improve self-concept.

surgery lose hair as part of the surgical preparation. Chemotherapy frequently results in some degree of hair loss. The speed of hair loss is unique to the child and can be as rapid as overnight or slower, with hair left on the pillow and in the hairbrush.

A second challenge to the child's body image is surgery. The scars of cranial and neck surgery are obvious, as are amputation and limb salvaging. Abdominal surgery for lymphoma is more easily concealed but is still a threat to the child's body image.

A third source of altered body image is the cushingoid features such as round and flushed face, prominent cheeks, double chin, and generalized obesity (Figure 50–5 ⊙) that result from the use of corticosteroids. As the child's weight increases, stretch marks similar to those of preg-

AS CHILDREN GROW

Children Need Help in Coping with Physical Effects of Cancer Treatment

Children of different ages experience differing threats to body image as a result of cancer treatment. A preschool girl may be most upset at hair loss, since she now looks like a boy. For many parents, especially of daughters, the loss of the child's hair can be devastating. Ask the parents and the child what the loss is like for them. Prepare them for the fact that it can be rapid or slow. Find out how they will plan to cope. Some children want the hair cut very short so its loss will not be as traumatic. Offer resources for wigs, hats, or other ideas. Put them in touch with children who have lost hair and with those who have now regrown it.

A school-age child has the most difficult time with changes that interfere with the developmental task of industry. Amputation, which decreases the child's ability to participate in activities such as sports, dancing, and school work, can be a major challenge during the school-age years. Assist children to adapt to new sports when they are able to do so. Partner with schools, coaches, and families to facilitate children's participation in activities they choose.

Teenagers are often most worried about changes like hair loss and cushingoid features, which cause them to look different from peers. Introducing adolescents to others of their own age who are coping with similar conditions can assist them in their developmental tasks.

FIGURE 50–5

The child with cushingoid changes frequently has a rounded face and prominent cheeks.

nancy may occur. These stretch marks often remain after the corticosteroids are decreased.

Body image disturbances occur when a child cannot integrate changes and continues to cling to old images despite their inconsistency with reality. Common means for assessing body image are drawings, colored pictures cut out by the child to form a collage, discussion, and observation. See Chapter 35 for further discussion of these and other assessment techniques that can be used with children. ∞

Stress and Coping. The diagnosis of cancer is a major stressor for both the child and the family. Although each child's prognosis and each family's coping mechanisms are unique, most families deal with the diagnosis in a manner similar to that of other families who have a child with a life-threatening illness (see Chapter 41 ∞). Assess the family (and child if old enough) for their understanding and acceptance of the diagnosis. Find out if the family has told the child and siblings about the diagnosis and if they need assistance in deciding how to do this (Ishibashi, 2001). Assess the level of anxiety during healthcare visits and scheduled treatments (Figure 50–6 ⊙). Evaluate the family's methods of coping, such as the ability to integrate relaxing and meaningful activities into family life, the use of support systems in the extended family and community, and the ability to alter expectations to take into account the child's health status. Concurrent stressors increase the difficulty of coping with childhood cancer. Evaluate the family for stressors such as illness or death of another family member, occupational changes, financial problems, relocation, and change in vacation plans. Evaluate the family's knowledge

of the U.S. Family Leave Act, which provides for parental use of sick time to treat an ill family member.

Knowledge. Anxious people tend to narrow their scope of attention and may read unintended messages into the behaviors of healthcare personnel. Anxiety also limits a person's ability to retain information.

Assess the child's knowledge of cancer and its treatment throughout the treatment period. As the child matures cognitively, reevaluate knowledge. Cancer and its treatment are complex topics. Parents are exposed to information in various forms, including written material, news reports, and Internet Web sites and resources. Evaluate their knowledge and information sources and provide them with opportunities to ask questions. Evaluate the learning style of the child and family in order to adapt approaches to meet their needs.

Support Systems. Cancer treatment generally occurs over a long time. The extended family is crucial in providing necessary support to the child, parents, and siblings. Identify key people in the family. They may be the parents, grandparents, or aunts and uncles. Support groups for children or other family members often help individuals and the family unit to meet the challenges of the disease. Thoroughly assess the coping strategies the family uses to meet the various challenges posed by the child's illness. This information helps to predict the success of interventions, such as home care with intravenous medications, and to decide when referrals for other supportive therapies are needed.

Assess family resources to identify support systems available to help the family during crises and if a child is expected to die. Extended supports include friends, jobs, insurance coverage, religious affiliations, cultural support systems, and the school system. Parents commonly lose

FIGURE 50–6

The child with cancer depends on parents and family members to provide support. Nurses can assist families and draw upon their strengths to help the child.

contact with close friends after the diagnosis of cancer in a child. This is an additional stressor for the family. Jobs are often a source of support because coworkers may have gone through the same experience. It may also be comforting for a parent to return to a job where he or she can feel a sense of security in tangible accomplishments. However, jobs can also be a source of stress if employers are unsympathetic to the demands of the child's hospitalization and clinic or office visits. The nurse caring for a child and family in the palliative care phase can best support family members by helping them to view the child's unique characteristics, conveying care and concern for the family, and continuing to have close contact with the dying child. Faith-based affiliations can be an important source of support. Evaluate whether such affiliations are meaningful for the family and, if so, plan for visits from the appropriate clergy. In some cultures, spiritual leaders are an important part of the family's support. Enable a healer to visit the child and conduct a healing ceremony if that will be supportive to the family and child.

The return to school may pose difficulties for the child with cancer or it may be a source of support to be connected again to peers. The child is encouraged to go to school, even if only for half a day per week, to stay connected to peers. Evaluate the school's ability to accept a medically vulnerable child into the classroom. Assess whether the other children and teachers have been prepared for the appearance and needs of the child with cancer. Nurses who work in the oncology department of the hospital or clinic can ask if the family would give consent to visit the school, meet with the school nurse, and plan together to meet the child's educational needs. Help the teacher devise a plan to prepare the children, and offer to visit the classroom to explain what the child with cancer is experiencing. Arrangements can be made for tutors to help the child keep up with schoolwork if he or she cannot attend school. An individualized education plan is needed. Parents need information about the legal right to this plan since the child is newly ill and they will likely not have been exposed to this in the past.

Developmental Assessment

Developmental assessment of children should be performed regularly during treatment for cancer at times when the child is feeling well so that results are accurate. Assessment of the child's physical and neurologic development helps determine the progress made during treatment and provides a baseline for evaluating the long-term effects of treatment. Children under 6 years of age who have cancer should receive regular developmental assessment with a standardized tool such as the Denver Screening Test (see Chapter 39 ∞). A home healthcare nurse can perform such testing, or it can be done by a nurse in the pediatric healthcare home (medical home) who sees the child for a general health supervision visit. Recommend referral to a neuropsychologist for testing early in treatment and if changes in developmental performance are noted. Observe developmental milestones at each contact with the child and refer for further assessment if regression has occurred. Performance in school and social activities with friends provides important information about expected developmental milestones in older children. If the parents have signed up for a clinical trial (research) treatment for the child, children should also give verbal or written assent when they have the cognitive maturity to do so.

Children who have received cranial radiation and intrathecal chemotherapy need regular scholastic evaluations. Impaired neurocognitive performance may be a long-term effect of treatment (Challinor, Miaskowski, Moore et al., 2000).

Assessment for Impact of Cancer Survival

Children with cancer have a variety of common psychologic and physiologic problems, regardless of their specific type of cancer. They and their families are dealing with a complex illness that influences their lives for years. The impact of this experience extends into all areas of function. Over the past 20 to 30 years, treatment for childhood cancers has been increasingly successful. About 1 in 1000 young adults is a survivor of childhood cancer. The success of new modalities and treatment combinations has, however, created special healthcare needs for many survivors (Figure 50–7 ⊙).

Surgery can have many results. Body organs may be removed and manipulated, leading to adhesions, intestinal obstruction, visual impairment, neurologic disruption, and sterility. Removal of the spleen can lead to serious infections. Amputation necessitates the need for prosthetic devices and physical rehabilitation.

Radiation has several long-term effects. It can impair the growth of bones and teeth, leading to conditions such as scoliosis, leg length discrepancy, or poor dental health. Hypothyroidism can be observed in those who have had head and neck radiation (Castellino & Hudson, 2002). Cardiotoxicity and pulmonary toxicity can result from mediastinal radiation. Delayed puberty and sterility can result from radiation effects to the cranium and spinal regions. Impaired neurocognitive performance may occur as long-term effects of treatment, especially with higher doses of radiation. Some studies have found lower behavioral and social competence in treated children (Challinor et al., 2000). Secondary cancers, most commonly solid tumors, occur in some survivors. **Secondary cancers** are also called second malignant neoplasm (SMN). They occur subsequent to the primary cancer and treatment but are of a different histologic type.

Chemotherapy can cause a wide variety of effects, both during its administration and for years afterward.

○ FIGURE 50–7

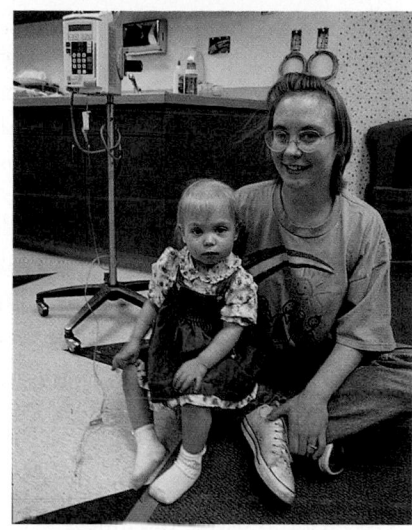

Survivors of childhood cancer. *A,* Nicole, 11 years old, is undergoing chemotherapy for Ewing's sarcoma. Her mother emphasizes, "It's our faith that has gotten us through this. The hardest part is how busy you are coming to treatments all the time. Nicole's younger brother sometimes feels neglected." *B,* According to Jesse, who is 10 years old and waiting for a bone marrow transplant, "The thing that has helped me the most [in dealing with acute lymphoblastic leukemia] is all the mail I got from my friends." His mother adds, "We're just really positive and think that everything will turn out all right." *C,* Cassie, 19 months old, has been diagnosed with neuroblastoma. At this age, it is hard for her to understand what is happening to her. Her mother has stayed with her each time she has come to the hospital, which has helped Cassie adjust to therapy. Her caregivers are confident that she will respond well to her treatment.

(See "Clinical Manifestations. Common Side Effects of Chemotherapy.") Cardiomyopathy can occur with some drugs, especially the anthracyclines. Temporary or permanent pulmonary toxicity and renal complications can develop. Neurologic effects of some drugs can lead to hearing loss (e.g., cisplatin and ifosfamide), cataracts, and paraplegia (e.g., intrathecal methotrexate for leukemia). Learning disabilities and change in intelligence quotient (IQ) occur in some children. Infertility may result (Castellino & Hudson, 2002). Although radiation is responsible for most secondary tumors, some chemotherapy drugs have also been implicated.

The diagnosis and stress of treatment, along with the risk of recurrence, are significant stressors for the child with cancer. Families may find it difficult to obtain full insurance coverage for the child who has had a prior cancer. Employment can be a potential problem for cancer survivors if employers have concerns about the earlier cancer diagnosis. Most people with cancer report fear of recurrence of the disease, which is a stressor. Depression, suicidal thoughts, and concerns about appearance are more common in survivors of childhood cancer (Recklitis, O'Leary, & Diller, 2003). However, hopefulness and the sense of having an added purpose in life can be positive outcomes for many cancer survivors. Some meet with others who have a recent diagnosis, or work on fund-raising events that financially support cancer research.

Nurses are involved with families when a diagnosis of cancer is made, during the therapy process, and in the years that follow. For a child who survives cancer, ongoing care is essential. Evaluate the child regularly with thorough physical, psychosocial, developmental, and cognitive assessments. Carefully monitor all body systems (e.g., cardiovascular; respiratory; musculoskeletal; eye, ear, nose, and throat; genitourinary). Record height and weight and general growth patterns. Ask about the child's interactions with peers and performance at school. Children who have received cranial radiation and intrathecal chemotherapy need regular scholastic evaluations. Impaired neurocognitive performance may occur as long-term effects of treatment, and appropriate interventions should be planned in these cases (Challinor et al., 2000). Be alert for signs and symptoms that could indicate a secondary tumor. Ask the parents about insurance coverage and other financial difficulties during ongoing care.

Plan care to assist the family to manage any long-term effects of cancer treatment. This may involve physical rehabilitation, support related to visual impairment, or treatment for cardiac or musculoskeletal abnormalities. Provide resources for information and support. Facilitate periodic evaluations in a healthcare agency so that serious outcomes of treatment can be identified early.

Children with cancer have a variety of common psychologic and physiologic challenges, regardless of their specific type of cancer. They and their families are dealing with a complex illness that influences their lives for years. The impact of this experience extends into all areas of function.

The accompanying "Nursing Care Plans" include several diagnoses that may be appropriate for the child with cancer who is receiving care in the hospital or at home. Among the many other diagnoses that may be appropriate for a child with cancer are the following:

- *Diarrhea* related to radiation therapy and toxins
- *Impaired Urinary Elimination* related to chemotherapy
- *Impaired Oral Mucous Membrane* related to chemotherapy and radiation therapy
- *Impaired Skin Integrity* related to altered nutritional state, effects of medication, radiation, and immobilization
- *Ineffective Individual Coping* related to situational crisis of chronic and acute illness
- *Disturbed Sleep Pattern* related to biochemical agents, anxiety, and unfamiliar surroundings
- *Deficient Diversional Activity* related to frequent lengthy treatments
- *Disturbed Body Image* related to chronic illness and treatments
- *Deficient Knowledge (Child or Parents)* related to lack of exposure to disease or treatments
- *Anticipatory Grieving* related to actual or potential loss

PLANNING AND IMPLEMENTATION

The nursing care of children newly diagnosed with cancer and their families includes immediate physiologic and psychologic support, along with anticipatory guidance about imminent and future medical interventions. Assist and support the family in making decisions about types of treatment that are appropriate for their child.

Nursing care of the hospitalized child with cancer and the child receiving ongoing therapy at home is summarized in the accompanying "Nursing Care Plans." These care plans are designed for the child who has progressed beyond cancer diagnosis and is receiving chemotherapy.

Physiologic care of the hospitalized child focuses on providing support during treatment. This includes ensuring optimal nutritional intake, administering medications, managing the multiple side effects of chemotherapy and radiation, ensuring adequate hydration, preventing infection, and managing pain during diagnostic procedures and treatment.

Ensure Optimal Nutritional Intake

Up to 30% of children with cancer are malnourished (Han-Markey, 2000). The high metabolic rate of cancer growth depletes the child's nutritional stores. Added to this is the catabolic effect of chemotherapy and radiation on normal cells, necessitating additional cellular replacement. The child needs increased nutritional intake at a time when nausea and vomiting are occurring as drug side effects, and when decreased activity and general health status result in diminished appetite. This often leads to extreme concern on the part of parents, and they may focus excessive attention on the child's intake.

Administer antiemetic drugs to lessen nausea from chemotherapy. Offer frequent, small meals. It may be helpful to offer the child's favorite foods at times when nausea

---

TEACHING HIGHLIGHTS

NUTRITION AND THE CHILD WITH CANCER

Because of the effects of cancer and chemotherapy or other treatment, the child often has a poor appetite. Mucosal sores lead to difficulty chewing and swallowing. Parents can enhance the nutritional intake of the child in a variety of ways:

- Provide frequent small feedings rather than three meals daily.
- Integrate the child's favorite foods into daily menus.
- Have nutritious snacks available for times when the child feels like eating.
- Sprinkle dried milk on top of cereals and other foods.
- Smooth, soft foods are usually preferred. Milkshakes with added peanut butter, puddings, and soft casseroles may be well tolerated. Try a variety of liquid protein-calorie supplements to find those the child likes.
- Avoid making food an area for disagreement. Do not force foods but rather, make them readily available.

- If the child is vomiting due to therapy, do not encourage food at that time. The child may develop food aversions to foods that are vomited.
- Administer antiemetics as ordered during therapy since they can prevent nausea and vomiting.
- Report weight loss and increased fatigue.
- Bring the child in for scheduled health visits so growth, development, and effects of therapy can be monitored.
- Some children need a temporary feeding tube to ensure adequate nutrition. Feedings at night can often increase intake and promote health. Occasionally a central line is inserted to provide total parenteral nutrition.
- Supplements and tube feedings will usually be covered by insurance if the provider writes an order for them.

NURSING CARE PLAN

HOSPITAL CARE OF THE CHILD WITH CANCER

Intervention	Rationale	Expected Outcome

1. Nursing Diagnosis: Pain related to tissue injury

Intervention	Rationale	Expected Outcome
NIC Priority Intervention: **Pain management:** Alleviation or reduction in pain to a level of comfort acceptable to patient		**NOC Suggested Outcome:** **Comfort level:** Feelings of physical and psychologic ease

Goal: The child will report reduced pain that is manageable.

Intervention	Rationale	Expected Outcome
■ Give analgesics as ordered. ■ Teach relaxation techniques, deep breathing, and distraction.	■ Adequate medications can reduce pain. ■ Nonpharmacologic methods work with the medication to reduce pain.	The child experiences pain reduced to the level that allows the child to interact appropriately and gain rest.

2. Nursing Diagnosis: Sleep Pattern Disturbed related to lack of sleep privacy

Intervention	Rationale	Expected Outcome
NIC Priority Intervention: **Sleep enhancement:** Facilitation of regular sleep/wake cycles		**NOC Suggested Outcome:** **Rest:** Extent and pattern of diminished activity for mental and physical rejuvenation

Goal: The child will sleep for hours appropriate to age. The child will report feeling rested.

Intervention	Rationale	Expected Outcome
■ Alter the environment to allow designated rest periods. ■ Plan care to reduce frequency of interruptions during normal rest and sleep times.	■ A quiet environment encourages relaxation needed for resting. ■ Reduced interruptions allow continuous sleep and rest.	The child rests and sleeps for an age-appropriate amount of time per day.

3. Nursing Diagnosis: Imbalanced Nutrition: Less than Body Requirements related to inability to ingest or digest food or absorb nutrients

Intervention	Rationale	Expected Outcome
NIC Priority Intervention: **Nutrition management:** Assistance with and provision of a balanced dietary intake		**NOC Suggested Outcome:** **Nutritional status:** Extent to which nutrients are available to meet metabolic needs

Goal: The child will maintain adequate nutritional intake. The child will experience reduced effects of chemotherapy (i.e., nausea and vomiting).

Intervention	Rationale	Expected Outcome
■ Offer small feedings. Encourage favorite foods. Refer to dietitian for special meals. Weigh daily. ■ Teach the child distraction and relaxation techniques. Give antiemetics according to orders.	■ Measures can increase caloric intake. Taste changes and mouth sores alter desire for food. ■ Pharmacologic and nonpharmacologic methods are effective in helping to reduce nausea.	The child maintains admission weight. The child has minimal side effects of nausea and vomiting.

4. Nursing Diagnosis: Risk for Constipation related to change in usual foods and eating patterns

Intervention	Rationale	Expected Outcome
NIC Priority Intervention: **Constipation management:** Prevention and alleviation of constipation		**NOC Suggested Outcome:** **Bowel elimination:** The ability of the gastrointestinal tract to form and evacuate stool effectively

Goal: The child will reestablish normal bowel pattern.

Intervention	Rationale	Expected Outcome
■ Record all output by size and description. Administer stool softeners. Test stool for guaiac. Report changes in stool to physician. Encourage adequate fluid intake.	■ Chemotherapy or tumor may create constipation, diarrhea, or blood in stool.	The child has normal bowel pattern.

5. Nursing Diagnosis: Fluid Volume Excess or Deficient related to medications

Intervention	Rationale	Expected Outcome
NIC Priority Intervention: **Fluid management:** Promotion of fluid balance and prevention of complications resulting from abnormal fluid levels		**NOC Suggested Outcome:** **Fluid balance:** Balance of water in the intracellular and extracellular compartments of the body

(continued)

HOSPITAL CARE OF THE CHILD WITH CANCER

Intervention	Rationale	Expected Outcome
Goal: The child will be adequately hydrated.		
■ Record all intake. Monitor intravenous rate and solution as appropriate. ■ Test specific gravity of urine daily.	■ Some drugs (e.g., cyclophosphamide) necessitate a high level of fluid intake to prevent complications. ■ Renal function may be affected by chemotherapy.	The child demonstrates adequate hydration. Mucous membranes are hydrated. Specific gravity remains within normal range.

6. Nursing Diagnosis: Risk for Infection related to immunosuppression, invasive procedures, malnutrition, or pharmaceutical agents

NOC Suggested Outcome: **Infection protection:** Prevention and early detection of infection in patient at risk		**NOC Suggested Outcome:** **Risk control:** Actions to eliminate or reduce health threats
Goal: The child will remain free of infection.		
■ Wash hands often. Maintain in isolation if needed. Transmission-based precautions may be needed to safeguard child. ■ Monitor temperature. Report elevation to physician.	■ Handwashing is effective to reduce organisms. Transmission-based precautions may be needed to safeguard child ■ Elevated temperature is a sign of infection.	The child remains infection-free. The child with an infection is effectively treated.
Goal: The child will return to normal, uninfected state.		
■ Administer intravenous antibiotics as ordered. Monitor temperature. Use cooling mattress as ordered. Report elevations over 38°C (101°F) to physician.	■ Multiple antibiotics are needed to deal with bacterial and fungal infections during neutropenia. Blood cultures may be taken to identify organism.	

7. Nursing Diagnosis: Ineffective Individual Coping related to situational crisis

NIC Priority Intervention: **Coping enhancement:** Assisting a patient to adapt to stressors which interfere with meeting life demands and roles		**NOC Suggested Outcome:** **Coping:** Actions to manage stressors that tax an individual's resources
Goal: The child will demonstrate normal adaptive coping methods.		
■ Encourage drawings and other therapeutic play for expression of feelings. Allow for expression of angry feelings, such as hitting dolls and throwing sponge balls. Discuss how to behave during treatments.	■ Expression of feelings helps identify avoidance coping for further intervention. Play is a normal way for child to express self and ideas. Misinterpretations can be corrected. Knowledge of appropriate and helpful behaviors supports self-esteem.	The child continues to use usual coping strategies expected for developmental stage.

8. Nursing Diagnosis: Ineffective Health Maintenance related to complex treatment, and lack of resources

NOC Suggested Outcome: **Health system guidance:** Facilitating use of health services		**NOC Suggested Outcome:** **Knowledge: Health behaviors:** Extent of understanding conveyed about promotion and protection of health
Goal: The child will state understanding of treatments and procedures.		
■ Use age-appropriate teaching methods. Content areas include child's cancer, medications (actions and side effects), how to deal with body changes, and how to deal with response of others to those changes. Correct misinterpretations. Anticipate upcoming events and teach the child and family about them.	■ Education helps by increasing understanding, removing fantasy, and clarifying fears. Education promotes the use of new learning in all areas of life.	The child demonstrates age-appropriate knowledge of the cancer, its treatments, and medications. The child has age-appropriate understanding of how to deal with changes in the body.

NURSING CARE PLAN

HOME CARE OF THE CHILD WITH CANCER

Intervention	Rationale	Expected Outcome

1. Nursing Diagnosis: Risk for Infection related to immunosuppression, chemotherapy, and presence of invasive lines

Intervention	Rationale	Expected Outcome
NIC Priority Intervention: **Infection protection:** Prevention and early detection of infection in child at risk		**NOC Suggested Outcome:** **Risk control:** Actions to eliminate or reduce health risks

Goal: The child will remain infection-free.

Intervention	Rationale	Expected Outcome
■ Educate the child and parents about meaning of blood counts. ■ Encourage parents/family members to use masks when they are ill. ■ Encourage good handwashing at all times. ■ Advise the child's teacher to tell parents if the child is exposed to communicable illness at school. ■ Clean vascular access site and inject heparin per protocol. Observe for signs of infection. Report infection to physician.	■ Knowledgeable parents and child can protect themselves. ■ Masks help decrease airborne infection if used properly. ■ Handwashing is best prevention. ■ Exposure can be reported to physician for possible use of antibiotics or antiviral drugs, or admission for treatment. ■ Use of heparin maintains an open access route by preventing clotting.	The child remains infection-free. All exposures are reported to physician immediately.

2. Nursing Diagnosis: Imbalanced Nutrition: Less than Body Requirements related to inability to ingest or digest adequate quantities of food or absorb adequate nutrients

Intervention	Rationale	Expected Outcome
NIC Priority Intervention: **Nutrition management:** Assistance with and provision of a balanced dietary intake		**NOC Suggested Outcome:** **Nutritional status:** Extent to which nutrients are available to meet metabolic needs

Goal: The child will maintain adequate nutritional intake.

Intervention	Rationale	Expected Outcome
■ Encourage small and frequent high-calorie meals. Encourage small bites of a variety of foods. ■ Promote good oral hygiene and use of nonalcohol mouthwashes. ■ Teach home enteral and parenteral nutrition if ordered.	■ Measures to increase caloric intake. Taste changes and favorite foods may no longer be preferred. ■ Mouth sores interrupt eating. Alcohol stings open sores. ■ Enteral or parenteral nutritional support may be used to enhance intake.	The child maintains normal weight for height.

3. Nursing Diagnosis: Ineffective Management of Therapeutic Regimen related to complex therapy

Intervention	Rationale	Expected Outcome
NIC Priority Intervention: **Family involvement:** Facilitating family participation in the emotional and physical care of the child		**NOC Suggested Outcome:** **Care management:** Family ability to manage complex therapy

Goal: The child will comply with oral medication regimen.

Intervention	Rationale	Expected Outcome
■ Educate parents and child about the importance of taking medication as prescribed. ■ Set up calendar with dates, times, and medications clearly labeled. ■ Reward the child for taking medications.	■ Understanding can assist parents and child in placing importance on medication intake. ■ Visual reminders can help them recall instructions. ■ Reinforcing desired behaviors through rewards is effective with children.	The child takes all medications according to prescription.

(continued)

NURSING CARE PLAN—continued

HOME CARE OF THE CHILD WITH CANCER

Intervention	Rationale	Expected Outcome
4. Nursing Diagnosis: Delayed Growth and Development related to serious illness		
NIC Priority Intervention: **Developmental enhancement:** Facilitating patient's caregivers to promote optimal growth and development of child		**NOC Suggested Outcome:** **Child growth and development:** Normal increase in body size and developmental skills
Goal: The child will demonstrate normal physical, emotional, and cognitive development.		
■ Encourage play appropriate to age. ■ Encourage the child to attend school. ■ Encourage seeing peers when unable to attend school. ■ Work with teachers to support reentry to school. Use puppets, videotape, and discussion with classmates.	■ Normal activities support self-esteem and self-knowledge. ■ School is the work of the child and promotes cognitive and social growth. ■ Peer contacts help the child in normal developmental tasks. ■ Classmates need to understand what has happened to their friend without asking the child directly.	The child continues to develop physically, emotionally, and cognitively at a normal pace.
5. Nursing Diagnosis: Fatigue related to disease state		
NIC Priority Intervention: **Energy management:** Regulating energy use to prevent fatigue and optimize function		**NOC Suggested Outcome:** **Energy conservation:** Extent of management of energy to initiate and sustain activity
Goal: The child will maintain energy levels necessary for normal activities.		
■ Problem-solve ways to save energy for play and school. ■ Plan with child for quiet activities during low-energy times.	■ The child and parents are assisted to see school and play as important. ■ The child is empowered to select and plan own activities.	The child plans use of time effectively to maintain energy for school and play. The child conserves energy during times of increased fatigue.
6. Nursing Diagnosis: Interrupted Family Processes related to situational crisis		
NIC Priority Intervention: **Family process maintenance:** Minimization of family process disruption events		**NOC Suggested Outcome:** **Family process:** Extent of maintenance of family support system
Goal: The child and family will demonstrate healthy adaptation.		
■ Encourage open communication. ■ Suggest that all family members develop support networks. ■ Parents should be proactive with siblings about their feelings and needs. ■ Encourage attendance of all family members at oncology camps.	■ Open discussion allows problem solving and ego support. ■ Networks expand support systems. ■ Siblings feel valued and problems are confronted early. ■ Oncology camps promote open discussion between peers for further support and fun.	Parents report better communication between themselves and the children. Family members report an increase in friends with whom they can share feelings. Family reports attending oncology camp and describes benefit of sharing with other families in same situation.

and vomiting are decreased. Ask the family what treatments they use to decrease the child's nausea and vomiting. Perform 24-hour dietary recalls to assess the child's intake, and evaluate height and weight regularly. Special nutritional products may be given orally, nasogastric or nasoduodenal tube feedings may be given, or total parenteral nutrition may be necessary.

Administer Medications

One of the most important interventions of the oncology nurse is administering medications safely. Most chemotherapeutic drugs are prescribed and calculated as dose per meter squared (dose/m^2), with m^2 calculated from the child's height and weight.

A number of chemotherapeutic drugs are commonly used in combinations. These drugs are prepared with special techniques under laminar flow devices to minimize potential toxic effects on healthcare providers. Gloves and other hazardous drug protocols are used. Care must be taken to avoid **extravasation** of intravenous drugs (leakage into the soft tissue around the infusion site), as permanent tissue damage can result.

In addition to chemotherapy drugs, the nurse administers other medications, such as antiemetics to control nausea, vitamin supplements, and antibiotics. Antiemetics such as ondansetron are given prophylactically when a cancer agent is administered that has known emetic effects. Ask parents about complementary therapy and medications they are obtaining from other sources and using at home. All medications must be safely administered and the child should be monitored for side effects. **Polypharmacy** (the use of several drugs at one time to treat multiple health conditions) can lead to multiple side effects and can challenge the body's ability to metabolize and excrete drugs.

Many children will receive fluids and medications at home via central lines. Consider referral to home healthcare infusion agencies for monitoring of these treatments and provision of supplies for home use.

Manage Treatment Side Effects

All cancer treatments affect some normal body cells as well as cancer cells, causing a wide variety of side effects. A frequent occurrence is **myelosuppression,** or suppression of blood cell production in the bone marrow. Be alert for signs of a decreased white blood cell count, such as infections. **Neutropenia** is present when the absolute neutrophil count (ANC) is <500 cells/mm^3 or if between 500 and 1000 cells/mm^3 when chemotherapy is being given and falling levels are anticipated. At these levels, children will be given a broad-spectrum antibiotic; granulocyte colony-stimulating factor (G-CSF) may be given (see Table 50–3) (Bryant, 2003). Take the child's temperature, isolate the child from others with infections, and perform serum laboratory studies as ordered. A colony-stimulating factor for white cell production may be administered, if necessary. A

treatment known as *leucovorin rescue* is used in conjunction with high-dose methotrexate chemotherapy. Leucovorin (citrovorum factor) is a form of folic acid that helps to protect normal cells from the destructive action of methotrexate. It is started within 24 hours of methotrexate administration and is given along with hydration therapy. Usual administration is q 6 hours X 72 hours or until serum methotrexate is at the desired level.

Protect the child from bruises and be alert for signs of bleeding such as petechiae or the presence of blood in vomit and urine. These are all effects of thrombocytopenia, or decreased platelets. When thrombocytopenia occurs, minimize needle sticks and other intrusive procedures. Be ready to deal with nosebleeds and watch for bleeding gums. Report any bleeding episodes to the physician. Be sure parents know that the child should avoid contact sports or other rough activities and that any healthcare provider, such as a dentist, should be informed of the child's treatment and condition (Bryant, 2003). Infusions to increase platelets are sometimes administered.

Inadequate red blood cell production can result in anemia. Encourage the child to eat iron-rich foods, and administer nutritional supplements as needed. Blood transfusions are sometimes needed to treat severe anemia.

Chemotherapy affects all rapidly growing cells in the body, but especially those of the mucous membranes. Provide good oral hygiene with a soft toothbrush, foam wand, or water irrigation device. Report oral breakdown promptly. See "Teaching Highlights: Oral Care" for common techniques to manage oral hygiene. Be alert for blood in vomitus and stool or dark colored stools, all of which can indicate bleeding in the gastrointestinal tract. Blood in the urine may also occur. Evaluate the effects of hair loss on the child. Know all side effects of specific drugs administered and monitor for them. Some side effects are late and may be seen after therapy is completed. Emphasize importance of all follow-up visits scheduled in the future for monitoring of late effects.

Radiation can cause burns to the skin. Examine the skin daily during hospitalization or weekly when making home visits. Leave the marks on the skin that outline the radiation target area. Avoid use of lotions, powders, and soaps on the target skin area. Some children may need to be anesthetized to ensure correct positioning for radiation; postanesthesia care will then be needed.

Ensure Adequate Hydration

Hydration management can be a challenge as the child may not be thirsty but is excreting large numbers of cell fragments and other substances as a result of treatment. Offer frequent small amounts of fluid. Include frozen ice pops or other fluid-containing foods such as Jell-O. Measure intake and output. To ensure adequate excretion, a number of

CLINICAL MANIFESTATIONS

COMMON SIDE EFFECTS OF CHEMOTHERAPY

SIDE EFFECT	CLINICAL MANIFESTATIONS	CLINICAL THERAPY
Bone marrow suppression	Evidence of suppression usually appears 7–10 days after administration of chemotherapy; recovery is usually complete within 3–4 weeks	Blood transfusions are administered when anemia is severe (Hgb < 7 g/dL) or platelets are very low Some institutions use a low-microbial diet to decrease the possibility that infectious organisms will colonize the intestine Septra is used for *Pneumocystis carinii* pneumonia prophylaxis; nystatin and oral vancomycin for antifungal and antibacterial prophylaxis Instruct the family and child about the importance of protecting the body from bruising during periods of mild to moderate thrombocytopenia (platelet count, < 5,000/mm^3) Careful handwashing is essential Encourage use of masks if family or staff have nasopharyngeal infections
Nausea and vomiting	Symptoms may occur immediately or 5–6 hours after administration of chemotherapy and may last 48 hours	Antiemetics, such as oldansetron, Kytril, Reglan, and Benadryl, are used to treat this side effect Teach relaxation techniques, hypnosis, and systematic desensitization (a hypnotic process that progressively reduces reactions to objects that cause strong emotional or physical responses) to help to decrease the child's symptoms Encourage mild exercise and change of diet (eating only easily digestible foods) 12 hours before chemotherapy
Anorexia and weight loss	May occur at any time	Hyperalimentation is necessary if dietary changes are unsuccessful in halting the child's weight loss Pay careful attention to changes in taste that affect food preferences Referral to a dietician may be helpful to achieve successful modification of the child's diet
Mouth sores	The oral mucositis resulting from chemotherapy usually occurs within 3–4 days and is often a contributing factor in anorexia	Antifungal agents, such as nystatin or clotrimazole, lessen the possibility of candidal infection Promote good oral hygiene, use soft foam wand or water irrigation to clean teeth; commercial mouthwashes are not recommended because they contain alcohol and increase drying of the oral cavity
Constipation	Can occur at any time in treatment but becomes more common as therapy progresses and dietary intake and physical activity decrease	Stool softeners and laxatives are used to treat this side effect Advise parents to increase fluids and fibrous foods in the child's diet
Pain	Pain can occur at any time and is best understood by subjective explanations of the child.	Acetaminophen, morphine, steroids, nonsteroidal anti-inflammatory drugs, and antidepressants may be used to manage pain Careful pain assessment is important; the location of the pain may provide a clue to its cause, for example, metastasis to the skull, infiltration of joints, or damage to soft tissue; pain associated with chemotherapy may also be related to oral mucositis, myalgia, or tumor embolization; painful polyneuropathy can follow treatment with vincristine or cisplatin Acetaminophen for pain can mask the presence of fever, which signals infection; careful and complete physical assessment is needed to identify infection Pharmacologic, nonhypnotic (deep breathing, self-control), and hypnotic methods of pain control may be used; the nonpharmacologic methods often prove helpful to children with pain from multiple etiologies

TEACHING HIGHLIGHTS

ORAL CARE

Since cancer treatment and poor nutritional status can adversely affect the oral status of children, families need help to plan and carry out prophylactic and treatment measures. Children continue to lose teeth, have new teeth erupt, and require nutrients to help in building teeth not yet erupted, even during cancer treatment. Some suggestions are:

- Provide a visit to the dentist early in treatment for assessment, treatment of dental disease, and to establish a prevention plan.
- Floss and brush teeth twice daily with a soft bristle brush and rinse with water.
- When granulocyte counts fall below 500/mm³ or platelets fall below 40,000/mm³, toothettes or gauze can be used to clean the teeth. Avoiding brushes will help to prevent bleeding and infection.
- Toothpaste can be used unless it causes discomfort.
- Medications may be used to prevent infection. They may include antibacterial mouthwash, nystatin, or fluconazole. Continue oral fluoride if it is not present in the drinking water.
- If bleeding, infection, or other oral care needs emerge, consult with the dentist and pediatric oncologist to develop a treatment plan.

(Chin, 1998; Gibson & Nelson, 2000)

chemotherapy drugs are given with intravenous fluids. It is important to administer fluids as ordered and ensure that the recommended urinary output excretion rate is maintained after drug administration.

Prevent and Treat Infection

Children with cancer have an altered immune system, both from the disease and from the effects of immunosuppressant drugs, and must be kept away from persons with known infections. Teach parents to avoid taking the child to places that attract large gatherings of people, such as department stores, once the child returns home. Teach administration of any drugs being used to prevent infection such as pentamidine or sulfa preparations for pneumocystis pneumonia prophylaxis. Emphasize the need to report any exposure to contagious diseases, especially chickenpox. Some drugs may mask signs of infection, so be alert for any signs of mild infection. Fever, malaise, and mild respiratory infection must all be reported promptly (see "Teaching Highlights: Reportable Events for Children Receiving Chemotherapy"). Keep the child's immunization record so immunizations that have not been given yet can be administered in regular clinic visits after therapy is complete, using Centers for Disease Control and Prevention (CDC) recommendations for timing after treatment. Follow recommendations for the immunization of children with cancer as published by the CDC

and the American Academy of Pediatrics. Usually, no immunizations are given to the child until 6 months after he or she has stopped receiving chemotherapy.

Management of infections is critical. Children are often hospitalized and central lines are used for antibiotic administration. Blood cultures and cultures of infected body parts help to establish the causative organisms. Due to lowered immune status, unusual agents are sometimes identified. Administer medication treatment on time and as ordered. Ensure standard precautions and transmission-based precautions are followed. Temperature, vital signs, and assessment of all body systems is performed at admission and at least every 4 hours.

Manage Pain

The child with cancer may experience pain from the disease itself and from the medical interventions, such as lumbar puncture, bone marrow aspiration, and frequent intravenous infusions and blood draws. Use all possible pain management techniques to keep the child comfortable, as this encourages cooperation throughout the long treatment period. Whenever possible, include the parents in comforting the child after painful procedures. (See Chapter 42 for

TEACHING HIGHLIGHTS

REPORTABLE EVENTS FOR CHILDREN RECEIVING CHEMOTHERAPY

Parents require verbal and written instructions about signs and symptoms to report to the child's oncologist while the child is receiving chemotherapy. Have parents report the following events to the child's oncologist if they occur while the child is receiving chemotherapy:

- Temperature above 38°C (101°F)
- Any bleeding, such as nosebleeds, blood in stool or urine, petechiae, bruising
- Pain or discomfort with urination or defecation
- Sores in the mouth
- Vomiting or diarrhea
- Persistent pain anywhere, including headache
- Signs of infection, such as cough, fever, runny nose, tugging at ears
- Signs of infection in central lines, such as redness, drainage, or tenderness
- Exposure to communicable diseases, especially varicella (chickenpox)

Parents should also inform dentists and other healthcare providers that the child is receiving chemotherapy prior to procedures. Prophylactic antibiotics should be given before and after dental care.

Adapted from Bindler, R. M., & Howry, L. B. (2005). Pediatric drug guide. Upper Saddle River, NJ: Prentice Hall Health.

suggestions on methods of pain management. ∞) (See "Complementary Care: Pain Management".)

Management of cancer pain has been the subject of an evidence-based practice report by the Agency for Health Care Research and Quality. The agency concluded that there is a lack of adequate studies on pain management, and there is limited application of existing work. These factors limit effective pain management in many patients with cancer (Agency for Healthcare Research and Quality, 2001a). Nurses must examine research on effective pain management for children and integrate findings into practice. See the Companion Website for relevant links.

Sedation for diagnostic and therapeutic procedures (see Chapter 42 ∞) may be used for pain management. Administer sedation as ordered for young children who are undergoing radiation. Coordinate other painful or intrusive tests so they can be done while the child is sedated for radiation.

Topical anesthetics such as EMLA cream may be used to numb the skin before an intravenous start, lumbar puncture, or bone marrow aspiration. Do not use EMLA on infants who are a gestational age of less than 37 weeks, who are under 20 kg, or who are under 12 months receiving treatment with methemoglobin-inducing agents. For all infants, be certain that parents realize the importance of limiting the area and duration as ordered and to keep the cream in a safe place to avoid ingestion by any children. Another local anesthetic, Numby Stuff, uses lidocaine 2% and epinephrine 1:100,000 application followed by electrical current to produce local anesthesia. Some fast-acting sprays are available for more minor anesthesia. Intradermal application of anesthesia with lidocaine is generally used for more painful and invasive procedures such as central line insertion. They may be combined with sedation to assist the child to relax.

COMPLEMENTARY CARE

PAIN MANAGEMENT

Children have many painful and invasive procedures during cancer treatment. In addition to use of medication, they will be helped by a variety of other pain management techniques. These include the following:

- Parent presence during procedures as a support person.
- Use of distraction and relaxation. Either a parent or healthcare provider can work with the child and integrate techniques, such as singing, counting, telling stories, and blowing bubbles. Children and teens can be taught to visualize positive scenes, use rhythmic breathing, or listen to music (Christensen & Fatchett, 2002).
- Hypnosis has been used successfully to manage both pain and nausea/vomiting during cancer treatment with children from 5 to 18 years (Liossi, 2000).

Provide Psychosocial Support

A diagnosis of cancer brings with it many emotions for the family. Initially parents experience shock and anger. They need basic information about the disease and the purpose of the tests that will be performed. Instructions often need to be repeated as parents may not process information the first time it is presented due to their increased stress levels. Help the parents plan how and when to tell the child the diagnosis. What the child needs to know is based on his or her developmental level and understanding.

Once the family has progressed from their initial state of shock about the diagnosis, they need to learn more about the disease. They may be interested in the pathophysiology, treatment, and expected outcome or the prognosis. Clarify their understanding of these areas and ask what questions they have. Provide verbal explanations and written material. Parents may talk with friends, purchase books, or search the Internet for information. Find out where they are getting information and provide additional resources when appropriate. Correct misconceptions and misinformation.

The family needs many strategies to deal with the challenge of long-term treatment for cancer. As the child experiences remissions and exacerbations or complications, the family feels alternately hopeful and discouraged. Identify the family's support systems and intervene as needed to enhance these systems. Facilitate contact with extended family members who might be of help, religious or spiritual connections, social service agencies, and other resources such as Internet and parent support groups. Assist parents who are concerned about job obligations and financial concerns. Help the parents to identify sources of financial assistance, respite from child care, and time for themselves.

Consider the impact on siblings when a child is being treated for cancer. They may alternately resent and feel guilty for the sibling's illness. They may not understand the treatments or disease. School progress may be slowed and teachers may not be aware of the sibling's stress. (See "Evidence-Based Nursing: Cancer and Stress.")

The child undergoing treatment for cancer needs support appropriate to his or her developmental stage and cognitive level. (See Chapters 33 and 40 for developmental levels and effective support strategies for children of different ages. ∞) Younger children primarily need support during painful procedures and separation from parents. Older children need intervention strategies to help work through feelings about treatments (Figure 50–8 ●). A major developmental task of adolescence is to attain independence and control, but cancer often interferes with adolescents' ability to achieve this task. Therefore, plan nursing strategies that empower adolescents as much as possible. Introduce them to other teens with similar diag-

EVIDENCE-BASED NURSING

CANCER AND STRESS

Clinical Problem

The family of a child with cancer experiences profound stress, and each member of the family needs to adjust his or her role. The needs of family members are often overlooked as the ill child becomes the center of treatment and attention. Family members often provide care for the child, which can be emotionally and physically draining, and can deplete family financial resources.

Evidence

In a study with 153 parents of children being treated at pediatric oncology facilities, nurses provided the Care of My Child with Cancer (CMCC) instrument. Six open-ended questions asked for information about the experience of caring for a child with cancer. Examples included "How does the difficulty of caring for your ill child impact on your ability to care for yourself?" and "What things have helped the most in caring for your ill child?" Results indicated that parent caregivers commonly report lack of caring for self. They have reduced sleep, altered nutrition, and feelings of stress and anxiety. Helpful behaviors by health professionals included prompt and accurate information about the child, with support, understanding, and offers to care for other children or household responsibilities (James et al., 2002).

In another study of 50 siblings of children with cancer, the Nurse-Sibling Social Support Questionnaire was administered. The tool asks siblings to write about things they wish nurses or parents would do to help them, and things that nurses or parents have done that were helpful. Siblings reported feeling left out and not being able to share feelings. They reported a need for emotional support and information, but also need to be with other children like themselves who understand the situation (Murray, 2002).

Implications

Being a family member when a child has cancer is a stressful event. Both parents and siblings express a need for information about the ill child's condition and treatment. Nurses should provide information at each health encounter and frequently ask what questions the family members have. Ask about siblings and include them in visits whenever possible. In addition to information, support is vital. Ask who the parents and siblings have told about the ill child. Who can they turn to when they want to talk? Who can the parents call upon for help at home? Who can the siblings invite to school performances and other events if the parents are unable to attend?

Critical Thinking

Refer back to Rasheed's situation at the chapter beginning. What information do you think his parents need to understand the connection between his enterocolitis and leukemia? Explain the infection and its treatment in terms they will likely understand. What support will his mother need as she returns to work and cannot stay full time with Rasheed during this hospitalization? Rasheed has a 7-year-old stepsister who comes to visit him in the hospital. She seems shy but interested in his care. How can you involve this younger sister in Rasheed's care and make her comfortable during her visit?

References

James, K., Keegan-Wells, D., Hinds, P. S., Kelly, K. P., Bond, D., Hall, B., et al., (2002). The care of my child with cancer. Parents' perceptions of caregiving demands. *Journal of Pediatric Oncology Nursing, 19,* 218–228.

Murray, J. S. (2002). A qualitative exploration of psychosocial support for siblings of children with cancer. *Journal of Pediatric Nursing, 17,* 327–337.

---

noses and allow them to make decisions and choices independent of parents when possible. An adolescent can decide which type of medication port would be best (e.g., an implantable port under the skin or a venous access device with tubing outside the body). Making this choice enables the teen to feel more in control of the disease and treatment.

Talk with the child's teachers before the return to school after treatment to explain the child's condition. Arrange for tutors if necessary to assist the child with school work during hospitalization and home care. Explore the option of summer camp for children with cancer. The Make-a-Wish Foundation strives to make dreams come true for ill children by sponsoring them for a desired activity or outing. Refer the child to this foundation if appropriate. See the Companion Website for links, as well as other resources.

The siblings of a child who has cancer can be stressed by the changes in the family. They may grieve over the ill brother or sister and may feel sad and depressed. They also can experience anger, guilt, or resentment and may have a lack of knowledge about the disease and treatment. Inquire about siblings and ask what they know about the child's condition. Find out who is caring for siblings and whether their teachers have been informed about the family situation. Include siblings in care when possible. Invite them to visit and to participate both during hospitalization and at home care visits. They can be involved in play therapy sessions and recreational activities with the ill child. Ask the parents if the siblings are demonstrating symptoms such as depression, behavioral changes, or decrease in school performance and suggest interventions as appropriate. They may benefit from speaking with a school counselor or can be referred to a support group for siblings of children with cancer. Some cancer summer camps welcome siblings as well as children with cancer.

The family of a child with cancer is faced with a life-threatening illness. Refer to Chapter 41 for strategies to assist the family in coping with this stressor. ∞ For some types of cancer, the child may experience a remission with treatment,

FIGURE 50-8

A child in a pediatric oncology clinic giving injections to a doll. This type of play therapy helps the child deal with fear, thus lowering her stress level.

but a recurrence of disease later as cancer cells grow again. The family may become angry or depressed about the relapse. Repeated treatments challenge the family's support systems. Waiting for the outcome of diagnostic tests can be an especially challenging time. Provide information as soon as possible. If the child's illness progresses, refer the family to hospice to help them care for the terminally ill child and work through the grieving process. Explore cancer support groups and information to share this information with families.

Discharge Planning and Home Care Teaching

Preparation for home care centers on creating a normal environment while supporting the child's physiologic and psychosocial responses to the cancer and treatments. Education is the primary focus of discharge planning. Teach the parents how to ensure adequate nutritional intake, to be alert for signs of infection, to protect the child from exposure to communicable diseases during times of neutropenia, to administer medications at home, and to handle vomiting and pain. Help the parents and child deal with any obstacles to normal development and functioning. Teach the parents and family about symptoms that need to be treated immediately.

Home management of a vascular access device or central line, such as a Broviac catheter, initially challenges parents (Figure 50-9). An implanted port may be used; it allows the child freedom to swim and engage in other activities. Parents will need information about whatever device the child has received. Demonstrate details about cleaning the site, instilling heparin in the line or reservoir, and other

needed care. After teaching the parents, observe them performing the procedure before the child is discharged.

Emphasize the need for the child and family to have fun and be as normal as possible. Play distracts the child and is essential in reducing fears. Children, parents, and siblings often benefit from participation in cancer support groups and cancer summer camps. These activities create additional support systems, build the child's self-esteem, and enhance coping skills through role modeling. (See "Teaching Highlights: Cancer Therapy.")

Make home visits to evaluate the family's strengths and needs in the home setting. Be sure that the family has adequate support from hospice and other end-of-life services when a child's condition is terminal.

Treatment for cancer is generally a long process. Most children are treated for a period of 2 to 3 years. Since normal developmental stages progress during this time, health promotion and health maintenance visits should still occur. Some usual care may have to be altered, but many of the same developmental concerns of all children should be addressed. Help parents to view the child as a "normal" child who is ill for a period of time, but still needs to have limits set on behavior, to develop healthy lifestyles, and to have environmental stimulation to learn to talk, read, or perform motor and cognitive tasks.

FIGURE 50-9

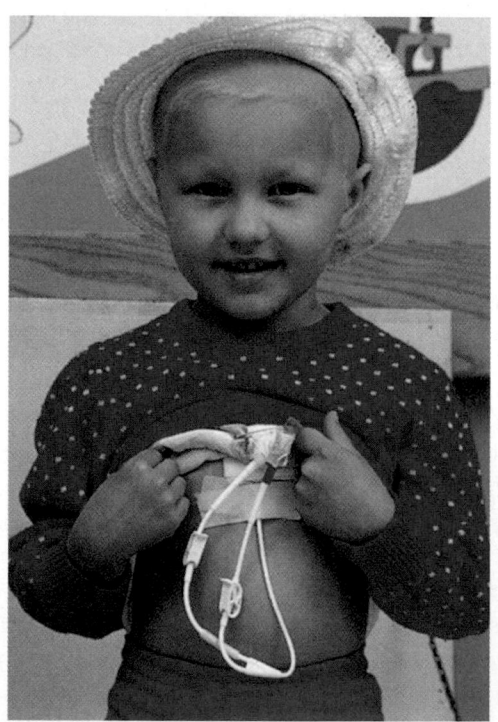

A vascular access device allows chemotherapeutic agents to be administered without the need for repeated "sticks" to the child.

HEALTH PROMOTION
Child Receiving Cancer Treatment

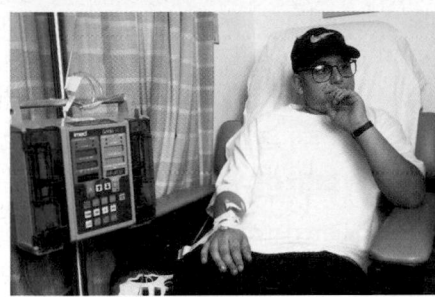

Cancer treatment often extends for several years, so the child needs to continue health promotion and health maintenance visits.

Growth and Development Surveillance

- The child is assessed for height, weight, and body mass index. This provides information about growth patterns which may be altered by cancer treatment. If indicated, 24-hour recalls and other assessments are performed.
- Teaching is provided about age-appropriate foods. Since appetite may be impaired during periods of treatment, the child may be lacking fruits, vegetables, or other foods, as well as the nutrients they include. Encourage parents to be sure the child has a well-balanced diet during periods of remission.
- Perform developmental screening of young children. Provide suggestions for parents about the stimulation that is appropriate for the child's age. Include quiet activities that can be used when the child is fatigued or receiving therapy. These might include reading books, listening to tapes and music, and working on a computer. Have the parent plan for these activities on days that the child goes for chemotherapy or other treatment.
- Ask about the school-age child's progress in school. Performance may be altered due to neurologic effects of treatment as well as missing school. Plan for the family to partner with the school personnel for provision of tutors, computer programs, or other needed assistance.
- Encourage continued social contact with peers when blood counts are adequate to prevent infection.

Physical Assessment and Screening

- Careful physical assessments are performed to identify any abnormalities that may result from cancer or its treatment. Cardiopulmonary and neuromuscular assessments are particularly important. Vision and hearing should be assessed prior to treatment and periodically throughout. Include measurements of fine and gross motor activity.

Elimination

- Toddlers may have an interruption in toilet training during periods when they do not feel well. Help parents to understand this regression and encourage them to start again when the child is feeling better.
- Some medications cause diarrhea or constipation so evaluate bowel patterns and provide guidance as needed. Skin care instruction may be needed if the child has diarrhea and is relatively immobile. Increasing fluids and fiber foods may be needed for constipation.
- Evaluate urinary output since many medications have effects on kidney function. Encourage adequate fluids for age to ensure elimination of medications.

Sleep and Fatigue

- Children undergoing treatment often have disturbed sleep patterns. Parents of young children may become exhausted working all day, getting the child to treatments, and having disturbed sleep at night. Assess both the child's sleep patterns and the family's experiences. Encourage plans for respite care to enable rest periods. Provide cots, rocking chairs, and other comfortable settings for child and family members during treatments.
- Both child and parents may not expect or understand the profound fatigue that occurs during cancer treatment (Davies, Whitsett, Bruce et al., 2002). They can be helped to plan for providing quiet times, and replenishing energy through naps, massage, relaxing baths, and spending time with family.

Physical Activity

- Since the child has periods of fatigue, patterns of physical activity may decrease. Emphasize the importance of integrating physical activity when the child feels well, since it is needed for learning gross motor skills, facilitating blood flow, improving mental status, and setting patterns for the future.

Disease and Injury Prevention Strategies

- The child with cancer has the same safety hazards as other children of the same age, and such topics as car safety seats, fire prevention, water safety, and violence prevention should be addressed.
- An important hazard for children with cancer is infection due to decreased immune response. Keep records of immunization status. Follow the recommendations of the CDC and AAP for other immunizations. Teach the hazards of large groups when the child's immune system is compromised. Teach care of central lines and other potential sources of infection. Have families report signs of infection and exposure to known illnesses promptly.

Mental and Spiritual Health

- Evaluate the child and family for signs of anxiety and depression. Ask how they are managing the cancer treatment and what poses the greatest challenges. Refer to other families with similar circumstances for support.
- Ensure that the child has contact with friends through childcare, school, or via phone, letters, and computer.
- Find out the impact of the child's cancer on the parent's jobs. Ask how the siblings have been coping, what changes there are in school performance, and whether teachers and others are aware of the stress the sibling may be experiencing.

Transitional Care

- As the child's treatment ends, instruct them about needed periodic follow-up with the oncologist. Continue to perform neurological examinations and ascertain school performance. Be alert for signs of secondary tumors.
- Ask about worries regarding the future. As teens grow older, have them take over more responsibility for informing care providers of their cancer history and assist them to transition to adult healthcare providers (Hobbie & Ogle, 2001).

EVALUATION

Expected outcomes of nursing care for the child with cancer relate to the specific disease, treatments, and responses. Some examples of outcomes include the following:

- Adequate intake to promote normal growth
- Hydration that supports body processes and ensures drug and cancer cell product elimination
- Prompt identification and treatment to minimize treatment side effects
- Management of pain to a level of comfort satisfactory to child and family
- Family use of resources to provide necessary support during hospitalizations and treatments
- Knowledge of management of treatment regimens
- Acceptance of prognosis and support of all family members

BRAIN TUMORS

Central nervous system or brain tumors are the most commonly occurring solid tumors in children and the second most common malignancy, after leukemia. Each year approximately 3000 children and adolescents are diagnosed with tumors of the brain and central nervous system, accounting for one in five childhood cancers (Ryan-Murray & Petriccione, 2002).

ETIOLOGY AND PATHOPHYSIOLOGY

While a few cases are associated with other diseases, the cause of most brain tumors is unknown. There may be an association between parental work in aircraft or agricultural industry, paints, solvents, radiation, and electromagnetic fields and higher incidence of brain tumors in children (Ryan-Murray & Petriccione, 2002). Brain tumors in children usually occur below the roof of the cerebellum and involve the cerebellum, midbrain, and brain stem (see "Pathophysiology Illustrated: Brain Tumors"). In contrast,

PATHOPHYSIOLOGY ILLUSTRATED

Brain Tumors

- Supratentorial tumors (cerebral astrocytoma, ependymoma, optic nerve gliomas)
- Tentorial notch tumors (pineal region tumors, hypothalamic glioma)
- Tentorial tumors
- Infratentorial tumors (brain stem gliomas, medulloblastoma, cerebellar astrocytoma, ependymoma)
- Foramen magnum tumors

- Supratentorial tumors
- Tentorial notch tumors
- Tentorial tumors
- Infratentorial tumors
- Foramen magnum tumors

Sites of brain tumors in children. Approximately 3000 children under the age of 15 years are diagnosed annually as having tumors of the brain and central nervous system. The four most common brain tumors in children are medulloblastoma, cerebral astrocytoma, ependymoma, and brain stem glioma.

brain tumors in adults are usually located above the areas between the cerebrum and cerebellum.

The most common brain tumors in children are medulloblastoma, cerebral and cerebellar astrocytoma, ependymoma (from ependymal cells lining the brain ventricles and spinal cord canal), and gliomas of the cerebrum or brain stem. Less common are supratentorial embryonal tumors and craniopharyngioma.

CLINICAL MANIFESTATIONS

Brain tumors in children can be manifested by behavioral and nervous system changes that occur either rapidly or more slowly and subtly. Some common symptoms include headache, nausea, vomiting, dizziness, change in vision or hearing, fatigue, and nonspecific signs. Nonspecific signs include slight behavior change, decreased school performance, or slight incoordination. Brain stem tumors can present with weight deficits, and may be mistakenly diagnosed as an eating disorder of infancy and childhood (failure to thrive). This may delay proper treatment (Lehman, Krishnamurthy, & Berlin, 2002). See "Clinical Manifestations of Brain Tumors" below for common manifestations of certain types of tumors.

Medulloblastomas are brain tumors in the external layer of the cerebellum. They account for 20% of childhood brain tumors, and commonly occur in children 5 to 6 years of age. Astrocytomas arise from glial cells and can be either above or below the area between the cerebrum and cerebellum. They account for 40% of childhood brain tumors. The presenting symptoms vary depending on the location of the tumor. Endocrine, vision, and behavioral changes are all possible, as well as increased intracranial pressure and seizures (Ryan-Murray & Petriccione, 2002).

Ependymomas commonly occur in the fourth ventricle of the posterior fossa and comprise 8% of childhood brain tumors. Impaired growth, hydrocephalus, seizures, and cranial nerve impairments are the most common manifestations. Brain stem gliomas are located in the pons and typically spread into the surrounding tissue. They account for 15% of childhood brain tumors (Conway, Asuncion, & DaRosso, 1999). Cerebral gliomas are another common cancer type in children.

CLINICAL THERAPY

Brain tumors are commonly diagnosed with computed tomography (CT), magnetic resonance imaging (MRI), myelography, positron emission tomography (PET), single-photon emission computed tomography (SPECT), myelography, and angiography. Neurophysiologic tests (electroencephalography and brain stem evoked potentials) are used to assess sensory pathway integrity and disease- or drug-related sensory dysfunction. Other tests that may be performed are tumor markers and cerebrospinal fluid cytology. Lumbar puncture identifies abnormal cells in the cerebrospinal fluid. Bone marrow aspiration and bone scans identify extracranial primary neoplastic growth, since cancers in other sites can metastasize to the brain.

Treatment depends on the type of brain tumor. Surgery is common. It may be performed to obtain a biopsy specimen, to debulk (reduce the tumor by partial removal) or excise the tumor, or to treat any hydrocephalus that may be present. During surgery, radiology images allow the neurosurgeon to see computerized images of the brain while stimulating nerves to determine their functioning. These techniques provide rapid feedback to the

CLINICAL MANIFESTATIONS

BRAIN TUMORS

TUMOR	ETIOLOGY	CLINICAL MANIFESTATIONS	CLINICAL THERAPY
Medulloblastoma	External layer of cerebellum	Headache, vomiting, ataxia	Surgery; chemotherapy with lomustine, vincristine, cisplatin, radiation
Astrocytomas	Glial cells, supratentorial or infratentorial	Seizures, visual disturbances, increased intracranial pressure, vomiting	Surgery; chemotherapy with vincristine, dactinomycin; radiation
Ependymoma	Fourth ventricle, posterior fossa	Hydrocephalus	Surgery, radiation
Brain stem gliomas	Pons	Cranial nerve (VI + VII) tract signs, nystagmus, ataxia, motor symptoms	Surgery, radiation

neurosurgeon. Laser surgery, which has delicate precise control and accuracy, is used when tumors are close to sensitive neural or vascular structures.

Use of radiation after surgery and chemotherapy has improved the survival of children with medulloblastoma and ependymoma. High-dose chemotherapy is often used, and this modality has improved the survival of children with central nervous system tumors (Conway et al., 1999). Low-dose chemotherapy can shrink and help manage some tumors. Intrathecal administration of chemotherapy is useful in some cases.

NURSING PRACTICE

The following drugs are used to treat brain tumors:

Cyclophosphamide	VP-16
Ifosfamide	Cisplatin
Lomustine	Carboplatin
Vincristine	

However, the blood–brain barrier reduces the effectiveness of chemotherapy for children with brain tumors. For example, when methotrexate is administered intrathecally (in the spinal canal), only a small amount crosses normal brain capillaries. Radiation is not used in children under 3 years because of resultant damage to brain cells. Hematopoietic stem cell transplantation is increasingly used.

Complications of treatment for children with brain tumors are significant. They include severe infections (associated with high-dose chemotherapy), seizure activity, sensorimotor defects, hydrocephalus, and growth problems. Care is taken to treat infections early and aggressively. If a cerebrospinal shunt is used, infection or blockage can occur (see Chapter 53 for further discussion of cerebrospinal shunts in children ∞). Anticonvulsants are commonly given prophylactically after surgery. Endocrine problems, such as growth hormone changes, hypothyroidism, and panhypopituitarism, may occur when the tumor is in the hypothalamic–pituitary area. Treatment may also lead to impaired cognitive function and emotional or behavioral problems in some children. Memory deficits and selective attention deficits are the most common problems.

Diabetes insipidus is a special consideration in children with midline brain tumors, such as those that compress the hypothalamus, pituitary stalk, or posterior pituitary gland. Manifestations of diabetes insipidus include voiding of large amounts of dilute urine with a specific gravity of less than 1.005 to 1.010 (see Chapter 52 ∞).

NURSING MANAGEMENT

NURSING ASSESSMENT AND DIAGNOSIS

The focus of physiologic assessment of the child with a brain tumor is determined by its presentation (Table 50–4). Presenting signs can be categorized as follows:

- Nonspecific signs related to increasing intracranial pressure
- Secondary signs related to displacement of intracranial structures
- Focal signs suggesting direct involvement of the brain and cranial nerves

Thorough neurologic examination before surgery is essential to provide a record of baseline functioning. The neurologic examination also allows the evaluation of the child's changing physiologic status before surgery. Ask if the child has manifested slow changes over time or has had quickly developing symptoms. Measurement of head circumference and assessment of the anterior fontanelle are necessary in children under the age of 18 months.

Perform developmental screening on young children using the Denver II or other developmental test (see Chapter 39 ∞). Ask about the child's social interactions, school performance, and any behavior changes that have occurred.

Several nursing diagnoses can be identified for the child with a brain tumor, depending on the type and location of the tumor. Some common examples follow:

- *Imbalanced Nutrition: Less than Body Requirements* related to loss of appetite
- *Impaired Physical Mobility* related to tumor pressure on coordination centers

---

TABLE 50–4 ❖ Physiologic Assessment of Brain Tumors

Clinical Manifestations	Assessment
Nonspecific signs: headache, morning vomiting, somnolence, irritability	Level of consciousness, pupil response, pupil shape and size
Secondary signs: disturbances of cranial nerves; other signs depend on site of tumor	All cranial nerves
Focal signs: truncal ataxia (midline brain tumors), general nystagmus, head tilting	Motor ability, head positions when watching television or looking at people (double vision, sixth cranial nerve involvement)

- *Delayed Growth and Development* related to effects of disability
- *Impaired Memory* related to neurologic disturbance
- *Acute Pain* related to diagnostic tests and treatment

PLANNING AND IMPLEMENTATION

The child with a brain tumor requires multidisciplinary care by, among others, a neurologist, neurosurgeon, pediatrician, dietitian, and social worker. Other specialists are also often needed. The nurse can act as a case manager to coordinate the complex care needed by the child.

For the nursing care of children immediately following surgery, refer to Chapter 43. ∞ In addition, close monitoring of neurologic status is needed postoperatively (refer to Chapter 53 ∞). Be especially alert for signs of increased intracranial pressure and infection. Observe for seizure activity. Administer drugs such as antibiotics and anticonvulsants as ordered.

Signs and symptoms of diabetes insipidus may occur following brain surgery (see Chapter 52 for a description of diabetes insipidus ∞). Nursing care includes hourly measurement of intake and output, measurement of serum sodium levels every 4 to 6 hours, accurate fluid replacement, and frequent assessment of neurologic status. An indwelling urinary catheter is useful for accurate measurement of urinary output. Both abnormally high or low urinary output can indicate problems and should be promptly reported.

Discharge Planning and Home Care Teaching

Teach the parents to watch for an increase in voiding of dilute urine. Be sure they can recognize the signs of infection and changes in the child's neurologic status. Once the child is ready for discharge, chemotherapy or radiation may begin; tell parents the reason and potential side effects of these treatments. Help the family get any special equipment they may need to care for the child at home, such as a wheelchair, bed rails, or dressings. The American Cancer Society is a potential resource for assistance with these needs. See the Companion Website for links. 🌐

Children with brain tumors, especially those who have received radiation, often have some permanent sequelae. They may have slowed development, incoordination, learning disabilities, or other effects. These sequelae are most common in children who are 3 years of age or younger at the time of radiation therapy. Perform accurate height and weight measures at each healthcare visit. Assess developmental milestones. Ask about progress in school and any special services that might be needed. Perform thorough neurologic assessments. Support the family as they learn to deal with unknown or changed

expectations for the child's performance (Freeman, O'Dell, & Meola, 2000).

EVALUATION

Expected outcomes of nursing care for the child with a brain tumor depend on the site of tumor, clinical therapy, and medical outcome. Some outcomes might include the following:

- Adequate nutritional intake to support growth and prevent malnutrition
- Maintenance of a safe environment
- Physical mobility allowed by developmental level and alterations of disease
- Provision of an environment to meet normal developmental milestones within capability of the child
- Management of pain to a comfort level
- Parental understanding of the diagnosis and treatment plan

NEUROBLASTOMA

Neuroblastoma is the solid tumor most commonly occurring outside the cranium of children. It is responsible for 8% of childhood cancers and 15% of cancer deaths in children. The average age at onset is 22 months. Prognosis varies, depending on the staging of the tumor (Table 50–5) and the age of the child, with more favorable outcomes in infants under 1 year of age and in presenting sites in the pelvis or thorax. Less favorable outcomes are associated with presence of N-myc oncogen amplification. Survival rates are 98% for stages 1 and 2, but drop to 22% for stage 4 (Dadd, 2002).

Neuroblastoma is commonly a smooth, hard, nontender mass that can occur anywhere along the sympathetic nervous system chain. A frequent location is the abdomen, although other sites are the adrenal, thoracic, and cervical areas. It is usually diagnosed in children under 5 years of age, with the median age at diagnosis being 2 years (McManus & Gilchrist, 2000).

ETIOLOGY AND PATHOPHYSIOLOGY

Neuroblastoma originates in primitive neurocrest cells that form the adrenal medulla, paraganglia, and sympathetic nervous system of the cervical sympathetic chain and the thoracic chain. Cervical, thoracic, or pelvic ganglia are origins in 30% of cases, with the remaining cases at various sites on the sympathetic chain (Ater, 2004). Metasteses to lymph nodes, bones, skull, liver, and skin are common.

The cause of neuroblastoma is unknown. Theories center on the possible effects of environmental factors such

TABLE 50-5 ❖ International Neuroblastoma Staging System

Stage	Description
1	Localized tumor confined to the area of origin; complete gross excision, with or without microscopic residual disease; identifiable ipsilateral and contralateral lymph nodes negative microscopically
2A	Unilateral tumor with incomplete gross excision; identifiable ipsilateral and contralateral lymph nodes negative microscopically
2B	Unilateral tumor with complete or incomplete gross excision; with positive ipsilateral regional lymph nodes; identifiable contralateral lymph nodes negative microscopically
3	Tumor infiltrating across the midline with or without regional lymph node involvement; or unilateral tumor with contralateral regional lymph node involvement; or midline tumor with bilateral regional lymph node involvement
4	Dissemination of tumor to distant lymph nodes, bone, bone marrow, liver, and/or other organs (except as defined in stage 4S)
4S	Localized primary tumor as defined for stage 1 or 2 with dissemination limited to liver, skin, and/or bone marrow

Data from Castleberry, R. P. (1997). Biology and treatment of neuroblastoma. *Pediatric Clinics of North America, 44*, 919-938.

as prenatal drug exposure from the mother and disturbed cellular nerve growth factors. Canada has recently noted a drop in neuroblastoma rates commensurate with fortification of flour with folate (French, Grant, Weitzman et al., 2003). A genetic defect found in many cases of neuroblastoma is a deletion of the short arm of chromosome 1 (1p del). Oncogenes are present in neuroblastoma cells in a DNA sequence known as N-myc. High levels of the N-myc oncogene are associated with rapid disease progression and a poorer prognosis.

CLINICAL MANIFESTATIONS

The location of the mass determines the symptoms. A retroperitoneal mass causes altered bowel and bladder function; characteristic signs are weight loss, abdominal distention, enlarged liver, irritability, fatigue, and fever. Dyspnea or infection may occur when the tumor is mediastinal. Neck and facial edema may result from vena cava syndrome if the tumor is mediastinal and large. Intracranial lesions may be present with periorbital ecchymosis. Malaise, fever, and a limp can occur if there has been metastasis to the bone. Bone marrow disease can manifest as **pancytopenia** (abnormal depression of all cellular blood

components) with neutropenia (causing infections) and anemia (causing fatigue). Metastatic spread can result in an array of symptoms affecting multiple organs.

CLINICAL THERAPY

The International Neuroblastoma Staging System (INSS) recommends different diagnostic and laboratory evaluations for diagnosis of the primary disease and of metastases (see Table 50–5). Biopsy of the tumor is used for initial diagnosis, and metastases are diagnosed by bone marrow biopsy, radiolabeled scanning, x-ray, CT, and MRI. Vanillylmandelic acid (VMA) and homovanillic acid (HVA) levels are usually elevated in the urine and blood (see Appendix B for normal values). They are used initially to diagnose the disease and later to follow its progress. Areas of necrosis and calcification are readily identifiable with radiologic tests. These tests also help in the staging of the disease by identifying metastases. Urinary catecholamines are increased.

Routine blood cell counts are needed, including CBC with differential. The test may reveal anemia and thrombocytopenia. There is no classic WBC response, although thrombocytopenia may occur in association with disseminated intravascular coagulation. **Leukocytosis** (higher than normal leukocyte count) and **leukopenia** (lower than normal leukocyte count) have been observed with bone marrow involvement. Serum electrolytes, liver function studies, lactic dehydrogenase (LDH), coagulation studies, and urinalysis are performed. Elevations in dopamine, ferritin, NSE (an enzyme in neural tissue), LDH, and GD2 (a sugar and lipid molecule on the surface of neural cells) are seen. All of these laboratory findings are used initially to diagnose the disease and later to follow its progress. A biopsy or surgical removal of the tumor will be followed by analysis of its type and genetic abnormalities. Areas of necrosis and calcification in major organs are readily identifiable with radiologic tests and MRIs. These tests also help in the staging of the disease by identifying metastases.

The stage of the tumor determines the treatment protocol. Surgical excision of the mass is performed, followed by chemotherapy with a combination of drugs. Baseline cardiac function is evaluated if doxorubicin will be used in treatment. (See Table 50–2 on page 1525.) Radiation is occasionally used. Bone marrow transplantation may be performed for advanced disease. HSCT may be performed for advanced disease, sometimes followed by the biological modifier *cis*-retinoic acid and fenretinide (to promote apoptosis). Studies are being conducted involving GD2, natural killer cells, and other treatments, as well as gene therapy to interrupt growth of abnormal cells (Dadd, 2002). Neuroblastoma is most responsive to treatment in children under 1 year of age.

NURSING MANAGEMENT

NURSING ASSESSMENT AND DIAGNOSIS

Assess the presenting site of the tumor, such as the neck or abdomen, by observation and inspection. Palpation is contraindicated. Carefully document related functioning, such as bowel and bladder function. Take vital signs to watch for elevated temperature and vital sign changes caused by a thoracic mass. Observe gait and coordination. Take weight and height and compare to earlier percentiles for the child. Specific assessments during treatment will depend on the treatment methods used (refer to the earlier discussions of chemotherapy and radiation treatment). Psychosocial assessment and emotional assessment of the family are needed.

A variety of nursing diagnoses may be appropriate for the child with neuroblastoma, depending on the location and extent of the presenting disease. Some common diagnoses might include the following:

- *Impaired Gas Exchange* related to ventilation-perfusion imbalance
- *Impaired Physical Mobility* related to neuromuscular impairment
- *Disturbed Sensory Perception (Visual)* related to altered sensory perception
- *Pain* related to tumor pressure and injury
- *Anticipatory Grieving (Family)* related to potential loss of significant person

PLANNING AND IMPLEMENTATION

The nursing management of the child with neuroblastoma can encompass the three phases of medical treatment: chemotherapy, surgery, and radiation. Specific postsurgical care depends on the size and site of the tumor. Normal postoperative care includes providing fluid support and respiratory care and preventing infection.

Nursing care during the chemotherapy phase includes minimizing side effects, preventing infection, teaching parents about the medications their child is receiving, and monitoring physical and emotional growth and development of the young child. When radiation is part of the treatment, use common nursing measures described earlier in the chapter.

Topics for parent and family teaching and discharge planning are presented in "Teaching Highlights: The Child with a Neuroblastoma." Ongoing support and connection to resources to assist in management of the child's treatment at home will be needed. When the prognosis is poor, parents may appreciate referrals to hospice, to other parents who have experienced similar child illnesses, and to other community resources. See Chapter 41 for additional nursing care for the end of life. ∞

EVALUATION

Expected outcomes of nursing care for the child with neuroblastoma include the following:

- Respiratory exchange to support daily activities
- Physical mobility to level possible considering developmental age

TEACHING HIGHLIGHTS

THE CHILD WITH A NEUROBLASTOMA

Surgery Phase
- Teach the parents to observe for signs of infection at the wound site and to take the child's temperature, if necessary.
- Assist the family to provide pain management including medication administration and various comfort measures.
- Teach the parents the importance of keeping accurate records of urine output and bowel movements and to notify the physician if the child does not have a bowel movement at least every 3 days.
- Continue with progression to a regular diet.

Chemotherapy Phase
The child frequently has a central line placed early in the chemotherapy phase. The central line greatly reduces the emotional trauma associated with chemotherapy and blood tests.

- Teach the child how to help the parents with cleaning of the central line.
- Teach the child how to protect the central line.
- Teach the parents how to clean and dress the site of the central line.
- Have the parents practice central line care with a model and then on the child before discharge to increase the parents' confidence.
- Give the parents written and illustrated information about care of a central line.
- Arrange for home care dressing supplies before discharge.
- Give the parents detailed chemotherapy information.
- Teach administration of any medications that the parent will perform via central line or other routes.
- Refer the family to the American Cancer Society for coloring books for children receiving chemotherapy.

- Management of sensory/perceptual alterations to provide for safety and sensory input
- Management of pain to level of comfort
- Acceptance and integration of diagnosis into lives of family members

WILMS' TUMOR (NEPHROBLASTOMA)

Nephroblastoma, an intrarenal tumor that is called Wilms' tumor, is a common abdominal tumor of childhood and accounts for 6% of all childhood tumors (Jaffe & Huff, 2004). Each year the incidence is approximately 8.1 cases per million children. Wilms' tumor occurs most frequently between 2 and 5 years of age, but may also occur in adolescents and adults (Drigan & Androkites, 2002).

ETIOLOGY AND PATHOPHYSIOLOGY

Wilms' tumor is associated with several congenital anomalies: aniridia (absence of the iris), hemihypertrophy (abnormal growth of one half of the body or a body structure), genitourinary anomalies, nevi, and hamartomas (benign, nodulelike growths). This connection suggests a genetic link; chromosome deletions at 11p13 and 11p15 (locations for WT1 and WT2 genes) have been associated with Wilms' tumor (Kline & Sevier, 2003). It has a high incidence in Beckwith-Wiedemann syndrome, which is characterized by macroglossia and hypoglycemia (McLorie, 2001). However, most children with Wilms' tumor have no other abnormalities. A tumor suppressor gene has been identified that acts to promote normal kidney development. This gene and others may be missing in children with Wilms' tumor (Jaffe & Huff, 2004). Wilms' tumor grows very quickly, doubling its size in 11 to 13 days. Such fast growth generally contributes to a large tumor by the time of diagnosis. However, there is usually good response to chemotherapy drugs (Scott, Britt, Juneau, & McKracken, 2001). Tissue type is associated with outcome, with anaplastic tumors having a less favorable prognosis.

CLINICAL MANIFESTATIONS

Wilms' tumor is usually an asymptomatic, firm, lobulated mass located to one side of the midline in the abdomen. Often a parent discovers the mass during the child's bath. Hypertension caused by increased renin activity related to renal damage is reported in 25% of cases. Hematuria is sometimes present. Bilateral Wilms' tumors occur in 5% to 10% of cases (Jaffe & Huff, 2004).

CLINICAL THERAPY

The diagnosis of Wilms' tumor is based on an ultrasound study of the abdomen and an intravenous pyelogram. CT scanning or MRI of the lungs, liver, spleen, and brain may be performed to identify any metastasis. This information is used in staging the tumor (Table 50–6). A complete blood count is obtained, as well as BUN and creatinine levels. Liver function tests are performed.

Treatment is multifaceted and increasingly successful; about 90% of early stages and 70% of metastic cases have long-term survivial (Pritchard-Jones, 2002). Surgery is performed to remove the affected kidney, to examine the opposite kidney, and to look for other sites of metastasis. Chemotherapy or radiation therapy, alone or in combination, is sometimes used before surgery to reduce the size of the tumor. Radiation, chemotherapy, or both may also follow surgery. Children whose tumors are almost completely

---

TABLE 50–6 ✛ National Wilms' Tumor Study Staging System

Stage	Description
I	The tumor is limited to the kidney and completely excised.
	The surface of the renal capsule is intact. The tumor is not ruptured before or during removal. No residual tumor is apparent beyond the margins of the excision.
II	The tumor extends beyond the kidney but is completely excised. Regional extension of the tumor is present i.e., penetration through the outer surface of the renal capsule into the perirenal soft tissues. Vessels outside the kidney substance are infiltrated or contain tumor thrombus. Biopsy may have been performed on the tumor, or local spillage of tumor confined to the flank has occurred. No residual tumor is apparent at or beyond the margin of excision.
III	Residual nonhematogenous tumor is confined to the abdomen. Any of the following may occur: ■ Lymph nodes on biopsy are found to be involved in the hilus, the periaortic chains, or beyond. ■ Diffuse peritoneal contamination by the tumor has occurred, such as by spillage of tumor beyond the flank before or during surgery, or by tumor growth that has penetrated through the peritoneal surface. ■ Implants are found on peritoneal surfaces. ■ The tumor extends beyond the surgical margins either microscopically or grossly. ■ The tumor is not completely resectable because of local infiltration into vital structures.
IV	Hematogenous metastasis: deposits are present beyond stage III (e.g., lung, liver, bone, and/or brain).
V	Bilateral renal involvement is present at diagnosis. An attempt should be made to stage each side according to the above criteria on the basis of extent of disease before biopsy.

Data from Green, D. M., Grigoriev, Y. A., Nan, B., Takashima, J. R., Norkool, P.A., D'Angio, G. J., & Breslow, N. E. (2001). Congestive heart failure after treatment for Wilms' tumor: A report from the National Wilms' Tumor study group. *Journal of Clinical Oncology, 19*, 1926-1934.

excised and who have a favorable prognosis do not require irradiation of the tumor bed.

Long-term complications of treatment include liver damage, portal hypertension, and mild cirrhosis, which may occur in children treated for right-sided Wilms' tumor. Radiation damage (such as thinning or weakening) of the skeleton, pelvis, and thorax has been reported. Kyphosis and scoliosis may occur from irradiation of vertebral bodies and the pelvis. Glomerular damage to the remaining kidney may also occur. Second malignancies in the original radiation field have occurred with orthovoltage radiation, but recent changes in radiation therapy have reduced this risk.

NURSING MANAGEMENT

NURSING ASSESSMENT AND DIAGNOSIS

Perform a thorough baseline assessment of the child. Do not palpate the abdomen because of the potential for spreading the cancerous cells. Monitor the child's blood pressure carefully as hypertension is a common finding that may require treatment.

Nursing diagnoses for a child with Wilms' tumor will differ depending on the phase of treatment. Some common nursing diagnoses might include the following:

- *Risk for Infection* related to inadequate defenses
- *Impaired Urinary Elimination* related to anatomic obstruction
- *Ineffective Cardiopulmonary Tissue Perfusion* related to hypertension caused by mechanical reduction of blood flow
- *Risk for Caregiver Role Strain* related to child's illness severity
- *Risk for Impaired Home Maintenance* related to child's disease

PLANNING AND IMPLEMENTATION

Nursing management can be divided into two phases: the postrenal surgery phase and the chemotherapy phase. (See Chapter 40 for general care of the child after surgery. ∞) Drawings and special teaching dolls with removable kidneys can be used to teach young children about the surgery. Although chemotherapy may occur at two different times, before and after surgery, nursing management considerations remain the same.

Nursing care during the postrenal surgery phase focuses on pain management and close monitoring of fluid levels. A large incision is necessary to remove the kidney, and the resultant postoperative shift of organs and fluid in the abdominal cavity may create discomfort for the child. Frequently reposition the child and use noninvasive and pharmacologic pain interventions to improve the child's comfort. Gentle handling is important. Monitor fluids closely following surgery to prevent hypovolemia and to assess the shift of fluids out of the third space and out of the body. Assess daily weight, intake and output (I&O), and urine specific gravity. Monitor the function of the remaining kidney. Take blood pressure frequently to watch for signs of shock and to assess the functioning of the remaining kidney.

During the chemotherapy phase, monitor the child for side effects of drugs, the potential for infection from the central line site, and the function of the remaining kidney. Advise parents about home care needs, administration of medications, and monitoring for drug side effects and ongoing needs for health monitoring. A long-term complication in children who received doxorubicin treatment is congestive heart failure, so ongoing periodic healthcare evaluations are needed. Be sure care is well coordinated among all healthcare providers.

EVALUATION

Desired outcomes for nursing care of the child with nephroblastoma include balanced intake and output, normal vital signs, recovery from surgery, and successful family management of postsurgical care and ongoing treatments.

BONE TUMORS

OSTEOSARCOMA

Osteosarcoma is a rare, malignant bone tumor that occurs predominantly in adolescent boys. Its peak incidence is during the rapid growth years. The tumor is usually located at the metaphysis of the distal femur, proximal tibia, or proximal humerus (Betcher, Simon, & McHard, 2002).

Etiology and Pathophysiology

Bone tissue produced by osteosarcoma never matures into compact bone. Although the cause of osteosarcoma is unknown, radiation exposure (either environmental or treatment related) is associated with its development. Survivors of retinoblastoma have a greatly increased incidence of osteosarcoma. An abnormality of gene p53 has been noted in some cases of this cancer, leading to oncogene malformations and possibly to an absence of tumor suppressor genes (Betcher et al., 2002).

Clinical Manifestations

The common initial symptoms are pain and swelling. The pain can be referred to the hip or back, which can delay diagnosis. Pulmonary metastasis occurs in 20% of cases. Other metastatic sites include kidney, adrenals, brain, and pericardium. When lung metastasis is the only site, lung resection may be successful for treatment. Disseminated metastases and bone lesions have poorer prognoses.

Clinical Therapy

Diagnosis is made through radiographic tests (radiographic studies of the affected area, bone scan, CT or MRI scans of involved bone), blood test for serum alkaline phosphatase (level may be elevated), and tumor biopsy (to confirm the diagnosis). Arteriography may be performed if limb-sparing surgery is contemplated.

Treatment involves both surgery and chemotherapy. The surgery is either a limb-salvage procedure or limb amputation. In limb-salvage procedures the tumor is removed and an internal prosthesis is inserted. A limb-salvage procedure is possible if bone growth has taken place and a neurobundle (area where several nerves converge) is not involved in the tumor. If these two criteria are not met, limb amputation is necessary. Physical rehabilitation will be needed after either amputation or limb-salvage procedure. Aggressive chemotherapy following surgery has improved the survival rate. At the time of diagnosis, most children have metastases (even though they may not be identifiable), so chemotherapy is needed. Chemotherapy is started before surgery to shrink the tumor, especially when limb-salvage surgery is planned. It is also given postoperatively to treat and prevent metastasis.

NURSING PRACTICE

The following drugs are used to treat osteosarcoma:
- Methotrexate with leucovorin rescue
- Doxorubicin
- Cisplatin
- Ifosfamide with mesna

EWING'S SARCOMA

Ewing's sarcoma is a malignant, small, round cell tumor usually involving the diaphyseal (shaft) portion of the long bones. The most common sites are the femur, pelvis, tibia, fibula, ribs, humerus, scapula, and clavicle, but any bone may be involved. Ewing's sarcoma occurs in two children per million, is most common in whites and Hispanics, and is rare in black and Asian-American children. The incidence is highest in children between the ages of 10 and 20 years (Betcher et al., 2002).

Translocations on chromosomes 11 and 22 have been identified in children with Ewing's sarcoma; these are t(11;22)(q24;q12). In addition, these tumors express a proto-oncogene, c-myc.

The symptoms are similar to those of osteosarcoma and may include pain, swelling, fever, an elevated WBC count, an elevated erythrocyte sedimentation rate, and elevated c-reactive protein. Some children present with a fracture of the affected bone. A tumor biopsy is necessary for diagnosis. Diagnostic tests are the same as those for osteosarcoma.

Initial treatment for Ewing's sarcoma is chemotherapy to reduce the tumor, followed by surgical removal of the entire bone or intensive high-dose irradiation of the entire bone. Limb-salvage procedures are now commonly performed rather than amputation. Surgery is preferred because of the possibility of a secondary cancer from radiation. Chemotherapy is always used after initial treatment, as undetectable metastases are nearly always present.

NURSING PRACTICE

The following drugs are used to treat Ewing's sarcoma:

Vincristine	Doxorubicin
Cyclophosphamide	Ifosfamide
Dactinomycin	Etoposide

NURSING MANAGEMENT

NURSING ASSESSMENT AND DIAGNOSIS

Physiologic assessment of the child with a bone tumor includes assessment of the site before surgery. Assess the child's pain or discomfort, mobility, and gait. Take careful vital signs, especially noting temperature and respirations. Psychologic assessments of the child and family are needed, especially if amputation is planned. Loss of a limb causes body image disturbances, particularly with school-age children and adolescents. Assess the child's understanding of the treatment and of care after surgery. Find out what support systems are available for assistance.

Observe the wound postoperatively for infection and hemorrhage. Assess circulation above and below the operative site. If edema is found, elevate the limb. If a limb-salvage procedure is performed, the child's extremity will remain, but it will not function as before because muscle insertion sites and mass have been removed with the tumor during surgery. Detailed charting of the condition of the surgical site and limb function is important.

If the limb has been amputated, assess the child for the following signs indicating a disturbed body image:

- Refusal to look at or touch the altered or missing body part
- Preoccupation with loss or change
- Feelings of shame or embarrassment, either verbalized or demonstrated
- Distorted perception of normal body (easily seen in the child's drawings of the body)
- Fears of rejection or unwanted attention from others
- Overexposure or hiding of the affected body part
- Actual or perceived change in the structure and function of the body or body parts

Psychosocial assessment of the child and family is discussed in more detail earlier in the general section titled "Childhood Cancer" (see pp. 1542–1544).

Nursing diagnoses for the child with a bone tumor are based on the treatment and needs of each child. The nursing diagnoses that might be appropriate include the following:

- *Risk for Infection* related to amputation or limb-salvage procedure
- *Impaired Skin Integrity* related to mechanical forces of prosthesis
- *Impaired Physical Mobility* related to musculoskeletal impairment
- *Impaired Adjustment* related to disability and lifestyle change
- *Disturbed Body Image* related to treatment and injury
- *Pain* related to physical injury of tissues

PLANNING AND IMPLEMENTATION

Care of the child after surgery involves general postoperative care (see Chapter 40 ∞). The child who has had an amputation has special needs regarding skin care and rehabilitation. Inspect the tissue at the surgical site, using sterile technique, and turn the child at least every 2 hours. The site needs to heal completely before chemotherapy can begin and a prosthesis can be made. Pain management is a major nursing care need. When amputation has occurred the adolescent will often experience phantom pain. This is pain that feels as if it is in the amputated extremity and is caused by trauma to the nerves in the area of the amputation. Acknowledge the pain as real since the nerve endings are intact and the patient is perceiving real discomfort. Medicate adequately and use additional pain control measures such as repositioning the limb using gentle movement, supporting the limb, and using distraction or deep breathing (Gilger, Groben, & Hinds, 2002).

Discuss insurance and other financial arrangements with the parents, as prosthetics can be costly. Physical therapy will be needed as well. Referral to a Shriners Hospital is an option for some families.

Implement plans to help the child deal with body image disturbance. Plan for a visit from another child who is well adjusted to a prosthesis. Help the child gradually learn how to care for the stump. Slow progress may be made as the child first looks briefly, then for longer periods, and finally is willing to touch the stump. Show the child how it is possible to continue with sports such as baseball, skiing, or biking with a prosthesis. A discussion group with others can be very useful for adolescents. Plan with the child how to tell friends about the surgery and what issues he or she may face upon return to school. Make plans for elevator access if needed and emergency evacuation procedures. Some children or adolescents may need referral for counseling to assist in dealing with body image disturbance.

The child will receive physical rehabilitation while hospitalized and after discharge. When the child is discharged, explain to the family the importance of bringing the child for outpatient chemotherapy and physical rehabilitation visits. Special arrangements may be needed at the child's school to accommodate a wheelchair, crutches, or ambulation with a new prosthesis. Call or visit the school to see whether there are buttons to open doors, wide doorways to facilitate passage, and any limitations of the building. Contact school personnel to plan the child's return.

Follow-up care is needed to monitor for progress and to be alert for signs of metastases. Fracture may be a sign of recurrent tumor. All body systems such as lungs, heart, kidneys, and liver are monitored for signs of recurrence.

EVALUATION

Expected outcomes of nursing care for the child with a bone tumor focus on the treatments required and adaptation to changes in lifestyle. Examples include the following:

- Healed surgical site with no signs of infection
- Adaptation to changes in mobility status
- Successful adjustment to changes required in school settings
- Maintenance of healthy skin

- Positive body image
- Management of pain to comfort level
- Successful integration of continuing medical therapy

LEUKEMIA

Leukemia is among the most commonly diagnosed pediatric malignancies in children under 14 years of age. A cancer of the blood-forming organs, leukemia is characterized by a proliferation of abnormal white blood cells in the body. Several types of leukemia are differentiated, depending on the blood cells affected. The main types are acute lymphoblastic leukemia, acute myelogenous leukemia, and the rare chronic leukemias of childhood.

The most common type of childhood leukemia is acute lymphoblastic leukemia (ALL), which accounts for 25% of all childhood cancer and 75% of leukemias in children. The peak age at onset is 2 to 4 years (Landier, 2001). ALL is more common in whites and in boys (Westlake & Bertolone, 2002). Subtypes of ALL are based on the French-American-British (FAB) system of classification. There are three types of ALL in the FAB system: L1, L2, and L3. Rasheed, who is described in the opening scenario, has ALL.

Acute nonlymphocytic leukemia (ANLL) refers to all leukemias from myeloid cells. About 17% of childhood leukemias are ANLL. ANLL is most common in children younger than 2 years of age and in adolescents. It is more common in males than females and in Asians/Pacific Islanders, Hispanics, and whites than in blacks (Landier, 2002; Reynolds, Von Behren, & Elkin, 2002). There are several subtypes of ANLL in the FAB classification:

M0 = acute nonlymphocytic leukemia without maturation

M1 = acute nonlymphocytic leukemia with poor maturation

M2 = acute nonlymphocytic leukemia with maturation

M3 = acute promyelocytic leukemia

M4 = acute myelomonocytic leukemia

M5 = acute monocytic leukemia

M6 = erythroleukemia

M7 = acute megakaryocytic leukemia

Because chronic leukemias such as chronic myelocytic, chronic myelomonocytic, and chronic lymphocytic leukemia are rare in children, the following discussion will focus on ALL and ANLL.

ETIOLOGY AND PATHOPHYSIOLOGY

The causes of leukemia are not well understood. Some investigators theorize that exposure to infectious agents can predispose children to leukemia (Kinlen & Balkwill, 2001). Genetic factors are believed to play a role in some types of the disease. For instance, children with chromosomal defects such as Down syndrome, neurofibromatosis type I, Bloom syndrome, and Shwachman syndrome have an increased incidence of ALL, and chromosomal abnormalities are present in most children with ALL (Westlake & Bertolone, 2002). Children with immune deficiency states, such as ataxia-telangiectasia, congenital hypogammaglobulinemia, and Wiskott–Aldrich syndrome, have an increased risk of ALL.

Ionizing radiation exposure when in utero and chemical agents such as treatment with chemotherapy for other cancers are thought to play some role in the development of ANLL. There are several chromosomal and genetic abnormalities associated with ANLL. For example, trisomy 8 is associated with all subtypes of the disease (Landier, 2002).

Leukemia occurs when the stem cells in the bone marrow produce immature WBCs that cannot function normally. These cells proliferate rapidly by cloning instead of normal mitosis, causing the bone marrow to fill with abnormal WBCs. The abnormal cells then spill out into the circulatory system where they steadily replace the normally functioning WBCs. As this occurs, the protective lymphocytic functions such as cellular and humeral immunity are reduced, leaving the body vulnerable to infections.

The malignant WBCs rapidly fill the bone marrow, replacing stem cells that produce erythrocytes (red blood cells) and other blood products such as platelets, thereby decreasing the amount of these products in circulation. The stem cells are replaced by leukemic clones, eventually resulting in anemia. Children with leukemia commonly experience abnormal bleeding because of the reduced amounts of platelets.

CLINICAL MANIFESTATIONS

Children with ALL and ANLL usually have fever, pallor, overt signs of bleeding, lethargy, malaise, anorexia, and large joint or bone pain. Petechiae, frank bleeding, and joint pain are cardinal signs of bone marrow failure. Enlargement of the liver and spleen (hepatosplenomegaly) and changes in the lymph nodes (lymphadenopathy) are common. If the leukemia has infiltrated the central nervous system (entered it by means of the circulatory or lymphoid system), the child may have signs such as headache, vomiting, papilledema, and sixth cranial nerve palsy (inability to move the eye laterally). These findings are caused by the leukemic cells massing and putting pressure on nerves. The testicles, spinal cord, and bone marrow are common sites for infiltration. The leukemic cells in the testicle become a mass that causes the testicle to enlarge, often painlessly.

MediaLink Video: Leukemia

CLINICAL THERAPY

Diagnosis is based initially on blood counts and bone marrow aspiration. Blood counts reveal anemia, **thrombocytopenia**, and neutropenia. Bone marrow aspiration reveals immature and abnormal lymphoblasts and hypercellular marrow and is the differential test. Percent of blast cells in marrow is measured and 25% lymphoblasts is definitive of disease (Westlake & Bertolone, 2002). Neutropenia, thrombocytopenia, and anemia are commonly noted. Other abnormal laboratory findings include elevated serum uric acid and elevated calcium, potassium, and phosphorus levels. New laboratory studies such as rapid flow cytometric assay are making the detection of even very small numbers of leukemic cells possible, so that treatment can improve prognosis in children with minimal residual disease (Coustan-Smith, Sancho, Hancock, et al., 2000). Leukemic cells are examined and classified by FAB type, and DNA analysis may provide clues about genetic changes; all of these considerations are used to establish the protocol for treatment. Cells of children with ALL are B cell or T cell; these classifications are also used to establish treatment protocols.

NURSING PRACTICE

Following are the laboratory values in leukemia:

	Usual	Common Values in Leukemia
Leukocytes	<10,000/µL	>10,000/µL
Platelets	150,000–400,000/µL	20,000–100,000/µL
Hemoglobin	12–16 g/dL	7–11 g/dL

Treatment of ALL involves radiation and chemotherapy. Radiation is used for central nervous system disease, in T cell leukemia, and for testicular involvement. Chemotherapy is organized into four phases: (1) induction, (2) consolidation, (3) delayed intensification, and (4) maintenance of remission. Additional drugs may be used for treatment of central nervous system involvement. Maintenance therapy may continue for 2 to 3 years, causing decreased resistance to infection for this prolonged period (Kanarek, 1998). Treatment of ANLL involves use of a wide variety of drugs during the induction and consolidation phases.

Maximum cell death occurs during the induction phase. The cells that remain after this period are more resistant to treatment. After 3 to 4 weeks, when a remission has occurred, central nervous system prophylaxis begins. Drugs are used in combination with cranial irradiation.

NURSING PRACTICE

The following drugs are used to treat acute lymphoblastic leukemia:

Induction phase

Prednisone	L-asparaginase
Vincristine	Daunorubicin

Central nervous system prophylaxis

Intrathecal methotrexate

Consolidation phase

L-asparaginase	Doxorubicin

Delayed intensification

Vincristine	Cyclophosphamide
Ara-C	

Maintenance phase

6-mercaptopurine or 6-thioguanine
Methotrexate

NURSING PRACTICE

The following drugs are used to treat ANLL:

Induction phase

Daunorubicin	Mitoxantrone
Doxorubicin	Cytarabine

Consolidation phase

Etoposide	Teniposide

During the consolidation phase, chemotherapy with l-asparaginase and doxorubicin is administered. Delayed intensification uses additional drugs to target the leukemic cells that have survived. Treatment during the maintenance phase is aimed at destroying the remaining leukemic cells. Combinations of active drugs are used to prevent resistance. Occasionally other drugs are added to the regimen, such as vincristine, prednisone, cyclophosphamide, intravenous methotrexate, cytosine arabinoside, or anthracyclines (See "Drug Guide" on the Companion Website).

The prognosis for children with leukemia is much improved with current therapy. However, several risk factors affect the long-term outcome. The most favorable findings are:

- Age at onset between 2 and 10 years.
- Initial hemoglobin level less than 10 g/dL.
- Low initial WBC count.
- Lack of B- or T-cell antigens.
- Absence of extramedullary (outside bone marrow or spinal cord) involvement.
- Rapid response to chemotherapy.

MEDIALINK Drug Guide: Methotrexate

The most important factor is the initial leukocyte count. The higher the leukocyte count (over 50,000/mm³) at diagnosis, the worse the prognosis. For children in the low-risk group, the probability of prolonged survival is as high as 90%. Infants under 12 months of age have a poor prognosis. Treatment methods and duration are adjusted for each child, depending on that child's risk factors. More aggressive treatment is undertaken for those in the higher risk groups.

Approximately 10% of children have a relapse within a year after completing treatment. Treatment for relapse consists of additional chemotherapy drugs. The prognosis is best if the relapse occurs late after the initial diagnosis and after the initial treatment is completed. Bone marrow transplantation is a treatment option for the child who has a relapse with ALL, who then achieves a second remission; the transplant is given when the child is in remission. Transplant is also used for children with ANLL; they do not need to be in remission for the transplant to be performed. Chemotherapy itself can create numerous complications, affecting all body organs. Central nervous system toxicity; damage to organs such as pituitary, liver, kidneys, heart, and lungs; and secondary malignancies sometimes occur.

NURSING MANAGEMENT

NURSING ASSESSMENT AND DIAGNOSIS

Thorough physical assessment is important to ensure prompt identification of problems without injuring the child who has deficient coagulation and immune function. Perform assessments every 8 hours or more often depending on the chemotherapy regimen. Observe carefully for bruising, other new sites of bleeding, and fever or other signs of infection. Once chemotherapy has begun, closely monitor renal functioning through specific gravity, I&O, and daily weight measurement. Monitor dietary intake, nausea, vomiting, and constipation. Observe for mucosal sores in the mouth. A central line is usually in place for intravenous infusion of medications, so carefully assess the line for proper functioning and for signs of infection. Ask the parents about any behavioral changes. Central nervous system infiltration can affect the child's level of consciousness, causing irritability, vomiting, and lethargy. However, chemotherapeutic drugs and antiemetics can also induce these nonspecific signs. Frequent venipunctures, bone marrow aspirations, and lumbar punctures require pain assessment and an evaluation of the level of knowledge and coping skills of child and family.

Leukemia causes many changes in the body, and confirmation of the disease is difficult for families to face. Among the many nursing diagnoses that might be appropriate for the child with leukemia are the following:

- *Imbalanced Nutrition: Less Than Body Requirements* related to inability to ingest food
- *Risk for Infection* related to altered immune system functioning
- *Risk for Injury* related to bleeding
- *Activity Intolerance* related to generalized weakness
- *Pain* related to chemotherapy and disease process
- *Disturbed Sleep Pattern* related to chemotherapy drugs and disease process
- *Anxiety (Child and Parent)* related to change in health status

PLANNING AND IMPLEMENTATION

Bone marrow suppression may necessitate transmission-based precautions. Instruct parents in the prevention of infection and use nursing care measures to prevent infection also. Perform careful handwashing; take temperature frequently; give mouth care with antibacterial mouth washes; inspect skin, mouth, rectal area, and central line site for any signs of infection. Care of mouth sores and other side effects of chemotherapy is presented in "Nursing Care Plan: Hospital Care of the Child with Cancer," earlier in this chapter.

Special attention to renal function is needed when the child receives cyclophosphamide. Gross hematuria is a side effect of this drug. Hydration with intravenous fluids to attain a specific gravity of less than 1.010 prevents or reduces the severity of hematuria. It also prepares the kidneys to manage products of tumor cell breakdown. To achieve the desired specific gravity, the child receives intravenous fluids at 1 1/2 times maintenance volume for at least 6 to 8 hours before and at least 1 1/2 hours after administration of the drug. Other chemotherapy drugs have different infusion times, while some do not require hydration prior to infusion. Check drug references carefully for recommendations with each drug. Evaluate the infusion site before and frequently during infusion. Although extravasation is not as common with central lines used in cancer treatment as in peripheral lines, it still can occur. Many chemotherapy agents are extremely toxic to tissues. In addition, lysis of the cancer cells can produce toxic side effects (see oncologic emergencies described earlier in the chapter). Careful monitoring of I&O is required to record the intravenous fluids, assess kidney functioning, and monitor excretion of by-products from destroyed tumor cells. Monitor specific gravity every 8 hours, as well as before and during administration of the drug, and when the intravenous fluids are reduced to maintenance volume levels. Daily weight measurements are important to assist in planning adequate hydration during chemotherapy, as well as to measure nutritional status.

Drug side effects may necessitate infusion of platelets or packed red blood cells. See the Skills Manual for techniques to be used in these situations. **SKILLS**

Many children are treated in an oncology clinic, staying in the hospital only on the day of intravenous drug administration and receiving oral medications at home. The time at the hospital is used to assess how the family is managing issues such as nutrition, sleep, medication administration, and obtaining psychosocial support. Careful teaching for the family is needed to ensure safe drug administration and identification of issues requiring further care.

Nurses play a key role in the long-term multidisciplinary treatment of children with leukemia. The impact of a diagnosis of leukemia and the long-term nature of treatment can severely stress the coping abilities of both the child and the family. Ongoing psychosocial assessment and emotional support are essential (see the general discussion of Psychosocial Assessment in the section on Childhood Cancer, pp. 1530–1532). Referral to support groups and social services may be beneficial. Help the family explore alternative therapies such as relaxation, imagery, and nutritional support that may aid the child. Be alert for any interactions that could occur between alternative therapies and the medical regimen.

TEACHING HIGHLIGHTS

CHEMOTHERAPY FOR LEUKEMIA

Physical Care
- Have rest periods each day.
- Avoid exposure to people with illnesses.
- Drink generous amounts of water.
- Eat a healthy diet, using frequent, small, and nutritious meals to obtain enough nutrients.
- Take medicines prescribed to decrease nausea.
- Maintain good oral hygiene with a soft toothbrush and water pick.
- Avoid sun exposure and check skin each day for any signs of bruises, pressure areas, cuts, or scratches.
- Allow time for and eat foods to promote bowel elimination.
- Promote bowel elimination through regular dietary and toileting practices.
- Report any signs of infection, changes in condition, or other concerns.

Emotional Care
- Be prepared for loss of hair with plans for hats, wigs, or other alternatives.
- Continue contact with friends via phone, Internet, and in person when possible.
- Try relaxation techniques to aid in sleep and management of treatments.
- Talk with clergy, teachers, parents, counselors, friends, or other supportive people about the experience of having leukemia.
- Keep a journal to record feelings and experiences.

COMPLEMENTARY CARE

ENHANCING CHEMOTHERAPY EFFECTIVENESS

Complementary medicine practices can often be easily integrated with and enhance effectiveness of chemotherapy. In a study of 20 children undergoing treatment for leukemia, parents were instructed to provide massage daily for 30 days. The children had an average age of 7 years. Parents and children completed anxiety and mood inventories, and children had blood studies as well. Those in the massage groups had lower anxiety scores and higher mood scores after the intervention. In addition the children had improved white blood cell count and neutrophil count. Massage therapy may be a useful addition to treatment regimens of young children for leukemia (Field, Cullen, Diego, et al., 2001). Nurses can suggest this intervention to families and arrange for them to obtain massage therapy training if they are interested.

EVALUATION

Expected outcomes for nursing care of the child with leukemia include the following:

- Prevention of infection
- Adequate hydration
- Normal urinary output
- Blood values within normal limits
- Successful family adaptation to parenting a child with chronic illness
- Adequate parental knowledge related to disease process

SOFT-TISSUE TUMORS

HODGKIN DISEASE

Hodgkin disease is a disorder of the lymphoid system. It usually arises in a single lymph node or an anatomic group of lymph nodes (see "Pathophysiology Illustrated: Hodgkin Disease"). There are approximately 3 cases per 100,000 people, with the peak occurrence in adolescent boys. Hodgkin disease has a childhood form but is rare in those under 14 years. Most cases involve a young adult form that affects those between 15 and 35 years of age, and an older adult form, usually seen in persons over 55 years of age (Thompson, 1999).

Etiology and Pathophysiology

Hodgkin disease occurs in clusters and has been reported in families. This suggests a possible genetic link as well as an infectious agent or environmental hazard. Some potential infectious agents may be herpes virus, cytomegalovirus, and Epstein-Barr virus.

PATHOPHYSIOLOGY ILLUSTRATED
Hodgkin Disease

Cervical nodes
Supraclavicular nodes
Lungs
Bone
Liver
Mesenteric nodes
Axilliary nodes
Mediastinal nodes
Spleen
Inguinal-femoral nodes

Lymph nodes and organs affected in Hodgkin disease in children.

TABLE 50–7 ✤ Staging System for Hodgkin Disease

Stage	Description
I	Disease within a single lymph node region
IE	Disease within a single extralymphatic organ
II	Disease within two or more lymph node regions on same side of diaphragm
IIE	Disease within extralymphatic organ, and of one or more lymph node regions on same side of diaphragm
III	Disease of lymph node regions on both sides of diaphragm
IIIE	Disease of lymph node regions on both sides of the diaphragm with involvement of extralymphatic organ
IIIS	As in III, plus disease within spleen
IIISE	As in III, plus disease in extralymphatic organs and spleen
IV	Disseminated disease within one or more lymphatic organs with or without lymph node involvement

Clinical Manifestations

The main symptom of Hodgkin disease is nontender, firm lymphadenopathy, usually in the supraclavicular and cervical nodes but occasionally in the mediastinal area. A mediastinal growth can cause respiratory difficulty because of pressure on the trachea or bronchi. Fever, night sweats, and weight loss occur in one third of children with Hodgkin disease and are associated with a more aggressive form of the disease. The leukocyte count and erythrocyte sedimentation rate (ESR) may be elevated.

Clinical Therapy

Diagnosis is based on lymph node biopsy; Reed-Sternberg cells (large cells with two nucleoli) are present. A staging classification is used to determine disease severity (Table 50–7). The basis for staging is data obtained from the history, physical examination, chest x-ray study (for metastasis), chest CT scan, CT or MRI scans of the retroperitoneal nodes, lymphangiogram if there is retroperitoneal involvement, laboratory studies (complete blood count, erythrocyte sedimentation rate, serum copper level, liver function tests), and a radionuclide scan with gallium. Bone marrow biopsy, bone scan, or a staging laparotomy may be performed if advanced disease is suspected. Increasingly, minimally invasive surgery can be used to biopsy or remove the spleen for diagnosis, avoiding the potential complications of major surgery (Kleinhaus & Boley, 1999).

Chemotherapy using a four-drug combination has been found to be the most effective drug treatment. Radiation is commonly added, with low doses for children who are still growing, and larger doses for those who are physically mature or those whose disease is more advanced at diagnosis. The 5-year survival rate is approximately 90%, depending on the stage of the disease at diagnosis.

NURSING PRACTICE

The following drugs are used to treat Hodgkin disease:

ABVD	Adriamycin + bleomycin + vinblastine + dacarbazine
ABVE	Adriamycin (doxorubicin) + bleomycin + vincristine + etoposide
ABVE-PC	Adriamycin (doxorubicin) + bleomycin + vincristine + etoposide + prednisone + cyclophosphamide
COPP	cyclophosphamide + Oncovin + procarbazine + prednisone
EBVP	etoposide + bleomycin + vinblastine + prednisone
MOPP	mechlorethamine + Oncovin (vincristine) + procarbazine + prednisone
OEPA	vincristine + etoposide + prednisone + Adriamycin (doxorubicin)
OPPA	Oncovin + procarbazine + prednisone + Adriamycin
VAMP	vinblastine + Adriamycin (doxorubicin) + methotrexate + prednisone
VEPA	vinblastine + etoposide + prednisone + Adriamycin (doxorubicin)

Bone marrow transplantation is a treatment option in children with advanced disease or relapse.

NON-HODGKIN LYMPHOMA

About 12% of pediatric cancers are lymphoma, and of these 40% to 45% are Hodgkin and 55% to 60% are non-Hodgkin. There are three types of pediatric non-Hodgkin lymphoma: (1) lymphoblastic lymphoma (30% to 40%), (2) small noncleaved cell (Burkitt) lymphoma (40% to 50%), and (3) large cell lymphoma ($\leq$15%) (Hussong, 2002). Lymphomas of all types are the third most common group of malignancies in children, following leukemia and brain tumors. Non-Hodgkin lymphomas are malignant tumors of lymphoreticular (internal framework of the lymph system) origin. The peak incidence for lymphomas occurs between the ages of 7 and 11 years, and they are three times more common in boys than in girls.

Lymphoblastic non-Hodgkin lymphomas are caused by T-cell abnormalities. These abnormal T cells are diffuse, highly malignant, and very aggressive and do not mature. T-cell lymphomas produced by these cells often occur in children with congenital or acquired immunodeficiency states, chronic immune stimulation, or autoimmune disease. Some lymphomas have B-cell abnormalities, most specifically Burkitt lymphoma; 8q24 chromosomal translocation may be found in these cases. Large cell lymphomas are variable in cell type affected and may also manifest chromosomal translocations (Hussong, 2002).

The incidence of lymphomas shows geographic variability. For example, a high incidence of Burkitt lymphoma is found in equatorial Africa, where it causes 50% of childhood cancer. Incidence in Hispanic children is higher than in whites, and blacks have the lowest incidence (Wilkinson, Fleming, MacKinnon et al., 2001). Males are affected more than females, and children with immune system compromise are most commonly affected. Epstein-Barr virus has been associated with Burkitt lymphoma.

Children with non-Hodgkin lymphoma frequently present with fever and weight loss. The lymph glands are usually enlarged or nodular, with the most frequent sites being the cervical, axillary, inguinal, and femoral nodes. However, the disease may be diffuse, without nodular glands. The anterior mediastinum is the primary site for T-cell lymphomas. Tumors that occur in this area may compress the airway (causing breathing difficulty) or superior vena cava (leading to swelling of the face, neck, or arms), and can cause pain. Jaw involvement is common in Burkitt lymphoma.

CBC is performed; additional blood tests include renal and liver function, electrolytes, uric acid, and LDH. Bone marrow aspiration and lumbar puncture are performed. Chest x-ray, bone scan, gallium scan, CT, and MRI can help to isolate affected body organs. Tissue biopsy confirms the diagnosis.

A staging system is used to describe the tumor mass and extension to other body areas (Table 50–8). Treatment is tailored to the type of cancer and its stage. Stages I and II may be treated with drugs such as vincristine, cyclophosphamide, prednisone, and methotrexate for several months. Intrathecal medication is added if head and neck cancers are present. Stages III and IV are treated with additional drugs (up to nine total) for longer periods (1 to 2 years). Radiation is uncommonly used and may be helpful to treat a tumor that is impinging on a body part. Surgery is used to biopsy the tumor mass and treat any complications caused by the cancer. HSCT is used for children with recurrent disease.

RHABDOMYOSARCOMA

Rhabdomyosarcoma is a soft tissue cancer common in children. It occurs most often in the muscles around the eyes (extraorbital), in the neck, and less commonly in the abdomen, genitourinary tract, and extremities. Among children under 15 years of age, rhabdomyosarcoma occurs more often in whites than in blacks or Asians (Kotsubo, 2002). It usually occurs in children under 5 years of age; however, it is uncommon in newborns, and if it presents in this age group, abdominal or pelvic sites are most common.

The cause of rhabdomyosarcoma is unknown. However, it is more common in children with neurofibromatosis and Li-Fraumeni syndrome. Mutations in tumor suppressor gene p53 are sometimes seen. Mothers of children with rhabdomyosarcoma are more likely to develop early breast cancer than other women (Ruymann & Grovas, 2000). The abnormal cells arise from mesenchyme that normally grows into muscle, fat, and bone (Kotsubo, 2002).

TABLE 50–8 ✣ St. Jude Children's Research Hospital Staging Classification for Non-Hodgkin Lymphoma

Stage	Description
I	Single tumor or node area involved; no tumor in abdomen or mediastinum
II	Single tumor with lymph node involvement; or two node areas or tumor on same side of diagphragm; or GI tumor in one site
III	Two tumors or node areas on different sides of diaphragm; or a primary mediastinal, intra-abdominal, or epidural tumor
IV	Any involvement with CNS or bone marrow metastases

Data from Hussong, M. R. (2002). Non-Hodgkin's lymphoma. In C. R. Baggott, K. P. Kelly, D. Fochtman, & G. V. Foley, *Nursing care of children and adolescents with cancer* (3rd ed., p. 539). Philadelphia: WB Saunders.

● **FIGURE 50–10**

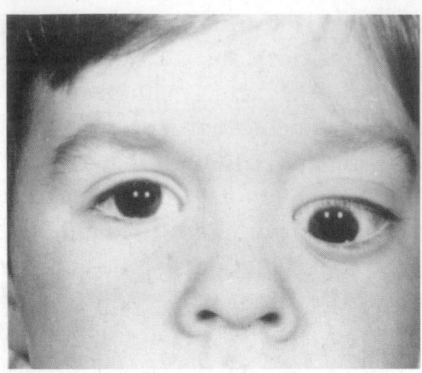

Rhabdomyosarcoma is characterized by ptosis and edema. Used with permission from Vaughn, D., Asbury, J., & Riordan-Eva, P. (1995). General ophthalmology (14th ed.). Norwalk, CT: Appleton: Lange.

Tumors close to the eye produce swelling, ptosis, visual disturbances, and eye movement abnormalities (Figure 50–10 ●). When the tumor occurs in the genitourinary tract, the result can be urinary obstruction, hematuria, dysuria, vaginal discharge, and a protruding vaginal mass. Rhabdomyosarcoma occurring in the abdomen may be asymptomatic. There is rapid metastasis to the lungs, bones, bone marrow, and distant lymph nodes.

Diagnosis is confirmed by CT, MRI, PET, bone marrow aspiration, and biopsy. CBC, renal and liver studies, and urinalysis are performed. Lumbar puncture may be used in head and neck tumors. A useful biologic marker, desmin, allows differentiation of rhabdomyosarcoma from other round cell tumors. Because 20% of children have metastatic disease at the time of diagnosis, chest and lung CT scans are performed.

Treatment includes surgical removal of the tumor when possible. However, if the tumor involves other structures, removal may not be possible. Many children have metastasis at the time of diagnosis, so the primary tumor may not be removed. Surgery is followed by wide-field radiation and chemotherapy with a combination of drugs. Some commonly used drugs include the following:

- Vincristine
- Actinomycin
- Cyclophosphamide
  (VAC therapy)

Prognosis depends on the site, staging (Table 50–9), and histologic findings, with about 70% of children surviving (Kotsubo, 2002).

RETINOBLASTOMA

Retinoblastoma is an intraocular malignancy of the retina. It may be bilateral (20% to 30%) or unilateral. In 40% of

TABLE 50–9 ✛ Classification of Rhabdomyosarcoma

Stage	Description
I	Localized, completely resected disease
II	Total gross resection with regional microscopic spread
III	Incomplete gross resection of biopsy
IV	Distant metastatic disease present

Data from Wexler, L. H., & Helman, L. J. (1997). Rhabdomyosarcoma and the undifferentiated sarcomas. In P. A. Pizzo & D. G. Poplack (Eds.), *Principles and practices of pediatric oncology* (3rd ed., p. 808). Philadelphia: Lippincott-Raven.

children, the disease is inherited by an autosomal dominant gene (Dulczak & Frothingham, 2002). Family history is therefore important to collect, although many cases occur with no family history of the cancer. The tumor arises from embryonic retinal cells. It may be a new mutation or may be passed on to offspring of affected individuals. The retinoblastoma gene, RB1, is on chromosome 13q.

The first sign of retinoblastoma is a white pupil, termed leukokoria or cat's-eye reflex (Figure 50–11 ●). The red reflex is absent, asymmetric, or of a differing color in the affected eye. Other symptoms may include a fixed strabismus (a constant deviation of one eye from the other), orbital inflammation, glaucoma, and heterochromia (irises of different colors).

Retinoblastoma is usually diagnosed when the child is between 1 and 2 years of age. The overall tumor-free sur-

● **FIGURE 50–11**

Retinoblastoma is characterized by leukokoria, a white reflection in the pupil. Used with permission from Hathaway, W. E., Hay, W. W., Jr., Grouthius, J. R., & Paisley, J. W. (1993). Current pediatric diagnosis and treatment (11th ed.). New York: McGraw-Hill Companies.

vival rate is 90%, 5 to 10 years after diagnosis. Children at risk for retinoblastoma due to family history can be tested for the RB1 gene. Diagnostic tests for the cancer include full ocular examination and CT or MRI scans of the eye orbit. All children with a history of retinoblastoma in the family should be examined by an ophthalmologist after birth, at 6 weeks, every 2 to 3 months until 2 years and then every 4 months until 3 years, and then annually (Dulczak & Frothingham, 2002; Pakakasama & Tomlinson, 2002) to aid in early diagnosis. Diagnostic tests include full ocular examination and CT or MRI scans of the eye orbit. Tumors are classified according to a staging system, from a very small localized tumor (group I) to tumors involving more than half the retina and with seeding into the vitreous (group V).

Treatment for retinoblastoma may include removal of the eye (enucleation) when there is permanent retinal damage or failure to respond to other treatment. Other surgical treatments involve cryotherapy or photocoagulation (argon laser therapy). Radiation is nearly always used, either as the sole treatment or before surgery to shrink the tumor. Chemotherapy is sometimes used but is frequently ineffective as the drugs often fail to penetrate sufficiently into the eye. Chemotherapy drugs include carboplatin, etoposide, vincristine, and cyclosporine. Multiple therapies are more commonly used in children with bilateral retinoblastoma. Children with retinoblastoma are at increased risk of developing a secondary tumor, including another retinoblastoma or a sarcoma, most commonly osteogenic sarcoma. However, most young children who have been treated for the disease have good health and normal mental abilities several years after treatment. The most common sequela of retinoblastoma is decrease in visual acuity (Ross, Lipper, Abramson et al., 2001).

NURSING MANAGEMENT

NURSING ASSESSMENT AND DIAGNOSIS

Physiologic Assessment

Physiologic assessment of the child with a soft-tissue tumor, such as Hodgkin disease, non-Hodgkin lymphoma, rhabdomyosarcoma, and other lymphomas, focuses on the child's general condition. Accurate height and weight measurements are essential to provide a baseline against which to measure the child's growth during treatment, as well as for calculation of chemotherapeutic drug dosages.

Observe the area of the tumor, such as the face, neck, and abdomen, and describe any changes. Monitor respiratory status if the tumor is in the face or neck. Report any changes in respiratory pattern to the physician. Avoid palpation of any tumor site or enlarged area; injudicious palpation and manipulation of a tumor site can influence metastasis. Notify the physician of a change in any lymph node or any other area of the body.

Gastrointestinal and genitourinary function can be altered by the presence of a tumor and by treatment such as chemotherapy and radiation. Careful measurement of the child's intake and output is essential. Abdominal tumors may affect defecation, so charting of all bowel movements is important. Explain to the family and child why keeping accurate records is necessary.

Observe wounds closely for lack of healing as a result of chemotherapy or radiation. Examine the mouth and extremities for wounds or ulcers. Nutritional changes caused by treatment will affect the body's ability to support healthy cells and heal wounds.

A thorough eye examination is warranted for any child who has a family history of retinoblastoma or has undergone treatment for a prior tumor. Assess color and position of the iris, eye movements, cover–uncover test, and other eye tests described in Chapter 35. ∞ Ask whether the child has been evaluated by an ophthalmologist.

Psychosocial Assessment

Assessment of the family's psychosocial status and coping mechanisms is an essential component of nursing care. Refer to the general discussion of psychosocial assessment under "Childhood Cancer," earlier in this chapter. Assessment of body image is needed when the child has a soft tissue tumor affecting appearance of the head and neck.

The location and type of soft-tissue tumor determine the specific nursing diagnoses for a particular child. Common nursing diagnoses might include the following:

- *Impaired Tissue Perfusion (Peripheral)* related to interruption of blood flow
- *Ineffective Breathing Pattern* related to effect of tumor deformity on neck or chest wall
- *Impaired Swallowing* related to acquired anatomic defect
- *Delayed Growth and Development* related to effects of treatment
- *Disturbed Body Image* related to illness and treatment
- *Disturbed Sensory Perception (Visual)* related to illness

PLANNING AND IMPLEMENTATION

Nursing management of children with soft-tissue tumors varies depending on the specific tumor. Children with lymphoma affecting the mediastinum may need respiratory support. Position the child so that the head is elevated. Administer chemotherapy drugs as ordered, maintaining adequate fluids to facilitate excretion of the resultant breakdown products. Monitor the central line used for chemotherapy administration, and teach parents care of the central line when the child is at home.

For the child with a rhabdomyosarcoma involving the bladder, monitor urinary output carefully. Report hematuria and painful urination. Monitor the changes that occur during therapy. For example, in children with eye tumors, observe for a decrease in ptosis, which may indicate successful treatment. Administer pain medications as needed and use distraction and other techniques to decrease the child's discomfort. Emphasize to parents the need for follow-up CT and MRI scans after completion of treatment.

When the child with retinoblastoma undergoes removal of the eye, the parents and child will need detailed instructions on postsurgical care. Demonstrate to the parents care of the socket and use of a conformer to maintain the eye socket shape. When healing is complete and the child receives a prosthetic eye, instruct parents about its insertion and care. The child can gradually be taught to take over this care when old enough. Encourage periodic healthcare visits to monitor for signs of a tumor in the other eye. Interventions to encourage normal developmental milestones are adapted if sensory alteration has resulted.

Pay attention to the body changes of the cancer and its treatment. Children and adolescents may need suggestions to deal with hair loss, disfigurement, and living with serious illness. Referral to other children and teens with similar concerns may be helpful. Parents of all children need help to encourage normal development in the child with cancer.

The child with a soft-tissue tumor often receives chemotherapy or radiation, or sometimes both modalities. Nursing management during chemotherapy and radiation is discussed earlier in this chapter in the general sections on these treatment measures (see pp. 1522-1526) and in "Nursing Care Plan: Hospital Care of the Child with Cancer." Generally, the family needs help to adjust to the diagnosis of a life-threatening disease and to the care of the ill child. Refer to Chapter 40 for a description of postsurgical care. ∞ Consult Chapter 46 for strategies to assist the child and family if the child has a visual impairment resulting from a retinoblastoma. ∞ Topics for parent and family teaching and discharge planning are similar to those previously presented. Referral resources to support the families of children with these types of cancer can be found on the Companion Website.

Nursing Care in the Community

Reinforce with families the importance of long-term follow-up after treatment for a soft-tissue tumor. Increased risk for secondary cancers for 2 to 3 decades is possible, and early identification can help with prompt diagnosis (Metayer, Lynch, Clarke et al., 2000). Partner with other healthcare providers to provide instructions to families as the child transitions from oncology treatment back to the pediatri-

TEACHING HIGHLIGHTS

CARE OF THE CHILD WITH A SOFT-TISSUE TUMOR

- Teach the family about the chemotherapy drugs and their side effects.
- Teach about the care of surgically placed venous access devices.
- Provide written and illustrated information about the chemotherapy protocol(s).
- Provide the family with radiation and surgery education specific to the tumor treatment.
- Refer the family to nutrition resources such as dietitians for ways to promote the child's adequate intake of food and fluid.

cian so they understand the importance of telling all care providers about the cancer and treatment. Establish oncology clinics to track and examine survivors. As children grow into teen and young adult years, help them to take over this important task in their care.

Some recommended annual examinations include the following:

- CBC
- Physical examination with special attention to skin, abdomen, and thyroid
- Monitoring for signs of hypo- and hyperthyroidism
- Neurologic and developmental examinations; monitoring of school performance
- First mammogram at 25 years in those with chest radiation
- Pap and pelvic examinations for teen and young adult women
- Mental status assessment

(Smith, 2002)

The following expected outcomes of nursing care for the child with a soft-tissue tumor are examples that illustrate the varied tumor presentations:

- Successful management of treatment side effects
- Healed surgical site with no signs of infection
- Adaptation to sensory loss
- Adaptation to altered self-image
- Growth and development to maximum potential
- Anticipatory grieving by parents in cases of terminal disease

Critical Concept Review

LEARNING OBJECTIVES

CONCEPTS

Describe the incidence, known etiologies, and common clinical manifestations of cancer.

1. Incidence:
   - Approximately 9,000 children in the United States were diagnosed with a form of cancer in 2004.
2. Etiology:
   - External stimuli.
   - Gene abnormalities.
   - Immune system and chromosomal abnormalities.
3. Common clinical manifestations:
   - Pain.
   - Cachexia.
   - Anemia.
   - Infection.
   - Bruising.
   - Neurologic symptoms.
   - Palpable mass.

Synthesize information about diagnostic tests and clinical therapy for cancer to plan comprehensive care for children undergoing these procedures.

1. Diagnostic tests:
   - Complete blood count.
   - Bone marrow aspiration and biopsy.
   - Lumbar puncture.
   - X-ray and CT.
   - MRI.
   - Ultrasound.
   - Biopsy of tumor.
2. Clinical therapy:
   - Surgery.
   - Chemotherapy.
   - Radiation.
   - Biotherapy.
   - Bone marrow transplantation.

Integrate information about oncologic emergencies into plans for monitoring all children with cancer.

1. Closely monitor complete blood count (CBC):
   - To prevent sepsis.
   - To prevent hemorrhage.
2. Monitor intake and output closely:
   - Encourage hydration to prevent hypercalcemia.
   - Observe for signs of water intoxication.
3. Observe for behavioral changes:
   - Space-occupying lesions may cause seizures or increased ICP.

Recognize the most common solid tumors in children, describe their treatment, and plan comprehensive nursing care.

Central nervous system and brain tumors are the most common solid tumors.
1. Treatment:
   - Surgery.
   - Chemotherapy; may be delivered intrathecally.
2. Nursing care:
   - Provide and refer for psychosocial support.
   - Closely monitor neurologic status.
   - Monitor for changes in ICP, seizure activity, and other neurological indicators.
   - Observe for signs and symptoms of diabetes insipidus, and other conditions arising from the tumor and treatment.
   - Assist parents with dealing with the behavioral and educational changes that may occur with their child.

LEARNING OBJECTIVES

CONCEPTS

Plan care for children and adolescents of all ages who have a diagnosis of leukemia.	1. Administer chemotherapy as ordered.
	2. Observe for signs and symptoms of bone marrow suppression:
	   ■ Anemia: encourage child to conserve energy.
	   ■ Leukopenia: encourage handwashing.
	   ■ Isolate child while counts are low; keep away from others with infection.
	   ■ Thrombocytopenia.
	3. Protect from injuries: no sports until counts increase.
	4. Nutrition: frequent small feedings when dealing with nausea.
	5. Monitor renal function.
	6. Provide psychosocial support for child and family.

Recognize the most common soft-tissue tumors in children, describe their treatment, and plan comprehensive care.	1. The most common soft-tissue tumors:
	   ■ Hodgkin Disease.
	   ■ Non-Hodgkin lymphoma.
	   ■ Rhabdomyosarcoma.
	   ■ Retinoblastoma.
	2. Treatment depends upon the tumor. May require:
	   ■ Surgery.
	   ■ Chemotherapy.
	   ■ Radiation.

Describe the impact of cancer survival on children and use this information to plan for ongoing physiological and psychosocial care in the children's futures.	1. Regular physical and laboratory examinations are needed. 2. Increased chance of development of other cancers due to original cancer treatment. 3. Encourage adolescents and young adults to manage their own care as much as possible. 4. Provide children, adolescents, and their families with educational and psychosocial support.

CRITICAL THINKING IN ACTION

View the **Critical Thinking in Action** video in Chapter 50 of the CD-ROM. Then, answer the questions that follow.

Seven-year-old Christina is brought to the hospital with an unusual rash, lethargy, and fever. Blood work is drawn, and the results are abnormal. The hematologist confirms that Christina has acute lymphoblastic leukemia (ALL), the most common childhood cancer. Her parents are in shock and disbelief about the news; she seems too young. Christina is immediately admitted to the hospital, and put on an IV with orders for more blood work.

Christina's blood work demonstrates the following: hemoglobin 9 g/dL, leukocytes 20,000/mm^3 and platelets 90,000/mm^3. Chemotherapy was initiated and precautions were taken to avoid infections. Recommendations for Christina include rest times daily, generous amounts of water, intake of healthy foods, and avoidance of sun exposure. The parents are happy when Christina comes home during the chemotherapy. The hemotologist advises them it is not uncommon to return to the hospital due to a chemotherapy complication. The parents are encouraged to remember to take care of themselves. This will help them deal with Christina's therapy more effectively.

1. What are some of the common side effects of chemotherapy?
2. Why is it important to check Christina's daily weights?
3. What symptoms should Christina's parents report to the doctor while she is on chemotherapy?
4. What are some developmentally-appropriate techniques you can encourage that will assist Christina to deal with her illness?

MEDIALINK

www.prenhall.com/london

CANCER CELL DIVIDING

■ NCLEX-RN® Review questions, case studies, and other interactive resources for this chapter can be found on the Companion Website at http://www.prenhall.com/london. Click on "Chapter 50" and "Begin" to select the activities for this chapter.

■ For tutorials including animations, more NCLEX-RN® Review questions, and an audio glossary, access the accompanying CD-ROM in this book.

REFERENCES

Agency for Healthcare Research and Quality. (2001b). *Management of cancer pain* (Evidence Report/Technology Assessment No. 35). Washington, DC: U.S. Department of Health and Human Services.

Agency for Healthcare Research and Quality. (2001a). *Uses of epoetin for anemia in oncology* (Evidence Report/Technology Assessment No. 30). Washington, DC: U.S. Department of Health and Human Services.

Alcoser, P. W., & Burchett, S. (1999). Bone marrow transplantation. *American Journal of Nursing, 99,* 26–31.

Alcoser, P. W., & Rogers, C. (2003). Treatment strategies in childhood cancer. *Journal of Pediatric Nursing, 18,* 103–112.

American Cancer Society. (2003). *National action plan for childhood cancer.* Retrieved February 16, 2004, from http://www.cancer.org.

American Cancer Society. (2004). *Statistics.* Retrieved February 16, 2004, from http://www. cancer.org.

Arceci, R. J., & Cripe, T. P. (2002). Emerging cancer-targeted therapies. *Pediatric Clinics of North America, 49,* 1339–1368.

Ater, J. L. (2004). Neuroblastoma. In R. E. Behrman, R. M. Kliegman, & H. B. Jenson. *Nelson textbook of pediatrics* (17th ed., pp. 1709–1711). Philadelphia: Saunders.

Baggott, C. R., Kelly, K. P., Fochtman, D., & Foley, G. V. (2002). *Nursing care of children and adolescents with cancer* (3rd ed.). Philadelphia: Saunders.

Baker, B. (1998). CNS tumors now most common cancer in children. *Pediatric News, 32(7),* 12.

Betcher, D. L., Simon, P. J., & McHard, K. M. (2002). In C. R. Baggott, K. P. Kelly, & D. Fochtman, *Nursing care of children and adolescents with cancer* (3rd ed., pp. 575–588). Philadelphia: WB Saunders.

Biggar, R. J., Frisch, M., & Goedert, J. J. (2000). Risk of cancer in children with AIDS. *Journal of the American Medical Association, 284,* 205–209.

Bindler, R. M., & Howry, L. B. (2005). *Pediatric drug guide.* Upper Saddle River, NJ: Prentice Hall Health (pp. 1275–1279).

Bleyer, A. (2004). Principles of diagnosis; principles of treatment. In R. E. Behrman, R. M. Kliegman, & H. B. Jenson, *Nelson textbook of pediatrics* (17th ed., pp 1684–1693). Philadelphia: Saunders.

Bryant, R. (2003). Managing side effects of childhood cancer treatment. *Journal of Pediatric Nursing, 18,* 113–125.

Castellino, S., & Hudson, M. M. (2002). Health issues in survivors of childhood cancer. *Southern Medical Journal, 95,* 977–984.

Cavusoglu, H. (2001). Depression in children with cancer. *Journal of Pediatric Nursing, 16,* 380–385.

Chaffee, S. (2001). Pediatric palliative care. *Primary Care, 28,* 365–370.

Challinor, J., Miaskowski, C., Moore, I., Slaughter, R., & Franck, L. (2000). Review of research studies that evaluated the impact of treatment for childhood cancers on neurorecognition and behavioral and social competence: Nursing implications. *Journal of the Society for Pediatric Nurses, 5,* 57–74.

Chase, S. (2000). St. John's Wort: Not so safe. *RN, 63,* 114.

Chin, E. A. (1998). A brief overview of the oral complications in pediatric oncology patients and suggested management strategies. *Journal of Dentistry for Children, 65,* 468–473.

Christensen, J., & Fatchett, D. (2002). Promoting parental use of distraction and relaxation in pediatric oncology patients during invasive procedures. *Journal of Pediatric Oncology Nursing, 19,* 127–132.

Conway, E. E., Asuncion, A., & DaRosso, R. (1999). Diagnosing and managing brain tumors: The pediatrician's role. Contemporary Pediatrics 16, 84–97.

Coustan-Smith, E., Sancho, J., Hancock, M. L., Boyett, J. M., Behm, F. G., Raimondi, S. C., et al. (2000). Clinical importance of minimal residual disease in childhood acute lymphoblastic leukemia. *Blood, 96,* 2691–2696.

Dadd, G. (2002). Neuroblastoma. In C. R. Baggott, K. P. Kelly, D. Fochtman, & G. V. Foley, *Nursing care of children and adolescents with cancer* (3rd ed., pp. 545–554). Philadelphia: Saunders.

Davies, B., Whitsett S. F., Bruce, A., & McCarthy, P. (2002). A typology of fatigue in children with cancer. Journal of Pediatric Oncology Nursing 19, 12–21.

Dean, R. (2000). *Alternative therapies may cause interactions in oncology patients.* American College of Clinical Pharmacology meeting, September 2000. Reported by Reuters. Retrieved September 25, 2000, from http://pediatrics.medscape.com/reuters/prof/2000/09/09.19/2000091prof003.html.

Drigan, R., & Androkites, A. L. (2002). In C. R. Baggott, K. P. Kelly, D. Fochtman, & G. V. Foley, *Nursing care of children and adolescents with cancer* (3rd ed., pp. 568–574). Philadelphia: Saunders.

Dulczak, S., & Frothingham, B. (2002). Retinoblastoma. In C. R. Baggott, K. P. Kelly, D. Fochtman, & G. V. Foley, *Nursing care of children and adolescents with cancer* (3rd ed., pp. 589–597). Philadelphia: Saunders.

Field, T., Cullen, C., Diego, M., Hernandez-Feir, M., Sprinz, P., Beebe, K., et al. (2001). Leukemia immune changes following massage therapy. *Journal of Bodywork and Movement Therapies, 5,* 271–274.

Freeman, K., O'Dell, C., & Meola, C. (2000). Issues in families of children with brain tumors. *Oncology Nursing Forum, 27,* 843–848.

French, A. E., Grant, R., Weitzman, S., Ray, J. G., Vermeulen, M. J., Sung, L., et al. (2003). Folic acid food fortification is associated with a decline in neuroblastoma. *Clinical Pharmacology Therapy, 74,* 288–294.

Gibson, F., & Nelson, W. (2000). Mouth care for children with cancer. *Paediatric Nursing, 12,* 18–22.

Gilger, E. A., Groben, V. J., & Hinds, P. S. (2002). Osteosarcoma nursing care guidelines: A tool to enhance the nursing care of children and adolescents enrolled on a medical research protocol. *Journal of Pediatric Oncology Nursing, 19,* 172–181.

Green, D. M., Grigoriev, Y. A., Nan, B., Takashima, J. R., Norkool, P. A., D'Angio, G. J., & Breslow, N. E. (2001). Congestive heart failure after treatment for Wilms' tumor: A report from the National Wilms' Tumor study group. *Journal of Clinical Oncology, 19,* 1926–1934.

Gurney, J. G., & Bondy, M. L. (2004). Cancer and benign tumors. In R. E. Behrman, R. M. Kliegman, & H. B. Jenson (Eds.), *Nelson Textbook of Pediatrics* (17th ed). Philadelphia: Saunders, p. 1680.

Han-Markey, T. (2000). Nutritional considerations in pediatric oncology. *Seminars in Oncology Nursing, 16,* 146–151.

Hendricks-Ferguson, V. L. (2000). Crisis intervention strategies when caring for families of children with cancer. *Journal of Pediatric Oncology Nursing, 17,* 3–11.

Hilden, J. M., Emanuel, E. J., Fairclogh, D. L., Link, M. P., Foley, K. M., Clarridge, B. C., et al., (2001). Attitudes and practices among pediatric oncologists regarding end-of-life care: Results of the 1998 American Society of Clinical Oncology survey. *Journal of Clinical Oncology, 19,* 205–212.

Hobbie, W. L., & Ogle, S. (2001). Transitional care for young adult survivors of childhood cancer. *Seminars in Oncology Nursing 17,* 268–273.

Hurwitz, C. A., Duncan, J., & Wolfe, J. (2004). Caring for the child with cancer at the close of life: "there are people who make it and I'm hoping I'm one of them. *JAMA, 292,* 2141–2149.

Hussong, M. R. (2002). Non-Hodgkin's lymphoma. In C. R. Baggott, K. P. Kelly, D. Fochtman, & G. V. Foley, *Nursing care of children and adolescents with cancer* (3rd ed., pp. 536–544). Philadelphia: Saunders.

Ishibashi, A. (2001). The needs of children and adolescents with cancer for information and social support. *Cancer Nursing, 24,* 61–67.

Jaffe, N., & Huff, V. (2004). Neoplasms of the kidney. In R. E. Behrman, R. M. Kliegman, & H. B. Jenson, *Nelson textbook of pediatrics* (17th ed, pp. 1711–1714). Philadelphia: Saunders.

James, K., Keegan-Wells, D., Hinds, P. S., Kelly, K. P., Bond, D., Hall, B., et al. (2002). The care of my child with cancer: Parents' perceptions of caregiving demands. *Journal of Pediatric Oncology Nursing, 19,* 218–228.

Kanarek, R. C. (1998). Facing the challenge of childhood leukemia. *American Journal of Nursing, 98,* 42–50.

Kelly, K. M., Jacobsen, J. S., Kennedy, D. D., Braudt, S. M., Mallick, M., & Weiner, M. A. (2000). Use of unconventional therapies by children at an urban medical center. *Journal of Pediatric Hematology/Oncology, 22,* 412–416.

Kemper, K. J., & Longwood Herbal Task Force. (1999). Shark cartilage, cat's claw, and other complementary cancer therapies. *Contemporary Pediatrics, 16,* 101–102, 105–106, 112, 115, 117–118, 121, 125–126.

Kinlen, L. J., & Balkwill, A. (2001). Infective cause of childhood leukemia and wartime population mixing in Orkney and Shetland, UK. *Lancet, 357,* 858.

Kleinhaus, S., & Boley, S. J. (1999). The latest news about minimally invasive surgery. *Contemporary Pediatrics, 16,* 125–134.

Kline, N. E., & Sevier, N. (2003). Solid tumors in children. *Journal of Pediatric Nursing, 18,* 96–102.

Kotsubo, C. Z. (2002). Rhabdomyosarcoma. In C. R. Baggott, K. P. Kelly, D. Fochtman, & G. V. Foley, *Nursing care of children and adolescents with cancer* (3rd ed., pp. 555–567). Philadelphia: Saunders.

Landier, W. (2001). Childhood acute lymphoblastic leukemia: Current perspectives. *Oncology Nursing Forum, 28,* 823–833.

Landier, W. (2002). Myeloid diseases. In C. R. Baggott, K. P. Kelly, D. Fochtman, & G. V. Foley, *Nursing care of children and adolescents with cancer* (3rd ed., pp. 491–502). Philadelphia: Saunders.

Lehman, R. A., Krishnamurthy, S., & Berlin, C. M. (2002). Weight and height deficits in children with brain stem tumors. *Clinical Pediatrics, 41,* 315–321.

Leonard, M. (2002). Diagnostic evaluations and staging procedures. In C. R. Baggott, K. P. Kelly, D. Fochtman, & G. V. Foley, *Nursing care of children and adolescents with cancer* (3rd ed., pp. 66–89). Philadelphia: Saunders.

Liossi, C. (2000). Clinical hypnosis in paediatric oncology: A critical review of the literature. *Sleep and Hypnosis, 5,* 268–274.

MacDonald, D. J., & Lessick, M. (2000). Hereditary cancers in children and ethical and psychosocial implications. *Journal of Pediatric Nursing, 15,* 217–225.

McLorie, G. A. (2001). Wilms' tumor (nephroblastoma). *Current Opinion in Urology, 11,* 567–570.

McManus, J., & Gilchrist, G. S. (2000). Neuroblastoma. In R. E. Behrman, R. M. Kliegman, & H. B. Jenson, *Nelson textbook of pediatrics* (16th ed., pp. 1552–1554). Philadelphia: WB Saunders.

Metayer, C., Lynch, C. F., Clarke, E. A., Glimelius, B., Storm, H., Pukkala, E., et al. (2000). Second cancers among long-term survivors of Hodgkin's disease diagnosed in childhood and adolescence. *Journal of Clinical Oncology, 18,* 2435–2443.

Moller, T. R., Garwicz, S., Barlow, L., Falck Winther, J., Glattre, E., Olafsdotti, G., et al., (2001). Decreasing late mortality among five-year survivors of cancer in childhood and adolescence: A population-based study in the Nordic countries. *Journal of Clinical Oncology, 19,* 3161–3181.

Murray, J. S. (2002). A qualitative exploration of psychosocial support for siblings of children with cancer. *Journal of Pediatric Nursing, 17,* 327–337.

National Cancer Institute (2005). National Cancer Institute research on childhood cancers. Retrieved November 1, 2005, from http://www.cancer.gov/ cancertopics/factsheet/sites-Types/childhood.

Occupational Safety and Health Administration (OSHA) (2003). Controlling Occupational exposure to hazardous drugs. Washington, D. C.: Office of Science and Technology Assessment.

Pakakasama, S., & Tomlinson, G. E. (2002). Genetic predisposition and screening in pediatric cancer. *Pediatric Clinics of North America, 49,* 1393–1413.

Pritchard-Jones, K. (2002). Controversies and advances in the management of Wilms' tumor. *Archives of Disease in Childhood, 87,* 241–244.

Recklitis, C., O'Leary, T., & Diller, L. (2003). Utility of routine psychological screening in the childhood cancer survivor clinic. *Journal of Clinical Oncology, 231,* 787–792.

Reiss, U., & Bolotin, E. (2002). New approaches to hematopoietic cell transplantation in oncology. *Pediatric Clinics of North America, 49,* 1437–1466.

Reynolds, P., Von Behren, J., & Elkin, E. P. (2002). Birth characteristics and leukemia in young children. *American Journal of Epidemiology, 155,* 603–613.

Ross, G., Lipper, E. G., Abramson, D., & Preiser, L. (2001). The development of young children with retinoblastoma. *Archives of Pediatric and Adolescent Medicine, 155,* 80–83.

Ross, J. A., Spector, L. G. Robison, L. L., & Olshan, A. F. (2005). Epidemiology of leukemia in children with Down syndrome. *Pediatric Blood Cancer ,44,* 8–12.

Ruymann, F. B., & Grovas, A. C. (2000). Progress in the diagnosis and treatment of rhabdomyosarcomas and related soft tissue sarcomas. Cancer Investigation 18, 223–241.

Ryan-Murray, J. & Petriccione, M. M. (2002). In C. R. Baggott, K. P. Kelly, D. Fochtman, & G. V. Foley, *Nursing care of children and adolescents with cancer* (3rd ed., pp. 503–523). Philadelphia: Saunders.

Scott, C. M., Britt, R. B., Juneau, C., & McKracken, K. (2001). Wilms' tumor: A primary care case study and differential diagnosis. *Internet Journal of Advanced Nursing, 5.* Retrieved January 20, 2004, from http://www.ispub.com.

Scott, J. T., Entwistle, V. A., Sowden, A. J., & Watt, I. (2003). Communicating with children and adolescents about their cancer. *Cochrane Library Issue 2,* 2003. Oxford: Update Software.

Smith, P. C. K. (2002). The role of the primary care advanced practice nurse in evaluating and monitoring childhood cancer survivors for a second malignant neoplasm. *Journal of Pediatric Oncology Nursing, 19,* 84–96.

Swerdlow, J. L. (2000). *Nature's medicine: Plants that heal.* Washington, DC: National Geographic Society.

Thompson, K. A. (1999). Detecting Hodgkin's disease. *American Journal of Nursing, 99,* 61–64.

Westlake, S. K., & Bertolone, K. L. (2002). Acute lymphoblastic leukemia. In C. R. Baggott, K. P. Kelly, D. Fochtman, & G. V. Foley, *Nursing care of children and adolescents with cancer* (3rd ed., pp. 466–490). Philadelphia: Saunders.

Wilkinson, J. D., Fleming, L. E., MacKinnon, J., Voti, L., Wohler-Torres, B., Peace, S., & Trapido, E. (2001). Lymphoma and lymphoid leukemia incidence in Florida children: Ethnic and racial distribution. *Cancer, 91,* 1402–1408.

Wolfe, J., Grier, H. E., & Klar, N. (2000). Symptoms and suffering at the end of life in children with cancer. *New England Journal of Medicine, 342,* 326–333.

Wolfe, J., Klar, N., Grier, H. E., Duncan, J., Salem-Schatz, S., Emanuel, E. J., & Weeks, J. C. (2000). Understanding of prognosis among parents of children who died of cancer. *Journal of the American Medical Association, 284,* 2469–2475.

Woodruff, T. J., Axelrad, D. A., Kyle, A. D., Nueke, O., Miller, G. G., & Hurley, B. J. (2004). Trends in environmentally related childhood illnesses. *Pediatrics, 113* (4 Suppl); 1133–1140.

The Child with Alterations in Gastrointestinal Function

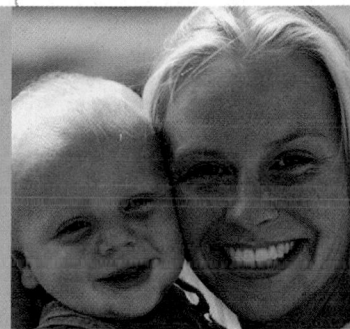

I was so worried when Jerome was born. He had no anal opening and his esophagus did not lead to his stomach. Now that he's had several surgeries, he is growing and doing pretty well, and I'm so happy to see him starting to smile. I can't wait until he is able to eat on his own instead of having tube feedings.

—*Mother of Jerome, 8 months old*

LEARNING OBJECTIVES

- Describe the general function of the gastrointestinal system.

- Discuss the pathophysiologic processes associated with specific gastrointestinal disorders in the pediatric population.

- Identify signs and symptoms that may indicate a disorder of the gastrointestinal system.

- Describe nursing management and plan care for disorders of the gastrointestinal system.

- Analyze developmentally appropriate approaches for nursing management of gastrointestinal disorders in the pediatric population.

- Discuss nursing management of the child with an injury (trauma or ingestion of injurious agent) to the gastrointestinal system.

MEDIALINK www.prenhall.com/london

CD-ROM

Skill 15-3: Administering a Gavage Feeding
Skill 16-3: Changing the Dressing for an Infant
  with an Ostomy
Skill 16-4: Changing an Ostomy Pouch for an
  Infant or Child
Animations:
  Lead Poisoning
Videos:
  Activated Charcoal
  Digestive System
  Stool Toileting: Refusals and Rewards
Nursing in Action: Changing an Ostomy Pouch
Audio Glossary
NCLEX-RN® Review

Companion Website

Thinking Critically
Case Study: The Child with a Cleft Palate
Care Plan: Managing Emesis in Pediatric Conditions
NCLEX-RN® Review
Case Study

MEDIALINK   Animation: Digestive System

What causes structural defects of the gastrointestinal tract such as the esophageal atresia and imperforate anus experienced by Jerome? What special care do children with gastrointestinal abnormalities need to promote growth and development during treatment for anomalies? This chapter discusses the care of infants who have structural defects and those with other common disorders of gastrointestinal functioning.

Through the gastrointestinal (GI) tract, a child ingests and absorbs the foods and fluids necessary to sustain life and promote growth. Most GI disturbances produce short-term symptoms that interfere with nutrition and fluid balance only briefly. Some disorders or severe defects lead to complications that prevent optimal nutrition and adequate growth. This chapter explores some common GI disorders in children. (See Chapter 43 for a discussion of specific fluid imbalances that may accompany GI disorders. ∞)

GI disorders can result from a congenital defect, acquired disease, infection, or injury. Structural problems may occur when development is altered or ceases in the first trimester of gestation. Because various parts of the GI system are developing at this point in gestation, it is not unusual for infants to have more than one structural defect of the GI system. This was the case with Jerome in the opening quote. Infections can cause an increase or decrease in motility and prevent proper absorption of nutrients. Interruption or destruction of the GI system can also result from trauma or ingestion of caustic substances. While reading this chapter, remember that any interruption or alteration in the GI system decreases the body's ability to obtain nutrients, thus impairing growth.

ANATOMY AND PHYSIOLOGY OF PEDIATRIC DIFFERENCES

Although the fetus makes sucking and swallowing movements in utero and ingests amniotic fluid, the GI system is immature at birth. The processes of absorption and excretion do not begin until after birth because the placenta provides nutrients and removes waste. Sucking is a primitive reflex that occurs whenever the lips or cheeks are stroked. The infant does not have voluntary control over swallowing until about 6 weeks of age.

The stomach capacity of the newborn is quite small, and intestinal motility (**peristalsis**) is greater than in older children. These characteristics explain the newborn's need for small, frequent feedings and the increased frequency and liquid consistency of bowel movements. Because of the relaxed cardiac sphincter, infants frequently regurgitate small amounts of feedings.

Digestion takes place in the duodenum. Infants have a deficiency of several enzymes: amylase (which digests carbohydrates), lipase (which enhances fat absorption), and trypsin (which catabolizes protein into polypeptides and some amino acids). Enzymes are usually not present in sufficient quantities to aid digestion until 4 to 6 months of age. Thus, abdominal distention from gas is common.

Liver function is also immature. After the first few weeks of life, the liver is able to conjugate bilirubin and excrete bile. The processes of **gluconeogenesis** (formation of glycogen from noncarbohydrates), plasma protein and ketone formation, vitamin storage, and **deamination** (removal of amino group from amino compound) remain immature during the first year of life.

By the second year of life, digestive processes are fairly complete. Stomach capacity increases to accommodate a three-meals-per-day feeding schedule. At about the same time, myelination of the spinal cord becomes complete and voluntary control over excretory functions can be achieved.

GROWTH AND DEVELOPMENT

Stomach capacity increases throughout early childhood:

Age	Capacity (mL)
Newborn	10 to 20
1 week	30 to 90
2 to 3 weeks	75 to 100
1 month	90 to 150
3 months	150 to 200
1 year	210 to 360
2 years	500

STRUCTURAL DEFECTS

Structural defects can involve one or more areas of the GI tract. These defects occur when growth and development of fetal structures are interrupted during the first trimester. This can leave the structure incomplete, resulting in atresia (absence or closure of a normal body orifice), malposition, nonclosure, or other abnormalities.

CLEFT LIP AND CLEFT PALATE

Cleft lip and cleft palate are two distinct facial defects that can occur singly or in combination (Figure 51–1 ○). Incomplete fusion of the lip occurs in approximately 1 in 700 births (Mitchell & Wood, 2000). It is more common in Native Americans and Asians than in whites, and less common in blacks. Incomplete fusion of the palate occurs in approximately 1 in 2000 births. Cleft lip and cleft palate are the fourth most common birth defect in the United States (Cleft Palate Foundation, 2004).

ETIOLOGY AND PATHOPHYSIOLOGY

Cleft lip with or without cleft palate results when the maxillary processes fail to fuse with the elevations on the frontal prominence during the sixth week of gestation. Normally union of the upper lip is complete by the seventh week. Fusion of the secondary palate occurs between 5 and 12 weeks of gestation. Failure of the tongue to move downward at the correct time prevents the palatine processes from fusing.

The intrauterine development of the hard and soft palates is completed in the first trimester. It is during this time that other major organ systems develop. Congenital defects such as tracheoesophageal fistula, omphalocele, trisomy 13, and skeletal dysplasias are associated with cleft lip and palate defects in 20% to 30% of cases. There is an increased incidence in families with a prior history of cleft lip or palate. The cause is believed to be multifactorial, involving a combination of environmental and genetic influences. When fortification of cereals and breads with folate

○ **FIGURE 51–1**

A

B

A, Unilateral cleft lip. **B,** Bilateral cleft lip.
Courtesy of Dr. Elizabeth Peterson, Spokane, WA.

MED ALINK

Case Study: The Child with a Cleft Palate

began in the United States in 1996 as a measure to decrease neural tube defects, the incidence of orofacial clefts also decreased. This may suggest that folate plays a role in formation of maxillary processes in the fetus (van Rooij, Vermeij-Keers, Kluijtmans et al., 2003).

CLINICAL MANIFESTATIONS

Cleft lip may be seen on ultrasound by 13 to 16 weeks' gestation (Mitchell & Wood, 2000). A cleft that involves the lip is apparent at birth. It may be a simple dimple in the vermilion border of the lip or a complete separation extending to the floor of the nose. The defect may be unilateral or bilateral and may occur alone or in combination with a cleft palate defect. Varying degrees of nasal deformity may also be present.

Cleft palate defects are less obvious when they occur without a cleft lip and may not be detected at birth. Clefts of the hard palate form a continuous opening between the mouth and nasal cavity and may be unilateral or bilateral, involving just the soft palate or both the soft and hard palate.

CLINICAL THERAPY

Cleft lip and palate are usually diagnosed at birth or during the newborn assessment. Medical management requires the combined efforts of a multidisciplinary team. Because speech, hearing, and dentition may be affected, coordinated care by specialists in plastic surgery, hearing, speech, and dentistry is necessary.

The cleft lip is usually repaired by about 2 to 3 months of age (Figure 51–2 ●). The lip is sutured together, and a

● FIGURE 51–2

A

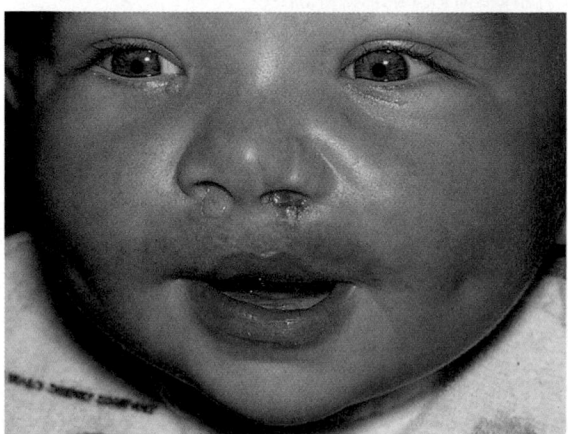

B

A, Repaired unilateral cleft lip (see Fig. 51-1A). *B,* Repaired bilateral cleft lip (see Fig. 51-1B).

Courtesy of Dr. Elizabeth Peterson, Spokane, WA.

Logan bow or other stabilizing device or dressing is put in place to prevent tension on the suture line. After surgery the infant's elbows are restrained to prevent flexion (see Skill 7–6). **SKILLS** To prevent injury to the suture line, the child is medicated to minimize crying.

Early closure of the lip enables the infant to form a better seal around the nipple for feeding. The sucking motion strengthens the muscles necessary for speech. Special feeding devices such as longer nipples with enlarged holes are available to help meet the infant's nutritional needs before surgical correction.

DEVELOPING CULTURAL COMPETENCE

CORRECTIVE SURGERY FOR CLEFT LIP AND PALATE

In many developing countries, infants do not have access to surgery for correction of cleft lip and palate. They may grow into childhood and adulthood with these abnormalities. Medical teams from the United States, Canada, and other countries sometimes travel to developing nations for short medical missions, performing surgery on the children and teaching local doctors surgical techniques. Are there medical missions in your area that perform these surgeries? What is the planning required for such trips to perform surgery safely and care for the children? What is the impact on the communities served?

Timing of the cleft palate repair varies among surgeons and depends on the size and severity of the cleft. Most surgeons perform closure operations when the infant is about 18 months old. This protects the formation of tooth buds and allows the infant to develop more normal speech patterns.

Infants with cleft lip and cleft palate are prone to recurrent otitis media, which can lead to tympanic membrane scarring and hearing loss. Antibiotics are prescribed to treat any infections that might lead to an ear infection. Because infants with chronic otitis media often have difficulty hearing, speech patterns may be altered. These infants require early, continuous intervention to prevent complications. (Refer to Chapter 46 for care of the child with chronic otitis media. ∞) The child who has had cleft palate repair requires orthodontic care. Early visits permit assessment of tooth eruption and the need for future orthodontic work.

NURSING MANAGEMENT

NURSING ASSESSMENT AND DIAGNOSIS

Physiologic Assessment

A cleft lip defect is observable at birth. A cleft palate defect is usually noted during the newborn assessment by palpation of the hard palate with the finger. A description of the location and extent of the defect helps the nurse determine the correct method of feeding. Thorough and complete physical assessment is needed since additional defects are sometimes present.

Psychosocial Assessment

Assessment of the family's reactions is an integral part of the overall nursing assessment. Physical deformities, especially of the face, can be devastating to parents. A poorly corrected defect can lead to low self-esteem in the older child. Assess the child's developmental level and social interactions with peers.

The accompanying "Nursing Care Plan" lists common nursing diagnoses for the infant with a cleft lip or palate. Other diagnoses that might be appropriate include the following:

- *Anxiety (Parent)* related to situational crisis and threat to self-concept
- *Ineffective Infant Feeding Pattern* related to anatomic abnormality
- *Risk for Caregiver Role Strain* related to complexity of caregiving tasks
- *Risk for Impaired Home Maintenance Management* related to infant's defect(s) and inadequate family support

PLANNING AND IMPLEMENTATION

Nursing care involves providing emotional support, performing postsurgical care, helping parents coordinate care and maintain a healthy home environment, and making appropriate referrals. See "Nursing Care Plan: The Infant with a Cleft Lip or Palate" for a summary of nursing care.

Provide Emotional Support

Parents may need assistance to view their infant as a whole person, rather than focusing solely on the physical defect. Promote parent–infant bonding by explaining the nature of the structural defect and the procedure for correction. Interact and speak to the infant in the parents' presence and point out positive attributes such as alertness, soft skin, or active movements. Self-blame is common among parents. Parents can also be referred to the American Cleft Palate Association for information about the disorder. (See the Companion Website for links to this resource. 🌐) Some plastic surgeons have photos of children before and after correction to show parents; this may reassure parents that their child can have a "normal" appearance (Uhrich & Mackin, 2001).

Parental anxiety is usual when children undergo surgery, and it is heightened when the surgery involves an infant. To minimize anxiety, give clear, concise explanations to parents. Allow sufficient time for parents to ask questions. Encourage parents to hold and cuddle the infant before surgery.

Provide Postoperative Care

Provide general postoperative care for the infant. (See "Nursing Care Plan: The Infant with a Cleft Lip or Palate" in this chapter and "Nursing Care Plan: The Child Undergoing Surgery" in Chapter 40. ∞) Assess vital signs frequently and maintain the infant's airway. Measure intake and output. When oral fluids with clear liquids are started, they are usually given through a dropper or a syringe. Position the infant in a sitting position for the feedings to avoid aspiration. The infant then progresses to half-strength formula or breast milk. After each feeding, clean the suture line with water or normal saline to avoid accumulation of feedings.

It is important to maintain the suture line to ensure healing. Position the infant in a supine or a side-lying position to avoid rubbing the suture line on the bedding. Keep elbows in soft restraints. Maintain the metal device or Steri-Strips placed over the incision. Place antibiotic body cream on the incision site as ordered. Medicate the infant regularly to control pain and to minimize crying and stress on the suture line. After cleft palate surgery, avoid the use of metal utensils or straws, which may disrupt the surgical site.

GROWTH AND DEVELOPMENT

An infant who has had a cleft lip repair needs stimulation to provide distraction. This approach will minimize crying, which can damage the suture line. Soft, colorful toys, mobiles, and other visual objects are helpful. Music also can be used to soothe the infant. Parental presence is comforting and reassuring.

Nursing Care in the Community

Identify and address home care needs well in advance of discharge. Discuss all aspects of the infant's care with the parents throughout hospitalization and after surgery. Involve parents in the infant's care to increase their comfort level before discharge and to promote bonding. Teach them feeding techniques, how to recognize signs of infection, how to position the infant, and how to care for the suture line. Breastfeeding is usually possible with some assistance from a lactation specialist, even if the mother pumps her breasts and milk is fed by a special nurser. Some infants may need a device placed in the mouth to enable them to establish suction. Several companies make special nursers that may be helpful for children with cleft lip or palate.

Management, especially in the first few months of life, involves many different healthcare professionals. In addition to hospital, clinic, and home health nurses, members

NURSING CARE PLAN

THE INFANT WITH A CLEFT LIP OR PALATE

Intervention	Rationale	Expected Outcome
Preoperative Care		

1. Nursing Diagnosis: Risk for Aspiration (breast milk, formula, or mucus) related to anatomic defect

Intervention	Rationale	Expected Outcome
NIC Priority Intervention: **Aspiration precautions:** Prevention or minimization of risk factors in the patient at risk of aspiration		**NOC Suggested Outcome:** **Airway maintenance:** Toleration of enteral feedings without aspiration

Goal: The infant will have no episodes of gagging or aspiration.

Intervention	Rationale	Expected Outcome
■ Assess respiratory status and monitor vital signs at least every 2 hours. ■ Position on side after feedings. ■ Feed slowly and use adaptive equipment as needed. ■ Burp frequently (after every 15–30 mL of fluid). ■ Position upright for feedings. ■ Keep suction equipment and bulb syringe at bedside.	■ Allows for early identification of problems. ■ Prevents aspiration of feedings. ■ Facilitates intake while minimizing risk of aspiration. ■ Helps to prevent regurgitation and aspiration. ■ Minimizes passage of feedings through cleft. ■ Suctioning may be necessary to remove milk or mucus.	The infant exhibits no signs of respiratory distress.

2. Nursing Diagnosis: Ineffective Family Coping related to birth of a child with a defect

Intervention	Rationale	Expected Outcome
NIC Priority Intervention: **Family involvement:** Facilitating family participation in the emotional and physical care of the child		**NOC Suggested Outcome:** **Positive coping:** Extent of coping mechanisms and ability to perform child's physical and emotional care

Goal: Parents will begin bonding process with the infant. The family's coping ability will be maximized. Parents will verbalize the nature and sequelae of the defect.

Intervention	Rationale	Expected Outcome
■ Help parents to hold the infant and facilitate feeding process. ■ Point out positive attributes of infant (hair, eyes, alertness, etc.). ■ Explain surgical procedure and expected outcome. Show pictures of other children's cleft lip repair. ■ Assess parents' knowledge of the defect, their degree of anxiety and level of discomfort, and the interpersonal relationships among family members. ■ Explore the reactions of extended family members. ■ Support open visitation. ■ Encourage parents to participate in caretaking activities (holding, diapering, feeding). ■ Provide information about the etiology of cleft lip and palate defects and the special needs of these infants. Encourage questions.	■ Contact is essential for bonding. ■ Helps parents see the child as a whole, rather than concentrating on the defect. ■ Eliminating unknown factors helps to decrease anxiety. ■ Helps to determine the appropriate timing and amount of information to be given regarding the child's defect. ■ Extended family is an important source of support for most parents of a newborn. Family members can often help promote acceptance and compliance with the treatment plan. ■ Allows parents to continue the bonding process. ■ Participation in infant care decreases anxiety and provides parents with a sense of purpose. ■ Concrete information allows parents time to understand the defect and reduces guilt.	Parents hold, comfort, and show concern for the infant. The family demonstrates improved coping ability before discharge. Parents receive necessary support to care for their infant.

NURSING CARE PLAN—continued

THE INFANT WITH A CLEFT LIP OR PALATE

Intervention	Rationale	Expected Outcome
2. Nursing Diagnosis: Ineffective Family Coping related to birth of a child with a defect *(continued)*		
■ Refer to parent support groups.	■ Support groups allow parents to express their feelings and concerns, to find people with concerns similar to their own, and to seek additional information.	
3. Nursing Diagnosis: Imbalanced Nutrition: Less than Body Requirements related to the infant's inability to ingest nutrients		
NIC Priority Intervention: **Nutrition management:** Provision of a balanced dietary intake of foods and fluids		**NOC Suggested Outcome:** **Nutrition status:** Amount of food and fluid taken over a 24-hour period
Goal: The infant will gain weight steadily.		
■ Assess fluid and calorie intake daily. Assess weight daily (same scale, same time, with infant completely undressed).	■ Provides an objective measurement of whether the infant is receiving sufficient caloric intake to promote growth. Using the same scale and procedure when weighing the infant provides for comparability between daily weights.	The infant maintains adequate nutritional intake and gains weight appropriately.
■ Observe for any respiratory impairment.	■ Any symptoms of respiratory compromise will interfere with the infant's ability to suck. Feedings should be initiated only if there are no signs of respiratory distress.	
■ Provide 100–150 cal/kg/day and 100–130 mL/kg/day of feedings and fluid. If the infant needs an increased number of calories to grow, referral to a nutritionist should be made. Formulas with higher calorie concentrations per ounce are available without increasing total fluids.	■ Provides optimal calories and fluids for growth and hydration.	
■ Facilitate breastfeeding.	■ Breast milk is recommended as the best food for an infant. The process of breastfeeding helps to promote bonding between mother and infant.	Successful breastfeeding is achieved if desired.
■ Hold the infant in a semisitting position.	■ Makes swallowing easier and reduces the amount of fluid return from the nose.	
■ Give the mother information on breastfeeding the infant with a cleft lip or palate such as plugging the cleft lip and eliciting a letdown reflex before breastfeeding.	■ Information and specific suggestions may encourage the mother to persist with breastfeeding.	
■ Contact the La Leche League for the name of a support person.	■ The La Leche League promotes breast-feeding for all infants. It can provide support people with experience who will aid the mother.	
■ If the mother is unable to breastfeed (or prefers not to), initiate bottle-feeding: Hold infant in an upright or semisitting position for feeding.	■ Facilitates swallowing and minimizes the amount of fluid return from the nose.	Feeding provides necessary nutrients and is a positive experience for parents and infant.
■ Place nipple against the inside cheek toward the back of the tongue. May need to use a premature nipple (slightly longer and softer than regular nipple with a larger opening) or a Brecht feeder (an oval bottle with a long, soft nipple).	■ Use of longer, softer nipples makes it easier for the infant to suck. A Brecht feeder decreases the amount of pressure in the bottle and makes the formula flow more easily.	

(continued)

NURSING CARE PLAN—continued

THE INFANT WITH A CLEFT LIP OR PALATE

Intervention	Rationale	Expected Outcome

3. Nursing Diagnosis: Imbalanced Nutrition: Less than Body Requirements related to the infant's inability to ingest nutrients (continued)

Intervention	Rationale	Expected Outcome
■ Feed small amounts slowly.	■ Small amounts and slow feeding do not tire the infant as quickly as do larger amounts given at a faster rate. They also decrease the calories used during feeding.	
■ Burp frequently, after 15–30 mL of formula has been given.	■ Frequent burping prevents the accumulation of air in the stomach, which can cause regurgitation or vomiting.	
■ Initiate nasogastric feedings if the infant is unable to ingest sufficient calories by mouth.	■ Adequate nutrition must be maintained. Use of a feeding tube allows the infant who has difficulty with oral feeding to receive adequate nutrition for growth.	

Postoperative Care

1. Nursing Diagnosis: Risk for Infection related to location of surgical procedure

NIC Priority Intervention:		NOC Suggested Outcome:
Infection control: Minimizing the acquisition and transmission of infectious agents		**Risk control:** Actions to eliminate or reduce actual, personal, or modifiable health risks

Goal: The infant's mucosal tissue will heal without infection.

Intervention	Rationale	Expected Outcome
■ Assess vital signs every 2 hours.	■ Elevated temperature may indicate infection.	The infant remains free of infection in the oral cavity. Tissues remain intact and pink.
■ Assess oral cavity every 2 hours or as needed for tenderness, reddened areas, lesions, or presence of secretions.	■ Aids in identifying infection.	
■ Cleanse suture line with normal saline or sterile water if ordered.	■ Helps decrease the presence of bacteria.	Healing process progresses without adverse events in postoperative period.
■ Cleanse the cleft areas by giving 5–15 mL of water after each feeding.	■ Prevents accumulation of carbohydrates, which encourage bacterial growth.	
■ If a crust has formed, use a cotton swab to apply a half-strength peroxide solution.	■ Helps loosen the crust, aiding in removal.	
■ Apply antibiotic cream to suture line as ordered.	■ Counteracts the growth of bacteria.	
■ Use careful handwashing and sterile technique when working with suture line.	■ Prevents the spread of microorganisms from other sources.	

2. Nursing Diagnosis: Ineffective Breathing Pattern related to surgical correction of defect

NIC Priority Intervention:		NOC Suggested Outcome:
Airway management: Facilitation of patency of air passages		**Vital signs status:** Temperature, pulse, respiration, and blood pressure within expected range for the infant/child

Goal: The infant will maintain an effective breathing pattern.

Intervention	Rationale	Expected Outcome
■ Assess respiratory status and monitor vital signs at least every 2 hours.	■ Allows for early identification of problems.	The infant shows no signs of respiratory infection or compromise.
■ Apply a cardiorespiratory monitor.	■ Enables early detection of abnormal respirations, facilitating prompt intervention.	
■ Keep suction equipment and bulb syringe at bedside. Gently suction oropharynx and nasopharynx as needed.	■ Gentle suctioning will keep the airway clear. Suctioning that is too vigorous can irritate the mucosa.	

NURSING CARE PLAN—continued

THE INFANT WITH A CLEFT LIP OR PALATE

Intervention	Rationale	Expected Outcome
2. Nursing Diagnosis: Ineffective Breathing Pattern related to surgical correction of defect (continued)		
■ Provide cool mist for first 24 hours postoperatively if ordered. ■ Reposition every 2 hours.	■ Moisturizes secretions to reduce pooling in lungs. Moisturizes oral cavity. ■ Ensures expansion of all lung fields.	
3. Nursing Diagnosis: Impaired Tissue Integrity related to mechanical factors		
NIC Priority Intervention: **Wound care:** Prevention of wound complications and promotion of wound healing		**NOC Suggested Outcome:** **Wound healing:** The extent to which cells and tissues have regenerated following intentional closure
Goal: Lip and/or palate will heal with minimal scarring or disruption.		
■ Position the infant with cleft lip repair on side or back only. ■ Use soft elbow restraints. Remove every 2 hours and replace. Do not leave the infant unattended when restraints are removed. ■ Maintain metal bar (Logan bow) or Steri-Strips placed over cleft lip repair. ■ Avoid metal utensils or straws after cleft palate repair. ■ Keep the infant well medicated for pain in initial postoperative period. Have parents hold and comfort the infant. ■ Provide developmentally appropriate activities (i.e., mobiles, music).	■ Prone position could cause rubbing on suture line. ■ Prevents the infant's hands from rubbing surgical site. Regular removal allows for skin and neurovascular checks. ■ Maintaining suture line will minimize scarring. ■ These devices may disrupt suture line. ■ Good pain management minimizes crying, which can cause stress on suture line. Increases bonding and soothes the child to decrease crying. ■ Soothes and keeps the infant calm.	Lip/palate heals without complications.
4. Nursing Diagnosis: Deficient Knowledge (Parent) related to lack of exposure and unfamiliarity with resources		
NIC Priority Intervention: **Teaching, disease process:** Assisting the parent to understand information related to cleft lip/palate		**NOC Suggested Outcome:** **Knowledge:** Extent of understanding conveyed about cleft lip/palate treatment
Goal: Before discharge, parents will verbalize home care methods for care of the infant with cleft lip and palate defect.		
■ Explain care and treatment (both short term and long term). Discuss potential complications. ■ Demonstrate feeding techniques and alternatives. Allow parents to demonstrate before discharge. ■ Provide written instructions for follow-up care arrangements. ■ Introduce the parents (if possible) to a primary care provider in the setting where the infant will receive follow-up care after discharge.	■ Assists the family to deal with the physical and psychosocial aspects of a child with a congenital defect. ■ Provides visual instructions. Redemonstration confirms learning. ■ Written instructions reinforce verbal instruction and provide a reference after discharge. ■ Continuity of care is important. Since the infant will require long-term follow-up, a contact with the new provider is helpful.	Parents accurately describe and demonstrate feeding techniques to facilitate optimal growth of the infant; describe interventions if respiratory distress occurs; and take the written instructions home with them on discharge.

(continued)

NURSING CARE PLAN—continued

THE INFANT WITH A CLEFT LIP OR PALATE

Intervention	Rationale	Expected Outcome
5. Nursing Diagnosis: Imbalanced Nutrition: Less than Body Requirements related to inability to ingest nutrients		
NIC Priority Intervention: **Nutrition management:** Promotion of a balanced dietary intake of foods and fluids		**NOC Suggested Outcome:** **Nutritional status:** Extent to which nutrients are available to meet metabolic needs
Goal: The infant will receive adequate nutritional intake.		
■ Maintain intravenous infusion as ordered. ■ Begin with clear liquids, then give half-strength formula or breast milk as ordered. ■ Use Asepto syringe or dropper in side of mouth. ■ Do not allow pacifiers. ■ Give high-calorie soft foods after cleft palate repair.	■ Provides fluid when NPO. ■ Ensures adequate fluids and nutrients. ■ Avoids suture line and resultant accumulation of formula in that area. ■ Sucking can disrupt suture line. ■ Rough foods, utensils, and straws could disrupt the surgical site.	The infant receives adequate nutritional intake. Infant resumes usual feeding patterns and gains weight appropriately.

of the healthcare team often include specialists such as the surgeon, speech specialist, geneticist, dentist, prosthodontist, audiologist, social worker, and pediatrician. The parents are the best coordinators of the child's care. Encourage them to keep a diary listing the professionals with whom they talk and the content of the discussions.

Discuss with the parents the financial implications of long-term care. Private insurance does not always cover all the costs of care necessary for the child. Refer parents to social services familiar with programs and financial aid for which the parents and child may be eligible. Relief of financial worries enables parents to concentrate on caring for the child.

Teach parents how to care for the child after discharge. If the child has siblings, emphasize that they will need preparation to accept the child. Sibling rivalry can be heightened when one child receives more attention in the home. Remind parents of the importance of setting limits and of spending time with each child. Determine whether additional family supports are necessary. Provide parents with information on support groups, physicians, social workers, Internet resources, and local services that can help maintain family continuity.

Discuss ways to prevent the infant from touching the suture line. Teach parents how to bundle an infant in a blanket with arms tucked inside the blanket. A front-sling baby carrier may also be used to immobilize the arms. Front-sling carriers provide the additional benefits of comforting the infant through contact with the parent and of

holding the infant upright, which aids in optimal positioning after feedings.

After surgical repair, parents need to be taught how to feed the infant and identify signs of complications (fever, vomiting, respiratory distress). Referral to a home healthcare agency for support may be helpful. Encourage follow-up visits with healthcare professionals (see "Health Promotion: The Child with Cleft Lip or Cleft Palate"). The child may need further evaluation of speech development, ear infections, or a recommendation for plastic surgery.

EVALUATION

Expected outcomes of nursing care in the preoperative period include the following:

■ Absence of respiratory distress and maintenance of normal respirations

■ Positive parent-infant bonding

■ Parental expression of support and comfort by family and community

■ Maintenance of normal weight by infant

■ Parental knowledge of defect, its correction, and infant needs

Expected outcomes of postoperative nursing care include the following:

■ Absence of infection

■ Clean healing of surgical area

HEALTH PROMOTION
The Child with Cleft Lip or Cleft Palate

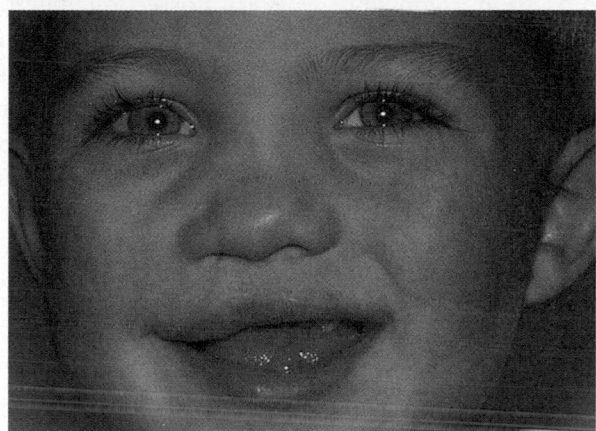

The child with cleft lip or cleft palate requires close monitoring and intervention to foster growth and development. The nurse can assist the child and family in many ways.

Growth and Development Surveillance
- Monitor the child's growth and developmental patterns.
- Monitor for developmental delays.
- Explain to parents that regression following surgery in the toddler or older child is normal.
- Ask the family about financial ability regarding speech therapy, dental care, and other services that may be required. Financial constraints can impede compliance to recommended therapies.

Nutrition
- Refer family to sources for nipples, nursers, and other special feeding devices.
- Assist mother with learning how to express breast milk and facilitate breastfeeding.
- Teach parents to avoid foods that can pose a choking hazard to the child.
- Teach parents to avoid straws, metal spoons, and other sharp utensils that may damage palate.
- Teach parents to feed the infant in an upright position and to burp the child frequently during feedings.

Physical Activity
- Activity for the child having surgical procedures to correct cleft palate is generally restricted for approximately 2 to 3 weeks to allow for healing.

- After healing has occurred, encourage the parents to promote the child's activities as they would any child without cleft lip or cleft palate.

Oral Health
- The child should be routinely screened for dental caries. Ask family about dental visits.
- Teach the parents to provide good dental hygiene to the child.
- Routine dental/orthodontic evaluation is necessary for the child with cleft palate.

Mental and Spiritual Health
- For uncorrected or poorly corrected cleft lip or palate, the child may experience poor self-esteem related to body image.
- Encourage family to adhere to treatment and surgical correction plan, including staged surgical corrections, dental care, and speech pathology assistance.
- Be alert for the child who has had experiences with teasing associated with articulation or physical appearance.
- Refer parents to Web sites such as Project Smile and other resources.
- Refer the child for counseling if indicated.

Relationships
- Evaluate the parents for parent–infant bonding.
- Promote bonding by encouraging the parents to participate in the infant's care, to hold the infant, and to recognize the infant's positive attributes.

Disease Prevention Strategies
- Teach family to recognize signs and symptoms of ear or other infections and to seek immediate evaluation. Treatment of acute otitis media by a specialist is necessary to prevent long-term effects of repeated infections.
- Emphasize to the parents the importance of audiology screening for children with cleft lip and palate to evaluate conductive hearing loss.

Injury Prevention Strategies (Safety)
- Assist parents to properly apply elbow restraints or to wrap child in mummy blanket to protect suture line in the postoperative period.
- Ask the parents about eating utensils the child uses.

- Absence of respiratory distress
- Effective pain management
- Fluid and electrolyte balance and adequate weight gain
- Parental description of infant care and feeding

ESOPHAGEAL ATRESIA AND TRACHEOESOPHAGEAL FISTULA

Esophageal atresia is a malformation that results from failure of the esophagus to develop as a continuous tube during the fourth and fifth weeks of gestation. Esophageal atresia with tracheoesophageal fistula occurs in approximately 1 in 4000 births, and about 30% of the infants are premature (Wyllie, 2004).

In esophageal atresia the foregut fails to lengthen, separate, and fuse into two parallel tubes (the esophagus and trachea) during fetal development. Instead the esophagus may end in a blind pouch or develop as a pouch connected to the trachea by a fistula (tracheoesophageal fistula) (see "Pathophysiology Illustrated: Esophageal Atresia and Tracheoesophageal Fistula"). Esophageal atresia is often associated with a maternal history of polyhydramnios. Associated anomalies may occur, including congenital heart defects, gastrointestinal or urinary tract anomalies, and musculoskeletal abnormalities. Jerome, described at the beginning of the chapter, had esophageal atresia as well as an imperforate anus.

Symptoms in the newborn include excessive salivation and drooling, often accompanied by cyanosis, choking, coughing, and sneezing. During feeding, the infant returns fluid through the nose and mouth. Aspiration places the infant at risk for pneumonia. Depending on the type of defect, the abdomen may become distended because of air trapping.

Diagnosis is usually confirmed by attempting to pass a 5 or 8 French nasogastric tube into the stomach. In most cases the tube meets resistance and can be advanced only minimally. Specific defects and associated anomalies are determined by x-ray examination. Echocardiogram and abdominal ultrasound are performed. Careful examination of the lungs is needed. A delay in diagnosis can be fatal because ingested fluid or secretions may enter the lungs.

A tube is inserted to suction the upper pouch. Intravenous antibiotics and fluids are begun. Surgery is performed as soon as possible. Surgical correction may be accomplished in several stages. The first stage usually involves ligation of the fistula and insertion of a gastrostomy tube. In the second stage, the two ends of the esophagus are reconnected, if possible. When surgical closure (anastomosis) is not possible, a gastrostomy tube must remain in place for use in feeding. Potential postoperative complications include gastroesophageal reflux, aspiration, and stricture formation. The prognosis is usually good with surgery.

NURSING MANAGEMENT

The nurse may recognize the signs and symptoms in the immediate newborn period. Assess for difficulty feeding and excessive drooling. Assess for the classic signs of choking, coughing, and cyanosis. Assess for respiratory distress and assess the lung sounds carefully.

Esophageal atresia is a surgical emergency. Preoperatively the infant requires close observation and intervention to maintain a patent airway. Suction should be readily available to remove any secretions that accumulate in the nasopharyngeal airway. Place the infant with the head of the bed slightly lowered to minimize aspiration of secretions into the trachea. Use continuous or low intermittent suction to remove secretions from the blind pouch. To confirm correct placement of the tube, aspiration of stomach contents and pH testing are required. Withhold oral fluids, and maintain the infant with intravenous fluids administered through an umbilical artery catheter.

After surgery, maintain gastrostomy drainage, and administer intravenous fluids and antibiotics. Total parenteral nutrition may be needed until gastrostomy or oral feedings are tolerated.

The parents require emotional support throughout the infant's hospitalization. Clearly explain all procedures. Encourage parents to bond with the infant by stroking and talking to the infant. Eliciting questions and allowing parents to participate in the infant's care, especially feeding (when permitted), can facilitate bonding and help to prepare parents for care of the infant after discharge.

Once enteral feedings have been established, the infant may be discharged from the hospital with a gastrostomy tube in place (Figure 51–3 ● and Skill 15–3). **SKILLS** Teach the parents about gastrostomy tube care and feeding, signs of infection, and how to prevent postoperative complications.

The outcomes of nursing care will depend on the extent of the defect and correction. Examples include the following:

- Adequate intake of fluids to promote hydration and growth

PATHOPHYSIOLOGY ILLUSTRATED
Esophageal Atresia and Tracheocsophageal Fistula

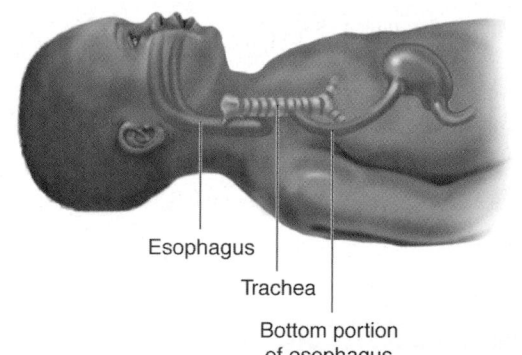

Esophagus

Trachea

Bottom portion
of esophagus

In the most common type of esophageal atresia and tracheoesophageal fistula, the upper segment of the esophagus ends in a blind pouch connected to the trachea; a fistula connects the lower segment to the trachea.

TEACHING HIGHLIGHTS

HOME CARE INSTRUCTIONS FOR THE CHILD REQUIRING GASTROSTOMY TUBE FEEDINGS AND CARE

Equipment
Prepared, prescribed feeding; enteral feeding pump; long-nosed syringe

Procedure
1. Wash hands.
2. Warm prescribed formula to room temperature.
3. Pour formula to run through the feeding bag.
4. Allow formula to run through the tubing to remove air. Close clamp.
5. Attach syringe to the end of the gastrostomy tube. Unclamp the gastrostomy tube.
6. Pull plunger back until resistance is felt. Check amount of formula in syringe. If more than half of the prescribed amount is withdrawn, refer to the section on problem solving (below). If less than the prescribed amount is withdrawn, push the formula gently back through the syringe.
7. Instill water through the tube.
8. Attach the feeding bag to the gastrostomy tube. Infuse at the prescribed rate.
9. Burp or bubble the infant throughout the feeding.
10. After feeding, flush the gastrostomy tube with water and clamp the tube.
11. Position the infant prone or side lying for 1/2 to 1 hour after feedings.

Psychosocial Needs
Hold and rock the infant or child during feedings.

Give a pacifier to an infant or a bottle or cup to a child to meet developmental needs.

Medication Administration
Use liquid medication whenever possible.

Crush only uncoated tablets.

Crush tablets to a fine powder and mix with water or juice

Flush tubing before and after medication administration.

Stoma Care
Wash the area around the stoma twice a day with soap and water.

Look for signs of infection, such as redness, swelling, and discharge.

Notify the physician if any signs of infection or leakage are present.

Problem Solving

PROBLEM	CAUSE	ACTION
Formula will not flow	Blocked tube (clamped, foreign material, viscous formula)	Check clamp. Reposition. Pull back on syringe. Instill water. Milk tube. Notify physician.
	Pump malfunction	Check pump. Call company. Give feeding by gravity.
Large volume of undigested formula removed before feeding	Delayed absorption	Reinfuse remaining formula. If more than half of feeding, subtract from amount given in the next feeding. Do not discard the residual.
Constipation	Decreased free fluids	Check for last bowel movement. Notify physician. Give water and juice between feedings as tolerated. Report bowel problems or hard stools to physician.
Diarrhea	Hyperosmolar formula	Dilute formula.
	Rapid rate of flow	Feed at a slower rate.
	Cold formula	Warm formula to room temperature before feeding.
	Bacterial contamination	Treat with antibiotics.
Dislodged tube	Inadequate stabilization	Bring child for emergency care
Skin irritation	Formula leakage	Skin care; barrier if needed

Note: From Borkowski, S. (1998). Pediatric stomas, tubes, and appliances. *Pediatric Clinics of North America, 45,* 1419-1435; and Young, C., & White, S. (1992). Preparing patients for tube feeding at home. *American Journal of Nursing, 92,* 46-53.

● FIGURE 51-3

A gastrostomy tube is used to feed the child with a gastrointestinal disorder such as esophageal atresia.

- Absence of respiratory distress
- Positive parent-infant bonding
- Absence of infection
- Parental use of support and information resources regarding the condition

PYLORIC STENOSIS

Pyloric stenosis is a hypertrophic obstruction of the circular muscle of the pyloric canal. Pyloric stenosis occurs in approximately 1 to 4 cases per 1000 live births, occurs 2 to 5 times more often in males than females, and is seen more in white children than in other races (Letton, 2001).

ETIOLOGY AND PATHOPHYSIOLOGY

The exact cause of pyloric stenosis is unknown, although frequently there is a family history of the disorder. Hypertrophy of the circular pylorus muscle results in stenosis of the passage between the stomach and the duodenum, partially obstructing the lumen of the stomach (see "Pathophysiology Illustrated: Pyloric Stenosis"). The lumen becomes inflamed and edematous, which narrows the opening until the obstruction becomes complete. At this time vomiting becomes more forceful. As the obstruction progresses, the infant becomes dehydrated and electrolytes are depleted, resulting in metabolic imbalances.

CLINICAL MANIFESTATIONS

Symptoms usually become evident 2 to 8 weeks after birth, although onset may vary. Initially the infant appears well or regurgitates slightly after feedings. The parents may describe the infant as a "good eater" who vomits occasionally. The symptoms in the early stages may be erroneously attributed to overfeeding, milk allergy, feeding intolerance, or gastroesophageal reflux (Morash, 2002). As the obstruction progresses, the vomiting becomes projectile. In **projectile vomiting,** the contents of the stomach may be ejected up to 3 feet from the infant. The vomitus is nonbilious and may become blood tinged because of repeated irritation to the esophagus. The infant is always hungry, appears irritable, fails to gain weight, and has fewer and smaller stools. Dehydration, alkalosis, and hyperbilirubinemia can occur.

CLINICAL THERAPY

On physical examination, visible peristaltic waves across the abdomen and an olive-sized mass in the left upper quadrant are often found. A sonogram is usually performed to confirm the diagnosis. This study is used to determine the diameter and length of the pyloric muscle. A thickened pylorus of >4 mm in diameter and length of >18 mm for the pyloric channel are diagnostic of pyloric stenosis (Blumer, Zucconi, Cohen et al., 2004). An upper gastrointestinal (UGI) study may be performed also, and reveals a narrowing of the pyloric channel, preventing the passage of the contrast medium.

Blood tests determine the degree of dehydration, electrolyte imbalance, and anemia (see Chapter 43 ∞); common findings are hypochloremia, metabolic alkalosis, and hyperbilirubinemia.

Surgical correction is the treatment of choice. Preoperatively the infant's condition is stabilized with intravenous fluids and electrolytes. A nasogastric tube is inserted to decompress the stomach. Surgery is performed as soon as possible after the infant's condition is stabilized. Open pyloromyotomy is performed through a periumbilical incision or through a small, transverse upper abdominal incision. Laparoscopic pyloromyotomy is currently used in many cases, and patients undergoing this surgical method reach full feeding sooner, have less emesis, and have a shorter hospital stay than those having an open procedure (Zitsman, 2003). With both procedures the circular muscle fibers are released to allow the passage of food and fluid.

The prognosis is good. The infant is usually taking fluids in 12 to 24 hours, and discharged on a regular diet by 36 to 48 hours after surgery.

NURSING MANAGEMENT

NURSING ASSESSMENT AND DIAGNOSIS

Observe the infant's abdomen for the presence of peristaltic waves. Bowel sounds are hyperactive on auscultation. Auscultate before palpating the abdomen since

PATHOPHYSIOLOGY ILLUSTRATED
Pyloric Stenosis

Muscular hypertrophy

Pyloric channel

In pyloric stenosis, the hypertrophied pyloric muscle causes symptoms of projectile vomiting and visible peristalsis.

palpation can cause a change in bowel patterns (see Chapter 35). ∞ Palpation reveals an olive-shaped mass in the right upper quadrant of the abdomen.

Assess skin turgor, fontanelles, urinary output, and mucous membranes to determine whether hydration is adequate. Measure vomitus and describe vomiting episodes. Be alert for signs of an electrolyte imbalance, particularly low levels of serum chloride, sodium, and potassium, and an elevated pH. (See Chapter 43 for a discussion of these electrolyte imbalances. ∞)

Assess the parents' level of anxiety related to the child's condition.

Among the nursing diagnoses that might be appropriate for the child with pyloric stenosis are the following:

- *Deficient Fluid Volume* related to active fluid volume loss
- *Imbalanced Nutrition: Less than Body Requirements* related to vomiting and inability to ingest nutrients
- *Disturbed Sleep Pattern* related to discomfort
- *Altered Family Processes* related to health status of family member

PLANNING AND IMPLEMENTATION

Nursing care centers on meeting the infant's fluid and electrolyte needs, minimizing weight loss, promoting rest and comfort, preventing infection, and providing supportive care for parents.

Meet Fluid and Electrolyte Needs

Because projectile vomiting will continue until the obstruction is relieved surgically, withhold oral feedings. Administer intravenous fluid therapy to correct fluid and electrolyte imbalances and to maintain adequate hydration. Because gastric fluid is high in potassium, hypokalemia can result (see Chapter 43 for a discussion of this electrolyte imbalance and the signs of its occurrence ∞). Monitor intake and output (including vomitus) and urine specific gravity. Inform parents that all diapers will be weighed to measure the infant's output of urine and stool.

Minimize Weight Loss

The infant loses weight because of frequent vomiting. Monitor weight daily both preoperatively and postoperatively. Begin small, frequent feedings of clear liquids within 4 to 6 hours postoperatively. If clear liquids are tolerated, advance the infant to formula or breast milk feedings.

Promote Rest and Comfort

During the preoperative period, the infant is hungry and cries often. Swaddle the infant to maintain warmth and provide comfort. Encourage the parents to hold and cuddle the infant. Provide a pacifier to meet the infant's need to suck.

Postoperatively the infant is uncomfortable because of the surgical incision. Instruct parents to avoid pressure on the incision. When diapering the infant, slide the diaper gently under the buttocks rather than lifting the legs. Swaddling, rocking, and use of a pacifier help to relax the infant. Acetaminophen or other analgesics can be administered to relieve discomfort as ordered. (See Chapter 42 for a discussion of pain management. ∞)

Prevent Infection

Postoperatively the incision is covered with collodion or Steri-Strips and should be kept clean and dry. Check the incision site for redness, swelling, or discharge. Monitor the infant's temperature every 4 hours. Auscultate lungs for clear respiratory sounds.

Provide Supportive Care

The need for hospitalization and surgery creates anxiety for parents. Encourage them to participate in the infant's care and to discuss their fears and concerns. Provide simple and

EVIDENCE-BASED NURSING

POSTOPERATIVE FEEDING METHODS FOLLOWING PYLOROMYOTOMY IN INFANTS

Problem

Postoperative feeding methods for infants following surgical correction (pyloromyotomy) of pyloric stenosis have remained unchanged for several decades. Conventional feeding methods include a prolonged NPO period following pyloromyotomy, with slow, incremental increases in volume and strength of feedings once feeding has resumed. Recent evidence indicates that a more liberal feeding method may prove beneficial, rather than harmful to the infant.

Evidence

Nurse researchers, in collaboration with a pediatric surgeon, conducted a 6-month retrospective study of 36 hypertrophic pyloric stenosis patients to compare conventional regimen feeds to ad lib feeds according to surgeon preference. The study revealed that the interval from the operating room to toleration of full feedings was less with the ad lib group as compared to the conventional regimen group. Additionally, discharges occurred sooner in the ad lib group.

Implications

The interval from the operating room to toleration of full feeds was significantly less with the ad lib fed infants compared to the conventionally fed infants. Significant decrease in length of stay was also noted. These findings led to practice changes at the hospital where the study was conducted.

Critical Thinking

How is feeding tolerance determined in the post-pyloromyotomy infant? If a surgeon prescribes conventional regimen feeding for post-pyloromyotomy infants, what collaborative approach could the nurse take to improve the feeding approach that is prescribed?

Reference

Morash, D. (2002). An interdisciplinary project that changed practice in feeding methods after pyloromyotomy. *Pediatric Nursing, 28*(2), 113–117.

---

clear explanations about the infant's condition and care. Advise parents that occasional vomiting after surgery may occur.

Discharge Planning and Home Care Teaching

Instruct parents to observe the incision for redness, swelling, or discharge and to notify the physician immediately if these occur or if the infant's temperature is higher than 38.5°C (101°F). To reduce the possibility of infection, advise parents to fold the infant's diaper so that it does not touch the incision. Provide instructions about feeding to ensure the infant's intake (see "Evidence-Based Nursing: Postoperative Feeding Methods Following Pyloromyotomy in Infants").

EVALUATION

Expected outcomes of care include pain control, intake of recommended fluid and food with absence of vomiting, and manifestation of normal growth patterns. See "Clinical Pathway: Pyloric Stenosis."

GASTROESOPHAGEAL REFLUX

Gastroesophageal reflux, the return of gastric contents into the esophagus, is the result of relaxation of the lower esophageal sphincter. Gastroesophageal reflux (GER) is one of the most common gastrointestinal disorders in children, affecting approximately 50% of healthy, full-term newborns (Jadcherla & Shaker, 2001). There is a higher incidence in premature infants, and males are affected three times more often than females. Children with neurologic

impairments, such as cerebral palsy, more commonly experience gastroesophageal reflux. The peak age of onset is 1 to 4 months of age. Some "spitting up" after feedings is considered normal in newborn infants, because of the weak cardiac sphincter of the stomach. However, regurgitation that continues and increases in frequency may be caused by GER and requires further investigation.

Gastroesophageal reflux disease (GERD) is a more serious manifestation of GER; it is a pathologic process in infants manifested by poor weight gain, esophagitis, neurobehavioral changes, and persistent respiratory symptoms or complications (Arguin & Swartz, 2004). Gastroesophageal reflux disease is diagnosed in approximately one in every 300 infants. Those children most at risk include those with esophageal atresia repair, neurologic disorders, hiatal hernia, bronchopulmonary dysplasia, asthma, and cystic fibrosis (Jung, 2001).

Postprandial regurgitation is the most common sign of gastroesophageal reflux in infants. The regurgitation ranges from spitting to forceful vomiting (Sondheimer, 2003). Children with gastroesophageal reflux are frequently hungry and irritable. They eat often but still lose weight. They have a history of vomiting and frequent upper respiratory infections. Reflux of stomach contents can lead to aspiration, resulting in frequent bouts of pneumonia, reactive airway disease, color changes during feeding, apnea, or hematemesis (Levy, 2001).

Diagnosis is confirmed by a thorough history of the child's feeding patterns and by diagnostic evaluation using contrast upper GI series, upper GI endoscopy, pH probe monitoring (insertion of a small catheter into the esophagus

CLINICAL PATHWAY

PYLORIC STENOSIS

CATEGORY	IMMEDIATE POSTOPERATIVE PERIOD	TRANSITION TO DISCHARGE	DISCHARGE TO HOME CARE
Daily outcomes	Client will: ■ have stable vital signs and be alert and responsive ■ have lungs clear to auscultation ■ have unlabored respirations and maintain oxygen saturation above 95% ■ have a clean, dry dressing ■ recover from anesthesia ■ have moist mucous membranes ■ have a urine specific gravity = 1.005–1.020 ■ demonstrate pain control Family displays effective coping with ongoing stressors Family verbalizes beginning understanding of expected postoperative course	Client will: ■ have stable vital signs and be alert and responsive ■ have lungs clear to auscultation ■ have unlabored respirations and maintain oxygen saturation above 95% ■ have a clean, dry wound with edges well approximated, healing by first intention ■ tolerate ordered diet without vomiting ■ have moist mucous membranes ■ have a urine specific gravity = 1.005–1.020 Family demonstrates understanding of home care instructions Family displays effective coping with ongoing stressors	Client is afebrile, has stable vital signs, and is alert and oriented Client has lungs clear to auscultation and unlabored respirations with an O_2 saturation >95% Client has clean, dry wound with edges well approximated Client has moist mucous membranes and urine specific gravity = 1.005–1.020 Family successfully plans for and transfers child home Client tolerates ordered diet without vomiting Family exhibits ability to cope with ongoing stressors
Assessments, tests, and treatments	Electrolytes Urine specific gravity q8hr Weight Vital signs and O_2 saturation and wound drainage assessment q15min × 4; q30min × 4; q1hr × 24 and prn Assess respiratory status q2–4hr and prn Level of consciousness Change position frequently Assess abdomen and bowel sounds q2–4hr Oxygen as ordered Strict intake and output Record and report vomiting Monitor temperature and provide warming measures as indicated Provide ongoing emotional support to family	Weight Urine specific gravity q8hr Vital signs, O_2 saturation, and dressing and wound drainage assessment q2–4hr and prn Assess respiratory status q4hr and prn Change position frequently Assess abdomen and bowel sounds q4hr Dressing change and wound assessment BID and prn Strict intake and output Observe responses to feeding and feeding technique Record and report vomiting Monitor temperature and provide warming or cooling measures as indicated	Weight Vital signs, O_2 saturation, and dressing and wound drainage assessment upon discharge Assess respiratory status Change position frequently Assess wound and apply dry sterile dressing every day and prn Assess abdomen and bowel sounds upon discharge Observe responses to feeding and feeding technique Record and report vomiting Monitor temperature and return for healthcare if needed
Knowledge deficit	Orient family to room and surroundings Provide simple, brief instructions Encourage family involvement in care Review specific postoperative care: turning, intravenous, pain management Evaluate understanding of teaching	Review plan of care Begin discharge teaching regarding wound care/dressing change and diet Review written discharge instructions with family Continue to encourage family participation in care Observe and coach family members regarding feeding Evaluate understanding of teaching	Complete discharge teaching to include wound care, diet, follow-up care and appointment, signs and symptoms to report, activity, and medication: name, purpose, dose, frequency, route, food interactions, and side effects Provide family with written discharge instructions regarding home care Evaluate understanding of teaching Provide telephone number/resource for questions

(continued)

CLINICAL PATHWAY—continued

PYLORIC STENOSIS

CATEGORY	IMMEDIATE POSTOPERATIVE PERIOD	TRANSITION TO DISCHARGE	DISCHARGE TO HOME CARE
Psychosocial	Assess anxiety related to surgery Encourage verbalization of concerns Assess coping status of family Provide emotional support to client and family Cuddle prn and encourage parents to cuddle child	Assess level of anxiety Encourage verbalization of concerns Assess coping status of family Provide emotional support to client and family Provide information and ongoing encouragement	Assess level of anxiety Encourage verbalization of concerns Assess coping status of family Provide emotional support to client and family Provide information and ongoing encouragement
Diet	NPO until feeding ordered	When fully awake, begin progressive diet as ordered Continue progressing diet as ordered Position on right side with head up after feedings Burp before feedings and frequently during feedings	Diet as ordered Position on right side with head up after feedings Burp before feedings and frequently during feedings Pacifier between meals if desired
Activity	Assess safety needs and provide adequate precautions	Maintain safety precautions	Maintain safety precautions
Medications	IV fluids Analgesics as ordered	Maintain IV line as ordered Analgesics as ordered; instruct parents in administration and assessment of results	Analgesics as ordered; document results D/C IV line
Transfer/ discharge plans	Establish discharge objectives with family Determine discharge needs Assess support system Begin home care instructions	Review progress toward discharge goals Make appropriate referrals Finalize discharge plans	Complete discharge instructions Ensure safe transfer home

Data from Beyea, S. C. (1996). *Critical pathways for collaborative nursing care.* Upper Saddle River, NJ: Prentice Hall-Health.

through the nose that is left in place for 18 to 24 hours to measure pH and thus determine number of reflux episodes), or gastroesophageal scintigraphy (radionuclide scanning to evaluate gastric emptying) (Jung 2001; Murray & Christie, 2000). Testing for cow's milk protein allergy, including cutaneous tests, eosinophil smears of the nasal mucosa, IgG anti-lactoglobulin levels, and intestinal biopsy, is generally performed since there is a high association between gastroesophageal reflux and cow's milk allergy (Arguin & Swartz, 2004).

Treatment depends on the severity of the condition. Mild cases may require only a modification of feeding habits, and usually resolve by 12 to 18 months (Murray & Christie, 2000). One to 4 teaspoons of rice cereal can be added to each 4 ounces of formula in the infant's bottle to thicken feedings. Commercial thickened formulas that are nutritionally balanced are available. Breast milk does not thicken with rice cereal addition, but the breastfeeding mother should be encouraged to continue and feed small amounts at a time with frequent burping; all infants should be positioned with

the upper body raised 30 degrees after feedings. Fatty foods and citrus juices are avoided. Medications (proton pump inhibitors, antacids, and histamine antagonists) may be prescribed to reduce the amount of stomach acid and lessen the child's discomfort (see Table 51–1).

Treatment for severe cases may include surgery to create a valve mechanism by wrapping the greater curvature of the stomach (fundus) around the distal esophagus (Nissen fundoplication). A gastrostomy tube is usually inserted during surgery and left in place for 6 weeks. Both infants with mild conditions and those undergoing surgical correction usually have decreased incidence of reflux. They may have episodes of mild reflux throughout life and may occasionally require medication for treatment.

NURSING MANAGEMENT

Nursing management focuses on obtaining a thorough history of the child's feeding patterns. Observe vomiting episodes and document amount, color, and consistency of emesis.

TABLE 51–1 ✤ Medications Used to Treat Gastroesophageal Reflux

Drug	Action
Antacid (aluminum hydroxide, aluminum carbonate)	Neutralizes refluxed material and decreases resultant discomfort
Histamine H₂ receptor antagonists Ranitidine (Zantac) Cimetidine (Tagamet) Famotidine (Pepcid)	Decreases gastric acid production
Cholinergic Metoclopramide (Reglan)	Increases esophageal motility and tone
Proton pump inhibitors Lansoprazole (Prevacid) Omeprazole (Prilosec)	Suppresses gastric acid production and secretion
Acetaminophen	Controls pain

Monitor the infant's weight daily and plot on a growth chart to note progress. Observe for any signs of respiratory distress, and keep the infant's nose and mouth clear of vomitus.

Adequate nutrition must be maintained. Infants receiving oral feedings should be given small, frequent feedings. Elevate the head of the bed to prevent aspiration if vomiting should occur. If the child has difficulty maintaining this position, a Tracy harness or reflux board may be used. The harness, which is pinned to the mattress, supports the infant in an upright position. The best position to place the postprandial infant with GERD is in the prone position with the head elevated. However, the prone position should not be used in the sleeping child due to the increased incidence of sudden infant death syndrome with this position. Caution parents to use the prone position only while the infant is awake and while being continuously observed by the parent (Arguin & Swartz, 2004). Parents are encouraged to hold their infant in an upright position for 20 to 30 minutes following feedings. Minimize seated positioning such as in an infant seat since this increases intra-abdominal pressure and promotes reflux.

If the child has a gastrostomy tube, it is important to maintain skin integrity around the stoma site. Secure the tube so the infant cannot dislodge or pull on it, and check daily to be sure the length is the same, indicating correct placement.

Discharge planning focuses on instructing parents in how to feed and position the infant, as well as providing comfort and emotional support. Encourage parents to hold and cuddle the infant during all feedings. Providing the infant with a pacifier helps to meet nonnutritive sucking needs. Teach parents how to suction the nose and mouth if vomiting occurs.

OMPHALOCELE AND GASTROSCHISIS

Omphaloceles are congenital malformations in which intra-abdominal contents herniate through the umbilical cord (Figure 51–4 ○). They result when the abdominal contents, such as intestines and liver, fail to return to the abdomen when the abdominal wall begins to close by the tenth week of gestation. The protrusion is covered by a translucent sac (peritoneum) into which the umbilical cord inserts. Omphalocele is often associated with other congenital anomalies such as cardiac defects; genitourinary anomalies; trisomy 13, 18, or 21; craniofacial abnormalities; and diaphragmatic abnormalities. Omphalocele with intestinal contents in the sac occurs in 1.25 in 5000 births, while those involving the liver and intestines are less frequent (Weir, 2003).

The size of the sac varies depending on the extent of the protrusion. Rupture of the sac results in evisceration of the abdominal contents. Treatment involves protecting the sac from injury, providing fluids and warmth, and surgical repair to replace the abdominal contents and close the abdominal wall. For smaller defects, primary closure is accomplished with one surgery. If the defect is severe, surgical correction may be performed in several steps. If an omphalocele occurs without associated defects, the child usually recovers from the surgery without incident and leads a normal life.

A related condition is gastroschisis, a congenital defect of the ventral abdominal wall, characterized by herniation of abdominal viscera outside the abdominal cavity through a defect in the abdominal wall to the side (most often to the right) of the umbilicus (Figure 51–5 ○). The most common abdominal organs involved are the small intestine and ascending colon, and, unlike omphalocele, no membrane covers the organs. Gastroschisis occurs in approximately 1 in 10,000 births, and has a survival rate of 92% (Weir, 2003).

Both gastroschisis and omphalocele are associated with elevation of maternal serum alpha-fetoprotein (MSAFP). Routine prenatal ultrasonography and determination of MSAFP levels permit early diagnosis and mobilization of the multidisciplinary team of obstetricians, geneticists, neonatologists, and pediatric surgeons needed to manage these congenital anomalies. Intensive care is needed to manage fluid status, temperature regulation, infection control, and vital signs. Surgical care is instituted as soon as possible. Current trends are to suture a prosthetic silo around a gastroschisis defect. The silo permits gradual return of the intestines to the abdominal cavity over 5 to 10 days as the cavity slowly enlarges (Weir, 2003).

● FIGURE 51-4

In omphalocele, the size of the sack depends on the extent of the protrusion of abdominal contents through the umbilical cord.

Used with permission from Rudolph, A. M., Hoffman, J. I. E., & Rudolph, C. D. (Eds.). (1991). Rudolph's pediatrics (19th ed., p. 1040). Stamford, CT: Appleton & Lange.

● FIGURE 51-5

The newborn with gastroschisis has abdominal contents located outside the abdominal wall.

Used with permission of the authors and the University of Iowa's Virtual Hospital®, http://www.vh.org

NURSING MANAGEMENT

Be alert for signs of associated congenital anomalies. (Refer to the discussions of tracheoesophageal fistula earlier in this chapter, of genitourinary anomalies in Chapter 52, and of congenital heart defects in Chapter 48. ∞)

Immediately after birth, follow physician protocol for maintaining the omphalocele sac, such as with sterile gauze soaked in normal saline solution covered with sterile plastic. Monitor vital signs at least hourly, paying close attention to temperature, as the infant can lose heat through the sac. The child should be in a warmer or isolette for maintenance of temperature control. Inspect the area for signs of infection.

Because the infant is NPO preoperatively, maintain fluid and electrolyte balance with intravenous fluids. Postoperative care includes measures to control pain, prevent infection, maintain fluid and electrolyte balance, and ensure adequate nutritional intake. Attainment of bowel motility and function varies and is often delayed for weeks after surgery; parenteral nutrition for the infant is used during this period (Ashburn, Pranikoff, & Turner, 2002).

Throughout the infant's hospitalization, parents need clear, accurate explanations about the infant's condition. To help the parents deal with the crisis of an acutely ill newborn, provide emotional support and encourage parents to express their feelings. When the child has multiple anomalies, parents need ongoing support for the lengthy treatment, numerous hospitalizations, and management of nutritional intake.

Expected outcomes of nursing care depend on the severity of the defect and its correction. Some examples include maintenance of normal vital signs, prompt identification of additional problems, healing of surgical site without signs of infection, pain control, proper intake of fluids, and establishment of an intake to support growth patterns.

INTUSSUSCEPTION

Intussusception occurs when one portion of the intestine prolapses and then invaginates or telescopes into another. It is one of the most frequent causes of intestinal obstruction during infancy, with an incidence of 1 to 4 in 1000 births. Most cases occur in boys between the ages of 3 months and 6 years (Wyllie, 2004). The etiology of intussusception is multifactorial, and direct causes cannot always be identified. Virus infection, use of medications that influence gut motility, and the body's inflammatory mediators such as cytokine, nitric oxide, and prostaglandins are all associated with increased rates of intussusception.

The most common site of intussusception is the ileocecal valve. Telescoping of the intestine obstructs the passage of stool. The walls of the intestine rub together, causing inflammation, edema, and decreased blood flow. This can lead to necrosis, perforation, hemorrhage, and peritonitis.

The onset is usually abrupt. A previously healthy infant or child suddenly experiences acute abdominal pain with vomiting and passage of brown stool. There may be periods of comfort between acute episodes of pain. As the condition worsens, painful episodes increase. The stools become red and resemble currant jelly because of the mix of blood and mucus. A palpable mass may be present in the upper right quadrant or mid-upper abdomen.

Diagnosis is made on the basis of the history and confirmed by radiographs and ultrasound of the abdomen; barium enema may be used (Orenstein, 2000). In some cases the hydrostatic pressure from the barium moves the bowel back into place. Oxygen, saline, and aqueous contrast material may also be used to reduce the intussusception. If these treatments are ineffective, surgical intervention to reduce the invaginated bowel and remove any necrotic tissue is necessary. Surgery usually corrects the problem.

NURSING MANAGEMENT

Nursing management focuses on maintaining or restoring fluid and electrolyte balance. Intravenous fluids are started immediately. Serum electrolyte monitoring is essential to correct imbalances.

Postoperative care focuses on monitoring for early signs of infection, managing the child's pain, and maintaining nasogastric tube patency. Assess vital signs, check for abdominal distention, and listen for bowel sounds every 4 hours. After normal bowel function returns, begin clear liquid feedings. Feedings are advanced to half-strength milk and other foods as the infant or child tolerates it.

Discharge usually occurs shortly after the infant or child begins taking full feedings. Instruct parents to watch for infection and to call the physician if symptoms recur, a fever develops, or appetite decreases.

HIRSCHSPRUNG DISEASE

Hirschsprung disease, also known as congenital aganglionic megacolon, is a congenital anomaly in which inadequate motility causes mechanical obstruction of the intestine. It is now known that the RET proto-oncogene is a major gene for the disease (Howard, 2001). The disease occurs in approximately one in every 5000 live births, and the incidence of transmitting this disease to offspring is approximately 3% (Swenson, 2002). Males are affected more commonly than females (Thompson, 2001). Hirschsprung disease can occur in combination with congenital heart defects, Down syndrome, and some other syndromes such as Smith-Lemli-Opitz syndrome and Waardenburg syndrome. It can be acute or chronic.

The absence of autonomic parasympathetic ganglion cells in the colon prevents peristalsis at that portion of the intestine, resulting in the accumulation of intestinal contents and abdominal distention. In contrast, another disorder known as chronic intestinal pseudo-obstruction (pseudo-Hirschsprung) is very rare and affects small bowel motility (Barr, 2000).

Clinical manifestations of Hirschsprung disease vary depending on the child's age at onset. In newborns, symptoms include failure to pass meconium, refusal to suck, abdominal distention, and bile-stained emesis. If Hirschsprung disease is not treated, the condition can lead to complete obstruction, respiratory distress, and shock.

In the older child, symptoms may include failure to gain weight and delayed growth. The child may have a history of abdominal distention, severe constipation alternating with **diarrhea** (frequent, watery stools), and vomiting. The stool may be normal size or have a ribbonlike appearance.

Diagnosis is made on the basis of the history, bowel patterns, anorectal manometry (reaction of the anal sphincter to distention of the rectum), radiographic contrast studies, and rectal biopsy for presence or absence of ganglion cells (Swenson, 2002). The rectum is small in size on palpation and does not contain stool.

Treatment in infancy involves surgical removal of the aganglionic bowel. In severe cases or in ill infants, a temporary colostomy is created. Closure of the colostomy and reanastomosis are performed about 3 to 6 months later (Rogers, 2001). For the child with a milder defect, management may involve dietary modification, stool softeners, and isotonic irrigations to prevent impaction until the child is toilet trained.

The return of normal bowel function depends on the amount of bowel involved. Some fecal incontinence and constipation may persist following surgery. A serious complication is enterocolitis (inflammation of the intestines), which is manifested by symptoms such as GI bleeding and diarrhea. Enterocolitis can occur before or after surgery, resulting in ischemia and ulceration of the bowel wall. Treatment may include total parenteral nutrition and a lactose-free diet.

NURSING MANAGEMENT

Nursing assessment in the newborn period includes careful observation for the passage of meconium. Because newborns are often discharged within 24 hours of birth, tell parents to notify the physician if no stool is passed or the abdomen becomes distended. When the disease is diagnosed later in infancy or in childhood, take a thorough history of weight gain, nutritional intake, and bowel habits.

Nursing management consists of carefully monitoring fluid and electrolyte balance and maintaining nutrition. Teach parents how to ensure regular bowel movements. Daily rectal irrigations with normal saline solution are necessary to promote adequate elimination and prevent obstruction. Teach parents how to prevent skin breakdown in the rectal area by changing diapers frequently, cleansing the area carefully, and applying protective ointment at each diaper change.

If surgical correction is necessary, nursing care includes monitoring for infection, managing pain, maintaining hydration, measuring abdominal circumference to detect any distention, and providing support to the child and family. Parents need instruction in ostomy care if the child has a colostomy (refer to the discussion later in this chapter). Provide appropriate referrals to an ostomy support group and enterostomal nurse specialist when indicated. Teach parents to be alert for and immediately report signs of complications. These include diarrhea and pelvic abscess from leakage of intestinal contents at the surgical site (characterized by fever and pain). Children occasionally develop constipation, and parents may need guidance to adapt the diet and fluid intake to manage this complication. Because some children develop malabsorption, be alert for signs of poor growth or malnutrition.

Expected outcomes of nursing care include prompt identification of obstruction, maintenance of normal bowel patterns, adequate hydration, and maintenance of clear skin.

ANORECTAL MALFORMATIONS

Malformations of the anus and rectum are common congenital anomalies. Minor anomalies occur in 1 in 4000 to 5000 births. They are often associated with abnormalities of the genitourinary tract, esophagus, duodenum, musculoskeletal system, craniofacial, and cardiovascular system, and with chromosomal abnormalities (Cho, Moore, & Fangman, 2001; Gereige & Frias, 2002). Chromosomal abnormalities such as trisomy 13, 18, or 21 may coexist, and some babies have VACTERL conditions. VACTERL refers to three or more anomalies of vertebral formation, anal atresia, congenital heart disease, tracheoesophageal fistula, reno-urinary anomalies, and radial limb defects (Davies, Creighton, & Wilcox, 2004).

Types of defects include anal stenosis (a thickened and constricted anal wall) and anal atresia (absence of anal opening). Diagnosis is usually made at birth or during the newborn assessment of anorectal structures and rectal patency. Failure to pass meconium may indicate a malformation high in the colon. Stool in the urine indicates a fistula between the colon and urinary tract. Ribbonlike stools may occur with some malformations. Ultrasound and lower GI radiographic studies confirm the diagnosis and demonstrate the extent of the anomaly. Higher defects are often less apparent at birth and involve more complicated treatment.

Medical management depends on the extent of the malformation. Some stenosed anal openings can be treated with dilation alone. An imperforate anal membrane is excised surgically, followed by daily manual dilations. More severe defects require reconstructive surgery. A temporary colostomy is sometimes performed to rest the bowel after reconstruction. The colostomy is generally closed between the age of 6 months and 1 year.

NURSING MANAGEMENT

During the initial newborn assessment, inspect the perineal area for a poorly developed anal dimple or sacral anomalies. Lubricate a rectal thermometer and insert it a short distance into the rectum to determine patency. Observation and recording of passage of meconium are essential.

Once the diagnosis has been made, intravenous fluids are initiated and a nasogastric tube is inserted to decompress the stomach. Monitor the child's intake and output and cardiorespiratory functioning. Provide emotional support to the parents and give them information about the upcoming surgery.

Postoperative care centers on preventing infection and respiratory complications from surgery, as well as maintaining hydration. Observe the incision for signs of infection, and provide careful wound care. Assess vital signs at least every 4 hours. Once the child's condition is stable, clear fluid oral intake is allowed, advancing to half- and full-strength formula or breast milk as tolerated. The infant will have a colostomy after surgery, and careful skin care around the stoma is essential to prevent breakdown of the fragile area. Colostomy care was a particular focus of nursing management for Jerome, described at the beginning of this chapter.

The child with associated abnormalities may need several surgeries and interventions to treat all of the conditions present. Partnering with families and the group of healthcare providers will assist in case management that facilitates the child's health and development. Health promotion and health maintenance that include support of family members, ensuring immunizations, and monitoring developmental status are important.

Discharge Planning and Home Care Teaching

Infants are increasingly discharged shortly after birth, so parents need clear instructions about normal newborn stools and what abnormalities to report.

After surgery, teach parents how to take the infant's temperature using the axillary route (see Skill 9–13). **SKILLS** Have them demonstrate the proper technique be-

---

THINKING CRITICALLY

ANAL ATRESIA AND ESOPHAGEAL ATRESIA

Jerome was born with both anal atresia and esophageal atresia. He has had several surgeries, and presently is 8 months of age. He has a colostomy for bowel elimination and a gastrostomy tube for feedings. What assessments will you perform of the colostomy site? How can you help Jerome's parents to manage the colostomy? What developmental milestones would you expect at Jerome's age? What suggestions do you have for the family about ways to stimulate Jerome's social, physical, and cognitive skills?

fore discharge. Explain the signs and symptoms of infection. Discuss feeding regimens and bowel habits necessary to maintain adequate nutrition for growth and development. Advise parents that children with anorectal malformations may have difficulty achieving bowel control. Patience in toilet training is important. When the child reaches an age appropriate for toilet training, encourage the family to speak with a healthcare provider to discuss the child's progress.

If a colostomy is performed, teach parents how to care for the ostomy site (see discussion of ostomies later in this chapter). Reassure parents that the colostomy will be closed in the future, and help them plan for that hospitalization. Refer them to ostomy support groups in the community or online. Discuss follow-up care and long-term management. Arrange follow-up visits and home care visits to evaluate the child's ostomy site and monitor growth.

Expected outcomes of nursing care include adequate fluid intake, normal bowel patterns, parental knowledge of ostomy or other treatment protocols, and eventual success with toilet training.

HERNIAS

A **hernia** is the protrusion or projection of an organ or a part of an organ through the muscle wall of the cavity that normally contains it. This protrusion may result from the failure of normal openings to close during fetal development or from weakness in the supporting musculature. When intra-abdominal pressure increases (as when the infant cries or strains to pass stool), the weakened area separates, causing a protrusion of underlying organs. Inguinal hernias are the most common type of hernia occurring in children (see Chapter 52 ∞). Other hernias that occur frequently in children are diaphragmatic and umbilical.

DIAPHRAGMATIC HERNIA

In a diaphragmatic hernia, abdominal contents protrude into the thoracic cavity through an opening in the diaphragm. Sites of herniation include the substernal space, the posterolateral region, and the esophageal hiatus. The posterolateral site (foramen of Bochdalek) is the most common location. The cause is a delay or failure in closure of the pleuroperitoneal musculature. The overall incidence of diaphragmatic hernia is 1 in 2500 live births (Singh, Bhende, & Kinnane, 2001). Associated anomalies, particularly cardiac defects, occur in some infants.

A diaphragmatic hernia is a life-threatening condition. Severe respiratory distress occurs shortly after birth. As the infant cries, abdominal organs extend into the thorax, decreasing the size of the thoracic cavity. The infant becomes dyspneic and cyanotic. Characteristic findings include a barrel-shaped chest and sunken abdomen.

Some cases of congenital diaphragmatic hernia are diagnosed in utero by ultrasound. If not identified prenatally, the condition is first identified postnatally by physical signs and symptoms; confirmation is made by chest radiologic examination. MRI is helpful in confirming the diagnosis and in determining the position of organs in the chest and abdomen (Hedrick, Crombleholme, Flake et al., 2004). Immediate respiratory support is essential. Extracorporeal membrane oxygenation (ECMO) may be used to provide cardiopulmonary bypass to rest the lungs. Alternatively, inhaled nitric oxide (iNO) and high-frequency oxygen ventilation (HFVO) preoperatively may improve survival outcomes and decrease concomitant morbidity (Bagolan, Casaccia, Crescenzi et al., 2004).

The infant is positioned with the head and thorax higher than the abdomen to facilitate downward movement of abdominal organs. A nasogastric tube is inserted to decompress the stomach. Ventilator support is necessary to manage respiratory compromise. Intravenous fluids are administered through an umbilical artery catheter.

Once the infant's condition is stabilized, the defect is corrected surgically. The prognosis is poor. Only 50% of infants survive, with death usually resulting from pulmonary hypoplasia. Even after surgery the infant may do well initially and then manifest severe respiratory decompensation.

NURSING MANAGEMENT

The infant with a diaphragmatic hernia is admitted to the neonatal intensive care unit (NICU) and requires continuous monitoring. Preoperative management centers on providing supportive care to the infant and parents. Note the infant's vital signs every 30 minutes on the cardiorespiratory monitor. Observe for worsening of respiratory compromise. Maintain intravenous fluid administration. Promote decreased stimulation to keep the infant calm and thus maintain low abdominal pressure. Keep parents informed about the infant's condition, and provide emotional support both before and after surgery.

Postoperative care includes positioning the infant on the affected side to facilitate expansion of the lung on the unaffected side, observing closely for signs of infection, maintaining respiratory support, and carefully monitoring fluid and electrolyte balance.

Before discharge, instruct parents in wound care, prevention of infection, and feeding techniques.

UMBILICAL HERNIA

An umbilical hernia results from a weak or imperfectly closed umbilical ring (Figure 51–6 ●). The condition is often associated with diastasis recti (lateral separation of

● **FIGURE 51–6**

The umbilical hernia of the newborn usually closes as the muscles strengthen in later infancy and childhood.

Used with permission from Zitelli, B., & Davis, H. (Eds.). (1994). Atlas of pediatric physical diagnosis *(2nd ed.). London: Mosby-Wolfe Publishing.*

the abdominal muscles). Umbilical hernia occurs in 1 out of every 6 children and is nearly 10 times more common in African-American children than white children. Umbilical hernias are also observed more frequently in females, infants with low birth weight, children with Down syndrome, and children with hypothyroidism (Katz, 2001).

The hernia appears as a soft swelling covered by skin. The herniated area protrudes with coughing, crying, or straining during a bowel movement. It is easily reduced by pushing the bowel back through the fibrous ring. The size of the defect may vary among individuals. Contents of the hernia include omentum or portions of the small intestine.

Most defects resolve spontaneously by 3 to 4 years of age. Surgery is indicated in cases of strangulation (closure of the umbilical ring around a portion of the bowel, preventing it from moving back into the abdomen), increased protrusion of the hernia after the age of 2 years, or little or no improvement in a large defect after the age of 4 years.

NURSING MANAGEMENT

Nursing management is generally supportive. Instruct parents not to apply tape, straps, or coins to reduce the hernia. This can cause strangulation of the hernia, necessitating immediate surgery. If surgery is required, it is usually performed in a short-stay unit. Postoperatively, teach parents how to care for the surgical site, to watch for bleeding, and

to recognize signs of infection. Reinforce the importance of returning for follow-up evaluation.

OSTOMIES

An intestinal **ostomy** is an opening, or **stoma,** into the small or large intestine that diverts fecal matter, providing an outlet when a distal surgical anastomosis, obstruction, or nonfunctioning structure prevents normal elimination. Depending on the integrity and function of anatomic structures, the ostomy may be temporary or permanent. Infants and small children with necrotizing enterocolitis, Hirschsprung disease, volvulus, or intussusception may require a temporary colostomy or ileostomy. Ostomies may also be indicated for children with inflammatory bowel disease, intestinal tumors, or abdominal trauma.

An ostomy may be elective or a surgical emergency. In all cases it affects a child's lifestyle, alters body image, causes anxiety, and increases the risk for alterations in physiologic processes (electrolyte imbalance, increased nutritional requirements). For adolescents, it may also result in dependence at a time when autonomy is a major developmental need (Figure 51–7 ●).

In assessing the family and child approaching ostomy surgery, it is important to determine their ability to understand and accept the physical changes that will occur. Parents may feel guilt and anger about the ostomy surgery when the child has a genetically transmitted disease, is injured, or has developed an obstruction from necrosis of the bowel. Encourage the parents and child to express their feelings, and correct any misunderstandings. Parents and

● **FIGURE 51–7**

Nursing strategies to address altered perceptions of body image and increased feelings of dependence are important when working with adolescents who have ostomies. Support groups or a visit from another teenager who has had an ostomy can facilitate positive coping, as demonstrated by this teenage girl.

MediaLink

Skills 16-3-16-4

older children may be referred for counseling and to support groups to help them deal with their feelings. Adolescents often benefit from a visit with an adolescent ostomate (someone who has an ostomy) who can answer questions about living with an ostomy.

PREOPERATIVE CARE

Preoperative education focuses on educating the child and family and preparing them for postoperative management. Discuss how the appliance will look, and explain the purpose of the pouch in developmentally appropriate terms. Encourage the parents and child to touch and manipulate all equipment. A younger child can be shown how to place a pouch on a doll. Older children can practice placing a pouch on their skin. These measures help relieve anxiety by providing information and increasing familiarity with the appliance.

GROWTH AND DEVELOPMENT

The preschooler has some manual dexterity and can help with some parts of the procedure for changing an ostomy appliance and cleaning the stoma. Teach the child using a doll or stuffed animal. Many school-age children are able to care for their ostomy independently. Teach them how to avoid leakage around the bag, which could be embarrassing. Adolescents are generally totally independent in their self-care of ostomies. However, they may need support to deal with the fact that they are different from their peers.

In addition to discussion of the appliance, preoperative education should include discussion of pain control and measures that will be used to prevent postoperative complications (turning, coughing, and breathing deeply). Gear the instructions to the child's developmental level. Encourage parental participation to promote compliance.

POSTOPERATIVE CARE

Postoperative care of a child with an ostomy is similar to that for any child who undergoes abdominal surgery. (See the discussion of nursing management for appendicitis later in this chapter and "Nursing Care Plan: The Child Undergoing Surgery" in Chapter 40. ∞) Management of the stoma may be done by an "ostomy nurse" or other nurses. Major interventions involve ensuring proper function of the stoma, identifying complications, and instituting daily stoma care. Assess the stoma, quality and amount of fecal matter, skin condition, and adherence of the pouch. Evaluate for the most common complications, which are prolapse, retraction, stenosis, and skin breakdown around the stoma. Evaluate the family's understanding and their ability to care for the ostomy.

Identify and address home care needs well in advance of discharge. Instructions include skin care, care of the stoma, appliance removal and application, and frequency of appliance changes (see Skills 16–3 to 16–4). **SKILLS** Begin teaching immediately after surgery with responsibility for care transferred gradually to the parents and child as they are ready. Discuss diet, activity level, hygiene, clothing, equipment, and financial considerations. Arrange for home visits to check periodically on the home management program.

Parents and children can be referred to the United Ostomy Association or a local ostomy group for information and support. Make referrals to social service, counseling, and a home health agency, if appropriate.

Expected outcomes of nursing care include successful adjustment to the ostomy, thorough evacuation of the bowel, absence of infection and other complications, intact skin, and formation of a positive self-image in the child.

NURSING PRACTICE

Avoid adhesive enhancers on the skin of newborns and premature infants. Their skin layers are so thin that removal of the appliance can strip off the skin. Remember also that adhesive contains latex and its constant use is not advised due to risk of latex allergy development (see Chapter 44∞).

INFLAMMATORY DISORDERS

Inflammatory disorders are reactions of specific tissues of the GI tract to trauma caused by injuries, foreign bodies, chemicals, microorganisms, or surgery. These disorders may be acute or chronic and may involve various segments of the GI tract.

APPENDICITIS

Appendicitis is an inflammation of the vermiform appendix, the small sac near the end of the cecum. The condition occurs most often in adolescent boys (10 to 19 years of age). Appendicitis is the most common cause for emergency abdominal surgery in children and adolescents in the United States (Kosloske, Love, Rohrer et al., 2004). Children account for 62,000 to 82,000 of the appendectomies performed every year in more than 250,000 Americans (Ziegler, 2004).

ETIOLOGY AND PATHOPHYSIOLOGY

Appendicitis almost always results from an obstruction in the appendiceal lumen. It can be caused by a fecalith (hard fecal mass), parasitic infestations, stenosis, hyperplasia of lymphoid tissue, or a tumor. Continued secretion of mucus following acute obstruction of the lumen increases pressure, causing ischemia, cellular death, and ulceration.

The appendix may perforate or rupture, resulting in fecal and bacterial contamination of the peritoneum. Peritonitis spreads quickly and if untreated can result in small bowel obstruction, electrolyte imbalances, septicemia, and hypovolemic shock.

CLINICAL MANIFESTATIONS

At onset, symptoms include periumbilical cramps, abdominal tenderness, and fever. In adolescent and young adult females, symptoms must be differentiated from those associated with ovulation (mittelschmerz), ruptured ectopic pregnancy, and pelvic inflammatory disease. As the inflammation progresses, pain in the right lower abdomen becomes constant. Pain is often most intense at McBurney's point, halfway between the anterior superior iliac crest and the umbilicus (see "Pathophysiology Illustrated: Appendicitis"). In 30% of children, however, the appendix is in a different location, so the pain may occur elsewhere. Symptoms progress to include guarding, rigid-

PATHOPHYSIOLOGY ILLUSTRATED
Appendicitis

McBurney's point is the common location of pain in children and adolescents with appendicitis.

ity, and rebound tenderness following palpation over the right lower quadrant. If the appendix ruptures, there is usually fever, sudden relief from abdominal pain, guarding and distention of the abdomen, rapid breathing, pallor, chills, and irritability.

Vomiting, diarrhea, or constipation may be present. As appendicitis progresses, the child remains motionless, usually in a side-lying position with knees flexed. Sudden relief of pain usually means that the appendix has ruptured.

CLINICAL THERAPY

Diagnosis of appendicitis in young children can be difficult because their pain may be less localized and their symptoms more diffuse than in the older child. Continuing evaluations over several hours are often needed to establish the diagnosis.

An elevated white blood cell count (above 15,000/mm^3) may occur. This leukocytosis occurs less often in young children than in teenagers. A history of abdominal pain, presence of a fecalith in the right lower abdomen on x-ray, and abdominal ultrasound help to confirm the diagnosis. Computerized tomography with contrast, C-reactive protein elevations, and urinalysis help to rule out other causes and establish the diagnosis.

Treatment involves immediate surgical removal (appendectomy), either through laparoscopic or open method (Vegunta, Ali, Wallace et al., 2004). Preoperatively the child is kept NPO. Intravenous fluids, electrolytes, and antibiotics are administered. A nasogastric tube may be inserted before or after surgery. Postoperatively the child has an abdominal incision, and intravenous antibiotics are administered to prevent infection. If the appendix has ruptured before surgery, a Penrose drain is inserted and the wound may not be completely sutured. Wound irrigations may be needed to help cleanse the peritoneum. Recovery is usually complete following uncomplicated removal of the appendix.

NURSING MANAGEMENT

NURSING ASSESSMENT AND DIAGNOSIS

Physiologic Assessment

A detailed assessment of the child's pain is necessary to differentiate appendicitis from other illnesses (see Chapter 42 ∞). Ask the child to point to the painful area and to describe the pain. Recognize that localizing the pain may be difficult for young children. Note onset, location, and intensity of pain; precipitating factors; and relief measures tried. During abdominal assessment, palpate last to avoid causing additional pain. Assess vital signs to determine baseline values, and monitor every 4 hours thereafter.

Psychosocial Assessment

Because appendicitis usually occurs in school-age children and adolescents, assessment of the child's coping skills is important. Adolescents, because of their preoccupation with body image, may be concerned about the surgical scar. Assess the parents' and child's anxiety about the sudden hospitalization and need for emergency surgery.

Among the nursing diagnoses that might be appropriate for the child with appendicitis are the following:

- *Acute Pain* related to inflammation and surgery
- *Risk for Deficient Fluid Volume Deficit* related to fluid volume loss and inadequate fluid volume intake
- *Anxiety/Fear* related to physical condition
- *Risk for Infection* related to bowel trauma
- *Risk for Ineffective Airway Clearance* related to retained secretions

PLANNING AND INTERVENTION

Nursing management focuses on promoting comfort, maintaining hydration, providing emotional support, supporting respiratory function, providing care of the surgical site, and monitoring for symptoms of infection.

Promote Comfort

A side-lying position with knees bent is usually the most comfortable. Administer analgesics as ordered, and note relief from pain. Manage postoperative pain in a similar manner. The child should be placed in a semi-Fowler or side-lying position on the right side. If the appendix has ruptured, lying on the right side helps the peritoneal cavity drain. Administer pain medication as ordered. Avoid a heating pad, which increases inflammation.

Maintain Hydration

Assess fluid volume status every 2 hours. Assess skin turgor, eyes, and mucous membranes for signs of dehydration. Monitor intake and output, and assess vital signs. An intravenous infusion is initiated preoperatively and continued until bowel function returns after surgery. Once bowel sounds return, offer water in small amounts and then other clear fluids.

Provide Emotional Support

For many children, this may be their first hospitalization and their first experience with healthcare personnel beyond their usual provider. The nurse must elicit a history, perform a physical examination, coordinate diagnostic tests, and prepare the child for surgery in a short period of time. Emotional support is essential for both child and parents. Good preoperative education can reduce anxiety. Answer any questions the child or parents may have. In the postoperative period, phone calls from friends or family members may be helpful.

Support Respiratory Function

General anesthesia during surgery compromises respiratory function. It is important for the child to turn, cough, and breathe deeply to prevent atelectasis. Encourage the child to splint the incision area with a pillow during coughing to decrease pain.

Recognize Symptoms of Infection

Assess vital signs and observe the abdominal incision every 4 hours for redness, edema, or drainage. If a drain is present, assess drainage for color, consistency, and amount. After the initial dressing has been changed, perform dressing changes frequently and keep the incision area clean and dry. Administer antibiotics as prescribed.

Discharge Planning and Home Care Teaching

The child is discharged once bowel function returns and he or she has a bowel movement. Give parents instructions on reestablishing a nutritious diet slowly and as tolerated. Teach parents to recognize the signs and symptoms of infection and to seek early treatment.

Normal activities can be resumed fairly quickly, but the child should avoid strenuous activities and contact sports in the immediate postoperative period. Parents should check with the child's physician before allowing the child to resume sports activities. Home tutoring may be needed for a short time so the child can keep up with schoolwork.

EVALUATION

Expected outcomes of nursing care include the following:

- Successful management of pain
- Absence of bodily infection
- Expressed knowledge and understanding by parent and child of the condition and treatment
- Clear respiratory sounds
- Adequate hydration
- Restoration of normal nutritional intake

NECROTIZING ENTEROCOLITIS

Necrotizing enterocolitis is a potentially life-threatening inflammatory disease of the intestinal tract that occurs primarily in premature infants. It affects from 4% to 13% of very low-birth-weight infants, and has up to a 40% mortality rate (Bell, 2005). It can be caused by several factors, among them intestinal ischemia, bacterial or viral infection (a result of the premature infant's decreased immune response and greater risk for infection), and immaturity of the gut (a result of the premature infant's decreased amount of gastric acid and proteolytic enzymes and underdeveloped protective intestinal mucin layer). The disease occurs most often in the terminal ileum and colon.

The infant may initially show signs of feeding intolerance (increased gastric residuals, vomiting, irritability, and abdominal distention). These signs are caused by inflammation and dilation of the bowel and accumulation of gas in the intestine. Bloody diarrhea may be present because of the hemorrhagic bowel. Signs of sepsis usually follow, and the infant's condition rapidly deteriorates.

Diagnosis is made on the basis of characteristic clinical findings and the presence of free peritoneal gas, dilated bowel loops, bowel distention, and bowel wall thickening on abdominal x-rays. Stools and emesis are monitored for occult blood. Laboratory data reveal anemia, leukopenia, leukocytosis, thrombocytopenia, electrolyte imbalance, and metabolic or respiratory acidosis. Blood cultures are positive for the organism present.

Necrotizing enterocolitis requires prompt intervention. Management begins with discontinuation of all enteral feedings. An orogastric tube is inserted to prevent gastric distention, and intravenous fluids are started. Total parenteral nutrition may be initiated through a central line. Antibiotics are administered prophylactically or to treat sepsis. Perforation or necrosis of the bowel necessitates surgical resection of the bowel. An ileostomy or colostomy may sometimes be performed. New treatments are being attempted with probiotics, live and beneficial microorganisms that promote normal gut flora. *Lactobacillus acidophilus* and *Bifidobacterium infantis* are examples of organisms that can be administered by special formula.

NURSING PRACTICE

Signs of sepsis include the following:

- Hypothermia or hyperthermia
- Jaundice
- Respiratory distress
- Hepatomegaly
- Abdominal distention
- Anorexia
- Vomiting
- Lethargy

All cases of necrotizing enterocolitis are treated with strict enteric precautions to prevent the spread of infection to other premature infants on the unit. Early aggressive enteral formula-feedings of premature infants is avoided because of the increased incidence of the disease in these cases. Human milk has been shown to protect against the disease; thus, breastfeeding or feeding the mother's expressed milk is the feeding method of choice for premature infants.

Long-term complications of necrotizing enterocolitis include short bowel syndrome, strictures, cholestasis, impaired nutrition and growth, and delayed developmental performance.

NURSING PRACTICE

Cholestasis is a disruption of bile flow. This is the most common problem in survivors of necrotizing enterocolitis. It is a complication of total parenteral nutrition (TPN) and commonly occurs 2 weeks after TPN therapy has been initiated. It is characterized by an elevated bilirubin (>2 mg/dL), hepatomegaly, and elevated serum transaminase.

NURSING MANAGEMENT

Nursing care centers on prevention and early detection of necrotizing enterocolitis to minimize bowel loss, and providing postoperative care. Watch for feeding intolerance by aspirating gastric residual (if the infant is receiving enteral feedings). Enteral feedings should progress slowly in preterm infants, by 2 to 8 mL/kg/day (Committee on Nutrition, American Academy of Pediatrics, 2004). Measure abdominal circumference in the premature or high-risk infant every 4 to 8 hours. Even minimal changes in circumference can indicate necrotizing enterocolitis; report them to the physician.

Maintaining fluid and electrolyte balance is essential. Provide comfort by holding and cuddling an infant who is NPO, and offer a pacifier to meet nonnutritive sucking needs. Careful assessment for infection and maintenance of skin integrity are essential. Gradually reestablish feedings once bowel function returns.

Parents need emotional support, reassurance, and help in bonding with their infant. They are coping with the birth of a critically ill infant. Because the symptoms of necrotizing enterocolitis do not appear until approximately 5 to 7 days after feedings are begun, parents may not be prepared for the infant's decline. The recovery of a premature infant is slow and can be complicated. Give clear explanations and encourage parents to ask questions and express their fears and concerns. If the infant's condition worsens, offer support for the parents of a child with life-threatening illness (see Chapter 41 ∞).

Once the child is discharged, frequent follow-up is needed. Encourage regular healthcare visits. Schedule home visits to help the family manage healthcare and normal developmental issues. If total parenteral nutrition is administered at home, the parents need to know how to administer it correctly and how to care for the central line. Carefully assess oral and enteral nutritional intake. Monitor the child's growth and compare it to previous findings. Several medications are likely to be used, and correct administration techniques must be reinforced. The infant requires regular and thorough physical assessments to identify any complications. Parents need to learn care of the ostomy if the child has one in place. Assess developmental progress by regular use of a test such as the Denver II (see Chapter 37 ∞).

Expected outcomes of nursing care for the child with necrotizing enterocolitis include successful treatment of infection, absence of signs of sepsis, management of fluid and electrolyte status, and provision of adequate nutrition. If surgery is performed, complete healing without infection or other complication is desired. If the infant is not successfully treated, support and comfort for the parents is a necessary outcome. When the child survives, long-term outcomes include normal developmental progression and nutrition to support growth.

MECKEL'S DIVERTICULUM

Meckel's diverticulum results when the omphalomesenteric duct, which connects the midgut to the yolk sac during embryonic development, fails to atrophy. Instead, an outpouching of the ileum remains, usually located near the ileocecal valve. The pouch contains gastric or pancreatic tissue, which secretes acid, causing irritation and ulceration. Meckel's diverticulum is the most common GI malformation and cause of lower GI bleeding in children; it occurs in 2% of the population, although many people are asymptomatic and do not know they have the disorder (Sadovsky, 2001).

Clinical manifestations usually appear by 2 years of age. The most common sign is painless dark or bright-red rectal bleeding, which results from the obstruction or ulceration. Often blood is passed without stool. Abdominal pain is uncommon, but when it occurs, it may resemble the pain of appendicitis. The child may have symptoms of intussusception, incarcerated hernia, volvulus, or intestinal obstruction. If untreated, diverticulitis may progress to perforation and peritonitis.

Diagnosis is based on the history. Contrast studies are usually not helpful because the diverticulum is often too small to visualize and may not fill with barium. Radionuclide imaging and scanning can usually detect the gastric tissue, confirming the diagnosis.

Treatment is surgical excision of the diverticulum and removal of any involved bowel. The prognosis is good following surgical excision.

NURSING MANAGEMENT

Preoperatively an intravenous infusion is initiated to correct fluid and electrolyte imbalances. Monitor intake and output. Observe for rectal bleeding, and test stools for **occult blood** (blood that is present in small quantities and is measurable only by laboratory testing). Keep the child on

bed rest. Assess vital signs every 2 hours, and monitor for signs of shock. Postoperative care is similar to that for an infant or child undergoing abdominal surgery. (See the earlier discussion of postsurgical nursing management of appendicitis and "Nursing Care Plan: The Child Undergoing Surgery" in Chapter 40. ∞)

At discharge, parents need instructions on caring for the surgical site, preventing infection, providing an adequate diet, and administering prescribed medications.

INFLAMMATORY BOWEL DISEASE

CROHN'S DISEASE AND ULCERATIVE COLITIS

Inflammatory bowel disease encompasses two distinct chronic disorders, Crohn's disease and ulcerative colitis, that have similar symptoms and treatment. Both diseases involve faulty regulation of the immune response of the intestinal mucosa in genetically predisposed people who have a genetic trigger (Gokhale, 2001). Inflammatory bowel disease differs from irritable bowel syndrome, which is discussed in the section on feeding and elimination disorders in Chapter 34. ∞

Crohn's disease is a chronic, inflammatory process. It can occur randomly throughout the GI tract, with the ileum, colon, and rectum the most common sites. A distinct feature of Crohn's disease is the development of enteric fistulas between loops of bowel or nearby organs. Mucosal ulcers begin in small locations, and then grow in size and depth into the mucosal wall. Submucosal inflammation can be severe. The etiology is unknown. There is strong evidence to support a genetic association. Crohn's disease is more common in whites and three to six times more prevalent in individuals of Jewish descent. It most often develops between 15 and 25 years of age, and has an incidence of 10 out of 100,000 children younger than age 18 years (Baron, 2002; Gokhale, 2001).

The onset of Crohn's disease is subtle. Crampy abdominal pain is usually reported first, followed by diarrhea. Other symptoms include fever, anorexia, growth failure or weight loss, general malaise, and joint pain. Diagnosis is based on laboratory evaluation (anemia is common; an elevated erythrocyte sedimentation rate, hypoalbuminemia, and thrombocytosis are other possible findings), diffuse abdominal tenderness, and radiologic and biopsy examinations.

Ulcerative colitis is a chronic recurrent disease of the colon and rectal mucosa of unknown etiology. Inflammation is limited to the mucosa and can involve the entire length of the bowel with varying degrees of inflammation, ulceration, hemorrhage, and edema. Emotional and other psychosocial factors may influence the presentation and course of the disease. It is more prevalent among persons of Jewish heritage. The disease develops before 20 years of age with peak onset at about 12 years.

CLINICAL MANIFESTATIONS

ULCERATIVE COLITIS AND CROHN'S DISEASE

	ULCERATIVE COLITIS	CROHN'S DISEASE
Type of lesions	Continuous, superficial involvement	Segmental, transmural (through the wall) involvement
Clinical manifestations		
Anal or perianal lesions	Rare	Common
Anorexia	Mild to moderate	Can be severe
Diarrhea	Often severe	Moderate
Growth retardation	Mild	Significant
Pain	Present	Common
Rectal bleeding	Present	Absent
Weight loss	Moderate	Severe
Risk of cancer	Slightly increased	Greatly increased

The first symptom of ulcerative colitis is usually diarrhea. Lower abdominal pain and cramping are present before and during a bowel movement and are relieved by the passage of stool and flatus. The stool is often mixed with blood and mucus. Weight loss or delayed growth, nutritional deficiencies, and arthralgias often occur as effects of the disease.

Diagnosis centers on evaluating the cause and identifying the extent of involved bowel and differentiating an infectious process (organisms such as *Shigella* and *Salmonella*) from ulcerative colitis. Endoscopy with biopsy is helpful to determine the extent and severity of the inflammatory process. Laboratory and bone age studies help to identify related nutritional, growth, and blood abnormalities. Common serum findings include elevated erythrocyte sedimentation rate, elevated C-reactive protein, hypoalbuminemia, thrombocytosis, and antineutrophil cytoplasmic antibodies (ANCA).

Crohn's disease and ulcerative colitis have periods of remission and exacerbation. Treatment for both diseases includes pharmacologic interventions (antibiotic, antiinflammatory, immunosuppressive, and antidiarrheal medications), nutrition therapy, and, in severe cases, surgery. Corticosteroids are given orally and as enemas to children with more severe disease. For children with milder disease, sulfasalazine decreases the number of relapses.

A nutritionist is part of the team treating the child. The goal of nutrition therapy is to provide adequate caloric intake and nutrients necessary for growth. Vitamin, iron, zinc, and folic acid supplementation is frequently required. Total parenteral nutrition (TPN) is often given to treat nutritional deficiencies and malnutrition, which accompany inflammatory bowel disease (see Skill 12–7). **SKILLS** A

NURSING PRACTICE

The following drugs are used in the treatment of inflammatory bowel disease:

Aminosalicylates
Sulfasalazine
Mesalamine
Olsalazine
Balsalazide

Corticosteroids
Prednisone
Methylprednisone
Hydrocortisone enema

Biologic Therapies
Tumor necrosis factor (TNFα)
Infliximab (Remicade)
Interleukin-10
Thalidomide

Immunosuppressants
6-Mercaptopurine (6-MP)
Azathioprine
Cyclosporine
Methotrexate
Tacrolimus (FK-506)

Antibacterials
Metronidazole
Ciprofloxacin

high-protein, high-carbohydrate, low-fiber diet with normal amounts of fat is recommended.

If other treatment measures fail to reduce inflammation, surgery is generally indicated. A temporary colostomy or ileostomy is performed to allow the bowel to rest. In Crohn's disease, however, ulcerations tend to recur elsewhere in the GI tract. Research is being done to see if intravenous infusion of antitumor necrosis factor antibody is successful in treating the disorder (Gokhale, 2001). In ulcerative colitis, removal of the diseased bowel provides a permanent cure.

NURSING MANAGEMENT

Nursing management occurs mainly in the community and home and focuses on helping the child and family adjust to the emotional impact of a chronic disease, administering medications and diet therapy, monitoring nutritional status, and providing appropriate referrals. Provide emotional support and counseling to help the child adjust to feeling "different" from peers. Inability to compete with peers and frequent absences from school can affect the child's self-esteem. Have the parents contact the school district to arrange for tutoring in case extended absences from school become necessary. Encourage the child who is not attending school regularly to maintain contact with friends through telephone calls, cards, and visits.

GROWTH AND DEVELOPMENT

Providing adequate stress reduction may be helpful in control of inflammatory bowel disease. Teach young children relaxation techniques, such as deep breathing, progressive tensing and relaxing of muscles, and visualization of favorite places. Encourage busy school age children and teens to have quiet and restful times each day, in addition to physical activity periods.

If the child is unable to eat or the intake of calories is insufficient to meet basic nutritional and metabolic needs, TPN is ordered (see Skill 12–7). **SKILLS** If the child is able to eat, parents need instructions about dietary needs. Frequently measure growth and assess nutrition.

TEACHING HIGHLIGHTS

DIET INSTRUCTIONS FOR INFLAMMATORY BOWEL DISEASE

- Several small feedings are usually better tolerated than three meals daily.
- Limiting fiber intake can help to decrease intestine motility and inflammation. Peel fruits and avoid large quantities of whole grains and nuts.
- If the child is not eating well, offer high-calorie meals. If lactose intolerance is not a problem for the particular child, cream soups, milkshakes, puddings, and custards can be offered.
- Liquid dietary supplements may be helpful to ensure protein and caloric requirements are met.
- Watch for foods that cause intestinal problems for the individual child, and avoid them in the future.
- Avoid having mealtime become a reason for family strife. Seek help of nurses and dietitians if needed.

Body image is a major concern for children and adolescents with inflammatory bowel disease. Corticosteroid therapy causes growth retardation and delayed sexual maturation. Encourage the child to discuss feelings about these side effects. If a permanent colostomy or ileostomy is required, help the child and family understand the need for surgical treatment. (See the discussion of ostomies earlier in this chapter.) Introduce the child and family to other children who have stomas.

Teach parents about medication administration and diet therapy. Reinforce to both the parents and child the importance of adhering to a strict medication regimen. Emphasize that medications should be continued even when the child is asymptomatic. Discuss the side effects of the drugs and what to do if any of these symptoms occur. When the child is taking systemic corticosteroids, immunizations are generally delayed until after the medication is discontinued.

Parents need instructions for TPN if this therapy is used, as well as information about care of a central venous catheter, including dressing changes, sterile and nonsterile techniques, signs of infection, how to handle infusion pumps and tubing, and how to measure the child's intake and output. Assist parents in obtaining equipment and supplies necessary for the child's care. Have parents demonstrate their mastery of care for the central venous catheter and their understanding of TPN techniques during home visits and appointments for healthcare.

Refer parents to social services, the visiting nurse association, and home healthcare agencies, if they are not receiving any of these services. For information about inflammatory bowel disease, refer families to the Crohn's and Colitis Foundation.

Expected outcomes of nursing care for the child with inflammatory bowel disease include the following:

- Normal growth and development
- Absence of gastrointestinal distress
- Successful management of medications without demonstration of side effects
- Freedom from infection due to TPN line
- Establishment of positive body image
- Integration of stress-lowering practices into daily life

PEPTIC ULCER

A peptic ulcer is an erosion of the mucosal tissue in the lower end of the esophagus, in the stomach (usually along the lesser curvature), or in the duodenum (gastric ulcer is the term sometimes used when the stomach mucosa is affected). Boys are more likely to have peptic ulcers than girls.

Peptic ulcers are much less common in children than in adults. African-American and Hispanic children are at greater risk for peptic ulcers (Simpson & Ivey, 2003).

Ulcers are classified as primary or secondary, depending on their etiology. Primary peptic ulcers occur in healthy children. Secondary (stress) ulcers occur in children with a preexisting illness or injury (often a burn) and in children receiving medications such as salicylates, corticosteroids, and nonsteroidal anti-inflammatory drugs. Diet usually is not a major factor in the development of peptic ulcers in children, although caffeine and alcohol consumption in adolescents may exacerbate the disease. Ulcers in both adults and children are often caused by *Helicobacter pylori*, a gram-negative rod. This organism is transmitted by the fecal–oral or oral–oral routes. Infections often occur in several members of a family, especially when the family's water supply is contaminated.

Clinical manifestations vary according to the age of the child and location of the ulcer. The most common symptom is abdominal pain (burning) associated with an empty stomach, which may awaken the child at night. Vomiting and pain after meals, anemia, occult blood in stools, and abdominal distention may also be present.

Diagnosis is based on the history and radiologic studies. *H. pylori* can be diagnosed by culture of the organism taken via gastroscopy, and by measuring urea in the urine and on the breath, since the organism hydrolyzes urea. The goals of medical management are to relieve discomfort and promote healing. When *H. pylori* is the causative agent, antimicrobial agents such as bismuth salts, tetracycline, and metronidazole combination are given. Other drug combinations, such as a combination of antacids in liquid form (Maalox, Mylanta) and histamine antagonists (ranitidine, cimetidine, and famotidine), are also used. Antibody titers are measured several times over 6 months to evaluate the effectiveness of therapy. The prognosis is usually good with early intervention.

NURSING MANAGEMENT

Nurses may identify children with peptic ulcer disease by looking for the symptoms and noting family history of *H. pylori* infection. Nursing care centers on interventions to promote adequate nutritional intake, promote healing, and prevent recurrences. Provide a nutritionally sound, age-appropriate diet. Omit foods only if they exacerbate the disorder.

DRUG GUIDE

RANITIDINE (ZANTAC)

Overview of Action

Ranitidine inhibits histamine action at the H_2 receptor sites of parietal cells, prohibiting basal and nocturnal secretion of gastric acid. It also suppresses the gastric acid secretion caused by food, insulin, amino acids, and pentagastrin. It is used for treatment of active GI hemorrhage or peptic ulcer disease, hypersecretory syndrome, and gastroesophageal reflux.

Routes, Dosage, Frequency

Modify dosage for renal impairment. Doses listed for duodenal ulcer, gastric ulcer, gastroesophageal reflux.

- **PO:** Child: 5 to 10 mg/kg/day in equally divided doses every 12 hours (maximum 300 mg/day); Adolescents and Adults: 150 mg BID or 300 mg at bedtime
- **IM, IV:** Newborns: 1.5 mg/kg/dose as loading dose, then 1.5 to 2 mg/kg/day in equally divided doses every 6 to 8 hours or 0.04 to 0.08 mg/kg/hour by continuous infusion; Infants and Children: 2 to 4 mg/kg/day in equally divided doses every 8 to 12 hours (maximum 150 mg/day); Adolescents and Adults: 50 mg every 6 to 8 hours (maximum daily dosage 400 mg or 6 mg/kg)

Nursing Implications

Assess: Assess amount and location of abdominal pain.

Administer: PO: Unaffected by food, usually given with or after meals. Syrup contains alcohol; peppermint flavored. Tablets can be crushed, mixed with small amounts of food and fluid. Effervescent preparations must be diluted in 80 to 240 mL just prior to ingestion.

IM: Do not use if discolored or has precipitate. Injection may cause burning. **IV:** For those over 12 years old: each 50 mg of drug must be diluted with at least 20 mL of 0.9% sodium chloride, 5% dextrose, or other compatible IV solutions; infuse slowly over at least 5 minutes maximum concentration 2.5 mg/mL. Rapid administration may cause bradycardia, tachycardia, or premature ventricular contractions. For intermittent infusion, dilution is 50 mg/100 mL (5 to 7 mL/min) infused over 15 to 20 min; continuous infusion over 24 hours preferred. Compatible with D5W, D10W, NS, LR.

Monitor: Assess for side effects. Side effects include malaise, dizziness, and vertigo; cardiac arrhythmia; bradycardia; constipation or diarrhea; hepatitis; hypersensitivity reaction. Monitor blood counts, renal and hepatic function during therapy.

Contraindications and Precautions: The drug is contraindicated in those with prior hypersensitivity to the drug; effervescent tablet is contraindicated in those with phenylketonuria. It is discontinued if liver abnormalities occur, and the dosage is lowered in renal disease.

Data from Bindler, R. M., & Howry, L. B. (2005). Pediatric drug guide with nursing implications. Upper Saddle River, NJ: Prentice Hall-Health.

Antibiotics must be given as scheduled. Emphasize the importance of continuing drug therapy. The family needs encouragement to continue the medications as ordered and to return for follow-up visits. Children who attend school may prefer to take antacids in the form of tablets, which are easier to carry than liquid preparations. A permission form to take medications at school needs to be filled out by the prescriber. Parents should check with the child's physician before giving any additional medication. Caution parents to avoid aspirin products, which irritate the gastric mucosa. If an antipyretic or pain medication is needed, acetaminophen should be given. Advise parents to read medication labels if they are unsure of product contents.

Because psychologic stress can contribute to peptic ulcer disease, help the parents and child identify sources of stress in the child's life. Assess coping mechanisms and provide referral for psychologic counseling, if appropriate. Teach relaxation techniques and recommend community classes on yoga or other stress reduction.

DISORDERS OF MOTILITY

Fluids are produced in large quantities as part of normal GI functioning. As food passes through the intestines, fluids are reabsorbed and moderately soft stool is formed and evacuated. In disorders such as diarrhea and constipation, fluid production is altered, causing either more or less fluid to be reabsorbed. This can severely alter the characteristics of the stool. Reabsorption of too little water produces diarrhea and can lead to fluid and electrolyte alterations. Reabsorption of too much fluid can cause constipation, which if untreated can lead to bowel obstruction.

GASTROENTERITIS (ACUTE DIARRHEA)

Gastroenteritis is an inflammation of the stomach and intestines that may be accompanied by vomiting and diarrhea. It can affect any part of the GI tract. Diarrhea is a common problem in children. It may be an acute problem, caused by viral, bacterial, or parasitic infections, or a chronic problem. Acute gastroenteritis affects approximately 30 million children per year in the United States (Reeves, Shannon, & Fleisher, 2002). Children under age 5 years average approximately two episodes of gastroenteritis each year. Infants and small children with gastroenteritis or diarrhea can quickly become dehydrated and are at risk for hypovolemic shock if fluid and electrolyte losses are not replaced (see Chapter 43 ∞).

ETIOLOGY AND PATHOPHYSIOLOGY

Diarrhea in children can have many different causes (Table 51–2). The specific etiology is not always identified. The common mechanism is a decrease in the ab-

TABLE 51–2 ❖ Causes of Diarrhea in Children

Etiology	Bowel Manifestations
Emotional stress (anxiety, fatigue)	Increased motility
Intestinal infection (bacteria [E. coli, Salmonella, Shigella], viral [human rotavirus, enteric adenovirus], fungal overgrowth)	Inflammation of mucosa; increased mucus secretion in colon
Food sensitivity (gluten, cow's milk)	Decreased digestion of food
Food intolerance (lactose, introduction of new foods, overfeeding)	Increased motility; increased mucus secretion in colon
Medications (iron, antibiotics)	Irritation and superinfection
Colon disease (colitis, necrotizing enterocolitis, enterocolitis)	Inflammation and ulceration of intestinal walls; reduced absorption of fluid; increased intestinal motility
Surgical alterations (short bowel syndrome)	Reduced size of colon; decreased absorption surface

sorptive capacity of the bowel through inflammation, decrease in surface area for absorption, or alteration of parasympathetic innervation. Children in childcare centers and those living in substandard housing with improper sanitation are at increased risk.

CLINICAL MANIFESTATIONS

Diarrhea may be mild, moderate, or severe. In mild diarrhea, stools are slightly increased in number and have a more liquid consistency. In moderate diarrhea the child has several loose or watery stools. Other symptoms include irritability, anorexia, nausea, and vomiting. Moderate diarrhea is usually self-limiting, resolving without treatment within 1 or 2 days. In severe diarrhea, watery stools are continuous. The child exhibits symptoms of fluid and electrolyte imbalance (see Chapter 43 ∞), has cramping, and is extremely irritable and difficult to console.

CLINICAL THERAPY

Diagnosis is based on the history, physical examination, and laboratory findings. A thorough history may help identify the cause. Ask parents about recent exposure to illnesses, use of antibiotics, travel, food and formula preparation, food sensitivities or allergies, and whether the child attends day care. Physical examination provides a guide to the severity of dehydration (see Chapter 43 ∞). The stool

MediaLink ● Care Plan: Managing Emesis in Pediatric Conditions can be examined for the presence of ova, parasites, infectious organisms, viruses, fat, and undigested sugars. Laboratory evaluation of serum and urine helps identify electrolyte imbalances and other deficiencies.

Medical management depends on the severity of the diarrhea and fluid and electrolyte imbalances. The goal of treatment is to correct the fluid and electrolyte imbalances. For mild to moderate dehydration, the child is rehydrated with oral rehydration therapy (see Chapter 43 ∞). This may be

CLINICAL MANIFESTATIONS

TREATMENT OF DEHYDRATION OF DIARRHEA

DEHYDRATION	CLINICAL THERAPY
None to minimal	Feed age-appropriate diet of breast milk, regular formula, bland foods <10 kg weight: Oral rehydration of 60–120 mL for each diarrheal stool or vomiting episode >10 kg weight: Oral rehydration of 120–240 mL for each diarrheal stool or vomiting episode
Mild (3%–5%) to moderate (6%–9%)	Oral rehydration with 50–100 mL/kg over 3–4 hours; continue with replacement of losses as described above
Severe (≥10%)	After rehydration, feed age-appropriate diet True emergency which causes shock or near-shock condition Bolus intravenous therapy with normal saline or Ringer's lactate, 20 mL/kg/hour until pulse and state of consciousness are normal Begin oral rehydration solution 100 mL/kg over 4 hours when level of consciousness improves or 5% dextrose ½ normal saline IV at twice maintenance fluid rate; continue with replacement of losses as described above; if unable to drink, administer through nasogastric tube or administer 5% dextrose ¼ normal saline with 20 mEq potassium IV After rehydration, feed age-appropriate diet

Adapted with permission from Morbidity and Mortality Weekly Report. (2003). Managing acute gastroenteritis among children. MMWR, 52 (RR-16), 1-16; and Committee on Nutrition (2004). Pediatric nutrition handbook (5th ed.). Elk Grove Village, IL: American Academy of Pediatrics.

accomplished at home or in the short-stay observation unit in a hospital with solutions such as Pedialyte, Ricelyte, or Lytren. Carbonated and very sugary beverages should not be given. Fermentation of sugar in the GI tract causes increased gas, abdominal distention, and an increased frequency of diarrhea.

For severe dehydration, rehydration is accomplished by intravenous infusion with a solution chosen to correct the specific imbalances. Isotonic fluid such as normal saline with glucose or Ringer's lactate are commonly used solutions (see Chapter 43 for further information about solutions to correct dehydration ∞). As soon as possible, clear liquids are introduced and then the child progresses to a regular diet. Foods generally are not withheld for more than 1 to 2 days.

If the diarrhea is caused by bacteria or parasites, antimicrobial therapy may be prescribed. Antiemetics and antidiarrheals are generally not used in young children since they can mask the signs and symptoms of more serious illness (Thielman & Guerrant, 2004).

NURSING MANAGEMENT

NURSING ASSESSMENT AND DIAGNOSIS

The nurse may encounter the child and family in the emergency department, urgent care center, clinic, or office. The child may be cared for over several hours at a clinic or urgent care center so that dehydration is treated with intravenous infusion, oral rehydration, or both, and then sent home with instructions for parents to care for the child. If the child is hospitalized, it is important to assess onset, frequency, color, amount, and consistency of stools. If the child is also vomiting, monitor the amount and type of vomitus. Initial and ongoing physical assessment of the child focuses on observing for signs and symptoms of dehydration, which reflect underlying fluid and electrolyte status. Evaluate urinary output and specific gravity. Weigh the infant or child on admission and daily thereafter. Monitor vital signs every 2 to 4 hours. A febrile child has increased water loss, contributing to the dehydration. Assess skin integrity, especially in the perineal and rectal areas, and note any breakdown or rashes. Avoid commercial baby wipes, which can promote additional skin irritation and breakdown.

"Nursing Care Plan: The Child with Gastroenteritis" lists common nursing diagnoses. Other diagnoses that might also be appropriate include the following:

- *Anxiety (Child and Parent)* related to change in health status
- *Disturbed Sleep Pattern* related to pain
- *Imbalanced Nutrition: Less than Body Requirements* related to inability to ingest sufficient nutrients

PLANNING AND IMPLEMENTATION

Nursing care focuses on providing emotional support, promoting rest and comfort, and ensuring adequate nutrition. See "Nursing Care Plan: The Child with Gastroenteritis" for a summary of nursing care.

Provide Emotional Support

The child may have been ill for several days or become suddenly ill a short time before seeking healthcare. The child and parents are usually anxious, so it is important to allow them to talk and ask questions. The child may require blood tests to help direct rehydration therapy. Using therapeutic play techniques, such as allowing the child to manipulate equipment, can reduce anxiety (see Chapter 34 ∞). To promote trust, be honest if a procedure will hurt. Encourage the child to express anger, fear, and pain.

Promote Rest and Comfort

Most children with gastroenteritis are quite ill and awaken frequently with periods of vomiting and diarrhea. Provide a quiet, restful environment. Darken the room and keep interruptions to a minimum. To reduce the child's anxiety, encourage parents to room-in. Place the child's favorite toys and comfort objects within reach. Keep the child's mouth moistened with a glycerine swab, a wet washcloth, or an occasional ice chip.

Ensure Adequate Nutrition

Offer liquids throughout the illness, even if an intravenous infusion is in place. Follow guidelines for oral rehydration therapy in Chapter 43. ∞ Find out what fluids the family uses at home. Small amounts of normal diet for age are provided. Infants are breastfed or given formula. The child's diet progresses based on tolerance for feedings, with a normal diet for age usually consumed in about 1 week.

Discharge Planning and Care in the Community

Discharge teaching should begin on arrival at the healthcare facility. Teach family members that handwashing is the most important measure that can be taken to prevent the spread of gastroenteritis. Tell parents what to expect as the child's GI system returns to normal. Teach the parents about the symptoms of dehydration and what to do if diarrhea recurs. Be sure that parents understand the recommended diet progression. Emphasize the necessity of good hygiene practices to prevent the spread of microorganisms that can cause gastroenteritis. If the child attends child care, have the parent inform the care center about the infection so the staff can be alerted to watch for other cases and can take steps to prevent the spread of infection.

COMPLEMENTARY CARE

CHILDREN AND HERBAL LAXATIVES

Herbal stimulant laxatives are used by some families as complementary therapies. The following are not recommended for use in children under 12 years:

- Aloe
- Buckthorn bark
- Cascara sagrada bark
- Senna leaf or pod
- Coffee
- Tea
- Cola nut
- Mate
- Ma huang

Question parents about the use of complementary therapy for their child's constipation. Educate them regarding avoiding the use of any therapies that are not recommended for children.

EVALUATION

Expected outcomes of nursing care for the child with gastroenteritis include the following:

- Correction of dehydration
- Adequate nutritional intake
- Return to normal bowel function
- Parental description of signs of dehydration
- Parental knowledge of importance of handwashing in decreasing transmission of infectious agents
- Maintenance of intact skin

CONSTIPATION

Constipation is a common complaint in the pediatric population and accounts for one quarter of all pediatric gastroenterology referrals (Coughlin, 2003). **Constipation** is characterized by a decrease in the frequency or passage of stools; the formation of hard, dry stools; or the oozing of liquid stool past a collection of hard, dry stool. Because stooling patterns vary among children, identification of an abnormal pattern is sometimes difficult. Infants usually have several bowel movements a day. For a young child, one bowel movement a day may be normal. As the child grows, however, three to four bowel movements a week may be a normal pattern. Constipation is characterized by pebble-like hard stools for a majority of bowel movements for at least 2 weeks, firm stools ≤2 times per week for at least 2 weeks, and no evidence of structural, endocrine, or metabolic disease (Lembo & Camilleri, 2003).

Constipation may be caused by an underlying disease, diet, or psychologic factor. It may result from defects in filling, or more commonly emptying, of the rectum. Pathologic causes of defective filling include ineffective colonic propulsive activity, caused by hypothyroidism or

NURSING CARE PLAN

THE CHILD WITH GASTROENTERITIS

Intervention	Rationale	Expected Outcome
1. Nursing Diagnosis: Diarrhea related to infectious process		
NIC Priority Intervention: **Diarrhea management:** Prevention and alleviation of diarrhea		**NOC Suggested Outcome:** **Fluid and electrolyte balance:** Balance of water and electrolytes in the intracellular and extracellular compartments of the body
Goal: The child's bowel function will be restored to normal.		
■ Obtain baseline vital signs and monitor every 2–4 hours. ■ Observe stools for amount, color, consistency, odor, and frequency. ■ Test stools for occult blood. ■ Monitor results of stool culture and sample for ova and parasites. ■ Wash hands well before and after contact with the child. ■ Isolate the child until the cause of the diarrhea is determined. ■ Assist the child with toileting and hygiene. ■ Administer prescribed oral rehydration and intravenous solutions. ■ Notify the physician if diarrhea persists, stool characteristics change, or other symptoms of dehydration electrolyte imbalance occur.	■ Fluid and electrolyte imbalances can alter vital body functions. ■ Aids in the diagnosis and in monitoring the child's status. ■ Frequent defecation and some infectious organisms can cause bleeding. ■ Rapid notification of the physician will facilitate treatment. ■ Helps prevent transmission of microorganisms. ■ Prevents exposure of other patients and staff. ■ The child may be weak, incontinent, physically impaired, or anxious and require assistance to use the bathroom. ■ Provides necessary fluids and nutrients. ■ Ensures early intervention.	The child's bowel function returns to normal.
2. Nursing Diagnosis: Deficient Fluid Volume related to active fluid volume loss		
NIC Priority Intervention: **Fluid monitoring:** Collection and analysis of patient data to regulate fluid balance		**NOC Suggested Outcome:** **Fluid and electrolyte balance:** Balance of water and electrolytes in the intracellular and extracellular compartments of the body
Goal: The child will remain hydrated and will begin to drink fluids within 24 hours of admission.		
■ Monitor intake and output. Be sure to document time of each voiding. ■ Compare admission weight to preadmission weight. Assess weight daily. ■ Assess level of consciousness, skin turgor, mucous membranes, skin color and temperature, capillary refill, eyes, and fontanelles every 4 hours. ■ Assess for vomiting. ■ Provide oral fluid and electrolyte replacement solution if able to tolerate.	■ Will determine if output exceeds input. Long periods of time without urine output can be an early indicator of poor renal function. A child should produce 1 mL of urine/kg/hr. ■ The degree of dehydration can be determined by the percentage of weight loss. Daily weights aid in determining progress toward rehydration. ■ Will determine degree of hydration and adequacy of interventions. ■ Vomiting frequently accompanies diarrhea and contributes to the child's fluid loss. ■ Less invasive than IV fluids. Provides for replacement of essential fluids and electrolytes.	The child has normal fluid and electrolyte balance as indicated by laboratory evaluation and physical examination.

NURSING CARE PLAN—continued

THE CHILD WITH GASTROENTERITIS

Intervention	Rationale	Expected Outcome
2. Nursing Diagnosis: Deficient Fluid Volume related to active fluid volume loss (continued)		
■ Provide and maintain IV replacement therapy, as ordered.	■ Use of IV replacement is based on the degree of dehydration, ongoing losses, insensible water losses, and electrolyte results.	
3. Nursing Diagnosis: Risk for Impaired Skin Integrity related to altered fluid status		
NIC Priority Intervention: **Skin surveillance:** Collection and analysis of patient data to maintain skin integrity		**NOC Suggested Outcome:** **Tissue integrity:** Structural intactness and normal physiologic function of skin
Goal: The child will remain free of skin breakdown and rashes.		
■ Assess skin of perineum and rectum for signs of skin breakdown or irritation. ■ Provide prevention or restorative care for infants as follows: **Preventive Care:** ■ Change diapers every 2 hours or as needed. ■ Use cloth diapers rather than disposable. ■ Wash diaper area after each soiling. ■ Apply A & D ointment. **Restorative Care:** ■ Place the infant prone and leave the buttocks open to air. ■ Notify the physician if the skin is severely broken or peeling or if a rash is present. ■ For toddlers and older children: Tub bathe at least daily (if condition allows) in tepid water. Pat the area dry. ■ Discourage the wearing of underwear if possible. ■ Apply A & D ointment at least four times daily.	■ Early assessment and intervention can prevent worsening of the condition. ■ Minimizes skin contact with chemical irritants from stool and urine. ■ Minimizes the mechanical and chemical irritation from disposables. ■ Removes traces of stool if present. ■ Provides a barrier and protects intact or reddened skin from becoming excoriated. ■ Promotes air circulation to the area. ■ Additional measures may be needed to ensure skin healing. ■ Helps loosen any fecal matter without scrubbing, which can cause additional irritation to the skin. ■ Allows air to circulate and prevents accumulation of moisture. ■ Provides a barrier and protects intact or reddened skin from becoming excoriated.	The child's perianal and rectal tissue remains pink and intact.

use of medication, and obstruction, caused by a structural anomaly (stricture or stenosis) or by an aganglionic segment (Hirschsprung disease). If the rectum fails to fill, stasis leads to excessive drying of the stools. Emptying of the rectum depends on the defecation reflex. Lesions of the spinal cord, weakness of the abdominal muscles, and local lesions blocking sphincter relaxation all may impede attempts to defecate.

Constipation during infancy is rare and is most often caused by mismanagement of diet. The transition from formula to cow's milk may cause a transient constipation because the bowel must adjust to the increased protein content of cow's milk. Constipation in young infants can usually be corrected by increasing the amount of fluids or

adding 2 oz of pear or apple juice to daily intake. In older infants, increasing the intake of cereals, fruits, and vegetables in the diet should correct the problem.

Constipation occurs most frequently in the toddler and preschool age groups. This increased incidence is often associated with learning to control body functions. Many children do not like the sensations of a bowel movement and may begin withholding stool, which accumulates in and dilates the rectum until the next urge to defecate. The increasingly hard and painful bowel movement reinforces the child's behavior, and a pattern develops. See Chapter 34 for a discussion of encopresis. ∞

Removing constipating foods (bananas, rice, and cheese) from the child's diet often decreases the constipation.

Increasing the child's intake of high-fiber foods (whole-grain breads, raw fruits and vegetables) and increasing fluids also promote defecation.

The school-age child may become constipated because time for toileting is limited. Busy school-age children may delay going to the bathroom. Children may also be hesitant to use an unfamiliar bathroom. Encouragement from parents and relaxation of bathroom privileges at school promote regularity and return of usual bowel patterns within a short time.

Diagnosis is based on a thorough history and physical examination. When constipation occurs along with growth failure, vomiting, or abdominal pain, further investigation is necessary to rule out other disorders. Dietary management is the treatment of choice for constipation that has no underlying pathologic cause. A single glycerin suppository or enema may be needed to remove hard stool, followed by dietary and fluid management.

Constipation may follow surgery, especially in children who are immobilized, such as by traction or a body cast. Stool softeners and a diet high in roughage and fluids prevent and treat constipation. Many families use herbal or other plant remedies to treat constipation.

NURSING MANAGEMENT

Take a diet history and obtain a description of bowel patterns from parents. Ask what the family does to treat constipation. Assessment of the child's food likes and dislikes may provide a clue to the cause of constipation. Nursing care focuses on teaching parents what constitutes normal bowel patterns in children and the importance of diet in maintaining normal bowel patterns. Regular bowel habits are encouraged by placing the child on the toilet 30 minutes after a meal or around the time defecation usually occurs. Providing positive reinforcement during toilet training helps prevent a withholding pattern.

Teach parents dietary measures to promote regularity of bowel movements. Children can be given a high-fiber diet that includes fruits and vegetables. Cut-up fresh fruits, dried fruits, and fruit juice can be offered as snacks. A glycerin suppository can be used periodically. This is a natural stimulant and lubricant of the bowel. Caution parents to avoid frequent use of laxatives, stool softeners, and enemas, since overuse can cause bowel dependency. Herbal stimulant laxatives are discouraged for children less than 12 years, whereas other intestinal motility aids are not generally harmful. Find out more about any herbs the family commonly uses.

INTESTINAL PARASITIC DISORDERS

Intestinal parasitic disorders occur most frequently in tropical regions. Outbreaks take place where water is not treated,

food is incorrectly prepared, or people live in crowded conditions with poor sanitation. In the United States, outbreaks of diseases caused by protozoa or helminths (worms) are increasing. Young children, especially those in day care, are most at risk of infection. Young children often lack good hygiene practices and are likely to put objects and their hands into their mouths. (See "Clinical Manifestations: Common Intestinal Parasitic Disorders.")

In addition, previously uncommon parasites are emerging in the United States. Included are *Cryptosporidium parvum, Dientamoeba fragilis, Blastocystis hominis,* and *Entamoeba coli.* The possibility of enteric infection should always be considered in children with continuing diarrhea or other intestinal symptoms (Cowden & Hotez, 2001).

Another common cause of young child infection is exposure to pets and wildlife. Pets should be checked for parasites and dewormed regularly. Public policies for cleanup of pet fecal material in parks can also decrease contamination. Sand and play boxes should be kept covered when not in use, and children should be taught good handwashing after exposure to their pets and not to approach or touch unfamiliar or wild animals (Kazacos, 2000).

NURSING PRACTICE

The following drugs are used in the treatment of intestinal protozoan infections:

Diloxanide furoate	Piperazine citrate
Furazolidone	Pyrantel pamoate
Iodoquinol	Tetracycline
Mebendazole	Thiabendazole
Metronidazole	Trimethoprim/sulfamethoxazole
Paromomycin	

Laboratory examination of stool specimens identifies the causative organism (protozoa, worms, larvae, or ova). Treatment usually involves an anthelmintic. Nursing care centers on preventive teaching. Emphasize the importance of good hygiene practices, especially careful handwashing, after toileting and when handling food. Instruct parents to give prescribed medications as directed even if the child's condition seems to be improved.

FEEDING DISORDERS

Feeding problems that interfere with a child's ability to ingest or tolerate formulas and foods usually become apparent during the first year of life. To prevent complications of poor nutrition, feeding methods or diet may need to be altered. The following discussion focuses on the common disorders of colic and rumination. See Chapter 31 ∞ for a discussion of food allergy and sensitivity and of feeding disorder of infancy

CLINICAL MANIFESTATIONS

COMMON INTESTINAL PARASITIC DISORDERS

PARASITIC INFECTION	TRANSMISSION, LIFE CYCLE, PATHOGENESIS	CLINICAL MANIFESTATIONS	CLINICAL THERAPY	COMMENTS
Giardiasis Organism: protozoan *Giardia lamblia* Giardia lamblia	Transmission is through person-to-person contact, unfiltered water, improperly prepared infected food, and contact with animals. Cysts are ingested and passed into the duodenum and proximal jejunum, where they begin actively feeding. They are excreted in the stool.	May be asymptomatic. *Infants:* diarrhea, vomiting, anorexia, failure to thrive *Older children:* abdominal cramps; intermittent loose, foul-smelling, watery, pale, and greasy stools.	Available medications include furazolidone and quinacrine. Furazolidone has fewer side effects than quinacrine but is more expensive. Metronidazole is also effective but is not licensed in the United States for treatment of giardiasis.	Most common intestinal parasitic organism in the United States. Infection may resolve spontaneously in 4–6 weeks without treatment. Parents or caregivers should wear gloves when handling diapers or stool of parasite-infected infant or child.
Enterobiasis (Pinworm) Organism: nematode *Enterobius vermicularis* Pinworm	Transmission is from discharged eggs inhaled or carried from hand to mouth. Eggs hatch in the upper intestine and mature in 15–28 days. Larvae then migrate to the cecum. After mating, the female migrates out of the anus and lays up to 17,000 eggs. Movement of worms causes intense itching. Scratching deposits eggs on the hands and under the nails.	Intense perianal itching, irritability, restlessness, and short attention span; in females, can migrate to the vagina and urethra to cause infection. Itching intensifies at night when the female comes to the anal opening to lay eggs.	Available medications include mebendazole, pyrantel pamoate, and piperazine citrate. The child and all household members should be treated at the same time. Treatment may be repeated in 2–3 weeks.	Most common helminthic infection in United States. Transmission is increased in crowded conditions such as housing developments, schools, and childcare centers.
Ascariasis (Roundworm) Organism: nematode *Ascaris lumbricoides* Roundworm	Transmission is from discharged eggs carried from hand to mouth. Adult lays eggs in small intestine. Eggs are excreted in stool, where they incubate for 2–3 weeks. Swallowed eggs hatch in the small intestine. Larvae may penetrate intestinal villi, entering the portal vein and liver, then moving to the lung. Larvae that ascend to upper respiratory tract are swallowed and proceed to the small intestine, where they repeat the cycle.	Mild infection may be asymptomatic. Severe infection may result in intestinal obstruction, peritonitis, obstructive jaundice, and lung involvement.	Available anthelminthic medications include mebendazole, pyrantel pamoate, or piperazine citrate. Stools should be examined 2 weeks after treatment and monthly for 3 months. Family members and contacts of the child should be treated if indicated. If the child has intestinal obstruction, treatment may include administering piperazine through a nasogastric tube and duodenal suction. Obstructing worms sometimes have to be surgically removed.	Most common in warm climates. Primarily affects children 1–4 years of age.

(continued)

CLINICAL MANIFESTATIONS—continued

COMMON INTESTINAL PARASITIC DISORDERS

PARASITIC INFECTION	TRANSMISSION, LIFE CYCLE, PATHOGENESIS	CLINICAL MANIFESTATIONS	CLINICAL THERAPY	COMMENTS
Hookworm disease Organism: nematode *Necator americanus* Hookworm	Transmission is through direct contact with infected soil containing larvae. Worms live in the small intestine and feed on villi, causing bleeding. Eggs are deposited in the bowel and excreted in feces. Eggs hatch in damp shaded soil. Larvae attach to and penetrate the skin, then enter the bloodstream, migrating to the lungs. Larvae then migrate to the upper respiratory passages and are swallowed.	In healthy individuals mild infection seldom causes problems. More severe infection may result in anemia and malnutrition. Presence of larvae on the skin may cause burning and itching, followed by redness and papular eruption.	Available medications include mebendazole and pyrantel pamoate. Stools should be examined 2 weeks after treatment and monthly for 3 months. Family members and contacts of the child should be treated if indicated.	Children should wear shoes when outdoors, although other unprotected areas of the skin may still come in contact with larvae.
Strongyloidiasis (Threadworm) Organism: nematode *Strongyloides stercoralis*	Transmission is from the ingestion of discharged larvae in the soil. Life cycle is similar to that of the hookworm, except the threadworm does not attach to the intestinal mucosa, and feeding larvae (rather than eggs) may be deposited in the soil.	Mild infection may be asymptomatic. Severe infection may result in abdominal pain and distention, nausea, vomiting, and diarrhea. Stools may be large and pale, with mucus. Severe infection may lead to a nutritional deficiency.	Available medications include thiabendazole or mebendazole. Treatment may need to be repeated if symptoms recur after treatment. Family members and contacts of the child should be examined and treated if indicated.	Most common in older children and adolescents.

Threadworm

PARASITIC INFECTION	TRANSMISSION, LIFE CYCLE, PATHOGENESIS	CLINICAL MANIFESTATIONS	CLINICAL THERAPY	COMMENTS
Visceral larva migrans (Toxocarlasis) Organism: nematode *Toxocara canis* or *T. catis*, commonly found in dogs and cats	Transmission is through the ingestion of eggs in the soil. Ingested eggs hatch in the intestine. Mobile larvae then migrate to the liver and eventually to all major organs (including the brain). Once migration is complete, they encapsulate in dense fibrous tissue.	Most cases are asymptomatic. Affected children may have a low-grade fever and recurrent upper airway diseases. Severe symptoms include hepatomegaly, pulmonary infiltration, and neurologic disturbances. In all cases there is a hypereosinophilia of the blood.	There is no specific treatment. Corticosteroids have been used in severe cases. Thiabendazole has been recommended but efficacy is not established (infection usually resolves spontaneously).	Most common in toddlers. Deworm household pets monthly if indicated. Keep children away from areas contaminated with animal droppings.

Note: Giardia lamblia courtesy of the Centers for Disease Control and Prevention, Atlanta, GA; pinworm (p. 718), roundworm (p. 714), hookworm (p. 719), and threadworm (p. 721) from Rudolph, A. M., Hoffman, J. I. E., & Rudolph, C. D. (1996). Rudolph's pediatrics (20th ed.). Stamford, CT: Appleton & Lange.

and childhood (failure to thrive). Chapter 36 has a discussion of the eating disorders anorexia nervosa and bulimia. ∞

COLIC

Colic is a feeding disorder characterized by paroxysmal abdominal pain of intestinal origin and severe crying. Approximately 5% to 28% of infants have colic during the first few months of life. The onset of colic is usually between the second and sixth weeks of life, and remission of symptoms generally occurs by 3 months of age (Miller, 2003). The etiology of colic is unknown. Proposed causes include feeding too rapidly and swallowing large amounts of air.

Characteristically the infant cries loudly and continuously, often for several hours. The infant's face may become flushed. The abdomen is distended and tense. Often the infant draws up the legs and clenches the hands. Episodes occur at the same time each day, usually in the late afternoon or early evening. Crying may stop only when the child is completely exhausted or after passage of flatus or stool. Carrying the child in the upright position is often helpful.

The symptoms initially may resemble intestinal obstruction or peritoneal infection. These conditions must be ruled out along with sensitivity to formula. Treatment is supportive. Usually by 3 months of age, the severity and frequency of symptoms decrease.

NURSING PRACTICE

Vomiting and feeding disorders can occur throughout childhood as well as in infancy. In older children, a pattern of **chronic vomiting** (low-grade nearly daily emesis) or **cyclic vomiting** (repeated severe vomiting of an episodic nature) can occur. These patterns differ from vomiting seen in colic or gastroesophageal reflux. Chronic vomiting is most often associated with peptic ulcer or irritable bowel, and cyclic vomiting is indicative of a syndrome known as abdominal migraine. Continuous vomiting of any nature should be evaluated (Li, 1996).

NURSING MANAGEMENT

Nursing care requires a thorough history of the infant's diet and daily schedule and the events surrounding episodes of colicky behavior. Assess the infant's feeding patterns and diet, including type, frequency, and amount of feeding (if breastfeeding, maternal diet history), and frequency of burping. Assess episodes of colic for onset, duration, and characteristics of cry. What measures are used to relieve crying? How effective are they? When possible, observe the feeding method. Parents of infants with colic are often tired and frustrated. They require frequent reassurance that they are not to blame for the infant's condition. Suggest ways of alleviating some of the infant's symptoms and discomfort.

TEACHING HIGHLIGHTS

SUGGESTIONS FOR ALLEVIATING COLIC

Provide Rhythmic Movement
Front-carrying sling carriers
Infant swing (battery-operated swing provides continuous motion)
Car ride

Alternate Positions
Swaddle infant in a soft, stretchy blanket with knees flexed up against abdomen or with legs straight
Place infant prone on parent's arm, supporting the body with one hand under the abdomen and cradling the head in the crook of the other arm

Reduce Environmental Stimuli
Respond to crying
Provide quiet, soothing music
Prevent sudden loud noises
Avoid smoking

Provide Various Tactile Stimuli
Offer a pacifier
Provide a warm bath
Massage abdomen

Alter Intake
Feed smaller amount and burp frequently
Use a bottle with a collapsible bag to prevent sucking air
Breastfeeding mothers: eliminate milk products and spicy or gas-producing foods
Hold upright for ½ hour after feeding

RUMINATION

Rumination is a rare and serious form of chronic regurgitation of recently ingested food into the mouth, followed by rechewing and reswallowing or expulsion of the material (Chial, Camilleri, Williams, et al., 2003). Chewing movements and mouthing of fingers often precede or accompany regurgitation. Close observation may reveal the infant actively initiating gagging with the tongue and fingers. The condition may lead to malnutrition and growth failure in infancy.

Rumination is most often associated with poor maternal–infant bonding. This kind of behavior is seen in infants deprived of tactile, visual, or auditory stimuli for long periods. The infant substitutes repetitive self-stimulation for the lack of appropriate external stimulation. (See the discussion of eating disorders of infancy and childhood in Chapter 34. ∞)

Diagnostic evaluation focuses on ruling out an organic cause and determining the degree and type of nutritional deficiencies. Treatment involves correcting the nutritional deficits and developing normal feeding patterns. An interdisciplinary approach with medical and nursing staff and social services is often needed to help parents meet the infant's nutritional and psychologic needs (see Chapter 34 ∞).

NURSING MANAGEMENT

Nursing care focuses on establishing a warm, caring relationship with the infant and the parents. Making eye contact with the infant, providing food regularly, and stimulating the infant through all the senses are ways to break the pattern of rumination.

Parents need to be included in the infant's care. Discuss proper nutrition and demonstrate feeding techniques and interactions that promote development. Determine the parents' support needs and make a referral to social service agencies as appropriate. A parent preoccupied with financial or other problems is less likely to attend to an infant's needs, resulting in continuation or recurrence of the pattern of rumination.

DISORDERS OF MALABSORPTION

Malabsorption occurs when a child cannot digest or absorb nutrients in the diet. Disorders of malabsorption include celiac disease, lactose intolerance, and short bowel syndrome. Cystic fibrosis, a common cause of malabsorption, is discussed in Chapter 47. ∞

CELIAC DISEASE

Celiac disease, or gluten-sensitive enteropathy, is a chronic malabsorption syndrome that is more common in Caucasian, European children and is uncommon in African-American or Asian children. It is also more common among members of the same family, so a genetic factor may play a role in etiology. About 1% to 4% of children with Down syndrome have celiac disease (Nehring, 2004). Current research is directed at locating the potential genetic abnormalities that occur in celiac disease, and using knowledge of genetics to carry out antibody titer level diagnostic testing (Hoffenberg, Bao, Eisenbarth, et al., 2000). Celiac disease is an immunologic disorder (Zelnik, Pacht, Obeid et al., 2004) characterized by an intolerance for gluten, a protein found in wheat, barley, rye, and oats. Inability to digest glutenin and gliadin (protein fractions) results in the accumulation of the amino acid glutamine, which is toxic to mucosal cells in the intestine. Damage to the villi ultimately impairs the absorptive process in the small intestine.

In the early stages, celiac disease affects fat absorption, resulting in excretion of large quantities of fat in the stools (steatorrhea). Stools are greasy, foul smelling, frothy, and excessive. As changes in the villi continue, the absorption of protein, carbohydrates, calcium, iron, folate, and vitamins A, D, E, K, and B$_{12}$ becomes impaired.

Symptoms usually occur when solid foods containing gluten are introduced to the child's diet (in the first 2 years of life), although celiac disease is sometimes first diagnosed in adulthood. The child exhibits chronic diarrhea, vomiting, irritability, malabsorption, abdominal pain, and failure to thrive (Zelnik et al., 2004) (Figure 51–8 ●). If diagnosis is delayed, the child begins to show evidence of protein deficiency (wasted musculature, abdominal distention), delayed dentition, and changes in bone density due to hypocalcemia.

Diagnosis is confirmed through measurement of fecal fat content, jejunal biopsy, and improvement with removal of gluten products from the diet. Serum antigliadin antibody (AGA) and reticulin antibody levels are elevated. IgA antiendomysial antibodies and IgA antitissue transglutaminase antibodies are commonly used in diagnosis (Murdock & Johnston, 2005).

Symptoms usually improve within a few days to weeks after dietary intervention. The intestinal villi return to normal in about 6 months. Growth should improve steadily, and height and weight should reach normal range within 1 year. Vitamin supplementation may be needed for a time if the child has become malnourished.

NURSING MANAGEMENT

Nursing care focuses on supporting the parents in maintaining a gluten-free diet for the child. Thoroughly explain the disease process to the parents. Emphasize the necessity of following a gluten-free diet. Help parents understand

● **FIGURE 51–8**

The child with celiac disease commonly shows failure to grow and wasting of extremities. The abdomen can appear large due to intestinal bloating and malnutrition.

Used with permission from Zitelli, B. J., & Davis, H. W. (Eds.). (1997). Atlas of pediatric physical diagnosis (3rd ed., p. 294, Figure 10–15a). St. Louis, MO: Mosby.

that celiac disease requires lifelong dietary modifications that should not be discontinued when the child is symptom-free. Discontinuation of the diet places the child at risk for growth retardation and the development of GI cancers in adulthood. All children with celiac disease should be seen by a dietitian several times during childhood. Nutritional assessment and continued teaching to maintain a gluten-free diet take place at these visits. Dietary management is made difficult by hidden gluten in many prepared foods, such as chocolate candy, prepared meats, ice cream, soups, condiments, and food starch.

An infant or toddler's diet is easily monitored at home. When the child enters school, however, ensuring adherence to dietary restrictions becomes more difficult. In addition to easily identified gluten based foods, such as bread, cake, doughnuts, cookies, and crackers, the child must also avoid processed foods that contain gluten as a filler. School-age children and adolescents are often tempted to eat these foods, especially when among peers. Emphasize the need for compliance while meeting the child's developmental needs.

The child's special dietary needs can place a financial burden on the family. Parents need to purchase prepared rice or corn flour products or make their own bread and bakery products. Advise parents that getting a dietary prescription enables them to deduct the cost of these ingredients and commercially prepared products as a medical expense.

Because the entire family must adapt to the diet, parents and siblings need support and management skills. For information and support, refer parents and children to several organizations, including the American Celiac Society, the Celiac Sprue Association/United States of America, and the Gluten Intolerance Group. Written materials are also available from Children's Memorial Hospital in Chicago.

Expected outcomes of nursing care include the following:

- Maintenance of normal dietary patterns
- Adequate absorption of essential nutrients as demonstrated by normal growth patterns and absence of deficiency symptoms
- Child and family knowledge of sources of dietary gluten

LACTOSE INTOLERANCE

Lactose intolerance is the inability to digest lactose, a disaccharide found in milk and other dairy products. It results from a congenital or acquired deficiency of the enzyme lactase. Congenital lactase deficiency of infancy is rare. See Chapter 34 for a general discussion of food intolerance. ∞ Abdominal pain, flatulence, and diarrhea occur shortly after birth when the infant is unable to hydrolyze lactose. The prevalence of secondary (acquired) lactase deficiency occurs in approximately 70% of African Ameri-

cans and Native Americans and more than 90% of Asian Americans (Barnard, 2003). Diarrhea develops rapidly after the child ingests milk and milk products. Some children can tolerate small ingestions of lactose but have symptoms when larger amounts are consumed. Incidence of lactose intolerance increases with advancing age throughout childhood.

Diagnosis is based on a thorough history and a hydrogen breath test, which measures the amount of hydrogen left after fermentation of unabsorbed carbohydrates. A lactose-free diet may eliminate the symptoms, confirming the diagnosis. Treatment for infants includes switching to a soy-based formula. For older children, eliminating lactose-containing foods is recommended. Enzyme tablets such as LactAid can be added to milk or sprinkled on foods to aid digestion.

NURSING MANAGEMENT

Nursing care is primarily supportive. Carefully explain dietary modifications to parents and discuss alternative sources of calcium (see Chapter 34 ∞). Discuss the need for supplementation of calcium and vitamin D to prevent deficiencies. Teach families how to read food labels to find hidden sources of lactose. For example, milk solids may be found in breads, cakes, candies, salad dressings, margarine, and processed food. Suggest lactase tablets for children who want to eat some dairy products.

SHORT BOWEL SYNDROME

Short bowel syndrome is a decreased ability to digest and absorb a regular diet because of a shortened intestine. Loss of intestine may result from extensive bowel resection for treatment of necrotizing enterocolitis or inflammatory disorders or from a congenital bowel anomaly such as intestinal malrotation, gastroschisis, or atresia.

The extent and location of the involved bowel determine the severity of the disorder. Because specific types of absorption occur primarily in certain parts of the bowel, the section lost determines which vitamins and other nutrients are inadequate. During the first 3 months after bowel resection, watery diarrhea is common. In the transition period, the remaining bowel usually increases its absorptive surface area and partially compensates for the absent intestine. At first, the infant or young child requires nutritional support to provide sufficient nutrients for growth and development. A combination of total parenteral nutrition via central line and oral fluids may be required. Once the bowel begins to recover, enteral feedings may be started. Careful management of enteral feedings includes a high-fat, low-carbohydrate diet with added stimulants for mucosal growth hormones (gastrin, insulin, enteroglucagon, and growth hormone). Careful management of nucleotide, glutamine, polyamine, and fatty acid components in enteral feedings can also encourage growth of normal intestinal mucosa (Committee on Nutrition, American Academy of Pediatrics, 2004).

NURSING MANAGEMENT

Nursing care focuses on meeting the child's nutritional and fluid needs and teaching parents how to care for the child at home. Establishing an adequate nutritional intake and bowel pattern is a lengthy process. TPN is provided initially until a feeding regimen can be established. Oral and enteral feedings are instituted gradually to allow the bowel time to compensate. Provide support to the family and child throughout this period. Teach parents how to prepare and administer total parenteral feedings and care for the central line (see Skill 12–7). **SKILLS** Once enteral or tube feedings are begun, teach management of the feeding pump and care of the feeding tube. Ensure regular bowel function and maintain skin integrity. Arrange home visits to monitor the child's growth and development, care of the central line and tube-feeding site, and any side effects such as fluid and electrolyte imbalance and diarrhea.

HEPATIC DISORDERS

The liver is one of the most vital organs in the body. Its essential functions include blood storage and filtration; secretion of bile and bilirubin; metabolism of fat, protein, and carbohydrates; synthesis of blood-clotting components; detoxification of hormones, drugs, and other substances; and storage of glycogen, iron, fat-soluble vitamins, and vitamin B_{12}. Thus, any inflammatory, obstructive, or degenerative disorder that affects liver function can be life threatening. The following discussion focuses on three common liver disorders in children: biliary atresia, viral hepatitis, and cirrhosis. A discussion of hyperbilirubinemia can be found in Chapter 31. ∞

BILIARY ATRESIA

Biliary atresia is the pathologic closure or absence of hepatic or common bile ducts at any point from the porta hepatis to the duodenum (Kotb, Kotb, Sheba et al., 2001). The disorder leads to cholestasis, fibrosis, and cirrhosis (Kelly, 2002). It is the most common pediatric liver disease necessitating transplantation and the most common cause of infant jaundice.

Initially the newborn is asymptomatic. Jaundice may not be detected until 2 to 3 weeks after birth. At that point bilirubin levels increase, accompanied by abdominal distention and hepatomegaly (see Appendix B and the CD-ROM for bilirubin levels and other liver function tests ∞). As the disease progresses, splenomegaly occurs. The infant experiences easy bruising, prolonged bleeding time, and intense itching. Stools have puttylike consistency and are white or clay colored because of the absence of bile pigments. Excretion of bilirubin and bile salts results in tea-colored urine. Failure to thrive and malnutrition occur as the destructive changes of the disease progress.

The cause of biliary atresia is unknown. Absence or blockage of the extrahepatic bile ducts results in blocked bile flow from the liver to the duodenum. This altered bile flow soon causes inflammation and fibrotic changes in the liver. In addition to blockage, the disease can also be caused by hepatocellular dysfunction. Lack of bile acids also interferes with digestion of fat and absorption of fat-soluble vitamins A, D, E, and K, resulting in steatorrhea and nutritional deficiencies. Without treatment the disease is fatal.

Diagnosis is based on the history, physical examination, and laboratory evaluation. Laboratory findings reveal elevated bilirubin levels, elevated serum aminotransferase and alkaline phosphatase values, prolonged prothrombin time, and increased ammonia levels. Ultrasound rules out other causes, and a liver biopsy is performed. Because liver damage develops rapidly in infants with biliary atresia, early diagnosis is essential.

Treatment involves surgery to attempt correction of the obstruction (hepatoportoenterostomy) and supportive care. In the hepatoportoenterostomy (Kasai procedure), a segment of the intestine is anastomosed to the porta hepatis. In most children this is a palliative treatment to promote bile drainage, maintain as much hepatic function as possible, and prevent the complications of liver failure. Supportive treatment is directed at managing the bleeding tendencies by administering oral vitamin K, preventing rickets through vitamin D supplementation; controlling itching and irritability with cholestyramine and antihistamines; and promoting adequate nutrition. Low-dose oral antibiotics are administered to prevent cholangitis (Kelly, 2002).

Although the hepatoportoenterostomy improves the prognosis, complications of liver disease continue to develop; liver transplantation is eventually needed. Donor shortage is the major factor limiting the use of liver transplantation (Tran, Nissen, Poordad et al., 2004). Advances in transplantation surgery now make it possible to perform partial liver transplants from living donor resections. This enables transplantation to be performed when the child is in optimal health, rather than waiting until an appropriate-size cadaver liver is available, and allows for donations from close family members who are often good tissue matches.

These advances, along with the development of cyclosporine and other immunosuppressants, have improved the first-year survival rate for children receiving liver transplantation to between 75% and 85% (SPLIT Research Group, 2001).

NURSING MANAGEMENT

Nursing care in the initial stages of biliary atresia is the same as that for any healthy newborn. As symptoms develop, the focus of nursing care becomes long-term management and support.

Diagnosis of this potentially fatal disorder can be devastating to parents. Provide emotional support and offer frequent explanations of tests during the initial diagnostic evaluation. As the disease progresses, the infant becomes irritable because of intense itching and the accumulation of toxins. Tepid baths may help to relieve itching and provide comfort. Dry skin by patting rather than rubbing to avoid further skin irritation. Promote rest by grouping nursing activities while the infant is awake. Care following a hepatoportoenterostomy is similar to that for a child undergoing abdominal surgery. (See the earlier discussion of postsurgical nursing management for appendicitis and "Nursing Care Plan: The Child Undergoing Surgery" in Chapter 40. ∞) Posttransplant care includes immunosuppressant drugs and close monitoring for vascular complications (see Table 51–3).

Discharge planning focuses on teaching parents how to care for the child's skin, provide for nutritional needs, administer medications, and monitor for increasing symptoms of liver disease. When the child has received a transplant, teach parents how to identify signs of rejection (nausea, vomiting, fever, and jaundice), as well as the administration and side effects of immunosuppressant medications. Refer parents to support groups, clergy, or social services if indicated. They will need ongoing visits from a home healthcare nurse to help them manage the child's complex care. The main expected outcomes of nursing care are the parent's ability to cope with the child's health status and to provide the necessary care. The child is expected to function at maximum potential considering the extent of disease.

VIRAL HEPATITIS

Hepatitis is an inflammation of the liver caused by a viral infection. It may be acute or chronic. Acute hepatitis is rapid in onset and if untreated may develop into chronic hepatitis. The most frequently diagnosed causative organ-

---

TABLE 51–3 ✣ Problems Encountered in Pediatric Liver Transplant

- **Lack of donors.** This problem is being solved by increasing use of split liver transplants when a partial transplant is provided by a family member, alleviating the need to wait for cadaver donations.

- **Immunosuppression.** Immunosuppressive therapies have been tested less in children than in adults and increased research is needed.

- **Morbidity and mortality of treatment.** Many of the drugs used after transplant have side effects of renal toxicity, malignancy, and other serious sequelae. The effects can be magnified in children who have decades of exposure to these drugs.

- **Recurrent and new diseases.** Diseases that may be caused by immunosuppression can occur, such as those caused by infectious agents. Other liver diseases such as cirrhosis and nonspecific hepatitis are seen in some children.

- **Influences on growth and development.** Drugs, liver disease, emotional strain, and disturbed nutritional intake and metabolism may all influence the growth, cognitive function, and developmental variation of children. Attention and consistent screening of development and family adaptation are needed.

Data from McDiarmid, S. V. (2000). Liver transplantation. The pediatric challenge. *Clinical Liver Disease, 4*, 879–927.

---

isms are hepatitis A virus (HAV), hepatitis B virus (HBV), hepatitis C virus (HCV), hepatitis D virus (HDV), and hepatitis E virus (HEV). Other types of non-A, non-B have been identified, such as hepatitis G. An estimated 136,000 cases of hepatitis occur annually in the United States, and one third of these are in children. Most cases are types A and B (Table 51–4).

ETIOLOGY AND PATHOPHYSIOLOGY

Hepatitis A is the most common form of acute viral hepatitis. It is highly contagious and traditionally has been called infectious hepatitis. Infection occurs primarily through the fecal–oral route. Transmission is by direct person-to-person spread or through ingestion of contaminated water or food (particularly shellfish). Hepatitis A frequently occurs in children in childcare settings where hygiene practices are poor. Food handlers can spread hepatitis A if not aware of their infection; it is a common cause of foodborne illness. The virus can live on surfaces for 1 month. Because the virus is transmitted in the early stages of the disease when individuals are often asymptomatic or only mildly ill, large numbers of people may be exposed before the diagnosis is confirmed (Table 51–5). Although a mild disease in many people, it may cause severe liver damage (Shovein, Damazo, & Hyams, 2000).

TABLE 51–4 ❖ Comparison of Hepatitis Types

Type	Incubation	% Icteric	% Who Become Chronic Carriers	Clinical Features
Hepatitis A				
Children < 5 years	4 weeks (10–50 days)	< 5	0	More acute onset; frequently subclinical in young
Adults		50–75	0	children
Hepatitis B				
Infants	1–6 months	< 5	> 90	Extrahepatic manifestations more common
Adults		20–60	5–10	
Hepatitis C				
All ages	6–7 weeks	20–30	≥ 60	Frequently anicteric; predisposes to hepatocellular carcinoma
Hepatitis D				
Coinfection with HBV	2–8 weeks	Unknown	< 5	Most common viral cause of fulminant hepatitis
Superinfection of HBV carrier			> 80	
Hepatitis E				
All ages	2–9 weeks	~10	0	Severe in pregnant women; high mortality and fetal loss

Data from Holst, B., & Ritter, D. (2001). Managing viral hepatitis. *Clinician Reviews, 11*, 51–62.

Hepatitis B, known traditionally as serum hepatitis, is a serious disease. Transmission is usually by the parenteral route through the exchange of blood or any body secretion or fluid. Other common transmission routes include sexual activity and transmission from mother to fetus in utero. Adolescents who use intravenous drugs and have unprotected sexual intercourse are at risk for contracting hepatitis B. Major sources for the spread of HBV are healthy chronic carriers. All body fluids of infected individuals are potentially contaminated with the virus.

The hepatitis C virus is transmitted primarily through blood and blood products, and blood banks now test for this virus. Infected children have commonly had repeated transfusions (as in sickle cell disease or hemophilia). Intra-

TABLE 51–5 ❖ Transmission, Immunization, and Prophylaxis for Hepatitis

Type	Primary Transmission	Immunization Available	Prophylaxis
Hepatitis A	Fecal-oral	Yes	Immune serum globulin Hepatitis A vaccine
Hepatitis B	Blood products Intravenous drug use In utero Sexual activity	Yes	Hepatitis B immune globulin Hepatitis B vaccine
Hepatitis C	Blood products Sexual activity Intravenous drug use	No	None
Hepatitis D	Blood products Intravenous drug use In utero Sexual activity	No	Hepatitis B vaccine
Hepatitis E	Fecal-oral	No	None

Data from Holst, B., & Ritter, D. (2001). Managing viral hepatitis. *Clinician Reviews, 11*, 51–62.

venous drug use, body piercing, and multiple sexual partners are also risk factors. Infected mothers may infect their children before birth or during breastfeeding (Estrada, 2000; National Institute on Drug Abuse, 2000).

Hepatitis D (delta virus) is a defective virus that can gain entry to a human only in connection with hepatitis B. This virus is suspected when someone diagnosed with hepatitis B has diminishing liver function, increasing jaundice, and deteriorating mental status.

Hepatitis E infection is primarily transmitted through contaminated water and is most common in developing countries. Outbreaks may occur in flooding and rainy seasons. A related infection transferred primarily through blood transfusion is hepatitis G (Holst & Ritter, 2001).

The liver's response to injury by the viruses that cause hepatitis is similar (see "Pathophysiology Illustrated: Viral Hepatitis"). Initially, invasion of the parenchymal cells by the virus results in local degeneration and necrosis. Subsequent infiltration of the parenchyma by lymphocytes, macrophages, plasma cells, eosinophils, and neutrophils causes inflammation that blocks biliary drainage into the intestine. Impaired bile excretion causes a buildup of bile in the blood, urine, and skin (jaundice). Structural changes in the parenchymal cells account for other altered liver functions. Regeneration of parenchymal cells occurs within 3 months, and most children recover completely.

In some children, however, a progressive and total destruction of the hepatic parenchyma known as acute fulminating hepatitis develops. Children with this form of the disease usually die of liver failure within 2 weeks of onset unless they receive a liver transplant. Another complication, chronic active hepatitis, may lead to scarring of the liver and progressive deterioration of liver function. The prognosis depends on the degree of liver involvement. In some people, especially those who develop chronic hepatitis, liver cancers and cirrhosis can develop.

CLINICAL MANIFESTATIONS

Acute hepatitis infection is characterized by two phases, the anicteric (absence of jaundice) phase and the icteric (jaundice) phase. The anicteric phase usually lasts 5 to 7 days. Signs and symptoms include nausea, vomiting, anorexia, malaise, fatigue, right upper quadrant pain, hepatosplenomegaly, and fever (see Table 51–4). The child becomes irritable, looks ill, and requires rest. In the icteric phase, signs and symptoms include darkening of urine, clay-colored stools, and the characteristic yellowing of the skin and sclera. Many children with hepatitis do not have jaundice, leading to difficulty in disease diagnosis and management. As the jaundice worsens, the child begins to feel better. This phase lasts approximately 4 weeks. Complete recovery with return of normal liver function and laboratory values may take 1 to 3 months.

PATHOPHYSIOLOGY ILLUSTRATED
Viral Hepatitis

Normal liver

HBV

Parenchymal cells

Hepatic artery branch

Portal vein branch

Bile duct

① Virus invades parenchymal cells, causing local degeneration and necrosis

Liver degenerated and inflamed

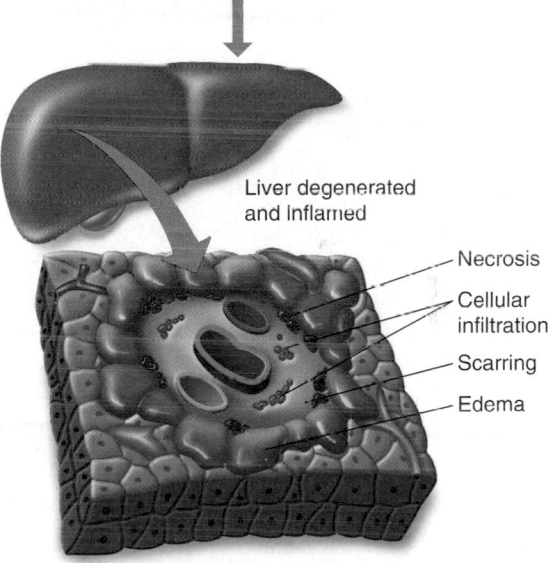

Necrosis

Cellular infiltration

Scarring

Edema

② Infiltration by lymphocytes, macrophages, and other white blood cells causes inflammation that blocks drainage

③ Structural changes occur in parenchymal cells, resulting in altered liver function:

Impaired bile excretion

Elevated ALT and alkaline phosphatase levels

Decreased albumin synthesis

The hepatitis virus causes degeneration and necrosis of the liver, which results in abnormal liver function and illness.

In some cases, hepatitis becomes chronic. A person with chronic hepatitis carries the virus, can transfer it to others, and may develop serious liver disease after several years.

CLINICAL THERAPY

Diagnosis is often made on the basis of a thorough history and physical examination. A history of exposure to persons with the disease is significant. Physical examination reveals a tender, enlarged liver, abdominal pain, and flulike symptoms. Laboratory evaluation includes serologic testing (to detect the presence of antigens and antibodies to HAV, HBV, HCV, or HDV) and liver function studies. Although a test for HEV has been developed, it is not available in developing countries, so diagnosis is usually based on the history.

The three goals of medical management are early detection to prevent complications, support and monitoring during the acute phase of the disease, and prevention of the spread of the disease. Early diagnosis is essential to follow the course of the illness and identify potential complications. Management includes bed rest during the flulike phase. If prothrombin times are increased, vitamin K is administered.

The spread of viral infections can be interrupted by elimination of the virus from the infected population, institution of proper hygiene, and passive or active immunization. To date, no antiviral agent has been developed to combat the hepatitis viruses. Prevention depends on breaking the cycle of infection. Active immunization for hepatitis A, a two-dose series, is recommended for all children at one year, certain individuals at risk of acquiring and transmitting the disease, and for children and childcare workers in certain states with endemic disease (see Chapter 45 ∞). People at risk include childcare staff and food handlers. Since childhood vaccination in high-risk areas was recommended, the overall hepatitis A rate has declined steadily, and in 2002, it was the lowest yet recorded (3.1/100,000) (Centers for Disease Control and Prevention [CDC], 2004).

Immunization for hepatitis B, a three-dose series, is recommended for all children and at-risk adults. The first dose is given within 12 hours of birth to the infant born of an infected mother (refer to the discussion of immunization in Chapter 45 ∞). A total of 7996 acute hepatitis B cases in the United States were reported in 2002, representing a greater than 65% decrease since 1990 (21,102 cases). This decline in hepatitis B rates coincides with the implementation of a national strategy to achieve the elimination of HBV infection. The rate among children 18 years of age and younger, the age group covered by the recommendation for routine childhood immunization, has declined by approximately 90% since 1990 (CDC, 2004).

Passive immunity to HAV can be achieved with standard pooled immune globulin. It must be administered within 2 weeks of exposure. Passive immunity to HBV can be achieved with hepatitis B immune globulin (HBIG). Used for one-time exposure and for infants of infected mothers, it is given within 12 hours of birth.

NURSING MANAGEMENT

NURSING ASSESSMENT AND DIAGNOSIS

The nurse usually encounters the child and family in an outpatient setting. In addition to observing the child for characteristic signs of hepatitis (jaundiced skin and sclera), assess for abdominal pain, anorexia, nausea and vomiting, malaise, and arthralgia. Also get a history of the child's contacts over the past 45 days for HAV and up to 180 days for HBV. For an infant, the hepatitis history of the mother and other family members is important.

Common nursing diagnoses for the child with acute hepatitis might include the following:

- *Risk for Imbalanced Nutrition: Less than Body Requirements* related to chronic illness
- *Fatigue* related to disease state
- *Risk for Deficient Diversional Activity* related to forced inactivity
- *Risk for Body Image Disturbance (Older Child)* related to jaundice
- *Anxiety (Parent and Child)* related to threat to health status
- *Pain* related to liver injury

PLANNING AND IMPLEMENTATION

Nursing care involves home and community considerations, as children are seldom admitted to the hospital for hepatitis treatment. The hospitalized child is placed in isolation. Prevention of the diseases is integrated into all healthcare by discussion of immunization and universal precautions. When hepatitis cases have occurred in the family or community, parents need additional detailed information about health precautions and infection control measures. In addition, teach parents the importance of checking with health professionals before administering any medications (even nonprescription medicines), maintaining adequate nutrition, promoting rest and comfort, and providing diversional activities.

Prevent Spread of Infection

Teach the parents and the child infection control measures to help prevent transmission of the virus. For parents, reinforce good hygiene practices, such as washing hands before and after toileting and proper disposal of soiled diapers. Siblings of a child with hepatitis B who have not already been immunized with the hepatitis B vaccine should be vaccinated immediately. Contacts of the child with hepatitis A should receive immune serum globulin and the first immunization in the hepatitis A series. Rifampin may be given in some cases. All health providers should receive the hepatitis B immunization series and use standard precautions at all times with everyone in healthcare. **SKILLS**

Maintain Adequate Nutrition

Initially, encourage the child to eat favorite foods. Once the anorexia and nausea have resolved, a high-protein, high-carbohydrate, low-fat diet is recommended. Increased protein helps maintain protein stores and prevent muscle wasting. Increased carbohydrates ensure adequate caloric intake and prevent protein depletion. Low-fat foods lessen stomach distention. Offer the child small, frequent feedings.

NURSING PRACTICE

Nurses in childcare centers can provide assessment of the center's procedures and teaching to prevent hepatitis A transmission. Help the center to set standards about:

- Handwashing after each diaper change
- Proper disposal of diapers
- Cleaning diaper-changing surfaces after each diaper change
- Never having food handlers perform diaper changes
- Instructing parents to keep children at home for at least 2 weeks after a diagnosis of hepatitis A
- Informing parents of other children when there is a case of hepatitis A and teaching them the symptoms of the condition

---

Promote Rest and Comfort

Bed rest is necessary only if the child has severe fatigue and malaise. However, most children voluntarily limit their activities during the initial phase of the disease. Keep the child quiet and comfortable. Offer comfort items such as favorite toys, blankets, and pillows.

Provide Diversional Activities

Hospitalized children with hepatitis are kept in isolation. Nonhospitalized children with hepatitis do not need to be isolated, but they should be kept at home for 2 weeks following the onset of symptoms. Parents who cannot take time off from work may need to arrange home sitters to stay with the child. Offer suggestions for diversional activities during this period. Young children can be given a new toy or favorite activities. Older children and adolescents can be given board games, puzzles, books or magazines, movies, or video games. Phone calls and short visits from friends help school-age children and adolescents maintain contact with peers.

EVALUATION

Expected outcomes of nursing care for hepatitis include the following:

- Prevention of new cases of the disease
- Full immunization coverage at recommended ages
- Restoration to normal liver function
- Reestablishment of nutritional intake to support growth
- Return to full energy and activity level
- Developmental progression during and after the disease
- Control of pain to level of comfort
- Absence of chronic liver disease

CIRRHOSIS

Cirrhosis is a degenerative disease process that results in fibrotic changes and fatty infiltration in the liver. It can occur in children of any age as the end stage of several disorders, including biliary atresia (Kelly, 2002). The diffuse destruction and regeneration of the hepatic parenchymal cells result in an increase in fibrous connective tissue and disorganization of the liver structure. The balance between destruction and regeneration determines the specific clinical presentation.

Clinical manifestations of cirrhosis vary. When the disease process results from obstruction, as in biliary atresia, jaundice is an initial sign that intensifies with progression of the disease. In other diseases that cause cirrhosis, jaundice may be a late sign, intermittent, or absent. Steatorrhea is frequently present and can lead to rickets, hemorrhage, and failure to gain weight. Anemia can occur as a result of chronic blood loss from the GI tract. Pruritus is common, particularly in children with biliary malformations. Clubbing of the digits and cyanosis are other common findings. Severe end-stage complications signaling hepatic failure can occur at any time and with little warning.

Diagnostic evaluation is based on the child's history of infection or disease with liver involvement. Physical examination may reveal jaundice, skin changes, ascites, and hemodynamic changes. Laboratory evaluation reveals abnormal liver function tests. A liver biopsy may help determine the extent of the parenchymal damage.

Medical management focuses on treating the child's symptoms and achieving optimal nutritional status and growth. See "Clinical Manifestations: Cirrhosis Complications" for a summary of treatment. Liver transplantation is

CLINICAL MANIFESTATIONS

CIRRHOSIS COMPLICATIONS

ETIOLOGY	CLINICAL MANIFESTATIONS	CLINICAL THERAPY
Fluid and electrolyte imbalance	Ascites	Restrict sodium, protein, and fluids. Administer diuretics (e.g., furosemide [Lasix]). Administer intravenous albumin.
Liver dysfunction	Hepatic encephalopathy	Restrict protein. Administer lactulose to control increased ammonia levels. Administer antibiotics. Correct any imbalances that can lead to coma (fluid and electrolyte imbalance).
Esophageal varices	Hemorrhage	Administer blood and blood products. Replace fluid and electrolytes. Administer vitamin B complex and vitamin K. Insert Sengstaken-Blakemore tube in cases of severe bleeding.

the most common treatment for biliary atresia and metabolic disorders and is the only treatment for end-stage liver disease.

NURSING MANAGEMENT

Nursing care focuses on monitoring physiologic and psychosocial changes to identify early signs of end-stage hepatic failure. Monitor vital signs every 2 to 4 hours. Measure weight daily to assess for fluid retention. Close monitoring of electrolytes and liver function test results helps determine the need for fluid replacement therapy.

Careful administration of medications and monitoring for side effects are necessary because drug metabolism is altered in liver disorders. If ascites is present, provide a low-sodium, low-protein diet and restrict fluids. Remove all water pitchers, glasses, and straws to minimize the child's desire to drink.

Parents of a child with cirrhosis are coping with a life-threatening disorder, and their anxiety and stress are high. The child may be awaiting a liver transplantation that represents the only hope for recovery. Support parents and encourage them to talk about their fears and concerns (see Chapter 37 ∞). Encourage parents to participate in the child's care. Referral to a support group or counseling may be beneficial.

INJURIES TO THE GASTROINTESTINAL SYSTEM

ABDOMINAL TRAUMA

The majority of abdominal injuries are caused by blunt trauma (85%), with penetrating trauma accounting for the remainder. Approximately half of blunt abdominal trauma is caused by motor vehicle crashes, in which children are struck by a vehicle or have lap belt injuries as a restrained passenger (Simone, 2003). Child abuse involving kicking or punching the abdomen is another major cause of blunt abdominal trauma. Penetrating trauma occurs due to impalement on an object, stabbing, or gunshot wounds. Children are more likely to have abdominal injuries because of the smaller amount of subcutaneous tissue surrounding organs, less developed abdominal muscle tone, and proportionately larger solid organs than in adults.

The kind of injury determines the extent of organ damage. High-velocity blunt trauma, which may occur in motor vehicle crashes, usually involves multiple organs. Solid organs such as the liver and spleen can be bruised or lacerated. The sudden increase in abdominal pressure that occurs with a lap belt injury causes hollow organs such as the stomach, intestines, and bladder to burst. Sports-related abdominal trauma is often associated with a direct blow to the abdomen, and a single organ is usually injured, such as when a child's abdomen strikes the handlebar of a bicycle.

NURSING PRACTICE

The child who is restrained in a motor vehicle with only a lap belt is at high risk for abdominal injury in a crash. As the car stops rapidly, the child's body is restrained and flexes around the lap belt. The sudden increase in abdominal pressure causes injury to hollow organs, and sometimes solid organs. Children no longer using car safety seats should sit in a booster seat so that a shoulder restraint is used in addition to the lap belt.

Clinical manifestations of abdominal injury include pain, abdominal distention, muscle guarding, decreased or absent bowel sounds, nausea and vomiting, hypotension, and shock. The external abdomen and back may have penetrating wounds, abrasions, bruising, or markings (e.g., tire tracks or lap belt marks) that provide a clue to injury beneath the skin surface. See Chapter 35 for techniques of abdominal assessment. ∞

The injured child is rapidly assessed for airway, breathing, and circulation, and is stabilized before examination of the abdomen is performed. A nasogastric tube is inserted to decompress the stomach and to detect the presence of blood. Plain abdominal x-rays may reveal air in the abdomen. An ultrasound can reveal free fluid in the abdomen. A CT scan assesses multiple organs for injury and for the presence of free fluid in the abdomen. Peritoneal lavage is used to identify hemorrhage in the abdomen of an unstable child (Simone, 2003). A rectal examination is performed to assess the bowel wall and to detect rectal bleeding. Baseline laboratory studies, including complete blood count, coagulation tests, blood type, and cross-match, are done. In addition, electrolytes and enzyme studies to detect liver, spleen, and pancreas injuries are obtained. A urinary catheter may be inserted to empty the bladder and to check for the presence of hematuria and bladder rupture.

Treatment of a liver or spleen injury takes place in the ICU and focuses on monitoring the child's physical status for hypovolemic shock, maintaining adequate fluid volume with IV fluids or blood products, and allowing the solid organ to heal without surgery in most cases. Pain management with opioids is initiated. Serial hematocrit levels are monitored to detect hemorrhage during this period. Parenteral or enteral nutrition may be initiated 24 to 48 hours to prevent infection and promote wound healing (Simone, 2003).

Exploratory laparotomy is performed to resect hollow organ injuries or to repair liver or spleen lacerations when bleeding is not controlled. The spleen is salvaged whenever possible to help maintain immune function. The child is usually discharged within 5 to 7 days. No strenuous activity is allowed for 6 to 8 weeks. The prognosis is generally good.

NURSING MANAGEMENT

Nursing care includes initial and ongoing assessments of the child's condition. Monitor vital signs every hour as warranted. Monitor the respiratory status as abdominal injuries may also have thoracic involvement. Abdominal distention, immobility, and pain may all affect the child's ability to take deep breaths. Measurement of abdominal circumference, intake and output monitoring, serial hematocrits, and auscultation of bowel sounds are also performed hourly. Notify the physician of any changes.

The child and parents are usually fearful and anxious when the child is admitted with a serious injury. If the injury was preventable, parents may have feelings of guilt or anger. Provide emotional support and avoid judgmental comments or statements that assign blame.

Once the child's condition is stabilized, the focus of nursing care shifts to preventive teaching. Parents should be taught safety measures to prevent future injuries. Discuss the use of car safety restraint devices for riding in an automobile (see Chapters 37 and 38 ∞). If the child's injury was the result of a bicycle fall or crash, discuss the importance of the proper bicycle size and safety measures such as use of a helmet and proper use of hand signals (see Chapter 36 ∞). Have the child practice safe biking habits at a bike rodeo sponsored by a local affiliate of SAFE KIDS USA.

POISONING

Poisoning is a common cause of death and injury in children between 1 and 4 years of age. About 1.2 million poisonings occur annually in the United States. Poisonings are the second leading cause of unintentional home-injury death and account for nearly one third of all unintentional home injuries (Home Safety Council, 2004a, 2004b). Young children are at risk for poisoning because they characteristically explore their environments (see Chapter 33 ∞). Infants and toddlers commonly place objects in their mouths. Some household items are non toxic and cause little harm. However, items that contain caustic agents or toxic chemicals can cause irreversible damage or death.

The Poison Prevention Packaging Act of 1970 mandates child-protective devices for all potentially toxic substances, such as household cleansers and medications. However, children still ingest many of them; analgesics and hydrocarbons remain the two most common causes of poisoning deaths (Powers, 2000). Many other items commonly found in the home are less obvious sources of toxins. The leaves, stems, or flowers of many common household and garden plants are poisonous. Examples include Boston ivy, poinsettia, philodendron, lily-of-the-valley, daffodil (bulbs), azalea, and rhododendron. Nail care products, mothballs, weed and bug killers, and rodent killers are other potential hazards. See "Clinical Manifestations: Commonly Ingested Toxic Agents" for treatments for several commonly ingested household toxins.

Most poisonings occur in the home (see Chapters 37 and 38 for health maintenance strategies related to poison prevention ∞). While 75% of poisons are ingested, other routes of contamination include dermal, inhalation, and ocular (Litovitz, Klein-Schwartz, White et al., 2001). Parents who suspect that their child has ingested a poison should immediately call the Poison Control Center (PCC). The PCC will advise parents about treatment to begin at home, and if the child needs treatment in the emergency department. If the child has vomited, the vomitus should be brought to the emergency department.

CLINICAL MANIFESTATIONS

COMMONLY INGESTED TOXIC AGENTS

TYPE	SOURCES	CLINICAL MANIFESTATIONS	CLINICAL THERAPY
Corrosives (strong acids and alkaline products that cause chemical burns of mucosal surfaces)	Batteries, household cleaners, Clinitest tablets, denture cleaners, bleach, toilet bowl cleaners	Severe burning pain in mouth, throat, or stomach; swelling of mucous membranes; edema of lips, tongue, and pharynx (respiratory obstruction); violent vomiting; hemoptysis; drooling; inability to clear secretions; signs of shock, anxiety, and agitation	*Do not induce vomiting!* Dilute toxin with water to prevent further damage. Give activated charcoal.
Hydrocarbons (organic compounds that contain carbon and hydrogen; most are distillates of petroleum)	Gasoline, kerosene, furniture polish, lighter fluid, paint thinners	Gagging, choking, coughing, nausea, vomiting, alteration in sensorium (lethargy), weakness, respiratory symptoms of pulmonary involvement, tachypnea, cyanosis, retractions, grunting	*Do not induce vomiting!* (Aspiration of hydrocarbons places child at high risk for pneumonia.) Use gastric lavage if severe central nervous system and respiratory impairment are present. Use of activated charcoal is controversial. Provide supportive care. Decontaminate skin by removing clothing and cleansing skin.
Acetaminophen	Many over-the-counter products	Nausea, vomiting, sweating, pallor, hepatic involvement (pain in upper right quadrant, jaundice, confusion, stupor, coagulation abnormalities)	Induce vomiting or perform gastric lavage, depending on amount ingested. Administer charcoal or NAC (concentrated form of Mucomyst), which binds with the metabolite, preventing absorption and protecting the liver.
Salicylate	Products containing aspirin	Nausea, disorientation, vomiting, dehydration, diaphoresis, hyperpnea, hyperpyrexia, bleeding tendencies, oliguria, tinnitus, convulsions, coma	Depends on amount ingested. Induce vomiting. Administer intravenous sodium bicarbonate, fluids, and vitamin K.
Mercury	Broken thermometers, chemicals, paints, pesticides, fungicides	Tremors, memory loss, insomnia, weight loss, diarrhea, anorexia, gingivitis	Similar to that for lead poisoning (see text discussion).
Iron	Multiple vitamin supplements	Vomiting, hematemesis, diarrhea, bloody stools, abdominal pain, metabolic acidosis, shock, seizures, coma	Induce vomiting. Administer intravenous fluids and sodium bicarbonate. Desferoxamine chelation therapy.

With older children, the possibility of intentional ingestion needs to be considered.

In the emergency department, the child's vital signs and level of consciousness are assessed and specific information about the poison is obtained from the parent. The goal of treatment is to prevent further absorption of the poison and to reverse or eliminate its effects. Management focuses on stabilizing the child's condition, identifying the toxic substance, reversing any undesirable effects, and eliminating the substance from the child's body. Table 51–6 summarizes emergency management for poisoning.

TABLE 51–6 ✤ Emergency Management for Poisoning

1. Stabilize the child. Assess ABCs (airway, breathing, and circulation). Provide ventilatory and oxygen support.
2. Perform a rapid physical examination, start an IV infusion, draw blood for toxicology screen, and apply a cardiac monitor.
3. Obtain a history of the ingestion, including substance ingested, where child was found, by whom, position, when, how long unsupervised, history of depression or suicide, allergies, and any other medical problems.
4. Reverse or eliminate the toxic substance using the appropriate method:
   a. *Antidotes and agonists*
      Mucomyst (for acetaminophen poisoning)
      Narcan (for opioid overdose)
      Romazicon (for benzodiazepine overdose)
   b. *Gastric lavage*
      - A gastric tube is inserted through the mouth.
      - Normal saline solution is instilled and aspirated until the return is clear. Reserved for children with central nervous system depression, diminished or absent gag reflex, or unwillingness to cooperate with other measures.
      - Contraindicated in children who have ingested alkaline corrosive substances, as insertion of the tube may cause esophageal perforation.
   c. *Activated charcoal*
      Used in children who have ingested acids to decrease continued damage and potential perforation of stomach and intestines.
      - Given to absorb and remove any remaining particles of toxic substances.
      - Usual dosage administration is 1 g/kg of body weight.
      - A commercial preparation of activated charcoal is administered orally or through a gastric tube.
   - Available as a ready-to-drink solution in an opaque container.
   - May be mixed with apple juice or soda if protocol allows to encourage consumption.
   - A covered cup and straw is used for oral ingestion to prevent the child from seeing the black liquid and to minimize spillage.
   - Activated charcoal is administered only after the child has stopped vomiting, because aspiration of charcoal is damaging to lung tissue.
   - Should not be administered for ingestion of caustic substances or hydrocarbons.
   d. *Cathartics*
      - Hasten excretion of a toxic substance and minimize absorption. The most commonly used cathartic is magnesium sulfate.
   Note: Syrup of ipecac. The use of ipecac is no longer recommended because it may not remove all poison and can be harmful in some situations. Encourage parents to remove it from their homes.
5. Other measures will depend on the child's condition, the nature of the ingested substance, and the time since ingestion. May include diuresis, fluid loading, cooling or warming measures, anticonvulsive measures, antiarrhythmic therapy, hemodialysis, or exchange transfusions.
6. The child's total condition is constantly evaluated to maintain airway, breathing, and circulation. Therapeutic management is adjusted as needed to treat evolving condition.
7. Consider the emotional status of the family. Provide information about the child, involve the child in care when possible, and arrange for support persons and services to be available to the child.

NURSING MANAGEMENT

Once immediate care has been provided, the focus of nursing care shifts to providing emotional support and preventing recurrence.

Provide Emotional Support

Wait until the child is out of immediate danger before questioning parents in detail about the incident. Encourage parents to express anger, guilt, or fear about the incident.

Prevent Recurrence

Discuss with parents the need to supervise infants and young children at all times. Ask parents how medicines and cleaning agents are stored and whether the house contains any plants. Teach proper methods of childproofing the home. They must contact the PCC (1-800-222-1222 in the United States and Puerto Rico) before administering this medication at home. Suggest ways to prevent recurrence of poisoning.

NURSING PRACTICE

The toll-free number for the American Association of Poison Control Centers (AAPCC) is 1-800-222-1222. This number can be accessed from anywhere in the United States and Puerto Rico, and the caller will be connected to the nearest PCC.

INGESTION OF FOREIGN OBJECTS

Approximately 80% of cases of ingestion of foreign objects occur in childhood. The majority of cases present in children between 6 and 36 months of age (Wahbeh, Wyllie & Kay, 2002). The most common object ingested is coins, accounting for 27% to 70% of cases. Pins, parts of toys, batteries, and bones from foods are some other commonly ingested objects. If the foreign body is lodged in the esophagus, they may present with substernal pain, drooling, and dysphagia. Some children may exhibit respiratory symptoms including

MediaLink

Animation: Activated Charcoal

TEACHING HIGHLIGHTS

AVOIDING CHILDHOOD POISONING

- Put the PCC phone number by every phone in the house (1-800-222-1222 in the United States and Puerto Rico).
- Place household cleaners, medications, vitamins, and other potentially poisonous substances out of the reach of children or in locked cabinets. Use warning stickers such as Mr. Yuk on all containers.
- Buy products with childproof caps.
- Store products in their original containers. Never place household cleansers or other products in food or beverage containers.
- Remove all house plants from the child's play areas.
- Use caution when visiting other settings that are not childproofed (e.g., grandparents' homes). Remember that visitors may have pills in their purses or pockets that are easily accessible.

wheezing or coughing. Serious complications can occur following foreign body ingestion. These complications include perforation of the intestinal tract, the most serious sequelae of foreign body ingestion.

Since approximately 60% to 90% of foreign bodies ingested in children are radio-opaque (Wahbeh et al., 2002), radiographs of the neck, chest, esophagus, and abdomen are useful tools in verifying ingestion and to identify the location of the object. Endoscopic examination and retrieval of the ingested foreign body may be necessary. Most (80% to 90%) foreign bodies pass spontaneously through the gastrointestinal system and are eliminated through stool. However, foreign bodies may become lodged in the esophagus and pose a significant risk to the child. Smooth, small, round objects that have passed into the stomach are generally allowed to pass through the bowel without intervention. Esophageal foreign bodies are removed or advanced into the stomach due to the risk for mucosal erosion and catastrophic perforation (Chen & Beierle, 2001).

NURSING MANAGEMENT

Nursing care centers on supporting the child, collaborative assistance in the identification and removal of the foreign body, and teaching the child and family measures to reduce reoccurrence. Partner with the family and assist them in establishing a safe home environment for the child. Encourage the family to keep all small items out of the child's reach and to ensure the child is monitored at all times. When the child has ingested an object, assess the child for drooling, wheezing, substernal pain, dysphagia, and coughing. Obtain a thorough history

from the family. Determine, if possible, what was ingested, when the ingestion occurred, and any symptoms that the child experienced. Assess breath sounds. Prepare the child for radiologic studies. Explain the procedures and reassure the child and family during the studies. Prepare for endoscopic examination and retrieval if necessary. Provide support, reassurance, and ongoing monitoring.

LEAD POISONING

Lead poisoning has been successfully prevented in many areas of the United States, with a substantial decline in lead levels from the mid-1970s. The average serum lead level for children is now 0.6 µg/dL, down from 15 µg/dL in 1976. Approximately 434,000 children in the United States have levels above the recommended level of 10 µg/dL. Many of these children are poor and live in older houses in inner cities (CDC, 2003). Even children with levels below 10 µg/dL may experience cognitive defects due to lead exposure. Lead in paint is the most common source of lead exposure for preschool children. Children are also exposed to lead when they ingest contaminated food, water, and soil or when they inhale dust contaminated with lead. Some major sources of lead include lead-based paint, soil and dust, food grown in contaminated soil, drinking water from lead-lined pipes or teapots, lead dust on parents' clothing from occupations like some artwork or construction, and air near smelters and battery-manufacturing plants.

Children are at greater risk for lead poisoning because they absorb and retain more lead in proportion to their weight than adults do. Lead is particularly harmful to children under the age of 7 years.

Lead interferes with normal cell function, primarily of the nervous system, blood cells, and kidneys, and adversely affects the metabolism of vitamin D and calcium. Clinical manifestations depend on the degree of toxicity. Neurologic effects include decreased IQ scores, cognitive deficits, impaired hearing, and growth delays. Impaired mental function can occur with blood levels even lower than 10 µg/dL. Lead ingestion by a woman during pregnancy can result in fetal malformations, reduced birth weight, and premature birth. Severe lead poisoning, which can result in encephalopathy, coma, and death, is now rare.

Once in the body, lead accumulates in the blood, soft tissues (kidney, bone marrow, liver, and brain), bones, and teeth. Lead absorbed by the bones and teeth is released slowly. Thus, exposure to even small doses, over time, can result in dangerously high levels of lead in the body.

The CDC now recommends screening children at high risk, with reduced screening for those at low risk. In addi-

CLINICAL MANIFESTATIONS

LEAD POISONING

MILD TOXICITY (10–15 µg/dL)	MODERATE TOXICITY (16–69 µg/dL)	SEVERE TOXICITY (>70 µg/dL)
Myalgia or paresthesia Mild fatigue	Arthralgia General fatigue	Paresis or paralysis Encephalopathy (may lead abruptly to seizures, changes in consciousness, coma, and death)
Irritability Lethargy Occasional abdominal discomfort	Difficulty concentrating Muscular exhaustibility Tremor Headache Diffuse abdominal pain Vomiting Weight loss Constipation Anemia	Lead line (blue-black) on gingival tissue Colic (intermittent, severe abdominal cramps)

Data from Agency for Toxic Substances and Disease Registry. (1990). *Lead toxicity, Case studies in environmental medicine* (p. 11). Atlanta: Author.

NURSING PRACTICE

Mercury is another heavy metal that can produce similar effects in the body to those seen in lead poisoning. Recent mercury levels measured in the National Health and Nutrition Examination Survey found that about 10% of women of childbearing age have had more mercury exposure than is recommended. The major source of mercury begins with pollution from power plants, waste incinerators, and industrial processes. Mercury is emitted into the air and falls to waters where it is ingested by fish. In most states, women of childbearing age and young children are warned to limit consumption of fish. Other sources of potential mercury contamination such as mercury thermometers should be eliminated (CDC, 2001).

tion, all children enrolled in Medicaid should be tested, with follow-up management and care (Advisory Committee on Childhood Lead Poisoning Prevention, 2000). A blood lead (Pb-B) level is the most useful screening and diagnostic test for lead exposure.

A Pb-B below 10 µg/dL is considered acceptable, although it may still not screen out all children with impaired development due to lead. An environmental history should be obtained for children with Pb-B levels between 10 and 19 µg/dL to identify removable sources of lead. Follow-up testing is required. Children with Pb-B levels between 20 and 69 µg/dL require a full medical evaluation, including a detailed environmental and behavioral history, physical examination, and tests for iron deficiency. Interventions to remove sources of lead from the child's environment are necessary. For levels above 25 µg/dL,

chelation therapy is also administered. Children with Pb-B levels greater than 70 µg/dL are critically ill from lead poisoning and require immediate chelation therapy and interventions to provide a lead-free environment.

Chelation therapy involves the administration of an agent that binds with lead, increasing its rate of excretion from the body. Calcium disodium ethylenediaminetetraacetate ($CaNa_2$ EDTA), dimercaprol (BAL), d-penicillamine, or succimer (DMSA) may be used. Children with Pb-B levels between 25 and 69 µg/dL receive $CaNa_2$ EDTA for 5 to 7 days, followed by a rest period and then a second chelation treatment. Children with Pb-B levels greater than 70 µg/dL are given both BAL and $CaNa_2$ EDTA, followed by a rest period and a second chelation treatment using $CaNa_2$ EDTA alone. Long-term follow-up of children receiving chelation therapy is essential. The child should never be discharged unless a lead-free home environment has been ensured.

NURSING MANAGEMENT

Nursing care centers on screening, education, and follow-up. Nurses often work with state and local health officials to plan screening for children at high risk of lead exposure. Ask parents about the child's development and eating habits and be alert for risk of lead exposure. Educate parents about sources of lead in the environment and techniques to reduce exposure. Emphasize the importance of housekeeping interventions to reduce exposure to lead dust. These interventions include damp mopping of hard surfaces, floors, window sills, and baseboards; washing the child's hands and face before meals; and frequent washing of toys and pacifiers.

DEVELOPING CULTURAL COMPETENCE

LEAD IN TRADITIONALLY USED SUBSTANCES

Traditional medicines and cosmetics may contain large amounts of lead. Examples include azarcon and greta, preparations that are used by Mexican Americans to treat empacho, a coliclike illness; chifong tokuwan, pay-loo-ah, ghasard, bali goli, and kandu, used by some Asian communities; and alkohl, kohl, surma, saoott, and cebagin, used by some Middle Eastern communities. Some candies from Mexico have been foound to have high lead levels.

Teach parents the importance of including foods high in iron and calcium in the child's diet to counteract losses of these minerals associated with lead exposure. The child should eat meals at regular intervals, since lead is absorbed more readily on an empty stomach.

Be sure that parents understand the importance of follow-up testing of lead levels. If the child is developmentally delayed, refer the family to an infant stimulation or child development program. Referral to social services and either a visiting nurse or home healthcare nurse may also be appropriate.

Expected outcomes of nursing care for the child with lead or other poisoning include the following:

- Normal growth and development, including cognition
- Adequate nutritional intake
- Removal of lead or other poisons from the child's environment
- Expressed understanding by family of measures to establish a safe environment for the child

Critical Concept Review

LEARNING OBJECTIVES

CONCEPTS

Describe the general function of the gastrointestinal system.	1. Ingestion, digestion, and absorption of fluids and nutrients. 2. Metabolism of needed nutrients. 3. Excretion of waste products.

Discuss the pathophysiologic processes associated with specific gastrointestinal disorders in the pediatric population.	1. Structural defects: occur when growth and development of fetal structures are interrupted in the first trimester:
	  ■ Cleft lip and palate.
	  ■ Esophageal atresia and tracheoesophageal fistula.
	  ■ Pyloric stenosis.
	2. Intussusception: occurs when one portion of the intestine prolapses and telescopes into another portion.
	3. Abdominal wall defects:
	  ■ Gastroschisis: vascular disruption of the fetal mesenteric vessels.
	  ■ Omphalocele: intra-abdominal contents herniate through the umbilical cord.
	4. Anorectal malformation: failure during fetal life for complete development of the anus and rectum.
	  ■ Anal stenosis.
	  ■ Anal atresia.
	  ■ Imperforate anus.
	5. Hernias: protrusion or projection of an organ through the muscle wall of the cavity that normally contains it, caused by failure to close during fetal development.
	  ■ Diaphragmatic hernia.
	  ■ Umbilical hernia.
	6. Disorders of motility:
	  ■ Gastroesophageal reflux: return of gastric contents into the esophagus caused by relaxation of the esophageal sphincter.
	  ■ Hirschsprung disease: congenital aganglionic megacolon.
	7. Inflammatory disorders:
	  ■ Peptic ulcers.
	  ■ Appendicitis.

LEARNING OBJECTIVES

CONCEPTS

Discuss the pathophysiologic processes associated with specific gastrointestinal disorders in the pediatric population.—*continued*

→

- ■ Necrotizing enterocolitis: caused by vascular compromise to the bowel of the newborn.
- ■ Meckel's diverticulum: failure of a fetal duct to atrophy.
- ■ Inflammatory bowel disease.
- 8. Disorders of malabsorption:
  - ■ Short bowel syndrome.
  - ■ Celiac disease.
- 9. Hepatic disorders:
  - ■ Hepatitis.
  - ■ Hyperbilirubinemia.
  - ■ Biliary atresia.

Identify signs and symptoms that may indicate a disorder of the gastrointestinal system.

→

1. Inability to gain weight or weight loss.
2. Vomiting, diarrhea, or constipation.
3. Lack of energy or lethargy.
4. Abdominal tenderness.
5. Abdominal distention.

Describe nursing management and plan care for disorders of the gastrointestinal system.

→

1. Assess abdominal girth.
2. Assess for presence of bowel sounds.
3. Begin oral feedings with frequent, small feedings of clear liquids, advance diet as tolerated.
4. Assess location and type of pain child is experiencing.
5. Determine if child is experiencing nausea or vomiting.
6. Determine stooling pattern.
7. Monitor intake and output.

Analyze developmentally appropriate approaches for nursing management of gastrointestinal disorders in the pediatric population.

→

1. Facilitate nipple- or breastfeeding in the child with a structural defect.
2. Instruct parents in the use of thickened formula for treatment of GER and GERD.
3. Assist children with hepatitis to make appropriate food choices that are palatable and conform to the restricted diet.
4. Encourage children with ostomies to take responsibility for own care.

Discuss nursing management of the child with an injury (trauma or ingestion of injurious agent) to the gastrointestinal system.

→

1. Promote hemodynamic stabilization:
   - ■ Fluid and blood replacement therapy.
   - ■ Frequent vital sign measurement.
   - ■ Strict measurement of intake and output.
2. Provide pre- and postoperative care.
3. Support the child and family.

CRITICAL THINKING IN ACTION

*View the **Critical Thinking in Action** video in Chapter 51 of the CD-ROM. Then, answer the questions that follow.*

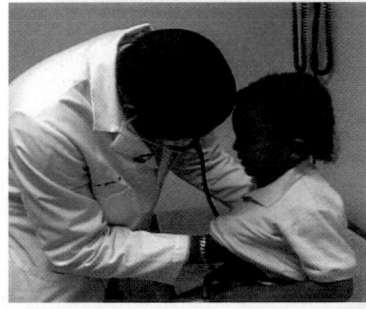

Ryan, a 3 year old, was last seen at 2 years of age, and appears today for a well-child check-up. He is in the 10th percentile for height (last visit was in the 25th percentile) and he is in the 5th percentile for weight (he was in the 10th percentile in the last visit). A development assessment shows that Ryan has only limited vocabulary; when asked to draw a circle, he only scribbles; and although he can run, his mother says he cannot kick a ball. The physical exam is unremarkable, except that he is found to be thin, but active. He will not make eye contact, and just seems to be generally uninterested. The mother says he has never been in the hospital or had surgery and is usually healthy. He has an easy gag reflex, tends to vomit frequently, and is often constipated. Past measurements for height and weight were usually in the fiftieth percentile. When asked about Ryan's environment, his mother tells you they moved into a house built prior to 1920 and have been doing some restoration, but recently had to stop because her husband lost his job and now they are on Medicaid.

The nurse practitioner performs some blood work and orders a CBC with differential, lead screening test, and sedimentary rate. The blood test results show Ryan has hemoglobin of 9 g/dL and a lead level of 30 µg/dL. The nurse practitioner recommends Ryan be taken to a specialist at the local university due to the high lead level and he is treated with chelation therapy. The public health department visits the home and finds high lead levels in the paint. The family is assisted to find alternative housing. After the lead level is lowered Ryan is referred to an early intervention program for treatment of development delays. Iron supplementation is started and the family is instructed in high iron foods.

1. What is the primary risk factor that Ryan has for lead poisoning?
2. What are some of the signs of lead poisoning Ryan is exhibiting?
3. What should Ryan's family be told regarding the role of the health department in treating the lead toxicity in Ryan?
4. How does chelation therapy alter lead levels?

MEDIALINK   www.prenhall.com/london

- NCLEX-RN® Review, case studies, and other interactive resources for this chapter can be found on the Companion Website at http://www.prenhall.com/london. Click on "Chapter 51" to select the activities for this chapter.

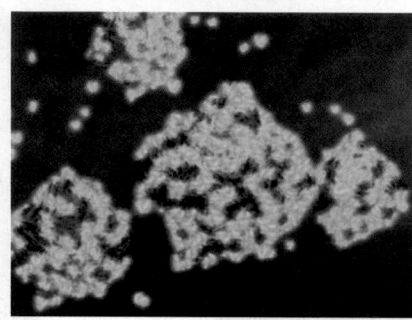

- For animations, more NCLEX-RN® Review questions, and an audio glossary, access the accompanying CD-ROM in this textbook.

REFERENCES

Advisory Committee on Childhood Lead Poisoning Prevention. (2000). Recommendations for blood lead screening of young children enrolled in Medicaid: Targeting a group at high risk. *Morbidity and Mortality Weekly Report, 49* (RR14), 1–13.

Arguin, A. L., & Swartz, M. K. (2004). Gastroesophageal reflux in infants: A primary care perspective. *Pediatric Nursing, 30,* 45–52.

Ashburn, D. A., Pranikoff, T., & Turner, C. S. (2002). Unusual presentations of gastroschisis. *American Surgeon, 68,* 724–727.

Bagolan, P., Casaccia, G., Crescenzi, F., Nahom, A., Trucchi, A., & Giorlandino, C. (2004). Impact of a current treatment protocol on outcome of high-risk congenital diaphragmatic hernia. *Journal of Pediatric Surgery, 39,* 313–318.

Barnard, N. D. (2003). The milk debate goes on and on and on! *Pediatrics, 112,* 448.

Baron, M. L. (2002). Crohn disease in children. *American Journal of Nursing, 102,* 26–34.

Barr, J. M. B. (2000). Chronic intestinal pseudo-obstruction: Pediatric case presentations and review of the literature. *Journal of the Society of Pediatric Nurses, 5,* 175–182.

Bell, E. F. (2005). Preventing necrotizing enterocolitis: What works and how safe? *Pediatrics, 115,* 173–175.

Blumenthal, M., Goldberg, A., & Brinckmann, J. (2000). *Herbal medicine, expanded commission E monographs.* Newton, MA: Integrative Medicine Communications.

Blumer, S. L., Zucconi, W. B., Cohen, H. L., Scriven, R. J., & Lee, T. K. (2004). The vomiting neonate: A review of the ACR appropriateness criteria and ultrasound's role in the workup of such patients. *Ultrasound Quarterly, 20*(3), 79–89.

Castiglia, P. T. (2001). Constipation in children. *Journal of Pediatric Health Care, 15,* 200–202.

Centers for Disease Control and Prevention. (2001). Blood and hair mercury levels in young children and women of childbearing age—United States, 1999. *Morbidity and Mortality Weekly Report, 50,* 140–143.

Centers for Disease Control and Prevention. (2003). Surveillance for elevated blood lead levels among children-United States, 1997–2001. *MMWR 52*(5510), 1–21.

Centers for Disease Control and Prevention. (2004). Summary of notifiable diseases, 2002. *Morbidity and Mortality Weekly, 51,* 1–84. http://www.cdc.gov.mmwr/preview/mmwrhtml/mm5153a1.htm. Retrieved 10/31/05.

Chen, M. K., & Beierle, E. A. (2001). Gastrointestinal foreign bodies. *Pediatric Annals, 30,* 736–742.

Chial, H. J., Camilleri, M., Williams, D. E., Litzinger, K., & Perrault, J. (2003). Rumination syndrome in children and adolescents: Diagnosis, treatment, and prognosis. *Pediatrics, 111,* 158–562.

Cho, S., Moore, S. P., & Fangman, T. (2001). One hundred three consecutive patients with anorectal malformations and their associated anomalies. *Archives of Pediatrics & Adolescent Medicine 155,* 587–591.

Cleft Palate Foundation. (2004). Retrieved June 26, 2004, from http://www.cleftline.org/aboutclp/

Committee on Nutrition, American Academy of Pediatrics. (2004). *Pediatric nutrition handbook* (5th ed.). Elk Grove Village, IL: American Academy of Pediatrics.

Connon, J. J. (1999). Celiac disease. In M. E. Shils, J. A. Olson, J. Shike, & A. C. Ross (Eds.), *Modern nutrition in health and disease* (9th ed., pp. 1163–1168). Baltimore: Williams & Wilkins.

Coughlin, E. C. (2003). Assessment and management of pediatric constipation in primary care. *Pediatric Nursing, 29,* 296–302.

Cowden, J. D., & Hotez, P. J. (2001). A field guide to emerging enteric protozoa. *Contemporary Pediatrics, 18,* 440–447.

Davies, M. C., Creighton, S. M., & Wilcox, D. T. (2004). Long-term outcomes of anorectal malformations. *Pediatric Surgery International, 20,* 567–572.

DerMarderosian, A. (Ed.). (2000). *Chamomile. The review of natural products: Facts and comparisons* [Monograph]. St. Louis, MO: Wolters Kluwer.

Estrada, B. (2000). Breast-feeding and vertical transmission of hepatitis C. *Infectious Medicine, 17,* 526–528.

Gereige, R. S., & Frias, J. L. (2002). Is it more than just constipation? *Pediatrics, 109,* 961–965.

Gokhale, R. (2001). Chronic abdominal pain: Inflammatory bowel disease and eosinophilic gastroenteropathy. *Pediatric Annals, 30,* 49–55.

Hedrick, H. L, Crombleholme, T. M., Flake, A. W., Nance, M. L., von Allmen, D., Howell, L. J., et al. (2004). Right congenital diaphragmatic hernia: Prenatal assessment and outcome. *Journal of Pediatric Surgery, 39,* 319–323.

Hoffenberg, E. J., Bao, F., Eisenbarth, G. S., Uhlhom, C., Haas, J. E., Sokol, R. J., et al. (2000). Transglutaminase antibodies in children with a genetic risk for celiac disease. *Journal of Pediatrics, 137*, 356–366.

Holst, B., & Ritter, D. (2001). Managing viral hepatitis. *Clinician Reviews, 11*, 51–62.

Home Safety Council. (2004a). Retrieved July 4, 2004, from http://www.homesafetycouncil.org/resource_center/resourcecenter.aspx Executive summary.

Home Safety Council. (2004b). *Poisonings second leading cause of unintentional injury deaths in American homes* (news release, Washington, DC: Home Safety Council, February 5, 2004). Retrieved July 4, 2004, from http://www.pr newswire.com

Howard, E. R. (2001). Hirschsprung's disease and allied disorders. *Gut, 49*(5), 741–742.

Jadcherla, S., & Shaker, R. (2001). Esophageal and upper esophageal sphincter motor function in babies. *American Journal of Medicine, 111*, 64–68.

Jakubik, L. D., Colfer, A., & Grossman, M. B. (2000). Pediatric short bowel syndrome: Pathophysiology, nursing care, and management issues. *Journal of the Society of Pediatric Nurses, 5*, 111–121.

Jung, A. D. (2001). Gastroesophageal reflux in infants and children. *American Family Physician, 64*, 1853–1860.

Katz, D. A. (2001). Evaluation and management of inguinal and umbilical hernias. *Pediatric Annals, 30*, 729–735.

Kazacos, K. R. (2000). Protecting children from helminthic zoonoses. *Contemporary Pediatrics*, (Suppl.), 1–24.

Kelly, D. A. (2002). Managing liver failure. *Postgraduate Medical Journal, 78*, 660–667.

Kosloske, A. M., Love, C. L., Rohrer, J. E., Goldthorn, J. F., & Lacey, S.R. (2004). The diagnosis of appendicitis in children: Outcomes of a strategy based on pediatric surgical evaluation. *Pediatrics, 113*, 29–34.

Kotb, M. A., Kotb, A., Sheba, M. F., & El Koofy, N. M. (2001). Evaluation of the triangular cord sign in the diagnosis of biliary atresia. *Pediatrics, 108*, 416–420.

Lembo, A., & Camilleri, M. (2003). Chronic constipation. *New England Journal of Medicine, 349*, 1360.

Letton, R. W. (2001). Pyloric stenosis. *Pediatric Annals, 30*, 745–750.

Levy, J. (2001). Gastroesophageal reflux and other causes of abdominal pain. *Pediatric Annals, 30*, 42–47.

Li, B. U. K. (1996). Cyclic vomiting: New understanding of an old disorder. *Contemporary Pediatrics, 13*, 48–62.

Litovitz, T. L., Klein-Schwartz, W., White, S., Cobaugh, D. J., Youniss, J., Omslaer, J. C., et al. (2001). 2000 annual report of the American Association of Poison Control Centers Toxic Exposure Surveillance System. *American Journal of Emergency Medicine, 19*, 337–395.

Lucassen, P. L., Assendelft, W. J., & Gubbels, J. W. (1998). Review: Some behavioral interventions, drugs, and dietary changes reduce infantile colic. *British Medical Journal, 316*, 1563–1569.

McDiarmid, S. V. (2000). Liver transplantation. The pediatric challenge. *Clinical Liver Disease, 4*, 879–927.

Miller, K. E. (2003). Colic: Prevalence, risk factors, and potential sequelae. *American Family Physician, 67*, 2005–2006.

Mitchell, J. C., & Wood, R. J. (2000). Management of cleft lip and palate in primary care. *Journal of Pediatric Health Care, 14*, 13–19.

Morash, D. (2002). An interdisciplinary project that changed practice in feeding methods after pyloromyotomy. *Pediatric Nursing, 28*, 113–117.

Murdock, A. M., & Johnston, S. D. (2005). *European Journal of Gastroenterology and Hepatology, 17*, 41–43.

Murray, K. F., & Christie, D. L. (2000). Vomiting in infancy: When should you worry? *Contemporary Pediatrics, 17*, 81–115.

National Institute on Drug Abuse. (2000). *Hepatitis C. Community drug alert bulletin* (NIH Publication No. 00–4663). Bethesda, MD: National Institutes of Health.

National Safety Council. (2000). *Injury facts.* Itasca, IL: Author.

Nehring, W. M. (2004). Down syndrome. In P. L. Allen & J. A. Vessey, *Primary care of the child with a chronic condition* (pp. 445–468). St. Louis, MO: Mosby.

O'Donnell, K. A., Glick, P. L., & Caty, M. G. (1998). Pediatric umbilical problems. *Pediatric Clinics of North America, 45*, 791–812.

O'Hara, M., Kiefer, D., Farrell, K., & Kemper, K. (1998). A review of 12 commonly used medicinal herbs. *Archives of Family Medicine, 7*, 523–536.

Orenstein, J. (2000). Update on intussusception. *Contemporary Pediatrics, 17*, 180–191.

Powers, K. S. (2000). Diagnosis and management of common toxic ingestions and inhalations. *Pediatric Annals, 29*, 330–343.

Reeves, J. J., Shannon, M. W., & Fleisher, G. R. (2002). Ondansetron decreases vomiting associated with acute gastroenteritis. *Pediatrics, 109*(4), e62.

Rogers, J. (2001). Hirschsprung's disease: Diagnosis and management in children. *British Journal of Nursing, 10*, 640–645.

Sadovsky, R. (2001). Meckel's diverticulum: Review and management. *American Family Physician, 64*, 2000–2001.

Shovein, J. T., Damazo, R. J., & Hyams, I. (2000). Hepatitis A: How benign is it? *American Journal of Nursing, 100*, 43–48.

Simone, S. (2003). Abdominal/genitourinary injuries. In P. A. Moloney-Harmon & S. J. Czerwinski, *Nursing care of the pediatric trauma patient* (pp. 227–247). Philadelphia: Saunders.

Simpson, T., & Ivey, J. (2003). Pediatric management problems. *Pediatric Nursing, 29*, 310.

Singh, S., Bhende, M., & Kinnane, J. M. (2001). Delayed presentations of congenital diaphragmatic hernia. *Pediatric Emergency Care, 17*, 269–271.

Snyder, J. (1997, July). Feeding during diarrhea: New AAP guidelines and innovations in oral rehydration solutions. *Contemporary Pediatrics Reporter, 6*.

Sondheimer, J. (2003). Gastroesophageal reflux. In W. Hay, A. Hayward, M. Levin, & J. Sondheimer

(Eds.), *Current pediatric diagnosis & treatment* (16th ed., pp. 614–615). New York: Lange Medical Books/McGraw-Hill.

SPLIT Research Group. (2001). Studies of pediatric liver transplantation (SPLIT): Year 2000 outcomes. *Transplantation, 72*, 463–476.

Swenson, O. (2002). Hirschsprung's disease. *Pediatrics, 109*, 914–918.

Thielman, N. M., & Guerrant, R. L. (2004). Acute infectious diarrhea. *New England Journal of Medicine, 350*, 38.

Thompson, J. (2001). Intussusception, pyloric stenosis and Hirschsprung's disease. *Community Practitioner, 74*, 312–313.

Tran, T. T., Nissen, N., Poordad, F. F., & Martin, P. (2004). Advances in liver transplantation: New strategies and current care expand access, enhance survival. *Postgraduate Medicine, 115*(5), 73–85.

Uhrich, K. S., & Mackin, A. L. (2001). Cleft lip and palate. *American Journal of Nursing, 101*, 24AA–FF.

van Rooij, I. A., Vermeij-Keers, C., Kluijtmans, L. A. J., Ocke, M. C., Zielhuis, G. A., Goorhuis-Brouwer, S. M., et al. (2003). Does the interaction between maternal folate intake and the methylenetetrahydrofolate reductase polymorphisms affect the risk of cleft lip with or without cleft palate? *Journal of Epidemiology, 157*, 583.

Vegunta, R. K., Ali, A., Wallace, L. J., Switzer, D. M., & Pearl, R. H. (2004). Laparoscopic appendectomy in children: Technically feasible and safe in all stages of acute appendicitis. *American Surgeon, 70*, 198–202.

Wahbeh, G., Wyllie, R., & Kay, M. (2002). Foreign body ingestion in infants and children. Location, location, location. *Clinical Pediatrics, 41*, 633–640.

Warner, B. W. (1996). Classification of congenital disorders of the anorectum. In A. M. Rudolph, J. I. E. Hoffman, & C. D. Rudolph (Eds.), *Rudolph's pediatrics* (29th ed., p. 1112). Stamford, CT: Appleton & Lange.

Weir, E. (2003). Congenital abdominal wall defects. *Canadian Medical Association Journal, 169*, 809.

West, L. (1997). Innovative approaches to the administration of activated charcoal in pediatric toxic ingestions. *Pediatric Nursing, 23*, 616–619.

Westerdahl, J. (1999). Botanicals in pediatrics. In P. Q. Samour, K. K. Helm, & C. E. Lang (Eds.), *Handbook of pediatric nutrition* (2nd ed., pp. 589–600). Gaithersburg, MD: Aspen.

Wyllie, R. (2004). Stomach and intestines; Ileus, adhesions, intussusception, and closed loop obstructions. In R. E. Behrman, R. M. Kliegman, & H. B. Jenson, *Nelson textbook of pediatrics* (17th ed., pp. 1228–1232, 1241–1243). Philadelphia: Saunders.

Young, C. & White S. (1992). Preparing patients for tube feeding at home. American Journal of Nursing, *92*, 46–53.

Zelnik, N., Pacht, A., Obeid, R., & Lerner, A. (2004). Range of neurological disorders in patients with celiac disease. *Pediatrics, 113*, 1672–1677.

Ziegler, M. M.(2004). The diagnosis of appendicitis: An evolving paradigm. *Pediatrics, 113*, 130–132.

Zitsman, J. L. (2003). Current concepts in minimal access surgery for children. *Pediatrics, 111*, 1239–1245.

The Child with Alterations in Genitourinary Function

Planning Terrell's day can be a challenge, because his treatment often interferes with his activities. We all hope that Terrell receives a kidney transplant soon so his growth will improve and he will not have to miss school during treatment.

—Aunt of Terrell

LEARNING OBJECTIVES

- Describe the pathophysiologic processes associated with genitourinary disorders in the pediatric population.

- Discuss the nursing management of a child with a structural defect of the genitourinary system.

- Develop a nursing care plan for the child with a urinary tract infection.

- Describe the growth and developmental issues for the child with chronic renal failure.

- Outline a plan to meet the fluid and dietary restrictions of a child with a renal disorder.

- Develop a nursing care plan for the child with acute and chronic renal failure on dialysis.

- List psychosocial issues for children of different ages who have surgery on the genitourinary system.

MEDIALINK www.prenhall.com/london

CD-ROM

Animations/Videos:
  Circumcision
  Renal Function
  Furosemide (Drug Animation)
  Sexually Transmitted Infections
Skill 16–1: Performing a Urinary Catheterization
NCLEX-RN® Review
Audio Glossary

Companion Website

NCLEX-RN® Review
Thinking Critically
Case Study
Audio Glossary
MediaLink Applications:
  Care Plan: A School-Age Child with Enuresis
  Case Study: A Child with Chronic Kidney Failure
  Care Plan: A Child with Kidney Failure
  Care Plan: A Child with Nephrotic Syndrome

any infections, structural disorders, and disease processes alter genitourinary function. Because the kidneys and other urinary system organs perform several essential body functions, including removing waste products and maintaining fluid and electrolyte balance, disorders that affect these organs pose a significant threat to the health of children.

Although the reproductive system is functionally immature until puberty, uncorrected structural defects and sexually transmitted diseases can have both psychologic and physiologic implications for the developing child.

ANATOMY AND PHYSIOLOGY OF PEDIATRIC DIFFERENCES

The genitourinary system is made up of the urinary and reproductive organs. The urinary system—kidneys, ureters, bladder, and urethra (Figure 52–1 ●)—excretes wastes and maintains acid-base and fluid and electrolyte balance. The reproductive system consists of internal and external organs that at maturity promote the conception and healthy development of a fetus.

URINARY SYSTEM

All of the nephrons that will make up the mature kidney are present at birth. The kidneys grow and the tubular system matures gradually during childhood, reaching full size by adolescence. Most renal growth occurs during the first 5 years of life. This increase in size is due primarily to enlargement of the nephrons. The efficiency of the kidney also increases with age. During the first 2 years of life, the kidneys are less efficient at regulating electrolyte and acid-base balance (see Chapter 43 ○○) and eliminating some drugs from the body.

● FIGURE 52–1

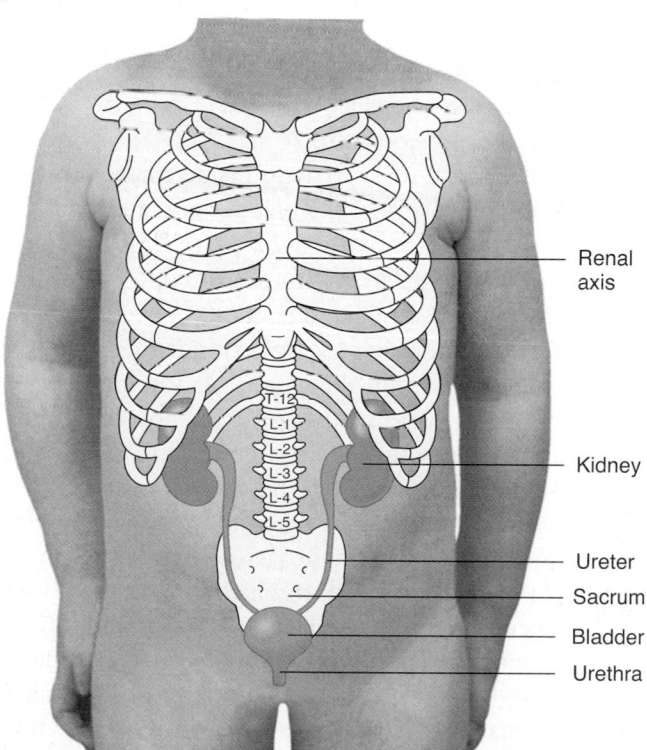

The kidneys are located between the twelfth thoracic (T12) and third lumbar (L3) vertebrae.

After the age of 2 years, the kidneys' efficiency increases markedly.

Bladder capacity increases with age from 20 to 50 mL at birth to 700 mL in adulthood. A child's bladder capacity (in ounces) can be estimated by adding 2 to the child's age (e.g., a 4-year-old has a bladder capacity of 6 ounces). Stimulation of "stretch receptors" within the bladder wall initiates urination. Simultaneous contraction of the detrusor muscle of the bladder and relaxation of the internal and external sphincters result in emptying of the bladder. Children less than 2 years of age cannot maintain bladder control because of insufficient nerve development.

GROWTH AND DEVELOPMENT

Urinary output per kilogram of body weight decreases as the child ages because the kidney becomes more efficient at concentrating urine. Expected output is as follows:

Infants	2 mL/kg/hr
Children	0.5 to 1 mL/kg/hr
Adolescents	40 to 80 mL/hr

Normal renal function requires the following: unimpaired renal blood flow, adequate glomerular ultrafiltration, normal tubular function, and unobstructed urine flow.

REPRODUCTIVE SYSTEM

The reproductive system in children is functionally immature until puberty. Throughout childhood the genitalia (with the exception of the clitoris in girls) enlarge gradually. The hormonal changes of puberty accelerate anatomic and functional development (see Chapter 35 for figures illustrating pubertal development ∞). In girls, the mons pubis becomes more prominent and hair begins to grow. The vagina lengthens, and the epithelial layers thicken. The uterus and ovaries enlarge, and the musculature and vascularization of the uterus also increase. In boys, downy hair begins to appear at the base of the penis, and the scrotum becomes increasingly pendulous. The penis grows longer and wider.

STRUCTURAL DEFECTS OF THE URINARY SYSTEM

BLADDER EXSTROPHY

Bladder exstrophy is a rare defect in which the posterior bladder wall extrudes through the lower abdominal wall (Figure 52–2 ●). Failure of the abdominal wall to close during fetal development results in eversion and protuberance of the bladder wall and a wide separation of the rec-

● **FIGURE 52–2**

This child has bladder exstrophy, noted by extrusion of the posterior bladder wall through the lower abdominal wall.

tus muscles and the symphysis pubis. The upper urinary tract is usually normal. The defect occurs in approximately 1 in every 400,000 live births and is more common in boys than girls (Sponseller, Jani, Jeffs et al., 2001). The bladder mucosa appears as a mass of bright-red tissue, and urine continually leaks from an open urethra. Females have a bifid (split) clitoris. Males have a short, stubby penis, and the glans is flattened with dorsal chordee and a ventral preduce. Epispadias (see page 1631) and bilateral inguinal hernias are also common.

Surgical reconstruction is performed in several stages. Primary closure of the bladder and abdominal wall is usually completed within 24 to 48 hours after birth. The wound and pelvis are immobilized to promote healing. An osteotomy (see Chapter 55 ∞) to rotate the innominate bones of the pelvis to approximate the symphysis pubis reduces tension on the closed bladder and abdominal wall. Epispadias repair is often performed at age 1 to 2 years or at the same time as the continence surgical procedure. Surgery to reconstruct the bladder neck and reimplant the ureters is performed when the bladder has achieved adequate capacity. The goals of surgical reconstruction are (1) bladder and abdominal wall closure; (2) urinary continence, with preservation of renal function; (3) creation of functional and normal-appearing genitalia; and (4) improvement of sexual functioning. Some children require permanent urinary diversion because a functional bladder cannot be reconstructed.

Because the bladder epithelium is abnormal, it is prone to neoplasms. Periodic examination and cystoscopy after the age of 20 years is recommended to detect malignancies.

NURSING MANAGEMENT

Preoperative nursing care centers on preventing infection and trauma to the exposed bladder. The bladder mucosa is covered in sterile plastic wrap to prevent trauma and irritation, and the surrounding area is cleaned daily and protected from leaking urine with a skin sealant.

Postoperatively the wound and pelvis are immobilized to facilitate healing. Internal and external immobilization techniques are used for pelvic closure (see Chapter 55 ∞). Avoid abduction of the infant's legs. Nursing care includes maintaining proper alignment, monitoring peripheral circulation, and providing meticulous wound and skin care.

Monitor renal function by assessing the adequacy of urine output and blood and urine chemistries to detect signs of renal damage. Observe for any signs of obstruction in the drainage tubes such as increased intensity of bladder spasms, decreased urine output, or urine or blood draining from the urethral meatus. Promote comfort and give antibiotics as ordered.

Parents need emotional support to help them cope with the disfiguring nature of the infant's defect and the uncertainty of complete repair. To promote parent–infant bonding, encourage parents to participate in all aspects of the infant's care, including bathing, feeding, and wound care. Discharge teaching should include instructions about dressing changes and diapering and the need to immediately report any signs of infection or change in renal function. Emphasize the need for routine follow-up visits after surgery to assess urinary function and to ensure that the next stages of surgery for continence control are performed at the appropriate time in the child's development. However, these children do not always achieve continence. Parents need help to promote the child's self-esteem and self-confidence with sexual identity and function. Psychologic counseling may help the child during adolescence.

HYPOSPADIAS AND EPISPADIAS

Hypospadias and epispadias are congenital anomalies involving the abnormal location of the urethral meatus in males (Figure 52–3 ●). Both defects result when the urethral folds fail to fuse completely over the urethral groove. The reported incidence of hypospadias is 1 in every 125 live male births (Stokowski, 2004).

With hypospadias, the urethral meatus can be located anywhere along the course of the anterior urethra on the ventral surface of the penile shaft, from the perineum to the tip of the glans. Most cases are mild, with the meatus slightly off center from the tip of the penis; in severe cases, the meatus is located on the scrotum. Hypospadias often occurs in conjunction with congenital *chordee*, a fibrous line of tissue that results in ventral curvature of the penile shaft.

In epispadias, the meatal opening is located on the dorsal surface of the penile shaft. Epispadias often occurs in conjunction with exstrophy of the bladder.

Diagnosis is made by prenatal ultrasound or by examination at birth. The infant should not be circumcised because the dorsal foreskin tissue may be used for surgical repair. The defects are corrected surgically, usually during the first year of life, to minimize psychologic effects when the child is older. Surgery is usually performed in a single operation, often as an outpatient procedure. The goals of surgical repair are (1) placement of the urethral meatus at the end of the glans penis with satisfactory caliber and configuration for a urinary stream (enabling the child to void in a standing position) and (2) release of chordee to straighten the penis (enabling future sexual function).

● **FIGURE 52–3**

Hypospadias and epispadias. **A,** In hypospadias the urethral canal is open on the ventral surface of the penis. **B,** In epispadias the canal is open on the dorsal surface.

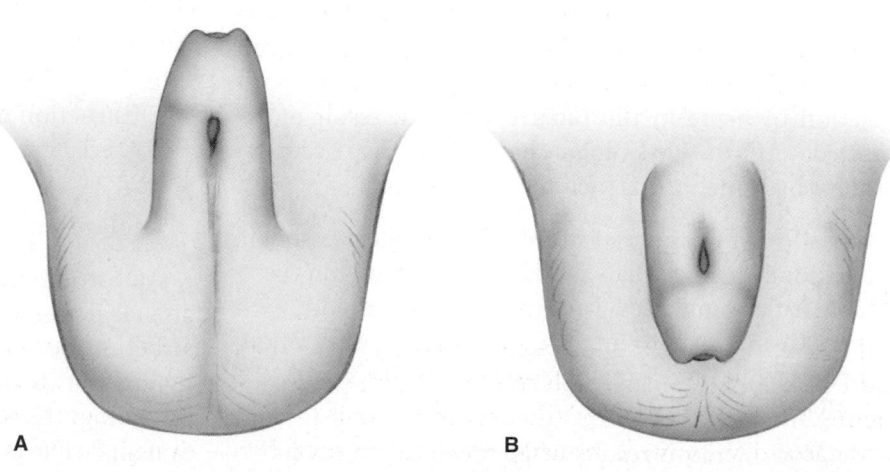

A   B

A caudal nerve block is often used for postoperative pain relief. Anticholinergic medications may be prescribed to relieve bladder spasms.

NURSING MANAGEMENT

It is important to address parents' concerns at the time of birth. Preoperative teaching can relieve some of their anxiety about the future appearance and functioning of the penis.

Postoperative care focuses on protecting the surgical site from injury. The infant or child returns from surgery with the penis wrapped in a simple dressing, and sometimes a urethral **stent** (a device used to maintain patency of the urethral canal) is placed to keep the new urethral canal open. Plan care to ensure that the stent does not get removed. Refer to the hospital's policy for the appropriate use of physical restraints in this situation.

Encourage fluid intake to maintain adequate urinary output and patency of the stent. Hourly documentation of intake and output is essential. Notify the physician if there is no urine drainage for 1 hour as this may indicate obstruction. Pain may be associated with bladder spasms. Anticholinergic medications such as oxybutynin or hyoscyamine may be prescribed. Acetaminophen may also be given for pain. Antibiotics are often prescribed until the urinary stent falls out.

Patients are often discharged the day of surgery. Discharge teaching should include instructions for parents about care of the reconstructed area, double-diapering to protect the stent, fluid intake, medication administration, and signs and symptoms of infection (see "Teaching Highlights: Caring for the Child after Hypospadias and Epispadias Repair" and Skill 16–2 in the *Clinical Skills Manual*). **SKILLS** Tell parents when the child needs to see the physician for dressing removal.

OBSTRUCTIVE UROPATHY

Obstructive uropathy refers to structural or functional abnormalities of the urinary system that interfere with urine flow. The pressure caused by urine backup compromises kidney function and often causes **hydronephrosis** (accumulation of urine in the renal pelvis as a result of obstructed outflow). Physiologic changes that may occur as a result of hydronephrosis include the following:

- Cessation of glomerular filtration when the pressure in the kidney pelvis equals the filtration pressure in the glomerular capillaries. To compensate, the blood pressure increases to increase the glomerular filtration pressure, but increasing pressure on the glomeruli leads to cell death.
- Metabolic acidosis results when the distal nephrons' ability to secrete hydrogen ions is impaired.

TEACHING HIGHLIGHTS

CARING FOR THE CHILD AFTER HYPOSPADIAS AND EPISPADIAS REPAIR

- Use double-diapering to protect the stent (the small tube that drains the urine). See Skill 16–2. **SKILLS**
- Restrict the infant or toddler from activities (e.g., playing on riding toys) that put pressure on the surgical site. Avoid holding the infant or child straddled on the hip. Limit the child's activity for 2 weeks.
- Encourage the infant or toddler to drink fluids to ensure adequate hydration. Provide fluids in a pleasant environment or using a special cup. Offer fruit juice, fruit-flavored ice pops, fruit-flavored juices, flavored ice cubes, and gelatin.
- Be sure to give the complete course of prescribed antibiotics to avoid infection.
- Watch for signs of infection: fever, swelling, redness, pain, strong-smelling urine, or change in flow of the urinary stream.
- The urine will be blood tinged for several days. Call the physician if urine is seen leaking from any area other than the penis.

A double-diapering technique protects the urinary stent after surgery for hypospadias or epispadias repair. The inner diaper collects stool; the outer diaper, urine.

- Impairment of the kidney's ability to concentrate urine results in polydipsia and polyuria.
- Obstruction results in urinary stasis, promoting bacterial growth.
- Restriction of urinary outflow causes progressive renal damage and chronic renal failure if untreated.

Obstructive uropathy may be caused by several congenital lesions such as ureteropelvic junction (UPJ) obstruction, posterior urethral valves (PUVs), and stenosis of hypoplasia of the ureterovesicular junction (see "Pathophysiology Illustrated: Obstruction Sites in the Urinary System"). The UPJ is the most common site of obstruction of the upper urinary tract in infants and children. PUVs

PATHOPHYSIOLOGY ILLUSTRATED

Obstruction Sites in the Urinary System

Kidney

Ureter

Bladder

Urethra

Stenosis of the
ureteropelvic valve

Stenosis of the
ureterovesicular junction

Stenosis of the
posterior urethral valve

Obstruction may occur in either the upper or lower urinary tract. Common sites of obstruction occur at the ureteropelvic valve, the ureterovesicular junction, or the posterior urethral valve. Why would damage from posterior urethral valves potentially be worse than other obstructions? Renal failure is most likely to occur when both kidneys are affected by hydronephrosis.

(abnormal folds of mucous in the male urethra) are the most common cause of anatomic bladder outlet obstruction, occurring in approximately 1 in 5000 to 8000 live male births (Vogt, 2002).

Prune-belly syndrome, also known as Eagle–Barrett syndrome, is another cause of hydronephrosis. In this congenital defect, the abdominal musculature fails to develop. The skin covering the abdominal wall is thin and resembles a wrinkled prune. Other characteristics include urinary tract anomalies, poor ureteral peristalsis, enlarged bladder, high risk for recurrent urinary tract infection, and bilateral cryptorchidism. Prune-belly syndrome occurs predominantly in males (95%), with an incidence of 1 in 35,000 to 50,000 births (Vogt, 2002).

Other conditions that can lead to hydronephrosis include myelomeningocele and neoplasms. Clinical manifestations vary, depending on the cause and location of the obstruction (see "Clinical Manifestations: Obstructive Lesions of the Urinary System").

Early diagnosis and treatment prevent kidney damage and deterioration of renal function. Prenatal ultrasound

may detect hydronephrosis and PUV. A diuretic enhanced radionuclide scan and voiding cytourethrogram are performed when UPJ or ureterovesicular obstruction is suspected. Table 52–1 lists diagnostic tests commonly used to identify urinary tract conditions.

The goals of surgical correction or diversion are to lower the pressure within the collecting system, which reduces renal damage, and to prevent stasis, which decreases the risk of infection. Surgical correction may necessitate **pyeloplasty** (removal of an obstructed segment of the ureter and reimplantation into the renal pelvis) or valve repair or reconstruction, depending on the cause of the obstruction. Urinary incontinence resulting from sphincter weakness is a common problem after surgery.

NURSING MANAGEMENT

Preoperative nursing care focuses on preparing the parents and child for the procedure and addressing parents' concerns about the postsurgical outcome. Give parents a

TABLE 52–1 ✛ **Diagnostic Tests for Urinary System Conditions**

Test	Use	Nursing Considerations
Urinalysis (see Skills 10-7—10-12) **SKILLS**	Detects specific gravity, presence of glucose, ketones, protein, blood cells, casts, crystals, and microorganisms.	Use a urine collection bag for infants and children who are not toilet trained. (See Skill 10-7.) Give fluids if unable to void.
Urine culture	Detects the presence of an infection in the urinary system.	Explain the process for cleaning the perineum and collecting the urine midstream in a sterile cup. Clean the perineum and collect a catheter specimen midstream in a sterile container. (See Skill 10-10.)
Voiding cystourethrogram or radionuclide cystography	Shows bladder structure and function, urethral anatomy, bladder masses. Detects vesicoureteral reflux.	Explain catheterization to child and that the bladder will be filled. (See Skill 16-1.) Provide coaching strategies for parents accompanying the child to help the child cope. Assess for allergies as contrast media is used.
Renal or bladder ultrasound	Identifies large renal scars, renal anomalies, obstruction, abscesses, masses, and hydronephrosis.	Noninvasive procedure. Fluids are administered as prescribed.
Intravenous pyelogram (intravenous urography)	Shows the kidney's collecting system, distal ureters, and bladder.	Assess for allergies as contrast medium is used. Infants and children are NPO prior to the study. An IV is started for injection of contrast.
Diuretic renogram	Helps distinguish between obstructive and nonobstructive lesions.	Hydrate the child before the exam. An IV is started and diuretic is infused. The child is catheterized to drain urine during the procedure.
Radionucleotide renal scan with $_{99m}$Tc dimercapto-succinic acid (DMSA)	Detects renal parenchymal lesions, renal atrophy, or scars. Differentiates between hydronephrosis caused by obstructive lesions, reflux, or a cyst.	Explain catheterization to child.
Renal biopsy	Determines presence and extent of renal involvement in specific disorders.	NPO 6 hours (or as prescribed) before biopsy. Prepare site and administer preprocedural sedation as prescribed. May require bowel evacuation before test.
Cystoscopy	Shows interior urethra and bladder.	Infants and children are NPO prior to the study. Sedation is administered. Children with cardiac anomalies need antibiotic prophylaxis. Fluids are forced after the procedure to detect problems with voiding.
CT (computed tomography)	Provides detailed visualization of structures of the urinary tract and major renal blood vessels.	Infant or child may be NPO and require bowel evacuation prior to study. Prepare child for size of equipment. Assess for allergies if contrast medium is used. Sedation may be needed.
MRI (magnetic resonance imaging)	Provides detailed visualization of structures of the urinary system.	Prepare child for sounds, size of equipment, and tunnel. Ensure that the child has no metallic implants. Sedation may be needed.

Data from Kraus, S. J. (2001). Genitourinary imaging in children. *Pediatric Clinics of North America, 48*(6), 1381-1423; Hanson, K.A. (2003). Diagnostic tests and tools in the evaluation of urologic disease, Part II. *Urologic Nursing, 23*(6), 405-415.

CLINICAL MANIFESTATIONS

OBSTRUCTIVE LESIONS OF THE URINARY SYSTEM

OBSTRUCTIVE LESION	CLINICAL MANIFESTATIONS
Ureteropelvic junction obstruction	In infants: abdominal mass (enlarged kidney), hypertension, urinary tract infection In children: hematuria, pain, intermittent nausea and vomiting
Posterior urethral valves	In infants: abdominal mass (enlarged kidney), distended bladder, poor urinary stream, urinary tract infection, sepsis, low specific gravity, polyuria, increased creatinine level, failure to thrive In children: urinary frequency and incontinence
Ureterovesicular junction obstruction	Urinary tract infection (recurrent or chronic), hematuria, pain, abdominal mass (enlarged kidney), enuresis

chance to discuss concerns about how the disorder will affect the child's long-term renal functioning.

Postoperative care involves monitoring vital signs and intake and output and observing for signs of urine retention, such as decreased output and bladder distention. Many children are discharged with stents or catheters. Teach parents how to change dressings, double-diaper, care for catheters, assess pain and give analgesics, and recognize signs of possible obstruction or infection. Parents should encourage the child to participate in age-appropriate activities. However, children should avoid contact sports because of their potential to injure the bladder.

URINARY TRACT INFECTION

A urinary tract infection (UTI) may be bacterial, viral, or fungal; it occurs in the urinary tract. Cystitis is a lower UTI that involves the urethra or bladder. Pyelonephritis is an upper UTI that involves the ureters, renal pelvis, and renal parenchyma. UTIs can be acute or chronic (the latter either recurrent or persistent).

UTIs are the second most common infections in children. What accounts for the high incidence of these infec-

tions? Among newborns and young infants, most infections occur in boys. They are usually associated with structural defects having a higher incidence in males (e.g., obstructive uropathy), which predispose the infant to infection. Among older infants and children, the incidence of UTIs is higher in girls. This is attributed to the shorter female urethra (2 cm [1 in.] in young girls) and its proximity to the anus and vagina, which increases the risk of contamination by fecal bacteria. An estimated 3% of females and 1% of males will have a UTI by age 11 years (National Kidney and Urological Diseases Information Clearinghouse, 2003).

ETIOLOGY AND PATHOPHYSIOLOGY

Many first UTIs are caused by *Escherichia coli*, a common gram-negative enteric bacterium. Other causative organisms include *Staphylococcus*, *Klebsiella*, *Proteus*, *Pseudomonas*, *Enterobacter*, and *Enterococcus*.

Urinary stasis enhances the risk of UTI. Stasis may be caused by abnormal anatomic structures or abnormal function (e.g., **neurogenic bladder** [interrupted nerve supply to the bladder leading to urinary tract obstruction, for example, from meningomyelocele or spinal cord trauma], common in children with myelomeningocele). Children normally void five to six times a day. Infrequent voiding, common in school-age children, results in incomplete emptying of the bladder and urinary stasis. Other factors associated with increased risk of UTI include an irritated perineum, constipation, masturbation, sexual abuse, and sexually active adolescent females.

Another cause of UTI is **vesicoureteral reflux**, the backflow of urine from the bladder into the ureters during voiding. This prevents complete emptying of the bladder and creates a reservoir for bacterial growth. Vesicoureteral reflux can also result from a structural anomaly in which the ureters insert in an abnormal position into the bladder.

Renal scarring can result from hydronephrosis or pyelonephritis due to the inflammatory and ischemic effects of the infection. Scars have been associated with hypertension, proteinuria, and kidney failure. The risk of kidney damage increases in the following instances:

- UTI in infant less than 1 year of age
- Delay in diagnosis and effective antibacterial treatment for an upper UTI
- Anatomic obstruction or nerve supply interruption
- Recurrent episodes of upper UTIs

CLINICAL MANIFESTATIONS

Symptoms depend not only on the location of the infection, but also on the age of the child. Symptoms in the newborn period tend to be nonspecific—unexplained fever, failure to thrive, poor feeding, vomiting and diarrhea, strong-smelling urine, and irritability. Any child under 2 years of age with a fever of unknown origin should be tested for a UTI. Not until the toddler years are the more "classic" symptoms of lower UTI seen as listed in the clinical manifestations table. About 40% of UTIs are asymptomatic.

CLINICAL THERAPY

A urine specimen is examined for the presence of bacteria. A dipstick leukocyte esterase test identifies white blood cells and pyuria. A nitrite dipstick detects bacteria. Using both dipsticks increases the sensitivity (88%) and specificity (93%) for diagnosing a UTI (Shaw & Gorelick, 1999). Diagnosis is confirmed with a urine culture collected by midstream clean-catch void, sterile catheterization, or suprapubic aspiration (see Skills 10–7 and 10–8). **SKILLS** Urine collection bags used on infants are reliable only when no pathogens are found as sterility of the specimen cannot be guaranteed. The diagnosis of infection is made from the number of colony-forming units (between 1000 and 100,000) depending upon the method of urine collection (Shaw & Gorelick, 1999). When the specimen is collected by sterile procedure, fewer organisms are needed to confirm infection. Antibiotic sensitivity for the specific organisms cultured is then determined.

Radiologic studies may be performed to detect structural abnormalities and renal scarring. A renal and bladder ultrasound is commonly performed soon after the diagnosis, and a voiding cystourethrogram (VCUG) is obtained to test for vesicoureteral reflux (Mahant, To, & Friedman, 2001). Renal and bladder sonography and a cystogram (either VCUG or radionuclide) are used to detect pyelonephritis and renal scarring (Kraus, 2001).

Antibiotic therapy is begun as soon as urine samples have been collected. The antibiotic is changed if necessary after culture sensitivity is determined. Follow-up cultures should be obtained 48 to 72 hours after drug therapy has started, at which time the urine should be sterile. Follow-up urine cultures should then be obtained monthly for 3 months, every 3 months for 6 months, and then annually. Subsequent infections may be asymptomatic. For children with vesicoureteral reflux or recurrent infections, a long-term, suppressive dose of an antibiotic may be ordered for prophylaxis, but there is limited evidence that this is effective (Williams, Lee, & Craig, 2001). Children with renal scarring should have their blood pressure monitored.

Children who appear ill and cannot tolerate oral antibiotics are often hospitalized because they need rehydration and parenteral antibiotic treatment. Infants may develop permanent kidney damage or generalized sepsis if the UTI is not treated aggressively. If a structural defect is identified, surgical correction may be necessary to prevent recurrent infections that could lead to renal damage.

NURSING MANAGEMENT

NURSING ASSESSMENT AND DIAGNOSIS

Physiologic Assessment

Take a history of urinary symptoms. Assess the infant for toxic (very ill) appearance, fever, and oral fluid intake. Measure the child's height and weight and plot on a growth curve to identify any change in growth pattern associated with a chronic illness. Take the infant's or child's blood pressure. Palpate the abdomen and suprapubic and costovertebral areas for masses, tenderness, and distention. Observe the urinary stream if possible and perform a urinalysis, including specific gravity. Proper collection of the urine specimen is essential. Get a clean-catch urine specimen if the child is able to cooperate. If not, get a catheterized sample (see Skills 10–7 and 10–8). **SKILLS** An early morning urine specimen is preferred because the urine is more concentrated.

CLINICAL MANIFESTATIONS

URINARY TRACT INFECTION CLINICAL MANIFESTATIONS AND THERAPY

TYPE OF UTI	CLINICAL MANIFESTATIONS	CLINICAL THERAPY
Lower UTI—cystitis	Frequency, dysuria, urgency, enuresis, strong-smelling urine, cloudy urine, hematuria, abdominal pain, fever	5- to 7-day course of trimethoprim or sulfamethoxazole or antibiotic matching organism sensitivity, encourage oral fluids, use an analgesic such as acetaminophen or pyridium
Upper UTI—pyelonephritis	High fever, chills, abdominal pain, flank pain, costovertebral angle tenderness, persistent vomiting, moderate to severe dehydration	Rehydration, antipyretics, IV antibiotics initially then transitioned to oral antibiotics matching organism sensitivity for a total of 7 to 10 days

Psychosocial Assessment

Sexually active adolescents may deny having symptoms because they fear disclosing their sexual activity to their parents. Careful questioning may be necessary to elicit these concerns. Be open and approachable and give the patient and family the chance to address their concerns.

Common nursing diagnoses for the child with a UTI include the following:

- *Impaired Urinary Elimination* related to recurrent urinary tract infections
- *Risk for Disproportionate Growth* related to chronic infection and renal damage
- *Urinary Retention* related to infrequent voiding habits or vesicoureteral reflux
- *Ineffective Therapeutic Regimen Management* related to lack of knowledge of preventive measures (adequate fluid intake, proper hygiene, signs, and prophylactic antibiotics)
- *Risk for deficient fluid volume* related to fever and inadequate intake

PLANNING AND IMPLEMENTATION

Nursing care for the hospitalized child with a complicated UTI centers on administering prescribed medications, promoting rehydration, assessing renal function, and teaching parents and older children how to minimize the risk of future infection.

Administer antibiotics and antipyretics as prescribed to maintain therapeutic drug levels and reduce fever. Encourage fluid intake to dilute the urine and flush the bladder. Frequent voiding minimizes urinary stasis. Document intake and output. Assess renal function by comparing the child's output to the expected measure of 1 mL/kg/hr and weigh the child daily.

Because bladder training is such an important milestone for young children, any disorder that affects voiding may have developmental implications. A toddler who has been toilet trained may regress and require diapers temporarily due to incontinence related to the UTI. An older child may develop enuresis after a prolonged period of being dry at night. A preschooler may perceive the infection as punishment for an imagined wrong such as masturbation. Reassure parents that this is normal and emphasize that they should offer the child support rather than disapproval.

Nursing Care in the Community

Children with UTIs are usually cared for at home. Teach parents that antibiotics must be taken for the full course and that they may be continued even after the infection has cleared to prevent a recurrence. Teach prevention through proper hygiene and avoidance of risk behaviors.

TEACHING HIGHLIGHTS

PREVENTION OF URINARY TRACT INFECTIONS

- Teach proper perineal hygiene. Girls should always wipe the perineum from front to back after voiding.
- Encourage the child to drink plenty of fluids and avoid long periods of "holding urine."
- Caution against tight underwear; children should wear cotton rather than nylon underwear.
- Encourage the child to void more frequently and to fully empty the bladder.
- Discourage bubble baths, bath oils, and hot tubs, which can irritate the urethra.
- Instruct sexually active adolescent girls to void before and after sexual intercourse to prevent urinary stasis and flush out bacteria introduced during intercourse.

Give parents specific guidelines for oral fluid intake. Make sure the amount of fluids recommended for a 24-hour period equals the maintenance fluids needed plus additional fluids required because of fever and diuresis to flush out pathogens. (See Chapter 43. ∞) Suggest that the parents avoid giving the child caffeinated and carbonated beverages as these may potentially irritate the bladder mucosa.

Encourage the child to void more frequently even after the infection has cleared. A wristwatch with an alarm may be a helpful reminder. The child with a neurogenic bladder needs to have clean intermittent catheterization performed several times a day to reduce urinary stasis and the potential for UTI.

Teach parents the signs and symptoms of recurrent infection and to seek care promptly.

EVALUATION

Expected outcomes of nursing care include:

- The child increases fluid intake and number of times voiding each day.
- Future UTIs are prevented.

ENURESIS

Enuresis is repeated involuntary voiding by a child old enough that bladder control is expected, usually about 5 to 6 years of age. (See Table 52–2 for bladder control milestones.) Enuresis can occur either at night (nocturnal), during the day (diurnal), or both night and day. Nocturnal enuresis accounts for approximately 50% of cases and occurs more often in boys than in girls, with a 3.5:1 ratio, whereas diurnal enuresis is more common in girls. Enuresis can be primary, intermittent, or secondary. In primary

TABLE 52–2 ✤ Milestones in the Development of Bladder Control

Age	Developmental Milestone
1½ years	Child passes urine at regular intervals.
2 years	Child announces when he or she is voiding.
2½ years	Child makes known need to void; can hold urine.
3 years	Child goes to the bathroom by himself or herself; holds urge if preoccupied with play.
2½–3½ years	Child achieves nighttime control.
4 years	Child shows great interest in going to bathrooms when away from home (shopping centers, movies).
5 years	Child voids approximately 7 times a day; prefers privacy; is able to initiate emptying of bladder at any degree of fullness.

enuresis the child has never had a dry night. It is thought to be due to a maturational delay and small functional bladder, not stress or a psychologic cause. In intermittent enuresis the child has occasional nights or periods of dryness. With secondary enuresis a child who has been reliably dry for 6 to 12 months begins bed-wetting. It is associated with stress, infections, and sleep disorders. Between 5 and 7 million children older than 5 years have primary nocturnal enuresis (Mercer, 2003).

Enuresis may result from neurologic or congenital structural disorders, illness, or stress. Nocturnal enuresis occurs frequently in children whose parents have a history of bedwetting. There is a 77% risk if both parents had enuresis, a 44% risk if one parent had enuresis, and a 15% risk if neither parent had enuresis (Tobias, 2000). In most children with primary enuresis, the bladder has a smaller functional capacity, and neuromuscular maturation of the inhibitory fibers is delayed. Often children with nocturnal enuresis are harder to arouse and may fail to respond to full bladder signals. Some children may produce more urine and exceed the functional bladder capacity due to a lack of circadian rhythm of vasopressin that helps concentrate the urine during sleep (Jalkut, Lerman, & Churchill, 2001). Minor abnormalities of the

🌸 GROWTH AND DEVELOPMENT

An estimated 15% to 20% of children who are partially toilet trained will continue to have wetting episodes after 5 years of age. An estimated 5% of 10-year-olds and 2% of 12- to 14-year-olds continue to have nocturnal enuresis (Issenman, Filmer, & Gorski, 1999).

bladder neck and urethra are also associated with enuresis. Some children are believed to have mild developmental delays. Children with obstructive sleep apnea have a higher rate of enuresis (Brooks & Topol, 2003). The majority of cases are not associated with structural or neurologic pathology.

Children with diurnal enuresis may have frequency, urgency, constant dribbling, and involuntary loss of control after voiding. Children with nocturnal enuresis have bed-wetting.

Diabetes mellitus or renal insufficiency should be ruled out in children with both enuresis and polyuria or oliguria. The child's lower spine is examined for fistulas, sacral dimples, or tufts of hair that could be signs of occult spina bifida. Prolonged hospitalization, family stressors, and preoccupation with school concerns also have been associated with secondary enuresis.

A thorough history can help identify potential causes of enuresis (see "Nursing Practice"). Enuretic children of-

☀ NURSING PRACTICE

QUESTIONS TO ASK WHEN TAKING AN ENURESIS HISTORY

Family History

Is there a family history of renal or urinary structural abnormalities?

Is there a family history of bed-wetting?

Family Management

How serious is the problem for the family?

What happens when the child wets? (Who gets up and changes sheets?)

How is the child treated? Is the child punished or blamed for wetting?

What remedies have been tried?

Toilet Training

Did the child have a difficult time with toilet training?

What method of toilet training did you use? When was toilet training initiated?

What are the child's current voiding and stooling patterns?

How long is the child's longest dry period, and when does it occur?

Does the child have a history of constipation or encopresis?

Stressors

How is the child doing in school? How are relationships with peers?

Are any new or chronic stressors present in the child's life?

How does the problem interfere with play and other activities?

Risk Factors

Diabetes

- Does the child void often or have urgency?
- Is the child frequently thirsty?

Urinary Tract Infection

- Does the child experience burning on urination?
- Has the child had a urinary tract infection before?

ten have a history of constipation. Rectal pressure on the posterior bladder wall stimulates the bladder to empty. Laboratory evaluation includes urinalysis and urine culture. Measurement of the child's functional bladder capacity may be performed. Bladder sonography to measure residual urine after voiding and uroflow (the rate of urine flow) measurement to identify a slow urine stream may be performed (Jalkut et al., 2001).

A multitreatment approach is usually most effective. Fluid restriction, bladder training, and enuresis alarms are common approaches (Table 52–3). A spontaneous cure happens in 15% of children each year, regardless of intervention or lack of intervention. Approximately one third of children with nocturnal enuresis are treated with medications. Imipramine, a tricyclic antidepressant, is often used but requires close monitoring because of its effects on mood and sleep-arousal patterns and the associated danger of overdoses. Desmopressin, given as a nasal spray or oral tablet, has an antidiuretic effect but is not used long term because of its expense. It is usually reserved for times when the child is away from home for a short period (e.g., sleepovers or camp). Relapse often occurs when medications are stopped. Avoiding foods believed to contribute to enuresis, such as those containing caffeine, milk, chocolate, and citrus, may be helpful (Tobias, 2000).

NURSING MANAGEMENT

Teach the child and parents about the physiologic development of bladder control and causes and treatment of enuresis. Explore feelings of guilt or blame. Make sure the parents are aware that the child cannot control the wetting. Psychosocial support is an essential part of care since stress is an important cause of secondary enuresis. Provide emotional support to the parents and child, and encourage the child's participation in the treatment plan. Refer the child for counseling or therapy if appropriate.

Assess the parents' and child's motivation and readiness for interventions. Before parents buy an enuresis alarm, suggest they use an alarm clock in the child's room for several nights to see if the child will arouse. Find out whether the child shares a room with others who will be disturbed by the alarm. Ask if the child and parents are willing to persist with an enuresis alarm, as it may take months to work. Evaluation of nursing care includes families choosing the intervention best for them, and an increase in the number of dry nights.

<table>
<tr><td colspan="2">**TABLE 52–3 ✤ Treatment Approaches for Enuresis**</td></tr>
<tr><td>**Approach**</td><td>**Description**</td></tr>
<tr><td>Fluid restriction</td><td>Fluid intake is limited in the evening and before the child goes to bed.</td></tr>
<tr><td>Bladder exercises</td><td>The child drinks a large amount and then holds urine as long as he or she can. The child practices stopping voiding midstream. Exercises should continue for at least 6 months.</td></tr>
<tr><td>Timed voiding</td><td>The child with diurnal enuresis is instructed to void every 2 hours and to use a double voiding pattern; this trains the bladder to empty completely and avoid overdistention.</td></tr>
<tr><td>Enuresis alarms</td><td>A detector strip is attached to the child's pants. The alarm sounds a buzzer that alerts the child when wetting occurs, so the child can get up and finish voiding in the bathroom. This works best for children over 7 years old, and takes 3 to 4 months for success.</td></tr>
<tr><td>Reward system</td><td>Set realistic goals for the child and reinforce dry days or nights with stars and stickers on a chart.</td></tr>
<tr><td>Medications</td><td>Imipramine is prescribed nightly for 2 to 4 months and then tapered over several months to reduce the rate of relapse. It is effective in 50% to 70% of children. Desmopressin is prescribed to children with nocturnal enuresis for special events such as camp or sleepovers. Oxybutynin is used for diurnal enuresis to relieve urgency and frequency from bladder irritability.</td></tr>
</table>

RENAL DISORDERS

NEPHROTIC SYNDROME

Nephrotic syndrome refers not to a specific disease, but rather to a clinical state characterized by edema, massive proteinuria, hypoalbuminemia, hypoproteinemia, hyperlipidemia, and altered immunity. Congenital nephrotic (CNF) syndrome, an autosomal recessive disorder, is extremely rare. The CNF gene is localized on the long arm of chromosome 19 (19q 13.1) (Goodyer & Kashtan, 1998). Primary nephrotic syndrome results from a disease that affects only the kidney, such as glomerulonephritis.

Approximately 85% of children with nephrotic syndrome have a type of primary disease called minimal change nephrotic syndrome (MCNS) (Huether, 2002). MCNS usually occurs in children between the ages of 2 and 7 years, with an incidence of 2 per 100,000 children, and it is more common in males than females. African-American and Hispanic children experience a greater incidence of nephrotic syndrome, and the disorder in these children is more virulent, progresses more rapidly to renal failure, and has a poorer prognosis (Robinson, Nahata, Mahan et al.,

2003). MCNS derives its name from the normal or only minimally changed appearance of the glomeruli on light microscopic evaluation. Because MCNS is the most common form of nephrotic syndrome, it is the focus of the following discussion.

ETIOLOGY AND PATHOPHYSIOLOGY

The cause of primary MCNS is unknown, but an immune system role is strongly suspected because an upper respiratory infection often precedes the onset of edema by 2 to 3 days (Robinson et al., 2003). The mechanism of increased glomerular permeability is unknown as the glomeruli appear normal; however, it may be related to the loss of a negative charge in the glomerular capillary wall (Huether, 2002). In MCNS increased permeability of the glomerular membrane permits large, negatively charged molecules such as albumin to pass through the membrane and be excreted in the urine. Proteinuria results in decreased oncotic pressure and edema, because fluid remains in the interstitial spaces instead of being pulled back into the vascular compartment (Robinson et al., 2003). Immunoglobulins are lost, resulting in altered immunity. Loss of protein in the urine, insufficient albumin production by the liver, and a decreased albumin concentration as a result of salt and water retention by the kidney contribute to hypoalbuminemia. Hypercoagulability occurs because of loss of antithrombin III in the urine and reduced levels of factors IX, XI, and XII. The liver, stimulated perhaps by hypoalbuminemia or decreased osmotic pressure, responds by increasing synthesis of lipoprotein, resulting in hyperlipidemia.

CLINICAL MANIFESTATIONS

In most children, edema develops gradually over several weeks. Children may have a history of periorbital edema on waking that resolves during the day as fluid shifts to the abdomen and lower extremities. Other signs include snug fit of clothing and shoes, pallor, hypertension, irritability, anorexia, hematuria, decreased urine output, and nonspecific malaise. The child's urine may be frothy or foamy. Parents often do not seek medical treatment until generalized edema develops on the child's extremities, abdomen, or genitals (Figure 52–4 ●). Respiratory distress from pleural effusion may occur in some cases.

Massive edema resulting in a dramatic weight gain and abdominal pain, with or without vomiting, may occur, depending on the amount of albumin lost and the amount of sodium ingested. The child becomes malnourished as a result of protein loss in the urine. The skin is pale and shiny with prominent veins, and the hair becomes more brittle. An increased risk of thrombosis is present.

● **FIGURE 52–4**

This boy has generalized edema, a characteristic finding in nephrotic syndrome.

CLINICAL THERAPY

Diagnosis is based on the history, characteristic symptoms, and laboratory findings. Serum albumin and sodium are decreased. Serum blood urea nitrogen (BUN), cholesterol, and electrolytes may be ordered. Urinalysis reveals massive proteinuria (50 mg/kg/day), the primary indicator of nephrotic syndrome. Microscopic hematuria may also be present. Renal ultrasound and a renal biopsy may be performed in some cases.

NURSING PRACTICE

A protein-to-creatinine (PR/CR) ratio of the first morning void is used to estimate protein excretion in children because of the challenges in obtaining 24-hour urines. Normal PR/CR ratios are less than 0.2 in children over 2 years and less than 0.5 in children 6 months to 24 months of age (Hogg, Furth, Lemley, et al., 2003).

Children may be hospitalized when severe edema or a major infection is present, but are usually treated as outpatients. Clinical therapy focuses on decreasing proteinuria, relieving edema, managing associated symptoms, improving nutrition, and preventing infection. A corticosteroid (such as prednisone) is prescribed to decrease proteinuria. In most children, urine protein levels fall to trace or negative values within 2 to 3 weeks of the start of therapy. Children who respond successfully to therapy continue to take corticosteroids daily for 6 weeks, and then 6 weeks of alternate-day treatment. Approximately 90% of children experience complete remission with corticosteroid therapy.

DRUG GUIDE

PREDNISONE

Overview of Action

Natural or synthetic, intermediate-acting glucocorticoid that has strong anti-inflammatory, immunosuppressant, and metabolic actions. Treats diseases such as renal, connective tissue, dermatologic, allergy, acute leukemia, and respiratory distress syndrome.

Routes, Dosage, Frequency

PO:

- 0.5 to 2 mg/kg/day in equally divided doses 4 times a day (maximum dose 80 mg/day).

- Nephrosis: 2 mg/kg/dose 1 to 3 times per day until urine is protein free for 5 days or for 28-day course (maximum of 80 mg/day). For persistent proteinuria may increase to 4 mg/kg/dose every other day for additional 28 days. Maintenance: 2 mg/kg/dose every other day for 28 days. To discontinue: taper over 4 to 6 weeks (Hogg, Portman, Milliner et al., 2000).

- Asthma: Acute: 1 to 2 mg/kg/day in 1 to 2 divided doses for 3 to 5 days, or under 1 year, 10 mg every 12 hours; 1 to 4 years, 20 mg every 12 hours; 5 to 13 years, 30 mg every 12 hours; over 13 years, 40 mg every 12 hours (maximum dose of 60 mg/day). Severe: 5 to 10 mg/day or 10 to 30 mg every other day, taper to aerosol corticosteroids.

    Note: Dosage is based on child's response to drug and severity of condition rather than strictly on weight or body surface.

    Contraindications: Hypersensitivity to the drug and systemic fungal infection.

    Side Effects: Usually dependent upon dosage and duration of treatment, but includes possible growth suppression, hypertension, hyperglycemia, peptic ulcer, congestive heart failure, psychotic behavior, increased appetite, impaired wound healing, and cushingoid features.

Nursing Implications

- *Assess:* Obtain baseline weight and height, blood pressure, intake and output ratio and pattern. Take the blood pressure twice a day during initial stabilization period and report an ascending pattern. Obtain a fasting glucose, electrolytes, and routine laboratory studies at regular intervals.

- *Administer:* PO: It is best to give a daily dose before 9 a.m. Alternate-day therapy is recommended to reduce growth-retarding effects. Give with food or milk to reduce gastrointestinal irritation. Tablets can be crushed and mixed with small amounts of food or fluid. Tablets are very bitter. If child is able to swallow capsules, they can be placed in a gelatin capsule. Follow with fluid of choice to cleanse child's palate.

- *Monitor:* Carefully assess child's response to drug to determine need for dosage adjustments. Observe for side effects, especially hypocalcemia, signs of adrenal insufficiency, symptoms of infection, or worsening of condition. Monitor blood pressure and daily weights; report any sudden weight gain to the physician. With long-term usage, monitor serum electrolytes, height (to evaluate impact of medication on growth), and bone density. Encourage a well-balanced diet low in sodium, and encourage good hygiene and dental care (possible oral fungal infections). To discontinue the medication, reduce the dose gradually, especially after long-term use, so it does not cause acute life-threatening adrenal insufficiency.

- *Patient Teaching:* Do not alter dose or stop medication abruptly as it could cause serious side effects or even death. Gradual tapering of dosage is necessary. Increasing the amount of medication will not speed the healing process. Monitor signs and symptoms of medication reactions, report signs of gastrointestinal distress, symptoms of adrenal insufficiency, or worsening of condition to physician. Obtain weekly weights; report a weight gain of 2 kg (5 lb) to physician. Stress importance of close medical supervision and follow-up. Get regular ophthalmologic examinations if on long-term therapy. Live vaccine immunizations should not be given when on high doses of corticosteroids. Inform any healthcare provider, including dentists, surgeons, or emergency care personnel, that child is on medication. Child should carry medical identification card. Observe for symptoms of infection. Do not use over-the-counter medications unless approved by the healthcare provider.

Data from Bindler, R. M., Howry, L. B., Wilson, B. A., et al. (2005). Pediatric drugs and nursing implications. Upper Saddle River, NJ: Prentice Hall-Health.

Relapses commonly happen with a respiratory infection or live virus immunizations; however, relapses become less frequent or stop during puberty. Children who have a relapse after drug therapy is discontinued get repeat therapy. Other medications used include diuretics, antihypertensive agents, and antibiotics. Alkylating agents (cyclophosphamide and chlorambucil) or cyclosporine may be used when nephrotic syndrome is resistant to corticosteroids. Since diuretics can precipitate hypovolemia, hyponatremia, and hypokalemia, electrolyte levels should be carefully monitored. Intravenous administration of albumin may occasionally be ordered in the child with massive edema who is resistant to diuretics (Robinson et al., 2003). Analgesics may be ordered for pain related to edema or flank pain from a urinary tract infection.

A normal diet for the child's age is recommended. No attempt should be made either to restrict or to increase protein intake. A "no added salt" diet is recommended during corticosteroid treatment as these children have an elevated total body sodium even though serum sodium concentrations are low (Hogg, Portman, Milliner et al., 2000).

NURSING MANAGEMENT

NURSING ASSESSMENT AND DIAGNOSES

Physiologic Assessment

Careful assessment of the child's hydration status and edema is essential. Carefully monitor intake and output. Weigh the child daily using the same scale, and measure abdominal girth to monitor changes in edema and ascites (see Skill 9–7 **SKILLS**). Monitor vital signs every 4 hours to watch for signs of respiratory distress, hypertension, or circulatory overload. Test urine for proteinuria and specific gravity at least once each shift. Assess for hypovolemia during periods of diuresis. Assess for skin breakdown.

Psychosocial Assessment

Children and parents are often fearful or anxious on admission. Because edema often develops gradually, parents may feel guilty if they did not seek medical attention immediately. School-age children with generalized edema are often concerned about their appearance. Careful questioning may be necessary to elicit these concerns. The child hospitalized for a recurrence of nephrotic syndrome may be frustrated or depressed. Assess individual and family coping mechanisms, support systems, and level of stress.

Common nursing diagnoses for the child with MCNS include the following:

- *Risk for Infection* related to immunosuppressive therapy
- *Risk for Impaired Skin Integrity* related to edema, lowered resistance to infection and injury, immobility, and malnutrition
- *Excess Fluid Volume* related to renal dysfunction and sodium retention
- *Imbalanced Nutrition: Less than Body Requirements* related to loss of appetite and protein loss in urine
- *Fatigue* related to fluid and electrolyte imbalance, albumin loss, altered nutrition, and renal failure
- *Deficient Diversional Activity* related to fatigue, immobility, and social isolation

PLANNING AND IMPLEMENTATION

Nursing care is mainly supportive and focuses on administering medications, preventing infection, preventing skin breakdown, meeting nutritional and fluid needs, promoting rest, and providing emotional support to the parents and child.

Administer Medications

It is important to give prescribed medications at the scheduled times. Watch for side effects of corticosteroids such as moon face, increased appetite, increased hair growth, abdominal distention, and mood swings, as well as adverse effects such as hypertension, nausea, and hyperglycemia. If the child is receiving albumin intravenously, monitor closely for hypertension or signs of volume overload caused by fluid shifts. If diuretics are used, observe for shock. The child may need to have albumin infused simultaneously with diuretics.

Prevent Infection

Children with MCNS are at risk for infection because of the loss of immunoglobulins in the urine and corticosteroid therapy. Careful handwashing is important. Use standard precautions. Strict aseptic technique is essential during invasive procedures. Monitor the child's white blood cell count when cytotoxic drugs are given as bone marrow suppression is a side effect. Monitor vital signs carefully to detect early signs of infection that may be masked by corticosteroid therapy. Decrease the child's social contacts during immunosuppressive treatment, and caution parents and children to avoid exposure to people with respiratory infections and communicable diseases. Emphasize the importance of avoiding shopping malls, sporting arenas, grocery stores, game stores, and other public areas where the risk of exposure to such infections is increased.

Prevent Skin Breakdown

Meticulous skin care is essential to prevent skin breakdown and potential infection. Assess the skin repeatedly, turn the child frequently, and use therapeutic mattresses (e.g., egg crate, airflow) to help prevent skin breakdown. Keep the skin clean and dry.

Meet Nutritional and Fluid Needs

Keep the child's food preferences in mind when planning menus. Encourage the child to eat by presenting attractive meals with small portions. Socialization during meals may improve the child's appetite. Fluids are not usually restricted except during severe edema.

Promote Rest

Provide opportunities for quiet play as tolerated, such as drawing, playing board games, listening to tapes, and watching videos. Adjust the child's daily schedule to allow rest periods after activities. Signs of fatigue may include irritability, mood swings, or withdrawal. Tell the parents and child about the importance of rest. Limiting visitors during the acute phase of the illness may be necessary. Telephone and computer contacts may be encouraged as an alternative to visitors. To provide a sense of control, encourage the child to set his or her own limits on activity.

Provide Emotional Support

Parents and children often need support to cope with this chronic disease. Thoroughly explain the child's disease and treatment regimen to parents. Parental anxiety in combination with the hospitalization may interfere with the child's independence. Help parents promote the child's independence by allowing the child to choose from the menu or to select the daily activity schedule. This gives the child some sense of control.

Children with MCNS may have a distorted body image because of sudden weight gain and edema. They may refuse to look in the mirror, refuse to participate in care, and take less interest in their appearance. Encourage children to express their feelings. Help them maintain a normal appearance by promoting normal grooming routines. Encourage children to wear their own pajamas rather than hospital gowns. Scarves or hats may be used to lessen the child's edematous appearance. Adolescents can be encouraged to write their feelings in a journal as a coping mechanism.

Discharge Planning and Home Care Teaching

Explain the disease process, prognosis, and treatment plan to parents and school-age children. Make sure parents know how to administer medications and can identify potential side effects. Inform parents about restricting fluid intake until the edema resolves. Instruct parents about the need to monitor urine daily for protein, and have them keep a diary to record results. Monitoring the child's weight each week may help identify early stages of fluid retention. This helps parents to spot a relapse before edema occurs.

Tutoring may be required for a short period after discharge. However, encourage parents to allow the child to return to normal activities once the acute episode has resolved. Emphasize the importance of avoiding contact with people with infectious diseases, because of the child's reduced immunity. Reinforce to parents that it is important to follow the "no added salt" diet as long as the child is receiving corticosteroid therapy or shows signs of MCNS. Warn them that steroids stimulate appetite, so they need to control the child's food intake and weight gain. No live immunizations should be given to the child who is relapsing or taking corticosteroid therapy. Withhold immunizations until 6 months after the completion of corticosteroid therapy. Although immunizations may trigger a relapse, pneumococcal vaccine and other immunizations are important to protect the child from serious preventable infections.

Most children do well with corticosteroid therapy; however, relapses are common. Even children with frequent relapses usually have a spontaneous resolution of MCNS before 30 years of age.

EVALUATION

Expected outcomes of nursing care include:

- The child responds to corticosteroid therapy.
- Dietary guidelines of "no added salt" are followed and food intake is controlled during corticosteroid therapy.
- Relapses are identified by parents before edema occurs.
- The child receives the additional recommended immunizations.

A discussion of Wilms' tumor can be found in Chapter 50. ∞

RENAL FAILURE

Renal failure, which may be acute or chronic, occurs when the kidney is unable to excrete wastes and concentrate urine. Acute renal failure occurs suddenly (over days or weeks) and may be reversible, whereas in chronic renal failure, kidney function diminishes gradually and permanently over months or years.

Both types of renal failure are characterized by **azotemia** (accumulation of nitrogenous wastes in the blood) and sometimes **oliguria** (urine output less than 0.5 to 1 mL/kg/hr), indicating the kidney's inability to excrete metabolic waste products. The degree of renal impairment is estimated by the glomerular filtration rate (Hogg, Furth, Lemley et al., 2003). **Uremia** occurs when there is an excess of urea and other nitrogenous waste products in the blood.

ACUTE RENAL FAILURE

Acute renal failure (ARF), in which kidney function abruptly diminishes, is characterized by a rapid rise in the BUN level. The kidneys are also unable to regulate extracellular fluid volume, sodium balance, and acid-base homeostasis. ARF is seen in 2% to 3% of children cared for in pediatric intensive care units, and up to 8% of infants cared for in neonatal intensive care units (Vogt & Avner, 2004). Potential causes include sepsis, poisoning, hemolytic uremic syndrome, hypovolemia, obstructive uropathy, and complication of cardiac surgery.

ETIOLOGY AND PATHOPHYSIOLOGY

ARF may be caused by prerenal or postrenal factors as well as actual kidney damage. Prerenal ARF is a result of decreased perfusion to an otherwise normal kidney in association with a systemic condition. Hypovolemia (hemorrhage or dehydration), septic shock, or cardiac failure may precipitate prerenal ARF. This is the most common type of ARF in infants and young children.

PATHOPHYSIOLOGY ILLUSTRATED
Acute Renal Failure

Ischemia (e.g., sepsis, trauma, hypotension)
Nephrotoxins (e.g., aminoglycosides)

Possible glomerular injury

Decreased permeability and decreased surface area

Tubular injury with sloughing of cells

Cast formation

Vasoconstriction

Tubular back leak

Obstruction

Proximal tubular reabsorption increased

Decreased intrarenal blood flow

Increased intraluminal pressure

Decreased GFR

Oliguria

The initial kidney injury is usually associated with an acute condition such as sepsis, trauma, and hypotension, or the result of treatment for an acute condition with a nephrotoxic medication. Injury to the kidney can occur because of glomerular injury, vasoconstriction of capillaries, or tubular injury. All consequences of injury lead to decreased glomerular filtration and oliguria.

ARF resulting from primary kidney damage (intrinsic) may be caused by infection, diseases such as hemolytic-uremic syndrome or acute glomerulonephritis, cortical necrosis, nephrotoxic drugs, or accidental ingestion of drugs or poisons. The structure most susceptible to damage is the kidney tubule. Injury to the tubule resulting in acute tubular necrosis is the most frequent cause of intrinsic renal failure in children.

Postrenal ARF is caused by obstruction of the urinary flow from both kidneys, such as occurs in posterior urethral valves or a neurogenic bladder. Children may have oliguria, or normal or increased urine output. Renal failure

NURSING PRACTICE

Nephrotoxic drugs include the following:

- Antimicrobials: aminoglycosides, cephalosporins, tetracycline, sulfonamides
- Radiographic contrast media with iodine
- Heavy metals: lead, barium, iron
- Nonsteroidal anti-inflammatory drugs: indomethacin, aspirin

without oliguria usually indicates a less severe renal injury. Children who recover from ARF may have residual kidney damage and compromised renal function.

CLINICAL MANIFESTATIONS

Characteristically, a healthy child suddenly becomes ill with nonspecific symptoms that indicate a significant illness or injury (e.g., nausea, vomiting, lethargy, edema, gross hematuria, oliguria, and hypertension). These symptoms are a result of electrolyte imbalances, uremia, and fluid overload. The child appears pale and lethargic. See the "Clinical Manifestations" tables for more information.

CLINICAL MANIFESTATIONS

ACUTE VERSUS CHRONIC RENAL FAILURE

TYPE OF RENAL FAILURE	CLINICAL MANIFESTATIONS
Acute renal failure	Gross hematuria, headache, edema, crackles, gallop heart rhythm, hypertension, hematuria, lethargy, nausea and vomiting, oliguria Mass in flank area if a cyst, tumor, or obstructive lesion is present
Chronic renal failure	Fatigue, malaise, poor appetite, nausea and vomiting, failure to thrive or short stature Headache, decreased mental alertness or ability to concentrate Secondary enuresis, chronic anemia, hypertension, edema Fractures with minimal trauma, rickets, valgus deformity

CLINICAL MANIFESTATIONS

ELECTROLYTE IMBALANCES IN ACUTE AND CHRONIC RENAL FAILURE

ELECTROLYTE IMBALANCE AND CAUSE	CLINICAL MANIFESTATIONS
Hyperkalemia Results from inability to adequately excrete potassium derived from diet and catabolized cells. In metabolic acidosis, potassium also moves from intracellular fluid to extracellular fluid.	- Peaked T waves, widening of QRS waves on ECG. - Dysrhythmias: ventricular dysrhythmias, heart block, ventricular fibrillation, cardiac arrest - Diarrhea - Muscle weakness
Hyponatremia In the acute oliguric phase, hyponatremia is related to the accumulation of fluid in excess of solute.	- Change in level of consciousness - Muscle cramps - Anorexia - Abdominal reflexes, depressed deep tendon reflexes - Cheyne-Stokes respirations - Seizures
Hypocalcemia Phosphate retention (hyperphosphatemia) due to impaired renal function depresses the serum calcium concentration. Calcium is deposited in injured cells. Hyperkalemia and metabolic acidosis may mask the common clinical manifestations of severe hypocalcemia.	- Muscle tingling - Changes in muscle tone - Seizures - Muscle cramps and twitching - Positive **Chvostek sign** (contraction of facial muscles after tapping facial nerve just anterior to parotid gland)

Hyperkalemia is the most life-threatening electrolyte disorder associated with ARF. Hyponatremia affects central nervous system function, resulting in symptoms that range from fatigue to seizures. Edema occurs as a result of sodium and water retention. (Refer to Chapter 43 for a discussion of these fluid and electrolyte alterations. ∞) Children with ARF are also more susceptible to infection because of depressed immune functioning.

CLINICAL THERAPY

Diagnosis of renal failure is based primarily on urinalysis and blood chemistry results, including BUN, serum creatinine, sodium, potassium, and calcium levels (Table 52–4). The kidneys are normal in size, and no signs of renal **osteodystrophy** (increased resorption of bone caused by chronic hyperparathyroidism) are found on x-ray. Various imaging studies to assess kidney structures, renal blood flow, and renal perfusion and function may be performed to determine whether the child has ARF or chronic renal failure. A renal biopsy may be required.

Treatment depends on the underlying cause of the renal failure. The goal is to minimize or prevent permanent renal damage while maintaining fluid and electrolyte balance and managing complications. Initial emergency treatment of children with fluid depletion focuses on rapid fluid replacement at 20 mL/kg of saline or lactated Ringer's solution given over 5 to 10 minutes and repeated as needed to ensure renal perfusion. Albumin may also be administered when blood loss is the cause of circulatory depletion. If oliguria persists after restoration of adequate fluid volume, intrinsic renal damage is suspected.

Children with fluid overload, like those with pulmonary edema, need diuretic therapy, and dialysis if they respond poorly to diuretics. Fluid requirements are calculated to maintain *zero water balance* (intake should equal output). Eliminate all potential sources of potassium intake until hyperkalemia is controlled (see Chapter 43 ∞). Other electrolyte imbalances are treated. Nutrition must be maintained with extra carbohydrate intake during the catabolic state. Antibiotics are prescribed for infection. Nephrotoxic antibiotics such as aminoglycosides are avoided (Table 52–5).

Children whose ARF is unresponsive to management require dialysis to correct severe electrolyte imbalances, manage fluid overload, and cleanse the blood of waste products. The clinical situation and age of the child determine whether hemodialysis or peritoneal dialysis is used. Refer to the "Renal Replacement Therapy" section on page 1653.

Prognosis depends on the cause of ARF. When renal failure results from drug toxicity or dehydration, the prognosis is generally good. However, ARF that results from diseases such as hemolytic-uremic syndrome or acute glomerulonephritis may be associated with residual kidney damage.

NURSING MANAGEMENT

NURSING ASSESSMENT AND DIAGNOSES

A complete history and physical examination are necessary to identify progression of symptoms and possible causes for renal failure.

Physiologic Assessment

Assess vital signs, level of consciousness, and other neurologic indicators to help identify clinical signs of electrolyte imbalance (see "Clinical Manifestations: Electrolyte Imbalances in Acute and Chronic Renal Failure" on page 1645). Measure the child's weight on admission to provide a baseline for evaluating changes in fluid status. Monitor urinalysis, urine culture, and blood chemistry studies. Inspect urine for color (Figure 52–5 ●). Cloudy urine may indicate infection; tea-colored urine suggests hematuria. Assess urine specific gravity and intake and output.

Psychosocial Assessment

The unexpected and acute nature of the child's hospitalization creates anxiety for both parents and child. Assess for feel-

TABLE 52–4 ✥ Diagnostic Tests for Renal Failure

Test	Normal Values	Findings in Renal Failure
Urinalysis		
pH	4.5–8	Lowered
Osmolarity	50–1400 mOsm/L	> 500 prenal < 350 intrinsic
Specific gravity	1.001–1.030	High: prerenal ARF Low: intrinsic ARF Normal: postrenal ARF
Protein	Negative	Positive
Blood Chemistry		
Potassium	3.5–5.8 mmol/L	Elevated
Sodium	135–148 mmol/L	Normal, low, or high, depends solely on the amount of water in the body
Calcium	2.2–2.7 mmol/L	Low
Phosphorus	1.23–2 mmol/L	High
Urea nitrogen	3.5–7.1 mmol/L	Increased
Creatinine	0.2–0.9 mmol/L	Increased
pH	7.38–7.42	Low acidic

ARF: acute renal failure

TABLE 52–5 ✣ Medications Used to Treat Complications of Acute Renal Failure

Complication	Medication	Action or Indication	Nursing Implications
Hyperkalemia (> 5.8 mmol/L)	Kayexalate Calcium gluconate 10%	Exchanges sodium for potassium Counteracts potassium-induced increased myocardial irritability	May require up to 4 hours to take effect. Monitor for ECG changes. Intravenous infiltration may result in tissue necrosis.
	Albuterol	Shifts potassium to the cells	Give by aerosol.
Metabolic acidosis	Sodium bicarbonate or sodium citrate	Helps correct metabolic acidosis by exchanging hydrogen for potassium	*Do not mix with calcium.* Complications include fluid overload, hypertension, and tetany.
Hypocalcemia (< 2.2 mmol/L)	Calcium gluconate 10%	Used in presence of tetany; provides ionized calcium to restore nervous tissue function to control serum phosphorus	Administer slowly to prevent bradycardia. Monitor for ECG changes.
Malignant hypertension (blood pressure > 95% for age, sex, and height percentile)	Sodium nitroprusside, nitroglycerin	Relaxes smooth muscle in peripheral arterioles	Administer by continuous intravenous infusion; fall in blood pressure is seen within 10–20 minutes.

● **FIGURE 52–5**

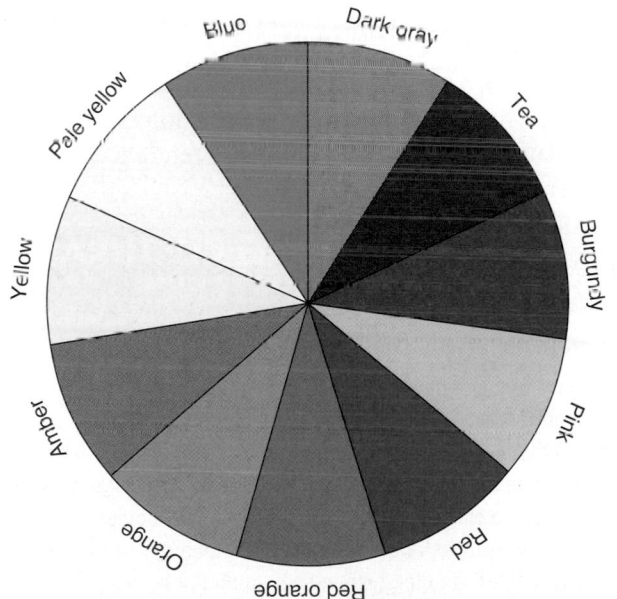

A color wheel, such as the one shown here, can be used as a guide in standardizing descriptions of urine color. Normal urine is pale yellow. Changes in urine color can indicate the following alterations: *yellow*—concentrated urine; *amber*—bile in urine; *orange*—alkaline or concentrated urine; *red-orange*—acid pH, medications; *red*—blood, menses; *pink*—dilute blood; *burgundy*—laxatives; *tea*—melanin, hematuria; *dark gray*—medications, dyes; *blues*—dyes, medications.

Used with permission from Cooper, C. (1993). What color is that urine specimen? American Journal of Nursing, 93, 37 Copyright © 1993 Connie Cooper, R.N., M.S.N.; graphics by Mike O'Grady, R.N., M.S.N.

ings of anger, guilt, or fear associated with the hospitalization. Such feelings are likely if ARF developed as a result of dehydration, a preventable injury, or poisoning. Assess coping mechanisms, family support systems, and level of stress.

Several nursing diagnoses may apply to the child with ARF, including the following:

- *Ineffective Renal Tissue Perfusion* related to hypovolemia, sepsis, or drug toxicity
- *Excess Fluid Volume* related to renal dysfunction and sodium retention
- *Imbalanced Nutrition: Less than Body Requirements* related to anorexia, nausea, vomiting, and catabolic state
- *Risk for Infection* related to invasive procedures and monitoring equipment, and diminished immune functioning
- *Compromised Family Coping* related to sudden hospitalization and uncertain prognosis of child

PLANNING AND IMPLEMENTATION

Nursing care focuses on preventing complications, maintaining fluid balance, administering medications, meeting nutritional needs, preventing infection, and providing emotional support to the child and parents.

Prevent Complications

Complications are best prevented by ensuring compliance with the treatment plan. Careful monitoring of vital signs,

MEDIALINK Care Plan: Child with Kidney Failure

intake and output, serum electrolytes, and level of consciousness can alert the nurse to changes that indicate potential complications. For example, if the serum sodium concentration rises and weight falls, insufficient fluids are being administered. If the serum sodium level falls and the weight increases, excessive fluids are being administered.

Maintain Fluid Balance

Estimate the child's fluid status by daily monitoring the weight (on the same scale at same time of day), intake and output, and blood pressure readings taken two or three times a day. Also monitor serum chemistry values, especially for sodium. The aim of maintaining fluid balance is to achieve a stable serum sodium concentration and a decrease in body weight by 0.5% to 1% a day.

If the child has oliguria, limit fluid intake, including parenteral nutrition, to replacement of insensible fluid loss (excreted by the lungs, skin, and gastrointestinal tract) which is about one third the daily maintenance requirements in afebrile children. If the child is febrile, fluid administration is increased by 12% for each centigrade degree of temperature elevation. The child with **renal insufficiency** (i.e., as the kidneys' ability to conserve sodium and concentrate the urine decreases) is at greater risk for fluid loss with illness. In cases of acute gastrointestinal illness, children are at greater risk for dehydration.

Administer Medications

Because the kidney's ability to excrete drugs is impaired in ARF, dosages of all medications should be adjusted. The actual dosage of the drug can be reduced or the time interval between doses may be increased. Check drug levels to monitor for drug toxicity. Know the signs of drug toxicity for each medication the child is receiving.

Meet Nutritional Needs

Children are at risk for malnutrition because of their high metabolic rate during ARF. Parenteral or enteral feeding may be used initially to minimize protein catabolism. The diet is tailored to the individual child's need for calories, carbohydrates, fats, and amino acids or protein hydrolysates. Depending on the degree of renal failure, sodium, potassium, and phosphorus may be restricted. Initiate oral feeding as soon as the child can tolerate it.

Prevent Infection

The child with ARF is extremely susceptible to nosocomial infections because of altered nutritional status, compromised immunity, and numerous invasive procedures. Thorough handwashing and standard precautions are imperative to decrease the risk of infection. Use sterile technique for all invasive procedures and when caring for lines. Drainage from catheter sites should be cultured to check for the presence of infectious organisms. Assess vital signs and lung sounds frequently.

Provide Emotional Support

The sudden onset of ARF presents parents with an unexpected threat to their child's life. Both the child and the parents experience anxiety because of the unexpected hospitalization and the uncertainty of the prognosis. Parents often feel guilty, regardless of the cause of renal failure. This guilt is intensified when renal failure is a result of dehydration or poisoning. Encourage parents to verbalize their fears and help them work through feelings of guilt. Explain procedures and treatment measures to decrease anxiety. Encouraging parents and older siblings to participate in the child's care can increase their sense of control.

Discharge Planning and Home Care Teaching

Encourage parental involvement early in the child's hospitalization. Be sure parents understand the importance of administering medications correctly. Teach family members proper technique for measuring blood pressure so they can monitor the child's hypertension, if ordered. Make sure the parents can identify signs of progressive renal failure (see the following chronic renal failure discussion).

Diet counseling is a key component of discharge planning and is usually performed by a renal dietitian. Depending on the degree of renal failure, the child's diet may include restrictions on protein, water, sodium, potassium, and phosphorus. The parents should be given written guidelines listing appropriate food choices to assist in menu planning. Ethnic and cultural preferences should be considered in listing menu options.

DEVELOPING CULTURAL COMPETENCE

REDUCING SODIUM IN THE CHILD'S DIET

Special effort is often needed to reduce the sodium in the diet of an Asian child. Sauces and seasonings for foods (soy sauce, mustards, monosodium glutamate, and garlic salt) are sodium rich even though the foods seasoned (rice, vegetables, shrimp, and chicken) are low in sodium. The child may ingest up to 18 grams of sodium a day with these added sauces and seasonings; 4 grams per day is the goal. The typical Mexican diet, high in sodium and potassium (avocados, tomatoes, beans), may also require significant modification. Individualized counseling and motivation are needed to encourage families to reduce the child's sodium intake and to use spices low in sodium when preparing meals.

Continued monitoring of renal function during follow-up examinations is critical as deterioration may occur over time. Referral to support groups can be helpful for both parents and children. The National Kidney Foundation is a source of numerous publications.

EVALUATION

Expected outcomes of nursing care include:

- The child's fluid status is balanced with edema-associated weight loss. Electrolyte and acid-base balance is restored.
- Nutritional needs are met.
- The child acquires no secondary infections.

CHRONIC RENAL FAILURE

Chronic renal failure (CRF) is a progressive, irreversible reduction in kidney function. The prevalence of CRF is approximately 18 per 1 million children (Vogt & Avner, 2004). Blacks have a higher rate of end-stage renal disease than whites by a ratio of 2.7:1 (Balinsky, 2000).

ETIOLOGY AND PATHOPHYSIOLOGY

In children, CRF usually results from developmental abnormalities of the kidney or obstructed urine flow and reflux, hereditary diseases such as polycystic kidney disease, infections such as hemolytic-uremic syndrome, and glomerulonephritis. (See discussions later in the chapter.)

The gradual, progressive loss of functioning nephrons ultimately results in **end-stage renal disease (ESRD)**. ESRD is characterized by minimal renal function (less than 10% of normal), uremic syndrome, anemia, and abnormal blood values. In ESRD, the kidneys can no longer maintain homeostasis and the child requires dialysis.

The kidneys excrete excess acid in the body and regulate the body's fluid and electrolyte balance. Renal failure disrupts this fluid and electrolyte balance. As renal failure progresses, metabolic acidosis occurs because the kidneys cannot excrete the acids that build up in the body. Retention of excessive sodium and water is a common cause of the elevated blood pressure associated with CRF. Insufficient calcium loss, phosphorus retention, and elevated parathyroid hormone levels lead to renal osteodystrophy. Osteodystrophy increases the child's risk for spontaneous fractures and rickets. Growth retardation is caused by disturbances in the metabolism of calcium, phosphorus, and vitamin D; decreased caloric intake; and metabolic acidosis. The kidneys also produce erythropoietin (the growth factor responsible for the production and maturation of red cells); lack of erythropoietin and progressive renal disease are the underlying causes of the anemia of CRF.

CLINICAL MANIFESTATIONS

Children with CRF frequently have no symptoms initially. Early renal failure with glomerular filtration rate (GFR) of 50% to 75% of normal has few or no clinical signs. As pro-

gression continues, renal insufficiency occurs with polyuria as the kidneys cannot concentrate the urine. Symptoms become more classic as CRF occurs with pallor, headache, nausea, and fatigue. Decreased mental alertness and ability to concentrate may be seen. The child may have anemia leading to tachycardia, tachypnea, and dyspnea on exertion. As the disease progresses, the child loses his or her appetite and has complications of renal impairment, including hypertension, pulmonary edema, growth retardation, osteodystrophy, delayed fine and gross motor development, and delayed sexual maturation. See the contrast with signs of acute renal failure on page 1645.

In ESRD, the most advanced form of CRF, renal failure adversely affects all body systems. As the severity of the clinical and biochemical disturbances resulting from progressive renal deterioration increases, uremic symptoms develop. Signs and symptoms of uremic syndrome include nausea and vomiting, progressive anemia, anorexia, dyspnea, malaise, uremic frost (urea crystals deposited on the skin), unpleasant (uremic) breath odor, headache, progressive confusion, tremors, pulmonary edema, and congestive heart failure.

CLINICAL THERAPY

Laboratory evaluation, including serum electrolytes, phosphate, BUN, and creatinine levels and pH, is used to confirm the diagnosis of CRF. An early morning urine sample is collected for culture, and to calculate the protein-to-creatinine ratio. The child's glomerular filtration rate is calculated from prediction equations using the serum creatinine level and the patient's height and gender. Imaging studies are performed to identify renal diseases that could be causing the renal failure. A renal biopsy may sometimes be performed.

CRF is irreversible. However, the course of the disease is variable. Some children progress quickly to renal failure, necessitating dialysis. Other children are managed with a combination of medication and diet therapy for some time before significant renal impairment occurs. Frequent modifications in the treatment plan are often necessary to address the child's changing status. The goals of treatment are to slow the progression of renal disease and to prevent complications.

Dietary management focuses on maximizing caloric intake for growth while limiting phosphorus, potassium, and sodium intake as needed to keep electrolytes in balance. Tube feedings or parenteral nutrition may be required to achieve optimal protein intake, especially in children under 1 year of age. When CRF is present, optimal intake of high-quality protein (meat, fish, poultry, and egg whites) for infants is 2 to 2.5 g/kg/day; for older children it is 1.5 to 2 g/kg/day. Vegetable oils, hard candy, sugar, honey, and jelly may be recommended to add calories to the child's diet.

Numerous medications are used to treat children with CRF. See Table 52–6.

MEDIALINK Case Study: A Child with Chronic Kidney Failure

TABLE 52–6 ✤ Medications Commonly Used by Children with Chronic Renal Failure

Medication	Action or Indication	Nursing Considerations
Vitamin and mineral supplement (Nephrocaps)	Add vitamins and minerals missing from heavily restricted diet	Only prescribed vitamins should be used, over-the-counter brands may contain elements that are harmful.
Phosphate binding agents: Calcium carbonate (Tums), calcium acetate (PhosLo), or sevelamer hydrochloride (Renagel)	Reduce absorption of phosphorus from the intestines	Ensure that phosphate binding agent is aluminum-free.
Calcitriol (Rocaltrol)	Replace the calcitriol that kidneys are no longer producing to keep calcium balance normal	Monitor serum calcium level. Ensure that calcium supplement is provided.
Epoetin alfa (Epogen, Procrit)	Stimulates bone marrow to produce red blood cells, treats anemia due to CRF	Given by IV or subcutaneous injection. Monitor blood pressure as hypertension is an adverse effect. Monitor hematocrit and serum ferritin level according to facility guidelines.
Iron supplementation	Treat iron deficiency when epoetin alfa is prescribed	May be administered orally or IV during hemodialysis.
Growth hormone (rhGH)	Used to stimulate growth in children with CRF	Record accurate height measurements at regular intervals.
Antihypertensive agents: Angiotensin-converting enzyme (ACE) inhibitor (enalapril, lisinopril) Loop diuretics	Used with proteinuric kidney disease as it slows the progression to ESRD Used when volume overload is present	Monitor renal function and electrolyte balance.

Children who progress to ESRD require renal replacement therapy. The timetable for dialysis or renal transplantation is different from that of adults; transplantation is the goal so the child has an optimal chance for a more normal childhood. Earlier initiation can prevent some complications of ESRD. In addition to the GFR, nonspecific signs such as uremic syndrome, poorly controlled hypertension, renal osteodystrophy, failure of head circumference measurement to increase normally, developmental delay, and poor growth are used in determining when to initiate therapy. (Refer to the "Renal Replacement Therapy" section in this chapter.) Infection is the most common morbidity in children receiving renal replacement therapy.

NURSING MANAGEMENT

NURSING ASSESSMENT AND DIAGNOSES

Nursing assessment focuses on identifying signs and symptoms of renal failure and associated complications, and assessing the psychosocial effects of renal failure on the child and family.

Physiologic Assessment

The initial and ongoing assessment of the child focuses on identifying complications of renal failure. Observe for signs of hypertension, edema, poor growth and development, osteodystrophy, and anemia. Assess vital signs to help identify electrolyte alterations (see page 1645).

Psychosocial Assessment

As renal disease progresses, the number of stressors on the child and family increases. Denial and disbelief are commonly the first reactions. A thorough family assessment can help to identify particular needs of the child and family (see Appendix H ∞). The development of ESRD is particularly challenging during childhood adolescence because of differences in appearance and social, psychologic, and physical issues. Nonadherence with treatments can endanger the adolescent's life.

Nursing diagnoses for the child with CRF are similar to those previously listed for ARF. Additional diagnoses might include the following:

- *Delayed Growth and Development* related to decreased protein and caloric intake and loss of protein in dialysate
- *Impaired Social Interaction* related to impaired immunity and hemodialysis schedule during school hours
- *Activity Intolerance* related to anemia and fatigue
- *Ineffective Therapeutic Regimen Management* related to complexity of care plan and economic difficulties

TABLE 52–7 ✤ Nutritional Information for the Child with Kidney Disease

Children with kidney disease have restricted diets, generally low in sodium, potassium, and phosphorus. A renal dietitian works with families of children with chronic renal failure to develop meal plans that fit a restricted diet. The nurse can help families remember that certain foods must be avoided or eaten in very small quantities by reviewing this table.

High-Sodium Content Foods	High-Potassium Content Foods	High-Phosphorus Content Foods
Soups and sauces: e.g., gravy, spaghetti and tomato sauce, barbeque sauce, steak sauce	*Fruit:* apricots, avocados, bananas, citrus fruits, fresh pears, nectarines, dates, figs, canteloupe and other melons, prunes, and raisins	*Dairy products:* milk, cheese, yogurt, custard, pudding, ice cream
Processed lunchmeats: e.g., bologna, ham, salami, hot dogs	*Vegetables:* celery, dried beans, lima beans, potatoes, leafy greens, spinach, tomatoes, winter squash	Dried beans, peas
Smoked meat and fish: bacon, chipped beef, corned beef, ham, lox	*Whole grains:* especially those containing bran	Nuts, peanut butter
Sauerkraut, pickles, and other pickled foods	Sardines, clams	Chocolate
Seasonings: horseradish, soy sauce, Worchestershire sauce, meat tenderizer, and monosodium glutamate (MSG)	Peanuts	Dark cola
	Dairy products: milk, ice cream, pudding, yogurt	Sausage, hot dog
	Potassium-containing salt substitutes	

■ *Disturbed Body Image* related to short stature and visible external catheter for dialysis

PLANNING AND IMPLEMENTATION

Hospital-Based Care

Children with CRF are usually hospitalized for one or more of the following reasons: initial diagnostic evaluation, dialysis treatment initiation, problems with the treatment plan, infection, or another problem. Nursing care for the hospitalized child with CRF focuses on monitoring for side effects of medications, preventing infection, meeting nutritional needs, and providing emotional support and anticipatory teaching.

Monitor for Side Effects of Medications

Watch for signs of electrolyte imbalance such as weakness, muscle cramps, dizziness, headache, and nausea and vomiting in children taking diuretics. Supervise the child's activities closely to prevent falls resulting from dizziness, especially at the beginning of diuretic therapy. If antihypertensive medications such as hydralazine are being administered, monitor the child's weight to detect excessive gain resulting from water and sodium retention.

Prevent Infection

The child with CRF is susceptible to infections. Be alert for signs of infection, such as elevated temperature; cloudy, strong-smelling urine; dysuria; changes in respiratory pattern; or productive cough. Emphasize to the child and family the importance of good handwashing practices. Make sure the child receives the 23-valent pneumococcal, and meningococcal vaccines in addition to usual childhood immunizations.

Meet Nutritional Needs

Maintaining adequate nutritional intake in a child with CRF who has dietary restrictions is challenging. Provide small, frequent feedings and present meals attractively to encourage the child to eat. A renal dietitian works with families of children with chronic renal failure to develop meal plans that fit a restricted diet. See Table 52–7 for foods that children with CRF should avoid.

Provide Emotional Support

Progressive CRF requires a total lifestyle change for the child and family. The parents and child need opportunities to express and work through their feelings related to the disease, prognosis, and treatment restrictions. Help children express their feelings through drawings or therapeutic play.

The need for ongoing dialysis treatments and the wait for a suitable donor kidney are stressful for both parents and child. Identify effective coping methods and family support systems to promote treatment compliance. The National Kidney Foundation and local support groups for kidney disease can give the family information or additional support. See the Companion Website for further information and links to these resources. 🌐

Discharge Planning and Home Care Teaching

Parents need to understand the necessity of long-term treatments and follow-up care. Help the family develop a schedule for medication administration that fits with their routine. Emphasize the importance of consistency in administration times. Teach parents how to recognize medication side effects and complications.

Appropriate referrals are made to home care nursing agencies as indicated. Home care nurses teach the parents of the child receiving peritoneal dialysis to perform the treatment and to identify complications, as well as provide necessary support and reassurance see page 1655.

Nursing Care in the Community

Children with CRF require frequent outpatient visits to monitor the progression of signs and symptoms, and to evaluate the effectiveness of current treatments. Blood and urine tests are performed to monitor renal function. Radiographs of the bones are often taken at 6-month intervals to assess changes caused by osteodystrophy.

When assessing the child, compare height, weight, and head circumference to age-specific norms to identify growth retardation and to plot progress. Assess developmental progress using the Denver II or another screening tool (see Chapter 37∞). Assess the adolescent for signs of delayed sexual maturation and, in girls, amenorrhea.

Promote good dentition and oral hygiene. Regular dental visits are important to reduce infections. Make sure the family understands the need for antibiotic prophylaxis before certain invasive procedures, including dental care (see Table 48–5 ∞). If possible, all immunizations should be provided before renal transplantation, as long-term immunosuppressive therapy will then be prescribed. Live vaccines should not be given to the child taking immunosuppressive agents.

Review any dietary restrictions with parents. Provide sample menus for meal planning to help parents incorporate dietary changes into daily meals. A renal dietitian usually helps the child make food selections and restrict fluids and sodium as necessary, taking into account the child's likes and dislikes and cultural background. High-caloric supplements may be needed because of anorexia. School-age children may not understand the consequences of nonadherence with dietary restrictions and may perceive these restrictions as punishment. Adolescents often resent the dietary restrictions and ongoing dialysis treatments, which pose a threat to their independence and evolving sense of self. Noncooperation, depression, and hostility are common responses. Discuss possible behavioral responses to dietary restrictions and limitations imposed by the treatment plan.

Encourage parents to register the young child for the Early Intervention Program to promote development and interaction with other children. The dialysis schedule for school-age children should enable the child to participate in school.

School-age children and adolescents are often embarrassed about being seen as different from peers. Ask the child how he or she feels about the need to follow a special diet, take medications, and undergo dialysis treatments. To minimize the psychologic consequences of coping with a chronic disease, encourage parents to promote the child's participation in age-appropriate activities. Attendance at school and contacts with peers promote normal growth and development. Work to promote the child's self-worth and a healthy self-esteem. Encourage adolescents to participate in a program that helps them transition to adult health services and job skill training. Begin teaching the child during early adolescence about the health condition, medications taken and their actions, how to access emergency help, and problems caused by nonadherence to treatment. As the adolescent ages, have the family begin giving more responsibility for self-care, such as making appointments for healthcare, obtaining prescription refills, and seeking out adult healthcare professionals and a dialysis program.

Give the parents timely information about the disease process, dialysis treatments, and issues related to renal transplantation, as the child's renal impairment progresses.

EVALUATION

Expected outcomes of nursing care include:

- The child is fully immunized with childhood and additional vaccines.
- The child's fluid status is maintained.
- The child eats foods that meet nutritional needs while adhering to dietary restrictions.

COMPLEMENTARY CARE

AVOIDING HERBAL SUPPLEMENTS IN CHILDREN WITH CHRONIC RENAL FAILURE

Herbal supplements should not be used in children with CRF as they may contain harmful minerals, such as potassium. The body of a child with CRF is unable to clear waste products. There is also the risk for interaction between the herbs and medications taken that could place the child at risk for rejection of a transplanted kidney (National Kidney Foundation, 2004).

RENAL REPLACEMENT THERAPY

Renal replacement therapy is the treatment for renal failure and includes both dialysis and renal transplantation. In 2002, 6982 children between birth and 19 years of age received some form of renal replacement therapy. Hemodialysis has emerged as the dominant form of dialysis when treatment is initiated. By the 18th month of ESRD treatment, transplant is the dominant treatment method (United States Renal Data System, 2004).

EVIDENCE-BASED NURSING

LIVING WITH END-STAGE RENAL DISEASE

Clinical Question (Problem)

End-stage renal disease is a serious chronic condition that requires significant adaptations in lifestyle and complex medical treatments that take a toll on the child and family. What is the impact of the condition on adolescents?

Evidence

A study of 35 adolescents, aged 13 to 18 years, was conducted to evaluate their perceptions of themselves and living with end-stage renal disease. Twenty-one of the adolescents provided responses that clustered into one of four groups:

- Normalization, $n=8$ (identified selves as independent and leading as normal a life as possible)
- Illness causes a barrier to normalcy, $n=5$ (the physical effects of the disease such as shortened stature affected how they looked and how they were treated by society), had psychologic effects
- Illness management was parent focused, $n=5$ (adolescents wished to be independent but perceived that they were dependent upon parents to help care for them)
- Illness management was self-focused, $n-3$ (perceived that ongoing treatment for renal disease was very hard, and they perceived that they were different from their peers)

The study group of adolescents was 65.7% white and 28.6% African American. They were predominantly from intact families and 68.6% had positive treatment outcomes due to renal transplants (Snethen, Broome, Bartels et al., 2001).

Implications

Children and adolescents who develop end-stage renal disease are expected to develop adaptive functioning skills as well as cope with the consequences of the disease (physical trauma and operative scars, corticosteroid side effects, dietary restrictions, growth failure, and responses of peers). Parents must modify lifestyles and their hopes and dreams for their children's future. Strategies for managing the disease differ for every family. Normalization is a coping process in which the family views the care of the child with a chronic condition as a "normal" part of life, rather than an inconvenience or something outside of their routine. They choose to focus on the normal aspect of the child's life and the family's life. In cases when normalization cannot be achieved or sustained, the adolescent's condition may have recently changed or another family stressor is present. Those families view their life and their child as different from other families because of the child's condition. Nurses can be effective in working with families by listening to the issues and offering suggestions. Often the opportunity to talk through the child's management plan will help the family consider different strategies that may be effective. The nurse may also provide linkages to community resources that may help the family.

Critical Thinking

Initiate a discussion with an adolescent with end-stage renal disease. Listen to the adolescent's description of living with the condition. Develop a nursing care plan to help the child take the next steps in self-management.

Reference

Snethen, J. A., Broome, M. E., Bartels, J., & Warady, B. A. (2001). Adolescent's perception of living with end-stage renal disease. *Pediatric Nursing, 27*(2), 159–167.

PERITONEAL DIALYSIS

In peritoneal dialysis the peritoneum of the abdomen is the membrane through which the body's waste products pass from the blood to the abdominal cavity. A catheter is inserted through the abdominal wall into the peritoneal cavity. The dialysis solution (**dialysate**) that enters the abdomen contains dextrose that pulls body wastes and extra fluid into the abdominal cavity. These wastes and extra fluid leave the body with the drained dialysate. This method of dialysis is beneficial to small children since it allows continuous removal of fluids and waste products, decreasing the toxic effects of waste products on the child's developing body. The child can ambulate and interact with the environment. Dietary and fluid restrictions are less severe. The timing of the treatment can be set to minimize the interruption of school, play, or other social events.

Two types of peritoneal dialysis are commonly used: continuous ambulatory peritoneal dialysis and automated peritoneal dialysis. Graduated cylinders are used to monitor the volume of fluid exchanged.

- Continuous ambulatory peritoneal dialysis (CAPD) uses gravity to instill prefilled bags of dialysate into the peritoneal cavity four or five times a day. The fluid remains in the cavity for 4 to 8 hours. An attached bag is folded under the child's clothes, permitting normal activity. After the allotted time, the dialysate is drained by hanging the bag lower than the pelvis. The repeated connections and disconnections with this method are time consuming for the child and family and increase the risk of infection.

- Automated peritoneal dialysis uses an automatic cycler to instill and drain the dialysate about five times over a 10-hour period, usually overnight. One additional exchange may be needed during the day. With this method the number of connections and disconnections is minimized, which reduces demands on the family as well as the risk of infection. This is the preferred peritoneal dialysis method since a more customized schedule can be developed to allow children to attend school (Verrina, Zacchello, Edefonti et al., 2001).

HEALTH PROMOTION
The Child with Chronic Renal Failure

Growth and Development Surveillance

- Compare the child's height, weight, and head circumference to age-specific norms to identify growth retardation and to plot progress.
- Assess developmental progress using the Denver II or another screening tool (refer to Chapter 37∞).
- Educate parents on normal developmental milestones and measures to promote achieving those milestones.
- Assess the adolescent for signs of delayed sexual maturation and, in girls, amenorrhea.

Nutrition

- Review the dietary restrictions with the child and parents.
- Partner with the family to assist the child to make food selections and to restrict fluids and sodium as necessary, taking into account the child's likes and dislikes and cultural background. Encourage the child and family to take a list of a few favorite foods to the dietitian to see if they can be integrated into the child's meal plan.
- Make meal time pleasant and make foods taste more appealing with permitted spices.
- Discuss possible behavioral responses by older children and adolescents to dietary restrictions and limitations imposed by the treatment plan. Involve the child and adolescent in discussions about dietary restrictions, and when possible integrate their recommendations for dietary restrictions and fluid management throughout the day.
- Emphasize to the school-age child that dietary and other restrictions are not punishment.
- Use enteral feeding at night to provide the needed calories for growth.
- Discuss a potential reward program that may be effective in motivating the child and adolescent to improve their nutritional habits and adherence to prescribed therapy (Ritz, 2002).

Physical Activity

- Encourage child to participate in developmentally appropriate activities as tolerated.

- Partner with the child to establish a routine plan for physical activity as tolerated that will help promote strong bones.

Oral Health

- Promote good dentition and oral hygiene.
- Schedule regular dental visits for examination and cleaning to reduce infections.
- Partner with the family to ensure they understand the need for antibiotic prophylaxis before certain invasive procedures, including dental care.

Mental and Spiritual Health

- Ask children how they feel about the need to follow a special diet, take medications, and undergo dialysis treatments. Ask what might make it easier for them to cope with the treatments, and integrate at least one idea into the care plan.
- Encourage parents to promote their child's participation in age-appropriate activities to minimize the psychologic consequences of coping with a chronic disease.
- Adolescents often resent the dietary restrictions and ongoing dialysis treatments, which pose a threat to their independence, evolving sense of self, and their need for independence. Noncooperation, depression, and hostility are common responses.
- In preparation for transitioning to adult healthcare, encourage adolescents to participate in a program that assists them with transition to adult health services and job skill training (Myers, 2002).

Relationships

- Attendance at school and contacts with peers promote normal growth and development.
- Work to promote the child's self-worth and a healthy self-esteem.
- Prepare the child for peer conflict.
- Ensure that parents understand the importance of encouraging normal socialization of their child.

Disease Prevention Strategies

- Partner with the child and family to establish plans to avoid large crowds, people with infections, or other risks that expose the child to infection.
- If possible, all immunizations should be provided before renal transplantation, as long-term immunosuppressive therapy will then be prescribed.
- Live vaccines should not be given to the child taking immunosuppressive agents.
- Encourage the family to maintain scheduled appointments for routine serum and urine diagnostic tests performed to monitor renal function.

TABLE 52–8 ✛ Complications of Peritoneal Dialysis

Complication	Cause
Peritonitis	
Cloudy dialysate, abdominal pain, tenderness, leukocytosis, fever (neonatal hypothermia), constipation	*Staphylococcus aureus, Staphylococcus epidermidis,* fungal infections, gram-negative rods (risk is proportional to duration of dialysis and inversely proportional to age)
Pain	
During inflow	Too rapid a rate of infusion, too large a volume of dialysate, encasement of catheter in a false passage, extremes in temperature of dialysate
During outflow at end of emptying	Omentum entering catheter at end of outflow
Leakage	
Fluid around catheter, edema of penis or scrotum secondary to leakage into abdominal subcutaneous tissue, fluid leakage to pleural spaces through diaphragm	Overfilling of abdomen, catheter that has migrated from peritoneal cavity
Respiratory symptoms	
Shortness of breath, decreased breath sounds in lower lobes, inadequate chest expansion	Abdominal fullness that compromises diaphragm movement, hole in diaphragm allowing dialysate into chest cavity

In children receiving peritoneal dialysis for ARF, a percutaneously placed catheter can be used for a few weeks. In children with CRF, a catheter is placed surgically for long-term use.

The primary complications of peritoneal dialysis are peritonitis and abdominal hernia (Table 52–8). Signs and symptoms of peritonitis associated with peritoneal dialysis include cloudy dialysate, fever, vomiting, diarrhea, abdominal pain, and tenderness. Chronic alterations in the peritoneal membrane transport capacity may result from peritonitis and may lead to peritoneal membrane failure (Warady, Schaefer, Holloway et al., 2000). Peritonitis is treated with antibiotics infused in the dialysate.

Teach the family to perform peritoneal dialysis and to use sterile technique when performing dialysis and when doing catheter care. Peritoneal dialysis is time consuming, and family members must be committed to managing this procedure daily. Help the family develop home routines that minimize disruptions to daily family life. For additional information, refer to "Nursing Care Plan: The Child Receiving Home Peritoneal Dialysis."

HEMODIALYSIS

In hemodialysis the blood flows through a machine with a special filter that removes body wastes and extra fluids. Blood is pumped out of the body and through a dialyzer, where waste products and extra fluids diffuse out across a semipermeable membrane. Dialysate is pumped in the direction opposite blood flow to promote waste extraction.

Differences in osmolarity and concentration between the child's blood and the dialysate alter the intravascular electrolyte concentration and reduce the intravascular volume. Hemodialysis is provided to children in the critical care setting and in a special center (Figure 52–6 ●). Treatment is usually performed three times a week, with each session lasting approximately 3 to 4 hours. Continuous renal replacement therapy (CRRT) is a form of continuous hemodialysis used when the child has acute renal failure, multiple organ failure, and hemodynamic instability.

In emergency hemodialysis and for infants, a double-lumen cannula is inserted into a large vein (e.g., the femoral, jugular, or subclavian vein). Children over 20 kg (44 lb) often have an artificial blood vessel, an arteriovenous shunt or fistula, created. Two needles are inserted into the arteriovenous fistula, one to carry blood to the dialyzer and the other to return cleaned blood to the body.

Hemodialysis is more efficient than peritoneal dialysis but requires close monitoring for symptoms related to hypotension or rapid changes in fluid and electrolyte balance. Uncommonly, a *disequilibrium syndrome* (rapid changes in the body's water and electrolyte balance during treatment) may occur during or soon after the dialysis procedure is initiated. Other complications include access thrombosis and infection. Heparin is used to achieve an active clotting time of 150%, which reduces the risk of thrombosis.

Nursing management focuses on care of the child during dialysis and teaching the child and family about the administration of heparin and the control of bleeding

NURSING CARE PLAN

THE CHILD RECEIVING HOME PERITONEAL DIALYSIS

Intervention	Rationale	Expected Outcome
1. Nursing Diagnosis: Imbalanced Nutrition: Less than Body Requirements related to poor appetite, feeling of fullness after a small amount, and loss of protein in dialysate		
NIC Priority Intervention: **Nutrition management:** Assistance with or provision of a balanced dietary intake of foods and fluids		**NOC Suggested Outcome:** **Nutrition status:** Food and fluid intake: Amount of food and fluid taken into the body over a 24-hour period
Goal: The child will obtain adequate nutrients each day.		
■ With a nutritionist, develop a diet plan to identify the amounts of essential nutrients needed. ■ Provide small, frequent meals of needed nutrients. ■ Make mealtimes pleasant and avoid battles over the child's intake. ■ Provide supplements by tube feeding if adequate oral intake is not possible.	■ Parents need concrete guidelines for food preparation. ■ The child will feel full with smaller amounts of food because of the dialysate. ■ The child will be more inclined to eat if there is less stress. ■ Adequate nutrition is important for growth and development, and must be supported if oral intake is inadequate.	The child's intake is adequate for an expected growth pattern to be maintained.
2. Nursing Diagnosis: Risk for Infection related to daily invasive procedure		
NIC Priority Intervention: **Infection control:** Minimizing the acquisition and transmission of infectious agents		**NOC Suggested Outcome:** **Risk control:** Actions to eliminate or reduce actual, personal, and modifiable health threats
Goal: The child will not develop peritonitis.		
■ Wash hands, use sterile gloves and aseptic technique for connection and disconnection of catheters. ■ Perform daily catheter site care.	■ Aseptic technique reduces chance of introducing bacteria into the abdomen. ■ Skin around the catheter site will have fewer organisms that could potentially cause infection.	The child does not develop peritonitis.
Goal: If peritonitis occurs, it will be treated appropriately.		
■ Observe for signs of infection (fever, abdominal pain, cloudy dialysate). ■ Report signs of infection to physician immediately.	■ Early identification of infection will reduce complications. ■ Rapid intervention may reduce need for hospitalization.	Hospitalization will not be needed for peritonitis due to early identification and prompt treatment.
3. Nursing Diagnosis: Caregiver Role Strain related to daily dialysis treatments		
NIC Priority Intervention: **Caregiver support:** Provision of necessary information, advocacy, and support to facilitate primary patient care by someone other than a healthcare professional		**NOC Suggested Outcome:** **Caregiver performance:** Direct care: Provision by family care provider of appropriate personal and healthcare for a family member or significant other
Goal: The family copes with daily demands for the child's dialysis treatments.		
■ Discuss the importance of daily, consistent dialysis treatments for the child's overall health status. ■ Collaborate with the family to identify strategies that could reduce the impact of dialysis on the family's life.	■ If parents understand the need for consistent dialysis treatments, they are more likely to adhere to guidelines. ■ When the family participates in planning care, adherence is more likely.	The family adheres to daily dialysis treatment guidelines.

NURSING CARE PLAN—continued

THE CHILD RECEIVING HOME PERITONEAL DIALYSIS

Intervention	Rationale	Expected Outcome
3. Nursing Diagnosis: Caregiver Role Strain related to daily dialysis treatments (continued)		
■ Refer the family to local support groups for emotional support, treatment strategies, and respite care.	■ Support groups may help the family develop effective coping strategies.	

4. Nursing Diagnosis: Disturbed Body Image related to small size and perception of being and looking different

NIC Priority Intervention:		**NOC Suggested Outcome:**
Body image enhancement: Improving a patient's conscious and unconscious perceptions and attitudes toward his/her body		**Psychosocial adjustment:** Life change: Psychosocial adaptation of an individual to a life change

Goal: The child will develop a sense of self-worth and self-esteem.

■ Identify and emphasize strengths the child has (e.g., interaction style, skills, or cognitive abilities) despite being smaller than peers.	■ Perception of personal strengths should increase self-esteem.	The child effectively interacts with peers and participates in age-appropriate activities.
■ Assist the child and family to identify popular clothing styles that hide the protuberant abdomen, dialysate bag, and catheter.	■ Clothing that conforms to current styles, but still hides dialysate, will help the child feel less different from peers.	
■ Increase the child's participation in self-care as appropriate for developmental age.	■ Ability to perform self care increases the child's sense of control.	
■ Promote participation in safe activities with peers.	■ Social interaction with peers helps reinforce similarities with others.	
■ Encourage the child to participate in support groups with other children receiving dialysis.	■ Interactions with other affected children provide a chance to express feelings and frustrations, and to develop successful coping strategies.	

5. Nursing Diagnosis: Ineffective Health promotion related to chronic condition

NIC Priority Intervention:		**NOC Suggested Outcome:**
Health system guidance: Facilitating a patient's location and use of appropriate health services		**Health-seeking behaviors:** Actions to promote optimal wellness, recovery, and rehabilitation

Goal: The child's routine health promotion visits will be integrated with the management of the chronic condition.

■ If a renal specialty team is not conveniently located and providing general healthcare, make sure the child has a primary care provider working in collaboration with the renal team.	■ A source of health promotion and acute minor illness care is important, especially if the family lives a distance from the tertiary care center.	The child is fully immunized at appropriate intervals and the family has a source of regular care in the community.
■ Assess the child regularly for height growth, developmental progress, and signs that the chronic condition is being managed effectively.	■ Routine assessments will allow potential complications to be identified earlier.	
■ Provide immunizations as recommended for the child with a chronic condition.	■ Immunizations may reduce the risk of potentially life-threatening infections in a child at high risk.	
■ Provide anticipatory guidance related to safety, developmental progress, appropriate physical activities, and behavior management.	■ Information will help the family support the child's health status and promote development.	

FIGURE 52–6

A   **B**

This child is undergoing hemodialysis. **A,** A surgically implanted vascular graft is being used here. One needle is placed in the arterialized end of the graft (red tubing), and one needle is placed in the venous end (blue tubing) for blood return. **B,** The child is able to draw or perform other quiet activities during dialysis treatment. Note that the child's blood pressure is monitored carefully throughout the treatment.

from minor trauma. Carefully monitor fluid balance in the child undergoing hemodialysis. Check vital signs and blood pressure every half hour. Monitor oral intake and urinary output every half hour when the child is on the dialysis equipment. Weigh the child before and after the dialysis to determine any fluid imbalances that must be adjusted in the next hemodialysis session.

THINKING CRITICALLY

THE CHILD ON HEMODIALYSIS

Terrell, who is now 5 years old, was born with posterior urethral valves, which caused damage to his kidneys. Despite undergoing surgery to correct the defect during infancy, his kidney function continued to deteriorate. End-stage renal disease was diagnosed 2 years ago, and dialysis treatment was initiated. Terrell requires a kidney transplant, but in the meantime he is being treated with hemodialysis. He visits the dialysis center three afternoons a week for treatments lasting approximately 3 to 4 hours. This schedule permits him to attend kindergarten classes in the morning.

At this visit Terrell has gained weight and is edematous. In talking with him, his primary nurse at the dialysis center discovers that Terrell has been drinking cokes and eating "junk food" at school. Terrell asks the nurse not to tell his mother because she will be mad, but that he just can't help eating and drinking what he isn't supposed to.

How does Terrell's growth and development level affect his adherence to the treatment regimen? What is the immediate intervention for the nurse to take with Terrell? What approach does the nurse take with discussing this nutritional issue with the family?

NURSING PRACTICE

Monitor the child receiving hemodialysis for complications that can occur suddenly.

- Hypotension—sudden nausea and vomiting, abdominal cramping, tachycardia, and dizziness
- Rapid fluid and electrolyte exchange—muscle cramping, nausea and vomiting, and dizziness
- Dysequilibrium syndrome—restlessness, headache, nausea and vomiting, blurred vision, muscle twitching, and altered level of consciousness

Because fluid and dietary limitations (foods containing reduced potassium, sodium, and phosphorus) are needed more often with hemodialysis than with peritoneal dialysis, make sure the family knows how to plan and provide for the child's daily nutritional needs. Review ways to reduce the risk of infection, including the daily care of the catheter site. Encourage showering rather than tub baths. Activities such as swimming may be discouraged.

KIDNEY TRANSPLANTATION

Kidney transplantation provides the only alternative to long-term dialysis for children with ESRD. It can normalize physiology and may let children grow normally. Because delaying transplantation has adverse effects on growth and development, children are given some priority over adults awaiting transplantation. Blood type compatibility between the donor and recipient is essential for a transplant to be successful. A human leukocyte antigen (HLA) system match also improves survival of the graft. A living relative donor kidney has a higher survival rate than a cadaver kidney. Children and their families are carefully screened prior to transplantation in an effort to identify problems that could lead to rejection of the kidney or infection that could be life threatening if the immune system is suppressed.

After transplantation, the child must take immunosuppressive medications such as corticosteroids, azathioprine, cyclosporine, and antilymphocyte antibodies to suppress rejection. Immunosuppression regimens use various combinations and sequences of these drugs to reduce the incidence of acute and chronic rejection. Signs of rejection include fever, increased BUN and serum creatinine levels, pain and tenderness over the abdomen, irritability, and weight gain.

Complications of immunosuppression therapy include opportunistic infection, lymphomas and skin cancer, and hypertension. Nonadherence to therapy is the primary cause of transplanted kidney loss (in 10% to 15% of pediatric kidney transplant recipients). Nonadherence is highest among families with instability, in adolescents, females, and in children with a previous kidney loss due to nonadherence (Griffin & Elkin, 2001). Adherence is higher in adolescents when their parents are knowledgeable and supportive, and when they promote the adolescent to become competent in self-care (Pool & Korus, 2002). Some primary kidney diseases, such as glomerulonephritis and hemolytic-uremic syndrome, can also recur in the transplanted kidney.

Nursing management includes teaching parents about the transplantation process before it occurs to help prepare them for the experience. Discuss all aspects of the child's care that will have an impact on the family's life, including follow-up appointments, medications, and general health promotion. Monitor adherence to immunosuppression treatment at each visit in an effort to identify issues early. Teach parents about the signs of acute rejection and infection, including when and how to notify the child's physician if immediate care is required.

POLYCYSTIC KIDNEY DISEASE

Polycystic kidney disease (PKD) is a genetic disorder that has autosomal recessive and autosomal dominant forms. Liver abnormalities are associated with both forms of the disease. The incidence of the autosomal recessive form is 1 per 20,000 live births, and it is most often detected in fetuses and infants (Guay-Woodford & Desmond, 2003). The autosomal dominant form is the most common inherited kidney disease, with a prevalence of 1 per 400 to 500 individuals. The autosomal dominant PKD results from mutations on the PKD1 locus on chromosome 16 and PKD2 on chromosome 4. The autosomal recessive gene (PKHD1) is located on chromosome 6 (National Kidney and Urologic Diseases Information Clearinghouse, 2004).

In PKD, cellular hyperplasia of the collecting ducts causes them to dilate. Fluid secreted into these ducts enables cyst sacs to form. Initially, cysts are usually less than 2 mm in size and do not obstruct urinary flow. As the child grows, however, the cysts become larger and fibrosis occurs. The cysts slowly replace much of the kidney's mass and reduce kidney function. Tubular atrophy may occur in some children, whereas others have minimal changes in renal function. PKD is associated with liver abnormalities that progress to fibrosis, portal hypertension, and biliary infection, becoming more severe with age.

Newborns with PKD may have enlarged kidneys, detected at birth. Those with the most severe form of the disease die shortly after birth of pulmonary hypoplasia. Clinical manifestations in infants with autosomal recessive PKD include Potter facies (low-set ears, small jaw, and a flattened nose). Hypertension develops early in infancy and is often severe. Infants may have expected urine output or oliguria. Polyuria and polydipsia develop with progressive renal insufficiency. Respiratory distress and feeding intolerance may develop from the enlarged kidneys. As uremia develops, infants and children develop renal osteodystrophy and progressive developmental delay and growth failure.

Sonogram or renal biopsy confirms the diagnosis. The disease is often diagnosed on prenatal ultrasound. Liver function tests are usually normal initially. A liver biopsy may also be performed. Other family members should be screened for subclinical cases of PKD.

Treatment is supportive. Medications such as diuretics are prescribed for hypertension. Fluid and electrolyte abnormalities are managed. Antibiotics treat urinary tract infection. Growth hormones may be used in some children to promote growth. Renal osteodystrophy is treated to suppress the parathyroid hormone. Many children develop

DEVELOPING CULTURAL COMPETENCE

RACE AND THE RENAL TRANSPLANT WAITING LIST

Access to the renal transplant waiting list differs depending on the patient's race. Black children are 12% less likely to be placed on the waiting list than whites at any point in time. It is unknown if these differences are due to physician bias in identifying transplant candidates, patient or family preference, or difference in the time to see a nephrologist (Furth, Garg, Neu et al., 2000).

ESRD by 10 years of age. Renal dialysis or a transplant prolong survival; however, liver problems may continue to complicate the child's health, even when the renal condition is well controlled. Up to 20% to 30% of children die by age 15 years (Davis & Avner, 2004).

NURSING MANAGEMENT

Nursing care is the same as that for the child with renal insufficiency and chronic renal failure. Observe the child for signs of progressive renal impairment. Make sure the family schedules follow-up appointments to assess growth, developmental progress, and the effectiveness of the treatment plan. Family teaching for home management focuses on medications, diet adequate in protein and calories to support growth, management of acute gastrointestinal illnesses, and care for the child with progressive renal insufficiency and a liver disorder. Since the disease is inherited, the family should be referred for genetic counseling.

HEMOLYTIC-UREMIC SYNDROME

Hemolytic-uremic syndrome (HUS) is an acute renal disease that is the most common cause of acute renal failure. HUS is an important cause of chronic renal failure. It occurs most often in children under age 4 years with a peak between 1 and 2 years. The syndrome has a classic triad of signs: (1) hemolytic anemia, (2) thrombocytopenia, and (3) ARF.

The development of HUS is often linked to enterohemorrhagic *Escherichia coli* strain 0157:H7, which produces a toxin that attaches to the glomeruli, collecting ducts, and distal tubules. Contaminated beef is the vector in more than half of cases. The toxin damages the lining of the glomerular arterioles, causing the endothelial cells to swell. In response, clotting mechanisms deposit fibrin in the renal arterioles and capillaries. This partial occlusion damages the red blood cells, resulting in hemolytic anemia. Platelets cluster in areas of vascular endothelial damage, causing thrombocytopenia. ARF develops from acute tubular necrosis as a consequence of blood clotting in the arterioles and the toxic effect of hemolyzed red blood cells on renal tubular cells. Autosomal recessive and autosomal dominant forms of HUS also exist, accounting for less than 5% of cases (Varade, 2000).

An episode of severe gastroenteritis with bloody diarrhea, upper respiratory infection, or UTI precedes the development of HUS by 1 to 2 weeks. Signs and symptoms of HUS include hemolytic anemia, hypertension, pallor and purpura, and neurologic involvement (irritability, seizures, altered level of consciousness, hallucinations, posturing, blindness), hematuria, proteinuria, oliguria or anuria, edema, and ascites. The child may also have hyperkalemia and metabolic acidosis as a result of renal failure. A peripheral blood smear with fragments of red blood cells, fibrin fragments, and a decreased platelet count (<140,000/μL[mm³]) confirms the diagnosis.

Treatment focuses on the complications of ARF and includes fluid restrictions and a high-calorie, high-carbohydrate diet that is low in protein, sodium, potassium, and phosphorus. Enteral nutrition is sometimes needed. The use of antibiotics is controversial. Medications may include calcium gluconate or calcium chloride, aluminum hydroxide gel to bind to phosphorus, Kayexalate to remove excess postassium, and antihypertensive agents. Treatment of diarrhea with antimotility medications is contraindicated because they increase the risk of progression from hemorrhagic colitis to HUS (Varade, 2000). Use of an oral toxin-binding agent was recently evaluated and found to have no benefit in children with diarrhea-associated HUS (Trachtman, Cnaan, Christen et al., 2003).

About 40% of children need dialysis, and approximately 3% to 5% of those affected will die (Trachtman et al., 2003). Peritoneal dialysis is preferred unless the child has severe colitis and abdominal tenderness. Some children may develop chronic renal failure. Transfusions of fresh packed red blood cells may be ordered to treat severe anemia. Platelets are given if the child is bleeding or if surgery is needed. Transfusions should be administered carefully to prevent hypertension caused by hypervolemia.

NURSING MANAGEMENT

Nursing care is the same as that for the child with ARF, described earlier. Careful monitoring of neurologic signs, laboratory values, fluid and electrolyte balance, and bleeding is essential. Monitor daily weights and assess intake and output. Assess the child for abdominal discomfort from diarrhea. Observe the child carefully for signs of progressive renal impairment. Discharge planning focuses on teaching parents about medications and dietary and fluid restrictions. Follow-up visits are necessary to evaluate the effectiveness of the treatment plan. Teach parents that HUS can be largely prevented by cooking of ground beef to 155°F throughout, meaning no more rare hamburgers. Teach them to wash hands carefully when handling raw ground meats, and to make sure utensils touching raw meat do not come into contact with cooked meats.

ACUTE POSTINFECTIOUS GLOMERULONEPHRITIS

Glomerulonephritis is an inflammation of the glomeruli of the kidneys. In children, it is most often a response to a group A beta-hemolytic streptococcal infection of the skin or pharynx. It is also caused by other organisms, including *Staphylococcus, Pneumococcus,* and *Coxsackie* viruses. The incidence of acute postinfectious glomerulonephritis

(APIGN) is highest in children who are 2 to 12 years of age, and the disorder is more common in boys than in girls (Lang & Towers, 2001). Early antibiotic therapy for streptococcal infection does not seem to prevent the development of APIGN (Patel & Bissler, 2001).

ETIOLOGY AND PATHOPHYSIOLOGY

The child with APIGN usually becomes ill after recovering from a strain of group A beta-hemolytic streptococcal infection of the upper respiratory tract or the skin that subsequently attacks the kidney. Signs of APIGN develop after 8 to 14 days.

Glomerular damage occurs as a result of an immune complex reaction that localizes on the glomerular capillary wall. Antibody–antigen complexes become lodged in the glomeruli, leading to inflammation and obstruction. Capillaries in the glomeruli are obstructed by damaged tissue cells, and the glomerular filtration rate is reduced. Vascular permeability increases, allowing red blood cells and red cell casts to be excreted. Sodium and water are retained, expanding the intravascular and interstitial compartments and resulting in the characteristic finding of edema.

CLINICAL MANIFESTATIONS

Many children are asymptomatic. In other children the onset is usually abrupt with flank or midabdominal pain, irritability, malaise, and fever. Microscopic hematuria is present in nearly all cases, and gross hematuria, resulting in tea-colored urine, is found in up to 50% of cases. Mild periorbital edema occurs early, but edema may progress in severity to cause dyspnea, cough, ascites, crackles, and a gallop rhythm (Lang & Towers, 2001). Acute hypertension may cause an encephalopathy that includes headache, nausea, vomiting, irritability, lethargy, and seizures. Oliguria may or may not be present.

CLINICAL THERAPY

The serum BUN and creatinine concentrations are elevated. Serum protein is decreased due to mild or moderate proteinuria. The white blood cell count and erythrocyte sedimentation rate may be elevated, and serum lipid levels are increased in about 40% of cases. An elevated antistreptolysin O (ASO) titer reflects the presence of antibodies from a recent streptococcal respiratory infection, but the ASO level associated with a recent skin infection is low. The anti-DNAse B titer is helpful for detecting antibodies associated with recent skin infections. Up to 90% of children have reduced serum C3. Urinalysis reveals hematuria, proteinuria, and red and white cell casts. Anemia is common in the acute phase, usually because extracellular fluid dilutes the serum. The hemoglobin level and hematocrit value may decrease during the late phase as a result of hematuria.

Treatment focuses on relief of symptoms and supportive therapy. Bed rest is a key component of the treatment plan during the acute phase. Hypertension can be managed with a combination of an antihypertensive medication (such as hydralazine) and a diuretic (such as furosemide). Mild to moderate hypertension should be treated with fluid and salt restriction. A course of antibiotics may be given to ensure eradication of the original infectious agent. Immediate emergency care is needed for severe hypertension with cerebral dysfunction; diazoxide or hydralazine is administered intravenously.

Fluid requirements are determined by careful monitoring of urinary output, weight, blood pressure, and serum electrolytes. Initially, only insensible losses are replaced until the status of renal function is known. The severity of edema determines the degree of dietary restriction. Sodium and potassium intake are restricted. With severe azotemia, protein intake may have to be limited.

The prognosis for over 95% of children with APIGN is good. Most children recover completely within a few weeks. Recurrences are unusual. Approximately 2% of children progress to end-stage renal disease (Lang & Towers, 2001).

NURSING MANAGEMENT

NURSING ASSESSMENT AND DIAGNOSES

Assess edema, which may be periorbital or dependent and shifts as the child's position is changed. Assess for circulatory congestion (crackles, dyspnea, and cough). Monitor blood pressure, which can rise as high as 200/120 mm Hg. With severe hypertension, assess for signs of central nervous system problems (headache, blurred vision, vomiting, decreased level of consciousness, confusion, and convulsions).

Nursing diagnoses may include the following:

- *Excess Fluid Volume* related to decreased glomerular filtration and increased sodium retention
- *Risk for Infection* related to renal impairment and corticosteroid therapy
- *Risk for Impaired Skin Integrity* related to tissue edema
- *Imbalanced Nutrition: Less than Body Requirements* related to loss of appetite and proteinuria
- *Activity Intolerance* related to fluid and electrolyte imbalance, infectious process, and altered nutrition
- *Effective Therapeutic Regimen Management* related to child's medication schedule and treatment regimen after discharge

PLANNING AND IMPLEMENTATION

As with other renal disorders, care of the child with APIGN requires careful monitoring of vital signs and fluid–electrolyte balance to evaluate renal functioning and identify complications. Bed rest is required during the acute phase. Nursing care focuses on monitoring fluid status, preventing infection, preventing skin breakdown, meeting nutritional needs, and providing emotional support to the child and family.

Monitor Fluid Status

Monitor vital signs, fluid and electrolyte status, and intake and output. Hypovolemia can occur as a result of fluid shifting from vascular to interstitial spaces despite the outward clinical signs of excess fluid retention. Monitor the degree of ascites by measuring abdominal girth. Document urine specific gravity. Make sure parents and visitors understand the need to limit fluids to prevent excessive intake.

Prevent Infection

Impaired renal function puts the child at risk for infection. Monitor for signs of infection, including fever, increased malaise, and an elevated white blood cell count. Instruct the family in good handwashing technique. Limit visitors, and screen for upper respiratory infections. Screen family members for the presence of streptococcal infection and refer for treatment if necessary.

Prevent Skin Breakdown

Dependent areas or areas prone to pressure are vulnerable to skin breakdown. Turn the child frequently. Pad bony prominences or susceptible areas with sheepskin, or protect skin with a transparent dressing. Make sure the child's bed is free of crumbs or sharp toys. Keep sheets tight and free of wrinkles.

Meet Nutritional Needs

A team approach (including the nurse, renal dietitian, parents, and child) is often needed to meet the child's nutritional needs. In most cases the child follows a "no added salt" and low-protein diet. Anorexia presents the greatest challenge to meeting daily nutritional requirements during the acute phase of the disease. To increase the child's appetite, encourage parents to bring the child's favorite foods from home, serve foods in age-appropriate quantities, and allow the child to eat with other children or with family members.

Provide Emotional Support

Parents of a child with APIGN commonly feel guilty. Parents may blame themselves for not responding more quickly to the child's initial symptoms or may believe they could have prevented the development of glomerular damage. Discuss the etiology of the disease and the child's treatment, and correct any misconceptions. Emphasize that APIGN develops in only a few children with streptococcal infection.

Discharge Planning and Home Care Teaching

Children are hospitalized for a few days, but it may take 3 weeks for hypertension and gross hematuria to resolve and longer for the disorder to resolve completely. Discharge planning focuses on teaching parents about the child's medication regimen, potential side effects of medications, dietary restrictions, and signs and symptoms of complications. Teach parents how to take the child's blood pressure and how to test urine for albumin, if ordered. Emphasize that it is important to avoid exposing the child to people with upper respiratory tract infections. Advise parents to allow the child to return to his or her normal routine and activities after discharge, with periods allowed for rest.

EVALUATION

Expected outcomes of nursing care are the following:

- The child receives appropriate fluid volume each day and maintains normal urine output of 0.5 to 1 mL/kg/hr.
- The child develops no areas of redness, abrasions, or skin breakdown over pressure points.
- The child's temperature remains within normal limits and the child is free of secondary infection.
- The child maintains preillness weight and tolerates daily intake that meets nutritional requirements.
- The parents administer medications as prescribed. The child's sodium and potassium levels reflect adherence to dietary restrictions.

STRUCTURAL DEFECTS OF THE REPRODUCTIVE SYSTEM

PHIMOSIS

In phimosis the foreskin over the glans penis cannot be pulled back, due to adhesions or infection. Circumcision, surgical removal of the foreskin, is often performed during the newborn period to prevent phimosis, for ease of proper male hygiene, and to prevent UTIs, balanitis (inflammation of the glans penis), and penile cancer (see Chapter 28 ∞). Betamethasone cream 0.05% applied twice daily for 4 to 8 weeks to the outer prepuce is an effective alternative to surgery (Ashfield, Nickel, Siemens et al., 2003).

CRYPTORCHIDISM

Cryptorchidism (undescended testes) occurs when one or both testes fail to descend through the inguinal canal into the scrotum. Normally, the testes descend during the seventh to ninth month of gestation.

Cryptorchidism may be the result of a testosterone deficiency, an absent or defective testis, or a structural problem such as a narrow inguinal canal, short spermatic cord, or adhesions. The disorder occurs in 3% of term male infants and in a higher rate of premature infants (Koo, 2001a). The higher temperature in the abdomen than in the scrotum results in morphologic changes to the testis that are apparent by 18 months of age. Lower sperm counts at sexual maturity may result (Koo, 2001b). Complications of uncorrected cryptorchidism include infertility, malignancy or torsion of the undescended testis, atrophy, and the psychologic effects of "empty" scrotum.

Cryptorchidism is usually detected during the newborn examination when palpation of the scrotum fails to reveal one or both testes. It is not unusual for boys with cryptorchidism to have an inguinal hernia as well. In a majority of cases, the testes descend spontaneously by 3 months of age. An undescended testis may be located in the inguinal canal, abdomen, perineum, or even the thigh. Ultrasound, CT scan, and MRI may be used to identify the location of the testes. A diagnostic laparoscope may also be needed to locate the testis. When neither testis can be palpated, hormonal or chromosomal evaluation may be performed to detect an intersex disorder.

An orchiopexy is performed at 1 year of age before further damage to the testes occurs. An incision is made at the location of the testis, either in the abdomen or in the inguinal area. Blood vessels are disentangled to allow the testis to reach into the lower scrotum. A second incision is made in the scrotum at the point where the testis is stitched to the inside wall to keep it in place. If the testis is defective or undeveloped, it may be removed surgically to decrease the risk of later malignancies and a prosthesis may be placed in the scrotum. The goals of surgery are repair of any hernia, enhanced fertility, and psychologic benefit. The orchiopexy also makes it easier to examine the testis for tumors. The risk of testicular cancer is 35 to 50 times greater in men with a history of cryptorchidism (Ferrer & McKenna, 2000).

NURSING MANAGEMENT

Preoperative nursing care includes preparing the parents and child for the procedure and addressing parents' concerns about the postsurgical outcome. Orchiopexy is often performed as an outpatient procedure. If the child is hospitalized, postoperative nursing care focuses on maintaining comfort and preventing infection. Encourage bed rest, and monitor voiding. Apply ice to the surgical area, and administer prescribed analgesics to relieve pain.

Discharge instructions should include demonstration of proper incision care. The diaper area should be cleaned well with each diaper change to decrease chances of infection. Teach parents to identify signs of infection such as redness, warmth, swelling, and discharge. Inform parents

to avoid straddling the infant across the hip and not to allow play on a riding toy for 2 weeks after surgery to promote healing and to prevent injury. Vigorous activity and rough play should also be avoided.

INGUINAL HERNIA AND HYDROCELE

An inguinal hernia is a painless inguinal or scrotal swelling of variable size that occurs when abdominal tissue such as bowel extends into the inguinal canal. A hydrocele is a fluid-filled mass in the scrotum. A hernia is found in 1% to 5% of term infants and up to 11% of preterm infants, more commonly in boys than girls (Burd & Burd, 2002).

During fetal development a peritoneal sac precedes the testicle's descent to the scrotum. The lower sac enfolds the testis to become the tunica vaginalis, and the upper sac atrophies before birth. Fluid may become trapped in the tunica vaginalis and cause the hydrocele. When the tunica vaginalis does not atrophy, an abdominal structure may move into it. In males the bowel is the most frequent tissue protruding into the groin, and in females an ovary or fallopian tube is a common finding (Katz, 2001).

Diagnosis is made by physical examination at birth or in early infancy. Palpation of the scrotum reveals a round, smooth, nontender mass. Transillumination helps determine whether the mass is a hernia or hydrocele (see Chapter 35 ∞). Parents may report an intermittent bulge in the groin or swelling in the scrotum. Swelling associated with a hernia may become more apparent with straining. Some hernias reduce in size during sleep.

Outpatient surgery is performed at an early age (usually after 3 months of age to reduce anesthesia risks) to avoid **incarceration** (hernia cannot be reduced and circulation is impaired), which is a medical emergency. A nerve block may be given in the operating room to reduce postoperative pain. The prognosis is generally excellent. Most hydroceles without inguinal hernia resolve spontaneously as the fluid reabsorbs by the time an infant is 1 to 2 years of age.

NURSING PRACTICE

Inguinal hernias can become incarcerated when a bit of bowel becomes trapped in the inguinal opening and the blood supply is constricted. The child has an acute onset of pain, abdominal distention, vomiting, and an irreducible mass. Other findings may include an edematous scrotum, poor feeding, and bloody stools (Burd & Burd, 2002). Efforts are made to reduce the hernia before surgery by placing the child in the Trendelenburg position and applying firm manual pressure on the affected side. The child needs surgery within 24 to 48 hours.

Nursing care for hydrocele and inguinal hernia includes explaining the disorder and its treatment and providing preoperative and postoperative teaching and care. Inform parents that the scrotum may be edematous and may appear bruised after surgery. Incision care involves careful cleaning of the diaper area. The incision is covered with a protective sealant rather than a dressing. Acetaminophen is provided for pain.

TESTICULAR TORSION

Testicular torsion is an emergency condition in which the testis suddenly rotates on its spermatic cord, cutting off its blood supply. The arteries and veins in the spermatic cord become twisted and interrupt the blood supply, leading to vascular engorgement and ischemia. Testicular torsion occurs in approximately 1 in 4000 males before 25 years of age, with the highest incidence at puberty (Sessions, Rabinowitz, Hulbert, et al., 2003; McAndrew, Pemberton, Kikiros, et al., 2002). Often the testicles are positioned horizontally in the scrotum, a congenital anomaly known as a bell clapper deformity, which predisposes the boy to this condition.

Manifestations include severe pain and erythema in the scrotum, nausea and vomiting, abdominal pain, and scrotal swelling that is not relieved by rest or scrotal support. The testes are tender on palpation and become edematous. The cremasteric reflex is absent. Symptoms generally start when the child is sleeping or inactive, but they can occur after trauma, sexual activity, or exercise. The testis is positioned higher in the scrotum than the unaffected testis because of the shortened vascular pedicle. A testicular scan or Doppler flow sonogram may be performed if immediately available; however, risk for delay in treatment and misdiagnosis with these procedures is possible (McAndrew et al., 2002).

Torsion must be reduced within 4 to 6 hours to save the testis. Manual reduction with an analgesic is sometimes attempted, but emergency surgery is more common. During surgery (orchipexy), the testis is untwisted and stitched to the side of the scrotum in the correct position. The procedure is usually performed bilaterally to prevent future torsion in the other testis.

Nursing management involves psychologic support for the child and family related to the need for emergency surgery and concern about the child's future fertility. Reassure parents that as only one testis is usually involved, fertility should not be affected. The child often goes home within a few hours of surgery; thus the child and family need to be taught about proper care of the incision and pain management. Explain to parents that the child should not lift heavy objects for 4 weeks or participate in strenuous activity for 2 weeks after surgery to promote healing. Teach the adolescent testicular self-examination.

See Chapter 5 for information on sexually transmitted infections.∞

Critical Concept Review

LEARNING OBJECTIVES

CONCEPTS

| Describe the pathophysiologic processes associated with genitourinary disorders in the pediatric population. | Genitourinary disorders in the pediatric population are usually caused by:
1. Incomplete organ development during fetal development.
2. Hydronephrosis.
3. Improper placement of ureters in bladder and urethra in penis.
4. Anatomic obstruction or incomplete nerve innervation.
5. Infections.
6. Genetic Disorders. |

| Discuss the nursing management of a child with a structural defect of the genitourinary system. | Nursing care focuses on:
1. Preventing infection and trauma:
  ■ Protection of exposed surfaces prior to surgery.
  ■ Maintenance of proper alignment and immobility after surgery.
2. Protecting surgical site from injury
3. Monitoring renal function:
  ■ Strict intake and output.
4. Providing pain management and comfort measures to infant. |

LEARNING OBJECTIVES

CONCEPTS

Discuss the nursing management of a child with a structural defect of the genitourinary system—continued	5. Providing emotional support to parents:
	  ■ Encourage parent-infant bonding.
	  ■ Instruct in discharge care.
	  ■ Emphasize need for follow-up care.
	  ■ Instruct parents in signs and symptoms of complications.
	6. Educating parents to care for child after surgery.

Develop a nursing care plan for the child with a urinary tract infection.	A nursing care plan for a child with a UTI includes: 1. Obtain a sterile urine specimen. 2. Begin and maintain antibiotic therapy. 3. Reinforce proper cleansing methods for girls (front to back). 4. Medicate child for fever and discomfort. 5. Reinforce need for completion of antibiotic treatment and follow-up urine specimen.

Describe the growth and developmental issues for the child with chronic renal failure.	1. Growth retardation. 2. Decreased mental alertness and ability to concentrate. 3. Fatigue. 4. Dyspnea on exertion. 5. Delayed fine and gross motor development. 6. Delayed sexual maturation.

Outline a plan to meet the fluid and dietary restrictions of a child with a renal disorder.	1 Restricted fluid needs:
	  ■ Make a visual display giving child exact amount of fluid allowed.
	  ■ Help child choose fluids high in calories and low in sodium.
	  ■ Separate fluids from meals
	2. Restricted dietary needs:
	  ■ Provide small, frequent feedings in a social atmosphere.
	  ■ Use high-calorie supplements.
	  ■ Instruct child and family on foods to avoid that are high in sodium, potassium, and phosphorus.
	  ■ Refer to renal dietician.

Develop a nursing care plan for the child with acute and chronic renal failure on dialysis.	Hemodialysis 1. Weigh child before and after dialysis. 2. Monitor fluid balance during therapy. 3. Check vital signs every half hour. 4. Monitor for any signs of bleeding from dialysis catheter. 5. Monitor PO intake and urinary output every half hour. 6. Provide distractions for child during therapy. Peritoneal dialysis 1. Teach family to perform peritoneal dialysis using sterile technique to connect and disconnect bags of dialysate. 2. Suggest clothing to help hide dialysate bags. 3. Educate parents about sings of peritonitis.

List psychosocial issues for children of different ages who have surgery on the genitourinary system	1. Preschool and school-age child:
	  ■ Embarrassment due to lack of continence.
	2. School-age child and adolescent:
	  ■ Embarrassment due to need for medications and doctor's visits.
	  ■ Development of self-esteem and self-confidence with sexual identity and function.

CRITICAL THINKING IN ACTION

View the **Critical Thinking in Action** video in Chapter 52 of the CD-ROM. Then, answer the questions that follow.

Kendra, a 2-year-old who appears ill, is brought into the urgent care center for a skin rash, fever, irritability, and edema. Her father is concerned she might also be dehydrated because she has had a decreased urine output. The doctor determines her skin rash does not blanche when pressure is applied and notes a purplish color. Last week Kendra was treated for an episode of abdominal pain, diarrhea, and vomiting. The doctor immediately admits her to the hospital and orders a urine culture, blood work, and stool tests. The stool comes back positive for the strain of E Coli usually found in contaminated hamburger meat. Kendra has Hemolytic Uremic Syndrome (HUS) and is in acute renal failure (ARF). She also has a low hemoglobin, elevated BUN and creatinine, hematuria, and electrolyte imbalances.

Kendra is given medication for her electrolyte imbalances, antihypertensive medications, and is placed on a high-calorie, high-carbohydrate diet with restrictions on protein, sodium, potassium, and phosphorus. You explain to her parents the extreme importance of adhering to her dietary and fluid restrictions to help keep her electrolytes and fluid level balanced. You educate them that in some cases children with HUS need dialysis and some children have long term kidney damage. You teach them how to take her blood pressure, and how to observe for edema so that Kendra can be monitored after she goes home.

1. How is drug administration adjusted for Kendra since she has ARF? What is an important nursing role when administering various medications to her?
2. What is the reason ARF develops in HUS?
3. What is one way Kendra's condition could have been prevented?
4. Renal failure is characterized by azotemia and oliguria. Describe what these are.

MEDIALINK

www.prenhall.com/london

- NCLEX-RN® Review, case studies, and other interactive resources for this chapter can be found on the Companion Website at http://www.prenhall.com/london. Click on "Chapter 52" and select the activities for this chapter.

audio
< play again

- For animations, more NCLEX-RN® Review questions, and an audio glossary, access the accompanying CD-ROM in this textbook.

REFERENCES

Ashfield, J. E., Nickel, K. R., Siemens, D. R., MacNeily, A. E., & Nickel, J. C. (2003). Treating phimosis with topical steroids in 194 children. *Journal of Urology, 169*(3), 1106–1108.

Balinsky, W. (2000). Pediatric end-stage renal disease: Incidence, management, and prevention. *Journal of Pediatric Health Care, 14*(6), 304–308.

Brooks, L. J., & Topol, H. I. (2003). Enuresis in children with sleep apnea. *Journal of Pediatrics, 142*(5), 515–518.

Burd, A. J., & Burd, R. S. (2002). Inguinal hernia in the premature infant: Management of a common problem. *Neonatal Network, 21*(7), 39–47.

Davis, I. D., & Avner, E. D. (2004). Anatomic abnormalities associated with hematuria. In R. E. Behrman, R. M. Kliegman, & H. B. Jenson, *Nelson textbook of pediatrics* (17th ed., pp. 1749–1750). Philadelphia: Saunders.

Ferrer, F. A., & McKenna, P. H. (2000). Current approaches to the undescended testicle. *Contemporary Pediatrics, 17*(1), 106–111.

Furth, S. L., Garg, P. P., Neu, A. M., Hwang, W., Fivush, B. A., & Powe, N. R. (2000). Racial differences in access to the kidney transplant waiting list for children and adolescents with end-stage renal disease. *Pediatrics, 106*(4), 756–761.

Goodyer, P., & Kashtan, C. (1998). The genetic basis of pediatric renal disease. *Seminars in Nephrology, 18*(3), 244–255.

Griffin, K. J., & Elkin, T. D. (2001). Nonadherence in pediatric transplantation: A review of the existing literature. *Pediatric Transplantation, 5*, 246–249.

Guay-Woodford, L.M., & Desmond, R. A. (2003). Autosomal recessive polycystic kidney disease: The clinical experience in North America. *Pediatrics, 111*(5), 1072–1080.

Hanson, K. A. (2003). Diagnostic tests and tools in the evaluation of urologic disease, Part II. *Urologic Nursing, 23*(6), 405–415.

Hogg, R. J., Furth, S., Lemley, K. V., Portman, R., Schwartz, G.J., et al. (2003). National Kidney Foundation's kidney disease outcomes quality initiative clinical practice guidelines for chronic kidney disease in children and adolescents: Evaluation, classification, and stratification. *Pediatrics, 111*(6), 1416–1421.

Hogg, R. J., Portman, R. J., Milliner, D., Lemley, K. V., Eddy, A., & Ingelfinger, J. (2000). Evaluation and management of proteinuria and nephrotic syndrome in children: Recommendation from a pediatric nephrology panel established at the National Kidney Foundation Conference on Proteinuria, Albuminuria, Risk, Assessment, Detection, and Elimination (PARADE). *Pediatrics, 105*(6), 1242–1249.

Huether, S. E. (2002). Alterations of renal and urinary tract function in children. In K. L. McCance & S. E. Huether, *Pathophysiology: The biologic basis for disease in adults and children* (4th ed., pp. 1217–1230), St. Louis, MO: Mosby.

Issenman, R. M., Filmer, R. B., & Gorski, P. A. (1999). A review of bowel and bladder control development in children: How gastrointestinal and urologic conditions relate to problems in toilet training. *Pediatrics, 103*(6), 1346–1352.

Jalkut, M. W., Lerman, S. E., & Churchill, B. M. (2001). Enuresis. *Pediatric Clinics of North America, 48*(6), 1461–1488.

Katz, D.A. (2001). Evaluation and management of inguinal and umbilical hernias. *Pediatric Annals, 30*(12), 729–735.

Koo, H. P. (2001a). Is it really cryptorchidism? *Contemporary Urology, 13*(1), 12–16, 31.

Koo, H.P. (2001b). Management of undescended testes. *Contemporary Urology, 13*(3), 20–26.

Kraus, S. J. (2001). Genitourinary imaging in children. *Pediatric Clinics of North America, 48*(6), 1381–1423.

Lang, M. M., & Towers, C. (2001). Identifying poststreptococcal glomerulonephritis. *Nurse Practitioner, 26*(8), 34–49.

Mahant, S., To, T., & Friedman, J. (2001). Timing of voiding cystourethrogram in the investigation of urinary tract infections in children. *Journal of Pediatrics, 139*(4), 568–571.

McAndrew, H. F., Pemberton, R., Kikiros, C. S., & Gollow, I. (2002). The incidence and investigation of acute scrotal problems in children. *Pediatric Surgery International, 18*, 435–437.

Mercer, R. (2003). Dry at night: Treating nocturnal enuresis. *Advance for Nurse Practitioners, 11*(2), 26–32.

Myers, P. S. (2002). Transitioning an adolescent dialysis patient to adult health care. *Nephrology Nursing Journal, 29*(4), 375–376.

National Kidney and Urological Diseases Information Clearinghouse. (2003). *Urinary tract infections in children* (NIH Publication No. 04-4246). Retrieved December 13, 2004, from http://www.kidney.niddk.nih.gov/kudiseases/pubs/utichildren/index.htm

National Kidney and Urological Diseases Information Clearinghouse. (2004). *Polycystic kidney disease* (NIH Publication No. 05-4008). Retrieved December 19, 2004, from http://www.kidney.niddk.nih.gov/kudiseases/pubs/polycystic/index.htm

National Kidney Foundation. (2004). *Use of herbal supplements in chronic kidney disease.* Retrieved December 23, 2004, from http://www.kidney.org/atoz/atozPrint.cfm?id=123

Patel, H. P., & Bissler, J. J. (2001). Hematuria in children. *Pediatric Clinics of North America, 48*(6), 1519–1537.

Pool, R., & Korus, M. (2002). Pediatric kidney transplantation: Growth, development, and nursing implications. *Progress in Transplantation, 12*(2), 129–135.

Ritz, S. (2002). Pediatric hemodialysis and peritoneal dialysis: Report rewards program. *Journal of Renal Nutrition, 12*(3), 199–204.

Robinson, R. F., Nahata, M. C., Mahan, J. D., & Batisky, D. L. (2003). Management of nephrotic syndrome in children. *Pharmacotherapy, 23*(8), 1021–1036.

Sessions, A. E., Rabinowitz, R., Hulbert, W. C., Goldstein, M. M., & Mevorach, R. A. (2003). Testicular torsion: Direction, degree, duration, and disinformation. *Journal of Urology, 169*(2), 663–665.

Shaw, K. N., & Gorelick, M. H. (1999). Urinary tract infection in the pediatric patient. *Pediatric Clinics of North America, 46*(6), 1111–1123.

Snethen, J. A., Broome, M. E., Bartels, J., & Warady, B. A. (2001). Adolescent's perception of living with end-stage renal disease. *Pediatric Nursing, 27*(2), 159–167.

Sponseller, P. D., Jani, M. M., Jeffs, R. D., & Gearhart, J. P. (2001). Anterior innominate osteotomy in repair of bladder exstrophy. *Journal of Bone and Joint Surgery, 83*(A-2), 184–193.

Stokowski, L. A. (2004). Hypospadias in the neonate. *Advances in Neonatal Care, 4*(4), 206–215.

Tobias, N. E. (2000). Management of nocturnal enuresis. *Nursing Clinics of North America, 35*(1), 37–60.

Trachtman, H., Cnaan, A., Christen, E., Gibbs, K., Zhao, S., Acheson, D. W et al. (2003). Effect of an oral Shiga toxin-binding agent on diarrhea-associated hemolytic uremic syndrome in children. *Journal of the American Medical Association, 290*(10), 1337–1344.

United States Renal Data System. (2004). *2004 Annual data report.* Retrieved December 13, 2004, from http://www.usrds.org/atlas.htm

Varade, W. S. (2000). Hemolytic uremic syndrome: Reducing the risks. *Contemporary Pediatrics, 17*(9), 54–64.

Verrina, E., Zacchello, G., Edefonti, A., Sorino, P., Rinaldi, S., et al. (2001). A multicenter survey on automated peritoneal dialysis prescription in children. *Advances in Peritoneal Dialysis, 17*, 264–268.

Vogt, B. A. (2002). A newborn with a urinary tract anomaly: What role for the general pediatrician? *Contemporary Pediatrics, 19*(10), 131–153.

Vogt, B. A., & Avner, E. D. (2004). Renal failure. In R. E. Behrman, R. M. Kliegman, & H. B. Jenson, *Nelson textbook of pediatrics* (17th ed., pp. 1767–1775). Philadelphia: Saunders.

Warady, B. A., Schaefer, F., Holloway, M., Alexander, S., Kandert, M., et al. (2000). Consensus guidelines for the treatment of peritonitis in pediatric patients receiving peritoneal dialysis. *Peritoneal Dialysis International, 20*(6), 610–624.

Williams, G., Lee, A., & Craig, J. (2001). Antibiotics for the prevention of urinary tract infections in children: A systematic review of randomized control trials. *Journal of Pediatrics, 138*(6), 868–874.

The Child with Alterations in Neurologic Function

It's so hard to watch your child experience a brain injury and lie in a coma. All we can do is be here every day for Antwan. We keep talking to him and trying to get him to respond to us. We keep hoping that he will fully recover.
—Mother of Antwan, 7 years old

LEARNING OBJECTIVES

- Describe the anatomy and physiology of the neurologic system.

- Describe the nursing assessment process and tools used for infants and children with altered levels of consciousness and other neurologic conditions.

- Differentiate between the signs of infants and children with epilepsy and status epilepticus, and describe appropriate nursing management for each condition.

- Differentiate between signs of bacterial meningitis, viral meningitis, encephalitis, Reye syndrome, and Guillain-Barré syndrome in infants and children.

- Describe the nursing care for the infant with myelodysplasia and hydrocephalus.

- Describe the focus of community-based nursing care for the child with cerebral palsy.

- Distinguish between the assessment findings of the child with a mild, moderate, and severe traumatic brain injury.

- Contrast the appropriate initial nursing management for mild and severe traumatic brain injury.

MEDIALINK www.prenhall.com/london

CD-ROM

Animations
   3-D Brain and Brainstem
   Coup-contrecoup Injury
   Diazepam
Videos:
   Seizure Disorders
   Living with Spina Bifida
Skill 9–5: Head Circumference
Skill 14–2: Oxygen Saturation: Pulse Oximetry
Skill 15–2: Inserting and Removing a Nasogastric Tube
Audio Glossary
NCLEX-RN® Review

Companion Website

Complementary Care: Music Therapy for Special
   Needs Children
Thinking Critically
Case Study: Post-Concussion for Return to
   Competitive Play
Critical Thinking: Traumatic Brain Injury Death
   Prevention
NCLEX-RN® Review
Case Study

ANATOMY AND PHYSIOLOGY OF PEDIATRIC DIFFERENCES

Knowledge of the anatomy of the nervous system makes neurologic symptoms easier to understand. The brain, spinal cord, and nerves are the major structures of the nervous system (Figure 53–1 ⊙). The spinal cord transmits impulses to and from the brain, conveying sensory information and relaying impulses that stimulate motor responses. Because the nervous system helps control and coordinate many body functions, alterations in neurologic function can have widespread effects on the body's metabolism.

Central nervous system (CNS) defects account for approximately one third of all apparent congenital malformations in live infants, and 90% of these are neural tube defects. CNS defects are responsible for 40% of infant deaths in the first year of life (Padgett, 2002).

At birth the nervous system is complete but immature. The infant is born with all the nerve cells he or she will have throughout life. However, the number of glial cells and dendrites, which enable receipt of nerve impulses, continues to increase until approximately 4 years of age. Myelination, which increases the speed and accuracy of nerve impulses, is also incomplete at birth. The myelination process accounts for the progressive acquisition of fine and gross motor skills and coordination during early childhood. This development proceeds in a cephalocaudal direction.

⊙ FIGURE 53–1

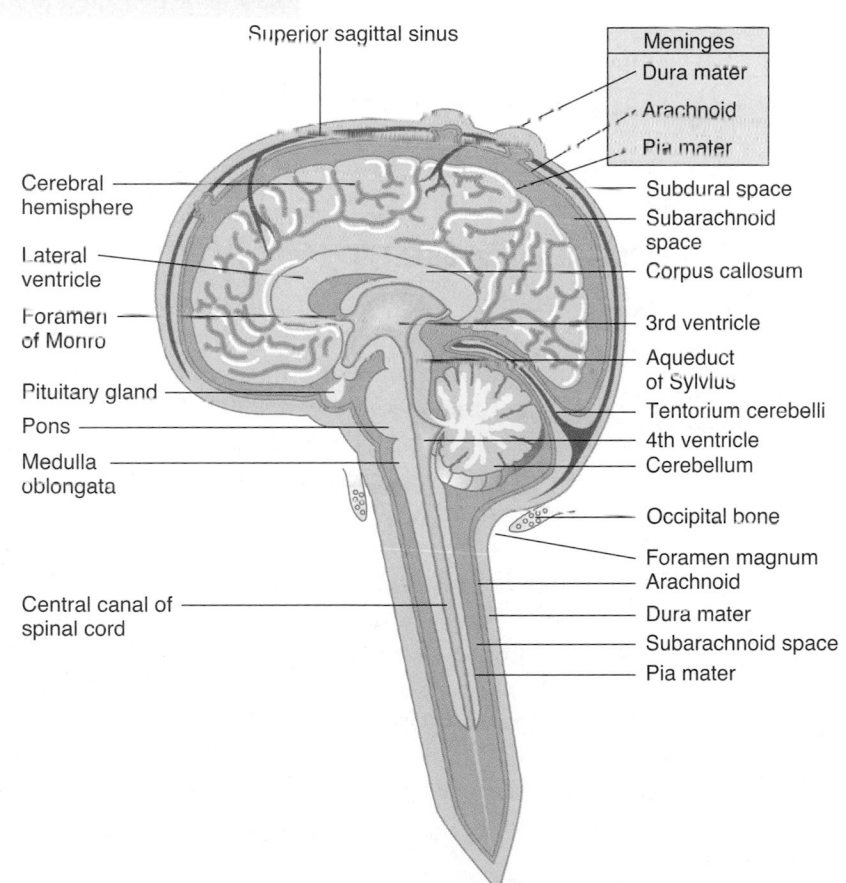

Transverse section of the brain and spinal cord. Knowledge of the anatomy of the brain is helpful in understanding the symptoms of neurologic dysfunction.

TABLE 53–1 ❖ **Summary of Anatomic and Physiologic Differences Between Children and Adults**	
Difference in Children	**Significance**
Top heavy; head is large in proportion to body; neck muscles not well developed	Prone to head injuries with falls; neck may not be able to support large head
Thin cranial bones that are not well developed; unfused sutures	Prone to fracture
Highly vascular brain; subarachnoid space small; dura firmly attached but can strip away from pericranium	Brain prone to hemorrhage; there is less cerebrospinal fluid to cushion the brain
Excessive spinal mobility; muscles, joint capsules, and ligaments of cervical spine immature	Greater risk for high cervical spine injury at C1–C2 level
Wedge-shaped, cartilaginous vertebral bodies; ossification of vertebral bodies incomplete	Greater risk for compression fractures of vertebrae with falls

The anatomic and physiologic differences between the nervous systems of children and adults help explain why children and adults have different neurologic problems (Table 53–1). For example, the skeletal structures of the skull and vertebrae protect the brain and spinal cord. In infants, however, the cranial bones and vertebrae are not completely ossified. The infant's brain and spinal cord are thus at greater risk for injury from trauma.

ALTERED STATES OF CONSCIOUSNESS

Level of consciousness (LOC) is perhaps the most important indicator of neurologic dysfunction. *Consciousness,* the responsiveness of the mind to sensory stimuli, has two components: *alertness,* or the ability to react to stimuli, and *cognitive power,* or the ability to process the data and respond either verbally or physically. *Unconsciousness,* on the other hand, is depressed cerebral function, or the inability of the brain to respond to stimuli. Altered levels of consciousness can be further categorized as:

- *Confusion:* disorientation to time, place, or person. The child may seem alert. Answers to simple questions may be correct, but responses to complex ones may be inaccurate.
- *Delirium:* state characterized by confusion, fear, agitation, hyperactivity, or anxiety.

- *Obtunded:* limited response to the environment; the child falls asleep unless given verbal or tactile stimulation.
- *Stupor:* response to vigorous stimulation only; the child returns to the unresponsive state when the stimulus is removed. For example, the child may react to a needlestick but not respond to a milder stimulus such as touching the skin.
- ***Coma:*** severely diminished response; the child cannot be aroused even by painful stimuli.

ETIOLOGY AND PATHOPHYSIOLOGY

Many conditions may alter the level of consciousness, including the following: trauma, hypoxia, infection, poisoning, seizures, endocrine or metabolic disturbances, electrolyte or acid-base imbalance, CNS pathology, and a congenital structural defect. Any of these pathologic processes can also cause increased **intracranial pressure** (force exerted by brain tissue, cerebrospinal fluid, and blood within the cranial vault). Decreased **cerebral perfusion pressure**, the amount of pressure needed to ensure that adequate oxygen and nutrients will be delivered to the brain, often results when the arterial blood flow to the brain is reduced due to increased intracranial pressure. Discovering the cause of the decreased level of consciousness is essential so that immediate treatment can begin, to prevent possible secondary effects of the illness or injury.

CLINICAL MANIFESTATIONS

Decline in a child's level of consciousness often follows a sequential pattern of deterioration. A child may first appear awake and alert, and may respond appropriately. Initial changes may be subtle: a slight disorientation to time, place, and person. The child may become restless or fussy, and actions that normally calm or soothe the child only increase irritability. As responsiveness decreases, the child may become drowsy but still respond to loud verbal commands and withdraw from painful stimuli. Keeping the child awake is sometimes difficult. Then response to pain progresses from purposeful to nonpurposeful. The child may exhibit decorticate or decerebrate **posturing**, the abnormal positions assumed after injury or damage to the brain (Figure 53–2 ●). Clinical manifestations of increased intracranial pressure are provided in Table 53–2.

Clinical Therapy

Clinical therapy focuses on early diagnosis of the cause of an altered level of consciousness and intervention to prevent further insult to the central nervous system. The Glasgow Coma Scale is used to quantify the level of consciousness,

● **FIGURE 53-2**

A

B

A, Decorticate posturing, characterized by rigid flexion, is associated with lesions above the brainstem in the corticospinal tracts. ***B,*** Decerebrate posturing, distinguished by rigid extension, is associated with lesions of the brainstem.

thus enabling future comparison of improvement or deterioration in the child's condition. Pediatric criteria take into account the child's developmental age for each category of the test (Table 53–3).

TABLE 53-2 ✛	**Signs of Increased Intracranial Pressure**
Timing of Signs	**Signs**
Early signs	Headache
	Visual disturbances, diplopia
	Nausea and vomiting
	Dizziness or vertigo
	Slight change in vital signs
	Pupils not as reactive or equal
	Sunsetting eyes
	Seizures
	Slight change in level of consciousness, restlessness
Infant has above signs plus:	Irritability
	Bulging fontanelle
	Wide sutures, increased head circumference
	Dilated scalp veins
	High-pitched, catlike cry
Late signs	Significant decrease in level of consciousness
	Cushing's triad
	■ Increased systolic blood pressure and widened pulse pressure
	■ Bradycardia
	■ Irregular respirations
	Fixed and dilated pupils

Laboratory tests include a complete blood cell count, blood chemistry, clotting factors, and blood culture; toxicology assessments of both blood and urine; and urinalysis with culture. A lumbar puncture may be performed to assess the cerebrospinal fluid for protein, glucose, or blood cells. An electroencephalogram (EEG) identifies damaged or nonfunctioning areas of the brain. Computed tomography (CT) or magnetic resonance imaging (MRI) is used to detect any lesions, structural abnormalities, vascular malformations, or edema. Skull x-ray studies are used to detect fractures or bony malformations.

The child is treated with oxygen, and assisted ventilation is provided when gas exchange is inadequate. Any metabolic, acid-base, or electrolyte imbalances are corrected. Antibiotics are initiated for suspected infection.

Efforts are made to maintain the cerebral perfusion pressure so that adequate oxygen and nutrients are supplied to brain tissue. In cases of hypovolemia, intravenous fluids are given. In cases of poor perfusion and fluid overload, dopamine or dobutamine is administered to increase cardiac output and perfusion of the brain. If the intracranial pressure is markedly increased and results from the accumulation of cerebrospinal fluid because of obstruction, a ventricular tap can be performed to decrease the pressure, relieving a life-threatening condition that can lead to coma.

NURSING MANAGEMENT

NURSING ASSESSMENT AND DIAGNOSIS

Initially assess the child's physiologic status, focusing on the child's responsiveness to the environment or stimuli,

TABLE 53–3 ✤ Glasgow Coma Scale for Assessment of Coma in Infants and Children

Category	Score	Infant and Young Child Criteria	Older Child and Adult Criteria
Eye opening	4	Spontaneous opening	Spontaneous
	3	To loud noise	To verbal stimuli
	2	To pain	To pain
	1	No response	No response
Verbal response	5	Smiles, coos, cries to appropriate stimuli	Oriented to time, place, and person; uses appropriate words and phrases
	4	Irritable; cries	Confused
	3	Inappropriate crying	Inappropriate words or verbal response
	2	Grunts, moans	Incomprehensible words
	1	No response	No response
Motor response	6	Spontaneous movement	Obeys commands
	5	Withdraws to touch	Localizes pain
	4	Withdraws to pain	Withdraws to pain
	3	Abnormal flexion (decorticate)	Flexion to pain (decorticate)
	2	Abnormal extension (decerebrate)	Extension to pain (decerebrate)
	1	No response	No response

Add the score from each category to get the total. The maximum score is 15, indicating the best level of neurologic functioning. The minimum is 3, indicating total neurologic unresponsiveness.

Used with permission from Teasdale, G., & Jennett, B. (1974). Assessment of coma and impaired consciousness. *Lancet, 2*, 81–84; and James, H. E. (1986). Neurologic evaluation and support in the child with acute brain insult. *Pediatric Annals, 15*(1), 17.

ability to maintain the airway, vital signs, and breathing patterns. Use the Glasgow Coma Scale to assess the child at specified intervals (see Table 53–3).

Assess the child's cranial nerves (see Table 35–20 in Chapter 35 ∞). The child's responses may differ significantly when stress and anxiety are reduced. Encourage the parents to take part in the examination to reduce the child's anxiety. In the unconscious child, cranial nerve assessment and interpretation are more challenging (Table 53–4).

Assess the child's respiratory effort and color. Monitor pulse oximetry and arterial blood gas measurements. Adequate air exchange to keep oxygen and carbon dioxide levels within normal ranges and maintaining acid-base balance are critical to reduce the risk of hypoxemia and increased intracranial pressure. If the child cannot maintain an adequate respiratory effort, mechanical ventilation will be necessary.

Among the nursing diagnoses that might be appropriate for the child with an altered level of consciousness or increased intracranial pressure are the following:

- *Ineffective Breathing Pattern* related to neuromuscular dysfunction associated with increased intracranial pressure
- *Risk for Aspiration* related to decreased level of consciousness
- *Risk for Impaired Skin Integrity* related to decreased level of consciousness and impaired mobility
- *Impaired Verbal Communication* related to physiologic condition of decreased level of consciousness
- *Interrupted Family Processes* related to care of a child with an acquired disability

GROWTH AND DEVELOPMENT

Following are developmentally appropriate cues in the Glasgow Coma Scale assessment:

- Eye opening. Note whether eye opening is spontaneous or occurs in response to stimuli.
- Verbal response. Crying in an infant is a positive response. The 2-year-old child who says "no" to each command is also responding in an age-appropriate way.
- Motor response. Motor score is probably the most critical aspect of this test, since the child cannot control reflexes. A fearful toddler may refuse to open his or her eyes or talk to strangers, but the child's reflexes should automatically respond to appropriate stimuli. Ask the child to reach for a finger puppet or doll rather than your hand. This makes the child feel less threatened, and the toy can be a reward.

PLANNING AND IMPLEMENTATION

Hospital-Based Nursing Care

Nursing care of the child with altered consciousness or increased intracranial pressure focuses on maintaining airway patency, monitoring neurologic status, performing routine care, providing sensory stimulation, and providing emotional support to parents. Nursing care for the child with increased intracranial pressure is described on page 1711.

TABLE 53–4 ✣ Assessment of Cranial Nerves in the Unconscious Child

Cranial Nerves	Reflex	Assessment Procedure and Normal Findings[a]
II, III	Pupillary	Shine a light source in eye. *Rapid, concentrically constricting pupils indicate intact cranial nerves, II, III.*
II, IV, VI	Oculocephalic	Should be performed with eyes held open (doll's eyes) and head turned from side to side. *Eyes gazing straight up or lagging slightly behind head motion indicate intact cranial nerves.* Precaution: Cervical spine injury must be ruled out before this assessment is performed.
III, VIII	Oculovestibular	Place the head in a midline and slightly elevated position. Inject ice water into ear canal. *Eyes deviating toward the irrigated ear indicate intact cranial nerves III, VIII.* Precautions: Cervical spine injury must be ruled out before this assessment is performed. Tympanic membrane must be intact; otherwise brain may be filled with bacteria-laden fluid. Note: This assessment is usually performed by a physician.
V, VII	Corneal	Cornea is gently swabbed with sterile cotton swab. *A blink indicates intact cranial nerves V, VII.*
IX, X	Gag	Pharynx is irritated with tongue depressor or cotton swab. *Gagging response indicates intact cranial nerves IX, X.*

[a]Italic indicates normal findings.

Make sure the child's airway is clear at all times. If the child is having difficulty managing secretions or does not have a gag reflex, intubation or a tracheostomy is performed. Frequent suctioning may be required (see Skill 15–4). **SKILLS** Keep suction apparatus with catheters, oxygen, resuscitation bag and mask, and extra tracheostomy tubes (if applicable) at the bedside. Perform pulse oximetry or arterial blood gas analysis at regular intervals to ensure that gas exchange is adequate. Mechanical ventilation may be required (see Skill 14–14). **SKILLS**

Perform routine neurologic checks. Evaluate pupil size and reactivity, eye movements, and motor function (Figure 53–3 ⊙). Monitor vital signs. Increased systolic blood pressure, a wide pulse pressure, and bradycardia indicate increased intracranial pressure. Observe for other signs of increased intracranial pressure listed in Table 53–2. Anticipate that seizures may occur. Raise and pad the side rails to protect the child from injury.

Perform routine nursing care. If the corneal reflex is absent, place artificial tears in the eyes and cover them with gauze, taping over so they remain closed. Perform routine mouth care by brushing the teeth and using swabs with water.

Provide adequate nutrition. Initially nutrients may be supplied intravenously. A nasogastric or gastrostomy tube may be inserted if the child remains unconscious or is not alert enough to take food by mouth (see Skill 15–2). **SKILLS** Prevent complications associated with immobility (muscle atrophy, contractures, and skin breakdown) as described in "Nursing Practice." Support physical therapy efforts with extra passive range of motion exercises.

Provide sensory stimulation. Because the child with a severely altered level of consciousness may still be able to hear, talking to him or her may be beneficial. Listening to music or tapes of family members talking or reading can soothe a child who has an altered level of consciousness

⊙ FIGURE 53–3

A

B

C

Pupil findings in various neurologic conditions with altered consciousness. *A,* A unilateral dilated and reactive pupil is associated with an intracranial mass. *B,* A fixed and dilated pupil may be a sign of impending brainstem herniation. *C,* Bilateral fixed and dilated pupils are associated with brainstem herniation from increased intracranial pressure.

NURSING PRACTICE

CARE OF THE IMMOBILE CHILD

- Help keep body in proper alignment with splints or rolls made of towels or blankets.
- Perform passive or gentle range of motion exercises three or four times per day according to physician's orders.
- Maintain skin integrity:
  - Change position every 2 hours.
  - Place child on foam or egg-crate mattress or sheepskin covering.
  - Massage child gently using lotion.

when family members cannot be present. Explain all procedures and actions.

When the child becomes more alert, orient the child to time, place, and person, depending on his or her age and level of understanding. Encourage parents to bring objects or toys from home to make the environment more familiar and promote a feeling of security.

Provide emotional support to the child and family. Explain the child's condition in simple terms. Encourage parents to take part in the child's care and therapy as much as possible. If the child's normal functioning has been permanently impaired, refer the family to the appropriate psychologic and social services for emotional support. (See Chapter 41 for more information about helping families cope with a child's life-threatening illness. ∞) Give family members chances to express their feelings.

Discharge Planning and Home Care Teaching

The child's transition from the hospital to home, a long-term care facility, or inpatient rehabilitation center must be planned well in advance of discharge. A case manager or social worker should be identified who can help plan the child's long-term care needs, including home health nursing, adaptation of the home, and the purchase of special equipment.

Nursing Care in the Community

Home care nurses play a vital role in the care of the child with an acquired neurologic dysfunction and prolonged altered consciousness. Teach the family how to care for the child with severe neurologic dysfunction and to perform routine procedures such as maintaining the airway, skin care, feeding, positioning, exercises, and stimulation. Regular follow-up visits are needed to assess the child's progress and to modify the treatment plan.

The child also needs to be linked with community rehabilitation services through an early intervention pro-

gram or school-based program. The home health nurse or case manager should help the family have an individual education plan developed for the child (see Chapter 39 ∞).

EVALUATION

Expected outcomes of nursing care include the following:

- The child's airway is maintained and the brain is adequately oxygenated.
- The family provides appropriate care to the child with prolonged altered consciousness to promote minimal long-term disabilities.

SEIZURE DISORDERS

Seizures are periods of abnormal electrical discharges in the brain that cause involuntary movement, and behavior and sensory alterations. They are a common neurologic disorder in children. Approximately 2% to 4% of children have one or more seizures during childhood from a variety of causes, most often during infancy. Epilepsy is a chronic disorder characterized by recurrent, unprovoked seizures secondary to a CNS disorder. Infants are susceptible to developing epilepsy in the first year of life with an incidence of 1 per 1000. The incidence decreases with age. The median age for the development of epilepsy is 5 to 6 years. In the United States, approximately 150,000 to 325,000 children between 5 and 14 years of age have epilepsy (Blair & Selekman, 2004).

ETIOLOGY AND PATHOPHYSIOLOGY

Seizures are believed to be the result of abnormal excessive concurrent electrical discharges from the cortical neuronal network of cells on the surface of the brain. Chemical changes within the neurons create an electrical negativity that enables the transfer of information between neurons. When an excessive number of these cells become excited, they discharge abnormally. These cells can be triggered by either environmental or physiologic stimuli such as emotional stress, anxiety, fatigue, infection, or metabolic disturbances. An acute insult such as a CNS infection, hypoxia, and brain trauma are the most common causes in children.

Some seizures are idiopathic, or not provoked by known stimuli. Genetic factors may lower the seizure threshold by making brain cells more vulnerable to abnormal electrical discharges. Acquired seizures may be caused by underlying pathologic conditions such as trauma, infection, hypoglycemia, endocrine dysfunction, toxins, tumors, or lesions that may be manifested at any time. See "Clinical Manifestations: Seizures."

Partial, or **focal**, seizures are caused by abnormal electrical activity in one hemisphere or a specific area of the cerebral cortex, most often the temporal, frontal, or parietal lobes. The symptoms depend on the region of the cortex affected.

In contrast, generalized seizures are the result of diffuse electrical activity that begins in both hemispheres of the brain simultaneously and spreads throughout the cortex into the brainstem. As a result, movements and spasms displayed by the child are bilateral and symmetric.

The length of a seizure, especially of a generalized seizure, is important because the airway may be compromised during the tonic phase. The basal metabolic rate rises during the peak of seizure activity. This change, in turn, increases the demand for oxygen and glucose. During a seizure the child may become pale or cyanotic as a result of hypoxia or hypoglycemia.

Febrile seizures are generalized seizures that usually occur in children as the result of rapid temperature rise above 39°C (102°F) in association with an acute illness. No evidence of intracranial infection or other defined cause is found. They are usually seen between 3 months and 5 years with a peak incidence between 17 to 24 months of age. There is often a family history of febrile seizures. In addition, children who have one febrile seizure have a 30% to 50% greater chance of having future seizures (Gill & Gieron-Korthals, 2002). The lower convulsive threshold of infants may explain this type of seizure.

CLINICAL MANIFESTATIONS

The symptoms of a seizure depend on the type and duration of the seizure. Seizures are classified into two types: *partial (focal) seizures* and *generalized seizures* of nonfocal origin. The specific characteristics of the various types of partial and generalized seizures are presented in "Clinical Manifestations: Seizures." Tonic–clonic seizures are the most common seizure type in children (Weinstein, 2002). The initial manifestations of the **tonic** phase of a generalized seizure are unconsciousness and continuous muscular contraction. The tonic phase is followed by the **clonic** phase, characterized by alternating muscular contraction and relaxation. During the **postictal period** following seizure activity, the level of consciousness is decreased. The length of the postictal period varies among children. An olfactory or visual aura may provide an early warning sign of a seizure. When the child recognizes the pattern of an aura, he or she may have time to avoid injury by getting to the floor.

Febrile seizures involve generalized tonic–clonic movements that last less than 15 minutes.

CLINICAL THERAPY

After the child's first seizure, it is essential that a thorough history be taken from the parent, primary caretaker, or witnesses to the event. The list of questions that should be asked is in "Nursing Practice." Details such as the descrip-

tion and length of the seizure, presence or absence of an aura, and whether the child lost consciousness should be noted. This information is used to identify the type of seizure according to the International Classification of Epileptic Seizures.

NURSING PRACTICE

QUESTIONS TO ASK ABOUT SEIZURES

- Did the child complain of not feeling well or feeling "funny" just before the seizure?
- Did the child complain of headache, nausea, muscle pain? Did the child vomit?
- Did the child suffer any trauma before the seizure?
- Did the child get into any medications or poisons before the seizure?
- Was the child sick or feverish before the seizure?
- What movements of the arms and legs were seen? On one side of the body or in one extremity only?
- Was the child's vision normal?
- Were the pupils dilated or the eyes deviated to one side?
- Was the child aware of surroundings? Could the child respond to questions?
- Was the child incontinent of urine or stool?
- How long did the episode last? When did the child begin to wake up?
- Was the child lethargic, weak, or uncoordinated upon arousal?
- Was the child injured during the convulsion?
- Did the child's color change (pale, red, blue)?

A complete physical and neurologic examination is performed. Laboratory tests that may be ordered include a complete blood cell count, blood chemistry, urine culture, and lumbar puncture. If the child is taking any anticonvulsants, the medication blood level is checked. An EEG is often performed at a follow-up visit between seizures. A lead level, toxicology screening, and radiologic tests such as CT scanning or MRI and angiography may be performed to identify a cerebral lesion or metabolic disorder in the brain.

Many convulsions are self-limiting and require no emergency intervention. Children with febrile seizures are usually not treated with an anticonvulsant at the time of the seizure because of their side effects. Long-term anticonvulsants are not recommended for simple febrile seizures (Shinnar & O'Dell, 2004). Instead, parents are taught to lower fevers by using antipyretics and keeping the child cool with light clothing, and to protect the child from injury if there is a future seizure.

Any child with a generalized seizure lasting longer than 10 minutes needs to be monitored for electrolytes, glucose, blood gases, increasing fever, and abnormal blood pressure. Anticonvulsants are given intravenously or rectally to control the seizure, as the longer the seizure lasts the harder it is to stop (Wheless, 2004). Monitor for continued motor activity and the potential for *status epilepticus* (a continuous seizure that lasts for more than 30 minutes or a series of seizures during which consciousness is not regained).

The postictal period ranges from 30 minutes to 2 hours. Management of the child in status epilepticus is described in Table 53–5.

Most seizure disorders are treated with anticonvulsants. A single medication (monotherapy) is preferred for seizure

CLINICAL MANIFESTATIONS

SEIZURES

TYPE OF SEIZURE AND CAUSE	CLINICAL MANIFESTATIONS
Partial Seizures ***Complex partial seizures*** (psychomotor seizures) Lesions, cysts, or tumors Perinatal trauma Focal sclerosis (i.e., scarring of the mediotemporal lobe from prolonged febrile seizures) Vascular anomalies (i.e., arteriovenous malformations) Brain trauma	*Onset:* 3 years of age to adolescence Consciousness is impaired immediately or gradually after a simple partial onset; lasts 30 seconds up to 5 minutes; postseizure amnesia or confusion May have abnormal motor activity, twitching, loss of tone, sensory changes such as tingling or numbness, may progress to a generalized seizure Aura frequently present, unusual taste or odor Feelings of anxiety, fear, or déjà vu (sensation that event occurred before) Abdominal pain Staring into space, mental confusion Posturing **Automatisms**—lip smacking, lip chewing, sucking
Simple partial seizures (focal seizures) Focal damage (e.g., with cerebral palsy) Tumors or lesions Arteriovenous malformation Brain abscesses	*Onset:* any age No loss of consciousness; lasts less than 30 seconds; no postseizure confusion No aura Motor responses may involve one extremity, part of extremity, or ipsilateral extremities with eyes and head turning in opposite direction Sensory responses involve paresthesias (decreased sensation or tingling); auditory, olfactory, or visual sensations; autonomic (sweating, papillary dilation) or psychic symptoms Motor and sensory involvement may be combined and progress to generalized seizure Jacksonian march (rare in children): tonic contractions of either fingers of one hand, toes of one foot, or one side of face become clonic or tonic-clonic movements; activity then "marches" up to adjacent muscles of either affected extremity or same side of body (such as face)
Generalized Seizures ***Tonic-clonic seizures*** (grand mal seizures) Cerebral damage from perinatal trauma, brain trauma, tumors, structural lesions, metabolic and neuromuscular degenerative disorders Genetic link Many are idiopathic	*Onset:* any age, rare before 6 months of age, strong familial incidence Abrupt onset seizure, 1–2 minute loss of consciousness, postseizure confusion (few minutes to hours) May or may not have aura Body becomes stiff and rigid when all muscles contract (tonic phase), followed by rhythmic jerking motions (clonic phase) Drooling or foaming at mouth as secretions are not swallowed Eyes roll upward or deviate to one side with pupils dilated Abdominal or chest wall rigidity with leg, head, and neck extended, and arms flexed or contracted Cry or grunt as air is forced out when diaphragm and chest muscles contract Urinary or bowel incontinence as muscles become flaccid during clonic phase Characterized by sleepiness, difficulty in arousal; hypertension; diaphoresis; headache, nausea, vomiting; poor coordination, decreased muscle tone; confusion, amnesia; slurred speech; visual disturbances; combativeness

CLINICAL MANIFESTATIONS—continued

SEIZURES

TYPE OF SEIZURE AND CAUSE	CLINICAL MANIFESTATIONS
Generalized Seizures *(continued)* ***Absence seizures*** (petit mal, or lapse seizures) Hyperventilation Genetic predisposition	*Onset:* age 3–12 years with remission in adolescence More prevalent in females May go on to develop other generalized seizures Hyperventilation or flashing lights may trigger a seizure Brief loss of consciousness, usually lasts 5–10 seconds, rarely exceeds 30 seconds, no postseizure confusion, lethargy, or sleepiness Frequent attacks (50–100 per day), may cluster, interfere with learning No aura Child may continue simple movements such as walking or looking, but ceases activities such as reading; slight increase or loss of muscle tone (head may droop, handheld objects may be dropped) Staring; usually a glazed eye appearance, episodes may be confused with daydreaming or inattentiveness Rolling of eyes, eye blinking, ptosis or fluttering of eyelids Amnesia
Myoclonic seizures Progressive or degenerative encephalopathy like Tay-Sachs disease	*Onset:* as early as 2 years, but more prevalent in school-age child or adolescent No loss of consciousness, child recovers in seconds, no postictal period Attacks occur most often upon falling asleep or awakening Quick involuntary muscle jerks, may appear to drop or throw object; sudden flexion and bending of upper torso and head, extremity, or body contractions, may be limited to one body part or whole body
Infantile spasms (myoclonic epilepsy of infancy, salaam seizures) Prenatal and perinatal encephalopathy Metabolic disorder Tuberous sclerosis Microcephaly Evolve into Lennox-Gastaut syndrome	*Onset:* begin at age 3 months and resolve by 2 years Positive history of gestational difficulties, developmental delays, or other neurologic abnormalities May occur with altered consciousness as part of a complex partial seizure Occur in clusters, 5 to 150 per day Episodes of abrupt flexor (jackknife seizures), extensor or mixed jerks occurring in flurries when infant is awakening or throughout wakefulness Eye rolling, either upward or downward Crying, pallor, or cyanosis Regression in development and irritability Seizure activity increases in intensity and severity over time
Akinetic or atonic seizures (drop attacks) Gray matter degenerative diseases and subacute seizures Sclerosing panencephalitis Many are idiopathic	*Onset:* first seen at 2 years, disappear by 6 years Momentary loss of consciousness Falls to ground with sudden loss of postural tone, inability to break fall, is limp for a period of time Quickly regains consciousness

control to minimize the side effects such as sleepiness, decreased attention and memory, difficulty with speech, ataxia, and diplopia. Monotherapy works for 60% to 70% of children with new-onset epilepsy (Blair & Selekman, 2004). See Table 53–6 for first and second line medications used. Serum drug levels are monitored to achieve therapeutic levels or when toxicity is possible. Therapeutic ranges of medications may be exceeded to control seizures when tolerated by the child. Medication dosage adjustments are often needed as the child grows. Approximately 25% to 30% of children have refractory or **intractable seizures**, seizures that continue to occur even with optimal medical management (Danielpour & Peacock, 2000). These children are often treated with multiple anticonvulsants. Regular blood

TABLE 53–5 ✤ Management of Status Epilepticus

Type of Care	Clinical Therapy
Emergency assessment and management	■ Maintain a patent airway. Muscle rigidity may compromise the airway. ■ Perform a jaw thrust maneuver if the airway is obstructed. ■ Keep suction equipment at the bedside in case secretions are excessive. ■ Give oxygen by mask, as increased metabolic demands deplete oxygen stores. ■ Monitor vital signs and circulation with pulse oximeter and cardiorespiratory monitor. ■ Assess neurologic level.
Ongoing urgent management	■ Establish an intravenous line to administer any necessary fluids or medications. ■ Administer glucose if the child is hypoglycemic; the physical stress of the seizure may result in declining glucose levels. ■ Insert a nasogastric tube. ■ Protect the child from injury. ■ Manage thermoregulation.
Medications	■ Administer benzodiazepines such as diazepam, lorazepam, or midazolam. If there is no response, the dose may be repeated. Phenytoin or phenobarbital may be necessary if seizure activity continues. Cumulative doses of drugs may produce apnea, so be prepared to assist ventilations.

testing is performed to identify any developing hematologic or liver problems, as well as to determine if therapeutic ranges of medications are maintained. *Families should be cautioned that herbal preparations with ginkgo may decrease the effectiveness of anticonvulsants.*

TABLE 53–6 ✤ Anticonvulsants Used to Treat Seizure Disorders

Emergency Medications	First Line Medications	Second Line Medications
Diazepam	Carbamazepine Ethosuximide Phenobarbital Phenytoin Primidone Valproic Acid	Clonazepam Felbamate Gabapentin Lamotrigine Tiagabine Topiramate

Surgery may occasionally be performed to remove a tumor, lesion, or portion of the brain that has been identified as causing the seizures, particularly when seizures are not responsive to medication. A vagal nerve stimulator is another option for children who are unable to tolerate multiple medications and are not candidates for surgery (Blair & Selekman, 2004).

A ketogenic diet is occasionally used for children under the age of 8 years with myoclonic and absence seizures. This diet involves a high intake of fat (90%), an adequate intake of protein (1 g/kg), and a very low intake of carbohydrates. Caloric intake is calculated at 75% and fluids are restricted to 80% of usual (Freeman, 2003). The ketosis caused by the diet is believed to produce anticonvulsant effects. The diet is customized to the child to maintain the ideal body weight, maximize ketosis, and achieve optimal seizure control. Family motivation must be high to maintain the diet for 2 to 3 years and to frequently monitor the child's urine ketone values (Katyal, Koehler, McGhee et al., 2000). The most common complications are constipation and kidney stones. Constipation is treated with medium chain triglycerides (MCT oil) and increasing fluids. Kidney stones are treated with increased fluid intake and alkalinizing the urine. Some children have discontinued the diet after 2 years with no seizures and no antiepileptic medications needed.

A trial of medication withdrawal is often attempted for children who have been seizure-free for at least 2 years. Approximately 60% to 70% of children are successfully weaned from antiepileptic medications and have no seizures (Blair & Selekman, 2004).

NURSING MANAGEMENT

NURSING ASSESSMENT AND DIAGNOSIS

Assess and monitor the child's physiologic status. Observe the specific seizure activity, level of consciousness, vital signs, and signs of hypoxia. During the postictal period, monitor the child's vital signs, perform neurologic checks, and keep the environment safe. Once the child is stable, a more definitive assessment can be made. Level of consciousness is one of the most important indicators of neurologic function. Remember that the child's lack of response may be the result of the postictal state.

Collect and analyze historical information about the seizure activity, clustering, aura, description of motor activity or changes in muscle tone, automatisms, and any changes in development or school performance to help determine the type of seizures the child has.

Assess the family's adaptation to the seizure disorder, including how well the family is coping with the uncertainty of when the next seizure will occur.

DRUG GUIDE

PHENYTOIN

Overview of Action
Inhibits seizure activity; reduces voltage, frequency, and spread of electrical discharges within the motor cortex. Used for control of tonic-clonic (generalized) and partial seizures with complex symptomatology, as well as seizures occurring before and after neurosurgery. May be used in status epilepticus, particulary in combination with diazepam.

Routes, Dosage, Frequency
PO or IV: For seizures
- Newborn: 15–20 mg/kg loading dose, then 12 hours later start 5 mg/kg in 2 to 3 equally divided doses.
- Infants/Children: 15–20 mg/kg loading dose, then 12 hours later start 5 mg/kg in 2 to 3 doses/day.

PO: For maintenance
- 6 mo–3 yr, 8–10 mg/kg/day in 2 to 3 doses; 4–6 yr, 7.5–9 mg/kg/day in 2 to 3 doses; 7–9 yr, 7–8 mg/kg/day in 2 to 3 doses; 10–16 yr, 6–7 mg/kg/day in 2 to 3 doses.

Contraindications: Hypersensitivity to the drug, seizures due to bradycardia, complete or incomplete heart block, pregnancy. Use with caution in impaired liver or kidney function, blood dyscrasias, diabetes mellitus, hyperglycemia, respiratory depression, and congestive heart failure.

Side Effects: Confusion, drowsiness, dizziness, headache, bradycardia, hypotension, photophobia, diplopia, blurred vision, hirsutism, thrombocytopenia, leukopenia, pancytopenia, hyperglycemia, weight gain, gingival hyperplasia, osteomalacia, Stevens-Johnson syndrome, lymphadenopathy.

Nursing Implications
Assess: **IV.** Continuously monitor vital signs and symptoms during IV infusion and for an hour afterwards. Observe for respiratory depression. **PO:** Periodic CBC, platelet count, liver function tests, serum glucose, serum calcium, serum magnesium. Serum levels of drug may be monitored.

Administer: Give the PO form with food or fluid to prevent gastric irritation. If given by feeding tube, dilute the solution with sterile water, D5W, or normal saline and flush tube with at least 20 mL after administration to avoid adherence to feeding tube. If given IV, give undiluted, slow infusion not to exceed 1–3 mg/kg/minute in infants and children (0.5 mg/kg/minute in newborns). Follow with sterile saline to decrease vein irritation. Do not use with solutions containing dextrose. Have emergency drugs and equipment available if given IV.

Monitor: CBC, liver function tests, and urinalysis are done monthly. Observe for side effects, especially gingival hyperplasia and rashes. Observe for and record seizure activity, neuropathy, and mental changes.

Patient Teaching: Inform the child and family that the drug may turn the urine pink or red-brown. If a measles-like rash or jaundice appears, discontinue the medication immediately and notify the physician. Do not otherwise suddenly stop the medications as seizures may occur. Do not accept changes in drug brand when refilling prescription without consulting the physician. Make sure sustained-release tablets are not chewed or crushed. Shake the suspension thoroughly before pouring. Folic acid, calcium, and vitamin D absorption may be decreased by the drug, so encourage adequate intake of calcium and vitamins. Good dental hygiene (brushing, flossing, and gum massage) and frequent dental visits are needed to reduce the severity of gingival hyperplasia. A medical alert band indicating seizures and phenytoin medication use should be worn. Avoid alcohol as it may increase phenytoin serum levels and cause toxicity. Mental alertness may be altered with this medication, so driving cars or other mechanical equipment should be avoided.

Adapted with permission from Bindler, R. M., Howry, L. B., Wilson, B. A., Shannon, M. T., & Stang, C. L. (2005). Pediatric drug guide nursing implications. Upper Saddle River, NJ: Prentice Hall.

DEVELOPING CULTURAL COMPETENCE

SEIZURES MAY BE VIEWED DIFFERENTLY
Seizures may have a special meaning by different cultural groups. For example, the Hmong believe the child is experiencing *quag dab peg* or "the spirit catches you and you fall down." Hmong view the condition as serious, but there is a sense of pride that the child has the condition. In 1997, Anne Fadiman wrote a compelling story about the cultural conflict between a Hmong family and healthcare providers over the treatment of their daughter's seizures, called *The Spirit Catches You and You Fall Down* (Fadiman, 1997; Spector, 2000).

Common nursing diagnoses for the child with a seizure disorder include the following:

- *Ineffective Breathing Pattern* related to neuromuscular dysfunction during the tonic phase of a seizure
- *Ineffective Airway Clearance* related to inability to control secretions during seizure
- *Risk for Trauma* related to seizure activity
- *Chronic Low Self-Esteem* related to refractory seizures and loss of bowel and bladder control during seizure activity
- *Anxiety* related to unpredictable nature of seizure disorder

■ *Ineffective Therapeutic Regimen Management* related to poor adherence with medications

■ *Readiness for Enhanced Family Processes* related to care of a child with a chronic disorder

PLANNING AND IMPLEMENTATION

Nursing care focuses on maintaining airway patency, ensuring safety, administering medications, and providing emotional support. Both acute care and long-term management are involved.

Maintain Airway Patency

Be sure that nothing is placed in the child's mouth during a seizure; loose teeth may be knocked out and aspirated. The child is placed on his or her side for secretions to drain. Monitor the child to ensure adequate oxygenation: the child's color should be pink, the heart rate at a normal or slightly above normal rate for age, and the pulse oximetry reading greater than 95%. Oxygen is usually given at SpO_2 levels below 95% (see Skill 14–2). **SKILLS**

Ensure Safety

Protect the child from self-harm during violent seizures (Figure 53–4 ●). If the child is in bed, the side rails should be padded to prevent injury. Children who have frequent, recurrent seizures should wear helmets to protect their heads in case they fall. All children with seizure disorders should wear some form of medical identification (e.g., a medical alert bracelet).

● **FIGURE 53–4**

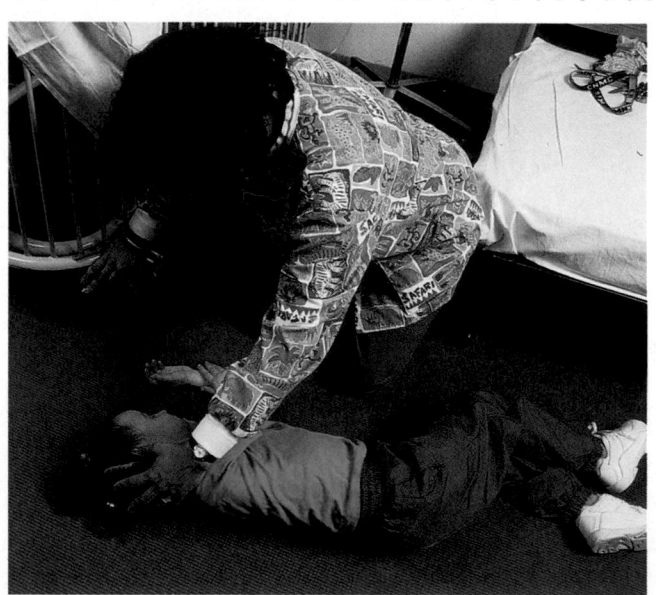

A child who has a seizure when standing should be gently assisted to the floor and placed in a side-lying position. Clear the area of any objects that might cause harm to the child.

Administer Medications

Take special precautions when administering intravenous medications (diazepam, lorazepam, fosphenytoin) for the emergency management of status epilepticus. Give these medications very slowly over several minutes to minimize the risk of respiratory or circulatory collapse.

Medications for the management of chronic seizures are given orally. Crushing pills and mixing them in a teaspoonful of applesauce, pudding, or other soft food make them more palatable and easier for the child to swallow.

When a child is NPO due to illness or on the day of surgery, seizure medications are usually given with a swallow of water. Obtain medication orders in these cases.

Provide Emotional Support

The loss of control of body movements and possible loss of consciousness make seizures frightening and difficult to accept for the child, parents, and other family members. Parents often feel guilty about the child's seizure disorder and compensate by not disciplining or restricting the child appropriately. Stress the need to treat the child as normally as possible. Refer the child and family to support groups and counseling services if indicated.

Discharge Planning and Home Care Teaching

Encourage parents to express their fears and anxieties. Answer their questions honestly, and refer them to organizations such as the Epilepsy Foundation of America, where they can get more information about the child's disorder. Be sure parents know how to administer medications and keep the child safe. Discuss with them whom to call with questions and when to return for follow-up.

Nursing Care in the Community

Educate the child and parents about medication regimens. Explain the purpose of each drug, its schedule for administration, and the importance of giving all doses. Explain the use of rectal diazepam (Diastat) for acute management of a seizure. Teaching the older child to take medications without parental intervention gives the child a feeling of control. Provide information about the side effects of medications ordered, and alert parents to the signs of toxic reactions or undermedication. Regular dental care is important because of the effect of phenytoin on the gingiva. Explain the importance of follow-up visits to healthcare providers so that medication blood levels and the effectiveness of the child's medications can be monitored.

The parents of children with recurrent febrile seizures should be taught how to give antipyretics in the proper dose. Parents need to know that antipyretics may not prevent a future febrile seizure associated with an acute illness.

EVIDENCE-BASED NURSING

SUPPORTING CHILDREN WITH EPILEPSY

Clinical Question (Problem)

Children who develop epilepsy during childhood are faced with many issues, such as making an adjustment to living with a chronic condition, managing their condition, and telling friends about the seizures. What information and support do school-age children need to live with epilepsy and how do they manage their lives?

Evidence

A scale developed to measure the psychosocial care needs of children with seizures was tested with a total of 63 children (average age of 10.5 years) at both 3 months and 6 months after the first seizure. Children were most satisfied with explanations they received from healthcare providers about their condition, but they were least satisfied with an opportunity to ask questions 3 months after the first seizure. Children wanted more information about activity restrictions, protection from injury, and handling future seizures. They also wanted to talk with other children their age with seizures and learn how to handle seizures at school (Austin, Dunn, Huster et al., 1998; McNelis, Musick, Austin et al., 1998). In another study, eight school-age children who had lived with epilepsy for at least a year were interviewed. They understood the need for medications and knew the medication name and dosage schedule, but six of the children did not like taking the medication or its side effects. Most of the children had found a way to educate their peers and to fit in with their peer group. Some of the children had identified warning signs of an impending seizure and took measures to prevent future seizures such as getting plenty of sleep, drinking adequate fluids, getting some exercise, staying out of the sun, and avoiding becoming angry (Hightower, Carmon, & Minick, 2002).

Implications

While the sample sizes for these studies are not large, information about living with epilepsy from the child's perspective is important. Learning about the child's understanding and perceptions helps the nurse to determine strategies that may help the child cope more effectively and to enhance development of self-esteem. As the child grows, self-management of the condition becomes increasingly important, along with preventive measures that can become part of the child's daily routine, such as sleep, hydration, nutrition, and avoiding certain types of stimulation.

Critical Thinking

Develop a teaching plan for a child between 10 and 12 years old with generalized seizures who is beginning to assume more responsibility for daily care. Be sure to include safety as well as self-esteem enhancement along with recognizing signs of seizures, nutrition, hydration, and medication administration.

References

Austin, J., Dunn, D., Huster, G., & Rose, D. (1998). Development of scales to measure psychosocial care needs of children with seizures and their parents. *Journal of Neuroscience Nursing, 30*(3), 155–160.

Hightower, S., Carmon, M., & Minick, P. (2002). A qualitative descriptive study of the lived experiences of school-aged children with epilepsy. *Journal of Pediatric Health Care, 16*(3), 131–137.

McNelis, A., Musick, B., Austin, J., Dunn, D., & Creasy, K. (1998). Psychosocial care needs of children with new-onset seizures. *Journal of Neuroscience Nursing, 30*(3), 161–165.

The potential toxicity of an anticonvulsant in a child with febrile seizures often outweighs the risk of the seizures, and parents can be reassured that complications from febrile seizures are rare.

Adolescent females need to be educated about the potential teratogenicity of some anticonvulsants, such as valproic acid and carbamazepine, that are associated with neural tube defects and heart defects. Contraception should be used when the adolescent is sexually active, until a planned pregnancy is desired. Anticonvulsants that reduce the risk for birth defects can be ordered at that time.

Teach families about safety guidelines for the child. Families of children with severe seizure disorders need to develop an emergency care plan so that emergency personnel know about their needs for care in advance (see Chapter 39 ∞).

Assist the family to develop an individual health plan so the child can receive medications during school hours, if necessary. Teachers and school administrators should know what to do if the child has a seizure and what information to report about the seizure. Parents may want to

TEACHING HIGHLIGHTS

SAFETY FOR THE CHILD WITH A SEIZURE DISORDER

Children with epilepsy have more injuries of all sorts, including burns and falls. Children are at increased risk for death due to drowning.

Planning for safety includes the following:

- Do not leave the child alone in the bathtub.
- Children who bathe alone should use the shower.
- A buddy and lifeguard should always be present when the child swims.
- A life vest should always be worn when boating.
- A child with frequent seizures should wear a helmet to protect the head in case of a fall.
- The child should not play or stand around open flames or outdoor grills.
- The child should avoid areas where fall risks are increased.
- A form of medical identification should be worn, such as a medical alert bracelet.

provide a towel and change of clothing for the child to use if incontinence occurs with the seizures.

Physical activity and exercise is important for all children. Encourage participation in sports when good supervision is provided. Activities such as rope climbing, rock or mountain climbing, tree climbing, snow skiing, scuba diving, and sky diving are more dangerous if seizures are not well controlled. Swimming and water sports require one-to-one supervision.

The child may be afraid of having a seizure in front of friends. Reassure the child and family that taking medications regularly should control seizures. Children need to be able to explain to peers what a seizure is and what to do if they are present when one occurs. Summer camps for children with seizures can be a safe and comfortable place for the child to enjoy outdoor activities. Tell parents to boost the child's self-image by emphasizing what the child can do, rather than focusing on contraindicated activities. Depending on state laws, most adolescents can drive after they have been seizure-free for at least 2 years.

EVALUATION

Expected outcomes of nursing management include the following:

- The child achieves good seizure control with medication, ketogenic diet, or surgical intervention.
- The child's self-esteem is enhanced through participation in well-supervised sports and activities.

INFECTIOUS DISEASES

BACTERIAL MENINGITIS

Meningitis, an inflammation of the meninges, can be caused by either bacterial or viral agents. Bacterial meningitis is more virulent than viral meningitis and is sometimes fatal. Newborns and infants are at greatest risk for bacterial meningitis. Infants and children who develop meningitis have the potential for acute complications and long-term morbidity.

ETIOLOGY AND PATHOPHYSIOLOGY

Meningitis may occur secondary to other infections such as otitis media, sinusitis, pharyngitis, cellulitis, pneumonia, or septic arthritis; brain trauma; or a neurosurgical procedure. Three organisms cause a majority of cases in children between 2 months and 12 years of age: *Haemophilus influenzae* type b, *Neisseria meningitidis*, and *Streptococcus pneumoniae*. The organisms causing

meningitis in newborns include these plus group B streptococcus (Prober, 2004). Fortunately, immunization of infants with the pneumococcal vaccine is reducing the incidence of meningitis caused by *Streptococcus pneumoniae* (Black, Shinefield, Baxter et al., 2004).

In many cases, bacteremia spreads the infectious agent to the CNS (see "Pathophysiology Illustrated: Central Nervous System Infection"). An inflammatory response follows. White blood cells accumulate, covering the surface of the brain with a thick, white, purulent exudate. The brain then becomes hyperemic and edematous. If the infection spreads to the ventricles, they can become obstructed and impede the flow of cerebrospinal fluid, causing increased intracranial pressure and hydrocephalus.

CLINICAL MANIFESTATIONS

Symptoms are variable and depend on the child's age, the pathogen, and the length of the illness before diagnosis. Onset may be sudden or the illness may develop over 1 to 2 days. Symptoms in the young infant may include fever, change in feeding pattern, vomiting, or diarrhea. The anterior fontanelle may be bulging or flat. The infant may be alert, restless, lethargic, or irritable. Rocking or cuddling, which normally calms a fussy infant, only irritates the infant with meningitis.

Older children are usually febrile; can have confusion, delirium, or impaired consciousness; can be irritable, lethargic, or confused; have vomiting; and complain of muscle or joint pain. A hemorrhagic rash, first appearing as petechiae and changing to purpura or large necrotic patches, may be seen in meningococcal meningitis. The child displays other symptoms consistent with meningeal irritation: headache (most often frontal), photophobia, esotropia, and *nuchal rigidity* (resistance to neck flexion). The child is comfortable only in an opisthotonic position (hyperextension of the head and neck to relieve discomfort (Figure 53–5 ●). The child may have a positive Kernig or Brudzinski sign, or both, on examination (Figures 53–6 and 53–7 ●).

Symptoms can progress to include seizures, apnea, cerebral edema, subdural effusion, hydrocephalus, disseminated intravascular coagulation (DIC), shock, and increased intracranial pressure.

CLINICAL THERAPY

Diagnosis is based on the history, clinical presentation, and laboratory findings. Laboratory tests include a complete blood count, blood cultures, serum electrolytes and osmolality, and clotting factors. Blood cultures usually identify the responsible bacteria causing meningitis. A lumbar puncture is performed to evaluate the cerebrospinal fluid for number of white blood cells and protein and glucose

PATHOPHYSIOLOGY ILLUSTRATED
Central Nervous System Infection

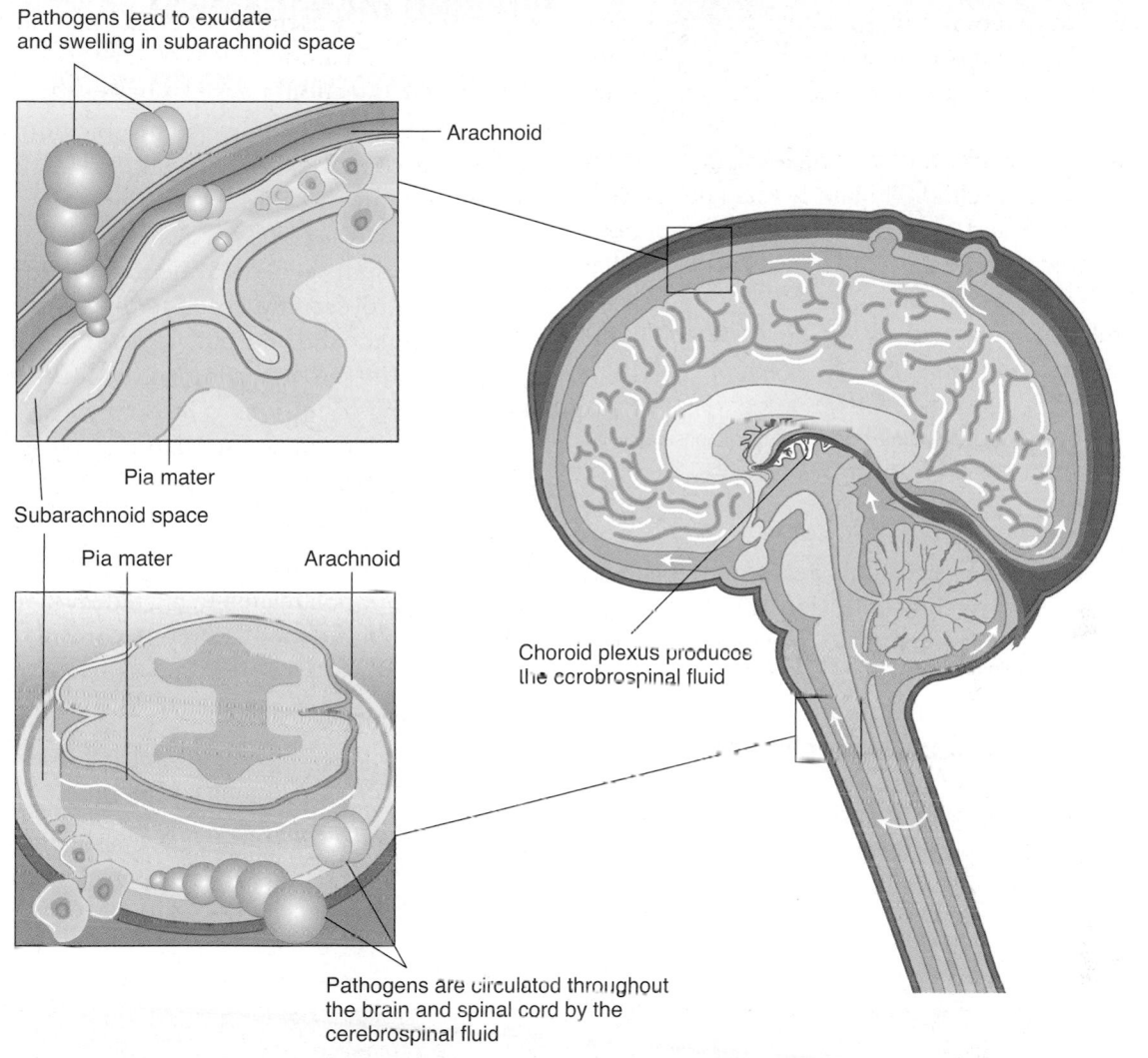

Pathogens lead to exudate and swelling in subarachnoid space

Arachnoid

Pia mater

Subarachnoid space

Pia mater

Arachnoid

Choroid plexus produces the cerebrospinal fluid

Pathogens are circulated throughout the brain and spinal cord by the cerebrospinal fluid

After bacteria reach the central nervous system, the pia mater, the arachnoid, and the cerebrospinal fluid–filled subarachnoid space become infected. The cerebrospinal fluid then circulates the pathogens throughout the brain and spinal cord.

levels. A Gram stain and culture are done on the cerebrospinal fluid. CT scanning may be performed when increased intracranial pressure or a brain abscess is suspected. Serum electrolytes and blood urea nitrogen are also tested.

Antibiotics are administered as soon as diagnostic tests are obtained. Antibiotics commonly used to treat bacterial meningitis include ampicillin, aminoglycosides, cefotaxime, ceftriaxone, and penicillin G. Antibiotics are often changed once culture and sensitivity results are known, especially as many organisms have resistance to certain antibiotics. These medications are administered intravenously for 7 to 21 days, depending on the organism and the child's clinical response. Depending on the causative organism, the disease may need to be reported to the local health department, and contacts may need to take prophylactic antibiotics, such as rifampin or ciprofloxacin. Corticosteroids (dexamethasone) are given as an adjunct to children over 6 weeks of age to reduce the risk of severe neurologic sequelae such as sensorineural hearing loss. In some cases, anticonvulsants and antipyretics are given (American Academy of Pediatrics, 2003a).

Infants and children receive nothing by mouth and are started on IV fluids. The IV fluids are initially restricted to two-thirds maintenance as careful monitoring for increased intracranial pressure and syndrome of inappropriate antidiuretic hormone (SIADH; see Chapter 56 ∞) is initiated. If

● FIGURE 53-5

The child with bacterial meningitis assumes an opisthotonic position, with the neck and the head hyperextended, to relieve discomfort.

the child is in shock, aggressive fluid resuscitation is performed to maintain the cerebral perfusion pressure.

Some infants and children who have had bacterial meningitis suffer neurologic damage despite early, aggressive management. The most common sequelae involve cranial nerves, especially the eighth, resulting in hearing loss. In addition, children may have seizures, hydrocephalus, subdural effusion, syndrome of insufficient antidiuretic hormone, developmental delay, learning problems, and behavior problems. Another potential complication is meningococcal

septicemia, characterized by high fever, hypotension, DIC, and multisystem organ failure (Harrison, 2001). See the discussion about meningococcemia in Chapter 49. ∞

NURSING MANAGEMENT

NURSING ASSESSMENT AND DIAGNOSIS

Assess the child's physiologic status, including vital signs and level of consciousness. Measure head circumference often in infants because of the potential for hydrocephalus. Be alert for signs of a change in the child's condition and response to treatment. Monitor the child's ability to control secretions and to drink sufficient fluids. Monitor intake and output. Assess for any sensory deficits. Identify parents' concerns about this potentially life-threatening condition.

Several nursing diagnoses that may apply to the child with bacterial meningitis are given in the accompanying "Nursing Care Plan." Additional nursing diagnoses might include the following:

- *Risk for Aspiration* related to altered level of consciousness and poor secretion control
- *Risk for Deficient Fluid Volume* related to poor oral fluid intake
- *Anticipatory Grieving (Parent)* related to the child's potentially life-threatening condition
- *Caregiver Role Strain* related to a hospitalized child and other family responsibilities

● FIGURE 53-6

To test for Kernig sign, raise the child's leg with the knee flexed. Then extend the child's leg at the knee. If any resistance is noted or pain is felt, the result is a positive Kernig sign. This is a common finding in meningitis.

● FIGURE 53-7

To test Brudzinski sign, flex the child's head while in a supine position. If this action makes the knees or hips flex involuntarily, a positive Brudzinski sign is present. This is a common finding in meningitis.

NURSING CARE PLAN

THE CHILD WITH BACTERIAL MENINGITIS

Intervention	Rationale	Expected Outcome
1. Nursing Diagnosis: Impaired Spontaneous Ventilation related to level of consciousness and respiratory muscle fatigue		
NIC Priority Intervention: **Respiratory monitoring:** Collection and analysis of patient data to ensure airway patency and adequate gas exchange		**NOC Suggested Outcome:** **Vital sign status:** Pulse, respiration, and blood pressure are within expected range for age
Goal: The child's respiratory failure does not progress to respiratory arrest.		
■ Place the child on a cardiorespiratory monitor with a 20-second alarm. ■ Have resuscitation equipment, including oxygen, resuscitation bag with mask, and suction apparatus, at the bedside. ■ Stimulate the child if apneic; if no response begin manual ventilations and call for emergency resuscitation. ■ Monitor heart rate and perform compressions if necessary.	■ The alarm on the monitor alerts staff that the child is having bradycardia or an apneic spell. ■ Equipment should be at the bedside in case of respiratory arrest. Bag-valve-mask ventilation is recommended as the child's respiratory secretions contain bacteria. ■ Stimulation may encourage spontaneous respirations; if not, ventilation is necessary. Calling for emergency resuscitation ensures help in managing the child in a timely manner. ■ The apneic child may have bradycardia resulting from cardiac hypoxia.	The child's respiratory failure is managed with assessment and prompt treatment.
2. Nursing Diagnosis: Ineffective Protection related to infection of cerebrospinal fluid and potential sequelae		
NIC Priority Intervention: **Neurologic monitoring:** Collection and analysis of patient data to prevent or minimize neurologic complications		**NOC Suggested Outcome:** **Neurologic status: Consciousness:** Extent to which an individual arouses, orients, and attends to the environment
Goal: The child will suffer minimal CNS injury secondary to infection.		
■ Administer prescribed antibiotics and corticosteroids as scheduled. ■ Note return of fever, nuchal rigidity, or irritability. Monitor vital signs, assess for signs of increased intracranial pressure, measure head circumference once or twice daily, note changes in responsiveness. Notify the physician immediately if any signs are detected.	■ Antibiotics help eradicate the pathogen and prevent cerebral edema. Corticosteroids diminish inflammatory response and reduce the chance of neurologic sequelae. ■ Watching for common sequelae such as subdural effusions or septic arthritis ensures prompt treatment.	The child's condition improves significantly within 48–72 hours (fever decreases and no signs of neurologic sequelae are detected).
Goal: The child will not develop cerebral edema as a result of water retention.		
■ Monitor for syndrome of inappropriate antidiuretic hormone secretion (SIADH) and watch for signs of increased intracranial pressure (ICP). ■ Perform strict intake and output measurements. Determine urine specific gravity. Check electrolytes and osmolality of both serum and urine. Weigh the child daily. Restrict fluids and give sodium chloride as ordered.	■ SIADH can be either avoided or quickly managed if recognized early. ■ Low urine output with a high specific gravity is a sign of fluid retention and SIADH. The child is maintained with lower fluids and provided sodium supplements to reduce the possibility for cerebral edema.	Cerebral edema does not develop. If SIADH or increased ICP occurs, the condition is treated promptly so effects are minimal.

(continued)

NURSING CARE PLAN—continued

THE CHILD WITH BACTERIAL MENINGITIS

Intervention	Rationale	Expected Outcome
Goal: The child will be free of injury resulting from DIC.		
▪ Be aware of needlesticks that continue to bleed and lesions that continue to ooze. Monitor clotting times. ▪ Administer blood products, vitamin K, or heparin as ordered.	▪ Prompt recognition leads to management of the coagulopathy. ▪ Prompt recognition allows for early initial treatment of DIC. The child may bleed to death if treatment is delayed.	The child does not sustain injury from DIC.
Goal: The child will be free of injury secondary to shock.		
▪ Monitor vital signs, including pulse, respirations, and blood pressure. Note perfusion (capillary refill, central versus proximal pulses). Check level of consciousness. Note urine output. ▪ Begin fluid resuscitation as ordered. ▪ Administer inotropes if ordered.	▪ Monitoring allows for prompt diagnosis of shock based on clinical signs. ▪ Intravenous fluid bolus may improve perfusion. ▪ Inotropes enhance perfusion when response to fluid challenge is minimal.	The child recovers from shock quickly with no complications. Prompt management of shock can enhance the child's recovery, since it prevents complications associated with poor perfusion (tissue acidosis and ischemia).

3. Nursing Diagnosis: Social Isolation related to decreased level of consciousness and hospitalization

NIC Priority Intervention:		NOC Suggested Outcome:
Socialization enhancement: Facilitation of the child's ability to interact with others		**Social involvement:** Frequency of an individual's social interaction behaviors
Goal: The child's social interaction will be near normal despite isolation.		
▪ Educate parents and other visitors to use proper infection control techniques. ▪ Encourage parents to help with daily activities such as feeding and bathing. ▪ Have age-appropriate games and toys in the room. Play with the child. When the child is feeling better, encourage watching television/videotape or listening to the radio/audiotape.	▪ Family members help fulfill the emotional and social needs of the ill and contagious child while the child is on isolation. ▪ Parental involvement in the child's care provides the child with a sense of security and emotional well-being. Parents have a sense of control and a feeling that they are doing something to enhance the child's recovery. ▪ Providing the child with toys and games as well as sensory stimulation helps the child achieve a sense of well-being.	The child's social and developmental needs are met by family members despite the child's illness and hospitalization.
Goal: The child with any degree of hearing loss will be identified.		
▪ Arrange for hearing assessment prior to discharge.	▪ Hearing loss is a common complication. Early intervention is needed to promote growth and development.	The child with identified hearing loss is referred to appropriate specialist or program for intervention.

4. Nursing Diagnosis: Acute Pain related to meningeal irritation

NIC Priority Intervention:		NOC Suggested Outcome:
Pain management: Alleviation of pain or reduction in pain to a level of comfort acceptable to patient		**Comfort level:** Feelings of physical and psychologic ease

NURSING CARE PLAN—continued

THE CHILD WITH BACTERIAL MENINGITIS

Intervention	Rationale	Expected Outcome
Goal: The child will be as comfortable as possible.		
■ Assess pain with age-appropriate pain scale. ■ Minimize tactile stimulation. ■ Allow the child to assume a comfortable position. ■ Keep the lights dim and maintain a quiet environment. ■ Provide pain medication as ordered.	■ Pain scales provide ability to quantify pain for future comparison. ■ Sensory stimulation increases discomfort. ■ The child determines the most comfortable position. Opisthotonic position, with the head and neck hyperextended, may be the most comfortable. ■ Dim lights reduce the discomfort from photophobia. Noise can disturb the child. ■ Round-the-clock pain management promotes comfort and healing.	The child is calm and expresses increased comfort.

5. Nursing Diagnosis: Risk for Infection (Family and Close Contacts) related to pathogens in the cerebrospinal fluid

NIC Priority Intervention:		NOC Suggested Outcome:
Infection control: Minimizing the acquisition and transmission of infectious agents		**Infection status:** Presence and extent of infection
Goal: Caretakers or family members will have no apparent evidence of infection.		
■ Explain rationale and dose schedule for taking rifampin or ciprofloxacin.	■ Rifampin and ciprofloxacin provide prophylaxis for many bacterial pathogens responsible for meningitis.	Family members and other close contacts complete rifampin or ciprofloxacin therapy and avoid becoming infected.

PLANNING AND IMPLEMENTATION

The "Nursing Care Plan" summarizes care for the child with bacterial meningitis. Nursing care begins with emergency treatment and continues as the child's condition stabilizes. Monitor respiratory and neurologic status, maintain hydration, administer medications, and prevent complications. Promote the child's comfort with reduced stimulation (dim lights, quiet room) and by placing in a side-lying position. Isolate the child and use standard and droplet precautions until the causative organism is identified and effective treatment is under way.

Monitor the child's response to antibiotic therapy. Observe for signs of gastrointestinal bleeding, which is a potential complication of corticosteroid use. Maintenance and replacement fluids are usually given to children with bacterial meningitis. However, it is important to monitor the serum sodium concentration and urine specific gravity because these children are at risk for SIADH. Fluids are restricted if SIADH is suspected. Sodium chloride, potassium, and acetate or lactate are administered intravenously to balance sodium excretion.

Respond to parents' concerns about their child's condition, explaining all measures to reduce the child's discomfort and treat the illness. Identify ways parents can help meet the child's comfort needs. Parents may also need help figuring out how to meet the needs of other children at home while spending time with the hospitalized child.

Discharge Planning and Home Care Teaching

Identify and address home care needs well in advance of discharge. Follow-up visits are important to monitor for complications and sequelae. Help parents deal with any physical requirements resulting from the child's illness and any emotional, social, and financial repercussions of the child's condition. Teach parents what to do if the child has a seizure.

Infants and toddlers with neurologic sequelae should be referred to an early intervention program. If the child has had a hearing loss, referral to an otolaryngologist and speech and language specialist should be made. Encourage early identification of other neurologic sequelae, such as learning problems. Children with hearing, learning, or attention disorders need individual education plans (see Chapter 39 ∞), and parents may need help planning for the child's special educational needs. Refer parents to the appropriate social service agencies for support and assistance.

Adolescents should be encouraged to get the meningococcal vaccine to prevent meningococcal meningitis.

EVALUATION

Expected outcomes of nursing care are provided in the "Nursing Care Plan."

VIRAL (ASEPTIC) MENINGITIS

Viral meningitis is an inflammatory response of the meninges characterized by an increased number of blood cells and protein in the cerebrospinal fluid. In the United States, an enterovirus is often the cause of more than 80% of viral meningitis cases (Prober, 2004).

Generally, the child with aseptic meningitis does not appear as ill as the child with bacterial meningitis. The child may be irritable or lethargic and usually has a fever. Other symptoms include general malaise, headache, photophobia, gastrointestinal distress, upper respiratory symptoms, and a maculopapular rash. The child may also show signs of meningeal irritation such as stiff neck, back pain, and positive Kernig and Brudzinski signs (see Figures 53–6 and 53–7). The infant may have a tense anterior fontanelle. Seizures are rare. Symptoms usually resolve spontaneously within 3 to 10 days.

The child with fever and meningeal signs is hospitalized. Blood, urine, and cerebrospinal fluid analyses are performed. Polymerase chain reaction testing helps detect viral meningitis. Until the diagnosis of aseptic meningitis is confirmed, the child is treated aggressively, as if he or she has bacterial meningitis. Treatment is supportive of symptoms.

NURSING MANAGEMENT

Initial nursing care focuses on providing supportive care as described for the child with bacterial meningitis. Give acetaminophen as ordered to reduce fever, headache, and muscle or joint pain. Keep the room dark and quiet (to decrease stimuli and meningeal irritation), give fluids either intravenously or orally, and promote comfort with proper positioning.

The child and family need information about the disease. Explain medical and nursing procedures in terms that the child and family can understand. Keep parents informed about the child's progress. Once the diagnosis of viral meningitis is made, immediately begin discharge planning and teaching for home care. Explain that recovery may take several weeks but that complete recovery is expected.

ENCEPHALITIS

Encephalitis is an inflammation of the brain usually caused by a viral infection. Inflammation of the meninges is also common.

Viruses are believed to cause most cases of encephalitis. Herpes simplex type I is the most common cause after the newborn period, and is associated with a high mortality rate. Those who survive often have significant neurologic sequelae (American Academy of Pediatrics, 2003a). Other viruses causing encephalitis include enteroviruses (poliovirus, echovirus, and coxsackievirus), adenoviruses and herpesviruses, arboviruses, measles, mumps, rubella, rabies, and hepatitis B.

Signs and symptoms depend on the causative organism and the location of the infection within the brain. An acute onset of a febrile illness with neurologic signs is the classic manifestation of encephalitis. Initially the child may have a severe headache, fever, signs of an upper respiratory infection, and nausea or vomiting. Meningeal irritation signs such as nuchal rigidity, photophobia, and positive Kernig and Brudzinski signs are common. Other neurologic signs vary. The child may be disoriented or confused, with behavioral or personality changes. Speech disturbances; motor dysfunction such as hemiparesis, ataxia, or weakness; cranial nerve deficits; or alterations in reflex response may be present. Focal or generalized seizures may occur, alternating with periods of screaming, hallucinating, and moving in a bizarre fashion. The child's level of consciousness may deteriorate from stupor to coma.

Diagnosis is based on history and laboratory findings. Information about recent immunizations, insect bites, or travel to areas where vectors are present should be obtained (e.g., cases of West Nile virus or eastern equine encephalitis). Cerebrospinal fluid analysis, blood serologic tests, and nasopharyngeal and stool specimens are evaluated to identify viral pathogens. Testing for virus specific immunoglobulin M antibodies with enzyme linked immunosorbent assay (ELISA) is performed after 5 days of acute illness. A CT scan, MRI, and EEG may also be performed. The nucleic acid detection test is used to assay for herpes DNA in the spinal fluid. Brain biopsy may be performed to diagnose herpes simplex and parasitic infections.

The child with encephalitis is at risk for seizures, respiratory failure, and increased intracranial pressure and should be cared for in an intensive care unit. Treatment is both pharmacologic and supportive. The child with a suspected bacterial infection should be treated with antibiotics until bacterial pathogens have been ruled out. Acyclovir may be used for herpes viral infections.

Children with encephalitis have many permanent neurologic sequelae. Although some children recover completely, many more are left with intellectual, motor, visual, or auditory deficits. The cardiovascular system, lungs, or liver may also be affected. Generally, the younger the child, the more serious the illness and the more severe the residual effects.

NURSING MANAGEMENT

Nursing care focuses on monitoring cardiorespiratory function, preventing complications resulting from immobility, reorienting the child, and teaching the parents about the child's condition.

Monitor the child's cardiorespiratory function. Check the child's airway and ability to handle secretions. Monitor respiratory status by observing color, pulse oximetry readings, and arterial blood gas values. Observe cardiopulmonary status by monitoring heart rate, blood pressure, capillary refill time, and urine output. Provide seizure precautions, and have appropriate equipment for managing seizures at the bedside. Prevent complications resulting from immobility as described on page 1674. Maintain skin integrity. Proper positioning with frequent turning is important. When indicated by the physician, perform chest physiotherapy to prevent pneumonia.

The child whose level of consciousness begins to improve may at first be confused and disoriented and may have residual effects of the disease. Orient the child to the hospital environment. Have the family help to reorient the child by bringing favorite stuffed animals or music from home. Engage in therapeutic play (refer to Chapter 40 for techniques ∞). Give the child age-appropriate toys to encourage a return to normal behavior.

Give the parents information about their child's condition and prognosis. If the child receives physical, occupational, or speech therapy, explain the treatment regimen to the parents.

Discharge Planning and Home Care Teaching

Encourage parents to take an active role in the child's physical and emotional care in the hospital, and give them written instructions about home care. Encourage the parents to learn specific physical, occupational, and speech therapies so they can work with their child at home between home care visits. Refer parents to home care, social services, family counseling, and support groups. Plan follow-up visits so the child can be evaluated for neurologic sequelae.

REYE SYNDROME

Reye syndrome is an acute **encephalopathy**, a cerebral dysfunction caused by a toxic, injury, inflammatory, or anoxic insult that may result in permanent tissue damage, although the dysfunction may improve over time. In 1980 an association was reported between the use of aspirin for a mild viral illness and subsequent development of Reye syndrome. Since most parents give children acetaminophen rather than aspirin for flulike symptoms and varicella, Reye syndrome has become rare with two reported cases per year between 1994 and 1997 (Belay, Bresee, Holman et al., 1999). The mortality rate for children who develop the condition is high.

The etiology of Reye syndrome is unclear. The disorder, an encephalopathy, usually develops after a mild viral illness, such as varicella or influenza. The disorder is characterized by cerebral edema and an enlarged, fatty, poorly functioning liver (due to an elevation of short chain fatty acid levels and hyperammonemia).

Reye syndrome begins with nausea and vomiting, mental status changes, seizures, and progressive unresponsiveness (Ressler & Nelson, 2000). The condition has five stages that indicate increasing signs of cerebral edema and neurologic dysfunction, as described in Table 53–7.

The diagnosis of Reye syndrome is based on an abrupt change in the child's level of consciousness and diagnostic laboratory tests. The child has often progressed to coma or stage III by the time of diagnosis. Liver enzyme and ammonia levels are elevated, blood glucose levels are below normal, and prothrombin time is prolonged. A liver biopsy is sometimes performed to confirm the diagnosis.

The child with Reye syndrome should be placed in a pediatric intensive care unit because of the potential for rapid deterioration. The goal of medical management is to provide supportive treatment and to prevent the secondary effects of cerebral edema and metabolic injury. Assisted ventilation is often needed once the child is comatose. Arterial and venous blood pressure monitoring is performed. The child is monitored for signs of increased intracranial pressure, which can be secondary to cerebral edema. Hypoglycemia is treated with intravenous glucose, and electrolytes, blood chemistry, and blood pH are monitored.

TABLE 53–7 ✢ Stages of Reye Syndrome

Stage	Clinical Manifestations
I	Vomiting; lethargy; appropriate responses to verbal commands; purposeful responses to pain; brisk pupillary reaction
II	Combativeness; stupor; inappropriate language; confusion; anxiety, fear; purposeful and nonpurposeful responses to pain; sluggish pupillary reaction; conjugate deviation with oculocephalic reflex; hyperactive reflexes; progresses to coma but interrupted by periods of screaming and ranting
III	Coma; decorticate rigidity; conjugate deviation with diminished oculocephalic reflex; sluggish pupillary reaction; decorticate posturing
IV	Coma with brainstem dysfunction; decerebrate rigidity; inconsistent or absent oculocephalic reflex; loss of corneal reflex; sluggish pupillary reaction; decerebrate posturing
V	Coma with seizures; flaccidity; loss of deep tendon reflexes; respiratory arrest

NURSING MANAGEMENT

Nursing care focuses on monitoring the child's physical status, providing emotional support, and teaching parents about disease prevention.

NURSING PRACTICE

Make sure all parents know not to give aspirin when the child has a viral illness such as chickenpox or influenza because aspirin is associated with the development of Reye syndrome. Instruct parents to check all over-the-counter medicines for the presence of aspirin compounds. Emphasize the importance of obtaining healthcare whenever a child's condition worsens at the end of a viral illness.

Check the child's respiratory and neurologic status frequently, and note any signs of improvement or deterioration. Orient the child who awakens from coma. Refer to the discussion of nursing management of altered states of consciousness at the beginning of this chapter for specific nursing interventions. Look for changes in laboratory values that indicate acidosis, an elevation of ammonia levels, or hypoglycemia. Monitor the child's intake and output. Correct imbalances by administering fluids, electrolytes, or medications as ordered. Prevent complications associated with immobility.

Provide emotional support to the parents, who may feel guilty because they did not seek medical attention sooner. Keep them informed about the child's condition, and prepare them for potential deterioration. Explain treatments to help reduce anxiety. Encourage the parents to participate in the child's care whenever possible.

Once the child is discharged, monitoring is needed to observe for sequelae of the illness. Developmental and neurologic deficits may occur and are more severe in children under 2 years of age. Arrange for home nursing visits during the recovery period so that developmental and neurologic status monitoring can be assessed. Be sure the parents know about community resources that can help them deal with the child's recovery.

GUILLAIN-BARRÉ SYNDROME (POSTINFECTIOUS POLYNEURITIS)

Guillain-Barré syndrome is an acute inflammatory demyelinating polyneuropathy. This condition may lead to deteriorating motor function and paralysis that progresses in an ascending pattern, as well as paresthesia and areflexia. It is the most common cause of acute flaccid paralysis in infants and children (Jones, 2000). Guillain-Barré syndrome is caused by an autoimmune response to an infectious organism, usually from a gastrointestinal or respiratory illness about 10 days prior to onset. It has also been associated with immunizations and cytomegalovirus (Jones, 2000).

Infants have an onset of rapidly progressive severe hypotonia, possible respiratory distress, and feeding difficulties. Older children have rapidly progressive symmetric weakness and muscle pain with varying degrees of distal paresthesia and numbness in the legs. This ascending weakness spreads to the upper extremities, trunk, chest, neck, face, and head. Deep tendon reflexes may be diminished or absent. The child may develop acute ataxia. Difficulty swallowing and facial weakness are signs of impending respiratory failure. Respiratory effort may be inadequate for proper ventilation. Cranial nerves may be affected, causing Bell's palsy, for example. A dysfunctional autonomic nervous system may cause such symptoms as hypertension, postural hypertension, sinus tachycardia or bradycardia, excessive diaphoresis, urinary and bowel incontinence, and facial flushing.

Diagnostic criteria of Guillain-Barré syndrome include progressive motor weakness (minimal weakness of the legs to total paralysis of all extremities), and areflexia of varying degrees. Cerebrospinal fluid analysis reveals twice the limit of normal protein levels, normal glucose level, and fewer than 10 white blood cells per cubic millimeter, a positive indicator of the condition (Sarnat, 2004). Electroconduction tests such as electromyography show acute muscle denervation.

Clinical therapy for Guillain-Barré syndrome is plasmapheresis or intravenous immune globulin when the child cannot ambulate. Guidelines for administration of intravenous immune globulin can be found in Chapter 44. ∞ Responses to intravenous immune globulin are dramatic, often within days. If the child can ambulate, physical therapy and supportive care are provided. The condition is rarely fatal.

NURSING MANAGEMENT

Nursing care focuses on monitoring respiratory status, meeting nutritional needs, managing autonomic nervous system dysfunction, preventing complications associated with immobility, providing emotional support, and teaching the parents how to care for the child after discharge.

Monitor Respiratory Status

Monitor the child's respiratory status closely, especially in the early phase of illness. Look for such signs as dyspnea, inability to handle secretions, inadequate respiratory effort, and color changes that may indicate the need for endotracheal intubation and mechanical ventilation.

Manage Autonomic Nervous System Dysfunction

Monitor the child's vital signs closely for episodes of tachycardia, bradycardia, and hypotension. Blood pressure fluctuations and autonomic instability are linked to fatal cardiac arrhythmias (Jones, 2000). Observe frequently for decreased responsiveness. Intervene promptly if these or other signs of autonomic nervous system dysfunction are noted.

Meet Nutritional Needs

Assess whether the child is having difficulty swallowing. If the child has no gag reflex, maintain nutritional needs with intravenous supplements or nasogastric tube feedings.

Prevent Complications

Prevent complications associated with immobility (see page 1674). Ensure good postural alignment, and turn the child every 2 hours. Maintaining skin integrity is also important.

Evaluate the child's muscle tone, strength, and symmetry. When the child's condition begins to improve, recovery of lost strength is the priority. Active exercise is emphasized in physical therapy. Encourage family members to participate in the child's care, especially during the recovery phase. They can help with the activities of daily living and reinforce what the child has learned in physical therapy.

Provide Emotional Support

Explain the progression of Guillain-Barré syndrome to the parents during the initial stages. Witnessing a rapid deterioration in their child's physical status can be frightening; therefore, preparation is essential to reduce their anxieties. Be honest when discussing recovery and prognosis for the child.

Have parents bring in favorite toys, dolls, or books to make the child feel more secure. Playing with or reading to the child can be comforting.

Discharge Planning and Home Care Teaching

Home care needs should be identified and addressed well in advance of discharge. Support the parents as they prepare for the child's return home. Provide referral to home care nurses who can manage all aspects of treatment, rehabilitation, and follow-up. Refer the parents to social workers who can help with financial arrangements and school considerations.

Nursing Care in the Community

Help the child to adjust to any residual effects of Guillain-Barré syndrome. Help the child practice exercises learned in physical therapy sessions, and encourage the child to perform activities of daily living, such as brushing the teeth or combing the hair. Refer the child to outpatient rehabilitation programs to promote recovery.

To promote a positive self-image, praise any effort the child makes to be self-sufficient. The child may be frustrated and angry. Allow the child to express these feelings in an appropriate way, either during play or in conversation.

HEADACHES

Children commonly experience headaches. They may be the cause of school absence, decreased extracurricular activity, and poor academic achievement. The majority of children experience a headache by late adolescence. Migraine headaches occur in 1% to 3% of children under 5 years of age, and 5% to 10% of children under 15 years (Rosenblum & Fisher, 2001).

Headaches have both benign (migraine, inflammatory, and tension) and structural causes. See "Clinical Manifestations: Causes of Headaches." Migraines may be triggered by stress; foods containing nitrates, glutamate, caffeine, tyramine, and salt; menses; oral contraceptives; fatigue; and hunger. Another family member often has similar headaches, so there may be a genetic predisposition.

- Tension headaches may be associated with stresses due to school, insecurity, or conflict in the family.

- Medication overuse (rebound) headaches are associated with the frequent use of medications for headaches, more than 2 to 3 times a week. Medications associated with this type of headache include acetaminophen, nonsteroidal anti-inflammatory drugs (NSAIDs), triptans, caffeine, opiates, benzodiazepines, barbiturates, and ergotamines (Reimschisel, 2003).

CLINICAL THERAPY

Clinical therapy involves taking a detailed history of the headache characteristics, onset, warning signs, duration, severity, and associated symptoms. The child is assessed for neurologic signs such as altered consciousness, abnormal cranial nerves, papilledema, and motor or sensory deficits. Radiologic studies (CT scan or MRI) are used only if a structural problem is suspected. Treatment includes relaxation techniques, analgesics, and anti-inflammatory medications. Food elimination diet trials are often used to identify foods that trigger headaches, but they are often unsuccessful. Medications to abort migraines (ergot or isometheptene) are used in children old enough to identify an aura, or warning. Adolescents may use sumatriptan in oral or nasal spray form to abort migraines. Cyproheptadine, beta-blockers, tricyclic antidepressants, and anticonvulsants (valproic acid, topiramate, and gabapentin) may be used prophylactically if headaches significantly interfere with usual activities (Lewis, Scott, & Rendin, 2002).

CLINICAL MANIFESTATIONS

CAUSES OF HEADACHES

TYPE OF HEADACHE AND CAUSE	CLINICAL MANIFESTATIONS	CLINICAL THERAPY
Migraine—vascular, acute recurrent	■ Unilateral or bilateral pulsatile throbbing pain lasting for hours or days ■ Pain often retro-orbital frontal and temporal region ■ Preschool-age children may have irritability, restlessness, malaise, head banging, head holding, and sensitivity to light and sound ■ Nausea and vomiting ■ Photophobia and phonophobia ■ Visual or motor aura several minutes before headache starts ■ Recurrent abdominal pain ■ Increased pain with activity ■ Relief with sleep	■ Food elimination trial to identify food triggers ■ Caffeine avoidance ■ Nose and light avoidance ■ Medications to abort migraine (ergot, isometheptene, sumatriptan) ■ Analgesic medication ■ Relaxation techniques and biofeedback
Tension—muscular contraction, acute recurrent or chronic nonprogressive	■ Dull, achy pain in band around head, in neck and shoulders that may last for days ■ Intermittent or constant pain with fluctuations in degree of pain ■ Nausea and vomiting are rare ■ Sensitive to light or sound ■ Pain not aggravated by increased physical activity	■ Relaxation techniques ■ Analgesic and anti-inflammatory medications ■ Ice pack ■ Rest
Medication overuse, acute recurrent	■ Dull, bilateral or unilateral pain in frontal area ■ Occur at least 2 to 4 times a week or daily ■ Can vary in character, location, and severity from time to time ■ Usually increases in frequency and severity over time, paralleling the increase in medication use ■ Recur with the abortive therapy or medication wears off	■ Discontinuation of all medications for headaches (caffeine, acetaminophen, NSAIDs, and triptans) ■ Clonidine may be used to treat withdrawal symptoms
Inflammatory—sinusitis or dental abscess, acute localized	■ Facial pain or tenderness over affected sinus ■ Dull, constant pressure ■ Severity of pain varies with head position ■ Fever	■ Analgesic, antipyretic, and anti-inflammatory medications ■ Antibiotic medications ■ Cold or heat application
Structural—space-occupying lesion, hemorrhage, increased intracranial pressure, chronic progressive	■ Pain that awakens child in morning ■ Pain worse in morning, with coughing, sneezing, or straining ■ Morning vomiting, no nausea ■ Worsening pain with exertion or position changes, increasing frequency ■ Abnormal neurologic signs within 2-6 months of headache onset (i.e., double vision, papilledema)	■ Surgery ■ Analgesic medications

NURSING MANAGEMENT

Nursing management involves assessing the child for potential neurologic signs associated with headaches and assisting the child and family to identify strategies for relieving the headaches. Encourage the child to keep a calendar or diary of headaches, including the events and stresses occurring at the time. Help the family and child implement the food elimination trial and gradually add foods to identify offending chemical triggers. Make sure the child learns to take the prescribed medications appropriately. Teach the child relaxation techniques (breathing control training, mental imagery, progressive relaxation, and biofeedback) to manage stress and the pain associated with the headaches. See Chapter 50 for care of the child with a brain tumor. ∞

STRUCTURAL DEFECTS

MICROCEPHALY

Microcephaly is a small brain with a head circumference below the third percentile on growth curves (Vannucci, 2002). It may be caused by chromosomal abnormalities, fetal insult, maternal infection, or destructive insult during infancy, such as infection, metabolic disorder, or anoxia. Children with microcephaly have cognitive impairments. See Chapter 54 for care of the child with mental retardation. ∞

HYDROCEPHALUS

Hydrocephalus is the body's response to an imbalance between the production and absorption of cerebrospinal fluid (CSF). The condition is often congenital and associated with other CNS malformations. The overall incidence is estimated to be 1 per 2000 births (Ditmyer, 2004). It is commonly associated with myelomeningocele, a spinal fluid–filled meningeal sac that contains a portion of the spinal cord and nerves protruding through a vertebral defect. Hydrocephalus can develop as a complication of illness or trauma.

ETIOLOGY AND PATHOPHYSIOLOGY

Hydrocephalus may be either communicating or noncommunicating, and congenital or acquired. In communicating hydrocephalus the CSF flows freely between normal channels and pathways, but absorption of the CSF in the subarachnoid space and the arachnoid villi is impaired. It can be acquired from postinfectious meningitis or intraventricular hemorrhage. It may be due to a congenital malformation in the subarachnoid spaces.

Noncommunicating hydrocephalus is responsible for most cases in children. It results from a blockage in the ventricular system that prevents CSF from entering the subarachnoid space (see "Pathophysiology Illustrated: Hydrocephalus"). Enlargement of one or more of the ventricles results. This obstruction can be caused by infection, hemorrhage, tumor, surgery, or structural deformity. Congenital structural defects include the Chiari II malformation (found in most children with myelomeningocele), aqueduct of Sylvius stenosis (a recessive X-linked cause of hydrocephalus), and the Dandy-Walker syndrome (a congenital communicating hydrocephalus malformation).

The Chiari II malformation involves a downward displacement of the cerebellum, brainstem, and fourth ventricle and herniation through the foramen magnum into the cervical spaces. Because these structures control respiration and the protective reflexes, as well as house the cranial nerves, the displacement can have varying effects such as sudden death, respiratory difficulty, swallowing difficulties, and the need for assisted ventilation. Signs and symptoms may occur at any time. Rapid surgical decompression is needed to reduce brainstem compression and to prevent death. Approximately 15% of children with this malformation die by the age of 3 years, and another third have permanent neurologic disability (Stevenson, 2004). A progression of clinical signs again occurs in adolescents and young adults (Lazzaretti & Pearson, 2004).

PATHOPHYSIOLOGY ILLUSTRATED

Hydrocephalus

Bulging fontanel

Lateral ventricle

Third ventricle

Aqueduct of Sylvius

Fourth ventricle

A   B

A, Normal size of ventricle. *B,* Enlarged ventricles, characteristic of hydrocephalus.

CLINICAL MANIFESTATIONS

The signs and symptoms of hydrocephalus vary with the age of the child (see "Clinical Manifestations: Hydrocephalus"). The predominant manifestation in infants is a rapidly increasing head circumference (Figure 53–8 ⊙). Older children show signs of increased intracranial pressure.

CLINICAL THERAPY

The diagnosis of hydrocephalus may be made prenatally by ultrasound or based on clinical manifestations and neuroimaging studies after birth. If hydrocephalus is detected in the fetus, sonography to detect other anomalies is performed, such as a neural tube defect. In the hospital setting, daily measurements of the infant's head circumference are critical in any infant at risk of developing hydrocephalus. In older children, signs of increased intracranial pressure are noted. CT scanning and MRI diagnose hydrocephalus, and in some cases reveal the anatomic cause. In the infant whose fontanelle is still open, ultrasonography or echoencephalography may be used to confirm the diagnosis. Severe congenital hydrocephalus combined with spina bifida is associated with a decreased survival rate of 20% to 46%, and a chance of normal intelligence in the survivors of 40% to 52% (Rudy, 2005).

Clinical therapy for hydrocephalus involves removing the obstruction (e.g., surgical removal of a tumor) or creating a new CSF pathway to divert excess CSF. A catheter or shunt is placed in the ventricle and passes the CSF to the

⊙ **FIGURE 53–8**

In communicating hydrocephalus, an excessive amount of cerebrospinal fluid accumulates in the subarachnoid space, producing the characteristic head enlargement seen here. When observing the child with hydrocephalus, look for a downward deviation of the eyes in which the lower half of the iris is hidden by the lower eyelid (sunsetting eyes). This finding occurs in severe hydrocephalus, but is not present in this child.

CLINICAL MANIFESTATIONS

HYDROCEPHALUS

CAUSE	CLINICAL MANIFESTATIONS

Congenital Structural Defect in Infancy
   Dandy-Walker syndrome
   Chiari II malformation
   Intraventricular hemorrhage
	Early signs
	Rapidly increasing head circumference; tense, bulging fontanelle, split sutures
	Bossing (protrusion) of frontal area, face is disproportionate for skull size
	Macewen's or "cracked-pot" sign
	Prominent, distended scalp veins, translucent scalp skin
	Sunsetting eyes (sclera visible above iris), sixth cranial nerve palsy
	Increased tone or hyperreflexia, Babinski sign
	Irritability or lethargy, poor feeding
	Decline in level of consciousness
	Difficulty holding head up
	
	Late signs
	Apnea
	Shrill, high-pitched cry
	Difficulty swallowing or feeding
	Vomiting
	Cardiopulmonary depression (severe cases)

Acquired Hydrocephalus in Older Child after Closure of Sutures
   Postinfectious
   Tumor
   Hemorrhage
	No head enlargement
	Headache upon arising with vomiting
	Fussiness, sleepiness, confusion, apathy, or altered level of consciousness
	Personality change, loss of interest in daily activities
	Poor judgment or verbal incoherence, worsening school performance, memory loss
	Ataxia, spasticity, or other alterations in motor development
	Visual defects secondary to pressure on second, third, and sixth cranial nerves
	Signs of increased intracranial pressure

O **FIGURE 53–9**

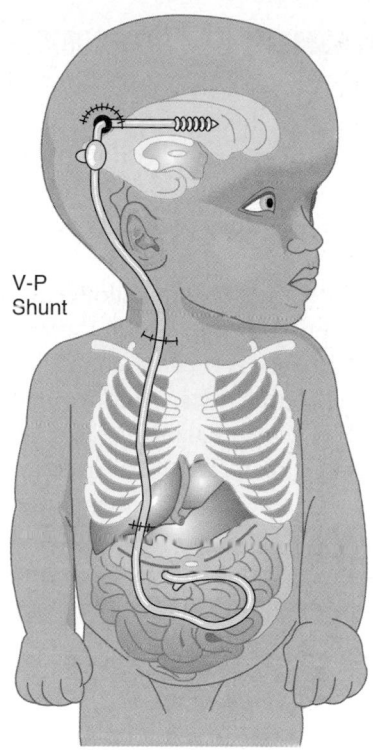

V-P Shunt

A ventriculoperitoneal shunt, commonly used to treat children with hydrocephalus, is usually placed at 3 to 4 months of age.

endoscopy procedure may be used in some patients in the future to avoid shunt placement (Ditmyer, 2004).

Mechanical complications may include blockage at either the proximal or the distal end of the catheter, kinking of the tubing, or valve breakdown. Infants or children with shunt failure show signs and symptoms of recurrent hydrocephalus and increased intracranial pressure. Shunt failure and ventricular size are confirmed by CT scanning or MRI. Shunt materials and systems continue to be refined in an attempt to reduce mechanical problems.

The most serious complication is shunt infection, which may occur at any time but is most prevalent in the first 2 months after placement. The infection rate is 4% per year, with infants under 6 months of age having the highest rates (Ditmyer, 2004). The infection may be confirmed by culture of the CSF obtained from the reservoir located in the burr hole (the hole through the skull through which the shunt is placed). Antibiotics are usually prescribed. The shunt is removed and an external drainage device is placed. A new shunt is inserted when the CSF cultures are sterile.

Some children, especially those with ventriculoatrial shunts, are placed on the same prophylactic antibiotic treatment regimen used for children with cardiac anomalies to reduce the risk of shunt infections (refer to Chapter 48 ∞).

peritoneal cavity, atrium of the heart, or the pleural spaces. Ventriculoperitoneal shunts (Figure 53–9 O) are commonly used, but a ventriculoatrial shunt may be used in older children. Shunt systems consist of four parts: a ventricular catheter, a pumping chamber or reservoir, a one-way pressure valve, and a distal catheter. Initial shunt placement is usually performed early in infancy. Adequate tubing is now inserted to accommodate the child's growth and reduce the need for future surgery. Researchers in neuroendoscopy are developing techniques to create a new pathway for CSF to flow between the ventricles and spinal cord in people with obstructive hydrocephalus. The new

NURSING MANAGEMENT

NURSING ASSESSMENT AND DIAGNOSIS

It is important for nurses to become familiar with the clinical manifestations of hydrocephalus to ensure prompt identification and treatment of children with this condition. Measure head circumference of all infants at each well-child visit to detect the condition at an early stage (see Skill 9–5). **SKILLS**

Assess the child with a ventriculoperitoneal shunt for signs and symptoms of shunt failure and infection. Important signs of infection include changes in responsiveness and irritability after fever is controlled. Other signs include low-grade fever, malaise, headache, and nausea. Measure the infant's head circumference daily when shunt failure is suspected. Report any abnormalities to the physician immediately.

Nursing diagnoses that might be appropriate for the child with hydrocephalus include the following:

- *Risk for Infection* related to presence of shunt
- *Impaired Physical Mobility (Level 2)* related to decreased muscle mass to lift the increased weight of head
- *Risk for Caregiver Role Strain* related to care of a child with a chronic condition or life-threatening illness
- *Anxiety (Parent)* related to repeated surgeries and life-threatening illness
- *Risk for Injury* related to potential shunt failure

PLANNING AND IMPLEMENTATION

Hospital-Based Nursing Care

Nursing care focuses on providing preoperative and postoperative care and providing emotional support.

Provide preoperative care. Position the child carefully; do not stretch or strain the neck muscles, since they must support the large head. Holding the child may be difficult because of the additional weight of the head. Provide good skin care. Reduce the chances for skin breakdown by placing sheepskin or a lamb's wool blanket under the head. Prevent any other complications associated with immobility (see page 1674).

Attend to the child's special nutritional needs. Because the infant is prone to vomiting, frequent small feedings with frequent burping are beneficial.

After surgery the child is usually placed in a flat position to prevent rapid CSF drainage. The head of the bed is elevated gradually. Take vital signs every 2 to 4 hours. Monitor the child carefully for any signs of shunt malfunction, increased intracranial pressure, or infection.

Support the parents and explain the child's condition and all procedures to be performed. Encourage parents

and family to help with the child's care in the hospital when appropriate. Be sympathetic and understanding, and allow parents to express their concerns. If hydrocephalus occurs during early infancy, the parents will be anxious about the impact of the chronic condition and subsequent surgical procedures. If hydrocephalus is secondary to neoplasm, however, the parents' anxieties are compounded by their child's life-threatening illness. Assure parents that most children with shunts lead normal lives, attending school and interacting with others no differently from their peers.

Discharge Planning and Home Care Teaching

Identify and address home care needs well in advance of discharge. Parents must learn how to care for a child with a shunt. Make parents and other family members aware of the signs and symptoms of both shunt failure (signs of increased intracranial pressure) and infection (changes in responsiveness, irritability, malaise, headache, nausea, and low-grade fever). Give them the telephone numbers of the pediatrician and the neurosurgeon, and make sure that they understand that they should contact a physician immediately if they suspect a problem. Inform parents that the child may develop a seizure disorder and how to care for the child if a seizure occurs. Refer families to the appropriate home care, social services, and support groups such as the Hydrocephalus Association. (See the Companion Website for links to such resources.)

Nursing Care in the Community

Infants and children need frequent monitoring to ensure proper shunt functioning. Head circumference is measured at each visit to monitor growth. Assess the child for visual problems and cognitive, speech, and motor developmental delays. Refer the child and family to an early intervention program to promote developmental progress. School-age children may need to have an individual education plan developed (see Chapter 39). ∞ Intellectual functioning outcomes may be associated with the cause of the hydrocephalus. For example, children with uncomplicated congenital causes do better than those with brain injury, infection, or intraventricular hemorrhage causes.

Parents seeking child care for their infant should be encouraged to use a setting with fewer children to decrease exposure to infection. Review the signs of shunt failure and infection with parents at each visit and make sure they have a plan to manage the emergency of a shunt failure.

Teach parents to protect the infant from injury. Infants with poor head control due to an enlarged head should not be placed in forward-facing car safety seats, regardless of their age. For these children, this position increases the risk of cervical spine injury and death in a car crash. As the child grows, encourage parents to avoid becoming over-protective and to allow the child to develop normally. Participation in sports with a high potential for head and abdominal impact should be discouraged.

EVALUATION

Expected outcomes of nursing care include the following:

- The child develops adequate neck muscle control to interact with the environment.

- Shunt infections and malfunctions are identified by the parents, and medical attention is sought quickly.

- The child's potential for growth and development is maximized by care and a stimulating environment.

NEURAL TUBE DEFECTS

The neural tube is the tissue that ultimately develops the CNS, including the brain and spinal cord. The incidence of neural tube defects is 0.7 to 1 per 1000 live births in the United States (Padgett, 2002). Types of neural tube defects include the following:

- **Anencephaly**—The brain does not develop above the brainstem.

- **Encephalocele**—A protrusion of meningeal tissue or meningeal-covered brain is observed through a defect in the skull.

- **Spina bifida occulta**—The posterior vertebral arches fail to fuse, most commonly at the fifth lumbar or first sacral vertebrae. The spinal cord and meninges lie entirely within the vertebral canal, and the condition is usually not visible externally. A tuft of hair, a dermoid cyst, or hemangioma may be found over the site. This is the mildest form of spina bifida.

- **Spina bifida cystica**—A defect occurs in closure of the posterior vertebral arch with protrusion through the bony spine.

- **Meningocele**—A spinal fluid–filled meningeal sac protrudes through a vertebral defect and is associated with no abnormalities of the spinal cord. The sac may be translucent or membranous. The spinal cord and spinal root are in normal position.

- **Meningomyelocele (spina bifida)**—A spinal fluid–filled meningeal sac containing a portion of the meninges, spinal cord, or nerve roots protrudes through a vertebral defect. Fluid leakage may also occur as the lesion is poorly covered with imperfect tissue.

MYELODYSPLASIA OR SPINA BIFIDA

Myelodysplasia (sometimes called meningomyelocele) refers to a malformation of the spinal cord and spinal canal, whereas spina bifida refers to a defect in one or more vertebrae through which spinal cord contents can protrude. The malformation can occur anywhere along the vertebral column, and it is most common at the lumbar or sacral portion of the spine. This is the most common developmental disorder of the CNS. The condition occurs in about 1 per 2000 births in the United States each year but varies by region of the country (Northrup & Volcik, 2000).

DEVELOPING CULTURAL COMPETENCE

RATES OF SPINA BIFIDA

The incidence of spina bifida varies with ethnicity and geographic location in the United States. Hispanic people, especially those in Texas, have the highest rate. The incidence in other ethnic groups in descending order are Caucasians, African Americans, and Asian Americans (Northrup & Volcik, 2000).

The cause of spina bifida is unknown, although environmental factors such as chemicals (excessive use of alcohol), medications (e.g., valproic acid and carbamazepine used for seizures, isotretinoin for acne), genetic factors, and maternal health conditions (type 1 diabetes mellitus, gestational diabetes, folic acid deficiency, and maternal obesity) have been implicated. The increased incidence of the condition in families indicates a possible genetic influence. Mandatory fortification of all enriched grain products with folate has resulted in a significant reduction in both spina bifida and anencephaly.

A saclike protrusion on the infant's back indicates meningocele or myelomeningocele (Figure 53–10 ●). The clinical manifestations seen depend on the location of the defect: the higher the defect, the greater the neurologic dysfunction:

- Sensory loss is more pronounced on the back of the legs. Sensory loss around the anus, genitalia, and feet is common.

- Thoracic or lumbar 1–2 level—paralysis of the legs; weakness and sensory loss in the trunk and lower body region.

- Lumbar 3 level—can flex hips and extend the knees. The ankles and toes are paralyzed.

- Lumbar 4–5 level—can flex hips and extend the knees; weak or absent ankle extension, toe flexion, and hip extension.

- Sacral level—mild weakness in ankles and toes; bladder and bowel function may be affected.

● FIGURE 53–10

Lumbosacral myelomeningocele is caused by a neural tube defect that results in incomplete closure of the vertebral column. As shown here, the meninges (and sometimes the spinal cord) protrude as a saclike structure. Observe for leakage of cerebrospinal fluid.

CLINICAL MANIFESTATIONS

MYELODYSPLASIA

CAUSE	CLINICAL MANIFESTATIONS
Interruption of the spinal cord at site of the spinal defect	Loss of motor and sensory function of the abdomen and lower extremities, dependent on defect level Scoliosis or kyphosis Incontinence of urine or urinary retention Incontinence of feces or constipation Sensory loss around genitalia
Muscle imbalance	Hip abnormalities, hip dysplasia Foot deformities, (e.g., clubfoot)

Chiari II malformation	Hydrocephalus
	Infants:
	  Difficulty swallowing
	  Apnea, respiratory difficulty, inspiratory stridor
	  Weak or poor cry
	  Sustained backward arching of the head (opisthotonos)
	Older children:
	  Choking, hoarseness, vocal cord paralysis
	  Disordered breathing during sleep
	  Stiffness or spasticity of arms and hands
	  Loss of feeling or sensation

Brain and spinal cord abnormalities	Learning problems, attention deficit disorder Problems with perceptual motor skills Memory and organization problems Problems with numerical reasoning

Bowel and bladder sphincters may be affected. Renal damage may result from neurologic impairment and urinary retention. Hydrocephalus is usually present in children with myelomeningocele because of the Chiari II malformation that is found in nearly all children with a defect above the sacral level. The range of potential problems for the child with spina bifida is listed in "Clinical Manifestations: Myelodysplasia."

Diagnosis is usually made prenatally, but after birth the lesion is examined and the neurologic status is evaluated. Radiologic imaging by ultrasonography, CT scan, MRI, and flat films of the spinal column can pinpoint the bony defect. Subsequent testing is performed to evaluate bowel and bladder function, neurologic and motor function, and cognitive function.

Surgery to close and repair the lesion usually occurs within 24 to 48 hours of the infant's birth to reduce infection. Depending upon the size of the defect, the excision area may be extensive. In some cases, uteromyelomeningocele repairs are performed. In cases of spina bifida occulta, surgical intervention is rarely needed.

Braces are used to support joint position and mobility. Assistive devices such as walkers, crutches, and wheelchairs are used to enhance mobility. To minimize the risk for osteoporosis, the diet should ensure adequate calcium and vitamin D, and weight-bearing activities should be encouraged.

Bladder interventions are initated early to prevent kidney damage and to maintain bladder function and urinary continence. Clean intermittent catheterization is used (see Chapter 52 ∞), but if it is not totally effective in promoting continence, surgical interventions may be performed. Stool softeners and glycerin or bisacodyl suppositories are prescribed for bowel evacuation.

Prognosis depends on the type of defect, the level of the lesion, and other complicating factors. Children need multiple surgeries and invasive procedures. A team of physicians, nurses, and therapists from the neurosurgery, orthopedic, urology, and physical medicine departments work with the child and family to form a comprehensive care plan.

NURSING PRACTICE

Between 18% and 40% of children with spina bifida have a latex allergy (see Chapter 44 ∞). Anaphylaxis caused by latex exposure in children has been reported. All children with latex allergy need to carry a kit with premeasured adrenaline for emergency treatment of anaphylaxis. Use nonlatex materials when providing care to the child in any setting. The Spina Bifida Association maintains an updated list of products containing latex and potential substitutes (see also Table 44–8). See the Companion Website for links to such resources.

NURSING MANAGEMENT

Hospital-Based Nursing Care

Nursing care focuses on providing preoperative and post-operative care, promoting mobility, and providing emotional support.

Cover the sac with a sterile saline dressing to protect its integrity and monitor for leakage of CSF. Place the infant in a prone position with hips slightly flexed and legs abducted to minimize tension on the sac. Maintain this position using towel rolls placed between the knees. Assess the infant regularly for motor deficits as well as bladder and bowel involvement. Frequently assess the vital signs and stay alert for signs of infection. The infant is difficult to handle before surgery. Feed the infant with the head turned to one side until surgery has been performed. Comfort the infant before surgery with tactile stimulation such as touching, patting, and cuddling.

Following surgery, monitor the infant's vital signs carefully. Watch closely for symptoms of infection, especially meningitis. If a ventriculoperitoneal shunt was placed, watch for hydrocephalus, increased intracranial pressure, or infection. Inspect the surgical site for CSF leakage. The infant should be placed in the prone or side-lying position, or in some cases may be held upright. Splints may be used to maintain extremity alignment.

Begin gentle range of motion exercises as soon as possible to prevent muscle contractures and atrophy. Extreme caution should be used because these children have brittle bones that fracture easily.

Support the parents by keeping them informed about their child's status. Allow them to express their frustrations and anger. As soon as parents are able to cope with the child's condition, encourage them to become involved in the child's care in the hospital.

The child with myelodysplasia may be hospitalized for surgery numerous times to correct deformities. Assess the child's vital signs, responsiveness, and level of pain. As the child may have decreased pain sensation in lower extremities, careful assessment is needed. Assess dressing sites for bleeding and drainage. Monitor the distal extremities for swelling and circulation. Use latex precautions with these children. See Chapter 44 for information about latex allergy. ∞

 GROWTH AND DEVELOPMENT

Treat older children according to their intellectual level, not their motor development. Encourage them to take responsibility for self-care, and recognize their need to control their body functions. Promote interaction with peers in the hospital and participation in activities. If children are hospitalized for an extended time, arrange schooling.

Discharge Planning and Home Care Teaching

Identify and address home care needs well in advance of discharge. Make sure family members understand how to care for the child at home. Help them get special devices such as splints, wedges, and rolls, if needed, to prevent complications. Instruct parents how to position, handle, feed, and perform range of motion exercises. Teach them the signs and symptoms of increased intracranial pressure, hydrocephalus, shunt infection or malfunction, and urinary tract infection. Home care nursing should be arranged, if necessary. The home care nurse reinforces the skills learned in the hospital setting and coordinates the numerous healthcare professionals working with the child and family. Refer parents to resource groups such as the Spina Bifida Association of America. (See the Companion Website for links to such resources.)

Nursing Care in the Community

To reduce complications and promote optimal development, children with myelodysplasia need comprehensive care planned and coordinated by a knowledgeable team of healthcare professionals. This care may be provided in partnership with the primary care physician.

Parents need to learn to catheterize the child and then at an appropriate age teach the child intermittent self-catheterization to prevent urinary tract infections and other renal complications. A Mitrofanoff procedure that creates a stoma for catheterizing the bladder from the abdominal wall and improves access for catheterization may be performed (Zickler & Richardson, 2004). Good nutrition planning is important to prevent obesity and to reduce constipation and complications such as fecal impaction. Bowel training is initiated to control bowel evacuation at appropriate times and places. A diet high in fiber helps ensure adequate stool. At a convenient time, a glycerin or bisacodyl suppository can be given. Consistency in time of day for bowel evacuation is important. Surgery to create a channel between the skin and bowel (Malone antegrade continence enema) is often performed in older children to improve the ease of bowel evacuation management (Zickler & Richardson, 2004).

Promote safety and independent mobility with proper use of braces, walkers, crutches, canes, and in some cases custom-designed wheelchairs and car safety seats (Figure 53–11 ●). For other safety guidelines, see "Teaching Highlights: Safety for the Child with Spina Bifida."

Parents are faced with the long-term financial issues of caring for the child who needs regular new adaptive equipment to match growth, as well as other medical supplies. At least 75% of children born with spina bifida generally survive to at least the early adult years (Bowman, McLone, Grant et al., 2001). Parents thus need to learn how to act as the child's case manager, or to work effectively with another person in this role.

FIGURE 53–11

A   B   C

Help determine the best assistive device for the child to gain the most independence for mobilizing and to promote development. The child may change devices in different settings to promote optimal independence. *A* and *B*, Braces and walkers may be best for young children to promote an upright posture that encourages a normal interaction with the environment. *C*, A motorized wheelchair can assist the child with a significant neurologic impairment to achieve independence and mobility.

TEACHING HIGHLIGHTS

SAFETY FOR THE CHILD WITH SPINA BIFIDA

Due to the loss of sensation in the lower extremities, injuries to the skin are not noticed by the child.

- Each day, check all skin surfaces and pressure points associated with sitting, braces, shoes, etc., for abrasions, scrapes, reddened areas, and other lesions.
- Keep all skin surfaces clean and dry.
- Use a gel-filled cushion and teach the child to shift position when in the wheelchair to avoid pressure sores.
- Avoid burns to the lower extremities by checking the temperature of bath water and car safety seats in a hot car.
- Take latex precautions as the child is at high risk for latex allergy. Inform all healthcare providers about the child's latex allergy.
- Use safe ambulation techniques with walkers, canes, and crutches.

CRANIOSYNOSTOSIS

Craniosynostosis is the premature closing of the cranial sutures during the first 18 months of life. This condition occurs in up to 1 in 2000 births (Renier, Lajeunie, Arnaud et al., 2000). Boys make up two thirds of all cases (McGee & Burkett, 2000). Most children have no family history of the condition, although 15% have autosomal dominant inherited syndromes such as Alpert syndrome and Crouzon syndrome (McGee & Burkett, 2000).

The cause of craniosynostosis is unknown. Closure of the sutures usually takes place at predetermined times during the child's development. Problems arise if one or more sutures close early. Bone growth continues in a direction parallel to the suture line, which leads to compensatory overgrowth at normal suture lines and the classic skull deformities associated with craniosynostosis (Figure 53–12 ◉). Sagittal synostosis accounts for 50% of cases. The infant typically has an elongated head and bilateral bossing on the frontal and occipital areas, facial symmetry, and flattened parietal bones. Bicoronal synostosis is associated with Alpert or Crouzon syndromes.

HEALTH PROMOTION
The Child with Myelodysplasia

Preventive Healthcare

- Provide all recommended immunizations. If the child has a seizure disorder, teach the parents that seizures may occur following immunizations.
- Perform all recommended routine screening procedures (vision, hearing, hematocrit, blood pressure).
- Obtain a urinalysis with culture in the newborn period and anytime there are signs of infection.
- Screen for scoliosis annually beginning at birth.

Growth and Development Surveillance

- Monitor the growth of the child (length or height, weight, head circumference) and plot on growth curves. Head circumference growth needs careful monitoring because of hydrocephalus.
- Assess developmental status regularly. Motor skills are often delayed.

Nutrition

- Teach families appropriate caloric intake and portion control to reduce the risk for obesity.
- Encourage increased fluids to reduce the risk for constipation and urinary tract infections.
- If the child has latex allergies, allergies to foods like bananas, avocados, papaya, kiwi, and other foods may occur.

Elimination

- Teach families to perform intermittent catheterization for bladder management and to reduce the risk for renal damage.
- Teach the child to perform self-catheterization and catheter care in preparation for school entry.
- Teach families to initiate bowel training so that a bowel regimen is established. A Malone antegrade continence enema surgical procedure may be performed to improve bowel control.

Sleep and Rest

- Position the child to prevent contractures. Change the child's position during the night to reduce pressure over skin surfaces.
- Teach parents to be alert for apnea spells or snoring that could be related to a Chiari II malformation.

Mental Health

- Be alert for psychosocial adjustment problems.
- Promote gradual independence in mobility and self-care.
- Encourage interaction with peers.

Family Assessment

- Assess family strengths and coping with care of the child, frequent hospitalizations, and surgeries.
- Assess family finances and ability to provide needed equipment and supplies for the child.

Positional *plagiocephaly* (a totally flat occiput) and *brachycephaly* (the skull is short in the anteroposterior dimension and wide between the parietal eminences) are seen increasingly in healthy infants because they are put to sleep on their back to prevent sudden infant death syndrome. Since the infant's sleep position does not change, the weight of the head flattens the skull. Congenital torticollis may also contribute to position preference when supine. It is speculated that infants who develop these skull shapes do not have enough supervised tummy time that

helps correct positional preference (Graham, Kreutzman, Earl et al., 2005).

Diagnosis is made by clinical appearance and measurement of the skull with metal calipers. Palpation of the skull reveals a bony ridge along a suture. Skull x-ray films, CT scan, and MRI confirm the diagnosis. The hands and feet should be carefully examined to detect any skeletal defect that could be associated with a syndrome (Renier et al., 2000).

Reconstructive surgery of the skull, the most common form of treatment for craniosynostosis, is performed to

● FIGURE 53–12

In craniosynostosis, the head shape is dependent upon which sutures are involved. Examples of different head shapes include those shown in **A,** sagittal synostosis and **B,** bicoronal synostosis.

A

B

protect mental development and vision. Many children need multiple procedures. Children having surgery before 1 year of age have a better outcome. After surgery, it is important for the incision to remain dry and intact. The nurse should also observe the child for symptoms of increased intracranial pressure (see Table 53–2). Explain to parents that surgery will improve the child's appearance. Assure them that most children with craniosynostosis are healthy, and that their brains develop normally.

A helmet device to correct severe cases of positional plagiocephaly or brachycephaly is most effective in infants under 9 months of age and when treatment is initiated at 6 months of age. The helmet is worn for 23 hours a day for 3 months. Remolding of the head shape continues after that treatment period because the infant spends more time awake and upright. Younger infants may be successfully treated with positioning and physical therapy for torticollis (Graham, Gomez, Halberg et al., 2005).

For information on neonatal substance abuse see Chapter 31. ∞

CEREBRAL PALSY

Cerebral palsy (CP) is a disorder of movement and posture that results from a nonprogressive abnormality of the immature brain occurring in the prenatal, perinatal, or postnatal (up to 2 years) period. CP is the most common chronic disorder of childhood, occurring in an estimated 2 to 3 per 1000 births (Nehring, 2004). Four types of motor dysfunction are seen with cerebral palsy—spastic, dyskinetic, ataxic, and mixed—related to the location of brain insult (see "Clinical Manifestations: Cerebral Palsy by Type of Insult"). Children with severe impairment of mobility and feeding skills have a greater risk of dying during childhood (Liptak & Accardo, 2004).

ETIOLOGY AND PATHOPHYSIOLOGY

Most CP cases are believed to be caused by congenital, hypoxic, ischemic, or infectious intrauterine insults to the CNS (McKearnan, Kieckhefer, Engel et al., 2004). The risk for CP is increased when intrauterine infection (chorioamnionitis) is documented (Van Eerden & Bernstein, 2003). Very premature infants are at high risk because of their immature central nervous systems and the measures taken at birth to promote their survival. CP related to prematurity is most often caused by injury to the white matter of the brain by conditions such as intraventricular hemorrhage. Birth asphyxia is believed to account for only 9% of the CP cases. No reduction of incidence of CP was noted since the use of electronic fetal heart rate monitoring was implemented (Van Eerden & Bernstein, 2003). Neonatal sepsis and hyperbilirubinemia place the infant at higher risk. In young children, CNS infection and head trauma are the major sources of acquired brain injury and subsequent motor dysfunction.

CLINICAL MANIFESTATIONS

Cerebral palsy is characterized by abnormal muscle tone and lack of coordination with spasticity found in the majority of cases (Table 53–8). Children have a variety of symptoms depending on their ages. See "Clinical Manifestations: Cerebral Palsy by Type of Insult." There is wide variability in symptoms depending on the area of the brain involved and the degree of anoxia. Children with cerebral palsy usually are delayed in meeting developmental milestones. For example, at 6 months of age, they may be unable to sit up, have persistent back arching, and have little spontaneous movement. They frequently have other problems, including visual defects such as strabismus, nystagmus, or refractory errors; hearing loss; language delay; speech impediment; or seizures. Feeding may be difficult because of oral motor involvement. Approximately 75% of children with CP have mental retardation or learning disabilities (Liptak & Accardo, 2004).

CLINICAL THERAPY

Diagnosis is usually based on clinical findings. CP is difficult to diagnose in the early months of life as it must be

TABLE 53–8 ✤ Clinical Characteristics of Cerebral Palsy

Clinical Characteristics	Definitions
Hypotonia	Floppiness, increased range of motion of joints, diminished reflex response

Hypertonia
  Rigidity
  Spasticity
	
	Tense, tight muscles
	Uncoordinated, awkward, stiff movements; scissoring or crossing of the legs; exaggerated reflex reactions

Athetosis	Constant involuntary writhing motions that are more severe distally
Ataxia	Irregularity in muscle coordination or action
Hemiplegia	Involvement of one side of the body with the upper extremities being more dysfunctional than the lower extremities
Diplegia	Involvement of all extremities, but the lower extremities are more affected than the upper, usually spastic
Quadriplegia	Involvement of all extremities with the arms in flexion and legs in extension

CLINICAL MANIFESTATIONS

CEREBRAL PALSY BY TYPE OF INSULT

CLASSIFICATION AND TYPE OF INSULT	CLINICAL MANIFESTATIONS
Spastic Cerebral cortex or pyramidal tract injury 75% of cases	Persistent hypertonia, rigidity Exaggerated deep tendon reflexes Persistent primitive reflexes Leads to contractures and abnormal curvature of the spine
Dyskinetic Extrapyramidal, basal ganglia injury 10% to 15% of cases	Impairment of voluntary muscle control Bizarre twisting movements Tremors, difficulty with fine and purposeful motor movements Exaggerated posturing Rigid muscle tone when awake and normal or decreased muscle tone when asleep Inconsistent muscle tone that may change hour to hour or day to day
Ataxic Cerebellar (extrapyramidal) injury 5% to 10% of cases	Abnormalities of voluntary movement involving balance and position of the trunk and limbs Difficulty controlling hand and arm movements during reaching Increased or decreased muscle tone Hypotonia in infancy Muscle instability and wide-based unsteady gait
Mixed Injuries to multiple areas	No dominant motor pattern Unique compensatory movements and posture to maintain control over specific neuromotor deficits Combination of characteristics from other types

distinguished from other neurologic conditions, and signs may be subtle. Suspicious findings include an infant who is small for age or who has a history of prematurity, low Apgar score (0 to 3 at 5 minutes), or inflammatory, traumatic, or anoxic event (Van Eerden & Bernstein, 2003). However, the majority of children who develop CP have normal Apgar scores at birth. Ultrasonography can be used to detect fetal and neonatal abnormalities of the brain, such as intraventricular hemorrhage. Neuromotor tests are used to evaluate the presence of normal movement patterns and absence of primitive reflexes and abnormal tone. Once CP is suspected, CT scans, MRI, and positron emission tomography may be performed.

It is not uncommon for children who are delayed in meeting developmental milestones or have neuromuscular abnormalities at 1 year of age to show gradual improvement in function. Half of the infants suspected to be at risk

for CP at 1 year of age are unimpaired neurologically by 2 years of age due to physical maturation (Pelligrino, 2002).

Clinical therapy focuses on helping the child develop to his or her maximum level of independence. Referrals are made for physical, occupational, and speech therapy, as well as special education to improve motor function and ability. Braces and splints, serial casting, and positioning devices (prone wedges, standers, and side-lyers) are used to promote range of motion, skeletal alignment, stability, and control of involuntary movements, and to prevent contractures.

Surgical interventions may be required to improve function by balancing muscle power and stabilizing uncontrollable joints. The Achilles tendon may be lengthened to increase range of motion in the ankle, which allows the heel to touch the floor and thus improves ambulation. The hamstrings may be released to correct knee flexion contractures. Other procedures may be performed to improve hip adduction or correct the natural position of the foot. A dorsal rhizotomy may be performed for spastic diplegia to cut the afferent fibers that contribute to spasticity; however, some muscle weakness may result from the procedure (Pelligrino, 2002). Physical therapy and occupational therapy promote optimal independent functioning.

Medications are given to control seizures, to control spasms (skeletal muscle relaxants, baclofen, and benzodiazepines), and to minimize gastrointestinal side effects (cimetidine or ranitidine). Baclofen is administered by intrathecal pump to decrease muscle tone and vasospasms when oral administration is ineffective or causes side effects (Pelligrino, 2002). See Figure 53–13 ●. Botulinum toxin injection into specific muscles is a relatively new therapy used to help control spasticity (Buck, 2003).

The prognosis for infants and children with cerebral palsy depends on the level of physical involvement and on

● **FIGURE 53–13**

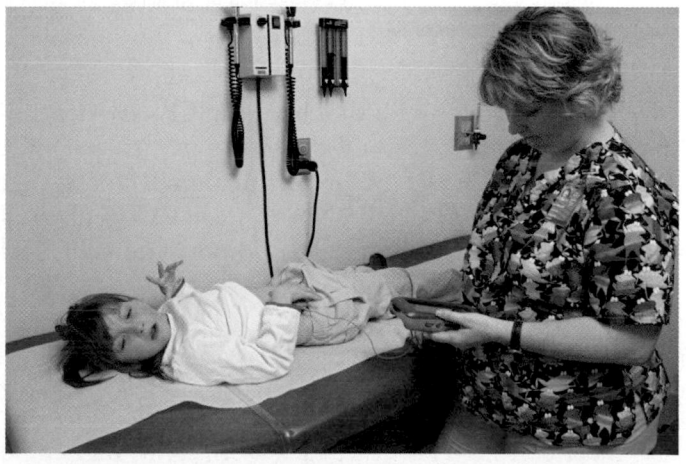

A child having a baclofen pump filled.

the presence of intellectual, visual, or hearing deficits. Many children with hemiplegia or ataxia show some improvement with maturation and are able to ambulate. Others need assistance with mobility and activities of daily living. They are usually cared for in their homes, but some receive care in long-term care facilities.

NURSING MANAGEMENT

NURSING ASSESSMENT AND DIAGNOSIS

Be alert for children whose histories indicate an increased risk for CP. Assess all children at each healthcare visit for developmental delays. Note any orthopedic, visual, auditory, or intellectual deficits. Assess for newborn reflexes, which may persist beyond the normal age in a child with cerebral palsy. Identify infants that appear to have an abnormal muscle tone or abnormal posture (arched back, becomes stiff when moving against gravity, neck or extremities have increased or decreased resistance to passive movement). Asymmetric or abnormal crawling by using 2 or 3 extremities indicates a motor problem. Hand dominance before the preschool years is another sign of a motor problem. Record dietary intake as well as height and weight percentiles for children suspected to have or diagnosed with the condition.

NURSING PRACTICE

Evaluate all infants who show symptoms of developmental delays, feeding difficulties caused by poor sucking, or abnormalities of muscle tone. Two simple screening assessments are:

- Place a clean diaper on the infant's face. The normal child will use two hands to remove it, but the infant with cerebral palsy will either use one hand or not remove the cloth at all.
- Turn the infant's head to one side. A persistent asymmetric tonic neck reflex (beyond 6 months of age) indicates a pathologic condition. Suspect cerebral palsy in any infant who has persistent primitive reflexes.

Nursing diagnoses for the child with CP vary, depending on the type of cerebral palsy, the particular child's symptoms and age, and the family situation. "Nursing Care Plan: The Child with Cerebral Palsy" includes several diagnoses that might be appropriate. Additional nursing diagnoses might include the following:

- *Risk for Constipation* related to low intake of fiber and fluids and insufficient physical activity
- *Impaired Tissue Integrity* related to decreased physical mobility and limited self-care ability
- *Impaired Verbal Communication* related to hearing and/or speech impairment

- *Impaired Home Maintenance Management* related to child's developmental disability and inadequate support system
- *Chronic Pain* related to spasticity and stretching exercises to prevent contractures
- *Delayed Growth and Development* related to lack of muscle strength or limited social interaction

PLANNING AND IMPLEMENTATION

The accompanying "Nursing Care Plan" summarizes care for the child with CP. Since the condition can range from mild to severe and involve numerous manifestations, interventions need to be adapted to the particular child and family. Nursing care focuses on providing adequate nutrition, maintaining skin integrity, promoting physical mobility, promoting safety, promoting growth and development, teaching parents how to care for the child, and providing emotional support.

Provide Adequate Nutrition

Children with CP require high-calorie diets or supplements to the diet because of feeding difficulties associated with spasticity. Many children have difficulty chewing and swallowing. Give the child small amounts of soft foods at a time. Utensils with large, padded handles may be easier for the child to use.

Maintain Skin Integrity

Take special care to protect the bony prominences from skin breakdown. Monitor the skin under splints and braces for redness.

Proper body alignment should be maintained at all times. Support the child with pillows, towels, and bolsters whether the child is in bed or in a chair. Support the head and body of a floppy infant. A spastic child with scissored, extended legs or an athetoid child who writhes constantly is difficult to carry and transport.

Promote Physical Mobility

Range of motion exercises are essential to maintain joint flexibility and to prevent contractures. Consult with the physical therapists who work with the child and help with recommended exercises. Refer parents to the appropriate resources for help getting adaptive devices (Figure 53–14 ●). Teach parents to position the child to foster flexion rather than extension so that the child can more easily interact with the environment (for example, by bringing objects closer to the face). Encourage parents to bring in the child's *adaptive appliances* (braces, positioning devices) for use during the hospitalization.

Consider the use of therapeutic massage or relaxation training to manage pain associated with spasticity and stretching exercises (McKearnan et al., 2004).

NURSING CARE PLAN

THE CHILD WITH CEREBRAL PALSY

Intervention	Rationale	Expected Outcome
1. Nursing Diagnosis: Impaired Physical Mobility related to decreased muscle strength and control		
NIC Priority Intervention: **Exercise therapy, joint mobility:** Use of active and passive body movement to maintain joint flexibility		**NOC Suggested Outcome:** **Joint movement—active:** Range of motion of joints with self-initiated movement
Goal: The child will attain maximum physical abilities possible.		
■ Perform development assessment and record age of achievement of milestones (e.g., reaching for objects, sitting). ■ Plan activities to use gross and fine motor skills (e.g., holding pen or eating utensils, toys positioned to encourage reaching and rolling over). ■ Allow time for the child to complete activities. ■ Perform range of motion exercises every 4 hours for the child unable to move body parts. Position the child to promote tendon stretching (e.g., foot plantar flexion instead of dorsiflexion, legs extended instead of flexed at knees and hips). ■ Arrange for and encourage parents to keep appointments with a rehabilitation therapist. ■ Teach the family to maintain appropriate brace wear.	■ Delayed development milestones are common with cerebral palsy. Once the child achieves one milestone, interventions are revised to assist in the next skill necessary. ■ Many activities of daily living and play activities promote physical development. ■ The child may perform tasks more slowly than most children. ■ Promotes mobility and increased circulation, and decreases the risk of contractures. ■ A regular and frequently reevaluated rehabilitation program assists in promoting development. ■ Adaptive devices are often necessary to maximize physical mobility.	The child reaches maximum physical mobility and all developmental milestones.
2. Nursing Diagnosis: Disturbed Sensory Perception (Visual or Auditory) related to cerebral damage		
NIC Priority Intervention: **Communication enhancement: Visual deficit:** Assistance with accepting or learning alternative methods for living with diminished vision		**NOC Suggested Outcome:** **Sensory function: Vision:** Extent to which visual images are sensed, with and without assistive devices
Goal: The child will receive and benefit from varied forms of sensory and perceptual input.		
■ Facilitate vision examinations by specialist. Promote the use of glasses and encourage recommended follow-up visits to specialists. ■ Maximize the use of intact senses (e.g., encourage touching of objects, provide auditory stimulation to enhance learning, use computers to promote communication).	■ Glasses often enhance sensory input. Assessment of vision as the child grows may identify needed prescription changes for glasses. ■ Other senses can compensate for those that are impaired.	The child receives adequate visual sensory/perceptual input to maximize developmental outcome.
3. Nursing Diagnosis: Imbalanced Nutrition: Less than Body Requirements related to difficulty in chewing and swallowing and high metabolic needs		
NIC Priority Intervention: **Nutrition management:** Assistance with or provision of a balanced dietary intake of foods and fluids		**NOC Suggested Outcome:** **Nutritional status: Nutrient intake:** Adequacy of nutrients taken into body

(continued)

NURSING CARE PLAN—continued

THE CHILD WITH CEREBRAL PALSY

Intervention	Rationale	Expected Outcome
Goal: The child will receive nutrients needed for normal growth.		
■ Monitor height and weight and plot on a growth grid. Perform hydration status assessment. ■ Teach the family techniques to promote caloric and nutrient intake: ■ Position the child upright for feedings. ■ Place foods far back in the mouth to overcome tongue thrust. ■ Use soft and blended foods. ■ Allow extra time for chewing and swallowing. ■ Obtain adaptive handles for utensils and encourage self-feeding skills. ■ Perform frequent respiratory assessment. Teach the family to avoid aspiration pneumonia. Teach care of gastrostomy and tube-feeding technique as appropriate.	■ Insufficient intake can lead to impaired growth and dehydration. ■ Special techniques can facilitate food intake. Adaptive handles may help the child better manage feeding self. ■ Aspiration pneumonia is a risk for the child with poor swallowing. Special feeding techniques may be needed.	The child shows normal growth patterns for height, weight, and other physical parameters.

4. Nursing Diagnosis: Ineffective Therapeutic Regimen Management: Family related to excessive demands made on family with child's complex care needs

NIC Priority Intervention: **Decision-making support:** Providing information and support for a patient who is making a decision regarding healthcare		**NOC Suggested Outcome:** **Compliance behavior:** Actions taken on the basis of professional advice to promote wellness, recovery, and rehabilitation
Goal: The family will adapt to growth and development needs of the child with cerebral palsy.		
■ Allow chances for parents to verbalize the impact of cerebral palsy on the family. Refer to other parents and support groups. ■ Explore community services for rehabilitation, respite care, child care, and other needs and refer family as appropriate. ■ During home and office visits, review the child's achievements and praise the family for care provided. ■ Teach the family skills needed to manage the child's care (e.g., medication administration, muscle stretching, physical rehabilitation, seizure management). ■ Teach case management techniques. ■ Involve siblings in the care for the child with cerebral palsy. Review for parents the needs of all children in the family.	■ The family needs a chance to explore the emotional and social impact of the child's care so they can integrate and grow from the experience. ■ Diverse services are available and will be needed due to the multiple impacts of cerebral palsy on the child. ■ The child's achievements are positive reinforcement of the family's efforts. ■ Complex skills must be learned before they can be performed efficiently. ■ The child requires care by many specialists. Many parents become case managers to coordinate care. ■ Siblings of the child with cerebral palsy may feel left out because of the care provided. Special efforts contribute to meeting the developmental needs of all family members.	The child demonstrates appropriate growth and developmental progress. The family successfully supports all of its members.

5. Nursing Diagnosis: Deficient Diversional Activity (Child) related to poor social skills

NIC Priority Intervention: **Recreation therapy:** Purposeful use of recreation to promote relaxation and enhancement of social skills		**NOC Suggested Outcome:** **Play participation:** Use of activities as needed for enjoyment, entertainment, and development by children

NURSING CARE PLAN—continued

THE CHILD WITH CEREBRAL PALSY

Intervention	Rationale	Expected Outcome
Goal: The child engages in activities that maximize growth and development.		
■ Refer the family to an early intervention program. Encourage contact with other children. When hospitalized, place the child in a room with other children whenever possible.	■ The child needs a variety of activities and contact with other children and adults to maximize development.	The child engages in activities to maximize development.
■ Work with the school to develop an individualized education plan that encourages interaction with peers and a variety of activities that support development.	■ The education system is obligated to work with families to provide methods to enhance learning, including social interactions.	
■ Investigate recreational programs for children with disabilities and share information with the parents.	■ Recreational programs for children with disabilities may promote social experiences and physical activity.	

Promote Safety

Safety belts should be used for children in strollers and wheelchairs (see Skills 8–1—8–3). **SKILLS** Determine if an adaptive car safety seat is needed so the child can be safely transported. A child with chronic seizures should wear a helmet to protect against further injury.

● **FIGURE 53–14**

A child with cerebral palsy has abnormal muscle tone and lack of physical coordination.

Promote Growth and Development

Remember that many children with CP are physically but not intellectually disabled. Use terminology appropriate for the child's developmental level. Help the child develop a positive self-image to ensure emotional health and social growth. Children with a hearing impairment may need referral to learn American Sign Language or other communication methods. Provide audio and visual activities for the child who is quadriplegic.

Adaptive and assistive technology may be needed to promote mobility and communication. **Assistive technology** is any item, equipment, or product customized for use to promote the functional capabilities and independence of an individual with disabilities. Examples include computers, adaptive utensils, and customized wheelchairs.

Foster Parental Knowledge

Teach parents about the disorder and arrange sessions to teach them about all of the child's special needs. Teach administration, desired effects, and side effects of medications prescribed for seizures. Make sure parents are aware of the need for dental care for children taking anticonvulsants.

Provide Emotional Support

Refer parents to individual and family counseling if appropriate. Listen to the parents' concerns and encourage them to express their feelings and ask questions. Explain what they can expect from future treatment. Work with other healthcare professionals to help families adjust to this chronic disease.

Nursing Care in the Community

Children with CP need continuous support in the community. A case manager such as the parent or nurse is often needed to coordinate care. Parents may need financial assistance to provide the care that the child needs and to obtain appliances such as braces, wheelchairs, or adaptive utensils. Children need new adaptive devices, ongoing developmental assessment and care planning, and possibly surgery as they grow. Although the brain lesion does not change, it manifests differently as the child grows. For example, once the child begins to walk, the extensor tone may cause Achilles cord tightening. Braces may decrease deformities, but surgery may eventually be needed.

Early intervention programs can help parents learn to meet their child's special needs, including physical, occupational, and speech therapy, as well as educational needs. The child often needs an individualized education plan to maximize learning potential (see Chapter 39 ∞). The nurse can be instrumental in helping parents meet the needs of the child with CP in preschools, schools, offices, clinics, and other settings. In addition the nurse makes referrals as appropriate to support groups and organizations such as the United Cerebral Palsy Association and Shriners Hospitals. Recreational activities may be identified through the National Association of Sports for Cerebral Palsy. An individualized transition plan developed during adolescence assists the family and adolescent with CP to develop plans for adult living. Vocational training options can be explored. See Chapter 39. ∞ The young adult (18 to 21 years) may be able to move into a group home or live independently if desired.

EVALUATION

Expected outcomes of nursing care for the child with CP are provided on the "Nursing Care Plan."

INJURIES OF THE NEUROLOGIC SYSTEM

TRAUMATIC BRAIN INJURY

A traumatic brain injury can be defined as any trauma involving the blunt force or penetration that causes a change in level of consciousness or an anatomic abnormality of the brain. Traumatic brain injury is the leading cause of death and disability among children (Blackman, 2005). On an annual basis in children under 15 years, there are 400,000 emergency department visits, 29,000 hospitalizations, and 3000 deaths (Centers for Disease Control, 2003). Children and adolescents with a moderate to severe injury may develop a permanent disability, such as epilepsy, cognitive

impairment, learning problems, and behavioral or emotional problems (Adekoya, Thurman, White, et al., 2002).

Young children with moderate and severe traumatic brain injury are at risk for long-term cognitive deficits. Most recovery occurs in the first 12 months after injury. Even if the child scores normal on intelligence tests, difficulties with learning skills such as short-term memory, problem solving, sequencing, concrete thinking, and visual-spatial organization are common. No new learning can occur before short-term memory returns (Blackman, 2005).

ETIOLOGY AND PATHOPHYSIOLOGY

Falls are a major cause of unintentional head injuries in young children. Infants fall from dressing tables, beds, and sofas and also tumble down stairs, especially in walkers (American Academy of Pediatrics, 2001). Child abuse, including shaken baby syndrome, accounts for a large number of traumatic brain injuries in children under 1 year old. Toddlers and preschool-age children lack good judgment, and they may run out into the street without looking where they are going, or they may lean out of windows and fall. School-age children may be injured in motor vehicle crashes, either as passengers or as pedestrians, and they may also be injured in bicycle, rollerblading, scooter, or skateboard mishaps. Adolescents are frequently the drivers in motor vehicle crashes; often alcohol or drugs are involved. Adolescents are also injured in sports-related incidents. An increasing number of traumatic brain injuries result from firearms.

Brain injuries can be categorized as either primary or secondary. Primary injuries occur at the time of the insult when the initial cellular damage takes place. These injuries result from either a direct blow to the head (coup injury) or from acceleration-deceleration movement of the brain within the skull (contrecoup injury; see "Pathophysiology Illustrated: Brain Injury"). At the time of impact, scalp injuries, skull fractures, contusions, and hematomas of brain tissue may occur.

The secondary phase of brain trauma is a biochemical and cellular response to the initial insult, and it can be manifested immediately or over hours, days, or weeks. Damage usually results from destruction of brain tissue secondary to hypoxia, hypotension, edema, change in the blood–brain barrier, or hemorrhage. The result is increased intracranial pressure, which further compounds brain injury by limiting the blood flow that delivers oxygen and nutrients as well as removes accumulated toxins from cell death.

CLINICAL MANIFESTATIONS

The signs and symptoms of brain injuries in children depend on the pathologic features and severity of the injury. The child with a mild brain injury may remain conscious or have brief loss of consciousness (seconds to a few min-

PATHOPHYSIOLOGY ILLUSTRATED

Brain Injury

Subdural vessels are torn

Contrecoup injury results from secondary impact as brain moves forward and then backward within skull

Coup injury results from initial impact

Bruising occurs as brain moves over skull floor

Brain injury can result from a direct blow to the head (coup injury) or the acceleration-deceleration movement of the brain (contrecoup injury)

utes). The child with a moderate brain injury loses consciousness for 5 to 10 minutes. A child with a severe brain injury is usually unconscious for more than 10 minutes and may rapidly show signs of increased intracranial pressure. See "Clinical Manifestations: Traumatic Brain Injury by Severity."

Unconsciousness may result from increased intracranial pressure, edema, hemorrhage, or parenchymal damage to both cerebral cortices or the brainstem. Post-traumatic seizures are common. Retinal hemorrhages are seen in 65% to 90% of children with inflicted traumatic brain injury (Schutzman & Greenes, 2001).

Vital signs are important indicators of brain injury. Changes in respiratory effort or periods of apnea can occur secondary to shock, injury to the spinal cord above C4, or damage to or pressure on the medulla. Heart rate and blood pressure are indices of brainstem function. Tachycardia can be a sign of blood loss, shock, hypoxia, anxiety, or pain. Cushing's triad, associated with increased intracranial pressure or compromised blood flow to the brainstem, is characterized by hypertension, increased systolic pressure with wide pulse pressure, bradycardia, and irregular respirations. Refer to the earlier discussion of altered states of consciousness for more information about increased intracranial pressure.

Reflexes may be hyporesponsive, hyperresponsive, or nonexistent. The child may assume a decorticate, decerebrate, **areflexic** (no response to verbal, sensory, or pain stimulation), or flaccid posture (see Figure 53–2).

CLINICAL THERAPY

Identifying the severity of a brain injury involves history, observation, examination, and diagnostic testing. Information should be obtained about how the injury occurred, the child's initial responses and current responses, any loss of consciousness, and the child's memory of the event.

NURSING PRACTICE

Any infant who arrives in the emergency department with seizures, failure to thrive, vomiting, lethargy, respiratory irregularities, or coma should be evaluated for child abuse (shaken child syndrome). The infant has a large head and relatively weak neck muscles. A frustrated adult can shake an infant and cause inertial injuries (acceleration and deceleration) to the head that tear nerve fibers in the brain.

Neurologic evaluation with the pediatric Glasgow Coma Scale is performed frequently to detect changes in the child's condition (see Table 53–3). Cranial nerves are

CLINICAL MANIFESTATIONS

TRAUMATIC BRAIN INJURY BY SEVERITY

TYPE OF BRAIN INJURY	CLINICAL MANIFESTATIONS
Concussion or mild brain injury	Low-grade headache that will not go away Slowness in thinking, acting, speaking, reading Memory problems Loss of balance, unsteady walking Difficulty paying attention or concentrating, change in performance at school Feeling tired all the time, change in sleeping pattern Change in eating patterns Increased sensitivity to lights, sounds, distractions Easily irritated Lack of motivation or interest in favorite toys
Moderate brain injury	Glasgow Coma Scale score of 9–12 Post-traumatic amnesia for 1–24 hours Loss of consciousness
Severe brain injury	Glasgow Coma Scale score of 8 or less Post-traumatic amnesia greater than 24 hours Coma Increased intracranial pressure

assessed (see Table 35-20 in Chapter 35 ∞ and Table 53–4). Review the discussion of altered states of consciousness at the beginning of this chapter for further details.

Laboratory tests include a complete blood cell count, blood chemistry, toxicology screening, and urinalysis. Radiologic examination identifies the specific injury. X-rays detect fractures of the skull and cervical vertebrae. A CT scan detects fractures, intracranial hemorrhage, swelling, and diffuse axonal injury. An MRI scan is used during recovery to determine the extent of brain damage. PET scans measure the blood flow in the brain. A fracture indicates a more serious injury. Many children with brain injuries have multiple other injuries. Even though cervical spine injuries are rare, all children with a brain injury should have a potential cervical spine injury ruled out by radiologic examination.

The initial management of a child with a brain injury is based on the child's physiologic status. The airway must be clear and stable, and hypoxia must be prevented. If indicated, the child is intubated, sedated, and chemically paralyzed to protect the airway and prevent aspiration. Hypoxia and hypercapnia have disastrous effects on cerebral function, as they can cause vasodilation and increased intracranial pressure. Assisted ventilation with 100% oxygen at the child's normal respiratory rate is often used for the first 24 hours after injury to maintain the oxygenation level (see Skill 14–14). **SKILLS** Hyperventilation may be used for a short period in cases of increased intracranial pressure, but prolonged use may cause cerebral ischemia (Adelson, Bratton, Carney, et al., 2003).

Perfusion of the brain must be maintained to ensure that it gets adequate oxygen and nutrients, and the accumulated neurotoxins are removed. Shock is treated aggressively with fluid boluses. Keep the head of the bed flat until adequate cerebral perfusion pressure is ensured. Fluids administration is then focused on maintaining the blood pressure.

Increased intracranial pressure must be controlled. Brain swelling can lead to worsening cerebral ischemia and **cerebral edema** (the increase in intracellular and extracellular fluid in the brain that results from anoxia, vasodilation, or vascular stasis). If unrelieved, brain contents begin shifting in the cranium, which can lead to **herniation** (protrusion of brain contents into the brain stem area). Diuretics such as mannitol or furosemide may be used to decrease intracranial pressure. A continuous infusion of hypertonic saline (3%) is sometimes used for control of increased intracranial pressure (Adelson, Bratton, Carney et al., 2003). Pain and sedation management promote comfort and help control intracranial pressure. Invasive procedures may be necessary to reduce increased intracranial pressure. Burr holes may be made or more extensive surgery may be performed to evacuate a lesion or hematoma. A ventricular catheter may be placed to drain CSF and to monitor pressure.

If there is no cervical spine injury, the head of the bed is elevated up to 30 degrees. The child's head is kept in the midline to promote venous (jugular) drainage. Hip flexion is avoided. The child's body temperature is kept within normal limits. The environment is kept as quiet as possible. Fluids may be restricted only after the child is hemodynamically stable. A urinary catheter is inserted to monitor output, and electrolytes should be checked frequently. Nutrition support should be started within 72 hours with total parenteral nutrition or enteral nutrition.

Aggressive support continues until the child regains consciousness and rehabilitation can be initiated. Physical therapists, occupational therapists, and speech therapists are members of the rehabilitation team. Disabilities that often result from a severe brain injury include motor and cognitive impairments, feeding disorders, hearing and vision impairments, and communication problems. Reliable predictions of outcome in the child who has suffered a severe brain injury cannot be made until 6 to 12 months postinjury.

NURSING MANAGEMENT

NURSING ASSESSMENT AND DIAGNOSIS

Assess the child's neurologic status frequently and compare to past findings, noting improvement, stability, or deterioration. Evaluate the child's level of consciousness using the pediatric Glasgow Coma Scale (see Table 53–3). Assess the pupils for size and reactivity, as well as cranial nerves. Monitor vital signs closely. Note decerebrate or decorticate posturing. If a ventricular catheter or bolt is inserted, monitor the actual pressure readings. Changes in these signs may indicate hypoxia, decreased perfusion, shock, or increased intracranial pressure (see Skill 9–17). **SKILLS** The cause of any deterioration must be quickly determined and appropriate interventions taken.

When the child has a decreased level of consciousness shortly after a brain injury, consider if a post-traumatic seizure occurred and if the child is still in the postictal state.

Suspect that the child with increased intracranial pressure is in pain, even when unresponsive. Observe for physiologic and behavioral signs of pain.

Nursing diagnoses that might be appropriate for the child with a brain injury include the following:

- *Ineffective Cerebral Tissue Perfusion* related to hypoventilation, hypovolemia, and/or reduction of arterial blood flow to the brain due to increased intracranial pressure
- *Risk for Aspiration* related to decreased level of consciousness and loss of protective reflexes
- *Risk for Imbalanced Fluid Volume* related to therapies for reducing intracranial pressure
- *Compromised Family Coping* related to life-threatening injury to child

PLANNING AND IMPLEMENTATION

Hospital-Based Nursing Care

Nursing care focuses on maintaining cardiopulmonary function, preventing complications, promoting recovery, and providing emotional support. Nursing management is based on prevention of secondary injury and return to an optimal level of function.

Maintain cardiopulmonary function. In the moderately injured child, observe breathing patterns and check color and level of consciousness. Check the pulse oximeter; the oxygen saturation should remain over 95%. Report any sign of decreased oxygenation or signs and symptoms of increased intracranial pressure to the physician immediately (see Table 53–2). Keep suction equipment at the bedside in case aspiration occurs.

THINKING CRITICALLY

Antwan, 7 years old, was injured when he was struck by a car and thrown several feet into the air. He was unconscious upon admission to the emergency department and showed some signs of increased intracranial pressure (dilated and fixed pupils). He was treated for shock, and his neurologic status and vital signs were frequently assessed. The initial evaluation revealed that Antwan had sustained several contusions of the brain, but no skull fracture. He was intubated and medicated to manage the increased intracranial pressure.

Antwan's intracranial pressure has now stabilized, but he still has not totally regained consciousness. He is restless and agitated, and unable to follow directions. His parents stay at his bedside and provide auditory and tactile stimulation, hoping he will eventually respond. Physical therapy has been initiated to prevent contractures and to maintain function. Long-term rehabilitation will be needed to help Antwan and his family achieve the best outcome possible after this injury.

What is the role of the nurse in acute care of the brain-injured child? What support does the family need to contribute to the child's care? How would you work with other healthcare professionals to coordinate care during the acute care phase? How would you help plan the long-term care for a child such as Antwan?

Reduce physiologic stresses on the body that could increase intracranial pressure. The nurse should minimize unpleasant stimuli when possible, keep the environment quiet, and avoid jarring the bed. Pain management and temperature control are important. Position the child to avoid excessive flexion of the hips and neck that could slow venous circulation. Monitor the effect of nursing procedures on level of intracranial pressure and determine if clustering procedures is better than spreading procedures over time. Encourage parents to talk to the child and provide comforting touch.

Administer medications as ordered. Provide oral care to keep mucous membranes moist and intact. Pad and cushion bony prominences, provide skin care, and change the child's position frequently. The eyes should be protected from corneal irritation with ophthalmic ointment and patching. Stool softeners and suppositories should be used as needed to prevent constipation. The side rails of the bed should be padded to protect the child if a seizure occurs.

Promote recovery and prevent physical deformities. Physical, occupational, and speech therapy should begin in the hospital. Work with these therapists to reinforce exercises and help teach parents the techniques so they can work with the child in the hospital and at home. Using toys, books, music, or games, provide stimulation based on the child's age and ability. Encourage parents to bring in favorite toys, stuffed animals, and tape recordings of the child's favorite music or of family members talking.

Provide emotional support to the family in collaboration with the social workers, physicians, psychologists, rehabilitation therapists, and members of the clergy caring for the child and family. All can help the family adjust to having a child with a new disability.

Discharge Planning and Home Care Teaching

Home care needs should be identified and addressed well in advance of discharge. Children with serious brain injuries benefit from inpatient or outpatient rehabilitation to promote optimal achievement of function. A case manager is often needed to coordinate services and resources during rehabilitation. Social services intervention may be needed when brain injury results from child abuse or shaken baby syndrome.

Give parents information about caring for children with mild or moderate brain injuries at home and possible behaviors to expect from the child. For children with disabilities, determine what adaptations and assistive technology are needed in the home to care for the child, such as a wheelchair, a walker, braces, or a special bed. Social work and home health agencies can often help the parents make special arrangements.

Nursing Care in the Community

Home care nursing may be important for the child with an acquired neurologic dysfunction and prolonged altered consciousness. The home care nurse can take over the case management for the disabled child and make sure the environment is safe. The nurse can teach the family to care for the child's needs, monitor the intake of fluids and foods, as well as position the child and perform range of motion exercises to reduce contractures. Many children with severe brain injuries qualify for Social Security Supplemental Security Income (SSI) benefits or the state program for children with special healthcare needs. Regular follow-up visits are needed to assess the child's recovery and to modify the treatment plan.

Even though the child looks normal within days of a mild or moderate brain injury, parents and teachers need to be aware that brain healing takes up to 6 weeks. Typical behaviors during this period may include any of the following: tiring easily, memory loss or forgetfulness, easy distractibility, difficulty concentrating, difficulty following directions, irritability or short temper, and needing help starting and finishing tasks. Educational assessment should be initiated if recovery takes longer than 6 weeks, and educational accommodations needed are often different from those needed by children with other learning disabilities. An individualized education plan is often needed. See Chapter 39. ∞ Children with moderate brain injuries often have problems with attention, problem solving, and speed of in-formation processing. The injury impairs new learning more than the retention of prior learning. Young children are at a special disadvantage because they have not had time to store knowledge and develop learning strategies.

The child or adolescent facing long-term rehabilitation needs support to adjust to the disability and to find the strength to maximize his or her abilities. Identify recreational opportunities for the child with disabilities to promote exercise and self-esteem. The adolescent may need to gain vocational skills and learn to live independently. Refer parents to the Brain Injury Association for further information. (See the Companion Website for links to such resources.)

Prevention of brain injury is another important role of the nurse. Encourage parents to obtain protective helmets and require children to use them for bicycling and skateboarding. Parents should be encouraged to wear a helmet themselves as role models. Encourage parents to monitor playgrounds for appropriate use of wood chips or cushioning tiles to reduce the severity of injuries associated with falls.

EVALUATION

Examples of expected outcomes of nursing care for the child with traumatic brain injury include the following:

- Cerebral perfusion pressure is maintained at an adequate rate to sustain oxygenation of the brain.
- Muscle function is maintained and physical deformities are prevented with range of motion exercises and splinting during the recovery stages of the brain injury.
- Parents are supported through the child's acute recovery phase and learn to provide care the child will need at home.
- The child's school performance is monitored and appropriate educational resources are provided to support the child's learning.

SPECIFIC HEAD INJURIES

SCALP INJURIES

Injuries to the scalp, which can be caused by falls, blunt trauma, or penetration of a foreign body, are usually benign. Although bleeding may be extensive, hypovolemia or shock is uncommon unless the patient is an infant.

Lacerations should be irrigated with copious amounts of sterile normal saline solution and inspected for bony fragments or depressions, CSF leakage with a dural tear, or debris. If the injury is simple, the laceration can be sutured and the child discharged from the emergency department. If not, a neurosurgeon should be consulted.

CONCUSSION

A concussion can involve transient impairment of consciousness that usually results from a direct blow to the head, face, neck, or elsewhere on the body with an "impulsive" force transmitted to the head (Cobb & Battin, 2004). It is secondary to stretching, compression, or shearing of nerve fibers. The injury is metabolic rather than gross structural damage or focal injury. The child has an alteration in mental status (e.g., amnesia, dizziness, memory or orientation impairment, unsteady gait), but not necessarily loss of consciousness. Concussions are categorized by three levels of severity (Table 53–9).

NURSING PRACTICE

Sports with a high risk for concussion include boxing, field hockey, football, ice hockey, lacrosse, martial arts, soccer, rodeo, wrestling, rugby, baseball, rollerblading, trampolining, and basketball. An estimated 62,800 high school athletes experience a concussion each year, and concussion related to football accounts for nearly 63% of these cases (Lovell, Collins, Iverson et al., 2003).

Treatment is supportive. Children are observed in the emergency department for several hours before being sent home with instructions to the parents to watch them closely for decreased responsiveness. Any child who is unconscious for more than 5 minutes or has amnesia of the event may be admitted to the hospital or observed in a short-stay unit to rule out other injury.

Pediatric concussive syndrome, which is believed to be caused by an injury to the brainstem, is seen in children who are less than 3 years old. Toddlers seem stunned at the time of injury, but they do not lose consciousness. Later, however, these children become pale, clammy, and lethargic, and they may vomit. They are usually brought to the hospital for treatment when these symptoms appear. These children may be placed in a short-stay unit for observation and usually recover within 24 hours.

Postconcussive syndrome, which is common in both children and adults, may occur anytime after the initial brain injury. Signs and symptoms can include headache, dizziness or vertigo, hearing loss, sleep disorders, fatigue, irritability, photophobia, subtle changes in personality, poor concentration, poor memory, and ataxia. Treatment is supportive. Symptoms usually disappear within several weeks but may last up to 6 months. Parents and teachers should be told to expect altered behavior in the child and encouraged to help the child maintain self-esteem.

Young athletes suffering a second concussion before complete recovery from the first develop *second impact syndrome*. This syndrome results in acute brain swelling, neurologic or cognitive deficits, and sometimes death from the cumulative effect of these concussions. Recommendations should be followed for the management of sports-related concussions to reduce the risk of disability and death. Removal from sports participation ranges from 1 week to the entire season, depending on the severity of concussion and neurologic symptoms (Guskiewicz, Weaver, Padua et al., 2000). High school athletes have a slower recovery time from brain injuries than college or adult athletes (Cobb & Battin, 2004). A postconcussive symptom scale is often used to provide uniform information about the actual recovery time from the concussion and to prevent athletes who try to minimize symptoms from returning to play too soon. Individuals with multiple concussions have a longer recovery time (Guskiewicz & McCrea, 2003).

SKULL FRACTURES

A fracture to any of the eight cranial bones is caused by a considerable force to the head. Any area of the skull with swelling or a hematoma should be evaluated for possible fracture. Diagnosis is made by visual inspection, palpation, radiologic study, or CT scan. Treatment should always include neurosurgical consultation.

Management of skull fractures depends on the type and extent of the injury (Table 53–10).

CEREBRAL CONTUSION

A cerebral contusion, or the bruising of brain tissue, is secondary to blunt trauma and can occur with either coup or contrecoup injuries (see "Pathophysiology Illustrated: Brain Injury"). Such injuries are rare in children less than 1 year of age. The temporal or frontal sections of the skull are the most common sites of this injury. Damage to the

---

TABLE 53–9 ❖ Levels of Concussion Severity

Grade 1

Transient confusion, no loss of consciousness, and a duration of mental status abnormalities of less than 15 minutes.

Grade 2

Transient confusion, no loss of consciousness, and a duration of mental status abnormalities of 15 minutes or longer.

Grade 3

Loss of consciousness, either brief (seconds) or prolonged (minutes or longer).

Adapted with permission from the Quality Standards Subcommittee, American Academy of Neurology. (1997). Practice parameters: The management of concussion in sports. *Neurology, 48*, 581–585.

MediaLink Case Study: Post-Concussion Return to Competitive Play

TABLE 53–10 ✤ Skull Fractures

Injury	Diagnosis and Clinical Therapy
Linear Fracture Results from impact to large area of the skull. Usually no symptoms. May have overlying hematoma or soft-tissue swelling. Such fractures in newborns may result from pressure from forceps or from maternal pelvic bones.	If fracture is on temporal bone or crosses sagittal suture line, a CT scan is performed to detect potential epidural hematoma. Consider the possibility of an inflicted injury. No treatment is commonly needed.
Depressed Fracture Break in skull itself or an area shattered into many fragments. Pieces of bone may be depressed into brain tissue with hematoma forming on top. This type of fracture in a newborn may be the result of a forceps injury.	Plain radiographic film or CT scan. Surgery to elevate bone fragments when depression is greater than 5 mm. Tetanus prophylaxis is given as needed. Many are associated with intracranial injury and post-traumatic epilepsy.
Compound Fracture Combination of a full-thickness scalp laceration and depressed skull fracture with the bone exposed, considered penetrating fractures if the dura is torn.	Visual diagnosis along with radiographic studies. Surgical debridement, a search for foreign bodies, and copious irrigation are performed. Parenteral antibiotics and tetanus prophylaxis are provided as needed.
Basilar Fracture Fracture at the base of the skull that may involve the frontal, ethmoid, sphenoid, temporal, or occipital bones. A dural tear may be present.	Diagnosis is confirmed by signs of blood behind the tympanic membranes, cerebrospinal fluid leakage from the nose or ears, periorbital ecchymosis (raccoon eyes), or bruising of the mastoid (Battle sign). Radiographic imaging locates the fracture site. Antibiotics may be prescribed. Surgical repair of the site of the cerebrospinal fluid lead is performed if the leak persists after 7–10 days. Transient or permanent cranial nerve injuries occur (e.g., hearing loss).

Data from Rosman, N. P. (1999). Acute head trauma. In J. A. McMillan, C. D. DeAngelis, R. D. Feigin, & J. B. Warshaw, *Oski's pediatrics: Principles and practice* (3rd ed., pp. 603–617). Philadelphia: Lippincott, Williams & Willkins.

parenchyma with tears in vessels or tissue, pulping, and subsequent areas of necrosis or infarction may occur.

The child may have focal symptoms depending on the area of injury. Altered levels of consciousness range from confusion and disorientation to being obtunded. A CT scan is used for diagnosis.

Treatment involves hospitalization for observation and to rule out other injuries. Surgical treatment is rarely necessary. Sequelae are focal and specific to the area of the brain that was injured. For example, an injury to the left temporal area may affect speech.

INTRACRANIAL HEMATOMAS

Intracranial hematomas are space-occupying lesions that expand rapidly or slowly, depending on whether they are arterial or venous in origin. They must be located quickly. Some lesions require evacuation as soon as possible to minimize the secondary effects of the injury. See "Clinical Manifestations: Intracranial Hematomas" for information on cause, symptoms, and clinical therapy.

PENETRATING INJURIES

Gunshot wounds to the head can damage tissue, bone, and vessels. Low-velocity bullets enter but do not exit the skull; instead they ricochet within the cranial vault, destroying brain tissue and vessels. Although the child may be conscious just after the injury, the level of consciousness quickly deteriorates because of the edema surrounding the penetration tract. High-velocity bullets, on the other hand, cause immediate, severe damage on impact. See Chapter 36 for a discussion of violence in childhood. ∞

CT scans evaluate gunshot trauma and pinpoint the location of bullet and bone fragments as well as parenchymal damage. Treatment involves surgical debridement of the tract, evacuation of any hematomas, and removal of accessible bone or bullet particles. Approximately 50% of children with gunshot wounds to the head die. Those who survive may suffer multiple focal deficits and seizures.

Impalement injuries frequently occur in children in association with lawn darts or dog bites. All objects must be left in place and removed in the operating room by a neurosurgeon. The child with an impalement injury is at high risk for focal injury and infection. After surgery, children with this type of injury are managed as with other postoperative brain injuries, with attention focused on level of consciousness, increased intracranial pressure, and infection control.

CLINICAL MANIFESTATIONS

INTRACRANIAL HEMATOMAS

TYPE OF HEMATOMA	CLINICAL MANIFESTATIONS	CLINICAL THERAPY
Subdural Hematoma Result of severe head trauma such as falls, assaults, motor vehicle crashes, or shaken child syndrome Occurs most frequently in children less than 1 year old Inertial forces cause laceration of the bridging veins; a venous hematoma forms beneath the dura and presses directly on brain	Symptoms (may not appear until 48–72 hours after the injury) include: ■ Change in level of consciousness (confusion, agitation, or lethargy) ■ Nausea or vomiting ■ Headache ■ Retinal hemorrhages in both eyes ■ Pupil on side of injury may be fixed and dilated ■ Seizures ■ Fever	Diagnosis confirmed by CT scan Hematoma is evacuated surgically Management of increased intracranial pressure; subdural taps may be necessary Morbidity and mortality rates are high Damage from the initial inertial injury is compounded by the hematoma The majority of surviving children develop seizures
Epidural Hematoma Rare in children, especially those less than 4 years of age Results from blunt trauma (most often falls), motor vehicle crashes, assaults, or baseball to temporal area Temporal and parietal areas are most common sites May be associated with linear skull fracture Arterial or venous bleeding occurs between the skull and the dura	Symptoms include: ■ Delayed onset, minimal or absent symptoms from initial impact ■ Rapid deterioration ■ Sleepiness or lethargy ■ Headache ■ Full fontanelle ■ Paresis of cranial nerves III and VI ■ Papilledema ■ Fixed and dilated pupil ■ Signs of increased intracranial pressure	Diagnosis confirmed by CT scan Treatment involves immediate surgical intervention; craniotomy is performed followed by evacuation of the hematoma Prognosis is good, although 25% of children have seizures May be fatal if bleeding is arterial
Intracerebral Hematoma Result of deep contusion or intracerebral laceration (secondary to foreign body, bony penetration, or impalement) Causes diffuse bleeding in parenchyma; there may be a hematoma with associated small areas of bleeding	Symptoms depend upon the size and location of the hematoma, as well as if size is increasing due to uncontrolled bleeding ■ Altered consciousness	Diagnosis confirmed by CT scan Surgical treatment not indicated Neurologic effects depend on size and location of lesion and whether bleeding can be controlled Hemiplegia or visual loss may result

SPINAL CORD INJURY

Less than 5% of spinal cord injuries occur in children under 16 years of age annually (Massagli, 2000). A high proportion of children under 15 years of age with spinal cord injury die immediately or within the first hour of injury. Even when the child survives the first hours, mortality rates are high (Moloney-Harmon & Adams, 2001).

Motor vehicle crashes are the leading cause of spinal cord injuries, either pedestrian-vehicular, bicycle-vehicular, passenger, or driver-related. Other causes of spinal injuries, especially in toddlers and young children, include falls and child abuse. Recreation or sports-related trauma accounts for more injuries as children grow older. Penetrating injuries such as stab and gunshot wounds are becoming more prevalent.

The mechanism of injury determines the type of lesion that occurs (Figure 53–15 ●). Hyperflexion injuries produce tears or avulsions and fractures of vertebral bodies, as well as subluxation and dislocation. Lateral flexion (rotation) may cause joint dislocations or unstable spinal fractures. Extension may result in the so-called hangman's fracture, ligament tears, avulsion fractures of vertebral bodies, as well as central

● FIGURE 53–15

A   B   C

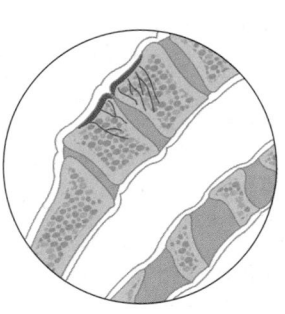

D

Mechanics of injury to the spinal cord. **A,** Hyperflexion. **B,** Lateral flexion. **C,** Extension. **D,** Compression.

or posterior spinal cord syndrome. Compression injuries cause anterior cord syndrome. Children are prone to specific kinds of spinal cord injuries because of the extreme mobility and flexibility of their spinal column. Table 53–11 describes the spinal cord injuries most common in children.

Spinal cord injuries are classified as complete or incomplete. Complete lesions are irreversible and involve a loss of sensory, motor, and autonomic function below the level of the injury. Incomplete lesions involve varying degrees of sensory, motor, and autonomic function below the level of injury. The higher the level of spinal cord injury, the more severe the neurologic damage. The child is often a victim of

GROWTH AND DEVELOPMENT

The vertebrae are incompletely ossified in children under 9 years. The facet joints are more shallow and horizontal. The young child's head is relatively large compared to the strength of the neck muscles. Atlanto-occipital dislocation (C1 to C3 level) occurs more frequently in infants and young children because of the flat articulation between the occiput and the top cervical vertebra, and the ligaments supporting this junction are underdeveloped and have more laxity (Steinmetz, Lechner, & Anderson, 2003). Children 9 to 15 years are more likely to have an injury at the C4 to C6 level (Massagli, 2000).

TABLE 53–11 ✤ Spinal Cord Injuries in Children

Spine Region	Injury Characteristics
Cervical	■ Site of 60% of spinal injuries in children under 10 years ■ Injury above C3 segment causes respiratory arrest and death without ventilatory support; many of these injuries are fatal ■ Diaphragm function is present when injury is at C5 level ■ Quadriplegia, some function of upper extremities when injury is at C6–C7 level ■ Loss of sphincter function ■ Sensory level lost below the sternum
Thoracic	■ Site of 20% of spinal injuries usually between 8 and 14 years ■ Full control of upper extremities including hands ■ Poor trunk balance
Thoracolumbar	■ Full control of muscles in abdomen and upper back ■ Good trunk balance
Lumbar	■ Most injuries occur at the L2–L4 level; second most common area of injury, probably a result of improperly placed lap belts ■ Below L3 may have functioning of muscles in upper leg ■ Loss of ankle and foot control

multiple trauma and may display signs of hypovolemic shock resulting from other injuries, increased intracranial pressure, or respiratory depression. Children can also experience neurogenic or spinal shock (see Chapter 48 ∞).

At the time of injury, the child is flaccid and areflexic below the lesion. There is loss of sensation because of spinal shock (hypotension, bradycardia, and hypothermia) due to autonomic dysfunction. Priapism (prolonged penile erection) may be present. Respiration may be compromised due to paralysis of the diaphragm.

As neurologic recovery begins, spinal reflex activity returns and increasing spasticity is seen below the level of the lesion. **Autonomic dysreflexia** is a condition in which hypertension, bradycardia, severe headaches, pallor below and flushing above the level of the spinal cord lesion, and seizures occur due to an impaired autonomic nervous system. This response can be triggered by a full bladder.

Diagnosis is made by observation, neurologic examination, and x-ray studies. X-ray studies include lateral cervical spine and anteroposterior and lateral views of the thoracic and lumbosacral spine. The child's immobilized position is unchanged until x-rays read by a radiologist have cleared the spine for injury. In addition, CT scanning, MRI, fluoroscopy,

or myelography may be performed. Up to 15% to 25% of children have spinal cord injury without radiographic abnormality (SCIWORA) because initial films or CT scans show no bony deformity. The child is believed to be free of injury; however, profound or progressive paralysis occurs immediately or within 48 hours. Developmental aspects of the vertebrae, muscles, ligaments, and soft tissues contribute to the lack of radiographic findings (Moloney-Harmon & Adams, 2001). An MRI can detect the injury.

Spinal injuries are managed aggressively. The child with a spinal cord injury may be placed in skeletal traction or a halo device. Surgery to reduce and internally fixate the fracture is performed for unstable fractures and dislocations. Decompression of the spinal cord and nerve roots may be performed if transaction is not complete.

To decrease neurologic sequelae, methylprednisolone is administered in high doses to children with motor deficits. Administration must be started within 8 hours of the injury. Atropine and norepinephrine may be given to manage spinal shock.

Complications of spinal cord injury include:

■ Impaired respiratory function due to a paralyzed diaphragm or diminished vital capacity.

■ Scoliosis if injury occurs before the skeleton is mature.

■ Hip instability due to poor acetabular development.

■ Pathologic fractures of the long bones due to immobilization hypercalcemia.

■ Pressure sores.

■ Deep vein thrombosis.

■ Autonomic dysreflexia.

An interdisciplinary approach is required to manage the rehabilitation and long-term care needs of the child and family.

NURSING MANAGEMENT

Hospital-Based Nursing Care

Nursing care focuses on monitoring vital signs, meeting nutritional needs, maintaining skin integrity, promoting independent functioning, encouraging therapeutic play, providing emotional support, and promoting rehabilitation.

Monitor vital signs and be alert for any changes, especially those that may signify increased respiratory difficulty or spinal shock (hypotension, bradycardia, and hypothermia), increased intracranial pressure (see Table 53–2), or autonomic dysreflexia. Monitor intake and output. Monitor bladder and bowel function.

Assess the cranial nerves as they may be affected by swelling around the spinal cord. Note the return of reflexes and change from flaccid tone to spasticity. Identify any changes in level of sensation or motor function.

Ensure adequate nutrition. A child with complete paralysis may require a gastrostomy tube. When the child begins to eat, feed soft foods slowly as the child may have some swallowing difficulties.

Prevent skin breakdown. See Chapter 57. ∞ Observe surgical sites for signs of infection or inflammation. Provide regular traction pin site care according to institutional guidelines.

Promote independent functioning by reinforcing the exercises and skills learned in physical and occupational therapy. Use supports, boots, footboards, splints, and braces as recommended by the therapists to prevent contractures (Figure 53–16 ●). If hand mobility is limited, explore options for independence. Encourage the child to be as independent as possible in a wheelchair. An important mobility goal is to achieve wheelchair transfer and to perform self-care. Identify adaptive equipment that make these goals possible.

Achieving bowel and bladder control may be difficult. Intermittent catheterizations may be necessary (see Skill 16–1). **SKILLS** Anticipate that constipation will occur and initiate bowel training with a diet high in fiber and the use of stool softeners.

Therapeutic play appropriate for the child's developmental level is an important part of the healing process. Provide as many normal activities for the child as possible, but do not give the child tasks that he or she will have difficulty completing. Child life teachers or tutors can help the child keep up with schoolwork.

Television, videotapes, and music can offer diversion for prolonged hospitalization. Paraplegic children can learn to use their arms and hands to play interactive games.

● **FIGURE 53–16**

Splints are often used to prevent contractures, thus maintaining optimal functioning of the child's hands or feet.

Devices can also be adapted so that the child can play video games or manipulate the television or radio.

Support the child emotionally. Encourage the child to meet small, short-term goals, including those that involve self-care. Encourage the child to express fears and frustrations.

Be compassionate and understanding. Encourage siblings to visit, answer their questions honestly, and help them to discuss their feelings. Involve the parents and siblings in the child's care as much as possible. When appropriate, encourage them to help with activities of daily living.

Discharge Planning and Home Care Teaching

Many children are discharged to inpatient rehabilitation facilities. Assist with arrangements for the transfer. Work closely with the child, parents, and other members of the healthcare team concerning placement. Home care needs, reintegration into educational programs, and safety issues should be identified and addressed well in advance of discharge from the rehabilitation facility. Refer families to social services, family counseling, and support groups if indicated.

The young child's ultimate functioning will be related to cognitive development, the amount of upper body strength, and the family's expectations (Massagli, 2000).

HYPOXIC-ISCHEMIC BRAIN INJURY (DROWNING AND NEAR-DROWNING)

Drowning is defined as death within 24 hours of a submersion incident. Near-drowning is survival for at least 24 hours after submersion. Over 90% of drownings occur in fresh water such as ponds and residential swimming pools (Zuckerman & Conway, 2000). Drowning is the second leading cause of injury-related deaths in children. Most pediatric victims are very young (under age 4 years) or in their teen years. Boys are five times more likely than girls to die from drowning.

 GROWTH AND DEVELOPMENT

Between 40% and 50% of children injured in drowning incidents are under 4 years of age, with peak incidence between ages 1 and 2 years. The majority (55%) of infant drownings are in bathtubs. The most common drowning locations for children 1 to 4 years old are artificial pools (56%) and other bodies of fresh water (26%). Among older children, 63% of drownings occur in natural bodies of fresh water (Brenner, Trumble, Smith et al., 2001).

A child can drown in as little water as it takes to cover the nose and mouth. The events preceding drowning follow a sequential pattern. The child trapped in water panics, struggles, tries to move using swimming motions, and holds his or her breath. Then the child swallows a small amount of fluid, vomits, and aspirates the vomitus. This leads to a brief period of laryngospasm, which lasts no more than 2 minutes. Because of the increasing panic and hypoxia, the child swallows more liquid. Then either the child goes into profound laryngospasm, becomes severely hypoxic, has a seizure, and dies (dry drowning), or the child becomes unconscious, the laryngospasm relaxes as reflexes are lost, and the child passively aspirates even greater amounts of water into the airway and stomach (wet drowning). Hypothermia may result because the child's body cools more quickly in water than air. See Chapter 57 for more information on hypothermia. ∞ As the child becomes hypoxic, the cardiac muscle becomes impaired and ultimately the heart stops.

Anoxia is the major insult associated with drowning. Anoxia leads to cerebral edema and increased intracranial pressure. Little can be done to resuscitate the brain, but with aggressive cardiopulmonary resuscitation, more severely brain-injured children are surviving in a permanent vegetative state. When the child is resuscitated, water in the lungs inactivates the surfactant. Pulmonary edema, acute respiratory distress syndrome, and pneumonia may develop.

The child who has been immersed exhibits a wide variety of signs and symptoms depending on the length of time underwater, the temperature of the water, the response to the episode, and the initial treatment performed at the scene. Children submerged for short periods have few symptoms and recover without complication. The child with a longer submersion can experience the following symptoms: decreased level of consciousness ranging from stupor to total unresponsiveness, cerebral edema, increased intracranial pressure, seizures, respiratory acidosis, irregular respirations, apnea, and gastric distention.

Medical intervention begins at the scene of the drowning with immediate ventilation and compressions, when indicated. The sooner cardiopulmonary resuscitation (CPR) is started, the better the child's prognosis. Children still requiring CPR upon arrival at the emergency department are most likely to die or have a significant neurologic impairment (American Academy of Pediatrics, 2003b). All near-drowning victims should be admitted to the hospital for at least 24 hours or observed in a short-stay observation unit for several hours, even when asymptomatic. Many life-threatening complications, including respiratory distress and cerebral edema, may not become evident for at least 12 hours after the incident.

Anoxic brain injury is the leading cause of mortality. Predictors of good outcome are submersion for less than 5 minutes and CPR for less than 10 minutes (Zuckerman & Conway, 2000).

NURSING MANAGEMENT

Nursing care of the child who survives a near-drowning focuses on monitoring the child's cardiopulmonary status and providing emotional support to the family.

Monitor the child's responsiveness, spontaneous respiratory efforts, oxygenation, and pulse. Check the pupils for reactivity. The child should be monitored for signs of complications such as respiratory distress and worsening mental status. Administer prescribed medications and position the child properly. Other nursing interventions, especially for the comatose child, can be found in the earlier discussion of altered states of consciousness.

Provide emotional support to the family. Be nonjudgmental and provide a forum for parents to express their feelings. Reassure parents who exhibit guilt reactions that their child is receiving all possible medical treatment. Parents may be faced with an unknown prognosis. Encourage them to seek assistance from social workers, members of the clergy, close friends, and relatives. Arrange for appropriate referrals.

Identify and address home care needs well in advance of discharge. Assist with arrangements for the child with minor deficits. Help the parents decide whether the comatose child will go home or to a long-term care facility.

Drowning can be prevented by education, legislation, and changes in the environment. Pool owners should erect climb-proof 5-foot fences around all four sides of the pool. Local ordinances may require such fences. Adolescents should learn the dangers of mixing alcohol and swimming. Five- and 10-gallon buckets should be kept empty when not in use. Emphasize the importance of closely supervising children when near or in the water, whether at pools, at the beach, or in the bathtub.

Critical Concept Review

LEARNING OBJECTIVES	CONCEPTS

Describe the anatomy and physiology of the neurologic system.

The major structures of the neurologic system are:
1. Brain.
2. Spinal cord: transmits impulses to and from the brain, conveying sensory information and relaying impulses that stimulate motor responses.
3. Nerves: the infant is born with all the nerve cells he or she will have throughout life. Myelination is immature and incomplete until age 4.

Describe the nursing assessment process and tools used for infants and children with altered levels of consciousness and other neurologic conditions.

1. Infants and children with altered levels of consciousness should be monitored for:
   - Responsiveness to environmental and sensory stimuli.
   - Pupil size and reactivity.
   - Movement of extremities.
   - Ability to maintain an airway.
   - Changes in vital signs.
   - Changes in breathing patterns.
   - Status of the cranial nerves.
2. Nurses should use the Glasgow Coma Score as well as cardiorespiratory monitors and pulse oximetry to monitor the child.

Differentiate between the signs of infants and children with epilepsy and status epilepticus, and describe appropriate nursing management for each condition.

1. Epilepsy:
   - Clinical manifestations depend upon type of seizure.
   - Last from 5 seconds to 1–2 minutes, depending upon type of seizure.
   - Signs range from momentary lapse of attention to unconsciousness with repetitive muscular contraction and relaxation.
   - Decreased level of consciousness during postictal period.
2. Nursing management of epilepsy:
   - Administer medications as ordered.
   - Protect child from injury
   - Instruct parents concerning importance of giving medications as prescribed to maintain blood levels of medications.
   - Instruct parents in management of seizures and when to call for emergency assistance.
3. Status epilepticus:
   - Continuous seizure that lasts longer than 30 minutes.
   - Series of seizures during which consciousness is not regained.
4. Nursing management of status epilepticus:
   - Maintain the airway of the child.
   - Establish IV access.
   - Monitor vital signs and oxygen saturation with pulse oximetry.
   - Administer medications as ordered.
   - Monitor for respiratory depression due to increased medication used.

Differentiate between signs of bacterial meningitis, viral meningitis, encephalitis, Reye syndrome, and Guillain-Barré syndrome in infants and children.

1. Bacterial meningitis:
   - Fever.
   - Lethargic and irritable.
   - Vomiting and diarrhea.
   - Hemorrhagic rash (meningococcal meningitis).
   - Nuchal rigidity, positive Kernig and Brudzinski signs.
   - Headache.
2. Viral meningitis:
   - Child appears less ill than child with bacterial meningitis.
   - Fever.
   - Irritable and lethargic.
   - Photophobia.
   - Upper respiratory symptoms.
   - Positive Kernig and Brudzinski signs.

LEARNING OBJECTIVES

CONCEPTS

Differentiate between signs of bacterial meningitis, viral meningitis, encephalitis, Reye syndrome, and Guillain-Barré syndrome in infants and children.—*continued*

3. Reye syndrome:
   - Irritability and lethargy.
   - Nausea and vomiting.
   - Seizures.
   - Progressive unresponsiveness and loss of reflexes.
4. Guillain-Barré syndrome:
   - Rapidly progressive severe hypotonia (infants).
   - Rapidly progressive ascending symmetric weakness (children).
   - Absent or diminished deep tendon reflexes.
   - Difficulty swallowing and facial weakness.
   - Respiratory difficulty.

Describe the nursing care for the infant with myelodysplasia and hydrocephalus.

1. Myelodysplasia:
   - Keep newborn in prone position.
   - Cover defect with sterile, saline dressing.
   - Monitor for signs of infection.
   - After surgery, monitor for wound healing and CSF leakage.
   - Measure head circumference daily.
   - Assess intake and output.
   - Avoid the use of latex products.
   - Assess neurologic status of the extremities.
   - Perform range of motion exercises and promote positioning for function.
2. Hydrocephalus:
   - Measure head circumference daily.
   - Observe for signs and symptoms of increased ICP.
   - Assess level of responsiveness.
   - Observe surgical site for signs of wound healing.
   - Position infant to aid in drainage of CSF.

Describe the focus of community-based nursing care for the child with cerebral palsy.

The nurse in the community assists in:
1. Coordination of multiple healthcare services and promoting health
2. Providing information to schools and other community agencies to meet the needs of the child.
3. Assuring access to adaptive equipment or assistive technology needed.
4. Planning the transition from adolescence to adulthood.

Distinguish between the assessment findings of the child with a mild, moderate, and severe traumatic brain injury.

1. Mild brain injury:
   - No loss (or very brief loss) of consciousness
   - Possible amnesia of event.
   - Mild headache unrelieved by medication.
   - Irritability.
   - Fatigue.
   - Possible changes in concentration and school performance.
2. Moderate brain injury:
   - Loss of consciousness.
   - Headache.
   - Nausea and vomiting.
   - Amnesia.
   - Glasgow Coma Score of 9–12.
3. Severe brain injury:
   - Prolonged period of unconsciousness.
   - Signs of increased ICP.
   - Glasgow Coma Score of 8 or less.
   - Amnesia lasting longer than 24 hours.

(continued)

LEARNING OBJECTIVES

CONCEPTS

Contrast the appropriate initial nursing management for mild and severe traumatic brain injury.

Nursing management of traumatic brain injury is as follows:
1. Mild injury:
   - Observe for changing levels of consciousness.
   - Instruct parents concerning signs and symptoms of increased ICP indicating need to return for immediate care.
2. Severe injury:
   - Assess airway, breathing, and circulation. Be prepared to assist ventilations.
   - Assess neurologic status frequently.
   - Monitor vital signs frequently.
   - Elevate head of bed if there is no neck injury.
   - Administer medications and IV fluids as ordered.
   - Monitor intracranial pressure if indicated.
   - Keep environment quiet.

CRITICAL THINKING IN ACTION

View the **Critical Thinking in Action** video in Chapter 53 of the CD-ROM. Then, answer the questions that follow.

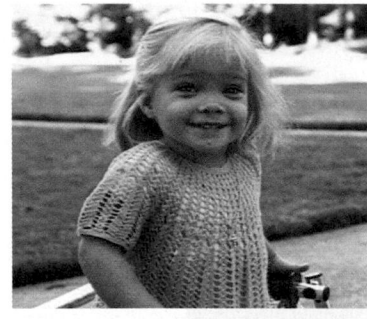

Abigail, a 3-year-old with myelodysplasia, is seen every few months with her parents in the multidisciplinary spina bifida clinic where you work. Her lesion is at the L3 level, so she can flex her hips and extend her knees, but her ankles and toes are paralyzed. She uses lower leg braces and a walker to mobilize and has minimal sensation in her lower legs and feet. Her bladder and bowel sphincters are also affected so Abigail and her parents have worked hard to establish bowel control with a high-fiber diet and by establishing specific times for bowel evacuation. Abigail's parents have learned to perform intermittent self-catheterization for bladder control to reduce the risk for kidney damage.

Her health history reveals she has experienced a case of otitis media since her last visit and responded well to antibiotics. Her legs are well protected by stockings to reduce rubbing by her braces. Her gait is becoming steadier with the walker, and her parents are encouraging exercise of her arms and upper trunk with swimming. You encourage Abigail's parents to promote her cognitive development with age-appropriate games and interaction with siblings.

1. What are the safety issues to discuss with Abigail's parents about spina bifida?
2. Describe spina bifida.
3. Identify important health promotion issues to discuss with Abigail's parents.
4. Describe the difference between meningocele and a myelomeningocele.

MediaLink

www.prenhall.com/london

- NCLEX-RN® Review, case studies, and other interactive resources for this chapter can be found on the Companion Website at http://www.prenhall.com/london. Click on "Chapter 53" to select the activities for this chapter.

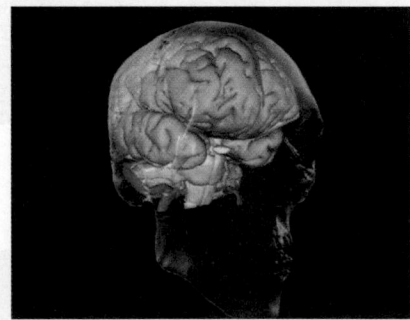

- For animations, more NCLEX-RN® Review questions, and an audio glossary, access the accompanying CD-ROM in this textbook.

REFERENCES

Adekoya, N., Thurman, D. J., White, D. D., & Webb, K.W. (2002). Surveillance for traumatic brain deaths—United States, 1989–1998. *Morbidity and Mortality Weekly Report, 51*(SS-10), 1–14.

Adelson, P. D., Bratton, S. L., Carney, N. A., Chestnut, R. A., du Coudray, H. E. M., Goldstein, B., and others. (2003). Threshold for treatment of intracranial hypertension: Guidelines for management of severe traumatic brain injury. *Pediatric Critical Care Medicine, 4*(Suppl. 3), S25–S27.

American Academy of Pediatrics Committee on Infectious Disease. (2003). *Red book: Report of the Committee on Infectious Disease* (26th ed.). Elk Grove Village, IL: Author.

American Academy of Pediatrics Committee on Injury and Poison Prevention. (2001). Injuries associated with infant walkers. *Pediatrics, 108*(3), 790–792.

American Academy of Pediatrics Committee on Injury, Violence, and Poison Prevention. (2003). Prevention of drowning in infants, children, and adolescents. *Pediatrics, 112*(2), 440–445.

Anderson, V., Catroppa, C., Morse, S., Haritou, F., & Rosenfeld, J. (2000). Recovery of intellectual ability following traumatic brain injury in childhood: Impact of injury severity and age at injury. *Pediatric Neurosurgery, 32*(6), 282–290.

Austin, J., Dunn, D., Huster, G., & Rose, D. (1998). Development of scales to measure psychosocial care needs of children with seizures and their parents. *Journal of Neuroscience Nursing, 30*(3), 155–160.

Belay, E. D., Bresee, J. S., Holman, R. C., Khan, A. S., Shahriari, A., & Schonberger, L. B. (1999). Reye's syndrome in the United States from 1981 through 1997. *New England Journal of Medicine, 340*(18), 1377–1382.

Black, S., Shinefield, H., Baxter, R., Austrian, R., Bracken, L., et al. (2004). Postlicensure surveillance for pneumococcal invasive disease after use of pneumococcal conjugate vaccine in Northern California Kaiser Permanente. *Pediatric Infectious Disease Journal, 23*(6), 485–489.

Blackman, J. A. (2005). Severe brain injury: Helping patient and family on the long road back. *Contemporary Pediatrics, 22*(1), 63–78.

Blair, J., & Selekman, J. (2004). Epilepsy. In P. J. Allen & J. A. Vessey (Eds.), *Primary care of the child with a chronic condition* (4th ed., pp. 469–497). St. Louis, MO: Mosby.

Bowman, R. M., McLone, D. G., Grant, J. A., Tomita, T., & Ito, J. A. (2001). Spina bifida outcome: A 25 year perspective. *Pediatric Neurosurgery, 34*(3), 114–120.

Brenner, R. A., Trumble, A. C., Smith, G. S., Kessler, E. P., & Overpeck, M. D. (2001). Where children drown, United States, 1995. *Pediatrics, 108*(1), 85–89.

Buck, M. L. (2003). Clinical applications for botulinum toxin type A in pediatric patients. *Pediatric Pharmacology, 9*(3). Retrieved April 18, 2003, from http://www.medscape.com/viewarticle/451626

Centers for Disease Control. (2003). *Traumatic brain injury incidence and distribution.* Retrieved February 25, 2004, from http://www.cdc.gov/ node/ do?id=0900f3ec8000dbdc&aspectId= A0400020&print=on

Cobb, S., & Battin, B. (2004). Second-impact syndrome. *Journal of School Nursing, 20*(5), 262–267.

Danielpour, M., & Peacock, W. J. (2000). Epilepsy surgery in children. *Clinical Neurosurgery, 47,* 400–421.

Ditmyer, S. (2004). Hydrocephalus. In P. J. Allen & J. A. Vessey (Eds.), *Primary care of the child with a chronic condition* (4th ed., pp. 543–560). St. Louis, MO: Mosby.

Fadiman, A. (1997). *The spirit catches you and you fall down.* New York: Farrar, Strauss, Giroux.

Freeman, J. M. (2003). What every pediatrician should know about the ketogenic diet. *Contemporary Pediatrics, 20*(5), 113–127.

Gill, J. K., & Gieron-Korthals, M. (2002). What pediatricians—and parents—need to know about febrile convulsions. *Contemporary Pediatrics, 19*(5), 139–144.

Graham, J. M., Gomez, M., Halberg, A., Earl, D. L., Kreutzman, J. T., Cui, J., & Guo, X. (2005). Management of deformational plagiocephaly: Repositioning versus orthotic therapy. *Journal of Pediatrics, 146*(2), 258–262.

Graham, J. M., Kreutzman, J., Earl, D., Halberg, A., Samayoa, C., & Guo, X. (2005). Deformational brachycephaly in supine-sleeping infants. *Journal of Pediatrics, 146*(2), 253–257.

Guskiewicz, K. M., & McCrea, M. (2003). Increased recovery time with multiple sports-related traumatic brain injuries. *Journal of the American Medical Association, 290,* 2549–2563.

Guskiewicz, K. M., Weaver, N. L., Padua, D. A., & Garrett, W. E. (2000). Epidemiology of concussion in collegiate and high school football players. *American Journal of Sports Medicine, 28*(5), 643–650.

Harrison, L. H. (2001, May). Meningococcal infection in adolescents and young adults. *Contemporary Pediatrics, 18* (Spring Supp.), 4–15.

Hightower, S., Carmon, M., & Minick, P. (2002). A qualitative descriptive study of the lived experiences of school-aged children with epilepsy. *Journal of Pediatric Health Care, 16*(3), 131–137.

Jones, H. R. (2000). Guillain-Barré syndrome: Perspectives with infants and children. *Seminars in Pediatric Neurology, 7*(2), 91–102.

Katyal, N. G., Koehler, A. N., McGhee, B., Foley, C. M., & Crumrine, P. K. (2000). The ketogenic diet in refractory epilepsy: The experience of Children's Hospital of Pittsburgh. *Clinical Pediatrics, 39*(3), 153–159.

Lazzaretti, C. C., & Pearson, C. (2004). Myelodysplasia. In P. J. Allen & J. A. Vessey (Eds.), *Primary care of the child with a chronic condition* (4th ed., pp. 630–643). St. Louis, MO: Mosby.

Lewis, D. W., Scott, D., & Rendin, V. (2002). Treatment of pediatric headache. *Expert Opinion in Pharmacotherapeutics, 3*(10), 1433–1441.

Liptak, G. S., & Accardo, P. J. (2004). Health and social outcomes of children with cerebral palsy. *Journal of Pediatrics, 145*(Suppl.), S36–S41.

Lovell, M. R., Collins, M. W., Iverson, G. L., Field, M., Maroon, J. C., et al. (2003). Recovery from mild concussion in high school athletes. *Journal of Neurosurgery, 98*(2), 296–301.

Massagli, T. L. (2000). Medical and rehabilitation issues in the care of children with spinal cord injury. *Physical Medicine and Rehabilitation Clinics of North America, 11*(1), 169–182.

McGee, S., & Burkett, K. W. (2000). Identifying common pediatric neurosurgical conditions in the primary care setting. *Nursing Clinics of North America, 35*(1), 61–85.

McKearnan, K. A., Kieckhefer, G. M., Engel, J. M., Jensen, M. P., & Labyak, S. (2004). Pain in children with cerebral palsy: A review. *Journal of Neuroscience Nursing, 36*(5), 252–259.

McNelis, A., Musick, B., Austin, J., Dunn, D., & Creasy, K. (1998). Psychosocial care needs of children with new-onset seizures. *Journal of Neuroscience Nursing, 30*(3), 161–165.

Moloney-Harmon, P. A., & Adams, P. (2001). Trauma. In M. A. Q. Curley & P. A. Moloney-Harmon, *Critical care nursing of infants and children* (2nd ed., pp. 947–979). Philadelphia: W. B. Saunders.

Nehring, W. M. (2004). Cerebral palsy. In P. J. Allen & J. A. Vessey (Eds.), *Primary care of the child with a chronic condition* (4th ed., pp. 327–346). St. Louis, MO: Mosby.

Northrup, H., & Volcik, K. A. (2000). Spina bifida and other neural tube defects. *Current Problems in Pediatrics, 30*(10), 317–331.

O'Hara, J., & Koch, T. K. (1998). Heading off headaches. *Contemporary Pediatrics, 15*(3), 97–116.

Padgett, K. (2002). Alterations in neurologic function in children. In K. L. McCance & S. E. Huether, *Pathophysiology: The biologic basis for disease in adults and children* (4th ed., pp. 566–596). St. Louis, MO: Mosby.

Pelligrino, L. (2002). Cerebral palsy. In M. L. Batshaw (Ed.), *Children with disabilities* (5th ed., pp. 443–466). Baltimore, MD: Paul H. Brooks Publishing Co.

Prober, C. G. (2004). Central nervous system infections. In R. E. Behrman, R. M. Kliegman, & H. B. Jepson, *Nelson textbook of pediatrics* (17th ed., pp. 2038–2047). Philadelphia: Saunders.

Reimschisel, T. (2003). Breaking the cycle of medication overuse headache. *Contemporary Pediatrics, 20*(10), 101–114.

Renier, D., Lajeunie, E., Arnaud, E., & Marchac, D. (2000). Management of craniosynostosis. *Children's Nervous System, 16,* 645–658.

Ressler, J. A., & Nelson, M. (2000). Central nervous system infections in the pediatric population. *Neuroimaging Clinics of North America, 10*(2), 427–443.

Rosenblum, R. K., & Fisher, P. G. (2001). A guide to children with acute and chronic headaches. *Journal of Pediatric Health Care, 15*(5), 229–235.

Rudy, C. (2005). Hydrocephalus. *Journal of Pediatric Health Care, 19*(2), 111, 127–128.

Sarnat, H. B. (2004). Guillain-Barré syndrome. In R. E. Behrman, R. M. Kliegman, & H. B. Jepson,

Nelson textbook of pediatrics (17th ed., pp. 2080–2081). Philadelphia: Saunders.

Scharff, L., & Kemper, K. J. (2003). For chronic pain, complementary and alternative medical approaches. *Contemporary Pediatrics, 20*(10), 117–141.

Schutzman, S. A., & Greenes, D. S. (2001). Pediatric minor head trauma. *Annals of Emergency Medicine, 27*(1), 65–74.

Shinnar, S., & O'Dell, C. (2004). Febrile seizures. *Pediatric Annals, 33*(6), 394–401.

Spector, R. E. (2000). *Cultural diversity in health and illness* (5th ed., p. 71). Upper Saddle River, NJ: Prentice Hall Health.

Steinmetz, M. P., Lechner, R. M., & Anderson, J. S. (2003). Atlantooccipital dislocation in children: Presentation, diagnosis, and management. *Neurosurgery Focus, 14*(2). Retrieved March 25, 2004, www.medscape.com/viewarticle/470602_print

Stevenson, K. L. (2004). Chiari type II malformations: Past, present, future. *Neurosurgical Focus, 16*(2). Retrieved March 29, 2004, from http://www.medscape,com/viewarticle/470602_print

Van Eerden, P., & Bernstein, P. S. (2003). Summary of the publications, "Neonatal encephalopathy and cerebral palsy: Defining the pathogenesis and pathophysiology" by the ACOG Task Force on Neonatal Encephalopathy and Cerebral Palsy. *Medscape OB/GYN & Women's Health, 8*(2). Retrieved July 10, 2003, from http://www.medscape.com/viewarticle/457882_

Vannucci, R. C. (2002). Disorders in the head size and shape. In A. A. Fanaroff & R. J. Martin, *Neonatal-perinatal medicine: Diseases of the fetus and infant* (7th ed., pp. 911–917). St. Louis, MO: Mosby.

Weinstein, S. (2002). Epilepsy. In M. L. Batshaw (Ed.), *Children with disabilities* (5th ed., pp. 493–523). Baltimore: Paul H. Brooks.

Wheless, J. W. (2004). Treatment of status epilepticus in children. *Pediatric Annals, 33*(6), 376–383.

Zickler, C. F., & Richardson, V. (2004). Achieving continence in children with neurogenic bowel and bladder. *Journal of Pediatric Health Care, 18*(6), 276–283.

Zuckerman, G. B., & Conway, E. E. (2000). Drowning and near-drowning: A pediatric epidemic. *Pediatric Annals, 29*(6), 360–366.

The Child with Alterations in Cognitive and Mental Health Function

We've been so worried about Cassandra. After being in the car crash, she has become so frightened of everything. She wakes up at night screaming and has lost interest in school and friends. We hope that her work with the therapist will help to decrease her fears and get her involved in all of her activities again.

—*Mother of Cassandra, 9 years old*

LEARNING OBJECTIVES

- Define mental health and describe major mental health disruptions in childhood.

- Discuss the clinical manifestations of the major mental health disorders of childhood and adolescence.

- Plan for the nursing management of children and adolescents with mental health disruptions in the hospital and community settings.

- Describe characteristics of common cognitive disorders of childhood.

- Plan nursing management for children with cognitive disorders.

- Establish and evaluate expected outcomes of care for the child with a cognitive disorder.

MEDIALINK www.prenhall.com/london

CD-ROM

Videos:
  ADD/ADHD
  Down Syndrome
Audio Glossary
NCLEX-RN® Review

Companion Website

Thinking Critically
Case Study: Calculating SSRI Dosage
Critical Thinking: Females and Post-traumatic Stress
  Disorder
Nursing Practice: Putting National Mental Health
  Goals into Community Practice
MediaLink Applications:
  Help Families to Evaluate Mental Health
    Information on the Internet
NCLEX-RN® Review
Case Study

This chapter will provide the knowledge and tools needed to provide appropriate care for children with alterations in mental health and cognition. Because much of mental healthcare is provided by psychiatric–mental health specialists, the nurse's role often centers on identification, support of the therapy, teaching, and referral. Cognitive conditions, on the other hand, are commonly managed by the family and the school personnel. The nurse also forms partnerships with families and school personnel to plan and evaluate care for the child with cognitive conditions such as mental retardation. A thorough knowledge of development is a prerequisite to understanding both mental health disruptions and cognitive conditions since developmental status is often altered in both mental health and cognitive conditions. Review Chapter 33 as needed to understand the relationships of development to the conditions described in the present chapter. ∞

Some cognitive/mental health conditions in children originate from a genetic or physiologic cause. Examples include mental retardation and childhood schizophrenia. Often the environments in which children live influence their characteristics and contribute to dysfunctions such as anxiety, depression, and post-traumatic stress disorder.

Most mental health conditions are treated in community settings, and nurses in these settings play an active role in the treatment and support of the child and family. Nurses may function as case managers, assisting a family to deal with all areas of the child's care. Occasionally a child is hospitalized for treatment of a significant mental health disruption, or a child hospitalized for another health problem requires continued mental health services.

MENTAL HEALTH ALTERATIONS OF CHILDREN AND ADOLESCENTS

Mental health is foundational to a sense of personal well-being. However, 25% of children in the United States suffer from mental illness that is severe enough to impair functioning at home or school, and only 30% of those children receive any mental health services (Melnyk, Brown, Jones et al., 2003; Melnyk, Feinstein, Tuttle et al., 2002). Further, some of the services received are not comprehensive or multidisciplinary, leading to unmet mental health needs (Navon, Nelson, Pagano et al., 2001). In other cases, the interventions used are not supported by theory and research (Hoagwood, Burns, Kiser et al., 2001).

The Surgeon General is leading an initiative to examine mental health in the United States and has identified a series of goals and steps toward improving mental healthcare for children (Department of Health and Human Services, 2000). From the ages of 10 to 21 years, mental health issues are among the top two leading causes of hospitalization in all age groups (see Chapter 1 ∞). This high rate of hospitalization suggests that children are not receiving mental health services early, when outpatient care is appropriate and prognosis is best. In order to confront this childhood mental health crisis, the Surgeon General's agenda includes promoting mental health as an essential part of child health, integrating mental health services into all health services provided to children, engaging families and youth in planning for mental healthcare, and developing and enhancing the infrastructure to support child and youth mental health services (Department of Health and Human Services, 2000). See Table 54–1 for a list of the goals established in the Surgeon General's report.

Nurses have been leaders in the field of pediatric mental healthcare. A recent initiative known as KySS (Keep your children/yourself Safe and Secure) was launched by nurses in 2001 and was the subject of a summit for health professional collaboration in 2003. The goals of the summit included

TABLE 54–1 ✤ Goals of the Surgeon General's National Action Agenda for Children's Mental Health

1. Promote public awareness of children's mental health issues and reduce stigma associated with mental illness.
2. Continue to develop, disseminate, and implement scientifically proven prevention and treatment services in the field of children's mental health.
3. Improve the assessment and recognition of mental health needs in children.
4. Eliminate racial/ethnic and socioeconomic disparities in access to mental healthcare.
5. Improve the infrastructure for children's mental health services, including support for scientifically proven interventions across professions.
6. Increase access to and coordination of quality mental health care services.
7. Train frontline providers to recognize and manage mental health issues, and educate mental health providers in scientifically proven prevention and treatment services.
8. Monitor the access to and coordination of quality mental health care services.

Courtesy of the Department of Health and Human Services, 2000.

identification of assessment, implementation, and dissemination strategies for promoting the mental health of children and teens in primary care and alternative care settings, and review of evidence-based practice to make recommendations for interventions and needed research areas (Melnyk, Moldenhauer, Tuttle et al., 2003).

During all health visits, mental health screening should be integrated into care so that disruptions can be identified. See Chapters 37 and 38 for specific questions to ask during health promotion and health maintenance visits. ∞ When a potential mental health condition exists, the child receives further assessment from a mental health specialist. A resource commonly used is the *Diagnostic and Statistical Manual,* which lists diagnostic criteria for known mental health conditions. The current edition is the DSM-IV-TR (American Psychiatric Association, 2000), and its criteria for several conditions are listed throughout this chapter.

Once a mental health problem is identified, the nurse assesses the child for related issues and conditions. Mental health is linked to development so developmental screening tests are administered. Mental health status can influence activity level, physiologic parameters, and risk for certain conditions. Therefore, height and weight, review of systems, vital signs, and medication/substance use history are important to perform. Family interactions, stressors, and methods of coping are assessed.

The primary treatment goal for children and adolescents with psychosocial disorders is to assist the child and family to achieve and maintain an optimal level of functioning through interventions designed to reduce the impact of stressors. Therapeutic interventions and communication are based on the principle that feelings motivate behaviors. Parents and others close to the child often fall into the habit of reacting to the child's behaviors rather than trying to find out what feelings may be precipitating the undesirable actions. While behaviors may be considered in treatment, feelings and life experiences are often explored to provide insight and to lead to behavior change. Medication may be used to enhance and support other therapy, or may be the major therapeutic measure.

When possible, mental health interventions should be founded on **evidence-based practice**, or a body of scientific knowledge. Such research knowledge is scant in pediatric mental health services, but is increasing due to healthcare research in this area. Nurses can include evidence-based practice and outcome measurement in mental healthcare whenever possible (Hoagwood, Burns, Kiser et al., 2001).

TREATMENT MODES

Three basic treatment modes are used: individual, family, and group therapy. The choice of treatment mode must take into account the child's age and developmental stage. Most therapists use several intervention strategies simultaneously. Different strategies are more or less effective and appropriate for children and adolescents in various stages of development. A thorough understanding of developmental needs, expectations, and abilities is therefore essential for mental health professionals.

Individual Therapy

Individual therapy involves only the child and the therapist. Treatment of specific emotional problems or disorders may involve various techniques such as play therapy, psychodrama, art therapy, and **cognitive therapy** (a technique used to help a person recognize automatic negative thinking). Individual therapy may be short term (four to six sessions) or long term (lasting for several years).

Family Therapy

Family therapy involves the exploration of a particular emotional problem and its manifestations among the family members. Family therapy is based on the idea that the emotional symptoms or problems of an individual are an expression of emotional symptoms or problems in the family. The focus is on the relationships among the family members, not the psychologic conflict within each individual member.

Group Therapy

Group therapy involves an ongoing or limited number of sessions in which several individuals participate. The emphasis is on the interpersonal styles of relating to one another in the group. Group therapy is particularly effective with adolescents because of the importance of the peer group at this age. An advantage of group therapy is that stimuli and feedback come from multiple sources (the group members) instead of just one person (the therapist).

THERAPEUTIC STRATEGIES

Play Therapy

Play is often called the language or work of the child. From a developmental perspective, children progressively learn to express feelings and needs through action, fantasy, and finally language. The special quality of play buffers children against the pressures and demands of daily life. Play helps children master developmental stages by strengthening physical and neurologic processes. Play also assists in cognitive learning, setting the stage for problem solving and creativity.

Play therapy is a technique that reveals problems on a fantasy level through the use of toys, dolls, clay, art, and other creative objects. It is often used with preschool and school-age children who are experiencing anxiety, stress, and other specific nonpsychotic mental disorders. Play therapy encourages the child to act out feelings such as anger, hostility, sadness, and fear. It also gives the therapist a chance to help the child understand, on a conscious or unconscious level, his or her own responses and behavior in a safe, supportive environment. This type of therapy was used for Cassandra, described in the opening quotation, who needed to gain some control over a frightening environment by acting out fears and trying solutions during play with a therapist. Play therapy is different from therapeutic play, which may be used with hospitalized children (see Chapter 40 ∞). Only a specialist is qualified to provide play therapy for mental health disorders.

Art Therapy

Children who may be apprehensive about playing can sometimes be encouraged to participate in art therapy, using brief drawing exercises. This technique is appropriate for children of all ages, including adolescents. The drawings can help the therapist gain information about the child, the family, and the interactions between the child and family. However, children's drawings should never be the only basis for a definitive diagnosis.

When used in conjunction with a thorough history and appropriate psychologic testing information, art therapy can guide the child's treatment. These drawing exercises provide an opportunity to help in the healing process. The therapist can assist the child to release feelings of anger, pain, or fear onto paper, where they can be examined objectively. (Figures 54–1 ● to 54–4 ● present several examples of this technique.)

● **FIGURE 54–1**

"Me." Drawn by a 14-year-old girl with major depression, anxiety, and school phobia who had experienced multiple losses over several years. Her mother had severe chronic lung problems and diabetes, and the girl had stopped attending school for fear that something would happen to her mother. This drawing represents the girl's obvious feelings of sadness and depression but also indicates a glimmer of hope (represented by the yellow mask coming from behind the dark mask of depression).

● **FIGURE 54–2**

"Self-Portrait." Drawn by a 15-year-old boy who was admitted through the emergency department after a failed suicide attempt by hanging. He had a psychiatric diagnosis of depression and polysubstance abuse (including inhalants and alcohol) and insisted that he was a member of a satanic cult in his hometown. Most of his drawings depicted a preoccupation with violence and suicide. The boy said that he always felt a "darkness" like a shadow that followed him around and wanted him dead. His family history was significant for depression and suicide on both his mother's and his father's side. His father also had a lengthy history of polysubstance abuse and alcoholism. The boy was discharged to a long-term residential treatment facility for adolescents.

● FIGURE 54-3

"An Activity." Drawn by an 8-year-old boy who was initially admitted to the medical-surgical floor of a pediatric hospital for dehydration resulting from vomiting and diarrhea. Psychiatric evaluation was ordered for extreme anxiety. These drawings, completed during the initial interview, led to further investigation, which revealed that the child had started a house fire in which his grandmother (his primary caretaker at the time) was killed. The family's home and all their belongings were lost. No one had known that the child had set the fire. Further sessions indicated that he had been setting neighborhood garage fires and watching them burn from a distance.

● FIGURE 54-4

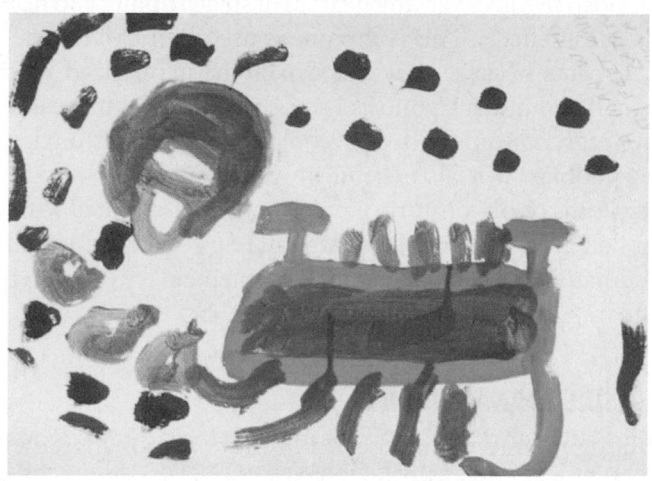

"A Family Activity." By the same boy who drew Figure 54-3. This drawing depicts a recurring incident of physical and emotional abuse by his mother's live-in boyfriend. It shows the family bathtub with feces and blood smeared on the floors and walls. The boy reported that when either he or his 3-year-old brother had a toileting accident the boyfriend would make them go into the bathroom and stand in the bathtub while he smeared the feces on the walls. He would then hit the children and make them clean up the mess. The boy had previously been removed from the mother's custody for neglect. He was transferred from the medical-surgical area to the inpatient children's psychiatric unit, where he received a diagnosis of depression, overanxious disorder, and child abuse (physical and emotional). Charges were filed against the mother's boyfriend and custody of both children was temporarily revoked.

Behavior and Cognitive Therapy

Behavior modification is a therapeutic technique that uses stimulus and response conditioning to alter inappropriate behaviors. It reinforces desirable behaviors, helping the child to replace maladaptive behaviors with more appropriate ones. This technique is based on the assumption that any learned behavior can be unlearned. Thus, if parents, nurses, teachers, and other adults consistently reinforce desirable behaviors, the child will eventually alter or discontinue undesirable behaviors.

Behavior modification may include (1) removing the child from the home to a more structured environment, such as a hospital, for a brief time, and (2) teaching the parents, teachers, and other appropriate adults to be agents of behavioral change. Several ongoing sessions may be required with the adults involved, using role play and other techniques. Consistency is the most important principle in the success of behavior modification.

Cognitive therapy teaches thinking patterns to change reactions to situations that cause anxiety or other undesirable conditions. The child is taught how his or her brain and body are working; this understanding assists the child in having control over the experience. Often a combination of cognitive and behavioral approaches is useful in treating children.

Visualization and Guided Imagery

The techniques of visualization and guided imagery begin with specific directions for progressive relaxation according to the child's ability. This form of therapy uses the child's own imagination and positive thinking to reduce stress and anxiety, decrease the experience of pain or discomfort, and promote healing. The techniques are especially useful for managing anxiety disorders and chronic pain. It is not easy for every child to use his or her imagination in this way, so the technique may not work or be appropriate for everyone.

DEVELOPING CULTURAL COMPETENCE

SPIRITUAL BELIEFS AND MENTAL HEALTH

In many cultures, care of the "spirit" is believed necessary to promote mental health. An identity with one's community and spiritual wholeness is promoted by storytelling, singing, rites of passage, and use of certain objects like bags of herbs. Asking about what the family believes and integrating practices into the plan of care will enhance the child's mental health.

Hypnosis

Hypnosis involves varying degrees of suggestibility and deep relaxation effects. This technique is useful for children and adolescents because they can usually be hypnotized more easily than adults. Hypnosis is especially helpful in treating physical symptoms with a psychologic component, anxiety, and phobias. It is also useful in managing severe physical symptoms or discomfort (pain or nausea) associated with a physiologic disorder or its treatment (e.g., cancer or juvenile rheumatoid arthritis). Refer to "Complementary Care: Hypnotherapy for Children" in Chapter 42. ∞

NURSING MANAGEMENT

Although many mental health disorders are managed effectively with therapy, medication, or both on an outpatient basis, some necessitate admission to an inpatient psychiatric setting. The nurse may encounter the child with a mental health disorder during hospitalization for a concurrent physiologic problem, or in a variety of community settings. If a child is hospitalized for a concurrent problem, assess the child's current level of functioning in relation to the mental health disorder.

Nursing assessment also focuses on identifying medications being taken, common abnormal behaviors (what triggers them, what reduces them), family interactions, and routines to maintain appropriate behaviors (Table 54–2). Then consider how to support the child within the hospital environment.

An important nursing intervention is to ensure safety of the child. Actions begin in the emergency department if a child is admitted for a mental health crisis. Remove or lock potentially dangerous material in the room such as medications, tubing, and sharps containers. A parent, guardian, or health professional should remain with the child at all times. Inform the family member of the need to stay with the child and how to immediately notify the nurse if the adult needs to leave or if the child's condition changes. Part of the initial care is to evaluate risk by asking if the child has tried to hurt himor herself or been thinking about that. Ask about recent stresses, thoughts of hurting someone else, and why the child thinks he or she has been brought to the emergency department (Meunier-Sham, 2003). If the child is admitted to the psychiatric unit, follow unit policies for ensuring safety for children who are at risk of hurting themselves or others.

Nursing care includes carrying out the prescribed treatment plan and administering psychotropic medications. Evaluate the child's medication regimen for administration schedule, dosage, side effects, and effectiveness. Inform the therapist of the child's hospitalization if the child has been hospitalized for a concurrent condition, and consult with the therapist about appropriate approaches for the child. Provide supportive care for the child and family.

Psychiatric hospitalization is a stressful event for all families, and both the family and child need supportive care. Continuation of family involvement is critical. (See "Evidence-Based Nursing: Family Needs During Hospitalization for Mental Healthcare.")

The nurse frequently is the liaison between the family and the therapist in making follow-up arrangements at the time of discharge. Be aware of the meaning of mental illness in various cultural groups and the treatments that may be commonly used. Integrate these complementary therapies into the care plan whenever safe. Families must feel that their responses and approaches to the child with a mental disorder are not judged by health professionals.

TABLE 54–2 ✛ Mental Health Assessment

The nurse gathers information about the child's mental health by asking questions and making observations. The following components may be helpful.

Appearance	Behavior	Development	Life Events	History
■ Clothing appropriate for age, setting, and developmental level ■ Facial expression and response to nurse ■ Body size and posture ■ Interactions with parents or others ■ Interest in surroundings	■ Level of consciousness and interaction with surroundings ■ Recent reported changes in behavior (e.g., sleep, eating patterns, communication with others, school performance, friendships, risky activities) ■ Problem behaviors identified by child or parent ■ Events associated with problem behaviors	■ Results of developmental testing ■ Progression of skills reported by family ■ Unusual capabilities or deficits ■ Progression in school and extracurricular activities	■ Recent stress or trauma ■ Changes in family structure ■ Chronic health conditions in family members	■ Prenatal events or birth trauma ■ Diagnosed mental health disorder in child or other family members ■ Neurologic injuries or diseases ■ Alterations in mental health function

DEVELOPING CULTURAL COMPETENCE

MENTAL HEALTH CAN BE DEFINED IN DIFFERENT WAYS

Various cultural groups define mental health in different ways. For most it is a sense of well-being, peace, and productive use of the mind. Various therapies are used to support and restore mental health. They may include healers, family and community support, relaxation or meditation, teas and other herbal products, and exorcism. Find out how individuals and groups define mental health and how they believe health is maintained. Be alert to learn if mental disorders are viewed as a negative stigma or are openly accepted and discussed.

The nurse in the community assesses how a child with a mental health disorder is functioning in each microsystem (see Chapter 33 ∞), such as home, day care, school, and with friends. Assess risk and protective factors of the child and family (see Chapter 36 ∞). Evaluate involvement in therapy sessions and ability to manage prescribed pharmacologic interventions.

DEVELOPMENTAL AND BEHAVIORAL DISORDERS

PERVASIVE DEVELOPMENTAL DISORDERS

It is estimated that 12% to 16% of children have a developmental or behavioral disorder. One of the most common sets of disorders is pervasive developmental disorders. **Pervasive developmental disorders (PDDs)** begin in early childhood and are characterized by impaired social interactions and communication, with restricted interests, activities, and behaviors (Baird, Charman, Cox, et al., 2001). These autistic spectrum disorders (ASDs) include autistic disorder (the most common type), Rett

EVIDENCE-BASED NURSING

FAMILY NEEDS DURING HOSPITALIZATION FOR MENTAL HEALTHCARE

Problem

Hospitalization for mental healthcare is always a stressful event. Families frequently do not understand treatment procedures or the child's condition and diagnosis. Treatment may last for several days to months, causing disruption in family roles and routines. Family stresses must be understood so that the nurse can adequately support both the child and the family.

Evidence

A nursing study involved interviews with 38 parents of 29 children who had recently been hospitalized for psychiatric illness. In this qualitative study, themes that emerged during the interviews were analyzed and categorized. Three major categories were identified (Scharer, 2002).

The first was a need for *information*. Parents often did not receive information about admission and unit procedures. Many felt that the physicians and other therapists were hard to reach and did not provide adequate information about the child's condition and treatment. Parents identified a need to have access to hospital records and the child's diagnosis. Such information was viewed as important to link to outpatient facilities where the child was also treated.

The second set of needs was for *instrumental support*. These items included reasonably priced lodging near the hospital, ready access to the hospitalized child, assistance with providing physical care for the hospitalized child, and improved physical environment of the hospital unit and rooms. Some parents voiced a lack of mental health services in their own communities, resulting in lack of care both before and after hospitalization.

The third need was for *emotional support*. Parents often felt isolated and did not know where to turn. They suggested that staff could provide additional emotional support, and that having a parent to call who had similar experiences would have been helpful.

Implications

The nurse in a psychiatric facility is in a unique position to offer support to the family of the child or adolescent. Information about the unit can be provided by videotape, tour, and written materials. Daily updates on the child's condition and treatment plan are needed. Families must be viewed as partners in the treatment, along with the child and health professionals. Provide an opportunity for parents to ask questions and be sure they understand the diagnosis and treatment.

Consider visiting hours and access to children. If they are limited to certain times, explain the reason to parents. Provide access to Ronald McDonald House or other low-cost facilities if the parent is from out of town. Provide assistance and instruction with any physical care the child needs. Consider changes that can be made to make the unit more welcoming and pleasant, such as color of walls, presence of posters and brochures, and general cleanliness.

Facilitate parent-to-parent communication. Ask parents each day about how they feel and what can be done for them. Use empathy and interest to convey support.

Critical Thinking

Why do you think that families find psychiatric facilities frightening or strange? How can you explain the need to remove items with which children could injure themselves or others? What questions will you ask early in the hospitalization to learn about facilities that are present in the home community that can be used for referral upon discharge? How could you locate available treatment options for a family from a community some distance from the hospital? How could support of the family influence the care and condition of their child or adolescent?

Reference

Scharer, K. (2002). What parents of mentally ill children need and want from mental health professionals. *Issues in Mental Health Nursing, 23,* 617–640.

syndrome, Asperger syndrome, childhood disintegrative disorder, and pervasive developmental disorder not otherwise specified. About two or more children in 1000 have autistic spectrum disorder, with about half of the cases consisting of autistic disorder (commonly called simply *autism*) (Committee on Children with Disabilities, 2001). This incidence represents an increase from formerly described levels. Before 1985, about 0.4 to 0.5 children in 1000 were diagnosed with autistic disorder (Hudson & Dixon, 2003). It is unclear whether there is a true increase in cases or simply improved techniques in making the diagnosis (Jick & Kaye, 2003). The disorder is about 4 times more common in males than females. Males frequently have mild forms of the disorder, and females commonly have associated mental retardation.

ETIOLOGY AND PATHOPHYSIOLOGY

The cause of autistic disorder is unknown. Genetic transmission, immune responses, and neuroanatomy are all being investigated as causes (Williams, Dalrymple, & Neal, 2000). Occurrence in siblings is 3% to 7%, leading to theories of genetic links (Committee on Children with Disabilities, 2001). Neurotransmitters such as dopamine, serotonin, and opioids are abnormal in some children and a focus of present research (Cade & Tidwell, 2001). Congenital rubella syndrome, fragile X syndrome, phenylketonuria, Down syndrome, and tuberous sclerosis are all associated with a higher than normal incidence (American Academy of Pediatrics, 2001a; Hudson & Dixon, 2003). Some earlier research studies suggested a relationship with measles-mumps-rubella vaccine (Kaye, Melero-Montes, & Jick, 2001), but more recent research has indicated that there is no connection between the vaccine and reported cases of the disorder (Bechtel, 2003; Dales, Hammer, & Smith, 2001).

CLINICAL MANIFESTATIONS

The essential features of the disorder typically become apparent by the time a child is 3 years of age. They involve impairments in the following three areas:

- Social reciprocity
- Communication
- Behavior (Towbin, Mauk, & Batshaw, 2002)

Children with autism are unable to relate to people as is normal for young children, or to respond to social and emotional cues. In addition, they engage in **stereotypy**, or rigid and obsessive behavior (see Figure 54–5 ●). Characteristically these repetitive behaviors in affected children include head banging, twirling in circles, biting themselves, and flapping their hands or arms. Frequently a child's behavior is self-stimulating or self-destructive. Responses to sensory stimuli are frequently abnormal and include an ex-

● **FIGURE 54–5**

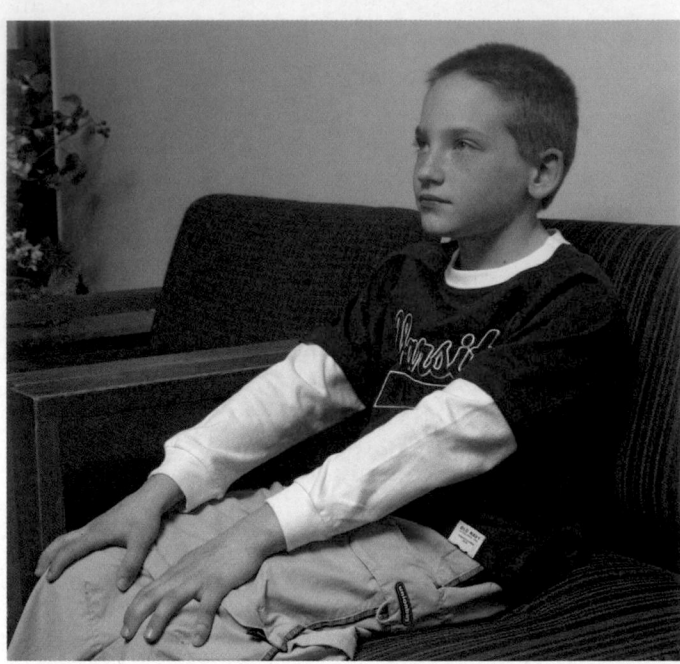

This child with autism sits stiffly in the chair and engages in rhythmic rocking behavior. He has a disengaged look and does not readily interact with other children or adults who are in his environment.

treme aversion to touch, loud noises, and bright lights. Emotional lability is common.

Difficulties or delays in speech and language are common communication problems, and are often the first symptoms that lead to diagnosis. Abnormal communication patterns include both verbal and nonverbal communication. Autistic children may eventually learn to talk, in some cases well, but their speech is likely to show certain abnormalities: use of *you* in place of *I;* **echolalia** (a compulsive parroting of what is heard); repeating questions rather than answering them; and fascination with rhythmic, repetitive songs and verses.

Behaviors of affected children show several differences from others. They do not commonly explore objects but have stereoptyped behaviors. They may line up objects, play with the same objects over and over, and have certain rituals that must be performed. They often become upset if these normal routines are disrupted. Rituals may involve eating only certain types or colors of foods or eating in specific patterns. Autistic children may manifest disturbances in the rate or sequence of development. They are frequently cognitively impaired but can demonstrate a wide range of intellectual ability and functioning. Cognitive impairment may become manifested early in life by slow developmental progression, particularly in social skills. Some children are impaired in particular areas of development, whereas others are above normal. Although 25% have microcephaly, most children have a normal appearance.

The specific differences in clinical manifestations of the types of autistic spectrum disorder are listed in "Clinical Manifestations: Autistic Spectrum Disorders (Pervasive Developmental Disorders)".

Clinical Therapy

Diagnosis is based on the presence of specific criteria, as described in the American Psychiatric Association's *Diagnostic and Statistical Manual of Mental Disorders,* 4th edition (DSM-IV), outlined in Table 54–3. Additional testing is done to rule out other causes of the child's behavior. Tests may include neuroimaging (CT scan or MRI), lead screening, DNA analysis, and electroencephalogram.

Early intervention helps maximize the child's potential and establish helpful support for parents. Treatment focuses on behavior management to reward appropriate behaviors, foster positive or adaptive coping skills, and facilitate effective communication. The goals of treatment are to reduce rigidity or stereotypy (repetitive, obsessive, machinelike movements) and other maladaptive behaviors. Often the child must be physically restrained from aggressive or self-destructive behaviors. Some parents choose to use complementary therapies such as vitamin supplements and dimethylglycine. Foods such as sugar, aspartame, milk products, and wheat are sometimes eliminated from the diet. Some families use medicines such as secretin (a pancreatic hormone) and antacids (Hyman & Levy, 2000). Vitamins A, C, or B may also be used by some as a complementary medicine approach.

The overall prognosis for autistic children to become functioning members of society is guarded. The extent of

CLINICAL MANIFESTATIONS

AUTISTIC SPECTRUM DISORDERS (PERVASIVE DEVELOPMENTAL DISORDERS)

DISORDER	CLINICAL MANIFESTATIONS	CLINICAL THERAPY
Autistic disorder	Impaired social, communicative, and behavioral development, usually noted in first year of life.	Early intervention is key to maximal performance. Interventions focus on improving behaviors and communication skills, providing physical and occupational therapy, structuring play interactions with other children, and educating parents about the child's needs.
Asperger syndrome	Impaired social interactions with normal language development for age; pitch, tone, and other speech characteristics may be abnormal. Verbal skills involving spelling and vocabulary are high with concept formation, language flexibility, and comprehension low.	Social interactions are focus of therapy.
Rett's disorder	Early development appears normal and symptoms emerge at 6–18 months. Ataxia, handwringing, intermittent hyperventilation, dementia, and growth retardation show progressive increase. Appears only in females as an X-linked dominant disorder; mutations occur in the gene MeCP2, affecting methyl-CpG-binding protein 2 which is important in brain development.	Early intervention in areas of abnormal behaviors.
Childhood disintegrative disorder	First 2–5 years of development appear normal followed by deterioration in many areas of functioning. Behaviors finally stabilize at some point without further deterioration.	Focus on areas of developmental function that show abnormality. Individualized education plans are needed in school to deal with communication, play, physical therapy, and teaching management skills to parents. Regression in toileting and other skills may occur.
Pervasive developmental disorder not otherwise specified	Severe social impairment without meeting DSM criteria for other types of autistic spectrum disorder.	Behavioral therapy focuses on building social skills.

TABLE 54–3 ✤ DSM-IV-TR Diagnostic Criteria for Autistic Disorder

A. A total of six or more items from 1, 2, and 3, with at least two from 1, and one each from 2 and 3:

1. Qualitative impairment in social interaction, as manifested by at least two of the following:
   a. Marked impairment in the use of multiple nonverbal behaviors such as eye-to-eye gaze, facial expression, body posture, and gestures to regulate social interaction
   b. Failure to develop peer relationships appropriate to developmental level
   c. A lack of spontaneous seeking to share enjoyment, interests, or achievements with other people
   d. Lack of social or emotional reciprocity

2. Qualitative impairments in communication as manifested by at least one of the following:
   a. Delay in, or total lack of, the development of spoken language (not accompanied by an attempt to compensate through alternative modes of communication such as gesture or mime)
   b. In individuals with adequate speech, marked impairment in the ability to initiate or sustain a conversation with others
   c. Stereotyped and repetitive use of language or idiosyncratic language
   d. Lack of varied, spontaneous make-believe play or social imitative play appropriate to developmental level

3. Restricted repetitive and stereotyped patterns of behavior, interests, and activities, as manifested by at least one of the following:
   a. Encompassing preoccupation with one or more stereotyped and restricted patterns of interest that is abnormal either in intensity or in focus
   b. Apparently inflexible adherence to specific, nonfunctional routines or rituals
   c. Stereotyped and repetitive motor mannerisms (e.g., hand or finger flapping or twisting, or complex whole-body movements)
   d. Persistent preoccupation with parts of objects

B. Delays or abnormal functioning in at least one of the following areas, with onset prior to age 3 years: (1) social interaction, (2) language as used in social communication, or (3) symbolic or imaginative play.

C. The disturbance is not better accounted for by Rett Syndrome or Childhood Disintegrative Disorder.

Used with permission from American Psychiatric Association. (2000). *Diagnostic and statistical manual of mental disorders* Text Revision (4th ed.). Washington, DC: Author. Copyright © 2000 American Psychiatric Association.

adequate adjustment varies greatly. Successful adjustment is more likely for children with higher IQs, adequate speech, and access to specialized programs.

NURSING MANAGEMENT

NURSING ASSESSMENT AND DIAGNOSIS

The nurse may encounter the autistic child when parents seek care for a suspected hearing impairment, speech diffi-

culty, or developmental delay. Early and frequent developmental screening of all children can help in referral for thorough assessment and identification of cases. Be alert to parental observations that the baby or young child does not look at them or provides other developmental or behavioral cues (Beauchesne & Kelley, 2004). Parents may report abnormal interaction such as lack of eye contact, disinterest in cuddling, minimal facial responsiveness, and failure to talk. Initial assessment focuses on language development, response to others, and hearing acuity (see Chapters 33 and 53 ∞). Specialized screening tests for autism are available online and are being evaluated for their usefulness.

When a child with a diagnosis of autistic disorder is hospitalized for a concurrent problem, obtain a history from the parents about the child's routines, rituals, and likes and dislikes, as well as ways to promote interaction and cooperation. Autistic children may carry a special toy or object that they play with during times of stress. Ask parents about these objects and their use.

Ask about the child's behaviors and observe them on admission. Obtain a history of acute and chronic illnesses and injuries. Ask about eating patterns and food restrictions. Inquire about complementary and alternative medicine treatments in a nonjudgmental and supportive manner.

Nursing diagnoses must be tailored to fit the individual needs of the child. Examples of nursing diagnoses that might be appropriate for autistic children include the following:

- *Impaired Verbal Communication,* related to psychologic condition
- *Impaired Social Interaction,* related to developmental disability
- *Disturbed Thought Processes,* related to mental disorder
- *Risk for Injury,* related to cognitive impairment
- *Risk for Caregiver Role Strain,* related to chronicity and demands of child's condition
- *Disabled Family Coping: Compromised,* related to having a child with prolonged disability

PLANNING AND IMPLEMENTATION

Nursing care focuses on stabilizing environmental stimuli, providing supportive care, enhancing communication, maintaining a safe environment, giving the parents anticipatory guidance, and providing emotional support.

Stabilize Environmental Stimuli

Autistic children interpret and respond to the environment differently from other individuals. Sounds that are not distressing to the average person may be interpreted by autistic children as louder, more frightening, and overwhelming. The child needs to be oriented to new settings such as a classroom or the hospital room and may adjust best to a small classroom or a hospital room with only one other child. Encourage parents to bring the child's favorite objects from home, and try to keep these objects in the same places, because the child does not cope well with changes in the environment.

Provide Supportive Care

Developing a trusting relationship with the autistic child is often difficult. Adjust communication techniques and teaching to the child's developmental level. Ask parents about the child's usual home routines, and maintain these routines as much as possible when the child is out of the home. Because self-care abilities are often limited, the child may need help meeting basic needs. School programs and individualized education plans (see Chapter 39 ∞) can help the child learn self-care skills. When possible, schedule daily care and routine procedures at consistent times to maintain predictability. Encourage parents to remain with the hospitalized child and to participate in daily care planning. Parents are integral parts of the treatment team when the child's learning goals are established in early intervention or school programs. Identify rituals for naptime and bedtime, and maintain them to promote rest and sleep. Establish patterns that help the child eat nutritious foods at mealtimes.

Enhance Communication

Since children with autism have impaired communication, nursing care focuses on using and improving communication with the child (Cade & Tidwell, 2001). Use speech when possible. When the child responds well to visual cues, pictures, computers, and other visual aids may form an important part of interactions. Some children use sign language.

Maintain a Safe Environment

Monitor autistic children at all times, including bathtime and bedtime. Close supervision is needed to ensure that the child does not obtain any harmful objects or engage in dangerous behaviors. Bicycle helmets and mittens are sometimes used to protect autistic children so that they can safely participate in activities.

Provide Anticipatory Guidance

Approximately half of all children with autistic disorder require lifelong supervision and support. This is especially true if the disorder is accompanied by mental retardation. Some children may grow up to lead independent lives, although they will have social limitations with impaired interpersonal relationships. Encourage parents to promote the child's development through behavior modification and specialized educational programs. The overall goal is to provide the child with the guidance, education, and support necessary for optimal functioning.

Nursing Care in the Community

Families need a great deal of support to cope with the challenges of caring for the autistic child. Help the family identify resources for child care, such as special toddler programs and preschools. The child will need an individualized education plan. The parent or primary caretaker often has a hard time getting respite care and may need assistance to find suitable resources. Siblings of the autistic child may need help explaining the disorder to their friends or teachers. Family support programs are available in some states to provide assistance to parents.

Offer the family genetic counseling. Parents need information on the need for immunizations since they may have heard about a potential connection between immunization and the disorder. Encourage parents to have the child immunized on the recommended schedule. Parents may have questions about where to find information on complementary and alternative therapies.

Local support groups for parents of autistic children are available in most areas. Parents can also be referred to the Autism Society of America for information. (See the Companion Website for links to such resources.)

EVALUATION

Expected outcomes of nursing care for the child with autism include the following:

- Management of behavioral symptoms
- Maximization of self-care
- Maintenance of safe environment
- Consistent developmental progression
- Successful communication strategies

ATTENTION DEFICIT DISORDER AND ATTENTION DEFICIT HYPERACTIVITY DISORDER

Attention deficit disorder (ADD) is a variation in central nervous system processing characterized by developmentally inappropriate behaviors involving inattention. When hyperactivity and impulsivity accompany inattention, the disorder is called attention deficit hyperactivity disorder (ADHD). The latter is the more common condition and affects from 4% to 12% of all school-age children, boys almost 4 times more commonly than girls (National Initiative for Children's Healthcare Quality, 2003). It is also known to affect adolescents and adults, and those with the disorder often continue to manifest at least some of the symptoms as they grow into adulthood. Hyperactivity and impulsivity may improve as the child nears adulthood, with inattentiveness the most persistent characteristic (McDonnell, Doyle, & Surman, 2003).

ETIOLOGY AND PATHOPHYSIOLOGY

Although a variety of physical and neurologic disorders are associated with ADHD, children with identifiable causes represent a small proportion of this population. Examples of known associations include exposure to high levels of lead in childhood and prenatal exposure to alcohol. There may be a deficit in the catecholamines dopamine and nor-epinephrine in some children, lowering the threshold for stimuli input. Genetic factors may be important, as well as family dynamics and environmental characteristics. Although ADHD occurs more commonly within families, a single gene has not been located and a specific mechanism of genetic transmission is not known. It is believed that a genetic predisposition interacts with the child's environment, so that both factors contribute to the appearance of the condition. Family stress, poverty, and poor nutrition may be contributing factors in some cases. Daily television exposure at ages 1 to 3 years is associated with attentional problems at 7 years (Christakis, Zimmerman, DiGiuseppe et al., 2004). Probably there are many types of attention deficit, resulting from several different mechanisms that involve interaction of genetic, biologic, and environmental risk factors (Gottesman, 2003).

CLINICAL MANIFESTATIONS

Children with ADD and ADHD have problems related to decreased attention span, impulsiveness, or increased motor activity. Symptoms can range from mild to severe. The disorders often coexist with various developmental learning disabilities. The child has difficulty completing tasks, fidgets constantly, is frequently loud, and interrupts others. Sleep disturbances are common. Because of these behaviors, the child often has difficulty developing and maintaining social relationships and may be shunned or teased by other children. This only increases the anxiety of the already compromised child, whose behavior is set on a downward-spiraling course.

Typically, girls with ADHD show less aggression and impulsiveness than boys, but far more anxiety, mood swings, social withdrawal, rejection, and cognitive and language problems. Girls tend to be older at the time of diagnosis. Children are frequently diagnosed with the disorder soon after beginning school, with its demands for attentive behavior (American Academy of Pediatrics [AAP], 2000b).

CLINICAL THERAPY

Children are usually brought for evaluation when behaviors escalate to the point of interfering with the daily functioning of teachers or parents. When children have learning disabilities or anxiety disorders, the problem is commonly misdiagnosed as ADHD without further evaluation of the child's symptoms. Therefore, obtaining an accurate diagnosis by a pediatric mental health specialist is important (AAP, 2000).

Specific diagnostic criteria (Table 54–4) must be applied to all children with the potential diagnosis. Behaviors both at home and school or child care must be evaluated, since abnormal patterns in two settings are needed for diagnosis. Based on the findings, desired outcomes are established for the child's performance and management of the disorder.

Treatment is established to meet the desired behavioral outcomes, and includes a combination of approaches, such as environmental changes, behavior therapy, and pharmacotherapy (AAP, 2001b). It is expected that treatment will be long term.

Children often benefit from environmental changes. Decreasing stimulation—for example, by turning off television, keeping the environment quiet, and maintaining an orderly and clutter-free desk or study area without distraction—may help the child to stay focused on the task at hand. Another relatively simple change is appropriate classroom placement, preferably in a small class with a teacher who can provide close supervision and a structured daily routine. Consistent limits and expectations should be set for the child. Children living in chaotic homes and communities may function better if the environment can be simplified. When aggressive behaviors occur, therapeutic approaches such as play and group therapy may be useful.

Behavior therapy involves rewarding the child for desired behaviors and applying consequences for undesirable behaviors. Children may be rewarded by praise or earn points toward a movie or other desired outing for staying seated during meals or quietly listening in a classroom.

Children with moderate to severe ADHD are treated with pharmacotherapy. Methylphenidate (Ritalin, Concerta) is most often prescribed. Usually a favorable response (a decrease in impulsive behaviors and an increase in the ability to sit still and attend to an activity for at least 15 minutes) is seen in the first 10 days of treatment and frequently with the first few doses. Other medications that may be used include dextroamphetamine (Dexedrine or Adderall), the tricyclic antidepressants desipramine and imipramine, and the antidepressant bupropion (Wellbutrin) (AAP, 2001b).

In addition to drug therapy, a variety of other treatments have been attempted for ADHD, and are commonly used by families. Chiropractic manipulation, biofeedback, visual or auditory therapy, and dietary interventions are examples of common complementary or alternative therapies. Some dietary interventions include elimination of dietary components, such as highly processed foods, sugar, aspartame, or yeast. Other therapies include supplements, such as iron, magnesium, zinc, and vitamin B_6. Herbs such as Pycnogenol, melatonin, and *Ginkgo biloba* are sometimes used (Arnold, Pinkham, & Votolato, 2000; Baumgaertel, 1999).

TABLE 54–4 ✣ DSM-IV-TR Diagnostic Criteria for Attention Deficit Hyperactivity Disorder

A. Either 1 or 2:

  1. Inattention: Six (or more) of the following symptoms of inattention have persisted for at least 6 months to a degree that is maladaptive and inconsistent with developmental level:

    a. Often fails to give close attention to details or makes careless mistakes in schoolwork, work, and other activities

    b. Often has difficulty sustaining attention in tasks or play activities

    c. Often does not seem to listen when spoken to directly

    d. Often does not follow through on instructions and fails to finish schoolwork, chores, or duties in the workplace (not due to oppositional behavior or failure to understand instructions)

    e. Often has difficulty organizing tasks and activities

    f. Often avoids, dislikes, or is reluctant to engage in tasks that require sustained mental effort (such as schoolwork or homework)

    g. Often loses things necessary for tasks or activities (e.g., toys, school assignments, pencils, books, or tools)

    h. Is often easily distracted by extraneous stimuli

    i. Is often forgetful in daily activities

  2. Hyperactivity-impulsivity: Six (or more) of the following symptoms of hyperactivity-impulsivity have persisted for at least 6 months to a degree that is maladaptive and inconsistent with developmental level:

    Hyperactivity

    a. Often fidgets with hands or feet or squirms in seat

    b. Often leaves seat in classroom or in other situations in which remaining seated is expected

    c. Often runs about or climbs excessively in situations in which it is inappropriate (in adolescents or adults, may be limited to subjective feelings of restlessness)

    d. Often has difficulty playing or engaging in leisure activities quietly

    e. Is often "on the go" or often acts as if "driven by a motor"

    f. Often talks excessively

    Impulsivity

    g. Often blurts out answers before questions have been completed

    h. Often has difficulty awaiting turn

    i. Often interrupts or intrudes on others (e.g., butts into conversations or games)

B. Some hyperactive-impulsive or inattentive symptoms that caused impairment were present before age 7 years.

C. Some impairment from the symptoms is present in two or more settings (e.g., at school [or work] and at home).

D. There must be clear evidence of clinically significant impairment in social, academic, or occupational functioning.

E. The symptoms do not occur exclusively during the course of a Pervasive Developmental Disorder, Schizophrenia, or other Psychotic Disorder and are not better accounted for by another mental disorder (e.g., Mood Disorder, Anxiety Disorder, Dissociative Disorder, or a Personality Disorder).

Used with permission from American Psychiatric Association. 2000. *Diagnostic and statistical manual of mental disorders* Text Revision (4th ed.). Washington, DC: Author. Copyright © 2000 American Psychiatric Association.

COMPLEMENTARY CARE

ALTERNATIVE TREATMENTS FOR ADHD

A variety of other treatments have been attempted for ADHD, and are commonly used by families. Chiropractic manipulation, biofeedback, and dietary interventions (both elimination diets and supplement use) are examples of common complementary or alternative therapies. Essential fatty acids (EFAs) have been studied for their beneficial effects on ADHD, specifically omega-3 and omega-6 fatty acids (Burgess, Stevens, Zhang et al., 2000; Kidd, 2000). Because the body does not manufacture EFAs, they must be obtained from the diet. Sources of omega-3 and omega-6 fatty acids include evening primrose oil, flaxseed oil, borage oil, and oils from coldwater fish such as cod and salmon. If parents wish to use this therapy, the oils can easily substitute for others in the diet and the fish can be part of a healthy diet. Be sure that excess intake of oils does not occur.

Although ADHD was once thought to be a disorder of childhood that gradually improved with age, it is now believed that symptoms continue into adulthood and that careful management in childhood helps lessen problems of social functioning later in life.

NURSING MANAGEMENT

NURSING ASSESSMENT AND DIAGNOSIS

The nurse often encounters the family who is concerned about the child's behavior before a diagnosis has been made. Ask about family and birth history and have the parents describe the child's behaviors. Perform developmental testing and look specifically for attention span and physical activity. Refer the family to their pediatric healthcare home for further assessment, and then to a mental healthcare specialist who is experienced in diagnosing ADHD.

Nurses may encounter the child with ADHD in the hospital when parents bring the child for treatment of an injury (e.g., fracture) or other problem. Explore the parent's report of the child's attention span in detail. Usually within a few minutes in an unstructured setting or waiting area, the child with ADHD becomes restless and searches for distraction. Gather information about the child's activity level and impulsiveness. Be alert for information that reveals a serious problem, such as hurting animals or other children. Find out about distractibility, attention deficit in activities of daily living, characteristic ways of reacting, and the extent of impulsiveness when the child is receiving medication. Find out how the family manages at home. Ask about a family history of the disorder, as that is a common finding among children with ADHD.

DRUG GUIDE

METHYLPHENIDATE HYDROCHLORIDE (RITALIN)

Overview of Action

Methylphenidate hydrochloride (Ritalin) is a derivative of piperidine that acts like an amphetamine. It causes CNS and respiratory stimulation and has some sympathomimetic activity. It may work by enhancing catecholamine effects in the reticular activating system, thereby affecting the cortex to improve attention span and task performance. It may also prevent flooding of sensory impulses into the cortex so that they enter in a more integrated manner. It is used to treat children with attention deficit hyperactivity disorder and adults with narcolepsy.

Routes, Dosage, Frequency

PO: For children 6 years or older: 2.5 to 5 mg before breakfast and lunch initially, increased in 2.5- to 5-mg increments weekly as needed or 0.25 mg/kg/day in 2 doses initially, increased by doubling weekly as needed; not to exceed 2 mg/kg/day or 60 mg/day. A sustained-release form is available so that children can take one pill in the morning and do not have to take more at school in the middle of the day; this can be used after the child is stabilized on the proper dose. The preparation called Concerta is dosed at 18 mg each morning, increased at weekly intervals as needed, with a maximum dose not to exceed 54 mg/day.

Side Effects: Insomnia, nervousness and agitation, palpitations, changes in blood pressure and pulse, blurred vision, anorexia and weight loss, hepatotoxicity, dermatitis

Contraindications: Tic syndromes, allergy to the drug, children under 6 years; do not give within 14 days of any MAO inhibitors

Nursing Implications

Measure height and weight and plot on growth grid. Take baseline vital signs. Do CBC and platelet count. Take history of previous drug therapy and reactions.

- *Administer:* Schedule II drug under Federal Controlled Substance Act. Do not give tablets late in afternoon or evening because doing so may interrupt sleep. Extended-release tablets are given once daily in early morning and should not be crushed or chewed.
- *Monitor:* Patient is seen in office for regular visits, when vital signs, height, weight, and CBC and platelet counts are performed. Observe for signs of bleeding and bruising. Question parents and teachers about child's behavior and ability to concentrate and perform tasks. If drug is to be effective, behavior change occurs within 1 month. Some drug-free holidays are recommended; monitor for behavior changes at these times. Supervise drug withdrawal carefully after prolonged use since severe depression and psychotic behavior have occurred.
- *Patient Teaching:* Take drug as directed. Do not withdraw quickly; tapering is recommended under supervision of prescriber. Measure child's weight weekly and report weight loss. Report signs of bleeding, fever, sore throat, or bruising. Report changes in child's ability to concentrate and general behavior. Store the medication out of reach of children. If the drug is taken during school hours, work with personnel to plan for safe administration.

Data from Bindler, R. M., & Howry, L. B. (2005). Pediatric drug guide with nursing implications. Upper Saddle River, NJ: Prentice Hall-Health.

Examples of nursing diagnoses that might be appropriate for a child with ADHD include the following:

- *Impaired Verbal Communication,* related to altered perceptions
- *Impaired Social Interaction,* related to chronic episodes of impulsive behavior
- *Chronic Low Self-esteem,* related to behaviors associated with ADD/ADHD
- *Risk for Injury,* related to high level of impulsiveness and excitability
- *Risk for Caregiver Role Strain,* related to management of child with unpredictable moods and high energy

PLANNING AND IMPLEMENTATION

Prevention can focus on discouraging regular television exposure for young children from 1 to 3 years and encouraging daily vigorous physical activity for all children. Nursing care of the hospitalized child with ADD/ADHD focuses on administering medications,

managing the child's environment, implementing behavioral management plans, providing emotional support to the child and family, promoting self-esteem, and ensuring ongoing care.

Administer Medications

Methylphenidate and other medications increase the child's attention span and decrease distractibility. Be alert for the common side effects of these medications, including anorexia, insomnia, and tachycardia. Administering medication early in the day helps to alleviate insomnia. Anorexia can be managed by giving medication at mealtimes. Careful monitoring of weight, height, and blood pressure is necessary.

Minimize Environmental Distractions

The child may need an environment with minimal distractions. When hospitalized, this may mean a room with only one other child. Keep potentially harmful equipment out of reach. Monitor and limit television and video game time. Use shades to darken the room at nap- or bedtime, and minimize noise. Teach parents to minimize distractions at home during periods when the child needs to concentrate; for example, when doing schoolwork. Visits to areas such as shopping malls and playgrounds may need to be limited. Plenty of daily exercise and minimal use of television and video games may help the child concentrate when needed for school work.

Implement Behavioral Management Plans

Behavior modification programs can help reduce specific impulsive behaviors. An example is setting up a reward program for the child who has taken medication as ordered or completed a homework assignment. The rewards may be daily as well as weekly or monthly, depending on the child's age. (For example, one completed homework assignment might be rewarded with 30 minutes of basketball or a bike ride; assignments completed for a week might be rewarded with an activity of the child's choice on the weekend.)

If punishment is necessary, the behavior should be corrected while simultaneously supporting the child as a person. Punishment is generally withdrawal of a privilege, and should follow the offense quickly as the child may not otherwise connect the punishment with the behavior.

Provide Emotional Support

Children with ADD or ADHD offer a special challenge to parents, teachers, and healthcare providers. Parents must cope simultaneously with managing the difficult needs and demands of a hard-to-handle child, obtaining appropriate evaluation and treatment, and understanding and accepting the diagnosis, even when the child exhibits different behaviors with different people. Family support is essential. Educate both the parents and the child about the importance of appropriate expectations and consequences of behaviors. Teach skills that will help as the child grows older: making lists of tasks to accomplish; having routines for eating, sleeping, recreation, and school work; minimizing stimuli in the environment when completing work; and asking teachers and friends to identify when behavior is inappropriate.

Promote Self-Esteem

Help the child understand the disorder at an appropriate developmental level, and facilitate a trusting relationship with healthcare providers. Assist the child with social skills through role-play, playing in small groups, and modeling. Promote the child's self-esteem by pointing out the positive aspects of behavior and treating instances of negative behavior as learning opportunities. Help the child to develop ego strengths (the consciousness to be able to screen outside stimuli and control internal demands), which will result in better impulse control and thus increase self-esteem over time.

NURSING PRACTICE

Many families who have a child with ADHD or another mental health disorder are embarrassed and feel shame because of the diagnosis. This may be especially true in certain cultures, such as some Asian groups, and in highly structured and highly achieving families. When taking histories from family members, it is best to be sensitive to the stigma some may feel. Ask questions in a private setting and ask about the family's feelings about a mental health disorder. Provide information in a nonjudgmental manner and if appropriate provide support from other families with similar experiences.

Nursing Care in the Community

Most children with ADHD are not hospitalized. Only occasionally will a child be hospitalized when needing care for another condition. Parents need support to understand the diagnosis and to learn how to manage the child. Emphasize the importance of a stable environment, at home as well as at school. At home the child may have difficulty staying on task. Parents need to consider age and developmental appropriateness of tasks, give clear and simple instructions, and provide frequent reminders to ensure completion. Routines in the evening can promote good sleep patterns.

The nurse can serve as a liaison to teachers and school personnel, or as the case manager for the child. An individualized education plan may be needed (see Chapter 39 ∞), with clear expected outcomes stated for the child's behaviors. Special classrooms or periods of instruction free from the distractions of the entire class may enable the child to improve school performance. Parents may have difficulty understanding the need for these approaches because the child often tests with above-average intelligence. Reinforce the importance of providing a structured environment free from unnecessary external stimuli. Be sure that parents understand behavioral approaches that will help the child, how to administer prescribed medications, and the importance of returning for healthcare visits to monitor for side effects. Medication should be locked safely away at home to keep it away from other children and prevent illegal use of this controlled substance. An individual school health plan may be needed for medication management.

Parents may have heard about ADHD in the media and often have many questions about its cause and management. Providing information about complementary and alternative treatments is a nursing role.

As the child grows older, explain the disorder and teach about techniques that will assist in dealing with problems. Emphasize the importance of doing homework or other tasks requiring concentration in a quiet environment without background noise from a television or radio. Encourage children with attention deficits to write down instructions from teachers and to use checklists to help them accomplish specific tasks.

EVALUATION

Expected outcomes of nursing care for the child with ADD or ADHD include the following:

- Understanding of disorder by parents and child
- Management of medication administration
- Increase in attentiveness and decrease in hyperactivity, impulsivity, and sleep disturbances
- Formation of positive self-image in the child
- Educational performance to maximum potential

MOOD DISORDERS

DEPRESSION

Depression is psychologic distress that can range from mild to severe. Only in recent years has depression in children been recognized as a clinical condition. Many children referred to child guidance centers and mental health professionals because of behavioral difficulties or poor achievement actually suffer from depression. The incidence of major depression is estimated to be about 2% in prepubertal children and about 4% to 8% in adolescents. Males and females are equally affected until adolescence when the incidence in girls rapidly increases until they are twice as commonly afflicted (Castiglia, 2000a, 2000b; Shugart & Lopez, 2002).

ETIOLOGY AND PATHOPHYSIOLOGY

Many theories have been proposed to explain the cause of depression in children and adolescents. Depression may be biologic in origin or a result of learned helplessness, cognitive distortion, social skills deficit, or family dysfunction. The physiologic theory focuses on monoamine neurotransmission. These amines include indolamine, serotonin, norepinephrine, and dopamine, and decreases are sometimes found in depression. Childhood depression sometimes occurs secondary to parental depression because the parental depression deprives the child of effective parenting. Abuse and neglect predispose children to depression, especially very young children. In about half of all children with depression, at least one other psychiatric diagnosis is made; these include conditions such as ADHD, anxiety disorder, or another personality disorder. Depressive disorders may contribute to other mental illness such as disturbed relationships, substance abuse, and suicide (Lyon & Morgan-Judge, 2000).

CLINICAL MANIFESTATIONS

Characteristic findings of major depression in children and adolescents include declining school performance; withdrawal from social activities; sleep disturbance (either too much or too little); appetite disturbance (too much or too little); multiple somatic complaints, especially headaches and stomachaches; decreased energy; difficulty concentrating and making decisions; low self-esteem; and feelings of hopelessness. There is much variation among children in the symptoms displayed, and they often have some but not all of the major criteria (Williamson, Birmaher, Brent et al., 2000).

CLINICAL THERAPY

Initial assessment is performed by a child psychologist or child psychiatrist. A variety of scales and techniques are used; however, very little guidance is available about evaluating children under 6 years of age. Examples of useful tools are the Children's Depression Inventory and the Revised Children's Manifest Anxiety Scale.

Treatment may include psychotherapy in combination with psychotropic medication. Often a combination of individual, family, and group therapy provides the greatest benefits for young children and adolescents. Involving parents and other family members in the treatment plan is essential. Group therapy is effective for adolescents because of the importance of peer group relationships during the teenage years. Cognitive therapy may be used with adolescents, and play therapy with younger children (see discussion of play therapy earlier in this chapter).

Antidepressant medications, most commonly the selective serotonin reuptake inhibitors (SSRIs), imipramine (Tofranil), desipramine (Norpramin), and amitriptyline (Elavil), may be prescribed (see Table 54–5). Studies of the tricyclic antidepressants (TCAs) have demonstrated their usefulness in adolescents but not in children (Hazell, O'Connell, Heathcote et al., 2003). The SSRIs act

GROWTH AND DEVELOPMENT

Symptoms of depression in children vary according to their developmental levels. Infants may fail to eat and grow, toddlers can show regressive behaviors in toileting and other activities, and school children may show a decrease in academic performance, increased or decreased activity, somatic complaints, and loss of friends. The adolescent can have a wide array of symptoms such as anxiety, decreased social contact, poor school performance, lack of prior involvement in activities, poor self-care, difficulty with parents and teachers, or focus on violence.

TABLE 54–5 ✣ Selective Serotonin Reuptake Inhibitor (SSRI) Drugs Used to Treat Depression

Medication	Pediatric Dose	Adolescent Dose	Selected Side Effects
Fluoxetine (Prozac)	2.5-40 mg daily or 0.5-1 mg/kg/day	10-60 mg daily	Restlessness, headaches, akathesia
Sertraline (Zoloft)	25-125 mg daily or 1.5-3 mg/kg/day	50-200 mg daily	Dry mouth, gastric upset
Paroxetine (Paxil)	5-40 mg daily or 0.25-0.7 mg/kg/day	20-40 mg daily	Dry mouth, weight gain
Fluvoxamine (Luvox)	50-100 mg bid or 1.5-4.5 mg/kg/day	50-300 mg daily	Dry mouth, gastric upset
Citalopram (Celexa)	Little data available	10-40 mg daily	Dry mouth, nausea, sleep disturbance

Data from Shugart, M. A., & Lopez, E. M. (2002). Depression in children and adults. *Postgraduate Medicine, 112,* 53–61; Walsh, K. H. (2002). Welcome advances in treating youth anxiety disorders. *Contemporary Pediatrics,* 19(9), 66–82.

Note: Although a variety of SSRIs are used in treatment of children and adolescents, the only approved U.S. FDA medication for major depressive disorder in this age group is Prozac, and the only approved FDA medications for OCD in pediatric age group are Prozac, Zoloft, Luvox, and Anafranil.

to block reuptake of serotonin in the synapse, so that serotonin (which influences mood) levels increase. Although the SSRIs are generally considered safer than some other antidepressants, their use in children has been limited, so side effects must be monitored. Fluoxetine is the only SSRI approved for use in children by the U.S. Food and Drug Administration (FDA); the other SSRIs have been used clinically but adequate research has not demonstrated their safety or efficacy in children. The major serious side effect is serotonin syndrome. This condition is characterized by agitation, muscle twitching, gastric upset, chills, fever, confusion, and dizziness. Generally the child is started with a low dose and it is increased slowly to minimize the chance of side effects. There have been some reports of children who developed suicidal thoughts and actually committed suicide while taking SSRIs. Because of these reports and the lack of efficacy evidence, the FDA has cautioned against use of paroxetine in children under 18 years (National Institute of Mental Health, 2004).

NURSING PRACTICE

Serotonin syndrome, the serious and life-threatening side effect of SSRIs, is caused by overstimulation of serotonin receptors. It is more likely to develop when the child or adolescent is also taking St. John's wort, other antidepressants, alcohol, diet pills, or drugs such as ecstasy and LSD (Lyon & Morgan-Judge, 2000). Be certain to ask questions in a nonjudgmental way about intake of any alternative therapies, other medications, or substance use to identify those most at risk.

Sudden cardiac death has occurred in several children on tricyclic antidepressants. Because of this risk, serum levels should be monitored and electrocardiograms (ECG)

are performed. Specific ECG changes along with a resting heart rate above 100, systolic blood pressure above 130 mm Hg, and diastolic blood pressure above 85 mm Hg necessitate immediate report to the prescriber.

NURSING PRACTICE

There have been reports of increased suicidal ideation and other behavioral changes in children and adolescents taking antidepressant medications. In both the United States and Canada, the medications are now accompanied by clear warnings for use in these age groups. Agencies in both countries have alerted healthcare providers and families of the risks, but leave decisions about medications to the prescribers and families since the risk of depressive illness in itself carries risk of harm to the individual. The U.S. Food and Drug Administration recommends that a Patient Medication Guide be provided to each patient, explaining the risks of the drug and precautions to take. Additional precautions are found in a boxed warning on the drug label. See Table 54–5 for further information about the approved drugs for use in children. Nurses must reinforce these important teaching points for all families when the child or adolescent receives medication, and emphasize the importance of follow-up visits and prompt reporting of any changes in the child or adolescent's behavior.

U.S. Food and Drug Administration. (2004). FDA Public Health Advisory, October 15, 2004.

NURSING MANAGEMENT

NURSING ASSESSMENT AND DIAGNOSIS

Take a thorough history and physical examination, including observation of behavior, at the time of admission. Assess the child for common risk factors for depression (Table 54–6).

TABLE 54–6 ✣ **Risk Factors for Child and Adolescent Depression**

Child	Family	School and Social Situations
■ Frequent feelings of sadness, sleep problems, loss of interest in activities ■ Increase in risk taking and impulsivity ■ Previous suicide attempt ■ Alcohol or substance abuse ■ Diagnosed psychotic disorder ■ Chronic illness and frequent hospitalization	■ Parental neglect, abuse, or loss ■ Dysfunctional family relationships ■ Family history of depression, suicide, substance abuse, alcoholism, other psychopathology	■ Academic pressures and underachievement ■ Stressful social relationships ■ Declining participation in social events

Several nursing diagnoses that might be appropriate for the child or adolescent hospitalized with depression are included in the accompanying "Nursing Care Plan." Other diagnoses might include the following:

■ *Imbalanced Nutrition: More than Body Requirements,* related to eating in response to internal cues other than hunger

■ *Powerlessness,* related to sense of helplessness

■ *Chronic Low Self-esteem,* related to negative self-evaluation

PLANNING AND IMPLEMENTATION

Nursing care of the child or adolescent hospitalized for depression includes administering medications and other therapy, and providing supportive care. Monitor vital signs of youth receiving antidepressant medications. Watch for common side effects of the agent(s) used. Carefully monitor for serious side effects of SSRIs and be aware that lower doses are used at initiation, with doses increasing slowly to the desired level. Monitor cardiovascular status, including hypertension and tachycardia, observe motor movement, and record dietary intake. Help parents to evaluate inpatient settings to be certain the care provided will best meet the needs of the child or adolescent. Refer to "Nursing Care Plan: The Child or Adolescent Hospitalized with Depression" for specific nursing interventions.

Discharge Planning and Home Care Teaching

When the child has been hospitalized and is returning home, teach parents to recognize signs and symptoms of worsening depression. Also teach them dosages and side effects of any prescribed medications. Refer the family to appropriate healthcare professionals and to support groups for family members dealing with depression.

Nursing Care in the Community

Most children with depression are cared for in the community. Maintain regular contact with the family through their healthcare visits to outpatient agencies and by making home visits. Monitor the child's affect, activity, and food intake. School teachers and counselors often are aware of the child's ability to perform in the school setting. Have the family schedule after-school care so young children are not left at home alone for extended periods. Assist the family in finding support for financial and emotional needs related to managing the child's depression. Major expected outcomes for nursing care of the child with depression are found on the accompanying "Nursing Care Plan."

BIPOLAR DISORDER (MANIC-DEPRESSION)

Bipolar disorder is a mental illness in which extreme changes in affect and energy are manifested. Moods most often alter

TEACHING HIGHLIGHTS

SELECTING RESIDENTIAL AND INPATIENT CARE FOR THE CHILD WITH MENTAL ILLNESS

Families need guidelines to help them evaluate inpatient facilities when a child with a mental disorder must be placed in an institution. You can refer them to the National Alliance for the Mentally Ill Web site. Provide questions for the families to ask:

■ What is the staff:youth ratio?

■ What are the guidelines for chemical and physical restraint?

■ Are children isolated when behaviors are inappropriate?

■ Are children constantly monitored visually when in restraint or when potentially dangerous to self or others?

■ Does the child have a full physical and psychologic evaluation by a specialist within 24 hours of entry to the facility?

■ What professionals review the plan of care and how often?

■ Who can the family speak to for regular updates on the child?

■ How often can the family visit?

■ What services will be covered by insurance?

■ What subjective feelings do the family members have as they visit the unit and facility?

■ What services will be offered on an ongoing basis upon discharge?

NURSING CARE PLAN

THE CHILD OR ADOLESCENT HOSPITALIZED WITH DEPRESSION

Intervention	Rationale	Expected Outcome

1. Nursing Diagnosis: Hopelessness related to long-term stress

NIC Priority Intervention: **Hope instillation:** Facilitation of the development of a positive outlook		**NOC Suggested Outcome:** **Hope:** Presence of internal state of optimism that is personally satisfying and life supporting

Goal: The child or adolescent will discuss feelings of hopelessness.

■ Encourage open expression of feelings. Explore hopeless, sad, or lonely feelings. Point out the connection between feelings and behavior. Assess the child or adolescent to identify the precipitating event when feelings of sadness arose. ■ Encourage the child or adolescent to take part in self-care and unit activities. Use routines to establish feelings of control. ■ Medicate as ordered and document results.	■ Expressing feelings may help to relieve sadness, loneliness, despair, and hopelessness. An accepting and nonjudgmental attitude must be maintained regarding any feelings expressed by the child. ■ An active role in self-care and treatment helps the child or adolescent to feel more in control. ■ Antidepressants modify mood to a more hopeful outlook.	By discharge, the child or adolescent expresses an interest in the future.

2. Nursing Diagnosis: Ineffective Individual Coping related to inadequate social support or disturbance in pattern of appraisal of throat

NIC Priority Intervention: **Coping enhancement:** Assisting a patient to adapt to perceived stressors, changes, or threats which interfere with meeting life demands and roles		**NOC Suggested Outcome:** **Coping:** Actions to manage stressors that tax an individual's resources

Goal: The child or adolescent will use effective coping skills.

■ Teach positive, effective coping strategies such as guided imagery and relaxation. Assist the child or adolescent to focus on strengths rather than weaknesses. ■ Assist the child or adolescent to identify friends, family members, and others who are positive and supportive.	■ Therapeutic techniques can help the child or adolescent to replace negative thoughts and images with more positive and effective beliefs and images. These interventions foster resilience. ■ Helps the child or adolescent to become aware that people can be caring and supportive (thus validating self-esteem).	The child or adolescent verbalizes and demonstrates ability to cope appropriately for his or her age.

3. Nursing Diagnosis: Impaired Social Interaction related to self-concept disturbance

NIC Priority Intervention: **Socialization enhancement:** Facilitation of ability to interact with others		**NOC Suggested Outcome:** **Social interaction skills:** An individual's use of effective interaction behaviors

Goal: The child or adolescent will participate in and initiate activities and conversation.

■ Assist the child or adolescent to identify topics and activities of interest. ■ Encourage interaction with peers and staff. ■ Facilitate visits from family and friends. ■ Provide guidance to family regarding interaction that promotes self-esteem.	■ The more the child or adolescent focuses on areas of interest, the less he or she will focus on internal anxiety and depression. ■ Each positive interaction reinforces feelings of success. Each success reinforces the desire for future social interaction. ■ Reinforces positive and rewarding relationships. ■ The family's existing interaction style is often negative.	By discharge, the child or adolescent initiates conversation and activities with staff and peers.

(continued)

NURSING CARE PLAN—continued

THE CHILD OR ADOLESCENT HOSPITALIZED WITH DEPRESSION

Intervention	Rationale	Expected Outcome
4. Nursing Diagnosis: Imbalanced Nutrition: Less than Body Requirements related to loss of appetite secondary to depression		
NIC Priority Intervention: **Nutrition management:** Assistance with or provision of a balanced dietary intake of foods and fluids		**NOC Suggested Outcome:** **Nutritional status:** Amount of food and fluid taken into the body over a 24-hour period
Goal: The child or adolescent's daily intake will be adequate to maintain optimal nutritional status.		
■ Offer nutritious finger foods, sandwiches, and high-calorie liquid supplements frequently throughout the day. ■ Offer easy-to-carry drinks that are high in vitamins, minerals, and calories. ■ Encourage daily vigorous physical activity of at least 30 minutes.	■ Convenient easy-to-eat foods encourage the child or adolescent to eat and maintain nutritional status. ■ These are a convenient method for meeting hydration and electrolyte needs. ■ Physical activity stimulates appetite.	The child or adolescent's daily intake will be adequate to maintain optimal nutritional status by discharge.

between mania and depression. Children often present with irritability or hyperactivity. About 1.5% of the total population and 1% of children have bipolar illness, although diagnosis and accurate numbers are difficult to obtain due to the frequency of accompanying additional mental illness and the lack of clear diagnostic criteria in childhood. Twenty percent of patients with bipolar disorder have the first manic episode in adolescence (Jellinek, Patel, & Froehle, 2002). About 10% to 20% of individuals with bipolar illness commit suicide. The average age for children to demonstrate bipolar disorder is 11 years, but a first manic episode at 5 years is not uncommon. Children may show mainly depressive symptoms, and then develop mania in adolescence, or may have episodes of both mania and depression in the same day.

The manic phase of bipolar illness is characterized by hyperactivity and high energy, irritability, aggression, and sometimes hallucinations. In the depressive phase, the child is sad, has alterations in sleep and eating patterns, and is socially withdrawn, similar to any depressive illness. The presence of comorbidities makes diagnosis difficult. Disorders that often present in the same children include conduct disorder, attention deficit hyperactivity disorder, depression, anxiety, autistic disorder, mental retardation, and Tourette's syndrome (Mohr, 2001).

Diagnosis and treatment of bipolar disorder should be performed by mental health specialists. Use of alcohol or illegal drugs should be ruled out as a cause of symptoms, even in children. Since the manic phase is often manifested by hyperactivity, the child may incorrectly be treated with stimulants (see treatment of ADHD earlier in this chapter), and the disease can be worsened. The treatment of bipolar disease involves a variety of drugs used to stabilize mood.

Lithium, valproate (Depakote), and carbamazepine (Tegretol) are most frequently used (Weller, Calvert, & Weller, 2003). Individual and family education and therapy can be helpful. The most important measure in preventing serious further illness is early recognition and treatment, so referral to mental health specialists is essential.

Nurses are instrumental in identifying children with the disorder, providing information to families, and monitoring the drugs and psychotherapy for the child. Nurses should observe for side effects to the specific drug regimen used and assist parents to find resources for healthcare since medications and other treatments may be costly. Parents and children need information about the disorder since it may recur several times during life. Nurses can assist the child to find social events and groups that build a sense of self-esteem.

ANXIETY AND RELATED DISORDERS

A large group of anxiety disorders can affect youth as well as adults. Some of the more common types seen in children and adolescents are described in the following sections, with detailed nursing management described after the last condition, post-traumatic stress disorder.

GENERALIZED ANXIETY

Anxiety is a subjective feeling of uncertainty and helplessness, usually accompanied by central nervous system signs, including restlessness, trembling, perspiration, and rapid pulse. Anxiety is second to only substance abuse (see

Chapter 36 ∞) in incidence for mental disorders and is a common mental disorder among children (Smoller, Finn, & White, 2000). Anxiety disorders are strongly linked to familial and genetic factors. They may coexist with other mental health disorders, or children sometimes have more than one type of anxiety (Walsh, 2002). Diagnosis is performed by a mental health specialist, and treatment is usually medication and individual therapy. While a variety of medications have been used to treat adults, studies are lacking in children. One medication that has been reported as safe and effective in children in at least one study is sertraline 50 mg/day (Rynn, Siqueland, & Rickels, 2001).

SEPARATION ANXIETY DISORDER

Separation anxiety disorder is characterized by an extreme state of uneasiness when in unfamiliar surroundings and often by refusal to visit friends' homes or attend school for at least 2 weeks. Approximately 75% of children with separation anxiety disorder refuse to attend school (see "School Phobia," to follow). Many children worry about losing a parent or significant other. They may have physical complaints, nightmares, and other sleep disturbance. This disorder occurs in approximately 4% to 5% of children and in twice as many girls as boys (Masi, Mucci, & Millepiedi, 2001). The peak age for occurrence is 7 to 9 years (Walsh, 2002). It may come and go and become worse at certain times.

Children with separation anxiety disorder tend to be perfectionistic, overly compliant, and eager to please. They appear to cling to the parent or caretaker. They may use physical complaints such as headaches, abdominal pain, nausea, and vomiting in an attempt to avoid being away from the parent. Depression frequently accompanies separation anxiety disorder. The resulting avoidant behaviors can interfere with personal growth and development, academic achievement, and social functioning.

Diagnosis is made by a mental health specialist. Treatment includes both child and parents. Parents learn about the disorder and how to structure the setting so that the child is expected to attend school. Consistency in expecta-

tions is needed since if the child is permitted to stay home some days or has missed school and other activities for longer periods, treatment is more difficult. Both parents and child work out the expectations for behavior for the child with the mental health therapist. Medication has occasionally been used if other therapy is not helpful. The SSRI fluoxetine has been used with a dose of 24 mg/day for children and 40 mg/day for adolescents (Walsh, 2002).

PANIC DISORDER

Panic disorder is the presence of recurrent, unexpected panic attacks. Panic attacks are periods of intense fear and discomfort in the absence of real danger. The risk of panic disorder ranges from 1.5% to 3.5% of the population (Smoller et al., 2000), with adolescence a common age for the onset of symptoms. The risk of panic disorder is 20 times more likely when there is a family history of the disorder (American Psychiatric Association, 2000).

Examples of the physical symptoms experienced are palpitations, sweating, chills, hot flashes, shaking, shortness of breath, choking, chest pain, nausea, and dizziness. The person describes feelings of danger or doom. Some people may have accompanying agoraphobia. **Agoraphobia** is an anxiety of being in places or situations from which escape may be difficult or embarrassing, or in which help may not be available. The attacks may be continuous or episodic, but generally are chronic.

Similar to anxiety, treatment may involve individual and family therapy, with use of medication in some cases. Nurses can help identify the disorder, refer for evaluation, and provide care in the community so that the child attends therapy sessions and takes medication as ordered (Carson, 2000).

OBSESSIVE-COMPULSIVE DISORDER

People with obsessive-compulsive disorder may be mildly or severely affected. One in about 200 children is affected, and there may be associated conditions such as tic disorders or attention deficit-hyperactivity (Leonard, Freeman, Barcia et al., 2001). Affected children have recurrent ritualistic thoughts or actions; these obsessions or compulsions interfere with daily life. Examples of behaviors and concerns are obsessions about dirt or germs, worries about harm, and sexual thoughts. Common behaviors are excessive handwashing, counting objects, and hoarding substances. These practices may take one hour or more of time each day. Children with OCD differ from adults in several ways. They have more aggressive obsessions, such as fears of catastrophe, more commonly hoard objects, and are more likely to have religious obsessions. The presence of additional mental health disorders is common (Geller, Biederman, Farone et al., 2001).

🌸 GROWTH AND DEVELOPMENT

The separation anxiety commonly experienced by a 2-year-old differs from the psychiatric disorder in age appropriateness, duration, and severity. Separation anxiety disorder affects children of preschool age or older, lasts for at least 2 weeks, and is characterized by excessive anxiety. In contrast, the separation anxiety experienced by the 2-year-old involves a single episode of separation from a familiar caretaker and is a characteristic response in toddlers.

The basal ganglia of the brain are affected and a genetic link is observed. Post-streptococcal autoimmune disorder may be a cause in some cases. Treatment may involve cognitive-behavioral therapy, where the feared occurrence is presented and the person learns that no harm will occur. Medications, particularly SSRIs, are effective in most children. Nurses can identify cases and refer for psychiatric evaluation. Families need instruction about medications and potential side effects.

NURSING PRACTICE

Pediatric autoimmune neuropsychiatric disorders (PANDAS) are characterized by obsessive-compulsive and/or tic disorder, childhood onset, association with Group A beta hemolytic streptococcal infection, and neurological abnormalities. It is believed that in certain children, the strep infection leads to a neural autoimmune response, resulting in the psychiatric disorder. Research continues to identify possible mechanisms, results, and treatments for this cause of OCD (March, 2004).

SCHOOL PHOBIA

School phobia (also called school avoidance or school refusal) is a persistent, irrational, or excessive fear of attending school. The child may fear being harmed or losing control. School phobia is common in children between 5 and 12 years of age, but can occur in children up to 16 years. The child's avoidance of school is often a manifestation of fear of leaving the parent or primary caretaker. Children commonly report that teachers and peers "pick on" them. Somatic complaints are similar to those in children with separation anxiety disorder. Characteristically, symptoms are present only on school days and not on weekends or holidays.

Treatment includes the family and child, and establishes firm limits for behavioral expectations and consequences. Antidepressant medications may sometimes be needed to help the child feel comfortable. The longer a child is out of school, the greater the likelihood that a chronic, treatment-resistant condition will result. Referral for psychiatric evaluation is indicated for persistent symptoms.

CONVERSION REACTION

Conversion reaction is a disorder in which a disturbance or loss of sensory, motor, or other physical functions suggests neurologic or other somatic disease. The disturbance or loss cannot be explained by any known pathophysiologic mechanism. Instead, psychologic factors are involved. About 3% of the population experiences conversion reactions at some time (American Psychiatric Association, 2000). Adolescence and early adulthood are common times for the onset to occur.

Conversion reactions develop in response to a catastrophic event such as threat, loss, or harm. Clinical manifestations include altered sensations such as blindness or deafness; paralysis or ataxia, including inability to stand or walk and loss of ability to speak (aphonia); involuntary movements, such as pseudoepileptic convulsions; and constant complaints of pain with no physical basis (psychogenic pain). Children under 10 years usually present with gait abnormalities or seizures. The onset of conversion symptoms is usually dramatic and sudden. Symptoms often appear to be neurologic, but on careful examination obvious discrepancies are found. The person is usually calm about the symptoms even though they are serious. Often the child or family members appear indifferent or unconcerned over what healthcare providers consider an overwhelming physical disability.

Children suspected of having a conversion reaction require a complete physical and neurologic evaluation to rule out any possible physiologic basis for the symptoms. Individual and family therapy is usually necessary to identify the source of the psychologic conflict, pain, or need resulting in the conversion symptoms.

POST-TRAUMATIC STRESS DISORDER

Post-traumatic stress victims have experienced or witnessed a life-threatening event with death or severe injury (Meltzer-Brody, Hidalgo, Connor et al., 2000). Although accurate statistics are not available on children, about 1% to 2% of children are probably affected, with increasing numbers as more children are exposed to war and other violence (Kessler, 2000). The child or adolescent with the disorder has feelings of fear, terror, and helplessness, and may relive the event frequently in thought and nightmares. The child may become emotionally numb in a subconscious attempt to protect the self, but may have a persistently increased state of arousal (Kent, Sullivan, & Rauch, 2000). Examples of events associated with post-traumatic stress include sexual or other child abuse, rape, car crash, fire, witnessing violence, and having experience in war. The events that occurred in the United States on September 11, 2001, are potential causes of post-traumatic stress in children who either had a family member involved, lived near the events, or in some other way were profoundly affected. Cassandra, described in the opening quotation of this chapter, was experiencing post-traumatic stress disorder (PTSD) due to a frightening car crash as she was driven to school. She was too young to describe her feelings verbally to her mother or school personnel; however, she manifested the sleep abnormalities and other complaints common in the disorder (Figure 54–6 ●). Even children of Holocaust victims experience PTSD, leading mental health professionals to believe that PTSD can be transmitted from parent to child (Yehud, Hallig, & Grossman, 2001). There

FIGURE 54–6

The psychologist uses play therapy to help Cassandra reenact her car crash. This helps her gain some control over the event so that it is not so frightening.

is a relatively high incidence of PTSD among incarcerated youth (Lamberg, 2001).

The disorder involves both a traumatic event and the child's reaction to this event. It is believed that brain changes occur in trauma, leading to neurobiologic alterations that cause dysfunction of memory. Female gender, having other psychiatric disorders, a family history of psychiatric illness, and severe or lengthy trauma are all risk factors. The incidence ranges from 1% to 9% (Meltzer-Brody et al., 2000).

The child with PTSD is often irritable, and has sleep problems and inattentiveness. There is a state of hypervigilance and exaggerated startle response, such as to touch or loud noises. The person feels detached from others and alone. Immediately after the event, the child may appear to have adapted and functions normally. However, after several weeks or even months, the symptoms of the disorder begin to appear.

A variety of antidepressants and SSRIs are used for pharmacologic treatment. Counseling and other mechanisms of care can help the victim deal with the events. Cassandra saw a clinical psychologist who used play therapy to help her communicate her fears related to a car crash. Once the fears are clearly communicated, they often lose their power over the person, so that normal behaviors can resume.

NURSING MANAGEMENT

Nurses often help identify PTSD victims so that they can get care. Ask about traumatic events in the past and how the child reacted. Inquire about recent changes in the child's behavior. Include school attendance, complaints of physical illness, sleep patterns, and rituals in behavior. A family history of mental disorders may be useful.

Nursing care for anxiety disorders focuses on behavioral and cognitive therapies to enhance coping skills. Mental health nurses may conduct group therapy sessions (Figure 54–7 ●). Group sessions for children often provide a forum for discussion of fears, an opportunity to enhance skills of working together, and an opportunity to learn coping skills. Being a member of a group with other children experiencing anxiety or trauma can remove the stigma and allow the child the freedom to explore the behavior and its causes. Several of the techniques described in the chapter, such as drawing pictures and discussing them or telling stories, are used by mental health nurses in child therapy groups.

FIGURE 54–7

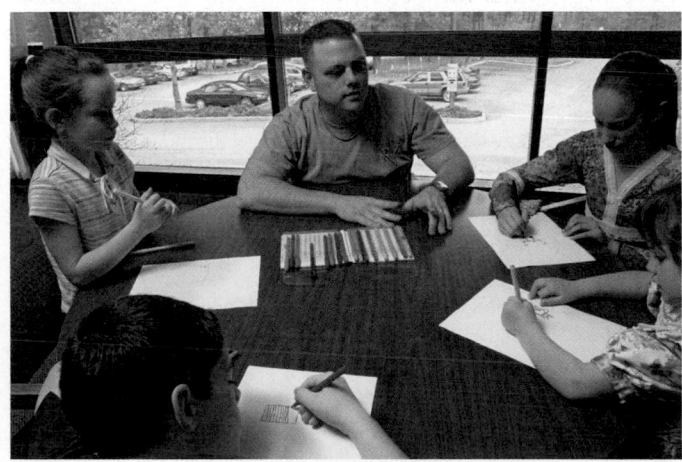

This nurse conducts a group therapy session for children who have experienced traumatic events and have resulting anxiety disorders. He is clearly engaged, has a positive rapport, and fosters exchanges among the children. Games and drawing are frequent techniques used in the group.

Children need to learn relaxation techniques and nurses may teach such techniques or recommend that the child consider participation in yoga or guided imagery classes. Inquire about alternative therapies that the child and family are using or have an interest in beginning, and refer as needed. Parents or other significant people should be included in the treatment program. Nurses often teach them basic information about the child's diagnosis and therapy. They should be in at least some therapy sessions with the child. Provide the family with resources that will assist with relief from worry about the child, guilt about causing an accident that triggered the child's symptoms, or other feelings related to the diagnosis.

Insurance companies may provide limited payment for mental health services. Help the family to see the importance of recommended therapy and assist them to find resources for care if needed. School personnel may need to know about the child's treatment. Partner with the families to provide needed information. Some schools have counselors that can be instrumental in carrying out treatment plans at school and acting as a resource in that setting. School personnel may be asked to provide feedback about the child's attendance, performance, and social skills as a measure of the success of therapy, and the community or school nurse can relay this information.

TEACHING HIGHLIGHTS

TALKING WITH CHILDREN ABOUT TRAUMATIC EVENTS

Whether a child or adolescent experiences trauma from a car crash, abuse, or environmental event, parents can help to decrease the effects of the stress and prevent the appearance of PTSD. Some suggestions for parents include:

- Be sure children feel free to ask parents, teachers, or others about the events and their feelings.
- Assure children that their feelings are normal and may return over time.
- Be honest and open in responses, without overloading children with more details than they need.
- Be prepared to repeat answers and discuss the same topics many times.
- Get help from counselors who can suggest how to talk with the child.
- Use communication methods appropriate at various ages, such as reading books, doing art projects, or drawing.
- Show children that they are loved by spending time and planning activities with them.
- Limit the television and other media time where the child is exposed to violence and traumatic events.
- Restore a sense of normal routines into the child's life.
- Be alert for increasing signs of distress and seek care from a professional if they occur.

Nurses often administer medications to children being treated for anxiety. Be alert for side effects and ensure the family knows how to safely administer the drugs. They should be kept locked securely. Have the child return for follow-up as needed since some medications may take several weeks to achieve effects, and close monitoring is essential. The child should have a medication alert tag for drugs being taken.

THINKING CRITICALLY

POST-TRAUMATIC STRESS DISORDER

Cassandra is a 9-year-old girl who has recently become fearful about attending school and has awakened crying at night. She is in the third grade at a school she has attended for 2 years. A few weeks ago, she was in a car crash as her mother drove her to school. She received only minor injuries and returned to school the next day. However, her mother believes that Cassandra's behavior has been worsening since the car crash. She spoke with the school nurse who is aware of no trauma at school, but did learn from the teacher that Cassandra has not been paying attention in class recently. Cassandra cannot explain why she does not want to go to school, only that her stomach aches or some other part of her body hurts.

Cassandra visited her pediatrician who ruled out any physical cause for her complaints, and referred her to a child psychologist. The psychologist has scheduled several sessions with Cassandra to help her learn to verbalize her fears and learn strategies to deal with them. She uses dolls in an attempt to help Cassandra act out her fears and gain some understanding. The psychologist communicates Cassandra's progress to you, the school nurse.

- How can you ensure Cassandra's attendance at school?
- What does the teacher need to know to support Cassandra in the classroom?
- What is your role as liaison between the psychologist, family, and school personnel?
- Parents often feel guilty when a child experiences a mental health disorder. What type of information and support do Cassandra's parents need?

SUICIDE

Suicide is the third leading cause of death in adolescents between 15 and 19 years of age. Over the past 40 years, teenage suicide has nearly tripled (Fish, 2000; National Strategy for Suicide Prevention, 2001). Suicide accounts for about 14% of deaths in teens. Nine percent of teens and 1% of prepubertal children have attempted suicide. Many more children have suicidal thoughts; 12% of 6- to 12-year-olds and 53% of adolescents have had suicidal thoughts (Horowitz, Wang, Koocher et al., 2001).

Boys die as a result of suicide four times more often than girls. This statistic is reversed for suicide attempts, perhaps because boys use lethal methods such as guns,

DEVELOPING CULTURAL COMPETENCE

SUICIDE AND ETHNICITY

Some ethnic groups have a high rate of suicide. For example, Native Americans and Alaskan Natives have a rate of suicide at 1.5 times the national average. Many youth in this group are suicide victims; it is the third major cause of death in Native American youth. The historic pain experienced by this ethnic group and lack of opportunities for many youth may be some of the reasons for a high suicide rate. Hispanic females have a higher rate of suicide than other gender and ethnic groups. White males have traditionally had highest rates of suicide, but recently blacks have had greatly increasing numbers of suicides (Rew, Thomas, Horner et al., 2001; Centers for Disease Control and Prevention, 2004a). *Healthy People 2010* goals focus on eliminating such health disparities by finding the causes, setting up prevention programs, and providing more support and opportunities for native populations.

TABLE 54–7 ✤ **Risk and Protective Factors for Suicide in Children and Adolescents**

Risk Factors	Protective Factors
History of previous attempted suicide	Emotional well-being
Friend committed or attempted suicide	Satisfactory school performance
School problems or changes in grades	Participation in sports or other group events
Pregnancy	Weight satisfaction
Drug use or abuse	Parent/family connectedness
Problems with a romantic relationship	Frequent discussions of important issues with family
Minority sexual practice	School connectedness
Loneliness, withdrawal	Safe school
Feelings of anxiety	Safe neighborhood
History of chronic family problems	Caring adult presence at school or elsewhere
Chronic illness	Availability of school counseling
Physical, emotional, or sexual abuse	School policies to limit and cope with fighting, bullying
History of suicide in a family member	
History of depression	
Chronic low self-esteem	
Change in behavior	
Change in weight	
Giving away special possessions	
Access to firearms and ammunition	

hanging, and jumping more often than girls, who use drug overdose and wrist cutting. Boys attempt suicide more often when depressed or in a challenging social situation, whereas girls more commonly attempt suicide as an impulsive act when in an unstable situation. It is not unusual for healthcare professionals and parents to label suicide attempts by children and adolescents "accidents." Up to half of childhood suicides may be recorded as accidents, suicide data for children under age 10 years are not maintained. Adults may have difficulty believing that young children, in particular, would have any reason to want to end their lives. Because of this, many children brought to the emergency department with indications of a suicide attempt are often classified as unintentional injury victims and released without arrangements for appropriate follow-up care.

Many risk factors for suicide exist in children and adolescents, while some protective factors are influential as well (Table 54–7). The most common precursor to adolescent suicide is depression (see earlier discussion). Common signs or symptoms of an underlying depression that could lead to suicide include boredom, restlessness, problems with concentration, irritability, lethargy, intentional misbehavior, preoccupation with one's own body or health, and excessive dependence on or isolation from others (especially adults or caregivers).

The child or adolescent at high risk for suicide may be admitted to a psychiatric unit for care or cared for in a community mental health facility. Treatment may include individual, group, or family therapy. Negotiating a "no suicide" contract is one method that may be used with a suicidal youth. In the contract, the child agrees not to attempt suicide during a specified time period. When a suicide attempt is made, the child or adolescent may be hospitalized for 24 hours, kept in a short-term monitoring unit, or sent home under close observation to ensure adequate assessment and monitoring. It is important to provide crisis intervention at the time of suicide attempt to minimize the opportunity for repeat attempts and begin a therapeutic treatment plan.

NURSING MANAGEMENT

The major nursing role is in prevention of suicide. Take all suicide threats seriously. Most suicides are committed with firearms present in the home. Ask at each healthcare visit if the family has firearms. Encourage parents to keep guns unloaded, with ammunition and firearms locked in separate locations. Be sure that children and adolescents do not have access to the keys for the locked firearms. Never underestimate the resourcefulness or abilities of a suicidal child or adolescent, regardless of age, IQ, or physical abilities.

Education in all school settings is appropriate to teach children about resources that can help them if they need it and to identify peers at risk. Be alert for children and adolescents at risk for suicide in any setting. Assess children and adolescents in schools, outpatient settings, and emergency departments for the possibility of suicidal behavior.

Report threats of suicide and depressive behavior. When a child or adolescent persists in threatening suicide after establishment of a "no suicide" contract, hospitalization is necessary to ensure safety. Recognize that when a child or adolescent has committed suicide, friends of the victim may be at increased risk. Teach students to report to teachers, nurses, or counselors about friends who have threatened suicide or seem depressed or display behaviors different from usual. Nurses often plan with mental health specialists to implement suicide prevention programs in schools and communities. Provide supportive services to family and friends whenever suicide occurs. Consult Web sites and refer parents as appropriate. The Suicide Prevention Resource Center has helpful regional offices to facilitate networks at national, state, territorial, community, and tribal levels.

Nursing care centers on taking appropriate precautions to ensure the child's safety. Monitor both the child and the hospital environment for any object that could be used for self-harm. Remove all potentially harmful objects, such as shoestrings, belts, pantyhose, and hair ribbons. Keep all personal care items (including toothbrush and shampoo) locked at the nursing station and monitor them constantly when used by the child.

Children or adolescents considered at high risk for suicidal behaviors are attended by a nursing staff member at all times, including while using the bathroom and sleeping. It may be necessary for the child to dress in a plain hospital gown, be kept in a visually monitored seclusion room, or (if seriously impaired and self-abusive) be medicated for restraint for a period of time. Restraints are used only when ordered by the physician and interdisciplinary team caring for the youth. Physical restraint is only a short-term approach to provide immediate safety if necessary. Chemical (medication) restraint may be needed to prevent self-injury by the suicidal person. See "Teaching Highlights: Selecting Residential and Inpatient Care for the Mentally Ill Child" for information to help families consider when choosing care for their suicidal child.

Hospitalization continues as long as the child's behavior is self-destructive. Children are referred for intensive individual and family therapy. Encourage parents to keep follow-up clinic appointments, to watch for self-destructive behaviors, and to administer any prescribed medications according to the treatment schedule. Arrange home visits and other community resources for families.

TIC DISORDERS AND TOURETTE SYNDROME

Tics are sudden, rapid, recurrent, nonrhythmic, and brief motor movements or vocalizations. They may involve movement of the head or upper body, blinking of eyes, or a variety of verbal noises. They may be worse during periods of stress or tiredness. Severe motor tics accompanied by verbal utterances are known as Tourette syndrome. The syndrome is often accompanied by other diagnoses such as attention deficit and learning disabilities (Kurlan, McDermott, Deeley et al., 2001). Many children have mild motor tics at some time which gradually disappear with no intervention. When the tics are severe or last over one year, they are considered chronic and may require attention from a mental health provider. This disorder is believed to be caused by dopamine abnormalities in the brain and can be successfully treated by haloperidol or other psychotropic medications. Children with Tourette syndrome may initially be incorrectly diagnosed with ADHD due to the increased motor activity. If they are medicated with a drug such as methylphenidate (Ritalin), their behaviors will worsen. Nursing care involves supporting parents and encouraging normal developmental progression for the child. Nurses should carefully monitor symptoms after medication is begun, minimize stress, and teach relaxation techniques.

SCHIZOPHRENIA

Schizophrenia is a psychotic disorder that is relatively rare in young children and adolescents, although it can occur in children as young as 5 years of age. The prevalence of schizophrenia increases after puberty and reaches adult levels by late adolescence. About 1 in 10,000 children develops schizophrenia (Lambert, 2001).

The cause of schizophrenia is unknown, but genetic predisposition or a neurovirus during pregnancy may play a role (Lambert, 2001). The brain is altered in the disease, with progressively enlarged ventricles and nervous system arousal. Impaired glucose metabolism is often present. The disorder most often manifests between 15 and 20 years of age. Onset is usually slow with increasing intensity. Most often the child demonstrates restlessness, poor appetite, and social withdrawal over several weeks to months. Behavioral problems, slowed development, and minor neurologic symptoms may occur.

The clinical manifestations of schizophrenia are the same in children as in adults. Characteristic behaviors include social withdrawal, impaired social relationships, flat **affect** (outward appearance of feeling or emotion), regression, loose associations (thought characterized by speech in which ideas shift from one subject to another that is unrelated), poor judgment and problem solving, anxiety, delusions, and hallucinations. Motor abnormalities may include rocking and arm flapping.

During adolescence, acute schizophrenia can occur suddenly while the teenager is making plans to leave home and family to attend college, marry, or work in another area. Onset of symptoms may be triggered by an important loss (death of a significant other, parent, child, or friend).

Clinical therapy for childhood schizophrenia is multifaceted, including individual psychotherapy, family therapy, and various psychotropic medications (antipsychotics such as haloperidol [Haldol], antianxiety agents such as lorazepam [Ativan], antidepressants such as imipramine [Tofranil], and newer antipsychotics such as clozapine, olanzapine, and risperidone). Drugs are only moderately effective at controlling hallucinations and delusions. Responses vary considerably, and children may have different responses than adults. Side effects determine what drugs are used and for how long. Antipsychotic medication is continued for at least 4 to 6 weeks before effectiveness can be determined. Medications often must be continued for several months or years after recovery from an acute schizophrenic episode, although medication-free trials may be tried in children who have not shown symptoms for 6 to 12 months (American Academy of Child and Adolescent Psychiatry, 2001).

Often, episodes of acute schizophrenia require inpatient hospitalization on a psychiatric unit for thorough diagnosis and beginning management. Treatment may include an intensive school-based program in a structured, supervised setting with specially trained professionals. The goal of initial treatment is to reduce or control psychotic episodes and provide a safe, structured environment for the child or adolescent, enabling the child to live each day at an optimal level of functioning. Outpatient care is provided in the community following initial diagnosis and establishment of a treatment regimen.

Most children require long-term treatment, including intermittent periods of hospitalization. Children or adolescents whose symptoms are difficult to control and who present a safety risk to themselves or others may require long-term residential treatment. Earlier age at diagnosis and delay in treatment lead to poorer prognosis.

NURSING MANAGEMENT

The nurse may encounter the child or adolescent with schizophrenia during hospitalization for an acute episode, for treatment of another problem, or while working with the individual in the community. Nursing care centers on providing for physical safety and psychologic care, and normal growth and development for the child.

Family education and involvement in the treatment plan are essential. Teach the family to monitor the child's symptoms and progression. Educating the child and parents about the risk of recurrence and methods to alleviate side effects of prescribed medications may increase compliance with the treatment plan. Assess the child for common medication side effects. For example, when excess weight is a potential side effect, frequent growth measure-

ments are made. Neurologic assessment and laboratory studies may be needed with some medications. Extrapyramidal side effects such as dystonia, Parkinson-like movement, and akathisia may occur with some drugs.

Help the family establish educational plans and integration within the school system. Communicate with school personnel to ensure understanding of the child's condition and ongoing management of the individualized education plan.

COGNITIVE DISORDERS

A wide array of cognitive conditions occur in childhood. Some are mild and not diagnosed until a child has difficulty in school, while others may be associated with physical signs that are visible at birth. Two common conditions, learning disabilities and mental retardation, are discussed in this section.

LEARNING DISABILITIES

Learning disabilities are a common problem of young children, affecting about 5% of school children. They involve neurologic conditions in which the brain cannot receive or process information in the normal manner. Often the impairment is only in one or two types of learning, making diagnosis difficult. Common types of learning disorders are listed in "Clinical Manifestations: Various Learning Disabilities."

Children may have difficulty in processing visual information which may be manifested in reading, writing, and mathematics performance. Others may have more difficulty with oral information, leading to problems in language development and reading (National Center for Learning Disabilities, 2004).

The causes of learning disorders are complex. Sometimes they are related to low birth weight or problems during the perinatal period. There may be a genetic component

CLINICAL MANIFESTATIONS

VARIOUS LEARNING DISABILITIES

DISORDER	CLINICAL MANIFESTATIONS
Dyslexia	Difficulty with writing, reading, spelling
Dyscalculia	Mathematics and computation problems
Dysgraphia	Difficulty with writing, spelling, and composition
Dyspraxia	Problems with manual dexterity and coordination

since their occurrence is more common when other family members are affected. Treatments involve learning how to compensate for the difficulties by using capabilities that are intact. Some children need to have all material written for them, and others need to have verbal presentations. Specific learning goals are established with the assistance of learning specialists. Children with learning disabilities should have individualized education plans (IEPs) established with realistic goals for school performance (see Chapter 39 for further information about IEPs ∞).

Nurses play a major role in identification of children with learning disabilities. They may be in contact with families during health promotion visits or in other settings when parents relay concern about the child's performance or difficulty in some aspect of school. Nurses should assess the child for the following developmental milestones which can indicate learning disability:

- Lack of ability to phrase sentences together by 2 1/2 years
- Inability to use speech that is understandable at least 50% of the time by 3 years
- Inability to ties shoes, button, hop, or cut by kindergarten
- Inability to sit for a short story by 3 to 5 years
(American Academy of Pediatrics, 2000a).

When a child may have a learning disability, the nurse should refer the family to the school or other testing resource. The nurse should partner with the family to plan for the child's learning needs, help the family to work closely with the child, suggest providing a setting at home to maximize potential for learning, and offer suggestions for building healthy self-esteem in the child. The nurse should assist the family to work with the school to establish annual goals for the child. Most children with learning disabilities can learn to perform well in their areas of strength and compensate for areas of difficulty. Early intervention is key to success and building a positive self-image regarding abilities.

MENTAL RETARDATION

Mental retardation is defined as significant limitation in intellectual functioning and adaptive behavior. It is mani-

fested in differences in conceptual, social, and practical life skills and begins before the age of 18 years (American Association of Mental Retardation, 2004). Events after that age that lead to limitations in function are generally referred to as brain injury. Intellectual functioning is generally characterized by an IQ below 70 to 75, and there are significant impairments in **adaptive functioning** (the ability to meet the standards expected for a cultural group). The child with mental retardation has adaptive deficits in at least two areas such as communication, self-care, home living, social/interpersonal skills, use of community resources, self-direction, functional academic skills, work, leisure, health, or safety. A low IQ score by itself does not necessarily correlate with an impaired ability to carry out adaptive skills. The child should be evaluated within the contexts of the individual cultural and community environment. The IQ score and the level of adaptive skills together determine the degree of severity of mental retardation.

Mental retardation is one type of developmental disability. A **developmental disability** is any of a variety of chronic conditions that are characterized by mental or physical impairments. Other examples include pervasive developmental disorder, cerebral palsy, and sensory loss. A developmental disability begins through the age of 21 years, and lasts throughout life (Centers for Disease Control and Prevention, 2004b).

ETIOLOGY AND PATHOPHYSIOLOGY

Mild retardation occurs in 3 to 6 per 1000 people, and mental retardation affects about 3% of the population (Baralle, 2001). The causes of mental retardation can be grouped into three general categories: prenatal errors in the development of the central nervous system, prenatal or postnatal changes in the person's biologic environment, and external forces leading to central nervous system damage. In each instance, the precipitating factor changes the form, function, and adaptation of the central nervous system. Table 54–8 provides examples of common conditions associated with mental retardation.

Three common conditions associated with retardation from prenatal life are Down syndrome, fragile X syndrome,

---

TABLE 54–8 ✤ Common Conditions Associated with Mental Retardation

Prenatal Conditions	Biologic Environment	External Forces
Down syndrome	Inborn errors of metabolism (e.g., phenylketonuria, hypothyroidism)	Traumatic brain injury (e.g., accident)
Fragile X syndrome		Poison ingestion (acute or chronic)
Fetal alcohol syndrome		Hypoxia/anoxic insult
Maternal infection (e.g., rubella, cytomegalovirus)		Infection (e.g., meningitis)
		Environmental deprivation

and fetal alcohol syndrome. About 1 in 1000 infants, or 4000 infants each year, are born with *Down syndrome* in the United States (Roizen, 2002). It is caused by an extra chromosome so the child has 47 rather than 46 chromosomes (see discussion of genetic transmission in Chapter 3 ∞). The most common chromosome affected is 21 so that the child often has "trisomy 21," or three instead of two copies of number 21 chromosome. In addition to mental retardation and physical signs, the child with Down syndrome is at higher risk of developing some other conditions such as cardiac defects, hearing loss, thyroid disease, and leukemia (Van Riper & Cohen, 2001).

Fragile X syndrome is caused by a single recessive gene abnormality on the X chromosome. A premutation to the X chromosome may occur in males or females. When a father or mother passes the faulty X chromosome to a daughter, it may remain as a premutation or may change into a true mutation. The daughter has two X chromosomes and therefore does not manifest this recessive disorder. However, she can pass the mutated X chromosome to her son who becomes affected with fragile X. The mutation of fragile X is on gene FMRP-1, which instructs cells to make a protein necessary for normal brain development (Bailey, Roberts, Mirrett et al., 2001).

Fetal alcohol syndrome (FAS) is caused by the effect of ethyl alcohol on the developing fetus. Alcohol ingestion by the pregnant woman can influence development of many body organs, and effects can range from mild to severe.

DEVELOPING CULTURAL COMPETENCE

FETAL ALCOHOL SYNDROME

Fetal alcohol syndrome is more common in groups with higher intake of alcohol. Since some Native-American tribes have a high rate of alcoholism, the federal government and some tribes have joined together to lower that risk among this ethnic group. On some reservations, such as the Yakama Nation in Washington State, alcoholic beverages are not sold and educational programs are in place.

For a discussion of phenylketonuria and hypothyroidism, two common biochemical causes of mental retardation, see Chapter 56. ∞ Other causes involve traumatic brain injury and infections of the central nervous system (see Chapter 53 ∞). Mental retardation is more common in children born prematurely.

CLINICAL MANIFESTATIONS

Mild mental retardation was originally described as an intelligence quotient (IQ) between 50 to 70, moderate retardation with IQ of 35 to 50, severe retardation for IQ 20 to 35, and profound retardation below 20. However, although an IQ below 70 is generally considered indicative of retardation, the functional assessment of the child is now considered a more accurate identification of children's performance and needs. Children who are mentally retarded manifest delays in all areas of development, including motor movement, language, and adaptive behavior. They usually achieve developmental milestones more slowly than the average child. These developmental delays may be the first indication to parents and care providers of the child's condition.

Mental retardation is sometimes accompanied by sensory impairment, speech problems, motor and orthopedic disabilities, and seizure disorders. Of children with mental retardation, 10% to 30% manifest one of these other disorders. Table 54–9 lists several physical characteristics associated with Down syndrome, fragile X syndrome, and fetal alcohol syndrome.

TABLE 54–9 ❖ **Characteristics Associated with Three Common Types of Mental Retardation**

Down Syndrome (see Figures 35–8 and 35–38B ◉)
Small head (microcephaly)
Flattened forehead
Wide, short neck
Epicanthal eye folds
White spots on eye iris (Brushfield spots)
Congenital cataracts
Flat nose
Small, low-set ears
Protruding tongue
Short broad hands
Simian line on palm
Wide space between first and second toes
Hearing loss
Increased incidence of diabetes, congenital heart defect, and leukemia
Hypotonia

Fragile X Syndrome
Long face
Prominent jaw
Large ears
Frequent otitis media
Large testicles
Epicanthal eye folds
Strabismus
High arched palate
Scoliosis
Pliable joints

Fetal Alcohol Syndrome (see Figure 33–4 ◉)
Flat midface
Low nasal bridge
Long philtrum with narrow upper lip
Short upturned nose
Poor coordination
Failure to thrive
Skeletal and joint abnormalities
Hearing loss

CLINICAL THERAPY

Mental retardation is diagnosed and initial treatment is planned in a multistep process, and by involving a multi-disciplinary team. The team may include a developmental specialist, physician, geneticist, nurse, teacher, language therapist, occupational therapist, and physical rehabilitation specialist. See Table 54–10 for a description of the DSM-IV-TR diagnostic criteria for mental retardation. Diagnosis begins with a comprehensive history and evaluation of the child's physical characteristics, developmental level, and intellectual and adaptive functioning. Laboratory tests such as chromosome analysis, blood enzyme levels, lead levels, or cranial imaging provide valuable information in some circumstances.

Developmental screening using a test such as the Denver II (see Chapters 33 and 37 ∞) can help identify children at risk. Intellectual and adaptive functioning are tested when mental retardation is suspected. A neurologic examination may indicate asymmetry of movement or strength, irritability or lethargy, or abnormal pitch to an infant's cry. Because mental retardation may be accompanied by physical abnormalities, it is important to observe the child for facial symmetry, distance between the eyes, level of the ears, hair growth, and palmar creases. These abnormalities may be clues to other health problems.

Based on the results of the evaluation, a multidisciplinary team plans the support needed to maximize the child's potential for development. Management focuses on early intervention to improve the degree of adaptive functioning. Associated physical, emotional, and behavioral problems are treated simultaneously. Depending on the child's condition, special education programs and physical or occupational therapy may be necessary (Figure 54–8 ●). The child may require supportive care and assistance with activities of daily living. The plans for intervention need to change as the child grows and the family situation alters.

TABLE 54–10 ✤ **DSM-IV-TR Diagnostic Criteria for Mental Retardation**

A. Significantly subaverage intellectual functioning: an IQ of approximately 70 or below on an individually administered IQ test (for infants, a clinical judgment of significantly subaverage intellectual functioning)

B. Concurrent deficits or impairments in present adaptive functioning (i.e., the person's effectiveness in meeting the standards expected for his or her age by his or her cultural group) in at least two of the following areas: communication, self-care, home living, social/interpersonal skills, use of community resources, self-direction, functional academic skills, work, leisure, health, and safety

C. The onset is before age 18 years

Used with permission from American Psychiatric Association. (2000). *Diagnostic and statistical manual of mental disorders* Text Revision (4th ed.). Washington, DC: Author. Copyright © 2000 American Psychiatric Association.

● **FIGURE 54–8**

Physical therapy is an important component of medical management for many children who are mentally retarded. *A,* This girl, who is severely retarded and uses a wheelchair, is being positioned in a mobile prone stander, which enables her to interact in a different manner with her therapists and the environment. *B,* Physical therapists also provide outpatient care in the community to children with varying degrees of disability.

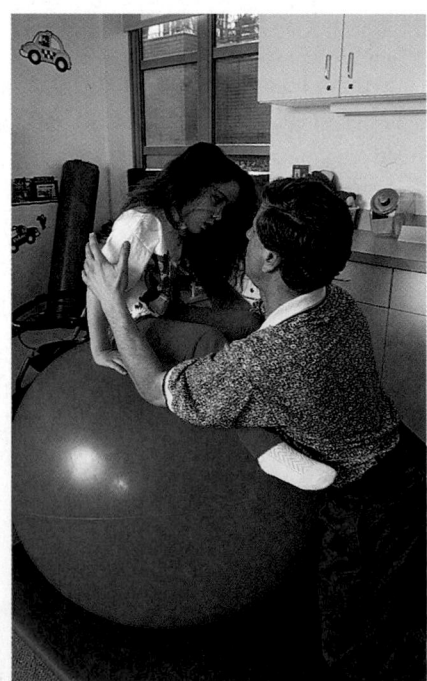

A   B

NURSING MANAGEMENT

NURSING ASSESSMENT AND DIAGNOSIS

Nurses can help to identify children with mental retardation through history taking, observation, and developmental screening during early childhood. The history should provide information about the mental and adaptive functioning of birth parents and other family members, as mental retardation may cluster in some families, and conditions such as fragile X syndrome are genetic. The pregnancy and birth history can provide important information about the mother's alcohol and drug use during pregnancy. Be alert for a history of difficult pregnancy and problems during birth. When genetic conditions in the family predispose family members to mental retardation, assess the child carefully. Children from deprived environments or those at risk because of environmental factors such as lead poisoning (see Chapter 51 ∞) are more likely to manifest mental retardation.

Many mentally retarded children are not diagnosed until they reach school age, particularly if the condition is mild or moderate. Early intervention, however, can help to enhance the child's functioning later. During home visits, during clinic appointments, in childcare centers, and during hospitalization, be alert for signs such as developmental delays, multiple (more than three) physical anomalies associated with a specific condition (see Table 54–9), or neurologic alterations. Developmental assessment should be part of each healthcare visit; see Chapters 37 and 38 for developmental surveillance recommended at each age. ∞

Once the diagnosis of mental retardation has been made, assess the adaptive functioning of the child and family. Perform a functional assessment of the child, including toileting, dressing, and feeding skills. Assess the child's language, sensory, and psychomotor functioning. Assess the home and community for safety hazards. Observe how the family is managing with the child. Ask about family activities that can include the child, and community and school attitudes and support. Assess the availability of services such as groups for parents and special education opportunities for children. Evaluate the coping skills of family members.

Several nursing diagnoses may be appropriate for the mentally retarded child, depending on the degree, cause, and outcome of the child's condition. Some of these diagnoses relate to impairments in adaptive functioning; others relate to the impact on the family. Examples include the following:

- *Delayed Growth and Development*, related to neonatal disease or condition
- *Imbalanced Nutrition: Less than Body Requirements*, related to inability to ingest sufficient food
- *Self-care Deficit: Dressing, Toileting, Bathing*, related to developmental disability
- *Impaired Verbal Communication*, related to developmental disability
- *Risk for Injury*, related to lack of understanding of environmental hazards
- *Compromised Family Coping*, related to the child's developmental variations

PLANNING AND IMPLEMENTATION

Nearly all children with mental retardation are cared for in the community. However, they may have conditions that require periodic hospitalization or frequent healthcare visits. Wherever nursing care occurs, it focuses on providing emotional support and information to family members, assisting the child with adaptive functioning, and fostering parental management of the child's activities. Whenever possible, the nurse uses preventive teaching to lower the risk of mental retardation. For example, nurses can integrate teaching into care for all women about the importance of avoiding all alcohol during any times when they might become pregnant. This helps prevent fetal alcohol syndrome, especially in early pregnancy when women may not know they are pregnant.

Provide Emotional Support and Information

Family members need empathy and support both at the time of diagnosis and in the ensuing years. Parents may be in an acute or chronic state of grief over the loss of the perfect child. Encourage them to verbalize their feelings. Introducing them to parents of other mentally retarded children may help and support them as they learn how to manage the child's needs. Discuss the availability of respite care to provide parents with a break from caretaking. Other family members such as grandparents and siblings may also feel grief or guilt and should be given an opportunity to talk about their feelings.

Parents need honest information and answers to their questions about the child's condition. Reinforce information provided by genetic counselors and other healthcare professionals. Parents need to know about community resources designed to assist children with mental retardation. The Education for All Handicapped Children Act, PL 94-142, provides free appropriate education to all handicapped children between 2 and 21 years of age. States and local communities may provide early intervention services for infants and toddlers with disabilities. Examples of programs include the Zero to Three project early intervention programs, special education preschools and schools, county health services, and respite care, among others. Ask parents if they have questions about individualized education plans and refer them to Internet sources if that may be helpful. Review federal and state laws and services that might be helpful to the family, and help them interpret information they find to analyze its strengths and limitations.

MediaLink   Help Families Evaluate Internet Information

Maintain a Safe Environment

The child with mental retardation requires close supervision because he or she may not understand common hazards. Ensure safety in the hospital. Assist parents to provide safety at home and school, and teach the child necessary skills such as pedestrian safety. Consider both physical and emotional safety. The child with mental retardation may be indiscriminately trusting and sometimes is at risk for physical or sexual abuse.

Provide Assistance with Adaptive Functioning

Encourage parents' efforts to maximize the child's areas of strength and identify needs related to adaptive behaviors. Refer them to resources to help with the child's impaired areas of adaptive functioning, such as communication, self-care, or social skills. During hospitalization, support parents' efforts to maintain the child's skills in toileting, dressing, and self-care by planning interventions to use the skills being taught at home.

Nursing Care in the Community

The child with mental retardation needs ongoing care throughout childhood; interventions must be adapted as the child develops and the family's needs evolve. Parents often act as case managers for the child's care. Assist parents as necessary to acquire the skills required to coordinate the child's plan of care. Evaluate the child's needs regularly and help parents with the treatment plan as necessary. Assist with plans for education and for services such as physical or speech therapy. Most children with mental retardation have an individualized education plan designed to meet their specific learning needs. Parents, nurses, and others such as teachers and language therapists are part of the team that establishes the child's individualized education plan. Promote optimal development and socialization. As the child reaches adolescence, education is directed toward a vocation, issues of sexuality, and the goal of independent living, when appropriate. Transition classes for adolescents with mental retardation can teach self-care skills that may enable some to live in group homes or other community settings. Parents need help planning for the child's future and their own retirement.

Specific guidelines for care are available for the child with Down syndrome. These guidelines suggest times for evaluation of hearing, growth, cardiac function, and other areas designed for early identification and treatment of associated disorders (Van Riper & Cohen, 2001). There are growth grids for children with Down syndrome, and specific topics to suggest for anticipatory guidance during healthcare visits (AAP, 2001c).

EVALUATION

The expected outcomes of nursing care depend on the child's needs and developmental level. Early in the diagnostic phase, desired outcomes may involve the family's understanding of the diagnosis and the child's special needs. Later outcomes may focus on the child's communication of self-help skills. Outcomes related to cognitive performance and adaptive skills may be developed during childhood.

Critical Concept Review

LEARNING OBJECTIVES

CONCEPTS

Define mental health and describe major mental health disruptions in childhood.

1. Mental health:
   - Successful engagement in activities and relationships and the ability to adapt to and cope with change.
2. Pervasive developmental disorders:
   - Impaired social interactions and communication with restricted interests, activities, and behaviors.
3. Attention deficit and attention deficit hyperactivity disorder:
   - Characterized by developmentally inappropriate behaviors involving attention.
4. Mood disorders:
   - Depression.
   - Bipolar disorder.
5. Anxiety disorders:
   - Group of disorders characterized by feelings of worry and uncertainty.
6. Tic disorders and Tourette syndrome.
7. Schizophrenia.

LEARNING OBJECTIVES

CONCEPTS

Discuss the clinical manifestations of the major mental health disorders of childhood and adolescence.

→

1. Pervasive development disorders:
   - Impaired social interaction and communication.
   - Restricted interests, social activities, and behaviors.
2. ADD and ADHD:
   - Decreased attention span.
   - Impulsiveness.
   - Increased motor activity.
3. Mood disorders:
   - Sadness.
   - Declining school performance.
   - Appetite and sleep disturbances.
   - Somatic complaints.
   - Extreme changes in affect and energy.
4. Anxiety disorders:
   - Restlessness.
   - Poor concentration.
   - Irritability.
   - Sleep disturbances.
   - Uneasiness in unfamiliar surroundings.
5. Tic disorders and Tourette syndrome:
   - Sudden, rapid recurrent, nonrhythmic, and brief motor movements and vocalizations.
6. Schizophrenia:
   - Social withdrawal.
   - Impaired social relationships.
   - Flat affect.
   - Regression.
   - Hallucinations.

Plan for the nursing management of children and adolescents with mental health disruptions in the hospital and community settings.

→

Hospital:
1. Assess child's current level of mental health functioning.
2. Continue prescribed treatments and medications.
3. Ensure child has no access to potentially dangerous materials and has adequate supervision.
4. Assess child's potential for self-harm.
Community settings:
1. Conduct ongoing assessment and evaluation of the child's mental health functioning.
2. Provide individual and group therapy sessions.
3. Refer families to mental health resources and support groups.

Describe characteristics of common cognitive disorders of childhood.

→

1. Learning disabilities:
   - Difficulty processing information by reading, writing, and math. Difficulty understanding oral information. Usually have normal IQ.
2. Down syndrome:
   - Hypotonia.
   - Epicanthal eye folds.
   - Simian crease on palm.
   - Flat nose.
   - Wide, short neck.
   - Mental retardation.
3. Fragile X syndrome:
   - Long face with prominent jaw and large ears.
   - Strabismus.
   - Aggressive behaviors.
   - Mental retardation.
4. Fetal alcohol syndrome:
   - Failure to thrive.
   - Flat midface with low nasal bridge.
   - Poor coordination.
   - Poor impulse control.
   - Low normal IQ to mental retardation.

LEARNING OBJECTIVES

CONCEPTS

Plan nursing management for children with cognitive disorders.

→

1. Assess for signs and symptoms of developmental delay.
2. Refer child for early intervention programs.
3. Refer parents to support groups.
4. Assist parents to obtain needed adaptive equipment.
5. Refer parents to programs that provide respite care.
6. When child is hospitalized, maintain home routine as much as possible.

Establish and evaluate expected outcomes of care for the child with a cognitive disorder.

→

Expected outcomes include:
1. The family will understand the child's diagnosis and the specific physical and developmental needs of the child.
2. The child will develop self-care skills appropriate to his or her developmental level.
3. The family will be able to access the necessary community and educational resources.

Evaluations include:
1. The family's ability to function and care for the child's needs.
2. The child's ability to perform self-help skills.
3. The family's ability to cope with changing needs of the child.

CRITICAL THINKING IN ACTION

*View the **Critical Thinking in Action** video in Chapter 54 of the CD-ROM. Then, answer the questions that follow.*

Douglas, a 5-year-old child with autism, comes into the office for his annual checkup and school immunizations of diphtheria tetanus acellular pertussis (DTaP), inactivated polio vaccine (IPV), and measles-mumps-rubella (MMR). He is very combative and it takes four people to help hold him and administer the vaccines. He will be attending a special school for children with autism and similar disorders. Diagnosed at 3 years old, he has never been in the hospital or had surgery. It is extremely difficult to examine him as he does not like to be touched. During prior visits in the office, Douglas has stood facing the wall and twisting his hands. He continues to be combative for most of the exam, even with the use of decreased stimuli, communication, and slow movements, but you are able to assess that his blood pressure is 95/53. He is in the 50th percentile for both height and weight and his temperature is 99°F.

You give her information about local support groups for children with autism and about local psychiatrists who can treat autism with types of medication to help control aggressive behavior. You also supply her with contact information for counselors in the area to help her deal with her own stress. She is appreciative of your help and support and looks forward to being able to send Douglas to school.

1. The mother has questions about the MMR vaccine and whether it causes autism. What can you tell her about that? Would you administer the vaccine today?
2. What can you tell the mother about safety issues with Douglas?
3. How can you enhance communication with Douglas when he comes into the office?

MEDIALINK

www.prenhall.com/london

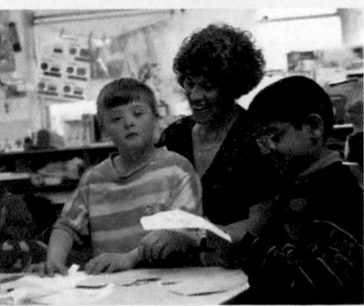

REFERENCES

American Academy of Child and Adolescent Psychiatry. (2001). The practice parameter for the assessment and treatment of children and adolescents with schizophrenia. *Journal of the American Academy of Child & Adolescent Psychiatry, 40(7),* 4S–23S.

American Academy of Pediatrics (2000a). Types of learning disabilities. Retrieved May 25, 2004, from www.medem.cfn/melb./article_detaillb_for printer.cfm?article_ID= ZZZ0Q5FNQ.

American Academy of Pediatrics, Committee on Quality Improvement, Subcommittee on Attention-Deficit/Hyperactivity Disorder. (2000b). Diagnosis and evaluation of the child with attention-deficit/hyperactivity disorder. *Pediatrics, 105,* 1158–1170.

American Academy of Pediatrics. (2001a). Diagnosis and management of autistic spectrum disorder. *Pediatrics, 107,* 1221–1226.

American Academy of Pediatrics, Committee on Quality Improvement, Subcommittee on Attention-Deficit/Hyperactivity Disorder. (2001b). Clinical practice guideline: Treatment of the school-aged child with attention-deficit/hyperactivity disorder. *Pediatrics, 108,* 1033–1044.

American Academy of Pediatrics, Committee on Genetics. (2001c). Health supervision for children with Down syndrome. *Pediatrics, 107,* 442–449.

American Association of Mental Retardation. (2004). *Definition of mental retardation.* Retrieved July 15, 2004, from http://www.aamr.org/Policies/faq_mental_retardation.html

American Psychiatric Association. (2000). *Diagnostic and statistical manual of mental disorders* (4th ed.): Text revision (DSM-IV-TR). Washington, DC: Author.

Arnold, L. E., Pinkham, S. M., & Votolato, N. (2000). Does zinc moderate essential fatty acid and amphetamine treatment of attention-deficit/hyperactivity disorder? *Journal of Adolescent Psychopharmacology, 10(2),* 111–117.

Bailey, D. B., Roberts, J. E., Mirrett, P., & Hatton, D. D. (2001). Identifying infants and toddlers with fragile X syndrome: Issues and recommendations. *Infants and Young Children, 14,* 24–33.

Baird, G., Charman, T., Cox, A., Baron-Cohen, S., Swettenham, J., Wheelwright, S., et al. (2001). Screening and surveillance for autism and pervasive developmental disorders. *Archives of Disease in Childhood, 84,* 468–475.

Baralle, D. (2001). Chromosomal aberrations, subtelomeric defects, and mental retardation. *Lancet, 358,* 7–8.

Baumgaertel, A. (1999). Alternative and controversial treatments for attention-deficit/hyperactivity disorder. *Pediatric Clinics of North America, 46,* 977–992.

Beauchesne, M. A., & Kelley, B. R. (2004). Evidence to support parental concerns as an early indicator of autism in children. *Pediatric Nursing, 30,* 57–67.

Bechtel, B. (2003, September). New research offers inroads to better understanding of autism. *Infectious Diseases in Children,* 14–16.

Bryden, K. E., Carrey, N. J., & Kutcher, S. P. (2001). Update and recommendations for the use of antipsychotics in early-onset psychosis. *Journal of Child and Adolescent Psychopharmacology, 11,* 113–130.

Burgess, J. R., Stevens, L., Zhang, W., & Peck, L. (2000). Long-chain polyunsaturated fatty acids in children with attention-deficit hyperactivity disorder. *American Journal of Clinical Nutrition, 71(1),* 327–330.

Cade, M., & Tidwell, S. (2001). Autism and the school nurse. *Journal of School Health, 71,* 96–100.

Carson, V. B. (2000). *Mental health nursing* (2nd ed.). Philadelphia: WB Saunders.

Castiglia, P. T. (2000a). Depression in adolescents. *Journal of Pediatric Health Care, 14,* 180–182. Retrieved July 15, 2004, from http://www.cdc.gov.ncipc.factsheets.suifacts.htm

Castiglia, P. T. (2000b). Depression in children. *Journal of Pediatric Health Care, 14,* 73–75.

Centers for Disease Control and Prevention. (2004a). *Suicide: Fact sheet.* Retrieved July 15, 2004, http://www.cdc.gov/ncbddd.dd.default.htm.

Centers for Disease Control and Prevention. (2004b). *Developmental disabilities.* Retrieved July 15, 2004, from http://www.cdc.gov.ncbddd.dd.default.htm

Christakis, D. A., Zimmerman, F. J., DiGiuseppe, D. L., & McCarty, C. A. (2004). Early television exposure and subsequent attentional problems in children. *Pediatrics 113,* 708–713.

Committee of Children with Disabilities, American Academy of Pediatrics. (2001). The pediatrician's role in the diagnosis and management of autistic spectrum disorder in children. *Pediatrics, 107,* 1221–1226.

Dales, L., Hammer, S. J., & Smith, N. J. (2001). Time trends in autism and in MMR immunization coverage in California. *Journal of the American Medical Association, 285,* 1183.

Department of Health and Human Services. (2000). *Report of the Surgeon General's conference on children's mental health: A national action agenda.* Washington, DC: U.S. Department of Health and Human Services.

Fish, K. B. (2000). Suicide awareness at the elementary school level. *Journal of Psychosocial Nursing, 38,* 20–23.

Geller, D. A., Biederman, J., Farone, S., Agranat, A., Cradock, K., Hagermoser, L., et al. (2001). Developmental aspects of obsessive compulsive disorder: Findings in children, adolescents and adults. *Journal of Nervous and Mental Disease, 189,* 471–477.

Gottesman, M. M. (2003). Helping parents make sense of ADHD diagnosis and treatment. *Journal of Pediatric Health Care, 17,* 149–154.

Hazell, P., O'Connell, D., Heathcote, D., & Henry, D. (2003). Tricyclic drugs for depression in children and adolescents (Cochrane Review). In *The Cochrane Library,* Issue 2. Oxford: Update Software.

Hoagwood, K., Burns, B. J., Kiser, L., Rindeisen, H., & Schoenwald, S. K. (2001). Evidence-based practice in child and adolescent mental health services. *Psychiatric Services, 52,* 1179–1189.

Horowitz, L. M., Wang, P. S., Koocher, G. P., Burr, B. H., Smith, M. F., Klavon, S., & Cleary, P. D. (2001). Detecting suicide risk in a pediatric emergency department: Development of a brief screening tool. *Pediatrics, 107,* 1133–1137.

Hudson, G. T., & Dixon, D. (2003). Autism: Challenges in diagnosis and treatment. *Clinician Reviews, 13,* 45–52.

Hyman, S. L., & Levy, S. E. (2000). Autistic spectrum disorders: When traditional medicine is not enough. *Contemporary Pediatrics, 17,* 101–116.

Jellinek, M., Patel, B. P., & Froehle, M. C. (2002). *Bright futures in practice: Mental health. Volume II. Tool kit.* Arlington, VA: National Center for Education in Maternal and Child Health.

Jick, H., & Kaye, J. A. (2003). Epidemiology and possible causes of autism. *Pharmacotherapy, 23,* 1524–1530.

Kaplan, E. L. (2000). PANDAS? Or PAND? Or both? Or neither? *Contemporary Pediatrics, 17,* 81–96.

Kaye, J. A., Melero-Montes, M. M., & Jick, H. (2001). Mumps, measles, and rubella vaccine and the incidence of autism recorded by general practitioners: A time-trend analysis. *British Medical Journal, 322,* 460–463.

Kent, J. M., Sullivan, G. M., & Rauch, S. L. (2000). The neurobiology of fear: Relevance to panic disorder and posttraumatic stress disorder. *Psychiatric Annals, 30,* 733–742.

Kessler, R. C. (2000). Posttraumatic stress disorder. *Journal of Clinical Psychiatry, 61*(Suppl. 15), 4–12.

Kidd, P. M. (2000). Attention deficit/hyperactivity disorder (ADHD) in children: Rationale for its integrative management. *Alternative Medicine Review, 5(5),* 402–428.

Kurlan, R., McDermott, M. P., Deeley, C., Como, P. G., Brower, C., Eapen, S., et al. (2001). Prevalence of tics in school children and adolescents associated with placement in special education. *Neurology, 57,* 1383–1388.

Lamberg, L. (2001). Psychiatrists explore the legacy of traumatic stress in early life. *Journal of the American Medical Association, 286,* 523–526.

Lambert, L. T. (2001). Identification and management of schizophrenia in childhood. *Journal of Child and Adolescent Psychiatric Nursing, 14,* 73–80.

Leonard, H. L., Freeman, J., Barcia, A., Garvey, M., Snider, L., & Swedo, S. E. (2001). Obsessive-compulsive disorder and related conditions. *Pediatric Annals, 30,* 154–160.

Lyon, D. E., & Morgan-Judge, T. (2000). Childhood depressive disorders. *Journal of School Nursing, 16(3),* 29–31.

March, J. S. (2004). Pediatric autoimmune neuropsychiatric disorders associated with streptococcal infection (PANDAS): Implications for clinical practice. *Archives of Pediatrics and Adolescent Medicine, 158,* 927–929.

Masi, G., Mucci, M., & Millepiedi, S. (2001). Separation anxiety disorder in children and adolescents: Epidemiology, diagnosis and management. *CNS Drugs, 15,* 93–104.

McDonnell, J. A., Doyle, R., & Surman, C. (2003). Current approaches to the management of ADHD: Diagnosis in adults is often overlooked. *Clinician Reviews, 13,* 110–117.

Melnyk, B. M., Brown, H. E., Jones, D. C., Kreipe, R., & Novak, J. (Eds.). (2003). Improving the mental/psychosocial health of US children and adolescents: Outcomes and implementation strategies from the National KySS Summit. *Journal of Pediatric Health Care, 17* (Suppl.), S1–S245.

Melnyk, B. M., Feinstein, N. F., Tuttle, J., Moldenhauer, Z., Herendeen, P., Veenema, T. G., et al. (2002). Mental health worries, communications, and needs of children, teens, and parents during the year of the nation's terrorist attack: Findings from the national KySS survey. *Journal of Pediatric Health Care, 16,* 222–234.

Melnyk, B. M., Moldenhauer, Z., Tuttle, J., Veenema, T. G., Jones, D., & Novak, J. (2003, February). Improving child and adolescent mental health: An evidence-based approach. *Advance for Nurse Practitioners,* 47–52.

Meltzer-Brody, S., Hidalgo, R., Connor, K. M., & Davidson, J. R. T. (2000). Posttraumatic stress disorder: Prevalence, health care use and costs, and pharmacologic considerations. *Psychiatric Annals, 30,* 722–730.

Meunier-Sham, J. (2003). Increased volume/length of stay for pediatric mental health patients: One ED's response. *Journal of Emergency Nursing, 29,* 229–239.

Mohr, W. K. (2001). Bipolar disorder in children. *Journal of Psychosocial Nursing & Mental Health Services, 39*(3), 12–23.

National Center for Learning Disabilities. (2004). *Learning disability.* Retrieved May 25, 2004, from http://www.ldanatl.org/

National Initiative for Children's Healthcare Quality. (2003). *Improving care for children with ADHD.* Boston: Author.

National Institute of Mental Health. (2004). *Antidepressant medications for children: Information for parents and caregivers.* Retrieved May 25, 2004, from http://www.nimh.nih.gov/press/StmntAntidepmeds.cfm?Output=Print.

National Strategy for Suicide Prevention. (2001). Suicide Prevention Facts. Retrieved November 5, 2001, from http://www.mentalhealth.org/suicideprevention.

Navon, M., Nelson, D., Pagano, M., & Murphy, M. (2001). Use of the pediatric symptom checklist in strategies to improve preventive behavioral health care. *Psychiatric Services, 52,* 800–804.

Rew, L., Thomas, N., Horner, S. D., Resnick, J. D., & Beuhring, T. (2001). Correlates of recent suicide attempts in a triethnic group of adolescents. *Journal of Nursing Scholarship, 33,* 361–167.

Roizen, N. J. (2002). Down syndrome. In M. L. Batshaw (Ed.), *Children with disabilities* (5th ed.). Baltimore: Paul H. Brookes.

Rynn, M. A., Siqueland, L., & Rickels, K. (2001). Placebo-controlled trial of sertraline in the treatment of children with generalized anxiety disorder. *American Journal of Psychiatry, 158,* 2008–2014.

Scharer, K. (2002). What parents of mentally ill children need and want from mental health professionals. *Issues in Mental Health Nursing, 23,* 617–640.

Shugart, M. A., & Lopez, E. M. (2002). Depression in children and adolescents. *Postgraduate Medicine, 112*(3), 53–61.

Smoller, J. W., Finn, C., & White, C. (2000). The genetics of anxiety disorders: An overview. *Psychiatry Annals, 30,* 745–753.

Towbin, K. E., Mauk, J. E., & Batshaw, M. L. (2002). Pervasive developmental disorders. In M. W. Batshaw. *Children with disabilities* (5th ed.). Baltimore: Paul H. Brookes.

Van Riper, M., & Cohen, W. I. (2001). Caring for children with Down syndrome and their families. *Journal of Pediatric Health Care, 15,* 123–131.

Walsh, K. H. (2002). Welcome advances in treating youth anxiety disorders. *Contemporary Pediatrics, 19*(9), 66–82.

Weller, E. B., Calvert, S. M., & Weller, R. A. (2003). Bipolar disorder in children and adolescents: Diagnosis and treatment. *Current Opinions in Psychiatry, 16,* 383–388.

Williams, P. G., Dalrymple, N., & Neal, J. (2000). Eating habits of children with autism. *Pediatric Nursing, 26,* 259–264.

Williamson, D. E., Birmaher, B., Brent, D. A., Bolach, L., Dahl, R. E., & Ryan, N. D. (2000). Atypical symptoms of depression in a sample of depressed child and adolescent outpatients. *Journal of the American Academy of Child and Adolescent Psychiatry, 39,* 1253–1259.

Yehud, R., Hallig, S. L., & Grossman, R. (2001). Childhood trauma and risk for PTSD: Relationship to intergenerational effects of trauma, parental PTSD, and cortisol excretion. *Developmental Psychopathology, 13,* 733–753.

The Child with Alterations in Musculoskeletal Function

When I got the call that Douglass was in the emergency room I was so scared. I guess we're lucky it was just a broken leg. I don't know what to do now, though—he broke his leg on a friend's trampoline. Should he go back to his friend's house? Should I tell him not to use the trampoline? It's hard to decide. And I never had a cast. What do you need to do with it?
—Mother of Douglass, 12 years old

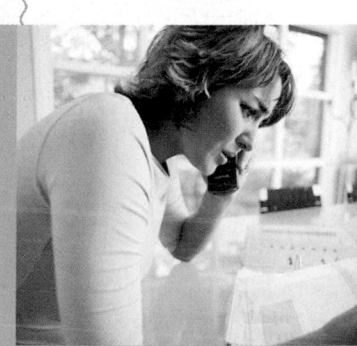

LEARNING OBJECTIVES

- Describe pediatric variations in the musculoskeletal system.

- Plan nursing care for children with structural deformities of the foot, hip, and spine.

- Recognize signs and symptoms of infectious musculoskeletal disorders and refer for appropriate care.

- Partner with families to plan care for children with musculoskeletal conditions that are chronic or require long-term care.

- Plan nursing interventions to promote safety and developmental progression in children who require braces, casts, traction, and surgery

- Provide nursing care for fractures, including teaching for injury prevention and nursing implementations for the child who has sustained a fracture.

MEDIALINK

www.prenhall.com/london

CD-ROM
Animation: Muscle Physiology
NCLEX-RN® Review
Audio Glossary

Companion Website
NCLEX-RN® Review
Thinking Critically
Case Study: Fracture Assessment
Care Plan: Home Care of an Infant in a Spica Cast
Audio Glossary

What concerns do parents and children have when a child has musculoskeletal conditions? Will the child need any special adaptations in the home and school? Can musculoskeletal injuries be prevented? The information in this chapter will answer these questions, and enable nurses to provide effective care for children who have musculoskeletal disorders.

The musculoskeletal system helps the body protect its vital organs, support weight, control motion, store minerals, and supply red blood cells. Bones provide a rigid framework for the body, muscles provide for active movement, and tendons and ligaments hold the bones and muscles together. Alterations in musculoskeletal functioning, therefore, can have a significant impact on a child's growth and development.

Musculoskeletal disorders may be congenital, such as clubfoot, or acquired, such as osteomyelitis. They may require short- or long-term management, and may be treated on an outpatient basis or require hospitalization. Many musculoskeletal disorders require surgical correction, casting, or braces.

Table 55–1 reviews several terms that will be used throughout this chapter in describing the positioning of a child's limbs.

ANATOMY AND PHYSIOLOGY OF PEDIATRIC DIFFERENCES

BONES

The bones of children and those of adults differ in several ways. Although primary centers of **ossification** (bone formation) are nearly complete at birth, a fibrous membrane still exists between the cranial bones (fontanelles) (see "As Children Grow: Sutures" in Chapter 35 ∞). The posterior fontanelle closes between 2 and 3 months of age. The anterior fontanelle does not close until approximately 18 months of age, allowing for growth of the brain and skull. In addition, the ends of the long bones (epiphyses) remain cartilaginous (Figure 55–1 ●). Long bone growth continues until approximately age 20 years, when skeletal maturation is complete.

Secondary ossification occurs as the long bones grow. Cartilage cells at the epiphyses are replaced by osteoblasts (immature bone cells), resulting in the deposition of calcium. Calcium intake during childhood and adolescence is essential to provide adequate bone density that will prevent osteoporosis and fractures in adulthood. See Chapter 34 for a discussion of inadequate calcium intake during school age and adolescence. ∞

The long bones of children are porous and less dense than those of adults. For this reason, children's bones can bend, buckle, or break as a result of a simple fall. Children and adolescents may suffer injuries to the musculoskeletal system from falls, car crashes, and sports. Fractures are one type of common injury. Because growth takes place at the epiphyseal plates, injuries to this portion of a long bone are of particular concern in young children.

In addition to the structural differences between the bones of children and adults, there are also functional differences in the skeletal system of children (see "As Children Grow: Children Are Not Just Small Adults" in Chapter 33 ∞). Before birth the thoracic and sacral regions of the spine are convex curves. As the infant learns to hold up the head, the cervical region becomes concave. When the child learns to stand, the lumbar region also becomes concave. Failure of the spine to assume these final curves results in an abnormal curvature of the spine (kyphosis or lordosis). The rapid bone growth

TABLE 55–1 ✜ **Musculoskeletal Positions**

Varus

An abnormal position of a limb that involves bending inward toward the midline of the body

Valgus

An abnormal position of a limb that involves bending outward away from the midline of the body

Adduction

Lateral movement of limbs toward the midline of the body

Abduction

Lateral movement of limbs away from the midline of the body

Inversion

Turning inward, usually more than normal

Eversion

Turning outward

Supination

Lying on the back or placing the hand so the palm faces upward

Pronation

Lying on the stomach or placing the hand so the palm faces downward

● **FIGURE 55-1**

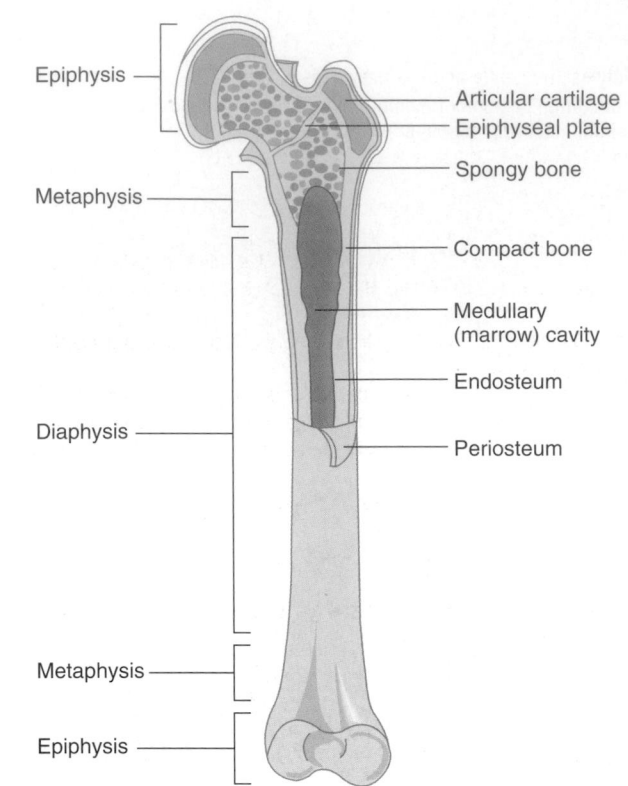

- Epiphysis
- Articular cartilage
- Epiphyseal plate
- Spongy bone
- Metaphysis
- Compact bone
- Medullary (marrow) cavity
- Endosteum
- Diaphysis
- Periosteum
- Metaphysis
- Epiphysis

The parts of long bones.

of childhood facilitates healing after fractures, but may also lead to "growing pains," as muscles are pulled when bones grow quickly.

MUSCLES, TENDONS, AND LIGAMENTS

The muscular system, unlike the skeletal system, is almost completely formed at birth. As a child grows, muscles do not increase in number, but rather in length and circumference. Until puberty, both ligaments and tendons are stronger than bone. When these structural differences are not recognized, a childhood fracture is sometimes mistaken for a **sprain**. A sprain is a tearing of ligaments, the structural support connecting bones, usually caused when a joint is twisted or otherwise traumatized. Tendons, which connect bones to muscles, grow in length and fibrous tissue as mechanical pressure is placed on them.

❋ DISORDERS OF THE FEET AND LEGS

METATARSUS ADDUCTUS

Metatarsus adductus, the most common congenital foot deformity, is characterized by an inward turning of the forefoot at the tarsometatarsal joints (Figure 55–2 ●). Of-

ten referred to as "intoeing," metatarsus adductus affects male and female infants equally and occurs in approximately 1 in 1000 births, with more common incidence among siblings. This condition is most likely caused by both intrauterine positioning and genetic factors (Ryan, 2001). Metatarsus adductus is differentiated from other causes of intoeing, such as internal tibial torsion (more common in children 12 to 18 months and learning to walk), and femoral anteversion (seen more often in preschool-age children).

Treatment depends on the degree of foot flexibility. If the foot can be readily maneuvered past the neutral position, simple exercises may correct the problem. Most cases resolve spontaneously by the time the infant is about 3 months of age. Serial casting is the treatment of choice for curvature angles greater than 15 degrees, or in cases that do not improve. The infant's feet are placed in a position as close to neutral as possible and are held secure with casts. Casts are changed weekly until the desired correction is achieved. Braces and orthopedic shoes may also be used to maintain correction after casting.

NURSING MANAGEMENT

Reassure parents that the child's condition can be corrected. If the child's deformity is mild, teach parents simple stretching exercises to perform at each diaper change. The foot is held securely by the heel, and the forefoot is moved outward from the body with the other hand. The position is maintained for 5 seconds, and repeated 5 times at each diaper change. If casting is necessary, provide cast care as

● **FIGURE 55-2**

Metatarsus adductus is characterized by convexity (curvature) of the lateral border of the foot. The child's right foot demonstrates the disorder. Note that the forefoot turns inward and appears out of alignment with the remainder of the foot.

TABLE 55–2 ✤ Nursing Care of the Child in a Cast

- A plaster cast takes anywhere from 24 to 48 hours to dry. When handling the wet cast, be gentle and use the palms of your hands, as fingertips can indent plaster and create pressure areas.
- After the cast is applied, elevate the extremity on a pillow above the level of the heart. Elevation helps reduce swelling and increases venous return.
- If the cast is applied after surgery, there may be drainage or bleeding through the cast material. Circle the stain and note the date and time on the cast to provide a way to assess the amount of fluid lost.
- Assess the distal pulses, and check the fingers and toes for color, warmth, capillary refill, and edema. Assess sensation as well as movement. Any deviation from normal may indicate nerve damage or decreased blood supply.
- During the first 24 hours, check the casted extremity every 15–30 minutes for 2 hours, then every 1–2 hours thereafter. The skin should be warm. It should blanch when slight pressure is applied and then return to its normal color within 3 seconds (**A**). For the next 2 days, assess the casted extremity at least every 4 hours.

- Check the edges of the cast for roughness or crumbling. If necessary, pull the inner stockinette over the edge of the cast and tape in place.
- The rough edges of the cast may also be alleviated by "petaling." This is done by securing adhesive tape to the inside of the cast and pulling it over the edge, covering the jagged or broken pieces of plaster, and securing it to the outer surface of the cast (**B, C, D**). Moleskin may be used on the cast as well.
- Keep the cast as clean and dry as possible. Cover the cast with a plastic bag or plastic wrap when the child bathes or showers.
- The skin under the cast may itch; however, do not use powders or lotions near the edges or under the cast as they can cause skin irritation.
- Be sure that children do not put small objects between the casts and their extremities; that can cause skin irritation as well as neurovascular compromise.

A

B

C

D

outlined in Table 55–2 and teach parents how to care for the child in a cast at home. If metatarsus adductus persists into childhood without correction, the challenge is to find shoes that accommodate the unusual shape of the foot.

CLUBFOOT

Clubfoot is a congenital abnormality in which the foot is twisted out of its normal position. It occurs in approximately 1 to 3 in 1000 births and affects boys nearly twice as often as girls and is bilateral in about half of cases (Gilmore & Thompson, 2003).

ETIOLOGY AND PATHOPHYSIOLOGY

The exact cause of clubfoot is unknown; however, several possible etiologies have been proposed. Some authorities believe abnormal intrauterine positioning causes the deformity. Others suspect neuromuscular or vascular problems as

causes. Yet other experts believe there is a genetic component, either at the chromosomal level or by the arrest of normal fetal development. A positive family history increases the chance of the deformity, and the incidence varies among ethnic groups. The condition is least common in Asian groups and Caucasians, with a higher incidence in groups from the Middle East, South Africa, and Mexico. It is most common in Polynesian groups (Blakeslee, 1997).

CLINICAL MANIFESTATIONS

A true clubfoot (talipes equinovarus) involves three areas of deformity: the midfoot is directed downward (**equinus**), the hindfoot turns inward (**varus**), and the forefoot curls toward the heel (adduction) and turns upward in partial supination. Muscles, tendons, and bones are all involved in the abnormality, and it cannot be corrected by exercise. Most children have this combination of findings. The foot is small with a shortened Achilles' tendon. Muscles in the

TEACHING HIGHLIGHTS

CARE OF THE CHILD WITH A CAST

Skin Care
- Check the skin around the cast edges for irritation, rubbing, or blistering. The skin should be clean and dry.
- You may cleanse the skin just under the cast edges and between the toes or fingers with a cotton-tipped applicator and rubbing alcohol. Avoid using lotions, oils, and powders near the cast as they may cause caking.
- Avoid poking sharp objects down inside the cast as this may result in sores.

Cast Care
- Keep the cast dry. Protect plaster with a cast shoe, thick sock, or sling.
- Allow a new, wet cast to air-dry for 24 hours.
- You may walk on a leg cast only if your physician has given you permission to do so.

Be Alert for Possible Complications
- Toes or fingers should be pink, not blue or white.
- Skin should be warm and the tips of the toes should blanch when pinched.
- Raise the casted arm or leg above heart level and rest it on pillows to prevent or reduce any swelling.

Notify Your Healthcare Provider If Any of the Following Occur
- Unusual odor beneath the cast
- Tingling
- Burning or numbness in the casted arm or leg
- Drainage through the cast
- Swelling or inability to move the fingers or toes
- Slippage of the cast
- Cast cracked, soft, or loose
- Sudden unexplained fever
- Unusual fussiness or irritability in an infant or child
- Fingers or toes that are blue or white
- Pain that is not relieved by any comfort measures (i.e., repositioning or pain medication)

Courtesy of Shriners Hospital for Children, Spokane, WA.

PATHOPHYSIOLOGY ILLUSTRATED
Clubfoot

Equinus

Varus

Supination

Bilateral clubfoot deformity. Parents of a child with clubfoot will have many questions. Can the condition be treated? Will the child be able to walk normally after surgery? Will they need help caring for the infant? How much will surgery and other care cost? Will any subsequent children have a clubfoot?

bones of the foot, which are primarily cartilaginous at birth, begin to ossify shortly thereafter. The foot is manipulated to achieve maximum correction first of the varus deformity and then of the equinus deformity. A long leg cast holds the foot in the desired position (Figure 55–3 ⊙). The cast is

⊙ **FIGURE 55–3**

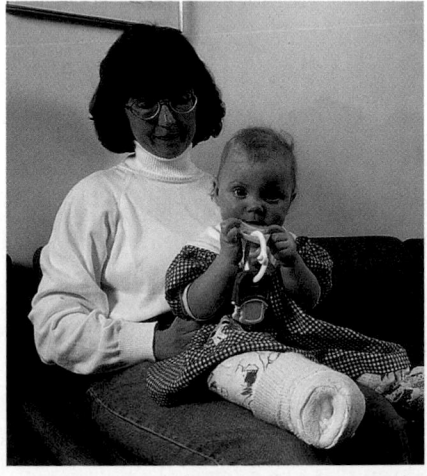

This girl has a long leg cast, which was applied after surgery to correct her clubfoot deformity.

lower leg are atrophied, but leg lengths are generally normal (see "Pathophysiology Illustrated: Clubfoot"). Clubhand is a rare occurrence that has characteristics similar to the foot deformity.

CLINICAL THERAPY

Diagnosis is made at birth on the basis of visual inspection. Radiographs are used to confirm the severity of the condition.

Early treatment is essential to achieve successful correction and reduce the chance of complications. Serial casting is the treatment of choice. Casting should begin as soon as possible after birth. Timing is critical because the short changed every 1 to 2 weeks. This regimen of manipulation and casting continues for approximately 8 to 12 weeks until maximum correction is achieved. If the deformity has been corrected, the child may begin wearing a splint or reverse last (shaped so that the foot turns outward away from the body instead of the normal inward turn) corrective shoes to maintain the correction (Gilmore & Thompson, 2003; Morcuende, Dolan, Dietz et al., 2004. If the deformity has not been corrected, surgery is required. Casting holds the foot in position until surgery is performed.

The age at which a child undergoes clubfoot surgery varies among surgeons. However, most children have surgery between 3 and 12 months of age. The one-stage posteromedial release procedure, which involves realignment of the bones of the foot and release of the constricting soft tissue, is most common. The foot is held in the proper position by one or more stainless steel pins. A cast is then applied with the knee flexed to prevent damage to the pin and to discourage weight bearing. Casting continues for 6 to 12 weeks. The child may then need to wear a brace or corrective shoes, depending on the severity of the deformity and the surgeon's preference.

More severe cases or those not corrected in infancy may require more than one surgery to correct the foot.

NURSING MANAGEMENT

NURSING ASSESSMENT AND DIAGNOSIS

Nursing assessment, which begins at birth and continues throughout the child's subsequent outpatient casting visits and hospitalization for surgery, includes taking a genetic and birth history, performing a physical examination (including position and appearance of the foot), and assessing the child's motor development and family's coping mechanisms. Because parents will need to bring the child for frequent cast changes, assess access to transportation and other arrangements needed for these visits.

Among the nursing diagnoses that might apply to the child with a clubfoot deformity are the following:

- *Impaired Physical Mobility* related to prescribed movement restriction of cast
- *Risk for Impaired Skin Integrity* related to cast
- *Altered Parenting* related to birth of a child with a physical defect
- *Health-Seeking Behaviors (Parental)* related to lack of information about deformity, treatment, and home care

PLANNING AND IMPLEMENTATION

Nursing management involves providing emotional support, educating the family about home care of the child in

a cast and the importance of keeping appointments at the outpatient facility for cast changes, preparing the family for the child's hospitalization if surgery is to occur, and providing postsurgical care.

Provide Emotional Support

Clubfoot affects both the child and the family. The child's foot deformity is upsetting to parents, and they need emotional support to allay their fears. Helping parents understand the condition and its treatment is essential.

Promote bonding by encouraging parents to hold and cuddle the child and to take an active role in the child's care. Explain that, with treatment, the child is expected to grow and develop normally.

Provide Cast and Brace Care

Routine cast care is outlined in Table 55–2 and is important to ensure skin and neurovascular integrity. After serial casting is complete, or after surgery, the child may progress to wearing a brace or special shoe for 6 to 12 months. Braces should fit snugly but should not interfere with neurovascular function. Before the child begins to wear a brace, check the skin for any areas of redness or breakdown. Give parents guidelines for brace wear. Emphasize that proper skin care is essential. If skin redness develops, arrange to have the fit of the brace evaluated and modified if necessary.

TEACHING HIGHLIGHTS

GUIDELINES FOR BRACE WEAR

- Braces should be as comfortable as possible and the child should have adequate mobility while wearing the brace.
- Begin wearing the brace for periods of 1 to 2 hours and then progress to 2 to 4 hours.
- Check the skin at 1- to 2-hour intervals initially, then lengthening to every 4 hours once skin has been clear for several days. If redness is apparent, leave the brace off and allow the skin to clear. If breakdown has occurred, the brace cannot be replaced until healing is complete. (See Chapter 57 for a discussion of pressure ulcers. ∞)
- Always have the child wear a clean white sock, T-shirt, or other thin white liner beneath the brace. Be sure the liner is wrinkle-free under the brace. Avoid using powders or lotions that can cause skin to break down. Toughen any sensitive areas using alcohol wipes.
- Reapply the brace when the skin returns to its normal color.
- Return to the physician or orthotic specialist if discomfort or red areas persist or if the brace needs adjustment or repair or is outgrown.
- Check the brace daily for rough edges.

Provide Postsurgical Care

Routine postoperative care after surgical correction includes neurovascular status checks every 2 hours for the first 24 hours and observing for any swelling around the cast edges (see Table 55–2). Apply ice bags to the foot, and keep the ankle and foot elevated on a pillow for 24 hours. This promotes healing and helps with venous return. Check for drainage or bleeding. Administer pain medication routinely for 24 to 48 hours. Popliteal or epidural blocks may be placed during surgery and used in the immediate post-surgical period for pain control. Monitor these blocks for effectiveness and any undesired effects (see Chapter 42 for detailed instructions on pain management ∞).

Discharge Planning and Home Care Teaching

Give parents written instructions for care of the child with a cast (see page 1766). In addition, assist them in the following ways:

- Demonstrate the use of a sponge bath to protect the cast from water breakdown.
- Discuss options for clothing that accommodate a cast, for example, one-piece snap suits or sweatpants.
- Discuss potential safety hazards that may result from awkward positioning. Be sure the child is properly situated in a car safety seat for the trip home.
- Provide resources for strollers and other equipment that will support the cast so it does not hang down during the baby's activities.
- Suggest that parents try to place toys within the child's reach, since the movements of a child in a cast may be slowed.

EVALUATION

Expected outcomes of nursing care include maintenance of skin integrity, recovery without complications after surgery, normal developmental progression of the child, and demonstrated parental knowledge of care of braces or casts, as needed.

GENU VARUM AND GENU VALGUM

Genu varum (bowlegs) is a deformity in which the knees are widely separated while the ankles are close together and the lower legs are turned inward (varus). In genu valgum (knock-knees), the knees are close together and the lower legs are directed outward (valgus) (Figure 55–4 ◉). Chapter 35 discusses the assessment of bowlegs and knock-knees in children. ∞

At certain stages of a child's development, the appearance of bowlegs or knock-knees is normal. Until 2 to 3 years

◉ FIGURE 55–4

A, Genu valgum, or knock-knees. Note that the ankles are far apart when the knees are together. *B,* Genu varum, or bowlegs. The legs are bowed so that the knees are far apart as the child stands.

of age, the knees are normally bowed, showing varus alignment, and by 4 to 5 years, some knock-knee or valgus alignment is common. However, the persistence of knock-knees beyond the age of 4 to 5 years necessitates further evaluation. The most common pathologic causes of bowed legs are Blount disease and rickets (see Chapter 35 ∞). Blount disease is characterized by abnormal growth on the medial side of the proximal tibia which causes an increasing varus deformity. It is believed to be due to increasing compression forces across the medial knee and is more common in overweight, black, and female children (Thompson, 2004b). Rickets is a result of inadequate bone mineralization, usually caused by a deficiency of calcium, vitamin D, or both. Since the bones are decalcified or softened, long bones such as those in the legs may bend into a bowed position. Occasionally rickets is congenital and is caused by an x-linked autosomal dominant or recessive gene with the chromosomal location Xp22.31-p21.3. It results in an enzyme deficiency of alkaline phosphatase which in turn leads to excessive inhibitors of bone mineralization. This type of rickets is rare and is called familial hypophosphatemic rickets (FHR).

Measurements, radiographs, arthrography (joint radiograph), magnetic resonance imaging (MRI), and computed tomography (CT) imaging may be used for accurate diagnosis. Braces are often used to correct mild deformities that could worsen as the child grows. Braces for bowlegs are worn at night; those for knock-knees both day and night. Duration of brace wear is determined by the severity of the deformity, which is usually evaluated by radiographs. If the deformity continues to worsen, surgery is necessary. Surgery is common in treatment of Blount disease. An **osteotomy** (cutting of the bone) is performed and the tibiofemoral angle surgically corrected. The child is then placed in a cast for approximately 6 to 10 weeks, or until completely healed. When dietary rickets is the cause of varus deformity, supplementation with calcium and vitamin D is needed. FHR is treated with calcium and phosphorus in 5 to 6 daily doses.

NURSING MANAGEMENT

Reassure parents that bowlegs and knock-knees are usually a normal part of a child's growth and development. These conditions often resolve on their own and need no treatment other than continued observation.

Nursing care focuses on educating the parents and child about the condition and its treatment. Give the child and family guidelines for brace wear and maintenance (see page 1767).

DISORDERS OF THE HIP

DEVELOPMENTAL DYSPLASIA OF THE HIP

Developmental dysplasia of the hip (DDH) refers to a variety of conditions in which the femoral head and the acetabulum are improperly aligned. These conditions include hip instability, **dislocation** (displacement of the bone from its normal articulation with the joint), **subluxation** (in this instance, a partial dislocation), and acetabular **dysplasia** (abnormal cellular or structural development) (American Academy of Pediatrics, 2000). In the past, DDH was referred to as congenital dislocated hip (CDH). The revised name of the disorder emphasizes that many cases of dislocation, subluxation, and dysplasia occur well after the neonatal period and involve more than a simple dislocation.

One in 100 newborns has hip instability, while dislocation occurs in 1 to 2 in 1000 births, and the condition affects girls four times as often as boys. It is unilateral in 80% of affected children, and the left hip is affected three times as often as the right (American Academy of Pediatrics, 2000).

ETIOLOGY AND PATHOPHYSIOLOGY

Although the exact cause of DDH is unknown, genetic factors appear to play a role. DDH is 20 to 50 times more common in first-degree relatives of an infant with the condition than in the general population. If one child of a set of identical twins has DDH, the other twin is affected 30% to 40% of the time. Some types of DDH are linked to early gestational events at 12 and 18 weeks' gestation, as the lower limbs rotate and surrounding muscles develop. On the other hand, milder cases may be influenced by mechanical forces in the last month of pregnancy such as

breech position or fetal size, and can occur after birth as the hip assumes an extended rather than flexed posture (Witt, 2003). The left hip is involved more often than the right hip as a result of intrauterine positioning of the left side of the fetus against the mother's sacrum. Maternal estrogen may cause laxity of the hip joint and capsule, leading to joint instability, especially in females who respond to these estrogen levels. DDH is more common in infants born in the breech position. Cultural factors may also be associated with DDH.

DEVELOPING CULTURAL COMPETENCE

DEVELOPMENTAL DYSPLASIA OF THE HIP

Infants who are positioned on cradleboards or traditionally swaddled, as in some Native American cultures, have a high incidence of developmental dysplasia of the hip (DDH). Canadian Indian babies have an incidence of 188/1000 births, and Navajo Indians in the southwestern United States have an incidence of 20/1000. Among cultures in which mothers carry infants on their hips or backs with the infants' legs abducted—as in Korean, Chinese, and some African groups—the incidence of DDH is very low and it rarely occurs (Witt, 2003).

CLINICAL MANIFESTATIONS

Common signs and symptoms of DDH include limited abduction of the affected hip, asymmetry of the gluteal and thigh fat folds, and telescoping or pistoning of the thigh (Figure 55–5 ●). The older child with untreated DDH walks with a significant limp, which results from telescoping of the femoral head into the pelvis. The longer the disorder goes untreated, the more pronounced the clinical manifestations become, and the worse the prognosis.

● **FIGURE 55–5**

The asymmetry of the gluteal and thigh fat folds is easy to see in this child with developmental dysplasia of the hip.

CLINICAL THERAPY

Physical examination reveals Allis' sign (one knee lower than the other when the knees are flexed) and positive Ortolani and Barlow maneuvers in babies under 8 to 12 weeks. Refer to Chapter 35 for a discussion of the assessment of hip dysplasia in newborns and infants. ∞ Radiographs are generally not reliable until approximately 4 months of age because the pelvis in a newborn is still primarily cartilaginous. Before 4 months of age, ultrasonography may be useful for diagnosis. After that age, radiographs are used for diagnosis.

Treatment plans vary according to the child's age. For infants younger than 3 months, the Pavlik harness is the most commonly used method for hip reduction (Figure 55–6 ●). The Pavlik harness is a dynamic splint— a splint that allows movement. It ensures hip flexion and abduction and does not allow hip extension or adduction. For infants older than 3 months of age, skin traction is used (Figure 55–7 ●). Correct positioning, which involves relocating the femoral head into the acetabulum while gently stretching the restrictive soft tissue, is essential. Surgery and a spica cast may be necessary. In children over 18 months of age, surgery and casting are usually necessary and bracing may also be required.

Early screening, detection, and treatment enable most affected children to attain normal hip function. Late diagnosis has lowered prognosis for full function.

● FIGURE 55–6

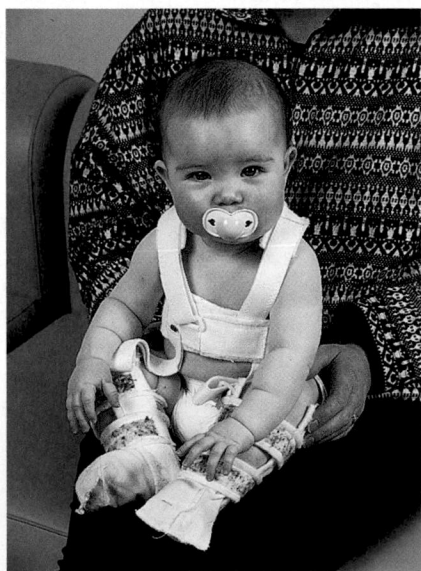

The most common treatment for DDH in a child under 3 months is a Pavlik harness. A shirt should be worn under the harness to prevent skin irritation. (It was omitted for clarity in this photograph.)

● FIGURE 55–7

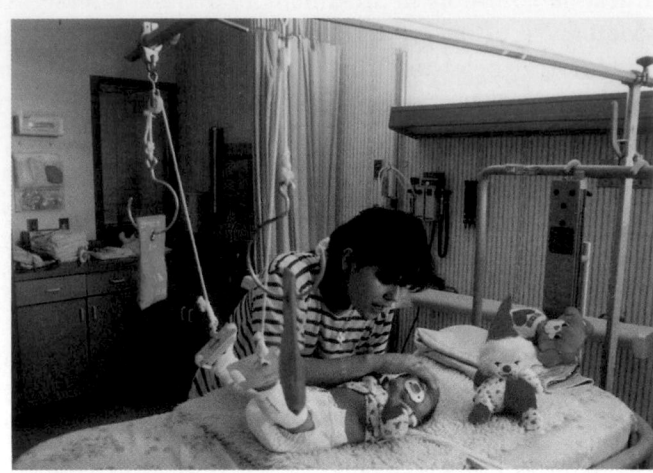

For infants older than 3 months of age, skin traction is commonly used for treatment of DDH.

NURSING MANAGEMENT

NURSING ASSESSMENT AND DIAGNOSIS

Assessment for DDH begins at birth and continues through all well-child checkups. The family history or birth data may indicate a high-risk infant. Instructions for performing the physical examination to assess the infant for DDH are given in Chapter 35. ∞ Once treatment begins, assessments are performed based on risks of the treatment. Assess the skin of the child in traction or a cast every few minutes in the immediate postoperative period, progressing to once or twice daily at home. Include respiratory and circulatory assessments when the child is immobilized. Ongoing assessment of the child's growth and development is needed. Weigh the casted child once the cast is dry so a baseline casted weight can be used for comparison while the cast remains in place.

Several nursing diagnoses that may apply to the child with DDH include the following:

- *Impaired Physical Mobility* related to prescribed movement restriction (Pavlik harness, traction, spica cast, brace)
- *Risk for Impaired Skin Integrity* related to irritation from harness straps or skin traction
- *Risk for Altered Urinary Elimination or Constipation* related to immobility caused by treatment
- *Risk for Impaired Nutrition* related to decreased appetite
- *Risk for Delayed Growth and Development* related to limited mobility and potential decreased exposure to stimulation

■ *Health-Seeking Behaviors (Parental)* related to lack of information about disease process and treatment

PLANNING AND IMPLEMENTATION

The infant with DDH is often cared for at home and in outpatient facilities. If surgery is performed, the child is hospitalized for surgery and the immediate postoperative period. Nursing care varies according to the medical treatment and the child's age. Management includes maintaining traction, if ordered; providing cast care; preventing complications resulting from immobility; promoting normal growth and development; and teaching parents how to care for a child in a cast, traction, or a Pavlik harness at home. Because treatment may interfere with the child's normal movement, the treatment plan should take into consideration the age and developmental stage of the child.

Maintain Traction

Bryant skin traction is the most common form of traction used in the treatment of DDH. (Types of traction are discussed later in the chapter.) Check the traction apparatus frequently to ensure proper alignment and healing. Traction may also be used in the home. The family needs careful instruction in how to care for the child in traction. In addition, a nurse should make several home visits to set up the traction apparatus and monitor the child's progress after discharge. The apparatus should be set up so that nuts and bolts are tight, knots are secure, weights are hanging free, and lines are straight. See Skill 17–6. **SKILLS**

Provide Cast Care

The principles of routine cast care presented in Table 55–2 apply to the care of spica casts. Special techniques should be used to help keep the cast clean and dry in children who are not toilet trained. Female and male urinals can be used for older children. Use a plastic lining to protect the cast edges during elimination for older children and use a small disposable diaper to cover the perineum in babies, tucking edges beneath the cast. Be sure to change the diaper frequently to prevent soiling of the cast.

Prevent Complications Resulting from Immobility

Immobilization from traction or a cast can cause alterations in physiologic functioning. To prevent complications:

■ Assess breathing patterns and lung sounds frequently for congestion or respiratory compromise.

■ Perform skin and neurovascular assessments approximately every 2 hours.

■ Use adequate padding and skin wrapping to avoid placing pressure on the popliteal space. Such pressure could lead to nerve damage.

■ For the child in a cast, change the child's position every 2 to 3 hours while awake to help avoid areas of pressure and promote increased circulation. The child can be placed either prone or supine or positioned on the floor and supported with pillows.

■ Help prevent skin irritation and breakdown in the child with a cast. Use moleskin to protect from rough edges. Place tape around the perineal opening of the cast to prevent soiling.

■ Increase fluids and fiber in the child's diet, as a change in bowel or bladder status is commonly associated with immobility.

■ If permitted by physician orders, release the child from traction for meals and daily care. The time out of traction should not exceed 1 hour per day. Encourage parents to hold and cuddle the child at this time to promote comfort and bonding.

Promote Normal Growth and Development

Engage the child in activities that stimulate the upper extremities and all five senses. Provide stimulating toys such as stacking blocks, brightly colored mobiles, soft balls, or musical toys. Position toys within the child's reach and interact with the child as much as possible.

Discharge Planning and Home Care Teaching

Teach parents how to care for a child in traction or a spica cast at home. Family members' active participation in the child's daily care during hospitalization gradually increases their confidence in their ability to provide care once home. Identify and address home care needs well in advance of discharge. Before discharge, be sure the parents have:

■ Information about general cast care (see page 1766), positioning, bathing, toileting, and age-appropriate diversional activities. Include body mechanics for the adults moving the child.

■ Knowledge of the importance of performing neurovascular checks and reporting any abnormalities immediately. Teach them circulation, motion, and sensitivity checks.

■ The parents should understand that the bar between the legs on the cast is not to be used for holding or turning the child. The bar is used to position the legs at the proper distance; using it to lift can cause the cast to fracture, weaken, or disintegrate.

■ Information on feeding the child.

- Safety teaching to minimize chance of injury to a casted child.

- Instruction about types of toys that are age-appropriate and measures to prevent them from being placed into the cast (a tee-shirt should be placed over the cast, covering its edges).

- Appropriate referrals for periodic assessment by a visiting nurse or home health nurse.

- Family resources to care for the child.

Before discharge, have parents demonstrate how to dress and feed a child in a spica cast. Ensure that safe travel arrangements have been made for the day of discharge. Help parents get an appropriate car safety seat in advance of discharge. Encourage parents to let the child interact with other children at home, and to provide the child in a cast with similar opportunities for play and social activities.

Nursing Care in the Community

Have parents of an infant in a Pavlik harness demonstrate proper application of the harness and care of the infant in the harness. Teach family members about daily care (bathing, dressing, and feeding) of the infant. Ideally, the harness is worn 23 hours per day and is removed only for skin checks and bathing. The hips and buttocks should be supported carefully when the infant is out of the harness. Demonstrate how to feed the infant in an upright position to maintain abduction and how to change a diaper without

TEACHING HIGHLIGHTS

TRANSPORTING THE CHILD WITH ORTHOPEDIC DEVICES

The American Academy of Pediatrics (1999) has established guidelines for transporting children with special healthcare needs.

- Riding in the rear seat is preferable.
- If the front seat must be used, the front passenger airbag should be disconnected.
- Use only car seat transport systems approved for use with special needs children.
- Install and use seats as instructed.
- Move a child from a wheelchair or other special device to the vehicle safety seat whenever this is reasonable.
- Pieces of medical equipment required during transportation (such as monitors or oxygen) or that are being transported with the child (such as wheelchair or walker) should be secured to the floor of the vehicle.
- If the child is transported by school bus, follow state and federal recommendations for school bus transportation of children with special needs.

TEACHING HIGHLIGHTS

GUIDELINES FOR PAVLIK HARNESS APPLICATION

1. Position the chest halter at nipple line and fasten with Velcro.
2. Position the legs and feet in the stirrups, being sure the hips are flexed and abducted. Fasten with Velcro.
3. Connect the chest halter and leg straps in front.
4. Connect the chest halter and leg straps in back.

All the straps are marked at the first fitting with indelible ink so they can be reattached easily after the harness is rinsed and dried.

removing the harness. Double-diapering may be recommended to support the hips.

Instruct the parents of an infant with a harness or a child in a cast to look for any reddened or irritated areas near the harness or cast edges and to check toes frequently for proper circulation. Frequent repositioning reduces the risk of pressure sores or circulatory compromise. The infant should wear an undershirt and socks under the harness to prevent rubbing of the skin.

Safety precautions are important as the child will not have normal mobility. Parents will need to use a specially designed car seat that accommodates the child with abducted hips. Strollers and cribs should provide sufficient room to protect the legs from injury and to prevent hip adduction.

EVALUATION

Expected outcomes for nursing care of the child with developmental dysplasia of the hip include the following:

- Maintenance of skin integrity
- Absence of complications due to immobility
- Knowledge by parents about the condition, treatment, and necessary home care
- Maintenance of a safe environment for the child

LEGG-CALVÉ-PERTHES DISEASE

Legg-Calvé-Perthes disease is a self-limiting condition in which there is avascular necrosis of the femoral head. The disease occurs in approximately 1 in 12,000 children and affects boys four times more often than girls. It usually occurs between the ages of 2 and 12 years, with an average age of 7 years at onset. The disease is bilateral in 20% of cases (Thompson, 2004a).

ETIOLOGY AND PATHOPHYSIOLOGY

The necrosis associated with Legg-Calvé-Perthes disease results from an interruption of the blood supply to the femoral epiphysis. How and why this occurs is not completely understood, but several predisposing factors have been identified. One theory is that a coagulation system disorder causes repeated vascular interruptions to the proximal femur (Eldridge, Dilley, Austin, et al., 2001). The incidence of Legg-Calvé-Perthes disease is up to 20% higher in families with a history of the disease than in the general population, which suggests that genetic factors may play a role. In one quarter of the cases, onset of the disease is preceded by a mild traumatic injury. Trauma may cause a subchondral fracture and resultant synovitis, which in turn causes pressure that occludes the blood supply. Children with Legg-Calvé-Perthes disease often have delayed skeletal maturation, increased thyroid levels, and low somatomedin C (insulin-like growth factor). It is more common in those with low birth weight, increased parental age, and exposure to environmental tobacco smoke (Roy, 1999).

CLINICAL MANIFESTATIONS

Legg-Calvé-Perthes disease progresses through four distinct stages after the original insult (usually unidentified)

occurs, over a period of 1 to 4 years. Early symptoms of Legg-Calvé-Perthes disease include a mild pain in the hip or anterior thigh and a limp, which are aggravated by increased activity and relieved by rest. The child favors the affected hip and limits hip movement to avoid discomfort (Davids, 1998).

As the disease progresses, range of motion becomes limited and weakness and muscle wasting develop. The affected thigh is 2 to 3 cm smaller than the unaffected thigh. Prolonged hip irritability may produce muscle spasms and increased pain. This period of the disease varies from 1 to 4 years. Gradually, revascularization begins and pain decreases.

CLINICAL THERAPY

Because the child's initial symptoms are so mild, parents often do not seek medical attention until symptoms have been present for several months. Diagnosis is made using standard anteroposterior and frog-leg radiographs. However, radiographs taken early in the course of the disease may be normal or show vague widening of the cartilage space. Bone scans and MRI may show the disease process

CLINICAL MANIFESTATIONS

LEGG-CALVÉ-PERTHES DISEASE

STAGE	CLINICAL MANIFESTATIONS
Prenecrosis	An insult causes loss of blood supply to the femoral head.
I—Necrosis	Avascular stage (3–6 months); the child is asymptomatic, bone radiographs are normal, and the head of the femur is structurally intact but avascular.
II—Revascularization	Period of 1–4 years characterized by pain and limitation of movement. Bone radiographs show new bone deposition and dead bone resorption. Fracture and deformity of the head of the femur can occur.
III—Bone healing	Reossification takes place; pain decreases.
IV—Remodeling	The disease process is over, pain is absent, and improvement in joint function occurs.

earlier than radiographs. Laboratory studies of the blood, such as white blood cell count, help to rule out inflammatory synovitis of the hip.

Medical management and prognosis depend on the degree of femoral involvement. Early detection is important. The desired outcome is a pain-free hip that functions properly. To promote healing and prevent deformity, the femoral head must be contained within the hip socket until ossification is complete. This can happen only if the hips remain in an abducted position. At the beginning of treatment, traction can be used to maintain the hips in an abducted and internally rotated position. Once abduction is accomplished, treatment consists of Petrie (leg abduction) casting, or surgical soft-tissue releases such as adductor tenotomy, followed by bracing. Toronto (Figure 55–8) and Scottish-Rite braces are most commonly used. Prognosis is good if the femoral head can be contained long enough for proper healing to occur. Severe disease may be treated by surgery to release adductor muscles, treat the acetabulum or femur, and restore range of motion. Children with untreated disease or those diagnosed late in the disease process occasionally develop osteoarthritis and hip dysfunction later in life (Roy, 1999).

NURSING MANAGEMENT

NURSING ASSESSMENT AND DIAGNOSIS

Suspect Legg-Calvé-Perthes disease in any child, especially a boy 2 to 12 years of age, who complains of hip discomfort accompanied by a limp. The school nurse may be the first person to observe the child with symptoms of Legg-Calvé-

◉ FIGURE 55–8

Although the Toronto brace may seem formidable for a child to wear, you can see by this photograph that, as usual, children adapt quite well to it.

Perthes disease. The child may complain of pain and have to rest during physical education classes. Refer the child to the healthcare provider immediately. Question the child who has an apparent limp about pain, and assess the child's range of motion. Ask if the child injured the hip at some time in the past.

Nursing diagnoses, which center on altered activities and compliance, might include the following:

- *Impaired Physical Mobility* related to restriction of brace or cast
- *Risk for Injury,* related to potential complications resulting from noncompliance with the treatment regimen
- *Risk for Noncompliance* related to duration of treatment
- *Deficient Diversional Activity* related to forced inactivity
- *Potential Disturbed Body Image* related to brace

PLANNING AND IMPLEMENTATION

Children with Legg-Calvé-Perthes disease often receive all of their treatment at home. Helping the child and family comply with the prescribed treatment plan may be challenging, because children develop the disease at an age when they are usually very active. The child, who may have little pain, often finds immobilization difficult.

Promote Normal Growth and Development

Give parents suggestions to help redirect the child's energy within the limitations in mobility imposed by treatment. A return to school promotes a feeling of normality. Coordinate the return to school by facilitating the child's use of an elevator or ramp as needed in that setting. Partner with the family to provide instruction for school personnel and other children to foster understanding of the child's condition and treatment. Activities that involve peers also help the child achieve developmental milestones. Help the child adjust to wearing a brace.

Nursing Care in the Community

Both the child and the family should be aware that treatment generally takes more than 2 years. Emphasize the importance of following the treatment plan to ensure adequate

GROWTH AND DEVELOPMENT

Legg-Calvé-Perthes disease primarily affects boys with an average age of 6 years. These school-age children are industrious and independent. Suggest activities that redirect energy and promote normal development. These may include horseback riding, which promotes hip abduction; swimming to increase mobility; handcrafts to promote fine motor skills; and computer activities to stimulate cognitive development.

hip containment and proper healing. Teach the family how to care for a child in traction and how to check the child's skin for breakdown (see Table 55–5 later in this chapter). Follow-up visits should be arranged at regular intervals, in addition to home care visits during the period of traction.

EVALUATION

Expected outcomes of nursing care are elimination of hip pain and discomfort, normal development during the period of immobilization, absence of complications, and parent and child knowledge of the treatment regimen.

SLIPPED CAPITAL FEMORAL EPIPHYSIS

Slipped capital femoral epiphysis (SCFE) occurs when the femoral head is displaced from the femoral neck. This condition is commonly seen during the adolescent growth spurt, between the ages of 12 to 15 years in boys and 10 to 13 years in girls. Boys are more often affected than girls. Blacks are affected more often than other ethnic groups. Children who are overweight are more likely to be affected as are those with sports injuries or other trauma, a history of radiation therapy, or endocrine disease (Acosta, Vade, Lomasney et al., 2001).

ETIOLOGY AND PATHOPHYSIOLOGY

The cause of SCFE is unknown. Predisposing factors include obesity, a recent growth spurt, and endocrine disorders such as hypothyroidism and hypogonadism. There may be a genetic predisposition to the development of the disorder (Acosta et al., 2001).

Slippage of the femoral head occurs at the proximal epiphyseal plate, and the femur displaces from the epiphysis (see "Pathophysiology Illustrated: Slipped Epiphysis"). Slippage is usually gradual (chronic), but may also result from acute trauma. The synovial membrane becomes inflamed, edematous, and painful. If untreated, callous formation occurs, resulting in a deformed hip with limited range of motion.

CLINICAL MANIFESTATIONS

Symptoms include limp, pain, and loss of hip motion. The condition is categorized as acute (sudden onset with less than 3 weeks' duration), chronic (longer than 3 weeks' duration), or acute-on-chronic (an additional slippage in a child with a chronic condition), depending on the onset and severity of symptoms. The child with an acute slip has sudden, severe pain and cannot bear weight. An acute slip may be associated with traumatic injury.

A chronic slip presents with persistent hip pain, which is generally aching or mild and can be referred to the

PATHOPHYSIOLOGY ILLUSTRATED
Slipped Epiphysis

Slipped epiphysis   Normal hip

In slipped capital femoral epiphysis, the femoral head is displaced from the femoral neck at the proximal epiphyseal plate.

thigh, knee, or both. A limp and decreased range of motion may also occur.

When the child has had a chronic slip and then sustains a traumatic incident that causes further slippage of the femoral head, an acute-on-chronic slip is said to have occurred. The child experiences sudden, severe pain.

CLINICAL THERAPY

A complete history provides information about risk factors and the development of the condition. Radiographs confirm the diagnosis. A bone scan, ultrasound, CT, and MRI may also be performed.

The goal of medical management is to stabilize the femoral head while keeping displacement to a minimum and retaining as much hip function as possible. Surgical treatment is usually necessary; this involves fixation of the epiphysis with screws or pins. If treated early, a single screw into the hip in an outpatient procedure is sufficient for stabilization; in more advanced cases, surgery becomes more complicated (Acosta et al., 2001). Medical treatment, which is occasionally used, includes a regimen of no weight bearing, bed rest, a spica cast, and Buck or Russell traction (see Table 55–4 later in this chapter).

Prognosis is related to the severity of the deformity and the occurrence of complications, such as avascular necrosis of the femoral head or **chondrolysis** (the breaking down and absorption of cartilage).

NURSING MANAGEMENT

NURSING ASSESSMENT AND DIAGNOSIS

The child usually presents with hip pain or referred pain to the groin, thigh, or knee, and limited mobility. A thorough history is needed to assess for injury as a cause. Assess the child's range of motion, pain, and limp, if apparent. Refer the child for treatment immediately if SCFE is suspected. This condition is considered to be an emergency, and it is essential that the child be treated immediately to keep weight off the affected joint.

Among the nursing diagnoses that may apply to the child with SCFE are the following:

- *Impaired Physical Mobility* related to treatment
- *Pain* related to hip injury
- *Risk for Disturbed Body Image* related to treatment
- *Risk for Delayed Growth and Development* related to mobility restrictions
- *Risk for Imbalanced Nutrition: More than Body Requirements* related to immobility
- *Ineffective Tissue Perfusion: Peripheral* related to traction, casting, and other treatments
- *Health-Seeking Behaviors (Child and Parental)* related to disease process and treatment

PLANNING AND IMPLEMENTATION

Nursing management involves caring for the child in traction or after surgery, administering medications and other pain-control interventions, maintaining mobility within the limits imposed by treatment, providing adequate nutrition, educating the child and family about the disorder, providing emotional support, and promoting compliance with the treatment plan.

Encourage Appropriate Nutritional Intake and Physical Activity

A growing adolescent needs increased amounts of proteins, carbohydrates, and calcium to promote skeletal healing. Provide written instructions about nutritional requirements to promote bone healing and maintain an ideal body weight. If a child is overweight, encourage weight loss by decreasing the percentage of fat and sugar in the diet and by increasing physical activity that is safe to do. Weight loss decreases pressure on the femoral epiphysis and can also lead to a more positive self-image. Incorporate upper body exercises into treatment, both to assist in weight control and to build muscle. A few visits to physical therapy may facilitate a program of upper body exercise and teach safe ways of increasing the total amount of physical activity.

Provide Emotional Support

Because the onset of SCFE is usually unexpected, the child and family may find themselves facing surgery with little warning. Explain the treatment plan simply and thoroughly. Reassure the child and family that with proper compliance, treatment should be successful.

Discharge Planning and Home Care Teaching

Help the family plan for the child's return to school. If attendance is not possible for a time due to traction or surgery, arrange for tutors and computer communication with school as needed. Follow-up visits are necessary until the child's epiphyseal plates close. It is not uncommon for SCFE to occur in the other hip. Make sure the child and family are aware of symptoms such as decreased range of motion or pain that could indicate onset of the disorder in the other hip. Tell parents to contact their healthcare provider immediately if these symptoms occur.

EVALUATION

Expected outcomes of nursing care for the child with slipped capital femoral epiphysis include maintenance of normal weight and recommended nutritional intake, absence of complications of immobility, successful adaptation to school following treatment, and family recognition of the need for ongoing monitoring for complications.

DISORDERS OF THE SPINE

SCOLIOSIS

Scoliosis is a lateral S- or C-shaped curvature of the spine that is often associated with a rotational deformity of the spine and ribs. Many people exhibit some degree of spinal curvature; curvatures of more than 10 degrees are considered abnormal. Curves are either structural or compensatory, as the spine curves to compensate for a structural deformity along its length. Idiopathic scoliosis occurs most often in girls, especially during the growth spurt between the ages of 10 and 13 years. Early onset of idiopathic scoliosis occurs before 10 years of age and comprises 15% of cases (Thompson, 2004a).

ETIOLOGY AND PATHOPHYSIOLOGY

The cause of scoliosis is complex. Structural scoliosis may be congenital, idiopathic, or acquired (associated with neuromuscular disorders such as muscular dystrophy or myelodysplasia, or secondary to spinal cord injuries).

In idiopathic structural scoliosis (the most common type), the spine for unknown reasons begins to curve later-

● FIGURE 55–9

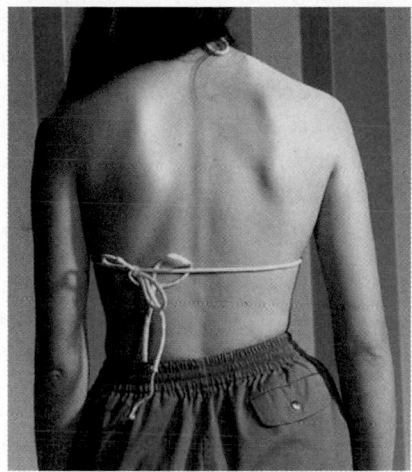

A child may have varying degrees of scoliosis. For mild forms, treatment will focus on strengthening and stretching. Moderate forms will require bracing. Severe forms may necessitate surgery and fusion. Clothes that fit at an angle, such as this teenage girl's shorts, and anatomic asymmetry of the back provide clues for early detection.

ally, with vertebral rotation. The most common curve is a right thoracic and left lumbar deformity. As the curve progresses, structural changes occur. The ribs on the concave side (inside of the curve) are forced closer together, while the ribs on the convex side separate widely, causing narrowing of the thoracic cage and formation of the rib hump. The lateral curvature affects the vertebral structure. Disk spaces are narrowed on the concave side and spread wider on the convex side, resulting in an asymmetric vertebral canal (Figure 55–9 ●).

Scoliosis can also occur in congenital diseases involving the spinal structure and in the musculoskeletal changes seen in conditions such as myelomeningocele, cerebral palsy (see Chapter 53 ∞), or muscular dystrophy. It can also be acquired after injury to the spinal cord.

CLINICAL MANIFESTATIONS

The classic signs of scoliosis include truncal asymmetry, uneven shoulders and hips, a one-sided rib hump, and a prominent scapula. The child does not complain of pain or discomfort.

CLINICAL THERAPY

Generally, observation and radiographic examination diagnose scoliosis. Additional diagnostic studies include MRI, CT, and bone scanning, which are used occasionally to assess the degree of curvature. The goal of medical management is to limit or stop progression of the curvature. Early detection is essential to successful treatment. Adequate treatment

and follow-up maximize the child's chances for proper spinal alignment. The treatment regimen chosen depends on the degree and progression of the curvature and the reaction of the child and family to medical management.

Treatment of children with mild scoliosis (curvatures of 10 to 20 degrees) consists of exercises to improve posture and muscle tone and to maintain, or possibly increase, flexibility of the spine. Emphasis is placed on bending strength toward the outside of the curve while stretching the inside of the curve. These exercises are not a cure, however, and the child should be evaluated by a physician at 3-month intervals, with radiographic evaluation every 6 months.

Medical management of moderate scoliosis (curvatures of 20 to 40 degrees) includes bracing with either a Boston or Milwaukee brace. The goal of wearing a brace is to maintain the existing spinal curvature with no increase. Brace wear begins immediately after diagnosis. To achieve maximum effectiveness, the brace should be worn 23 hours per day. Brace treatment is lengthy and requires a high degree of compliance, which can be difficult for adolescents, for whom body image or sports involvement is often important.

Children with severe scoliosis (curvatures of 40 degrees or more) require surgery, which involves spinal fusion. The majority of spinal fusions are performed using instrumentation with Luque wires, Coutrel-Dubosset (CD) instrumentation, Texas Scottish Rite Hospital system, and Moss-Miami system (Slote, 2002). These treatments stabilize the spine well during surgery, may be accompanied by bone grafting to the spine, and require no long-term therapy. Following surgery with wires or instrumentation, the child is on bed rest during a recovery period and then is generally fitted with anteroposterior plastic shells (also called thoracolumbar sacral orthotics) that are worn for several months to provide stability for the spine. The wires will remain in the back permanently.

NURSING MANAGEMENT

NURSING ASSESSMENT AND DIAGNOSIS

School nurses often screen children for scoliosis, generally in the fifth and seventh grades. Several states mandate this screening. When abnormalities are noted, refer the child to an orthopedic center for further evaluation. Children should be examined every 6 to 9 months thereafter. If scoliosis is detected, the child's brothers and sisters should be examined and observed closely. Scoliosis screening involves the following.
From the front:

■ Is the head midline?
■ Are the shoulders at the same height?

■ Is there the same amount of space between the arms and body on each side?

From the back:

■ Is the head midline?
■ Are the shoulders at the same height?
■ Are the scapulae equally prominent and at the same height?
■ Is the spine straight?
■ Is there the same amount of space between the arms and body on each side?
■ Are the hips at the same height?

With the adolescent holding hands together and bent over slightly:

■ Are the scapula humps even?

With the adolescent holding hands together and bent over toward the floor:

■ Are the flank humps even?
■ Is the spine straight?
■ Is there a marked roundness when viewed from the side? (evidence of kyphosis)

Once scoliosis has been identified, the focus becomes education and follow-up. Any child with scoliosis should have a comprehensive neurologic, cardiac, and respiratory examination, since the rib cage deformity can influence the functioning of these systems.

The following nursing diagnoses may apply to the child with scoliosis who is not having surgery:

■ *Risk for Noncompliance* with exercise program related to duration and intensity of exercise
■ *Impaired Physical Mobility* related to brace
■ *Risk for Impaired Skin Integrity* related to brace
■ *Health-Seeking Behaviors (Child and Parental)* related to unfamiliarity with disease process
■ *Disturbed Body Image* related to deformity and brace wear

Common nursing diagnoses for the child having surgery can be found in the accompanying "Nursing Care Plan".

PLANNING AND IMPLEMENTATION

An important aspect of nursing care is patient education. Patient acceptance is critical to the success of treatment. Children and their families need to understand the condition and the stages of treatment. This is particularly true for adolescents undergoing treatment for scoliosis. Children or adolescents facing surgery require education, reas-

surance, and support. Teach about pain control and the patient-controlled analgesia (PCA) pump. Often the child donates some of his or her own blood prior to surgery, and the family may also donate so blood transfused in surgery is the child's or family's. Teach the child the safety that this ensures. The adolescent will benefit from learning about deep breathing, positioning, surgical incision, and all other aspects of postoperative care. The "Nursing Care Plan" summarizes nursing care for the child undergoing surgery for scoliosis.

Promote Acceptance of the Treatment Plan

Provide instructions about exercises that will help to decrease the severity of the spinal curvature. Demonstrate the exercises, and explain their purpose (i.e., to strengthen back muscles). Help the child adjust to wearing a brace. Adolescents, in particular, may be reluctant to wear an external device such as a brace. To promote a sense of control, allow the adolescent to choose when to exercise and when to be out of the brace, within the treatment guidelines. Provide reassurance and encouragement and promote interaction with peers. Suggesting that the adolescent work with a peer support person who is being treated for scoliosis or has had the condition in the past may be beneficial. Provide information about fashionable clothing that can be worn with the brace and facilitate visits to department stores that will help the teen shop for clothing.

THINKING CRITICALLY

ADOLESCENT SELF-IMAGE AND BRACES

A comparison of 150 adolescents wearing a brace for scoliosis with 150 adolescents without scoliosis showed that those wearing the brace had poorer perception of self-image when completing the Piers-Harris scale "How I feel about myself." In addition, only 5% of youth with scoliosis had opportunities to discuss their feelings with health professionals, and 90% stated that they wanted more opportunities to do so (Sapountzi-Krepia, Valavanis, Panteleakis, et al., 2001). The findings that adolescents are concerned with body image is not surprising, considering the teens' developmental stage that focuses on appearance and fitting in with others. It is surprising that this is not acknowledged and discussed during healthcare. Health professionals should realize that wearing a brace can be difficult for adolescents and provide a chance for youth to discuss how they feel about the diagnosis and treatment. Consider interventions that aid in improving body image. What measures can you suggest to enhance the body image of a teen in an upper body brace? How can the adolescent find clothes that allow for wearing of the brace but meet contemporary fashions? What other interventions can enhance the teen's body image? How can you assess body image during visits in a clinic, office setting, or school?

NURSING CARE PLAN

THE CHILD UNDERGOING SURGERY FOR SCOLIOSIS

Intervention	Rationale	Expected Outcome
1. Nursing Diagnosis: Deficient Knowledge (Child and Parents) related to lack of information about surgery		
NIC Priority Intervention: **Teaching disease process and preoperative:** Assisting the patient to understand information and mentally prepare for surgery and postoperative recovery		**NOC Suggested Outcome:** **Knowledge:** Extent of understanding conveyed about scoliosis treatment
Goal: The child and parents will verbalize understanding of the disease, its treatment, and the surgical procedure.		
■ Teach the child and family about the course of the disease, its signs and symptoms, and treatment. Provide appropriate handouts. Encourage the child and parents to ask questions. ■ Begin preoperative teaching at the time of admission. Orient the child to hospital and postoperative procedures. Before surgery, have the child demonstrate log-rolling, range of motion exercises, and the use of an incentive spirometer. Discuss pain management.	■ Understanding and involvement increase motivation and compliance while reducing fear. ■ Preoperative teaching and familiarity with hospital procedures reduce the stress related to surgery and postoperative complications.	The child and family accurately verbalize knowledge about the disease and its treatment. The child and family ask appropriate questions about postoperative care.
2. Nursing Diagnosis: Ineffective Breathing Pattern related to hypoventilation syndrome		
NIC Priority Intervention: **Airway management and respiratory monitoring:** Facilitation of patency of air passages and analysis of patient data		**NOC Suggested Outcome:** **Respiratory status ventilation:** Movement of air in and out of the lungs
Goal: The child will show no signs of respiratory compromise.		
■ Monitor respiratory status, especially after the administration of analgesics. Apply pulse oximeter. ■ Administer oxygen if ordered ■ Have the child use an incentive spirometer. ■ Monitor intake and output. ■ Reposition the child at least every 2 hours.	■ Evaluation of the child's respiratory condition anticipates and avoids complications. Analgesics such as morphine may increase or potentiate respiratory compromise. ■ Oxygen increases peripheral oxygen saturation to 95%–100%. ■ Spirometry increases lung expansion and aeration of the alveoli. ■ Good hydration promotes loose secretions and helps prevent infection. ■ Repositioning ensures inflation of the lung fields.	The child has normal respiratory patterns.
3. Nursing Diagnosis: Risk for Injury related to neurovascular deficit secondary to instrumentation		
NIC Priority Intervention: **Injury prevention:** Instituting special precautions with patient at risk		**NOC Suggested Outcome:** **Risk control:** Actions to eliminate or reduce modifiable health risks
Goal: The child's neurovascular system will remain intact as evidenced by circulation, sensation, and motor checks. The child will feel no numbness or tingling.		
■ Monitor the child's color, circulation, capillary refill, warmth, sensation, and motion in all extremities. Perform neurovascular checks every 2 hours for the first 24 hours and then every 4 hours for the next 48 hours. Record presence of pedal and distal tibial pulses every hour for 48 hours. Report changes and abnormal findings immediately.	■ When the spinal column is manipulated during surgery, altered neurovascular status, thrombosis formation, and paralysis are possible complications. Postoperative risks include loss of bowel or bladder control, weakness or paralysis, and impaired vision or sensation.	The child exhibits only temporary alteration (pale skin, faint pulse, and edema occur but then resolve within the initial postoperative phase). The child returns to the preoperative baseline state by discharge.

(continued)

NURSING CARE PLAN—continued

THE CHILD UNDERGOING SURGERY FOR SCOLIOSIS

Intervention	Rationale	Expected Outcome
3. Nursing Diagnosis: Risk for Injury related to neurovascular deficit secondary to instrumentation *(continued)*		
■ Have the child wear antiembolism stockings until ambulatory. The stockings may be removed for 1 hour 2–3 times daily. ■ Check for any pain, swelling, or a positive Homans' sign in the legs. Record any evidence of edema. ■ Monitor input and output. ■ Encourage and assist the child with range of motion exercises, both passive and active.	■ Antiembolism stockings prevent blood clots and promote venous return. Thrombus formation is a postoperative risk. ■ Swelling may indicate a tight dressing and tissue damage. A positive Homans' sign and pain may indicate thrombus formation. ■ Abnormalities may indicate a fluid shift problem. ■ Activity promotes mobility and reduces risk of thrombus formation.	

4. Nursing Diagnosis: Pain related to spinal fusion with instrumentation

Intervention	Rationale	Expected Outcome
NIC Priority Intervention: **Pain management:** Alleviation of pain or a reduction of pain to a level of comfort acceptable to the patient		**NOC Suggested Outcome:** **Pain level:** Amount of reported or demonstrated pain

Goal: The child will verbalize an adequate level of comfort or show absence of pain behavior within 1 hour of a specific nursing intervention.

Intervention	Rationale	Expected Outcome
■ Assess the level of pain and initiate pain management strategies as soon as possible. Use patient-controlled analgesia if ordered. ■ Administer pain medication around-the-clock to help ensure pain relief, especially during the first 48 hours. Monitor epidural blocks and patient-controlled analgesia or other methods used for pain control. ■ Use nonpharmacologic pain management techniques, such as imagery, relaxation, touch, music, application of heat and cold, and reduced environmental stimulation to supplement medications (see Chapter 42 ∞). ■ Document pain assessment interventions and the child's reactions. ■ Reassure the child that some discomfort is expected and that a variety of measures can be tried to reduce discomfort.	■ Adequate pain management allows for faster healing and a more cooperative patient. Patient-controlled analgesics may be effective. ■ Medicating around-the-clock helps to maintain comfort. Monitoring ensures patient safety. ■ Alternative treatments also interrupt the pain stimulus and provide relief. Nonpharmacologic methods can be an effective adjunct to pain management. ■ Proper documentation guides the selection of the most effective means of pain control. ■ Realistic expectations decrease anxiety and give the child a sense of control.	The child experiences pain relief early in the postoperative period.

5. Nursing Diagnosis: Impaired Physical Mobility related to movement restrictions and pain

Intervention	Rationale	Expected Outcome
NIC Priority Intervention: **Positioning and ambulation:** Moving the patient to provide comfort and promote healing, assist with walking		**NOC Suggested Outcome:** **Ambulation:** Ability to walk from place to place

Goal: The child will maintain proper body alignment and progress with activity as ordered by the physician. If no anteroposterior shell bracing is required, the child will have active mobility by the third to fifth postoperative day.

Intervention	Rationale	Expected Outcome
■ Reposition the child every 2 hours using the log-roll technique. Support the back, feet, and knees with pillows.	■ Proper positioning prevents twisting or turning the spine.	The child is as mobile as appropriate for condition within 3–5 days after surgery.

NURSING CARE PLAN—continued

THE CHILD UNDERGOING SURGERY FOR SCOLIOSIS

Intervention	Rationale	Expected Outcome
5. Nursing Diagnosis: Impaired Physical Mobility related to movement restrictions and pain (continued)		
■ Have the child do passive and active range of motion exercises every 2 hours for 48 hours and then every 4 hours while awake. Have the child dangle his or her legs at the bedside by the second to fourth postoperative day. Begin ambulation by the third to fifth postoperative day. Note any complaints of dizziness, pallor, etc. Proceed slowly.	■ Exercises help maintain strength, circulation, and muscle tone. If the spine is stable and the physician has ordered no external support, the child may progress to full ambulation as tolerated. If the spine is not stable, great care must be taken until external supportive devices are used.	

6. Nursing Diagnosis: Risk for Disturbed Body Image related to treatment

NIC Priority Intervention: **Body image enhancement:** Improving conscious and unconscious perceptions toward the body		**NOC Suggested Outcome:** **Body image:** Positive perception of own appearance and body

Goal: The child will verbalize feelings about body image and self-esteem in relation to the disease and its treatment. The child will be informed about available support services and use them as needed.

■ Encourage independence in daily activities within allowable limits. Use positive reinforcements. Encourage the child to participate in community activities, if possible. Involve the child in scoliosis support groups. ■ Provide contact with a peer resource person who has undergone treatment for scoliosis.	■ Involvement in activities demonstrates that a "normal" life is realistic. ■ Peers are an effective means of support.	The child has a positive self-image and is involved in community activities or support groups.

7. Nursing Diagnosis: Risk for Deficient Knowledge (child and parents) related to lack of information about home care

NIC Priority Intervention: **Teaching: prescribed treatment:** Preparing family to understand and perform prescribed treatment		**NOC Suggested Outcome:** **Knowledge:** Extent of understanding conveyed about postoperative treatment and follow-up care

Goal: The child and family will verbalize reduced anxiety about home care. The child will demonstrate knowledge of self-care and permitted activities.

■ Teach cast or brace care as appropriate (see pages 1766 and 1767). Provide oral and written instructions and a list of activity limitations. Have the child and family demonstrate adequate knowledge. ■ Arrange for follow-up appointments as ordered by the physician. Encourage the child and family to notify the nurse or physician if they have any questions or concerns.	■ Providing education decreases anxiety and increases compliance with treatment plan. Demonstration reinforces the learning process. ■ Follow-up visits help the nurse and physician evaluate the effectiveness of the treatment plan and patient compliance.	The child and family demonstrate home care and implementation of discharge teaching.

Discharge Planning and Home Care Teaching

Identify and address home care needs well in advance of discharge after spinal surgery. The child will need to adapt to a new set of body mechanics. Show the child how to do simple tasks without bending or twisting the torso. Have the child demonstrate the ability to perform activities of daily living before discharge from the hospital. Partner with physical therapy/rehabilitation personnel to plan for the youth's needs related to safe and effective movement with the brace.

Activities for the child who has had spinal surgery are commonly limited for a period of time. The child can usually walk and perform physical activity such as gentle swimming, but lifting heavy loads, bending or twisting at the waist, or engaging in activities such as skiing, rollerblading, bicycle riding, and many other sports may not be allowed. Restrictions usually should be followed for 6 to 8 months, depending on the type of surgery and the surgeon. Emphasize to both the child and the family the importance of compliance. Give written discharge instructions to the child and family. Follow-up visits are important. The child should be examined 4 to 6 weeks after discharge, then every 3 to 4 months for 1 year, and every 1 to 2 years thereafter. The metal hardware in the back necessitates that after surgery the teen must carry a written physician explanation since the hardware will set off metal detectors at airports.

Several organizations provide information and assistance to families of children with scoliosis. Make referrals as appropriate.

EVALUATION

Expected outcomes of nursing care for the child with scoliosis treated by brace are maintenance of intact skin and compliance with prescribed therapy. Expected outcomes after surgical correction are listed on the accompanying "Nursing Care Plan."

TORTICOLLIS, KYPHOSIS, AND LORDOSIS

Torticollis is tilt of the head caused by rotation of the cervical spine. The cause is generally an injury sustained to the sternocleidomastoid muscle at the time of birth or to a cervical spine abnormality. Stretching exercises or surgical lengthening of the sternocleidomastoid muscle are usual treatments. Occasionally the cause of torticollis is visual impairment, leading to constant turning in one direction to see with the better eye.

Kyphosis (hunchback) and lordosis (swayback) are two other types of spinal curvature that may occur in children. Clinical therapy depends on the cause and degree of the curvature, and the age of the child at onset. Nurses can

GROWTH AND DEVELOPMENT

Postural lordosis is a characteristic finding in toddlers but should disappear by the school-age years.

perform thorough musculoskeletal assessments of children (see Chapter 35 ∞) and refer any children with abnormalities for further evaluation.

ADDITIONAL DISORDERS OF THE BONES AND JOINTS

OSTEOPOROSIS AND OSTEOPENIA

Osteoporosis, a condition in which there is decreased density and mass of bone, promotes the risk of fractures and is commonly associated with aging. However, children can have osteoporosis (also known as metabolic bone disease or a bone mineral density more than 2.5 standard deviations below the norm) related to imbalanced nutrition or other pathologic conditions. Osteoporosis is preceded by osteopenia or low bone mass, which is between 1 and 2.5 standard deviations below the norm (Bowman & Russell, 2001; Chan & Bishop, 2002).

ETIOLOGY AND PATHOPHYSIOLOGY

Very-low-birth-weight infants who are premature often have osteopenia of prematurity because much of bone mass is usually acquired in the latter weeks of pregnancy. In addition, they may have other health problems after birth and be unable to ingest enough nutrients to meet metabolic needs for bone growth. Prematures are often less active than other infants, which decreases the amount of mechanical loading on their bones, a factor known to increase bone resorption and decrease bone mass (Abad-Sinden, Verbrugge, & Buck, 2001; Moyer-Mileur, Brunstetter, McNaught et al., 2000).

A group of children who may show signs of osteoporosis are those who have decreased mechanical loading. Children with spina bifida or cerebral palsy, conditions that interfere with ambulation, have limited pressure on bones and resultant lowered bone mass in affected extremities and spine. Some other conditions are associated with lower bone mass, including Turner syndrome, growth hormone deficiency, osteogenesis imperfecta, juvenile rheumatoid arthritis, and diabetes. Children who are treated for disorders or injuries with casting and bracing are also at high risk of osteoporosis due to immobilization.

Lastly, adolescence is a period when adequate intakes of calcium and vitamin D are needed to maximize bone

CLINICAL MANIFESTATIONS

KYPHOSIS AND LORDOSIS

CONDITION	CLINICAL MANIFESTATIONS	DIAGNOSTIC TESTS AND CLINICAL THERAPY	NURSING MANAGEMENT
Kyphosis Excessive convex curvature of the cervical thoracic spine	Visible hunchback or rounded shoulders; shortness of breath or fatigue; abdominal creases and tight hamstrings in severe cases	*Diagnostic tests:* Spinal curvature is assessed by having the child bend 90 degrees at the waist and looking at the scapular area from side. Diagnosis is confirmed by radiograph. *Clinical therapy:* Exercises are prescribed for mild condition; bracing is commonly used; surgery is performed in severe cases.	Provide support. Encourage exercises and diligent brace wear. Help the child to deal with the psychologic stress of altered body image.
Lordosis Excessive concave curvature of the lumbar spine with an angle of more than 60 degrees; most common in prepubescent girls and African Americans	Presence of swayback; prominent buttocks; hip flexion contractures; tight hamstrings	*Diagnostic tests:* Spinal curvature is assessed by looking at the standing child from the side. Lumbar lordosis is confirmed by visualizing the spine on standing, lateral radiograph. *Clinical therapy:* Treatment focuses on exercises and postural awareness. Bracing and surgery are rarely prescribed.	Provide support. Reassure the child and family that the condition is often outgrown as the child matures. Encourage physical conditioning exercises and follow-up examinations on a yearly basis.

formation and prevent osteoporosis later in life. Adolescents, particularly females, often do not meet the recommended daily allowance (RDA) for these nutrients and are at risk for osteoporosis even though it may not be manifested for years. Other lifestyle patterns of youth that decrease bone formation are smoking, alcohol use, excessive soda intake, and keeping weight at a very low level (Durst, 2000). Those with anorexia nervosa are clearly at risk for osteoporosis.

CLINICAL MANIFESTATIONS

Osteoporosis is a silent disease, as is its precursor osteopenia; those who have the disorders are often without signs or symptoms for years. It may become apparent when a baby or child has a fracture and radiologic studies make the problem evident.

CLINICAL THERAPY

Bone mineral content and density are measured by single-photon absorptiometry (SPA), dual-photon absorptiometry (DPA), and dual-energy x-ray absorptiometry (DEXA). Although uncommonly used, serum studies such as bone-specific alkaline phosphatase, phosphorus, and type-I collagen can be used to measure osteoblastic and osteoclastic activity. Over 90% of the body's calcium is stored in bone so serum calcium is not reflective of bone density.

Premature newborns at risk of osteopenia of prematurity need collaborative management by neonatologists, neonatal nutritionists, and neonatal nurses. Breast milk is enhanced by adding special fortifiers; premature formula should be used rather than regular baby formula. When babies need enteral or parenteral feedings, calcium-to-phosphorus ratios are carefully balanced to enhance osteoblastic activity. Extremity range of motion for very-low-birth-weight newborns can decrease bone loss in the period after birth (Litmanovitz, Dolfin, Friedland et al., 2003).

For older children at risk of developing osteoporosis, calcium and vitamin D intake is encouraged and oral supplements may be given. Standing therapy for those who are nonambulatory can provide mechanical weight and enhance bone density (Caulton, Ward, Alsop et al., 2004). Bisphosphonates, calcitonin, fluoride, and parathyroid hormone have been used but there are no clear data to indicate their effectiveness in children (Chan & Bishop, 2002). When a cast or other immobilizing device is removed from a child, a gradually increasing program of exercise in collaboration with physical rehabilitation professionals promotes bone strengthening and lowered risk for fractures or related sequelae.

NURSING MANAGEMENT

NURSING ASSESSMENT AND DIAGNOSIS

Nurses identify newborns, children, and adolescents at risk of developing low bone mass and density. This is accomplished by identifying diseases putting the child at risk. Ask about exercise and activity patterns, and physical therapy for children who are nonambulatory. Dietary intake is measured periodically for all youth at health promotion visits, and RDAs for calcium, phosphorus, and vitamin D are compared to intake.

Nursing diagnoses that may apply to the child with osteoporosis include the following:

■ *Imbalanced Nutrition* related to inability to consume essential nutrients

■ *Risk for Injury to Bones* related to decreased bone mass and density

■ *Ineffective Health Maintenance* related to inadequate dietary intake

PLANNING AND IMPLEMENTATION

Perform a dietary analysis of children at risk (see Chapter 34 for detailed methods for diet assessment ∞). Refer children at risk to nutritionists and physicians for further education and diagnosis. Suggest referrals to physical rehabilitation to recommend weight-bearing exercise. Administer nutritional supplements when prescribed, and teach families how to give these medications. Partner with families to provide therapy that stimulates weight bearing for nonambulatory children. Teach parents how to recognize fractures in children who may not have normal sensation and are unable to report them. Swelling, unusual shape of a limb, fussiness of the child, and falls should be reported promptly.

When osteoporosis is due to immobility, many other symptoms occur as well. Be alert for these problems and integrate physical activity into care as much as possible to minimize their effects.

EVALUATION

Expected outcomes of nursing care for the child with a potential for osteoporosis include adequate intake of recommended amounts of nutrients, absence of fractures, and normal findings on studies of bone mineral content and density.

OSTEOMYELITIS

Osteomyelitis is an infection of the bone, most often one of the long bones of the lower extremity. It may be acute or chronic and may spread into surrounding tissues. Although osteomyelitis may occur at any age, it is most common in children between the ages of 1 and 12 years. Boys are affected two to three times as often as girls, primarily because they have a greater incidence of trauma (Carek, Dickerson, & Sack, 2001).

ETIOLOGY AND PATHOPHYSIOLOGY

Osteomyelitis is caused by a microorganism, usually bacterial but possibly viral or fungal. *Staphylococcus aureus* is the most common causative pathogen, followed by *Escherichia coli*, group B streptococci, *Streptococcus aureus*, *Streptococcus pyogenes*, and *Haemophilus influenzae*. Common sources of infection are upper respiratory infection, trauma to the bone, and surgery.

The infecting organism spreads through the bloodstream or through a penetrating injury to the bone, where it becomes established. Most infections in children begin in the metaphysis (see Figure 55–1), which has a sluggish blood supply. Eventually the infection may penetrate the bone cortex and periosteum. Inflammation and abscess formation can interrupt the blood supply to the underlying bone, affect the surrounding soft tissue, and, if the infection is left untreated, lead to necrosis.

CLINICAL MANIFESTATIONS

Symptoms include pain and tenderness with swelling, decreased mobility of the infected joint, and fever. Redness over the area may occur. The child may refuse to walk or may limp. The onset of acute osteomyelitis is generally rapid and is therefore sometimes misdiagnosed as a sports injury (Fernandez, Carrol, & Baker, 2000).

CLINICAL THERAPY

A history suggestive of osteomyelitis includes an upper respiratory infection or blunt trauma followed by pain at the area of a growth plate. Laboratory evaluation shows leukocytosis and an elevated erythrocyte sedimentation rate (ESR) and C-reactive protein (Carek et al., 2001). The degree of ESR elevation is directly related to the severity of the infection. Radiographs and bone scans may identify the area of involvement. A needle aspiration of the site or a blood culture can confirm the diagnosis and provide a culture of the causative organism.

GROWTH AND DEVELOPMENT

Osteomyelitis in a newborn is of great concern, as before 18 months of age the blood vessels cross the growth plates. This creates a higher risk of epiphyseal involvement with resultant limb length discrepancy.

Medical management begins with the intravenous administration of a broad-spectrum antibiotic, even before culture results are available. Since *S. aureus* is a common cause of infection, the antibiotic should be effective against this organism. Treatment is influenced by the possibility of methicillin-resistant *S. aureus* (MRSA), so beginning antibiotics are usually vancomycin or clindamycin, drugs effective against MRSA. Once the culture results are obtained, the antibiotic may be altered. Oral antibiotics are given once an adequate response has occurred. However, extended intravenous home therapy may be used. Antibiotic therapy continues for about 3 to 6 weeks. The cause of infection is not always identified from culture so ESR and C-protein are followed carefully in these cases to identify if treatment is successful. Some clinicians treat with antibiotics until the ESR is <25–30 mm/hour (Givner & Kaplan, 2003). When an adequate response is not obtained within 2 to 3 days, the area may be aspirated again, or surgically drained. Intravenous fluids may be administered to ensure adequate hydration. In children with extensive orthopedic surgery, or in those with immunosuppression, a short course of prophylactic antibiotic may be administered after surgery.

Prompt diagnosis and treatment usually completely resolve the infection. The prognosis is related to the initiation of therapy—the earlier treatment begins, the better the outcome. Long-term unfavorable outcomes include disruption of the growth plate, which can interrupt growth, and damage to the joints from septic arthritis.

NURSING MANAGEMENT

NURSING ASSESSMENT AND DIAGNOSIS

A thorough history, including information about the onset of symptoms and a history of recent infections or puncture wounds, is essential. Ask about immunization status, especially tetanus vaccine. Assess the affected area for signs of redness, swelling, pain, and decreased range of motion. Measure vital signs; increased temperature and pulse in particular may provide clues about worsening infection. When osteomyelitis is possible, all cultures of blood or wound must be taken before antibiotic therapy is started.

Among the nursing diagnoses that may apply to the child with osteomyelitis are the following:

- *Acute Pain* related to biologic injury
- *Impaired Physical Mobility* related to discomfort
- *Risk for Infection (Sepsis)* related to spread of infection
- *Risk for Imbalanced Nutrition: Less than Body Requirements* related to loss of appetite
- *Health-Seeking Behaviors (Child and Parental)* related to lack of information about disease process

PLANNING AND IMPLEMENTATION

Nursing management focuses on administering antibiotics, protecting the child from spread of the infection, and encouraging a well-balanced diet. Use standard precautions, with transmission-based precautions for any drainage from the site of infection.

Obtain Cultures and Blood Work

Blood cultures and cultures of any open wound must be performed before the first dose of antibiotic when osteomyelitis is suspected. Obtain continuing blood samples as needed to monitor ESR and C-reactive protein. See Skill 10–5. **SKILLS**

Administer Fluids and Medications

Administer intravenous fluids as ordered to maintain the child's hydration status. Antibiotics are administered intravenously, at first, then orally. Monitor the intravenous site and provide care for the central line, if one is used. See Skill 12 5. **SKILLS**

In the early stages of the infection, analgesics are prescribed to relieve the associated pain and joint tenderness.

Protect from the Spread of Infection

Strict aseptic technique and transmission-based precautions should be used during all dressing changes. Children and family members should avoid direct contact with any dressings or drainage. Teach good hygiene practices, including handwashing, to maintain infection control. Take vital signs and evaluate the child frequently for symptoms indicating the spread of infection (e.g., increasing pain, difficulty breathing, increased pulse rate, fever).

Encourage a Well-Balanced Diet

Educate both the child and the parents about healthy dietary choices that promote healing. A high-protein diet and extra vitamin C will contribute to this process. Encourage increased fluid intake to provide adequate hydration and circulation.

Discharge Planning and Home Care Teaching

Emphasize the importance of completing the full course of antibiotic therapy, especially for children who have had an abscess or lesion surgically drained. Some children may be discharged on intravenous antibiotics if the family is willing to learn the procedure for medication administration and care of the central line. Several sessions of demonstration and return demonstration are needed to ensure safe administration. If the family is unable to perform antibiotic therapy, a home infusion company may be available to come to the home and administer the medication. Explain that failure to follow the prescribed antibiotic therapy may result in chronic infection. Emphasize the importance of returning for blood analysis to monitor progression of healing.

Consider the child's age and developmental level and partner with the family to plan quiet activities and access to school work. Provide suggestions for the family if the child will be immobilized at home.

NURSING PRACTICE

If the child needs to remain home for a period of time during treatment for osteomyelitis, help the family plan for completion of school tasks.

- Contact the school and ask that work be sent home.
- Arrange for a tutor if needed.
- Facilitate computer communication between child, teacher, and other students.
- Help the family plan for help at home to monitor the child when they need to be at work or performing other tasks.
- Refer families to financial resources as appropriate for the services the child needs.
- Suggest activities that the child can do at home that foster developmental progress.

EVALUATION

Expected outcomes of nursing care for the child with osteomyelitis include the following:

- Absence of signs of infection or sepsis
- Completion of prescribed course of antibiotics
- Prevention of infection in contacts
- Adequate intake of fluids and nutrients
- Absence of pain
- Return to normal activities of daily living

SKELETAL TUBERCULOSIS AND SEPTIC ARTHRITIS

Skeletal tuberculosis (Figure 55–10 ●) and septic arthritis are two infections that, although infrequent, may affect chil-

● **FIGURE 55–10**

This boy from Kenya had surgery to correct severe kyphosis and scoliosis, caused by tuberculosis of the spine. A Risser cast has been applied to maintain stability of the spine and thoracic cage during healing. Notice the area cut out of the cast to allow for auscultation of the abdomen, as well as to facilitate the child's comfort and adequate intake of food.

dren and adolescents. See "Clinical Manifestations: Skeletal Tuberculosis and Septic Arthritis" for diagnostic tests and medical and nursing management for these infections.

ACHONDROPLASIA

Dwarfism is a genetic condition usually resulting in an adult height of 58 inches or less. The most common cause of dwarfism is achondroplasia which causes short arms and legs. The torso and head are approximately normal size, but decreased growth of long bones causes short stature. This is known as disproportionate short stature. Achondroplasia is caused by an abnormal gene of chromosome 4 and occurs in 1 in 26,000 births (March of Dimes, 2004). The gene is coded to produce proteins called fibroblast growth factor receptors. When less receptors are produced the cells cannot respond normally to signals from growth factors. Achondroplasia may occur as a new genetic mutation with no previous family history or can occur when one or both parents are also dwarfs. There are other less common forms of dwarfism with about 200 identified types.

Children with achondroplasia have short legs and arms, short fingers with a separation between middle and ring fingers, and a large, prominent forehead. Hydrocephalus sometimes occurs in children with achondroplasia (see Chapter 53

CLINICAL MANIFESTATIONS

SKELETAL TUBERCULOSIS AND SEPTIC ARTHRITIS

CONDITION	CLINICAL MANIFESTATIONS	DIAGNOSTIC TESTS AND CLINICAL THERAPY	NURSING MANAGEMENT
Skeletal Tuberculosis Rare microbacterial infection that can be very destructive. The spine is the most frequent site of infection (Pott's disease), with joints and other sites sometimes affected.	Depending on the site, pain, limp, severe muscle spasms, kyphosis, muscle atrophy, "doughy" swelling of joints, decreased joint motion, changes in reflexes, low-grade fever	*Diagnostic tests:* Diagnostic studies include tuberculosis skin test, complete blood count, synovial fluid analysis, and radiographs of affected limb or joint. *Clinical therapy:* Antibiotic therapy (using a combination of drugs) for 6–9 months is the treatment of choice. The affected site is immobilized. Disease may become resistant to these drugs, and additional drug therapy may be necessary.	Educate the child and family about the disorder and stress the importance of complying with long-term antibiotic therapy. Test all members of the family for tuberculosis. Report the disease to the local health department. Facilitate the immobilization and physical therapy of the child at home.
Septic Arthritis Joint infection of the synovial space most often caused by *Haemophilus influenzae*, *Staphylococcus,* and *Streptococcus*. The most common site of infection is the knee, followed by the hip, ankle, and elbow.	Fever, pain and local inflammation, joint tenderness, swelling, loss of spontaneous movement	*Diagnostic tests:* Diagnosis is made based on joint aspiration findings. Radiographic changes may not be evident until later in the disease process. *Clinical therapy:* This is a medical emergency requiring prompt treatment to avoid permanent disability. Treatment involves joint aspiration, open drainage, and irrigation, followed by intravenous antibiotic therapy for 3–4 weeks and then oral antibiotics. If the full course of antibiotic treatment is not completed, the child risks recurrent infection and further degeneration of the infected joint.	Educate the child and family about the disorder and emphasize the importance of proper antibiotic therapy. Carefully position the painful joint.

for a description of hydrocephalus ∞). Most children with the disorder inherit the gene from one parent. Since only one faulty gene must be present for manifestation of the disorder, it is a dominant characteristic. When a child inherits two copies of the gene from two affected parents, a fatal form of achondroplasia occurs which is characterized by a small thorax, respiratory failure, and death in infancy.

Children with the disorder are diagnosed at birth or shortly after. When there is a family history, genetic testing before or after birth identifies the presence of the faulty gene. Characteristics common in the growth disorder include frequent otitis media, dental malocclusion, bowing of legs, and sleep apnea. Marked lordosis can be present during childhood. Low back and leg pain are common as the child grows into adulthood. Perhaps the greatest challenge for families is helping the child to establish a positive self-image in a society that values greater height.

There is no treatment for the disorder at this time. Gene therapy and human growth hormone therapy are being explored as possible future treatments. Some children and adults with dwarfism have undergone limb-lengthening procedures such as that described later in this chapter (see page 1799).

Other orthopedic intervention may be needed to treat back pain or bone problems. For those children who develop hydrocephalus, insertion of a shunt to divert excess fluid may be needed. Treatment of conditions such as otitis media and malocclusion of teeth is provided.

NURSING MANAGEMENT

Nurses play an important role in helping families when a child is diagnosed with achondroplasia. If a parent is a dwarf or there is a positive family history of dwarfism, genetic counseling should be offered prenatally. Explain findings of testing and provide assistance with decision making about pregnancy if needed. Nurses assist parents who have a child with achondroplasia to adjust to the diagnosis, particularly if the parents have had no previous experience with the condition. They may feel guilt and anxiety; contact with other families who have children with achondroplasia can be a supportive intervention.

Nurses help the child with achondroplasia to develop a positive self-concept during childhood. Many resources such as the Little People of America Web site provide suggestions about how to foster a positive self-concept, adjust the home to facilitate the dwarf, and assist the child with adjustments in school settings. Partner with school nurses to ensure the child's successful inclusion in all school facilities. While some families decide to explore limb-lengthening procedures, most organizations state that focus should be placed on development of a healthy self-image rather than encouraging limb lengthening.

Nurses provide careful assessments of children throughout childhood. Head circumference is especially important in early childhood to identify hydrocephalus if it should occur. Carefully evaluate growth with specialized growth grids for achondroplasia, evaluate dental health at each visit, and perform developmental assessment with special emphasis on gross motor skills. Suggest activities such as swimming and biking that provide activity with little stress on bones. Assist the family by providing resources that assist with planning for car safety seats, methods of adjusting the home, and partnering with the school to provide a supportive atmosphere for the child. Some helpful organizations include Little People of America, Dwarf Athletic Association of America, Human Growth Foundation, Magic Foundation for Children's Growth and Related Adult Disorders, and March of Dimes. Refer for care for otitis media and provide postoperative care if ear tubes are inserted (see Chapter 46 ∞). Refer to dentists and orthodontists and encourage regular dental care.

MARFAN SYNDROME

Marfan syndrome is another example of a condition inherited in an autosomal dominant manner. About 1 in 5000 children are affected with the syndrome which manifests with several conditions of connective tissue. The most common problems are cardiac (mitral valve prolapse, aortic regurgitation, abnormal aortic root dimensions), skeletal (pectus excavatum, long arms and digits, scoliosis, elongated head, high arched palate), ocular (lens subluxation), and respiratory (pneumothorax) (Yetman, Huang, Bornemeier et al. 2003). The average age for diagnosis is 3 years, with a heart murmur the usual finding. Careful assessment identifies additional characteristics of the condition along with a positive family history.

There is no treatment for the syndrome, which causes abnormal formation of fibrillin matrix in connective tissue. However, early diagnosis can be successful in treating the cardiac abnormalities with medication or surgery to prevent dissection of the aorta, the major cause of death (Holcomb, 2000). Surgery may be needed to correct scoliosis, pectus excavatum, or pneumothorax. Careful monitoring throughout life is needed to prevent and treat abnormalities associated with the disorder.

Nursing management of Marfan syndrome begins with identification of infants and children with symptoms of the disorder. Once diagnosed, collaboration with a cardiologist, ophthalmologist, and orthopedist is needed throughout the child's life. The child may require surgery for one or more conditions, can require antibiotics during elective procedures or dental care if the mitral valve is affected, and needs echocardiogram and other cardiac studies regularly. The nurse may need to explain the disorder to the family and provide referrals for genetic counseling. The child needs support during childhood to learn about the disorder and to manage the medication and monitoring required.

 THINKING CRITICALLY

AUTOSOMAL DOMINANT DISORDERS

Both achondroplasia and Marfan syndrome are autosomal dominant disorders. Does this mean that the child needs one or two genes to manifest the disorders? If one parent has the disorder, what is the chance that a pregnancy will result in an affected child? Will there ever be a carrier who does not manifest the disease? See Chapter 3 for further information about autosomal dominant inheritance. ∞

OSTEOGENESIS IMPERFECTA

Osteogenesis imperfecta, also known as brittle bone disease, is a connective tissue disorder that primarily affects the bones. Children with this condition have fragile bones that are more likely to fracture. The major type of osteogenesis imperfecta occurs in 1 in 30,000 live births and affects boys and girls equally. Clinical manifestations include multiple and frequent fractures; blue sclerae; thin, soft skin; increased joint flexibility; enlargement of the anterior fontanelle; weak muscles; soft, pliable, brittle bones; and short stature. Conductive hearing loss can occur by adolescence or young adulthood (Paterson, Monk, & McAllion, 2001).

The underlying disorder is a biochemical defect in the production of collagen. The disease is genetically transmitted, generally in an autosomal dominant inheritance pattern, although some types are transmitted in a recessive pattern. The most common types are caused by mutations on the COLIA 1 or COLIA 2 genes on chromosomes 17 and 7 (Astrom & Soderhall, 2002).

The disease is classified into four types. In type I disease, the most common form, children have fragile bones, blue sclerae, weakened tooth dentin, and possible hearing loss that manifests in adolescence. In type II disease, the ribs and skeleton are extensively involved; most children with this form of the disease die in utero or shortly after birth. Type III disease is identified in the newborn period or in infancy when the child sustains numerous fractures and manifests blue sclerae. Severe bone fragility and kyphoscoliosis are observed. Type IV disease is characterized by fractures without other symptoms of the disease. Bowing of the legs and other structural deformities can occur; however, the incidence of fractures decreases beginning in puberty (Osteogenesis Imperfecta Foundation, 2003).

Improved knowledge about the genetic transmission of this disease means that some cases of osteogenesis imperfecta can be identified before birth using ultrasound or collagen analysis of chorionic villus cells. In many cases, however, diagnosis of osteogenesis imperfecta is made only when the child has a delay in walking or sustains a fracture. Radiographic evaluation may detect old as well as new fractures. This may lead to an erroneous diagnosis of child abuse. Tests such as DEXA can be used to measure bone density. Serum alkaline phosphatase may be elevated; other measures of bone metabolism such as serum osteocalcin, procollagen 1 C-terminal peptide, collagen 1 teleopeptide, and urine deoxypyridinoline may be performed occasionally to measure effects of experimental medication.

There is no cure for osteogenesis imperfecta. Medical management consists primarily of fracture care and prevention of deformities. The goal is to maximize the child's independence and mobility while minimizing the risk of fractures. Treatment includes physical therapy; casting, bracing, or splinting; surgical stabilization; nutritional management with high vitamin D and calcium; and bisphosphonate medication such as pamidronate (Gonzalez, Pavia, Ros et al., 2001). Bone marrow transplant has been used successfully in some children with severe osteogenesis

imperfecta and is under further research (Horwitz, Prockop, Gordon et al., 2001).

NURSING MANAGEMENT

Nursing care is primarily supportive and focuses on educating the parents and child about the disease and its treatment. The family may have been suspected of child abuse before the disease was diagnosed; explain the similar presenting symptoms of these cases. Ask about favorite activities of the child since these will need to be integrated into plans for physical activity and developmental progression. Perform careful growth measurements and developmental screening.

To prevent fractures, children with osteogenesis imperfecta must be handled gently. Support the trunk and extremities using a blanket whenever moving the child. Such tasks as bathing and diapering may cause fractures and should be performed carefully. Never pull the legs upward during diaper changes, but slip a hand gently under the hips to raise them.

Children usually have several or many fractures during childhood. The period of immobility and casting causes further bone breakdown due to decreased weight bearing, further increasing the chance of fracture. The child should have a well-balanced diet with additional vitamin C, vitamin D, and calcium to encourage healing and bone growth. Calories should be limited to maintain weight at recommended levels since immobility can lead to overweight and the child is generally short for his or her age. Partner with parents if the child is receiving experimental bisphosphonate medication, so that doses are properly administered and serum/urine samples are obtained for monitoring.

When the child needs a fracture stabilized in surgery, or is having rods inserted to strengthen bones, surgical care management is important. Assess the child's vital signs and growth measurements. Obtain accurate weight before surgery and again after with the cast in place. Administer fluids and use pain control techniques such as medication and other comfort measures. Be alert for signs of infection such as osteomyelitis, or respiratory or urinary tract infection. Begin fluids and perform dietary teaching before discharge to promote intake that fosters healing. Follow activity orders precisely to minimize safety hazards for the family. Partner with physical and occupational rehabilitation professionals to plan for the child's return home and to school and to ensure the family can perform range of motion exercises and other therapies. Ensure that the family has an approved car safety seat to transport the child.

Emphasize the importance of maintaining normal patterns of growth and development. Help toddlers explore and interact safely in their environment. Socialization is essential during the school-age and adolescent years. Encourage exercise, such as swimming, to improve muscle tone and prevent obesity. Adaptive equipment and motorized wheelchairs promote independent functioning. Maintenance of function can depend on proper rehabilitation services. Arrange and manage such services for the family.

The Osteogenesis Imperfecta Foundation provides information about the disease and can put families in touch with others who have the disease. See the Companion Website for links to these resources. Parents should receive genetic counseling. For parents who have a child with type II or III osteogenesis imperfecta, the terminal nature of the condition necessitates psychologic support, linkage to potential resources, and assistance with managing other tasks of family life (see Chapter 41 for management of end-of-life care ∞). The siblings and extended family will need support to understand the disease and deal with their feelings and the affected child.

MUSCULAR DYSTROPHIES

The muscular dystrophies are a group of inherited diseases characterized by muscle fiber degeneration and muscle wasting. These disorders can begin early or late in life, and onset can be at birth or gradual. They are all terminal disorders but the progression can vary from a few to many years.

Many kinds of muscular dystrophies affect children and adults. The most common form of childhood muscular dy-

CLINICAL MANIFESTATIONS

MUSCULAR DYSTROPHIES OF CHILDHOOD

TYPE OF DYSTROPHY	CLINICAL MANIFESTATIONS	CLINICAL THERAPY
Duchenne Muscular Dystrophy X-linked recessive disorder seen in boys (on Xp21 gene); however, 30%–50% of affected children have no family history Onset: within the first 3–4 years of life	Delayed walking; frequent falls; easily tired when walking, running, or climbing stairs; toe walking, hypertrophied calves; waddling gait; lordosis; positive Gowers' maneuver; mental retardation frequently seen	Supportive care; physical therapy and braces to help maintain mobility and prevent contractures Most children are wheelchair bound by 12 years of age; death usually occurs during adolescence from respiratory or cardiac failure
Becker Muscular Dystrophy X-linked recessive disorder Onset: usually after 5 years	Symptoms are similar to those of Duchenne muscular dystrophy, but milder and delayed; child is mobile until late teens; normal intelligence; congestive heart failure; contractures	Supportive care, same as for Duchenne muscular dystrophy Slow progression (same as for Duchenne muscular dystrophy); death usually occurs from the third to the fifth decade of life
Facioscapulohumeral Muscular Dystrophy Autosomal dominant disorder (on 4q35 chromosome) Onset: later childhood and adolescence	Face, shoulder girdle, lower limbs affected; unable to raise arms over head; lordosis; cannot close eyes, whistle, smile, or drink from a straw because of inability to move face; characteristic appearance includes facial weakness, winging of the scapula, thin arms, well-developed forearms	Physical therapy Slow progression; confined to wheelchair as older adult, but usually attains normal life span
Emery-Dreifuss Muscular Dystrophy X-linked recessive disorder (on Xq28 gene) Onset: childhood	Early onset of contractures followed by weakness; Achilles' tendon, elbow, and spine affected; muscle weakness in upper body follows, with lower body weakness occurring later; cardiac conduction defect may occur	Physical therapy Surgery Pacemaker insertion
Congenital Muscular Dystrophies Autosomal recessive group of disorders Onset: present at birth	Muscle weaknesses present at birth; motor development delay; contractures and joint deformities; hypotonia	Correction of skeletal deformity (orthosis or surgery) Usually nonprogressive

strophy is Duchenne muscular dystrophy (pseudohypertrophic), which occurs in 1 in 3500 live male births. **Pseudohypertrophy** refers to enlargement of the muscles as a result of their infiltration with fatty tissue. The gene for Duchenne muscular dystrophy was identified in 1987; it is carried in the Xp21.2 region of the chromosome and is either absent or deleted in affected children. This area codes for a protein called dystrophin which is needed as a muscle membrane stabilizer. A cascade of cellular events occurs, leading to necrosis in the fibers and their replacement by connective tissue and fat (Papazian & Alfonso, 2002). Since this is an X-linked disorder, it is seen only in males. There is similar incidence in various ethnic groups.

Becker muscular dystrophy is also X-linked and affects 1 in 20,000 males. Although the gene mutation is similar to

Duchenne, it is milder in form. Other rare muscular dystrophies manifest in infancy, later childhood, or adolescence. There are a variety of genetic mutations ranging from X-linked to autosomal.

Diagnosis and classification are most often based on clinical signs and the pattern of muscle involvement. Children with muscular dystrophy have generalized muscle weakness. They compensate for weak lower extremities by using the upper extremity muscles to raise themselves to a standing position (Gowers' maneuver) (Figure 55–11 ⊙). Biochemical examinations such as serum enzyme assay, muscle biopsy, and electromyography confirm the diagnosis. Serum creatine kinase (CK) is elevated early in the disease. Muscle biopsy can measure dystrophin, the muscle protein that is deficient in muscular dystrophy. Genetic

⊙ **FIGURE 55–11**

A

B

C

D

E

Since the leg muscles of children with muscular dystrophy are weak, these children must perform the Gowers' maneuver to raise themselves to a standing position. **A** and **B,** The child first maneuvers to a position supported by arms and legs. **C,** The child next pushes off the floor and rests one hand on the knee. **D** and **E,** The child then pushes himself upright.

HEALTH PROMOTION

The Child with Muscular Dystrophy

The child with muscular dystrophy needs close monitoring and intervention to foster growth and development in spite of a chronic and terminal disease. The nurse in health promotion can assist the child and family in many ways.

Growth and Development Surveillance
- Perform developmental screening of the young child.
- Refer to early intervention programs that establish educational plans to foster development.
- Provide resources and ideas for the parents based on the child's status rather than expected age norms.
- Measure growth at each healthcare visit and plot on growth grids. Be alert for the child who is gaining weight due to decreased activity in order to avoid overweight.

Nutrition
- Perform 24-hour analysis and evaluate for all essential nutrients. Base the analysis on the child's height and weight rather than chronological age.
- Ask about appetite and food likes and dislikes.
- Encourage adequate fluid, whole grains, fruits, and vegetables to maintain bowel function.
- For the infant with muscular dystrophy, evaluate intake carefully; gavage feeding or nutritional supplementation such as with high-calorie formula may be needed.

Physical Activity
- Carefully monitor physical ability at each visit. Observe for decreases in movement, difficulty ambulating, or a history of falls.
- Partner with physical therapists to ensure range of motion and proper positioning of extremities.
- Explore activities that the child can do as mobility decreases. Swimming and upper body exercise may be good options.
- If the child is using a wheelchair, evaluate fit, safety, and ability to move the chair by arm controls.
- Physical activity should be regular and daily. Ensure that the family has resources to accomplish this need.

Activities of Daily Living
- Partner with occupational therapy to evaluate the child's ability to feed, bathe, dress, and provide own oral care. Provide adaptive devices as needed.
- Encourage the family to provide time for the child to perform own self-care as much as possible.
- Make a home visit or discuss with the family adaptations that could make it easier for the child to be independent in activities of daily living. Low drawers for clothing, or open shelves that do not require pulling out to get items are examples of important adaptations.

Mental and Spiritual Health
- Inquire about the child's general mood.
- Ask the parents what is best and worst about their lives at this time. Use the information to establish a list of their meaningful activities and to identify the areas most in need of support.
- Ask about sources of support such as a group for parents of a child with muscular dystrophy, family participation in faith-based activity, and extended family or neighbors.
- Be alert for signs of depression in child or family (see Chapter 34 ∞).
- Assist the family to establish activities to increase self-esteem in the youth. The youth should be able to make choices appropriate for developmental age.
- If the child was diagnosed at a younger age, ask what the parents have now told him or her about the disease. Provide support and role-playing opportunities for parents who wish to tell the child about the terminal nature of the disorder.
- Refer for services such as genetic counseling, grief counseling, or other supportive interventions.

Relationships
- Ask about siblings and their relationship with the child with muscular dystrophy.
- Inquire about the child's participation in early intervention or school programs, and community groups. Refer the family to resources that encourage the child's interactions with peers. This is particularly important for teens.
- Ask the parents if and how often they are able to spend time with other adults.

Disease Prevention Strategies
- Immunize the child at recommended times. If the child is ill and immunization is delayed, be sure to call the family back promptly so that infectious diseases can be avoided. Annual influenza vaccine is needed. If the child is treated with steroids for the disease, follow recommendations for immunization of children on steroids.
- Teach the family to avoid crowds and known infectious persons. The child may need to be out of school for a few days or weeks if there is influenza or other diseases in the school population.
- Teach the family signs of infection, especially of the respiratory tract. Have them report these symptoms promptly.
- Monitor effects of antibiotics when administered for infection.
- Encourage daily activities that encourage deep breathing. Swimming, blowing into an incentive spirometer, or playing with a pinwheel are examples.

Injury Prevention Strategies
- Inquire about whether the family has an emergency evacuation plan for the child in case of house fire or other emergency. Assist them to develop a plan.
- If the child is using oxygen, teach about fire safety.
- When mechanical ventilation is used at home, help the family establish emergency backup systems for power outage, such as portable generators.
- Assist the family to learn proper body mechanics to safely transfer and provide care for the child.

testing establishes the specific abnormality and type of disease present. Testing of newborns may be offered to families who have one child with the disease since this helps some families to adapt and prepare for the care the child will need (Parsons, Clarke, Hood et al., 2002). Respiratory function is measured periodically with pulmonary function tests and overnight pulse oximetry (Sobus, Horan, & Warren, 2000).

There is no effective treatment for childhood muscular dystrophy. Research is being directed at several techniques to repair mutations by gene therapy (Takeda & Miyagoe-Suzuki, 2001). The steroids prednisone and deflazacort may preserve muscle function, preserving walking for a longer period (Biggar, Gingras, Feblings et al., 2001).

Progressive weakness and muscle deformity result in chronic disability (Figure 55–12 ◉). The goal of medical management is to provide support and prevent complications such as infection or spinal deformities. The team ap

◉ FIGURE 55–12

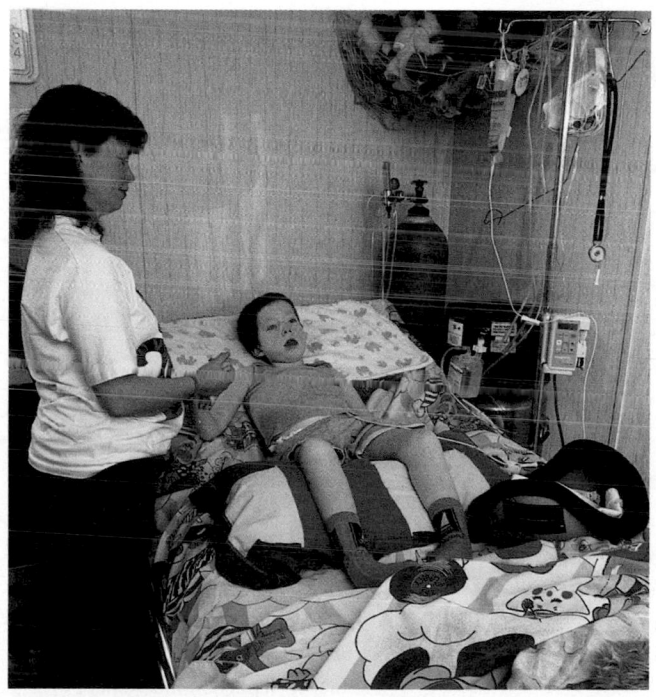

This young boy with muscular dystrophy needs to receive tube feedings and home nursing care. He attends school when possible and is able to use an adapted computer.

proach to managing the child with muscular dystrophy ensures a comprehensive management plan. Team members should include physicians (pediatrician, orthopedic surgeon, neurologist), nurses, physical and occupational therapists, a nutritionist, and a social worker.

NURSING MANAGEMENT

Nursing care focuses on promoting independence and mobility and providing psychosocial support that helps the child and family deal with this progressive, incapacitating disease. Nearly all body systems become involved in the disease, and emotional care is important as well for child and family.

Monitor cardiac and respiratory functioning frequently. Administer oxygen or respiratory therapy as ordered. Perform periodic developmental and nutritional assessments, and give parents suggestions for encouraging the child's development. Meet with teachers to evaluate the child's learning needs and functioning in the classroom.

Encourage the child to be independent for as long as possible. Concentrate on what the child can accomplish, and do not ask the child to complete tasks that may prove frustrating. Reading books to the child, listening to tapes, and watching television offer the child stimulation during hospitalization. Exercise as tolerated contributes to muscle strength. Physical therapy helps the child ambulate and prevents joint contractures. It is important to provide good back support and posture by keeping the child's body in alignment when confined to a wheelchair.

Parents may feel guilty and hopeless. Encourage parents to express their feelings. Genetic counseling is recommended for the entire family, and it is especially important to identify women who are carriers of one of the X-linked disorders. Siblings may feel neglected because their brother or sister is receiving so much attention. They may be concerned that they will develop the disease, and in some families, this indeed occurs. Encourage the parents to involve siblings in the child's care to reassure them of their importance.

Refer family members to resource and support groups such as the Muscular Dystrophy Association. The Companion Website contains such resources. Provide ongoing support during hospitalizations, management of home care, and the child's changes in condition.

INJURIES TO THE MUSCULOSKELETAL SYSTEM

Musculoskeletal injuries are classified according to the mechanism, the location, and the force of the injury. Strains, sprains, dislocations, and fractures are the most common musculoskeletal injuries in children. Distinguishing among these injuries is often difficult. See the clinical manifestations table below. See "Evidence-Based Nursing" for a discussion of backpack use by children. A detailed discussion of fractures follows.

FRACTURES

A fracture is a break in a bone that occurs when more stress is placed on the bone than the bone can withstand. Fractures may occur at any age; they are frequent in children because their bones are less dense and more porous than those of adults (see "Pathophysiology Illustrated: Classification and Types of Fractures").

ETIOLOGY AND PATHOPHYSIOLOGY

Fractures in children may result from direct trauma to a bone (falls, sports injuries, abuse, motor vehicle crashes) or

CLINICAL MANIFESTATIONS

STRAINS, SPRAINS, AND DISLOCATIONS

CONDITION	CLINICAL MANIFESTATIONS	CLINICAL THERAPY
Strain ■ Stretching or tearing of either a muscle or a tendon, usually from overuse (example: back strain resulting from improper or overly heavy lifting).	■ Vary according to the type and severity of the strain. Pain can be acute or chronic.	■ Rest and support of the injured part until the muscle or tendon heals and normal activity can occur.
Sprain ■ Stretching or tearing of a ligament, usually caused by falls, sports injuries, or motor vehicle crashes.	■ Edema, joint immobility, and pain.	■ For the first 24–36 hours: **R**est **I**ce **C**ompression **E**levation ■ After the first 24–36 hours, mobility is gradually increased.
Dislocation ■ Complete displacement of an articular joint surface, usually associated with falls, sports injuries, or motor vehicle crashes. Although almost any joint may be dislocated, most dislocations occur in the shoulder, knee, and hip.	■ Pain and tenderness, swelling and obvious deformity, and instability of the joint.	■ Varies according to the site and severity of the injury, and consists of: Shoulder: Open or closed reduction followed by the application of a sling. Knee: Closed reduction with gentle traction, then immobilization with a splint. Hip (posterior): Immediate closed reduction or possibly open reduction, traction, or hip spica cast. Hip (anterior): Immediate closed reduction, extension traction, and hip spica cast.

EVIDENCE-BASED NURSING

DO HEAVY BACKPACKS CAUSE BACK PAIN?

Problem

Many children wear backpacks that are heavy and are carried for large parts of the day. Low back, neck, and shoulder pain seem to be increasing in children and a possible connection with backpacks has been suggested.

Evidence

Several studies have now investigated the relationships between backpack use and complaints of pain. In one study, 1126 youth from 12 to 18 years completed a questionnaire about backpack use and their health, and had physical measurements completed. Almost 75% of the youth had back pain, and the pain was associated with poorer general health, being overweight, being female, and carrying heavier backpacks (Sheir-Neiss, Kruse, Rahman et al., 2003). In another study of 745 adolescents, 45% had back pain, and severe neck and shoulder pain was suffered by 6%. The weight of backpacks was not associated with incidence of pain reports in this study (van Gent, Dols, de Rover et al., 2003).

Implications

A clear association between backpack use and weight and complaints of pain is not evident. Therefore, nurses should ask about backpack use at health promotion visits and advise on how to wear them. The American Academy of Pediatrics (http://www.pediatrics.org) lists recommendations for backpack use:

- Have wide, padded shoulder straps and wear the pack on both shoulders, close to the body.
- Use a padded back and waist strap.
- Be sure the backpack is lightweight (no more than 10% to 20% of the youth's weight) or consider a rolling pack if it is heavy.
- Practice back-strengthening exercises and learn to bend at the knees.

Critical Thinking

How will you partner with youth who are in sports after school to plan how to carry school items and sports gear safely? What exercises can you plan to help strengthen the back and thighs for carrying a pack?

References

Sheir-Neiss, G. I., Kruse, R. W., Rahman, T., Jacobsen, L. P., & Pelli, J. A. (2003). Association of backpack use and back pain in adolescents. *Spine, 28,* 922–930.

Van Gent, C., Dols, J. J., de Rover, C. J., Hira Sing, R. A., & de Bet, H. C. (2003). The weight of schoolbags and the occurrence of neck, shoulder, and back pain in young adolescents. *Spine, 28,* 916–921.

---

bone diseases that result in weakening of the bone (osteogenesis imperfecta). Trauma may be caused by an acute injury, or direct and forceful impact, or by overuse such as in chronic and repetitive activities (Eiff & Hatch, 2003).

CLINICAL MANIFESTATIONS

Signs and symptoms of fractures vary depending on the location, type, and nature of the causative injury. Fractures are generally characterized by pain, abnormal positioning, edema, immobility or decreased range of motion, ecchymosis, guarding, and crepitus. Childhood fractures most often involve the clavicle, tibia, ulna, and femur, with distal forearm fractures the most common type. Douglass, described in the opening vignette, had a fracture of his tibia. Fractures to the pelvis are often associated with motor vehicle crashes. Epiphyseal (growth plate) injuries are common in children. These injuries are described using the Salter-Harris classification system (Figure 55–13).

CLINICAL THERAPY

Radiographs are useful for determining the exact location and type of the fracture. Medical management consists of two basic steps: (1) reduction to realign displaced or frag-

GROWTH AND DEVELOPMENT

Stress fractures are becoming more common in adolescents who limit their intake of calories and calcium in an attempt to remain lean for sports such as distance running or gymnastics. These fractures may present with chronic pain that changes in intensity. Be alert to this possibility when teenagers' diets and athletic activities place them at risk.

mented bones, and (2) immobilization so that healing can take place.

A closed reduction aligns the bone by manual manipulation or traction. Conscious sedation or pain management

GROWTH AND DEVELOPMENT

The risk of bone fractures in adolescent females who drink carbonated beverages is three times higher than in those who do not drink these beverages. It is thought that the high phosphorus content of carbonated beverages fosters bone loss and that these beverages displace milk, a major calcium source, in the diet (Wyshak, 2000).

PATHOPHYSIOLOGY ILLUSTRATED

Classification and Types of Fractures

CLASSIFICATION	TYPE
Complete (transverse) fracture	**Spiral fracture**
Break across entire section of a bone at a right angle to the bone shaft resulting in two or more fragments	Associated with twisting force; fracture coils around the bone
Open fracture	**Closed fracture**
Broken bone protrudes through the skin leaving a path to the fracture site; high risk of infection exists	Broken bone does not protrude through the skin
Greenstick fracture	**Comminuted fracture**
Caused by compression force; often seen in young children	Associated with high-impact forces; bone breaks into three or more segments

Additional types of fractures include: incomplete, in which the break occurs in only one side of the cortex; oblique, in which the fracture slants across the long axis of the bone; compression, in which two bones are jammed together (usually occurs in spinal area); and compacted, in which one bone fragment is wedged into another.

may be used during closed reduction. An open reduction requires surgical alignment of the bone, often using pins, plates, wires, or screws. For open fractures, surgery must also be performed for debridement, to remove dead tissue and clean the wound. Casting is the most common external method of immobilization. Casts may be placed on extremities (short or long leg or arm cast), the upper body to immobilize the spine, or from chest to legs to stabilize pelvis or hips (spica cast). Leg casts may be walking or nonwalking casts. Cast material is either plaster or a synthetic fabric. Other external methods of stabilization include traction and splinting (see Table 55–4 later in this chapter for types of traction). Pins may be inserted to stabilize the fracture, and can be used with or without casts or traction. A child with multiple fractures following a car crash or other trauma may need a combination of treatments (Frye & Luterman, 1999).

Healing of fractures is influenced by factors including age, size of the involved bone, and fracture site. Fractures heal more quickly in children than in adults. Immobilization is essential for the bone-healing process. If a fracture is properly reduced, complications should be minimal (Table 55–3). Fractures involving the epiphyseal growth plate must be treated properly to minimize the chance for limb length discrepancy, joint incongruity, and angular deformities.

○ FIGURE 55-13

The Salter-Harris classification system is based on the angle of the fracture in relation to the epiphysis.

Type I
Common
Growth plate undisturbed
Growth disturbances rare

Type II
Most common
Growth disturbances rare

Type III
Less common
Serious threat to growth
    and joint

Type IV
Serious threat to growth

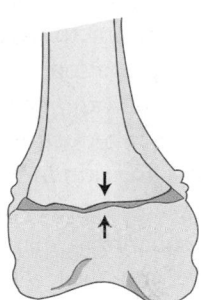

Type V
Rare
Crush injury causes cell death in growth plate,
    resulting in arrested growth and limited
    bone length
If growth plate is partially destroyed, angular
    deformities may result

NURSING MANAGEMENT

NURSING ASSESSMENT AND DIAGNOSIS

When dealing with an injured child, be alert to the signs and symptoms of fractures before moving the child. When in doubt about the type of injury, apply a splint to immobilize the joints above and below the injury. Try to identify the cause of the injury by asking the child, parents, or other family members what happened. Evaluate pain, swelling, and any abnormal positioning of the injured area. When a child is admitted to the emergency department or hospital, nursing assessment includes the extent of the injury, the degree of pain, and the child's vital signs (respiratory status, pulse, and blood pressure). Monitor all systems since infection, fat emboli, and other problems can emerge during the treatment period.

Several nursing diagnoses may apply to the child with a fracture. They include the following:

- *Pain* related to injury
- *Risk for Impaired Skin Integrity* related to treatment

TABLE 55-3 ✤ Complications of Fracture Reduction

Complication	Clinical Therapy

Infection
  Acute (may occur with open
  fractures)
  Chronic (osteomyelitis)
	Debridement, drainage, culture,
	  and treatment with antibiotics

Neurovascular injury resulting from physical nerve damage	Nerve repair
Vascular injury	Vascular repair, amputation, tendon lengthening

Malunion (undesired healed
  alignment of bone) or
  delayed union
	Corrective osteotomy; prolonged
	  immobilization

Nonunion	Surgical intervention; internal fixation
Leg length discrepancy	Shoe lift

- *Risk for Infection* related to open fracture or trauma
- *Impaired Physical Mobility* related to treatment
- *Health-Seeking Behaviors* related to lack of information about treatment and expected outcome

PLANNING AND IMPLEMENTATION

Nurses may be in community settings when children experience a fracture and may need to provide emergency care and arrange for transport. Inform emergency personnel of the assessment data to provide for safe care. In addition, be aware that repeated fractures in the same child can be a sign of other healthcare conditions. Young children may have osteogenesis imperfecta, an older child may be experimenting with risky behavior, and child abuse may have occurred if there are several fractures in various states of healing or if the parental explanation does not match the clinical presentation. Nursing care focuses on care of the child before and after fracture reduction, encouraging mobility as ordered, maintaining skin integrity, preventing infection, and teaching the parents and child how to care for the fracture. If conscious sedation or pain blocks are used, nursing care for these procedures is needed. See Skill 13–4. **SKILLS** When caring for a child who has undergone fracture reduction, it is important to know the signs of complications. Notify the physician immediately if these signs occur. The major serious complication is **compartment syndrome**, or a condition of increased pressure in a limited space such as the soft tissue of an extremity, which compromises circulation and nervous innervation (Harvey, 2001).

Maintain Proper Alignment

Immobilization maintains proper alignment of the fracture. Casts and traction are methods used for immobilizing an injured child. Cast care guidelines are included in Table 55–2, earlier in this chapter.

Different types of traction are used, depending on the location and type of fracture (Table 55–4). Nursing care for the child in traction is described in Table 55–5.

Monitor Neurovascular Status

Neurovascular assessment is used for early detection of compartment syndrome. Compartment syndrome may occur with a crush injury or when a fracture is reduced. The swelling of inflammation reduces blood flow to the affected area, and casting causes further constriction of blood flow. Douglass, who was described in the chapter opener quote, had a splint applied for several days, with casting later, to allow swelling to decrease and to minimize risk for compartment syndrome. Monitor the child's sensation to touch, temperature, movement, strength of the pulse, and capillary refill time in the extremity distal to the injury. Monitor every 15 minutes after the cast is applied for at least 2 hours

and then every 1 to 2 hours, depending on the facility's policy and the child's condition. Keep the cast elevated above heart level to minimize edema. Report symptoms of compartment syndrome immediately as permanent damage to nerves and circulatory system can occur.

Promote Mobility

The amount of mobility the child is allowed is ordered by the physician; restrictions depend on the extent and site of the fracture. Fractures of the hip or pelvis may involve body casts; wheeled carts make mobility possible. Children with leg fractures can sometimes bear weight on the cast, but if they cannot, they move around with crutches, walkers, or wheelchairs. See Skill 17–7. **SKILLS**

Discharge Planning and Home Care Teaching

Most fractures can be easily managed at home. Activities are generally limited for approximately 8 weeks. Teach the parents and child cast care, activity restrictions, and how to identify problems that should be reported (see page 1766). Help parents to identify any modifications that may be needed at home and school. The child who has to manage steps at home or school may need special training with crutches or a temporary ramp. Refer parents to home health nurses or home teaching services if indicated. Provide pertinent teaching to prevent future injuries. Reinforce the need for protective gear for many sports (see Chapter 37).

CLINICAL MANIFESTATIONS

COMPARTMENT SYNDROME

Clinical manifestations begin about 30 minutes after tissue ischemia starts. Major manifestations are:

- Paresthesia (tingling, burning, loss of 2-point discrimination)
- Pain (unrelieved by medication, characterized by crying in the young child)
- Pressure (skin is tense, cast appears tight)
- Pallor* (pale, gray or white skin tone)
- Paralysis* (weakness or inability to move extremity)
- Pulselessness* (weak or absent pulse)

* = late sign

Check extremities for:

- Color
- Temperature
- Capillary refill
- Peripheral pulses
- Edema
- Sensation
- Motor ability
- Pain

Document results and report changes or abnormal results immediately. Changes are a medical emergency.

TABLE 55–4 ✣ Types of Traction

Skin Traction

Pull is applied to the skin surface, which puts traction directly on the bones and muscles. Traction is attached to the skin with adhesive materials or straps, or foam boots, belts, or halters.

Dunlop Traction (can be either skeletal or skin)

Used for fracture of the humerus. The flexed arm is suspended horizontally with straps placed on both the upper and lower portions for pull from both sides.

A   B

Bryant Traction (A)

Used specifically for the child under 3 years of age and weighing less than 35 pounds (17.5 kg), who has developmental dysplasia of the hip or a fractured femur. This bilateral traction is applied to the child's legs and kept in place by wrapping the legs from foot to thigh with elastic bandages. The hips are flexed at a 90-degree angle, with knees extended. This position is maintained by attaching the traction appliance to weights and pulleys suspended above the crib. The buttocks do not rest on the mattress, but are slightly elevated off the bed.

Buck Traction (B)

Used for knee immobilization; to correct contractures or deformities; or for short-term immobilization of a fracture. It keeps the leg in an extended position, without hip flexion. Traction is applied to the extremity in one direction (straight line) with a single pulley system.

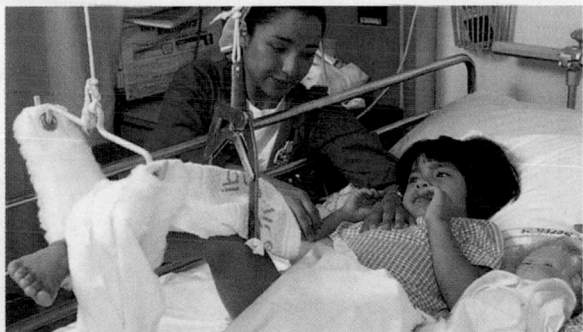

D

90–90 Traction (D)

Used for fractures of the femur or tibia. A skeletal pin or wire is surgically placed through the distal part of the femur, while the lower part of the extremity is in a boot cast. Traction ropes and pulleys are applied at the pin site and on the boot cast to maintain the flexion of both the hip and knee at 90 degrees. This traction can also be used for treatment of an upper extremity fracture.

Skeletal Traction

Pull is directly applied to the bone by pins, wires, tongs, or other apparatus that have been surgically placed through the distal end of the bone.

Skeletal Cervical Traction

Used for cervical spine injuries to reduce fractures and dislocations. Crutchfield, Gardner-Wells, or Vinke tongs are placed in the skull with bur holes. Weights are attached to the apparatus with a rope and pulley system to the hyperextended head.

Halo Traction

Used to immobilize the head and neck after cervical injury or dislocation. Also used for positioning and immobilization after cervical injury.

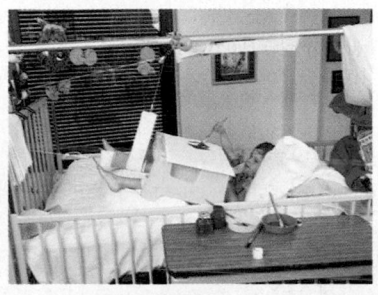

C

Russell Traction (C)

Used for fractures of the femur and lower leg. Traction is placed on the lower leg while the knee is suspended in a padded sling. The slightly flexed hips and knees are immobilized. One force is applied by a double pulley to the foot and another force is applied upward using a sling under the knee and an overhead pulley.

E

External Fixators (E)

These devices can be used in the treatment of simple fractures, both open and closed; complex fractures with extensive soft tissue involvement; correction of bony or soft tissue deformities; pseudoarthroses; and limb length discrepancy. They are attached to the extremity by percutaneous transfixing of pins or wires to the bone. When used to lengthen an extremity, the device can be "distracted" or turned as ordered by the surgeon for a very small amount several times daily. This separates the bone and allows new growth, gradually lengthening the extremity.

TABLE 55–5 ✣ Care of the Child with Traction or External Fixator

1. Assess the child in traction by first checking the equipment. Make sure that the equipment is in the proper position. Observe both the body appliance and the attached weights and pulleys. Make certain that the child's body is in proper alignment.
2. Assess the skin under the straps and pin insertion sites for any signs of redness, edema, or skin breakdown.
3. Assess the extremity by checking neurovascular status frequently (check warmth, color, distal pulses, capillary refill time, movement, sensation).
4. Provide pin care when ordered using sterile technique. Clean the area surrounding the pin with cotton-tipped applicators saturated with normal saline or half-strength hydrogen peroxide. Clean the area again with sterile water or more saline. Apply an antibacterial ointment, if ordered, using another cotton-tipped applicator.
5. When the traction equipment can be removed, skin care should be performed every 4 hours.
6. Place a sheepskin pad under the child's extremity if orders permit.

SPORTS INJURIES

Sports injuries are the most common type of injury in youth from 13 to 19 years. Football, wrestling, soccer, and gymnastics are the sports most commonly associated with injury (Stracciolini & Metzl, 2000). Fractures, which were described earlier, are common sports injuries of young athletes. Douglass in the opening scenario is a good example of this type of injury. However, a variety of other injuries that affect the musculoskeletal system are common in sports. Children and adolescents have characteristics that put them at risk for injury. These include:

- Vulnerability of growth plates to injury, especially the distal tibia and fibula.

- Increased joint mobility from lax tendons and ligaments, leading to injury of the knee, ankle, and hip.

- Softer bones, leading to fractures and to more common injury to underlying organs.

- Lack of experience in the sport and inadequate training.

- Lack of acceptance of protective gear.

- Impatience with taking the time to heal after injury.

- Vulnerability to spinal injury related to high impact sports and recreation such as diving in unsupervised locations.

Some of the common sports injuries are listed in Table 55–6. Treatment for sprains, strains, dislocations, and fractures is described in the preceding sections. Head and neck injuries are discussed in Chapter 53 ∞ and dental emergencies in Chapter 46. ∞ A few general approaches to minimize and treat injuries for youth athletes follow.

Athletes can benefit from teaching that enhances performance of their sports and also minimizes chance of injury. They should receive instruction in correct techniques from a person qualified to coach and supervise children. Nurses should encourage youths to gradually increase time and intensity at a sport, rather than immediately playing a new sport for long periods of time. Parents should be encouraged to inquire about the coach's experience and also verify that the coaching staff is prepared in emergency care.

TABLE 55–6 ✣ Common Sports Injuries

Sport	Type of Injuries
Baseball	▪ Hand and finger fractures and sprains ▪ Contusions and sprains of upper or lower extremities; wrists, elbows, knees, and ankles are common sites ▪ Injury to body parts when hit by a ball, (e.g., broken teeth, face, head, eye, and chest injuries)
Football	▪ Head and neck injury such as skull or cervical vertebrae fracture ▪ Pulled muscles or dislocations in shoulders and legs
Gymnastics	▪ Wrist and elbow fractures and strains ▪ Tendonitis in elbows and ankles/legs
Hockey (ice and inline)	▪ Dental injury ▪ Leg fractures ▪ Head and neck injuries
Soccer	▪ Head and neck injury ▪ Strains and fractures of legs
Wrestling	▪ Fractures and dislocations of upper and lower extremities

The nurse should be alert for sports injuries during contacts with children and adolescents in health promotion visits. The nurse should ask about sports participation for all youths, but especially when there are complaints of sore muscles, edema of body parts, and bruises. Neurovascular assessment of extremities, including color, temperature, capillary refill time, edema, pulses, sensation, and pain, should be performed. Questions should be phrased so that sports such as skateboarding or snowboarding, which may not be performed under supervision or in organized sports programs, can be identified. Youths may not consider these "sports."

Youngsters should be taught to warm up for 10 to 15 minutes before participation and to cool down for a corresponding period at the end of activity. They should be instructed to wear recommended gear for the sport, including equipment such as a well-fitted protective helmet, face masks, eye protection, mouth guards, elbow and wrist guards, gloves, knee pads, and shin pads. Parents may need assistance to learn about the recommended equipment and resources for purchase. Frequent updates are needed as the child grows. The child should be taught not to ignore pain.

Injuries such as muscle strains should be treated promptly. They involve several steps:

- Resting the injury for 24 to 48 hours, applying ice for 20 minutes 4 times daily, compression with an elastic wrap to provide comfort and decrease edema, and elevating the part affected above heart level
- Gradually increasing motion to the part
- Adding flexibility and resistance or strengthening exercises
- Returning gradually to the sport, usually in 2 to 3 weeks after injury (Harper, 2002)

The nurse should partner with the child, family, and other health professionals to plan for activity whenever an injury has occurred. It is important to praise the family and youth for physical activity, an important part of a healthy lifestyle. Community resources should be provided to foster sports participation.

AMPUTATIONS

Amputation—the complete absence of a body extremity—can be either congenital or acquired. Approximately two thirds of amputations in children are congenital and one third are acquired. Congenital amputations can be caused by constrictive amniotic bands, drugs, or irradiation. Acquired amputations are generally associated with trauma or the result of a disease or disorder.

The child with an absent limb should be fitted with a prosthesis as soon as feasible. This fosters a positive body image, independence, and self-confidence and also ensures that motor skills develop as normally as possible. The prosthetic device should be reevaluated as the child progresses physically and developmentally. Children with traumatic amputations may need frequent stump reconstructions because as children grow, so do their bones, and the skin tends to adhere to the bone. Bone may need to be cut and soft tissue added to keep the stump rounded. Joint fusions or stump lengthenings may also be needed to allow the effective use of a prosthesis.

NURSING MANAGEMENT

Nursing care focuses on providing emotional support regarding altered body image, managing pain, maintaining skin integrity, and encouraging maximal independent functioning.

Recovering from the loss of a limb is one of the most difficult challenges facing a child. Emphasize what the child can do rather than what he or she cannot do. Good listening skills are important.

The child who has had surgery or a traumatic injury experiences pain. Many techniques discussed in Chapter 42 are useful interventions. ∞ After surgery, an epidural may be the treatment of choice. Oral analgesics are used during the period of adaptation to a prosthesis if the stump is tender. Children may have "phantom" limb pain in the lost extremity although this phenomenon is less common in children than in adults (Ray, 2000).

The child usually begins wearing the prosthetic device for 1- to 2-hour intervals. Check the skin for any redness or breakdown. If redness or breakdown develops, leave the prosthesis off and allow the skin to clear before reapplying. Have the prosthesis adjusted if necessary, and increase wearing time as tolerated by the child.

Children with amputated limbs quickly learn how to accommodate to the prosthetic device. Use physical therapy programs specifically designed to help the child perform activities of daily living.

Discharge Planning and Home Care Teaching

Answer any questions the family has about how to care for the prosthetic device and how to perform skin checks. Encourage parents to allow the child to participate in physically and emotionally challenging peer activities. Sporting activities that enable the child to participate using modified equipment are a good way to build self-confidence and motivation. For example, ski centers may offer programs that teach children with physical disabilities how to ski, or the paraolympics may be motivating for some children. Assess the need for counseling and offer referrals as appropriate.

THINKING CRITICALLY

THE CHILD WEARING A CAST

Douglass was admitted to the clinic today for application of a short leg cast. He broke his leg nearly a week ago when he was on a trampoline with three friends, trying to see who could jump the highest. Douglass slipped and his leg hit the frame on the side. His friends helped him off the trampoline and found someone to transport Douglass to the emergency department. They then reached his mother by phone, who rushed to the hospital when she heard the news.

His mother states that he is now 12 years old and in middle school. He has been going to a friend's house nearly every day after school and spending time on activities such as the trampoline and rollerblading, as well as watching television and playing video games. She felt this was safer than him being at home alone during her work hours, but is now starting to wonder about whether to allow Douglass to engage in activities with his friend.

A splint has provided support for several days and has allowed the swelling to decrease before today's cast application. Douglass has been non–weight bearing on his leg and has been using crutches. He returned to school yesterday for part of the day and found it was hard to get to all of his classes.

- What concerns will Douglass have once his cast is in place?
- What teaching should you provide to help him keep the cast intact and to ensure his safety?
- What signs or symptoms might indicate infection or loss of circulation and need to be reported immediately?
- Will any special adaptations be needed in his home and school?
- Is there any way his injury could have been avoided? What teaching does he need now to avoid further injuries?

Critical Concept Review

LEARNING OBJECTIVES

CONCEPTS

Describe pediatric variations in the musculoskeletal system.	1. A fibrous membrane exists between the cranial bones to allow for skull growth. 2. Ends of the long bones remain cartilaginous. 3. Long bones are porous and less dense. 4. Bones can bend, buckle, or break due to a simple fall. 5. Muscles increase only in length and circumference.
Plan nursing care for children with structural deformities of the foot, hip, and spine.	Foot: 1. Instruct parents in simple stretching exercises. 2. Provide cast care and instruct parents in cast care. Hip: 1. Provide frequent assessment of the skin and neurovascular status of the affected leg or legs after surgery, or if placed in cast or harness. 2. Maintain traction, if ordered. 3. Increase fluids and fiber in the child's diet. 4. Instruct parents in the use of the Pavlik harness and have them return demonstration of application. Spine: 1. Support self-image if placed in brace. 2. Instruct in exercises to strengthen muscles of spine. 3. Monitor respiratory and circulatory status after fusion surgery. 4. Provide adequate pain medication and instruct in use of PCA. 5. Instruct family in use of brace postoperatively.
Recognize signs and symptoms of infectious musculoskeletal disorders and refer for appropriate care.	Signs and symptoms of infection include: 1. Pain and tenderness with swelling of affected extremity. 2. Decreased mobility of infected joint. 3. Fever. 4. Redness over the area.

LEARNING OBJECTIVES

CONCEPTS

Partner with families to plan care for children with musculoskeletal conditions that are chronic or require long-term care.

→

1. Help child establish a positive self-image.
2. Assist parents in locating support groups.
3. Provide resources to assist with safety issues such as car seats and home adjustments.
4. Instruct parents in identifying signs and symptoms of complications.
5. Assist parents in dealing with changing condition of the child (for example, with muscular dystrophy).
6. Collaborate with multiple providers who care for child.

Plan nursing interventions to promote safety and developmental progression in children who require braces, casts, traction, and surgery.

→

1. Position child on side (casts and braces), or with head slightly elevated for feeding.
2. Provide age-appropriate toys.
3. Monitor neurovascular and skin status.
4. Promote mobility as allowed.
5. Instruct parents in cast and brace care.

Provide nursing care for fractures, including teaching for injury prevention and nursing implementations for the child who has sustained a fracture.

→

1. Immobilize site of fracture until casted or surgically corrected.
2. Keep extremity elevated.
3. Use palms to handle cast until dry.
4. Monitor neurovascular status of the extremity frequently.
5. Provide pain medication as needed.

Injury prevention instruction should include:
1. Warm-up before beginning exercise.
2. Use protective equipment.
3. Treat sprains and strains promptly.

CRITICAL THINKING IN ACTION

View the **Critical Thinking in Action** video in Chapter 55 of the CD-ROM. Then, answer the questions that follow.

Peter, now 7 years old, was diagnosed at 5 years with Duchenne muscular dystrophy. His parents are well-informed about the disease since they had on alder son who died of the disorder at 19 years. At the present time he walks on his toes but is able to ambulate well with leg braces. Today, Peter is visiting the specialty clinic for children with muscular dystrophies. His braces will be checked for fit and performance, physical therapy will be performed, and he will attend a group session with other school age children. During these visits, the parents also meet in a support group with other families and receive instruction and resources to help them with Peter's health management. As a nurse in the clinic you perform a physical and mental assessment on Peter. All findings are within normal limits, although he has had some constipation and several upper respiratory infections. You learn that he has an individualized education plan (IEP) in place at school that allows for periods of rest and physical therapy; the parents report that he is at grade level and excels at computer modeling.

1. What are the main roles of the nurse working with Peter in the specialty clinic?
2. Children with muscular dystrophy often get to a standing position by mainly using arm muscles. What is the name of the manuever?
3. What are some of the tests performed to see if a child has muscular dystrophy, and what are the expected results?
4. Who can Peter expect to meet with on the days he goes to the specialty clinic for muscular dystrophy?

REFERENCES

Abad-Sinden, A., Verbrugge, K. C., & Buck, M. L. (2001). Assessment, prevention and management of metabolic bone disease in very low birthweight infants: The role of the neonatal nutritionist. *Nutrition in Clinical Practice, 16,* 13–19.

Acosta, K., Vade, A., Lomasney, L. M., Demos, T. C., & Bielski, R. (2001). Radiologic case study. *Orthopedics, 24,* 737–745.

American Academy of Pediatrics, Committee on Injury and Poison Prevention. (1999). Transporting children with special health care needs. *Pediatrics, 104,* 988–992.

American Academy of Pediatrics, Committee on Quality Improvement and Subcommittee on Developmental Dysplasia of the Hip. Clinical practice guideline: Early detection of developmental dysplasia of the hip. (2000). *Pediatrics, 105,* 896–905.

Astrom, E., & Soderhall, S. (2002). Beneficial effect of long term intravenous bisphosphonate treatment of osteogenesis imperfecta. *Archives of Disease in Childhood, 86,* 356–361.

Biggar, W. D., Gingras, M., Feblings, D. L., Harris, V. A., & Steele, C. A. (2001). Deflazacort treatment of Duchenne muscular dystrophy. *Journal of Pediatrics, 138,* 45–50.

Blakeslee, T. J. (1997). Congenital talipes equinovarus (clubfoot). *Clinics in Podiatric Medicine and Surgery, 14,* 9–55.

Bowman, B. A., & Russell, R. M. (2001). *Present knowledge of nutrition* (8th ed.). Washington, DC: International Life Sciences Institute.

Carek, P. J., Dickerson, L. M., & Sack, J. L. (2001). Diagnosis and management of osteomyelitis. *American Family Physician, 63,* 2413–2420.

Caulton, J. M., Ward, K. A., Alsop, C. W., Dunn, G., Adams, J. E., & Mughal, M. Z. (2004). A randomized controlled trial of standing programme on bone mineral density in non-ambulant children with cerebral palsy. *Archives of Disease in Childhood, 89,* 131–135.

Chan, Y. Y., & Bishop, N. J. (2002). Clinical management of childhood osteoporosis. *International Journal of Clinical Practice, 56,* 280–286.

Davids, J. R. (1998). Limping. In L. T. Staheli (Ed.), *Pediatric orthopedic secrets* (pp. 195–199). Philadelphia: Hanley & Belfus.

DeBaun, B. J. (1998). Prevention of infection in the orthopedic surgery patient. *Nursing Clinics of North America, 33,* 671–684.

Durst, E. S. (2000). The A, B, C's of bone building in adolescence. *Journal of the American Academy of Nurse Practitioners, 12,* 135–140.

Eiff, M. P., & Hatch, R. L. (2003). Boning up on common pediatric fractures. *Pediatrics, 20*(11), 30–59.

Eldridge, J., Dilley, A., Austin, H., El-Jamil, M., Wolstein, L., Doris, J., et al. (2001). The role of protein C, protein S, and resistance to activated protein C in Legg-Perthes disease. *Pediatrics, 107,* 1329–1334.

Fernandez, J., Carrol, C. L., & Baker, C. J. (2000). Discitis and vertebral osteomyelitis in children: An 18-year review. *Pediatrics, 105,* 1299–1304.

Frye, K. E., & Luterman, A. (1999). Burns and fractures. *Orthopaedic Nursing, 18*(1), 30–35.

Gilmore, A., & Thompson, G. H. (2003). Common childhood foot deformities. *Consultant for Pediatricians, 2,* 63–71.

Givner, L. B., & Kaplan, S. L. (2003). Bone and joint infections: Pediatrics. Presented at the 40th annual meeting of the Infectious Diseases Society of America. As reported in *Infectious Diseases in Children* (February 2003), p. 82.

Gonzalez, E., Pavia, C., Ros, J., Villaronga, M., Valls, C., & Exxcola, J. (2001). Efficacy of low dose schedule pamidronate infusion in children with osteogenesis imperfecta. *Journal of Pediatric Endocrinology and Metabolism, 14,* 529–533.

Harper, R. S. (2002, December). Back in the game: Preventing and treating athletic injuries in adolescents. *Advance for Nurse Practitioners,* 55–66.

Harvey, C. (2001). Compartment syndrome: When it is least expected. *Orthopaedic Nursing, 20*(3), 15–26.

Holcomb, S. S. (2000). Marfan syndrome: A review. *Dimensions of Critical Care Nursing, 19*(4), 22–24.

Horwitz, E. M., Prockop, D. J., Gordon, P. L., Koo, W. W., Fitzpatrick, L. A., Neel, M. D., et al. (2001). Clinical responses to bone marrow transplantation in children with severe osteogenesis imperfecta. *Blood, 97,* 1227–1231.

Kautz, S. M., & Skaggs, D. L. (1998). Getting an angle on spinal deformities. *Contemporary Pediatrics, 15,* 111–128.

Kunkler, C. E. (1999). Neurovascular assessment. *Orthopaedic Nursing, 18*(3), 63–71.

Litmanovitz, I., Dolfin, T., Friedland, O., Arnon, S., Regev, R., Shainkin-Kestenbaum, R., et al. (2003). Early physical activity intervention prevents decrease of bone strength in very low birth weight infants. *Pediatrics, 112,* 15–19.

March of Dimes. (2004). *Achondroplasia.* Retrieved June 1, 2004, from http://www.marchofdimes.com/professionals/681_1204.asp. 3

Morcuende, J. A., Dolan, L. A., Dietz, F. R., & Ponseti, I. V. (2004). Radical reduction in the rate of extensive corrective surgery for clubfoot using the Ponseti method. *Pediatrics, 113,* 376–380.

Moyer-Mileur, L. J., Brunstetter, V., McNaught, T. P., Gill, G., & Chan, G. M. (2000). Daily physical activity program increases bone mineralization and growth in preterm very low birth weight infants. *Pediatrics, 106,* 1088–1092.

Osteogenesis Imperfecta Foundation. (2003). An Introduction to Osteogenesis Imperfeta for Medical Professionals, Individuals, and Families. Retrieved November 10, 2005, from http://www.oif.org

Papazian, O., & Alfonso, I. (2002). Adolescents with muscular dystrophies. *Adolescent Medicine, 13,* 511–532.

Parsons, E. P., Clarke, A. J., Hood, K., Lycett, E., & Bailey, D. M. (2002). Newborn screening for Duchenne muscular dystrophy: A psychosocial study. *Archives of Disease in Childhood, 86,* F91–F95.

Paterson, C. R., Monk, E. A., & McAllion, S. J. (2001). How common is hearing impairment in osteogenesis imperfecta? *Journal of Laryngology and Otolaryngology, 115,* 280–282.

Ray, R. L. (2000). Complications of lower extremity amputations. *Topics in Emergency Medicine, 22*(3), 35–43.

Roy, D. R. (1999). Current concept in Legg-Calvé-Perthes Disease. *Pediatric Annals, 28,* 748–754.

Ryan, D. J. (2001). Intoeing: A developmental norm. *Orthopaedic Nursing, 20*(2), 13–18.

Sapountzi-Krepia, D. S., Valavanis, J., Panteleakis, G. P., Zangana, D. T., Vlachojiannis, P. C., & Sapkas, G. S. (2001). Perceptions of body image, happiness and satisfaction in adolescents wearing a Boston brace for scoliosis treatment. *Issues and Innovations in Nursing Practice, 35,* 683–690.

Sheir-Neiss, G. I., Kruse, R. W., Rahman, T., Jacobsen, L. P., & Pelli, J. A. (2003). Association of backpack use and back pain in adolescents. *Spine, 28,* 922–930.

Slote, R. J. (2002). Psychological aspects of caring for the adolescent undergoing spinal fusion for scoliosis. *Orthopedic Nursing, 21,* 19–32.

Sobus, K. M. L., Horan, S. M., & Warren, R. H. (2000). Respiratory management of neuromuscular diseases in children. *Physical Medicine and Rehabilitation, 14,* 285–299.

Stracciolini, A., & Metzl, J. D. (2000). Pediatric sports emergencies. *Physical Medicine and Rehabilitation Clinics of North America, 11,* 961–979.

Takeda, S., & Miyagoe-Suzuki, Y. (2001). Gene therapy for muscular dystrophies: Current status and future prospects. *Biodrugs, 15,* 635–644.

Thompson, G. H. (2004a). The spine. In R. E. Behrman, R. M. Kliegman, & H. B. Jenson, *Nelson textbook of pediatrics* (17th ed., pp. 2280–2287). Philadelphia: Saunders.

Thompson, G. H. (2004b). Torsional and angular deformities. In R. F. Behrman, R. M. Kliegman, & H. B. Jenson, *Nelson textbook of pediatrics* (17th ed., pp. 2261–2269). Philadelphia: Saunders.

Van Gent, C., Dols, J. J., de Rover, C. J., Hira Sing, R. A., & de Bet, H. C. (2003). The weight of schoolbags and the occurrence of neck, shoulder, and back pain in young adolescents. *Spine, 28,* 916–921.

Witt, C. (2003). Detecting developmental dysplasia of the hip. *Advances in Neonatal Care, 3,* 65–75.

Wyshak, G. (2000). Teenaged girls, carbonated beverage consumption, and bone fractures. *Archives of Pediatrics and Adolescent Medicine, 154,* 610–613.

Yetman, A. T., Huang, P., Bornemeier, R. A., & McCrindle, B. W. (2003). Comparison of outcome of the Marfan syndrome in patients diagnosed at age ≤ 6 years versus those diagnosed at 6 years of age. *American Journal of Cardiology, 91,* 102–103.

The Child with Alterations in Endocrine Function

I am really worried about how Anthony is going to learn to manage all these aspects of diabetes care. Learning to check his blood sugar is pretty easy compared to counting calories and figuring out how much insulin to take and when to take it. I hope we have some time to get into a routine with his diabetes management before he gets sick. We have to work hard to keep the diabetes under control.

—*Mother of Anthony, 12 years old*

LEARNING OBJECTIVES

- Identify the function of important hormones of the endocrine system.

- Identify signs and symptoms that may indicate a disorder of the endocrine system.

- Describe differences in pathophysiology between primary and nephrogenic diabetes insipidus.

- Identify all conditions for which short stature is a sign.

- Develop a nursing care plan for each type of acquired metabolic disorder.

- Develop a family education plan for the child that needs lifelong cortisol replacement.

- Distinguish between the nursing care of the child with type 1 and type 2 diabetes.

- Develop a nursing care plan for the child with an inherited metabolic disorder.

MEDIALINK www.prenhall.com/london

CD-ROM

Animations:
  Physiology of Diabetes
  Responding to Hypoglycemia
Video
  Adolescent Diabetes and Quality of Life
Skills 9-1 through 9-7
NCLEX-RN® Review
Audio Glossary

Companion Website

Objectives
NCLEX-RN® Review
Case Study: Diabetic Risk Factors
Thinking Critically
Case Study: Child with Type 1 Diabetes Returning to
  Elementary School
MediaLink Applications:
  Identify Strategies to Help Girls Understand Early
    Pubertal Development
  Develop a Peer Strategy: Child with Inborn Errors
    of Metabolism and Diet

The endocrine system controls the cellular activity that regulates growth and body metabolism through the release of hormones. Hormones are chemical messengers secreted by various glands that exert controlling effects on the cells of the body. Overlapping with all body systems, the general functions of the endocrine system include the following:

- Differentiation of the reproductive and central nervous systems in the fetus
- Regulation of the pace of growth and development in concert with the central nervous system throughout childhood and adolescence
- Coordination of the male and female reproductive systems, enabling sexual reproduction
- Maintenance of an optimal level of hormones for body functioning
- Maintenance of homeostasis, a healthy internal environment, in the presence of a constantly changing external environment

Inborn errors of metabolism—inherited biochemical abnormalities of the urea cycle and amino acid and organic acid metabolism—often have a significant impact on the endocrine system's ability to support growth and development. Some chromosomal abnormalities also result in disturbances in growth and sexual development.

Endocrine disturbances result in alterations in metabolism, growth and development, and behavior that may have significant implications for children. If not diagnosed and treated early, these conditions can result in delays in growth and development, mental retardation, and, occasionally, death. However, treatment, which usually consists of supplementation of missing hormones, adjustment of hormone levels, or dietary measures, allows most children to live a normal life.

ANATOMY AND PHYSIOLOGY OF PEDIATRIC DIFFERENCES

The hypothalamic-pituitary axis produces a number of releasing and inhibiting hormones that regulate the function of many endocrine glands, including the thyroid, adrenal, and male and female reproductive glands. In addition, hormones originating from this axis regulate growth. Other endocrine glands include the parathyroid glands, and islets of Langerhans in the pancreas (Figure 56–1 ⊙). All of these glands secrete hormones into the bloodstream, which carries them to target organs or tissues. Most hormones exert their influence through interaction with receptors in the target cells of specific tissues (Table 56–1).

The regulation of hormone secretion occurs through a *negative feedback* mechanism that functions to maintain an optimal internal environment in the body. Negative feedback occurs when an endocrine gland or secretory tissue receives a message that the target cells have received an adequate amount of hormone. In response, further secretion is inhibited. Secretion is resumed only when the secretory tissue receives another message indicating that levels of the hormone are low.

The endocrine system is responsible for sexual differentiation during fetal development and for stimulating growth and development during childhood and adolescence. This includes stimulating development of the reproductive system in both sexes.

Puberty (sexual maturation, lasting 2 to 3 years) occurs when the gonads secrete increased amounts of the sex hormones estrogen and testosterone. At the average age of 10 years in girls and 11 years in boys, the hypothalamus produces increased amounts of *gonadotropin-releasing hormone*. This hormone stimulates the anterior pituitary gland to increase the production of

● **FIGURE 56-1**

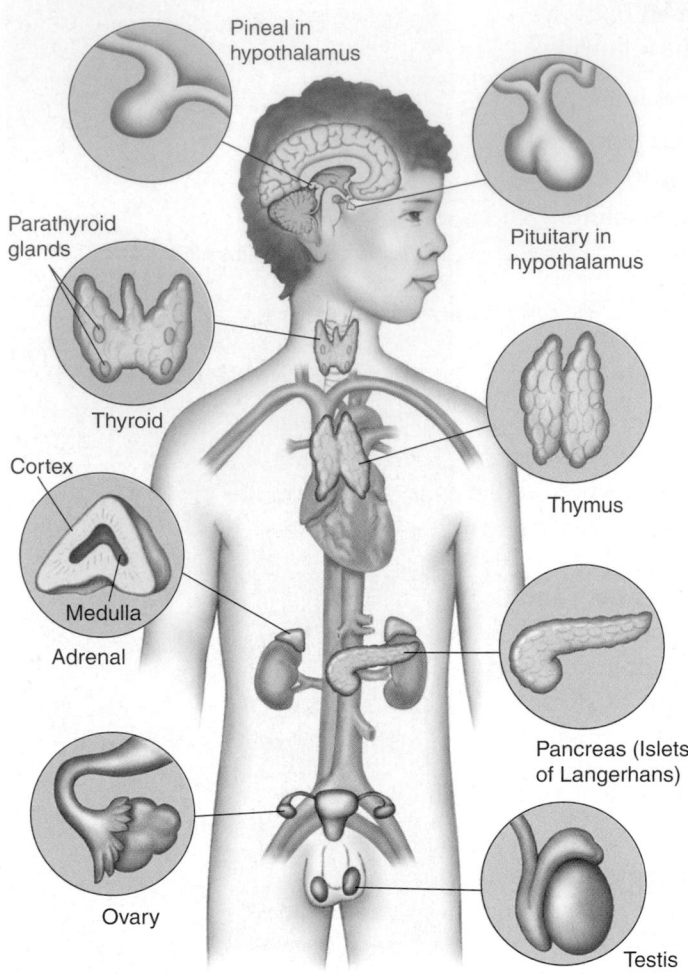

Major organs and glands of the endocrine system.

luteinizing hormone (LH) and follicle-stimulating hormone (FSH). These hormones in turn stimulate the gonads to secrete more sex hormones (Figure 56-2 ●), resulting in the development of primary and secondary sex characteristics.

DISORDERS OF PITUITARY FUNCTION

GROWTH HORMONE DEFICIENCY (HYPOPITUITARISM)

Growth hormone deficiency (GHD) is a disorder caused by decreased activity of the pituitary gland. Because most children with this disorder secrete inadequate amounts of growth hormone, the term *growth hormone deficiency* is often preferred to *hypopituitarism*. The disorder is diagnosed more often in males than females since males are more often referred for evaluation of short stature.

The release of growth hormone from the anterior pituitary gland is controlled by the hypothalamus, which secretes releasing and inhibitory factors. Growth hormone stimulates linear growth and bone mineral density, as well as the growth of all body tissues. It also stimulates the synthesis of proteins in the liver, among them the somatomedins or insulin-like growth factors (IGFs), which promote glucose use by the cells and cell proliferation.

Infarction of the pituitary gland (related to sickle cell disease), central nervous system infection, disease, tumors of the pituitary gland or hypothalamus (primarily craniopharyngiomas and gliomas), other brain tumors, cranial irradiation, brain trauma, chemotherapy, and psychosocial deprivation may cause GHD by interfering with the production or release of growth hormone. Dominant or recessive inheritance or a genetic mutation may cause deficiency of growth hormone or abnormalities of hormone receptors (Witchel & Finegold, 2002). Other major causes of short stature include familial short stature, hypothyroidism, Turner syndrome, *constitutional growth delay* (delayed pubertal hormone secretion causes a late pubertal growth spurt), chronic renal failure, Cushing syndrome, inborn error of metabolism, and severe cardiac, pulmonary, or gastrointestinal disease. Psychosocial dwarfism is a syndrome of emotional deprivation

● **FIGURE 56-2**

Feedback mechanism in hormonal stimulation of the gonads during puberty.

TABLE 56–1 ✛ Endocrine Glands and Their Functions

Gland/Hormone	Function
Anterior Pituitary	
Growth hormone (somatotropin)	Stimulates growth and metabolism of all body tissues
Thyroid-stimulating hormone (TSH)	Stimulates thyroid hormone secretion
Adrenocorticotropic hormone (ACTH) (corticotropin)	Stimulates secretion of glucocorticoids and androgens
Follicle-stimulating hormone (FSH) (a gonadotropin)	Stimulates secretion of estrogen, stimulates follicle maturation in ovaries; also critical for sperm production in males
Luteinizing hormone (LH) and interstitial cell-stimulating hormone (ICSH) (male analogue) (a gonadotropin)	Stimulates secretion of androgens in males and progesterone in females
Prolactin-releasing hormone	Stimulates secretion of prolactin that stimulates the secretion of milk during lactation
Melanocyte-stimulating hormone (MSH)	Stimulates skin pigmentation
Posterior Pituitary	
Antidiuretic hormone (ADH) (vasopressin)	Promotes water reabsorption back into the blood, decreasing urine output
Oxytocin	Stimulates uterine contractions and breast milk letdown reflex
Beta endorphins	May regulate body temperature, food and water intake
Thyroid	
Thyroxine (T_4) and triiodothyronine (T_3)	Regulates metabolic rate of all cells, body heat production; protein, fat, and carbohydrate catabolism in all cells
Thyrocalcitonin	Stimulates bone ossification and development
Parathyroid	
Parathyroid hormone	Regulates serum calcium levels and excretion of phosphorus
Adrenal	
Aldosterone	Conserves sodium and excretion of potassium
Androgens	Stimulates bone development and secondary sexual characteristics
Cortisol	Stimulates anti-inflammatory reactions, protects from stress
Epinephrine	Activates sympathetic nervous system; stimulates increase in blood pressure and blood glucose levels
Pancreas (Islets of Langerhans)	
Insulin	Facilitates cellular glucose utilization
Glucagon	Increases blood glucose
Somatostatin	Stimulates inhibition of insulin and glucagon secretion; may prevent excess insulin secretion
Ovaries	
Estrogen	Stimulates development of breasts and ova
Progesterone	Stimulates breast glandular development; acts to maintain pregnancy
Testes	
Testosterone	Stimulates production of sperm, development of secondary sexual characteristics, and closure of epiphysis

that causes suppression of pituitary hormone production, resulting in adrenocorticotropic hormone (ACTH).

Children with GHD have normal birth weights and lengths. By the age of 1 year, however, they are below the third percentile on the growth chart. They characteristically grow at a rate of less than 5 cm (2 in.) per year. Other characteristic findings in infants include hypoglycemic seizures, hypona- tremia, neonatal jaundice, pale optic discs, micropenis, and undescended testicles. Children with GHD tend to be over- weight and to have youthful facial features, higher pitched voices, delayed dentition, "ripply" abdominal fat, decreased muscle mass, delayed skeletal maturation, delayed sexual mat- uration, and hypoglycemia. Slipped capital femoral epiphysis has been associated with GHD (Halec & Zimmerman, 2004a).

TABLE 56–2 ✤ Diagnostic Tests for Short Stature

Test	Purpose Related to Short Stature
IGF-1 and IGF-BP3	Excludes GHD if normal, hormones directly related to skeletal growth
Radiographic views of the sella turcica (site of the pituitary gland) by radiograph, CT, or MRI	Demonstrates size of the sella turcica or a tumor
Karyotype (girls)	Detects Turner syndrome (see page 1843)
Thyroid function studies	Detects hypothyroidism (see page 1814)
ACTH and cortisol levels	Detects other pituitary hormonal deficiencies
Urine creatinine, pH, specific gravity, urea nitrogen, electrolytes	Detects chronic renal failure (see Chapter 52 ∞)
Bone age	Identifies other potential causes of delayed growth
Complete blood count and erythrocyte sedimentation rate	Screens for inflammatory bowel disease with anemia
Antigliadin antibodies	Screens for celiac disease

IGF-1 = Insulin-like growth factor 1, IGF-BP3 = Insulin-like growth factor binding protein 3, GHD = growth hormone deficiency, ACTH = adrenocorticotropic hormone

Data from D'Ercole, A. J., & Underwood, L. (1996). Anterior pituitary gland and hypothalamus. In A. M. Rudolph, J. I. E. Hoffman, & C. D. Rudolph (Eds.), *Rudolph's pediatrics* (20th ed., p. 1692). Stamford, CT: Appleton & Lange; Parks, J. S. (2004). Disorders of the hypothalamus and pituitary gland. In R. E. Behrman, R. M. Kliegman, & H. B. Jenson (Eds.), *Nelson textbook of pediatrics* (17th ed., pp. 1845–1853). Philadelphia: Saunders.

Any child whose height is 2 to 3 standard deviations below the mean height for age or whose measurement is falling off the normal growth chart should be evaluated for short stature (Table 56–2). A child whose screening tests reveal low levels of IGF-1 requires further evaluation by a pediatric endocrinologist. A careful history, physical examination, assessment of pubertal development and unusual facies, and radiologic studies are necessary to identify possible causes of short stature. A radiograph of the bones of the wrist is used to evaluate the stage of bone ossification, and thus the **bone age** of the child. Using standardized norms for bone ossification, it can be determined if the child's chronologic and bone ages match. A significantly delayed (less than the child's age) or advanced (greater than the child's age) bone age indicates the possibility of a systemic chronic disease or hormone

abnormality. Provocative growth hormone testing, in which various medications (arginine, clonidine, glucagon, insulin, L-dopa) are administered to stimulate release of growth hormone, may be used to confirm growth hormone deficiency.

Treatment depends on the cause of the deficiency. Brain tumors must be treated effectively before growth hormone therapy can be considered. See Chapter 50. ∞ Uses for growth hormone therapy that have been approved by the U.S. Food and Drug Administration (FDA) include GHD, chronic renal insufficiency and pretransplantation, Turner syndrome, small-for-gestational-age child who has not achieved normal height by age 2 years, Prader-Willi syndrome, idiopathic short stature unlikely to catch up in height, adults with GHD, and adults with AIDS wasting (Wilson, Rose, Cohen et al., 2003). Most indications for growth hormone (GH) replacement require daily or alternate day injections. The child usually experiences increased growth velocity for the first year of treatment, followed by a gradual decrease in growth for subsequent months or years. Growth should progress at least at the normal growth rate for age while maintained on GH treatment. Replacement therapy is continued until either the child achieves an acceptable height or growth velocity drops to less than 2 cm (1 in.) per year. Close monitoring of growth and endocrinology visits every 3 to 4 months are needed. If growth is slower than anticipated, improper preparation and administration of GH and adherence to therapy must be considered (Halec & Zimmerman, 2004a). In some cases the onset of puberty is delayed with gonadotropin-releasing hormone analogues to provide more time for growth hormone therapy to stimulate growth.

NURSING MANAGEMENT

Nursing care consists of monitoring growth, teaching the child and family about the disorder and its treatment, and providing emotional support. Carefully measure the child's height and weight and plot them on a growth chart (see Appendix C and Skills 9–1 to 9–7). **SKILLS**

Teach the parents and child about the GH replacement therapy, preparation and administration of subcutaneous injections, rotating injection sites, potential side effects, and actions to take if noticed. Provide the parents with ideas about how to minimize the child's stress associated with daily injections. Give parents educational resources, such as information from the Magic Foundation, the Human Growth Foundation, and the Short Stature Foundation. Since replacement therapy is expensive (approximately $35,000 per year) and may not be covered by insurance, parents may need financial assistance that is sometimes available from the growth hormone manufacturers.

Children with GHD, especially those due to tumors and trauma from radiation or surgery, may have academic problems because of acquired learning disabilities. Before the child enters or returns to school, a comprehensive evaluation should be performed to identify potential problems.

The best results occur when treatment is begun at an early age, before the psychologic effects of short stature become apparent and when attainment of near-normal height can be reached. People often treat short children on the basis of their size rather than their age, and such children experience social prejudice about height. Teasing is a common problem. The teenage years may be particularly stressful because of adolescents' characteristic preoccupation with body image.

Encourage parents and teachers to treat the child in an age-appropriate manner. The child should dress in clothing that reflects chronologic age. Emphasize the child's strengths, support independence, and encourage participation in age-appropriate activities to aid in the development of a positive self-image. Suggest that the child take part in sports in which ability does not depend on size (e.g., swimming, gymnastics, wrestling, ice skating, and martial arts). Identifying positive role models, short people who accomplish their goals, also promotes a positive image. Refer the child for counseling if appropriate.

HYPERPITUITARISM

Hyperpituitarism, a disorder in which excessive secretion of growth hormone increases the growth rate, is rare in children. Oversecretion of growth hormone is usually caused by a pituitary adenoma. If combined with precocious puberty, a tumor of the hypothalamus may be present. Affected children can grow to 7 or 8 feet in height when oversecretion occurs before closure of the epiphyseal plates. If the disorder occurs after closure of the epiphyseal plates, acromegaly occurs.

Because tall stature is valued in our society, assessment of children (particularly boys) with accelerated linear growth is often delayed. Any child whose predicted height exceeds that consistent with parental height should be evaluated for possible growth problems and underlying pathologic conditions.

A complete history is obtained, and physical examination and laboratory testing are performed. Increased levels of IGF-1 establish the diagnosis of hyperpituitarism. A bone age radiologic examination is performed to determine if the epiphyseal plates have begun to fuse. Radiologic studies are used to detect a tumor. Thorough evaluation is required to differentiate hyperpituitarism from familial tall stature.

Treatment depends on the cause of the excessive growth and may involve surgical removal of a tumor or pituitary gland (hypophysectomy), radiation therapy, or radioactive implants. High doses of sex steroids are given to close the epiphyseal plates. The child may need lifelong pituitary hormone replacement following surgery.

NURSING MANAGEMENT

Tall stature, like short stature, can be stressful for children. Tall children are often treated as if they are older than their chronologic age. Tall adolescents may have problems with self-image, and girls in particular may worry about their appearance.

Nursing care focuses on teaching the parents and child about the disorder and its treatment, providing emotional support, and, if surgery is required, providing preoperative and postoperative teaching and care (see Chapter 40 ∞).

DIABETES INSIPIDUS

Two forms of diabetes insipidus (DI) exist: true (or central) antidiuretic hormone (ADH) deficiency and familial nephrogenic diabetes insipidus. Both disorders involve ADH, a hormone secreted by the posterior pituitary gland. ADH facilitates concentration of the urine by stimulating reabsorption of water from the distal tubule of the kidney. When ADH is inadequate, the tubules do not resorb, leading to **polyuria** (passage of a large volume of urine in a given period). Plasma osmolarity, or the concentration of solutes in the blood, is an important factor in ADH secretion.

DI can occur at any age and results from ADH or vasopressin deficiency (central DI) or inability of the renal collecting tubules to respond to the ADH. Primary brain tumors account for 50% of central DI (Saborio, Tipton, & Chan, 2000). Other neurogenic causes of DI include central nervous system trauma, infection, electrolyte imbalances, hypoxic brain damage, vascular anomalies, or infiltrative diseases like leukemia. Most cases of nephrogenic DI are genetic, either an X-linked or an autosomal recessive form. It may also be acquired from drug toxicity or adverse drug reaction (Parks, 2004).

Polyuria and **polydipsia** (excessive thirst) are the cardinal signs of DI. See "Clinical Manifestations: Diabetes Insipidus." In infants symptoms may include failure to thrive, poor feeding, and irritability. Diapers are saturated. Although the onset of symptoms is usually sudden, diagnosis is often delayed. Children who can quench their thirst may not complain to parents about symptoms. The child may be obese due to an excessive intake of high-caloric fluids.

In all forms of diabetes insipidus, the urine cannot be concentrated, no matter how dehydrated the child becomes. Dehydration usually precipitates diagnosis. Serum sodium concentration and osmolality increase rapidly to pathologic levels. Seizures may occur in response to extreme electrolyte imbalances. Often an unconscious child is admitted to the emergency department with dehydration and hypernatremia.

Urine osmolality is decreased (< 200 mOsm/kg), urine specific gravity is decreased (< 1.005), serum

CLINICAL MANIFESTATIONS

DIABETES INSIPIDUS

CAUSE	CLINICAL MANIFESTATIONS	CLINICAL THERAPY
True Diabetes Insipidus ADH deficiency Familial or idiopathic	Polyuria, polydipsia Nocturia, enuresis Thirsty at night, irritable if fluids withheld Constipation, fever, dehydration	Desmopressin acetate
Nephrogenic Diabetes Insipidus Familial, decreased responsiveness of kidneys to ADH	Polyuria, polydipsia Hypernatremia in neonatal period Dehydration, fever, vomiting Mental status changes	Diuretics High fluid intake Salt and protein restricted diet

sodium is elevated (>145 mEq/L), and serum osmolality is elevated (> 285 mOsm/L) (Trimarchi, 2001). Diagnosis is confirmed by measuring the plasma arginine vasopressin (AVP) level before and during a fluid deprivation test, which is usually conducted in the hospital or in a carefully controlled outpatient setting for up to 8 hours. Fluid intake is prohibited during the procedure. Weight, urine output, specific gravity, and osmolality are measured every 2 hours. The specific gravity will remain less than 1.005 even after dehydration rather than urine concentration. A dose of aqueous vasopressin is given after several hours. A decreased urine output and increased urine concentration confirm the diagnosis of central DI. No response to vasopressin is seen in cases of nephrogenic DI. An MRI may be ordered to visualize the pituitary gland.

NURSING PRACTICE

During the fluid deprivation test, advise parents that the child will be frustrated and irritable from thirst. No one should drink in front of the child during the testing period. Monitor the child's vital signs and intake and output carefully. The test is stopped if the child loses 3% to 5% of body weight and develops a fever and hypotension (Dveirin & Tunnessen, 2000).

Treatment of central ADH deficiency consists of the subcutaneous, intranasal, or oral desmopressin acetate (DDAVP) with an effect lasting 8 to 12 hours. DDAVP reduces urinary output, enabling the child to live a more normal life with a decrease in thirst, urinary output, and nocturia. The dose of DDAVP must be titered for suffi-

cient coverage of metabolic needs. Nephrogenic DI is treated with thiazide diuretics, which promote sodium excretion and stimulate the proximal tubule to reabsorb water. Prostaglandin inhibitors (indomethacin) may also be prescribed to have an additive effect on decreased water excretion. A high fluid intake and a low sodium diet are also ordered (Cheetham & Baylis, 2002). The child's sodium and potassium levels must be carefully monitored to prevent hypernatremia and hypokalemia (see Chapter 43 ∞).

NURSING MANAGEMENT

Nursing care centers on administering medications and teaching parents how to manage the condition and recognize signs of altered fluid status. Educate parents about DDAVP administration, obtaining and recording daily weights, measuring intake and output, and recognizing signs of inadequate fluid intake (see Chapter 43 ∞). The child should consume fluids equal to the amount of output. The child's fluid intake should be adjusted to prevent dehydration during an illness. Infants usually need fluid intake even during the night. Many infants have coexisting brain damage and need nasogastric or gastrostomy feeding to maintain adequate hydration and nutrition. When excessive fluid is consumed, the child will not be able to excrete the excess water load with DDAVP treatment.

When the child with nephrogenic diabetes insipidus has an acute illness, the child's physician should be notified immediately because the increased metabolic activity may cause dehydration and hypernatremia that can cause mental retardation, seizures, and cerebral calcification. Additional fluids are needed to prevent dehydration.

SYNDROME OF INAPPROPRIATE ANTIDIURETIC HORMONE (SIADH)

SIADH results from an excessive amount of serum ADH. It is seen in children with central nervous system infections such as meningitis or pneumonia, and in children receiving positive pressure ventilation. It is caused by hypoxic or traumatic brain injury, and by diseases of the hypothalamus, pituitary stalk, or posterior pituitary. Some medications, including diuretics and chemotherapy, have been associated with SIADH.

Failure of normal feedback mechanisms from the hypothalamus, pituitary gland, and kidney results in excessive secretion of ADH, leading to water reabsorption despite the presence of a low serum osmolality. ADH secretion causes increased permeability of the distal renal tubules and collecting ducts, resulting in water reabsorption, increased intravascular volume, and decreased urine output (Trimarchi, 2001). Elevated ADH also causes suppression of the renin-angiotensin mechanism and sodium excretion. The outcome is **water intoxication** (an abnormal proportion of water to sodium in the extracellular fluid), hyponatremia, and cellular edema.

Signs include elevated blood pressure, distended jugular veins, crackles in lung fields, weight gain without edema, fluid and electrolyte imbalance, and concentrated urine with decreased urine output. As serum sodium levels continue to fall, lethargy, confusion, headache, altered level of consciousness, seizures, and coma occur due to cerebral edema.

Laboratory findings include a high urine osmolality (> 1200 mOsm/kg), elevated specific gravity (> 1.032), low serum osmolality (< 275 mOsm/kg), low serum sodium (< 135 g/Eq/L), and decreased BUN and hematocrit. Fluids are restricted to prevent further dilution of the blood. Medications include diuretics, demeclocycline to block action of ADH at the renal collecting tubules, and hypertonic saline IV fluids.

NURSING MANAGEMENT

Nursing care focuses on preventing injury, monitoring fluid balance, and monitoring nutritional intake. Monitor for level of consciousness, headache, and seizure activity. Implement seizure precautions. Monitor intake and output, serum sodium, urine osmolality, and specific gravity. Educate the parents about the hidden sources of water and fluids in foods, avoiding excessive fluid intake, and the importance of weighing the child daily and reporting weight gain that could indicate fluid retention. Lifelong medication may be required depending upon the cause of the disorder. Emphasize the importance of follow-up as the drug has nephrotoxic side effects. Medical alert identification should be worn.

PRECOCIOUS PUBERTY

Puberty normally occurs between 8 and 13 years of age in girls and between 9 1/2 and 14 years of age in boys. Precocious puberty is defined as the appearance of any secondary sexual characteristics before 8 years of age in girls and 9 years of age in boys.

> ## DEVELOPING CULTURAL COMPETENCE
>
> ### ONSET OF PUBERTY
>
> Differences exist by race in the onset of puberty and secondary sexual characteristics. African-American girls begin puberty between 8 and 9 years of age. Caucasian girls begin puberty by 10 years of age (Herman-Giddens, Slora, Wasserman et al., 1997; Lalwani, Reindollar, & Davis, 2003).

Early secretion of the normal hormones responsible for pubertal changes usually is not associated with abnormalities. However, a benign hypothalamic tumor may be present. Other causes include brain injury; brain tumor; postinfectious encephalitis or meningitis; congenital adrenal hyperplasia; tumors of the ovary, adrenal gland, or testicle; and exogenous sources or androgens (i.e., anabolic steroids). In males gonadotropin-dependent precocious puberty is usually the result of a CNS disorder such as an intracranial tumor, and in females it is usually idiopathic (Traggiai & Stanhope, 2003). Other disorders with isolated signs of premature sexual development usually require no treatment: premature **thelarche** is breast development, premature menarche is vaginal bleeding without other signs of sexual development, and premature **adrenarche** is development of pubic and axillary sexual hair before 8 years of age in girls and 9 years in boys.

Children with precocious puberty have an advanced bone age (premature skeletal maturation) and may appear unusually tall for their age. Their growth ceases prematurely, however, as the hormones stimulate closure of the epiphyseal plates, resulting in short stature. Behavior changes may include mood swings and emotional lability.

Serum diagnostic studies include LH, FSH, testosterone, or estradiol. Provocative testing includes gonadotropin-releasing hormone (GnRH) stimulation to confirm the diagnosis. Radiologic imaging may be performed. CNS tumors require surgery, radiation, chemotherapy, or a combination of these. If the condition begins before age 6 years in girls, treatment is initiated immediately with a gonadotropin-releasing hormone analogue (GnRHa), usually leuprolide acetate (Lupron) injections once a month or nafarelin acetate (Synarel) intranasally twice a day. For older girls, growth patterns are monitored. There are no definitive criteria for beginning treatment in children over age 6 years (Tato, Savage, Antoniazzi et al., 2001).

NURSING MANAGEMENT

Nursing care centers on teaching the child and parents about the condition, administering medication, and providing emotional support. Inform the child in age-appropriate terms that the physiologic changes are normal but are occurring at an earlier than usual age. Reassure the child that friends will go through the same stages of development eventually. Remember that the child's social, cognitive, and emotional development matches his or her age, even though the physical development is advanced. Determine the family's ability to manage the cost of treatment, about $6000 to $10,000 a year. Financial assistance may be available through pharmaceutical companies.

Children with precocious puberty become self-conscious as body changes occur. Parents should be advised to dress the child in a manner appropriate to his or her chronologic age, even though the child may look older. Looser clothing may help hide some of the body changes that are occurring. Provide privacy during examinations. Encourage the child to express his or her feelings about the changes. The child may need to practice role-playing as a coping mechanism to manage teasing by other children. Parents should be advised that they may need to discuss issues of sexuality with the child at an earlier age than normal. Refer the child for counseling if appropriate.

DISORDERS OF THYROID FUNCTION

HYPOTHYROIDISM

Hypothyroidism is a disorder in which levels of active thyroid hormones are decreased. It may be congenital or acquired. Congenital hypothyroidism occurs in approximately 1 in 4000 live births and is twice as common in girls as in boys (Palma Sisto, 2004). It is less prevalent in African-American infants but more frequent in infants of Asian and Hispanic origin (1 in 2000 births). It also occurs more commonly in children with Down syndrome. Acquired hypothyroidism is more common in girls than in boys.

ETIOLOGY AND PATHOPHYSIOLOGY

Thyroid hormones are important for growth and development and for metabolizing nutrients and energy. When these hormones are not available to stimulate other hormones or specific target cells, growth is delayed and mental retardation develops.

Congenital hypothyroidism is usually caused by a spontaneous gene mutation, an autosomal recessive genetic transmission of an enzyme deficiency, hypoplasia or aplasia of the thyroid gland, failure of the CNS–thyroid feedback mechanism to develop, or iodine deficiency. Mental retardation (cretinism) is irreversible if the disorder is not treated.

Acquired hypothyroidism can be idiopathic or result from autoimmune thyroiditis (Hashimoto thyroiditis), late-onset thyroid dysfunction, isolated thyroid-stimulating hormone (TSH) deficiency due to pituitary or hypothalamic dysfunction, or exposure to drugs or substances such as lithium that interfere with thyroid hormone synthesis. A genetic predisposition to autoimmune thyroiditis and an autosomal dominant inheritance of thyroid antibodies has been identified (Roberts & Ladenson, 2004).

CLINICAL MANIFESTATIONS

Infants with congenital hypothyroidism have few clinical signs of the disorder in the first weeks of life. In untreated infants the characteristic cretinoid features (thickened protuberant tongue, thick lips, dull appearance) appear during the first few months of life. Other signs include prolonged neonatal jaundice, hypotonia, macroglossia, respiratory distress, bradycardia, decreased pulse pressure, cool extremities, mottling, umbilical hernia, a posterior fontanelle larger than 1 cm in diameter, difficulty feeding, lethargy, constipation, and a hoarse cry.

Children with acquired hypothyroidism have many of the same signs as adults: decreased appetite, dry, cool skin, thinning hair or hair loss, depressed deep tendon reflexes, bradycardia, constipation, sensitivity to cold temperatures, abnormal menses, and a **goiter** (a nontender enlarged thyroid gland). Manifestations unique to children include change in past normal growth patterns with a weight increase, decreased height velocity, delayed bone and dental age, muscle hypertrophy with muscle weakness, and delayed or precocious puberty.

CLINICAL THERAPY

Congenital hypothyroidism is usually detected during newborn screening of thyroxine (T_4) and TSH levels, which is mandatory in all states. An elevated TSH level indicates that the disease originated in the thyroid, not the pituitary. Two tests are frequently performed so that the disorder is identified, before the newborn leaves the hospital and at the first healthcare visit at 1 to 2 weeks of age. Rapid response from the laboratory testing the samples is important to reduce the time to diagnosis and the effects of hypothyroidism on the infant's development.

If the T_4 level is below normal and the TSH level is increased, the synthetic thyroid hormone levothyroxine

(Synthroid) is prescribed. The dose is increased gradually as the child grows to ensure a **euthyroid** (normal thyroid) state. A pediatric endocrinologist monitors treatment. Periodic evaluation of T_4 and TSH serum levels, bone age, and growth parameters is necessary to assess for signs of excess or inadequate thyroid hormone.

Antithyroid antibodies are measured in children with a goiter and suspected Hashimoto thyroiditis, as increased titers of antithyroglobin and antimicrosomal antibodies are often found.

To ensure an adequate growth rate and prevent mental retardation, the hormone must be taken throughout life. Children with congenital hypothyroidism that are diagnosed before 3 months of age have the best prognosis for optimal mental development. Treated children with the most severe form of congenital hypothyroidism lose 6 to 15 IQ points, while less severely affected children have an IQ similar to their siblings (Van Vliet, 2001). Children with acquired hypothyroidism usually have normal growth following a period of catch-up growth. Many adolescents with Hashimoto thyroiditis have a spontaneous remission.

NURSING MANAGEMENT

NURSING ASSESSMENT AND DIAGNOSIS

Routine neonatal screening is performed before discharge from the hospital and is often repeated at the infant's first health visit to evaluate levels of circulating thyroid hormones (see Skill 10–2). **SKILLS**

Record the length or height and weight at each follow-up visit and plot on a growth curve. The child is assessed for signs of inadequate growth to determine if the dose of thyroid hormone needs to be adjusted and to monitor compliance with medication. Conduct developmental screening to detect delays in developmental milestones.

Among the nursing diagnoses that might be appropriate for the child with hypothyroidism are the following:

- *Imbalanced Nutrition: Less than Body Requirements* related to loss of appetite
- *Risk for Delayed Development* related to delayed initiation of thyroid replacement therapy
- *Risk for Disproportionate Growth* related to poor adherence to thyroid hormone therapy
- *Constipation* related to decreased bowel motility
- *Fatigue* related to inadequate dose of thyroid medication

PLANNING AND IMPLEMENTATION

Nursing care focuses on teaching the parents and child about the disorder and its treatment and monitoring the child's growth rate. Explain how to administer thyroid hormone (e.g., tablets can be crushed and mixed in a small amount of formula or applesauce). Advise parents that the child may experience temporary sleep disturbances or behavioral changes in response to therapy. Teach the parents how to assess for an increased pulse rate, which could indicate the presence of too much thyroid hormone, and advise them to report problems such as fatigue, which could indicate an improper drug dose that needs to be adjusted.

Caution parents to dress the child appropriately for the season to prevent hypothermia. Modify the child's diet by increasing the amount of fruits and bulk if constipation is a problem.

Reassure the family that the child will develop normally with hormone replacement therapy. Reinforce the importance of follow-up visits to assess growth rate and response to therapy and to regulate drug dosages as the child grows. Periodic assessments of educational achievement are needed. Even with good control, adolescents have persistent visual-spatial deficits, and memory and attention problems. Those with more severe disease or who take longer to get to euthyroid status have the poorest academic achievement and more behavior problems (Rovet & Ehrlich, 2000). Parents should be informed that therapy will be lifelong and is needed to promote the child's mental development. When the cause is genetic, make a referral for genetic counseling.

EVALUATION

Expected outcomes of nursing care of the child with hypothyroidism include the following:

- The child maintains adequate growth of height and weight, following a percentile curve throughout childhood.
- The child's diet contains adequate fruits and bulk to prevent constipation.
- The child's cognitive development is appropriate for age.

HYPERTHYROIDISM

Hyperthyroidism, a disorder of excessive levels of circulating thyroid hormones, is rare in children and adolescents. It is most common in adolescent girls and is almost always due to Graves disease (Nebesio, Siddiqui, Pescovitz et al., 2002). The disorder may present in the preschool years, but has an increased incidence in adolescence.

ETIOLOGY AND PATHOPHYSIOLOGY

Graves disease is an autoimmune disorder in which the body produces antibodies that attack the cells of the thyroid gland. It has a high familial incidence. Immunoglobulins produced by the B lymphocytes stimulate oversecretion of thyroid hormones, resulting in the clinical symptoms.

Other more unusual forms of hyperthyroidism result from thyroiditis and thyroid hormone–producing tumors, including thyroid adenomas and carcinomas, and pituitary adenomas. Congenital hyperthyroidism can occur in infants of mothers with Graves disease because of transplacental transfer of immunoglobulins.

CLINICAL MANIFESTATIONS

Signs and symptoms are caused by hyperactivity of the sympathetic nervous system. Characteristic findings include an enlarged, nontender thyroid gland (goiter), prominent eyes (exophthalmos) (Figure 56–3 ●), eyelid lag, tachycardia, nervousness, restlessness or irritability, increased appetite with weight loss, emotional lability, heat intolerance, diaphoresis, insomnia, tremor, and muscle weakness. The thyroid gland may be slightly enlarged or grow to three to four times its normal size; feel warm, soft, and fleshy; and have an auditory bruit on auscultation. Onset is subtle, and the condition often goes unrecognized for 1 to 2 years.

Children with Graves disease usually have behavioral problems and declining performance in school. They become easily frustrated in the classroom and overheated and fatigued during physical education class. It is difficult for them to relax or sleep. These symptoms usually prompt parents to seek medical treatment for them.

● **FIGURE 56–3**

Exophthalmos and an enlarged thyroid in an adolescent with Graves disease.

Used with permission from Zitelli, B., & Davis, H. (Eds.). (1997). Atlas of pediatric physical diagnosis (3rd ed., p. 271). St. Louis, MO: Mosby-Wolfe.

CLINICAL THERAPY

Diagnostic studies include laboratory evaluation of serum TSH, T_3 (triiodothyronine), and T_4 levels, and a thyroid scan. T_3 and T_4 levels are markedly elevated while the TSH level is decreased. Serum studies to detect autoantibodies specific for the various thyroid disorders are performed.

The goal of clinical therapy is to inhibit excessive secretion of thyroid hormones. Treatment may include antithyroid drug therapy, radiation therapy, or surgery. Drug therapy is most often the initial treatment, but compliance is often a problem because of drug side effects. Methimazole (Tapazole) and propylthiouracil (PTU) are given to inhibit thyroid hormone secretion. PTU therapy can cause temporary side effects, including skin rashes, urticaria, and lymphadenopathy. If rash, fever, or sore throat develops, a healthcare professional should perform hematologic studies. Treatment continues for 18 months to 2 years or until the thyroid decreases in size, and remission occurs (Ginsberg, 2003). Symptoms usually improve within weeks of starting treatment. Beta-adrenergic blocking agents such as propranolol may be given to relieve symptoms of tremors, tachycardia, and restlessness.

If drug therapy is ineffective, radiation therapy using oral radioactive iodine (131I) is the next treatment choice. Current data do not indicate a relationship between radioactive iodine and cancer or leukemia. It also does not appear to increase the risk of birth defects in future offspring in those treated (Ginsberg, 2003). Thyroidectomy provides immediate cure, and avoids radiation and possible long-term complications of radioactive iodine (Boger & Perrier, 2004). Manipulation of the parathyroid gland during surgery may result in excess release of parathyroid hormone, leading to hypercalcemia. Severe **thyrotoxicosis** or thyroid "storm" may occur when thyroid hormone is suddenly released into the bloodstream during surgery. The child experiences fever, diaphoresis, tachycardia, hypertension, and tremors, progressing to shock and, if untreated, death. Treatment includes antithyroid drugs and propranolol.

NURSING MANAGEMENT

NURSING ASSESSMENT AND DIAGNOSIS

Assess the child's vital signs, as blood pressure and pulse may be elevated. Keep a record of food intake. Accurate measurement and recording of height and weight are important to establish baselines and identify patterns of growth. Observe the child's behavior, activity, and level of fatigue.

Common nursing diagnoses for the child with hyperthyroidism include the following:

- *Ineffective Thermoregulation (Elevated)* related to illness and excessive activity of the sympathetic nervous system

- *Imbalanced Nutrition: Less than Body Requirements* related to high metabolic needs

- *Disturbed Body Image* related to changes caused by illness (prominent eyes, excessive perspiration, and tremors)

- *Fatigue* related to hypermetabolic state and sleep deprivation

PLANNING AND IMPLEMENTATION

Nursing care focuses on teaching the child and parents about the disorder and its treatment, promoting rest, providing emotional support, and, if the child needs surgery, providing preoperative and postoperative teaching and care. Promote increased caloric intake by providing five or six moderate meals per day. Encourage the child and family to express their feelings and concerns about the disorder. Pointing out even slight improvements in the child's condition increases adherence with therapy.

Children with hyperthyroidism are easily fatigued. Rest periods should be scheduled at school and home and physical activities kept to a minimum until symptoms resolve. Encourage parents to provide a cool environment and allow the child to wear fewer clothes until symptoms subside.

Children who have partial or total removal of the thyroid gland receive antithyroid drugs, such as iodine, for approximately 2 weeks before surgery. Teach the child and parents about drug therapy and instruct parents to watch for side effects of antithyroid drugs, including fever, urticaria, and lymphadenopathy. Provide preoperative teaching (see Chapter 40 ∞). Young children, in particular, may be fearful about having their throat "cut."

Postoperatively, elevate the head of the bed to 30 degrees and assess the child for bleeding, hoarseness, difficulty breathing, and thyrotoxicosis. A tracheostomy kit, suction supplies, and IV calcium gluconate should be immediately available for emergency treatment of hypercalcemia and respiratory distress.

Teach the family about the need for lifelong thyroid hormone replacement if radiation or surgery is performed. The child should wear a medical alert bracelet. Make sure the child is monitored regularly to ensure that the T_4 level is adequate to sustain growth.

EVALUATION

Expected outcomes of nursing care for the child with hyperthyroidism include the following:

- The child regains lost weight and maintains the previously established growth curve because the T_4 level remains appropriate.

- The child participates in daily activities without experiencing fatigue.

DISORDERS OF THE PARATHYROID

Children usually have four parathyroid glands located posterior to the thyroid gland. Their primary function is to work in conjunction with vitamin D to regulate total body calcium.

HYPERPARATHYROIDISM

Primary hyperparathyroidism, rare during childhood, is most often the result of a tumor (adenoma) which secretes the hormone without proper regulation (Doyle & DiGeorge, 2004). Secondary hyperparathyroidism is due to disease outside of the parathyroid gland, leading to excessive secretion of parathyroid hormone (Rudock, 2002). This is commonly seen in chronic renal failure when the kidneys are unable to reabsorb calcium, causing low serum calcium levels and stimulating continual secretion of parathyroid hormone to maintain normal serum calcium levels. See Chapter 52. ∞

At any age, symptoms of primary hyperparathyroidism may include bone pain, nephrolithiasis (kidney stones), and pathologic bone fractures. Hypercalcemia may cause symptoms of muscle weakness, peptic ulcer disease, fatigue, volume depletion, and subtle mental disturbance (Viera, 2002). Abdominal pain may be present and may indicate pancreatitis.

There is often a delay between development of symptoms and diagnosis. Elevated serum calcium and PTH levels are diagnostic (Kollars, Zarroug, van Heerden et al., 2005). Radiographic images may reveal signs of rickets. For primary hyperparathyroidism, surgical parathyroid exploration is performed to remove the adenoma. Surgical cure rate is estimated to be 90% (Viera, 2002). Treatment of secondary hyperparathyroidism focuses on prevention of hypercalcemia utilizing vitamin D replacement and phosphorus binders.

NURSING MANAGEMENT

Nursing care centers on fluid management and electrolyte monitoring. In children who require surgery, assess for respiratory distress and a potential airway obstruction due to edema and a potential hematoma in the pretracheal space. Monitor for signs of infection.

Following surgery, educate the child and parents to recognize signs of hypocalcemia and to provide appropriate amounts of calcium supplementation. After diagnosis or after surgical intervention, follow-up is important to monitor serum calcium and phosphorus levels.

HYPOPARATHYROIDISM

Primary hypoparathyroidism is rare, but it may result from congenital disorders (parathyroid aplasia, DiGeorge syndrome), surgical removal of the parathyroid glands, disease processes destroying the parathyroid glands (Wilson disease, hemochromatosis), or medications (i.e., aluminum, asparagine, doxorubicin, cytosine, arabinoside). The primary result is hypocalcemia and hyperphosphatemia.

Infants may display hyperirritability, muscle rigidity, seizures, vomiting, abdominal distention, apneic episodes, intermittent cyanosis, or twitching. Muscle pain and cramps may progress to numbness, stiffness, and tingling of the hands and feet. A positive **Chvostek sign** (spasm of facial muscles after tapping facial nerve) reveals hyperreflexia. Life-threatening tetany and convulsions may occur with severe hypocalcemia (Doyle & DiGeorge, 2004).

Serum calcium and PTH levels are low and serum phosphorus is elevated. Radiographs often demonstrate increased bone density. A 12-lead ECG may demonstrate a prolonged QT interval. In emergencies intravenous calcium and calcitriol are administered to treat seizures, tetany, life-threatening hypotension, and cardiac arrhythmias. Oral calcitriol and calcium are given for an indefinite period of time (Palma Sisto, 2004). Foods with high phosphorus content (dairy products and eggs) are limited.

NURSING PRACTICE

Dilute intravenous calcium per hospital protocol. Infiltration of IV calcium can cause extravasation and tissue sloughing. Always check the patency of the IV prior to administration.

NURSING MANAGEMENT

Assess and stabilize the airway, breathing, and circulation. In the acute care setting, children should be placed on a cardiorespiratory monitor. Maintain seizure precautions until normal serum calcium levels are attained. Obtain intravenous access and administer calcium supplementation as ordered.

Partner with the family to ensure their understanding of the need for calcium supplementation and reduced intake of phosphorus. Teach the family that periodic monitoring of calcium levels is important. Inform the family that hypoparathyroidism may require lifelong therapy.

DISORDERS OF ADRENAL FUNCTION

CUSHING SYNDROME

Cushing syndrome, also called adrenocortical hyperfunction, is characterized by a group of symptoms resulting from excess levels of glucocorticoids (especially cortisol) in the bloodstream. It is uncommon in children and the true incidence is unknown. During infancy and childhood, most cases of endogenous Cushing syndrome are due to malignant adrenal or pituitary tumor that causes adrenal cortex hyperfunction (Levine & White, 2004). Another cause is hyperplasia of one or both adrenal glands. The increased secretion of cortisol alters metabolism.

The initial sign in most children is gradual excessive weight gain and growth retardation. It generally takes up to 5 years for the child to develop the characteristic "cushingoid" appearance, which includes a moon face (chubby cheeks and a double chin) and fat pads over the shoulders and back (buffalo hump). The most common reasons for cushingoid features in children are excessive doses of corticosteroids and prolonged use of corticosteroids as treatment for other diseases in which signs may develop in a shorter time. Corticosteroids suppress adrenal function when given long term. These children do not have Cushing syndrome. See "Clinical Manifestations: Cushing Syndrome." Other signs include mental changes and delayed puberty.

Diagnosis is based on characteristic physical findings and laboratory values, including increased 24-hour urinary levels of free cortisol, and 17-hydroxycorticosteroid (17-OHCs); and elevated nighttime salivary cortisol level. The child has chronic hyperglycemia and an elevated glycosylated hemoglobin concentration. See Appendix B for lab values.

The adrenal suppression test with an 11 P.M. dose of dexamethasone reveals that adrenal cortisol output is not suppressed overnight as would occur in healthy children. Computed tomography (CT) and magnetic resonance imaging (MRI) detect tumors in the adrenal and pituitary glands.

Surgical removal is the current treatment of choice for adrenal tumors or pituitary adenomas. Lifelong cortisol replacement is required when both adrenal glands are removed. The prognosis for children with malignant adrenal tumors is poor.

NURSING MANAGEMENT

The nurse usually encounters a child with Cushing syndrome when the child is hospitalized for diagnostic evaluation or surgery. Nursing assessment includes monitoring the child's vital signs and fluid and nutritional status, and assessing muscle strength and endurance during hospital play activities.

CLINICAL MANIFESTATIONS

CUSHING SYNDROME

CAUSE	CLINICAL MANIFESTATIONS
Catabolism of protein	Muscle weakness and wasting, capillary weakness and bruising, growth failure with delayed bone age, fatigue
Decreased absorption of calcium from the intestines	Demineralization of bones, osteoporosis
Increased appetite	Weight gain primarily on the trunk, striae on the abdomen, buttocks, thighs
Salt-retention	Increased blood volume and hypertension

Teach the child and family about the disorder and its treatment. For children undergoing surgery, provide preoperative and postoperative teaching and care. Answer any questions the child and family may have and explain all laboratory and diagnostic tests. Explain to parents that the child's cushingoid appearance is reversible with treatment. Refer to Chapter 50 for general nursing care of the child with cancer. ∞ Provide nutritional guidance or refer the child and parents to a nutritionist to promote maintenance of an appropriate weight.

For children who need cortisol replacement therapy because both adrenal glands were surgically removed, administering the drug early in the morning or every other day causes fewer symptoms than daily administration and mimics the normal diurnal pattern of cortisol secretion. Cortisol replacement in the postoperative period must be explained carefully to parents. Hydrocortisone (Cortef, Solu-Cortef, cortisone acetate) comes in liquid, tablet, or injectable form. The oral preparations of cortisone have a bitter taste and can cause gastric irritation. Giving the dose at mealtimes and using antacids between meals helps reduce these side effects. Teach parents how and when to administer the injectable form, usually when the child is vomiting or has diarrhea, or cannot take the oral medication. Failure to give medication when the child is ill may lead to severe illness and cardiovascular collapse.

NURSING PRACTICE

Signs of acute adrenal insufficiency may include increased irritability, headache, confusion, restlessness, nausea and vomiting, diarrhea, abdominal pain, dehydration, fever, loss of appetite, and lethargy. If untreated, the child will go into shock. In newborns, the symptoms include failure to thrive, weakness, vomiting, and dehydration. Hyponatremia and hyperkalemia are key signs.

Teach parents to be alert to signs of acute adrenal insufficiency during the withdrawal of corticosteroid therapy, and to inform all healthcare providers of the child's condition and medication. The child should wear a medical alert bracelet at all times.

CONGENITAL ADRENAL HYPERPLASIA

Congenital adrenal hyperplasia (CAH), sometimes called adrenogenital syndrome, adrenocortical hyperplasia, or congenital adrenogenital hyperplasia, is an autosomal recessive disorder that causes a deficiency of one of the enzymes necessary for the synthesis of cortisol and aldosterone. The defective gene CYP21 is located on the short arm of chromosome 6. It occurs in 1 in 14,000 live births, and males and females are affected equally (Pang, 2003). The incidence is highest in Native Alaskans (American Academy of Pediatrics, 2000).

ETIOLOGY AND PATHOPHYSIOLOGY

More than 90% of children with CAH have partial or complete 21-hydroxylase enzyme deficiency in which deficient aldosterone synthesis leads to excessive renal excretion of salt (salt losing). This form has an autosomal recessive inheritance pattern. About 10% of children have 11-hydroxylase deficiency. The remainder have deficiencies involving five other enzymes. In its most severe form, the disorder can be life threatening. Of the two classic forms of the disorder, 75% are salt-losing, caused by aldosterone deficiency, and 25% are non-salt-losing, or simple **virilization** (the production of masculine secondary sexual characteristics in females). In all forms, increased secretion of ACTH occurs in response to diminished cortisol levels.

During fetal development the lack of cortisol triggers the pituitary to continue secretion of ACTH. This in turn stimulates overproduction of the adrenal androgens. Virilization of the female external genitalia begins in week 10 of gestation. If untreated, the overproduction of androgens results in accelerated height, early closure of the epiphyseal plates, and premature sexual development with both pubic and axillary hair.

CLINICAL MANIFESTATIONS

Congenital adrenal hyperplasia is the most common cause of **pseudohermaphroditism** (ambiguous genitalia) in newborn girls. The female infant is born with an enlarged clitoris and partial or complete labial fusions. The vagina usually has a common opening with the urethra (Figure 56–4 ●). Severely virilized females may be mistaken for males with cryptorchidism, hypospadias, or micropenis. The uterus, ovaries, and fallopian tubes are normal. The male infant may look normal at birth or may have a slightly enlarged penis and hyperpigmented scrotum. The boy may have tall stature and an adult-sized penis by school age, but the testes are appropriately sized for age. Partial enzyme deficiency produces less obvious symptoms. Precocious puberty, tall stature for age, acne, and excessive muscle development may be noted in both males and females as the child grows. Due to early epiphyseal fusion, adult stature is shorter.

Signs of adrenal insufficiency may be the first indication of the disorder. Recurrent vomiting, dehydration, metabolic acidosis, hypotension, and hypoglycemia are characteristic signs of the salt-wasting form of the disorder. Hypertension with hypokalemic alkalosis is alternately found in children with 11-hydroxylase deficiency.

CLINICAL THERAPY

Diagnosis in infants and children is usually confirmed by laboratory evaluation of serum 17-hydroxyprogesterone

● **FIGURE 56–4**

Newborn girl with ambiguous genitalia.
Courtesy of Patrick C. Walsh, MD.

(17-OHP) level. Routine newborn screening for CAH is performed in 29 states (Lashley, 2002). Prenatal screening is available. In instances of ambiguous genitalia, a **karyotype** (a microscopic chromosome study in which the 46 chromosomes of the child are lined up in pairs from largest to smallest to detect errors in chromosome number, shape, and size) determines the infant's gender. Ultrasonography may be used to visualize pelvic structures.

In the salt-wasting form of the disorder, the child may have hyponatremia, hyperkalemia, a high urine sodium level, and low serum and urinary aldosterone levels. Serum concentrations of testosterone in girls and androstenedione in boys and girls are elevated in affected infants. Elevated ACTH with measurement of serum cortisol and 17-OHP levels are necessary to confirm the diagnosis (American Academy of Pediatrics, 2000). Diagnosis may be delayed in the non-salt-losing form until 3 to 7 years.

The goal of treatment is to suppress adrenal secretion of androgens by replacing deficient hormones. This is accomplished by the lifelong use of oral glucocorticoids (dexamethasone, prednisone, or hydrocortisone). The glucocorticoid replacement reduces secretion of ACTH which had overstimulated the adrenal cortex. As a result, excessive adrenal androgen production is suppressed. The dose is individualized by monitoring growth parameters, bone age, and hormone levels. If the infant has the salt-wasting form of the disorder, salt is added to the infant's formula, and a mineralocorticoid (Florinef) is given to replace the missing hormone. Hormone dosage must be doubled or tripled during acute illnesses or injury and for surgery. Injectable hydrocortisone is used for severe stress. Adrenalectomy is recommended only in cases when medical therapy is ineffective (Pang, 2003).

Reconstructive surgery of the enlarged clitoris is often performed on girls during the first year of life. Vaginal reconstruction is performed later.

NURSING MANAGEMENT

NURSING ASSESSMENT AND DIAGNOSIS

Assess the infant and child for signs of dehydration, electrolyte imbalance, and hypovolemic shock in the salt-wasting form of the disease (see Skill 9–22). **SKILLS** Monitor the airway, breathing, circulation, and responsiveness. Assess vital signs and assess peripheral perfusion (capillary refill, distal pulses, color and temperature of the extremities) frequently to detect early changes in condition.

Assess the parents' emotional response to a child with ambiguous genitalia and a chronic condition. Explore their values and beliefs regarding gender roles and sexuality while awaiting results of the karyotype.

Nursing diagnoses for the child with congenital adrenal hyperplasia might include the following:

- *Risk for Impaired Parenting* related to a child with undetermined gender identity
- *Caregiver Role Strain* related to care of a child with a chronic, potentially life-threatening condition
- *Risk for Deficient Fluid Volume* related to failure of regulatory mechanisms and excess excretion of salt by the kidneys
- *Risk for Disproportionate Growth* related to accelerated growth and premature closure of epiphyseal plates

PLANNING AND IMPLEMENTATION

Nursing care of the newborn with CAH focuses on teaching parents about the disorder and its treatment, providing emotional support, and preoperative and postoperative teaching for parents of infants undergoing reconstructive surgery. The administration of glucocorticoids and mineralocorticoids must be carefully controlled.

It is often difficult for parents to accept that their infant, whose genitalia look male, is really female. With medication and surgery, the genitalia assume a female appearance and all organs necessary for future childbearing are usually functional. Several surgeries may be performed before 2 years of age and then during adolescence to dilate the vagina. Because of the risk for adrenal insufficiency, the child will most likely be hospitalized for surgery rather than having outpatient surgery.

Nurses can assist parents in educating the child's siblings, grandparents, other family members, and childcare workers about the condition. In the newborn nursery, the infant should be referred to as "your beautiful infant," not "your son" or "your daughter," until gender identity is confirmed.

Inform parents that genetic counseling should be provided for the child during adolescence. Parents considering a future pregnancy should also be informed that prenatal testing may detect congenital adrenal hyperplasia in the fetus. Refer the family for counseling if indicated.

Nursing Care in the Community

Teach parents about the special problems that develop in the salt-wasting form of the disease during acute illness. Explain the medication regimen and help the family develop an emergency care plan. The child should wear a medical alert bracelet. Teach parents how to administer intramuscular injections of hydrocortisone. If injectable hydrocortisone is not available, the child needs urgent treatment in an emergency department. The child may become dehydrated quickly and need intravenous fluid and electrolyte replacement in addition to higher doses of hydrocortisone.

TEACHING HIGHLIGHTS

HYDROCORTISONE ADMINISTRATION

Teach the family the following tips regarding hydrocortisone administration:

- Always give the medication on time since the prescribed schedule follows the body's normal cortisol release pattern.
- Never abruptly discontinue the medication.
- If the child has vomiting or diarrhea and is unable to take the medication by mouth, administer the injections as instructed.
- Always have injectable hydrocortisone available at home and school and everywhere the child travels. An emergency kit should be available at all times to supply cortisol to the child during acute illnesses and stressful situations.

EVALUATION

Expected outcomes of nursing care for congenital adrenal hyperplasia include the following:

- Parents learn to give glucocorticoids appropriately when the child is ill and prevent episodes of adrenal crisis.
- Families effectively cope with the virilized appearance of the child's genitalia and bond with the child.

ADRENAL INSUFFICIENCY (ADDISON DISEASE)

Adrenal insufficiency, also known as Addison disease, is a rare disorder in childhood characterized by a deficiency of glucocorticoids (cortisone) and mineralocorticoids (aldosterone). It may be acquired after trauma; with tuberculosis, AIDS, meningococcemia, or fungal infections that destroy the adrenal glands; or as the result of an autoimmune process. The lack of glucocorticoids affects the body's ability to handle stress (Gance-Cleveland, 2003).

Adrenal insufficiency usually develops slowly as the adrenal glands deteriorate. The early signs may not be noticed but include weakness with fatigue, lethargy and emotional lability, anorexia and salt craving, and poor weight gain or weight loss. Skin changes include hyperpigmentation on pressure points, lip borders, gingival margins, nipples, palms, soles, body creases, and scarred areas of the body, as well as generalized bronzing of the skin or freckling without tan lines even in winter months. Additional signs include abdominal pain, nausea and vomiting, diarrhea, and symptomatic hypoglycemia. If the child experiences a stressful period (illness, injury, or surgery), acute adrenal insufficiency may occur. Signs of an adrenal crisis include weakness, fever, abdominal pain, hypoglycemia with seizures, hypotension, dehydration, shock, and coma.

Serum cortisol and urinary 17-hydroxycorticoid levels are measured in the early morning. Low levels of serum cortisol are associated with adrenal insufficiency. The ACTH stimulation test is used to detect adrenal gland reserve. Electrolyte values generally reveal low serum sodium, elevated serum potassium, and low fasting blood glucose levels. CT may be used to visualize the adrenal glands.

Treatment involves replacement of the deficient hormones. Oral hydrocortisone is given in the lowest therapeutic dose to control symptoms and promote normal growth. Fludrocortisone acetate (Florinef) replaces the missing mineralocorticoid in children with aldosterone deficiency. Adrenal crisis is treated by fluid and electrolyte resuscitation, treatment of the precipitating illness or injury, adequate doses of glucocorticoid, and maintenance doses of mineralocorticoid.

NURSING MANAGEMENT

Nursing management focuses on educating the child and parents about the disorder, providing emotional support, and caring for the child during acute episodes. See the earlier discussion of congenital adrenal hyperplasia for further detail.

PHEOCHROMOCYTOMA

Pheochromocytoma is a tumor of the adrenal gland, but it may be extra-adrenal with no anatomic connection. In most cases these tumors are benign and curable. They can occur in a familial pattern (autosomal dominant trait) with a 3:2 male to female ratio. The incidence is 1 to 500,000 children, and most tumors are diagnosed in children between the ages of 6 and 14 years (Reddy, O'Neill, Holcomb et al., 2000). Pheochromocytomas occur in 1% to 2% of patients with neurofibromatosis, an autosomal dominant genetic disorder in which tumors grow along nerves.

The tumor causes an excessive release of catecholamines epinephrine and norepinephrine leading to hypertension. Clinical manifestations include labile hypertension with a systolic reading that may reach 250 mm Hg, tachycardia, arrhythmias, palpitations, profuse sweating with cool extremities, flushing, headache, abdominal pain, nausea and vomiting, weight loss, visual disturbances, weakness, polydipsia, and polyuria. The classic triad of signs includes new-onset hypertension, new or worsening diabetes mellitus, and hypertensive crisis. Because release of catecholamines (norepinephrine and epinephrine) from the tumor is not continuous, these symptoms occur intermittently. Attacks may occur daily or monthly and generally last minutes to an hour (Failor & Capell, 2003). In some cases the condition may be silent until a stressor such as surgery causes a hypertensive crisis.

Diagnosis is based on 24-hour urine studies to detect the presence of urinary catecholamines and vanilmandelic acid (VMA) levels (see Appendix B). CT, PET scan, MRI, and ultrasound studies are required to locate the tumor in preparation for surgery. Most are located on the adrenal gland, but they may also be located in the chest, bladder, head, and neck (Failor & Capell, 2003). The treatment of choice is surgical removal of the tumor; however, the procedure is dangerous and may result in pheochromocytoma crisis, manifested by seizures, shock, altered level of consciousness, disseminated intravascular coagulation, rhabdomyolysis (skeletal muscle destruction), and acute renal failure. Alpha- and beta-adrenergic blocking agents to control hypertension, tachycardia, and catecholamine release are given for 10 to 14 days before surgery (Harris & Fawcett, 2002). Plasma catecholamines are used to measure the effectiveness of the preoperative adrenergic blockade. Postoperatively, for several days, a 24-hour urine collection is measured for catecholamines to determine if all tumor sites were removed. With successful removal of all tumor sites, the prognosis is generally good. Follow-up is important to assess for recurrence.

NURSING MANAGEMENT

Nursing care is mainly supportive. Provide preoperative and postoperative teaching and care (see Chapter 40 ∞). Preoperatively, monitor vital signs and observe for signs of complications associated with pheochromocytoma crisis. Administer antihypertensives and watch for any signs of hyperglycemia (see page 1839). Postoperatively, the child may be managed initially in an intensive care unit. Monitor blood pressure, and observe for neurologic signs, respiratory distress, and signs of shock. Lifelong follow-up care with screening for hypertension and increased urinary catecholamine levels is required as symptoms recur in up to 20% of patients 2 to 7 years after surgery (Reddy et al., 2000).

DISORDERS OF PANCREATIC FUNCTION

DIABETES MELLITUS

Diabetes mellitus, the most common metabolic disease in children, is a disorder of carbohydrate, protein, and fat metabolism. There are two main types of diabetes. Most children have immune-mediated type 1 diabetes, formerly called insulin-dependent diabetes mellitus or juvenile diabetes. However, a disturbingly large number of children are being diagnosed with type 2 diabetes, formerly called noninsulin-dependent diabetes.

TYPE 1 DIABETES

In the United States, the prevalence of type 1 diabetes among all children 19 years of age and younger is 1.7 per 1000 (Centers for Disease Control and Prevention, 2004). Each year approximately 13,000 children under age 18 years are diagnosed with type 1 diabetes (American Diabetes Association, 2004a). Peak incidence occurs in childhood at 5 to 7 years and again at puberty, but it may present at any age (Alemzadeh & Wyatt, 2004). Caucasians experience a higher incidence of type 1 diabetes than other racial groups. Boys and girls are equally affected.

Etiology and Pathophysiology

Type 1 diabetes is thought to be caused by a genetic component, environmental influences, and an autoimmune response that damages the pancreatic beta cells (Alemzadeh & Wyatt, 2004). Type 1 diabetes has familial tendencies but does not show any specific pattern of inheritance. Inheritance of the DR3 and DR4 markers on the human leukocyte antigen (HLA) complex on chromosome 6 increases the likelihood of developing type 1 diabetes. If the child inherits one marker, the child's risk is 2 to 3 times higher. If both markers are inherited, the child's risk is 7 to 10 times higher (Alemzadeh & Wyatt, 2004). The child inherits a susceptibility to the disease rather than the disease itself.

Insulin helps transport glucose into the cells so that the body can use it as an energy source. It also prevents the outflow of glucose from the liver to the general circulation. Environmental factors such as enteroviruses or toxins are believed to lead to an autoimmune destruction of the beta cells in the islets of Langerhans (see "Pathophysiology Illustrated"). Antigens are generated that lead to production of antibodies that indicate ongoing destruction of the islet cells. As the destruction continues, the child develops glucose intolerance.

The preclinical stage may last up to 13 years as the autoimmune process begins early in life (Silverstein & Rosenbloom, 2000). Lack of insulin results in a rise in blood glucose level and a decrease in the glucose level inside the cells. When the renal threshold for glucose (180 mg/dL) is exceeded, **glycosuria** (abnormal amount of glucose in the urine) occurs as a result of osmotic diuresis (Alemzadeh & Wyatt, 2004). Fluids follow the highly osmotic glucose and are excreted in large volumes (polyuria).

When glucose is unavailable to the cells for metabolism, free fatty acids provide an alternate source of energy. The liver metabolizes fatty acids at an increased rate, producing acetyl coenzyme A (CoA). The by-products of

acetyl CoA metabolism (ketone bodies) accumulate in the body, resulting in a state of metabolic acidosis, or ketoacidosis. (Refer to Chapter 43 for discussion of metabolic acidosis. ∞)

Clinical Manifestations

The classic signs of type 1 diabetes are polyuria, polydipsia, and **polyphagia** (excessive appetite) with significant weight loss. See "Clinical Manifestations: Diabetes by Type." Unexplained fatigue or lethargy, headaches, stomachaches, and occasional enuresis may also occur in a previously toilet-trained child. Adolescent girls may have vaginitis caused by *Candida,* which thrives in the hyperglycemic tissues. Symptoms develop gradually and insidiously but have usually been present less than a month. In severe cases diabetic ketoacidosis (DKA), a type of metabolic acidosis, may develop. This condition is discussed in more detail on p. 1837. See "Nursing Practice" for information about cystic fibrosis–related diabetes.

NURSING PRACTICE

Cystic fibrosis–related diabetes (CFRD) has similar features of types 1 and 2 diabetes; however, it is considered a separate condition. In cystic fibrosis, the pancreas does not produce sufficient insulin (as in type 1 diabetes), which is referred to as insulin deficiency. Another mechanism of CFRD is insulin resistance, in which the body fails to utilize insulin normally, requiring more insulin for metabolism. Insulin deficiency and insulin resistance combined in the patient with cystic fibrosis can lead to the development of diabetes more frequently than those in the general population (Cystic Fibrosis Foundation, 2002).

Clinical Therapy

Diagnosis is based on the presence of classic symptoms and plasma glucose levels as follows (American Diabetes Association, 2004b):

- Fasting plasma glucose ≥ 126 mg/dL (7 mmol/L), no caloric intake for at least 8 hours
- Two-hour plasma glucose ≥ 200 mg/dL (11.1 mmol/L) during an oral glucose tolerance test
- Plasma glucose concentration ≥ 200 mg/dL (11.1 mmol/L) taken at any time of day regardless of time of last meal

Other laboratory tests for known autoantibodies that can indicate an autoimmune attack against the insulin-producing beta cells of the pancreas may be ordered such as glutamic acid decarboxylase (GAD-65), insulin autoantibodies, and islet cell cytoplasmic autoantibodies. A careful history is necessary to rule out a stress-related illness, corticosteroid use, fracture, acute infection, cystic fibrosis,

PATHOPHYSIOLOGY ILLUSTRATED

Mechanism of Diabetes Mellitus

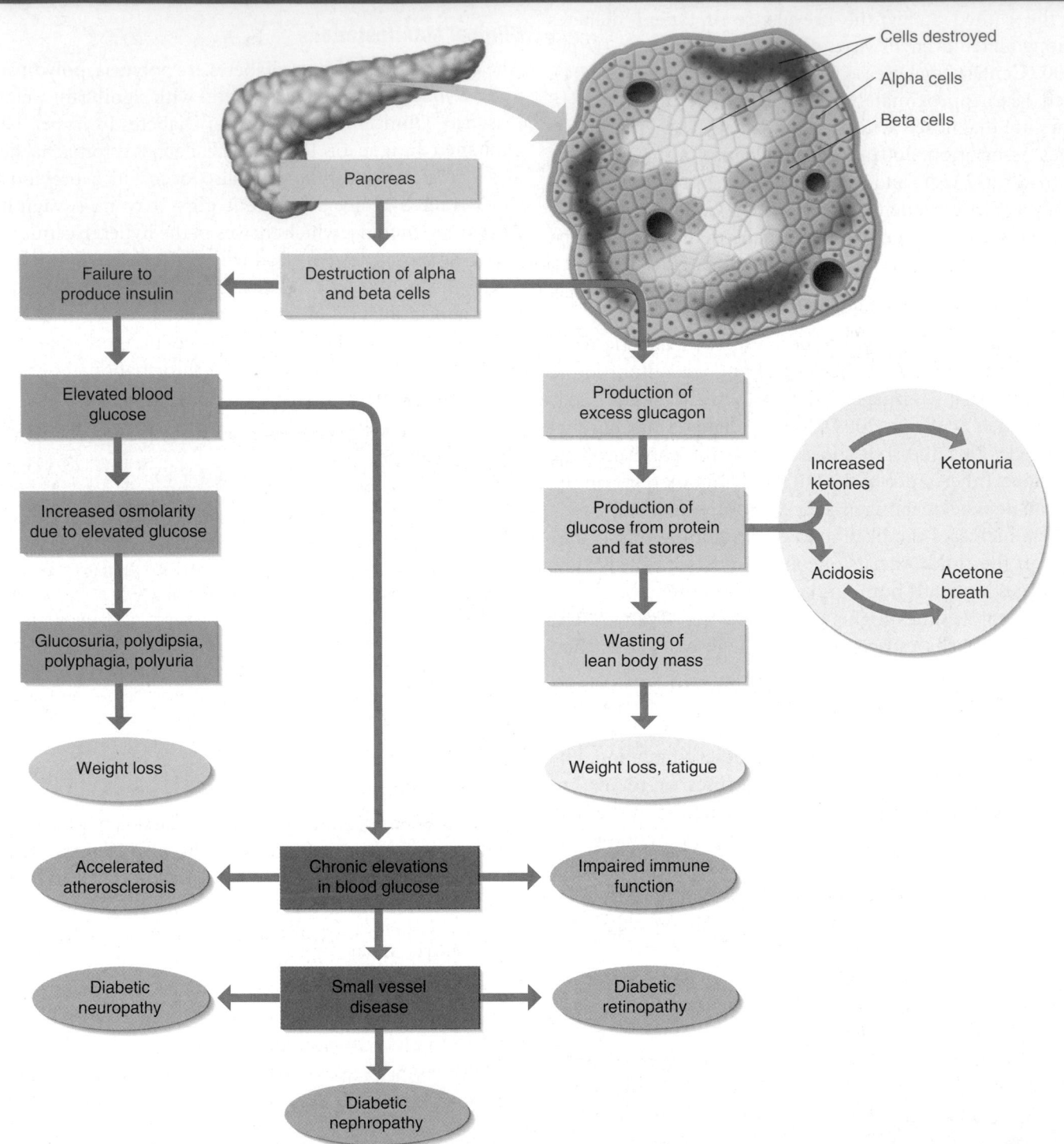

Destruction of the alpha and beta cells in the islets of Langerhans produces multiple metabolic changes. Acute signs and symptoms are followed by short-term and long-term complications if the disease is not well managed.

CLINICAL MANIFESTATIONS

DIABETES BY TYPE

CAUSE	CLINICAL MANIFESTATIONS	CLINICAL THERAPY
Type 1—immune mediated, insulin deficiency due to pancreatic beta cell destruction	Polyuria, polydipsia Recent weight loss, but may be overweight Ketoacidosis on initial presentation in 30% to 40% of cases, at continued risk for ketoacidosis Short duration of symptoms Ketosis Initial period of decreased insulin requirement, then need insulin for survival	Blood glucose monitoring Insulin Dietary management, balancing carbohydrate intake to insulin Exercise
Type 2—insulin resistance with relative insulin secretory defect	Obese, little or no weight loss, or may have significant weight loss Acanthosis nigricans Long duration of symptoms Polyuria, polydipsia, may be mild or absent Glycosuria without ketonuria in 33% of cases on initial presentation Ketoacidosis on initial presentation in 5% to 25% of cases Lipid disorders Hypertension Androgen-mediated problems such as acne, hirsutism, menstrual disturbances, polycystic ovary disease Excessive weight gain and fatigue due to insulin resistance	Diet with decreased calories and low-fat foods Decrease sedentary activity time or increase routine physical activity Blood glucose monitoring Oral medication (metformin) to improve insulin sensitivity

pancreatitis, or liver disease. See "Nursing Practice" for laboratory values associated with pre-diabetes.

NURSING PRACTICE

The American Diabetes Association considers a fasting glucose of 100–125 mg/dL (5.6–6.9 mmol/L) to be an *impaired fasting glucose,* and a 2-hour postload glucose of 140–199 mg/dL to be an *impaired glucose tolerance.* Individuals with impaired fasting glucose or impaired glucose tolerance are now referred to as having "pre-diabetes," indicating that they have a relatively high risk for development of diabetes (American Diabetes Association, 2004b).

Clinical therapy for type 1 diabetes combines insulin, nutrition management to support growth and maintain blood glucose at near-normal levels, an exercise regimen, and psychosocial support.

Insulin Therapy. Multiple approaches to insulin therapy for children and adolescents are available, and an approach that works for the child and family should be selected. The American Diabetes Association (2004b) recommends that blood glucose levels be normalized using basal-bolus therapy for children and adolescents. Research reveals that the risk for developing retinopathy, microalbuminuria, albuminuria, and clinical neuropathy is significantly lower with basal-bolus therapy over more conventional regimens.

The goal of initial basal-bolus therapy is to lower blood glucose levels, stabilize glucose levels, and eliminate ketones. Insulin doses are adjusted according to frequent serum glucose monitoring, at least four times a day. Insulin can be administered by an insulin pump (continuous subcutaneous insulin infusion [CSII]) or by multiple daily injections (MDI). The goal of insulin therapy is to maintain serum glucose levels from 80 to 120 mg/dL before meals and 100 to 140 mg/dL at bedtime

DRUG GUIDE

INSULIN

Overview of Action

Insulin is an endogenous hormone, secreted by the beta cells of the pancreas, that enhances the transmembrane passage of glucose across cell membranes. Insulin lowers the blood glucose level by stimulating glucose passage across cell membranes and uptake into the cells. It also promotes the conversion of glucose to glycogen and inhibits hepatic glucose production from glycogen. It is used as a regular management of type 1 and type 2 diabetes, and for emergency care of diabetic ketoacidosis. Insulin human injection is extracted from beta cells of pork pancreas or synthesized by recombinant DNA technology.

Routes, Dosage, Frequency

Insulin is usually provided in a concentration of 100 units/mL. Diluted insulin may be prepared by a pharmacist. Doses are individualized. Factors such as stress, activity, dietary intake, and status of health cause variations in the insulin dose. The following recommendations can be used for initiating therapy:

IV: Diabetic ketoacidosis (DKA): IV: 0.1 unit/kg bolus, then 0.1 unit/kg/hour continuous drip depending on glucose levels, degree of acidosis, and patient's clinical condition.

SC: 2–4 units regular insulin 15–30 minutes before meals and at bedtime. Regular doses are adjusted as needed when other intermediate and long-acting insulins are added to the regimen.

PUMP: Take 90% of the usual daily insulin dose given by injection as the number to calculate the total daily pump dose. Take 50% of the total pump dose and divide it by 24 to obtain the hourly basal pump dose. Then use the other 50% and divide it into 4 daily doses that are given by bolus at mealtimes. For example, 20% may be given with breakfast, 10% for midday meal, 15% for evening meal, and 5% for evening snack.

Side Effects: Skin reactions such as hives, wheal, induration, or hypertrophy; hypoglycemia; allergic reaction.

Nursing Implications

Assessment: Assess for symptoms of hyperglycemia or hypoglycemia, including urine and blood glucose levels. History of events leading to onset of symptoms, time, and amount of last insulin dosage, illness, exercise, stress, or dietary intake. Assess child's level of growth and development, attitude, and understanding of disease and treatment, and family dynamics and interactions. If newly diagnosed, assess diabetic family and child's level of acceptance, willingness to learn, and ability to grasp large amount of information.

Administer: Use only insulin ordered and carefully read label to prevent giving incorrect insulin. Do not switch brands, strengths, type, species, or purity because it may affect dosage adjustment. Do not give cold insulin as lipodystrophy, reduced absorption, or local discomfort can result. Rotate sites using SC tissue of upper arms, thighs, upper back, buttocks, and stomach. Insulin pump injections are given into the abdomen.

Monitor: Monitor blood glucose levels several times daily. Monitor for symptoms of hypoglycemia, hyperglycemia, and Somogyi reactions (rebound hyperglycemia), as well as for presence of glycosuria. Identify peak action times for insulin used, as that is when hypoglycemia is most likely to occur. Observe child for clammy skin and restlessness. Give child sucrose or glucose PO and check blood level immediately.

Patient Teaching: Learn correct technique for SC or insertion of needles for pump. Respond promptly to signs of hypoglycemia with 4 oz fruit juice or sweetened beverage, followed by complex carbohydrate and protein food. Carry simple sugar source at all times and ensure child has access to them at school. Notify healthcare provider of blood glucose level < 80 and > 120 mg/dL. Insulin may be stored at room temperature but do not expose to excessive heat or sunlight. Do not freeze. Discard opened refrigerated vials after 28 days, and unrefrigerated vials after 14 days.

(American Diabetes Association, 2002). Glycemic goals for children younger than 6 years old are generally less tight since they lack the cognitive capacity to recognize and respond to hypoglycemic symptoms (American Diabetes Association, 2004b).

With basal-bolus therapy, basal insulin is administered once a day (Lantus or glargine), or twice daily (Humulin or Ultralente). Then a bolus of rapid-acting insulin is administered with each meal and snack based on the carbohydrate grams consumed. The goal of basal-bolus insulin therapy is to maintain a blood glucose level as close to the target range as possible and to minimize episodes of hyperglycemia and hypoglycemia (see pages 1839). Several forms of insulin are available as identified in Table 56–3.

NURSING PRACTICE

Insulin is usually provided in prepackaged doses of 100 units/mL. Diluted insulin prepared by a pharmacist may be used for infants and toddlers who require a small insulin dosage. Insulin cartridges, disposable pens, and other devices are available, making insulin easy to carry by adolescents for frequent insulin injections during the day.

Basal-bolus therapy for type 1 diabetes includes:

- Monitoring blood glucose four to eight times a day and once a week at midnight and 3 A.M.

TABLE 56–3 ✛ Insulin Action (Subcutaneous Route)

Type	Onset	Peak	Duration
Rapid Acting			
Lispro/Humalog	5–15 min	1 hr	2–4 hr
Insulin aspart	10–20 min	1–3 hr	3–5 hr
Short Acting			
Regular	½–1 hr	2–4 hr	6–8 hr
Intermediate Acting			
NPH	1–2 hr	6–12 hr	18–26 hr
Lente	1–2 hr	6–12 hr	24–26 hr
Long Acting			
Ultralente	4–8 hr	10–20 hr	16–24 hr
Lantus/insulin glargine	1–2 hr	none/slight	24 hr

Note: Intermediate-acting insulin mixed with short- or rapid-acting insulin (e.g., 70% NPH/30% regular, 50% NPH/50% regular, and 75% NPH/25% insulin lispro) is also available.

- Consistent carbohydrate counting.
- Anticipating exercise in the routine.

Basal-bolus therapy can be achieved with three or more insulin injections a day or a continuous subcutaneous insulin infusion (CSII) by an insulin pump. CSII by insulin pump has recently been found to lower the HbA$_{1c}$ and improve metabolic control in youth with type 1 diabetes (Doyle, Weinzimer, Steffen et al., 2004). Stress, infection, and illness may either increase or decrease insulin needs. In addition, increased insulin doses are often required during growth and at puberty. See Table 56–4 for criteria for selecting insulin pump therapy. Advantages and disadvantages of an insulin pump are outlined in Table 56–5.

For some children, conventional insulin therapy may be used, requiring two or three insulin injections a day. One example of conventional insulin therapy consists of daily administration of a combination of a short-acting (regular) insulin and an intermediate-acting (NPH or Lente) or long-acting (Ultralente) insulin before breakfast and before the evening meal (Figure 56–5 ⬤). Older children may use a regimen of tighter control that includes two injections a day of intermediate or long-acting insulin and an injection of rapid-acting insulin with each meal to match carbohydrate intake. Advantages of rapid-acting insulin (Lispro) in therapy to achieve tight glucose control include:

- Decreased number of nocturnal hypoglycemic episodes.
- Meal coverage for toddlers who have unpredictable food consumption.
- Flexibility for adolescents concerned about weight gain who do not want to eat a midmorning snack.

Insulin therapy is evaluated every 3 months with a hemoglobin A$_{1c}$ (HbA$_{1c}$) level, an objective measurement of glycemic control. It represents the amount of glucose irreversibly attached to the hemoglobin molecule over an extended period (the life span of the red blood cell, approximately 120 days), therefore predicting an index of glucose control over the prior 6 to 8 weeks (Haller, Stalvey, & Silverstein, 2004). The HbA$_{1c}$ is below 6.2% for individuals

TABLE 56–4 ✛ Criteria for Selecting Insulin Pump Therapy in Children of Different Ages

Toddlers and Young Children	Children Over 10 Years
Problems during therapy ■ Recurrent episodes of moderate and severe hypoglycemia ■ Persistent HbA$_{1c}$ ≥ 9% even with changes in insulin dosing ■ Unexplained erratic changes in blood glucose levels not resolved with insulin dosing changes ■ Recurrent diabetic ketoacidosis or severe hyperglycemia Parents or caregivers available to provide constant supervision ■ Understand pump functioning ■ Able to adjust basal and bolus doses ■ Monitor blood glucose levels 4 times daily ■ Have collaborative working relationship with healthcare providers Child can tolerate catheter and infusion set and refrain from touching the catheter and pump	Disease management readiness ■ 3–6 months of intensive insulin therapy, including 3 or more shots per day ■ 3–6 months of monitoring and recording blood glucose levels at least 4 times per day ■ 3–6 months of carbohydrate counting ■ Ability to give abdominal injections and no fear of needles ■ Diabetes identification medallion ■ Ability to make small adjustments in treatment regimen appropriately between visits ■ Evidence of diabetes team contact in emergency situations Psychosocial readiness ■ Child/adolescent responsible for majority of diabetes self-care

Adapted from Litton, J., Rice, A., Friedman, N., Oden, J., Lee, M. M., & Freemark, M. (2002). Insulin pump therapy in toddlers and preschool children with type 1 diabetes mellitus. *Journal of Pediatrics, 141,* 490–495; Cogen, F. R., Streisand, R., & Sarin, S. (2002). Selecting children and adolescents for insulin pump therapy: Medical and behavioral considerations. *Diabetes Spectrum, 15*(2), 72–75.

TABLE 56–5 ✤ Advantages and Disadvantages of an External Insulin Infusion Pump

Advantages	Disadvantages
■ Delivers a continuous infusion of insulin to match the basal rate needed plus an insulin bolus at mealtime ■ Helps maintain blood glucose control between meals ■ Decreases HbA_{1c} ■ Improves growth in children ■ Reduces number of injections ■ Allows child to eat with less adherence to a schedule ■ Reduces number of injection sites, so variation in absorption decreases ■ More closely simulates normal pancreatic function, exact dosing of insulin since basal rates can be changed every ½ hour ■ Frequency of severe hypoglycemia has been decreased and fewer incidences of DKA ■ More flexible lifestyle is permitted	■ Requires highly motivated child and supportive parents and healthcare professionals ■ Requires willingness to live connected to a device (can be disconnected for short periods by removing or clamping the catheter; however, DKA can occur within hours of interruption of insulin flow) ■ The site must be changed every 2–4 days, at least 1 inch from the last site ■ Necessitates more time and energy to monitor blood glucose levels, nutritional intake, and insulin bolus calculation ■ Involves changing syringe, catheter, and skin setup every 2–3 days ■ Infections can occur at the injection site ■ Weight gain is common when blood glucose control improves

Data from Saudek, C. D. (1997). Novel forms of insulin delivery. *Endocrinology and Metabolism Clinics of North America, 26*(3), 599–610; Maniatis, A. K., Klingensmith, G. J., Slover, R. H., Mowry, C. J., & Chase, H. P. (2001). Continuous subcutaneous insulin infusion therapy for children and adolescents: An option for routine diabetes care. *Pediatrics, 107*(2), 351–356; and Miller, M. M. (2003). Insulin pump therapy. *Advance for Nurse Practitioners, 11*(11), 61–66.

without diabetes, and the goal for children with diabetes is 7.5% to 8% depending on age and healthcare provider preferences. It is also important to determine if the HbA_{1c} matches recorded blood sugars.

Exercise Program. Physical activity is associated with increased insulin sensitivity. Regular exercise and fitness improves glucose control, reduces cardiovascular risk factors, contributes to weight loss, and improves overall well-being. Blood lipid levels are also positively affected. However, the child must have an adequate caloric intake to prevent hypoglycemia. Excessive exercise associated with sports requires careful planning and management.

Nutrition Therapy. Consideration of the child and family's culture, lifestyle, and finances is important in developing an individualized nutrition plan. Daily caloric requirements are individualized for each child according to his or her needs to support growth and development and for disease management.

Carbohydrate counting provides flexibility in meal planning and is simple for children and adolescents to use.

One carbohydrate choice equals 15 grams of carbohydrates. Younger school-age children can consume two to four carbohydrate choices per meal, while older children and adolescents can consume four to six. Additional carbohydrate choices are necessary for more physically active children. Between-meal snacks generally consist of one to two carbohydrate choices, depending on the type of insulin used (Evert, 2004). One unit of insulin covers 8 grams of carbohydrates, making insulin dosage calculation for meal coverage relatively easy. If additional carbohydrates are eaten at a meal or snack, the number of insulin units can also be adjusted providing further flexibility. A high-fiber diet is also recommended for improved control of blood glucose.

Many new developments for diabetes management are being evaluated. Studies of the effectiveness of inhaled insulin for administration before meals also are being conducted (Quattrin, Belanger, Bohannon et al., 2004). Noninvasive or continuous glucose monitoring techniques are being investigated and have been approved by the FDA for adults (Silverstein & Rosenbloom, 2000). Pancreatic

● FIGURE 56–5

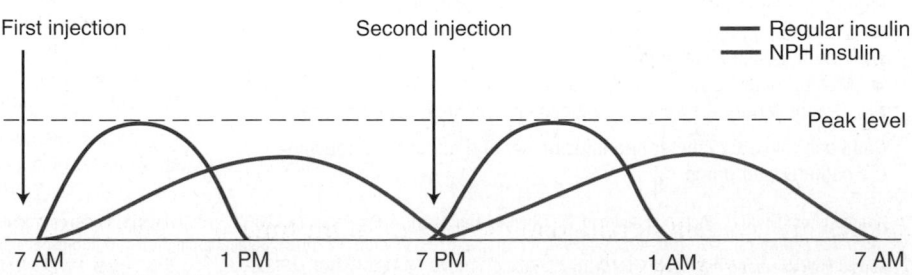

Conventional therapy. Insulin levels vary over a 24-hour period in relation to injections and mealtimes.

THINKING CRITICALLY

MANAGING ADOLESCENT DIABETES

Anthony, 12 years old, has just been diagnosed with diabetes mellitus. His parents took him to their family physician after Anthony complained of being constantly thirsty and hungry for over a week. Despite this he lost 5 pounds. They note that he had a viral illness about 1 month ago but seemed to recover from it. His mother says that Anthony seemed lethargic for several days.

Anthony and his family must now learn to manage his diabetes using the combination of a food plan, exercise, and insulin therapy. Monitoring his blood glucose level is important in determining how much insulin he will need every day. Anthony and his mother will need to learn to schedule his meals and snacks; to have appropriate amounts of protein, fat, and carbohydrates at each meal; and to count carbohydrates. Anthony's meals and activity will need to be coordinated with the insulin doses. Anthony and his parents will need to watch closely for signs of hypoglycemia. Develop a teaching plan that includes the following information:

- What causes diabetes?
- What potential problems need prompt treatment?
- What does Anthony need to monitor for when he gets sick?
- Intensive therapy will be a goal of Anthony's treatment—how can you help Anthony and his family decide if this should be accomplished with insulin injections or an insulin pump?
- What are some strategies to help an adolescent actively participate in his disease management and maintain optimal diabetic control?

transplantation for patients requiring a kidney transplant is now performed with evidence of improved short-term outcomes (Eisenbrath, Polonsky, & Buse, 2003). Isolated pancreatic transplant is not performed because immunosuppression therapy is destructive to the islet cells.

Complications of type 1 diabetes (retinopathy, heart disease, renal failure, and peripheral vascular disease) result from long-term hyperglycemic effects on the blood vessels. Without careful management, children with diabetes may develop renal failure and loss of vision in adulthood. Intensive therapy is expected to reduce the risk for or delay the development of these complications. Risk may be further reduced if the adolescent does not begin smoking and if the blood pressure is controlled.

NURSING MANAGEMENT

NURSING ASSESSMENT AND DIAGNOSIS

Physiologic Assessment

Children are generally admitted to the hospital at the time of diagnosis. Assess the child's physiologic status, focusing on vital signs and level of consciousness. Assess hydration

by checking mucous membranes, skin turgor, and urine output. Blood initially is collected hourly to monitor blood gases, glucose, and electrolytes. Once the child is stable, assess dietary and caloric intake and the ability of the child or family to manage care.

Psychosocial Assessment

Parents may feel guilty at the time of diagnosis if they waited to seek care until the child began to experience symptoms of DKA. Assess coping mechanisms, ability to manage the disease, and educational needs of both the child and parents. Examples of questions to use in assessing the family's strengths and limitations in the child's disease management include:

- Do both parents or the single parent work? What hours?
- Who else is involved in the child's care?
- What is the child's usual daily schedule? Does the schedule vary on the weekend or any other days of the week?
- Does the child have health insurance? What coverage exists for diabetes education, treatment, and home management?
- Does the child have any cognitive, behavioral, motor, or visual problems coexisting with this condition?
- What other family stressors coexist with the diagnosis?

Developmental Assessment

Assess the child's developmental level, particularly fine motor skills and cognitive level. The child will need to learn how to obtain and read a blood glucose sample and how to inject insulin (see Skill 10–3). **SKILLS** Children can usually perform some of these tasks with supervision by 6 to 8 years of age.

Adolescents perceive type 1 diabetes as a disability and often deny having the disease so they can be like their peers when eating and exercising. Talk with the adolescent and assess problem-solving skills associated with daily condition management, and the ability to manage special circumstances such as illness or changes in exercise. Self-management is the eventual goal, and the child's responsibilities are gradually increased.

Several diagnoses that may apply to the child newly diagnosed with type 1 diabetes are provided in the accompanying "Nursing Care Plans." Additional diagnoses that may be appropriate include the following:

- *Risk for Deficient Fluid Volume* related to active fluid loss associated with hyperglycemia
- *Ineffective Breathing Pattern* related to neuromuscular dysfunction associated with metabolic acidosis
- *Ineffective Denial* related to inability to admit impact of disease on lifestyle

MEDIALINK

Video: Adolescent Diabetes and Quality of Life

PLANNING AND IMPLEMENTATION

Nursing care focuses on teaching the child and parents about the disease and its management, managing dietary intake, providing emotional support, and planning strategies for daily management in the community. Refer to the accompanying "Nursing Care Plans," which summarize nursing care for the child who is hospitalized with newly diagnosed type 1 diabetes, and the child who is receiving care in the community. Some hospitals have developed clinical pathways to streamline and standardize diabetes care.

Provide Education

The nurse is an important member of the management team (physician, nurse, nutritionist, and social worker) and is usually responsible for educating the child and family. An advanced-practice nurse or diabetic nurse educator in the clinic setting often does this teaching, since children may be hospitalized only briefly following diagnosis.

The timing and amount of information provided are especially important in the first days following diagnosis. Both the child and parents are very tired, and they are often in a state of shock and disbelief. Information presented during this period needs to be repeated. Use this time to assess learning needs and to answer the family's questions. Initial teaching focuses on the survival skills necessary for home management (insulin administration, blood glucose testing, record keeping, dietary management, and the recognition and treatment of both hypoglycemia and hyperglycemia).

Explain the goals of insulin therapy. Teach the child and parents how to administer insulin and perform blood glucose tests (Figure 56–6 ⬤). Rotating the injection sites is im-

⬤ **FIGURE 56–6**

This mother is being taught how to test her child's blood glucose level.

portant to decrease the chances of *lipoatrophy,* loss of subcutaneous tissue, or hypertrophy in which collagen is replaced by fat cells (Figure 56–7 ⬤). The absorption rate of insulin varies by the site used. Insulin is usually absorbed most rapidly from the abdomen; however, insulin absorption is increased in the extremities with exercise. An understanding of the different types of insulin and their actions is essential.

Once the child and parents demonstrate understanding of this information, teach guidelines for managing episodes of hyperglycemia during acute illness and using a sliding scale. A sliding scale indicates specific insulin dosages appropriate for a particular blood glucose level. The family also needs to learn "sick day" care guidelines to prevent diabetic ketoacidosis.

☀ ## TEACHING HIGHLIGHTS

SICK DAY GUIDELINES

When the child with diabetes is sick, parents need to be extra attentive to the child's glycemic control. The following recommendations should be followed (Boland & Grey, 2004):

- Seek medical attention for fever or other signs of infection.
- Monitor the blood glucose levels more often than routine (every 1 to 4 hours).
- Test urine ketones when the blood glucose level is greater than 200 mg/dL.
- The usual dose of insulin may be increased for high blood glucose levels.
- Do not skip doses of insulin.
- Maintain a large fluid intake (more than 8 oz hourly) even if the child cannot eat to maintain food and fluid intake. Seek medical attention if this is not possible. Fluids should have carbohydrates to maintain the child's usual caloric intake.

NURSING CARE PLAN

THE CHILD HOSPITALIZED WITH NEWLY DIAGNOSED TYPE 1 DIABETES MELLITUS

Intervention	Rationale	Expected Outcome

1. Nursing Diagnosis: Deficient Knowledge (Child and Parents) related to lack of exposure to diabetic management in the newly diagnosed child

NIC Priority Intervention:		NOC Suggested Outcome:
Individual teaching: Planning, implementing, and evaluating a teaching program designed to address a patient's particular need		**Knowledge:** Extent of understanding conveyed about treatment regimen

Goal: The child and parents will acquire survival skills for home management.

■ Assess the child's developmental level and select an educational approach and self-care activities to match. ■ Teach blood glucose monitoring, drawing up and injecting insulin, urine testing for ketones, record keeping, survival food guidelines, and when to call the healthcare provider. ■ Use demonstration/return demonstration until the child and family are comfortable with procedures.	■ Learning goals for the child must match knowledge and skill expectations appropriate for developmental stage. ■ Diabetic management survival skills are needed for initial home management until more extensive education can be completed that permits more independent management. ■ Evaluation permits positive reinforcement and guidance for modification of techniques.	The child and parents demonstrate proper technique for blood glucose monitoring, urine testing for ketones, drawing up insulin doses and injection, and record keeping.

Goal: The child and parents will recognize signs and symptoms of hypoglycemia and hyperglycemia.

■ Teach signs and symptoms of hypoglycemic and hyperglycemic reactions. ■ Teach the child to test blood glucose when feeling different than usual, and record the reading and symptoms felt.	■ Recognition of and treatment of poor glucose control will prevent progression of symptoms. ■ Permits child to learn his/her specific symptoms of hyper- and hypoglycemia.	The child and family can describe symptoms of hypoglycemia and hyperglycemia.

2. Nursing Diagnosis: Risk for Injury related to periods of hypoglycemia and diabetic ketoacidosis

NIC Priority Intervention:		NOC Suggested Outcome:
Hypoglycemia monitoring: Instituting special precautions with patient at risk for injury		**Risk control:** Actions to eliminate or reduce actual, personal, and modifiable health threats

Goal: The child will experience few episodes of hypoglycemia during hospitalization.

■ Assess the child at least every 2 hours for signs of hypoglycemia. If signs are present, check blood glucose to verify and administer source of quick sugar. ■ When the child is NPO for a special procedure, verify with physician when food, fluids, and insulin are to be given, or if an intravenous infusion with dextrose is to be given. ■ Have glucose paste or 50% dextrose solution readily available.	■ Hypoglycemia commonly occurs during hospitalization because of change in diet, lack of food intake, or illness. ■ Giving insulin without food intake can lead to hypoglycemia. Intravenous dextrose and insulin can be used when the child must be NPO. ■ Dextrose is used for emergency intravenous treatment of severe hypoglycemia. Glucose paste is used for oral treatment.	The child and staff manage episodes of hypoglycemia without a crisis developing.

(continued)

NURSING CARE PLAN—continued

THE CHILD HOSPITALIZED WITH NEWLY DIAGNOSED TYPE 1 DIABETES MELLITUS

Intervention	Rationale	Expected Outcome
Goal: The child's condition is treated slowly to gradually reverse hyperglycemia and ketoacidosis and to prevent cerebral edema.		
▪ Assess the child's mental status for improvement or deterioration. ▪ Check blood glucose and urine ketones frequently to confirm reduction in blood glucose level and ketosis and to identify the insulin dose for administration. ▪ Monitor and control IV fluid intake. Measure output. ▪ Have insulin doses checked by a second nurse.	▪ Improvement in mental status may indicate successful treatment. Deterioration may indicate onset of cerebral edema. ▪ Frequent blood glucose and ketone level determination helps assess progress in treating ketoacidosis. ▪ The child with ketoacidosis will be dehydrated. IV fluid intake needs to be carefully controlled to prevent cerebral edema. ▪ Doses are frequently small, and the possibility of error is great.	The child's hyperglycemia and ketoacidosis resolves without additional complications.
Goal: The child and parents will demonstrate emergency management of hypoglycemia.		
▪ Identify sources of glucose to give in case of hypoglycemic reaction. Tell the child and parent to carry glucose tablets or paste with them at all times.	▪ Access to sources of glucose and its rapid administration are important for emergency care.	The child and family can identify several glucose sources for emergencies. The child and family have a source of glucose with them at each visit.
Goal: The child and parents will demonstrate management of sick days.		
▪ Teach the child and family to test blood glucose and urine for ketones with acute symptoms and notify the healthcare provider.	▪ When the child is ill, hyperglycemia needs special management to prevent progression to ketoacidosis.	The child's hyperglycemic episodes do not progress to ketoacidosis.
3. Nursing Diagnosis: Imbalanced Nutrition: Less than Body Requirements related to glycosuria		
NIC Priority Intervention: **Nutrition management:** Assistance with or provision of a balanced dietary intake of foods and fluids		**NOC Suggested Outcome:** **Nutritional status:** Extent to which nutrients are available to meet metabolic needs
Goal: The child will eat a well-balanced diet and maintain normal height and weight proportions.		
▪ Encourage and serve meals and snacks with consistent carbohydrates at the same time each day. ▪ Provide a calorie nonrestricted diet.	▪ Keeps blood glucose levels stable during initial disease management stages. ▪ Enables weight lost during onset of diabetes to be regained.	The child regains weight lost and demonstrates normal growth and stable blood glucose levels.
Goal: The child and parents will state understanding of dietary management of diabetes mellitus.		
▪ Make an appointment with a nutritionist who can assess the child's favorite foods and promote their integration into the child's diet. Reinforce the dietary information taught. ▪ Provide sample menus and teach the use of carbohydrate counting.	▪ The nutritionist can develop dietary recommendations that fit the specific needs of the child and include favorite foods, thereby increasing compliance with the diet. ▪ Assists the family and adolescent with diet planning.	The child and parents describe nutritional needs of the child and select the dietary management best suited to the family's and child's eating habits.

NURSING CARE PLAN

THE CHILD WITH PREVIOUSLY DIAGNOSED TYPE 1 DIABETES BEING CARED FOR AT HOME

Intervention	Rationale	Expected Outcome
1. Nursing Diagnosis: Imbalanced Nutrition: Less than Body Requirements related to chronic illness (diabetes mellitus)		
NIC Priority Intervention: **Weight management:** Assistance with or provision of a balanced dietary intake of foods and fluids		**NOC Suggested Outcome:** **Nutritional status: Nutrient value:** Adequacy of nutrients taken into body
Goal: The child will eat a well-balanced diet that maintains weight proportional to height.		
■ Assess height and weight regularly and plot on growth chart. ■ Make an appointment with a nutritionist who can assess the child's favorite foods and integrate them into a food plan that controls caloric intake. Encourage the child to keep a food diary.	■ Assesses change in body mass index to identify potential weight problem early. ■ Inclusion of child's favorite foods helps child adapt to changes in the food plan.	Diet records indicate meals and snacks have the appropriate distribution of carbohydrates, protein, and fats, and daily caloric intake goals are met.
2. Nursing Diagnosis: Readiness for Enhanced Family Processes related to management of a chronic disease		
NIC Priority Intervention: **Family process maintenance:** Minimization of family process disruption effects		**NOC Suggested Outcome:** **Family functioning:** Ability of family to meet the needs of its members through developmental transitions
Goal: The child and family will manage the food plan, exercise, blood glucose monitoring, and medications regimen.		
■ Assess the family's lifestyle and attempt to fit the child's care needs into the family's schedule. ■ Discuss the family's routines for special occasions and vacations. Identify ways to modify the child's management for these occasions.	■ Fitting the care to the family's lifestyle promotes adherence with the regimen. ■ It is important for the child to participate in special events with the family and peers as a normal child to promote psychologic development.	The child and family make minimal changes in usual lifestyle while managing the type 1 diabetes.
3. Nursing Diagnosis: Ineffective Coping (Individual) related to inadequate level of confidence in ability to cope		
NIC Priority Intervention: **Coping enhancement:** Assisting a patient to adapt to perceived stressors, changes, or threats which interfere with meeting life demands and roles		**NOC Suggested Outcome:** **Coping:** Actions to manage stressors that tax an individual's resources
Goal: The child will demonstrate enhanced coping skills.		
■ Ask how the child has solved problems in the past. Review possible problems the child may encounter. Together evaluate the effectiveness of solutions. Suggest other solutions to consider.	■ Children's success in mastering maturational conflicts and daily psychosocial problems will influence their pattern of coping.	The child demonstrates enhanced coping skills and expresses positive attitude toward self. The child displays warmth and affection toward family.
Goal: The child will develop positive self-esteem.		
■ Role-play ways to talk about diabetes with friends and teachers. Encourage the child to express feelings about diabetes to those he or she trusts. ■ Encourage the child to attend diabetes camp. ■ Encourage the child to continue previous social activities and hobbies.	■ Sharing information about the condition helps others understand changes in lifestyle needed by the child. Expressing feelings decreases anxiety. ■ Learning and support networks developed at camp can promote self-esteem. ■ Increased social interaction, especially in group sessions, improves self-esteem.	The child demonstrates confidence in interactions with peers and maintains social network.

(continued)

NURSING CARE PLAN—continued

THE CHILD WITH PREVIOUSLY DIAGNOSED TYPE 1 DIABETES BEING CARED FOR AT HOME

Intervention	Rationale	Expected Outcome
4. Nursing Diagnosis: Health-Seeking Behaviors (Child) related to learning self-management of chronic disorder		
NIC Priority Intervention: **Self-modification assistance:** Reinforcement of self-directed change initiated by the patient to achieve personally important goals		**NOC Suggested Outcome:** **Health promotion:** Actions to sustain or increase wellness
Goal: The child will develop independent ability to manage diabetes care.		
■ Allow the child to perform as many self-care procedures as possible at each developmental stage. ■ Encourage the child to make decisions regarding care. Review decisions and discuss possible alternative solutions. Role-play possible scenarios. ■ Encourage parents to stay involved even when the adolescent takes primary responsibility for care. ■ Provide 24-hour access to physician or diabetes nurse educator. Encourage the child to seek help early.	■ Normal growth and development are ensured if the child is encouraged to participate in care from the beginning. ■ Trust develops when children sense that their decisions are respected or at least considered by others. ■ The child's diabetic control is likely to be better when the parents continue to show interest and supervise care. ■ The child needs to overcome concerns about calling for guidance, and thus maintain better control.	The child is able to perform as many diabetic care techniques as possible for age.

Caution parents to check the blood glucose level of a toddler who is extremely sleepy or irritable, as these can be signs of either hypoglycemia or hyperglycemia.

● FIGURE 56–7

Insulin injection sites. Give all morning insulin in one site (e.g., arms) and all evening insulin in another (e.g., legs) because of different rates of absorption from these sites. Space injections about 1/2 inch (1.25 cm) apart.

Manage Food Intake

The preferred diet for children with type 1 diabetes is a low-saturated-fat, low-sodium food plan. The child needs adequate calories to reach or maintain a desirable body weight. The meal plan should consist of 55% carbohydrates, 30% fat, and 15% protein. The Food Guide Pyramid (see page 929 in Chapter 34 ∞) may be used to teach the child and family the correct portions and which foods are considered carbohydrates, fats, and proteins. A variety of simple and complex carbohydrates should be eaten. An increased ratio of polyunsaturated fats should be eaten to reduce serum lipid levels. Eating at consistent intervals is important for glycemic control, whether counting calories or following a conventional treatment plan (three meals a day and three snacks a day). Although the child with diabetes is not restricted from eating any food, certain foods need to be balanced by extra insulin. A nutritionist can help the family integrate preferred ethnic foods into the child's diet. Nonnutritive sweeteners such as aspartame and saccharin may be used in moderation. The child and family should understand how to read food labels.

Provide Emotional Support

The diagnosis of type 1 diabetes often comes as a shock to the family. If there is a familial history, parents may feel guilty about having caused the disease. The diagnosis of a chronic disease that requires daily management can be difficult to accept. Give parents information about diabetes education programs, put them in touch with other parents of diabetic children, and help them to learn the role they can play in managing the disease.

Support for the child depends on age and developmental stage. Encourage the child to express feelings about the disease and its management. The adolescent may benefit from contact with other adolescents who have diabetes.

Discharge Planning and Home Care Teaching

Home care needs should be identified and addressed before discharge. Initial survival skills described earlier are taught with the plans for ongoing outpatient education.

Make every effort to incorporate the diabetic regimen (insulin administration, food plan, blood glucose monitoring, and exercise) into the family's present lifestyle. The fewer changes the family has to make, the greater the chance of adherence.

The family and child newly diagnosed with diabetes should be made aware of the "honeymoon phase." This is a period during new-onset diabetes when the child has some residual beta-cell function, which reduces exogenous insulin requirements. The child and family may assume this is an indication that the diabetes "is better." However, insulin requirement does eventually return. The duration of this phase varies among individuals.

Provide written materials and refer parents to books and other materials they can use in teaching the child about diabetes. The Juvenile Diabetic Research Foundation and the American Diabetes Association are good sources of information. See the Companion Website for links to these resources.

Nursing Care in the Community

During follow-up visits, ask the child or parents about signs indicating problems of diabetic control. Questions to ask that could help identify problems in diabetic control include:

- Is the child hungry at meals? Between meals?
- How much fluid is the child drinking?
- Has the child been going to the bathroom frequently or had episodes of bed-wetting?
- Does the child have dry skin?
- Are there sores on the feet? Do scratches or scrapes take a long time to heal?
- Has the child had any skin infections?
- Does the child have changes in mood (depression, unexplained sadness, irritability) or energy level from day to day or throughout the day?
- Have there been any changes in vision?

Record growth measurements and vital signs in the child's chart. Review the child's typical dietary intake and exercise regimens. Assess the child's sexual development using Tanner staging guidelines (see Chapter 35 ∞). Puberty may be delayed if diabetic control is inadequate. Evaluation for the potential complications of diabetes should be performed annually, including blood for lipid levels, blood pressure, liver and renal function, urine for albumin, an ophthalmologic examination for retinopathy, and a neurologic examination of the extremities for neuropathies.

Education is ongoing, especially for children who develop diabetes at a young age. As they grow and assume more responsibility for their care, they need to learn more about the pathophysiology of the disease and the rationale for its management.

Continually work with the child to help him or her assume responsibility for self-care, and with parents to promote the child's self-care (Figure 56–8 ●). The child's developmental stage and cognitive level influence his or her readiness to take on responsibility for self-care. Summer camps and other programs for children with diabetes are often helpful in providing education and support.

The preschool child's need for autonomy and control can be met by allowing the child to choose snacks or to pick which finger to stick for glucose testing and by helping parents to gather necessary supplies. School-age children can learn to test blood glucose, administer insulin, and keep

● **FIGURE 56-8**

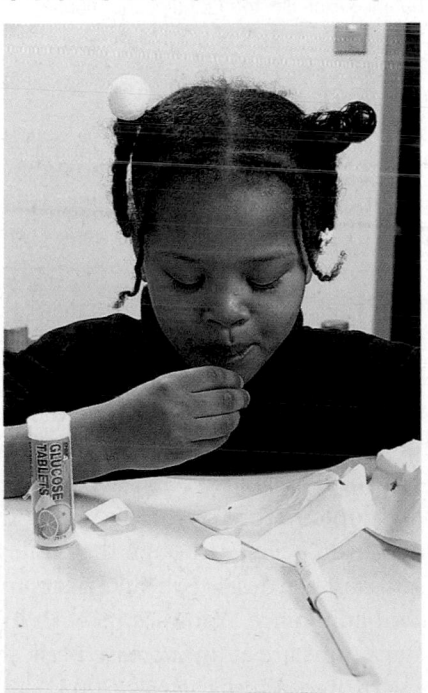

This girl is old enough to understand the need to take glucose tablets or another form of a rapidly absorbed sugar when her blood glucose level is low.

HEALTH PROMOTION
The Child with Diabetes Mellitus

Growth and Development Surveillance
- Compare the child's height, weight, and head circumference to age-specific norms to determine if growth is meeting expectations for age.
- Assess developmental progress using the Denver II or another screening tool (refer to Chapter 37 ∞). Assess school performance.
- Assess for delays in development of sexual secondary characteristics and pubertal changes.

Nutrition
- Promote adherence to nutrition guidelines by including the child's personal preferences in the food plan.

Physical Activity
- Encourage regular physical activity and educate the child to modify insulin dosage or food intake for extra physical activity periods.
- Encourage the child to participate in sports when interested and work to balance exercise, food intake, and insulin dosage.

Oral Health
- Promote good dentition and oral hygiene.
- Regular dental visits are important to reduce risk of infections.
- The child with poorly controlled diabetes is at risk of gingivitis and cavities.

Mental and Spiritual Health
- Provide the child and adolescent an opportunity to discuss feelings regarding diabetes.
- Assess the adolescent for evidence of depression.

Relationships
- The child should attend school or childcare as any other child.
- Encourage the development of special friends who can be informed about the child's disorder and seek help when needed.

Disease Prevention Strategies
- Encourage family to maintain the child's active immunization status.
- Children with diabetes should receive an annual influenza vaccine.
- Refer the child for an annual ophthalmologic examination.
- Maintain appointments for regular evaluation of $HgbA_{1c}$ to monitor glycemic control.

Injury Prevention Strategies
- Encourage the child to wear a medical identification tag.
- Encourage daily inspection of feet and foot care.
- Provide the family with strategies for safe disposal of needles and syringes.

---

records. They should be taught how to select foods and portion sizes appropriate for dietary management and how to plan food intake for an exercise program. School-age children need to learn to recognize the signs of hypoglycemia and hyperglycemia, and understand the importance of carrying a rapidly absorbed sugar product.

Although adolescents understand explanations about the potential complications of diabetes, they are present-time oriented and may rebel against the daily regimen of insulin injections, the food plan, and the exercise plan. Successful self-care depends in part on the adolescent's adjustment to the chronic nature of the disease and feelings of being different from peers. Although the adolescent is able to manage self-care, the desire to be like peers may interfere with treatment adherence. Adolescents with high levels of depressive symptoms are at an increased risk for hospitalization (Stewart, Rao, Emslie, et al., 2005). Talk with the adolescent to assess mood and to evaluate motivation to manage the meal plan, exercise regimen, blood glucose monitoring, and insulin therapy. Discuss how carbohy-

drate counting and insulin dose adjustment may provide the flexibility to participate in activities with peers. Collaborate with the adolescent in preparation to assume care, and assist parents in accepting the growing independence from adult supervision. A discussion of the hazards associated with having diabetes and the use of alcohol, drugs, and tobacco should occur.

The child with diabetes should be treated as any other child without a chronic condition, including limit setting and consistent discipline for unacceptable behavior. Children with type 1 diabetes may learn maladaptive behaviors, using their disease to obtain something they want. Teach parents to be alert to signs of maladaption, such as helpless, demanding, or whining behaviors, and any evidence of poor coping. Additional behaviors may include skipping blood glucose testing and losing or damaging equipment. Food may become a battleground for toddlers who are picky eaters, but must eat enough for the insulin dose. Referral for counseling may be appropriate for some families.

TEACHING HIGHLIGHTS

TREATING HYPOGLYCEMIC EPISODES

- If the child shows signs of hypoglycemia (pallor, sweating, tremors, dizziness, numb lips or mouth, confusion, irritability, altered mental status), test the blood glucose level.
- Assist the child to do the test, as skills needed to get an accurate reading deteriorate with altered mental status.
- If the blood glucose reading is ≤ 70 mg/dL, give glucose rapidly. Use one of the following:
    - 1/2 cup orange juice
    - 3/4 cup of sugar-sweetened beverage
    - 1 small box raisins
    - 3 to 4 glucose tablets
- Wait 15 minutes and recheck the blood glucose level. Repeat the glucose if it is still ≤ 70/mg/dL. Recheck the blood glucose level in another 15 minutes.
- Once blood sugar has returned to at least 80 mg/dL, give a more substantial snack such as cheese and crackers if the next meal will be more than 30 minutes later or an activity or exercise is planned.
- If the child is unconscious, administer glucagon IM or subcutaneously.

The child with type 1 diabetes may develop circulatory and neurologic changes over time. Emphasize the importance of good foot care from an early age, for example, wearing clean cotton socks; changing socks and shoes when they are damp; washing, drying, and powdering feet; and keeping toenails short.

Explain to parents that the child should wear some type of medical alert identification. Help them have an individualized school health plan developed (see Chapter 39 ∞) to ensure that school administrators and teachers can identify the signs of hypoglycemia or hyperglycemia and provide emergency management.

Evaluation

Expected outcomes of nursing care for children with type 1 diabetes can be found in the "Nursing Care Plans."

DIABETIC KETOACIDOSIS

Diabetic ketoacidosis (DKA) is the common and potentially life-threatening condition that occurs in children with type 1 diabetes when the body must burn fat for energy because no insulin is available to metabolize glucose. DKA is associated with severe metabolic, electrolyte, and fluid imbalances.

Potential causes of DKA include incorrect or missed insulin doses or administration just under the skin, an illness, trauma, or surgery. Most have no clinical evidence of infection (Flood & Chiang, 2001). Insulin deficiency is accompanied by a compensatory increase in hormones (epinephrine, norepinephrine, cortisol, growth hormone, and glucagon) which are released when inadequate glucose is delivered to

EVIDENCE-BASED NURSING

ADOLESCENT WITH DIABETES AND QUALITY OF LIFE

Clinical Question
How do adolescents with diabetes in different age groups view their quality of life?

Evidence
A descriptive correlational study exploring the quality of life for 69 adolescents with type 1 diabetes versus 75 healthy adolescents revealed that adolescents with diabetes expressed lower life satisfaction and health perception controls. The mean age for both groups was 15 years. The adolescents with diabetes experienced psychologic and physiologic turmoil while attempting to balance their treatment regimen. Additionally, Caucasian middle adolescents (aged >15 years and <17 years) had lower life satisfaction than the younger (>13 years and <15 years) and older adolescents (>17 years and <19 years). Differences in level of metabolic control were not associated with worries of life satisfaction among youth with diabetes (Faulkner, 2003).

Implications
Developmental tasks of adolescents focus on development of self-concept and self-esteem, an important consideration when working with them. Adolescents with type 1 diabetes must also cope with the in-creasing responsibility for complex self-management, including insulin administration, blood glucose testing, exercise, and nutrition. In addition they are experiencing all the normal psychologic and physiologic changes that occur during this period while trying to make decisions about their future. Self-esteem and self-concept often become linked with the disease as peers react to the differences noted. Life satisfaction, perceived control, and worries associated with having diabetes are important considerations when counseling the teenager and family about diabetic management.

Critical Thinking
What are some possible reasons for adolescents in the middle age range to perceive a lower life satisfaction than younger or older adolescents? How will you address quality of life issues with adolescents in different age groups? What options can you explore with the adolescent and family that may improve the adolescent's view of quality of life?

Reference
Faulkner, M. S. (2003). Quality of life for adolescents with type 1 diabetes: Parental and youth perspectives. *Pediatric Nursing, 29*(5), 362–368.

the cells. The muscle cells break down protein into amino acids that are then converted to glucose by the liver, leading to hyperglycemia. The adipose tissue releases fatty acids that are transformed by the liver into ketone bodies. Their accumulation leads to ketoacidosis. The hyperglycemia causes an osmotic diuresis resulting in dehydration, acidosis, and hyperosmolality. Altered consciousness occurs as symptoms progress (Hafeez & Vuguin, 2000).

Characteristic signs of DKA include dehydration, weight loss, tachycardia, flushed ears and cheeks, Kussmaul respirations, acetone breath, altered level of consciousness, and hypotension. Hyperglycemia, glycosuria, and ketonuria are also present. In response to metabolic acidosis, children complain of abdominal or chest pain, nausea, and vomiting. The disorder may progress to electrolyte disturbances, arrhythmias, altered consciousness, shock, and death if untreated. Cerebral edema is a life-threatening complication, thought to be related to hyperosmolality. Signs and symptoms include headache, lethargy, tachycardia or bradycardia, and widening pulse pressure.

DKA is present with the following findings: blood glucose level greater than 300 mg/dL, serum ketones, acidosis (pH less than or equal to 7.3 and bicarbonate less than 15 mEq/L), glycosuria, and ketonuria. Electrolyte disorders also occur (hyperkalemia, hyperchloremia, hyponatremia, hypophosphatemia, hypocalcemia, and hypomagnesemia). The blood urea nitrogen (BUN) and creatinine are elevated due to dehydration. Diabetic coma occurs when the serum osmolality exceeds 350 mOsm/kg. Normal serum osmolality is 275 to 295 mOsm/kg. The child with ketoacidosis is usually hospitalized. Medical management includes intravenous fluids and electrolytes for dehydration and acidosis. Regular insulin is given by continuous infusion pump to decrease the serum glucose level at a rate not to exceed 100 mg/dL/hr. Faster reduction of hyperglycemia and serum osmolality increases the risk for cerebral edema. Mannitol is kept on standby for treatment of neurologic deterioration. Bicarbonate is no longer used for treatment of DKA as it places the child at risk for increased acidosis and hyperosmolality. As insulin is administered, potassium shifts to the cells, resulting in hypokalemia. Potassium supplementation is given only after confirmation of renal function.

Cerebral edema occurs in about 3% of children with DKA, but it accounts for 30% of DKA deaths and 20% of the overall childhood diabetes mortality (Felner & White, 2001). See Chapter 53 for information about cerebral edema. ∞

NURSING MANAGEMENT

Continuously monitor the child's vital signs, respiratory status, perfusion, and mental status. Assess for changes in neurologic status, respiratory pattern, blood pressure, and heart rate. Attach a cardiac monitor and observe for ar-

rhythmias associated with hypokalemia. Frequently monitor the electrolytes and acid-base status, the blood glucose levels, and the urine ketone levels. Monitor intake and output and assess for dehydration.

Give intravenous fluids in boluses of 10 to 20 mL/kg rapidly over 5 minutes if the child is in shock. See Chapter 48. ∞ Give enough fluids to reverse the fluid deficit. Replace electrolytes as needed. The insulin infusion must be carefully maintained to control the gradual reduction in hyperglycemia. Wean the child off intravenous insulin and transition to subcutaneous insulin when clinically stable. Oral feeding is introduced when the child is alert and the glucose level is stabilized.

NURSING PRACTICE

Insulin binds to IV tubing. Let 50 to 100 mL run through new IV tubing to saturate all the binding sites. This ensures that the full dose of insulin reaches the child from the outset.

The prevention of future episodes of DKA is important. The parents and child need to learn strategies to keep hyperglycemic episodes from progressing to DKA. For example, the child's urine should be tested for ketones if three or four consecutive blood glucose readings are higher than 200 mg/dL, or if the child is sick. If the child has a high blood glucose and moderate or large amounts of ketones, treatment with extra insulin and fluids can be initiated. This monitoring is especially important when the child has significant stressors such as an illness. It is important for the child and family to know that insulin is needed even when the child is not eating to counter the hormones secreted in response to the stressor.

TEACHING HIGHLIGHTS

PREVENTING DKA

Call the child's healthcare provider if the child has the following signs (Kaufman & Halvorson, 1999; Boland & Grey, 2004):

- Vomiting more than two times or for longer than 4 hours
- More than five diarrheal stools
- Sick and cannot eat
- An altered mental status
- Temperature over 102°F (38.9°C)
- Blood glucose >400 mg/dL on two separate readings, or >200 mg/dL and moderate to large ketones
- Large ketones, acetone breath
- Evidence of a bacterial infection
- Trouble breathing
- Decreased urine output, dysuria, or signs of urinary tract infection

HYPOGLYCEMIA

Hypoglycemia can develop within minutes in children with type 1 diabetes mellitus. The symptoms outlined in "Clinical Manifestations: Hypoglycemia and Hyperglycemia" may occur when blood glucose levels suddenly drop or fall below 70 mg/dL. Children are at risk of hypoglycemia due to their rapid growth rates and unpredictable eating habits and physical activity. Common causes include an error in insulin dosage, errors in injection technique, inadequate calories because of missed meals, or exercise without a corresponding increase in caloric intake.

Hypoglycemia can be diagnosed on the basis of the sudden onset of signs and symptoms. A blood glucose reading should be taken to confirm the diagnosis, since signs of hyperglycemia and hypoglycemia may be difficult to distinguish. Give glucose immediately but only in the form of a low-fat carbohydrate-containing snack or drink, sugar gel, glucose tablets, or glucose paste. The fat in frost-ing, candy bars, and other higher fat snacks prevents the sugar from working quickly. In the hospital, administer an intravenous infusion of dextrose to prevent progression of symptoms. If the child becomes unconscious, sugar gel or glucose paste can be squeezed onto the gums or a glucagon injection can be given.

NURSING MANAGEMENT

Teach parents and children to recognize the signs of hypoglycemia and take appropriate action. Teach parents to give an intramuscular or subcutaneous dose of **glucagon** (a hormone produced by the pancreas that helps release stored glucose from the liver) for severe cases of hypoglycemia. Reinforce the importance of balancing dietary intake, insulin, and exercise every day. Since the effects of glucose, dextrose, and glucagon are temporary, additional snacks or a meal is provided once the child is alert. Monitor the child continually for several hours after treatment.

CLINICAL MANIFESTATIONS

HYPOGLYCEMIA AND HYPERGLYCEMIA

CAUSE	CLINICAL MANIFESTATIONS	CLINICAL THERAPY
Hypoglycemia ■ Insulin dose too high for food eaten ■ Insulin injection into muscle ■ Too much exercise for insulin dose ■ Too long between meals/snacks ■ Too few carbohydrates eaten ■ Illness, stress	Rapid onset Irritability, nervousness, tremors, shaky feeling, difficulty concentrating or speaking, behavior change, confusion, repeating something over and over Unconsciousness, seizure, shallow breathing, tachycardia Pallor, sweating Moist mucous membranes, hunger Headache, dizziness, blurred vision, double vision, photophobia Numb lips or mouth	If conscious, give 15 grams of carbohydrate. Wait 15 minutes and recheck blood glucose level. Give another 15 grams of carbohydrate if ≤ 70 mg/dL. Recheck the blood glucose level in 15 minutes. If unconscious, give glucagon by injection.
Hyperglycemia ■ Insulin dose too low for food eaten ■ Illness or injury, stress ■ Too many carbohydrates eaten ■ Meals/snacks too close together ■ Insulin injected just under skin or injected into hypertrophied areas ■ Decreased activity	Gradual onset Lethargy, sleepiness, slowed responses, or confusion Deep, rapid breathing Flushed skin, dry skin Dry mucous membranes, thirst, hunger, dehydration Weakness, fatigue Headache, abdominal pain, nausea, vomiting Blurred vision Shock	Additional insulin given at usual injection time. Sliding scale insulin doses for specific blood glucose levels when ill or injured. Extra injections if hyperglycemia and moderate to large ketones. Increased fluids.

TYPE 2 DIABETES

Type 2 diabetes is a disease associated with **insulin resistance** (an alteration of the insulin receptor that signals the presence of insulin in the interior of cells). It may be connected with an insulin secretory defect in the pancreas (caused by a decrease in the beta cell weight and number) and insulin deficiency (Gungor & Arslanian, 2004). The single most important risk factor for type 2 diabetes is obesity, and approximately 80% of children with type 2 diabetes are overweight (American Diabetes Association, 2004a). Other significant risk factors include low physical exercise, a diet high in fat, minority race, polycystic ovary syndrome, and type 2 diabetes in a first-degree relative (Alemzadeh & Wyatt, 2004). Between 74% and 100% of children with type 2 diabetes have a first- or second-degree relative with the same type of diabetes (American Diabetes Association, 2000). The peak age of onset in children is at the time of puberty, and females are affected more than males with a 1.7:1 ratio (Pinhas-Hamiel & Zeitler, 2001).

The increasing number of children being diagnosed with type 2 diabetes has caused significant concern in the healthcare community. Up to 45% of children with a new diagnosis of diabetes have type 2. The increasing rate of obesity among children is thought to be a contributing factor (American Diabetes Association, 2004a).

ETIOLOGY AND PATHOPHYSIOLOGY

Type 2 diabetes is a complex metabolic disorder in which the child has insulin resistance, and insulin fails to transfer glucose into the cells. With the increased weight, the visceral fat produces a cytokine hormone (tumor necrosis factor) that desensitizes the insulin receptor to insulin. The pancreatic cells produce more insulin in an attempt to facilitate glucose transfer and overcome the insulin resistance. This results in **hyperinsulinemia** (elevated insulin levels in the blood). The child maintains a balance between hyperinsulinemia and insulin resistance and a nor-

mal glycemic state. As insulin resistance worsens, the islet of Langerhans beta cells fail in their ability to hypersecrete insulin. This leads to impaired glucose tolerance, and overt diabetes develops. The growth hormone secretion may have a role during puberty in promoting insulin resistance.

CLINICAL MANIFESTATIONS

Signs and symptoms of type 2 diabetes upon initial presentation are very different from type 1. Onset is more insidious, and a history of polydipsia and polyuria is uncommon (Alemzadeh & Wyatt, 2004). **Acanthosis nigricans**, hyperpigmentation and thickening of the skin with velvety irregularities in the skin folds of the neck, axillae, elbows, knees, groin, and abdomen, is a common finding associated with chronic hyperinsulinemia (see Figure 56–9 ●). The child is usually obese, usually with truncal (or central) adiposity. The child may present in diabetic ketoacidosis. Other clinical manifestations can be found on page 1825.

CLINICAL THERAPY

Obesity and the presence of acanthosis nigricans on physical examination are clues to the diagnosis. Blood glucose levels $\geq$ 200 mg/dL without fasting, or a fasting glucose $\geq$ 126 mg/dL are diagnostic of diabetes. Hemoglobin A_{1c} provides an accurate indicator of the average serum glucose level for the past 120 days (life of a red blood cell). Urine is tested and ketones are found in about 50% of children. Islet

● **FIGURE 56–9**

Acanthosis nigricans.

Used with permission of Audrey Austin, M.D., Children's National Medical Center, Washington, D.C.

DEVELOPING CULTURAL COMPETENCE

TYPE 2 DIABETES

Children of African-American, Native American, and Hispanic origin are at greater risk for developing type 2 diabetes (American Diabetes Association, 2004a). The disease in children appears to be following the same racial and ethnic distribution as found in adults (Brosnan, Upchurch, & Schreiner, 2001). Particularly affected are members of some American Indian tribes that historically had a high level of exercise and had hunter-gatherer types of diet. In some groups, such as the Pima Indians of the Southwest, the majority have diabetes and face complications from the disease.

cell autoantibodies, insulin levels, glutamic acid decarboxylase autoantibody test (GAD-65), and fasting C-peptid level are used to differentiate between type 1 and type 2 diabetes. The child with type 2 diabetes has higher insulin and fasting C-peptid levels than the child with type 1 diabetes. Islet cell and GAD-65 autoantibodies will not be present. A fasting lipid profile is obtained since dyslipidemia (primarily elevated LDL-C and triglycerides) is usually present. Elevated fasting insulin levels are present (see Appendix B ∞).

The goal of clinical therapy is normal physical and emotional development, control of hypo- and hyperglycemia, and minimization of long-term complications. Insulin is occasionally required at the time of diagnosis to gain glycemic control or when the child presents in DKA. Thereafter insulin may only be needed for periods of increased stress.

Nutrition education and weight loss make up the major therapy. The child needs to have gradual sustained weight loss, metabolic control of blood glucose levels, exercise, and emotional support. Oral medication is used when diet and exercise efforts are inadequate to control hyperglycemia. Metformin enhances insulin sensitivity, slows the gastrointestinal absorption of glucose, and reduces the hepatic and renal glucose production. It can be used when there is normal liver and kidney function and no ketosis. If additional medication is needed, sulfonylurea or meglitinides may be used; however, they are not approved for use in children in the United States due to liver toxicity (Alemzadeh & Wyatt, 2004). The adolescent may ultimately need insulin for glycemic control.

NURSING MANAGEMENT

NURSING ASSESSMENT AND DIAGNOSIS

Because the child does not often have an acute onset, assess any child with a body mass index (BMI) greater than 85th percentile for age and sex for signs of insulin resistance (acanthosis nigricans, hypertension, and dyslipidemia). Family history of diabetes in an overweight child is a reason to begin screening for the condition. Once the child has been diagnosed, monitor the child's blood glucose levels and blood pressure. Assess the child's diet and activity patterns to determine appropriate changes for disease management. Consider evaluating the siblings for diabetes. Nursing diagnoses that may apply to the child with type 2 diabetes include the following:

- *Imbalanced Nutrition: More than Body Requirements* related to obesity and ethnic and cultural norms
- *Activity Intolerance* related to sedentary lifestyle and disease state (insulin resistance)
- *Fatigue* related to disease state (insulin resistance)

- *Ineffective Therapeutic Regimen Management (Family and Individual)* related to family conflict over changing eating patterns
- *Situational Low Self-esteem* related to situational crisis associated with diagnosis of new-onset chronic illness

PLANNING AND IMPLEMENTATION

The child with type 2 diabetes may be hospitalized at the time of diagnosis because of ketoacidosis. However, the nurse in an inpatient setting is more likely to encounter this child when hospitalized for another condition or during visits for healthcare in clinics or schools. Nursing care focuses on managing the child's blood glucose levels and hypertension during the hospitalization, assessing growth and dietary intake, evaluating goals for weight loss and exercise programs, and reviewing the child's knowledge about diabetes and strategies for management at home.

Nursing Care in the Community

Since the child is initially diagnosed and managed on an outpatient basis, nursing care focuses on teaching the child and parents about the disease and its management, managing dietary intake, providing emotional support, and planning strategies for daily management in the community.

Educate the child and family about the disease and lifestyle changes required for effective management of the condition. Focus on the need to increase activity with routine exercise of at least 30 to 60 minutes daily and by decreasing sedentary activity time, such as computer and television viewing time to no more than 2 hours daily. Customize the activity strategy for each child with motivation to develop a regular routine.

Work with the family to substitute high-calorie and high-fat foods with a meal plan sensitive to the family's resources and ethnic preferences. Suggestions include limiting fast food, and snacking on fruits and vegetables rather than foods high in fat and sugar. Assess the child's height, weight, and BMI on each visit, and plot on the appropriate growth curve for age and sex on each visit. A gradual sustained weight loss or decrease in BMI is the goal. If the child is going through a growth height spurt, maintenance of weight rather than weight loss is the goal. Make sure the child takes a multivitamin daily because of dietary restrictions. Encourage the entire family to make dietary changes, especially since other family members are also at risk for the condition.

Teach the child and family to perform home blood glucose testing to monitor glycemic control. This will let the child and family know that efforts to manage the disease are successful. Take HbA_{1c} levels at each visit to determine the average blood glucose level for the past 3 months. A HbA_{1c} level of 7% or less is the goal. When dietary control and exercise are not successful in reducing blood glucose levels, teach the child and family about the prescribed oral medication.

Give the child and family chances to talk about the impact of the disease on their lives. Identify resources for information about strategies that have worked for other families. Identify local support groups and peer groups for the family and child. Visit the Companion Website for links to such resources.

Make sure the child gets annual evaluations for potential complications of diabetes. The tests to be performed include blood for lipid levels, blood pressure, liver and renal function, urine for albumin, an eye examination for retinopathy, and a neurologic examination of the extremities for neuropathies. The child with type 2 diabetes has the same risk for developing long-term vascular complications as the child with type 1 diabetes when hyperglycemia is poorly controlled.

EVALUATION

Examples of expected outcomes of nursing care include the following:

- The child decreases sedentary activity time to under 2 hours a day.
- The child's daily intake of fruits and vegetables increases to 5 to 8 servings daily, and total fat intake decreases to less than 30% of total calories.
- The child's body mass index slowly and consistently decreases.

DISORDERS OF GONADAL FUNCTION

GYNECOMASTIA

Gynecomastia is the presence of unilateral or bilateral enlarged breast tissue in males. It is a common finding during adolescence and is sometimes confused with subcutaneous fat pads in obese boys. Gynecomastia occurs when the ratio of estrogen to testosterone is greater than the usual male ratio. It is also associated with drugs that increase the circulating concentration of prolactin such as marijuana, tricyclic antidepressants, and calcium channel blockers. The amount of breast tissue varies among boys. The condition usually disappears in 1 to 2 years.

Nursing care focuses on reassuring the boy and his parents that gynecomastia is common and transient. Because of the body image concerns common during adolescence, embarrassment is a frequent problem. Recommend clothing styles and other methods to camouflage the enlarged breasts.

AMENORRHEA

Amenorrhea, or lack of menstruation, may be primary or secondary. Criteria for primary amenorrhea include absence of menarche by age 14.5 years in association with no growth or development of secondary sexual characteristics, or absence of menses by age 16 when secondary sexual characteristics and growth are present.

Secondary amenorrhea is the cessation of menstrual periods 6 months or 3 cycles after menstruation has begun; it is characterized by an absence of spontaneous bleeding for at least 120 days. Pregnancy is the most common cause of secondary amenorrhea in adolescents. It is common for adolescents to have irregular menstrual cycles and duration of the menstrual period for 1 to 2 years after menarche. A large number of cycles are anovulatory for the first 2 years after menarche.

Primary amenorrhea is most often caused by structural defects of the reproductive system; chromosomal abnormalities (such as Turner syndrome); or hypothalamic or pituitary tumors, thyroid dysfunction, or polycystic ovary syndrome. No underlying pathologic condition is found in some adolescents. Primary or secondary amenorrhea may be found in competitive athletes.

A thorough history (including sexual activity), physical examination, and laboratory evaluation are required to determine the cause of amenorrhea. The history focuses on asking questions about recent excessive weight loss or gain; excessive physical activity or sports training; chronic illness; use of illegal drugs, birth control pills, or phenothiazines; emotional problems; and age of the mother at menarche. The physical examination focuses on evaluating the adolescent's stage of sexual development and assessing for hirsutism (see Chapter 35 ∞). A vaginal examination is performed to determine vaginal patency and if the vaginal mucosa is estrogenized. A pregnancy test is performed. A bone age and hormone levels are evaluated (estrogen, LH, FSH, and prolactin).

GROWTH AND DEVELOPMENT

Girls competing in sports such as gymnastics, ballet, and long-distance running need to maintain a low weight and a perfect body type. The inadequate nutrition and strenuous activity may cause the hypothalamus to inhibit gonadotropin-releasing hormone and to increase corticotropin secretion. Low serum estradiol levels result (Sanfilippo, 2004). Amenorrhea or oligomenorrhea and bone demineralization often result. This, in turn, may increase the girl's risk of fractures and osteoporosis in young adulthood. See Chapter 55. ∞

Treatment of amenorrhea depends on the specific cause. The most common approach is to give birth control pills containing both estrogen and progesterone. Athletic teenagers are encouraged to eat a well-balanced, high-calorie diet. Calcium supplements may be ordered. Estrogen with progesterone in low doses may be prescribed for athletes to reduce the risk for osteoporosis. Nursing management centers on patient education and emotional support. The goal is to maintain normal growth and development.

See Chapter 4 for information on dysmenorrhea. ∞

DISORDERS RELATED TO SEX CHROMOSOME ABNORMALITIES

TURNER SYNDROME

Turner syndrome is the most common sex chromosome abnormality in females. Affected girls have a missing, partially absent, or abnormal X chromosome. It occurs in approximately 1 in 2000 to 5000 live female births (Halec & Zimmerman, 2004b). The cause of the chromosomal error is unknown. Approximately 99% of fetuses with the disorder are spontaneously aborted. In the absence of one X chromosome, the oocytes in the ovaries disappear and are nearly all gone by age 2 years. Other specific clinical manifestations are related to specific genes missing.

Characteristic clinical findings include significant short stature (less than 5th percentile); a short, webbed neck with a low posterior hairline; cubitus valgus (increased angle at the elbow); scoliosis; broad chest with widely spaced nipples; lymphedema; hyperconvex fingernails; dark, pigmented nevi; delayed puberty; amenorrhea; and infertility (Figure 56–10 ●). Few girls have all of these features.

Among the conditions that may be associated with Turner syndrome are congenital heart disease; coarctation of aorta; hypertension; structural abnormalities of the kidney; congenital lymphedema; hypothyroidism or Hashimoto thyroiditis; chronic or recurrent otitis media; ptosis, myopia, or amblyopia (lazy eye); inflammatory bowel disease; idiopathic hypertension; and scoliosis.

Growth usually proceeds at a normal rate for the first 2 to 3 years of life and then slows. Breast tissue, which begins to bud at about 10 to 12 years, fails to develop fully. Only in rare instances does a girl with Turner syndrome menstruate spontaneously or become able to conceive. Without treatment, final height is approximately 56 inches.

Characteristic physical findings may alert healthcare providers to suspect Turner syndrome. Some infants, however, have few of these characteristics. In some instances diagnosis is made only when short stature and delayed puberty become apparent in the teenage years. The condition is diagnosed definitively by a karyotype, which reveals the classic 45,XO chromosome pattern or 46,XX pattern with one misshapen X chromosome. Prenatal diagnosis includes triple maternal marker screening of alpha-

● **FIGURE 56–10**

What characteristic physical manifestations of Turner syndrome can you identify in this girl?

Used with permission from Zitelli, B. J., & Davis, H. W. (Eds.). (1997). Atlas of pediatric physical diagnosis (3rd ed., p. 14, Fig. 1–19a). St. Louis, MO: Mosby.

fetoprotein, estradiol, and human chorionic gonadotropin (HCG); maternal progesterone; and inhibin A levels.

Treatment involves carefully monitoring the child's growth. A growth chart made especially for girls with Turner syndrome is available from the Turner Syndrome Society. Growth hormone therapy may be prescribed to promote growth during childhood, and therapy can begin at age 2 years (Halec & Zimmerman, 2004b). Low-dose estrogen therapy is usually begun at about 15 years of age, with dosage increases over the next 2 to 3 years. Waiting until 15 years gives the girl the opportunity to achieve her maximum height before hormones cause the growth plates to close. This treatment produces pubertal changes such as breast development and pubic hair. Progesterone is added to the estrogen therapy to initiate menstrual periods.

NURSING MANAGEMENT

Nursing assessment is focused on monitoring growth rates and observing for signs of cardiac, renal, gastrointestinal, vision, hearing, musculoskeletal, or thyroid dysfunction. Carefully measure the child's height and plot on the growth curve. Teach the family the correct administration of growth hormone and potential side effects.

The lack of growth and sexual development associated with Turner syndrome presents problems not only for physical growth but also for psychosocial development. The girl's perception of her body and how she differs from peers affects self-image, self-consciousness, and self-esteem. In the United States, cultural values place importance on attaining normal to tall stature. Short children tend to be treated according to their size rather than their age. Emphasis is also placed on sexual maturity. Encourage parents to treat the child by her chronologic age rather than size. The nurse can be instrumental in helping the child adapt to the condition and gain self-esteem. Be an active listener and reinforce abilities and skills that the girl exhibits. Encourage parents to provide support. The Turner Syndrome Society can provide additional information about the disorder for parents and adolescents.

Even though their intelligence is generally normal, they have a higher incidence of learning problems because of visual–spatial deficits that affect performance on mathematical and manual dexterity tasks (Ranke & Saenger, 2001).

KLINEFELTER SYNDROME

Klinefelter syndrome is a genetic condition that occurs in boys who have an extra X chromosome (usually 47,XXY). It occurs in approximately 1 in 600 to 800 male births. It is the single most common chromosomal abnormality in humans (Visootsak, Aylstock, & Graham, 2001) and is the single most common cause of hypogonadism (decreased secretory activity of the gonad) and infertility in males.

Most infants appear normal at birth. The condition is usually diagnosed during the school-age years when the boy's behavior becomes a problem in the classroom. Boys with Klinefelter syndrome may have emotional problems because of delayed language development and auditory processing problems that are frustrating to the child. Intelligence quotient (IQ) scores are often 10 to 15 points below those of unaffected siblings, and IQs below 80 are not uncommon. Boys with Klinefelter syndrome are tall and thin, with overly long arms and legs. The arm span to height ratio is normal. The onset of puberty may be delayed with an abnormal progression. Testicular size is decreased at all ages. Less facial and body hair may develop. Gynecomastia is a characteristic finding. Associated conditions that occur with Klinefelter syndrome include cardiac anomalies, pulmonary disease, dental abnormalities, and scoliosis.

Chromosomal analysis revealing one or more extra X chromosomes confirms the diagnosis. Diagnosis is often delayed until behavior problems occur in the school setting or delayed puberty is investigated. The goal of treatment is to stimulate masculinization and the development of secondary sex characteristics when adolescence is delayed. Testosterone replacement is begun when the boy is 11 or 12 years of age. Depo-Testosterone

is given by intramuscular injection every 3 to 4 weeks to maintain serum testosterone levels within the normal range. The dose is increased gradually until an adult dose is reached between 15 and 17 years of age; however, this does not improve fertility. Hormone treatment helps improve behavior, concentration, and learning ability (Visootsak et al., 2001). It also helps to promote normal body proportions and prevent gynecomastia.

NURSING MANAGEMENT

Nursing care consists of educating the parents and child about the syndrome, evaluating the child's and family's coping mechanisms, assisting with school problems, and reinforcing the child's strengths. Encourage parents to channel their son's energy into areas that will provide opportunities for success and productive experiences. Emphasize the importance of rewarding the boy's successes in school, sports, or hobbies. Make genetic counseling available to adolescents, if indicated, because sexual functioning and fertility may be impaired.

INBORN ERRORS OF METABOLISM

Inborn errors of metabolism are inherited biochemical abnormalities of the urea cycle, amino acid, and organic acid metabolism. Therefore, protein, carbohydrate, fat, electrolyte, blood, and respiratory metabolism can be affected. Individually they are rare disorders; however, as a group they are a significant health problem in infancy.

The biochemical defect usually causes an abnormal chemical by-product to accumulate in the blood, urine, or tissues or results in a decreased amount of normal enzymes. Most disorders are associated with protein intolerance, and symptoms develop shortly after formula or breast milk feedings are begun.

Clinical manifestations usually occur within days or weeks of birth. Signs and symptoms may include lethargy and poor feeding, persistent vomiting, abnormal muscle tone and seizures, apnea and tachycardia, and an unusual urine or body odor (musty, sweet odor of maple syrup or burnt sugar, or cheesy or sweaty feet).

In many states, neonatal screening is used to detect several of these conditions before symptoms develop. Four million newborns are screened each year for metabolic disorders (e.g., phenylketonuria), hematologic disorders (e.g., sickle cell anemia), and endocrinopathies (e.g., hypothyroidism) (Centers for Disease Control and Prevention, 2001).

However, most inborn errors of metabolism are not detected until signs and symptoms are present. Initial laboratory tests include measurement of serum glucose, electrolytes, blood gases, and serum ammonia. Test results make it possible to classify the disorder by the presence of hypoglycemia, metabolic acidosis, hyperammonemia, or liver dysfunction. Further diagnostic laboratory tests are then performed.

Treatment, when available, focuses on replacing or reducing the amount of the substance causing the biochemical abnormality.

Four of the more common inborn errors of metabolism—phenylketonuria, maple syrup urine disease, galactosemia, and fatty acid oxidation defects—are presented here. Congenital hypothyroidism and congenital adrenal hyperplasia, also considered inborn errors of metabolism, were discussed earlier in this chapter.

PHENYLKETONURIA

Phenylketonuria (PKU) is an autosomal recessive inherited disorder of amino acid metabolism that affects the body's use of protein. It is caused by a mutation of the phenylalanine hydroxylase gene. The incidence is 1 in 17,000 live births per year in the U.S. population. PKU is rare in African-American, Latin-American, Ashkenazi Jewish, and Japanese populations (Read & Charbonneau, 2004).

DEVELOPING CULTURAL COMPETENCE

PHENYLKETONURIA

Phenylketonuria is rare in African, Jewish, and Japanese populations. It is more commonly found in isolated communities with numerous intermarriages between families over several generations.

Children with PKU have a deficiency of the liver enzyme phenylalanine hydroxylase that normally breaks down the essential amino acid phenylalanine into tyrosine. As a result, phenylalanine accumulates in the blood, causing a musty or mousey body and urine odor, irritability, vomiting, hyperactivity, hypertonia, hyperreflexive deep tendon reflexes, seizures, and an eczema-like rash (Rezvani, 2004). Persistence of elevated phenylalanine leads to disruption of cellular processes of myelination and protein synthesis, and results in a seizure disorder and untreatable mental retardation.

Infants appear normal at birth except for lighter skin complexion than their nonaffected siblings. If diagnosis is delayed, a mousy or musty body odor is noted and mental retardation may be severe. Microcephaly, prominent maxilla and widely spaced teeth, enamel hypoplasia, and growth retardation are other common findings in untreated children (Rezvani, 2004).

Screening for PKU is required by state law in all 50 states. For best results the newborn should have begun formula or breast milk feeding before specimen collection. Early hospital discharge places newborns at risk for false-negative screening tests if screened within 24 hours of birth. Screening needs to occur no sooner than 48 hours after birth, or the test should be repeated at 1 to 2 weeks of age. If the test shows elevated levels of plasma phenylalanine, a repeat quantitative test is performed. If the second test is positive, the family is referred to an outpatient treatment center. Serum phenylalanine should be measured periodically throughout life. Levels greater than 15 mg/dL are considered dangerous.

PKU is treated using special formulas (e.g., Lofenalac, Minafen, and Albumaid XP) and a diet low in phenylalanine to keep plasma phenylalanine levels between 2 and 6 mg/dL. The diet must also meet the child's needs for optimal growth. Breastfeeding is possible if phenylalanine levels are monitored. High-protein foods (meats and dairy products) and aspartame are avoided because they contain large amounts of phenylalanine. Elemental medical foods (modified protein hydrosylates in which the phenylalanine has been removed) are used instead. The low-phenylalanine diet should be maintained throughout life. If dietary control is lost before 6 years of age, there is a significant impact on IQ. If adults go off the diet, there is no change in their IQ, but they may perform less well on tasks requiring attention and processing speed (National Institutes of Health, 2000). The low phenylalanine diet is especially important for adolescent females and women prior to conception and during pregnancy to prevent congenital anomalies (low birth weight, mental retardation, microcephaly) in the fetus.

NURSING MANAGEMENT

Nursing care is mainly supportive and focuses on teaching parents about the disorder and its management. The low-phenylalanine diet is a rigid, strict diet that excludes many foods. Educate the family about sources of phenylalanine, and refer the family to a nutritionist to establish an appropriate meal plan. Parents and children need a great deal of support to promote compliance. The formula and elemental medical food costs are relatively high. The formula is usually reimbursed by insurance, but negotiations with health plans may help parents obtain some support for medical foods. Like children with diabetes mellitus, children with PKU may rebel against the dietary limitations in an effort to be like their peers. Reinforcement of education is important during this time. The current recommendation is for all patients to remain on the phenylalanine restricted diet for life (Rezvani, 2004).

Refer parents of an affected child who are considering a future pregnancy and adolescents with the disorder for genetic counseling.

GALACTOSEMIA

Galactosemia, a disorder of carbohydrate metabolism, has an autosomal recessive inheritance pattern. It occurs in 1 in 50,000 live births (Larsson & Therrell, 2002).

Galactosemia results from a deficiency of the liver enzyme galactose 1-phosphate uridyltransferase (GALT), one of three enzymes needed to convert galactose to glucose. The lack of enzyme leads to an accumulation of galactose metabolites in the eyes, liver, kidney, and brain, rapidly damaging the organs and causing life-threatening problems. Children become susceptible to gram-negative sepsis.

Early signs include poor sucking, failure to gain weight due to vomiting followed by diarrhea, hypoglycemia, and an enlarged liver. Later signs include mental retardation, jaundice, ascites, sepsis, lethargy, seizures, hypotonia, cataracts, and coma. Babies may die within 1 month of birth without treatment, usually due to sepsis. When diagnosis is not made at birth, damage to the liver (cirrhosis) and brain (mental retardation) become progressively more severe and irreversible.

Routine newborn screening for galactosemia is performed in almost all U.S. newborn screening programs (Larsson & Therrell, 2002). (See Skill 10–2.) **SKILLS** Infants not initially screened are identified once they become symptomatic. The diagnosis is based upon history, physical examination, and laboratory tests (galactose, SGOT, and SGPT are abnormally high). Urine specimens are checked for reducing substances (the Clinitest is positive and the Clinistix is negative) in several specimens while the infant is receiving breast milk or formula with lactose.

Treatment involves placing infants on a lactose- or galactose-free formula (e.g., Nutramigen, a meat-based or soybean formula), which remains the child's milk substitute for life. Improvement in the infant's condition is generally seen within 24 hours. A galactose-free diet (no milk or cheese products, including foods with dry milk prod-

ucts) is prescribed when the infant is ready for solids. In spite of compliance with the diet, complications (learning disabilities, speech defects, ovarian failure, and neurologic syndromes) develop in many children.

Nursing management focuses on educating the parents and child about the disorder and required diet, assessing coping abilities, and providing emotional support. Refer the family to a nutritionist for diet counseling. Families must learn to screen foods for added milk solids and to avoid medications, such as antibiotics, that have lactose fillers. Calcium supplementation may be needed. Advise parents that several galactose-free cheeses are sold commercially. Because the disorder is inherited, refer the family for genetic counseling.

DEFECTS IN FATTY ACID OXIDATION

Mitochondrial oxidation of fatty acids is an energy-producing pathway that becomes essential during periods of starvation, when the body fuel converts from carbohydrate to fat. Gene defects can occur in nearly every stage in the fatty acid oxidation pathway resulting in many subclasses of fatty acid oxidation defects. All of these defects are autosomal recessive traits that occur in both males and females. Most patients have a northwestern European ancestry (Venditti & Stanley, 2004).

Screening has revealed that fatty acid oxidation disorders are among the most common inborn errors of metabolism. Some of these defects include medium-chain acyl-CoA dehydrogenase (MCAD) deficiency (most common), long-chain acyl-CoA dehydrogenase (LCHAD) deficiency, and plasma carnitine deficiency. If undiagnosed, these disorders can lead to serious complications affecting the heart, liver, eyes, and muscular system, and even death.

The most common presentation is an acute-onset life-threatening coma and hypoglycemia induced by a period of fasting. Other manifestations often include cardiomyopathy, hepatomegaly, and muscle weakness. Infants and children can be asymptomatic except for times during fasting or stress.

Diagnosis can occur during routine newborn screening when laboratories use mass spectrometry. Most cases are identified during an acute presentation of symptoms when laboratory evaluation may include blood gases, electrolytes, hepatic profile, plasma lactate, plasma amino acids, urine organic acids, acylcarnitine profile, quantitative carnitine levels, and urine for ketones. Hypoglycemia is usually present and ketone levels are unusually low. Liver function tests demonstrate elevated transaminases, urea, and ammonia. Plasma and tissue concentrations of total carnitine are reduced. Skin biopsies are often obtained for fibroblast analysis. Physical examination may reveal hepatomegaly due to fatty infiltration.

Treatment of acute illnesses with 10% dextrose is needed to suppress lipolysis. Chronic therapy is to avoid fasting, ensuring that no more than 10 hours passes before food is eaten. Carnitine supplementation may be required in some disorders as it is useful in preventing low blood sugar and assists in removing metabolic waste from cells.

Nursing management involves educating parents about the importance of frequent feedings and avoidance of fasting. These children should go no longer than 8 to 12 hours without food. Infants should be fed around the clock every 2 to 4 hours. If the infant or child is unable to sustain oral intake during an acute illness, he or she must be referred to the hospital for intravenous dextrose supplementation. Even simple infections such as an ear infection or influenza can become life threatening for these children. Several snack foods and meals of low-fat and high-carbohydrate foods (i.e., cereal, pasta) are recommended throughout the day. Genetic counseling should be offered to the family. If one child in the family is diagnosed with the disorder, the siblings should also be tested, even if they are asymptomatic.

MAPLE SYRUP URINE DISEASE

Maple syrup urine disease (MSUD), a disorder of amino acid metabolism, has an autosomal recessive inheritance pattern. It is rare—found in 1 in 225,000 live births—but has a high incidence in some Pennsylvania Mennonites (1 in 380 live births) (Robinson & Drumm, 2001).

In MSUD, three essential amino acids (leucine, isoleucine, and valine) cannot be broken down because of absent or defective enzyme branched-chain alpha-ketoacid dehydrogenase. This results in alpha ketoacidosis. All three amino acids are essential to form normal structures such as the hair, skin, and muscle. Leucine has the potential to build up in the brain and cause cerebral edema, progressive neurologic impairment, and death.

Within 3 to 7 days of life, the newborn develops symptoms of poor appetite, lethargy, vomiting, variable muscle tone, irritability, seizures, high-pitched cry, and a sweet odor of maple syrup in the body fluids. The symptoms may quickly progress to coma and death if not treated (Larsson & Therrell, 2002).

Not all states require newborn screening for this condition. Diagnosis is made with laboratory tests of the urine for positive ketones and blood tests for elevated leucine, isoleucine, alloisoleucine (a stereoisomer of isoleucine not normally found in the blood), and valine.

Treatment during the acute stage involves removal of the branched-chain amino acids and their metabolites from the tissues and body fluids. Some critically ill infants may require dialysis to remove these compounds as renal clearance is poor. Lifelong treatment with specially designed medical formulas and foods rich in amino acids, calories, vitamins, minerals, and other nutrients is required. These special medical foods have the three amino acids removed. The child needs special low-protein foods that are adequate for growth with enough calories to support twice the child's basal metabolic rate. Daily urine testing is required to determine if ketones are being excreted, an indication that the body is in a catabolic state. A liver transplant has been performed in a few affected children who were subsequently able to tolerate a normal diet (Rezvani & Rosenblatt, 2004). Long-term prognosis of affected children is guarded as severe ketoacidosis, cerebral edema, and death may occur during stressful situations such as infection and surgery.

Nursing care includes educating the family about the disorder and special dietary requirements. The parents need to learn how to mix the child's special formula with a natural protein source, amino acid supplements, and water. The child needs formula even when ill; provide a sick day plan to prevent ketoacidosis. The child should be permitted moderate exercise only to prevent increases in leucine levels. Help families identify sources of information or support groups who can share recipes and tips for managing the child's condition. See the Companion Website for links to such resources.

When the child starts child care or school, it is important for teachers and other care providers to know foods the child should avoid and a list of snacks that can be used for special occasions. The child should have formula and other supplements available to ensure a steady intake of calories during the day. An individualized school health plan should be developed with the school nurse so that teachers and other school personnel are informed.

Critical Concept Review

LEARNING OBJECTIVES

CONCEPTS

Identify the function of important hormones of the endocrine system.

1. Gonadotropin-releasing hormone:
   - Stimulates anterior pituitary to produce LH and FSH.
2. Growth hormone:
   - Regulates linear bone growth and growth of all tissues.
3. Antidiuretic hormone:
   - Regulates urine concentration by the kidneys.
4. Thyroid hormone:
   - Regulates metabolism of cells and body heat production.
5. Parathyroid hormone:
   - Regulates serum calcium levels and phosphorus excretion.
6. Insulin:
   - Regulates glucose utilization by the cells.

Identify signs and symptoms that may indicate a disorder of the endocrine system.

1. Delayed or accelerated growth.
2. Impaired metabolism.
3. Mental retardation.
4. Delayed or accelerated sexual development.
5. Polyuria and polydipsia.
6. Cushingoid features.

Describe differences in pathophysiology between primary and nephrogenic diabetes insipidus.

1. Primary diabetes insipidus:
   - Most cases are caused by brain tumors or CNS trauma.
   - Diagnosis of primary DI confirmed if urine output decreases and concentration increases after a dose of vasopressin.
2. Nephrogenic diabetes insipidus:
   - Most cases are genetic or caused by drug toxicity or an adverse drug reaction.
   - There will be no reaction to a dose of vasopressin.

Identify all conditions of which short stature is a sign.

1. Growth hormone deficiency.
2. Familial short stature.
3. Constitutional growth delay.
4. Hypothyroidism.
5. Precocious puberty.
6. Turner syndrome.
7. Chronic renal failure.
8. Cushing syndrome.
9. Inborn error of metabolism.
10. Severe cardiac, pulmonary, and GI disease.

Develop a nursing care plan for each type of acquired metabolic disorder.

1. Diabetes insipidus:
   - Monitor intake and output and daily weight.
   - Replace fluids orally or by IV to match output.
   - Administer DDAVP as ordered.
   - Instruct child and parents in use of medication.
2. Hyperpituitarism:
   - Teach parents and child about disorder.
   - Support a positive self-image.
   - Provide pre- and postoperative nursing care as needed.
3. SIADH:
   - Monitor fluid balance and avoid excess fluid intake.
   - Monitor for changes in behavior or level of consciousness.

LEARNING OBJECTIVES

CONCEPTS

Develop a nursing care plan for each type of acquired metabolic disorder.—*continued*	■ Implement seizure precautions.
	■ Monitor laboratory work for serum sodium, urine osmolality, and specific gravity.
	■ Weigh child daily.
	4. Precocious puberty:
	   ■ Teach parents and child about condition and how to treat the child according to chronological age.
	   ■ Provide emotional support.
	   ■ Teach parents to administer medication.
	5. Hyperthyroidism:
	   ■ Carefully assess vital signs.
	   ■ Teach parents and child about disorder.
	   ■ Promote rest.
	   ■ Provide increased calories in 5–6 small meals.
	   ■ Provide a cool environment.
	   ■ Provide pre- and postoperative care as needed.
	6. Hyperparathyroidism:
	   ■ Manage fluid and electrolytes.
	   ■ Assess for respiratory distress and airway obstruction.
	   ■ Monitor for signs of infection.
	   ■ Monitor the serum calcium and phosphorus levels.
	   ■ Provide pre- and postoperative teaching and care.
	   ■ Teach parents and child the signs of hypocalcemia.
	7. Adrenal insufficiency:
	   ■ Educate parents and child about disorder and need for cortisol replacement.
	   ■ Administer replacement medication.
	   ■ Instruct parents in use of replacement cortisol.
	8. Pheochromocytoma:
	   ■ Provide pre- and postoperative teaching and care.
	   ■ Closely monitor vital signs.
	   ■ Administer antihypertensives as needed.
	   ■ Postoperatively, observe for neurologic signs, respiratory distress, and signs of shock.
	   ■ Instruct parents in need for lifelong follow-up care.

Develop a family education plan for the child that needs lifelong cortisol replacement.	1. Administer medication early in the morning:
	   ■ May be given every other day to reduce side effects.
	2. Give medication at mealtimes:
	   ■ May use antacids between meals if medication causes GI side effects.
	3. Teach parents how to inject medication:
	   ■ Instruct in the reasons why the injectable form may be needed.
	4. Assist parents to understand serious complications that can occur if medication is not given.
	5. Instruct parents in signs and symptoms of acute adrenal insufficiency.
	6. Instruct parents to inform all healthcare providers about the child's condition.
	7. Instruct parents to have child wear a medical alert bracelet.

Distinguish between the nursing care of the child with type 1 and type 2 diabetes.	Type 1 diabetes: 1. Teach child and parents about the disease. 2. Monitor blood glucose levels frequently. 3. Administer insulin three or more times a day, or teach the use of an insulin pump. 4. Teach parents and the child meal planning with carbohydrate counting or other diet plan. 5. Teach child and parents how to administer insulin injections. 6. Encourage a balance of diet, activity, and insulin to maintain blood glucose level. 7. Provide simple sugars followed by a complex carbohydrate for symptoms of hypoglycemia. 8. Instruct child and family about symptoms of both hypo- and hyperglycemia. 9. Instruct family concerning sick day rules for the child. Type 2 diabetes: 1. Monitor child's blood glucose and blood pressure. 2. Teach child and family how to check blood glucose at home. 3. Assess diet and activity pattern. 4. Administer medication to control hyperglycemia. 5. Help child and parent to plan nutritious meals that encourage weight loss. 6. Assist child to increase activity and weight loss.

(continued)

LEARNING OBJECTIVES

CONCEPTS

Develop a nursing care plan for the child with an inherited metabolic disorder.

1. Perform newborn screening test as indicated by state law.
2. Administer special diet or medication prescribed for child.
3. Instruct parents in use of special formula and preparation of special diets.
4. Refer to a nutritional counselor.
5. Assess coping abilities of parents.
6. Support emotional status of parents.

CRITICAL THINKING IN ACTION

View the **Critical Thinking in Action** video in Chapter 56 of the CD-ROM. Then, answer the questions that follow.

A 14-year-old, Amanda, is admitted to the hospital with newly diagnosed type 1 diabetes mellitus. She had initially been taken to her doctor's office for enuresis, polyphagia, polydipsia, and lethargy, but when assessed, her urinalysis had glucose and ketones, and she had a weight loss of 15 pounds.

Upon admission to the hospital where you work, a full assessment is performed and the following vital signs are documented: weight 115 pounds, temperature 98.8°F, respiratory rate 40 breaths per minute, heart rate 90 beats per minute, and blood pressure 106/63. She has dry mucous membranes, but skin turgor is brisk. Blood is drawn immediately and will continue to be drawn every hour until she is stable.

After determining Amanda's developmental level, you decide she is able to understand the nutritional guidelines associated with type 1 diabetes and how to, under adult supervision, perform blood glucose monitoring as well as how to draw up and administer insulin. Amanda and her parents spend most of the time in the hospital learning survival skills for managing her diabetes. Daily education and monitoring will occur in the diabetes clinic until the family is confident about taking care of Amanda. Regular follow-up visits will be scheduled with the diabetes nurse educator and endocrinologist.

1. What is the most likely blood work done on Amanda when admitted to the hospital for type 1 diabetes?
2. How should the family be told to manage hypoglycemic episodes?
3. What should the parents be told about preventing diabetic ketoacidosis in Amanda?
4. How often should blood glucose monitoring be performed once the condition is stabilized?

MEDIALINK

www.prenhall.com/london

■ NCLEX-RN® Review, case studies, and other interactive resources for this chapter can be found on the Companion Website at http://www.prenhall.com/london. Click on "Chapter 56" to select the activities for this chapter.

■ For animations, more NCLEX-RN® Review questions, and an audio glossary, access the accompanying CD-ROM in this textbook.

REFERENCES

Alemzadeh, R., & Wyatt, D. T. (2004). Diabetes mellitus in children. In R. E. Berhman, R. M. Kliegman, & H. B. Jenson (Eds.), *Nelson textbook of pediatrics* (17th ed., pp. 1947–1972). Philadelphia: W. B. Saunders.

American Academy of Pediatrics Committee on Bioethics. (2001). Ethical issues with genetic testing in pediatrics. *Pediatrics, 107*(6), 1451–1455.

American Academy of Pediatrics Section on Endocrinology and Committee on Genetics.

(2000). Technical report: Congenital adrenal hyperplasia. *Pediatrics, 106*(6), 1511–1518.

American Diabetes Association. (2000). Type 2 diabetes in children and adolescents. *Diabetes Care, 23*(3), 381–389.

American Diabetes Association. (2002). Clinical practice recommendations. *Diabetes Care, 25*(1).

American Diabetes Association. (2004a). *Diabetes statistics for youth.* Retrieved February 1, 2005, from http://www.diabetes.org/utils/printthispage.jsp?PageID-STATISTICS_233184

American Diabetes Association. (2004b). *Clinical practice recommendations.* Retrieved February 1, 2005, from http://www.diabetes.org/for-health-professionals-and-scientists/cpr/jsp

Boger, M. S., & Perrier, N. D. (2004). Advantages and disadvantages of surgical therapy and optional extent of thyroidectomy for the treatment of hyperthyroidism. *Surgical Clinics of North America, 84,* 849–874.

Boland, E. A., & Grey, M. (2004). Diabetes mellitus (types 1 and 2). In P. J. Allen & J. A. Vessey (Eds.), *Primary care of the child with a chronic condition* (4th ed., pp. 426–444). St. Louis, MO: Mosby.

Brosnan, C. A., Upchurch, S., & Schreiner, B. (2001). Type 2 diabetes in children and adolescents: An emerging disease. *Journal of Pediatric Health Care, 15*(4), 187–193.

Bryant, K. G., Horns, K. M., Longo, N., & Schiefelbein, J. (2004). A primer on newborn screening. *Advances in Neonatal Care, 4*(5), 306–317.

Centers for Disease Control and Prevention. (2001). Using tandem mass spectrometry for metabolic disease screening among newborns: A report of a work group. *Morbidity and Mortality Weekly Report, 50*(RR-31), 1–34.

Centers for Disease Control and Prevention. (2004). *Diabetes projects.* Retrieved December 10, 2004, from http://www.cdc.gov/diabetes/projects/cda2.htm

Cheetham, T., & Baylis, P. H. (2002). Diabetes insipidus in children. *Pediatric Drugs, 4*(12), 785–796.

Cogen, F. R., Streisand, R., & Sarin, S. (2002). Selecting children and adolescents for insulin pump therapy: Medical and behavioral considerations. *Diabetes Spectrum, 15*(2), 72–75.

Cystic Fibrosis Foundation. (2002). *Nutrition: Cystic fibrosis: Changes through life.* Retrieved February 1, 2005, from http://www.cff.org

Doyle, D. A., & DiGeorge, A. M. (2004). Disorders of the parathyroid. In R. E. Behrman, R. M. Kliegman, & H. B. Jenson (Eds.), *Nelson textbook of pediatrics* (17th ed., pp. 1890–1898). Philadelphia: W. B. Saunders.

Doyle, E. A., Weinzimer, S. A., Steffen, A. T., Ahern, J. H., Vincent, M., & Tamborlane, W. V. (2004). A randomized prospective trial comparing the efficacy of continuous subcutaneous insulin infusion with multiple daily injections using insulin glargine. *Diabetes Care, 27*(7), 1554–1558.

Dveirin, K., & Tunnessen, W. W. (2000). A 14-month-old with polyuria and polydipsia: Searching for buried treasure. *Contemporary Pediatrics, 17*(10), 23–30.

Eisenbrath, G. S., Polonsky, K. S., & Buse, J. B. (2003). In P. R. Larsen, H. Kronenberg, S. Melmed, & K. Polonsky (Ed.), *Williams textbook of endocrinology* (10th ed., pp. 1485–1504). Philadelphia: Saunders.

Evert, A. B. (2004). Tools and techniques for working with young people with diabetes. *Diabetes Spectrum, 17*(1), 8–14.

Expert Committee on the Diagnosis and Classification of Diabetes Mellitus. (1999). Report of the expert committee on the diagnosis and classification of diabetes mellitus. *Diabetes Care, 22* (Suppl. 1), S5–S19.

Failor, R. A., & Capell, P. T. (2003). Hyperaldosteronism and pheochromocytoma: New tricks and tests. *Primary Care: Clinics in Office Practice, 30*(4), 801–820viii.

Faulkner, M. S. (2003). Quality of life for adolescents with type 1 diabetes: Parental and youth perspectives. *Pediatric Nursing, 29*(5), 362–368.

Felner, E. I., & White, P. C. (2001). Improving management of diabetic ketoacidosis in children. *Pediatrics, 108*(3), 735–740.

Flood, R. G., & Chiang, V. W. (2001). Rate and prediction of infection in children with diabetic ketoacidosis. *Journal of Emergency Medicine, 19*(4), 270–273.

Gance-Cleveland, B. (2003). Adaptation to Addison's disease in a child: A case study. *Journal of Pediatric Health Care, 17*(6), 301–310.

Ginsberg, J. (2003). Diagnosis and management of Graves' disease. *Canadian Medical Association Journal, 168*(5), 575–585.

Gungor, N., & Arslanian, S. (2004). Progressive beta cell failure in type 2 diabetes mellitus of youth. *Journal of Pediatrics, 144*(5), 656–659.

Hafeez, W., & Vuguin, P. (2000). Managing diabetic ketoacidosis: A delicate balance. *Contemporary Pediatrics, 17*(6), 72–83.

Halec, I., & Zimmerman, D. (2004a). Managing growth hormone treatment in pediatric patients. *Pediatric Annals, 33*(3), 183–190.

Halec, I., & Zimmerman, D. (2004b) Coordinating care for children with Turner syndrome. *Pediatric Annals, 33*(3), 189–196.

Haller, M. J., Stalvey, M. S., & Silverstein, J. H. (2004). Predictors of control of diabetes: Monitoring may be the key. *Journal of Pediatrics, 144*(5), 660–661.

Harris, G. D., & Fawcett, G. F. (2002). Hypertensive endocrine disorders. *Clinics in Family Practice, 4*(3), 585–600.

Herman-Giddens, M. E., Slora, E. J., Wasserman, R. C., Bourdony, C. J., Bhapkar, M. V., Koch, G. G., et al. (1997). Secondary sexual characteristics and menses in young girls seen in office practice: A study from the pediatric research in office settings network. *Pediatrics, 99*(4), 505–512.

Ismail, A. A. A., & Barth, J. H. (2001). Endocrinology of gynecomastia. *Annals of Clinical Biochemistry, 38*(6), 596–607.

Kaufman, F. R., & Halvorson, M. (1999). The treatment and prevention of diabetic ketoacidosis in children and adolescents with type 1 diabetes. *Pediatric Annals, 28*(9), 576–582.

Kollars, J., Zarroug, A. E., van Heerden, J., Lteif, A., Stavlo, P., et al. (2005). Primary hyperparathyroidism in pediatric patients. *Pediatrics, 115*(4), 974–980.

Lalwani, S., Reindollar, R. H., & Davis, A. J. (2003). Normal onset of puberty: Have the definitions changed? *Obstetrics and Gynecology Clinics, 30*(2), 279–286.

Larsson, A., & Therrell, B. L. (2002). Newborn screening: The role of the obstetrician. *Clinical Obstetrics and Gynecology, 45*(3), 697–732.

Lashley, F. R. (2002). Newborn screening: New opportunities and new challenges. *Newborn and Infant Nursing Reviews, 2*(4), 228–242.

Levine, L. S., & White, P. C. (2004). Disorders of the adrenal glands. In R. E. Behrman, R. M. Kliegman, & H. B. Jenson (Eds.), *Nelson textbook of pediatrics* (17th ed., pp. 1898–1921). Philadelphia: W. B. Saunders.

Litton, J., Rice, A., Friedman, N., Oden, J., Lee, M. M., & Freemark, M. (2002). Insulin pump therapy in toddlers and preschool children with type 1 diabetes mellitus. *Journal of Pediatrics, 141,* 490–495.

Miller, M. M. (2003). Insulin pump therapy. *Advance for Nurse Practitioners, 11*(11), 61–66.

National Institutes of Health. (2000, October 16–18). *Phenylketonuria: Screening and management* (NIH Consensus Statement), *17*(3), 1–33.

Nebesio, T. D., Siddiqui, A. R., Pescovitz, O. H., & Eugster, E. A. (2002). Time course to hypothyroidism after fixed-dose radioblation therapy of Graves' disease in children. *Journal of Pediatrics, 141*(1), 99–103.

Palma Sisto, P. A. (2004). Endocrine disorders in the neonate. *Pediatric Clinics of North America, 51*(4), 1141–1168.

Pang, S. (2003). Newborn screening for congenital adrenal hyperplasia. *Pediatric Annals, 32*(8), 516–523.

Parks, J. S. (2004). Disorders of the hypothalamus and pituitary gland. In R. E. Behrman, R. M. Kliegman, & H. B. Jenson (Eds.), *Nelson textbook of pediatrics* (17th ed., pp. 1845–1853). Philadelphia: W. B. Saunders.

Pinhas-Hamiel, O., & Zeitler, P. (2001). Type 2 diabetes: Not just for grownups anymore. *Contemporary Pediatrics, 18*(1), 102–125.

Quattrin, T., Belanger, A., Bohannon, N. J. V., & Schwartz, S. L. (2004). Efficacy and safety of inhaled insulin (Exubera) compared with subcutaneous insulin therapy in patients with type 1 diabetes. *Diabetes Care, 27*(11), 2622–2627.

Ramchandani, N. (2004). Type 2 diabetes in children. *American Journal of Nursing, 14*(3), 65–68.

Ranke, W. B., & Saenger, P. (2001, July 28). Turner's syndrome. *Lancet, 358,* 309–314.

Read, C. Y., & Charbonneau, R. M. (2004) Phenylketonuria. In P. J. Allen & J. A. Vessey (Eds.), *Primary care of the child with a chronic condition* (4th ed., pp. 667–681). St. Louis, MO: Mosby.

Reddy, V. S., O'Neill, J. A., Holcomb, G. W., Neblett, W. W., Pietsch, J. B., & Morgan, W. M. (2000). Twenty-five year surgical experience with pheochromocytoma in children. *American Surgeon, 66*(12), 1085–1091.

Rezvani, I. (2004). Defects in metabolism of amino acids. In R. E. Behrman, R. M. Kliegman, & H. B. Jenson (Eds.), *Nelson textbook of pediatrics* (17th ed., pp. 398–402). Philadelphia: W. B. Saunders.

Rezvani, I., & Rosenblatt, D. S. (2004). Valine, leucine, isoleucine and related organic acidemias. In R. E. Behrman, R. M. Kliegman, & H. B. Jenson (Eds.), *Nelson textbook of pediatrics* (17th ed., pp. 409–421). Philadelphia: W.B. Saunders.

Roberts, C .G. P., & Ladenson, P. W. (2004). Hypothyroidism. *Lancet, 363*(9411), 793–803.

Robinson, D., & Drumm, L. (2001). Maple syrup urine disease: A standard of nursing care. *Pediatric Nursing, 27*(3), 256–264, 270.

Rovet, J. F., & Ehrlich, R. (2000). Psychoeducational outcome in children with early-treated congenital hypothyroidism. *Pediatrics, 105*(3), 515–522.

Rudock, A. S. (2002). Secondary hyperparathyroidism—current concepts and controversies. *Clinics in Family Practice, 4*(3), 639–642.

Rudy, C. (2004). Jessica's summer growth spurt. *Journal of Pediatric Health Care, 18*(5), 254, 267–268.

Saborio, P., Tipton, G. A., & Chan, J. C. M. (2000). Diabetes insipidus. *Pediatrics in Review, 21*(4), 122–129.

Sanfilippo, J. S. (2004). Gynecologic problems of childhood. In R. E. Behrman, R. M. Kliegman, & H. B. Jenson (Eds.), *Nelson textbook of pediatrics* (17th ed., pp. 1827–1844). Philadelphia: W. B. Saunders.

Saudek, C. D. (1997). Novel forms of insulin delivery. *Endocrinology and Metabolism Clinics of North America, 26*(3), 599–610.

Silverstein, J. H., & Rosenbloom, A. L. (2000). New developments in type 1 (insulin dependent) diabetes. *Clinical Pediatrics, 39*(5), 257–266.

Skidmore-Roth, L. (2001). *Mosby's handbook of herbs and natural supplements.* St. Louis, MO: Mosby.

Stewart, S. M., Rao, U., Emslie, G. J., Klein, D., & White, P. C. (2005). Depressive symptoms predict hospitalization for adolescents with type 1 diabetes mellitus. *Pediatrics, 115*(5), 1315–1319.

Tato, L., Savage, M. O., Antoniazzi, F., Buzi, F., DiMaio, S., et al. (2001). Optimal therapy of pubertal disorders in precocious/early puberty. *Journal of Endocrinology & Metabolism, 14,* 985–995.

Traggiai, C., & Stanhope, R. (2003). Disorders of pubertal development. *Best Practice & Research Clinical Obstetrics and Gynecology, 17*(1), 41–56.

Trimarchi, T. (2001). Endocrine critical care problems. In M. A. Q. Curley & P. A. Moloney-Harmon (Eds.), *Critical care nursing of infants and children* (2nd ed., pp. 805–819). Philadelphia: W. B. Saunders.

Van Vliet, G. (2001, July 14). Treatment of congenital hypothyroidism. *Lancet, 358,* 86–87.

Venditti, C. P., & Stanley, C. A. (2004). Defects in metabolism of lipids. In R. E. Behrman, R. M. Kliegman, & H. B. Jenson (Eds.), *Nelson textbook of pediatrics* (17th ed., pp. 433–438). Philadelphia: W. B. Saunders.

Viera, A. J. (2002). Hyperparathyroidism. *Clinics in Family Practice, 4*(3), 627–638.

Visootsak, J., Aylstock, M., & Graham, J. M. (2001). Klinefelter syndrome and its variants: An update and review for the primary pediatrician. *Clinical Pediatrics, 40*(12), 639–651.

Wilson, T. A., Rose, S. R., Cohen, P., Rogol, A. D., Backeljauw, P., et al. (2003). Update of guidelines for the use of growth hormone in children: The Lawson Wilkins Pediatric Endocrinology Society Drug and Therapeutics Committee. *Journal of Pediatrics, 143*(4), 415–421.

Witchel, S. F., & Finegold, D. N. (2002). Endocrinology. In B. J. Zitelli & H. W. Davis. *Atlas of pediatric physical diagnosis* (4th ed., pp. 315–336). St. Louis, MO: Mosby.

Yensel, C. S., Preud'Homme, D., & Curry, D. M. (2004). Childhood obesity and insulin-resistant syndrome. *Journal of Pediatric Nursing, 19*(4), 238–246.

The Child with Alterations in Skin Integrity

> *I didn't know that soup could cause such a bad injury. The hardest thing for me to deal with is all the pain Sherray has with each dressing change.*
> —*Mother of Sherray, 6 years old*

LEARNING OBJECTIVES

- Identify the characteristics of different skin lesions by their cause, including those caused by irritants, drug reactions, mites, infection, and injury.

- Describe the stages of wound healing.

- Identify the skin conditions that have a hereditary cause or hereditary predisposition.

- Describe a nursing care plan for a child with alterations in skin integrity, including dermatitis, infectious disorders, and infestations.

- Develop an education plan for adolescents with acne to promote self-care.

- Describe the process to measure the extent of burns and burn severity in children.

- Develop a nursing care plan for the child with a full-thickness burn injury.

- Identify preventive strategies to reduce the risk of injury from bites and stings.

MEDIALINK

www.prenhall.com/london

CD-ROM

Animations:
   Integumentary Repair
   Layers of the Skin
Nursing in Action: Topical Medication: Burn Wound Care
Skill 13–3: Sedation Monitoring
Skill 16–1: Performing a Urinary Catheterization
Audio Glossary
NCLEX-RN® Review

Companion Website

Thinking Critically
   Care Plan: Atopic Dermatitis
MediaLink Applications:
   Adolescents and Acne Management
   Develop a Community Education Program: Dog
     Bite Reduction
   Scald Burn Reduction in Children
NCLEX-RN® Review
Case Study

MediaLink   Animation: Layers of the Skin

The skin is the largest organ in the body and performs several essential functions. The skin protects underlying tissues from invasion by microorganisms and from trauma. The nerves in the skin enable the perception of pain, heat, and cold. The body regulates its temperature by dilation or constriction of blood vessels and sweat glands that act under the control of the central nervous system. The skin also supplements the body's intake of vitamin D by synthesizing this vitamin from ultraviolet light. The sweat glands secrete a solution of water, electrolytes, and urea, thus helping to rid the body of toxins.

ANATOMY AND PHYSIOLOGY OF PEDIATRIC DIFFERENCES

The skin has three distinct layers: the epidermis, the dermis, and the subcutaneous fatty layer that separates the skin from the underlying tissue (Figure 57–1 ⊙). The epidermis is the thin, outermost layer of skin that grows rapidly and contains the melanocytes. Within the dermis are nerves, muscles, connective tissue, hair follicles, sebaceous and sweat glands, lymph channels, and blood vessels. The subcutaneous layer contains the hair, sebaceous glands, eccrine and apocrine sweat glands, and a layer of fat to help insulate the body from cold temperatures.

⊙ **FIGURE 57–1**

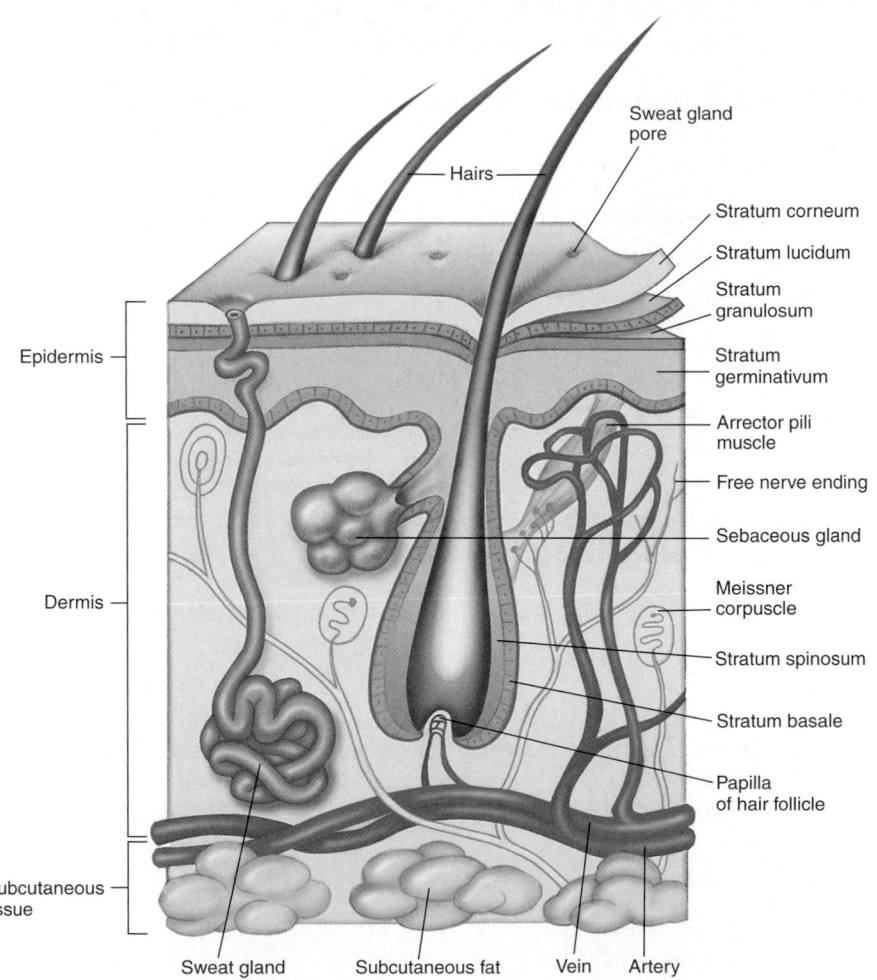

Layers of the skin with accessory structures.

The infant's skin is thin, with little underlying subcutaneous fat. Because of this the infant loses heat more rapidly, has greater difficulty regulating body temperature, and becomes more easily chilled than an older child or an adult. The thinner skin also leads to increased absorption of harmful chemical substances. The infant's skin contains more water than an adult's and has loosely attached cells. As the infant grows, the skin toughens and becomes less hydrated, making it less susceptible to bacteria. See changes in skin characteristics in "As Children Grow: Integumentary System Changes."

Sebaceous glands function at birth, although somewhat immaturely. They vary in size and appear all over the body except on the hands and soles of the feet. Sebum, a lipid substance produced and secreted into the hair follicle or directly onto the skin, lubricates the skin and hair.

Eccrine glands, located in the dermis, open onto the skin surface. They secrete an odorless, watery fluid, primarily in response to emotional stress. They also respond to changes in body temperature. As body temperature increases, the glands increase production of sweat; its evaporation cools the body. Because the eccrine sweat glands usually are not fully functional until middle childhood, infants and young children cannot regulate temperature as effectively as older children and adults.

Apocrine glands, located mainly in the axillary and genital areas, do not function until puberty. Decomposition of the fluid secreted by these glands leads to body odor. Their biologic function, however, is unknown.

SKIN LESIONS

Skin lesions vary in size, shape, color, and texture characteristics. The two major types of skin lesions are primary lesions and secondary lesions. Primary lesions arise from previously healthy skin and include macules, patches, papules, nodules, tumors, vesicles, pustules, bullae, and wheals (see "Pathophysiology Illustrated" in Chapter 35 ∞). Secondary

AS CHILDREN GROW

Integumentary System Changes

Newborns
Skin is very thin
Epidermis is loosely bound to the dermis, friction can cause separation of the layers with blistering
Eccrine sweat glands function, produce sweat in response to heat and emotional stimuli
Apocrine sweat glands are small and nonfunctional
Less melanin is present at birth so skin is lighter colored

Adolescents
Skin thickens
Epidermis and dermis are tightly bound, increasing resistance to infection and irritation
Eccrine sweat glands achieve full function, after puberty males sweat more than females
Apocrine sweat glands mature during puberty
Melanin is at adult levels, determining skin color and serving as a shield against ultraviolet radiation

The structures of the skin mature during childhood, reaching adult function at puberty.

TABLE 57-1 ✣ Common Secondary Skin Lesions and Associated Conditions

Lesion Name	Description	Example
Burrow	A narrow, raised irregular channel caused by a parasite	Scabies
Comedone	A plug of sebaceous and keratin material in a hair follicle	Acne
Crust	Dried residue of serum, pus, or blood	Impetigo
Erosion	Loss of superficial epidermis; moist but does not bleed	Ruptured chickenpox vesicle
Excoriation	Abrasion or scratch mark	Scratched insect bite
Fissure	Linear crack in skin	Tinea pedis (athlete's foot)
Keloid	Overdevelopment or hypertrophy of scar that extends beyond wound edges and above skin line due to excess collagen	Healed skin area following traumatic injury
Lichenification	Thickening of skin with increased visibility of normal skin furrows	Eczema (atopic dermatitis)
Scale	Thin flake of exfoliated epidermis	Dandruff, psoriasis
Scar	Replacement of destroyed tissue with fibrous tissue	Healed surgical incision
Telangiectasia	Dilated, superficial blood vessels	Birthmark
Ulcer	Deeper loss of skin surface; bleeding or scarring may ensue	Chancre

lesions result from changes in primary lesions. They include crusts, scales, **lichenification** (thickening of the skin), scars, keloids, excoriation, fissures, erosion, and ulcers (Table 57–1). It is important for the nurse to be able to identify and describe the primary and secondary skin lesions and understand their underlying cause and treatment. See "Complementary Care: Skin Lesions."

WOUND HEALING

Wound healing occurs in three overlapping phases: inflammation, reconstruction, and maturation (see "Pathophysiology Illustrated: Phases of Wound Healing") (Valencia, Falabella, & Schachner, 2001).

Inflammation, the initial response at the injury site, lasts approximately 3 to 5 days. This phase prepares the injury site for the repair process. The blood coagulates as platelets, red blood cells, and fibrin gather to form a clot. This seals the wound, preventing bacterial invasion and joining the wound edges. Vasodilation, which occurs shortly after injury, allows leukocytes to travel to the injury site, where they ingest bacteria and debris.

Reconstruction or **epithelialization** (the process by which epithelial cells grow into the wound from surrounding healthy tissue), the second phase, may last from 5 days to 4 weeks, depending on the extent of the injury. Capillary

budding to reestablish the blood flow and natural **debridement** (enzyme action to clean the lesion and dissolve the clot or scab) occur. The wound contracts. Fibroblasts multiply, producing collagen and granulation tissue

COMPLEMENTARY CARE

SKIN LESIONS

CONDITION	COMPLEMENTARY THERAPY	USE
Poison ivy	Aloe, calendula, oatmeal (topical)	Relief from itching
Atopic dermatitis	Evening primrose oil (oral)	Decreases excoriations and lichenification. Decreases need for antihistamines for itching
Accelerated wound healing, burns, abrasions	Aloe vera gel (topical)	Antimicrobial effects, bacteriostatic, bacteriocidal
Skin inflammation	Chamomile (topical)	Wound drying, antimicrobial properties
Acne	5% tea tree oil (topical)	Antibiotic, decreases open and closed comedones

Used with permission from Gardner, P., Coles, D., & Kemper, K. J. (2001). The skinny on herbal remedies for dermatologic disorders. *Contemporary Pediatrics, 18*(7), 103–114.

PATHOPHYSIOLOGY ILLUSTRATED
Phases of Wound Healing

Inflammation (3–5 days)

Clot formation that seals the wound with fibrin and trapped cells and platelets

Increased blood flow to area carrying exudate with phagocytes and lymphocytes to the site

Increased capillary permeability, causing swelling

Dilute toxic products released by dying cells

Phagocytosis

Inflammation

- Swelling/inflammation
- Clotting and wound sealing
- Neutrophils and monocytes (phagocytosis)
- Increased capillary permeability

A

Wound healing occurs in three overlapping phases.

Data from Rote, N. S. (2002). Inflammation. In K. L. McCance & S. E. Huether (Eds.), Pathophysiology: The basis for disease in adults and children (4th ed., pp. 197–226). St. Louis: Mosby.

Reconstruction (4 days to 2 weeks)

Debridement or cleanup of the site, fibrinolytic enzymes dissolve the fibrin clots

Regeneration of destroyed cells if injury is minor

Collagen production for scar formation occurs when tissue is too injured to regenerate

Epithelialization with granulation tissue that includes capillary budding and becomes scar tissue

Wound contraction, inward movement of the wound edge

Reconstruction

- Epithelialization
- Collagen production
- Fibroblast migration
- Capillary budding

B

Maturation (Months to 2 Years)

Remodeling of the site as scar tissue forms

Scar formation and strengthening

Capillary disappearance from scar tissue

Maturation

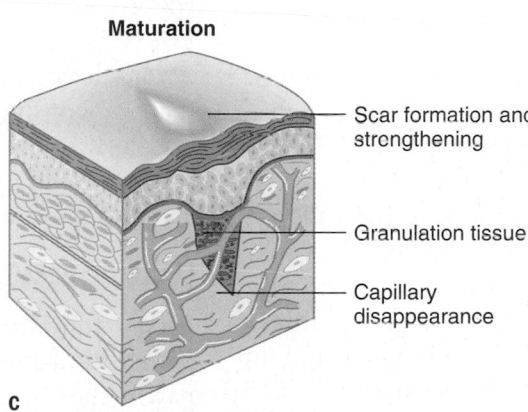

- Scar formation and strengthening
- Granulation tissue
- Capillary disappearance

C

to fill the wound to skin level. A fine layer of epithelial cells forms over the site.

Maturation or remodeling, the third phase, involves continued collagen production for scar production. Although the scar gradually strengthens and devascularizes, it will never be as strong as normal skin. Maturation can take months to years, depending on the extent of the injury.

Formation of a **keloid**, a scar that extends beyond the original boundaries of the wound, is due to an imbalance between collagen synthesis and collagen breakdown. The cause is unknown, but there is a familial tendency.

DERMATITIS

Many skin inflammations occur in early childhood. Most are easily treated and do not have long-term consequences. Dermatitis is a condition in which the skin changes in response to external stimuli. The four most common types of dermatitis in infants, children, and adolescents are contact dermatitis, diaper dermatitis, seborrheic dermatitis, and eczema (atopic dermatitis). It is important to understand that these skin disorders bring emotional problems for the family and child. Be sympathetic and remember that the family and child can see the skin condition and need to be reassured that the child is not infectious.

CONTACT DERMATITIS

Contact dermatitis is an inflammation of the skin that occurs in response to direct contact with an allergen or irritant. Up to 35% of the infant population is affected, most commonly between 9 and 12 months of age (Kazaks & Lane, 2000). At least 20% of children are at risk for allergic contact dermatitis (Weston & Bruckner, 2000).

When contact dermatitis is caused by an external irritant, an inflammatory response occurs, but there is no immune response. Common irritants include soaps, detergents, fabric softeners, bleaches, lotions, urine, and stool. Sweating and friction enhance the absorption of the allergen or irritant. Photodermatitis can result when the child has contact with citrus rinds and juice or fig leaves followed by sun exposure. The child develops erythema and blistering at the site of the exposure that then becomes hyperpigmented. The hyperpigmentation fades over time (Friedlander, 1998).

In allergic contact dermatitis, an antigen is absorbed from the skin surface during the initial sensitization phase, and an immune memory is created. Generally, repeated exposures or a long-term exposure is required to cause the immune response and the dermatitis. Common allergens include poison ivy, poison oak, lanolin, neomycin, rubber, chemicals in shoe leather, nickel, fragrances, and latex. Children may have both irritant and allergic reactions to latex, found in many types of hospital equipment and supplies, as well as in products in the home and community (see Chapter 44 ∞).

The allergic contact dermatitis is characterized by erythema, edema, pruritus, vesicles, or bullae that rupture, ooze, and crust. The rash is usually limited to the area of contact. Symptoms of allergic contact dermatitis can develop within 12 to 24 hours after exposure, and peak in 3 to 5 days (Weston & Bruckner, 2000). Symptoms can last up to 3 to 4 weeks without treatment. In contrast, irritant contact dermatitis is a discrete area of redness that corresponds to the exposure location. The rash usually develops within

TABLE 57–2 ✤ Distribution of Lesions by Type of Allergen

Distribution of Lesion	Allergen
Linear	Plant exposure
Earlobes, neck	Nickel
Dorsal aspects of toes and feet	Rubber or leather chemical in shoes
Face, eyelids	Cosmetics
Subumbilical	Snaps on pants
Axillary	Deodorants

Adapted with permission from Weston, W. L., & Bruckner, A. (2000). Allergic contact dermatitis. *Pediatric Clinics of North America, 47*(4), 897–907.

a few hours of contact, peaks within 24 hours, and quickly resolves with removal of the irritant. The distribution of the lesions provides clues about the source and identity of the allergen. See Table 57–2.

Treatment involves removing the offending agent (e.g., clothes, plant, soap). Calamine lotion can be applied to the affected skin. Cool compresses with aluminum acetate (Burow's solution) promote drying. Wet dressings and colloidal oatmeal soaks relieve itching. Antihistamines may be given for a sedative effect when the child is too irritable to sleep. Acute allergic contact dermatitis is managed with medium potency topical corticosteroids when less than 10% of the body surface area is affected. The topical corticosteroids are applied to the affected area twice a day for 2 to 3 weeks. Stopping the treatment too soon can cause rebound dermatitis. Reactions to poison ivy covering more than 10% of the body surface area require treatment with oral corticosteroids for 7 to 14 days and a tapered dose for 7 to 10 additional days. See Chapter 52 for information about prednisone. ∞

NURSING MANAGEMENT

Patient education for home care management focuses on care of the skin and prevention of future exposures. Teach parents how to apply topical corticosteroids and to keep using the ointment for 2 to 3 weeks even when the skin shows signs of healing. When oatmeal soaks are used, caution parents that the tub will be slippery, and to pat the child dry to leave the oatmeal film in place. Wet dressings may be soothing and help loosen crusts. Burow's or Domeboro solution applied to blistered or oozing lesions for 20 minutes daily helps dry lesions (Allen, 2004). Familiarize parents with the symptoms of infection in the affected area (i.e., increased redness, oozing, fever) and tell them when to return for follow-up care.

Teach parents to avoid exposure to allergens or irritants. Advise parents to wash all clothes before the first wearing and to rinse clothes an extra time to remove all the soap. Mild soap should be used to clean the skin. Place a barrier between the irritant (e.g., metal, shoe leather) and the skin. If a nickel allergy exists, avoid use of nickel jewelry and belt buckles.

DIAPER DERMATITIS

Diaper dermatitis, a common cause of irritant contact dermatitis, occurs in approximately one third of young children, usually in a mild form. It is most common in infants from 4 to 12 months of age. Diaper dermatitis is a primary reaction to urine, feces, moisture, or friction. Urine and feces interact with the skin to cause dermatitis. The urine increases the wetness and pH of the skin, increasing abrasion and its permeability to irritants and microbes. Fecal organisms provide more irritants. Breastfed babies' stools have a lower pH, and this helps reduce their incidence of diaper rash (Kazaks & Lane, 2000).

Candida albicans, a secondary infection, is a common complication of diaper dermatitis or antibiotic therapy for another condition. It is frequently the underlying cause of severe diaper rash. Diaper candidiasis often occurs simultaneously with oral candidiasis (see later discussion).

The rash is characterized by glazed red plaques over skin in contact with the diaper area. Usually the perineum, genitals, and buttocks are affected, and the skinfolds are spared. In severe cases, the infant develops a rash that is fiery red, raised, and confluent. Pustules with tenderness can also be present (Figure 57–2 ●). When a secondary infection with *Candida albicans* occurs, the rash has bright-red scaly plaques with sharp margins in the skinfolds. Small papules and pustules may be seen, along with satellite lesions.

Mild diaper dermatitis is treated with a barrier or protective sealant such as zinc oxide, Desitin, or Balmex. Treatment for moderate or severe diaper dermatitis involves application of low or moderate potency (0.25% or 1%) hydrocortisone cream with each diaper change for 5 to 7 days and good basic hygiene. The cream must be applied before any protective sealant is used. Diaper candidiasis is treated with alternating applications of 1% hydrocortisone cream and antifungal creams (clotrimazole or nystatin) applied to the affected areas at diaper change. An oral antifungal agent may be given to clear the candidiasis from the intestines. Fluorinated topical corticosteroids should not be used because of the higher rate of absorption through damaged skin.

NURSING MANAGEMENT

Severe diaper dermatitis can be a major source of stress for parents who must deal with a child in constant discomfort. Instruct parents to change the diaper as soon as the infant is wet, or at least every 2 hours during the day and once during the night.

Encourage parents to use superabsorbent disposable diapers, which tend to reduce the frequency and severity of diaper dermatitis. When wet, these diapers form a gel that

● **FIGURE 57–2**

Diaper dermatitis. Note the skinfold that is free of inflammation.
Courtesy of the Centers for Disease Control, Atlanta, GA.

keeps the skin drier than cloth diapers. However, this should not be an excuse for waiting until the diaper is saturated to change it. Tell parents to avoid using tight diapers and waterproof pants. A & D ointment, zinc oxide, Desitin, and Balmex can be used to protect the skin from urine and stool. Mineral oil may be helpful in removing pastes.

Advise parents to wash the perianal area with warm water and a mild soap (such as Dove or Tone) or a cleanser not needing water (Aquanil HC lotion or Cetaphil) only after a bowel movement. Advise parents to use soft paper towels with water or babywipes without alcohol at other times. Talcum powder is abrasive and offers no protection (Atherton, 2004).

Exposing the diaper area to air helps aid healing; for example, parents could allow the child to go without a diaper while lying on an absorbent pad or cloth. Watch for signs of infection since the skin is damaged and can allow infectious organisms to grow. If this occurs, additional treatment will be needed.

SEBORRHEIC DERMATITIS

Seborrheic dermatitis is a recurrent inflammatory skin condition thought to be caused by an overgrowth of *Pityrosporum* yeast, commonly found in areas of sebaceous gland activity. The condition is influenced by hormones and associated with an oily complexion. The rash is found over the areas of the body where the sebaceous glands are most plentiful: scalp (cradle cap), forehead, and postauricular and periorbital areas. It may also occur on the skin of the eyelids, inguinal area, or nasolabial folds. The condition is frequently seen in infants up to 3 months of age and in adolescents.

Common symptoms are pruritus and a mildly erythematous, adherent, waxy scaling of the scalp (or "dandruff"). Yellow-red patches with greasy scaling may be present, typically on the scalp and nasolabial folds on the face, behind the ears, on the upper chest, and sometimes on the **intertriginous** (skin folds of the neck, axillae, antecubital fossa) areas (Figure 57–3 ●). The rash itches less than atopic dermatitis.

Treatment for seborrheic dermatitis consists of daily shampooing with a medicated shampoo (e.g., Selsun or Head and Shoulders). An emollient is left on the scalp for about 20 minutes to soften the crusts. The scales are removed by brushing with the fingertips, a baby hairbrush, or a soft toothbrush. The hair is then rinsed thoroughly. Lesions on the body can be treated with shampoos containing selenium sulfide or salicylic acid. Use baby shampoo to wash lesions on the eyelids and eyelashes. Treatments are continued for several days after the lesions disappear. Topical corticosteroids are used to treat seborrhea that is not on the scalp.

● **FIGURE 57–3**

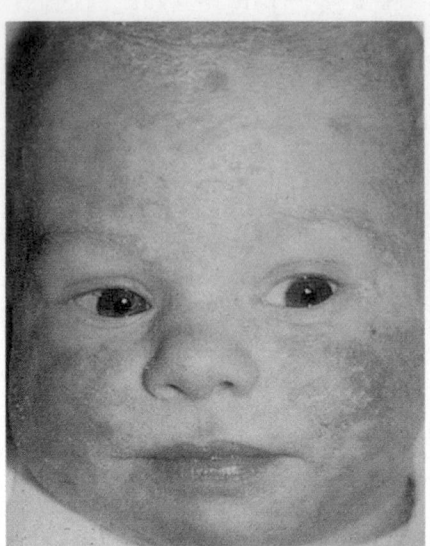

Seborrheic dermatitis.

NURSING MANAGEMENT

Teach new parents to wash the infant's hair regularly with each bath. Reassure parents that gentle cleansing will not harm the infant's "soft spot." Demonstrate bathing to show them the proper technique, if necessary. Follow-up is seldom necessary, as the condition resolves with treatment. Advise adolescents that emotional distress may trigger future flare-ups and to initiate treatment promptly when symptoms begin.

ECZEMA (ATOPIC DERMATITIS)

Eczema, also called atopic dermatitis, is a chronic, superficial inflammatory skin disorder characterized by intense pruritus. The condition affects infants, children, and adolescents. It is common, and is believed to affect up to 20% of young school children (Dohil & Eichenfield, 2005). Up to 75% of children who develop the condition do so during the first 6 months of life, and most of the remainder who have the condition develop it by 5 years of age (Nicol, 2000). An increasing prevalence has been noted in developed countries that also exhibit an increased rate of asthma, demonstrating the allergic tendency for this condition (Raimer, 2000).

ETIOLOGY AND PATHOPHYSIOLOGY

The etiology of eczema is unknown, but an immune disorder of the skin is influenced by a genetic predisposition, and external triggers may be involved. Children have T-cell activation and excessive production of IgE (Paller, 2001). See Chapter 44 for a discussion of IgE. ∞ The disorder tends to occur in children with hereditary allergic tendencies (**atopy**). If one parent has allergies (e.g., hay fever, asthma, or contact dermatitis), the child has a 60% greater chance of having allergies. This increases to 80% if both parents have allergies (Cheigh, 2003). Food allergens are an important cause in young infants. Several factors exacerbate the condition: triggers (house mites, animal dander, pollens), food allergies, irritants (soaps, detergents, chemicals, solvents, abrasive clothing), hormonal changes, and emotional stress.

Children with eczema have **xerosis**, generally dry skin that is more likely to crack and fissure. The barrier function of the skin is impaired leading to increased water loss from the epidermis and decreased elasticity. When the skin is chronically dry, irritants have a greater chance to penetrate, and the child is more susceptible to infection.

CLINICAL MANIFESTATIONS

Acute eczema is characterized by pruritus and erythematous patches with vesicles, exudate, and crusts (Figure 57–4 ◉). Subacute eczema is characterized by scaling with erythema and excoriation. Some patches may weep. There are often postinflammatory pigment changes. Symptoms of chronic eczema are pruritus, dryness, scaling, and lichenification (thickening of the skin with increased visibility of normal skin furrows). Inflammation usually occurs on the face, upper arms, back, upper thighs, and back of the hands and feet. Skinfolds such as the antecubital and popliteal areas are often affected. The itching interferes with sleep and causes irritability. The child moves so much due to itching discomfort that a perception of hyperactivity may occur. Exacerbations of eczema are related to factors such as allergies, dry skin, high and low ambient temperatures, perspiring, scratching, anxiety, stress, and skin irritants (e.g., detergents, wool, other rough fabrics). Erythema and warmth may indicate a secondary bacterial infection.

◉ **FIGURE 57–4**

Chronic eczema.

Eczema occurs in three forms: infantile (ages 2 months to 2 years), childhood (ages 2 years to puberty), and adolescent. Children typically have numerous relapses. See "Clinical Manifestations: Eczema."

CLINICAL THERAPY

Eczema is distinguished from other forms of dermatitis by its history and clinical manifestations. No laboratory tests are diagnostic. Diagnostic criteria for eczema include an itching skin condition with three of these factors (Raimer, 2000):

- History of flexural dermatitis (knees, ankles, neck, or cheeks) if less than 4 years old
- History of asthma or hay fever in a child, or in a first-degree relative if less than 4 years old
- History of dry skin in past year
- Skin rash occurring before 2 years of age
- Visible flexural dermatitis; dermatitis on cheeks, forehead, and outer limbs if less than 4 years old

As there is no cure, the goals of treatment are to hydrate and lubricate the skin, reduce pruritus, minimize inflammatory changes, and try to determine what triggers flare-ups. The cardinal principle of topical therapy for oozing or weeping is "wet on wet." If lesions are weeping, wet compresses (cotton cloths) soaked in aluminum acetate solution sometimes are used. The skin is lubricated by applying occlusive topical ointment after bathing to trap moisture and prevent drying. Moisturizing ointments and creams (Eucerin cream, Aquaphor ointment, Vanicream, Cetaphil cream, SBR-Lipocream, and white petrolatum) should be applied three to four times a day or whenever the skin feels dry.

Topical corticosteroids reduce inflammation. Ointments are preferred over creams because of their occlusive effect, which ensures a stronger barrier and absorption into the skin. Hydrocortisone 1% to 2.5% or triamcinolone 0.1% is usually the drug of choice; however, many different preparations and strengths exist. Corticosteroids are used two times daily for 2 weeks and must be applied before the skin moisturizer is used. Newer corticosteroid ointments such as fluticasone propionate and mometasone furoate are effective for once-daily use (Dohil & Eichenfield, 2005). Lower potency ointments are used for thinner skin areas, such as the face, diaper area, and skin folds. A more potent ointment is used for flare-ups, with tapering to lower potency as the dermatitis improves. When the dermatitis resolves, topical corticosteroids are tapered in frequency of application and potency and then discontinued. Topical steroids are not used on healthy skin to reduce the risk for steroid side effects. Oral corticosteroids may be used for an acute exacerbation; however, there is often a rebound effect

CLINICAL MANIFESTATIONS

ECZEMA

TYPE	CLINICAL MANIFESTATIONS	OUTCOME
Infantile (2 months to 2 years)	Exudative, crusty, papulovesicular, and erythematous lesions on cheeks, scalp, forehead, neck, trunk, and extensor surfaces of extremities Diaper area spared because skin is damp and the diaper protects the area from scratching Intensely pruritic, child wiggles to rub and scratch areas out of reach Lichenification after the child can scratch at about 2 months of age	50% of cases resolve by age 2 to 3 years
Childhood (2 years to puberty)	Erythematous, dry, scaly or weeping, well-circumscribed, papular, more thickened and lichenified lesions on flexor surfaces of extremities, neck, and retroauricular folds Once toilet trained, buttocks are affected	Subacute and chronic 75% of cases have no recurrence after adolescence
Adolescent (puberty and onward)	Much the same as childhood eczema but generalized form is less acute Localized areas affected may include eyelids, where earlobe touches the face, fingertips, toes, nipple, and the vulvar area	May recur as it is more often a chronic inflammation

(i.e., after the medication is discontinued, the rash returns). Complementary therapy may also be beneficial.

NURSING PRACTICE

The percentage following the topical corticosteroid preparation is not an indication of its strength. The strength is based upon the type of preparation (ointment, lotion, or cream), and whether it is fluorinated. Avoid the use of fluorinated corticosteroids on the face, genitalia, and skin folds where absorption of the medication is increased because of how thick the skin is. Occlusive dressings, such as may occur with a tight-fitting diaper, further increase the potential absorption. The lowest concentration of topical corticosteroids should also be used in these areas. Posterior cataracts and glaucoma are a potential adverse effect of topical corticosteroid use around the eyes. Other adverse effects may include skin atrophy due to decreased collagen synthesis and striae after 3 to 4 weeks of therapy.

Topical antibiotics are used to treat excoriated, open lesions and those that appear infected. Oral antibiotics are often given to reduce the *Staphylococcus aureus* population as these organisms can trigger an immune cascade that increases pruritus. Oral and topical antibiotics are often used in 7- to 10-day intervals rather than continuously to reduce the risk of drug-resistant organisms getting established (Shwayder, 2003). Superinfections with herpes simplex may be treated with acyclovir.

Immunomodulator ointments (tacrolimus and pimecrolimus) are increasingly used as a second-line treatment for some children, but they may be too expensive for some families. The medication has been approved by the U.S. Food and Drug Administration (FDA) for children over 2 years of age for short-term or intermittent treatment who are not responsive to conventional therapy. Recent warnings of increased risk for lymphoma and skin cancer associated with duration of use may be of concern to parents (FDA, 2005).

Antihistamine agents such as diphenhydramine (Benadryl) or hydroxyzine (Vistaril and Atarax) have a limited effect on itching, but the sedative effect may help promote sleep. Methods to reduce pruritus include environmental controls, such as humidification in the winter and air conditioning in the summer. A humidifier counteracts dryness of the surrounding air, minimizing loss of skin moisture.

COMPLEMENTARY CARE

CHINESE MEDICAL HERBS FOR ATOPIC DERMATITIS

One or more of the components of Zemaphyte, a mixture of plant extracts based on Chinese herbal therapy, has been found effective in treatment of children with atopic dermatitis (Latchman, Xu, Poulter et al., 2002).

The mixture contains 10 primary herbs that are ground, placed in teabags, and boiled for 90 minutes. The herbs include the following: Ledebouriella seseloides, Potentilla chinensis, Clematis armandii, Rehmannia glutinosa, Paeonia lactoflora, Lophatherum gracile, Dictamnus dasycarpus, Tribulus terrestris, Glycyrrhiza uralensis, and Schizonepeta tenuifolia.

Children should not eat food 1 hour prior to drinking the warm mixture. If the liquid is too unpleasant tasting to drink, it can be freeze-dried into granules to put into a capsule. Significant improvements in skin lesion severity were noted in children who completed a year of treatment without significant adverse effects.

Air conditioning limits unnecessary sweating that can exacerbate inflamed areas.

Breast milk is hypoallergenic, and exclusive breastfeeding for the first 3 months of life may be associated with a lower incidence of eczema in infants with a positive family history. Introduction of solid foods at a later age, after 4 months, can result in decreased eczema during the first 4 years of life. In some children, avoidance of highly allergenic foods such as eggs, wheat, milk, and peanuts from the diets of infants and lactating mothers may improve the skin condition (Cheigh, 2003). When regular therapy does not result in improvements in skin condition, an allergy specialist may help identify food and other environmental allergens that trigger the eczema. See Chapter 44. ∞

NURSING MANAGEMENT

NURSING ASSESSMENT AND DIAGNOSIS

Take a thorough history, including any family history of allergy, environmental or dietary factors, and past exacerbations. Note distribution and type of lesions.

Identify the impact that the skin disorder is having on the child and family. Do the child, siblings, or other family members have disturbed sleep? Is the child's self-esteem disturbed? What other stresses has the child's skin disorder placed on the family?

Common nursing diagnoses that may be appropriate for the child with eczema include the following:

- *Impaired Tissue Integrity* related to chemical irritants and mechanical factors (abrasive clothing)
- *Disturbed Sleep Pattern* related to prolonged physical discomfort (itching)
- *Risk for Infection* related to breaks in skin barrier
- *Chronic Low Self-Esteem* related to chronic illness and peer reaction to visible skin lesions
- *Ineffective Therapeutic Regimen Management (Families)* related to excessive demands made on the family to keep the condition under control

PLANNING AND IMPLEMENTATION

Nursing management focuses on education and emotional support. Although it has no "cure," eczema can be controlled. Advise parents that the lesions are not contagious and will not usually result in scarring. Help parents and adolescents deal with the frustration of the acute flare-ups of the condition by reinforcing that remissions do occur with good home care.

Teach parents or adolescents to avoid using harsh or perfumed soaps or bubble bath. Bathing with tepid water once or twice a day with a mild soap (e.g., Dove or Tone) is recommended. Washing clean skin with soap and hot water only dries it out and may increase itching. Pat the skin dry or air-dry. Moisturizers should be applied within 3 minutes of exiting the bath to help promote absorption and retention of moisture, once or twice daily. Use wet wraps for severely affected skin to replace moisture. Wool clothing and clothing washed in harsh laundry detergents should be avoided because it can increase skin irritation and pruritus. Encourage loose cotton clothing.

Teach parents and adolescents how to apply topical ointments or creams. A thin layer over the entire area should be applied twice a day. The medication should be rubbed in gently and completely. Treatment should continue until the skin clears. Instruct parents to place clean cotton gloves or socks over the infant or young child's hands and to keep the child's fingernails cut short to decrease scratching and reduce the chance of secondary infection.

Eczema produces visible changes that can affect a child's self-confidence and self-esteem. Identify activities that the child can participate in to improve self-esteem. Even though humidity and sweating can make eczema worse, have the child shower after a sporting event or strenuous activity to clean the skin. Needed medications and lubricants can then be applied.

Eczema that is difficult to manage is more stressful and has a more profound effect on the child's and family's quality of life. The use of immunomodulators in children with moderate or severe eczema significantly improves the quality of life in children and adults as measured by daily activities, feelings, relationships, and sleep (Drake & Prendergast, 2001; Whalley, Huels, McKenna et al., 2002).

Once the condition is under control, counsel the parents about how to introduce a food that was previously eliminated when an allergen cause of eczema was suspected (see Chapter 44 ∞). Emphasize that increased itching within hours of eating a food may be associated with an eczema flare-up. Teach parents how to control the skin inflammation that results, as described. Once a specific food allergy has been identified, refer the parents to a nutritionist for counseling about alternative food options that will fulfill daily nutritional requirements. Tell parents that food allergies can change, so foods connected with eczema can sometimes be safely eaten later in life. Different food sensitivities may also develop. Refer the family to the Food Allergy Network. (See the Companion Website for links to such resources.)

EVALUATION

Expected outcomes of nursing care include the following:

- Control of the child's eczema is maintained and no infection occurs.
- Parents identify triggers of the child's eczema and avoid or eliminate them.
- The child's sleep is minimally disturbed by itching.

DRUG REACTIONS

Adverse reactions to over-the-counter or prescription medications are relatively common. Children with drug allergies usually have reactions after ingestion (e.g., aspirin, antibiotics, sedatives), injection (e.g., penicillin), or direct skin contact with medications. Drug sensitivities may result from variations in an individual's ability to tolerate a particular drug or concentration of a drug or from allergic responses. (See Chapter 44 for a description of allergic reactions. ∞)

Sensitivity reactions to a drug not previously administered may take up to 7 days to develop. If the child has been sensitized to a drug, the reaction is almost immediate. The most common reactions in children are erythematous macules and papules or urticaria, which may be pruritic. Drugs most likely to cause maculopapular eruptions, urticaria, and pruritus include the following: amoxicillin, ampicillin, cephalosporins, erythromycin, penicillin G, semisynthetic penicillins, sulfamethoxazole, and trimethoprim (Vanderhooft, 1998). Some drug reactions can be life threatening. Be alert to the possibility of serious drug reactions that may become a medical emergency. See "Clinical Manifestations: Drug Reactions."

The treatment of choice for most drug sensitivity reactions is discontinuation of the causative drug. In some cases, a drug may be continued with careful monitoring when the child has a sensitivity reaction because it is the best treatment choice. Supportive measures should be

taken to decrease the intensity of the reaction. An antihistamine may be used to block the release of histamine, which causes the rash. Topical corticosteroids, cool compresses, and baths may also be prescribed for pruritus. For some severe drug reactions, the child must be hospitalized and treated on a burn unit.

NURSING MANAGEMENT

Teach parents to be alert for the signs of drug sensitivity reactions. Obtain a careful history of the child's past reactions to medications before starting new therapies. If a reaction occurs, discontinue the medication until the physician is notified.

NURSING PRACTICE

Children with a true drug allergy (having a past serious systemic reaction) should never be treated with that drug again. Prominently mark the child's records so that all allergies are easily identified. The child should wear a medical alert bracelet.

ACNE

Acne is a chronic inflammatory disorder of the pilosebaceous hair follicles on the face and trunk. It is the most common skin disorder in the pediatric population. It is triggered by the increased androgen production of puberty and the overproduction of sebum. The prevalence in adolescents 12 to 16 years of age is estimated to approach 50% to 85% (Rudy, 2003). Acne is found in all ethnic groups and is present equally in males and females. Acne may also occur in newborns in response to maternal androgen hormones. This form of acne usually develops between 2 and 4 weeks of age and resolves by 4 to 6 months of age.

ETIOLOGY AND PATHOPHYSIOLOGY

Acne is caused by the interaction of several factors: an overgrowth of residential bacteria on the skin, increased sebum production, and abnormal follicular shedding of skin cells that are more adherent than normal. The extra sebum caused by androgen secretion mixes with the shed skin cells and causes them to clump together. The keratin and sebum that usually flow to the skin surface are obstructed in the follicular canal, causing **comedones** (whiteheads and blackheads). The sebum behind the comedone is an ideal environment for the anaerobic *Propionibacterium acnes,* and this bacterium metabolizes the sebum, causing an inflammatory reaction. When the inflammatory reaction is close to the surface, a papule or pustule develops. If the inflammatory reaction is deeper, a larger papule or nodule develops. Although acne follows familial trends, data to

CLINICAL MANIFESTATIONS

DRUG REACTIONS

TYPE OF REACTION	CLINICAL MANIFESTATIONS	CLINICAL THERAPY
Allergic drug reaction Most commonly caused by sulfonamides, tetracyclines, NSAIDs, oral contraceptives, barbiturates, and phenolphthalein.	Erythematous macules and papules. Pruritus. Urticaria, may move among body parts. A fixed drug reaction may commonly involve the face, genitals, sacrum. Recurrent localized target lesions may be seen with repeated exposure. Healing with hyperpigmentation of the center may be seen (Cohen, 2002).	Remove offending drug. Topical antipruritics. Oral antihistamines. Lubricate skin when scaly. Systemic corticosteroids if no response to other treatment.
Stevens-Johnson syndrome (erythema multiforme major) Hypersensitivity reaction to the drug (sulfonamides, anticonvulsants, and NSAIDs) or reaction to an infectious agent.	Prodrome of an upper respiratory infection for 1 to 7 days with cough, coryza, sore throat, fever, malaise, headache, muscle aches, joint pain. Vomiting and diarrhea may be seen. Skin lesions are blistering and crusting on the mucous membranes and redness in the eyes. Blisters may spread to the entire skin surface. Red macules may then progress to edematous papules, target lesions with vesicular dusty centers. Pruritus.	Remove offending drug. Balance intake and output. Gentle debridement of crusts. Oral antihistamines. Topical antipruritics. Nutritional support. Ophthalmic consultation. Corticosteroid and IV immune globulin use is controversial as no studies have demonstrated effectiveness.
Toxic epidermal necrolysis Potentially life-threatening hypersensitivity reaction to NSAIDs, sulfa, antibiotics, and anticonvulsants.	Rash similar to Stevens-Johnson syndrome. Appearance of tender skin, then bullae or erosions occur over more than 20% of body surface area. Full-thickness epidermis peels off in sheets easily with tangential pressure (Nikolsky's sign). Respiratory tract may have mucosal sloughing. Causes hypopigmentation in children with dark skin, but hyperpigmentation in children with white skin. Hyperpigmentation fades over time. Signs of sepsis.	May be cared for in a burn center, see page 1864. Debridement of blisters and necrotic epidermis. Gentle cleaning with saline or Burow's solution (aluminum acetate) compresses. Topical antibiotic ointment, but no creams with sulfa as this may be original cause of toxicity. Sterile nonadherent dressings. Wounds may be covered with biosynthetic dressing, human allografts to reduce infection and pain. IV immunomodulators have shown some success, but prospective studies are needed. Intensive nutritional support. Ophthalmic consultation and eye care. No corticosteroids.

(continued)

CLINICAL MANIFESTATIONS—continued

DRUG REACTIONS

TYPE OF REACTION	CLINICAL MANIFESTATIONS	CLINICAL THERAPY
Erythema multiforme minor Hypersensitivity reaction to anticonvulsants, penicillin, salicylates, sulfa antibiotics, barbiturates, and phenytoin; infectious agents.	Prodromal symptoms of a mild respiratory infection (malaise, fever, weakness, sore throat, cough). Target lesions with dusky centers (papules, vesicles, or bullae in a pale ring with an erythematous border). Lesions may or may not be present on the mucosa, common on palms and soles. Edema. Burning, pruritus, or tenseness of the skin.	Remove offending drug. Oral antihistamines. Topical antipruritics. Analgesics. Cool compresses or baths. Topical corticosteroids are sometimes prescribed.

Data from Vanderhooft, S. L. (1998). Is the rash really an adverse drug reaction? Contemporary Pediatrics, 15(5), 118–137; Valencia, I. C., Falabela, A. F., & Schachner, L. A. (2001). New developments in wound care for infants and children. Pediatric Annals, 30(4), 211–218; Schmidt, C. E. (2003). A 12-month-old girl with maculopapular lesions and lower extremity edema. Journal of Emergency Nursing, 29(3), 204–207; Cohen, B. A. (2002). Plaques: Oval, itchy, and red: What's your diagnosis? Contemporary Pediatrics, 19(4), 36–41.

define a pattern of inheritance are not conclusive. Medications associated with the appearance of acne lesions include androgens, corticosteroids, phenytoin, lithium, and isoniazid (Rudy, 2003). Other factors that can trigger acne include friction of the skin from hairbands, helmets, and hats, as well as oil-based cosmetics.

CLINICAL MANIFESTATIONS

Noninflammatory acne involves a follicular plug (comedone) that precedes inflammatory acne lesions. There are three main types of acne: comedonal (characterized by open and closed comedones), papulopustular (characterized by papules and pustules) (Figure 57–5 ●), and cystic (characterized by nodules and cysts). Closed comedones are flesh-colored papules with tiny follicular openings, called whiteheads. Open comedones are found when the follicular plug has enlarged and dilated the follicular opening, called blackheads. Lesions occur most often on the face, upper chest, shoulders, and back. Scars form when the surrounding dermis is damaged. Types of scars may include the following: ice pick (small, deep, punched out pits), atrophic macules, hypertrophic scars or keloids, or broad sloping depressions (Woodard, 2002).

CLINICAL THERAPY

Diagnosis is based upon the examination of the skin. The goal of treatment is to suppress lesions until the condition is outgrown, thus preventing infection and scarring, and minimizing psychologic distress. The severity of skin le-

● FIGURE 57–5

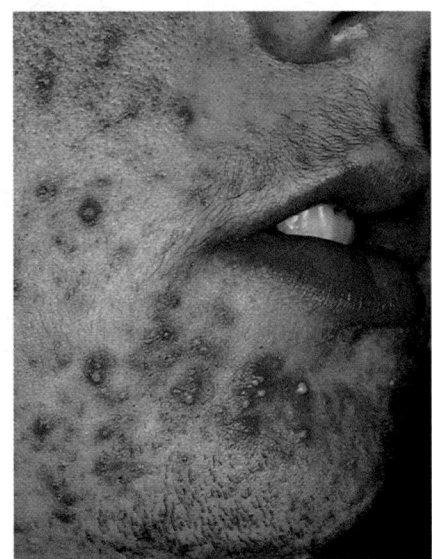

Pustular acne can have a significant effect on an adolescent's self-esteem.

Used with permission from Habif, T. P. (1990). Clinical dermatology: A color guide to diagnosis and therapy (2nd ed., p. 113). St. Louis, MO: Mosby-Year Book.

sions is graded, and treatment is customized to the severity level. See Table 57–3.

Topical keratolytics are used, such as benzoyl peroxide that has both a bacteriostatic action and effect on follicular hyperkeratosis. Other topical keratolytics include azelaic acid 20%, salicylic acid, and sulfur. Topical antibiotics help to reduce the colonization of bacteria and to reduce inflammation.

Topical retinoids (tretinoin, adapalene, tazarotene) slow desquamation and decrease the adherence of shed cells within the follicles leading to reduced follicular plugging. Dryness and scaling of the skin are typical after several days of treatment. It may seem as if the condition is worsening in the first 1 to 3 weeks of treatment, but with continued treatment, the skin adapts (Rudy, 2003). Adolescents with more dry and sensitive skin should use creams, while those with more oily skin should use gels.

Oral antibiotics are used for moderate or severe acne. Generally 3 months are needed for medication to be effective. After a good response to oral antibiotics and topical acne medications, the antibiotic dose is tapered to the lowest dose that maintains acne control when used in combination with topical medications. Increasing numbers of cases of bacterial resistance to antibiotics have been noted. A recurrence or flare-up of acne after it has been controlled may indicate that the bacteria have developed resistance to the antibiotic. The antibiotic may need to be replaced to find one that is effective. Isotretinoin (Accutane) is reserved for the most serious cases that are not responsive to other therapies.

Oral contraceptives with norgestimate and ethinyl estradiol are FDA approved for the treatment of acne (Sidbury & Paller, 2000). Spironolactone is sometimes prescribed due to its action in decreasing sebum production, and when prescribed with oral contraceptives, its action is enhanced (Woodard, 2002).

NURSING MANAGEMENT

NURSING ASSESSMENT AND DIAGNOSIS

Physical assessment should include documentation regarding distribution, type, and severity of acne lesions. Assess the adolescent's and parents' knowledge about the cause and treatment of acne. Also explore the amount of emotional distress the acne is causing the adolescent.

Common nursing diagnoses are presented in "Nursing Care Plan: The Adolescent with Acne."

PLANNING AND IMPLEMENTATION

Nursing care for the adolescent with acne is summarized in the accompanying "Nursing Care Plan." Nursing management focuses on educating the child and parents about acne and its treatment. Advise adolescents to wash their hands before touching affected areas and to avoid picking or squeezing the lesions. Remind them that the inflammation occurs with the rupture of lesions below the skin surface, which picking and squeezing may cause. In addition, advise them to avoid using any cleansing products that have a greasy base, to shampoo hair regularly (to treat seborrhea that can accompany acne), to expect flare-ups despite treatment, and to eat a well-balanced diet.

Topical medications should be spread in a thin film over the skin, according to directions. Emphasize that treatment is often long term. Significant improvement may not be seen until at least 6 to 12 weeks after the start of treatment.

Correct misconceptions about dietary causes. Although no food has been found to cause acne or an increase in severity of lesions, good nutrition is important. Teach parents and children that increased sweating, as well as heat and humidity, may exacerbate acne. Emotional stress may increase adrenal androgen production, resulting in increased sebum production and acne flare-ups.

TABLE 57–3 ❖ Treatment Protocols for Acne

Appearance	Treatment
Grade I Comedonal acne (comedones only)	Tretinoin (Retin-A) 0.025% cream daily, in the evening, salicylic acid, adapalene, tazarotene
Grade II Papulopustular acne (red papules, pustules)	2.5% benzoyl peroxide gel, Tretinoin (Retin-A) in evening, topical clindamycin and erythromycin, topical tetracycline, azaleic acid cream twice a day
Grade III Cystic acne (red papules, many pustules, cysts)	Tretinoin (Retin-A) and benzoyl peroxide twice a day, with oral antibiotics (tetracycline, minocycline, or doxycycline)
Grade IV Pustulocystic nodular (severe, resistant to other treatment)	Isotretinoin (Accutane)

Data from Sidbury, R., & Paller, A. S. (2000). The diagnosis and management of acne. *Pediatric Annals, 29*(1), 17–24.

NURSING CARE PLAN

THE ADOLESCENT WITH ACNE

Intervention	Rationale	Expected Outcome
1. Nursing Diagnosis: Effective, Individual Therapeutic Regimen Management related to hygiene and skin care		
NIC Priority Intervention: **Health education:** Developing and providing instruction and learning experiences to facilitate voluntary adaptation of behavior conducive to health in individuals, families, groups, or communities		**NOC Suggested Outcome:** **Symptom control behavior:** Personal actions to minimize perceived adverse changes in physical and emotional functioning
Goal: The adolescent will verbalize proper hygiene, nutrition, and treatment of acne. The adolescent will verbalize understanding of treatment regimen.		

■ Teach good skin care:
  ■ Wash skin with mild soap and water twice a day.
  ■ Do not use astringents.
  ■ Avoid vigorous scrubbing.
■ Praise good habits.
 	
■ Advise the adolescent to wash hair with antiseborrheic shampoo, avoid oil-based cosmetics or lotions.
 	
■ Encourage a balanced diet, adequate fluids, exercise, and adequate rest.
■ Encourage the adolescent to keep a diary of health and diet habits.
 	
■ Educate the adolescent about medications (action, side effects, dosage, method of application).
■ Encourage application of tretinoin at night. Encourage use of nonoil sunscreens of at least SPF 15.
■ Educate the adolescent about time needed for response and importance of daily compliance.
	■ Good hygiene and appropriate skin care reduce surface oils and bacteria, which intensify inflammatory reactions.
	
	■ Positive reinforcement encourages continued effort.
	■ Treats seborrhea, which frequently accompanies acne. Oil-based preparations can obstruct sebaceous glands, exacerbating acne.
	■ Adequate nutrients, water, and exercise promote healthy skin.
	■ A record may help identify associations with flare-ups that can be avoided in the future.
	■ Proper application of medication enhances healing of lesions.
	
	■ Helps reduce sensitivity to sun and avoid sunburn.
	
	■ May take up to 3 months for significant improvement to occur. The adolescent needs a reason to continue with the care plan.
		The adolescent exhibits good hygiene habits.
		
		The adolescent implements the treatment regimen as outlined, resulting in a noticeable reduction in lesions.

2. Nursing Diagnosis: Disturbed Body Image related to biophysical factors (visible facial lesions)		
NIC Priority Intervention: **Self-esteem enhancement:** Assisting a patient to increase his or her personal judgment of self-worth		**NOC Suggested Outcome:** **Self-esteem:** Personal judgment of self-worth
Goal: The adolescent will demonstrate increased self-confidence and self-esteem.		
■ Establish a rapport with the adolescent. ■ Provide education about the condition and therapy modalities. ■ Encourage the adolescent to be responsible for treatment and follow-up, and give positive reinforcement. ■ Encourage the adolescent to become involved with school activities and peers.	■ A trusting relationship promotes verbalization of concerns and fears. ■ Providing information better enables the adolescent to take control of the condition. ■ Responsibility reinforces sense of self-esteem. ■ Involvement in activities helps enhance self-esteem and allows the adolescent to explore new experiences and friendships.	The adolescent freely discusses concerns and fears. The adolescent demonstrates active involvement in own care. The adolescent shows increased confidence, as demonstrated by involvement in extracurricular activities.

DRUG GUIDE

ISOTRETINOIN (ACCUTANE)

Action

Isotretinoin acts on the skin by reducing sebaceous gland size and thus decreasing sebum secretion. The drug blocks follicular keratinization and has antiacne properties.

Routes, Dosage, Frequency

PO: 0.5 mg/kg/day in 2 divided doses

A single 5-month course of therapy is effective in many patients. Improvement is permanent in 70% to 75% of patients treated. A second course of therapy may be used for some patients.

Nursing Management

Assessment: Assess extent and severity of skin lesions. Basic lipid levels and liver function tests are performed at beginning of treatment, and adolescent females need two negative pregnancy tests before starting on isotretinoin.

Administration: Because of its teratogenicity and potential adverse reactions, the U.S. Food and Drug Administration requires individuals taking isotretinoin to sign informed consent about teratogenicity, monthly blood testing, and the potential for depression or suicide ideation (Woodard, 2002). A recent study examining the association between isotretinoin (Accutane) and mental health problems found no increased risk for depression, suicide, or other psychologic problems (Jick, Kremers, & Vasilakis-Scaramozza, 2000). However, press reports have linked isotretinoin to depression and suicide.

Monitor: Because of potential adverse reactions of hepatotoxicity and increased levels of triglycerides, monthly laboratory monitoring of liver function, cholesterol, and triglycerides is also required. A monthly pregnancy test is required during treatment.

Patient Education:

- Adolescents are educated about the requirement to use two forms of contraception when taking isotretinoin (Buck, 2001). Contraception must be used 1 month prior to treatment, during, and 1 month after therapy is completed. A 1-month supply of isotretinoin is provided to promote compliance.
- Encourage the adolescent to continue taking the medication during the first few weeks, even when acne appears to be getting worse. This may indicate a response of deep unseen lesions.
- Do not self-medicate with vitamins that contain vitamin A which may enhance isotretinoin toxicity.
- Restrict use of alcohol and dietary fat intake to help prevent hyperlipidemia.
- Avoid exposure to sun and sunlamps because of photosensitivity.

Caution patients using tretinoin that this medication is **phototoxic** (a rapid nonimmunologic reaction of the skin when exposed to sunlight), resulting in sunburn with even minimal exposure. Teach correct procedures for taking other prescribed drugs, such as tetracycline and isotretinoin (Accutane), and discuss possible side effects. Emphasize the importance of return visits to the adolescent's healthcare provider to monitor medication side effects.

Psychologic support is an important aspect of care. Because adolescents are preoccupied with their body image and peer relationships, they often find having acne embarrassing. Encourage them to express their feelings and refer for counseling, if necessary.

EVALUATION

Expected outcomes of nursing care can be found in "Nursing Care Plan: The Adolescent with Acne."

TEACHING HIGHLIGHTS

CARING FOR ACNE

- Wash the hands frequently and avoid touching the face to reduce the transfer of oils (e.g., from greasy foods) and bacteria to the face. Avoid picking and squeezing pimples.
- Use gentle cleansers to wash the face twice a day. Do not use abrasive sponges or cloths. Wait 20 minutes until the skin is thoroughly dry before applying topical medications.
- Avoid the use of astringents and aftershaves that contain alcohol and may further dry the skin.
- Avoid hats or gear that can cause friction and occlusion of the skin.
- Limit the use of pomades or petrolatum-based hair products. Keep hair spray and other hair products away from the face.
- Use noncomedonic (for acne-prone skin) moisturizers.
- Use oil-free or water-based makeup. Avoid waterproof makeup.
- Use noncomedonic sunscreen or protective clothing even on cloudy days.
- Continue daily therapies, even when acne has improved significantly, so acne does not return.

INFECTIOUS DISORDERS

BACTERIAL INFECTIONS

IMPETIGO

Impetigo is a highly contagious, superficial (epidermal) infection caused by streptococci, staphylococci, or both. The most common sites are the face, around the mouth, the hands, the neck, and the extremities. It is the most common bacterial skin condition in children.

Minor skin abrasions, lacerations, insect bites, burns, and dermatitis provide the portal for the infectious agent commonly present in the environment. *Group A beta-hemolytic streptococcus* and *Staphylococcus aureus* are usually responsible. *Staphylococcus aureus* colonizes on the skin and mucous membranes, particularly in the nose and throat. This infection occurs more commonly in children who are in close physical contact with others, such as in childcare settings, or who have poor hygiene.

Impetigo lesions begin as a vesicle or pustule surrounded by edema and redness, usually at a site that has been injured. This progresses to an exudative and crusting stage. The initially serous vesicular fluid becomes cloudy, and the vesicle ruptures, leaving a honey-colored crust covering an ulcerated base. Common sites include the intertriginous areas, skinfolds such as in the neck, axillae, or diaper area. The rash may spread to the face and extremities by self-innoculation. In bullous impetigo, vesicles stimulated by a toxin enlarge into bullae with straw-colored fluid and then rupture (Figure 57–6 ●). A thin honey-colored crust forms when the bullae rupture. When the crust is removed, a moist, erythematous lesion with a collar of skin around the erosion is seen. These lesions occur more commonly in moist skinfold areas.

Impetigo is diagnosed by a Gram stain and bacterial culture. Local treatment involves removal of the crusts and application of a topical antibiotic. Crusts are soaked in warm water and gently scrubbed off with an antiseptic soap. A topical bactericidal ointment (such as bacitracin or mupirocin) is applied for 5 to 7 days. If there is no response to topical antibiotics, a skin culture and systemic antibiotic (e.g., dicloxacillin or erythromycin) may be needed. Methicillin-resistant *Staphylococcus aureus* is becoming more common and identifying the appropriate antibiotic to which it is sensitive is important. In children with bullous impetigo, an oral antibiotic may be used. The infection is communicable for 48 hours after antibiotic ointment treatment is begun.

If the child has a history of recurrent impetigo, determine if a person in contact with the child is a nasal carrier of *Staphylococcus aureus*. The carrier can be effectively treated with topical mupirocin ointment applied to the nares four times daily (Mancini, 2000).

Nursing Management

Advise parents that they must continue oral or topical medications for the full number of days prescribed. Tell the parents to observe all close contacts and family members for lesions. Caution them that an infected child should not share towels or toiletries with others and that all linens and clothing used by the child should be washed separately with detergent in hot water. Fingernails should be kept short and clean to prevent spreading infection by scratch-

● **FIGURE 57–6**

A

B

Bullous impetigo.

A, Courtesy of the Centers for Disease Control, Atlanta, GA. B, Courtesy of Dr. William H. Sorey, University of Mississippi Medical Center.

ing. Inform the childcare center about the infection, so staff can sanitize toys and surfaces.

Increased cases of methicillin-resistant *Staphylococcus aureus* have been reported among athletes in high school, particularly when skin trauma occurs or when items are shared. Educate parents, adolescents, coaches, and teachers about the importance of a regular schedule for cleaning equipment and showers with soap and water after all practice sessions, discouraging sharing of towels and clothing, covering wounds, and recognizing infections that need treatment (Centers for Disease Control, 2003a).

FOLLICULITIS

Folliculitis is a superficial inflammation of the pilosebaceous follicle caused by infection, trauma, or irritation. The causative organism is usually *Staphylococcus aureus*. The condition is common in children and teenagers because of increased sweat production. Folliculitis may be associated with *Pseudomonas aeruginosa* exposure in a poorly chlorinated pool or hot tub.

Symptoms include tenderness, localized swelling, and the formation of tiny dome-shaped, yellowish pustules and red papules at follicular openings with surrounding erythema. Individual lesions may become deeper and form an abscess (furuncle). Lesions are usually seen in clusters on the face, scalp, trunk, and extremities. Ruptured lesions heal with hyperpigmentation and no scarring. Some children have fever, aching, and flulike symptoms. If associated with *Pseudomonas* exposure in a pool or hot tub, lesions may develop on areas covered by bathing suits.

Treatment of inflamed follicles consists of washing the affected area with a topical antibiotic cleanser and water, followed by application of hot compresses for 20 minutes, four times a day. A benzoyl peroxide gel or wash or another drying agent will also help clear the infection. Complications are rare. If lesions do not resolve within a week, the child may need systemic antibiotics (e.g., cephalexin or dicloxacillin) and, if the infection is deep, incision and drainage.

Nursing Management

Nursing management focuses on educating the parents and child about prevention. Advise children to shower daily and shortly after exercise, to cleanse with an antibacterial soap, and to wear loose cotton clothing. Talk with parents about the importance of maintaining the correct pH level and chlorine concentration in swimming pools and hot tubs. Bathing suits of affected children should be laundered and well dried before the next use.

CELLULITIS

Cellulitis is an acute inflammation of the dermis and underlying connective tissue characterized by red or lilac, tender, warm, edematous skin that may have an ill-defined, nonelevated border. The condition usually occurs on the face and extremities as a result of trauma or a compromised skin barrier.

Etiology and Pathophysiology

Children with cellulitis often have a history of trauma, impetigo, folliculitis, or recent otitis media. Common causative organisms are *Staphylococcus aureus*, *Streptococcus pneumoniae*, *Haemophilus influenzae*, and beta-hemolytic and group A *streptococcus*. The condition may also result from a nearby abscess or sinusitis. Onset is usually rapid.

Clinical Manifestations

Children with cellulitis have a rapid onset and they appear ill. Classic signs and symptoms include erythema, edema of the face or infected limb, and warmth and tenderness around the infected site (Figure 57–7 ⦿). Other symptoms include fever, chills, malaise, and enlargement and tenderness of regional lymph nodes. Lymphangitis may be present. In some cases, a rapidly progressive lesion may result in septicemia.

Clinical Therapy

Blood studies may show an increase in white blood cells. Cultures are taken by needle aspiration, if possible, to identify the causative organisms. Blood cultures are taken if the child has a toxic (very ill) appearance (see Skill 10–5). **SKILLS**

⦿ **FIGURE 57–7**

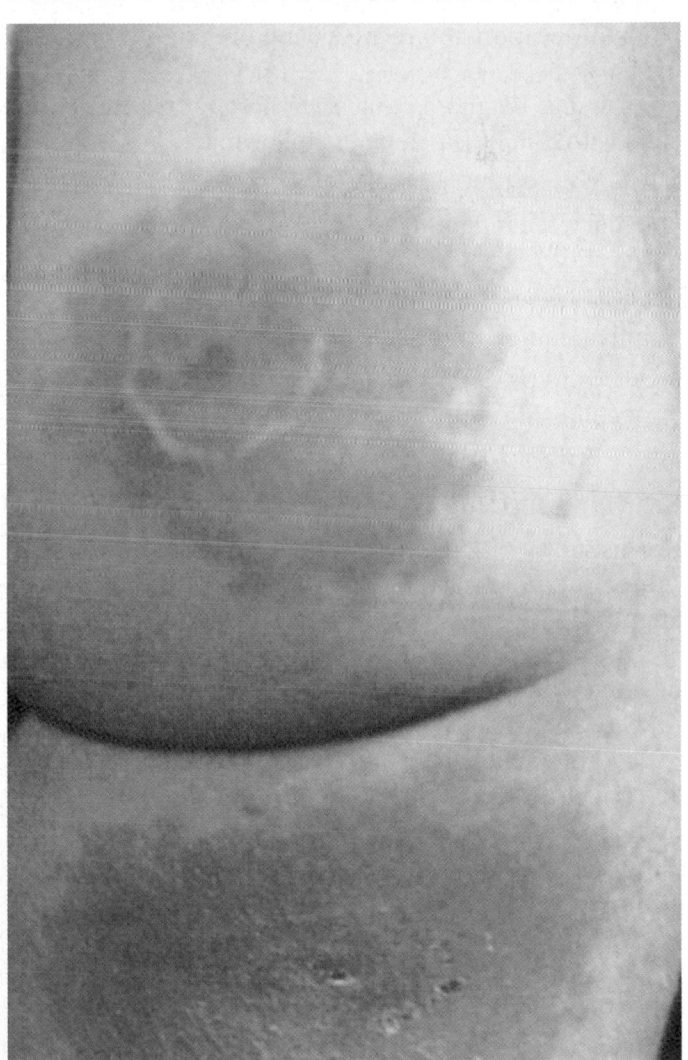

Characteristic appearance of cellulitis.

Used with permission from Ben-Amitai, D., & Ashkenazi, S. (1993). Common bacterial skin infections in children. Pediatric Annals, 22(4), 226. Photograph courtesy of Dr. Aryeh Metzker.

If the face is involved, antibiotic therapy is administered to avoid serious complications. (Periorbital cellulitis is discussed in Chapter 46. ∞) Children with severe cases or a large affected surface area are treated with systemic antibiotics and analgesics in the hospital to prevent sepsis. Children with cellulitis on the trunk, limbs, or perianal area may be treated on an outpatient basis with oral antibiotics. Recovery begins within 48 hours, but therapy should continue for at least 10 days. Untreated cellulitis or cellulitis that does not respond to treatment can lead to osteomyelitis, arthritis, or serious systemic infection.

NURSING MANAGEMENT

NURSING ASSESSMENT AND DIAGNOSIS

Assessment centers on recognition of infection, documentation of location and related symptoms, and monitoring of vital signs.

Nursing diagnoses that may be appropriate for the child with cellulitis include the following:

- *Impaired Skin Integrity* related to mechanical factors (injury, the inflammatory process, and presence of infection)
- *Acute Pain* related to injury agents (swelling and inflammation of the skin)
- *Interrupted Family Processes* related to home care needs of child with acute illness

PLANNING AND IMPLEMENTATION

Because of the risk of sepsis, cellulitis is managed carefully. Administer prescribed oral or IV antibiotics as scheduled. Supportive care includes warm compresses to the affected area four times daily, elevation of the affected limb, and bed rest. Outpatient follow-up is crucial to ensure response to therapy.

Advise parents about possible complications, such as abscess formation. Instruct parents of children treated at home to contact their healthcare provider if the child has any of the following signs:

- Spread of the infected area in the 24- to 48-hour period after the start of treatment
- Temperature over 38.3°C (101°F)
- Increased lethargy

Reinforce to parents the importance of compliance with the treatment regimen and the seriousness of the possible complications.

EVALUATION

Expected outcomes of nursing care include pain control, adherence with administration of antibiotics, and resolution of the infection without progression to systemic infection.

VIRAL INFECTIOUS DISORDERS

MOLLUSCUM CONTAGIOSUM

Molluscum contagiosum is a skin infection caused by a poxvirus. It is transmitted by direct contact, by contact with contaminated objects, or by sexual contact. The individual lesions are pearl-like, skin-colored smooth papules about 1 to 5 mm in size. The lesion has a central depression, and a plug of cheesy material can be expressed when punctured. Lesions may appear anywhere on the body, but tend to be seen more commonly on the face, trunk, and extremities. In adolescents, lesions are more common on the inner thighs, genitals, and pubic areas. The palms and soles are not involved. Children may have few to hundreds of lesions. Immunosuppressed and immunodeficient children often have larger and more numerous lesions. Children with atopic dermatitis treated with topical corticosteroids may have more numerous lesions. The lesions often disappear spontaneously in 6 to 18 months, but the condition can continue for several years.

In mild cases, no intervention is needed (Smolinski & Yan, 2005). Clinical therapy may involve the daily application of tretinoin to irritate the skin and stimulate the immune system to respond to the viral condition. Curettage after topical anesthesia or **cryotherapy** (freezing each lesion with liquid nitrogen) may be performed by dermatologists. Scarring may result from clinical therapy. Secondary infections are treated with topical or oral antibiotics.

NURSING MANAGEMENT

Nursing education focuses on reducing disease transmission. Infected children should avoid public swimming pools, hot tubs, and other joint bathing as the virus is more easily transmitted when the skin is wet. Towels and sponges should not be shared.

The skin should be washed daily with gentle fragrance-free cleansers, followed by application of a hypoallergenic moisturizer or emollient to the entire skin surface. If tretinoin is selected as a therapy, educate the parents how to apply the lotion. Teach parents to recognize potential secondary infections.

When intervention such as curettage or cryotherapy is performed, inform the child about what will happen, and then provide distraction during the procedure to reduce anxiety. Ensure that the child has adequate topical anesthetic to minimize any pain from the intervention.

WARTS (PAPILLOMAVIRUS)

Several types of human papillomavirus infect epithelial cells and cause warts. Various types of warts are found in children: common warts that appear on any skin surface and plantar warts found on the feet. The human papillomavirus is commonly transmitted by direct skin to skin contact or mucous membrane contact. The virus also survives on various surfaces, and transmission can occur with contact, such as plantar warts from locker room floors. The incubation period may be 2 to 6 months; however, a latency period may exist in some cases. Children with immune compromise are more susceptible and often have numerous warts.

Common warts appear as skin-colored, rough, scaly papules and nodules on exposed skin surfaces. Individual and multiple warts may be seen, or large plaques may form if autoinoculation occurs. Warts usually cause no pain or itching unless in skin surface areas or creases that become irritated. Plantar warts appear as papules and plaques on the bottom of feet that grow inward and cause pain. Small black dots result from thrombosed vessels on the surface of the warts caused by weight bearing.

No intervention may be recommended as warts often resolve spontaneously over a couple of years. Application of duct tape that is changed every 1 to 3 days over a couple of months is often effective (Smolinski & Yan, 2005). Clinical therapy usually involves some form of destructive therapy, such as cryotherapy, application of caustic substances or peeling agents, electrocautery, and laser therapy. Treatment is not always successful and may result in scarring.

Nursing Management

Educate the parents and child about the application of peeling agents and caustic substances when prescribed for home use. If the reaction to the substance is painful, encourage the parents to reduce the frequency of the treatment until the pain subsides and then to resume the original treatment schedule. Successful treatment may take several months, and parents may need encouragement to continue the therapy and remain optimistic.

Other viral skin conditions are described in Chapter 45. ∞

FUNGAL INFECTIONS

ORAL CANDIDIASIS (THRUSH)

Oral candidiasis (moniliasis or thrush) is a fungal infection that occurs as an acute condition in newborns (usually acquired during birth from the vaginal canal of an infected mother) and a chronic condition in young children who have an immune disorder, regularly use a corticosteroid inhaler, or are receiving antibiotics which have disturbed the normal flora, allowing the growth of the fungus.

Oral thrush is characterized by white patches that look like coagulated milk on the oral mucosa and may bleed when removed (Figure 57–8 ●). Milk residue can be removed from the oral mucosa with gentle swabbing. With candidiasis, however, attempts at gentle removal are unsuccessful. The infant may refuse to nurse or feed because of discomfort and pain. The infant may also have diaper dermatitis superinfection with candidiasis. Fever is usually not present.

Treatment involves oral nystatin suspension or clotrimazole, which is applied to the mouth and tongue after feedings. Fluconazole or itraconazole may be used for immunocompromised patients with oropharyngeal candidiasis. If infection is severe, occurs in the esophagus, or invades other body systems, oral fluconazole or intravenous amphotericin B may be prescribed for a minimum of 21 days.

Nursing Management

Educate parents to give the oral medication to infants. Parents should use a swab to apply the suspension to the buccal mucosa and tongue surfaces, allowing the infant to swallow the remaining suspension. Older children should be told to swish the solution around in the mouth before swallowing it.

To prevent a reinfection, educate parents about sterilizing bottle nipples and pacifiers. A commercial antiseptic spray may be used on toys that cannot be autoclaved, but follow directions carefully so the child does not ingest any

● FIGURE 57–8

Thrush, an acute pseudomembranous form of oral candidiasis, is a common fungal infection in infants and children.

Used with permission from Zitelli, B. J., & Davis, H. W. (Eds.). (1997). Atlas of pediatric physical diagnosis (3rd ed., p. 104, Fig. 4–50a). St. Louis, MO: Mosby.

harmful residue. Teach parents and older children with asthma to rinse the mouth well with water after using a corticosteroid inhaler to prevent candidiasis. If a spacer is used, it should also be rinsed with water after use.

DERMATOPHYTOSES (RINGWORM)

Dermatophytoses are fungal infections that affect the skin, hair, or nails. Children of all ages may be affected. Dermatophytoses may be spread from person to person, from animal to person, or by contact with an inanimate object (e.g., clothing or linens) belonging to an infected individual. The most common infections are tinea capitis, tinea corporis, tinea cruris, and tinea pedis. See "Clinical Manifestations: Tinea Infections."

Diagnosis is confirmed through microscopic examination of the hair and scale scrapings using a potassium hydroxide (KOH) wet mount to reveal rows and chains of spores within the hair shaft. A fungal culture can also be taken from a scalp lesion by rubbing a cotton-tipped applicator across the scalp and placing it in a throat culture tube. A Wood's lamp is also useful in identifying some forms of tinea that fluoresce under ultraviolet light. However, *Trichophyton tonsurans,* the most common cause of tinea capitis, does not fluoresce with a Wood's lamp (Brodell & Vescera, 2002). Tinea caused by a microsporum infection fluoresces a brilliant green under the Wood's lamp (American Academy of Pediatrics, 2003). An oral antifungal agent (e.g., griseofulvin) is usually prescribed for tinea capitis, but resistance is developing. As the medication is still effective in higher doses, it remains the drug of choice. See "Clinical Manifestations: Tinea Infections" for clinical therapy information.

Nursing Management

All members of the family and household pets should be assessed for fungal lesions. Since person-to-person transmission is common, personal contact with hair and sharing hair accessories, brushes, and hats should be avoided. In some cases, there may be an asymptomatic carrier in the family, in which case everyone should be treated. Teach parents and older children or teenagers that fungi are found in soil and animals and are transmitted through direct contact.

DEVELOPING CULTURAL COMPETENCE

TINEA CAPITIS

While tinea capitis can occur in any racial or ethnic group, it is most prevalent in African-American children. This is believed due to immunologic factors, genetic factors, or hair care practices. For this reason, any African-American child with scaling in the scalp should be screened for tinea capitis (Elewski & Krowchuk, 2001).

Advise parents to give oral griseofulvin with fatty foods such as whole milk or peanut butter to enhance absorption. The medications must be used for the entire prescribed period, even if the lesions are gone, to prevent recurrence of the infection. For children with tinea cruris, encourage loose-fitting undergarments to promote dryness. With tinea pedis, feet should be kept clean and dry and nails clipped short. Encourage the use of 100% cotton socks that wick moisture away from the skin. Encourage children to wear shower shoes in public showers and locker rooms.

Parents of children with tinea capitis should be told that hair regrowth is slow and may take 6 to 12 months. In some cases hair loss is permanent, which can be particularly stressful for older children or adolescents. Provide emotional support.

INFESTATIONS

PEDICULOSIS CAPITIS (LICE)

Pediculosis capitis is a lice infestation of the hair and scalp. Infestation occurs among children of all socioeconomic levels. Parents or teachers may be the first to notice lice, or healthcare providers may spot them during routine examination (see Chapter 35 ∞). Outbreaks occur periodically among preschool and school-age children, particularly those in day care and elementary school.

Head lice live and reproduce only on humans and are transmitted by direct hair-to-hair contact or indirect contact such as sharing of hair accessories, brushes, hats, towels, and bedding. Lice do not fly or jump, but they can crawl quickly. The female louse lays her eggs (nits) on the hair shaft, close to the scalp (see Figure 35–4 in Chapter 35 ∞). The incubation period for eggs to hatch is 8 to 10 days.

Clinical manifestations include intense pruritus and complaints of "dandruff" that sticks to the hair (actually the nits) and "bugs" in the hair. Nits look like silvery white, yellow, or darker 1-mm teardrops adhering to one side of the hair shaft. Secondary effects of scratching include inflammation, pustules, and bacterial infection. Nits are found most commonly behind the ears and at the base of the head. Lice are wingless insects about the size of a sesame seed. They move quickly away from light and are not often seen. Posterior cervical nodes are frequently palpable.

Treatment involves a pediculicide shampoo, such as pyrethrum with an enzymatic lice egg remover, or an ovicidal rinse, such as permethrin (Nix). Permethrin cream rinse is applied to washed and towel-dried hair. The preparation is applied, left in place for 10 minutes, and then rinsed. The hair is towel-dried, and the nits are removed with a fine-toothed comb. A second treatment is needed in 7 days as the neurotoxin is not effective on nits. Permethrin resistance has been reported, but a 5% concentration is effective. Lindane

TINEA INFECTIONS

SITE, INCIDENCE, AND COMMON DERMATOPHYTE	CLINICAL MANIFESTATIONS	CLINICAL THERAPY
Tinea capitis (scalp) *Trichophyton tonsurans* *Trichophyton violaceum* *Trichophyton soudanense* *Trichophyton verrucosum* *Microsporum canis* Usually prepubertal children between 1 and 10 years 	Circumscribed hair loss Broken hairs; black, dotted stubbed appearance where weakened hair has broken off Diffuse fine scaling, may appear as seborrhea with yellow greasy scales Many scaly pustular bald areas with indistinct margins Mild itching **Kerion**—large purulent tender boggy mass on scalp with drainage Papules, pustules, and crusting on scalp Suboccipital or posterior cervical nodes	Griseofulvin orally for 6 to 8 weeks, or 2 weeks after symptoms disappear Selenium sulfide shampoo 2 to 3 times weekly, leave on for 10 minutes before rinsing to help eliminate scalp spores Alternative antifungal agents used when children do not tolerate or respond to griseofulvin include fluconazole, itraconazole, and terbinafine (not approved by FDA for children < 12 years of age)
Tinea corporis (trunk) *Trichophyton tonsurans* *Trichophyton rubrum* *Microsporum canis* *Epidermophyton floccosum* Children and adolescents 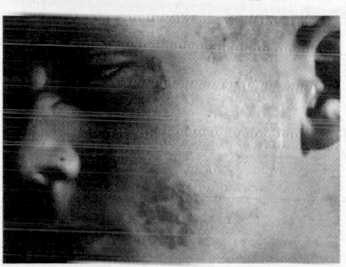	Pink, scaly circular patch with an expanding border, may be scaly or erythematous throughout Slightly raised borders with a clearing center Usually acquired from contact with infected humans, cats, dogs, or horses (Monroe, 2005)	Topical cream (e.g., clotrimazole, miconazole, ketoconazole, naftifine, or terbinafine) twice a day for 4 weeks Wash body with selenium sulfide shampoo An oral antifungal agent may be needed for extensive lesions, hair follicle involvement, or no response to topical therapy
Tinea cruris ("jock itch") *Epidermophyton floccosum* *Trichophyton rubrum* Rare before adolescence	Annular lesions Scaly, erythematous eruption symmetric bilaterally, may spread to abdomen, buttocks, and upper thighs, usually spare penis and scrotum May have elevated lesions, papules, or vesicles Tinea pedis may have been spread by hand to groin area	Topical antifungal agent such as imidazole for 2 weeks or butenafine, naftifine, or terbinafine for 1 week Wash body with selenium sulfide shampoo Decrease moisture and occlusion to area
Tinea pedis ("athlete's foot") *Trichophyton rubrum* *Trichophyton mentagrophytes* *Epidermophyton floccosum* Children and adolescents	Vesicles or erosions on instep or between toes (fissures, red scaly) Peeling maceration and fissures in lateral toe web spaces (indicate secondary bacterial involvement) Dry scaly patches or plaques with mild erythema on plantar and lateral surfaces of foot Itching	Broad-spectrum topical antifungal agent that has antibacterial properties, (e.g., econazole or ciclopirox) Keep feet dry with absorbent talc Allow to air-dry Use 100% cotton socks, change twice daily

Photographs of tinea capitis and tinea corporis courtesy of the Centers for Disease Control and Prevention, Atlanta, GA.

TABLE 57–4 ✤ Medications and Preparations for Head Lice

Name of Medication/Preparation	Nursing Considerations
Insecticide-Free	
Lice B Gone	Apply all products to *dry hair.*
Lice Away Enzyme Shampoo	
Hair Clean 1-2-3	
Oil, petrolatum jelly, mayonnaise	Cover with shower cap overnight.
Distilled white vinegar used as a rinse	Used as a rinse to loosen nits.
Formic acid used as a rinse	Used as a rinse to loosen nits.
First-Line Pesticide Treatment	
Permethrin 1% Crème Rinse—Nix	Should be applied to *dry hair and scalp.* Massage into the hair one section at a time. Wet hair dilutes the product and may contribute to treatment failure.
Pyrethrin shampoo (0.17% to 0.33%) or Piperonyl butoxide (2% to 4%)—Rid, A-200, R&C, Triple X, Pronto, Tegrin-LT, InnoGel Plus	
Second-Line Pesticide Treatment	
Malathion 0.5%—Ovide lotion	Apply to *dry scalp and hair* until soaked and allowed to dry naturally. Leave on for 8–12 hours. Do not expose the child to electric heat sources as the malathion treatment contains flammable alcohol.
Lindane 1% or "lindano"—Kwell, limited effectiveness due to resistance	
Non-FDA Approved	
Trimethoprim/sulfamethoxazole Ivermectin—antiparasitic	Drug in bloodstream is ingested by louse, destroys bacterial flora in louse intestine. Does not treat the nits.

shampoo is not recommended because of lice resistance and toxicity (Angel, Nigro, & Levy, 2000). See Table 57–4 for products used to treat lice. Tests of home remedies (vinegar, isopropyl alcohol, olive oil, mayonnaise, melted butter, and petroleum jelly) revealed that only petroleum jelly caused significant louse mortality and allowed only 6% of eggs to hatch. None of the home remedy products were effective means of louse control (Takano-Lee, Edman, Mullens et al., 2004).

NURSING MANAGEMENT

Carefully assess children who have been exposed to head lice using a bright light and magnifying glass (see Chapter 35 ∞). To avoid potential reinfestation of other children, change gloves frequently when assessing several children in a classroom setting.

Infestation with lice can be upsetting for both the child and family. Emphasize to the family that anyone can get lice. Thorough interventions and education are essential for effective treatment. All contacts of the child should be examined for infestation and should be treated as necessary. Tell parents that children infested with lice should not return to child care or school until after the first pediculicide treatment is completed. Teach the child not to share clothing, headwear, or combs.

Explain to parents that the shampoo and rinses prescribed are pesticides and must be used for the time specified and as directed. An extra bottle of shampoo may be needed if the child has extra long hair. Keep these products out of the eyes and mouth of the child during their use as they will irritate mucous membranes.

To remove nits, use a small-toothed comb, tweezers, and a basin filled with water or isopropyl alcohol to dip and clean the comb and tweezers. Comb 1-inch sections from the scalp outward and pin these out of the way when done. Nits adhere to the hair shaft and must be manually pulled down the shaft with the comb, tweezers, or fingernails. All nits should be removed. Have blunt-nosed scissors available to cut a hair shaft below the level of the nit when the nit cannot be removed. Put the child under a bright light and use distractions such as a video to keep the child entertained during the procedure. An alternative therapy for boys is to cut off the hair in a close buzz cut. A shorter hair cut for girls may help with nit removal.

Although lice can survive for only about 3 days away from a human host, shed nits may hatch 8 to 10 days later. For this reason, the child's bedding and clothing should be changed daily, laundered in hot water with detergent, and dried in a hot dryer for 20 minutes. Nonessential bedding and clothing can be stored in a tightly sealed bag for 2 to 3 weeks and then washed. Hair accessories, brushes, and combs should be discarded or soaked in hot soapy water (54.4°C [130°F]) for 10 minutes. Vacuum furniture and carpets and treat them with a hot iron when possible. Use of an insecticide in the home to kill the lice on carpets, furniture, and other items with which young children and pets come into contact is not recommended. Seal toys and other personal items that cannot be washed or dry-cleaned in a plastic bag for 2 weeks.

SCABIES

Scabies is a highly contagious infestation caused by the mite *Sarcoptes scabiei*. It is spread by skin-to-skin contact. Children of all ages and both sexes can be affected. The highest prevalence is in children under 2 years of age (Angel et al., 2000).

The female mite burrows into the outer layer of the epidermis (stratum corneum) to lay her eggs, leaving a trail of debris and feces. The larvae hatch in approximately 2 to 4 days and proceed toward the surface of the skin. The cycle is repeated 14 to 17 days later. Hypersensitivity to the ova and mite feces causes irritation and intense pruritus approximately 1 month after infestation. Nodules, which can persist for weeks after effective treatment, develop as a granulomatous response to the dead mite antigens and feces. Because the mite usually takes at least 45 minutes to burrow into the skin, transient contact is unlikely to cause infestation.

Symptoms include a rash with various types of lesions, severe pruritus that worsens at night, and restlessness. Lesions are usually located in the webs of the fingers, in the intergluteal folds, around the axillae, or on the palms, wrists, head, neck, legs, buttocks, chest, abdomen, and waist (Figure 57–9 ●). In infants the palms, insteps of the feet, and scalp and face can be affected. Lesions may appear as linear, threadlike, grayish burrows 1 to 10 cm in length, which may end in a pinpoint vesicle. The lesion may have been obliterated by the child's scratching and secondary infection.

Diagnosis is confirmed by examination under the microscope of scrapings from a burrow, which reveals actively moving mites, fecal pellets, eggs, or nits. Treatment involves application of a scabicide, such as 5% permethrin lotion, over the entire body from the chin down. Apply scabicide only to the scalp and forehead of infants. The lotion can be applied to the face of older children if lesions are present. Precipitated sulfur in petrolatum for three successive nights is used to treat scabies in infants under 2 months of age who should not be exposed to the more toxic scabicide lotions (Metry & Hebert, 2000). It is malodorous and messy and stains the bedding and clothing, so parents do not like using it.

Application of 5% permethrin lotion or malathion (Ovide) is preceded by a warm soap and water bath. Lindane is no longer recommended for full-body application in infants and young children because of toxicity (Angel et al.,

Diffuse scabies in an infant. The lesions are most numerous around the axillae, chest, and abdomen.

Used with permission from Habif, T. P. (1990). Clinical dermatology: A color guide to diagnosis and therapy (2nd ed., p. 298). St. Louis, MO: Mosby-Year Book.

2000). The skin must be cool and dry before the lotion is applied. The lotion is left in place for 8 to 12 hours (overnight) before washing it off. A second treatment is used 1 week later. Topical and oral ivermectin is a new antiparasitic product with FDA approval for children over 5 years of age. All members of the household and childcare contacts should be treated at the same time, even if they have no symptoms.

Itching may persist for 1 to 2 weeks after treatment. An oral antihistamine (e.g., Benadryl, Atarax) may be prescribed to help relieve itching. Antibiotics may be needed when a secondary infection occurs.

NURSING MANAGEMENT

Advise parents that scabies is transmitted by close contact and is very contagious. All clothing, bedding, and pillowcases used by the child should be changed daily, washed with hot water, and ironed before reuse. Nonwashable toys and other items should be sealed in plastic bags for 5 to 7 days.

Family members who are not infected should avoid touching the affected child until after treatment is completed. If they do, they should wash their hands well. Inform the parents about signs of secondary infections and that itching and nodules may persist for weeks after effective treatment. Encourage the use of emollients as the treatment dries the skin.

Scabies, like pediculosis, can be embarrassing or upsetting for the child and family. Educate the child and parents about the condition, its spread, and treatment measures to prevent recurrence.

VASCULAR TUMORS (HEMANGIOMAS)

Vascular tumors or hemangiomas occur in 1% to 3% of all newborns; however, by the age of 1 year, approximately 10% of infants are affected. An increased incidence has been noted in girls and preterm infants weighing less than 1500 g. The head and neck are common sites. The risk for a hemangioma is greater in children of women who had chorionic villus sampling during pregnancy (Dinehart, Kincannon, & Geronemus, 2001).

Vascular tumors are neoplasms of endothelial cells and increased numbers of small blood vessels that undergo rapid growth and proliferation during the first 6 to 10 months of life that may lead to ulceration. This phase is followed by a slow **involution** (process of decreasing in size) that is completed in 95% of children by adolescence (Cohen, 2004). Hemangiomas may be superficial (located in the epidermis), deep (located in the dermis or subcutaneous tissue), or mixed superficial and deep. Multiple hemangiomas or a large facial hemangioma is associated with hemangiomas in major organs, such as the liver. Complications caused by the rapid growth and pressure against or obstruction of vital structures (e.g., airway, eye, or ear canal) may occur.

Superficial hemangiomas are bright-red vascular cutaneous plaques that resemble strawberries. Deep hemangiomas appear as bluish tumors covered with normal-appearing epidermis. Mixed hemangiomas have features of both superficial and deep tumors. The lesions, appearing any place on the body, are minimally compressible and have no bruit or thrill. As the hemangioma involutes, signs of tissue atrophy, wrinkles, telangiectasias, and hypopigmentation may be noted.

Initial diagnosis is by physical examination and monitoring the growth of the vascular tumor. When a vital organ could become obstructed, ultrasound, computed tomography, or magnetic resonance imaging may be performed. Systemic corticosteroids are used during the proliferation phase for infants with extensive facial hemangiomas. Oral prednisone is given once a day for 7 to 10 days when a response is noted, and the dose is then tapered to the lowest effective dose for a 4- to 6-week course of treatment. This is followed by a 2- to 4-week rest period between courses of corticosteroid treatment (Dinehart et al., 2001). Treatment often continues throughout the proliferative phase so that rebound growth does not occur (Drolet, Esterly, & Frieden, 1999). Injections of corticosteroids into small localized hemangiomas are sometimes performed. Pulsed dye laser treatment at 2- to 3-week intervals is used for superficial hemangiomas during the proliferative phase. The hemangioma will darken for 1 to 2 weeks, the darkness will fade to red, and eventual lightening of the treated skin surface occurs. Recombinant interferon alpha may be used to treat life-threatening hemangiomas that fail to respond to corticosteroids.

NURSING MANAGEMENT

Assess the distribution of the hemangioma and consider the potential for complications as it goes through a rapid growth stage. Monitor the child for signs of any complications, such as ulceration or stridor that could be associated with compression on the airway. Assess the parents' response to the infant's appearance and how they are managing interactions with friends and family about the infant's changing appearance. Take photos of the infant at each visit so that parents have a record of improvements once therapy is initiated.

Teach the parents about the type of vascular lesion and potential treatment options. When corticosteroids are prescribed, teach the parents about administration, the need to take the full course as prescribed, and potential side effects. Inform parents about the possible ulceration of a rapidly growing hemangioma, what signs to expect, and how to protect the skin until the infant is seen by the physician.

Talk with parents about comments received about the infant's appearance and provide some possible responses that parents can make. To promote attachment, help the parents see the infant's positive characteristics, such as responsiveness and smiling. Show photos of other children with similar lesions who have completed therapy to show that improvements in appearance are gradual, but possible.

Teach parents to protect the skin surface from trauma after pulsed dye laser treatments and to keep the infant's nails short to prevent scratching. Cleanse the area treated with water and pat it dry. Inform parents to avoid sun exposure for several weeks after the treatments, and to use sunscreen in the future.

INJURIES TO THE SKIN

PRESSURE ULCERS

More and more children with disabilities are cared for in hospital, community, and home care settings. Many are at risk for skin breakdown and pressure ulcers. Children at greatest risk are those with limited mobility or high activity, sensory deficits, the inability to change positions, or incontinence (Table 57–5).

Soft tissues may be compressed between a bony prominence and another surface. Tissue ischemia occurs when high pressure is maintained over a short period of time or low pressure is maintained over a prolonged time. The cells

TABLE 57–5 ✤ Sites and Potential Causes of Pressure Ulcers

Sites	Potential Causes
Occipital region of scalp	Inability to lift head
Sacrum and buttocks	Confinement to bed or wheelchair
Legs and feet	Orthotics, leg braces, casts
Spine and neck	Scoliosis brace
Knees and elbows	Rubbing against bed sheet

are deprived of oxygen and nutrients, and metabolic waste products accumulate, injuring the soft tissue. Without appropriate intervention, the injury progresses rapidly and a pressure ulcer forms (see "Pathophysiology Illustrated: The Four Stages of Ulcer Formation").

The earliest sign of skin damage is an area of redness that does not go away within 30 minutes of removing the pressure or skin irritant. Children with dark skin may have persistent red, blue, or purple discoloration. As the injury progresses, the skin looks rubbed or raw like an abrasion or blister. Damage then extends through the epidermis and dermis, forming an ulcer. The ulcer then deepens to underlying muscles, bone, or connective tissue unless treated.

Initial treatment for early stages of skin damage involves removing pressure from the affected site until the skin has healed. Children who use leg braces for alignment and mobility are often put in wheelchairs. Children who use wheelchairs are often put on bed rest on a pressure-reducing surface. Frequent repositioning is needed. A transparent film may be applied to affected red skin to minimize friction. Pressure ulcers are treated with dressings, such as hydrocolloids, gels or hydrogels, and calcium alginates.

NURSING MANAGEMENT

Carefully inspect the dependent skin surfaces of all infants and children confined to bed at least three times in each 24-hour period. Evaluate the risk for skin damage based on factors that can contribute to skin breakdown. Identify the size (diameter and depth) and character of the skin lesion. Note any signs of infection, the appearance of wound edges, type of tissue at the wound base, and drainage.

 GROWTH AND DEVELOPMENT

The site of greatest pressure in infants and young children is the occiput. Older children have increased pressure on the sacral and occipital areas.

Follow guidelines for pressure ulcer prevention such as increased ambulation, frequent position changes, pressure-reducing surfaces, and moisture barriers. If the child is incontinent, change the diaper frequently to keep the skin clean and dry. Provide wound care and dressing changes according to agency guidelines. These guidelines may include saline irrigation, debridement, and a dressing appropriate for the wound condition (see Skill 17–1). **SKILLS** Avoid using tape to hold dressings in place unless a protective skin barrier is used.

Teach parents of children with braces to inspect the skin under the braces every day for irritation (redness or blisters). Help the child to use a mirror with a long handle to inspect skin on the bottom and sides of the feet, behind the knees, and on the lower legs. Check all edges of the braces for roughness or breakage that can pinch or scrape the skin. If any skin irritation is seen and redness does not go away within 30 minutes, do not put the brace back on until the skin heals. Inform the child's physician so that treatment can be started immediately. To prevent braces from rubbing on bare skin, have the child wear cotton socks under the braces and make sure the shoes are large enough to accommodate the brace, socks, and the foot. Advise parents to return to a prosthetist regularly for brace refitting as the child grows.

Children who use a wheelchair are at risk for skin breakdown on the buttocks and lower back from the pressure of sitting for hours. A wheelchair cushion can distribute and shift the child's weight when sitting in the chair. Teach the child to change position frequently by doing wheelchair push-ups or by shifting the weight (leaning to the side or forward) for several minutes every 10 to 15 minutes. Make sure the child wears a safety belt when sitting in the wheelchair. Teach school personnel about the child's recommended protocol so they can provide opportunities in school to change positions and reinforce the routine.

BURNS

Burns are the third leading cause of injury deaths (after motor vehicle crashes and drowning) in children between 1 and 14 years of age (Forum on Child and Family Statistics, 2004). Boys between the ages of 1 and 4 years are twice as likely as girls to be burned. The national average age of pediatric burn patients is 32 months. In 1999, 99,500 children less than 15 years of age were treated in U.S. emergency departments for burns (Perry, 2003).

There are four main types of burns: thermal, chemical, electrical, and radioactive. Thermal burns, the most common in children, result from flames, scalds (such as coffee or grease), or contact with hot objects (such as a wood stove or curling iron). Chemical burns occur when children touch or ingest caustic agents. Electrical burns are caused

PATHOPHYSIOLOGY ILLUSTRATED
The Four Stages of Ulcer Formation

A, Stage 1, nonblanchable erythema of intact skin. *B,* Stage 2, blister or abrasion, partial-thickness loss with damage through epidermis, dermis, or both. **C,** Stage 3, full-thickness loss with exposure of subcutaneous tissue. *D,* Stage 4, full-thickness loss that extends to muscle, bone, or supporting tissues.

Courtesy of Sandra Quigley, Children's Hospital, Boston, MA.

by direct or alternating current in electrical wires, appliances, or high-voltage wires. Radiation burns result from exposure to radioactive substances or sunlight. About 10% of all burns in children are due to child abuse (Rodgers, 2000). See Chapter 36 for a description of child abuse. ∞

ETIOLOGY AND PATHOPHYSIOLOGY

Children at different developmental stages are at risk for different types of burns.

- Infants are most often injured by thermal burns (scalding liquids, house fires) (Figure 57–10 ◉).
- Toddlers are at risk for thermal burns (pulling hot liquids or grease onto themselves), electrical burns (biting electrical cords) (Figure 57–11 ◉), contact burns, and chemical burns (ingesting cleaning agents and other substances) associated with exploring the environment.
- Preschool-age children are most often injured by scalding or contact with hot appliances (curling irons, ovens).
- School-age children are at risk for thermal burns (playing with matches, fireworks), electrical burns (climbing high-voltage towers, climbing trees, and contact with electrical wires), and chemical burns (combustion experiments) associated with their curiosity and interest in experimentation.
- Adolescents also experience thermal, chemical, and electrical burns.

● **FIGURE 57-10**

Thermal (coald) burns are the most common burn injury in infancy.

Immediately after the burn, intense vasoconstriction occurs in response to substances released by the injured cells. Ischemia due to vasoconstriction may increase the depth of the burn injury. Then vasoactive hormones are released, which increases capillary permeability. This permits fluid and plasma to shift into the interstitial spaces, causing edema and decreased volume circulating in the blood vessels. Capillary integrity is not restored for 18 to 36 hours after the burn injury. The child loses increased water and heat through the injured epidermis. The child's metabolic

● **FIGURE 57-11**

Electrical burn caused by biting on electrical cord. The burn is caused when the current arcs through the lips, often causing a full-thickness injury through the mucosa, muscle, nerves, and blood vessels. The labial artery may be injured and cause significant bleeding once the eschar falls off after 2 to 3 weeks.

Courtesy Dr. Lezley McIveen, Department of Dentistry, Children's National Medical Center, Washington, DC.

rate and need for calories increase in the attempt to maintain body temperature.

CLINICAL MANIFESTATIONS

Burns are classified by depth. Burn depth may be defined as partial thickness or full thickness. Partial-thickness burns, in which the injured tissue can regenerate and heal, may be either first- or second-degree. Full-thickness burns, in which the injured tissue cannot regenerate, are also known as third-degree burns. The depth of the burn depends upon the temperature and duration of the heat application, and on the ability of tissues to dissipate the transferred energy. See "Pathophysiology Illustrated: Classification of Burns by Depth" for clinical manifestations by burn depth.

NURSING PRACTICE

A full-thickness burn can occur in adults after only 2 seconds' immersion in water with a temperature of 65°C (149°F). The amount of time for a burn to occur increases to 10 minutes when water temperature is 50°C (122°F). Because infants and children have more sensitive skin, they need less time to receive a serious burn (Stewart, 2000).

Signs of infection include purulent drainage, focal areas of necrosis, edema, erythema, discoloration of wound margins, and conversion from partial-thickness to full-thickness injury depth (Rodgers, 2000).

CLINICAL THERAPY

Assessment of Burn Severity

Burn severity is determined by the depth of the burn injury, percentage of body surface area (BSA) affected, and involvement of specific body parts. A Lund and Browder chart with BSA distributions for various body parts at different ages is used to calculate the area affected by the burn injury (Figure 57–12 ●). The palm of a child's hand (without fingers and thumb) is 1% of his or her body surface area and can be used to make a quick estimate of the burn size. Once the affected BSA is calculated, the burn can be classified as minor, moderate, or major (Table 57–6). Children with moderate and major burns require hospitalization, and those with major burns will usually be transferred to a burn center.

The involvement of specific body parts or specific burn distributions increase the burn severity, regardless of the percentage of BSA affected. Burns to the face, hands, feet, or perineal area are treated as major injuries because of the potential for cosmetic and functional impairment. **Circumferential** burns (injury completely surrounding the

PATHOPHYSIOLOGY ILLUSTRATED

Classification of Burns by Depth

Superficial Partial Thickness (first degree)

Damages only outer layer of skin; burn is painful and red; heals in a few days (e.g., sunburn)

Erythema, blanches on pressure, no bullae, peeling after a few days due to premature cell death

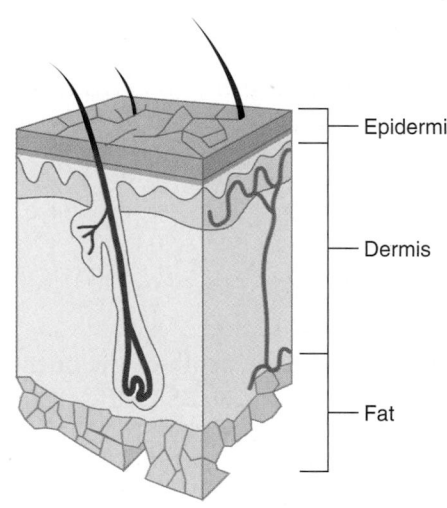

- Epidermis
- Dermis
- Fat

Partial Thickness (second degree)

Involves epidermis and upper layers of dermis; may have sparing of sweat glands and sebaceous glands; heals in 10–14 days

Blisters or bullae, erythema, blanches on pressure, pain and sensitivity to cold air, minimal scar formation

Full Thickness (third degree)

Involves all of epidermis and dermis; may also involve underlying tissue; nerve endings usually destroyed; requires skin grafting

Skin may appear brown, black, deep cherry red, white to gray, waxy or translucent; usually no pain, injured area may appear sunken

thorax or an extremity), anterior chest burns, and smoke inhalation are also classified as major burns.

Initial Treatment

The first step is to ensure that the child has an airway, is breathing, and has a pulse. Then stop the burning process by removing jewelry and clothing. Moist soaks or ice (if a small surface area is affected) is used to stop the burning process and to relieve pain. A tetanus vaccine booster is given if more than 5 years have passed since the last vaccine, or when the child has not completed the full vaccine series.

Treatment of Major Burns

The goals of treatment include decrease burn fluid losses, prevent infection, control pain, promote nutrition, and salvage all viable tissue. Fluid replacement is necessary to maintain the cardiovascular and renal systems and to prevent hypovolemic shock in cases of major burn injury. Fluid shifts from the vasculature to the interstitial spaces (third spacing) soon after the burn. Fluid replacement for the first 24 hours after the injury is based on a fluid volume formula calculated from the child's body weight, affected BSA, and normal maintenance needs. The

Parkland and Galveston formulas are two examples used for this calculation. Lactated Ringer's or normal saline solution is the preferred fluid. Hypotonic intravenous solutions such as D5W increase the risk of hyponatremia, cerebral edema, and seizures (Stewart, 2000). Half of the total volume calculated for the 24-hour period is infused over the first 8 hours, starting at the time of the burn rather than arrival time in the emergency department. The remainder is distributed evenly over the next 16 hours. Fluid volume is reduced after 24 to 48 hours once the capillary integrity is restored. Efforts are focused on maintaining the child's temperature because heat is lost rapidly through burned skin.

Fever is a normal, expected outcome of any significant burn injury, but it is not always a sign of infection. Treatment may include analgesics, ice packs, cooling blankets, or cool hydrotherapy sessions. Infection is a frequent complication, and can cause the burn depth to increase (Rodgers, 2000). Wounds are cultured to identify specific organisms for antibiotic therapy rather than routinely giving prophylactic antibiotic treatment (Sheridan, 2005).

Continuous enteral feedings are often begun within 6 hours of the burn injury to support the child's increased nutritional requirements, due to the increased metabolic rate needed to support healing and the body's stress response to injury (Herndon & Spies, 2001). Burned children often need nearly twice the basal metabolic caloric re-

quirements and nearly 2 g/kg body weight of protein (Smith, 2000).

Aggressive pain management with intravenous opioids is needed around the clock and for all procedures. The

TABLE 57–6 ✤ Classification of Burn Severity in Children

Minor

Can usually be treated as an outpatient	Partial thickness < 10% BSA
	Full thickness < 2% BSA

Moderate

Can be treated in burn unit or general hospital	Partial thickness 10%–20% BSA
	Full thickness 3%–10% BSA

Major

Should be treated in a specialized burn center	Partial thickness >20% BSA
	Full thickness ≥10% BSA
	All burns involving face, eyes, ears, hands, feet, and perineum that may result in cosmetic or functional impairment
	All burns complicated by inhalation injury, major trauma, and preexisting chronic conditions

Adapted with permission from Perry, C. M. (2003). Thermal injuries. In P. A. Moloney-Harmon & S. J. Czerwinski (Eds.), *Nursing care of the pediatric trauma patient* (p. 279). St. Louis: Saunders.

● FIGURE 57–12

Relative Percentages of Areas Affected by Growth

	Age in years					
Area	0	1	5	10	11	Adult
A = 1/2 of head	9 1/2	8 1/2	6 1/2	5 1/2	4 1/2	3 1/2
B = 1/2 of one thigh	2 3/4	3 1/4	4	4 1/2	4 1/2	4 3/4
C = 1/2 of one lower leg	2 1/2	2 1/2	2 3/4	3	3 1/4	3 1/2

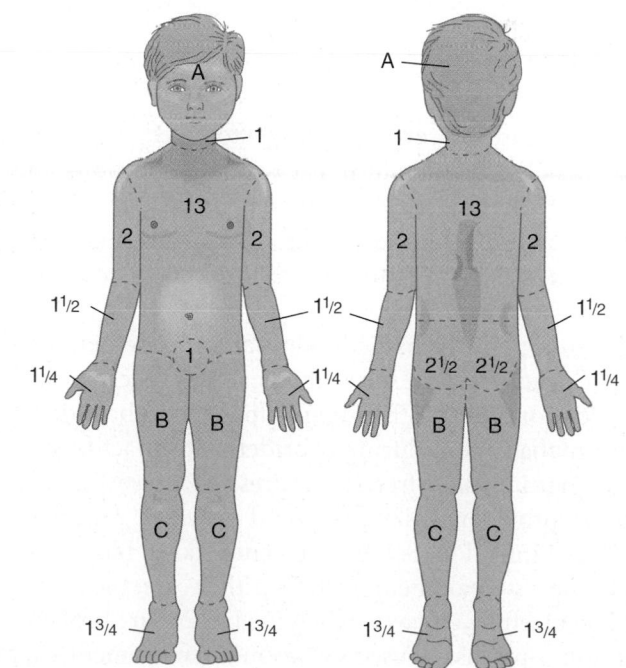

Lund and Browder chart for determining percentage of body surface areas in pediatric burn injuries.

Adapted with permission from Artz, C. P., & Moncrief, J. A. (1969). The treatment of burns (2nd ed.). Philadelphia: Saunders.

burns cause a significant emotional overlay that increases the perception of pain. See Chapter 42 for pain management information. ∞ Cimetidine or other H₂ blockers may be ordered to prevent a burn stress ulcer.

Special consideration is needed when burns involve certain areas of the body:

- Deep partial-thickness and full-thickness burns develop **eschar** (the tough leathery scab that forms over severely burned areas) with no elasticity. When the burn is circumferential, blood flow can become restricted due to edema and cause tissue hypoxia. Assess for an increase in cyanosis, deep tissue pain, and capillary refill time, and a decreased pulse distal to a circumferential burn. If you detect these signs, notify the physician immediately. An **escharotomy** (incision into the constricting tissue) may be necessary to restore peripheral circulation.

- Facial burns usually cause significant edema. Care must be taken to ensure airway patency. An ophthalmologist should be consulted for burns to the eye to assess damage and prescribe treatment. If the lips are burned, an infant may be unable to suck.

- Burns of the hands require careful management to maintain function. Special splinting and physical therapy are usually necessary.

- Perineal burns are at higher risk for infection because of frequent contamination with urine and stool. Frequent dressing changes are required. A urinary catheter is usually inserted but is removed once hydration status is stable to minimize the risk of urinary tract infection.

Wound Management

Burn wound care has several goals: (1) to speed wound debridement, (2) to maintain moist wound conditions and adequate circulation, (3) to conserve body heat and fluids, (4) to protect from infection, and (5) to control scarring and prevent scar contracture. Several treatment regimens are used to achieve these goals.

The entire body is bathed to initiate debridement (removal of dead tissue to speed the healing process). Conscious sedation and anesthesiology support may be ordered for pain management during debridement. Intact blisters provide a natural, pain-free, sterile dressing; however, some healthcare providers believe the fluid provides a medium for bacterial infection. Some burn centers keep blisters intact and others break them open. In either case, the tissues should be carefully cut away when the blisters are broken.

Various options are used for wound management after debridement. Traditional burn care for a partial-thickness injury involves the use of antibacterial agents, such as silver sulfadiazine (Silvadene), Sulfamylon, or bacitracin after ini-

THINKING CRITICALLY

THE CHILD WITH A PARTIAL-THICKNESS BURN

Sherray, 6 years old, was admitted to the hospital with a deep partial-thickness burn after dropping a bowl of soup on her leg. By her second day in the hospital, it is clear that Sherray's burn is not full thickness and that no skin grafting is needed. She will be discharged the next day.

Sherray's treatment includes a bath with wound debridement and dressing changes twice a day. Although pain medication is provided, the debridement and dressing changes cause a lot of anxiety and pain. Sherray needs a high-protein, high-calorie diet to promote wound healing. She has a hard time extending her leg and walking because movement stretches the burned skin, so she needs assistance to get out of bed and participate in child life activities.

Sherray's mother is rooming in, and remains at her side during the dressing changes. Her greatest concern right now is to help Sherray deal with the burn injury and to reduce the chance of infection. Over the next couple of days, Sherray's mother will take more responsibility for the dressing changes in anticipation of continuing her daughter's care at home.

- What signs of infection must you watch for?
- What is the procedure Sherray's mother will need to use to provide care to the wound at home?
- What are some suggestions for pain management during wound care that could be used at home?
- What suggestions can you make to help Sherray extend and use her leg, despite the pain movement causes?
- What are some foods that Sherray's mother can prepare at home to provide the high-protein and high-calorie diet needed for healing?

tial cleansing. Dressings are added to cover the burned area and changed once or twice daily. These dressing changes are often painful. When the old dressing is removed, a layer of eschar is also debrided. (See Skill 17–2.) **SKILLS**

Hydrotherapy (whirlpool) baths may be given twice daily to cleanse the wound before debridement, to increase vasodilation and circulation, and to speed healing. The water loosens exudate, topical medications, and dead tissue. As a rule, tap water is used for debridement. Gentle washing is necessary to protect new epithelial cells. Granulation tissue forms as a result of daily debridement. Superficial second-degree burns reepithelialize within 3 weeks.

Skin grafting is necessary with any deep second- or third-degree burn. Often a temporary skin substitute or **allograft** (cadaver skin from a skin bank) is used to cover a second-degree burn until healing occurs. An allograft also covers and improves the condition of a deep second- and third-degree burn until **autografting** (use of healthy skin taken from a nonburned area of the child's body) can be performed. The graft is placed after the wound is debrided

○ FIGURE 57–13

A

B

A, Trans-Cyte, a temporary skin substitute, prior to application. **B,** Application of Trans-Cyte after debridement of a scald burn.

Courtesy of Martin R. Eichelberger, M.D., Children's National Medical Center, Washington, D.C.

in the operating room to reveal healthy, bleeding tissue. This forms a protective barrier over the wound surface to decrease infection risk and to protect against fluid loss. An autograft is permanent. The donor site (where the autograft was harvested) is a new wound, causing pain and requiring close monitoring for signs of infection.

Trans-Cyte is a temporary skin substitute bioengineered from newborn foreskin tissue that is approved for use by the FDA. It forms a protective barrier over the wound surface to decrease infection risk and to protect against fluid loss. Research conducted in children indicates that it promotes healing more rapidly than Silvadene, decreases infection risk, avoids painful burn dressings, and reduces length of hospital stay (Figure 57–13 ○) (Lukish, Eichelberger, Newman et al., 2001; Wiebelhaus & Hansen, 2001). It is applied with a surgical adhesive or staples and covered with a bulky dressing or pressure dressing.

During the rehabilitation stage, Jobst or pressure garments are used to reduce development of hypertrophic scarring and contractures. Such garments are worn 24 hours a day for 6 to 8 months to shorten the time of scar maturation and to reduce the thickness of the scars (Perry, 2003). Cosmetic surgery may be needed to improve the child's appearance.

NURSING MANAGEMENT

NURSING ASSESSMENT AND DIAGNOSIS

Emergency assessment is based on the ABCs of basic life support (airway, breathing, and circulation). Assessment of the airway is necessary, especially when there are signs of smoke inhalation or burns to the face and neck. Other potential injuries are important to identify when the mechanism of injury also includes a fall or explosion. Identify signs of respiratory distress and any potential bleeding source. A weak, thready pulse, tachycardia, and pallor are important signs of early shock that may provide clues to an internal injury.

Obtain information about the type of burn (e.g., thermal, electrical, chemical) and a complete history. If a burn injury was preventable, parents may be emotionally stressed by feelings of guilt. Take care to avoid sounding accusatory when questioning parents about the injury. Be alert to signs of child abuse (e.g., glove and stocking burns, burns that spare flexor surfaces, contact burns from cigarettes or irons, and zebra burn lines from contact with a hot grate) (Figure 57–14 ○). Child neglect can be a factor in the burn of an inadequately supervised child. When taking a burn history, carefully document type of injury, time of injury, people present at the time of the injury, first aid administered, and history of other unusual injuries or emergency department visits.

Physical assessment should be thorough, including frequent monitoring of vital signs, pain control, and daily weight measurement. Monitor the child's circulatory and respiratory status to identify signs of hypovolemia in the first 24 hours or fluid overload as capillary integrity is restored. Perform a head-to-toe assessment at the beginning of every shift followed by system-specific assessments, depending on clinical findings and changes in the child's status. Be alert to signs of infection such as purulent drainage

MEDIALINK ○ Nursing in Action: Topical Medication: Burn Wound Care

● **FIGURE 57–14**

A

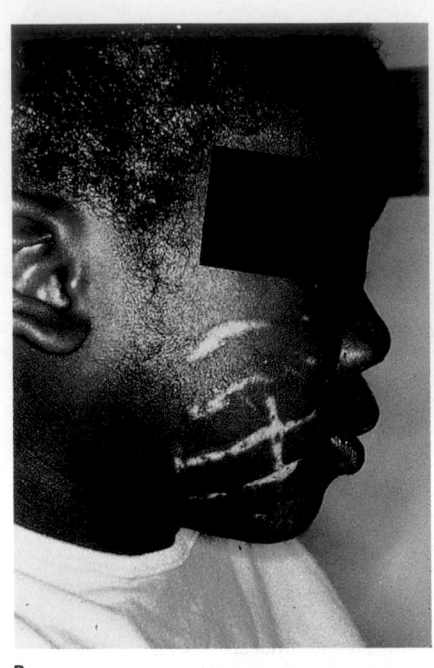

B

Burn injuries associated with child abuse. **A,** Burns of the hands or feet that are distributed like gloves or stockings. **B,** Zebra burns from a grate.

Used with permission from American Academy of Pediatrics, Elk Grove Village, IL, and the Kempe Children's Center, Denver, CO.

and edematous, red, or discolored wound margins. Intake and output must be monitored closely. A urinary catheter may be inserted to enable close monitoring of urine output (see Skill 16–1). **SKILLS**

Assess the child's concerns over appearance and the stress of hospitalization. Determine if the child has memories or nightmares about the burn and arrange psychologic support as needed.

Common nursing diagnoses for the child with a major burn injury are included in the accompanying "Nursing Care Plan." Additional nursing diagnoses for the child with a major burn might include the following:

■ *Impaired Physical Mobility* related to movement prescriptions (limb immobilization) and pain

■ *Disturbed Body Image* related to burn injury

■ *Anxiety* related to situational crisis and threat of death or disfigurement

PLANNING AND IMPLEMENTATION

Nursing care focuses on performing burn care, preventing complications, and providing emotional support. Care of the burned child involves various treatments designed to promote healing and prevent complications. These include

dressing changes, hydrotherapy, antibiotic therapy, analgesic support, physical therapy, play therapy, and possibly skin grafting.

Begin pain management as soon as possible. Soak charred clothing off with sterile saline and clip any hair within 2 inches of the burn to keep it out of the burn site. Cleanse the burn with mild soap and water and remove any foreign matter. If a chemical is the burning agent, remove the clothing and wash with lots of water. Elevate burned extremities. See "Nursing Care Plan: The Child with a Major Burn Injury."

Severe morbidity is likely with major burns. Significant scarring may occur regardless of autografting. Contractures and loss of function are also possible. Inadequate fluid replacement may lead to irreversible renal damage or cardiac damage, necessitating close follow-up unrelated to the actual burn injury. Children with major burns require comprehensive follow-up, sometimes involving repeated hospitalizations for surgery to release burn contractures, perform new grafting, or provide scar revision.

Prevent Complications

Severe complications of burns include infections, pneumonia, and renal failure, as well as possible irreversible loss of function of the burned area. The healthcare team's goal

NURSING CARE PLAN

THE CHILD WITH A MAJOR BURN INJURY

Intervention	Rationale	Expected Outcome
1. Nursing Diagnosis: Acute Pain related to physical injury agents		
NIC Priority Intervention: **Pain management:** Alleviation of pain or a reduction in pain to a level of comfort that is acceptable to the patient		**NOC Suggested Outcome:** **Comfort level:** Feelings of physical and psychologic ease
Goal: The child will verbalize adequate relief from pain and will be able to perform activities of daily living (ADLs).		
■ Assess the level of pain frequently using pain scales (see Chapter 42 ∞). ■ Cover burns as much as possible. ■ Change the child's position frequently. Perform range of motion exercises. ■ Encourage verbalization about pain. ■ Provide diversional activities. ■ Promote uninterrupted sleep with use of medications. ■ Use analgesics before all dressing changes and burn care.	■ Pain scale provides objective measurement. Pain is always present, but changes in location and intensity may indicate complications. ■ Temperature changes or movement of air causes pain. ■ Reduces joint stiffness and prevents contractures. ■ Provides outlet for emotions and helps the child cope. ■ Helps lessen focus on pain. ■ Sleep deprivation can increase pain perception. ■ Helps to reduce pain and decreases anxiety for subsequent dressing changes.	The child verbalizes adequate relief from pain and is able to perform ADLs.
2. Nursing Diagnosis: Risk for Infection related to trauma and destruction of skin barrier		
NIC Priority Intervention: **Infection protection:** Prevention and early detection of infection in a patient at risk		**NOC Suggested Outcome:** **Risk control:** Actions to eliminate or reduce actual, personal, and modifiable health threats
Goal: The child will be free of infection during healing process.		
■ Take vital signs frequently. ■ Use standard precautions (gown, gloves, mask) when wounds of a major burn are exposed. Limit visitors (no one with an upper respiratory infection or other contagious disease). ■ Clip hair around burns. ■ Keep biosynthetic burn dressing dry. ■ Do not place the IV in any burned area. ■ Administer oral or IV antibiotics for diagnosed infections as prescribed.	■ Increased temperature is an early sign of infection. ■ Reduces risk of wound contamination. ■ Hair harbors bacteria. ■ Helps reduce the number of bacteria introduced to the burned site. ■ Reduces risk of wound contamination. ■ Antibiotics administered as prescribed help to clear the infection quickly.	The child either stays free of secondary infection, or has infection diagnosed and treated early.
3. Nursing Diagnosis: Risk for Deficient Fluid Volume related to loss of fluids through wounds and to subsequent excess fluid intake		
NIC Priority Intervention: **Fluid management:** Promotion of fluid balance and prevention of complications resulting from abnormal or undesired fluid levels		**NOC Suggested Outcome:** **Fluid balance:** Balance of water in the intracellular and extracellular compartments of the body.

(continued)

NURSING CARE PLAN—continued

THE CHILD WITH A MAJOR BURN INJURY

Intervention	Rationale	Expected Outcome
Goal: The child will maintain adequate urine output.		
■ Monitor vital signs, central venous pressure, capillary refill time, pulses. ■ Administer IV and oral fluids as ordered. ■ Estimate insensible fluid losses. ■ Monitor intake and output. ■ Weigh child daily. ■ Insert urinary catheter. ■ Monitor for hyponatremia and hypercalcemia (see Chapter 43 ∞).	■ The child is initially at risk for hypovolemic shock and needs fluid resuscitation (see Chapter 48 ∞). ■ Careful calculation of fluid needs and ensuring proper intake helps keep the child properly hydrated. ■ Losses are increased during the first 72 hours after burn injury; may need replacement. Plasma is lost through burn site because of capillary damage. ■ The child is at risk for fluid overload during hydration, and for edema in the tissues at the burn site. ■ Significant weight loss or gain can help determine fluid imbalances. ■ Helps maintain accurate output measurement during critical care stage. ■ Sodium is lost with burn fluid and potassium is lost from damaged cells, causing electrolyte imbalances.	The child maintains normal urine output and burn site edema is not excessive.

4. Nursing Diagnosis: Ineffective Peripheral Tissue Perfusion related to mechanical reduction of venous and/or arterial blood flow (edema) of circumferential burns

NIC Priority Intervention:		NOC Suggested Outcome:
Circulatory care: Promotion of arterial and venous circulation		**Tissue perfusion (peripheral):** Extent to which blood flows through the small vessels of the extremities and maintains tissue function

Goal: The child will maintain adequate perfusion in burned extremities.		
■ Elevate extremities. Check distal pulse hourly. Notify the physician of decreased or absent pulses. ■ Check eschar.	■ Elevation helps to reduce dependent edema by promoting venous return. Dependent edema can constrict peripheral circulation. ■ Eschar can constrict peripheral circulation in edematous extremity.	The child has no episodes of poor perfusion in the burned extremity.

5. Nursing Diagnosis: Ineffective Breathing Pattern related to respiratory muscle fatigue due to smoke inhalation and airway edema

NIC Priority Intervention:		NOC Suggested Outcome:
Respiratory monitoring: Collection and analysis of patient data to ensure airway patency and adequate gas exchange		**Vital signs status:** Temperature, pulse, respiration, and blood pressure within expected range for the individual

Goal: The child will maintain or demonstrate improvement in breathing pattern.		
■ Closely monitor quality of respirations, breath sounds, mucus secretions, pulse oximetry. ■ Provide thorough pulmonary care. ■ Elevate head of bed. Keep intubation tube at bedside. ■ Administer corticosteroids, as prescribed.	■ Excess fluid replacement can cause pulmonary edema; toxins from burning products can cause airway inflammation. ■ Pulmonary care assists in removal of secretions to prevent infection. ■ Dyspnea, nasal flaring, and air hunger (respiratory distress) may develop. ■ Reduces airway edema.	The child has regular and unlabored breathing pattern.

NURSING CARE PLAN—continued

THE CHILD WITH A MAJOR BURN INJURY

Intervention	Rationale	Expected Outcome

6. Nursing Diagnosis: Impaired Physical Mobility related to joint stiffness due to burns

Intervention	Rationale	Expected Outcome
NIC Priority Intervention: **Exercise therapy, joint mobility:** Use of active or passive body movement to maintain or restore joint flexibility		**NOC Suggested Outcome:** **Joint movement (active):** Range of motion of joints with self-initiated movement

Goal: The child will maintain maximum range of motion.

Intervention	Rationale	Expected Outcome
■ Arrange physical and occupational therapy twice daily for stretching and range of motion exercises. Splint as ordered. Encourage independent ADLs.	■ Good positioning, range of motion exercises, and alignment prevent contractures.	The child maintains maximum range of motion without contractures.

7. Nursing Diagnosis: Imbalanced Nutrition: Less than Body Requirements related to high metabolic needs

Intervention	Rationale	Expected Outcome
NIC Priority Intervention: **Nutrition management:** Assistance with or provision of balanced dietary intake of foods and fluids		**NOC Suggested Outcome:** **Nutritional status:** Extent to which nutrients are available to meet metabolic needs

Goal: The child will maintain weight and demonstrate adequate serum albumin and hydration.

Intervention	Rationale	Expected Outcome
■ Provide an opportunity to choose meals. Offer a variety of foods. Provide snacks. ■ Encourage the child to have meals with other children. ■ Provide a multivitamin supplement. ■ Substitute milk and juices for water. ■ Provide nasogastric feedings as needed. ■ Weigh the child daily.	■ Encourages intake. General malaise and anorexia lead to poor healing. ■ Socialization improves intake. ■ Vitamin C aids zinc absorption; zinc aids in healing. ■ A child with a burn greater than 10% of BSA cannot usually meet nutrition requirements without assistance. ■ Provides objective evaluation.	The child maintains weight, adequate hydration, normal serum albumin.

8. Nursing Diagnosis: Anxiety (Child) related to threat to or change in health status

Intervention	Rationale	Expected Outcome
NIC Priority Intervention: **Anxiety reduction:** Minimizing apprehension, dread, foreboding, or uneasiness related to an unidentified source of anticipated danger		**NOC Suggested Outcome:** **Coping:** Actions to manage stressors that tax an individual's resources

Goal: The child will verbalize reduced anxiety.

Intervention	Rationale	Expected Outcome
■ Provide continuity of care providers. ■ Encourage parents to stay with the child; calls from home; pictures from classmates. ■ Group tasks and activities.	■ Helps to build a trusting relationship. ■ Familiar surroundings, people, and items encourage relaxation. ■ Reduces overstimulation and encourages rest.	The child expresses and shows signs of reduced anxiety.

9. Nursing Diagnosis: Anxiety (Parent) related to situational crisis

Intervention	Rationale	Expected Outcome
NIC Priority Intervention: **Coping enhancement:** Assisting a patient to adapt to perceived stressors, changes, or threats which interfere with meeting life demands and roles		**NOC Suggested Outcome:** **Anxiety control:** Ability to eliminate or reduce feelings of apprehension and tension from an unidentified source

(continued)

NURSING CARE PLAN—continued

THE CHILD WITH A MAJOR BURN INJURY

Intervention	Rationale	Expected Outcome
Goal: Parents will verbalize decreased anxiety.		
■ Provide educational materials about healing, grafting, dressing changes, and course of action. ■ Be flexible when teaching parents about wound care. ■ Refer to social services or parent support group.	■ Knowledge reduces anxiety. ■ Adults learn in many different ways. ■ Allows for venting of fears and guilt feelings, and provides exchange of ideas on dealing with hospitalization and long-term care.	Parents state decreased anxiety, and describe plans and solve problems related to care of the child at home.

is to prevent complications. Parents need to be involved in their child's care and to learn how to change dressings, assess for infection and dehydration, and perform range of motion exercises to aid in the child's recovery.

Wound Care

When a synthetic skin cover such as Trans-Cyte is used, protect the area from moisture and ointments, as these interfere with adherence. Since Trans-Cyte is transparent, the site can be monitored for signs of infection and wound healing, and regular dressing changes are not needed. Assess the skin covering for air bubbles or fluid, and aspirate or drain as ordered. If the covering is used over a joint, a splint will be used to prevent movement. When the burn heals, the synthetic skin covering loosens, permitting it to be trimmed.

Provide Emotional Support

Burned children have received a profound insult to their body and their self-image. Fear and anxiety about disfigurement and scarring are common, especially among adolescents. The shock and pain of the injury cause increased stress, as do the unfamiliar surroundings and presence of healthcare providers.

An attitude of genuine interest and concern by the nurse is essential. Orient the child to his or her surroundings frequently and give ample preparation for procedures, when possible. Continuity of care providers is important in developing a trusting relationship with the child and family. Encourage the child and parents to voice concerns, and show understanding and support.

Play therapy is encouraged for children, even if they can only observe initially. Play therapy serves several purposes for the child with a major burn:

■ It provides an outlet for frustration, independence, and creativity.

■ It promotes activities that challenge range of motion.

■ It normalizes the child's daily routine.

■ It encourages the child, who sees the progress other children make day by day.

Families are at risk for emotional stress. Forewarn them about the expected edema and the changes in the child's body. Parents often feel guilty and responsible for the child's injury. Help parents focus on recovery rather than past actions. Fear usually results from lack of knowledge about the severity of the burn and the child's status, especially in the early stages of burn care and admission to the hospital ICU. Include the family in the child's care whenever possible. The family needs information and frequent updates. This promotes trust between the family and the healthcare team.

Autografting procedures enable the child to recover from major burns, but the operation leaves visible scarring. Psychologic support is therefore essential to the child's recovery. Social workers, chaplains, art therapists, child life specialists, and play therapists are all trained to help the child and family deal with the stressors of recovery. Make appropriate referrals to ensure that the child and family receive necessary services.

Discharge Planning and Home Care Teaching

Identify and address home care needs well in advance of discharge. Thorough assessment is necessary to identify the family's needs related to the child's discharge home or to a rehabilitation facility. Discharge planning may include instructing parents in nutrition and diet needs, safety in the home, burn wound care, use of pressure garments, and range of motion exercises to prevent contractures.

Provide support and encouragement to parents as they learn how to care for the burned child. Many parents find it difficult to perform dressing change procedures they know will inflict pain to their child. Provide pain medication for dressing changes along with guidelines for how soon before the dressing change to give the medication. Specific guidelines for dressing changes should be outlined so that parents and healthcare team members have the same focus. Parents should first observe care being performed and then provide repeat demonstrations until competent.

Nursing Care in the Community

Care of the child with a burn requires long-term therapy and rehabilitation. Nurses in clinic and home care settings continue the care provided during hospitalization. Long-term care commonly occurs in the home, with frequent visits to healthcare professionals. In some cases, children regularly return to the hospital clinic for dressing changes. Children with extensive burns or with burns in locations where scarring may limit function must often wear a pressure (Jobst) garment, and sometimes a face mask if the face was burned. The pressure garment may present a threat to the child's body image, but it is an important way to decrease scarring. Scarring may also be managed through drug injections or surgery (i.e., revision, grafting, or Z-plasty). Help families understand the need for the special garments and masks and how to clean and care for them.

Continued physical therapy and occupational therapy are often needed to increase strength and dexterity in performing self-care skills and to prevent contractures. Emphasis is placed on returning to normal activities of daily living as soon as possible, such as returning to school. Some children have home tutors or computer connections to school for a time to ensure opportunities for learning while decreasing their risk of exposure to infection.

School reentry is often a traumatic experience, especially for older children and adolescents, because of the fear of rejection, decreased self-esteem, and impaired body image. The child's primary nurse, social worker, and child life specialist may visit the school of a child with a burn injury before the child returns to school—bringing photographs of the child, pressure garments, or other items—to inform classmates and allow them to explore their feelings about the child's burn injury. Several communities offer support groups for families and children with burn injuries. Referral to these groups may be beneficial.

A major role of nurses in the community is prevention. Provide burn prevention information to parents at each health promotion visit. Become involved with a Safe Kids coalition or local firefighters to help educate families and caregivers about ways to prevent scald burns and house fires.

Management of Minor Burns

Many children with minor burns are cared for at home after an initial visit to the emergency department or urgent care clinic. Discuss home remedies for minor burn care.

TEACHING HIGHLIGHTS

CARING FOR MINOR BURNS

- Place burn under cool, running water to stop the burning process and to help reduce pain.
- Do not use ice as it can cause more damage to the injured skin.
- Remove all clothing and jewelry from the burned area.
- Apply a topical antibiotic such as Neosporin to the burned area on the face.

For superficial burns covering a small area, use moist soaks to stop the burning process and to relieve pain. Any open blisters are debrided, and a thin layer of silver sulfadiazine is applied over the burn. Do not place this medication close to the eyes or mouth. Bacitracin is often used for burns on the face. The burn is then covered with one or two layers of gauze. Burn dressings should be changed twice daily. This involves cleaning the burn and reapplying antibiotic cream.

Tell parents to increase the child's fluid intake to compensate for loss of fluid through damaged skin. A high-calorie, high-protein diet is necessary to meet the increased nutritional requirements of healing. Acetaminophen (Tylenol) with codeine is often given, especially before dressing changes. Infection is a common complication. Educate the parents to observe for signs of infection (inflammation extending under the dressing, bad odor, excessive exudates, and fever), and notify the physician immediately if noticed. The child should be seen within 48 hours of treatment to monitor progress. Reinforce to parents the importance of follow-up appointments.

Moisturizing creams can be used after healing to relieve residual drying. The healed skin is very sensitive to sunburn, so cover the area or use a sunscreen. Sunscreen also helps prevent hyperpigmentation after burn healing.

DEVELOPING CULTURAL COMPETENCE

LITARGIRIO USE

When taking a history about methods used to treat minor burns in children, inquire about the use of "litargirio." This is a traditional remedy used for burn and wound healing and as a deodorant and foot fungicide in the Dominican Republic. The powder is sold in small packets at specialty stores that cater to Spanish-speaking populations. It contains up to 79% lead and can cause lead toxicity in children (FDA, 2005).

MEDIALINK Scald Burn Reduction in Children

SUNBURN

Sunburn is a burn injury to the outer layer of skin caused by excess sun exposure, or sun exposure after taking phototoxic drugs (acne medication, chlorpheniramine, diphenylhydramine, sulfonamides, tetracycline) (Laughlin-Richard, 2000). It occurs more often in children with red or blond hair and fair skin that freckles easily. These children have less **melanin** (skin pigment) to protect their skin against harmful ultraviolet rays. Repeated sunburns during childhood correlate strongly with the development of moles during childhood and adolescence, and with the development of skin cancer (basal cell carcinoma, squamous cell carcinoma, and melanoma) in adulthood. Melanoma is the most common cancer in individuals less than 30 years of age (Centers for Disease Control, 2002). Avoiding sunburn during childhood is believed to be more important than protecting skin during adulthood.

NURSING PRACTICE

An estimated 80% of a person's lifetime exposure to sunburns occurs before 21 years of age, while the epidermis is relatively thin (Centers for Disease Control, 2002). Melanin is also present in low levels during infancy and childhood (Laughlin-Richard, 2000). For these reasons, children should use a sunscreen with an SPF of 15 or higher during all outdoor activities. However, the use of sunscreen does not ensure that sunburn will be prevented, especially during lengthy sun exposure.

Erythema and skin tenderness usually develop between 30 minutes and 4 hours after exposure to sunlight. Increased vasodilation and vascular permeability result in the extravasation of fluid to the tissues and white blood cell migration to the damaged skin. The erythema peaks at 24 hours. Prolonged exposure can result in edema, vesiculation, bullae, or ulceration. Systemic complaints include malaise, insomnia (because of skin tenderness), fatigue, headaches, and chilling (because of rapid heat loss).

Treatment is generally supportive. Pain can be relieved by cool compresses followed by application of a low-potency topical corticosteroid (on unblistered skin). Children with severe sunburn may need nonsteroidal anti-inflammatory drugs (NSAIDs) for pain relief and to reduce inflammation. See Chapter 42 for information on NSAIDs. ∞

NURSING MANAGEMENT

Educate parents and children about preventing sunburn. Advise them that repeated sunburns may lead to permanent skin damage, skin cancer, cataracts, and premature aging of the skin. Recommend to parents that children use sunscreens, use a sun block such as zinc oxide, wear pro-

tective clothing, and limit the amount of time they spend in the sun. Children should also wear sunglasses with 99% ultraviolet blockage. See "Teaching Highlights: Preventing Sunburn."

HYPOTHERMIA

Hypothermia is a condition in which the core body temperature falls below 35°C (95°F). This occurs when the heat produced by the body is less than the heat lost. Hypothermia is a life-threatening emergency that can occur in any season and any geographic location. Infants and young children are at risk because of immature temperature regulatory mechanisms, thinner skin, limited subcutaneous fat, and high skin surface area to body mass ratio. Adolescents are at risk due to risk-taking behaviors such as drug and alcohol use and engaging in remote outdoor activities without proper equipment.

Hypothermia is associated with near-drowning episodes because body heat is lost quickly in water, as compared with air. As the core body temperature falls, the body

---

TEACHING HIGHLIGHTS

PREVENTING SUNBURN

- Keep children out of direct sunlight as much as possible, especially the midday sun. Avoid scheduling outdoor activities during the hours of maximum exposure (10 a.m. to 2 p.m.).
- When outdoors, minimize exposed areas by wearing hats and long-sleeves, closely woven cotton clothing and pants; wear T-shirts while swimming. Special sun protection clothing is now available from some manufacturers.
- Be aware that water, concrete, and sand reflect sunlight and increase exposure up to 90% by reflecting up to 85% of the ultraviolet rays.
- Use sunscreen with at least 15 SPF. For optimal protection, apply as thickly as directed to all exposed areas 30–45 minutes before sun exposure. Reapply every 2 hours as needed, or sooner if swimming, toweling off, or perspiring heavily.
- Use a waterproof sunscreen when swimming; this provides protection in water for approximately 60–80 minutes. Then reapply. Avoid placing waterproof sunscreen in the eyes as it causes severe pain and a chemical burn. Call the poison control center immediately for guidance.
- Avoid using sunscreens in infants less than 6 months of age because of the possibility of absorption of the chemicals through their skin.
- Remember that a child can be burned even on a cloudy day. Up to 80% of ultraviolet rays can penetrate the cloud cover.
- If the child is taking any medications, check with the healthcare practitioner before exposure (some medications cause hypersensitivity to sunlight).

EVIDENCE-BASED NURSING

EDUCATION TO PREVENT SUNBURN

Clinical Question (Problem)

Excessive exposure to ultraviolet (UV) radiation during childhood and adolescence is associated with the development of skin cancer during adulthood. Which prevention strategies successfully promote reduced sun exposure in children and adolescents to help reverse the dramatic increase in skin cancer attributed to UV radiation exposure?

Evidence

The parents of 77 children seen in a medical clinic in Florida were surveyed about attitudes and practices related to sun protection for their children. Less than 50% of parents reported regular use of sun protection for their children despite some knowledge of sun protection measures and consequences of sun exposure. Their children were outside 1 to 4 hours a day. Sunscreen was the most common sun protection measure used, but half of the parents felt it was okay to stay outside longer when sunscreen was used. This practice potentially increased the overall sun exposure for these children (Johnson, Davy, Boyett et al., 2001). When these same parents were asked about sun protection counseling received from the child's physician, those who received enthusiastic counseling perceived that sun protection was important for their children. Of the 21 parents who received enthusiastic sun protection counseling, more than 40% reported increased sun protection habits, and they were more likely to teach their child safe sun habits (Davy, Boyett, Weathers, et al., 2002). A national telephone survey of 651 parents of children ages 5 to 12 years was conducted to assess the parent's skin cancer knowledge, sun protection behavior, and perceived risk of skin cancer, as well as the child's sun protection behavior, and the parents' and child's vigilance in sunscreen use. Results indicated that children were more likely to get sunburns when parents also got sunburns. When both parents and children were vigilant in using sunscreen, children were less likely to get sunburns (O'Riordan, Geller, Brooks et al., 2003). A 1-to 2-hour sun exposure education program for children between 5 and 15 years was developed by the Environmental Protection Agency and evaluated in 85 schools across the country. When compared to children in schools that did not receive the education, study children were more likely to report a change in attitude about the healthier look with a suntan, and intentions to play in the shade more frequently. There were no changes in plans to wear sunscreen, sunglasses, or protective clothing (Geller, Rutsch, Kenausis et al., 2003).

Implications

Successful strategies to reduce exposure to UV radiation have not yet been identified. Information about sun protection behaviors indicates a need for education and behavior change by parents and children. Parents are also important role models for their children in sun protection behavior. Regularly wearing a hat and sunglasses, covering skin, and staying in the shade should also be encouraged. Since an effective education strategy has not been identified, an alternative strategy, such as policy changes to reduce sun exposure in childcare and school settings, may be more effective.

Critical Thinking

Develop guidelines that a childcare center could use for the reduction of UV radiation exposure by enrolled infants and children.

References

Johnson, K., Davy, L., Boyett, T., Weathers, L., & Roetzheim, R. G. (2001). Sun protection practices for children: Knowledge, attitudes, and parent behaviors. *Archives of Pediatric and Adolescent Medicine, 155*(8), 891–896; Davy, L., Boyett, T., Weathers, L., Campbell, R. J., & Roetzheim, R. B. (2002). Sun protection counseling by pediatricians. *Ambulatory Pediatrics, 2*(3), 207–211; O'Riordan, D. L., Geller, A. C., Brooks, D. R., Zhang, Z., & Miller, D. R. (2003). Sunburn reduction through parental role modeling and sunscreen vigilance. *Journal of Pediatrics, 142,* 67–72; and Geller, A., Rutsch, L., Kenausis, K., & Zhang, Z. (2003). Evaluation of the SunWise school program. *Journal of School Nursing, 19*(2), 93–99.

---

tries to conserve the core temperature at the expense of the extremities. Increased muscle tone and an increased metabolic rate occur. Shivering is the body's attempt to rewarm the blood before it returns to the core of the body. Other causes of hypothermia include exposure to a cold environment, ingestion of alcohol or barbiturates, trauma or a brain disorder that interferes with temperature regulation, and overwhelming sepsis.

Symptoms of mild hypothermia include slurred speech, poor coordination, poor judgment and inappropriate behavior, and shivering. Symptoms of moderate hypothermia include depressed respirations, slow pulse, low blood pressure, pale or cyanotic color, shivering, lethargy, hallucinations, and coma. Profound hypothermia (body temperature below 29°C [84°F]) may result in absence of respirations and pulse, ventricular fibrillation, dilated and unresponsive pupils, and coma.

Clinical therapy focuses on resuscitation, if necessary, and gradual core body rewarming. The child who has been immersed in cold water for a long time (up to 30 to 45 minutes) should receive CPR until the body temperature returns to normal because the hypothermia may have preserved vital organs. Warmed IV fluids are needed to expand blood volume and promote cardiac output. Assess body temperature with a rectal probe inserted about 15 cm. Aggressive rewarming is performed with warmed IV fluids, warmed oxygen, and warm packs to the trunk of the body.

For mild hypothermia (temperature above 35°C [95°F]), external heat lamps, immersion in warm water, and an electric blanket may be all that are necessary. More aggressive techniques are required for profound hypothermia. These may include humidified, warm oxygen; warmed intravenous fluids; hemodialysis; or application of warmth to core circulation areas (axilla, groin, and posterior neck).

NURSING MANAGEMENT

Monitor vital signs and urine output during rewarming. Prevention is geared toward educating parents to layer children's clothing in cold climates, recognize signs of hypothermia, decrease time of exposure to cold, and know how to treat mild hypothermia. Teach school-age children and adolescents who go on camping and hunting trips how to recognize and manage hypothermia in themselves and others. Teach preventive techniques such as avoiding riding snowmobiles or walking on ice that is not known to be deep enough to support the weight.

If a child becomes hypothermic during an outing such as a camping trip, a warm person should get into a sleeping bag (or under the blankets) next to the child. This action will warm the child and prevent further heat loss. First aid for hypothermia includes moving the child to a dry area and removing any wet clothing. Replace with warm, dry clothing, and encourage the child to drink a warm, high-calorie liquid, if able.

FROSTBITE

Frostbite is a cold injury that results from overexposure of the skin cells to temperatures low enough to cause crystal formation. Frostbite develops in tissues exposed to temperatures below freezing for more than an hour when environmental protection is inadequate. Areas of the body at high risk for frostbite include the hands, feet, cheeks, nose, and ears. Ice crystallizes in the tissues, resulting in dehydration of the cells and ischemic damage.

Clinical manifestations depend on the severity and depth of the cellular damage (von Heimburg, Noah, Sieckmann et al., 2001):

- Superficial skin affected—pallor and waxy skin with a spongy texture, decreased sensation.

- Full-thickness skin affected—erythema, vesicle formation with clear or pink fluid, numbness.

- Full-thickness and subcutaneous skin affected—local edema, grayish blue discoloration.

- Deeper cold injury—deep cyanosis, no vesicles or local edema, necrosis of subcutaneous tissue or lower, possibly involving the muscles or tendons.

The skin at first appears pale and is numb. Rapid rewarming causes a flush and the sensation of tingling, burning, or prickling in the affected area. The erythema and mild swelling develop into bullae. The extent of injury usually is not initially apparent.

NURSING MANAGEMENT

If frostbite is suspected, get the child to a warmer environment, loosen all constricting clothing, and remove any wet clothes. Because the frostbitten area is numb, extreme caution is needed to protect it from any trauma. Obtain healthcare as soon as possible. Rewarming is done slowly to decrease the chance of cellular damage. Immerse the affected part for 10 to 15 minutes in water warmed to between 38°C and 40°C (100.4°F and 104°F). Analgesics may be given to manage pain. Gently clean the affected skin with saline. Cover the exposed skin with sterile dressings. As the extent of the cold injury is gradually revealed, the ruptured vesicles and eschar are debrided. Whirlpool and physical therapy treatment are important to improve circulation and maintain function. Amputation may be needed when circulation is not restored.

As with hypothermia, the goal of management is prevention. Teach parents to layer children's clothing for warmth and to pack extra blankets and clothing if cold temperatures are expected during outdoor activities. Teach adolescents how to avoid frostbite during hunting and other cold weather expeditions. Wet clothing should be changed quickly. Early care is instrumental in minimizing permanent injury. Severe frostbite requires hospitalization, fluid management, dressing changes, and careful attention to diet. Provide emotional support to the child and family while they wait to learn the full extent of injury and disability.

BITES

ANIMAL BITES

Approximately 154,625 dog bites occurred among children under 14 years of age in 2001 and required treatment in the emergency department, with injury rates highest among children between 5 and 9 years of age (Centers for Disease Control, 2003b). Other animals that may bite include cats, birds, turtles, and wild animals such as bats, squirrels, and raccoons. Children, especially those less than 8 years old, are at higher risk for animal bites, and boys are bitten more than twice as often as girls (Bernardo, Gardner, O'Connor et al., 2000). Most dogs are known by the child. Bites are often associated with the child's inappropriate behavior, such as teasing, playing, or interfering with feeding.

Dog bites tend to be crushing, rather than clean, sharp lacerations. Cat bites tend to be puncture wounds. Assessment includes noting the location and number of puncture wounds, abrasions, lacerations, and crushing injuries; redness or swelling at entry sites; redness extending out from site (possible cellulitis); and any drainage related to the bite. The nurse should check for nerve, muscle, tendon, or vascular damage and carefully document findings. Head and neck bites require radiographic examination to rule out any associated injury, such as trauma to the airway or breathing structures or a depressed skull fracture.

To decrease infection, initial treatment involves wound irrigation, removal of devitalized tissue, and a clean dressing. Conscious sedation and pain management may be needed for some children. Small wounds may be closed with adhesive strips rather than suturing because of the potential for infection. Severe bites sometimes require surgical closure or reconstruction. Wounds over joints should be immobilized and elevated. Puncture wounds should not be irrigated or sutured. The major complication of bites is infection such as cellulitis. Cat bites can result in septic arthritis and osteomyelitis if a bone or joint is punctured. Antibiotics and early treatment can greatly decrease these complications.

Dog bites should be reported and the dog should be observed for 10 days for signs of rabies. Cat bites are also dangerous as fewer cats are immunized against rabies. Bites by wild animals in areas with endemic rabies require rabies prophylaxis. Human rabies immune globulin (HRIG) or human diploid cell rabies vaccine (HDCV) should be given to all children bitten by wild animals in which rabies cannot be excluded, as well as to children bitten by domestic animals (cats and dogs) suspected or proven to be rabid. See Chapter 45 for a description of rabies treatment. ∞

HUMAN BITES

Human bites are more common than most people realize. They usually occur in toddlers and young children. Because the mouth harbors many bacteria, infection is fairly common. The nurse should assess the risk for hepatitis B and HIV infection. Antibiotics may be prescribed to prevent systemic complications. Initial treatment includes irrigating with sterile saline and debridement. Parents should be instructed about how to care for the wound. Follow-up is important to watch for infection.

Nursing Management

If a child is bitten by an animal, take a complete and accurate history that includes the following information: extent of the injury, circumstances surrounding the attack, present location of the animal, and attempts to assess the animal's health.

Wound care is important. To decrease infection, high-pressure wound irrigation with large quantities of sterile saline or lactated Ringer's solution is performed rather than scrubbing. A 19-gauge needle on a 60-mL syringe may be used. Apply a clean dressing and elevate the affected body part to reduce bleeding. Check the child's immunization record to determine whether a tetanus booster is necessary. Teach parents how to care for the wound and signs of infection that indicate a need to return for care.

Educate parents about preventing animal and human bites and the importance of teaching children appropriate behavior around other children and animals. When these bites occur in a childcare or school setting, inform parents

TEACHING HIGHLIGHTS

PREVENTING ANIMAL BITES

General guidelines for pets in the home
- Never leave a young child alone with an animal.
- Do not buy or adopt a pet unless you are confident of your child's ability to respect it.
- Spay or neuter the pet to reduce aggression.

If an animal (wild or unknown) is sick or acting strangely, notify the health department.

Teach children the following rules
- Avoid all unfamiliar animals and report them to a parent.
- Avoid contact with all wild animals.
- Do not touch an animal when it is eating, sleeping, or nursing.
- Never overexcite an animal, even in play. Do not rough house or play games that stimulate aggressive behavior.
- Never tease or throw objects at an animal.
- Never put your face close to an animal. Seek permission before hugging or petting an animal.
- If approached by a dog, stay calm, stand still, talk softly, and back away slowly until the dog loses interest; do not run.
- If attacked, pretend to be a tree or a log and protect the face.

about the human bite so they can discuss potential risks and follow up with a healthcare provider.

As children with bites are often cared for at home, teach the parents about the normal healing process, proper wound care, and the signs and symptoms of infection.

INSECT BITES AND STINGS

Insect bites and stings occur frequently in children and usually are not a cause for concern. Exceptions include bites or stings by insects that carry parasites or communicable diseases (ticks, mosquitos), those of venomous insects (spiders), and those that produce an allergic reaction. About 4% of the population is sensitized to bee stings (White, Stewart, & Murdock, 2001). See "Clinical Manifestations: Insect Bites and Stings." (For a discussion of Lyme disease and Rocky Mountain spotted fever, see Chapter 45. ∞)

Nursing Management

The goal of nursing care is prevention. Become familiar with the harmful insects in your area, so you can identify them and recognize their effects. Children should be taught to avoid spiders and other biting or stinging insects. Many commercial repellents (OFF, Cutter's, Deep Woods OFF) are available. Most products contain DEET (diethyltoluamide) and are effective against many insects, including mosquitos, fleas, ticks, and chiggers. However, DEET does not repel stinging insects. Wash DEET off the skin with

MEDIALINK Dog Bite Reduction

CLINICAL MANIFESTATIONS

INSECT BITES AND STINGS

TYPE	CLINICAL MANIFESTATIONS	CLINICAL THERAPY
Mosquitoes and Fleas Local inflammation results from injected foreign protein or chemicals.	Local reactions: ■ Discrete, red papules and edema at the bite site with itching, burning, pain, and hives; minimal discomfort ■ Pruritic wheals and bullae tend to develop with repeat exposure Systemic reactions: ■ Wheezing, urticaria ■ Laryngeal edema ■ Shock	Local reactions ■ Cold compresses or ice applied to the site ■ Antihistamine medication Systemic reactions need emergency medical treatment
Bee or Wasp Sting Venoms contain enzymes that affect vascular tone and permeability.	Local reaction: ■ Mild, local pain ■ Erythema and edema Systemic reaction: ■ Generalized urticaria, flushing, angioedema, pruritis ■ Wheezing ■ Anaphylaxis is rare	Local reactions: ■ Remove stinger as soon as possible ■ Ice or cold compresses and elevate extremity ■ A dash of meat tenderizer (papain powder) and a drop of water massaged into the skin for 5 minutes relieves the pain ■ Antihistamine medication Systemic reactions are treated with glucocorticoids and antihistamines or epinephrine Desensitization for severe reactions
Fire Ants Venom is hemolytic and neurotoxic, causing a histaminelike response.	■ A black center at the point of the bite, or trial of lesions across skin ■ Initial wheal becomes a vesicle in a few hours; in 24 hours the fluid is cloudy, and the vesicle has a red halo ■ Pruritis, erythema, edema, induration Systemic and anaphylactic reactions can occur	Local reactions: ■ Ice or cold compresses ■ Antihistamine medication ■ Elevate extremity Systemic reactions—same as bees and wasps
Black Widow Spider Venom is neurotoxic.	■ Stinging sensation at time of bite ■ Localized edema and erythema, two fang marks, petechiae branching from site Systemic reaction in 1–3 hours, symptoms peak in 3–12 hours, diminish in 72 hours ■ Muscle rigidity of torso and abdomen, priapism, muscle cramps near the bite ■ Malaise, sweating, nausea, vomiting, dizziness, restlessness, insomnia ■ Hypertension and arrhythmias ■ Oliguria	Ice Diazepam and opioids Antihistamine medication Hydrocortisone may decrease the inflammatory response Antivenom IV is used in severe reactions after negative skin test for hypersensitivity to horse serum
Brown Recluse Spider Venom contains proteolytic enzymes and sphingomyelinase D, a cytotoxic factor.	■ Itching, pain, and erythema at bite site in first 6–12 hours; evolves to purple bull's eye lesion that signals beginning of necrosis; reddish blisters; a white ring is surrounded by an irregular erythematous ring (Zeglin, 2005) ■ Severe progressive reactions may occur in 12–72 hours, including fever, chills, restlessness, malaise, joint pain, and nausea and vomiting	Ice Cleanse the wound and good wound care Analgesics Oral anti-inflammatory agent Antibiotics for secondary infection Excision and skin grafting in cases of severe necrosis

soap and water once the child is back indoors. Caution parents to avoid overuse of products containing DEET, especially with infants and small children. Cases of toxic encephalopathy have been reported following repeated use on children's bedding and clothing (Metry & Hebert, 2000). It is believed that a combination of DEET with sunscreens may decrease the effectiveness of the sunscreen, so limit the sun exposure for these children.

Warn parents against using heavily perfumed shampoos, powders, soaps, or lotions, or dressing children in bright clothing when outdoors, as these may attract insects. Avoid eating sweet foods and beverages outdoors as these will attract bees and wasps. Pour beverages into a cup rather than drinking from a can to prevent stings to the mouth and lips.

Household pets may be a source of fleas or ticks. Encourage frequent inspection of pets and preventive treatments against fleas and ticks before pets are allowed prolonged contact with children.

When a known allergy to Hymenoptera has occurred, the child should wear a medical alert identification and carry an emergency kit with epinephrine. Teach parents and school personnel how to administer epinephrine. Desensitization injections may be given.

SNAKE BITES

Venomous snakes are found in most areas of the country. During warm months, snakes are active and likely to bite if disturbed. Fortunately, many bites are dry, delivering no venom. Fatalities are rare. Rattlesnake, copperhead, and cottonmouth venom is composed of enzymes that break down tissue, neurotoxins, cardiotoxins, and other components that cause hemolysis and vascular permeability (Cordasco, Jones, & Lindell, 2001). Coral snake venom causes neuromuscular paralysis.

Puncture marks, white wheal, and burning sensation appear at the site of the bite. Erythema, bruising, and edema rapidly develop and extend from the site for up to 24 hours. Systemic signs include dizziness, tachycardia, nausea, vomiting, diarrhea, sweating, and chills. Children may receive a higher concentration of venom for body mass than adults and have a more severe response to the bite. Such a severe response may include hypotension, altered consciousness, and bleeding from multiple sites (disseminated intravascular coagulation), pulmonary edema, and renal failure.

Clinical therapy involves immobilization of the extremity and a cold compress to slow the spread of the venom. Tourniquets and excision of the bite are no longer recommended. Laboratory studies include complete blood count, platelet count, coagulation studies, electrolytes, and renal function. Attempts to identify the

snake causing the bite should be made to determine if it is poisonous. The poison control center is contacted to obtain treatment guidelines. Specific antivenom is usually administered within 4 to 6 hours. CroFab®, a newer antivenom used for cottonmouth, copperhead, and rattlesnake bites, is available, but limited data on use in children exist (Schmidt, 2005). Because antivenom contains a hyperimmune horse serum product, anaphylaxis or delayed serum sickness may develop. A skin test may be performed first to detect hypersensitivity. Antihistamines are often given in anticipation of a hypersensitivity reaction. A tetanus booster is given if vaccination status is unknown or the tetanus series is incomplete.

Nursing Management

Nursing care involves assessing the child for initial and progressive signs of the venom's effect. First aid involves immobilizing the extremity, keeping it in a dependent position to slow the spread of venom, and cold compresses. Rings or constricting items should be quickly removed from the injured extremity. Clean the wound with germicidal soap and water. Keep the child quiet and calm to slow the circulation. Help the child identify the snake from pictures of snakes common to the area; however, keep in mind that other venomous snakes may be kept as exotic pets.

The antivenom is diluted in saline and slowly administered intravenously as ordered. Help locate additional antivenom if the hospital does not have an adequate supply. Monitor the child for progressive signs of venom effect, and for hypersensitivity responses to antivenom. Provide skin care for the swollen and tense skin to prevent abrasions and to prevent additional injury. Monitor the site for necrosis and secondary infection. Provide emotional support to the child and family. Teach children and their families to avoid future snakebites.

CONTUSIONS

Contusions are soft-tissue injuries that have a variety of causes. Often it is difficult to assess whether an injury has caused underlying tissue damage. An injury does not have to break the skin to result in internal damage. Radiographic examination may be necessary to rule out broken bones or further tissue damage. Signs and symptoms that indicate a need for treatment include swelling that does not subside within 72 hours, intense pain, inability to move the injured part, and infection.

Elevate the injured extremity and apply ice as soon as possible after injury. This can reduce inflammation and swelling in the area.

FOREIGN BODIES

Many skin injuries result from penetration of foreign particles. Common substances include gravel from abrasions, bee stingers, and splinters. Treatment of superficial foreign bodies involves irrigating the wound to try to forcibly dislodge the debris. A deeply embedded foreign body is best removed under medical supervision to avoid permanent injury or scarring.

LACERATIONS

Lacerations are caused by cuts or tears to the skin. In many cases the cut is minor and can be managed at home with gentle cleansing, antibiotic ointment, and a bandage. More extensive lacerations and those on the face or over joints often need suturing to promote healing and reduce scarring. Laceration repair is performed after wound cleansing and appropriate local analgesia to control pain. Sutures are usually removed about 7 days later.

Critical Concept Review

LEARNING OBJECTIVES	CONCEPTS
Identify the characteristics of different skin lesions by their cause, including those caused by irritants, drug reactions, mites, infection, and injury.	1. Irritant skin lesions: ■ Papulovesicular lesions. ■ Very pruritic. ■ Erythematous. ■ Well circumscribed. 2. Drug reactions: ■ Erythematous macules and papules. ■ Pruritic. ■ Urticaria. 3. Mites: ■ Intense pruritus. ■ Papular, pustular, and vesicular lesions. 4. Infection: ■ Edema. ■ Erythema. ■ Papular and vesicular lesions. 5. Injuries: ■ Pressure ulcers and burns: loss of tissue in stages beginning with epidermis and progressing through the muscular layer. ■ Animal bites: usually cause puncture wounds.
Describe the stages of wound healing.	1. Inflammation (3–5 days): ■ Preparation of the injury site for repair. ■ Coagulation occurs. ■ Vasodilation allows white blood cells to reach the injured tissue. 2. Reconstruction/epithelialization (4 days to 2 weeks): ■ Blood flow is reestablished. ■ Wound edges grow toward each other. ■ Collagen and granulation tissue are produced. 3. Maturation (months–2 years): ■ Continued collagen production for scar formation.
Identify the skin conditions that have a hereditary cause or hereditary predisposition.	1. Dermatitis: ■ Eczema (atopic dermatitis). ■ Contact dermatitis. 2. Epidermolysis bullosa.

LEARNING OBJECTIVES

CONCEPTS

Describe a nursing care plan for a child with alterations in skin integrity, including dermatitis, infectious disorders, and infestations.

1. Obtain a complete family history of allergies and skin lesions.
2. Eliminate possible allergens from the child's environment.
3. Cleanse skin as ordered.
4. Apply appropriate topical medications.
5. Treat infestation sites of body with appropriate medication.
6. Provide medications to decrease itching.
7. Provide cool soaks to skin.
8. Treat all clothing, linens, and toys that have been in contact with the child with infestation.
9. Keep child's fingernails short to prevent damage from scratching.

Develop an education plan for adolescents with acne to promote self-care.

1. Inform parents and adolescents that acne does not have a dietary cause.
2. Inform adolescents that excessive perspiration and emotional stress may increase the number of acne lesions.
3. Instruct the adolescent in a recommended skin cleansing routine.
4. Teach the adolescent and parents concerning medication administration (both oral and topical) including side effects.
5. Caution the adolescent that some acne medications increase the skin's sensitivity to the sun.
6. Emphasize the importance of returning to the healthcare provider for scheduled follow-up appointments.

Describe the process to measure the extent of burns and burn severity in children.

1. Assessment of burn severity includes:
   - Depth of the burn injury.
   - Percentage of body surface area affected.
   - Involvement of specific body parts.
2. Burns to the hands, feet, face, or perineal area are treated as major injuries because of the potential for functional and cosmetic appearance.

Develop a nursing care plan for the child with a full-thickness burn injury.

1. Maintain adequate fluid volume:
   - Monitor vital signs.
   - Administer volume-expanding IV fluids as ordered
   - Monitor intake and output.
2. Observe for any respiratory difficulties.
3. Maintain sterile technique when changing dressing.
4. Provide adequate pain relief.
5. Promote functional use of joints and extremities.
6. Provide optimum nutrition for healing.
7. Assist child in the use of guided imagery and distraction during dressing changes.

Identify preventive strategies to reduce the risk of injury from bites and stings.

1. Parents should apply appropriate commercial insect repellent to exposed skin and clothes of children.
2. Parents should inspect child's skin for ticks after playing outside.
3. Children should wear long pants and sleeves, and pants should be tucked into boots to avoid tick bites.
4. Instruct children to stay calm when near stinging insects.
5. Wear light-colored clothes and avoid eating sweetened foods and beverages when outside.
6. Inspect and treat pets for fleas and ticks.

CRITICAL THINKING IN ACTION

*View the **Critical Thinking in Action** video in Chapter 57 of the CD-ROM. Then, answer the questions that follow.*

Twelve-year old Rebecca is admitted to the burn unit after being scalded by spilling boiling spaghetti water on her chest, abdomen, and legs when attempting to carry the pot to the sink. The burn is classified as moderate with a mixture of partial thickness and full thickness covering a BSA of 12%. IV fluids are started in the emergency department and a continuous infusion of morphine is given for pain. Her temperature is 101°F. The initial debridement of the burns is performed in the operating room so that Rebecca is anesthetized and does not feel pain from the procedure. Following debridement, Rebecca is put on a high calorie, high protein diet to help meet her increased nutritional requirements. Her parents are encouraged to bring in foods that they can encourage Rebecca to eat. Wound care is performed twice a day so the burn sites can be inspected for signs of infection and for development of eschar. Pain medication for wound care is provided through the IV. After the burn sites are cleaned, antibiotic cream and a dressing is applied. Rebecca's nutritional intake and urine output are carefully monitored while she is hospitalized. Physical therapy is initiated to maintain range of motion and to prevent contractures. The nurse talks with Rebecca and her family about what to expect as the burns heal. Education of the family includes signs and symptoms of infection and the expected need for skin grafts over the full-thickness burn sites. After a few days in the hospital, Rebecca is discharged with daily follow-up in the burn clinic for wound care.

1. What is the most likely type of IV fluids started on Rebecca in the hospital and why?
2. What is the reason it is important to monitor Rebecca's urine output?
3. What is the reason Rebecca needed her extremities elevated and distal pulses checked frequently?
4. What are the goals of burn wound care for Rebecca?
5. Why is it important to monitor burns that have eschar?

MEDIALINK

www.prenhall.com/london

- NCLEX-RN® Review, case studies, and other interactive resources for this chapter can be found on the Companion Website at http://www.prenhall.com/london. Click on "Chapter 57" and select the activities for this chapter.

Damaged and Bleeding Dermal Blood Vessels

◄ ▬ ↻ ❚❚ ►

- For animations, more NCLEX-RN® Review questions, and an audio glossary, access the accompanying CD-ROM in this textbook.

REFERENCES

Allen, P. L. J. (2004). Leaves of three, let them be: If it were only that easy! *Pediatric Nursing, 30*(2), 129–135.

American Academy of Pediatrics Committee on Infectious Disease. (2003). *Red book, report of the Committee on Infectious Disease* (26th ed). Elk Grove Village, IL: Author.

Angel, T. A., Nigro, J., & Levy, M. L. (2000). Infestations in the pediatric patient. *Pediatric Clinics of North America, 47*(4), 921–935.

Atherton, D. J. (2004). A review of the pathophysiology, prevention and treatment of irritant diaper dermatitis. *Current Medical Research and Opinion, 20*(5), 645–649.

Bernardo, L. M., Gardner, M. J., O'Connor, J., & Amon, N. (2000). Dog bites in children treated in a pediatric emergency department. *Journal of Society of Pediatric Nurses, 5*(2), 87–95.

Brodell, R.T., & Vescera, G. (2002). Black-dot tinea capitis. *Postgraduate Medicine, 111*(4), 123–126.

Buck, M. L. (2001). Isotretinoin: Improving patient education and reducing risk. *Pediatric Pharmacology, 7*(7), 1–6.

Centers for Disease Control and Prevention. (2002). Guidelines for school programs to prevent cancer. *Morbidity and Mortality Weekly Report, 51* (RR-4), 1–18.

Centers for Disease Control and Prevention. (2003a). Methicillin-resistant *Staphylococcus aureus* infections among competitive sports participants—Colorado, Indiana, Pennsylvania, and Los Angeles County, 2000–2003. *Morbidity and Mortality Weekly Report, 52*(33), 793–795.

Centers for Disease Control and Prevention. (2003b). Nonfatal dog bites—Related injuries treated in hospital emergency departments—United States, 2001. *Morbidity and Mortality Weekly Report, 52*(26), 605–610.

Cheigh, N. H. (2003). Managing a common disorder in children: Atopic dermatitis. *Journal of Pediatric Health Care, 17*(2), 84–88.

Cohen, B. A. (2002). Plaques: Oval, itchy, and red: What's your diagnosis? *Contemporary Pediatrics, 19*(4), 36–41.

Cohen, B. A. (2004). Another baby and another cutaneous lesion—and more on efficient recognition and management. *Contemporary Pediatrics, 21*(10), 39–57.

Cordasco, R., Jones, W., & Lindell, W. (2001). Treatment of the pediatric snakebite victim. *Air Medical Journal, 20*(2), 32–34.

Davy, L., Boyett, T., Weathers, L., Campbell, R. J., & Roetzheim, R. B. (2002). Sun protection counseling by pediatricians. *Ambulatory Pediatrics, 2*(3), 207–211.

Dinehart, S., Kincannon, J., & Geronemus, R. (2001). Hemangiomas: Evaluation and treatment. *Dermatologic Surgery, 27*(5), 475–485.

Dohil, M. A., & Eichenfield, L. F. (2005). A treatment approach for atopic dermatitis. *Pediatric Annals, 34*(3), 201–210.

Drake, L., & Prendergast, M. (2001). The impact of tacrolimus ointment on health-related quality of life of adult and pediatric patients with atopic dermatitis. *Journal of American Academy of Dermatology, 44*, S65–S72.

Drolet, B. A., Esterly, N. B., & Frieden, I. J. (1999). Hemangiomas in children. *New England Journal of Medicine, 341*(3), 173–181.

Elewski, B. E., & Krowchuk, D. P. (2001, September). Update on tinea capitis: Reaching consensus. *Contemporary Pediatrics, 18*, S11–S14.

Food and Drug Administration. (2005). *FDA public health advisory: Elidel (pimecrolimus) and Protopic (tacrolimus) ointment.* Retrieved April 3, 2005, from http://www.fda.gov/cder/drug/advisory/elidel_protopic.htm

Forum on Child and Family Statistics. (2004). America's Children 2004. Retrieved February 9, 2005, from http://childstats.gov/ac2004/tables/health7b.asp.

Friedlander, S. F. (1998). Contact dermatitis. *Pediatrics in Review, 19*(5), 166–170.

Gardner, P., Coles, D., & Kemper, K. J. (2001). The skinny on herbal remedies for dermatologic disorders. *Contemporary Pediatrics, 18*(7), 103–114.

Geller, A., Rutsch, L., Kenausis, K., & Zhang, Z. (2003). Evaluation of the SunWise school program. *Journal of School Nursing, 19*(2), 93–99.

Herndon, D. N., & Spies, M. (2001). Modern burn care. *Seminars in Pediatric Surgery, 10*(1), 28–31.

Jick, S. S., Kremers, H. M., & Vasilakis-Scarmozza, C. (2000). Isotretinoin use and risk of depression, psychotic symptoms, suicide, and attempted suicide. *Archives of Dermatology, 136*(10), 1231–1236.

Johnson, K., Davy, L., Boyett, T., Weathers, L., & Roetzheim, R. G. (2001). Sun protection practices for children: Knowledge, attitudes, and parent behaviors. *Archives of Pediatric and Adolescent Medicine, 155*(8), 891–896.

Kazaks, E. L., & Lane, A. T. (2000). Diaper dermatitis. *Pediatric Clinics of North America, 47*(4), 909–919.

Latchman, Y. E., Xu, X. J., Poulter, L. W., Ruston, M. H. A., & Brostoff, J. (2002). Chinese medical herbs in the treatment of atopic dermatitis. *ACI International, 14*(1), 4–9.

Laughlin-Richard, N. (2000). Sun exposure and skin cancer prevention in children and adolescents. *Journal of School Nursing, 16*(2), 20–26.

Lukish, J. R., Eichelberger, M. R., Newman, K. D., Pao, M., Nobuhara, K., Keating, M., et al. (2001). The use of a bioactive skin substitute decreases length of stay for pediatric burn patients. *Journal of Pediatric Surgery, 36*(8), 1118–1121.

Mancini, A. J. (2000). Acne vulgaris: A treatment update. *Contemporary Pediatrics, 17*(12), 122–133.

Metry, D. W., & Hebert, A. A. (2000). Insect and arachnid stings, bites, infestations, and repellents. *Pediatric Annals, 29*(1), 39–48.

Monroe, J. R. (2005). All that is round is not fungal. *Clinician Reviews, 15*(2), 46–53.

Nicol, N. H. (2000). Managing atopic dermatitis in children and adults. *Nurse Practitioner, 25*(4), 54–76.

O'Riordan, D. L., Geller, A. C., Brooks, D. R., Zhang, Z., & Miller, D.R. (2003). Sunburn reduction through parental role modeling and sunscreen vigilance. *Journal of Pediatrics, 142,* 67–72.

Paller, A. S. (2001). Use of nonsteroidal topical immunomodulators for the treatment of atopic dermatitis in the pediatric population. *Journal of Pediatrics, 138*(2), 163–168.

Perry, C. M. (2003). Thermal injuries. In P. A. Maloney-Harmon & S. J. Czerwinski (Eds.), *Nursing care of the pediatric trauma patient* (pp. 277–294). St. Louis, MO: Saunders.

Raimer, S. S. (2000). Managing pediatric atopic dermatitis. *Clinical Pediatrics, 39*(1), 1–14.

Rodgers, G. L. (2000). Reducing the toll of childhood burns. *Contemporary Pediatrics, 17*(4), 152–173.

Rote, N. S. (2002). Inflammation. In K. L. McCance & S. E. Huether (Eds.), *Pathophysiology: The biologic basis for disease in adults and children* (4th ed., pp. 197–226). St. Louis, MO: Mosby.

Rudy, S. J. (2003). Overview of the evaluation and management of acne vulgaris. *Pediatric Nursing, 29*(4), 287–293.

Schachner, L., Field, T., Hernandez-Ruif, M., Duarte, A. M., & Krasnegor, J. (1998). Atopic dermatitis symptoms decreased in children following massage therapy. *Pediatric Dermatology, 15*(5), 390–395.

Schmidt, C. E. (2003). A 12-month-old girl with maculopapular lesions and lower extremity edema. *Journal of Emergency Nursing, 29*(3), 204–207.

Schmidt, J. M. (2005). Antivenom therapy for snakebites in children: Is there evidence? *Current Opinion in Pediatrics, 17,* 234–238.

Sheridan, R. L. (2005). Sepsis in pediatric burn patients. *Pediatric Critical Care Medicine, 6*(3, Suppl.), S112–S119.

Shwayder, T. (2003). Five common skin problems—and a string of pearls for managing them. *Contemporary Pediatrics, 20*(7), 34–54.

Sidbury, R., & Paller, A. S. (2000). The diagnosis and management of acne. *Pediatric Annals, 29*(1), 17–24.

Smith, M. L. (2000). Pediatric burns: Management of thermal, electrical, and chemical burns and burn-like dermatologic conditions. *Pediatric Annals, 29*(6), 367–378.

Smolinski, K. N., & Yan, A. C. (2005). How and when to treat molluscum contagiosum and warts in children. *Pediatric Annals, 34*(3), 211–221.

Stewart, C. (2000). Emergency care of pediatric burns. *Pediatric Emergency Medicine Reports, 5*(10), 101–112.

Takano-Lee, M., Edman, J. D., Mullens, B. A., & Clark, J. M. (2004). Home remedies to control head lice: Assessment of home remedies to control the human head louse, *Pediculus humanus capitis* (Anoplura: Pediculidae). *Journal of Pediatric Nursing, 19*(6), 393–398.

Valencia, I. C., Falabella, A. F., & Schachner, L. A. (2001). New developments in wound care for infants and children. *Pediatric Annals, 30*(4), 211–218.

Vanderhooft, S. L. (1998). Is the rash really a drug reaction? *Contemporary Pediatrics, 15*(5), 118–137.

Von Heimburg, D., Noah, E. M., Sieckmann, U. P. F., & Pallua, N. (2001). Hyperbaric oxygen treatment in deep frostbite of both hands in a boy. *Burns, 27,* 404–408.

Weston, W. L., & Bruckner, A. (2000). Allergic contact dermatitis. *Pediatric Clinics of North America, 47*(4), 897–907.

Whalley, D., Huels, J., McKenna, S. P., & van Assche, D. (2002). The benefit of pimecrolumus on parents' quality of life in the treatment of pediatric atopic dermatitis. *Pediatrics, 110*(6), 1133–1136.

White, G. L., Stewart, J. S., & Murdock, R. T. (2001). Hymenoptera stings: Treatment and prevention. *Physician Assistant, 25*(2), 15–23.

Wiebelhaus, P., & Hansen, S. L. (2001). Another choice for burn victims. *RN, 64*(9), 34–37.

Williams, J. V., Godfrey, J. C., & Friedlander, S. F. (2003). Superficial fungal infections: Confronting the fungus among us. *Contemporary Pediatrics, 20*(1), 58–80.

Woodard, I. (2002). Adolescent acne: A stepwise approach to management. *Topics in Advanced Practice Nursing eJournal, 2*(2). Retrieved September 24, 2003, from http://www.medscape.com/viewarticle/430534

Zeglin, D. (2005). Brown recluse spider bites. *American Journal of Nursing, 105*(2), 64–68.

Appendices

Appendix A

Selected Maternal-Newborn Laboratory Values

✤ Normal Maternal Laboratory Values

Test	Nonpregnant Values	Pregnant Values
Hematocrit	37%–47%	32%–42%
Hemoglobin	12–16 g/dL**	10–14 g/dL**
Platelets	150,000–350,000/mm³	Significant increase 3–5 days after birth (predisposes to thrombosis)
Partial thromboplastin time (PTT)	12–14 seconds	Slight decrease in pregnancy and again in labor (placental site clotting)
Fibrinogen	250 mg/dL	400 mg/dL
Serum glucose		
Fasting	70–80 mg/dL	65 mg/dL
2-hour postprandial	60–110 mg/dL	Less than 140 mg/dL
Total protein	6.7–8.3 g/dL	5.5–7.5 g/dL
White blood cell total	4500–10,000/mm³	5000–15,000/mm³
Polymorphonuclear cells	54%–62%	60%–85%
Lymphocytes	38%–46%	15%–40%

**At sea level

✤ Normal Term Neonatal Cord Blood Laboratory Values

Test	Normal Values
Hematocrit	43%–63%*
Hemoglobin	14–20 g/dL
Platelets	150,000–350,000/mm³
Reticulocyte	3%–7%
White blood cell total	10,000–30,000/mm³
White blood cell differential	
Polymorphonuclear (segs)	40%–80%
Lymphocytes	20%–40%
Monocytes	3%–10%
Serum glucose	45–96 mg/dL*
Serum electrolytes	
Sodium	126–166 mEq/L*
Potassium	5.6–12.0 mEq/L*
Chloride	98–110 mEq/L*
Carbon dioxide	13–29 mmol/L
Bicarbonate	18–23 mEq/L
Calcium	8.2–11.1 mg/dL
Total protein	4.8–7.3 g/dL

Note: Adapted from Fanaroff, A. A., & Martin, R. J. (Eds.). (2002). *Neonatal-perinatal medicine* (7th ed.). St. Louis, MO: Mosby.

*All laboratory values are approximate. Consult your local laboratory for guidelines as to normal values.

Appendix B
Selected Pediatric Laboratory Values

All laboratory value ranges listed are approximate. Consult your local laboratory for guidelines as to normal values for the specific testing procedures used.

NORMAL VALUE RANGES: BLOOD
Albumin (S)[1]

1 month–1 year: 2.8–4.8 g/dL
1–18 years: 3.2–4.7 g/dL

Alkaline Phosphatase (S)[1]

Age	Male Units/L	Female Units/L
1-30 days	75-316	48-406
1-3 years	104-345	108-317
4-6 years	93-309	96-297
7-9 years	86-315	69-325
10-12 years	42-362	51-332
13-15 years	74-390	50-162
16-18 years	52-171	47-119

Blood Chemistry
Chloride (S, P)[1]

< 1 year: 96–111 mmol/L
1–17 years: 102–112 mmol/L

Glucose (S, P)[1]

54–117 mg/dL (3–6.49 mmol/L)

Magnesium (P, S)[1]

1.6–2.5 mg/dL (0.7–1 mmol/L)

Osmolality (S)[1]

280–300 mOsm/kg

Potassium (S, P)[1]

3.3–4.7 mmol/L

Sodium (P, S)[1]

132–141 mmol/L

Urea Nitrogen (S, P)[1]

1–13 years: 4–17 mg/dL (1.1–4.6 mmol/L)
14–19 years: 7–21 mg/dL (1.9–5.7 mmol/L)

KEY for type of specimen: S = serum; B = whole blood; P = plasma.

Blood Gases
Carbon Dioxide, Partial Pressure (Pco_2) (B)[1]

Infant: 27–41 mmHg (3.6–5.5 kPa)
Children: 32–48 mmHg (4.3–6.4 kPa)

Oxygen, Partial Pressure (Po_2) (B)[1]

> 1 day: 83–108 mmHg (11–14.4 pKa)

Bicarbonate, Actual (P)[2]

Calculated from pH and $Paco_2$
Newborns: 17.2–23.6 mmol/L
Children: 18–25 mmol/L

pH (B)[1]

0–6 months: 7.18–7.5
6–12 months: 7.27–7.49

Base Excess (B)[1]

Infant:	−7 to −1 mmol/L
Child:	−4 to +2 mmol/L
Thereafter:	−3 to +3 mmol/L

Oxygen Saturation (B)[1]

Newborns: 85–90%
Thereafter: 95–99%

Cholesterol (S)[3]
Total Cholesterol

Borderline > 170 mg/dL
Elevated > 200 mg/dL

High-Density Lipoprotein

< 35 mg/dL

Low-Density Lipoprotein

Borderline > 110 mg/dL
Elevated > 130 mg/dL

Triglycerides

< 150 mg/dL

C-Reactive Protein (CRP) (P, S)[1]

86–10,406 mcg/L

Hemoglobin A_{1c} (B)[1]

Normal: 4–7%
Stable diabetic patients: 8–10%

Hemoglobin Electrophoresis (B)[2]

A_1 hemoglobin: 96–98.5% of total hemoglobin
A_2 hemoglobin: 1.5–4% of total hemoglobin

Hematology Values (B)

Values for children 2 to 12 years

Red Blood Cell (RBC)[1]

$3.89–4.96 \times 10^{12}/L$

Hemoglobin (HGB)[1]

10.2–13.4 g/dL

Hematocrit (HCT)[1]

31.7–39.3%

Mean Corpuscular Volume (MCV)[1]

72.7–86.5 micrometer^3

Mean Corpuscular Hemoglobin (MCH)[1]

24.1–29.4 picograms

Mean Corpuscular Hemoglobin Concentration (MCHC)[1]

32.4–35.3%

Reticulocyte Count[1]

0.8–2.2%

Sedimentation Rate (Micro)[2]

<2 years: 1–5 mm/hr
>2 years: 1–8 mm/hr

White Blood Cell (WBC)[1]

$5.4–11.0 \times 10^9/L$

Differential[1]

Neutrophils	34.3-72.9%
Eosinophils	2.4-4.8%
Basophils	1%
Lymphocytes	13.5-52.8%
Atypical Lymphocytes	2.6-5.6%
Monocytes	3.5-13.4%

Iron-Related Values

Ferritin (P, S)[1]

1–6 months: 47–449 ng/mL
Thereafter: 47–110 ng/mL

Iron (S, P)[1]

5–11 am: 20–105 mcg/dL (3.6–18.8 micromol/L)

Iron-Binding Capacity (S, P)[1]

1–5 years: 268–441 mcg/dL (48–79 micromol/L)
6–9 years: 240–508 mcg/dL (43–91 micromol/L)
10–19 years: 290–575 mcg/dL (52–103 micromol/L)

Lead (B)[1]

0–15 years: <5 mcg/dL

Thyroid Hormones

Thyroid-Stimulating Hormone (TSH) (P, S)[1]

Age	Males	Females
1–30 days	0.52-16 mUnit/mL	0.72-13.1 mUnit/mL
1 month–5 years	0.55-7.1 mUnit/mL	0.46-8.1 mUnit/mL
6–18 years	0.37-6 mUnit/mL	0.36-5.8 mUnit/mL

Thyroxine (T_4) (S, P)[1]

Age	Males	Females
1–30 days	5.9-21.5 mg/dL	6.3-21.5 mg/dL
1–6 years	6.1-13.1 mg/dL	7.1-14.1 mg/dL
7–12 years	6.7-13.4 mg/dL	6.1-12.1 mg/dL
13–15 years	4.8-11.5 mg/dL	5.8-11.2 mg/dL
16–18 years	5.9-11.5 mg/dL	5.2-13.2 mg/dL

Thyroxine, "Free" (Free T_4)(S, P)[1]

1–12 months: 0.76–2 ng/dL
1–5 years: 0.90–1.72 ng/dL
6–18 years: 0.81–1.68 ng/dL

Thyroxine-Binding Globulin (TBG) (P)[1]

0–6 years: 16.2–33.8 mg/L
7–12 years: 15–29.2 mg/L
13–18 years: 13.4–28.7 mg/L

Triiodothyronine (T_3) (S)[1]

0–11 years: 90–260 ng/dL
12–18 years: 100–210 ng/dL

NORMAL VALUE RANGES: URINE

Addis Count[2]

Red cells (12-hr specimen): <1 million
White cells (12-hr specimen): <2 million
Casts (12-hr specimen): <10,000
Protein (12-hr specimen): <55 mg

Catecholamines (Norepinephrine, Epinephrine)[1]

Values in mmol/mol creatinine

Age	Norepinephrine	Epinephrine
<1 year	0.017–0.207	0–0.232
1–4 years	0.017–0.194	0–0.051
4–10 years	0.018–0.072	0.003–0.057
10–18 years	0.003–0.07	0.001–0.027

Chloride[2]

Infants: 1.7–8.5 mmol/24 hr
Children: 17–34 mmol/24 hr
Adults: 140–240 mmol/24 hr

Creatine[1]

3–8 years: 0.11–0.68 g/24 hr
9–12 years: 0.17–1.41 g/24 hr
13–17 years: 0.29–1.87 g/24 hr

Creatinine[1]

3–8 years: 0.11–0.68 g/24 hr
9–12 years: 0.17–1.41 g/24 hr
13–17 years: 0.29–1.87 g/24 hr
Adults: 0.63–2.5 g/24 hr

Osmolality[3]

Infants: 50–600 mOsm/L
Older children: 50–1400 mOsm/L

Phosphorus, Tubular Reabsorption[2]

78–97%

Potassium[2]

26–123 mmol/L

Specific Gravity

1.01–1.03

NORMAL VALUE RANGES: SWEAT

Electrolytes[1]

Normal: <40 mmol/L for both sodium and chloride
Patients with cystic fibrosis: >60 mmol/L for both sodium and chloride

NORMAL VALUE RANGES: CEREBROSPINAL FLUID

Protein[1]

< 1 month: 15–153 mg/dL
< 3 months: 15–93 mg/dL
>3 months: 15–45 mg/dL

Glucose[1]

All ages: 60–80% of blood glucose

Adapted from:
[1] Soldin, S. J., Brugnara, C., & Wong, E. C. (2003). *Pediatric reference ranges* (4th ed.). Washington, DC: AACC Press.
[2] Hay, W. W., Hayward, A. R., Levin, M. J., Sondheimer, J. M., and Associate Authors. (2003). *Current pediatric diagnosis and treatment* (16th ed.) New York, Lange Medical Books/McGraw-Hill
[3] Kavey, R. W., Daniels, S. R., Lauer, R. M., Atkins, D. L., Hayman, L. L., & Taubert, K. (2003). American Heart Association guidelines for primary prevention of atherosclerotic cardiovascular disease beginning in childhood. *Journal of Pediatrics, 142,* 368–372.

● FIGURE C–1

Birth to 36 months: Boys
Length-for-age and Weight-for-age percentiles

NAME _____

RECORD # _____

Revised April 20, 2001.
SOURCE: Developed by the National Center for Health Statistics in collaboration with
the National Center for Chronic Disease Prevention and Health Promotion (2000).
http://www.cdc.gov/growthcharts

Physical growth percentiles for length and weight—boys: birth to 36 months.

From CDC, 2001. www.cdc.gov/growthcharts

● **FIGURE C-2**

Birth to 36 months: Boys
Head circumference-for-age and
Weight-for-length percentiles

NAME _____

RECORD # _____

SOURCE: Developed by the National Center for Health Statistics in collaboration with
the National Center for Chronic Disease Prevention and Health Promotion (2000).
http://www.cdc.gov/growthcharts

CDC

Physical growth percentiles for head circumference, weight for length—boys: birth to 36 months.

From CDC, 2001. www.cdc.gov/growthcharts

FIGURE C-3

Physical growth percentiles for length and weight—girls: birth to 36 months.

From CDC, 2001. www.cdc.gov/growthcharts

● FIGURE C–4

Birth to 36 months: Girls
Head circumference-for-age and
Weight-for-length percentiles

NAME _____

RECORD # _____

SOURCE: Developed by the National Center for Health Statistics in collaboration with
the National Center for Chronic Disease Prevention and Health Promotion (2000).
http://www.cdc.gov/growthcharts

Physical growth percentiles for head circumference, weight for length—girls: birth to 36 months.

From CDC, 2001. www.cdc.gov/growthcharts

FIGURE C–5

Physical growth percentiles for stature and weight according to age—boys: 2 to 20 years.

From CDC, 2001. www.cdc.gov/growthcharts

● FIGURE C–6

2 to 20 years: Boys
Body mass index-for-age percentiles

NAME _____

RECORD # _____

Date	Age	Weight	Stature	BMI*	Comments

*To Calculate BMI: Weight (kg) ÷ Stature (cm) ÷ Stature (cm) x 10,000
or Weight (lb) ÷ Stature (in) ÷ Stature (in) x 703

AGE (YEARS)

BMI values: 35, 34, 33, 32, 31, 30, 29, 28, 27, 26, 25, 24, 23, 22, 21, 20, 19, 18, 17, 16, 15, 14, 13, 12

Percentile curves: 97, 95, 90, 85, 75, 50, 25, 10, 3

kg/m²   kg/m²

Age axis: 2 3 4 5 6 7 8 9 10 11 12 13 14 15 16 17 18 19 20

SOURCE: Developed by the National Center for Health Statistics in collaboration with
the National Center for Chronic Disease Prevention and Health Promotion (2000).
http://www.cdc.gov/growthcharts

Physical growth percentiles for body mass index according to age—boys: 2 to 20 years.

From CDC, 2001. www.cdc.gov/growthcharts

● FIGURE C–7

Weight-for-stature percentiles: Boys

NAME _____

RECORD # _____

Date	Age	Weight	Stature	Comments

STATURE

SOURCE: Developed by the National Center for Health Statistics in collaboration with
the National Center for Chronic Disease Prevention and Health Promotion (2000).
http://www.cdc.gov/growthcharts

Physical growth percentiles for weight for stature—boys: 2 to 20 years.

From CDC, 2001. www.cdc.gov/growthcharts

FIGURE C–8

Physical growth percentiles for stature and weight according to age—girls: 2 to 20 years.

From CDC, 2001. www.cdc.gov/growthcharts

● FIGURE C-9

2 to 20 years: Girls
Body mass index-for-age percentiles

NAME _____

RECORD # _____

Date	Age	Weight	Stature	BMI*	Comments

*To Calculate BMI: Weight (kg) ÷ Stature (cm) ÷ Stature (cm) x 10,000
or Weight (lb) ÷ Stature (in) ÷ Stature (in) x 703

AGE (YEARS)

SOURCE: Developed by the National Center for Health Statistics in collaboration with
the National Center for Chronic Disease Prevention and Health Promotion (2000).
http://www.cdc.gov/growthcharts

Physical growth percentiles for body mass index according to age—girls: 2 to 20 years.

From CDC, 2001. www.cdc.gov/growthcharts

FIGURE C-10

Weight-for-stature percentiles: Girls

NAME _____

RECORD # _____

Date	Age	Weight	Stature	Comments

SOURCE: Developed by the National Center for Health Statistics in collaboration with
the National Center for Chronic Disease Prevention and Health Promotion (2000).
http://www.cdc.gov/growthcharts

Physical growth percentiles for weight for stature—girls: 2 to 20 years.

From CDC, 2001. www.cdc.gov/growthcharts

Appendix D
Conversions and Equivalents

❖ Temperature Conversion

(Fahrenheit temperature − 32) × 5/9 = Centigrade temperature
(Centigrade temperature × 9/5) + 32 = Fahrenheit temperature

❖ Selected Conversion to Metric Measures

Known Value	Multiply by	To Find
inches	2.54	centimeters
ounces	28	grams
pounds	454	grams
pounds	0.45	kilogram

❖ Selected Conversion from Metric Measures

Known Value	Multiply by	To Find
centimeters	0.4	inches
grams	0.035	ounces
grams	0.0022	pounds
kilograms	2.2	pounds

❖ Conversion of Pounds and Ounces to Grams

							OUNCES									
	0	**1**	**2**	**3**	**4**	**5**	**6**	**7**	**8**	**9**	**10**	**11**	**12**	**13**	**14**	**15**
0	–	28	57	85	113	142	170	198	227	255	283	312	340	369	397	425
1	454	482	510	539	567	595	624	652	680	709	737	765	794	822	850	879
2	907	936	964	992	1021	1049	1077	1106	1134	1162	1191	1219	1247	1276	1304	1332
3	1361	1389	1417	1446	1474	1503	1531	1559	1588	1616	1644	1673	1701	1729	1758	1786
4	1814	1843	1871	1899	1928	1956	1984	2013	2041	2070	2098	2126	2155	2183	2211	2240
5	2268	2296	2325	2353	2381	2410	2438	2466	2495	2523	2551	2580	2608	2637	2665	2693
6	2722	2750	2778	2807	2835	2863	2892	2920	2948	2977	3005	3033	3062	3090	3118	3147
7	3175	3203	3232	3260	3289	3317	3345	3374	3402	3430	3459	3487	3515	3544	3572	3600
8	3629	3657	3685	3714	3742	3770	3799	3827	3856	3884	3912	3941	3969	3997	4026	4054
9	4082	4111	4139	4167	4196	4224	4252	4281	4309	4337	4366	4394	4423	4451	4479	4508
10	4536	4564	4593	4621	4649	4678	4706	4734	4763	4791	4819	4848	4876	4904	4933	4961
11	4990	5018	5046	5075	5103	5131	5160	5188	5216	5245	5273	5301	5330	5358	5386	5415
12	5443	5471	5500	5528	5557	5585	5613	5642	5670	5698	5727	5755	5783	5812	5840	5868
13	5897	5925	5953	5982	6010	6038	6067	6095	6123	6152	6180	6209	6237	6265	6294	6322
14	6350	6379	6407	6435	6464	6492	6520	6549	6577	6605	6634	6662	6690	6719	6747	6776
15	6804	6832	6860	6889	6917	6945	6973	7002	7030	7059	7087	7115	7144	7172	7201	7228
16	7257	7286	7313	7342	7371	7399	7427	7456	7484	7512	7541	7569	7597	7626	7654	7682
17	7711	7739	7768	7796	7824	7853	7881	7909	7938	7966	7994	8023	8051	8079	8108	8136
18	8165	8192	8221	8249	8278	8306	8335	8363	8391	8420	8448	8476	8504	8533	8561	8590
19	8618	8646	8675	8703	8731	8760	8788	8816	8845	8873	8902	8930	8958	8987	9015	9043
20	9072	9100	9128	9157	9185	9213	9242	9270	9298	9327	9355	9383	9412	9440	9469	9497
21	9525	9554	9582	9610	9639	9667	9695	9724	9752	9780	9809	9837	9865	9894	9922	9950
22	9979	10007	10036	10064	10092	10120	10149	10177	10206	10234	10262	10291	10319	10347	10376	10404

POUNDS

Appendix E
Actions and Effects of Selected Drugs During Breastfeeding*

ANTICOAGULANTS
Coumarin derivatives (warfarin, dicumarol): Relatively safe to use; only small amount in breast milk; check PTT.
Heparin and derivatives (Lovenox): Does not cross into breast milk; check PTT.

ANTICONVULSANTS
Phenytoin (Dilantin), phenobarbital: Generally considered safe; if high doses of phenobarbital are ingested, may cause drowsiness; short-acting phenobarbiturates (secobarbital) preferred, because they appear in lower concentration in milk.
Magnesium sulfate: Lactogenesis may be delayed.

ANTIDEPRESSANTS
SSRI class
Fluoxetine (Prozac), fluvoxamine: Effect on newborn unknown but may be of concern.
Tricyclic antidepressants (doxepin): Sedation, potential respiratory arrest in infant.

ANTIHISTAMINES
Diphenhydramine (Benadryl), Claritin, Allegra: May cause decreased milk supply; infant may become drowsy or irritable.
Clemastine (Tavist): Contraindicated.

ANTIHYPERTENSIVES
β adrenergic blockers:
Atenolol, acebutolol: Cyanosis.
Tenormin: Hypotension, bradycardia.

ANTIMETABOLITES
Unknown, probably long-term anti-DNA effect on the infant; potentially very toxic.

ANTIMICROBIALS
Aminoglycosides: May cause ototoxicity or nephrotoxicity if given for more than 2 weeks.
Ampicillin: Skin rash, candidiasis; diarrhea.
Azithromycin: No risk to newborn.
Chloramphenicol (rarely used): Possible bone marrow suppression; too low a dose for Gray syndrome; refusal of breast.
Erythromycin: Accumulates in breast milk, idiopathic hypertrophic pyloric stenosis.
Methacycline: Possible inhibition of bone growth; may cause discoloration of the teeth; use should be avoided.
Metronidazole (Flagyl): Possible neurologic disorders or blood dyscrasias; delay breastfeeding for 12 hours after dose.

Penicillin: Possible allergic response; candidiasis.
Quinolones (synthetic antibiotics): Can cause arthropathies.
Sulfonamides: May cause hyperbilirubinemia; use contraindicated until infant is over 1 week old.
Tetracycline: Long-term use and large doses should be avoided; may cause tooth staining or inhibition of bone growth.

ANTITHYROIDS
Thiouracil: Contraindicated during lactation; may cause goiter or agranulocytosis.
Propylthiouracil: Safe; monitor infant thyroid function.

BARBITURATES
Phenothiazines: May produce sedation.

BRONCHODILATORS
Aminophylline: May cause insomnia or irritability in the infant.
Leukotriene inhibitors (Zyflo, Accolate): Potential tumorigenicity.

CAFFEINE
Excessive consumption may cause jitteriness or wakefulness.

CARDIOVASCULAR
Clonidine (Catapres): Reduces milk volume.
Methyldopa: Increases milk volume.
Propranolol (Inderal): May cause hypoglycemia; possibility of other blocking effects, especially if infant has renal or liver dysfunction.
Quinidine: May cause arrhythmias in infant.
Reserpine (Serpasil): Nasal stuffiness, lethargy, or diarrhea in infant.

CORTICOSTEROIDS
Adrenal suppression may occur with long-term administration of doses greater than 20 mg/day.

DIURETICS
Furosemide (Lasix): Not excreted in breast milk.
Thiazide diuretics (Esidrix, HydroDIURIL, Oretic): Safe but can cause dehydration, reduce milk production.

HEAVY METALS
Gold: Potentially toxic; gold salts—compatible with breastfeeding.
Lead: Excreted in breast milk; high maternal levels can affect neuropsychologic development.
Mercury: Excreted in the milk and hazardous to infant.

HORMONES

Androgens: Suppress lactation.

Thyroid hormones: May mask hypothyroidism.

LAXATIVES

Peri-Colace, Dulcolax: Relatively safe.

Milk of magnesia, Metamucil: Relatively safe.

NARCOTIC ANALGESICS

Codeine: Accumulation may lead to neonatal depression.

Meperidine: Avoid use. May lead to neonatal depression.

Morphine: Long-term use may cause newborn addiction.

NONNARCOTIC ANALGESICS, NSAID

Acetaminophen (Tylenol): Relatively safe for short-term analgesia.

Ibuprofen (Motrin): Safe.

Propoxyphene (Darvon): May cause sleepiness and poor breastfeeding in infant.

Salicylates (aspirin): Safe after first week of life; monitor PTT.

ORAL CONTRACEPTIVES

Combined estrogen/progestin pills: Significantly decrease milk supply; may alter milk composition; may cause gynecomastia in male infants.

Progestin only (DMPA, Norplant): Safe if started after lactation is established.

RADIOACTIVE MATERIALS FOR TESTING

Gallium citrate (67G): Insignificant amount excreted in breast milk; no breastfeeding for 2 weeks.

Iodine: Contraindicated; may affect infant's thyroid gland.

^{125}I: Discontinue breastfeeding for 24 hours.

^{131}I: Breastfeeding should be discontinued until excretion is no longer significant; may be resumed after 10 days.

Technetium-99m: Discontinue breastfeeding for 24 hours (half-life = 6 hours).

SEDATIVES/TRANQUILIZERS

Diazepam (Valium): May accumulate to high levels; may increase neonatal jaundice; may cause lethargy, weight loss, and poor suck.

Lithium: Contraindicated; may cause neonatal flaccidity and hypotonia.

SMOKING CESSATION

Nicotine patch (Nicoderm, Nicotrol): Irritability, abnormal sleep patterns, poor feeding.

Bupropion (Zyban, Wellbutrin): No effect on breastfeeding.

SUBSTANCE ABUSE

Alcohol: Potential motor developmental delay; mild sedative effect.

Amphetamines: Controversial; may cause irritability, poor sleeping pattern.

Cocaine, crack: Extreme irritability, tachycardia, vomiting, apnea.

Marijuana: Drowsiness.

Heroin: Tremors, restlessness, vomiting, poor feeding.

Nicotine (smoking): Shock, vomiting, diarrhea, decreased milk production.

*Based on data from Riordan, J., & Auerbach, K. J. (2005). Breastfeeding and human lactation *(3rd ed., pp. 146–166). *Boston: Jones & Bartlett; Briggs, G. G., Freeman, R. K., & Yaffe, S. J. (2005). Drugs in pregnancy and lactation *(7th ed.). *Baltimore: Williams & Wilkins; Hale, T. (2004). Medications and mothers' milk *(11th ed.). *Amarillo, TX: Pharmasoft Publishing; Committee on Drugs, American Academy of Pediatrics. (2001). The transfer of drugs and other chemicals into human milk. *Pediatrics, 108 *(3), 776.

Appendix F
Common Abbreviations in Maternal-Newborn and Women's Health Nursing

AC	Abdominal circumference
accel	Acceleration of fetal heart rate
AFAFP	Amniotic fluid alpha-fetoprotein
AFI	Amniotic fluid index
AFP	Alpha-fetoprotein
AFV	Amniotic fluid volume
AGA	Average for gestational age
AI	Amnioinfusion
AMOL	Active management of labor
AOP	Apnea of prematurity *or* Anemia of prematurity
ARBOW	Artificial rupture of bag of waters
AROM	Artificial rupture of membranes
ART	Artificial reproductive technology
BAT	Brown adipose tissue (brown fat)
BBOW	Bulging bag of water
BBT	Basal body temperature
BL	Baseline (fetal heart rate baseline)
BOW	Bag of waters
β-hCG	Beta-human chorionic gonadotropin
BPD	Biparietal diameter *or* Bronchopulmonary dysplasia
BPP	Biophysical profile
BRB	Bright red bleeding *or* Breakthrough bleeding
BR CA	Breast cancer
BSE	Breast self-examination
BSST	Breast self-stimulation test
CC	Chest circumference *or* Cord compression
CEI	Continuous epidural infusion
C–H	Crown-to-heel length
CID	Cytomegalic inclusion disease
CLD	Chronic lung disease
CM	Certified midwife
CMV	Cytomegalovirus
CNM	Certified nurse-midwife
CNP	Certified nurse practitioner
CNS	Clinical nurse specialist
CP	Chest pain
CPAP	Continuous positive airway pressure
CPD	Cephalopelvic disproportion *or* Citrate-phosphate-dextrose
CRL	Crown-rump length
CRNP	Certified registered nurse practitioner
C/S	Cesarean section (or C-section)
CST	Contraction stress test
CT	Chlamydia
CVA	Costovertebral angle
CVS	Chorionic villus sampling
D&C	Dilatation and curettage
D&E	Dilatation and evacuation
decels	Deceleration of fetal heart rate
DFMR	Daily fetal movement response
dil	Dilatation
DTR	Deep tendon reflexes
DV	Domestic violence
EAB	Elective abortion
ECMO	Extracorporeal membrane oxygenator
EDB	Estimated date of birth
EDC	Estimated date of confinement
EDD	Estimated date of delivery
EFM	Electronic fetal monitoring
EFW	Estimated fetal weight
EIA	Enzyme immunoassay
ELF	Elective low forceps
ELISA	Enzyme-linked immunosorbent assay
EP	Ectopic pregnancy
epis	Episiotomy
FAD	Fetal activity diary
FAE	Fetal alcohol effects
FAS	Fetal alcohol syndrome
FBD	Fibrocystic breast disease
FBM	Fetal breathing movements
FBS	Fetal blood sample *or* Fasting blood sugar test
FCC	Family-centered care

FECG	Fetal electrocardiogram
FeSO$_4$	Ferrous sulfate (iron supplement)
FHR	Fetal heart rate
FHT	Fetal heart tones
Fhx	Family history
FL	Femur length
FMC	Fetal movement count
FMR	Fetal movement record
FPG	Fasting plasma glucose test
FSE	Fetal scalp electrode
FSH	Follicle-stimulating hormone
FSHRH	Follicle-stimulating hormone-releasing hormone
FSPO$_2$	Fetal arterial oxygen saturation
G or grav	Gravida
GC	Gonorrhea
GDM	Gestational diabetes mellitus
GIFT	Gamete intrafallopian transfer
GnRF	Gonadotropin-releasing factor
GnRH	Gonadotropin-releasing hormone
GTD	Gestational trophoblastic disease
GTPAL	Gravida, term, preterm, abortion, living children; a system of recording maternity history
HA	Head-abdominal ratio or headache
HAI	Hemagglutination-inhibition test
HC	Head compression
hCG	Human chorionic gonadotropin
hCS	Human chorionic somatomammotropin (same as hPL)
HIV	Human immunodeficiency virus
HMD	Hyaline membrane disease
hMG	Human menopausal gonadotropin
hPL	Human placental lactogen
HPV	Human papilloma virus
HRT	Hormone replacement therapy
HSV	Herpes simplex virus
ICSI	Intracytoplasmic sperm injection
IDM	Infant of a diabetic mother
IPG	Impedance phlebography
ISAM	Infant of a substance-abusing mother
IU	International units
IUD	Intrauterine device

IUFD	Intrauterine fetal death
IUGR	Intrauterine growth restriction
IUPC	Intrauterine pressure catheter
IUS	Intrauterine system
IVF	In vitro fertilization
LADA	Left-acromion-dorsal-anterior
LADP	Left-acromion-dorsal-posterior
LBC	Lamellar body count
LBW	Low birth weight
LDR	Labor, delivery, and recovery room
LGA	Large for gestational age
LH	Luteinizing hormone
LHRH	Luteinizing hormone-releasing hormone
LMA	Left-mentum-anterior
LML	Left mediolateral (episiotomy)
LMP	Last menstrual period *or* Left-mentum-posterior
LMT	Left-mentum-transverse
LOA	Left-occiput-anterior
LOF	Low outlet forceps
LOP	Left-occiput-posterior
LOS	Length of stay
LOT	Left-occiput-transverse
L/S	Lecithin/sphingomyelin ratio
LSA	Left-sacrum-anterior
LSP	Left-sacrum-posterior
LST	Left-sacrum-transverse
MAS	Meconium aspiration syndrome
mec	Meconium
mec st	Meconium stain
MLE	Midline episiotomy
MSAFP	Maternal serum alpha-fetoprotein
MUGB	4-methylumbelliferyl quanidinobenzoate
multip	Multipara
NEC	Necrotizing enterocolitis
NGU	Nongonococcal urethritis
NP	Nurse practitioner
NSCST	Nipple stimulation contraction stress test
NST	Nonstress test *or* Nonshivering thermogenesis
NSVD	Normal sterile vaginal delivery
NTD	Neural tube defect
NTE	Neutral thermal environment
OA	Occiput anterior

OC	Oral contraceptive
OCPs	Oral contraceptive pills
OCT	Oxytocin challenge test
OF	Occipitofrontal diameter of fetal head
OFC	Occipitofrontal circumference
OGTT	Oral glucose tolerance test
OM	Occipitomental (diameter)
OP	Occiput posterior
p	Para
Pap smear	Papanicolaou smear
PCA	Patient-controlled analgesia
PDA	Patent ductus arteriosus
PEEP	Positive end-expiratory pressure
PG	Phosphatidylglycerol or Prostaglandin
PID	Pelvic inflammatory disease
Pit	Pitocin
PKU	Phenylketonuria
PMS	Premenstrual syndrome
PNV	Prenatal vitamins
PPHN	Persistent pulmonary hypertension
Premie	Premature infant
primip	Primipara
PROM	Premature rupture of membranes
PSI	Prostaglandin synthesis inhibitor
PUBS	Percutaneous umbilical blood sampling
RADA	Right-acromion-dorsal-anterior
RADP	Right-acromion-dorsal-posterior
RDS	Respiratory distress syndrome
REM	Rapid eye movements
RIA	Radioimmunoassay
RLF	Retrolental fibroplasia
RMA	Right-mentum-anterior
RMP	Right-mentum-posterior
RMT	Right-mentum-transverse
ROA	Right-occiput-anterior
ROM	Rupture of membranes
ROP	Right-occiput-posterior or Retinopathy of prematurity
ROT	Right-occiput-transverse
RRA	Radioreceptor assay
RSA	Right-sacrum-anterior
RSP	Right-sacrum-posterior
RST	Right-sacrum-transverse
SAB	Spontaneous abortion
SET	Surrogate embryo transfer
SGA	Small for gestational age
SIDS	Sudden infant death syndrome
SMB	Submentobregmatic diameter
SOB	Suboccipitobregmatic diameter or Shortness of breath
SPA	Sperm penetration assay
SRBOW	Spontaneous rupture of bag of waters
SROM	Spontaneous rupture of membranes
STD	Sexually transmitted disease
STI	Sexually transmitted infection
STS	Serologic test for syphilis
SVE	Sterile vaginal examination
TAB	Therapeutic abortion
TC	Thoracic circumference
TCM	Transcutaneous monitoring
TDI or THI	Therapeutic donor insemination (H designates mate is donor)
TET	Tubal embryo transfer
TOL	Trial of labor
TORCH	Toxoplasmosis, rubella, cytomegalovirus, herpesvirus hominis type 2
TSS	Toxic shock syndrome
u	Umbilicus
UA	Uterine activity
UAC	Umbilical artery catheter
UAU	Uterine activity units
UC	Uterine contraction
UPI	Uteroplacental insufficiency
US	Ultrasound
VBAC	Vaginal birth after cesarean
VDRL	Venereal Disease Research Laboratories
VIP	Voluntary interruption of pregnancy
VLBW	Very low birth weight
VVC	Vulvovaginal candidiasis
WIC	Special Supplemental Nutrition Program for Women, Infants, and Children
ZIFT	Zygote intrafallopian transfer

ACTH	Adrenocorticotropic hormone
ADD	Attention deficit disorder
ADH	Antidiuretic hormone
ADHD	Attention deficit hyperactivity disorder
AFB	Aspirated foreign body
AI	Adequate intake
ALL	Acute lymphoblastic leukemia
ALTE	Apparent life-threatening event
ANLL	Acute nonlymphocytic leukemia
AOP	Apnea of prematurity
APIGN	Acute postinfectious glomerulonephritis
ARF	Acute renal failure
AS	Aortic stenosis
ASD	Atrial septal defect
ASO	Antistreptolysin-O
BMI	Body mass index
BPD	Bronchopulmonary dysplasia
BSA	Body surface area
CBC	Complete blood count
CF	Cystic fibrosis
CHD	Congenital heart defect *or* Congenital heart disease
CHF	Congestive heart failure
CHIP	Child health insurance program
COA	Coarctation of aorta
CP	Cerebral palsy
CRF	Chronic renal failure
CSHCN	Children with special healthcare needs
CT	Computerized tomography
dB	Decibel
DDAVP	Desmopressin acetate
DDH	Developmental dysplasia of hip
DKA	Diabetic ketoacidosis
DRI	Dietary Reference Intake
DSM	Diagnostic and Statistical Manual of Mental Disorders
DTaP	Diphtheria, tetanus toxoid and acellular pertussis immunization
DTRs	Deep tendon reflexes
EAR	Estimated average requirement
EEG	Electroencephalogram
EMLA	Eutectic mixture of local anesthetics

ESRD	End stage renal disease
FTT	Failure to thrive
GC	Gonorrhea
GCS	Glasgow Coma Scale *or* Glasgow Coma Score
H&H	Hematocrit and hemoglobin
HIB	*Haemophilus influenzae* immunization
HIV	Human immunodeficiency virus
HOME	Home Observation for Measurement of the Environment
HUS	Hemolytic uremic syndrome
Hz	Hertz
IEP	Individualized Education Plan
IGF	Insulin-like growth factor
IHP	Individualized Health Plan
IVIG	Intravenous immunoglobulin
IPV	Inactivated poliovirus vaccine
IVP	Intravenous pyelogram
JRA	Juvenile rheumatoid arthritis
LOC	Level of consciousness
LTB	Laryngotracheobronchitis
MCNS	Minimal change nephrotic syndrome
MDI	Metered dose inhaler
MMR	Measles, mumps, rubella immunization
MR	Mental retardation
MRI	Magnetic resonance imaging
NEC	Necrotizing enterocolitis
NSAIDs	Nonsteroidal anti-inflammatory drugs
OFC	Occipital frontal circumference
PCA	Patient-controlled analgesia
PCV	Heptavalent Pneumococcal Conjugate immunization
PDA	Patent ductus arteriosus
PEFR	Peak expiratory flow rate
PGE$_1$	Prostaglandin E$_1$
PICU	Pediatric intensive care unit

PKU	Phenylketonuria	**TANF**	Temporary Assistance for Needy Families
PPD	Purified protein derivative (TB test)	**TB**	Tuberculosis
PS	Pulmonic stenosis	**TEF**	Tracheoesophageal fistula
		TGA	Transposition of the great arteries
RAST	Radioallergosorbent test	**TPN**	Total parenteral nutrition
RBC	Red blood cell	**TSH**	Thyroid stimulating hormone
RDA	Recommended dietary allowance	**Tx**	Traction
RDS	Respiratory distress syndrome		
RSV	Respiratory syncytial virus	**UA**	Urinalysis
		UI	Upper intake
S_1	First heart sound	**UTI**	Urinary tract infection
S_2	Second heart sound		
SCID	Severe combined immunodeficiency disease	**VSD**	Ventricular septal defect
SIDS	Sudden infant death syndrome	**WBC**	White blood cell
STI	Sexually transmitted infection	**WIC**	Special Supplemental Nutrition Program for Women, Infants, and Children
SVT	Supraventricular tachycardia		

The following form is shortened for ease in assessing a family. If you are not sure what data should be covered in each of the assessment areas below, please refer to the original reference where more detailed questions/areas are presented.

   Before using the following guidelines in completing family assessments, note that not all areas included below will be germane for each of the families visited. The guidelines are comprehensive and allow depth when probing is necessary. Do not feel that every subarea needs to be covered when the broad area of inquiry poses no problems to the family or concern to the health worker. Second, by virtue of the interdependence of the family system, one will find unavoidable redundancy. The assessor should try not to repeat data, but to refer the reader back to sections where this information has already been described.

IDENTIFYING DATA

1. Family Name
2. Address and Phone
3. Family Composition: The Family Genogram
4. Type of Family Form
5. Cultural (Ethnic) Background
6. Religious Identification
7. Social Class Status
8. Social Class Mobility

DEVELOPMENTAL STAGE AND HISTORY OF FAMILY

9. Family's Present Developmental Stage
10. Extent of Family Developmental Tasks Fulfillment
11. Nuclear Family History
12. History of Family of Origin of Both Parents

ENVIRONMENTAL DATA

13. Characteristics of Home
14. Characteristics of Neighborhood and Larger Community
15. Family's Geographical Mobility
16. Family's Associations and Transactions with Community

FAMILY STRUCTURE

17. Communication Patterns
    Extent of Functional and Dysfunctional Communication (types of recurring patterns)
    Extent of Emotional (Affective) Messages and How Expressed
    Characteristics of Communication Within Family Subsystems
    Extent of Congruent and Incongruent Messages
    Types of Dysfunctional Communication Processes Seen in Family
    Areas of Closed Communication
    Familial and Contextual Variables Affecting Communication

18. Power Structure
    Power Outcomes
    Decision-making Process
    Power Bases
    Variables Affecting Family Power
    Overall Family System and Subsystem Power (Family Power Continuum Placement)

19. Role Structure
    Formal Role Structure
    Informal Role Structure
    Analysis of Role Models (optional)
    Variables Affecting Role Structure

20. Family Values
    Compare the family to American core values or family's reference group values and/or identify important family values and their importance (priority) in family.
    Congruence Between the Family's Values and the Family's Reference Group or Wider Community
    Disparity in Value Systems
    Presence of Value Conflicts in Family
    Effect of the Above Values and Value Conflicts on Health Status of Family

FAMILY FUNCTIONS

21. Affective Function
    Mutual Nurturance, Closeness, and Identification
    Separateness and Connectedness
    Family's Need–Response Patterns

22. Socialization Function
    Family Childrearing Practices
    Adaptability of Childrearing Practices for Family Form and Family's Situation
    Who Is (Are) Socializing Agent(s) for Child(ren)?
    Value of Children in Family
    Cultural Beliefs That Influence Family's Childrearing Patterns
    Social Class Influence on Childrearing Patterns
    Estimation About Whether Family Is at Risk for Childrearing Problems and if so, Indication of High-Risk Factors
    Adequacy of Home Environment for Children's Needs to Play

23. Health Care Function
    Family's Health Beliefs, Values, and Behavior
    Family's Definitions of Health–Illness and Its Level of Knowledge
    Family's Perceived Health Status and Illness Susceptibility
    Family's Dietary Practices
    Adequacy of family diet (recommended 3-day food history record)
    Function of mealtimes and attitudes toward food and mealtimes.
    Shopping (and its planning) practices.
    Person(s) responsible for planning, shopping, and preparation of meals.
    Sleep and Rest Habits
    Physical Activity and Recreation Practices
    Family's Therapeutic and Recreational Drug, Alcohol, and Tobacco Practices
    Family's Role in Self-care Practices
    Medically Based Preventive Measures (physicals, eye and hearing tests, immunizations, dental care)
    Complementary and Alternative Therapies
    Family Health History (both general and specific diseases—environmentally and genetically related)
    Health Care Services Received
    Feelings and Perceptions Regarding Health Services
    Emergency Health Services
    Source of Payments for Health and Other Services
    Logistics of Receiving Care

FAMILY STRESS, COPING, AND ADAPTATION

24. Family Stressors, Strengths, and Perceptions
    Stressors Family Is Experiencing
    Strengths That Counterbalance Stressors
    Family's Definition of the Situation

25. Family Coping Strategies
    How the Family Is Reacting to the Stressors
    Extent of Family's Use of Internal Coping Strategies (past/present)
    Extent of Family's Use of External Coping Strategies (past/present)
    Dysfunctional Coping Strategies Utilized (past/present; extent of use)

26. Family Adaptation
    Overall Family Adaptation
    Estimation of Whether Family Is in Crisis

27. Tracking Stressors, Coping, and Adaptation Over Time

Used with permission from Friedman, M. M., Bowden, V. R., Jones, E. G. (2003). *Family nursing: Research, theory, and practice,* (5th ed.). Upper Saddle River, NJ: Prentice Hall.

1. First, remember that it requires trust on the part of the client to allow nonsigning caregivers and an interpreter into her life.
2. It is important to use a registered interpreter. Medical interpreters are registered with the Registry of Interpreters for the Deaf. Although family members and friends may offer to interpret, it is best to use registered medical interpreters because they are required to translate the clients' and nurses' words accurately without adding in any other opinion.
3. Greet the client and family with a handshake and body posture that indicates welcome. You may point to your name tag and use the American Sign Language (ASL) alphabet cards to spell out your name. The client may wish to select cards to indicate her name. It is especially important as you work together to make the effort to provide a greeting as you would with speaking clients; greetings help develop rapport.
4. Once the interpreter is present, continue to look at the client and speak directly to her. There will be a temptation to look at the interpreter, and it will help to remember that you are speaking to the client.
5. Avoid phrasing your words as if you are talking to the interpreter (e.g., "Can you tell her ?"). Instead, phrase your questions as you do with speaking clients (e.g., "I'm going to ask you some questions now.").
6. Depend on the deaf client to ask questions.
7. Look at the client's face for signs of difficulty in understanding. Deaf clients have a behavior of "gesturing" that involves shaking their heads as if to indicate "yes" even when they do not understand. If the client is nodding "yes," ask her to repeat the directions you have just given.
8. Be as direct as possible. Keep to what you want to know or what you want to convey. Speak in short sentences, using nontechnical words. Avoid colloquial or slang words. Be sure to explain what you want to do before you do it. For instance, tell her you want to start an IV and explain the equipment. Then, with her permission, start the IV.
9. Be aware that deaf clients may have difficulty understanding when to take medications. It will be helpful to associate taking medications or completing some treatment or activity with meals. (For instance, while showing her the two capsules she is to take when she goes home, tell her to take the two capsules at breakfast and another two capsules at bedtime.) Avoid saying "take two capsules at 8:00 A.M., 2:00 P.M., and 12:00 A.M."
10. The difference in interpreting time may also affect obtaining a history. It is best to begin with a specific event in the past and work forward.

WHAT TO DO UNTIL THE INTERPRETER ARRIVES

1. Role-play as much as possible.
2. Demonstrate what you want the client to do or what you want to do.
3. Be resourceful.
4. Remember that some deaf clients can read lips. Some may read written language, but use care in assuming the client understands.

WHAT TO DO TO PREPARE FOR WORKING WITH A DEAF CLIENT

1. Contact local agencies that work with deaf clients to see what resources are available. Ask about classes in ASL. Being able to use some basic signs will be very helpful while waiting for an interpreter to arrive.
2. Read to learn more about the deaf culture. Contact your local agency or the National Information Center on Deafness, Silver Spring, Maryland, to get suggestions on books you might read.
3. Investigate your health facility. What is available to assist you? Look for videos used for teaching in the maternal-child unit and note if they have captions. Remember that many deaf clients do not read written language, so it will be important to review the content of the video with an interpreter present.

Prepared with the kind assistance of Mr. Gerald Dement, Interpreter Coordinator, Pikes Peak Center on Deafness, Colorado Springs, Colorado.

Appendix J
Dietary Reference Intakes

	Age	Vitamin A (mcg/d)	Vitamin D (mcg/d)	Vitamin E (mg/d α-tocopherol)	Vitamin K (mcg/d)	Vitamin C (mg/d)	Thiamin (mg/d)	Riboflavin (mg/d)	Niacin (mg/d)	Vitamin B$_6$ (mg/d)
Infants	0–6 months	400*	5*	4*	2.0*	40*	0.2*	0.3*	~0.2*	0.1*
	7–12 months	500*	5*	5*	2.5*	50*	0.3*	0.4*	~0.4*	0.3*
Children	1–3 years	300	5*	6	30*	15	0.5	0.5	6	0.5
	4–8 years	400	5*	7	55*	25	0.6	0.6	8	0.6
Males	9–13 years	600	5*	11	60*	45	0.9	0.9	12	1.0
	14–18 years	900	5*	15	75*	75	1.2	1.3	16	1.3
Females	9–13 years	600	5*	11	60*	45	0.9	0.9	12	1.0
	14–18 years	700	5*	15	75*	65	1.0	1.0	14	1.2

*Values are Adequate Intakes (AI) rather than Recommended Dietary Allowances (RDAs). All other values on chart are RDAs. See Chapters 12, 29, and 34 for discussion of nutrient requirements.

Note: All data from Institute of Medicine. (1997–2004). Dietary Reference Intakes. Washington, DC: National Academy Press. Available also at http://www.nas.edu/Iam

	Age	From Food	From Beverages	Total
Infants	0–6 months	0	0.7	0.7*
	7–12 months	0.2	0.6	0.8*
Children	1–3 years	0.4	0.9	1.3*
	4–8 years	0.5	1.2	1.7*
Males	9–13 years	0.6	1.8	2.4*
	14–18 years	0.7	2.6	3.3*
Females	9–13 years	0.5	1.6	2.1*
	14–18 years	0.5	1.8	2.3*

*Values are Adequate Intakes.

APPENDIX J 1929

Folate (mcg/d)	Vitamin B$_{12}$ (mcg/d)	Calcium (mg/d)	Phosphorus (mg/d)	Magnesium (mg/d)	Iron (mg/d)	Zinc (mg/d)	Iodine (mcg/d)	Selenium (mcg/d)	Potassium (g/d)	Sodium (g/d)
65*	0.4*	210*	100*	30*	0.27*	2.0*	110*	15*	0.4*	0.12*
80*	0.5*	270*	275*	75*	11	3	130*	20*	0.7*	0.37*
150	0.9	500*	460	80	7	3	90	20	3*	1*
200	1.2	800*	500	130	10	5	90	30	3.8*	1.2*
300	1.8	1300*	1250	240	8	8	120	40	4.5*	1.5*
400	2.4	1300*	1250	240	11	11	150	55	4.5*	1.5*
300	1.8	1300*	1250	410	8	8	120	40	4*	1.5*
400	2.4	1300*	1250	360	15	9	150	55	4.7*	1.5*

TABLE J-3 ❖ Recommended Dietary Allowances

	Age	Protein	Carbohydrate	Polyunsaturated Fatty Acids n-6	Polyunsaturated Fatty Acids n-3	Total Fat	Fiber
Infants	0–6 months	9.1 g/d or 1.52 g/kg/d*	60 g/d*	4.4 g/d	0.5 g/d	31 g/d	NE
	7–12 months	1.5 g/kg/d	95 g/d*	4.6 g/d	0.5 g/d	30 g/d	NE
Children	1–3 years	1.1 g/kg/d or 13 g/d	130 g/d	7 g/d (linoleic)	0.7 g/d (α-linolenic)	NE	19 g/d
	4–8 years	0.95 g/kg/d or 19 g/d	130 g/d	10 g/d (linoleic)	0.9 g/d (α-linolenic)	NE	25 g/d
Males	9–13 years	0.95 g/kg/d or 34 g/d	130 g/d	12 g/d (linoleic)	1.2 g/d (α-linolenic)	NE	31 g/d
	14–18 years	0.85 g/kg/d or 52 g/d	130 g/d	16 g/d (linoleic)	1.6 g/d (α-linolenic)	NE	38 g/d
Females	9–13 years	0.95 g/kg/d or 34 g/d	130 g/d	10 g/d (linoleic)	1.0 g/d (α-linolenic)	NE	26 g/d
	14–18 years	0.85 g/kg/d or 46 g/d	130 g/d	11 g/d (linoleic)	1.1 g/d (α-linolenic)	NE	26 g/d

*Values are Adequate Intakes (AIs) rather than Recommended Dietary Allowances (RDAs). All other values on charts are RDAs.

NE = not established

All data from Institute of Medicine. (2002). *Dietary Reference Intakes.* Washington DC: National Academy Press. www.nap.edu/iom

♣ Recommended Dietary Allowances

	Age	Vitamin A (µg/d)	Vitamin D (µg/d)	Vitamin E (mg/d d α-tocopherol)	Vitamin K (µg/d)	Vitamin C (mg/d)	Thiamin (mg/d)	Riboflavin (mg/d)	Niacin (mg/d)	Vitamin B6 (mg/d)	Folate (µg/d)	Vitamin B12 (µg/d)	Calcium (mg/d)	Phosphorus (mg/d)	Magnesium (mg/d)	Iron (mg/d)	Zinc (mg/d)	Iodine (µg/d)	Selenium (µg/d)
Females	9–13 y	600	5*	11	60*	45	0.9	0.9	12	1.0	300	1.8	1300*	1250	240	8	8	120	40
	14–18 y	700	5*	15	75*	65	1.0	1.0	14	1.2	400	2.4	1300*	1250	360	15	9	150	55
	19–30 y	700	5*	15	90*	75	1.1	1.1	14	1.3	400	2.4	1000*	700	310	18	8	150	55
	31–50 y	700	5*	15	90*	75	1.1	1.1	14	1.3	400	2.4	1000*	700	320	18	8	150	55
	50–70 y	700	10*	15	90*	75	1.1	1.1	14	1.5	400	2.4	1200*	700	320	8	8	150	55
	> 70 y	700	15*	15	90*	75	1.1	1.1	14	1.5	400	2.4	1200*	700	320	8	8	150	55
Pregnancy	≤ 18 y	750	5*	15	75*	80	1.4	1.4	18	1.9	600	2.6	1300*	1250	400	27	12	220	60
	19–30 y	770	5*	15	90*	85	1.4	1.4	18	1.9	600	2.6	1000*	700	350	27	11	220	60
	31–50 y	770	5*	15	90*	85	1.4	1.4	18	1.9	600	2.6	1000*	700	360	27	11	220	60
Lactation	≤ 18 y	1200	5*	19	75*	115	1.4	1.6	17	2.0	500	2.8	1300*	1250	360	10	13	290	70
	19–30 y	1300	5*	19	90*	120	1.4	1.6	17	2.0	500	2.8	1000*	700	310	9	12	290	70
	31–50 y	1300	5*	19	90*	120	1.4	1.6	17	2.0	500	2.8	1000*	700	320	9	12	290	70

*Values are Adequate Intakes (AI) rather than Recommended Dietary Allowances (RDAs). All other values on chart are RDAs.

STANDARDS FOR PROFESSIONAL NURSING PRACTICE IN THE CARE OF WOMEN AND NEWBORNS

Standards of Care for Nurses in the Care of Women and Newborns include:

- Collecting health data.
- Analyzing the assessment data in determining diagnoses.
- Identifying expected outcomes individualized to the woman or newborn.
- Developing a plan of care that prescribes interventions to attain expected outcome.
- Implementing the interventions identified in the plan of care.
- Evaluating the patient's progress toward outcomes.

Standards of Professional Performance in the Care of Women and Newborns include:

- Systematically evaluating the quality and effectiveness of nursing practice.
- Evaluating his/her own nursing practice in relation to professional practice standards and relevant statutes and regulations.
- Acquiring and maintaining current knowledge in nursing practice.
- Contributing to the professional development of peers, colleagues, and others.
- Making nursing decisions and actions on behalf of patients that are determined in an ethical manner.
- Collaborating with the patient, significant others, and health care providers in providing patient care.
- Using research findings in practice.
- Considering factors related to safety, effectiveness, and cost in planning and delivering patient care.
- Contributing to the environment of care delivery within the practice setting.
- Being professionally and legally accountable for his/her practice.

PROFESSIONAL PRACTICE FOR NEONATAL NURSING

Standards of Practice for Neonatal Nursing include:

- Collecting comprehensive data on the healthcare needs of the infant and family.
- Formulating diagnoses based on analysis and synthesis of assessment data.
- Identifying expected individualized outcomes of care based on the needs of the infant and family.
- Developing a plan of care that prescribes intervention to attain expected outcomes.
- Implementing the plan of care:
  - Coordination of care
  - Health teaching and health promotion
  - Consultation
  - Prescriptive authority and treatment
- Evaluating the progress of the infant and family toward the attainment of established, expected outcomes.

Standards of Performance for Neonatal Nursing include:

- Systematically evaluating the quality and effectiveness of nursing practice.
- Acquiring and maintaining current knowledge and competency in nursing practice.
- Evaluating one's own nursing practice in relation to professional practice standards and guidelines, relevant statutes, rules, and regulations.
- Interacting with, and contributing to the professional development of, peers, other healthcare providers, and team members as colleagues.
- Collaborating with the family or caregiver and others in the conduct of nursing practice.
- Deciding and acting on behalf of infants and their families or caregivers in all areas of practice in an ethical manner.
- Integrating research findings into practice.
- Considering factors related to safety, effectiveness, cost, and impact on practice in the planning and delivering of nursing services.
- Providing leadership in the professional practice setting and the profession.

PROFESSIONAL PRACTICE STANDARDS FOR PEDIATRIC NURSING PRACTICE

Standards of Care for the Pediatric Nurse include:

- Collecting health data.
- Analyzing the assessment data in determining diagnoses.
- Identifying expected outcomes individualized to the child and family.
- Developing a plan of care that prescribes interventions to attain expected outcomes.
- Implementing the interventions identified in the plan of care.

Standards of Performance for the Pediatric Nurse include:

- Systematically evaluating the quality and effectiveness of pediatric nursing practice.
- Evaluating own nursing practice in relation to professional practice standards and relevant statutes and regulations.

- Acquiring and maintaining current knowledge and competence in pediatric nursing practice.
- Interacting with and contributing to the professional development of peers, colleagues, and other healthcare providers.
- Making assessments and recommendations and taking action on behalf of children and their families in an ethical manner.
- Collaborating with the child, family, and other healthcare providers in providing patient care.
- Contributing to nursing and pediatric healthcare through the use of research methods and findings.
- Considering factors related to safety, effectiveness, and cost in planning and delivering care.

Used with permission from American Nurses Association & the Society of Pediatric Nurses. (2003). *Scope and standards of pediatric nursing practice.* Washington, DC: nursebooks.org. American Nurses Association, 600 Maryland Ave SW, Suite 100W, Washington, DC 20024-2571.

NOMOGRAM

Note: Nomogram modified from data of E. Boyd by C. D. West; from Behrman, R. E., Kliegman, R. M., & Jenson, H. B. (Eds.). (2004). *Nelson textbook of pediatrics* (17th ed.). Philadelphia: W. B. Saunders.

NOMOGRAM

Pediatric doses of medications are generally based on body surface area (BSA) or weight. To calculate a child's BSA, draw a straight line from the height (in the left-hand column) to the weight (in the right-hand column). The point at which the line intersects the surface area (SA) column is the BSA (measured in square meters [m²]). If the child is of roughly normal proportion, BSA can be calculated from the weight alone (in the enclosed area).

Index

Withdrawal:
  alcohol, 308
  as contraceptive method, 77
  opioid
    in infant of a drug-abusing mother, 799,
      800t
    signs and symptoms, 1218t

Photo Credits

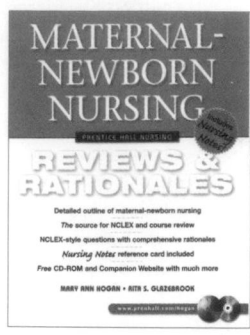